Primary Care
Medicine

FOURTH EDITION

ALLAN H. GOROLL, M.D.
Physician
Massachusetts General Hospital
Associate Professor of Medicine
Harvard Medical School
Boston, Massachusetts

ALBERT G. MULLEY, JR., M.D., M.P.P.
Chief, General Internal Medicine Unit
Massachusetts General Hospital
Harvard Medical School
Boston, Massachusetts

With 65 contributors

Primary Care Medicine

Office Evaluation and Management of the Adult Patient

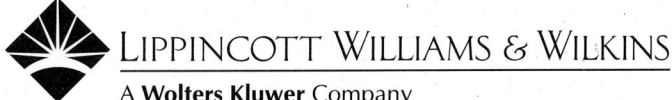

LIPPINCOTT WILLIAMS & WILKINS
A **Wolters Kluwer** Company

Philadelphia • Baltimore • New York • London
Buenos Aires • Hong Kong • Sydney • Tokyo

Acquisitions Editor: Richard Winters
Developmental Editor: Delois Patterson
Production Editor: W. Christopher Granville
Manufacturing Manager: Colin Warnock
Cover Designer: Patricia Gast
Compositor: Graphic World Inc.
Printer: Quebecor World

Library of Congress Cataloging-in-Publication Data

Primary care medicine: office evaluation and management of the adult patient / [edited by] Allan H. Goroll, Lawrence A. May, Albert G. Mulley, Jr.; with 65 contributors.–
4th ed.
    p. ; cm.
  Includes bibliographical references and index.
  ISBN 0-7817-1248-3
  1. Family medicine. 2. Ambulatory medical care. I. Goroll, Allan H. II. May, Lawrence A. III. Mulley, Albert G.
  [DNLM: 1. Primary Health Care. 2. Ambulatory Care. W 84.6 P94916 2000]
RC46 .G56 2000
616–dc21

                                                            00-027376

Care has been taken to confirm the accuracy of the information presented and to describe generally accepted practices. However, the authors, editors, and publisher are not responsible for errors or omissions or for any consequences from application of the information in this book and make no warranty, expressed or implied, with respect to the currency, completeness, or accuracy of the contents of the publication. Application of this information in a particular situation remains the professional responsibility of the practitioner.

The authors, editors, and publisher have exerted every effort to ensure that drug selection and dosage set forth in this text are in accordance with current recommendations and practice at the time of publication. However, in view of ongoing research, changes in government regulations, and the constant flow of information relating to drug therapy and drug reactions, the reader is urged to check the package insert for each drug for any change in indications and dosage and for added warnings and precautions. This is particularly important when the recommended agent is a new or infrequently employed drug.

Some drugs and medical devices presented in this publication have Food and Drug Administration (FDA) clearance for limited use in restricted research settings. It is the responsibility of the health care provider to ascertain the FDA status of each drug or device planned for use in their clinical practice.

10 9 8 7 6 5 4 3 2

TO ALEXANDER LEAF, M.D. for his foresight, encouragement, and support

Contents

15. Psychiatric and Behavioral Problems 1147

16. Allied Fields 1227

Contributors

Ernie-Paul Barrette, M.D.
Assistant in Medicine
Department of Medicine
Instructor
Department of Medicine
Harvard Medical School
Boston, Massachusetts

Michael J. Barry, M.D.
Chief
General Medicine Unit
Massachusetts General Hospital
Associate Professor
Department of Medicine
Harvard Medical School
Boston, Massachusetts

Arthur J. Barsky III M.D.
Director of Psychosomatic Research
Department of Psychiatry
Brigham and Women's Hospital
Professor
Department of Psychiatry
Harvard Medical School
Boston, Massachusetts

J. Andrew Billings, M.D.
Director
Palliative Care Service
Massachusetts General Hospital
Co-Director
Center for Palliative Care
Harvard Medical School
Boston, Massachusetts

Stephen L. Boswell, M.D.
Executive Director
Fenway Community Health Center
Instructor in Medicine
Infectious Disease Unit
Massachusetts General Hospital
Harvard Medical School
Boston, Massachusetts

Robert J. Boyd M.D.
Visiting Orthopaedic Surgeon
Massachusetts General Hospital
Assistant Clinical Professor of Orthopedics
Harvard Medical School
Boston, Massachusetts

David C. Brewster, M.D.
Division of Vascular Surgery
Massachusetts General Hospital
Clinical Professor of Surgery
Harvard Medical School
Boston, Massachusetts

M. Cornelia Cremens, M.D.
Assistant in Psychiatry and Medicine
Massachusetts General Hospital
Instructor in Psychiatry and Medicine
Harvard Medical School
Boston, Massachusetts

Carolyn J. Crimmins-Hintlian, M.D.
Business Manager/Nutritionist
Massachusetts General Hospital
Associate in Ambulatory Care and Prevention
Harvard Medical School
Boston, Massachusetts

Benjamin Davis, M.D.
Assistant Physician
Department of Infectious Disease
Massachusetts General Hospital
Instructor in Medicine
Harvard Medical School
Boston, Massachusetts

Thomas Delaney, M.D.
Chief, Department of Radiation Oncology
Massachusetts General Hospital
Boston, Massachusetts

Jules L. Dienstag, M.D.
Physician
Gastrointestinal Unit
Massachusetts General Hospital
Associate Professor of Medicine
Department of Medicine
Harvard Medical School
Boston, Massachusetts

Linda L. Emanuel, M.D., Ph.D.
Professor of Medicine
Director, Interdisciplinary Program in Professionalism and
    Human Rights
Northwestern Medical School
Chicago, Illinois

Leslie S. -T. Fang, M.D.
Clinical Director
Medical Services Associates
Massachusetts General Hospital
Boston, Massachusetts

Mason W. Freeman, M.D.
Unit Chief, Lipid Metabolism
Medical Director, Lipid Clinic
Co-Director, Lipid Assay Laboratory
Director, Lipid Metabolism Laboratory
Massachusetts General Hospital
Boston, Massachusetts

Lawrence S. Friedman, M.D.
Physician, Gastrointestinal Unit
Chief, Walter Bauer Firm (Medical Services)
Massachusetts General Hospital
Associate Professor of Medicine
Harvard Medical School
Boston, Massachusetts

Nancy J. Gagliano, M.D.
Clinical Director
Women's Health Associates
Associate Medical Director
MGPO
Massachusetts General Hospital
Boston, Massachusetts

Paul J. Gethner, M.D.
Clinical Associate Professor of Medicine (Dermatology)
University of California, Los Angeles
School of Medicine
Los Angeles, California

Ellie J.C. Goldstein, M.D.
Director
RM Alden Research Lab
Santa Monica - UCLA Medical Center
Santa Monica, California
Clinical Professor of Medicine
University of California, Los Angeles
School of Medicine
Los Angeles, California

John D. Goodson, M.D.
Staff Physician
Department of Medicine
Massachusetts General Hospital
Associate Professor of Medicine
Harvard Medical School
Boston, Massachusetts

Todd E. Gorman, M.D.
Assistant Professor of Medicine
University of Vermont Medical School
Fletcher Allen Health Center
Burlington, Vermont

Allan H. Goroll, M.D.
Physician
Department of Medicine
Massachusetts General Hospital
Associate Professor of Medicine
Harvard Medical School
Boston, Massachusetts

Elizabeth S. Gould, O.D.
Optometrist
Ophthalmic Consultants of Boston
Boston, Massachusetts

David A. Greenberg, M.D.
Executive Director
Chicago Eye Institute
Chicago, Illinois

A. Julianna Gulya, M.D.
Clinical Professor
Department of Otolaryngology Head and Neck Surgery
George Washington University
Washington, DC

Eleanor Z. Hanna, Ph.D.
Psychologist
Department of Psychiatry
Massachusetts General Hospital
Instructor
Department of Psychiatry
Harvard Medical School
Boston, Massachusetts

Gale S. Haydock, M.D.
Associate Physician
Department of Medicine
Massachusetts General Hospital
Instructor in Medicine
Department of Medicine
Harvard Medical School
Boston, Massachusetts

Robert A. Hughes, M.D.
Medical Director
Anticoagulant Therapy Unit
Massachusetts General Hospital
Assistant Professor
Department of Medicine
Harvard Medical School
Boston, Massachusetts

Elaine M. Hylek, M.D.
Assistant Physician
Department of Medicine
Massachusetts General Hospital
Instructor in Medicine
Department of Medicine
Harvard Medical School
Boston, Massachusetts

Michael A. Jenike, M.D.
Associate and Chief
Department of Psychiatry
Massachusetts General Hospital
Professor of Psychiatry
Department of Psychiatry
Harvard Medical School
Boston, Massachusetts

Jesse B. Jupiter, M.D.
Director, Hand Surgery
Department Orthopaedic Surgery
Massachusetts General Hospital
Professor
Department of Orthopaedic Surgery
Harvard Medical School
Boston, Massachusetts

John P. Kelly, D.M.D., M.D.
Chief
Division of Oral and Maxillofacial Surgery
Long Island Jewish Medical Center
New Hyde Park, New York
Chair and Associate Professor
Oral and Maxillofacial Surgery
School of Dental Medicine
SUNY at Stony Brook
Stony Brook, New York

Linda A. King, M.D.
Assistant Professor in Medicine
Division of General Internal Medicine
Section of Palliative Care and Medical Ethics
University of Pittsburgh School of Medicine
Pittsburgh, Pennsylvania

William A. Kormos, M.D., M.P.H.
Assistant in Medicine
Department of Medicine
Massachusetts General Hospital
Instructor in Medicine
Department of Medicine
Harvard Medical School
Boston, Massachusetts

Eric Kortz, M.D.
Private Pracatice
Englewood, California

Eric L. Krakauer, M.D., Ph.D.
Associate Director
Palliative Care Service
Massachusetts General Hospital
Instructor
Department of Medicine and Social Medicine
Harvard Medical School
Boston, Massachusetts

Richard R. Liberthson, M.D.
Physician and Pediatrician
Department of Cardiology
Massachusetts General Hospital
Associate Professor
Department of Pediatrics
Harvard Medical School
Boston, Massachusetts

Patrick L. Lillard, M.D.
Clinical Director, Addiction Services
Department of Psychiatry
Massachusetts General Hospital
Professor of Psychiatry
Harvard Medical School
Boston, Massachusetts

Alice Y. Liu, M.D., Ph.D.
Senior Resident in Dermatology
The Combined UCLA - VA West Los Angeles
    Dermatology Residency Program
Los Angeles, California

Nicholas J. Lowe, M.D.
Professor of Dermatology
University of California, Los Angeles
School of Medicine
Director
Skin Research Foundation of California
Santa Monica, California

Charles J. McCabe, M.D.
Associate Chief
Emergency Services
Massachusetts General Hospital
Associate Professor of Surgery
Harvard Medical School
Boston, Massachusetts

William E. Minichiello, M.D.
Associate Director, OCD Institute
Massachusetts General Hospital
Associate Professor
Department of Psychiatry
Harvard Medical School
Boston, Massachusetts

Albert G. Mulley, Jr., M.D., M.P.P.
Chief, General Internal Medicine Unit
Massachusetts General Hospital
Associate Professor
Department of Medicine
Harvard Medical School
Boston, Massachusetts

Samuel R. Nussbaum, M.D.
Professor of Clinical Medicine
Washington University School of Medicine
St. Louis, Missouri

L. Christine Oliver, M.D.
Associate Physician
Department of Medicine
Massachusetts General Hospital
Assistant Professor
Department of Medicine
Harvard Medical School
Boston, Massachusetts

Susan Oliverio, M.D., M.P.H.
Assistant in Medicine
Department of Medicine
Massachusetts General Hospital
Instructor in Medicine
Harvard Medical School
Boston, Massachusetts

Amber Owen, M.D.
Clinical Research Fellow
Clinical Research Specialists
Santa Monica, California

Amy A. Pruitt, M.D.
Staff Neurologist
Department of Neurology
Hospital of the University of Pennsylvania
Associate Professor
Department of Neurology
University of Pennsylvania Medical Center
Philadelphia, Pennsylvania

Scott L. Rauch, M.D.
Chief of Psychiatry
Massachusetts General Hospital
Associate Professor of Psychiatry
Department of Psychiatry
Harvard Medical School
Boston, Massachusetts

Claudia U. Richter, M.D.
Associate Surgeon
Department of Ophthalmology
Massachusetts Eye and Ear Infirmary
Assistant in Ophthalmology
Department of Ophthalmology
Harvard Medical School
Boston, Massachusetts

James M. Richter, M.D.
Medical Director
Massachusetts General Physicians Organization
Assistant Professor of Medicine
Department of Medicine
Harvard Medical School
Boston, Massachusetts

Nancy A. Rigotti, M.D.
Director
Tobacco Research and Treatment Center
Massachusetts General Hospital
Associate Professor
Departmental Medicine
Harvard Medical School
Boston, Massachusetts

David Ring, M.D.
Department of Orthopaedic Surgery
Massachusetts General Hospital
Instructor
Department of Orthopaedic Surgery
Harvard Medical School
Boston, Massachusetts

Lawrence J. Ronan, M.D.
Director, Combined Program in Medicine/Pediatrics
Massachusetts General Hospital
Instructor, Department of Pediatrics
Harvard Medical School
Boston, Massachusetts

Edward T. Ryan, M.D.
Director
Travelers' Advice and Immunization Center
Director
Tropical and Geographic Medicine
Division of Infectious Diseases
Massachusetts General Hospital
Instructor in Medicine
Harvard Medical School
Boston, Massachusetts

Linda C. Shafer, M.D.
Psychiatrist
Department of Psychiatry
Massachusetts General Hospital
Instructor in Psychiatry
Department of Psychiatry
Harvard Medical School
Boston, Massachusetts

William V. R. Shellow, M.D.
Chief, Department of Dermatology
West Los Angeles VA Healthcare Center
Professor of Medicine (Dermatology)
University of California, Los Angeles
School of Medicine
Los Angeles, California

Harvey B. Simon, M.D.
Physician
Department of Medicine
Massachusetts General Hospital
Associate Professor of Medicine
Harvard Medical School
Health Sciences Technology Faculty
Massachusetts Institute of Technology
Boston, Massachusetts

Arthur J. Sober, M.D.
Associate Chief
Department of Dermatology
Massachusetts General Hospital
Professor
Department of Dermatology
Harvard Medical School
Boston, Massachusetts

Roger F. Steinert, M.D.
Surgeon
Massachusetts Eye and Ear Infirmary
Boston Eye Surgery and Laser Center
Ophthalmic Consultants of Boston
Associate Clinical Professor
Department of Ophthalmology
Harvard Medical School
Boston, Massachusetts

John D. Stoeckle, M.D.
Physician
Department of Medicine
Massachusetts General Hospital
Professor of Medicine, Emeritus
Department of Medicine
Harvard Medical School
Boston, Massachusetts

Katharine K. Treadway, M.D.
Physician
Department of Medicine
Massachusetts General Hospital
Assistant Professor
Department of Medicine
Harvard Medical School
Boston, Massachusetts

Jeffrey B. Weilburg, M.D.
Associate Medical Director
Massachusetts General Physician Organization
Associate Professor of Psychiatry
Department of Psychiatry
Harvard Medical School
Boston, Massachusetts

Debra F. Weinstein, M.D.
Director of Graduate Medical Education
Massachusetts General Hospital
Instructor in Medicine
Department of Medicine
Harvard Medical School
Boston, Massachusetts

William R. Wilson, M.D.
Chief
Department of Otolaryngology/Head and Neck Surgery
The George Washington University Medical Center
Professor
Otolaryngology/Head and Neck Surgery
The George Washington University
Washington, DC

John J. Worthington III, M.D.
Staff Psychiatrist
Department of Psychiatry
Massachusetts General Hospital
Instructor
Department of Psychiatry
Harvard Medical School
Boston, Massachusetts

Preface

We celebrate the new millenium with the fourth edition of *Primary Care Medicine*. In the twenty years since publication of the first edition, the primary care agenda has expanded from the modernization of generalism to reform of health care delivery. Propelled by its emphasis on comprehensive care and coordination, primary care has moved from the periphery of medicine to center stage. With this move comes ever-increasing pressure to ensure that care is not only personalized and high-quality, but also cost-effective. Such responsibilities and expectations pose both the challenge and promise of modern primary care, which the fourth edition is designed to help learners master and practitioners fulfill.

Those who have used the book in the past will recognize our continued commitment to a terse yet thoughtful, problem-based style. A comprehensive index plus well-marked chapter sections, subsections, and chapter cross-references facilitate quick, easy location of desired information. Emphasis is placed on key clinical data essential to decision-making and on critical use of tests and therapies that truly add value to overall management. Practical recommendations that incorporate the best available evidence, expert consensus guidelines, clinical judgment, and everyday common sense are put forward at the end of every chapter (often in bulleted form). Each chapter includes an annotated bibliography that highlights and encourages the reading of the best available studies and analyses; over 2,000 new references have been added for this edition.

Like previous editions, this edition represents a major rewriting. Every chapter has been revised and many extensively rewritten to incorporate the important advances in medicine that have taken place over the last 5 years. Major changes in the approach to such conditions as HIV infection, diabetes, syncope, coronary disease, heart failure, peptic ulcer disease, osteoporosis, menopause, hepatitis, rheumatoid arthritis, inflammatory bowel disease, and asthma are covered in depth. New sections on chronic pain, domestic violence, ethical challenges of managed care, adolescent medicine, and alternative/complementary medicine have been added, reflecting further expansion of the primary care role and new treatment modalities. The best evidence on safety and efficacy of alternative/complementary therapies is provided to facilitate patient education and rational choice of therapy. Moreover, the chapters on estimating and communicating risk and prognosis and on interpreting evidence of therapeutic efficacy are designed to help provide the thoughtful advise and effective counsel patients expect and appreciate from their primary care physician, even in this era of "surfing the net."

We continue to be deeply moved and humbled by the enthusiastic responses to each new edition of *Primary Care Medicine*. The editors and our colleagues have worked hard to make this edition the best one yet and hope it will prove useful for learning and patient care. In keeping with its pioneering tradition (e.g., first textbook in the field), *Primary Care Medicine* is about to become the first "living" textbook of primary care, to be continuously updated and made available on the internet as new advances emerge from the scientific literature. See you on the Web!

Allan H. Goroll, M.D.
Albert G. Mulley, Jr., MD., M.P.P.

Acknowledgments

Readers familiar with previous editions of *Primary Care Medicine* will note the absence from this edition of our fellow editor and friend, Dr. Lawrence May, who departs because he has assumed a senior management position in industry. Dr. May was a founding editor and continued through the third edition. His insights and initiative contributed significantly to the original content, style and format of the book. His combination of rigorous training, sound clinical judgement and decades of experience as a community-based primary care physician helped ensure that *Primary Care Medicine* address the realities of daily front-line clinical practice. Dr. May remains an Associate Clinical Professor at UCLA School of Medicine and continues in clinical practice. We want to acknowledge his important contributions to previous editions and honor him as an *Editor Emeritus*.

Although this is a book written predominantly by primary care physicians for primary care physicians, we are nonetheless most grateful for and dependent upon the contributions of our subspecialty colleagues. Special mention goes to Dr. William Shellow, Professor of Dermatology, UCLA, and Dr. Amy Pruitt, Associate Professor of Neurology, Univ. of Pennsylvania, both of whom took major responsibility for important sections of the book. Also our thanks to Dr. James M. Richter, Associate Professor of Medicine, Harvard Univ., for authoring many of the gastroenterology chapters, and Dr. Roger Steinert, Professor of Ophthalmology, Harvard Univ., and Dr. Claudia Richter of Harvard Univ. for their ophthalmology contributions.

Over the years and 3 previous editions, many individuals have participated in the writing or revision of many chapters. Listing all is not possible here, but those who contributed to a chapter in the 3rd edition, but not in the fourth are acknowledged here because of the usefulness of their contributions to the collective effort of preparing the 4th edition. These persons and the chapters they worked on include Dr. Harvey B. Simon for prior work on Chapters 6, 49, 50, 51, 52, 124, 141, 219, 220; Dr. Gregory B. Curfman for prior work on Chapters 31, 36; Dr. Deborah F. Weinstein for prior work on Chapter 63; Dr. Frederick W. Ruymann for prior work on Chapter 73; Dr. Jerry Younger for prior work on Chapters 89, 90; Dr. Samuel B. Nussbaum for prior work on Chapters 96, 98, 102, 144, and 164; Dr. Anne W. Moulton for prior work on Chapters 114, 115, 116, 117; Dr. Karyn M. Montgomery for prior work on Chapters 116, 117; Dr. Elaine Carlson for prior work on Chapters 114, 115; Drs. Flora Treger and Jennifer Jeremiah for prior work on Chapter 121; Dr. Robert Boyd for prior work on Chapters 151, 152; Dr. Stephen J. Friedman for prior work on Chapters 178, 184, 195, 197; Dr. Ellie Goldstein for prior work on Chapters 190, 196; Dr. Ronald M. Reisner for prior work on Chapter 185; and Dr. Jeffrey E. Galpin for prior work on Chapters 192, 193; Dr. Jerrold F. Rosenbaum for prior work on Chapter 226; and Dr. Steven E. Hyman for prior work on Chapter 227.

The dedication and commitment to quality of our publishing colleagues at Lippincott, Williams and Wilkins, especially Mr. Richard Winters, the publishing editor, and Delois Patterson, managing editor, continue to be extraordinary and greatly valued. They are but a few of the many Lippincott publishing professionals who have contributed to the success of *Primary Care Medicine* and to whom we are most indebted.

Primary Care
Medicine

1

Principles of
Primary Care

1

The Practice of Primary Care

Part 1: The Tasks of Primary Care

JOHN D. STOECKLE

DEFINITION OF PRIMARY CARE

Primary care is coordinated, comprehensive, and personal care, available on both a first-contact and a continuous basis. It incorporates several tasks: medical diagnosis and treatment, psychological assessment and management, personal support, communication of information about illness, prevention, and health maintenance.

This book addresses the clinical problems encountered by primary care physicians in the office practice of adult medicine. In this setting, the physician's responsibilities and tasks extend beyond the narrow technologic confines of medical diagnosis and treatment. Although a great deal of effort must be focused on accurate diagnosis and technically sound therapy, the other clinical tasks that complete the very definition of primary care also assume major importance.

Alongside this clinical definition of primary care stands a plethora of other definitions; these derive from organizational, functional, professional, and academic perspectives. For example, policy planners have defined primary care as a *level of medical services*, one that is provided outside the hospital. Presumably, primary care (community-based services) is, then, a less technical practice in comparison with secondary care (consultant or specialty services) and tertiary care (hospital services). This organizational definition provides a scheme for the allocation of public resources among these health services, each of which has a distinct professional, economic, institutional, and political structure. For another definition, Alpert and Charney have looked at important *patient care functions* of doctors—namely, to provide access, continuity, and integration. Although this view is useful in describing the functions performed by practitioners for their patients within organized health services, it does not define the content of their clinical work. From the standpoint of professionalism, primary care has been defined as a *specialty* concentrating on general medicine practiced outside the hospital but devoid of the special procedures and technology that typically characterize specialization. This definition has been useful in organizing general internal medicine, general

pediatrics, and family practice and in designing a new curriculum for the education and training of doctors. From the university comes still another definition of primary care as an *academic discipline* concerned with the expansion of knowledge unique to primary practice and personal care, a definition that contains the promise of a departmental position for primary care in the medical school.

Although each of these definitions presents a particular perspective about primary care and serves some special purpose, none explains the primary care physician's day-to-day work with patients.

From the perspective of the doctor's practice, primary care can be defined by several tasks: (a) medical diagnosis and treatment; (b) psychological diagnosis and treatment; (c) personal support of patients of all backgrounds, in all stages of illness; (d) communication of information about diagnosis, treatment, prevention, and prognosis; (e) maintenance of patients with chronic illness; and (f) prevention of disability and disease through detection, education, behavioral change, and preventive treatment. These tasks comprise the clinical work of doctors providing primary care. They not only restate medicine's central mandate of patient care but also constitute a clinical definition of primary care to which the information in this text is applied.

TASKS AND THEIR RATIONALE

Except for medical diagnosis and treatment, the tasks that define primary care may seem merely vocational—that is, practical but not scientifically based. However, social science research has provided a logical and rational basis for the clinical work of primary care. Attention to the skillful conduct of these tasks appears to improve outcomes and reduce the risk that patients will file malpractice claims. The data derived from these studies concern the patient's *illness* rather than the doctor's definition of *disease*; they are contained in the cognitive, communicative, and behavioral processes by which the patient defines

1

being ill; and they are found in the clinical and social science literature on such topics as the patient's emotional reactions, personality, expectations, requests, attributions, views of treatment, and social networks, to mention but a few. Knowledge concerning such aspects of care in conjunction with statistical thinking contributes a rational framework for the tasks of primary care.

Medical Diagnosis and Treatment remain central tasks, although they are by no means the end point of care. As the patient's first contact with medical services, the primary doctor not only must be knowledgeable about disease but also must exercise critical judgment in determining the scope, site, and pace of the medical workup and management. In organizing diagnosis and management, the physician needs to know the clinical presentation and natural history of illness, the uses and limits of the laboratory, and the indications for and shortcomings of invasive tests and therapeutic measures. In continuing care, the issues are the same. The doctor's critical attitude toward the use of technology and the referral of patients for special therapies or diagnostic techniques remains essential. Methods developed in clinical epidemiology and decision analysis that help the clinician rationally choose among a sometimes bewildering array of diagnostic and therapeutic options are discussed in Chapter 2 and 5.

Psychological Diagnosis and Treatment and Personal Support complement the medical components of care. Studies documenting the relationship between emotional reactions and illness, coupled with surveys showing a high frequency of such reactions in office practice, underscore their importance in patients seeking medical help. The recognition of anxiety, depression, sexual dysfunction, personality disturbance, and psychosis is necessary for the interpretation of bodily complaints, the communication of personal feelings, and the joint decision of doctor and patient regarding acceptable and effective treatment plans.

The recognition of emotional reactions alone is insufficient. The doctor's response to the normal patient's psychological defenses is essential to securing cooperation and relieving anxiety. Understanding the patient's defenses and personality style allows the clinician to provide meaningful support and respond appropriately to the patient's emotional needs. The care rendered is then likely to be perceived as personal and psychologically acceptable. Much of this analysis of the psychological aspects of clinical practice derives from classic case studies by Kahana and Bibring, Lipsett, Balaint, and Zaborenko et al. on the emotional reactions and personality traits of patients with medical disorders. More recent qualitative surveys of medical practice populations document the importance of emotional states, especially depression, in the outcome of treatment. Written exercises involving emotional expression have been shown in randomized trials to increase subjective well-being, decrease care-seeking behavior, and improve outcomes of some chronic conditions.

Eliciting and Addressing Patient Expectations and Requests are also important. *Expectations* often play a major part in seeking help, complying with treatment, and feeling satisfied with care. In their studies of illness behavior and patients' use of doctors, Zola and Mechanic viewed expectations as explanations of patients' decisions to see a doctor. In health centers in Israel, Shuval et al. found specific expectations of visits to doctors: status enhancement in seeing socially important professionals; catharsis of grief, anger, and despair; sanctioning of failure to cope; and understanding and control of illness through medical

"scientific" explanations. This brief list is by no means complete, for along with these so-called latent expectations are traditional or "real" medical ones—for example, that the doctor is a healer of disease and possesses techniques for its control, relief, or cure. Such expectations not only explain the decision to seek medical care but also are, in fact, elements of the clinical tasks of personal support and communication of information about illness.

Newer clinical studies by Lazare and colleagues have separated *requests* from expectations. Requests are specific and concrete helping actions and behaviors identified by patients. These studies identified some 14 requests and demonstrated that their prompt recognition and negotiation benefited both patient and doctor. The doctor's interest in ascertaining what treatment the patient wants indicates a reciprocity that is associated with greater satisfaction and adherence to medical advice. These efforts are part of the task of personal support and management. Still other elements of the management task, such as decisions about continued care, referral, and discharge, are also realized through an understanding of requests; thus, physicians need both to elicit and to respond to them.

Communication of Information about Illness. The need to inform, explain, reassure, and advise patients is essential to primary care. This task often depends on a knowledge of the patient's attributions (i.e., what the patient thinks is the cause of illness). If the patient's *attributions* differ from the doctor's and are not uncovered, the patient's anxieties may not be relieved, nor will the doctor's explanation be accepted. Knowing how and what to tell the patient about an illness is often difficult, especially if the patient's interpretation of the illness has not been elicited.

Mechanic, for example, suggests that patients with bodily complaints may go to the primary care doctor not for relief of physical discomfort but rather to learn what is causing their complaints and sometimes to obtain reassurance that the causes of their complaints are less serious than they may have thought. Such confirmation or correction of the patient's attributions is a kind of "attribution therapy." From a broader perspective, Kleinman assigns to attributions a major function in all medical care systems—namely, the control of illness through the explanation of its cause. In effect, the doctor's clinical or scientific explanations of illness provide labels, names, and models so that the patient feels the illness can be understood and controlled, regardless of its technical treatment. In essence, the patient's beliefs about illness need to be elicited so that they can be used in explanation, education, and reassurance (see appendix).

Maintenance of the Chronically Ill requires continuous, long-term treatment and is a distinct task of primary care. Here, obtaining patient compliance is essential because most long-term treatment now takes place without daily medical supervision, and most of that treatment requires the self-administration of drugs. To improve adherence to therapy, it has become increasingly important to learn about the *patient's views of treatment* and actual self-treatment. So far, the record on adherence to treatment has not been good. A wide discrepancy between what is prescribed and what is done typifies the literature of "following the doctor's orders," and the problem seems to be as much the doctor's as the patient's.

Knowledge about patients' views and behaviors can be used to design more effective therapeutic regimens and to alter therapeutic directions. Moreover, the act of eliciting information may improve communication between doctor and patient, thus strengthening their relationship and further promoting therapeutic efforts. More studies of patient views of treatment and of the dynamics of the doctor–patient relationship should provide new knowledge that can be used to enhance compliance.

Prevention of Disease and Disability, an essential task of primary care, emphasizes screening and the assessment of risk and function. With early intervention through health education, behavioral change, and preventive treatment, some of the expected morbidity, disability, and mortality may be delayed—if not prevented—and costly technologic interventions and therapies avoided. The primary physician needs to know which conditions and risk factors are worth screening for and how best to detect and effectively manage them (see Chapter 3).

A less commonly considered but no less important aspect of prevention involves attention to the patient's *social network* because illness is often precipitated by a disruption of interpersonal relationships. For example, Parkes and others have noted an increased mortality and morbidity among recent widows, and Zola has reported that interpersonal crises are among the most frequent of five common circumstances that motivate patients to seek medical attention. Knowledge of patients' social situations can help in the prevention of illness and visits to the doctor by focusing attention on stresses that might be precipitants. Attention to social networks is important for personal treatment. If significant loss or separation occurs, a major part of treatment can involve helping the patient reestablish a social network, thus lessening dependence on professional help from the doctor, nurse, or social worker. Patient illness narratives and doctors' clinical experiences illustrate that much of the work of care is done by patients themselves, their families, and their informal networks. Helping patients to share the preventive work with others can be of major benefit.

THE PROMISE OF PRIMARY CARE MEDICINE

So far, the clinical tasks of primary care have been proposed as a perspective from which readers can view the information in this text. In addition, the tasks also promise changes in our ideas about standards of treatment, doctor–patient relations, professional relations, organization, prevention, clinical excellence, and clinical effectiveness.

Treatment. The ideal of personal treatment is revived and reemphasized. Although it is not entirely dead, the increasing size, specialization, and organization of practice often make personal, patient-oriented treatment a luxury rather than a medical care necessity. Patient-centered treatment also means that specific therapeutic regimens must be not only technically correct but also designed to be acceptable to patients, especially because more patients than ever are being cared for on an outpatient basis.

Doctor–Patient Relationship. Patient-centered treatment in primary care practice implies a doctor–patient relationship in which the doctor acts out several behaviors that will enhance the patient's participation in care and treatment:

1. Making the relationship more democratic by eliciting and responding to patients' preferences in decisions regarding the scope of diagnosis and alternatives of treatment.
2. Developing patient participation by transmitting appropriate information so that patients can make intelligent choices.

3. Attending to patients' feelings about illness and treatment with regard, genuine concern, and empathy.
4. Providing helping actions that are person-centered by eliciting, acknowledging, and responding to patients' own perspectives of their illness and care.
5. Responding by negotiation to patients' choices, decisions, and requests; similarly, acknowledging and negotiating conflict, even if in the relationship itself.
6. Promoting health education, self-help, and preventive behaviors by communicating information about diagnosis, treatment, and prevention.
7. Conveying respect for the person of the patient without regard to the patient's gender, race, ethnicity, age, or social class.

Social Change and the Doctor–Patient Relationship. Changes in our patient population, practice organization, and information technologies require changes in the uses of the relationship to continue the improvement of care. Interpreters for the interview, assessments of the aged, advocacy for patients' treatment, and skill in the use of information technologies for patient education are needed.

Today, our patient population is older and more multicultural, trends that are predicted to continue as the United States remains an open society and longevity increases with better control of chronic disease. Patient care now requires understanding varied cultural backgrounds and performing functional assessments of older patients. The doctor in the clinical interview often needs the skills of a trained interpreter, not just the help of a family member. With older patients, there is the need to assess visual, auditory, vocal, and cognitive functions to help overcome or cope with communication barriers.

In a market economy of health care, practice organizations are becoming larger, incorporated, managed, and often commercialized. In incorporated practices, more physicians are employees. The doctor's shared decision making with the patient is often monitored and sometimes restricted, depending on health care plans and insurers. In the managed care setting, patients look upon the doctor to be their advocate and protect their interests.

With modern information technologies (especially through the Internet and Worldwide Web), patients can access and receive more information and instruction on disease management and obtain more mutual support and personal advice than ever before. Such improved access to information, if facilitated and guided by the primary care physician, can promote better patient understanding, compliance, and self-care.

Organization. The ambulatory practice organizations outside the hospital (offices, health centers, group practices, health maintenance organizations) have become essential sites for the delivery of primary care services. Because the goals of primary care include not only cure but also prevention and health maintenance, the ambulatory setting emerges as the major organizational locus for the delivery of primary care services. The move to outpatient care has been greatly facilitated by the direct availability to the primary physician of the major technologies for screening, diagnosis, and treatment. Even the management of chronic illness, one of society's major health problems, is now largely conducted in the outpatient setting.

Prevention. The ideal of prevention in practice has been to deal with the individual patient seeking help. Primary care medicine also examines the epidemiology of the entire practice, and even its community base, to institute a program of effective preventive intervention.

Clinical Excellence and Ethics. Skills in medical diagnosis and treatment have often been the only measure of clinical excellence. The ideal of excellence is now expanded to include all the tasks of primary care, the communicative as well as the technical. In making decisions about the use of technologies, new ethical considerations are also required. For the public accountability of medical practice, the primary physician must support professional group efforts that scientifically examine the appropriate use of medical technologies. These are now being conducted as outcome, clinical effectiveness, technology, and evidence-based assessments. In the care of individual patients, the primary physician must continue to elicit preferences and exercise discretionary decisions regarding the personal needs and benefit of each patient.

Clinical Effectiveness. The usual objective criteria for efficacy of diagnosis and treatment have been derived from the standards of clinical science. Consideration of subjective parameters, such as patient acceptance and a sense of well-being, is mandatory in the primary care setting and must be added to the assessment of clinical efficacy.

These themes on the clinical tasks and promises of primary care run through the chapters that follow, sometimes explicitly, sometimes latently; however, they are always central to providing personalized care to patients.

ANNOTATED BIBLIOGRAPHY

Alpert JJ, Charney E. The education of physicians for primary care. DHEW Publication No 74-31B. Washington, DC: US Government Printing Office, 1975. (*One of the original functional definitions of primary care.*)

Balaint M. The doctor, the patient and the illness. New York: International Universities Press, 1957. (*A classic study of the British general practitioner's negotiations with patients about diagnosis and treatment.*)

Kahana RJ, Bibring GL. Personality types in medical management. In: Zinberg NE, ed. Psychiatry and medical practice in a general hospital. New York: International Universities Press, 1965: 108. (*Classic discussion of the use of defense mechanisms derived from personality assessment in treatment.*)

Kanfert JM, Dutsch RW. Communication through interpreters in health care: ethical dilemmas arising from differences in class, culture, language, and power. J Clin Ethics 1994;8:71. (*Addresses the problems that language and cultural differences bring to the patient care setting.*)

Kasl SV, Cobb S. Health behavior, illness behavior and sick role behavior. I: Health and illness. Arch Environ Health 1966;12:245. (*A thorough review of sociological and psychiatric studies on the factors that lead to a decision to seek help.*)

Kleinman AM. Toward a comparative study of medical systems: an integrated approach to the study of the relationship of medicine and culture. Sci Med Man 1973;1:55. (*A study that examines the specific and general significance of attributions.*)

Kravitz RL, Cope OW, Bhrany V, et al. Internal medicine patients' expectations for care at office visits. J Gen Intern Med 1994;9:75. (*Rapid evolution in requests and needs.*)

Lazare A, Cohen F, Mignone R, et al. The walk-in patient as a customer: a key dimension in evaluation and treatment. Am J Orthopsychiatry 1972;42:872. (*Classic article introducing the concept of the patient as "customer."*)

Lindemann E. Symptomatology and management of acute grief. Am J Psychiatry 1944;101:141. (*A classic article on the symptoms in medical patients.*)

Levinson W, Roter DL, Mullooly JP, et al. Physician–patient communication: the relationship with malpractice claims among primary care physicians and surgeons. JAMA 1997;227:555. (*An examination of interview behavior. Less-rushed visits, the use of humor, and providing an orientation to the visit were independent predictors of less likelihood to be sued; the use of facilitation showed a trend to lowering the risk of law suits.*)

Lipsett D. Medical and psychological characteristics of "crocks." Psychiatr Med 1970;15:293. (*Classic description of the patient who needs to have bodily complaints; suggests management taking this need into account.*)

McKinlay JB. Social networks, lay consultation and help-seeking behavior. Social Forces 1973;51:275. (*Uses networks to explain differences in help-seeking behavior.*)

McWhinney IR. General practice as an academic discipline. Lancet 1966;1:419. (*Defines primary care from an academic perspective.*)

Mechanic D. Medical sociology. New York: Free Press, 1968. (*A classic text detailing the interaction of social factors and illness.*)

Mechanic D. Social psychologic factors affecting the presentation of bodily complaints. N Engl J Med 1972;286:1132. (*A sociologic study that examines the factors influencing a patient's decision to seek medical help.*)

Mulley AG. Applying effectiveness and outcomes research to clinical practice. In: Heitoff HA, Lohr KM, eds. Effectiveness and outcomes in health care. Washington, DC: National Academy Press, 1990. (*A very useful overview.*)

Parkes CM. Effects of bereavement on physical and mental health—a study of medical records of widows. Br Med J 1964;2:274. (*One of a number of studies documenting increased morbidity and mortality among widows shortly after the death of their husbands.*)

Quill TE, Brody H. Physician recommendations and patient autonomy: finding a balance between physician power and patient choice. Ann Intern Med 1996;125:763. (*Provides recommendations that promote collaboration.*)

Shuval JT, Antonovsky A, Davies AM. Social function of medical practice: doctor–patient relationship in Israel. San Francisco: Jossey-Bass, 1970. (*An analysis of the rates and reasons for medical visits; provides a typology of the uses of medical visits.*)

Smyth JM, Stone AA, Hurewitz A, et al. Effects of writing about stressful experiences on symptom reduction in patients with asthma or rheumatoid arthritis. JAMA 1999;281:1304. (*In this randomized trial, patients with asthma and rheumatoid arthritis who were asked to write about their most stressful experience demonstrated clinically important improvement in outcomes after 4 months.*)

Stewart AL, Greenfield S, Hays RD, et al. Functional studies and well-being of patients with chronic conditions. JAMA 1989;262:907. (*A demonstration of the usefulness of expanded outcomes measures that include emotional and functional elements.*)

Stoeckle JD. Reflections on modern doctoring. Milbank Q 1988; 66:79. (*A discussion of some of the organizational, professional, and ethical issues involved in the contemporary practice of medicine.*)

Stoeckle JD, Zola IK, Davidson GE. On going to see the doctor. The contributions of the patient to the decision to seek medical aid. J Chronic Dis 1963;16:975. (*An analysis of patients' expectations in medical practice.*)

Stoeckle JD, Zola IK, Davidson GE. The quality and significance of psychological distress in medical patients. J Chronic Dis 1964;17:959. (*A review of studies of the psychological distress of medical patients.*)

Waitzkin H, Stoeckle JD. The communication of information about illness: clinical, sociological and methodological considerations. In: Lipowski ZJ, ed. Advances in psychosomatic medicine: psychosocial aspects of physical illness. Basel: S Karger, 1972:180 (vol 8). (*The role of communication in the patient–doctor relationship and a review of the research on communication in medical practice.*)

Woloshin S, Bickell NA, Schwartz LM, et al. Language barriers in medicine in the US. JAMA 1995;273:724. (*Reviews the scope of language in medical encounters.*)

Xuegin G, Henderson G. Rethinking ethnicity and health care. Springfield: Charles C Thomas Publisher, 1999. (*Comprehensive discussion of the increasingly important role of ethnicity in patient care.*)

Zaborenko RN, Zaborenko L, Hengea RA. The psychodynamics of physicianhood. Psychiatry 1970;33:102. (*An illustration of the importance of understanding patients' defenses and personalities and the uses this knowledge may have in the treatment relationship.*)

Zola IK. Studying the decision to see a doctor. In: Lipowski ZJ, ed. Advances in psychosomatic medicine: psychosocial aspects of physical illness. Basel: S Karger, 1972:216 (vol 8). (*Describes the typology of decisions and their dynamics.*)

Appendix: Approaches to Encouraging Compliance

That 20% to 80% of patients do not comply with medical advice is repeatedly quoted. Such dismal statistics are derived from a rigid definition of compliance as patients' all-or-nothing adherence to medical instructions, whereas their treatment behaviors are far more variable, ranging from the optimal cooperative response to the ritualistic, retreatist, and innovative. Regardless of the extent and variability of noncompliance, patients' adherence to medication regimens is critical in effectively treating medical disorders, as is their adoption and learning of appropriate behaviors (in regard to eating, exercise, smoking, drinking, relaxation, and use of drugs) for preventing disease.

Explanations and theories of noncompliance have focused on patients' beliefs, attitudes, expectations, and feelings that interfere with their "taking pills" or "changing habits." Even if such factors do interfere, they can be changed. Compliance can be improved by practitioner–patient communication that responds to patient views and develops the patient's ability to adhere to medical advice through education and the learning of new behaviors. By making the clinical decision a "shared" process, the physician empowers the patient and fosters a partnership that enhances compliance and outcomes.

Specific Strategies

The education/communication strategies and techniques helpful in facilitating compliance begin with the doctor–patient relationship. A positive, mutually respectful doctor–patient relationship is important in making the patient "ready" to receive patient education and negotiate the goals and means of treatment. Moreover, the physician's explanations and educational efforts, in turn, contribute to that relationship. Specific strategies utilize persuasion, medical advice, feedback, and monitoring.

Persuasion, or Why Do It?

1. Describe immediate and long-term treatment benefits along with health risk and cost. If possible, present treatment options and acknowledge if the rationale differs from the views of the patient.

2. Assist patients in clarifying their priorities (requests) for treatment (e.g., patients presenting with pain may request an explanation rather than medication).

3. Use your expertise, experience, and relationship to assert your own expectations for patient compliance in supporting the patient's treatment choice and capacity to carry it out.

Medical Advice, or What to Do

1. Adapt instructions to the patient's language and knowledge level, responding to any misconceptions about treatment.

2. Make directions explicit, simple, personalized, and operational (how many, what kind, and when to take "pills"; organizing "pill taking" into the routine of the patient's everyday life).

3. Use multiple modes of communication, both verbal and written instructions, and, when available, audiovisual materials that reinforce general knowledge about treatment. Enlist other members of the clinical team in providing instructions; also recruit family in the educational process.

Feedback, or What Advice Was Negotiated?

1. Have the patient repeat the medical advice given and the rationale for it.

2. Have the patient rehearse how medical advice will be carried out.

3. Jointly plan return visits, phone calls, and additional reviews with clinical team (nurse practitioners, physician assistants) if needed.

Monitoring Compliance, or What Have You Done?

1. At return visits, review the patient's compliance by direct questioning, again eliciting the rationale along with the problems the patient has experienced in treatment.

2. Use information to reexplain or redesign treatment, reinforce behaviors, and reward the patient.

3. Encourage and organize the patient's self-monitoring of treatment (e.g., blood pressure measurements).

In general, these educational strategies and tactics are not systematically carried out in practitioner–patient communication. Their use in patient education should result in greater compliance with medical advice.

ANNOTATED BIBLIOGRAPHY

Kaplan SH, Greenfield S, Gandek B, et al. Characteristics of physicians with participatory decision-making styles. Ann Intern Med 1996;124:497. (*Documents the qualities and benefits of participatory decision making.*)

Quill TE, Brody H. Physician recommendations and patient autonomy: finding a balance between physician power and patient choice. Ann Intern Med 1996;125:763. (*Provides recommendations that promote collaboration.*)

Sackett DL, Snow JC. The magnitude of compliance and non-compliance. In: Haynes R, Sackett D, eds. Compliance in health care. Baltimore: Johns Hopkins University Press, 1979. (*One of many useful chapters in this book devoted to both academic and practical aspects of the compliance issue.*)

Stimson GV. Obeying the doctor's orders: a view from the other side. Soc Sci Med 1974;8:97. (*A study detailing what patients think after they have left the doctor's office.*)

Part 2: Approaches to Common Ethical and Legal Issues in Primary Care Practice
LINDA L. EMANUEL

Being a patient's primary physician necessitates the skillful management of several key ethical and legal issues. These include maintenance of confidentiality, provision of informed consent, assistance in developing a health care proxy and living will, and determination of patient incompetence. The advent of managed care and new incentive schemes raise a host of ethical problems that need to be addressed. Timely and skillful attention to the basics in these areas can greatly facilitate care and minimize problems later on for both patient and physician.

CONFIDENTIALITY

Trust—the *sine qua non* of the patient–doctor relationship—requires that patients' confidences be kept by the physician. This precept is well articulated in the Hippocratic Oath. It is also honored in the law as part of the constitutional right to privacy. Physicians should be able to reassure the patient who is concerned about confidentiality of the primacy and privacy of the patient–doctor relationship. However, there are some limits to this confidentiality, and these should be clarified and discussed with the patient at the earliest relevant moment.

Limits to Confidentiality. Confidentiality is limited by the imperative *to protect third parties from harm*, as may occur, for example, when a patient reveals to a psychiatrist a plan to murder someone. In everyday primary care practice, balancing obligations to the patient with obligations to a third party depends on an assessment of relative harms. This can be a difficult judgment. One such example is the reporting of a venereal disease or AIDS to the patient's sexual contact(s). State requirements vary. Persuading the patient to reveal the information directly to the third party often allows the discharge of all obligations to the third party with minimal damage to the patient–doctor alliance. Occasionally, confidentiality must be breached when it is *in the best interests of the patient*, although this rule should be used sparingly. The physician should reveal the minimum that is necessary in such situations.

Sometimes, the *physician's role* or *responsibility* limits the ability to keep a patient's confidence. A physician employed by a company, school, military unit, or court has split allegiances, which the patient must be made aware of at the outset. Medical information must be reported to insurance companies in many cases, but not all, and the consent of the patient is always required before this can occur. More subtle constraints on confidentiality can arise when *medical records* are readily accessed by other employees, such as those in a billing office. Policies and procedures for affording extra protection to patients who may be known to employees are indicated. Physicians may receive *court subpoenas*, in response to which they must appear in court with the appropriate information. A patient's privilege to bar the physician from testifying may be invoked but certainly can be overruled by the court.

Sharing of Information within the Limits of Confidentiality. Sharing of information about a patient among members of the health care team is rarely problematic. However, the risk of losing sight of the confidential nature of the relationship with the patient rises as the number of persons included in the health care team increases; this is a problem that needs to be guarded against. Patient information used for teaching rounds or publication should be carefully edited to remove any identifying features.

Involving family or friends in a patient's care is often in the best interests of the patient, but sharing patient information with them must be preceded by the patient's explicit permission. When family members reveal information relevant to the patient that they ask the physician to withhold from the patient, the request cannot be honored, and the family should be made aware of this obligation ahead of time if possible. The conflict may be resolved by persuading the family of the inadvisability of such secrecy.

Patient Data in Large Electronic Systems. With the use of computer-based records and central support systems has arisen the issue of how to maintain the proper confidentiality of patient records in large electronic systems. Among other concerns, protective measures must still allow the desirable use of information—for example, for systematic quality improvement or approved research activities. The issue is largely an institutional policy matter, and quality improvement and research information in many cases can be pursued without a breach of patient confidentiality by the use of only de-identified, aggregate data. However, individual physicians should be sure that the institution in which they work provides suitable confidentiality protection in the electronic medium, and that physicians and others abide by the protective measures. These should include the use of personal identification codes for access to computers that hold patient information. If a physician has concerns about the inappropriate use of information, even after working to improve the system, possibly separate personal computers (with user codes and frequent backup to prevent loss of data) or paper-only files may be an appropriate option.

Improperly Motivated Requests for Confidentiality. Such requests may be encountered from patients with seductive, suicidal, hostile, or criminal intentions. The physician should immediately involve another colleague, either as chaperone or consultant, and document the encounter. These steps will serve to protect the physician from such charges as sexual misconduct, harboring a fugitive, or facilitating a suicide. They also help to preserve good judgment and justified levels of confidentiality, and they free the physician from the intimidating nature of the secret.

FINANCIAL INCENTIVES

Medicine is a profession with its own standards for handling financial matters. Major medical ethics codes all note the need to avoid financial exploitation of patients, many of whom are in situations such that they would spend unfair amounts of money in the hope of securing their health.

Reasonable and Honest Charges. Physicians should charge or help ensure that their institutions charge fees that are not exorbitant. In addition, physicians should avoid charging for services, such as referral, that involve minimal work and for services provided by other colleagues, as the other colleague will bill for these services. Reimbursement claims should honestly describe the service rendered and should avoid claiming for subcomponents of the service for the purpose of securing a higher reimbursement rate. If the physician feels unable to secure needed services for patients within a set of billing or reimbursement standards, attempts should be made openly and honestly to bring changes to the system.

Fee-splitting Arrangements. Self-employed and group practice physicians working within fee-for-service systems need to avoid arrangements such as "self-referrals" and "kickbacks." Such arrangements include those in which physicians refer patients to facilities in which the physician has a financial interest or to other physicians who pay the referring physician a referral fee, and those in which physicians receive payment from a drug company for each prescription written for a specified drug. These arrangements can influence a physician to recommend actions that are not so much in the patient's interest as in the physician's financial interest.

Incentives. Physicians employed in a managed care environment often face incentives that are in place to influence their treatment decisions. Although some argue that physician incentives are a good thing if they are aligned with patient interests, others note that they encourage physicians to follow their personal interests when instead professionalism requires that physicians be altruistic and serve patient needs. Either way, individual physicians working in a system that uses incentives should be sure that the incentives are (a) a relatively small proportion of a physician's income, (b) paid relatively infrequently, (c) shared by a group of physicians rather than applied to individuals, and (d) designed in such a way that they foster good patient care. A useful rule of thumb may be to ask the following question: Would the physician be embarrassed to disclose the incentive arrangement to the patient? These standards may minimize the inappropriate influence of incentives. If incentive systems deviate from professional standards, physicians can work within the institution to effect change and if necessary can also decline to receive inappropriate incentives.

INFORMED CONSENT

Informed consent is much more than a legal document. In fact, a signed document in the absence of a valid discussion with the physician is unlikely to be of legal benefit. Informed consent is a continuing part of the patient–physician relationship and involves the giving and interpretation of information, deliberation, and joint decision making. As such, informed consent represents an integral part of the continuing therapeutic alliance.

Informed consent is required for most nonemergent decisions, whether routine or major.

Required Components of Information Giving and Consent. Laws and legal opinions have defined the following required components of information giving: The patient must receive a description of the *nature of the treatment*, the associated risks (both major and frequent), and their expected time of occurrence. It is neither reasonable nor appropriate for the physician

to furnish an exhaustive catalogue of risks; the physician's role here is to provide relevant information and judgment. The *expected benefits* and *alternative treatments* should also be reviewed relative to the recommended action.

Each component of informed consent can be pursued to varying levels of intensity. The courts initially adopted a *"standard of practice"* criterion in which the physician was expected to provide information according to the standards of current practice in the community. Later, the criterion shifted toward providing what a hypothetically *"reasonable person"* would want to know. Presently, a mixed standard is in general use. In practice, valid consent is most likely to be given when information giving is tailored to suit the needs of the individual patient.

Consent also has required components. First, there must be an *understanding of the information* by the patient. A practical means of assessing understanding is to ask the patient about concerns and expectations; the responses can guide further information giving. Second, the decision must be *voluntary*. However, persuasion is fully appropriate, and physicians need not feel constrained from expressing their best medical judgment.

Consent to Research. Consent by a patient to participate in a research protocol requires that particular attention be paid to the patient's sense of volunteerism and understanding. The design of the study protocol must be fully understood. Randomized, controlled trials require patients to take the chance of receiving the standard treatment instead of what may be the desired treatment. In some trials, patients also take the chance of receiving placebo treatment, and in double-blind studies, the patient's physician will not know which treatment the patient is receiving. The benefit to patients in the control arm may be limited to improved monitoring.

Patients must understand that the physician may have conflicting interests. For example, there may be a gain in collegiality, career advancement, or even material benefit. Many of these interests are inevitable and acceptable, but they must be fully disclosed and discussed with the patient. Reassurance of a true primary commitment by the physician to the patient should be possible. If such a primary commitment to the patient is lacking, the patient should be transferred to another physician for care or should not participate in the research protocol.

ADVANCE DIRECTIVES FOR HEALTH CARE: LIVING WILLS, PROXY DECISION MAKERS, AND COMPREHENSIVE DIRECTIVES

The term *advance directives* refers to provisions made by patients to direct their health care in case of future incompetence. Advance directives are written statements and can include a living will and the designation of a proxy decision maker (sometimes referred to as *durable power of attorney for health care*). Ideally, advance directives combine both modalities. They are inactive until such time as incompetence occurs.

The Office Discussion. For the sake of clear communication, advance directives should be completed in the context of a discussion with the patient and witnessed by the person who will be the designated proxy decision maker. Outpatients have been found to be very receptive to advance planning, often expecting physicians to take the initiative. When structured around the completion of an advance directive document, the core discussion can be expected to take about 15 to 30 minutes. Interval follow-up discussions are appropriate and particularly relevant at times of a significant change in the patient's health or personal circumstances. Although it is common to undertake advance planning for the elderly and seriously ill, planning for the young and healthy can be quite worthwhile. Planning discussions can be regarded as a good investment of time in that they can make subsequent difficult decisions more efficient. Moreover, they help build a quality relationship of shared decision making around the patient's goals and the physician's expertise and efforts at health promotion.

As important as any other components of advance care planning are the education and sense of readiness provided to the patient, proxy, and physician. These discussions foster a sense of participation and consensus and consign documents and legalities to their proper role as necessary but peripheral components.

Choosing the Document. Using a standardized, worksheet-type document or the outline of a document can be very helpful. A well-designed worksheet facilitates discussion. Many facilities have recommended documents available, and some generic documents have been designed to be binding in all states. Usually, there are separate documents for a written statement of preferences and for the designation of a proxy, although more efficient documents combining the two exist. If a patient has a document already drawn up, the physician should review it with the patient. It is helpful to include scenarios in the document, and they should cover a range of prognoses, disabilities, and treatment choices, so that the patient's threshold for withholding or withdrawing treatment can be ascertained. Patients should be advised that advance directives can elect for intervention as well as withdrawal or withholding of treatment, depending on the situation. Treatment decisions should be as specific as possible and linked to statements regarding the goals of intervention and general values of health care.

Legal Considerations. Federal law requires that patients be informed of hospital policy regarding living wills at the time of admission and be asked whether they have any advance directives already drawn up. This information must be entered into the medical record. Advance directives must be honored under constitutional law as a statement of the patient's autonomous wishes. Rarely, there may be a conflict between a patient's wishes and local statutes. For example, some states restrict the withdrawal of nutrition and hydration to terminally ill patients, which potentially prevents withdrawal from hopelessly but not terminally ill patients, such as those in a persistent vegetative state. The patient should be informed if conflict exists. Conflicts related to differences in values between the patient and physician should be discussed fully so that they can be resolved before problematic decisions arise. An inability to resolve the conflict is cause for asking the patient to agree to transfer of care should the circumstances in question arise.

PATIENTS WHO ARE CONFUSED OR REFUSE CARE

Many treatment refusals arise from fear, perceived loss of control, distrust, or anger. Discussing patient concerns in a receptive, respectful manner that also offers the patient some choices and a sense of control often suffices to reverse the refusal. Treatment refusal may be a result of patient incompetence, but other refusals may be well reasoned and valid.

Right to Refuse Treatment. The right to refuse medical care is strongly endorsed by the law as part of a constitutional right to privacy. The Supreme Court has affirmed that this right exists for competent patients, incompetent patients with explicit preferences, and even incompetent patients without explicit preferences (although the right is more difficult to implement in this circumstance). Treatments that have been determined in case law to be terminable range from mechanical respiration to artificial nutrition and hydration. The Patient Self-determination Act of 1990 requires that patients be reminded on enrollment in or admission to a health care facility of their right to accept or refuse medical treatment.

However, the right to refuse care is *not absolute*. It can be limited by opposing interests. Some states invoke their interest in preserving life to restrict withholding or withdrawing of life-sustaining treatments from incompetent patients unless they are terminally ill or, in some states, in a hopeless or persistent vegetative state. The protection of minors may limit a competent patient's right to refuse treatment.

Declaring and Determining Incompetence. If a patient's refusal of care appears related to mental or psychological incompetence(s), the patient can be declared incompetent and the refusal can be overridden. Incompetence is commonly declared by the physician, sometimes with the help of a consulting psychiatrist. Review by an institutional ethics committee or even the judiciary should be considered if (a) a question arises about who should be the surrogate decision maker for the patient; (b) legal action is current or anticipated; or (c) the case involves the termination of life-sustaining treatment in the absence of a valid advance directive to that effect.

Determining incompetence involves assessing inability to make the individual decision at hand. Competence is not an all-or-nothing state. A patient may be competent for some decisions but incompetent for others. There are four minimum standards of competence: The patient must (a) be able to *communicate a choice*; (b) have an adequate *factual understanding* of information relevant to the decision (e.g., be able to paraphrase the information); (c) *appreciate the implications* of the decision; and (d) be able to *manipulate relevant information rationally*. Rational manipulation refers to the ability to understand, for example, not only that nontreatment of a gangrenous limb may result in death, but also that death means the end of life.

If incompetence is determined, a proxy decision maker should be appointed promptly. Generally, this person should be someone other than the physician and will be responsible for speaking with the physician on behalf of the patient.

SEXUAL BOUNDARIES AND THE PATIENT–PHYSICIAN RELATIONSHIP

The intimacy of the patient–physician encounter and the trust required for the therapeutic encounter together require that personal boundaries be clear and well maintained. One such boundary concerns sexual behavior. A unanimous standard throughout major traditions in medicine is that physicians should not engage in sexual relations with their patients. Variations in opinion tend to relate to matters of definition—what exactly constitutes a sexual touch, for instance—and to questions such as whether or not the prohibition applies to former patients.

In general, physicians should stay well away from sexual behavior in the professional context and avoid behavior that tests any fine distinctions. One allegation of sexual misconduct can end an entire medical career. If any concerns arise—for instance, if the physician's instincts suggest that such feelings exist on either side and certainly if a patient makes sexual overtures—some of the following steps may help. Involve a chaperone, especially during the physical examination of any sexual region of the anatomy. Ask a colleague on your team for additional insight; a nurse may be able to provide important feedback about patient perceptions. Consult a physician colleague; apart from receiving helpful advice, shared information is less likely to become a coercive secret. Spend enough quality time with friends and family to be secure in your personal life. Consider displaying evidence of personal commitment, such as photographs of loved ones on your desk, a code of ethics on the wall, and so forth.

ANNOTATED BIBLIOGRAPHY

American College of Physicians. Ethics manual: fourth edition. Ann Intern Med 1997;128:576. (*Practical guide to clinical practice from a leading professional organization.*)

American Medical Association. Education for physicians in end-of-life care (EPEC) curriculum. Chicago: American Medical Association, 1999. (*A 16-module instructional text on end-of-life care, including a discussion of advance care planning.*)

Applebaum PS, Lidz CW, Meisel A. Informed consent: legal theory and clinical practice. New York: Oxford University Press, 1987. (*An excellent resource for theory, relevant case law, and clinical guidance regarding informed consent.*)

Dunn PM, Levinson W. Discussing futility with patients and families. J Gen Intern Med 1996;11:689. (*A practical approach to this difficult conversation.*)

Emanuel LL, Barry MJ, Stoeckle JD, et al. Advance directives for medical care: a case for greater use. N Engl J Med 1991;324:889. (*Scenario-based advance planning in a reasonable amount of office time.*)

Emanuel EJ. A review of the ethical and legal aspects of terminating medical care. Am J Med 1988;84:291. (*Discusses issues of competence, use of advance directives, and types of care terminated.*)

Gramelspacher GP, Xiao-Hua Z, Hanna MP, et al. Preferences of physicians and their patients for end-of-life care. J Gen Intern Med 1997;12:346. (*Explores the differences and areas of concurrence.*)

Johnson SH. Judicial review of disciplinary action for sexual misconduct in the practice of medicine. JAMA 1993;270:1596. (*The problem from the judicial perspective.*)

Kassirer JP. Managed care and the morality of the marketplace. N Engl J Med 1995;333:50. (*An editorial on the market-driven approach to health care reform and its moral implications.*)

Singer PA, Martin DK, Lavery JV, et al. Reconceptualizing advance care planning from the patient's perspective. Arch Intern Med 1998;158:879. (*A slightly different perspective is provided, with an emphasis on the role of relationships in the advance planning exercise.*)

Tsevat J, Cook F, Green ML, et al. Health values of the seriously ill. Ann Intern Med 1995;122:514. (*Prospective, longitudinal, multicenter study showing wider variations than surrogates believed.*)

2
Selection and Interpretation of Diagnostic Tests

Laboratory investigations are often essential to patient care. Although the history and physical examination remain the foundation of a clinical database and sometimes suffice, the limits to what we can know about a patient are continually expanding with the addition of new diagnostic tests. These tests have many uses: to make a diagnosis in a patient known to be sick; to provide prognostic information for a patient with known disease; to identify a person with subclinical disease or at risk for subsequent development of disease; and to monitor ongoing therapy. The ultimate objective is to reduce morbidity and mortality and increase satisfaction and the sense of well-being. If the physician and patient are to reach these objectives, they must avoid some pitfalls along the way that can result from misuse or misinterpretation of laboratory tests.

Pitfalls are more likely to be avoided if the physician appreciates the inherent uncertainty and probabilistic nature of the diagnostic process and understands the relationship between the characteristics of a diagnostic test and those of the patient(s) being tested. Sometimes, a diagnosis is evident when a patient presents with a pathognomonic constellation of signs and symptoms. In most cases, however, presenting signs or symptoms are not specific. Rather, they can be explained by a number of diagnoses, each with distinctly different implications for the patient's health. On completion of the history and physical examination, the clinician considers a list of conditions, referred to as the *differential diagnosis*, that might explain the findings. The diagnoses can then be ranked to reflect an implicit assignment of probabilities to each. Such a ranking can be thought of as the physician's index of suspicion for each condition, based on knowledge and past experience with similar patients. The purpose of subsequent laboratory testing is to refine the initial probability estimates and, in the process, to revise the differential diagnosis. The probability of any particular disease on the revised list will depend on its probability of being present before testing and the validity of the information provided by test results.

VOCABULARY OF DIAGNOSTIC TEST INTERPRETATION

Terminology is important in diagnostic test interpretation. Clinical pathologists often focus on a test's accuracy and precision. *Accuracy* is the degree of closeness of the measurement made to the true value, measured by some alternative "gold standard" or definitive test. *Precision* is a test's ability to give nearly the same result in repeated determinations. Clinicians are more concerned with the ability of a test result to discriminate between persons with and persons without a given disease or condition; this discriminating ability can be characterized by a test's sensitivity and specificity. *Sensitivity* is the probability that a test result will be positive when the test is applied to a person who actually has the disease. *Specificity* is the probability that a test result will be negative when the test is applied to a person who actually does not have the disease. A perfectly sensitive test can rule out disease if the result is negative. A perfectly specific test can rule in disease if the result is positive. Because most tests are neither perfectly sensitive nor perfectly specific, the result must be interpreted probabilistically rather than categorically.

Although sensitivity and specificity are important considerations in selecting a test, the probabilities they measure are not in themselves what ordinarily concern the physician and the patient after the test result has returned. Both are concerned with the following questions: If the result is positive, what is the probability that disease is present? If the result is negative, what is the probability that the patient is indeed disease-free? These probabilities are known respectively as the *predictive value positive* and the *predictive value negative*. They are determined not only by the sensitivity and specificity of the test, but also by the probability of the disease being present before the test was ordered.

Relationships between sensitivity and specificity and positive and negative predictive values can be better understood by referring to a two-by-two table (Fig. 2.1). The two columns indicate the presence or absence of disease (note that a gold standard of diagnosis is assumed), and the two rows indicate positive or negative test results. Any given patient with a test result could be included in one of the four cells labeled a, b, c, or d. Definitions of sensitivity, specificity, predictive value positive, and predictive value negative can be restated by using these labels. It is important to note that each of these four ratios has a

Disease

		Present	Absent	
Test	Positive	a	b	$a+b$
	Negative	c	d	$c+d$
		$a+c$	$b+d$	$a+b+c+d$

Definitions

Sensitivity:	$\dfrac{a}{a+c}$	False negative rate:	$\dfrac{c}{a+c}$
Specificity:	$\dfrac{d}{b+d}$	False positive rate:	$\dfrac{b}{b+d}$
Predictive value positive:	$\dfrac{a}{a+b}$	False alarm rate:	$\dfrac{b}{a+b}$
Predictive value negative:	$\dfrac{d}{c+d}$	False reassurance rate:	$\dfrac{c}{c+d}$

FIG. 2.1. The two-by-two table clarifies relationships between test characteristics (sensitivity and specificity) and the predictive values of positive and negative test results. Clinicians, interpreting a diagnostic test, can fill in the table if they are aware of the sensitivity and specificity of the test and a patient's (population's) pretest probability (prevalence) of disease. The pretest probability is $(a+c)$ and $(1 - $ the pretest probability) is $(b+d)$. Multiplying $(a+c)$ by the sensitivity provides the value for a, and multiplying $(b+d)$ by the specificity provides the value for d. Values for cell c and cell b can be determined by simple subtraction. With the cells filled in, the predictive value of a negative or positive test result can be calculated easily. It is worth noting that this calculation method is precisely equivalent to Bayes' theorem of conditional probability.

complement. The complement of sensitivity (1 − sensitivity) is referred to as the *false-negative rate*, whereas the complement of specificity (1 − specificity) is referred to as the *false-positive rate*. These terms are often used ambiguously in the medical literature; the false-negative rate is confused with the complement of the predictive value negative, which is *best* termed the *false-reassurance rate*; the false-positive rate is confused with the complement of the predictive value positive, which is *best* termed the *false-alarm rate*.

INTERPRETING TEST RESULTS: REVISING DIAGNOSTIC PROBABILITIES

When clinicians interpret test results, they usually process the information informally. Rarely is a pad and pencil or calculator used to revise probability estimates explicitly. However, sometimes the revision of diagnostic probabilities is counterintuitive; for instance, it has been shown that most clinicians rely too heavily on positive test results when the pretest probability or disease prevalence is low.

Attention to the two-by-two table indicates why predictive values are crucially dependent on disease prevalence. This is particularly true when one is using a test to screen for a rare disease. If a disease is rare, even a very small false-positive rate (which is, remember, the complement of specificity) is multiplied by a very large relative number—that is, $(b + d) \times (a + c)$. Therefore, b will be surprisingly large relative to a, and the predictive value positive will be counterintuitively low. Examples of this effect are evident in Table 2.1.

Consider the example of a noninvasive test to detect coronary disease applied to a 40-year-old man with a history of atypical chest pain. Based on test evaluations reported in the literature, the sensitivity and specificity of the test can be estimated at 80% and 90%, respectively. Based on symptoms and risk factors, the clinician estimates that the patient's pretest probability of coronary disease is 0.20. (This is the same as saying that the prevalence of coronary disease in a population of similar patients would be 20%.)

According to Fig. 2.1, with a pretest probability of 0.20, $a + c = 0.20$ and $b + d = 0.80$. Multiplying 0.20 by 0.8 (the sensitivity) gives us a value of 0.16 for a (subtraction gives us a value of 0.04 for c). Multiplying 0.80 by 0.9 (the specificity) gives us a value of 0.72 for d (again, subtraction gives us 0.08 for b). The predictive value positive, then, is 0.16/0.24, or 0.67. The predictive value negative is 0.72/0.76, or 0.95.

Clinicians can use another method to revise probabilities quickly to test their intuition. It requires an understanding of *odds* as well as probability. If p is the probability that a particular disease is present, the ratio of p to $(1 − p)$, or $p/(1 − p)$, is called the *odds favoring that disease*. The *odds against that disease* being present are represented by $(1 − p)/p$. Just as one can estimate the pretest probability of disease before diagnostic tests are performed, one can express that estimate as the pretest odds.

Pretest odds can be revised simply by multiplying a ratio called the *likelihood ratio*, which is the relative occurrence of the test result among persons with and without disease—that is, the probability of the result (either positive or negative or a particular range of values) given the presence of disease divided by the probability of that result given the absence of disease. Note that the positive likelihood ratio is nothing more (or less) than the ratio of sensitivity to the false-positive rate (i.e., 1 − speci-

Table 2.1. Effect of Prior Probability (Prevalence)
on Predictive Value of Positive Test Results

PRIOR PROBABILITY (PREVALENCE) (%)	PREDICTIVE VALUE OF POSITIVE TEST RESULT (%)		
	SENSITIVITY 90% SPECIFICITY 90%	SENSITIVITY 95% SPECIFICITY 95%	SENSITIVITY 99% SPECIFICITY 99%
0.1	0.9	1.9	9.0
1	8.3	16.1	50.0
2	15.5	27.9	66.9
5	32.1	50.0	83.9
50	90.0	95.0	99.0

ficity). The negative likelihood ratio is the ratio of the false-negative rate (i.e., 1 − sensitivity) to the specificity. Likelihood ratios therefore include all the information contained in estimates of sensitivity and specificity. When the pretest odds of a disease are multiplied by the likelihood ratio, the result—sometimes termed the *posttest odds*—represents the odds favoring disease given the test result.

Returning to the example, the patient with atypical chest pain could have his chances of having coronary disease expressed as odds rather than a probability. A probability of 0.20 is equivalent to odds of 1/4 (0.20/0.80). The likelihood ratio for a test with a sensitivity of 0.8 and a specificity of 0.9 is 8 [0.8/ (1 − 0.9)]. The pretest odds can be converted to posttest odds following a positive test result simply by multiplying by the positive likelihood ratio: 1/4 × 8 = 2. Note that the posttest odds ratio of 2:1 is equivalent to the posttest probability of 0.66.

For some, it is easier to revise probabilities in the clinical setting by using likelihood ratios. A nomogram can be helpful until one gets used to converting from probabilities to odds and back again (Fig. 2.2). Likelihood ratios also have the advantage of capturing more clinical data from the patient's particular test results. Whereas estimates of sensitivity and specificity usually rely on a dichotomous positive–negative result threshold, different likelihood ratios can be determined for different ranges of test results. For example, a very high creatine phosphokinase (CPK) level will have a higher positive likelihood ratio than a moderate elevation. The degree of elevation will then be reflected in the revised probability of myocardial infarction.

WHERE DOES THE INFORMATION COME FROM?

One of the reasons clinicians are reluctant to take a quantitative approach to diagnostic test interpretation is that such an approach suggests a precision that belies our uncertainty about pretest probabilities and about sensitivity and specificity of even commonly used tests. The estimation of pretest probability hinges on epidemiologic information about the incidence and prevalence of various diseases, modified on the basis of patient characteristics and presenting symptoms. This kind of information is all too rarely presented in the medical literature. Estimates are necessarily uncertain.

There is also uncertainty about the sensitivity and specificity of tests. Rarely are these values presented in medical texts, and test evaluations in the medical literature can sometimes be misleading. The clinician should be familiar with some of the reasons why a test rarely performs as well in general use as it does during the evaluation study that appears in the medical journal.

False-positive Rate and Pretest Probability: Overestimating Predictive Values

The importance of the pretest probability of disease in an individual patient (or the prevalence of disease in a population of such patients) for determining the predictive values of a test is often not fully appreciated and may lead to disappointment in the clinical performance of the test. Consider how, during its evaluation, the sensitivity and specificity of a test are estimated. Two groups of patients are assembled. One consists of patients known to have the disease in question as defined by some gold standard (represented by $a + c$ in Fig. 2.1). The other consists of persons without disease based on the same gold standard (represented by $b + d$). The test being evaluated is then applied to both populations. The proportion of those with disease who have

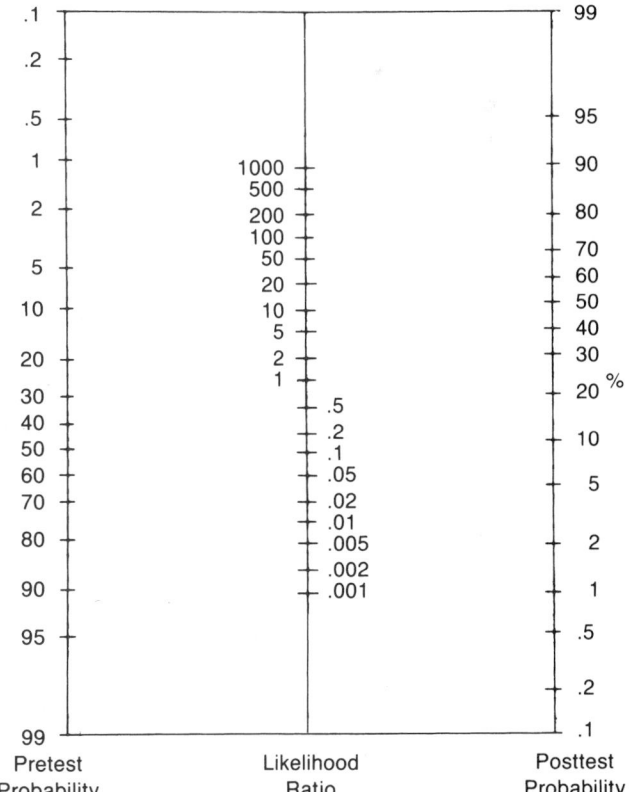

FIG. 2.2. A nomogram for applying likelihood ratios. [Adapted from Fagan TJ. Nomogram for Bayes' theorem [Letter]. N Engl J Med 1975;293:257, with permission. (Sackett DL, Haynes RB, Tugwell P. Clinical epidemiology, 1985.)]

a positive result [$a/(a + c)$] provides us with an estimate of the test's sensitivity. The proportion of those without the disease who have a negative result [$d/(b + d)$] gives us an estimate of the test's specificity. Our confidence that these estimates of sensitivity and specificity are accurate increases with the number of people in each group tested. The investigator can most efficiently maximize confidence in the estimates of both sensitivity and specificity by applying the test to disease and nondisease groups of equal size. It is not surprising, therefore, that tests are often evaluated by applying them to populations in which disease and nondisease occur with equal frequency, or nearly so.

If sensitivity, specificity, and predictive values are sufficiently high in such an evaluation study, the test is proposed for general use. What happens when the test is adopted and applied in a general population in which the disease is much less likely to be present than nondisease? The sensitivity and specificity should remain the same, but the predictive value positive will necessarily fall, and its complement, the false-alarm rate, will necessarily increase. This phenomenon is most important when the disease in question is rare, as is evident in Table 2.1.

Defining Disease for Diagnostic Test Evaluation: The Gold Standard Problem

To evaluate a diagnostic test, an investigator must be able to distinguish between persons with and without disease by some alternative method. Often, this gold standard test is more invasive or more expensive than the newer, proposed test being evaluated. (The newer test would not be worth evaluating if it did not confer some advantage for patient or clinician.) Sometimes, a gold standard is not readily available. If the disease is one with a short, predictable, natural history (e.g., pancreatic cancer), an investigator may resort to follow-up, defining the absence of disease by morbidity-free survival during a specified period. But if the disease has a highly variable natural history (e.g., coronary disease and most rheumatologic disorders), the follow-up approach becomes impractical. Instead, the investigator must rely on more arbitrary and often more subjective criteria to define disease, including combinations of tests, signs, and symptoms. Herein lies a potential pitfall that can affect the accuracy of the estimates of sensitivity and specificity. If the diagnostic criteria are not assessed independently of the test being evaluated, the sensitivity, specificity, or both will be overestimated.

The problem occurs in its most obvious form when a positive test result leads the investigator to a more extensive search for disease than was applied to those with a negative test result. A related problem occurs when the test and the diagnostic criteria are very similar biologic measures. This will result in overly optimistic estimates of sensitivity and specificity. For example, to the extent that false-negative isoenzyme results are correlated with false-negative enzyme results, the sensitivity of the test will be overestimated. To the extent that false-positive results are correlated with false-positive results, the specificity of the new test will be overestimated.

The Narrow Spectrum Problem: Overestimating Sensitivity When the "Disease" Group Is Too Sick

When investigators assemble a group known to have the disease in question by means of some gold standard, they may choose patients with unequivocal diagnostic (gold standard) findings. In doing so, they may select a severely ill group that is not representative of the disease in the general population—that is, they will focus on too narrow a spectrum of disease.

Consider a group of investigators evaluating a noninvasive test for coronary artery disease, such as an electrocardiographically monitored exercise tolerance test. To be sure that they are dealing with true coronary disease, the investigators include only people with unequivocal prior myocardial infarction or with classic angina symptoms. By using their chosen criteria for a positive test result, they determine that the sensitivity of the test is 90%. What they (and the readers of their report) may not realize is that the test is more sensitive when coronary disease is extensive (two- or three-vessel disease rather than single-vessel disease) or severe (99% stenosis rather than 80% stenosis) and that their gold standard criteria have selected for patients with extensive or severe disease. When the test is used to detect less extensive disease producing more equivocal symptoms in the general population, its sensitivity will prove disappointing. Recognize that the sensitivity estimate provided by the evaluation is accurate for the narrow spectrum of disease severity found in the test population. The disappointment comes when that estimate is generalized inappropriately to include those with less severe disease.

The Comorbidity Problem: Overestimating Specificity When the "No Disease" Group Is Too Well

In the same way that investigators can assemble a "disease" group that is sicker than the population to which the test will eventually be applied, they can assemble a "no disease" group that is too healthy. Many tests will perform better when used to discriminate between "disease A" and "no disease" than when used to discriminate between disease A, on the one hand, and diseases B through Z, on the other. Consider the fledgling investigator who wishes to estimate the sensitivity and specificity of guaiac testing as a screening test for colonic cancer. The investigator knows about the spectrum problem and has included in the "disease" group people with early cancers. For the "no disease" group, medical school students have been selected. It should be clear that this choice of controls will provide an estimate of specificity that is higher than could be expected when the test is generally applied to a population including older individuals more likely to have a nonmalignant source of occult bleeding. Obviously, the controls should not have the target disease (i.e., colon cancer). However, if all comorbid conditions that the test might confuse with the disease (e.g., peptic ulcer disease, diverticular disease) are also excluded from the control population, the investigator's estimate of specificity will be too optimistic.

Investigators can guard against such disappointments by drawing their "disease" and "no disease" populations from the target population in which the test will eventually be used. The spectrum of disease that should be detected in the target population should be represented in the "disease" group. Comorbid conditions that might be confused with that disease should be included in the "no disease" control group. Such an effectiveness evaluation of a diagnostic test might be preceded by a simpler study comparing very sick with completely well persons. If the test cannot discriminate between the very sick and the very well in such an efficacy study, the more difficult effectiveness trial need not be undertaken. The clinician can guard against being misled by reports of a test's efficacy by carefully considering the populations in which a test has been evaluated and not generalizing the results inappropriately to larger, more heterogeneous groups.

How Does the Test Compare with Others?

A final reason for disappointment with the application of apparently promising tests is failure to consider adequately a test's potential role in the constellation of tests that is already available. Does the new test provide new information? Does it obviate the need for more invasive or more expensive tests? If the answer to these questions is no, the worth of the test and its evaluation are in obvious doubt.

WHICH TESTS SHOULD WE USE?

Perfect tests are rare. Clinicians must choose among tests with imperfect sensitivity and specificity. The physician frequently has some choice about the sensitivity and specificity of a test. Obviously, alternative tests—usually those that are more costly or invasive—may be more sensitive and more specific. A new technology or an improved skill in interpretation may improve both measures. Often, however, the physician can increase specificity only by accepting a decrease in sensitivity. The most graphic examples of this principle involve tests that provide quantitative results, such as the measurement of serum prostate-specific antigen when the diagnosis of prostate cancer is being considered. The general case is illustrated in Fig. 2.3. Note that the "normal" values for the test results are all too often derived from frequency distributions of results among apparently well persons; the potential trade-off between sensitivity and specificity is not considered.

Which is more important, sensitivity or specificity? In general, the answer depends on the cost—which includes patient inconvenience, morbidity, and mortality as well as dollars—of false-negative results compared with that of false-positive re-sults, and the benefits of true-negative and true-positive results. Sensitive tests or less stringent criteria for disease and the resulting low false-negative rate should be favored when effective treatment for the condition exists and the cost of lost opportunity is great. High specificity or more stringent criteria for disease and the resulting low false-positive rate are most important when a positive diagnostic result does not significantly influence therapy or outcome and may be a burden for the patient.

Clinicians who are mindful of the purpose of making a particular diagnosis, who consider the natural history of a disease in addition to the prognostic and therapeutic implications of the diagnosis, are likely to make efficient use of the laboratory while maximizing health benefits for their patients.

A.G.M.

ANNOTATED BIBLIOGRAPHY

Griner PF, Mayewski RJ, Mushlin AI, et al. Selection and interpretation of diagnostic tests and procedures: principles and applications. Ann Intern Med 1981;94[4 Pt 2]:557. (*A very well-presented primer with many good examples.*)

Griner PF, Panzer RJ, Greenland P. Diagnostic strategies for common medical problems. Philadelphia: American College of Physicians, 1991. (*A superb resource. Includes information about prior probabilities and sensitivity and specificity of tests, and recommends well-reasoned strategies.*)

Jaeschke R, Guyatt G, Sackett DL, for the Evidence-Based Medicine Working Group. Users' guide to the medical literature. III. How to use an article about a diagnostic test. A. Are the results of the study valid? B. What are the results and will they help me in caring for my patients? JAMA 1994;271:389, 703. (*Part of an updated series designed to provide practical applications of clinical epidemiology for the practitioner.*)

Ransohoff DF, Feinstein AR. Problems of spectrum and bias in evaluating the efficacy of diagnostic tests. N Engl J Med 1975;299:926. (*Reviews problems in disease definition and population selection that may affect evaluations of diagnostic tests.*)

Reid MC, Lane DA, Feinstein AR. Academic calculations versus clinical judgments: practicing physicians' use of quantitative measures of test accuracy. Am J Med 1998;104:374. (*Clinicians in this telephone survey avoided any quantitative approaches to interpretation of diagnostic tests.*)

Sox HC Jr. Common diagnostic tests: use and interpretation, 2nd ed. Philadelphia: American College of Physicians, 1990. (*An excellent volume with introductory chapters on diagnostic reasoning and probability theory followed by 16 chapters on specific tests.*)

Vecchio TJ. Predictive value of a single diagnostic test in unselected populations. N Engl J Med 1966;274:1171. (*Early article pointing out the importance of prevalence to predictive value.*)

Woolf SH, Kamerow DB. Testing for uncommon conditions. Arch Intern Med 1990;150:2451. (*A reasoned and careful analysis of the sometimes irrational drive to find the zebra, often at great cost to patients and society.*)

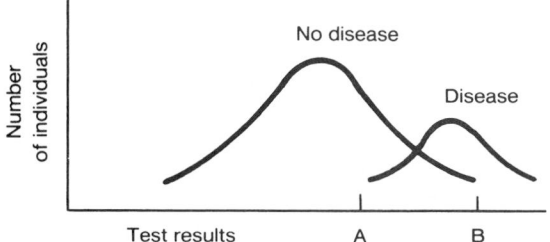

FIG. 2.3. Hypothetical distribution of test results among patients with and without disease. Because the distributions overlap, the test is far from perfect. If all patients with values to the right of *A* are said to have "positive" results, the test will be 100% sensitive but will have a low specificity. If only those patients with values to the right of *B* are said to have "positive" results, the test will be 100% specific but will have a low sensitivity. The choice of a cutoff value between *A* and *B* should depend on the relative importance of true- and false-positive and true- and false-negative results.

3
Health Maintenance and the Role of Screening

Public interest in health maintenance or, more positively, health enhancement has grown dramatically in recent years. Many Americans have demonstrated their interest in exercise, good dietary habits, maintenance of appropriate body weight, and stress reduction. Increased enthusiasm stems from the growing awareness of associations between elements of lifestyle and health. Despite reliable evidence and public acceptance of these associations, however, many people continue to indulge in self-destructive habits such as smoking, overeating, and alcohol abuse. Efforts to alter such behavior are often frustratingly ineffective. Patients who seek reassurance from physician visits that include routine screening procedures often persist in behavior that greatly increases their risk of morbidity.

Physicians must acknowledge their primary role in prevention as that of educators. Accurate information regarding risk factors is most likely to reinforce health-enhancing behavior and alter self-destructive behavior. Physicians must appreciate the potential for behavior modification and familiarize themselves with local resources. Routine screening for specific diseases, the health maintenance activity most closely identified with the physician, should be performed selectively. The limits of screening tests as well as their potential health benefits should be clearly understood by every primary care physician.

Specific risk factors and screening tests are discussed in subsequent chapters. This chapter focuses on the question, What makes a disease or risk factor worth screening for? The relationship between prevalence and the predictive value of a test is particularly important in the screening situation (see Chapter 2). Because the physician is more interested in improving health outcomes for patients than in simply providing them with diagnoses, elements of the natural history of the disease and of the effectiveness of therapy are critically important.

CRITERIA FOR SCREENING

Whether or not a screening policy results in improved health outcomes depends on the characteristics of the disease(s), the test(s), and the patient population. These are summarized in Table 3.1.

NATURAL HISTORY OF THE DISEASE AND EFFECTIVENESS OF THERAPY

Screening tests are performed to identify asymptomatic disease. The alternative is to wait until the patient presents with symptoms and then make a diagnosis. The question then is, What makes a disease worth diagnosing early? The practical objective of screening is prevention of morbidity and mortality—not simply early diagnosis. There is little benefit to the patient, and perhaps considerable harm, in advancing the time of

Table 3.1.   Criteria for Screening

Characteristics of the disease
Significant effect on quality or length of life
Prevalence sufficiently high to justify costs
Acceptable methods of treatment available
Asymptomatic period during which detection and treatment significantly reduce morbidity and mortality
Treatment in the asymptomatic phase yields a better therapeutic result than treatment delayed until symptoms appear

Characteristics of the test
Sufficiently sensitive to detect disease during the asymptomatic period
Sufficiently specific to provide acceptable predictive value positive
Acceptable to patients

Characteristics of the population screened
Sufficiently high disease prevalence
Accessibility
Compliance with subsequent diagnostic tests and necessary therapy

diagnosis of a disease for which earlier treatment does not influence outcome.

The importance of the natural history of the disease and the effectiveness of therapy can be illustrated by considering Fig. 3.1. As it shows schematically, some variable time after the biologic onset of a disease, a diagnosis is possible with the use of a screening test. This is followed by another variable time period, during which the patient has no symptoms. Usually, a short time after symptoms appear, the clinical diagnosis is made. Eventually, after the course of therapy has been selected and completed, there is an identifiable clinical outcome that can range from cure and complete health to death.

Often, outcome depends somewhat on the point during the natural history of the disease at which therapy is initiated. This is clearest in the case of localized versus metastatic cancer. Many tumors can be readily excised, and the patient cured of the disease, during early stages. The opportunity for cure is often lost when tumor spread makes excision or other local therapy impractical. The "escape from cure" may not be as dramatic as the point of tumor metastasis; a disease may simply become more refractory to therapy, which increases the likelihood of morbid complications. The practical purpose of screening is to advance the time of the diagnosis to a point in the natural history of the disease when a relative or absolute "escape from cure" is less likely to have occurred.

Although the natural history of any disease varies a great deal among persons afflicted, some generalizations are worthwhile. If an "escape from cure" generally occurs at point A in Fig. 3.1 or at any point before available screening tests can detect the disease in question, the value of screening must be questioned. The most common result will be bad news sooner for the patient but no difference in outcome. If "escape from

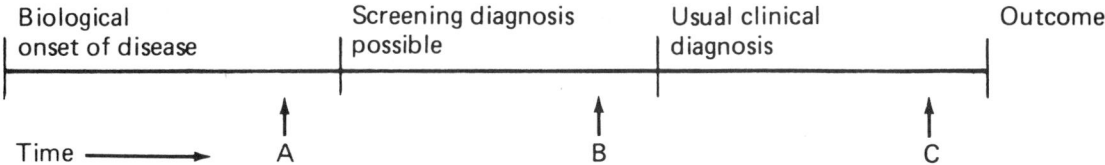

"Escape from cure" at point A: Screening may not affect outcome

"Escape from cure" at point B: High priority for screening

"Escape from cure" at point C: Education and improved access to
care may be more efficient than
screening tests

FIG. 3.1. Relationships between screening and natural history of disease.

cure" routinely occurs after symptoms appear (e.g., at point C), screening may be valuable but can likely be supplanted by patient and professional education programs aimed at ensuring early presentation and prompt diagnosis. Diseases in which "escape from cure" generally occurs after the disease is detectable but while it remains asymptomatic (e.g., at point B) are the most appropriate targets of screening efforts.

Several points about the evaluation of screening programs can also be made with reference to Fig. 3.1. Critics of indiscriminate screening point out that the benefits of a screening program can easily be overestimated if the relationship between time of diagnosis and natural history is not understood. One fallacy results from neglecting the importance of *lead time* when evaluating the effect of screening on subsequent survival. Because screening has the potential to advance the time of diagnosis from one point in the natural history to another and because survival is, by necessity, measured from the time of diagnosis rather than from the time of onset, the survival of patients whose diseases are detected by screening should be expected to be longer than that of patients who present symptomatically. Extensive follow-up data on many patients allow approximation of the average length of time by which the diagnosis is advanced by screening. This illusory gain in survival, the lead time, can then be subtracted from any measured difference in survival duration to learn the true benefits of the screening program.

The second fallacy that can lead to overestimation of screening benefits depends on the variability in natural history among individual cases of the same disease. Patients who have less aggressive disease and so spend more time in a detectable but asymptomatic stage are, other things being equal, more likely to have their disease detected by a screening test than are patients with more aggressive disease. If patients with indolent, asymptomatic disease are more likely to have an indolent clinical course after diagnosis, patients with disease diagnosed by screening should be expected to have longer survival rates than patients who present symptomatically. Arguments about the impact of such biologic determinism versus that of advancing the time of diagnosis have most frequently been raised with regard to breast and prostate cancers, but they apply generally to all screening. This potential bias toward prolonged survival among patients with disease detected by screening tests has been called *time-linked bias sampling.*

Neither of these arguments is meant to deny the value of screening for treatable disease. They simply advise caution in interpreting apparently favorable results based on unsophisticated measures of effectiveness.

VALIDITY OF AVAILABLE SCREENING TESTS AND POPULATIONS SCREENED

Diseases worth identifying usually have a relatively low prevalence in the asymptomatic population. As a result, the specificity of the diagnostic test used is the principal determinant of the predictive value positive of the test. Tests that may be very useful in diagnosis when the prior probability of disease is 10% or 20% may produce an unacceptable number of false-positive results when used in a screening situation. Such nonspecificity has been referred to as the *cost of a screening test.* The costs, including morbidity and patient concern, of diagnostic evaluations among patients with false-positive screening results can far outweigh other costs of a screening program. The sensitivity and specificity of the screening test, costs, and patient acceptability are critical considerations in the decision to screen for disease.

The importance of disease prevalence in determining the predictive value positive is one basis for the use of risk factors in screening policy. By limiting screening to a high-risk population, the physician in effect increases the prevalence of the disease in the population tested (and alternatively increases the prior probability of the disease in any individual patient), thereby increasing the predictive value positive and decreasing the false-alarm rate and the number of false-positive results.

HEALTH MAINTENANCE—WHAT IS APPROPRIATE?

Periodic health evaluation has been recommended with varying degrees of enthusiasm throughout the 20th century. Many patients believe in its value; the majority of Americans feel that more health resources should be expended on preventive efforts. However, the value of periodic examinations and specific preventive measures has been questioned. Evidence regarding the effectiveness of periodic examinations, measured in terms of decreased morbidity and mortality, is fragmentary. Supporters of periodic evaluation argue that the additional benefits of regular physician contact result in a greater sense of well-being. Such contact provides opportunities for appropriate patient education.

Table 3.2. Conditions that Warrant Periodic Evaluation in All Patients of Appropriate Age and Gender

DISEASE	COMMENTS
Hypertension	See Chapters 14, 19, and 26.
Hyperlipidemia	See Chapters 5 and 27.
Smoking	See Chapter 54.
Colon cancer	See Chapter 56.
Breast cancer	See Chapter 106.
Cervical cancer	See Chapter 107.
Alcoholism	See Chapter 228.

Routine examinations should be tailored to the individual patient. Although the importance of the characteristics of the patient, the diseases, and the test in determining appropriate prevention strategies must be recognized, summary recommendations can be useful. A number of reviews, each applying the criteria discussed in this chapter, have offered recommendations for preventive health care. The recommendations of the American Cancer Society, the American College of Physicians, the Canadian Task Force on the Periodic Health Examination, and the U.S. Preventive Services Task Force have received the most attention. Relatively few conditions have received general endorsement as targets for screening among *asymptomatic* persons *without* specific *risk factors*. These are summarized in

Table 3.3. Conditions that Warrant Periodic Evaluation in Selected Patients

CONDITION	RISK FACTORS	COMMENTS
Rubella susceptibility	Anticipated pregnancy and risk-group membership; occupation (health care worker)	See Chapter 6.
Human immunodeficiency virus infection	Anticipated pregnancy and risk-group membership; blood transfusions 1978–1985	See Chapter 7.
Endocarditis susceptibility	Valvular heart disease	See Chapter 16.
Rheumatic fever susceptibility	Rheumatic fever history	See Chapter 17.
Tuberculosis (PPD reactivity)	Occupational exposure	See Chapters 38 and 49.
Occupational lung disease	Occupational exposure	See Chapter 39.
Susceptibility to hepatitis B virus	Male homosexual Exposure Occupation (health care worker)	See Chapter 57.
Anemia	Pregnancy	See Chapter 77.
Sickle cell trait	African-American of childbearing age	Genetic counseling must be acceptable; see Chapter 78.
Thyroid cancer	Radiation of head and neck	See Chapter 94.
Diabetes	Pregnancy; family history of diabetes; obesity; or history of gestational diabetes	See Chapter 93.
Endometrial cancer	Exogenous estrogens	See Chapter 109.
Vaginal cancer	*In utero* diethylstilbestrol exposure	See Chapter 110.
Syphilis	Male homosexual Pregnancy Other sexually transmitted disease	See Chapter 124.
Chlamydial genitourinary infection	Other sexually transmitted disease Women of childbearing age	See Chapter 125.
Bacteriuria	Pregnancy Kidney stones	See Chapter 127.
Lower urinary tract cancer	Occupational exposure to aromatic amines (e.g., dyestuffs, leather tanning, rubber)	See Chapter 128.
Testicular cancer	Cryptorchidism	See Chapters 131 and 143.
Osteoporosis	Early menopause	See Chapter 144.
Cerebrovascular disease	Advanced age, TIA history	See Chapter 171.
Skin cancer	Fair skin, sun exposure Family history	See Chapter 177.
Glaucoma	Family history Advanced age	See Chapter 198.
Oral cancer	Alcohol Tobacco	See Chapter 211.
Decreased hearing	Advanced age, excessive noise	See Chapter 212.

PPD, purified protein derivative; TIA, transient ischemic attack.

Table 3.2. The rationales for these recommendations are presented in the subsequent chapters noted in the table.

Table 3.3 provides a summary of recommendations that have been made for other preventive services that are warranted in selected patients. Again, the rationales for these recommendations are presented in subsequent chapters. It should be noted that uncertainty about both the natural history and the effectiveness of therapy, the importance of specific risk factors, and the sensitivity and specificity of potential screening tests rarely, if ever, allow proof of the effectiveness of a screening procedure. Some conclusions and recommendations, necessarily based on speculative data, remain controversial. The clinician must also be mindful of the potential to help patients avoid preventable morbidity and early death by taking the time to provide advice and counsel about behavior and life-style. Patients often need specific advice, not only about the use of alcohol, tobacco, and harmful substances, but also about diet, exercise, sexual practices, and injury prevention. Such discussions have the potential to produce a far greater effect on health and longevity than do specific screening tests and procedures.

A.G.M.

ANNOTATED BIBLIOGRAPHY

Canadian Task Force on the Periodic Health Examination. Canadian guide to clinical preventive healthcare. Ottawa: Canada Communications Group, 1994. (*A compendium of evidence-based recommendations.*)

Feinleb M, Zelen M. Some pitfalls in the evaluation of screening programs. Arch Environ Health 1969;19:412. (*Classic review of problems with predictive value positive, lead time, and time-linked bias sampling.*)

Hayward RS, Steinberg EP, Ford DE, et al. Preventive care guidelines: 1991. Ann Intern Med 1991;114:758. (*Reviews the history of preventive care guidelines as well as explanations for the different recommendations from different consensus groups. Includes encyclopedic comparisons of recommendations—made by the American College of Physicians, both Canadian and American task forces, and others—for many conditions and procedures, including immunization and chemoprophylaxis.*)

Medical Practice Committee, American College of Physicians. Periodic health examination: a guide for designing individualized preventive health care in the asymptomatic patient. Ann Intern Med 1981;95:729. (*Succinct summary of recommendations.*)

Sox HC Jr. Preventive health services in adults. N Engl J Med 1994;330:1589. (*Succinct summary of issues and recommendations by the chairman of the US Preventive Services Task Force.*)

US Preventive Services Task Force. Guide to clinical preventive services, 2nd ed. Washington, DC: US Department of Health and Human Services, 1996. (*Superb summary of evidence for 70 selected conditions. Strong emphasis on counseling patients about harmful or risky behavior.*)

4

Estimating and Communicating Risk and Prognosis

Diagnosis is a process of classification. A constellation of symptoms, signs, and test results is given a label, and the patient who presents with those characteristics is implicitly grouped with other patients who have presented with similar findings. What makes the classification process and the resulting label so significant for both patient and clinician is what it implies about the future. Will symptoms persist, get worse, or resolve spontaneously? What other health outcomes can be expected? Will therapeutic interventions improve chances for a good outcome?

Similar questions arise when a patient is found to have a risk factor that increases the likelihood of future disease. How great is the risk? What are the chances of avoiding the anticipated bad outcome, either because of efforts to lower risk or by good fortune? To answer such questions, the primary care physician must understand the methods by which valid information about prognosis and risk is derived from the experience of previous patients. Doctor–patient dialogues about the future implications of an illness or risk factor are often momentous for patients. Information about an uncertain future must be communicated with clarity, compassion, and an appreciation for the uniqueness of each patient's needs.

RISK AND PROGNOSIS: PREDICTING THE PATIENT'S FUTURE

The source for information about the future of any particular patient is the collective experience of previous patients with the same condition. The accuracy of the information so derived depends on the manner in which that experience is collected and recorded and on the degree of similarity between the patient at hand and past patients who have been followed over time.

Theoretically, the best mechanism for studying prognosis would be to characterize patients carefully at the time of diagnosis (or when a risk factor is identified) with regard to disease stage and severity, presence or absence of any comorbid conditions, and other factors that could be expected to have an impact on outcome. Because such factors are often systematically influenced by the pattern of patient referral, the setting in which patients are seen and the manner in which they happened to be there would be described. All patients would be examined with the same level of scrutiny at the time they entered the *cohort* and during subsequent follow-up examinations. Relevant outcomes, and criteria by which they would be measured, would be specified in advance. Those conducting follow-up examinations would be unaware of baseline differences among patients so as not to be influenced by expected associations between these variables and outcomes. All patients would be followed, and their status with regard to outcomes would be known at the time the experience was analyzed. The impact of different baseline characteristics on relevant outcomes would be examined by reporting experience for different subgroups or developing statistical models. The predictive validity of these models would be tested in separate samples of patients.

Rarely, if ever, is it possible to meet all these methodologic objectives. As a result, much of the research that clinicians rely on for information about risk and prognosis is potentially misleading. To avoid being misled and misleading patients, clinicians must understand the biases that can be introduced when suboptimal methods are used to gather information to help predict the future.

When the outcomes of interest are rare events, it may not be feasible to assemble a cohort large enough, and follow it long enough, to accumulate sufficient experience to provide useful estimates of prognosis or risk. Alternatively, patients who have already experienced the outcome can be identified as cases and their past histories examined to identify events or *exposures* that may have conferred risk and may be of prognostic value. *Control* patients without the outcome of interest can also be questioned about the same exposures. Comparison of the rates of exposure among cases and controls can produce an estimate of the degree of risk associated with the exposure. The *odds ratio* is an estimate of the *relative risk* that is very accurate when the disease or outcome in question is rare. This retrospective case–control approach places a heavy burden on the investigator and sources of information to ensure that similar degrees of scrutiny are applied to the histories of cases and controls. Selective recollection of the past, often with greater vigilance stimulated by the outcome of interest, can produce misleading estimates of risk and prognosis.

Even if patients with a particular risk factor or diagnosis are identified prospectively and followed forward in time, biases that can lead to faulty conclusions may be introduced. Perhaps the most important bias for primary care physicians to recognize has been termed *referral filter bias*. It occurs frequently as a result of the fact that patients in many published reports have been described because they have been referred to academic centers. Such patients often have complicating characteristics and exhibit a worse prognosis than do patients who are drawn from an entire population or a representative sample of a population. Similar problems arise when patients are selected for study based on particular test results. Patients with more worrisome signs and symptoms may be more likely to be tested and more likely to fare poorly over time. Alternatively, patients who are tested may have better access to medical care and fare better than average as a result.

Differences in the ways patients are followed over time can also introduce important biases. Patients lost to follow-up may be different from those who remain in the cohort. A conservative approach to estimating prognosis when some patients are lost to follow-up before the relevant outcome has occurred is to assume that all lost patients experienced the outcome, and then to assume that no lost patients experienced it. The first assumption produces an *upper bound estimate*, with lost patients included in both numerator and denominator; the second produces a *lower bound estimate*, with lost patients included only in the denominator.

Even when patients are successfully followed over time, biases can be introduced by the selective use of tests and other outcome measures or by the expectations of clinicians who are aware of patient characteristics that may or may not have real prognostic significance. Statistical models that have not been validated on independent samples may mistake random variations among characteristics and outcomes for important prognostic associations.

DESCRIBING THE RISK OF FUTURE DISEASE

People are generally very interested in the risk of untoward events and ways to reduce risks. Despite the high level of interest, there is a great deal of confusion about the meaning of quantitative expressions of risk. This confusion often carries over to conversations between doctors and patients. An important source of confusion is the distinction between *relative* and *absolute* risk. The effect of risk factors is usually expressed as a relative risk or risk ratio—that is, the incidence of disease among people with the risk factor divided by the incidence among people without the factor (often estimated as the odds ratio from a case–control study). However, for the individual patient with the risk factor, the incidence of disease, the absolute risk of the outcome, may be more useful. For example, a patient may have a 20- or 30-fold increased risk for a rare disease but still face less than a 1% absolute risk for development of that disease in his or her lifetime. Another way of conveying the implications of a risk factor is to cite the attributable risk, which is the difference between the incidence among exposed people and the incidence among those who are not exposed.

Such distinctions are also important in weighing the harms and benefits of interventions designed to reduce risk. Treating hypertension may well reduce the risk of stroke by 40% (the relative risk reduction). However, doctor and patient should also understand that the baseline risk of stroke during the next 10 years may be as low as 1% for some patients with mild hypertension. This means that the benefit of risk reduction, or the risk difference attributable to the untreated mild hypertension, is the difference between 1.0% and 0.6%, or 0.4%. Another approach to summarizing this kind of data is to cite the number of patients one would need to treat to have the desired effect in a single patient. Returning to the hypertension example, treating 1,000 patients would reduce the number of strokes from 10 to 6, so 250 people with mild hypertension would have to be treated to avoid one stroke.

DESCRIBING OUTCOMES DURING AN UNCERTAIN FUTURE

The diagnosis of a particular condition is generally much more predictive of future outcomes than the identification of risk factors. Outcomes are more frequent and are often described as simple rates. The proportion of people with a particular condition who eventually die of that disease is the *case fatality rate*. Some indication of the duration of survival may be included by describing survival at a point in time after diagnosis (e.g., the 5-year survival rate). Simple rates have the advantage of being easy to remember and communicate. However, valuable information is lost when prognosis, the distribution of uncertain events over time, is summarized by a single rate. The more complete picture of prognosis is captured in a *survival curve*. Survival curves are often used to display the proportion of a cohort surviving over time, but the same technique can be used to display the occurrence, or lack thereof, of other events, such as onset of symptoms or recurrence of disease. Survival curves are constructed by plotting sequentially calculated probabilities of survival (or freedom from events) over time. The decrease in the height of the curve at any time period depends on the proportion of the remaining cohort who experience the event during that period, with patients lost to follow-up excluded from the denominator. Sometimes, the proportion of people who experience events, rather than the proportion who are event-free, is plotted on the vertical axis. Such *cumulative incidence curves* convey the same information.

It is important to remember that survival curves display serial estimates that are based on the experience of fewer and fewer people as events and loss to follow-up deplete the denominator. Therefore, the clinician can be more confident in the estimates displayed on the left part of the curve than on the right. The distant future is more uncertain than the near term. However, when a new diagnosis of serious disease is made, it is often the near term that is of greatest interest to the patient. A cumulative recurrence risk of 30% may be frightening to the woman with early-stage breast cancer, and this may be a case in which use of the simple rate to express prognosis is a disservice. The more complete picture presented by a survival curve, including attention to the low annual incidence of recurrence in the near term, may be more helpful to the patient.

THE UNIQUENESS OF EACH PATIENT

Descriptions of risk and prognosis should be provided to patients with an appreciation for the uniqueness of each person and his or her predicament. Different people respond differently to the same risk. A 1% risk for stroke during a 5- or 10-year period may be threatening to some but inconsequential to others. This can be explained by the very real competing risks that different people face because of other medical conditions or the environment in which they live. Similarly, different people have different attitudes about trade-offs between the present or near future and the distant future. Putting up with side effects or inconvenience now for some *possible* benefit in the future

makes good sense to some but little sense to others. Again, competing risks explain some of these differences. Another important difference among patients relates to their desire for information about the future. Many demand such information. Others would rather not know details about prognosis, even when that means that they must defer to the clinician for important decisions. As in other aspects of patient education, respect for the patient's autonomy and personal values during the communication of information about illness and its implications for the future requires a negotiated approach to patient care.

A.G.M.

ANNOTATED BIBLIOGRAPHY

Concato J, Feinstein AR, Holford TR. The risk of determining risk with multivariable models. Ann Intern Med 1993;118:201. (*Reviews principles and standards for application of multivariable statistical methods in general medical literature.*)

Fletcher RH, Fletcher SW, Wagner EH. Clinical epidemiology: the essentials, 2nd ed. Baltimore: Williams & Wilkins, 1988. (*A good general reference, with careful treatment of risk and prognosis in Chapters 5 and 6.*)

Laupacis A, Sackett DL, Roberts RS. An assessment of clinically useful measures of the consequences of treatment. N Engl J Med 1988;318:1728. (*An analysis of alternative approaches to summarizing effectiveness data, including the number needed to treat, or NNT.*)

Laupacis A, Wells G, Richardson WS, et al., for the Evidence-Based Medicine Working Group. Users' guide to the medical literature. V. How to use an article about prognosis. JAMA 1994;272:234. (*A systematic approach to practical application of the literature.*)

Sackett DL, Haynes RB, Guyatt GH, et al. Clinical epidemiology: a basic science for clinical medicine, 2nd ed. Boston: Little, Brown, 1991. (*Very well written from the perspective of the clinician who wants to be a critical appraiser of published experience relevant to prognosis.*)

Wasson JH, Sox HC, Neff RK, et al. Clinical prediction rules: applications and methodological standards. N Engl J Med 1985;313:793. (*Provides a checklist for methodological standards for studies that purport to define prognostic variables.*)

5

Choosing among Treatment Options

Although discerning diagnosis and accurate prognosis are essential to effective patient care, the process of choosing among treatment options can have the greatest impact on relief of suffering and prolongation of life. The right choice depends on accurate information about the effects of various treatment strategies on health outcomes. Will symptoms be relieved or at least reduced? Will serious complications of disease be averted by timely intervention, or will treatment side effects or complications decrease the quality or length of life? Treatment choices also depend on patients' preferences for different possible health outcomes and on their attitudes toward risks or their willingness to endure morbidity now for some possible future benefit. And, as noted in Chapter 4, different patients have different preferences and attitudes toward risks and time trade-offs. Effective therapeutic decision making therefore requires both a strong clinical knowledge base and the communication skills necessary to gain an empathic understanding of the individual patient's wants and needs.

WHAT WE KNOW ABOUT TREATMENT EFFECTIVENESS

The cumulative knowledge base about the effectiveness of treatments of human disease is prodigious. And yet, the use of the vast majority of therapeutic interventions in clinical practice is not supported by evidence derived from clinical trials. Clinicians often rely on their own experience with similar patients, supplemented by published case series, to estimate the likelihood of relevant health outcomes with alternative treatments. This less-than-rigorous approach produces different opinions about treatment effectiveness that lead to wide variations in clinical practices for ostensibly similar patients. Because of less stringent regulatory control, the knowledge gaps are generally greater with devices and surgical procedures than with drugs. For example, diskectomy for lumbar disk disease was first described in 1934. Nevertheless, the first and only randomized trial was published in 1983 and included only 60 surgical patients. The collective experience of the millions of patients who have undergone diskectomy worldwide contributes relatively little to our knowledge. Similarly, transurethral prostatectomy represented the standard of care for benign prostatic hyperplasia for 40 years before publication of a clinical trial.

RANDOMIZED CLINICAL TRIALS AND TREATMENT EFFECTIVENESS

Even when randomized trials are performed, uncertainty remains about the effectiveness of treatment for a specific patient. This in part reflects the methods used in clinical trials to measure the isolated effects of the experimental treatment. Explicit inclusion and exclusion criteria are applied to ensure that the study population is homogeneous, which minimizes the impact of patient-specific variables on outcomes. Patients with severe disease or important comorbid conditions are often excluded. Others may be excluded because of age or sex. Patients who meet criteria are then randomized to one of two or more carefully defined treatment strategies. Barriers are erected to discourage patients from switching from one treatment to another, and other steps are taken to preserve the integrity of the treatments.

The course of patients in randomized trials is carefully monitored, with equal attention given to patients regardless of treatment, and their outcomes are determined by means of explicit, predefined measures. Ideally, both patients and those who measure outcomes are unaware of the treatment assignment, even if this requires the use of placebos or sham procedures. Otherwise, expectations may have a real effect on perceived treatment outcomes and be interpreted as specific effects of treatment.

All these steps serve to protect the validity of the trial as a test of the hypothesis that the treatments compared in the trial have different effects on outcome. However, these same steps often limit the applicability, or generalizability, of the study findings to patients for whom the study treatment might be considered. The clinician must be concerned both about the internal validity of the trial as a test of the effectiveness hypothesis, and about its external validity—that is, the extent to which results are applicable to the different patients seen in practice.

All too frequently, individual trials may not be large enough to provide definitive answers to clinical questions. Increasingly, data from multiple trials are being combined in metaanalyses to allow careful systematic interpretation of the evidence.

OTHER STUDIES OF TREATMENT EFFECTIVENESS

Randomized trials are not always necessary. When a new treatment has unprecedented or dramatic effects, such as penicillin for pneumococcal pneumonia or pacemaker insertion for life-threatening bradycardia, a trial is neither possible nor desirable. When results of trials would be helpful because treatment effects are more equivocal, they are often not available. Randomized trials are costly, time-consuming, and poorly accepted by many clinicians and patients. Sometimes, a trial is obsolete before it is completed because the experimental treatment is modified or replaced altogether by a newer approach or technology.

For all these reasons, clinicians must rely on data from observational studies as well as randomized trial results. However, great caution must be used in the application of conclusions of observational studies to patient care. Differences in patient characteristics among alternative treatment groups may lead to erroneous conclusions about treatment effectiveness. Although there have been important advances in the use of statistical methods to control for such different prognostic factors in an attempt to isolate the treatment effect, the investigator can control only for those factors that are anticipated and measured. Observational studies complement randomized trials. They can be used to design efficient and targeted trials and to assess the generalizability of trial results. However, the clinician should be mindful of the quality of evidence when making treatment choices, and there is no substitute for a well-conducted randomized trial.

The Impact of Patients' Expectations on Outcomes

There is ample evidence demonstrating that patients' expectations regarding the effectiveness of treatment has a profound influence on the outcome of treatment. It is not at all unusual for patients receiving inactive agents (placebos) or sham surgical procedures to report an improvement in symptoms. For example, as much as two thirds of the symptom improvement appreciated by patients taking finasteride for benign prostatic hyperplasia was reported by those assigned to placebo in double-blind randomized trials. Furthermore, improvement in objective outcomes, such as mortality rates, have been reported following use of placebo agents or sham surgical procedures. There are also examples of studies in which patients who have sufficiently high expectations to comply faithfully with a prescribed regimen do better than patients who do not. These "compliance effects" occur regardless of whether the regimen includes an active agent or actual procedure. It is likely that the effect of patients' expectation plays a substantial role in the perceived effectiveness of many interventions, including those termed "complementary" or "alternative" because they are outside the mainstream of what is taught in medical schools. An important task of primary care is to teach patients the rules of evidence that are critical to the scientific basis of health services.

TREATMENT CHOICE AND PATIENT VALUES

Even if the probabilities of outcomes contingent on alternative treatment choices can be estimated precisely, there is still much work to be done to ensure a wise treatment choice for a particular patient. Consider the predicament of the 75-year-old man who is bothered by nocturia and urinary frequency resulting from benign prostatic hyperplasia. He can live with his symptoms, but this means accepting a diminished quality of life. He may choose to try a medical approach, such as finasteride or an α-blocker, with hope of modest relief of symptoms. Alternatively, surgical therapy offers a good chance of more dramatic symptom relief but also confers a small but real risk of a catastrophic event that could result in death. Surgery also puts the patient at risk for complications, such as incontinence or impotence, that can diminish the quality of life as much as or more than nocturia and frequency.

The probabilities of these outcomes are critically important to the decision. Equally important, however, is how the patient feels about the outcomes. Different men feel differently about trade-offs between urinary function and sexual function, and they have different attitudes toward the small risk of perioperative death. These personal value judgments are as important in determining the "right" choice as are the probabilities that are derived from clinical research. The right choice, therefore, requires careful communication between clinician and patient about what the possible outcomes will mean for that patient's quality of life.

A.G.M.

ANNOTATED BIBLIOGRAPHY

Bero LA, Jadad AR. How consumers and policy makers can use systematic reviews for decision making. Ann Intern Med 1997;127:37. (*Strategies for optimizing the information value of systematic reviews in clinical and policy decision making.*)

The Cochrane Library, Issue 4. Update software: 1998. Oxford, England. (*A remarkable compendium of medical evidence available as a searchable compact disk and on the Internet.*)

Guyatt GH, Sackett DL, Cook DJ, for the Evidence-Based Medicine Working Group. Users' guide to the medical literature. II. How to use an article about therapy or prevention. A. Are the results of the study valid? B. What were the results and will they help me in caring for my patients? JAMA 1994;270:2598 and 271:59. (*Practical application of clinical epidemiology to better understand evidence of therapeutic effectiveness.*)

Eisenberg DM, Davis RB, Ettner SL, et al. Trends in alternative medicine use in the United States, 1990–1997. JAMA 1998;280:1569. (*A substantial increase in use of alternative medicine during the nineties—more than 40% of the U.S. population.*)

Guyatt G, Sackett D, Taylor DW, et al. Determining optimal therapy—randomized trials in individual patients. N Engl J Med 1986; 314:889. (*Persuasive argument for blinded, placebo-controlled, crossover trials in individual patients to evaluate the specific effects of medical treatments more critically.*)

Mulley AG. Assessing patients' utilities: can the ends justify the means? Med Care 1989;27:S269. (*A somewhat technical discussion of the role of patients' preferences and their measurement in clinical decision making.*)

Oxman AD, Cook DJ, Guyatt GH, for the Evidence-Based Medicine Working Group. Users' guide to the medical literature. VI. How to use an overview. JAMA 1994;272:1367. (*More practical advice about how to use the literature—in this case, by interpreting increasingly prevalent systematic overviews.*)

6

Immunization

EDWARD T. RYAN

Immunization is the most cost-effective means of preventing disease. Immunizations are grouped into five major categories: (a) routine vaccinations of childhood, (b) routine vaccinations of adulthood (Table 6.1), (c) postexposure prophylactic immunizations, (d) travel-related immunizations, and (e) work-related/special circumstance immunizations. Of these, administration of vaccines during childhood has been most successful; fewer than 100 children die each year of vaccine-preventable illnesses in the United States. In comparison, 50,000 to 70,000 adults die each year in the United States of vaccine-preventable illnesses.

Compared with responses in young adults or children, responses are often lower in elderly or immunocompromised persons; however, vaccines still induce clinically meaningful protective immunity in most adult populations. Vaccine administration in adults is safe; most adverse reactions occur at the injection site and include induration, erythema, and tenderness; low-grade fever and mild constitutional symptoms may also occur. Severe complications such as anaphylactic shock occur in fewer than 1 in 1 million inoculations. Individuals with a high likelihood of having severe reactions can usually be identified before the administration of a specific agent. Although most people born in the United States receive standard immunizations during childhood, approximately 1 in 25 persons currently living in the United States was born in another country. Many of these people have been incompletely immunized.

GENERAL PRINCIPLES OF IMMUNIZATION

Types of Immunization

Immunizations can be either *active* or *passive*.

Active Immunization entails the administration of a *vaccine* (live attenuated microorganisms, killed microorganisms, or purified proteins or polysaccharides of microorganisms) or a *toxoid* (a deactivated toxin). Active immunization often provides long-term (lasting for years or, less frequently, for life) protective immunity; however, meaningful immunity is often not achieved until 2 to 4 weeks after vaccination. Vaccines that are live attenuated versions of an infectious agent are usually more efficacious and provide more long-lasting immunity than do nonliving vaccines. Similarly, polysaccharide-based vaccines are in general less immunogenic than protein-based vaccines; however, the coupling of polysaccharide antigens to "carrier" proteins can markedly increase immunologic responses against polysaccharide components.

Passive Immunization entails the administration of preformed antibody (such as immunoglobulin). Passive immunization results in immediate protective immunity, but such immunity is short-term (usually lasting for only 3 to 6 months).

Administration

A host of strategies are available for administration.

Table 6.1.   Summary of Recommendations for Routine Adult Immunizations[a]

VACCINE NAME	FOR WHOM RECOMMENDED
• **Influenza** *"Flu shot"* • Give IM.	• Adults who are 65 years of age or older. • People 6 months to 65 years of age with medical problems such as heart disease, lung disease, diabetes, renal dysfunction, hemoglobinopathies, immunosuppression; people living in long-term care facilities. • People 6 months of age or older working or living with at-risk people. • All health care workers and those who provide key community services. • Healthy pregnant women who will be in their second or third trimesters during the influenza season. • Pregnant women who have underlying medical conditions should be vaccinated before the flu season, regardless of the state of pregnancy. • Anyone who wishes to reduce the likelihood of becoming ill with influenza. • Persons traveling to areas where influenza activity exists or among people from areas of the world where there is current influenza activity.
• **Pneumococcal** • Give IM or SQ.	• Adults who are 65 years of age or older. • People 2 to 65 years of age who have chronic illness or other risk factors, including chronic cardiac or pulmonary diseases, chronic liver disease, alcoholism, diabetes mellitus, CSF leaks, and persons living in special environments or social settings (including Alaska natives and certain American Indian populations). Those at highest risk of fatal pneumococcal infection are persons with anatomic or functional asplenia (including sickle cell disease); immunocompromised persons, including those with HIV infection, leukemia, lymphoma, Hodgkin's disease, multiple myeloma, generalized malignancy, chronic renal failure, or nephrotic syndrome; those receiving immunosuppressive chemotherapy (including corticosteroids); and those who have received an organ or bone marrow transplant.
• **Hepatitis B** (Hep-B) • Give IM. • Brands may be used interchangeably.	• High-risk adults, including household contacts and sex partners of Hb$_s$Ag-positive persons; users of illicit injectable drugs; heterosexuals with more than one sex partner in 6 months; men who have sex with men; people with recently diagnosed STDs; patients in hemodialysis units and patients with renal disease that may result in dialysis; recipients of certain blood products; health care workers and public safety workers who are exposed to blood; clients and staff of institutions for the developmentally disabled; inmates of long-term correctional facilities; certain international travelers. *Note:* Prior serologic testing may be recommended depending on the specific level of risk or likelihood of previous exposure. • All adolescents. • *Note:* In 1997, the NIH Consensus Development Conference, a panel of national experts, recommended that hepatitis B vaccination be given to all persons infected with hepatitis C virus. • *Editor's note: Perform serologic screening for people who have emigrated from endemic areas. When Hb$_s$Ag-positive persons are identified, offer them appropriate disease management. In addition, screen their household members and intimate contacts and, if found susceptible, vaccinate.*
• **Hepatitis A** (Hep-A) • Give IM. • Brands may be used interchangeably.	• People who travel outside the U.S. (except for northern and western Europe, new Zealand, Australia, Canada, and Japan). • People with chronic liver disease, including people with hepatitis C virus infection, people with hepatitis B who have chronic liver disease, illicit drug users, men who have sex with men, people with clotting factor disorders, people who work with hepatitis A virus in experimental lab settings (this does not refer to routine medical laboratories), and food handlers when health authorities or private employers determine vaccination to be cost-effective. • *Note:* Prevaccination testing is likely to be cost-effective for persons over 40 years of age as well as for younger persons in certain groups with a high prevalence of hepatitis A virus infection.
• **Td** (Tetanus, diphtheria) • Give IM.	• All adolescents and adults. • After the primary series has been completed, a booster dose is recommended every 10 years. Make sure your patients have received a primary series of three doses. • A booster dose as early as five years later may be needed for the purpose of wound management, so consult ACIP recommendations.
• **MMR** (Measles, mumps, rubella) • Give SQ.	• Adults born in 1957 or later who are 18 years of age or older (including those born outside the U.S.) should receive at least one dose of MMR if there is no serologic proof of immunity or documentation of a dose given on or after first birthday. • Adults in high-risk groups, such as health care workers, students entering colleges and other educational institutions after high school, and international travelers, should receive a total of two doses. • All women of childbearing age (i.e., adolescent girls and premenopausal adult women) who do not have acceptable evidence of rubella immunity or vaccination. • *Note:* Adults born before 1957 are usually considered immune, but proof of immunity may be desirable for health care workers.

[a]Detailed Advisory Committee on Immunization Practices (ACIP) recommendations can be found at www.cdc.gov/nip.

CSF, cerebrospinal fluid; Hb$_s$Ag, hepatitis B surface antigen; STD, sexually transmitted disease; IPV, inactivated poliomyelitis vaccine.

Adapted from the Advisory Committee on Immunization Practices by the Immunization Action Coalition *ad hoc* team (August 1999), with additions.

SCHEDULE	CONTRAINDICATIONS AND PRECAUTIONS (MILD ILLNESS NOT A CONTRAINDICATION)
• Given every year. • In the temperate Northern Hemisphere, October through November is the optimal time to receive an annual flu shot to maximize protection, but the vaccine may be given at any time during the influenza season (typically December through March) or at other times when the risk of influenza exists. • May be given anytime during the influenza season. • May be given with all other vaccines but at a separate site.	• Previous anaphylactic reaction to this vaccine, to any of its components, or to eggs. • Moderate or severe acute illness.
• Routinely given as one-time dose; administer if previous vaccination history is unknown. • One time revaccination is recommended 5 years later for people at highest risk of fatal pneumococcal infection or rapid antibody loss (e.g., renal disease) and for people older than 65 years if the first dose was given before age 65 and 5 years or more have elapsed since previous dose. • May be given with all other vaccines but at a separate site.	• Previous anaphylactic reaction to this vaccine or to any of its components. • Moderate or severe acute illness.

• Three doses are needed on a 0, 1, 6 months schedule.
• Alternate timing options for vaccination include
    0, 2, 4 months
    0, 1, 4 months
• There must be 4 weeks between doses #1 and #2, and 8 weeks between doses #2 and #3. Overall, there must be at least 4 months between doses #1 and #3.
• Schedule for those who have fallen behind: If the series is delayed between doses, do not start the series over. Continue from where you left off.
• May be given with all other vaccines but at a separate site.
	• Previous anaphylactic reaction to this vaccine or to any of its components.
	• Moderate or severe acute illness.

• Two doses are needed. • The minimum interval between doses #1 and #2 is 6 months. • If dose #2 is delayed, do not repeat dose #1. Just give dose #2. • May be given with all other vaccines but at a separate site.	• Previous anaphylactic reaction to this vaccine or to any of its components. • Moderate or severe acute illness. • Safety during pregnancy has not been determined, so benefits must be weighed against potential risk.

• Booster dose every 10 years after completion of the primary series of three doses.
• **For those who have fallen behind:** The primary series is three doses:
  • Give dose #2 four weeks after #1.
  • Dose #3 is given 6 to 12 months after #2.
• May be given with all other vaccines but at a separate site.
	• Previous anaphylactic or neurologic reaction to this vaccine or to any of its components.
	• Moderate or severe acute illness.

• One or two doses are needed. • If dose #2 is recommended, give it no sooner than 4 weeks after dose #1. • May be given with all other vaccines but at a separate site. • If varicella vaccine and MMR (or other live viral vaccines such as yellow fever vaccine) are needed and are not administered on the same day, space them at least 4 weeks apart.	• Previous anaphylactic reaction to this vaccine or to any of its components. (Anaphylactic reaction to eggs is no longer a contraindication to MMR.) • Pregnancy or possibility of pregnancy within 3 months. • HIV positivity is *not* a contraindication to MMR except for those who are severely immunocompromised. • Immunocompromise caused by cancer, leukemia, lymphoma, and immunosuppressive drug therapy, including high-dose steroids or radiation therapy. • If blood products or immune globulin have been administered during the past 11 months, consult the ACIP recommendations regarding time to wait before vaccinating. • Moderate or severe acute illness. • *Note:* MMR is *not* contraindicated if a PPD test has been done recently. PPD should be delayed for 4 to 6 weeks after an MMR has been given.

(continued)

Table 6.1. Summary of Recommendations for Routine Adult Immunizations[a] (Continued)

VACCINE NAME	FOR WHOM RECOMMENDED
• **Varicella** (Var) *"Chickenpox shot"* • Give SQ.	• All susceptible adults and adolescents should be vaccinated. Make special efforts to vaccinate susceptible persons who have close contact with persons at high risk for serious complications (e.g., health care workers and family contacts of immunocompromised persons) and susceptible persons who are at high risk of exposure (e.g., teachers of young children, day care employees, residents and staff in institutional settings such as colleges and correctional institutions, military personnel, adolescents and adults living with children, nonpregnant women of childbearing age, and international travelers who do not have evidence of immunity). • *Note:* People with reliable histories of chickenpox (e.g., self-report or parental report of disease) can be assumed to be immune. For adults who have no reliable history, serologic testing may be cost-effective because most adults with a negative or uncertain history of varicella are immune.
• **Polio** (IPV) • Give IM or SQ.	• Not routinely recommended for persons 18 years of age or older. • *Note:* Adults living in the U.S. who never received or completed a primary series of polio vaccine need not be vaccinated unless they intend to travel to areas where exposure to wild-type virus is likely. Previously vaccinated adults should receive one booster dose if traveling to polio endemic areas.
• **Lyme Disease** • Give IM.	• Consider for persons 15 to 70 years of age who reside, work, or play in areas of high or moderate risk and who engage in activities that result in frequent or prolonged exposure to tick-infested habitat. • Persons with a history of previous uncomplicated Lyme disease who are at continued high risk for Lyme disease (see description in the first bullet). • See ACIP statement for a definition of high and moderate risk.

[a]Detailed Advisory Committee on Immunization Practices (ACIP) recommendations can be found at www.cdc.gov/nip.

CSF, cerebrospinal fluid; Hb$_s$Ag, hepatitis B surface antigen; STD, sexually transmitted disease; IPV, inactivated poliomyelitis vaccine.

Adapted from the Advisory Committee on Immunization Practices by the Immunization Action Coalition *ad hoc* team (August 1999), with additions.

Technique. With a few exceptions, most vaccines can be administered simultaneously. An adult can usually tolerate the administration of up to four vaccines (two vaccines administered separately in each deltoid area) in a given appointment. Adults should be vaccinated in the *deltoid area* of their upper extremities. Because of unreliable absorption, inoculations (other than certain immunoglobulin preparations) should not be administered in the gluteal region. A new syringe and needle should be used for each vaccination/immunization. If more than one live attenuated viral vaccine (e.g., measles, mumps, and rubella; varicella; yellow fever) is indicated, the vaccines should be administered on the same day (at different injection sites) or at least 30 days apart. When live vaccines are administered on different days sooner than 30 days apart, immunologic responses decrease. For similar reasons, inoculations with the cholera vaccine (rarely, if ever, indicated) and the yellow fever vaccine should be separated by at least 3 weeks.

Combining Passive and Active Immunization. Immunoglobulin preparations (and immunoglobulin-containing blood products) should not be administered with live vaccines when the immunoglobulin preparation contains antibodies directed against such viruses. If a patient requires both an immunoglobulin preparation and a live viral vaccine, the viral vaccine should be administered at least 2 weeks before the immunoglobulin preparation (if possible). If the immunoglobulin preparation is administered first, 3 to 11 months (usually 3 to 6) should elapse before the live viral vaccine is administered. Simultaneous administration of immunoglobulin preparations,

the oral polio vaccine, and all or any of the nonliving vaccines is not problematic. Persons with immunoglobulin A deficiency should not receive immunoglobulin preparations unless the risk of illness clearly outweighs the risk of anaphylaxis.

Allergic Reactions

A person who has an anaphylactic reaction to *eggs* or *egg proteins* should not receive vaccines grown in chick egg embryos or cell cultures. For special circumstances, vaccine desensitization protocols are available. Gastric or intestinal discomfort after eating eggs is not a contraindication to receiving these vaccines. Vaccines sometimes contain low levels of antibiotics that can trigger an allergic reaction. No vaccine that is available in the United States contains penicillin, so an allergy to penicillin does not contraindicate the use of any vaccine in the United States. However, the measles, mumps, and rubella (MMR), varicella, and inactivated polio virus (IPV) vaccines do contain low levels of *neomycin*; individuals with a history of anaphylactic reactions to neomycin should not receive these vaccines. IPV should also not be administered to individuals with a history of anaphylactic reactions to *polymyxin B* or *streptomycin*. Similarly, the oral polio vaccine should not be administered to individuals with a history of anaphylactic reactions to *streptomycin*.

If an individual has a history of a reaction to any vaccine, the repeated administration of that vaccine should be carefully weighed against the risk and severity of the illness in that individual and the severity of the previous reaction.

SCHEDULE	CONTRAINDICATIONS AND PRECAUTIONS (MILD ILLNESS NOT A CONTRAINDICATION)
• Two doses are needed. • Dose #2 is given 4 to 8 weeks after dose #1. • May be given with all other vaccines but at a separate site. • If varicella vaccine and MMR (or other live viral vaccines such as yellow fever vaccine) are needed and are not administered on the same day, space them at least 4 weeks apart. • If the second dose is delayed, do not repeat dose #1. Just give dose #2.	• Previous anaphylactic reaction to this vaccine or to any of its components. • Pregnancy or possibility of pregnancy within 1 month (manufacturer recommends 3 months). • Immunocompromise caused by malignancies and primary or acquired cellular immunodeficiency, including HIV/AIDS. *Note:* For those on high-dose immunosuppressive therapy, consult ACIP recommendations regarding delay time. • If blood products or immune globulin have been administered during the past 5 months, consult the ACIP recommendations regarding time to wait before vaccinating. • Moderate or severe acute illness. • *Note:* Manufacturer recommends that salicylates be avoided for 6 weeks after administration of varicella vaccine because of a theoretical risk of Reye's syndrome.
• Refer to ACIP recommendations regarding unique situations, schedules, and dosing information. • May be given with all other vaccines but at a separate site.	• Refer to ACIP recommendations.
• Three doses are needed. Give at intervals of 0, 1, and 12 months. Schedule dose #1 (given in year 1) and dose #3 (given in year 2) to be given several weeks before tick season. See ACIP statement for details. • Safety of administering Lyme disease vaccine with other vaccines has not been established. • ACIP says if it must be administered concurrently with other vaccines, give it at a separate site.	• Previous anaphylactic reaction to this vaccine or to any of its components. • Pregnancy. • Moderate or severe acute illness. • Treatment-resistant Lyme arthritis. • There are not enough data to recommend Lyme disease vaccine to persons with these conditions: immunodeficiency, diseases associated with joint swelling (including rheumatoid arthritis) or diffuse muscular pain, chronic health conditions resulting from Lyme disease.

Vaccination during Pregnancy and Breast-feeding

As a general rule, live attenuated vaccines should not be administered to pregnant women (Table 6.2). Similarly, a woman who receives a live attenuated viral vaccine should be advised to avoid pregnancy for 3 months. Pregnancy in a household contact is not a contraindication to vaccine administration (except to varicella vaccine if the pregnant woman is herself not immune to varicella/chickenpox). Breast-feeding is not a contraindication to vaccine administration (only the rubella vaccine has been reported to be transmitted through breast milk, and this attenuated virus has not been known to be harmful to neonates or infants).

Vaccination of Immunocompromised Persons

Severely immunocompromised persons should not receive vaccines of *live attenuated viruses* (Tables 6.3 and 6.4). Moreover, an individual with an immunocompromised household contact should not receive the live oral polio vaccine or the varicella vaccine because person-to-person transmission can occur. The MMR vaccine, however, may be administered to individuals infected with the human immunodeficiency virus who are not severely immunocompromised. All vaccines of *inactivated viruses* can be safely administered to immunocompromised individuals, although immune responses may be less than optimal. Anecdotal reports associate administration of the tetanus-diphtheria (Td) vaccine with organ rejection in transplant recipients, but conclusive data are lacking.

Misconceptions about Contraindications

Mild or moderate *local reactions* to a previous vaccination (including tenderness, redness, or swelling at the injection site, or a low-grade fever) are not contraindications to subsequent vaccination. Neither are mild respiratory, intestinal, or *flulike illnesses*, *low-grade fever*, or a history of a recent illness contraindications to vaccine administration. Current antibiotic therapy is a contraindication only to the administration of the oral typhoid vaccine (an attenuated bacterial strain that is killed by antibiotics); all other vaccines can be administered to an individual receiving antibiotics. With the exception of allergies to neomycin, streptomycin, or polymyxin B, allergies to antibiotics are not a contraindication to vaccine administration. Moreover, a history of seizures is not a contraindication to vaccine administration, nor is a history of a non–vaccine-associated chronic demyelinating condition (such as multiple sclerosis or Guillain-Barré syndrome); many such individuals are at increased risk for a number of vaccine-preventable illnesses.

Record Keeping

The National Childhood Vaccine Injury Act of 1988 requires that all health care providers who administer MMR vaccines (in any combination), polio vaccines, or diphtheria, pertussis, and tetanus vaccines (in any combination) maintain immunization records and contact the Centers for Disease Control and Prevention (CDC) and the Food and Drug Administration (FDA) if an adverse reaction occurs. This is true

Table 6.2. Vaccination During Pregnancy

VACCINE	TYPE	INDICATIONS FOR VACCINATION DURING PREGNANCY
Live virus vaccine[a]		
Measles Mumps Rubella	Live attenuated	Contraindicated. May give immunoglobulin for exposure.
Yellow fever	Live attenuated	Contraindicated except if exposure to yellow fever virus is unavoidable.
Poliomyelitis	Trivalent live attenuated (OPV)	Persons at substantial risk of exposure. ACIP has recommended use in outbreak. Many would use IPV (see below).
Varicella	Live attenuated	Contraindicated. If exposure and susceptible, give VZIG.
Inactivated virus vaccines Hepatitis A	Killed virus	Data on safety in pregnancy are not available. Should weigh theoretical risk of vaccination against risk of disease.
Hepatitis B	Recombinant produced purified hepatitis B surface antigen	Pregnancy is not a contraindication. Preexposure and postexposure prophylaxis can be administered if indicated.
Influenza	Inactivated type A and type B virus vaccines	Women who will be in second or third trimester during flu season. All high-risk pregnant women.
Japanese encephalitis	Killed virus	Should reflect actual risks of disease and probable benefits of vaccine.
Poliomyelitis	Killed virus (IPV)	May be preferred over OPV because of risk of vaccine-associated paralysis.
Rabies	Killed virus Rabies IG	Substantial risk of exposure. Pregnancy is not a contraindication for postexposure prophylaxis.
Live bacterial vaccines Typhoid (Ty21a)	Live bacterial	Avoid on theoretical grounds (see below).
Tuberculosis (BCG)	Live bacterial	Contraindicated.
Inactivated bacterial vaccines Typhoid	Heat/phenol-inactivated	Avoid because of systemic reactions and febrile responses (see below).
Plague	Killed bacterial	Selective vaccination of exposed persons.
Meningococcal	Polysaccharide	Only in unusual outbreak situations or high-risk persons.
Pneumococcal	Polysaccharide	Only for high-risk persons.
Haemophilus b conjugate	Polysaccharide-protein	Only for high-risk persons.
Typhoid (Vi capsular polysaccharide vaccine)	Polysaccharide	Use if indicated. Preferred over Ty21a and heat/phenol-inactivated vaccine in pregnancy.
Toxoids Tetanus-diphtheria (Td)	Combined tetanus-diphtheria toxoids, adult formulation	Safe. Indication: lack of primary series, or no booster within past 10 years.
Immune globulins, pooled or hyperimmune	Immune globulin or specific globulin preparations	Exposure or anticipated unavoidable exposure to measles, hepatitis A, hepatitis B, rabies, tetanus, or varicella.

[a]Delay pregnancy for three months following MMR, yellow fever vaccine or varicella vaccine. (ACIP recommends at least one month delay after varicella vaccine; manufacturer recommends three month delay).

OPV, oral polio vaccine; BCG, bacille Calmette-Guérin; IPV, inactivated polio vaccine; IG, immune globulin; VZIG, varicella zoster immune globulin.

Adapted from Centers for Disease Control and Prevention, *Health Information for International Travel 1996–1997,* DHHS, Atlanta, GA, with additions. See also *Guidelines for Vaccinating Pregnant Women,* ACIP (Advisory Committee on Immunization Practices) Recommendations, October 1998, available at www.immunize.org/genr.d/pregguid.htm.

even if a vaccine is administered to an adult. Records should include the date, name of the vaccine, manufacturer, lot number, inoculation site, route of administration, and name of the person administering the vaccine. Federal law also requires the distribution of vaccine information statements (VIS) to persons (even adults) receiving certain vaccines (MMR, polio, diphtheria, pertussis, and tetanus vaccines in any combination). VIS can be accessed at www.cdc.gov/nip/far.htm or www.immunize.org/vis (VIS sheets are available in 18 languages).

Table 6.3. Summary of ACIP Recommendations on Immunization of Immunocompromised Persons

VACCINE	ROUTINE (NOT IMMUNO-COMPROMISED)	HIV INFECTION/AIDS	SEVERELY IMMUNOCOMPRO-MISED (NON-HIV-RELATED)[a]	AFTER SOLID ORGAN TRANSPLANT ON CHRONIC IMMUNOSUPPRESSIVE THERAPY	ASPLENIA	RENAL FAILURE	DIABETES	ALCOHOLISM AND ALCOHOLIC CIRRHOSIS
Td	Recommended	Recommended	Recommended	Recommended[e]	Recommended	Recommended	Recommended	Recommended
MMR (MR/M/R)	Use if indicated	Recommended/considered[b]	Contraindicated	Contraindicated	Use if indicated	Use if indicated	Use if indicated	Use if indicated
Hepatitis B	Use if indicated	Use if indicated	Use if indicated	Use if indicated	Use if indicated	Recommended[c]	Use if indicated	Use if indicated
Hib	Not recommended	Considered[d]	Considered	Considered	Recommended	Use if indicated	Use if indicated	Use if indicated
Pneumococcal	Recommended if ≥65 years of age or high-risk	Recommended	Recommended	Recommended	Recommended	Recommended	Recommended	Recommended
Meningococcal	Use if indicated	Use if indicated	Use if indicated	Use if indicated	Recommended	Use if indicated	Use if indicated	Use if indicated
Influenza	Recommended if ≥65 years of age or high-risk	Recommended	Recommended	Recommended	Recommended	Recommended	Recommended	Recommended

[a]Severe immunosuppression can be the result of congenital immunodeficiency, HIV infection, leukemia, lymphoma, generalized malignancy, or therapy with alkylating agents, antimetabolites, radiation, or large amounts of corticosteroids.

[b]See discussion of MMR. Would avoid if severely immunocompromised.

[c]Patients with renal failure on dialysis should have their anti-Hb$_s$ response tested after vaccination, and those found not to respond should be revaccinated.

[d]In some areas, HIV-infected individuals may have a higher incidence of infection with *H. influenzae* b, not routinely recommended.

[e]Anecdotal reports of organ transplant rejection after vaccination with Td.

Td, tetanus, diphtheria; Hib, *Haemophilius influenzae* type b; MMR, measles, mumps, rubella; Hb$_s$, hepatitis B surface antigen.

Adapted with permission from MMWR 1993; 42(RR-4):1, with additions.

Table 6.4. Summary of ACIP Recommendations on Immunization of Immunocompromised Persons

VACCINE	NOT IMMUNOCOMPROMISED	HIV INFECTION/AIDS	SEVERELY IMMUNOCOMPROMISED (NON—HIV-RELATED)[a]	AFTER SOLID ORGAN TRANSPLANT OR LONG-TERM IMMUNOSUPPRESSIVE THERAPY	ASPLENIA, RENAL FAILURE, DIABETES, ALCOHOLISM, AND ALCOHOLIC CIRRHOSIS
Live vaccines					
BCG	Use if indicated[c]	Contraindicated	Contraindicated	Contraindicated	Use if indicated[c, d]
OPV	Use if indicated[c, d]	Contraindicated	Contraindicated	Contraindicated	Use if indicated[c, d]
Varicella	Use if indicated[c]	Contraindicated[f]	Contraindicated	Contraindicated	Use if indicated[c, d]
Typhoid, Ty21a[e]	Use if indicated[c]	Contraindicated[f]	Contraindicated	Contraindicated	Use if indicated[c, d]
Yellow fever[b]	Use if indicated[c]	Contraindicated[f]	Contraindicated	Contraindicated	Use if indicated[c, d]
Killed or inactivated vaccines					
IPV	Use if indicated	Use if indicated	Use if indicated	Use if indicated	Use if indicated
Cholera	Use if indicated	Use if indicated	Use if indicated	Use if indicated	Use if indicated
Hepatitis A	Use if indicated	Use if indicated	Use if indicated	Use if indicated	Use if indicated
Typhoid (nonliving)[e]	Use if indicated	Use if indicated	Use if indicated	Use if indicated	Use if indicated
Rabies	Use if indicated	Use if indicated	Use if indicated	Use if indicated	Use if indicated
Japanese encephalitis	Use if indicated	Use if indicated	Use if indicated	Use if indicated	Use if indicated

[a]Severe immunosuppression can be the result of congenital immunodeficiency, HIV infection, leukemia, lymphoma, aplastic anemia, generalized malignancy, or therapy with alkylating agents, antimetabolites, radiation, or large amounts of corticosteroids.

[b]Yellow fever vaccine should be considered for immunocompromised patients when exposure to yellow fever cannot be avoided (see text).

[c]See text.

[d]Generally avoid.

[e]Vi capsular polysaccharide vaccine preferred.

[f]If asymptomatic HIV infection, probably safe. Avoid if severely immunocompromised.

BCG = bacille Calmette-Guérin; OPV = oral polio vaccine; ACIP = Advisory Committee on Immunization Practices; IPV = inactivated Polio Vaccine.

Adapted with permission from MMWR 1993;42(RR-4):1, with additions.

SPECIFIC IMMUNIZATION PROGRAMS

Tetanus

Despite the fact that almost half of all individuals older than 60 years of age lack protective levels of serum antitetanus toxin antibodies, fewer than 100 cases of tetanus occur each year in the United States. Almost all cases of tetanus reported in the United States occur in adults who did not complete a primary tetanus immunization series or who did not receive appropriate treatment for a tetanus-prone wound. Prevention of tetanus should, therefore, concentrate on primary vaccination and proper postexposure immunization (Table 6.5); immigrants and elderly persons are most likely not to have received a primary immunization series.

The tetanus vaccine can be administered as a *monovalent vaccine* (T) or in combination with the *diphtheria vaccine* (Td). The tetanus and diphtheria vaccines are based on formaldehyde-treated toxoids (detoxified toxins). Td should be administered rather than tetanus toxoid alone because the diphtheria toxoid does not increase the rate of adverse events and diphtheria is reemerging as an infectious disease problem worldwide. The more common reactions to Td vaccine include erythema, induration, and tenderness at the inoculation site. It is recommended that all adults receive a Td vaccine every 10 years, although some authorities suggest that a one-time tetanus booster at age 50 may suffice for individuals who have received a full primary series. Appropriate postexposure prophylaxis is required regardless of vaccination regimen.

Adults who require a primary Td series should receive two doses IM 4 weeks apart, and a third dose 6 to 12 months after the second inoculation. There is no need to repeat doses if the schedule is interrupted.

Diphtheria

In the United States, diphtheria in adults is rare (fewer than 10 cases per year), especially among adults who have received a complete primary series, even if it has been more than 10 years since the administration of a diphtheria booster. More than half of American adults lack protective levels of antidiphtheria toxin antibodies. Worldwide, there has been a resurgence of diphtheria in several countries, including the states of the former Soviet Union. Travelers to such countries should receive Td vaccine if it has been longer than 10 years since their last booster. Diphtheria antitoxin of equine origin may be used to treat respiratory diphtheria.

Pertussis

Because the pertussis vaccine is associated with frequent adverse events in older children and adults, its administration is restricted to children younger than 7 years. Many adults are not immunized and therefore susceptible. Adults presenting with a severe, persistent cough should be suspected of having pertussis infection (see Chapter 52). The new acellular pertussis vaccine is associated with a lower side effect profile but is approved only for use in children.

Table 6.5. Wound Management After Exposure: Tetanus

Patients with three or more previous tetanus toxoid doses:
1. Give Td[a] for clean, minor wounds only if more than 10 years since last dose.
2. For other wounds,[b] give Td if more than 5 years since last dose.

Patients with fewer than three or unknown number of prior tetanus toxoid doses:
1. Give Td for clean, minor wounds.
2. Give Td and TIG (tetanus immune globulin 250 U IM) for other wounds.

[a]Tetanus and diphtheria toxoids, adsorbed.

[b]Such as, but not limited to, wounds contaminated with dust, feces, soil, and saliva; puncture wounds; convulsions; wounds resulting from missiles, crushing, burns, frost bite.

Adapted with permission from MMWR Morb Mortal Wkly Rep 1991;40(RR-10):1 and from *Tetanus and Diphtheria Toxoids 7/28/98* at www.cdc.gov/nip.

Measles, Mumps, and Rubella

Measles, measles and rubella (MR), and measles, mumps, and rubella (MMR) vaccines are available. Individuals immune to one or more components of the combination vaccines can still receive MMR vaccine. The MMR vaccines (in any combination) should not be administered to pregnant women or to severely immunocompromised persons; women of child-bearing age should be cautioned to avoid pregnancy for 3 months after vaccination. Individuals with a history of severe allergic reaction to eggs should not receive vaccines containing measles or mumps components, nor should the vaccine be administered to individuals with anaphylactic reactions to neomycin. Individuals who have received immunoglobulin preparations or blood/blood products in the preceding 3 to 11 months may not generate adequate immune responses to vaccination.

Measles. In most circumstances, use of the MMR vaccine is preferred. Persons born before 1957 are assumed to be immune to measles because of the very high likelihood of exposure; such persons do not require serologic evaluation for antibody. In the United States, measles is almost eradicated; most cases that currently occur are associated with international travel or educational institutions. After a single inoculation of the live attenuated measles vaccine (in any combination), protective antibody levels develop in approximately 90% to 95% of individuals. The remaining 5% to 10% remain at risk for measles. A second dose of the vaccine will result in protective immunity in almost all of these individuals. Those immunized between 1963 and 1967 may have received an inactivated measles vaccine and should receive the live viral vaccine.

Preexposure Immunization. Because of a resurgence of measles, it is now recommended that persons born after 1956 who are attending *postsecondary educational institutions*, who are *health professionals*, or who are *traveling to a foreign country* receive two doses of live attenuated MMR vaccine (or measles monovalent vaccine), separated by at least 1 month, unless they have a physician-documented case of measles or serologic confirmation of measles antibody. Many secondary schools now require documentation of two vaccinations against measles. It is more cost-effective to administer the two doses of the vaccine to all individuals than to screen patients for a serologic response after a single vaccination.

Postexposure Prophylaxis. A susceptible individual exposed to someone with measles should receive IM *immunoglobulin* (0.25 mL/kg, maximum of 15 mL) followed 6 months later by live measles vaccine. Immunoglobulin can prevent or modify infection if given within 6 days of exposure. The vaccine itself may afford some protection if administered within 72 hours of exposure. Postexposure immunoglobulin should also be administered to severely immunocompromised individuals exposed to active measles (regardless of immunization history). Because measles vaccination can temporarily suppress tuberculin reactivity, any tuberculosis skin testing should be performed on the day of vaccination or at least 4 to 6 weeks later.

Mumps. Because lifelong protective immunity develops in almost all individuals after immunization with a single inoculation of the live attenuated mumps vaccine, routine immunization with MMR results in adequate protection of almost all individuals. A mumps vaccination is indicated for individuals born after 1956 who have not received at least one live mumps vaccine, have not had a physician-documented case of mumps, or who lack serologic evidence of immunity. Administration of immunoglobulin after exposure to mumps has not been documented to be of clinical efficacy.

Rubella. Protective immunity develops in almost all individuals after a single vaccination with a live attenuated rubella vaccine. Routine vaccination with MMR is sufficient in almost all cases. Because rubella causes considerable morbidity if acquired during pregnancy, special emphasis should be placed on identifying susceptible women of childbearing age (especially among immigrant populations). Susceptible women should receive the rubella vaccine before they become pregnant or after they have delivered. Health care workers with antibody evidence of immunity should also be immunized. The vaccine is well tolerated, although mild and transient arthralgias or arthritis can occur.

Polio

In the United States, parenterally administered *inactivated polio vaccine* (IPV) is replacing the live *oral polio vaccine* (OPV) because the approximately 5 to 10 cases of poliomyelitis that occur each year in the United States are caused by OPV (risk in recipients or household contacts of recipients is 1 per 500,000 first doses administered). IPV does not cause poliomyelitis. There are now few indications for use of OPV: mass vaccination during outbreaks of poliomyelitis; vaccination of unimmunized children traveling in fewer than 4 weeks to areas of the world with endemic or epidemic poliomyelitis; and, vaccination of individuals who refuse IPV. Although the World Health Organization (WHO) has targeted polio for eradication, it is still active in a number of regions of the world (especially South Asia and sub-Saharan Africa). As such, paralytic poliomyelitis could recur in epidemic fashion in the United States if population-based immunity is allowed to wane.

Routine polio vaccination of adults in the United States is not recommended. Individuals planning to travel to *Africa*, *Asia*, the *Middle East*, and some areas of *Eastern Europe* should receive a booster dose of IPV if more than 10 years has elapsed since primary vaccination. The clinical efficacy of additional boosters is unknown; some recommend repeated boost every 10 years for ongoing travel to endemic areas. *Laboratory workers* and *health care professionals* who are exposed to wild-type polio virus should also be vaccinated. A three-vaccine primary series of IPV can be administered to an adult at 0 and at 4 to 8 weeks, and at least 4 weeks (preferably 6 to 12 months) after the second inoculation.

Contraindications. The polio vaccine should never be administered to an *immunocompromised* individual, to anyone with a household contact who is immunocompromised, or to a person with a history of an anaphylactic reaction to *streptomycin*. IPV should not be administered to individuals with a history of anaphylactic reactions to streptomycin, polymyxin B, or neomycin. A prior episode of polio (caused by one strain of polio virus) is not a contraindication to receiving IPV (protective against three strains of polio virus).

Influenza

Approximately 20,000 people die of influenza each year in the United States. Most of these deaths occur in persons 65 years of age or older, with those having cardiopulmonary conditions at greatest risk. The vaccine is composed of inactivated viruses formulated yearly to include two influenza viral type A strains and one type B strain. Contrary to popular belief, the vaccine does not cause influenza. In young adults, the vaccine is quite effective at reducing the severity of clinical illness and time lost from work. In older persons, there is a 30% to 40% reduction in overall clinical illness and a decrease in pneumonia, hospitalization, and deaths from influenza. Despite these benefits, vaccination rates fall short.

Indications and Timing. Individuals with chronic cardiopulmonary disorders (including asthma), women who will be in their second or third trimesters of pregnancy during the flu season, high-risk women who will be pregnant at any point during the flu season, residents of long-term care facilities or nursing homes, immunocompromised individuals, those who care for elderly or immunocompromised persons, health care workers, and individuals over the age of 65 should receive the vaccine. Some groups recommend that the vaccine be administered to all individuals 50 years of age or older. The vaccine should be offered to anyone who wishes to avoid the flu. In the continental United States, administration should be between October and mid-November, but the vaccine can be administered at any time during the flu season. Although the influenza season is usually well defined in the temperate United States, influenza outbreaks occur at different times throughout the world. Protection begins 1 to 2 weeks after inoculation and continues for 6 months. The duration of protective immunity in frail, elderly, or immunocompromised individuals may be shorter. During a community outbreak of influenza, drugs effective against influenza viruses have a useful adjunctive role (see Chapter 52).

Side Effects and Contraindications. Transient low-grade fever, myalgia, and malaise can occur after immunization. Individuals with a history of influenza vaccine–associated Guillain-Barré syndrome should not receive the influenza vaccine. The risk of the vaccine in individuals with a history of Guillain-Barré syndrome not associated with influenza vaccination is controversial. Such persons may be at high risk for severe influenza.

Pneumococcal Pneumonia

Approximately 500,000 cases of pneumonia and 40,000 deaths are caused by *Streptococcus pneumoniae* each year in the United States. In addition, pneumococcal disease accounts for an estimated 3,000 cases of meningitis and 50,000 cases of bacteremia, annually. The current vaccine contains capsular polysaccharide components of 23 pneumococcal types; these account for approximately 80% to 90% of invasive pneumococcal infections and include the six serotypes most frequently associated with antibiotic resistance. Because antibiotic resistance is rapidly rising, immunization is of increasing importance.

Efficacy. The vaccine reduces the incidence of pneumococcal bacteremia and pneumonia among younger individuals and among older individuals who are able to generate a good antibody response. Overall, the vaccine is 60% to 80% effective at preventing invasive disease. Efficacy in immunosuppressed individuals is less well defined.

Indications. Severe disease is most likely to develop in persons more than 65 years of age and those with cardiopulmonary disease, immunocompromise, diabetes, alcoholism, or hepatic or renal failure, and they should receive the vaccine. The vaccine should be administered at least 2 weeks before elective splenectomy or immunosuppression (if possible). Alaskan natives, African-American adults, and certain American Indian populations are also at increased risk. Fewer than 20% of members of target populations have received the vaccine, and only 45% of the elderly have been vaccinated.

Because not all persons manifest a full antibody response on first vaccination and because antibody levels may decline with time, some recommend a booster vaccination if 5 or more years has elapsed since first vaccination, although the utility of booster vaccination has not been definitively established.

Safety. The pneumococcal vaccine is safe; most reactions are minor and occur at the inoculation site. Severe allergic reactions are rare but might become more frequent with subsequent immunizations. Pneumococcal and influenza vaccines can be administered at separate inoculation sites during a single office visit. A new pneumococcal 7 valent diphtheria CRM 197 protein conjugate vaccine has recently been approved for use in children, but has not been approved for use in adults.

Haemophilus influenzae Infection

Before the introduction of the *H. influenzae type b conjugate vaccine (Hib)*, most cases of invasive disease in children were caused by *H. influenzae* capsular type b, but with the application of Hib vaccine, most cases now represent non–type b disease. A number of Hib vaccines are available, all linking a polysaccharide molecule (polyribosylribotol phosphate, or PRT) to a carrier protein to increase immunogenicity. The vaccine is often administered to individuals with functional or anatomic asplenia or immunoglobulin deficiencies because such persons have a higher incidence of invasive disease caused by encapsulated organisms. However, definitive benefit has not been established, perhaps because many such individuals already have humoral immunity against *H. influenzae* type b.

Meningococcal Disease

Meningococcal disease is endemic throughout the world, and large epidemics can occur globally. Information on meningococcal disease activity is available at www.cdc.gov. In the United States, meningococcal infection is usually caused by *Neisseria meningitidis* serogroup B or C and occurs as isolated cases or as small outbreaks. A meningococcal polysaccharide vaccine that is quadrivalent for serogroups A, C, Y, and W-135 is available in the United States. Routine administration is not recommended, but persons with anatomic or functional asplenia and those with defective complement should be given the vaccine. Additionally, the vaccine should be recommended for travelers who visit certain areas of the world during "meningitis season" (e.g., the Sahel region of sub-Saharan Africa during the dry winter months (December through June). Controversy currently exists on whether the vaccine should be administered to college-age students in the United States. The low incidence of meningococcal disease in this population argues against routine administration of the vaccine. Some experts, however, recommend that the vaccine be administered to college freshmen who will reside in a dormitory. The vaccine is well tolerated; most adverse reactions are mild and local. The need for booster vaccination is not well documented, and a booster vaccination is not required within 3 to 5 years of primary inoculation. Saudi Arabia requires documentaion of meningococcal vaccination from all pilgrims.

Rabies

Rabies is a potentially fatal viral infection transmitted in the saliva of animals, usually through a bite. More rarely, cases result from the contamination of wounds with saliva of a rabies-infected animal; aerosol transmission occurs in special circumstances (e.g., research laboratories, bat-infested caves). Although dog bites account for the majority of rabies cases throughout the world, dog bites account for a minority (38%) of human rabies cases in the United States (and in 50% of such cases, the dog bite occurred overseas). Most rabies in the United States occurs in nondomesticated animals, especially bats, skunks, foxes, coyotes, raccoons, and woodchucks. Rabies should be considered in any case of *rapidly progressive encephalitis*, even in individuals who do not have a history of an animal bite. Therapy is preventive in nature and should be administered as either preexposure or, more commonly, postexposure prophylaxis.

Indications. Persons bitten by infected animals should receive *postexposure prophylaxis*. The risk of transmission of rabies through a ferret bite approximates that associated with a dog or cat bite. Because bat bites can be small, may not be recalled, and can be missed on physical examination, rabies postexposure prophylaxis is recommended for individuals who have a bat exposure and cannot exclude a bat bite. Such situations might include an individual who awakens in a room with a bat, someone who is unresponsive in a room with a bat (unconscious or intoxicated), or a person in a room with a bat who cannot report an exposure (a small child).

Postexposure prophylaxis consists of three crucial steps (Table 6.6):

- First, the wound should be immediately and thoroughly *cleaned* and extensively *irrigated* with soap and water. Cleaning the wound with iodine or alcohol is not sufficient.
- Second, 20 IU of *rabies human immunoglobulin* (HRIG) per kilogram should be administered to individuals with an exposure who have not received the rabies vaccine within the previous 2 years. The entire HRIG dose should be instilled directly into the animal bite. If the entire HRIG dose cannot be instilled into the wound, as much of the dose that can be administered should be locally instilled and the remainder inoculated IM at a site distinct from the vaccine inoculation. If there is more than one animal bite, the HRIG dose should be divided equally among sites.
- Third, all individuals should receive *rabies vaccine* (a 1-mL dose of any of the rabies vaccines administered IM in the deltoid). If an individual has received a rabies primary vaccine series approved in the United States within the previous 2 years (or a booster dose after a primary series within the previous 2 years), that individual should receive two rabies boosters (days 0 and 3). Individuals who have not received such rabies vaccines within the previous 2 years should receive five doses (days 0, 3, 7, 14, and 28). HRIG and rabies vaccine should never be administered at the same site or with the same syringe.

Vaccine Preparations and Administration. Currently, three rabies vaccines are approved in the United States, the HDCV (human diploid cell rabies vaccine; Imovax, Pasteur Merieux Connaught), the RVA (rabies vaccine adsorbed, SmithKline Beecham), and the PCEC rabies vaccine (purified chick embryo cell culture; RabAvert, Chiron). An intradermal 0.1-mL dose (approved for use with HDCV for preexposure prophylaxis) should never be used for postexposure prophylaxis. When postexposure prophylaxis is administered, no more than the recommended dose of HRIG should be administered (because HRIG can partially suppress the antibody response to rabies vaccine). Tetanus prophylaxis should be considered.

Adverse Effects. Most reactions to rabies vaccine are local and mild. Serum sickness–type reactions can occur, especially with multiple boosting doses of HDCV or RVA; the PCEC vaccine is rarely associated with such reactions. The PCEC rabies vaccine can be used for booster vaccination regardless of the identity of the primary vaccination series. HRIG available in the United States appears to be safe. The safety of antirabies immunoglobulin preparations (human and rabbit) manufactured overseas has not been formally evaluated. Because rabies is a fatal illness, pregnancy should not be considered a contraindication to postexposure prophylaxis if it is indicated.

Preexposure Prophylaxis. Individuals who may be at risk for rabies should consider receiving preexposure prophylaxis, including those who work with animals, laboratory researchers who work with rabies virus, travelers who plan on spending a prolonged period of time in endemic areas, and possibly short-term travelers who will be in rabies-endemic areas without access to medical care. Preexposure rabies vaccination consists of three 1-mL dose immunizations administered IM in the deltoid on days 0, 7, 21 *or* 28. The HDCV is approved as an intradermal injection of 0.1 mL; however, intradermal HDCV and malaria chemoprophylaxis (with chloroquine or mefloquine) should not be simultaneously administered. Antibody levels should be regularly checked in persons with ongoing exposure to rabies, and booster vaccinations should be administered as needed (Table 6.6). Further information can be obtained from the CDC (telephone 404-639-3111) or from the local department of public health, which may have an "on-call" rabies specialist.

Varicella

The complication rate of varicella infection (*chickenpox*) is higher in adults than in children; pneumonitis, hepatitis, encephalitis, and death are more frequent. Approximately 5% of American adults are not immune; the rate is higher among those born outside the United States. Since the varicella vaccine became a routine vaccine of childhood, the incidence of varicella infection has been falling rapidly. The varicella vaccine is a live attenuated viral vaccine that is most immunogenic in children (who need only a single inoculation). The vaccine is administered twice to adults, the second inoculation 4 to 8 weeks after the first. The vaccine is not completely protective, but a 70% re-

Table 6.6.   Rabies Immunization

I. PREEXPOSURE IMMUNIZATION.   Preexposure immunization consists of three doses of HDCV, PCEC, or RVA, 1.0 mL, IM (i.e., deltoid area), one each on days 0, 7, and 21 or 28. ONLY HDCV may be administered by the intradermal (ID) dose/route (0.1 mL ID on days 0, 7, and 21 or 28). If traveler will be taking chloroquine or mefloquine for malaria chemoprophylaxis, the three-dose series must be completed before antimalarials are begun. If this is not possible, the IM dose/route should be used. Administration of routine booster doses of vaccine depends on exposure risk category as noted below. Preexposure immunization of immunosuppressed persons is not recommended.

RISK CATEGORY	NATURE OF RISK	CRITERIA FOR PREEXPOSURE IMMUNIZATION IN TYPICAL POPULATIONS[a]	PREEXPOSURE REGIMEN
Continuous	Virus present continuously, often in high concentrations. Specific exposures likely to go unrecognized. Bite, nonbite, or aerosol exposure.	Rabies research lab workers.[a] Rabies biologics production workers.	Primary course. Serologic testing every 6 months; booster vaccination if antibody titer is below acceptable level.[b]
Frequent	Exposure usually episodic with source recognized, but exposure may also be unrecognized. Bite, nonbite, or aerosol exposure possible.	Rabies diagnostic lab workers,[a] spelunkers, veterinarians and staff, animal control and wildlife workers in rabies-epizootic areas.	Primary course. Serologic testing every 2 years; booster vaccination if antibody titer is below acceptable level.[b]
Infrequent (greater than that of population at large)	Exposure nearly always episodic with source recognized. Bite or nonbite exposure.	Veterinarians and animal control and wildlife workers in areas with low rabies rates. Veterinary students. Travelers visiting areas where rabies is enzootic and immediate access to appropriate medical care, including biologics, is limited.	Primary course. No serologic testing or booster vaccination.
Rare (population at large)	Exposure always episodic, with source recognized. Bite or nonbite exposure.	U.S. population at large, including individuals in rabies-epizootic areas.	No preexposure immunization necessary.

II. POSTEXPOSURE IMMUNIZATION.   All postexposure treatment should begin with immediate thorough cleansing of all wounds with soap and water.
Persons not previously immunized: RIG, 20 IU/kg body weight, infiltrated at bite site (if possible), remainder IM; five doses of HDCV, PCEC, or RVA, 1.0 mL IM (i.e., deltoid area), one each on days 0, 3, 7, 14, and 28.
Persons previously immunized[c]**:** Two doses of HDCV, PCEC, or RVA, 1.0 mL, IM (i.e., deltoid area), one each on days 0 and 3. RIG should not be administered.

[a]Judgment of relative risk and extra monitoring of vaccination status of laboratory workers is the responsibility of the laboratory supervisor (see U.S. Department of Health and Human Service's *Biosafety in Microbiological and Biomedical Laboratories, 1984*).

[b]Preexposure booster immunization consists of one dose of HDCV, PCEC, or RVA, 1.0 mL/dose, IM (deltoid area) or HDCV, 0.1 mL ID (deltoid). Minimum acceptable antibody level is complete virus neutralization at a 1:5 serum dilution by the rapid fluorescent focus inhibition test. A booster dose should be administered if titer falls below this level.

[c]Preexposure immunization with HDCV, PCEC, or RVA; prior postexposure prophylaxis with HDCV, PCEC, or RVA; or persons previously immunized with any other type of rabies vaccine *and* a documented history of positive antibody response to the prior vaccination.

HDCV, human diploid cell vaccine; RVA, rabies vaccine adsorbed; RIG, rabies immune globulin; PCEC, purified chick embryo cell culture.

Adapted from Centers for Disease Control and Prevention, *Health Information for International Travel 1999-2000*, DHHS, Atlanta, GA.

duction in the expected number of cases is achieved. When the vaccine is administered to adults who have a high frequency of exposure (through a household contact), approximately 27% of adults report breakthrough chickenpox, but of a mild nature. The efficacy of the vaccine for protection against the complications of chickenpox (including encephalitis, hepatitis, and pneumonitis) has not been assessed, but it may well be protective. The need for booster vaccination has not been established.

Indications. The vaccine should be administered to all susceptible adults and adolescents with a high risk of exposure (health care workers, day care workers, teachers, institutional care workers, those involved in postsecondary school educational institutions, military personnel, and travelers, among others) and to all susceptible persons who would be at risk for severe complications of varicella (nonpregnant women of childbearing age, family members of immunocompromised individuals). The majority of adults who do not report a history of chickenpox have serologic evidence of a previous episode of varicella. The serum of adults who deny a previous episode

of chickenpox should be screened for antivaricella antibodies. The vaccine should not be administered to immunocompromised individuals or pregnant women. The manufacturer recommends that vaccinated women avoid pregnancy for 3 months after inoculation. Individuals who have received immunoglobulin preparations or blood/blood products within the previous 3 to 11 months may not adequately respond to the vaccine. The vaccine should not be administered to individuals with an anaphylactic reaction to neomycin. The vaccine requires storage at a temperature below −15°C.

Adverse Effects. The vaccine is well tolerated by most individuals. Common reactions are local in nature: A temperature of 37.7°C (100°F) or higher will develop in approximately 10% of individuals after the first or second vaccination; 25% to 30% will complain of local erythema, tenderness, and swelling at the inoculation site; in 3%, a *localized varicella-like rash* will develop at the injection site after the first inoculation, and such a rash will develop after the second inoculation in approximately 1%. Rashes occur 1 to 3 weeks after inoculation. A *generalized* *varicella-like rash* can occur in 5% after the first inoculation and in 1% after the second. The median number of lesions in such individuals is five.

Precautions. The vaccine strain of the virus has been *transmitted* to susceptible contacts. Persons receiving vaccine should avoid contact with immunocompromised individuals who lack immunity to varicella and should avoid contact with susceptible pregnant women. The manufacturer advises that such precautions be taken for 6 weeks after inoculation and that vaccinated individuals avoid contact with newborn infants of mothers who lack a documented history of chickenpox or laboratory evidence of prior varicella. The manufacturer also advises that *salicylate products* not be administered for 6 weeks after vaccination because of the theoretical risk of *Reye's syndrome*. In a number of individuals who have received the varicella vaccine, *herpes zoster infection* (shingles) has subsequently developed. In some of these cases, viral cultures disclosed the presence of wild-type varicella virus, demonstrating the incomplete protective efficacy of the vaccine.

Postexposure Prophylaxis. If susceptible pregnant or immunocompromised individuals are exposed to varicella, they should receive IM *varicella zoster immunoglobulin* (VZIG; 125 U/10 kg; maximum dose, 625 U). For susceptible individuals who are neither immunocompromised nor pregnant, postexposure use of the varicella vaccine is worth considering. The varicella vaccine appears effective in preventing chickenpox and in reducing the severity of the disease if used within 3 and possibly up to 5 days after exposure. The vaccine should not be administered concomitantly with varicella immunoglobulin.

Lyme Disease

Lyme disease is transmitted by *Ixodes* ticks. The causative agent of Lyme disease, the spirochete *Borrelia burgdorferi*, is usually transmitted when a nymphal tick feeds, usually during the late spring and summer. (Feeding of adult ticks occurs during the fall, winter, and early spring and is less likely to transmit *B. burgdorferi*.) OspA (outer surface protein A) is a *B. burgdorferi* antigen that the spirochete expresses only when it is within the digestive system of the tick vector. The first vaccine against *B. burgdorferi* is now available (LYMErix vaccine, SmithKline Beecham). Others are under development. It induces anti-OspA antibody responses. Vaccine efficacy is believed to be related to the transfer (during a blood meal) of a vaccine recipient's serum anti-OspA antibody into the tick's intestinal system; the antibody attacks the organism while it is still within the tick.

Efficacy. Vaccine efficacy appears to be directly related to the titer of serum anti-OspA antibody and is maximized by frequent vaccine administration/boosting. When administered between January and April (immediately preceding the occurrence of nymphal feeding) as two monthly doses, the vaccine demonstrates efficacy of approximately 50%. Efficacy increases to 75% to 80% with an additional booster given at 1 year. Efficacy is reportedly near 100% for protection against asymptomatic Western blot seroconversion. To achieve the maximal 80% protection against definitive disease achieved in trials, three properly timed doses of the vaccine given during a 12-month period are required. Preliminary evidence suggests that similar protection may also be achieved with an accelerated vaccine schedule (0, 1, and 2 months).

Indications. The transmission of Lyme disease is very focal, with the overwhelming majority of Lyme disease cases in the United States occurring in focal areas of the Northeast and upper Midwest. Risk is related to exposure to infected ticks during outdoor activities, particularly in grassy and wooded areas. Individuals who should consider receiving the vaccine include those with (a) *intense and sustained* occupational or recreational *outdoor exposure* in tick-infested areas endemic for Lyme disease; (b) *long-term residents* of highly endemic areas (the yearly risk for such individuals is cumulative); (c) individuals with a history of *antibiotic-responsive Lyme disease* who have a recurrent or ongoing risk for acquiring Lyme disease (secondary infections can occur). The LYMErix vaccine is approved for use in individuals between the ages of 15 and 70 years.

Individuals with short-term exposures outdoors (<3 months) in highly endemic areas are at low risk for acquiring Lyme disease (risk approximately 0.1% to 1.0%). This risk can be markedly diminished with simple antitick measures, which include using insect repellents, wearing long trousers, and checking routinely for adherent ticks. These measures need to be continued even by persons who receive the vaccine because they will still be at risk for other tick-borne illnesses, such as babesiosis, tularemia, ehrlichiosis, and Rocky Mountain spotted fever. Administration of the vaccine to this population should be handled on an individual basis.

Contraindications. Those who should not receive the vaccine include (a) individuals with a history of *antibiotic-refractory (treatment-resistant) Lyme arthritis* (such arthritis is possibly related to anti-OspA immunologic responses); (b) *children* under 15 years of age (safety and efficacy not yet established); (c) *elderly persons* over 70 years of age (safety not yet established); (d) those with immunologically mediated *inflammatory joint disease* (anti-OspA antibodies could possibly worsen the arthritis—see below). Data are insufficient regarding use in persons with multiple sclerosis or demyelinating neurologic conditions, diffuse muscular pain, or chronic health conditions. The vaccine has also not been studied in pregnant or nursing women. Immunosuppressed individuals may have a less-than-optimal immune response.

Adverse Effects. The long-term safety of the anti-OspA antibody response induced by the vaccine is unknown. Anti-OspA antibodies may be related to the *immunologically mediated* joint disease that sometimes complicates Lyme disease (so-called antibiotic-resistant Lyme arthritis). Whether stimulating the production of such antibodies will increase the frequency of immunologically mediated joint injury remains to be seen and continues to be at least a theoretical concern.

The stimulation of Osp A antibody by Lyme vaccine may *interfere with serologic testing* for Lyme infection. Some enzyme-linked immunosorbent assays (ELISAs) test for OspA antibody and may produce a false-positive reading in an immunized person. In addition, an OspA band can appear on the more definitive Western immunoblot test. Although the screening ELISA will often be read as positive, the 31-kD anti-OspA band should not interfere with Western blot interpretation if strict CDC guidelines for interpretation are used.

Tuberculosis

Bacille Calmette-Guérin (BCG) is a live attenuated strain of *Mycobacterium bovis* that is used in *children* throughout the world to prevent tuberculosis. Vaccine trials in *adults* have yielded conflicting results. Overall, the vaccine may be approximately 30%-50% effective. Most immigrants to the United

States will have received the BCG vaccine as children. A positive tuberculin skin test result, however, should not be ascribed to BCG vaccination in any individual, regardless of the country of origin. In the United States, where the prevention of tuberculosis rests on the proper identification and treatment of exposed individuals, BCG is rarely administered to protect individuals against tuberculosis (see Chapter 49). The vaccine may be considered for individuals exposed to multiple drug–resistant tuberculosis, including health care workers who practice in certain prison settings or in certain overseas clinics. It may also be useful for those who cannot receive preventive therapy but have close contact with an individual with active, untreated disease or with disease that is ineffectively treated or multiple drug–resistant. The vaccine is administered intradermally; ulceration and prolonged discharge at the site of vaccination, regional adenitis, and osteitis occur in up to 20%. Disseminated BCG can develop in immunocompromised individuals who receive the vaccine.

Hepatitis B

Hepatitis B vaccines contain recombinant, noninfectious hepatitis B surface antigen. Two hepatitis vaccines are available in the United States: Engerix-B (SmithKline Beecham) and Recombivax HB (Merck). They can be used interchangeably, even in a primary inoculation. Three doses induce protective antibodies in more than 90% of healthy young adults. Antibody responses decline with increasing age and are lower in immunocompromised individuals.

Indications. Because it has been difficult to carry out vaccination among many high-risk groups, the hepatitis B vaccine has been introduced as a *standard childhood vaccine*. Nonetheless, high-risk persons should still be offered vaccination, especially individuals likely to comply, such as those with occupational or other exposure to blood or body fluids and the household and sexual contacts of hepatitis B virus carriers. Other high-risk groups include intravenous drug users, those with multiple sexual partners, male homosexuals, and individuals with a recent history of a sexually transmitted disease. The hepatitis B vaccine should be considered for long-term overseas travelers, especially for those who may be exposed to blood or bodily secretions through employment or sexual contact. The prevalence of hepatitis B infection is much higher, and the carrier state and chronic active hepatitis are much more frequent, in Asia, Africa, and Latin America than in the Unites States.

Postexposure Prophylaxis should be administered to individuals with mucous membrane or percutaneous exposure to blood or bodily secretions of individuals known or suspected of being acutely infected with hepatitis B or of being a hepatitis B carrier. IM hepatitis B immunoglobulin (HBIG; 0.06 mL/kg) should be administered immediately after exposure, ideally within 6 days. The vaccine series should also be started.

Administration. The vaccine can be administered to adults in three doses (0, 1, and 6 months), although other vaccination regimens can be employed. The Engerix-B vaccine can also be administered at 0, 1, 2 and 12 months; this accelerated regimen results in a more rapid increase in the serum anti-hepatitis B response. The hepatitis B vaccine should routinely be administered IM in adults in the deltoid muscle; injection in the buttock has been associated with a lower antibody response.

Postimmunization Serologic Testing for hepatitis B surface antibody should be performed in individuals who are immuno-

compromised, 30 years of age or older when they receive the vaccine, or at high risk for ongoing exposure to hepatitis B. Those who do not respond to the vaccine should repeat the complete three-dose inoculation series (rebooting); serum should then be rechecked for antibody. Those who remain serologically negative after administration of six hepatitis B vaccines should be considered "nonimmune." Such persons may be chronically infected with hepatitis B, and their serum should be tested for hepatitis B surface antigen. Routine rebooting or serologic evaluation of individuals who respond to the vaccine is not recommended.

Adverse Effects. The vaccine is well tolerated, with a mild local reaction at the injection site being the most common adverse event. The risk for Guillain-Barré syndrome or multiple sclerosis is not increased.

Hepatitis A

Indications for vaccination against hepatitis A infection are increasing in the United States. The vaccine is most frequently administered before travel to countries other than the major industrialized nations, but vaccination should also be considered for high-risk groups (e.g., male homosexuals, users of illegal drugs, those regularly receiving clotting factor transfusions, and persons with chronic liver disease). Food handlers and day care workers should also consider vaccination. The Advisory Committee on Immunization Practices (ACIP) recommends that the vaccine be administered routinely to children living in communities and states with the highest rates of infection (>20 cases per 100,000 population) and considered in areas with somewhat lower rates (>10 cases per 100,000). Many communities in the Western United States have such incidence levels of hepatitis A.

Preparations and Administration. Two versions of the vaccine are currently available in the United States: HAVRIX (SmithKline Beecham) and VAQTA (Merck). The vaccines are administered to adults in a two-dose primary series at 0 and 6 to 12 months (HAVRIX) or at 0 and 6 months (VAQTA). A three-dose series for children and adolescents is also available. Protective antibody levels that persist for 6 to 12 months are achieved in more than 95% of recipients after a single dose. Protective levels that last for more than 10 years can be induced with the second immunization.

Individuals who require immediate and full protection should receive *immunoglobulin* IM (0.02 mL/kg if short-term protection of 1 to 2 months is required, and 0.06 mL/kg if long-term protection of 3 to 5 months is required). Hepatitis A vaccine and immunoglobulin can be administered simultaneously at distinct inoculation sites. Individuals who have been exposed to a person with hepatitis A (e.g., close household or sexual contact of an individual with active hepatitis A, restaurant outbreak) should receive *postexposure prophylaxis* with IM immunoglobulin (0.02 mL/kg). Immunoglobulin prophylaxis given more than 2 weeks after exposure is unlikely to be of benefit and is not indicated. A combination hepatitis A and hepatitis B vaccine (three doses: 0, 1, 6 months) has recently been approved for use in the United States (Twinrix, SmithKline Beecham).

Typhoid

Because most cases of typhoid reported in the United States each year are acquired abroad, typhoid vaccine use is targeted for travelers to areas endemic for *Salmonella typhi* infection, especially when long-term nonhotel stays are planned. Currently, three typhoid vaccines are available.

The oldest is a heat/phenol-inactivated vaccine, approved for children 6 months to 2 years of age. A two-dose vaccine series confers immunogenicity; the second inoculation is administered at least 4 weeks after the first dose. Adverse effects include fever and pain with induration and erythema at the injection site. Two newer vaccines are better tolerated. A recombinant vaccine comprised of purified capsular polysaccharide Vi antigen (Typhim Vi, Pasteur Merieux Connaught) is approved for individuals 2 years of age or older. It is administered as a single dose and provides approximately 60% to 75% protection for 2 years.

An oral typhoid vaccine, based on a live attenuated strain of *Salmonella typhi* (Ty21a), is also available (Vivotif Berna vaccine; Swiss Serum and Vaccine Institute, Berne, Switzerland). The oral vaccine can be used in individuals 6 years of age or older and is administered as a single pill every other day for four doses (days 0, 2, 4, and 6). It provides approximately 60% to 75% protection for 5 years and is well tolerated by most individuals.

Patients should be reminded to keep their vaccine refrigerated between doses. Mild intestinal upset is the most common adverse event. The oral vaccine should be taken with cool liquid 1 hour before a meal. Immunocompromised individuals and those with chronic inflammatory bowel disease should not receive the oral vaccine, nor should persons taking antimicrobial agents (antibiotics or antimalarial agents).

Japanese Encephalitis

Japanese encephalitis (JE) is a mosquito-borne viral infection that exists throughout eastern, southeastern, and southern Asia. In most individuals who become infected, encephalitis or severe illness does not develop, but when it does, the death rate is 25% and the rate of severe neurologic sequelae is 50%. The disease occurs in rural environments and is transmitted by a mosquito vector that normally feeds on pigs and birds. Individuals from the United States at highest risk are those staying longer than 30 days in rural areas (usually in an Asian locale with extensive rice farming and pig husbandry) during the appropriate mosquito season (May through October in many areas of Asia, but year-round in endemic tropical areas). The overall risk to a traveler is approximately 1 in 1 million; however, this risk may increase to more than 1 in 20,000 per week for high-risk travel. Risk can be markedly decreased through the use of protective clothing and insect repellents, especially at dusk.

The JE vaccine (a formalin-inactivated product derived from infected mouse brains) is administered in a three-dose primary series (days 0, 7, and 14 or 30). Booster inoculation may be administered every 2 years. The most common adverse effects are local, but mild constitutional symptoms may develop in up to 10%. In 0.6% of recipients, the vaccine can cause *urticaria, angioedema, respiratory distress, hypotension,* and *anaphylaxis.* Most allergic reactions can be treated with antihistamines and corticosteroids; epinephrine and supportive care may be required. Severe reactions usually occur within a day of vaccination but have occurred as long as 2 weeks after administration of any of the three inoculations. Individuals with a history of severe allergic reactions, angioedema, or urticaria are at highest risk for severe reactions. Individuals should be observed in the office for approximately 30 minutes after admin-

istration, and those who receive the vaccine should have access to medical care for at least 10 days after completion of the vaccine series. Consequently, the vaccine series needs to be started at least 24 days before departure if the accelerated vaccination course of 0, 7, and 14 days is employed.

Yellow Fever

Yellow fever is a mosquito-borne hemorrhagic viral illness that can be severe; it is endemic in sub-Saharan Africa and tropical Latin America. The live attenuated virus vaccine is the only immunization legally required for crossing some international borders. Contraindications include allergy to eggs, immunocompromise, and pregnancy. Women who receive the vaccine should be advised not to become pregnant for 3 months after vaccination. The vaccine can be administered only through WHO-approved centers. State departments of public health keeps a list of such sites. Individuals who require yellow fever vaccination should be directed to a yellow fever vaccination center. Immunized individuals will receive a WHO vaccination certificate. The vaccination record becomes "acceptable" to immigration officers 10 days after the vaccine has been administered. The vaccine is effective for 10 years. Vaccination is recommended for individuals traveling to or living in endemic areas. Countries may require documentation of yellow fever vaccination, even from individuals who only pass through endemic areas. Countries reporting yellow fever are posted by the WHO and the CDC; a listing can be accessed at www.cdc.gov.

Most reactions to yellow fever vaccine are local in nature. More rarely, systemic symptoms may develop, usually 5 to 10 days after vaccination. Because of the risk for vaccine-associated encephalitis, the vaccine should never be administered to children 4 months of age or younger, and rarely to children 4 to 9 months of age. If an individual is proceeding to an endemic yellow fever area and the vaccine is contraindicated, a yellow fever waiver certificate can be issued from the WHO yellow fever vaccination center. Immunocompromised individuals and pregnant women who will live long-term in a highly endemic yellow fever area of the world should carefully weigh the risk of vaccination versus the risks of illness. A desensitization protocol is available for individuals with a history of a severe allergy to eggs. The injectable cholera vaccine and the yellow fever vaccine should not be administered within 3 weeks of each other. The effectiveness of the yellow fever vaccine is not affected by the administration of immunoglobulin.

Cholera

The risk of cholera for routine travelers is extremely low; the food and water that transmit *Vibrio cholerae* usually have to be heavily and grossly contaminated, and simple food and water precautions effectively eliminate any real risk of contracting cholera. Individuals who die of cholera die of dehydration, not of the infection itself. In the extremely unlikely event that a traveler does contract cholera, simple rehydration therapy will prevent death. The only cholera vaccine currently available in the United States is an injectable phenol-killed *Vibrio cholerae* vaccine. The vaccine is minimally protective and is associated with a very high rate of adverse events. These factors combine to limit the utility of cholera vaccination in the United States. The WHO has removed the cholera vaccine from its list of vaccines for travelers. During outbreaks, local governments may require documentation of vaccination against cholera from some travelers. If used, the vaccine is administered in two doses at least 1 week apart and, preferably, 1 month or more apart. Boosters are required every 6 months. Oral vaccines are available for use outside the United States.

Smallpox

In the United States, the smallpox vaccine is currently administered only to certain laboratory researchers and to individuals in the Armed Services. The vaccine contains a live attenuated virus and can result in disseminated vaccinia in individuals who are immunocompromised. Because of the risk for the reemergence of smallpox resulting from a bioterrorist act, the vaccine is once again being formulated.

Other Conditions

Vaccines exist for a number of other infections, including *anthrax*, *typhus*, and *plague*. Vaccines are usually administered to individuals at high risk for these disorders (usually through employment-related exposures) or to military personnel.

ANNOTATED BIBLIOGRAPHY

American College of Physicians. Guide for adult immunization, 3rd ed. ACP Task Force on Adult Immunization and Infectious Diseases Society of America. Philadelphia: American College of Physicians, 1994. (*Summary statements on immunization of adults. Excellent office reference. New edition in preparation.*)

Atkinson WL. The pink book: epidemiology and prevention of vaccine preventable diseases, 5th ed. Atlanta, GA: Centers for Disease Control and Prevention, 1999. (*Practical vaccine information. Telephone number is 800-418-7246. Also available online at* www.cdc.gov/nip/far.htm.)

Centers for Disease Control and Prevention. Health information for international travel 1999–2000 (the yellow book). Atlanta, GA: Department of Health and Human Services. Available free online at www.cdc.gov. (*The standard reference from the CDC on travel-related immunizations. Fax information service at 888-232-3299.*)

Jenson HB. Pocket guide to vaccination and prophylaxis. Philadelphia: WB Saunders, 1999. (*Easy-to-use pocket summary for all vaccines and immunizations, including postexposure prophylaxis. Excellent office resource.*)

Peter G, ed. The 1997 red book: report of the committee on infectious diseases, 24th ed. Elk Grove Village, IL: American Academy of Pediatrics, 1997. (*Overview of infectious diseases considers incubation periods, clinical manifestations, and preventive measures, including immunization and postexposure prophylaxis. New edition in preparation.*)

Websites/Internet Resources

www.cdc.gov
Main site for immunization-related resources and information.

www.cdc.gov/nip
National Immunization Program website.

www.cdc.gov/nip/far.htm
Excellent central resource page of the National Immunization Program/CDC. Includes VIS; ACIP recommendations; the pink book; vaccine safety information; tabular summaries of recommendations for adults, adolescents, and children; other resources.

www.cdc.gov/nip/vacsafe
Vaccine safety website.

www.cdc.gov/od/nvpo
National Vaccine Program office website.

www.cdc.gov/travel
Review of travel-related vaccines. Includes the complete yellow book online.

www.cdc.gov/nip/publications/ACIP-list.htm
Up-to-date ACIP statements that review immunizations against infectious diseases. ACIP statements can also be accessed by e-mail at nipinfo@cdc.gov or by calling the CDC immunization information hotline at 800-232-2522.

www.cdc.gov/mmwr
Morbidity and Mortality Weekly Report online (free). Vaccine updates and recommendations are published here.

www.nfid.org/ncai
Website of the National Coalition for Adult Immunization.

www.who.int/
WHO. Lists infectious disease outbreaks and immunization recommendations.

www.immunize.org
Site maintained by the Immunization Action Coalition (IAC), a nonprofit organization; the site includes/accesses many immunization-related resources (patient education resources, policy statements, contact numbers for each state's immunization program office, links to other sites). The IAC also produces two newsletters that cover immunization-related updates and developments: Needle Tips *and* Vaccinate Adults. *These publications are free. All materials are reviewed by the CDC. The IAC can be contacted at 1573 Selby Avenue, Suite 234, St. Paul, MN 55104-6328. Telephone: 651-647-9008/9; e-mail:* admin@immunize.org.

www.immunize.org/genr.d/pregguid.htm
Includes CDC guidelines for vaccinating pregnant women. Also available from the CDC at 404-639-8226.

2

Systemic Problems

7

Screening for HIV-1 Infection
STEPHEN L. BOSWELL

Knowledge of the status of human immunodeficiency virus (HIV) infection in the asymptomatic period permits infected persons to seek potentially beneficial medical treatment in a timely fashion, including antiretroviral agents and other medications that decrease the risk for the development of opportunistic infections (see Chapter 13). These measures delay the onset of the acquired immunodeficiency syndrome (AIDS) and prolong survival. In addition, early identification of HIV-1 infection can increase the effectiveness of tuberculin skin testing and thus improve tuberculosis screening and prophylaxis (see Chapter 49). Appropriate counseling, an essential part of screening for HIV-1 infection, may help prevent some individuals from transmitting HIV-1 by modifying their behavior. However, indiscriminate testing, especially among patients at very low risk for HIV-1 infection, raises the chance of a false-positive result and its attendant psychosocial morbidity. The primary care physician should know how best to advise the patient who asks about HIV-1 testing and whom to recommend for testing.

ASSESSING THE RISK FOR HIV-1 INFECTION

In the United States, it is estimated that between 800,000 and 900,000 people are infected with HIV-1. A related retrovirus, HIV-2, can also cause immune dysfunction, although it is generally less pathogenic than HIV-1. HIV-2 is distributed primarily in West Africa, but a few cases have been identified in the United States. Those at highest risk for infection with HIV-1 are men with a history of homosexual or bisexual activity (approximately 50% of those infected); intravenous drug users and their sexual contacts (approximately 25% of those infected); the sexual contacts of homosexual or bisexual men; persons who received blood and blood products between 1978 and 1985; and children born to infected women. The risk for directly acquiring HIV-1 infection through processed blood or selected blood products (plasma and clotting factor concentrates) has dramatically decreased since 1985 as a consequence of the widespread screening of those who donate blood and plasma, the use of serologic tests for HIV, and the viral inactivation of various plasma products.

Knowledge of the epidemiology of HIV-1 infection is necessary to estimate the pretest probability of HIV-1 infection in the person for whom screening is being considered. Attention to the pretest probability estimate is important to the decision to screen. Placing too much weight on the high sensitivity and specificity of HIV-1 antibody testing and ignoring the pretest probability is a common error (see Chapters 2 and 3).

The pretest probability of HIV-1 infection in a given patient is a function of the patient's previous risk behavior and the geographic location of the behavior. The testing setting, too, may be helpful in assessing the likelihood of infection. Settings characterized by high seroprevalence include sexually transmitted disease clinics, psychiatric hospitals, homeless shelters, alcohol rehabilitation facilities, and inner city emergency departments. These factors should be weighed when the need for HIV-1 testing is assessed.

When the behavioral risk factors for acquiring HIV-1 infection are being assessed in an individual patient, the following questions are particularly useful in clinical practice. Has the patient

- had sex with someone known to have HIV-1 infection or AIDS?
- had a history of sexually transmitted diseases?
- had sex with many men or women or had sex with someone who has had sex with many men or women?
- had sex with someone who has used needles to take drugs?
- shared needles to take drugs?
- had a history of receiving blood transfusions or clotting factor between 1978 and 1985?

If the answer to any of these questions is yes, then the patient and physician should give serious consideration to having HIV-1 antibody testing performed.

In addition, the Centers for Disease Control and Prevention recommends counseling and early diagnosis of HIV-1 infection for the following persons:

- Persons who consider themselves at risk for infection,
- Persons attending sexually transmitted disease clinics and drug abuse clinics
- Women seeking family planning services
- Patients with tuberculosis

TESTING FOR HIV-1 INFECTION

Viral Dynamics and the Immunologic Response to HIV-1

After transmission of HIV-1, usually a 2- to 8-week period elapses before the acute retroviral syndrome develops. This flu-like illness occurs in 50% to 90% of infected individuals, lasts 2 to 4 weeks, and resolves spontaneously. Coincidentally with the acute illness, high-grade viremia develops; titers of 50 to 100 million particles per milliliter have been reported. Viral titers begin to fall 2 to 3 weeks after the onset of acute symptoms, usually before an HIV-1 antibody response can be detected. This observation suggests that a response other than HIV-1 antibody formation may be responsible for the initial control of virus replication. Recent evidence suggests a central role for HIV-1–specific cell-mediated immunity in the control of virus replication during primary HIV-1 infection. Serial measurement of proliferative responses to HIV-1 antigens with the use of CD4+ lymphocytes from acutely infected individuals demonstrated a strong inverse correlation between the generation of HIV-specific CD4+ lymphocyte helper cells and plasma HIV-1 RNA levels. Similarly, among long-term nonprogressors, the highest HIV-specific proliferative responses were associated with the lowest plasma HIV-1 RNA levels.

Although the presence of symptoms is common among those who are acutely infected, symptoms often go unrecognized in the primary care setting because of their similarity to those of other common illnesses. Physicians should maintain a high level of suspicion for HIV infection in all patients presenting with a compatible syndrome. A careful evaluation of the patient's risk behaviors during the 3-month period before presentation should be obtained for all such patients. When appropriate, laboratory testing should be performed. This testing may include measurement of HIV RNA by HIV polymerase chain reaction or HIV branched-chain DNA and detection of HIV antibody. Although determination of HIV RNA is the preferred method of testing, a test for p24 antigen can be used when RNA testing is not readily available. A negative p24 antigen test result does not rule out acute infection, however. The information regarding the treatment of acute HIV infection is very limited, but the available data generally support antiretroviral treatment.

HIV-1 Antibody Assays

The diagnosis of HIV-1 infection is most frequently accomplished by detection of specific antibodies against viral antigens in serum. Recently, diagnostic testing of saliva and urine has been developed. Enzyme immunoassays (EIAs) for HIV-1 detection were first developed in 1985. Although EIAs are easily automated, inexpensive, and well suited for testing large numbers of samples, they can nonspecifically bind antibodies and produce false-positive results in patients exposed to other infections or vaccines. The assays have improved; first-generation tests used viral lysates as a source of viral antigens, whereas the current third-generation tests use recombinant DNA proteins coated on paper strips, beads, and microplate wells. The most advanced assays have a reported sensitivity and specificity of greater than 99.9% in serum from subjects with known HIV-1 infection and uninfected controls.

Rapid serologic screening tests have been developed for office use, including HIV antigen–coated gelatin or latex particle agglutination assays. These tests can be performed quickly (in some cases within 10 minutes), but they still require Western blot confirmation. Data suggest that some particle agglutination assays may be slightly less sensitive and specific than EIA is in moderate- or high-titer samples. Additional rapid screening assays based on the use of dipsticks and other technologies are available. When EIA is compared with several of these rapid assays, data suggest that the rapid assays can be significantly less sensitive in the testing of samples with a low titer of antibodies. This may be a particular problem during primary HIV-1 infection, when antibodies against selected antigens may not yet be present or may be present at very low titer. In general, EIA with confirmatory Western blot is the preferred screening test.

An important limitation of the HIV-1 screening assays used in the United States is that they primarily detect a single subtype of HIV-1. HIV-1 displays significant genetic variability. It can be categorized into a major group (M) and outlier groups (O). Group M can be further divided into subtypes or clades A through J. These clades show significant geographic variability. Many conventional assays for HIV-1 screening were developed by using a group M, subtype B virus, the predominant clade in the United States and Europe. Consequently, their ability to detect geographically diverse subtypes is limited. Several manufacturers are attempting to address this issue by adding non-subtype B peptides to their assays, but it should be remembered that the geography of HIV-1 acquisition can affect the accuracy of HIV-1 screening.

Body fluids other than blood can be used to determine a person's HIV-1 status. Oral fluids and urine may contain antibodies against HIV-1. Recently, the United States Food and Drug Administration approved several tests in which these fluids are used. The *OraSure* test, developed by Epitope, collects oral mucosal transudate via a cotton swab that is inserted into the mouth for 2 minutes. The swab is then packaged and sent to a reference laboratory for standard EIA and Western blot confirmation. This test has demonstrated 99.99% sensitivity and specificity in comparison with standard Western blot confirmation. The *Calypte* urine EIA test identifies urine HIV-1 immunoglobulin G antibody. The sensitivity and specificity of this test are comparable with those of serum EIA. However, Western blot testing of blood is required for confirmation of results.

In an effort to widen testing options further, kits specifically designed to be used in the home have been developed. With one such kit, *Home Access System*, developed by the Home Access Health Corporation, blood is collected by means of a lancet. The blood is blotted onto a test card, mailed to a reference laboratory, and tested by standard EIA and confirmatory Western blot. Within a week, the person undergoing testing may retrieve results by calling an automated system that stores results by a specific number assigned to each kit. A counselor is available to discuss a negative result, if desired. A call for a positive result is connected immediately to a telephone counselor, who will discuss the results with the caller.

A positive EIA test result should be confirmed by Western blot testing. Relative to EIA, the Western blot is slower, more labor-intensive, and much more expensive, but it is able to measure specific HIV-1 antibodies and so enhance the specificity of testing. It detects antibodies directed at specific HIV-1 proteins (core, envelope, and polymerase) after their separation by gel electrophoresis.

For the licensed Western blot, the interpretation of reactive and nonreactive test results is based on data from clinical studies submitted to the Food and Drug Administration for licensure. A test result is considered positive with this Western blot if antibodies to multiple virus-specific protein bands are present (i.e., p24, p31, and either gp41 or gp160). If fewer bands are present, the test is considered indeterminate; it is interpreted as negative only if no bands are present on the blot. When these criteria are used for interpreting test results, the probability of either a false-positive or a false-negative result is extremely small. It should be noted, however, that as many as 15% to 20% of tests on persons at low risk for HIV-1 infection may be described as indeterminate. Sera from persons recently infected with HIV-1 also may produce an indeterminate Western blot pattern. For such persons, a repeated Western blot on a second specimen obtained after the initial specimen often yields a positive blot pattern within 6 months. Conversely, follow-up testing of uninfected persons whose serum had an indeterminate blot pattern on initial testing usually will show no change in the banding pattern. Serum from some HIV-infected persons who have advanced immunodeficiency may have an indeterminate pattern because of a loss of antibodies to non-envelope proteins.

Despite the existence of a licensed Western blot test, many laboratories continue to use unlicensed tests because of cost and the stringent criteria required for interpreting the licensed test. The performance characteristics of the unlicensed tests have not been uniformly subjected to the same rigorous scrutiny required for licensure by the Food and Drug Administration. Although recommendations for standardization have been published, the extent to which these are followed is unknown. Information about production standards, variability between lots, or validation of criteria used for interpretation often is not available. The absence of standardization and appropriate quality controls may result in a lower sensitivity or specificity and therefore a higher probability of inaccurate results.

Other Tests

Tests for virus and viral components are now readily available in the United States. These tests include virus culture, p24 antigen assays, polymerase chain reaction assays, and signal amplification assays. In general, these assays are not used for the initial diagnosis of HIV-1 infection in adults.

Virus culture is time-consuming, costly, difficult to standardize, and relatively insensitive. Assays for p24 antigen are hampered by the low prevalence of antigen during the asymptomatic phase of HIV-1 infection. Polymerase chain reaction and signal amplification assays have a high false-positive rate and are not suitable for screening in most circumstances.

Surrogate markers do not test directly for virus and antibody. The most common is the CD4+ lymphocyte count, which is useful for assessing prognosis and therapeutic decision making but should not be used as an indirect method of determining whether a patient is infected with HIV-1.

Test Interpretation: Minimizing False-positive and False-negative Results

In testing for the presence of HIV-1 antibodies and interpreting the results, it is necessary to consider the timing of antibody responses to HIV-1 infection (Fig. 7.1), the sensitivity and specificity of the enzyme-linked immunosorbent assay (ELISA) and Western blot tests, and the pretest probability of the person being tested. For example, a negative ELISA result in a patient with a pretest probability of 0.1% (1 in 1,000) virtually rules out the diagnosis of HIV-1 infection. However, the same test result in a person with a 50% pretest probability of HIV-1 infection does not lower the posttest probability to zero (in biologic terms, it is possible that the patient is being tested before the appearance of antibody). Conversely, a positive ELISA result in a person with a low pretest probability (0.1%) produces a posttest probability of only 40%, which necessitates confirmatory testing.

A major objective is to limit the risk for a false-positive result and its potentially adverse psychological and social consequences. Pretest counseling is especially important for low-risk persons, who need to be informed of the risk for a false-positive result. It is often advisable to repeat an ELISA if a positive result is found in someone with no identifiable risk factor or has been obtained from a site that performs anonymous testing. There is always the finite possibility of laboratory error or sample mislabeling. Confirmatory testing with Western blot is essential and is a standard procedure in most laboratories.

A negative Western blot result in the setting of a positive ELISA and a small pretest probability of HIV-1 rules out HIV-1 infection. A positive Western blot result following a positive ELISA virtually rules in the diagnosis of HIV-1 infection, even among persons with a low pretest probability, but an "indeterminate" result can be problematic.

Despite the enhanced specificity afforded by adding the Western blot to the testing sequence, a small but important proportion (15% to 20%) of individuals with a positive ELISA result will have an "indeterminate" Western blot result. The most frequent cause of this is the presence of a single band of antibody, usually against p24. In high-risk individuals, this may reflect ongoing seroconversion. Low-risk persons with this result are virtually never infected. Testing should be repeated

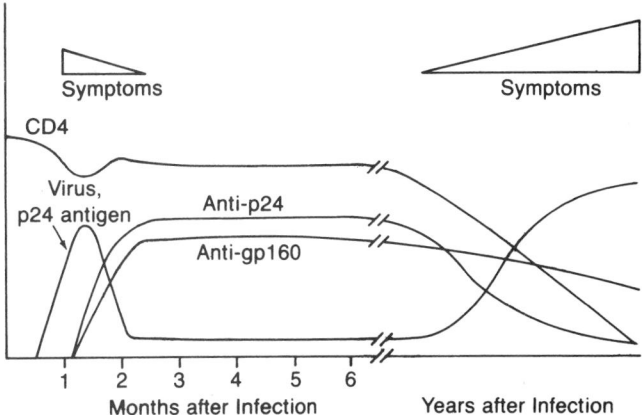

FIG. 7.1. Natural history of HIV-1 infection. Adapted from Clark SJ, Saag MS, Decker WD, et al. N Engl J Med 324:951.

Table 7.1. Centers for Disease Control
Recommendations for HIV Serologic Testing

- Persons who have sexually transmitted diseases.

- High-risk individuals: intravenous drug users, sexually active gay and bisexual men, hemophiliacs, regular sexual partners of persons in these categories and persons with known HIV infection; lower-incidence groups include prostitutes and persons who received transfusions during 1978–1985.

- Persons who consider themselves at risk or request the test.

- Women at risk who are of childbearing age or who are pregnant. Women at increased risk include IV drug users; prostitutes; women who have had male sexual partners who are IV drug users, bisexual, or HIV-infected; women living in communities or born in countries with a high prevalence in women; and women who received blood transfusion between 1978 and 1985.

- Individuals with clinical or laboratory findings suggesting HIV infection. These include generalized lymphadenopathy; unexplained dementia; chronic, unexplained fever or diarrhea; unexplained weight loss; or diseases that commonly complicate HIV, such as chronic or generalized herpes, thrush, recurrent or refractory vaginal candidiasis, oral hairy lukopakia, and "opportunistic" tumors, including Kaposi's sarcoma and B-cell lymphoma.

- Patients with active tuberculosis.

- Recipient and source of blood and body fluid exposures. Body fluids besides blood considered at risk include semen, vaginal secretions, cerebrospinal fluid, synovial fluid, pleural fluid, peritoneal fluid, pericardial fluid, amniotic fluid, and any bloody body fluid. Body fluids not considered at risk are feces, nasal secretions, sputum, saliva, sweat, tears, urine, and vomitus unless they contain visible blood.

- Health care workers who perform exposure-prone invasive procedures.

- Patients who are 15 to 55 years of age and who are admitted to a hospital at which the seroprevalence rate is 1% or higher or where AIDS patients account for more than 1 in 1,000 discharges.

- Donors of blood, semen, and organs.

From MMWR Morb Mortal Wkly Rep 1993; 42(RR-2):1, with permission.

within 2 to 6 months of the initial indeterminate result. If the individual is infected with HIV-1, a positive ELISA result will usually be accompanied by two or more positive bands on the Western blot. Among low-risk persons, the single band will frequently persist. In general, low-risk individuals with indeterminate test results should be reassured that HIV-1 infection is unlikely.

False-negative test results most frequently occur when testing is performed during the "window period"—usually within 6 months after viral transmission. Alternative methods of identifying HIV-1 infection are available in cases in which further clarification is desirable. These include polymerase chain reaction, viral culture, and detection of p24 antigen. These tests should not be used in place of antibody testing, but occasionally they may be useful.

Repeated Screening

Repeated screening at 6- to 12-month intervals is indicated for those who continue to practice high-risk behavior. An essential part of HIV-1 testing is the provision of HIV-1 counseling. All persons should be carefully instructed regarding how to minimize the risk for HIV-1 transmission.

RECOMMENDATIONS

- Patients at high risk for HIV-1 disease should be screened (Table 7.1).

- High-risk patients whose test results are negative but who continue high-risk behavior should be rescreened every 6 to 12 months.

- Patients at low risk who are donors of blood, semen, or organs should also be screened.

- Low-risk donors and low-risk persons who desire to know their HIV-1 status should be counseled about the possibility of a false-positive result, especially about an indeterminate Western blot result after a positive ELISA result.

- The interpretation of test results must take into account pretest probability, sensitivity and specificity of testing methods, and timing of the testing in relation to time of possible infection.

- Patient education regarding HIV-1 transmission and HIV-1 risk reduction should be part of every screening effort.

- Once a diagnosis of HIV-1 infection is established, the patient should be referred to a clinician with expertise in its management.

- Whenever possible, HIV-1 testing should be conducted in an anonymous fashion.

- Clinicians should be alert to the possibility of the acute retroviral syndrome when evaluating patients with a compatible symptom complex.

ANNOTATED BIBLIOGRAPHY

Anonymous or confidential HIV counseling and voluntary testing in federally funded testing sites—United States, 1995–1997. MMWR Morb Mortal Wkly Rep 1999;48(24):509. (*Documents the importance of anonymous and confidential testing opportunities.*)

Cardo DM, Culver DH, Ciesielski CA, et al. A case–control study of HIV seroconversion in health-care workers after percutaneous exposure. Centers for Disease Control and Prevention Needlestick Surveillance Group. N Engl J Med 1997;337:1485. (*The average risk of HIV infection after occupational percutaneous exposure is 0.3%, but it increases with volume of blood.*)

Centers for Disease Control and Prevention. Recommendations for HIV testing services for inpatients and outpatients in acute care hospital settings. MMWR Morb Mortal Wkly Rep 1993;42(RR-2):1. (*Delineates the responsibilities of hospitals toward HIV testing.*)

Centers for Disease Control and Prevention. Technical guidance on HIV counseling. MMWR Morb Mortal Wkly Rep 1993;42(RR-2):11. (*Best available information.*)

Clark SJ, Saag MS, Decker WD, et al. High titers of cytopathic virus in plasma of patients with symptomatic primary HIV-1 infection. N Engl J Med 1991;324:954. (*Natural history of infection.*)

Frank AP, Wandell MG, Headings MD, et al. Anonymous HIV testing using home collection and telemedicine counseling. A multicenter evaluation. Arch Intern Med 1997;157:309. (*Documents effectiveness of home testing when process includes careful counseling.*)

Henrard DR, Daar E, Farzadegan H, et al. Virologic and immunologic characterization of symptomatic and asymptomatic primary HIV-1 infection. J Acquir Immune Defic Syndr Hum Retrovirol 1995;9:305. (*Suggests that those with acute symptomatic HIV infection may progress more rapidly to AIDS.*)

Higgins DL, Galavotti C, O'Reilly KR, et al. Evidence for the effects of HIV antibody counseling and testing on risk behaviors. JAMA 1991;266:2419. (*Behavior improves.*)

HIV Counseling and Testing—United States, 1993. MMWR Morb Mortal Wkly Rep 1995;44(9):169. (*An examination of variations in the rates of use of private and public HIV CT sites by state.*)

Horsburgh CR Jr., Ou CY, Jason J, et al. Duration of human immunodeficiency virus infection before detection of antibody. Lancet 1989;2:637. (*Window period defined.*)

Ho DJ, Dondero TJ, Rayfield MA, et al. The emerging genetic diversity of HIV. The importance of global surveillance for diagnostics, research, and prevention. JAMA 1996;275:210. (*Details the implications of HIV mutation for testing effectiveness.*)

Jackson JB MacDonald KL, Cadwell J, et al. Absence of HIV infection in blood donors with indeterminate Western blot tests for antibody to HIV-1. N Engl J Med 1990;322:217. (*The meaning of an indeterminate result.*)

Kessler HA, Blaauw B, Spear J, et al. Diagnosis of human immunodeficiency virus infection in seronegative homosexuals presenting with an acute viral syndrome. JAMA 1987;258:1196. (*May be seronegative in early phase of illness. Results of repeat testing are usually positive.*)

Kuun E, Brashaw M, Heyns AD. Sensitivity and specificity of standard and rapid HIV-antibody tests evaluated by seroconversion and non-seroconversion low-titre panels. Vox Sang 1997;72:11. (*Suggests some potential problems with currently available rapid HIV-antibody tests.*)

Lafeuillade A, Poggi C, Tamalet C, et al. Effects of combination of zidovudine, didanosine, and lamivudine on primary human immunodeficiency virus type 1 infection. J Infect Dis 1997;175:1051.

O'Brien TR, George JR, Epstein JS, et al. Testing for antibodies to human immunodeficiency virus type 2 in the United States. MMWR Morb Mortal Wkly Rep 1992;41(RR-12):1. (*Type 2 is rare in the United States but is relevant in cases with a significant travel history, such as to West Africa.*)

O'Gorman MR, et al. Interpretive criteria of the Western blot assay for serodiagnosis of human immunodeficiency virus type 1 infection. Arch Pathol Lab Med 1991;115:26. (*Criteria for positive, negative, and indeterminate results; published erratum appears in Arch Pathol Lab Med 1991;115:783.*)

Quinn TC. Screening for HIV infection: benefits and costs. N Engl J Med 1992;327:486. (*An editorial focusing on testing patients at time of hospital admission.*)

Rosenberg ES, Caliendo AM, and Walker BD. Acute HIV infection among patients tested for mononucleosis [Letter]. N Engl J Med 1999;340:969. (*About 1% of those who tested negative for mononucleosis had acute HIV in this series of more than 500 patients.*)

US Public Health Service. Recommendations for human immunodeficiency virus counseling and voluntary testing for pregnant women. MMWR Morb Mortal Wkly Rep 1995;44(RR-7):1. (*Defines risk sufficient to recommend testing, as summarized in Table 7.1.*)

Update: HIV counseling and testing using rapid tests—United States, 1995. MMWR Morb Mortal Wkly Rep 1998;47(11):211. (*Evaluation of rapid testing strategies from a public health perspective.*)

8
Evaluation of Chronic Fatigue

Chronic fatigue ranks as one of the most common complaints in primary care practice, with a reported frequency in excess of 20%. It can also be one of the more frustrating problems to assess because it is a sensitive but nonspecific indicator of underlying medical or psychological pathology. Regardless of cause, the patient typically reports a lack of energy, listlessness, and being too tired to participate in family, work, or even leisure activities. Many speculate that they have a vitamin or mineral deficiency and self-treat accordingly before coming for evaluation. Others fear an underlying malignancy, endocrine disorder, or serious infection (e.g., HIV infection, tuberculosis, hepatitis, "chronic mono") and request extensive testing.

Most patients bothered by chronic fatigue come to the primary physician looking for an organic cause, especially those with a rather abrupt onset of symptoms. Although most studies of chronic fatigue find the vast majority of cases to have a psychological basis (e.g., depression), few patients initially report psychological symptoms, and if they do, they view such symptoms as secondary to a medical illness. Attempts by the physician to address psychological issues may be misinterpreted by the patient as not being taken seriously. Thus, the primary physician has the difficult tasks of sorting through a vast number of potential etiologies and patient concerns, determining what proportion of the problem is physiological and what part

is psychological, and helping the patient to understand and deal effectively with the underlying condition and its consequences.

PATHOPHYSIOLOGY AND CLINICAL PRESENTATIONS

Almost all illnesses are capable of causing fatigue; however, a few are noteworthy for the prominence of the symptom in the clinical presentation.

Psychological Etiologies. As just noted, fatigue is an important somatic symptom of *depression*, often coexisting with early morning awakening, appetite and sexual disturbances, and multiple bodily complaints. Abnormalities of central nervous system neurotransmitter metabolism and function are believed to play a major role in the pathogenesis of depression (see Chapter 227). *Chronic anxiety* may result in generalized fatigue, in part because it interferes with obtaining adequate physical and psychological rest. Patients report trouble falling asleep and a host of associated bodily complaints. Many maintain their neck muscles in a constantly tensed state, which gives rise to occipital–nuchal headaches. Seemingly unprovoked episodes of palpitations, difficulty breathing, and chest tightness may occur, especially in those whose anxiety is accompanied by a panic disorder (see Chapter 226).

Patients in whom somatization represents an underlying *personality disorder* may complain of chronic fatigue, often accompanied by a host of other refractory symptoms. Such individuals have a lifelong history of bodily complaints that elude diagnosis and treatment. Their symptoms are a cross they bear in a crude attempt to achieve a modicum of self-esteem (see Chapter 230).

Medications. Many of the medications used to treat anxiety, depression, and insomnia have substantial sedating effects. When used in excess, they may actually worsen the patient's symptoms and sense of fatigue rather than alleviate them. Of the antidepressants, *amitriptyline*, *doxepin*, and *trazodone* are among the more sedating, which makes them useful when agitation is a problem, but they can also lead to a feeling of being "knocked out" (see Chapter 227). Long-term use of *hypnotics* and withdrawal from them may exacerbate difficulty in falling asleep (see Chapter 232). Excessive use of *minor tranquilizers* can cause tiredness, especially when daily doses are sufficient to produce high serum levels of the drug and its active metabolites (see Chapter 226).

Antihypertensives that penetrate the central nervous system (e.g., *reserpine*, *methyldopa*, *clonidine*, *propranolol*) may precipitate depression or fatigue. Reserpine can cause depression when used in doses exceeding 0.5 mg daily, especially in patients with a prior history of depression. The same is true for β-blockers, although fatigue is the more common side effect (see Chapter 26) and a major reason for discontinuing the medication. *Antihistamines* used for allergic rhinitis are another common pharmacologic precipitant of fatigue, especially those that penetrate the central nervous system (e.g., *diphenhydramine*, *chlorpheniramine*).

Endocrine Disturbances are important, treatable precipitants. Dysfunction of the thyroid, adrenal, pituitary, parathyroid, or endocrine pancreas can be subtle in onset, starting out inconspicuously as fatigue, perhaps accompanied by more specific symptoms. For example, *hypothyroidism* may present as fatigue, perhaps in association with weight gain, dry skin, mild hoarseness, or cold intolerance (see Chapter 104). In the elderly, hyperthyroidism may take an atypical form (*apathetic hyperthyroidism*), characterized by fatigue, marked weight loss, apathy, and otherwise unexplained atrial fibrillation (see Chapter 103).

Patients with *Addison's disease* manifest an insidious onset of fatigue in conjunction with weight loss, vague gastrointestinal upset, postural hypotension, and eventually hyperpigmentation. *Panhypopituitarism* from postpartum hemorrhage or a tumor of the sellar region can cause fatigue. The postpartum patient fails to lactate or resume menstruation; lassitude, decreased libido, and loss of axillary and pubic hair ensue. Later, symptoms of hypothyroidism may develop. The patient with a pituitary tumor may note galactorrhea and amenorrhea (see Chapter 100).

Poorly controlled *diabetes mellitus* may present as fatigue accompanied by polyuria when glycosuria is severe enough to produce caloric wasting and volume depletion (see Chapter 102). Similarly, fatigue may be the initial symptom of *hyperparathyroidism* and other causes of hypercalcemia.

Metabolic Disturbances. *Chronic renal failure* may present inconspicuously with fatigue and few localizing symptoms or signs aside from laboratory findings of azotemia, mild anemia, impaired renal concentrating ability, and an abnormal urinary sediment (see Chapter 142). *Hepatocellular failure* is an important source of lassitude. Jaundice, ascites, petechiae, asterixis, spider angiomata, and other signs of hepatic insufficiency usually contribute to the clinical picture. However, in anicteric hepatitis and mild forms of chronic hepatitis, jaundice may be minimal or absent while fatigue is prominent; the same holds for the prodromal phase of acute viral hepatitis (see Chapters 70 and 71).

Hematologic and Oncologic Etiologies. *Iron deficiency* is often blamed for fatigue, although the correlation between iron deficiency anemia and fatigue is poor, especially when the anemia is mild (see Chapter 79). In a double-blind study of menstruating women with mild anemia resulting from iron deficiency, no significant difference was noted between the effects of iron and of placebo on fatigue. The relation between severe anemia (hematocrit <20) and fatigue is more direct. Lassitude prevails, at times in association with exertional dyspnea or with postural hypotension when blood loss is acute.

Occult malignancy is a much feared etiology. Although fatigue and lassitude accompany most cancers, *pancreatic carcinoma* is the archetypal example of a tumor that may present initially as marked fatigue with few localizing symptoms. Severe weight loss, depression, and apathy may also dominate the clinical picture before other manifestations of the malignancy become evident. Malignancies causing hypercalcemia (e.g., breast cancer, myeloma) may present with fatigue, although usually the hypercalcemia is a late development.

Cardiopulmonary Disease. The hallmark of fatigue associated with cardiopulmonary disease is a history of exertional dyspnea. Fatigue sometimes dominates the clinical presentation of patients with *chronic congestive heart failure* or *chronic lung disease*, especially when patients with heart failure are treated aggressively for symptoms of pulmonary congestion (see Chapters 32 and 47). Disturbed sleep resulting from *sleep apnea* is an often overlooked cause of chronic fatigue. Daytime sleepiness, excessive snoring, irregular breathing, disturbed sleep, and hemoglobin desaturation are characteristic. If untreated, sleep apnea may progress to pulmonary hypertension (see Chapter 46).

Infectious Diseases. Profound fatigue, low-grade fever, and lymphadenopathy are the hallmarks of a number of much feared infectious etiologies, including *mononucleosis*, *viral hepatitis*, and *HIV disease*. Other viral illnesses, such as *cytomegalovirus infection* and the possibly virus-triggered *chronic fatigue syndrome* (see below), may also present in this way. *Tuberculosis* and *subacute bacterial endocarditis* are important infectious etiologies of fatigue in which few localizing symptoms may be present. A history of cough, night sweats, HIV infection, or exposure is sometimes elicited from the patient with tuberculosis (see Chapter 49). Recent dental work, a heart murmur, and IV drug abuse are risk factors for subacute bacterial endocarditis. *Lyme disease* is noteworthy for fatigue accompanied by joint complaints, headache, and low-grade fever (see Chapter 160).

Connective Tissue Disease and Other Forms of Immune Dysfunction. Marked fatigue may dominate the initial clinical presentation of most *rheumatoid diseases*, before characteristic inflammatory connective tissue manifestations become evident (see Chapter 156).

Chronic Fatigue Syndrome (CFS) is an idiopathic condition characterized by new onset of persistent or relapsing fatigue lasting at least 6 consecutive months in patients with no prior history of such fatigue. Associated symptoms may include migratory arthralgias, myalgias, sore throat, tender lymph nodes, new generalized headache, unrefreshing sleep, postexertional malaise, and impaired memory or concentration. The initial presentation may be flulike, but unlike the typical symptoms of postviral fatigue, these symptoms persist far beyond 1 to 2 months. CFS accounts for about 5% to 10% of all cases of chronic fatigue. Peak prevalence is among persons ages 20 to 50 years; women outnumber men by 3 to 1.

Etiology. The etiology of CFS remains unknown. The most consistent finding of CFS etiologic studies has been the inconsistency of results. Early, uncontrolled studies revealed intriguing suggestions of *Epstein-Barr virus* (EBV) *reactivation, immunologic dysfunction,* and even *chronic candidal infection.* The findings encouraged early etiologic designations such as "chronic mononucleosis," "chronic fatigue and immune dysfunction syndrome" (CFIDS), and "chronic candidiasis." Attempts at treatment with antiviral agents, immunoglobulin injections, and systemic antifungal agents proved ineffective when studied in controlled fashion. Moreover, subsequent controlled studies found many CFS patients with no evidence of EBV infection/reactivation, immunologic dysfunction, or chronic candidal infection. Still, some investigators continue to explore the relation between stress (a known risk factor for CFS), immune modulation, and reactivation of latent viruses, with an eye toward these conditions triggering neuroendocine responses.

Current research focuses on *neuroendocrinologic mechanisms.* Interest derives from the observation that *neurally mediated hypotension* occurs with increased frequency in CFS patients; however, questions remain as to whether this is a cause or an effect of the deconditioning that occurs in CFS patients. An association with *fibromyalgia* has been noted, but it is unclear whether this represents a common pathophysiology or overlapping diagnostic criteria (see also Chapter 159).

Some view CFS as predominantly a *psychiatric condition,* given the high prevalence of concurrent psychiatric disease, particularly *somatization disorder,* found in CFS patients subjected to detailed psychiatric study (range, 20% to 70%). Some wonder whether this association is a consequence of the original diagnostic criteria for CFS, which had many features overlapping with those of somatization disorder (see below). Nonetheless, there is a trend toward an increased risk of suicidality and a high prevalence of major depression, but no higher than that found in patients with other chronic disabling disease. In addition, the physical manifestations noted above are atypical for such psychiatric disorders as depression and anxiety, and the anhedonia, guilt, and low motivation that characterize depression are infrequent in CFS. In fact, these patients are highly motivated and work hard to deal with their illness.

DIFFERENTIAL DIAGNOSIS

Although the list of conditions that may present with fatigue is extensive, most cases have a strong overlay of anxiety, depression, or both, even when the cause is medical. Fatigue, of course, may accompany any illness, but those listed in Table 8.1 are notable for the prominence of lassitude in the clinical presentation. Depression and associated psychiatric conditions account for about two thirds of cases of persistent fatigue subjected to comprehensive medical and psychological evaluation. Another one fourth of cases remain idiopathic, having some but not enough features to qualify as CFS. About 5% meet the Centers for Disease Control and Prevention (CDC) criteria for chronic fatigue syndrome, and 3% turn out to be previously unrecognized medical disorders.

WORKUP

In most instances, the evaluation of fatigue can be conveniently performed in the office. Two or three visits may be needed to establish the underlying etiology; at times, the patient may insist that medical illness be ruled out before agreeing to discuss psychosocial matters.

Table 8.1. Some Conditions Presenting as Chronic Fatigue

Psychological	Infectious
Depression	Endocarditis
Anxiety	Tuberculosis
Somatization disorder	Mononucleosis
	Hepatitis
Pharmacologic	Parasitic disease
Hypnotics	HIV infection
Antihypertensives	Cytomegalovirus infection
Antidepressants	
Tranquilizers	Cardiopulmonary
Drug abuse and drug withdrawal	Chronic congestive heart failure
	Chronic obstructive pulmonary disease
Endocrine–metabolic	
Hypothyroidism	Connective tissue disease–immune hyperreactivity
Diabetes mellitus	Rheumatoid disease
Apathetic hyperthyroidism of the elderly	Chronic fatigue syndrome
Pituitary insufficiency	
Hyperparathyroidism or hypercalcemia of any origin	Disturbed sleep
Addison's disease	Sleep apnea
Chronic renal failure	Esophageal reflux
Hepatocellular failure	Allergic rhinitis
	Psychological etiologies (see above)
Neoplastic–hematologic	
Occult malignancy (e.g., pancreatic cancer)	
Severe anemia	

History. The inquiry should begin with a thorough *description of the fatigue* to be sure that the patient is not confusing focal neuromuscular disease with generalized lassitude. Because *depression* underlies many cases of fatigue, it is essential to check for its somatic manifestations, such as early morning awakening, alteration of appetite, and multisystem functional complaints. It is also important to ask about significant losses, low self-esteem, and occurrence of crying spells and suicidal thoughts. *Anxiety* is suggested by unresolved conflict, persistent nervousness, recurrent bouts of excessive uneasiness, and trouble falling asleep. A lifelong history of *refractory bodily complaints* that defy diagnosis and treatment should raise suspicion of a personality disturbance.

Any abuse of *hypnotics* or *tranquilizers* needs to be ascertained and considered as a cause of disturbed sleep and resultant fatigue. Fatigue in the elderly patient should not be ascribed to age; an underlying psychogenic or medical illness is likely.

A history of *fever*, *sweats*, *weight loss*, and *adenopathy* points toward smoldering infection and occult neoplasm. Symptoms suggesting a metabolic or endocrinologic cause include *polyuria*, polydipsia, changes in skin pigmentation and texture, hoarseness, *cold intolerance*, nausea, and *abnormal menses*. Symmetric *joint pain* and morning stiffness are clues to underlying rheumatoid disease.

Checking into factors that might disturb sleep can lead to detection of treatable etiologies such as *sleep apnea* (see Chapter 46), *esophageal reflux* (see Chapter 61), and *allergic rhinitis* (see Chapter 222).

The *past medical history* should be investigated for anemia, rheumatic fever, mononucleosis, heart murmur, recurrent urinary tract infection, proteinuria, liver disease, alcohol and drug abuse, and depression. *Epidemiologic considerations* ought to include exposure to tuberculosis, mononucleosis, and hepatitis; any risk factors for AIDS are important to note (see Chapter 13). *Travel* to areas where parasitic infections are endemic, work in meat-packing industries or on a farm, and a sudden common source outbreak of illness are other potentially important epidemiologic clues.

A full listing of all the patient's *medications* should be obtained. Often overlooked are over-the-counter antihistamines that patients use for sleep, allergies, and colds. Most centrally acting antihypertensive agents are capable of causing fatigue, and their use should be noted, as should that of all psychotropic agents.

Physical Examination. Vital signs including *postural pulse* and *blood pressure*, *temperature*, and *weight* should be determined. If no fever is noted on examination in the office but it is suggested by history, then a 10 p.m. reading at home is indicated. *Skin* is assessed for change in pigmentation, purpura, dryness, rash, jaundice, and pallor. Endocarditis may first be suggested by the finding of splinter hemorrhages or petechiae. *Funduscopic examination* may reveal Roth's spots, diabetic retinopathy, or even, in rare instances, a tuberculoma. The *sclerae* are observed for icterus. If examination of the *pharynx* reveals petechiae at the junction of the hard and soft palate, mononucleosis ought to be considered. The *thyroid* is checked for goiter.

Careful examination of all *lymph nodes* is essential; size, degree of tenderness, and distribution should be noted. Diffuse adenopathy suggests malignancy and infection and is sometimes a sign of HIV infection (see Chapter 12). *Breasts* should be checked for masses, as breast cancer and its attendant hypercalcemia may present as fatigue. The *lungs* are examined for rales, consolidation, and effusion, and the *heart* for murmurs, rubs, gallops, and rhythm disturbances. Unexplained atrial fibrillation in the elderly may be a manifestation of apathetic hyperthyroidism.

The *abdomen* is palpated for organomegaly, masses, ascites, and hepatic tenderness. The *rectal examination* includes a look for masses, prostatic pathology, and occult blood. The *genitalia* should be checked for masses suggestive of malignancy and tenderness indicative of infection. The *joints* are assessed for signs of inflammation. A complete *neurologic examination* is necessary to be sure that the patient's fatigue is not really a manifestation of neuromuscular disease. Any tenderness, atrophy, focal weakness, or fasciculations in the muscles are noted. Deep tendon reflexes that have a slow relaxation phase are suggestive of hypothyroidism. Even visual field testing is important, for a pituitary lesion may produce a bitemporal hemianopsia. *Mental status assessment* is critical, including observation of affect, thinking, judgment, and memory. Formal testing for suicidality is indicated (see Chapter 227) because of the high prevalence of depression in this patient population.

Laboratory Tests. In the overtly depressed patient with an otherwise completely normal history and physical examination, there is no need to proceed with an extensive laboratory workup for occult medical illness. A *complete cell blood count* (CBC) and *erythrocyte sedimentation rate* (ESR) are often ordered for screening purposes. The CBC, particularly if accompanied by a look at the peripheral smear and differential, may provide important clues to underlying infection, inflammatory disease, hepatocellular failure, or malignancy. Unfortunately, the ESR has not proved to be sensitive or specific enough to help in detecting or ruling out occult illness. Consequently, many physicians no longer order the ESR, whereas others continue to use it with the intent of acting on it only if the result is markedly elevated (e.g., >75 mm/h).

A particularly difficult situation is the patient with no evidence of depression as a primary cause and an unrevealing history and physical examination. Here, a few extra serum chemistries (*calcium*, *albumin*, *blood urea nitrogen*, *creatinine*, *glucose*, and *transaminase-aminotransferase*) are warranted to help rule out clinically subtle conditions that may present as fatigue, such as hypercalcemia, mild renal failure, early diabetes mellitus, and anicteric hepatitis. A *thyrotropin* (TSH) test is worth considering because thyroid disease represents a very treatable cause that can have a very subtle presentation, and the improved TSH assay is very sensitive for the detection of most forms of hyperthyroidism and hypothyroidism. The elderly fatigued patient with weight loss and unexplained atrial fibrillation is a prime candidate for a TSH determination. Other thyroid indices add little and should not be obtained unless the TSH level is abnormal (see Chapters 103 and 104).

Patients with recent onset of persisting fatigue and adenopathy should undergo a *heterophile* test for acute mononucleosis. However, *viral antibody titers* (with the exception of testing for *viral hepatitis* and *HIV infection*) are of no known utility in patients with undiagnosed chronic fatigue. Ordering a battery of viral antibody titers was popular when CFS was thought to be caused by chronic EBV infection or reactivation of other viruses. Without a proven etiologic role for viruses in CFS, viral titers proved to be useless and sometimes misleading, especially when results were "positive" in a patient with severe depression who refused to accept a psychiatric diagnosis. The same holds true for *Candida* and *fungal testing*. *Lyme titers* are also of little use in the absence of other evidence suggestive of Lyme disease, such as polyarthritis, history of tick bite, or erythema chronicum migrans (see Chapter 160). Testing for viral hepatitis is clearly indicated in those with a transaminase elevation, and HIV testing is appropriate when diffuse adenopathy or a history of high-risk behavior is present.

Neuroimaging studies have been used investigationally in persons with CFS to assess regional brain function. Positron emission tomography (PET) and single-photon emission computed tomography (SPECT) have demonstrated areas of brain hypometabolism and hypoperfusion, respectively, in CFS patients. Because the specificity and pathophysiologic significance of these findings remain to be determined, these imaging techniques are not indicated at present for the workup of chronic fatigue or diagnosis of CFS.

Diagnosis of Chronic Fatigue Syndrome. No test or set of tests is diagnostic for CFS. Diagnosis is based on clinical findings and the ruling out of other etiologies. A *working case definition* was developed by the CDC in 1988 to provide a more uniform basis for identifying and studying patients with CFS. Patients had to fulfill two major criteria, plus either six symptom criteria and two physical criteria or eight symptom criteria (Table 8.2).

Despite the development of a case definition, studies continued to produce unacceptably inconsistent results, suggesting that the case definition was producing too much heterogeneity in CFS populations and too much overlap with somatization disorders. In 1994, the CDC sponsored a revision of the case definition (Table 8.2). Two major criteria were eliminated: (a) more than 50% reduction in activity, because it is too difficult to quantify, and (b) absence of any psychiatric disease, because nonpsychotic depression and anxiety are frequent in CFS. In addition, the number of minor criteria was reduced from eight to four (Table 8.2) to reduce overlap with somatization disorder.

Subgroup classifications were recommended to facilitate identification for the study of patients who might have similar prognoses and responses to therapy. Subgroupings criteria include comorbid conditions, severity of fatigue, duration, and current level of physical function. Finally, a designation of *idiopathic chronic fatigue* was proposed for the substantial number of persons with unexplained fatigue meeting some but not all of the criteria for chronic fatigue syndrome.

Clinicians need to keep in mind that case definitions are only consensus views intended to facilitate research. Although such definitions can be used for clinical diagnosis, they are not based on scientifically established criteria and remain somewhat arbitrary, requiring clinical judgment for proper use in patient care. Until the etiology of CFS is better understood, these shortcomings will have to be taken into consideration when the working definition is used for diagnostic purposes. (The reader is urged to watch the literature closely for further developments.)

Table 8.2. Centers for Disease Control Case Definition Criteria for Chronic Fatigue Syndrome

	1988 CRITERIA	1994 CRITERIA
Major criteria		
New onset	+	+
No previous history	+	+
Duration >6 months	+	+
Does not improve with bed rest	+	+
All other illnesses excluded	+	+
Activity reduction >50%	+	−
All psychiatric illnesses excluded	+	+/−
Minor criteria	Need 8 of 14	Need 4 of 8
Sore throat	+	+
Painful lymph nodes	+	+
Muscle discomfort	+	+
Prolonged fatigue after exercise	+	+
Generalized (new) headache	+	+
Migratory arthralgias	+	+
Impaired concentration or memory	+	+
Unrefreshing sleep	+	+
Low-grade fever	+	−
Generalized weakness	+	−
Acute onset	+	−
Documented low-grade fever	+	−
Documented nonexudative pharyngitis	+	−
Documented palpable or tender lymph nodes	+	−
Subclassifications		
Presence of comorbid conditions (depression)	None	Yes
Current level of fatigue	None	Yes
Duration of fatigue	None	Yes
Current level of physical function	None	Yes

From Levine PH. Chronic fatigue syndrome comes of age. Am J Med 1997; 105:35, with permission.

PATIENT EDUCATION

It is often useful to determine patients' views of their illness before proceeding with patient education, so that the explanation will address patient concerns and perspectives. Patients who have a medical view of their condition are more receptive to a biologic explanation for their symptoms, even if the cause is psychogenic. However, one must be careful not evoke a misleading medical explanation, such as "viral infection" or "immune dysfunction," especially in the setting of a suspected or possible psychogenic etiology, because this might cause a patient to delay or refuse psychiatric intervention. Patients with evidence of underlying psychogenic disease need an especially thorough review of the evidence for their diagnosis and a careful explanation of their symptoms because many come to the physician thinking they have a medical problem. For example, reviewing the diagnostic criteria for depression and describing the neurochemical mechanisms by which depression leads to fatigue (see Chapter 227) can be helpful.

The attention given to CFS in the lay press often necessitates addressing the issue of its likelihood and some of its purported, although unfounded, causes (e.g., EBV infection, yeast infection, immune dysfunction). Many patients with a psychogenic etiology prefer to cling to this diagnosis as an acceptable explanation of their psychophysiologic symptoms rather than face a diagnosis of depression, anxiety, or somatization disorder. In addition to a careful workup, a respectful, sympathetic, open-minded approach is essential (see Chapter 230).

The Patient with Chronic Fatigue Syndrome. In addition to the measures noted above, the physician should emphasize the legitimacy of the patient's symptoms and summarize the workup, its rationale, and findings. Also useful is a review of the idiopathic nature of the illness, its generally self-limited course, and often favorable response to simple measures (see below). Establishing a partnership with the patient is key to successful management. Certain beliefs and behaviors known to perpetuate disability and lead to a worse outcome in CFS must be addressed, particularly the view that a purely physical disease mechanism is present that is unresponsive to intervention and that exercise is harmful. Such beliefs and associated behaviors contribute to resignation, anxiety, and depression and exacerbate deconditioning and the feeling of fatigue. At times, referral for formal *cognitive behavior therapy* is worth pursuing to achieve the educational and behavioral goals so important to recovery (see below). It is important that any new symptoms or signs be investigated thoroughly and not simply attributed to CFS.

SYMPTOMATIC RELIEF

When the cause of fatigue is endocrinologic, metabolic, or infectious, treatment needs to be specific and aimed at the underlying condition. Malignancy is often accompanied by a reactive depression that can be helped by development of a strong, supportive *doctor–patient relationship* (see Chapter 87). The fatigue of endogenous depression can be treated with support and tricyclic *antidepressants*; imipramine may be less sedating than amitriptyline (starting dose is 25 to 50 mg at bedtime, increased by 25 to 50 mg at a time). The sleep disorder caused by depression may respond well to small doses, with the fatigue dissipating as the patient gets a good night's sleep.

Affective changes may not occur at low doses (see Chapter 227).

Anxiety-related fatigue can be difficult to treat. Prescribing antianxiety agents can lead to excessive use and worsening of symptoms (see Chapter 226); however, a brief and limited trial of *benzodiazepine* therapy at bedtime is worth an attempt. For example, 5 mg of chlordiazepoxide can help the patient to fall asleep and get much-needed rest. There is no evidence that any one benzodiazepine is superior to any other for sleep, although flurazepam is widely promoted and prescribed, often in conjunction with another benzodiazepine. (This can sometimes lead to excessive benzodiazepine intake). Once symptomatic control of anxiety is accomplished, work can begin on helping the patient to deal with his or her problems.

If fatigue results from sleep disturbed by sleep apnea, reflux, or allergic rhinitis, then treatment should be directed toward the underlying pathophysiology (see Chapters 46, 61, and 222).

Approach to the Patient with Chronic Fatigue Syndrome. Some of the best results to date have been achieved with *cognitive behavior therapy*, a nonpharmacologic treatment that focuses on identifying and reversing beliefs and coping mechanisms that perpetuate disability and block recovery. More than 75% of patients experience a return to normal daily activity by 12 months, in comparison with 25% randomized to standard medical care alone. Although this approach does not directly address the underlying etiology of CFS (which remains unknown), it does seek to deal with ideas and behaviors that encourage passivity and hinder self-help and symptomatic improvement. Treatment begins by elucidating the patient's beliefs about the illness and by exploring the behaviors that follow from these beliefs. Those marked by helplessness and passivity are targeted for change during a series of sessions in which the therapist works in partnership with the patient. The goal is to have the patient regain a sense of control and active participation in recovery. Although most studies of cognitive behavior therapy in CFS involve formally trained therapists, there is no theoretical reason why the primary care physician cannot personally conduct the basic steps of the program (Table 8.3).

A basic part of the cognitive behavior program is a gentle, graded *exercise program*. Some have even speculated that exercise is the key element, but exercise in the absence of a cognitive component leads to a high dropout rate. Those bothered by disordered sleep may benefit from *low-dose antidepressant therapy* (e.g., 25 mg of nortriptyline at bedtime, 10 to 20 mg of doxepin at bedtime, or 10 mg of paroxetine every morning). Higher doses do not appear to confer better results. *NSAIDs* provide symptomatic relief in patients bothered by myalgias, arthralgias, or headache.

Table 8.3.   Basic Steps in
Cognitive Behavioral Therapy

1. Problem assessment and formulation
2. Identification of beliefs and coping behaviors that perpetuate illness-related disability
3. Development of more adaptive beliefs and coping behaviors
4. Patient testing of new approach to the illness and adopting it if it works
5. Consolidating gains and planning further self-help

From Sharpe M. Cognitive behavior therapy for chronic fatigue syndrome: efficacy and implications. Am J Med 1998;105:104S, with permission.

A host of enthusiastic reports from uncontrolled studies have appeared claiming marked benefit from *liver extract, antifungal therapy, antiviral drugs, vitamins, immunoglobulin infusions, fatty acids, fludrocortisone,* and so on. Almost without exception, none has proved beneficial when subjected to randomized, double-blind, placebo-controlled study. Definitive etiologic therapy will have to await a better understanding of CFS pathophysiology. Fortunately, it appears that symptoms are self-limited, often improving or even clearing within 12 to 18 months. A strong *patient–doctor alliance* is essential, not only for providing support, but also for protecting the patient from unnecessary testing and unproven therapies.

A.H.G.

ANNOTATED BIBLIOGRAPHY

Aurbach G, Mallette L, Patten B, et al. Hyperparathyroidism: recent studies. NIH conference. Ann Intern Med 1973;79:566. (*Fatigue headed the list of symptoms reported in 57 cases of primary hyperparathyroidism; 24% reported the problem.*)

Croog SH, Levine S, Testa A, et al. The effects of antihypertensive therapy on the quality of life. N Engl J Med 1986;314:1657. (*The incidence of fatigue was about 5% in persons taking the antihypertensive agents methyldopa and propranolol.*)

Dismukes WE, Wade JS, Lee JY, et al. A randomized, double-blind trial of nystatin therapy for the candidiasis hypersensitivity syndrome. N Engl J Med 1990;323:1717. (*Strong evidence against yeast infection as the cause of the chronic fatigue syndrome.*)

Freeman R, Komaroff AL. Does the chronic fatigue syndrome involve the autonomic nervous system? Am J Med 1997;102:357. (*Evidence supporting autonomic dysfunction, but not distinguishing between deconditioning and an autonomic neuropathy.*)

Fukuda K, Straus SE, Hickie I, et al. The chronic fatigue syndrome: a comprehensive approach to its definition and study. Ann Intern Med 1994;121:953. (*The current CDC consensus working definition of the syndrome and recommendations for evaluation and study.*)

Gold D, Bowden R, Sixbey J, et al. Chronic fatigue: a prospective clinical and virologic study. JAMA 1990;264:48. (*Isolated EBV was no more frequent in patients with chronic fatigue than it was in healthy controls, and improvement in patients with chronic fatigue was not associated with any change in EBV levels.*)

Goldenberg DL, Simms RW, Geiger A, et al. High frequency of fibromyalgia in patients with chronic fatigue syndrome seen in a primary care practice. Arthritis Rheum 1990;33:381. (*An interesting association, but significance unclear.*)

Holmes GP, Kaplan JE, Gantz NM, et al. Chronic fatigue syndrome: a working case definition. Ann Intern Med 1988;108:387. (*The original working case definition of CFS.*)

Kaslow JE, Rucker L, Onishi R. Liver extract–folic acid–cyanocobalamin vs. placebo for chronic fatigue syndrome. Arch Intern Med 1989;149:2501. (*A double-blind, placebo-controlled, crossover study showing no benefit.*)

Kendell RE. Chronic fatigue, viruses, and depression. Lancet 1991;337:160. (*An editorial summing up the evidence. Favors the view that most have depression and a few might have some kind of postviral syndrome.*)

Kroenke K, Wood DR, Mangelsdorff, et al. Chronic fatigue in primary care. JAMA 1988;260:929. (*Documents a high prevalence of persistence and functional impairment.*)

Manu P, Lane TJ, Mathews DA. The frequency of the chronic fatigue syndrome in patients with symptoms of persistent fatigue. Ann Intern Med 1988;109:554. (*The prevalence was only 5%, which indicates that the condition is actually quite uncommon among those presenting with fatigue.*)

Sharpe M. Cognitive behavior therapy for chronic fatigue syndrome: efficacy and implications. Am J Med 1998;105(3A):104s. (*Best summary of the approach; nearly 75% achieve a return to normal daily activity by 12 months.*)

Sox HC, Liang MH. The erythrocyte sedimentation rate. Ann Intern Med 1986;104:515. (*A critical review arguing the test is not a useful screening procedure in most instances.*)

Thomas F, Mazzaferri E, Skillman T. Apathetic thyrotoxicosis: a distinctive clinical and laboratory entity. Ann Intern Med 1970;72:679. (*A classic article identifying the condition; patients are typically elderly and depressed, and they exhibit marked weight loss and otherwise unexplained atrial fibrillation.*)

*Vollmer-Conna U, Hicki I, Hadzi-Pavlovic D, et al. Intr*avenous immunoglobulin is ineffective in the treatment of patients with chronic fatigue syndrome. Am J Med 1997;103:38. (*A randomized, double-blind study showing no benefit.*)

Wood M, Elwood P. Symptoms of iron deficiency anemia: a community survey. Br J Prev Soc Med 1966;20:117. (*Correlation between hemoglobin concentration and symptoms was poor; iron therapy produced no statistically significant improvement in symptoms.*)

9

Evaluation of Weight Loss

Involuntary weight loss is a sensitive, although nonspecific, complaint frequently encountered in primary care practice. Reports of prevalence range as high as 10% to 20%, with frequency greatest among the elderly. Unexplained weight loss often suggests the presence of serious pathology, yet a substantial fraction of patients turn out to be free of organic illness. For example, in a series of patients with involuntary weight loss followed for 1 year, 50% either died or deteriorated during the course of the study; however, another 35% were well at the time of follow-up. Involuntary weight loss in excess of 2.5 kg is usu-

ally considered a reasonable threshold for evaluation, as more than 95% of patients with an organic etiology will have lost at least that much weight. However, unless extreme, the amount of weight loss is not predictive of an organic etiology. In many cases of weight loss, accompanying symptoms readily suggest the cause, but when a marked fall in weight is the sole or predominant complaint, the assessment can be difficult. The primary physician needs to determine at the time of initial presentation who requires an extensive medical evaluation and who can be followed expectantly.

PATHOPHYSIOLOGY AND CLINICAL PRESENTATION

Pathophysiology

When the number of calories available for utilization falls below daily needs, weight is lost; 1 lb of fat is consumed for every 3,500-calorie deficit. The principal mechanisms resulting in caloric deficits are reduced food intake, malabsorption, excess nutrient loss, and increased caloric requirements. Loss of fluid will also register as a fall in weight, with about 1 kg (2.2 lb) lost for every liter removed. Although more than one mechanism may be operating in a given case, each mechanism has a few characteristic clinical features. Anorexia or disinterest in food typifies causes of *reduced intake*. Foul-smelling, bulky, greasy stools are seen in the later stages of *malabsorption*; subtle changes in stool consistency and frequency are noted earlier (see Chapter 64). Recurrent vomiting, profuse diarrhea, polyuria, or fistulous drainage can lead to *excessive loss*. Increased food intake, hyperactivity, and fever are prominent in cases of *increased demand*.

Clinical Presentation

Although many causes of weight loss are readily evident, some conditions may be clinically subtle and present as unexplained weight loss. These deserve special elaboration.

Major depression is the leading cause of unexplained weight loss, especially in the elderly, in whom the condition accounts for up to 30% of cases. As frequent as it is, depression is often overlooked unless specifically considered. Somatic manifestations include appetite disturbance, early morning awakening, multiple bodily complaints, and fatigue; anhedonia, low self-esteem, feelings of guilt, and suicidal thoughts are among the characteristic psychological features. The death of a loved one, social isolation, and poverty are important psychosocial precipitants (see Chapter 227).

Eating disorders may involve covert behaviors. The patient suffering from *anorexia nervosa* may deny any disturbance of appetite yet persist in restricting food intake to the point of cachexia. Prevalence is highest among adolescent girls and young women. They decide to diet to an extreme degree, are preoccupied with a phobic concern about being fat, and are motivated by a relentless pursuit of thinness. Dieting persists because its psychological gratifications outweigh those derived from the intake of food. Paradoxically, the patient often reports feeling well and initially appears bright and undisturbed by the weight loss; anorexia is usually denied. At times, a few specific foods are the only ones consumed (e.g., vegetable juices). Amenorrhea is invariable and appears shortly after weight loss begins. A variant of anorexia nervosa consists of surreptitiously induced vomiting following engorgement with food; hypokalemic alkalosis results (see Chapter 234).

Carcinoma of the pancreas is the prototypical neoplasm associated with dramatic weight loss. The mean age of onset is 55; men outnumber women 2 to 1. There are about 9.5 cases per 100,000 population. Weight loss is found in 79% to 90% of patients at the time of diagnosis and averages 15 to 20 lb. The degree of weight loss does not seem to correlate with size, location, or extent of disease. For example, in a series of 100 cases, eight patients had resectable tumors; of the eight, two had weight loss of 25 and 40 lb, respectively. Aversion to food is more typical of this malignancy than is true anorexia. In many instances, weight loss precedes all other symptoms; once jaundice and abdominal pain supervene, the tumor is usually far advanced. Many other gastrointestinal malignancies follow a similar clinical course.

Most patients with *HIV infection* come to experience weight loss, and the spectrum of causes is wide. One may be inadequate intake resulting from dysphagia, depression, or medication. Early satiety is another mechanism that can result from gastrointestinal invasion by lymphoma, Kaposi's sarcoma, or *Mycobacterium avium-intracellulare* infection. Weight loss in the setting of adequate caloric intake suggests disseminated infection by *Mycobacterium avium-intracellulare* or *cytomegalovirus* as well as occult malignancy. Often, the later stages of *AIDS* are characterized by a *wasting syndrome*, which includes loss of more than 10% of baseline weight, recurrent fever, and persistent diarrhea in the absence of alternative explanations (see Chapter 13).

Marked weight loss is a late sign of *malabsorption*, but modest reductions can occur in the early stages of illness, when stools are noted to be a bit softer and more frequent than usual. Steatorrhea, abdominal discomfort, bloating, and pain accompany more dramatic falls in weight when disease is further advanced. Early *Crohn's disease* in adolescents has been noted on occasion to begin inconspicuously with anorexia predominating. For example, in a small series of 11 adolescent girls labeled as having anorexia nervosa, three were shown to have Crohn's disease when barium studies were obtained. *Blind loop syndrome* and *giardiasis* may also have indolent presentations with weight loss and vague abdominal discomfort; however, changes in stools are usually present also, with patients reporting mushy, foul-smelling bowel movements (see Chapter 58).

Increased caloric demand resulting from hyperthyroidism is usually obvious; however, *apathetic hyperthyroidism* of the elderly may be mistaken for malignancy because weight loss is profound and the patient appears listless. The typical symptoms of excess thyroid hormone are absent, and unexplained atrial fibrillation is often present (see Chapter 103).

Although *diabetes mellitus* is commonly found in overweight adults, it may be the cause of weight loss when substantial wasting of calories occurs because of poorly controlled glycosuria. Young male insulin-dependent diabetic patients are sometimes plagued by diarrhea, which exacerbates fluid and nutrient losses; true malabsorption has been noted in a few (see Chapter 102).

Patients with an *underlying medical cause* for their weight loss usually present with symptoms and signs that strongly suggest organic illness. In a Veterans Administration study of 91 patients with involuntary weight loss, the cause in the overwhelming majority was readily diagnosed on the basis of the initial history and physical examination; only one patient had a truly occult malignancy (see below).

DIFFERENTIAL DIAGNOSIS

The extensive number of causes of weight loss can be grouped pathophysiologically. Decreased intake, impaired absorption, increased loss, and excess demand are the principal mechanisms around which the differential can be organized (Table 9.1). Almost any illness can cause involuntary weight loss; the table emphasizes those conditions seen in the ambulatory setting that may present as unexplained loss of weight.

Studies from primary care practices find depression to be the leading cause of unexplained weight loss, with prevalence reported in the range of 15% to 30%. Among the elderly, psychosocial factors such as loss of a spouse, social isolation, and

Table 9.1. Some Important Causes of Weight Loss

Decreased Intake
HIV infection, AIDS
Depression, bereavement
Anxiety
Poor dentition, loss of taste
Esophageal disease
Gastrointestinal disease worsened by food (e.g., peptic ulcer)
Drugs (e.g., digitalis excess, quinidine, amphetamines, NSAIDs, antitumor agents)
Hypercalcemia
Alcoholism
Prodrome of viral hepatitis
Hypokalemia
Uremia
Malignancy
Chronic congestive heart failure
Chronic inflammatory disease
Anorexia nervosa
Social isolation, poverty
Dementia

Impaired Absorption
Cholestasis
Pancreatic insufficiency
Postgastrectomy
Small-bowel disease
Parasitic infection (e.g., giardiasis)
Blind loop syndrome
Drugs (e.g., cholestyramine, cathartics)
AIDS

Increased Nutrient Loss
Uncontrolled diabetes mellitus
Persistent diarrhea
Recurrent vomiting
Drainage from a fistulous tract

Excess Demand
Hyperthyroidism
Fever
Malignancy
Emotional states (e.g., manic disease)
Amphetamine abuse

poverty can exacerbate inadequate food intake resulting from depression. Occult malignancy, although much feared in the elderly, is usually a distant runner-up, with half the prevalence of depression. In some series, therapeutic diets, particularly those for hyperlipidemia and diabetes, also rank high in the list of causes, followed by uncontrolled diabetes and oropharyngeal problems. In the elderly, immobility, poor dentition, dementia, side effects of medication, and a decrease in sense of taste are additional causative factors that require consideration.

WORKUP

Increased attention to the detection of depression and a strategy of close follow-up have reduced the percentage of idiopathic cases from about 25% to 7%. Because extensive testing for unexplained weight loss can be arduous and expensive, it is helpful, when possible, to recognize first by history and physical examination those patients unlikely to have a medical cause. The probability of serious medical illness is low and the prognosis is good for persons with a history and physical examination devoid of evidence for organic pathology. Screening laboratory studies add little to the determination. Those deemed to have a low probability of medical illness might be more productively assessed for underlying depression and psychosocial factors leading to poor caloric intake. Subjecting them at the

outset to extensive diagnostic testing in search of an occult malignancy is likely to be wasteful and of low yield when the pretest probability of cancer is low. The overall strategy is to conduct a clinical assessment that focuses on defining the underlying mechanism of weight loss so that any laboratory investigation can proceed in a logical and parsimonious fashion.

History

The first task is to document that weight loss has indeed occurred and to determine its extent. In some settings, almost half of patients do not prove to have lost weight once available records have been checked. In the absence of recorded weights, meaningful historical data include a change in clothing size, the ability to report an exact weight change, and confirmation of the history by a family member.

The history can be used to help identify the mechanism(s) responsible for the decline in weight by obtaining the details of daily food intake (including calorie count) and inquiring into the presence of any appetite disturbance, dysphagia, odynophagia, steatorrhea, diarrhea, vomiting, polyuria, or symptoms of a hypermetabolic state.

When *decreased intake* is suspected, one needs to inquire into the somatic and affective symptoms of depression (see Chapter 227). Other areas of questioning should include checking for nausea and vomiting, abdominal pain, melena, early satiety, excessive use of alcohol (see Chapter 228), exposure to and risk factors for hepatitis, poor dentition, oral candidiasis, aphthous ulcers, discomfort induced by eating, medication use, history of renal or liver disease, and anxiety. Risk factors for HIV infection should also be explored (see Chapter 13). If the patient is a young woman, anorexia nervosa should be considered, and a gentle inquiry into eating habits, self-image, and attitudes about weight is indicated (see Chapter 234). Family members should also be questioned.

In the elderly, questions about social isolation, bereavement, physical impairment, poor dentition, and poverty can be of critical importance in identifying impediments to adequate food intake. A review of drug use in the elderly is also essential because of the large number of medications prescribed and their potential for inducing anorexia and gastrointestinal upset. Additionally, patients should be checked for a loss of taste, which is sometimes responsible for poor intake in the elderly.

When *impairment of absorption* is suspected, inquiries are made into previous gastrointestinal surgery, the character of the stools, jaundice, history of pancreatitis, travel to an area known for giardiasis or other parasites, symptoms of inflammatory bowel disease (see Chapter 73), easy bruising, paresthesias, and sore tongue. Increased nutrient loss is assessed historically by ascertaining the quality and quantity of material lost in addition to the frequency and duration of the condition. Of major importance is checking for symptoms of diabetic enteropathy (diarrhea in conjunction with polyuria and polydipsia).

When *excess demand* is under consideration, the patient needs to be questioned about fever, malignancy, symptoms of hyperthyroidism, amphetamine abuse (see Chapter 235), chronic anxiety (see Chapter 226), manic states, and HIV disease (see Chapter 13).

Physical Examination

The examination should begin with an accurate weight determination, followed by the notation of any wasting, apathetic appearance, fever, tachycardia, pallor, ecchymoses, jaundice, stigmata of hyperthyroidism or hepatocellular failure, or signs of Kaposi's sarcoma. Next, the head and neck are examined for glossitis, stomatitis, poor dentition, goiter, and lymphadenopathy. The lungs and heart are examined for crackles, wheezes, consolidation, effusion, cardiomegaly, murmur, and a third heart sound. The abdomen is studied for surgical scars, organomegaly, hyperactive bowel sounds, focal tenderness, distention, ascites, and masses. The rectum is examined for masses, tenderness, discharge, blood, and the appearance of the stool. The neurologic examination includes a check for signs of vitamin B_{12} deficiency suggestive of terminal ileal disease (see Chapter 79) as well as any tremor, manic or depressive affect, or signs of dementia.

Laboratory Testing

Because the number of potential investigations is enormous, laboratory testing should be selective to avoid being wasteful, burdensome, and misleading. The history and physical examination will usually identify the basic mechanism(s) of weight loss and suggest specific causes that can be confirmed or ruled out by further investigation. As noted earlier, patients with perfectly normal physical examination findings and a history devoid of any symptoms suggestive of serious underlying medical illness are at low risk. It is reasonable to watch them for a month, focus on psychosocial determinants, and not immediately initiate an extensive laboratory workup. They should be given nutritional advice and a follow-up appointment at 4 weeks and asked to keep a diary of food intake and weight. Those with clinical evidence suggesting an important underlying mechanism can proceed to a focused laboratory workup if the diagnosis remains unconfirmed by history and physical examination.

Decreased Intake. When decreased intake is manifested by a markedly reduced appetite accompanied by nausea, it is worth obtaining a few selected serum chemistries, including measurement of *calcium*, *potassium*, *creatinine*, *transaminase*, and *amylase*, to check for a possible gastrointestinal or metabolic precipitant. Patients with such symptoms who are taking a digitalis preparation, quinidine, or any other drug that can cause gastrointestinal upset at toxic levels should have a *serum drug concentration* determined. If NSAIDs are being taken, they should be stopped. Those not taking an NSAID should be considered for endoscopic or radiologic evaluation of the upper gastrointestinal tract and *Helicobacter* testing (see Chapter 68). In the HIV-infected patient, endoscopy may be indicated to search for upper gastrointestinal mucosal erosion (see Chapter 13).

Impaired Absorption. Stool should be obtained for gross and microscopic examination and guaiac testing performed. A *qualitative stool fat* examination, in which fecal material is stained for neutral fat, is a basic step in the workup of suspected malabsorption. If doubt persists, a 72-hour stool collection for *quantitative stool fat* provides more precise information, with values of less than 8 g/d ruling out malabsorption. The *serum carotene* level is another useful marker of fat absorption. Its absorption is independent of pancreatic function, so that a normal level in the setting of malabsorption suggests pancreatic dysfunction. Similarly, the D-*xylose* test can help distinguish pancreatic dysfunction from small bowel disease, because D-xylose absorption also does not require pancreatic enzyme activity

(see Chapter 74). An elevated *serum amylase* or the radiologic demonstration of *pancreatic calcification* indicates pancreatitis (see Chapter 72), but a *secretin stimulation test* may be necessary to assess pancreatic exocrine function better. Sprue and blind loop syndrome are the most common forms of small-bowel pathology responsible for malabsorption. A small-bowel radiologic *contrast study* might be suggestive, but a *small-bowel biopsy* is necessary for the diagnosis of sprue; an abnormal *carbon 14 glycolate breath test* will help document bacterial overgrowth, although usually the test is unnecessary.

For the diagnosis of *giardiasis*, a *stool sample for ova and parasites* suffices in many instances. Because parasites are passed intermittently, three or more stools on alternate days should be examined. Because the cysts are hardy, a fresh stool specimen is not required. Trophozoites are more likely to be found in acute cases. Examination of a duodenal aspirate or jejunal biopsy specimen is resorted to when suspicion is high but stool findings are negative. Although these tests are more productive, they are cumbersome; some clinicians instead advocate a diagnostic trial of an antigiardial drug such as metronidazole.

Increased Nutrient Loss. Any patient suspected of diabetes mellitus should have a *urinalysis* for glycosuria. Marked glycosuria should be present in the patient with weight loss caused by diabetes.

Excess Demand. Suspicion of hyperthyroidism necessitates a *thyrotropin* (TSH) determination, especially in the elderly, apathetic patient with unexplained atrial fibrillation and weight loss (see Chapter 103). In the febrile HIV patient with adequate caloric intake, the weight loss likely represents excessive demand; *cultures* of blood and stool for *acid-fast bacilli* and of blood and urine for *cytomegalovirus* are required.

One of the most difficult diagnostic issues encountered in the workup of weight loss concerns the possibility of *occult malignancy*. Deciding when to embark on a search for tumor requires an estimate not only of the likelihood of finding a malignancy but also of the chances that it will be treatable. Unfortunately, by the time weight loss has occurred, most gastrointestinal malignancies are rather far advanced. When weight loss is the only symptom, pancreatic carcinoma may still be resectable if no other symptoms have appeared. *Abdominal ultrasonography* and *computed tomography* have improved case detection in some settings but not in others. Impact on survival remains to be realized (see Chapter 76). In a primary care study of elderly patients with undiagnosed weight loss, the yield of computed tomography was very low in the absence of clinical evidence of an underlying lesion.

SYMPTOMATIC THERAPY

The first task is to be sure food is available to the patient, particularly the elderly person who may be too isolated, impoverished, infirm, or depressed to take in adequate calories. It is estimated that the intake of 10% to 15% of elderly persons is below 1,000 kcal/d. Ensuring at least one hot meal per day is essential and can usually be arranged with the help of local social service agencies.

Most medical causes of weight loss must be corrected and cannot be readily treated symptomatically. However, there are important exceptions to this generalization. Sometimes, the severe anorexia associated with malignancy or use of antitumor agents can be overcome by pharmacologic means (see Chapter 91). The poor intake seen with hepatitis can be improved by providing small, frequent feedings, especially in the morning, when nausea is less severe (see Chapter 70). Appetite disturbances associated with depression are often amenable to tricyclic therapy (see Chapter 227). Maldigestion resulting from pancreatic insufficiency can be compensated for by the use of oral pancreatic enzyme preparations (see Chapter 72). The bacterial overgrowth of blind loop syndrome responds to oral broad-spectrum antibiotic therapy (e.g., 250 mg of tetracycline four times daily or 250 mg of amoxicillin three times daily), given for multiple 10-day courses or for 3 or 4 days each week indefinitely. Caloric supplements in the form of medium-chain triglyceride and dextrose preparations can provide marked improvement when severe fat and carbohydrate maldigestion or malabsorption is present. Initially, 3 oz is given with each meal; gradually this is increased to 6 oz, including supplements between meals. If sprue is suspected, a gluten-free diet can be tried empirically.

Fat-soluble vitamin supplements are also needed in cases of malabsorption to prevent malnutrition, even though caloric intake may be replenished. The fat-soluble vitamins A, D, and K are the most likely to be depleted. Dosage requirements in such cases are 25,000 to 50,000 U daily for vitamin A, 30,000 U for vitamin D, and 4 to 12 g for oral vitamin K. Monthly vitamin B_{12} injections of 1,000 mu are needed for terminal ileal disease presenting with megaloblastic anemia (see Chapter 82). Methods to control excessive vomiting and diarrhea are discussed in Chapters 59 and 64, respectively.

INDICATIONS FOR REFERRAL AND ADMISSION

Anyone with a weight loss in excess of 15 kg is likely to have a life-threatening condition and requires prompt hospitalization. The AIDS patient with unexplained weight loss may also benefit from some form of inpatient care while undergoing further evaluation. Any person with substantial weight loss who is suspected of having anorexia nervosa should be hospitalized and seen by a psychiatrist experienced in dealing with anorexia because this too can be a life-threatening condition (see Chapter 234). When malabsorption is documented by 72-hour stool fat assessment, consultation with a gastroenterologist should coincide with proceeding to further assessment. HIV patients with weight loss can certainly be evaluated by their primary care physician provided that the physician is familiar with the evaluation of such patients. Otherwise, referral is indicated.

A.H.G.

ANNOTATED BIBLIOGRAPHY

Bach MC, Howell DA, Valenti AJ. Aphthous ulceration of the gastrointestinal tract in patients with AIDS. Ann Intern Med 1990;112:465. (*An important cause of decreased intake resulting from odynophagia and dysphagia.*)

Greene JB. Clinical approach to weight loss in the patient with AIDS. Gastroenterol Clin North Am 1988;17:573. (*A very useful algorithm for guiding the potentially complex workup in the AIDS patient.*)

Health and Public Policy Committee, American College of Physicians. Eating disorders: anorexia nervosa and bulimia. Ann Intern Med 1986;105:790. (*A thoughtful position paper outlining the role of the primary physician in the care of patients with eating disorders.*)

Marton KI, Sox HC, Krupp JR. Involuntary weight loss: diagnostic and prognostic significance. Ann Intern Med 1981;5:568. (*A prospective study attempting to identify predictors of serious pathology and poor prognosis.*)

Morley JE, Silver AJ, Fiatarone M, et al. Nutrition and the elderly. J Am Geriatr Soc 1986;34:823. (*A review of critical factors that are often overlooked.*)

Ryan ME, Olsen WA. A diagnostic approach to malabsorption syndromes. Clin Gastroenterol 1983;12:533. (*A pathophysiologic approach.*)

Schiffman SS, Warwick ZS. Flavor enhancement of foods for the elderly can reverse anorexia. Neurobiol Aging 1988;9:24. (*A very practical idea.*)

Thomas FB, Mazzaferri EL, Skillman TG. Apathetic thyrotoxicosis: a distinctive clinical and laboratory entity. Ann Intern Med 1970;72:679. (*Classic article describing this syndrome, which is characterized by marked weight loss, apathy, and unexplained atrial fibrillation in the elderly.*)

Thompson MP, Morris LK. Unexplained weight loss in the ambulatory elderly. J Am Geriatr Soc 1991;39:497. (*A study of patients from seven primary care centers; depression the most common cause; malignancy next; many cases remained undiagnosed; CT low in yield.*)

Wilson M-M G, Vaswani S, Liu D, et al. Prevalence and causes of undernutrition in medical outpatients. Am J Med 1998;104:56. (*A population study from primary care practice; prevalence 11% in patients 65 years and older, 7% in younger persons; leading causes in the elderly include depression, poorly controlled diabetes, and occult cancer; etiology often unrecognized although readily identifiable.*)

10
Evaluation of Overweight and Obesity

Overweight and obesity have become major health concerns in modern postindustrial societies, affecting an estimated 55% of Americans over the age of 20. The personal and social costs are enormous—approaching $100 billion annually when medical complications, lost wages, and expenditures for weight reduction efforts are taken into account, not to mention the accompanying emotional pain, social stigmatization, and discrimination that may ensue. Excessive weight is a major risk factor for cardiovascular disease, type II diabetes mellitus, and hypertension, and it is also associated with impaired pulmonary function (including sleep apnea), surgical risk, osteoarthritis, gallbladder disease, and a risk for some cancers.

The tasks for the primary physician in the evaluation of patients with excess weight include not only an attempt to identify etiologic factors, but also a careful assessment of weight status and fat distribution as risk factors for major disease. This chapter focuses on the diagnostic evaluation; see Chapter 233 for the approach to treatment.

PATHOPHYSIOLOGY AND CLINICAL PRESENTATION

Definitions. The currently preferred definitions of overweight and obesity are based on *body mass index* (BMI) determinations, which approximate total body fat content and correlate with disease risk (Table 10.1). *Overweight* is defined as a BMI of 25 to 29.9 kg/m². *Obesity* is defined as a BMI greater than 30 kg/m², and *morbid obesity* by a BMI greater than 40 kg/m².

Physiology. Caloric intake and energy expenditure are linked through hypothalamic regulation of appetite and metabolism. The hypothalamus integrates a complex and redundant set of afferent signals, including *leptin* released from adipose tissue; *norepinephrine* from the autonomic nervous system; *epinephrine*, *insulin*, *androgens*, *glucocorticoids*, *peptide YY*, *progesterone*, and *estrogens* from endocrine glands; *glucagon, cholecystokinin, bombesin peptides, neurotensin, growth hormone–releasing hormone, somatostatin*, and *glucose* from the gastrointestinal tract; and *dopamine, τ-amino butyric acid, galanin, opioids, growth hormone–releasing factor, somatostatin*, and *serotonin* from the central nervous system. The efferent output from the hypothalamus controls energy expenditure and appetite by the release of *norepinephrine, serotonin, neuropeptide Y, glucagon-like peptide I*, and *corticotropin-releasing hormone*, which act on the autonomic nervous system and the thyroid gland.

Pathophysiology. Obesity is often the consequence of physical inactivity in persons with an underlying disturbance in metabolism, appetite control, or dietary composition. In most instances, the etiology is multifactorial, although one factor may predominate. Susceptibility is influenced by genetic determinants that were once advantageous in regard to evolution, such as those that reduce energy expenditure or encourage the intake of energy-rich foods. However, such inherited traits can be counterproductive to good health in postindustrial societies, in which physical demands are greatly reduced and high-calorie food is plentiful and inexpensive.

Physical inactivity emerges as a leading cause of obesity in modern society, underscored by the increasing prevalence of obesity despite a decline in average daily caloric intake. When daily life makes few physical demands, caloric needs drop precipitously, which leads to an epidemic of excess weight, even among those without major genetic susceptibility to weight gain. Some genetic variability in the propensity for exercise has been described, which may contribute to inactivity in some.

Metabolic factors are important, genetically determined contributors to excessive weight and include resting energy expenditure, thermic effect of food, and exercise-induced energy expenditure. Among these, a reduction in energy utilization with exercise correlates the most strongly with risk for weight gain. Ninefold to 30-fold variations have been observed. Because exercise-induced energy expenditure accounts for about 30% of total energy demand, any genetic propensity for reduced energy expenditure with exertion could substantially increase the risk for obesity.

Dietary composition actually plays a much smaller role than might be expected. In most persons, changing the percentages of dietary fat, protein, and carbohydrate *without* changing the number of calories consumed has little or no influence on the development of obesity. Diets high in fat contribute to obesity mostly because they are rich in calories, not because they are rich in fat. Despite claims to the contrary by those promoting weight loss diets, there is no evidence that dietary composition alone is a major determinant of obesity for the vast majority of persons. Almost all weight loss diets work by restricting total calories (see Chapter 233). The *timing of food intake* may contribute modestly to obesity; eating once daily, particularly before going to bed, predisposes to the accumulation of adipose tissue in some persons.

Appetite disturbances have long been suspected as a cause of obesity. Many obese individuals appear to eat without satiety. In some, there appears to be resistance to normal appetite controls, such as the appetite suppressant leptin, serum levels of which actually increase in obese subjects. Moreover, the effects of appetite suppressants can be overcome in some animals by providing easy access to palatable, energy-rich foods.

Genetic factors, as noted earlier, play a substantial role by influencing energy utilization, appetite, food preferences, and even propensity for physical activity. The importance of genetic factors is underscored by findings from studies of twins, families,

Table 10.1. Definition and Classification of Excess Weight

CLASS	BMI (KG/M²)	WAIST CIRCUMFERENCE[a]	RELATIVE RISK[b]
Normal	18.5–24.9	Normal	Normal
		Increased	Increased
Overweight	25.0–29.9	Normal	Increased
		Increased	High
Obese	30.0–34.9	Normal	High
		Increased	Very high
	35.0–39.9	Normal	Very high
		Increased	Very high
Obese, morbid	40.0+	All are increased	Extremely high

[a]Increased, >102 cm (40 in) in men, >88 cm (35 in in women).

[b]For diabetes type 2, hypertension, coronary artery disease.

BMI, body mass index.

Adapted from Expert Panel on the Identification, Evaluation, and Treatment of Overweight and Obesity in Adults. Executive summary of the clinical guidelines on the identification, evaluation, and treatment of overweight and obesity in adults. Arch Intern Med 1998;158:1855, with permission.

and adoptees, which reveal a strong relation between weight class of adoptees and their biologic parents, but none between adoptees and their adopted parents. Parental obesity doubles the risk for adult obesity in obese and nonobese children under the age of 10 years. Obese children under the age of 3 years who have an obese parent have a very high risk for adult obesity, but they experience no increase in risk if neither parent is obese. Genetic factors are estimated to account for nearly 50% of the risk of becoming overweight, and even more for becoming obese.

Developmental and environmental factors, manifested by parenteral influences and childhood environment, contribute to the development of adult obesity. As the age of the child increases, the influence of environment increases. Over the age of 10 years, heredity becomes a less dominant determinant of adult obesity, and environment increases in importance.

Psychological and behavioral factors have long been thought important; however, there is no known psychological explanation for why reactive hyperphagia develops in some persons as a response to emotional stress, whereas anorexia is the reaction of others. Considerable research has been unable to determine any particular personality organization or cluster of psychological defense mechanisms clearly linked to obesity. Nonetheless, psychological problems frequently contribute to the onset and perpetuation of obesity-inducing behavioral changes. For example, some individuals characteristically overeat in response to stress, loss, or frustration. Those with the *night eating syndrome*, characterized by insomnia, massive late-evening "refrigerator raids," and morning anorexia, also experience particular emotional distress when they try to reform their eating behaviors. Usually, coinciding social stresses are present as well. The appetite disturbance associated with *major depression* may lead to either an increase or decrease in weight.

Social factors are key determinants of the frequency and nature of feasts, timing of meals, role and meaning of food, types of foods consumed, and norms of appearance. In our society, excess weight occurs far more frequently among the socioeconomically disadvantaged than among others. Whether this difference represents dietary preference, socially motivated behavior, or interactional factors is unclear. In certain occupations, such as wrestling, obesity is a help, not a hindrance. In former times, corpulence was a sign of prosperity and was cultivated by bankers and businessmen.

Clinical Presentation. Most cases of overweight and obesity occur independently of an underlying medical condition, although they may exacerbate or lead to illness. However, in 5% to 10% of cases, an underlying medical condition or medication that affects energy expenditure, fuel utilization, appetite, or physical activity may be responsible. Often, the mechanism is an effect on one of the substances involved in regulating energy intake or expenditure (see above).

Pharmacologic agents prescribed for clinical conditions other than obesity may cause weight gain. *β-Blockers* and *central sympatholytics* (e.g., clonidine) can decrease metabolic rate and energy expenditure. *Glucocorticosteroids* cause hypertrophic obesity in a characteristic truncal pattern. *Antidepressants*, such as the *tricyclics* and *selective serotonin reuptake inhibitors*, and some *antihistamines* (e.g., cyproheptadine) act as appetite stimulants. Weight gain is also common with oral contraceptive use.

Endocrine disturbances are more often the result rather than the cause of excess weight. However, *hypothyroidism* (see Chapter 104) has been found to account for up to 5% of cases in some series. *Cushing's syndrome* is a rare cause and is usually accompanied by characteristic features of truncal obesity and peripheral muscle wasting. *Stein-Leventhal syndrome*—polycystic ovaries, absent menses, and moderate hirsutism (see Chapter 112)—often goes unrecognized as an endocrinologic form of obesity; the precise mechanism of the obesity is unknown. *Eunuchism* and *hyperinsulin states* may also be associated with obesity.

Neurologic causes of obesity are usually not cryptic; they mostly result from *hypothalamic injury*, as occurs with craniopharyngiomas, encephalitis, or trauma. Visual field defects or headaches are usually present. Two rare types of neurologic disease without obvious central nervous system symptoms have been described. Kleine-Levin syndrome consists of periodic hyperphagia and hypersomnia. A second syndrome is characterized by preoccupation with food and accompanying electroencephalographic abnormalities that respond to phenytoin.

Mental illness may heralded by weight gain. The appetite disturbance of *major depression* is one of the cardinal manifestations of the condition and may be a presenting complaint (see Chapter 227).

DIFFERENTIAL DIAGNOSIS

The causes of obesity can be primary or secondary, with the latter being medical conditions that result in obesity. Some forms of secondary weight gain are a consequence of salt retention and fluid overload rather than an increase in fat cell mass. Among the important causes of sodium retention are congestive heart failure, severe hepatocellular disease, and renal failure (see Chapters 32, 71, and 142). Primary forms of obesity can be classified by their underlying pathophysiology. The vast majority of cases are primary in nature. An etiologic/pathophysiologic diagnosis is essential to the design of an effective management program (Table 10.2).

WORKUP

A principal objective of the overweight/obesity evaluation is to determine how much risk the weight problem confers. The risk assessment begins with an estimate of the amount and distribution of fat, followed by a consideration of other risk factors and underlying conditions that add to morbidity and mortality risks; it concludes with estimates of relative and absolute risk. Additional components of the workup pertinent to management include elucidation of the underlying mechanism(s) responsible for the patient's weight problem, detection of any underlying illnesses presenting as weight excess, and assessment of the patient's motivation to lose weight.

Weight Assessment. To establish whether an individual has a weight problem that poses a health risk, an estimation of the *amount* and *distribution* of fat is required. Both are independent determinants of disease risk. Fat distribution is particularly important, even among persons who are not obese.

Measurement of Body Fat. This is best accomplished by calculating the *BMI*:

$$BMI = \frac{\text{Body Weight (kg)}}{\text{Height (m}^2)}$$

Table 10.2.   Important Causes of Obesity

Primary

Psychological factors
 Depression
 Anxiety
 Frustration

Biologic factors
 Reduced thermogenesis
 Increased fat cell mass
 Autonomic dysfunction
 Altered hypothalamic set point
 Single large daily meal taken before bedtime
 Decreased energy expenditure
 Drugs (e.g., tricyclic antidepressants, oral contraceptives,
  corticosteroids, phenothiazines)

Genetic Influences
 Familial obesity

Social and occupational factors
 Lower socioeconomic class
 Social/occupational situation

Secondary

Endocrine disease
 Hypothyroidism
 Stein-Leventhal syndrome
 Cushing's syndrome

Neurologic disease
 Hypothalamic injury (e.g., trauma, encephalitis, craniopharyngioma)

The BMI determination assumes that weight is measured with shoes and heavy clothing removed. If weight is obtained with shoes and all clothing on, then 5 lb should be subtracted for men and 3 lb for women. The BMI is calculated by taking the weight in kilograms and dividing it by the square of the height in meters (or by multiplying by 703 the weight in pounds divided by the square of the height in inches). This ratio of weight to height actually calculates total body mass rather than fat mass, but it correlates highly with the amount of body fat and its associated health risks except in very muscular individuals, who might be falsely labeled as overweight with use of the BMI. The BMI range of 20 to 24.9 is classified as "normal" because no actuarial increase in disease mortality is noted within it. Mortality begins to increase as the BMI exceeds 25, and it is here that health professionals should be concerned. Most expert consensus panels recommend that health professionals adopt the BMI as the preferred measure for evaluating weight status because it provides the best estimate of disease risk (Fig. 10.1 and Table 10.1).

Height and weight tables have the advantage of simplicity. However, there are serious limitations to their use. Standard charts typically list "ideal" or desired weights based on actuarial data, yet it is not weight *per se* that minimizes morbidity or the incidence of disease. The person having a significant percentage of lean body mass, such as a physical laborer, may well exceed "ideal" body weight yet not be obese. On the other hand, some individuals may be within the ideal range but have non–insulin-dependent diabetes mellitus, hypertension, or other conditions that would benefit from weight reduction. The Metropolitan Life Insurance Company has published revised reference weights in an attempt to isolate the effect of weight alone on longevity; individuals with major diseases, such as cancer, diabetes, or heart disease, were omitted from the study

(Table 10.3). Life tables, based only on mortality, ignore possible nonfatal risks associated with increased weight.

Height and weight formulas are sometimes used to determine ideal body weight and estimate the degree of obesity, but they provide only the crudest of estimates and should not be used to set goals for weight reduction. They are provided here only because they are sometimes referred to. (Appropriate weight goals for patients can be determined only by a thorough analysis of their medical history and physical findings, supplemented by appropriate laboratory evaluation.)

Female weight: Allow 100 lb for first 5 ft of height plus 5 lb for each additional inch.

Male weight: Allow 106 lb for first 5 ft of height plus 6 lb for each additional inch.

The measurement of *skinfold thickness* is used by some to quantify adiposity. Calipers are used to measure skinfold thickness in the triceps and subscapular regions. However, reliability can be a problem when skinfold measurements are used because body fat increases with age, grossly obese patients are difficult to measure, and results vary among providers using the calipers.

Bioelectric impedance analysis is sometimes used to measure body fat. Electrodes are applied to one arm and leg, and the impedance is measured. Impedance is proportional to the aqueous composition of the body. Formulas are used to estimate the

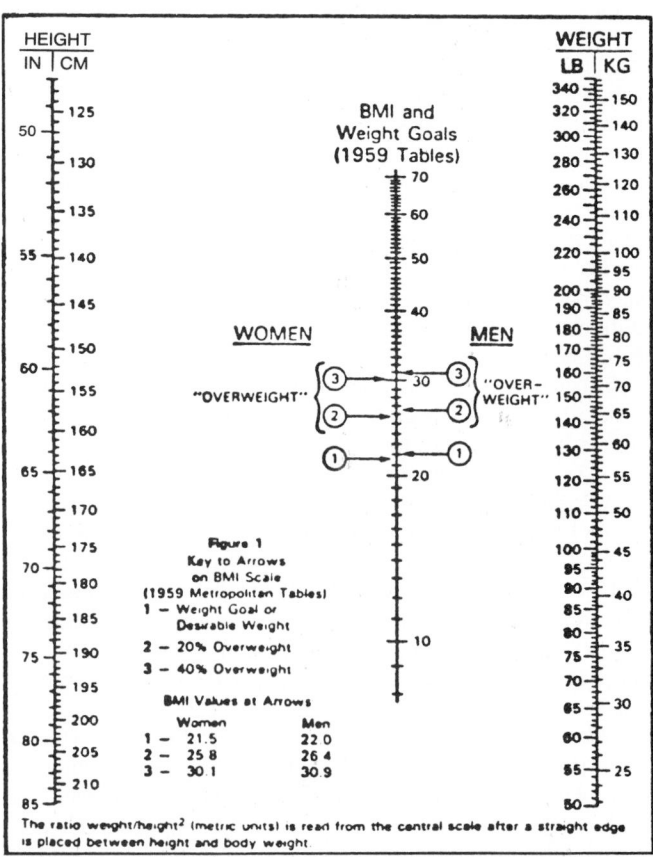

FIG. 10.1.   Nomogram for body mass index (kg/m²). Weights and heights are without clothing. With clothes, add 5 lb (2.3 kg) for men and 3 lb (1.4 kg) for women. Add 1 in (2.5 cm) in height for shoes. (New weight standards for men and women. J Am Diet Assoc 1985;85:1119, with permission. Stat Bull Metropolitan Life Insurance Company 1959;40:1.)

Table 10.3. Optimal Weights,[a] in Pounds, for Adults Ages 25 and Over (Light Clothing)

HEIGHT (IN SHOES)	SMALL FRAME	MEDIUM FRAME	LARGE FRAME
Men			
5 ft 2 in	112–120	118–129	126–141
5 3	115–123	121–133	129–144
5 4	118–126	124–136	132–148
5 5	121–129	127–139	135–152
5 6	124–133	130–143	138–156
5 7	128–137	134–147	142–161
5 8	132–141	138–152	147–166
5 9	136–145	142–156	151–170
5 10	140–150	146–160	155–174
5 11	144–154	150–165	159–179
6 0	148–158	154–170	164–184
6 1	152–162	158–175	168–189
6 2	156–167	162–180	173–194
6 3	160–171	167–185	178–199
6 4	164–175	172–190	182–204
Women			
4 10	92–98	96–107	104–119
4 11	94–101	98–110	106–122
5 0	96–104	101–113	109–125
5 1	99–107	104–116	112–128
5 2	102–110	107–119	115–131
5 3	105–113	110–122	118–134
5 4	108–116	113–126	121–138
5 5	111–119	116–130	125–142
5 6	114–123	120–135	129–146
5 7	118–127	124–139	133–150
5 8	122–131	128–143	137–154
5 9	126–135	132–147	141–158
5 10	130–140	136–151	145–163
5 11	134–144	140–155	149–168
6 0	138–148	144–159	153–173

[a]Weights associated with the lowest mortality rates (derived from actuarial data, Metropolitan Life Insurance Company).

percentage of fat in the body. Although accurate, this method is expensive and not readily available.

The old-fashioned *"eyeball test"* remains a mainstay of assessment: If a person looks fat, he or she is likely to be fat. However, quantification and correlation with risk are crude with this common sense method.

Measurement of Fat Distribution. The other independent determinant of health risk associated with excess weight is fat distribution, which can be quantified by measuring *waist circumference*. The circumference of the waist is obtained at the narrowest area above the umbilicus. Measurements in excess of sex-specific cutoffs (>102 cm, or 40 in, in men and >88 cm, or 35 in, in women) confer an increased relative risk of disease morbidity and mortality (Table 10.3). The effect of fat distribution on risk is so strong that waist circumference is important even in persons who are not technically overweight. However, in morbidly obese patients, waist circumference is always exceeded and the measurement confers no additional risk.

The *ratio* of *waist* or *abdominal circumference* to *hip* or *gluteal circumference* provides an even more precise quantitative index of regional fat distribution. The hip circumference is measured at the maximal gluteal protrusion. Individuals with excess upper body fat (android obesity) are at higher risk for diabetes, atherosclerosis, and stroke than are those who have more adipose tissue in the hips, buttocks, and thighs (gynecoid

obesity). In quantitative terms, individuals with waist-to-hip ratios greater than 0.8 for women and 1.0 for men have an increased risk for coronary disease.

Estimation of Disease Risk. One begins with determinations of total body fat and fat distribution, represented respectively by BMI and waist circumference. These parameters correlate well with *relative risk*, especially among persons under the age of 65 years (Table 10.3). Relative risk from obesity is greatest among younger persons and declines somewhat with advancing age.

Determination of the *absolute risk* associated with obesity requires checking for underlying *coronary heart disease* (see Chapter 20), *type 2 diabetes mellitus* (see Chapter 93), *noncoronary atherosclerotic disease* (see Chapters 23 and 171), *hypertension* (see Chapter 19), and *sleep apnea* (see Chapter 46), in addition to the end-organ injuries that may result from them (see Chapters 26, 30, 102, 35, and 46). The cardiovascular risk assessment is enhanced by screening for principal risk factors such as *hyperlipidemia* (see Chapter 15), *hypertension* (see Chapter 14), *smoking* (see Chapter 54), and premature coronary disease in first-degree relatives. Calculations of absolute risk are possible from a consideration of these factors (see Chapters 26 and 27). Searches for *osteoarthritis* (see Chapter 146), *cholelithiasis* (see Chapter 69), and *stress incontinence* also help predict risk of weight-related consequences.

Assessment of Etiology and Consequences. As important as risk assessment is, etiologic factors and health consequences deserve attention because they are relevant to the approach to management.

History. An extensive weight history should include age of onset of obesity, weight status of parents and siblings, and any identifiable circumstances associated with the onset of obesity. Although dietary composition *per se* is not a risk factor for obesity, dietary composition and quantity need to be ascertained to determine total caloric intake. A high-fat diet is likely to provide excessive calories. Because physical inactivity is a major precipitant of excess weight, the patient's daily activities should be elucidated in detail to estimate daily energy requirements. Proclivity toward exercise should also be ascertained. A careful review of ongoing psychological and situational stresses is essential and should include screening for depression (see Chapter 227). Any recent attempts at smoking cessation should be reviewed for effect on weight. The social and cultural dimensions of the history should be explored for their possible contribution to weight gain.

Even in a patient without obvious medical pathology, a workup that screens for underlying endocrinologic and neurologic diseases is essential, as is a check for drug-induced causes. The history requires a thorough neuroendocrine review of symptoms: fatigue, unexplained weight gain, cold intolerance, hoarseness, change in skin and hair texture, amenorrhea, hirsutism, easy bruising, weakness, visual disturbances, and headache. Medications are reviewed for agents that may stimulate appetite or affect metabolism, such as antidepressants, oral contraceptives, corticosteroids, phenothiazines, antithyroid medications, β-blockers, and insulin.

A review of systems for the consequences of obesity should include inquiry into chest pain, shortness of breath, polyuria, polydipsia, impotence, numbness, limb pain or coldness, transient neurologic deficits, daytime sleepiness, apneic periods at night, and pain in weight-bearing joints.

The Physical Examination includes a check for such etiologic clues as moon facies, hirsutism, dry and thickened skin, coarse hair, truncal obesity, pigmented striae, goiter, adnexal masses, lack of secondary sex characteristics, delayed relaxation of ankle jerks, and visual field deficits. The physical examination should include a search for the consequences of obesity, including blood pressure elevation, diabetic retinopathic changes, carotid bruits, obstruction of soft tissues in the upper airway, cor pulmonale, rales, cardiac enlargement, degenerative changes in the hips and knees, and signs of peripheral arterial insufficiency and peripheral neuropathy.

Laboratory Testing includes two components: the diagnosis of an underlying medical etiology and the detection of metabolic consequences. A strategy of routinely testing for all possible medical causes in the absence of suggestive clinical findings adds to expenses and increases the risk of generating a high percentage of false-positive results (see Chapter 2). Nonetheless, some clinicians routinely screen for hypothyroidism with a *thyrotropin* determination because the test is sensitive, the condition has a relatively high frequency, and the clinical presentation of hypothyroidism can be very subtle (see Chapter 104).

The laboratory evaluation is most productive when directed at causes suggested by the history and physical examination. For example, the obese patient suspected of having Cushing's syndrome because of truncal obesity, peripheral wasting, and pigmented striae is a reasonable candidate for an overnight *1-mg dexamethasone suppression test*. If headaches accompanied by a visual field disturbance are present, then *computed tomography* of the sella turcica is needed to check for the possibility of a pituitary tumor (see Chapter 100).

Testing for the metabolic consequences of obesity is straightforward and includes a random serum glucose measurement and lipid profile (see Chapter 15). These results help determine overall cardiovascular risk. Patients bothered by daytime sleepiness and a history of excessive snoring and disturbed sleep resulting from irregular breathing should be considered for an evaluation of sleep apnea (see Chapter 46). At the present time, measures of energy expenditure, thermogenesis, autonomic function, fat cell count, and set point are relegated to the research laboratory, but in time they may become part of the clinical evaluation.

INDICATIONS FOR REFERRAL

Patients who are morbidly obese and demonstrate such adverse sequelae as marked respiratory compromise, disabling arthritis, or symptomatic coronary disease require consultation for consideration of a very low-calorie diet under the supervision of persons experienced in its implementation (see Chapter 233). Referral for consideration of surgical approaches to treatment may also be indicated in such persons. Obstructive sleep apnea in patients with mild to moderate obesity may not require such extreme measures, but pulmonary consultation in conjunction with a weight loss program is indicated (see Chapter 46).

PATIENT EDUCATION

Most patients come for evaluation out of concern for an underlying medical condition. The vast majority have no such cause and need to know that inactivity is the principal reason for their weight gain. Although they may have genetically determined risk factors, such as a proclivity for high-fat food and a reduced exercise-related energy expenditure, they will benefit when the physician reemphasizes the overwhelming importance of exercise and an active life-style to weight control (see Chapter 233). The occasional patient whose obesity is driven predominantly by heredity (both parents obese, onset before age 3 years) appreciates knowing that the weight problem is not a consequence of defective character. For the vast majority, the education process begins by drawing attention away from diets, medical conditions, and "metabolism problems" and to the importance of exercise. The goals are to provide the patient with an estimate of the disease risk posed by the excessive weight and an assessment of the factors contributing to it.

RECOMMENDATIONS

- Begin the weight assessment by determining amount of body fat and fat distribution, which independently correlate with the relative risk associated with excess weight.
- Estimate body fat content by calculating the BMI (body weight in kilograms divided by the square of the height in meters).
- Determine fat distribution by measuring the waist circumference at the narrowest area above the umbilicus.
- Estimate the relative risk of cardiovascular disease, type 2 diabetes, and hypertension from these determinations.
- Search for major cardiovascular risk factors and for evidence of end-organ damage to determine the absolute risk of cardiovascular morbidity and mortality.
- Check the history and physical examination for etiologic factors, ranging from familial propensity and early age of onset to dietary excess, physical inactivity, and underlying medical and psychological conditions.
- Use laboratory testing only to test etiologic hypotheses suggested by the history and physical examination or to screen for cardiovascular risk factors (e.g., hypercholesterolemia, diabetes).
- Provide the patient with an estimate of the disease risk posed by the excessive weight and an assessment of the factors contributing to it.

A.H.G.

ANNOTATED BIBLIOGRAPHY

Expert Panel on the Identification, Evaluation, and Treatment of Overweight and Obesity in Adults. Executive summary of the clinical guidelines on the identification, evaluation, and treatment of overweight and obesity in adults. Arch Intern Med 1998;158:1855. (*Latest evidence-based consensus panel recommendations.*)

Hubert HB, Feinleib M, McNamara PM, et al. Obesity as an independent risk factor for cardiovascular disease: a 26-year follow-up of participants in the Framingham Heart Study. Circulation 1983;67:968. (*Classic study establishing obesity as a risk factor.*)

Kuczmarksi RJ, Carrol MD, Flegal KM, et al. Varying body mass index cutoff points to describe overweight prevalence among US adults: NHANES III (1988–1994). Obes Res 1997;5:542. (*The epidemiologic data documenting prevalence and risk.*)

Liebel RL, Hirsch J, Appel BE, et al. Energy intake required to maintain body weight is not affected by wide variation in diet composition. Am J Clin Nutr 1992;55:350. (*Best evidence that what you eat is less important than the total number of calories.*)

Manson JE, Willett WC, Stampfer MJ, et al. Body weight and mortality among women. N Engl J Med 1995;333:677. (*Follow-up data at 16 years from the prospective Nurses' Health Study showing a striking relation between all-cause mortality and excess weight in middle-aged women.*)

Rexrode KM, Carey VJ, Hennekens CH, et al. Abdominal adiposity and coronary heart disease in women. JAMA 1998;280:1843. (*Data from the Nurses' Health Study showing increased waist circumference to be an independent risk factor for coronary disease, even in persons who have a normal BMI.*)

Rosenbaum M, Leibel RL, Hirsch J. Obesity. N Engl J Med 1997;337:396. (*Review of physiology and pathophysiology of weight control.*)

Senie RT, Rosen PP, Rhodes P, et al. Obesity at diagnosis of breast carcinoma influences duration of disease-free interval. Ann Intern Med 1992;116:26. (*Obesity reduced rate of disease-free survival by more than 25%.*)

Stevens J, Cai J, Pamuk ER, et al. The effect of age on the association between body-mass index and mortality. N Engl J Med 1998;338:1. (*An epidemiologic study; overweight increased all-cause mortality and cardiovascular mortality, but less so with advancing age.*)

Weinsier RL, Hunter GR, Heini AF, et al. The etiology of obesity: relative contributions of metabolic factors, diet, and physical activity. Am J Med 1998;105:145. (*An analysis of available data arguing that physical activity appears to be the most important determinant in postindustrial societies.*)

11
Evaluation of Fever
HARVEY B. SIMON

Since antiquity, fever has been recognized as a cardinal manifestation of disease. Indeed, people identify fever as a sign of illness more readily than they recognize the importance of most other symptoms. In addition to causing concern, the presence of fever usually raises high therapeutic expectations. Even in the era before antibiotics, John Milton observed that "the fever is to the Physitians, the eternal reproach" (1641). In the popular mind today, fever is equated with infection, and infections are expected to respond to the administration of "wonder drugs." As a result, the physician is faced with the challenge of defining the cause of the fever, instituting appropriate therapy, and explaining the reasons for limiting antibiotic use to bacterial infections.

PATHOPHYSIOLOGY AND CLINICAL PRESENTATION

"Normal" Body Temperature. Popular lore notwithstanding, 98.6°F (37°C) is *not* normal body temperature. In fact, there is no single normal value; like so many other biologic phenomena, body temperature displays a circadian rhythm. In healthy individuals, mean rectal temperatures vary from a low of about 97°F (36.1°C) in early morning to a high of about 99.3°F (37.4°C) in late afternoon. In children, the normal range may be even greater. Moreover, physiologic factors such as exercise and the menstrual cycle can further alter body temperature. In practical terms, understanding the diurnal rhythm of body temperature is important for two reasons. First, many patients have been unnecessarily subjected to extensive workups and even psychologically incapacitated in the erroneous quest for a cause of deviation from the mythical "normal" temperature of 98.6°F. Second, the fever of disease states is superimposed on the normal cycle, so that fevers are generally highest in the evenings and lowest in the mornings. As a result, frequent temperature recordings throughout the day are required to monitor fever in sick patients. The absence of fever in a single office visit does not exclude a febrile illness.

Clinical Manifestations of Fever. The presenting complaints of the febrile patient may be explained by the underlying disease process or by the fever itself. The signs and symptoms of fever vary tremendously. Some patients are asymptomatic; more often, they have a sensation of warmth or flushing. Malaise and fatigue are common. The hypothalamus, acting through somatic efferent nerves, increases muscle tone to generate heat and raise body temperature; many febrile patients experience *myalgias* as a result.

These same factors account for one of the most dramatic manifestations of fever: the *shaking chill* or *rigor*. It is taught that rigor is a manifestation of bacteremia, but in fact any stimulus that raises the hypothalamic set point rapidly may produce a rigor. Patients experiencing a rigor exhibit uncontrolled violent shaking and trembling, and they characteristically heap themselves with blankets even as their temperatures are shooting up. This phenomenon also has a physiologic basis. Despite their high central or core temperature, these patients subjectively feel cold because their surface temperature is reduced. To generate fever in response to hypothalamic stimuli, cutaneous vasoconstriction occurs, skin temperature falls, and cold receptors in the skin sense this as cold. Quite the reverse occurs during defervescence; body temperature falls in response to cutaneous vasodilation, and drenching sweats typically terminate an episode of fever.

Other manifestations of temperature elevation include central nervous system symptoms that range from a mild inability to concentrate to *confusion*, *delirium*, or even stupor, especially in the elderly or debilitated patient. High fevers (104° to 106°F) may produce *convulsions* in infants and young children without any primary neurologic disorder. Increased cardiac output is an invariable consequence of fever, and *tachycardia* typically accompanies fever. Tachycardia is so usual that its absence should lead one to suspect uncommon problems such as typhoid fever, in which relative bradycardia is typical (for unknown reasons), drug fever, and factitious fever. Patients with underlying heart disease may respond to the high-output stress of fever with angina or heart failure.

Another sign of fever is the so-called fever blister—*labial herpes simplex*. The problem is probably not precipitated by fever *per se*, for it is much more common in some infections, such as pneumococcal pneumonia and meningococcal meningitis, than in other febrile states.

Because fever accompanies infection so frequently, numerous investigators have tried to determine if fever has any protective or beneficial role. There are a few circumstances, such as central nervous system syphilis, in which elevations of body temperature may exceed the thermal tolerance of the infectious agent. In fact, induced fever was once a form of therapy for syphilis. In several animal models, fever enhances recovery from experimental infections; however, there is no such proven clinical benefit from fever in humans.

Consequences of Fever. Is fever detrimental? Most otherwise healthy individuals can tolerate temperatures up to 105°F (40.5°C) without ill effects, although even in these individuals symptoms often warrant therapy. In children, high fevers should be suppressed because convulsions may occur. Patients with heart disease should also receive antipyretic therapy. Each increase of 1°F in temperature increases the basal metabolic rate by 7%, which results in increased demands on the heart, so that myocardial ischemia, failure, or even shock can ensue. In addition, extreme hyperthermia beyond 108°F (42.1°C) may cause direct cellular damage. Vascular endothelium seems particularly susceptible to such damage, and disseminated intravascular coagulation frequently accompanies extreme hyperthermia. Other structures that may be directly damaged are brain, muscle, and heart. Finally, metabolic derangements such as hypoxia, acidosis, and sometimes hyperkalemia can result from extreme pyrexia and, in turn, further contribute to coma, seizures, arrhythmias, or hypotension, which can be lethal. Nevertheless, patients have survived temperatures of up to 108°F without demonstrable organ damage, although mortality in this temperature range is appreciable. Body temperatures as high as 113°F have been demonstrated in humans, but these have been uniformly lethal.

DIFFERENTIAL DIAGNOSIS

Many inflammatory, infectious, neoplastic, and hypersensitivity processes can produce fever. Most *acute fevers* encountered in the office setting are of obvious causes such as upper respiratory or urinary tract infection. Viral illnesses, drug allergy (especially to antibiotics), and connective tissue disease are other important precipitants.

Recurrent or *intermittent* fever is most characteristic of infectious conditions with cyclic features, such as malaria, hepatitis B, leptospirosis, brucellosis, and disseminated fungal infection. Migration of intraluminal parasites (as in schistosomiasis, amebiasis, and trypanosomiasis) can lead to intermittent fever, as can cell lysis by intracellular parasites (e.g., *Bartonella* and *Ehrlichia*). A cyclic pattern of high fevers for 1 to 2 weeks alternating with afebrile periods suggests the pathognomonic *Pel-Ebstein fever* of Hodgkin's disease.

Unexplained persistent fever can be a major diagnostic challenge. "Fevers of unknown origin" (FUOs) are defined as those persisting for 3 weeks, exceeding temperatures of 101°F, and

Table 11.1. Causes of Fever of Undetermined Origin

"The Big Three"
I. Infections: 20–40%
   A. Systemic
      1. Tuberculosis (miliary)
      2. Infective endocarditis (subacute)
      3. Miscellaneous infections: cytomegalovirus infection, toxoplasmosis, brucellosis, psittacosis, gonococcemia, chronic meningococcemia, disseminated mycoses
   B. Localized
      1. Hepatic infections (liver abscess, cholangitis)
      2. Other visceral infections (pancreatic, tuboovarian, and pericholecystic abscesses; empyema of gallbladder)
      3. Intraperitoneal infections (subhepatic, subphrenic, paracolic, appendiceal, pelvic, and other abscesses)
      4. Urinary tract infections (pyelonephritis, renal carbuncle, perinephric abscess, prostatic abscess)
II. Neoplasms: 7–20%. Especially lymphomas, leukemias, renal cell carcinoma, atrial myomas, and cancers metastatic to bone or liver
III. Collagen-vascular and other multisystem disease: 15–25%. Including temporal arteritis and juvenile rheumatoid arthritis as well as systemic lupus erythematosus, rheumatoid arthritis, polyarteritis nodosa, Wegener's granulomatosis, mixed connective tissue disease, sarcoidosis

Less Common Causes: 5–15%
I. Noninfectious granulomatous diseases (e.g., granulomatous hepatitis)
II. Inflammatory bowel disease
III. Pulmonary embolization
IV. Drug fever
V. Factitious fever
VI. Hepatic cirrhosis with active hepatocellular necrosis
VII. Miscellaneous uncommon diseases (familial Mediterranean fever, Whipple's disease)
VII. Undiagnosed

Modified from Jacoby GA, Swartz MN. Fever of unknown origin. N Engl J Med 1973;289:1407, with permission.

Table 11.2. Fever of Unknown Origin in Patients with HIV Infection or Cancer

HIV Patients
Infection (75% of cases)
   Mycobacterial infection (*M. tuberculosis, M. avium* complex)
   Cytomegalovirus infection
   Toxoplasmosis
   Pneumocystis infection
   Cryptococcal infection
   Salmonella infection
   Aspergillosis
   Herpes zoster
   Underlying HIV infection
Noninfectious (10%)
   Lymphoma (non-Hodgkin's)
   Drug fever
Unexplained (15%)

Cancer Patients
Infection (50%), usually as a consequence of neutropenia
   Gram-negative bacilli
   Fungi
Malignancy
   Extension and widespread dissemination of underlying malignancy

Adapted from Hirschman JV. Fever of unknown origin in adults. Clin Infect Dis 1997;24:291, with permission.

eluding 1 week of intensive diagnostic study. In both community and referral centers, infection (localized and systemic), neoplasms, and collagen vascular diseases account for more than 75% of cases (Table 11.1). Most of these represent unusual presentations of common diseases rather than rare conditions. In the community setting, intraabdominal abscesses and lymphomas account for nearly a third of cases. The spectrum of FUO disease has evolved in the past two decades. HIV infection raises a whole new set of diagnostic possibilities [e.g., *Pneumocystis* pneumonia, *Mycobacteria avium* infection (see Chapter 13 and Table 11.2)] as does immunosuppression from cancer chemotherapy, intravenous drug abuse, and the increasing use of prosthetic devices. Newly discovered infectious etiologies, such as Lyme disease, also add to the list.

WORKUP

The acutely febrile patient presents a common but demanding problem in differential diagnosis. In most cases, a careful history and physical examination will reveal the diagnostic clues, so that laboratory studies can be used selectively. The evaluation of persistent fever can be more demanding. The initial office evaluation should help determine the proper pace of diagnostic testing and need for therapeutic intervention. If the illness is insidious in onset and only slowly progressive, or if the patient is nontoxic and clinically stable, one may proceed with the workup in a deliberate manner on an ambulatory basis, utilizing serial clinical observations and time as key diagnostic tools. On the other hand, if the patient is a compromised host or is acutely ill and toxic, several immediate diagnostic studies are mandatory, and treatment may be required even before all the results are available; hospitalization is usually necessary in such cases. Table 11.3 lists some factors that should prompt an aggressive approach to diagnosis and therapy.

Febrile illnesses are most commonly acute processes that are either readily diagnosed and treated (common bacterial infections) or self-limited despite the lack of a specific diagnosis (viral infections, allergic reactions). However, patients will occasionally present with undiagnosed fevers, fulfilling the classic criterion for FUO. In both situations, the keys to diagnosis are a careful history and a meticulous physical examination, which almost always suggest the diagnosis and guide the rational use of imaging studies and other diagnostic modalities.

Table 11.3. Febrile Patients Who Require Special Attention

Vulnerable Hosts
Age (very young or very old)
Corticosteroid or immunosuppressive therapy
Serious underlying diseases (neutropenia, sickle cell anemia, diabetes, cirrhosis, advanced chronic obstructive pulmonary disease, renal failure, malignancies, AIDS)
Implanted prosthetic devices (heart valves, joint prostheses)
Intravenous drug abuse
Toxic Patients
Rigors, prostration, extreme pyrexia
Hypotension, oliguria
Central nervous system abnormalities
Cardiorespiratory compromise
New significant cardiac murmurs
Petechial eruption
Marked leukocytosis or leukopenia

History

The infectious disease history should stress several items not routinely emphasized: (a) host factors, (b) epidemiology, (c) symptomatology, and (d) drug history.

Host Factors. One should determine if patients are basically healthy or if they have an underlying disease that may render them unusually susceptible to infection. Patients taking *corticosteroids* or other *immunosuppressive agents* are especially vulnerable to infection. Patients with hematologic and other *malignancies, HIV infection, chronic liver disease, diabetes mellitus, neutropenia,* or *sickle cell anemia* may become infected with unusual opportunistic pathogens or may fail to respond normally to common infectious agents. Individuals with implanted *prosthetic devices,* such as artificial heart valves or hip prostheses, are also at increased risk for serious infection. Finally, patients with a *past history* of certain infectious processes, such as pyelonephritis, may be prone to relapses or recurrences of similar problems.

Epidemiology. Epidemiologic inquiry is often very productive. Inquiry is necessary about *high-risk sexual activity* in screening for HIV infection, *travel* in determining exposure to parasitic infections, and *intravenous drug abuse* for estimating risk of endocarditis and viral hepatitis. Less obvious factors, such as *animal contacts,* may be of great importance. Vectors of infection can be found even among household pets, such as cats (cat-scratch disease and *Pasteurella multocida* cellulitis from bites or scratches, toxoplasmosis from fecal contamination), parakeets (psittacosis), and turtles (salmonellosis). A history of *bites* by stray dogs, skunks, or bats may suggest the possibility of rabies. Animal contacts can also provide exposure to insect vectors such as *ticks. Homelessness* places patients at great risk for a host of infectious etiologies, including tuberculosis, HIV infection, viral hepatitis, right-sided endocarditis from intravenous drug abuse, and even louse-borne infections such as the one caused by *Bartonella quintana,* the notorious organism responsible for trench fever in World War I.

An inquiry into what is "going around" in the *community* may be helpful. A very localized outbreak of a flulike illness or atypical pneumonia may be a clue to *Legionella* infection (see Chapter 52). Being exposed to or part of a *population with a high incidence* of tuberculosis (see Chapter 49), HIV infection (see Chapter 13), or viral hepatitis (see Chapter 70) raises the risk of contracting the infection. Intravenous drug abusers are at notoriously high risk for such conditions, in addition to bacterial endocarditis. The patient's *occupation* is also sometimes revealing. For example, abattoir workers may be exposed to brucellosis, leather workers to anthrax, and gardeners to sporotrichosis.

Symptomatology may serve to pinpoint the site of infection. *Localizing symptoms* should be sought. They include rash, headache, cranial tenderness, sinus discomfort, ear pain, toothache, sore throat, tender thyroid gland, breast mass or tenderness, pleuritic chest pain, cough, dyspnea, abdominal pain, flank pain, dysuria, vaginal discharge, pelvic pain, anorectal or perineal discomfort, testicular pain, bone pain, joint swelling, joint stiffness or pain, calf or vein tenderness, neck stiffness, focal neurologic deficit, and alteration in consciousness. The *pattern of fever* can be useful diagnostically; periodicity suggests parasitic etiologies and Hodgkin's disease.

Medications. A full review of all drug use and any substance abuse (see Chapter 235) is essential. Is the patient taking any medications that may be responsible for fever as a manifestation of hypersensitivity? Does the patient have any drug allergies? Has the patient been taking antibiotics, which can alter susceptibility to infection by favoring drug-resistant organisms or mask infection by rendering the patient culture-negative? Is there an underlying problem (e.g., renal failure) that may alter the choice of therapeutic agents and lead to the use of a less common agent?

Physical Examination

Vital signs should be determined in all cases. Fever is an important but nonspecific sign of infection; some patients with infections are afebrile, whereas others may have a fever resulting from noninfectious causes, such as hypersensitivity states and lymphoreticular malignancies. The shaking chill or rigor may suggest bacteremia, but it is also not specific. In the neonate or in occasional adults with overwhelming sepsis, hypothermia may be present. Respiratory distress may signal pulmonary infection or septic shock, and hypotension may be the presenting finding leading to a diagnosis of sepsis.

The *skin and mucous membranes* may provide crucial information. To cite a few examples: Petechial eruptions on the skin suggest meningococcemia or Rocky Mountain spotted fever, and those at the junction of the hard and soft palate occur with infectious mononucleosis. Pustular lesions raise the question of gonococcemia (see Chapter 137) or staphylococcal endocarditis. Splinter hemorrhages and conjunctival petechiae herald endocarditis. Ecthyma gangrenosa is a hallmark of *Pseudomonas* septicemia. Macular or vesicular eruptions occur with viral infections, and bullae with *Vibrio vulnificus* infection. Erythema chronicum migrans is an important sign of Lyme disease.

The *sinuses* should be percussed for tenderness and transilluminated for evidence of sinusitis. In the elderly, the *scalp* is palpated for the tender arteries of cranial arteritis. The optic *fundi* are examined for the retinopathy of connective tissue disease (see Chapter 146), the Roth spots of endocarditis, and the choroidal tubercles of miliary tuberculosis and *Candida* septicemia. The *tympanic membranes* should be examined for effusion and erythema, and the oral cavity for tonsillar pathology, tooth abscess, and salivary gland tenderness. The *neck* is checked for thyroid gland tenderness and local adenopathy. Careful examination of all the *lymph nodes* for enlargement may provide a very important clue to etiology, as might the distribution of the adenopathy (see Chapter 12).

The *breasts* are examined for masses, tenderness, and nipple discharge. The *chest* is noted for rubs and signs of consolidation and effusion. A careful *heart* examination for murmurs and rubs is essential. The *abdomen* is checked for organomegaly, masses, tenderness, guarding, rebound, and tenderness of the costovertebral angle.

The *genitorectal area* is all too frequently overlooked, yet it is often a source of key information. The woman without an obvious source of fever must have a careful pelvic examination with a search for cervical discharge, adnexal tenderness, and mass lesions (see Chapter 114). In men, the prostate and testicles need to be checked gently for tenderness and masses and the penis for discharge and rash (see Chapter 136). The rectal examination should include evaluation for discharge, tenderness, and masses (see Chapter 66), and the stool should be tested for occult blood.

Musculoskeletal examination may suggest inflammation or infection of the bone or joints if swelling, increased warmth, or tenderness is present. The *lower extremities* are examined for evidence of phlebitis (asymmetric swelling, calf tenderness, palpable cord). The *neurologic evaluation* should include a look for signs of meningeal irritation, the presence of focal deficits, and disturbances in mentation.

Laboratory Studies

If the history and physical examination findings provide strong indications of an infectious process, laboratory studies can be used selectively to confirm or refute the clinical diagnosis. For example, in the patient with an obvious viral upper respiratory infection, no studies are necessary. In patients with bronchitis, a sputum smear and culture may be all that is required, but if pneumonia is a possibility, a chest radiograph and complete blood cell count (CBC) are minimal additional requirements (see Chapter 52). In the patient with probable lower urinary tract infection, a urinalysis and perhaps a culture may suffice, but if there is concern about upper tract infection, especially as a complication of obstruction, then renal function tests, blood cultures, renal ultrasonography, and intravenous pyelography deserve serious consideration (see Chapter 133).

In other patients, however, more extensive tests are needed to establish a diagnosis when the cause of fever remains unknown. Although such studies must be individualized, the approach to the diagnosis of an obscure fever should include the following.

Complete Blood Cell Count, Differential, and Sedimentation Rate. Leukocytosis and a "shift to the left" suggest but do not prove bacterial infection. Toxic granulations, Döhle's bodies, and vacuoles in polymorphonuclear leukocytes are suggestive of bacterial sepsis but are not entirely specific. In most instances, the erythrocyte sedimentation rate (ESR) lacks the sensitivity and specificity needed for it to serve as an adequate means of detecting or ruling out such causes of fever as tumor, connective tissue disease, and infection. Although a very elevated ESR is an invitation to additional testing and may be a clue to a specific process such as temporal arteritis (see Chapter 161), many elevations are a consequence of trivial conditions unrelated to the cause of fever. The ESR should be ordered and interpreted cautiously and not viewed as a screening test for "disease."

Urinalysis. Pyuria strongly suggests urinary tract infection. Gram's stain of the unspun urine specimen can be diagnostic (see Chapter 127). Isolated hematuria may be a clue to an underlying glomerular disease or urinary tract malignancy, such as hypernephroma, which is notoriously difficult to diagnose early and a classic FUO etiology.

Radiographic Studies. *Chest radiographs* may detect infiltrates, effusions, masses, or nodes even in the absence of abnormalities on physical examination, whereas *kidney–ureter–bladder* (KUB) and upright abdominal films can disclose air–fluid levels in the bowel. *Ultrasonographic* or *computed tomographic* (CT) study may be needed if a mass lesion is suspected, such as an abscess or tumor (see below). *Plain films of bone* will show diagnostic changes of osteomyelitis after 10 to 14 days; for earlier diagnosis, consider *radionuclide bone scanning* and *magnetic resonance imaging* (MRI).

Blood Chemistries. The blood sugar determination is helpful in a search of previously unsuspected diabetes mellitus. The test is also important in evaluating the significance of the sugar concentration in various body fluids. Liver function tests are useful in helping to define obscure sources of fever. For example, transaminase elevation suggests hepatitis, and isolated rises in alkaline phosphatase point to infiltration of the liver.

Examination of Body Fluids. If there is any possibility of meningitis, a lumbar puncture is mandatory. Aspiration and study of pleural effusions, ascitic fluid, or joint effusions may be diagnostic. Such specimens should be examined directly by cell counts and stains (see below). Sugar and protein determinations help differentiate etiologies; in general, bacterial, mycobacterial, and fungal infections produce low sugar and high protein levels in body fluid.

Cultures. If the patient has a heart murmur or a prosthetic heart valve or other implantable device, or if the patient appears seriously ill, *blood cultures* should be obtained. Having three sets of two blood cultures from separate venipunctures maximizes test sensitivity. Most patients should have cultures taken of *urine* (clean catch or catheterized specimen) and *sputum*. If other body fluids are obtainable, they should likewise be cultured. Special mycobacterial and fungal media are required for culturing if the patient is a compromised host or has undergone prolonged antibiotic therapy. Anaerobic cultures are important when one is dealing with a possible abscess or other infection of the pulmonary, gastrointestinal, or pelvic regions.

Microscopic Evaluation. Any body fluid that can be obtained should be examined by the *Gram's stain* technique. Sputum, urine, wound exudates, cerebrospinal fluid, pleural fluid, ascitic fluid, and joint fluid often reveal the cause of infection on Gram's stain. Even Gram's stains of the stool may be helpful in certain specific situations, such as acute diarrhea (see Chapter 64). The presence of bacteria in a specimen of body fluid that is normally sterile is presumptive evidence of infection. This is particularly true when one is examining the spun sediment obtained from cerebrospinal fluid. Likewise, bacteria are not found in normal ascitic, joint, or pleural fluid. The presence of bacteria in unspun urine correlates well with significant urinary tract infection. However, Gram's stains must be examined and interpreted with a certain amount of caution. For example, if one sees epithelial cells in a sputum specimen, one can be certain that the specimen contains mouth organisms and is not representative of conditions in the tracheobronchial tree. In such instances, one should obtain a better sputum sample. In the presence of bacterial pneumonia, the sputum usually contains many polymorphonuclear leukocytes and a large number of bacteria. *Acid-fast stains* are required to visualize mycobacteria (see Chapter 49), and specially stained *wet mounts* of body fluids can be useful in uncovering numerous types of fungal infections.

Immunologic Studies. In selected instances, serologic testing for evidence of infection can be of great help. Examples include suspected HIV infection [*enzyme-linked immunosorbent assay* (ELISA) and *Western blot testing* (see Chapter 13)], rheumatic fever and other streptococcal infections (*anti-DNAase B titers*), infectious mononucleosis (*heterophile test*), and salmonella (*Widal titers*). Skin tests (especially the *tuberculin test*) can provide confirmatory evidence and need to be considered when clinical findings are suggestive. Testing for *antinuclear antibody* and *rheumatoid factor* may help in the diagnosis of a suspected vasculitis or rheumatoid disease. The presence of rheumatoid factor or immune complexes can be clues to "culture-negative" endocarditis or underlying connective tissue disease (see Chapter 146). In the diagnosis of obscure fevers, it is often useful to freeze and save an "acute-phase serum" for later comparison with a "convalescent serum."

The Febrile Patient without a Diagnosis

Although an enormous number of studies are available for the evaluation of undiagnosed febrile illnesses, it is important to proceed with these in a logical, step-by-step fashion instead of subjecting the patient to a random series of expensive, time-consuming, uncomfortable, or even hazardous studies. The first step in the subsequent workup is to *document fever* by measuring rectal temperatures every 4 hours. If fever is documented, further evaluation should be directed to the most common causes of FUO, listed in Table 11.1. The history remains the best source of clues to the diagnosis. Although MRI and CT can confirm suspected etiologies, blindly ordering such expensive imaging studies is usually unnecessary and wasteful. In a study from the community hospital setting, the history, physical examination, and basic laboratory studies supplemented by serologic testing revealed the diagnosis in more than 85% of instances. In the United States and Europe, malignancy, infection, and connective tissue disease each account for a quarter to a third of cases. In developing nations, infection is the predominant cause. About 8% of cases are without a diagnosis after workup, but the cause is usually identified after a period of close follow-up.

Radiographic and Invasive Studies may be revealing, but they require careful selection. At times, a contrast study or radionuclide scan will reveal a source of fever. *Ultrasonography* is useful for noninvasively identifying pathology in the liver, gallbladder, pancreas, kidneys, and pelvis. *Abdominal CT* helps visualize a suspected source of fever in the retroperitoneum (e.g., lymphoma), upper abdomen (e.g., pancreatic or liver cancer), and large bowel (e.g., diverticular abscess). *Bone scan* or *MRI* may localize an abscess or malignancy that has invaded bone; MRI is the more sensitive test to detect early disease. *Bone marrow* or *liver biopsy* may detect a granulomatous or neoplastic process. A *lumbar puncture* is unlikely to help unless nuchal rigidity or neurologic abnormalities are present. A blind *laparotomy* is not performed unless clear clues to intraabdominal abnormalities are present that cannot be evaluated with less invasive procedures.

Therapeutic Trials. Only in the acutely ill, toxic patient is it necessary to begin broad antibiotic coverage before the diagnosis is established. It is essential, although commonly forgotten, to obtain cultures of blood, urine, and other pertinent fluids before treatment is initiated, so that rational decisions can be made later concerning therapy. In the nontoxic patient with an acute febrile illness and in the person with a true FUO, blind therapeutic trials are rarely helpful and are often confusing or even harmful. In this context, it is useful to remember one definition of empiric therapy: what the ignorant do to the helpless. In occasional patients with FUO, therapeutic trials may be necessary. If it has not already been done, the simplest trial is to halt all but the most essential of medications. Other trials include administration of IV antibiotics for suspected culture-negative endocarditis, combined chemotherapy for occult tuberculosis, or salicylates or steroids for noninfectious inflammatory disease. Such trials should always be conducted with a specific end point or time limit in mind, carefully planned observations, patient consent, and a mixture of humility and trepidation.

The Second Look. Despite the array of sophisticated technology available for the study of febrile illnesses, the history and physical examination remain the keys to diagnosis in most cases. Time can be a most valuable diagnostic tool. Unless the patient is progressively deteriorating, it may be advisable to interrupt the workup for a period of clinical observation, possibly with the aid of symptomatic therapy such as antipyretics. A second look, beginning with the history and physical examination, may then be fruitful.

Unexplained Fever in High-risk Patients (with HIV Infection or Cancer). The risk for infection is markedly increased in patients with HIV infection (especially when CD4+ cell counts fall below $100/cm^3$) and in those with cancer complicated by neutropenia. Opportunistic organisms dominate the list of causes (Table 11.2). A careful history and physical examination remain the cornerstone of assessment. When the cause remains unclear, laboratory testing should include blood cultures for bacteria, fungi, and mycobacteria. If blood cultures are negative but the suspicion of mycobacterial and fungal infection persists, then liver and bone marrow biopsies with cultures are indicated. Serum cryptococcal antigen testing provides a sensitive means of identifying disseminated infection. In cancer patients, unexplained fever also suggests dissemination of malignancy. Chest CT with contrast can be useful when intrathoracic spread (including involvement of mediastinal lymph nodes) is a concern, and abdominal CT with contrast can help detect spread to the liver and retroperitoneal nodes. Lymph node enlargement should trigger consideration of node biopsy.

SYMPTOMATIC THERAPY

The best therapy is obviously to treat the underlying cause. However, antipyretic therapy may provide comfort and prevent complications. The first issue, of course, is to determine if fever should be treated. An elevated temperature itself does not necessarily call for therapy. However, if unpleasant symptoms are present, the patient has a limited cardiac reserve, or the complications of fever are imminent, antipyretics should be administered. Antipyretic therapy depends on the use of both chemical agents and physical methods. The most effective antipyretic drugs are the *salicylates* and *acetaminophen*; both appear to act on the hypothalamus to lower the thermal set point. Although parenteral salicylates are available, oral or rectal administration of either aspirin or acetaminophen is preferable. Doses of up to 1.2 g of either drug may be given to adults to initiate antipyretic therapy. In addition to their intrinsic toxicities, it must be remembered that both aspirin and acetaminophen occasionally produce an exaggerated response, with hypothermia and even dangerous hypotension. Patients with typhoid fever or Hodgkin's disease and elderly and debilitated patients seem to be at somewhat greater risk for this uncommon complication.

Physical cooling is also extremely effective. At the simplest level, undressing and exposing the patient to a cool ambient temperature will allow cooling by radiation; a bedside fan will promote cooling by convection also. Sponging with cool water or alcohol is helpful and promotes evaporation. With extreme elevations (>106°F), more drastic measures are necessary and hospitalization is urgent. *Immersion in an ice water bath* is the most efficient of these methods and may be indicated in hyperthermic emergencies, such as heat stroke. All methods of physical cooling present the risk for hypothermic overresponse and should therefore be discontinued when the body temperature begins to fall below critical levels.

Hyperthermic emergencies are rare, but fever is common and most often presents as an unpleasant symptom rather than a medical crisis. It seems appropriate, therefore, to conclude with a comment about patient comfort. Although fever causes discomfort in most patients, physical cooling produces discomfort in virtually all of them; often, the treatment is remembered as far worse than the illness itself. As a result, these measures should be employed only when fever itself presents medical problems. The same is true to a lesser extent of aspirin and acetaminophen. In particular, many patients find rapid rises and falls of temperature very distressing; therefore, administering antipyretics every 4 hours for the first day or two of treatment may be preferable to waiting for the fever to spike.

INDICATIONS FOR ADMISSION

The very toxic or vulnerable patient (Table 11.2) should be admitted promptly for aggressive study, monitoring, and consideration of means to lower temperature. In cases of weight loss and debilitation, early hospitalization should also be considered. Moreover, when fever remains elevated above 101°F for weeks and ambulatory diagnostic efforts have been unsuccessful, it is often beneficial to bring the patient into the hospital for closer evaluation and documentation of fever; the advice of an infectious disease consultant can be helpful.

PATIENT EDUCATION

Whenever fever is suspected in the ambulatory setting, the patient should be instructed to keep a record of temperatures, preferably rectal, taken each evening, when elevations are most likely to occur. The patient needs to be reassured that there is nothing abnormal about temperatures in the range of 97.0°F to 99.3°F.

ANNOTATED BIBLIOGRAPHY

DiNubile MJ. Acute fevers of unknown origin. Arch Intern Med 1993;153:2525. (*A plea for restraint in the empiric use of antibiotics when etiology is unknown.*)

Drancourt M, Mainardi JL, Brouqui P, et al. *Bartonella (Rochalimaea) quintana* endocarditis in three homeless men. N Engl J Med 1995;332:419. (*An example of the impact of social situation on the cause of fever; this louse-borne organism caused trench fever in World War I and has now been found among the homeless.*)

Hirschman JV. Normal body temperature. JAMA 1992;267:414. (*A discussion of patients who claim their normal temperature is less than 98.6°F.*)

Hirschman JV. Fever of unknown origin in adults. Clin Infect Dis 1997;24:291. (*Updated review of the problem, extending the classic approach of earlier writers and incorporating newer diagnostic approaches.*)

Jacoby GA, Swartz MN. Fever of undetermined origin. N Engl J Med 1973;289:1407. (*A still-useful review of the etiologies that should be considered in the patient with fever of unknown origin.*)

Kazanjian PH. Fever of unknown origin: review of 86 patients treated in community hospitals. Clin Infect Dis 1992;15:968. (*Unlike most series, which derive from referral centers, this one reports on etiologies seen in community settings.*)

Kearney RA, Eisen HJ, Wolf JE. Nonvalvular infections of the cardiovascular system. Ann Intern Med 1994;121:219. (*Very useful discussion of the risk factors, clinical presentation, diagnosis, and treatment of these often difficult-to-detect causes of unexplained fever.*)

Knockaert DC, Vanneste LJ, Vanneste SB, et al. Fever of unknown origin in the 1980s. Arch Intern Med 1992;152:51. (*An update of the diagnostic spectrum, which includes HIV-related diseases.*)

Kumar KL, Reuler JB. Drug fever. West J Med 1986;144:753. (*Superb review of drug fever, especially of clinical presentations.*)

Larson EB, Featherstone HJ, Petersdorf RG. Fever of undetermined origin: diagnosis and follow-up of 105 cases. Medicine (Baltimore) 1982;61:269. (*An update of the original 1961 review; cancer was the leading cause.*)

Lew DP, Waldvogel FA. Osteomyelitis. N Engl J Med 1997;336:999. (*Recent review of this important etiology of persistent fever, with 62 references.*)

Marantz PR, Linzer M, Feiner CJ, et al. Inability to predict diagnosis in febrile intravenous drug abusers. Ann Intern Med 1987;106:823. (*Initially difficult to determine risk of serious underlying illness.*)

Petersdorf RG. Fever of unknown origin: an old friend revisited. Arch Intern Med 1992;154:21. (*An editorial commenting on the changing pattern of etiologies cited in the Knockaert study.*)

Petersdorf RG, Beeson PB. Fever of unexplained origin: report on 100 cases. Medicine (Baltimore) 1961;40:1. (*The classic article on fever of unknown origin; it details a logical diagnostic approach that is still useful today.*)

Simon HB. Current concepts: hyperthermia. N Engl J Med 1993;329:483. (*Review of noninfectious causes of fever.*)

Sox HC, Liang MH. The erythrocyte sedimentation rate. Ann Intern Med 1986;104:515. (*A critical review of the test, arguing that it is not a useful screening procedure.*)

Styrt B, Sugarman B. Antipyresis and fever. Arch Intern Med 1990;150:1589. (*A thoughtful consideration of the evidence concerning the need to treat temperature elevations.*)

Young EJ, Fainstein V, Musher DM. Drug-induced fever. Rev Infect Dis 1982;4:69. (*Antibiotics were responsible for most cases.*)

12
Evaluation of Lymphadenopathy
HARVEY B. SIMON

Of the nearly 600 lymph nodes throughout the body, only a few are normally palpable, including small nodes in the submandibular, axillary, and inguinal regions. Nevertheless, lymphadenopathy is a very common presenting symptom. Most often, adenopathy indicates benign, self-limited disease; this is particularly true in children and young adults, who are more prone to reactive lymphatic hyperplasia. Despite this, patient concern is often substantial because of worry about serious infectious processes (e.g., AIDS) on the one hand and neoplastic diseases on the other. A systematic evaluation of lymphadenopathy will provide both reassurance and a correct diagnosis. A critical decision for the primary physician is when to refer the patient for a lymph node biopsy.

PATHOPHYSIOLOGY AND CLINICAL PRESENTATION

Localized Adenopathy. Small lymph nodes in the neck, axilla, and groin may be palpable in normal individuals. Palpable nodes in other regions or any node exceeding 1 cm in size should be regarded as potentially abnormal. Inflammation and infiltration are responsible for pathologic enlargement. Although size alone is not itself diagnostic, nodes *larger than 3 cm* suggest neoplastic disease. Localized lymphadenopathy may represent spread of disease from an area of drainage. Of particular importance are palpable supraclavicular nodes. The left one, sometimes referred to as the *"sentinel" node*, is in contact with the thoracic duct, which drains much of the abdominal cavity. The right supraclavicular node drains the mediastinum, lungs, and esophagus.

Hilar Adenopathy. Bilateral hilar adenopathy encountered as an incidental finding on a chest radiograph in an otherwise asymptomatic patient is likely to be caused by *sarcoidosis*. In about 80% of such cases, the adenopathy will resolve spontaneously. In areas endemic for fungal infection, asymptomatic bilateral hilar adenopathy may result from *coccidiomycosis* or *histoplasmosis*. *Lymphoma* and *bronchogenic carcinoma* can cause bilateral hilar adenopathy, but the patient is rarely asymptomatic at the time of presentation. The same pertains, although to a lesser degree, to primary *tuberculosis*.

Unilateral hilar adenopathy is most often a manifestation of lymphoma or bronchogenic carcinoma, although granulomatous diseases may also present in this fashion.

Generalized Lymphadenopathy results from systemic processes, such as infection, malignancy, hypersensitivity, and sometimes even metabolic disease with node infiltration. The adenopathy associated with infection may be caused by the disease itself (e.g., *HIV* infection) or to secondary infection (e.g., with *cytomegalovirus*). It may result from an illness that first produces localized adenopathy (e.g., *cat-scratch disease*). At the intersection of neoplastic and reactive lymphadenopathy is *Castleman disease*, a rare idiopathic atypical lymphoproliferative disease that can be localized or multicentric. Its clinical presentation can mimic that of lymphoma and HIV disease. Localized disease has a benign clinical course, but multicentric disease produces disseminated lymphadenopathy, systemic symptoms, and an increased risk for infection and cancer.

Other Lymphatic Abnormalities. In addition to lymphadenopathy, abnormalities of the lymphatic system may present in other ways. *Lymphangitis*, appearing as red, warm streaks along the course of superficial lymphatic networks, suggests an acute inflammatory response to pyogenic infection in the drainage area; staphylococci and streptococci are frequently responsible. *Lymphadenitis*, presenting as a tender, warm, soft, rapidly enlarging node, has a similar significance and often reflects acute pyogenic infection of the node itself. An idiopathic variant, necrotizing lymphadenitis (*Kikuchi's disease*), causes self-limited tender cervical adenopathy. *Lymphedema* results from the interruption of lymphatic drainage; surgical node dissection, radiotherapy, or fibrosis caused by chronic infections such as filariasis or lymphogranuloma venereum are causes of lymphedema.

DIFFERENTIAL DIAGNOSIS

The causes of lymphadenopathy can be conveniently considered in terms of location of the enlarged nodes (Table 12.1). In children and young adults, most adenopathy is a result of reactive hyperplasia and is less likely to represent serious pathology than it is in adults. In persons under the age of 30, the cause proves to be benign in 80% of cases; in persons over age 50, the rate of benign disease falls to 40%.

WORKUP

History and Physical Examination

A number of basic questions arise in the evaluation of lymphadenopathy that can be readily addressed by a careful history and physical examination:

1. Is the palpable mass indeed a lymph node? A variety of other structures, including enlarged parotid glands, cervical hygromas, thyroglossal and branchial cysts, hemangiomas, abscesses, lipomas, and other tumors, may on occasion be confused with lymphadenopathy.
2. Is the lymphadenopathy acute or chronic? Clearly, lymph node enlargement resulting from acute viral or pyogenic infection becomes less likely as the days and weeks pass, and granulomatous inflammation (sarcoidosis, tuberculosis, fungal infection) and neoplastic disease become greater worries. Even so, chronicity alone is not always a harbinger of serious disease, for on occasion reactive hyperplasia can persist for many months.
3. What is the character of the enlarged node itself? Tender, mobile nodes most often reflect lymphadenitis or lymphatic hyperplasia in response to acute inflammation. Firm, rubbery, nontender nodes may be found in lymphoma. Painless, stone-hard, fixed, matted nodes suggest metastatic carcinoma.
4. Is the adenopathy localized or generalized? Numerous systemic processes that include *infections* (e.g., infectious mononucleosis and other viral infections, toxoplasmosis, secondary syphilis), *hypersensitivity reactions* [serum sickness, reactions to phenytoin (Dilantin) and other drugs, and vasculitis, including systemic lupus erythematosus and rheumatoid arthritis], *metabolic diseases* (hyperthyroidism and various lipidoses), and *neoplasia* (especially leukemia) can produce generalized lymphadenopathy. However, Hodgkin's disease is usually unicentric in origin and spreads to contiguous regional nodes, so that generalized adenopathy is rare except in very advanced disease. Although certain non-Hodgkin's lymphomas may be multicentric, generalized adenopathy is also a late finding and is usually asymmetric, unlike the earlier and more symmetric adenopathy of some leukemias, such as chronic lymphocytic leukemia.

Generalized adenopathy, particularly if accompanied by weight loss, fever, or other constitutional symptoms, should raise the question of *AIDS* or HIV infection. Male homosexuals, IV drug abusers, hemophiliacs and other multiply transfused individuals, and Haitians are at particular risk (see Chapter 13).

Localized adenopathy should raise additional possibilities, depending on the area involved. For example, *submandibular* lymphadenopathy, which is perhaps the most common type of adenopathy, frequently results from pharyngitis (viral, streptococcal, gonococcal) or head and neck or intraoral infection. Although these benign processes vastly predominate, it should be remembered that patients with Hodgkin's disease most often present with cervical lymphadenopathy. *Preauricular* adenopathy may be a component of "occuloglandular fevers" resulting from adenoviral conjunctivitis, sarcoidosis, tularemia, cat-scratch disease, and other processes. *Posterior auricular* or *posterior cervical* adenopathy frequently reflects infections of the scalp but may also be prominent in systemic processes, such as rubella or toxoplasmosis.

Whereas *anterior cervical* lymphadenopathy often results from head and neck infections, isolated supraclavicular node enlargement is more indicative of metastatic malignancy; the *right supraclavicular* nodes drain the mediastinum, esophagus, and thorax, and *left supraclavicular* adenopathy (Virchow's node) is suggestive of primary intraabdominal neoplasia. *Axillary* nodes become enlarged in response to infection of the upper extremities, but breast cancer must also be considered. Although enlarged *epitrochlear* nodes are traditionally associated with secondary syphilis, this finding reflects generalized lymphadenopathy in lues; epitrochlear lymphadenopathy can be seen in many other systemic processes and in response to hand infections. Inguinal lymphadenopathy is much more common. Inguinal nodes are palpable in most normal individuals, but they can enlarge substantially in infections of the genitalia or perineum, and in infections of the lower extremities.

Bilateral hilar adenopathy in an asymptomatic patient raises the possibilities of sarcoidosis and fungal exposure. Unilateral hilar disease suggests lymphoma, cancer, and granulomatous disease, as does bilateral disease in a symptomatic patient or one with abnormal physical examination findings.

5. Are there associated systemic or localizing symptoms or signs? Fever, rash, weight loss, sore throat, dental pain, genital inflammation, and infections of the extremities are clues that may be particularly helpful. Of these symptoms, night sweats and weight loss are suggestive of granulomatous and neoplastic disease. Ear, nose, and throat symptoms suggest reactive lymphatic hyperplasia secondary to viral or localized bacterial infection.

A careful examination of the skin for a primary inoculation site may provide the clue to a diagnosis of cat-scratch disease or tularemia. A check for scalp infections, dermatophytes, and scabies is also needed. The liver and spleen are carefully examined; organomegaly may be an important clue for mononucleosis, sarcoidosis, or malignancy. Sternal tenderness may be present in leukemia.

Table 12.1.   Important Causes of Lymphadenopathy

GENERALIZED LYMPHADENOPATHY	LOCALIZED LYMPHADENOPATHY
Infections Mononucleosis AIDS AIDS-related complex (ARC) Toxoplasmosis Secondary syphilis	**Anterior Auricular** Viral conjunctivitis Trachoma, posterior auricular Rubella Scalp infection
Hypersensitivity Reactions Serum sickness Phenytoin and other drugs Vasculitis (lupus, rheumatoid arthritis)	**Submandibular or Cervical (unilateral)** Buccal cavity infection Pharyngitis (can be bilateral) Nasopharyngeal tumor Thyroid malignancy
Metabolic Disease Hyperthyroidism Lipidoses	**Cervical Bilateral** Mononucleosis Sarcoidosis Toxoplasmosis Pharyngitis
Neoplasia Leukemia Hodgkin's disease (advanced stages) Non-Hodgkin's lymphoma	**Supraclavicular, Right** Pulmonary malignancy Mediastinal malignancy Esophageal malignancy
	Supraclavicular, Left Intrabdominal malignancy Renal malignancy Testicular or ovarian malignancy
	Axillary Breast malignancy or infection Upper extremity infection
	Epitrochlear Syphilis (bilateral) Hand infection (unilateral)
	Inguinal Syphilis Genital herpes Lymphogranuloma venereum Chancroid Lower extremity or local infection
	Any Region Cat-scratch fever Hodgkin's disease Non-Hodgkin's lymphoma Leukemia Metastatic cancer Sarcoidosis Granulomatous infections
	Hilar Adenopathy, Bilateral Sarcoidosis Fungal infection (histoplasmosis, coccidioidomycosis) Lymphoma Bronchogenic carcinoma Tuberculosis
	Hilar Adenopathy, Unilateral Lymphoma Bronchogenic carcinoma Tuberculosis Sarcoidosis

6. Are there unusual epidemiologic clues? To cite a few examples, in patients exposed to cats, cat-scratch disease or toxoplasmosis, which can also result from eating poorly cooked meat, may develop. Travel to the southwestern United States may suggest the possibility of plague. An appropriate travel history or exposure to bird droppings may suggest fungal infection, as may lacerations sustained during gardening in the case of sporotrichosis. Contact with wild rodents can result in tularemia, as can tick bites. A history of exposure to tuberculosis may be an important clue to scrofula. More commonly, community outbreaks can provide clues to the diagnosis of streptococcal pharyngitis or rubella, whereas a history of sexual exposure may raise the question of gonorrhea, syphilis, genital herpes, or lymphogranuloma.

Laboratory Studies

Laboratory studies need not be very elaborate. A *complete blood cell count* with *differential* often provides useful information and is almost always indicated. For example, atypical lymphocytosis suggests mononucleosis, other viral infections, and toxoplasmosis; granulocytosis is indicative of pyogenic infection; eosinophilia raises the question of a hypersensitivity reaction; pancytopenia is consistent with marrow suppression by tumor and HIV infection.

Other studies are based on the clinical presentation of the lymphadenopathy. A variety of blood chemistries may help in selected cases. Elevations of *uric acid* may reflect lymphoma or other hematologic malignancies. *Serum liver chemistries* (especially the *alkaline phosphatase* level) provide objective parameters to follow. Although such abnormalities are nonspecific, they do suggest liver involvement, which can be further evaluated by biopsy.

Localized Adenopathy. If pharyngitis and cervical or submandibular adenopathy are present, a *throat culture* is mandatory. It should be remembered that although these specimens are routinely processed for streptococci, a special Thayer-Martin medium also must be used if gonococci are suspected. *Urethral* or *cervical cultures* and smears should also be obtained if gonorrhea is a potential cause of inguinal lymphadenopathy. *Blood cultures* are indicated in the rare cases of suspected plague, tularemia, or brucellosis or if the clinical picture suggests staphylococcal or streptococcal lymphadenitis. Biopsy may be necessary to rule out lymphoma and Hodgkin's disease if the adenopathy is progressive and the remainder of the workup is unrevealing (see below).

On occasion, lymphomatous retroperitoneal or intraabdominal nodes may enlarge enough to present as an abdominal mass. When lymphoma is a serious possibility, or when staging is necessary in known lymphoma or Hodgkin's disease, *abdominal computed tomography* (CT) can be used to detect enlargement of the retroperitoneal nodes; *bone marrow biopsy* may provide a tissue diagnosis (see Chapter 84).

Generalized Adenopathy. Serologic tests can be of great value. The *heterophile test* and *serologic tests for syphilis* are obvious examples. In addition, a serum sample from the acute phase of the illness can be frozen to be submitted with a later, convalescent-phase serum specimen for antibody titers against viruses, fungi, and toxoplasmosis. Brucellosis can also be diagnosed serologically. Serologic tests, including those for *antinuclear antibodies* and *rheumatoid factor*, may suggest a noninfectious process, such as collagen vascular disease.

Hilar Adenopathy. *Tuberculin skin testing* with purified protein derivative (PPD) and the *angiotensin-converting enzyme* (ACE) determination can facilitate the assessment. If the results of both are negative and the patient is white, then bronchoscopy and mediastinoscopy may be necessary to rule out lymphoma. If the patient is ACE-positive and PPD-negative, then the probability is very high that sarcoidosis is the cause, and there is little need for further evaluation. If the patient is ACE-negative and PPD-positive, then primary tuberculosis is likely. Reliable skin tests are also available for coccidioidomycosis and tularemia. On the other hand, cutaneous anergy may suggest sarcoidosis or lymphoma, but this is a nonspecific finding. Skin testing can be very helpful in the diagnosis of cat-scratch disease, but, as with the Kveim test, the necessary antigen is available only on a research basis in selected centers.

Among radiologic studies, the *chest radiograph* is particularly valuable because hilar adenopathy may be present in patients with enlargement of peripheral nodes. Hilar adenopathy may also be detected on chest radiograph in the absence of peripheral lymphadenopathy. Sarcoidosis, lymphoma, fungal infection, tuberculosis, or metastatic carcinoma (particularly from a lung primary) should be among the diagnostic considerations. *CT* can provide additional definition. *Mediastinoscopy* may be required for tissue diagnosis, although not in asymptomatic patients with bilateral hilar adenopathy and clear lung fields, who most likely have sarcoidosis or a fungal exposure.

Lymph Node Biopsy should be considered as the most direct approach to the diagnosis of lymphadenopathy. Although the majority of such procedures are technically easy and can be accomplished under local anesthesia, this is an invasive test that can sometimes prove nondiagnostic. It should be employed only when simpler approaches have failed to give a diagnosis and suspicion of a therapeutically important cause remains (e.g., tuberculosis, lymphoma, cancer, sarcoidosis, cat-scratch disease). Sometimes, careful *observation* for a period of time may be diagnostically useful before biopsy is undertaken. In many cases of benign lymphadenopathy, the nodes will regress spontaneously even if no etiologic diagnosis has been made. However, some lymphomas may regress transiently and simulate a more benign etiology.

If undiagnosed adenopathy persists during a period of weeks to months, especially if the nodes are enlarging or if neoplastic disease remains a concern, then consideration of node biopsy is indicated. In one retrospective study, weight loss, night sweats, nodes larger than 2 cm, and abnormal chest radiographic findings were the strongest predictors of important disease before biopsy. In the case of fluctuant nodes, *needle aspiration* can be used to diagnose infectious processes in some cases.

The node to be sampled should be selected with care; if generalized adenopathy is present, it is best to avoid inguinal or axillary nodes if possible because reactive hyperplasia in these areas may make interpretation difficult. In general, enlarged *supraclavicular nodes* have the highest diagnostic yield. When possible, *excisional biopsy* is preferred. At the time of biopsy, tissue should be submitted for appropriate bacteriologic smears and cultures in addition to histologic study. Touch preparations may be useful. Special stains for bacteria, mycobacteria, and fungi may be helpful, as may specific stains for unusual processes, such as periodic acid–Schiff (PAS) stains for Whipple's disease or lipidosis and Congo red stains for amyloid. The interpretation of lymph node pathology can be quite difficult and requires careful study by experienced observers. With such study, benign processes such as toxoplasmosis or cat-scratch disease can be suspected histologically, and detailed analysis of serial sections may reveal lymphomas that are not diagnosed with less intensive pathologic study. Finally, if pathologic study reveals reactive hyperplasia or is nondiagnostic, patients should be followed carefully, as up to 25% may eventually exhibit an illness responsible for the lymphadenopathy, most often lymphoma.

Evaluation of Lymphadenopathy in the HIV-infected Patient. In most patients who are HIV-positive, the lymphadenopathy represents follicular hyperplasia in response to HIV infection. However, the list of possible causes includes lymphoma, mycobacterial and viral infections, Kaposi's sarcoma, and other cancers (see Chapter 13). The principles for evaluation and biopsy are similar to those for the non-HIV patient, with the proviso that the probability of serious underlying pathology is increased. Suggested criteria for lymph node biopsy in these patients include a diameter greater than 2 cm, rapidly enlarging or asymmetric adenopathy, constitutional symptoms, and intrathoracic adenopathy on chest radiograph. When these rather restrictive criteria are used and needle aspiration is the mode of biopsy, yields of less than 50% have been reported, with most patients having follicular hyperplasia.

INDICATIONS FOR REFERRAL

Any patient suspected of harboring a malignancy should have a consultation with an oncologist or oncologic surgeon to consider further the need for biopsy and to determine the best approach to obtaining a tissue diagnosis. Simply arranging for the biopsy of an accessible node may fail to achieve a diagnosis and will subject the patient to an unnecessary invasive procedure. Consultation may also be useful if one is thinking about a period of observation and wants to be sure that this represents a reasonable approach.

ANNOTATED BIBLIOGRAPHY

Greenfield S, Jordan MC. The clinical investigation of lymphadenopathy in primary care practice. JAMA 1978;240:1388. (*A still-useful algorithm for the workup of peripheral lymphadenopathy in the ambulatory setting.*)

Herrad J, Cabanillas F, Rice L, et al. The clinical behavior of localized and multicentric Castleman disease. Ann Intern Med 1998;128:657. (*Best review of this idiopathic condition, which has both reactive and neoplastic characteristics and can mimic lymphoma.*)

Schroer KR, Fransilla KO. Atypical hyperplasia of lymph nodes: a follow-up study. Cancer 1979;44:115. (*Of patients with nondiagnostic lymph node biopsies, 6% to 25% were found within a few months to have lymphoma, cancer, connective tissue disease, or infection. Emphasizes importance of follow-up.*)

Slap GB, Brooks JSJ, Schwartz JS. When to perform biopsies of enlarged peripheral lymph nodes in young patients. JAMA 1984;252:1321. (*A retrospective study of 123 patients up to the age of 25 who underwent lymph node biopsy. A predictive model was developed to determine before biopsy which patients were likely to have "treatable" causes of adenopathy.*)

Slap GB, Connor JL, Wigton RS, et al. Validation of a model to identify young patients for lymph node biopsy. JAMA 1986;255:2768. (*Follow-up study testing the above model found that it performed well.*)

Tompkins DC, Steigbigel RT. *Rochalimaea*'s role in cat-scratch disease and bacillary angiomatosis. Ann Intern Med 1993;118:388. (*Editorial useful for its terse review of the criteria for diagnosis of cat-scratch disease, an important infectious cause of localized and diffuse lymphadenopathy.*)

13
Approach to the Patient with HIV-1 Infection
STEPHEN L. BOSWELL

Despite the fact that a cure remains elusive, the management of the person infected with human immunodeficiency virus (HIV-1) has improved significantly in recent years. Most care is now conducted in the outpatient setting, even for patients with the acquired immunodeficiency syndrome (AIDS). Intervention in the asymptomatic period, new therapies, and innovative strategies to prevent secondary infections have significantly decreased morbidity and increased survival. With the shift in management to the outpatient setting, primary care physicians have assumed an increasingly central role in the comprehensive care of the patient infected with HIV-1; they are responsible for initial diagnosis, counseling, prevention of spread, initiation of antiviral and prophylactic therapies, outpatient treatment of secondary infection, determination of need for hospitalization, and provision of supportive care in the late stages of illness. This requires that the primary care physician be knowledgeable about HIV-1 risk behaviors, disease manifestations, laboratory techniques, current therapy, and prophylaxis strategies. It is recommended that an expert be involved in the care of all those who are infected with HIV-1. This can be accomplished by an expert primary care clinician or by an expert consultant.

CASE DEFINITION AND EPIDEMIOLOGY OF HIV-1 INFECTION AND AIDS

Case Definition. The Centers for Disease Control and Prevention (CDC) criteria for *HIV-1 infection* in patients older than 13 years of age include the following:

- repeatedly reactive results on screening tests for HIV-1 antibody, with specific antibody identified by the use of supplemental tests, *or*
- direct identification of virus in host tissues by virus isolation, *or*
- detection of HIV-1 antigen, *or*
- a positive result on any other highly specific licensed test for HIV-1.

In 1993, the CDC revised the criteria for the *definition of AIDS* to incorporate clinical presentations in women and heterosexuals and advances in understanding the significance of counts of CD4+ lymphocytes (also known as helper T lymphocytes or CD4 cells). This CDC surveillance definition of AIDS requires the following:

- a CD4+ T-lymphocyte count below 200/mm^3 and laboratory evidence of HIV-1 infection, *or*

- presence of an AIDS-indicator disease, *or*
- presence of pulmonary tuberculosis, recurrent pneumonia, or invasive cervical cancer in a patient with laboratory evidence of HIV-1 infection, *and*
- absence of another reason for immune impairment.

Epidemiology. HIV-1 infection is a pandemic. It has become the world's leading infectious cause of death, a position previously held by tuberculosis. In 1998 alone, an estimated 2.3 million people died of AIDS-related causes worldwide. It has moved to this position from relative obscurity when five cases of AIDS were reported in Los Angeles in 1981. HIV-1 is spreading most rapidly in Asia, with more than 5 million cases estimated. The epidemic continues to expand in South America but appears to have slowed significantly in North America and Europe. In developing countries, the virus is spread primarily through heterosexual contact and affects males and females on a more equal basis than in Western countries.

In the United States, between 800,000 and 900,000 Americans are now infected with HIV-1, and the numbers continue to rise. Despite this fact, the death rate from AIDS has dropped significantly in most Western countries in the past several years. This is attributable to significant improvements in medical treatment. The African-American and Hispanic communities are increasingly affected. The epidemic appears to have plateaued in the gay population. The incidence of HIV-1 infection continues to rise in injection drug users, women, and persons who have acquired HIV-1 through heterosexual contact.

In the United States, those at highest risk for infection are men with a history of *homosexual* or *bisexual* activity; *IV drug users* and their sexual contacts; the *sexual contacts* of homosexual or bisexual men; persons who received *blood and blood products before 1985*; and *children* born to infected women. The risk for directly acquiring HIV-1 infection through processed blood or selected blood products (plasma and clotting factor concentrates) has dramatically decreased since 1985 as a consequence of the widespread screening of those who donate blood and plasma, the use of serologic tests for HIV-1, and the viral inactivation of various plasma products.

AIDS is only part of the much larger epidemic of HIV-1 infection. For every person who is living with AIDS in the United States, four to five people are infected with HIV-1 but have minimal or no symptoms. They often present to health care providers for problems related to high-risk activity (e.g., IV drug use), unaware they are carrying HIV-1. These encounters provide a critical opportunity to teach about HIV-1 infection.

PATHOPHYSIOLOGY, CLINICAL PRESENTATION, AND COURSE

Pathophysiology

The *human immunodeficiency virus* is an RNA retrovirus that includes a core protein (p24), a reverse transcriptase, an HIV-1 protease, and envelope glycoproteins. Isolates of HIV-1 differ genetically and antigenically, particularly in regard to envelope proteins (a feature that has complicated the development of an effective vaccine).

HIV-1 is transmitted through *sexual contact, parenteral exposure* to blood and selected blood products, and *maternal transmission* (via breast milk and perinatal transmission). Once the virus enters the body, it attaches to the surface of *CD4+ T lymphocytes*. These helper T lymphocytes are the target of HIV-

1, by virtue of the affinity of the virus for receptors on their surface. Once attached, the virus enters the lymphocyte and uncoats. Its RNA is transcribed to DNA by reverse transcriptase. The DNA may remain in the cytoplasm or become integrated into the host cell genome, where it can remain latent until some stimulus triggers replication of virus.

Ten billion viral particles are produced in an infected person each day. Most of these viral particles are produced by activated CD4+ lymphocytes, which are killed when the virus enters the lytic stage of infection. These cells are central to maintaining immunocompetence. With damage to the CD4-cell population, patients are at increased risk for clinical manifestations directly associated with the disease, including HIV encephalopathy and HIV-1–associated wasting. As HIV-1 infection progresses, the risks for opportunistic infections and neoplasm increase. Death occurs most frequently because of wasting, opportunistic infection, or neoplasm.

Clinical Presentations and Course

HIV-1 infection in humans is a continuum that can be crudely broken into four phases: (a) primary HIV-1 infection, (b) asymptomatic infection, (c) symptomatic HIV infection, and (d) AIDS. The rate of disease progression varies from person to person and appears to depend on both viral and host factors. In general, the use of antiretroviral therapy and chemoprophylaxis of opportunistic infection have a profound effect on the pace of disease progression.

Primary Infection. The first, brief phase of the illness is a *mononucleosis-like syndrome*. In the initial years of the epidemic, the syndrome was not recognized, but after the development of serologic tests, it became possible to link it to HIV-1. The syndrome consists of fever, sweats, lethargy, malaise, myalgias, arthralgias, headaches, photophobia, diarrhea, sore throat, lymphadenopathy, and a truncal maculopapular rash. It is of sudden onset and lasts 3 to 14 days. More than 50% of individuals infected with HIV-1 experience one or more of these symptoms. Less frequently, neurologic signs and symptoms occur, such as those of meningoencephalitis, myelopathy, peripheral neuropathy, and Guillain-Barré syndrome. The most common neurologic symptoms in primary HIV-1 infection are headache and photophobia. The symptoms that most markedly differentiate seroconversion subjects from control subjects are *swollen lymph nodes*, truncal or generalized *rash*, *depression*, irritability, anorexia, *weight loss*, and *retroorbital* pain. Unfortunately, these symptoms are not specific for primary HIV-1 infection.

Asymptomatic Seropositivity. The second phase of HIV-1 infection is the longest of the four phases and also the most variable. It typically lasts *4 to 7 years* and is distinguished by the lack of overt evidence of HIV-1 infection.

Symptomatic Seropositivity (Pre-AIDS). The onset of the third phase of HIV-1 infection ushers in the first physical evidence of immune system dysfunction. *Persistent generalized lymphadenopathy* is often an early sign of this phase. *Localized fungal infections* of the toes, fingernails, and mouth frequently occur. Among women, recalcitrant *vaginal yeast* and *trichomonal infections* often recur. *Oral hairy leukoplakia*, one of the most commonly missed signs of HIV-1 infection, is very prevalent and typically found on the tongue. Cutaneous manifestations of this phase of illness include widespread *warts*, *molluscum contagiosum*, exacerbations of *psoriasis*, and *seborrheic dermatitis*. Multidermatomal *herpes zoster* and an increased severity or frequency of *herpes simplex* infections can occur. Constitutional symptoms, including *night sweats*, *weight loss*, and *diarrhea*, are often seen. Without treatment, the duration of this phase is typically *1 to 3 years*.

Symptomatic Seropositivity (AIDS) is characterized by significant immune suppression, which leads to the development of disseminated opportunistic infections and unusual malignancies. Pulmonary, gastrointestinal, neurologic, and systemic symptoms are common.

Pneumocystis carinii pneumonia (PCP) is among the most common infections in AIDS patients, with an attack rate of almost 80% in patients not receiving primary prophylaxis (see below). Fever, night sweats, malaise, and weight loss typically precede the onset of pulmonary symptoms by days to weeks. A dry cough may be the first pulmonary manifestation, followed by shortness of breath. Diffuse infiltrates on chest radiographs, a widening alveolar–arteriolar oxygen gradient (>30 mm Hg), and a low partial pressure of oxygen (<50 mm Hg) are associated with reduced survival.

Pulmonary and disseminated forms of invasive fungal infection with *Cryptococcus neoformans*, *Histoplasma capsulatum*, and *Coccidioides immitis* are other hallmarks of AIDS. Cryptococcal infection occurs throughout the United States and often presents subtly, with headache, fever, and malaise. Altered mentation and stiff neck are absent in most cases. At times, pulmonary complaints dominate the clinical picture of cryptococcal infection. Pulmonary and systemic complaints are prominent in patients with histoplasmosis or coccidioidomycosis. Infiltrates on the chest film of a patient living in an endemic area suggest the diagnosis; splenomegaly can be marked in histoplasmosis.

Mycobacterial infections, both pulmonary and disseminated, are consequences of falling CD4-cell counts. HIV-1–seropositive patients with latent tubercular infection are at increased risk for reactivation and dissemination. Meningeal involvement is the most common form of disseminated disease. Many strains isolated from AIDS patients demonstrate multiple-drug resistance (see Chapter 49). *Mycobacterium avium–intracellulare* infection is an accompaniment of very advanced disease. The clinical presentation is one of wasting, fever, sweats, diarrhea, and weight loss. Blood cultures are often positive.

Recurrent bacterial pneumonia (two or more episodes per year) is a more recently appreciated manifestation of AIDS. The presentations and organisms are typical of bacterial pneumonia, with positive sputum cultures and infiltrates on chest radiograph. Such cases of pneumonia are 20 times more common in HIV-1 patients with low CD4-cell counts (<200/mm³) than in those with normal counts. The recurrent development of such cases of pneumonia represents significant immunosuppression.

Cytomegalovirus (CMV) infection, often a reactivation of latent disease, is common in AIDS. *Retinitis*, presenting as unilateral visual loss or floaters and, if untreated, progressing to bilateral disease and blindness, afflicts about 5% to 10% of AIDS patients. Exudates and hemorrhages are noted on funduscopic examination. Esophagitis, gastritis, and colitis also may develop.

Enteric infections cause considerable morbidity in AIDS patients and typically present as weight loss, cramping pain, and large-volume diarrhea. *Salmonella*, *Shigella*, and *Campylobacter* are the leading causes, infection with the latter two more characteristically presenting with bloody diarrhea and leukocytes on Wright's stain of a fecal smear. *Cryptosporidium*, a protozoan, is an important cause of diarrhea in AIDS patients in undeveloped areas.

HIV-1 wasting syndrome is characterized by the profound involuntary loss of more than 10% of body weight in conjunction with either chronic diarrhea (two or more stools per day for more than 1 month) or fever and persistent weakness for a similar period in the absence of another cause.

Neurologic injury from HIV-1 infection ranges from mild *peripheral neuropathy* causing paresthesias to *encephalopathy* with debilitating dementia. The virus appears to be neurotropic, causing significant neurologic injury in up to 30% of AIDS patients. *AIDS dementia complex* results from direct injury to neurons from HIV-1 invasion of the central nervous system (CNS). Early on, there may be only minor impairment of cognitive or motor function, but in later stages, frank dementia and disabling motor disturbances ensue. Neuroimaging studies may show diffuse atrophic changes.

Opportunistic CNS infections also occur. *Toxoplasmosis* is one of the most common. Most *Toxoplasma gondii* disease represents reactivation of latent infection. About one third of those who are seropositive for immunoglobulin G experience reactivation. CNS involvement can cause symptoms both of a mass lesion (discrete deficits, headache) and of encephalitis (fever, altered mental status). The images on scanning by computed tomography (CT) or magnetic resonance imaging (MRI) are characteristic: multiple (more than three) contrast-enhanced mass lesions in the basal ganglia and subcortical white matter.

Syphilis is of increased likelihood in HIV-1 patients with a history of high-risk sexual behavior, and it may take an atypical or accelerated course, including CNS spread.

Malignancies are a consequence of the reduction in cellular immunity. *Kaposi's sarcoma*, non-Hodgkin's lymphoma, and primary CNS lymphoma occur with greatly increased frequency in the setting of HIV-1 infection and serve to define the onset of AIDS. Kaposi's sarcoma is characterized by raised, violaceous, nonblanching plaques or nodules on the skin or mucous membranes. Visceral involvement may occur, presenting as hematemesis, melena, or hematochezia. A mass lesion on a neuroimaging study may represent a *primary CNS lymphoma*, especially in a patient free of the encephalopathic findings that occur with toxoplasmosis of the CNS. Such lymphomas are rare except in the context of HIV-1 infection. The incidence of *cervical dysplasia* is increased 10-fold in HIV-1–seropositive women. The development of *invasive cervical cancer* is indicative of severe immune compromise.

Skin problems in addition to Kaposi's sarcoma are an important source of morbidity. They range from cellulitis to drug eruptions and increase in frequency with worsening of immune function. Drug reactions are particularly common, with trimethoprim/sulfamethoxazole, dapsone/trimethoprim, and aminopenicillins most often implicated.

Prognosis. The prognosis strongly correlates with the CD4-cell count and is inversely related to the HIV load. Asymptomatic HIV-1–seropositive patients with CD4-cell counts above 500/mm³ and a low viral load may remain otherwise healthy without treatment for many years. However, as HIV-1 infection progresses, patients are at increased risk for clinical manifestations directly associated with the disease (see above). Most frequently, death is caused by opportunistic infection or malignancy. Earlier intervention in HIV-1 infection postpones the onset of AIDS and improves overall survival and quality of life (see below).

DIAGNOSIS

The Diagnosis of HIV-1 Infection is usually made serologically, by the presence of persistent HIV-1 antibody positivity. Alternative diagnostic methods include virus isolation and HIV-1 antigen detection. The very sensitive *ELISA* method (enzyme-linked immunosorbent assay) is used for HIV-1 antibody screening, with positive tests subjected to the more specific *Western blot analysis* for confirmation. The sensitivity and specificity of the ELISA are in the range of 99% for patients at high risk, but the predictive value of a positive test result falls in patients at low risk. Occasionally, it is necessary to attempt direct detection of the virus (with such methods as viral culture, polymerase chain reaction, branched-chain DNA, or p24 antigen) when clinical suspicion is high but standard screening test results are normal.

The Diagnosis of AIDS has little bearing on the clinical management and is useful primarily for historical and epidemiologic reasons. When the HIV epidemic was first recognized, the diagnosis of AIDS was predominantly a clinical one, based on the identification of an *indicator condition*. However, the initial AIDS definition emphasized conditions seen in HIV-1–infected gay men and omitted attention to the CD4-cell count and to presentations in other populations, such as women and heterosexuals. These shortcomings were addressed in the newest CDC surveillance definition of AIDS (see above), which expands the list of indicator conditions to include *pulmonary tuberculosis*, invasive *cervical cancer*, and *recurrent pneumonia* in patients who are HIV-1–seropositive. In addition, the importance of immune status is acknowledged in the these diagnostic criteria, with HIV-1–seropositive patients having a *CD4-cell count* below 200/mm³ now included among those considered to have AIDS.

WORKUP

Once a diagnosis of HIV-1 infection is made, the goals of the workup are to identify the stage of illness, determine prognosis, and promptly identify complications of immune incompetence. Progression of immune system damage is a major concern. Patients with falling CD4-cell counts and high viral loads (>100,000 copies per milliliter) are at particularly high risk and should be treated promptly and followed closely.

History

The initial interview of the HIV-1–infected patient should seek information about *infections*, *malignancies*, and *exposures* that may indicate ongoing immune dysfunction or the potential for future difficulty.

Past Medical History is carefully reviewed for a previous diagnosis of herpetic infections; aseptic meningitis; recurrent sinusitis; skin problems such as folliculitis, staphylococcal infections, psoriasis, molluscum contagiosum, warts, persistent tinea, or seborrhea; recurrent bacterial pneumonia caused by encapsulated organisms (*Haemophilus influenzae*, pneumococci); oral and vaginal candidiasis; abnormal Papanicolaou smear findings; sexually transmitted diseases (if there is a history of syphilis, the details of treatment and serologic titers should be carefully documented); hepatitis B infection or vaccination; hepatitis C infection; tuberculosis (including history of skin testing, exposures, chest radiographs, vaccination, prophylaxis, and treatment); and gastrointestinal infections with parasitic organisms or more common bacterial pathogens. A travel history may be useful in assessing the risk of exposure to histoplasmosis and coccidioidomycosis.

Review of Systems. Because HIV-1 infection is usually a multisystem disease, the review of systems takes on particular importance. It begins with inquiry into *systemic symptoms* (fever, chills, drenching night sweats, fatigue, weight loss), which may be manifestations of acute infection or more advanced disease. *Skin* complaints should be reviewed, particularly reports of violaceous nodules or plaques, pustules, petechiae, groin rashes, or herpetic lesions. Moving to the *HEENT* (head, ears, eyes, nose, throat) review, it is important to ask about sinus pain and any purulent drainage, sore throat, coated tongue, and white patches in the pharynx. Inquiry into *lymphadenopathy* may prove informative.

The *pulmonary* review includes a check for dyspnea, persistent dry or productive cough, and hemoptysis. A nonproductive cough of recent onset in conjunction with dyspnea on exertion should raise suspicion for *Pneumocystis* pneumonia. Patients should be asked about *gastrointestinal* symptoms, especially odynophagia (painful swallowing suggestive of fungal esophagitis), abdominal pain, nausea, vomiting, diarrhea, melena, hematochezia, hematemesis, tenesmus, and perianal pain. Diarrhea and tenesmus suggest large-bowel pathology. Cramping periumbilical pain, diarrhea, and increased flatus point to a small-bowel process. Early satiety, anorexia, and weight loss may be manifestations of gastrointestinal lymphoma. Genitourinary involvement is screened by inquiry into abnormal vaginal bleeding or discharge, dyspareunia, urinary frequency, dysuria, and hematuria.

The *neurologic* review is critical. Unilateral headache becoming more generalized in conjunction with a stiff neck suggests spread of a parameningeal focus of infection into the CNS. New onset of lateralized weakness or numbness, especially if accompanied by a worsening unilateral headache, raises the question of a mass lesion (lymphoma, toxoplasmosis, brain abscess). Monocular visual field disturbances and floaters are characteristic complaints in patients with CMV retinitis. Diplopia and homonymous hemianopsia may indicate a CNS infection or malignancy. Numbness or tingling in the fingers or toes points to a peripheral neuropathy or myelopathy.

Neuropsychiatric difficulties raise the question of AIDS dementia complex. Suggestive symptoms include cognitive problems, difficulty with concentration, memory loss, insomnia, apathy, social isolation, and alterations in mood, especially depression. When accompanied by fever and delirium, they are more likely to be the consequence of an encephalopathy, but such difficulties may also occur as a consequence of a reactive depression. Distinguishing among these conditions can sometimes be difficult and may require neuropsychiatric testing and other diagnostic tests.

Physical Examination

The physical examination is directed toward signs of immunocompromise and its consequences. It includes a careful inspection of the skin, sinuses, eyes, oral cavity, lymph nodes, chest, abdomen, pelvis, and central and peripheral nervous systems. In addition, vital signs should be obtained and carefully recorded. Subtle but persistent unintended weight loss occurs frequently in HIV-1 infection and can be one of the earliest manifestations of disease progression, secondary infection, or malignancy.

Skin is one of the most frequently affected organs. Kaposi's sarcoma (especially prevalent in gay men), warts, molluscum contagiosum, psoriasis, seborrheic dermatitis, and fungal infections of the toes and nails are especially common. A painless, persistent, raised purple lesion, especially if there is more than one such lesion, may be Kaposi's sarcoma and warrants biopsy. Facial seborrhea, scars from recurrent herpetic infections, and premature graying are among the more subtle signs of immunocompromise.

HEENT. The sinuses are noted for tenderness, failure to transilluminate, and purulent discharge. Funduscopic examination may reveal retinal exudates, hemorrhages, or cotton–wool spots suggestive of CMV infection. The exudate is typically pale and associated with hemorrhage; it usually begins peripherally and may be difficult to visualize during routine funduscopic examination.

Careful examination of the oral cavity is essential, with a search for signs of oral hairy leukoplakia, thrush, mucosal petechiae, stomatitis, gingivitis, and Kaposi's sarcoma. Thrush is an important indicator of disease progression. The most common form is *pseudomembranous candidiasis*, removable white plaques on any oral mucosal surface. *Atrophic oral candidiasis* appears as smooth red patches on the hard or soft palate, buccal mucosa, or dorsal surface of the tongue. These may be easily missed without careful inspection. Rarely, candidiasis can occur in a leukoplakia-like form consisting of white lesions that cannot be wiped off but regress with prolonged antifungal therapy. This form of *Candida* infection can easily be confused with oral hairy leukoplakia and is distinguished primarily by its response to therapy (biopsy is rarely warranted). *Angular cheilitis* caused by *Candida* can appear as erythema, cracks, and fissures at the corner of the mouth. This may require the addition of a topical antifungal cream for adequate treatment. Mucosal petechiae can be the sole evidence of HIV-1–associated thrombocytopenia. *Kaposi's sarcoma* often produces oral lesions on the hard and soft palate and gingivae. Aphthous stomatitis may be easily confused with stomatitis associated with herpes simplex or CMV infections. Biopsy may be required to distinguish them. Lymphoma may appear as a mass or ulcer(s), most commonly seen in the peritonsillar region.

Lymph Nodes are checked periodically, as adenopathy may be an important sign of disease progression. If lymphadenopathy occurs in two or more noncontiguous extrainguinal sites and persists for longer than 3 months, and if no cause other than HIV-1 can be found, the condition is referred to as *persistent generalized lymphadenopathy*. Occasionally, *splenomegaly* may be found in association with persistent generalized lymphadenopathy. Asymmetric, large, firm, tender nodes may be evidence of malignancy or secondary infection and often require biopsy.

Chest, Abdomen, Rectum, and Genitalia. The lungs are examined for signs of consolidation, pleural inflammation, and ef-

fusion. The heart is checked for murmurs and rubs. The abdomen is noted for enlargement of the liver or spleen and for localized tenderness. Genital and rectal examinations are essential in all patients. Although evidence suggests that Papanicolaou test sensitivity may be reduced among HIV-1–infected women, it is currently recommended that it be performed semiannually because of the greatly increased risk for invasive cervical cancer. Lymphoma, squamous cell carcinoma, CMV infection, and acyclovir-resistant herpes simplex infections are examples of unresponsive anorectal lesions that may require biopsy for diagnosis. Anoscopy or sigmoidoscopy may be necessary to diagnose rectal or colonic lesions or diarrhea.

Neurologic Examination should be conducted regularly and include a careful assessment for meningeal irritation, focal neurologic deficits, and changes in mental status. Evidence for peripheral neuropathy, myelopathy, and myopathy should be sought because these are common and often treatable abnormalities. A detailed mental status examination may aid in the early detection of AIDS dementia complex.

Laboratory Testing

Laboratory testing plays an essential role, not only in workup and monitoring but also in deciding on the nature and timing of therapy. Testing is used to identify those patients who might benefit from special interventions (e.g., hepatitis B vaccine for those who are negative for both hepatitis B surface antibody and hepatitis B core antibody). In other instances, it may reveal hidden medical problems that can be treated (e.g., interferon-α for the treatment of chronic hepatitis C infection). Decisions regarding the initiation of antiretroviral therapy and PCP prophylaxis are largely based on the results of laboratory tests, especially the CD4-cell count (see below). Increasingly, the effectiveness of antiretroviral therapy is being measured by the CD4-cell count and HIV load.

Initial Testing of the Patient Seropositive for HIV-1. A *complete blood cell count* and *platelet count* are essential (Table 13.1). Anemia of chronic disease, lymphopenia, and thrombocytopenia are common among HIV-1–infected patients, especially those with advanced disease. Idiopathic thrombocytopenia is sometimes seen in the acute phase of HIV-1 infection. Macrocytic anemia occurs in patients receiving zidovudine. Marrow suppression with pancytopenia may develop in the context of invasion by lymphoma or disseminated fungal infection. Proper workup may require measurement of serum iron, ferritin, folate, and vitamin B_{12} concentrations (see Chapter 79). When the cause of anemia is being assessed, it should be recognized that the measurement of mean corpuscular volume may be confounded by the macrocytosis that commonly occurs when patients are taking zidovudine and stavudine.

Before any drug therapies are initiated, baseline *serum chemistries* (electrolytes, blood urea nitrogen, creatinine, transaminase, alkaline phosphatase) may help to identify drug toxicities and comorbid conditions such as HIV- or drug-related renal insufficiency and liver damage associated with alcohol abuse or viral hepatitis.

Serologic testing for syphilis is essential because of its high prevalence among HIV-1–infected individuals. False-positive test results are not uncommon and can be excluded with a

Table 13.1.   Laboratory Testing

TEST	INDICATION FOR BASELINE TEST	TEST FREQUENCY
HIV serology	All patients without written documentation of positive serology	Baseline only
CBC count/diff/plt	All patients	As necessary
Chemistry	All patients	As necessary
CD4+ T-cell count	All patients	Every 3 to 4 months
HIV RNA (viral load)	All patients	Every 1 to 4 months
RPR or VDRL	All patients	Yearly
PPD	All patients without history of (+)PPD, TB treatment or prophylaxis	Consider yearly PPD for those at high risk
Toxoplasma IgG	All patients	As indicated
Varicella IgG	All patients	Baseline only
CMV IgG	All patients	Baseline only
HAA	All patients	Baseline only
HB_sAg	All patients	Baseline and as indicated
HB_sAb and/or HB_cAb	All patients	Baseline
Anti-HCV	All patients	Baseline and as indicated
G-6-PD	Nonwhite patients	Baseline only
Pap smear	All women	Yearly
CXR	All patients	As indicated

CBC, complete blood cell; diff, differential; plt, platelet; RPR, rapid plasma reagent; VDRL, Venereal Disease Research Laboratory; PPD, purified protein derivative; IgG, immune globulin G; CMV, cytomegalovirus; HAA, hepatitis A antibody; HB_sAg, hepatitis B surface antigen; HB_sAb, hepatitis B surface antibody; HB_cAb, hepatitis B core antibody; HCV, hepatitis C virus; G-6-PD, glucose-6-phosphate dehydrogenase; CXR, chest x-ray.

confirmatory fluorescein *Treponema* antibody (FTA) test. The natural history of syphilis may be altered by HIV-1 infection, and therefore careful attention to a history and prior treatment for syphilis is essential. If a history of syphilis cannot be documented or if a positive result is accompanied by neurologic signs or symptoms, further workup, including a lumbar puncture, is advocated by most authorities (see Chapters 124 and 141). Patients who experience therapeutic failure or who cannot receive standard therapy with benzathine penicillin should undergo lumbar puncture also. Interpretation of cerebrospinal fluid results may be difficult, however. Cerebrospinal fluid VDRL (Venereal Disease Research Laboratory) testing is insensitive, and mononuclear pleocytosis and elevated cerebrospinal fluid protein are frequent in HIV infection without neurosyphilis.

Immunoglobulin G serology for *T. gondii* may be helpful in identifying those individuals who would benefit from chemoprophylaxis to prevent reactivation. This prophylaxis is recommended in guidelines on opportunistic infection prevention released by the U.S. Public Health Service and the Infectious Disease Society of America. Estimates have placed the risk for development of toxoplasmic encephalitis in an HIV-infected *Toxoplasma*-seropositive patient at between 20% and 50%. Seropositive patients should receive prophylaxis against toxoplasmosis when the CD4+-lymphocyte count drops below $100/mm^3$.

Culturing for CMV has little role in managing the HIV-1–seropositive asymptomatic patient. However, CMV serology should be obtained. Patients who are CMV-seronegative should be given CMV-negative or leukocyte-reduced cellular blood products only.

All HIV-1–seropositive patients should have an *intermediate-strength purified protein derivative* (PPD) tuberculin skin test unless they have previously been documented to be PPD-positive, have a history of tuberculosis, or have received the bacille Calmette-Guérin (BCG) vaccine. The test result should be interpreted as positive if the area of induration is *greater than 5 mm* (modified Mantoux test). Routine anergy testing is no longer recommended because of its poor predictive value and because prophylaxis in anergic individuals has been relatively ineffective.

Screening for hepatitis B (see Chapter 57) should be performed to determine the need for immunization. *Hepatitis C screening* may help to identify patients who might benefit from therapy. *Hepatitis A* vaccine can be safely given in HIV-infected patients and should be considered in patients without evidence of prior exposure.

Periodic screening of *vitamin B_{12}* levels should be conducted because vitamin B_{12} deficiency is extremely common, especially among those patients with advanced HIV-1 disease and chronic diarrhea.

Glucose-6-phosphate dehydrogenase (G-6-PD) deficiency is a genetic condition that predisposes individuals to hemolysis when they are exposed to oxidant drugs. Dapsone, primaquine, and sulfonamides are examples of oxidant drugs that are frequently used in HIV-1–infected patients. The most common variants of G-6-PD deficiency occur in two forms. The first, Gd^{A-}, occurs in approximately 10% of black men and 1% to 2%

of black women. The second, Gd^{med}, occurs in men from the Mediterranean regions, India, and Southeast Asia. The hemolysis associated with Gd^{med} can be life-threatening, whereas that associated with Gd^{A-} is milder and more self-limited. Individuals at risk should be screened either at baseline or before therapy is initiated with an oxidant drug.

Formal *neuropsychiatric testing* may be needed to document AIDS dementia complex and is best conducted by a technician experienced in the assessment of HIV-1–infected patients.

Women infected with HIV-1 have an elevated risk for pelvic inflammatory disease, *Candida* vaginitis, and cervical dysplasia. This later condition may progress more rapidly as immunodeficiency progresses and can lead to invasive cervical carcinoma. All HIV-1–infected women should have a baseline pelvic examination with Papanicolaou smear. The use of routine colposcopy is controversial, but the test should be performed in women with abnormal Papanicolaou smear results or a history of vaginal condylomata. It should be repeated at least annually in asymptomatic women. More frequent evaluations are recommended in women with abnormalities and with more advanced disease.

Assessing the Degree of Immunocompromise and Prognosis. The *CD4-cell count* is the best single indicator of risk for disease progression. AIDS develops within 1 year in approximately 30% of patients with a CD4-cell count lower than 200/mm^3 if they are left untreated. AIDS develops within 3 years in 50% of patients with a count between 200 and 400. The risk for development of AIDS in untreated individuals with CD4-cell counts above 400 is 15% within 3 years. The CD4-cell count is used to determine when to initiate antiretroviral therapy and PCP prophylaxis. Finally, the CD4-cell count is useful in assessing the response to antiretroviral therapy. The primary care physician must be aware of factors that can affect the CD4-cell count. These include diurnal variation, use of corticosteroids, intercurrent illness, variations between and within laboratories, coinfection with human T-cell lymphotropic virus type I (HTLV-I), and variation in the components of the white blood cell count. The *CD4 percentage* is less subject to variation than is the absolute CD4 cell count and may be a more suitable measure of immune status. A CD4-cell count greater than 500 is believed to be equivalent to a CD4 percentage greater than 29; a count between 200 and 499 is equivalent to a percentage of 14 to 28, and a count lower than 200 is equivalent to a percentage lower than 14.

Quantitative virology (often referred to as *viral load*) is a critical part of the evaluation of an HIV-infected individual. *Plasma HIV-1 RNA levels* provide complementary prognostic information to the CD4+ count. In addition, they are essential in determining the response to antiretroviral therapy. Viral load assays are of several types and include HIV RNA polymerase chain reaction, branched-chain DNA (HIV bDNA), and the nucleic acid sequence-based amplification (NASBA). Commercially available assays can now detect viral loads as low as 20 to 50 copies per milliliter. In general, viral loads are highest (>100,000 copies per milliliter) during the acute retroviral syndrome and during advanced disease. They are often lowest (100 to 100,000 copies per milliliter) during the asymptomatic phase of HIV infection. Many factors can influence viral loads, including intercurrent illness and recent vaccination. In these circumstances, viral load measurement should be deferred for several weeks or months.

Changes in HIV RNA level at the initiation of therapy correlate strongly with prognosis. A threefold change in viral load is necessary to be clinically significant. A more than 10-fold reduction in RNA level is associated with a significant reduction in risk for disease progression. Failure to obtain such a reduction within 8 weeks of initiation should trigger consideration of modifying the regimen. Viremia should continue to decline and will usually reach its nadir by week 16. The speed of viral load decline is affected by the baseline CD4-cell count, initial viral load, potency of the regimen, medication adherence, prior exposure to antiretrovirals, and the presence of opportunistic infections. These individual differences should be considered when the effect of therapy is being monitored. Optimal antiretroviral therapy will push the viral load below 400 to 500 copies per milliliter by 6 months.

Plasma HIV RNA levels and the CD4-cell count should be measured at the time of diagnosis and every 3 to 4 months thereafter. Less frequent evaluation may be reasonable in those with a high CD4-cell count, whereas more frequent evaluation may be reasonable in those with more advanced disease and in whom therapy is being changed.

Other tests have been studied for value in assessing prognosis (*infectious HIV-1 titers*, *syncytium-inducing viral phenotype*, *ratio of CD4 to CD8 lymphocytes*, β_2-*microglobulin*, *neopterin*, and HIV *p24 antigen*). None has proved as useful as the CD4+ and HIV-1 RNA determinations.

Diagnosis of Conditions Indicative of AIDS. As noted earlier, the diagnosis of AIDS depends principally on the identification of an indicator condition or on finding in an HIV-1–seropositive patient a CD4-cell count lower than 200. Although clinical findings help in making a presumptive diagnosis of an indicator condition, a definitive diagnosis depends on laboratory confirmation. Diagnostic modalities include histologic or cytologic study, culturing, serologic study, neuroimaging, and endoscopy.

A few comments are warranted. Candidiasis is diagnosed by direct observation or microscopy, not from culture, because *Candida* is a common contaminant. The diagnosis of HIV encephalopathy is one of exclusion and requires examination of cerebrospinal fluid and neuroimaging to rule out other causes. HIV wasting syndrome is another diagnosis of exclusion, and a search for cancer, tuberculosis, cryptosporidiosis, and other specific forms of enteritis is necessary before HIV wasting syndrome can be diagnosed.

PRINCIPLES OF MANAGEMENT

The major components of therapy are vaccination, antiretroviral agents, prophylaxis and treatment of opportunistic infections, and counseling. Each plays a major role. Although the disease remains invariably fatal pending development of curative therapy, a comprehensive and humanely administered treatment program can do much to preserve quality of life and reduce suffering.

Vaccination

An HIV-1–seropositive adult, especially one whose CD4-cell count is above 200/mm^3, should be vaccinated to the degree possible. However, no live-virus vaccines should be used because

Table 13.2.   Immunizations

VACCINE	INDICATION	FREQUENCY
Pneumovax	All patients without history of prior vaccination	Consider repeat after 5 to 6 years
Hepatitis A vaccine	All patients negative for HAA, especially those with chronic hepatitis B and hepatitis C infections	One series only
Hepatitis B vaccine	Patients negative for HB$_s$Ab or HB$_c$Ab	One series only
Tetanus booster	Patients without tetanus booster in previous 10 years	Every 10 years
Flu vaccine	All patients as clinically appropriate	Yearly

HAA, hepatitis A antibody; HB$_s$Ab, hepatitis B surface antibody; HB$_c$Ab, hepatitis B core antibody.

the patient may already be immunocompromised. All HIV-1–seropositive individuals should receive the *pneumococcal polysaccharide* vaccine, the *influenza vaccine* (yearly), and the *hepatitis B vaccine* (if not already antibody-positive). In addition, a *tetanus—diphtheria* booster should be given to any patient who has not received one within the last 10 years. The immunogenicity of these vaccines in HIV-1 patients has been called into question, especially in more advanced disease (CD4-cell count < 200/mm³). Consequently, vaccination should be conducted as early in HIV-1 infection as possible (Table 13.2).

Initial Antiretroviral Therapy

Candidates for Treatment. Antiretrovitral therapy should be initiated in a patient who exhibits any one of the following characteristics: (a) *signs* or *symptoms* that are attributable to HIV-1 infection; (b) an absolute *CD4-cell count below 500/μL*; or (c) *plasma HIV-1 RNA* concentration (viral load) *above 10,000 copies per mL*. For those HIV-1–infected individuals who have no symptoms attributable to HIV-1, have an absolute CD4-cell count above 500/μL, and a plasma HIV-1 RNA concentration below 10,000 copies per milliliter, antiretroviral therapy may be deferred. However, many experienced clinicians would offer treatment to any HIV-1–seropositive patient with *detectable viremia*. If treatment is deferred, the patient should be carefully followed, with reevaluation of plasma HIV-1 RNA concentration and CD4-cell count every 3 to 6 months. Significant increases in plasma HIV-1 RNA concentration or drops in CD4-cell count should precipitate the initiation of antiretroviral therapy.

Some experienced clinicians believe that all HIV-1–seropositive individuals should be offered antiretroviral therapy regardless of plasma HIV-1 RNA concentration or CD4-cell count. If this approach is taken, careful attention must be paid to assisting the patient in maintaining adherence. This can be a particularly difficult problem if the patient feels healthy before therapy is initiated. The problem is further exacerbated by the complicated regimens currently in use. These regimens can involve taking more than 20 pills per day and may cause multiple side effects. Individuals embarking on antiretroviral therapy must un-

derstand that adherence to the regimen is essential to the ultimate success of therapy.

Choice of Initial Regimen should be based on the goal of reducing and maintaining the plasma HIV-1 RNA concentration as low as possible. This will forestall the development of viral resistance, drug failure, and disease progression. One should bear in mind that the *higher the plasma HIV-1 RNA* concentration before the initiation of therapy, the more potent the antiretroviral regimen must be to suppress it.

Triple-drug regimens involving two nucleoside analogues and at least one protease inhibitor or efavirenz will most likely be required to suppress very high plasma HIV-1 RNA concentrations (>100,000 copies per milliliter) to undetectable levels (currently, <400 to 500 copies per milliliter). In tailoring antiretroviral therapy to individual patients, the clinician should consider several factors. Among these are *overlapping toxicities*, *pharmacokinetic interactions*, *absence of cross-resistance*, and *drug sequencing* that preserves future antiretroviral options.

The most studied *three-drug regimens* used as initial therapy involve *two nucleoside reverse transcriptase inhibitors* (NRTIs) and either a *non-nucleoside reverse transcriptase inhibitor* (NNRTI) or a *protease inhibitor* (PI) (Table 13.3). If a patient's disease is advanced or the plasma HIV-1 RNA concentration is very elevated, a highly active regimen comprising at least one potent PI or efavirenz should be used. If *lamivudine* is used as one of the NRTIs, it should be part of a regimen that will decrease the plasma HIV-1 RNA concentration to a level below detection. Lamivudine resistance mutations develop quickly in the presence of virus replication to cause significant cross-resistance with other NRTIs, including didanosine and zalcitabine. Similarly, nevirapine, delavirdine, and efavirenz, if used as part of an initial regimen, should be used in combinations that will decrease the plasma HIV-1 RNA concentration

Table 13.3.   Recommended Antiretroviral Agents for Treatment of Established HIV Infection

	Column A (PI or NNRTI)	Column B (NRTI)
Preferred	Indinavir	ZDV + ddI
	Nelfinavir	d4T + ddI
	Ritonavir	ZDV + ddC
	Saquinavir-SGC	ZDV + 3TC
	Ritonavir + saquinavir-SGC	d4T + 3TC
	Efavirenz	ddI + 3TC
Alternative	Nevirapine or delavirdine + 2 NRTIs (see above)	
	Abacavir + ZDV + 3TC	
Not generally recommended	2 NRTIs	
	Saquinavir-HGC + 2 NRTIs	
Not recommended	D4T + ZDV	
	ddC + ddI	
	ddC + d4T	
	ddC + 3TC	

PI, protease inhibitor; NRTI, nucleoside reverse transcriptase inhibitor; NNRTI, non-nucleoside reverse transcriptase inhibitor; ZDV, zidovudine; ddI, didanosine; ddC, zalcitabine.

below detection. Resistance to these drugs develops quickly if significant viral replication occurs in their presence.

The NRTI abacavir, in combination with zidovudine and lamivudine, can suppress the viral load to undetectable levels in the majority of antiretroviral therapy-naive patients. This regimen spares the patient the initial use of PIs and NNRTIs with their attendant side effects. However, abacavir is associated with a serious hypersensitivity syndrome, and the durability of viral load suppression associated with its use in a triple-NRTI regimen is uncertain. For these reasons, the Panel on Clinical Practices for Treatment of HIV Infection convened by the Department of Health and Human Services and the Henry J. Kaiser Family Foundation has recommended that PI-containing and efavirenz-containing regimens be considered the preferred regimens.

Subsequent Antiretroviral Therapy

Changes in Antiretroviral Therapy may be necessary because of treatment failure, drug toxicity, or nonadherence. Treatment failure occurs when the viral load significantly increases or the desired reduction is not achieved, when the CD4-cell count decreases significantly, or when clinical progression occurs. If a new regimen fails to achieve a threefold to sixfold reduction in viral load by 4 weeks, or less than a 10-fold reduction by 8 weeks, a change in therapy should be considered. If a regimen achieves the 4- and 8-week goals but fails to suppress the viral load to undetectable levels by 4 to 6 months, the patient's regimen should be reevaluated carefully.

Failure may be for several reasons, including viral resistance to one or more antiretroviral agents, altered absorption or metabolism of one or more agents, altered pharmacokinetics resulting from drug interactions, and poor patient adherence to a regimen. Before antiretroviral therapy is changed, it is important to understand the reason(s) for the failure of the current regimen. This understanding will improve the likelihood of success with future regimens.

Table 13.4 provides representative options for subsequent antiretroviral regimens. When a change in antiretrovirals is being considered, a distinction between drug failure and drug

Table 13.4. Antiretroviral Options for Patients Who Have Failed Therapy

PRIOR REGIMEN	NEW REGIMEN
2 NRTIs +	2 new NRTIs +
nelfinavir	RTV; or IDV; or SQV + RTV; or NNRTI + RTV; or NNRTI + IDV; or APV
ritonavir	SQV + RTV; NFV + NNRTI; or NFV + SQV; or APV
indinavir	SQV + RTV; NFV + NNRTI; or NFV + SQV; or APV
saquinavir	RTV + SQV; or NNRTI + IDV
2 NRTIs + NNRTI	2 new NRTs + a protease inhibitor
2 NRTIs	2 new NRTIs + a protease inhibitor 2 new NRTIs + RTV + SQV 1 new NRTI + 1 NNRTI + a protease inhibitor 2 protease inhibitors + NNRTI
1 NRTI	2 new NRTIs + a protease inhibitor 2 new NRTIs + NNRTI 1 new NRTI + 1 NNRTI + protease inhibitor

RTV, ritonavir; IDV, indinavir; SQV, saquinavir; NVP, nevirapine; NFV, nelfinavir; DLV, delavirdine; APV, amprenavir; NRTI, nucleoside reverse transcriptase inhibitor; NNRTI, non-nucleoside reverse transcriptase inhibitor.

toxicity is essential. In the case of drug toxicity, it is appropriate to substitute one or more antiretrovirals of the same potency and from the same class of agents as the agent suspected of causing the toxicity. In the case of drug failure, a detailed history of current and past antiretroviral agents is essential. In this situation, agents with as little overlapping resistance as possible should be sought. In a three-drug regimen, at least two and preferably three new agents should be used. As the patient becomes more "drug-experienced," the task of minimizing overlapping resistance becomes more difficult, and one must rely extensively on plasma viral load and CD4-cell count to inform drug choices.

Evaluating Drug Resistance. Viral genotyping or phenotyping may prove useful when drug choices are made in initial therapy or treatment failure. However, these technologies have significant technical limitations and are not widely available for clinical use. They assess only the predominant viral quasispecies circulating in plasma. Resistant variants selected by drug pressure may quickly contract to a level below the threshold of detection in plasma when selective pressure is removed. Resistant variants remain and will return to detectable levels quickly if selection pressure is reapplied.

The value of viral resistance testing in the clinical management of HIV infection has yet to be fully established. Each assay and assay service requires standardization and validation. The interpretation of resistance assays requires expert input.

Special Considerations

Several situations warrant specific comment with regard to the use of antiretroviral therapy: primary infection, postexposure prophylaxis, and perinatal transmission.

Primary Infection may represent an opportunity to alter the course of HIV-1 disease significantly for an infected individual. Short-term improvements in viral load and CD4-cell count have been reported when antiretroviral therapy is given during primary infection, but these data are limited. Many experts recommend antiretroviral therapy for all patients who demonstrate laboratory evidence of primary infection. This evidence includes detectable HIV RNA in plasma by either the polymerase chain reaction or the branched-chain DNA method together with a negative or indeterminate result of an HIV antibody test. If a clinical trial for acute infection is unavailable or is declined by the patient, a regimen may be selected from the options available for treating established infection (Table 13.3). This regimen should be maintained indefinitely pending the availability of further information.

Postexposure Prophylaxis. The use of antiretroviral agents to prevent transmission resulting from high-risk exposures in the *occupational setting* has been widely accepted for several years. Guidelines governing the use of these agents for this purpose should be followed. The risk for seroconversion is very low. In a survey of 1,103 health care workers with documented percutaneous exposure, only four (0.36%) had undergone seroconversion, and none of those with nonintact skin or mucous membrane exposure had undergone seroconversion. About one third of exposed persons took zidovudine after exposure; seroconversion occurred in one despite zidovudine prophylaxis. No data from placebo-controlled, randomized trials are available.

In their absence, a consensus treatment protocol has been established as part of a multicenter open study. Data are pending.

In the absence of definitive data, the decision to administer antiretroviral prophylaxis must be individualized and shared with the patient. In counseling the patient, one should take into account the severity of the exposure, the very low risk for seroconversion, the fact that such therapy does not provide absolute protection, the high incidence of drug side effects, and the need for frequent monitoring.

Antiretroviral prophylaxis for *high-risk sexual exposures* is being studied. No guidelines for the use of antiretrovirals in this setting are currently available. However, the CDC is developing recommendations. Information pertaining to the effectiveness, safety, and tolerability of regimens used for postexposure prophylaxis is limited.

Preventing Perinatal Transmission. Zidovudine and nevirapine have been shown to decrease the likelihood of HIV-1 transmission significantly in the perinatal setting. At the present time, no other antiretrovirals have been demonstrated to reduce the likelihood of vertical HIV-1 transmission. Therefore, zidovudine, nevirapine, or both should be included as a component of any antiretroviral regimen used during pregnancy whenever possible.

Opportunistic Infection: Prophylaxis and Treatment

Prophylaxis and prompt treatment of opportunistic infection can significantly lessen disease morbidity and the need for hospitalization. Several of the most common infections will be discussed here. These include PCP, tuberculosis, toxoplasmosis, and candidiasis.

Pneumocystis carinii. **Pneumonia** is the most common infection in HIV-1–infected adults. Adults with CD4-cell counts below 200 (or <14% of total lymphocytes) or a history of oropharyngeal candidiasis should receive PCP prophylaxis. Several prophylaxis regimens are available. *Trimethoprim/sulfamethoxazole* (TMS) is the preferred agent. One double-strength tablet per day is recommended. However, one single-strength tablet per day is also effective and may be better tolerated. TMS at a dose of one double-strength tablet per day confers cross-protection against *T. gondii* and some common respiratory bacterial pathogens. For most patients, it is well tolerated, but a substantial proportion of patients expereince adverse reactions, primarily fever and rash, so that desensitization or consideration of an alternative means of PCP prophylaxis is necessary. Desensitization to TMS can be employed successfully in up to 70% of patients who experience these reactions.

Dapsone (50 to 100 mg once daily) is an effective prophylactic agent for PCP. This is a very inexpensive drug with a long half-life. Less frequent dosing may be effective, but such dosing schemes may decrease overall adherence.

Aerosolized pentamidine (300 mg once every 4 weeks via a Respirgard II nebulizer) has also been shown to be effective in preventing PCP, although not quite to the same degree as TMS. When breakthroughs occur, the upper lobe is predominantly affected. The dissemination of *Pneumocystis carinii* to other tissues has been reported. Individuals with active tuberculosis should not receive aerosolized pentamidine because it greatly increases the risk for tuberculosis among health care providers administering the therapy.

Atovaquone (1,500 mg each day) is comparable to aerosolized pentamidine in effectiveness but is substantially more expensive.

Workup for an HIV-1 patient with a CD4-cell count below 200 and new respiratory symptoms includes a *chest radiograph* and an *induced sputum*. The sputum should be sent for *Gram's stain*, routine *culture*, *mycobacterial stain* and *culture*, *fungal wet preparation* and *culture*, and *immunofluorescent stain* for *Pneumocystis carinii*. *Oximetry* and *arterial blood gases* may provide additional information. If the radiograph reveals a bilateral interstitial infiltrate and the sputum Gram's stain is not diagnostic of a specific etiology, the patient should be treated presumptively for PCP pending the results of immunofluorescent stains. If the patient appears clinically stable and is not in respiratory distress, treatment can be initiated on an outpatient basis. Careful follow-up is essential.

Effective *oral therapies* for PCP include *TMS, dapsone/trimethoprim, atovaquone,* and *clindamycin/primaquine*. One of the most effective and easily tolerated of these regimens is dapsone (75 to 100 mg/d in an average-sized adult) combined with trimethoprim (15 mg/kg daily in three or four divided doses). TMS (15 mg/kg daily by trimethoprim content in three or four divided doses) is effective but causes more adverse reactions than does dapsone/trimethoprim. Clindamycin/primaquine may be used in patients who are unable to tolerate dapsone/trimethoprim or TMS. G-6-PD–, Gd^{med}-deficient patients should not receive dapsone, TMS, or primaquine. Effective IV therapies include TMS, trimetrexate, and *pentamidine*.

Oral corticosteroid therapy should be used when a significant alveolar–arterial oxygen gradient (>30 mm Hg) is present, provided it is started within 72 hours of initiating antibiotic treatment. Later therapy has not been shown to improve outcome. If a patient is in respiratory distress or has a significant alveolar–arterial gradient, hospitalization should be considered.

Tuberculosis and Atypical Mycobacteria. All seropositive individuals whose PPD status is unknown should have a *5-TU (tuberculin units) PPD* planted. The test result is considered positive in HIV-1 individuals if *5 mm or more of induration* develops (see Chapter 38). Several regimens may be used for prophylaxis of tuberculosis in this setting. These include *isoniazid* (300 mg each day with 50 mg of pyridoxine for 9 months, or 900 mg with 100 mg of pyridoxine given twice weekly for 9 months) and *rifampin* (600 mg given with 20 mg of pyrazinamide per kilogram daily for 2 months). Many authorities suggest that anergic individuals with a history of PPD positivity also should receive a course of isoniazid.

As noted above, the use of aerosolized pentamidine may induce coughing and thereby facilitate transmission of undiagnosed pulmonary tuberculosis from HIV-1–infected patients to persons sharing the same breathing space during or after treatment. The potential for transmission of tuberculosis depends on the prevalence of tubercular infection in the HIV-1–infected population being served and on such factors as room ventilation, the number of infectious droplet nuclei generated by the patient, and duration of exposure. Specially ventilated facilities are required for the drug to be delivered safely.

The development of *active tuberculosis* in the HIV patient is a problem made even more serious because of the associated risk for *multiple drug-resistant strains*. Such patients require very careful attention to respiratory precautions (see Chapter 49).

Prophylaxis of *Mycobacterium avium* complex (MAC) infection should be instituted for those with CD4-cell counts below 50/mm³. *Clarithromycin* (500 mg each day) and *azithromycin* (1,200 mg given once each week) are the preferred prophylactic agents. In addition to their prophylactic activity against MAC, clarithromycin and azithromycin may provide protection against respiratory bacterial infections.

Treatment of MAC infection requires multiple drugs. One of the most effective regimens comprises clarithromycin (500 mg given every 12 hours) and ethambutol (15 mg/kg of body weight given daily) with or without rifabutin (300 mg daily). Azithromycin may be substituted for clarithromycin at a dose of 500 to 600 mg daily.

Toxoplasmosis. TMS (*one single-strength tablet each day or one double-strength tablet three times each week*) or *dapsone/pyrimethamine* (50 mg of *dapsone* per day + 50 mg of *pyrimethamine* per week + 25 mg of *folinic acid* per week, or 200 mg of *dapsone* per week + 75 mg of *pyrimethamine* per week + 25 mg of *folinic acid* per week) appears to provide effective chemoprophylaxis in patients seropositive for *T. gondii* who have CD4-cell counts below 100/mm³. For those individuals who are not seropositive, thorough cooking of meat and careful hand washing after contact with raw meat should be emphasized. Further, cat owners should clean litter boxes while wearing gloves and practice careful hand washing afterward or have another person perform this chore. Patients who are gardeners should be encouraged to use gloves while enjoying this pastime. Patients with encephalitis require hospitalization for the initiation of sulfadiazine, pyrimethamine, and leukovorin (100- to 200-mg loading dose of *pyrimethamine*, then 50 to 100 mg daily + 10 mg of *folinic acid* daily PO + 4 to 8 g of *sulfadiazine* or *trisulfapyrimidine* daily for at least 6 weeks). Alternative regimens involving the use of *pyrimethamine* and *folinic acid* with either *clindamycin, azithromycin, clarithromycin,* or *atovaquone* can also be used.

Candida infection occurs frequently in HIV-1–infected individuals, especially as the CD4-cell count drops below 200/mm³. Thrush, esophageal candidiasis, and vaginitis are the most common forms of this infection. Although prophylaxis of thrush is not routinely recommended, occasionally long-term maintenance therapy is required to stem recurrent infections. Topical agents for *oral candidiasis* are effective and well tolerated. One 10-mg *clotrimazole troche* held in the mouth for 15 to 30 minutes three times each day is effective. *Chlorhexidine gluconate* may be useful, especially among patients with significant gingivitis and periodontitis. *Nystatin* is available in either an oral suspension or a pastille. Nystatin oral pastilles (200,000 U, one pastille taken three times each day) or nystatin suspension (100,000 U/mL, swish-and-swallow 15 mL six times a day) can also be used.

Esophageal candidiasis is treated with systemic therapy. *Fluconazole* (200 mg given once daily for 2 to 3 weeks) is one of the most effective therapies. *Itraconazole* (100 to 200 mg given twice daily, or a 100- to 200-mg oral suspension given once daily) may also be used for this purpose. Amphotericin B with or without *flucytosine* may be required for infections unresponsive to either fluconazole or itraconazole.

Vulvovaginal candidiasis is a common problem for HIV-1–infected women. It tends to occur earlier in HIV-1 infection than does oral candidiasis. Again, several agents are available for *prophylaxis*: intravaginal *miconazole* suppository (200 mg taken for 3 days or 2% cream taken for 7 days), *clotrimazole* (1% cream taken for 7 to 14 days, 100-mg tablets taken daily for 7 days, 100-mg tablets taken twice daily for 3 days, or 500 mg taken once), and *fluconazole* (150-mg tablet given orally once). Maintenance therapy may be required to prevent frequent relapse (100 mg of *ketoconazole* given daily, 50 to 100 mg of *fluconazole* given daily, or 200 mg of *fluconazole* given weekly).

Cytomegalovirus. *Ganciclovir, foscarnet, cidofovir,* and *fomivirsen* are the drugs approved for the treatment of *CMV retinitis. Foscarnet (60 mg/kg IV every 8 hours or 90 mg/kg IV every 12 hours for 14 to 21 days)* has been shown to be superior to *ganciclovir* in patients with normal renal function. For patients with impaired renal function, *ganciclovir* (5 mg/kg IV twice daily for 14 to 21 days) is preferred. However, granulocyte counts have to be monitored closely because both cause granulocytopenia. It should be noted that data suggest that alternating or combining *ganciclovir* and *foscarnet* may be less toxic and more active against CMV than giving foscarnet alone. An intraocular *ganciclovir* release device (*Vitrasert*) can also be used for local treatment. *Cidofovir* (5mg/kg IV once weekly for 2 weeks followed by 5 mg/kg IV every 2 weeks; 2 g of probenecid should be given 3 hours before each dose and 1 g PO at 2 and 8 hours after each dose) and *fomivirsen* (330 mg by intravitreal injection on day 1 and day 15, then monthly) may also be used but should not be considered as first-line therapy.

Extraocular CMV disease may be treated with *ganciclovir* and *foscarnet* at doses similar to those used for ocular disease. In general, induction therapy is generally given for a longer period (3 to 6 weeks) in extraocular disease. Maintenance therapy should be considered, especially after reinduction and relapse.

Counseling

Counseling the HIV-1–infected patient involves many aspects, including personal, psychosocial, and financial issues. Assisting patients in understanding and accepting the changes in their sense of self and in life plans and goals is essential to successful care. It is particularly important to educate individuals as much as possible about the disease and its treatment; this helps them regain some sense of control. It is particularly helpful to focus on what patients can do rather than on what is out of their control. Giving accurate information on current estimates of *prognosis* is essential and can be done without destroying hope, especially in view of the advances in therapy and survival.

The *risk for suicide* is increased 30- to 60-fold in HIV-1 patients, especially early in the illness when the diagnosis is first known and in the very late stages of the disease when delirium may be present. Most patients who eventually commit suicide talk of it beforehand to friends and health care workers. Prevention through careful patient preparation at the time of diagnosis and screening for suicidality (see Chapter 227) should be an intrinsic part of the counseling and supportive effort.

It is essential to review *measures for safe sex* with HIV-1–seropositive individuals and their partners. These steps are useful in preventing transmission not only of HIV-1 infection but also of other sexually transmitted diseases. This is extremely important for the HIV-1–infected individual.

Understanding the patient's existing *support network* and helping the patient develop additional supports can be very important. It is often helpful if the patient can link up with infected peers to share experiences and concerns; this helps to minimize isolation, loneliness, and fear.

In many cities, special *community resources* are now available to aid HIV-1–infected patients with legal, social, and financial issues pertaining to the infection. It is important for every physician who cares for such patients to identify these resources.

Finally, it is essential to *discuss death* and *dying* with each patient in an open manner. Often, these issues are shunned by others in the patient's support network. The value of being able to obtain honest and direct answers about death and dying from one's physician cannot be underestimated. During these discussions, the physician and patient should strive to come to a common understanding of the patient's wishes regarding this very important issue.

INDICATIONS FOR ADMISSION AND CONSULTATION

Although outpatient care is preferred for many elements of HIV-1 management, in several instances, prompt hospitalization is essential. The patient with signs or symptoms suggestive of significant pulmonary, CNS, or disseminated infection (especially severe *Pneumocystis* pneumonia, tuberculosis, atypical mycobacterial infection, syphilis, toxoplasmosis, histoplasmosis, coccidioidomycosis, cryptococcosis, or CMV infection) requires prompt hospital admission and infectious disease consultation. Outpatient treatment may be possible later, even for administration of parenteral therapy, but treatment should be initiated in the hospital. Also requiring immediate hospitalization is the suicidal patient, particularly one who admits to having made specific plans for suicide. Urgent psychiatric consultation is essential. When appropriate, referral for *hospice care* should be considered. At this stage of illness, hospital admissions should be kept to a minimum except as needed for purposes of providing comfort.

ANNOTATED BIBLIOGRAPHY

Buehler JW, Ward JW. A new definition for AIDS surveillance. Ann Intern Med 1993;118:390. (*An editorial on the implications of the expanded surveillance definition.*)

Carpenter CCJ, Fischl MA, Hammer SM, et al. Antiretroviral therapy for HIV infection in 1996: recommendations of an international panel. International AIDS Society—USA. JAMA 1996;276:146. (*Recommendations for initiation of antiviral therapy, including issues related to acute infection, maternal-to-infant transmission, and occupational exposure.*)

Carpenter CCJ, Fischl MA, Hammer SM, et al. Antiretroviral therapy for HIV infection in 1997: updated recommendations of the International AIDS Society—USA Panel. JAMA 1997;277:1962. (*Presents a stronger rationale for earlier initiation of antiviral therapy.*)

Cohen M. Natural history of HIV infection in women. Obstet Gynecol Clin North Am 1997;24:743. (*Phases of the natural history of HIV infection in women are reviewed, including opportunities for prevention, acute infection, pathogenesis, therapeutic plans, and terminal care.*)

Connor EM, Sperling RS, Gelber R, et al. Reduction of maternal-fetal transmission of human immunodeficiency virus type 1 with zidovudine treatment. N Engl J Med 1994;331:1173. (*Risk reduced by two thirds.*)

Coopman SA, Johnson RA, Platt R, et al. Cutaneous disease and drug reactions in HIV infection. N Engl J Med 1993;328:1670. (*Very high incidence of cutaneous reactions noted, especially drug reactions, and these increase as immune function worsens.*)

Guidelines for use of antiretroviral agents in HIV-infected adults. MMWR Morb Mortal Wkly Rep 1998;47(RR-05). (*Authoritative recommendations.*)

Ho DD, Neumann AU, Perelson AS, et al. Rapid turnover of plasma virions and CD4 lymphocytes in HIV-1 infection. Nature 1995;373:123. (*Documents exponential decrease in viral load and increase in CD4-cell count with PIs.*)

Hollander H. Neurologic and psychiatric manifestations of HIV disease. J Gen Intern Med 1991;6(1S):S24. (*Helpful summary and review.*)

Hughes MD, Johnson VA, Hirsch MS, et al. Monitoring plasma HIV-1 RNA levels in addition to CD4+-lymphocyte count improves assessment of antiretroviral therapeutic response. Ann Intern Med 1997;1126:929. (*Documents impact of HIV-1 RNA measurement.*)

Imrie A, Beveridge A, Genn W, et al. Transmission of human immunodeficiency virus type 1 resistant to nevirapine and zidovudine. J Infect Dis 1997;175:1502. (*Notable case report.*)

Mellors JW, Rinaldo CR Jr., Gupta P, et al. Prognosis in HIV-1 infection predicted by the quantity of virus in plasma. Science 1996;272:1167. (*Documents superiority of viral load over CD4-cell counts for predicting prognosis.*)

Navia BA, Jordan BD, Price RW. The AIDS dementia complex. I: Clinical features. Ann Neurol 1986;19:517. (*An important and debilitating accompaniment of advanced disease that must be distinguished from more treatable forms of CNS deterioration.*)

O'Brien WA, Hartigan PM, Martin D, et al. Changes in plasma HIV-1 RNA and CD4+ lymphocyte counts and the risk of progression to AIDS. N Engl J Med 1996;334:426. (*Treatment-induced changes in HIV-1 RNA and CD4-cell counts are valid predictors of prognosis.*)

Pierce M, Crampton S, Henry D, et al. A randomized trial of clarithromycin as prophylaxis against disseminated *Mycobacterium avium* complex infection in patients with advanced acquired immunodeficiency syndrome. N Engl J Med 1996;335:384. (*This randomized clinical trial was stopped when infection developed in 16% of control subjects and 6% of those receiving clarithromycin.*)

Prevention and treatment of tuberculosis among patients infected with human immunodeficiency virus: principles of therapy and revised recommendations. MMWR Morb Mortal Wkly Rep 1998;47(RR-20). (*Authoritative recommendations.*)

Public Health Service guidelines for the management of health-care worker exposures to HIV and recommendations for postexposure prophylaxis. MMWR Morb Mortal Wkly Rep 1998;47(RR-07). (*Authoritative recommendations.*)

Report of NIH panel to define principles of therapy of HIV infection. MMWR Morb Mortal Wkly Rep 1998;47(RR-05). (*Authoritative recommendations.*)

Revised classification system for HIV infection and expanded surveillance case definition for AIDS among adolescents and adults, 1993. MMWR Morb Mortal Wkly Rep 1992;41(RR-17):1. (*Current CDC criteria for the diagnosis and classification of HIV infection and AIDS.*)

Schafer A, Friedman W, Mielke M, et al. The increased frequency of cervical dysplasia—neoplasia in women infected with the human immunodeficiency virus is related to the degree of immunosuppression. Am J Obstet Gynecol 1991;164:593. (*An example of a unique presentation of AIDS in women and its relation to CD4-cell counts.*)

Schneider MM, Hoepelman AI, Eeftinck Schattenkerk JK, et al. Controlled trial of aerosolized pentamidine or trimethoprim-sulfamethoxazole as primary prophylaxis against *Pneumocystis carnii* pneumonia in patients with human immunodeficiency virus infection. N Engl J Med 1992;327:1836. (*TMS proved superior but was not always well tolerated.*)

Studies of Ocular Complications of AIDS Research Group, in collaboration with the AIDS Clinical Trials Group. Mortality in patients with the acquired immunodeficiency syndrome treated with either foscarnet or ganciclovir for cytomegalovirus retinitis. N Engl J Med 1992;326:213. (*Foscarnet is more effective but not as well tolerated.*)

The National Institutes of Health/University of California Expert Panel for Corticosteroids as Adjunctive Therapy for Pneumocystis Pneumonia. Consensus statement on the use of corticosteroids as adjunctive therapy for *Pneumocystis* pneumonia in the acquired immunodeficiency syndrome. N Engl J Med 1990;323:1500. (*Worthwhile if used within the first 72 hours.*)

Tokars JI, Marcus R, Culver DH, et al. Surveillance of HIV infection and zidovudine use among health care workers after occupational exposure to HIV-infected blood. Ann Intern Med 1993;118:913. (*Risk for seroconversion with percutaneous exposure was 0.36%, with mucous membrane exposure zero, and with skin exposure zero; zidovudine was not fully protective.*)

USPHS/IDSA guidelines for the prevention of opportunistic infections in persons infected with human immunodeficiency virus, 1997. MMWR Morb Mortal Wkly Rep 1997;46(RR-12).

Volberding PA, et al. Zidovudine in asymptomatic human immunodeficiency virus infection. A controlled trial in persons with fewer than 500 CD4-positive cells per cubic millimeter. N Engl J Med 1990; 322:941. (*Found safe and effective, although effect on survival is not addressed.*)

3

Cardiovascular Problems

14
Screening for Hypertension
KATHARINE K. TREADWAY

Hypertension can justifiably be considered the most significant condition the practitioner concerned with health maintenance will meet in clinical practice. The size of the affected population is staggering—20% of adults in the United States have systolic pressures greater than 160 mm Hg or diastolic pressures greater than 95 mm Hg. Among the elderly, the prevalence is even greater. Excess morbidity and mortality caused by hypertension have been well documented. Over the past 30 years, efforts to educate both physicians and the general public about the importance of identifying and treating high blood pressure and the improved options for treatment have resulted in improved blood pressure control and a significant decrease in morbidity and mortality from cardiovascular disease and stroke. Despite this, the percentage of Americans who are aware of and who are adequately treated for their hypertension has actually declined during this decade.

Evaluation and management of the identified hypertensive patient are presented in Chapters 19 and 26. This chapter reviews the epidemiology of high blood pressure, its importance as a risk factor, its measurement, and the evidence for the effectiveness of therapy.

EPIDEMIOLOGY AND RISK FACTORS

Depending on the definition of hypertension used, 15% to 25% of the U.S. population is considered hypertensive. Of those who are hypertensive, approximately 70% fall into the so-called stage I category (see below). Most estimates of the prevalence of hypertension derive from the National Health and Nutrition Examination Surveys of the early 1960s and late 1970s. Subsequent smaller surveys have both substantiated its prevalence and confirmed that age, race, and sex significantly affect prevalence.

Age. Systolic and diastolic blood pressures rise steadily with age into the fifth and sixth decades, when the increase levels off. By then, the prevalence of hypertension approaches 50%. The complication risk also rises steadily with age. The prevalence of hypertension (systolic at least 160 mm Hg or diastolic at least 95 mm Hg) among persons aged 25 to 34 is approximately 5%. By age 55 to 64, it has risen to 35% to 40%. Using the definitions proposed by the Joint National Committee on Detection, Evaluation and Treatment of High Blood Pressure's sixth report, the prevalence is considerably higher.

Gender. Males in all age groups have a higher prevalence of hypertension than females. In the third and fourth decades, it is more than twice as common among men as among women. The ratio decreases with advancing age, so that by age 60 there is only a slight male predominance. Men have substantially higher complication rates than women. The Framingham Study demonstrated that for the major complications of hypertension, risk in mildly hypertensive women equals that of normotensive men. The postulated mechanisms for this reduced risk in women include the beneficial effects of estrogen on vasculature and the different hemodynamic profile of premenopausal hypertensive women, which includes a lower peripheral resistance and higher cardiac output. After menopause, estrogen levels fall, the hemodynamic profile shifts to one of high peripheral resistance and normal cardiac output, and by age 70 the incidences of stroke and coronary disease in women approach those of men.

Race. There is a marked *increase* in prevalence of hypertension among *African-Americans*. Compared with whites, the overall prevalence ratio is 2:1; it is higher in young adults and lower in the elderly. Severe hypertension occurs nearly five times more often than in whites. In addition, the complication rate for any given blood pressure is significantly higher. For example, compared with white hypertensives, African-Americans have an 80% higher mortality from stroke, a 50% higher mortality from heart disease, and a 320% higher incidence of end-stage renal failure. Whether this represents as yet undefined differences in the underlying physiology of hypertension in African-Americans or whether this represents inadequate access to medical care is unclear, although it is likely that both factors play a role.

Obesity. Prevalence increases in obese patients, as does the prevalence of hyperlipidemia and type 2 diabetes mellitus. The association of these three conditions has been attributed to the presence of relative insulin resistance, which may cause hypertension in some patients (see Chapter 19). Data from the Nurses' Study demonstrates that women who gain more than 20 pounds after age 18 have a fivefold increase in the risk of developing hypertension compared with those who did not gain weight. Conversely, women who were at higher body mass index levels at age 18 and lost 5 to 10 pounds had about half the risk of developing hypertension.

Other Risk Factors. Hypertension is more likely to occur in patients with a *positive family history*. It is increasingly clear that hypertension may be caused by a variety of genetic mutations and that there are probably several different genetic forms of hypertension. In addition, there is undoubtedly significant interplay with the environment. *Increased salt intake* correlates with increased prevalence in large populations, though not in individuals. This suggests differing individual susceptibilities to the effects of high salt intake, and indeed there are clearly salt-sensitive hypertensives, although at present we have no simple way of identifying them. An individual's prior or current salt intake, per se, is not a predictor of blood pressure level. *Alcohol* intake in excess of 2 ounces per day is linked to hypertension. The mechanism of *alcohol-induced hypertension* appears to be related to alcohol's ability to stimulate the release of corticotropin-releasing factor from the hypothalamus, which in turn increases central nervous system sympathetic activity and causes a rise in blood pressure. *Sedentary life-style* has been associated with an increase in the risk of developing hypertension. The role of *psychological stress* and its concomitant sympathetic stimulation appears to be variable and possibly a function of underlying differences in susceptibility. *Cigarette smoking*, an important risk factor in its own right, is not positively associated with increased blood pressure, but hypertensive smokers are at significantly greater risk to develop cardiovascular complications than are hypertensive nonsmokers.

HYPERTENSION AS A RISK FACTOR FOR CARDIOVASCULAR MORBIDITY AND MORTALITY

The complications of hypertension may be divided into *hypertensive risks*—those that result directly from the presence of high blood pressure—and *atherosclerotic risks*—those for which hypertension is one of several risk factors. The major hypertensive complications are *stroke, congestive heart failure, renal failure, and left ventricular hypertrophy*. The atherosclerotic complications are coronary artery disease, cerebrovascular disease, and peripheral vascular disease. Although the risk of all these complications rises gradually over all levels of blood pressure, increasing by about 30% for every 10 mm Hg rise in pressure, the risk in a given individual for developing atherosclerotic complications varies enormously, depending on what other risk factors are present. It is important to understand that diastolic and systolic pressures are equally predictive of risk.

Although hypertension remains one of the principal atherosclerotic risk factors for development of coronary artery disease, the additive effects from smoking, hypercholesterolemia, glucose intolerance, and left ventricular hypertrophy are also extremely important (see Chapters 15, 54, and 93). For example, the chance of a 40-year-old man with moderate hyperten-

sion alone developing ischemic heart disease over an 8-year period is about 5%, but it rises to 70% if all coronary risk factors are present. The Framingham study has also shown hypertension to be the dominant predictor of congestive heart failure, with a sixfold increase in incidence among hypertensives.

NATURAL HISTORY OF HYPERTENSION AND EFFECTIVENESS OF THERAPY

Natural History. With rare exceptions, hypertension is an *asymptomatic* disease. The natural history is one of *insidious* damage that is most often clinically silent for a decade or more. It typically begins between the ages of 35 and 55, often preceded by a period of lability. Those patients with blood pressures at the high end of normal (135 to 140/85 to 90) are far more likely to develop hypertension than those with lower pressures. About 70% of hypertensives will fall into stage I, although this group accounts for something over 50% of the excess cardiovascular mortality attributable to hypertension. About 20% of stage I hypertensives will progress to higher stages if left untreated and about 1% will go on to develop malignant hypertension. About 15% to 30% will become spontaneously normotensive, although we have no way to identify in which patients this will occur.

Effectiveness of Treatment. Convincing evidence for vigorous *early treatment* of hypertension began to appear 25 years ago with publication of the landmark Veterans Administration Cooperative Study, the first large-scale, placebo-controlled, randomized, prospective study. It involved patients with *moderate to severe hypertension* and found that rates of major nonfatal events and cardiovascular death fell with treatment more than 10-fold among those with severe hypertension and 3-fold among those with moderate pressure elevations. Treatment was most effective in reducing risks of stroke and congestive heart failure.

Later randomized studies expanded these initial findings, and meta-analyses of such studies confirmed the efficacy of treatment and expanded the spectrum of illness to those with mild to moderate hypertension. A meta-analysis of nine observational studies estimated that for each 5-mm Hg increase in blood pressure, the risk of stroke increases approximately 34% and the risk of coronary disease by about 21%. In a companion meta-analysis of 14 randomized controlled trials of antihypertensive therapy, in which blood pressure was lowered in the treatment group by about 5 to 6 mm Hg more than in the control group, the incidence of stroke was reduced by 42% and that of coronary disease by 14%. The reason for the less than predicted benefit in reducing the incidence of coronary events is not clear, although many theories have been proposed. One suggestion, that the trials lasted too short a time to demonstrate full benefit in the reduction of coronary disease, has gained some credence with improved benefit demonstrated in the MRFIT trial after 10 years.

Findings from other studies indicate that benefit from blood pressure reduction increases with severity of blood pressure elevation, African-Americans and those older than 50 years of age benefit most, and young white women benefit least. This difference in benefit can be explained by the lower level of overall cardiovascular risk in young white women. Treating *systolic hypertension* in the elderly significantly lowers the risk of stroke and coronary disease. Finally, lowering blood pressure also reduces the incidence of congestive heart failure and reduces the progression of renal disease.

Although the benefits of treating hypertension appear clear, it is interesting to note that mildly hypertensive patients whose blood pressure spontaneously reverts to normal seem to do even better than those whose pressure is lowered by medication. This finding was first noted in the landmark Australian study of mild hypertensives, in which almost half of the placebo group became spontaneously normotensive over the 5-year period of the study. Such patients had fewer complications than those who achieved a similar level of blood pressure with medication.

In sum, the benefit of lowering blood pressure is real and particularly important as regards incidence of stroke. Reduction in rate of coronary events is also achieved, though to a lesser extent. In most studies, the *benefit* from treatment of hypertension appears *within 2 to 3 years of initiation of therapy*.

Decision to Treat. The decision to initiate pharmacologic therapy is based on an estimate of *overall cardiovascular risk*. Such an estimate requires consideration not only of blood pressure but also of age, race, sex, smoking, hypercholesterolemia, diabetes, and family history of hypertensive or cardiac complications and the presence or absence of target-organ damage. The costs from medical therapy are weighed against the expected benefits, an especially important determination in young patients with mild uncomplicated disease (see Chapter 26).

SCREENING METHODS

Measurement of Blood Pressure. Blood pressure should be measured at each health encounter. Although the process of identifying patients with hypertension seems relatively straightforward, there are numerous pitfalls and chances for error in measuring blood pressure that can be avoided by proper screening protocol. All personnel responsible for recording blood pressures should be aware of the sources of measurement error. Effective screening technique includes having the patient *rest for 5 minutes* before measurement is made. The pressure should be taken in both arms while the patient is *seated comfortably with back and arm supported. Two or more readings* are taken, separated by 2 minutes. If these readings differ by more than 5 mm Hg, then *additional readings* should be taken. Patients should refrain from smoking or drinking a caffeinated beverage at least 30 minutes before a determination. Note should be made if the patient is cold, anxious, has a full bladder, or has recently exercised, smoked, or had caffeine, because any of these factors may transiently elevate pressure.

Reliable equipment and its proper use are is important. *Mercury bulb manometers* are best; *aneroid manometers*, if used, should be checked and recalibrated regularly. The cuff should be placed as high on the arm as possible and the arm supported and positioned at *heart level* while the pressure is taken. *Cuff size* must be adequate to avoid falsely elevated readings. The *width* of the cuff's inflatable bladder should be greater than *two thirds* the arm width and its *length* greater than *two thirds* the arm *circumference*. Using a standard size cuff in a muscular or obese adult will result in a reading that is as much as 10 mm Hg higher than the true blood pressure. To avoid this error, a large adult-sized cuff should be used in such patients. Although most auscultate using the diaphragm of the stethoscope, the *bell* is recommended for its superior transmission of the low-pitched sounds that characterize the last of the Korotkoff sounds (see Chapter 19).

Systolic pressure is defined as the point at which sound is first heard (Korotkoff 1). *Diastolic pressure* is taken at the point at which sound *disappears* (Korotkoff 5) rather than when it changes in quality (Korotkoff 4). The *averages* of two successive measurements in each arm are recorded. Variability of blood pressure may be related to recent physical activity, emotional state, or body position. Although such factors must be kept in mind, the predictive value of the "casual" blood pressure determination has been validated. Nonetheless, the diagnosis of hypertension must never be made on the basis of a single reading but rather should be based on multiple determinations taken over several visits. A check of the blood pressure should be a routine component of every patient visit, regardless of the presenting complaint (see Chapter 19).

CONCLUSIONS AND RECOMMENDATIONS

- Hypertension is an extremely common condition and the strongest predictor of subsequent cardiovascular and cerebrovascular morbidity and mortality. It is usually asymptomatic, with insidious damage to target organs occurring.
- A large segment of the hypertensive population will benefit from treatment, showing significant reductions in rates of stroke, congestive heart failure, renal failure, and coronary disease. Absolute risk reduction from treatment is a function of pretreatment risk.
- Detection is simple, reliable, and inexpensive. All adults should be screened for hypertension. Its detection and treatment are among the foremost responsibilities of the primary care physician (see also Chapter 19 for diagnostic evaluation and Chapter 26 for treatment).

ANNOTATED BIBLIOGRAPHY

Collin R, Peto R, MacMahon S, et al. Blood pressure, stroke, and coronary disease. Part 2. Short-term reductions in blood pressure: overview of randomized drug trials in their epidemiological context. Lancet 1990;335:827. (*Important meta-analysis of randomized trials demonstrating significant reductions in risk of stroke and coronary disease.*)

Freis ED. Should mild hypertension be treated? N Engl J Med 1982;307:306. (*Reviews the evidence and recommends treatment for patients with borderline or mild hypertension and other risk factors, but withholding of drug therapy from those without other risk factors.*)

Frohlich ED, Grim C, Labarthe DR, et al. Report of a special task force appointed by the Steering Committee, American Heart Association: recommendations for human blood pressure determinations by sphygmomanometers. Hypertension 1988;11:209A. (*Consensus panel recommendations on technique.*)

Gueyffier F, Boutitie F, Boissel J, et al. Effect of anti-hypertensive drug treatment on cardiovascular outcomes in men and women. Ann Intern Med 1997;126:761. (*Major meta-analysis of randomized controlled trials; treatment benefit the same for men and women and a function of pretreatment cardiovascular risk.*)

Huang Z, Willet WC, Manson J, et al. Body weight, weight change and risk for hypertension in women. Ann Intern Med 1998;128:81. (*Obesity is a major risk factor.*)

Hypertension Detection Follow-Up Program Cooperative Group. The effect of treatment on mortality in "mild" hypertension. N Engl J Med 1982;307:976. *(Classic paper; 20% lower 5-year mortality was found in patients with diastolic blood pressures between 90 and 104 mm Hg who were treated intensively with stepped care compared with similar patients who were simply referred to their usual source of care for treatment.)*

Joint National Committee on Prevention, Detection, Evaluation, and Treatment of High Blood Pressure. Sixth report of the Joint National Committee on Detection, Evaluation and Treatment of High Blood Pressure (JNC VI). Arch Intern Med 1997;157:2413. *(A major consensus report.)*

Kannel WB, Wolf PA, McGee DL. Systolic blood pressure, arterial rigidity, and risk of stroke. JAMA 1981;245:1225. *(Classic paper. Subjects with isolated systolic hypertension experienced two to four times as many strokes as did normotensive persons in the Framingham study.)*

Lerman CE, Brody DS, Hui T, et al. The white-coat hypertension response: prevalence and predictors. J Gen Intern Med 1989;4:226. *(Prevalence was 39% and most common in the elderly and those on more medication.)*

MacMahon S, Peto R, Cutler J, et al. Blood pressure, stroke, and coronary heart disease. Part 1. Prolonged differences in blood pressure: prospective observational studies corrected for the regression dilution bias. Lancet 1990;335:765. *(Major meta-analysis documenting that risk of stroke and coronary disease correlates closely with level of blood pressure over the range of 70 to 110 mm Hg diastolic.)*

Maxwell MH, Waks AU, Schroth PC, et al. Error in blood pressure measurement due to incorrect cuff size in obese patients. Lancet 1982;2:8288. *(The standard adult size cuff results in readings of about 10 mm Hg in excess of the true pressure in obese patients. A large cuff is needed.)*

Medical Research Council Working Party. MRC trial of treatment of mild hypertension: principal results. BMJ 1985;291:97. *(Documents reduction in strokes by treatment of patients with mild disease.)*

Messerli FH, Garavaglia GE. Disparate cardiovascular findings in men and women with essential hypertension. Ann Intern Med 1987;107:158. *(Best documentation of the differences.)*

Systolic Hypertension in the Elderly Program (SHEP) Cooperative Research Group. Prevention of stroke by antihypertensive drug treatment in older persons with isolated systolic hypertension. JAMA 1991;265:3255. *(Treatment of isolated systolic hypertension reduced risk of stroke in the elderly.)*

Veterans Administration Cooperative Study Group on Antihypertensive Agents. Effects of treatment on morbidity in hypertension. I. Results in patients with diastolic blood pressures averaging 115 through 129 mm Hg. JAMA 1967;202:1028.

Veterans Administration Cooperative Study Group on Antihypertensive Agents. Effects of treatment on morbidity in hypertension. II. Results in patients with diastolic blood pressure averaging 90 through 114 mm Hg. JAMA 1970;213:1143.

Veterans Administration Cooperative Study Group on Antihypertensive Agents. Effects of treatment on morbidity in hypertension. III. Influence of age, diastolic pressure, and prior cardiovascular disease. Further analysis of side effects. Circulation 1972;45:901. *(These three studies are the original randomized prospective trials that established the benefit of treating hypertension.)*

15

Screening for Hyperlipidemia

GALE S. HAYDOCK
MASON W. FREEMAN

Coronary heart disease (CHD) is the single largest cause of death in American men and women, making identification and treatment of its risk factors a major health care priority. The common dyslipidemias (elevated low-density-lipoprotein [LDL] cholesterol, low and high-density-lipoprotein [HDL] cholesterol) rank among the major established CHD risk factors. Other dyslipidemias that may contribute to risk include hypertriglyceridemia and increased lipoprotein (a) (Lp[a]). Twenty percent of all adults older than 20 years of age have a total serum cholesterol concentration in excess of 240 mg/dL, a level associated with an accelerating risk of CHD. Fifty percent of the adult population has total cholesterol levels exceeding 200 mg/dL, the level considered desirable.

Patient and professional awareness of the importance of hypercholesterolemia has contributed to a modest (8%) reduction in mean total cholesterol over the past two decades, but the problem remains widespread. Screening for hyperlipidemia is a key element in the primary and secondary prevention of CHD. Proper screening is the responsibility of all primary care physicians and requires attention to several questions: Which lipid abnormalities truly increase coronary risk? To what degree will lowering them reduce such risk? How are they best measured? At what age should screening be initiated and for how long?

RISK FACTORS FOR HYPERLIPIDEMIA

Age. Cholesterol levels increase with age. Total cholesterol increases, on the average, more than 2 mg/dL per year during early adulthood and continues increasing but at a lesser rate until age 65, after which it declines slightly.

Gender. Men have higher total cholesterol levels than women until age 50 and an approximately twofold higher risk of developing CHD. Women carry a higher proportion of cholesterol in the form of HDL cholesterol (primarily HDL_2). At the onset of menopause, women lose the protective effect of estrogen, resulting in a net increase in cholesterol and an increased risk of CHD. As women move into their mid-sixties and beyond, their risk of developing CHD approaches that of men of the same age.

Genetic Factors. Primary lipid disorders arising from a *monogenic* (single gene) abnormality account for only a small fraction of patients with hyperlipidemia. These relatively uncommon genetic disorders are, however, frequently responsible for the most severe hyperlipidemias. These are, in turn, associated with the most aggressive forms of coronary artery disease. Because these disorders are more likely to affect the immediate relatives of an affected patient than are complex polygenic conditions, family screening should be performed in the relatives of patients suspected of harboring these genetic mutations.

Diet. A diet high in *saturated fatty acids* raises total and LDL cholesterol. Total and LDL cholesterol are also increased by dietary *cholesterol*, but the effect is smaller than that of saturated fatty acids. *Caloric excess* resulting in obesity has more of an effect on triglycerides than on cholesterol. *Alcohol* has little effect on total cholesterol levels, but it can cause an acute rise in triglycerides among people with hypertriglyceridemia. Moderate alcohol ingestion also causes a rise in HDL levels.

Medications. Antihypertensive agents that adversely affect lipid levels can compromise the effort to reduce CHD risk. *Thiazides* increase LDL cholesterol, at least temporarily, when taken in full doses. The effect is hypothesized to account for the shortfall in reduction in mortality found among hypertensives treated with thiazides (see Chapter 26). *Beta-blockers* cause modest reductions in HDL cholesterol. *Exogenous estrogens* increase HDL$_2$ and can cause extreme triglyceride increases in patients with hypertriglyceridemia. *Corticosteroids* and HIV *protease inhibitors* can also dramatically elevate serum lipids.

Exercise, Weight, Smoking, and Concurrent Diseases. Activity increases HDL cholesterol; inactivity and obesity appear to decrease it. A reduction in HDL cholesterol occurs with *smoking*. *Diabetes* is associated with elevations in triglycerides, which is frequently accompanied by low HDL cholesterol levels. *Hypothyroidism, nephrotic syndrome, and obstructive liver disease* are important causes of secondary hypercholesterolemia, characterized by increases in total and LDL cholesterol levels.

HYPERLIPIDEMIA AS A RISK FACTOR FOR CORONARY HEART DISEASE

Total Cholesterol. Both epidemiologic and prospective studies have demonstrated that hypercholesterolemia is an independent risk factor for the development of CHD in persons younger than 65 years of age. Coronary risk increases curvilinearly with increasing total cholesterol levels, even within the "normal" range. Over the usually encountered range of total cholesterol values (180 to 300 mg/dL), risk increases by an average of four- to fivefold. Risk begins to accelerate more sharply when the total cholesterol level exceeds 240 mg/dL. Levels lower than 200 mg/dL are considered desirable, although epidemiologic data can still demonstrate an increasing risk for CHD in the interval between 160 and 200 mg/dL.

Low-Density Lipoprotein (LDL) Cholesterol. The positive relationship between total cholesterol and CHD risk derives mainly from the atherogenic LDL cholesterol component. Because the LDL cholesterol accounts for about two thirds of the total cholesterol in the typical patient, the total cholesterol concentration is generally used as a proxy for LDL cholesterol. LDL cholesterol serum levels in excess of 160 mg/dL are associated with significant increases in CHD risk.

Lp(a), consisting of LDL attached to a protein of variable size, called "apoprotein little a," appears in most (but not all) studies to contribute independently of LDL cholesterol to CHD risk. The lack of an accurate inexpensive test, some uncertainty as to the exact risk relationship, and the absence of any studies demonstrating that a reduction in Lp(a) levels results in improve clinical outcomes has kept this marker from being routinely assayed.

High-Density Lipoprotein (HDL) Cholesterol. The relation of the HDL cholesterol level to CHD risk is an inverse one. HDL cholesterol exerts a protective effect that is at least as strong as the atherogenic effect of LDL. For every 10-mg/dL increment in HDL cholesterol concentration, there is a 50% decrease in coronary risk. An HDL cholesterol level lower than 35 mg/dL has come to be recognized as a major independent risk factor for CHD. A level in excess of 60 mg/dL is considered a "negative" risk factor (see Chapter 27). A low HDL cholesterol increases CHD risk across the full range of total and LDL cholesterol concentrations. A patient with a low total cholesterol level is still at increased risk of CHD if HDL cholesterol is low. Conversely, it is possible for a person with an elevated total cholesterol to be at low risk for CHD by virtue of having a very high HDL cholesterol (60 to 100 mg/dL). The determination of a *total-to-HDL cholesterol ratio* helps to distinguish such low-risk individuals from others with elevated total cholesterol. The Framingham Study showed that the ratio was a strong predictor of risk. A ratio of 5 approximates the average or standard risk, with ratios of 10 and 20 denoting double and triple the risk. A ratio of 4.5 or less is considered desirable.

Subfractions of HDL (e.g., HDL$_2$, HDL$_3$) and subcomponents (e.g., *apolipoprotein A1*) also appear protective and inversely predictive of CHD risk. However, they are difficult to measure, and their contribution to estimation of CHD risk does not appear additive to that provided by measurement of the total HDL cholesterol level.

Triglycerides. The importance of *hypertriglyceridemia* to cardiovascular risk remains controversial. In univariate analysis, it is consistently associated with increased CHD risk, but in multivariate analysis, most of this risk is lost when the contribution of HDL cholesterol is factored out. Because high serum levels of triglycerides may causally contribute to lowered HDL levels, one cannot conclude that hypertriglyceridemia is unimportant. Data from the Framingham Heart Study suggest that the high triglyceride/low HDL syndrome is a more important risk factor for women than men, some of which may be due to the association of this lipid profile with insulin resistance or frank glucose intolerance.

Lipid-related Coronary Heart Disease Risk Among the Young and the Elderly. The importance of hypercholesterolemia as a predictor of coronary disease is best established in middle-aged men and postmenopausal women. In the young and the elderly, the relationship is less well established due to a paucity of data.

For young men (under age 35) and premenopausal women, elevated total and LDL cholesterol levels increase *long-term risk* of developing CHD. However, *short-term* CHD risk among those with even moderately high LDL cholesterol levels (160 to 220 mg/dL) but no other CHD risk factors remains relatively low. However, the presence of additional CHD risk factors, particularly diabetes or family history of early CHD, appears to increase short-term risk, as does development of a very high LDL cholesterol level (220 mg/dL).

CHD risk due to hypercholesterolemia in the *elderly* is also incompletely defined. The relative risk of CHD observed in men 60 to 79 years of age with marked hypercholesterolemia is about 1.5. This relative risk is lower than that in comparably hypercholesterolemic patients younger than 60 years of age. The difference is believed to be related to the high prevalence of already established CHD, hypertension, and diabetes in this age group. Among hyperlipidemic elderly patients with established CHD, the relative risk of a new coronary event is just as high as in younger patients. Because the elderly have the highest rates of coronary disease in the population (85% of individuals dying of CHD are 65 years or older), the aggressiveness with which to screen older individuals is a topic of heated debate in the prevention field.

EFFECTIVENESS OF TREATMENT

Nonpharmacologic Measures. Decreases in intake of cholesterol and saturated fat in controlled settings can *reduce total and LDL cholesterol* levels by 30% or more, but this magnitude of reduction is rarely achieved in clinical practice. LDL cholesterol levels are lowered by an average of 10% when reasonably intensive diets are used in the outpatient setting. Dietary measures may also produce a small (approximately 5%) reduction in HDL cholesterol concentration, though the overall total-to-HDL ratio still improves. Weight loss (if obese), aerobic exercise, and smoking cessation can raise the HDL cholesterol level and facilitate the dietary lowering of LDL cholesterol. These measures also reduce CHD risk by decreasing blood pressure and glucose intolerance. Caloric and fat restrictions and control of diabetes lower triglyceride levels, an effect added to by prohibition of alcohol. Reductions in CHD risk follow from cholesterol lowering and amelioration of other risk factors.

Addition of Pharmacologic Measures. Adding drug therapy to a diet and exercise program enhances the lipid-lowering effort. Reductions two to three times greater (25% to 35%) than those achieved by dietary measures alone are attainable and associated with a further lowering of CHD risk. The reduction is most evident among patients with established CHD—a *secondary prevention* effect—with CHD mortality reduced by over 40% and all-cause mortality by 30%. In addition, a halt to plaque progression and a modest amount of *plaque regression* have been demonstrated in patients with established CHD treated aggressively with medical therapy. Pharmacologic therapy for hypercholesterolemic persons without clinically evident CHD (so-called *primary prevention*) also reduces CHD risk. Reductions of approximately 30% in rates of nonfatal infarction, death from CHD, and death from all forms of cardiovascular disease have been achieved in medically treated men and women with moderate increases in their LDL cholesterol levels (LDL levels of 150 to 190 mg/dL). The cardiovascular benefit of these interventions with the HMG CoA reductase inhibitor class of drugs ("statins") has not been associated with any increase in noncardiac deaths (an earlier concern, not borne out in large-scale prospective clinical trials).

SCREENING METHODS

Determinations of total cholesterol, LDL cholesterol, and HDL cholesterol levels would allow reasonable estimates of CHD risk. Decisions about which test(s) to order in screening a particular patient require consideration of test accuracy, cost, availability, significance, and presence of other CHD risk factors.

Measurement of Cholesterol and Choice of Method. The total blood cholesterol is the sum of the cholesterol concentrations contained in the three major circulating lipoproteins (HDL, LDL, and very-low-density lipoproteins [VLDL]). Thus, total cholesterol = LDL cholesterol + HDL cholesterol + VLDL cholesterol. Most laboratories measure total cholesterol and HDL cholesterol directly, calculate the VLDL concentration by dividing the triglyceride concentration by 5 (as long as triglyceride is less than 400 mg/dL), and then mathematically derive the LDL cholesterol concentration.

The accuracy of determinations of total cholesterol and its fractions can vary considerably. The popular *finger-stick method* using a capillary tube and *desktop analyzer* has demonstrated false-negative rates ranging from 12% to 47% for detection of lipid elevations. The best results with finger-stick measurements are for nonfasting total cholesterol, which most closely approximate those obtained by *venous sampling and laboratory processing* (which average 3% to 5% higher). HDL cholesterol measurement by desktop analyzers is less accurate. The finger-stick technology has improved since its inception, but in one recent study, the error rate of a desktop analyzer fell outside of the National Cholesterol Education Program (NCEP) guidelines for three of the four standard lipid measurements. Because this study was conducted in a speciality lipid clinic with experienced technical personnel, the error rates observed may underestimate what would be seen in a busy clinical office practice.

Not all laboratories ensure accuracy of results. Acceptable laboratories are those with instruments calibrated to the standards of the Centers for Disease Control and Prevention, with a margin of error (coefficient of variation) of 3% for a total cholesterol measurement. If finger-stick screening methods reveal a total cholesterol elevation, the determination should be repeated by a proper laboratory before deciding to initiate lipid-lowering therapy (see Chapter 27).

Fasting is unnecessary when screening by measurement of the total cholesterol level, because it is not markedly affected by immediate food intake. However, chronic stress or serious illness might cause the level to fall significantly. Thus, it is best to measure lipid levels in patients when they have recovered from any acute infections, illnesses that results in tissue necrosis, or surgical procedures. A significant drop in total cholesterol and triglyceride levels has been demonstrated when a patient assumes a recumbent position, usually within 5 minutes, and it reaches a maximum of 10% to 12% within 20 to 30 minutes.

Selection of Persons for Screening. The approach to screening lipid levels in patients has been controversial, with the American College of Physicians (ACP) promulgating screening guidelines that differ substantially from those recommended by the NCEP. The differences largely reflect a greater emphasis on cost effectiveness in the ACP guidelines than in those issued by the NCEP. Importantly, both the NCEP guidelines and the ACP recommendations were issued before publication of the most recent statin trials, which show marked reductions in cardiovascular and all-cause mortality and no increase in noncardiovascular disease in hypercholesterolemic patients treated with statins. (Preliminary studies raised concerns about increases in noncardiovascular morbidity and mortality in individuals treated with cholesterol-lowering agents.)

The results of these studies favor the more aggressive screening program suggested by the NCEP. The decision to treat with cholesterol-lowering drugs, however, should still take into consideration the absolute risk for the development of coronary disease that any given patient has. Treating moderately hypercholesterolemic young individuals with costly drugs for several decades before they are statistically likely to experience any CHD events may not be a wise use of health care resources, even if some benefit can be shown. This decision is a matter of judgment and philosophy, and it is likely to be one in which considerable practice variability can be expected. Nevertheless, nonpharmacologic treatments of hyperlipidemia can be both effective and inexpensive and are more likely to be adopted by patients who are aware of their hyperlipidemia.

The *NCEP guidelines* recommended measuring a *total and HDL cholesterol* in all adults 20 years of age and older *every 5 years*. Additional testing is determined by the results of those screens. For those without evidence of CHD, if the total cholesterol is less than 200 mg/dL and the HDL cholesterol is at least 35 mg/dL, the screening is repeated in 5 years. For individuals with total cholesterol levels more than 240 mg/dL or between 200 and 240 with multiple risk factors present, a complete lipoprotein profile is recommended. This includes measurement of triglyceride levels and a calculation of the LDL. NCEP treatment guidelines (see Chapter 27) are then triggered by the LDL value and the presence or absence of risk factors. For those with evidence of CHD, a complete lipoprotein profile is done initially.

The issue of cholesterol screening in the *elderly* also remains somewhat unsettled. It is clearly indicated for those at high risk for CHD (multiple CHD risk factors, established CHD, other clinically evident atherosclerotic disease) who are otherwise well. Screening lower risk healthy persons older than 70 years of age is of unknown value but likely to be beneficial, given the high prevalence of silent CHD in the population. The subgroup analyses that have been done in the over 65 population enrolled in the statin trials demonstrate clear benefits to treatment, although the number of older patients that have been studied remains small. At what point an elderly person is beyond the age where primary prevention of CHD should be considered is a topic that is little informed by any data.

What to Screen. A nonfasting determination of total and HDL cholesterol suffices for patients with no other cardiovascular risk factors. For those with CHD or other CHD risk factors as outlined above, total cholesterol, HDL cholesterol, and serum triglycerides should be measured only after fasting for more than 12 hours. This permits the LDL level to be calculated, if the triglycerides are less than 400 mg/dL, and allows the physician to make any treatment decisions based on the LDL cutpoints contained in the NCEP guidelines.

LDL cholesterol, triglycerides, VLDL cholesterol, and lipoprotein electrophoresis are not indicated for screening purposes. The use of other measurements in assessing risk, such as Lp(a), homocysteine, and C-reactive protein levels (a potential marker of inflammation in the artery wall), are not yet estab-lished as worthwhile screening tools in the assessment of patients with CHD.

CONCLUSIONS AND RECOMMENDATIONS

- Hypercholesterolemia is a problem of substantial proportions in the United States and a major risk factor for CHD.
- Elevations in levels of total cholesterol or LDL cholesterol and reduction in HDL cholesterol are strongly positive independent risk factors for the development of CHD in persons younger than 65 years of age.
- Diet, exercise, smoking cessation, and drug therapy are effective measures for treatment of lipid abnormalities associated with CHD risk.
- Reductions in CHD morbidity and mortality have been demonstrated with treatment, particularly in high-risk hyperlipidemic patients such as those with established CHD, but also in hyperlipidemic men and women without clinical evidence of CHD.
- Random serum total and HDL cholesterol measurements should be performed at least every 5 years in persons older than 20 years of age. Those at increased risk of CHD because of smoking, diabetes, hypertension, family history of premature CHD, or symptomatic noncoronary atheromatous disease require more frequent screening.
- Elderly persons are reasonable candidates for cholesterol screening, provided their overall clinical condition would warrant treatment of hypercholesterolemia.
- An HDL cholesterol determination should be part of the screening profile, provided the technology for performing the measurement is available. Results from desktop analyzers using finger-stick blood samples are often erroneous.
- The ratio of total cholesterol to HDL cholesterol should be calculated. A ratio lower than 4.5 is desirable.
- Determination of LDL cholesterol level is not necessary for screening purposes.
- Neither a triglyceride determination nor a lipoprotein electrophoresis is indicated for screening.
- The value of measuring biologically important risk factors such as Lp(a) and certain apolipoproteins is yet to be demonstrated.
- If the finger-stick screening serum total cholesterol is greater than 200 mg/dL, then a repeat determination using venipuncture and laboratory techniques is indicated for confirmation. Further testing and treatment are based on the patient's age and risk factor profile (see Chapter 27).

ANNOTATED BIBLIOGRAPHY

Brown G, Albers JJ, Fisher LD, et al. Regression of coronary artery disease as a result of intensive lipid-lowering therapy. N Engl J Med 1990;323:1289. *(Significant plaque regression is documented in coronary arteries in this angiographic study of intensive therapy.)*

Criqui MH, Heiss G, Cohn R, et al. Plasma triglyceride level and mortality from coronary heart disease. N Engl J Med 1993;328:1220. *(No independent association with CHD risk found.)*

Expert Panel on Detection, Evaluation, and Treatment of High Blood Cholesterol in Adults. Summary of the second report. JAMA 1993;269:3015. *(Major consensus panel recommendations, revising those of 1988 report; more emphasis on total CHD risk, on importance of HDL.)*

Hunninghake DB, Stein EA, Dujovne CA, et al. The efficacy of intensive dietary therapy alone or combined with lovastatin in outpatients with hypercholesterolemia. N Engl J Med 1993;328:1213. *(Diet alone provided only a 5% LDL reduction; medication added another 27%.)*

Kafonek SD, Donovan L, Lovejoy KL, et al. Biologic variation of lipids and lipoproteins in fingerstick blood. Clin Chem 1996;42:2002. *(Biologic variability in serum lipids is greater than the analytic variability, but desktop analyzer accuracy still falls somewhat short of the guidelines suggested by the NCEP.)*

Kannel WB. High-density lipoproteins: epidemiologic profile and risks of coronary artery disease. Am J Cardiol 1983;52:9B. *(Classic epidemiologic study establishing the contribution of the individual values and ratios of total cholesterol, HDL cholesterol, and LDL cholesterol toward predicting cardiovascular risk.)*

Klag KJ, Ford DE, Mead LA, et al. Serum cholesterol in young men and subsequent cardiovascular disease. N Engl J Med 1993;328:313. *(Strong association found between serum cholesterol level in early life and CHD in midlife.)*

Lipid Research Clinics Program. The Lipid Research Clinics Coronary Primary Prevention Trial. JAMA 1984;251:351. *(A significant reduction was observed in the incidence of coronary heart disease by lowering the total cholesterol and LDL cholesterol in asymptomatic middle-aged men with primary hypercholesterolemia.)*

National Cholesterol Education Program. Report of the expert panel on detection, evaluation, treatment of high blood cholesterol in adults. Arch Intern Med 1988;148:36. *(Consensus panel report; urges screening all adults for total cholesterol every 5 years.)*

National Cholesterol Education Program Adult Treatment Panel. Prevalence of high blood cholesterol among US adults. JAMA 1993;269:3009. *(20% of Americans have cholesterol ≥240 mg/dL; 50%, ≥200 mg/dL; best available epidemiologic data.)*

Rubin SM, Sidney S, Black DM. High blood cholesterol in elderly men and the excess risk for coronary heart disease. Ann Intern Med 1990;113:916. *(Relative risk was 1.5, indicating that cholesterol is an independent risk factor for cardiovascular mortality.)*

Scandinavian Simvistatin Survival Study Group. Randomized trial of cholesterol lowering in 4444 patients with coronary heart disease: the Scandinavian Survival Study. Lancet 1994;344:1383. *(A major randomized study of the efficacy of secondary prevention showing 42% reduction in CHD mortality and no increased risk of noncardiac death.)*

Shepherd J, Cobbe SM, Ford I, et al. Prevention of coronary heart disease with pravastatin in men with hypercholesterolemia. N Engl J Med 1995;333:1301. *(A randomized, placebo-controlled, prospective trial of men without CHD examining the efficacy of statin therapy for primary prevention; finds approximately 30% reductions in rates of nonfatal infarction, CHD death, and cardiovascular death.)*

Sox HC Jr. Screening for lipid disorders under health system reform. N Engl J Med 1993;328:1269. *(An editorial reviewing recommendations for screening from a cost-effectiveness perspective.)*

Stampfer MJ, Sacks FM, Salvini S, et al. A prospective study of cholesterol, apolipoproteins, and the risk of myocardial infarction. N Engl J Med 1991;325:373. *(HDL cholesterol was important in predicting risk for myocardial infarction; the ratio of total to HDL cholesterol was especially useful. A one unit change in the ratio was associated with a 53% change in risk.)*

Wilson PWF, D'Agostino R, et al. Prediction of coronary heart disease using risk factor categories. Circulation 1998;97:1837. *(Using data from the Framingham Heart Study, the authors generated prediction algorithms that permit a more quantitative assessment of coronary artery disease risk to be made.)*

16
Bacterial Endocarditis Prophylaxis

Once universally fatal, bacterial endocarditis remains a serious disease, with a mortality rate of about 25 percent. The pathogenesis of endocarditis suggests that individual infections might be prevented by judicious use of prophylactic antibiotics, yet the incidence of this infection has not changed much despite the widespread availability of antibiotics. Recent data even question the effectiveness of prophylaxis, at least among patients undergoing dental procedures. The primary care provider must understand the evidence for benefit and accurately assess individual risk in order to properly apply recommendations for prophylaxis. Patient education is essential to ensure compliance.

EPIDEMIOLOGY AND RISK FACTORS

During the past several decades, there has been a shift in the incidence of endocarditis to older age groups; the current mean age is about 50 years. Men predominate in those over 50; under 50, the gender ratio is more nearly equal.

Risk Factors. Individual risk of endocarditis is typically viewed as a function of cardiac and procedural risk factors (see Tables 16.1, 2, 3). However, up to 30% of cases of endocarditis occur in the absence of underlying heart disease, and spontaneous transient bacteremia confers greater cumulative risk among susceptible individuals than do procedures. Clearly, all individuals have some finite risk of developing endocarditis. Because of the difficulty in predicting who is most susceptible and when, it has been estimated that no more than 6 % of endocarditis cases can be prevented. Nonetheless, the morbidity and mortality of endocarditis are sufficient justification to advocate preventive measures for patients at substantial risk.

Cardiac. In the preantibiotic era, chronic rheumatic heart disease was the underlying lesion in up to 90 % of endocarditis cases. Now prosthetic cardiac valves, previous endocarditis (recurrence rate as high as 10%), complex congenital heart disease, and surgically constructed pulmonary shunts are the high-risk cardiac lesions (see Table 16.1). Moderate risk is associated with other cardiac anomalies (see Table 16.2). How-

Table 16.1. Cardiac Risk Factors for Endocarditis

1. **High Risk**
   a. Prosthetic heart valve(s)
   b. History of endocarditis
2. **Moderate Risk**
   a. Rheumatic or other acquired valvular disease
   b. Congenital heart disease (excluding atrial septal defect of the secundum type)
   c. Idiopathic hypertrophic subaortic stenosis
3. **Probable Moderate Risk**
   a. Mitral valve prolapse
   b. Undiagnosed murmurs

ever, as noted, endocarditis can occur without known predisposing cardiac disease. Prosthetic-valve endocarditis may be early, usually associated with surgery and most often involving nosocomial pathogens (eg, staphylococci). Late disease occurs after procedures that induce bacteremia and typically involves bacteria of low virulence that are rarely able to infect damaged natural valves. Prosthetic valve endocarditis is a serious condition; overall mortality is substantial, even with antibiotics and valve replacement.

Procedural. Data on incidence of bacteremia with procedures are fragmentary at best, but risk appears greatest with dental procedures. Tooth extraction and periodontal surgery have incidence rates of about 50 percent; other dental procedures approach that figure. Endocarditis risk is minimal with coronary artery bypass graft surgery or placement of pacemakers or implanted defibrillators. Some nondental procedures also have a substantial incidence of subsequent bacteremia, but others have little (see Tables 16.2, 3).

NATURAL HISTORY OF ENDOCARDITIS AND EFFECTIVENESS OF THERAPY

Natural History. Untreated endocarditis is uniformly fatal. Current mortality rates are approximately 10 percent with natural valves and 25 percent to 65 percent with prosthetic valves. Death often follows congestive heart failure, arterial emboli, myocardial infarction, myocardial abscesses, or other complications.

Table 16.2.   Common Events Predisposing to Bacteremia

EVENT	INSTANCES IN WHICH BACTEREMIA OCCURS (%)
Dental extraction	75
Tooth brushing, flossing, or irrigation	
Normal gingiva	20
Gingivitis	50
Bronchoscopy	
Fiberoptic	<1
Rigid	15
Fiberoptic endoscopy	10
Sigmoidoscopy	5
Barium enema	10
Liver biopsy	5
Transurethral resection of prostate	
Sterile urine	10
Infected urine	50

Table 16.3.   Other Events and Procedures

Respiratory tract
  Tonsillectomy and/or adenoidectomy
  Surgical operations that involve respiratory mucosa
  Bronchoscopy with a rigid bronchoscope
Gastrointestinal tract
  Sclerotherapy for esophageal varices
  Esophageal stricture dilation
  Endoscopic retrograde cholangiography with bilary obstruction
  Biliary tract surgery
  Surgical operations that involve intestinal mucosa
Genitourinary tract
  Prostatic surgery
  Cystoscopy
  Urethral dilation

Effectiveness of Therapy. The best estimates of protective efficacy for antibiotic therapy derive from case-control studies and range from 48% to 91%. There are no data from prospective trials, in part because of the very large number of patients needed and difficulties in identifying patients at risk and detecting transient bacteremias. Most recommendations for prophylactic antibiotic regimens are based primarily on experience with experimental animal models.

RISK OF PROPHYLACTIC THERAPY

For penicillin prophylaxis, the risk of serious reaction is very small in patients without previous allergy or a history of rheumatic fever–about 1 to 4 per 100,000. The risk of death caused by serious penicillin reaction has been estimated at 1 to 2 per 100,000 patients receiving the drug. Less information is available concerning risks associated with other prophylactic antibiotics, including amoxicillin, which is now recommended because it is better absorbed from the gastrointestinal tract and provides higher and more sustained serum levels. Surveys have identified very few serious reactions to other oral regimens, including clindamycin. Even with parenteral regimens including aminoglycosides, there is little toxicity when the drug is given for the brief period necessary for adequate prophylaxis.

IDENTIFYING PATIENTS AT RISK

An individual's risk of procedure-related endocarditis can be estimated by checking for important heart disease (see Table 16.1) and taking into account the likelihood of a procedure-related bacteremia (see Tables 16.2, 3). A history of congenital or rheumatic heart disease and presence of a murmur indicative of hemodynamically significant disease indicate substantial risk. Echocardiographic documentation of hypertrophic cardiomyopathy or the presence of valve calcification can also be considered an indication for prophylaxis.

The most difficult cases are those where risk appears to be intermediate, as with mitral valve prolapse or with an isolated systolic murmur without a helpful history or other cardiac findings (see Chapter 21). Bacterial endocarditis prophylaxis for this group is controversial. Risk-benefit analyses suggest that expected morbidity and mortality associated with penicillin therapy outweigh the benefits of prevention. Nevertheless, many clinicians continue to recommend prophylaxis. The American Heart Association currently recommends prophylaxis for patients with mitral valve prolapse only if there is evidence of significant valvular regurgitation.

Endocarditis prophylaxis is recommended for those in the high and moderate-risk categories (see Table 16.1). It is not recommended for those in the negligible-risk category (no greater risk than the general population). It should be kept in mind that the absolute risk of endocarditis, even for the high-risk patient is extremely low (eg, <1 case per 1000 tooth extractions).

CONCLUSIONS AND RECOMMENDATIONS

Clinical effectiveness of endocarditis prophylaxis is difficult to demonstrate definitively. However, when the serious morbidity and mortality associated with the disease are weighed against the small risk associated with prophylaxis, vigorous preventive efforts have been considered justified. Identifiable risk varies with the type of heart abnormality and the event responsible for bacteremia, as summarized in Table 16.1, Table 16.2, and Table 16.3.

Consensus recommendations for prophylactic regimens have been revised to maximize compliance and efficacy (see Tables 16.4 and 16.5). The absence of evidence for an association between dental procedures and subsequent endocarditis will likely stimulate reconsideration of these recommendations.

As in all preventive efforts, patient education is extremely important. All patients with identifiable risk should be urged to maintain a high level of oral health to minimize the potential for recurrent bacteremia. Patients receiving rheumatic fever prophylaxis must understand that their continuous therapy will not protect them from endocarditis.

A.G.M.

ANNOTATED BIBLIOGRAPHY

Clemens JD, Horwitz RI, Jaffe CC et al. A controlled evaluation of the risk of bacterial endocarditis in persons with mitral valve prolapse. N Engl J Med 1982;307:776. (*Odds ratio of 8.2 for endocarditis for people with mitral valve prolapse.*)

Dajani AS, Bawdon RE, Berry MC. Oral amoxicillin as prophylaxis for endocarditis: What is the optimal dose? Clin Inf Dis 1994; 18:157.(*Adequate serum levels with single 2.0 g dose.*)

Dajani AS, Taubert KA, Wilson W, et al. Prevention of bacterial endocarditis. Recommendations by the American Heart association. JAMA 1997;277:1794. (*Latest recommendations; simplified approach designed to increase compliance and reduce adverse effects.*)

Devereux RB, Frary CJ, Kramer-Fox R, et al. Cost-effectiveness of infective endocarditis prophylaxis for mitral valve prolapse with or without a mitral regurgitant murmur. Am J Cardiol 1994;74:1024. (*Cost-effectiveness maximized when prophylaxis restricted to those with mitral murmurs.*)

Doyle EF, Spagnuolo M, Taranta A, et al. The risk of bacterial endocarditis during antirheumatic prophylaxis. JAMA 1967; 201:807. (*Sixteen cases were reported during 3615 patient-years of antirheumatic prophylaxis.*)

Durack DT. Prevention of infective endocarditis. N Engl J Med 1995; 332:38. (*Sound, concise review of the rationale and supporting literature.*)

Everett ED, Hirschman JV. Transient bacteremia and endocarditis prophylaxis. A review. Medicine (Baltimore) 1977;56:61. (*Review of incidence data for bacteremia associated with relevant clinical procedures.*)

Imperiale TF, Horwitz RI. Does prophylaxis prevent postdental infective endocarditis? A controlled evaluation of protective efficacy. Am J Med 1990;88:131. (*A 91% protective efficacy for antibiotic prophylaxis estimated.*)

Table 16.4. Prophylactic Regimens for Dental, Oral, Respiratory Tract, or Esophageal Procedures

SITUATION	AGENT	REGIMEN*
Standard general prophylaxis	Amoxicillin	Adults: 2.0 g; children: 50 mg/kg orally 1 h before procedure
Unable to take oral medications	Ampicillin	Adults: 2.0 g Intramuscularly (IM) or intravenously (IV); children: 50 mg/kg IM or IV within 30 min before procedure
Allergic to penicillin	Clindamycin or	Adults: 600 mg; children: 20 mg/kg orally 1 h before procedure
	Cephalexin† or cefadroxil† or	Adults: 2.0 g; children; 50 mg/kg orally 1 h before procedure
	Azithromycin or clarithromycin	Adults: 500 mg; children: 20 mg/kg orally 1 h before procedure
Allergic to penicillin and unable to take oral medications	Clindamycin or Cefazolin	Adults: 600 mg; children: 20 mg/kg IV within 30 min before procedure Adults: 1.0 g; children: 25 mg/kg IM or IV within 30 min before procedure

*Total children's dose should not exceed adult dose.

†Cephalosporins should not be used in individuals with immediate-type hypersensitivity reaction (uticaria, angioedema, or anaphylaxis) to penicillins.

Table 16.5. Prophylactic Regimens for Genitourinary Gastrointestinal (Excluding Esophageal) Procedures

SITUATION	AGENT*	REGIMEN†
High-risk patients	Ampicillin plus Gentamicin	Adults: ampicillin 2.0 g Intramuscularly (IM) or intravenously (IV) plus gentamicin 1.5 mg/kg (not to exceed 120 mg) within 30 min of starting the procedure; 6 h later, ampicillin 1 g IM/IV or amoxicillin 1 g orally Children: ampicillin 50 mg/kg IM or IV (not to exceed 2.0 g) plus gentamicin 1.5 mg/kg within 30 min of starting the procedure; 6 h later, ampicillin 25 mg/kg IM/IV or amoxicillin 25 mg/ kg orally
High-risk patients allergic to ampicillin/amoxicillin	Vancomycin plus Gentamicin	Adults: vancomycin 1.0 g IV over 1-2 h plus gentamicin 1.5 mg/kg IV/IM (not to exceed 120 mg); complete injection/infusion within 30 min of starting the procedure Children: vancomycin 20 mg/kg IV over 1-2 h plus gentamicin 2.0 g IM/IV; complete injection/ infusion within 30 min of starting the procedure
Moderate-risk patients	Amoxicillin or Ampicillin	Adults: Amoxicillin 2.0 g orally 1 h before procedure, or ampicillin 2.0 g IM/IV within 30 min starting the procedure Children: amoxicillin 50 mg/kg orally 1 h before procedure, or ampicillin 50 mg/kg IM/IV within 30 min of starting the procedure
Moderate-risk patients allergic to ampicillin/amoxicillin	Vancomycin	Adults: vancomycin 1.0 g IV over 1-2 h; complete infusion within 30 min of starting the procedure Children: vancomycin 20 mg/kg IV over 1-2 h; complete infusion within 30 min of starting the procedure

*Total children's dose should not exceed adult dose.

†No second dose of vancomycin or gentamicin is recommended.

Ivert TS, Dismukes WE, Cobbs CG et al. Prosthetic valve endocarditis. Circulation 1984;69:223. *(High risk of both early and late endocarditis with prosthetic valves, especially mechanical prostheses and prior native valve endocarditis.)*

Madlon-Kay DJ. Endocarditis prophylaxis in a primary care clinic. J Fam Pract 1991;32:504. *(One of many studies that document poor compliance with AHA recommendations.)*

Spirito P, Rapezzi C, Betocchi S, et al. Infective endocarditis in hypertrophic cardiomyopathy: prevalence, incidence, and indications for antibiotic prophylaxis. Circulation 1999;99:2132. *(Risk greatest in those with obstructive lesions.)*

Strom BL, Abrutyn E, Berlin JA, et al. Dental and cardiac risk factors for infective endocarditis. Ann Intern Med 1998;129:761. *(Dental treatment is not a risk factor for endocarditis but cardiac valvular abnormalities are strong risk factors.)*

Van der Meer JT, Van Wijk W, Thompson J, et al. Efficacy of antibiotic prophylaxis for prevention of native-valve endocarditis. Lancet 1992;339:135. *(A 49% protective efficacy found.)*

17
Rheumatic Fever Prophylaxis

Despite a decline in incidence that began before the availability of antibiotics, rheumatic fever and rheumatic heart disease remain significant causes of preventable morbidity. Localized resurgences occurred in the United States during the early 1990s and equally affected adults and children and the well-to-do and the disadvantaged. Primary prevention depends on appropriate diagnosis and effective treatment of group A streptococcal pharyngitis (see Chapter 220). Vaccination against streptococcal infection may be possible in the future, but current preventive measures depend on discriminating antibiotic use.

The prophylactic use of antibiotics has been shown to be effective for primary prevention during epidemics among closed populations. The major role of antibiotic prophylaxis, however, is in prevention of second attacks. The risk of recurrence after streptococcal infection is especially high in patients with evidence of carditis. Continuous streptococcal prophylaxis in patients with prior rheumatic fever is the major means of preventing the cardiac sequelae of rheumatic fever recurrences. It is the task of the primary physician to identify patients who would benefit from such prophylaxis and to provide the instruction necessary for long-term adherence.

EPIDEMIOLOGY AND RISK FACTORS

The epidemiology of rheumatic fever parallels that of streptococcal infection. Rare in children younger than 5 years of age, it is most common in older children and adolescents. Incidence decreases after adolescence; cases after age 40 are very rare. There is no clear predilection for either sex.

Although a genetic predisposition has not been proven, an association between certain human leukocyte antigens and rheumatic diseases has been identified, at least among white patients. Heterogeneity in the immune response to a specific streptococcal cell-wall antigen, the group A carbohydrate, has been demonstrated, but predictors of the hyperimmune response associated with the clinical sequelae of rheumatic fever have not been identified.

Racial differences in the incidence of rheumatic fever exist but disappear when socioeconomic status is considered; crowded living conditions is an important variable. Crowding may also explain the high incidence in cold climates and during winter months in temperate climates.

All demographic risk factors are heavily outweighed by a previous history of rheumatic fever. The likelihood of an attack after streptococcal infection is at least five times higher among individuals with previous rheumatic fever.

NATURAL HISTORY OF RHEUMATIC FEVER AND EFFECTIVENESS OF THERAPY

Rheumatic fever follows between 0.5% and 3.0% of ineffectively treated cases of group A streptococcal upper respiratory infections. Diagnosis and appropriate antibiotic therapy will prevent rheumatic fever in the individual case, but such efforts cannot be expected to eliminate rheumatic disease because of the high proportion of streptococcal infections that are subclinical. Approximately one third of patients with primary rheumatic fever have no history of preceding respiratory infec-

Table 17.1.   Risk of Recurrent Rheumatic Fever After Group A Streptococcal Infection

	RECURRENCES OF STREPTOCOCCAL INFECTION (%)
Interval Since Onset of Last Rheumatic Episode	
Up to 2 yr	28
2–5 yr	15
5 yr and over	10
Number of Previous Attacks of Rheumatic Fever	
2 or more	27
1	14
Rheumatic Heart Disease	
Not present	13
Present	26

Modified from Spagnuolo M, Pasternack B, Taranta A, et al. Risk of rheumatic fever recurrences after streptococcal infections. N Engl J Med 1971;285:641.

Table 17.2. Prophylaxis and Attack Rates of Streptococcal Infection and Rheumatic Fever Recurrences

	ORAL SULFADIAZINE (1 G/D)	ORAL PENICILLIN G (200,000 UNITS DAILY)	IM BENZATHINE PENICILLIN G (1.2 MILLION UNITS EVERY 4 WK)
Number of patient-years	576	545	560
Number of streptococcal infections	138	113	34
(rate/100 patient-years)	(24.0)	(20.7)	(6.1)
Number of rheumatic fever recurrences	16	30	2
(rate/100 patient-years)	(2.8)	(5.5)	(0.4)

Modified from Wood H, Feinstein AR, Tarant A, et al. Rheumatic fever in children and adolescents III. Comparative effectiveness of three prophylaxis regimens in preventing streptococcal infections and rheumatic recurrences. Ann Intern Med 1964;60:31.

tions. Another one third have symptoms but do not seek medical care. The remainder are ineffectively diagnosed or treated.

Among all patients with group A streptococcal infection and a history of previous rheumatic fever, the recurrence rate is 15%. More specific rates can be estimated for subgroups depending on the number of previous rheumatic attacks, the interval since the last attack, and whether or not there was evidence of carditis. Specific attack rates are summarized in Table 17.1.

Because of these high secondary attack rates and the ubiquity of the streptococcus, *continuous* antibiotic prophylaxis of streptococcal infection is the only feasible method of preventing rheumatic fever recurrences. Three antibiotic regimens have gained general acceptance:

1. Benzathine penicillin G, 1,200,000 units IM every 3 or 4 weeks;
2. Sulfadiazine, 1 g/d PO (500 mg for patients weighing less than 60 pounds);
3. Penicillin G, 250 mg PO twice a day.

Although the effectiveness of erythromycin (250 mg PO twice a day) has not been studied, it is recommended for the rare patient allergic to both penicillin and sulfonamides. The classic study comparing the effectiveness of these three regimens in preventing streptococcal infection and rheumatic fever is summarized in Table 17.2. Some reports suggest that failure rates may be higher when benzathine penicillin injections are administered every 4 weeks rather than every 3. Because adherence is more difficult with the greater frequency, some have suggested doses of 1,800,000 units or even 2,400,000 units depending on weight, but further study is needed.

There are no firm guidelines regarding the duration of continuous antibiotic prophylaxis after an episode of rheumatic fever. Factors that influence the likelihood of rheumatic recurrence after infection have already been reviewed. Within limits, the physician can estimate the risk of exposure of a particular patient to streptococcal infection. For example, parents of young children, teachers and other school personnel, health care providers, and military personnel are at high risk.

RISKS OF ANTIBIOTIC PROPHYLAXIS

The risks of penicillin administration are discussed in Chapter 16 on endocarditis prophylaxis. It should be emphasized that, in a large series, reactions after parenteral administration were no more common than those after oral therapy.

CONCLUSIONS AND RECOMMENDATIONS

- Primary prevention of rheumatic fever depends on accurate diagnosis and treatment of symptomatic streptococcal upper respiratory infections. Prevention of rheumatic fever recurrences depends on continuous streptococcal prophylaxis of the patients at risk.
- Injections of benzathine penicillin G (1,200,000 units IM) every 3 or 4 weeks provide the most effective prophylaxis and are recommended in patients with a high risk of both streptococcal exposure and a rheumatic recurrence after infection. Acceptable oral regimens in patients at lower risk include sulfadiazine, 1 g/d PO; *or* penicillin G, 250 mg PO twice daily; *or* erythromycin, 250 mg PO twice daily (in patients allergic to both penicillin and sulfa drugs).
- The duration of prophylaxis should be based on the risk incurred by the particular patient.
- All patients with rheumatic fever should be treated until age 25 or for 5 years after an episode (whichever is longer). In those with two or more previous attacks or with rheumatic heart disease, therapy should be continued until age 40 or for 10 years after the last episode. Prophylaxis in patients with rheumatic heart disease at high risk of streptococcal exposure should be continued indefinitely.

A.G.M.

ANNOTATED BIBLIOGRAPHY

Ayoub EM. The search for host determinants of susceptibility to rheumatic fever: the missing link. Circulation 1984;69:197. (*Reviews evidence for genetic markers and immune hyperresponsiveness to streptococcal antigens among people predisposed to rheumatic fever.*)

Berrios X, del Campo E, Guzman B, et al. Discontinuing rheumatic fever prophylaxis in selected adolescents and young adults. A prospective study. Ann Intern Med 1993;118:401. (*Documents relatively low risk of recurrence, 0.7 cases per 100 person-years, when prophylaxis was discontinued in selected patients in Chile.*)

Bland EF. Rheumatic fever: the way it was. Circulation 1987;76:1190-1195. (*Reflections of an astute clinical leader in the field.*)

Breese BB, Disney FA. Penicillin in the treatment of streptococcal infections. A comparison of effectiveness of five different oral and one parenteral form. N Engl J Med 1958;259:57. (*No difference was found in reaction rates between IM and PO use.*)

Currie BJ. Are currently recommended doses of benzathine penicillin G adequate for secondary prophylaxis of rheumatic fever? Pediatrics 1996;97:989. (*Because failure rates may be higher with*

1,200,000 units every 4 weeks compared with every 3 weeks, suggests higher doses if 8 three week injection is used.)

Dajani DA, Taubert K, Ferrieri P, et al. Treatment of acute streptococcal pharyngitis and prevention of rheumatic fever: a statement for health professionals. Committee on Rheumatic Fever, Endocarditis, and Kawasaki Disease of the Council on Cardiovascular Disease in the Young, the American Heart Association. Pediatrics 1995;96:758. *(Update of the recommendations previously issued in 1988.)*

Holmberg SD, Faich GA. Streptococcal pharyngitis and acute rheumatic fever in Rhode Island. JAMA 1983;250:2307. *(Of patients receiving throat cultures, nearly 90% were given antibiotic therapy before the culture results were known and nearly 40% continued antibiotic therapy for 10 days regardless of results. Only three definite cases of rheumatic fever were identified during a 5-year period.)*

International Rheumatic Fever Study Group. Allergic reactions to long-term benzathine penicillin prophylaxis for rheumatic fever. Lancet 1991;337:1308. *(Risk found to be very low.)*

Land MA, Bisno AL. Acute rheumatic fever: a vanishing disease in suburbia. JAMA 1983;249:895. *(A retrospective analysis in Memphis-Shelby County detecting a 0.64 case per 100,000 population annual incidence of acute rheumatic fever. An accompanying editorial ponders explanations for the dramatic fall in acute rheumatic fever incidence in the United States.)*

McFarland RB. Reactions to benzathine penicillin. N Engl J Med 1958;259:62. *(Reaction rate of 1.3% after single injection in 12,858 naval recruits.)*

Rammelkamp CH, Wannamaker LW, Denny FW. The epidemiology and prevention of rheumatic fever—1952. Bull NY Acad Med 1997;74:119. *(The classic article reprinted for its historical interest.)*

Schwartz RH, Wientzen RL, Pedreira F, et al. Penicillin V for group A pharyngeal tonsillitis. JAMA 1981;246:1790. *(A randomized control trial demonstrating a treatment failure rate of 31% for patients treated for 7 days compared with 18% for those treated for 10 days.)*

Spagnuolo M, Pasternack B, Taranta A. Risk of rheumatic fever recurrences after streptococcal infections. N Engl J Med 1971;285:641. *(Data are reviewed in Table 17.1.)*

Stollerman GH. Variation in group A streptococci and the prevalence of rheumatic fever: a half-century vigil. Ann Intern Med 1993;118:467. *(Editorial that provides historical perspective on rheumatic fever and its prevention.)*

Wood HF, Feinstein AR, Taranta A, et al. Rheumatic fever in children and adolescents. III. Comparative effectiveness of three prophylaxis regimens in preventing streptococcal infections and rheumatic recurrences. Ann Intern Med 1964;60:31. *(Data are reviewed in Table 17.2.)*

18

Exercise for Prevention of Cardiovascular Disease

HARVEY B. SIMON

When performed regularly and properly, exercise has a powerful protective effect against coronary artery disease, effective for both primary prevention and secondary prevention. Exercise also provides significant benefits for many of the chronic diseases that affect American society, including hypertension, stroke, type 2 diabetes, osteoporosis, and common cancers (e.g., colon, breast, female reproductive tract). Despite these benefits, only about 22% of American adults exercise at recommended levels. Sedentary living imposes a relative risk of dying from coronary artery disease of 1.9. The magnitude of this excess relative risk approaches that of smoking (2.5), elevated cholesterol (2.4), and hypertension (2.1). Because sedentary living is to two to three times more prevalent than any of these other risk factors, it can be argued that physical inactivity is the single largest contributor to the epidemic of coronary artery disease. About 250,000 excess deaths in the United States each year can be attributed to lack of exercise.

The primary care physician can have a powerful motivating effect on patients by educating them about the benefits and approaches to exercise. One needs to identify those patients at risk for exercise-induced complications and prescribe a personalized exercise program that is safe and effective. Also important is identification, initial treatment, and appropriate referral of exercise-related problems.

PHYSIOLOGY AND CLINICAL EFFECTS OF EXERCISE

Physiology

Physical work may involve either *aerobic* or *anaerobic* metabolism, and it may rely on either isotonic or isometric muscular activity. Energy must be generated continuously during exercise, because the total amount of stored ATP in muscles can sustain only 10 seconds of maximal exertion. The production of new ATP requires metabolism of muscle glycogen. The availability of oxygen determines whether this metabolism will be aerobic or anaerobic. When oxygen supply is adequate, metabolism is aerobic and glycogen is completely metabolized to pyruvate and then to water and CO_2 through the Krebs cycle.

With increasing exercise intensity, the ability of the lungs to take up oxygen and of the heart and blood vessels to deliver it to muscle cells is exceeded, and metabolism becomes anaerobic. The costs of anaerobic metabolism are substantial. Anaerobic metabolism is inefficient; it generates only one third as much energy from each gram of glycogen, and it increases production of lactic acid, resulting in muscle cramps, fatigue, and dyspnea. Lactic acid is buffered by bicarbonate, resulting in increased CO_2 production and hyperventilation. Clinically, an abrupt rise in respiratory rate indicates that the anaerobic threshold has been crossed. Endurance training can be expected to increase the anaerobic threshold, thus allowing more work to be performed under favorable aerobic conditions.

Aerobic and Anaerobic Exercise. The goal of training is to improve cardiovascular function and muscular efficiency. The type of exercise is critical. Although maximal exertion (used in anaerobic training) is beneficial to certain competitive athletes, the cornerstone of training for fitness is endurance or *aerobic exercise* using large muscle groups in continuous rhythmic activity for prolonged periods. *Jogging and brisk walking* are ideal for this. Other good training activities include *bicycling, swimming, cross-country skiing, rowing,* and *rope jumping.* These activities provide *isotonic exercise* whereby skeletal muscle fibers shorten in length with little change in tension. Heart rate and cardiac output increase, but peripheral vascular resistance falls.

In contrast, sports that depend on very brief bursts of intense activity, such as weight lifting, provide *isometric exercise* in which muscle tension increases with little change in fiber length. Such exercise produces a marked increase in peripheral vascular resistance and blood pressure with little increase in cardiac output. Aerobic power does not increase with isometric exercising, and the hypertensive response can be hazardous to patients with cardiovascular disease. Because arm work has a greater tendency to produce tachycardia and hypertension than does an equivalent degree of leg work, it is particularly important to limit the resistance level in arm exercises for patients with hypertension or heart disease.

Sports that allow prolonged periods of inactivity, such as baseball or golf, are poor for cardiopulmonary conditioning. Similarly, although activities providing sustained but gentle muscular effort, such as yoga, can be important parts of a fitness program because they are excellent for promoting flexibility and strength, they are poor tools for attaining cardiopulmonary fitness.

Effects of Exercise

The effects of regular exercise can be classified in terms of cardiovascular, musculoskeletal, metabolic, and psychological functions. Regular endurance-type exercise improves cardiovascular performance and tends to lower blood pressure, body fat, weight, and serum triglycerides while elevating serum high-density lipoproteins. Physical fitness may also assist in the psychological response to stress.

Cardiovascular. The most thoroughly documented results of aerobic exercise concern changes in cardiovascular performance. Exercise requires an increase in the body's oxygen consumption, which is made possible by increased oxygen uptake by pulmonary ventilation, increased oxygen delivery by the heart and the peripheral circulation, and increased oxygen extraction by muscle. Endurance training enhances the efficiency of these processes by both central and peripheral mechanisms. At rest and at submaximal work loads, the fit individual has a slower heart rate than does the untrained person. Stroke volume is increased so that cardiac output for a given work load is unchanged. Although the achievable maximum heart rate is not increased by training, the maximum cardiac output and maximum oxygen consumption are greatly enhanced so that the

well-trained individuals can both attain higher work loads and sustain them for longer periods before becoming exhausted.

Although there is little firm evidence that exercise increases myocardial oxygen supply or produces collateral vascularization in humans, *myocardial oxygen demand* for a given work load *decreases.* This diminution in myocardial oxygen consumption is made possible by the lower heart rate and lower systolic blood pressure that accompany exercise in the fit individual. This can be of particular benefit to the patient with angina, as this "double product" of heart rate × blood pressure determines the angina threshold (see Chapter 30). In addition, animal studies have demonstrated increased coronary artery cross-sectional area, increased myocardial capillary density, and myocardial hypertrophy in rats and dogs forced to exercise.

The peripheral effects of repetitive isotonic exercise are also of great importance in endurance training. *Capillary blood flow* to muscle is increased. Muscle fibers increase in volume, and muscle strength and endurance are enhanced. Muscle mitochondria increase in size and number, and respiratory enzymes increase. As a result, muscle oxygen extraction is improved. Training also improves neuromuscular coordination and musculoskeletal efficiency.

Another important cardiovascular effect of exercise is on *blood pressure.* Systolic pressure normally increases during aerobic exercise, but this rise tends to be slightly less in the fit individual. More important, total peripheral resistance decreases as a result of improved muscle blood flow and decreased circulating catecholamine levels. The net result in trained individuals is lower blood pressure, both during exercise and at rest. Because this effect is actually more prominent in hypertensive subjects, endurance training can be an important nonpharmacologic treatment for the control of mild to moderate hypertension (see Chapter 26).

Less well-established cardiovascular benefits of exercise training include a possible *diminution of arrhythmias,* perhaps because of lower catecholamine levels. In addition, exercise increases *fibrinolytic activity* and decreases platelet adhesiveness; these hematologic effects may, to some degree, protect against atherogenesis. In these areas, too, the data are preliminary. The effects on cardiovascular morbidity and mortality can be marked (see below).

Metabolic. The metabolic benefits of exercise are well documented. *Weight control* is an important motivating factor for many runners. An average jogger can be expected to consume about 600 calories in an hour of running. Other endurance activities have similar effects (Table 18.1). Although exercise alone will produce only a slow reduction in total body weight, the percentage of body fat decreases more rapidly, resulting in visible increases in muscle tone. Perhaps most important, fit people often become motivated to adhere to dietary patterns that will permit sustained weight control.

Another metabolic effect of great interest is that of regular exercise on the blood lipids. In many runners, serum *triglyceride* levels fall dramatically without changes in the dietary intake of fats or carbohydrates. The total *cholesterol* level changes less predictably, but *high-density lipoprotein* levels are reliably increased by aerobic exercise, and these higher levels correlate with a lower risk for coronary artery disease (see Chapter 15).

Table 18.1. Approximate Metabolic Expenditures Associated with Selected Activities[a]

AVERAGE ENERGY OUTPUT	ACTIVITY
1 met	Rest
1½–2 mets 2–2½ kcal/min	Desk work Standing Strolling (1 mile/h)
2–3 mets 2½–4 kcal/min	Level walking (2 miles/h) Level biking (5 miles/h) Golf (power cart)
3–4 mets 4–5 kcal/min	Walking (3 miles/h) Bicycling (6 miles/h) Badminton Housework
4–5 mets 5–6 kcal/min	Golf (carrying clubs) Dancing Tennis (doubles) Raking leaves Calisthenics
5–6 mets 6–7 kcal/min	Walking (4 miles/h) Bicycling (10 miles/h) Skating Shoveling garden soil Average sexual activity
6–7 mets 7–8 kcal/min	Brisk walking (5 miles/h) Tennis (singles) Snow shoveling Downhill skiing Water skiing
7–8 mets 8–10 kcal/min	Jogging (5 miles/h) Bicycling (12 miles/h) Basketball Canoeing Mountain climbing Ditch digging Touch football
8–9 mets 10–11 kcal/min	Jogging (6 miles/h) Cross-country skiing Squash or handball (recreational)
Over 10 mets Over 11 kcal/min	Squash or handball (competitive) Running 6 miles/h: 10 mets 8 miles/h: 13½ mets 10 miles/hd: 17 mets

[a]Energy outputs are expressed in mets. One met is the energy expended at rest and equals 3.5 mL O_2/kg body weight/min. (Calorie consumption values are a 70-kg person.)

(Modified from Fox SM, Naughty JP, Gorman DA. Physical activity and cardiovascular health. III. The exercise prescription; frequency and type of activity. Mod Concepts Cardiovasc Dis 1972;41:6.)

Several population studies demonstrate that sedentary living increases the risk of developing *glucose intolerance* and *type 2 diabetes* and that good cardiorespiratory fitness reduces risk. The risk associated with lack of exercise appears independent of other known risk factors.

Psychological. Most individuals who engage in regular exercise develop an *improved self-image*. This can be of great importance in the rehabilitation of patients with ischemic heart disease (see Chapter 31) and can also be used to help motivate healthy individuals to modify other risk factors by following a prudent diet and discontinuing smoking. The recreational aspects of exercise tend to lessen anxiety and depression. Run-

ning is being studied as a tool for the treatment of depression, and early results in small groups of patients are encouraging. Nevertheless, the so-called runner's high proves elusive or illusionary for many joggers. Although exercise has many psychological benefits, it is hardly a panacea. Patients can be encouraged to exercise for both psychological and physical gains, but they must have realistic expectations.

Morbidity and Mortality. Because of its amelioration of many cardiovascular risk factors, it would seem reasonable to expect regular exercise to *reduce risk of cardiovascular morbidity and mortality*. Although there are no data from prospective, randomized, controlled studies to allow a definitive conclusion about cause and effect, numerous observational and epidemiologic studies carefully quantifying exercise, documenting cardiovascular fitness, and controlling for most confounding factors demonstrate an inverse relationship between amount of physical activity and cardiovascular morbidity and mortality. However, such studies cannot rule out the possibility that *genetic factors* and *self-selection* might account for some of the benefit observed, that is, if healthy people tend to exercise more, then the reduced mortality in active people may related to underlying factors rather than to the exercise per se.

The best *evidence* against genetic factors and self-selection as the predominant causes for the observed benefit of exercise derive from epidemiologic studies. The Finnish Twin Cohort study revealed a reduction in mortality risk of 34% for occasional exercisers and of 56% for conditioned exercisers compared with their genetically identical twins who were sedentary. In a study of Harvard alumni that included those who participated in varsity sports, sedentary men were at a 64% higher risk for a first myocardial infarction than were classmates who expended at least 2,000 kcal/wk in exercise. Varsity sports participation (a marker of initial fitness and genetic endowment) conferred no protective effect unless exercise was continued in later years.

Maintaining a physically active life-style can be expected to reduce the risk of myocardial infarction by 35% to 70%. Whereas exercise is most effective when commenced early in life, physical activity confers benefit even if initiated later in life. In the Harvard alumni study, men who began to exercise in middle age enjoyed a 23% reduction in mortality compared with their peers who remained sedentary. British investigators noted that the initiation of even light to moderate exercise can reduce all cause mortality by 45%, even after adjusting for potential confounders. Among adult residents of Kings County, Washington, gardening for more than 60 minutes a week was associated with a 68% lower risk of primary cardiac arrests and walking with a 73% risk reduction as compared with sedentary individuals. Among elderly men, walking more than 2 miles a day reduces the mortality rate by nearly 50% compared with those who walk less than 1 mile per day.

Most data regarding the benefits of exercise pertain to men. The best data pertaining to the effects of exercise for primary prevention of coronary events in women derive from the Nurses' Health Study, involving over 72,000 female nurses aged 40 to 65 years who were free of coronary disease and followed for 8 years. There were 645 coronary events (death or nonfatal infarction), with an inversely progressive relationship found between amount of exercise (expressed as energy expenditure) and age-adjusted relative risk of coronary events. Compared with those in the lowest exercise quintile, the range of relative risk was 0.77 to 0.46, with the later figure for those in the highest exercise quintile. Those who engaged in moderate exercise (walking 20 min/mile for 3 or more hours per week) had the same degree of risk reduction (about 35%) as those who engaged in more vigorous forms of exercise. Persons who were previously sedentary and became active in middle adulthood reduced their relative risk.

Although these studies concentrate on the role of exercise in the *primary prevention* of cardiovascular disease, attention is also being directed to the role of physical training in the treatment of patients with established atherosclerotic heart disease (*secondary prevention*). Independent meta-analyses of prospective trials of exercise in the treatment of coronary artery disease demonstrated a 20% to 25% decrease in overall mortality in the exercise group; fatal reinfarction and total cardiovascular deaths were also significantly reduced in the exercise group, but nonfatal reinfarctions were no different in the exercise and control groups.

Other Benefits. Although the greatest protective effect of exercise is on the cardiovascular system, reducing the risk of heart attack, sudden cardiac death, stroke, and hypertension, there are other important benefits of habitual exercise. Women who begin exercising in early adulthood experience nearly a 50% reduction in their lifetime risk of *breast and reproductive cancer*. Physically active men have a significantly lower risk of *colon cancer*. Exercise increases bone density, helping to prevent *osteoporosis*. Patients with *chronic obstructive lung disease* and *peripheral vascular disease* report symptomatic and functional improvements.

MEDICAL SCREENING OF POTENTIAL EXERCISERS

Medical screening of the prospective participant and prescription of an appropriate exercise program are essential for the person who has been inactive. In addition, we recommend that all adults planning to engage in vigorous activity (including young persons who want to participate in competitive athletics) screened for underlying heart disease before beginning. The goal is to reduce the risk of sudden cardiac death. Any decision to restrict a young person from engaging in competitive sports or other vigorous activity should be based on firm evidence, because of the potentially devastating social and psychological impacts the restriction may have. A cardiac consultation is warranted for young persons the primary care physician deems in need of restriction.

The initial screening effort does not need to entail elaborate laboratory testing, but a careful and detailed *cardiovascular history* and *physical examination* are essential. The value of the *resting electrocardiogram* (ECG) for detection of coronary disease in asymptomatic healthy persons is nil, but the test is warranted in asymptomatic young persons who plan to engage in competitive athletics for its ability to detect conduction, rhythm, voltage, and repolarization anomalies that might be tip-offs to important underlying myocardial disease. Even *exercise stress testing* for detection of silent coronary disease is of limited utility in healthy asymptomatic persons but should be considered in those with coronary risk factors (see below).

What to Look For

Silent coronary disease is obviously the major concern for men over the age of 45 years and for menopausal women seeking to start an exercise program (see Chapter 30). When evaluating younger persons who seek to engage in competitive athletics, it is important to check not only for the *major valvular diseases* (e.g., *aortic stenosis, mitral stenosis,* and *mitral valve prolapse,* see Chapters 21 and 33) and rhythm disturbances (see Chapter 25), but also for *hypertrophic cardiomyopathy* and *arrhythmogenic right ventricular cardiomyopathy*, two uncommon often unsuspected conditions that are important causes of sudden death in competitive athletes. The presence of any one of these conditions may be relatively silent or heralded by such findings as palpitations on exertion, syncope or near syncope, lightheadedness, exertional dyspnea chest discomfort, a family history of heart disease or of sudden cardiac death, voltage and ST- and T-wave abnormalities on ECG, and atrial or ventricular premature beats or frank dysrhythmias. A high index of suspicion is warranted.

Hypertrophic cardiomyopathy may be mistaken for the "*athlete's heart,*" seen in persons who engage in strenuous anaerobic exercise. However, a history of effort syncope or near syncope, a family history of cardiac sudden death, a systolic heart murmur that increases with maneuvers that decrease left ventricular volume (see Chapter 21), and marked increase in voltages, prominent Q waves, and deep negative T-waves on resting ECG should make one suspicious of hypertrophic disease. Cardiac ultrasound is required. Diagnostic findings differentiating this condition from athlete's heart include asymmetric wall thickening, involvement of the right and left ventricular, total wall thickness greater than 13 mm, and outflow tract obstruction. Heavy exertion should be restricted and a cardiac consultation obtained.

Arrhythmogenic right ventricular cardiomyopathy is rare but as noted above has been found to be an important cause of arrhythmogenic death in younger persons who engage in competitive sports. Suggestive findings include a family history of sudden cardiac death, palpitations on exertion, inverted T-waves in the right precordial leads on ECG, and ventricular premature beats with a left-bundle-branch pattern.

Anomalous origin of coronary artery is another leading cause of sudden death in athletes. It is typically asymptomatic and difficult to detect premorbidly.

History. The first step in medical screening is obtaining a detailed personal and family history. Each patient should be carefully questioned about symptoms that suggest cardiovascular disease, including chest pain, palpitations, dyspnea, undue fatigue, syncope, and claudication. It is very important to review health habits in detail, with special attention to previous exercise patterns, smoking, diet, and the use of oral contraceptive agents. Of particular importance in the family history is the presence of coronary heart disease, peripheral vascular disease, hypertension, stroke, diabetes, or sudden death.

Physical Examination. A complete physical examination is also vital to the medical screening of the prospective exerciser. Height and weight should be recorded, and it may be useful to calculate the body mass index or to measure the percent body fat (see Chapter 10). The blood pressure is taken at rest with the patient supine and standing, and the heart rate and pressure are recorded after mild exercise (stair climbing or sit-ups are satisfactory for this purpose). The chest is examined for rales, wheezes, and rhonchi and the heart for cardiomegaly, gallops, murmurs, and rhythm disturbances. The peripheral pulses and abdomen should be palpated to exclude atherosclerotic disease and an aortic aneurysm. The musculoskeletal system should be evaluated both to exclude significant pathology and to determine whether specific flexibility or strengthening exercises are required as part of the training program.

Laboratory Studies. Several laboratory studies are helpful in the screening process. Screening for atherosclerotic risk factors is essential (glucose, lipid profile). Also useful are checks of serum hemoglobin and creatinine. For patients older than 40 years of age (especially those with cardiac risk factors or a family history of heart disease), a *resting ECG* is helpful to check for ischemia, left ventricular hypertrophy, and disturbances of rate and rhythm. Young persons who are going to engage in competitive athletics and who have a history of heart murmur, palpitations, dyspnea, undue fatigue, syncope, lightheadedness, or a family history of sudden death, premature heart disease, or dysrhythmias might also benefit from a resting ECG.

If any of these screening procedures discloses evidence suggesting heart disease, then *exercise stress testing* is mandatory before an exercise program is initiated. Even if preliminary screening reveals no evidence of heart disease, stress testing may be helpful for asymptomatic patients with multiple cardiac risk factors, especially if they have been sedentary. Some argue that stress testing may be a prudent precursor in men older than 50 years of age and in women older than 60 years of age who are considering a vigorous exercise program, even if they are asymptomatic and apparently healthy, because atherosclerotic heart disease is so prevalent in our society. However, it must be remembered that stress testing has a very low predictive value in persons with a low pretest probability of coronary artery disease (see Chapter 36). In persons with a history of palpitations or symptoms of lightheadedness, stress testing and *Holter monitoring* may be useful for uncovering exercise-induced arrhythmias and hypotension. Other uses of stress testing are to evaluate the individual's exercise capacity and establish the maximal and target heart rates for use in the exercise prescription. *Echocardiography* is indicated if there is a heart murmur on physical examination (see Chapter 21).

In special cases, additional studies may be desirable, such as forced expiratory volume in 1 second, vital capacity, and arterial blood gases in patients with subjective dyspnea or suspected pulmonary disease. Specialized ergometric testing can determine maximal oxygen consumption, total work capacity, and other physiologic parameters.

Classification. Medical screening and exercise testing allow the physician to assign each patient to one of three categories:

1. *No restrictions, no supervision*: Individuals with normal studies who can undertake an exercise program without medical supervision. Even in these healthy people, individualized exercise prescriptions and guidance regarding training techniques and safety precautions will be of great value.
2. *Some restrictions, some supervision*: Patients with ischemic heart disease, moderate hypertension, or moderate chronic obstructive lung disease will benefit from graded exercise programs, but they should be referred to a specialized exercise rehabilitation program that can provide medical supervision and facilities for emergency treatment. However, if structured rehabilitation is not available, milder forms of exercise without medical supervision can still be recommended (e.g., walking, stationary bicycling) with appropriate precautions.
3. *Marked restrictions or exclusion, marked supervision*: Physical exertion is contraindicated in the presence of uncontrolled congestive heart failure, ventricular irritability, uncontrolled hypertension, unstable diabetes, or uncontrolled epilepsy, although patients with these conditions can sometimes be enrolled in supervised programs if they respond to medical therapy. Patients with left ventricular or aortic aneurysms or hemodynamically significant aortic valve disease should be excluded from exercise programs.

EXERCISE PRESCRIPTION

Role of the Primary Physician. People can exercise for recreation, for health, or for fitness and sports competition. The primary care physician has an important role in encouraging and counseling exercise. The objective is to help the patient find a form and amount of exercise that will be safe, beneficial, enjoyable, and carried out over a prolonged period of time. Imposing a program of exercise is much less effective in achieving sustained compliance than finding out what the patient is willing and interested in doing. Helping the patient to incorporate an exercise program into a busy life-style is critical. Whereas formal workouts are essential for optimal fitness and physical performance, modest levels of physical activity during daily life have important health benefits (see above). Life-style interventions appear to be as effective as formal exercise programs of similar intensity in improving cardiovascular fitness, blood pressure, and body fat composition.

Primary care physicians should encourage all patients who are capable of physical activity to exercise nearly every day; simply walking for 30 to 45 minutes can reduce cardiovascular risk significantly. For patients who are interested and capable, the physician should be prepared to prescribe a program of fitness training.

Fitness Program. The basic elements include frequency, intensity, and duration of exercise.

A *frequency* of three exercise sessions per week are required to develop and maintain fitness, and five sessions per week probably provide near maximum benefit. Hence, the exercise prescription should call for at least three workouts each week. Many individuals prefer a routine of daily activity; this is an excellent program, but it is advisable to schedule easier and harder workouts on alternate days to prevent injuries and allow the muscles to recover.

The *intensity and duration* of training are closely related. Equal degrees of fitness can be attained through less intense exercise sustained over a longer period or through more vigorous effort for shorter periods. Maximum cardiopulmonary fitness can be attained by 15 to 60 minutes of continuous aerobic exercises that are strenuous enough to raise the heart rate to 60% to 80% of maximum or the oxygen uptake to 50% to 85% of maximum. However, as pointed out by the results of the

Nurses' Health Study, maximum reductions in coronary risk need do not necessarily require attainment of maximum cardiopulmonary fitness. Moderate degrees of exercise appear to provide the same degree of protection as vigorous activity, at least in middle-aged women.

Optimal fitness goals must be attained very slowly and gradually, and the physician's exercise prescription should provide a practical means of attaining them. Both the starting point and the rate of progression depend on the health, age, and fitness of the participant. As a rule of thumb, the beginner should plan to exercise aerobically for 10 to 12 minutes at a pace sufficient to increase heart rate to 60% to 80% of maximum without producing breathlessness.

Each aerobic workout session begins with a 5- to 10-minute *warm-up period*. At the beginning of exercise, even the well-conditioned athlete experiences some degree of dyspnea due to anaerobic metabolism. It takes 45 to 90 seconds for cardiac output to increase enough to meet the new work load and provide the "second wind." A warm-up period will minimize this initial anaerobic period and also allow muscles to loosen and stretch out, which prevents many injuries. For the runner, the warm-up period should consist of stretching exercise, calisthenics, and a gradual progression from walking to slow jogging to running.

The actual *training period* should initially consist of a total of 10 to 12 minutes of exercise. At first, it is best to alternate periods of effort with periods of recovery. This is easily accomplished by alternating full intensity exercise with low intensity exercise. For example, an unfit or older individual might alternate 1 minute of full exercising with 1 minute of gentle exercise, repeating this cycle 10 to 12 times during each training day. When this can be accomplished with comfort—perhaps at the end of 10 to 20 sessions over 2 to 3 weeks—the schedule can be advanced to 2 minutes of full exercise alternating with 2 minutes of gentle exercise, with six cycles in each session. After this is mastered, the exercise ritual can be extended to 3 or 4 minutes with only 1 or 2 minutes of rest for three or four cycles and then to two 6-minute runs with 1 or 2 minutes of walking in between. By the end of 1 or 2 months, most individuals can expect to be able to exercise for 10 to 20 minutes continuously.

Although the young and athletic person will progress more rapidly than the older or unfit one, it is important to urge restraint. One of the most common causes of orthopedic injuries is attempting too much too quickly. Once a base of 10 to 20 minutes of exercise is well established, further progress can be encouraged. It is reasonable to increase time or distance by a rate of about 10% per week. This can be accomplished by extending one or two sessions while preserving some short distance days or by gradually extending each session. At the end of 4 to 6 months, 3 to 4 miles of jogging or equivalent exercise 3 to 5 days per week will provide maximum conditioning. This level must be maintained to sustain the cardiopulmonary benefits of exercise. Feelings of accomplishment and well-being usually provide motivation for sustained participation, often at even higher levels. As little as 20 minutes of aerobic exercise three times per week is beneficial, but 3 to 4 hours of exercise per week provides the maximum longevity benefits.

In addition to the duration of exercise, the *intensity or pace* of exercise requires consideration. The most precise readily available measure of intensity is the *heart rate*. Patients should work at a pace sufficient to raise the pulse to 60% to 80% of maximum. If exercise testing has been performed, an observed maximal heart rate can be used for this calculation. In the absence of such data, the maximal heart rate can be estimated for healthy individuals by subtracting the age from 220. As a rough guide, the target of 60% to 80% of this maximum translates to 130 to 150 beats per minute for younger persons and to 110 to 125 beats per minute for older ones. Patients can be taught to count their carotid or radial pulse just before and immediately after exercise and to adjust their pace to attain and maintain the target heart rate. It can be very helpful to have patients keep a daily record of these figures together with the time and approximate distance covered. As training progresses, a more rapid pace will be required to achieve the target heart rate.

Many people find it difficult or unpleasant to take their pulse. For such persons, intensity of effort can be roughly gauged by the *"talking" pace*—the intensity sufficient to feel one is working hard while still able to talk to a companion without feeling dyspneic.

The *cool-down period* completes the exercise prescription. A period of 5 to 10 minutes of walking and stretching exercises is desirable. This prevents the marked vasodilatation for dissipation of heat from causing hypotension and hypoperfusion. Very hot or very cold showers should be avoided.

PATIENT EDUCATION

Motivating the Patient. Patient need to know that next to smoking, hypertension, and hypercholesterolemia, inactivity is one of the most important treatable cardiac risk factors. Many do not appreciate that exercise not only can help them to look, feel, and work better, but it can reduce overall coronary morbidity and mortality. Also helpful is emphasizing that even modest amounts of activity (including informal exercise such as gardening) can provide substantial health benefits and that moderate exercise (e.g., walking at a moderate pace) can be as effective in reducing coronary risk as vigorous activity. This helps patients find enjoyable activities that can be incorporated into their daily life and facilitates motivation. The goal is to have them take up and sustain a program of endurance-type activity. Most important to success is choosing a form of exercise that is enjoyable and readily incorporated into daily living.

Focusing on Safety. Exercise is not without risk, and patients need to know what to look for and how to respond. There is no question that exercise can precipitate cardiac arrhythmias and myocardial ischemia in persons with underlying *heart disease*. Sudden death is a tragic, though infrequent, complication of exercise. Careful medical screening of potential exercisers (see above) and design of an appropriate individualized exercise prescription are essential to patient safety. In addition, detailed review of cardiac warning signs (chest pressure, dizziness, lightheadedness, dyspnea, palpitations, unusual fatigue, nausea, diaphoresis) is critical along with advice to stop exercising immediately if such symptoms develop. One must be sure the patient will not continue exercising or rationalize the symptoms away by misattributing them to such harmless causes as "indigestion" or "gas." Meticulous supervision of high-risk individuals and use of closely controlled conditioning programs have enabled survivors of myocardial infarctions to engage safely in aerobic exercise, even marathon running.

Some exercisers encounter exercise-induced *asthma*, particularly during cold weather. Advising use of a face mask that warms inspired air often suffices; sometimes prophylactic treatment with inhaled cromolyn, albuterol, or montelukast is necessary and helpful (see Chapter 48). Extreme environmental conditions may also produce thermal stress ranging from frostbite to heat stroke. Here too, prevention is the best therapy. The physician should be able to advise the exerciser about appropriate fluid intake, clothing, acclimatization, and safe duration of exposure and exercise. Similar advice prevents dehydration and electrolyte depletion.

Musculoskeletal injuries are very common and result from overuse, inflexibility, and muscle imbalance (see Chapters 152 and 154). Overuse is prevented by gradual increases in exercise; inflexibility and imbalance are avoided by stretching and strengthening (see below). Providing advice about equipment and technique can also help lessen the risk of injury (see below).

PRACTICAL ADVICE FOR THE BEGINNING EXERCISER

Food and Fluid Intake. It is best to avoid exercise within 2 hours of a substantial meal. Despite many claims to the contrary, no specific dietary programs are required for exercise. The obese person should restrict calories to reduce, whereas the lean individual may require increased caloric intake to maintain weight. Competitive athletes believe that increased carbohydrate intake during the 3 days before a competitive endurance event helps improve performance, and there is some experimental evidence suggesting that such "carbohydrate loading" does increase muscle glycogen content. Adequate fluid intake is essential, particularly in warm weather, because the sensation of thirst lags behind volume depletion. It is best to begin drinking small amounts before thirst becomes overt. Water is excellent, though some athletes prefer balanced electrolyte solutions or even carbonated beverages.

Climate. Thermal stress presents a potentially serious threat. When confronted with an abrupt change in climate, the exerciser should sharply reduce distance and speed for several days until acclimatization is achieved. In warm humid weather, outdoor exercise should be confined to early morning or evening hours or shady locations, distances and speed should be reduced, fluids should be taken at frequent intervals during the run, and clothing should be light colored and lightweight. Environmental temperatures between 50°F and 60°F are ideal for exercising in shorts and T shirts. Between 40°F and 50°F, a warmup suit is generally sufficient; below 40°F, gloves or mittens and a hat are important. Multiple layers of thin flexible clothing are better than a single bulky garment. Woolen fabrics are ideal, but a soft cotton layer should be next to the skin. An extra layer of thermal underwear is vital for temperatures below 30°F, and if winds are strong or temperatures drop below 15°F, an additional layer such as a turtleneck, extra shorts, and possibly a ski mask are required. Again, distances should be reduced in bitter cold, and it is particularly important to avoid wet conditions, which can lead to frostbite, especially of the feet.

Air pollutants may cause irritation of the upper and lower respiratory tract, and carbon monoxide can impair oxygenation and precipitate angina. One should avoid jogging or biking on heavily traveled roads, during rush hours, and on days when temperature inversions increase air pollution.

Safety. Safety is of utmost importance. The runner and walker should run facing the flow of cars. Sidewalks are preferred; although country roads are appealing, it is desirable to stay with a companion in isolated areas in case of injury. Daytime exercise is safer both because one is more visible to cars and can see road hazards more easily. Bright-colored clothing should be encouraged, and at night reflectorized vests are mandatory. Dogs are best avoided by means of an impromptu detour, but if this is not possible, they can generally be intimidated by a firm command to "go home" or by the threat of a stick or stone.

Equipment. One of the advantages of jogging and walking is that elaborate equipment is not required; however, good athletic *shoes* are essential. Many excellent shoes are available; the choice should be dictated by fit, comfort, and support rather than by endorsements or ratings. The toe box should provide enough room for dorsiflexion during take-off, the sole should be flexible and provide adequate cushioning, and the heel should be fairly snug without exerting pressure on the Achilles tendon. Most good athletic shoes are costly but are durable and useful for reducing the risk of injury. Good shoes are important; other items ranging from stopwatches to designer sweat suits are optional to say the least.

Orthotics and other orthopedic devices are sometimes helpful for refractory problems. Patients with overuse injuries who fail to limit their activity may require a splint or cast to enforce inactivity, even if immobilization is not actually necessary for healing. The use of such devices requires referral to an orthopedist or podiatrist skilled in treating runners' musculoskeletal problems.

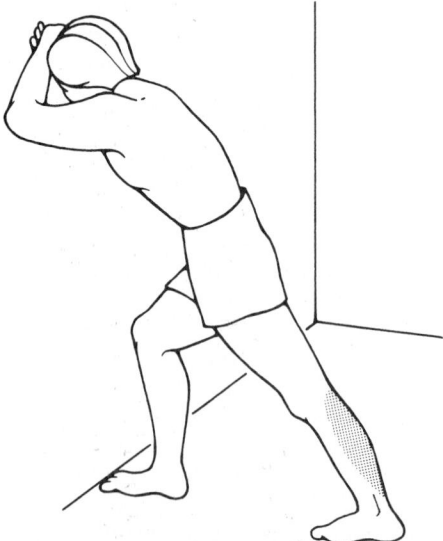

Figure 18.1. Calf, Achilles, and soleus stretch. Stand 3 feet from a wall with one foot forward, leaning forward to support your upper body by resting your forearms against the wall. Bend the forward leg at the knee. Keep the rear leg straight with the heel on the floor, and slowly press your hips forward until you feel the calf stretch. Hold for 15 seconds. Relax and then repeat with the rear knee slightly bent so that you feel the Achilles stretch. Repeat with the other leg forward.

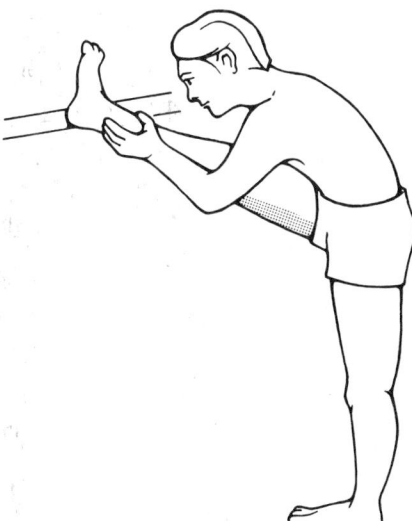

Figure 18.2. Hamstring stretch. Rest one leg on a sturdy table or desk. Keeping both legs straight, slowly bend forward at the waist so that you feel the hamstring stretch. Hold for 30 seconds. Repeat with the other leg up.

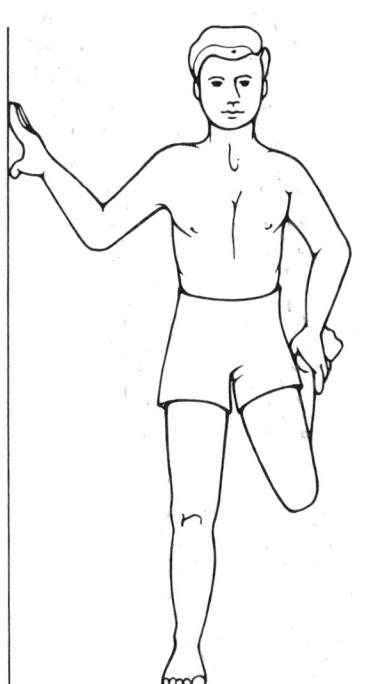

Figure 18.3. Quadriceps stretch. Stand at arm's length from a wall with your feet parallel to the wall. Rest your hand on the wall for support. Hold your ankle in your free hand, and pull the foot back and up until the heel touches the buttocks, while leaning slightly forward from the waist. Repeat with the other leg.

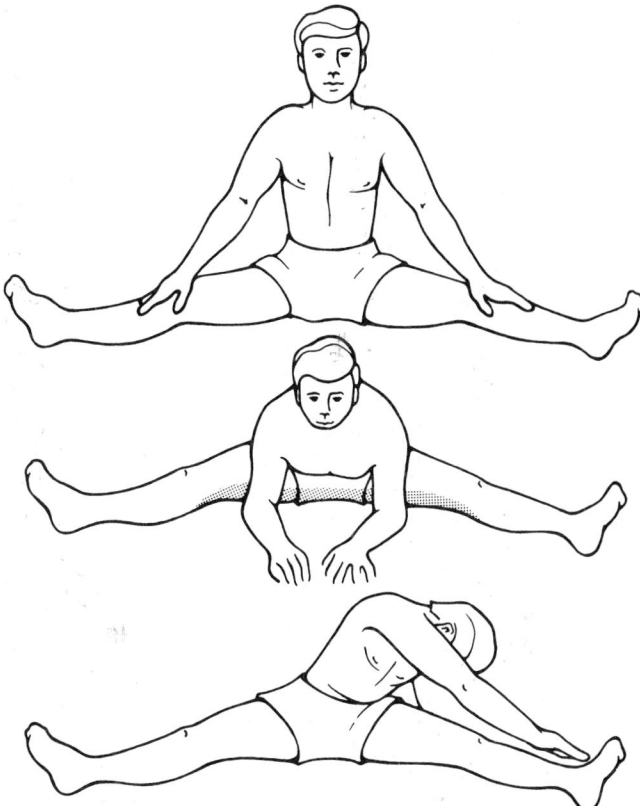

Figure 18.4. Hip and side stretch. Sit on the floor and spread your legs as far apart as possible. With your legs and back straight, bend forward from the waist until you feel a stretch at the inner thighs. Hold for 20 seconds. Relax, then twist at the waist, and lean to touch your right hand to your left foot. Hold for 20 seconds. Repeat on the other side.

Stretching. Aerobic exercise programs may produce asymmetric muscular development. In runners, the calf, hamstring, and Achilles tendon can become overdeveloped and/or shortened and tight. Hill running and sprinting may produce similar effects on the quadriceps and hip flexors. A regular program of stretching exercises is essential to promote flexibility and balanced muscular development. These exercises are ideal for the warm-up and cool-down periods before and after exercise.

Stretching routines are almost as numerous and varied as runners themselves. Four exercises are of particular value: the Achilles and soleus stretch (Fig. 18.1), the hamstring stretch (Fig. 18.2), the quadriceps stretch (Fig. 18.3), and the hip and side stretch (Fig. 18.4).

With increased training, more stretching will be necessary. In addition to flexibility, balanced muscular strength can be important. Bent-knee situps are particularly valuable in strengthening abdominal muscles and preventing "side stitches." Upper extremity strength is surprisingly important; push-ups are the simplest upper extremity exercise. For older persons, low-resistance high-repetition weight training is extremely helpful for maintaining muscle mass and bone density during the aging progress.

Exercise is not a panacea, but it has many cardiopulmonary, metabolic, and psychological benefits. The physician has a crucial role in motivating, screening, and preventing problems. Periodic return visits may be necessary for dealing with various running-related problems. These visits afford the opportunity for the physician to counsel patience and persistence. Joggers who get through the difficult 2 or 3 months at the beginning of training are likely to develop running habits that are both enjoyable and healthful.

RECOMMENDATIONS

- Encourage all persons to engage regularly in physical activity that provides aerobic exercise.
- Help the individual choose an activity program that is medically appropriate, enjoyable, and readily incorporated into daily living. The program does not need to be one of formal exercise; even gardening and modest daily informal activity can provide a survival benefit. Life-style interventions appear to be as effective as formal exercise programs of similar intensity in improving cardiovascular fitness, blood pressure, and body fat composition.
- For the person who is not interested in structured training, design a program of life-style change that provides regular aerobic activity (e.g., walking more, riding less; climbing stairs instead of taking elevators).
- For individuals interested in a formal fitness program, screen first for underlying cardiopulmonary disease, predominantly by a careful history and physical examination. Those with risk factors, symptoms, or signs of heart disease are candidates for additional cardiac studies to help determine the safe limits of their exercise program.
- For persons medically appropriate for fitness training, prescribe a program of aerobic exercise, three times per week. Start with 5 minutes for warm up, 10 to 12 minutes for exercise, and 5 minutes for cooling down. As a rule of thumb, the beginner should plan to exercise aerobically for 10 to 12 minutes at a pace sufficient to increase heart rate to 60% to 80% of maximum without producing breathlessness.
- Design the program so that the optimal fitness goals are attained very slowly and gradually. The intensity target should be at a comfortable level (e.g., the "talking" pace—the intensity sufficient to feel one is working hard while still able to talk to a companion without feeling dyspneic).
- Increase intensity gently and duration gradually (e.g., by 10% each week). Avoid too much too soon. Set both the starting point and the rate of progression according to the health, age, and fitness of the participant.
- Set for those who desire maximum cardiopulmonary fitness a goal of exercising continuously for 15 to 60 minutes, performing aerobic exercises that are strenuous enough to raise the heart rate to 80% of maximum (maximum rate in beats per minute = $[220 - \text{age}] \times 0.8$). Equal degrees of fitness can be attained through less intense exercise sustained over a longer period or through more vigorous effort for shorter periods.
- Consider a program of moderate exercise for those who desire a near maximum reduction in risk of coronary disease without achieving maximum cardiopulmonary fitness. For example, recommend for middle-aged women a program of walking at a moderate pace (20 min/mile) for 3 or more hours a week. One does not need to prescribe vigorous exercise to maximize coronary risk reduction. Those who have not been active previously should be encouraged to begin a program of moderate exercise, with walking an excellent and practical suggestion.
- For persons engaged in a program of fitness training, recommend a minimum of three sessions per week to develop and maintain fitness; recommend five sessions per week for those interested in maximum benefit.
- For those who prefer a routine of daily activity, recommend easier and harder workouts on alternate days to prevent injuries and allow the muscles to recover.
- Review cardiac warning signs (chest pressure, dizziness, lightheadedness, dyspnea, palpitations, unusual fatigue, nausea, diaphoresis). Teach all exercisers to stop activity immediately if such symptoms develop and call for assistance.

ANNOTATED BIBLIOGRAPHY

American College of Sports Medicine. The recommended quantity and quality of exercise for developing and maintaining cardiorespiratory and muscular fitness and flexibility in healthy adults. Med Sci Sports Exerc 1998;30:975. *(Position paper of the ACSM.)*

Berlin JA, Colditz GA. A metaanalysis of physical activity in the prevention of coronary heart disease. Am J Epidemiol 1990;132:612. *(Sedentary living increases the risk of coronary artery disease; relative risk 1.9.)*

Burke AD, Farb A, Malcom GT. Plaque rupture and sudden death related to exertion in men with coronary disease. JAMA 1999;281:921. *(Important insight into the mechanism of sudden death during exercise.)*

Dunn AL, Marcus BH, Kampert JB. Comparison of the lifestyle and structured intervention to increase physical activity and cardiorespiratory fitness: a randomized trial. JAMA 1999;281:327. *(Lifestyle interventions and structured training are both effective in promoting fitness and reducing risk factors.)*

Blair SN, Kohl HW, Paffenbarger RS Jr, et al. Physical fitness and all-cause mortality: a prospective study of healthy men and women. JAMA 1989;262:2395. *(Exercise reduces mortality from coronary artery disease, cancer, and all causes; even modest exercise exerts a protective effect.)*

Cooper KH, Pollock ML, Martin RP, et al. Physical fitness levels vs. selected coronary risk factors. A cross-sectional study. JAMA 1976;236:116. *(A classic prevalence study of nearly 3,000 men showing an inverse relationship between physical fitness and resting heart rate, blood pressure, body weight, percent body fat, and serum levels of cholesterol, triglycerides, and glucose.)*

Corrado D, Basso C, Schiavon M, et al. Screening for hypertrophic cardiomyopathy in young adults. N Engl J Med 1998;339:364. *(An epidemiologic study of a community-based screening program; findings suggest that lives can be saved, especially when there is an effort to detect hypertrophic cardiomyopathy.)*

Curfman GD. Is exercise beneficial—or hazardous—to your health? N Engl J Med 1993;329:1730. *(The answer is "both.")*

Curfman GD. The health benefits of exercise: a critical reappraisal. N Engl J Med 1993;328:574. *(An editorial examining the quality of the data supporting the health benefits of exercise; notes most data are observational.)*

Curfman GD, Thomas GS, Paffenbarger RS Jr. Physical activity and primary prevention of cardiovascular disease. Cardiol Clin 1985;3:203. *(Part of a superb symposium on preventive cardiology.)*

Hakin AA, Petrovitch H, Burchfiel CM. Effects of walking on mortality among nonsmoking retired men. N Engl J Med 1998;338:94. *(Walking works.)*

Kelemen MH, Effron MB, Valenti SA, et al. Exercise training combined with antihypertensive drug therapy. JAMA 1990;263:2766. *(A prospective randomized trial of 52 hypertensive men demonstrating that exercise training can control moderate hypertension as effectively as propranolol or diltiazem.)*

Kujcla UM, Kaprio J, Sarna S. Relationship of leisure-time physical activity and mortality. JAMA 1998;275:440. *(The Finnish Twin Cohort Study; physical activity associated with reduced mortality even after genetic and other familial factors are taken into account.)*

Lane NA, Bloch DA, Hubert HB, et al. Running, osteoarthritis, and bone density: initial 2-year longitudinal study. Am J Med 1990;88:452. *(Running increases bone density without producing osteoarthritis.)*

Lemaire RN, Siscovick DS, Ragnonathan TE, et al. Leisure-time physical activity and the risk of primary cardiac arrest. Arch Intern Med 1999;159:686. *(Even modest activity appears to reduce the risk of sudden cardiac death.)*

Maron BJ. Cardiovascular risks to young persons on the athletic field. Ann Intern Med 1998;129:379. *(A review of sudden death in athletes with current American recommendations for screening.)*

Manson JE, Hu FB, Rich-Edwards JW, et al. A prospective study of walking as compared with vigorous exercise in the prevention of coronary heart disease in women. N Engl J Med 1999;341:651. *(A prospective epidemiologic study from the Nurses' Health Study database; moderately paced walking 3 hours per week reduced coronary risk to the same degree as more vigorous exercise.)*

Mittleman MA, MacClure M, Tofler GH, et al. Triggering of acute myocardial infarction by heavy exertion: protection against triggering by regular exertion. N Engl J Med 1993;329:1677. *(The title summarizes the findings.)*

Paffenbarger RS Jr, Hyde RT, Wing AL, et al. The association of changes in physical activity level and other lifestyle characteristics with mortality among men. N Engl J Med 1993;328:538. *(Beginning moderately vigorous sports activity independently lowered all-cause and coronary heart disease mortality.)*

Sandvik L, Erikssen J, Thaulow E, et al. Physical fitness as a predictor of mortality among healthy, middle-aged Norwegian men. N Engl J Med 1993;328:533. *(A high level of fitness was associated with lower all-cause mortality; fitness was an independent predictor of cardiovascular mortality.)*

Simon HB. Patient-directed nonprescription approaches to cardiovascular disease. Arch Intern Med 1994;154:2283. *(A review of lifestyle and nonprescription interventions.)*

Siscovick DS, Ekelund LG, Johnson JL, et al. Sensitivity of exercise electrocardiography for acute cardiac events during moderate and strenuous physical activity. Arch Intern Med 1991;151:325. *(A submaximal electrocardiographic exercise stress test was not sensitive in asymptomatic hypercholesterolemic men.)*

Wannamethee SG, Shaper AG, Walker M. Changes in physical activity, mortality, and incidence of coronary heart disease in men. Lancet 1998;315:1603. *(Maintaining or initiating light or moderate physical activity reduces mortality in older men with and without diagnosed cardiovascular disease.)*

Wei M, Gibbons LW, Mitchell TL, et al. The association between cardiorespiratory fitness and impaired fasting glucose and type 2 diabetes mellitus in men. Ann Intern Med 1999;130:89. *(A population-based prospective study in middle-aged white men showing low fitness to be an independent risk factor for type 2 diabetes after correcting for known risk factors.)*

19

Evaluation of Hypertension

KATHARINE K. TREADWAY

High blood pressure, if unrecognized or untreated, significantly increases the morbidity and mortality associated with coronary disease, heart failure, renal failure, and stroke. Risk further increases dramatically in the presence of smoking, glucose intolerance, hyperlipidemia, left ventricular hypertrophy (LVH), male gender, African-American race, or increasing age. Treatment of hypertension—even if only partial—can greatly reduce its morbidity and mortality risks.

Upon encountering blood pressure elevation, the first priority for the primary physician is to *confirm the diagnosis*. After confirmation, the evaluation focuses on three major tasks. The first is to rule out any *secondary causes*. Although about 95% of patients have primary disease (no clearly definable underlying cause), a search for a secondary etiology is important, because if such a cause is present, treatment will need to be etiologic to be effective. The second is to assess the *severity of disease*, because risk and type of treatment program derive from the degree of pressure elevation and amount of target-organ (end-organ) damage. The third is to identify any concurrent *cardiovascular risk factors*, because their presence will affect the threshold for initiating therapy and the nature of the treatment program. As of yet, attempts to determine the principal underlying pathophysiology have proven elusive, though when it becomes feasible to do so, the results should facilitate diagnosis and further rationalize treatment.

DEFINITION AND CLASSIFICATION OF HYPERTENSION

Definition. The definition of hypertension is arbitrary (it even varies from country to country). Actuarial data have shown that morbidity and mortality related to complications of hypertension increase linearly with increasing levels of either systolic (SBP) or diastolic blood pressure (DBP). Hence, no critical level of blood pressure exists beyond which risk becomes highly magnified. Most definitions of hypertension refer to a level of blood pressure associated with a substantial risk of complications. A major consensus report, the Sixth Report of the Joint National Committee on Detection, Evaluation, and Treatment of High Blood Pressure (JNC VI) recommends a *SBP greater than or equal to 140 mm Hg and a DBP of 90 mm Hg or more* for the definition of hypertension.

The definition of hypertension must be *individualized* for each patient. The diagnosis derives not only from the absolute level of blood pressure but also from the presence or absence of other *cardiovascular risk factors*. Factors besides hypertension identified by the Framingham study as significant contributors to cardiovascular risk include cigarette smoking, elevated serum cholesterol, glucose intolerance, and electrocardiographic evidence of LVH with strain. In addition, African-American race, male gender, and age greater than 50 need to be taken into account. The patient with borderline hypertension, a moderately elevated serum cholesterol level, and a history of

Table 19.1. Classification of Blood Pressure for Adults Aged 18 Years and Older[a]

CATEGORY	SYSTOLIC (mm Hg)	DIASTOLIC (mm Hg)
Normal[b]	<130	<85
High normal	130–139	85–89
Hypertension[c]		
Stage 1 (mild)	140–159	90–99
Stage 2 (moderate)	160–179	100–109
Stage 3 (severe)	≥180	≥110

[a]Not taking antihypertensive drugs and not acutely ill. When systolic and diastolic pressure fall into different categories, the higher category should be selected to classify the individual's blood pressure status. For instance, 160/92 mm Hg should be classified as stage 2, and 180/120 mm Hg should be classified as stage 4. Isolated systolic hypertension is defined as a systolic blood pressure of 140 mm Hg or more and a diastolic blood pressure of less than 90 mm Hg and staged appropriately (e.g., 170/85 mm Hg is defined as stage 2 isolated systolic hypertension). In addition to classifying stages of hypertension on the basis of average blood pressure levels, the clinician should specify presence or absence of target-organ disease and additional risk factors. For example, a patient with diabetes and a blood pressure of 142/94 mm Hg, plus left ventricular hypertrophy should be classified as having "stage 1 hypertension with target-organ disease (left ventricular hypertrophy) and with another major risk factor (diabetes)." This specificity is important for risk classification and management.

[b]Optimal blood pressure with respect to cardiovascular risk is less than 120 mm Hg systolic and less than 80 mm Hg diastolic. However, unusually low readings should be evaluated for clinical significances.

[c]Based on the average of two or more readings taken at each of two or more visits after an initial screening.

From Sixth Report of the Joint National Committee (JNC VI) on Detection, Evaluation, and Treatment of High Blood Pressure. Arch Intern Med 1997;137:2413.

smoking has a fivefold higher risk of incurring cardiovascular disease than the patient with borderline hypertension alone.

Classification. The JNC VI recommendations include eliminating the traditional designations of "*mild*," "*moderate*," and "*severe*" hypertension to avoid the misleading notion than mild hypertension is not a significant health risk. Instead, they designate three stages:

- *Stage I*—DBP 90 to 99 mm, SBP 140 to 159 mm;
- *Stage II*—DBP 100 to 109 mm, SBP 160 to 179 mm;
- *Stage III*—DBP more than 110 mm, SBP more than 180 mm.

In addition, a "high-normal" category (DBP 85 to 89, SBP 135 to 139) is designated to highlight the increased risk of developing sustained hypertension in this group (Table 19.1).

PATHOPHYSIOLOGY AND CLINICAL PRESENTATION
Pathophysiology

Control of blood pressure and the pathophysiology of hypertension are still incompletely understood. It has become increasingly clear that hypertension is a polygenic disorder with probable variable penetrance and phenotype in which environment may play a modifying role. Thus, it represents a complex interaction of multiple genetic and environmental factors playing varyingly significant roles in particular patients. Because there is a strong familial predisposition to hypertension, much of the pathophysiology is likely to be an expression of inherited defects in the regulation of blood pressure. There are probably several mechanistic subtypes of "primary" hypertension. It is also likely that several abnormal mechanisms are present in any one individual. It is unlikely that single gene mutations will be found to be responsible except in rare instances. As of yet, it is usually not possible to identify specific etiologic mechanisms in a given case. Nonetheless, several elements deserve elaboration and provide a rational basis for evaluation and therapy.

Primary determinants of blood pressure are *cardiac output* and *peripheral resistance*. Each is affected by a variety of factors, which, in turn, have multiple control points (Fig. 19.1).

Sodium. Several lines of evidence continue to implicate sodium. Population studies demonstrate a relationship between high blood pressure and high sodium intake. In cultures where salt intake is low, hypertension is exceedingly rare. When members of those same cultures migrate into cultures in which salt intake is high, approximately 25% to 30% will develop hypertension. Sodium restriction, as well as use of diuretics, has long been known to reduce blood pressure in a subset of hypertensives. However, sodium intake is a poor predictor of hyperten-

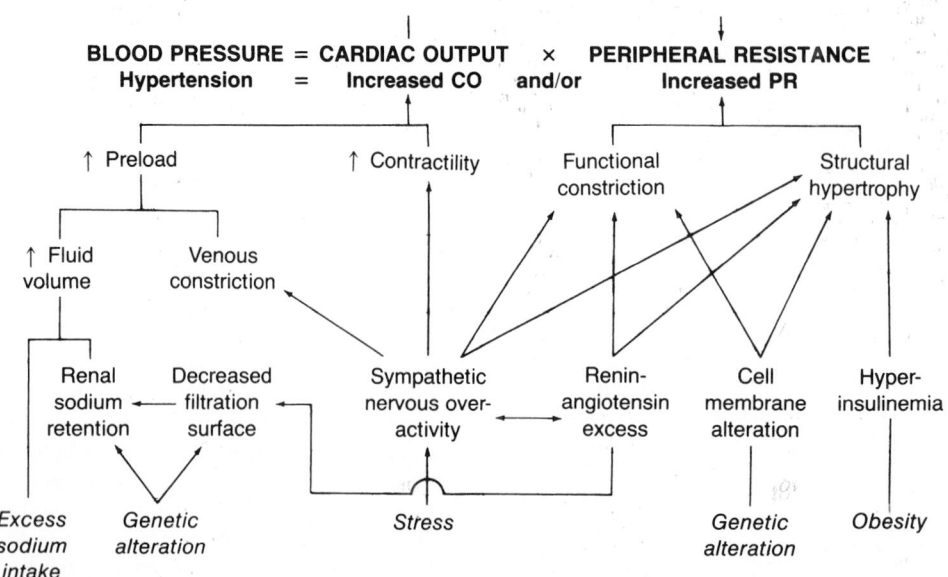

Fig. 19.1. Factors involved in control of blood pressure. (From Kaplan NM. Clinical hypertension, 5th ed. Baltimore: William & Wilkins, 1990:57, with permission.)

sion in a given individual, suggesting that susceptibility depends on many other factors, probably both genetic and environmental. It is postulated that many hypertensives have an inherited defect in the ability of the kidney to excrete excess sodium. This leads to an increase in intravascular volume that is corrected by an as yet unidentified factor—the putative "natriuretic hormone"—that inhibits the Na$^+$/K$^+$-ATPase pump. The net result is an increase in intracellular sodium, which raises *free intracellular calcium*. The rise in intracellular calcium heightens vascular tone and elevates blood pressure. Natriuresis is effected at the cost of a higher resting pressure. Additionally, in salt-sensitive patients, a high sodium intake has been associated with higher levels of norepinephrine and an increased responsiveness to norepinephrine.

Catecholamines. Catecholamines affect blood pressure regulation both centrally via the vasomotor centers in the brain and peripherally through the action of the sympathetic nervous system. Catecholamines elevate blood pressure both by increasing peripheral resistance and increasing cardiac output. Sympathetic hyperactivity has been suggested as playing a primary role in the development of hypertension in some patients. *Pheochromocytoma* provides a model for secondary hypertension based on excessive catecholamines. Studies on patients with borderline hypertension have allowed clear identification of subgroups in which a defect in autonomic nervous system controls exists, resulting in excessive sympathetic and reduced parasympathetic activity. An exaggerated pressor response to external stressful stimuli has been demonstrated in some hypertensive patients and in their normotensive offspring. Also described are "hyperkinetic" hypertensives, who are generally young and present with tachycardia and elevated cardiac output. Their hypertension may reflect the interaction of an underlying predisposition and various environmental stimuli.

Renin-Angiotensin System. Renin is secreted by the juxtaglomerular apparatus in response to a number of stimuli, including a decrease in intravascular volume, decreased perfusion pressure, β-adrenergic stimulation, and hypokalemia. Renin acts on angiotensinogen (a decapeptide produced in the liver) to form *angiotensin I*, a substance with no known biologic activity. Angiotensin I is converted in the lung to *angiotensin II* by *angiotensin-converting enzyme*. Angiotensin II is a potent vasoconstrictor that also acts on the adrenal cortex to release aldosterone, which increases sodium and water reabsorption in the distal tubule of the nephron.

Renin production is inversely proportional to effective blood volume. Anything that increases effective blood volume suppresses renin and anything that decreases effective blood volume stimulates renin. For example, in *primary hyperaldosteronism*, autonomous production of the salt-retaining hormone aldosterone by an adrenal adenoma results in intravascular volume expansion and renin suppression. Conversely, in *renal artery stenosis*, decreased renal perfusion on the affected side is perceived by that kidney as decreased effective blood volume. In renin studies of patients with primary hypertension, about 15% have a high renin, the remainder showing normal or low levels. It is still not clear how much of a role this system plays in the pathogenesis of primary hypertension. One theory suggests that in patients with hypertension, a "normal" renin may in fact be inappropriately high due to a relative insensitivity to the adrenal cortical effects of angiotensin II. In addition, in about 50% of hypertensives with normal or elevated renin levels, there is a defect in the normal modulation of responsiveness to angiotensin II based on sodium intake, so-called nonmodulators. In these patients, the defect can be reversed by the use of angiotensin-converting enzyme inhibitors.

At present, we have no way to identify such patients, but this offers a glimpse of the potential of eventually being able to accurately diagnose the underlying etiology of hypertension in a given patient and adjust therapy specifically. Finally, there are local renin-angiotensin systems within the brain, heart, kidney, and placenta. It is possible that locally derived angiotensin II may play a significant role in the development of hypertension and in some of its consequences.

Insulin. The increased frequency of hypertension in patients with type II diabetes has stimulated search for a common mechanistic link. Elevations in serum insulin have been found capable of increasing plasma catecholamines and stimulating sodium reabsorption in the kidney, both of which are capable of raising blood pressure. In addition, insulin enhances the pressor responses to angiotensin II and serves as a potent growth factor for vascular smooth muscle, which could lead to hypertrophy and increased peripheral resistance. Insulin levels are higher in obese nondiabetic hypertensives than in their normotensive counterparts, suggesting a mechanism linking obesity with hypertension. Relative insulin resistance has also been identified in nonobese hypertensive patients and in nonhypertensive nonobese offspring of hypertensive parents, suggesting that elevated insulin levels may occur as part of a genetic defect and are not necessarily secondary to obesity.

Calcium. Increased intracellular calcium appears to increase vascular tone. Alteration in calcium binding at the cellular level may lead to increased levels of free intracellular calcium with a resultant increase in vascular tone.

Alteration of Cell Membrane Function. A variety of abnormalities in cellular sodium transport has been demonstrated to occur in some hypertensive patients. These include the Na$^+$-Li$^+$ countertransport system, the Na$^+$-H$^+$ exchange, the Na$^+$-K$^+$ ATPase pump and the Na$^+$-K$^+$-Cl$^-$ cotransport systems, among many others. The result of these abnormal transport systems is to increase intracellular sodium.

Clinical Presentations

Primary or "essential" hypertension accounts for at least 95% of cases. Onset is usually between ages 30 and 50, except for *isolated systolic hypertension*, which is typically a disease of the elderly. Often, a family history of hypertension can be elicited. For 80% of patients, the onset is gradual and the severity mild. Patients with uncomplicated disease are asymptomatic. Although some patients report fatigue, headache, lightheadedness, flushing, or epistaxis, the correlation between symptoms and blood pressure is poor, except in patients with dangerous elevations in pressure. The rare syndrome of *hypertensive encephalopathy* occurs in the setting of malignant hypertension, where DBP rises rapidly above 130 mm Hg, accompanied by symptoms and signs of increased intracranial pressure (restlessness, confusion, somnolence, blurred vision, nausea, vomiting, blurred disc margins, retinal hemorrhages) and heart failure (dyspnea, rales, third heart sound).

Most patients remain asymptomatic unless end-organ damage develops, causing symptoms of congestive failure, renal failure, cerebrovascular insufficiency, peripheral vascular disease, or ischemic heart disease.

Labile hypertension is blood pressure that intermittently rises above the normal levels for each given age group and sex. Established hypertension has been shown to develop more commonly in such patients.

"White-coat hypertension" is a term used to describe blood pressure elevations that occur in the doctor's office but not in the home or work environment. The condition is seen in both hypertensive and normotensive patients. Persons who manifest this condition typically have SBP and DBP at least 10 mm Hg greater in the office than at home but do not have greater blood pressure reactivity in the ambulatory setting. They tend to be older and are more likely to receive more antihypertensive medication than their peers, because they seem to be refractory.

Pseudohypertension occurs in elderly persons with very stiff brachial arteries secondary to fibrosis and atherosclerotic change. The vessel walls resist compression by the blood pressure cuff, resulting in sphygmomanometer readings for systolic pressure that markedly exceed the true intraarterial pressure and may simulate very high levels of hypertension. Suggestive clinical findings that differentiate this form of pressure elevation from true systolic hypertension of the elderly include absence of target organ changes (no signs of retinopathy, ventricular hypertrophy, nephropathy) despite the marked elevation in blood pressure. *Osler's maneuver* (inflating the cuff above the measured SBP and seeing if a nonpulsatile radial artery can be palpated) is purported to be helpful in confirming the condition, but its efficacy is unproven.

Pseudorefractory hypertension, a form of apparently refractory disease, has been described in patients who manifest a marked vasoconstrictor response to blood pressure determinations performed with an arm cuff. Their predominant elevation is in DBP, compared with the white-coat hypertensive, who responds with a rise in SBP. Such patients are apt to be mistaken for truly refractory hypertensives because pressures may remain elevated both in the office and at home. The tipoff to this condition is the absence of end-organ damage (e.g., normal fundi, normal cardiac ultrasound) despite apparent persistence of hypertension.

Secondary hypertension has a definable etiology (Table 19.2), occurs within a wide age range, and is often abrupt in on-

set and severe in magnitude; family history is commonly negative. Certain forms of secondary hypertension may be heralded by specific symptoms. For example, leg claudication may be a manifestation of *coarctation* of the aorta, causing lower extremity ischemia. The patient with *Cushing's syndrome* may complain of hirsutism or easy bruising. Almost all patients with *pheochromocytoma* report paroxysms of excessive perspiration, headaches, or palpitations; about half have sustained hypertension in addition to the paroxysmal symptoms. Hypokalemia ensues from *primary aldosteronism* and may trigger muscle cramps, weakness, and polyuria.

DIFFERENTIAL DIAGNOSIS

About 95% of new hypertensive patients encountered in primary care practice have primary or essential disease. Secondary causes account for the remainder, with one large study showing renal failure accounting for 2.4%, renovascular disease for 1.0%, primary aldosteronism for 1.0%, drugs for 0.8%, pheochromocytoma for 0.2%, and Cushing's syndrome for 0.1%. Coarctation of the aorta is usually detected earlier in life and rarely presents as unexplained adult-onset hypertension (Table 19.3).

WORKUP

As noted earlier, the goals of the evaluation include firmly establishing the diagnosis; ruling out secondary causes; and determining the severity of the pressure elevation, the degree of target-organ damage, and the degree of overall cardiovascular risk.

Establishing the Diagnosis

Use of proper technique for measurement of the blood pressure is essential (see Chapter 14 and below). Except in patients with severely elevated blood pressure, the diagnosis of hypertension should almost always be based on *multiple determinations* of blood pressure, preferably not only on different visits but by different personnel and in different settings. As noted above, there is a tendency for blood pressures to be higher when

Table 19.2.   Primary versus Secondary Hypertension: Specific Screening Protocols

CAUSE (PREVALENCE, %)[a]	SCREEN	CONFIRMATION
Coarctation (NA)	Arm and leg blood pressure, chest radiograph	Eccocardiography or CT
Cushing's Syndrome (0.1)	Cushingoid appearance; 1-mg dexamethasone suppression test	
Drug-Induced Syndrome (0.8)	History: amphetamines, oral contraceptives, estrogens, corticosteroids, licorice, thyroid hormone	
↑ Intracranial Pressure (NA)	Neurologic evaluation	
Pheochromocytoma (0.2)	History of paroxysmal hypertension, headache, perspiration, palpitations *or* fixed diastolic ≥130 mm Hg; 24-hour urinary metanephrine or VMA	Catecholamine levels, angiography CT
Primary Aldosteronism (Conn's or idiopathic) (0.1)	Serum K+, serum aldosterone; plasma renin ≥50 to 1	Inhibition and stimulation of aldosterone and renin secretion
Renal Disease (2.4)	History of congenital disease, diabetes, proteinuria, pyelonephritis, obstruction; urinalysis; BUN or creatinine	Creatinine clearance, IVP, ultrasound, biopsy
Renovascular Disease (1.0)	Clinical prediction rule, captopril renal scan and/or MRA (see Table 19.3).	Angiography and differential renal vein renins

[a]From Danielson M, Dammstrom B. The prevalence of secondary and curable hypertension. Acta Med Scand 1981;209:451.

NA, not available; VMA, zanill-mandelic acid ; PRA, plasma renin activity; BUN, blood urea nitrogen; CT, computed tomography; MRA; magnetic resonance angiography.

taken by a physician than when taken by a nurse or other medical worker. Repeating the blood pressure at the end of the visit can also be informative, because pressures are likely to be less elevated at the end of a visit than at the beginning. Studies comparing the correlation of LVH with pressures obtained in the physician's office, at home, and at work show that *work-site readings* correlate best with degree of LDH.

Teaching the patient to check one's pressure at home and at work can greatly facilitate diagnosis and management, but *home determinations* should be viewed as an adjunct, not as a replacement for office-based measurements. Home determinations are diagnostically useful when there is concern the office reading might represent "white-coat" hypertension caused by patient anxiety. Home determinations are usually lower than those obtained in the office. Readings in excess of 138/85 mm Hg are considered elevated. If home determinations are to be undertaken, the patient's technique and equipment should be checked and calibrated during an office visit, comparing their readings taken in the office with those obtained by the physician using a mercury bulb manometer. In general, the mechanical aneroid manometers are simple, inexpensive, and accurate but need to be checked frequently. Finger monitors are convenient and easy to use, but they are not accurate and not recommended. If home monitoring proves to be sufficiently accurate, one can consider using such determinations to facilitate management (see Chapter 26).

When there is a marked discrepancy between home and office pressures or a wide variation in pressures obtained throughout the day, *24-hour ambulatory monitoring* may be useful, though usually it is unnecessary and quite expensive. Such monitoring appears to be the most accurate way to assess blood pressure, with no regression to the mean and better correlation with left ventricular mass than casual blood pressures. Under study conditions, patients who undergo ambulatory monitoring and adjustment of therapy based on its findings need less intensive therapy, but costs are not reduced due to the expense of the monitoring. It is still not clear how to best use this information in a cost-effective manner other than to resolve discrepancies in readings if they occur.

Conducting the Basic Workup

The basic diagnostic evaluation consists of ruling out *secondary causes* and determining the severity of the pressure elevation, the degree of *target-organ damage*, and the presence of *cardiovascular risk factors*.

History. It is best to begin by eliciting the patient's hypertensive history: date of onset or last previously normal blood pressure, level at time of onset, any medications taken, and response to therapy. Such information facilitates determination of etiology and helps guide workup. For example, sudden onset at a young age, very high pressure, no family history, and refractoriness to treatment suggest a secondary cause (see below). In addition, the history is checked for contributing factors, such as prior *renal disease, salt* and *alcohol excess,* and recent *weight* gain. Noting any associated modifiable cardiovascular risk factors (*smoking, hypercholesterolemia, diabetes, and obesity*) facilitates assessment of total coronary risk. Evidence of cardiovascular and neurologic complications such as a history of prior myocardial infarction or stroke and symptoms suggestive of angina, congestive heart failure, claudication, or transient ischemic attacks should be sought. It is important to inquire about the use of medications that may exacerbate hypertension such as amphetamines, oral contraceptives, corticosteroids, thyroid hormone (in excess), over-the-counter sympathomimetic decongestants, and, in the elderly, chronic use of nonsteroidal antiinflammatory agents. In addition, excessive alcohol use and cocaine abuse may elevate blood pressure.

Awareness of the *symptoms* associated with *secondary etiologies* is essential. Complaints such as hirsutism, easy bruising, paroxysms of palpitations and sweats, weakness, muscle cramps, and leg claudication should all suggest a secondary form of hypertension. Other clues to a secondary cause—especially renovascular disease—are onset at the extremes of age, rapid and severe course, and refractoriness to medication (see below).

Physical Examination. Coffee intake and smoking should be halted at least 30 minutes before taking the pressure. Blood pressure is properly measured in *both arms* while the patient is seated comfortably and after resting for 5 minutes. The cuff should be placed on the bared upper arm, which is supported by the examiner at heart level. The Korotkoff sounds are best listened for by using the stethoscope *bell* rather than the diaphragm; the bell better transmits the low-pitched sounds of diastole. The average of two successive measurements in each arm is recorded. *Diastolic pressure* is taken at the point at which *sound disappears* (Korotkoff 5) rather than when it changes in quality (Korotkoff 4). *Cuff size* must be adequate to avoid falsely elevated readings (cuff width greater than two thirds of arm width, length of inflatable portion greater than two thirds of arm circumference). In the elderly, the pressure should also be taken standing to detect any postural changes. Any *auscultatory gap* (loss and reappearance of the Korotkoff sounds) should be noted because it correlates with arterial stiffness and carotid atherosclerosis, known predictors of prognosis.

The remainder of the examination focuses on *weight* and *pulse* measurements; the *skin* for stigmata of Cushing's syndrome, chronic renal failure, or neurofibromatosis; *fundoscopy* for arteriolar narrowing, increased vascular tortuosity, arteriovenous nicking, or hemorrhages; the *thyroid* for enlargement or nodularity; *carotid pulses* for bruits or diminution of pulse; *lungs* for signs of heart failure; *heart* for left ventricular lift and S_4 and S_3 heart sounds; *peripheral vasculature* for pulses, bruits, and abnormalities in bilateral arm and leg pressure measurements and simultaneous radial and femoral pulse palpation; *abdomen* for masses and bruits; and the *neurologic exam* for focal deficits.

Basic Laboratory Studies. The laboratory evaluation of high blood pressure has three purposes: to ascertain the degree of end-organ damage resulting from hypertension, to identify patients at high risk for the development of cardiovascular complications, and to screen for secondary possibly reversible forms of the disease. Despite the wide array of sophisticated diagnostic techniques now readily available, there is increasing evidence that the diagnosis of secondary hypertension can be made accurately and economically by the alert physician on the basis of a careful history, a physical examination, and only a few simple diagnostic tests. Extensive laboratory evaluation of patients with high blood pressure is unwarranted.

The basic laboratory investigation of hypertension for detection of secondary causes and end-organ damage and for determination of cardiovascular risk needs to include little more than a *complete blood count, urinalysis, blood urea nitrogen, creati-*

nine, potassium, calcium (with albumin), *fasting blood sugar, total and high-density lipoprotein cholesterol,* and *electrocardiogram* (ECG). The urinalysis provides evidence of primary renal disease. The extent of renal compromise due to renal disease or secondary to the hypertension itself is indicated by the blood urea nitrogen, creatinine, and urinalysis. Fasting blood sugar, serum cholesterol, and ECG supply data regarding cardiovascular risk and presence of left atrial enlargement and ventricular hypertrophy. Serum potassium is a valuable screening test for primary aldosteronism and should be known before diuretic therapy is instituted. Total cost of these determinations is reasonable. In most patients, evaluation can and should stop here.

More extensive routine laboratory evaluation of patients with high blood pressure has come under a great deal of criticism. The yield in the absence of clinical evidence for a secondary cause is low, and such testing is not cost effective. It was hoped that *renin profiling* would help identify the underlying pathophysiology in patients with primary disease, guide workup for secondary causes, and rationalize selection of therapy. However, the renin assay continues to suffer from difficulties with accuracy and reliability, except in certain research laboratories. Moreover, most hypertensives have normal renin levels, undermining the value of widespread testing. Finally, when renin profiling has been used to guide choice of therapy, benefit has been hard to demonstrate.

Echocardiography for detection of LVH has been useful in research studies, with presence of LVH associated with an increased risk of cardiovascular complications. However, its routine use rarely adds much to the assessment, except in the setting of refractory hypertension where definitive evidence of end-organ hypertrophy helps one distinguish between true and apparent refractoriness to therapy (see Chapter 26). When the need to search for LVH is less pressing (e.g., in the patient with newly encountered blood pressure elevation), the ECG can provide a reasonable though less sensitive estimate. Of interest, however, is the finding from the Framingham data that the presence of LVH on ECG confers higher risk than that found only on echocardiogram.

Evaluation of Suspected Secondary Causes of Hypertension

Patients at somewhat higher risk for *secondary hypertension* include those with abrupt onset (especially if female and younger than 35 years of age, without a family history of hypertension, or older than age 50 and with evidence of diffuse atherosclerosis), with severe hypertension (DBP more than 120 mm Hg), or with failure to respond to maximum medical therapy despite full compliance. Fortunately, in most patients at high risk for secondary hypertension, a specific diagnosis will be suggested by history and physical examination, supplemented by a few well-chosen laboratory studies (Table 19.1).

Cushing's syndrome is often heralded by its characteristic clinical features (e.g., truncal obesity, facial plethora, violaceous abdominal striae, proximal muscle thinning and weakness, "buffalo hump"), but the presentation may be more subtle. The initial test of choice is the 24-hour *urinary free cortisol*. A finding in excess of 250 μg/d is virtually diagnostic; a level above the upper limit of normal (65 μg/d) in a person with characteristic clinical features strongly supports the diagnosis, but a reading below it rules out the condition. Persons with suspected disease need an assessment of corticotropin (ACTH) dependence, which can be performed by simultaneous late p.m. determinations of *plasma ACTH* and *cortisol*. An elevated cortisol and an inappropriately normal or elevated ACTH indicates an ACTH-producing source; an elevated cortisol and a suppressed ACTH level (less than 5 pg/mL) suggests an autonomous adrenal or ectopic source. Alternatively, an overnight 1 mg *dexamethasone suppression test* can be performed (1 mg is taken at midnight and an 8 a.m. plasma cortisol is obtained). A cortisol level more than 5 μg/dL is suggestive of an autonomous gland, but false-positives are common (due to obesity, stress, depression, alcohol excess).

Coarctation of the aorta is suggested by the presence of reduced pulses in the lower extremities in a person with elevated arm pressures. The suspicion is enhanced by finding reduced blood pressure measurements in the lower extremities and a delay in pulse transmission on simultaneous palpation of radial and femoral pulses. In severe cases, a flow murmur may be audible over the anterior chest or back. A chest radiograph may show rib notching. Confirmation can be obtained by echocardiography or chest computed tomography (CT).

Pheochromocytoma is suggested by a story of *paroxysmal sympathetic discharge* (sweats, palpitations, tachycardia). The *24-hour urine* assay for *catecholamines, VMA,* or *metanephrines* is a sensitive screening test for pheochromocytoma, especially when collected the same day that the patient reports symptoms and processed using the more sensitive liquid chromatography assay. Two normal 24-hour urines performed while the patient is symptomatic virtually rules out the diagnosis. Two positive urines have a high predictive value for the presence of pheochromocytoma. Methyldopa can falsely elevate metanephrines. Although *combination studies* are often ordered (i.e., urinary catecholamines plus metanephrines or VMA), they add little to the power of testing because their sensitivities and specificities are nearly identical. *Plasma* determinations of *catecholamines* and *metanephrines* are available and touted as more sensitive and specific, but sensitivity and specificity are not yet well established. If urinary screening for pheochromocytoma is positive, then one can proceed to *CT of the adrenal glands*—sensitivity is about 90% for lesions larger than 1 cm in diameter. Use of the CT should be limited to patients whose urines test positive and should never be used as a screening test for pheochromocytoma, because innocent adrenal masses having nothing to do with hypertension are common.

Primary hyperaldosteronism is usually suggested by otherwise unexplained *hypokalemia* or excessive potassium requirements in a person taking diuretics. Untreated hypertensive patients with primary hyperaldosteronism demonstrate an inappropriately high ratio (more than 20) of *plasma aldosterone* to *plasma renin*. Measuring the ratio is a reasonable screening test for suspected primary hyperaldosteronism. Confirmation requires measurements of aldosterone secretion in the setting of sodium loading and sodium depletion, which are best performed by referral to an endocrinologist.

Renovascular hypertension should be considered when blood pressure elevation is of new onset, hard to control, or associated with worsening renal function (see Table 19.3). The definitive test remains *renal arteriography* in combination with *renal-vein renin* determinations. Angiographic study with renin sampling not only identifies the anatomic and physiologic im-

Table 19.3.   Clinical Features Suggestive of Renal Artery Stenosis

Highly Suggestive Features:
- Deteriorating control in compliant, long-standing hypertensive patient (atherosclerotic disease)
- Deterioration in renal function during ACE inhibitor therapy (bilateral disease)
- Abrupt onset of hypertension in a young woman with no family hx (fibromuscular hyperplasia)

Additionally Predictive Features (for added diagnostic sensitivity and specificity)
- Advancing age
- Abdominal bruit
- Increasing serum creatinine
- Currrent or former smoking
- Concurrent atherosclerotic disease
- Recent onset of hypertension
- Elevated serum cholesterol

Based on Krijnen P, van Jaarsveld BC, Steyerberg EW, et al. Ann Intern Med 1998;129:705.

pairments, but also allows for immediate therapeutic angioplasty. However, the study has several disadvantages, including its invasiveness, risk of embolic complications, high expense, and risk of dye-induced renal injury. These risks necessitate careful case selectionn. The best noninvasive approach(es) to screening for hemodynamically significant renal artery stenosis continue to be explored.

A potentially useful *clinical prediction* rule was developed for screening those with drug-resistant disease or rising serum creatinine during ACE-inhibitor therapy. Using multivariate analysis, key clinical features predictive of renal artery stenosis in such patients were identified (see Table 19.3). Sensitivity and specificity for this prediction rule are about 70% and 90% respectively.

The *captopril renal scan* (using radionuclide scintigraphy performed 1 hour after a dose of captopril) is another means of screening. Captopril enhances differences in glomerular filtration between normal and hypoperfused kidneys. While the test shows adequate specificity (.90 to .95), it is expensive and its sensitivity is disappointing (.6 to .7). Sensitivity is especially impaired by the scan's nondiagnostic readings in the setting of bilateral stenosis and stenosis-related complications, such as azotemia or a small poorly functioning kidney. *Magnetic resonance angiography (MRA)* offers a more sensitive and very specific contrast-free noninvasive means of identifying anatomically significant renal artery stenosis (sensitivity approaches 90%, specificity over 95%); however, the test is extremely expensive and, unlike captopril scanning, does not provide physiologic information.

The ultimate contributions to blood pressure control of prediction rules and these noninvasive studies singly or collectively remain to be determined. The literature should be followed for emerging data. Prediction rules have been used successfully to determine response to treatment. The younger the patient, the more recent the onset of hypertension, and the lower the systolic pressure, the greater the probability of response to revascularization for renal artery disease.

Risk Stratification

Incorporating the findings of the workup for cardiovascular risk factors, clinically overt cardiovascular disease, and target-organ damage into a risk profile helps to guide therapy (see Chapter 26). The most important factors predicting cardiovascular risk include the presence of *diabetes mellitus,*

clinical cardiovascular disease, and *target-organ damage.* Damage to target organs (manifested by hypertensive retinopathic changes, signs of LVH with remodeling, and proteinuria or renal insufficiency) indicates significant risk of subsequent cardiovascular morbidity and mortality. Similarly, manifestations of overt cardiovascular disease (e.g., angina, claudication, congestive heart failure, stroke, carotid bruit) portend poor outcome if hypertension remains untreated. The JNC VI identifies three risk categories of increasing severity (A, B, and C) based on these determinants that can be used to guide clinical decision making:

- *Risk Group A* (no additional risk): No cardiovascular risk factors; no clinical cardiovascular disease or target-organ damage;
- *Risk Group B* (moderate addition risk): At least one risk factor, not including diabetes, clinical cardiovascular disease, or target-organ disease;
- *Risk Group C* (marked additional risk): Clinical cardiovascular disease or target-organ disease or diabetes, with or without other risk factors.

Combining these risk categories with the stage of hypertension provides a rational guide to the urgency of therapy and the intensity of the treatment program (see Chapter 26).

RECOMMENDATIONS

- Upon encountering blood pressure elevation, *confirm the diagnosis* but do not test for underlying pathophysiology (except in cases of suspected secondary hypertension), because such testing is not yet sufficiently accurate to aid in clinical decision making.
- Check for and rule out any clinically suggested *secondary causes.*
- Assess the *severity* of the blood pressure elevation.
- Identify any *target-organ (end-organ) damage.*
- Identify any and all concurrent *cardiovascular risk factors,* including clinically overt cardiovascular disease.
- Combine these risk determinations into an *overall estimate of cardiovascular risk.*

ANNOTATED BIBLIOGRAPHY

American College of Physicians. Automated ambulatory blood pressure and self-measured blood pressure monitoring devices: their role in the diagnosis and management of hypertension. Ann Intern Med 1993;118:889. (*A position paper suggesting these methods have an adjunctive role in selected situations but cannot be recommended for widespread use.*)

Baker RH, Ende J. Confounders of auscultatory blood pressure measurement. J Gen Intern Med 1995;10:223. (*Very practical review; 65 references.*)

Bakker J, Beck FJ, Beutler JJ, et al. Renal artery stenosis and accessory renal arteries: accuracy of detection and visulization with gadolinium-enhanced breath-hold MR angiography. Radiology 2000;214:373-380. (*High degree of sensitivity and specificity found; best study design to date, but still some short comings.*)

Bravo EL. Plasma or urinary metanephrines for the diagnosis of pheochromocytoma? That is the question. Ann Intern Med 1996;125:331. (*Editorial addressing available tests, finding that urinary metanephrines remain an excellent choice when done properly and a sensitive assay is used.*)

Cavallini MC, Roman MJ, Blank S, et al. Association of the auscultatory gap with vascular disease in hypertensive patients. Ann Intern Med 1996;124:877. (*Presence of a gap associated with carotid plaque and peripheral arterial stiffness, suggesting it might be a useful predictor of prognosis.*)

Ferguson RK. Cost and yield of the hypertensive evaluation: experience of a community-based referral clinic. Ann Intern Med 1975;82:761. (*The conclusions first expressed in this paper 25 years ago are still valid today; emphasizes that secondary hypertension can be detected on the basis of a careful examination and only a few simple diagnostic tests.*)

Frohlich ED, Grim C, Labarthe DR, et al. Report of a special task force appointed by the Steering Committee, American Heart Association. Recommendations for human blood pressure determinations by sphygmomanometers. Hypertension 1988;11:209A. (*The most critical review of technique.*)

Ganguly A. Primary aldosteronism. N Engl J Med 1998;339:1828. (*Best review of hyperaldosteronism, including the approach to its diagnosis.*)

Joint National Committee on Detection, Evaluation, and Treatment of High Blood Pressure. Sixth report of the Joint National Committee on Detection, Evaluation, and Treatment of High Blood Pressure (JNC VI). Arch Intern Med 1997;157:2413. (*The consensus report.*)

Krijnen P, van Jaarsveld BC, Steyerberg EW, et al. A clinical prediction rule for renal artery stenosis. Ann Intern Med 1998;129:705. (*A well-designed effort that provides a set of clinical criteria as sensitive and specific as scintigraphy.*)

Lerman CE, Brody DS, Hui T, et al. The white-coat hypertension response: prevalence and predictors. J Gen Intern Med 1987;4:226. (*Thirty-nine percent of the study sample was found to manifest this response; the elderly and those with the least hostility on psychological testing were most likely to show it.*)

Mejia AD, Egan BM, Schork NJ, et al. Artifacts in measurement of blood pressure and lack of target organ involvement in the assessment of patients with treatment-resistant hypertension. Ann Intern Med 1990;112:270. (*Identifies three types of artifacts in the measurement of blood pressure in patients who appear refractory to treatment.*)

Messerli FH. Osler's maneuver, pseudohypertension, and true hypertension in the elderly. Am J Med 1986;80:906. (*Addresses the problem of accurately measuring blood pressure in older persons with stiff brachial arteries.*)

Staessen JA, Byttebier G, Buntinx F, et al. Antihypertensive treatment based on conventional or ambulatory blood pressure measurement. JAMA 1997;278:1065. (*Adjustment of antihypertensive treatment based on ambulatory monitoring allowed less intensive treatment with no compromise of blood pressure control or inhibition of left ventricular hypertrophy, but no reduction in cost either.*)

Weiss NS. Relation of high blood pressure to headache, epistaxis, and selected other symptoms. N Engl J Med 1972;287:631. (*Classic paper; no clear relation was shown between these symptoms and the level of blood pressure; emphasizes that all but malignant hypertension is usually asymptomatic.*)

Wilcox CS. Screening for renal artery stenosis: are scans more accurate than clinical criteria? Ann Intern Med 1998;129:738. (*The answer is "no"; thoughtful editorial reviewing the sensitivity and specificity of available screening approaches.*)

Working Group on Renovascular Hypertension. Detection, evaluation, and treatment of renovascular hypertension. Arch Intern Med 1987;147:820. (*A consensus panel's recommendations regarding this difficult problem.*)

20
Evaluation of Chest Pain

The patient who presents with chest pain in the outpatient setting poses a diagnostic challenge. The spectrum of diagnostic possibilities ranges from life-threatening cardiac, pulmonary, and aortic etiologies to esophageal and musculoskeletal causes. Harmless conditions may mimic more serious disease. Atypical chest pain can be especially problematic. The primary physician must be skilled in quickly and accurately differentiating the patient who requires immediate hospitalization from the person who can be safely evaluated in the outpatient setting. Initial decision making depends predominantly on a careful assessment of the history supplemented, when possible, by checking for a few key physical and electrocardiographic findings. Further testing must be selected judiciously to avoid generating false-positive results.

PATHOPHYSIOLOGY AND CLINICAL PRESENTATION

Chest pain may arise from chest wall, intrathoracic, abdominal, or even psychophysiologic sources.

Chest Wall. Pain originating in the chest wall is usually due to musculoskeletal pathology, although occasionally nerve injury is responsible. Typically, the pain can be pinpointed by the patient, being somatic in nature. It is aggravated by deep inspiration, cough, direct palpation, and movement. Common sites of involvement are the costochondral and chondrosternal junctions. Duration ranges from a few seconds to several days and quality from sharp to dull or aching. Sometimes the patient complains of tightness. Vigorous and unaccustomed exertion can lead to muscular and ligamentous strain, which may account for some cases. Others are due to *costochondritis* (Tietze's syndrome), which is an inflammatory condition that causes localized swelling, erythema, warmth, and tenderness at the costochondral or chondrosternal junction. *Rib fracture* may produce a similar picture, although location is different, and there is a history of antecedent trauma or metastatic cancer. Of interest, there is an increased frequency of musculoskeletal pain in patients with angina, which causes a potentially confusing clinical presentation.

Nerve injury due to a recrudescence of *herpes zoster* infection can be very painful, with a dermatomal distribution being characteristic. The pain may precede the typical rash (prosaically described as "dew drops on a rose petal"; see Chapter 193) by 3 to 5 days. Neurologic complaints range from hypoesthesia to dysesthesia and hyperesthesia. In the elderly, the pain may persist for months, long after the rash resolves.

Nerve injury from *cervical root compression* (see Chapter 148) due to cervical spine disease or a *thoracic outlet syndrome* can produce pain in the chest and upper arm, superficially resembling angina. In the outlet syndrome, a cervical rib may compress part of the brachial plexus, resulting in motor and sensory deficits in an ulnar distribution at the same time that there is discomfort in the chest and upper arm (see Chapter 167).

Lungs and Pleura. *Inflammation or distention of the pleura* produces true "pleuritic pain," which is worsened by deep inspiration and cough but relatively unaffected by movement or palpation. A host of causes can trigger the inflammatory process, including infection, pulmonary infarction, neoplasm, uremia, and connective tissue disease. The more florid the inflammation, the greater the pain. An infectious origin is more likely to cause pain than is a low-grade serositis associated with connective tissue disease. Stretching of the pleura after a *spontaneous pneumothorax* results in acute onset of pleuritic pain and dyspnea. The condition occurs in young persons and those with emphysema, in which there can be rupture of a bleb. If the pneumothorax is large, deviation of the trachea may be observed.

Pleurodynia is a self-limited source of pleuritic pain, most common in children and young adults and associated with a respiratory viral infection, such as that due to coxsackie virus B. A typical viral syndrome precedes the acute onset of chest pain. Chest pain in the setting of a viral upper respiratory infection may also occur from cough-initiated injury to the chest wall or from bronchospasm. Young healthy persons sometimes note a sudden sharp pleuritic episode relieved by taking a deep breath, referred to as the *precordial-catch syndrome.* Its mechanism is unclear, but a transient folding of the pleura on itself is hypothesized.

Most diseases of the *pulmonary parenchyma* do not cause chest pain unless they extend to a pain-sensitive structure (e.g., vessel wall, pleura). Consequently, the chest pain occurring in the context of *pneumonia, pulmonary tuberculosis,* or *pulmonary embolization* will be pleuritic and represent extensive disease. It is estimated that fewer than 10% of embolic episodes trigger chest pain. The most common manifestations of embolization are dyspnea, tachypnea, and tachycardia, which are nearly universal but may be short-lived. Pleural rub, effusion, fever, and hemoptysis suggest the presence of pulmonary infarction and pleural reaction.

Heart and Pericardium. *Coronary artery disease* impairing myocardial blood supply and presenting as *angina pectoris* is the most important cardiac source of chest pain. Coronary perfusion may be similarly compromised by critical *aortic stenosis* leading to angina (see Chapter 33). The classic hallmarks of angina are its sudden onset with exertion, emotional stress, or eating (usually a very large meal) and its relief within minutes by rest or nitroglycerin. Patients usually describe their chest pain as a squeezing, heaviness, or pressure, although it may be burning or sharp. The quality of the pain is not diagnostic, and many patients state the sensation is more a "discomfort" than a true pain. Radiation to the jaw, neck, shoulder, arm, back, or upper abdomen is common and may present in the absence of chest symptoms. At times, the arm is reported to feel numb or tingling. Autonomic epiphenomena such as diaphoresis and nausea may accompany the episode, as may dyspnea if there is transient pump failure or marked anxiety. Episodes last 2 to 20 minutes. Prompt response to nitroglycerin is characteristic; relief is usually obtained within 5 minutes.

Gender and racial differences in presentation have been explored. The clinical presentation of myocardial ischemia in *women*, particularly women under the age of 60 years, can differ from that in men. Chest pain is more likely to be absent or atypical (see below) and may be overshadowed by exertional fatigue, shortness of breath, diaphoresis, arm tingling, jaw discomfort, nausea, or other epiphenomena of ischemia that are easy to dismiss as "noncardiac." Diabetes mellitus is a major risk factor for early onset of ischemic heart disease in women. As regards the effect of race on presentation, acute chest pain presentations appear to be similar among whites and African-Americans.

Unstable angina is one of the *acute coronary syndromes*, along with *non–Q wave myocardial infarction* and *Q-wave myocardial infarction.* All are important causes of coronary chest pain and result from acute plaque rupture that triggers platelet activation, thrombin clot formation, and active vasoconstriction. The clinical presentations of unstable angina include onset of new chest pain within the past 2 months severe enough to inhibit activity; established angina now increasing in frequency, severity, and duration (*crescendo angina*) and occurring with progressively less provocation; and development of *rest pain* or *nocturnal angina* in a person with a previously stable anginal pattern. Immediate mortality risk is high (up to 4%) but declines after 1 to 2 weeks. Clinical features associated with greatest risk include rest pain in excess of 20 minutes, signs of pump failure (hypotension, rales, S_3), new or worsening mitral regurgitation, and 1 mm or more of ST segment change with pain.

Women with unstable angina are less likely than men to present with acute ST segment elevation indicative of vessel-occluding infarction. Compared with men presenting with unstable angina, they are older; more likely to have diabetes, hypertension, and prior heart failure; and typically present hours later into the episode.

Myocardial infarction is typically heralded by chest pain exceeding that of unstable angina, but the presentation is often more subtle or even silent, particularly in diabetics, the elderly, and women. Bad prognostic signs include heart failure, hypotension, mitral regurgitation, ST segment elevation, and a new left bundle branch block. Onset of *postinfarction angina* is also associated with high risk.

Variant angina, as originally described by Prinzmetal, refers to anginal pain occurring exclusively at rest in conjunction with transient ST segment elevation on electrocardiogram (ECG). Classically, this syndrome was associated with coronary artery spasm at the site of high-grade proximal fixed stenosis. However, other forms of coronary disease may produce a similar clinical picture, and coronary vasospasm may present in ways other than Prinzmetal's description. *Cocaine abuse* can trigger ischemia by precipitating coronary vasoconstriction, increasing myocardial oxygen demand, and enhancing platelet aggregation. It may present as angina in a young person with no other coronary heart disease (CHD) risk factors.

Atypical angina (atypical chest pain) is a term used to denote angina-like chest pain that differs in location, quality, or other characteristics from more typical angina yet is still suggestive by virtue of similar precipitants, timing, or other features. Some define the term more precisely, indicating presence of any two of angina's three cardinal features (substernal location, exercise precipitation, prompt relief by rest or nitroglycerine). As many as 50% of such patients who come to angiography prove to have coronary disease. Among the remainder, there appear to be increased incidences of panic disorder, major depression, esophageal disease, and coronary microcirculatory dysfunction. The mechanisms for many of these causes are not well understood, but recent interest has focused on the coronary microcirculation. *Coronary microvascular dysfunction* has been noted, characterized by abnormal responses to autonomic and biochemical stimuli. Normally, vasodilatory endothelial stimuli such as acetylcholine fail to lower arterial resistance. These patients exhibit increased microvascular resistance and reductions in perfusion. Such microvascular dysfunction has been found with increased frequency among patients with atypical angina who exhibit an ischemic response to exercise stress testing yet have entirely normal coronary angiograms. The terms "*microvascular angina*" and "*syndrome X*" have been applied to such persons. The significance of these findings is still is unclear and requires much more study, but they suggest a possible explanation for the chest pain of patients with *hypertrophic cardiomyopathy*.

Mitral valve prolapse is notorious for its association with atypical chest pain. The commonly held view of a link between the two has been challenged by recent studies controlling more stringently for selection bias. Some argue the apparent association is due to an increased frequency of underlying psychopathology, such as panic disorder (see below), that may trigger chest pain. Symptoms of autonomic dysfunction (e.g., palpitations, sweating, dizziness) may sometimes accompany the chest pain and simulate an ischemic attack.

Pericarditis may present with pleuritic pain, resulting from spread of the inflammatory process from the relatively insensitive pericardium to the adjacent pain-sensitive parietal pleura. The pain is sharp, aggravated by respiratory activity, and sometimes precipitated by swallowing if the posterior aspect of the heart is involved. When the diaphragmatic surface of the pericardium is involved, pain will be referred to the tip of the shoulder. Change in position may alter the pain. Patients often note lessening of pain on sitting up and leaning forward. Pericarditis can also produce a second type of pain that mimics angina. Its most diagnostic physical finding is a two- or three-component friction rub.

A vexing pericardial problem is the development of chest pain after coronary bypass surgery. The return of typical angina raises the specter of graft occlusion, but pleuritic pain suggests the *postpericardiotomy syndrome*.

Aorta. *Aortic dissection* is a must-not-miss cause of chest pain. Almost invariably (70% to 90% of cases), it begins with sudden onset of severe chest or interscapular pain, maximal from the start, and tearing or ripping in quality. If it begins in the chest, it may radiate to the interscapular region, neck, jaw, lower back, or even down into the legs. Associated symptoms include neurologic deficits from cutoff of blood supply to the brain, spinal cord, or limb. Loss or diminution of a major peripheral pulse is a key physical finding, as are new onset of aortic insufficiency and pericardial tamponade due to dissection into the aortic root.

Esophagus. Esophageal pain can be the great mimicker of anginal chest pain, producing chest discomfort that can resemble angina in quality, location, radiation, and even precipitants (e.g., exposure to cold, exertion). Unlike angina, esophageal chest pain is more likely to persist as a dull sensation for several hours after an acute attack and may occur with swallowing. The pain sometimes radiates to the interscapular region. The chest pain may occur spontaneously or in the context of meals or *acid reflux* (manifested by retrosternal burning that may be brought on by a large meal, lying down, or bending over and relieved by antacids). Some patients report *dysphagia* as an accompanying symptom. In some instances, studies of esophageal function reveal *motor dysfunction* (e.g., nonpropulsive contractions or "spasm") and acid reflux from the stomach. Nitrates and calcium-channel blockers may provide relief in such cases, as they do for angina. Some patients with atypical chest pain and normal coronary angiograms manifest both esophageal spasm and microcirculatory dysfunction, raising the intriguing possibility of a generalized disorder of smooth muscle reactivity.

About half of patients with noncardiac (i.e., angiogram-negative) angina-like chest pain report no concurrent dysphagia or heartburn and manifest no signs of reflux or motor dysfunction on detailed esophageal testing. In the past, such chest pain was labeled as "*noncardiac chest pain of unknown etiology*"; however, controlled studies using impedance planimetry reveal esophageal *hypersensitivity, hyperreactivity, and stiffness* in a large proportion of previously undiagnosed patients. These findings suggest a *sensory* or "*nociceptive*" etiology to much noncardiac chest pain. It appears that, in such patients, normal degrees of esophageal distention result in exaggerated perceptions of pain and in hyperreactivity.

Other Gastrointestinal Tract Sources. An attack of acute *cholecystitis* may resemble angina by producing substernal discomfort that responds to nitrates, which reduce cystic duct spasm. On rare occasions, *pancreatitis or peptic ulcer* disease produces substernal chest pain. Even a patient with gaseous distention of the bowel in the area of the splenic flexure may complain of precordial discomfort.

Psyche. Dramatic chest pain presentations are common among patients with underlying psychopathology. In addition to presentations that may be clinically indistinguishable from angina, patients with *anxiety* or *depression* often describe feelings of chest heaviness or tightness that can last for hours to days, unrelated to exertion and unrelieved by rest. In patients with anxiety disorders, this sensation may be accompanied by a feeling of inability to take in a deep breath. When there is associated hyperventilation, the resulting hypocapnia leaves the patient lightheaded and the extremities tingling.

Cardiac neurosis may lead to reports of chest pain mimicking angina. At other times, the patient misinterprets a noncardiac chest sensation. Patients with a *personality disorder* and *somatization* may describe almost any form of chest pain, including some suggestive of angina. A life-long pattern of multiple refractory bodily complaints is characteristic (see Chapter 230). *Malingering* represents a conscious effort to feign illness for secondary gain. The hallmark is inconsistency of the story. Although other forms of psychogenic chest pain may bring secondary benefits to the patient, there is no premeditated attempt to deceive.

Patients with atypical chest pain related to an underlying depression or panic disorder tend to be younger, more often female, more apt to have a higher number of accompanying autonomic symptoms, more bothered by phobias, and more likely to describe an atypical form of chest pain than those with chest pain and a positive coronary angiogram.

DIFFERENTIAL DIAGNOSIS

The differential diagnosis of chest pain can be organized along anatomic lines, as outlined in Table 20.1. Must-not-miss diagnoses include CHD, critical aortic stenosis, aortic dissection, pneumothorax, cholecystitis, pericarditis, and pleuritis from pneumonia, embolization, or cancer. Underdiagnosis and delay in diagnosis of CHD is a problem in women under the age of 60 years, because their clinical presentations may be atypical or ignored. A high index of suspicion is warranted in such persons, especially when there is preexisting diabetes, a major risk factor for early development of CHD in women. Underdiagnosis of CHD is also a problem for African-Americans presenting with chest pain.

WORKUP

The first priority is to determine the *need for emergent hospitalization*. This requires estimating the likelihood of myocardial ischemia, aortic dissection, and pulmonary embolization, conditions that place the patient at high risk for a potentially life-threatening complication. Timeliness of the assessment is of the utmost importance, because outcome often depends on prompt intervention. In many instances, the decision to immediately hospitalize will need to be made by history alone, often on the basis of a telephone call by the patient. Delaying hospitalization is a major cause of poor outcome. Delays tend to be particularly prevalent among women and African-Americans. Postmenopausal women presenting with ischemic chest pain are one third less likely to be admitted to the hospital than men with the same degree of cardiac risk.

An efficient triage strategy for initial decision making is one that determines and stratifies chest pain risk on the basis of pre-

Table 20.1. Differential Diagnosis of Chest Pain

I. **Chest Wall**
   A. Muscular disorders
      1. Muscle spasm (precordial-catch syndrome)
      2. Pleurodynia
      3. Muscle strain
   B. Skeletal disorders
      1. Costochondritis (Tietze's syndrome)
      2. Rib fracture
      3. Metastatic disease of bone
      4. Cervical or thoracic spine disease
   C. Neurologic disorders
      1. Herpes zoster infection or postherpetic pain
      2. Nerve root compression
II. **Cardiopulmonary**
   A. Cardiac disorders
      1. Pericarditis
      2. Myocardial ischemia
      3. Prolapsed mitral valve
   B. Pleuropulmonary disorders
      1. Pleurisy of any origin
      2. Pneumothorax
      3. Pulmonary embolization with infarction
      4. Pneumonitis
      5. Bronchospasm
III. **Aortic**
   A. Dissecting aortic aneurysm
IV. **Gastrointestinal**
   A. Esophageal disorders
      1. Reflux
      2. Spasm
   B. Others
      1. Cholecystitis
      2. Peptic ulcer disease
      3. Pancreatitis
      4. Splenic flexure gas
V. **Psychogenic**
   A. Anxiety (with or without hyperventilation)
   B. Cardiac neurosis
   C. Malingering
   D. Depression

senting history supplemented by physical examination, ECG, and on occasion chest x-ray (if available and deemed necessary). Predictions of risk based on this approach have proven to be extremely powerful and can be used to determine who will benefit most from prompt hospitalization and aggressive testing. Extensively testing low-probability patients for ischemia, dissection, and embolization is not only wasteful, it leads to a high false-alarm rate with its attendant adverse consequences. Although there may be psychological pressure to proceed to elaborate diagnostic studies in all patients with chest pain, only those with at least a modest pretest probability (e.g., at least 20%) of serious pathology benefit from such testing (see Chapter 2). The provision of meaningful reassurance does not usually require exhaustive testing, but it is aided by a careful clinical assessment (see Patient Education, below).

History

Estimating Probability of Coronary Disease by History. A careful chest pain description is critical. The prevalence of angiographically confirmed CHD approaches 90% in persons with a classic story for angina (see above). Prevalence declines to less than 15% in those coming to catheterization who have nonanginal chest pain. In the Framingham study, patients presenting with new onset of definite angina had a relative risk of a coronary event over 2 years of 3.7 for men and 5.9 for women. Relative risk fell for those with possible angina to 3.0 for men and 2.9 for women and to 1.3 for men and 0.8 for women with nonanginal chest pain.

Among the features of the chest pain description with the greatest discriminant value are its *timing* in relation to *precipitating* and *alleviating factors*. Quality, location, radiation, and intensity of pain are notoriously nonspecific. Precordial pain radiating down the left arm can occur with almost any cause of chest pain. A common pitfall in taking the history is to provide classic descriptions of chest pain to the patient who cannot give a quick crisp account of his or her chest pain. Under the duress of the physician's interrogation, the patient may agree to one of these neat descriptions, leading to a false-positive diagnosis. The initial vagueness may have been more useful.

Past medical history is reviewed for major *cardiac risk factors* (e.g., hypertension, diabetes, smoking, hypercholesterolemia, and obesity). Inquiry into cocaine use is essential, especially in young persons presenting with ischemia-like chest pain. *Family history* is checked for *premature coronary disease*. Note is also taken of patient *age and gender*. Postmenopausal women with coronary artery disease have an especially poor prognosis. Awareness of the potential biasing effects of gender and race on clinical thinking is critical to avoiding them. Race and gender have been found to be independent determinants of how patients are assessed. Because there are no differences in acute chest pain presentations among whites and African-Americans, the chest pain presentation can be evaluated without need to adjust for race. However, differences in CHD presentation between sexes need to be kept in mind. Women are often underdiagnosed, in part because the story may be atypical or vague (e.g., exertional fatigue, arm tingling, nausea, shortness of breath). A high index of suspicion for CHD is required in women under the age of 60 years presenting with chest pain, especially if they have preexisting diabetes (which negates the beneficial effects of estrogen).

Checking for an Acute Coronary Syndrome. Any person with angina-like pain and cardiac risk factors should be asked if the pain is of *greater than 20 minutes'* duration, *crescendo* in pattern, now occurring at *rest* or at *night* and with exertion, of *new onset* (especially if severe enough to limit activity), or associated with *dyspnea*. An answer of "yes" to any of these questions on telephone triage should prompt immediate hospitalization by ambulance, because risk of an acute coronary syndrome is sufficiently high and time is of the utmost importance. If evaluated in the office, the patient needs only a brief physical examination and ECG (only if immediately available; see below) to complete the initial assessment.

Consideration of Noncardiac Etiologies in Persons with Angina-like Pain. Some elements of the history suggestive of coronary disease are also important for the other causes they suggest. *Pain brought on by exertion and relieved by rest* is certainly indicative of angina, but psychogenic disease and even esophageal spasm may behave in similar fashion, necessitating at least consideration of these alternative diagnoses. A check for anxiety, depression, panic episodes, headache, nervousness, weakness, fatigue, and life-long history of multiple bodily complaints may help identify a psychogenic origin. Heartburn, dys-phagia, symptoms associated with meals, and an absence of CHD risk factors raise the possibility of esophageal disease. Recurrent episodes that last hours to days provide further evidence of a noncardiac origin. *Prompt response to nitroglycerin* is another characteristic feature of CHD, but esophageal spasm, coronary microvascular disease, cystic duct spasm, and even some psychogenic etiologies may also respond to nitrates. *Chest pain brought on by eating* may be due to angina, but in the absence of other risk factors for CHD, one needs to consider gastroesophageal or pancreaticobiliary pathology. As noted earlier, response to nitroglycerin is not necessarily helpful in differentiation.

Checking for Aortic Dissection. Attention to onset, radiation, and associated symptoms are critical for early identification of aortic dissection. One checks for *sudden* onset; *maximum* intensity from the start (often described as a catastrophic presentation of tearing or searing pain); radiation into the *interscapular* region, *jaw*, neck, or down into the lower back or legs; and any accompanying *new neurologic deficit or syncopal episode*. Such a presentation should strongly suggest acute dissection of the thoracic aorta and warrant consideration of immediate hospitalization. Past medical history is reviewed for atherosclerotic risk factors, existing vascular disease, blunt trauma to the chest, and connective tissue disease (e.g., Marfan's syndrome). Although many less serious conditions can cause chest pain that radiates into the back (esophageal pathology being the most common), the seriousness of aortic dissection mandates a careful review of the history and risk factors. Seventy percent to 90% of cases exhibit the characteristically dramatic presentation, but 10% to 30% are more subtle in their manifestations, necessitating a high index of suspicion for the condition.

Evaluating Pleuritic Pain. *Pain worsened by deep inspiration or cough* is a hallmark of pleural irritation, but such pain is also suggestive of pericarditis and chest wall pathology. Even aortic dissection may cause pain worsened by movement due to respiration. Focal *chest wall tenderness* worsened by movement quickly narrows the differential to a chest wall origin. In the absence of focal chest wall pain, one needs to search promptly for evidence of intrathoracic pathology. Inquiry is needed into fever, cough, sputum production, tuberculosis exposure, hemoptysis, smoking, HIV exposure or high-risk behavior, unilateral leg edema, calf tenderness, shortness of breath, past history of embolization, recent orthopedic surgery, and oral contraceptive use. Pneumothorax should come to mind when pleuritic pain is *sudden* in onset and accompanied by *dyspnea* in a young patient with a previous history of pneumothorax or when the patient has long-standing bullous emphysema. Precordial-catch syndrome is suggested by brief self-limited episodes in an otherwise healthy young person. Pleuritic pain worsened by turning but relieved by *sitting up and leaning forward* is indicative of pericarditis, which can be further assessed by physical examination. Attention to *the context* of the patient's pleuritic pain often suggests the diagnosis. Onset in a person with known metastatic cancer may be due to a pathologic fracture, pleural metastasis, or pulmonary embolization. The same pain in an otherwise healthy young person with new onset of a dry cough, low-grade fever, and myalgias is consistent with viral-

Table 20.2.   Estimating Clinical Pretest Probability of Pulmonary Embolization

PRETEST PROBABILITY	CLINICAL FEATURES
Low	"Typical" clinical features, but alternative diagnosis as or more likely than pulmonary embolization and no risk factors; or "Atypical" clinical features and alternative diagnosis as or more likely, regardless of presence or absence of risk factors; or "Atypical" clinical features, alternative diagnosis less likely, but no risk factors
Intermediate	"Typical" clinical features, alternative diagnosis less likely, no risk factors; or "Typical" clinical features, alternative diagnosis as or more likely, but with risk factors; or "Atypical" clinical features, alternative diagnosis less likely, but with risk factors; or "Severe" clinical features, alternative diagnosis as or more likely
High	"Typical" clinical features, alternative diagnosis less likely, risk factors; or "Severe" clinical features, alternative diagnosis less likely

"Typical" clinical features for pulmonary embolization—at least two of the following (dyspnea or acute worsening of dyspnea, pleuritic chest pain, noncardiac chest pain, hemoptysis, pleural rub, and $SaO_2 < 92\%$) plus heart rate > 90, leg symptoms, low-grade fever, or abnormal chest x-ray.

"Atypical" clinical features for pulmonary embolization—some of the "typical" findings but not enough to meet criteria for "typical."

"Severe" clinical features for pulmonary embolization—"typical" findings plus either syncope, heart rate > 100 or systolic blood pressure < 90 mm Hg, requirement for O_2 supplementation > 40%, or signs of acute right heart failure (elevated jugular venous pressure (JVP), new $S_1Q_3T_3$, RBBB); or signs of acute right-heart failure plus any of the other features.

Risk factors—surgery within 12 weeks, complete bed rest for at least 3 days in the prior 4 weeks, strong family history of deep vein thrombosis (DVT) or Pulmonary embolism (PE) (two or more family members or a first-degree relative), ongoing cancer, postpartum, or lower extremity paralysis.

From Wells PS, Ginsberg JS, Anderson DR, et al. Use of a clinical model for safe management of patients with suspected pulmonary embolism. Ann Intern Med 1998;129:997, with permission.

induced pleurodynia and muscle soreness from coughing. A critical task is *estimating the pretest probability of pulmonary embolization*, which is aided by attention to key historical features and presence of risk factors (Table 20.2).

Physical Examination

In cases of acute chest pain where the history is very suggestive of unstable angina, pulmonary embolization, or aortic dissection, the decision to immediately hospitalize can be made on the basis of history alone. There is no reason to delay admission. In the setting of less acute chest pain or a more ambiguous story, the physical examination can provide important evidence pertinent to the differential diagnosis and the assessment of risk.

General appearance and vital signs can be telling. Tachypnea and tachycardia in a person with acute pleuritic pain are suggestive of pulmonary embolization, whereas an anxious, sighing, hyperventilating individual who complains of constant chest tightness is likely to be suffering from an anxiety disorder. Blood pressure is noted for elevation (an important risk factor for cardiovascular disease), for hypotension (a bad prognostic sign in acute coronary syndromes), and for asymmetry (a sign of aortic dissection). The *skin* is noted for cyanosis, herpetic rash, pallor, jaundice, and xanthomata. Examination of the *fundi* may provide evidence of atherosclerotic, diabetic, or hypertensive disease. The *carotid pulse* is palpated for delay in upstroke, suggesting hemodynamically significant aortic stenosis, and checked for its loss in the person with possible aortic dissection. The *jugular venous pressure* is noted; it may be transiently elevated during an ischemic episode or newly elevated from acute right heart strain due to acute pulmonary embolization.

The *chest wall* is examined carefully in the person reporting "pleuritic" pain, beginning with inspection for signs of trauma and the *rash of herpes zoster* and palpation for swelling and focal tenderness. If pain is elicited, it is important to be sure the pain on palpation is identical to the patient's presenting complaint. One should next listen to the *lungs for a pleural friction rub* during inspiration and expiration and note any signs of consolidation or effusion. *Hyperresonance*, absent breath sounds, and *tracheal deviation* suggest a significant pneumothorax that requires immediate attention. Checking for *rales* (crackles) in the patient with angina assesses the possibility of ischemic left ventricular dysfunction (another sign of pump failure and poor prognosis).

On examination of the *heart*, the left ventricular impulse is observed and noted for signs of hypertrophy (indicative of significant aortic stenosis, long-standing hypertension, or a hypertrophic cardiomyopathy). Signs of ischemic myocardial dysfunction, such as *loss of physiologic splitting* of the second heart sound, development of an S_4, and presence of an S_3 are sought; they may be transient, occurring only during chest pain, but their presence suggests considerable myocardium at risk. Listening for the *systolic ejection murmur* of aortic stenosis should not be forgotten in the patient with angina nor should the *systolic regurgitant murmur* of mitral regurgitation due to papillary muscle ischemia. If the chest pain is pleuritic, then carefully listening for the two- to three-component *pericardial friction rub* is indicated. Although the relation between mitral valve prolapse and chest pain is questionable, listening briefly for a mid-systolic click and late systolic murmur completes the examination.

The *abdomen* is checked for epigastric and right upper quadrant tenderness (especially when evidence suggests gastric or hepatobiliary disease) and for masses (particularly an abdominal aneurysm in the context of suspected dissection). The *legs* require careful examination for unilateral edema and other signs of phlebitis (see Chapter 22), a potential source of pulmonary embolization in the person presenting with pleuritic pain. All *peripheral pulses* are checked, noting any absences and evidence of acute ischemia, which might occur with an aortic dissection. The *spine* is palpated for areas of tenderness along the cervical and thoracic segments, and the *neurologic* examination needs to include a check for new focal deficits, another possible clue to dissection.

Laboratory Studies

Outpatient Testing versus Immediate Hospitalization. Although laboratory studies can be helpful, *one should not delay the decision to urgently hospitalize when the clinical picture suggests unstable angina or pulmonary embolization.* In fact, any delay brought about by taking time to obtain a "nice-to-have" but not essential diagnostic study in the office could be life threatening. Only those studies that are essential to immediate decision making should be considered. Even an ECG may be superfluous in the face of a reasonable story for unstable angina, because a normal study would not change the decision to hospitalize immediately.

Whom to Test. For patients who are deemed appropriate for outpatient evaluation, test selection should focus on conditions for which there is *at least a low-intermediate pretest probability* (e.g., more than 20%). Using such a probability threshold minimizes the risk of generating an unacceptably high proportion of false-positive results (see Chapter 2), which can lead to unwarranted disability and unnecessary invasive interventions. Because physician responses to the chest pain presentation sometimes differ by patient gender or race, it is important to keep the possibility of bias in mind so that the diagnostic assessment is not unduly influenced by it. African-American women are 60% less likely to be referred for cardiac catheterization than white men with the same pretest risk of coronary disease.

Suspected Coronary Heart Disease. The approach to laboratory workup for coronary disease is determined by the condition's pretest probability and an appreciation for the sensitivity, specificity, and cost of available tests (see Table 20.3).

Clinically High Probability—Unstable Angina. As noted above, the very-high-probability patient (multiple CHD risk factors, history very suggestive of *unstable angina*) requires *immediate hospitalization* without delay. Additional outpatient testing is unwarranted. Once the patient arrives in the emergency room, a *resting ECG* is critical to initial decision making, used in most critical pathways for optimal emergency room triage of chest pain patients. Any ST- or T-wave changes indicative of ischemia are an indication for prompt consideration of therapy, be it thrombolytic or revascularization. Proceeding directly to *coronary angiography* is more cost effective than stress testing in such very-high-probability patients.

A normal ECG is not by itself sufficient evidence for discharge of the high-probability patient, but a shortened period of observation (e.g., 6 hours) followed by *stress testing* is being ap-

plied in some centers to safely minimize length of stay for patients with no ECG changes and normal serum levels of myocardial *creatine phosphokinase and troponin I.* Exclusionary criteria for early stress testing include ongoing chest pain, signs of heart failure, and elevations in creatine phosphokinase or troponin levels. Considerable debate continues as to the most cost-effective approach to initial inpatient evaluation of such patients.

Clinically High Probability—Stable Angina. The patient with CHD risk factors and a clinical presentation that is classic for *stable angina* does not need any testing to establish the diagnosis of coronary disease (the pretest probability is already in excess of 90%). Rather, the role of testing is to *estimate prognosis and stratify risk,* which inform selection of initial treatment (i.e., revascularization vs. medical therapy; see Chapter 30). A well-recognized prognostic determinant is *amount of myocardium at risk,* which can be assessed by electrocardiographic, radionuclide, or echocardiographic stress testing (see below and Chapters 30 and 36). A less well-recognized risk factor is prior silent myocardial infarction, which may be detected by *resting ECG* (new Q waves or new ST- or T-wave changes since last ECG) or *cardiac ultrasound* (segmental wall akinesis). Postinfarction angina is a sign of potentially severe coronary disease, especially in persons with prior silent infarction (16-fold increase in mortality risk).

Clinically Intermediate Probability—Unstable Angina. The initial approach to this patient is the same as for the high-probability patient (i.e., immediate emergency room assessment; see above).

Clinically Intermediate Probability—Stable Angina. Patients in this category typically have a single cardiac risk factor and give a history of atypical chest pain that is noncrescendo in pattern. In such persons, a *resting ECG* may be helpful, but nonemergent *stress testing* is needed if the resting ECG is nondiagnostic. Several modalities are available for stress testing (see also Chapter 36).

Exercise electrocardiography provides excellent sensitivity and specificity for detection of high-risk coronary disease (i.e., left main, left main equivalent, or three-vessel disease) at low cost, but false-positives occur in younger women, sensitivity is lower in the setting of less serious forms of coronary disease, and the test cannot be interpreted adequately unless the resting ECG is normal.

Stress echocardiography can be performed by bicycle exercise or dobutamine stimulation; cost is somewhat higher than with ECG, but sensitivity and specificity are better.

Radionuclide imaging with thallium or technetium sestamibi uses planar scanning and, more recently, *single-photon*

Table 20.3.   Sensitivity, Specificity, and Costs of Stress Tests for the Detection of Coronary Disease

TEST TYPE	SENSITIVITY	SPECIFICITY	SENSITIVITY FOR THREE-VESSEL/LEFT-MAIN DISEASE	RELATIVE COST
Electrocardiographic	0.68	0.77	0.86	1.0
Echocardiographic	0.76	0.88	0.94	2.5
Thallium imaging, planar only	0.79	0.73	0.93	2.0
SPECT scanning	0.88	0.77	0.98	4.0
PET scanning	0.91	0.82	?	14.0

SPECT, single-photon emission computed tomography; PET, positron emission tomography.

From Garber AM, Solomon NA. Cost-effectiveness of alternative test strategies for the diagnosis of coronary artery disease. Ann Intern Med 1999, 130:719, with permission.

emission computed tomography (SPECT), which enhances sensitivity and specificity by providing three-dimensional views. It can be performed by treadmill exercising or adenosine injection, which causes a steal phenomenon and enhances differences in uptake. Increased sensitivity is achieved with radionuclide imaging but at increased cost. *Positron emission tomography* (PET) is the most sensitive and specific of tests for coronary insufficiency but also the most expensive and still limited in availability. *Ambulatory electrocardiographic monitoring* is not recommended because specificity is low and the false-positive rate is high.

Sensitivity for detection of coronary disease ranges from 0.68 for ECG to 0.91 for PET. All are very sensitive for detection of left main, left main equivalent, and three-vessel coronary disease, with sensitivities ranging from 0.86 for ECG stress testing to 0.98 for SPECT. Electrocardiographic stress testing is by far the lowest in *cost* but also slightly less sensitive and specific than other modalities. Cost-effectiveness analyses identify ECG and echocardiographic stress testing as the most cost effective for diagnosis of coronary disease in chest pain patients with an intermediate pretest probability of coronary disease. SPECT may also be cost effective in settings where its cost is lower than average. The increased sensitivity and specificity associated with PET scanning are insufficient at the present time to overcome its very high cost (see Chapter 36).

Clinically Low Probability. The patient with clearly nonanginal chest pain, no CHD risk factors and a normal cardiac examination has such a low probability of CHD that testing is likely to generate only negative or false-positive results and excessive medical bills. Even a CHD test with high sensitivity and specificity will perform poorly and produce an excessive proportion of false-positive results if applied to a person with a very low pretest probability of CHD (see Chapters 2 and 36).

Occasionally, a *resting ECG* is obtained to reassure the very anxious low-risk patient. Performing this low-cost test has been found to speed resumption of normal activity in the overly concerned patient without greatly increasing cost. This approach should not be used unless there is strong patient need for some "objective" reassurance and the patient is warned beforehand that a positive result is most likely to be a false-positive. As lay knowledge of testing modalities for coronary disease increases, requests among low-risk patients for stress testing are likely to escalate but should be rebuffed because such testing will only increase cost without improving diagnostic accuracy.

Suspected Esophageal Disease. The obvious case of esophageal disease (retrosternal burning, difficulty swallowing) requires no testing unless symptoms are refractory, in which case a search for malignancy is indicated (see Chapter 60). More problematic diagnostically is the patient with angina-like pain, a normal cardiac evaluation (including angiography), and no esophageal symptoms. As many as 20% of patients with pain suspicious enough to warrant coronary angiography have been shown to have esophageal disorders. A convincing diagnosis of esophageal disease might save the patient a cardiac catheterization.

A host of provocative tests and esophageal function studies are available, including *manometry*, 24-hour *pH monitoring,* *edrophonium* provocation, and *acid perfusion* (see Chapter 60 for details). Although initial reports promoted their usefulness in the evaluation of chest pain, more carefully controlled study has failed to detect differences in esophageal function, either between periods of pain and no pain or between asymptomatic healthy control subjects and patients. In about 25% of patients, edrophonium chloride or acid provocation will trigger pain in patients and not in control subjects, but there is no difference in motor response. Either motor dysfunction is not the etiology in most esophageal cases or the tests of motor function are not very good. In either case, there seems to be little rational for their routine application. Recent reports suggest that measuring the response to *esophageal distention* better differentiates patients from control subjects. Distention testing is still a research tool and not available for clinical use, but the future trend in diagnosis of esophageal chest pain is likely to be toward identification of altered nociception and a heightened sensory response.

Pleuritic Chest Pain—Suspected Pulmonary Embolization. Just as for coronary disease, cost-effective test selection for embolization requires attention to its *pretest probability.* A validated model developed by Canadian investigators for estimating pretest probability uses *history and physical examination* supplemented by *chest x-ray and ECG* (Table 20.2). The most frequent radiographic finding in cases of embolization is a unilateral effusion. The utility of an ECG in patients with suspected embolus is marginal. The electrocardiographic findings of acute right heart strain ($S_1Q_3T_3$) are helpful if present, but sensitivity is low and a normal ECG certainly does not rule out the diagnosis. The most common electrocardiographic abnormality is inverted T waves in leads V*1-4* (representing posterior ischemia due to right coronary artery compression from right heart overload). *Arterial blood gases* are insensitive and often of little help in identifying patients with pulmonary emboli, but *arterial oxygen saturation* can add to the estimate of pretest probability.

Pulmonary Angiography. This study remains the gold standard for diagnosis of pulmonary embolism and should be used when definitive diagnosis is essential, urgent, and not available from noninvasive testing. Angiography without prior scanning is urged by some experts, especially if the risk of anticoagulant therapy is high for the patient and a definitive diagnosis is needed before commencing treatment. Nonetheless, rational use of noninvasive approaches to testing can greatly reduce the need for invasive study in most instances.

Ventilation-Perfusion Scanning. The test is widely used in patients with suspected embolization. As demonstrated in the landmark Prospective Investigation of Pulmonary Embolism Diagnosis (PIOPED), a normal or nearly normal scan in a patient with a low pretest clinical probability of embolization effectively rules out the diagnosis (negative predictive value, 96%). Likewise, a "high-probability" scan rules in the diagnosis if the patient has a high pretest probability (positive predictive value, 96%). Ventilation-perfusion (V/Q) scanning by itself can reduce the need for angiography in the 40% of cases where the pretest probabilities are strong and the scan results are concordant with these probabilities.

Unfortunately, the V/Q scans of a large proportion of patients produce either equivocal results or findings that are discordant with pretest probabilities. High false-positive rates are especially prevalent in those with preexisting lung disease and in the elderly. The addition of ventilation scanning has not solved the problem of false-positives. In the PIOPED, 40% of patients with a "low-probability" scan and a high pretest probability proved to have pulmonary embolization by angiography.

Forty-four percent of patients with a high-probability scan and a low pretest probability had no embolization by angiography. The largest single group of patients were those with scans of "intermediate" probability, in whom embolization could be neither ruled in or out. These high rates of false-positives and false-negatives among selected groups of patients and the large number of indeterminate scans reflect shortcomings in the sensitivity and specificity of the test. Assuming any abnormality on scan to be a positive test, sensitivity would still be only about 90% and specificity just 10%. V/Q scanning remains widely used as a screening test for pulmonary embolism, but additional testing is needed in many patients.

D-Dimer Testing. This test provides a promising approach to noninvasive screening for pulmonary embolism. D-dimer is a degradation product of cross-linked fibrin. Its formation occurs in the context of ongoing thrombosis and fibrinolysis, making its measurement a potentially sensitive indicator of active venous thrombosis and thromboembolization. Reports of sensitivity in the setting of pulmonary embolism range from 85% to 100%, depending on the assay used. Specificity is not high (40% to 68%); D-dimer acts as an acute phase reactant and its levels rise in response to any event that induces fibrinolysis, such as inflammation, cancer, or trauma. Because D-dimer testing lacks specificity, confirmatory testing is needed when a result is "positive" (i.e., more than 0.5 μg/dL).

These characteristics make the D-dimer test most useful for ruling out pulmonary embolization, especially in chest pain patients with a low pretest probability. In such patients, the negative predictive value of a normal D-dimer level (less than 0.5 μg/dL) is 99%, effectively ruling out embolization and obviating the need for V/Q scanning or venous ultrasound testing. The test is also useful as a supplementary test in persons with a moderate pretest probability of embolization who have a nondiagnostic V/Q scan. A normal D-dimer in this setting provides a negative predictive value of 95%; if there is also a negative venous ultrasound, the negative predictive value of a normal D-dimer approaches 100%.

The original ELISA assay required testing on plasma and took 3 to 4 hours. Newer assays provide nearly equivalent sensitivity and can be performed in minutes on whole blood. Of concern are reports of unsatisfactory performance of the whole blood assay in cancer patients, where a negative result has not been found to reliably exclude DVT.

Venous Ultrasound of the Lower Extremities. Compression venous ultrasound provides some of the specificity lacking in V/Q scanning and D-dimer testing. Venous ultrasound is very specific and sensitive for detection of symptomatic deep vein thrombosis in the proximal veins (sensitivity 95%, specificity 96%). Because almost all pulmonary thromboemboli originate from the deep proximal veins of the legs, venous ultrasound has been proposed as a means to improve noninvasive diagnosis of embolization. However, the sensitivity of a single study is limited, because up to 40% of patients with embolism have no deductible clot remaining in the proximal venous system after initial embolization. To overcome this limitation, serial studies are done over 1 to 2 weeks. In most instances, a clot needs to reform in the leg before reembolization. Thus, sensitivity of the test for risk of embolization can be greatly enhanced by performing serial ultrasound studies. Even if the diagnosis of embolism cannot be confirmed initially, the risk of reembolization can be estimated by serial study. Using serial ultrasound in conjunction with V/Q scanning and pretest probability for embolism, Canadian investigators made an accurate diagnosis in over 96% of cases for suspected embolism; the false-negative rate was only 0.6%, with angiography needed in only 3.7% of cases.

Application of serial ultrasound has been found especially useful in patients with a moderate pretest probability and indeterminate V/Q scan findings. In this setting, a normal serial ultrasound rules out the diagnosis or at least obviates the need for immediate anticoagulation or angiography; a positive study rules it in, again obviating the need for angiography. Ultrasound in combination with D-dimer determination has been found effective in excluding embolism in patients with a low clinical suspicion for embolism.

Helical (Spiral) Computed Tomography. This new technology is designed to detect emboli-induced pulmonary filling defects by means of a two-dimensional volumetric image of the lung. Although rapid to perform (about 30 seconds), the test requires intravenous contrast and is expensive. Some have proposed it as an alternative to V/Q scanning or angiography. Although helical computed tomography (CT) test shows promise for use in the evaluation of patients with poor pulmonary reserve who have a nondiagnostic lung scan plus a negative venous ultrasound and in those with a very high pretest probability, available data are inadequate to determine what the best application(s) of this technology may be and how it may contribute to diagnosis and decision making. Prospective trials are needed.

Approach to Testing. Pretest probability of pulmonary embolization should be used to guide test selection (Table 20.2).

Low pretest probability patients can be screened by application of a sensitive noninvasive test such as D-dimer assay or V/Q scan, with selection dependent on availability and local expertise. A completely normal V/Q scan or D-dimer study rules out clinically significant pulmonary embolism in low-probability patients (negative predictive value well in excess of 95% in major prospective studies). A normal D-dimer can obviate the need for the more expensive V/Q scan. A nondiagnostic V/Q scan or a D-dimer level more than 0.5 μg/dL necessitates additional testing, such as venous Doppler ultrasound; if the initial ultrasound is negative and the patient is in no cardiopulmonary distress, then withholding anticoagulation and testing serially is a reasonable strategy.

High pretest probability patients should be admitted and have anticoagulation started pending the results of testing. V/Q scanning can then proceed, followed by ultrasound if the result is indeterminate. If ultrasound is positive, the diagnosis is confirmed; if negative or equivocal, then angiography is indicated, because noninvasive testing remains insufficiently sensitive at this time to rule out embolization in a patient with a high pretest probability.

Intermediate pretest probability patients should start with a V/Q scan. A normal V/Q scan rules out the diagnosis. An indeterminate V/Q result does not and should be followed by venous ultrasound and D-dimer testing, which if negative rules out embolism. If D-dimer testing is not available, then serial ultrasound testing is a reasonable substitute to ensure absence of DVT and risk of embolization.

Pleuritic Chest Pain—Suspected Pulmonary Infection and Other Nonembolic Etiologies. The *chest x-ray* is the initial test of choice. Pneumococcal pneumonia and tuberculosis often present with acute pleuritic chest pain and may be mistaken clinically for pulmonary embolism. Consequently, any patient with pleuritic pain, sputum production, and an infiltrate of chest film should also have both *Gram's and acid-fast stains* made. A pleural effusion may also be detected on chest film. Any non-loculated pleural effusion of unknown etiology should be tapped, gram-stained, cultured, examined microscopically, and sent for cell count, glucose, lactic dehydrogenase, and protein determinations (see Chapter 43). *Suspicion of pneumothorax* is also an indication for a chest film, but if radiography is not immediately available and the patient is in respiratory distress, decompression should not be delayed.

When *pericarditis* is under consideration, an ECG is essential. However, the ECG changes of early repolarization, a harmless finding seen in young men, may closely resemble those of acute pericarditis. The presence of concave ST segment elevations in both limb and precordial leads and the presence of PR segment depressions in the precordial leads, if they occur in the limb leads, distinguish pericarditis from early repolarization. *Cardiac ultrasonography* may reveal a pericardial effusion. An antinuclear antibody, blood urea nitrogen, and tuberculin skin test are indicated when the cause of pericarditis is not readily evident.

Suspected Aortic Dissection. A *chest x-ray*, which may demonstrate a widened mediastinum (especially in traumatic aortic rupture), is sometimes performed for screening purposes, but if dissection is truly suspected on clinical grounds, then emergency admission for aortic angiography is indicated. Delaying admission to obtain a chest film is unwise. Patients with traumatic aortic dissection may also be well served by *transesophageal ultrasonography* preferred to *transthoracic ultrasonography*, which is less sensitive for detecting disease in the aortic arch. *CT with contrast* is useful when the aortogram is not available or is negative, yet clinical suspicion remains high. Many now proceed directly to CT because it is less invasive and can be done on shorter notice than angiography. *Magnetic resonance imaging* can also detect dissection and provides another noninvasive alternative to contrast angiography.

Other Conditions. Only a few *musculoskeletal* disorders require chest radiography: suspected rib fractures and cervical or thoracic spine disease. If a *gastrointestinal* cause is suspected, a contrast study may be in order. The ECG may show T-wave depression in cholecystitis and pancreatitis and may mistakenly be interpreted as evidence of coronary disease.

The anxious patient with *psychogenic* pain may find a chest radiograph and/or ECG reassuring. In most instances, however, a thorough history and careful physical examination combined with a detailed explanation should suffice. Repeating tests "just to be sure" may begin to undermine the patient's confidence in the physician's explanation and even heighten anxiety, especially if there are repeat studies.

It is important to realize that as many as 10% to 15% of cases remain undiagnosed, even after careful and thorough evaluation. Nevertheless, in such instances it is still possible to rule out the presence of an acutely serious etiology. Most patients with chest pain that initially eludes diagnosis can be followed expectantly for the time being.

SYMPTOMATIC RELIEF

Relief of pain must be based on an etiologic diagnosis. To simply suppress the pain with analgesics or sedatives before a diagnosis is made may hide important clues and endanger the patient. However, musculoskeletal forms of chest pain may benefit from analgesia, especially if the patient is splinting and not ventilating adequately. When the diagnosis of costochondritis is certain, local injection with lidocaine into the point of maximal tenderness can provide dramatic relief. An antacid regimen or H_2-blocker therapy in conjunction with other antireflux and acid-reducing measures are helpful in patients with esophagitis. Nitrates and calcium channel blockers are sometimes of benefit to patients with esophageal spasm (see Chapter 61). Patients with depression or panic disorder require specific therapy directed at the underlying psychopathology; failure to treat etiologically may result in prolonged refractory disability from the chest pain (see Chapters 226 and 227).

PATIENT EDUCATION AND INDICATIONS FOR REFERRAL

Teaching Recognition of Acute Coronary Syndromes. The availability of effective early interventions for acute coronary syndromes and the risk of delay necessitate that patients are taught to recognize the symptoms and to call for help immediately. Those with multiple cardiac risk factors or known heart disease deserve top priority for such an educational intervention. Knowledge of key symptoms, especially duration in excess of 20 minutes; new rest pain; and epiphenomena of ischemia (e.g., diaphoresis, nausea, jaw or neck pain, lightheadedness) is weak, particularly among socioeconomically disadvantaged groups, minorities, the elderly, and younger patients. Patients should be instructed to call for an ambulance and not delay. Delay has been documented in up to 50% of cases and often compromises outcome. The importance of minimizing delay in presentation makes patient education and telephone triage important tools. Practices should be organized to handle chest pain telephone calls with no delay.

Providing Explanation and Meaningful Reassurance. A detailed review of clinical findings and their meaning is as essential to the effective evaluation of chest pain as is a correct diagnosis. When a harmless etiology is identified, it is not enough to dismiss the chest pain as "nothing to worry about," because the symptom is associated with too many fears for such words to suffice. Meaningful reassurance requires eliciting patient concerns about their chest pain and addressing these concerns by specifically reviewing the pertinent clinical findings. Failure to do so may lead to unnecessary activity restrictions (e.g., fear to engage in sexual relations, favorite sports, or important work activities) or trigger requests for otherwise unnecessary testing. Patients making repeated visits, asking for referrals, or requesting elaborate testing usually harbor unexplored concerns. The effort taken to provide meaningful explanation is usually well worth the time in terms of patient appreciation, cost containment, and risk management.

Indications for Admission and Referral. As noted earlier, immediate referral to the nearest emergency room is essential to achieving the best possible outcome for the patient with any clinical or laboratory evidence for an acute coronary syndrome, pulmonary embolization, aortic dissection, or large pneumothorax. Key features include a story of unstable angina, sudden onset of severe tearing or searing chest pain with radiation into the back, new pleuritic chest pain in a patient with risk factors for pulmonary embolization or pneumothorax, severe dyspnea, signs of respiratory or hemodynamic compromise, and ischemic ECG changes with pain. For the chest pain patient who presents to the office with evidence of postinfarction angina or ECG findings of prior silent infarction, plans should be made for prompt hospital admission and cardiac consultation—such patients are at high risk. Acute chest pain in the context of cocaine use is also an indication for immediate hospitalization, even in a young person with no other cardiac risk factors. Referral for drug counseling should not be overlooked; it too is critical to a successful outcome (see Chapter 235). Patients at risk for a life-threatening chest pain etiology should be taught to recognize key symptoms and instructed to call 911 first if symptoms are acutely severe, even before calling the primary care physician.

Outpatient workup is reasonable for the patient with low to intermediate probability of pulmonary embolization, provided there are no signs of respiratory or hemodynamic compromise and the appropriate initial testing (e.g., D-dimer determination, V/Q scan, venous ultrasound) can be completed within 2 to 3 hours. For the patient with pleuritic chest pain due to pneumonia, knowledge of the clinical features predictive of a complication is necessary to determine candidacy for admission (see Chapter 52). The utility of referral for esophageal function testing appears limited, but endoscopy or barium swallow should be considered if there is refractory reflux or dysphagia. The patient with panic disorder or depression severe enough to cause disabling chest pain symptoms will benefit from psychiatric referral (see Chapters 226 and 227).

RECOMMENDATIONS

- Identify the high-risk chest pain patient who requires immediate hospitalization by performing a triage history focusing on evidence for acute coronary syndrome, significant pulmonary embolization, aortic dissection, and acute cardiopulmonary compromise. Avoid common biases based on patient age, gender, and race.
- If the story is strongly suggestive, admit by ambulance; minimize delay.
- If the initial history is not strongly indicative of one of these etiologies, evaluate promptly in the office with a more detailed history and careful physical examination, supplemented, where appropriate, by ECG and chest x-ray.
- Formulate the initial differential diagnosis from these data; include a pretest estimate of myocardial ischemia, pulmonary embolization, and aortic dissection, because immediate decision making and the optimal locus and approach to further workup of these conditions heavily depends on such probability estimates.
- Select the appropriate testing strategy based on the pretest probability for the condition in question.

For Suspected Coronary Artery Disease

- Low pretest probability: Explain why the chest pain is unlikely to be of cardiac origin and consider obtaining a resting ECG if it will help reassure the patient.
- Intermediate pretest probability: If the presentation is suggestive of unstable angina, proceed to immediate hospitalization and emergency room triage protocols. If the presentation is one of "stable" (i.e., noncrescendo) chest pain, proceed on a nonemergent basis to stress testing. Obtain either exercise ECG (if the resting ECG is normal) or exercise echocardiography; both are reasonably cost effective; if other noninvasive modalities (e.g., radionuclide stress testing) are available locally at lower cost or with enhanced sensitivity and specificity, then their use may also be cost effective and should be considered.
- High pretest probability: If the presentation is very suggestive of unstable angina, proceed to immediate hospitalization and emergency room triage protocols. For those with ECG changes on arrival in the emergency room, immediate angiography without prior noninvasive testing appears to be the more cost-effective diagnostic approach. For those whose presentation is indicative of stable angina, proceed to nonemergent stress testing for determination of amount of myocardium at risk (see Chapter 36 for test selection).
- To minimize delay in hospitalization, teach the high-risk patient and family the symptoms of acute coronary syndromes and instruct them to call 911 immediately if such symptoms occur.
- Reduce requests for unnecessary testing by eliciting patient concerns about their chest pain, performing a detailed history and physical examination, obtaining an ECG, and addressing their concerns by a careful review of clinical findings.
- Omit routine use of esophageal studies in assessment of chest pain in patients who rule out for coronary disease.

For Suspected Pulmonary Embolization

- Low pretest probability: Screen by ordering a sensitive test noninvasive test, such as D-dimer assay or V/Q scan, with selection dependent on availability and local expertise. A nondiagnostic V/Q scan or a D-dimer level in excess of 0.5 μg/dL necessitates additional testing, with serial venous ultrasound a reasonable choice.
- Intermediate pretest probability: Begin with V/Q scanning. A normal V/Q scan rules out the diagnosis. A nondiagnostic V/Q result does not and should be followed by D-dimer or serial ultrasound, which if negative rules out embolism.
- High pretest probability: Admit to the hospital and begin anticoagulation, pending the results of testing. Start with V/Q scanning, followed by ultrasound if the result is indeterminate. If ultrasound is positive, the diagnosis is confirmed; if negative or equivocal, then angiography is indicated, because noninvasive testing remains insufficiently sensitive at this time to rule out embolization in a patient with a high pretest probability.

A.H.G.

ANNOTATED BIBLIOGRAPHY

Becker DM, Philbrick JT, Bachhuber TL, et al. D-dimer testing and acute venous thromboembolism. A shortcut to accurate diagnosis? Arch Intern Med 1996;156:939. (*A detailed evaluation of the original assay for D-dimer testing and its clinical application.*)

Daton W, Hall ML, Russo J. Chest pain: relationship of psychiatric illness to coronary arteriographic results. Am J Med 1988;84:1. (*Greatly increased incidence of major depression and panic disorder in patients with angiographically negative chest pain.*)

DeSanctis RW, Dorochazi RB, Austen WG, et al. Aortic dissection. N Engl J Med 1987;317:1060. (*A superb review, with emphasis on clinical features; 83 references.*)

Diamond GA, Forrester JS. Analysis of probability as an aid in the clinical diagnosis of coronary artery disease. N Engl J Med 1979;300:1350. (A classic paper on the importance of pretest probability in diagnosis of coronary disease.)

Dracup K, Alonzo AA, Atkins JM, et al. The physician's role in minimizing prehospital delay in patients at high risk for acute myocardial infarction: recommendations from the National Heart Attack Alert Program. Ann Intern Med 1997;126:645. (Strategies for minimizing delay in hospitalization.)

Egashira K, Inouile T, Hirooka Y, et al. Evidence of impaired endothelium-dependent coronary vasodilatation in patients with angina pectoris and normal coronary angiograms. N Engl J Med 1993;328:1659. (Evidence for microvascular dysfunction in patients with angina and normal angiography.)

Epstein SE, Gerber LH, Borer JS. Chest wall syndrome. JAMA 1979;241:2793. (Best description of the condition and the physical maneuvers that might elicit the pain associated with it.)

Feldman RL. Ambulatory electrocardiographic monitoring: the test for ischemia? Ann Intern Med 1988;109:608. (An editorial urging caution in the use of the technology for detection of ischemia, pointing out the many problems in interpreting ST segment depression on Holter monitoring.)

Frobert O, Funch-Jensen P, Bagger JP. Diagnostic value of esophageal studies in patients with angina-like chest pain and normal coronary angiograms. Ann Intern Med 1996;124:959. (A controlled study finding no difference between patients and controls in 24-hour esophageal monitoring studies and or provocation testing; authors argue that routine use of such testing is of questionable value in patients with noncardiac chest pain.)

Garber AM, Solomon NA. Cost-effectiveness of alternative test strategies for the diagnosis of coronary artery disease. Ann Intern Med 1999;130:719. (A meta-analysis combined with a cost-effectiveness study suggesting that echocardiography and in some instances SPECT are the most cost-effective approaches to testing in persons with an intermediate pretest probability; immediate angiography is best for those with a high pretest probability.)

Ginsberg JS, Wells PS, Kearon C, et al. Sensitivity and specificity of a rapid whole-blood assay for D-dimer in the diagnosis of pulmonary embolism. Ann Intern Med 1998;129:1006. (Large prospective cohort study demonstrating a sensitivity of 85% and a specificity of 68% for this very practical rapid assay of that can be performed in the outpatient setting.)

Hochman JS, Tamis JE, Thompson TD, et al. Sex, clinical presentation, and outcome in patients with acute coronary syndromes. N Engl J Med 1999;341:226. (Data from the GUSTO IIb study showing gender-based differences in presentation and outcomes.)

Isner JM, Mark Estes NA, Thompson PD, et al. Acute cardiac events temporally related to cocaine abuse. N Engl J Med 1986;315:1438. (Documents this serious cause of cardiac chest pain in young patients.)

Kayser HL. Tietze's syndrome—a literature review. Am J Med 1956;21:982. (Points out the often epidemic nature of the illness; still the best review.)

Kearon C, Ginsberg JS, Hirsh J. The role of venous ultrasonography in the diagnosis of suspected deep venous thrombosis and pulmonary embolism. Ann Intern Med 1998;129:1044. (Reviews the evidence for the efficacy of the test in the diagnosis of pulmonary embolization.)

Kirshenbaum HD, Ockene IS, Alpert JS, et al. The spectrum of coronary artery spasm. JAMA 1981;246:354. (Emphasizes the variability of clinical presentation of coronary artery spasm and the difficulty of diagnosis.)

Kuntz KM, Fleischmann KE, Hunink MGM, et al. Cost-effectiveness of diagnostic strategies for patients with chest pain. Ann Intern Med 1999;130:709. (One of the best available decision analyses to date; ECG and echo stress testing proved the most cost-effective in persons with intermediate pretest probability of coronary disease.)

Lee AYY, Julian JJ, Levine MN, et al. Clinical utility of a rapid whole-blood D-dimer assay in patients with cancer who present with suspected acute deep vein thrombosis. Ann Intern Med 1999;131:417. (Negative test unable to reliably exclude DVT in cancer patients.)

The PIOPED Investigators. Value of the ventilation/perfusion scan in acute pulmonary embolism: Results of the Prospective Investigation of Pulmonary Embolism Diagnosis (PIOPED). JAMA 1990;263:2753. (Best study of sensitivity and specificity of V/Q scanning.)

Pryor DB, Shaw L, McCants CB, et al. Value of the history and physical in identifying patients at increased risk of coronary disease. Ann Intern Med 1993;118:81. (Clinical assessment effectively predicted CHD risk and need for further study.)

Rao SSC, Gregersen H, Hayek B, et al. Unexplained chest pain: the hypersensitive, hyperreactive, and poorly compliant esophagus. Ann Intern Med 1996;124:950. (Using the investigative method of esophageal impedance planimetry, investigators find that the esophagus of patients with noncardiac chest pain of unknown etiology has a reduced threshold for pain, reduced compliance, and enhanced reactivity to distention compared to controls.)

Rathbun SW, Raskob GE, Whitsett TL. Sensitivity and specificity of helical computed tomography in the diagnosis of pulmonary embolism: a systematic review. Ann Intern Med 2000;132:227. (Critical analysis of available data revealing inadequate information to determine appropriate use of this new technology.)

Robin ED. Overdiagnosis and overtreatment of pulmonary embolism. Ann Intern Med 1977;87:775. (A classic discussion of the shortcomings of lung scans and arterial blood gases.)

Schulman KA, Berline JA, Harless W, et al. The effect of race and sex on physicians' recommendations for cardiac catheterization. N Engl J Med 1999;340:618. (A videotape study of simulated patients that controlled for cardiac risk; race and sex were powerful independent predictors of risk assessment and management recommendations by participating physicians.)

Sigurdsson E, Thorgeirsson G, Sigvaldason H, et al. Unrecognized myocardial infarction: epidemiology, clinical characteristics, and prognostic role of angina pectoris: the Reykjavik Study. Ann Intern Med 1995;122:96. (A population-based prospective study of men; angina in persons with silent myocardial infarction was associated with a 16-fold increase in mortality.)

Wells PS, Ginsberg JS, Anderson DR, et al. Use of a clinical model for safe management of patients with suspected pulmonary embolism. Ann Intern Med 1998;129:997. (A multicenter prospective cohort study demonstrating efficacy and safety of combining clinical assessment of pretest probability, V/Q scanning and venous ultrasound to evaluate persons for pulmonary embolization.)

Wexler L. Studies of acute coronary syndromes in women—lessons for everyone. N Engl J Med 1999;341:275. (An editorial summing up what is known about the differences between men and women and the implications of these differences for treatment of all patients.)

21
Evaluation of the Asymptomatic Systolic Murmur

In the outpatient setting, systolic murmurs are often noted incidentally in otherwise asymptomatic patients. Although many asymptomatic murmurs are due to conditions of no prognostic significance, the absence of symptoms does not rule out the presymptomatic phase of potentially serious pathology, such as tight aortic stenosis. The primary physician should be able to conduct an effective clinical assessment in the office that differentiates the harmless murmur from one that requires additional investigation. Early detection of clinically silent but prognostically important disease is critical to optimizing outcomes and to identifying patients who require close follow-up. Routinely ordering a cardiac ultrasound examination on every patient discovered to have a systolic heart murmur is both expensive and unnecessary, but close follow-up and serial testing are essential in selected cases. This chapter focuses on clinical assessment of the asymptomatic patient (see Chapters 20, 24, 25, 33, and 40 for detailed discussions of evaluation and management of symptomatic patients with structural heart disease).

PATHOPHYSIOLOGY AND CLINICAL PRESENTATION (SEE ALSO CHAPTER 33)

Systolic murmurs can be divided into two broad categories: ejection and regurgitant. *Ejection murmurs* result from turbulent flow of blood across the ventricular outflow tracts during systole. They are characteristically crescendo-decrescendo, medium to low pitched, and heard best at the base of the heart, beginning after the first heart sound and ending before the second. *Regurgitation murmurs* represent backflow of blood due to incompetence of the mitral or tricuspid valve or the ventricular septum. They are typically higher in pitch, heard best at the apex or midsternal border, holosystolic or mid to late systolic in timing, and, like ejection murmurs, crescendo-decrescendo in pattern (unless rheumatic in origin, where the intensity is constant).

Ejection murmurs are common and often occur in the absence of heart disease. However, absence of symptoms does not mean absence of important underlying pathology. Regurgitant murmurs are associated with some abnormality of the mitral or tricuspid valve apparatus, valve ring, or septum, but the underlying lesion is not always of clinical significance.

Ejection Murmurs

"Physiologic" murmurs occur when there is increased ejection velocity across a normal valve creating turbulence. Causes of increased velocity include fever, anemia, pregnancy, hyperthyroidism, exercise, and conditions associated with a large stroke volume (e.g., aortic regurgitation, bradycardia, atrial septal defect [ASD]). Dilation of the aorta, as in hypertension or aging, may also produce a flow murmur by causing turbulent flow in the dilated segment.

"Innocent" murmurs occur in normal hearts under resting conditions. The origin of such murmurs is a subject of debate, with recent evidence pointing to the aortic root. Because there is no obstruction in the outflow tract, the murmur reflects the normal ejection pattern of blood from the ventricles and is early systolic and crescendo-decrescendo. Because chamber pressures are normal, there is normal splitting of heart sounds. Valves are normal; there are no adventitious sounds or other murmurs.

Early *aortic* and *pulmonic valve disease* may produce murmurs identical to physiologic ones, except that the former are often accompanied by an early systolic *ejection click*. In *pulmonic stenosis*, the murmur increases with inspiration, and the pulmonic component of the second sound is delayed as the disease progresses, widening the splitting of the second heart sound. With increasing stenosis, ejection murmurs usually become louder and more prolonged, with peak intensity occurring later in systole. In hemodynamically significant aortic stenosis, a sustained left ventricular heave develops, the carotid upstroke becomes delayed and lower in amplitude (the *parvus et tardus* pattern), and the second heart sound becomes softer and single as the aortic closing sound decreases.

Calcific aortic stenosis is the most common cause of aortic stenosis in the elderly. Onset is in the fourth decade if the underlying valve is bicuspid and in the sixth to eighth decades if the valve is an otherwise normal tricuspid one. Most patients present with symptoms of advanced disease (angina, heart failure, syncope), because the condition often goes unrecognized in the asymptomatic phase. Early diagnosis is often made difficult by the speed of disease progression and the deceptively subtle and atypical physical findings in elderly persons with hemodynamically significant disease. Valve calcification can progress rapidly, leading to hemodynamically significant outflow tract obstruction in as little as 1 to 2 years. Unlike other forms of aortic stenosis, the murmur at the base may reappear at the apex as a higher pitched sound and simulate mitral regurgitation (*Gallavardin's phenomenon*). In addition, the left ventricular lift associated with hemodynamically significant disease may be less prominent due to myocardial decompensation, and the carotid upstroke may be normal if the carotid artery is stiff due to age.

Hypertrophic cardiomyopathy (*idiopathic hypertrophic subaortic stenosis*) produces an ejection quality murmur by dynamically obstructing the left ventricular outflow tract. Displacement of the mitral valve may also occur dynamically and cause regurgitation. The ejection murmur is affected by the size of the left ventricular cavity and contractility. Maneuvers that decrease cavity size (e.g., Valsalva) increase obstruction and intensify the murmur. When there is marked obstruction, the murmur lasts through most of systole and its peak is delayed beyond mid-systole. Some patients are prone to tachyarrhythmias. The electrocardiogram (ECG) shows high voltage.

ASDs produce physiologic murmurs due to increased right ventricular stroke volume. However, unlike other physiologic murmurs, there is often wide and fixed splitting of the second sound due to left-to-right shunting of blood and a delay in right ventricular ejection.

Patients with physiologic or innocent murmurs are generally asymptomatic from a cardiac standpoint and usually have no previous history of heart disease. Patients with mild varieties of aortic or pulmonic stenosis, hypertrophic cardiomyopathy, or a small ASD may be asymptomatic as well. In patients with aortic stenosis, onset of symptoms (e.g., angina, dyspnea, postural lightheadedness) is usually a late development indicating advanced disease (see Chapter 33).

Regurgitant Murmurs

Regurgitant murmurs of the arterioventricular valves may be *holosystolic* or *late systolic*, depending on the anatomy and function of the compromised valve apparatus. The holosystolic regurgitant mitral murmurs are seen with causes that render the valve incompetent throughout systole, such as *rheumatic mitral valve disease, endocarditis,* severe cases of *dilated cardiomyopathy, papillary muscle rupture,* and *endocardial fibrosis* of the valve surface from *phentermine/fenfluramine* use (see below). Mid-late systolic murmurs are characteristic of regurgitation due to *mitral valve prolapse* (MVP) and *papillary muscle dysfunction*, where valve incompetence develops as systole progresses.

The murmur of *tricuspid regurgitation* is similar in quality and timing to that of mitral regurgitation but heard best along the left sternal border and characteristically increasing with inspiration. Valve injury and right ventricular dilatation are the principal causes. A *ventricular septal defect* (VSD) may also produce a holosystolic murmur at the left sternal border, caused by left-to-right shunting of blood. It is differentiated from tricuspid regurgitation by maneuvers that increase afterload (see below).

The most common cause of an asymptomatic mitral regurgitant murmur in the outpatient setting is *MVP*. In the Framingham study, the prevalence was as high as 17% among young women, 4% among young men. Overall, 5% of the population had echocardiographic evidence of MVP, with 4% manifesting a murmur of grade 2/6 or louder. MVP, with its late systolic murmur, is often preceded by a click as the redundant mitral valve leaflets prolapse into the atrium during late systole. Most patients with MVP have no other signs or symptoms of heart disease, although an important minority experience atypical chest pain, dysrhythmias, or dyspnea. In a few instances, hemodynamically significant mitral regurgitation occurs. Asthenic builds in both men and women have been associated with MVP, as has small breast size in women. Nonspecific T-wave changes, particularly inferior lead T-wave inversion, have been described. Diagnosis is confirmed by finding prominent late systolic prolapse on M-mode echocardiography or definite prolapse on the mitral valve leaflets in the parasternal long-axis view on two-dimensional ultrasound study.

The widespread use of the diet-pill combination *phentermine/fenfluramine* in the mid-late 1990s (see Chapter 234) was associated with reports of new onset of clinically significant incompetence of mitral, tricuspid, and aortic valves. The valves of persons who came to surgery were characterized by striking fibrosis of the endocardial surface identical to that seen in carcinoid syndrome, leading some to speculate that this might be the consequence of excessive seratonergic effects on valve endocardial metabolism. Patients at greatest risk appeared to be those taking the combination program at maximal doses for prolonged periods, but the true magnitude of the risk has been hard to determine. Because of concern over valve injury, both drugs have been withdrawn from the market.

DIFFERENTIAL DIAGNOSIS

The differential diagnosis can be listed according to the underlying pathophysiology. Thus, systolic ejection murmurs can be classified as innocent, physiologic, aortic, and pulmonic. Regurgitant murmurs may be caused by incompetence of the mitral or tricuspid valves or by a VSD (Table 21.1).

WORKUP

Differentiating Systolic Regurgitant Murmurs from Ejection Murmurs

Making the distinction early in the evaluation helps focus the workup and narrow the differential diagnosis (Table 21.1). The murmur's *timing, quality,* and *location* are among the most important differentiating features. As noted earlier, ejection quality murmurs are typically harsh, best heard with the bell, usually loudest at the base, and radiate into the neck and down to the apex. In elderly patients with calcific aortic stenosis, the murmur may be higher pitched and maximal at the apex, mimicking mitral regurgitation. The systolic regurgitant murmurs of mitral and tricuspid regurgitation are characteristically high pitched, well localized to the apex or left sternal border (unless

Table 21.1.   Differential Diagnosis of Systolic Ejection Murmur

1. **Innocent Murmurs**
2. **Physiologic Murmurs**
   a. Exercise or emotion
   b. Fever
   c. Anemia
   d. Hyperthyroidism
   e. Conditions with large stroke volumes: atrial septal defect, aortic regurgitation, bradycardia
   f. Pregnancy
3. **Aortic Murmurs**
   a. Aortic stenosis
   b. Hypertrophic cardiomyopathy
   c. Sub- and supravalvular fixed stenoses
4. **Pulmonic Murmurs**
   a. Pulmonic stenosis
5. **Mitral Regurgitation Murmurs**
   a. Rheumatic mitral insufficiency
   b. Mitral valve prolapse syndrome
   c. Congenital mitral valve disease
   d. Rupture of chordae tendineae
   e. Papillary muscle dysfunction
   f. Left atrial myxoma
   g. Dilated mitral valve ring
6. **Tricuspid Regurgitation Murmurs**
   a. Rheumatic tricuspid insufficiency
   b. Dilated tricuspid valve ring
7. **Ventricular Septal Defect**

very loud), and pansystolic or late systolic (and sometimes preceded by a click). All ejection murmurs and most regurgitant murmurs (except for those of rheumatic origin) have a crescendo-decresendo pattern, making this feature of little use in differentiation. Similarly, finding of electrocardiographic evidence of hypertrophy does not rule out a regurgitant etiology, because some degree of eccentric hypertrophy often develops in compensated mitral regurgitation.

A few additional murmur characteristics and responses to *maneuvers* can be helpful diagnostically. Ejection murmurs change in intensity with heart *rate* and length of the cardiac cycle, becoming softer with increases in rate and louder as rate decreases. Regurgitant murmurs change little if at all with heart rate. *Handgrip* and other maneuvers that increase systolic pressure (e.g., *transient arterial occlusion* by inflation of blood pressure cuffs applied to both arms) markedly augments the intensity of the regurgitant murmurs of mitral regurgitation and VSD. Right-sided heart murmurs can be differentiated from left sided ones by the augmentation in intensity that occurs with quiet *inspiration*.

Assessment of Ejection Murmurs

Separating Harmless Causes from More Serious Pathology. Attention to *timing, quality, intensity, and location* are helpful. *Innocent and physiologic murmurs* are usually mid-range in frequency, less than 3/6 in intensity, peak in early systole, stop long before S_2, and are heard best at the base, although they can radiate to neck and apex. Valsalva and standing decrease their intensity. The second sound is normally split and of normal intensity; there are no clicks, heaves, S_3S_4, or other murmurs. The *ECG* and *chest radiograph* are normal. Signs of anemia, fever, hyperthyroidism, and anxiety should be sought.

The murmurs resulting from *ASD* and hemodynamically *insignificant aortic and pulmonic stenoses* may resemble physiologic murmurs. However, in most cases of ASD there is widened and fixed splitting of S_2, and in more than 90% of cases there is a conduction defect of the *right bundle branch* type, producing a QRS and lead V_1 with an RSR prime configuration. A normal ECG and normal splitting of S_2 make an ASD unlikely. When one is in doubt, an echocardiogram can be used to look for abnormal septal motion and right ventricular enlargement; a normal study rules out the diagnosis. *Mild aortic stenosis* in the young patient may be impossible to distinguish from a physiologic murmur; the presence of an ejection click is an important clue to the former.

Estimating Severity of Aortic Stenosis. As aortic stenosis progresses and becomes more hemodynamically significant, the murmur typically gets louder and peaks later in systole, the second heart sound decreases in intensity (becoming equal to or less intense than the first sound at the base), a left ventricular lift develops, a thrill may be palpable, and the carotid upstroke becomes delayed. Evidence of left ventricular hypertrophy may appear on ECG (e.g., increased voltage, strain pattern), although the test is not a sensitive indicator.

A high index of suspicion is necessary both for the detection of *calcific aortic stenosis in the elderly* and the estimation of its severity. One needs to remember to listen at the apex and at the base and not to be lulled into a false sense of security by the softness of the murmur, the absence of a vigorous left ventric-

ular heave, or the normality of the carotid upstroke. Its presentation as a medium- to high-pitched muscial murmur, heard best at the apex, may lead to confusion with mitral regurgitation. Helping to differentiate it from mitral regurgitation is the decrease in the murmur's intensity with increase in heart rate; in mitral regurgitation, there is no change in the murmur with heart rate.

Confirmation of suspected valvular and subvalvular obstruction to left ventricular outflow and accurate estimation of its severity can be accomplished noninvasively by *cardiac ultrasound* performed in conjunction with a continuous-wave *Doppler study*. For aortic stenosis, reasonably accurate estimates can often be obtained of valve area and pressure gradient across the valve. Severe stenosis is defined as a mean gradient in excess of 40 mm Hg with a calculated valve area less than 0.75 cm^2. A valve area in the range of 0.76 to 1.1 cm^2 and a gradient in the range of 15 to 39 mm Hg defines moderate disease. Overestimates of severity can occur in the setting of low flow. The degree of valve calcification noted on echocardiography corresponds to the severity of stenosis. The test is also diagnostic of hypertrophic cardiomyopathy and essential to estimation of its severity.

Clinical Recognition of Idiopathic Hypertrophic Subaortic Stenosis. Several maneuvers help differentiate the systolic ejection murmur associated with this type of cardiomyopathy from other ejection murmurs. Most distinctive are the murmur's responses to *squatting*, passive *leg elevation*, and *Valsalva*, maneuvers that affect left ventricular chamber size through their effects on venous return. A lessening of venous return decreases chamber size and increases obstruction to outflow by the hypertrophic heart muscle. This is why Valsalva (bearing down against a closed glottis) results in an increase in the intensity of the murmur. With passive leg elevation and with change from standing to squatting, the murmur of hypertrophic disease characteristically *decreases* as venous return rises. Although sometimes the murmur may not change substantially with increasing venous return, any clearcut increase in the murmur under such circumstances rules out hypertrophic cardiomyopathy. The murmur peaks around mid-systole, which helps distinguish it from those innocent murmurs that peak earlier. Other features of the murmur include maximal intensity along the left sternal border and a brisk *carotid upstroke* that is sometimes *bisferiens* (bifid) in quality.

Clinical Recognition of Pulmonic Stenosis. Hemodynamically significant pulmonic stenosis is suggested by a prolonged and loud murmur (greater than 3/6) that characteristically increases with *inspiration*, wide splitting or absence of the pulmonic component of the second heart sound, an ejection click that decreases with inspiration, a right ventricular lift, evidence of pulmonary artery dilation on chest film, and prominent R wave in V_1 indicative of right ventricular hypertrophy. A normal ECG and an early systolic murmur rule out significant pulmonic stenosis. Mild hemodynamically insignificant pulmonic stenosis may be indistinguishable from an innocent murmur, but usually no therapy is indicated and therefore misdiagnosis is of little consequence.

Summary. The key components of the initial evaluation of the systolic ejection murmur in the asymptomatic patient include attention to carotid upstroke; left and right ventricular impulses; second heart sound; clicks; the quality, timing, intensity, and location of the murmur; and the effects of provocative maneuvers that affect venous return, heart rate, and systemic resistance. ECG and chest radiograph may be helpful. Cardiac ultrasound examination, in conjunction with Doppler study, are indicated if there is clinical suspicion of hemodynamically significant disease or the diagnosis remains in doubt and there are adverse consequences to not identifying the lesion.

Assessment of Regurgitant Murmurs

The *timing* and *location* of the regurgitant murmur are among the most helpful features diagnostically. The response to a number of simple bedside maneuvers can also provide useful information.

Holosystolic Murmurs. A holosystolic murmur suggests rheumatic or cardiomyopathic *mitral insufficiency, tricuspid insufficiency,* or a *VSD.* The murmur of classic mitral insufficiency is best heard at the apex and radiates laterally into the axilla; it varies little with cycle length or with respiration but increases markedly with *handgrip* and other maneuvers that transiently increase systemic resistance (e.g., bilateral blood pressure cuff inflation). With chronic increase in volume load, there is likely to be palpable enlargement of the left ventricle. Because multivalve involvement is the rule and heart failure may occur, a careful listening for other murmurs and a check for signs of heart failure (e.g., rales, third heart sound) are in order. However, a third heart sound is quite common in mitral regurgitation and not as predictive of systolic dysfunction as it is in other forms of heart disease.

Differentiating Tricuspid from Mitral Insufficiency. One notes the effect of *respiration* on the murmur. The systolic regurgitant murmur of tricuspid insufficiency increases with quiet inspiration and sustained abdominal pressure (applied to the right upper quadrant to compress the liver). Moreover, it is usually loudest at the lower left sternal border, but when the right ventricle is very large, it may be heard at the apex. It does not radiate well to the axilla. Intensity is strongly influenced by respiration, increasing at the beginning of inspiration and fading during early expiration. The presence of *hepatojugular reflux* is very suggestive and should be checked.

Identifying Ventricular Septal Defect. The holosystolic murmur of *VSD* can be heard best at the sternal border and does not radiate to the axilla. Intensity does not vary with respiration, but like mitral regurgitation, it is increased with Valsalva, handgrip, and blood pressure cuff application. The murmur often has some mid-systolic accentuation and may be confused with an ejection murmur. Like mitral regurgitation, intensity of the murmur increases markedly with handgrip and other maneuvers that increase systemic resistance.

Late Systolic Murmurs. *MVP* is characterized by a mid- to late-systolic murmur preceded by a mid-systolic click. Some forms of *papillary muscle dysfunction* will also result in a mitral regurgitant murmur of similar timing, usually in the setting of anteroseptal ischemia. Suspicion of MVP is reinforced by hearing a mid-systolic click, which tends to move toward the first heart sound with standing (a maneuver that reduces left ventricular volume and softens the murmur). The MVP murmur may occur in the absence of a click. The intensity of the suspected MVP murmur should be noted. The louder the murmur, the more hemodynamically significant the regurgitation, and the greater the risks of endocarditis and other cardiovascular complications. Handgrip or Valsalva maneuver may increase the intensity of the murmur. Increasing duration of the murmur is a sign of worsening prolapse. Development of a holosytolic murmur without a systolic click in a person with known MVP is associated with an increased risk of an adverse event.

Testing for Mitral Valve Prolapse. An *echocardiogram* can confirm MVP when uncertainty persists. Minor degrees of valve prolapse are normal. One should insist that ultrasound criteria are met before giving the patient a diagnosis of MVP. The major criterion is *systolic displacement* of one or both valve leaflets into the left atrium beyond the plane of the mitral annulus in the parasternal long-axis view on two-dimensional ultrasound study. *Valve thickening* and *redundancy* are other features, but a *nonclassic form of MVP* has been described in which there is no thickening, little risk for endocarditis, and little hemodynamically significant regurgitation. Ultrasound can differentiate the two and thus may help with cardiac risk stratification, although a very small risk of embolic stroke is similar in both forms.

Indiscriminate use of echocardiography is to be avoided. Searching for "silent" MVP in the patient with vague chest pains and an entirely normal cardiac examination is of no value. Use of ultrasound in suspected MVP can facilitate diagnosis, but the contribution to outcome remains to be demonstrated. In most instances, the change in management engendered involves initiation of endocarditis prophylaxis (see Chapter 16). However, Doppler echocardiographic studies suggest that audible, and especially loud, systolic regurgitant murmurs are very likely to represent hemodynamically significant disease. An ultrasound examination is indicated when such a murmur is encountered.

PATIENT EDUCATION AND INDICATIONS FOR REFERRAL

Patient Education

When the murmur is determined to be innocent or hemodynamically insignificant after careful evaluation, it is essential to provide detailed explanation as part of the delivery of meaningful reassurance. Marked concern and even distrust may be precipitated by a perfunctory explanation that "it's harmless and nothing serious," especially if detailed auscultation continues to be conducted on subsequent visits. Concern about a murmur that is left incompletely explained can lead to unnecessary self-restriction of activity. Reassurance should include a discussion of the cause of the murmur, its significance, and prognosis. Informing the patient of other possible causes considered and ruled out is particularly helpful to the well-educated or medically curious patient and can obviate the demand for unnecessary testing or referral. The patient with a harmless murmur should be specifically told there is no need to restrict activity or undergo further evaluation at the present time.

Aortic Stenosis. Asymptomatic persons found to have aortic stenosis (especially the elderly) should be informed of the importance of regular follow-up examinations and taught to watch for the symptoms of hemodynamically significant disease (i.e., postural lightheadedness, angina, exertional dyspnea), with instructions given to report immediately should they occur. (Also see Chapter 33).

Mitral Valve Prolapse. Counseling is particularly important for the patient with insignificant *MVP*. Patients should be informed that MVP is a heterogeneous condition, with most at no increased risk for cardiac complications. Those with readily audible MVP regurgitant murmurs should be advised about the need for endocarditis prophylaxis (see Chapter 16).

Indications for Referral

The person with hemodynamically significant aortic stenosis (valve area less than 0/9 cm²) needs close follow-up, annual echocardiography, and consideration of cardiac consultation if stenosis continues to progress, even in the absence of symptoms. Onset of symptoms makes the referral urgent (see Chapter 33). Worsening exertional dyspnea in the patient with rheumatic, ischemic, or cardiomyopathic mitral regurgitation is also an indication for prompt cardiac consultation, because it suggests the left ventricle is decompensating (see Chapter 33). Annual echocardiography has been recommended for asymptomatic persons with hemodynamically significant mitral regurgitation, with referral indicated if there is progressive enlargement of the left ventricle or a fall in ejection fraction below 60%. Referral is also needed for the patient with tricuspid regurgitation and worsening hepatojugular reflux and other signs of right-sided failure.

Those with particularly loud murmurs of MVP suggestive of hemodynamically significant disease should be referred for cardiac consultation after undergoing ultrasound examination for confirmation. Most can be reassured that they are at no increased risk and that progression to more serious disease is very rare. Prompt referral is indicated for the rare MVP patient with complex ventricular irritability, prolonged QT intervals, a family history of sudden death, or a transient ischemic event.

RECOMMENDATIONS

- Begin by determining whether the systolic murmur is regurgitant or ejection in quality by attention to the murmur's location, quality, and timing.
- Differentiate right-sided from left-sided pathology by observing response of the murmur to inspiration.
- If the murmur is ejection in quality, distinguish between innocent/physiologic murmurs and those due to structural heart disease.
- For left-sided ejection murmurs, distinguish between aortic stenosis and hypertrophic cardiomyopathy.
- If aortic stenosis is suspected, estimate clinical severity by physical examination and obtain Doppler cardiac ultrasound in those persons with physical findings suggestive of hemodynamically significant disease.
- Follow patients with calcific aortic stenosis closely and repeat ultrasound examination periodically.
- If there is evidence of hypertrophic cardiomyopathy (idiopathic hypertrophic subaortic stenosis) by physical examination, order Doppler cardiac ultrasound to confirm.
- For holosystolic murmurs, differentiate by physical examination between arteriovenous valve regurgitation and VSD; if

arteriovenous valve regurgitation is suspected, determine whether the murmur is mitral or pulmonic. Obtain Doppler ultrasound if there is clinical evidence of hemodynamically significant regurgitation.
- For late systolic murmurs, differentiate between MVP and valve regurgitation due to papillary muscle dysfunction. If hemodynamically significant MVP is suspected, obtain Doppler ultrasound to confirm.
- Refer for cardiac consultation any patient found to have severe aortic stenosis or any other hemodynamically significant lesion with poor prognosis (e.g., hypertrophic cardiomyopathy, mitral regurgitation with falling ejection fraction).
- Provide detailed reassurance to patients with harmless lesions to minimize demand for unneccesary testing, and make clear to patients with hemodynamically significant disease the need for close follow-up.

A.H.G.

ANNOTATED BIBLIOGRAPHY

Brenner SJ, Duffy CI, Thomas JD. Progression of aortic stenosis in 394 patients. J Am Coll Cardiol 1995;25:305. (*A serial Doppler ultrasound study with a 3-year mean duration of follow-up; documents speed with which progression can occur in elderly patients.*)

Carabello BA, Crawford FA. Valvular heart disease. N Engl J Med 1997;337:32. (*Excellent review that emphasizes pathophysiology and timely detection of clinically important disease.*)

Connolly HM, Crary JL, McGoon MD, et al. Valvular heart disease associated with fenfluramine-phentermine. N Engl J Med 1997;337:581. (*Major report on valvular damage associated with use of this once popular diet-pill combination.*)

Coughlin HC. Mitral valve prolapse: is echocardiography yielding too little or too much information to the practicing physician? Am J Med 1989;87:367. (*A strong plea for viewing MVP as a heterogeneous disorder and using ultrasound selectively.*)

Craige E. Should auscultation be rehabilitated? N Engl J Med 1988;318:1611. (*An editorial urging reemphasis on physical diagnosis.*)

Devereaux RB, Kramer-Fox R, Kligfield P. Mitral valve prolapse: causes, clinical manifestations, and management. Ann Intern Med 1989;111:305. (*Comprehensive review; 172 references.*)

Etchells E, Bell C, Robb K. Does this patient have an abnormal systolic murmur? JAMA 1997;277:564. (*A comprehensive literature review of the evidence for the accuracy and precision of clinical findings in the diagnosis of systolic murmurs.*)

Etchells E, Glenns V, Shadowitz S, et al. A bedside clinical prediction rule for detecting moderate or severe aortic stenosis. J Gen Intern Med 1998;13:699. (*A cross-sectional study confirming the efficacy of physical examination in identifying and ruling out hemodynamically significant aortic stenosis.*)

Finegam RE, Gianelly RD, Harrison DC. Aortic stenosis in the elderly: relevance of age to diagnosis and treatment. N Engl J Med 1969;281:1261. (*An important classic paper; physical findings such as carotid upstroke and quality and location of the murmur may be misleading in assessing aortic stenosis in the elderly.*)

Folland ED, Kriegel BJ, Henderson WG, et al. Implications of third heart sounds in patients with valvular heart disease. N Engl J Med 1992;327:458. (*Indicative of failure in aortic stenosis but not necessarily in mitral regurgitation.*)

Heckerling PS, Wiener SL, Moses VK, et al. Accuracy of precordial percussion in detecting cardiomegaly. Am J Med 1991;91:328. (*Not often performed but found surprisingly useful.*)

Hershman WY, Moskowitz MA, Marton KI, et al. Utility of echocardiography in patients with suspected mitral valve prolapse. Am J Med 1989;87:371. *(Diagnosis changed in 56%, treatment in 27%, but significance unclear.)*

Lembo NJ, Dell'Italia LJ, Crawford MH, et al. Bedside diagnosis of systolic murmurs. N Engl J Med 1988;318:1572. *(One of the few studies providing sensitivity and specificity data on diagnostic maneuvers.)*

Lombard TJ, Selzer A. Valvular aortic stenosis. Ann Intern Med 1987;106:292. *(Clinical presentations of 397 patients, with emphasis on disease in the elderly.)*

Maisel AS, Atwood JE, Goldberger AL. Hepatojugular reflux: useful in the bedside diagnosis of tricuspid regurgitation. Ann Intern Med 1984;101:781. *(Specificity 100%, sensitivity of 66% in detecting tricuspid regurgitation; increase in murmur intensity with deep inspiration was as specific and more sensitive.)*

Maron BJ, Bonow RO, Cannon RO 3rd, et al. Hypertrophic cardiomyopathy: interrelations of clinical manifestations, pathophysiology, and therapy. Parts 1 and 2. N Engl J Med 1987;316:844. *(Best discussion of correlations between pathophysiology and clinical findings.)*

Nishimura RA, McGoon MD, Shub C, et al. Echocardiographically documented mitral valve prolapse: long-term follow-up of 237 patients. N Engl J Med 1985;313:1305. *(Identifies a low-risk subgroup.)*

Rothman A, Goldberger AL. Aids to cardiac auscultation. Ann Intern Med 1983;99:346. *(Critical review of maneuvers.)*

Stein PD, Sabbah H. Aortic origin of innocent murmur. Am J Cardiol 1977;39:665. *(Presents extensive data for an aortic origin.)*

22
Evaluation of Leg Edema

Leg edema can be a bothersome complaint and an initial symptom of serious underlying disease. Acute onset of unilateral swelling raises the question of deep vein thrombophlebitis (DVT), which must be addressed promptly. Bilateral disease is particularly common in the elderly and often a manifestation of chronic venous insufficiency, congestive heart failure, or venodilating medications; however, pulmonary hypertension may account for as much as a fifth of cases and usually goes unrecognized. Noninvasive methods, particularly venous and cardiac ultrasound, have greatly facilitated evaluation, but clinical estimation of pretest probability is essential to optimal test selection and interpretation. Especially important to the pretest assessment of unilateral edema is knowledge of the incidence, risk factors, symptoms, and signs of DVT. In bilateral edema, awareness of the potential contributions from often overlooked etiologies (such as pulmonary hypertension and use of nonsteroidal antiinflammatory drugs [NSAIDs]) can inform the clinical assessment and guide workup.

PATHOPHYSIOLOGY AND CLINICAL PRESENTATION

Edema is defined as an increase in extracellular volume. It develops if hydrostatic pressure exceeds colloid oncotic pressure, capillary permeability increases, or lymphatic drainage becomes impaired. Hydrostatic pressure is a function of intravascular volume, blood pressure, and venous outflow. Colloid oncotic pressure depends on the serum albumin concentration.

Decreased oncotic pressure is usually due to *hypoalbuminemia*, which can occur secondary to malnutrition, hepatocellular failure, or excess renal or gastrointestinal loss of albumin. The resultant fall in intravascular volume from excessive transudation of fluid stimulates salt retention. This compensatory effort to maintain adequate intravascular volume leads to further edema formation because the underlying oncotic deficit remains. Edema sets in when the serum albumin concentration falls below 2.5 g/100 mL. Leg swelling due to hypoalbuminemia is typically bilateral, pitting, and sometimes accompanied by edema of the face and eyelids (especially on awakening).

Increased hydrostatic pressure may result from excessive *fluid retention* (such as is seen with congestive heart failure or drugs [NSAIDs, corticosteroids]), *impairment of venous outflow* from DVT, or *pulmonary hypertension* (which may be a consequence of sleep apnea, left heart failure, or chronic obstructive lung disease). Venodilating drugs (such as *nifedipine*) may lead to an increase in hydrostatic pressure as blood pools in the lower extremities. A localized increase in hydrostatic pressure develops in the legs during prolonged standing, especially if the valves in the leg veins are incompetent. Increased hydrostatic pressure due to fluid retention produces bilaterally symmetric edema, whereas swelling due to venous insufficiency may be asymmetric and accompanied by varicosities and other signs of venous disease, such as stasis dermatitis, ulcers, and brawny induration.

DVT may have a very subtle presentation, with acute onset of *unilateral or asymmetric leg edema* as the only manifestation. Such textbook findings as calf tenderness, palpable cord, and positive Homan's sign are often absent. The findings most predictive of significant DVT are swelling of the entire leg, asymmetric leg edema (more than 3 cm difference in calf circumferences), pitting edema of the involved leg, tenderness along deep veins, and prominent collateral superficial veins. Most clots due to thrombophlebitis form in the small veins of the calf; 20% to 30% propagate proximally into the popliteal and femoral veins of the knee and thigh. Clot below the knee poses little risk of pulmonary embolization, but extension above the knee markedly increases its chances. Unilateral lower leg edema can also result from venous compression by a *popliteal (Baker's) cyst*. A stroke that causes paresis in one leg may result in unilateral edema due to reductions in vascular tone and venous and lymphatic drainage; thrombophlebitis may ensue. In addition to paralysis, the independent predictors of DVT include active cancer, recent plaster cast/prolonged immobilization, and recent major surgery (especially of the hip or knee). Hypercoagulability increases risk and occurs with estrogen use and with resistance to activated protein C. The latter is seen in patients with *factor V Leiden mutation*, affecting 2% to

3% of white populations, producing a relative risk for DVT of 3.3, and accounting for about 5% of cases.

Increased capillary permeability is another mechanism of leg edema associated with immunologic injury, infection, inflammation, or trauma. A permeability defect is also believed to be responsible for *idiopathic edema*, a poorly understood but common problem seen almost exclusively in women. Although some patients report a periodicity to the problem that seems to parallel the menstrual cycle, careful studies have failed to find sufficient evidence to warrant the label "*cyclic edema*." The condition is especially aggravated by hot weather and standing, more so than occurs with venous insufficiency. Transient abdominal distention is common, and weight may fluctuate several pounds over the course of the day. The disorder is not progressive, but it can cause considerable discomfort. It is often accompanied by headache, fatigue, anxiety, and other functional symptoms. Some patients are bothered by nocturia.

Lymphatic obstruction hinders reabsorption of interstitial fluid. The swelling usually starts in the feet and progresses upward; often the problem is unilateral. The edema of lymphatic obstruction tends to have a brawny quality and evidences little pitting, except in its early stages. Recumbency provides only minor relief compared with edema from other causes.

DIFFERENTIAL DIAGNOSIS

The differential diagnosis of edema can be organized according to clinical presentations and pathophysiologic mechanisms (Table 22.1). The list of etiologies for bilateral edema is particularly extensive. In primary care practice, the leading causes of bilateral disease include venous insufficiency, heart failure, pulmonary hypertension, and hypoalbuminemia; pulmonary hypertension is the most commonly missed diagnosis. Certain infiltrative conditions may be mistaken for edema, such

Table 22.1.   Important Causes of Leg Edema

I. Unilateral or Asymmetric Swelling
  A. Increased hydrostatic pressure
    1. Deep vein thrombophlebitis
    2. Venous insufficiency
    3. Popliteal (Baker's) cyst
  B. Increased capillary permeability
    1. Cellulitis
    2. Trauma
  C. Lymphatic obstruction (local)
II. Bilateral Swelling
  A. Decreased oncotic pressure
    1. Malnutrition
    2. Hepatocellular failure
    3. Nephrotic syndrome
    4. Protein-losing enteropathy
  B. Increased hydrostatic pressure
    1. Congestive heart failure
    2. Renal failure
    3. Use of salt-retaining drugs (e.g., corticosteroids, estrogens)
    4. Venous insufficiency
    5. Pulmonary hypertens
ion and premenstrual state
    6. Pregnancy
  C. Increased capillary permeability
    1. Systemic vasculitis
    2. Idiopathic edema
    3. Allergic reactions
  D. Lymphatic obstruction (retroperitoneal or generalized)

as pretibial myxedema and lipedema (a familial bilateral deposition of excess fat).

WORKUP

Diagnosis of leg edema can be challenging. The initial clinical impression often undergoes revision upon laboratory testing, underscoring the difficulty in making an accurate diagnosis on the basis of history and physical examination alone. In a study from primary care practice, venous insufficiency was overdiagnosed clinically and heart failure and pulmonary hypertension markedly underdiagnosed. Nonetheless, attention to clinical features is critical to making the best possible pretest probability assessment, which is essential to test selection and interpretation.

History. The distribution of the swelling should be ascertained, because it helps to focus the differential diagnosis. If edema is reported to be predominantly *unilateral or asymmetric*, the patient ought to be questioned about the major risk factors for DVT, including active malignancy, recent paralysis or plaster casting, prolonged immobilization, major surgery (especially of the hip or knee), estrogen use, and family history of DVT (suggestive of an inherited hypercoagulable state). Any report of tenderness along deep veins, swelling of the entire leg, and marked asymmetry of the swelling should be noted and confirmed by physical examination (see below). If the edema is reportedly *bilateral and symmetric*, then it is important to check for a history of venous insufficiency, but also for dyspnea on exertion; orthopnea; paroxysmal nocturnal dyspnea; severe snoring; daytime sleepiness; interrupted sleep; chronic productive cough; a history of cardiac, pulmonary, renal, or hepatic failure; malnutrition; and use of such drugs as nifedipine, other vasodilators, NSAIDs, and corticosteroids. A report of acute facial swelling suggests an allergic reaction or hypoalbuminemia if the swelling is more chronic.

Physical Examination. The first priority is to confirm the distribution of the problem. Careful measurements of calf and thigh diameters is also very helpful.

In *unilateral edema*, if the swelling is predominantly limited to one leg, the limb ought to be examined for tenderness, redness, increased warmth, varicosities, and a palpable thrombosed vein. Unfortunately, the often-cited classic signs of DVT (i.e., calf tenderness, palpable cord, positive Homan's sign) are neither very sensitive nor specific; unilateral edema may be the only clue aside from a history of risk factors. Nonetheless, a difference in calf circumferences of more than 3 cm is an independent predictor of DVT, as is tenderness along deep veins, swelling of the entire leg, pitting edema, and prominence of collateral superficial veins. Encountering three or more of these findings in a patient with risk factors for DVT is associated with a pretest probability for DVT of about 75%. If edema is prominent but pitting is only minimal, it suggests that lymphatic obstruction might be the cause.

The patient with *bilateral leg edema* should have the blood pressure measured for hypertension, which might be a sign of renal failure. The skin is checked for evidence of chronic cardiopulmonary disease (cyanosis, clubbing) and for signs of hepatocellular failure (jaundice, spider angiomata, ecchymoses); the jugular veins for distention; the chest for rales, wheezes, and effusion; the heart for signs of pulmonary hypertension (a right ventricular heave or right ventricular S_3, increased prominence of P_2, widened splitting of S_2) and signs of heart failure (S_3, abnormal splitting of S_2); and the abdomen for hepatojugular reflux and ascites. Any lymphadenopathy should be noted.

Laboratory Studies. The patient with new onset of unilateral or asymmetric leg edema needs diagnostic testing to address the question of DVT, because of the high false-positive and false-negative rates based on clinical findings alone. Only 20% to 40% of patients thought to have DVT on clinical grounds prove to have clot on further testing. Testing is also critical in bilateral leg edema, because underlying cardiopulmonary disease is often inapparent from the history and physical examination alone.

Unilateral or Asymmetric Leg Edema. Risk stratification can help guide the approach to test ordering and interpretation. Although the diagnosis of DVT cannot be made clinically, reasonable estimates of pretest probability for DVT can be made by attention to clinical features found to be independent predictors of DVT (Table 22.2). Using this probability estimate in conjunction with the results from noninvasive testing helps to determine who requires anticoagulation, further testing, or no anticoagulation. For example, a person at high or intermediate risk with a positive study should be immediately anticoagulated. A person at low risk with a normal ultrasound has the diagnosis ruled out. A person at intermediate risk with an initially normal study needs serial testing; if repeatedly negative at 2 weeks, then the diagnosis is ruled out; if positive, the diagnosis is ruled in.

Particularly important is detection of DVT above the knee, because clot here is associated with a high risk of pulmonary embolization. Below the knee, the risk of embolization is only about 3%. Ruling out clot above the knee is the major objective of testing in the patient with unexplained leg edema. High test sensitivity and specificity are required in this setting, not only to rule out DVT but also to provide sufficient positive predictive value to justify initiation of anticoagulant therapy. A number of noninvasive approaches have replaced venography as the initial test of choice.

Table 22.2. Model for Clinical Prediction of Deep Vein Thrombophlebitis[a]

CLINICAL FEATURE	SCORE
History	
Active cancer	1
Paralysis, recent plaster cast	1
Recent immobilization or major surgery	1
Physical Examination	
Tenderness along deep veins	1
Swelling of entire leg	1
>3 cm difference in calf circumference	1
Pitting edema	1
Collateral superficial veins	1
Clinical Assessment	
Alternative diagnosis likely	−2

[a]Pretest probability of deep vein thrombosis: high if score of 3 points or greater; intermediate if score of 1–2 points, and low if score of 0 or less.

From Wells PS, Anderson DR, Bormanis J, et al. Value of assessment of pretest probability of deep vein thrombosis in clinical management. Lancet 1997;350:1795, with permission.

Venous ultrasound study involving the combination of B-mode or two-dimensional *ultrasonography* and color-flow *Doppler* ultrasound (so-called triplex scanning) has proven practical and highly sensitive and specific. Failure of the vein to compress during ultrasound scanning is highly correlated with DVT. At times, direct visualization of clot is possible. Doppler measures blood flow, helping to identify the vein and any reduction in flow due to clot. Doppler alone is highly technician dependent. Computerized color enhancement of Doppler data facilitates test performance and interpretation. For detection of thrombophlebitis above the knee, sensitivity and specificity of triplex scanning range from 97% to 99%. For thrombophlebitis below the knee, sensitivity and specificity fall to 80%, because as many as 40% of calf vein studies are technically unsuccessful due to poor sound penetration. Successful below-the-knee studies have the same sensitivity and specificity as those above the knee. Duplex ultrasound (triplex minus the color enhancement) is becoming the minimum standard for noninvasive testing for DVT.

A technically satisfactory study that is negative for clot above the knee virtually rules out the diagnosis of worrisome DVT in a person with a low pretest risk. If pretest probability is intermediate and initial testing is negative, then serial testing every 2 to 3 days over 1 to 2 weeks is indicated while anticoagulation is held. A positive study has a very high predictive value, sufficient to warrant initiating anticoagulation. Persistently negative test results rule out the diagnosis. If clinical suspicion is high for DVT and the initial study is negative, serial study or immediate venography is indicated.

Impedance plethysmography remains a widely used noninvasive approach to the diagnosis of DVT. It detects changes in leg volume that follow respiration and inflation and deflation of a thigh blood pressure cuff. In DVT, the normal pattern is altered and detectable by plethysmography. Most reports of test sensitivity range from 83% to 93% and specificity from 83% to 97%, but some figures are in the 65% to 70% range for tests performed in outpatients. The test is somewhat technician dependent, accounting for some of the variation in test performance figures reported. Calf-vein and nonobstructing thrombi are not well detected. Sensitivity can be enhanced by serial studies, which are obtained if there is suspicion of propagation. The test is useful for detection of recurrent thrombophlebitis, because an abnormal test usually reverts to normal 3 months after initiation of anticoagulant therapy. When specificity in a particular laboratory is less than 90%, then the predictive value of a positive test for DVT in a patient with unilateral leg edema will be in the range of 75% to 80%, not high enough to justify anticoagulation without further confirmatory testing. A negative test in a patient suspected on clinical grounds to have DVT should be followed either by a venogram or by serial plethysmography studies 2 and 4 days after the initial study.

D-dimer is a degradation product of cross-linked fibrin. Its formation occurs in the context of ongoing fibrinolysis, making its measurement a potentially sensitive indicator of active thrombosis. D-dimer testing provides a promising approach to quickly screening for DVT without the need to repeat noninvasive testing if the initial noninvasive study is negative but clinical suspicion persists. A quick ruling out of DVT is especially important in the context of suspected pulmonary embolism, the setting in which D-dimer testing for DVT is most frequently applied. Reports of sensitivity range from 85% to 100%, depending on the assay used and the cutoff level for a positive test. Specificity is poor (40% to 68%), because D-dimer acts as an acute phase reactant and its level rises in response to any event that induces fibrinolysis, such as inflammation, cancer, or trauma. The combination of high sensitivity and low specificity make the test most useful as a means of ruling out DVT. The test can be used alone in low probability patients to rule out DVT and in conjunction with ultrasound or plethysmography in patients with a higher pretest probability. If both D-dimer and one of the noninvasive studies are normal, then the probability of DVT is extremely low and serial testing can usually be omitted. Because D-dimer testing lacks specificity, confirmatory testing with ultrasound or plethysmography is necessary when a "positive" (i.e., more than 0.5 μg/dL) test result is obtained.

Venography remains the definitive test for the detection of acute deep vein occlusion. When performed and interpreted by an experienced radiologist, it is nearly 100% sensitive and specific. However, it is invasive, expensive, often painful, requires considerable expertise to perform and interpret, and includes a small (2% to 3%) risk of inducing thrombosis or a hypersensitivity reaction to the contrast medium. Moreover, as many as 25% of patients who are candidates for venography have unsuccessful studies. Hospitalization is usually required. These disadvantages plus the advent of sensitive noninvasive methods have relegated venography to a backup role in the evaluation for DVT, mostly for cases where noninvasive study is technically difficult (e.g., after knee or hip replacement). In the case of suspected lymphedema, venography is the test of first choice for detecting a cause of lymphatic obstruction and should be obtained before lymphangiography is attempted. Severe lymphatic obstruction may interfere with attaining a satisfactory lymphangiogram.

Testing for underlying etiology and hypercoagulable state of DVT is essential to determining the risk of recurrence and the proper duration of anticoagulation (see Chapter 35).

Bilateral Leg Edema. The patient with more generalized edema involving both legs should have a *chest film* in search of heart failure and pleural fluid, a *urinalysis* for detection of albuminuria, a check of the serum *albumin*, and determinations of the serum *creatinine and blood urea nitrogen* for evidence of renal insufficiency. If the serum albumin is low, then measurements of the prothrombin time and liver function testing are indicated for further documentation of hepatocellular failure (see Chapter 71). If the serum albumin is low and protein is detected in the urine, a *24-hour urine* collection for albumin and creatinine is indicated (see Chapter 130).

When the diagnosis of bilateral leg edema remains inapparent, consideration of underlying cardiopulmonary disease is indicated and a *cardiac ultrasound with Doppler* should be considered, especially in persons over the age of 45. The test provides an excellent noninvasive approach to detection of heart failure, be it due to systolic or diastolic dysfunction and to identification of pulmonary hypertension that might not be otherwise apparent. If pulmonary hypertension is suggested by cardiac ultrasound, then consideration of sleep apnea is indicated, because of its high prevalence among adults and the subtlety of its presentation (see Chapter 46).

PATIENT EDUCATION AND SYMPTOMATIC THERAPY

When edema is due to increased hydrostatic pressure or decreased oncotic pressure, a number of simple measures can provide the patient some symptomatic relief. The patient should be advised to *restrict salt* intake, avoid prolonged standing or prolonged sitting with the legs dependent, elevate the legs whenever possible, and avoid wearing garments that might restrict venous return (e.g., garters and girdles). Proper *support stockings* might provide some added benefit. If possible, use of salt-retaining drugs should be discontinued or minimized. Severe edema may require *diuretic* therapy (see Chapter 35 for details on therapy of venous insufficiency). Lymphatic obstruction and increased capillary permeability do not respond well to these measures.

Patients with idiopathic edema are sometimes helped by salt restriction, support hose, elevation, and diuretic use in the early evening. In addition to diuretics, other drugs have been reported to be useful, including propranolol and captopril. It is important to reassure the patient with this condition that the edema poses no threat to health. Furthermore, idiopathic edema often runs a self-limited course, subsiding spontaneously over a few months to several years.

Patients with chronic leg edema should be instructed to call the physician at the first sign of unilateral increase in swelling or pain, because they are at increased risk of thrombophlebitis.

RECOMMENDATIONS

For Unilateral or Markedly Asymmetric Leg Edema

- Review history for risk factors for DVT (e.g., active malignancy, recent paralysis or plaster casting, prolonged immobilization, recent major surgery [especially of the hip or knee], current estrogen use, family history of DVT).
- Check physical examination for key signs of DVT (e.g., difference in calf circumferences of more than 3 cm, tenderness along deep veins, palpable cord, pitting edema of the entire leg, prominence of collateral superficial veins).
- Estimate pretest probability of DVT based on history and physical examination.
- Obtain compression Doppler venous ultrasound or plethysmography of the involved limb in all patients. If a negative result is obtained but clinical suspicion persists, then repeat within 3 to 5 days.
- Use combination of pretest probability and tests result to determine need for further testing. When pretest probability is intermediate and initial noninvasive study is negative, either repeat the noninvasive study every 3 days for up to 2 weeks or obtain a D-dimer determination; if these are not available, then proceed directly to venography.

For Bilateral Leg Edema

- Review history for symptoms of venous insufficiency, heart failure, and chronic pulmonary disease, especially sleep apnea. Also check for a history of renal or hepatic disease, malnutrition, and use of such drugs as nifedipine, NSAIDs, and corticosteroids.
- Check serum albumin; if normal and no other etiology evident, obtain cardiac ultrasound for detection of subclinical heart failure and pulmonary hypertension.

A.H.G.

ANNOTATED BIBLIOGRAPHY

Anderson DR, Lensing AWA, Wells PS, et al. Limitations of impedance plethysmography in the diagnosis of clinically suspected deep-vein thrombosis. Ann Intern Med 1993;118:25. *(A study in outpatients; reports lower sensitivity than widely quoted.)*

Becker DM, Philbrick JT, Bachhuber TL, et al. D-dimer testing and acute venous thromboembolism. A shortcut to accurate diagnosis? Arch Intern Med 1996;156:939. *(A detailed evaluation of the original assay for D-dimer testing and its clinical application.)*

Bettmann MA, Robbins A, Braun SD, et al. Contrast venography of the leg: diagnostic efficacy, tolerance, and complication rates with ionic and nonionic contrast media. Radiology 1987;165:113. *(Critical review of the methodology.)*

Blankfield RP, Finkelhor RS, Alexander JJ, et al. Etiology and diagnosis of bilateral leg edema in primary care. Am J Med 1998;105:192. *(A study from primary care practice showing marked underrecognition of heart failure and pulmonary hypertension as causes of bilateral leg edema; argues for more use of cardiac ultrasonography in the workup.)*

Cranley JJ, Canos AJ, Sull WJ. The diagnosis of deep vein thrombosis, fallibility of clinical symptoms and signs. Arch Surg 1976;111:34. *(Classic signs of deep vein thrombosis occurred with approximately equal frequency in people with and without deep vein thrombosis.)*

Ginsberg JS, Kearon C, Kouketis J, et al. The use of D-dimer testing and impedance plethysmographic examination in patients with clinical indications of deep vein thrombosis. Arch Intern Med 1997;157:1077. *(Using the new whole-blood assay, the combination of tests had a negative predictive value of 98.5%.)*

Huisman MV, Buller HR, Tencate JW, et al. Serial impedance plethysmography for suspected deep venous thrombosis in outpatients. N Engl J Med 1986;314:823. *(Sensitivity enhanced by serial studies; especially useful for detection of propagating clot.)*

Kahn SR. The clinical diagnosis of deep venous thrombosis. Arch Intern Med 1998;158:2315. *(A scholarly but also useful review of studies on clinically predicting probability of DVT.)*

Lee AYY, Julian JA, Levine MN, et al. Clinical utility of a rapid whole-blood D-dimer assay in patients with cancer who present with suspected acute deep venous thrombosis. Ann Intern Med 1999;131:417. *(A negative test did not reliably rule out DVT in this population.)*

Lensing AWA, Prandoni P, Brandjes D, et al. Detection of deep-vein thrombosis by real-time B-mode ultrasonography. N Engl J Med 1989;320:342. *(Sensitivity 100%, specificity 99% for clot above the knee; both fall to 80% for clot below the knee.)*

Philbrick JT, Becker DM. Calf deep venous thrombosis. A wolf in sheep's clothing? Arch Intern Med 1988;148:2131. *(Twenty percent to 30% of patients with calf-vein thrombosis have proximal propagation.)*

Rodeghiero F, Tosetto A. Activated protein C resistance and factor V Leiden mutation are independent risk factors for venous thromboembolism. Ann Intern Med 1999;130:643. *(These hypercoagulable states account for up to 15% of cases of DVT, making attention to these states of potential importance in evaluation of DVT, especially that which is recurrent.)*

Rose SC, Zwiebel WJ, Nelson BD, et al. Symptomatic lower extremity deep venous thrombosis: accuracy, limitations, and role of color duplex flow imaging in diagnosis. Radiology 1990;175:639. *(Accuracy 99% for DVT above the knee but only 81% below the knee.)*

Streeten DHP. Idiopathic edema: pathogenesis, clinical futures and treatment. Metabolism 1978;27:353. *(Comprehensive review; concludes that upright posture is an important contributor to excess transudation of fluid in more than 30%.)*

Wells PS, Anderson DR, Bormanis J, et al. Value of assessment of pretest probability of deep vein thrombosis in clinical management. Lancet 1997;350:1795. *(Best available prediction model for guiding test ordering and interpretation in patients suspected of DVT.)*

White RH, McGahan JP, Daschbach MM, et al. Diagnosis of deep-vein thrombosis using duplex ultrasound. Ann Intern Med 1989;111:297. *(A review of available studies; combined figures for sensitivity and specificity in the range of 95% for DVT above the knee; 51 references.)*

23

Evaluation of Arterial Insufficiency of the Lower Extremities

DAVID C. BREWSTER

Peripheral arterial disease of the lower extremities is usually a manifestation of systemic atherosclerosis. It is more common in men and increases in prevalence with age. The condition affects a large segment of the elderly population, many of whom are asymptomatic during the early stages of their illness. With progression, intermittent claudication ensues, experienced by about 5% of the U.S. population more than 55 years of age and by over 20% of those more than 75 years of age. Atherosclerotic occlusive disease is by far the most common cause of arterial insufficiency, although lower extremity ischemia may also be caused by embolism, arterial dissection, trauma, thrombosis of an aneurysm, or Buerger's disease.

Proper clinical management requires the physician first to recognize the manifestations of ischemic disease and carefully evaluate its severity. Many patients with mild to moderate vascular insufficiency can be managed conservatively, whereas others with acute ischemia or more severe chronic ischemia that threatens to cause tissue necrosis require more intensive investigation and often surgery (see Chapter 34).

The primary physician must be able to differentiate between patients with arterial insufficiency and those with exertional limb pain due to other causes (e.g., radiculopathy, spinal stenosis). Moreover, one needs to know the indications for and limitations of the newer noninvasive techniques for evaluating blood flow and the indications for arteriography and referral for consideration of revascularization.

PATHOPHYSIOLOGY AND CLINICAL PRESENTATION

Risk Factors and Associated Conditions. The major risk factors for peripheral arterial disease are those for atherosclerosis, with cigarette smoking and diabetes mellitus making the greatest contributions. Adding to risk are low high-density lipoprotein cholesterol, high triglycerides, and high homocysteine levels. Such risk factors are the same as those for *coronary artery disease* and *cerebrovascular disease*, which have increased prevalences in persons with peripheral artery disease. The probability of encountering symptomatic cardiovascular disease in patients with peripheral artery insufficiency is about 30%; more than 60% prove to have underlying cardiovascular disease when subjected to diagnostic testing. Peripheral artery disease is an independent risk factor for development of atherosclerotic disease elsewhere.

Reduction in Flow. Occlusive disease generally becomes symptomatic by gradual reduction of blood flow to the involved extremity or organ. Symptoms finally occur when a critical arterial stenosis is reached. Pressure and blood flow are not significantly diminished until at least 75% of the cross-sectional area of the vessel lumen is obliterated by the disease process. This is approximately equivalent to a 50% reduction in lumen diameter. More severe stenoses or even total occlusions may remain essentially asymptomatic as long as collateral circulation maintains sufficient blood flow around a lesion to satisfy the metabolic demands of the distal limb at rest and during exercise. Development of ischemic symptoms in the leg implies either inadequate collateral circulation or additional occlusive disease distal to the particular collateral bed. Thus, lesions in the aortoiliac segment may cause little difficulty unless, as is commonly the case, there is associated disease in the femoropopliteal arterial territory.

Distribution of Disease. Arteriosclerotic plaques producing stenosis or occlusion of the arterial lumen are often segmentally distributed, with a predilection for arterial bifurcations. The infrarenal abdominal aorta and aortic bifurcation are common sites of disease, as are the iliac and femoral artery bifurcations. Diabetic patients seem prone to onset of arteriosclerosis at an earlier age and often have a more distal distribution of occlusive arterial lesions involving the more distal infrapopliteal, tibial, and small runoff vessels.

Early Manifestations. The first sign of impaired arterial circulation is usually *intermittent claudication* (from the Latin *claudicare*, to limp), a manifestation of reduced arterial blood flow that remains adequate at rest but inadequate during exercise. During exercise, the metabolic demands of skeletal muscle in the legs require a 5- to 10-fold increase in blood flow and oxygen delivery. In patients with occlusive disease of major conduit vessels, the requisite increase in blood flow cannot be achieved and a supply-and-demand mismatch occurs, resulting in muscle ischemia and pain. With cessation of activity, metabolic demand quickly returns to baseline and symptoms abate.

Patients report pain or discomfort in the lower extremity brought on by walking and relieved by stopping. Discomfort is usually described as a cramping or aching that steadily increases in severity as distance or speed of walking increases and is frequently worse when walking up an incline. Most characteristically, it involves the calf muscles as a result of disease in the superficial femoral artery, the most common location of lower extremity obliterative disease. However, claudication may also be noted in more proximal muscle groups of the hip, thigh, and buttock area when there is aortoiliac involvement.

Later Manifestations. As the severity of the occlusive process worsens, blood flow becomes inadequate for tissue needs even at rest, resulting in the manifestations of more severe arterial insufficiency: *ischemic rest pain* and tissue *necrosis* (ischemic ulceration or gangrene). Rest pain typically occurs at night from leg elevation associated with lying in bed. Patients classically describe ischemic rest pain as an "ache," "pain," "numbness," or "squeezing," most often in the toes and arch of the foot. It may awaken them from sleep and ease when the leg is placed in a dependent position (e.g., dangling the leg over the bedside or standing and walking about). Simple gravitational effects improve arteriolar flow and lessen ischemia.

Ischemic ulcers are painful and appear as punched out lesions on the dorsum or lateral aspect of the foot. A hallmark of ischemic ulceration is intense pain associated with the lesion.

Clinical Variants. Peripheral arterial insufficiency has three basic anatomic variations, though any number may be present in a given patient. Aortoiliac disease is most common in patients who smoke or have hypercholesterolemia. Claudication in the buttock or thigh is characteristic. The femoral pulses are absent or diminished, but pedal pulses may be intact. *Femoropopliteal disease* accounts for two thirds of cases and presents as calf pain with exertion. Femoral pulses may be preserved, but popliteal and pedal pulses are absent or diminished. *Tibioperoneal occlusion* is a disease of diabetics and older patients. Skin ulcers and atrophic skin changes are common.

Clinical Course and Prognosis. The natural history and associated clinical course of peripheral arterial disease is quite variable and often favorable. In the Framingham study population, only one third of those developing claudication went on to have persistent symptoms; the remainder experienced remission or transient symptoms. However, 15% of those presenting with severe disease required amputation over the ensuing 2 years. Persistent smokers and diabetics have the worst prognoses.

Any consideration of prognosis for this atherosclerotic disease has to include the substantial risks of *cardiovascular morbidity* and *mortality*, which are increased fivefold compared with persons without peripheral arterial disease.

DIFFERENTIAL DIAGNOSIS

Lower extremity ischemia may also be caused by arterial embolism, dissection, trauma, thrombosis of an aneurysm, or thromboangiitis obliterans (Buerger's disease). Other nonvascular conditions may mimic the symptoms of claudication or ischemic rest pain. Pain in the hip, thigh, or knee region with walking is frequently a result of *degenerative disc disease, osteoarthritis* of the hip or knee, or *Paget's disease.* Sciatic or other radicular pain may cause confusion. Various other neurologic or musculoskeletal disorders may be at fault. *Cauda equina compression* by disc, tumor, or spinal canal stenosis produces a well-known *"pseudoclaudication"* syndrome. Such nonvascular causes of pain may be suspected when pain is not clearly related to a predictable amount of exercise and is not promptly relieved by cessation of activity. *Nocturnal leg cramps* are commonly mistaken for ischemic pain, being localized to the calf but differing in that they are exclusively a night-time phenomenon.

Diabetic neuropathy can be difficult to differentiate from ischemic rest pain, particularly in a patient with diminished or absent pulses. In both conditions, a burning constant ache is often present in the forefoot and toes. The presence of paresthesias in addition to pain suggests a neurologic source. True ischemic rest pain is usually worse with elevation and frequently is relieved somewhat by dependency of the limb. Such features may be used in differentiation. In all such instances, noninvasive studies during exercise may be of substantial help in the differential diagnosis.

WORKUP

The diagnosis of peripheral vascular disease and an accurate assessment of its level and severity may be made by a careful history and physical examination to an extent not usually possible in many other disease states. The availability of effective treatment for peripheral vascular disease makes it mandatory that early and accurate diagnosis be established before end-stage problems develop and threaten limb loss.

History. *Intermittent claudication* is the hallmark of vascular insufficiency and, by multivariate analysis, an independent predictor of the disease. A reliable story for its presence can be pathognomonic in a person with atherosclerotic risk factors (Table 23.1). The patient who describes a cramp or ache in the calf or thigh muscles that is reproducibly brought on by *walking a predictable distance* should be suspected, especially if the discomfort is relieved within minutes by simply stopping. The location of the pain may help to localize the occlusive process. In some instances of proximal disease, the pain may be located principally in the hip or buttock region, causing confusion with other neuroorthopedic conditions such as spinal stenosis and

lumbar radiculopathy. If the walking distance required to produce the pain varies considerably from day to day or if the patient must sit or lie down for more than several minutes to obtain relief, the physician should suspect a nonvascular cause, such as spinal stenosis. Weightbearing and other activities that extend the lumbar spine will aggravate the pain of spinal stenosis. Similarly, the pain should involve the same areas consistently and not different portions of the leg from day to day. Crampy pain occurring in the calf at rest, particularly at night, rarely signifies a vascular problem. The triad of discomfort brought on by exercise, relief achieved within 2 to 5 minutes by stopping, and ability to walk the same distance again once the discomfort ceases is strongly suggestive of vascular insufficiency.

Complaints of *pain at rest* and with exercise suggest more advanced ischemia. A history of prior claudication is almost always obtained in such patients unless the distribution of the occlusive process is quite distal or in small vessels only. Ischemic rest pain typically involves the toes or forefoot, not the calf or thigh. It is usually improved with dependency of the limb and therefore is worse at night. Pain that is not confined to the distal foot, that is better with elevation, or that occurs in a patient without intermittent claudication should alert the physician to look for other possible causes, such as diabetic neuropathy or a neuroorthopedic problem.

Symptoms of tissue necrosis will usually be quite apparent. Peripheral *gangrene* without prior symptoms should raise the possibility of embolic disease or small vessel occlusions due to conditions other than chronic arteriosclerosis. In patients with leg ulceration, historical clues suggesting a traumatic, dermatologic, or venous origin should also be sought; many leg and foot ulcers are not ischemic in origin.

A complete history should include questioning for sexual difficulties. Erectile *impotence*, long associated with severe aortoiliac occlusive disease, has been termed the *Leriche syndrome* after the French surgeon who first reported its significance in 1923. Finally, it is of utmost importance to note the existence of known risk factors for arteriosclerosis (e.g., family history, smoking, diabetes mellitus, hypertension, lipid disorders) and related problems in the coronary and cerebrovascular systems indicative of the systemic nature of the atherosclerosis.

Physical Examination. Exam can help confirm, localize, and establish the severity of the arterial lesion. Findings that independently predict disease include abnormal pedal pulses and femoral artery bruits.

Palpation of peripheral pulses is the keystone of the examination. Palpation of the abdomen for the aortic pulsation and of both extremities for femoral, popliteal, posterior tibial, and dorsalis pedis pulses should be routine in all patients. Reduced or absent pulses in the symptomatic region are characteristic of arterial insufficiency. In one study, the absence of the posterior tibial pulse was the best predictor of peripheral arterial disease. Local factors such as edema or marked obesity may hinder palpation. Abnormally prominent pulsations suggest aneurysmal disease. *Auscultation* of the aortic and groin regions should also be performed, with the finding of *bruits* further supporting the possible existence of arterial occlusive disease. Simple exercise of the patient at the bedside may greatly intensify femoral bruits, and this is occasionally a useful maneuver. The absence of a bruit, however, has little meaning, because marked reduc-

Table 23.1. Differentiating True Claudication from Pseudoclaudication

CLINICAL FEATURE	CLAUDICATION	PSEUDOCLAUDICATION
Character of discomfort	Cramping, tightness, tiredness, aching	Same, tingling, weak, clumsy
Location	Buttock, hip, thigh, calf, foot	Same
Exercise-induced	Yes	Yes
Distance to pain	Same each time	Variable
Occurs with standing	No	Yes
Relief	With cessation of walking	With sitting or position change

Adapted from Krajewski LP, Olin JW. In: Young JR, Olin JW, Bartholomew JR, eds. Peripheral vascular disease, 2nd ed. St. Louis: Yearbook, 1996:208, with permission.

tion of flow in a severely stenotic or occluded vessel will not produce a bruit.

Other useful findings are abnormal pallor on elevation of the legs, *rubor on dependency*, and *prolonged capillary filling time* (especially when one leg is compared with the other). Temperature differences and atrophic skin and nail changes are less reliable indicators of chronic arterial insufficiency. Careful spine, hip, knee, and neurologic examinations are important to rule out nonvascular causes of exertional lower extremity pain.

Laboratory Studies. History and physical examination are usually sufficient to establish the diagnosis and provide a rough estimate of severity. In patients with mild-to-moderate disease free of limb-threatening ischemia or unacceptable activity limitations, no further investigation is necessary other than evaluation for potential *risk factors* such as hypertension, hyperlipidemia, smoking, and diabetes (see Chapters 14, 15, 54, and 93, respectively). Blood sugar determination may detect a previously undiagnosed diabetic, but there is still no firm evidence that tight control of the serum glucose level prevents or ameliorates macrovascular disease (see Chapter 102).

In patients with premature atherosclerotic disease but no evident precipitants, the possibility of *hyperhomocysteinemia* deserves consideration. The relation between this inborn error of metabolism and vascular disease has now been established. Diagnosis is suggested by elevated serum homocysteine levels after overnight methionine loading.

Noninvasive vascular laboratory studies are indicated if the diagnosis or degree of impairment is uncertain or if the disease appears clinically severe enough to warrant consideration of surgical correction. A host of noninvasive testing methods is available, ranging from segmental blood pressure measurements to Doppler and two-dimensional ultrasound techniques. These methods are becoming widely available and are relatively simple to use, inexpensive compared with angiography, and without risk or discomfort to the patient. Such tests may be extremely helpful in establishing a vascular etiology for complaints of pain in the leg and in quantifying clinical impressions, which are often somewhat imprecise. Because they can be used repeatedly, such tests are also particularly helpful in evaluating improvement or deterioration of the patient's condition over time and in assessing the benefit of various forms of treatment or operation.

It should be emphasized that these methods are not meant to replace or lessen the value of a good history and physical examination but rather to supplement them and provide such additional information as site and severity of stenosis.

Segmental blood pressure measurements are taken at the arm, upper thigh, above and below the knee, and above the ankle with the patient supine. A *Doppler* device measures systolic pressure in each location. Normally there is an increase in pressure as the pressure wave moves distally. A reduction in pressure suggests arterial occlusion. Sensitivity and specificity are maximized by determining the *ankle/brachial ratio or index* (a ratio of the systolic pressure found in the posterior tibial–dorsalis pedis arteries divided by the pressure in the brachial artery). An index of less than 0.9 has a 95% sensitivity in patients with angiographically proven disease and a 100% specificity in normals. Segmental pressures can be used as a screening test for further evaluation and in gauging severity. A ratio of less than 0.8 correlates with moderate disease, 0.6 with severe

or multilevel disease, and less than 0.4 with severe disease and a high risk of complications. The test is not reliable in patients with calcified vessels (e.g., diabetics).

Pulse-volume recordings are particularly useful for assessment of distal vascular disease, especially in patients with stiff vessels. Doppler and plethysmographic methods are used. The patient with stiff vessels and distal disease may have a normal ankle pressure, but the normally sharp pulse-volume wave form becomes blunted with obstruction. Sensitivity is improved when treadmill exercise is added to the examination. Diabetics, who tend to have stiff vessels and distal disease, are good candidates for pulse-volume recording.

Duplex ultrasonic scanning combines two-dimensional (B-mode) real-time ultrasound with pulsed Doppler to provide more precise anatomic and flow data than are available from other methods. The ultrasound probe is placed over specific vessels to measure velocity of flow. B-mode ultrasound identifies the site and nature of the stenosis. Adding *color-flow enhancement* (triplex scanning) improves test performance. Triplex scanning has a sensitivity of 88% and a specificity of 95%; the figures for duplex scanning are 82% and 92%, respectively. Although such examinations are somewhat time consuming and require an experienced examiner, they are likely to play an increasing role in noninvasively assessing peripheral vascular disease.

Preoperative Studies. When surgery is being contemplated, one needs to determine the precise anatomy of the occlusive disease. Although *contrast arteriography* has little place in the initial diagnostic evaluation of arterial insufficiency, its contribution is essential in the assessment of the patient who is being considered for surgical intervention (see Chapter 34). The procedure is generally regarded as indispensable for precise localization of the disease process and proper selection of the most appropriate invasive procedure. A major disadvantage and risk associated with arteriography is acute *dye-induced renal failure*. Patients with peripheral vascular disease commonly have concurrent renal vascular disease or renal dysfunction, making them especially vulnerable to acute renal failure upon exposure to a large iodinated contrast load. Arteriography should also be used with caution in persons with other forms of underlying renal disease and in persons with a history of allergy to iodine or iodinated radiologic contrast agents.

Magnetic resonance angiography (MRA) provides a noninvasive alternative to contrast arteriography for imaging the peripheral arterial circulation without risk of dye-induced acute renal failure or allergic reaction. It is particularly helpful in patients with a history of severe allergic reactions to iodinated contrast, renal insufficiency, or other contraindications to conventional catheter arteriography. Further advances in MRA using noniodinated contrast hold promise for providing an even more effective diagnostic alternative to conventional contrast arteriography in patients being considered for surgery.

INDICATIONS FOR REFERRAL AND ADMISSION

Although most patients with mild to moderate lower extremity occlusive disease can be well managed conservatively (see Chapter 34), those with pain that markedly limits daily activities and significantly impairs life-style may benefit from referral for consultation with an experienced vascular surgeon to

Table 23.2. Criteria for Surgical Referral

- Severe (disabling) intermittent claudication; ankle systolic pressure < 50 mm Hg after exercise; cannot complete standard 5-min treadmill exercise study
- Persistent ischemic rest pain; resting ankle systolic pressure < 50 mm Hg
- Ischemic ulceration or gangrene of foot/toes

review available treatment options, including revascularization. Those with evidence of more advanced disease (ischemic rest pain, nonhealing ischemic ulcerations) need prompt referral for revascularization due to the high likelihood of amputation and limb loss without revascularization. The noninvasive vascular laboratory may be very helpful in providing objective data to help define patients with critical ischemia and the need for prompt revascularization (Table 23.2). Patients with gangrenous lesions of the lower extremities or an infected ischemic ulcer require prompt hospital admission, particularly if they are diabetic.

ANNOTATED BIBLIOGRAPHY

Cambria RP, Brewster DC, Kaufman JA, et al. Magnetic resonance angiography in the management of lower extremity arterial occlusive disease: a prospective study. J Vasc Surg 1997;25:380. (*Evaluation of the utility and accuracy of MRA.*)

Clarke R, Daly L, Robinson K et al. Hyperhomocysteinemia: an independent risk factor for vascular disease. N Engl J Med 1991; 324:1149. (*Documents this condition to be an independent and important risk factor for premature vascular disease.*)

Criqui MH, Fronek A, Klauber MR, et al. The sensitivity, specificity, and predictive value of traditional clinical evaluation of peripheral arterial disease: results from noninvasive testing in a defined population. Circulation 1985;71:240. (*Lack of a posterior tibial pulse was the single best predictor of peripheral vascular disease.*)

Kohler TR, Nance DR, Cramer MM, et al. Duplex scanning for diagnosis of aortoiliac and femoropopliteal disease: a prospective study. Circulation 1987;76:1074. (*Well-designed study showing a favorable comparison between duplex scanning and conventional arteriography in the diagnosis of peripheral vascular disease.*)

McGee SR, Boyko EJ. Physical examination and chronic lower-extremity ischemia. Arch Intern Med 1998;158:1364. (*A critical literature review identifying those features of the examination most useful in determining presence and distribution of ischemia.*)

Polack JF, Karmel MI, Mannick JA, et al. Determination of the extent of lower extremity peripheral arterial disease with color-assisted duplex sonography: comparison with angiography. AJR Am J Roentgenol 1990;1550:1085. (*Description of the methodology; sensitivity 88%, specificity 95%.*)

Weitz JI, Byrne Clagett GP, et al. Diagnosis and treatment of chronic arterial insufficiency of the lower extremities: a critical review. Circulation 1996;94:3026. (*A useful and informative review relative to the incidence, natural history, and outcomes of treatment.*)

24
Evaluation of Syncope

Syncope and near-syncope are among the most difficult of conditions to evaluate, especially when recurrent and not accompanied by readily identifiable precipitants. Often contributing to the diagnostic difficulty are vague descriptions of the event, an unrevealing physical examination, and initial laboratory studies that are unremarkable. When confronted with a report of loss of consciousness, the primary physician first needs to check for an underlying cardiovascular or seizure disorder, for these may require prompt attention. In about 50% of cases, the cause of syncope will not be evident on initial evaluation, necessitating consideration of a more extensive workup. A detailed knowledge of important clinical clues and a thorough understanding of the indications for and limitations of available testing modalities are essential for a cost-effective evaluation of this difficult problem.

PATHOPHYSIOLOGY AND CLINICAL PRESENTATIONS

Basic Mechanisms. Syncope may ensue from inadequate cerebral perfusion, seizure activity, severe metabolic derangement, or psychological disturbance. The pathophysiologic common denominator of many cases is inadequate cerebral perfusion. Contributing mechanisms include sudden decrease in peripheral vascular resistance, inadequate cardiac output, failure of vasoconstrictive reflexes, and functional or anatomic cerebral vascular occlusion. Any number may be operative in a given case. Metabolic disturbances, such as hypoglycemia, hypocarbia, and hypoxia, usually do not result in syncope unless profound, although they may alter consciousness. Generalized seizure activity that spreads to the brainstem will rapidly lead to loss of consciousness. Most psychogenic precipitants of syncope operate by the neurocardiovascular mechanisms noted above, with the exception of hysteria, in which there may not be a true loss of consciousness.

Neurocardiogenic syncope, also referred to as *"vasodepressor"* or *"vasovagal"* syncope, accounts for a large number of cases, especially those occurring in otherwise healthy young persons. Although the precise mechanistic details are still being elucidated, its hallmarks are inappropriate bradycardia and vasodilation. The normal compensatory responses to standing up are vasoconstriction, tachycardia, withdrawal of vagal tone, and release of vasoconstricting and volume-retaining hormones (renin and vasopressin). In persons with neurocardiogenic syncope, there is interruption of these sympathetic reflex responses and an increase in vagal activity. The result is *bradycardia, vasodilation*, and marked falls in systemic blood pressure and cerebral perfusion. Among the explanations advanced to account for the phenomenon are excessive vagal tone, excessive initial sympathetic stimulation producing very vigorous contractions that overstimulate intracardiac parasympathetic mechanoreceptors, and hypersensitivity of these receptors. Beta-blockers and disopyramide have been found helpful. The myocardium and conduction system are normal—an important reason why prognosis is excellent.

Clinical presentations range from the common "simple faint" associated with emotional distress to the near-syncopal episode of a trained athlete in the midst of competition. Distention of a viscus (as occurs in performing an esophagoscopy, pleural tap, or bladder puncture) may also trigger an episode.

The patient experiences *premonitory symptoms* of sweating, epigastric queasiness, lightheadedness, and pallor. Dilation of the pupils, blurring of vision, yawning and sighing, or hyperventilation may occur. The patient feels restless and unable to concentrate. At the outset, the heart rate may be rapid, but it slows markedly as the process unfolds. The onset of premonitory symptoms usually helps prevent a drop attack and resultant injury. After several minutes, full consciousness is regained, though weakness, sweatiness, and nausea may persist. Control of bladder and bowels is never lost.

The presence of *pallor* and *diaphoresis* is paradoxical, but both may be prominent and reflect the high circulating levels of epinephrine found in this state of otherwise marked sympathetic inhibition. Such features make for a very distressing clinical presentation, mimicking serious cardiovascular disease.

Sometimes the hypotension and hypoperfusion that occur are so profound that cerebral hypoxia and seizure activity (*convulsive syncope*) ensue. This convulsive syncope is distinct from loss of consciousness that accompanies a generalized seizure disorder and does not respond to antiseizure medication.

Tilt-table study can reproduce the symptoms in susceptible persons. Many patients report a prodrome of blurred vision, vertigo, tinnitus, and nausea when tested on a tilt table (see below).

Autonomic insufficiency is another cause of reduced cerebral perfusion pressure, and it is particularly important in the setting of a fall in intravascular volume from dehydration or acute blood loss. On standing, the patient experiences *orthostatic hypotension*, because reflex vasoconstriction and increase in heart rate fail to occur. Hypotension progresses over seconds to a few minutes, until perfusion is inadequate for maintenance of consciousness. During the presyncopal period, there is no increase in heart rate or other signs of autonomic response, such as pallor, nausea, or sweating. The period of syncope is brief, and consciousness returns promptly. Near-syncope is common among these patients, as are impotence and bladder and bowel disturbances.

Postprandial hypotension is a form of postural hypotension analogous to autonomic insufficiency. It is defined as a 20-mm Hg decrease in systolic pressure within 2 hours of beginning a meal. Prevalence is greatest among elderly hypertensive patients. Postulated mechanisms range from inadequacies in sympathetic response and baroreceptor function to excessive insulin-induced and vasopeptide-induced vasodilatation and splanchnic pooling. Consequences may be serious and include falls, syncope, angina, and stroke.

Carotid sinus hypersensitivity can cause marked *reflex bradycardia* and a fall in arterial resistance. Most patients with this condition are elderly and have underlying atherosclerotic heart disease manifested by ischemic changes on electrocardiogram (ECG). Massage of the carotid sinus often results in long asystolic pauses. Digitalis administration seems to aggravate the condition. Carotid sinus syncope may also cause a vasodepressor form of syncope in which heart rate remains unchanged. Minor events can trigger symptoms; wearing a tight collar, turning the head, or shaving may cause lightheadedness, sweating, pallor, and nausea, followed by fainting. When the predominant mechanism is asystole, the loss of consciousness can be precipitous.

Posttussive syncope is characterized by loss of consciousness that follows a prolonged bout of forceful coughing. Men with chronic bronchitis are most often affected. The mechanism is believed to involve decreased cardiac output due to decreased venous return, increased cerebral vascular resistance secondary to hypocapnia, and compression of cerebral vessels by an increase in cerebrospinal fluid pressure. Prolonged Valsalva maneuvers have a similar effect; the increase in intrathoracic pressure impedes venous return and decreases cardiac output.

Postmicturition syncope takes place in the context of emptying a distended bladder. The typical setting involves a male who has gotten up at night to urinate after consuming considerable amounts of alcohol. Consciousness is lost without much warning. Drainage of ascitic fluid or a distended bladder may produce a similar effect. The mechanism is unknown. Valsalva maneuver and reflex vasodilation have been implicated. Valsalva plays an important role in *postdefecation syncope*, in which straining decreases venous return and consequently cardiac output.

Cerebrovascular disease leads to syncope if there is vertebrobasilar insufficiency of the midbrain affecting the reticular activating system or in the rare instance of total or near-total occlusion of the major vessels supplying the brain. Lesser degrees of obstruction may contribute to minor lightheadedness on standing and can be aggravated by use of antihypertensive agents and volume depletion. Patients with substantial cerebrovascular disease often have evidence of previous strokes manifested by focal neurologic deficits. A *transient ischemic attack* involving the vertebrobasilar circulation may lead to syncope by temporarily depriving the brainstem's reticular activating system of adequate perfusion. Brainstem neurologic deficits typically accompany or precede the loss of consciousness.

Subclavian steal syndrome results from occlusion of the proximal subclavian artery, leading to reversal of flow in the adjacent vertebral artery. When vascular resistance in the arm falls, for example, during exercise, flow is redirected away from the brain and ischemic symptoms may ensue.

Effort syncope occurs in the setting of underlying *valvular heart disease*. Exercise induces peripheral vasodilation, but cardiac output cannot be increased adequately and syncope results. *Severe aortic stenosis* and marked *hypertrophic cardiomyopathy* obstruct the ventricular outflow tract to a degree sufficient to limit cardiac response to exercise (see Chapter 33). Total blockade of the mitral orifice from an *atrial myxoma* and *pulmonary hypertension* can have similar consequences. Loss of consciousness comes with little warning.

Cardiac dysrhythmias may precipitate sudden loss of consciousness with none of the premonitory manifestations of neurocardiogenic syncope. Important dysrhythmias associated with syncope include *complete heart block* (Stokes-Adams attacks) and *ventricular tachycardia* (see Chapter 29). Occasionally, a supraventricular tachycardia with a very rapid ventricular response rate will sufficiently compromise cardiac output to result in near-syncope (see Chapter 28). Once effective systoles have ceased, fewer than 5 seconds of consciousness remain. Palpitations are sometimes reported, and loss of consciousness can occur while the patient is supine. Common precipitants of these dysrhythmias include acute ischemia, sick sinus syndrome, digitalis toxicity, and the preexcitation syndromes. Patients with chronic bifascicular and trifascicular block are more likely to have syncopal attacks, but those with syncope have not been found to have an increased risk of sudden death.

Seizures differ from other causes of syncope in that aura, postictal symptoms, incontinence, and tonic-clonic movements often dominate the clinical picture. However, akinetic petit mal attacks have few of these features, although normal blood pressure and pulse help distinguish them from seizures having cardiovascular causes (see Chapter 170). As noted above, convulsions may occur in the setting of vagally mediated cerebral hypoperfusion in the absence of an underlying seizure disorder.

Psychiatric Disease. Psychiatric causes are becoming increasingly appreciated as etiologic factors in syncope of unknown origin. *Generalized anxiety disorder, panic disorder,* and *depression* are frequently found in populations of such patients who have no evidence of heart disease. Their fainting spells often resolve with treatment of the underlying psychopathology. Prevalence is greatest in younger persons with frequent syncopal episodes, in those who never sustain injury from their loss of consciousness, and in patients who present with multiple somatic and psychiatric symptoms, such as fear, anxiousness, nausea, lightheadedness, and numbness. Reproduction of symptoms by 2 to 3 minutes of open-mouth hyperventilation is characteristic. *Hysteria* may result in apparent loss of consciousness; the spell is a *conversion reaction* characterized by graceful fainting to the floor or couch; frequent presence of an audience; normal pulse, skin color, and blood pressure; and an emotionally detached description of the episode.

Metabolic factors (e.g., hypoxia, hypocarbia, hypoglycemia) are more likely to alter consciousness than to cause actual syncope. Restlessness, confusion, and anxiety are prominent and precede loss of consciousness. When hyperventilation is responsible, the patient first complains of a smothering or suffocating feeling in conjunction with paresthesias in the limbs and circumorally (see Chapter 226). Syncope may take place while the patient is sitting or lying down. Hypoglycemia rarely causes loss of consciousness (see Chapter 97).

DIFFERENTIAL DIAGNOSIS

Important causes of syncope are listed in Table 24.1. In a series of 176 ambulatory patients evaluated for syncope, 9% had a cardiac etiology, 45% had some form of vasomotor instability, 1% had seizures, 6% had other causes, and 39% were unexplained. With the addition of tilt-table testing and psychiatric assessment, at least half of the unexplained cases demonstrate evidence of a neurocardiogenic (vasovagal) mechanism and many of the remainder have a psychiatric etiology (generalized anxiety, panic disorder, depression). In the elderly, the prevalence of cardiac disease among patients presenting with syncope increases to about 33%.

Table 24.1.   Important Causes of Syncope

1. **Cardiac**
   a. Arrhythmias (sick sinus syndrome, ventricular tachycardia, very rapid supraventricular tachycardia)
   b. Heart block (Stokes-Adams attacks)
   c. Aortic stenosis, severe
   d. Asymmetric septal hypertrophy, severe
   e. Primary pulmonary hypertension
   f. Atrial myxoma
   g. Prolapsed mitral valve
2. **Vascular-Reflex**
   a. Neurocardiogenic (vasovagal, vasodepressor)
   b. Orthostatic hypotension (ganglionic blocking agents, diabetes, old age, prolonged bedrest)
   c. Carotid sinus hypersensitivity
   d. Cerebral vascular disease, severe
   e. Subclavian steal syndrome
   f. Posttussive syncope
   g. Valsalva syncope
   h. Postmicturition syncope (emptying distended bladder)
   i. Postprandial syncope
3. **Psychologic-Neurologic**
   a. Seizures
   b. Hysteria
   c. Generalized anxiety disorder
   d. Depression
   e. Panic disorder
4. **Metabolic**
   a. Hyperventilation
   b. Hypoxia
   c. Hypoglycemia (rarely)

The prognosis for syncope due to underlying cardiac disease is much worse (1-year mortality rates of 18% to 33%) than that for noncardiac or unexplained syncope (1-year mortality rates of 6% to 12%). In the elderly with unexplained syncope, the mortality rate nearly doubles. However, recurrence rates are similar for both categories (about 33%), and recurrence is not a risk factor for adverse outcome.

WORKUP

Evaluation Strategy

Initial Workup. The principal task initially is to differentiate between cardiac and noncardiac etiologies, because prognosis is poorest for those with underlying heart disease. A *detailed history, focused physical examination*, and the resting 12-lead *ECG* are the most valuable elements of the initial evaluation. These elements alone provide a diagnosis in at about 50% of cases and suggest the diagnosis in many others. The physician and patient should appreciate that routinely ordering a battery of "syncope tests" is not only wasteful and ineffective but also more likely to produce false-positive results than true-positive ones when ordered in the context of a low pretest probability for the condition in question.

Subsequent Testing. For the 50% of patients who remain undiagnosed after the initial history, physical, and ECG, the evaluation proceeds according to the clinical presentation and probability of underlying heart disease. In persons with known or strongly suspected heart disease, the key task is detection of a serious dysrhythmia or conduction disturbance, for which *Holter monitoring and electrophysiologic study* (EPS) are the tests of choice. *Continuous-loop electrocardiographic recording* is useful in those who have no evidence of structural heart disease but report palpitations and have frequent syncopal episodes. Persons free of organic heart disease who have infrequent syncopal episodes and suspected neurocardiogenic (vasovagal) syncope are the best candidates for *tilt-table testing. Psychiatric evaluation* is indicated for patients with frequent events, no heart disease, and no injury from their spells.

This approach results in a diagnosis in most patients. Fortunately, the prognosis for patients with a single unexplained episode of syncope is excellent. Nonetheless, a detailed search for underlying heart disease is essential and a major priority in the evaluation.

History

The differentiation of cardiac and neurologic disease from less worrisome etiologies begins with a *thorough description* of the syncopal event and its surrounding circumstances. The absence of premonitory symptoms in the presyncopal period is consistent with a sudden fall in cardiac output or the abrupt onset of generalized seizure activity. Nausea, diaphoresis, pallor, and lightheadedness are more typical of reflex and vascular causes. If recall of premonitory details is sketchy, one should be careful about interrogating the patient too vigorously with leading questions, for the absence of associated or prodromal symptoms may have important diagnostic meaning. Although a seizure disorder may present with sudden loss of consciousness and no warning, more typically there are some vague premonitory symptoms and the characteristic tonic-clonic movements and sphincter incontinence.

Identification of precipitants requires asking about emotional upsets, crowded hot surroundings, sudden standing (especially in elderly hypertensive patients after a meal), prolonged and forceful coughing, Valsalva maneuvers, micturition, vigorous exercise, hyperventilation, and symptoms of acute blood loss. Effort syncope raises the question of hemodynamically significant ventricular outflow tract obstruction. Exertional chest pain is another important clue of underlying organic heart disease. Position just before syncope is worth noting, because loss of consciousness while recumbent argues against a reflex or vascular mechanism. A check of medications is always in order and especially productive in the assessment of the elderly person presenting with syncope.

The *past medical history* should be searched for prior infarction, heart murmur, and use of cardioactive medications. A history of diabetes, stroke, use of antihypertensive agents, prolonged bedrest, impotence, and bladder and bowel incontinence should be checked for when the patient reports lightheadedness or syncope on standing.

Reports from witnesses should be sought whenever possible. Activity, position, complaints, and appearance before syncope and duration of the episode, associated motor activity, and behavior on regaining consciousness deserve attention. Some observers will even report pulse and respirations. A seizure disorder is usually not difficult to distinguish from cardiac syncope because of the preceding aura, motor activity, incontinence, and postictal symptoms of confusion, drowsiness, and paresis. However, when there are no motor manifestations, as in akinetic petit mal seizures, the differentiation may be impossible to make by history alone.

It is important not to mistake other conditions for true loss of consciousness. Vertigo (see Chapter 166), neuroglycopenic symptoms (see Chapter 97), and the lightheadedness associated with an anxiety and other psychiatric conditions (see Chapters 226 and 227) are sometimes confused with syncope or nearsyncope. On the other hand, reports of the combination of psychiatric and somatic symptoms (e.g., lightheadedness, anxiousness, numbness, nausea) in a patient with otherwise unexplained loss of consciousness should suggest an underlying psychiatric etiology.

Physical Examination

The emphasis is again on the cardiovascular system. *Postural signs* provide essential information. *Blood pressure* and *pulse* are first measured in both arms with the patient lying supine for about 5 minutes and again on standing up. Most patients who demonstrate a postural fall in blood pressure will do so within 30 to 60 seconds of assuming the standing position. However, it may be necessary to wait as long as 5 minutes. Recent studies have found that 95% of cases with postural hypotension will be detected within 2 minutes of standing and most within 30 to 60 seconds. The skin is checked for pallor and ecchymoses (the latter, a sign of trauma from a seizure). Torso and head, including the tongue, require scrutiny for signs of trauma sustained during a motor seizure.

Carotid pulses are auscultated for bruits and gently palpated for volume and carotid upstroke (see Chapter 33). If there is no evidence of carotid artery disease, one can *massage* the carotid and observe for reflex bradycardia (asystole of more than 3 seconds) and hypotension. The maneuver is indicated when a hypersensitive carotid sinus reflex is suspected, as in elderly patients with unexplained falls. However, because it may also cut off blood supply and cause syncope when there is severe cerebral occlusive disease, it should not be attempted in such patients.

The neck veins are noted for distention and the chest for rales and rhonchi. The *heart* is palpated for heaves and thrills and is auscultated for clicks and murmurs with the patient in the supine, decubitus, and sitting positions. Systolic murmurs should be evaluated for evidence of aortic stenosis, asymmetric septal hypertrophy, and mitral valve prolapse (see Chapter 21). A variable diastolic murmur raises the question of atrial myxoma. Neurologic assessment includes a search for focal deficits indicative of prior stroke.

Provocative maneuvers are particularly helpful in identifying conditions that alter consciousness but do not cause syncope. Asking the patient to voluntarily hyperventilate or spin around may reproduce symptoms and confirm a clinical suspicion. Exercising the arm is worthwhile if subclavian steal syndrome is suspected.

Laboratory Studies

As noted earlier, routinely ordering a battery of "syncope tests" is wasteful and ineffective. Although one does not want to miss an underlying cardiac etiology, test selection should still reflect consideration of the pretest probability of heart disease. Test yield in patients with a very low pretest probability of heart disease is extremely low, and risk of false-positives is high (see Chapter 2).

Electrocardiogram. Most patients should have an ECG performed at the time of initial evaluation, because detection of underlying heart disease remains a major priority of the diagnostic workup. One needs to check not only for ischemic changes, heart block, and tachyarrhythmias but also for subtle clues such as a short PR interval, delta waves, or new onset of bundle branch block. However, neither an ECG nor other laboratory studies is necessary when the history strongly suggests a harmless faint brought on by emotional factors, the physical examination is normal, and the patient has no risk factors for organic heart disease.

Holter Monitoring. If the ECG is unrevealing but an arrhythmia transient heart block or other form of underlying heart disease is still suspected on clinical grounds (e.g., sudden loss of consciousness without warning, effort syncope, chest pain), then a *24-hour ambulatory ECG recording (Holter monitor)* deserves consideration. Holter monitoring has become an almost routine part of the syncope workup, especially in patients who remain undiagnosed after initial history, physical examination, and resting ECG. Yet the correlation between findings on Holter monitoring and symptoms is poor, with arrhythmia-related symptoms occurring in only 2% of patients studied and syncope or presyncope occurring without an associated arrhythmia in 15%.

Although the correlation between symptoms and Holter findings is not strong, Holter findings do provide an independent assessment of risk for underlying heart disease and sudden death. Syncopal patients with frequent premature ventricular contractions (more than 10 an hour), repetitive premature ventricular contractions (32 in a row), or sinus pauses (more than 2 seconds) on Holter monitoring have an increased risk of sudden death and overall mortality that is independent of other factors. Patients with these findings constitute a high-risk subgroup that deserved further cardiac evaluation. There may be an increase in yield of arrhythmias detected if Holter monitoring is extended to 48 hours, but many arrhythmias are asymptomatic and of unclear significance.

Continuous-loop (event) recording for detection of symptomatic arrhythmias is made feasible with *patient-activated intermittent recorders*. By virtue to their *continuous loop* technology, these recorders can capture the previous several minutes of cardiac rhythm and detect a symptom-producing dysrhythmia shortly after it has occurred, provided the patient is capable of activating the unit. Continuous-loop recording is useful in persons with relatively frequent syncopal episodes who have little likelihood of serious underlying heart disease (and thus are at low risk for a life-threatening dysrhythmia). Yield is highest in those who report palpitations (range, 27% - 45%).

Exercise stress testing may bring out arrhythmias not found during Holter monitoring, but even more useful is the test's sensitivity for the diagnosis of ischemic heart disease (see Chapter 36). Patients who report chest pain before syncope, effort syncope, or have an abnormal resting ECG suggestive of ischemic disease are prime candidates for stress testing. However, those with effort syncope should not be subjected to stress testing until tight aortic stenosis and other forms of critical ventricular outflow tract obstruction have been excluded by echocardiography, because there is the risk of sudden death with stress testing in such patients. Routine use of stress testing to rule out "silent" heart disease in the absence of clinical or electrocardiographic evidence yields little and increases cost.

Echocardiography can provide key diagnostic information in patients suspected of valvular or structural heart disease because of effort syncope, chest pain, palpitations, systolic ejection murmur, systolic click, abnormal carotid upstroke with transmitted bruit, or an abnormal ECG. It is also the noninvasive test of choice if a left atrial myxoma is suspected. In the absence of evidence for heart disease, routine echocardiography contributes little to the assessment. Syncope patients who are going to have a stress test should be subjected to echocardiogram before stress testing if there is any suggestion clinically of obstruction to the left ventricular outflow tract (e.g., systolic ejection murmur).

EPS has been advocated to detect arrhythmogenic causes of syncope, particularly *ventricular tachycardia*, because of the limited specificity of Holter monitoring results described above. The value of EPS in the assessment of patients with structural heart disease and fixed conduction defects is well documented, but its sensitivity and specificity for identifying transient rhythm disturbances, especially *bradyarrhythmias*, in patients with unexplained syncope has been disappointing.

The detection of ventricular tachycardia and hemodynamically significant bradycardia are the principal reasons for performing EPS. Consequently, prime candidates are those with an increased risk of such an arrhythmia (e.g., persons with previous myocardial infarction, ischemic heart disease, or congestive heart failure). To improve EPS performance, criteria for better patient selection have been sought. In the largest study to date, patients with evidence of underlying organic heart disease and frequent premature ventricular contractions on resting ECG were at increased risk for sustained ventricular tachycardia during EPS. Those with first-degree arterioventricular block, bundle branch block, or sinus bradycardia on resting ECG were at increased risk of a hemodynamically significant bradyarrhythmia during EPS. Overall, 87% of those with at least one of these clinical risk factors had an important outcome on EPS, whereas the EPS was normal in 95% of those with none of these risk factors. Holter findings may also prove predictive, but data are limited.

Although invasive and very expensive (requiring cardiac catheterization), EPS may be preferred to outpatient Holter monitoring in elderly persons with syncope and conduction disease on ECG, because another episode might result in serious injury. Another reason for consideration of EPS is presence of preexcitation (short PR interval, less than 0.12 seconds) on ECG. Such patients are at increased risk of sustained rapid supraventricular tachycardia with hypotension. Patients with unexplained syncope but no evidence of structural heart disease and a normal ECG are not likely to benefit from EPS. The test should not be considered a routine part of a syncope-of-unknown origin workup.

Upright Tilt-Testing. The growing appreciation of neurocardiogenic mechanisms of syncope has stimulated interest in provocative maneuvers such as upright tilt testing. The best candidates are those in whom heart disease has been ruled out and a vasovagal mechanism is suspected on the basis of the clinical history (e.g., premonitory nausea and flushing). The test is predicated on the hypothesis that in susceptible persons the decrease in venous return from placement on a tilt table brought up to 60 degrees elevation will trigger the potent reflex responses that lead to neurocardiogenic syncope (see above). *Isoproterenol* infusion is added to enhance sensitivity and speed the test if tilting without isoproterenol produces no response after 15 minutes.

Criteria for a positive test vary and include hypotension and bradycardia, but reproduction of the patient's syncope and associated symptoms is the *sine qua non* of a diagnostic study.

Sensitivity ranges from about 65% to 80%, enhanced by isoproterenol infusion. *Specificity* is 90% without isoproterenol and decreases to 75% when it is infused, because of false-positive responses, particularly in young healthy persons. Most authorities recommend first performing the tilt test without isoproterenol infusion, reserving it for patients with a negative initial study who have premonitory symptoms suggestive of a vasovagal mechanism. In older patients, tilt testing with isoproterenol can be conducted safely, but prior stress testing is recommended to rule out underlying ischemia, which might be exacerbated by isoproterenol infusion.

Tilt-table testing is sometimes helpful in uncovering underlying psychopathology, such as a conversion reaction, in which the apparent loss of consciousness occurs during testing but without hypotension or bradycardia.

Other Studies. The *electroencephalogram* has repeatedly been shown to be of little use in evaluating syncope in the absence of either a history suggestive of seizure or neurologic deficits. Even when a seizure disorder is present, the routine electroencephalogram has a sensitivity of only 50%. Sleep studies and photic stimulation may improve sensitivity to 80% (see Chapter 170). Similarly, neuroimaging studies (computed tomography, magnetic resonance imaging) should generally be reserved for patients with focal seizures or defects on neurologic examination (in one study, 7 of 20 patients with and none of 17 patients without such findings had abnormalities detected on computed tomography).

Random *blood sugar* determinations are of little use in documenting hypoglycemia; a blood sugar at the time of symptoms is better (see Chapter 97). Arterial *blood gases* can detect hypocarbia when hyperventilation is suspected and hypoxia when ventilation/perfusion mismatching is of concern. However, such testing is usually unnecessary because the etiologies responsible for such blood gas abnormalities are usually self-evident.

Patients with Unexplained Syncope

When the above evaluation ends without an answer other than the absence of evidence for serious underlying cardiac or neurologic pathology, then a period of watchful waiting can be considered. Patients with a fully negative evaluation are at low risk for an occult life-threatening etiology and sudden death. Those with a rare event can be reassured and followed expectantly.

Patient with Frequent Recurrences. Frequent syncopal attacks of unknown etiology are difficult to manage with a watchful-waiting approach. Recurrent episodes beg an explanation. Patients with unexplained disease despite a full assessment benefit from close follow-up and careful reassessment for new clues by careful history and physical examination at the time of recurrences. *Hospitalization* for observation in persons with very frequent syncopal attacks may help guide further evaluation by providing the opportunity to directly observe an episode.

Assessment for a psychiatric etiology (e.g., generalized anxiety disorder, panic disorder, depression) should be considered in younger persons with frequent episodes, in those who never sustain injury from their loss of consciousness, and in those with multiple bodily complaints and symptoms of anxiousness (e.g., numbness, nausea, constant lightheadedness, fearfulness).

Screening instruments for anxiety and depression (see Chapters 226 and 227) are useful for initial assessment, as is the *hyperventilation maneuver*, in which the patient breathes rapidly and deeply with mouth open for 2 to 3 minutes. The development of syncope or near-syncope in response to hyperventilation has a positive predictive value of over 50% for a psychiatric etiology. *Tilt-table testing* for persons with suspected hysteria (in which syncope represents a conversions reaction) may reveal the characteristic apparent loss of consciousness in the absence of changes in vital signs.

Elderly Patient with Unexplained Syncope. In many instances the etiology is not one single factor but a combination (e.g., blunted autonomic responsiveness, medications, dehydration, underlying heart disease). A review of current medications is always in order as are the circumstances of each syncopal event (e.g., standing after a meal, urination, or a bowel movement). Because the prevalence of cardiovascular disease is high in this age group, reconsideration of the common etiologies (e.g., coronary disease, heart failure, conduction system disease, other dysrhythmias) and less common etiologies (e.g., calcific aortic stenosis, carotid sinus hypersensitivity) is in order (see above). If not already performed, carotid sinus massage should be carried out, provided there is no evidence of ongoing cardiovascular or cerebrovascular disease, such as recent myocardial infarction, carotid bruit, recent stroke, or ventricular arrhythmias. The rationale for performing carotid massage is that persons with a positive test (asystole greater than 3 seconds in response to massage) appear to benefit from implantation of a demand pacemaker.

SYMPTOMATIC THERAPY AND PATIENT EDUCATION

The most effective therapies are those that are etiologic, particularly treatments that address serious underlying cardiac pathology (e.g., see Chapters 28, 29, 30, 32, and 33). A number of symptomatic measures help patients with less-threatening conditions, which are still important to treat because of their impact on the quality of daily life.

Orthostatic Hypotension. The first priority is to review all medications and reduce or eliminate those that are likely to exacerbate the problem (e.g., diuretics, vasodilators, beta-blockers, hypnotics). A number of simple measures deserve emphasis. One teaches the patient to avoid abrupt postural changes by sitting on the edge of the bed in the morning before getting up and to elevate the head of the bed at night to counter the reflex hypertension that occurs when supine. Girdles, garters, and other constricting garments should not be worn if they decrease venous return, but elastic stockings may be helpful. One can advise the patient to avoid prolonged standing and to contract the calf muscles when standing to increase venous blood flow. Liberalization of salt intake is useful; *fludrocortisone* (0.1 to 1.0 mg daily) may be necessary. Patients with severe orthostatic hypotension due to multiple system failure or pure autonomic dysfunction may require additional treatment. Agents to be considered include *phenylpropanolamine* in low doses, *midodrine, indomethacin, and yohimbine*. Careful testing is required, because responses are very idiosyncratic.

Postprandial Hypotension. Simple measures include smaller more frequent meals, liberalized salt intake, adequate fluid intake, reduction in carbohydrate content of meals, patient education regarding the risk of falling up to 90 minutes after eating, avoidance of prolonged sitting, avoidance of standing still after a meal, encouraging a walk after eating, and avoidance of alcohol before or with meals. In addition, the above measures for management of orthostatic hypotension can be implemented. α-Agonists (e.g., phenylephrine every 6 to 12 hours) are sometimes used but of questionable safety in elderly persons. Caffeine is of little benefit. The somatostatin analogue octreotide (50 μg SC a half hour before meals) can be considered, but only for the most seriously affected persons because a painful injection is required to administer the substance.

Neurocardiogenic Syncope. Patients with confirmed neurocardiogenic disease may be candidates for a trial of a *betablocker* (e.g., metoprolol) or *disopyramide*. The role of *demand pacing* in such cases is unresolved; some nonrandomized studies suggest a benefit in up to one fourth of patients, but there are no randomized trials. Loosening the collar is sometimes helpful for the person with a *hypersensitive carotid sinus* reflex; demand pacing can be considered if simpler measures fail. A demand pacemaker is indicated only when heart block or severe bradycardia has been proven responsible for syncope. Empiric pacing in patients with undiagnosed recurrent episodes is to be discouraged.

Underlying Psychiatric Illness. The treatment of any underlying anxiety disorder, depression, or panic disorder results in a significant reduction in syncopal episodes and is strongly recommended (see Chapters 226 and 227).

Patient Education. The patient without evidence of underlying cardiac or neurologic disease can be reassured, even if syncopal episodes continue. Mortality does not increase with recurrent episodes, as long as there continues to be no evidence of underlying cardiac or neurologic disease. The value of a thoughtful workup in conjunction with thorough explanation should not be underestimated in helping patients with unexplained syncope to remain active. If serious heart and neurologic diseases have been ruled out, further evaluation can safely proceed on an outpatient basis even though the cause may remain undetermined. Family members and close friends should be instructed to take careful note of all events surrounding the syncopal period, including appearance, position, activity, complaints, and behavior. They might even be taught to palpate the radial or femoral pulse to provide data on heart rate and rhythm during an episode.

INDICATIONS FOR ADMISSION

It is safest to hospitalize patients with syncope who have any clinical evidence suggesting underlying heart disease, including those with a history of effort syncope, chest pain, known coronary or valvular disease, systolic ejection murmur, abnormal resting ECG, or severe postural drop in blood pressure. Similarly, persons with evidence indicating the possibility of cerebrovascular disease or a seizure disorder (e.g., carotid bruit, prior stroke, witnessed seizure activity, or suggestive symptoms) are best served by hospitalization. Although many elderly patients benefit from an inpatient evaluation because of the increased probability of underlying cardiovascular disease, not all do, especially when the circumstances are clearly situa-

tional (e.g., postprandial, postmicturition). Admission to the hospital for observation of the obscure case is a difficult decision, but, as noted above, is most useful if episodes are frequent enough to provide opportunity for observing one.

RECOMMENDATIONS*

- Begin the evaluation with a comprehensive history and focused physical examination that emphasizes detection of underlying heart disease; obtain a resting ECG.
- Base further test selection on the pretest likelihood of underlying heart disease.

For Intermediate to High Pretest Probability of Serious Underlying Heart Disease

- Conduct the initial evaluation in the hospital and include Holter monitoring or EPS (if high suspicion of ventricular tachycardia), supplemented by stress testing and/or echocardiography.

For Low Pretest Probability of Serious Underlying Heart Disease

- Conduct the assessment in the outpatient setting and include continuous-loop event monitoring (especially for persons with structurally normal hearts, a history of palpitations, and frequent episodes), psychiatric testing (especially for younger persons with frequent episodes in the absence of evidence for heart disease, for those with multiple somatic and psychiatric symptoms, and for those with no injury from syncopal episodes), tilt-table testing (especially for persons with infrequent episodes who have no evidence of underlying heart disease and a story suggestive of neurocardiogenic [vasovagal] syncope or conversion reaction).
- Also consider conducting the initial evaluation on an inpatient basis for persons suspected of having a seizure disorder or stroke and for the frail elderly person who sustains a serious injury from a first syncopal episode.

A.H.G.

ANNOTATED BIBLIOGRAPHY

Abboud FM. Neurocardiogenic syncope. N Engl J Med 1993; 328:1117. (*A very concise and excellent summary of pathophysiology, plus an editorial on the clinical implications.*)

Almquist A, Goldenberg IF, Milstein S, et al. Provocation of bradycardia and hypotension by isoproterenol and upright posture in patients with unexplained syncope. N Engl J Med 1989;320:346. (*Tilt-testing and isoproterenol reproduced symptoms in patients who otherwise had unexplained syncope after exhaustive evaluation.*)

Atkins D, Hanusa B, Sefcik T, et al. Syncope and orthostatic hypotension. Am J Med 1991;91:179. (*Orthostatic hypotension was found to be very common in patients with syncope, and present in most within 2 minutes of standing; those with greater degrees of orthostasis tended to have fewer syncopal recurrences.*)

*Adapted from the Clinical guidelines proposed by Linzer M, Yang EH, Estes M III, et al. Diagnosing syncope. Part 1. Value of history, physical examination, and electrocardiography. Ann Intern Med 1997;126:989, with permission.

Barron SA, Rogovski Z, Hemli Y. Vagal cardiovascular reflexes in young persons with syncope. Ann Intern Med 1993;118:943. *(High level of vagal tone found.)*

Benditt DG, Petersen M, Lurie KG, et al. Cardiac pacing for prevention of recurrent vasovagal syncope. Ann Intern Med 1995;122:204. *(A systematic review of the evidence, finding many gaps, but some indication of benefit in selected patients.)*

Brignole M, Menozzi C, Gianfranchi L, et al. Carotid sinus massage, eyeball compression, and head-up tilt test in patients with syncope of uncertain origin and in healthy control subjects. Am Heart J 1991;122:1644. *(Data supporting the utility of carotid sinus massage in elderly persons with syncope.)*

Calkins H, Byrne M, El-Atassi R, et al. The economic burden of unrecognized vasodepressor syncope. Am J Med 1993;95:473. *(Much unnecessary testing greatly increases the cost of evaluation.)*

Fujimura O, Yee R, Klein GJ. The diagnostic sensitivity of electrophysiologic testing in patients with syncope caused by transient bradycardia. N Engl J Med 1989;321:1703. *(Sensitivity and specificity were disappointingly low in patients with proven bradyarrhythmic syncope.)*

Gibson TC, Heitzman MR. Diagnostic efficacy of 24-hour electrocardiographic monitoring for syncope. Am J Cardiol 1984;53:1013. *(Of 1,512 patients referred for Holter monitoring because of syncope, 15 had an episode of syncope, of which 7 were related to an arrhythmia, and 241 reported presyncope, of which 24 were arrhythmia related.)*

Grubb BP, TemesyArmos P, Hahn H, et al. Utility of upright tilt-table testing in the evaluation and management of syncope of unknown origin. Am J Med 1991;90:6. *(The test proved valuable in a highly selected group of patients with unexplained syncope; false-positive rate was zero in six control subjects. Treatment halted episodes in those who were positive.)*

Jansen RWMM, Lipsitz LA. Postprandial hypotension: epidemiology, pathophysiology, and clinical management. Ann Intern Med 1995;122:286. *(A literature review finding such hypotension to be very common in the elderly and a potential cause of falls and syncope.)*

Joran J, Shannon JR, Biaggioni I, et al. Contrasting actions of pressor agents in severe autonomic failure. Am J Med 1998;105:116. *(A placebo-controlled trial comparing the effects of phenylpropanolamine, midodrine, caffeine, idomethacin, and yohimbine.)*

Kapoor WN. Evaluation and management of the patient with syncope. JAMA 1992;268:2553. *(Very useful review, especially for its critical look at yields of laboratory studies; 74 references.)*

Kapoor WN. Back to the basics for the workup of syncope. J Gen Intern Med 1994;10:695. *(An editorial emphasizing the value of the history, physical examination, and limited testing.)*

Kapoor WN, Brant N. Evaluation of syncope by upright tilt testing with isoproterenol. Ann Intern Med 1992;116:358. *(A controlled study in young persons showing the test had a low specificity, with high rates of positive responses in both syncopal patients and controls; dampens enthusiasm for the test.)*

Kapoor W, Cha R, Peterson JR, et al. Prolonged electrocardiographic monitoring in patients with syncope. Am J Med 1987;82:20. *(Patients with syncope and frequent or repetitive ventricular premature beats or sinus pauses had an increased risk of overall mortality and sudden death.)*

Kapoor W, Karpf M, Levy GS. Issues in evaluating patients with syncope. Ann Intern Med 1984;100:755. *(An editorial describing emphasis on meticulous history, physical examination, and electrocardiogram with discriminating use of additional tests in evaluation of patients with syncope.)*

Kapoor WN, Karpf M, Wieand S, et al. A prospective evaluation and follow-up of patients with syncope. N Engl J Med 1983;309:197.

(Patients with a cardiovascular cause for syncope face much higher risk than those with noncardiovascular or unknown causes.)

Kapoor WN, Peterson J, Wieand HS, et al. Diagnostic and prognostic implications of recurrences in patients with syncope. Am J Med 1987;83:700. *(Recurrences are common but not a predictor of mortality, sudden death, or etiology.)*

Kapoor WN, Smith M, Miller NL. Upright tilt-table testing in evaluating syncope: a comprehensive literature review. Am J Med 1994;97:78. *(Finds the test useful when it can reproduce symptoms in persons who have had cardiac causes ruled out.)*

Kapoor W, Snustad D, Peterson J, et al. Syncope in the elderly. Am J Med 1989;80:419. *(They have an increased risk of underlying heart disease and overall mortality.)*

Kwoh CK, Beck JR, Pauker SG. Repeated syncope with negative diagnostic evaluation. Med Decis Making 1984;4:351. *(A sophisticated decision analysis approach to the question of whether or not to pace, including a well-structured review of the literature.)*

Lee RT, Cook EF, Day SC, et al. Long-term survival after transient loss of consciousness. J Gen Intern Med 1988;3:337. *(Patients with a cardiac, neurologic, drug, or metabolic etiology had a worse prognosis; 7-year follow-up.)*

Linzer M, Prystowsky EN, Divine GW, et al. Predicting outcomes of electrophysiologic studies of patients with unexplained syncope. J Gen Intern Med 1991;6:113. *(Identifies predictors of a positive EPS study and thus selection criteria for those who should be studied.)*

Linzer M, Yang EH, Estes M III, et al. Diagnosing syncope. Part 1. Value of history, physical examination, and electrocardiography. Ann Intern Med 1997;126:989. *(A literature review and position paper outlining a clinical guideline in which history, physical examination, and ECG are recommended as the core the evaluation.)*

Linzer M, Yang, EH, Estes M III, et al. Diagnosing syncope. Part 2. Unexplained syncope. Ann Intern Med 1997;127:76. *(A literature review and position paper on approaches to testing the 50% of patients who remain undiagnosed after history, physical examination and ECG.)*

Lipsitz LA. Syncope in the elderly. Ann Intern Med 1983;99:92. *(An extensive clinical review stressing the selective use of diagnostic tests in evaluating syncope as well as attention to drug effects and treatment of symptomatic abnormalities.)*

McIntosh SJ, Lawson J, Henry RA. Clinical characteristics of vasodepressor, cardioinhibitory, and mixed carotid sinus syndrome in the elderly. Am J Med 1993;95:203. *(A cause of unexplained falls in the elderly.)*

Novak V, Novak P, Opfer-Gehrking TL, et al. Clinical and laboratory indices that enhance the diagnosis of postural tachycardia syndrome. Mayo Clin Proc 1998;73:1141. *(An approach to better characterization of this syndrome.)*

Onrot J, Goldenberg MR, Hollister AS, et al. Management of chronic orthostatic hypotension. Am J Med 1986;80:454. *(An excellent review of therapeutic measures based on an etiologic formulation; 71 references.)*

Silverstein MD, Singer DE, Mulley AG, et al. Patients with syncope admitted to medical intensive care units. JAMA 1982;248:1185. *(Among this intensive care unit population, those with cardiovascular syncope had a 19% 1-year mortality rate, whereas those with noncardiovascular or unexplained syncope had a 6% rate. The authors conclude that patients discharged with unexplained syncope do not face increased risk of death during the subsequent year.)*

Spitzer RL, Williams JB, Kroenke K, et al. Utility of a new procedure for diagnosing mental disorder in primary care. The PRIME 1000 study. JAMA 1994;272:1749. *(The evidence for usefulness of hyperventilation and screening instruments in testing for psychiatric disorders.)*

Palpitations are disconcerting and often incite fear, although most cases seen in the office occur among persons with no serious underlying heart disease. The patient with palpitations reports a disquieting awareness of one's heartbeat, which may be described as a pounding, racing, skipping, flopping, or fluttering sensation. The primary physician must be able to differentiate the high-risk person in need of an intensive evaluation from the low-risk individual who can be reassured after a screening assessment. Ambulatory monitoring techniques and electrophysiologic study have improved detection of arrhythmias; their indications and limitations need to be understood.

PATHOPHYSIOLOGY AND CLINICAL PRESENTATION

Most healthy individuals are unaware of their resting heartbeat. Sudden change in rate or rhythm, increase in stroke volume or contractility, and unusual cardiac movement within the thorax may cause awareness of the heartbeat. Acute changes in heart rate or rhythm may be noted, but chronic dysrhythmias often go unnoticed. Patients with depression and other somatization disorders have excessive health concerns and a heightened awareness of normal bodily sensations that can make even the normally imperceptible heartbeat of daily life an unpleasant experience that they report as palpitations. For most other patients, palpitations represent an acute disturbance of the heartbeat.

Premature Atrial or Ventricular Contractions. Awareness of a premature beat derives from the pause and vigorous beat that follows the premature contraction. The delay allows for prolonged ventricular filling, which triggers an increase in contractility and stroke volume. The excessive motion of the heart may be felt as a "turning over" or "flopping." The sensations are isolated and tend to be most noticeable when the heart rate is slow and the patient is lying in bed supine or in the left lateral decubitus position. If there is atrioventricular dissociation and atrial contraction against a closed arterioventricular valve (as may occur in ventricular premature contractions), then a "pounding in the neck" or a sudden bulging of the neck veins (jugular *cannon venous A waves*) may be the presentation. Some patients with frequent jugular cannon A waves may report inability to catch one's breath, although they deny frank dyspnea.

In the absence of underlying heart disease, ventricular premature beats (even when frequent or complex) have no adverse effect on prognosis. Only in the context of heart disease does the presence of PVCs connote an unfavorable prognosis (see below). Similarly, atrial premature beats are harmless in the absence of heart disease, but may be a harbinger of more compromising atrial dysrhythmias when they occur in the setting of cardiac pathology.

Sinus Tachycardia. Excess adrenergic stimulation results in increased contractility and sinus tachycardia, which may pres-ent as palpitations with a fast regular rhythm. Onset can be abrupt; resolution is usually more gradual. A constant rapid pounding at rest is felt by patients with *hyperkinetic states* (e.g., fever, severe anemia, hyperthyroidism, anxiety, agitated depression) due to the catecholamine-induced increase in contractility and stroke volume. Patients with anxiety-induced palpitations often have an underlying *panic disorder* (see Chapter 226); typically, they have difficulty telling whether the palpitations or the anxiety came first. Unappreciated is the high frequency of other supraventricular dysrhythmias in this group of patients (see below). An uncommon variant of sinus tachycardia, *inappropriate sinus tachycardia*, is believed to represent a hypersensitivity to catecholamine stimulation. *Hyperthyroidism* may have a palpitation presentation similar to that of anxiety (see Chapter 103); it may also cause atrial fibrillation (see below). In rare instances, the source of adrenergic outpouring is a *pheochromocytoma*. Its incidence is less than 0.1%, with about half of cases presenting as paroxysms of palpitations, hypertension, perspiration, tremor, nervousness, and other signs of adrenergic stimulation. Episodes are often spontaneous in origin but may be triggered by emotion and thus mimic an anxiety attack. An *insulin reaction* can produce a similar clinical picture (see Chapter 102), driven by an outpouring of catecholamines. A regular rhythm without tachycardia is noted in cases of valvular disease accompanied by large stroke volumes, as in *aortic regurgitation.*

Supraventricular Tachycardias. Attacks of palpitations that are regular in rhythm and rapid in rate may also be due to paroxysmal *supraventricular tachycardia* (SVT), sometimes referred to as *paroxysmal atrial tachycardia*. There are two basic mechanisms. *In atrioventricular nodal tachycardia*, the most common SVT, there are two functionally distinct conduction pathways in the nodal area that enable a reentrant circuit to develop, producing ventricular response rates as high as 160 to 180 beats/min. If the atria in this rhythm disturbance are unaffected by the nodal rhythm disturbance, there can be arterioventricular nodal dissociation manifested as rapid regular pounding in the neck. The condition is considerably more common in women than men and occurs in a wide variety of patients, including those with normal hearts, sick-sinus syndrome, mitral valve prolapse and other forms of valvular disease, coronary artery disease, and cardiomyopathy. Onset may occur in the setting of emotional stress (e.g., panic attack). Some patients note that standing up after bending over may bring on an episode that can be terminated by lying down.

In the second form of SVT with a regular rhythm, *atrioventricular reciprocating tachycardia*, there is a large macrorentrant circuit that involves the atrium, the arterioventricular node, an accessory pathway (e.g., Bundle of Kent or James), and the ventricle. The *preexcitation syndromes* (so-called because of their short electrocardiographic PR intervals), *Wolff-Parkinson-White* (WPW) and *Lown-Ganong-Lown*, operate by the reciprocating mechanism. An electrocardiographic hallmark of WPW is the delta wave at the beginning of the QRS, indicative of aberrant conduction through the accessory bundle; the QRS may be widened considerably during a run of SVT and mimic a ventricular dysrhythmia, especially when WPW is complicated by a very rapid ventricular response rate, as in atrial flutter or atrial fibrillation (see below). Any SVT with a very rapid ventricular response rate may seriously compromise cardiac output in a patient with underlying heart disease and cause chest pain, dyspnea, profound weakness, or even loss of consciousness.

Onset of SVT is characteristically sudden and may be precipitated by excess *alcohol, emotional upset,* or strenuous *exertion.* Caffeinated beverages are less of a risk factor. SVTs may be initiated by the occurrence of premature beats that alter conduction in the normal pathway. Paroxysms cease when the conducting properties of the reentrant circuit are disturbed by changes in vagal tone, hence the report by patients of ability to terminate attacks by Valsalva. Resolution is typically abrupt. Syncope is uncommon, but may occur at the outset if the rate is very rapid and/or there is acute vasodilation.

Some of the conditions associated with SVT are responsible for other dysrhythmias as well. For example, almost half of patients with *sick sinus syndrome* experience *heart block* or marked *bradycardia* in addition to bouts of SVT.

Paroxysmal Atrial Fibrillation. Sudden onset of palpitations with an irregularly irregular rhythm and rapid rate typifies *paroxysmal atrial fibrillation,* which occurs in a host of settings including *acute alcohol excess* ("holiday heart"), *infection, hyperthyroidism, sick-sinus syndrome, WPW syndrome, cardiomyopathy,* and acute worsening of *ischemia or congestive heart failure*; the condition is also found among otherwise healthy young people ("lone" *atrial fibrillation*). High levels of circulating catecholamines may trigger atrial fibrillation, especially in someone with underlying organic heart disease. A common precipitant is exercise or the termination of exercise with its surge of vagal tone. Chronic atrial fibrillation usually does not produce palpitations. An irregularly irregular tachycardia may also be seen if there are runs of *multifocal atrial tachycardia* (MAT), which takes place in the context of severe pulmonary disease, particularly when there is an acute fall in Po_2 or pH. Frequent atrial or ventricular premature contractions can lead to a similarly irregular rhythm and rapid rate.

Ventricular Tachycardia. Ventricular tachycardia is among the most worrisome of dysrhythmias related to palpitations, being associated in some instances with risk of sudden death. Nonetheless, not all ventricular tachycardia represents life-threatening disease. *Nonsustained ventricular tachycardia* (NSVT) may occur in otherwise normal persons (*idiopathic ventricular tachycardia*) and in those with underlying heart disease. In idiopathic disease, the ventricular arrhythmia most often arises from the right ventricular outflow tract; the heart appears structurally normal. Onset is typically in the second or third decades of life and may present as palpitations, near-syncope, or even true loss of consciousness. In normal subjects, NSVT is not associated with an increased risk of sudden death; however, any NSVT that compromises cardiac output may lead to dizziness, near syncope, or loss of consciousness.

More worrisome are runs of nonsustained or sustained ventricular tachycardia occurring in the context of underlying heart disease. Patients with such a presentation have an increased risk of sudden death, especially those with *ischemia,* prior myocardial infarction with *scar* formation, *dilated cardiomyopathy, hypertensive heart disease* with left ventricular remodeling, or hemodynamically significant *valvular disease.* The clinical picture may be dominated by manifestations of the underlying heart disease, but more subtle forms of heart disease (e.g., *hypertrophic cardiomyopathy and prolonged QT syndrome*) also may trigger ventricular tachycardia and result in sudden death.

Hypertrophic cardiomyopathy is a hereditary condition featuring asymmetric hypertrophy, right ventricular involvement, outflow tract obstruction, prominent septal Q waves in the anteroapical leads of the electrocardiogram (ECG), and a wall thickness on ultrasound of more than 13 mm. A characteristic finding on physical examination is a systolic ejection murmur along the left sternal border that increases with Valsalva and decreases with passive leg elevation (see Chapter 21).

Prolonged QT syndrome is a disorder of repolarization that increases susceptibility to potentially lethal polymorphic ventricular tachycardias (*"torsades de pointes"*). Hereditary and acquired forms have been described. In the hereditary form, there is a strong family history of sudden death below the age of 30 and congenital deafness. Ten-year mortality rates after onset of syncope approach 50%. Precipitants include severe emotional stress and very vigorous exercise. On ECG, prolongation of the QT interval, bradycardia, T-wave alternans, and notched T waves are characteristic. In the much more common acquired form, QT prolongation occurs as a result of medications or clinical conditions. Medications with this potential include the commonly used antihistamines such as *terfenadine and astemizole,* usually when taken in excess or concurrently with a drug that inhibits its metabolism (e.g., cimetidine) or causes QT prolongation itself (e.g., the *macrolide antibiotics, ketoconazole, itraconazole*). Other pharmacologic precipitants include the *class IA antiarrhythmics* (e.g., quinidine, procainamide, disopyramide), *class III antiarrhythmics* (e.g., sotalol), *tricyclic* antidepressants, and *phenothiazines.* Clinical conditions that prolong the QT interval include *hypokalemia, hypomagnesemia, hypocalcemia, hypothyroidism, starvation* and *liquid protein* diets.

Patients with underlying heart disease have a lowered threshold for ventricular tachycardia. In addition to the factors associated with prolonged QT interval, *digitalis toxicity* is an important precipitant of ventricular tachycardia. Digitalis toxicity is associated with ventricular tachycardia, atrial fibrillation, ventricular bigeminy, and junctional tachycardias. Concurrent hypokalemia and hypomagnesemia lower the threshold for development of "dig-toxic" rhythm disturbances (see Chapters 28, 29). The *methylxanthines* (e.g., theophylline) have a narrow therapeutic range, which when exceeded increases the risk of serious rhythm disturbances, including ventricular tachycardia, especially in persons with underlying heart disease.

DIFFERENTIAL DIAGNOSIS

The causes of palpitations can be listed in terms of their clinical presentation (Table 25.1).

Table 25.1. Important Causes of Palpitations

1. **Isolated Single Palpitations**
   a. Premature atrial or ventricular beats
   b. The beat after a blocked beat
   c. The beat after a compensatory pause
2. **Paroxysmal Episodes with Abrupt Onset and Resolution (rate usually rapid)**
   a. Rhythm irregular
      1. Paroxysmal atrial fibrillation
      2. Paroxysmal atrial tachycardia with variable block
      3. Frequent atrial or ventricular premature beats
      4. Multifocal atrial tachycardia
   b. Rhythm regular
      1. Supraventricular tachycardias with constant block 1:1 conduction
3. **Paroxysmal Episodes with Less Abrupt Onset or Resolution (rhythm usually regular, rate rapid)**
   a. Exertion
   b. Emotion
   c. Drug side effect (e.g., sympathomimetics, theophylline compounds)
   d. Stimulant use (coffee, tea, tobacco)
   e. Insulin reaction
   f. Pheochromocytoma
4. **Persistent Palpitations at Rest with Regular Rhythm (rate normal, slow, or rapid)**
   a. Aortic or mitral regurgitation
   b. Large ventricular septal defect
   c. Bradycardia
   d. Severe anemia
   e. Hyperthyroidism (may also cause atrial fibrillation)
   f. Pregnancy
   g. Fever
   h. Marked volume depletion
   i. Anxiety neurosis

WORKUP

Although determining the nature of the heartbeat disturbance helps to identify etiology and prognosis, the key determinant of prognosis is the presence, type, and severity of underlying heart disease. Consequently, a search for cardiac pathology is a high priority.

History. Eliciting a complete *description* of the patient's palpitations is essential, including its mode of onset, frequency, rate, rhythm, duration, termination, associated symptoms, and precipitants and alleviating factors. Unfortunately, many patients are unable to give an accurate or detailed account of their symptoms. The relation of the onset of symptoms to exertion can aid in separating the anxious individual, whose symptoms may occur at rest and are usually not worsened by exertion, from the patient with heart disease and impaired exercise tolerance. Identification of precipitants such as emotional upset, stimulant intake, fever, pregnancy, volume depletion, and severe anemia is essential, because their recognition can contribute to design of proper therapy. Inquiry into symptoms of an insulin reaction (see Chapter 102) and hyperthyroidism (see Chapter 103) may also prove productive.

The more hypochondriacal or somatizing the patient, the poorer the correlation between symptoms and Holter monitoring results; however, reports of fluttering, stopping, or beating irregularly are predictive of finding an arrhythmia. Any isolated thumping or flip-flopping in the chest suggests an atrial or ventricular premature beat. Associated pounding in the neck is indicative of arterioventricular dissociation, as seen with ventric-

ular premature beats or arterioventricular nodal tachycardia. Sudden onset and sudden cessation of rapid regular heartbeats are characteristic of nodal and reentrant SVT and NSVT, whereas more gradual onset and cessation characterize sinus tachycardia. Palpitations brought on by exercise or emotional stress point to idiopathic ventricular tachycardia, atrial fibrillation, other SVTs, prolonged QT interval, and inappropriate sinus tachycardia. Onset in conjunction with a panic attack is indicative not only of sinus tachycardia but also of nodal reentrant tachycardia, as is onset with standing up after bending over and cessation with lying down.

Inquiries into concurrent dyspnea, chest pain, lightheadedness, near-syncope, and syncope are essential both for etiology and assessment of hemodynamic severity. Syncope suggests ventricular tachycardia or a very fast SVT with vasodilatation. Chest pain and dyspnea may also be signs of marked hemodynamic compromise. Additionally useful are questions about risk factors for coronary disease (smoking, diabetes, hypertension, hyperlipidemia, positive family history of early onset syncope or sudden death before age 30) and prior cardiac history (heart murmur, rheumatic fever, myocardial infarction, other forms of cardiac illness, family history of heart disease). Although one should not mistake symptoms of anxiety, such as chest tightness and air hunger at rest, for evidence of organic heart disease, the presence of anxiety symptoms does not rule out an arterioventricular nodal tachycardia. Nonetheless, assessment is not complete without specific inquiry into symptoms of panic and somatization disorders (see Chapters 226 and 230).

Use of all cardiotonic drugs should be detailed, including antiarrhythmics, digitalis preparations, theophylline compounds, sympathomimetics, and anticholinergics. Also to review are drugs associated with QT prolongation: antiarrhythmics, terfenadine, astemizole, macrolide antibiotics, ketoconazole, itraconazole, phenothiazines, and tricyclic antidepressants. Many over-the-counter decongestants and diet pills contain catecholamines or theophylline derivatives; their abuse may be responsible for symptoms. The history should include inquiry into alcohol abuse (see Chapter 228), a common precipitant of paroxysmal SVT. Family history of early-onset syncope can be a clue to hereditary prolonged QT syndrome or hypertrophic cardiomyopathy.

Physical Examination. Important observations include determination of the blood pressure for elevation, marked postural change, and widened pulse pressure. The apical pulse is noted for rate and rhythm disturbances; relying on the peripheral pulse may be misleading when there is a pulse deficit, as occurs in atrial fibrillation or premature beats. The temperature should be recorded. The skin is examined for pallor and signs of hyperthyroidism and anemia; the eyes for exophthalmos; the neck for goiter; the carotid pulse for upstroke; the jugular venous pulse for distention and cannon A waves; the chest for rales, rhonchi, wheezes, and dullness; the heart for heaves, thrills, clicks, murmurs, rubs, and third heart sound; and extremities for edema and calf tenderness. The finding of a systolic ejection murmur along the left sternal border should be followed by examining its response to Valsalva maneuver; an increase in intensity suggests hypertrophic cardiomyopathy. Response to modest exercise should also be noted, because a number of dysrhythmias may be triggered by it. Finally, the mental status examination should include checking for manifestations of anxiety, depression, panic disorder, and substance abuse (see Chapters 226 to 228, 230, and 235). In addition to possibly providing important diagnostic information, the careful unhurried physical examination can be of considerable use in reassuring the worried patient.

Laboratory Studies. A few basic hematologic and chemistry studies contribute to the assessment of etiology and risk. Patients with signs of a hyperkinetic state require a *hemoglobin* determination to rule out a significant anemia and a *thyrotropin* test to rule out hyperthyroidism. Patients with underlying heart disease should have a check of the serum *potassium, calcium,* and magnesium, especially if taking a digitalis preparation; a serum cardiac glycoside level (e.g., for *digoxin*) is equally important to rule out toxic accumulation of the drug. A fingerstick *blood glucose* can be diagnostic in the setting of a suspected insulin reaction triggering hypoglycemia (see Chapter 102). When there is sufficient clinical evidence to warrant consideration of pheochromocytoma, a 24-hour *urine for VMA* can be helpful (see Chapter 26). Most of the remainder of the laboratory workup is directed toward identifying the rhythm disturbance and detecting underlying heart disease.

Resting Electrocardiogram. Most if not all patients with palpitations should have a resting 12-lead ECG. Even if physical examination is completely normal and no disturbances of rate or rhythm are noted on the ECG, one might detect a manifestation of underlying heart disease. Specifically, the ECG needs to be studied for axis shift, short PR interval (less than 0.12 seconds), abnormal P-wave morphology including signs of atrial enlargement, QRS widening, increase in QRS voltage, prominent septal Q waves, prolonged QT interval, delta waves, and ST- and T-wave changes. If a dysrhythmia is noted, it is worth obtaining a 2-minute rhythm strip to better characterize the rhythm disturbance. The anxiety-laden person often insists on having an ECG and finds comfort in a normal result; unfortunately, in many cases the reassurance is only transient.

Ambulatory Electrocardiographic Monitoring. Patients whose palpitations are accompanied by evidence of *underlying heart disease* are the best candidates for ambulatory monitoring, because they are at increased risk of having a clinically significant arrhythmia. So long as they are not experiencing syncope, near-syncope, heart failure, or angina in association with their palpitations, they can undergo an outpatient evaluation that includes ambulatory monitoring. The utility of ambulatory monitoring in otherwise healthy patients who complain solely of palpitations remains less clear, although the reassurance value can be considerable if typical episodes occur in the presence of a normal ECG recording.

The most cost-effective approach to ambulatory monitoring is use of an *event recorder* rather than *Holter monitoring*, because most episodes of palpitations are relatively infrequent. A 2-week monitoring period using a continuous-loop event recorder yields more diagnoses at lower cost than does 48-hour Holter monitoring or 4 weeks of event recording. The only drawback to the continuous-loop event recorder is that it requires patient activation, which can be a problem if the dysrhythmia incapacitates the patient. Although monitoring may be continuous, preservation of the ECG record is usually limited to a few minutes about the time of activation. Most units use continuous-loop recording technology, although more advanced storage technologies are under development. Some permit telephone transmission of the rhythm disturbance. Intermittent ECG recorders allow prolonged monitoring at reasonable cost in patients with relatively infrequent episodes of palpitations. Ambulatory monitoring has been disappointing as a method for detecting ischemia.

The yield from Holter monitoring is greatest in patients with daily symptoms. Patients are asked to keep a diary to ascertain the relationship between symptoms and rhythm disturbances. Because atrial and ventricular premature beats and short runs of SVT are common in normal asymptomatic patients, a positive test requires a clear-cut correlation between symptoms reported in the patient log and ECG findings. Most studies of Holter monitoring show a very high incidence of recorded "abnormalities" but a very poor correlation between ECG findings and reported symptoms. The patient who experiences typical symptoms but no concurrent rhythm disturbances during the Holter monitoring can be reassured. The patient who fails to have a symptomatic episode during Holter monitoring—a common occurrence—may be scheduled for a repeat study; however, yield is low in patients whose initial Holter study is normal and frequency of episodes is low. The cost of repeat Holter monitoring can be high.

One of the more disconcerting findings on event monitoring is a *wide QRS tachycardia*. Although not usually encountered in the outpatient setting, it may be found on an event monitoring and needs to be addressed to determine whether it represents a rather harmless *SVT with aberrancy* or a more ominous *ventricular tachycardia*. Findings associated with a ventricular origin include a history of heart disease, evidence of an old myocardial infarction on a resting ECG, arterioventricular dissociation (which is often absent but can be diagnostic if present), a QRS duration of more than 160 ms if there is a right bundle branch pattern or more than 140 ms if the pattern is left bundle, a combination of left bundle branch block and right axis deviation, extreme left axis deviation (less than -90 to $+180$ degrees), and a different QRS pattern during tachycardia than on resting ECG in patients with preexisting bundle branch block. The combination of these findings provides reasonable sensitivity and specificity; most single findings are relatively weak discriminants.

Exercise Stress Testing. Although Holter monitoring is more likely to detect ventricular irritability than is stress testing, stress testing will sometimes uncover ventricular tachycardias that do not appear on Holter or event monitoring, suggesting to some that the studies might be complementary. The best candidates for exercise stress testing are those who report palpitations occurring during or immediately after exercise. SVTs, atrial fibrillation, and idiopathic ventricular tachycardia are commonly triggered by exercise or its termination and may be detected by the test. Alternatively, one can ask the patient to exercise during ambulatory monitoring. Stress testing is also indicated if palpitations occur in the context of angina-like chest pain, suggesting either an ischemic mechanism or sufficient hemodynamic compromise to result in ischemia (see Chapters 20 and 36). To ensure patient safety, one needs to rule out hemodynamically significant aortic stenosis, hypertrophic cardiomyopathy, and QT prolongation before proceeding with exercise testing, because they are associated with an increased risk of an adverse event with stress testing.

Echocardiography. Patients suspected of having valvular or cardiomyopathic disease on the basis of history, physical examination, or ECG should undergo echocardiography for confirmation and determination of severity of disease (see Chapters 21 and 33). Routine ordering of cardiac ultrasound in the absence of clinical suspicion is of little utility and only increases the cost of evaluation.

Electrophysiologic Study. Palpitations leading to syncope or near-syncope raise the question of a major rhythm disturbance (e.g., very rapid SVT, ventricular tachycardia, complete heart block). When occurring in the context of underlying organic heart disease, such arrhythmias have an especially poor prognosis (see Chapters 28 and 29). Electrophysiologic study (EPS) can help uncover such arrhythmias and their pathologic mechanisms. The search for a focus of malignant arrhythmogenicity also helps guide treatment. The value of EPS in syncopal patients who have significant organic heart disease is well documented, but sensitivity and specificity for identifying important arrhythmias or conduction system disturbances in syncopal patients without signs of underlying heart disease have been disappointing. EPS remains an important diagnostic modality in the evaluation of patients with suspected ventricular tachycardia or documented heart block. Careful patient selection is essential (see Chapters 24 and 29). EPS is very expensive and not without risk, because it includes induction of potentially dangerous dysrhythmias. The study requires cardiac catheterization, sophisticated equipment, and a highly trained and experienced staff.

PATIENT EDUCATION AND SYMPTOMATIC RELIEF

Providing Reassurance. When palpitations prove to be no more than a manifestation of excessive bodily concern or a harmless dysrhythmia with no adverse consequences, efforts should be made to provide meaningful reassurance. Failure to do so is likely to lead to unnecessary limitation of activity and demands for additional testing or referrals to specialists. Hasty or perfunctory words of comfort are worthless. A careful history and physical examination, combined with eliciting and responding directly to patient concerns, views, and requests (within reason), must take place before the patient can be told the palpitations are harmless. Such reassurance may be all that is needed, especially when combined with advice to increase physical activity and cut down on alcohol, smoking, and stress. Ambulatory monitoring or exercise stress testing may have a role in helping to reassure the overly anxious patient. Directly addressing any underlying psychopathology may be required (see Chapters 226, 227, and 230).

Symptomatic Management. Proper management of dysrhythmias in patients with underlying heart disease is treatment of the underlying pathology. For patients with no underlying heart disease who find their symptoms intolerable, a few simple measures are worth considering.

Atrial and Ventricular Premature Beats. If the palpitations persist and are bothersome, a trial of beta-blocker therapy may be beneficial symptomatically. Often as little as 25 to 50 mg/day of atenolol or the equivalent decreases the frequency of atrial or ventricular premature beats to the point where they are tolerable. Patients with idiopathic chronic ventricular bigeminy causing fatigue or exertional near-syncope because of a slow ef-

fective heart rate might benefit from consideration of radioablation if they do not respond to beta-blockade. All nonessential drugs capable of causing palpitations should be stopped.

The role of *caffeine* in precipitating cardiac arrhythmias and the usefulness of restricting its intake in symptomatic patients has been debated for decades. Available data show benefit only for restricting excessive intake (more than five cups a day), unless the patient reports caffeine-induced symptoms.

Supraventricular Tachycardia and Sinus Tachycardia. Detailed discussion of treatment for SVT is presented in Chapter 28, but a few simple measures are worth noting. *Vagal maneuvers* are often effective in halting SVT. *Valsalva* and *carotid sinus massage* (in the absence of carotid disease) can be taught to the patient and suggested as the first line of therapy after the onset of an attack. Prophylaxis of SVT attacks can be accomplished by avoiding known precipitants, such as alcohol and stimulants. If a panic attack disorder is the cause of episodes of palpitations, one can consider beta-blockade, a minor tranquilizer, or an antidepressant (see Chapter 226).

Symptomatic treatment of sinus tachycardia necessitates correcting the underlying precipitant (e.g., anemia [see Chapter 82], volume depletion, hyperthyroidism [see Chapter 103], fever [see Chapter 11]), and congestive failure [see Chapter 32]). Patients with hypoglycemic episodes need an adjustment in their insulin regimen and/or dietary program (see Chapter 102). Treatment of MAT requires correction of the underlying pulmonary problem rather than use of antiarrhythmic drugs. Improvement in oxygenation and pH status is essential.

Ventricular Tachycardia. Episodes that cause syncope require attention even when there is no threat of sudden death associated with them (see Chapter 29).

INDICATIONS FOR ADMISSION AND REFERRAL

Admission. Patients with palpitations associated with syncope, near-syncope, angina-like chest pain, or true dyspnea are candidates for prompt inpatient evaluation, especially if they have evidence of underlying organic heart disease. Hospitalization is also indicated if a patient with known heart disease demonstrates runs of ventricular tachycardia, even if these are not sustained or hemodynamically compromising; mortality risk is high. Patients with SVT who manifest hemodynamic compromise (e.g., fall in blood pressure, dyspnea, angina, near-syncope) also need prompt hospital admission.

Referral. Patients with underlying heart disease and palpitations leading to syncope, near-syncope, chest pain, or dyspnea require cardiac consultation for consideration of electrophysiologic study, as do those with underlying heart disease and episodes of ventricular tachycardia (sustained or nonsustained), whether hemodynamically compromising or not. All such patients are at high risk and likely to benefit from EPS both diagnostically and often therapeutically (see Chapters 28 and 29).

A.H.G.

ANNOTATED BIBLIOGRAPHY

Akhtar M, Shenasa M, Jazayeri M, et al. Wide QRS complex tachycardia. Ann Intern Med 1988;109:905. *(The vast majority proved to be ventricular in origin; good discussion of criteria for distinguishing between supraventricular and ventricular sources.)*

Barnett PA, Peter CT, Swan HJC, et al. The frequency and prognostic significance of electrocardiographic abnormalities in clinically normal individuals. Prog Cardiovasc Dis 1981;23:299. *(Normals have a high incidence of arrhythmias; provocative discussion on what constitutes "normal.")*

Barsky AJ, Clearly PD, Barnett MC, et al. The accuracy of symptoms reporting by patients complaining of palpitations. Am J Med 1994;97:214. *(The more hypochondriacal or somatizing the patient, the poorer the correlation between symptoms and Holter monitoring results; however, reports of fluttering, stopping, or beating irregularly were predictive of an arrhythmia.)*

Barsky AJ, Cleary PD, Coeytaux RR, et al. Psychiatric disorders in medical outpatients complaining of palpitations. J Gen Intern Med 1994;9:306. *(Panic disorder accounted for palpitations in nearly 20% of patients.)*

Cohen EJ, Klatsky AL, Armstrong MA. Alcohol use and supraventricular arrhythmia. Am J Cardiol 1988;62:971. *(Alcohol excess precipitates a host of SVTs.)*

DiMarco JP, Philbrick JT. Use of ambulatory electrocardiographic (Holter) monitoring. Ann Intern Med 1990;113:53. *(A comprehensive and critical review focusing on advantages and limitations of Holter monitoring; 139 references.)*

Kapoor WN, Cha R, Peterson JR, et al. Prolonged electrocardiographic monitoring in patients with syncope. Am J Med 1987;82:20. *(Patients with syncope and frequent or repetitive ventricular premature beats or sinus pauses had an increased risk of overall mortality.)*

Kennedy HL, Whitlock JA, Sprague MK, et al. Long-term follow-up of symptomatic healthy subjects with frequent and complex ventricular ectopy. N Engl J Med 1985;312:193. *(No increased risk of cardiac morbidity or mortality.)*

Kinlay S, Leitch JW, Neil A, et al. Cardiac event recorders yield more diagnoses and are more cost-effective than 48-hour Holter monitoring in patients with palpitations: a controlled clinical trial. Ann Intern Med 1996;124:16. *(A randomized crossover study; the title says it all.)*

Krol RB, Morady F, Flaker S, et al. Electrophysiologic testing in patients with unexplained syncope: clinical and noninvasive predictors of outcome. J Am Coll Cardiol 1987;10:358. *(Predictors include previous myocardial infarction, low ejection fraction, and conduction abnormalities on ECG.)*

Lessmeier TJ, Gamperlin D, Johnson-Liddon V, et al. Unrecognized paroxysmal supraventricular tachycardia: potential for misdiagnosis as panic disorder. Arch Intern Med 1997;157:537. *(Panic disorder was very common among patients with EPS-proven SVT.)*

Lowenstein SR, Gabow PA, Cramer J, et al. The role of alcohol in new onset atrial fibrillation. Arch Intern Med 1983;143:1882. *(Among 40 cases of new onset atrial fibrillation, alcohol caused or contributed to approximately two thirds; 90% of these converted spontaneously to sinus rhythm within 24 hours.)*

Myers MG. Caffeine and cardiac arrhythmias. Ann Intern Med 1991;114:147. *(Reviews the evidence for and against a causative role; moderate intake appears to have little effect, even in patients with heart disease.)*

Ryan M, Lown B, Horn H. Comparison of ventricular ectopic activity during 24-hour monitoring and exercise testing in patients with coronary heart disease. N Engl J Med 1975;292:224. *(Monitoring proved better in exposing ventricular irritability, but there were instances when ectopic activity was detected only by stress testing.)*

Shen WK, Holmes DR, Hammill SC. Transtelephonic monitoring: documentation of transient cardiac rhythm disturbances. Mayo Clin Proc 1987;62:109. *(Another method for capturing infrequent but potentially important episodes.)*

Simetbaum PJ, Kim KY, Josephson ME, et al. Diagnostic yield and optimal duration of continuous-loop event monitoring for the diagnosis of palpitations. Ann Intern Med 1998;128:890. *(A prospective cohort study; yield found to drop off markedly after 2 weeks.)*

Tan HL, Hou CJ, Lauer MR, et al. Electrophysiologic mechanisms of the long QT syndromes and torsade de pointes. Ann Intern Med 1995;122:701. *(Excellent review of the condition.)*

Varma N, Josephson ME. Therapy of "idiopathic" ventricular tachycardia. J Cardiovasc Electrophysiol 1997;8:104. *(Includes good descriptions of pathophysiology and clinical presentations.)*

Weber BE, Kapoor WN. Evaluation and outcomes of patients with palpitations. Am J Med 1996;100:138. *(Although psychiatric disorders are common, true arrhythmic etiologies need to be ruled out.)*

Appendix: Evaluation of Atrial Fibrillation in the Outpatient Setting

Atrial fibrillation (AF) is one of several dysrhythmias that can produce an irregularly irregular heartbeat. It is often a manifestation of underlying heart disease but sometimes is discovered in a patient with no overt cardiac pathology. Many patients tolerate the arrhythmia well and can be evaluated thoroughly and safely in the outpatient setting, although the etiology does not necessarily need to be harmless. The primary care physician needs to determine if it is safe to conduct the assessment in the office setting and how to carry out a cost-efficient evaluation.

PATHOPHYSIOLOGY

The postulated electrophysiologic mechanisms of AF include focal automaticity and a complex form of reentry. Factors that may precipitate or perpetuate AF include increased atrial size, increased atrial pressure, varying repolarization times of neighboring areas of atrial myocardium, and occurrence of atrial premature beats during the vulnerable period of an atrial cycle. Increases in circulating catecholamines may precipitate atrial premature beats and AF. Ischemia and disease of the sinoatrial nodes also predispose to atrial dysrhythmias by suppressing the SA node and allowing other atrial foci to fire. Epidemiologic data from the Framingham study reveal that heart failure and rheumatic heart disease are the most powerful predictors of AF and hypertension the most commonly associated condition, suggesting that myocardial damage and left atrial dilatation are important precursors of the condition.

CLINICAL PRESENTATIONS

The hallmarks of AF are the characteristic electrocardiographic findings of an *irregularly irregular ventricular rhythm* and *atrial fibrillatory waves*. The fibrillatory waves range in appearance from fine irregular undulations of the baseline to very coarse waves. The QRS duration is usually normal but may widen with aberrant conduction and simulate ventricular tachyarrhythmias. The ST segments and T waves may be abnormal in appearance if there is rapid ventricular response, underlying heart disease, or use of digitalis.

AF can present as a paroxysmal or chronic dysrhythmia, both with and without evidence of underlying heart disease. Its incidence in community settings is about 2% over 20 years. The overwhelming majority of AF patients have underlying heart disease at the time of onset. AF is often a sign of advanced heart disease; onset is associated with a twofold increase in mortality.

Some patients with incidentally discovered AF are asymptomatic; however, if the AF is paroxysmal or the ventricular rate is very rapid, *palpitations* may be reported. If cardiac output falls precipitously, symptoms of *heart failure* may occur. Rapid rate may also lead to myocardial *ischemia* in patients with underlying coronary artery disease. Systemic *embolization* may be the first sign of AF and present as an acute neurologic or peripheral vascular event. An increasingly common cause of transient AF is *coronary artery bypass graft* surgery. Usually, the AF is self-limited and resolves during the recovery period.

A number of acute noncardiac conditions can precipitate AF in the absence of clinically apparent heart disease; these include acute *alcohol intoxication*, decompensated *chronic obstructive lung disease, pneumonia, and pulmonary embolization.* However, AF does not always occur in the context of overt heart disease or an acute event such as sudden pulmonary decompensation. The entities associated with seemingly isolated bouts of AF deserve particular attention because detection is sometimes difficult and therapy is different from most other causes of AF.

Lone Atrial Fibrillation. "Lone" AF (LAF) is used to denote AF in patients without clinically evident heart disease. In about two thirds of cases, the condition presents as isolated or recurrent episodes of paroxysmal AF; in the remainder, the AF is chronic. Studies of military recruits found its prevalence to be about 1 in 10,000. LAF is a harmless condition in young people; they characteristically experience episodes precipitated by emotional stress, alcohol, use of stimulants, or smoking. Detailed investigations have failed to reveal underlying heart disease, chamber enlargement, or risk of embolization. The prognosis in young patients is excellent, with no increased risk of stroke. In those with LAF over the age of 60, there is a moderate increase in stroke risk, believed due to silent progression of atherosclerotic disease. Older LAF patients with hypertension have high stroke risk and should probably not be designated as having LAF but rather as having AF with underlying hypertensive heart disease.

Alcoholic Cardiomyopathy. The early stages of alcoholic cardiomyopathy may present as paroxysms of AF triggered by binge drinking. The distinction between this condition and lone fibrillation triggered by alcohol ("*holiday heart*") may be difficult but is suggested by the finding of cardiomegaly even in the absence of heart failure. Abstinence can halt or even reverse the condition, but continued drinking leads to progression and, in some, chronic AF.

Tachycardia-Bradycardia Syndrome. Also known as *sick sinus syndrome*, this is an important and sometimes subtle cause of AF. The exact cause of this condition is unknown but is believed to be related to diffuse degeneration of conducting system tissue. Patients exhibit sinus node dysfunction, often in conjunction with arterioventricular nodal disease and lack of an adequate escape mechanism. Atrial tachyarrhythmias may alternate with symptomatic bradycardia and sinus arrest. Clinical presentations include palpitations, lightheadedness, and syncope. At times, the first manifestation may be a paroxysm of AF. Identification is most important, because treatment directed only toward the AF may worsen the bradyarrhythmia (see Chapter 28). Paroxysmal AF due to sick sinus syndrome is associated with an increased risk of thromboembolism.

Wolff-Parkinson-White Syndrome. WPW is a preexcitation syndrome that produces a host of supraventricular and ventricular dysrhythmias, particularly paroxysms of AF associated with a very rapid ventricular response rate. In fact, a ventricular rate greater than 200 beats/min in the absence of another cause for AF should make one suspicious of WPW. The condition is believed to be at least partially congenital in nature and characterized by rapid atrioventricular conduction over an accessory pathway (*the Kent bundle*). This anomalous conduction pathway bypasses the arterioventricular node and produces preexcitation, manifested by the characteristic baseline ECG findings of a *shortened PR interval* (less than 0.12 seconds) and *delta waves* at the onset of the QRS. Some WPW patients have normal baseline ECGs and show anomalous conduction only during tachyarrhythmias, making electrocardiographic identification difficult. During rapid AF, there may be a widening of the QRS, mimicking ventricular fibrillation. The reported incidence of AF among patients with WPW ranges from 11% to 39%. WPW is an important cause of AF to recognize, because the AF may actually worsen with digitalis therapy (see Chapter 28) and has the potential to degenerate into ventricular tachycardia and fibrillation.

Apathetic Hyperthyroidism of the Elderly. AF that appears to occur in the absence of underlying heart disease may be due to hyperthyroidism, especially in the elderly. In the most florid form of this presentation, patients may manifest marked apathy suggesting depression or impressive weight loss that may simulate occult malignancy (see Chapter 103). Sometimes, AF is the predominant manifestation. The usual signs and symptoms of thyrotoxicosis are absent. The AF is difficult to control with standard modes of antiarrhythmic therapy but usually reverts to sinus rhythm with correction of the hyperthyroid state (see Chapter 28).

DIFFERENTIAL DIAGNOSIS

AF is only one of a number of dysrhythmias that present as an irregularly irregular pulse. Frequent atrial premature beats, MAT, SVTs with variable block, sinus arrhythmia, and frequent ventricular premature beats all may produce an irregularly irregular rhythm.

The most common cause of AF in the community setting is hypertensive heart disease; however, only those hypertensive patients with evidence of left ventricular hypertrophy are likely to develop AF. The major causes of AF are listed in Table 25.2.

WORKUP

The diagnosis of AF is based on the characteristic *ECG findings* of an irregularly irregular ventricular response and atrial fibrillatory waves. These fibrillatory waves range from barely perceptible irregular undulations of the ECG baseline to very coarse waves. The standard lead best suited for detection of atrial activity is lead V_1, followed by leads II, III, and AVF. Occasionally, the routine 12-lead ECG will show no atrial activity; in such instances, one can check lead V_3R for evidence of atrial

Table 25.2.   Important Causes of Atrial Fibrillation

Paroxysmal Atrial Fibrillation
"Lone" fibrillation
Acute ischemia
Alcohol intoxication and early alcoholic cardiomyopathy
Sick sinus syndrome
Wolff-Parkinson-White syndrome
Acute pulmonary embolization
Acute pericarditis
Acute pulmonary decompensation
Acute heart failure
Any cause of chronic atrial fibrillation

Sustained Atrial Fibrillation
Advanced rheumatic mitral valve disease
Chronic congestive heart failure
Advanced aortic valve disease
Advanced hypertensive heart disease
Coronary artery disease
Advanced cardiomyopathy
Congenital heart disease
Apathetic hyperthyroidism of the elderly
Sick sinus syndrome
"Lone" fibrillation
Constrictive pericarditis
Digitalis toxicity (rarely)

activity or infer the diagnosis of AF based on the characteristic ventricular response pattern and a QRS of normal duration. MAT, paroxysmal atrial tachycardia, atrial flutter with variable block, frequent atrial premature beats, and sinus arrhythmia all produce rhythms that can resemble AF, but the presence of P waves or flutter waves on ECG separate them from AF. If the ventricular response rate is too rapid to reveal atrial activity, *vagal maneuvers* and gentle *carotid sinus massage* can be attempted (provided there is no evidence of carotid artery disease) to slow the rate and uncover any hidden fibrillatory or P waves.

History. The young patient with a paroxysm of AF should be questioned about a prior history of such episodes, excess intake of stimulants and alcohol, emotional stress, fever, heart murmur, and chest pain. Older patients should be queried about preexisting heart disease, hypertension, chest pain, dyspnea, cough, calf pain, leg edema, fever, lightheadedness, near-syncope, loss of consciousness, weight loss, depression, history of heart murmur or rheumatic fever, and any prior attacks of palpitations. A careful drug history should be taken with emphasis on alcohol abuse (see Chapter 228). Any use of digitalis should be noted; however, digitalis toxicity only rarely results in AF. A long-standing history of attacks dating from young adulthood suggests WPW syndrome. The presence of marked weight loss and depression in an elderly patient with unexplained AF points to apathetic hyperthyroidism. The older patient with episodes of altered consciousness may suffer from sick sinus syndrome.

Physical Examination. In addition to noting heart rate, blood pressure, respiratory rate, jugular venous pulse, and other signs of hemodynamic status, the patient should be checked for apathetic appearance, evidence of marked weight loss, cyanosis, goiter, wheezes, friction rub, heart murmur, calf tenderness, asymmetric leg edema, and signs of alcohol intoxication. The most common cause of "silent" mitral valve disease is failure to listen specifically for the murmurs of mitral stenosis and mitral regurgitation. Placing the patient in the left lateral

decubitus position may be necessary to appreciate the murmurs. Only in rare instances are the murmurs of mitral valve disease truly inaudible (see Chapter 33).

Laboratory Studies. The *ECG* often provides useful information beyond identification of the arrhythmia. A ventricular response rate greater than 200 beats/min suggests WPW syndrome, as does a widened QRS due to aberrant conduction; delta waves may be seen within some of the aberrantly conducted beats. The appearance of the fibrillatory waves on ECG provides some hints of etiology. Coarse fibrillatory waves are most typical of AF resulting from rheumatic heart disease and other causes of marked left atrial enlargement, whereas fine fibrillatory waves are more common in cases due to atherosclerotic and hypertensive heart diseases. The ST and T wave segments should be checked for evidence of ischemia, strain, digitalis effect, and pericarditis (see Chapter 20). Advanced valvular and hypertensive forms of heart disease are suggested by finding ECG evidence of left ventricular hypertrophy.

A cardiogram taken after return to sinus rhythm should be checked for a shortened PR interval and delta waves diagnostic of WPW syndrome. Occasionally, preexcitation is concealed on the resting ECG, so that the ECG of some WPW patients appears normal; in such instances, the diagnosis of WPW syndrome can be difficult. Other clues to WPW syndrome include a ventricular response rate during AF of greater than 200 beats/min and delta waves distorting the QRS complex.

A rhythm strip sometimes reveals sinus node disease, but often a 24-hour *Holter monitor* will be needed to detect the episodes of bradycardia and tachycardia that characterize the sick sinus syndrome. *Chest radiograph* is the best simple test for determining heart failure, cardiomegaly, and intrapulmonary pathology. Cardiomegaly may be the only evidence of an underlying cardiomyopathy. *Echocardiogram* provides an excellent noninvasive means of further evaluating suspected valvular, congenital, cardiomyopathic, and pericardial forms of heart disease. However, the cost effectiveness of ordering an echocardiogram routinely in the workup of AF to search for an occult high-risk cause such as mitral stenosis remains a subject of debate. The elderly apathetic patient with unexplained AF requires measurement of *thyrotropin* level to rule out hyperthyroidism (see Chapter 103). Although AF is a very uncommon manifestation of digitalis toxicity, a serum *digoxin level* is probably worth checking when no other cause is apparent and the patient is known to be taking the drug.

In summary, the evaluation can be performed on an outpatient basis if the patient is tolerating the rhythm well and there is no evidence of failure, ischemia, or embolization. A careful history and physical examination, supplemented by ECG, chest radiograph, and, in selected instances, an echocardiogram complete the evaluation in most patients. Patients with AF of unknown cause should be studied further for evidence of sick sinus syndrome, apathetic hyperthyroidism, alcoholic cardiomyopathy, and WPW syndrome.

INDICATIONS FOR ADMISSION

Once the diagnosis of AF is established, one needs to determine if workup can proceed on an outpatient basis. Prompt hospital admission is needed for the patient with evidence of acute congestive heart failure, ischemia, embolization, hypotension, or a very rapid ventricular response rate (more than 150 to 170 beats/min). If there is no hemodynamic compromise, an outpatient workup can commence.

A.H.G.

ANNOTATED BIBLIOGRAPHY

Brand FN, Abbott RD, Kannel WB, et al. Characteristics and prognosis of lone atrial fibrillation: 30-year follow-up in the Framingham Study. JAMA 1985;254:3449. *(A fourfold increase in stroke risk was noted, but patients were older and had more cardiovascular risk factors than patients in other studies of lone AF.)*

Campbell RWF, Smith RA, Gallagher JJ, et al. Atrial fibrillation in the preexcitation syndrome. Am J Cardiol 1977;40:514. *(AF due to preexcitation syndromes can cause very rapid and aberrantly conducted ventricular responses; ventricular dysrhythmias can sometimes result.)*

Culler MR, Boone JA, Gazes PC. Fibrillatory wave size as a clue to etiologic diagnosis. Am Heart J 1983;66:425. *(Coarse atrial fibrillatory waves found most frequently in patients with mitral valve disease and left atrial enlargement; also noted in "lone" AF and hyperthyroidism.)*

Desbiens NA. Should all patients with atrial fibrillation be screened with echocardiography? J Gen Intern Med 1992;7:131. *(A decision-analysis study on the efficacy of routinely screening AF patients by echocardiography for unrecognized mitral stenosis; the benefit was small and screening was not recommended.)*

Engel TR, Luck JC. Effect of whiskey on atrial vulnerability and "holiday heart." J Am Coll Cardiol 1983;1:816. *(Alcohol enhanced vulnerability to AF in patients without clinical evidence of cardiomyopathy or heart failure.)*

Ettinger PO, Wu DF, De La Cruz C Jr, et al. Arrhythmias and the "holiday heart": alcohol-associated cardiac rhythm disorders. Am Heart J 1978;895:955. *(Paroxysmal AF may be a sign of early alcoholic cardiomyopathy and be induced by binge drinking.)*

Forfar JC, Miller HC, Toft AD. Occult thyrotoxicosis: a correctable cause of "idiopathic" atrial fibrillation. Am J Cardiol 1979;44:9. *(Ten of 75 patients presenting with AF of unknown cause were hyperthyroid.)*

Hanson HH, et al. Auricular fibrillation in normal hearts. N Engl J Med 1949;240:947. *(Classic paper describing the entity of "lone fibrillation.")*

Kannel WB, Abbott RD, Savage DD, et al. Epidemiologic features of chronic atrial fibrillation: the Framingham Study. N Engl J Med 1982;306:1018. *(A major epidemiologic study; heart failure and rheumatic heart disease were the most powerful predictive precursors of chronic AF; chronic AF was associated with a doubling of overall and cardiovascular mortality.)*

Kopecky SL, Gersh BJ, McGoon MD, et al. The natural history of lone atrial fibrillation: a population-based study over three decades. N Engl J Med 1987;317:669. *(A retrospective study of patients under the age of 60 showing that lone AF was associated with a very low risk of stroke.)*

Kopecky SL, Gersh BJ, McGoon MD, et al. Lone atrial fibrillation in elderly persons: a marker for cardiovascular risk. Arch Intern Med 1999;159:1118. *(Population-based study in Olmsted County; risk of stroke increased in patients over the age of 60.)*

Mathew JP, Parks R, Savino JS, et al. Atrial fibrillation following coronary artery bypass graft surgery: predictors, outcomes, and resource utilization. JAMA 1996;276:300. *(Occurred in 27% of patients underling coronary artery bypass graft; self-limited but increased length of stay; risk factors identified.)*

Shlofmitz RA, Hirsch BE, Meyer BR. New onset atrial fibrillation. J Gen Intern Med 1986;1:139. *(A retrospective study showing that urgent hospitalization is rarely necessary.)*

26
Management of Hypertension
KATHARINE K. TREADWAY

Hypertension is one of the few conditions in medicine that can be readily detected and effectively treated in the asymptomatic period before irreparable harm is done. It ranks as a leading risk factor for cardiovascular disease and as a major reason for office visits and prescription of medication. Cardiovascular disease is the leading cause of death in the United States. Of these deaths, 83% are caused by myocardial infarction and 17% are from stroke. There has been a steady decline in cardiovascular death over the last three decades, at least some of which is attributable to the lowering of blood pressure in the general population. The frequency and importance of hypertension demand that the primary physician be expert in its management and capable of designing a regimen that is safe, effective, and well tolerated.

PRINCIPLES OF MANAGEMENT

The first tasks are to confirm the diagnosis and estimate overall cardiovascular risk. This guides program design, which includes nonpharmacologic and pharmacologic interventions.

Confirming the Diagnosis and Estimating Overall Cardiovascular Risk

Confirming the Diagnosis. Because treatment of hypertension is likely to be lifelong, it is essential that the diagnosis be well established before committing the patient to therapy. Initiation of antihypertensive treatment should be preceded by a careful evaluation that not only confirms the diagnosis but also rules out secondary causes, identifies any additional cardiovascular risk factors, and assesses presence and degree of target-organ damage (see Chapters 14 and 19).

Classification. The Sixth Joint National Committee (JNC VI) recommendations include eliminating the traditional designations of "mild," "moderate," "severe," and "very severe" hypertension to avoid the misleading notion than mild hypertension is not a significant health risk. Instead, they designate three stages:

- *Stage 1*—diastolic blood pressure (DBP) 90 to 99 mm, systolic blood pressure (SBP) 140 to 159 mm.

- *Stage 2*—DBP 100 to 109 mm, SBP 160 to 179mm
- *Stage 3*—DBP ≥ 110 to 119 mm, SBP ≥ 180 to 209 mm

In addition, a *"high-normal"* category (DBP 85 to 89, SBP 135 to 139) is designated to highlight the increased risk of developing sustained hypertension in this group.

Estimating Total Cardiovascular Risk. Because the goal of antihypertensive therapy is to reduce cardiovascular morbidity and mortality, the treatment program must address the patient's *total cardiovascular risk*, not just the elevation in blood pressure. The degree of total cardiovascular risk will determine the pace, intensity, and scope of treatment. Consequently, estimation of total cardiovascular risk becomes the first priority in program design. The task requires determining the *degree* of *blood pressure elevation* and identifying any other *cardiovascular risk factors* (e.g., smoking, diabetes, hypercholesterolemia, concurrent cardiovascular or peripheral vascular disease, age, gender) and any manifestations of *target-organ disease* (e.g., left ventricular hypertrophy [LVH], retinopathy, nephrosclerosis; see Chapter 19). Although benefits of antihypertensive drug treatment differ in men and women, in meta-analytic study the differences appear to be due to mostly differences in individual cardiovascular risk than to gender differences, underscoring the importance of a personalized risk assessment.

For any level of blood pressure elevation, the presence of such features dramatically accelerates the risk from hypertension. For example, the risk of a 40-year-old man developing coronary disease in the next 10 years with stage 1 to 2 hypertension (formerly known as mild to moderate disease) is about 15%. If that same 40-year-old also has elevated cholesterol, a low high-density lipoprotein (HDL), diabetes, LVH on electrocardiogram, and smokes, risk increases to about 60% (see Appendix).

Even modest elevation in blood pressure greatly increases risk, a very important fact from a population perspective. Most excess cardiovascular mortality from hypertension in the United States derives from patients with stage 1 disease (formerly called mild), accounting for almost 80% of the hypertensive population and almost 60% of the excess cardiovascular mortality attributable to hypertension. Blood pressures in this range are not benign.

Nonpharmacologic Measures (See Fig. 26.1)

The principal nonpharmacologic measures for treatment of hypertension include *salt restriction, reduction of excess weight* (see Chapter 223), *exercise* (see Chapter 18), and use of a *diet low in saturated fat and rich in fruits and vegetables.* These proven measures should be the foundation of every treatment program and also serve as an excellent means of primary prevention. Additional measures include elimination of excess alcohol intake and ensuring adequate dietary potassium, magnesium, and calcium. Behavioral therapies may make a modest contribution to reduction in pressure but do not appear sufficient as the sole means of therapy in most patients. All nonpharmacologic measures should continue even if drug therapy needs to be instituted, because they enhance its effectiveness and allow for use of fewer medications at lower doses.

Salt restriction still ranks as one of the mainstays of nonpharmacologic therapy for all hypertensive patients, regardless of underlying pathophysiology, although the degree of benefit is rather modest when examined by meta-analysis of randomized trials (i.e., 3 to 5 mm Hg for SBP, 2 to 3 mm Hg for DBP). Although it is clear that individuals vary in their degree of salt sensitivity, *African-Americans* and the *elderly*, who tend to have low-renin volume-expanded hypertension, appear to respond particularly well to sodium restriction. Because we currently do not have effective ways to identify those most likely to respond to sodium restriction, all patients should be instructed in either a *no-added-salt diet* (4 g sodium/d) or a *low-sodium diet* (2 g/d), depending on their volume status. Not only may salt restriction alone provide adequate control in some mild cases, but it can profoundly affect the efficacy of pharmacologic therapy. Patients receiving diuretics who had an unrestricted salt intake showed a blood pressure reduction of 4% compared with a 15% reduction for those restricting their sodium intake.

Weight reduction achieves significant decreases in blood pressure, even if ideal weight is not reached. The effect is independent of salt intake. All patients who are more than 15% above their ideal body weight should be urged to lose weight. In the TAIM study, patients receiving placebo who lost 4.5 kg or more of weight had the same reduction in pressure as those who maintained their usual diet and were treated with chlorthalidone or atenolol. The relation between obesity and blood pressure is particularly strong among young to middle-aged adults. In addition, weight loss is important in patients with central adiposity (hip to waist ratio more than 0.85 in women and more than 0.95 in men). Such patients have a higher incidence of hypertension, diabetes, and hyperlipidemia and a higher risk of cardiovascular disease. Weight loss in this group will therefore reduce multiple risk factors simultaneously.

Reduction in Excess Alchol Consumption. Epidemiologic data indicate a relationship between excess alcohol consumption and risk of hypertension. More than 2 oz of alcohol per day significantly increases the risk of becoming hypertensive. Small scale studies suggest that a daily alcohol intake of less than 1 oz may result in a modest decrease in blood pressure. Excessive alcohol intake is a frequent cause of "refractory" hypertension.

Exercise of the aerobic variety helps to reduce weight, improves cardiovascular conditioning and lipid profile, and may help in patients with mild uncomplicated hypertension (see Chapter 18). Patients with mild hypertension given an exercise program of aerobic and circuit weight training three times per week for 10 weeks showed pressure reductions comparable with those achieved with beta-blocker or calcium channel blocker therapy and obviated the need for chronic drug treatment. Candidates for a vigorous exercise program should undergo cardiac stress testing first (see Chapter 18).

Other Dietary Measures. In addition to salt restriction, *other dietary measures* include a *low-saturated-fat* diet rich in *fruits, vegetables,* and *low-fat dairy products,* which can reduce blood pressure significantly in persons with mild hypertension taking no medications. Such diets provide full daily requirements of calcium, potassium, and magnesium, factors believed to contribute to blood pressure control. The landmark Dietary Approaches to Stop Hypertension study demonstrated reductions of 11.4 mm Hg in SBP and 5.5 mm Hg in DBP in mildly hypertensive patients put on such a diet. These benefits were achieved in the context of modest sodium restriction (3 g/d), limitation of alcohol intake, and no weight reduction, indicating that a restricted-fat diet rich in fruits, vegetables, and low-fat dairy products makes an independent contribution to treatment and to prevention. This dietary approach appears to be more effective than prescribing supplementation of individual elements. Meta-analysis of randomized clinical trials of dietary calcium supplementation shows a statistically significant but not clinically significant decrease (1 to 2 mm Hg) in SBP only.

Behavioral therapies such as *relaxation* techniques and *biofeedback* programs have gained popularity in recent years. Small-scale studies suggested a modest benefit, especially in those with mild pressure elevations, but a rigorous meta-analysis of available studies found little specific benefit. Although behavioral techniques were superior to no therapy, they provided no more benefit than self-monitoring or sham techniques.

Pharmacologic Therapy—Basics Issues (Fig. 26.2)

When to Initiate Medication. As note above, treatment is guided by estimate of overall cardiovascular risk. Persons with stage III (severe) hypertension, target-organ damage, or multiple cardiovascular risk factors (especially diabetes) should begin pharmacologic therapy at the outset. For others, pharmacologic treatment can usually be deferred for weeks to months while the life-style modifications enumerated above are instituted. If blood pressure does not normalize within 6 months, pharmacologic therapy should be initiated. Patients at the lowest level of increased risk (e.g., age less than 50 years, stage 1 disease, and no other cardiovascular risk factors or signs of target-organ involvement) can probably delay pharmacologic therapy for 6 to 12 months while nonpharmacologic measures are tried.

Elderly patients with *isolated systolic hypertension* have a significant risk of cardiovascular disease and should be treated. The Systolic Hypertension in the Elderly Program study found a significant reduction in fatal and nonfatal strokes and a lesser reduction in fatal and nonfatal myocardial infarction when the SBP was lowered to *less than 160 mm Hg*. Data in younger patients are scarce, but isolated systolic hypertension is less of a problem in younger age groups.

Goals, Efficacy, and Duration of Treatment. As noted earlier, the reduction in overall cardiovascular risk to prevent heart attack and stroke requires not only reducing blood pressure but also attending to the other cardiovascular risk factors amenable to treatment (e.g., smoking, lipids, hyperglycemia, LVH; see Chapters 54, 27, and 102). Blood pressure should be lowered to least 140/90 mm Hg, with 135/85 mm Hg the minimum goal in persons at greatest risk. The Hypertension Optimal Treatment study found the optimal DBP for reducing cardiovascular risk in middle-aged hypertensive men to be 83 mm Hg and lower for those with diabetes and increased risk of hypertensive stroke. When following patients with home monitoring devices, home blood pressures should generally be less than 135/85 mm Hg, which takes into account any underestimates of true pressure by home readings.

Because there is no cure for essential hypertension, drug treatment has often been viewed as lifelong. Some patients with very mild hypertension may be able to stop medication, provided they continue nonpharmacologic measures and successfully control other risk factors. Even patients with substantial hypertension who require multidrug regimens may be candidates for a reduction in drug therapy. Patients with stage 1 disease whose blood pressure is well controlled with pressures in the 120/80 range for some months may be gradually weaned off medication with the caveat that they should continue to be monitored biyearly for some time as pressures can slowly rise months after stopping therapy.

Selection of Drugs. *JNC VI* recommends that *thiazide diuretics and beta-blockers* are considered in most instances the preferred first-line agents for pharmacologic treatment of hypertension. These agents are the only drugs to date demonstrating significant reductions in cardiovascular morbidity and mortality in large-scale, prospective, randomized, controlled trials. Not only are they of proven efficacy, but their cost is low. Regardless of medical regimen selected, all nonpharmacologic measures should be continued, because they enhance the effectiveness of drug therapy and allow for use of fewer medications at lower doses.

Large scale randomized controlled trials are currently ongoing to determine whether other drugs currently recommended as alternative first-line agents by JNC VI (i.e., *angiotensin-converting enzyme inhibitors* [ACEIs], *calcium channel blockers and alpha-blockers*) are as effective as beta-blockers and thiazides in achieving the desired outcomes. The CAPP Trial has revealed comparable ethicasy for Captopril in reducing cardiovascular morbidity and mortality. The ALLHAT Study suggests that alpha-blocker use may be associated with an increased risk of heart failure. These interim findings suggest that all inhabitors are likely to be confirmed first line agents but that alpha-blockers are not.

Sequencing. The traditional *"stepped-care"* approach of *adding* an additional pharmacologic agent for control has been modified. Like the original approach, a first-line agent is started and *increased* in dose as tolerated, as long as there is a partial response to initial therapy. The dose may be further increased or a low dose of an agent from another first-line class can be added. However, if there is no response to the initial dose, then *switching* to another first-line agent of a different class is recommended rather than adding a second agent. Monotherapy suffices in about 60% to 80% of cases. If the first drug is not a thiazide, it should almost always be the second drug because it enhances the effectiveness of all other antihypertensive agents.

Cost Containment. Without attention to cost, the financial burden of a pharmacologic program can easily become so great that patients fill only part of a prescription or cut frequency or dose, compromising compliance and threatening blood pressure control. The advent of ACEIs, angiotensin II blockers, new calcium channel blockers, and the newer α- and β-blocking agents has greatly improved efficacy and convenience and reduced side effects and adverse reactions, but not without increasing cost in many instances. Until cost is reduced by market pressures and expiration of patent protection, expense is

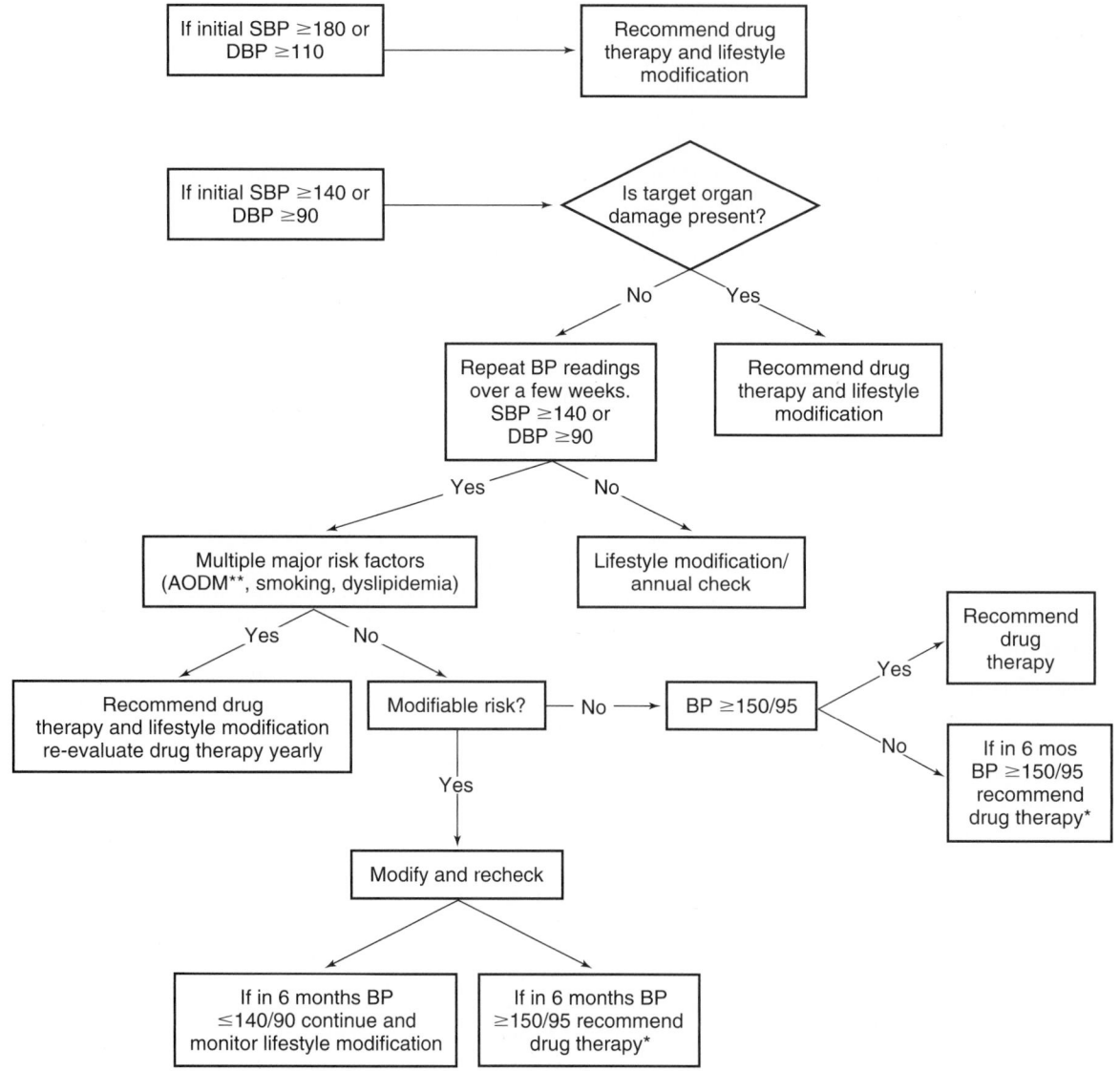

Fig. 26.1. Approach to the patient with stage 1 ("mild") hypertension. (From World Health Organization. Recommendations for management of mild hypertension. J Hypertens 1989;7:689, with permission.)

likely to remain a barrier to use. Primary care physicians must consider affordability in the design of the modern antihypertensive regimen. Thiazides and generic beta-blockers (e.g., propranolol or atenolol) are effective inexpensive drugs that provide a very reasonable alternative to the more expensive antihypertensive preparations. In addition to their proven effectiveness in lowering cardiovascular mortality, they are by far the most cost-effective approach to pharmacologic therapy (Table 26.1).

Additional approaches to minimizing cost include use of a *generic* preparation when available, substituting a *sustained-release preparation* if it is less expensive than a multidose regimen, staying with a less expensive older antihypertensive agents if reasonably effective and well tolerated, and attempting to reduce dose to the minimum necessary. If a second first-line agent must be added, one should always consider prescribing a *thiazide* diuretic, which is capable of markedly enhancing program efficacy at very little additional cost.

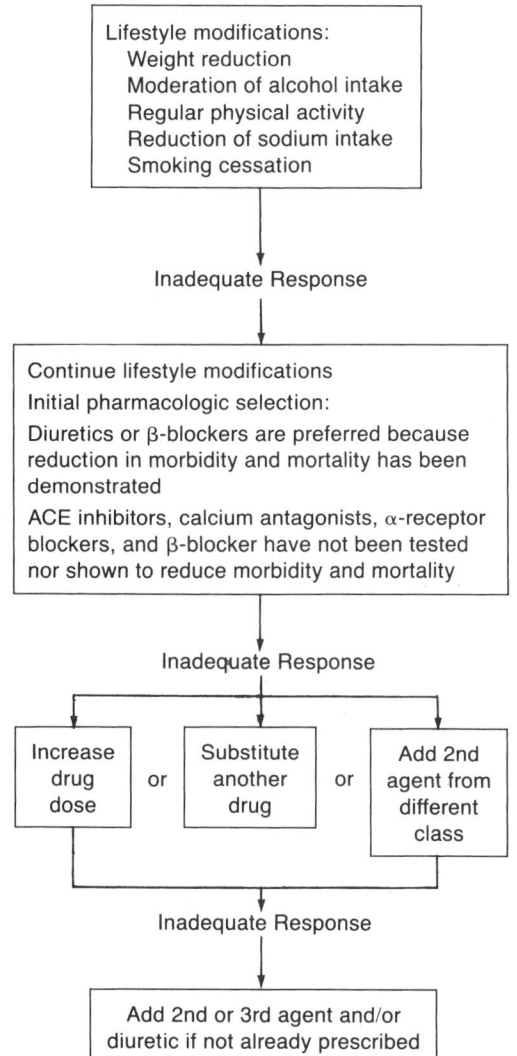

Fig. 26.2. Treatment algorithm for pharmacologic therapy of high blood pressure. (From the Joint National Committee. The fifth report of the Joint National Committee on Prevention, Detection, Evaluation, and Treatment of High Blood Pressure. Arch Intern Med 1995;155:5, with permission.)

Pharmacologic Therapy—First-line Agents

The first-line agents are the drugs of choice because of efficacy and minimal side effects. They may be used singly or in combination. Several, but not all, have been shown to reduce cardiovascular morbidity and mortality. Cost ranges from modest to very expensive.

Thiazide Diuretics. As noted, these continue to be recommended as first-line agents for most patients, being low in cost and of proven efficacy in reducing cardiovascular morbidity and mortality. Compared with other first-line agents for the treatment of stage I hypertension, they produce comparable reductions in blood pressure and LVH. When used at low doses, thiazides remain a safe, well-tolerated, very inexpensive, and effective means of treatment (Table 26.1).

Nonetheless, their use had been declining until recently over concerns raised by a 1990 meta-analysis showing less survival

benefit than expected from the blood pressure reductions achieved. To explain this discrepancy in predicted and actual outcomes, several authorities invoked the known potentially adverse thiazide side effects of hypokalemia, elevation in low-density lipoprotein (LDL) cholesterol, and glucose intolerance. Of note, these side effects occur principally with high-dose therapy (e.g., 50 to 100 mg/d hydrochlorothiazide) and can be avoided by restricting use to modest doses (e.g., hydrochlorothiazide, 12.5 to 25.0 mg/d). Because there is little sacrifice in control by restricting doses to these levels, such doses have now become the standard for thiazide use.

Mechanism of Action. Thiazides enhance sodium excretion, resulting in a reduced intravascular volume and reduced peripheral resistance (presumably by lowering intracellular sodium in vascular smooth muscle cells). Potassium excretion is increased, and uric acid and calcium excretions are decreased.

Adverse Effects. *Potassium wasting* is a consequence of the drug's effect on the distal tubule and is exacerbated by high salt intake. Clinically significant *hypercalcemia* is exceedingly rare, although a decrease in calcium excretion does occur and can be beneficial in patients with osteoporosis or calcium-containing renal stones (see Chapter 135). *Hyperglycemia* is usually mild and infrequent at the low doses currently recommended. Mild *hyperuricemia* may occur but usually not to the degree that necessitates discontinuation of therapy. A transient increase in *LDL cholesterol* has been noted. Thiazides may cause rash, especially a photo-sensitizing type, and rarely may precipitate pancreatitis. Most adverse metabolic effects can be minimized or eliminated by restricting dose to the equivalent of 25 mg/d or less of hydrochlorothiazide.

Monitoring. Checking the serum *potassium* regularly and correction of even mild hypokalemia are essential in a person with underlying cardiac disease, particularly one bothered by dysrhythmias or taking digoxin (see Chapters 29 and 32). Hypokalemia can be prevented by concomitant salt restriction, increased dietary potassium, and, when necessary, the addition of potassium-sparing agents or supplements (see Chapter 32). Potassium levels should be maintained in the normal range. Severe degrees of hypokalemia may cause muscle weakness. The serum *glucose* requires close monitoring when thiazides are used in a diabetic, and the *uric acid* should be watched if the patient has clinical gout. There is no need to monitor LDL cholesterol or serum calcium.

Beta-Blockers. These are highly effective in reducing cardiovascular morbidity and mortality, generally well tolerated, and relatively low in cost. In addition, they are the only class of antihypertensive medication that provides secondary prevention following a myocardial infarction.

Mechanism of Action. Exactly how these agents lower blood pressure remains unclear. They decrease cardiac output, renin release, central sympathetic activity, catecholamine release, and peripheral resistance. Any or all of these may be involved in the means by which they lower blood pressure.

Adverse Effects. Adverse effects include *bradycardia, fatigue, impotence, depression, decreased exercise tolerance, nightmares, and increased airway resistance.* As such, these agents should be used with great care if at all in patients with asthma, severe chronic obstructive pulmonary disease (COPD), or serious depression. Their cautious use in heart failure may actually be beneficial (see Chapter 32). They may modestly in-

Table 26.1. Antihypertensive Drugs

CLASS	DRUG	INITIAL/MAXIMUM DOSE (mg/D)	FREQUENCY	RELATIVE COST
Diuretics	Thiazide-type			
	Hydrochlorothiazide (generic)	12.5/50	qd/bid	1
	Esidrix			4
	Microzide			12
	Chlorthiazide (generic)	125/500	qd/bid	1.5
	Diuril			4
	Chlorthalidone (generic)	12.5/50	qd	1
	Hygroton			22
	Indapamide (generic)	1.25/5	qd	11
	Lozol			26
	Metolazone (generic)	1.25/5	qd	17
	Mykrox	0.5/1		22
	Potassium sparing			
	Triamterene (Dyrenium)	50–150	qd/bid	11
	Spironolactone	12.5–100	qd/bid	10
	Aldactazide			13
	Amiloride	5–10	qd/bid	11
	Midamor			15
	Combination			
	Hydrochlorothiazide 25/ triamterene 37.5		qd/bid	7
	Dyazide			14
	Maxide			15
	Hydrochlorothiazide 50 amiloride 5 mg		qd	2
	Moduretic			18
	Hydrochlorothiazide 25/ spironolactone 25		qd/bid	10
	Aldactazide			14
	Loop			
	Furosemide	20/320	qd/tid	1
	Lasix			5
	Ethacrynic acid (Edecrin)	25/100	qd/tid	10
	Bumetanide	0.5/5	qd/tid	4
	Torsemide (Demadex)	5–20	qd/bid	15
Beta-Blockers	Atenolol	25–100	qd/bid	1
	Tenormin			31
	Betaxolol (Kerlone)	5–40	qd	26
	Bisoprolol (Zebeta)	5–20	qd	32
	Metoprolol	50–200	qd/bid	2
	Lopressor			19
	Toprol XL	50–400	qd	16
	Nadolol	20–240	qd	14
	Corgard			36
	Propranolol	40–240	bid	1
	Inderal			32
	Inderal LA			28
	Timolol	10–40	bid	31
	Blocadren			28
Beta-blockers with Intrinsic Sympathetic Activity	Acebutolol	200–1,200	qd/bid	24
	Sectral			35
	Carteolol	2.5–10	qd	31
	Penbutolol (Levatol)	20	qd	37
	Pindolol	10–60	bid	8
	Visken			59
Alpha-beta-blockers	Carvedilol (Coreg)	12.5–50	bid	92
	Labetalol (generic)	200–1,200	bid	28
	Normodyne			33
	Trandate			33
Angiotensin Converting-Enzyme Inhibitors	Benazpril (Lotensin)	10–40	qd/bid	23
	Captopril (generic)	12.5–150	bid/tid	1
	Capoten			26
	Enalapril (Vasotec)	2.5–40	qd/bid	24
	Fosinopril (Monopril)	10–40	qd/bid	26
	Lisinopril (Prinivil)	5–40	qd	26
	(Zestril)			26
	Moexipril (Univasc)	7.5–30	qd/bid	17
	Quinapril (Accupril)	5–80	qd/bid	28
	Ramipril (Altace)	1.25–20	qd/bid	22
	Trandolapril (Mavik)	1–4	qd	20

Table 26.1.   (Continued)

CLASS	DRUG	INITIAL/MAXIMUM DOSE (mg/D)	FREQUENCY	RELATIVE COST
Antiotension-Receptor Antagonists	Candesartan cilexetil (Atacand)	8–32	qd	36
	Irbesartan (Avapro)	150–300	qd	36
	Losartan (Cozaar)	25–100	qd/bid	37
	Telmisartan (Micardis)	40–80	qd	38
	Valsartan (Diovan)	80–320	qd	36
	Side effects: same as ACEIs but do not cause cough			
Calcium-Channel Blockers	Dihydropyridines			
	Amlodipine (Norvasc)	2.5–10	qd	40
	Felodipine (Plendil)	2.5–10	qd	29
	Extended release			
	Isradipine (DynaCirc CR)	5–10	qd	37
	Nicardipine (Cardene SR)	60–120	bid	40
	Nifedipine (Adalat CL)	30–90	qd	31
	(Procardia XL)			42
	Nisoldipine (Sular)	10–60	qd	27
	Nondihydropyridines	120–360	bid	48
	Diltiazem (extended release)			
	Cardizem SR			54
	Cardizem CD	120–360	qd	35
	Dilacor XR	120–480	qd	35
	Diltia XT	120–480	qd	27
	Tiamate	120–480	qd	52
	Tiazac	120–480	qd	28
	Verapamil (extended release)	120–480	qd/bid	35
	Calan SR			32
	Isoptin SR			32
	Verelan			37
	Covera HS	180–480	qd	35
Alpha-blockers	(1st dose at bedtime)			
	Prazosin (generic)	1–20	bid/tid	2
	(Minipress)			14
	Terazosin (Hytrin)	1–20	qd	51
	Doxazosin (Cardura)	1–16	qd	30
Sympatholytics (central)	Clonidine	0.1–0.6	bid/tid	1
	Catapres			20
	Catapres TTS	1 patch weekly		
	(transdermal)	0.1–0.3		32
	Guanabenz	4–64	bid	12
	Wytensin			24
	Guafacine (Isurelim)	1–3	qd	19
	Tenex			32
	Methyldopa	250–2000	bid	4
	Aldomet			18
Sympatholytics (peripheral)	Guanethidine (Ismetlin)	10–50	qd	18
	Guanadrel (Hylorel)	10–75	bid	22
	Reserprine	0.05–01	qd	1
Vasodilator (direct)	Hydralazine	40–200	bid/qid	3
	Apresoline			30
	Minoxidil	2.5–40	qd/bid	3
	Loniten			17
Combination Preparations (Selected)				
ACEIs/diuretics	Benazepril 5, 10, 20/HCTZ 6.25, 12.5 or 25		qd	24
	Lotensin HCT			
	Captopril 25 or 50/HCTZ 15 or 25		qd	22
	Capozide			28
	Enalapril 5 or 10/HCTZ 12.5 or 25			
	Vaseretic			33
	Lisinopril 10 or 20/HCTZ 12.5 or 25			
	Prinzide			31
	Zestoretic			29
	Moexipril 7.5 or 15/HCTZ 12.5 or 25			
	Uniretic			17
Angiotension-II-Receptor Antagonists and Diuretics	Losartan 50 or 100/HCTZ 12.5 or 25			
	Hyzaar			37
	Valsartan 80–160/HCTZ 12.5			
	Diovan HCT			36

crease insulin resistance and slightly reduce HDL cholesterol, side effects that do not seem to cancel their beneficial effects on hypertension and its associated risks.

The degree of *lipid solubility* has been linked theoretically to the degree of central nervous system (CNS) penetration and the likelihood of neuropsychiatric side effects, such as depression, lethargy, sexual dysfunction, and nightmares. The elderly are particularly susceptible to such side effects. Atenolol and nadolol are the most lipid insoluble, whereas propranolol and metoprolol are among the most lipid soluble. Studies testing these theoretic concerns have shown little difference clinically for lipophilic and lipophobic preparations. However, sexual dysfunction and depression appear to be more common with lipophilic agents than lipophobic ones, although still occurring on occasion with use of the latter.

Preparations. All appear to be equally effective for treatment of hypertension, though differences in their cardioselectivity, lipid solubility, and intrinsic sympathomimetic activity can be used to advantage. *Cardioselectivity* is characterized by greater effect on β_1-adrenergic receptors of the heart than on the β_2-receptors of blood vessels and bronchi. A cardioselective preparation is preferred in patients with COPD or asthma because it reduces the chances of inducing bronchospasm. However, cardioselectivity is a relative quality that declines as dose increases. Furthermore, even cardioselective beta-blockers are not well tolerated in asthmatics and COPD patients with active bronchospasm. *Atenolol* and *metoprolol* are examples of the commonly used cardioselective beta-blockers.

Some beta-blockers have *intrinsic sympathomimetic activity*. Those with such action tend to cause less bradycardia and less disruption of lipid and carbohydrate metabolism. They help maintain cardiac output with exercise, allowing cardiac conditioning. They are comparable with other beta-blockers in ability to lower blood pressure. Examples include *pindolol, acebutolol,* and *carvedilol*.

The beta-blocker *labetalol* is unique in that it has both α- and β-*blocking* actions, with about one fourth the potency of propranolol and one sixth the potency of phentolamine. Its rapid onset of action has made it useful for use in hypertensive emergencies—especially when given parenterally—but its chronic oral use has been limited by tendencies to cause orthostatic hypotension, sexual dysfunction, and hepatocellular injury.

Angiotensin-converting Enzyme Inhibitors. ACEIs are the class of choice in patients with type 1 or type 2 diabetes, because of their demonstrated protective effect on the kidney. In addition, they have been shown to reduce cardiovascular mortality in patients with heart failure and in those with myocardial infarction complicated by systolic dysfunction.

Mechanism of Action. These drugs block the conversion of renin-activated angiotensin I to angiotensin II, a potent vasoconstrictor that also stimulates the production of aldosterone. In addition, they inhibit the breakdown of bradykinin, itself a vasodilator, which also stimulates the production of vasodilatory prostaglandins. At least some of the effects of these drugs are related to their effect on local angiotensin systems in key organs (e.g., heart and kidney).

Adverse Effects. The most troublesome side effect is an annoying *dry cough* that occurs in about 10% of patients. It is mostly nocturnal, described as an irritation in the throat, and

believed to be linked to the effect of the drug on bradykinins. About half of patients who experience the cough find it severe enough to warrant discontinuation of the medication. Switching to another ACEI rarely solves the problem.

Because the ACEIs block the production of aldosterone, they can lead to *hyperkalemia* when used in conjunction with a potassium-sparing diuretic, potassium supplementation, or nonsteroidal antiinflammatory drugs. Potentially fatal hyperkalemia has been reported in diabetic patients with hyporeninemic/hypoaldosteronemic hypertension. Close monitoring of the serum potassium is indicated in such situations.

Although ACEIs preserve renal function in hypertensive diabetics, they can cause *renal failure* in the setting of significant bilateral renal artery stenosis. The originally reported *glomerular injury* and *agranulocytosis* are very rare, except at the extremely high doses used in early clinical trials. However, patients with renal failure are still at risk for glomerular injury when large doses are used, necessitating careful monitoring of renal function. Uncommon side effects include rash, taste disturbances, and *angioedema*.

The blockade of the local renin-angiotensin system in the placenta is thought to be responsible for the adverse effects these drugs have on the developing fetus, presumably by impairing *placental blood flow*.

Preparations. There are a large number of ACEIs on the market, differing predominantly in cost and duration of action. Generic captopril is the least expensive, but needs to be taken at least twice daily, compared with many other preparations that require only once-daily dosing (Table 26.1).

Angiotensin II Receptor Antagonists. This relatively new class of drugs blocks the angiotensin II receptor, thus inhibiting the vasoconstictive effects of angiotensin II and the associated stimulation of aldosterone production. These agents have no effect on bradykinin metabolism, which probably accounts for their being free of the cough that may accompany ACEI therapy. Aside from the lack of cough, their side effects resemble those of ACEIs. No data are yet available on the ability of these medications to reduce cardiovascular morbidity and mortality; consequently, drugs in this class should be reserved for patients intolerant to ACEIs because of cough or angioedema.

Calcium-Channel Blockers. These are generally well tolerated and effective in lowering blood pressure, making them popular antihypertensive agents. Still, there is no evidence from prospective, randomized, controlled trials showing their use associated with reduced cardiovascular morbidity and mortality. To the contrary, this class of antihypertensives has been the subject of significant controversy since publication of retrospective data suggesting an increased incidence of myocardial infarction and sudden death associated with their use. The data pertain primarily to the short-acting preparations (especially nifedipine and its congeners), with speculation that their rapid onset and offset of effect may result in wide swings in blood pressure, increasing sympathetic tone and ultimately myocardial oxygen demand. Currently, the short-acting versions of these drugs are not recommended. Whether these adverse effects extend to the long-acting preparations has yet to be settled, and studies are currently ongoing to try to answer this question. Until then, the long-acting preparations should be used with caution and not as a preferred choice for first-line use, a position they once occupied.

Mechanism of Action. These drugs impede the entry of calcium in heart and vascular smooth muscle cells, resulting in a decreased cellular calcium concentration that reduces vascular smooth muscle contraction and lowers peripheral resistance. These agents also have a mild natriuretic effect, making them potentially useful in patients with sodium retention (e.g., the elderly and African-Americans). None adversely effects lipids or insulin sensitivity, and all reduce LVH.

Preparations and Adverse Effects. There is considerable variation in action and side effects among the classic calcium channel blockers (nifedipine, diltiazem, and verapamil; Table 26.1).

Nifedipine and its dihydropyridine congeners (e.g., *nicardipine, isradipine, felodipine*) are potent vasodilators but cause little net reduction in inotropy. Their main drawbacks are *reflex tachycardia and peripheral edema*, secondary to venodilating effects. As noted above, the reports of increased risk of *myocardial infarction and cardiac sudden death* are associated with use of their short-acting formulations, which trigger reflex sympathetic activation. Occasionally, headache and flushing may be troublesome. In a small number of patients, *esophageal reflux* can become a problem secondary to relaxation of the lower esophageal sphincter.

Verapamil's main disadvantages are *negative inotropy* and *conduction system disturbances* leading to arterioventricular nodal block and bradycardia; the drug should not be used in patients with heart failure or suspected conduction system disease. Leg edema is usually not a problem unless heart failure worsens, but *constipation, headache,* and *dizziness* can be problematic.

Diltiazem falls between nifedipine and verapamil, having mildly negative effects on inotropy and conduction but less likely than nifedipine to cause leg edema. Efficacy is enhanced by addition of a small dose of thiazide diuretic.

Newer agents in this class have been developed and promoted as more "cardiofriendly" (e.g., *amlodipine*); they produce little reflex tachycardia, negative inotropy, or peripheral edema. As noted above, most of the reports of cardiac morbidity and mortality have involved use of short-acting formulations, leading some to speculate that the *longer-acting* preparations and the newer agents may be safer. Definitive data on the relative and absolute safety of the calcium channel blockers and how they compare with other antihypertensive agents will have to await the completion of several large-scale, randomized, prospective trials underway.

Alpha-Blockers. These drugs act peripherally at vascular postsynaptic α-adrenergic receptors, causing arteriolar and venous dilation. Because they affect both the arterial and venous systems, they cause less reflex tachycardia than pure arterial vasodilators (see below). With some of the older alpha-blockers (e.g., *prazosin, terazosin*), profound *postural hypotension* leading to *syncope* occurred 1 to 3 hours after the initial dose, especially in elderly patients and those taking diuretics. This can be avoided by starting with a low dose at bedtime and instructing the patient to stay supine for at least 3 hours. The newer preparations such as *doxazosin* are longer acting and appear less likely to cause first-dose syncope. Postural lightheadedness is still a problem, affecting about one fifth of patients and more

likely as dose is increased above 1 mg/d. These drugs have no adverse effects on lipids; in fact, they mildly raise HDL cholesterol and slightly reduce LDL (both on the order of 3% to 5%). In addition, they reverse LVH. Although useful these agents may increase the rise of heart failure and should not be considered prime first line agents in elderly hypertensive men with symptomatic prostatism(see Chapter 138).

Pharmacologic Therapy—Second-line Agents

The second-line agents are worth considering when the list of first-line agents has been exhausted; however, most have features that make them less desirable. Consequently, they should not take precedence over a first-line drug. Second-line agents are generally reserved for patients who are refractory to combinations of first-line agents or who have special underlying conditions such as renal failure. They include the loop diuretics, distal tubular diuretics, centrally acting sympatholytics, and the older peripheral vasodilators.

Loop and Potassium-sparing Diuretics. Loop diuretics (*furosemide, ethacrynic acid, and bumetanide*) are reserved for patients with evidence of renal insufficiency (creatinine clearance less than 30% of normal) or with allergy to thiazides. They are typically used in conjunction with *minoxidil* (see below).

Distal tubular diuretics (e.g. *spironolactone, triamterene, amiloride*) are weak antihypertensive agents used predominantly in combination with thiazides to spare potassium loss. The combination preparations are widely promoted, but it is best to avoid starting with such a fixed combination until the necessary thiazide dose has been established. Hypertensive patients who must avoid hypokalemia (e.g., those taking digitalis, experiencing ventricular irritability, or suffering from organic heart disease) are the best candidates. Other indications are mineralocorticoid hypertension, thiazide hypersensitivity, and severe gout. These drugs must be used with extreme *caution* in patients with renal insufficiency, ACEI use, or insulin-dependent diabetes with renin deficiency, where risk of serious *hyperkalemia* is substantial. The tendency of spironolactone to cause gynecomastia limits its use in hypertension to patients with primary hyperaldosteronism.

Centrally Acting Sympatholytics. α-*Methyldopa, clonidine, and guanabenz* are centrally acting sympatholytics that reduce blood pressure by stimulating central α-adrenergic receptors, which in turn reduce sympathetic outflow to the heart and vasculature. Because they cause secondary *sodium retention* and generally require the use of a diuretic, they should be considered as second-line agents. Although all these agents frequently cause drowsiness, fatigue, and impotence, lower doses are often quite well tolerated, even in the elderly. α-Methyldopa occasionally causes fever, acute or chronic hepatitis, and a Coombs'-positive hemolytic anemia. *Clonidine* (and sometimes methyldopa) are more likely to cause sedation, dry mouth, and *rebound hypertension* with abrupt cessation of therapy. A slow-release transdermal clonidine patch is available and convenient but very expensive and commonly irritating to the skin. Low-dose clonidine (0.1 mg) given as a once-daily dose before bed is well tolerated in the elderly. Guanabenz and guanfacine are similar to clonidine in action and side effects.

Reserpine is one of the oldest antihypertensive agents, acting as a postganglionic adrenergic antagonist. Its advantages are low cost, good efficacy, and once-daily dose. Significant side effects include *severe depression*, nightmares, drowsiness, nasal congestion, gastrointestinal disturbances, and bradycardia.

Older Arterial Vasodilators. These drugs are rarely used because of the availability of better tolerated and more effective agents. The older arterial vasodilators (e.g., *hydralazine, minoxidil*) act directly to relax arterial smooth muscle. Disadvantages include reflex tachycardia, sodium and water retention and short duration of action necessitating frequent doseing. *Hydralazine* is typically used as a third-line agent in combination with a beta-blocker and a diuretic agent. It can cause headache, dizziness, and a lupuslike syndrome, especially in doses exceeding 200 mg/d. Reflex tachycardia may exacerbate angina. *Minoxidil* is an extremely potent vasodilator that should be used only in patients with moderately severe hypertension uncontrolled by other medications (see below). Both a beta-blocker and a loop diuretic must be used with it. Salt and water retention may be marked, requiring high doses of furosemide. Hypertrichosis is common and has led to the drug's topical use for hair loss. Rare adverse effects include pericardial effusion and even cardiac tamponade.

Special Situations

Refractory Hypertension. Patients are considered "refractory" if they fail to achieve target blood pressure reductions despite full doses of a three-drug regimen.

Etiologies. The most common causes are *poor compliance, alcohol excess, and obesity*. Worrisome etiologies include *renal failure, renovascular disease*, and other secondary causes of hypertension (see Chapter 19). Use of over-the-counter decongestants containing sympathomimetics, nonsteroidal anti-inflammatory agents, and exogenous estrogens are among the pharmacologic causes. At times, the cause is a treatment regimen that contains an irrational combination, such as two agents within the same class, or an *inadequate amount of diuretic* for the degree of salt intake and sodium retention present. Occasionally, the *anxiety* of the office visit results in pseudo-refractoriness, so-called "white-coat" hypertension (see Chapter 19).

Assessment. Medication compliance, weight gain, salt and alcohol excess, and use of other drugs should be observed. Pill counts are the best compliance check. A history of nocturia or ankle edema is suggestive of volume overload, from excessive salt intake or deterioration of cardiac or renal function. Physical examination is performed to check for signs of secondary etiologies (see Chapter 19), target organ damage, and volume overload. If white-coat hypertension is suspected, blood pressures should be taken by the patient at home and at work, after checking patient's technique in the office. *Continuous ambulatory monitoring* may also be of use in this situation (see Chapter 19).

If there is no clinical evidence of a secondary cause, then a check of the serum sodium, potassium, blood urea nitrogen, and creatinine should suffice. The *echocardiogram*, a sensitive measure of target-organ disease, can help differentiate between true refractoriness and pseudo-refractoriness.

Empiric Therapy. If workup fails to reveal a definite cause, the patient should be placed on a 2-g/d sodium/reduced-calorie diet, restricted to 1 oz of alcohol per day, and prescribed an exercise program. A maximal three-drug regimen should be continued (including an adequate diuretic dose). The patient is instructed to monitor pressure at home and should be followed closely. If these measures fail, then before escalating the medication program, one should consider consultation with a hypertension specialist for further consideration of possible causes (e.g., renal artery stenosis; see Chapter 19). Patients who are truly refractory yet free of a serious underlying etiology may respond to the combination of *minoxidil, a loop diuretic, and a beta-blocker*.

Hypertension Associated with Estrogen Use. Elevation of SBP and DBP occurs in most patients receiving estrogen therapy over prolonged periods. Five percent of patients become outright hypertensive, and approximately one half of these remain hypertensive after hormonal therapy has been discontinued. Factors that predispose to the development of hypertension include family history or past history of high blood pressure, chronic renal disease, and hypertension with a previous pregnancy. A patient should be started on oral contraceptive or estrogen replacement therapy only after a careful history has excluded these predisposing factors. Once therapy has begun, continued blood pressure monitoring is required for the duration of treatment. The development of hypertension should prompt cessation of therapy.

Hypertension in Pregnancy. Hypertension that develops during pregnancy may represent either *preexisting hypertension* or *preeclampsia*.

Preexisting Hypertension. Pressure elevations that appear before 20 weeks are almost always due to preexisting disease. Some preexisting hypertension improves during pregnancy because of the hemodynamic changes that occur. Such patients may terminate therapy for the duration of their pregnancy, but pressures should be followed closely as should the urinalysis for early development of proteinuria (a powerful predictor of adverse outcomes). Others require continuation of treatment. The goal of lowering blood pressure in those with preexisting disease is the safety of the mother. There is no fetal benefit to blood pressure reduction; antihypertensive drugs do not cure or reverse preeclampsia.

The usual threshold for initiating antihypertensive medication is a DBP exceeding 100 mm Hg. For DBPs between 90 and 100 mg Hg, *modest sodium restriction* and increased *rest* often suffice. If they do not and blood pressure continues to rise, then beginning *methyldopa or hydralazine* is safe and effective in pregnancy. *Beta-blockers* should be avoided in the first trimester due to risk of growth retardation, but they may be used in low doses later. *ACEIs are contraindicated* due to the dependence of placental blood flow on intrauterine renin angiotensin. *Diuretics* taken before pregnancy may be continued, as may *alpha-blockers and calcium channel blockers*, although recommendations regarding their use remain to be fully formulated.

Preeclampsia. Blood pressure of 140/90 mm Hg or higher, *edema*, and *proteinuria* all appear in the *third trimester*. The typical patient is a very young primagravida, but multiple births, diabetes, and hydatidiform mole contribute to risk. At 17 to 20 weeks of gestation, a resting blood pressure more than 110/75 mm Hg (sitting) or more than 100/65 mm Hg (left lateral decubitus position) suggests an increased risk of developing preeclampsia, because normally the pressure is lower at this time of pregnancy. If DBP rises above 90 mm Hg, *bedrest* is initiated and hospitalization considered.

Most antihypertensive medications safe for use in pregnancy are appropriate for treatment of preeclampsia. Low-dose aspirin does not prevent preeclampsia. *Nitroprusside* is given in severe cases that require hospitalization. The use of volume expansion remains controversial. *Diuretics and salt restriction are to be avoided*, because these patients usually are intravascularly volume constricted. Such treatment might aggravate the condition by further stimulating the renin-angiotensin-aldosterone axis. *Magnesium sulfate* is still the treatment of choice for prevention of seizures associated with eclampsia.

Hypertension in the Elderly. *Isolated systolic hypertension* (SBP more than 160 mm Hg), a common finding in the elderly, significantly increases the risk of cardiovascular morbidity and mortality in persons over the age of 65 years. In fact, SBP is among the most powerful of predictors; treatment lowers the risk. The goals of therapy are to reduce SBP to less than 160 mm Hg and DBP to less than 90 mm Hg.

Nonpharmacologic Therapy. The elderly tend to have low-renin volume-overload hypertension and exhibit considerable sensitivity to salt intake. For those with very modest pressure elevations, one can begin with *salt restriction*, a gentle exercise program, and *weight reduction*, if overweight. Many elderly patients respond well to a 2-g/d low-sodium diet. Reduction of excess *alcohol* intake to no more than 1 oz/d is also important and occasionally overlooked. Nonpharmacologic measures can lower pressure by as much as 10 mm Hg.

Pharmacologic Therapy. When drug treatment is necessary, a *thiazide* diuretic is the drug of choice for initial therapy. It is best to start with a low dose (e.g., hydrochlorothiazide 12.5 to 25.0 mg/d) and increase dose gradually. Increments should be small to avoid rapid lowering of pressure and postural hypotension, which can lead to lightheadedness and falls. In general, the elderly do not tolerate aggressive diuretic therapy or *beta-blockers* as well as younger patients. A review of 10 beta-blocker trials in the elderly found their use often failed to achieve adequate control or reductions in cardiovascular risk. Other drugs likely to cause marked postural hypotension (e.g., alpha-blockers) or daytime sedation (centrally acting sympatholytic agents, e.g., methyldopa, clonidine) are also less desirable. JNC VI recommends use of a thiazide or a long-acting *calcium channel blocker* in elderly patients. Cardiovascular risk reduction with use of calcium channel blockers has been demonstrated in elderly diabetics with systolic hypertension; results in nondiabetics is less impressive.

The African-American Patient. Hypertension is more prevalent in African-Americans (38.2%), more commonly of the low-renin salt-sensitive variety, and more likely to be accompanied by target-organ damage than in whites. The high prevalence of obesity, smoking, and salt excess contribute, as does decreased access to medical care. African-Americans show twice the risk of developing renal insufficiency, even when treated. They respond particularly well to *thiazides, sodium restriction, weight loss,* and *smoking cessation. Calcium channel*

blockers have shown very promising results, though their use greatly increases cost of treatment, which, in turn, might compromise long-term compliance. *ACEIs* and *beta-blockers* are somewhat less effective, perhaps because of the low-renin physiology prevalent in this population.

The Diabetic Patient. Control of hypertension is particularly important in diabetics, because there are risks of stroke, cardiovascular disease, and renal failure are particularly high. *ACEIs* are the class of choice because they decrease proteinuria and slow the progression of diabetic nephropathy. *Calcium channel blockers* also may be protective of the kidney and are tolerated and effective, demonstrating cardiovascular risk in elderly diabetics with systolic hypertension. Although *thiazide* diuretics may slightly worsen glucose intolerance and hyperlipidemia, these adverse effects can be minimized or avoided by using small doses (e.g., 12.5 to 25 mg/d of hydrochlorothiazide). *Beta-blockers* are not contraindicated in patients taking insulin, but a relatively cardioselective preparation (e.g., atenolol or metoprolol) is preferred, because it is less likely to mask catecholamine-induced hypoglycemic symptoms.

The Patient with Renal Failure. Hypertension can lead to renal injury and exacerbate it. Blood pressure control is essential in the setting of renal parenchymal disease. A *reduced protein diet* (40 to 45 g/d) and *salt restriction* (2 g/d) helps preserve renal function and control of blood pressure in patients with azotemia. When the serum creatinine rises above 2.5 mg/dL, sodium retention occurs, which can lead to exacerbation of blood pressure. *Furosemide, metolazone,* and other potent diuretics can help counter this sodium retention and reduce pressure. *ACEIs* reduce proteinuria and can be helpful in the setting of renal failure, unless the cause is renal artery stenosis, in which case they may aggravate renal dysfunction. *Beta-blockers, vasodilators,* and *calcium channel blockers* are also effective. *Minoxidil,* in combination with a loop diuretic and a beta-blocker, may be necessary in refractory cases.

The Stroke Patient. Control of hypertension reduces the risk of recurrent stroke. The main pitfalls of treatment are reductions in pressure that are too rapid or too vigorous, leading to cerebral hypoperfusion. Gradual gentle pressure reductions that preserve CNS perfusion and avoid postural hypotension are the objective.

PATIENT EDUCATION

Patient education is essential to ensuring *compliance*. Being a silent condition, hypertension does not always command the full attention of patients. High cost of medication, high frequency of doses, and drug side effects further compromise compliance. Nonetheless, some educational and behavioral efforts can enhance patient cooperation. Educationally, one needs to review the cardiovascular consequences of untreated hypertension and the ability of treatment to greatly reduce risk. Knowledge of the importance of nonpharmacologic measures is also critical and reassuring to many. That weight reduction, smoking cessation, and decrease in sodium intake may allow reduction or even elimination of antihypertensive medication can serve as a powerful motivating force.

One of the best approaches to improving compliance is to have the patient monitor blood pressure at home. Teaching the patient to perform *home blood pressure determinations* can foster considerable interest in blood pressure control and greatly stimulate adherence to a treatment program. Effective home monitoring may even decrease the need for some office visits.

Medication side effects need to be addressed. Sexual dysfunction, fatigue, and depression have long bothered hypertensive patients who require drug therapy and lead many to stop their medication, often without notifying the physician. It is essential to specifically inquire about potential side effects, including symptoms of sexual dysfunction (see Chapter 229) and depression (see Chapter 227), before and after initiation of a medical regimen and to incorporate the findings into design of the patient's program. Patients may be reluctant to raise these issues themselves. Use of a medication that does not interfere with sexual capacity or mental function (e.g., an ACEI such as captopril) may be indicated (see above).

INDICATIONS FOR REFERRAL AND ADMISSION

Immediate hospitalization is indicated for patients with evidence of *malignant hypertension* (DBP more than 130 mm Hg, retinal hemorrhages, papilledema, mental status changes, heart failure). Referral may be useful for patients with refractory hypertension of unknown etiology (see above), a suspected secondary cause, or worsening renal failure in the setting of adequate control.

THERAPEUTIC RECOMMENDATIONS

For All Patients

- Prescribe a no-added salt diet (3 to 4 g/d) that is low in saturated fat and rich in fruits, vegetables, and low-fat dairy products; consider greater sodium restriction in persons likely to have volume-overload hypertension (e.g., African-Americans, the elderly).
- Advise weight reduction (especially if more than 15% above ideal weight).
- Limit alcohol intake to 1 oz/d.
- Insist on complete smoking cessation (see Chapter 54).
- Prescribe an exercise program (see Chapter 18).

For Patients with Stage 1 Hypertension (DBP 90 to 99 mm Hg, SBP 140 to 159 mm Hg), No Additional Cardiovascular Risk Factors, and No Signs of Target Organ Disease

- Institute full nonpharmacologic measures.
- Repeat blood pressure determinations regularly over the next 6 months.
- If improvement noted (DBP less than 90, SBP less than 140), then continue nonpharmacologic measures and monitor blood pressure every 3 months.
- If no improvement after 6 to 12 months of nonpharmacologic therapy or if it fails to lower the blood pressure (DBP less than 90, SBP less than 140), then add a first-line antihypertensive agent to the nonpharmacologic program.

For Patients with Stage 1 Hypertension Plus Additional Cardiovascular Risk Factors or Signs of Target Organ Disease

- Immediately institute a full nonpharmacologic program.
- Repeat blood pressure determinations regularly over 3 months.
- If blood pressure is not normalized after 3 months, then add a first-line antihypertensive agent to the nonpharmacologic program.

For Patients with Stage 2 Hypertension (DBP 100 to 109 mm Hg, SBP 160 to 179 mm Hg), Especially if Accompanied by Cardiovascular Risk Factors or Target-Organ Damage

- Immediately institute a full nonpharmacologic program.
- If blood pressure not normalized after 1 to 2 months, then add a first-line antihypertensive agent to the nonpharmacologic program and advance pharmacologic program as needed.
- Monitor blood pressure closely.

For Patients with Stage 3 Disease (DBP 110 to 119 mm Hg, SBP 180 to 209 mm Hg)

- Immediately institute full doses of a first-line agent and consider early use of a second first-line agent if necessary.
- If pressure improved but not normalized within 1 week, add the second first-line agent.
- If no response to initial first-line agent within a few days, begin a second first-line agent from a different class at full doses and consider adding a second drug at the same time.
- Prescribe a full nonpharmacologic program.
- Follow closely.

For Patients with Stage 4 Disease (DBP greater than 120 mm Hg, SBP greater than 210 mm Hg)

- Consider emergency hospitalization, especially if there is evidence of acute target-organ injury (e.g., papilledema, retinal hemorrhages, heart failure, altered mental status).
- Patients with a similarly elevated pressure, but no evidence of target organ involvement, can be given oral labetalol in the office to acutely reduce pressure, started on a two- or three-drug regimen, and followed up in a few days.

Initiation and Advancement of Pharmacologic Therapy

- Begin pharmacologic therapy with a first-line agent, preferably a diuretic or beta-blocker.
- Choose agent based on consideration of patient's overall clinical situation (see below) and start with a modest dose (Table 26.1). In most cases this will be a diuretic.
- If pressure does not improve within 1 month of initiating drug therapy, increase dose and recheck in 4 weeks.
- If there is no response despite increasing dose, then switch to another first-line drug from a different class.
- If there is only a partial response, then the choice is either to further increase dose or to add a low dose of another first-line drug from a different class (e.g., add hydrochlorothiazide, 12.5 to 25 mg/d or a beta-blocker).

- Once pressure normalizes, recheck blood pressure at 3- to 6-month intervals.
- If a two-drug regimen using two first-line agents from different classes does not suffice, select a third drug from a new class. A particularly effective three-drug regimen is an ACEI, a thiazide diuretic, and a beta-blocker.
- Consider a sustained-release formulation if it is likely to increase compliance and reduce cost of a daily dose.

First-line Agents: Recommendations for Use

- *Thiazides:* Consider for almost all patients, but especially useful in those likely to have volume-overload hypertension (e.g., the elderly, African-Americans, persons with nocturia or leg edema); provides effective low-cost therapy and enhances antihypertensive effects of beta-blockers, calcium channel blockers, and ACEIs. Limit doses to modest amounts (e.g., 12.5 to 25 mg/d of hydrochlorothiazide) to minimize adverse metabolic effects, particularly in patients with marked hypercholesterolemia, poorly controlled diabetes, symptomatic gout, cardiac arrhythmias, or severe underlying coronary disease. For monotherapy, use no more than moderate doses (e.g., 25 to 50 mg/d of hydrochlorothiazide). Regularly monitor serum potassium in persons with underlying heart disease.
- *Beta-blockers:* Consider for most patients and preferred in those with concurrent coronary artery disease or high cardiovascular risk; not as effective or as well tolerated in the elderly; among the most cost effective. Choose a relatively cardioselective preparation with low CNS penetration (e.g., atenolol) to minimize CNS effects. If some degree of sedation is deemed desirable, consider an agent with some CNS preparation (e.g. atpronol). Prescribe generic formulations (e.g. atroponal, atenolol) to keep costs low. Avoid in patients with severe bronchospasm or nonischemic heart failure. Add a small dose of thiazide if fluid retention develops or if enhanced pressure control is desired.
- *ACEIs:* Consider for most patients; preferred agent for those with diabetes or heart failure; useful choice in those with volume overload, underlying sexual dysfunction, depression, and intolerance to CNS effects of other antihypertensive agents. May be used alone or in combination with a diuretic or a beta-blocker, which enhance their effectiveness; contraindicated in pregnancy and in bilateral renal artery stenosis. Monitor renal function and serum potassium, especially in those with underlying renal dysfunction. Consider generic captopril to minimize expense of use.
- *Calcium-Channel Blockers:* Until more data on safety and efficacy are available, use these agents with caution and not as a preferred class for hypertension. Consider as an alternative to thiazides and ACEIs in patients with volume overload hypertension (e.g., elderly, African-Americans) and in diabetics. Avoid use of short-acting preparations, because of concerns about increased risk of myocardial infarction and cardiac sudden death. Use cautiously in patients with conduction defects, especially if already taking a beta-blocker. Avoid if possible in patients bothered by peripheral edema; short-acting agents contraindicated in heart failure. If use unavoidable, consider an agent with the least known adverse peripheral vascular and cardiovascular effects (e.g., amlodipine). Prescribe a sustained-release preparation to minimize cost and cardiac risk and switch from a short-acting preparation to a long-acting preparation if patient already taking a calcium channel blocker. Obtain cardiac consultation regarding use in persons with known coronary artery disease.

ANNOTATED BIBLIOGRAPHY

Allender PS, Cutler JA, Follmann D, et al. Dietary calcium and blood pressure: a meta-analysis of randomized clinical trials. Ann Intern Med 1996;126:825. (*Statistically but not clinically significant decrease in SBP with calcium supplementation.*)

ALLHAT Officers and Coordinators for the ALLHAT Collaborative Research Group. Major cardiovascular events in hypertensive patients randomized to doxazosin vs. chlorphalidone: the Antihypertensive and Lipid-lowering Treatment to Prevent Heart Attack Trail (ALLTHAT). JAMA 2000;283:1967. (*Major randomized prospective controlled trial; compared to other first line agents studied, doxazosin fails to reduce CHF risk.*)

Appel LJ, Moore TJ, Ovarzanek E, et al. A clinical trial of the effects of dietary patterns on blood pressure. N Engl J Med 1997;336:1117. (*A randomized trial in normotensive and mildly hypertensive patients; a diet rich in vegetables and fruits and low in saturated fat can significantly reduce blood pressure.*)

Christlieb AR. Treatment selection considerations for the hypertensive diabetic patient. Arch Intern Med 1990;150:1167. (*ACEIs lead as the drug class of choice; some possible benefit with calcium channel blockers as well; 78 references.*)

Collins R, Peto R, MacMahon S, et al. Blood pressure, stroke, and coronary disease. Part II. Short-term reductions in blood pressure. Lancet 1990;335:827. (*A major meta-analysis documenting efficacy of blood pressure reduction in reducing risk, especially of stroke but also of coronary disease.*)

Croog SH, Levine S, Testa MA, et al. The effects of antihypertensive therapy on the quality of life. N Engl J Med 1986;314:1657. (*A multicenter randomized double-blind study showing that ACEIs were the best tolerated.*)

Cunningham FG, Lindheimer MD. Hypertension in pregnancy. N Engl J Med 1992;326:927. (*An excellent review; 61 references.*)

Dimsdale JE, Newton RP, Joist T. Neuropsychological side effects of beta-blockers. Arch Intern Med 1989;149:514. (*A review of 55 studies on the issue; concluding there is little evidence for a difference in CNS effects of the lipophilic and lipophobic preparations.*)

Dzau VJ. Renin and myocardial infarction in hypertension. N Engl J Med 1991;324:1128. (*An editorial summarizing the uses and problems with renin profiling, especially as it regards predicting risk of infarction.*)

Edelson JT, Weinstein MC, Tosteson AN, et al. Long-term cost-effectiveness of various initial monotherapies for mild to moderate hypertension. JAMA 1990;263:407. (*Propranolol was best, followed by hydrochlorothiazide.*)

Eisenberg DM, Delbanco TL, Berkey CS, et al. Cognitive behavioral techniques for hypertension: are they effective? Ann Intern Med 1993;118:964. (*A meta-analysis incorporating data from the limited number of available well-designed studies; found no benefit over placebo.*)

Eisenberg DM, Landsberg L, Allred EN, et al. Inability to demonstrate physiologic correlates of subjective improvement among patients taught the relaxation response. J Gen Intern Med 1991;6:64. (*Blood pressure did not go down in this study of patients with borderline or labile hypertension.*)

Estacio RO, Jeffers BW, Hiatt WR, et al. The effect of nisoldipine as compared with enalapril on cardiovascular outcomes in patients with non-insulin-dependent diabetes and hypertension. N Engl J

Med 1998;338:645. *(Data from the Appropriate Blood Pressure Control in Diabetes trial showing ACEI use far superior to calcium channel blocker therapy as regards cardiovascular morbidity and mortality.)*

Farnett L, Mulrow CD, Linn WD, et al. The J-curve phenomenon and the treatment of hypertension. JAMA 1991;265:489. *(An analysis of 13 major studies; diastolic reduction below 85 mm Hg increased risk of an adverse cardiac event, though stroke risk continued to decline.)*

Freis ED, et al. Veterans Administration cooperative study group on antihypertensive agents. I. Effects of treatment on morbidity in hypertension: results in patients with diastolic blood pressures averaging 115 through 129 mm Hg. JAMA 1967;202:1028.

Freis ED, et al. Veterans Administration cooperative study group on antihypertensive agents. II. Results in patients with diastolic blood pressure averaging 90 through 114 mm Hg. JAMA 1970; 213:1143. *(The classic studies demonstrating that treatment of hypertension reduced morbidity and mortality from heart failure, renal failure, and stroke.)*

Graudal NA, Galloe AM, Garred P. Effects of sodium restriction on blood pressure, renin, aldosterone, catecholamines, cholesterols, and triglyceride. JAMA 1998:279:1383. *(A meta-analysis showing significant but modest benefit [3 to 5 mm Hg for SBP and 2 to 3 mm Hg for DBP].)*

Grimm RH, Neaton JD, Elmer PJ, et al. The influence of oral potassium chloride on blood pressure in hypertensive men on a low-sodium diet. N Engl J Med 1990;322:569. *(Supplemental potassium was not sufficient to eliminate the need for antihypertensive therapy in men on a sodium-restricted diet.)*

Gueyffier F, Boutitie F, Boissel J-P, et al. Effect of antihypertensive drug treatment on cardiovascular outcomes in women and men: a meta-analysis of individual patient data from randomized, controlled trials. Ann Intern Med 1997;126:761. *(A major meta-analysis examining the differences in benefits from treatment in men and women; most differences are due to underlying individual risks rather than gender differences.)*

Houston MC. New insights and new approaches for the treatment of essential hypertension: selection of therapy based on coronary heart disease risk factor analysis, hemodynamic profiles, quality of life, and subsets of hypertension. Am Heart J 1989;117:911. *(Excellent discussion of the factors that should guide design of the treatment program.)*

Huang Z, Willet WC, Manson JE, et al. Body weight, weight change, and risk for hypertension in women. Ann Intern Med 1998;128:81. *(Data from the Nurses' Health Study showing weight to be an important risk factor, even modest weight gain, and its loss associated with reduced risk.)*

Joint National Committee. The sixth report of the Joint National Committee on Prevention, Detection, Evaluation, and Treatment of High Blood Pressure. Arch Intern Med 1997:157:2413. *(Latest report of this authoritative consensus group.)*

Kannel WB, Wolf PA, McGee DL. Systolic blood pressure, arterial rigidity, and risk of stroke. JAMA 1981;245:1225. *(The classic paper from the Framingham Study on increased risk of stroke with isolated systolic hypertension.)*

Kaplan NM. Maximally reducing cardiovascular risk in the treatment of hypertension. Ann Intern Med 1988;109:36. *(Redirects attention from level of blood pressure to overall cardiovascular risk; recommends ACEIs, calcium channel blockers, and alpha-blockers from this perspective.)*

Kelemen MH, Effron MB, Valenti SA, et al. Exercise training combined with antihypertensive drug therapy. JAMA 1990; 263:2766. *(Exercise was just as effective as drug therapy and obviated the need for medication in mildly hypertensive patients.)*

Langdon CG. Doxazosin: a study in a cohort of patients with hypertension in general practice. Am Heart J 1991;121:268. *(This alpha-blocker was remarkably well tolerated and improved the lipid profile of hyperlipidemic hypertensive patients.)*

MacMahon SW, Norton RN. Alcohol and hypertension. Ann Intern Med 1986;105:124. *(An editorial summarizing the evidence linking the two conditions and recommending a limit of less than 2 oz/d.)*

MacMahon SW, Peto R, Cutler J, et al. Blood pressure, stroke, and coronary heart disease. Part 1. Prolonged differences in blood pressure: prospective observational studies corrected for the regression dilution bias. Lancet 1990;335:765. *(A meta-analysis of data from nine population-based studies showing a continuous relation between blood pressures between 70 and 110 mm Hg and risks of stroke and coronary disease.)*

Medical Research Council Working Party. Stroke and coronary heart disease in mild hypertension: risk factors and value of treatment. Br Med J 1988;296:1565. *(Excellent benefit analysis of treating mild hypertension; concludes that treatment is worthwhile.)*

Mejia AD, Egan BM, Schork NJ, et al. Artifacts in measurement of blood pressure and lack of target organ involvement in the assessment of patients with treatment-resistant hypertension. Ann Intern Med 1990;112:270. *(Identifies artifactual causes of elevated office blood pressure in patients who seem refractory to three-drug therapy.)*

Messerli FH, Grossman E, Goldbourt U. Are beta-blockers efficacious as first-line therapy for hypertension in the elderly? A systematic review. JAMA 1998;279:1903. *(A systematic review of 10 major studies; finds the answer is a qualified "no.")*

Mosterd A, D'Agostino RB, Silbershatz H, et al. Trends in the prevalence of hypertension, antihypertensive therapy, and left ventricular hypertrophy from 1950 to 1989. N Engl J Med 1999;340:1221. *(Major epidemiologic investigation of data from the Framingham Study showing that the widespread application of antihypertensive treatment is associated with lowered prevalences of hypertension and LVH.)*

National Heart Foundation of Australia Study. Treatment of mild hypertension in the elderly. Med J Aust 1981;2:398. *(Elderly patients with DBPs greater than 95 mm Hg benefited from therapy.)*

National High Blood Pressure Education Program Working Group. Report on high blood pressure in pregnancy. Am J Obstet Gynecol 1990;163:1689. *(Comprehensive consensus report and excellent review of the issue.)*

National High Blood Pressure Education Program Working Group. Report on primary prevention of hypertension. Arch Intern Med 1993;153:186. *(Major review of nonpharmacologic measures; 327 references.)*

Neaton JD, Grimm RH, Prineas RJ, et al. Treatment of mild hypertension study: final results. JAMA 1993;270:713. *(Drugs plus nonpharmacologic measures better than nonpharmacologic measures alone.)*

Oparil S. Antihypertensive therapy—efficacy and quality of life. N Engl J Med 1993;328:959. *(An editorial reviewing the importance of this issue to the successful treatment of hypertension.)*

Packer M, O'Conner CM, Ghali JK, et al. Effect of amlodipine on morbidity and mortality in severe chronic heart failure. N Engl J Med 1996;335:1107. *(A randomized prospective study in patients with ejection fraction less than 0.3, showing no association with worsening failure, life-threatening dysrhythmias, or sudden death.)*

Perez-Stable E, Coates TJ, Baron RB, et al. Comparison of a lifestyle modification program with propranolol use in the management of diastolic hypertension. J Gen Intern Med 1995;10:410. *(A randomized placebo-controlled trial with a 2 × 2 factorial design showing drug therapy superior to life-style modification; patients did not comply with the life-style changes.)*

Preston RA, Materson BJ, Reda DJ, et al. Age-race subgroup compared with renin profile as predictors of blood pressure response to antihypertensive therapy. JAMA 1998;280:1168. *(From the VA Cooperative Study; consideration of age and race better predicted response to treatment than renin profile, underscoring the importance of these factors in choice of agent.)*

Radack K, Deck C. Do nonsteroidal antiinflammatory drugs interfere with blood pressure control in hypertensive patients? J Gen Intern Med 1987;2:108. *(A critical review of available studies, concluding some evidence of impairment, but better data are needed.)*

Rutan G, Kuller LHJ, Wentworth DN, et al. Mortality associated with diastolic hypertension and isolated systolic hypertension among men screened for the Multiple Risk Factor Intervention Trial. Circulation 1988;77:504. *(The MRFIT study, showing an overall survival benefit but increased risk of sudden cardiovascular death in thiazide-treated patients with baseline electrocardiographic abnormalities.)*

Saunders E, Weir MR, Kong BW, et al. A comparison of the efficacy and safety of a beta-blocker, a calcium-channel blocker, and an ACE inhibitor in hypertensive blacks. Arch Intern Med 1990;150:1707. *(The calcium channel blocker was the most effective, but response rates to the others exceeded 50%; all were well tolerated.)*

Schmieder RE, Rockstroh JK, Messerli FZ. Antihypertensive therapy: to stop or not to stop? JAMA 1991;265:1566. *(A review of the evidence for cessation of therapy; 80 references.)*

Schoenberger JA, Testa M, Ross AD, et al. Efficacy, safety, and quality of life assessment of captopril antihypertensive therapy in clinical practice. Arch Intern Med 1990;150:301. *(Reports the experience in 30,000 patients, with mean pressure reduction of 15 mm Hg, efficacy across all age and racial groups, few side effects, and no adverse effects on quality of life.)*

Sibai BM, Lindheimer M, Hauth J, et al. Risk factors for preeclampsia, abruptio placentae, and adverse neonatal outcomes among women with chronic hypertension. N Engl J Med 1998:339:667. *(Appearance of proteinuria early in pregnancy was a strong predictor of adverse outcomes in these hypertensive women.)*

Stewart EM, Deckro JP, Mamish ME, et al. Nonpharmacologic treatment of the elderly hypertensive patients. Circulation 1989;80[Suppl II]:189. *(Nondrug therapies lowered pressures by an average of 9.0 mm Hg; salt restriction was especially effective.)*

Systolic Hypertension in the Elderly Cooperative Research Group. Prevention of stroke by antihypertensive drug treatment in older persons with isolated systolic hypertension. JAMA 1991;265:3255. *(The landmark SHEP study; treatment of isolated systolic hypertension does indeed significantly reduce risk of stroke.)*

Testa MA, Anderson RB, Nackley JF, et al. Quality of life and antihypertensive therapy in men—a comparison of captopril with enalapril. N Engl J Med 1993;328:907. *(Captopril was the better tolerated.)*

Townsend RR, Holland OB. Combination of converting enzyme inhibitor with diuretic for the treatment of hypertension. Arch Intern Med 1990;150:1175. *(The case for an ACEI plus low-dose diuretic.)*

Tuomilehto J, Rastenyte D, Birkenhager WH, et al. Effects of calcium-channel blockade in older patients with diabetes and systolic hypertension. N Engl J Med 1999;340:677. *(A post-hoc analysis of data from the Systolic Hypertension in Europe Trial showing reductions in cardiovascular morbidity and mortality with use of long-acting dihydropyridine calcium channel blocker.)*

Wassertheil Smoller S, Blaufox D, Oberman A, et al. Effect of antihypertensives on sexual function and quality of life: the TAIM study. Ann Intern Med 1991;114:613. *(Treatment with low-dose thiazide or atenolol did not to impair quality of life; sexual function problems occurred only in thiazide-treated patients.)*

Working Group on Management of Patients with Hypertension and High Blood Cholesterol. National Education Program's working group report on the management of patients with hypertension and high blood cholesterol. Ann Intern Med 1991;114:224. *(Provides an integrated approach to treating these major risk factors when they occur concurrently.)*

World Health Organization. Recommendations for management of mild hypertension. J Hypertens 1989;7:689. *(Important consensus view of treatment goals for mild disease.)*

Appendix.   Coronary Heart Disease Risk Factor Prediction Chart

1. FIND POINTS FOR EACH RISK FACTOR

AGE (IF FEMALE)				AGE (IF MALE)				HDL Cholesterol	Pts.	Total Cholesterol	Pts.	Systolic Blood Pressure		Other	Pts.
Age	Pts.	Age	Pts.	Age	Pts.	Age	Pts.								
30	−12	47–48	5	30	−2	57–59	13	25–26	7	139–151	−3	98–104	−2	Cigarettes	4
31	−11	49–50	6	31	−1	60–61	14	27–29	6	152–166	−2	105–112	−1	Diabetic-male	3
32	−9	51–52	7	32–33	0	62–64	15	30–32	5	167–182	−1	113–120	0	Diabetic-female	6
33	−8	53–55	8	34	1	65–67	16	33–35	4	183–199	0	121–129	1	ECG-LVH	9
34	−6	56–60	9	35–36	2	68–70	17	36–38	3	200–219	1	130–139	2		
35	−5	61–67	10	37–38	3	71–73	18	39–42	2	220–239	2	140–149	3	0 pts for each NO	
36	−4	68–74	11	39	4	74	19	43–46	1	240–262	3	150–160	4		
37	−3			40–41	5			47–50	0	263–288	4	161–172	5		
38	−2			42–43	6			51–55	−1	289–315	5	173–185	6		
39	−1			44–45	7			56–60	−2	316–330	6				
40	0			46–47	8			61–66	−3						
41	1			48–49	9			67–73	−4						
42–43	2			50–51	10			74–80	−5						
44	3			52–52	11			81–87	−6						
45–46	4			55–56	12			88–96	−7						

2. SUM POINTS FOR ALL RISK FACTORS

_____ + _____ + _____ + _____ + _____ + _____ + _____ = _____
    Age   HDL-C   Total-C   SBP   Smoker   Diabetes   ECG-LVH   Point Total

NOTE: *Minus Points Subtract From Total.*

3. LOOK UP RISK CORRESPONDING TO POINT TOTAL

Pts.	Probability 5 Yr.	10 Yr.	Pts.	Probability 5 Yr.	10 Yr.	Pts.	Probability 5 Yr.	10 Yr.	Pts.	Probability 5 Yr.	10 Yr.
≤1	<1%	<2%	10	2%	6%	19	8%	16%	28	19%	33%
2	1%	2%	11	3%	6%	20	8%	18%	29	20%	36%
3	1%	2%	12	3%	7%	21	9%	19%	30	22%	38%
4	1%	2%	13	3%	8%	22	11%	21%	31	24%	40%
5	1%	3%	14	4%	9%	23	12%	23%	32	25%	42%
6	1%	3%	15	5%	10%	24	13%	25%			
7	1%	4%	16	5%	12%	25	14%	27%			
8	2%	4%	17	6%	13%	26	16%	29%			
9	2%	5%	18	7%	14%	27	17%	31%			

4. COMPARE TO AVERAGE 10-YEAR RISK

Age	Probability Women	Men
30–34	<1%	3%
35–39	−1%	5%
40–44	2%	6%
45–49	5%	10%
50–54	8%	14%
55–59	12%	16%
60–64	13%	21%
65–69	9%	30%
70–74	12%	24%

These charts were prepared with the help of William B. Kannel, M.D., Professor of Medicine and Public Health, and Ralph D'Agostino, Ph.D., Head, Department of Mathematics, both at Boston University; Keaven Anderson, Ph.D., Statistician, NHLBI, Framingham Study; Daniel McGee, Ph.D., Associate Professor, University of Arizona. Framingham Heart Study. ©1990. American Heart Association.

ECG = electrocardiogram; Pts. = points; HD = high-density lipoprotein; SBP = systolic blood pressure; LVH = left ventricular hypertension.

27
Approach to the Patient with Hypercholesterolemia
MASON W. FREEMAN

Over the last several years, evidence has accumulated demonstrating that treatment of hypercholesterolemia can reduce atherosclerosis and its attendant cardiovascular complications (see Chapter 15). These findings have heightened physician and patient awareness of the importance of hypercholesterolemia. The primary care physician needs to be capable of evaluating hypercholesterolemia and of designing and implementing a treatment program that effectively uses dietary treatment, exercise, weight loss, and, when necessary, cholesterol-lowering drugs.

PATHOPHYSIOLOGY

The production of atherogenic lipoproteins and the induction of atheromatous plaques by those lipoproteins involve distinct pathways. The presence of an elevated serum cholesterol level does not, by itself, guarantee the development of atherosclerotic lesions that will become clinically important any more than a normal cholesterol concentration ensures plaque-free coronary arteries. The formation and subsequent rupture of atherosclerotic lesions, leading to the acute coronary syndromes of unstable angina and myocardial infarction, depend on complex cellular and metabolic interactions. Serum lipids, inflammatory cells recruited to the sites of lipid deposition, the normal cellular constituents of the artery wall, and components of the blood coagulation system all contribute to the pathogenesis of atherosclerosis and its clinical consequences.

Lipoproteins

An understanding of lipoproteins and their metabolism helps guide physicians in evaluating and treating lipid disorders. To circulate in the aqueous environment of the blood, nonpolar lipids such as cholesterol and triglyceride are complexed with proteins and the more polar phospholipids into spheres called *lipoproteins*. The protein components of the lipoproteins are known as *apoproteins*, which play both structural and functional roles in the metabolism of lipid particles. Genetically inherited mutations in either the structure of apoproteins or the receptors that bind them account for many of the most severe forms of hyperlipidemia. The lipoproteins are usually divided into four major classes based on particle density, which is a reflection of their relative protein and lipid content: *chylomicrons, very-low density lipoproteins (VLDLs); low-density lipoproteins (LDLs); and high-density lipoproteins* (HDLs). There are also subdivisions and minor classes of lipoproteins (Table 27.1).

Chylomicrons derive from dietary fat and carry triglycerides throughout the body. They have the lowest density of all lipoproteins and will float to the top of a plasma specimen left in the refrigerator overnight. The chylomicron itself is probably not atherogenic, but the role of the triglyceride-depleted chylomicron remnant remains uncertain. Triglyceride makes up most of the chylomicron and is removed by the action of lipoprotein lipase. Patients deficient in this enzyme or its cofactors (insulin and apolipoprotein CII) have very high serum triglyceride levels and increased risk of acute pancreatitis.

VLDLs are also triglyceride rich and are acted on by lipoprotein lipase. Their function is to carry triglycerides synthesized in the liver and intestines to capillary beds in adipose tissue and muscle, where they are hydrolyzed. After removal of their triglyceride, VLDL remnants can be further metabolized to LDL. The atherogenicity of native VLDL is controversial, but the metabolism of VLDL to atherogenic lipoproteins is not in doubt. VLDLs serve as acceptors of cholesterol transferred from HDL, possibly accounting in part for the inverse relation between HDL cholesterol and VLDL triglyceride. The serum enzyme cholesterol ester transfer protein mediates the process.

LDLs are the major carriers of cholesterol in humans, responsible for supplying cholesterol to the tissues, and the lipoproteins most clearly implicated in atherogenesis. LDL levels are increased in persons who consume large amounts of saturated fat and/or cholesterol, have defects in the LDL re-ceptor (familial hypercholesterolemia), have defects in the structure of LDL apoprotein B, or have a polygenic form of increased LDL. When serum LDLs exceed a threshold concentration, they traverse the endothelial wall and can become trapped in the arterial intima. There, they may undergo oxidation or other modification, may be taken up by macrophages, and may stimulate atherogenesis. The association of serum total cholesterol with coronary heart disease (CHD) is predominantly a reflection of the role of LDL, because LDL cholesterol constitutes the bulk of serum cholesterol in most humans. Many well designed studies demonstrate that lowering the LDL cholesterol can dramatically reduce subsequent coronary events and all-cause mortality in hypercholesterolemic patients.

HDLs are believed to function in peripheral tissues as an acceptor of free cholesterol that has diffused out of cellular membranes. The cholesterol is esterified and stored in the central core of the HDL and may be further metabolized. This reverse transport system may explain why patients with very high HDL levels have a reduced risk of developing CHD, even if their LDL levels are elevated. *Apolipoprotein AI* is the major apoprotein of HDL, and its level also inversely correlates with the risk of CHD. Women have higher levels of HDL cholesterol than men, in part because of their higher estrogen levels. Exercise increases HDL, whereas obesity, hypertriglyceridemia, and smoking lower HDL. The HDL cholesterol concentration is the single most powerful lipid predictor of CHD risk, but treatments designed to raise HDL cholesterol levels are limited and the significance of such interventions on coronary disease outcomes remains uncertain.

Dietary Influences

Dietary fat and cholesterol have a substantial influence on serum and LDL cholesterol levels. Saturated fat intake has a greater effect on serum cholesterol than does dietary cholesterol intake. For each increase in percentage of total calories contributed by saturated fats, serum cholesterol increases by a factor of 2.16, whereas the serum cholesterol increase is only 0.068 for each percentage increase in dietary cholesterol. This relationship is summarized in the equation of Hegsted:

$$\text{Change in total cholesterol} = 2.16 \, \text{delta S} - 1.65 \, \text{delta P} + 0.068 \, \text{delta C}$$

where delta S, delta P, and delta C are the changes in the percentage of total calories contributed by saturated fats, polyunsaturated fats, and cholesterol, respectively. Fats are characterized by their constituent fatty acid composition. The fatty acids are characterized as saturated, polyunsaturated, or monounsaturated. The state of saturation refers to the number of carbon–carbon double bonds contained in the fatty acid.

Table 27.1. Lipoprotein Composition

LIPOPROTEIN	PROTEIN	CHOLESTEROL	CHOLESTEROL ESTER %	PHOSPHOLIPID	TG
VLDL	10.4	5.8	13.9	15.2	53.4
IDL	17.8	6.5	22.5	21.7	31.4
LDL	25.0	8.6	41.9	20.9	3.5
HDL$_2$	42.6	5.2	20.3	30.1	2.2
HDL$_3$	54.9	2.6	16.1	25.0	1.4
Chylomicrons	1–2	1–3	2–4	3–8	80–95

Values are % composition by weight. VLDL = very low density lipoprotein; IDL = intermediate density lipoprotein; LDL = low density lipoprotein; HDL = high density lipoprotein; TG = trygliceride.

Saturated Fatty Acids can raise LDL cholesterol, in part by altering the LDL receptor's catabolic activity. The long-chain saturated fatty acids common to the American diet—lauric (12 carbons), myristic (14 carbons), palmitic (16 carbons), and stearic (18 carbons)—have no double bonds and are not essential for human growth and development. Not all saturated fatty acids trigger rises in LDL cholesterol. For example, stearic acid and some shorter chain fatty acids (caproic and caprylic) do not. In the typical American diet, about one third of the saturated fat content of the diet derives from *meat* and meat products, whereas another third comes from *dairy products* and eggs, and 10% from baked goods. Vegetable oils also may contain saturated fat (see Appendix I), especially the so-called "*tropical oils*" (coconut and palm) and cocoa butter, which are commonly used in commercial food preparation. Even when unsaturated oils (see below) are used in processed foods, they usually undergo "*partial hydrogenation*," which adds back hydrogens to the carbon–carbon bonds, eliminating some double bonds and making the fatty acids more saturated. This saturation process is performed to make these oils more solid at room temperature, but it also makes them more hypercholesterolemic.

Monounsaturated Fatty Acids are present in all animal and vegetable fats. The most common dietary form is *oleic acid*, plentiful in peanuts, almonds, olives, and avocados. Oils derived from these sources neither raise nor lower LDL cholesterol by themselves, although cholesterol and CHD risk fall if they are used as substitutes for saturated fat. Mediterranean diets rich in *olive oil* and other sources of monounsaturated fatty acids appear to be relatively nonatherogenic, even though they are not low in fat.

Polyunsaturated Fatty Acids (PUFAs), unlike saturated and monounsaturated fatty acids, are not synthesized by the body. They must be present in the diet and are referred to as *essential fatty acids*. The location of the first double bond from the methyl end of the molecule determines the nomenclature of the PUFAs. The major dietary fatty acids contain either an n-6 or n-3 first double bond. *Linoleic* and *arachidonic acids* are the common Ω-6 PUFAs, found in considerable quantities in *liquid vegetable oils* (sunflower, safflower, corn, and soybean). The Ω-3 fatty acids are represented by linoleic acid (found in canola oil and leafy vegetables) and the *omega-3 fish oils* (eicosapentanoic and docosahexanoic acids). The latter attracted considerable interest when epidemiologic studies found a link between their consumption and reduced rates of CHD mortality.

When vegetable oils rich in PUFAs are subjected to *partial hydrogenation* in commercial food processing, not only do some of their double bonds get converted to single bonds, but others shift from the "*cis*" configuration into the "*trans*" configuration, which increases their atherogenicity and associated CHD risk. Intake of such substances increases LDL cholesterol, lipoprotein(a) (LPa), and triglycerides and reduces HDL cholesterol. Data from The Nurses' Health Study suggest that replacing *trans* unsaturated fats in the diet with polyunsaturated fats can reduce CHD risk by nearly 60%, a much greater reduction than even that achieved by reducing overall fat intake.

Cholesterol. As the Hegsted formula indicates, dietary cholesterol has a much smaller effect than saturated fatty acids on raising total cholesterol. For every additional 100 mg of dietary cholesterol consumed per day, the serum cholesterol will rise by about 8 to 10 mg/dL. However, *organ meats* (e.g., brain, kidney, heart, sweetbreads) and *egg yolks* are concentrated sources of dietary cholesterol (see Appendix II) and can have a substantial impact on serum cholesterol levels. Although *shellfish* contain moderate amounts of cholesterol, they have relatively small amounts of saturated fat and are sources of Ω-3 PUFAs. Cholesterol is absent from food derived from plants. Plant sterols can actually block cholesterol absorption in the intestine, and a commercially available margarine containing the plant sterol sitostanol is now available as a cholesterol-lowering agent. It reduces serum cholesterol levels by up to 10% to 15%.

Other dietary factors. *Low-fat high-carbohydrate diets* can *reduce HDL* cholesterol and *increase triglycerides*. Especially in obese persons, increased total caloric intake may induce overproduction of VLDL triglycerides while reducing HDL cholesterol levels. Data from The Nurses' Health Study suggest that substituting carbohydrate for saturated fat in the diet may reduce CHD risk by about 15% but substituting carbohydrate for polyunsaturated fat may increase CHD risk by over 50%. There is no evidence that either *dietary carbohydrate* (whether simple sugars or complex ones) or *protein* significantly affects LDL cholesterol.

The *fiber* content of food has generated much interest. *Insoluble fiber* (typically cellulose found in wheat bran) has no cholesterol-lowering effect, although it is beneficial for lowering the risk of diverticular disease and colon cancer (see Chapter 65). *Soluble fiber* (pectins, certain gums, psyllium) has received much attention in the lay press stimulated by claims about *oat bran*, which contains the gum beta-glycan. Initial studies were encouraging, but subsequent data suggested the cholesterol decreases observed were no greater than those found with use of insoluble fiber and probably resulted from replacement of dietary fat in the diet rather than from a direct effect on lipid metabolism. When studied in patients already taking a low-fat diet, high soluble fiber intake appeared to lower serum cholesterol by a modest amount (3% to 7%).

WORKUP

Diagnosis. The diagnosis of hypercholesterolemia should always be based on *repeat measurements* of serum lipids, because combined analytic and biologic variations in serum lipids range from 10% to 20%. A single measurement should never be viewed as sufficient for a diagnosis of hypercholesterolemia. A *venous sample* processed in a laboratory meeting Centers for Disease Control and Prevention standards for cholesterol determination (see Chapter 15) is recommended.

Once an elevated (more than 200 mg/dL) total cholesterol level is confirmed, then follow-up and further investigation are based on degree of elevation and presence of other CHD risk factors. Patients considered appropriate for lipoprotein analysis are those with a *total cholesterol level higher than 240 mg/dL* or a total cholesterol level of 200 to 239 mg/dL plus established CHD or two other CHD risk factors (Table 27.2). In such individuals, a *fasting* venous sample for determination of serum cholesterol, *HDL cholesterol,* and *triglycerides* is necessary for characterization of the lipid disorder and design of therapy.

Table 27.2. Initial Classification and Recommended Follow-up Based on Total Cholesterol

Classification, mg/dL

<200	Desirable blood cholesterol
200–239	Borderline-high blood cholesterol
≥240	High blood cholesterol

Recommended Follow-Up

Total cholesterol, <200 mg/dL	Repeat within 5 yr
Total cholesterol, 200–239 mg/dL	
Without definite CHD or two other CHD risk factors (one of which can be male sex)	Dietary information and recheck annually
With definite CHD or two other CHD risk factors (one of which can be male sex)	Lipoprotein analysis; further action based on LDL cholesterol level
Total cholesterol ≥ 240 mg/dL	

CHD, coronary heart disease; LDL, low-density lipoprotein.

From Report of the National Cholesterol Education Program. Expert Panel on Detection, Evaluation, and Treatment of High Blood Cholesterol in Adults. Arch Intern Med 1988;148:36, with permission.

Some patients present with HDL cholesterol having already been measured as part of the lipid-screening effort. The growing appreciation of a low HDL cholesterol (less than 35 mg/dL) as a CHD risk factor has led to recommendations for including it in lipid screening (see Chapter 15). Only if the measurement was performed in a manner ensuring its accuracy (see Chapter 15) should it be used in the initial determination of CHD risk.

Otherwise, it is best to wait until the HDL cholesterol is remeasured as part of the formal lipoprotein evaluation.

With measurement of total and HDL cholesterol and triglyceride levels, it is possible to *estimate the VLDL* level and *calculate the LDL cholesterol* concentration using the formula:

LDL cholesterol = total cholesterol − [HDL cholesterol + triglyceride/5]

The TG/5 factor represents a close estimate of VLDL cholesterol and derives from the observation that VLDL cholesterol is usually 20% of the serum triglyceride value. The validity of this formula for estimating LDL cholesterol has been confirmed by direct LDL cholesterol measurement and remains fairly accurate so long as the total triglyceride is less than 400 mg/dL. A *fasting* sample is required for accurate results, because chylomicrons appearing in the blood after a meal do not contain the same ratio of triglyceride to cholesterol found in VLDL. If the triglyceride level is greater than 400 mg/dL, the LDL cholesterol can be determined accurately only by methods available to a lipid research laboratory, although direct LDL assays of varying quality have recently become available for use on routine chemical autoanalyzers.

Excluding Secondary Causes. Before embarking on a treatment plan, one must exclude conditions that might secondarily lead to hyperlipidemia. The most important are *hypothyroidism, nephrotic syndrome,* and *diabetes* (Table 27.3), best screened for by a serum thyroid-stimulating hormone, urine dipstick for protein, and serum glucose, respectively (see Chapters 93, 104,

Table 27.3. Classification of Lipoprotein Disorders

NAME	PRIMARY DISORDER	SECONDARY DISORDER	LIPOPROTEIN INVOLVED	XANTHOMAS
Increased Triglycerides and Cholesterol				
Combined hyperlidemia	Unknown	Hypothyroidism	LDL and VLDL	None
Remnant hyperlipidemia	Familial dysbetalipoproteinemia	Hypothyroidism SLE	IDL	Tuberous, Palmar Tuboeruptive
Increased Cholesterol				
Familial hypercholesterolemia	LDL receptor defects		LDL	Tendon
Combined hyperlipidemia	Unknown	Hypothyroidism Nephrotic syndrome	LDL	
Polygenic hypercholesterolemia	Unknown	Hypothyroidism	LDL	
Familial hyperalphalipoproteinemia	Unknown		HDL	
Increased Triglycerides				
Exogenous hypertriglyceridemia	Lipoprotein lipase (LPL) deficiency Apo C-II deficiency LPL inhibition	SLE	Chylomicrons	Tuboeruptive
Endogenous hypertriglyceridemia (hyper TG)	Familial hypertriglycidemia	Diabetes Dysglobulinemia Uremia Nephrotic syndrome Lipodystrophies Steroids Alcohol Estrogen Hypothyroidism	VLDL	Usually None
Mixed hypertriglyceridemia	Familial hyperTG LPL deficiency Apo C-II deficiency	(Same as for endogenous hypertriglyceridemia)	VLDL and chylomicrons	Tuboeruptive

IDL-intermediate density lipoprotein

Table 27.4.   CHD Risk Associated With Lipoprotein Cholesterol Abnormalities[a]

LIPOPROTEIN-CHOLESTEROL	LEVEL (MG/DL)	ESTIMATED CHD RISK
LDL cholesterol	<130	Low
	130–159	Moderate
	≥160	High
HDL cholesterol	>65 (and total cholesterol/HDL ratio > 4.5)	Low
	<35 (and total cholesterol/HDL ratio > 4.5)	Moderate-high
VLDL cholesterol	50–100 (or fasting triglycerides 250–500)	Low
	>100 (or fasting triglycerides > 500)	?

[a]Presence of additional CHD risk factors greatly increase risk for any level of lipoprotein cholesterol.

and 130). Drugs can affect lipid levels as well, with LDL elevations occurring with *thiazide* use and triglyceride levels rising with *beta-blockers*. Postmenopausal *estrogen replacement* lowers LDL and increases HDL and triglyceride.

Classification. The original *Fredrickson classification* scheme is of limited utility now that a better understanding of the genetics of these diseases has emerged. However, no unified classification of comparable simplicity has replaced it. For most clinical purposes, it is probably simplest to separate patients into three broad categories: those with *elevated cholesterol, elevated cholesterol and triglyceride, or elevated triglyceride only*. Table 27.3 summarizes the likely diagnoses under these broad categories. The possibility of a genetic disorder should be considered if extremes of any lipid level are encountered or if there is a history of premature CHD in the patient or family. Classification by risk stratification is also helpful for both patient and physician (see below and Tables 27.4 and 27.5).

PRINCIPLES OF MANAGEMENT

The goals are to reduce coronary morbidity and mortality. Both *primary prevention* (reducing risk of having a first coronary event) and *secondary prevention* (reducing risk of a new coronary event in a person with established CHD) are sought.

Table 27.5.   CHD Risk Factors and CHD Risk Status

Risk Factors Other Than Elevated LDL Cholesterol Level
Age > 45 for male; >55 or premature menopause for female without estrogen replacement
Family history of premature CHD (definite myocardial infarction or sudden death in first-degree male relative before age 55 or before 65 in female first-degree relative)
Current cigarette smoking
Hypertension (systolic >140 or diastolic >90)
Low HDL cholesterol (<35 mg/dL)
Diabetes mellitus

CHD Risk Status
Highest
 Clinically evident CHD or other atherosclerotic disease (peripheral arterial insufficiency, symptomatic carotid artery disease)
 No CHD but two or more CHD risk factors in addition to hypercholesterolemia
 No CHD and fewer than two other CHD risk factors in addition to hypercholesterolemia
 No CHD, no risk factors
Lowest

Adapted from Summary of the Second Report of the National Cholesterol Education Program Expert Panel on Detection, Evaluation, and Treatment of High Blood Cholesterol in Adults. JAMA 1993;269:3015, with permission.

The most impressive reductions in risk are achieved in patients at greatest risk (see below).

The growing appreciation for the importance of lipid abnormalities and for the efficacy of treatment have stimulated the National Institutes of Health to sponsor a National Cholesterol Education Program (NCEP). It convened an expert panel, which has formulated consensus treatment recommendations, many of which are included below. The approach to treatment of hyperlipidemia is guided by an *assessment of total CHD risk*, not just the lipid abnormality. For a given degree of LDL cholesterol elevation, the threshold for initiation of therapy decreases and the intensity of therapy increases with increasing CHD risk. Dietary modification, complemented by exercise and weight reduction, is the core of the lipid treatment program, with pharmacologic therapy reserved for those at higher risk and for persons failing behavioral therapies.

Risk Assessment as a Guide to Selection of Therapy

With benefit from treatment of hypercholesterolemia closely linked to the degree of pretreatment CHD risk, a careful assessment of that risk is imperative to deciding whom to treat, when to treat, and how aggressively to treat. The CHD risk assessment should be a comprehensive one, extending beyond lipid levels to include consideration of *blood pressure, smoking, diabetes, family history of premature CHD, age, sex, and presence of established CHD or other atherosclerotic disease* (e.g., peripheral arterial insufficiency, symptomatic carotid disease). The increasing awareness of elevated HDL cholesterol as a factor in reducing CHD risk has led to its designation as a "negative risk factor." Conversely, an *HDL cholesterol serum level less than 35 mg/dL* comes onto the list of positive risk factors (Table 27.5).

A gradient of CHD risk has been defined by the NCEP expert panel, taking into account degree of LDL elevation and presence of other CHD risk factors (Tables 27.4 and 27.5). For a given elevation in LDL cholesterol level, patients considered at highest risk are those with established CHD or other atherosclerotic disease. Next come patients without CHD who have two or more CHD risk factors, followed by those having no CHD and fewer than two CHD risk factors.

The NCEP treatment recommendations follow directly from the degree of estimated CHD risk. Dietary modification is the sole mode of therapy for patients at the lower end of the CHD risk spectrum, whereas pharmacologic measures are reserved for patients at higher risk or for those who fail dietary intervention (Table 27.6). Additional considerations include possible adverse effects of long-term pharmacologic therapy (an issue when deal-

Table 27.6. Treatment Recommendations

PATIENT CATEGORY	INITIAL LDL LEVEL (mg/dL)	LDL GOAL (mg/dL)
	Dietary Therapy	
No CHD, <2 risk factors	>160	<160
No CHD, ≥2 risk factors	>130	<130
With CHD	>100	<100
	Add Drug Treatment	
No CHD, <2 risk factors	>190	<160
No CHD, ≥2 risk factors	>160	<130
With CHD	>130	<100

Adapted from Summary of the Second Report of the National Cholesterol Education Program Expert Panel on Detection, Evaluation, and Treatment of High Blood Cholesterol in Adults. JAMA 1993;269:3015, with permission.

ing with young persons) and appropriateness of the patient for treatment (an issue in the frail elderly and seriously ill).

Dietary Modification, Exercise and Weight Loss

Dietary modification remains the cornerstone of treatment, effective for both treatment and prevention of hypercholesterolemia. As suggested by the Hegsted equation (see above), the greatest contributor to hypercholesterolemia is the consumption of saturated fat, with excess cholesterol contributing to a lesser extent. *Reductions in total fat, saturated fat, partially hydrogenated unsaturated fatty acids,* and dietary *cholesterol* are recommended for all adults. Not only is it important to reduce total fat in the diet, but perhaps even more critical is *substituting* foods that provide *polyunsaturated and monounsaturated fats* for those rich in saturated and *trans* unsaturated fat.

In conjunction with exercise and weight loss (which contribute to reductions in lipid levels and ameliorate other cardiac risk factors), dietary modification provides an excellent nonpharmacologic means of improving the patient's lipid profile and reducing CHD risk. The adverse effects are nil, making it the safest of treatments for hypercholesterolemia and especially well suited for persons with only a modest increase in CHD risk (e.g., hypercholesterolemic young men and premenopausal women with no other CHD risk factors). Even for high-risk patients, diet is central to the treatment program, having an additive effect.

Efficacy. Decreases in intake of cholesterol and saturated fat in controlled settings can reduce total and LDL cholesterol by 15% to 30%, but the reductions average about 10% when similarly intensive dietary programs are prescribed for outpatient use. Although reductions in total and saturated fat are important, substituting polyunsaturates and monounsaturates for saturated and unsaturated fats appear to be as or even more important in reducing CHD risk by dietary intervention. Data from the Nurses' Health Study provide the best available estimates of expected changes in CHD risk from various dietary substitutions:

- Substituting polyunsaturated fat for saturated fat: 42% *decrease* in CHD risk (for every 5% of total calories);
- Substituting polyunsaturated fat for *trans* unsaturated fat: 57% *decrease* in CHD risk (for every 2% of total calories);
- Substituting carbohydrate for saturated fat: 17% *decrease* in CHD risk;
- Substituting carbohydrate for polyunsaturated fat and monounsaturated fat: 20% to 60% *increase* in CHD risk.

Note that not all substitutions are beneficial. Simply substituting carbohydrate for all fat might not be the best dietary strategy for reducing CHD, because beneficial polyunsaturates would also be eliminated as well.

The net effects of various dietary substitutions are related in part to their effects on CHD risk factors, including HDL cholesterol, LDL cholesterol, triglycerides, lipoproteins, and platelets and clotting factors. For example, substituting total fat intake with carbohydrate may produce a small (approximately 5%) reduction in HDL cholesterol, although the overall total-to-HDL cholesterol ratio still improves. Caloric and fat restrictions are also effective in lowering triglyceride levels, an effect enhanced by prohibition of alcohol. Reductions in CHD risk parallel the degree of cholesterol lowering and reduction of other risk factors.

Response to dietary modification is determined to some extent by the etiology of the hypercholesterolemia. When the phase I diet (see below) is prescribed for outpatient use in patients other than those with monogenic hypercholesterolemia, the total and LDL cholesterol levels fall by 5% to 15%. Typically, the total serum cholesterol level will fall to 140 to 160 mg/dL in normal individuals consuming a very low-fat (5% to 10% of total calories) diet. More modest but still useful reductions can be expected from less stringent diets. In the setting of metabolic ward study, there is wide variability in the magnitude of LDL cholesterol reductions achieved by lowering saturated fat intake, ranging from less than 5% to over 50%. Patients with severe monogenic hypercholesterolemias rarely respond to diet alone, whereas other individuals consuming a high-fat diet may demonstrate marked benefit.

Phased Approach to Dietary Modification. The phased approach, as exemplified by the American Heart Association's three-phase dietary plan, maximizes adherence. Total fat, saturated fat, and cholesterol intake are gradually reduced with partial replacement by polyunsaturated fats (which by the Hegsted equation have a modest cholesterol-lowering effect). Excess dietary saturated and trans unsaturated fats are supplanted by use of polyunsaturated and monounsaturated fats and by complex carbohydrates (fruits, vegetables, cereals, pasta, grains, and legumes).

Given the high prevalence of undesirable cholesterol levels in the U.S. population, it is recommended that all Americans adopt the *phase I diet* (Table 27.7):

- *Total fat* as a percentage of total calories is *reduced to 30%* from an average 40% to 45%;
- *Saturated fat is reduced* to 10% of total calories;
- *Polyunsaturated fat is increased* to 10% of calories;
- *Dietary cholesterol intake is reduced* from 500 to 300 mg/d;
- *Protein* is held constant;
- The *Ω*-6 PUFAs found in vegetable oils should not exceed 10% of calories, because they may lower HDL cholesterol.

Table 27.7. American Heart Association Three-Phase Dietary Plan

	AVERAGE U.S. DIET	PHASE I	PHASE II	PHASE III
Total fat (as % total calories)	40–45	30	25	20
Saturated	17	10	~6	~3
Monounsaturated	18	10	~9	~7
Polyunsaturated	7	10	~10	~10
Protein (as % total calories)	15–20	15	15	15
Carbohydrate (as % total calories)	40–45	55	60	65
Dietary cholesterol, mg	500	300	200–250	100–150

The phase I diet usually does not require a dramatic alteration in one's eating habits and can be readily adopted by most persons. It is important to note that much of the polyunsaturated fat found in "low-cholesterol low-fat" processed food products is usually partially hydrogenated, converting otherwise beneficial vegetable oils into the undesirable trans unsaturated configuration. Such processed food products should not be considered a substitute for saturated fat but neither should saturated fat be considered a healthier alternative to such products and trigger reverting back to lard-based or tropical oil-based processed foods.

The *phase II diet* (Table 27.7) entails more effort, because it goes beyond eliminating the obvious sources of fat and cholesterol. It is indicated for patients who do not achieve adequate results with a phase I diet and for patients at highest CHD risk (e.g., established CHD).

If just the phase I dietary interventions were widely implemented, the overall incidence of CHD in the population would probably drop significantly. The recommended percentages of fat intake in the diet must be translated into real menus and food recommendations if good compliance with these recommendations is to be realized. The counsel of a dietitian is often beneficial, particularly if a phase II diet is indicated. A good working knowledge of the fat content of common foods is essential for patient, family, and health care team (see Appendix III). A number of "heart healthy" cookbooks are on the market to help patients in their food choices and preparation. The use of faddish cholesterol cookbooks should be discouraged because these often do not promote sustainable healthy eating habits. Increasingly, restaurants are offering low-fat menu choices, and patients should be encouraged to select them.

Nonprescription dietary supplements are no substitute for dietary reduction in total fat, saturated fat, and cholesterol. Nonetheless, they are popular with patients, even though they can be expensive. Preliminary data from prospective studies of *omega-3 fish oil* supplements are encouraging, but they are too limited to serve as the basis for dietary recommendations. Impairment of clotting has been noted with use of high doses.

The *antioxidant vitamins* (C, E, and beta-carotene) do not lower cholesterol levels; however they are purported to increase. LDL resistance to oxidative change and thus reduce risk of arterial wall injury. Data from small-scale human studies of vitamin E suggested a possible reduction in CHD risk but emerging events from perspective large scale randomized trials failed to confirm a significant benefit. However, these studies are not definitive; the first of a number of ongoing large-scale trials failed to show a significant benefit of vitamin E. The typical dose of vitamin E used in these studies is 400 to 800 IU/d. There is no evidence that beta-carotene reduces CHD events; its use for CHD prevention is not recommended. More data on vitamin E and C will be forthcoming and should be informative.

Garlic (one half to one clove a day) may produce a modest (5%) reduction in serum cholesterol, but powder and oil preparations have not demonstrated consistent significant benefit. Use of fiber preparations such as *psyllium* (10 g/d) also provide modest benefit, as does the soluble fiber in oat-containing cereals.

Exercise and Weight Loss. The Second Report of the NCEP places renewed emphasis on exercise and weight reduction as complements to dietary therapy and as essential components of a comprehensive nonpharmacologic program. They are helpful not only in correcting lipid abnormalities but also in reducing other CHD risk factors and total CHD risk. For example, exercise will raise the level of HDL cholesterol, decrease blood pressure, and increase efficiency of peripheral oxygen extraction (see Chapter 18). Weight loss efforts can lower fat intake, reduce risk of diabetes mellitus, and decrease myocardial work.

Drug Therapy

Dietary modification is not uniformly effective in achieving target reductions in LDL cholesterol or desired increases in HDL cholesterol. Addition of drug therapy to a diet and exercise program should be considered in high-risk patients whose lipid abnormalities remain inadequately controlled despite intensive dietary efforts. More widespread application of drug therapy remains controversial, with concerns persisting as to its cost effectiveness and risk-to-benefit ratio in patients at the lower end of the risk spectrum. Nevertheless, several recent studies of cholesterol-lowering drugs have shown impressive reductions in CHD morbidity and mortality in patients without established coronary disease (i.e., primary prevention studies) providing increased impetus for pharmacologic treatment of hyperlipidemias.

Effectiveness and Safety. The addition of drug therapy to a diet and exercise program can greatly enhance lipid-lowering results and lead to significant reductions in *nonfatal* and *fatal cardiac events* (i.e., myocardial infarction, revascularization, cardiac death). Reductions in *all-cause mortality* have also been demonstrated in lipid-lowering drug trials, particularly in higher risk populations. With intensive drug therapy, the rate of plaque progression falls, and modest *plaque regression* can be demonstrated in major coronary vessels and systemic arteries. There is now evidence that lipid-lowering medication (statins) also can reduce *risk of stroke* in persons with atherosclerotic carotid disease.

The reductions in CHD events have been noted in patients with established atherosclerotic disease (*secondary prevention*), who experience 30% to 40% reductions in coronary morbidity and mortality. In addition, benefit also accrues to persons with no clinical CHD and only moderate increases in CHD risk, whose reductions in rates of fatal and nonfatal coronary events with use of pharmacologic therapy (*primary prevention*) are on the order of 20% to 30%.

An early concern about an increased risk of cancer and violent deaths with use of some lipid-lowering agents has failed to materialize in major prospective, randomized, placebo-controlled studies. In four of the largest such trials conducted to date, collectively involving tens of thousands of patients (the 4S-Scandinavian, West of Scotland, AFCAPS/TexCAPS, and LIPID studies), no increase in rates of cancer or noncardiac deaths were observed. However, each class of drug therapies has important adverse effects that need to be taken into account when considering pharmacologic intervention (see below).

Candidacy for Pharmacologic Therapy. The risk-to-benefit ratio for pharmacologic therapy appears most favorable in patients at greatest CHD risk and least favorable in those at lowest risk. Because most data derive from studies involving *middle-aged men* and *postmenopausal women* with *established CHD* or *multiple CHD risk factors*, one must extrapolate to estimate effects in other populations. Treatment recommendations by NCEP are based on total CHD risk that includes lipid profile and associated cardiac risk factors.

In the *elderly*, high CHD risk is common. One might reasonably expect the benefit noted in high-risk middle-aged patients to accrue also to elderly persons at similar risk. Duration of therapy is less likely to be very prolonged, lessening risk of an adverse effect from long-term effect. These expectations remain to be proven, but important emerging data (e.g., from the AFCAPS/TexCAPS trial) argue in favor of applying pharmacologic treatment to elderly patients.

Young men (age less than 35) and *premenopausal women* with no CHD risk factors other than hypercholesterolemia are best considered for nonpharmacologic therapy, because their short-term risk of CHD is low and the safety of long-term drug therapy is not established. For young persons at greater CHD risk (e.g., LDL cholesterol more than 220 mg/dL, potent CHD risk factors such as diabetes mellitus or strong family history of premature CHD), the potential gain from use of lipid-lowering medication may outweigh the risk, but there are no outcomes data yet available to confirm this. Again, the exercise of good clinical judgment is essential.

Available Agents. Design of a pharmacologic regimen must take into account the patient's degree of *CHD risk,* the nature of the *lipoprotein abnormality,* and the drugs' *mechanisms of action* and *side effects*. The best program is one that addresses and fits well into the patient's overall clinical state. A large degree of individualization is necessary. The range of available drugs is extensive, varying greatly in cost, effect on cholesterol fractions, efficacy, and side effects (Table 27.8).

HMG-CoA Reductase Inhibitors (the Statins). These agents have become first-line drug therapy because of their effectiveness, patient acceptability, and increasingly favorable safety record. They block the rate-limiting enzyme for cholesterol synthesis, HMG-CoA reductase. This inhibition decreases intracellular cholesterol and increases *clearance of LDL*. Serum LDL levels fall by 20% to 60%, depending on dose and preparation. They affect plaque regression, even when used alone. HDL levels generally stay the same or increase slightly. Statins also influence thrombotic and inflammatory mechanisms, effects whose importance remains to be elucidated, but may account for some of the surprising efficacy seen in persons with lesser degrees of increased CHD risk (see below).

Table 27.8.   Drugs Used to Treat Hyperlipidemia

NAME	INDICATIONS	EFFECTS	DOSAGE	SIDE EFFECTS	RELATIVE COST (STARTING DOSE)*
Bile and Sequestrants (cholestyramine, colestipol)	↑ LDL	↓ LDL ↓ or no change HDL	Cholestyramine 8–24 g/d Colestipol 10–30 g/d	Constipation, heartburn, bloating	Cholest: 14.2 Colest: 12.3
HMG-CoA Reductase inhibitors	↑ LDL; ↑ HDL	↓ LDL; ↑ HDL; ↓ VLDL (minor)		↑ Transaminases; myositis	
Atorzastatin			10-80 mg/d		7.2
Cerivastatin			0.3-0.4 mg/d		5.1
Fluvastatin			20-40 mg/d		4.8
Lovastatin**			20-80 mg/d		9.0
Pravestatin			20-80 mg/d		8.3
Simvastatin			10-80 mg/d		14.7
Niacin (nicotinic acid)	↑ LDL ↓ HDL, VLDL	↓ LDL ↑ HDL ↓ VLDL	1.5–8 g/d	Flushing, pruritus, PUD, hyperglycemia, rashes	1.0
Gemfibrozil	↑ VLDL	↓ VLDL ↑ HDL ↑ LDL (if triglycerides high)	600–1,200 mg/d	? + gallstones potentiates warfarin	4.3
Fish oils (Ω-3 fatty acids)	↑ VLDL	↓ VLDL ↑↓ LDL	? 2–3 g or more of Ω-3 fatty acids/d	Platelet inhibition	0.5

*initial dose

**cost is for non-generic formulation; generic formulation should be considerably less expensive when it becomes available.

Cost and cost effectiveness are important considerations in selecting statin therapy, because all these agents are expensive and use is likely to be measured in years. Although fluvastatin and cerivastatin are generally the least expensive and pravastatin and simvastatin the most expensive, cost often depends on specific pricing contracts with large payors, making generalizations difficult. The statins differ principally in cost and potency, which parallel one another. The least potent, *fluvastatin*, is also the least expensive, followed by *lovastatin* and *pravastatin*, which are similar in terms of cost and potency. *Cerivastatin* is similar to the latter two in its ultimate LDL cholesterol–lowering effect, but is more potent on a milligram basis. *Simvastatin* and *atorvastatin* give the greatest cholesterol reductions at U.S. Food and Drug Administration–approved dosing levels, with atorvastatin having modestly greater efficacy at its maximum dose.

Although the major drawback to statin use is cost, cost savings from reduced rates of cardiac events, time lost from productive work, and premature death at least partly offset the high cost of treatment. Formal cost-effectiveness analyses are now appearing in the literature. Data from the Scandinavian Simvastatin Survival Study ("4S") examined cost per year of life gained and found statin therapy cost effective in men and women over a broad spectrum of ages and cholesterol ranges. The cost per year of life gained was less than half of that for other cost-effective preventive measures such as mammography.

Dosing. Starting dose for all these agents is 10 to 20 mg/d, except for cerivastatin, which is 0.3 mg/d. The maximum dose is currently 80 mg/d for lovastatin, simvastatin, and atorvastatin and 40 mg/d for fluvastatin and pravastatin. The shorter acting agents are best taken at night, the time of peak cholesterol synthesis, but all drugs work well even if taken once daily in the morning.

Adverse Effects: Asymptomatic *hepatocellular dysfunction* manifested by an increase in serum levels of hepatocellular enzymes (e.g., aspartate and alanine aminotranferases) is the most common adverse effect. Incidence ranges from about 3% for any elevation to less than 1% for elevations greater than three times the upper limit of normal. All such increases are reversible with cessation of therapy, which should be considered when liver enzyme levels continue to rise or reach more than three times the upper limit of normal. Transaminase monitoring is strongly recommended, with initial measurements made after 1 to 2 months of therapy, and follow-up measurements made at 6 months and 1 year. The lack of new onset of liver toxicity after 1 year of therapy has led many to advocate limited monitoring after 1 year.

Harmless elevations in *muscle enzymes* (e.g., creatine phosphokinase less than 10 times the upper limit of normal) occur in about 0.6% of cases and require no action. Myalgias without creatine phosphokinase elevations also occur with statin use, making routine monitoring of creatine phosphokinase of limited value. Symptomatic *myositis* is rare, but risk is increased when *niacin* is used in conjunction with statin therapy. In the setting of concurrent *gemfibrozil* use, *rhabdomyolysis* has occurred. Thus, joint use of a statin and a fibrate (either gemfibrozil or fenofibrate) should be done only with great caution and probably only by a lipid specialist. Because of an FDA warning against this combination, pharmacists will often not fill a prescription that places a patient on both drugs without first calling the physician.

As noted earlier, initial concerns about an increase in non-CHD mortality (e.g., from cancer, suicide, or violence) were raised by early meta-analyses, but large-scale prospective studies of statins show no evidence for such adverse effects.

Choice of Agent. Although most experts believe that all of the statins will reduce coronary events in proportion to their efficacy in lowering LDL cholesterol, not all statins have been proven to do so. To date only simvastatin, pravastatin, and lovastatin have been shown in prospective studies to reduce coronary events and/or all-cause mortality. Not surprisingly, the drugs for which outcomes studies have been conducted are also generally priced higher than those for which data are not available. Whether this difference warrants their selection over the lower cost drugs remains a judgment call. Patients who require modest reductions in LDL cholesterol (less than 25%) can be started on any of the statins with the expectation that the reduction will be achieved. Those with marked LDL elevations and high overall CHD risk require more intensive therapy (more than 30% reductions) and are better served if started on a more potent statin such as simvastatin or atorvastatin.

Niacin. This agent is an effective and inexpensive first-line cholesterol-lowering drug. Its exact mechanism of action remains unknown, although it does affect fatty acid mobilization, *lowers LDL* and VLDL levels, and *raises HDL* levels. These changes can be dramatic, although the average LDL reduction is about 15% to 20%. Data from the Coronary Drug Project demonstrated decreased rates of new infarction and mortality in niacin-treated men with a prior myocardial infarction. Also, reduction in all-cause mortality appears to result from use in patients with established CHD. The combination of niacin plus colestipol has produced documented regression of atheromatous plaque in coronary arteries. Being a B-complex vitamin (nicotinic acid), niacin is available over the counter in nonprescription and in prescription formulations.

Adverse Effects: Niacin's principal adverse effects include a litany of side effects, resulting from the *large doses* required. Niacin can exacerbate *gout* and *diabetes*, elevate *liver enzymes*, and produce *rashes, nausea,* and *vomiting*. It also triggers acute prostaglandin-mediated vasodilation that can result in flushing and even postural lightheadedness. *Pretreatment with aspirin* mitigates this reaction. Dry skin and occasionally acanthosis nigricans may accompany niacin use. Lanolin cream helps the former, and prompt cessation clears the latter. Side effects can be minimized by starting with a dose of 100 mg three times daily, taken with meals. A gradual escalation of the dose to 1.5 to 3.0 g/d may be needed to achieve the desired results. Some studies have used niacin at doses as high as 8 g/d, but the frequency and severity of side effects would not be acceptable in clinical practice.

Preparations: Niacin is available in regular and *time-release* preparations, with the latter more expensive but much more convenient and better tolerated except for a higher incidence of *hepatic toxicity*. One should find a brand of niacin that is inexpensive and reliable, and it is suggested that patients take only that form. Transaminases (aminotransferases) should be monitored regularly, as well as glucose and uric acid levels. A new formulation of niacin that can be taken once a day and that induces significantly less flushing is available by prescription (Niaspan). It is significantly more expensive than the available nonprescription formulations.

Bile Acid Sequestrants (Cholestyramine and Colestipol). These nonabsorbable agents have been first-line pharmacologic therapy for many years, with an established record of safety.

They are very useful for patients who are not at great CHD risk but in whom diet alone fails to lower LDL cholesterol to target levels. Though not as cost effective as the statins or niacin, they are very effective when used in combination with them to treat high-risk patients with severe hypercholesterolemia. They bind bile acids in the gut and interrupt their normal enterohepatic circulation. The resultant shunting of cholesterol in the liver to bile acid production leads to a fall in total and LDL cholesterols.

Adverse Effects: The bile sequestrants are nonabsorbable resins whose major *side effects* are gastrointestinal—*constipation, bloating, heartburn,* and *nausea.* A high-fiber diet or psyllium supplement and use of these agents just before a meal will usually ameliorate the gastrointestinal upset. The potential to *impede absorption of certain drugs* (e.g., digoxin, thyroxin, warfarin, tetracycline, phenobarbital) necessitates that bile sequestrants not be taken until at least 1 hour after or 4 hours before these other drugs. In rare instances, steatorrhea and malabsorption of the fat-soluble vitamins (A, D, E, and K) can occur. The usual starting dose is one scoop of the powdered form of the drug (4 g of cholestyramine, 5 g of colestipol) in a large glass of water twice a day. Dose can be increased to a total of three scoops twice daily. A newer formulation of cholestyramine, which is significantly less gritty (Lo-Cholest), can be tried if the texture of the generic drug formulation should prove unacceptable.

Estrogens. In postmenopausal women, estrogen replacement therapy is effective in *lowering* the levels of *LDL cholesterol* and *raising* those of *HDL cholesterol*, with attendant reductions in CHD risk. Because of the risk of endometrial cancer associated with unopposed estrogen use (see Chapter 118), a progestin is usually prescribed as well. The addition of progestin does not appear to significantly reduce the CHD benefit of estrogen replacement therapy, but confirmation by prospective randomized trial is needed. The HERS study showed no benefit of such hormone replacement therapy (HRT) on cardiovascular outcomes in women with established CHD. There was an increase in adverse events in the period of initiation of HRT, although in later stages there was a trend toward improved outcomes. Overall, no benefit was noted. This well-designed prospective study raises serious questions about the efficacy of HRT in protecting women against the complications of coronary artery disease. Most experts would not stop HRT in women with coronary disease, but far fewer would intiate it for this reason as a result of the HERS trial. The study did not address the issue of HRT in women without CHD, and data on this issue are still several years away. Data are also not available on the newer "designer estrogens" such as raloxifene, which also have a favorable effect on lipid profiles.

Fibrates (Gemfibrozil and Fenofibrate)

Because these drugs lower LDL cholesterol much less effectively than the statins, they are not considered first-line drugs for the treatment of hypercholesterolemia. Nonetheless, they do have specific uses. They *decrease VLDL* synthesis and enhance its clearance. They also *raise HDL cholesterol*, most prominently in those who have concomitant *triglyceride elevations.* The effect on LDL cholesterol is variable, although an 8% to 15% reduction can be seen in patients who do not have markedly elevated VLDL levels.

Both fibrate agents are generally well tolerated, but they can increase bile cholesterol content, raising the risk of gallstone formation and potentiating the effect of warfarin. The FDA has issued a warning about their use in combination with statins, because *rhabdomyolysis* has occurred when gemfibrozil and a statin are used concurrently. An earlier drug in this class, clofibrate, was taken off the market because of reports of *increased mortality* associated with its use. Although the FDA has approved both fibrates, these agents have yet to demonstrate a reduction in all-cause mortality. A VA gemfibrozil study of men with low HDL cholesterol did show improvement in coronary outcomes; HDL cholesterol rose, triglycerides fell, and LDL cholesterol stayed the same.

Probucol. This agent was formerly used as an LDL cholesterol-lowering drug, but it is no longer marketed for this purpose because more effective agents are now available. It is also not listed as a major drug for treatment of hypercholesterolemia. It *lowers LDL* cholesterol about 15% but frequently *decreases HDL* by 20% to 30%. The net effect is a more atherogenic lipid profile. However, probucol is an effective *LDL antioxidant* and decreases LDL uptake by macrophages, which theoretically could inhibit atherogenesis independent of any effect on LDL concentration.

Treatment Thresholds For Drug Therapy, Goals, and Monitoring

Treatment Thresholds. Current guidelines derive from the consensus views of the NCEP panel, but they predate recent recent studies demonstrating benefit to persons without CHD who have cholesterol levels lower than the currently recommended thressholds for drug therapy (e.g., LDL cholesterol 150 mg/dL). Thus, the current guidelines should be considered rather conservative. For those with *two or more CHD risk factors,* the NCEP recommends initiating drug therapy if the *LDL cholesterol remains above 160 mg/dL* after life-style modifications have been made. For those with *fewer than 2 CHD risk factors,* drug therapy is recommended for *LDL cholesterol above 190 mg/dL.*

Although epidemiologic data show a strong inverse relation between HDL level and CHD risk, there are no data yet from large-scale, randomized, prospective clinical trials showing that raising HDL cholesterol in itself significantly reduces CHD mortality. However, treatment does seem to lower CHD morbidity. Generally healthy middle-aged and elderly persons with *low HDL cholesterol* and *"normal" LDL* cholesterol demonstrate a significant reduction in risk of a first acute major coronary event (e.g., myocardial infarction, unstable angina) when treated with a statin drug (e.g., the AFCAPS/TexCAPS trial). Such findings suggest that even persons with modest increases in CHD risk—as manifested by advancing age and an isolated low HDL cholesterol—might benefit from pharmacologic therapy. The mechanism of the benefit may be other than the effect on HDL cholesterol, because in the AFCAPS/TexCAPS study, HDL cholesterol rose only 6%.

In view of recent data, lowering the threshhold for drug therapy below that recommended by the NCEP guidelines could be justified on the basis of recent outcome studies, but the cost effectiveness of such an approach remains to be established. Results are typically reported in terms of reduction in relative risk. Absolute risk becomes an issue in younger patient populations, where a 20% to 30% reduction in relative risk may represent only a modest clinical achievement if the absolute risk of having a CHD event over the next 10 years is only 2% (absolute risk falls to 1.6%).

Treatment Goals. The ultimate treatment goal is *reduction in CHD risk*; the immediate one is reduction of LDL cholesterol. Target levels have been lowered, reflecting the improvement in outcomes associated with lower lipid levels. For *primary prevention* (no established CHD), the NCEP target is an *LDL cholesterol level less than 130 mg/dL. For secondary prevention* (established CHD), the goal is an LDL cholesterol level *less than 100 mg/dL.*

Monitoring. This is performed by measurement of the LDL cholesterol level, beginning about 6 to 8 weeks after initiation of therapy and then every 3 to 4 months until control is established. Afterward, every 6 to 12 months is usually sufficient. More frequent monitoring for development of abnormalities in serum chemistries (e.g., liver enzymes) is indicated when using certain pharmacologic agents (see above).

Treatment in the Elderly

Prevalence of hypercholesterolemia is greatest in those older than 65 years of age. As in other age groups, elevations in total and LDL cholesterol are predictive of increased cardiovascular risk. However, the statistical risk relationship is not as strong as in younger patients, due in part to the frequent occurrence of other important risk factors in the elderly (e.g., diabetes, hypertension). Elderly patients may have other advanced diseases, making prevention of coronary disease appear irrelevant to their overall quality of life. But, in those who are vigorous and have a considerable life expectancy, primary and secondary prevention of CHD can be very important.

Several factors favor treatment. The coronary disease of women may be less advanced than that of men due to the protective effects of estrogens before menopause or due to use of postmenopausal estrogen replacement therapy. In addition, the benefits from secondary prevention of coronary disease by lowering of cholesterol exceed even the benefits of primary prevention. With the advent of better tolerated cholesterol-lowering medication, the risks of adverse effects and their negative impact on quality of life are declining. All these factors combine to recommend treatment of hypercholesterolemia in elderly patients.

Dietary Measures. Dietary therapy of hypercholesterolemia in the elderly is similar to that for all adults and should be carried out as the first step in treatment, though dietary measures do not always suffice by themselves. Carbohydrate should not replace most fat in the diet, rather polyunsaturates and monounsaturates should be increased. The Ω-6 polyunsaturated fatty acids found in vegetable oils should not exceed 10% of calories. For the elderly, modifications of the usual low-saturated-fat diet are needed to ensure adequate calcium intake for prevention of osteoporosis. Use of skim milk and low-fat and nonfat yogurts are examples of ways to *maintain calcium* intake while cutting down on saturated fat. Maintaining *adequate protein intake* is also essential, meaning that lean cuts of red meat ought to be allowed in addition to fish and skinless chicken to ensure palatability of the diet. *High fiber* is essential for good bowel function and cannot hurt the cholesterol-lowering effort.

Pharmacologic Therapy. Because dietary therapy alone frequently fails to achieve the goal of an LDL cholesterol lower than 130 mg/dL, drug treatment must often be considered.

Statin therapy is indicated when aggressive lowering of LDL cholesterol is needed. The statins have also proven useful for primary prevention in elderly persons with low HDL cholesterol and average LDL cholesterol. These drugs are well tolerated in the elderly, with minor diarrhea, myalgias, and occasional sleep disturbances being the most common problems. Minor transaminase elevations are common; they are usually asymptomatic and not a cause for discontinuation unless they reach three times normal. However, regular transaminase monitoring is required throughout the course of therapy. As noted earlier, initial concerns about an increased risk of malignancy have proven unfounded in large-scale, prospective, long-term, follow-up studies. Statins are recommended as first-line drug therapy for hypercholesterolemia in the elderly.

The *bile sequestrants* are safe but can cause considerable gastrointestinal upset, especially constipation. Increasing dietary fiber helps. Because sequestrants can impair drug absorption, their use in elderly patients must include instruction to take other medications at least 1 hour before or 4 hours after sequestrant use. Among the drugs that might be affected by sequestrants are warfarin, propranolol, digitalis preparations, thyroxin, and antibiotics. Low-dose sequestrants are a reasonable first choice for pharmacologic therapy.

Niacin is effective, although not always well tolerated. Its advantages over statins are its ability to also raise HDL cholesterol and its low cost. The incidence of side effects in the elderly is high, with flushing, gastrointestinal upset, dry mouth, and dry eyes being particularly annoying. The drug may exacerbate peptic ulcer disease, elevate transaminases, and trigger arrhythmias and hypotension. Multiple daily doses are usually required.

PATIENT EDUCATION

Regarding Diet and Exercise. The importance of patient education in the management of hyperlipidemia cannot be overemphasized, because treatment starts with alterations in the patient's eating and exercise habits (see Chapters 18 and 233). The first step in therapy should be a careful review of the rationale for treating hypercholesterolemia, followed by a discussion of basic dietary principles for lowering cholesterol. Consultation with a dietitian can be very helpful. Many patients are surprised to learn that dietary fat is more atherogenic than dietary cholesterol itself (witness the patient who eats his cholesterol-free potato chips with abandon). Reviewing the saturated fat and trans fat content of foods regularly consumed by the patient is quite worthwhile. At times, simply removing a few grossly offending foods from the diet (e.g., processed snack foods, cheese, grossly fatty meats, cold cuts, fried food) will ensure a good start to a change in eating habits. More comprehensive diet planning can be aided by discussion with the nurse or dietitian, facilitated by written material such as that produced by the American Heart Association. Periodic visits to check diet, weight, and cholesterol are excellent, although often overlooked, means of facilitating compliance and providing reinforcement.

Regarding Medications. Patients need to understand the rationale for their medical program and the details of its proper use and side effects. Some mistakenly believe their drug program is curative and stop treatment after a few months of therapy. Others harbor exaggerated concerns about adverse drug effects and stop medication prematurely. Cost is another factor that often limits compliance, necessitating a strategy that takes into account the patient's insurance coverage for medication. However, careful studies find that adequacy of insurance does not by itself explain the nearly 40% fall off in compliance that occurs over 5 years among patients prescribed lipid-lowering medication. Choice of agent, comorbidity, and socioeconomic status also play important roles, underscoring the importance of comprehensive and ongoing patient education.

INDICATIONS FOR REFERRAL

To the Dietician. Patients prescribed a dietary program should have a consultation with a *dietitian* if they are unclear about the food choices they should make or if compliance with the diet is problematic. Dieticians can provide educational materials, food preparation advice, and the periodic feedback that patients often need to permanently change their eating habits.

To the Lipid Specialist. Patients with high-risk lipid profiles who do not respond to diet plus one or two first-line drugs, those with extremes of any lipoprotein level, or a family history of premature coronary disease (before age 55 years) should be considered for referral to a physician expert in diagnosis and treatment of lipid disorders. Some genetic disorders are particularly refractory to standard therapies, and patients with these conditions will benefit from consideration of genetic links and more complex treatment regimens that are the province of a lipid specialist. Identification of affected family members can also be accomplished. Lipid research laboratories can often categorize specific genetic abnormalities through testing not routinely available in most clinical laboratories. Ultracentrifugation of lipoproteins, polymerase chain reaction amplification of DNA, and cell-based receptor and enzymatic assays can be used to help pinpoint the cause and screen other family members for the problem. Although these more sophisticated tests may not yet translate into different therapeutic options, they often help clarify family questions about the risks of CHD in related individuals and are likely to influence therapeutic options in the years ahead.

THERAPEUTIC RECOMMENDATIONS

Effective reduction of CHD risk requires identifying and aggressively treating all CHD risk factors responsive to medical intervention, including smoking, hypertension, diabetes, and obesity (see Chapters 26, 54, 102, and 233). Focusing on hyperlipidemia alone is insufficient. In treating hypercholesterolemia, one should determine total CHD risk (see Tables 27.4 and 27.5) and treat accordingly (see Table 27.6).

High Risk (Established CHD; LDL Cholesterol 160 mg/dL plus Two Risk Factors or LDL Cholesterol 190 mg/dL and No Other CHD Risk Factors)

- Start with dietary restriction of total fat intake to no more than 20% of calories, substituting polyunsaturated and monounsaturated fats for saturated fat, partially hydrogenated unsaturated fat, and cholesterol. Highly motivated individuals may avoid the need for life-long medication by strict adherence to phase II or phase III dietary programs, achieving LDL reductions of 40 to 80 mg/dL. Allow 4 to 6 months for implementation of dietary life-style changes. Even if dietary change does not bring LDL cholesterol down to desired levels, diet will enhance the effect from lipid-lowering therapy.

- Initiate pharmacologic therapy if goals for LDL cholesterol reduction have not been met by diet alone. For most patients, a statin preparation is the drug of first choice.

- Minimize cost of statin therapy by matching statin preparation with degree of LDL cholesterol reduction needed. For example, if an LDL cholesterol reduction of 30% to 40% is required, consider starting simvastatin or atorvastatin 20 mg/d (see above); if an LDL cholesterol reduction of less than 25% is needed, then any of the statins can be used and cost should determine choice.

- Consider niacin (average dose, 1.5 to 3.0 g/d) as an alternative choice, if LDL cholesterol elevation is accompanied by a low HDL cholesterol (less than 35 mg/dL). In postmenopausal women with this lipid profile, estrogen replacement therapy is an alternative to niacin.

- Consider adding a second agent in those with high CHD risk who fail to adequately respond to diet plus maximal doses of a single agent. The bile resins (e.g., cholestyramine or colestipol, one to two scoops twice daily) are well suited to combination programs. One should generally avoid the combination of a statin plus gemfibrozil because of the increased risk of rhabdomyolysis and the combination of a statin plus full doses of niacin because of increased risk of myositis.

- Aim for LDL cholesterol of less than 100 mg/dL for those with established CHD and less than 130 mg/dL for all others.

Moderate Risk (LDL Cholesterol 130 to 159 mg/dL plus Two CHD Risk Factors or LDL Cholesterol 160 to 189 mg/dL and No Other CHD Risk Factors)

- Begin with dietary therapy. In patients with large intakes of saturated fat and cholesterol, the phase I diet can produce sufficient reductions in cholesterol of 20 to 40 mg/dL. More aggressive dietary fat restriction (phase II diet) may be needed in those who do not respond adequately. PUFAs should be increased moderately but to no more than 10% of total calories. The minimum goal is a reduction of LDL cholesterol to less than 130 mg/dL in those with two or more CHD risk factors and to well under 160 mg/dL in those with fewer than two risk factors.

- Drug therapy is usually not necessary but should be considered in those who fail to respond to dietary measures.

Modest Risk (Isolated Low HDL Cholesterol [Less than 35 mg/dL]; LDL Cholesterol Not Elevated)

- Prescribe nonpharmacologic measures that can increase HDL cholesterol, including aerobic exercise, smoking cessation, and weight loss if obese. Such actions can increase HDL by 5 to 15 mg/dL.

- Prescribe a phase I diet, in which saturated fat, cholesterol, and partially hydrogenated vegetable oils are restricted and replaced by monounsaturated and polyunsaturated fats.

- Use clinical judgment in considering pharmacologic treatment if nonpharmacologic measures prove insufficient.

- Although the NCEP does not yet recommend pharmacologic correction of an isolated HDL cholesterol, pay attention to total CHD risk. In those with multiple cardiac risk factors and a low HDL cholesterol consider statin therapy for middle-aged and elderly persons; consider estrogen replacement therapy for the postmenopausal women; consider niacin as an additional option, especially for younger persons who tolerate the drug better than do the elderly; and always take into account HDL cholesterol level when designing a pharmacologic program for persons with LDL cholesterol elevation.

Elevated Triglycerides (Fasting Triglycerides More than 250 mg/dL)

- Because no consensus exists on need for treatment, exercise clinical judgment.
- Consider treatment in persons with elevated triglycerides in the setting of low HDL cholesterol (less than 35 mg/dL), as the latter may rise substantially with use of triglyceride-lowering drugs.
- To accomplish this goal, consider gemfibrozil (600 mg twice daily) or fenofibrate (67 to 201 mg/d).
- Such drugs can also be used to reduce the risk of pancreatitis in persons with very high triglyceride levels (more than 800 mg/dL).

All Patients

- Fully explain the condition and the rationale for the treatment program to ensure compliance; emphasize the importance of dietary modification, exercise, and compliance with any drug program that might be necessary. Customize the patient-education and treatment programs to the needs and capabilities of the patient.
- Address patient concerns, especially those regarding long-term use of lipid-lowering medications or dietary modifications. Enlist the services of a dietician if there are concerns or questions regarding dietary changes.
- Consider for referral to a lipid specialist patients with high-risk lipid profiles who do not respond to diet plus one or two first-line drugs, those with extremes of any lipoprotein level, or a family history of premature coronary disease (before age 55 years).

ANNOTATED BIBLIOGRAPHY

Avorn J, Monette J, Lacour A, et al. Persistence of use of lipid-lowering medications: a cross-national study. JAMA 1998;279:1458. (*A cohort study involving well-insured patients from New Jersey and Quebec finding that choice of agent, comorbidity, and socioeconomic status were important contributors to noncompliance.*)

Bradford RH, Shear CL, Chremos AN, et al. Expanded clinical evaluation of lovastatin (EXCEL) study results. Arch Intern Med 1991;151:43. (*Detailed data on efficacy and safety; found to be highly effective and safe, especially when used in low doses in combination with a dietary program.*)

CashinHemphill L, Mack WJ, Pogoda JM, et al. Beneficial effects of colestipol niacin on coronary atherosclerosis: a 4-year follow-up. JAMA 1990;264:3013. (*A report from the Cholesterol Lowering Atherosclerosis Study documenting decreased progression and increased regression of coronary atherosclerosis.*)

Criqui MH, Heiss G, Cohn R, et al. Plasma triglyceride level and mortality from coronary heart disease. N Engl J Med 1993;328:1220. (*No independent association with CHD risk found, but relation to low HDL noted.*)

Denke MA, Grundy SM. Hypercholesterolemia in the elderly: resolving the treatment dilemma. Ann Intern Med 1990;112:780. (*A detailed review of the risks and benefits; favors treatment of high-risk patients; 83 references.*)

Downs JR, Clearfield M, Weis S, et al. Primary prevention of acute coronary events with lovastatin in men and women with average cholesterol levels: results of AFCAPS/TexCAPS. JAMA 1998;279:1615. (*The AFCAPS/TexCAPS study; prospective, randomized, placebo-controlled trial of lovastatin for primary prevention of CHD in 6,500 otherwise healthy middle-aged and elderly patients with low HDL and normal LDL; 37% reduction in CHD risk demonstrated over 5 years of follow-up.*)

Expert Panel on Detection, Evaluation, and Treatment of High Blood Cholesterol in Adults. Summary of the second report of the National Cholesterol Education Program. JAMA 1993;269:3015. (*Major report from this consensus panel.*)

Goldman L, Weinstein MC, Goldman PA, et al. Cost-effectiveness of HMG-CoA reductase inhibition for primary and secondary prevention of coronary heart disease. JAMA 1991;265:1145. (*Lovastatin found very cost effective for secondary prevention, less so for primary prevention, except in very high-risk groups.*)

Grodstein F, Stampfer MJ, Colditz GA, et al. Postmenopausal hormone therapy and mortality. N Engl J Med 1997;336:1769. (*Ongoing analysis of data from Nurses Health Study showing that current users of postmenopausal hormone replacement therapy had a lower risk of death than did subjects that had never taken hormones but that a longer duration of use was associated with a declining benefit. In addition, this study suggested that those with the highest risk of coronary disease derived the most benefit from the hormone therapy.*)

Henkin Y, Oberman A, Hurst DC, et al. Niacin revisited: clinical observations on an important but underutilized drug. Am J Med 1991;91:239. (*Makes the case for more use of this effective inexpensive drug; but notes dose-related toxicities.*)

Hu FB, Stampfer MJ, Manson JE, et al. Dietary fat intake and the risk of coronary heart disease in women. N Engl J Med 1997;337:1491. (*Largest and longest running prospective epidemiologic study of the relation of diet to coronary disease risk; finds that replacing saturated and trans unsaturated fats with polyunsaturated fat produced a greater reduction in coronary disease risk than reducing overall fat intake.*)

Hulley S, Grady S, Bush T, et al. Randomized trial of estrogen plus progestin for secondary prevention of coronary heart disease in postmenopausal women. JAMA 1998;280:605. (*This randomized trial demonstrated no benefit of hormone replacement therapy on survival in women with established coronary disease. This is the first large-scale prospective study of its kind, and the results were the opposite of those most retrospective studies would have predicted. Women without coronary disease were not included in this study, so the value of hormone replacement therapy in that group is still uncertain.*)

Hunninghake DB, Stein EA, Dujovne CA, et al. The efficacy of intensive dietary therapy alone or combined with lovastatin in outpatients with hypercholesterolemia. N Engl J Med 1993;328:1213. (*Diet alone provided only a 5% LDL reduction; medication added another 27%.*)

Isaacsohn JL, Moser M, Stein EA, et al. Garlic powder and plasma lipids and lipoproteins: a multicenter, randomized, placebo-controlled trial. Arch Intern Med 1998;158:1189. (*Garlic powder was given at a dose of 900 mg/d for 12 weeks; no significant differences noted compared to the group prescribed placebo.*)

Jenkins DJA, Uolever TMS, Venketshwer R, et al. Effect on blood lipids of very high intakes of fiber in diets low in saturated fat and cholesterol. N Engl J Med 1993;329:21. (*Foods rich in soluble fiber can lower cholesterol.*)

Johannesson M, Jonsson B, Kjekshus J, et al. Cost effectiveness of simvastatin treatment to lower cholesterol levels in patients with coronary heart disease. N Engl J Med 1997;336:332. (*Data from the 4S study showing simvastatin treatment is cost effective in men and women over a wide range of ages and cholesterol elevations.*)

Klag KJ, Ford DE, Mead LA, et al. Serum cholesterol in young men and subsequent cardiovascular disease. N Engl J Med 1993;328:313. (*Strong association found between serum cholesterol level in early life and CHD in midlife.*)

LIPID Study. Prevention of cardiovascular events and death with pravastatin in patients with coronary heart disease and a broad range of initial cholesterol levels. The Long-Term Intervention with Pravastatin in Ischaemic Disease Study Group. N Engl J Med 1998;339:1349. (*A study involving more than 9,000 patients with results quite similar to those of the CARE study. Treatment of modestly elevated LDL cholesterol levels with pravastatin improved cardiovascular mortality by 24% and overall mortality was reduced 22%. No increase in breast cancer was noted.*)

Mensink RP, Katan M. Effect of dietary trans fatty acids on high-density and low-density lipoprotein cholesterol levels in healthy subjects. N Engl J Med 1991;323:439. (*Distressing data indicating that the partially hydrogenated unsaturated fatty acids found in processed foods promote undesirable lipid levels as much or more than the saturated fatty acids they were intended to replace.*)

Pearson TA, Patel RV. The quest for a cholesterol-decreasing diet. Should we subtract, substitute, or supplement. Ann Intern Med 1993;119:627. (*An editorial arguing for reduction in fat intake as the primary therapy; good review of dietary supplements.*)

Pierce LR, Wysowski DK, Gross TP. Myopathy and rhabdomyolysis associated with lovastatin-gemfibrozil combination therapy. JAMA 1990;264:71. (*Documents this serious complication; the combination is generally to be avoided.*)

Pitt B, Waters D, Brown WV, et al, for the Atorvstatin vs. Revasculazation Treatment Investigators. Aggressive lipid-lowering therapy compared angioplasty in stable coronary artery disease. N Engl J Med 1999;341:70. (*Atronstation at least as effective as angioplasty for reducing rate of coronary events.*)

Rubins HB, Robins SJ, Collins D, et al, For the Veterans Affairs high-density lipoprotein cholesterol intervention trial study group. Gemfibrozil for the secondary prevention of coronary heart disease in men with low levels of high-density lipoprotein cholesterol. N Engl J Med 1999;341:410. (*The VA-HIT trial; reduction in risk of infarction or death demonstrated.*)

Sacks FM, Pfeffer MA, Moye LA, et al. The effect of pravastatin on coronary events after myocardial infarction in patients with average cholesterol levels. N Engl J Med 1997;335:1001. (*An important extension of the Scandinavian Simvastatin Study in that patients with much lower LDL cholesterol values were chosen for cholesterol lowering. Improved cardiovascular mortality was seen in the pravastatin-treated group. The later LIPID study also showed a reduction in overall mortality using the same drug.*)

Scandinavian Simvastatin Survival Study Group. Randomized trial of cholesterol lowering in 4444 patients with coronary heart disease: the Scandinavian Survival Study. Lancet 1994;344:1383. (*The first major, randomized, prospective study of the efficacy of cholesterol lowering in patients with CHD showing a 42% reduction in CHD mortality and a 30% reduction in all cause mortality with no increased risk of noncardiac death.*)

Schaefer EJ, Lamon-Fava S, Ausman LM, et al. Individual variability in lipoprotein cholesterol response to NCEP step 2 diets. Am J Clin Nutr 1997;65:823-830. (*A metabolic ward study of a step 2 diet showing an impressive reduction in serum cholesterol levels in the whole study group on average, but the variability between individuals was quite substantial.*)

Shepherd J, Cobbe SM, Ford I, et al. Prevention of coronary heart disease with pravastatin in men with hypercholesterolemia. N Engl J Med 1995;333:1301. (*The West of Scotland Study; a randomized, placebo-controlled, prospective trial of men without CHD examining the efficacy of statin therapy for primary prevention in persons with moderately high risk of CHD; finds approximately 30% reductions in rates of nonfatal infarction, CHD death, and cardiovascular death.*)

Sprecher DL, Harris BV, Goldberg AC, et al. Efficacy of psyllium in reducing serum cholesterol levels in hypercholesterolemic patients on high or low-fat diets. Ann Intern Med 1993; 119:545. (*A 5% to 10% lowering achieved in both groups.*)

Appendix I. Fatty Acid Composition of Commonly Consumed Foods
(as Percentage of Total Fatty Acids)

FOOD	SATURATED	MONOUNSATURATED	POLYUNSATURATED
Butter, cream, milk	65	30	5
Beef	46	48	6
Bacon and pork	38	50	12
Lard	42	45	13
Chicken	33	39	28
Fish	29	31	40
Coconut oil	92	6	2
Palm kernel oil	86	12	2
Cocoa butter	63	34	3
Olive oil	15	76	9
Peanut oil	20	48	32
Cottonseed oil	27	20	53
Soybean oil	16	24	60
Corn oil	13	26	61
Sunflower seed oil	11	22	67
Safflower seed oil	10	13	77

Appendix II.   Cholesterol Content of Common Foods

FOOD	AMOUNT OF FOOD	CHOLESTEROL CONTENT (mg)	FOOD	AMOUNT OF FOOD	CHOLESTEROL CONTENT (mg)
Brains	3.5 oz (100 g)	>2,000			
Liver, chicken	3.5 oz	555	Beef	3.5 oz	65
Kidney	3.5 oz	375	Pork	3.5 oz	62
Liver, beef	3.5 oz	300	Clams	3.5 oz	50
Caviar	1 tbsp	>300	Flounder	3.5 oz	50
Egg yolk	1	252	Oysters	3.5 oz	50
Shrimp	3.5 oz	150	Ice cream (regular)	1 cup	40
Crab	3.5 oz	100	Butter	1 tbsp	35
Mackerel	3.5 oz	95	Scallops	3.5 oz	35
Lobster (cooked)	3.5 oz	85	Milk, whole	1 cup	14
Cheese, cheddar	3.5 oz	84	Milk, 2%	1 cup	9
Veal	3.5 oz	70	Milk, skim	1 cup	2
Chicken, breast	3.5 oz	67	Margarine	1 tbsp	0

Appendix III.   Fat Content of Meats, Poultry, Fish, and Other Protein Sources, 3-Ounce Portions

	TOTAL FAT (G)	SATURATED FAT (G)	CALORIES	CHOLESTEROL (mg)
Red meat				
Veal top round (roasted)	2.9	1.0	127	88
Pork tenderloin (roasted)	4.1	1.4	133	67
Beef top round (broiled)	4.2	1.4	153	71
Beef eye of round (roasted)	4.2	1.5	143	59
Pork sirloin chop, boneless (broiled)	5.7	1.5	156	78
Pork loin roast, boneless (roasted)	6.4	2.4	160	66
Lamb leg (roasted)	6.6	2.3	162	78
Pork loin chop, bone in (broiled)	6.9	2.5	165	70
Beef tenderloin (broiled)	8.5	3.2	179	71
Frankfurter, beef and pork (boiled)	24.8	9.1	272	42
Pork sausage, country style (cooked)	26.5	9.2	314	71
Poultry				
Turkey breast, skinless (roasted)	2.7	0.9	133	59
Chicken breast, skinless (roasted)	3.0	0.9	140	72
Turkey thigh, skinless (roasted)	6.1	2.1	159	72
Chicken thigh, skinless (roasted)	9.3	2.6	178	81
Chicken breast, skin on (fried)	11.2	3.0	221	72
Duck, skin on (roasted)	24.1	8.2	286	71
Fish and seafood				
Lobster meat (cooked)	0.5	<0.1	83	61
Scallops, bay or sea (raw)	0.6	<0.1	75	28
Cod (broiled)	0.7	0.1	89	47
Shrimp (moist heat cooked)	0.9	0.2	84	166
Flounder (broiled)	1.3	0.3	99	58
Crab, Alaska king (steamed)	1.3	0.1	82	45
Oysters (eastern, raw)	2.1	0.5	59	47
Tuna, white (canned in water)	2.1	0.6	116	36
Trout, rainbow (broiled)	3.7	0.7	128	62
Tuna, light (canned in oil)	7.0	1.3	168	15
Salmon, sockeye (broiled)	9.3	1.6	184	74
Other				
Tofu/bean curd	4.1	0.6	65	0
Eggs (hard boiled)	9.5	2.8	134	466
American cheese food (pasteurized process)	20.9	13.1	279	54
Cheddar cheese	28.2	17.9	343	89
Peanuts (roasted in shell)	41.4	7.3	495	0
Peanut butter	43.5	7.2	502	0

Sources: United States Department of Agriculture, Composition of Foods. Handbooks 8–1, 8–5, 8–7, 8–10, 8–12, 8–13, 8–15, 8–16, 8–17; HVH–CWRI Nutrient Data Base.

28
Outpatient Management of Atrial Fibrillation

Atrial fibrillation (AF) usually presents in the office setting without hemodynamic compromise, making it amenable to outpatient management by the primary care physician. The first tasks are to ensure adequate rate control and identify and attend to underlying precipitants and etiologies (see Chapter 25). Subsequent tasks are to determine the risk of embolization and to design a safe cost-effective program appropriate to the degree of risk. The principal treatment options are institution of chronic antithrombotic therapy in combination with pharmacologic rate control and proceeding to cardioversion followed by chronic antiarrhythmic therapy to maintain sinus rhythm. Because data from randomized prospective studies comparing these very different approaches with treatment are not yet available and because there is a wide spectrum of disease and stroke risk associated with AF, considerable clinical judgment and attention to the specific needs of the individual patient are required to manage AF safely and effectively. Regardless of approach taken, attention to stroke prevention is a critical priority that is too often inadequately addressed.

CLINICAL PRESENTATION AND COURSE

AF may be paroxysmal or chronic. Paroxysms typically occur in patients with lone atrial fibrillation, sick sinus syndrome, or Wolff-Parkinson-White (WPW) syndrome and during exacerbations of cardiomyopathic, valvular, and ischemic forms of organic heart disease. Advanced forms of these conditions often result in chronic AF. AF may also be triggered by hyperthyroidism. Although chronic fibrillation may be a manifestation of serious organic heart disease and represent an increase in overall risk, chronicity is not the prime determinant of embolic risk; the prime determinants are the presence of underlying heart disease and risk factors for thrombus formation.

Lone Atrial Fibrillation. Lone AF is characterized by the occurrence of atrial fibrillation in the absence of clinically evident heart disease or cardiovascular risk factors. In about two thirds of cases, the condition presents as isolated or recurrent episodes of paroxysmal AF; in the remainder, the AF is chronic. Survival rates and stroke risks are similar regardless of whether the lone AF episodes are paroxysmal or chronic. Lone AF may be annoying and sometimes frightening, but the key question is the risk of embolization that it confers. In patients younger than 60 years, survival and embolic risk are no different than that of a population of similar age; however, in patients older than 60 years there is nearly a fourfold increase in relative risk of stroke, probably due to the increased probability of underlying cardiovascular risk factors in older patients with seemingly "lone" AF. Thus, lone AF appears to pose little risk, but only if the patient is relatively young and has no other cardiovascular risk factors.

Apathetic Hyperthyroidism of the Elderly. Clinically inapparent hyperthyroidism may be mistaken for lone AF, because there may be little evidence of organic heart disease and the typical symptoms and signs of hyperthyroidism can also be absent. Sometimes, the clinical presentation more closely resembles depression or occult malignancy, with significant weight loss, marked apathy, and unexplained AF dominating the clinical picture. Diagnosis is made by ruling out underlying organic heart disease and finding the thyrotropin to be undetectable and the free thyroxin index or total triiodothyronine substantially elevated (see Chapters 8 and 103). Treatment directed at the hyperthyroidism usually terminates the AF. Although uncommon, this eminently treatable form of AF should not be missed. Stroke risk is minimal if there is no accompanying organic heart disease.

Underlying Heart Disease. Patients with AF in the context of underlying heart disease have a much more serious problem. Not only is the risk of embolization significantly increased, but the AF may also lead to hemodynamic compromise. Chronic atrial fibrillation in such patients usually reflects serious cardiac pathology. In the Framingham study, onset of atrial fibrillation and *heart failure* were closely linked. Furthermore, the development of chronic AF corresponded with a doubling of cardiovascular mortality.

Some conditions that cause AF also manifest concurrent disease of the conducting system, further increasing risk. For example, patients with the *tachycardia-bradycardia (sick sinus) syndrome* have sinus node dysfunction, often in conjunction with arterioventricular nodal disease and lack of an adequate escape mechanism. Characteristic presentations include episodes of atrial fibrillation with a slow ventricular response rate and bouts of severe bradycardia leading to syncope or near-syncope.

Paroxysms of rapid AF and other supraventricular tachycardias are characteristic of *WPW syndrome*. In this condition, an accessory connection between the atrium and the ventricle (e.g., the Kent bundle) leads to preexcitation (short PR interval, delta waves) and a host of supraventricular dysrhythmias. The AF may be associated with a very fast ventricular response rate facilitated by rapid antegrade conduction over the accessory conduction pathway. There may be a widening of the QRS, mimicking ventricular fibrillation. In rare instances, the rapid ventricular response can degenerate into true ventricular fibrillation and sudden death. Fortunately, the risk of such serious ventricular dysrhythmias is very low in previously asymptomatic WPW patients, in part because the accessory pathways tend to lose antegrade conductivity over time.

An episode of AF in a patient with preexisting heart disease may be precipitated by such factors as *acute heart failure, ischemia, fever, infection, hypoxia,* or *hypovolemia.* Correction of the precipitant often results in at least a temporary return to sinus rhythm. If there is a *valvular, cardiomyopathic,* or *ischemic process* that continues unabated, the paroxysms of AF may become more frequent and prolonged, culminating in chronic AF. AF is particularly common in patients with mitral valve disease, due to rather early onset of increased left atrial pressure and size. AF is much less common in disease of the aortic valve; when it does occur, it signifies very severe advanced disease (see Chapter 33).

Alcohol has been implicated as a major precipitant of AF. Binge drinking may induce paroxysms of AF and ventricular dysrhythmias (so-called "*holiday heart*" disease). Although there may be no overt evidence of underlying heart disease, there is some debate as to just how normal the hearts really are of patients who experience alcohol-induced arrhythmias. Chronic alcohol abuse can lead to *alcoholic cardiomyopathy*, which may present as paroxysmal AF during binge drinking. As drinking continues, the cardiomyopathy progresses and the AF becomes more established. The condition is potentially reversible with total abstinence.

Systemic Embolization and Stroke. Both epidemiologic and prospective studies have documented an increased risk of systemic embolization and stroke in patients with AF. It used to be thought that increased risk applied only to patients with AF caused by *rheumatic mitral valve disease* (relative risk increased nearly 15-fold), but community-based studies have identified lesser but still significant increases (e.g., four- to five-fold) in stroke risk for *all* AF patients with *underlying heart disease*. Independent predictors of high risk for stroke or systemic embolization in nonrheumatic AF patients include *clinical congestive heart failure or systolic dysfunction, previous thromboembolism, systolic hypertension* (more than 160 mm Hg), and *age older than 75 years if female*. Prospective transthoracic echocardiographic study confirms that left ventricular dysfunction is an independent predictor of stroke risk, and transesophageal echocardiographic (TEE) studies find that *thrombus* in the *left atrium* or *left atrial appendage* also powerfully predicts embolic risk.

Atherosclerotic risk factors (e.g., *diabetes, hypertension*) markedly increase the risk of systemic embolization and stroke in persons with AF, perhaps by contributing to development of *complex atherosclerotic plaque* in the transverse portion of the thoracic *aorta*, found in TEE studies to be an independent risk factor for embolic stroke.

Data from the Framingham study suggest that risk of stroke is greatest at the onset of AF, with more than 25% of AF-associated strokes occurring shortly after onset. In addition, patients with AF have twice the likelihood of having a recurrence of stroke within the first 6 months compared with patients with stroke and no AF.

Reduction in Cardiac Output: Risk of Death. The decrease in ventricular filling and loss of atrial contraction that result from AF lead to a fall in cardiac output and a rise in pulmonary capillary wedge pressure. When these are substantial, shortness of breath and reduced exercise tolerance may ensue. Rapid AF is especially likely to trigger hemodynamic compromise and heart failure. Cardiomyopathic changes are sometimes a consequence of rapid AF, further compromising cardiac output and exacerbating symptoms. Overall, AF increases the risk of death by as much as twofold.

PRINCIPLES OF MANAGEMENT

The first priorities are assessment of hemodynamic state and establishment of rate control, which requires identification and treatment of precipitants and underlying etiology. Then attention turns to determining the risk of systemic embolization and selecting an appropriate approach to stroke prophylaxis, be it chronic anticoagulation/rate control or cardioversion/chronic antiarrhythmic therapy or any combination thereof.

Assessment of Hemodynamic State and Establishment of Rate Control

Heart rate is an important determinant of hemodynamic state and myocardial oxygen demand. If there is any evidence of significant hemodynamic compromise (e.g., hypotension, congestive heart failure, ischemia), the patient must be immediately *hospitalized* and, in most instances, *urgently cardioverted*. Patients exhibiting no such compromise can be treated as outpatients. The goal is a ventricular response rate at rest of less than 85 beats/min and less than 110 beats/min after mild exercise (e.g., 10 situps or standing up 10 times from a chair). Heart rate may appear well controlled at rest when there is little adrenergic stimulation but rise markedly with mild effort; one needs to evaluate control both at rest and on exertion. For rate control, the drugs most often used in the outpatient setting are beta-blockers, calcium channel blockers, and digoxin.

Digoxin. Although still useful in properly selected patients (such as those with AF due to systolic dysfunction; see Chapter 32), digoxin should no longer be considered the cornerstone of pharmacologic therapy for AF, because the drug has several important shortcomings. It tends to be *ineffective* in slowing heart rate when vagal tone is low and adrenergic stimulation is high, as during *exercise, stress, fever, hypovolemia, hyperthyroidism, ischemia,* or *hypoxia*. Control may be fine at rest but inadequate in the setting of sympathetic drive. Moreover, in the absence of heart failure, digoxin neither restores *sinus rhythm* nor *maintains sinus rhythm* and does little to reduce the frequency and severity of paroxysmal AF episodes. This lack of efficacy is believed related to the drug's dependence on *vagal tone* for full effect and the high level of adrenergic stimulation common to situations that trigger paroxysms of AF or worsen rate control. Electrophysiologic studies show the drug actually shortens the atrial refractory period and may contribute to persistence of AF. By facilitating conduction through the bypass tract and shortening its refractory period, digoxin may exacerbate AF due to WPW syndrome. Careful case selection and close monitoring of therapy are critical to safe effective digoxin use (see Chapter 32).

Adverse Effects. The narrow therapeutic index for digoxin also discourages its use. Subtle dysrhythmic manifestations of digitalis toxicity in the setting of AF include *regularization* of AF, a manifestation of *junctional tachycardia*, and frequent *ventricular premature beats*. The latter should not be confused on electrocardiogram with the widened QRS complexes caused by the *Ashmann phenomenon* (prolonged relative refractory period in the beat after a long RR interval). Although ventricular response rate provides a "bioassay" of digitalis effect and makes frequent sampling of digoxin levels unnecessary, watching for changes in rhythm can be very informative. Whenever there is suspicion of digitalis toxicity, digoxin should be held and a serum level checked.

Beta-Blockers. Beta-blocking agents and calcium channel blockers have supplanted digoxin as the drugs of choice for rate control in AF, largely because of their superior efficacy in settings of high adrenergic stimulation. Beta-blockers slow ventricular response by increasing the refractoriness of the atrioventricular node and blocking the β-adrenergic effect of catecholamines on heart rate. Unlike digoxin, they do not require vagal tone to slow ventricular response rate, making them particularly useful when exercise, situational stress, hyperthyroidism, fever, hypoxemia, or ischemia is responsible for the tachyarrhythmia. Although negatively inotropic, beta-blockers may even be used with benefit (albeit cautiously) for AF in the setting of congestive heart failure (see Chapter 32).

Calcium-Channel Blockers. Like beta-blockers, a number of calcium-channel blockers have proven useful for AF rate control. *Verapamil* is the prototypical calcium-channel blocker used in AF; its ability to prolong the refractory period and the conduction time of arterioventricular nodal tissue reduces the ventricular response rate. *Diltiazem* acts similarly although not quite as potently; it is also less negatively inotropic. Unlike digoxin, calcium channel blockers do not require vagal tone to be maximally effective and consequently they control AF under circumstances that ordinarily would be refractory to digoxin (i.e., high sympathetic tone). Caution is required when using these calcium channel blockers in patients with underlying conduction system disease (e.g., sick sinus syndrome), because they may exacerbate heart block. The drug is contraindicated in WPW syndrome, due to its ability to enhance conduction through the accessory pathway (see below). Use of short-acting preparations in the setting of congestive heart failure is associated with an increased risk of cardiac death (see Chapter 32). In general, sustained-release formulations appear to be better tolerated than short-acting ones (see Chapter 26).

Etiologic Approach to Rate Control. Selection of the proper agent for rate control requires an etiologic diagnosis (see Chapter 25). Empiric therapy without regard for the underlying pathophysiology risks hemodynamic worsening. The importance of this principal is underscored by the approaches required to establish rate control in WPW syndrome, sick sinus syndrome, and hyperthyroidism.

WPW syndrome requires special mention because of the small but important risk of hemodynamic compromise associated with the disorder and standard approaches to rate control. WPW patients with very rapid ventricular rates and hemodynamic deterioration during an attack of AF should be hospitalized, promptly referred to a cardiologist, and treated with urgent *electrical cardioversion.* WPW patients with occasional bouts of AF that are well tolerated and self-limited require no treatment so long as the shortest RR interval during an attack is greater than 180 ms—a shorter interval is associated with an increased risk of ventricular fibrillation. No restrictions on activity are necessary. *Digoxin* and *calcium channel blockers should not be used*, because they encourage conduction through the accessory pathway by blocking conduction through the arterioventricular node. Future episodes of AF are prevented by the

use of antiarrhythmic agents such as *amiodarone* or *radiofrequency ablation.* Inpatient electrophysiologic testing is used to help judge which agent is most likely to provide optimal control of ventricular rate during AF. *Beta-blockers* are sometimes helpful in protecting against recurrent episodes of AF but should also be subjected to electrophysiologic study before being used in patients with potentially serious attacks of AF. Cardiac consultation is essential.

Tachycardia-Bradycardia (Sick Sinus) Syndrome. Patients with the tachycardia-bradycardia form of *sick sinus syndrome* pose a therapeutic dilemma: Although their AF usually responds well to *beta-blockade, verapamil,* or *digoxin,* these therapies may seriously exacerbate episodes of bradycardia by further suppressing conduction through the arterioventricular node. Consequently, *pacemaker implantation* is often necessary for patients with symptomatic tachycardia-bradycardia syndrome.

Hyperthyroidism. AF caused by *hyperthyroidism* responds best to beta-blockade, although definitive treatment of the underlying thyroid disease (see Chapter 103) is essential to successful prevention of future episodes of AF. At times, elective cardioversion (see below) is necessary to restore sinus rhythm after successful treatment of the hyperthyroidism.

Assessment of Risk for Systemic Embolization and Approaches to Prophylaxis

Prevention of systemic embolization and stroke is a key therapeutic priority. Although there is agreement that AF increases the risk of stroke, there remains considerable variation of opinion about the best way to reduce stroke risk. A large-scale, prospective, randomized, clinical trial (the Atrial Fibrillation Follow-up Investigation of Rhythm Management) comparing cardioversion/maintenance of sinus rhythm with chronic anticoagulation/AF rate control is underway and should help provide guidance. In the meantime, considerable clinical judgment is required. Cost-effectiveness studies and decision analyses have tried to provide some guidance, but these studies are limited by their basic assumptions. Nonetheless, an emerging approach to treatment focuses on degree of stroke risk, with stratification helping to identify an appropriate set of therapeutic modalities. Also important are the patient's cardiovascular status, likelihood for successful cardioversion and maintenance of sinus rhythm, and ability to comply with and tolerate antiarrhythmic or anticoagulant programs.

Assessment of Stroke Risk. The *history, physical exam,* and pertinent laboratory studies (particularly *echocardiography*) are reviewed for important risk factors (see below) to help stratify the patient's degree of risk. Although not yet validated by prospective studies, such stratification has the potential to rationalized selection of treatment modality. It is also important to remember that embolic stroke risk is not solely a function of AF but also related to overall atherosclerotic risk, as manifested by complex plaque formation in the aortic arch.

High risk (more than 8%/yr) is a reasonable categorization for persons with *mitral stenosis* or other forms of *rheumatic valvular heart disease* and for those with *nonrheumatic heart disease* accompanied by *prior embolization* or *stroke* or evidence of marked *systolic dysfunction,* severe *congestive heart failure*, significant *left atrial mural thrombus*, or *female sex plus age more than 75 years.*

Moderate-to-high risk (5% to 8%/yr) might be the appropriate designation for those with less severe degrees of underlying heart disease and for those with *marked left atrial enlargement (more than 6.0 cm)* or other independent risk factors for stroke such as *diabetes, hypertension,* or *hypercholesterolemia.*

Moderate risk (3% to -5%/yr) has been suggested as a designation for patients with no risk factors other than *systolic hypertension* (more than 160 mm Hg). *Lone fibrillators older than 60 years* of age might also be grouped in this category, because they manifest a similar degree of risk.

Low-to-moderate risk (1% to 3%/yr) has been confirmed by prospective study in AF patients treated with aspirin who manifest no evidence of congestive heart failure, systolic dysfunction, previous thromboembolism, systolic blood pressure more than 160 mm Hg, or age older than 75 years.

Low risk (less than 1%) might be the designation for those whose risk is similar to that of patients without AF, as occurs in *lone fibrillators younger than 60 years of age* truly devoid of any stroke risk factors or underlying heart disease.

Warfarin Anticoagulation. The demonstrated relationship between thrombus in the left atrium and risk of thromboembolism in AF provides a strong rationale for anticoagulation therapy. Several large-scale, prospective, randomized, controlled trials with long-term follow-up have demonstrated that warfarin anticoagulation significantly reduces the risk of systemic embolization and stroke not only in persons with rheumatic AF but also in those with nonrheumatic heart disease. Risk is lowered by nearly two thirds with application of warfarin anticoagulation. Modern well-monitored oral anticoagulation programs help ensure safety and minimize risk of major hemorrhage (see Chapter 83). Long-term warfarin anticoagulation represents one of the few well-established evidence-based approaches to stroke prophylaxis in AF. TEE studies suggest the mechanism is prevention of clot formation and resolution of preexisting clot.

Despite the important association between thrombus formation and stroke risk, oral anticoagulation is not the most potent of prophylactic measures in AF, falling short of cardioversion in many settings, but superior to aspirin. Consequently, although warfarin may be essential to prophylaxis in certain situations (e.g., previous embolization, cardioversion failure, inability to tolerate antiarrhythmics), it often does not suffice as monotherapy and may not be the treatment of first choice in many high-risk situations. In persons over the age of 75 years, oral anticoagulation becomes problematic, because its use is associated with an increased risk of hemorrhagic stroke that nearly cancels its prophylactic benefit. A low-dose warfarin program (PT INR less than 1.2 to 1.5) plus aspirin is not as effective as adjusted-dose warfarin that achieves a greater degree of anticoagulation (PT INR 2.0 to 3.0).

Short-term warfarin anticoagulation is prescribed for *elective cardioversion* to reduce the modest risk of embolization associated with the procedure. Treatment is usually begun 3 to 4 weeks before cardioversion (which allows for dissolution of any thrombus that is present and prevention of new thrombus formation) and continued for 4 weeks after cardioversion (which limits the risk of late embolization due to atrial instabil-ity and slow return of full atrial contractility). Patients with a very high risk of stroke are treated chronically with warfarin prophylaxis after cardioversion (those with lesser risk are given aspirin). The indications, optimal intensity, proper duration, and cost effectiveness of long-term postcardioversion anticoagulation remain to be determined. *TEE* can be used to detect left atrial thrombus and better determine need for a month of oral anticoagulation. TEE is especially useful in persons who have a relative contraindication to oral anticoagulation and also can obviate the need for delay in cardioversion. Persons with no thrombus on TEE have a very low risk of embolization; they require only a brief period of heparinization at the time of cardioversion. Although expensive and requiring skilled operators, the study may be worth performing to better estimate embolic risk in the patient with a relative contraindication to warfarin therapy.

Aspirin. Low-moderate risk patients with nonvalvular AF treated with aspirin (325 mg/d) experience a very low rate of embolic events, approaching that of patients without AF. Because aspirin is less likely to cause cerebral hemorrhage than warfarin, it is preferable in the low-risk setting. However, when used in higher risk patients, even in combination with low-dose warfarin, aspirin does not provide the same protection as does standard-dose warfarin. Some physicians use aspirin for stroke prophylaxis after cardioversion in persons of low-moderate moderate or low stroke risk, because of the high probability AF recurring.

Elective Cardioversion. An increasingly practical and safe approach to management of AF is to restore and maintain normal sinus rhythm. Not only can stroke risk be reduced in many AF patients by eliminating left atrial stasis, but the adverse hemodynamic effects of AF are also reversed, and exercise tolerance may improve as restoration of atrial contractility enhances cardiac output. Before the advent of safe effective means of cardioversion and maintenance of sinus rhythm, cardioversion followed by chronic antiarrhythmic therapy was fraught with a high risk of relapse and adverse proarrhythmic effects from drugs used to sustain sinus rhythm. As noted earlier, the relative efficacy of cardioversion compared with chronic anticoagulation remains unknown.

Candidacy. Patients experiencing *exercise intolerance* from the hemodynamic compromise associated with loss of atrial contraction should be considered for cardioversion. Other determinants of candidacy are degree of stroke risk and likelihood of remaining in sinus rhythm. A recent cost-effectiveness analysis found cardioversion superior to chronic anticoagulation when there was high or moderate-to-high embolic risk. The best predictors of successful cardioversion and sustained maintenance of sinus rhythm are *duration of AF* and *age*. AF of recent onset due to an acute stress (e.g., alcohol binge, pneumonia) often reverts spontaneously. At the other end of the spectrum, AF of more than 1 year is unlikely to cardiovert and hold as sinus rhythm, probably because of atrial fibrosis that occurs over time. Fibrosis is also believed to be at least part of the reason why age is a predictor of outcome. *Atrial size* is associated inversely with outcome, but often size appears to be more a reflection of AF duration than an independent predictor of success or failure. Nonetheless, a normal left atrial size is associated with a high probability of successful cardioversion and maintenance of sinus rhythm, whereas a left atrial diameter of more than 60 mm retains independent predictive value as a sign of poor outcome. Other factors that have been identified as predictors of poor outcome include advanced *mitral stenosis,* other forms of rheumatic heart disease, and chronic *congestive heart failure;* however, with the exception of these conditions, etiology is usually not a powerful predictor of responsiveness to cardioversion.

Mode of Cardioversion. Cardioversion may be electrical or chemical. *Electrical cardioversion* is the procedure of choice for urgently converting AF to sinus rhythm. It also has the highest success rate of any modality for restoring normal sinus rhythm. Pretreatment with antiarrhythmic agents is usually unnecessary and not deemed desirable because of its negative effect on atrial contractility. Anesthesia is often recommended. Any digoxin being used is withheld for 2 days before cardioversion, because there is an increased risk of ventricular dysrhythmias when the heart is countershocked in the presence of high digoxin levels. As noted above, the risk of embolization is a function of duration of AF and can be minimized by precardioversion oral anticoagulation and a month of warfarin after cardioversion (see above). Although many patients experience a prompt increase in cardiac output, up to a third do not because of chronic atrial changes associated with AF that may take up to a month to revert back toward normal.

Chemical cardioversion is a reasonable consideration for patients with recent onset of AF (less than 1 week), especially when there is no significant underlying myocardial disease. Single doses of a modern *class IC antiarrhythmic (e.g., flecainide 300 mg or propafenone 600 mg)* can restore sinus rhythm in over 75% of such patients. Because class IC antiarrhythmics may convert AF to very rapid atrial flutter with 1:1 conduction and cause acute hemodynamic compromise, chemical cardioversion is often supplemented with an arterioventricular nodal blocking drug such as a beta-blocker. Because class IC antiarrhythmics can suppress sinoatrial node function, patients may actually feel worse immediately after chemical cardioversion. As the suppressant effect wears off, cardiac output improves and patients begin to feel better. The newer class IC agents (flecainide, propafenone) have largely replaced *quinidine* for cardioversion, because single-dose therapy often suffices and these agents are more effective, although still associated with proarrhythmic risk (e.g., polymorphic ventricular tachycardias such as torsades de pointes). Moreover, they are negatively inotropic and should be used with caution if at all in persons with underlying myocardial or valvular impairment.

Maintenance of Sinus Rhythm. Because of the high likelihood of recurrence of AF (50% to 70%/yr), chronic antiarrhythmic therapy is often prescribed in persons at high risk of relapse (e.g., those with previous relapse, marked left atrial enlargement, advanced underlying heart disease, high voltage required for cardioversion). Of available agents, *amiodarone* is among the most effective (20% recurrence rate vs. 50% recurrence with most other drugs) and safest, with little to no proarrhythmic effect, no increased risk of sudden death, and no impairment of contractility. Low doses of the drug (e.g., 100 to 200 mg once daily) often suffice, and the agent can be used in the setting of heart failure. Side effects are numerous but usually not severe enough to warrant termination of therapy. Important adverse effects include *pulmonary toxicity* (interstitial changes related to total dose), *thyroid suppression* (due to the iodine in amiodarone), *acute gastrointestinal upset, chronic constipation, corneal cysts,* and *neurologic dysfunction* (tremor, ataxia, peripheral neuropathy). The drug *potentiates* the effect of *warfarin* and may cause minor *abnormalities in liver function tests,* but frank hepatocellular injury is rare.

Amiodarone has relegated previously used agents such as *quinidine* and *disopyramide* to secondary roles for maintenance of sinus rhythm. The proarrhythmic and gastrointestinal side effects of quinidine, as well as its suboptimal efficacy (50% relapse rate), discourage its use. Of greatest concern is quinidine's propensity to cause *QT prolongation* and polymorphic ventricular tachycardias (e.g., *torsades de pointes*), which are associated with increased risks of *syncope* and *sudden death.* Although amiodarone also increases the QT interval, it does not trigger torsades nearly as readily as the older drugs. Disopyramide has also been displaced as a first-line agent because of its disappointing efficacy, negative inotropy, and anticholinergic side effects. The newer class IC antiarrhythmics (e.g., *flecainide* and *propafenone*) are being explored for their possible role in maintenance of sinus rhythm, but they are negatively inotropic and have proarrhythmic effects, making them less than ideal for persons with underlying heart disease.

Beta-blockers are helpful for maintenance of sinus rhythm in cases where marked adrenergic stimulation is associated with precipitation or persistence of AF. Persons with underlying ischemic heart disease may be especially good candidates (see Chapter 30), and even persons with congestive heart failure may benefit when small doses are used in conjunction with close monitoring.

Atrial pacing and implantable atrial defibrillation have been proposed as nonpharmacologic approaches to maintenance of sinus rhythm in persons who are unresponsive to other measures and tolerate AF poorly. Persons with sick sinus syndrome, who may already be candidates for pacemaker therapy, appear to be promising candidates for atrial pacing as a means of preventing recurrent AF. More prospective study is needed.

Ablation of the atrial reentrant circuit causing AF has been performed both surgically (the *maze procedure*) and by radiofrequency techniques during electrophysiologic study. Safety and long-term efficacy have yet to be established, but such procedures could conceivably prove useful in patients with frequent recurrences who tolerate their AF poorly and do not respond to other measures.

PATIENT EDUCATION

The young patient with paroxysmal AF who is free of underlying heart disease needs to be fully reassured to prevent cardiac neurosis and the unnecessary restriction of activity. Such patients should be instructed to quit smoking, avoid sleep deprivation, and limit use of alcohol and stimulants. They often will benefit from use of relaxation techniques (see Chapter 226) at times of stress. WPW patients whose episodes of AF are brief, infrequent, and well tolerated can also be reassured and encouraged to remain fully active. Patients with AF secondary to alcohol abuse and evolving cardiomyopathy need to be informed of the risk of alcoholic cardiomyopathy and strongly urged to abstain from alcohol. In addition, patients at risk for AF from any other cause should be advised to use caution in their social drinking, because excess intake may increase vulnerability to AF (see Chapters 25 and 228).

It is important to teach AF patients and family members to watch for signs of hemodynamic compromise, such as rapid heart rate, unexplained weight gain, worsening dyspnea on exertion, and decreased exercise tolerance. Patients often fear that long-term digoxin therapy will be habit forming or injurious to the heart; reassurance and education about its use are often much appreciated. However, they need to be aware of the symptoms and signs of digitalis toxicity (see Chapter 32) so that correction of the problem is not unnecessarily delayed.

INDICATIONS FOR ADMISSION AND REFERRAL

Patients unable to tolerate their AF due to congestive heart failure or ischemia should be immediately hospitalized. The same is true if the ventricular response rate is extremely rapid (more than 170 beats/min). Electrical cardioversion may be urgent. Hospitalization is also indicated for patients refractory to medical therapy and those with new onset of embolization. Patients who are candidates for elective cardioversion need at least a temporary stay, even if only for the day.

Referral is indicated for patients with refractory AF, suspicion of WPW syndrome, sick sinus syndrome, or AF resulting in hemodynamic compromise. Patients deemed possible candidates for elective cardioversion also should be referred for cardiac consultation.

THERAPEUTIC RECOMMENDATIONS

Rate Control

- Admit for consideration of urgent cardioversion any patient with evidence of hemodynamic compromise (i.e., acute or worsening congestive failure, ischemia, or acute embolization) or a very rapid ventricular response rate (more than 150 beats/min).
- Conduct a careful workup for identification and treatment of precipitants and underlying etiologies (see Chapter 25).
- Begin therapy for rate control if ventricular response rate at rest is more than 85 beats/min or more than 110 beats/min after mild exercise. Unless there is concurrent heart failure, start with a modest dose of a beta-blocker (e.g., atenolol 25 mg/d) or a calcium channel blocker (e.g., diltiazem, 30 mg four times a day, switching to a sustained-release formulation once an effective dose is established). In the setting of left ventricular systolic dysfunction, consider digoxin or very cautious low-dose use of a beta-blocker and avoid calcium channel blockers (see Chapter 32).
- In the setting of WPW and other preexcitation syndromes, refer for consideration of electrophysiologic study and ablative therapy; do not treat with digoxin or calcium channel blockers because of their tendency to enhance conduction through accessory pathways. Young patients with brief and infrequent bouts of AF due to WPW need not be treated if episodes are well tolerated and the shortest RR interval is greater than 180 ms.
- In the setting of sick sinus syndrome, use considerable caution in initiation of rate-control therapy because such patients are especially susceptible to symptomatic bradycardia; if marked bradycardia occurs upon initiation of such therapy, then refer for consideration of pacemaker implantation.

- If rate control is difficult to achieve, recheck for failure, ischemia, fever, hypovolemia, hypoxia, recurrent pulmonary embolization, hyperthyroidism, and WPW syndrome. Treatment should be directed at the underlying condition. Hospitalize and cardiovert if the AF is not well tolerated.

Stroke Prophylaxis

- For patients with underlying heart disease and AF of less than 48 hours' duration, consider immediate referral for elective cardioversion (either pharmacologic or electrical); precardioversion warfarin anticoagulation is not necessary so long as cardioversion is carried out within 48 hours of onset.
- For all patients with underlying heart disease and AF of more than 48 hours' duration or of unknown duration, begin oral anticoagulant therapy with warfarin as early as possible, unless there is a serious contraindication to warfarin therapy (see Chapter 83). Prescribed an adjustable-dose warfarin program that achieves a prothrombin time of 2.0 to 3.0 INR.
- For those at high risk for systemic embolization (e.g., prior embolization or stroke, systolic dysfunction, clinical congestive heart failure, significant left atrial mural thrombus, or female sex plus age more than 75 years), consider elective cardioversion. Also consider for elective cardioversion those with exercise intolerance or fatigue due to AF, intolerable symptomatic palpitations, or inability to take long-term oral anticoagulation. Screen out those with a high probability of unresponsiveness or relapse (e.g., AF more than 1 years' duration, marked left atrial enlargement, rheumatic etiology).
- Before elective cardioversion in persons with AF of more than 48 hours' duration, prescribe 3 to 4 weeks of adjusted-dose warfarin anticoagulation (to achieve a PT INR of 2.0 to 3.0).
- If it is deemed desirable to proceed directly to elective cardioversion without waiting 3 to 4 weeks for oral anticoagulation, then obtain a TEE to enhance determination of stroke risk. If no thrombus is detected in the left atrium or left atrial appendage, then it is reasonable to proceed directly to cardioversion.
- After cardioversion, whether preceded by warfarin or not, prescribe adjusted-dose warfarin for at least 4 weeks after restoration of sinus rhythm.
- After cardioversion in those with a high risk of AF recurrence (e.g., marked left atrial enlargement, advanced age, high amount of energy required for cardioversion), consider chronic adjusted-dose warfarin prophylaxis, especially if the patient has clinical features conferring high stroke risk. Alternatively, consider chronic antiarrhythmic therapy with low-dose amiodarone (e.g., 100 to 200 mg/d); monitor liver function tests and thyrotropin every 6 months.
- Refer those with frequent recurrences of AF that occur despite antiarrhythmic therapy for consideration of interventional approaches (e.g., atrial ablation, pacing, or defibrillator placement), especially if recurrences are not well tolerated hemodynamically.
- For those with clinical characteristics that make them poor candidates for elective cardioversion (e.g., AF more than 1 years' duration, advanced rheumatic valvular disease, marked left atrial enlargement), consider long-term adjusted-dose warfarin anticoagulation, especially if they have clinical features predictive of high risk for stroke.

- For AF patients with a low-to-moderate risk of embolic stroke (i.e., no congestive heart failure or significant systolic dysfunction, no previous thromboembolism, systolic pressure less than 160 mm Hg, and age less than 75 years), consider chronic aspirin therapy (e.g., 325 mg/d). Those with concurrent atherosclerotic risk factors are likely to benefit the most.
- Consider chronic aspirin therapy also for those who cannot take or refuse oral anticoagulation.
- Advise patients with paroxysms of AF from whatever cause to use alcohol only in moderation and avoid bouts of acute intoxication, because such bouts increase vulnerability for AF.

A.H.G.

ANNOTATED BIBLIOGRAPHY

Atrial Fibrillation Investigators. Echocardiographic predictors of stroke in patients with atrial fibrillation: a prospective study of 1066 patients from 3 clinical trials. Arch Intern Med 1998;158:1316. (*Identifies left ventricular dysfunction as an independent predictor.*)

Boston Area Anticoagulation Trial for Atrial Fibrillation Investigators. The effect of low-dose warfarin on the risk of stroke in patients with nonrheumatic atrial fibrillation. N Engl J Med 1990;323:1505. (*One of several major randomized trials demonstrating benefit in patients with chronic or paroxysmal AF.*)

Brand FN, Abbott RD, Kannel WB, et al. Characteristics and prognosis of lone atrial fibrillation: 30-year follow-up in the Framingham Study. JAMA 1985;254:3449. (*A fourfold increase in stroke risk was noted, but patients were older and had more cardiovascular risk factors than patients in other studies of lone AF.*)

Catherwood E, Fitzpatrick D, Greenberg ML, et al. Cost-effectiveness of cardioversion and antiarrhythmic therapy in nonvalvular atrial fibrillation. Ann Intern Med 1999;130:625. (*This analysis supports cardioversion supplemented by amiodarone over warfarin monotherapy for high-risk patients.*)

Engel TR, Luck JC. Effect of whiskey on atrial vulnerability and "holiday heart." J Am Col Cardiol 1983;1:816. (*Alcohol enhanced vulnerability to AF in patients without clinical evidence of cardiomyopathy or heart failure.*)

Falk RH. Proarrhythmia in patients treated for atrial fibrillation or flutter. Ann Intern Med 1992;117:141. (*A review of the potential for dysrhythmias from drugs used to treat AF.*)

Falk RH, Leavitt JI. Digoxin for atrial fibrillation: a drug whose time has gone? Ann Intern Med 1991;114:573. (*A review critical of digoxin that emphasizes its shortcomings in the treatment of AF; 22 references.*)

Gage BF, Cardinalli AB, Albers GW, et al. Cost-effectiveness of warfarin and aspirin for prophylaxis of stroke in patients with nonvalvular atrial fibrillation. JAMA 1995;274:1839. (*Data supporting the cost-effectiveness of warfarin.*)

Go AS, Hylek EM, Borowsky LH, et al. Warfarin use among ambulatory patients with nonvalvular atrial fibrillation: the AnTicoagulation and Risk Factor in Atrial Fibrillation (ATRIA) Study. Ann Intern Med 1999;131:927. (*A cross-sectional study of an HMO population; documents marked underutilization of warfarin in ideal candidates.*)

Grace AA, Camm AJ. Quinidine. N Engl J Med 1998;338:35 (*Excellent modern review of this long prescribed drug; addresses its uses and limitations in AF; 105 references.*)

Kannel WB, Abbott RD, Savage DD, et al. Epidemiologic features of chronic atrial fibrillation: the Framingham Study. N Engl J Med 1982;306:1018. (*A major epidemiologic study; heart failure and rheumatic heart disease were the most powerful predictive precursors of chronic AF; chronic AF was associated with a doubling of overall and cardiovascular mortality.*)

Klein AL, Grimm RA, Black IW, et al. Cardioversion guided by transesophageal echocardiography: the ACUTE Pilot Study. A randomized controlled trial. Ann Intern Med 1997;126:200. (*Initial data suggesting that TEE can identify patients appropriate for early cardioversion.*)

Kopecky SL, Gersh BJ, McGoon MD, et al. The natural history of lone atrial fibrillation: a population-based study over three decades. N Engl J Med 1987;317:669. (*A retrospective study of patients under the age of 60 showing that lone AF was associated with a very low risk of stroke.*)

Manning WJ, Silverman DI, Gordon SPF, et al. Cardioversion from atrial fibrillation without prolonged anticoagulation with use of transesophageal echocardiography to exclude presence of atrial thrombi. N Engl J Med 1993;328:750. (*Preliminary data suggesting this technology may make possible early cardioversion in many patients.*)

Meyers DG, Gonzalez ER, Nelson WP. The role of prophylactic anticoagulation in cardioversion of atrial fibrillation. Cardiovasc Rev Rep 1985;6:647. (*A critical review of the available evidence presented in pooled form. Argues that few conclusions can be drawn from available data and that prospective randomized studies are needed.*)

Podrid PJ. Amiodarone: reevaluation of an old drug. Ann Intern Med 1995;122:689. (*Excellent review that includes considerable data on utility of the drug in AF; 109 references.*)

Rawles JM, Metcalfe MJ, Jennings K. Time occurrence, duration and ventricular rate of paroxysmal atrial fibrillation: the effect of digoxin. Br Heart J 1990;63:225. (*Digoxin was observed in this Holter monitoring study to have little effect on preventing recurrences, slowing rate at the onset of a paroxysm, or terminating episodes.*)

Singer DE. Randomized trials of warfarin for atrial fibrillation. N Engl J Med 1992;327:1451. (*A fine editorial tersely summarizing the known and unknown.*)

Stollberger C, Chnupa P, Kronik G, et al. Transesophageal echocardiography to assess embolic risk in patients with atrial fibrillation. Ann Intern Med 1998;128:630. (*A multicenter observational study identifying important risk factors for embolic stroke in AF, including thrombus in the left atrium, hypertension, previous stroke, and advancing age.*)

The Stroke Prevention in Atrial Fibrillation Investigators. Predictors of thromboembolism in atrial fibrillation. Ann Intern Med 1992;116:1. (*A two-part study; recent congestive heart failure, hypertension, previous embolism, left ventricular dysfunction, and left atrial enlargement were independent predictors of stroke risk.*)

The Stroke Prevention in Atrial Fibrillation Investigators. Adjusted-dose warfarin versus low-intensity, fixed-dose warfarin plus aspirin for high-risk patients with atrial fibrillation: Stroke Prevention in Atrial Fibrillation III randomized clinical trial. Lancet 1996;348:633. (*SPAF III, finding that adjusted-dose therapy was superior to low-intensity therapy plus aspirin.*)

The Stroke Prevention in Atrial Fibrillation Investigators. Transesophageal echocardiographic correlates of thromboembolism in high-risk patients with nonvalvular atrial fibrillation. Ann Intern Med 1998;128:639. (*A prospective observational study finding that left atrial thrombus and complex aortic atherosclerotic plaque detected by TEE are highly correlated with risk of subsequent thromboembolism.*)

The Stroke Prevention in Atrial Fibrillation Investigators. Patients with nonvalvular atrial fibrillation at low risk of stroke during treatment with aspirin: Stroke Prevention in Atrial Fibrillation III Study. JAMA 1998;279:1273. (*Prospective cohort study identifying AF patients at low-risk for subsequent embolic complications.*)

Weigner MJ, Caulfield TA, Danias PG, et al. Risk for clinical thromboembolism associated with conversion to sinus rhythm in patients with atrial fibrillation lasting less than 48 hours. Ann Intern Med 1997;126:615. *(A prospective observational study finding that cardioversion-related risk was nil.)*

Wolf PA, Kannel WB, McGee DL, et al. Duration of atrial fibrillation and imminence of stroke: the Framingham Study. Stroke 1983;14:664. *(Important epidemiology data; risk of embolic stroke found to be maximal at onset of AF, independent of other risk factors for stroke, and substantial, even in AF patients without rheumatic mitral disease; recurrence was twice as likely in patients with AF.)*

29

Management of Ventricular Irritability in the Ambulatory Setting

The discovery of ventricular ectopy in the outpatient setting raises concerns about serious underlying heart disease and the possibilities of cardiac arrest and sudden death. At issue is how much danger the ventricular irritability poses, a critical determination because treatment is also fraught with risk. In some instances, pharmacologic suppression of ventricular irritability may actually increase risk of sudden death rather than reduce it. Management of ventricular ectopy is shifting from reliance on antiarrhythmic drugs to implantation of cardioverter-defibrillators, which have demonstrated promising results in preventing cardiac arrest and sudden death. Determining the optimal approach to management in this period of change requires close consultation with a cardiologist experienced in treating ventricular dysrhythmias. The primary care physician's principal tasks are to identify high-risk patients, arrange timely cardiac consultation, help patients choose the treatment option best suited to their needs, and monitor therapy. Knowledge of the relative benefits of antiarrhythmic drugs and implantable defibrillators is essential to therapeutic decision making. Close monitoring and long-term follow-up by the primary physician help to ensure safe and effective management.

CLINICAL PRESENTATION AND COURSE

Premature ventricular contractions (PVCs) are ubiquitous and commonly found among patients both with and without underlying heart disease. In studies of the general population, at least one PVC per routine electrocardiogram (ECG) was found in 1% of Air Force recruits, 4% of life insurance applicants, 7% of men older than 34 years of age, and 40% to 75% of normal persons subjected to 24 to 48 hours of continuous ambulatory (Holter) monitoring. The incidence and prevalence of PVCs increase with age and with exercise.

In the ambulatory setting, ventricular irritability usually presents in one of several ways: as an incidental finding on routine examination or ECG; as an ECG finding in a patient being evaluated for palpitations, dizziness, or syncope; or as a complication of underlying heart disease noted on resting ECG, exercise stress test, or Holter monitoring. *Frequent PVCs* are defined as more than 60 ectopic beats/h; *complex ventricular ectopy* is characterized by multiforms, repetitive forms, bigeminy, or R on T. *Ventricular tachycardia* (VT) refers to three or more PVCs in a row; in the *monomorphic* type, all QRS complexes are identical; in *polymorphic* VT (e.g., torsades de pointes), the QRS complexes are all different. *Nonsustained VT* refers to brief self-limited runs of VT; *sustained VT* persists in the absence of intervention. Prognosis is a function of the presence and severity of any underlying heart disease and the nature of the ventricular ectopic activity.

Benign Ventricular Arrhythmias

Initially, prospective studies of large populations of ambulatory men were thought to have shown a correlation between PVCs on routine ECG and subsequent sudden death; however, when these results were reexamined controlling for other cardiac risk factors, PVCs were not found to be an independent determinant of cardiac death in the general population. *Asymptomatic healthy* subjects, even those with frequent or complex PVCs, showed *no increased mortality* on long-term follow-up. Regardless of the presence and persistence of worrisome ventricular irritability, such patients have prognoses no different from those of other healthy people; there is no increased risk of cardiac death.

Other natural history surveys also emphasized that in the absence of hypertension, angina, history of myocardial infarction, heart failure, cardiomegaly on chest x-ray, or ECG signs of ischemia, left ventricular (LV) hypertrophy, or bundle branch block, people with PVCs are at no greater risk for cardiac death than the general population.

Potentially Adverse Ventricular Arrhythmias

In comparison with patients free of underlying heart disease, the situation is more worrisome for patients with a variety of cardiac problems, such as those recovering from a *recent myocardial infarction*. In the Coronary Drug Project study of over 2,000 survivors of myocardial infarction, the occurrence of even a *single PVC* on a routine ECG taken 3 months or more after the infarct was associated with a *doubling* of the *mortality rate* during the 3-year follow-up period. The features most predictive of mortality are *high frequency* of PVCs (more than 30/h over a 24-hour period) and presence of *complex* ventricular ectopy, especially repetitive beats (33 consecutive complexes). Prognosis is particularly poor in the setting of a *failing left ventricle* (ejection fraction less than 0.4). For patients with recent myocardial infarction, reduced ejection fraction, and nonsustained VT, the rate for cardiac arrest or sudden death approaches 20% at 2 years and exceeds 30% at 5 years.

In patients with a history of *remote myocardial infarction*, the frequency and complexity of PVCs also influence prognosis. The absence of ventricular irritability on a 1-hour ECG recording performed 3 to 9 months postinfarction is associated with a 6% risk of sudden cardiac death over 5 years, compared with 12% in patients with unifocal PVCs and 25% in those with complex ventricular ectopy. *Complex ventricular ectopy* (e.g., multifocal PVCs, nonsustained VT) has the strongest influence on risk for sudden cardiac death in this population (see below).

The situation is similar for patients with *other forms of heart disease* that cause myocardial scarring and abnormal wall motion. Patients with hypertrophic or congestive *cardiomyopathy*, hemodynamically significant *valvular disease, congenital heart disease* with ventricular hypertrophy, hypertensive *LV hypertrophy*, and revascularization or valve surgery have been found to be at significantly increased risk of sudden death if experiencing frequent or complex PVCs, especially in the context of a *reduced ejection fraction*. The ventricular ectopy is not merely a manifestation of the underlying heart disease but an independent predictor of prognosis.

Malignant Ventricular Arrhythmias

Nonsustained VT is a worrisome arrhythmia characterized by runs of VT that spontaneously revert to sinus rhythm within several beats. Unless there is hemodynamic compromise, nonsustained VT may be asymptomatic. In the context of *chronic coronary artery disease and LV dysfunction*, it represents a malignant form of electrical instability that is an independent risk factor for sudden death, increasing risk fivefold to 30% at 2 years. It has a more benign form, found in young patients with *no demonstrable heart disease* and characterized by resolution with exercise, no associated symptoms, and a regular relatively slow rate (less than 150 beats/min) with uniform cycle length and QRS morphology.

Recurrent sustained VT is a very dangerous ventricular arrhythmia, especially when it occurs in the context of *LV dysfunction*. Untreated, the 1-year mortality rate is about 40%; prognosis is poorest in symptomatic patients with compromised LV function. The arrhythmia is characterized by repeated episodes of VT, some of which may persist for up to several hours. Many patients become symptomatic due to a fall in cardiac output, which can lead to syncope, near-syncope, angina, or dyspnea. Coronary artery disease and cardiomyopathy account for almost 90% of cases. About 1% of postinfarction patients experience this arrhythmia during the first year of follow-up.

Torsades de pointes is a rapid polymorphic VT that often deteriorates into ventricular fibrillation. The characteristic feature is a QRS axis that twists about the ECG baseline, going from positive to negative and back again. The arrhythmia occurs in the context of *QT interval prolongation*, be it congenital or acquired. This is a very malignant ventricular dysrhythmia most commonly seen as an *acquired* condition in patients with electrolyte abnormalities (especially hypokalemia, hypo-

magnesemia) and use of drugs that prolong the QT interval, including antiarrhythmics (e.g., procainamide, quinidine, disopyramide), antifungal agents (e.g., ketoconazole, itraconazole), antibiotics (e.g., macrolides), antihistamines (e.g., terfenadine, astemizole), and prokinetic agents (e.g., cisapride). Risk is increased when an electrolyte abnormality occurs during antiarrhythmic therapy or when several potentially etiologic agents are being used concurrently (e.g., an antihistamine and an antibiotic). In the *congenital form* of QT prolongation, patients are young and have no evidence of structural heart disease but may have a family history of early (before age 30) sudden death in first-degree relatives, a personal history of prior syncope (especially in the setting of stress) or deafness, and ECG findings of QT prolongation, T-wave alternans, and notched T waves in at least three leads.

In sum, the main determinants of adverse prognosis in patients with ventricular ectopy are the presence of underlying heart disease and a failing left ventricle. Each of these factors is an independent predictor of survival. The complexity of the ventricular ectopy is also a determinant of prognosis, especially in patients with heart disease and LV failure, where VT portends an especially high risk of cardiac sudden death.

Probability of Occult Heart Disease in Asymptomatic Persons with Premature Ventricular Contractions

As long as the asymptomatic patient with PVCs has no evidence of underlying heart disease, the prognosis appears fine, but what is the probability of occult heart disease in an otherwise apparently healthy patient presenting with frequent or complex PVCs? The best approximation is that risk is not high. In a study of such patients subjected to coronary catheterization and angiography, only one fourth were found to have significant coronary artery disease (defined as more than 50% luminal narrowing). The characteristics of the ventricular ectopy did not differentiate those with coronary disease from those without it. These asymptomatic patients were treated with modest doses of beta-blocking agents and had normal survival rates after 5 years of follow-up. On the other hand, patients with syncope of unknown origin who manifest complex ventricular irritability and signs of underlying heart disease have a high risk of further syncope and cardiac death, especially if they demonstrate inducible sustained VT on electrophysiologic study.

PRINCIPLES OF MANAGEMENT

The approach to management is undergoing a fundamental change as treatment shifts from traditional reliance on class I antiarrhythmic drugs (Table 29.1) to use of implantable car-

Table 29.1. Classes of Antiarrhythmic Drugs and Their Effects

CLASS (AGENTS)	ACTIVITY	ELECTROCARDIOGRAPHIC EFFECT	PROARRHYTHMIC
IA (quinidine, procainamide, disopyramide)	↓PVC ↓VT rate	↑QRS ↑QT	Yes (torsades)
IB (mexiletine, tocainide)	↓PVC	Nil	Yes
IC (flecainide, moricizine)	↓PVC ↓VT rate	↑QRS	Yes (VT, VF)
II (beta-blockers)	Improved survival	↑PR and QRS	No
III (amiodarone, sotalol)	↓VT	↑PR and QT	Yes (torsades)

Adapted from Nattel S, Singh B. Evolution, mechanisms, and classification of antiarrhythmic drugs. Am J Cardiol 1999[Suppl]84:11R, with permission.
PVC, premature ventricular contraction; VT, ventricular tachycardia; VF, ventricular fibrillation.

dioverter-defibrillators, beta-blockers, and class III antiarrhythmics. This shift derives, in part, from well-designed trials (e.g., Cardiac Arrhythmia Suppression Trial [CAST]; see below) revealing a paradoxical increase in risk of sudden death with use of antiarrhythmic agents, presumably a consequence of proarrhythmic drug effects. Equally important, prospective randomized trials find implantable cardioverter-defibrillators superior to antiarrhythmic agents in reducing rates of cardiac arrest and sudden death in very high-risk patents. Confirmation of these findings is still required as is clearer definition who benefits most from a cardioverter-defibrillator, but these findings have stimulated increasing reliance on defibrillator implantation in high-risk patients. Combination strategies are also being explored, such as cardioverter-defibrillator implantation supplemented by beta-blockade and a pharmacologic strategy of beta-blockade plus a class III antiarrhythmic agent.

During this period of flux in the treatment of ventricular irritability, it is essential that the primary care physician follow the literature for results of ongoing prospective trials and work closely with a cardiologist skilled in the management of ventricular dysrhythmias to ensure effective safe management. Because all therapies for serious ventricular ectopy are fraught with risk, it is essential to select carefully for treatment only those patients likely to benefit from intervention.

Candidacy for Treatment

Despite the increased risk of cardiac sudden death in patients with underlying heart disease manifest complex ventricular irritability, only those at highest risk appear to profit from antiarrhythmic measures. To date, prospective randomized trials of cardioverter-defibrillator implantation (e.g., MADIT, Antiarrhythmics versus Implantable Defibrillators [AVID] investigators, MUST) have demonstrated reductions in rates of cardiac arrest and sudden death in persons with;

- Resuscitation from near-fatal ventricular fibrillation;
- Sustained VT with syncope;
- Sustained VT plus a reduced ejection fraction (less than 0.40) and symptoms of hemodynamic compromise with VT (e.g., near-syncope, angina, dyspnea);
- Recent myocardial infarction associated with an ejection fraction less than 0.40, a history of asymptomatic nonsustained VT, and sustained VT on electrophysiologic study (EPS).

Of note, those with a reduced ejection fraction (less than 0.36), an abnormal signal-averaged ECG (a measure of increased risk for VT), and significant coronary disease showed no gain from defibrillator implantation (i.e., the CABG Patch study).

The spectrum of patients qualifying for treatment has been narrowed considerably by the finding that both antiarrhythmic agents (especially class I drugs) fail to reduce cardiac morbidity and mortality and may even increase risk of cardiac sudden death (see below). No longer are patients with underlying heart disease and complex ventricular irritability considered appropriate candidates for antiarrhythmic drug therapy if they are asymptomatic and have preserved LV function. Beta-blockade may be appropriate for such individuals, especially if they have coronary artery disease, but antiarrhythmic therapy is considered problematic. Under study is the combined use of beta-

blockers (which do reduce mortality) and the class III antiarrhythmic agent amiodarone (which has very little proarrhythmic activity) for relatively high-risk patients with coronary disease who are not candidates for defibrillator implantation.

Some authorities rank inherited conditions associated with a high risk of life-threatening ventricular dysrhythmias and sudden death as indications for prophylactic treatment. *Congenital prolonged QT syndrome* and *hypertrophic cardiomyopathy* are the most important of these conditions. Common clinical features include a family history of cardiac sudden death or cardiac arrest in a first-degree relative under the age of 30 years and a history of stress-induced syncope. Reduction in mortality with prophylactic therapy remains to be established prospectively.

In sum, the realization that risk of sudden death may be exacerbated by pharmacologic antiarrhythmic therapy and that implantable cardioverter-defibrillators do not work for everyone with high-risk disease has greatly increased the threshold for treatment. At present, only patients with the most malignant forms of ventricular dysrhythmic disease (e.g., prior cardiac arrest; symptomatic or inducible sustained VT, especially in the context of recent myocardial infarction; and reduced ejection fraction) should be considered candidates for prophylactic treatment.

Identification of Candidates for Treatment

Clinical Features. Patients who present in the outpatient setting with complex ventricular irritability, especially nonsustained VT, should be evaluated thoroughly for *underlying heart disease and LV dysfunction* (see Chapter 25), because these features increase risk of cardiac sudden death. Conversely, those patients with heart disease and a reduced ejection fraction should be checked for clinical features suggestive of *VT*, because of VT's potentially significant contribution to risk. Finding a history of syncope or near-syncope in a postinfarction patient can be a particularly important clue to VT, especially when the syncopal episode occurs with less than 5 seconds of warning, is accompanied by other symptoms of pump dysfunction (angina, dyspnea), and there are no major residual symptoms during recovery (a characteristic of less serious causes of syncope). Family history of sudden death before age 30 or stress-related syncope should raise suspicion of congenital prolongation of the QT interval and hypertrophic cardiomyopathy.

Electrophysiologic Study. EPS is an invasive procedure, requiring formal cardiac catheterization and an experienced staff. Inducibility of sustained VT correlates well with risks of clinically sustained VT, cardiac arrest, cardiac sudden death, and benefit from cardioverter-defibrillator implantation. Consequently, the study is often performed to identify candidates for defibrillator implantation. At present, those who should be referred for consideration of EPS include patients with asymptomatic nonsustained VT who have evidence of *underlying heart disease* and a *reduced ejection fraction* (less than 0.40). Nearly 40% of such patients will demonstrate inducible sustained VT and improved survival from defibrillator implantation. Others in whom EPS facilitates decision making are those with syncope of unknown origin who manifest clinical findings suggestive of a cardiac etiology (see above). Less compelling is the need for EPS in those with documented VT accompanied by *hemodynamic compromise* (syncope, near-syncope, angina, dyspnea). Studies are undergoing to better determine the indications for this very expensive and invasive procedure and simpler alternatives to predict outcome and benefit from therapy.

Ambulatory Monitoring. The importance of detecting VT has stimulated some to consider ambulatory monitoring to screen all potentially high-risk patients (i.e., those with recent myocardial infarction, hypertrophic cardiomyopathy, or congestive heart failure). However, except for those with syncope or a family history of early sudden death, such screening has not changed outcomes and is not recommended at this time.

Selection and Initiation of Therapy

Choice of Treatment. As alluded to earlier, implantation of a *cardioverter-defibrillator* is emerging as the best available approach to management of high-risk patients with life-threatening ventricular dysrhythmias. Emerging data from initial prospective, randomized, controlled trials (e.g., MAVID, MUST, AVID) that compare cardioverter-defibrillator implantation to *pharmacologic suppression* consistently find cardioverter-defibrillator implantation the superior treatment for reducing rates of cardiac arrest and sudden death. Although additional large-scale randomized trials directly comparing these two modes of therapy are needed to confirm initial findings, the observed benefits of are on the order of a 25% reduction in relative risk and a 7% reduction in absolute risk of cardiac arrest or sudden death at 5 years. All-cause mortality declines by a similar amount. Compared with patients treated pharmacologically, relative risk decreases by nearly 75% with cardioverter-defibrillator implantation. In some studies, all the treatment benefit observed was attributable to implantation therapy.

Implantable Cardioverter-Defibrillators. Currently available technology involves implantation of a pacemaker-sized device using procedures similar to those for pacemakers (e.g., subclavian or cephalic vein insertion, subcutaneous or submuscular left pectoral generator implantation). A complex right ventricular lead is used for sensing and pacing; a coiling of this lead delivers any needed shock. The unit discharges a high-voltage shock in response to detecting ventricular fibrillation or rapid VT and begins pacing when slower monomorphic VT is detected. Maximum output is up to 30 joules; amount needed for defibrillation is between 5 and 15 joules. Dual-chamber models better discriminate between ventricular and supraventricular tachyarrhythmias and allow dual-chamber pacing. Implantation

is associated with a small risk of infection (2%); perioperative morality is less than 1%. Inappropriate shocks from mistaking supraventricular tachyarrhythmias for VT are the most common operational complication, occurring in about 20% of patients. Inappropriate firing can be terminated by placing a magnet over the device box, which should be done during any resuscitation efforts. Battery depletion is rare; battery life ranges from 5 to 9 years depending on the amount of discharging required. After implantation, there is no increased risk of endocarditis and no need for endocarditis prophylaxis.

Indications and Contraindications. Implantation is used both for primary and secondary prevention of life-threatening ventricular dysrhythmias (Table 29.2). The indications are in a state of evolution as the full scope of benefit continues to be updated by the results of ongoing prospective randomized trials. *Contraindications* include use for dysrhythmias triggered by a *self-limited event* (e.g., acute myocardial infarction, electrolyte or metabolic disturbances) and refractory disease necessitating frequent shocks in a person with less than a year of life expectancy.

Effect on Quality of Life. Most patients adapt well, but the shock can be uncomfortable, described as similar to putting one's hand in an electrical socket. Frequent shocks can be very demoralizing and upsetting, necessitating additional measures (e.g., reprogramming, addition of pharmacologic therapy). About 15% experience brief syncope due to delay in cardioversion. The risk of a recurrence decreases with time, reaching a nadir 6 months after an episode. Consequently, most authorities recommend that patients who have a defibrillator implanted for primary prophylaxis do not drive for the first 6 months after implantation and for 6 months after every shock. A permanent ban on driving is absolute for those who drive commercially.

Precautions. Some forms of *electromagnetic exposure* are contraindicated, such as *magnetic resonance imaging*. Microwave ovens pose no hazard nor do airport security gates or brief passes of a handheld wand to detect metal objects, but security staff should be informed on the device's presence before passing through. Cellular digital phones do not interfere with operation of the device, but it is recommended that they are not carried or placed within 6 inches of the unit.

Concurrent Drug Therapy. Beta-blockers are widely used in patients with implantable defibrillators to reduce frequency of dysrhythmia- and tachycardia-induced shocks, especially in persons with underlying ischemic heart disease. Some cardiologists use *antiarrhythmics* to reduce the frequency of triggering arrhythmias, but use of these agents can cause drug-induced arrhythmias and raise the threshold voltage necessary to pace or defibrillate.

Table 29.2.   Indications for Cardioverter-Defibrillator Implantation for Ventricular Dysrhythmias

Primary Prevention
- Nonsustained VT plus inducible sustained VT in persons with underlying coronary heart disease and reduced ejection fraction (<0.4).
- Presence of an inherited condition with a high-risk for life-threatening ventricular dysrhythmias (e.g., prolonged QT syndrome, hypertrophic cardiomyopathy), especially if accompanied by a history of syncope or family history of sudden death or cardiac arrest at an early age.

Secondary Prevention
- History of ventricular fibrillatory arrest and resuscitation without a self-limited cause.
- History of sustained VT with hemodynamic compromise in the absence of a self-limited cause.
- Unexplained syncope plus inducible sustained VT.

Adapted from Pinski SL, Fahy GJ. Implantable cardioverter-defibrillators. Am J Med 1999;106;446, with permission.

VT, ventricular tachycardia.

Beta-Blockade. Beta-blocking agents increase the fibrillatory threshold and reduce the risk of ventricular fibrillation and sudden death. These agents—sometimes referred to as *class II* antiarrhythmics—are safe and especially useful when the ventricular dysrhythmia is caused by underlying ischemic heart disease. They are among the few drugs proven to reduce mortality in patients with coronary artery disease (see Chapter 30). Not only do they reduce risk of sudden death, they also reduce overall mortality. Unlike other drugs with antiarrhythmic properties, the beta-blockers have no proarrhythmic effects. They are also useful for suppression of symptomatic ventricular irritability related to digitalis toxicity, exercise, emotional stress, prolonged QT interval syndromes, and tricyclic antidepressants.

These features make beta-blockers ideal for prevention of sudden death in patients with malignant ventricular irritability due to coronary artery disease and other conditions that respond to beta-blockade. At least some of the benefit associated with class III antiarrhythmics has been attributed to their adrenergic-blocking activity (see below). As noted above, beta-blockers are also being used in persons with cardioverter-defibrillators to reduce the number of shocks by suppressing the rate of VT and episodes of SVT. Combined use of a class III antiarrhythmic (e.g., amiodarone) with a beta-blocker is promising and currently being explored in prospective trials.

Antiarrhythmic Drugs. Although all antiarrhythmic drugs can suppress ventricular ectopy, their net effect on survival has been disappointing. At best, a slight reduction in overall mortality has been found (as with amiodarone in very high-risk patients), but more commonly the result is no benefit over placebo or even an increase in mortality (as found in CAST with use of class IC drugs). Consequently, drug therapy is increasingly relegated to a second-line role for prevention of cardiac arrest and sudden death in favor of cardioverter-defibrillator implantation. In addition, the practice of testing for and seeking to eliminate observable or inducible ventricular irritability is being abandoned because it does not correlate with outcomes.

At the same time, new approaches to antiarrhythmic therapy are being explored. Use in combination with cardioverter-defibrillator implantation is being investigated as a means of reducing the number of shocks and improving survival. Advances in understanding the basic pathophysiology of malignant ventricular irritability and clinical data from prospective randomized trials are stimulating a shift from use of class I agents (e.g., quinidine, procainamide, disopyramide) to class III drugs (e.g., amiodarone, sotalol). There is exploration of combination drug regimens (e.g., amiodarone plus a beta-blocker) in which complementary modes of action are sought.

Indications for Therapy. Patients who present with symptomatic sustained VT or prior ventricular fibrillation arrest who cannot undergo or refuse cardioverter-defibrillator implantation are reasonable candidates for antiarrhythmic therapy. For asymptomatic patients with preserved LV function and frequent or complex PVCs or nonsustained VT, there is no evidence of survival benefit with use of antiarrhythmic agents. Patients unnerved by their PVCs (actually by the forceful compensatory beats), but otherwise asymptomatic, might be made more comfortable by beta-blockade or low-dose amiodarone. Drug therapy to suppress ventricular dysrhythmias may also be helpful in persons with implanted defibrillators who experience frequent

shocks, but safety and impact on outcomes remains to be established. Pharmacologic treatment of ventricular irritability remains in considerable flux, necessitating close monitoring of the literature for results of long-term prospective trials currently underway to determine the best use of drug therapy.

Choice of Agent. Ability to suppress malignant ventricular ectopy used to be the principal criterion for choice of drug. The standard of care was to subject high-risk patients to EPS to see if a given drug could suppress inducible sustained VT. Only those agents demonstrating ability to do so were deemed appropriate for long-term use. The finding in the CAST study that suppressibility does not correlate with outcomes has led to abandonment of EPS study for choice of agent. In its place is empirical therapy, limited to well-tolerated agents proven to reduce rates of cardiac sudden death and all-cause mortality. Currently only the *beta-blockers* and the class III antiarrhythmic drug *amiodarone* meet these efficacy criteria, largely replacing the *class I agents (e.g., quinidine, procainamide, disopyramide)* as first-line drugs for life-threatening ventricular dysrhythmias. The class I drugs are now relegated mostly to supporting roles, such as reducing the frequency of shocks in persons with implantable cardioverter-defibrillators.

Amiodarone, a class III antiarrhythmic, blocks a number of cellular ionic channels and also exerts noncompetitive antiadrenergic effects. When used in high-risk patients, the drug demonstrates a significant reduction (29%) in risk of arrhythmic sudden death and a more modest reduction (13%) in overall mortality. Empiric amiodarone therapy prescribed for cardiac arrest survivors has been shown capable of reducing mortality from 50% to 20% at 2 years. Despite being well tolerated, amiodarone has a number of adverse effects, most of which are dose and duration related. An important one is *pulmonary fibrosis,* usually preceded by a reversible patchy pneumonitis. Another complication is *corneal deposits*; these usually do not interfere with vision and disappear with discontinuation of the drug. *Gastrointestinal upset* (including constipation) is common as are minor increases in liver enzymes, but clinically significant *hepatitis* occurs in 4% of patients. Ataxia and tremor may also develop. The drug contains an iodinated segment that can interfere with thyroid metabolism and may lead to *hypothyroidism. Drug–drug interactions* are substantial: Amiodarone increases the serum levels of *digoxin, quinidine,* and *procainamide* and potentiates the effect of *warfarin.* Dose adjustments are necessary when amiodarone is used. Amiodarone prolongs the *QT interval,* and there is a small (1%) risk of torsades de pointes associated with its use. This rate is about a tenth of that seen with other antiarrhythmic agents. Effect on inotropy is minimal. Overall, the drug is reasonably well tolerated when used carefully by experienced clinicians.

Sotalol has a combination of nonselective beta-blocking affects and electrophysiologic features common to class III antiarrhythmics. These features make it a theoretically attractive agent, and indeed, it is effective in suppressing serious ventricular ectopy. However, at high doses it prolongs the QT interval, subjecting patients to the risk of torsades de pointes, especially if accompanied by hypokalemia or hypomagnesemia. The risk of torsades accounts for the failure of the drug to reduce mortality in some controlled trials.

Quinidine use, and most other class I agents, often continues in patients whose initiation of therapy for ventricular ectopy predates current standards; it does not prolong survival. Its association with *prolongation of the QT interval*, usually as a result of excessive dosing but occasionally as an idiosyncratic reaction to a single dose, increases the risk of serious VT (especially *torsades de pointes*), which can lead to ventricular fibrillation. "*Quinidine syncope*" is probably a manifestation of torsades de pointes. The drug *reduces digoxin clearance* and can double its serum concentration, necessitating reduction in digoxin dose when both are used simultaneously. The most common side effects are gastrointestinal (*nausea, vomiting, and diarrhea*). Other common side effects include *tinnitus* and *vertigo*. Hypersensitivity reactions are occasionally encountered; *rash, thrombocytopenia, hepatitis,* or *hemolytic anemia* may result.

Disopyramide has many of the same electrophysiologic properties as quinidine plus a rather pronounced *negative inotropic effect*. Although disopyramide is relatively free of the troublesome gastrointestinal side effects associated with quinidine, it does have substantial anticholinergic activity, which commonly produces *urinary retention, constipation, blurred vision,* and *dry mouth.*

Procainamide acts similarly to quinidine and disopyramide. In addition, the drug can cause *arterioventricular block.* Chronic use of procainamide is associated with appearance of *antinuclear antibodies* in about 80% of patients; 20% to 30% of these patients develop a slowly reversible *lupuslike syndrome.* Rate of development of this syndrome is a function of acetylator phenotype; patients who slowly acetylate the drug are at greater risk. Concurrent use of amiodarone, ranitidine, or trimethoprim can increase the serum procainamide level.

Mexiletine and tocainide are orally active *analogues of xylocaine.* Although they can suppress ventricular dysrhythmias refractory to other agents, their antiarrhythmic potency in crossover studies is about the same as quinidine, and like other class I agents, they occasionally worsen ventricular irritability. Of the two, mexiletine is the more negatively inotropic and also has modest suppressive effect on atrioventricular nodal conduction. Side effects are dose related and include tremor, ataxia, confusion, dizziness, nausea, and anorexia. Tocainide causes bone marrow suppression, with *agranulocytosis* reported in 0.2%. Rare instances of pulmonary fibrosis and pneumonitis have occurred.

Flecainide and moricizine are potent oral class IC (local anesthetic type) antiarrhythmic agents capable of suppressing sustained ventricular arrhythmias. However, randomized, prospective, controlled, clinical trials (CAST I and II) found these agents also had marked proarrhythmic effects, leading to increased rates of cardiac sudden death. These findings underscore the point that *suppression of ventricular arrhythmias does not predict increased survival*, at least in patients with prior myocardial infarction. The clinician should keep this fact in mind when reviewing claims of efficacy for antiarrhythmic drugs. The current role for these drugs is to reduce the frequency of shocks in persons with implantable defibrillators.

Radiofrequency Catheter Ablative Therapy. Catheter ablation is most successful in persons with VT who have no evidence of underlying structural heart disease (90% cure rate) and in those with VT involving a reentrant mechanism. Persons with VT due to coronary disease have a much lower response rate (less than 50%). The mapping component of the procedure can only be performed when there is hemodynamic stability during the induction of VT, a situation that is infrequent in persons with structural heart disease.

Diet and Exercise. There is no evidence that moderate intake of *caffeinated beverages* is harmful to patients with serious ventricular irritability. Although restriction of caffeine may cut down on the frequency of minor ventricular irritability, there is no evidence caffeine restriction has any effect on important outcomes. Promising data suggest a diet rich in *omega-3 fatty acids* may have an electrically stabilizing effect on myocardial cells; whether this translates into reduced risk of sudden death in high-risk persons is under study. In some forms of dysrhythmic heart diseases (e.g., severe ischemia, congenital form of QT prolongation), extreme exertion should be restricted because it increases the risk of symptomatic VT and cardiac sudden death.

Monitoring Therapy

For Patients Treated with a Cardioverter-Defibrillator. Monitoring such patients is relatively simple, because the devices have built-in monitoring and storage capacity. At the time of a visit to the cardiologist, the memory can be downloaded for study. The patient should be questioned about the number of shocks experienced and the number and type of any other symptomatic events. The device is "interrogated" for assessment of battery status and lead function.

For Patients Treated Pharmacologically. For patients taking antiarrhythmic agents, there are no clearcut guidelines for monitoring therapy. The previous standard of regularly repeated *EPS* or *ambulatory monitoring* has been invalidated by the lack of correlation between suppression of ventricular irritability and outcomes. Those taking pharmacologic therapy for control of bothersome symptoms related to VT (e.g., syncope, near-syncope, dyspnea, angina) should be asked to keep a diary of such symptoms and considered for transtelephonic continuous-loop ambulatory monitoring only if there is concern about the frequency or severity of episodes.

Even though pharmacologic treatment of ventricular irritability is still largely problematic, the primary physician can do much to ensure safety and minimize iatrogenic complications. Monitoring *serum potassium* and *magnesium* and maintaining normal levels of these electrolytes are essential for reducing the proarrhythmic risk of torsades de pointes. When a digitalis preparation is used, it too needs careful monitoring in the setting of antiarrhythmic use. Renal and hepatic function determinations (*blood urea nitrogen, creatinine, transaminase*) bear watching, because they represent the principal routes of antiarrhythmic excretion. Drugs with potential for bone marrow suppression (e.g., tocainide) necessitate periodic checking of the *complete blood count.* Thyroid indices (e.g., *thyroid-stimulating hormone*) bear watching in patients taking amiodarone. Measurement of *serum drug levels* is an important aid to safe use of these antiarrhythmic agents. Proper interpretation of the data requires that levels be drawn long enough after the last dose so that one is not mistaking a peak serum level for a steady state one.

Monitoring the *ECG* for evidence of excessive dose and idiosyncratic reactions is also essential. Quinidine, procainamide, and disopyramide and some of the other class I agents can substantially *prolong the PR, QRS, and QT intervals* when serum levels are in the toxic range. Modest QT interval prolongation is to be expected and is a sign of therapeutic effect, but marked prolongation is an important sign of excessive dose and a need to withhold further medication. Marked prolongation of the QT interval also can occur idiosyncratically at the very onset of therapy in some patients taking quinidine; it should be checked. QT prolongation also needs to be watched for with use of class III agents, especially sotalol.

INDICATIONS FOR REFERRAL AND ADMISSION

Any patient found to have sustained VT complicated by symptoms of hemodynamic compromise (dyspnea, near-syncope, angina) should be emergently admitted to the hospital and referred to a cardiologist skilled in performing EPS and treating life-threatening ventricular irritability. The same pertains to a patient with acute syncope who presents with features suggestive of a serious cardiac rhythm disturbance (i.e., syncopal episode with less than 5 seconds of warning, other symptoms of pump dysfunction, no major residual symptoms during recovery). A bit less urgent is the case of asymptomatic nonsustained VT, but risk is still very high, and referral for consideration of EPS is indicated when there is a history of recent myocardial infarction and evidence of LV dysfunction. Asymptomatic patients with normal LV function who manifest complex ventricular ectopy other than VT are not candidates for treatment and do not require admission or referral, although cardiac consultation may be done for reassurance.

PATIENT EDUCATION

Patients and their families need to know the prognostic meaning of the ventricular irritability so that they can respond appropriately. Putting the problem in context avoids over- and underresponding. Any fears regarding a potentially serious arrhythmia can be lessened by reviewing available therapies and their ability to reduce the risk of sudden death. Full disclosure improves compliance by reinforcing the importance of therapy; patients are also more willing to put up with annoying side effects from the drugs and cardioverter-defibrillators. Those with cardioverter-defibrillators need to be fully informed about driving, cell phone use, and other precautions regarding electromagnetic interference (see earlier).

Patient education is also crucial to patients with harmless forms of ventricular irritability. Knowing that the palpitations and abnormal ECG have no implications for long-term survival is tremendously reassuring and can prevent development of a cardiac neurosis and unnecessary restriction of activity.

CONCLUSIONS AND THERAPEUTIC RECOMMENDATIONS

- The main independent determinants of prognosis in patients with ventricular ectopy are the presence of underlying heart disease and a failing left ventricle. The complexity of the ventricular ectopy is also a determinant of prognosis, especially in patients with heart disease and LV failure; VT portends an especially high risk of cardiac sudden death.

- Patients presenting with ventricular ectopy should be evaluated for underlying heart disease and LV dysfunction.
- Patients presenting with nonsustained VT in the setting of recent myocardial infarction and reduced ejection fraction should undergo EPS to test for inducible sustained VT, an indication for prophylactic measures.
- Patients presenting with syncope and clinical evidence suggesting a cardiac etiology are also candidates for EPS to test for inducible sustained VT.
- The principal goals of therapy are prevention of symptomatic sustained VT, cardiac arrest, and sudden death.
- Cardioverter-defibrillator implantation has become the treatment of choice for attainment of treatment goals in very high-risk patients.
- Evidence-based indications for treatment (Table 29.2) remain rather narrow, limited to specific groups of patients at extremely high risk of sudden death.
- Beta-blocker therapy is indicated for all patients with malignant ventricular irritability due to underlying coronary artery disease, especially for persons who have had a myocardial infarction.
- Antiarrhythmic drug therapy has been largely relegated to a second-line position because of its proarrhythmic potential and failure in most instances to achieve significant reductions in sudden death and all-cause mortality; best results have been found with use of class III agents manifesting antiadrenergic activity (e.g., amiodarone).
- High-risk patients who refuse or are not candidates for cardioverter-defibrillator implantation might be considered for amiodarone therapy.
- Because drug therapy is fraught with many potentially adverse effects, it should be undertaken only in conjunction with cardiac consultation. EPS testing for ability to suppress inducible VT is no longer recommended because results do not correlate with outcomes.
- Patients with symptomatic VT without structural heart disease are potential candidates for catheter radioablation.
- Under investigation are combination strategies such as cardioverter-defibrillator implantation plus an antiarrhythmic agent and beta-blocker use in conjunction with an antiarrhythmic agent.
- Patients with underlying heart disease, LV dysfunction, and sustained VT are at very high risk of sudden death and require prompt admission and cardiac consultation, especially if they experience arrhythmia-induced symptoms of hemodynamic compromise. Treatment is indicated for these patients and is best initiated in the inpatient setting, in collaboration with a cardiologist skilled in treating malignant ventricular arrhythmias. Outpatient assessment and initiation of therapy may be possible in asymptomatic persons with nonsustained VT, but prompt cardiac consultation is warranted.
- Monitoring should include checking for hemodynamic compromise (near-syncope, dyspnea, angina), number of shocks (in persons with defibrillators), ECG for QT interval prolongation and new dysrhythmias, and serum levels for potassium, magnesium, creatinine, transaminase, and drug concentrations (especially if taking antiarrhythmic drugs).
- Detailed patient education is essential to maximize compliance, safety, and quality of life.

A.H.G.

ANNOTATED BIBLIOGRAPHY

Amiodarone Trials Meta-Analysis Investigators. Effect of prophylactic amiodarone on mortality after acute myocardial infarction and in congestive heart failure: meta-analysis of individual data from 6500 patients in randomized trials. Lancet 1997;350:1417. (*Detects a significant reduction [29%] in risk of arrhythmic sudden death and a more modest reduction [13%] in overall mortality.*)

Antiarrhythmics versus Implantable Defibrillators (AVID) Investigators. A comparison of antiarrhythmic-drug therapy with implantable defibrillators in patients resuscitated from near-fatal ventricular arrhythmias. N Engl J Med 1997;337:1576. (*In this group of very high-risk patients, survival was enhanced by defibrillator therapy but not by antiarrhythmic drugs in terms of survival.*)

Bigger JT. Definition of benign versus malignant ventricular arrhythmias. Am J Cardiol 1983;52:47C. (*A excellent review of the various forms of ventricular irritability and the degree of risk associated with each of them.*)

Bigger JT. Prophylactic use of implanted cardiac defibrillators in patients at high risk for ventricular arrhythmias after coronary-artery bypass graft surgery. N Engl J Med 1997;337:1569. (*The CABG PATCH study, a randomized trial showing no benefit in survival for persons with a reduced ejection fraction and an abnormal resting ECG.*)

Bikkina M, Larson MG, Levy D. Prognostic implications of asymptomatic ventricular arrhythmias: the Framingham Heart Study. Ann Intern Med 1992;117:990. (*Important epidemiologic data; increased risk of myocardial infarction or death from coronary disease.*)

Boutitie F, Boissel JP, Connolly SJ, et al. Amiodarone interaction with beta-blockers: analysis of the merged EMIAT and CAMIAT databases. Circulation 1999;82:91. (*A subgroup analysis combining data from two large prospective trials suggesting a synergistic effect with improved survival in postinfarction patients.*)

Buxton AE. Antiarrhythmic drugs: good for premature ventricular complexes but bad for patients? Ann Intern Med 1992;116:420. (*An editorial; reviews the disappointing results with class IC antiarrhythmics; more proarrhythmic than suppressive; good discussion of the implications.*)

Buxton AD, Lee KL, Fisher JD, et al. A randomized study of the prevention of sudden death in patients with coronary artery disease. N Engl J Med 1999;341:1882. (*A randomized controlled trial; implantable defibrillator reduced risk of sudden death, but antiarrhythmic pharmacotherapy did not in these patients with NSVT, heart failure, inducible VT, and recent infarction.*)

Cairns JA, Connolly SJ, Roberts RS, et al. Randomized trial of outcome after myocardial infarction in patients with frequent or repetitive premature depolarizations: CAMIAT. Lancet 1997;349. (*Risk of sudden death significantly reduced with amiodarone use, but only a trend toward reduction in total mortality in this major Canadian trial.*)

Cardiac Arrhythmia Suppression Trial II Investigators. Effect of the antiarrhythmic agent moricizine on survival after myocardial infarction. N Engl J Med 1992;327:227. (*The CAST II results with moricizine were as disappointing as for flecainide and encainide; see next reference. All had proarrhythmic effects and increased mortality, despite showing powerful ability to suppress inducible sustained VT; strong evidence against relying on EPS testing for drug selection.*)

Echt DS, Liebson PR, Mitchell B, et al. Mortality and morbidity in patients receiving encainide, flecainide, or placebo: the Cardiac Arrhythmia Suppression Trial. N Engl J Med 1991;324:781. (*CAST I, a major randomized controlled study of class I antiarrhythmic therapy in mildly symptomatic patients with complex ventricular ectopy, coronary artery disease, and reduced ejection fraction; demonstrates an excessive incidence of arrhythmic deaths in patients randomized to antiarrhythmic therapy.*)

Kendall MJ, Lynch KP, Hjalmarson A, et al. Beta-blockers and sudden cardiac death. Ann Intern Med 1995;123:358. (*A systematic review finding marked benefit, greater than with any other treatment modality.*)

Kennedy HL, Pescarmona J, Bouchard RJ, et al. Coronary artery status of apparently healthy subjects with frequent and complex ventricular ectopy. Ann Intern Med 1980;92:179. (*One fourth of apparently healthy patients being followed for complex and frequent VEA were found to have significant coronary stenosis; no clinical features of the ectopy that differentiated them.*)

Kennedy HL, Whitlock JA, Sprague MK. Long-term follow-up of asymptomatic healthy subjects with frequent and complex ventricular ectopy. N Engl J Med 1985;312:1983. (*Important study; regardless of the presence of frequent and complex ventricular irritability, there was no increase in mortality among these healthy patients; mean follow-up of 6.5 years.*)

Marchlinski FE, Zada ES, Deely MP, et al. Concomitant device and drug therapy: current trends, potential benefits, and adverse interactions. Am J Cardiol 1999;84[Suppl]:69R. (*A review of the current state of concomitant use; some data, much interest, a number of concerns; a good paper for coming attractions.*)

Mason JW, et al. A comparison of electrophysiologic testing with Holter monitoring to predict arrhythmic drug efficacy for ventricular tachycardias. N Engl J Med 1993;329:445. (*Holter monitoring was more predictive of efficacy in this first large prospective randomized trial of the two methods; however, very narrow spectrum of patients and both methods failed to predict the 50% recurrence rate of VT at 2 years.*)

McLenachan JM, Henderson E, Morris KI, et al. Ventricular arrhythmias in patients with hypertensive left ventricular hypertrophy. N Engl J Med 1987;317:787. (*Documents increased frequency of complex ventricular irritability in such patients.*)

Meinertz T, et al. Significance of ventricular arrhythmias in idiopathic dilated cardiomyopathy. Am J Cardiol 1981;53:902. (*Ventricular irritability was a determinant of increased risk in these patients.*)

Meyers MG. Caffeine and cardiac arrhythmias. Ann Intern Med 1991;114:147. (*Critical literature review; no evidence that moderate intake of caffeine increases the frequency or severity of dysrhythmias in normals or those with heart disease, even those with preexisting serious VEA.*)

Minardo JD, Heger JJ, Miles WM, et al. Clinical characteristics of patients with ventricular fibrillation during antiarrhythmic drug therapy. N Engl J Med 1988;319:257. (*Ventricular fibrillation occurred early and was most likely in patients with LV dysfunction and concomitant digitalis and diuretic therapy.*)

Nattel S, Singh B. Evolution, mechanisms, and classification of antiarrhythmic drugs. Am J Cardiol 1999[Suppl]84:11R. (*Excellent review and summary.*)

Pinski SL, Fahy GJ. Implantable cardioverter-defibrillators. Am J Med 1999;106:446. (*Very useful and practical review of evidence for the noncardiologist; 102 references.*)

Podrid PJ. Amiodarone: reevaluation of an old drug. Ann Intern Med 1995;122:689. (*Excellent review that includes considerable data on utility of the drug in VT/ventricular fibrillation; 109 references.*)

Powell AC, Gold MR, Brooks R, et al. Electrophysiologic response to moricizine in patients with sustained ventricular arrhythmias. Ann Intern Med 1992;116:382. (*Another of the promising class IC antiarrhythmics proves ineffective in suppressing VT and manifests proarrhythmic activity; failure of suppressibility to predict outcome.*)

Ruberman W, et al. Ventricular premature complexes and sudden death after myocardial infarction. Circulation 1981;64:297. *(Frequent and complex ventricular irritability in postmyocardial infarction patients was associated with increased risk of sudden death.)*

Ruskin J. Ventricular extrasystoles in healthy subjects. N Engl J Med 1985;312:238. *(An editorial summarizing current knowledge and pinpointing areas of continued uncertainty.)*

Singh BN. Current antiarrhythmic drugs: an overview of mechanisms of action and potential clinical utility. J Cardiovasc Electrophysiol 1999;1:283. *(A detailed and useful review linking basic science and clinical use.)*

Stanton MS, Prystowsky EN, Fineberg NS, et al. Arrhythmogenic effects of antiarrhythmic drugs. J Am Coll Cardiol 1989;14:209. *(A review of over 1000 drug trials; risk was highest in patients with a low ejection fraction and a history of VT.)*

Tan HL, Hou CJY, Laurer MR, et al. Electrophysiologic mechanisms of the long QT interval syndromes and torsades de pointes. Ann Intern Med 1995;122:701. *(Excellent basic science review.)*

Zimetbaum PJ, Josephson ME. The evolving role of ambulatory arrhythmia monitoring in general clinical practice. Ann Intern Med 1999;120:848. *(A detailed review that includes evidence showing little benefit as a screening test for VT in asymptomatic patients with underlying heart disease.)*

30

Management of Chronic Stable Angina

Several million Americans suffer from coronary heart disease (CHD), and more than 600,000 die each year from the condition and its complications. Even for patients with chronic stable angina—the form of CHD most commonly encountered in the office setting—the risk of death is high (2% to 12% annually). The array of treatment modalities is extensive, ranging from nitrates, beta-blocking agents, and calcium channel blockers to aspirin, angioplasty, and coronary bypass surgery. These medical and surgical approaches are complemented by aggressive treatment of underlying cardiovascular risk factors. The goals of therapy include symptom relief, improved exercise capacity and quality of life, prevention of infarction, and, ultimately, improved survival.

One must understand the limitations and indications for the vast array of therapeutic options. Design of the basic medical regimen and determining when interventional measures need consideration are among the important responsibilities of the primary care physician. Although long-term management of stable angina usually falls to the primary physician, a good working relationship with a consulting cardiologist is often helpful.

PATHOPHYSIOLOGY

Angina is a symptomatic manifestation of *myocardial ischemia*, occurring when oxygen demand exceeds available vascular supply. Most cases of chronic stable angina are related to fixed *atherosclerotic lesions* narrowing the major coronary vessels. A series of step-wise thrombotic events is believed to account for much of the atherosclerotic occlusion that occurs in the large epicardial arteries. These lesions may develop as a consequence of episodes of acute *thrombosis*, in which activated *platelets* and other elements of the clotting system appear to play major roles, triggered by reactive endothelial injury in areas of cholesterol deposition. Many, if not most, episodes of *acute coronary insufficiency (unstable angina) and infarction* are associated with acute thrombosis, often occurring at an ulcerated, eccentrically located, or ruptured plaque, not necessarily at a site of severe stenosis.

Restriction of coronary blood supply may also ensue from *coronary vasospasm*, believed related to loss of normal endothelial vasoregulatory activity. The coronary endothelium appears to cease production of vasoactive peptides and prostaglandins, leaving vascular smooth muscle unopposed and susceptible to spasm. It has been documented in patients both with and without underlying atherosclerotic disease and sometimes presents as *variant angina* (rest pain, ST-segment elevation). Prevalence is about 3% in patients undergoing coronary angiography with ergonovine stimulation, but the true prevalence is estimated to be far greater. Spasm is suspected of playing a role in acute myocardial infarction and triggering anginal episodes. *Cigarette smoking* and *hyperlipidemia* appear to interfere with normal endothelial activity. Precipitants include stress, cold, α-adrenergic stimulation in the setting of beta-blockade, abrupt nitrate withdrawal, ergonovine, cocaine use, and direct mechanical irritation from cardiac catheterization.

Aortic stenosis can lead to angina when hemodynamically significant valvular stenosis or calcific obstruction of a coronary ostia results in inadequate coronary perfusion (see Chapter 33).

Coronary microvascular dysfunction, characterized by inappropriately vasoconstrictive responses to autonomic and biochemical stimuli, can increase total resistance and reduce myocardial perfusion. The significance of these findings is still unclear, but they have been found with increased frequency among patients with the combination of atypical angina, an ischemic response to exercise stress testing, and a normal coronary angiogram. The terms *"microvascular angina"* and *"syndrome X"* have been applied to such persons. More study is needed, but the findings suggest a possible explanation for the ischemic chest pain of patients with *hypertrophic cardiomyopathy*. Diabetics with hyperinsulinism may also be at increased risk for microvascular disease.

There is a growing appreciation for the frequency and importance of *silent myocardial ischemia*, defined as objectively documented ischemia occurring in the absence of symptoms. On the basis of results from exercise stress testing and ambulatory monitoring, it is estimated that more than half of patients with chronic stable angina experience episodes of silent ischemia. Contrary to common belief, controlled studies find that the incidence in diabetics is no greater than in nondiabetics. Mechanism remains a subject of investigation, but it does not appear to be the result of less severe or less extensive ischemia.

Regardless of etiology, ischemic episodes are often triggered or aggravated by conditions that increase myocardial oxygen demand (e.g., *hyperthyroidism, fever*) or decrease oxygen supply (e.g., *severe anemia, respiratory insufficiency*). A *circadian susceptibility* to ischemic events has been identified, with the morning hours being the time of greatest risk. Mechanism(s) remains unknown, but the phenomenon can be blocked by beta-blockers or aspirin.

NATURAL HISTORY

Although the clinical course of some patients may extend over 15 to 20 years, most patients with chronic stable angina are at considerably increased risk of cardiovascular death. Among the factors strongly affecting prognosis are the *number* and *location* of *stenoses*. Combined angiographic data obtained before widespread use of bypass surgery reveal that patients with significant disease in one vessel have a mean annual mortality rate of 2.2%. This increases to a rate of 4.5% to 7.0% if the lesion involves the *left main* coronary artery. High-grade proximal stenosis of the left anterior descending artery has a prognosis similar to that of left-main disease and is sometimes referred to as a "*left-main equivalent*" lesion. With stenosis of two vessels, the mean annual mortality rate is 6.8%; the rate rises to 11.4% for *three-vessel disease*.

Prognosis also closely correlates with *severity of ischemia*, as measured by radionuclide or echocardiographic imaging and by electrocardiographic changes during exercise stress testing (see Chapter 36), regardless of whether the disease is symptomatic or silent. Other major independent determinants of increased risk are *left ventricular (LV) dysfunction* (see Chapter 32), *ventricular ectopy* (see Chapter 29), an intercurrent ischemic event within the last 6 months, and cigarette smoking. The onset of angina in a patient with hemodynamically significant aortic stenosis reduces mean survival to about 2 to 3 years (see Chapter 33).

Many *CHD risk factors* are powerful independent determinants of prognosis. *Smoking, diabetes mellitus, hypertension, hypercholesterolemia, low high-density lipoprotein cholesterol,* and *age* (45 years in men, 55 years in women) are well documented for their effect on prognosis in patients with stable angina due to atherosclerotic coronary artery disease. *Hyperhomocysteinemia* is emerging from epidemiologic studies as another potentially significant prognostic factor; however, a causal relationship between elevations in homocysteine and progression of atherosclerotic disease remains to be established.

The natural history of *coronary artery spasm* is highly variable, reflecting the heterogeneity of patients with this condition. An important variable is the presence of underlying atherosclerotic disease. If spasm occurs in the absence of fixed stenoses, the prognosis is relatively good (e.g., no mortality, 39% remission over 6 years). Some investigators even suggest that spasm may be a temporary condition; however, myocardial infarction, heart block, and malignant arrhythmias have been documented. The prognosis of patients with spasm in the setting of underlying coronary stenosis is a function of the coronary anatomy; patients with multivessel disease are at greatest risk. Whether risk is significantly enhanced by the presence of spasm is not yet known.

Risk Stratification. Patients can be classified as low, moderate, or high risk on the basis of stress testing and echocardio-

graphic findings (Table 30.1) (see Chapters 21 and 36). Although individual patients may fall into the gray zones between categories, such risk stratification can help focus and guide treatment decisions.

PRINCIPLES OF MANAGEMENT

The ultimate goals are to reduce the risks of infarction and death. In patients with CHD, identification and aggressive treatment of atherosclerotic risk factors—*hypertension* (see Chapter 26), *hypercholesterolemia* (see Chapter 27), *smoking* (see Chapter 54), and perhaps *diabetes* (see Chapter 102)—can reduce cardiovascular morbidity and mortality. Under study is the effect of normalizing *homocysteine* on outcomes (see Chapter 31). The magnitude of risk reduction from such *secondary prevention* efforts can be impressive, exceeding that associated with primary prevention (see Chapter 31), although such efforts are often overlooked or mistakenly viewed as not productive. *Beta-blockers* and *bypass surgery* also provide effective secondary prevention in high-risk individuals, as does *aspirin* and *aggressive lipid-lowering* (see below).

The more immediate objectives are to control symptoms and enhance exercise capacity, which entail *improving blood supply* and *reducing oxygen demand*. Although drug therapy and interventional methods are the most heavily used treatment modalities (see below), attention also needs to be paid to conditions that increase oxygen demand and reduce oxygen availability. Among the former are *heart failure* (see Chapter 32) and *hyperthyroidism* (see Chapter 103). The latter include severe *anemia* (see Chapter 82), *chronic obstructive pulmonary disease* (see Chapter 47), and *interstitial lung disease* (see Chapter 46). An exercise program helps reduce peripheral oxygen demand (see Chapters 18 and 31). For patients with angina caused by hemodynamically significant aortic stenosis, *correction of the outflow tract obstruction* is indicated (see Chapter 33).

An effective management strategy needs to address the full spectrum of risk factors and precipitants and the relative benefits of medical therapy versus revascularization. To maximize patient safety, the aggressiveness of intervention should be proportional to the patient's degree of risk (Table 30.1). Knowledge of the treatment and outcome characteristics of available modalities is essential to program design. Often the choices are stated as if they are mutually exclusive, but even if revascularization is chosen, aggressive medical treatment of

Table 30.1. Risk Stratification for Patients with Stable Angina

Low Risk
  No angina currently or minimal angina
  Normal left ventricular function (normal ejection fraction)
  Small amount of myocardium at risk (probable single-vessel disease)

Moderate Risk
  Moderate angina
  Normal left ventricular function (normal ejection fraction)
  Moderate amount of myocardium at risk (probable two-vessel or proximal left anterior descending artery disease)

High Risk
  Severe angina
  Extensive amount of myocardium at risk (probable three-vessel, left-main, or "left-main equivalent" disease)
  Impaired left ventricular function (ejection fraction <0.40)

CHD risk factors remains the foundation of CHD management.

Medical Therapy: Nitrates

Although they have little demonstrable impact on survival, nitrates continue to be one of the cornerstones of CHD management. Their principal contributions are symptomatic relief and prevention of anginal episodes. Nitrates are vasodilators that work by releasing nitric oxide, which stimulates guanyl cyclase conversion of GTP to cyclic GMP, resulting in vascular smooth muscle relaxation. They act predominantly on the *venous capacitance vessels*, though they have a lesser effect on the *arterial bed*. Nitrates have no direct chronotropic or inotropic effects but decrease myocardial oxygen demand predominantly by *reducing preload* through a lowering of LV filling pressure and end-diastolic volume. Nitrates also have a favorable but lesser effect on *afterload*, modestly reducing systemic blood pressure. Regional myocardial perfusion may be improved by the ability of nitrates to *dilate epicardial coronary arteries* (including stenotic segments) and collateral vessels, but there is little effect on the smaller resistance arteries, thus preventing a steal phenomenon from developing (as seen with short-acting dihydropyridine calcium channel blockers). Nitrates are moderately effective in lessening coronary vasospasm. *Tolerance* to nitrates can develop if dosing intervals are too short (see below). Because nitrates and β-adrenergic blocking agents have complementary effects on myocardial oxygen demand, they are often used together (see below).

There is little question as to the efficacy of nitrates for relief of anginal pain and improvement in exercise tolerance in patients with stable coronary artery disease. In addition, nitrates remain the drug of first choice in patients with variant angina due to coronary vasospasm. However, the effect of nitrates on prognosis remains unknown. Most studies of survival involve multiple-drug regimens combining nitrates with beta-blocking agents; such studies do document improved survival in postinfarction patients, but most of the benefit appears attributable to beta-blockade.

Sublingual nitroglycerin (TNG) tablets provide short-term (up to 30 minutes) relief of anginal pain and improvement in exercise tolerance when taken prophylactically. Advantages include low cost, rapid onset of action (30 seconds to 3 minutes), safety, and proven efficacy for symptomatic relief. The drawback is its short duration of action. TNG must be taken sublingually because oral doses are denitrified and hepatically inactivated on the first pass through the portal circulation. Because the drug is volatile, it is best kept in a tightly capped amber vial, stored in a cool place. Once a bottle of TNG is opened, the contents remain maximally effective for up to 6 months. After that, it is best to assume the TNG has lost some of its potency and to prescribe a fresh bottle. Often, the patient using old TNG will notice less benefit and fewer of the usual side effects accompanying use of TNG (headache, burning under the tongue). Before concluding that a patient's failure to respond to TNG is due to disease progression or nitrate resistance (see below), it is important to be sure that "fresh" TNG is being used.

Aerosolized TNG spray delivers 0.4 mg of TNG to the surface of the tongue from a metered-dose aerosol canister; the drug is rapidly absorbed transmucosally. Onset and duration of action and efficacy of a single dose are similar to those of a 0.4-mg sublingual TNG tablet. Each canister contains about 200 doses. Canister-stored TNG will retain efficacy for up to 3 years. Cost per dose is substantially greater than for TNG tablets, but prolonged shelf life helps to reduce total cost to the patient. The spray is a reasonable alternative in patients who wear dentures or have dry mucous membranes. Proper use requires holding the canister close to the tongue, directing the spray at the tongue, not inhaling the spray, and closing the mouth after each dose.

Isosorbide dinitrate was developed to provide more sustained nitrate activity and better *anginal prophylaxis*. Single oral doses of 20 to 40 mg significantly improve hemodynamic parameters and exercise tolerance, and the effect persists up to 4 hours. Onset of action is 15 to 30 minutes and clinical duration of action, 4 to 8 hours. The optimal *dosage schedule* is two or three times a day, with an *eccentric pattern* (e.g., early morning, midafternoon) to minimize risk of nitrate tolerance (see below). Such eccentric schedules appear to strike the best balance between avoidance of tolerance and control of angina. A sustained-release form of isosorbide dinitrate with a 12-hour serum half-life is available but not recommended because of highly variable intestinal absorption and risk of nitrate tolerance (unless used only once daily).

Both *chewable* and *sublingual* isosorbide preparations are available and provide a more rapid onset of action (5 to 15 minutes), but duration of action falls to about 2 hours. It remains to be seen whether the faster onset shorter acting forms of isosorbide are so much better than sublingual TNG as to warrant their added expense.

Isosorbide mononitrate provides longer acting nitrate than isosorbide dinitrate. When given twice daily, it can provide up to 12 hours of antianginal activity. A large once-daily dose of the sustained-release formulation can give up to 12 hours of relief. Isosorbide mononitrate offers no significant advantage over generic isosorbide dinitrate for control of chronic stable angina, except convenience. The mononitrate costs 10 times more per day than the generic dinitrate preparation. The heavily promoted feature of reduced risk of nitrate tolerance with mononitrate use is probably true, but less expensive means of accomplishing this objective are available (see below).

Nitroglycerin ointment has been rediscovered as an effective method for providing long-acting anginal prophylaxis. Improved exercise tolerance and hemodynamic effects persist for up to 6 hours. Because the ointment can be messy and irritating to the skin if applied to the same area around the clock, it is best suited for nocturnal use.

Transdermal nitroglycerin patches can deliver nitroglycerin for 24 hours in a convenient-to-use form. Serum nitrate levels approach the peak level obtained with sublingual nitroglycerin. Initial round-the-clock improvements in symptoms and exercise tolerance decline after 7 to 10 days of continuous patch use, because the sustained high nitrate levels lead to *nitrate tolerance* (see below). Proper use requires a 10- to 12-hour period of *nitrate washout*, having the stable angina patient put the patch on in the morning and remove it in the evening. Continued use of the patch is reasonable in those patients who show definite clinical benefit. If there is none, then the patch should be discontinued. In patients who have been using patches for months to years, termination is best conducted in a tapering fashion to avoid precipitation of a nitrate withdrawal syndrome.

Initiation of Nitrate Therapy. Determining the *proper dose* of a long-acting nitrate is achieved by monitoring the effect of the agent on heart rate, blood pressure, and exercise tolerance. Long-acting nitrate therapy should be introduced gradually; starting with too large a dose produces severe vascular headaches that force many patients to stop their medication. Beginning with a low-dose program (e.g., 5 mg of isosorbide three times a day) and advancing it slowly over 1 to 2 weeks, one can achieve substantial nitrate doses without significant headache. Patients with migraine headaches may be very intolerant of nitrates; combining nitrate therapy with a beta-blocking agent can often overcome this difficulty, especially if the beta-blocker is started first.

Dosage is increased until customary activity can be undertaken without pain, the heart rate at rest rises by 10 to 15 beats/min, or blood pressure falls to the point of causing postural lightheadedness. The development of headache is not a reliable therapeutic end point, because this side effect usually disappears with continuation of therapy.

Prevention of Nitrate Tolerance. *Nitrate tolerance* refers to the loss of hemodynamic benefit associated with continuous nitrate use over prolonged periods. It is believed to be related to sulfhydryl depletion in vascular endothelial cells. Tolerance is both dose and time dependent. In the outpatient setting, nitrate tolerance is seen after 7 to 10 days of continuous 5-mg transdermal TNG patch use and with as little as 30 mg of isosorbide given four times daily. The common denominator is insufficient time for adequate nitrate washout. Onset can be as rapid as 12 to 24 hours with use of intravenous TNG. Tolerance develops to both the peripheral and coronary vasodilator effects of nitrates. Prevention of tolerance appears to require a regimen that provides for rapid increases and decreases in nitrate levels over the course of the day and a daily nitrate-free period. A daily period of 10 to 12 hours off nitrate therapy is recommended to minimize the risk of nitrate tolerance. The least expensive approach is to prescribe an *"asymmetric"* *dosing* schedule for isosorbide dinitrate (e.g., 8 a.m., 2 p.m., 8 p.m.) in place of the standard "symmetric" program of every 6 or 8 hours. Alternatively, a once-daily dose of isosorbide mononitrate or applying a transdermal nitroglycerin patch for only 12 hours might achieve the same objective, but the cost is considerably greater.

β-Adrenergic Blocking Agents

Beta-blockers reduce the frequency of *angina* (especially that which is exercise induced) and improve *exercise tolerance*. These agents are among the few treatment modalities proven to prevent *cardiac sudden death* and prolong *survival* in patients surviving myocardial infarction, with 45% reductions in sudden death and 20% reductions in all-cause mortality demonstrated in long-term prospective trials. In patients with stable coronary disease, beta-blockers appear to reduce the frequency of silent ischemia and other coronary events. The benefits of beta-blockade are attributed to their lowering of myocardial oxygen consumption—they reduce *contractility, blood pressure*, and *heart rate*—and their raising of the *ventricular fibrillatory threshold*. In addition, a slower heart rate provides more time for *myocardial perfusion*, which occurs predominantly during diastole.

Despite these proven benefits, beta-blockers continue to be underused especially the elderly.

Categorization. Beta-blockers can be categorized according to their relative cardioselectivity, lipid solubility, intrinsic agonist activity, and alpha-blocking capacity.

Cardioselectivity refers to the degree of preferential affinity for β_1-receptors, which predominate in the heart and are the principal target of antianginal therapy. Beta-blockers that lack cardioselectivity are more likely at low doses to cause side effects associated with β_2-blockade (bronchospasm, peripheral vasoconstriction, and inhibition of glycogenolysis; see below). Cardioselectivity fades as doses increase. At low to intermediate doses, cardioselectivity is demonstrated by *atenolol, metoprolol, acebutolol, betaxolol,* and *bisoprolol.*

Lipid solubility affects absorption, metabolism, serum half-life, and degree to which an agent crosses the blood–brain barrier. The more lipid soluble an agent is, the more rapid its absorption, the shorter its half-life, and the more likely its entry into the central nervous system (CNS). Lipid-soluble preparations are, for the most part, hepatically metabolized. The most lipid-soluble beta-blockers included propranolol, followed by metoprolol, and then pindolol; the least lipid soluble include atenolol and nadolol. Although it used to be thought that lipid solubility predicted degree of CNS side effects (depression, psychomotor retardation), this quality appears less important than cardioselectivity. An intriguing observation is that those beta-blockers best studied and proven to lower risk of sudden death are the lipid-soluble agents, suggesting to some that central adrenergic inhibition might play an important role in reducing the risk of sudden death.

Agonist activity is an intrinsic characteristic of *pindolol, acebutolol, carteolol, labetalol,* and *penbutolol.* At low doses, these drugs show some sympatholytic action and tend to cause less reduction in heart rate, contractility, and conduction than other beta-blockers. Consequently, they are worth considering in patients who develop symptomatic bradycardia with use of standard beta-blockers. However, as doses increase, these agonist effects are overpowered by the underlying beta-blocking activity.

Alpha-blocking activity is a feature of *labetalol* and *carvedilol.* This characteristic makes these agents useful in situations where potent afterload reduction is desired, as in hypertension and congestive heart failure. Labetalol combines nonselective beta-blockade with agonist activity and alpha-blocking action; it is used predominantly in hypertensive patients. Adverse effects include greater degrees of postural hypotension and sexual dysfunction than seen with most other beta-blockers. Carvedilol offers nonselective beta-blockade in conjunction with alpha-blockade; in addition, it prevents up-regulation of cardiac beta-receptors, reduces cardiac norepinephrine, and demonstrates antioxidant effects. The drug is U.S. Food and Drug Administration (FDA)-approved for use in heart failure, where it has been shown to reduce morbidity and mortality (see Chapter 32).

Adverse effects are directly attributable to the consequences of beta-blockade on a host of organ systems that require β-stimulation for normal functioning. Risk is greatest when there is underlying organ-system dysfunction. Heart failure, heart block, and severe bronchospasm are among the most worrisome of potential adverse effects, but risk can be minimized by careful prescribing and monitoring. In most instances, some degree of beta-blockade can be instituted, especially if cardioselective agents are used. Abrupt withdrawal of beta-blocker therapy can lead to rebound adrenergic stimulation and its attendant adverse consequences.

Heart failure may develop or worsen in patients with preexisting LV dysfunction. Not all patients with a reduced ejection fraction necessarily worsen; those with heart failure due to coronary disease may actually improve (see Chapter 32), but careful monitoring is essential. Concurrent use of other negatively inotropic drugs (e.g., verapamil, disopyramide) should be eliminated or at least minimized.

Heart Block. Patients with underlying conduction system disease may experience symptomatic *bradycardia* or *heart block* due to slowing of the sinoatrial node and atrioventricular conduction; sinus arrest may ensue in such patients. A preparation with some intrinsic β-agonist activity may be preferred if a beta-blocker is to be used in the setting of underlying conduction system disease. Close monitoring is critical to safe use in persons with underlying conduction system disease.

Coronary vasoconstriction is a theoretical concern in patients with coronary disease, especially in those with atherosclerotic disease complicated by vasospasm and in those with purely vasospastic disease. Clinically, it is rarely a problem. In fact, beta-blockers have actually proved useful in patients with variant angina, although they are usually prescribed in conjunction with coronary vasodilators such as nitrates or calcium channel blockers. The observed benefit of beta-blockers in settings of suspected coronary vasoconstriction is believed related to their favorable effects on platelet aggregation, oxygen demand, and other factors contributing to vasospasm or angina.

Peripheral vasoconstriction can occur with beta-blocker therapy, particularly in patients who suffer from vasospastic Raynaud's disease. However, as long as a low-dose cardioselective program is used, the Raynaud's patient can usually tolerate beta-blocker treatment. Similarly, patients with peripheral atherosclerotic arterial disease rarely suffer a compromise in limb perfusion when taking a beta-blocker (see Chapter 34).

Bronchospasm. By blocking β_2-receptors, nonselective beta-blockers (and all preparations when used in full doses) may trigger bronchospasm, the most serious side effect of beta-blocker use. Bronchospasm may occur in any patient with a history of bronchospastic disease, even if asymptomatic at the time of initiating therapy. Many regard asthma as a relative contraindication to beta-blocker use, but careful use is possible in patients with inactive or well-controlled bronchospastic disease, so long as doses are kept low and a cardioselective agent is used. Nonetheless, caution and careful monitoring of flow rates are advised, because even low doses of a relatively cardioselective agent can worsen bronchospasm in a patient with asthma.

Hypoglycemia. Beta-blockers will *blunt the adrenergic response* to hypoglycemia. This may impair patient recognition of a hypoglycemic episode in patients taking insulin or potent oral agents and, in theory, prolong the duration of hypoglycemia by inhibiting catecholamine-induced glycogenolysis and glucose mobilization. In actual practice, prolongation of hypoglycemia is rare, and diabetics have a very high risk of cardiovascular morbidity and mortality that is markedly reduced by beta-blocker therapy. Consequently, beta-blocker use is not contraindicated in diabetics, even in those taking insulin, but careful dosing and cardioselectivity are required as are detailed

patient education and careful program design (see Chapter 102).

CNS Effects and Depression. The CNS effects of beta-blockers are of considerable concern to patients and often a cause for discontinuation of therapy. Anecdotal reports of *cognitive problems, depression, sexual dysfunction, altered sleep, nightmares,* and *fatigue* appeared soon after propranolol became widely available. Their frequency is particularly high in the elderly with use of propranolol, but much less so with cardioselective agents. Some suggest that the incidence of CNS side effects could be substantially reduced by use of lipid-insoluble preparations (e.g., atenolol, nadolol, timolol), though the relative advantage of using lipid-insoluble beta-blockers remains a subject of debate. More important to avoidance of CNS effects appears to be use of a cardioselective agent. The issue of an increased *risk of depression* with beta-blocker use also remains unresolved, pending data from prospective, randomized, placebo-controlled trials. In one of the few well-designed studies—comparing atenolol to nifedipine in elderly hypertensive patients—atenolol was found to impair neither cognition nor mood. Pending further data, it appears that depression or other forms of CNS dysfunction are contraindications to beta-blocker therapy. Use of a cardioselective lipid-insoluble preparation is probably preferable in such patients, provided there is careful monitoring of mood, sleep pattern, and sexual and cognitive functioning.

Rebound. Abrupt *withdrawal* of beta-blockade can precipitate an exacerbation of *angina, acute coronary insufficiency,* or even *infarction.* It has been hypothesized that an *"upregulation" of beta-adrenergic receptors* results from long-term blockade and makes these patients more sensitive to unopposed β-adrenergic stimulation. Onset is characteristically within 2 to 6 days after abrupt cessation of therapy. Concern about withdrawal often occurs in the perioperative setting, where medications might have been held for surgery. About 10% of stable anginal patients experience a serious *rebound* in symptoms when beta-blockade is suddenly terminated. Infarction and death may occur. Those at greatest risk are patients on large doses who have achieved much benefit from beta-blockade. Withholding beta-blockers for up to 48 hours can be done without risking any increase in angina. Patients who experience an exacerbation usually do so 2 to 6 days after abrupt discontinuation of therapy. Tapering therapy over the course of 1 to 2 weeks can minimize a withdrawal reaction.

Lipids. Although beta-blocker use (especially of nonselective agents) may cause a modest increase in serum triglycerides and a small reduction in serum HDL cholesterol, there is no evidence that these effects are clinically significant. Moreover, both animal and human studies demonstrate beta-blocker inhibition of serum factors and vessel wall stresses important to atherogenesis.

Choice of Agent. The choice of agent should be based predominantly on cost, need for cardioselectivity, and duration of action. Generically available formulations (e.g., propranolol, metoprolol, atenolol) are one tenth to one thirtieth the cost of brand-name beta-blockers. Cardioselectivity deserves consideration in patients with asthma, peripheral vascular disease, or neuropsychiatric problems. Duration of action becomes important for maximizing compliance, which is facilitated by use of agents that can be administered on a once-daily or twice-daily basis. The combination of low cost, cardioselectivity, and prolonged duration of action make generic preparations of *metoprolol* and *atenolol* the preferred beta-blockers for most patients with coronary disease. An agent with some intrinsic β-agonist activity (e.g., generic *pindolol*) may be worth considering in anginal patients with conduction system disease or sinus node dysfunction bothered by symptomatic bradycardia when taking a beta-blocker without such activity. The presence of heart failure does not need to be a contraindication to beta-blocker use; both long-acting metoprolol and carvedilol have demonstrated ability to improve survival in patients with heart failure (see Chapter 32).

Initiation of beta-blocker therapy requires titration of dose against the *resting* and *exercise heart rates*. Lowering the resting heart rate to about 60 beats/min is usually considered evidence of sufficient beta-blockade but may not be a reliable indicator in elderly patients. A subset of patients do not achieve adequate control of their angina at this level of beta-blockade. Further increases in dosage (and a slower resting heart rate) may be necessary to prevent chest pain. Such bradycardia is often well tolerated hemodynamically. Typical target heart rates are 50 to 60 beats/min at rest, with an increase to 70 to 80 with moderate exercise and to no more than 100 with vigorous exercise. The true measures of adequate therapy remain the suppression of angina and improvement of exercise tolerance. Times of maximum diurnal adrenergic activity (early morning and early evening) are the ones most important to cover with beta-blockade, because they are times when risks of cardiac events are greatest.

Angiotensin-Converting Enzyme Inhibitors

Angiotensin-converting enzyme (ACE) inhibition is emerging as an essential component of CHD management, not only in patients with *impaired LV function* but also in those with ejection fractions that are not reduced. In addition to inhibiting angiotensin-induced vasoconstriction, ACE inhibitors have shown ability to limit vascular smooth muscle proliferation, plaque rupture, and LV hypertrophy and to improve vascular endothelial function and fibrinolysis. Postinfarction patients with ejection fractions less than 0.4 achieve significant reductions in cardiac morbidity and mortality with ACE inhibitor use (see Chapter 32).

Now evidence is accumulating that even in the *absence of LV dysfunction*, ACE inhibition can significantly reduce cardiovascular *morbidity* and *mortality* independent of its effect on blood pressure. In the first large-scale randomized controlled trial to test this hypothesis (the Heart Outcomes Prevention Evaluation [HOPE]), reductions of 20% to 30% in relative risk were achieved in primary cardiovascular morbidity and mortality end points such as death, infarction, and stroke. The observed benefits were independent of aspirin use, beta-blockers, lipid-lowering agents, and antihypertensive drugs, suggesting a unique mode of action. Interestingly, there was no effect on rate of unstable angina. Although more data are needed to confirm these important findings, clinicians should consider ACE inhibition in patients with substantial CHD risk, even if LV function is preserved. Patients already taking ACE inhibitors should certainly continue with them in addition to any other medications prescribed for control of angina.

About 10% of patients experience an intolerable *dry cough* with ACE inhibitor use, which often leads to discontinuation of therapy. *Angiotensin II receptor antagonists* (e.g., losartan) are sometimes substituted; their effect on cardiovascular morbidity and mortality in CHD patients is unknown. Also unknown is the significance of any interaction between *aspirin* and ACE inhibitors, which are likely to be used concurrently in CHD patients; none was reported in the HOPE study. Surveys of primary care practices reveal considerable underuse of ACE inhibitors in CHD patients with LV dysfunction. The attention that is likely to be given to ACE inhibition because of the HOPE study is likely to change this behavior and extend the spectrum of ACE inhibitor use if confirmed by other large-scale randomized trials.

Calcium-Channel Blockers

Drugs in this class remain popular among many clinicians and patients for treatment of chronic stable angina, because they are generally well tolerated and effective for control of symptoms. They reduce the frequency of anginal episodes, prolong exercise tolerance, and decrease the need for nitroglycerin. They are especially useful in persons with coronary vasospasm. Although symptomatically beneficial, calcium channel blockers have yet to demonstrate any reduction in rates of myocardial infarction, need for revascularization, cardiac sudden death, or overall mortality. In addition, concerns have arisen about the safety of the short-acting preparations. Recent findings from several retrospective, prospective, and meta-analytic studies suggest increased risks (relative risk, 1.5 to 1.6) of myocardial infarction and cardiac death in patients taking short-acting calcium channel blockers. Moreover, risk of cardiac death is significantly increased when calcium channel blockers are used in the setting of LV failure (see Chapter 32). In fact, many of these agents are contraindicated when coronary disease is complicated by chronic heart failure. Pending the results of randomized trials of long-acting calcium channel blockers, many authorities currently recommend that calcium channel blockers are relegated to a secondary role in management of chronic stable angina. They suggest that use should be limited to patients who cannot tolerate beta-blockers or beta-blockade or who fail to achieve adequate control of symptoms with nitrates and beta-blockade.

Mechanisms of Action. These agents typically inhibit calcium transport via the "slow" or "L-type" calcium channels of the cellular membranes in myocardial, vascular, and nonvascular smooth muscle tissues. In the heart, calcium channel blockade reduces *inotropy* and slows *conduction*; in vascular tissue, the result is *vasodilation*, which may be accompanied by *reflex tachycardia*. Responses of vascular smooth muscle to angiotensin II and catecholamines are blunted. The net effects range from coronary and systemic vasodilation to decreases in myocardial contractility and conductivity. Coronary vasodilation improves perfusion in patients prone to coronary vasospasm. In most stable anginal patients, symptomatic benefit is believed to derive from a reduction in myocardial oxygen demand brought about by reductions in contractility, filling pressure (preload), and systemic blood pressure (afterload).

Classification. The different classes of calcium channel blockers are distinguished by their binding site within the L-channel and by their relative clinical effects on myocardial, conducting system, and vascular functions. They all cause vasodilation and a lowering of blood pressure, but the degree of pressure reduction varies as does the net effect on contractility and conduction.

Dihydropyridines. Nifedipine is the prototypical agent of this class. Those approved for use in stable angina include nifedipine, *nicardipine,* and *amlodipine.* At present, only amlodipine and the long-acting formulation of nifedipine are recommended for use, because of the concerns regarding safety of short-acting calcium channel blockers. Nifedipine is the most active vasodilator of all the calcium-channel blockers. Its main effect is arterial. Both coronary and peripheral arterial dilatation result, making this agent especially useful for patients with coronary vasospasm and hypertension (see Chapter 26). Although nifedipine is negatively inotropic, its net effect on LV function is minimal because the drug induces a strong β-adrenergic reflex response to its arterial vasodilation. In some patients, a *reflex tachycardia* occurs with use of the short-acting preparation. Its potent vasodilating effects produce a higher incidence of *flushing, hypotension, dizziness, leg edema,* and *headache* than occurs with other drugs in its class. Also, unlike the others, nifedipine has no clinically significant suppressant effect on the sinoatrial or atrioventricular nodes, making it safe for use in patients with underlying conduction system disease. Nifedipine has been shown to be effective for symptomatic treatment of chronic stable angina and variant angina. Because of concerns about increased risk of sudden cardiac death and marked reflex tachycardia with use of short-acting dihydropyridines, only the sustained-release preparation of nifedipine is currently recommended for use.

Second-generation dihydropyridines (e.g., nicardipine, isradipine, felodipine, nisoldipine) are marketed predominantly as antihypertensive agents and promoted for their "vascular selectivity" because they do not affect atrioventricular or sinoatrial node activity. They are available in sustained-release formulations but are not FDA-approved for use in chronic stable angina. Like nifedipine, these induce arterial dilation and an initial reflex tachycardia, often necessitating concurrent use of a beta-blocker. Side effects are similar to those of nifedipine (flushing, peripheral edema, headache, lightheadedness). They are less negatively inotropic than earlier calcium-channel blockers, but they are still contraindicated in the setting of concurrent chronic heart failure. Amlodipine, promoted as the most "cardiofriendly" of the dihydropyridines, has the least effect on contractility, conductivity, and neurohumoral reflexes (no reflex tachycardia) and appears safe for use in the setting of LV dysfunction (see below).

Phenylalkylamines. Verapamil is the prototype in this class, which has the most pronounced net effects on myocardial contractility and atrioventricular conduction. Even though they effectively reduce afterload, they can precipitate heart failure in patients with underlying LV dysfunction and cause heart block in patients with conduction system disease, contraindicating their use in patients with severe LV failure or marked conduction system disease. This potent ability to slow atrioventricular conduction has made verapamil extremely useful for acute treatment of supraventricular tachycardias (see Chapter 28). Constipation and leg edema are conse-

quences of its dilating effect on gastrointestinal and venous smooth muscle.

Benzothiazepines. Diltiazem is the prototype and among the better tolerated of the calcium channel blockers. Although it more closely resembles verapamil than nifedipine, its pharmacologic profile is unique. Compared with verapamil, it causes greater slowing of the sinoatrial node but has less influence on the atrioventricular junction, contractility, and vascular tone. In studies of its effects on mortality and reinfarction in post-myocardial infarction patients, there was no overall improvement in either mortality or reinfarction; those with LV dysfunction showed increased rates of adverse outcomes, suggesting that any possible benefit is limited to those with preserved LV function.

T-type Calcium-Channel Blockers. Mebefradil blocks not only the L-type calcium channel but also the T-type (transient) calcium channel. T-type channels are found in vascular smooth muscle and conduction system tissue but not in ventricular myocardium. The result is coronary and peripheral vascular dilatation, but no impairment of myocardial contractility. Mebefradil is effective for treatment of stable angina, but whether it will prove safe for use in the setting of concurrent heart failure remains to be established.

Adverse Effects. As noted earlier, increased risks of myocardial infarction and cardiac death have been reported in patient populations taking short-acting calcium channel blockers. The extent of risk remains to be defined. Proposed mechanisms include increased myocardial oxygen demand from reflex tachycardia and decreased coronary perfusion from acute drop in filling pressure. Calcium-channel blocker use also increases the risks of worsening heart failure, life-threatening arrhythmias, myocardial infarction, and death when used in patients with chronic LV dysfunction. The mechanisms responsible for these cardiac complications remain poorly understood. It was thought that the reflex tachycardia and negative inotropic effects of many of these agents were responsible, but even the use of sustained-release preparations and agents with little effect on the left ventricle have not lowered the risk. As noted, *heart block* and *sinoatrial node suppression* may occur with use of verapamil- and diltiazem-like agents.

Use and Choice of Calcium-Channel Blockers. Given the inability of calcium-channel blockers to reduce cardiac risk and ongoing concerns regarding their safety, the use of these agents should be limited to long-acting preparations in persons who fail to achieve adequate symptomatic control with beta-blockade and nitrates. Although all classes of calcium channel blockers have antianginal activity, selection of an individual agent needs to take into account cost, convenience, and the status of the patient's left ventricle and conducting system.

Cost and Convenience. From a cost-effectiveness perspective, calcium channel blockers do not rank highly. Even the generic sustained-release formulations are as much as 5 times the cost of generic beta-blockers; brand-name formulations are 10 to 25 times more expensive. The availability of many different sustained-release preparations facilitates compliance but at the expense of increased cost.

Use in the setting of LV dysfunction is discouraged, given the increased risk of sudden death and other adverse cardiac outcomes noted earlier. Negatively inotropic agents (e.g., verapamil, diltiazem) are especially important to avoid, but even agents without much negative inotropic effect have produced poor outcomes. Only *amlodipine* appears reasonably well tolerated in anginal patients with severe chronic LV dysfunction (ejection fraction less than 30%). Why it should be the best tolerated of the calcium channel blockers remains unclear, although it is among the least negatively inotropic. However, amlodipine does not improve survival and carries a 5% risk of inducing pulmonary edema, probably because of pulmonary vasodilation. Moreover, its cost is high. An *ACE inhibitor* (see above) might better contribute to outcome in this setting.

Use in the setting of conduction-system disease necessitates avoiding agents that suppress conduction system and/or sinus node function (e.g., verapamil and diltiazem respectively). Nifedipine and the second-generation dihydropyridines (e.g., amlodipine) are preferred. Moreover, their marked effects on noncardiac smooth muscle result in the highest incidence among calcium channel blockers of extracardiac side effects such as peripheral edema, flushing, and postural hypotension.

Antiplatelet Therapy and Oral Anticoagulation

With the increasing appreciation for the roles of platelets, clotting factors, and vascular reactivity in coronary artery disease comes renewed interest in the benefits of inhibiting platelet function and thrombus formation.

Antiplatelet Therapy. Of the conventional platelet inhibitors (e.g., aspirin, dipyridamole, sulfinpyrazone), only aspirin has proven effective in reducing cardiac risk. Aspirin prolongs survival in patients with *unstable angina* and reduces the risk of myocardial infarction in persons with *chronic stable angina*. In The Physicians' Health Study, participants with chronic stable angina demonstrated an 87% reduction in risk of myocardial infarction and a trend toward reduced risk of death from infarction; however, there was also a trend toward an increase in risk of hemorrhagic stroke. Aspirin therapy did not prevent the onset of angina.

New antiplatelet therapies are emerging. A promising approach for acute settings is use of *monoclonal antibodies* that block platelet *glycoprotein IIb/IIIa receptors*, which are important to platelet aggregation and thrombus formation. Initial studies show a 50% reduction in periprocedural infarction when used with angioplasty and reduced rates of infarction in the setting of unstable angina when added to a program of aspirin and heparin. Use in stable angina is not established; results of initial studies show results similar to those for aspirin.

Oral Anticoagulation. Meta-analysis of major randomized controlled trials of warfarin therapy in patients with CHD reveals significant reductions in myocardial infarction, stroke, and cardiovascular death with high-intensity (INR 2.8 to 4.5) oral anticoagulation. Risks of infarction and stroke are reduced with moderate intensity (INR 2.0 to 3.0) therapy. The benefits of high and moderate intensity anticoagulation approximate those seen with use of aspirin, but risk of bleeding is increased in proportion to the intensity of oral anticoagulation. Combining aspirin use with moderate intensity oral anticoagulation appears promising but remains to be confirmed.

Treatment of Cardiovascular Risk Factors and Precipitants

Risk Factors. An essential component of the management program is attention to cardiovascular risk factors. Patients with coronary disease have five times the risk of a coronary event. Secondary preventive efforts can improve quality of life, reduce risk of coronary events, obviate the need for revascularization, and prolong survival, especially those that address *hypercholesterolemia* (see Chapter 27), *hypertension* (see Chapter 26), *smoking* (see Chapter 54), *diabetes* (see Chapter 102), *exercise* (see Chapters 18 and 31), and *emotional stress* (see below and Chapters 31 and 226). The value of treating *hyperhomocysteinemia* remains to be established, and there continues to be much debate about the benefit of *hormone replacement* (see Chapter 31).

Risk factor reduction can be just as important to outcomes as properly implemented medical and surgical therapies, as evidenced by a randomized trial of aggressive lipid-lowering therapy compared with angioplasty in patients with mild-to-moderate stable angina. Lipid lowering was equal to if not better than angioplasty with regards to reducing frequency of future cardiac events (Atorvastatin versus Revascularization Treatment study).

Precipitants. *Smoking* and *hypertension* are not only CHD risk factors but also potentially important precipitants of angina. The absorbed nicotine increases blood pressure and heart rate, thus increasing myocardial oxygen demand. Nicotine may also cause vasospasm, and the rise in carboxyhemoglobin from smoke inhalation cuts down on oxygen delivery. Even passive smoking (from being in a smoke-filled room) can reduce exercise tolerance in patients with stable angina. Cessation of smoking can be psychologically stressful and physically uncomfortable, but the immediate and long-term benefits greatly outweigh the short-term discomfort. The development of symptomatic coronary disease may provide a potent stimulus to smoking cessation; the effort often succeeds when the physician takes a strong interest in achieving it (see Chapter 54). Hypertension can exacerbate angina by raising myocardial oxygen demand through its effect on afterload.

Psychological stress is well recognized as an important precipitant, but only recently has it been appreciated how common stress-induced ischemia is in patients with coronary artery disease. Episodes of silent ischemia and symptomatic ischemia have been documented in stressful situations. Public speaking and difficult mental tasks can induce as much symptomatic and silent ischemia as exertion in patients with coronary artery disease. High levels of life stress and social isolation are independent predictors of death from coronary disease. The role of personality style, such as so-called type A behavior, remains a subject of debate, although the evidence from studies of mental stress suggests that coronary patients who have a low tolerance for frustrating circumstances might be expected to have an increased likelihood of ischemic stress responses.

Addressing the psychosocial stresses that the anginal patient encounters is critical. An adequate evaluation includes a thorough psychosocial history with emphasis on those factors contributing to stress and social isolation. Urging the hard-driving impatient person to change their personality style is counterproductive, but counseling them on means of coping with frustration and introducing them to simple *relaxation techniques* (see Appendix of Chapter 226) may be better appreciated. If acute anxiety or situational stress is known to predictably precipitate severe chest pain or significant silent ischemia, occasional prophylactic use of a *minor tranquilizer* may be warranted. However, frequent benzodiazepine use in the absence of a true anxiety disorder is strongly discouraged because it can lead to tolerance and even addiction (see Chapter 226); furthermore, tranquilizer use is no substitute for an adequate medical regimen. *Beta-blocker* therapy can be quite effective in limiting the adverse cardiac effects of anxiety by blocking the attendant adrenergic discharge.

Depression and *anxiety* are common responses to the diagnosis of coronary disease; they can impair not only the patient's psychological sense of well-being but also the physical responses to medical and interventional therapies. Moreover, anxiety is a risk factor for cardiac sudden death, and depression is more powerful predictor of heart disease than personality style. After a year of proper therapy for angina, any untreated anxiety or depression correlates more closely with exercise capacity and functional status than the severity of the underlying coronary disease. Despite receiving and complying with proper antianginal regimens, patients with these psychological states manifest more physical incapacity than patients free of active depression or anxiety. The close link between these states and functional status makes it imperative to check for and treat anxiety and depression (see Chapters 226 and 227) at the time of initial CHD workup and again during implementation of the antianginal program. Patients who fail to respond to what seems to be a properly instituted cardiac regimen should be evaluated for an underlying affective disorder.

Other precipitants that should be checked for and addressed include severe *anemia* (see Chapter 82), *hyperthyroidism* (see Chapter 103), *heart failure* (see Chapter 32), and *hypoxemia* due to lung disease (see Chapters 46 and 47). All are capable of worsening both symptomatic and silent myocardial ischemia in the context of underlying coronary disease. Neither *coffee* nor *caffeine* consumption has been shown to increase the risk of coronary disease, although an oft-quoted epidemiologic study found a minor trend toward increased risk in patients consuming more than four cups of decaffeinated coffee per day.

Exercise can significantly improve functional status and directly and indirectly improve important outcomes by improving skeletal muscle efficiency, decreasing heart rate and blood pressure, and enhancing moral well-being (see Chapters 18 and 31).

Designing the Medical Regimen

Criteria for Inclusion. With such a vast array of available medical therapies, the first priority is to ensure that the medical program includes those measures proven to enhance major outcomes. The goal is not only to eliminate anginal pain but also to reduce the risks of myocardial infarction, need for revascularization, and cardiac death. Consequently, *beta-blockade, aspirin,* and *aggressive control of cardiovascular risk factors* should be incorporated whenever possible into the medical regimen. In persons with LV dysfunction (and possibly in those with preserved LV function), an *ACE inhibitor* is essential to maximizing survival. In addition, any *precipitating factors* must be identified and addressed, because they can have major effects on response to treatment. The program should include

an *exercise program* to enhance functional status. Surveys of CHD patients in primary care practices often find underuse of therapies with proven benefit (e.g., beta-blockers, ACE inhibitors). A common error is to focus on relief of angina and ignore overall cardiovascular risk; patients are prescribed nitrates and calcium channel blockers, but not beta-blockers, ACE inhibitors, aspirin, and treatment that aggressively reduces cardiovascular risk factors.

Evidence to guide selection of treatment modalities for patients with stable angina suffers from the tendency of investigators to concentrate their efforts on postinfarction populations. A number of recommendations for patients with stable angina are extrapolations from postinfarction studies (e.g., the mortality benefit of beta-blockers). More long-term studies using cardiac events and mortality as outcomes are needed to validate these recommendations for anginal patients who have not infarcted. Pending such data, it seems reasonable to extrapolate the medical recommendations to this population, especially because most measures are well tolerated, relatively inexpensive, and safe. To withhold them might risk losing an opportunity to improve outcomes. Extrapolation of revascularization recommendations is not another story, because the risks associated with interventional therapy are much higher (see below).

Commonly Used Combinations of Antianginal Agents. Combining *nitrates* with *beta-blockers* usually achieves good symptomatic control at low cost and takes advantage of the positive contribution of beta-blockers to major outcomes. In general, *calcium channel blockers* should be relegated to a second-line role and avoided in the setting of LV dysfunction. Nonetheless, they may add a degree of symptomatic relief when added to a program of beta-blockade in persons free of conduction disturbances and LV dysfunction (most calcium channel blockers are contraindicated in heart failure; see Chapter 32).

The combination of *nitrates plus a calcium channel blocker* is occasionally worth considering in very symptomatic patients who cannot tolerate beta-blockade (e.g., those with severe bronchospastic disease). The calcium channel blocker should be one that blunts reflex tachycardia (e.g., diltiazem, verapamil). Such a program may be particularly effective in patients with stubborn vasospastic disease, but it must be undertaken with care because of the potential for hypotension and worsening angina.

Adding a *calcium channel blocker* to a program of *beta-blockade* and *long-acting nitrates* is sometimes useful, especially in persons with suspected vasospasm or a need to decrease doses of the other agents due to bothersome side effects.

Combined use of a beta-blocker and a calcium channel blocker often requires reduced doses of both agents due to the risks of adversely affecting contractility, chronotropy, conduction, and blood pressure. Concurrent use of potent arterial vasodilators (e.g., alpha-blockers, centrally acting vasodilators) is to be avoided due to the risk of serious hypotension. Care is also required when combination therapy is used in conjunction with digoxin, because of potential for further suppression of conduction through the atrioventricular node.

Revascularization

Revascularization provides the opportunity to improve coronary blood flow, control of angina, and exercise tolerance. In high-risk patients, risk of infarction is reduced and long-term survival is enhanced. The principal revascularization modalities are *percutaneous transluminal angioplasty* (PTCA) and *coronary artery bypass graft* (CABG) surgery. Both procedures have become among the most commonly performed invasive therapies in the nation, with over 500,000 performed annually. Considerable debate has surrounded the indications for their use, because of widespread uncritical use before randomized study. The indications for CABG have become much clearer with completion of major multicenter studies of long-term survival. Meanwhile, the indications for PTCA continue to expand as the technology improves and controlled data emerge. Outcomes from *directional atherectomy* remain disappointing because of unacceptably high complication rates due to debris and endothelial damage associated with the procedure.

Angioplasty. PTCA was developed as an alternative to surgical revasculariztion for patients who remain unacceptably symptomatic despite medical therapy yet do not have high-risk disease (Table 30.1), which is an absolute indication for CABG. Angioplasty involves passing a balloon catheter into a stenosed vessel and inflating the balloon at the site of the narrowing to widen the lumen. It requires coronary angiography and, when performed on a critical artery, surgical standby, given the risk of sudden vessel occlusion from manipulation leading to infarction. A *high-grade proximal stenosis* (70%) that is smooth, concentric, less than 0.5 cm in length, and noncalcified is considered the lesion most amenable to PTCA treatment. The immediate success rate for PTCA in patients with favorable lesions is in excess of 85%. The insertion of a wire-mesh *stent* with PTCA improves patency and reduces the risk of restenosis. Rapid advances in stent technology have led to their widespread application; well over a half-million stenting procedures are being done annually, both for initial treatment of stenoses and for restenosed vessels. Although PTCA with stenting has become commonplace, its cost effectiveness and long-term impact on cardiovascular morbidity and mortality remain to be established. Of note, use of medical therapy does not appear to decline after PTCA, despite a decline in angina.

Benefits. Symptomatic low-risk patients receiving PTCA demonstrate better symptomatic relief and exercise tolerance at 6 months of follow-up than do those treated medically, although there is a small risk of periprocedural myocardial infarction. Patients randomized to PTCA versus CABG achieve nearly equivalent outcomes for cardiac morbidity and mortality at 5 years (86.6% vs. 89.3%), but over half of those treated with PTCA require a repeat revascularization within 1 to 3 years; up to one third eventually come to bypass surgery. Risk of Q-wave infarction is higher for CABG in the short run, but equals out over time. Among subgroups, diabetics may do better with CABG compared with PTCA.

The long-term safety, efficacy, and cost effectiveness of PTCA compared with medical therapy and bypass surgery remain to be defined. The literature should be followed closely, as there will be much data forthcoming, especially on use of PTCA with stenting in higher risk patients such as those with left-main and left-main-equivalent disease. Sorely needed are large-scale, randomized, controlled trials comparing PTCA, CABG, and medical therapy with regards to long-term cardiovascular morbidity and mortality. To date, the end points of many studies have been limited to symptom relief, exercise tolerance, quality of life, and short-term risks of restenosis, complications, and cardiac events; more data are needed on long-term outcomes. The hope is that the technologic advances afforded by PTCA with stenting will result in superior outcomes and expand its indications. Whether this mode of revasculariztion will prove a cost-effective alternative to surgery and to medical therapy remains to be demonstrated. The currently high rates of restenosis (see below) make repeat revascularization procedures more likely; this needs to be factored into the calculation of relative costs and benefits and discussed with patients as they choose between treatment alternatives.

Risks. The risk of *restenosis* with PTCA alone is substantial (e.g., 25% to 40% at 6 months) but can be reduced by nearly 50% by stent use. Because stent placement can trigger *acute thrombosis* (heralded by angina) or *subacute thrombosis* (manifested by acute infarction or death), the procedure is followed immediately by 2 to 4 weeks of potent antiplatelet therapy. Currently prescribed regimens include *aspirin* plus *ticlopidine*, *clopidogrel* (which lacks the marrow-suppression risk of ticlopidine), and *abciximab* (which blocks platelet glycoprotein IIb/IIIa receptors). Trials are ongoing to determine the optimum program. With antiplatelet therapy, the rates of stent-related acute and subacute thrombosis are markedly reduced (e.g., less than 0.5% and less than 1.5%, respectively). Other periprocedural risks include *bleeding* and *vascular injury* that require urgent surgical repair (1%), coronary *artery perforation* (less than 1%), *infection* (rare), and contrast-induced nephropathy (0 to 44% depending on presence of underlying kidney disease).

After 6 months of patency, the reappearance of angina usually represents progression of another lesion that was not dilated rather than late restenosis. Nonetheless, in-stent restenosis (more than 50% reduction in lumen diameter) remains a concern and can occur in up to 20% to 30% of patients. Most patients remain asymptomatic, but those that do redevelop angina pose a difficult challenge because treatment is problematic. Intimal neoproliferation is believed to be a contributing factor; methods to minimize it are being sought (e.g., local application of radiation).

Costs. Angioplasty represents a multibillion dollar health care expenditure in the United States annually. Per patient, total costs of PTCA plus stenting can reach thousands of dollars. Although the cost of a PTCA-plus-stenting procedure remains a fraction of that for CABG, it still represents a substantial expenditure, especially if it needs to be repeated. Moreover, medical therapies that prolong survival are often continued, negating major cost savings from reduction in medication use. Cost-effectiveness data are needed.

Indications. For those anginal patients who have unacceptably symptomatic *single- or two-vessel disease without LV dysfunction*, PTCA represents a reasonable *alternative* to medical therapy and to bypass surgery. At present, *moderate-risk patients* with considerable angina are typically offered PTCA as the *initial treatment* because it can be more effective than medical therapy for relief of anginal symptoms; *low-risk patients* can be offered PTCA if they *fail medical therapy*. For patients with preserved LV function who respond well to medical therapy and demonstrate good exercise tolerance, medical therapy is currently preferred, given the good prognosis it affords, especially in conjunction with aggressive lipid lowering.

Contraindications. In addition to local anatomic considerations (stenosis near a branch point, diffuse occlusive disease of a vessel, involvement of a smaller vessel), there are a number of other settings in which PTCA does not appear successful. In patients with *left-main* or *three-vessel disease*, the risk of PTCA is greater than that of CABG, which remains the treatment of choice in patients who can undergo surgery (see below). As with bypass surgery, high rates of restenosis have occurred in patients with *variant angina*, making this form of revascularization ill advised in patients with vasospastic disease.

Coronary Artery Bypass Graft Surgery. Surgical revascularization is the treatment of choice in persons with *high-risk disease* (Table 30.1). It not only improves symptoms and functional status but prolongs survival and reduces risk of infarction.

Benefits. Three landmark studies established CABG as the treatment choice for high-risk patients. In the Veterans Administration (VA) study of bypass surgery in patients with stable angina, those with *left-main disease* randomized to surgery experienced significant improvements in rates of *infarction* and *survival* (average annual mortality fell from more than 10% to 3%). Also benefiting were markedly symptomatic patients with *three-vessel disease* and *LV dysfunction* but not those with normal LV function and disease limited to two vessels. The Coronary Artery Surgery Study included patients with less serious illness (no left-main disease or severe angina); again, only high-risk patients—those with three-vessel disease and LV dysfunction—showed a statistically significant improvement in rates of infarction and cardiac death. The European Coronary Artery Surgery Study confirmed improved survival in patients with left-main disease and found that benefit also accrued to those having *three-vessel disease* with *preserved LV function* and to those with *two-vessel disease* that included a high-grade proximal stenosis of the left anterior-descending coronary artery ("*left-main equivalent*" anatomy). *Late graft occlusion* has reduced some of the apparent advantages of surgical therapy that were noted enthusiastically in earlier reports. Use of the left internal mammary artery for grafting reduces the rate of late graft occlusion to 15% at 10 years. Risk factor modification remains important, even after bypass surgery.

Patients with less severe multivessel disease (Table 30.1) do not experience a survival benefit with revascularization but may achieve *symptom relief* when medical therapy proves inadequate. At issue is whether surgery or angioplasty is the preferred approach to revascularization in such patients. Meta-analyses find the rates of survival and cardiac events to be similar (except for diabetics, who do better with CABG), as are the effects on symptoms, but PTCA patients are nearly 10 times much more likely (risk approaching 50%) to require a repeat revascularization procedure within 3 to 5 years.

Risks. In major centers, the perioperative complication rates for elective CABG in high-risk patients include mortality (2%), infarction (2.5%), arrhythmia (10%), major bleeding requiring reoperation (2%), stroke (1%), and embolization (1%). Higher complication rates are found in hospitals that do relatively fewer bypass procedures per year.

Indications. In sum, bypass surgery is superior to medical therapy for prevention of infarction and prolongation of survival in stable high-risk anginal patients (i.e., those with significant *left-main, proximal left-anterior descending,* or *three-vessel disease*, especially if accompanied by *LV dysfunction*). Patients at less risk who continue to be limited by their angina despite a full medical regimen and aggressive treatment of risk factors are also reasonable candidates for revascularization. CABG is the preferred revascularization procedure for diabetics and those patients who are reluctant to undergo a repeat revascularization procedure within the next 5 years.

Contraindications. Most studies of surgical therapy for patients with *coronary spasm* show disappointing results (e.g., higher rates of mortality and nonfatal infarction). In such patients, surgical therapy should be considered only when medical therapy has failed and spasm has been documented in or about an area of fixed critical stenosis and not in other vessels or distally.

Identifying Candidates. Exercise stress testing and *echocardiography* are the best noninvasive means of screening and identifying potential candidates for revascularization (see Chapters 20 and 36). Those demonstrating a large amount of myocardium at risk and/or a reduced ejection fraction are candidates for *angiography*.

Overall Strategy: Choosing between Initial Medical Therapy and Revascularization

A practical management strategy supported by currently available evidence assigns the patient to initial medical therapy or revascularization on the basis of estimated risk and degree of incapacity as determined by stress testing, echocardiography, and severity of symptoms:

- *Low-risk patients* (mild-moderate angina, normal ejection fraction, small amount of myocardium at risk, probable single-vessel disease): Medical therapy, with revascularization reserved for those incapacitated by angina despite full medical therapy and aggressive risk factor reduction.
- *Moderate-risk patients* (moderate severity of angina, moderate amount of myocardium at risk, probable two-vessel disease, normal ejection fraction): Initial revascularization (PTCA or CABG) if very symptomatic; if not, a trial of medical therapy and aggressive risk factor reduction.
- *High-risk patients* (moderate to severe angina; large amount of myocardium at risk; three-vessel, left-main, or left-main-equivalent disease; reduced ejection fraction): CABG plus ACE inhibitor therapy.

Regardless of the initial mode of therapy, all patients require aggressive treatment of CHD risk factors, because of the major contribution to outcome that accrues with smoking cessation, control of hypertension, and reduction of lipids.

Patient Education

Patient education is pivotal, both to ensure proper compliance with what can be a rather complex medical regimen and to maximize functional status. An understanding of the rationale behind the medical regimen will facilitate its effective use. Counseling about prognosis and allowable activity can prevent unnecessary restriction of activity, relieve fear, and improve life-style. Of particular concern to many patients is the safety of engaging in *sexual intercourse*. The issue should be addressed openly and directly, even if the patient does not take the initiative to raise the subject. Failure to do so can lead to marital problems, depression, and a worsening of symptoms. Guidelines for engaging in sexual activity are similar to those for any other form of physical exertion. The oxygen demands of intercourse among married middle-aged partners are about the same as those for climbing a flight of stairs. If intercourse takes place among unaccustomed partners, the physical and emotional stress may be considerably greater and the oxygen requirements increased substantially. If patients have serious concerns as to how much activity they can safely tolerate, an exercise test may be of value for reassurance, especially if they are needlessly limiting themselves.

With advances in medical therapy and revascularization technology, patients now have an expanded choice of treatment options. In circumstances where outcomes are similar, the advantages and disadvantages of PTCA versus CABG versus medical therapy need to be reviewed so that a treatment program well tailored to the patient's needs and preferences can be designed. Many of the racial differences noted in rates of revascularization among whites and blacks in the United States appear to be a function of familiarity rather than preference. Patient education is essential to ensuring that there is not inappropriate underutilization. Despite obtaining cardiac consultation, many patients will ask the independent opinion of their primary care physician whom they view as knowing them best. This role necessitates keeping well informed on the risks and benefits of treatment options for stable angina.

Indications for Admission and Referral

Admission is required when the anginal pattern is increasing in frequency or severity or is becoming harder to control. Episodes that are starting to last more than 15 minutes and beginning to occur at rest and with exertion suggest progression to *unstable angina*, with its attendant increase in risk of acute infarction. Hospitalization may also be of benefit to judge the adequacy of a medical regimen and to check on compliance when a patient with stable angina reports insufficient relief of symptoms. Referral to a cardiologist for consideration of coronary angiography and angioplasty is indicated when maximum medical therapy has failed to control symptoms and when leftmain or severe three-vessel disease is suspected. The same is true if tight aortic stenosis is a consideration (see Chapter 33).

THERAPEUTIC RECOMMENDATIONS

General Measures for All Patients (including Those Undergoing Revascularization)

- Identify and aggressively treat all major CHD risk factors, particularly hypertension (see Chapter 26), hyperlipidemia (see Chapter 27), and smoking (see Chapter 54).
- Check for and correct any concurrent precipitating or aggravating factors, such as heart failure (see Chapter 32), severe anemia (see Chapter 82), hyperthyroidism (see Chapter 104), hypoxemia (see Chapter 47), and critical aortic stenosis (see Chapter 33).
- Screen for and treat psychosocial factors that can adversely effect outcomes, including anxiety (see Chapter 226), depression (see Chapter 227), situational stress, and social isolation.
- Begin low-dose enteric-coated aspirin (81 mg/d).
- Consider ACE inhibitor therapy; initiate if the patient has a reduced ejection fraction (less than 0.4) (see Chapter 32), consider for the CHD patient with preserved LV function and multiple CHD risk factors (e.g., diabetes, hypertension).

- Determine patient's prognosis and degree of CHD risk by ascertaining amount of myocardium at risk through stress testing (see Chapter 36) and by assessing LV function through echocardiography or radionuclide scanning (see Chapters 32 and 36). Use the risk categorization to guide further program design.
- Thoroughly review with patient and family the rationale and proper use of therapies; encourage monitoring response to treatment; counsel on allowable activity, encourage exercise as tolerated, and help avoid self-imposed unnecessary limits on activity.
- Begin a gentle exercise program (e.g., walking 20 minutes three times a week) and a more intensive program for the highly motivated; obtain an exercise stress test first (see Chapter 31).
- Promptly admit any patient with unstable angina or markedly worsening LV dysfunction and obtain cardiac consultation.

Low-risk Patients (Mild-to-Moderate Angina, Normal Ejection Fraction, Small Amount of Myocardium at Risk, Probable Single-vessel Disease)

- Prescribe as needed TNG, 0.4 mg, for symptomatic relief of anginal episodes; instruct the patient to rest at the time of pain and to take a second and a third TNG if the pain does not resolve within 5 minutes of each TNG dose. Advise maintaining a fresh supply of TNG and discarding any bottle that has been open for more than 6 months or any tablets that fail to cause sublingual burning or head throbbing.
- Prescribe prophylactic use of sublingual TNG if angina is predictable and short-term (less than 30 minutes) protection will suffice (e.g., before carrying bundles, climbing stairs or a hill).
- Begin beta-blockade with a generic formulation of a long-acting cardioselective agent (e.g., atenolol 25 to 50 mg/d or metoprolol 25 mg twice daily); adjust dose to ensure adequate beta-blockade (heart rate less than 60 beats/min at rest, less than 100 beats/min with vigorous exertion). If beta-blockade must be terminated, do so only in a tapering fashion over 1 to 2 weeks; have the patient reduce activity during this time.
- If anginal control is not sufficient with the above measures but the patient responds well to TNG, then add a long-acting nitrate to the program (e.g., isosorbide dinitrate, beginning with 5 mg three times a day and advancing slowly over 1 to 2 weeks in increments of 5 mg per dose); dose in asymmetric fashion (8 a.m., 2 p.m., 8 p.m.) to minimize risk of nitrate tolerance.
- Consider a trial of calcium channel blocker therapy (e.g., long-acting diltiazem 90-120 mg/d, amlodipine 5 mg/d) only if the patient continues to be unacceptably symptomatic despite full doses of nitrates and beta-blockers. Use only a long-acting formulation. Monitor conduction and LV function, especially when using in combination with a beta-blocker. With the exception of amlodipine, do not use if there is underlying heart failure or clinically significant conduction system disease.
- Consider referral for angiography and possible revascularization only if the patient continues to be unacceptably limited by angina despite full compliance with the above medical regimen plus aggressive treatment of CHD risk factors.

Moderate-risk Patients (Moderate Angina, Moderate Amount of Myocardium at Risk, Probable Two-Vessel Disease, Normal Ejection Fraction)

- Give trial of full medical regimen as outlined for patients with low-risk disease. If it provides adequate control of symptoms, then continue indefinitely in conjunction with very aggressive and comprehensive treatment of CHD risk factors and precipitants.
- If exercise tolerance and functional status remain impaired, then refer for angiography and determination of candidacy for revascularization.
- If candidate for revascularization, assess patient's preference for PTCA vs CABG.

High-risk Patients (Moderate-to-Severe Angina; Large Amount of Myocardium at Risk; Suspected Three-Vessel, Left-Main, or Left-Main-Equivalent Disease; Reduced Ejection Fraction)

- Refer immediately for angiography and consideration of CABG.
- Recommend CABG for those found to have left-main, left-main equivalent, or three-vessel disease, especially if complicated by LV dysfunction. (Some proximal LAD lesions might be suitable for PTCA plus stenting.)

A.H.G.

ANNOTATED BIBLIOGRAPHY

Abernethy DR, Schwartz JB. Calcium-antagonist drugs. N Engl J Med 1999;341:1447. *(Detailed review of calcium channel blockers that includes discussion of use in coronary disease; 102 references.)*

Anand SS, Yusuf S. Oral anticoagulant therapy in patients with coronary artery disease: a meta-analysis. JAMA 1999;282:2058. *(Finds that high- and moderate-intensity anticoagulation reduces rates of infarction and stroke to the same degree as aspirin; also notes promising data suggesting that moderate-intensity anticoagulation plus aspirin may be superior to aspirin alone.)*

Bonow RO, Kent KM, Rosing DR, et al. Exercise-induced ischemia in mildly symptomatic patients with coronary artery disease and preserved left ventricular function: identification of subgroups at risk of death during medical therapy. N Engl J Med 1984;311:1339. *(Mildly symptomatic patients with three-vessel disease who have a fall in ejection fraction with exercise had a poor prognosis.)*

Burris JF. β-Blockers, dyslipidemia, and coronary disease. Arch Intern Med 1993;153:2085. *(Addresses the question of adverse effect; finds no proof.)*

The Bypass Angioplasty Revascularization Investigation (BARI) Investigators. Chronic stable angina: angioplasty versus bypass surgery for patients with multivessel disease. N Engl J Med 1996;335:217. *(No difference found in 5-year survival in this randomized multicenter trial; however, over half of angioplasty patients required a second revascularization procedure.)*

CASS Principal Investigators. Myocardial infarction and mortality in the Coronary Artery Surgery Study (CASS) randomized trial. N Engl J Med 1984;310:750. *(One of the landmark randomized studies on the efficacy and indications for bypass surgery. Neither prolongation of life nor prevention of infarction was demonstrated in mildly symptomatic patients.)*

Cohn PF. Silent myocardial ischemia. Ann Intern Med 1988;109:312. *(Excellent terse review; includes discussion of mechanisms, detection, prognosis, and treatment; 61 references.)*

Cohn PF. Concomitant use of nitrates, calcium channel blockers, and beta-blockers for optimal antianginal therapy. Clin Cardiol 1994;17:415. *(Improved control with triple therapy in difficult cases.)*

DeCesare N, Bartorelli A, Fabbiocchi F, et al. Superior efficacy of propranolol versus nifedipine in double-component angina, as related to different influences on coronary vasomotility. Am J Med 1989;87:15. *(Interestingly, propranolol produced no important vasoconstriction, whereas nifedipine's effect was variable, ranging from vasodilation to vasoconstriction.)*

Dimsdale JE, Newton RP, Joist T. Neuropsychological side effects of beta-blockers. Arch Intern Med 1989;149:514. *(A review of 55 studies; concludes there is little evidence for a difference in CNS effects between the lipophilic and lipophobic preparations.)*

Elkayam U. Tolerance to organic nitrates: evidence, mechanisms, clinical relevance, and strategies for prevention. Ann Intern Med 1991;114:667. *(Among the best reviews of nitrate tolerance; 134 references.)*

The EPISTENT Investigators. Randomized, placebo-controlled and balloon-angioplasty-controlled trial to assess safety of coronary stenting with use of platelet glycoprotein-IIb/IIIa blockade. Lancet 1998;352:87-92. *(Platelet receptor blockade significantly reduced the risk of procedure-related adverse outcomes.)*

Erbel R, Haude M, Hopp HW, et al. Coronary-artery stenting compared with balloon angioplasty for restenosis after initial balloon angioplasty. N Engl J Med 1998;339:1672. *(Stenting reduced the rate of restenosis by about 40% and improved event-free survival at 250 days by about 12% but at a cost of subacute thrombosis to 3.9%.)*

Francis GS. ACE inhibition in cardiovascular disease. N Engl J Med 2000;342:201-202. *(An editorial summarizing the mechanisms of action and clinical studies indicating a major role for ACE inhibitor use in CHD.)*

Gersh BJ, Kronmal RA, Schaff HV, et al. Comparison of coronary artery bypass surgery and medical therapy in patients 65 years of age or older. N Engl J Med 1985;313:217. *(A subgroup analysis of the CASS study; benefit demonstrated in the elderly.)*

Gottlieb SS, McCarter RJ, Vogel RA. Effect of beta-blockade on mortality among high-risk and low-risk patients after myocardial infarction N Engl J Med 1998;339:489. *(A large-scale observational study of over 200,000 patients suggesting that high-risk patients benefit as much if not more than low-risk patients.)*

Grobbee DE, Rimm EB, Giovannucci E, et al. Coffee, caffeine, and cardiovascular disease in men. N Engl J Med 1990;323:1026. *(An epidemiologic study of 45,000 men; no increase in risk of coronary disease.)*

Hasdai D, Lerman A, Grill DE, et al. Medical therapy after successful percutaneous coronary angioplasty. Ann Intern Med 1999;130:108. *(A retrospective cohort study showing that use of antianginal medication does not decrease after successful angioplasty that reduces angina.)*

The Heart Outcomes Prevention Evaluation Study Investigators. Effects of an angiotensin-converting-enzyme inhibitor, ramipril, on death from cardiovascular causes, myocardial infarction, and stroke in high-risk patients. N Engl J Med 2000;342:145. *(The HOPE Study, a multicenter, randomized, controlled trial that included CHD patients with normal LV function; found significant [20% to 30%] reductions in CHD morbidity and mortality.)*

Houston MC, Hodge R. Beta-adrenergic blocker withdrawal syndromes in hypertension and other cardiovascular diseases. Am Heart J 1988;116:515. *(Documents that withdrawal is usually mild, but of 338 patients developing withdrawal, 15 infarcted and 8 died.)*

Kendall MJ, Lynch KP, Hjalmarson A, et al. Beta-blockers and sudden cardiac death. Ann Intern Med 1995;123:358. *(A systematic review documenting the survival benefit of beta-blockade.)*

Kotler TS, Diamond GA. Exercise thallium-201 scintigraphy in the diagnosis and prognosis of coronary artery disease. Ann Intern Med 1990;113:684. *(Authoritative review serving as the basis of a policy statement by the American College of Physicians in the same issue; 193 references.)*

Luchi RJ, Chahine RA, Raizner AE. Coronary artery spasm. Ann Intern Med 1979;91:441. *(Excellent review of pathophysiology and its clinical implications; 118 references.)*

Manson JE, Grobbee DE, Stampfer MJ, et al. Aspirin in the primary prevention of angina pectoris in a randomized trial of United States physicians. Am J Med 1990;89:772. *(A report from the Physicians' Health Study indicating that alternate-day aspirin failed to reduce the incidence of symptomatic coronary disease.)*

Mark DB, Shaw L, Harrell FE Jr, et al. Prognostic value of a treadmill exercise score in outpatients with suspected coronary artery disease. N Engl J Med 1991;325:849. *(Demonstrates ability of the electrocardiographic stress test to distinguish high- from low-risk patients.)*

Morrow K, Morris CK, Froelicher VF, et al. Prediction of cardiovascular death in men undergoing noninvasive evaluation for coronary artery disease. Ann Intern Med 1993;118:689. *(Data on predictive value of noninvasive testing.)*

Muller JE, Tofler GH, Stone PH. Circadian variation and triggers of onset of acute cardiovascular disease. Circulation 1989;79:733. *(The morning hours are the time of greatest risk.)*

The Multicenter Diltiazem Postinfarction Trial Research Group. The effect of diltiazem on mortality and reinfarction after myocardial infarction. N Engl J Med 1988;319:385. *(A major, randomized, multicenter study. Patients with normal LV function showed improved survival and lower rates of infarction; those with LV dysfunction showed reduced survival and increased rates of infarction; overall, the net effect was nil.)*

The Norwegian Multicenter Study Group. Timolol-induced reduction in mortality and reinfarction in patients surviving acute myocardial infarction. N Engl J Med 1981;304:801. *(This landmark trial demonstrated a 45% reduction in sudden death among postmyocardial infarction patients attributable to beta-blockade with timolol.)*

O'Meara JJ, Dehmer GJ. Care of the patient and management of complications after percutaneous coronary angioplasty. Ann Intern Med 1997;127:458. *(Excellent review of what can go wrong and how to respond to it.)*

Packer M. Combined beta-adrenergic and calcium-entry blockade in angina pectoris. N Engl J Med 1989;320:709. *(A critical review of studies on this approach to anginal treatment; finds the data support its use only in patients with preserved LV function who fail full doses of single agent therapy; 128 references.)*

Packer M, O'Connor CM, Ghali JK, et al. Effect of amlodipine on morbidity and mortality in severe chronic heart failure. N Engl J Med 1996;334:1107. *(A randomized multicenter controlled trial of 1,153 patients finding no increase in risk of cardiovascular morbidity or mortality with amlodipine use in patients with severe heart failure.)*

Parisi AF, Folland ED, Hartigan P, et al. A comparison of angioplasty with medical therapy in the treatment of single-vessel coronary artery disease. Veterans Affairs ACME Investigators. N Engl J Med 1992;326:10. *(A randomized multicenter study; PTCA was superior to medical therapy for relief of pain and exercise tolerance at 6 months, but there was an increased risk of acute infarction.)*

Parker JD, Parker JO. Nitrate therapy for stable angina pectoris. N Engl J Med 1998;338:520. *(Best current review by leading experts on nitrate use; 97 references.)*

Parker JO, Amies MH, Hawkinson RW, et al. Intermittent transdermal nitroglycerine therapy in angina pectoris: clinically effective without tolerance or rebound: Minitran Efficacy Study Group. Circulation 1995;91:1368. *(Data on the importance of a patch-free period.)*

Parker JO, Farrell B, Lahey KA, et al. Effect of intervals between doses on the development of tolerance to isosorbide dinitrate. N Engl J Med 1987;316:1440. *(A placebo-controlled study in patients with chronic stable angina; onset of tolerance found with four times a day but not three times a day or twice daily dosing.)*

Parker JO, Van Koughnett KA, Farrell B. Nitroglycerin lingual spray: clinical efficacy and dose-response relation. Am J Cardiol 1986;57:1. *(Efficacy and dosing are nearly identical to sublingual TNG.)*

Peterson ED, Shaw LK, DeLong ER, et al. Racial variation in the use of coronary-revascularization procedures. N Engl J Med 1997;336:480. *(Rate of usage decreased among blacks, even after adjusting for clinical indications.)*

Pitt B, Waters D, Brown WM, et al. Aggressive lipid-lowering therapy compared with angioplasty in stable coronary artery disease. N Engl J Med 1999;341:70. *(Stable anginal patients randomized to high-dose atorvastatin had a 13% rate of ischemic events compared with a 21% rate for those treated with angioplasty.)*

Pryor DB, Shaw L, Harrell FE Jr, et al. Estimating the likelihood of severe coronary disease. Am J Med 1991;90:553. *(Describes a validated scoring system based on simple clinical findings that identifies high-risk patients; a potentially useful low-cost alternative.)*

Ridker PM, Manson JE, Gaziano JM, et al. Low-dose aspirin therapy for chronic stable angina: a randomized, placebo-controlled clinical trial. Ann Intern Med 1991;114:835. *(The Physicians' Health Study; risk of a first infarction reduced by 87%; survival did not improve significantly, and risk of stroke trended upward.)*

Rozanski A, Bairey CN, Krantz DS, et al. Mental stress and the induction of silent myocardial ischemia in patients with coronary artery disease. N Engl J Med 1988;318:1005. *(A controlled study; personally relevant stress was just as potent an inducer of ischemia as exertion.)*

Serruys PW, de Jaegere P, Kiemeneij F, et al. A comparison of balloon-expandable-stent implantation with balloon angioplasty in patients with coronary artery disease. BENESTENT Study Group. N Engl J Med 1994;331:489. *(Stents found effective for preventing abrupt vessel closure and restenosis.)*

Siegel D, Grady D, Browner WS, et al. Risk factor modification after myocardial infarction. Ann Intern Med 1988;109:213. *(Substantial reduction in CHD risk can be achieved with modest reduction in risk factors.)*

Silber S, Vogler AC, Krause KH, et al. Induction and circumvention of nitrate tolerance applying different dosage intervals. Am J Med 1987;83:860. *(An eccentric schedule that allowed 10 to 12 hours of washout was most effective.)*

Sim I, Gupta M, McDonald K, et al. A meta-analysis of randomized trials comparing coronary artery bypass grafting with percutaneous transluminal coronary angioplasty in multivessel coronary artery disease. Am J Cardiol 1995:76:1025. *(Similar efficacy and similar rates of cardiac morbidity and mortality but marked increase in need for repeat revascularization with PTCA.)*

Skinner MH, Futterman A, Morrissette D, et al. Atenolol compared with nifedipine: effect on cognitive function and mood in elderly hypertensive patients. Ann Intern Med 1992;116:615. *(One of the few randomized, controlled, double-blinded, crossover studies on the CNS effects of a beta-blocker; no adverse effect on mood or cognitive function detected.)*

Solomon AJ, Gersh BJ. Management of chronic stable angina: medical therapy, percutaneous transluminal coronary angioplasty, and coronary artery bypass graft surgery. Lessons from the randomized trials. Ann Intern Med 1998;128:216. *(A systematic review; concludes that in low-risk patients, medical therapy is the preferred initial modality; in moderate risk patients, revascularization is worth considering; in high risk patients, CABG provides the best outcomes.)*

Strauss WE, Fortin T, Hartigan P. A comparison of quality of life scores in patients with angina pectoris after angioplasty compared with after medical therapy: outcomes of randomized clinical trials. Veterans Affairs ACME Investigators. Circulation 1995;92:1710. *(Quality of life improved with PTCA in persons with proximal LAD lesions.)*

Sullivan MD, LaCroix AZ, Baum C, et al. Functional status in coronary artery disease: a one-year prospective study of the role of anxiety and depression. Am J Med 1997;103:348. *(Anxiety and depression proved to be important determinants of functional status.)*

Sytkowski PA, Kannel WB, D'Agostino RB. Changes in risk factors and the decline in mortality from cardiovascular disease: the Framingham Study. N Engl J Med 1990;322:1635. *(Documents a 40% decline in mortality, most attributed to risk factor control.)*

Varhaskas E. Twelve-year follow-up of survival in the randomized European coronary surgery study. N Engl J Med 1988;319:332. *(A late follow-up report of one of the three major randomized studies of bypass surgery; confirms survival benefit for patients with left-main, three-vessel, and "left-main equivalent" disease.)*

Veterans Administration Coronary Artery Bypass Surgery Cooperative Study Group. Eleven-year survival in the Veterans Administration randomized trial of coronary bypass surgery for stable angina. N Engl J Med 1984;311:1333. *(Landmark study. Only those with a very high risk of dying [left-main disease, very severe three-vessel disease] demonstrated a benefit from surgery at 11 years of follow-up; earlier benefits found at 7 years disappeared by year 11.)*

Viscoli CM, Horwitz RI, Singer BH. Beta-blockers after myocardial infarction: influence of first-year clinical course on long-term effectiveness. Ann Intern Med 1993;118:99. *(Benefit appears greatest in those whose clinical course is characterized by recurrent ischemic events, congestive heart failure, arrhythmias, or severe comorbidity.)*

Whittle J, Conigliaro J, Good CB, et al. Do patient preferences contribute to racial differences in cardiovascular procedure use? J Gen Intern Med 1997;12:267. *(The answer was maybe, but not as much as familiarity with the procedure.)*

Willard JE, Lange RA, Hillis LD. Use of aspirin in ischemic heart disease. N Engl J Med 1992;327:175. *(Comprehensive review; 86 references.)*

Yusuf S. Calcium antagonists in coronary artery disease and hypertension: time for reevaluation? Circulation 1995;92:1079. *(Retrospective review raising concern about safety.)*

31
Cardiovascular Rehabilitation and Secondary Prevention of Coronary Heart Disease

The major goals of cardiovascular rehabilitation and secondary prevention of coronary heart disease (CHD) (i.e., prevention in patients with established disease) are to improve functional capacity, reduce the risks of future cardiac events (e.g., infarction, revascularization, cardiac arrest), and prolong survival. The results of major long-term randomized controlled trials indicate that these goals can be achieved cost effectively through concerted application of preventive therapies. Some modalities are medical (e.g., aspirin, beta-blockers, angiotensin-converting enzyme [ACE] inhibitors), and others are interventional (e.g., revascularization). Those that address risk factors have the unique capacity to stabilize and even induce regression of the atherosclerotic process, yielding some of the greatest reductions in risk when applied aggressively.

Because some interventions require changes in the patient's life-style, the influence of the primary physician is critically important. One needs to know what interventions are effective and how to tailor a secondary prevention program to the needs and capabilities of the individual patient. Upon experiencing a myocardial infarction (MI) or receiving a diagnosis of coronary artery disease, most patients become highly motivated to live a more healthy life-style, providing an excellent opportunity to effect important changes in diet and exercise as part of a comprehensive program of risk reduction through secondary prevention.

CARDIAC REHABILITATION: EXERCISE AND LIFE-STYLE MODIFICATION PROGRAMS

Goals. A program of cardiovascular rehabilitation usually begins in the hospital at the time of a acute cardiac event and continues in outpatient setting after discharge. The major goals of the *inpatient phase* include prevention of physical deconditioning, patient education regarding coronary risk factors, and interventions aimed at preventing psychological disability resulting from the anxiety and depression that frequently follow an acute coronary event. In the *early outpatient convalescence phase*, the goal is to return the patient to the level of physical conditioning that existed before the cardiac event. The *late convalescence/physical training phase* is designed to enhance the patient's physical conditioning. The goal of the maintenance or follow-up phase is to encourage life-long adherence to good health habits. The rehabilitation effort combines an exercise program with dietary modification and aggressive treatment of risk factors.

Phase I: Early Rehabilitation. This phase begins *during hospitalization* for an acute coronary event. Physical deconditioning is avoided by initiating a program of low-level activity as soon as possible after clinical stability has been achieved. In practice, low-level activity can begin safely as soon as the third day after admission for an uncomplicated MI, as soon as symptoms have been controlled in patients admitted for medical therapy of angina, and as soon as the patient who has undergone coronary artery bypass surgery can walk. Initial activity should consist of *slow walking* (60 to 80 steps a minute); the heart rate should not exceed 15 to 20 beats/min above the resting level (or 10 to 15 beats/min above the resting value in patients receiving β-adrenergic blocking agents). An alternative low-level activity program can be initiated during hospitalization with a *stationary bicycle ergometer* in the free-wheeling mode, where the systemic oxygen consumption is only 1.3 times resting oxygen consumption. This low level of activity is comparable in intensity with slow walking and is quite safe for most patients. Either mode effectively prevents skeletal muscle deconditioning and atrophy. Low-level activity also improves morale; patients believe they are contributing positively to the recovery process. Before hospital discharge, most patients should be observed by their physician while *climbing a flight of stairs*. This will provide confidence that such tasks can be performed safely and will often uncover specific questions about what should and should not be done during the first weeks at home.

Submaximal exercise testing before hospital discharge has been recommended and is performed routinely in many centers. A treadmill exercise test to a 5-met level has been found to be safe even when performed within 10 days of an uncomplicated MI. Successful completion of an exercise test before discharge from the hospital helps to restore patient confidence and suggests that the recovery process is proceeding smoothly. The information obtained has prognostic implications and may be useful in patient management. A negative submaximal test predicts an excellent prognosis during the subsequent year, whereas a test that is positive for ischemic electrocardiographic changes with or without anginal symptoms predicts a poorer outcome. In the latter instance, a more aggressive medical approach, coronary angioplasty, or coronary artery bypass surgery may be indicated (see Chapter 30). Exercise testing can also be effective in exposing latent ventricular dysrhythmias and may help in selecting patients whose long-term prognosis may benefit from β-adrenergic blocker therapy (see Chapters 29 and 30). In addition, the procedure helps in deciding which patients can safely undergo early discharge. Radionuclide scintigraphy in conjunction with submaximal exercise testing may sharpen risk stratification after MI, especially if the resting electrocardiogram is abnormal, prohibiting an electrocardiographic stress test (see Chapter 36).

Phase II: Early Convalescence. It begins at the time of hospital discharge and continues for 3 to 6 weeks. Because evidence from experimental animal models suggests that high-level physical activity soon after MI may promote infarct expansion and possible ventricular aneurysm formation, the prescribed activity level remains relatively low during phase II. Exercise intensity is regulated by monitoring peak heart rate, which should not exceed the level achieved during the predischarge submaximal exercise test. If the predischarge exercise test disclosed ischemic electrocardiographic changes, anginal symptoms, or ventricular dysrhythmias, then the heart rate during exercise training sessions should be maintained below the heart rate at which any of these pathologic events was observed. The exercise training modalities used during phase II, as in phase I, usually consist of *walking* and *stationary bicycling*. The process of educating the patient and the family about coronary risk factors is an important component of phase II (see below).

Phase III: Late Convalescence/Physical Training. The program is designed to increase the patient's level of physical conditioning. Based on a *maximal exercise test* performed 3 to 6 weeks after discharge, the exercise prescription is rewritten to provide a greater *physiologic training* effect. This test allows the patient's heart rate and blood pressure responses to exercise to be quantified and provides another screening test for latent myocardial ischemia and ventricular dysrhythmias. The exercise training modalities used during phase II can be broadened during phase III to establish a balanced exercise program that will have long-term patient appeal. Upper extremity conditioning may be added, especially in patients for whom upper extremity work is important to daily activity. During phase III, efforts to modify risk factors continue. These include *dietary interventions* to lower the total serum cholesterol and low-density-lipoprotein cholesterol concentrations, raise high-density-lipoprotein cholesterol concentration, and achieve ideal body weight (see below and Chapters 27 and 233). *Hypertension control* (see Chapter 26) and *smoking cessation* (see Chapter 54) are critically important. *Management of psychological stress* and *depression* should also be addressed (see Chapters 226 and 227), particularly as the patient returns to work. A well-balanced cardiac rehabilitation program attends to all these factors and should involve the patient's family as well.

Phase IV: Maintenance/Follow-up. The goal is to encourage life-long adherence to the healthy habits established during phase III. Follow-up visits at 6- to 12-month intervals are important. Blood pressure and pulse measurement, serum lipid levels, and even repeat maximal exercise tolerance tests can provide useful feedback to the patient and indicate areas that may require life-style change to minimize coronary risk. Further research is needed to improve our understanding about the most effective methods of achieving permanent life-style modification.

Mechanisms of Benefit from Exercise. Regular physical exercise may benefit patients with coronary artery disease by a number of mechanisms. Among these is the "*physiologic training effect*." Because of the increase in peripheral oxygen extraction by working skeletal muscles and the increase in cardiac stroke volume that constitute the training effect, the cardiovascular system of the trained subject is able to deliver a given quantity of oxygenated blood to the peripheral tissues at a lower heart rate. Because systemic arterial pressure also tends to be somewhat lower during exercise in the trained state, the rate-pressure product (heart rate $\times$ systolic arterial pressure), which correlates closely with myocardial oxygen consumption under most physiologic conditions, is often substantially lower than in the untrained state. The benefit to the patient with ischemic heart disease is obvious; it becomes possible for the trained patient to exercise to a higher level before reaching the critical rate-pressure product at which myocardial ischemia develops. β-Adrenergic blockers benefit patients with angina pectoris in a similar fashion, by reducing heart rate and blood pressure during exertion. Unlike exercise training, however, beta-blocking agents also tend to *reduce the maximal cardiac output* that can be achieved during exertion and thereby also decrease maximal oxygen consumption and exercise capacity.

Exercise training may benefit patients with cardiovascular disease by other physiologic mechanisms as well. Aerobic exercise training results in *dilatation of large coronary arteries*, and this effect may diminish the hemodynamic compromise from existing coronary artery lesions. Some evidence also suggests that exercise training may improve collateral blood flow to ischemic zones. Coronary blood flow under conditions of maximal coronary vasodilation may also be increased. Whatever the mechanism, myocardial perfusion has been observed to increase by 25% to 50%. Another important beneficial effect is an *increase in high-density-lipoprotein cholesterol* concentration (see Chapter 15). Potentially important protective mechanisms of aerobic exercise include an *increase in fibrinolytic response* to occlusive stimuli in the trained state and an *increase in the myocardial ventricular fibrillation threshold*, rendering it less vulnerable.

Effects of Programs on Morbidity, Mortality, and Quality of Life. Cardiac rehabilitation programs for secondary prevention reduce all-cause mortality, cardiovascular mortality, and fatal reinfarction by 20% to 25%. The best effect is on sudden death, which declines by over 35%. Quality of life also increases as patients regain confidence and develop a better sense of physical well-being. Because the data derive from comprehensive exercise rehabilitation programs that also incorporate such efforts as smoking cessation, dietary modification, and stress reduction, it is difficult to know the precise proportion of benefit due to exercise alone.

Cost Effectiveness. Cardiac rehabilitation programs are cost effective. Their cost effectiveness is achieved by reductions in rates of rehospitalization, length of stay, and charges per hospitalization.

Program Design: How Much and What Type of Exercise? *Motivating the Patient.* Views about the amount of exercise needed to reduce cardiovascular risk are undergoing considerable change. The classic assumption was that one must achieve a physiologic training effect to obtain health benefits and that such a training effect requires *aerobic (endurance) exercise* (running, jogging, fast walking, cycling, rowing, cross-country skiing, swimming) performed at least *four times a week for at least 30 minutes a session*, resulting in a heart rate of 70% to 85% of a predicted maximum. However, significant reductions in coronary risk do not require attainment of maximum cardiopulmonary fitness. Moderate degrees of exercise may provide nearly equivalent results. Persons with low baseline levels of activity demonstrate the greatest improvement in outcomes with exercise training, even if exercising only moderately (e.g., walking 3 to 4 miles/h). Epidemiologic data suggest that simple informal exercise carried out as part of everyday life (e.g., walking, stair climbing, working in the yard) confers survival benefit. The current consensus recommendation for the inactive person is to *accumulate a total of 30 minutes* of moderate exertion over the course of the day rather than to put in 30 minutes of exercise at a single session.

The *traditional approach* to determining the proper intensity of exercise for a cardiac rehabilitation program is to *calculate 70% to 85% of a measured maximal heart rate*. The measured maximal heart rate is usually based on the results of an exercise stress test. The mode of exercise used for exercise testing should be specific to the type of exercise planned for the training program (e.g., treadmill testing for a walking/jogging program, bicycle ergometer testing for a cycling program). Some authorities suggest other methods of calculating the target heart rate, but in practice, the traditional calculation is generally the most efficient. This exercise intensity translates to approximately 60% to 80% of maximal oxygen consumption. The relationship between heart rate and oxygen consumption is not influenced by β-adrenergic blockade. This point is important in cardiac rehabilitation, because many patients receive a beta-blocking agent as part of their post-MI therapeutic regimen (see Chapter 30). Such patients require a formal graded exercise test under the influence of a beta-blocker if they are going to be taking a beta-blocker while engaged in an exercise training program.

The current consensus regarding the approach to exercise is shifting from an emphasis on maximizing intensity to *maximizing compliance*. For previously inactive patients, this translates into a program of a *moderate degree of exercise*, usually prescribed as starting with *walking at a rate of 3 to 4 miles/h* for 30 minutes each day. This more practical and sustainable approach to exercise training is designed to increase long-term complacence and extend participation in exercise programs beyond the meager 25% who currently engage in them for cardiac rehabilitation.

Program Implementation. Only a fraction of coronary patients who would benefit from a well-designed exercise/rehabilitation program actually undergo it. Part of this results from most programs being institutionally based, requiring travel to and from the site. The original basis for this "on-site" requirement was concern about cardiac events during exercise and the need for on-site medical supervision. Although the rate of sudden death in medically supervised programs is extremely low, home programs supplemented by occasional institutional visits and regular nurse follow-up by can also be carried out safely, provided there is careful patient selection (e.g., no ischemia or dysrhythmias on stress testing, good functional capacity, frequent exercising, good reliability). Those who should be closely supervised are those who exercise infrequently and manifest poor functional capacity at baseline. Physician enthusiasm, provision of close supervision, and adoption of a moderate exercise program rather than one that stresses more intensive exertion all help the patient to get started and continue. Most important to compliance is design of a program that the patient likes to do and finds doable (see Chapter 18).

RISK FACTOR REDUCTION

As noted earlier, exercise is but one important component of a comprehensive program of secondary prevention of coronary artery disease. The benefits to survival from aggressive risk factor reduction are as large as any intervention in secondary prevention of coronary disease. Unlike other modalities of secondary prevention, they directly address the atherosclerotic process.

Risk Factor Reductions of Proven Benefit. Effective treatment of *hypertension* (see Chapter 26), *hypercholesterolemia* (see Chapter 27), and *smoking* (see Chapter 54) can reduce cardiovascular morbidity and mortality by 25% to 50%. In many instances, atherosclerotic progression can be halted, and in about 25% of cases, plaque regression may be observed, particularly with aggressive lipid-lowering efforts. Control of *obesity* (see Chapter 233) and diabetes (see Chapter 102), although not directly proven to reduce cardiovascular risk in themselves, are critical to effective control of key CHD risk factors (e.g., lipids, blood pressure). Stress management and treatment of underlying *anxiety* and *depression* can markedly decrease event rates and mortality from sudden death by up to 50% and improve functional status (see Chapters 226 and 227).

Risk Factor Reductions of Potential Benefit. There is considerable interest in the contributions of *homocysteine reduction* and *hormone replacement* therapy (HRT) to the secondary prevention of CHD.

Homocysteine Reduction. Epidemiologic data indicate a dose-dependent association between plasma homocysteine and risk of cardiovascular disease. To date, the association appears independent of other cardiovascular risk factors; however, it remains to be proven by prospective randomized trials that decreasing homocysteine levels will reduce cardiovascular risk. Despite the absence of a proven benefit, many physicians currently screen for and treat CHD patients with homocysteine elevations, even moderate ones, because treatment is safe and simple. *Folic acid* supplementation with or without *vitamins B_6 and B_{12}* will lower homocysteine levels by nearly 25% in 2 to 6 weeks, even in persons who are not deficient in these vitamins. The higher the pretreatment homocysteine level and the lower the folate stores, the greater the reduction in homocysteine.

Doses of folate more than 0.4 mg/d usually provide no additional benefit, but lower doses are not very effective. Folate given to a B_{12}-deficient patient can aggravate the B_{12} deficiency, mask its hematologic features, and lead to neurologic impairment (see Chapter 79). Such consequences lead many to add oral B_{12} (0.5 mg/d) to the daily program or to check serum B_{12} level before beginning folate therapy. Vitamin B_6 is safe to use so long as the daily dose (which averages 25 to 50 mg/d) does not exceed 400 mg/d, a dose associated with sensory neuropathy.

Relatively inexpensive *measurement* of plasma homocysteine is becoming available; accuracy is facilitated by fasting, and sensitivity is enhanced by methionine loading, which stresses the involved metabolic pathways. Ongoing prospective trials should help determine the usefulness of lowering homocysteine and the need for screening CHD patients for this condition. At this time, screening and treatment of homocysteine elevation cannot yet be recommended in persons with CHD.

Hormone Replacement Therapy. Because *menopause* is a risk factor for CHD, HRT has been examined as a possible means of achieving primary and secondary prevention of CHD events in women. Although epidemiologic data suggested a strong association between HRT use in postmenopausal women having CHD and reduced risk of further coronary events (nonfatal infarction and cardiac death), a disappointing landmark prospective study of the question (the Heart and Estrogen/Progestin Replacement Study) failed to confirm this benefit. Conse-

quently, initiating a program of estrogen plus progesterone in older postmenopausal women with CHD for secondary prevention of CHD is not recommended at the present time. However, there is little harm to continuing HRT in such women who have been taking it for years for prevention of osteoporosis and other noncardiac complications of menopause. Moreover, the same randomized study suggested the possibility of a late benefit after several years of such therapy, but this trend remains to be confirmed.

MEDICAL THERAPIES

Besides risk factor reduction, one needs to consider pharmacologic interventions that can enhance survival and reduce rates of cardiac events. Evidence-based modalities include beta-blockade, ACE inhibition, and antiplatelet therapy. Some dietary interventions appear very promising.

Beta-Blockade. β-Adrenergic blockade significantly reduces the total mortality rate and the incidences of recurrent infarction and sudden death in patients who have had a recent MI. Rates of reduction in mortality range from 26% to 39%; reinfarction rates fall by 23% to 28%. Concerns for adverse effects often factor into prescribing decisions and probably contribute to the low rates of postinfarction beta-blocker utilization (30% to 60%) seen in community-based practice. Underutilization is especially common in elderly patients. The major trials excluded individuals at increased risk for adverse effects of beta-blockade, such as patients with severe pulmonary disease, marked congestive heart failure, insulin-requiring diabetes mellitus, and the elderly. Observational studies find no increased risk from use in such "high-risk" patients and no compromise in benefit. In fact, high-risk groups actually demonstrate a higher absolute reduction in risk because of a higher baseline mortality rate. Pending data from randomized prospective studies, it is recommended that all postinfarction patients are given a trial of beta-blocker therapy shortly after infarction and that those with relative contraindications to such therapy have the trial conducted under close supervision, starting at low doses (e.g., 12.5 to 25 mg/d of atenolol) and titrating upward as tolerated until beta-blockade is achieved. Because early morning and early evening are times of greatest adrenergic stimulation and cardiac risk, it is important that a beta-blocker program ensure adequate beta-blockade during these critical periods.

Angiotensin-Converting Enzyme Inhibition. ACE inhibition is emerging as a major approach to reducing CHD mortality and reinfarction risks in postinfarction patients. Initially found effective in postinfarction patients with left ventricular dysfunction (ejection fraction less than 0.4), ACE inhibitor use has more recently demonstrated clinically significant reductions (20% to 30%) in morbidity and mortality for CHD patients with preserved left ventricular function (Heart Outcomes Prevention Evaluation [HOPE] study), including those who have not suffered infarction. Not only is survival improved, but so are the rates of infarction, stroke, and need for revascularization. Proposed mechanisms of action include not only inhibition of the angiotensin-renin-aldosterone system, but also the ability to limit vascular smooth muscle proliferation, plaque rupture, and left ventricular hypertrophy and to improve vascular endothelial function and fibrinolysis. All CHD patients should be considered for ACE inhibitor therapy. Choice of ACE inhibitor and optimal dose have not been established, but there appears to be little difference among ACE inhibitors, suggesting that benefit may be attained with any drug in this class, starting at a modest dose (e.g., generic captopril 25 mg bid, generic lisinopril 10 mg/d; the HOPE study used ramipril 10 mg/d). It is unknown whether angiotensin-II-receptor antagonists will provide the same protection.

Antiplatelet Agents and Oral Anticoagulants. Modest but significant reductions (20%) in death and reinfarction are achieved with *long-term aspirin* therapy in CHD patients. Aspirin has also been found efficacious in preventing MI among patients with unstable angina. Long-term prophylactic therapy with aspirin should be strongly considered for patients with acute MI and unstable angina.

Therapy with warfarin is not routinely prescribed in postinfarction patients, because although results may be slightly better than with aspirin, there is an increased risk of major bleeding. The Anticoagulants in the Secondary Prevention of Events in Coronary Thrombosis trial demonstrated a 50% reduction in risk of reinfarction; however, intensive anticoagulation was required (INR 2.8 to 4.8), raising the risk of hemorrhagic complications. Combination therapy with lower dose warfarin plus aspirin is being studied.

Antiarrhythmic Therapy. There is no evidence for a protective effect with use of antiarrhythmic drugs; the marked proarrhythmic effects of potent class I agents appear to negate their ability to suppress malignant ventricular irritability. Only *beta-blockers* and *implantable defibrillators/cardioverters* have demonstrated a clearcut beneficial effect in reducing risk of sudden death in high-risk patients. Whether class III antiarrhythmics such as amiodarone when used alone or in conjunction with other agents will prove useful remains unknown (see also Chapter 29).

DIETARY MEASURES AND SUPPLEMENTS

Diet. The role of a *low-saturated-fat low-cholesterol diet* is well established for CHD prevention. It remains an essential part of a lipid-control program essential to aggressive risk factor reduction (see Chapter 27). Of increasing interest for CHD prophylaxis is a diet rich in omega-3 fatty acids. A 30% reduction in overall mortality has been observed in MI survivors who twice weekly consumed fish rich in these fatty acids. Although most believe omega-3 fatty acids improve CHD prognosis by their effects on atherosclerosis and clotting mechanisms—indeed, daily intake of a 1.5-g fish oil capsule can slow progression of vessel plaques—others find a stabilizing effect on myocardial cell membrane channels that appears to raise the threshold for dysrhythmias, perhaps accounting for the association between reduced rates of sudden death and fish consumption. More study is needed to test the validity of these initial findings, but a once- or twice-weekly serving of salmon or other oily fish seems like a reasonably pleasant approach to secondary prevention. There is no evidence that restriction of *caffeinated beverages* is necessary.

Vitamin Supplements. Being "natural," these substances are currently very popular among patients, stimulated by enthusi-

astic reports in the lay press of their possible "antioxidant" benefits in atherosclerosis. In addition to *folic acid* and *vitamins B_6 and B_{12}* for treatment of *homocysteine* elevations (see above), *vitamins E, beta-carotene,* and *C* have all received mention as possibly beneficial agents, supported by initial epidemiologic data.

Vitamin E has received the most attention because of suggestive epidemiologic data; however, findings from randomized placebo-controlled trials have failed to confirm a significant benefit. In one such study of 400 or 800 IU of vitamin E daily for up to 2 years, there was a statistically significant reduction in nonfatal MI, but the incidence of cardiovascular death and all-cause mortality was higher in those taking vitamin E than among control subjects taking placebo. Similar findings of no difference in total CHD risk was found in a randomized trials of Finnish smokers. Vitamin E cannot be recommended at this time.

With *beta-carotene*, again, epidemiologically suggestive data were followed by failure to demonstrate any reduction on the incidence of CHD events; there was an increase in incidence of lung cancer among smokers. When used in combination with vitamin A, beta-carotene has been found to increase the incidence of cardiovascular mortality and all-cause mortality.

With *vitamin C*, epidemiologic data suggest a reduction in CHD, but prospective studies are needed to confirm these findings

REVASCULARIZATION

Surgical revascularization (coronary artery bypass and graft) produces long-term reductions in risks of reinfarction and CHD mortality that approach 40% in patients with *high-risk disease* (moderate-to-severe angina; large amount of myocardium at risk; suspected three-vessel, left-main, or left-main-equivalent disease; reduced ejection fraction).

For patients with *lesser degrees of risk*, coronary artery bypass and graft does not reduce risk compared with medical therapy but does improve functional status and quality of life in patients who remain unacceptably symptomatic despite full medical management. *Angioplasty* is replacing bypass surgery as the preferred means of revascularization for anginal control in such cases (see Chapter 30). Although enthusiastically embraced by the interventional cardiology community for treatment of CHD, it remains to be demonstrated by prospective randomized controlled trials what impact angioplasty will have on rates of reinfarction, cardiac arrest, and death.

Even after successful revascularization that eliminates angina, most patients continue to use antianginal medications at nearly the same rate or greater than they did before revascularization, negating some of the cost benefit to be expected from revascularization. Perhaps this is out of fear of stopping a seemingly successful program. Those agents that do improve prognosis (e.g., beta-blockers, aspirin, ACE inhibitors) should certainly be continued; however, drugs such as nitrates and calcium channel blockers that are taken for symptomatic relief yet have no demonstrably beneficial effect on cardiovascular morbidity or mortality should be phased out.

In some centers, patients with acute non-Q-wave infarctions are sent routinely for immediate angiography and prompt revascularization. However, such patients who have no clinical or laboratory evidence of ongoing ischemia or heart failure can be managed just as successfully with regular medical therapy, reserving angiography and revascularization for those who develop ischemia or failure or who later manifest evidence of high-risk disease by stress testing. In fact, mortality 1 year postinfarction is lower with conservative therapy than with immediate revascularization. Even after 2 years of follow-up, no survival advantage for immediate revascularization can be found.

PATIENT EDUCATION

The patient who has suffered an acute coronary event is among those in greatest need of health education and individualized life-style counseling. Patient and family are apt to be depressed and frightened by the diagnosis of "coronary disease," believing the prognosis to be grim and fearing invalidism, especially if an infarction has occurred. They need to be informed that in the vast majority of uncomplicated cases, a return to job and regular activity is the rule rather than the exception and that there is much that they can do to greatly improve their prognosis.

Prognosis is a major concern of the patient and family and should be reviewed, not only with the intent of being accurate and realistic but also with an eye toward communicating the significant improvements in prognosis that are achievable by a comprehensive program of secondary prevention. Most published survival rates derive from prospective epidemiologic studies and do not reflect the effects of secondary-prevention programs. Average annual mortality in the Framingham Study was 5% for men and 7% for women. Patients at greatest risk for late cardiac death were those with persistent "malignant" ventricular irritability (see Chapter 29), azotemia, previous infarction, persistent congestive failure, angina, or advanced age. Once congestive heart failure ensued, 50% were dead within 5 years. Risk of postinfarction angina in the Framingham Study was 2.9% for men and 9.6% for women. Risk of heart failure was 2.3%. Many complications of infarction are a function of the degree of myocardial damage. This is consistent with the observation that prognosis correlates with extensiveness of disease, a finding also supported by angiographic studies (see Chapter 30). As noted above, 1-year survival can be estimated from a limited treadmill exercise test done before discharge.

In reviewing prognosis, it is essential to review the reductions in risk associated with implementation of secondary preventive measures (Table 31.1). On average, each element of the program has the potential to reduce risk by 25% to 50%, providing a very substantial improvement in outcomes if implemented. This is a very important and highly motivating message that needs to be conveyed and goes far beyond the common perception that revascularization is the only thing that can be done. In reality, revascularization has a relatively small role in improving prognosis for most patients.

Counseling needs to begin in the predischarge period. Realistic concerns and excessive fears of incapacitation may dramatically alter self-image and diminish self-respect. The most effective way of dealing with such fears is to specifically elicit and address the patient's and the family's concerns and discuss the plan for recovery and rehabilitation and its impact on quality of life and survival. Specific statements concerning *exercise capacity* can be based on graded treadmill stress testing during the recovery period. Knowing what one should and should not do during various stages of the recovery process can help reduce some of the anxiety that accompanies having heart disease.

Activity guidelines should be given. Unsupervised activities during the first month after an MI should require no more than 3 mets (Table 18.1). By the time 6 to 8 weeks have passed, tasks requiring up to 5 mets will be safe for most patients, provided a gradual increase in activity has not been interrupted by symptoms or complications. Specific guidelines, tailored to the patient's personal occupational and recreational interests, are essential.

Some concerns may not always be verbalized by the patient. One such concern is the safety of resuming *sexual activity*. Often, there is fear of sudden death during intercourse. The safety of sexual activity should be routinely discussed with the patient and spouse, even if the topic is not initially raised by them. Sexual intercourse with a familiar partner requires about 3 to 5 mets. Thus, sexual activity can be safely resumed by most patients as early as 4 weeks post-MI. During the early return to full sexual activity, the patient should be advised to avoid coital positions that require sustained isometric exercise, such as upper torso weight-bearing with the arms.

The period after an acute coronary event is also a time when patients are particularly receptive to counseling about changes in *life-style* that reduce coronary risk, such as smoking cessation (see Chapter 54) and dietary change (see Chapter 27). The primary physician is ideally suited to take advantage of this opportunity. A balanced cardiac rehabilitation program offers a very positive response to a very frightening event. In many instances, the results are extremely gratifying, with a patient who is healthier and more fit than before the acute coronary event.

A.H.G.

Table 31.1. Effect of Secondary Prevention Measures on Risk of CHD Events (New Infarction, Cardiac Arrest, Cardiac Death)*

MEASURE	REPORTED REDUCTION IN CHD MORBIDITY/ MORTALITY (%)
Lipid lowering	7–76
Exercise	20–25
Smoking cessation	50
Hypertension control	8–38
Stress management	10–65
Aspirin	25
Beta-blockade	20
Coronary artery bypass (in high-risk patients)	39
Angiotensin-converting enzyme inhibition	20–30
Angioplasty	0–?

*Adapted from Merz CNB, Rozanski A, Forrester JS. Am J Med 1997;102:572, with permission.
CHD, coronary heart disease.

ANNOTATED BIBLIOGRAPHY

Albert CM, Hennekens CH, O'Donnell CJ, et al. Fish consumption and risk of sudden cardiac death. JAMA 1998;279:23. (*Epidemiologic data suggesting a relationship between omega-3 fatty acid intake and reduced rates of sudden death.*)

American College of Physicians. Guidelines for risk stratification after myocardial infarction. Ann Intern Med 1997;126:556. *(An evidence-based consensus, focusing on risk assessment before discharge after acute MI.)*

Anderson RE, Blair SN, Cheskin LJ, et al. Encouraging patients to become more physically active: the physician's role. Ann Intern Med 1997;127:395. *(An excellent essay on getting patients started, designing the exercise prescription, and maintaining activity.)*

Beta Blocker Heart Attack Trial Research Group. A randomized trial of propranolol in patients with acute myocardial infarction. JAMA 1982;247:1707. *(This large-scale randomized trial among men and women with one prior MI demonstrated a reduction in total mortality from 9.8% to 7.2% and in cardiovascular mortality from 8.5% to 6.2%.)*

Blumenthal JA, Babyak MA, Krantz DS, et al. Stress management and exercise training in cardiac patients with myocardial ischemia. Arch Intern Med 1997;157:2213. *(A randomized trial showing a marked reduction in cardiac events with a program of stress reduction and exercise.)*

Boden WE, O'Rourke RA, Crawford MH, et al. Outcomes in patients with acute non-Q-wave myocardial infarction randomly assigned to an invasive as compared with a conservative management strategy. N Engl J Med 1998;338:1785. *(A multicenter VA study of men demonstrating a short-term worsening of outcomes and no long-term benefit from early angiography and revascularization compared with medical management and consideration of revascularization only when new evidence of ischemia develops.)*

Brown G, Alpers JJ, Fisher LD, et al. Regression of coronary artery disease as a result of intensive lipid-lowering therapy in men with high levels of apolipoprotein B. N Engl J Med 1990;323:1289. *(Intensive lipid-lowering therapy reduced the frequency of progression of coronary lesions, promoted regression, and reduced the frequency of cardiovascular events.)*

Curfman GD. Shorter hospital stay for myocardial infarction. N Engl J Med 1988;318:1123. *(A summary of available data, indicating safety of shortened stay for patients with uncomplicated infarction.)*

Echt DS, Liebson PR, Mitchell LB, et al. Mortality and morbidity in patients receiving encainide, flecainide, or placebo. The Cardiac Arrhythmia Suppression Trial. N Engl J Med 1991;324:781. *(In patients with asymptomatic ventricular arrhythmia after MI, antiarrhythmic therapy resulted in poorer survival.)*

Eikelboom JW, Lonn E, Genest J Jr, et al. Homocyst(e)ine and cardiovascular disease: a critical review of the epidemiologic evidence. Ann Intern Med 1999;131:363. *(A systematic review finding strong epidemiologic evidence for an association, but no proof that treatment lowers CHD risk.)*

EPSIM Research Group. A controlled comparison of aspirin and oral anticoagulants in prevention of death of myocardial infarction. N Engl J Med 1982;307:701. *(No difference in mortality or reinfarction was noted.)*

Frasure-Smith N, Prince R. The ischemic heart life stress monitoring program: impact on mortality. Psychosom Med 1985;47:431. *(Large-scale randomized program of stress management achieving a 63% reduction in sudden death; cessation of program resulted in disappearance of the mortality benefit in 6 months.)*

Giri S, Thompson PD, Kiernan FJ, et al. Clinical and angiographic characteristics of exertion-related acute myocardial infarction. JAMA 1999;282:1731. *(Prospective observational cohort study finding that habitually inactive patients are at greatest risk for exertion-related MIs.)*

Gottlieb SS, McCarter RJ, Vogel RA. Effect of beta-blockade on mortality among high-risk and low-risk patients after myocardial infarction. N Engl J Med 1998;339:489. *(A large-scale observational study of over 200,000 patients suggesting that high-risk patients benefit as much if not more than low-risk patients.)*

Grobbee DE, Rimm EB, Giovannucci E, et al. Coffee, caffeine, and cardiovascular disease in men. N Engl J Med 1990;323:1026. *(An epidemiologic study of 45,000 men; no increase in risk of coronary disease.)*

Hasdai D, Lerman A, Grill DE, et al. Medical therapy after successful percutaneous coronary angioplasty. Ann Intern Med 1999;130:108. *(A retrospective cohort study showing that use of antianginal medication does not decrease after successful angioplasty that reduces angina.)*

The Heart Outcomes Prevention Evaluation Study Investigators. Effects of an angiotensin-converting-enzyme inhibitor, ramipril, on death from cardiovascular causes, myocardial infarction, and stroke in high-risk patients. N Engl J Med 2000;342:145. *(The HOPE study, a multicenter, randomized, controlled trial that included CHD patients with normal left ventricular function; found significant [20% to 30%] reductions in CHD morbidity and mortality.)*

Hennekens CH, Buring JE, Sandercock P, et al. Aspirin and other antiplatelet agents in the secondary and primary prevention of cardiovascular disease. Circulation 1989;80:749. *(A good summary of the role for antiplatelet therapy.)*

Hulley S, Grady D, Bush T, et al. Randomized trial of estrogen plus progestin for secondary prevention of coronary heart disease in postmenopausal women. Heart and Estrogen/Progestin Replacement Study (HERS) Research Group. JAMA 1998;280:605. *(A large-scale, randomized, placebo-controlled trial averaging 4.1 years of follow-up failing to confirm observational reports that HRT is effective for secondary prevention of CHD events [nonfatal infarction and cardiac death] in postmenopausal women with documented coronary disease.)*

Krumholz HM, Radford MJ, Ellerbeck EF, et al. Aspirin for secondary prevention after acute myocardial infarction in the elderly: prescribed use and outcomes. Ann Intern Med 1996;124:292. *(Despite clearcut evidence of benefit, 24% not prescribed aspirin.)*

Krumholz HM, Radford MJ, Wang Y, et al. Early beta-blocker therapy for acute myocardial infarction in elderly patients. Ann Intern Med 1999;131:648. *(Evidence for the underutilization of beta-blockade; 51% of patients did not receive this proven treatment.)*

Kujala UM, Kaprio J, Sarna S, et al. Relationship of leisure-time physical activity and mortality. The Finnish Twin Cohort. JAMA 1998;279:440. *(Even leisure-time physical activity was associated with a significant reduction in mortality.)*

Lau J, Altman EM, Jimenez-Silva J, et al. Cumulative meta-analysis of therapeutic trials for myocardial infarction. N Engl J Med 1992;327:248. *(Summarizes data on the efficacy of cardiac rehabilitation in secondary prevention after myocardial infarction.)*

Lewis HD, Davis JW, Archibald DG, et al. Protective effects of aspirin against acute myocardial infarction and death in men with unstable angina. N Engl J Med 1983;309:396. *(Men treated for 12 weeks with buffered aspirin had a 51% lower incidence of death from acute infarction compared with placebo controls.)*

Malinow MR, Duell PB, Hess PB, et al. Reduction of plasma homocyst(e)ine levels by breakfast cereal fortified with folic acid in patients with coronary disease. N Engl J Med 1998;338:1009. *(Fortified breakfast cereal can reduce plasma homocysteine modestly, a purported risk factor for coronary mortality.)*

Merz CNB, Rozanski A, Forrester JS. The secondary prevention of coronary artery disease. Am J Med 1997;102:572. *(Very useful review of the evidence on benefits of a secondary prevention program; 140 references.)*

Muller JE, Tofler GH, Stone PH. Circadian variation and triggers of onset of acute cardiovascular disease. Circulation 1989;79:733. *(The morning hours are the time of greatest risk.)*

NIH Consensus Development Panel on Physical Activity and Cardiovascular Health. Physical activity and cardiovascular health. JAMA

1996;276:241. (*Useful summary of current knowledge presented as answers to basic questions.*)

Norwegian MultiCenter Study Group. Timolol-induced reduction in mortality and reinfarction in patients surviving acute myocardial infarction. N Engl J Med 1981;304:801. (*A landmark study of beta-blockade demonstrating a 45% reduction in sudden death among post-MI patients.*)

NygArd O, Nordrehaug JE, Refsum H, et al. Plasma homocysteine levels and mortality in patients with coronary artery disease. N Engl J Med 1997;337:230. (*Some of the strongest epidemiologic data suggesting that homocysteine elevation is a potent and independent predictor of mortality.*)

O'Connor GT, Buring JE, Yusuf S, et al. An overview of randomized trials of rehabilitation with exercise after myocardial infarction. Circulation 1989;80:234. (*An important meta-analysis; efficacy of cardiac rehabilitation after MI when exercise rehabilitation was linked with modification of other coronary risk factors.*)

Pfeffer MA, Braunwald E, Moye LA, et al. Effect of captopril on mortality and morbidity in patients with left ventricular dysfunction after myocardial infarction. Results of the survival and ventricular enlargements trial. N Engl J Med 1992;327:669. (*Compared with placebo, treatment with captopril improved long-term outcome.*)

Shaw LW. Effects of a prescribed supervised exercise program on mortality and cardiovascular morbidity in patients after myocardial infarction. Am J Cardiol 1981;48:39. (*Results of the National Exercise and Heart Disease Project, which examined the effects of a formal exercise program on prognosis.*)

Siegel D, Grady D, Browner WS, et al. Risk factor modification after myocardial infarction. Ann Intern Med 1988;109:213. (*Substantial reduction in CHD risk can be achieved with modest reduction in risk factors.*)

Smith P, Arnesen H, Holme I. The effect of warfarin on mortality and reinfarction after myocardial infarction. N Engl J Med 1990;323:147. (*Beneficial effects noted.*)

Stephens NG, Parsons A, Schofield PM, et al. Randomised controlled trial of vitamin E in patients with coronary disease. Cambridge heart antioxidant study. Lancet 1996;347:781. (*Randomized placebo-controlled trial finding a reduction in nonfatal MI but increases in CHD and all-cause mortality.*)

Theroux P, Waters DD, Halphen C, et al. Prognostic value of exercise testing soon after myocardial infarction. N Engl J Med 1979;301:341. (*Demonstrates both the safety and usefulness of such testing.*)

Van Camp SP, Peterson RA. Cardiovascular complications of outpatient cardiac rehabilitation programs. JAMA 1986;256:1160. (*Documents very low risk of cardiac events associated with supervised programs.*)

Viscoli CM, Horwitz RI, Singer BH. Beta-blockers after myocardial infarction: influence of first-year clinical course on long-term effectiveness. Ann Intern Med 1993;118:99. (*Benefit appears greatest in those whose clinical course is characterized by recurrent ischemic events, congestive heart failure, arrhythmias, or severe comorbidity.*)

Yusuf S, Zucker D, Peduzzi P, et al. Effect of coronary artery bypass graft surgery on survival: overview of 10-year results from randomized trials by the Coronary Artery Bypass Graft Surgery Trialists Collaboration. Lancet 1994;334:563. (*Meta-analysis demonstrating nearly a 40% reduction in mortality in high-risk patients at 10 years of follow-up.*)

32
Management of Chronic Congestive Heart Failure

Chronic congestive heart failure (CHF) ranks among the most serious of cardiac problems encountered in office practice. Advances in the understanding of CHF's pathophysiology and the advent and timely application of increasingly effective therapies now provide the primary physician with the opportunity to significantly reduce the cardiac morbidity and mortality associated with the condition. The growing appreciation of both systolic and diastolic dysfunction and their respective roles in CHF have led to more precisely targeted therapy. Diuretics, angiotensin-converting enzyme (ACE) inhibitors, and digitalis are the cornerstones of treatment, with ACE inhibitors markedly improving prognosis when used in timely fashion. Primary care physicians need to ensure that their CHF patients are prescribed ACE inhibitors, a practice that remains only partially implemented.

A carefully designed program tailored to the patient's underlying pathophysiology helps to maximize outcomes and prevent such complications as prerenal azotemia, drug- or electrolyte-induced dysrhythmias, and dehydration. Successful management of CHF in the outpatient setting also requires identification and correction of treatable underlying causes and elimination of precipitating factors. Because multidrug regimens are often necessary, thorough patient and family education are essential to limit complications and prevent unnecessary hospitalizations that result from poor compliance or drug toxicity.

PATHOPHYSIOLOGY, CLINICAL PRESENTATION, AND COURSE

Pathophysiology. The "congestive" manifestations of CHF—leg edema, orthopnea, paroxysmal nocturnal dyspnea, rales, jugular venous distention—represent elevations in right or left ventricular filling pressures. Traditionally, filling pressure elevations have been viewed as a consequence of *systolic dysfunction* producing a backup of blood into the pulmonary and systemic venous systems. The hallmark of systolic dysfunction is a *reduced ejection fraction*.

An increasing appreciation for the role of *diastolic dysfunction* in CHF has emerged. As many as 40% of patients presenting with congestive failure appear to have reasonably well-preserved systolic function (ejection fraction more than 0.45) but suffer from diastolic dysfunction, manifested by increased resistance to diastolic ventricular filling. Diastolic dysfunction has been demonstrated in the setting of valvular, hypertrophic, ischemic, and cardiomyopathic diseases. Mechanisms include impairment of diastolic myocardial relaxation, valvular dysfunction, loss of myocardial dispensability, ventricular remodeling, and intracellular calcium overload. Diastolic dysfunction has also been noted in the setting of volume overload.

Heart failure triggers a number of compensatory neurohumoral mechanisms, which ultimately become troublesome. The initial fall in cardiac output activates the *renin-angiotensin-aldosterone axis*, leading initially to *fluid retention and sympathetic discharge*, which temporarily help preserve cardiac output but at the cost of an increase in preload and afterload. Abnormalities in release of atrial natriuretic peptide, prostaglandin metabolism, and neurohumoral regulation contribute to volume overload. Eventually, the resultant venous hypertension and increased left ventricular work affect the failing heart, which cannot tolerate such increases in work, and cardiac output drops. Normal hearts respond to increased venous return via the Frank-Starling mechanism to increase cardiac output, but not the failing heart. The result is increased pulmonary and systemic hypertension and no improvement in cardiac output. The progressive decrease in cardiac output and rise in venous pressure trigger further neurohumoral activity, and a vicious cycle is established. Late changes effected by these compensatory mechanisms include myocardial and vascular *remodeling* and *fibrosis*.

Clinical Presentation. Regardless of etiology, the clinical manifestations of CHF are quite stereotyped and reflect the magnitude of the fall in cardiac output and the rise in pulmonary and systemic venous pressures. Initially and in mild cases, the patient may complain of *fatigability, dyspnea on exertion,* or unexplained *weight gain.* There may be few overt physical signs of failure, but chest x-ray often shows *redistribution* of pulmonary venous flow to the upper lung fields and/or *cardiomegaly. Fatigue* becomes increasingly prominent as cardiac output falls. As pulmonary congestion increases, dyspnea worsens, *orthopnea* is noted, and *paroxysmal nocturnal dyspnea* may be reported. At this stage, *rales* become evident on auscultation of the lungs, but their absence does not rule out the presence of CHF. Sometimes failure-induced *bronchospasm* dominates the pulmonary examination. In severe cases, the chest film will show *interstitial pulmonary edema.* In chronic CHF, right-sided or bilateral *pleural effusions* are common. *Ankle edema, jugular venous distention,* and *hepatojugular reflux* are indicative of elevated systemic venous pressure; if CHF is predominantly left-sided, these findings may not be present. An *S_3 gallop* is among the most specific physical signs of failure, but it is often difficult to hear. If left ventricular dilation becomes very marked, a *mitral regurgitant murmur* may become evident. Pedal edema is one of the least specific signs of CHF; in the elderly, isolated pedal edema is more likely to be a result of venous insufficiency (see Chapter 22).

Partially treated CHF may present with atypical manifestations. For example, potent diuretic therapy may eliminate most congestive manifestations, whereas pump function remains depressed. Dyspnea, orthopnea, leg edema, rales, and even radiologic signs of CHF (see below) may be absent, and fatigue might dominate the clinical picture.

Clinical Course. Because congestive failure is not a single disease, it does not have a uniform natural history. Clinical course and response to therapy depend on the nature of the underlying etiology and the state of the myocardium at the time of presentation. For example, the appearance of CHF in a patient with aortic stenosis is an ominous prognostic sign associated with a mean survival of no more than a year or two. However, if the valve is replaced before irreversible myocardial decompensation has occurred, the prognosis is altered dramatically (see Chapter 33). Cases of CHF caused by alcohol abuse, thiamine deficiency, hypertensive heart disease, and hyperthyroidism also have favorable outcomes if detected and treated early. However, if uncorrected, they lead to cardiomyopathic changes and accelerated mortality.

The Framingham Study has provided interesting epidemiologic data concerning CHF in the community setting before the advent of echocardiography and vasodilator therapy. The annual incidence rate for development of failure was 2.3 per 1,000 for men and 1.4 per 1,000 for women. The major causes were hypertension in one third of the patients, hypertension in combination with coronary disease in another one third, isolated coronary disease in about 10%, and valvular disease in another 10%. Sixty percent of patients had a serious noncardiac illness along with CHF. Five-year survival rates, regardless of cause, were only 50%. Later studies have shown significantly improved survival rates associated with the use of ACE inhibitors, even in patients with advanced disease (see below).

Several factors have been examined for their correlation with prognosis. In an important study, *plasma norepinephrine* levels were found by multivariate analysis to correlate strongly with mortality risk and were superior to such catheterization data as pulmonary wedge pressure, cardiac index, mean arterial pressure, and heart rate. The higher the plasma norepinephrine level, the poorer the prognosis. The high catecholamine level represents autonomic compensation for falling cardiac output, though such a compensatory mechanism is not without its own risks, especially for patients with underlying ischemic or hypertensive disease who cannot tolerate the increase in afterload.

DIAGNOSIS AND MONITORING OF HEART FAILURE

Heart failure is frequently a mistaken diagnosis. Because many of its manifestations are due to compensatory mechanisms, the typical clinical findings may be nonspecific and misleading. A common error is to attribute ankle edema or dyspnea to CHF. In a study of patients on digitalis for supposed CHF, 40% did not fulfill basic diagnostic criteria for the condition. Right-sided heart failure is easier to document than left-sided heart failure.

Clinical Diagnosis

Right-sided heart failure is defined clinically as a right atrial pressure greater than 6 cm H_2O, manifested by a *jugular venous pressure less than 6 cm H_2O.* The presence of ankle edema in the absence of jugular venous distention does not constitute a diagnosis of right heart failure. On the other hand and as noted earlier, the absence of ankle edema and jugular venous distention do not necessarily rule out right-sided heart failure, especially in the patient taking diuretics.

Left-sided heart failure is more difficult to diagnose solely on clinical grounds. By themselves, most findings on history and physical examination are neither very sensitive nor specific, but in conjunction with other evidence they can be quite helpful. A story of orthopnea and paroxysmal nocturnal dyspnea is suggestive, as are *basilar rales* on pulmonary examination. The finding of a *third heart sound (S_3)* is among the more specific of signs for systolic dysfunction, but it is often difficult to elicit and is sometimes present in elderly hypertensive patients with a normal ejection fraction. In the absence of definitive radiologic evidence of pulmonary edema, the diagnosis of left-sided heart failure is best supported by the finding of upper zone redistribution and one of the other historical, physical, or laboratory findings just noted. In the absence of upper zone redistribution, the presence of any three other findings (e.g., S_3, cardiomegaly, and basilar rales) constitutes reasonable evidence for the diagnosis.

Laboratory Diagnosis

Identification of Congestive Heart Failure. The *chest x-ray* remains an excellent readily available test for diagnosis of CHF. Characteristic findings include upper zone flow redistribution, cardiomegaly, prominent interstitial markings, Kerley "B" lines, and perihilar haziness. Patients who develop CHF only during exertion may not show interstitial changes on a chest film done at rest, although cardiomegaly and upper zone redistribution may be present. The *electrocardiogram* can be useful for detection of left atrial enlargement, which in conjunction with cardiomegaly by chest film has diagnostic value as do the electrocardiographic findings of left ventricular hypertrophy and ischemia.

Cardiac ultrasound has become the test of choice for assessment of clinically suspected CHF. The test allows for measurements of *ejection fraction* and *chamber size* and for detection of *valvular* and *wall abnormalities*, extending information obtained by clinical assessment and chest x-ray. The finding of left ventricular dilatation in persons without myocardial infarction is an independent risk factor for CHF and the detection of subclinical disease. The ultrasound is also essential to identification of the patient's underlying pathophysiology.

Determining the Underlying Pathophysiology. *Echocardiography* with *Doppler* assessment of flow allows for detection of both systolic and diastolic dysfunction. In CHF patients with systolic dysfunction, the ejection fraction is reduced (less than 0.45), whereas the ejection fraction is preserved (more than 0.45) in the setting of diastolic dysfunction. Doppler techniques help confirm the diagnosis of diastolic dysfunction by identifying abnormal diastolic flow across the mitral valve. The ability of the cardiac ultrasound study to detect left ventricular hypertrophy, hypertrophic and restrictive cardiomyopathic changes, ischemia, and pericardial disease makes the study an excellent choice for etiology of diastolic dysfunction.

Monitoring

Once the diagnosis of heart failure is made and its underlying pathophysiology determined, assessment shifts to monitoring. Simple measures often suffice, including patient weight, symptoms (particularly exercise tolerance), physical examination, blood urea nitrogen (BUN), creatinine, and chest x-ray. Repeated use of elaborate diagnostic technology for monitoring is usually unnecessary, raising the cost of care without improving outcomes.

PRINCIPLES OF MANAGEMENT

Searching for and treating a reversible underlying etiology is the first task of management. All too often, many cases are encountered at the time irreversible myocardial damage has occurred, but when a treatable cause is present and detected early, there is an opportunity for definitive measures to bring about a successful outcome. *Coronary artery disease* (see Chapter 30), *valvular disease* (see Chapter 33), *alcohol excess* (see Chapter 228), *hypertension (see Chapter 26), hyperthyroidism* (see Chapter 103), *and hypothyroidism* (see Chapter 104) are examples of conditions requiring etiologic therapy. A stereotypic approach to treatment that ignores etiology may lead to loss of a unique therapeutic opportunity and even be counterproductive.

Attending to precipitating factors is another priority. Acute *ischemia* (see Chapter 30), *severe anemia* (see Chapter 82), *high fever* (see Chapter 11), *atrial fibrillation* and other *supraventricular tachycardias* (see Chapter 28), *pneumonia* (see Chapter 52), *pulmonary embolization* (see Chapter 35), *excess salt intake, marked obesity* (see Chapter 233), *and excess exertion or emotional stress* may worsen or precipitate failure in patients with decreased myocardial reserve. Excessive doses of beta-blockers (see Chapter 30) or other negatively inotropic agents (e.g., *verapamil, disopyramide*) may also bring on CHF. A careful search for these factors is essential.

Treating Pathophysiologically. Loop diuretics directly address volume overload. ACE inhibition counters the dysfunctional response of the angiotensin-renin-aldosterone system to poor systemic perfusion, reducing both preload and afterload; digoxin provides an inotropic boost to hearts manifesting systolic dysfunction. Combination therapy utilizing a loop diuretic, ACE inhibitor, with or without digoxin has become the standard of treatment. When properly applied, such therapy has the potential to reduce cardiac morbidity and mortality across a wide range of patients. Beta-blockade and spironolactone have promising adjunctive roles: Selective use of beta-blockers blunts excessive sympathetic stimulation, and small doses of spironolactone inhibit the marked aldosterone effects of severe disease.

Diastolic dysfunction requires attention first to its underlying etiology (e.g., hypertension, left ventricular outflow tract obstruction, ischemia, valvular regurgitation, myocardial disease, pericardial disease). Supportive therapy includes maintenance of normal sinus rhythm, rate control if the patient is in atrial fibrillation, and careful use of diuretics and ACE inhibitors, avoiding too precipitous a fall in preload that might compromise cardiac output. Nitrates are sometimes used in place of ACE inhibition. Beta-blockers may also contribute, particularly in patients with underlying ischemic heart disease or hypertrophic cardiomyopathy; venodilating calcium channel blockers are sometimes considered, but their use in heart failure can be problematic (see below).

Systolic dysfunction also requires addressing the underlying cause (e.g., ischemia, hypertension, cardiomyopathy, valvular disease). The combination of diuretics, ACE inhibitors, and digitalis serve as first-line agents, improving contractility, reducing afterload, and eliminating excess volume. Low doses of a beta-blocker may actually improve the ejection fraction, and spironolactone helps reverse the adverse physiology of advanced heart failure by inhibiting aldosterone.

Diuretics

Rationale for Use as Initial Therapy. Diuretics are an important *initial therapy* when there is evidence of volume overload. The degree of compensatory fluid retention in CHF is typically excessive, leading to pulmonary congestion and/or peripheral edema. In patients with mild to moderate CHF, symptoms of volume overload respond best acutely to diuretic therapy compared with ACE inhibition. However, diuretic therapy alone is usually insufficient for chronic treatment of CHF, in part because it stimulates the renin-angiotensin system and raises serum catecholamines, leading to increased afterload, reduced cardiac output, and further sodium retention. Although diuretics may be effective in controlling peripheral edema and pulmonary congestion, they do little to prevent the progression of heart failure or improve prognosis. Consequently, diuretics emerge as important treatment for relief of congestive symptoms, but they are insufficient for altering prognosis, especially in patients with a failing left ventricle.

Overzealous use of diuretics may acutely worsen the situation by producing prerenal azotemia or a dangerous fall in filling pressure (as in critical aortic stenosis). Moreover, escalating diuretic therapy in mitral or aortic valve disease may inappropriately delay the timing of surgical therapy (see Chapter 33).

Selection of Agent and Initiation of Therapy. When symptoms are slight (mild exertional dyspnea, minor ankle edema) or when the patient is asymptomatic but showing weight gain or x-ray findings indicative of early CHF, then diuretic therapy can be initiated with a *thiazide* (e.g., 50 mg/d hydrochlorothiazide). The degree of dyspnea on exertion and weight change are the simplest clinical parameters to follow for gauging response to therapy in mild cases.

Increasing severity of symptoms is an indication for switching to a *loop diuretic* (e.g., *furosemide or ethacrynic acid*). Small doses of loop diuretics may also benefit patients with mild to moderate failure that cannot be adequately controlled by thiazides. Caution is warranted when treating a patient for the first time with a loop diuretic, because a marked diuresis may be evoked, particularly with use of a parenteral dose but sometimes with an oral dose. If a thiazide had been used previously, it should be stopped rather than continued in conjunction with the loop diuretic, because the two agents are very potent when used together (see below). The mercurials have dropped from use because of the need to administer them parentally.

The *potassium-sparing diuretics* (amiloride, triamterene) are relatively weak agents used mainly in conjunction with thiazides and loop diuretics to prevent potassium depletion. Their onset of action is slow; full effect may take up to a week to become evident and they should be used with caution if at all in persons taking ACE inhibitors, because of the risk of hyperkalemia. *Spironolactone* is also a weak diuretic with potassium-sparing effects and of little use for acute reduction in volume; however, small doses may be useful in patients with severe CHF (see below).

Use in Later Stages of Congestive Heart Failure. In severe CHF, absorption of oral loop diuretics declines, which accounts for the oft-noted reduction in efficacy during an exacerbation of heart failure. The maximal effect of a loop diuretic can be achieved by using a *large, single, daily dose* rather than divided doses. Parenteral administration of the drug or high-dose oral therapy is required to achieve diuresis. At times, supplementing oral therapy with an occasional *parenteral dose* in the office will suffice to counter worsening failure refractory to oral therapy. *Adding a thiazide* to the diuretic program may be useful in failure refractory to large doses of the loop diuretic alone. For patients with renal impairment, *metolazone* can be useful as the adjunct. It is similar in potency to the thiazides but more effective in the setting of azotemia.

Spironolactone, the aldosterone-receptor antagonist, can reduce cardiac morbidity and mortality when added to standard maximal medical therapy in persons with severe CHF. The purported mechanism entails inhibition of excessive aldosterone stimulation, a pathophysiologic feature of advanced CHF. Small doses (25 to 50 mg/d) added to a program of ACE inhibitor, loop diuretic, and digoxin improve survival by nearly 30%. If spironolactone is added to the standard maximal program, monitoring for hyperkalemia is essential and potassium supplementation should be limited to persons who manifest a serum potassium of less than 3.5 mg/dL.

Monitoring Diuretic Therapy. Monitoring *postural signs, BUN,* and *creatinine* are essential to avoid excess volume depletion and severe prerenal azotemia. When a potassium-wasting diuretic is being used in conjunction with digitalis therapy, it is critical to carefully monitor the *serum potassium* (see Appendix). The incidence of digitalis toxicity rises appreciably in the setting of hypokalemia. *Magnesium depletion* may also be triggered by diuretic therapy and contribute to digitalis sensitivity and refractory hypokalemia. Use of a potassium-sparing drug necessitates watching for hyperkalemia and discontinuing chronic potassium supplementation once hypokalemia is corrected.

Diuretic Preparations

Thiazides are sulfonamide derivatives, believed to inhibit sodium reabsorption in the cortical tubule. Although the number of thiazide preparations is large, they differ only in cost and duration of action. *Hydrochlorothiazide* is the least expensive and is available generically. Thiazides cause modest potassium depletion, which can be clinically important if there is underlying heart disease, especially in the setting of ventricular irritability, ischemia, or use of digitalis. Under such circumstances, careful monitoring for hypokalemia and assiduous potassium supplementation or use of a potassium-sparing diuretic may be needed. Mild hyperglycemia and hyperuricemia may result but are usually of little clinical significance (see Chapters 102 and 155). During the first 7 to 10 days of therapy, the serum calcium may rise, but it will stay elevated indefinitely only in patients with underlying hyperparathyroidism. Absorption from the gastrointestinal tract is rapid; onset of action is 1 hour, and half-life 12 to 24 hours.

Metolazone, another sulfonamide diuretic similar to the thiazides in site of action, possesses a longer half-life and is more effective in patients with impaired renal function. The effective half-life is 24 to 48 hours, compared with 12 to 24 hours for the thiazides. Being a sulfonamide, it shares many of the same side effects, such as hypokalemia, hyperglycemia, and hyperuricemia. The maximum daily dose is 10 to 20 mg. Metolazone can be combined with a loop diuretic for use in very refractory cases in which volume overload is a major problem.

Loop diuretics are potent agents that act at the loop of Henle. Examples include *furosemide, ethacrynic acid,* and *bumetanide.* Absorption is rapid, as is onset of diuretic action (30 to 60 minutes); effects last 4 to 8 hours. Caution must be exercised with their use, because serious volume depletion may occur. Frequent urination is a common complaint; evening doses should be avoided if possible. Starting dose of furosemide is 20 to 40 mg/d. Prerenal azotemia (manifested by a BUN–creatinine ratio of more than 20:1), postural hypotension, lightheadedness, and fatigue are clues to marked hypovolemia. Hypokalemia is the most serious metabolic consequence, necessitating careful monitoring of the serum potassium and supplementation should it fall to less than 3.5 mg/dL. Mild hyperglycemia and hyperuricemia may also occur. Ethacrynic acid is potentially ototoxic, especially when used in combination with an aminoglycoside antibiotic such as kanamycin. Audiograms should be obtained if ethacrynic acid is to be given for a prolonged period.

The potassium-sparing diuretics (e.g., *triamterene, ameloride*) are weak diuretics used predominantly to help preserve potassium. *Spironolactone,* the aldosterone-receptor antagonist, is also potassium sparing but has a unique role in severe CHF by helping to counter aldosterone excess. Serious hyperkalemia may occur with the use of these agents, particularly in treatment programs that include ACE inhibition or potassium supplementation. Frequent serum potassium determinations and discontinuation of potassium supplementation with onset of their use is essential. These drugs should not be used in renal failure, because life-threatening hyperkalemia may ensue. Spironolactone can cause gynecomastia and breast pain in chronic users; there is also a question of increased risk of carcinogenesis with long-term use based only on animal data.

Fixed combinations containing a potassium-sparing diuretic and a thiazide are heavily promoted and expensive (see Chapter 21), although they are convenient and facilitate compliance. Before prescribing such a preparation, the proper dose of each agent should be determined separately. The combination preparation is reasonable to use only if it can provide the exact dosages desired. Many combinations contain subtherapeutic thiazide doses.

Angiotensin-Converting Enzyme Inhibitors

Rationale. Advances in understanding the effects of preload and afterload on cardiac output in the failing heart have added a new dimension to the treatment of CHF. Agents have been sought that would act safely both on the arterial bed (to reduce impedance to the ejection of blood from the left ventricle) and on the venous bed (to decrease preload and reduce pulmonary and systemic venous congestion). The goal was to address both systolic and diastolic dysfunction. Initially, no single agent sufficed, but the combined use of hydralazine for arterial dilation and isosorbide for venodilation achieved significant afterload

and preload reductions, symptomatic improvement, and a 20% to 30% reduction in mortality in patients with mild to moderate heart failure.

With the advent of ACE inhibitors (e.g., captopril, enalapril, lisinopril) came the opportunity to achieve both goals with a single agent and in a more physiologically advantageous manner than previously achievable. These agents act on both the arterial and venous sides of the circulation, decreasing left ventricular filling pressure and increasing cardiac output. They bind to a receptor on the ACE, preventing the formation of angiotensin II—a potent vasoconstrictor and stimulant of renin and aldosterone secretion. Conventional vasodilator therapy triggers neurohumoral counterregulatory mechanisms that result in reflex vasoconstriction, adrenergic stimulation of the heart, and sodium retention; the ACE inhibitors do not set off such counterregulatory forces. In addition, their suppression of the renin-angiotensin-aldosterone axis helps prevent the harmful myocardial and vascular fibrosis and remodeling that result from long-term activation of this system.

Unlike digitalis (whose efficacy is confined to patients with significant systolic dysfunction), ACE inhibitors have been found effective in most CHF patients, whether they are suffering from mild, moderate, or severe disease. Several landmark studies (e.g., CONSENSUS, SOLVD) have documented this broad spectrum of efficacy, demonstrating significant reductions in cardiac *mortality* and *morbidity* from progressive heart failure compared with therapy that included use of other vasodilators and diuretics and digoxin. Reductions in heart size, symptoms, and need for other medications were also found.

Randomized controlled trials (e.g., the Vasodilator–Heart Failure Trial) have established that ACE inhibitor therapy is superior to combination use of nonspecific vasodilators such as hydralazine-isosorbide in patients with chronic CHF, probably in part by not triggering potentially harmful neurohumoral counterregulatory mechanisms.

Choice of Agent. Debate continues as to optimal choice of ACE inhibitor. Cost and convenience are two major determinants. Generic captopril is probably the least expensive at present but has the disadvantage of requiring administration three times daily compared with the once daily proprietary preparations (e.g., lisinopril). In the few randomized controlled studies directly comparing ACE inhibitors for treatment of chronic CHF, both longer and shorter-acting preparations proved similarly effective, although the long-acting agents tended to have a greater propensity to cause prolonged hypotension, especially when used in high doses. Quality-of-life study comparing captopril with enalapril in hypertensive patients suggested that captopril may be the better tolerated, causing less sexual dysfunction. The patents on many of the proprietary ACE inhibitors are soon to expire, which should lead to reductions in cost and make less necessary a choice between cost and convenience/compliance.

Initiating Therapy and Minimizing Adverse Effects. ACE inhibitor therapy should be considered if diuretics alone fail to control congestive symptoms. It is important to inquire into exercise tolerance; patients may note improvement at rest with use of diuretics but still have exercise intolerance. To achieve maximum long-term benefit, treatment should not be delayed until the later stages of CHF. Persons with mild to moderate CHF (NYHA class II disease) experience significant reductions in morbidity and mortality with addition of ACE inhibitor treatment.

Because *hypotension* is common at the onset of therapy (especially in the elderly), it is recommended to start with *small doses* (e.g., as little as 6.25 mg of captopril, 2.5 to 5.0 mg of lisinopril) and *reduce concurrent diuretic therapy*. The dose is then increased gradually to the doses associated with a survival benefit (e.g., captopril 50 mg three times a day, lisinopril 20 mg/d). Monitoring *blood pressure* is important not only to ensure adequate renal perfusion but also to minimize dizziness and falls. Most CHF patients are elderly and can be very susceptible to even mild degrees of cerebral hypoperfusion. Continuous blood pressure monitoring is needed, because onset of hypotension may be delayed a few weeks yet persist.

Renal Dysfunction. Patients with preexisting bilateral renal artery stenosis and those receiving very large ACE inhibitor doses are at greatest risk for renal impairment, limiting use under such circumstances. Monitoring of renal function (BUN, creatinine, urinalysis) is indicated. Any otherwise inexplicable deterioration in renal function should result in considering a reduction in dose, which may suffice. Rarely is discontinuation of therapy necessary, although there have been case reports of proteinuria and membranous glomerulopathy linked to ACE inhibitor therapy that resolved only with cessation of therapy. Early reports of frequent renal dysfunction with use of these agents were due to the very high doses given.

Because ACE inhibitors reduce aldosterone levels, the *serum potassium* may rise and should be monitored, particularly in patients receiving potassium supplementation or a potassium-sparing agent as part of their diuretic therapy. In many instances, such supplementation or use of a potassium-sparing agent can be discontinued or at least reduced.

Other adverse effects are mostly idiosyncratic and include a dry irritant cough (affecting as many as 10%), *neutropenia* (usually within the first 3 months and only with captopril, due to its sulfhydryl group), loss of taste, and rash (including necrotizing vasculitis). *Angioedema* has also been reported. The cough is believed due to the agent's effect on kinins and can be very irritating, interfering with sleep and causing the patient to stop taking the drug.

Alternatives in Patients Intolerant to Angiotensin-converting Enzyme Inhibitor Therapy.
Patients who cannot tolerate ACE inhibitor therapy because of incapacitating cough or worsening of renal function clearly attributable to the drug can be switched to an *angiotensin II receptor blocker* (e.g., *losartan*) or to combination vasodilator therapy consisting of *hydralazine* and *isosorbide*. Although expensive and not yet proven to have the same morbidity and mortality benefits as ACE inhibitors, the angiotensin II receptor blocker agents also target the angiotensin system and appear to have similar hemodynamic effects without inducing cough. They are well tolerated and a reasonable alternative, especially in elderly patients.

Although ACE inhibitors replaced the combination vasodilator program of *hydralazine* and *isosorbide*, this program still has sufficient survival and hemodynamic benefits to warrant its consideration as an alternative in patients who cannot tolerate ACE inhibition.

Digitalis

Rationale. Digitalis remains a cornerstone of treatment for CHF in persons with systolic dysfunction (ejection fraction less than 40%) by virtue of its ability to increase contractility in the failing heart (mediated through an increase in intracellular calcium by inhibiting the myocyte sodium pump). Other beneficial effects include reduction in neurohumoral responses, vasodilation, increased baroreceptor responsiveness, and increased vagal tone. Although symptomatic and physiologic improvements have been found across the spectrum of patients with systolic dysfunction, the best results have been demonstrated in those with *severe systolic dysfunction* (NYHA class III and IV disease, ejection fraction less than 0.25, audible third heart sound S_3, marked left ventricular dilation). In fact, the presence of an S_3 is a strong predictor of marked response to cardiac glycoside therapy. When added to a program of diuretics and ACE inhibitors in appropriately selected patients, digoxin significantly reduces the rate of hospitalization due to worsening heart failure and shows a strong trend toward reducing cardiac mortality (as in the DIG study). However, patients with CHF in the presence of preserved systolic function and sinus rhythm do not appear to benefit.

Patient Selection. In patients with significant systolic dysfunction (ejection fraction less than 0.40) who remain unacceptably symptomatic despite a program of loop diuretic and ACE inhibitor therapy, digitalis treatment should be seriously considered. Highest priority should be given to those with severe systolic dysfunction (NYHA class III and IV disease, ejection fraction less than 0.25, audible third heart sound S_3, marked left ventricular dilation), but even those with less degrees of pump failure may benefit. The drug can be safely used for systolic dysfunction in patients who have suffered recent myocardial infarction; there is no excess mortality.

Digitalis also remains the drug of choice for heart failure induced by *rapid atrial fibrillation* and some other supraventricular tachycardias (see Chapter 28). The drug is also of use acutely in patients with CHF resulting from *uncontrolled hypertension* or *severe aortic stenosis* but is no substitute for blood pressure reduction (see Chapter 26) or for valve surgery when the aortic stenosis is critical (see Chapter 33). Digitalis is of little use in heart failure resulting from hypertrophic cardiomyopathies, be they idiopathic or due to long-standing hypertension (a common etiology among outpatients, especially women). Patients with idiopathic hypertrophic subaortic stenosis may develop worsening outflow tract obstruction with use of digitalis.

Digitalis is also of no proven benefit in cases of mitral stenosis, as long as the patient is in sinus rhythm, and is of no use in patients with episodes of CHF due to recurrent transient ischemia. The efficacy of digitalis in *cor pulmonale* is in question; the drug is occasionally beneficial, but the results are not impressive and the risks of toxicity are increased in the setting of hypoxia.

Choice of Preparation and Initiation of Therapy. *Digoxin* is the preparation of choice in most patients (see below). Those who are stable can be started on an oral *maintenance dose* without resorting to a loading dose. Using a daily digoxin maintenance dose of 0.25 mg, one can achieve therapeutic serum levels in 5 to 7 days. If the patient is less stable, but not so compromised as to require hospitalization, then an oral *loading dose* of 1.0 to 1.25 mg can be prescribed in divided doses over 24 hours.

The decision to initiate digitalis therapy should not be made casually. Digitalis toxicity is common and can be deadly. Digitalis therapy should be instituted only *after* before a program of loop diuretic therapy and ACE inhibition has been fully instituted and proven insufficient. Use of serum concentration measurements helps limit the incidence of digitalis toxicity as does careful monitoring and maintenance of serum potassium. However, one cannot depend on serum levels alone for the diagnosis of digitalis toxicity, because there is considerable overlap in serum concentrations among those with and without evidence of toxicity.

Digitalis Preparations. Numerous digitalis preparations are available; the physician should become familiar with one or two, learn their pharmacokinetics, and use them predominantly. *Digoxin* is the most widely used. In the past, some variations in bioavailability had been noted among different brands; this has been corrected. Half-life of digoxin is 36 hours; onset of action is 1 to 2 hours when taken orally; absorption from the gastrointestinal tract ranges from 50% to 75% complete. Excretion is renal and decreases significantly with reduction in creatinine clearance. Higher doses are not needed in obese patients; their nonlipid extracellular fluid volume is normal.

If a patient presents taking a digitalis preparation other than digoxin, it is best to leave them on the drug they are used to. The exception to this generalization concerns patients taking *digitalis leaf.* Because of its variable and unpredictable composition of digoxin and digitoxin, digitalis leaf should be discontinued, and one of the preparations containing only a single active ingredient should be used instead. *Digitoxin* may be beneficial when digitalis must be given to a patient with renal failure, because elimination of digitoxin is not dependent on renal function. However, a major disadvantage with digitoxin is its long half-life of 4 to 6 days, making for serious problems if toxic levels occur. Digoxin can be used safely in renal failure as long as renal function and serum levels are frequently checked and necessary dosage adjustments made.

Monitoring Therapy. Digitalis therapy requires careful monitoring. *Serum levels* should be measured at least three or four times per year, more frequently if there are changes in the patient's renal or volume status. Monitoring should help reduce the incidence of digitalis toxicity. A sample should be drawn at least 6 hours after the last dose, because there is a 4- to 6-hour rise in serum level after an oral dose. In most instances, it is best to have the patient omit the day's dose when coming to the office for a serum determination.

A number of factors can affect serum concentration, including renal function when digoxin is being used and hepatic function in digitoxin therapy.

Absorption of digitalis from the gut remains adequate in CHF but may fall in severe cases of malabsorption. Thyroid status can affect digitalis metabolism; hypothyroidism prolongs the half-life, and hyperthyroidism shortens it. Treatment of thyroid disease needs to be accompanied by an adjustment of dose.

The serum level of digitalis is not in itself diagnostic of *toxicity*, because there is considerable overlap in serum concentra-

tions among those with and without evidence of toxicity, but if the *digoxin level* is *greater than 2.0 ng/mL*, the probability of encountering toxicity increases considerably. In one series, 80% of patients without evidence of toxicity had a digoxin level below 2.0 ng/mL; in 87% of those with toxicity, the level was above 2.0 ng/mL.

To avoid *digitalis toxicity*, even when the dose is closely followed, the physician needs to monitor factors that increase the "sensitivity" of the myocardium to the toxic effects of the drug. Such factors include *hypokalemia*, abnormalities in serum *calcium* and *magnesium*, organic heart disease, and pulmonary disease with acute *hypoxia*.

Digitalis Toxicity. Symptoms of digitalis toxicity can be divided into noncardiac and cardiac manifestations. Anorexia, nausea, vomiting, diarrhea, visual disturbances including yellow halos around lights, and in rare instances delirium have been described since Withering's time. Arrhythmias are the predominant cardiac manifestation of toxicity. Digitalis can cause any type of rhythm and/or conduction disturbance because it affects automaticity of myocardial tissues and the conduction system. *Ventricular irritability* (especially bigeminy), *paroxysmal atrial tachycardia* with block, and *junctional tachycardia* are particularly characteristic of digitalis excess.

The unexplained onset of an arrhythmia in a patient on digitalis raises the possibility of drug-related toxicity. The drug should be withheld; a serum level obtained; potassium, calcium, and magnesium levels checked; and serious consideration given to immediate hospitalization for monitoring and parenteral antiarrhythmic therapy. The high incidence and mortality rate of this preventable and often treatable condition call for vigilance.

Pitfalls in Digitalis Use. A few pitfalls in the use of digitalis are worth repeating. Digitalis should not be used unless there is genuine evidence of severe chronic systolic dysfunction or atrial fibrillation. An all-too-common error is to assume that ankle edema in the elderly patient is a sign of CHF and an indication for starting digitalis. The ankle edema may be due to venous insufficiency; even if due to congestive heart failure, it may be a manifestation of diastolic dysfunction and respond better to diuretics or ACE inhibitors. Digitalis should not be discontinued unless a reversible cause of pump failure has been fully corrected or there is no basis for using the drug in the first place. Patients who respond to digitalis need the drug chronically; they have been shown to deteriorate clinically and hemodynamically when the drug is withdrawn in experimental circumstances, even in the context of ACE inhibitor use. Digitalis-induced ST-T wave changes on the electrocardiogram have no correlation with optimal or toxic dose levels and cannot be used for such determinations. Serum drug levels are necessary.

Alternatives to Digitalis to Enhance Contractility: Phosphodiesterase Inhibitors. These agents are potent enhancers of contractility, but experimental results have been marred by increased rates of cardiac death. Early reports noted impressive clinical improvement with such agents as *milrinone, flosequinan,* and *vesnarinone,* but follow-up revealed unacceptable rates of cardiac morbidity and mortality—flosequinan had to be recalled after receiving U.S. Food and Drug Administration

(FDA) approval. Vesnarinone improves survival and functional status when used in doses too small to affect phosphodiesterase, but in larger doses, cardiac mortality rises markedly. Such results underscore the importance of factors other than contractility in determining the outcome of CHF. Demonstrating improved contractility does necessarily predict improved outcome. Neurohumoral activation is believed to be a causative factor affecting CHF mortality.

Beta-Blockers

Although the traditional view has been that beta-blockade will worsen outcomes in CHF, there is emerging evidence that it may be helpful as an adjunct to standard therapy, possibly slowing disease progression. Sympathetic stimulation is one of the major neurohumoral responses to heart failure, increasing with severity of disease and serving as an independent predictor of mortality. Some believe that it may play a role in disease progression. A few large-scale, randomized, placebo-controlled trials of both cardioselective and nonselective beta-blockers (e.g., metoprolol-XL, bisoprolol, and carvedilol) in CHF have shown improvements in symptoms, ejection fraction, rates of hospitalization for heart failure, and, in some instances, survival. *Carvedilol* (a nonspecific beta-blocker that also blocks α receptors, prevents upregulation of cardiac beta receptors, reduces cardiac norepinephrine, and demonstrates strong antioxidant effects) has received FDA approval for use in CHF, showing benefit when added to standard therapy in persons with moderately severe CHF (NYHA class II and III). Definitive evidence for a long-term mortality benefit and safety in persons with severe CHF (NYHA class IV) remains to be demonstrated. Moreover, there is concern about a short-term increase in risk with use of such agents.

Until more data are forthcoming, beta-blockers should be considered only as a possible adjunct to standard therapy, not as a replacement. Cardiac consultation is recommended, both to facilitate case selection and initiation of therapy. Patients may worsen clinically during the first weeks of beta-blocker treatment. Doses at first should be small (e.g., metoprolol-XL 25 mg/d, carvedilol 3.25 mg/d) and titrated upward slowly. The immediate goal is a resting heart rate of 50 to 60 beats/min. An increase in diuretic dose may be necessary due to fluid retention, which is common in the early phases of beta-blocker therapy.

Oral Anticoagulation

Although the presence of CHF is not, per se, an indication for warfarin anticoagulant therapy, it does increase the risk of thromboembolic disease in a patient with an underlying predisposition for an embolic event. For example, the CHF patient who is put to bed rest is at increased risk of deep vein thrombophlebitis and deserves consideration for anticoagulation (see Chapter 35). The same holds true for the patient in atrial fibrillation who develops CHF (see Chapter 28). The initiation and monitoring of oral anticoagulant therapy require considerable attention to detail (see Chapter 83).

Concurrent Drug Use

Use of medications that might depress left ventricular function or alter neurohumoral regulatory mechanisms should be undertaken with extreme care and only after the potential risk is weighed. For example, *beta-blocking agents* (see above), *disopyramide*, and such calcium channel blockers as *verapamil* are myocardial suppressants; they are relatively contraindicated for use in CHF. In a study of the role of prostaglandins in CHF, it was discovered that use of prostaglandin inhibitors, such as the *nonsteroidal antiinflammatory agent* indomethacin, caused a worsening of CHF in patients with advanced disease complicated by hyponatremia; patients without hyponatremia were unaffected.

Fortunately, some important medications are not contraindicated in CHF. For example, the *tricyclic antidepressants* do not cause a reduction in left ventricular performance; they are relatively well tolerated, although they occasionally cause postural hypotension in CHF patients. A study of the effects of *acute intake of alcohol* on patients with functional class III or IV CHF found no deleterious effect on cardiac function; in fact, a modest reduction in afterload was noted, although the authors hastened to add that they were not recommending alcohol as a vasodilator.

Calcium Channel Blocker Use in Congestive Heart Failure. Many patients with heart failure have underlying ischemic heart disease or hypertension and may already be taking a calcium channel blocker for control of anginal symptoms or blood pressure. One needs to be aware that randomized, prospective, controlled studies have documented a significant increase in the risks of worsening heart failure, life-threatening arrhythmias, myocardial infarction, and death with the use of calcium channel blocker therapy when calcium channel blockers are used in persons with heart failure. These risks have prompted many authorities to advise against prescribing calcium channel blocker therapy for patients with coronary disease complicated by severe chronic heart failure.

The mechanisms responsible for these cardiac complications remain poorly understood. It was thought that the reflex tachycardia and negative inotropic effects of many of these agents were responsible, but even the use of sustained-release preparations and agents with little effect on the left ventricle have not lowered the risk. Of the calcium channel blockers, only *amlodipine* has proven safe for use in anginal patients with severe chronic left ventricular dysfunction (ejection fraction less than 30%). Of the drugs in its class, it appears to have the least effect on contractility, conductivity, and neurohumoral reflexes. Why it should be the best tolerated of the calcium channel blockers remains unclear, although it appears to be among the least negatively inotropic. However, amlodipine does not improve survival and carries a 5% risk of inducing pulmonary edema, probably because of pulmonary vasodilation. Moreover, its cost is high. All drugs in this class should be used with caution, if at all, in patients with clinical evidence of chronic CHF. Cardiac consultation is indicated.

Nonpharmacologic Measures

Salt restriction has traditionally occupied an important place in supportive therapy. It is probably most helpful in preventing unnecessary exacerbations of failure. Patients are placed on a *no-added-salt diet*, which provides about *4 g sodium/d*. The patient and family are instructed to prepare and serve meals without addition of salt and to avoid foods with large salt content, including canned ham (which is packed in salt water), bacon, catsup, canned soups, and other processed foods. Rarely is extreme salt restriction (e.g., 1 to 2 g sodium diet) urged on the patient, because it is often unrealistic and unpalatable, leading to poor caloric intake and depression. Fluid restriction is reserved for severe cases that are complicated by hyponatremia.

The activity prescription has an important function in minimizing myocardial work demands while maintaining the patient's ability to live as fully as possible. The level of allowable activity needs to be tailored to the patient's medical status, lifestyle, and responsibilities. Patients with symptoms of failure on moderate exertion (NYHA class II disease) can continue to work as long as reasonable limits are placed on emotional and physical demands. It may be more stressful psychologically (and consequently physically) to have to quit one's job than to continue working in a somewhat more limited capacity. In most instances, the amount of allowable activity can be determined from an office visit by a careful history that elicits the degree of exertion that precipitates symptoms. At times, symptoms may be out of proportion to physical findings; taking a walk up a flight of stairs with the patient can provide helpful data regarding exercise tolerance. Treadmill testing is sometimes necessary to gauge exercise capacity, especially if the patient has coronary disease and it is unclear whether it is failure or ischemia that is limiting the patient. Regardless of etiology, a daily rest period and reduction of psychological stress are key means of lessening myocardial work in the patient with failure.

If weight is increasing, orthopnea worsening, and dyspnea on exertion more severe and brought on by less exertion, activity should be further restricted. A few days of bedrest are often beneficial and may obviate the need for hospitalization. The patient with failure who is put to bed should use a footboard or get out of bed periodically to avoid prolonged venous stasis and thrombus formation.

PATIENT EDUCATION

Because the medical program is often complex and the need for compliance is great, the physician must take the time to discuss with patient and family the rationale behind therapy and to set with them the guidelines for activity, diet, and use of medication. In this way they can become valuable partners in the treatment effort.

Patients should be instructed to weigh themselves each morning before breakfast and to keep a *weight record*. If their clinical status, weight, and medication program are stable, less frequent recordings are necessary. Patients are advised to call their physician if weight increases suddenly by more than 2 or 3 pounds, because this may be the earliest sign of increasing CHF and a forerunner of more severe symptoms. Reliable intelligent patients may be instructed to adjust their diuretic doses according to weight. Debilitated or uncooperative individuals should have a family member or visiting nurse obtain weight recordings. Weight is among the most helpful parameters to follow in outpatient management of failure.

Patients and their families must know the identity of the medication being used. It is easy for the patient to become confused, because multiple-drug regimens are common and many of the pills are similar in appearance. Medication booklets are invaluable. Each tablet is taped to the page alongside its generic and brand names, dose schedule, indication for use, and warning signs of toxicity. For patients with poor eyesight, a family member or visiting nurse should set aside the pills to be taken each day.

INDICATIONS FOR REFERRAL AND ADMISSION

Patients with markedly worsening or refractory failure should be considered for hospital admission and cardiac consultation. For the patient with stubbornly persistent disease, hospitalization provides the opportunity for valuable observation under controlled conditions that ensure compliance with the medical regimen. Moreover, hospitalization provides opportunity to initiate additional therapy under close supervision and to search for a treatable underlying etiology that may have initially eluded detection. Cardiac consultation is also indicated when considering some of the newer adjunctive therapies such as beta-blockade or aldosterone inhibition with spironolactone. Relatively young patients failing maximal medical therapy may be appropriate for consideration of transplantation, provided renal, pulmonary, hepatic, and central nervous system functions are preserved. Other indications for admission include evidence of digitalis toxicity, renal failure, hypotension, and inadequate support and supervision at home.

THERAPEUTIC RECOMMENDATIONS

- Identify the etiology of the CHF (e.g., dysrhythmia, hypertension, valvular disease, ischemia, cardiomyopathy) and any precipitating factors (e.g., fever, anemia, atrial fibrillation, infection, salt excess); treat these specifically if they are amenable to therapy rather than relying solely on symptomatic measures to ameliorate the CHF.
- Identify the underlying pathophysiology, particularly the degree to which there is systolic and/or diastolic dysfunction, and tailor the treatment program to the patient's pathophysiology.

Mild Disease (NYHA Class I)

- Initiate a no-added-salt diet (4 g sodium) but do not restrict water intake unless dilutional hyponatremia ensues.
- Begin diuretic therapy if there is evidence of volume overload or pulmonary venous congestion. If symptoms are mild, begin with a thiazide (e.g., hydrochlorothiazide 50 to 100 mg/d).
- If thiazides do not suffice, switch to a loop diuretic (e.g., furosemide 20 to 40 mg once or twice daily). Be alert for a very brisk diuresis in patients who have never before received a loop diuretic. Exercise particular caution with use of potent diuretics in situations that require a high filling pressure (e.g., critical aortic stenosis).
- In initial stages of loop diuretic use, divide daily dose to minimize the inconvenience of a large diuresis in the morning or evening that might interfere with activity. Avoid giving an evening dose if sleep is being interrupted by nocturia.
- If patient does not respond adequately to a loop diuretic dose that is being given in divided fashion, try combining the entire daily dose into one administration of the drug, before increasing total daily dose.

Mild to Moderate Disease (NYHA Class II to III)

- If moderate doses of diuretic therapy do not suffice to relieve congestive symptoms, then add an ACE inhibitor, starting at a low dose to minimize the risks of hypotension and hypoperfusion (e.g., 6.25 mg captopril three times a day or 5.0 mg lisinopril/d). Monitor blood pressure, potassium, BUN, and creatinine, and decrease diuretic dose if blood pressure falls or prerenal azotemia develops.
- Gradually advance ACE inhibitor therapy to improve exercise tolerance and relieve congestive symptoms while continuing to monitor blood pressure, potassium, and renal function. If tolerated, advance to doses associated with best outcomes (e.g., captopril 50 mg three times a day; lisinopril, 10 to 20 mg/d).

Moderate to Severe Disease (NYHA Class III to IV)

- In patients with moderate to severe heart failure due to worsening systolic dysfunction (low ejection fraction, S_3, left ventricular dilation), add a digitalis preparation to the program of a loop diuretic and an ACE inhibitor.
- Use digoxin as the digitalis preparation of choice, except in the setting of severe renal failure, where digitoxin or markedly reduced doses of digoxin are indicated.
- If the candidate for digitalis is relatively stable, begin therapy with an oral maintenance dose (e.g., digoxin 0.25 mg/d), checking the serum level in 1 week and making any needed dose adjustments on the basis of clinical response and serum level.
- If the digitalis candidate has worsening heart failure but does not require immediate hospitalization, then start digitalis therapy with a loading dose of 1.0 to 1.25 mg of digoxin orally, given in four divided doses over 24 hours. Dose is then adjusted as above.
- If volume overload persists, advance loop diuretic therapy to full doses (e.g., 80 to 120 mg/d of furosemide), given once daily to achieve maximum effect; add a thiazide or metolazone (if there is azotemia) if additional diuresis is desired. Monitor for prerenal azotemia and halt advancement of diuretic program if it becomes marked.
- Be sure full doses of an ACE inhibitor are being prescribed and taken (e.g., captopril 50 mg three times a day; lisinopril, 10 to 20 mg/d). For patients unable to tolerate an ACE inhibitor because of development of an irritant dry cough, consider switching to an angiotensin II antagonist (e.g., losartan 50 mg/d).

Refractory Disease: Adjunctive Programs, Hospitalization, and Transplantation

- Consider addition of low-dose spironolactone (25 mg/d) in persons with severe disease who are still unacceptably symptomatic. Cease any potassium supplementation and monitor potassium levels closely; use with extreme caution, if at all, in the setting of worsening renal function (creatinine more than 2.5 mg/dL).
- Consider adding a low dose of beta-blocker therapy (e.g., carvedilol 3.25 mg/d or metoprolol-XL 12.5 to 25 mg/d) for patients with moderate disease and suboptimal response to standard therapy. Obtain cardiac consultation to facilitate

case selection and initiation of therapy. In most instances, resting heart rate should be in excess of 70 to 80 beats/min and systolic blood pressure more than 100 to 110 mm Hg. Titrate dose slowly upward to achieve a resting heart rate of 50 to 60 beats/min. Monitor patient closely for fluid retention and clinical worsening, especially in the first 2 months of treatment; adjust diuretic dose upward if necessary.
- Consider hospitalization for patients with severe refractory disease for full review of disease status, precipitants, aggravating factors, compliance, and initiation of any adjunctive therapies. Also admit for markedly worsening CHF, suspected digitalis toxicity, or inadequate support and supervision at home.
- Refer for consideration of transplantation the relatively young patient with end-stage myocardial disease but preserved renal, hepatic, pulmonary, and neurologic function.

Monitoring and Adjusting Therapy

- Advise patient and family to check weight regularly, measuring it before breakfast and calling if there is an unexplained weight gain of more than 2 to 3 pounds since the last reading.
- Monitor potassium, BUN, and creatinine regularly and, in persons taking digitalis therapy, follow the serum digoxin level. Avoid having the serum digoxin level drawn sooner than 6 hours after the last dose, because there is a transient increase in serum level after an oral dose.
- Monitor serum potassium particularly closely in those taking digitalis plus potent diuretics or an ACE inhibitor plus a potassium-sparing diuretic or potassium supplementation. Correct any potassium abnormality promptly to minimize risk of a serious dysrhythmia.
- If prerenal azotemia develops or worsens, adjust the diuretic program; for those taking digoxin, obtain a serum digoxin level and reduce the dose until a serum digoxin level is available to guide further administration or estimate the required dose from available nomograms.
- Monitor heart rate and rhythm; if a cardiac dysrhythmia is noted, investigate and treat promptly, especially in persons taking a digitalis preparation who manifest paroxysmal atrial tachycardia with block, ventricular irritability (especially bigeminy), junctional tachycardia, or severe bradycardia.
- Use oral potassium supplements and potassium-sparing diuretics with extreme caution, if at all, in patients taking ACE inhibitors and only if the serum potassium falls to less than 3.5 mg/dL. If a potassium-sparing diuretic is used, chronic oral potassium supplementation should be stopped.
- Monitor serum magnesium in patients taking digitalis and those with refractory hypokalemia. Diuretic-induced hypomagnesemia is common and may impair potassium repletion; it also enhances sensitivity to the toxic effects of digitalis.

Additional Measures and Precautions

- Initiate oral anticoagulant therapy for CHF patients if prolonged bedrest, atrial fibrillation, or severe congestive cardiomyopathy ensue (see Chapter 83).
- Avoid, if possible, large doses and combinations of cardiac drugs with negative inotropic effects such as verapamil, disopyramide, and beta-blockers. If beneficial, use smallest dose possible and prescribe in conjunction with cardiac con-

sultation (see above). Consider discontinuation of calcium channel blockers in patients with chronic CHF, especially those with ejection fractions less than 0.3. Of available calcium channel blockers, only amlodipine is not associated with increased risk of worsening failure, life-threatening dysrhythmias, and sudden death. Obtain cardiac consultation if continued use is believed essential.

- Provide patient and family with thorough instruction on the purpose and proper use of medications prescribed for CHF.
- Advise bedrest for exacerbations of CHF, but discourage major reorganization of a patient's life-style unless symptoms are severe and refractory. A gentle exercise program may actually improve exercise tolerance once the exacerbation has cleared.

A.H.G.

ANNOTATED BIBLIOGRAPHY

Braunwald E. ACE inhibitors—a cornerstone of the treatment of heart failure. N Engl J Med 1991;325:351. *(An editorial summarizing the evidence for the central role of these drugs in treatment of CHF.)*

Chakko S, Woska D, Martinez H, et al. Clinical, radiographic, hemodynamic correlations in chronic congestive heart failure: conflicting results may lead to inappropriate care. Am J Med 1991;90:353. *(Critical look at methods for diagnosis of CHF.)*

Cohn JN, Goldstein SO, Greenberg BH, et al. A dose-dependent increase in mortality with vesnarinone among patients with severe heart failure. N Engl J Med 1998;339:1810. *(A large, prospective, randomized trial; short-term benefit outweighed by the long-term mortality risk.)*

Cohn JN, Johnson G, Ziesche S, et al. A comparison of enalapril with hydralazine–isosorbide dinitrate in the treatment of chronic congestive heart failure. N Engl J Med 1991;325:303. *(Enalapril proved superior to hydralazine-isosorbide, though mechanisms of action differed and suggested possible complementarity.)*

The CONSENSUS Trial Study Group. Effects of enalapril on mortality in severe congestive heart failure. N Engl J Med 1987;23:1429. *(Adding enalapril to conventional therapy reduced mortality and improved symptoms in this prospective, randomized, multicenter study of patients with severe heart failure.)*

The Digitalis Investigation Group. The effect of digoxin on mortality and morbidity in patients with heart failure. N Engl J Med 1997;336:525. *(Multicenter, randomized, controlled trial in persons with all levels of CHF; significant reduction in rate of hospitalization for heart failure and strong trend toward reduction in cardiovascular mortality; best results in persons with severe left ventricular dysfunction.)*

Fleg JL, Hinton PC, La Katta EG, et al. Physician utilization of laboratory procedures to monitor outpatients with congestive heart failure. Arch Intern Med 1989;149:393. *(High cost of monitoring documented among those using diagnostic studies for monitoring.)*

Grossman W. Diastolic dysfunction in congestive heart failure. N Engl J Med 1991;325:1557. *(Excellent basic science review of diastolic dysfunction that is clinically useful.)*

Jaeschke R, Oxman AD, Guyatt GH. To what extent do congestive heart failure patients in sinus rhythm benefit from digoxin therapy? A systematic overview and meta-analysis. Am J Med 1990;88:279. *(A meta-analytic study indicating that patients with severe systolic dysfunction do best.)*

Lee DC, Johnson RA, Bingham JB, et al. Heart failure in outpatients: a randomized trial of digoxin versus placebo. N Engl J Med 1982;306:699. *(Only CHF patients with an S_3 and other signs of severe systolic dysfunction showed benefit from long-term digoxin therapy.)*

MERIT-HF Study Group. Effect of metoprolol CR/XL in chronic heart failure: metoprolol CR/XL randomized intervention trial in congestive heart failure (MERIT-HF). Lancet 1999;353:2001. *(One of the first large-scale studies to demonstrate survival benefit with beta-blocker use in CHF; nearly 50% reduction in mortality in persons with mild to moderate heart failure.)*

Packer M. The search for the ideal positive inotropic agent. N Engl J Med 1993;329:201. *(An editorial addressing the significance of the increase in mortality seen with use of many positively inotropic agents.)*

Packer M, Bristow MR, Cohn JN, et al. The effect of carvedilol on morbidity and mortality in patients with chronic congestive heart failure. N Engl J Med 1996;334:1349. *(Large randomized control trial demonstrating promising but not definitive results for use of this beta blocker in CHF.)*

Packer M, Gheorghiade M, Young JB, et al. Withdrawal of digoxin from patients with chronic heart failure treated with angiotensin-converting-enzyme inhibitors. N Engl J Med 1993;329:1. *(Withdrawal of digoxin associated with an increased risk of worsening in patients with systolic dysfunction.)*

Packer M, Lee WH, Yushak M, et al. Comparison of captopril and enalapril in patients with severe chronic heart failure. N Engl J Med 1986;315:847. *(Both were effective, but enalapril use was more likely to cause hypotension and renal dysfunction; unfortunately, only very large doses were used.)*

Packer M, O'Conner CM, Ghali JK, et al. Effect of amlodipine on morbidity and mortality in severe chronic heart failure. N Engl J Med 1996;335:1107. *(A randomized prospective study in patients with ejection fraction less than 0.3, showing no association with worsening failure, life-threatening dysrhythmias, or sudden death.)*

Pitt B, Zannad F, Remme WM, et al. The effect of spironolactone on morbidity and mortality in patients with severe heart failure. N Engl J Med 1999;341:709. *(The RALES trial, a randomized, double-blind, placebo-controlled trial of spironolactone in persons with severe heart failure [ejection fraction less than 0.35; NYHA class III or IV disease] already taking maximal medical therapy; demonstrated significant reductions in mortality and morbidity.)*

Smith TW. Digoxin in heart failure. N Engl J Med 1993;329:51. *(An editorial summarizing evidence for efficacy.)*

The SOLVD Investigators. Effect of enalapril on survival in patients with reduced left ventricular ejection fractions and congestive heart failure. N Engl J Med 1991;325:293. *(Enalapril reduced mortality and hospitalization in this important randomized, prospective, multicenter trial of patients with mild to moderate heart failure.)*

Spirito P, Maron BJ. Doppler echocardiography for assessing left ventricular diastolic function. Ann Intern Med 1988;109:122. *(A review of the technique for diagnosis of diastolic dysfunction; 70 references.)*

Testa MA, Anderson RB, Nackley JF, et al. Quality of life and antihypertensive therapy in men—a comparison of captopril with enalapril. N Engl J Med 1993;328:907. *(Captopril was the better tolerated.)*

Whang R. Magnesium deficiency: pathogenesis, prevalence, and clinical implications. Am J Med 1987;82[Suppl 3A]:24. *(A terse review of this important problem, especially in patients taking digitalis and diuretics.)*

Appendix: Potassium Supplementation in Congestive Heart Failure

Indications and Precautions. Patients with heart failure have considerable underlying heart disease and often take digitalis and diuretics, putting them at greatly increased risk for hypokalemia-induced arrhythmias. Prompt correction and prevention of hypokalemia are essential. However, because ACE inhibitor therapy has become a standard part of the CHF treatment regimen, the use of potassium supplements and potassium-sparing diuretics must be undertaken with caution and careful monitoring of the serum potassium. The risk of hyperkalemia is substantial, particularly in the setting of renal failure.

Individual responses to potassium-wasting diuretics and ACE inhibitors vary widely as do requirements for potassium replacement, necessitating regular monitoring of the serum potassium level, which is not an exact measure of total body potassium but rather a rough guide. Potassium supplementation should not be undertaken unless the serum potassium falls below 3.5 mg/dL.

Approaches to Supplementation. Potassium may be taken in the form of dietary additions or potassium-containing preparations. The amount needed is usually determined empirically, ranging from 0 to 60 mEq/d over and above normal dietary potassium intake.

Dietary Measures. For patients on thiazides, dietary replacement often suffices. When a loop diuretic is used, the potassium loss may be greater, necessitating a potassium preparation (unless a potassium-sparing agent is used). *Dietary measures* are the most palatable way to provide potassium. There are 15 mEq in a 10-oz glass of orange, pineapple, or grapefruit juice; a medium-sized banana; a baked potato; or two oranges. Tomato juice has almost twice the potassium content of orange juice, but most brands have added salt to enhance taste.

Salt substitutes contain potassium chloride (KCl), but some are also 50% sodium chloride. Even those that are pure KCl do not provide sufficient potassium to serve effectively as a supplement.

Patients who need to maintain normokalemia but cannot do so by dietary means require a *potassium preparation*. There is a plethora of these on the market. Oral supplements combine potassium with any of a number of different anions. Only the chloride form is effective in correcting the hypokalemic alkalosis that results from diuretic use. However, any form will prevent potassium depletion unless there is concurrently severe sodium chloride depletion.

Potassium chloride elixir remains the safest and least expensive. The 10% solution contains 20 mEq of potassium per tablespoon (15 mL). It is most easily taken in orange juice; some find it unpalatable, even when mixed in fruit juice. However, when faced with the high cost of alternatives, many patients who complain of its taste are willing to reconsider using it. Its safety, chloride content, and ability to deliver more potassium per dose than most other preparations strongly recommend it. Citrus-flavored *effervescent* tablets dissolved in water provide an alternative to the elixir preparation but at greater cost and without much improvement in taste.

Potassium Chloride Tablets. The earliest preparations caused a high incidence of mucosal injury, leading to gastrointestinal ulceration, bleeding, obstruction, and perforation. A second generation of tablet preparations was devised by encoating them in a *wax matrix* to slow release and reduce mucosal injury. Examples include Slow-K, Kaon-Cl, Klotrix, K-Tab, and others. Encoating decreases the risk of gastrointestinal complications but does not entirely eliminate it. Complications continue to occur, often in unpredictable fashion.

Microencapsulation represents another release strategy. KCl is prepared in small crystals, each coated with a polymer permeable to water, theoretically helping to disperse the potassium while minimizing locally high concentrations. Endoscopic data suggest some improved safety over other tablet forms, but cost is almost 10 times that of the elixir for an equivalent dose. Moreover, because each tablet contains only 8 mEq of potassium, multiple tablets are needed each day to provide the 15 to 45 mEq usually required.

Potassium gluconate and bicarbonate preparations are available, some in the form of liquids, others as effervescent tablets. Although they tend to be more palatable, disadvantages include high cost and absence of chloride to counter alkalosis.

Potassium-sparing Diuretics. If all attempts at potassium supplementation fail, then a potassium-sparing diuretic is indicated. Combinations with a thiazide are now available in generic formulation and may provide a reasonable and inexpensive alternative to diuretic plus potassium supplementation in patients requiring both a thiazide and tight potassium control. As noted above, use of a potassium-sparing diuretic in persons taking an ACE inhibitor should be undertaken only with great caution and close monitoring for hyperkalemia, particularly in the setting of worsening renal function.

Refractory hypokalemia requires checking for hypomagnesemia (see above) and hyperaldosteronism (see Chapter 19).

A.H.G.

ANNOTATED BIBLIOGRAPHY

Micro-K potassium supplement. Med Lett Drugs Ther 1982;24:71. *(This KCl preparation may be safer than previously available slow-release preparations but at greatly increased cost.)*

Slow-release potassium. Med Lett Drugs Ther 1978;20:29. *(Small bowel ulceration reported in patients using these preparations.)*

33
Management of Valvular Heart Disease
RICHARD R. LIBERTHSON

As a result of increased physician awareness and improvements in noninvasive diagnostic techniques, the diagnosis of valvular heart disease is being made earlier in the course of illness. Such techniques also reveal cardiomyopathies that may contribute to valvular dysfunction or simulate it by causing outflow-tract obstruction (see Chapter 21). Outpatient management of valvular heart disease has become commonplace because symptoms are frequently absent or mild at the time the condition is discovered. Although consultation with a cardiologist is often obtained, the responsibility for long-term care usually falls on the primary physician. Proper management requires that the primary physician is familiar with the natural history of valvular disease, the early warning signs of hemodynamic deterioration, and the indications for medical and surgical therapies. Skill in application of anticoagulation (see Chapter 83) and antibiotic prophylaxis (see Chapter 16) is essential as is ability to manage the early phases of heart failure (see Chapter 32) and atrial fibrillation (see Chapter 28). Of major importance is the proper timing of referral for consideration of valve repair. Also important is the early recognition and proper management of the common cardiomyopathies that cause left ventricular outflow tract obstruction (see Appendix).

NATURAL HISTORY

Mitral Stenosis

Most cases of mitral stenosis are *rheumatic* in origin, even though as many as 50% of patients cannot give a history of rheumatic fever. The symptom-free interval averages about 10 years (range, 3 to 25 years). In most instances, symptoms develop gradually over a decade, roughly paralleling the progression of stenosis; however, some people remain relatively free of complaints until stenosis becomes severe. Left atrial and pulmonary venous pressures increase substantially as valve area falls below 1.5 cm², and at this point patients typically experience *dyspnea on exertion*. Any stimulus that rapidly increases blood flow or decreases the time available for diastolic filling can precipitate a sudden increase in pulmonary congestion and result in acute shortness of breath. Strenuous activity, fever, emotion, and onset of atrial fibrillation are often responsible for acute dyspnea.

Progressive narrowing of the valve orifice is accompanied by worsening exercise tolerance and increasing dyspnea. In patients with tight stenosis (valve area less than 1.0 cm²), the period from onset of symptoms to incapacity averages 7 years, but the decline can be precipitous with the onset of atrial fibrillation or pneumonia. Chronic marked increase in pulmonary venous pressure often leads to fixed *pulmonary hypertension*. Cardiac output usually falls with onset of severe pulmonary hypertension, and fatigue may become a prominent symptom. The right ventricle hypertrophies in response to the rise in pulmonary artery pressure, and *right-sided heart failure* and death ensue

unless intervention occurs; deterioration may be rapid at this stage.

Atrial fibrillation complicates 40% to 50% of cases of symptomatic mitral stenosis. The correlation between development of atrial fibrillation and the severity of stenosis is slight and not due solely to the degree of left atrial enlargement. The loss of atrial systole and the increase in heart rate that characterize atrial fibrillation markedly reduce flow across the mitral valve and boost left atrial pressure. Premature atrial contractions and paroxysmal atrial fibrillation often precede sustained atrial fibrillation due to mitral stenosis.

Systemic embolization occurs in 10% to 20% of patients with mitral stenosis. Age and presence of atrial fibrillation are the major determinants of risk; severity of stenosis is not a determinant, and in fact, embolization may be a presenting symptom of mitral stenosis.

In sum, there is typically a symptom-free period of about 10 years. Patients then begin to note dyspnea on exertion over the next 10 years, which progresses in many instances in the following decade. Once symptoms are present on minimal exertion, survival becomes markedly reduced. Patients with New York Heart Association class IV disease (symptoms at rest) have been found to have a 5-year mortality rate of 85%. Some patients have disease that may remain stable for many years. In another subset of patients, symptoms do not develop until late in the illness.

Mitral Regurgitation

Rheumatic mitral regurgitation can remain asymptomatic for many years, because the left ventricle dilates and adjusts well to the increase in volume load. Onset of dyspnea and fatigue may not occur for decades. Symptoms take an average of 10 years to progress to the point of disability and need for surgery. It is not until very *late* in the course of the disease that myocardial reserve falters. Once the left ventricle fails, patients note *progressive dyspnea* and *fatigue*; symptoms become present at rest (functional class IV disease). If pulmonary hypertension develops, signs of right-sided heart failure will ensue. Prognosis is poor at this stage.

Atrial fibrillation is found in more than 75% of cases, but the abrupt episodes of pulmonary congestion that typify mitral stenosis complicated by atrial fibrillation are less frequent in mitral regurgitation, although rupture of one of the chordae tendineae can result in sudden deterioration.

Nonrheumatic forms of chronic mitral regurgitation are commonly encountered in the outpatient setting. Etiologies include mitral valve prolapse, papillary muscle dysfunction, and calcified mitral valve annulus. The widespread use of the diet-pill combination *phentermine/fenfluramine* in the mid-late 1990s (see Chapter 234) was associated with reports of new onset of clinically significant incompetence of mitral, tricuspid, and aortic valves. The valves of persons who came to surgery were characterized by striking fibrosis of the endocardial surface identical to that seen in carcinoid syndrome, leading some to speculate that this might be the consequence of excessive seratonergic effects on valve endocardial metabolism. Patients at greatest risk appeared to be those taking the combination program at maximal doses for prolonged periods (more than 4 months), but the true magnitude of the risk has been hard to determine. Because of concern over valve injury, both drugs have been withdrawn from the market.

Mitral valve prolapse (MVP) is one of the most common valvular disorders, with a community prevalence of 2.5%, which is less than the previous estimate of 5% that resulted from data skewed by referral bias. Only patients with truly redundant and thickened mitral leaflets on B-mode (two-dimensional) cardiac ultrasound should be considered to have MVP. These patients have myxomatous proliferation of the spongiosa and elongation of the chordae. Many patients with normal mitral valve leaflets appearing bowed or saddle-shaped on certain echocardiographic views have been mistakenly labeled as having MVP and approached as if they have its attendant risks.

Although patients with true MVP are at increased risk for valvular incompetence, endocarditis, systemic embolization, and dysrhythmias, the prognosis for most is excellent, and most are entirely asymptomatic and at only minimal risk. Many MVP patients do not experience hemodynamically significant regurgitation or an increase in regurgitant flow with time, but there is a subset that do, particularly those with an initial left ventricular diastolic dimension in excess of 60 mm. The associated valvular insufficiency can cause *chronic volume overload,* leading to *left-ventricular dysfunction* and sometimes necessitating mitral valve replacement. Because the initial phases of decline may not be accompanied by symptoms or major fall in ejection fraction, serial echocardiographic examination is required for timely detection of left ventricular dysfunction.

There is a slight increase in risk of *bacterial endocarditis,* especially in those with clinically evident valvular incompetence (regurgitant murmur evident on examination) or a markedly redundant and thickened valve on echocardiogram. The American Heart Association suggests endocarditis prophylaxis for those with MVP who have evidence of mitral insufficiency. Patients with normal variants have little or no increase in risk of endocarditis and do not require antibiotic prophylaxis (see Chapter 16).

Stroke risk is also much less than previously estimated, due to stricter criteria and better precision in diagnosis of MVP. Among younger persons with embolic stroke, there is no increase in prevalence of MVP, suggesting that risk is minimal in the absence of other embolic risk factors. A very small group of MVP patients have *malignant ventricular arrhythmias*; overall risk of sudden death is extremely low in most patients with MVP but heightened in those with a history of syncope, prior ventricular tachyarrhythmias, or a family history of sudden death. Risk appears related to degree of myxomatous changes but not to degree of valve incompetence or left ventricular dysfunction.

Some have raised the question of a relation between *panic disorder* and MVP, because of paniclike symptoms occurring in a small percentage of patients with MVP. Indeed, a small percentage of MVP patients do suffer from *autonomic dysfunction* and complain of palpitations, atypical chest pain, orthostatic dizziness, near-syncope, cold extremities, throbbing headaches, and neurasthenia and manifest tachyarrhythmias, orthostatic hypotension, and peripheral vasoconstriction. However, careful studies have found no causal link between MVP and autonomic dysfunction or panic disorder.

Papillary muscle dysfunction is responsible for as many as 10% of mitral regurgitation cases found clinically. Causes include ischemic injury, left ventricular dilatation, and cardiomyopathy. Ischemic heart disease is the most frequent etiology, with 40% of posterior infarcts and 20% of anterior infarcts accompanied by the development of papillary muscle dysfunction. The amount of regurgitant flow is highly variable. Severe mitral regurgitation and marked pulmonary congestion can occur, even in the context of only a minimal reduction in left ventricular ejection fraction. However, prognosis does depend on left ventricular systolic performance.

Calcification of the mitral annulus occurs in older people, often in conjunction with calcification of the aortic valve. The mitral lesion is usually not of hemodynamic significance, but heart block can develop if calcification extends into the ventricular septum.

Mixed Mitral Disease

Mortality is increased when significant stenosis and regurgitation occur simultaneously. In one large series of patients managed medically, the 10-year survival rate from the time of diagnosis was 33%.

Aortic Stenosis

Because of the marked ability of the left ventricle to hypertrophy and compensate for the pressure load, patients with aortic stenosis can remain symptom-free for many years, even with tight stenosis (valve area less than 0.7 cm^2). This is especially true in young patients. However, it must be remembered that sudden death can occur in previously asymptomatic individuals with critical aortic stenosis. Onset of *angina* and *effort syncope* suggest a hemodynamically critical lesion that is limiting cardiac output, although in as many as 30% to 60% of aortic stenosis patients with angina, there coexists significant occlusion of a coronary vessel. Survival averages 3 years from the onset of angina or effort syncope. The development of *congestive failure* is an ominous sign, for it signals the inability of the myocardium to continue tolerating the severe pressure load; survival averages 2 years from the time failure is first noted. More than half of patients with aortic stenosis die of congestive failure. Sudden death accounts for another 20%. The mean age of death for patients dying suddenly is 60 years; the mechanism of death in these cases is believed to be a dysrhythmia triggered by myocardial ischemia, although debate continues. The rate of stenosis is unpredictable and can progress rapidly over a few years, especially as the patient enters their sixties. Figures for survival are only averages; the range is wide, and many patients die soon after the onset of symptoms.

Age at clinical onset of aortic stenosis is dependent in part on the underlying etiology. Significant aortic stenosis appearing in a patient younger than 30 years of age is congenital in origin, due most often to a *bicuspid* valve. In approximately 15% of such patients, obstruction is caused by a discrete *subaortic membrane.* Patients presenting between ages 30 and 70 have either a bicuspid valve or a valve damaged by *rheumatic fever.*

Those who present with significant aortic stenosis caused by rheumatic fever average 10 to 15 years older than patients who present with rheumatic mitral stenosis, due to the more gradual progression of the illness when it involves the aortic valve. Nevertheless, the course can be one of rapid deterioration.

Aortic stenosis developing in the *elderly* is usually due to *primary degenerative calcification* of a normal aortic valve. Unlike aortic stenosis caused by rheumatic disease with its fusion of valve commissures, *calcific aortic stenosis* results from calcific thickening of the valve leaflets and their loss of mobility. Patients with calcification of a bicuspid valve may present as early as the sixth decade; those with senile calcification of a tricuspid aortic valve present with stenosis in the eighth and ninth decades. By 80 years of age, half of the population has a systolic ejection murmur; in a small percentage, hemodynamically significant stenosis ensues.

Calcific aortic stenosis of the elderly now accounts for most new aortic stenosis cases. Unlike rheumatic aortic stenosis with its fixed valve orifice, the degree of stenosis in calcific aortic stenosis varies with the strength of the left ventricle. The weaker its contraction, the less the valve will open and the greater the outflow obstruction. A failing left ventricle may cause a rapid downhill course. Thus, the contractile state of the left ventricle is a critical determinant of the clinical course of calcific aortic stenosis. Also, the degree of calcification may progress.

Aortic sclerosis in the elderly, even in the absence of hemodynamically significant stenosis, is associated with a 50% increase in morbidity and mortality from coronary artery disease. As such, it serves as a marker for atherosclerotic disease but is not necessarily a pathologic lesion of significance to valvular function.

Aortic Regurgitation

Rheumatic fever accounts for the largest number of aortic regurgitation cases. Most patients live for decades with little incapacity, as the left ventricle dilates to accommodate the extra volume load. The latent period from occurrence of rheumatic fever to onset of clinical manifestations is about 10 years. During the next decade, symptoms appear and progress. The onset of symptoms is typically gradual, with *palpitations* being among the earliest changes noted by the patient, followed by *dyspnea on exertion* and *fatigability*. Appearance of *left ventricular hypertrophy* with strain and progressive *left ventricular dilation* are associated with a markedly increased risk of heart failure and death within 5 years. If exertional dyspnea worsens, other manifestations of congestive failure are likely to follow and signal the beginning of a rapidly declining phase of the disease due to left ventricular decompensation. At this stage, deterioration is rapid, with death occurring within 1 to 2 years of the onset of congestive failure. *Angina* is common, reported by almost 30% of patients; unlike the angina of aortic stenosis, it typically takes place *at rest* rather than on exertion. Angina becomes more frequent when there is worsening heart failure. *Sudden death* may also occur in patients with severe aortic regurgitation.

Nonrheumatic Causes. About 5% of persons with a *bicuspid aortic* valve also have aortic regurgitation as may those with other less common anomalies (e.g., supracrystal ventricular

septal defect and discrete subaortic membranes). Other causes of aortic regurgitation include *syphilis*, myxomatous degeneration, bacterial endocarditis, and connective tissue disease. Aortic regurgitation secondary to untreated syphilis appears about 15 to 25 years after the initial infection and often has a more rapid downhill course than aortic regurgitation caused by rheumatic fever. *Myxomatous degeneration* has been found in 10% to 15% of cases of aortic regurgitation studied pathologically. The process is progressive and becomes clinically evident between the ages of 30 and 60. Although *bacterial endocarditis* can damage a tricuspid aortic valve, particularly one that is fibrotic or calcific, it is far more likely to occur with a bicuspid valve.

Ankylosing spondylitis is complicated by aortic regurgitation in about 3% of cases. The severity of the lesion is highly variable, and conduction defects are frequent. Aortic regurgitation may appear before the onset of other symptoms, but in most instances it follows the appearance of arthritic symptoms by 10 to 20 years. The presence of severe aortic regurgitation shortens the otherwise normal life expectancy of patients with ankylosing spondylitis. *Reiter's syndrome* is associated with the development of aortic regurgitation in 5% of cases, typically in those with florid manifestations of the disease such as iritis, mucocutaneous changes, and extensive sacroiliac inflammation. Onset of aortic regurgitation occurs an average of 15 years after the disease is first noted, often preceded by conduction disturbances. The severity and course of the aortic regurgitation are highly variable.

Use of the appetite-suppressant combination *phentermine/ fenfluramine* in the mid-late 1990s (see Chapter 234) was also associated with reports of new onset of aortic insufficiency. Risk appeared greatest for those using the combination rather than a single agent and for use in excess of 4 months. The precise magnitudes of the relative and absolute risks remain controversial, and the natural history of the lesion is unknown.

Mixed Aortic Valve Disease. Many patients with aortic stenosis have some degree of aortic regurgitation, and vice versa. Whenever the gradient across the aortic valve is greater than 25 mm Hg in the context of significant regurgitation, there begins to develop a substantial pressure load and an increased volume load on the left ventricle. The clinical course is similar to that for isolated aortic stenosis of the same degree, although some clinicians believe there is an earlier onset of symptoms.

Combined Aortic and Mitral Disease. The etiology is mostly rheumatic; in fact, most cases of rheumatic fever produce some degree of multiple valve damage, though disease of one valve often dominates the clinical picture. Mitral stenosis may be overlooked in the setting of concurrent heart failure, pneumonia, or aortic valvular disease. In a study of 152 patients with echocardiographically significant mitral stenosis, 15% of mitral stenosis cases were unrecognized before ultrasound examination, yet most had an audible murmur on reexamination. The most common combination is aortic regurgitation in conjunction with mitral disease. Atrial fibrillation and systemic embolization are more frequent than in isolated aortic regurgitation, as is the severity of pulmonary symptoms. Less common is the coexistence of aortic stenosis and mitral stenosis. Symptoms and signs of aortic stenosis are blunted by significant mitral stenosis, such that pulmonary symptoms, atrial fibrillation, and systemic embolization may dominate the presentation, but there may be more angina and syncope than expected from isolated mitral stenosis. Course is dictated by the severity of the individual lesions, but mitral stenosis can delay the appearance of some of the manifestations of advanced aortic stenosis.

ESTIMATING SEVERITY OF DISEASE

Mitral Stenosis

Symptoms provide crude indications of the severity of stenosis. *Dyspnea* correlates with increase in left atrial pressure and development of *pulmonary venous congestion*, but the relationship between degree of stenosis and elevation of left atrial pressure is variable. *Fatigue* occurs most often in the context of *pulmonary hypertension*, but the nonspecific nature of the symptom lessens its utility in estimating severity. *Hemoptysis* is related to pulmonary *venous hypertension* but does not necessarily imply severe stenosis. Thus, history alone may fail to detect severe stenosis that is unaccompanied by marked pulmonary congestion; however, a worsening of dyspnea and a decline in exercise tolerance suggest hemodynamic deterioration and require further investigation.

On *physical examination*, the interval between the second heart sound and the opening snap, referred to as the S_2-OS interval, and the duration and timing of the diastolic murmur provide additional clues of severity. The S_2-OS interval is a function of the elevation in left atrial pressure. The greater the pressure, the shorter the interval. Unfortunately, the degree of mitral stenosis is not the only determinant of left atrial pressure; the interval can be affected by factors other than valve area, such as heart rate and left ventricular pressure. Moreover, the valve must be mobile to snap; in advanced disease, the valve may calcify and the snap becomes inaudible. Nevertheless, the S_2-OS interval is useful because it can be determined at the bedside and does provide data that may help in judging severity when considered in the context of other findings. Perhaps the most precise use of the interval is in separating hemodynamically insignificant disease from moderate and severe mitral stenosis. An interval of greater than 0.11 seconds at rest with a heart rate of 70 to 80 beats/min argues against a significant lesion (although there are exceptions). Patients with moderate to tight stenosis usually demonstrate intervals less than 0.08 seconds, which shorten with exercise. Proper estimation of the S_2-OS interval takes considerable practice.

The intensity of the *diastolic murmur* does not correlate with severity of stenosis, but its duration through diastole does. However, development of pulmonary hypertension may decrease cardiac output from the right side of the heart, result in a diminution of flow across the mitral valve, and consequently shorten the duration of the murmur.

Chest x-ray provides important evidence of severity. The earliest radiologic sign of mitral stenosis is dilation of the left atrium, which is best seen on a lateral view in conjunction with a barium swallow to outline the esophagus. The finding is not a very reliable manifestation of severity. A better sign is redistribution of pulmonary venous blood flow, producing dilation of the upper zone pulmonary veins. Upper zone redistribution becomes prominent at a left atrial pressure of 25 mm Hg and parallels severity of stenosis. This change in pulmonary venous flow is very sensitive to changes in left atrial pressure, but it is not unique to mitral stenosis. Radiologic evidence of pulmonary hypertension (dilation of the right pulmonary artery to 15 to 18 mm, rapid tapering of vessels, and right ventricular enlargement) strongly suggests advanced mitral stenosis, although again the findings are not specific for mitral stenosis. Presence of Kerley B lines, perihilar haze, and other manifestations of interstitial edema are seen in patients with severe dyspnea due to mitral stenosis; the absence of interstitial edema on chest film does not rule out tight mitral stenosis, but a patient with dyspnea at rest should always show these changes on chest x-ray; otherwise, one must question the etiology of the shortness of breath. In sum, no single radiologic finding is specific for severe mitral stenosis, but x-ray data can provide important supporting evidence.

The *electrocardiogram* (ECG) is of limited utility for estimation of severity. The best ECG sign appears to be the QRS axis; a rightward shift to greater than +60 is associated with a valve area of less than 1.3 cm^2 in more than 85% of cases. The absence of the rightward shift in axis means little. The greater the pulmonary artery pressure, the more likely right ventricular hypertrophy will appear on ECG.

Cardiac ultrasound (echocardiography) is the most sensitive noninvasive method for evaluating mitral stenosis. *One-dimensional (M-mode)* echocardiography readily identifies mitral valve thickening, calcification (when present), and the degree of limitation of valvular movement or excursion. *Two-dimensional (B-mode)* echocardiography provides definitive assessment by allowing direct visualization of the entire valve and its supporting apparatus, measurement of the valve orifice, left atrial and left ventricular chamber dimensions, and assessment of abnormality of other cardiac valves. The addition of *Doppler ultrasound* techniques—including *continuous-wave* Doppler and *color-flow* study—to the ultrasound examination provides detailed delineation of valve anatomy, blood flow, and magnitude of obstruction. A scoring system based on ultrasound data helps to stratify risk and identify candidates for transcatheter balloon dilation of the stenotic valve.

Transesophageal ultrasound is useful when there is concern about intracavity thrombosis (as in atrial fibrillation; see Chapter 28) or valvular vegetations (as in endocarditis). *Cardiac catheterization* is indicated when symptoms are progressive and cardiac surgery or balloon valvuloplasty is being considered (see below).

Mitral Regurgitation

A reasonable estimate of the severity of mitral insufficiency can be obtained by history and physical examination. *Dyspnea on exertion* and *fatigability* are early symptoms of hemodynamically significant regurgitation, although the absence of such symptoms does not rule out severe disease. On physical examination, severe mitral regurgitation produces *left ventricular enlargement* with a hyperdynamic, slightly diffuse, apical impulse displaced to the left but of normal timing and duration. In addition, there is a pansystolic murmur (its loudness does not correlate directly with severity), a loud *third heart sound* (S_3), often a mid-diastolic rumble from increased flow across the mitral valve, and at times wide splitting of the second sound due to shortening of left ventricular systole and early aortic valve closure. In contrast to other forms of valvular disease, a third heart sound may sometimes be audible in a mitral regurgitation patient in the absence of other signs of severe mitral regurgitation and need not represent a failing left ventricle.

In patients with advanced disease, cardiomegaly and left atrial enlargement are pronounced on *chest film*. A normal heart on chest x-ray and absence of an apical pansystolic murmur rule out significant mitral regurgitation. The *ECG* reflects both left atrial and left ventricular enlargement but is hardly specific for mitral regurgitation. *B-mode cardiac ultrasound* is useful for identifying the specific process causing the mitral regurgitation, be it rheumatic fever, prolapse, a ruptured chordae tendineae, or endocarditis. Also readily ascertained are such important items as left atrial and left ventricular size and ejection fraction. In addition, the severity of disease can be ascertained by *Doppler study* that includes color-flow mapping.

Cardiac catheterization is indicated in patients with progressive symptoms and rapidly increasing heart size who are being considered for surgery. One needs to estimate degree of regurgitation, assess ventricular function, and check for the presence and severity of associated valvular and coronary disease.

Mitral Valve Prolapse. In patients with mitral regurgitation due to MVP, severity of regurgitation increases with *age, male gender, duration* of the murmur, degree of *valve leaflet thickening,* and degree of *posterior leaflet prolapse*. Only patients with truly redundant and thickened mitral leaflets are at risk for complications from MVP (e.g., valvular incompetence, endocarditis, systemic embolization, and dysrhythmias). Those with mild bowing and normal leaflets should be considered to have a variant of the normal mitral valve and not true MVP. Those with true MVP and associated valvular insufficiency are at risk for chronic volume overload leading to left ventricular dysfunction; there may be no premonitory symptoms or fall in the ejection fraction.

Aortic Stenosis

There are numerous pitfalls in the clinical estimation of severity of aortic stenosis, especially in the elderly. Nevertheless, careful history and physical examination can provide important clues. Effort *syncope, angina*, and symptoms of congestive *heart failure* point to advanced disease with markedly reduced chances of 5-year survival. At times, it is impossible to tell clinically if these worrisome symptoms are due to aortic stenosis, because of the high prevalence of coexisting coronary disease. The presence of angina must be interpreted cautiously; cardiac catheterization and coronary angiography are generally necessary.

Delay in carotid artery upstroke is one of the most helpful physical signs of significant aortic stenosis, especially in the young. A normal upstroke in a patient younger than 60 years of age is strong evidence against important stenosis; however, upstroke may appear normal in the elderly patient with severe stenosis because of a stiff noncompliant carotid artery. Particularly when there are prominent transmitted carotid thrills, the *brachial arteries* may better reflect the severity of aortic stenosis and should also be assessed by palpation. When coincidental aortic regurgitation is present, the upstroke may also appear normal in the presence of marked stenosis. A misleading delay in carotid upstroke can occur from the combination of systemic hypertension and congestive heart failure. Elevation of systolic blood pressure does not rule out hemodynamically significant aortic stenosis, though a pressure greater than 200 mm Hg and a pulse pressure in excess of 80 mm Hg are unusual when stenosis is marked.

In young patients, the *intensity* of the *murmur* often correlates with severity; however, although it is generally true that critical aortic stenosis is unlikely in a young ambulating person who has less than a 3/6 systolic ejection murmur, rare exceptions do occur. In patients with far advanced disease and a failing left ventricle, the murmur may decrease in intensity and appear insignificant as flow across the valve diminishes. In general, the longer the murmur takes to reach peak intensity, the greater the stenosis. Unfortunately, the *timing of maximal intensity* may not be delayed in some cases of severe stenosis, but if the murmur does peak after mid-systole, the stenosis is usually significant. Because the murmur of aortic stenosis in the elderly may lose its characteristic qualities, it is best to judge severity on the basis of symptoms and other findings. Aortic stenosis in the elderly in the absence of evidence of significant outflow tract obstruction suggests *aortic sclerosis*.

A delay in the aortic component of the *second heart sound* (S_2) is another sign of significant aortic stenosis. S_2 may be single or paradoxically split. Calcification and increased rigidity of the valve will often diminish the intensity of the aortic closing sound; it may become inaudible. A forceful *left ventricular impulse* noted on palpation of the precordium is a reliable indication of secondary left ventricular hypertrophy due to significant outflow obstruction.

The *ECG* can contribute to the evaluation by showing signs of left ventricular *hypertrophy* (increased voltage and a strain pattern in the precordial leads V_5 and V_6). The likelihood of finding a strain pattern (i.e., ST and T wave depression in the apical and lateral leads) increases with the increase in gradient across the aortic valve. These ECG changes also identify patients at increased risk of sudden death, as fewer than 10% of patients succumbing to sudden death demonstrate a normal ECG. In children, the ECG is less helpful; even severe aortic stenosis may not produce left ventricular hypertrophy and a strain pattern.

Cardiac ultrasound has become essential for assessment of aortic stenosis, capable of determining degree of calcification, valve anatomy, chamber size, and left ventricular contractility. In the elderly, the *degree of valvular calcification* correlates with severity of stenosis. The absence of significant calcification in a patient older than 60 years of age greatly reduces the probability of important valvular stenosis. Poststenotic dilation of the aorta suggests aortic valvular stenosis but does not have quantitative meaning. The findings of thickening and decreased mobility of the aortic valve leaflets suggest advancing disease. Echocardiography can help distinguish valvular from subvalvular stenosis and, if subvalvular, whether the stenosis is secondary to a discrete membrane, a fibromuscular bar, or a hypertrophic myocardium as in *hypertrophic cardiomyopathy*. In the young patient with normal left ventricular function, the echocardiogram can provide an indirect estimate of the magnitude of the obstructive gradient. The echocardiogram also delineates the magnitude of left ventricular wall thickening and any associated valvular abnormality, particularly rheumatic valve disease. The addition of Doppler techniques to the echocardiographic evaluation provides an accurate determination of valve area and helps detect any accompanying aortic regurgitation. The finding of mitral regurgitation, especially if progressive on serial studies, correlates with severity and progression of aortic stenosis.

Cardiac catheterization is indicated in the young asymptomatic patient with evidence of severe stenosis, as well as in any patient with known aortic stenosis who begins to develop symptoms of angina, heart failure, or syncope. Elderly patients who are deemed healthy enough to be candidates for surgery should also have *coronary angiography* performed to identify significant occlusive disease that may be the source of symptoms or may limit chances of surviving surgery without correction at the time of valve replacement.

Aortic Regurgitation

Severity of aortic regurgitation can usually be well assessed clinically in cases of isolated valvular insufficiency. Marked regurgitation that is long-standing produces dyspnea, a loud diastolic murmur that extends beyond mid-diastole, an S_3, a bounding pulse, and a widened pulse pressure. The absence of a wide pulse pressure does not rule out hemodynamically significant aortic regurgitation nor does the degree of widening necessarily correlate quantitatively with severity. Changes in peripheral resistance alone can cause large variations in pulse pressure. ECG and x-ray evidence of left ventricular hypertrophy and enlargement are indicative of long-standing significant regurgitation and suggest worsening left ventricular function if they progress.

The *echocardiogram* with *Doppler* enhancement can determine left ventricular size and contractility and delineate the specific disease process in aortic regurgitation—be it rheumatic, annular dilation, or advanced luetic destruction. Signs of left ventricular dysfunction by ultrasound study often precede symptoms and help determine the optimal time for consideration of surgery (see below). Doppler has a sensitivity approaching 100% for diagnosis of aortic regurgitation, especially when *color-flow* techniques are used, far superior to physical examination or B-mode echocardiography. Color-flow techniques can provide an excellent noninvasive estimate of regurgitant severity that is within 10% of that found at cardiac catheterization. *Transesophageal echocardiography* is worth considering when endocarditis is a concern.

When aortic regurgitation occurs in the presence of coexisting aortic stenosis, mitral stenosis, or heart failure, the estimation of severity can be very difficult to judge on clinical grounds alone. Consultation with a cardiologist and *catheterization* are often needed.

PRINCIPLES OF MANAGEMENT

Therapeutic Objectives and Timing of Interventions. The principal objectives are to preserve exercise capacity, life-style, and life expectancy and to minimize the chances of endocarditis and systemic embolization. Proper timing of intervention is essential to successful treatment. A common management error is to inappropriately delay surgery or valvuloplasty, allowing irreversible myocardial decompensation to develop; this increases the risk of operation and reduces the postoperative benefit. A physician can be lulled into a false sense of security by continuing to control symptoms through repetitive escalations of medical therapy. The need for progressive increases in med-

ication suggests worsening ventricular function and the need for interventional therapy. By ignoring the significance of such developments, the physician may miss the optimal opportunity for the best possible surgical outcome, long-term improvement, and survival.

Roles of Medical and Surgical Interventions. Early in the course of illness, therapy is predominantly medical, directed at minimizing pulmonary venous congestion (see Chapter 32) and preventing potentially dangerous complications, such as arrhythmias (see Chapters 28 and 29), bacterial endocarditis (see Chapter 16), and systemic embolization (see Chapter 83). Most people can be well managed on an outpatient basis for many years with a mild diuretic regimen supplemented by an angiotensin-converting enzyme inhibitor or digitalis (see Chapter 32) before the need for interventional therapy. However, inappropriately escalating and prolonging medical therapy beyond the optimal time for surgery is a common mistake that must be avoided if the best surgical outcome is to be obtained.

More advanced stages of disease may require invasive intervention. Life expectancy and quality of life are clearly improved by properly timed intervention. Advances in valvuloplasty technique, prosthetic valve design, and operative technique have produced substantial reductions in interventional mortality. At present, mortality rates for patients undergoing valve surgery in major centers average less than 1% for mitral valvulotomy and less than 5% for mitral or aortic valve replacement. Operative mortality increases sharply when patients with advanced disease (e.g., functional class IV) undergo surgery. However, patients with severe disease should not be denied an operation if they have sufficient myocardial reserve and thus a chance for meaningful survival.

The 5-year life expectancy rate for patients with class IV disease who live through valve replacement is usually less than 50%, but this figure is much better than the less than 5% rate for similar patients managed medically. Thus, even when surgery is inordinately delayed, it may still offer the patient some opportunity for prolonging survival. Contraindications to valve surgery include serious coexisting noncardiac illness that would compromise survival and the existence of end-stage myocardial decompensation that would make surgery for naught.

Percutaneous balloon angioplasty is being used effectively and safely for relief of severe mitral valvular stenosis in carefully selected patients. For young patients with valvular aortic stenosis, it has also proved to be efficacious, but in the elderly with severe aortic stenosis, results have been disappointing (high short-term rates of stroke, aortic insufficiency, and mortality). Balloon angioplasty has proven most useful as a palliative short-term measure for patients who are too ill to tolerate the risk of open heart surgery; long-term efficacy is limited.

Postsurgical Management. It is important to emphasize that patients who undergo valve surgery still have a "cardiac problem" after surgical correction, be it a prosthetic valve with a variable and still unknown late course, a need for anticoagulation and endocarditis prophylaxis, or an associated cardiac abnormality such as coronary, myocardial, or conduction system disease. All too often this is forgotten after the patient undergoes valve repair. Such patients need continued close follow-up and will always remain "cardiac patients."

THERAPEUTIC RECOMMENDATIONS AND INDICATIONS FOR REFERRAL AND ADMISSION

- Monitor all patients by periodic assessment of exercise tolerance, cardiopulmonary examination, chest x-ray, and cardiac ultrasound examination (including Doppler study).
- All patients with any form of valvular heart disease should receive prophylaxis for bacterial endocarditis (see Chapter 16).
- Patients younger than 35 years of age with previous rheumatic fever should be considered for rheumatic fever prophylaxis (see Chapter 17), particularly if they have frequent β-streptococcal infections or exposure to young children.
- Onset of atrial fibrillation with a rapid ventricular response rate accompanied by acute hemodynamic deterioration is an indication for immediate hospital admission and treatment. Patients with slower rates who tolerate the atrial fibrillation can be digitalized on an outpatient basis (see Chapter 28).
- Occurrence of systemic embolization is an indication for urgent admission and intravenous anticoagulant therapy followed by long-term oral anticoagulant treatment (see Chapter 83). Some clinicians argue that valve surgery should be considered if embolization occurs; most concur that surgery is indicated if embolization happens repeatedly.

Mitral Stenosis

- Asymptomatic patients with mild to moderate stenosis need no restriction of activity. Those with evidence of tight stenosis and relatively few symptoms should be advised of the risk of precipitating symptoms by extreme exertion or pregnancy.
- Patients with mild dyspnea that occurs only on exertion can be started on a mild diuretic program (e.g., hydrochlorothiazide 50 to 100 mg/d) and advised to follow a no-added-salt diet. Digitalis is of no benefit in isolated mitral stenosis unless there is atrial fibrillation. Extremely vigorous exertion and emotional upset should be avoided to prevent precipitating symptoms.
- Chronic warfarin oral anticoagulation is indicated for the patient with mitral stenosis, particularly when there is atrial fibrillation (see Chapter 28).
- The development of tight mitral stenosis (as evidenced by a short S_2-OS interval, prolonged diastolic murmur, left atrial enlargement and upper zone redistribution on chest x-ray, and narrowed valve orifice and reduced flow on ultrasound) necessitates referral to a cardiologist for consideration of invasive intervention, be it surgery or balloon angioplasty, even if few symptoms are reported. Consultation is also needed for worsening dyspnea that is inadequately controlled by a mild diuretic program and salt restriction.
- Young patients with evidence of isolated tight mitral stenosis with a pliable noncalcified valve should be considered for interventional therapy early in the course of their illness, even before symptoms are disabling, because transcatheter or surgical valvulotomy can be performed. Both procedures provide long-lasting hemodynamic improvement.
- Early referral for cardiologic assessment is advisable, because percutaneous balloon mitral valvulotomy is an increasingly attractive alternative to surgical mitral commissurotomy in appropriately selected patients.

- Older patients with fibrotic valves (absent opening snap, heavy valve calcification, and limited motion) must undergo valve replacement if surgery is needed. Because surgical mortality and complications are greater for valve replacement than for valvulotomy, surgery need not be advised until symptoms are more disabling. However, surgery should not be delayed until symptoms occur at rest or on minimal exertion, because operative risk and long-term mortality increase substantially. A walk with your patient down a corridor or up a flight of stairs may be of great help in convincing both you and the patient that the time for surgery has arrived.
- Cardiac consultation for consideration of catheterization is indicated in the patient being considered for surgery when there is a question of mixed mitral disease or involvement of multiple valves or when symptoms are out of proportion to objective evidence of disease.

Mitral Regurgitation

- Asymptomatic young patients need no restriction of activity.
- Onset of fatigue and dyspnea can be treated with initiation of a gentle diuretic program (e.g., 50 to 100 mg/d hydrochlorothiazide) in conjunction with a no-added-salt diet. A modest diuretic program that adequately controls symptoms may suffice for years in patients with mild to moderate mitral regurgitation and is not an indication for surgery.
- The development of any increase in dyspnea that requires escalation of diuretic therapy is an indication for cardiac consultation concerning valve replacement. Progressive deterioration in clinical status and increasing heart size suggest presence of myocardial decompensation; prompt referral is indicated; medical therapy is no substitute for valve surgery.
- Refractory congestive failure due to mitral regurgitation is not a contraindication to surgery, though risk is increased. Before surgery, symptoms may be lessened by vasodilator therapy, particularly angiotensin-converting enzyme inhibitors (e.g., captopril 25 to 50 mg three times daily; see Chapter 32), which can diminish the magnitude of regurgitant flow by decreasing afterload. Use of vasodilators can benefit the inoperable patient.
- Patients with incapacitating dyspnea and pulmonary congestion thought to be caused by papillary muscle dysfunction should be referred to the cardiologist for catheterization to determine if valve replacement will be of benefit. In one series, those with ejection fractions above 0.35 had the best surgical survival. If there is coexisting coronary disease, it should be treated (see Chapter 30).
- Valve reconstruction is becoming an increasingly frequent option in mitral regurgitation, obviating the need for an artificial valve and its attendant risks in many cases.
- Patients with a prolapsed mitral valve rarely require treatment other than endocarditis prophylaxis (see Chapter 16). Dyspnea is uncommon and digitalis, diuretics, and salt restriction are unnecessary, because the magnitude of the regurgitation is usually insignificant and rarely progressive. However, those with a dilated left ventricle and marked regurgitation should be followed with serial cardiac ultrasonography for early detection of left ventricular dysfunction, a sign of poor prognosis and an indication for consideration of repair. The rare patient with a history of syncope or ventricular tachycardia or a family history of sudden

death requires consideration of treatment for malignant ventricular dysrhythmias (see Chapter 29); those with isolated palpitations do not. There is no evidence that prophylaxis for systemic embolization is needed in the absence of concurrent risk factors.

- Patients with calcification of the mitral valve annulus should be followed for development of heart block. Regurgitant flow is usually small; consequently, dyspnea and pulmonary congestion are not major problems.
- Chronic anticoagulation is indicated in mitral regurgitation patients with atrial fibrillation, especially when accompanied by marked left atrial and left ventricular enlargement.

Aortic Stenosis

- Patients with aortic sclerosis are at no increased risk from their valvular disease, but the sclerosis is a marker of increased atherosclerotic risk, which should be attended to (see Chapters 26, 27, 30, and 31).
- Asymptomatic patients with mild aortic stenosis do not require restriction of activity.
- Young asymptomatic patients with evidence of tight stenosis should be advised against heavy physical exertion (e.g., competitive sports) and referred to a cardiologist for consideration of catheterization and valvuloplasty or valve replacement. Cardiac catheterization is needed.
- Many young patients with tight aortic stenosis may benefit from transcatheter aortic balloon valvuloplasty. Results in appropriately selected young patients are comparable with those achieved with surgical valvuloplasty.
- In elderly patients, especially those with fibrotic, calcified valves, and associated aortic incompetence, balloon valvuloplasty is appropriate only as a palliative measure in those unfit for surgery.
- Onset of angina, effort syncope, or congestive heart failure dictates prompt referral for consideration of valve surgery. These are signs of critical stenosis and predict a poor prognosis unless definitive therapy is undertaken. Such patients are at risk for sudden death. Medical therapy is no substitute.
- Congestive failure can be treated symptomatically on a temporary basis by prescribing digitalis and a moderate diuretic program (e.g., cautious use of furosemide 20 to 40 mg/d; see Chapter 32). Such therapy may help reduce pulmonary congestion and sustain cardiac output temporarily, but the need for a high diastolic filling pressure must be kept in mind; overzealous diuretic therapy can cause a precipitous fall in cardiac output; afterload reduction may also be dangerous in severe aortic stenosis.
- Angina can be treated symptomatically but cautiously with nitrates pending surgery (see Chapter 30); beta-blockers are contraindicated due to their negative inotropic effects. Coronary angiography is required at the time of cardiac catheterization to determine if there is coexisting significant coronary artery disease and the need for a bypass procedure at the time of valve replacement.
- Advanced age is not an absolute contraindication to valve replacement. Survival from surgery is predominantly a function of the patient's myocardial reserve. Consequently, even patients in their eighties need not be denied surgery if they are otherwise reasonable surgical candidates and demonstrate an adequate ejection fraction, even in the setting of severe aortic stenosis.

- Because calcification of the aortic valve can progress rapidly over a few years, patients with aortic stenosis should have careful longitudinal care and regular follow-up, even when disease appears hemodynamically insignificant and the patient is asymptomatic.

Aortic Regurgitation

- No activity restrictions are necessary in young asymptomatic patients with mild regurgitation.
- Assess severity with an initial cardiac ultrasound examination that includes Doppler study and follow patients having evidence of severe regurgitation with serial ultrasound examinations in addition to regular office assessments.
- Asymptomatic patients with moderately severe disease may be treated with afterload reduction (e.g., lisinopril 10 mg twice daily), which appears capable of reducing left ventricular end-systolic and end-diastolic pressures and perhaps slowing disease progression.
- Patients with evidence of worsening left ventricular function (left ventricular hypertrophy) with a strain pattern on ECG, increasing cardiomegaly on chest film, falling ejection fraction, and increasing left ventricular end-systolic dimension on ultrasound examination) should be referred to a cardiologist for consideration of surgery, even in the absence of symptoms. Patients with a declining left ventricle have an increased risk of ventricular tachycardia and an increased 5-year mortality rate. Early identification of high-risk patients is suggested in the hope of correcting aortic regurgitation before the development of irreversible myocardial decompensation, which may have already started by the time symptoms occur.
- Onset of mild symptoms of pulmonary congestion (dyspnea on climbing more than one flight of stairs) in the absence of evidence of significant left ventricular dysfunction can be treated medically with digitalization, a mild diuretic (50 to 100 mg hydrochlorothiazide), or afterload reduction (e.g., lisinopril 10 mg twice daily), but close clinical follow-up and frequent serial ultrasound examinations are essential to prevent inappropriate delay of surgery. Progression of dyspnea to onset after climbing less than one flight of stairs or worsening of left ventricular function on follow-up ultrasound examination indicates the need for prompt cardiac consultation and consideration of surgery.
- Patients with dyspnea prompted by minimal exertion, orthopnea, or paroxysmal nocturnal dyspnea require prompt referral for surgery, because life expectancy is less than 1 year without surgery. Medical therapy with digitalis and diuretics may provide some symptomatic relief temporarily but must not be used in place of valve surgery at this stage of illness.

PATIENT EDUCATION

By far, the most essential elements of patient education are teaching the importance of endocarditis prophylaxis (see Chapter 16) and self-monitoring for early symptoms of cardiac decompensation. The patient with rheumatic heart disease also requires instruction in prophylaxis against group A β-streptococcal infection (see Chapter 17). The chances of compliance are certain to improve if time is taken to explain the rationale for prophylaxis and self-monitoring. Patients and their families should also be fully briefed on allowable activity, to avoid both unnecessary restriction and the risk of sudden death in the high-risk patient (e.g., the young person with critical aortic stenosis). If the safety of unlimited activity is in doubt, then a cardiac consultation may be helpful.

The patient's functional status and the proper timing of interventional therapy can be optimized by close regularly scheduled follow-up and instructions to promptly report early symptoms of cardiac decompensation (e.g., onset of exertional dyspnea). Patient confidence and a sense of partnership care are fostered by such follow-up. It is helpful to inform the patient of the treatability of this condition and its excellent prognosis when therapy is properly selected and timed. This provides the rationale for careful self-monitoring. If the patient cannot be depended on to relate symptoms accurately, then a family member or friend needs to be recruited to watch for early manifestations of worsening disease and monitor therapy. Detailed review of the medical program with all concerned cannot be overemphasized, given the very serious consequences from misuse of diuretics, digitalis, and anticoagulants in valvular disease. Of particular importance is warning against unauthorized self-escalation of the medical program when symptoms worsen.

ANNOTATED BIBLIOGRAPHY

Biem HJ, Detsky AS, Armstrong PW. Management of asymptomatic chronic aortic regurgitation with left ventricular dysfunction: a decision analysis. J Gen Intern Med 1990;5:394. (*Strongly favors surgical intervention at the first signs of significant left ventricular dysfunction, even though the patient may remain asymptomatic.*)

Brady ST, Davis CA, Kussmal WG, et al. Percutaneous aortic balloon valvuloplasty in octogenarians: morbidity and mortality. Ann Intern Med 1989;110:761. (*Hemodynamics improved but overall short-term mortality was very high [32%].*)

Brener SJ, Duffy CI, Thomas JD, et al. Progression of aortic stenosis in 394 patients. J Am Coll Cardiol 1995;25:305. (*An echocardiographic study demonstrating significant yearly progression; left ventricular hypertrophy and mitral regurgitation were risk factors for the greatest increases in gradient; mitral regurgitation was associated with reduction in left ventricular function.*)

Brunnen PL, Finlayson JD, Short D. Serious mitral stenosis with slight symptoms. Br Med J 1964;1:1958. (*Classic paper; symptoms may be slight, but young patients with tight stenosis are at risk for sudden deterioration; pregnancy was a major precipitant.*)

Chen JTT, Beliar VS, Morris JJ, et al. Correlation of roentgen findings with hemodynamic data in pure mitral stenosis. AJR Am J Roentgenol 1968;102:280. (*Another classic; prominent upper-zone redistribution and pulmonary artery dilation correlated closely with severity.*)

Choudhry NK, Etchells EE. Does this patient have aortic regurgitation? JAMA 1999;281:2231. (*Best review of the physical findings and the evidence supporting their significance.*)

Collins JJ Jr. The evolution of artificial heart valves. N Engl J Med 1991;324:624. (*A still useful editorial and terse but detailed review for the general reader.*)

Folland ED, Kriegel BJ, Henderson WG, et al. Implications of third heart sounds in patients with valvular heart disease. N Engl J Med 1992;327:458. (*Indicative of failure in aortic stenosis but not in mitral regurgitation.*)

Fowler NO, Van Der BelKahn JM. Indications for surgical replacement of the mitral valve. Am J Cardiol 1979;44:148. (*A still pertinent review that emphasizes timing of surgical therapy; 41 references.*)

Freed LA, Levy D, Levine RA, et al. Prevalence and clinical outcome of mitral-valve prolapse. N Engl J Med 1999;341:1. (*Best available community-based data; show lower prevalence and lower risk of adverse sequelae than previous reports.*)

Fukada N, Oki T, Iuchi A, et al. Predisposing factors for severe mitral regurgitation in idiopathic mitral valve prolapse. Am J Cardiol 1995;76:503. (*Severity of regurgitation correlated with age, male gender, duration of the murmur, degree of valve leaflet thickening, and presence of posterior leaflet prolapse.*)

Goldschlager N, Pfeifer J, Cohn D, et al. Natural history of aortic regurgitation. Am J Med 1973;54:577. (*Long symptomatic period, but once symptoms occur, irreversible myocardial changes may have already taken place.*)

Graboys TB, Cohn PF. Prevalence of angina and abnormal coronary arteriograms in severe aortic stenosis. Am Heart J 1977;93:683. (*20% had at least one significant luminal stenosis.*)

Hammermeister KE, Sethi GK, Henderson WG, et al. Comparison of outcomes in men 11 years after heart-valve replacement with a mechanical valve or bioprosthesis. N Engl J Med 1993;328:1289. (*Useful data for selection of prosthesis.*)

Jick H, Vasilakis C, Weinrauch LA, et al. A population-based study of appetite-suppressant drugs and the risk of cardiac valve regurgitation. N Engl J Med 1998;339:719. (*Marked increased in risk documented, especially in those taking more than 4 months' of treatment.*)

Lee RT, Bhatia SJS, St John Sutton MG. Assessment of valvular heart disease with Doppler echocardiography. JAMA 1989; 262:2131. (*Excellent review of this very important technologic addition to the assessment of valvular disease; 30 references.*)

Libethson RR. Sudden death from cardiac causes in children and young adults. N Engl J Med 1996;334:1039. (*Review of high-risk etiologies, including aortic stenosis and hypertrophic cardiomyopathy.*)

Lieberman EB, Bashore TM, Hermiller JB, et al. Balloon aortic valvuloplasty in adults: failure of procedure to improve long-term survival. J Am Coll Cardiol 1995;26:1522. (*No improvement over the natural history of the disease; 6% event-free survival at 3 years.*)

Lin M, Chiang HT, Liu SL, et al. Vasodilator therapy in chronic asymptomatic aortic regurgitation: enalapril versus hydralazine therapy. J Am Coll Cardiol 1994;24:1046. (*Afterload reduction with enalapril was superior to vasodilator therapy with hydralazine.*)

Marks AR, Choong CY, Sanfilippo AJ, et al. Identification of high-risk and low-risk subgroups of patients with mitral-valve prolapse. N Engl J Med 1989;320:1031. (*Those with valve thickening and redundancy were at greatest risk of complications.*)

Nishimura RA, McGoon MD. Perspectives on mitral-valve prolapse. N Engl J Med 1999;341:48. (*An editorial providing an excellent summary of case definition and risk for complications.*)

Oh JK, Taliercio CP, Holmes DR, et al. Prediction of the severity of aortic stenosis by Doppler aortic valve area determination. J Am Coll Cardiol 1988;11:1227. (*A prospective study of 100 patients coming to catheterization; excellent correlation found between Doppler and catheterization results.*)

Otto CM, Lind BK, Kitzman DW, et al. Association of aortic-valve sclerosis with cardiovascular mortality and morbidity in the elderly. N Engl J Med 1999;341:142. (*Its presence was associated with a 50% increase in coronary morbidity and mortality even when there was no stenosis, suggesting it can serve as a marker of atherosclerotic disease.*)

Palacios IF. Farewell to surgical mitral commissurotomy for many patients. Circulation 1998;97:223. (*Update on the status of balloon dilatation.*)

Reyes VP, Raju BS, Wynne J, et al. Percutaneous balloon valvuloplasty compared with open surgical commissurotomy for mitral stenosis. N Engl J Med 1994;331:961. (*In persons less than 30 years of age, percutaneous balloon valvuloplasty was superior.*)

Selzer A. Changing aspects of the natural history of valvular aortic stenosis. N Engl J Med 1987;317:91. (*Most of the aortic stenosis now being encountered is due to calcific degenerative disease of the elderly; excellent review of its presentation and clinical course and how it differs from rheumatic aortic stenosis; 116 references.*)

Sherrid M, Goyal A, Delia E, et al. Unsuspected mitral stenosis. Am J Med 1991;90:189. (*Hemodynamically significant disease detected by ultrasound was missed clinically due to concurrent aortic stenosis, heart failure, pneumonia, or just a low index of suspicion; most cases had an audible mitral stenosis murmur on reexamination.*)

Siemienczuk D, Greenberg B, Morris C, et al. Chronic aortic insufficiency: factors associated with progression to aortic valve replacement. Ann Intern Med 1989;110:587. (*Measurement of left ventricular size and function were predictive of need for valve replacement.*)

Taylor AA, Davies AO, Mares A, et al. Spectrum of dysautonomia in mitral valvular prolapse. Am J Med 1989;86:287. (*Dysautonomic responses occurred irrespective of the presence of MVP; refutes the purported etiologic link between these responses and MVP.*)

Vohra J, Sathe S, Warren R, et al. Malignant ventricular arrhythmias in patients with mitral valve prolapse and mild mitral regurgitation. Pacing Clin Electrophysiol 1993;16:387. (*Characteristics of patients at high risk for serious dysrhythmias.*)

Appendix: Management of Hypertrophic Cardiomyopathy

Hypertrophic cardiomyopathy (HCM) with left ventricular outflow tract obstruction (also referred to as *idiopathic hypertrophic subaortic stenosis* [IHSS]) has many clinical features that resemble valvular aortic stenosis. Noteworthy differences include absence of an ejection sound in early systole and absence of poststenotic dilatation of the ascending aorta. Patients with IHSS have an increase in the intensity of their murmur with Valsalva (absent in those with HCM and no outflow tract obstruction). IHSS and other forms of HCM are generally but not always *familial*, usually transmitted as an autosomal dominant trait. Because of the potential for high frequency in family members, familial screening is essential. Transthoracic ultrasound is diagnostic; cardiac catheterization is rarely necessary.

The most serious consequence of IHSS is *sudden cardiac death*. Those at greatest risk have a history of prior syncope and ventricular tachyarrhythmias and a family history of sudden death. Such high-risk persons require warning about engaging in strenuous exercise; bacterial endocarditis prophylaxis is indicated. Those who develop atrial fibrillation are at risk for embolization and need oral anticoagulation (see Chapters 28 and 83). *Beta-blockade* is recommended for most individuals—the decrease in contractility reduces the degree of outflow tract obstruction. Treatment of hypertension has particular merit. Data from community-based study suggest that the prognosis is not quite as serious as originally suspected from referral center investigations. Most patients do quite well, but there appears to be a subset at increased risk.

ANNOTATED BIBLIOGRAPHY

Maron BJ, Casey SA, Poliac LC, et al. Clinical course of hypertrophic cardiomyopathy in a regional United States cohort. JAMA 1999;281:650. (*A retrospective cohort study that avoids referral bias showing HCM not to be a major risk factor for premature death or shortened life expectancy; data helps puts the condition in perspective.*)

Wigle ED, Rakowski H, Kimball BP, et al. Hypertrophic cardiomyopathy: clinical spectrum and treatment. Circulation 1995;92:1680. (*Major review of diagnosis and management.*)

34
Management of Peripheral Arterial Disease

DAVID C. BREWSTER

Treatment of peripheral arterial insufficiency has undergone a quiet revolution. Plaque regression has now been demonstrated with aggressive lipid-lowering therapy (see Chapter 27), and in properly selected patients, percutaneous transluminal angioplasty (PTA) with or without intraluminal stenting produces results that approach those of bypass surgery. In addition, great progress has been made in arterial reconstructive surgery for severe cases, making possible the salvage of limbs that would otherwise require amputation. The wealth of available therapeutic options and a relatively favorable natural history provide the symptomatic patient with substantial opportunity for improvement. The primary physician needs to know the natural history of arterial occlusive disease so as to optimize the timing and intensity of therapy; the techniques, efficacies, and indications for conservative therapy, including risk factor modification, and the indications for angioplasty and bypass surgery. With so many treatment modalities available, the primary physician has to be skilled in the timing, selection, implementation, and coordination of care.

NATURAL HISTORY OF PERIPHERAL ARTERIAL DISEASE

The *prognoses* for the *limb* and for *symptoms* in patients presenting with claudication are quite good. The worst clinical courses occur among patients manifesting ischemic ulcers or rest pain, especially if they suffer from long-standing diabetes mellitus or persist in smoking. Even before the advent of surgical reconstruction, only 3% of patients with peripheral artery disease came to amputation within 5 years if the sole manifestation of their disease was claudication, and none of these persons required amputation if they ceased smoking, but over 10% who continued to smoke lost a limb. In the angiographic era, nearly 80% remain stable or improve, and only about 6% come to amputation. Not surprisingly, prognosis parallels severity of disease as measured by distance walked before onset of claudication. Most amputations occur in the high-risk group, but even in severe cases, nearly 70% stay the same or improve and only 15% come to amputation, underscoring the fact that progression to loss of limb is hardly inevitable. After 5 years from onset of symptoms, about half of patients remain symptomatically stable or improved. In the Framingham Study, only a third of patients presenting with intermittent claudication still had persistent symptoms 4 years later. In essence, prognosis is rather good, especially if major atherosclerotic risk factors can be brought under control.

Although prognosis for the limb is favorable, *mortality* rates—both overall and cardiovascular—are high. The risk of dying from a cardiovascular cause is sixfold greater in those with peripheral arterial disease than in those of similar age, sex, and lipid profile without it. All-cause mortality increases threefold, due almost entirely to the increase in cardiovascular risk. Combined mortality rates are in the range of 30%, 50%, and 70% at 5, 10, and 15 years after onset of symptoms, respectively—a relative risk about three times that for patients of similar age and gender. Concurrent disease of the coronary arteries, cerebrovasculature, or aorta accounts for most of the increased mortality, underscoring the systemic nature of atherosclerosis and its adverse effect on prognosis. The prevalence of systemic atherosclerosis in patients with peripheral arterial insufficiency should not be surprising, given that up to 80% give a history of smoking, 40% have hypertension, 30% have lipid abnormalities, and 20% have diabetes.

PRINCIPLES OF MANAGEMENT

Clinical Assessment (see also Chapter 23)

In the patient with diabetes who presents with an ischemic ankle or foot ulceration, the history and physical examination supplemented by a Doppler flow study have been shown to be predictive of outcome and can help direct management. Physicians encountering a diabetic with a foot ulcer should inquire into previous amputation and painful skin ulceration. If there has been previous amputation, the likelihood ratio for an adverse action is 4.0 and the patient should be considered for aggressive therapy (e.g., revascularization). If there is neither previous amputation nor tender ulceration, risk is reduced (likelihood ratio 0.33) and an initial conservative (medical) approach is reasonable. If the ulcer is painful but there is no history of amputation, then referral for Doppler study would be indicated. An audible Doppler posterior-tibial pulse in a person with a painful ulcer is associated with an excellent outcome (relative risk of adverse outcome 0.4) and candidacy for conservative therapy.

In the patient with atherosclerosis who presents with claudication, a full review of atherosclerotic risk factors is essential, as is a detailed history and physical examination for findings indicative of poor prognosis (e.g., rest pain, dependent rubor, cold extremity, painful ulceration, necrotic tissue). Patients with evidence of worrisome disease should be referred promptly for exercise Doppler study to identify candidates for angiography and surgical intervention (see Chapter 23). Because evidence of peripheral vascular disease is a strong predictor of concurrent cardiovascular disease with its attendant morbidity and mortality, a thorough cardiac assessment is essential, especially if surgical intervention is being contemplated (see below).

Medical Management

The basic objectives of medical management are to control or limit disease progression, increase exercise tolerance, and minimize risk of complications.

Smoking Cessation. The most important methods for achieving these objectives are cessation of cigarette smoking, regular daily exercise, and meticulous foot care. Smoking hastens progression of atherosclerosis and may further impair blood flow by inducing vasoconstriction. *Smoking cessation* ranks as a major priority for the patient with peripheral arterial disease. Cessation can reduce rest pain, claudication, risk of amputation, and need for bypass surgery. The risk of repeat occlusion after angioplasty or bypass falls by over two thirds in those who quit. Moreover, quitting decreases cardiovascular morbidity and mortality. The chances of successfully quitting are greatest when a smoker becomes symptomatic from a complication of smoking; the physician's influence is considerable in this context. Nicotine gum or transdermal patch serves as a useful cessation aid by minimizing nicotine withdrawal, although nicotine may induce vasospasm (see Chapter 54). Because vasospasm usually does not play a major role in claudication, nicotine therapy is probably not contraindicated in these patients, but care is advised if used.

Exercise. Daily exercise remains a cornerstone of the treatment program, even though it now appears unlikely that it increases skeletal muscle blood flow or development of collaterals in the ischemic limb. Suggested mechanisms include improvements in muscle metabolism, peak oxygen consumption, red cell movement, and pain threshold. Whatever the reason, physical training significantly increases the pain-free walking distance, which emphasizes that claudication is not strictly a symptom of abnormal hemodynamics. The programs showing the best results are those that combine supervised *group walking sessions* with additional sessions performed daily at home. The best candidates are those with stable intermittent claudication who are free of rest pain, ulceration, unstable angina, congestive heart failure, and severe lung disease or arthritis. Although group results are excellent, predicting outcome in an individual patient is difficult. Most who achieve benefit report it within 3 months of initiating an exercise program. Regularity of exercise is more important than intensity or duration, although at least 30 min/d of continuous leg exercise appears necessary. Any form of dynamic leg exercise will suffice, including stationary bicycling, stair climbing, and walking. An exercise program can also reduce cardiovascular risk (see Chapter 29).

Foot Care. Careful attention to foot care is vital to prevention of limb loss. It has been estimated that up to 80% of amputations required in diabetics are attributable to poor foot care. Feet need to be inspected daily, especially in diabetics with peripheral neuropathy that limits protective sensation. As little as an hour of patient education has been shown to reduce the amputation and ulceration rate by two thirds.

Atherosclerotic Risk Factors. Aggressive treatment of *hyperlipidemia* can reduce or halt atherosclerotic plaque progression in peripheral vessels; modest plaque regression has also been demonstrated. Some decrease in risk and severity of symptomatic peripheral ischemic disease can be expected, but the most important benefit stems from the marked reductions in cardiovascular morbidity and mortality. Because patients with peripheral arterial disease are at high risk for life-threatening cardiovascular complications, they stand to gain considerably from aggressive lipid-lowering therapy (see Chapter 27).

If *hypertension* is present, it too deserves attention (see Chapter 26). The effect of blood pressure reduction on progression of peripheral vascular disease remains unknown, but treatment clearly reduces morbidity and mortality from stroke and cardiovascular disease. Choosing an agent on the basis of its effect on peripheral vascular tone does not appear to be critical, although some patients complain of worsening symptoms on beta-blocker therapy. Controlled studies have failed to confirm an adverse effect with beta-blockers. Antihypertensive agents with vasodilating potential (e.g., calcium channel blockers) do not materially improve claudication symptoms. Angiotensin-converting enzyme inhibitors are contraindicated if there is co-existing renal artery stenosis.

Weight reduction can be helpful by lessening work load and reducing metabolic demands of the extremities. In addition, weight reduction may also help lower lipid levels, glucose intolerance, and cardiovascular risk (see Chapter 10).

Control of diabetes (see Chapter 102) is essential to limb preservation, mostly by reducing risk of neuropathy. To date, there is no evidence that "tight" control of diabetes improves the clinical course of large-vessel peripheral arterial disease. Perhaps that is because diabetic peripheral vascular disease begins earlier and progresses more rapidly than that of other patients. Moreover, large vessels can remain relatively patent, whereas small vessels become occluded. Foot care is essential.

Hyperhomocysteinemia may be responsible in patients who present with extensive premature peripheral arterial disease (occurring before age 50). Elevated homocysteine levels respond to use of folate supplements plus vitamins B_6 and B_{12} (see Chapter 31).

Pharmacologic Therapy. *Antiplatelet agents* hold some promise. Although there is no evidence that aspirin improves claudication symptoms per se, many clinicians use the drug in peripheral artery disease patients to reduce their risks of stroke and cardiovascular events (see Chapters 30, 31, and 171). Moreover, there is some angiographic evidence of an inhibitory effect on progression of peripheral atherosclerosis. *Dipyridamole* may have similar effects on the peripheral vasculature, but its use is limited by its adverse effects on the ischemic heart (increased risk of cardiac events believed due to a steal phenomenon). *Ticlopidine*, a potent antagonist of platelet adenosine diphosphate, has demonstrated a modest benefit in claudication symptoms, but its use is limited by risks of neutropenia and thrombotic thrombocytopenic purpura. *Clopidogrel*, a similarly potent antiplatelet agent without the associated hematologic risks, has not been evaluated for efficacy in improving claudication symptoms but may be considered as an alternative to aspirin in patients unable to tolerate salicylates. Oral anticoagulants (e.g., warfarin) provide no benefit in chronic management of peripheral arterial disease.

Cilostozol, which possesses antiplatelet, antithrombotic, and vasodilating properties, is approved by the U.S. Food and Drug Administration for symptomatic treatment of intermittent claudication. Although the exact mechanism(s) of action responsible for benefit remains uncertain, the drug does modestly increase walking distances (by 28% to 54%) in comparison with placebo and pentoxyphylline in patients with mild-to-moderate claudication. Onset of action can be slow, ranging from 2 to 12 weeks. Side effects include headache, which can be severe, and tachycardia; ventricular ectopy has been noted. The drug is contraindicated in persons with congestive heart failure. There is concern about long-term use, based on reports of cardiovascular injury in animals exposed to the drug more than 52 weeks. *Pentoxifylline*, an agent that appears to increase erythrocyte deformability and blood viscosity and reduce platelet activity, has been promoted as a potentially useful drug for treatment of symptomatic peripheral arterial disease. In placebo-controlled trials, benefit is nil to modest. High cost, nausea, and dizziness further limit pentoxiphylline's appeal.

Gene therapy and *angiogenesis* are exciting areas of intense investigation. Work is ongoing with growth factors for vascular endothelial cells and fibroblasts in an attempt to stimulate angiogenesis. The hope is to stimulate capillary proliferation and collateral blood vessel formation in ischemic tissues. Such arterial gene therapy holds promise, especially for patients with nonreconstructible disease by conventional angioplasty or surgery. Agents that block specific inducers of atherosclerosis are also under investigation, including *omega-3 fatty acids* and *prostaglandin E analogues*.

Chelation therapy and *vasodilators* are heavily promoted but provide no demonstrable benefit to symptoms or clinical course when tested in placebo-controlled, double-blind, randomized trials. The failure of vasodilator therapy reinforces the view that vasoconstriction plays little role in claudication. Although vasodilators may not be helpful, vasoconstrictors can be harmful and should be used with caution, if at all, in patients with severe disease, especially in those with ulcers or rest pain. *Ergot derivatives* are a classic example; *alpha-blockers* also may aggravate ischemic symptoms and impede healing of skin lesions. *Beta-blockers* do not compromise perfusion or worsened symptoms, despite anecdotal reports.

Interventional Therapies

Candidacy. Patients who continue to have disabling symptoms despite implementation of a full medical regimen (smoking cessation, exercise program, control of cardiovascular risk factors) are potential candidates for interventional therapy. With the advent of angioplasty and improvements in surgical technique, the threshold for invasive therapy has been lowered, but the decision to consider such treatment should not be taken lightly or made prematurely. The relatively favorable natural history of peripheral vascular disease and the excellent responses to medical measures argue for resorting to interventional therapy only after other approaches have failed and the patient is incapacitated or a limb is at risk. Persisting inability to walk two blocks and carry out activities of daily living are typical functional criteria for consideration of interventional therapy. Rest pain and a nonhealing ulcer are even more compelling reasons.

Before referring the patient for interventional therapy, a full set of noninvasive studies (including *Doppler ultrasound* scanning and *segmental blood pressures*) should be ordered to more precisely document the location and severity of disease (see Chapter 23). The best candidates for interventional measures are those with proximal disease and preserved distal runoff. Patients who prove to have predominantly small vessel disease (e.g., diabetics) do not benefit much from interventional therapy unless there is concurrent proximal disease that can be alleviated. *Angiography* will be necessary to make the final determination, but detailed noninvasive study can help screen patients and minimize unnecessary angiography, with its attendant risks of intimal dissection, groin hematoma, and dye-induced renal failure.

Percutaneous Transluminal Angioplasty and Stenting. PTA has emerged as a cost-effective and less invasive alternative to bypass surgery, especially for the patient with segmental stenosis of the aortoiliac or femoral artery. In patients with lesions amenable to angioplasty, PTA produces short- and long-term results similar to those of surgery. The cost of PTA is one fifth that of surgery; however, durability of result is moderately less, reducing but not eliminating the cost differential.

The procedure is typically performed at the time of angiography, using a balloon catheter inserted percutaneously at a remote site, usually the femoral artery, and manipulated fluoroscopically within the diseased segment of artery. With balloon inflation, the obstructing plaque is cracked and vessel lumen enhanced.

Results are best for short segmental stenoses in proximal vessels. Patency rates, both immediate and long-term, are a function of location. Aortoiliac procedures average a 90% immediate success rate, and 80% are patent at 5 years; for a femoral lesion, the rates average 75% and 50%, respectively. Risks include groin hematoma, dissection, renal ischemia, and distal embolization. The overall complication rate averages 10%, with about 2% to 5% being serious enough to warrant surgical intervention. Mortality is less than 0.5%. As expected, experienced teams in centers performing large numbers of PTAs have the best results and the fewest complications.

PTA is suitable for about 30% of patients being considered for interventional therapy. The remainder tend to have more widespread or distal occlusive disease. PTA has a lower morbidity and mortality than standard surgery, making it an especially attractive option in patients who are bad surgical risks because of severe underlying disease. In addition, it may be combined with surgery (e.g., correcting a proximal iliac stenosis by balloon angioplasty and bypassing a more distal lesion with a femoropopliteal graft). Poor candidates for PTA include those with a complete occlusion, a stenotic lesion greater than 10 cm in length, multiple serial stenoses, calcified or eccentric plaque, or poor distal runoff.

Stenting is used to improve results of PTA when there is elastic recoil or localized plaque dissection that compromises the vessel lumen. Whether routine initial use of stents with PTA is a better overall strategy than selective use of stenting remains under study. Available data suggest that selective stenting is more cost effective. Advances in stent technology are encouraging increasingly aggressive use of PTA to treat more extensively diseased arterial segments.

Recanalization Techniques. Because angioplasty cannot be performed on a totally occluded vessel, there has been considerable interest in *recanalization techniques.* *Laser* methods and *mechanical arthrectomy* devices have been applied to allow percutaneous catheter-based opening of atherosclerotic arteries. The initial enthusiasm and commercial promotion of such devices have proven premature; these techniques are rarely used as sole therapy in current practice. With current technology, these techniques can sometimes serve as an *adjunct* to conventional balloon angioplasty, carving out a small channel in a limited area of total occlusion so that a standard PTA balloon catheter may traverse the lesion. The literature should be followed for well-designed studies of this emerging technology.

Surgical Therapy. In patients with *claudication alone*, surgery should be considered only in those who are so severely disabled that their ability to earn a living is compromised, their desired life-style is intolerably limited, and their vascular lesions are not amenable to PTA. The role of arterial reconstruction for claudication alone remains controversial. In general, the physician must attempt to determine the significance of ischemic symptoms in each patient. The patient's age, work requirements, social circumstances, and general state of health must all be considered. When doubt exists, referral for a surgical opinion is often useful.

Surgical referral is clearly indicated in patients with *advanced ischemia* resulting in *ischemic rest pain*, nonhealing *ischemic ulcerations*, or *gangrene*. Such limbs are clearly at risk, and arterial reconstruction is indicated, if feasible, to maximize chances of limb salvage. In such circumstances, patients should be referred for surgical investigation as soon as possible, before tissue necrosis or infection become too extensive. The morbidity and mortality of common revascularization procedures is in many instances less than that associated with major amputation. For poor-risk patients, various "extraanatomic" reconstructions are also available, which may be done with even more safety.

Many patients with significant arterial insufficiency that requires surgery also have underlying coronary disease that is hemodynamically critical. The coronary disease may be clinically silent due to the exercise restrictions stemming from severe claudication. Such patients have high rates of perioperative morbidity and mortality. *Stress testing* before surgery helps to identify high-risk patients who would benefit from coronary revascularization before peripheral vascular surgery (see Chapter 36).

Great progress has been made in the surgical management of arterial insufficiency. With an experienced surgeon, careful preoperative cardiac evaluation, and good anesthetic and postoperative management, the patient may anticipate successful correction of aortoiliac occlusive disease, with a mortality risk of only 1% to 2% and excellent long-term patency of approximately 85% to 90% at 5 years. Femoropopliteal or tibial artery bypass may be done with even greater safety, although long-term patency is somewhat less, with approximately 70% to 75% of saphenous vein grafts still patent at 5 years. If the saphenous vein is unavailable for use, a number of suitable alternative prosthetic grafts have been developed within recent years. With improvement of direct reconstructive methods, lumbar sympathectomy is rarely considered a primary mode of treatment.

PATIENT EDUCATION

Patient education is vital, because a favorable outcome requires strong patient participation in the treatment program (cessation of smoking, daily exercise, foot care, risk factor reduction). Compliance is facilitated by the patient's understanding the atherosclerotic basis of the problem, the factors that may aggravate the severity of symptoms, and the rationale behind the measures recommended. Many patients come to the physician with reluctance to walk and fear of limb loss. The benefits of exercise, the likelihood of improvement, and the low risk of limb loss are usually of great comfort and reassurance to the patient and family. The importance for foot care must be repeatedly emphasized, especially in the diabetic. A single hour of detailed foot care instruction can greatly reduce the risk of limb loss. Also important to stress is that even the most trivial foot injury or lesion requires prompt attention. Specific instructions for an appropriate exercise program are essential; recommending such a program can provide a considerable psychological boost.

The psychologic management of the patient is essential in preventing depression and invalidism. Emphasis should be on the generally favorable prognosis and the patient's ability to improve his or her own condition. Frequent follow-up in the early stages of the treatment program is reassuring and helps maximize compliance. The patient with new claudication should be seen at least every 2 to 3 months to assess exercise tolerance and inspect the feet for potential pressure points and ulcers.

INDICATIONS FOR REFERRAL AND ADMISSION

Patients with disabling claudication who fail to respond to conservative therapy and have noninvasive evidence of proximal disease should be referred for consideration of PTA. Patients needing direct referral for consideration of bypass surgery are those with such severe disease (rest pain, nonhealing ulcers, early gangrene) that they are at risk for losing the limb. Urgent hospitalization is indicated for the patient with early gangrenous changes or signs of infection in an ischemic extremity. Those with refractory claudication whose life-style or livelihood are *intolerably* compromised by the inability to walk distances and who appear by noninvasive testing to have disease too distal or too diffuse for PTA are also potential candidates for surgery. The final determination regarding candidacy for angioplasty or surgery requires angiography, but noninvasive screening can maximize the appropriateness of the referral.

THERAPEUTIC RECOMMENDATIONS

- *Cessation of smoking.* Total cessation is essential, both to limit disease progression and to prevent reocclusion after interventional therapy. The patient must be firmly told that he or she must stop smoking completely. Smoking as little as five cigarettes per day can compromise a limb. The physician must be unequivocal about this, because patients often interpret half-hearted advice as only a suggestion (see Chapter 54).
- *Exercise.* In the patient with claudication, the best exercise is daily walking. Patients are advised to walk to the point of discomfort, stop briefly, and then resume walking. At least 30 minutes of relatively continuous walking each day is recommended. A weekly group session can be extremely useful. An exercise bicycle can be used as an alternative mode of exercise. It is important to emphasize to the patient that pain does not indicate harm or damage to the leg and that exercise can help rather than aggravate the condition. Any tendency to restrict activity, sometimes to the point of invalidism or confinement to the home, should be avoided, unless severe ischemia is present. Consideration of the patient's cardiac status is important in the design of the exercise program (see Chapters 18 and 31).
- *Elevating the head of the bed.* Patients with advanced ischemia and rest pain at night may benefit from raising the head of the bed on 6- to 8-inch blocks so that the feet and legs are made slightly dependent; gravity may aid blood flow enough to allow more comfortable sleep.
- *Foot care.* This aspect of preventive medicine is of extreme importance, particularly in the diabetic patient who often lacks protective sensation due to neuropathy and who may be more susceptible to infection. Because there is often a great deal of confusion about what is meant by "foot care," its components require elaboration:

  1. *Inspection.* The feet should be inspected daily for any scratches, cuts, fissures, blisters, or other lesions, particularly around the nail beds, between the toes, and on the heels.
  2. *Washing.* The feet should be washed daily with mild soap and lukewarm (never hot) water. Rinse thoroughly and dry gently but completely, particularly between the toes. Excessive soaking, leading to maceration, should be avoided.
  3. *Lanolin.* A moisturizing cream such as lanolin or Eucerin should be applied to the skin of the foot and heel but not between the toes. A light film, well rubbed in, will prevent drying and cracking of the skin, which is often the genesis of a lesion, particularly on the heel. The cream should not be applied thickly or allowed to "cake" on the foot.
  4. *Lambswool.* A small amount of lambast or dry cotton or gauze may be placed between the toes to prevent lesions, which may occur if toes are allowed to rub together, particularly if orthopedic deformities of the toes are present.
  5. *Powder.* An antifungal powder, such as nystatin, should be applied between the toes if excessive moisture or maceration is a problem.
  6. *Proper footwear.* Properly fitting shoes with ample space in the forefoot are essential. Special shoes are rarely necessary.
  7. *Podiatry.* Nails should be cut with extreme care, in good light, and only if vision is normal. They should be cut straight across and even with the end of the toe, never close to the skin or into the corner of the nailbed. Any abnormality of the nails and any corns or calluses should be treated by the physician or podiatrist.
  8. *Avoidance of trauma.* Never use adhesive tape on the skin (paper tape is better) or any strong antiseptic solution. Avoid heating pads, hot packs, heat lamps, and scalding hot water. Never walk barefoot.

- *Patient education.* It is the physician's responsibility to educate patients in these points of foot care and to urge them to call at the first sign of difficulty; delay can lead to limb loss if gangrene and/or osteomyelitis ensues.

- *Weight reduction* (see Chapter 233).
- *Aggressive control of major atherosclerotic risk factors* (e.g., hypertension [see Chapter 26], hyperlipidemia [see Chapter 27], and smoking). Aggressive control can halt disease progression and may promote plaque regression. It also lowers the associated cardiovascular morbidity and mortality (see Chapters 30 and 31). In patients with premature disease, test for homocysteine elevation and treat with folate and vitamins B_6 and B_{12} if positive (see Chapter 31).
- *Medications.* Consider aspirin for its generally beneficial effects on cardiovascular risk. Consider a short course (less than 3 months) of cilostazol if symptoms are interfering with ability to engage in an exercise program; avoid longer term use and use in persons with heart failure or ventricular dysrhythmias.
- *Referral for Consideration of Revascularization.* In patients with claudication alone, PTA is worth considering if the pain is disabling and refractory to a full trial of medical therapy and noninvasive study suggests only focal proximal disease. Referral for consideration of surgery is indicated only in patients who have failed medical therapy, have disease that appears amenable to surgery but not PTA, and are so significantly disabled by claudication that their livelihood or life-style is intolerably compromised by their inability to walk distances. Final decision requires angiography, but noninvasive study to screen for appropriate candidates is essential. In patients with more severe disease, those with rest pain, nonhealing ulcers, or early gangrene who have a limb that is in jeopardy should be considered for operation with some urgency. Conduct preoperative stress testing to identify patients with high cardiac risk who might need further cardiac evaluation and possibly cardiac revascularization prior to peripheral vascular surgery.

ANNOTATED BIBLIOGRAPHY

Brewster DC, Cambria RP, Darling RC, et al. Long-term results of combined iliac balloon angioplasty and distal surgical revascularization. Ann Surg 1989;210:324. *(Good long-term results for combined interventional therapy.)*

Byrne J, Darling RC, Change BB, et al. Infrainguinal arterial reconstruction for claudication: is it worth the risk? An analysis of 409 procedures. J Vasc Surg 1999;29:259. *(Results data emphasizing benefit and safety in most patients with claudication.)*

Coffman JD. Intermittent claudication—be conservative. N Engl J Med 1991;325:577. *(Editorial stressing relatively benign natural history of the condition.)*

Criqui MH, Langer RD, Fronek A, et al. Mortality over a period of 10 years in patients with peripheral arterial disease. N Engl J Med 1992;326:381. *(Relative risk of all-cause mortality was 3.0, due mostly to a sixfold increase in risk of cardiovascular death.)*

Dawson DL, Cutler BS, Meissner MH, et al. Cilostozol has beneficial effects in treatment of intermittent claudication. Results from a multicenter randomized, prospective, double-blind trial. Circulation 1998;98:678. *(Short-term safety and modest efficacy demonstrated.)*

Duffield RGM, Lewis B, Miller NE, et al. Treatment of hyperlipidemia retards progression of symptomatic femoral atherosclerosis. Lancet 1983;2:639. *(Early evidence that aggressive lipid lowering could markedly slow disease progression.)*

Ernst E, Fialke V. A review of the clinical effectiveness of exercise therapy for intermittent claudication. Arch Intern Med 1993;153:2357. *(A supervised high-intensity program of at least 2 months works best.)*

Hiatt WR, Regensteiner JG, Wolfel EE, et al. Effect of exercise training on skeletal muscle histology and metabolism in peripheral arterial disease. J Appl Physiol 1996;81:780. *(Possible mechanisms of benefit.)*

Hirsch AT, Treat-Jacobson D, Lando HA, et al. The role of tobacco cessation, antiplatelet, and lipid-lowering therapies in the treatment of peripheral arterial disease. Vasc Med 1997;2:243. *(Good review of conservative treatment measures.)*

Isner JM, Walsh K, Symes J, et al. Arterial gene therapy for therapeutic angiogenesis in patients with peripheral arterial disease. Circulation 1995;91:2687. *(Pioneering work and promising early results.)*

Krupski WC. The peripheral vascular consequences of smoking. Ann Vasc Surg 1991;3:291. *(A thorough review of the vascular effects and possible mechanisms by which tobacco usage causes or aggravates atherosclerotic disease.)*

Malone JM, Snyder M, Anderson G, et al. Prevention of amputation by diabetic education. Am J Surg 1989;158:520. *(A single 1-hour educational program on foot care resulted in a marked decrease in the amputation rate.)*

Radack K, Wyderski RJ. Conservative management of intermittent claudication. Ann Intern Med 1990;113:135. *(Review of the evidence for efficacy of walking, smoking cessation, and pentoxiphylline; 99 references.)*

Regensteiner JG, Steiner JF, Hiatt WR. Exercise training improves functional status in patients with peripheral arterial disease. J Vasc Surg 1996;23:104. *(Objective outcomes measures demonstrating significant benefit.)*

Reiber GE, Pecoraro RE, Koepsell TD. Risk factors for amputation in patients with diabetes mellitus. Ann Intern Med 1992;117:97. *(Identifies important clinical features that were predictive.)*

Tetteroo E, van der Graaf Y, Bosch JL, et al. Randomized comparison of primary stent placement versus primary angioplasty followed by selective stent placement in patients with iliac-artery occlusive disease. Dutch Iliac Stent Trial Group. Lancet 1998;351:1153. *(Suggests that routine stenting is not necessary or beneficial; selective stenting saved expense as well.)*

Wilson SE, Wolf GL, Cross AP. Percutaneous transluminal angioplasty versus operation for peripheral arteriosclerosis. Report of a prospective randomized trial in a selected group of patients. J Vasc Surg 1989;9:1. *(In a group of patients with lesions amenable to PTA, short- and long-term success rates were similar for both surgery and PTA.)*

Wong T, Detsky A. Preoperative cardiac risk assessment for patients having peripheral vascular surgery. Ann Intern Med 1992;116:743. *(High risk of infarction makes preoperative assessment essential; good review of the data.)*

35

Management of Peripheral Venous Disease

DAVID C. BREWSTER

Problems of the peripheral venous system (varicose veins, venous insufficiency, and phlebitis) are extremely prevalent, especially among the elderly. Many physicians do little for the more mundane complaints referable to the venous system because of lack of knowledge and confusion about pathophysiology and proper management. Such attitudes are unfortunate, because neglected venous problems can cause considerable disability and place the patient at serious risk. The primary management of venous diseases is still largely nonoperative, and great benefit is possible with well-conceived office care.

PATHOPHYSIOLOGY AND CLINICAL PRESENTATION

The high frequency of venous disorders of the lower extremities is unique to humans and reflects the consequences of an upright posture and gravity. To return blood from the periphery to the right heart, the venous system in the legs must work against the force of gravity without the aid of organs specifically designed for this purpose. A number of factors work to lessen venous pressure in the leg and propel blood toward the heart. These include the *"muscular pump"* effect of the exercising calf musculature, the negative intrathoracic pressure created by the *"bellows effect"* of the chest wall with respiration, and the presence of multiple valves in both superficial and deep venous systems. The last prevents reflux of blood and serves to reduce pressure in the veins that would otherwise equal the weight of an uninterrupted column of blood from the heart to the foot (approximately 100 mm Hg).

A knowledge of basic anatomy of the venous system is vital to evaluation and management of lower extremity venous problems. The existence of two venous systems, superficial and deep, is well known. A third system linking the superficial and deep systems, the communicating or perforating veins, is less well recognized but of great importance. Valves also exist in the communicating veins, permitting flow from the superficial to the deep system but preventing retrograde flow.

When functioning properly, these three systems work in coordinated fashion. The deep system, composed of paired anterior and posterior tibial and peroneal veins, popliteal veins, and superficial and deep femoral veins, handles approximately 80% to 90% of venous return, whereas the superficial network of greater and lesser saphenous systems is much less important in this respect.

Clinical disorders of the venous system usually stem from obstruction to venous return due to thrombosis of the vein lumen or from incompetent venous valves that allow reflux of blood and persistent elevation of venous pressure in the leg and foot.

Varicose Veins

Pathophysiology. The superficial veins lie in the subcutaneous tissue and lack the support afforded by muscle and fascial compartments, making them most prone to difficulty. Varicose veins are extremely common and probably affect some 10% to 20% of the adult population to some degree. They are more common in women, who also seem more likely to consult a physician for advice. A family history of varicosities is present in most patients and lends support to the concept of a hereditary or congenital etiology. It is unclear whether the primary problem is a congenital *incompetence of valves* or a *weakness* of the venous wall itself, which causes dilation of the vein lumen and subsequent valve inadequacy. In any event, a self-perpetuating cycle ensues of venous reflux leading to further vein dilation and valve failure.

In time, the poorly supported superficial veins widen, elongate, and become tortuous. In a smaller percentage of patients, the initial defect may be in the communicating veins, where poorly functioning valves allow abnormal flow toward the superficial system, causing eventual overdistention. In other patients, acquired factors such as old *trauma* or venous *thrombosis* may play a role. Factors that raise intraluminal vein pressure, such as repeated *pregnancies, obesity*, or wearing of *tight garments* that constrict the thigh, may be of importance. The final common pathway remains valvular incompetence.

Clinical Presentation. Varicosities most commonly involve the veins of the greater saphenous system and its tributaries and therefore occur principally in the medial and anterior thigh, calf, and ankle regions. The lesser saphenous system may also be involved, producing varicosities of the posterior calf and lateral ankle region. The exact distribution of involved branches is of real importance only when considering surgical correction.

The presenting symptoms of varicose veins are extremely variable and often seem to bear little relationship to the apparent severity of the varicosities. Complaints are more frequent in women, particularly young women at the time of the menstrual period. Clearly, hormonal factors that favor fluid retention may aggravate venous distention, but in many such patients the main concern is over the cosmetic appearance of minor varicosities.

Typically, patients complain of local aching or burning pain in the area of the varicosities, particularly at the end of the day after having been on their feet at work. *"Tiredness," "heaviness,"* or a *"bursting"* sensation are commonly reported. *Itchiness* due to a stasis dermatitis may occur in the region of a severe and chronic varix, especially in the region of an incompetent perforating vein. Mild *swelling* of the ankle region may occur; however, this is relatively unusual with uncomplicated varicose veins. Similarly, ulceration attributable solely to varicose veins is rare. Severe swelling or recurrent ulceration almost always implies problems with the deep venous system (see below).

Large varices may be subject to trauma and bleeding. Much more commonly, however, the distended vein with sluggish blood flow may thrombose, leading to *superficial phlebitis*.

Chronic Venous Insufficiency

Pathophysiology. Chronic venous insufficiency, also called the *postphlebitic syndrome*, is a common chronic disorder that is particularly disabling if stubborn venous ulcers develop. Although the superficial venous system may be secondarily involved with varicose veins, the principal defect lies in the deep venous system. A documented history of *deep venous thrombosis* (DVT) can be obtained in fewer than one half of patients with chronic venous insufficiency, but it is believed to be the underlying etiology in most instances. DVT can often be clinically silent, as documented by prospective ^{125}I-fibrinogen scanning studies in postoperative patients. Despite subsequent recanalization of deep venous occlusions, the phlebitic inflammatory process deforms or destroys venous valves in the deep system, and their incompetence results in reflux and increased venous pressure. Communicating veins undergo similar changes through valvular damage or simply by exposure to chronically elevated pressure from the deep venous system.

Some authorities believe *congenital valvular incompetence* may also play a role, similar to varicose veins of the superficial system. Regardless of cause, high venous pressure generated by muscular contraction forces blood through damaged valves in communicating veins toward the superficial system, resulting in "ambulatory venous hypertension."

Such venous hypertension results in *edema*, usually most prominent in the calf and ankle region. Indeed, swelling is one of the hallmarks of chronic venous insufficiency and usually differentiates the problem from simple varicose veins. Swelling of the thigh may occur, denoting valvular incompetence at the iliofemoral level as well. Generally, this is less severe and less troublesome than the edema of the lower leg.

Venous hypertension leads not only to interstitial fluid accumulation but also to extravasation of plasma proteins and red blood cells into subcutaneous tissues. In time, this results in *brawny induration* of the skin and *pigmentation* of the thickened but fragile tissue. The presence of edema and continual high venous pressure results in reduced local capillary flow and relative hypoxia, which further increase the likelihood of tissue breakdown and subsequent healing difficulties. Eventually these processes and accompanying infection lead to damage of the lymphatics, aggravating swelling and local tissue breakdown.

Clinical Presentation. The presenting complaints of patients with chronic venous insufficiency usually center around swelling or ulceration of the lower leg. Chronic recurrent *swelling* causes a sensation of tightness or bursting and heaviness or aching of the limb. This is often worst at the end of the day and may largely disappear overnight. With chronicity, brawny *induration, hyperpigmentation*, and skin *ulceration* may ensue.

Superficial Thrombophlebitis

The cause of acute thrombus formation in the venous system is often unclear, but in most instances factors contributing to *intimal damage, stasis,* and *hypercoagulability* (Virchow's triad) comprise the pathophysiologic determinants of venous thrombophlebitis. The condition almost always arises in varicose veins and is clearly a result of static blood flow in these channels. Trauma may occasionally be implicated. In the upper extremity, the cause is most often iatrogenic after intravenous cannulation, but when it occurs in several locations over a short time span, it suggests *migratory superficial phlebitis*. The latter occurs in the context of occult malignancy, especially carcinoma of the pancreas, presumably due to a hypercoagulable state induced by the tumor. On examination of the patient with superficial thrombophlebitis, there will be pain, tenderness, and erythema along the course of the vein, which may also be palpated as a tender cord or knot.

Deep Vein Thrombophlebitis

Pathophysiology. As in superficial thrombophlebitis, there is usually some combination of *intimal damage, stasis,* and *hypercoagulability*. In about half of instances, the immediate cause is an identifiable self-limited event (e.g., recent surgery, new onset of paralysis, stasis, trauma, pregnancy) or some other acquired factor; in the other half of cases, no clinical precipitant is evident, leading to the designation "*idiopathic*." A host of risk factors have been identified (Table 35.1). The emerging pathophysiologic view of idiopathic DVT is that many cases occur in the context of underlying chronic hypercoagulability

Table 35.1. Causes of "Idiopathic" Deep Vein Thrombophlebitis

RISK FACTOR	RISK[a]	PERCENT OF CASES OF IDIOPATHIC DISEASE
Hereditary Causes		
Factor V Leiden mutation	+	20% first DVT, up to 50% recurrent
Deficiency in protein S or C or antithrombin III	++	7% first DVT, up to 20% recurrent
Homocysteinemia	++	?
Prothrombin gene mutation	++	6% first DVT, up to 18% recurrent
Acquired Causes		
Adenocarcinoma	+++	8% first DVT, up to 17% recurrent
Antiphospholipid antibodies	+++	5% first DVT

[a]Risk increased markedly when present in combination with factor V Leiden mutation.
DVT; deep vein thrombophlebitis.

(either hereditary or acquired) and that a supervening clinical or subclinical event exacerbates the hypercoagulability or causes venous stasis or endothelial injury, triggering acute thrombophlebitis. This view of idiopathic DVT as a *chronic disease* has important implications for therapy (see below) and is supported by the high frequency of recurrent disease, often occurring in a previously unaffected limb.

Hereditary Factors. A number of hereditary risk factors have been identified in the past few years. Mutation in the gene controlling factor V synthesis leads to production of *factor V Leiden*, which is resistant to inactivation by the endogenous anticoagulant, activated protein C. The factor V variant can be found in 25% to 50% of persons with idiopathic DVT and is particularly prevalent among persons of European decent. Although not an extremely powerful risk factor by itself, factor V Leiden confers an independent degree of risk that may rise substantially in the context of other risk factors, such as estrogen use. The *prothrombin gene mutation* is found in only about 5% to 10% of cases, but its presence increases risk by about two to four times more than does factor V Leiden. Deficiencies in the production of proteins that limit clotting to the site of vascular injury (*proteins S and C and antithrombin III*) are found in about 20% of persons with recurrent DVT. Most patients are heterozygotes for the deficiency, which is a potent risk factor for DVT.

Acquired Factors. Major *trauma, recent surgery* (within 3 months), *pregnancy, estrogen use, immobilization,* and *congestive heart failure* are among the powerful readily apparent precipitants of acquired causes of DVT (Table 35.1). Less evident is the production of antiphospholipid antibodies, which are believed to induce thrombosis by causing vascular injury or by interacting with other abnormal clotting factors to induce a hypercoagulable state. Two classes of antiphospholipid antibodies have been identified: *anticardiolipin* and *lupus anticoagulant*. Both appear to develop in response to prior infection. A *secondary antiphospholipid syndrome* is seen in persons with systemic lupus erythematosus. Low titers of antiphospholipid antibody can be found in a small proportion of normal persons and in up to 25% of pregnant woman by the end of the first trimester. A sevenfold increase in risk is associated with production of antiphospholipid antibodies, especially the lupus anticoagulant variety, making this a potent acquired risk factor for DVT. *Malignancy,* especially adenocarcinoma originating in the lung, gastrointestinal tract, or urogenital system, substantially increases the risk of DVT (presumably by inducing hypercoagulability). Less appreciated is the relationship of *occult malignancy* to DVT. Among patients presenting with a first case of idiopathic DVT, more than 10% have been found to have an underlying occult malignancy. The risk of developing clinically evident cancer within 2 years of an episode of idiopathic DVT is estimated at about 8% for a first attack and 17% for recurrent DVT.

Clinical Presentation. DVT is notoriously variable and often subtle in its clinical presentation. Classically, the patient complains of pain in the limb, worse with motion, walking, or dependency and better with rest or elevation of the extremity. Leg edema below the level of the clot, pain on compression of the knee, a *Homan's sign* (calf pain produced by dorsiflexion of the foot), and a palpable cord are cited as the classic physical findings. With extensive DVT, a dusky cyanosis may appear.

Engorged or prominent superficial veins are also suggestive of deep venous obstruction. Unfortunately, most classic findings have proven to be disappointingly low in sensitivity and specificity. A patient reporting little or no pain and showing no calf tenderness may harbor extensive deep venous clots, whereas another with impressive pain, calf tenderness, and an apparently positive Homan's sign may be clot-free. *Unilateral leg edema* may be the only finding; it stands out as the most sensitive indicator of DVT.

EVALUATION

Varicose Veins

On physical examination one should note the extent and location of the varicosities and, more importantly, look for signs suggesting pathology in the deep venous system: thrombophlebitis, stasis changes, ulceration, or swelling. Such findings are unusual in patients with only superficial venous pathology but commonly found in those with involvement of both superficial and deep systems. Complaints of leg pain should be carefully evaluated to rule out other possibilities, such as arterial insufficiency, orthopedic or joint disorders, or neurologic problems. Severe varicosities occurring at a young age suggest a congenital arteriovenous malformation, whereas varicosities appearing after trauma should always raise the question of an arteriovenous fistula, which also may produce a bruit.

Venous Insufficiency

Venous insufficiency needs to be distinguished from other causes of leg edema such as lymphatic obstruction, hypoalbuminemia, and DVT (see Chapter 22). Any accompanying leg ulcers must be differentiated from those due to arterial insufficiency, which tend to be more "punched out" in appearance and localized to the dorsum or lateral aspect of the foot or ankle. A history of claudication, rest pain relieved by dependency, absent pulses, bruits, dependent rubor, and atrophic skin changes also helps distinguish arterial disease from venous insufficiency. Noninvasive studies can be helpful (see Chapter 23).

Superficial Thrombophlebitis

Physical examination should strive to exclude other diagnoses that may be confused with superficial thrombophlebitis, such as cellulitis or lymphangitis. In the latter two, one notes the absence of a palpable thrombosed vein, widespread distribution of erythema and swelling beyond the course of a vein, and identification of a possible focus of infection. Musculoskeletal and neurologic causes of pain and tenderness should be sought, such as a Baker's cyst in the popliteal fossa (see Chapter 152), or radicular pain (see Chapter 147). Swelling of the extremity should also be carefully noted, as isolated superficial phlebitis should not contribute to generalized edema.

Deep Vein Thrombophlebitis

The initial evaluation of the patient who complains of unilateral leg edema (more than 3 cm difference in calf diameter)—with or without calf pain—must include consideration of DVT (see Chapter 22). Prompt detection of deep vein thrombophlebitis is critical; undetected and untreated, it may lead to pulmonary embolization, with its substantial risk of major cardiopulmonary morbidity and mortality. Identification of DVT in the absence of obvious precipitants raises the question of underlying hypercoagulability and occult malignancy, which needs to be addressed.

History and Physical Examination. Truly unilateral swelling, particularly extending above the knee, makes venous thrombosis more likely, but cellulitis and lymphedema must also be considered. Pain alone is an unreliable symptom. The findings of calf tenderness and a "positive" Homan's' sign are by no means conclusive. Numerous studies have demonstrated the relative inaccuracy of diagnosis by history and physical examination alone (which is incorrect in up to 50% of cases) and the importance of laboratory testing. Nonetheless, a careful review of the history and physical examination for *DVT risk factors* (e.g., previous DVT, major trauma, recent surgery or pregnancy, current estrogen use, congestive heart failure, limb paralysis, concurrent adenocarcinoma, nephrotic syndrome, systemic lupus) helps to estimate risk. History should also be reviewed for a *family history of recurrent DVT*, which if present suggests a hereditary hypercoagulable state such as factor V Leiden or deficiency in proteins S and C or antithrombin III.

Laboratory Studies for Deep Vein Thrombosis (See also Chapter 22). Noninvasive studies have made a great contribution to the evaluation of patients with possible DVT. The cost savings alone related to patients found to be free of DVT, in whom venography, anticoagulation, and hospitalization are avoided, are enormous. The necessity of firmly establishing the diagnosis by means other than history or physical examination cannot be overemphasized.

Compression venous ultrasound has emerged as the most sensitive and specific of available noninvasive methods for diagnosis of DVT, especially when standard two-dimensional ultrasound ("*duplex scanning*") is enhanced by color-flow *Doppler* technology (so-called "*triplex scanning*"). Sensitivity and specificity for DVT above the knee—where risk of embolization is greatest—exceed 97%, especially with serial testing. Doppler ultrasound is considerably less sensitive (about 60%) for DVT below the knee, but this lack of sensitivity is not clinically important because risk of embolization associated with clot below the knee is negligible (about 3%). Nonetheless, vigilance is indicated in a patient at risk for DVT, because 20% to 30% of clots below the knee propagate above it. If propagation is suspected (e.g., worsening leg edema that extends above the knee) or the first test result is negative but clinical suspicion remains high, then repeat scanning every 2 to 3 days for 1 to 2 weeks is indicated. In some settings the test performs less well, such as in asymptomatic persons who have recently undergone orthopedic surgery, where test sensitivity can be as low as 62%. Drawbacks of duplex and triplex scanning include high equipment costs and required technician time and expertise. Nonetheless, the technology is widely available and clearly the diagnostic procedure of choice in most instances.

Impedance plethysmography remains in widespread use as a noninvasive alternative to Doppler ultrasound. Sensitivity for detection of DVT above the knee approaches 90% to 95% for the test when serial studies are performed, but specificity can be disappointing, producing a high rate of false positives.

Because sensitivity is very high (in excess of 95%) but specificity is not (48% to 65%), D-*dimer testing* (see Chapter 22) is best applied in conjunction with noninvasive vascular study to rule out DVT. The test contributes to assessment by serving as a means of ruling out DVT at the time of initial presentation in patients with a low or low-to-intermediate pretest probability. Its use can obviate the need for repeated noninvasive vascular study when the initial ultrasound is negative (see Chapter 22). In low-probability patients, a negative D-dimer test provides strong presumptive evidence against the diagnosis of DVT and may suffice for ruling out the condition.

Contrast venography remains the gold standard for diagnosis of DVT, but several disadvantages render it undesirable as an initial test. Not only can venography be quite uncomfortable, but it occasionally induces phlebitis (1% to 3%). Moreover, it is costly and technically unsuccessful in up to 20% of candidates. The study involves considerable expertise for both its performance and interpretation and usually requires hospitalization. Nonetheless, it continues to be an important diagnostic modality for use when the results of noninvasive study are inconclusive and the clinical situation mandates additional testing (e.g., suspected iliac-vein occlusion, worrisome disparity between clinical and laboratory findings, symptomatic postphlebitic patient whose chronic venous disease makes noninvasive study difficult to interpret).

Test Interpretation. Patients with an *intermediate-to-high pretest probability* of DVT and a positive Doppler ultrasound test result can be considered to have DVT above the knee and anticoagulated without venography. If the test is nondiagnostic, then either repeat ultrasound every 2 to 3 days for the next 1 to 2 weeks or immediate venography is indicated, depending on the degree of clinical urgency. Patients with a *low or low-to-intermediate pretest probability* and a negative ultrasound result can be confidently observed without anticoagulation. If symptoms worsen, then repeat testing can be performed. When the initial study is negative and pretest probability is low to intermediate, then anticoagulation can be held, but noninvasive testing should be repeated in 48 to 72 hours.

Assessment for Hypercoagulability. Cases in which there is no apparent acute risk factor for DVT—so-called "*idiopathic*" *DVT*—manifest a high prevalence (approaching 40%) of underlying hypercoagulability (Table 35.1) and a high rate of recurrence (e.g., up to 27% per patient-year). Such figures argue for careful consideration of *hereditary* and *acquired* causes of hypercoagulability (Table 35.1).

Acquired Conditions. Among the important acquired etiologies of idiopathic disease is the *antiphospholipid antibody syndrome*, characterized by thrombosis and elevated titers of antiphospholipid antibody (i.e., *lupus anticoagulant* or *anticardiolipin antibody*). In less than half of such cases, the patient has clinically active systemic lupus or a lupuslike syndrome (*secondary antiphospholipid syndrome*); in the remainder, there is no evidence of active lupus, although the antinuclear antibody test may be positive (*primary antiphospholipid syndrome*). Some patients report a history of fetal loss. Those at greatest risk of thrombosis manifest high antibody titers, thrombocytopenia, Raynaud's phenomenon, and livido reticularis. The antiphospholipid antibody syndrome confers significant risk of recurrent venous thrombosis and arterial clot formation and should be considered in idiopathic and recurrent cases of DVT, especially if the patient has active lupus (see Chapter 146), a positive antinuclear antibody test, or a history of fetal loss. Identification of antiphospholipid antibodies is achieved by serologic testing that includes activated partial thromboplastin time, Russell vipor venom time, and dilutional studies.

Idiopathic cases, especially if recurrent, also raise the specter of *occult malignancy*. The frequency of occult cancer in idiopathic disease is just high enough—about 10% in initial cases and close to 20% in recurrent idiopathic cases—to justify a malignancy workup, focusing on detection of potentially curable cancers (e.g., skin, breast, colon, prostate, bladder, lymph nodes, testes, uterus) and those that at least respond to treatment (e.g., small cell cancer of the lung, ovarian carcinoma). Standard screening procedures for curable malignancies (e.g., stool testing for occult blood, sigmoidoscopy, Papanicolaou smear, mammography) are reasonable, but routine computed tomography of the lung and abdomen is of no proven value. The optimal laboratory investigation for underlying malignancy in patients with idiopathic DVT remains to be determined; available data suggest some utility for basic of studies, such as the complete blood count, urinalysis, serum albumin, and chest x-ray. The approach to additional testing should be based primarily on initial clinical findings. Patients not found to have cancer after a careful initial workup have a very low risk of presenting with cancer at a later date. Although such patients need to be followed closely, they require no special additional testing in the absence of new clinical findings.

Hereditary Conditions. Most hereditary hypercoagulable states (e.g., *factor V Leiden, deficiency in protein S or C, or antithrombin III*) represent gene mutations that by themselves confer only modest increases in hypercoagulability. However, when combined with an acquired risk factor for DVT, they appear to greatly increase the likelihood of thrombus formation. This could explain why some patients develop thrombophlebitis and others do not when exposed to the same external risk factors. Although some hereditary hypercoagulable states are rather common (e.g., factor V Leiden can be found in 20% of whites with idiopathic DVT), it remains to be demonstrated that routine screening for these conditions is cost effective. Testing should be considered when the results would substantively affect treatment decisions (e.g., duration of anticoagulation).

Hyperhomocysteinemia, leading to vessel wall injury and increased risks of venous thrombosis and premature atherosclerosis, may be hereditary (enzyme mutation, homozygous) or acquired (folate deficiency). Plasma homocysteine levels in excess of 18.5 nmol/mL (normal, 4 to 15 nmol/mL) confer a fourfold increase in risk of DVT. Screening for homocysteine elevation is appropriate for those with recurrent idiopathic DVT.

MANAGEMENT

Varicose Veins

Conservative Measures. Management of varicose veins can very often be satisfactorily accomplished by nonoperative means, based on appreciation of the principal problem of valve incompetence and poor soft tissue support. Untreated, most varicose veins will slowly worsen and may lead to increasing difficulty and disability. All patients will benefit from proper *elastic support* of medium weight, together with periodic *elevation* of the extremity at intervals during the day. Elastic support is best achieved by a properly fitted surgical stocking obtained from a hospital or commercial surgical company. The various stockings sold in department or drug stores are usually of too lightweight and improper fit. Ace wraps are cumbersome and often applied improperly, creating a "tourniquet" effect at the knee level. A below-knee stocking is preferred, because proper compression is difficult to achieve in the thigh, above-the-knee stockings are difficult to keep up, and patient compliance is considerably less. Fortunately, varicosities in the thigh are much less often associated with symptoms or complications.

In addition, obese patients are urged to *lose weight*, and women are reminded to *avoid* the use of *tight garters* or panty girdles, which will constrict superficial venous return at the thigh level. *Prolonged standing* should be avoided as much as feasible.

Sclerotherapy has some enthusiasts but is not generally recommended. The technique involves injection of a sclerosing agent into the vein lumen followed by application of a pressure dressing maintained for several weeks. An inflammatory reaction causing eventual fibrosis and obliteration of the vein lumen is hoped for. Although occasionally used for small isolated varices or so-called spider veins, sclerotherapy is rarely beneficial for the primary treatment of significant varicose veins.

Surgery. Indications for surgical referral include persistently symptomatic varicose veins (particularly if a conservative approach has been tried), cosmetic dissatisfaction, or recurrent episodes of superficial thrombophlebitis. The option of surgical therapy should probably be discussed initially, because some patients, particularly young women, will prefer this to chronic use of elastic support. In most instances of primary varicose veins, an excellent result can be expected from surgery with extremely low morbidity and a hospitalization of only 2 to 3 days. In experienced hands, the "recurrence" rate of varicose veins should be less than 10%. Often, successful treatment can be achieved with small incisions and so-called "stab-avulsion" techniques; formal stripping of the saphenous vein may not be necessary.

Venous Insufficiency

Management before Ulceration. Treatment of venous insufficiency is best initiated before the occurrence of venous ulceration, which will follow in many untreated cases. An understanding of the pathophysiology again emphasizes the importance of elastic support and periodic elevation of the extremity. *Patient education* is essential, because compliance is poor otherwise. A *knee-length heavyweight elastic stocking* is prescribed and must be worn religiously from the moment the patient gets out of bed until retiring at night. The leg is best elevated on a pillow or by raising the entire foot of the bed at night. *Periodic elevation* during the day is essential in most patients; it must be emphasized to the patient that the leg should be above the level of the heart for this to be effective. This must be done as often as necessary to prevent formation of edema.

Mild diuretic therapy (e.g., hydrochlorothiazide 50 mg/d) may be of some help in stubborn edema. The chronic and incurable nature of the problem must be made clear to the patient, with reassurance given that symptoms and problems are controllable and preventable by strict adherence to the above program.

Management after Ulceration. Progression to the point of ulceration creates a much more troublesome problem. The ulcers may occur with even minor and unrecalled trauma because of atrophic vulnerable skin and subcutaneous tissues. Most ulcers develop just above the medial malleolus, usually overlying an incompetent communicating vein. These lesions will be refractory to all methods of care as long as venous hypertension from the incompetent deep system continues to be transmitted to the superficial tissues. Secondary infection is common, further impairing any chance for local tissue repair.

Management at this stage is much more difficult, time consuming, and often expensive. Preferred treatment is an extended period of *bedrest* with *elevation* of the involved extremity well above heart level at all times, combined with *wet to dry saline dressings* to the ulceration, applied three times daily (see also Chapter 197). Hopefully such a program can be carried out at home by the family, perhaps with the help of a visiting nurse. Healing may be anticipated over a 2- to 4-week period. Hospitalization is generally not necessary unless dictated by social circumstances. Any infection should be cultured and treated appropriately with oral antibiotics; staphylococci and gram-negative rods are common. The patient should be urged to exercise the calf muscles repeatedly while in bed, ideally against a footboard, to minimize the occurrence of acute deep venous thrombosis.

Alternatively, particularly for patients who cannot afford extensive time off their feet, an *Unna paste venous boot* may be used. Properly applied, this medicated bandage can supply good compression, does not require much patient cooperation, and allows the patient to remain ambulatory. Such boot dressings are best changed every 7 to 10 days. With some experience, many venous ulcers may be successfully handled in this manner. Once healed, chronic use of a heavyweight elastic stocking is resumed.

Surgical referral is advisable for recurrent or nonhealing ulcerations, because surgical interruption of incompetent communicating veins underlying these areas, together with stripping and ligation of associated superficial varicosities, may be indicated. In recent years, some surgeons have reported good results with direct repair of incompetent venous valves or interposition of a competent valve from an arm vein into the deep venous system of the leg. Insufficient long-term experience exists, however, to ascertain the usefulness of such surgical therapy at this time.

Superficial Thrombophlebitis

Superficial thrombophlebitis in the lower leg is best managed by a combination of *local heat* and *compression* with a good elastic stocking. Antiinflammatory agents such as *aspirin* or one of the other nonsteroidal drugs may be useful. Antibiotics have no role. Women taking birth control pills should probably discontinue their use. The patient should avoid sitting or standing but remain ambulatory to minimize the chance of developing any associated clot in the deep venous system. Pain and inflammation usually resolve within 1 to 2 weeks.

If superficial phlebitis extends above the knee, consideration of anticoagulation or ligation of the saphenous vein at the level of the saphenofemoral junction in the groin may be indicated, and surgical consultation should be considered. This is particularly true if the process has ascended while under treatment and observation. The rationale is the increased risk of extension of thrombus into the deep system.

Deep Vein Thrombophlebitis

Initial Therapy: Heparinization (Unfractionated versus Low-Molecular-Weight). DVT above the knee is associated with a high risk of thromboembolization. Standard therapy of acute DVT involves prompt *hospitalization* for immediate intravenous treatment with *unfractionated heparin* and initiation of *oral anticoagulation* with *warfarin*. Heparin and warfarin are continued until the prothrombin time (as measured by INR) has been in therapeutic range for 3 to 4 days (see Chapter 83), at which time heparin is stopped, warfarin is continued, and the patient is discharged.

The advent of *low-molecular-weight heparin* provides the opportunity for outpatient treatment of acute DVT. Its principal mechanism of action (accelerating formation of irreversible complexes between antithrombin III and activated factor X) is the same as for unfractionated heparin, but there is reduced interaction with platelets and thrombin, making possible equivalent efficacy with less risk for bleeding. Bioavailability is enhanced and half-life is longer because there is little binding to plasma proteins, red cells, or vascular endothelium. Prospective randomized studies show low-molecular-weight heparin to be at least as effective as unfractionated heparin in preventing thromboembolic events, as safe or safer with regards to major bleeding complications, and superior with respect to survival (reduced all-cause mortality at 6 months). The efficacy, safety, and ease of use (standardized dose, twice-daily dosing, no need for partial thromboplastin time monitoring or intravenous access) enable anticoagulation to proceed much earlier on an outpatient basis. For patients with uncomplicated acute DVT, the length of hospital stay needed to initiate anticoagulation has been reduced from nearly a week to 3 days or less. In selected low-risk cases with a good home environment, hospitalization can be reduced to less than 24 hours or even obviated. These features make low-molecular-weight heparin the emerging treatment of choice for initial management of acute DVT uncomplicated by pulmonary embolization. Although low-molecular-weight heparin costs much more per dose than conventional heparin therapy, it is more cost effective by virtue its ability to markedly reduce length of hospital stay without increasing risk of bleeding or thromboembolization.

Low-molecular-weight heparin preparations include dalteparin, enoxaparin, nadroprin, reviparin, and tinzaprin. Although they differ with respect to protein binding and other qualities, none stands out as clearly superior with regards to safety or efficacy. Dalteparin and enoxaparin are the most commonly prescribed preparations in the United States for outpatient use. They are administered twice daily by subcutaneous injection of a fixed weight-adjusted dose (e.g., dalteparin 100 units/kg twice daily or enoxaparin 1 mg/kg twice daily). The two drugs appear to be clinically equivalent, but dalteparin is about one third lower in cost. Treatment is continued for approximately a week until oral anticoagulation with warfarin (usually started on day 2) is in therapeutic range (INR 2.0) for at least 2 days—same as with unfractionated heparin. The patient must be medically stable, reliable, and have a supportive home environment and available visiting nurse services. The major clinical contraindications to outpatient heparinization are preexisting bleeding difficulties and marked hypercoagulability (e.g., recent surgery, trauma, cancer). The patient should be medically and hemodynamically stable. Monitoring requirements are minimal, but platelet counts and prothrombin times on days 3 and 7 are suggested to check for heparin-induced thrombocytopenia and to assess oral anticoagulation (see Chapter 83).

Oral Anticoagulation. Heparinization is continued while oral anticoagulation with *warfarin* is initiated (see Chapter 83). Heparin is stopped after the prothrombin time reaches an INR more than 2.0 for at least 24 to 48 hours (the time needed for previously synthesized prothrombin to clear the serum).

Duration of warfarin therapy for prophylaxis of recurrent DVT is a function of underlying etiology and number of episodes. A *3-month course* usually suffices for a first episode of DVT occurring in the setting of a clearcut *self-limited* precipitant, such as surgery or trauma. Considerably more than 3 months of treatment are needed for patients with an initial episode of *idiopathic disease*, because their risk of recurrence can exceed 5% per year. The optimum duration of therapy for patients with idiopathic disease has yet to be defined, but most authorities consider 6 months a minimum for a first episode. Risk of recurrence is greatest (approaching 25%/yr) in those with a circulating *lupus anticoagulant*. Other hypercoagulability risk factors do not appear to confer nearly as much risk, but even persons with idiopathic disease and no identifiable determinants of hypercoagulability manifest increased risk of recurrent thrombosis. Long-term anticoagulation should be considered in patients with idiopathic disease, especially if there is a recurrence, persistent lupus anticoagulant, or if the degree of thrombosis was severe or complicated by pulmonary embolization. Chronic anticoagulation is also indicated in other persons with a history of recurrent DVT or DVT in the context of concurrent cancer.

The *intensity* of chronic oral anticoagulation that optimizes DVT prophylaxis while minimizing bleeding complications also remains to be established. The standard intensity of oral anticoagulation for a 3-month course is that which achieves an INR of 2 to 3. However, the prospect of long-term programs of treatment begs the question of optimal intensity. Under study conditions, maintaining an INR between 2.0 and 3.0 dramatically reduces risk of DVT recurrence, whereas increasing risk of major bleeding by only 3% per patient-year. Observational studies put the risk of major bleeding a bit higher at 5% to 7% per patient-year. Data from randomized studies comparing chronic standard and low-dose warfarin programs for primary prophylaxis of DVT suggest that a low-dose regimen (INR 1.5 to 2.0) may minimize bleeding complications without sacrificing efficacy (see Chapter 83). Whether such an approach can be extrapolated to persons with previous DVT remains to be established. For now an INR of 2.0 to 3.0 is recommended for secondary prevention, but the literature should be followed closely.

Thrombolytic therapy (streptokinase, tissue plasminogen activator) deserves consideration in patients with *proximal DVT*,

especially of the *iliofemoral* system. The objective is to minimize the chances of developing postphlebitic syndrome by instituting clot-lysis therapy. The best results have been achieved in patients with proximal vein DVT of the femoral or iliac system treated within 3 days of onset of symptoms; most studies have used streptokinase. Clot lysis occurs in about 50% of instances. Because there is an increased risk of major bleeding, particularly cerebral hemorrhage, prompt referral to a vascular specialist is indicated to facilitate case selection. Contraindications include recent surgery, trauma, recent or active hemorrhage, any bleeding diathesis, pregnancy, and intracranial disease.

DVT below the knee poses little risk of embolization so long as the clot does not propagate up into the thigh. Risk of propagation ranges from 10% to 30%. Risk of embolization from a clot that stays below the knee is small (short-term risk, 0.3% to 1.0%). Outpatients suspected of having DVT, but without evidence of extension above the knee, do not require immediate anticoagulation; however, they should be followed closely with serial evaluation for evidence of propagation. Those who require the closest monitoring are patients with multiple risk factors for DVT. Repeat noninvasive study, using Doppler ultrasound or plethysmography, is indicated (see above).

INDICATIONS FOR ADMISSION AND REFERRAL

Admission. Among patients with peripheral venous disease, those with DVT are at greatest risk acutely and most in need of consideration for immediate hospitalization. Although urgent evaluation is definitely in order, hospitalization is no longer inevitable for patients with DVT above the knee. As long as there is no evidence suggesting pulmonary embolization, iliofemoral extension, or hemodynamic instability and as long as the patient is reliable and the home situation is supportive, heparinization can proceed safely and effectively at home with administration of low-molecular-weight heparin.

Referral. Surgical consultation is indicated for the patient with superficial phlebitis that extends above the knee, because saphenous vein ligation at the level of the saphenofemoral junction in the groin may be indicated if the process has ascended while under treatment and observation. Surgical referral is also advisable for recurrent or nonhealing ulcerations due to chronic severe venous insufficiency. Consideration of surgery is reasonable for the patient with persistently symptomatic varicose veins (particularly if a conservative approach has failed), cosmetic dissatisfaction, or recurrent episodes of superficial thrombophlebitis.

ANNOTATED BIBLIOGRAPHY

Anderson DR, Lensing AW, Wells PS, et al. Limitations of impedance plethysmography in the diagnosis of clinically suspected deep-vein thrombosis. Ann Intern Med 1993;118:25. *(The sensitivity and specificity were less than in most reports, pointing out limitations of the technology.)*

The Columbus Investigators. Low-molecular-weight heparin in the treatment of patients with venous thromboembolism. N Engl J Med 1997;337:657. *(Randomized prospective study comparing low-molecular-weight heparin with conventional heparin therapy;*

safety and efficacy similar for both approaches to heparinization.)

Cornuz J, Pearson SD, Creager MA, et al. Importance of findings on the initial evaluation for cancer in patients with symptomatic idiopathic deep venous thrombosis. Ann Intern Med 1996;125:785. *(Of 142 patients presenting with DVT, 12% were found to have a cancer on comprehensive initial clinical evaluation; none of those who had no evidence on initial evaluation were found to have cancer later.)*

Cranley JJ, Canos AJ, Sull WJ. The diagnosis of deep venous thrombosis: fallibility of clinical symptoms and signs. Arch Surg 1976;111:34. *(Classic paper documenting the inaccuracy of clinical diagnosis.)*

Gould MK, Dembitzer AD, Sanders GD, et al. Low-molecular-weight heparins compared with unfractionated heparin for treatment of acute deep venous thrombosis: a cost-effectiveness analysis. Ann Intern Med 1999;130:789. *(A decision model study finding low-molecular-weight heparin to be highly cost effective when used in inpatient care and cost saving when even a few patients can be treated on an outpatient basis.)*

Heijber H, Buller HR, Lensing AWA, et al. A comparison of real-time compression ultrasonography for the diagnosis of deep-vein thrombosis in symptomatic outpatients. N Engl J Med 1993;329:1365. *(Ultrasound proved superior, with a higher positive predictive value: 94% versus 83%.)*

Hull RD, Raskob GE, Pineo GF, et al. Subcutaneous low-molecular-weight heparin compared with continuous intravenous heparin in the treatment of proximal vein thrombosis. N Engl J Med 1992;326:975. *(One of the original reports demonstrating safety and efficacy.)*

Kearon C, Fent M, Hirsh J, et al. A comparison of three months of anticoagulation with extended anticoagulation for a first episode of idiopathic venous thromboembolism. N Engl J Med 1999;340:901. *(A double-blind, randomized, prospective study demonstrating 95% reduction in rate of recurrent DVT with prolonged anticoagulation and only a 3% per patient-year risk of major bleeding; all patients with idiopathic disease were at risk for recurrence, not just those with identifiable risk factors for hypercoagulability.)*

Khamashta MA, Cuadrado MJ, Mujic F, et al. The management of thrombosis in the antiphospholipid-antibody syndrome. N Engl J Med 1995;332:993. *(Long-term oral anticoagulation at an INR more than 3 proved most effective in this retrospective analysis.)*

Markel A, Manzo RA, Strandness DE. The potential role of thrombolytic therapy in venous thrombosis. Arch Intern Med 1992;152:1265. *(A review concluding that while lytic therapy may have potential, use is often limited by concomitant clinical contraindications.)*

Price DT, Ridker PM. Factor V Leiden mutation and the risks for thromboembolic disease: a clinical perspective. Ann Intern Med 1997;1217:895. *(Good discussion of this recently described though very common mutation and its contribution to hypercoagulability.)*

Rodeghiero F, Tosetto A. Activated protein C resistance and factor V Leiden mutation are independent risk factors for venous thromboembolism. Ann Intern Med 1999;130:643. *(These hypercoagulable states account for up to 15% of cases of DVT, making attention to these states of potential importance in evaluation of DVT, especially that which is recurrent.)*

Rogers LQ, Lutcher CL. Streptokinase therapy for deep vein thrombosis: a comprehensive review of the English literature. Am J Med 1990;88:389. *(Concludes that streptokinase can be of value in properly selected patients, namely those with proximal DVT treated within 7 days of onset of symptoms; 76 references.)*

Schulman S, Granqvist S, Holmstrom M, et al. The duration of oral anticoagulant therapy after a second episode of venous thromboembolism. N Engl J Med 1997;336:393. *(Risk of recurrence was high and markedly reduced by chronic anticoagulation in this prospective randomized trial; slight increase in risk of major bleeding noted.)*

Simioni P, Prandoni P, Lensing AWA, et al. The risk of recurrent venous thromboembolism in patients with an Arg 506 to Gln mutation in the gene for factor V (factor V Leiden). N Engl J Med 1997;336:399. *(Original report identifying increased risk of DVT in persons with this common gene mutation.)*

Strandness DE, Langlois Y, Kramer M, et al. Long-term sequelae of acute venous thrombosis. JAMA 1983;250:1289. *(Long-term sequelae including hyperpigmentation, pain, and swelling were not uncommon and were associated with occluded or incompetent distal deep veins.)*

Wells PS, Lensing AWA, Davidson BL, et al. Accuracy of ultrasound for the diagnosis of deep venous thrombosis in asymptomatic patients after orthopedic surgery: a meta-analysis. Ann Intern Med 1995;122:47. *(Sensitivity decreases to 62% when used to screen for DVT in this setting.)*

Weitz JI. Low-molecular-weight heparins. N Engl J Med 1997;337:688. *(Excellent review of practical and scientific issues; with comparisons; 100 references.)*

36

Stress Testing

The cardiac stress test plays a central role in the evaluation of suspected and known coronary heart disease (CHD) by providing a noninvasive means of detecting ischemia and determining prognosis. Electrocardiographic (ECG), radionuclide, and echocardiographic approaches present the clinician with an array of study options, which include pharmacologic stressing for patients who cannot exercise. The choices can be daunting. Design of a cost-effective workup for CHD (see Chapters 20, 30, and 31) benefits from attention to the performance characteristics, costs, advantages, and disadvantages of available stress-testing modalities.

PHYSIOLOGIC BASIS OF THE TEST

Stress testing assesses the ability of the coronary circulation to meet the enhanced myocardial oxygen requirements of exercise- or drug-induced stress. Because the rate of oxygen extraction by the heart is relatively fixed, increased oxygen demand must be met by an increase in coronary blood flow. When coronary artery stenosis critically limits blood supply, oxygen demand may so exceed supply that myocardial ischemia ensues, manifested by transient changes in ECG ST segments, ventricular wall motion, and radionuclide distribution. In addition, the patient may experience abnormal blood pressure and heart rate responses, angina, or an anginal equivalent such as severe dyspnea.

The demand placed on the coronary circulation can be quantified: The product of heart rate times systolic blood pressure closely parallels the measured myocardial oxygen consumption during isotonic exercise and is designated in "*metabolic equivalents*" (METS), where 1 MET = 3.5 mL O_2 consumed/kg/min. Heart rate alone provides a good approximation of oxygen consumption. Because known quantities of work are being performed, the exercise stress test can also provide a measure of exercise capacity and aid in the detection, quantification, and localization of coronary disease.

APPROACHES TO STRESS TESTING

The stress test may use exercise or pharmacologic measures to challenge the capacity of the coronary circulation. Exercise remains the simplest means, usually achieved by treadmill or stationary bicycle activity. Pharmacologic approaches stress the coronary circulation by inducing either reflex tachycardia or intracardiac vasodilation.

Exercise-based Testing. Exercise testing for the detection of coronary disease uses dynamic (isotonic) rather than sustained-contraction (isometric) exercise. Isotonic exercise permits smooth increases in the rate-pressure product to be accomplished, allowing the patient's ischemic threshold to be approached gradually. Nevertheless, isometric exercise testing (e.g., by sustained handgrip) can be of use in special situations, such as in assessing the safety of isometric activities in patients with known coronary disease.

Testing protocols for isotonic exercise testing are divided into maximal and submaximal types, depending on the level of exercise achieved during the test.

A maximal test is defined as one in which systemic oxygen consumption reaches a plateau before exercise is terminated. Maximal effort is usually approximated by exercising the individual to an age-adjusted predicted maximal heart rate. Values for maximal predicted heart rate can be obtained from standardized tables or regression formulas, but the value *220 minus age in years for men or 210 minus age for women* provides a reasonable approximation of the true maximal heart rate. Tests terminated before maximum predicted heart rate has been achieved are less sensitive for diagnosis of CHD. In general, it is best to continue the test to the predicted maximum heart rate or to maximum perceived effort or until angina, ischemia, arrhythmia, or hypotension occurs. If a patient is receiving a β-adrenergic blocking agent, the end point of heart rate is supplanted by having the patient exercise to exhaustion. If perceived effort is "very hard" (19 or 20 on the Borg scale) at the termination of the test, it can be reasonably assumed that maximal exertion has been closely approximated.

A submaximal exercise test is by definition one in which maximal systemic oxygen consumption is not achieved. The test may be terminated prematurely by design (at a certain percentage of predicted maximal heart rate or at a given level of systemic oxygen consumption) or it may be terminated because of the appearance of angina, marked ischemic ECG changes, cardiac arrhythmias, severe hypertension, or hypotension. Submaximal testing has proved useful and safe for early determination of prognosis shortly *after myocardial infarction*. When conducted within 2 weeks of infarction, a submaximal exercise test to a 5-MET level identifies patients at increased risk for subsequent coronary events and death. Many cardiologists prefer to perform a symptom-limited exercise test 1 month after myocardial infarction in lieu of an earlier submaximal test.

Most exercise tests are "*staged*," meaning graded amounts of work are performed in a progressively increasing manner. The rationale for graded exercise is to obtain the greatest increase in heart rate before musculoskeletal fatigue limits the amount of exercise that the patient can performed. Onset of muscle fatigue before achievement of maximum heart rate reduces test sensitivity. Currently, the *treadmill* and *bicycle ergometer* are the most popular devices used for exercise testing. Slightly higher values for maximal oxygen consumption can usually be obtained on the treadmill than on the bicycle ergometer, because a somewhat larger muscle mass is called on during treadmill exercise.

Many different exercise protocols are available for the treadmill and bicycle. Although the staged *Bruce protocol* is very popular and widely used, it has the disadvantages of unequal changes in work load between stages and a very abrupt increase in work load at stage IV, which is too vigorous for many cardiac patients. Walking protocols are generally preferred over protocols that require running for diagnostic purposes in unfit populations. Bicycle ergometer protocols usually consist of 2- to 3-minute stages in which workload is increased by 10 to 30 watts per stage, depending on the level of physical conditioning of the subject. For both treadmill and bicycle tests, it is best to select a protocol that will allow the patient to reach maximal exertion within a 10- to 12-minute period. A longer test may be limited by the subject's endurance, and a shorter test usually increases the workload too rapidly.

Electrocardiographic Monitoring. Continuous *ECG monitoring* is used during exercise testing, as is periodic determination of blood pressure and symptoms. Multilead systems have replaced the traditional single modified V_5 ECG lead (CM_5). Sensitivity is greatly enhanced by use of multiple leads, especially for detection of inferior ischemia. At present, 12-lead monitoring is commonly performed multiple times during the test and three to six leads are monitored continuously; adding another three leads over the right-precordium appears to enhance detection of ischemia due to right coronary or left circumflex disease (see below). The ST segments are assessed for change with exercise. The depth, configuration, and extent of any ST-segment depressions correlate with presence and severity of coronary disease (see below and Fig. 36.1), as do blood pressure responses and time to development of symptoms. Because ischemic changes may not occur on the ECG until after exercise, monitoring is continued for at least 5 to 7 minutes into the recovery phase.

Radionuclide Imaging. Radioisotopes can be administered as part of exercise testing to help image myocardial perfusion. *Technesium sestamibi* and *thallium-201* are the two radionuclides in most widespread use. Their regional distribution in the myocardium is proportional to regional coronary blood flow; underperfused areas will take up less of the isotope and will ap-

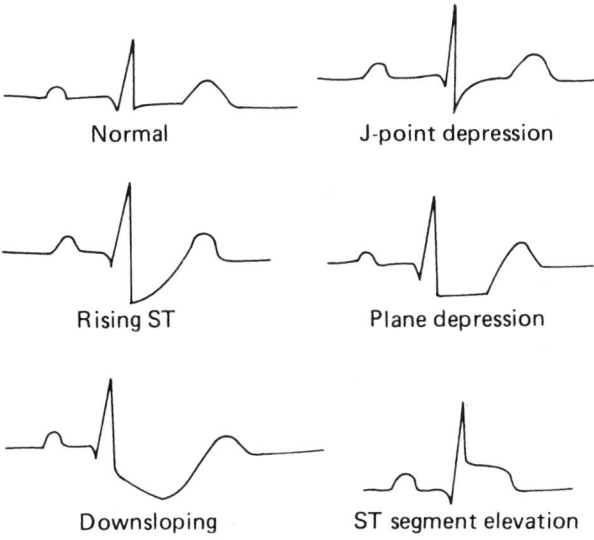

Normal   J-point depression

Rising ST   Plane depression

Downsloping   ST segment elevation

Figure 36-1. Exercise-induced ST segment changes.

pear as "cold" spots on the perfusion scan. Areas of viable but ischemic myocardium will appear underperfused during exercise but will "fill in" at rest. Therefore, sequential scanning during exercise and at rest are required to diagnose hemodynamically significant coronary stenoses and distinguish them from areas of previous infarction.

Sestamibi testing requires a 2-day protocol, with a 1-hour resting scan on day 1 and a 2-hour exercise and imaging session on day 2. Thallium study is done all in one day but requires 2 hours for exercise imaging and a 3-hour wait before a 1-hour imaging session at rest. Sestamibi administration allows for determination of ejection fraction. Thallium provides images of pulmonary uptake, which parallel pulmonary capillary wedge pressure and correlate with prognosis. *Single-photon emission computed tomography* (SPECT) is replacing *planar scanning* technology for image production because it provides better sensitivity.

Echocardiographic Imaging. Stress echocardiographic study provides information on global ventricular function in response to exercise (by measuring change in ejection fraction and end-systolic volume) and on segmental myocardial perfusion (by comparing regional ventricular wall motion at rest and during or just after maximal exercise). Ischemic manifestations include failure to increase ejection fraction with exercise and new regional wall-motion abnormalities. Compared with radionuclide testing, there is less time required, no radiation exposure, and lower cost; in addition, results are immediately available. Test sensitivity for ischemia is reduced by presence of resting wall-motion abnormalities.

Pharmacologic Stress Testing. Patients who cannot exercise are potential candidates for pharmacologic approaches to testing the adequacy of the coronary circulation, be it by inducing reflex tachycardia or coronary vasodilation. Because the sensitivity of ST-segment changes associated with pharmacologic stress testing is low, cardiac imaging (either radionuclide or echocardiographic) is required.

Adenosine or Dipyridamole with Radionuclide Scanning. These agents rapidly induce coronary vasodilation when given by intravenous infusion, usually over 4 to 6 minutes. Normal coronary arteries respond by dilating and markedly increasing regional myocardial blood flow. Diseased vessels are unable to respond in such fashion. The net result is a steal phenomenon, in which blood flow is diverted away from the areas of myocardium supplied by the stenosed vessels, exacerbating the differences in regional perfusion. Radionuclide (thallium or technesium sestamibi) is administered in conjunction with the vasodilator infusion to provide images of regional myocardial perfusion and detect any significant differences suggestive of clinically important coronary disease. Adenosine is the shorter acting of the two vasodilators (half-life 10 seconds vs. 20 minutes) and preferred by many because adverse effects (e.g., flushing, nausea, headache, chest tightness, hypotension) are shorter lived, though more common, than with dipyridamole. Methylxanthines (e.g., theophylline, caffeine) block the actions of these agents and should be withheld for up to 3 days before testing.

Dobutamine with Echocardiography. Dobutamine is a relatively selective β-agonist that is used to stress coronary circulatory capacity by inducing an increase in myocardial oxygen demand through simulative effects on heart rate and myocardial contractility. Underperfused areas show up on ultrasound as thickened hypokinetic myocardium. Sometimes, the muscarinic blocking agent atropine is infused in addition to dobutamine if at least 85% of the maximum predicted heart rate is not achieved by dobutamine alone. Side effects of dobutamine include chest pain, palpitations, dysrhythmias, and blood pressure changes. They usually resolve quickly with cessation of the infusion. Test safety is similar to that for exercise.

Dipyridamole with Positron Emission Tomography. Positron emission tomography (PET) involves administration of the vasodilator dipyridamole along with rubidium-82. The isotope's myocardial uptake is measured by PET, providing a very sensitive and specific, albeit expensive, means of imaging ischemia.

TEST SENSITIVITY, SPECIFICITY, AND PREDICTIVE VALUE FOR CORONARY DISEASE

Gold Standard, Workup Bias, and Test Limitations. The gold standard for the diagnosis of CHD remains the *coronary angiogram*. A significant stenosis is defined as an angiographic narrowing of the vessel lumen by 50% or greater. Stress-test performance characteristics (sensitivity and specificity) are determined by comparing test results against angiographic findings. However, the figures cited in the literature for sensitivity and specificity may be subject to "*workup bias*" that derives from preferential enrollment of study patients likely to have coronary disease and therefore willing to undergo angiography. The consequence of such bias is an exaggeration of test sensitivity and underestimation of test specificity. Workup bias always needs to be considered when interpreting published studies of sensitivity and specificity (see Chapter 2).

Another limitation of stress testing is that it does not identify lesions that may become the cause of sudden death; it only detects impaired blood flow. Most patients who die suddenly from coronary disease do not succumb from a chronic flow-limiting atherosclerotic plaque. Rather, they may die from the acute rupturing and thrombosis of a nonoccluding plaque. Exercise testing does not help to identify such non–flow-limiting lesions, although it can provide an estimate of prognosis by determining extent and severity of disease, which correlates with overall risk (see below). Direct identification of dangerous plaques remains an area of active investigation.

Predictive Value for Coronary Heart Disease and the Importance of Pretest Probability in Test Performance. With an emphasis in the stress-test literature on test performance characteristics (i.e., sensitivity and specificity), it is easy to confuse them with predictive value (the probability of CHD, given a "positive" stress test). The latter is the relevant probability for the clinician caring for the patient with suspected coronary disease and necessitates considering not only test sensitivity and specificity but also the patient's pretest probability for CHD. Figures for the predictive accuracy of the exercise stress test have varied greatly from series to series and between men and women, often because of wide differences in the prevalence of underlying coronary disease in the populations studied. The predictive accuracy of any diagnostic test is directly related to the *prevalence* of the disease in the population examined (see Chapter 2).

A stress test will have a low predictive accuracy when disease prevalence is low, regardless of how sensitive and specific the test is. Proper test interpretation necessitates knowing not only the sensitivity and specificity of the test but also the patient's pretest likelihood of CHD. A positive test in a person with a low pretest probability is far more likely to be a false-positive than a true-positive. Careful estimation of the patient's pretest probability of CHD (see Chapter 20) is essential to proper stress-test interpretation. Prevalence of coronary disease has been found to be 16% in patients with nonanginal chest pain, 50% in those with atypical pain, and 89% when typical angina is present.

High Pretest Probability. The predictive value of a positive stress test for diagnosis of CHD is mathematically greatest in patients with *typical angina* and *multiple coronary risk factors*; however, in such instances the history of classic angina (pretest probability for CHD, about 90%) is about as good for diagnosis as the test's predictive value (about 90%). Thus, performing a stress test adds little to diagnosis beyond that which is already known from the history. In such patients, the value of stress testing is confined to estimating prognosis and assessing need for revascularization (see below and Chapter 30).

Intermediate Pretest Probability. Stress testing may be of considerable diagnostic help in patients with *atypical chest pain,* as long as the criteria for atypical pain are rather rigid (e.g., at least two characteristics of classic angina [see Chapter 20] must be present along with a risk factor or two). In this context, a positive exercise test would substantially increase the posttest likelihood of underlying coronary disease and a negative test would substantially reduce it. In general, exercise testing makes its greatest diagnostic contribution to those whose pretest likelihood of having coronary disease is intermediate.

Low Pretest Probability. In the setting of *noncardiac chest pain* and *no risk factors*, the stress test is not likely to perform well. Although a negative test can be very reassuring to the pa-

tient, the specificity of stress testing is not high enough to eliminate the risk of a false-positive result. The ratio of false-positives to true-positives in the setting of a low pretest probability is likely to be high, making it necessary to warn the patient that a positive test result in this setting is not tantamount to a diagnosis of coronary disease. In trying to reassure a nervous patient who does not have coronary disease by performing a stress test, one might actually make matters worse. Careful thought and patient preparation are needed before going ahead with stress testing such patients. The same considerations and high risk of false-positives also limit the usefulness of stress testing as a screening procedure for detection of CHD in *asymptomatic patients.*

Electrocardiographic Testing. Although not very sensitive for detection of single-vessel coronary disease (sensitivity, 35% to 61%), the standard ECG study approaches other forms of stress testing for detection of more serious anatomy such as left-main or three-vessel disease (sensitivity, 75% to 93%; see below). Overall, the mean sensitivity for detection of coronary disease is about 68% and specificity, 77%. When adjusted for workup bias, the figures are 45% and 85%, respectively. The wide ranges cited for ECG sensitivity and specificity have to do with differences in diagnostic criteria and approaches to testing and monitoring.

Diagnostic Criteria and Other Factors Affecting Test Sensitivity and Specificity. A major factor affecting sensitivity and specificity is the magnitude of *ST segment depression* used as a diagnostic criterion for ischemia. Lowering the ST-segment criterion from at least 2.0 mm of ST depression to 1.0 mm increases sensitivity by nearly threefold but reduces specificity by 10 percentage points. The *configuration of the ST segment* (Fig. 36.1) is also important to specificity. A downsloping ST-segment criterion produces a specificity of 99%; horizontal or plane depression is associated with a specificity of 85%; and a slowly upsloping ST segment (at least 1.5 mm ST depression at 0.08 seconds after the J point) produces a specificity of 68%. Taking into account not only *ST-segment* changes but also any abnormal *blood pressure* or *heart rate* responses and any *angina* or severe *dyspnea* can raise relative sensitivity by over 20%. The occurrence of typical angina during exercise confers, by itself, a sensitivity of 51% and specificity of 90%, about the same diagnostic significance as ST-segment changes.

The *type of exercise protocol* and the *number and location of ECG leads* affect sensitivity. Submaximal protocols are much less sensitive than maximal ones. A 12-lead study is more sensitive than one using fewer leads. The addition of 3 right-precordial leads to a standard 12-lead study markedly improves test sensitivity for single-vessel disease, particularly that involving either the right coronary artery or the left circumflex. With such multilead testing, sensitivity and specificity approach that of radionuclide scanning.

False-Positives. The specificity of ST segment changes is limited by the fact that ST segment depression is not unique to coronary disease. Patients with *valvular* or *hypertensive* disease, nonischemic myocardial disease, and *preexcitation* syndromes may demonstrate ST segment depression during exercise in the absence of ischemia. In addition, left ventric-

Table 36.1. Sensitivity, Specificity, and Costs of Stress Tests for the Detection of Coronary Disease

TEST TYPE	SENSITIVITY	SPECIFICITY	SENSITIVITY FOR THREE-VESSEL/LEFT-MAIN DISEASE	RELATIVE COST
Electrocardiographic	0.68	0.77	0.86	1.0
Echocardiographic	0.76	0.88	0.94	2.5
Thallium imaging, planar only	0.79	0.73	0.93	2.0
SPECT	0.88	0.77	0.98	4.0
PET[a]	0.91	0.82	?	14.0

SPECT, single-photon emission computed tomography; PET, positron emission tomography.

[a]Sensitivity and specificity as reported from nonresearch center settings.

Adapted from Garber AM, Solomon NA. Cost-effectiveness of alternative test strategies for the diagnosis of coronary artery disease. Ann Intern Med 1999;130:719, with permission.

ular *hypertrophy*, recent *glucose* ingestion, *hypokalemia*, and *sedatives* may produce false-positive results. *Digitalis* glycosides are notorious for their ability to cause deviations in ST segments. If possible, it is best to discontinue digitalis for at least 48 hours before testing. If this is not feasible, then exercise-associated ischemia should not be diagnosed until at least 2 minutes of ST segment depression is observed. Studies have also suggested that false-positive responses may be more common in middle-aged *women* than in men by a factor as high as 3, but this may be more a reflection of the low pretest probability of CHD in this population than of a problem with the test. Simple *J-point depression* with a rapidly upsloping ST segment is a nonspecific finding and not diagnostic of ischemia.

Asymptomatic patients with few or *no CHD risk factors* who are subjected to exercise testing and demonstrate "ischemic" changes are, as noted earlier, less likely to have underlying coronary disease and more likely to have a false-positive test. Therefore, asymptomatic subjects with an abnormal stress test should be screened carefully for possible causes of a false-positive response. In asymptomatic populations, abnormal ST segment responses should be viewed as a "risk factor" for coronary disease rather than as definite evidence of the disease. In these individuals, the incidence of coronary disease is modest (about 6%) but doubles by the sixth decade.

Radionuclide Scanning. Stress-test sensitivity is enhanced by radionuclide scanning. With use of planar scanning, overall test sensitivity for detection of coronary disease rises from 68% for ECG to 79% when planar scanning is used and to 88% with SPECT. Specificity is about the same as for ECG testing. Sensitivity for three-vessel and left-main disease rises from 86% for ECG to 93% and 98% for planar scanning and SPECT, respectively. Use of radionuclide scanning has proved especially valuable in patients who have resting repolarization abnormalities on the ECG or left bundle branch block, both of which render interpretation of the standard exercise test difficult. Scanning is also useful in patients whose ECG stress-test results are suspected to be false-positive or false-negative. Test performance characteristics are about the same for exercise and pharmacologic methods of radionuclide stress testing. Test sensitivity is reduced by image attenuation due to obesity or large breasts.

Echocardiography. Echocardiographic assessment has a reported mean sensitivity of 76% for detection of coronary disease and a specificity of 88% (Table 36.1). Mean sensitivity for three-vessel or left-main disease is 94%. Results are similar for exercise and dobutamine-stimulated testing, provided the same increase in heart rate is achieved. Reported figures are from centers where there is major expertise in the performance of the study. Test performance is very operator dependent, and local results may be quite different from those reported in the literature if the operator is inexperienced. Obesity and emphysema may impair performance of the test.

Positron Emission Tomography. Test sensitivity and specificity in research settings often exceed 95%, but when the test is applied in community settings, test performance drops into the 85% range.

STRESS TESTING FOR ASSESSMENT OF CORONARY HEART DISEASE PROGNOSIS

Stress testing represents a useful noninvasive means of screening for predictors of poor CHD prognosis, including left-main, three-vessel, and left-main-equivalent disease and left ventricular dysfunction. Assessment of prognosis of patients in the early postinfarction period also may be aided by exercise testing.

Electrocardiogram. Whereas ECG stress testing is relatively insensitive for detection of single-vessel disease, it compares rather favorably with radionuclide and echocardiographic studies for detection of high-risk anatomy (mean sensitivities 86%, 93% to 98%, and 94% respectively; Table 36.1) and poor prognosis. Stress test findings indicative of worrisome disease include marked ST-segment depression, multilead ST-segment depression, early onset of ST changes, persistence of ST-segment depression past 8 minutes into the recovery period, downward sloping ST configuration, hypotensive response at low workloads, impairment of heart rate response to exercise, and development of angina. The occurrence of both angina and ischemic changes during exercise has been reported to predict an increased likelihood of multivessel disease.

The *Duke exercise treadmill score* is a widely used and well-validated prognostic formula that incorporates easily measured stress-test parameters identified by multivariate analysis as independently predictive of CHD prognosis. It is calculated as follows: exercise time − (5 times the ST deviation in mm) − (4 times the treadmill angina index), where exercise time is in minutes of the Bruce treadmill protocol; ST deviation is the largest ST displacement in mm in any lead; and angina index is scored 0 for no angina, 1 for typical angina during the test, and 2 for angina that halts the test. A score of −11 or less indicates "high risk" (5-year mortality more than 25%), whereas a score of +5 or more predicts "low risk" (5-year mortality less than 6%). Patients at high and moderate-to-high risk require consideration of coronary angiography for identification of high-risk coronary disease and determination of candidacy for bypass surgery (see Chapter 30). Even in the presence of resting ST-segment abnormalities, the ECG stress test retains its ability to risk-stratify patients with CHD by means of the Duke treadmill score.

Although ECG stress testing can help determine prognosis and guide need for angiography, the study does not localize the site of ischemia. Most patients with a positive ECG stress test have ST-segment changes in the anteroapical leads irrespective of the location of their ischemia. More diffuse involvement only indicates increased probability of high-risk coronary anatomy. Coronary angiography is required when considering revascularization.

Submaximal ECG stress testing is very helpful prognostically in the *postinfarction period*. The greater the workload tolerated, the better the prognosis. Patients who develop angina on a limited exercise test conducted just before hospital discharge have twice the rate of postinfarction angina. Those with no ST-segment changes have a very low 1-year mortality (about 2%), compared with a 25% mortality for those who develop ST-segment depression during exercise testing.

Radionuclide Scanning. Unlike ECG testing, thallium and technesium images identify the location and extent of underperfused myocardium (sometimes referred to as the "*amount of myocardium at risk*"). Diffuse ischemia suggests high-risk coronary disease (three-vessel or left-main stenosis) and the need to consider coronary revascularization (see Chapter 30). *Pulmonary uptake* of thallium is a sign of left ventricular dysfunction, another independent indicator of poor prognosis. First-pass resting sestamibi images provide an estimate of ejection fraction and aid in assessment of left-ventricular function.

Echocardiography. Stress echocardiography supplies information on extent and location of ischemia by its 16-segment analysis of left ventricular wall motion. The greater the number of segments manifesting wall motion abnormalities, the greater the probability of multivessel or left-main disease. Resting wall-motion abnormalities reduce predictive accuracy. Echocardiography provides an accurate estimate of left ventricular ejection fraction, an important prognostic determinant.

OTHER ROLES FOR STRESS TESTING

Determination of Exercise Capacity. The patient is made to perform known quantities of work under direct observation and continuous ECG monitoring. This determination is essential for designing a safe cardiac rehabilitation program and may help to reassure the patient who is unnecessarily restricting activity out of fear of sudden death or infarction. The work level achieved during the test can be used to define the degree of incapacity (when it is in question) and provide guidelines for establishing safe levels of daily activity for the patient.

Detection of Dysrhythmias. Assessment of atrial and ventricular rhythm disturbances can sometimes be facilitated by exercise testing, especially if the dysrhythmia is believed to be exercise induced. Ambulatory monitoring should be obtained in conjunction with an exercise test if the objective is optimal detection of dysrhythmias; electrophysiologic study may also be indicated (see Chapters 25, 28, and 29).

SAFETY AND CONTRAINDICATIONS

Reported mortality in a multicenter study involving 170,000 exercise tests was 0.01%. There was no relationship to the type of test or to exercise intensity. Morbidity requiring hospitalization was 0.2%. Safety is enhanced by a preexamination history, a physical examination, and a resting ECG. Patients with unstable angina, uncompensated congestive failure, severe anemia, high-grade heart block, severe aortic stenosis, cor pulmonale, or severe hypertension should not undergo testing. A physician should be present throughout, and a defibrillator and other resuscitation equipment should be in the room. The test should be terminated if blood pressure or heart rate falls suddenly during exercise or if exhaustion, angina, faintness, marked ST changes, severe hypertension, or serious arrhythmias (ventricular tachycardia, heart block, etc.) occur. When performed by experienced personnel, exercise testing is very safe and is one of the most useful noninvasive tests for evaluating cardiovascular function and disease.

The safety of pharmacologically induced stress testing is similar to that for exercise-induced studies. Contraindications to adenosine or dipyrimadole stress testing include severe COPD, asthma, and significant carotid or aortic stenosis. Contraindications to dobutamine stress testing include cardiac dysrhythmias and uncontrolled hypertension.

TEST SELECTION FOR CORONARY HEART DISEASE DIAGNOSIS AND PROGNOSIS

The *ECG stress test* remains a very cost-effective diagnostic option for the patient with a normal resting ECG. Although the standard test is rather insensitive for identification of single-vessel disease, its sensitivity for high-risk coronary disease and correlation with prognosis are very high, approaching those of the much more expensive radionuclide studies (Table 36.1). Moreover, use of right-precordial leads holds promise for enhancing sensitivity for single-vessel disease. Even in the setting of nonspecific resting ECG abnormalities, the ECG stress test retains its prognostic utility when using the Duke treadmill score.

Echocardiographic stress testing represents another cost-effective option for CHD diagnosis. Sensitivity and specificity when performed by expert operators are similar to that for radionuclide scanning, and like the more expensive scans, information is provided on left ventricular function and regional perfusion.

Radionuclide scanning is very sensitive and specific for diagnosis of coronary disease and extremely useful when resting ECG abnormalities preclude ECG stress testing for identification of CHD. However, isotopic imaging is many times more expensive than ECG testing and only marginally better for detection of high-risk disease and determination of prognosis (Table 36.1). These factors limit its cost effectiveness.

For patients unable to exercise, infusion of a vasodilator (*adenosine* or *dipyrimadole*) in conjunction with radionuclide scanning is a reasonable option; dobutamine echocardiography is another. *PET* cannot be recommending at this time, because its cost is extremely high and test performance in the community setting is no better than that of radionuclide imaging.

A.H.G.

ANNOTATED BIBLIOGRAPHY

Bartel AG, Behar US, Peter US, et al. Graded exercise stress tests in angiographically documented coronary artery disease. Circulation 1974;49:348. *(Classic paper demonstrating that the depth of ST-segment depression correlated with severity and extent of coronary disease.)*

Bruce RA. Methods of exercise testing. Am J Cardiol 1974;33:715. *(Another classic paper providing a concise and thorough discussion of the differences in various methods of stress testing by one of the pioneers in the field.)*

DeBusk RF. Specialized testing after recent myocardial infarction. Ann Intern Med 1989;110:470. *(Reviews exercise testing and other diagnostic tests for risk stratification after acute myocardial infarction.)*

Epstein SE, Quyyumi AA, Bonow RO. Sudden cardiac death without warning: possible mechanisms and implications for screening asymptomatic populations. N Engl J Med 1989;321:320. *(An interesting discussion of the pitfalls of using exercise testing to screen asymptomatic persons for coronary disease.)*

Froelicher VF, Lehmann KG, Thomas R, et al. The electrocardiographic exercise test in a population with reduced workup bias: diagnostic performance, computerized interpretation, and multivariable prediction. Ann Intern Med 1998;128:965. *(A prospective multicenter study designed to minimize workup bias; found increased specificity but slightly reduced sensitivity for detection of coronary disease.)*

Gill JB, Ruddy TD, Newell JB, et al. Prognostic importance of thallium uptake by the lungs during exercise in coronary artery disease. N Engl J Med 1987;317:1485. *(Finds lung uptake to be an independent predictor of poor prognosis.)*

Hunink MGM, Kuntz KM, Fleischmann ED, et al. Noninvasive imaging for the diagnosis of coronary artery disease: focusing the development of new diagnostic imaging. Ann Intern Med 1999;131:673. *(A decision-analysis cost-effectiveness study indicating that new imaging techniques such as magnetic resonance imaging or electron-beam computed tomography would have to be relatively inexpensive and extremely sensitive and specific to be more cost effective than currently available modalities.)*

Kuntz KM, Fleischmann KE, Hunink MGM, et al. Cost-effectiveness of diagnostic strategies for patients with chest pain. Ann Intern Med 1999;130:709. *(A cost-effectiveness analysis finding exercise ECG and echocardiography cost effective in patients with mild to moderate risk of CHD.)*

Kwok Y, Kim C, Grady D, et al. Meta-analysis of exercise testing to detect coronary disease in women. Am J Cardiol 1999;83:660. *(Finds ECG, thallium, and stress echocardiography only moderately sensitive and specific for diagnosis of coronary disease in women.)*

Kwok JMF, Miller TD, Christian TF, et al. Prognostic value of a treadmill exercise score in symptomatic patients with nonspecific ST-T abnormalities on resting ECG. JAMA 1999;282:1047. *(An inception cohort study with 7 years of follow-up showing that the Duke treadmill score retains its prognostic value despite resting ECG abnormalities.)*

Leppo JA, Boucher CA, Okada RD, et al. Serial thallium-201 myocardial imaging following dipyridamole infusion. Circulation 1982;66:649. *(One of the original papers of describing the utility pharmacologic stress testing in lieu of exercise stress testing.)*

Mark DB, Hlatky MA, Harrell FE, et al. Exercise treadmill score for predicting prognosis in coronary artery disease. Ann Intern Med 1987;1106:793. *(The Duke treadmill scoring system; incorporates elements identified by multivariate analysis, such as exercise duration, ST-segment change, and the occurrence of angina, into a single predictive index.)*

Mark DB, Shaw L, Harrell FE, Jr, et al. Prognostic value of a treadmill exercise score in outpatients with suspected coronary artery disease. N Engl J Med 1991;325:849. *(A prospective study validating the Duke criteria for risk stratification based on ECG stress test findings.)*

Martin CM, McConahay DR. Maximum treadmill exercise electrocardiography. Circulation 1972;46:956. *(Provides data on the changes in test sensitivity and specificity with changes in ST-segment criteria.)*

Mayo Clinic Cardiovascular Working Group on Stress Testing. Cardiovascular stress testing: a description of the various types of stress tests and indications for their use. Mayo Clin Proc 1996;71:43. *(Excellent, terse review for the generalist reader.)*

Michaellides AP, Psomadaki ZD, Dilaveris PE, et al. Improved detection of coronary artery disease by exercise electrocardiography with use of right precordial leads. N Engl J Med 1999;340:340. *(Sensitivity increased from 66% to 92% for detection of coronary artery disease; a major advance for ECG stress testing if it can be confirmed.)*

Morrow K, Morris CK, Froelicher VF, et al. Prediction of cardiovascular death in men undergoing noninvasive evaluation for coronary artery disease. Ann Intern Med 1993;118:689. *(Data on use of a predictive rule utilizing clinical findings and results from exercise stress testing.)*

Nallamothu N, Ghods M, Heo J, et al. Comparison of thallium-201 single-photon emission computed tomography and electrocardiographic response during exercise in patients with normal resting electrocardiographic results. J Am Coll Cardiol 1995;25:830. *(SPECT found more sensitive than ECG for detection of CHD.)*

Philbrick JT, Horowitz RW, Feinstein AR. Methodological problems of exercise testing for diagnosis of coronary artery disease: groups, analysis, and bias. Am J Cardiol 1987;106:793. *(The effect of "workup bias" on test performance explored.)*

Rifkin RD, Hood WB. Bayesian analysis of electrocardiographic exercise stress testing. N Engl J Med 1977;297:681. *(Argues that the results of the stress test should be viewed as a probability statement, rather than as "positive" or "negative.")*

Sox HC Jr, Littenberg B, Garber AM. The role of exercise testing in screening for coronary artery disease. Ann Intern Med

1989;110:456. *(A cost-effectiveness analysis of exercise testing as a screening test for coronary disease.)*

Tavel ME, Shaar C. Relation between the electrocardiographic stress test and degree and location of myocardial ischemia. Am J Cardiol 1999;84:119. *(Degree of ST depression and extent of these changes correlated with extent of disease but did not localize it.)*

Theroux PT, Waters DD, Halphen C, et al. Prognostic value of exercise testing soon after myocardial infarction. N Engl J Med 1979;301:341. *(Performance of a limited treadmill test just before hospital discharge provided useful prognostic information.)*

Weiner DA, McCabe C, Heuter DC, et al. The predictive value of anginal chest pain as an indicator of coronary disease during exercise testing. Am Heart J 1978;96:458. *(The occurrence of anginal pain during exercise was found to be as predictive as ischemic ECG changes.)*

Weiner DA, Ryan TJ, McCabe CH, et al. Exercise stress testing. N Engl J Med 1979;301:230. *(A detailed study of data from the Coronary Artery Surgery Study examining the influence of the prevalence of coronary artery disease on the diagnostic accuracy of stress testing.)*

4
Respiratory Problems

37
Screening for Lung Cancer

Lung cancer is the most common fatal malignancy among men and women in the United States. In recent years, it has claimed the lives of as many men as have tumors of the colon and rectum, prostate, pancreas, and stomach combined. The incidence of lung tumors in men has been rising dramatically since 1930. More recently, a dramatic increase among women has occurred. Approximately 10% of American men and 5% of American women alive today will have lung cancer during their lifetime; of these, more than 85% will die of the disease.

Most people are aware of the epidemic proportions of the lung cancer problem. Many have lost friends or relatives and know the grim prognosis of the disease. The screening of asymptomatic persons who are at high risk can offer little reassurance. Efforts to improve the prognosis by early detection have been thwarted by the insensitivity of available tests, poor compliance with screening programs among patients at high risk, and the aggressive natural history of most lung tumors. Without an understanding of these limitations, the primary care provider may expend resources that produce little more than exaggerated fear in some patients and inappropriate reassurance in others. Knowledge of the risk factors for and natural history of this disease, and of the validity of available diagnostic tests, provides the basis for a reasoned approach to many pulmonary symptoms (see Chapters 40-44).

EPIDEMIOLOGY AND RISK FACTORS

The epidemiology of lung cancer is dominated by its association with smoking. The dramatic increase in cancer death rates among men and the more recent increase among women can be attributed to increases in cigarette consumption. A dose–response relationship between duration and intensity of cigarette smoking and risk for lung cancer has been documented in men and women. In comparison with the risk for lung cancer among nonsmokers, the risk is increased 5, 10, and 20 times for men who smoke less than half a pack, one-half to one pack, and one to two packs per day, respectively. A decrease in risk has been demonstrated in smokers who are able to stop and in those who smoke filter-tipped cigarettes. A decrease in the prevalence of smoking among adults since 1965 should be followed by a declining incidence of lung cancer. Cigar and pipe smokers incur much less risk, but again a dose–response relationship has been documented (see Chapter 54).

The association between smoking and cancer is strongest for the epidermoid (squamous cell) and small-cell undifferentiated (oat cell) tumors. The relationship is less certain for adenocarcinoma (alveolar cell) and large-cell undifferentiated (anaplastic) histologic types.

The observation that lung cancer occurs in men far more often than in women can be explained for the most part by differences in smoking patterns. In fact, lung cancer without a smoking history is more common among women. A slight apparent excess of lung cancer cases also occurs in urban areas and among low-income groups. The presence of polycyclic organic matter in urban pollution and in some occupational environments (see Chapter 39) may provide a partial explanation. Exposure to asbestos, chromate, nickel, uranium, or radon gas has also been associated with significantly increased rates of lung cancer. The combined effect of such exposures and smoking is generally more than additive. For example, smokers exposed to asbestos have a 90-fold greater risk for lung cancer than do unexposed nonsmokers.

NATURAL HISTORY OF LUNG CANCER AND EFFECTIVENESS OF THERAPY

The rapidly progressive and usually inexorable course of lung cancer frustrates screening efforts. The 5-year survival rate is between 5% and 10%. At the time of symptomatic presentation, 75% of patients have lesions that are clearly unresectable. Of the remainder, 60% prove to be unresectable because of mediastinal involvement, discovered by further evaluation or at thoracotomy. Five-year survival rates after resection in the relatively few remaining patients vary from about 10% for patients with oat cell tumors to 30% for patients with squamous cell tumors.

Reports of 5-year survival rates based on the symptoms present at the time of diagnosis are more relevant to the question of early detection. In a group of patients with an overall 5-year survival of 7%, the 6% with disease discovered before the appearance of symptoms had an 18% survival rate, compared with 10% to 15% for patients with local symptoms and 6% for those with systemic symptoms. Nearly one third of the patients had symptoms of metastatic disease; all died within 5 years.

Higher survival rates have been reported in patients after resection of *in situ* lung cancer diagnosed by means of chest radiography or sputum cytology followed by bronchoscopy, but these may represent little more than selection of slow-growing or otherwise benign lesions. Some highly speculative estimates of growth rate suggest that squamous cell carcinomas and adenocarcinomas take as long as 10 and 25 years, respectively, to reach a size likely to be detected by radiography. If such estimates are accurate and if the natural history is widely variable, overestimation of the benefits of early detection are likely a consequence of the problems of lead time and time-linked bias sampling (see Chapter 3).

SCREENING AND DIAGNOSTIC TESTS

Chest Radiography. In a controlled British study of semiannual chest radiography in more than 29,000 men, 101 lung tumors were detected during a 3-year period. Seventy-six were detected in a control population of 25,000. The overall 5-year survival rates among cancer patients from the screened and control groups were 15% and 6%, respectively. Of the 101 cancers in the screened group, only 65 were detected by routine chest radiography; the remainder presented symptomatically during screening intervals.

The value of chest radiographic screening was also addressed by the Philadelphia Pulmonary Neoplasm Project, which attempted to screen more than 6,000 male volunteers older than 45 years with semiannual radiographic examinations. Lung cancer developed in 121 patients during a 10-year period, with an ultimate mortality rate of 92% at 5 years. The poor results were attributed to poor patient compliance with screening, patient and physician delay, advanced age or concomitant illness contraindicating surgical therapy, and inadequate sensitivity of the screening method.

Three additional randomized trials of lung cancer screening were conducted by members of the Cooperative Early Lung Cancer Group. Separate studies at the Mayo Clinic, Memorial Sloan-Kettering Cancer Center, and Johns Hopkins Hospital each enrolled more than 10,000 male smokers. In the Mayo study, those randomized to close surveillance were screened with both sputum cytology and chest radiographic examination every 4 months, whereas control patients were advised, but not reminded, to have such studies annually. At Memorial Sloan-Kettering and Johns Hopkins, patients were randomized to undergo either annual chest radiography and sputum cytology every 4 months or annual chest radiography alone. The findings of these studies indicate that screening, particularly sputum cytology, may advance the time of diagnosis, with more cancers detected in an earlier stage. However, no difference in survival was found between screening groups at Memorial Sloan-Kettering and at Johns Hopkins, which suggests that no benefit is derived from the addition of cytology to annual radiographic screening. Furthermore, in the Mayo study, no significant difference was noted in lung cancer mortality rates between the screened and control groups despite the fact that more than twice as many postsurgical stage I lung cancers were found in the screened group as among controls.

It should be kept in mind that false-positive chest radiographic findings engender considerable fear in addition to the morbidity associated with confirmatory diagnostic tests. Although the specificity of radiographic screening has been shown to be in the range of 90% to 97%, it is still too low to provide an acceptable predictive value. A Veterans Administration study of lung cancer screens found 438 false-positive radiographic readings, compared with 97 true-positive readings, for suspected neoplasm. In the Memorial Sloan-Kettering study described above, 10,040 persons were screened with both chest radiography and cytology. Approximately 10% had abnormal chest radiographic findings that led to additional studies to rule out cancer. The predictive value of such a positive finding in this and other recent studies has been in the range of 1% to 5%.

Cytologic Screening. The sensitivity of cytologic screening varies with the cell type and location of the tumor and the methods of specimen collection. It used to be thought that a single cytologic specimen would detect about 70% of squamous cell lesions and that three specimens would increase sensitivity to 90%. However, data from recent large, randomized trials indicate that cytologic examination is much less sensitive. Only 10% of cancers in the Memorial Sloan-Kettering study and 13% of those in the Mayo study were detected initially by cytology alone. Presumably, these disappointing findings can be explained by the spectrum problem—that is, decreased sensitivity for early- rather than late-stage tumors (see Chapter 3). The low sensitivity can also be explained by the relatively low proportion of cancers that were of the squamous cell type, which is the histologic type most likely to be detected by cytologic examination. The specificity of sputum cytologic examination is high, in the range of 98% to 99%. In the Memorial Sloan-Kettering prevalence screen of 10,040 men, only seven screenees had cytology findings classified as marked atypia or cancer before they were found not to have cancer. Although rare, such false-positive findings are highly problematic and often require meticulous bronchoscopic examination to sixth- and seventh-generation bronchi.

It should be noted that as *diagnostic* tests, chest radiography and cytologic examination are complementary. In a Veterans Administration study, cytology alone had an overall screening sensitivity of 33% and a specificity of 98%; radiographic screening had a sensitivity of 42% and specificity of 98%; the sensitivity for combined radiographic and cytologic examination was 63%. Radiographic examination is more sensitive for peripheral lesions, whereas cytologic examination is more sensitive for central squamous cell tumors.

Low-dose Computed Tomography. Computed tomography techniques have been adapted in an effort to detect early lung cancer in the general population and among asymptomatic high-risk persons. Population-based screening in Japan has demonstrated greater sensitivity than has chest radiography. One study found lung cancer in 0.5% of those screened, but specificity was limited and the predictive value of a positive screen result was less than 10%. Prevalence screening among long-term smokers detected cancers among 2.7%, a percentage four times higher than was detected with concurrent chest radiography. Nearly all the detected cancers were resectable, and most were stage I. However, the impact of computed tomographic screening on mortality awaits further study.

SUMMARY AND CONCLUSIONS

- Lung cancer is a major cause of morbidity and mortality, especially among men. The incidence is increasing among women.

- Smoking is the overwhelming risk factor for lung cancer. Occupational exposures also are relevant.
- Little is known about the presymptomatic natural history of lung cancer. It is presumed to be highly variable. The 5-year survival despite all forms of therapy is 5% to 10%. Survival is slightly better when an asymptomatic lesion is detected.
- Cytologic examination of the sputum and chest radiography are complementary diagnostic tests. However, neither is sensitive nor specific enough to serve as a screening test.
- Large-scale early detection programs have demonstrated little benefit. Such efforts to improve prognosis have been thwarted by the usually rapid course of lung cancer, the characteristics of the patients at risk, and the relative insensitivity of available tests.

A.G.M.

ANNOTATED BIBLIOGRAPHY

(Additional references concerning the relationship of lung cancer to smoking appear in the annotated bibliography following Chapter 54.)

Berlin NI, Buncher CR, Fontana RS. Results of the initial screen (prevalence). Early lung cancer detection: introduction. Am Rev Respir Dis 1984;130:549. (*This introduction is followed by three articles describing prevalence screen results of studies performed at Johns Hopkins, the Mayo Clinic, and Memorial Sloan-Kettering.*)

Boucot KR, Weiss W. Is curable lung cancer detected by semiannual screening? JAMA 1973;224:1361. (*Reviews the data of the Philadelphia Pulmonary Neoplasm Project, in which the 5-year survival of men offered semiannual radiographic screening was only 8%.*)

Eddy DM. Screening for lung cancer. Ann Intern Med 1989;111:232. (*Well-reasoned analytic review that includes a discussion of the Johns Hopkins, Mayo, and Memorial Sloan-Kettering studies.*)

Flehinger BJ, Kimmel M, Melamed MR. The effect of surgical treatment on survival from early lung cancer. Implications for screening. Chest 1992;101:1013. (*Analysis of the Hopkins, Mayo, and Sloan Kettering data, with a focus on outcomes for patients with stage I cancer.*)

Fontana RS, Sanderson DR, Woolner LB, et al. Screening for lung cancer. A critique of the Mayo Lung Project. Cancer 1991;67:1155. (*A review of the Mayo Clinic trial, including the results of follow-up for 5 years beyond the 6-year study period.*)

Hammond EC, Selikoff IJ, Seidman H. Asbestos exposure, cigarette smoking and death rates. Ann N Y Acad Sci 1979;330:473. (*Includes data from 18,000 insulation workers: relative risks of 90 and 50 for two-pack and half-pack smokers, respectively, in comparison with unexposed nonsmokers.*)

Henschke CI, McCauley DI, Yankelevitz DF, et al. Early lung cancer action project: overall design and findings from baseline screening. Lancet 1999;592. (*Preliminary findings of prevalence screening among high-risk persons with chest radiography and low-dose computed tomography. Noncalcified nodules were found in 23%, and malignancies were found in 2.7%.*)

Hubbell FA, Greenfield S, Tyler JL, et al. The impact of routine admission chest x-ray films on patient care. N Engl J Med 1985;312:209. (*The impact of routine admission chest radiography on the care of 742 consecutive patients admitted to a Veterans Administration hospital was negligible; in only one case was a new pulmonary malignancy detected, and outcome was unaffected.*)

Kubik A, Parkin DM, Khlat M, et al. Lack of benefit from semiannual screening for cancer of the lung: follow-up report of a randomized controlled trial on a population of high-risk males in Czechoslovakia. Int J Cancer 1990;45:26. (*Chest radiography and sputum cytology twice each year for 3 years produced no measurable benefit.*)

Melamed MR, Flehinger BJ, Zaman MB, et al. Screening for lung cancer: results of the Memorial Sloan-Kettering study in New York. Chest 1984;86:44. (*Addition of sputum cytology to chest radiography was ineffective.*)

38
Tuberculosis Screening and Prophylaxis

BENJAMIN DAVIS
HARVEY B. SIMON

Active tuberculosis (TB) remains relatively uncommon in ambulatory practice, although its prevalence is beginning to increase again in some populations, especially patients infected with HIV, immigrants from countries where TB is endemic, and the urban poor. Being a contagious yet potentially treatable condition, TB is always an important consideration in patients presenting with hemoptysis (see Chapter 42), chronic cough (see Chapter 41), or fever and weight loss (see Chapters 9 and 10). Tuberculin reactivity remains prevalent. On a daily basis, the primary physician faces the questions of whether to test for reactivity and how to respond when it is present.

EPIDEMIOLOGY AND RISK FACTORS

Until the mid 1980s, the number of reported TB cases in the United States was declining at an annual rate of about 6%, with most new cases occurring among the institutionalized elderly, who represented a remaining pool of latent endogenous infection. The prevalence of tuberculin skin test positivity in this population has been estimated at 20% and the prevalence of active disease at 2.4%. In 1985, the incidence of active TB began to grow for the first time in half a century, in part because of the HIV epidemic, but also because of cutbacks in funding for the public health clinics responsible for treating and preventing TB. Federal resources were returned to state and local TB-control programs in the early 1990s. Since 1992, the rates of TB have fallen annually, and in 1996, a rate of eight cases per 100,000 represents the lowest seen since national reporting began in 1953. TB remains a problem for patients infected with HIV, the foreign-born, and the urban poor. Compared with persons uninfected with HIV, whose risk for development of active TB after infection is *10% per lifetime*, HIV-infected persons have a risk for development of active disease of *10% per year*. Other population groups with a disproportionately high incidence of TB include alcoholics; IV drug users; patients with diabetes, malnutrition, or end-stage renal disease; persons who have undergone gastrectomy; and patients who take immunosuppressive drugs.

NATURAL HISTORY OF TUBERCULOSIS AND EFFECTIVENESS OF THERAPY

Natural History

Mycobacterium tuberculosis is transmitted by way of fresh droplet nuclei expelled by a person with cavitary disease. It cannot be spread by hands, utensils, or other fomites, although organisms can be cultivated from room dust. Although inoculation can occur via the gastrointestinal tract, the vast majority of infections in the United States begin in the lung (see Chapter 49). Until the HIV epidemic, it was rare for primary infection to result in early progressive disease; young children were at greatest risk for this complication. However, among HIV-positive patients, the risk for rapid progression to active disease is substantial, with some studies showing a rate of 30% and a mean incubation period of only 80 days. Based on polymerase chain reaction and molecular epidemiology studies, it is now felt that 40% of all active TB cases in urban centers like New York City represent newly acquired infection rather than reactivation of latent disease.

Approximately 5% to 15% of new tuberculous infections eventually progress to serious disease. Risk is greatest during the years immediately following infection. Late reactivation occurs in only 3% to 5% of patients without clinical disease 5 years after infection.

Effectiveness of Therapy

Three strategies may be used in the prevention of clinical infection: (a) biologic prophylaxis of uninfected persons with bacille Calmette-Guérin (BCG) vaccine; (b) chemoprophylaxis of newly or recently infected persons with isoniazid (INH); and (c) INH chemoprophylaxis of selected persons with latent infection.

Biologic Prophylaxis with BCG vaccine is widely practiced in countries where TB is prevalent. The vaccine is used for prevention in uninfected persons; it is of no value in infected persons. BCG vaccine contains a live, attenuated strain of *Mycobacterium bovis*, which has little virulence in humans. It should not be administered to patients who react positively to the purified protein derivative (PPD) tuberculin skin test. BCG itself may cause a positive PPD test result in the first 2 to 3 years following vaccination. After this period, however, a positive PPD test result should not be ascribed to vaccination with BCG, nor should prior BCG vaccination be considered a reason not to perform skin testing, if it is otherwise indicated. The vaccine has been in clinical use since 1922, but its role remains controversial. Early trials demonstrated that BCG could prevent TB in up to 80% of recipients, but subsequent trials on the Indian subcontinent failed to demonstrate efficacy. Even though recent studies in Great Britain and Canada suggest that the vaccine may be up to 60% effective, BCG is not currently recommended for routine use in the United States. The relatively low incidence of new tuberculous infections in the United States

still makes case finding and INH prophylaxis a more effective approach (see below).

Chemoprophylaxis appears to reduce significantly the risk for progression from latent infection to active disease. In patients who have not received chemotherapy, a positive skin test result implies the presence of a few dormant but viable tubercle bacilli, which have the potential for reactivation. It has been demonstrated that the administration of *INH* daily for 6 to 12 months reduces the risk for reactivation by up to 80%. Because the risk for progressive disease is greatest soon after infection, recent converters to tuberculin reactivity are most likely to benefit from such therapy.

Current guidelines for INH chemoprophylaxis depend on the patient's *age*, the *strength of the tuberculin reaction*, and the presence of *other risk factors*. The following groups should be considered candidates *regardless of age*:

- Patients with known or suspected HIV infection (5 mm).
- Close (especially household) contacts of patients with known active pulmonary TB (5 mm). *Children and adolescent contacts of a person with TB should be offered INH regardless of PPD status until a PPD test can be repeated at 12 weeks.*
- Patients with fibronodular disease on chest radiography compatible with old, healed TB (5 mm).
- Patients with documented PPD conversion within the preceding 2 years (10 mm).
- IV drug users uninfected with HIV (10 mm).
- Patients with medical conditions predisposing to active TB, such as malnutrition, diabetes, end-stage renal disease, silicosis, gastrectomy, or use of immunosuppressive drugs (10 mm).

The following groups should be considered candidates for INH chemoprophylaxis if less than 35 years old:

- Foreign-born patients from countries where TB is endemic (10 mm).
- Native-born patients from medically underserved low-income areas, especially if homeless (10 mm).
- Patients residing in long-term care facilities such as nursing homes, correctional facilities, and mental institutions (10 mm).

Persons without risk factors for acquiring TB and without medical conditions predisposing to active TB should be considered candidates for INH only *when they are younger than 35 years and when the PPD test shows at least 15 mm of induration.*

When INH is used for prophylaxis, it should be administered *daily* for *6 months*, except in the case of *HIV-positive* persons and those with *old TB* according to radiographic criteria; the latter require *12 months* of INH. INH may also be given twice weekly via directly observed therapy (DOT). Enthusiasm for INH prophylaxis must be tempered by the significant side effects of the drug, particularly hepatotoxicity. Liver injury is quite rare in patients younger than 20 years and occurs in no more than 0.2% of those between ages 20 and 34. On the other hand, INH-induced liver disease may develop in more than 2% of patients older than 50 (see Chapter 49). *INH alone should never be given to a patient with active TB.* A chest radiograph and a clinical encounter designed to uncover subtle signs and symptoms of active TB are mandatory before INH chemoprophylaxis is initiated. *If any doubt exists*, INH should be deferred pending the results of sputum cultures or the resolution of ambiguous symptoms.

The Centers for Disease Control and Prevention (CDC) has recommended that a *2-month regimen of rifampin (RIF) and pyrazinamide (PZA)* be used as an alternative to 12 months of INH in *HIV-infected persons*. It is anticipated that this recommendation will be extended to HIV-negative patients in the near future. Although its shorter duration will increase adherence, the two-drug regimen is more likely to cause side effects.

SCREENING AND DIAGNOSTIC TESTS

The tuberculin skin test is the most useful test for the diagnosis of past or present tuberculous infection. The Mantoux test with use of an intradermal injection of Tween 80–stabilized *PPD* is more reliable than multiple-puncture tests, such as the Tine Test. PPD is available in three strengths: the *"first strength"* contains *1 tuberculin unit (TU)*; the *"intermediate strength,"* *5 TU*; and the *"second strength,"* *250 TU*. Only the *5-TU strength should be used for screening*.

The tuberculin skin test result should be interpreted 48 to 72 hours after injection; the diameter of *induration* (not erythema) determines the interpretation. Until recently, a single standard was used to interpret the tuberculin skin test in all people: 0 to 4 mm was "negative," 5 to 9 mm was "doubtful," and 10 mm or more was "positive." As noted above, authorities such as the CDC now recommend that different skin test criteria be applied to different population groups, to provide a more accurate assessment of risk.

The current CDC *criteria for skin test positivity* include the following:

- Induration of *5 mm* for patients who are HIV-positive and for patients who are very likely to have TB, such as close contacts of documented cases and patients with chest x-ray films that strongly suggest TB (see Chapter 49)
- Induration of *10 mm* for members of high-incidence populations or for patients with medical conditions predisposing to active TB
- Induration of *15 mm* for persons with no identifiable risk factors

Repeated tuberculin skin tests can produce a *booster effect*, but only among patients already infected with TB. Among hospital employees or other populations who may undergo repeated skin testing, a booster effect can be mistaken for tuberculin conversion. Confusion can be avoided by repeated testing of persons with negative or doubtful skin test results 1 week later; any increase in the diameter of induration can be attributed to the booster effect. In contrast, increased reactivity that occurs at 1 year, but not at 1 week, should be attributed to newly acquired infection.

False-negative reactions (anergy) have been documented in up to 20% of patients with TB, particularly those who are immunocompromised by HIV infection, overwhelming or advanced disease, malnutrition, or debility. Approximately 50% of patients with clinical AIDS may have false-negative PPD test results in the setting of active TB. The lowering of the criterion for a positive skin test result in HIV-positive patients to a 5-mm induration is an attempt to improve test sensitivity. The CDC no longer recommends the use of *Candida*, mumps, or tetanus toxoid antigens as "controls" for anergy because anergic HIV-positive patients do not benefit from INH chemoprophylaxis.

In addition to immunologic incompetence of the host, other causes of false-negative skin test results are mishandling of the antigen and faulty injection technique. Tuberculin should never be transferred from one container to another, and skin tests should be administered as soon as possible after the syringe is filled. Subcutaneous rather than intradermal injection may result in false-negative reactions. Because tuberculin sensitivity develops 2 to 10 weeks after initial infection, results of early skin tests may be negative in newly infected persons.

Although tuberculin skin testing is highly specific, false-positive reactions may also occur, usually because of cross-reactivity with atypical mycobacterial antigens acquired environmentally. This may cause intermediate skin test reactions in people who have not been exposed to *M. tuberculosis*—hence the requirement for larger areas of induration when a low-risk population is screened.

RECOMMENDATIONS AND CONCLUSIONS

- As long as the tuberculin skin test and INH remain useful for case finding and prophylaxis, respectively, biologic prophylaxis with BCG for PPD-negative patients is not recommended.
- PPD testing should be performed *annually in all HIV-infected patients*. Other high-risk persons should also be tested, including IV drug abusers, homeless persons, immigrants from countries with a high incidence of TB, prisoners, residents of long-term care facilities, and persons who are immunosuppressed or have chronic illnesses known to increase the risk for active TB.
- Healthy persons with a high risk for exposure to TB, such as those in the health care professions, should undergo tuberculin testing on an annual basis so long as they remain PPD-negative.
- INH prophylaxis should be considered for tuberculin-positive persons based on the strength of the PPD reaction, the presence of risk factors, and age. Positive reactors require 6 months of daily INH prophylaxis (300 mg/d); those at highest risk (HIV-positive, old TB on chest x-ray films) require 12 months of daily prophylactic treatment. Care must be taken to ensure compliance to prevent the emergence of drug-resistant strains, and twice-weekly DOT may be appropriate.
- Treatment with RIF and PZA for 2 months is as effective as treatment with INH alone for 12 months in HIV-infected patients, although side effects are more common.
- Active TB must be excluded before INH chemoprophylaxis is begun.

ANNOTATED BIBLIOGRAPHY

American Thoracic Society/Centers for Disease Control. Diagnostic standards and classification of tuberculosis. Am Rev Respir Dis 1990;142:725. (*Standards for the administration and interpretation of the tuberculin skin test.*)

American Thoracic Society. Treatment of tuberulosis and tuberculous infection in adults and children. Am J Respir Dis 1994;149:1359. (*Current standards for the treatment of TB and the administration of INH chemoprophylaxis.*)

Boyd JC, Marr JJ. Decreasing reliability of acid-fast smear techniques for detection of tuberculosis. Ann Intern Med 1975;82:849. [*Misleading title but very useful article pointing out high specificity of smears (99%) but low predictive value (45%) because of low prevalence; sensitivity 22%.*]

Centers for Disease Control. Anergy skin testing and preventive therapy for HIV-infected persons: revised recommendations. MMWR Morb Mortal Wkly Rep 1997;46:RR-15. (*Revised recommendations against use of "anergy panel" or control antigens for patients with or without HIV infection.*)

Centers for Disease Control. Guidelines for preventing the transmission of tuberculosis in health-care settings, with special focus on HIV-related issues. MMWR Morb Mortal Wkly Rep 1990;39:RR-17. (*Important advice on preventing nosocomial infection; items germane to outpatient care included.*)

Centers for Disease Control. Prevention and treatment of tuberculosis among patients infected with HIV: principles of therapy and revised recommendations. MMWR Morb Mortal Wkly Rep 1998;47:RR-20. (*Two-month regimen of RIF and PZA is as effective as 12 months of INH alone.*)

Centers for Disease Control. Progress towards elimination of tuberculosis—United States, 1998. MMWR Morb Mortal Wkly Rep 1999;48:732. (*The 1998 rate of 6.8 cases per 100,000 population was 35% lower than the 1992 rate. Also appears in JAMA 1999;282:1125.*)

Centers for Disease Control, Advisory Committee for the Elimination of Tuberculosis. Screening for tuberculosis and tuberculous infection in high-risk populations, and the use of preventive therapy for tuberculous infection in the United States. MMWR Morb Mortal Wkly Rep 1990;39:RR-8. (*Recommends aggressive testing and treatment.*)

Centers for Disease Control, Advisory Committee for the Elimination of Tuberculosis. Use of BCG vaccines in the control of tuberculosis. MMWR Morb Mortal Wkly Rep 1989;37:663. (*CDC guidelines for BCG prophylaxis.*)

Dooley SW, Jarvis WR, Martone WJ, et al. Multidrug-resistant tuberculosis. Ann Intern Med 1992;117:257. (*A terse summary of this worrisome condition and means of prevention.*)

Dye C, Scheele S, Dolin P et al. Global burden of tuberculosis: estimated incidence, prevalence, and mortality by country. JAMA 1999;282:677. (*In 1997, 8 million new cases and nearly 2 million deaths.*)

Frieden TR, Sterling T, Pablos-Mendez A, et al. Emergence of drug-resistant tuberculosis in New York City. N Engl J Med 1993;328:521. (*High prevalence among HIV-positive persons, IV drug abusers, and those previously treated.*)

Gourevitch MN, Hartel D, Selwyn PA, et al. Effectiveness of isoniazid chemoprophylaxis for HIV-infected drug users at high risk for active tuberculosis. AIDS 1999;13:2009. (*Among tuberculin reactors, rates of active TB were 0.5/100 and 2.0/100 person-years in those completing and not completing prophylaxis, respectively.*)

Graham MH, Nelson KE, Solomon L, et al. Prevalence of tuberculin positivity and skin test anergy in HIV-1-seropositive and -seronegative intravenous drug users. JAMA 1992;267:369. (*Finds a high rate of anergy in HIV-positive patients, especially those with low CD4-cell counts, in addition to reductions in the diameter of response; suggests that the criterion for positivity be reduced to 2 mm.*)

International Union against Tuberculosis Committee on Prophylaxis. Efficacy of various durations of isoniazid preventive therapy for tuberculosis: 5-year follow-up of the IUAT trial. Bull World Health Organ 1982;60:555. (*In a cooperative European study of 27,830 tuberculin-positive adults with fibrotic pulmonary lesions, 52 weeks of INH therapy produced a 75% reduction in TB, and 24 weeks of treatment provided a 65% reduction. Hepatitis occurred in 0.5% of the INH recipients and in 0.1% of the placebo recipients. For the 52-week regimen, the benefit–risk [TB averted–INH hepatitis induced] ratio was 2.1; for 24 weeks the ratio was 2.6.*)

Selwyn PA, Hartel D, Lewis VA. A prospective study of the risk of tuberculosis among intravenous drug abusers with HIV infection. N Engl J Med 1989;320:545. (*Documents a very high risk for infection, even in those who are PPD-negative.*)

Stead WW, Lofgren JP, Warren E, et al. Tuberculosis as an endemic and nosocomial infection among the elderly in nursing homes. N Engl J Med 1985;312:1483. (*A study of 25,000 elderly nursing home residents showing a high prevalence of tuberculin reactivity and active disease; risk for new infection was great.*)

Thompson NJ, Glassrath JL, Snider DE Jr, et al. The booster phenomenon in serial tuberculin testing. Am Rev Respir Dis 1979;119:387. (*A good discussion of the booster phenomenon, with guidelines for serial skin testing in high-risk population groups.*)

Wadhawan D, Hira S, Mwansa N, et al. Isoniazid prophylaxis among patients with HIV-1 infection. In: Proceedings of the Seventh International Conference on AIDS, Florence, Italy, 1991 (abst WB 2261). (*INH prophylaxis reduced the risk for progression from infection to active disease in these high-risk patients.*)

39

Evaluation and Prevention of Occupational and Environmental Respiratory Disease

L. CHRISTINE OLIVER
JOHN D. STOECKLE

Occupational lung disease, one of the 10 leading causes of work-related health problems in the United States, results from the inhalation of organic and inorganic dusts, irritant vapors and gases, and toxic fumes, which adversely affect both the upper and lower respiratory tracts. Although the true scope of occupational respiratory illness and disease is unknown, some estimates can be given. In the United States, about 15% of newly diagnosed cases of asthma in adults are the consequence of occupational exposures. It has been estimated that approximately 65,000 men in the United States have clinically identifiable asbestosis; moreover, it is predicted that 19,000 cases of malignant mesothelioma and 55,000 cases of lung cancer will occur by the year 2009 in men with a history of occupational exposure to asbestos. Persons permanently disabled by respiratory disease resulting from previous exposure to cotton dust number about 30,000; active cotton mill workers who are partially disabled number about 85,000. Ten percent of active coal miners and 20% of retired miners have coal worker's pneumoconiosis (CWP). The U.S. Department of Labor has estimated that more than 1 million workers are exposed to silica and that approximately 60,000 have silicosis.

Nevertheless, these figures underestimate the extent of occupational pulmonary disease. The reasons are several. First, because the clinical findings in patients with work-related respiratory disease resemble those in persons with respiratory disease that is not occupationally related, the diagnosis is often missed. Second, the latency period between exposure and the subsequent development of disease may be long, which obscures the causal relationship. Third, physicians often underdiagnose because they have inadequate training in occupational medicine. Fourth, occupational disease is underreported by health care personnel. Further, the estimates do not include the "paraoccupational" lung disease that results from bystander exposure, household contact with toxins carried home on work clothes, and neighborhood exposure. Asbestos-related disease has been reported in family members of asbestos workers and in persons living in close proximity to shipyards and asbestos manufacturing plants. Chronic beryllium disease has resulted from residence in the neighborhood of beryllium plants, and asthma from residence near grain elevators.

It is critical that the primary care physician be familiar with occupational lung diseases and their diagnosis if unnecessary morbidity is to be avoided. Because respiratory symptoms caused by toxic exposures are nonspecific, recognizing their relationship to the toxic agent or agents is essential to proper diagnosis and treatment. Continued exposure may result in needless, irreversible functional abnormalities and the development of chronic and even fatal respiratory disease.

PATHOPHYSIOLOGY AND CLINICAL PRESENTATION

Inhaled dusts, gases, and fumes exert their effects on the respiratory tract in several ways. The first is *direct irritation* and *inflammatory response*. Symptoms include excessive mucous secretion, cough, airways hyperreactivity, chest tightness or pain, wheeze, and dyspnea. Asthma, chemical pneumonitis, or pulmonary edema may develop. Irritation is associated with an inflammatory response involving chemosensitive neurons and the release of vasoactive and chemotactic mediators. Clinical manifestations may be delayed, as after exposure to the irritant gases nitrogen dioxide and phosgene, when a delay of 12 to 24 hours may precede the onset of pulmonary edema.

Second, dusts such as silica and asbestos may be retained in the lungs and provoke a *fibrotic* or *granulomatous response*. To reach the lower respiratory tract, substances must have a particle size of 5 μm or less. The latency between onset of exposure and the clinical manifestation of disease may be as long as 20 to 25 years and is often related to the intensity of exposure.

Third, an *immunologic response* with *development of hypersensitivity* may play a role in occupational lung disease. Hypersensitivity is important etiologically in hypersensitivity pneumonitis, certain types of occupational asthma, and pulmonary beryllium disease. Increased circulating levels of immunoglobu-

lins, rheumatoid factor, antinuclear antibody, and α_1-antitrypsin have been observed in persons with asbestosis. Peripheral blood T-lymphocyte abnormalities appear to be related to the duration of asbestos exposure and radiographic outcome. Elevated titers of circulating antinuclear antibody and rheumatoid factor are seen in association with silicosis. Persons with beryllium disease are reported to have alterations in circulating T lymphocytes and a high rate of blast transformation of lymphocytes in peripheral blood and bronchoalveolar lavage specimens.

Fourth, *other host factors* are important. Asbestos acts synergistically with cigarette smoke to increase the risk for lung cancer. The prevalence of bronchitis and airways obstruction is increased in welders and coal miners who smoke in comparison with their nonsmoking co-workers.

Finally, *social* and *economic factors* often determine the geographic proximity of home to industrial sources of air pollution, and *work practices* affect the likelihood that family members will bring workplace toxins home on work clothes.

Occupational respiratory disease can be classified clinically as airways disease, interstitial disease, or cancer (Table 39.1).

Airways Disease

Work-related airways disease may be acute or chronic and reversible or irreversible. Airways obstruction may or may not be present. The nature of the exposure and duration of exposure after development of symptoms are important variables in determining outcome.

Occupational Asthma is the most common occupational lung disease in developed countries. Of cases of work-related lung disease reported in the United Kingdom and British

Table 39.1. Classification of Occupational Respiratory Disease

Airways Disease
Occupational asthma
  Causal agents: toluene diisocyanate (TDI) and other isocyanates, phthalic anhydride, nickel, chromium, platinum salts, formaldehyde, *Bacillus subtilis* proteolytic enzyme, grains, animal products, epoxy resins, Western red cedar, mahogany, oak, and irritant gases, vapors, fumes
Byssinosis
  Causal agents: cotton, flax, hemp
Multiple chemical sensitivity
  Causal agents: chemical irritants such as isocyanates, ammonia, acetone, sodium hypochlorite, solvents, sulfuric and hydrochloric acids
Industrial bronchitis
  Causal agents: diesel exhaust, high level of nonspecific dust (e.g., construction site), welding fumes, coal dust, sulfur dioxide, vanadium pentoxide

Pulmonary Fibrosis
  Causal agents: asbestos, silica, beryllium, coal dust, talc, kaolin, and organic dusts such as thermophilic actinomycetes, *Aspergillus*, animal proteins

Cancer
  Causal agents: asbestos, silica (with silicosis), diesel exhaust, arsenic trioxide, hexavalent chromium, nickel, bischloromethyl ether (BCME), chloromethylmethyl ether (CMME), vinyl chloride monomer, radiation, uranium (radon daughters), radon

Noncardiogenic Pulmonary Edema
  Causal agents: oxides of nitrogen, phosgene, chlorine, ammonia, sulfuric acid

Columbia, 26% and 52%, respectively, were occupational asthma. Inhalation of substances in the workplace can cause or exacerbate reversible airways hyperreactivity, with or without airways obstruction. Preexisting asthma that is exacerbated by occupational exposures is diagnosed as occupationally aggravated asthma.

At least 250 agents have been reported to cause occupational asthma. These substances have most recently been classified on the basis of their association with latency, and those with similar latency are further subdivided on the basis of molecular weight. Asthma that is associated with exposure to high-molecular-weight substances is mediated by immunoglobulin E and is similar etiologically to "allergic" asthma that is not related to work. The mechanism in the case of low-molecular-weight (<1,000 D) substances is less clear. An example of such substances is the class of chemicals known as isocyanates, which are in widespread use in the manufacture of rigid and flexible foams, products used in floor refinishing, sealant materials, wood varnishes, and packaging and thermal insulation materials. They cause asthma through either or both of two mechanisms: (a) direct irritation of bronchial mucosa and (b) sensitization through an immunologic mechanism that is not yet clearly defined. Once sensitized, persons are at risk for severe and even fatal attacks of asthma on repeated exposure. Substances that induce asthma without latency include irritant vapors, gases, and fumes.

Occupational asthma occurs in persons both with and without atopy. Symptoms include chest tightness, wheezing, dyspnea, and cough. Lung function tests may reveal small-airways dysfunction and an obstructive defect that is partially reversible following administration of bronchodilators. Temporal associations between work and decline in lung function, measured by peak expiratory flow (PEF) or forced expiratory volume in 1 second (FEV_1), may be observed during the work shift or more gradually during the work week. A fixed level of obstruction may ultimately develop. The longer the duration of exposure after onset of symptoms, the more likely is the development of irreversible changes.

Byssinosis is characterized by respiratory symptoms and obstructive airways disease and follows exposure to cotton, flax, and hemp dust. It is seen most commonly in the United States among cotton textile workers. Symptoms of chest tightness and dyspnea, with reduction in rates of air flow, initially appear on the first day of the work week after a 2-day absence from work. These abnormalities may become persistent and result in chronic, irreversible disease if exposure is continued. The bract of the cotton plants is thought to contain the causal agent.

Airways Disease and Multiple Chemical Sensitivity may occur together following an acute inciting event and subsequent exposure to multiple, often unrelated chemicals. The occurrence of airways disease as one of the manifestations of multiple chemical sensitivity is a logical outcome of a postulated physiologic mechanism for chemical sensitivity—namely, irritation of respiratory tract epithelium followed by an inflammatory response with release of mediators, effects on epithelial chemosensitive neurons, and alteration in the permeability of respiratory tract epithelium. Causal workplace exposures often occur in the service sector and affect white collar professionals.

Industrial Bronchitis is a nonspecific manifestation of airway irritation and inflammation. It is characterized by cough and the production of sputum and results from the inhalation of particulates and irritants. Acute bronchitis is self-limited. Chronic bronchitis is defined as cough and sputum production on most days for 3 months or more per year, in two or more consecutive years. It may be associated with the development of irreversible airways obstruction. Causal agents include coal dust and silica, irritant gases such as sulfur dioxide, diesel exhaust, and welding fumes. Industrial bronchitis is also associated with exposure to high levels of nonspecific dust (e.g., in the construction industry).

Interstitial Lung Disease

Interstitial lung disease associated with exposure to dust (pneumoconiosis) was at one time the most commonly recognized form of occupational lung disease. In 1950, the International Labor Organization developed a system for classifying interstitial fibrosis of the lung resulting from exposure to silica and coal dust; the system was updated in the 1970s to include exposure to asbestos. The most common of the pneumoconioses are described below.

Asbestosis is fibrosis of the lung parenchyma or pleura as a result of asbestos exposure. Fibrosis of the pleura may take one of two forms—circumscribed pleural plaques or diffuse pleural thickening. Pleural plaques may contain calcium. The severity of asbestos-related pulmonary fibrosis is related to both total dose and latency. In epidemiologic studies, parenchymal asbestosis is more closely associated with dose, and pleural asbestosis with latency. Respiratory symptoms are nonspecific and depend on the extent of disease. Physical examination may reveal characteristic dry end-inspiratory crackles at the lung bases. Physiologic abnormalities include restrictive mechanics and impaired gas exchange. Small-airways dysfunction, probably resulting from peribronchiolar fibrosis, may be an early finding.

Radiographic changes on posterior–anterior views of the chest include irregular, small opacities in the lower lung zones and pleural plaques. Lateral views of the chest are useful in detecting *calcified hemidiaphragmatic plaques*, a hallmark of asbestos exposure. The value of oblique views in detecting pleural plaques is inversely related to risk for development of disease. Extensive pleural thickening has been associated with respiratory failure; the presence of pleural plaques has been associated with increased risk for subsequent development of lung cancer and malignant mesothelioma. The full effect of exposure to asbestos in asbestos-containing materials in schools and other public buildings remains to be determined. Asbestosis has been reported in school custodians, and malignant mesothelioma in custodians and building occupants.

Silicosis results from exposure to silicon dioxide (SiO_2) or quartz, which is fibrogenic. Silica exposure occurs in a wide variety of occupational settings. Particularly important is bystander exposure. For example, sand blasters are often provided with respiratory protection while workers around them are not. Silicosis may occur in a simple nodular form or in a "complicated" form with progressive massive fibrosis (PMF). Latency and severity of disease are directly related to level of dust exposure. Fulminant silicosis may develop after 1 to 2 years of high-level exposure. It may be complicated by mycobacterial or fungal infection. Radiographic abnormalities characteristically precede functional abnormalities and initially occur as small, rounded opacities involving the upper lung zones. Hilar lymph nodes may become enlarged with "eggshell" calcifications. Physiologic abnormalities reflect the peribronchiolar location of the silicotic nodules and include small-airways dysfunction and impaired gas exchange in the early stages. With PMF, obstruction, restriction, or a mixed pattern may develop.

Coal Worker's Pneumoconiosis results from the deposition of coal dust in peribronchial tissues, with the formation of dust macules and the distention of terminal bronchioles. The occurrence and extent of disease depend on both the level of dust exposure and the rank of the coal, with anthracite being more fibrogenic than bituminous coal. CWP occurs in two forms: "simple" pneumoconiosis, characterized by the presence of small dust nodules, usually less than 5 μm in diameter, and "complicated" pneumoconiosis, or PMF, characterized by large masses of dust and collagen tissue. The most prevalent respiratory symptom is chronic bronchitis, which is unrelated to the radiographic appearance of the lungs and is more common in miners who smoke. Physiologic abnormalities on lung function testing are variable and, with the exception of the single-breath diffusing capacity for carbon monoxide (D_{LCO}), unrelated to the radiographic appearance in simple CWP. A reduced D_{LCO} is associated with category p opacities (<1.5 mm in diameter) in simple CWP and with advanced PMF. Airway obstruction may be seen in PMF and in association with chronic bronchitis.

Acute and Chronic Beryllium Disease results from the inhalation of beryllium oxide. At risk are workers engaged in the manufacture of beryllium-containing products and in the electronics and aircraft industries. Acute disease follows the inhalation of relatively high concentrations of beryllium. Its irritant effect on the respiratory tract may produce nasopharyngitis, tracheobronchitis, or clinical pneumonitis. Chronic beryllium disease is a systemic granulomatous disorder that is often confused with sarcoidosis. The chest radiograph typically reveals a diffuse reticulonodular infiltrate, with hilar lymphadenopathy in about 40% of patients. Lung function tests may reveal obstruction or restriction and impaired gas exchange. The angiotensin$_1$-converting enzyme level is elevated in about 50% of persons with active sarcoidosis, a finding that may be useful in distinguishing this entity from chronic beryllium disease. Elevated levels of beryllium in urine or tissue suggest the diagnosis and provide definitive evidence of exposure. The blast transformation of pulmonary lymphocytes on *in vitro* exposure to beryllium salts confirms the diagnosis.

Hypersensitivity Pneumonitis (Extrinsic Allergic Alveolitis) occurs following exposure to organic dust. Causal agents include thermophilic actinomycetes, *Aspergillus*, and serum and urine protein from animals and fish. Clinical disorders include farmer's lung, bird fancier's lung, bagassosis, humidifier fever, and animal handler's lung. Both acute and chronic reactions may occur. The chest radiograph may reveal miliary or larger discrete opacities in the middle and lower lung zones. Repeated exposure may result in recurrence of symptoms and ultimately in the development of chronic disease, with interstitial fibrosis on the chest radiograph and impaired lung function on physiologic testing. The acute phase may be mild and pass relatively unnoticed. Antigen-specific precipitins appear in about 90% of cases.

So-called "benign" pneumoconioses occur following exposure to certain inert dusts. The chest radiograph reveals interstitial opacities. Lung function generally remains intact. These pneumoconioses follow exposure to iron oxide (siderosis), tin oxide (stannosis), barium (baritosis), and zirconium.

Cancer

Occupational and environmental exposures causally associated with cancer of the respiratory tract include *asbestos*, *radon*, *diesel exhaust*, arsenic, chromium (hexavalent), nickel, vinyl chloride monomer, radiation, and possibly fumes from the welding of stainless steel. Radon daughters of uranium and the chemicals bischloromethyl ether and chloromethylmethyl ether have been shown to cause *small-cell carcinoma*. Of the environmental concerns, asbestos and radon are the two most closely linked to cancer.

Asbestos causes both *bronchogenic carcinoma* and *malignant mesothelioma*, a tumor of the pleura and peritoneum. Asbestos and cigarette smoke act synergistically to increase the risk for lung cancer 50 to 70 times, whereas asbestos alone increases the risk by a factor of three to five. Smoking does not affect the risk for malignant mesothelioma. The risk appears to be greater with exposure to processed asbestos than with exposure to mined asbestos because processing breaks up the bundles into shorter thinner fibers that can reach the lung more readily.

Radon is a naturally occurring gas emanating from uranium-containing rock and soil that is ubiquitous in the United States. Radon itself is harmless, but its daughter products emit α-particles, a potential source of radiation-induced injury to the tracheobronchial tree when attached to dust particles that are inhaled during many years. It is estimated that up to 10% of homes in the United States are built on soils sufficiently radon-rich to produce indoor radon concentrations of concern (>4 pCi/L as established by the Environmental Protection Agency). The actual risk to persons is unknown, but long-term exposure is probably required. The estimated risk derives from experience with uranium miners and is of the magnitude of 5,000 to 50,000 lung cancers per year in the United States. The Environmental Protection Agency recommends that homes in radon-rich areas be tested and remediation efforts undertaken if the level exceeds 4 pCi/L. Remediation, which is not expensive, involves venting the gas in the soil under the home away from the foundation.

NATURAL HISTORY OF DISEASE AND EFFECTIVENESS OF CONTROL

Although much remains to be learned about the natural history of most occupational lung diseases, practical control steps can be taken. It is worthwhile to distinguish agents commonly causing acute symptoms from those producing disease that becomes evident only after an asymptomatic latent period. Continued exposure to a causal agent increases the likelihood of chronic, irreversible, and more severe disease. This is true whether symptoms are manifested acutely or only after a long latency. The difference is that for those diseases with a short latency or none at all, the cause should be more easily recognized and exposures reduced or eliminated altogether.

Occupational asthma is an example of an acute disease that may be reversible if its association with the causal agent is recognized and addressed. With continued exposure, it can progress to chronic, irreversible disease. Other examples are byssinosis and disorders caused by organic dusts (farmer's lung) and toxic metals (beryllium), in which acute and then chronic symptoms are related to the level and duration of exposure.

Diseases such as CWP and asbestosis become clinically manifest only after a long and asymptomatic latent period. Clinical findings of CWP usually follow 10 years of exposure. Similarly, 10 to 20 years of asbestos exposure is typically required to produce detectable pulmonary asbestosis. Silicosis also has a long latent period unless exposure is intense. Despite improved methods of dust control, elimination of exposure altogether is advised for people with identifiable pneumoconiosis. Disease once manifested continues to progress even after cessation of exposure. Moreover, continued exposure to a substance that is also a carcinogen increases the risk for development of related lung cancer.

DIAGNOSIS

Eliciting the *occupational history* is the most important step in the diagnosis of occupational respiratory disease. Although a chronologic lifetime work history is ideal, it is often unnecessary in the primary care setting. Three questions will usually suffice: (a) What is your current job? (b) What was your previous job? and (c) What is your usual job—that is, the one you have worked at the longest? It is important to obtain not only a job title but also a job description. Specific information about the type, level, and duration of exposure is needed. Material safety data sheets for chemicals in use in the workplace and the results of industrial hygiene surveys of the workplace are often useful sources of exposure information. It is important to characterize the temporal relationship of symptoms and disease to work, and to inquire about similar illness in co-workers and family members. A screening environmental history is also important, including exposure to possible air pollutants and radon.

Lung function tests and other laboratory tests provide valuable diagnostic information. A reduced DLCO may be the only abnormality in developing pulmonary fibrosis. Small-airways dysfunction may be an early sign of interstitial or obstructive lung disease. Preshift and postshift *PEF* or *spirometry* is often useful in the diagnosis of occupational asthma. If the history and clinical findings suggest a diagnosis of pneumoconiosis, then a *chest radiograph* should be interpreted according to the International Labor Organization system of classification, developed for purposes of standardization and more specific radiographic characterization and quantification of pneumoconiosis. *Bronchial provocation* by inhalation under carefully controlled conditions can be a useful tool in the diagnosis of occupational asthma.

Thorough documentation is essential, not only to design a treatment program but also to determine disability and compensation.

RECOMMENDATIONS FOR PREVENTION

- Include an occupational/environmental history as a routine part of the screening medical examination in all patients.
- Recommend testing when exposure is suggested by the history.
- Consider obtaining a DLCO determination if pulmonary fibrosis is a concern, a chest radiograph if pneumoconiosis is suspected, and prework and postwork spirometry supplemented by bronchial provocation testing if occupational asthma is a possibility.
- If the diagnosis is confirmed, inform the patient and explain its possible relation to any occupational or environmental causes. Ascertaining patient understanding is important because of statutes of limitation associated with legal remedies, such as workers' compensation.
- Work with the patient, employer, and community if possible to develop a reasonable approach to the reduction or elimination of the causal exposure.
- Inform the employee and a regulatory agency, such as the Occupational Safety and Health Administration or Environmental Protection Agency, of any serious or potentially life-threatening hazards to the patient, co-workers, or other citizens to facilitate an evaluation of the workplace and environment and elimination of the toxic exposure.
- Encourage patients to abstain from habits, such as smoking, that are inherently toxic to the lungs and exacerbate respiratory effects of workplace and environmental exposures.
- Institute appropriate medical surveillance for the subsequent development of other exposure-related pulmonary disease, such as lung cancer.
- Elimination of exposure through the use of rigorous engineering and environmental controls is the ultimate goal in prevention. Removal from the job or home should be a last resort.

ANNOTATED BIBLIOGRAPHY

Banks DE. Respiratory effects of isocyanates. In: Rom WN, ed. Environmental and occupational medicine. New York: Lippincott–Raven Publishers, 1998:537. (*Review of clinical manifestations and pathoyphysiology of isocyanate-induced asthma.*)

Bascom R. Multiple chemical sensitivity: a respiratory disorder? Toxicol Ind Health 1992;8:221. (*Discussion of link between exposure-related alteration in function of respiratory mucosa and multiple chemical sensitivity.*)

Becklake MR. Asbestos-related diseases of the lung and other organs: their epidemiology and implications for clinical practice. Am Rev Respir Dis 1976;114:55. (*Comprehensive review.*)

Bouhuys A, Heapty LJ, Schilling RSF, et al. Byssinosis in U.S. N Engl J Med 1967;277:170. (*Chronic irreversible disease occurs mainly in reactors, those with acute reversible symptoms.*)

Chan-Yeung M, Malo JL. Occupational asthma. N Engl J Med 1995;333:107. (*Very useful discussion for the general reader.*)

Goodman LR. Radiology of asbestos disease. JAMA 1983;249:644. (*Succinct, illustrated summary of characteristic findings.*)

Hammond EC, Selikoff IJ, Seidman H. Asbestos exposure, cigarette smoking and death rates. Ann N Y Acad Sci 1979;330:473. (*Study of independent and interactive contributions of asbestos exposure and cigarette smoking to death from lung cancer in 17,800 asbestos insulation workers.*)

Kriebel D, Sprince NL, Eisen EA, et al. Beryllium exposure and pulmonary function: a cross-sectional study of beryllium workers. Br J Ind Med 1988;45:167. (*Detailed documentation of associated physiologic changes.*)

Kreiss K, Newman LS, Mroz MM, et al. Risks of beryllium disease related to work processes at a metal, alloy, and oxide production plant. Occup Environ Med 1997;54:605. (*Discussion of job-related beryllium exposures and subsequent physiologic and immunologic response.*)

Landregan PL. Asbestos—still a carcinogen. N Engl J Med 1998;338:1618. (*An editorial addressing the risks associated with various forms of asbestos, after a recent study suggested the risk in mining communities is not as high as originally thought.*)

National Research Council: Biologic Effects of Ionizing Radiation (BEIR). Health risks of radon and other internally deposited alpha emitters. Washington, DC: National Academy Press, 1987. (*Comprehensive and authoritative report on the risk associated with exposure to radon.*)

Oliver LC, Sprince N, Greene R. Asbestos-related disease in public school custodians. Am J Ind Med 1991;19:303. (*Reports increased risk associated with building exposures.*)

Oliver LC. Occupational and environmental asthma: legal and ethical aspects of patient management. Chest 1990;98:220S. (*Two very difficult issues in the care of these patients.*)

Parkes WR. Occupational lung disorders. Boston: Butterworth-Heineman, 1994. (*Chapters 12, 13, 20, and 21 provide a detailed discussion of silicosis, CWP, hypersensitivity pneumonitis, and occupational asthma; exceptional photography.*)

Stoeckle JD, Hardy HL, Weber AL. Chronic beryllium disease: a report of 60 cases and selective review of the literature. Am J Med 1969;46:545. (*Exposures occurred primarily during the manufacture of fluorescent lamps. Cor pulmonale was the usual cause of death.*)

Wilkinson P, Hansell DM, Janssens J, et al. Is lung cancer associated with asbestos exposure when there are no small opacities on the chest radiograph? Lancet 1995;345:1074. (*Study documenting increased risk for lung cancer in the absence of radiographic evidence of asbestosis, with general discussion.*)

40
Evaluation of Chronic Dyspnea

Dyspnea is the subjective sensation of difficult or uncomfortable breathing. Patients commonly complain of "shortness of breath" to describe their respiratory difficulty. *Acute dyspnea* is most often a manifestation of sudden left ventricular dysfunction (see Chapter 32), bronchospasm (see Chapter 48), pneumonia (see Chapter 52), pulmonary embolization (see Chapter 20), or anxiety (see Chapter 226). The patient often presents in the urgent care setting. Patients with chronic dyspnea, even when severe, are more likely to come to the office for care. Longstanding dyspnea can be evaluated safely in the outpatient setting.

Heart and lung diseases account for most cases of chronic dyspnea. At times, the differentiation can be difficult; moreover, these causes often coexist. In such instances, diagnosis requires determining which one is predominant. In evaluating the chronically dyspneic patient, one needs to check for precipitants and reversible components, in addition to ascertaining the cause. Also important are an assessment of functional status, severity of deficits, and prognosis.

PATHOPHYSIOLOGY AND CLINICAL PRESENTATION

The pathophysiology of dyspnea is multifactorial and complex. In most instances, dyspnea results from cardiac or pulmonary decompensation and is provoked by the stimulation of receptors responsive to metabolic changes, pulmonary interstitial stretch, respiratory muscle tension, and central respiratory command. Shortness of breath is experienced when ventilatory demand exceeds the actual or perceived capacity of the lungs to respond. The work of breathing may be increased by altered chest wall mechanics, decreased lung compliance, airway obstruction, increased ventilatory requirements, or exogenous factors such as obesity.

Dyspnea occurs in several important clinical settings. *Congestive heart failure* (CHF) can cause dyspnea as pulmonary capillary pressure rises and fluid accumulates in the interstitium, leading to a fall in pulmonary compliance and a sense of difficulty breathing. The earliest symptom is often dyspnea on exertion. More severe failure is manifested by orthopnea and finally paroxysmal nocturnal dyspnea. Basilar crackles (rales) and a third heart sound (S_3) are important signs of left-sided heart failure and pulmonary venous hypertension; the S_3 is one of the most specific signs of CHF. Peripheral edema and jugular venous distention are common manifestations of right-sided heart failure, but these findings, particularly leg edema, are very nonspecific, (see Chapter 22). Contributing and precipitating factors include fever, acute ischemia, excessive dietary sodium intake, dysrhythmias, concurrent use of agents that are negatively inotropic (e.g., β-blockers, disopyramide, verapamil), and poor compliance with medical regimen (see Chapter 32).

Besides CHF, a number of other causes of pulmonary venous hypertension result in increased pulmonary capillary pressure and dyspnea. *Mitral stenosis* is the most important in this class of conditions.

Airway obstruction at any level of the respiratory tract can lead to difficulty breathing. *Tracheal stenosis* resulting from intrinsic disease or extrinsic compression is characterized by dyspnea in conjunction with stridor and inspiratory retraction of the supraclavicular space. *Chronic obstructive pulmonary disease* (COPD) (see Chapter 47) is the leading cause of airway obstruction. *Chronic bronchitis* is a subcategory of COPD that is defined as cough and sputum production persisting for 3 months or more in two consecutive years. Characteristically, these patients have a long history of smoking, productive cough, and a slowly progressive decline in exercise capacity. In advanced stages, they may become plethoric and cyanotic and cough incessantly; the term "blue bloater" has been applied to such patients. Tobacco-stained fingers, wheezes, coarse rales, rhonchi, and a prolonged expiratory phase of respiration are often present on examination. Signs of cor pulmonale (right ventricular heave, jugular venous distention, leg edema) are late findings indicative of severe, advanced disease.

Another group of COPD patients are those with *emphysema*. Sputum production is minimal compared with that in patients with bronchitis, and mismatching of ventilation and perfusion is less pronounced; consequently, hypoxia and cyanosis are less prominent. Gradual deterioration in exercise capacity takes place through many years. Patients with advanced emphysema appear thin and barrel-chested. They may purse their lips during expiration to keep their poorly supported airways from collapsing. The chest is hyperresonant, breath sounds are distant, and a few end-expiratory wheezes may be noted; expiration is prolonged.

Patients with COPD and *bronchiectasis* have a clinical presentation similar to that of patients with chronic bronchitis, except that their physical findings are more localized, the clinical course is punctuated by more frequent episodes of pneumonia, and their sputum tends to be more copious and sometimes bloody.

Asthma is another of the obstructive airway diseases. It usually produces attacks of acute dyspnea, but airway obstruction may persist for a prolonged period after an acute episode and result in more chronic respiratory complaints, including exercise intolerance, cough, and sputum production. At times, sputum production may be the predominant early symptom and mistaken for infection. Diffuse wheezes are commonly noted on examination; severe cases are characterized by use of accessory muscles, retraction, and pulsus paradoxus. Exercise-induced asthma is common in young people and may contribute to recurrent dyspneic episodes (see Chapter 48).

Diffuse *interstitial lung disease* alters pulmonary compliance and may lead to a disturbance in the balance between ventilation and perfusion. The process is usually very gradual, and often patients have few symptoms when pulmonary involvement is mild or even moderate; however, tachypnea and cyanosis ensue in severe cases. Diffuse, "dry" midexpiratory crackles are often heard on auscultation. As the interstitial process progresses, dyspnea and hypoxia worsen and exercise tolerance deteriorates (see Chapter 46).

Kyphoscoliosis is the major chest wall deformity capable of seriously impairing pulmonary musculoskeletal mechanics. Advanced cases can even terminate in cor pulmonale and respiratory failure. Among the extrapulmonary conditions hindering lung mechanics are severe *obesity*, marked *ascites* (see Chapter 71), and large *pleural effusions* (see Chapter 43). Dyspnea is often the chief complaint in such patients.

Pulmonary hypertension represents a serious cause of chronic dyspnea and has a poor prognosis. It may be primary or secondary and is characterized by a fixed elevation in pulmonary artery pressure and resultant strain on the right side of the heart strain. Common physical findings include an accentuated pulmonic component of S_2, a right ventricular S_3, the murmur of tricuspid regurgitation, and peripheral edema.

Secondary pulmonary hypertension occurs with conditions that chronically elevate pulmonary artery pressure, such as *recurrent pulmonary embolization*, *chronic hypoxemia*, *pulmonary parenchymal disease*, and *left-sided heart failure*.

Some forms of secondary disease have subtle presentations and can easily be mistaken for primary disease. For example, pulmonary hypertension resulting from recurrent pulmonary embolization typically occurs in patients with few symptoms of embolization. Except for recalling perhaps a single episode of pleuritic chest pain and acute dyspnea, most patients report few symptoms before the onset of pulmonary hypertension. In those with symptomatic, recurrent embolization, significant pulmonary hypertension rarely develops. The reason for this paradox remains unclear. The source of emboli is believed to be the proximal deep veins of the legs.

Primary pulmonary hypertension is a diagnosis of exclusion. It occurs most commonly in women between the ages of 20 and 40. The mean age is about 35, and the ratio of women to men is 1.7:1. Dyspnea is the most frequently reported symptom, followed by fatigue, near-syncope, and Raynaud's phenomenon. An immunologic basis for the condition is suspected because of the high frequency of antinuclear antibody seropositivity in many of these patients, especially women. Immunologically mediated endothelial damage is postulated. Hyperventilation may result and be mistakenly attributed to anxiety.

Anxiety attacks are often confused with more serious conditions because the patient may appear to be in severe respiratory distress. Patients often report chest tightness or claim that they cannot take in enough air. The florid, acute case is represented by the hyperventilation syndrome (see Chapter 226), but more common is a less dramatic, chronic feeling of dyspnea and fatigue that is affected little by exertion. Frequent sighing, multiple bodily complaints, nervousness, and normal physical examination findings are typical of such patients.

DIFFERENTIAL DIAGNOSIS

The causes of chronic dyspnea encountered in the office setting are listed in Table 40.1.

WORKUP

History remains the single most useful diagnostic modality. In studies of dyspnea, the diagnosis is established by the history in about 75% of instances. However, differentiating dyspnea caused by cardiac disease from that caused by pulmonary pathology can be a challenge. For example, exertional dyspnea occurs in both cardiac and pulmonary disease. A frequent mis-

Table 40.1. Common Causes of Chronic Dyspnea

Cardiac
Congestive heart failure
Other causes of pulmonary venous congestion (mitral stenosis, mitral regurgitation)

Pulmonary
Chronic obstructive pulmonary disease
Pulmonary parenchymal disease (including interstitial diseases)
Pulmonary hypertension
Severe kyphoscoliosis
Exogenous mechanical factors (ascites, massive obesity, large pleural effusion)
Chronic asthma

Psychological
Anxiety

Hematologic
Severe chronic anemia

conception is that paroxysmal nocturnal dyspnea is unique to heart failure. Excessive airway secretions from chronic obstructive lung disease often pool at night and lead to airway obstruction, causing dyspnea and forcing the patient to sit up to clear the airway. Wheezing is a nonspecific manifestation of large-airway bronchospasm, whether it is caused by heart failure or obstructive lung disease.

In general, a history dominated by chronic cough, sputum production, recurrent respiratory infection, occupational exposure, or heavy smoking suggests lung disease rather than a cardiac origin. However, unless a strong history of previous lung disease or substantial sputum production is present, it may be very hard to distinguish a cardiac from a pulmonary source on the basis of history alone. Moreover, both may coexist concurrently. Physical findings and laboratory studies are often necessary for a better differentiation (see below).

Dyspnea that is a manifestation of a chronic anxiety state may superficially mimic cardiopulmonary disease and cause some confusion. Onset at rest in conjunction with a sense of chest tightness, suffocation, or inability to take in air are characteristic features of the history. Also, little evidence of significant heart or lung disease is present, although the patient may fear it greatly. Multiple bodily complaints, a history of emotional difficulties, an absence of activity limitations, and a lack of exacerbation on exercising argue for a psychogenic cause. Unfortunately, patients with pulmonary hypertension may have episodes that can resemble anxiety-induced bouts of dyspnea; sometimes, a young patient with primary pulmonary hypertension is incorrectly labeled "neurotic."

It is helpful to define as precisely as possible the degree of activity that precipitates the sensation of dyspnea, estimate the severity of disease, determine the extent of disability, and detect changes over time. One means of achieving these objectives is to relate symptoms to the patient's daily activities and interpret the degree of restriction in terms of the expected endurance of a patient of similar age.

Factors that may contribute to the occurrence or worsening of dyspnea should be documented, including cigarette smoking, occupational exposure, excessive salt intake, weight gain, and increasing sputum production. The occupational history is particularly important, as the relationships between exposures and lung disease are becoming increasingly evident (see Chapter 39).

The patient should be asked about hemoptysis; the symptom raises the possibilities of bronchiectasis, endobronchial malignancy, embolization with infarction, and pneumonia. If embolization is suspected, the physician must inquire about pleuritic chest pain, leg edema, and other symptoms of deep vein thrombophlebitis (see Chapter 22), in addition to such risk factors as chronic venous insufficiency, inactivity, and—in young women—the use of oral contraceptives and pregnancy. Careful inquiry for historical evidence of recurrent pulmonary embolization is particularly important if pulmonary hypertension is encountered.

Physical Examination should begin with a check for tachycardia, tachypnea, fever, and hypertension. Weight increase must not be forgotten, for it may be an early sign of worsening CHF (see Chapter 32). The patient's respiratory efforts need to be observed carefully to obtain an estimate of the amount of work expended in breathing; contractions of the accessory muscles of respiration suggest severe difficulty. Retraction of the

supraclavicular fossa implies tracheal stenosis that has become critical. Pursed-lip breathing and a prolonged expiratory phase are signs of significant outflow obstruction. The best way to observe air flow obstruction is to have the patient take a deep breath and blow out as hard and as fast as possible. The chest is examined for increased anterior–posterior diameter (suggestive of COPD) and deformity resulting from kyphoscoliosis or ankylosing spondylitis. Retraction of the intercostal muscles on inspiration is characteristic of emphysema.

The chest should be percussed for dullness and hyperresonance and auscultated for wheezes, crackles, and quality of breath sounds. Unfortunately, eliciting wheezing on maximal forced exhalation has proved neither sensitive nor specific for the diagnosis of asthma and cannot be recommended as a technique for uncovering underlying airway hyperreactivity. Crackles suggest fluid in the airway, as occurs with bronchitis, pneumonitis, and CHF. Normal findings on lung examination do not rule out pulmonary pathology but do lessen its probability and the likelihood that it is severe. The cardiac examination should focus on signs of left-sided heart failure (see Chapter 32), detection of left-sided heart murmurs (see Chapters 21 and 33), and signs of pulmonary hypertension and its consequences (accentuated and delayed pulmonic valve component of S_2, right ventricular heave, right ventricular S_3, right-sided systolic regurgitant murmur of tricuspid insufficiency, jugular venous distention, and peripheral edema). It is important to recognize that many of the signs of right-sided heart failure may be a consequence of longstanding pulmonary disease and therefore are not specific for a cardiac etiology. The abdomen is examined for ascites and hepatojugular reflux; the legs are checked for edema and other signs of phlebitis (see Chapters 16 and 30). Finally, the patient's mental status is checked for manifestations of an anxiety disorder; particularly germane is excessive sighing.

Laboratory Studies. The *chest radiograph* is essential to evaluation and should be studied for pulmonary venous redistribution, effusions, interstitial changes, hyperinflation, infiltrates, enlargement of the pulmonary arteries (indicative of pulmonary hypertension), cardiac chamber enlargement, and valve calcification. Upper zone redistribution of pulmonary blood flow is among the earliest radiographic findings of CHF (see Chapter 32); however, redistribution may also occur in COPD because of destruction of vessels in the lower lung fields. The radiographic diagnosis can be made with a high degree of accuracy if any two of the following criteria are met: depression and flattening of the diaphragm with blunting of the costophrenic angles on posterior–anterior film; irregular lucency of the lung fields; abnormally enlarged retrosternal space; diaphragmatic flattening or concavity on the lateral film. Chest radiography is sometimes useful for the detection of interstitial lung disease because physical findings may be minimal. However, radiographic findings may also be unimpressive, so that further study is necessary (see below). When an infiltrate is present, *Gram's stain* of the *sputum* and *culture* are often informative, especially when the patient is febrile, is coughing more than usual, or reports a change in sputum.

Sputum cytology is indicated under similar circumstances, particularly if hemoptysis has developed. A *Ziehl-Neelsen stain* for acid-fast bacilli and *sputum culture for tuberculosis* are also important components of the workup when an infiltrate is detected (see Chapter 49).

Simple *pulmonary function tests* can be reliably performed in the office on an inexpensive spirometer. *Forced expiratory volume in 1 second* (FEV₁) and *vital capacity* are the most informative of these measurements for detecting obstructive and restrictive defects and determining their severity. The ratio of FEV₁ to vital capacity is markedly reduced in clinically important obstructive disease. In restrictive disease, the ratio is close to 1.0, but the vital capacity is significantly reduced. An FEV₁ determination can also provide prognostic information. A reading of less than 1.0 L/s is associated with a poor 5-year survival rate among patients with COPD (see Chapter 47). Patients suspected of having tracheal stenosis may require *flow–volume studies* to identify the lesion and determine its severity; referral is indicated.

Arterial blood gas determinations are not routinely available in most office settings, but they are worth obtaining when deteriorating ventilation is suspected. Hospitalization should be considered when the carbon dioxide tension (Pco_2) is inappropriately elevated for the respiratory rate and repeated determinations reveal further increases in Pco_2. Measuring arterial blood gases before and after exercise is helpful in assessing the severity of diffuse interstitial disease. A fall in oxygen tension (Po_2) is evidence of a significant degree of interstitial disease. When use of accessory muscles is noted and the patient's condition appears to be worsening, prompt hospital admission should be arranged without time taken to determine arterial blood gases in the office.

A reduction in *single-breath carbon monoxide diffusing capacity* (DLCO) may be the earliest sign of interstitial fibrosis. The test is particularly useful in the evaluation of dyspnea associated with suspected occupational interstitial disease (see Chapters 39 and 46).

Sometimes, the combination of history, physical examination, chest radiography, and pulmonary function testing is not sufficient to determine the relative contributions of heart disease and lung disease to a case of dyspnea. When findings are equivocal, it may be helpful to order a *cardiac ultrasonographic* examination, a readily available, noninvasive means of determining chamber size, valvular anatomy, and left ventricular function. The ejection fraction will be reduced in the setting of left ventricular dysfunction and relatively preserved in patients with predominantly pulmonary disease. Cardiac ultrasonography in conjunction with *Doppler* study is an excellent means of detecting important treatable causes of pulmonary hypertension, such as tight mitral stenosis (see Chapter 33) and sometimes pulmonary embolization. An old-fashioned but occasionally useful parameter, the *circulation time*, is prolonged by 4 seconds or more beyond the upper limit of normal (16 seconds) in patients with CHF.

The neurotic patient with anxiety-induced dyspnea often benefits from undergoing chest radiography and simple pulmonary function testing; the confirmation of a well-functioning respiratory system may provide some reassurance and lessen concern over bodily symptoms. At times, a *walk with the patient* up and down a few flights of stairs is just as convincing for both physician and patient. Climbing stairs with a patient complaining of dyspnea is also useful if cardiopulmonary disease is suspected, as exercise tolerance can be quantified in terms of the number of flights climbed and the heart and respiratory rates attained.

Evaluation of Pulmonary Hypertension. Finding evidence suggestive of pulmonary hypertension (dyspnea, signs of right-sided heart strain on physical examination and electrocardio-gram, prominent main pulmonary artery and hilar vessels in conjunction with decreased peripheral vessels on chest x-ray film) necessitates consideration of its treatable causes, such as recurrent pulmonary embolization, sleep apnea (see Chapter 8), and mitral stenosis (see Chapter 33). Although pulmonary hypertension is typically quite advanced by the time the diagnosis is made, efforts at earlier recognition and identification of treatable causes are imperative if the prognosis is to be improved.

Echocardiography has shown considerable promise in the noninvasive diagnosis of cor pulmonale and pulmonary hypertension and their antecedent conditions. The *perfusion lung scan* has proved to be a safe, noninvasive means of screening for recurrent pulmonary embolization and differentiating it from primary pulmonary hypertensive disease. In primary disease, the scan findings may be normal, or the scan may show a subsegmental or diffuse patchy peripheral distribution of labeled albumin. In secondary disease resulting from recurrent pulmonary emboli, the scan shows multiple segmental or large subsegmental defects. Any segmental or large subsegmental perfusion defect in a patient with pulmonary hypertension is an indication for consideration of *pulmonary angiography*. Ventilation scanning usually does not add enough specificity to the evaluation in this context to obviate the need for angiography.

SYMPTOMATIC MANAGEMENT AND PATIENT EDUCATION

The relief of dyspnea requires attention to *exacerbating factors* in addition to the underlying etiology. Symptomatic management begins with correcting reversible forms of airway obstruction (see Chapters 47 and 48) and precipitants of left ventricular dysfunction (see Chapter 32). Any concurrent respiratory tract infection requires treatment (see Chapter 52). If a large pleural effusion (see Chapter 43), a severe anemia (see Chapter 82), or an acute situational stress (see Chapter 226) is present, it too should receive prompt attention. Environmental irritants ought to be eliminated (see Chapter 39). All patients with dyspnea should be advised to stop smoking; often, the onset of even mild dyspnea is a sufficient stimulus to quit, especially when combined with the physician's urging (see Chapter 54).

Attention to the underlying cause cannot be overemphasized, whether it is heart disease (see Chapters 30, 32, and 33), lung disease (see Chapters 47, 48, and 52), a mechanical factor such as massive obesity (see Chapter 233), or an anxiety disorder (see Chapter 226). Dyspneic patients with such disorders greatly appreciate knowing the cause of their discomfort and its prognosis, especially when it differs from what their perception has been.

Many patients with chronic dyspnea request *home oxygen therapy*. Such requests are reasonable if the patient has a condition causing chronic hypoxemia, provided that no evidence of carbon dioxide retention, with its attendant risk of suppression of respiratory drive, is present. Nocturnal oxygen therapy is particularly useful in preventing pulmonary hypertension in patients with chronic hypoxemia, but it must be used with care (see Chapter 47). Patients without significant hypoxemia—even those with chronic emphysema—do not benefit from oxygen therapy.

Selected patients with lung or heart disease may benefit from an *exercise program*; exercise tolerance often improves, although the effect on survival remains unproven (see Chapters 18, 30, 31, and 47). It is important that patients be reminded to note the level of activity that they can tolerate and report any decrease. Precipitants of worsening exercise tolerance should also be monitored.

The use of *anxiolytics* is helpful only in patients whose dyspnea is a manifestation of a severe anxiety disorder. Even then, extreme caution must be exercised in the long-term use of such medications (see Chapter 226). Prescribing tranquilizers for a patient with heart or lung disease who is anxious because of trouble with breathing is more likely to exacerbate the respiratory problem than to help it.

INDICATIONS FOR REFERRAL AND ADMISSION

For patients with underlying heart or lung disease who experience a worsening of their chronic dyspnea, prompt hospital admission should be considered, especially if the change is rapid. It may represent acute left ventricular decompensation, ventilatory failure, or hypoxemia. Acute anxiety can superficially mimic cardiopulmonary decompensation and needs to be ruled out (see above) before hospitalization is authorized. Pulmonary consultation may be helpful in the patient with suspected pulmonary hypertension, both for design of the diagnostic assessment and for selection of the treatment plan if a secondary cause is identified. For the patient found to have pulmonary hypertension secondary to recurrent pulmonary embolization, referral to a surgeon experienced in performing thromboendarterectomy should be considered.

A.H.G./A.G.M.

ANNOTATED BIBLIOGRAPHY

Baumstark A, Swensson RG, Hessel SJ, et al. Evaluating the radiographic assessment of pulmonary venous hypertension in chronic heart disease. Am J Radiol 1984;142:877. (*Suggests that the assessment can be quite accurate, with a sensitivity of 0.75 and a specificity of 0.88.*)

Come PC. Echocardiographic recognition of pulmonary arterial disease and determination of its cause. Am J Med 1988;84:384. (*Provides evidence for the utility of ultrasonography in the identification and differential diagnosis of pulmonary hypertension.*)

D'Alonzo GE, Bower JS, Dantzker DR. Differentiation of patients with primary and thromboembolic pulmonary hypertension. Chest 1984;85:457. (*The pattern on perfusion lung scan is different.*)

Enright PL, McClelland RL, Newman AB, et al. Underdiagnosis and undertreatment of asthma in the elderly. Cardiovascular Health Study Research Group. Chest 1999;116:603. (*Asthma was both underdiagnosed and undertreated in this community-based sample of nearly 5,000 people age 65 or older.*)

Hull RD, Hirsch J, Carter CJ, et al. Pulmonary angiography, ventilation lung scanning, and venography for clinically suspected pulmonary embolism with abnormal perfusion lung scan. Ann Intern Med 1983;98:891. (*Details the indications for each; angiography remains the definitive test.*)

King DK, Thompson BT, Johnson DC. Wheezing on maximal forced exhalation in the diagnosis of atypical asthma. Ann Intern Med 1989;110;451. (*Wheezing proved neither sensitive nor specific.*)

Lee DC, Johnson RA, Bingham JB, et al. Heart failure in outpatients. N Engl J Med 1982;306:699. (*Includes a discussion of clinical findings indicative of the diagnosis and predictive of response to therapy.*)

Jones NL. Exercise testing in pulmonary evaluation: clinical application. N Engl J Med 1975;293:647. (*Describes the use of exercise pulmonary function tests in evaluating dyspnea; article on page 341 of same issue details methods and physiology of exercise testing.*)

Liss HP, Grant BJB. The effect of nasal flow on breathlessness in patients with chronic obstructive lung disease. Am Rev Respir Dis 1988;137:1285. (*Nasal cannular delivery of room air provided as much relief of dyspnea as did cannular delivery of oxygen.*)

Man GCW, Hsu K, Sproule BJ. Effect of alprazolam on exercise and dyspnea in patients with chronic obstructive lung disease. Chest 1986;90:832. (*No benefit was found in patients who had normal Po_2 values.*)

Morgan WC, Hodge HL. Diagnostic evaluation of dyspnea. Am Fam Physician 1998;57:711. (*Effective review of dyspnea attributable to cardiac, pulmonary, and other causes.*)

Mulrow CD, Lucey CR, Farnett LE. Discriminating causes of dyspnea through clinical examination. J Gen Intern Med 1993;8:383. (*Accuracy of clinical assessment was 70%.*)

Pratt PC. Role of conventional chest radiography in diagnosis and exclusion of emphysema. Am J Med 1987;82:998. (*A review arguing that a high degree of accuracy can be achieved if validated criteria are used; 40 references.*)

Raffin TA. Indications for arterial blood gas analysis. Ann Intern Med 1986;105:390. (*A critical review of uses of blood gas determinations; 76 references.*)

Rich S, Levitsky S, Brundage BH. Pulmonary hypertension from chronic pulmonary embolism. Ann Intern Med 1988;108:425. (*A review exploring the often confusing relationship between these two conditions; 87 references.*)

Rich S, Dantzker DR, Ayers SM, et al. Primary pulmonary hypertension: a national prospective study. Ann Intern Med 1987;107:216. (*Findings from a national registry; best available data on clinical and epidemiologic features.*)

Tobin MJ. Dyspnea: pathophysiologic basis, clinical presentation, and management. Arch Intern Med 1990;150:1604. (*Useful review, with emphasis on pathophysiology; includes a good discussion of hyperventilation syndrome; 97 references.*)

41
Evaluation of Chronic Cough

A chronic cough (one lasting longer than 3 weeks) poses a challenging evaluation problem because the list of causes ranges from the trivial to the life-threatening. Patients present because they fear that "something is wrong"; AIDS, cancer, tuberculosis (TB), and pneumonia lead the list of concerns. Relief from symptoms is another reason for patient presentation. The primary physician must keep in mind more worrisome causes (e.g., bronchogenic carcinoma and TB) and be aware that cough may be an important although atypical presentation of such common conditions as asthma and gastroesophageal reflux. The objective is to conduct a complete yet efficient evaluation that avoids both unnecessary testing and excessive delay.

PATHOPHYSIOLOGY AND CLINICAL PRESENTATION

The physiologic function of cough is to remove foreign substances and mucus from the respiratory tract. It is a three-phase mechanical process that involves a deep inspiration, increasing lung volume, muscular contraction against a closed glottis, and sudden opening of the glottis. The maneuver produces and sustains a high linear air velocity to expel material from the respiratory tree.

Cough is a reflex response that is mediated by the medulla but is subject to voluntary control. The afferent limb may involve receptors in the larynx, respiratory tree, pleura, acoustic duct, nose, sinuses, pharynx, stomach, or diaphragm. The receptors respond to mechanical, inflammatory, or irritant stimuli. The trigeminal, glossopharyngeal, phrenic, and vagus nerves can carry the afferent signal. The efferent limb of the cough reflex involves the recurrent laryngeal, phrenic, and spinal motor nerves, which innervate the respiratory muscles.

The most common cause of chronic cough is *cigarette smoking*, which may trigger the cough reflex by direct bronchial irritation; alternatively, smoking may induce inflammatory changes and the production of mucus, which stimulates a self-propagating productive cough. Chronic bronchitis may ensue. Chronic cough and decreased flow rates have been observed in adolescents after only 3 to 5 years of smoking. Pipe and cigar smoking cause lesser degrees of difficulty.

Environmental Irritants play a major role in the production of cough in patients living in industrialized urban areas. Pollutants that are frequently involved are heavy smog, sulfur dioxide, nitrous oxide, and industrial gases such as ammonia. In Britain, the relationship between air quality and production of cough has been documented. The dusts and particulate matter that are capable of producing pneumoconioses contribute to the problem (see Chapter 39). The excessive drying of normal airway moisture that takes place in centrally heated homes (humidity may fall below 10% unless a humidifier is utilized) can result in a persistent dry cough during the winter months.

Carcinoma of the Lung may present with cough in its early stages, particularly when an endobronchial lesion is present. Often, the cigarette smoker notes a change in the pattern of a chronic "cigarette cough." *Hemoptysis* is noted in about 5% to 10% of early cases. Other clues are localized wheezing and purulent sputum suggestive of obstruction. In later stages, cough is present in conjunction with weight loss, anorexia, and dyspnea. In some instances, a systemic syndrome (e.g., inappropriate secretion of antidiuretic hormone, hypertrophic pulmonary osteoarthropathy, dermatomyositis, peripheral neuropathy) may precede the appearance of tumor.

Asthma. Cough may be the predominant manifestation. Studies of asthmatic patients have emphasized that cough can occur in the absence of wheezing or abnormalities on routine pulmonary function testing. The cough is characteristically worse at night and can be triggered or exacerbated by exposure to environmental irritants, allergens, or cold. Exercise is a common stimulant. In such cases, the bronchorrheal component of asthma predominates, but methacholine or carbachol challenge will often unmask the obstructive manifestations (see Chapter 48).

Inflammation anywhere along the upper or lower respiratory tract is capable of producing cough; receptors capable of transmitting impulses that stimulate cough are believed to be distributed throughout the respiratory system. The greater the inflammatory stimulus, the larger the white cell response and the more purulent the sputum. (The green coloration of very purulent sputum is caused by the degeneration of white cells.) A number of patients experience a dry, persistent cough after an upper respiratory infection; the cough may last more than 8 weeks and is unrelated to postnasal drip or airway hyperreactivity. The pathophysiology of this cough is believed to be related to airway epithelial damage.

Chronic Bronchitis is among the most common causes of chronic cough and sputum production. The condition is defined clinically as the presence of a productive cough that persists for at least 3 months for two consecutive years. A morning cough is often prominent, and bronchospasm is a frequent accompaniment (see Chapter 47). *Bronchiectasis* is also characterized by cough and sputum production, but it differs clinically from bronchitis in that repeated bouts of hemoptysis and pneumonia are more likely to occur. Copious amounts of purulent sputum are often produced. Chronic cough and sputum production commonly persist between episodes of pneumonia. Focal destruction of supporting lung tissue leads to dilation of bronchi and focal findings of rhonchi and wheezes on physical examination. A history of suppurative pneumonia in childhood is sometimes elicited.

Nasal and Otic Problems are often overlooked as sources of chronic cough. *Chronic allergic rhinitis* (see Chapter 222) with resultant postnasal drip ranks as one of the leading causes of chronic cough productive of clear sputum. The nasal mucosa may be edematous and the pharyngeal mucosal "cobblestoned" in appearance. Similarly, *sinusitis* (see Chapter 219) may be associated with a persistent cough and sputum production secondary to excessive retropharyngeal drainage of mucus. It accounts for up to a third of patients with postnasal drip. Sinus tenderness and purulent nasal drainage are typical manifestations, but they may be absent even in the presence of significant mucosal thickening on sinus films. Even impacted cerumen and external otitis have been implicated in stimulating the cough reflex (see Chapter 218).

Interstitial Lung Disease and Extraluminal Compression may stimulate mechanical receptors and result in a nonproductive cough. Fibrotic diseases of the interstitium and pulmonary edema are examples of intrapulmonary causes, and hilar adenopathy, aortic aneurysm, and neoplasm are important extraluminal mass lesions. *Chronic interstitial pulmonary edema* is associated with nocturnal cough because venous return is increased at night, which worsens heart failure (see Chapter 32). When failure is severe, frothy pink or blood-tinged sputum may be noted.

Psychogenic Cough is more prevalent in children but may occur in adults; characteristically, it is nonproductive, occurs at times of emotional stress, and ceases during the night.

Gastroesophageal Reflux sometimes leads to chronic cough. In fact, it is among the three most common causes identified in case series of patients with persistent chronic cough. Mechanisms include (a) esophageal irritation with stimulation of an esophageal–tracheobronchial reflex and (b) nocturnal aspiration of gastric juices. Cough may be the only presenting symptom.

The advent of *angiotensin-converting enzyme inhibitors (ACE)* inhibitors has been associated with an unexpectedly high incidence of dry nocturnal cough, with reports of 10% to 15% of patients being affected. First reported with use of enalapril, the cough has been associated with most long-acting ACE inhibitor preparations. Patients complain of an irritated feeling. The cough usually does not respond to a switch to another ACE inhibitor, although reducing the dose may help. In about 50% of instances, the cough is so annoying that ACE inhibitor therapy must be terminated.

DIFFERENTIAL DIAGNOSIS

The common causes of chronic cough are listed in Table 41.1. In a series of 139 consecutive cases of chronic cough encountered in the community setting, the cause was hyperactive airway disease in 21%, postnasal drip in 19%, postinfectious status in 9%, chronic bronchitis in 4%, gastroesophageal reflux in 4%, and, in a few cases, occupational lung disease and psychiatric illness. In a referral setting study, a postnasal drip syndrome accounted for 41% of cases, asthma for 24%, esophageal reflux for 21%, and chronic bronchitis for 5%. Cough was the sole presentation of asthma in 28% of asthmatic patients and of reflux in 43% of patients with reflux. In a fourth of cases, more than one cause was identified. Sinusitis accounted for 38% of cases of postnasal drip. Rarer causes of chronic cough include irritation of the pleura, diaphragm, or pericardium. Osteophytes of the cervical spine and pacemaker malfunction have been reported as truly rare causes of cough.

WORKUP

Although in some cases the cause of a chronic cough is readily apparent, presentations of even the common underlying

Table 41.1. Important Causes of Chronic or Persistent Cough

Environmental Irritants
Cigarette smoking (cigar and pipe smoking to a lesser degree)
Pollutants (sulfur dioxide, nitrous oxide, particulate matter)
Dusts (all agents capable of producing pneumoconioses)
Lack of humidity

Lower Respiratory Tract Problems
Lung cancer
Asthma (including variant asthma)
Chronic obstructive lung disease (especially bronchitis)
Interstitial lung disease
Congestive heart failure (chronic interstitial pulmonary edema)
Pneumonitis
Bronchiectasis

Upper Respiratory Tract Problems
Chronic rhinitis
Chronic sinusitis
Disease of the external auditory canal
Pharyngitis
Angiotensin-converting enzyme inhibitors

Extrinsic Compressive Lesions
Adenopathy
Malignancy
Aortic aneurysm

Psychogenic Factors

Gastrointestinal Problems
Reflux esophagitis

conditions may be subtle, so that careful investigation is necessary. During the initial workup, the physician should consider serious causes (cancer, TB, heart failure) while checking for the much more common treatable causes (asthma, esophageal reflux, postnasal drip). In a detailed study of workup for chronic cough, history offered the highest yield, with 70% of patients having a true-positive finding; physical examination was second, with 49%, and laboratory studies were third, with an average of 22% of patients having true-positive findings.

History. A careful history and description of the cough, combined with a review of aggravating and alleviating factors and any associated symptoms, can provide useful information, although presentations overlap to a considerable degree. A cough that worsens when the patient lies down suggests postnasal drip, esophageal reflux, bronchiectasis, bronchitis, and heart failure. One accompanied by the production of clear sputum is consistent with a hypersensitivity mechanism, whereas persistent purulence suggests chronic infection (e.g., chronic sinusitis, bronchiectasis, or TB), and bloody sputum raises the specter of cancer, TB, and bronchiectasis (see Chapter 42). Associated symptoms of orthopnea, dyspnea on exertion, and paroxysmal nocturnal dyspnea implicate heart failure; dyspnea may also reflect pneumonitis or asthma. By definition, chronic bronchitis is diagnosed by the history of a chronic productive cough 3 months of the year for two consecutive years. The diagnosis is reinforced by a reduction in coughing with cessation of smoking or avoidance of environmental irritants.

Although postnasal drip, throat clearing, and nasal discharge are characteristic of conditions causing a postnasal drip syndrome, some of these symptoms may also occur in patients with asthma or even esophageal reflux. Chronic throat clearing is also consistent with a psychogenic etiology. Although heartburn or a sour taste in the mouth are reported by most patients whose cough is caused by reflux, as many as 40% of those whose cough proves to be linked to reflux do not report these symptoms. Hoarseness is usually indicative of tracheobronchial disease with laryngeal involvement but may represent a tumor impinging on the recurrent laryngeal nerve.

The history should also detail smoking habits, environmental and occupational exposures, and use of ACE inhibitors and should include a review for previous allergies, asthma, sinusitis, recent respiratory infection, and TB exposure.

Physical Examination should emphasize the upper respiratory tract, chest, and cardiovascular system. The physician needs to examine the skin for cyanosis and clubbing; the pharynx for postnasal discharge, mucosal edema, and tonsillar enlargement; the nose for polyps, discharge, and obstruction; the sinuses for tenderness; and the ears for impacted cerumen or otitis. The trachea is palpated for position and the neck for masses and adenopathy. Auscultation and percussion of the lungs (including the apices) are performed to detect wheezing, crackles, and signs of consolidation or effusion. Generalized wheezing is associated with obstruction from asthma or bronchitis, but localized wheezing may be a sign of tumor. Wheezing only on maximal forced exhalation was found to be neither sensitive nor specific for the diagnosis of variant asthma. During cardiac examination, the physician should evaluate the jugular venous pulse for elevated systemic venous pressure, palpate for chamber enlargement, and listen for a third heart sound, all indicative of heart failure.

Laboratory Studies. Testing can very often be held to a minimum when a careful history is taken and a thorough physical examination performed. For example, when the history is suggestive of chronic rhinitis causing a postnasal drip, one can proceed directly to a diagnostic trial of antihistamines and decongestants without resorting to laboratory testing. Alternatively, a topically active corticosteroid nasal spray may be used for the trial. Similarly, the patient with suspected asthma may be given a diagnostic trial of inhaled steroids (see Chapter 48). In most cases of chronic cough, only a few, well-chosen studies are usually necessary. *Chest radiography* is essential when historical or physical evidence raises the question of carcinoma, pneumonitis, tuberculosis, heart failure, or bronchiectasis. However, the test is overused and not necessary in the nonsmoker who presents with a persistent cough after a recent upper respiratory infection and whose physical examination findings are normal. The chest film may be used to provide reassurance, but a careful explanation and follow-up in 4 to 6 weeks should suffice. The search for pneumonitis should be reserved for patients with a history of disease related to HIV infection or findings suggestive of ongoing infection (persistent production of purulent sputum, night sweats, fever, respiratory rate >25/min, rales, asymmetric respirations, increased vocal fremitus).

Sinus films are usually unnecessary when the history is positive for postnasal drip. In fact, the correlation between the appearance on films and symptoms considered typical of sinusitis may be poor. In rare instances, a patient who has eluded diagnosis may have an occult sinusitis identified by sinus films, with mucosal thickening of more than 6 mm identified on radiographic study. However, routine sinus films are unnecessary.

When purulent sputum is present or an infiltrate has been identified on chest x-ray films, every effort should be made to obtain *sputum for examination.* Patients with a history of producing purulent sputum in conjunction with cough, but who cannot raise sputum at the time of examination, should be instructed to drink a few glasses of water and remain a while to see if sputum can be raised. Inducing sputum by use of a saline spray may also be helpful. A surprisingly common omission in evaluating a cough productive of purulent sputum is failure to obtain and examine the sputum.

An important component of the sputum examination is the *Gram's stain.* In persons at high risk for TB (e.g., recent immigrants, immunocompromised hosts), an *acid-fast stain* for tubercle bacilli is needed. *Culturing* the sputum is also important, especially when TB is a possibility, because the acid-fast examination is not very sensitive and the diagnosis cannot be ruled out with certainty until three early-morning sputum samples have failed to produce growth by 4 to 6 weeks (see Chapters 38 and 49).

Sputum cytology—in which three early-morning sputum samples are obtained—can be a useful screening test for pulmonary neoplasm (see Chapters 37, 42, and 53) when clinical findings raise suspicion (history of smoking, hemoptysis, nodule on chest x-ray film). Pulmonary histiocytes must be demonstrated on each specimen to prove that the sample of pulmonary secretions is adequate. A "negative" test result in the absence of histiocytes is the source of many false-negative readings.

Because sputum cytology is not a particularly sensitive test, it cannot be used to rule out lung cancer. When tumor remains in the differential diagnosis, *fiberoptic bronchoscopy* should be considered. It is also helpful in the evaluation of obstructing lesions and infiltrates that elude diagnosis, as biopsy specimens, washings, and cultures can be taken. However, if the chest radiographic findings are normal and no hemoptysis or history of smoking is present, then the yield from bronchoscopy is very low, and further workup for cancer is unlikely to be productive.

Cough of Obscure Cause. When the cause remains elusive despite the extensive workup described above, *postnasal drip syndrome, variant asthma,* and *gastroesophageal reflux* should be considered. These conditions account for a substantial proportion of hard-to-diagnose cases of chronic cough. As noted earlier, the history and physical examination may not reveal the symptoms and signs typically associated with them. Starting empiric therapy with decongestants, first with bronchodilators and then histamine₂ antagonists, is a reasonable approach. If testing is to be effective and a false-positive diagnosis avoided, a knowledge of test accuracy in identifying these conditions in patients with chronic cough is necessary. Traditional *spirometry* with *bronchodilator administration* was found in one study to have only a 50% positive predictive value in patients with chronic cough because of a high false-positive rate (33%), although its sensitivity was excellent (approaching 100%). *Methacholine challenge* to induce bronchospasm has a similarly high degree of sensitivity but a lower false-positive rate (22%), so that it has a slightly better positive predictive value (60%). Both tests rule out asthma if results are normal. A positive test result needs to be confirmed by a response to bronchodilator therapy.

The diagnosis of esophageal reflux is harder to make in the absence of typical symptoms. Whereas a history of retrosternal burning traveling upward has a predictive value of more than 90% for gastroesophageal reflux, its absence does not rule it out. Prolonged *monitoring* of *esophageal pH* has proved to be the most effective test for esophageal reflux in patients with chronic cough. In the best study of its efficacy, the test had a positive predictive value of more than 95%, with few false-positive and false-negative results. Monitoring of pH was far superior to barium swallow, which had a high false-negative rate. As noted above, an alternative to pH monitoring is a *diagnostic trial of therapy with a histamine₂ blocker* (see Chapter 61). However, 1 to 2 months of therapy may be necessary to demonstrate a definitive reduction in cough. Thus, pH monitoring may be the most rapid means of diagnosis of reflux-induced cough. Patients with reflux symptoms do not need radiologic study or endoscopy unless cancer or obstruction is a concern (see Chapter 61).

SYMPTOMATIC THERAPY AND PATIENT EDUCATION

The most effective means of stopping the cough is to identify and treat the underlying cause (see Chapters 47, 49, 61, and 222). An empiric trial of an etiologic therapy can be highly effective in providing a diagnosis as well as relief of symptoms (see above); however, certain etiologic therapies should not be used empirically—especially antibiotics in the absence of proven infection. Symptomatic management is distinguished from empiric etiologic therapy. It is directed at eliminating precipitants and suppressing the cough. The goal is to prevent the complications that may result from prolonged forceful coughing, such as sleeplessness, musculoskeletal pain, rib fractures, pneumothorax, exhaustion, pneumomediastinum, posttussive syncope (see Chapter 24), and rupture of subconjunctival or nasal veins. The occurrence of any of these complications may be a reason for occasionally suppressing a cough that has not been completely diagnosed.

The first priority and simplest manipulation is to remove or reduce irritants. Of paramount importance is *cessation of smoking* and passive exposure to cigarette smoke; this alone eliminated cough in 77% and reduced it in another 17% of patients within a month. Second, an appropriate *humidity* should be maintained. If a humidifier is used, it should be kept clean because it can become colonized with bacteria or fungi and cause infection or hypersensitivity pneumonitis. Third, adequate internal *hydration* should be encouraged, with at least 1,500 mL of fluid consumed daily. These simple measures alone may abolish cough in many patients.

The patient with a chronic cough secondary to established underlying lung disease requires careful education. The patient must be informed that sputum should be expectorated when possible. Patients with chronic bronchitis or bronchiectasis can be taught how to cough with quiet, forceful expirations and how to perform *postural drainage* to promote removal of mucus from the bronchioles. Postural drainage is best performed before meals and at bedtime. *Ipratropium* is sometimes helpful in reducing nighttime cough in the patient with chronic obstructive pulmonary disease (see Chapter 47).

Patients with chronic cough often request *temporary cough suppression* to allow uninterrupted sleep; such suppression is also required when complications of cough arise. A wide variety of agents have been used to treat cough. The most effective are the *narcotic antitussives*, which act centrally to suppress the medullary cough center. Other preparations are expectorants or mucolytic agents, which merely help to mobilize sputum. They can also have a mild placebo effect, although it is not impressive. When cough significantly interferes with sleeping or eating, a narcotic cough suppressant should be used. *Codeine* is the drug of choice. It should be given in relatively small doses of 8 to 15 mg at intervals of 3 to 4 hours, according to the patient's needs. In many instances, a dose before bedtime will suffice. Liquid and tablet preparations are equally effective. If a small dose does not suppress the cough, doses of up to 60 mg every 3 to 4 hours may be tried. It is worth noting that many patients expect to use a syrup for cough suppression; prescribing the drug in syrup form may provide some psychological benefit. Patients for whom a narcotic antitussive is prescribed should be given small quantities and followed closely to ensure that the cough resolves and excessive use does not result. The obvious exception to this precaution is the patient with incurable lung cancer, who should receive the doses necessary to provide relief from the discomfort of persistent cough.

Non-narcotic antitussives lack addiction potential but are not as effective as codeine. The most popular and effective over-the-counter cough suppressant is *dextromethorphan*, which has a mild suppressant effect. Many over-the-counter preparations contain *alcohol, sympathomimetics,* and *antihistamines*. The mucolytic effects of alcohol are minimal. The sympathomimetics are of little use except in patients whose cough derives from chronic vasomotor rhinitis (see Chapter 222). The antihistamines are most useful for patients with allergic upper airway disease (see Chapter 222) and are a helpful adjunct for inducing sleep when taken at bedtime. Some over-the-counter agents dull the peripheral sensory receptors; this is the rationale for putting mild topical anesthetics in sprays, syrups, and cough lozenges. They are of questionable utility.

Expectorants are heavily consumed. More than 60 preparations containing guaifenesin are available; terpin hydrate is another popular expectorant. These agents are often combined with an effective cough suppressant and, as such, produce a beneficial effect, but by themselves they have no proven effect and represent an unnecessary expense. They are given when the patient insists on something for cough but clear indications for cough suppression are lacking, or when the patient believes expectorants will help.

Patients with cough secondary to asthma respond to inhaled topically active *corticosteroids* and *bronchodilators* (see Chapter 48). Topical steroid therapy may also help in allergic rhinitis (see Chapter 222). Patients with persistent cough after a recent respiratory tract infection and no signs of pneumonitis may benefit from a short course of inhaled steroid therapy, which presumably lessens residual inflammatory changes. Time is another effective therapy.

Patients with suspected reflux should respond to a course of antireflux therapy with *antacids* and *histamine₂* blockers (see Chapter 61), although, as noted above, the benefits may not become apparent for several weeks.

INDICATIONS FOR REFERRAL

Although endobronchial cancer is feared, it is not a common cause of chronic cough in the absence of other findings, especially in the patient with normal chest radiographic findings. However, the patient without a diagnosis who has risk factors for cancer (smoking, occupational exposure) requires a consultation for consideration of bronchoscopy, particularly if the chest radiographic findings are abnormal. The patient with a normal chest radiographic findings and no risk factors can be followed expectantly without resort to bronchoscopy because the likelihood of a positive study result is small.

A.H.G./A.G.M.

ANNOTATED BIBLIOGRAPHY

Bloustine S, Langston L, Miller T, et al. Ear cough (Arnold's reflex). Otol Rhinol Laryngol 1976;85:406. (*A clinical survey of 688 patients revealed an incidence of 1.74% for ear cough reflex, a reminder to examine the ear.*)

Corrao W, Braman SS, Irwin RS. Chronic cough as the sole presenting manifestation of bronchial asthma. N Engl J Med 1979;300:633. (*Six patients with cough as the presenting symptom of asthma; they had no prior history of wheezing.*)

Diehr P, Wood RW, Bushyhead J, et al. Prediction of pneumonia in outpatients with acute cough—a statistical approach. J Chron Dis 1984;37:215. (*A study of nearly 2,000 patients presenting with cough with or without radiographic evidence of pneumonia. A discriminate analysis scoring system is presented.*)

Ing AJ, Ngu MC, Breslin ABX. Chronic persistent cough and clearance of esophageal acid. Chest 1992;102:1668. (*Acid reflux is an important cause; impaired clearance of acid found.*)

Irwin RS, Corrao WM, Pratter MR. Chronic persistent cough in the adult: the spectrum and frequency of causes and successful outcome of specific therapy. Am Rev Respir Dis 1981;123:413. (*Intensive study of a series of 49 patients revealed 12 with asthma; 14 with postnasal drip; nine with asthma plus postnasal drip, usually following upper respiratory infection; six with bronchitis; five with esophagitis; and one each with cough of malignant, cardiac, or interstitial origin.*)

Irwin RS, Curley FJ, French CL. Chronic cough: the spectrum and frequency of causes, key components of the diagnostic evaluation, and outcome of specific therapy. Am Rev Respir Dis 1990;141:640. (*A prospective study of a systematic anatomic diagnostic evaluation protocol; asthma, postnasal drip, and esophageal reflux accounted for a large percentage of cases; detailed data on utility of various diagnostic modalities.*)

Irwin RS, Curley FJ. The treatment of cough. Chest 1991;99:1477. (*A comprehensive review of symptomatic therapies; 68 references.*)

Irwin RS, French CT, Smyrnios NA, et al. Interpretation of positive results of a methacholine inhalation challenge and one week of inhaled bronchodilator use in diagnosing and treating cough-variant asthma. Arch Intern Med 1997;157:1981. (*Response to specific asthma therapy not associated with dose of methacholine required to reduce forced expiratory volume in 1 second.*)

King DK, Thompson BT, Johnson DC. Wheezing on maximal forced exhalation in the diagnosis of atypical asthma. Ann Intern Med 1989;110:451. (*The maneuver proved neither sensitive nor specific for the diagnosis of asthma.*)

Israeli ZH, Hall WD. Cough and angioneurotic edema associated with angiotensin-converting enzyme inhibitor therapy. Ann Intern Med 1992;117:234. (*A review of pathophysiology and clinical presentation.*)

Laudon RG. Smoking and cough frequency. Rev Respir Dis 1976;114:1033. (*Article confirms that smokers cough more frequently than nonsmokers.*)

Lawler WR. An office approach to the diagnosis of chronic cough. Am Fam Physician 1998;58:2015. (*Reasoned approach emphasizing empiric therapy.*)

McFadden FR Jr. Exertional dyspnea and cough as preludes to acute attacks of asthma. N Engl J Med 1975;292:555. (*Wheezing may be absent as an early manifestation of an acute attack, and cough may dominate the clinical picture.*)

McGarvey LP, Heaney LG, Lawson JT, et al. Evaluation and outcome of patients with chronic nonproductive cough using a comprehensive diagnostic protocol. Thorax 1998;53:738. (*Asthma, gastroesophageal reflux disease, and postnasal drip syndrome equally common and responsive to therapy in this series.*)

Metlay JP, Stafford RS, Singer DE. National trends in the use of antibiotics by primary care physicians for adult patients with cough. Arch Intern Med 1998;158:1813. (*Cough-related visits and proportion receiving antibiotics increased from 1980 to 1994; overall, 66% received antibiotics!*)

Palombini BC, Villanova CA, Araujo E, et al. A pathogenic triad in chronic cough: asthma, postnasal drip syndrome, and gastroesophageal reflux disease. Chest 1999;116:279. (*The five most important causative factors were asthma, postnasal drip syndrome, gastroesophageal reflux disease, bronchiectasis, and tracheobronchial collapse.*)

Patrick H, Patrick F. Chronic cough. Med Clin North Am 1995;79:361. (*Excellent review.*)

Poe RH, Harder RV, Israel RH, et al. Chronic persistent cough: experience in diagnosis and outcome using an anatomic diagnostic protocol. Chest 1989;95:723. (*Irwin's protocol does not work as well in the community setting; in about 14% of cases, the underlying condition remains undiagnosed.*)

Pratter MR, Bartter T, Akers S, et al. An algorithmic approach to chronic cough. Ann Intern Med 1993;119:977. (*Describes a sequential workup with use of response to antihistamine–decongestant medication.*)

Smyrnios NA, Irwin RS, Curley FJ, et al. From a prospective study of chronic cough: diagnostic and therapeutic aspects in older adults. Arch Intern Med 1998;158:1222. (*Causes among older adults the same as among younger: postnasal drip, gastroesophageal reflux disease, and asthma predominate.*)

Thiadens HA, de Bock GH, Dekker FW, et al. Identifying asthma and chronic obstructive pulmonary disease in patients with persistent cough presenting to general practitioners: descriptive study. BMJ 1998;316:1286. (*Of those presenting with persistent cough, 39% were found to have asthma and 7% chronic obstructive pulmonary disease.*)

42
Evaluation of Hemoptysis

Because of its well-known associations with cancer and tuberculosis, hemoptysis is an alarming symptom for both patient and physician. Hemoptysis is the coughing up of either blood-tinged or grossly bloody sputum. In the office, the primary physician is usually confronted with a patient who has noted sputum streaked with blood. Most patients prove to have inconsequential lesions, but a thorough evaluation is necessary because the seriousness of the underlying cause does not correlate with the amount of blood coughed up.

PATHOPHYSIOLOGY AND CLINICAL PRESENTATION

Inflammation of the tracheobronchial mucosa accounts for many cases of hemoptysis. Minor mucosal erosions can result from *upper respiratory infections* and *bronchitis*; blood-streaked sputum is often noted, especially if coughing has been vigorous and prolonged. Patients with *bronchiectasis* are more subject to recurrent episodes of grossly bloody sputum because necrosis of the bronchial mucosa can be quite severe. Up to 50% of patients with bronchiectasis experience hemoptysis. In the United States, hemoptysis occurring with *tuberculosis* (TB) is usually caused by mucosal ulceration, although potentially fatal bleeding can occur when a blood vessel adjacent to a cavitary lesion ruptures. About 10% to 15% of patients with TB report some form of hemoptysis; most of these episodes are minor and involve sputum tinged with small amounts of blood. Endobronchial inflammatory injury from granuloma formation is the mechanism of hemoptysis associated with *sarcoidosis*;

small amounts of blood-streaked sputum are occasionally noted.

Mucosal injury can also be a consequence of *bronchogenic carcinoma*. Disruption of endobronchial tissue may be minor and cause little more than minimal hemoptysis from time to time; hemorrhage is rare. Between 35% and 55% of patients with proven bronchogenic carcinoma report at least one episode of hemoptysis during the course of their illness; it is the presenting symptom in about 10% of cases. The amount of bleeding can vary considerably and need not be impressive. For example, in one study, malignancy was the cause in 25% of patients with minimal hemoptysis. However, most patients have a positive smoking history and abnormal chest radiographic findings.

Carcinoma metastatic to the lung rarely results in hemoptysis. *Bronchial adenomas* are quite vascular, and they are commonly central and endobronchial in location; as a consequence, they frequently bleed, and recurrent episodes of hemoptysis are reported in about half of cases.

Injury to the pulmonary vasculature is an important source of hemoptysis. *Lung abscess* may result in damage to adjacent vessels and frequently presents with bloody and purulent sputum. *Necrotizing pneumonias*, such as those produced by *Klebsiella*, can cause substantial vascular disruption; 25% to 50% of patients cough up tenacious, bloody sputum referred to as "currant jelly." *Aspergillomas* are also capable of causing vascular injury; hemoptysis is the most common symptom of the condition. The patient with an aspergilloma is typically a compromised host with prior cavitary disease from TB, bronchiectasis, or the like. *Pulmonary infarction* secondary to embolization is characterized by the sudden onset of pleuritic pain in conjunction with hemoptysis; embolization without infarction does not cause hemoptysis. Pulmonary contusion resulting from blunt *chest trauma* may present with hemoptysis following a nonpenetrating blow to the thorax.

Marked elevations in pulmonary capillary pressure can cause vascular injury and extravasation of red cells. The pink, frothy sputum of *pulmonary edema* is a manifestation of this process. More grossly bloody sputum sometimes occurs in severe mitral stenosis when a dilated pulmonary–bronchial venous connection ruptures. Vasculitic injury is responsible for the hemoptysis found in *Wegener's granulomatosis* and *Goodpasture's syndrome*. Hematuria often accompanies both conditions. Hereditary vascular malformations are subject to recurrent bleeding. *Arteriovenous malformations* may be accompanied by an audible bruit on auscultation of the lung. In *hereditary hemorrhagic telangiectasia*, a family history of bleeding problems is often present, or prior episodes of bleeding from multiple sites have been noted; telangiectases may be visible in the buccal cavity and on the skin. Bleeding into the interstitium characterizes *idiopathic pulmonary hemosiderosis*. This rare disease, uncommon in adults, is manifested by diffuse interstitial infiltrates, anemia, and hemoptysis.

Hemoptysis may be the first sign of a *bleeding disorder* or *excessive anticoagulant therapy*; however, an underlying bronchopulmonary lesion is usually also present.

DIFFERENTIAL DIAGNOSIS

Acute and chronic bronchitis are the most common causes, followed by bronchogenic carcinoma, TB, pneumonia, and bronchiectasis. Most prevalence figures are obtained from

chest clinics and inpatient units serving preselected populations of patients with either abnormal chest radiographic findings or unexplained hemoptysis; therefore, they cannot be readily extrapolated to the primary care setting. In everyday office practice, the nasal mucosa and oropharynx are more often the source of blood-tinged sputum than is the lower respiratory tract. The high incidence of pulmonary infections associated with HIV, the more widespread use of fiberoptic bronchoscopy, and increases in cigarette smoking and lung cancer in women also must be kept in mind when data from published clinical series that are more than 10 years old are being interpreted. In a fiberoptic bronchoscopy study performed in a general hospital setting that included both inpatients and outpatients, bronchitis accounted for 37% of cases, bronchogenic carcinoma for 19%, TB for 7%, and bronchiectasis for only 1%. The briskness of bleeding did not correlate with the cause. In a review of studies comprising a total of nearly 1,000 patients with hemoptysis and normal chest radiographic findings, lung cancer was eventually diagnosed in 5.4%. Most cancers that cause hemoptysis are endobronchial, but about 15% are parenchymal. The more common and important causes of hemoptysis are listed in Table 42.1.

WORKUP

As noted earlier, most cases of blood-tinged sputum encountered in the primary care setting, especially during the winter, originate in the upper respiratory tract. Such cases do not require further investigation. To avoid unnecessary workup for a pulmonary cause, the history and physical examination should first focus on the nasal and oropharyngeal mucosa. Only in the absence of an upper respiratory source of bleeding need further workup proceed in the manner detailed in the following paragraphs.

History. Evaluation of the patient with a suspected lower respiratory source of hemoptysis should begin with considera-

Table 42.1. Important Causes of Hemoptysis

Gross Hemoptysis
Tuberculosis (with cavitary disease)
Bronchiectasis
Bronchial adenoma
Bronchogenic carcinoma (uncommon)
Aspergilloma
Necrotizing pneumonia
Lung abscess
Pulmonary contusion
Arteriovenous malformation
Hereditary hemorrhagic telangiectasia
Bleeding disorder or excessive anticoagulant therapy
Mitral stenosis (with rupture of a bronchial vessel)
Immune alveolar disease

Blood-Streaked Sputum
Any of the causes of gross hemoptysis
Upper respiratory tract infection
Chronic bronchitis
Sarcoidosis
Bronchogenic carcinoma
Tuberculosis
Pulmonary infarction
Pulmonary edema
Mitral stenosis
Idiopathic pulmonary hemosiderosis
Immune alveolar disease

tion of the epidemiology of the serious underlying causes. Concern about pulmonary neoplasm should be highest in the older man with a long history of heavy smoking or asbestos exposure. The elderly patient with evidence of old disease on chest x-ray films should be presumed to have reactivated TB infection. The adolescent with hemoptysis may have a new infection resulting from recent TB exposure. The compromised host with previous cavitary disease is at risk for an aspergilloma.

The patient's description of the sputum associated with hemoptysis can be of some diagnostic help. Pink sputum is suggestive of pulmonary edematous fluid; putrid sputum is indicative of a lung abscess; material resembling currant jelly points to a necrotizing pneumonia; copious amounts of purulent sputum mixed with blood are consistent with bronchiectasis. The commonly described blood-streaked sputum is nonspecific.

The patient should be asked about previous episodes of bleeding, any family history of hemoptysis, hematuria, concurrent pleuritic chest pain, known heart murmur or history of rheumatic fever, lymph node enlargement, blunt chest trauma, symptoms of heart failure (see Chapter 32), and use of anticoagulant drugs. Determining the amount of blood produced is not particularly helpful for diagnostic purposes. As noted above, it is important to be certain that the patient has no history of a coexisting nasopharyngeal problem or a source of gastrointestinal bleeding that may be mistaken for true hemoptysis.

Physical Examination is directed at detecting nonpulmonary sources of bleeding in addition to evidence of chest and systemic disease. The vital signs should be checked for fever and tachypnea, the skin for ecchymoses and telangiectases, and the nails for clubbing. Clubbing is associated with neoplasm, bronchiectasis, lung abscess, and other severe pulmonary disorders (see Chapter 45). Nodes are examined for enlargement, which is suggestive of sarcoidosis, TB, and malignancy (see Chapters 12 and 51). The neck is noted for jugular venous distention, consistent with heart failure and severe mitral disease. Examination of the chest should include a search for bruits, signs of consolidation, wheezes, crackles, and chest wall contusion.

The history and physical findings can be used to determine the pace at which workup should proceed, in addition to the selection and sequence of laboratory tests. Patients with minimal hemoptysis may be evaluated on an outpatient basis as long as they are given explicit advice to return immediately if severe bleeding ensues. The patient with a suspected bleeding diathesis should not be sent home.

Laboratory Studies. *Chest radiography* is essential to assessment. As alluded to earlier, the vast majority of patients with hemoptysis resulting from bronchogenic carcinoma have abnormal chest radiographic findings. In addition to uncovering a mass lesion, chest films may reveal an abscess, infiltrate, interstitial change (see Chapter 46), hilar adenopathy, signs of congestive failure (see Chapter 32), or evidence of significant mitral stenosis (see Chapter 33). Less common radiologic findings include peribronchial cuffing, indicative of bronchiectasis, and a crescentic radiolucency surrounding a coin lesion, characteristic of an aspergilloma. However, in most instances, the appearance of the chest film is normal, and consideration of further study is warranted.

A *sputum Gram's stain* is essential if the sputum appears grossly purulent or the patient is febrile. An *acid-fast stain* for tubercle bacilli is also essential, not only for diagnosis but for a rough assessment of infectivity (see Chapter 49). The sensitivity of the acid-fast smear depends on the diligence with which the search for pathogenic organisms is made. In one series, only 20% of culture-positive samples were identified in advance by acid-fast smear. It should be noted that despite the very high specificity of a positive smear, its predictive value may be as low as 50% when the sputum specimens of low-risk patients are examined. A *tuberculin skin test* should be performed if the patient's PPD (purified protein derivative) reactivity status is not known. However, approximately 7% of all adults (25% of adults over age 50) will have positive reactions (see Chapters 38 and 49).

Sputum cytologies should be obtained in all patients without a clear diagnosis. It used to be thought that the sensitivity of a single sputum cytology examination was about 70% in the detection of squamous cell lesions, and that three consecutive cytologic examinations increased the sensitivity to 90%. However, data from the large screening trials suggest a lower sensitivity, at least for early cancers. The specificity of sputum cytology is greater than 99% when the specimen is reviewed by an experienced cytopathologist.

Fiberoptic bronchoscopy can be extremely helpful for diagnosis when used thoughtfully. Its most common indication is to exclude the possibility of tumor. However, the test should not be viewed as a routine part of the evaluation for hemoptysis because the yield is extremely low in situations in which the risk for malignancy is very low (e.g., a nonsmoker under the age of 50 with normal chest radiographic findings). Bronchoscopy enhances the sensitivity of cytologic and bacteriologic studies when washings for specimens are obtained during the procedure, and the test has proved capable of detecting otherwise occult endobronchial cancers in patients at increased risk for lung malignancy (e.g., older than 50 years, male gender, history of smoking), even if the chest radiographic findings are nonlocalizing. Patients with a high-risk profile, "positive" or "suspect" cytology, or a radiologic abnormality are appropriate candidates for bronchoscopy. Subjecting low-risk patients to bronchoscopic examination is wasteful and unlikely to affect management or outcome. Moreover, the cost and morbidity associated with bronchoscopy are not trivial.

Serious complications are rare with fiberoptic bronchoscopy, but they do occur. In a review of 48,000 procedures, fewer than 100 life-threatening cardiovascular or respiratory complications were reported, most often in older persons with chronic obstructive pulmonary disease and coronary disease. Hypoxia occurs commonly following bronchoscopy.

Bronchoscopy is mandatory in all patients with massive hemoptysis who are being seriously considered for surgery, to localize the site of bleeding. Rigid bronchoscopy is preferred in this situation.

Chest computed tomography (CT) may better define a suspect lesion seen on chest x-ray films and may be indicated for some patients with normal chest radiographic findings to increase the sensitivity for parenchymal lesions. CT will also identify endobronchial tumors with a sensitivity of approximately 80%. However, the specificity of CT-visualized endobronchial lesions for cancer is somewhat limited (approximately 65%).

Parameters of bleeding, such as the prothrombin time (PT), partial thromboplastin time (PTT), platelet count, and bleeding time, should be determined if more than one site of bleeding is noted.

Cryptogenic Hemoptysis is hemoptysis occurring in patients with normal or nonlocalizing chest radiographic findings and nondiagnostic findings on fiberoptic bronchoscopy. What to do in such a situation can be perplexing. The prognosis appears to be favorable, with more than 90% of these patients experiencing resolution of their hemoptysis by 6 months and no cases of cancer, active TB, or other serious pathology emerging after the initial evaluation. A careful history and physical examination, in combination with chest radiography and the proper use of bronchoscopy, appear to exclude cancer, active TB, and other must-not-miss diseases effectively, so that repeated bronchoscopy, pulmonary angiography, CT, and bronchography are of little use in these patients. In one study, bronchial inflammation (bronchitis) was the most common cause, followed by the sequelae of old tuberculous disease.

A.G.M.

INDICATIONS FOR REFERRAL AND ADMISSION

Patients with hemoptysis who are believed to be at increased risk for an underlying malignancy (abnormal chest radiographic findings, male sex, older than 50, smoking history) are candidates for bronchoscopy. Patients with brisk bleeding require urgent hospitalization.

ANNOTATED BIBLIOGRAPHY

Adelman M, Haponik EF, Bleecker ER, et al. Cryptogenic hemoptysis: clinical features, bronchoscopic findings, and natural history in 67 patients. Ann Intern Med 1985;102:829. (*Prognosis was excellent, and no cancer, TB, or other serious causes were missed by a careful history and physical examination combined with chest radiography and bronchoscopy.*)

Colice GL. Detecting lung cancers as a cause of hemoptysis in patients with a normal chest radiograph. Chest 1997;111:877. (*Review of the literature and decision analysis concluding that bronchoscopy, with or without initial sputum cytology, is the most efficient diagnostic strategy.*)

Fontana RS, Sanderson DR, Woolner LB, et al. Screening for lung cancer. A critique of the Mayo Lung Project. Cancer 1991;67:1155. (*Includes late follow-up of the Mayo trial with information about the sensitivity and specificity of chest radiography and sputum cytology.*)

Leatherman J, Davies SF, Hoidal JR. Alveolar hemorrhage syndromes: diffuse microvascular lung hemorrhage in immune and idiopathic disorders. Medicine (Baltimore) 1984;63:343. (*Comprehensive review.*)

Johnston H, Reisz G. Changing spectrum of hemoptysis. Arch Intern Med 1989;149:1666. (*A study of bronchoscopy in both inpatients and outpatients in the general hospital setting. Emphasizes that bronchiectasis is waning as a cause of hemoptysis; bronchitis is first, followed by cancer and tuberculosis.*)

McGuinness G, Beacher JR, Harkin TJ, et al. Hemoptysis: prospective high-resolution CT/bronchoscopic correlation. Chest 1994; 105:1155. (*Fifty-seven patients underwent both studies: CT had a sensitivity of 84% and a specificity of 68%.*)

Millar AB, Boothroyd AE, Edwards D, et al. The role of computed tomography in the investigation of unexplained hemoptysis. Respir Med 1992;86:39. (*Unusually large proportion of parenchymal cancers in this study.*)

Nelson JE, Forman M. Hemoptysis in HIV-infected patients. Chest 1996;110:737. (*Most cases attributable to infection, usually bacterial.*)

Poe RH, Israel RH, Marin MG, et al. Utility of fiberoptic bronchoscopy in patients with hemoptysis and a nonlocalizing roentgenogram. Chest 1988;93:70. (*Utility was greatest in male patients older than 50 who had a history of smoking.*)

Santiago S, Tobias J, Williams AJ. A reappraisal of the causes of hemoptysis. Arch Intern Med 1991;151:2449. (*Bronchogenic carcinoma, bronchitis, and idiopathic disease were the leading causes.*)

Set PAK, Flower CDR, Smith IE, et al. Hemoptysis: comparative study of the role of CT and fiberoptic bronchoscopy. Radiology 1993;189:677. (*CT had a low false-positive rate for endobronchial lesions.*)

Surratt PM, Smiddy JF, Gruber B. Deaths and complications associated with fiberoptic bronchoscopy. Chest 1976;69:747. (*In nearly 50,000 procedures, 52 severe respiratory complications and 27 severe cardiovascular complications.*)

43
Evaluation of Pleural Effusions

Most pleural effusions encountered in the office are discovered as incidental findings, and they often pose a diagnostic challenge because the cause is frequently unclear. Of major concern are the possibilities of tumor and infection. Outpatient evaluation of a pleural effusion requires that the physician be skilled in performing a diagnostic thoracentesis in the office and in differentiating a transudate from an exudate. The primary physician should be able to carry out the initial evaluation of a pleural effusion safely in the ambulatory setting, provided the patient's respiratory status is satisfactory and no evidence of serious acute illness is present.

PATHOPHYSIOLOGY AND CLINICAL PRESENTATION

The pleural cavity normally contains a small volume of serous fluid that serves as a lubricant. About 17 mL of such fluid is formed each day by transudation from the parietal pleural surface and is reabsorbed predominantly by the visceral pleura through lymphatic stomata into the lymphatic system. When the transudation of fluid is excessive or an exudative process involving the pleural surfaces is present, an effusion forms. Once more than 200 mL is formed, the effusion becomes visible radiographically. Effusions are classified pathophysiologically as transudates or exudates. Clinically, the distinction is based on pleural fluid protein and lactate dehydrogenase (LDH) concentrations. An effusion is *transudative* if any two of the following three criteria are met: (a) the ratio of *pleural fluid protein to serum protein is less than 0.5*, (b) the ratio of *pleural fluid LDH concentration to serum LDH concentration is less than 0.6*, and (c) the *pleural fluid LDH concentration is less than two-thirds the upper limit of normal for the serum LDH concentration*. If these ratios or levels are exceeded, the effusion is exudative.

Transudates

Increased hydrostatic pressure in the pulmonary interstitium and decreased colloid oncotic pressure produce transudates. Increased hydrostatic pressure below the diaphragm, as occurs in ascites or peritoneal dialysis, can also result in a transudative pleural effusion. Because transudates are rarely associated with pleural inflammation, they are not usually accompanied by pleuritic pain, but they may lead to shortness of breath if they are large enough to interfere with respiratory mechanics. They may be unilateral but are often bilateral. Physical examination of the lung reveals dullness and diminished breath sounds. If the effusion has produced some atelectasis, bronchial breath sounds and increased vocal fremitus above the effusion may be present. Most transudates have a protein concentration of less than 3.0 g/100 mL, but chronic transudates may show higher concentrations and mimic an exudative process.

Congestive Heart Failure is among the most common causes of transudative effusions. Left-sided heart failure increases the pulmonary capillary pressure (see Chapter 32), which forces excess fluid into the interstitium. Right ventricular failure contributes by raising central venous pressure, which elevates the hydrostatic force in the capillaries of the parietal pleura and diminishes fluid reabsorption. Most effusions associated with congestive failure are *bilateral*, but at times an *isolated right-sided* effusion is seen; isolated left-sided effusions resulting from congestive failure are rare. The reason for the right-sided preference is unknown. Symptoms and signs of congestive failure (see Chapter 32) are usually evident. In more than 85% of effusions resulting from heart failure, the protein concentration is less than 3.0 g/100 mL. The concentration may be greater if the effusion is chronic or the patient has recently been undergoing a brisk diuresis. The pleural fluid is usually clear, but it may be bloody with red cell counts in excess of 5,000/mL.

Pulmonary Embolization is accompanied by pleural effusion in up to 50% of cases. The effusions are usually small and do not depend on the occurrence of pulmonary infarction. Cell count, differential, and protein concentration vary considerably. The transudative effusion associated with a pulmonary embolus may result from localized interstitial edema. The effusions that result from infarction are more likely to be bloody. Bilateral effusions can be seen when emboli affect both lungs. A small effusion on chest x-ray films in a patient with pleuritic chest pain can be an important clue (see Chapter 20).

Other Causes of Transudation. In the *nephrotic syndrome*, a similar but more generalized interstitial edema may ensue and lead to effusion. *Overexpanded extracellular volume* as a consequence of severe *hypoalbuminemia* or *salt retention* can produce a transudative effusion, but edematous fluid first collects in parts of the body where hydrostatic pressures are greatest (e.g., lower extremities) before fluid appears in the pleural space. Cardiomegaly may be in evidence, but overt signs of congestive failure are usually absent. Generalized edema is rare before the serum albumin level falls below 2.0 to 2.5 g/100 mL.

Intraabdominal diseases are occasionally responsible for transudative effusions. A *right-sided* pleural effusion develops in between 5% and 10% of patients with *ascites* resulting from *cirrhosis*; the composition of the effusion resembles that of the ascitic fluid. In cases of *pancreatitis* or a *subphrenic abscess*, a *"sympathetic effusion"* with the characteristics of a transudate sometimes forms; it soon changes into an exudate.

Pleural effusions are common after *coronary bypass graft surgery* and do not imply serious pathology. The same holds for the postpartum patient. Transudates may form in the setting of *pericardial disease*, *myxedema*, and *sarcoidosis*; the mechanism(s) remain unknown.

Exudates

Exudates result from inflammatory or infiltrative disease of the pleura and its adjacent structures; damage occurs to capillary membranes, and protein-rich material accumulates in the pleural space. Obstruction to lymphatic flow can also produce an exudative effusion. Because most exudates form as a consequence of pleural injury, they are often accompanied by pleuritic chest pain, especially in the acute phase, when a friction rub may be heard before much fluid accumulates. The fluid is initially free-flowing but may become walled off and loculated when a marked inflammatory response develops. The protein content is usually greater than 3.0 g/100 mL. The fluid is typically deep yellow or cloudy in appearance. The leukocyte count is often above 1,000/mL; a count above 10,000/mL is suggestive of an empyema, particularly if most of the cells are neutrophils.

Neoplasms are often responsible for the development of effusions. Most pleural fluid accumulations caused by malignancies have the characteristics of exudates, although at times the protein concentration is less than 3.0 g/100 mL. Mechanisms of exudate formation include pleural metastasis with increased permeability and obstruction of lymphatic outflow. The formation of a malignant effusion is often a poor prognostic sign, particularly if the pH of the fluid is less than 7.3 and the glucose level is less than 60 mg/dL, which indicates extensive pleural involvement with tumor.

Bronchogenic carcinoma is the tumor most frequently associated with a pleural effusion. Fluid collects in most instances as a direct result of pleural invasion; unilateral effusions are the rule. Patients report dyspnea when the effusion is large and occasionally complain of pleuritic chest pain. The pleural fluid is usually clear and straw-colored, but it may be bloody and the glucose level may be very low. The white cell count is typically around 2,500/mL, with most cells being lymphocytes. Malignant cells are found in about 60% of instances. Unfortunately, the disease and its effusions are progressive; thoracentesis is followed by rapid reaccumulation.

Pleural effusions caused by *metastatic carcinoma* are more likely to be bilateral than are those associated with bronchogenic carcinoma because they occur as a consequence of lymphatic obstruction or diffuse seeding of the pleura. When effusions are caused by seeding, results of cytologic examination of the pleural fluid are positive in up to 90% of cases. Carcinoma of the *breast* is the leading metastatic tumor producing pleural effusions, accounting for 25% of all malignant effusions. The characteristics of the pleural fluid are similar to those of effusions caused by bronchogenic carcinoma. *Lymphoma* is another major cause of malignant bilateral pleural effusions, responsible for up to 20% of cases. The formation of a large effusion is a sign of advanced disease; evidence of pleural, parenchymal, and lymph node involvement is often present by the time a significant effusion appears. The pleural fluid may be a transudate or an exudate; most of the cells are lymphocytes. Cough and dyspnea accompany parenchymal involvement, but pleuritic pain is rare.

Mesotheliomas have become an increasingly important source of effusion as the incidence of *asbestos exposure* has increased. Only malignant mesotheliomas produce important pleural fluid accumulations. The latent period for mesothelioma formation ranges from 20 to 40 years after asbestos exposure; the degree of exposure may appear inconsequential (see Chapter 39). Chest pain, cough, and shortness of breath result from extensive pleural disease and large effusions. The fluid may be bloody and often contains malignant cells, but they are sometimes hard to identify cytologically, so that chromosomal analysis is necessary. The fluid may be high in *hyaluronic acid*. Because the tumor is only locally invasive, no signs of extrathoracic disease are present.

Impressive effusions can form as a consequence of *benign ovarian neoplasms (Meigs' syndrome)*. The tumor produces ascites, and fluid tracks across the diaphragm and into the thorax. The effusion is typically on the right but may be left-sided or even bilateral; it is exudative in quality, free of malignant cells, and similar in composition to the ascitic fluid from which it derives. Removal of the ovarian tumor results in prompt resolution of the effusion.

Infections are an important source of exudative pleural effusions, but effusions are uncommonly associated with the *acute bacterial pneumonias* encountered in ambulatory patients. For example, an effusion develops in only about 5% of patients with *pneumococcal pneumonia*, and it is usually small and transient. Such effusions are termed *parapneumonic* to imply that bacteria need not have entered the pleural space to cause the effusion. The term *empyema* is reserved for cases in which organisms are recovered from the pleural fluid, either by Gram's stain or culture. Empyema is a rare but worrisome event, seen in fewer than 1% of the cases of pneumococcal pneumonia that present in the outpatient setting; most cases occur when proper antibiotic therapy is delayed. Cough, sputum production, fever, chills, and pleuritic pain may be prominent. Early on, the pleural fluid appears serous and may be sterile, but it quickly turns purulent and positive for organisms when empyema develops. In some instances, the pleural fluid offers the only opportunity for recovery of the causative organism. Characteristics of the pleural empyema fluid include a white cell count in excess of 5,000 to 10,000/mL, with neutrophils predominating. The concentration of glucose is typically less than 20 mg/100 mL. Pleural scarring may be substantial if the empyema fluid is allowed to remain.

Viral pneumonitis and *mycoplasmal pneumonia* are sometimes associated with pleural effusions in the course of illness, but the effusions are small, transient, and of little consequence (see Chapter 52).

The effusion caused by postprimary tuberculosis (TB) represents a delayed hypersensitivity reaction to spillage of organisms into the pleural space during early bacteremia or subclinical parenchymal disease (see Chapter 49). The effusion is almost always unilateral. The patient may be relatively free of symptoms or exhibit lethargy, fever, and weight loss; at times, the clinical picture is dominated by acute onset of pleuritic pain and fever. Cough and sputum are conspicuously absent. The chest radiograph may show little more than an isolated effusion, but the result of an intermediate-strength tuberculin skin test is usually positive. The pleural fluid has the qualities of an exudate; the glucose concentration may be low. The white cell count averages 1,000 to 2,000/mL; lymphocytes predominate; mesothelial cells are scarce (<2%). Neutrophils may be seen early in the course of the illness. Organisms are rarely found on acid-fast stain of the fluid and can be cultured from the fluid in only 25% of cases. Most of these effusions resolve spontaneously within a few months and leave little or no residual; however, symptomatic pulmonary parenchymal involvement eventually develops in more than half of such patients (see Chapter 47).

Rheumatoid Diseases, particularly systemic lupus erythematosus, can produce transient pleuropericardial inflammation during their course, usually after other signs and symptoms have appeared. There may be a brief period of pleuritic pain. On occasion, pleural involvement may be the initial clinical presentation of the disease. In most instances, the pleural fluid has the characteristics of a exudate and may demonstrate low glucose and serum complement levels.

Rheumatoid arthritis is much less likely to produce a pleural effusion than is lupus, but the fluid often persists. Fewer than 5% of patients experience pleuropericardial involvement; these people usually have a history of extraarticular manifestations and joint symptoms. Occasionally, the effusion is the first manifestation of rheumatoid disease. The effusion is an exudate, with a predominance of lymphocytes and a very low (<20 mg/100 mL) glucose concentration. Although the fluid may contain rheumatoid factor, its presence is not unique to this disease.

Intraabdominal Pathology can lead to the production of an exudative pleural effusion, particularly when recent abdominal surgery, intestinal perforation, or hepatobiliary disease is complicated by development of a *subdiaphragmatic abscess*. In addition to gastrointestinal symptoms, pleuritic pain, fever, weight loss, and malaise may be present. Often, the symptoms are nonspecific, so that patients put off the decision to seek medical help. The diaphragm on the involved side (which is the right in two thirds of cases) is elevated and moves poorly on fluoroscopy. A pathognomonic subdiaphragmatic air–fluid level may be present on chest film. The pleural fluid is usually sterile, although it may have a high leukocyte count. If the diaphragm has been perforated, an empyema can form. The pleural effusion associated with *pancreatitis* may begin as a transudate but usually becomes exudative. The effusions are most often on the left but may be bilateral or right-sided. The fluid characteristically has a *high amylase* concentration and is blood-tinged in one third of cases.

DIFFERENTIAL DIAGNOSIS

Although the causes of pleural effusion can be conveniently divided into those conditions that produce transudates and those that result in exudates (see Table 43.1), it is important to keep in mind that a number of conditions can cause both. In

Table 43.1. Important Causes of Pleural Effusions

Transudates
Congestive heart failure
Hypoalbuminemia, severe
Salt-retention syndromes
Ascites secondary to cirrhosis
Early phases of a sympathetic effusion
Neoplasm (on occasion)
Peritoneal dialysis
Postpartum
Cardiac bypass graft surgery

Exudates
Neoplasms
   Bronchogenic carcinoma
   Breast cancer
   Lymphoma
   Mesothelioma
   Meigs' syndrome
Infections
   Tuberculosis (and atypical myobacteria in AIDS patients)
   Bacterial pneumonia (including empyema)
   Viral pneumonitis
   Mycoplasmal pneumonia
   Pneumocystis pneumonia
Pulmonary embolization
Connective tissue disease
   Rheumatoid arthritis
   Systemic lupus erythematosus
Intraabdominal disease
   Subphrenic abscess
   Pancreatitis
Idiopathic

such conditions, the initial effusion is transudative but turns exudative as the disease process continues. Chronic congestive heart failure is the most frequently encountered such condition in the ambulatory population. Neoplasms account for the majority of cases seen in referral populations. In a series reported from the Mayo Clinic, bronchogenic carcinoma was the leading cause of malignant pleural effusion, accounting for 30% of cases, followed by breast carcinoma (25%) and lymphoma (20%). Infection is the third most common cause of accumulation of fluid in the pleural space, with TB still accounting for a substantial proportion of effusions subjected to full evaluation. Bloody effusions are most often caused by neoplasms but are also seen in congestive heart failure, pulmonary embolization with infarction, TB, and pancreatitis. About 15% of effusions remain unexplained; most idiopathic effusions are exudates.

Among AIDS patients, infections cause more than two thirds of effusions, with bacterial, mycobacterial, and *Pneumocystis* pneumonias accounting for most. Hypoalbuminemia is the leading noninfectious cause of effusion among patients with advanced HIV disease.

WORKUP

The diagnosis of pleural effusion is usually suggested by the findings of dullness and diminished breath sounds upward from the lung base and confirmed by chest radiography. The first task after identifying the effusion is to assess the degree, if any, of respiratory compromise associated with the effusion. The vital signs should be checked for tachypnea and tachycardia, the skin should be checked for cyanosis, and the chest should be checked for use of accessory muscles of respiration. Patients with objective evidence of substantial respiratory compromise

should be admitted to the hospital for further workup. Those who are comfortable can be assessed on an outpatient basis. Although radiologic features may suggest a diagnosis, the history and physical examination complemented by examination of the pleural fluid are essential to an accurate assessment.

History. The patient should be asked about the presence of fever, cough, sputum production, chest pain, dyspnea, edema, and abdominal pain; prior history of malignant, hepatic, renal, or HIV disease; exposure to TB or asbestos; and symptoms of rheumatoid disease (see Chapter 146). Cough, fever, and sputum production in conjunction with pleuritic chest pain suggest pneumonitis with pleural involvement. Pleuritic pain is also consistent with embolization, malignancy, and pleural inflammation with adjacent pericarditis resulting from connective tissue disease. Dyspnea may be induced by the effusion alone, but the symptom is indicative of congestive heart failure when accompanied by orthopnea and paroxysmal nocturnal dyspnea. A history of peripheral edema raises the possibilities of hypoalbuminemia, volume overload, and congestive failure. A history of alcohol abuse, recent abdominal surgery, or abdominal pain or distention points to a source below the diaphragm.

Physical Examination. In addition to the assessment for respiratory compromise, the vital signs are checked for fever and weight change. The integument is inspected for petechiae, purpura, spider angiomata, jaundice, clubbing (see Chapter 45), manifestations of rheumatoid disease (see Chapter 146), and rashes. The neck is noted for jugular venous distention and tracheal deviation, the lymph nodes are checked for enlargement, and the breasts are checked for masses. On lung examination, the level of the effusion and extent of involvement are determined. It is worth noting any compression of adjacent lung, suggested by egophony and bronchial breath sounds heard above the effusion. A pleural friction rub may be audible but is usually lacking when a considerable amount of fluid has accumulated. The heart should be checked for a third sound, indicative of pump failure, and a three-component friction rub, suggestive of pericarditis. The abdomen is examined for signs of ascites, organomegaly, focal tenderness, and peritonitis (see Chapter 58). A pelvic examination is performed to rule out the presence of an ovarian mass, and the extremities are noted for edema, calf tenderness, and signs of joint inflammation.

Laboratory Evaluation. The centerpieces of the laboratory workup are the chest radiograph and pleural fluid analysis. The *chest radiograph* should be studied for pleura-based densities, infiltrates, signs of congestive heart failure (see Chapter 32), hilar adenopathy, coin lesions, and loculation of fluid (detection of which requires lateral decubitus views). The elevation of a hemidiaphragm and the presence of a subdiaphragmatic air–fluid level are important radiologic signs of a subphrenic abscess. The location of the effusion may be helpful. Among transudative effusions caused by cardiac failure, unilateral effusions tend to be right-sided, and bilateral effusions usually are asymmetric with more fluid on the right side. On the other hand, effusions associated with pericarditis or pancreatitis tend to be left-sided.

When a cause is not readily evident from the history, physical examination, and chest film, then a *diagnostic thoracentesis* is indicated. In some instances, of course, a thoracentesis need not be performed on the first visit. Such instances include the afebrile patient with clinical evidence of congestive heart failure, the postpartum woman who is otherwise well, the patient who has undergone bypass graft surgery, and the young patient with a small effusion in conjunction with a viral or mycoplasmal pneumonia. These patients can be followed expectantly with repeated chest films; failure of the effusion to clear with resolution of the presumptive cause is an indication for thoracentesis.

A diagnostic thoracentesis can be performed safely and comfortably in the office on patients who have free-flowing effusions confirmed by lateral decubitus films. Ultrasonography has been increasingly used to help guide thoracentesis, but it has not been shown to enhance the safety or yield of the procedure except in situations of very small effusions. Thoracentesis for loculated effusions is more difficult and is associated with a greater risk for pneumothorax; it is best not to tap such effusions in the office.

A few pitfalls in thoracentesis technique must be avoided. A common error is for the examiner to enter the chest too far below the meniscus of the effusion, thereby risking penetration of the diaphragm or entry into the diaphragmatic sulcus, which is likely to be sealed off from the effusion by lung tissue. To define the proper entry point, the lung fields should be percussed and auscultated to determine the upper border of the effusion. Because pleural fluid rises in a meniscus where it comes in contact with the parietal pleura, the needle should be passed into the chest one interspace *above* the upper border of the effusion as determined by examination. A few millimeters of penetration into the pleural space at the level of the meniscus allows full drainage without the complications of a low entry. Injury to the neurovascular bundle along the inferior surface of the rib is avoided by aiming the needle just above the *superior* margin of the rib, which is accomplished by "walking the needle" over the anesthetized surface of the rib. Pneumothorax is minimized by withdrawing or changing the needle position as soon as air bubbles begin to appear or one feels the visceral pleura contacting the needle tip; the onset of coughing is common at this stage. The patient should be advised to resist the impulse to cough because during coughing the lung may become impaled on the needle. Use of a large-bore Intracath (14 or 16 gauge) minimizes the risk for needle injury to the lung. A chest x-ray film should be obtained after thoracentesis to be sure that a significant pneumothorax has not been produced.

The laboratory analysis of pleural fluid should begin with determination of the *protein* and *LDH concentrations*. A simultaneous serum sample should also be sent for protein and LDH levels. As noted earlier, the three most useful findings to distinguish a pleural exudate from a transudate are a *pleural fluid LDH level above 200 U*, a *pleural-to-serum LDH ratio above 0.6*, and a *pleural-to-serum protein ratio above 0.5*. Fulfillment of any two of these three criteria has a sensitivity in excess of 90% and a specificity of 99%. If this first step indicates that the effusion is a transudate, no further laboratory analysis of the fluid is indicated. In fact, because of the poor specificity of white and red blood cell counts, glucose and amylase levels, and even bacterial cultures (as a consequence of contamination), such tests performed on transudates may be misleading.

If any of the criteria for an exudate are met, the laboratory analysis should include a *differential cell count*, *bacterial culture* (including cultures for anaerobes and mycobacteria), and *cytologic examination*. Although a high white blood cell count

may indicate infection, it is a nonspecific finding. A lymphocyte predominance is suggestive of TB or malignancy but does not help in distinguishing between the two. The sensitivity of cytologic examination depends on the mechanism of the malignant effusion and extent of disease; it may be as high as 95% in advanced disease with extensive pleural involvement, but as low as 50% in early disease. However, a positive result of cytology are highly specific when reported by an experienced pathologist.

In certain circumstances, other tests may be useful. A *low pleural fluid glucose level* (<60 mg/dL) is associated with TB, other serious infections, and advanced pleural involvement with malignancy. A *low pleural fluid pH* (<7.30) has a similar meaning. Conversely, when the pleural fluid pH is low, the result of the pleural fluid cytologic examination is likely to be positive if an underlying cancer is present. Very low glucose levels (<30 mg/dL) are most consistently associated with the effusion of rheumatoid arthritis. An elevated *amylase* level may point to pancreatitis as the cause of effusion, but it can also be seen in malignant effusion. Specific tumor markers have not proved useful, except in the case of *chromosomal analysis* for identifying malignant mesothelioma. Similarly, measurement of *complement levels* (CH_{50}, C3, and C4) should be reserved for the rare instance when it is necessary to confirm that an exudative effusion in a patient with rheumatoid disease is caused by the underlying disorder and not another condition. Pleural fluid antinuclear antibody (ANA) measurement may be useful in further establishing the diagnosis of lupus pleuritis.

In about 15% of cases, the cause of an exudative effusion is not evident after complete laboratory analysis of the pleural fluid from an initial thoracentesis. If malignancy is still suspected, repeated thoracentesis is indicated. Sensitivity approaches 90% with submission of fluid specimens from three separate pleural taps in patients with underlying malignancy. Test sensitivity is particularly high in cases of advanced pleural involvement by tumor, as suggested by a pleural fluid pH of less than 7.30 and a glucose level below 60 mg/dL. *Pleural biopsy* alone may be less sensitive than cytologic examination of pleural fluid in detecting malignancy, but the two tests are complementary, with a sensitivity in excess of 90% when used together. Pleural biopsy is most useful in detecting TB, having a sensitivity of 60% to 80%. Again, the biopsy information is complementary; fluid culture or examination of pleural tissue (or both) will yield a diagnosis of TB in up to 95% of those with the disease. Both pleural tissue and pleural fluid should be submitted for mycobacterial culture.

When pleural biopsy is contemplated, it should be anticipated that most specimens will disclose only nonspecific inflammatory changes. Although the diagnosis of malignant effusion will eventually be made in as many as 20% of such patients, in most cases the effusion will resolve spontaneously without serious sequelae. When a history of hemoptysis is present or a pulmonary abnormality is noted on chest radiography, *fiberoptic bronchoscopy* may prove useful.

INDICATIONS FOR ADMISSION AND REFERRAL

The patient with respiratory discomfort is best evaluated on an inpatient basis, especially if HIV-positive; inpatient evaluation is also indicated when embolization, severe congestive failure, acute empyema, or an intraabdominal crisis is likely. Few of these patients present to the physician in the office; however, the patient with a chronic but enlarging collection of pleural fluid is apt to be encountered. The person who appears to be tolerating the effusion without much discomfort can be evaluated and managed on an outpatient basis as long as no evidence suggests an empyema or a subphrenic abscess, conditions that require surgical attention. Referral is appropriate when malignancy or TB is suspected and pleural biopsy or fiberoptic bronchoscopy is deemed necessary.

SYMPTOMATIC MANAGEMENT

The patient can be made comfortable before a diagnosis is established. Pleuritic pain often responds to indomethacin; the drug has an advantage over narcotics in that it does not produce any suppressive effect on respiration. Removal of fluid is indicated when the effusion is compromising respiratory efforts. Usually, no more than a liter should be removed at one time to avoid intravascular volume depletion on reequilibration. Malignant pleural effusions are notoriously difficult to treat in the setting of advanced disease with marked pleural involvement (pleural fluid pH <7.30 and glucose level <60 mg/dL). Comfort measures are preferable to repeated attempts at sclerosing therapy under such circumstances (see Chapter 92).

A.H.G./A.G.M.

ANNOTATED BIBLIOGRAPHY

Chang SC, Perng RP. The role of fiber optic bronchoscopy in evaluating the causes of pleural effusions. Arch Intern Med 1989;149:855. (*Useful in patients with hemoptysis or a pulmonary abnormality on chest radiography.*)

Fine NL, Smith LR, Sheedy PF. Frequency of pleural effusions in mycoplasma and viral pneumonias. N Engl J Med 1970;283:790. (*Small transient effusions are common in these conditions, but large effusions are rare.*)

Frist B, Kahan AV, Koss LG. Comparison of the diagnostic value of biopsies of the pleura and cytologic evaluation of pleural fluids. Ann Intern Med 1972;77:507. (*Among 106 patients with malignant effusion, 97% had positive findings on fluid cytology and 38% had positive findings on pleural biopsy; together, the tests had a sensitivity approaching 100%.*)

Heffner JE, Brown LK, Barbieri CA. Diagnostic value of tests that discriminate between exudative and transudative pleural effusions. Primary Study Investigators. Chest 1997;111:970. (*Critical meta-analysis of studies of nearly 1,500 patients with pleural effusion.*)

Hughson WG, Friedman PJ, Feigin DS, et al. Postpartum pleural effusion: a common radiologic finding. Ann Intern Med 1982;97:856. (*In a small prospective study, a majority of asymptomatic women had a pleural effusion within 24 hours after delivery.*)

Hunder GG. Pleural fluid complement in systemic lupus erythematosus and rheumatoid arthritis. Ann Intern Med 1972;76:356. (*Complement levels are low.*)

Joseph J, Strange C, Sahn SA. Pleural effusions in hospitalized patients with AIDS. Ann Intern Med 1993;118:856. (*Although this was not a study of outpatients, the findings suggest causes to consider when an HIV-positive patient is encountered, especially one with AIDS.*)

Light RW. Pleural diseases. Dis Mon 1992;38:261. (*Comprehensive review.*)

Light RW. Useful tests on the pleural fluid in the management of patients with pleural effusions. Curr Opin Pulm Med 1999;5:245. (*Succinct expert review.*)

Light RW, Ball WC. Glucose and amylase in pleural effusion. JAMA 1973;225:259. (*Tuberculosis and malignant effusions were not universally associated with low glucose values.*)

Light RW, MacGregor MI, Ball WC Jr, et al. Cells in pleural fluid. Their value in differential diagnosis. Arch Intern Med 1973;132:854. (*In a review of the diagnostic significance of cell counts, the authors conclude that the finding of many mesothelial cells is incompatible with TB; red cell counts above 10,000/mL suggest neoplasm, infarction, or trauma; a predominance of lymphocytes is consistent with tuberculosis and neoplasm.*)

Light RW, MacGregor MI, Luchsinger PC, et al. Pleural effusions: the diagnostic separation of transudate and exudate. Ann Intern Med 1972;77:507. (*A classic article that details rigorous criteria for the separation of transudates from exudates.*)

Lossos IS, Breuer R, Intrator O, et al. Differential diagnosis of pleural effusion by lactate dehydrogenase isoenzyme analysis. Chest 1997;111:648. (*Algorithm based on LDH isoenzyme alone had a positive predictive value of 83%.*)

Peterman TA, Speicher CE. Evaluating pleural effusions. JAMA 1984;252:1051. (*Advocates a two-stage procedure for identifying exudates based on rapid determination of protein and LDH values, which eliminates the need to order additional tests for transudates.*)

Poe RE, Israel RH, Vtell MJ, et al. Sensitivity, specificity, and predictive values of closed pleural biopsy. Arch Intern Med 1984;144:325. (*Sensitivity was 68% for malignant disease.*)

Sahn SA. The pleura. Am Rev Respir Dis 1988;138:184. (*An exhaustive review of pleural pathophysiology and pleural effusion.*)

Sahn SA, Good JT Jr. Pleural fluid pH in malignant effusions. Ann Intern Med 1988;108:349. (*A pH below 7.30 correlated with advanced pleural involvement by tumor and a very poor prognosis.*)

Weiss JM, Spodick DH. Association of left pleural effusion with pericardial disease. N Engl J Med 1983;308:696. (*Patients with pericarditis tend to have unilateral, left-sided pleural effusions or bilateral effusions that are larger on the left; this is in contrast to the right-sided dominance seen in congestive heart failure.*)

44
Evaluation of the Solitary Pulmonary Nodule

Solitary nodules are found at a rate of one to two per 1,000 routine chest radiographs. The discovery is a worrisome finding because it raises the possibilities of primary lung cancer and solitary metastasis from a nonpulmonary source. The patient is usually asymptomatic and undergoing chest radiography for either an unrelated issue or screening. Granulomas and hamartomas account for the majority. About 30% prove to be malignant. Pulmonary malignancies with the greatest potential for cure present as solitary nodules. Consequently, thorough assessment is of the utmost importance. On the other hand, the majority of these lesions are not cancers, and to subject all patients to invasive studies and excision can lead to much unnecessary morbidity. The primary physician needs to determine the likelihood of malignancy on the basis of clinical and radiologic findings and identify the patient who requires referral for consideration of bronchoscopy, percutaneous needle biopsy, or thoracotomy. Workup can be performed on an outpatient basis.

PATHOPHYSIOLOGY AND CLINICAL PRESENTATION

Solitary pulmonary nodules characteristically appear in the middle or lateral lung fields, surrounded by normal lung and unaccompanied by satellite lesions. They have smooth contours and are usually round ("coin" lesions) or oval. Neoplastic, granulomatous, vascular, and cystic processes are the principal pathologic mechanisms responsible for nodule formation. The nodule displaces normal aerated lung parenchyma and does not cause symptoms unless airway obstruction, pleural invasion, interference with respiratory mechanics, or involvement of blood vessels or nerves occurs. Inflammatory lesions double in volume in less than 5 weeks, malignancies take between 1 and 18 months to double, and benign nodules take longer. A solitary nodule that does not change in size for 2 years is benign. The older the patient, the greater the chances that the nodule is malignant; the probability is less than 2% below age 30 and increases by 10% to 15% with each succeeding decade. A history of smoking greatly increases the probability that the nodule is malignant, as does concurrent weight loss, headache, or bone pain.

Benign and malignant solitary lung nodules may have a similar appearance on chest x-ray films. However, the distribution *patterns of calcification* are different and of diagnostic utility. Benign lesions tend to have calcium deposited in central, peripheral, concentric, "popcorn," or homogeneous patterns, whereas eccentric patterns of calcification are more characteristic of malignancies (see below and Fig. 44.1).

Among lung cancers, adenocarcinomas tend to be located peripherally; squamous and small-cell cancers are usually more central in location. However, squamous cell cancers that are located peripherally tend to show cavitation.

DIFFERENTIAL DIAGNOSIS

Healed infectious granulomas account for the majority of solitary nodules. In most series, 20% to 40% prove to be cancers. Of these, more than 75% are *primary lung cancers*, and the remainder are *metastatic lesions*. Tumors of the *breast*, *colon*, and *testicles* are particularly prone to metastasize to the lung. Of the 60% to 80% of solitary pulmonary nodules that prove to be benign, 85% to 90% are granulomas; most are *tuberculous*, but in endemic areas, *histoplasmosis* and *coccidioidomycosis* are important considerations. Benign pulmonary tumors such as *hamartomas* account for about 5% of benign nodules. The remainder are *bronchogenic cysts*, *hydatid cysts*, *pseudolymphomas*, *arteriovenous malformations*, and *bronchopulmonary sequestrations*. Extrapulmonary lesions, such as skin lesions, moles, nipples, chest wall and rib lesions, and pleural plaques, may be confused with solitary lesions of lung parenchyma.

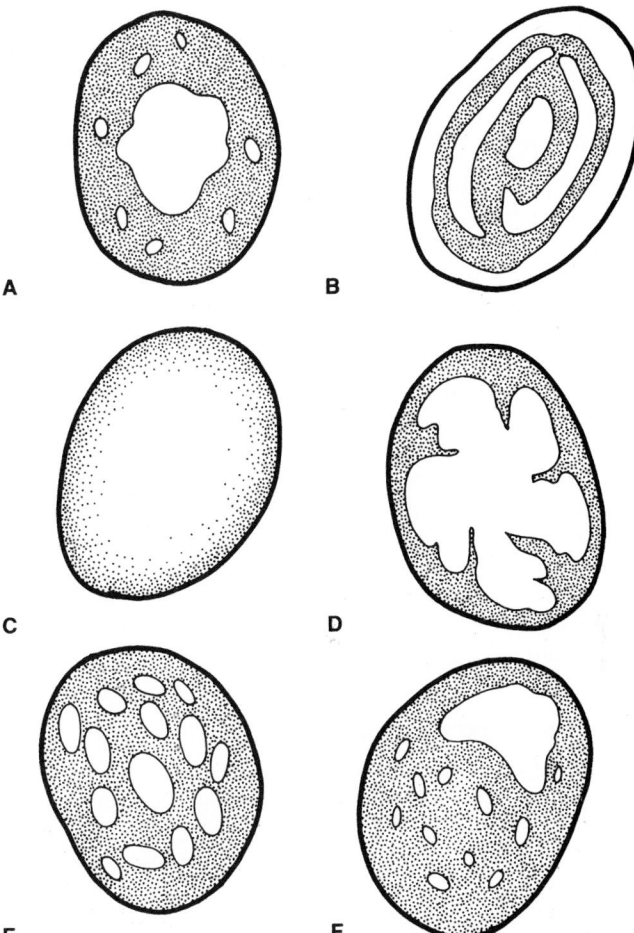

FIG. 44.1. Patterns of calcification in solitary pulmonary nodules include central (**A**), laminated (**B**), diffuse (**C**), "popcorn" (**D**), stippled (**E**), and eccentric (**F**). A through D are virtually always benign; E and F may be benign or malignant.

WORKUP

The major issue posed by a solitary nodule is the chance of an early resectable lung cancer. Many surgeons argue that the risk of thoracotomy is small and the potential benefit considerable, as resection of a nodule that proves to be an early primary lung cancer may provide the patient with a chance for cure. They note that for resected bronchogenic carcinomas and solitary lung metastases presenting as solitary nodules, average 5-year survivals are 60% and 35%, respectively. On the other hand, pulmonologists have argued that lesions that possess many of the criteria of benignity can be managed conservatively, and that definitive tissue diagnosis can be approached by bronchoscopy or needle biopsy without resorting to early thoracotomy, which has a surgical mortality ranging from 1% to 10%. A review of the literature reveals passionate advocates on both sides. Conclusive data taking into account morbidity and mortality of both approaches are still lacking.

The task of the primary care physician is to make the best possible clinical estimate of cancer risk based on history, physical examination, and appearance of the nodule on chest x-ray films and computed tomography (CT), with the possible addition of positron emission tomography (PET). Proper patient selection is the best means of maximizing the yield from invasive study and surgical intervention and minimizing the rate of false alarms and unnecessary morbid procedures.

History

The age of the patient and a history of smoking are important determinants of cancer risk. The likelihood ratio for malignancy in men increases markedly with age, estimated at 0.1 for those below age 35 to 5.7 for those over 70. Likelihood ratios for smoking range from 0.15 for those who have never smoked to 3.9 for those currently smoking more than two packs per day. The probability of cancer is 50% for patients in their 60s but less than 2% for those under 30. Although symptoms are often absent, it is worth inquiring into bone pain, headache, weight loss, and other symptoms suggestive of malignancy. A history of hemoptysis, even if minimal (see Chapter 42), and of known previous breast, bowel, or testicular cancer also increases the likelihood of malignancy. A history of exposure to tuberculosis (TB) or residence in an area in which histoplasmosis or coccidioidomycosis is endemic raises the possibility of a granulomatous etiology but does not rule out malignancy. A family history of hemorrhagic telangiectasia can be a valuable clue.

Physical Examination

The physical examination is generally unrevealing, but the presence of a breast or testicular mass, occult blood in the stool, clubbing (see Chapter 45), cutaneous or mucosal telangiectasia, or an audible bruit over the chest wall (suggestive of a vascular etiology) should be excluded. Perhaps the most important part of the physical examination is careful palpation of lymph nodes, particularly those in the supraclavicular and axillary regions. If enlarged, such nodes can be sampled by biopsy, which may eliminate the need for thoracotomy or other invasive procedures.

Laboratory Studies

Chest Radiography. *Appearance* of the lesion and its *doubling time* are among the most useful data for determining the chances of malignancy. An assessment of doubling time—the period during which the tumor doubles in volume—can be especially helpful, but this is possible immediately only if *previous chest films* are available. It is important to keep in mind that doubling refers to volume, not diameter. In doubling, the diameter of the lesion need increase by only 28%, not 100%. A doubling time of more than 2 years or less than 30 days makes malignancy unlikely.

Every effort should be made to locate old chest x-ray films before further studies are undertaken. If no old films are available and it is determined reasonable to follow the patient expectantly (see below), then serial films should be obtained, the first one 3 weeks after the time of initial evaluation and then others at intervals of 3 to 6 months for the next year. The interval can be decreased to every 6 to 12 months thereafter.

If previous films are unavailable, careful evaluation of the *radiologic appearance* of the nodule is indicated. A most helpful sign is the presence of *calcification*. Laminated or concentric calcification is specific for granulomas. Central, diffuse, or homogeneous patterns of calcification are, with rare exceptions,

also associated with benign lesions. However, radiographically visible calcium in stippled or eccentric patterns can occur in both malignant and benign lesions. Moreover, a primary cancer may engulf a preexisting calcified granuloma or scar; eccentricity of the calcium in the nodule should raise this possibility (Fig. 44.1).

The *location*, *size*, and *shape* of the nodule on a chest x-ray film are less valuable distinguishing signs. Both cancers and tuberculous granulomas are more common in the upper and middle lobes than in the lower lobes. Small lesions are more likely to be benign or, if they are malignant, are still at a stage when detection and definitive diagnosis may have the greatest positive impact. Ill-defined borders suggest a primary malignancy, as does lobulation of the margin of the nodule. However, smooth borders are also seen with metastatic lesions. Cavitation occurs with nearly equal frequency in cancers and granulomas.

Computed Tomography has become the imaging technique of choice for evaluation of the solitary pulmonary nodule. It provides much better definition of the lesion and pattern of calcification than does chest radiography and reduces the false-negative rate associated with reliance on chest radiographic appearance alone. What appears to be a single nodule on plain film may actually be one of several lesions on CT and indicative of metastatic disease. CT is useful for guiding needle biopsy and allows assessment of the mediastinum, which is useful in staging lesions suspected to be malignant (although its sensitivity and specificity for staging have been found wanting in patients with lesions smaller than 3 cm; see Chapter 53).

Taking thin sections (high-resolution CT) or using iodinated contrast can sometimes uncover calcification not visible by standard CT, can better confirm hamartomas and arteriovenous malformations, and can enhance the appearance of malignant nodules.

Positron Emission Tomography with ^{18}F-2-fluoro-2-deoxy-D-glucose (FDG) has been shown to add useful discriminating information for nodules deemed indeterminate based on radiographic appearance. Studies suggest a sensitivity of 90% to 95% and specificity of 85% to 90%. Decision analysis suggests that a CT plus an FDG-PET strategy may be most effective and may actually be cost-saving among patients for whom the probability of cancer is between 0.12 to 0.69.

Magnetic Resonance Imaging is inferior to CT for imaging solitary pulmonary nodules. It does not detect calcification well but reveals the mediastinum better than does CT, and it is useful for imaging chest wall invasion, aortopulmonic window adenopathy, and superior sulcus tremors.

Ancillary Studies. An intermediate-strength *tuberculin skin test* should be implanted (see Chapter 38). If sputum is available, it should be stained for *acid-fast organisms* and *cultured for TB*. In endemic areas, *fungal cultures* and histoplasmin complement fixation titers may be of importance.

Sputum cytologic examination is the least invasive means of identifying a malignancy. Three first morning samples should be obtained on consecutive days. Yield is highest when the sample contains pulmonary histiocytes (a sign of a deep sample) and the lesion is in the upper lobes, centrally located, communicating with a bronchus, or larger than 2 cm in diameter (see Chapter 37). Although the specificity of the test is high in experienced hands, its sensitivity has been found wanting in many studies, with figures ranging from 13% to 77%. Thus, a negative study does not rule out the diagnosis. Moreover, because of the importance of distinguishing a small-cell carcinoma from cancers of other cell types (see Chapter 53), it is often necessary to obtain tissue for diagnosis. Because of these shortcomings, some have argued that sputum cytology is not worth the effort, except in patients who are too ill to undergo invasive study.

Diagnostic Approach

Conservative Approach to further evaluation is reasonable in patients determined to have little chance of cancer by noninvasive evaluation. Withholding invasive study is a legitimate management option in patients with lesions that have not enlarged in 5 years and in young, nonsmoking patients with radiologic evidence that suggests benignity (central, laminated, diffuse, or "popcorn" pattern of calcification; sharp borders). Careful follow-up with serial chest films taken according to the schedule noted above is essential because some malignancies can be slow-growing.

Invasive Diagnostic Measures deserve consideration if malignancy is still considered possible after noninvasive evaluation. Thoracotomy with resection represents the most direct and definitive means of diagnosis (and treatment), but it is associated with a perioperative mortality risk of 1% to 10% and considerable morbidity (see Chapter 53). Less morbid options include bronchoscopy with transbronchial biopsy and needle aspiration biopsy under fluoroscopic or CT control.

Fiberoptic bronchoscopic examination with bronchial brushing and biopsy may yield a diagnosis if a bronchus appears to enter the lesion on CT, but the sensitivity is substantially lower (10% to 30%) when nodules are small (<2 cm) and well circumscribed. *Transthoracic needle aspiration* is a far more valuable approach to diagnosis. Sensitivity for detection of malignancy approaches 95% when the nodule is accessible to the transthoracic approach. Accurate pathologic diagnosis is facilitated by using a large-bore needle rather than a "skinny" one and by taking multiple samples. Specific histologic types of malignant lesions can often be identified.

Mediastinoscopy and *thoracotomy* are indicated when the pre-procedure probability of an early resectable primary lung cancer is high (see Chapter 53) and the patient is a good operative risk. Patients with severe obstructive or restrictive disease should first undergo formal pulmonary function testing.

Choice of Diagnostic Approach depends on the estimated probability of malignancy, location of the lesion, ability and willingness of the patient to tolerate the event (or the uncertainty, if watchful waiting is a consideration), and availability of the needed technical expertise.

The high-probability patient who can tolerate surgery and whose lesion has been determined to be resectable (see Chapter 53) should undergo thoracotomy and resection. Patients with an intermediate probability of malignancy might be best approached by transthoracic needle biopsy if it appears technically feasible. Patients with a very low risk are reasonable candidates for careful follow-up by serial radiographic study.

In sum, the optimal approach to evaluation of the patient with a solitary pulmonary nodule remains problematic because outcome data are lacking. It appears that a conservative approach to evaluation is justified in patients judged to be at low risk for malignancy based on epidemiologic, historical, physical, and radiographic criteria. Patients at high risk for malignancy require a tissue diagnosis. Improvements in noninvasive evaluation techniques are reflected in the lower number of surgical procedures being performed for solitary nodules and the higher proportion of malignancies found among those that are sampled or resected. However, in a significant number of cases, substantial ambiguity remains after noninvasive evaluation. Formal clinical prediction rules have been developed based on elements of history (age, smoking, and prior cancer) and radiologic appearance (nodule diameter, presence of spicules, and upper lobe location), but they do not yield better results than does a clinician who considers these and other factors. Patients for whom the probability of malignancy is neither low enough for them to be followed conservatively nor high enough for them to undergo surgery face a dilemma. The uncertainty and possible outcomes of alternative approaches should be shared with these patients so that a satisfactory plan can be devised.

PATIENT EDUCATION AND INDICATIONS FOR REFERRAL

Patients suspected on clinical and radiologic grounds of having a malignancy should be referred for tissue diagnosis. Decisions regarding the need for and type of invasive procedure should be made in conjunction with surgical and radiologic consultants. When the probability of malignancy is unclear, the patient needs to be informed about the lack of diagnostic certainty provided by noninvasive study, and about the nature of further tests that might be undertaken. Patients who cannot emotionally tolerate the uncertainty should be advised to undergo a definitive procedure to end the constant worry about the possibility of malignancy. The patient who can live with such uncertainty and is reluctant to undergo a thoracotomy or biopsy might be followed with serial chest films at 3- to 6-month intervals for 2 years.

A.H.G./A.G.M.

ANNOTATED BIBLIOGRAPHY

Becker GL, Whitlock WL, Schaefer PS, et al. The impact of thoracic computed tomography in clinically staged T1, N0, M0 chest lesions. Arch Intern Med 1990;150:557. (*Did not find CT to be helpful for staging the suspected lesion in patients with lung nodules smaller than 3 cm.*)

Cummings SR, Lillington GA, Richard RJ. Estimating the probability of malignancy in solitary pulmonary nodules. Am Rev Respir Dis 1986;134:449. (*Utilizes prevalence, diameter of nodule, age, smoking history, calcification pattern, and type of edge; very useful.*)

Fulkerson WJ. Fiberoptic bronchoscopy. N Engl J Med 1984;311:511. (*Reviews the indications, contraindications, complications, and diagnostic yield of fiberoptic bronchoscopy and endobronchial biopsy.*)

Gupta NC, Maloof J, Gunel E. Probability of malignancy in solitary pulmonary nodules using fluorine-18-FDG and PET. J Nucl Med 1996;37:943. (*Sensitivity and specificity of 93% and 88%, respectively, in this study.*)

Khouri NF, Stitik FP, Erozan YS, et al. Transthoracic needle aspiration biopsy of benign and malignant lung lesions. Am J Roentgenol 1985;144:281. (*Diagnostic yield well in excess of 80% and helped by use of wide aspiration needle, which facilitates diagnosis of benign lesions.*)

MacDougall B, Weinerman B. The value of sputum cytology. J Gen Intern Med 1992;7:11. (*Sensitivity and specificity were found lacking, and the test was of limited use in the workup of suspected lung cancer.*)

Nathan MH. Management of solitary pulmonary nodules: an organized approach based on growth rates and statistics. JAMA 1974; 227:1141. (*A very conservative approach is advocated—observation of the nodule with serial roentgenograms to calculate the doubling time.*)

Rubins JB, Rubins HB. Temporal trends in the prevalence of malignancy in resected solitary pulmonary lesions. Chest 1996;109:100. (*Increasing proportion of procedures result in a diagnosis of malignancy, independently of age and lesion size, reflecting better noninvasive discrimination.*)

Swenson SJ. Solitary pulmonary nodule: CT evaluation of enhancement with iodinated contrast material. Radiology 1992;182:343. (*Improved detection of malignancy suggested.*)

Swenson SJ, Jett JR, Payne WS, et al. An integrated approach to evaluation of the solitary pulmonary nodule. Mayo Clin Proc 1990;65:173. (*A critical review of diagnostic studies; 79 references.*)

Swenson SJ, Silverstein MD, Edell ES, et al. Solitary pulmonary nodules: clinical prediction model versus physicians. Mayo Clin Proc 1999;74:319. (*Clinicians performed as well as prediction rule utilizing three elements of history and three radiographic features.*)

Toomes H, Delphendahl A, Manke HG, et al. The coin lesion of the lung: a review of 955 resected coin lesions. Cancer 1983;51:534. (*A useful series for statistics on types of lesions identified.*)

45
Evaluation of Clubbing

The term *clubbing* refers to enlargement and sponginess of the nail beds of the fingers and toes and reduction in the angle created by the nail and the dorsum of the distal phalanx. Clubbing is sometimes accompanied by a chronic subperiosteal osteitis, *hypertrophic osteoarthropathy*. Patients rarely complain of clubbed fingers; it is the physician who detects this abnormality as an incidental finding on physical examination. Because clubbing or hypertrophic osteoarthropathy may be the first clinical sign of a serious underlying condition, such as a pulmonary neoplasm, it is important for the primary physician to recognize these findings and investigate their possible causes.

PATHOPHYSIOLOGY AND CLINICAL PRESENTATION

Hypotheses explaining the pathogenesis of clubbing and osteoarthropathy implicate autonomic influences, arteriovenous shunting, and blood-borne substances. The precise pathophysiology remains uncertain, but it is known that intrathoracic vagotomy can abolish clubbing and osteoarthropathy, as can correction of an arteriovenous shunt or removal of a pulmonary tumor.

The pathologic examination of clubbed fingers reveals increased vascularity. In hypertrophic osteoarthropathy, the periosteum is found to be edematous, hyperemic, and infiltrated by mononuclear cells. Periosteal elevation, new bone formation, and endosteal resorption in the distal ends of long bones, metacarpals, and metatarsals are all present. Soft-tissue swelling in the distal ends of the fingers and toes may lead to clubbing.

Clubbing is usually asymptomatic. Patients with hypertrophic osteoarthropathy may have pain in the wrists, ankles, hands, and feet; erythema and effusions are sometimes noted. Hypertrophic osteoarthropathy may precede clubbing or occur without it, but generally the two appear together. Clubbing often takes place in the absence of osteoarthropathy. Either finding may develop before the clinical presentation of one of the conditions associated with it.

Idiopathic hypertrophic osteoarthropathy, sometimes referred to as pachydermoperiostosis, is a benign condition that must be distinguished from hypertrophic osteoarthropathy secondary to systemic disease. These patients show periosteal new bone formation, swelling of the joints, and thickened and furred skin in addition to clubbing. The benign syndrome can be differentiated from secondary hypertrophic osteoarthropathy by development in adolescence, slow growth, a paucity of joint symptoms, and the absence of concurrent hepatic or pulmonary disease.

DIFFERENTIAL DIAGNOSIS

Clubbing and hypertrophic osteoarthropathy occur in 2% to 12% of patients with *lung cancer*, developing with equal frequency in patients with large-cell cancer, squamous cell cancer, or adenocarcinoma, but rarely in the setting of small-cell cancer. Clubbing alone may be more frequent, and the prevalence depends on the sensitivity of the diagnostic criteria used to designate digits as "clubbed." A recently proposed, sensitive, standardized measure identified clubbing in 37% of those with lung cancer and found no difference in prevalence among patients with squamous cell cancer, adenocarcinoma, or small-cell cancer. Metastatic lung tumors are rarely responsible for such changes. With the decline in the incidence of *chronic pulmonary infectious* diseases (such as tuberculosis, lung abscess, and bronchiectasis), carcinoma of the lung has emerged as the leading cause of hypertrophic osteoarthropathy. Clubbing and osteoarthropathy are seen in patients with cyanotic congenital heart disease with *right-to-left shunts*, subacute bacterial *endocarditis*, and *cystic fibrosis*. Clubbing is a classic sign of chronic *hypoxemia* in patients with chronic obstructive lung disease. In addition, there are *hereditary* or idiopathic forms of clubbing and hypertrophic osteoarthropathy that have no clinical significance. Unilateral clubbing is associated with impairment of the vascular supply to the arm that occurs with aortic, subclavian, or innominate artery lesions. Clubbing may develop in jackhammer operators.

Clubbing has also been described in a number of nonpulmonary conditions, including inflammatory bowel disease and chronic liver disease. Case reports of clubbing in association with a myriad of diseases have been published. Some of these include esophageal cancer, early HIV infection, and antiphospholipid antibody syndrome. Each of these reports includes disclaimers about the presence of comorbid pulmonary disease. Nonetheless, it is difficult to judge their significance.

Clubbing must be differentiated from a number of other phalangeal conditions that resemble it. In many normal people, particularly African-Americans, curvature of the nails is increased. Infections of the terminal phalanges, such as felon and chronic paronychia, may be confused with clubbing, as may thyroid acropachy.

WORKUP

The evaluation of clubbing should begin with confirmation of the characteristic physical findings: *loss of the angle* made by the nail and *increase* in the *ballotability* of the nail bed. Hypertrophic osteoarthropathy is identified by *radiography of the long bones*; the typical changes are increase in periosteal thickness and new bone formation at distal ends. Once it is clear that clubbing or hypertrophic osteoarthropathy is present, evaluation for an underlying cause can commence.

History. Before an elaborate search for a serious illness is undertaken, it should be established whether clubbing has been lifelong and is present in other family members, which would be indicative of the harmless familial variety. Symptoms such as cough, sputum production, hemoptysis, and dyspnea point to a respiratory problem and may have already triggered an evaluation of the lungs (see Chapters 40 through 42). The patient should be questioned about history of a heart murmur and exercise intolerance, and about prior liver disease, cramping lower abdominal pain, diarrhea, bloody stools, and joint problems. Smoking and other risk factors related to the development of lung cancer (see Chapter 37) should be assessed. Exposure to tuberculosis also needs to be ascertained (see Chapter 38).

Physical Examination requires a check for fever, tachypnea, tachycardia, cyanosis, tobacco stains, jugular venous distention, barrel chest, wheezes, rhonchi, rales (crackles), signs of consolidation or effusion, heart murmur, skin lesions of hepatocellular disease, and signs of cirrhosis. Lymph nodes should be palpated for enlargement, and joints should be checked for hypertrophic changes and signs of inflammation.

Laboratory Studies. The only mandatory laboratory study is a *chest radiograph*, as early pleural, pulmonary, or mediastinal neoplasm may be asymptomatic. A complete blood cell count and stool examination for occult blood may be of help. Further evaluation of the liver, thyroid, heart, or bowel should be undertaken only if symptoms or physical findings suggest disease in these areas. Patients with new onset of clubbing and a long history of smoking should be followed for the develop-

ment of pulmonary neoplasm; periodic examinations including sputum cytology and chest radiography are appropriate.

Differentiating Osteoarthropathy from Rheumatoid Disease can be difficult. An extensive review of patients with clubbing and lung cancer showed that the symptoms of osteoarthropathy were often mistaken for arthritis and predated the diagnosis of neoplasm by a mean of 4.9 months. Frequent complaints of bilateral joint discomfort in the small joints, such as the wrists and hands, and an adequate response to aspirin or nonsteroidal agents tended to persuade physicians that they were dealing with rheumatologic disease. Also noteworthy were the findings of acute elevation in acute-phase reactants and the presence of rheumatoid factor in 1 of 14 and antinuclear antibody in 5 of 12. The symmetric involvement of small peripheral joints and the tendency to development of synovitis present a significant diagnostic dilemma, with some patients having a syndrome indistinguishable from that of an inflammatory arthritis.

SYMPTOMATIC MANAGEMENT AND PATIENT EDUCATION

No symptomatic therapy is available for clubbing. It is an innocuous cosmetic disturbance. Discomfort in the bones and joints secondary to hypertrophic osteoarthropathy can be treated with aspirin. Rarely, joint symptoms are disabling; these may require extreme therapies such as corticosteroids or intrathoracic vagotomy. Resection of the underlying lung cancer may reduce joint pain and swelling of the fingers. Such therapeutic options should be undertaken in consultation with a specialist familiar with the problem.

Patient education is important in any condition in which the physician discovers a potential sign of disease that is not obvious to the patient. It is likely that patients will be disturbed by the investigation and by the possibility of serious disease. The physician must take time to inform the patient that clubbing can be a harmless finding in addition to a helpful guide to the early diagnosis of disease. The patient who smokes should be strongly advised to quit (see Chapter 54).

A.H.G./A.G.M.

ANNOTATED BIBLIOGRAPHY

Baughman RP, Gunther KL, Buchsbaum JA, et al. Prevalence of digital clubbing in bronchogenic carcinoma by a new digital index. Clin Exp Rheumatol 1998;16:21. (*Proposed new measure of clubbing yielded positive results in 37% of patients with cancer; no difference in prevalence among those with squamous cell cancer, adenocarcinoma, or small-cell cancer.*)

Boonen A, Schrey G, Van der Linden S. Clubbing in human immunodeficiency virus infection. Br J Rheumatol 1996;35:292. (*Case report of two patients in whom clubbing appeared shortly after seroconversion.*)

Coutts II, Gilson JC, Kerr IH, et al. Significance of finger clubbing in asbestosis. Thorax 1987;42:117. (*Clubbing not associated with degree of asbestos exposure but with severity of functional disease and fibrosis.*)

Kitis G, Thompson H, Allan RN. Finger clubbing in inflammatory bowel disease: its prevalence and pathogenesis. Br Med J 1979;2:825. (*Clubbing found in 38% of patients with Crohn's disease and in 15% of those with ulcerative colitis.*)

Pineada CJ, Fonseca C, Martinez-Lavin M. The spectrum of soft tissue and skeletal abnormalities of hypertrophic osteoarthropathy. J Rheumatol 1990;17:626. (*Detailed description of characteristic findings.*)

Segal AN, Mackenzie AH. Hypertrophic osteoarthropathy: a ten-year retrospective analysis. Semin Arthritis Rheum 1985;12:220. (*Authoritative review with extensive study of 16 patients who had hy-*pertrophic osteoarthropathy; the differentiation from rheumatoid disease can sometimes be difficult.*)

Stenseth JH, Clagett OT, Woolner LB. Hypertrophic pulmonary osteoarthropathy. Dis Chest 1967;52:62. (*Review of 888 pulmonary neoplasms revealed a 9.2% incidence of hypertrophic osteoarthropathy.*)

46

Approach to the Patient with Sleep Apnea

Obstructive sleep apnea is estimated to affect up to 2% to 4% of middle-aged men and women and even greater proportions of the elderly. Despite its high prevalence, the condition is often overlooked because its symptoms (e.g., daytime tiredness, snoring) may be mistaken for normal phenomena of everyday life. Insufficient recognition in primary care practice continues despite the growing appreciation of the frequency and potentially serious consequences of this condition (e.g., motor vehicle accidents and deaths, cardiovascular morbidity and mortality, pulmonary hypertension). The primary care physician needs to be cognizant of the early and varied manifestations of sleep apnea so that a timely workup can commence and treatment can be instituted before the onset of potentially life-threatening consequences.

PATHOPHYSIOLOGY AND CLINICAL PRESENTATION

Definitions. *Sleep apnea* is defined as five or more episodes of apnea or hypopnea per hour of sleep; more than 20 episodes per hour is classified as clinically significant disease because it correlates with an increased risk for adverse outcomes. Sleep apnea may result from *central suppression of* respiration (as occurs with congestive heart failure and carbon dioxide retention) or from *upper airway obstruction*. In the former condition (*central sleep apnea*), air flow ceases because of the loss of central respiratory drive; in the latter (*obstructive sleep apnea*), air flow ceases because of obstruction despite chest and abdominal respiratory efforts during apnea. Obstructive sleep apnea is the most common form of sleep apnea encountered in the office setting. *Upper airway resistance syndrome* is an intermediate category, in which air flow is maintained by increased respiratory effort despite partial airway obstruction.

Mechanisms. Obstructive sleep apnea occurs when the patency of the nasopharyngeal airway become insufficient during sleep. Anatomic risk factors include nuchal obesity (cricothyroid neck circumference >17 inches for men, >16 inches for women), deviated septum, nasal polyps, enlarged uvula and soft palate, small chin with deep overbite, enlarged tonsils, and hypertrophy of the lateral pharyngeal musculature. Although obesity appears to be a major factor (causing fat deposition in the tongue and pharyngeal tissues), persons who are not obese are also at risk if they manifest other anatomic risk factors. In addition to being anatomically predisposed, patients with obstructive sleep apnea appear to be unable to sustain sufficient oropharyngeal muscle dilator activity during sleep to prevent airway collapse during the negative pressure of inspiration. The suppressive effects of alcohol and sedatives on such neuromuscular function may explain their role in exacerbating obstructive sleep apnea. Hypothyroidism may be a risk factor.

When the obstruction is mild and not physiologically disturbing, *snoring* is the only manifestation, and sleep is not interrupted. With increasing degrees of obstruction, snoring becomes louder and compensatory respiratory efforts are triggered, causing electroencephalographically detectable *arousals from sleep*. Frequent arousals during the night disrupt normal sleep "architecture" and result in *daytime sleepiness*. In the upper airway resistance syndrome, near-normal air flow is maintained by compensatory respiratory efforts, but at the cost of sleep arousals. More severe degrees of obstruction can lead to *hypopnea* (50% reduction in air flow with oxygen desaturation ≥4%) or *apnea* (cessation of air flow for at least 10 s). The more severe and more prolonged the obstruction, the more likely and more severe are blood *oxygen desaturation* and *hypoxemia*, consequences of ventilation–perfusion mismatching as a result of the perfused lung not being adequately ventilated.

The adverse cardiovascular consequences of sleep apnea are related to hypoxemia. The decline in arterial oxygen increases pulmonary vascular resistance; when severe and chronic, it can lead to sustained *pulmonary hypertension* and ultimately *cor pulmonale*, particularly in persons with underlying chronic obstructive pulmonary disease or morbid obesity. Airway obstruction, episodes of apnea, and hypoxemia trigger compensatory increases not only in ventilatory effort but also in sympathetic tone, which may explain the association between severe degrees of sleep apnea and *systemic hypertension*, *cardiac arrhythmias*, and increased *cardiovascular morbidity* and *mortality*. Sleep apnea is an independent risk factor for hypertension. Severe degrees of obstructive sleep apnea can also lead to hypercarbia and *central suppression* of respiration, as seen in persons with the *obesity–hypoventilation (pickwickian) syndrome*. *Dysmenorrhea* and *amenorrhea* are consequences in women of reproductive age.

The disturbance in sleep caused by obstructive sleep apnea may impair *cognition* and *psychomotor performance*. In severe sleep apnea, hypersomnolence develops, markedly increasing the risk for injuries during work and driving. The risk ratio for *traffic accidents* increases to 6.3 and appears independent of other risk factors.

Clinical Presentations. Often, the patient presents at the insistence of a bed partner who is bothered or worried by *loud* *and intermittent snoring, disturbed* or *restless sleep,* periods of *irregular* or *halted breathing,* and *choking* or *gasping.* Patients presenting with obstructive sleep apnea typically complain of excessive *daytime sleepiness*; they may note falling asleep at work or at a meeting. Women are somewhat more likely to report *chronic fatigue.* Patients find they awaken not feeling refreshed and may have a morning *headache. Work performance* may be suffering, and the history of a work-related or automobile *accident* resulting from sleepiness may be elicited. Family and friends may note a *personality change. Obesity* is common but is not a necessary part of the clinical presentation; nearly half of premenopausal women with disordered nocturnal breathing are thin but have another contributing anatomic feature, such as a *severe overbite* or a *high hard palate.* A positive *family history* is noted, usually in persons with a contributing anatomic factor or obesity.

DIFFERENTIAL DIAGNOSIS

Because obstructive sleep apnea may present as daytime tiredness, it must be differentiated from other causes of chronic fatigue (see Chapter 8). In patients who present with interrupted sleep, other sleep disturbances deserve consideration (see Chapter 232). In those whose presentation is predominantly one of difficulty in breathing at night, heart failure (see Chapter 32), chronic obstructive lung disease (see Chapter 47), and other causes of snoring (see Chapter 223) should be considered.

WORKUP

History. A high index of suspicion is appropriate when a patient, whether obese or not, presents with symptoms of excessive daytime sleepiness, tiredness, or fatigue. A history of very loud intermittent snoring, irregular respiratory activity with spells of gasping or choking that interrupt sleep, or witnessed episodes of apnea is strongly suggestive. Also worth noting are any accidents, job performance difficulties, and personality changes or cognitive difficulties, especially if occurring in the context of daytime sleepiness. Risk factors that help in identifying patients with obstructive sleep apnea include marked obesity (body mass index >28 kg/m²), increasing age, obstructive upper airway abnormalities, regular use of sedatives or alcohol, and hypothyroidism.

Physical Examination. The blood pressure should be checked for elevation and the integument noted for any cyanosis, clubbing, or signs of hypothyroidism (see Chapter 104). The upper airway is examined for overbite, a high hard palate, other potentially obstructing nasopharyngeal lesions (e.g., nasal polyps, tonsillar hypertrophy, large uvula), and nasopharyngeal narrowing. The neck circumference should be measured to document any nuchal obesity. In persons with suspected severe obstructive sleep apnea, one should check for signs of pulmonary hypertension and cor pulmonale (e.g., right ventricular heave, loud pulmonic component of the second heart sound, jugular venous distention, leg edema).

Laboratory Studies. Currently, the definitive and most cost-effective diagnostic procedure in symptomatic patients clinically suspected of obstructive sleep apnea is a formal *polysomnographic study,* which includes overnight monitoring of the electroencephalogram, eye movements, muscle activity, chest movements, air flow, and blood oxygen saturation. Although such testing is expensive, it is nevertheless the most cost-effective of the available diagnostic modalities at present; the high sensitivity and specificity minimize both false-positive results (which generate unnecessary, expensive long-term therapy) and false-negative results (which lead to the failure to treat disease and the risk for considerable morbidity and mortality).

Home-monitoring methods for diagnosis are improving, but they still lack the sensitivity and specificity of polysomnography. Although the sensitivity and specificity of the most sophisticated home methods are reported to exceed 95%, and although the positive predictive value of a positive result can be high (approaching 99% in patients in whom obstructive sleep apnea is strongly suspected clinically), the negative predictive value and false-negative rate of these tests remain disappointing (77% and 23%, respectively). Based on these performance characteristics, some health care systems recommend screening with a high-quality home-monitoring method (simple periodic oximetry is insufficient), with referral to formal polysomnography reserved for those in whom obstructive sleep apnea is strongly suspected clinically but whose home-monitoring test results are negative. The cost-effectiveness of such a two-step strategy in comparison with polysomnographic testing of all patients with suspected obstructive sleep apnea remains to be determined.

Few routine laboratory studies are of value. A *thyroid-stimulating hormone* (TSH) determination is indicated if clinical evidence of hypothyroidism is present. Unless the patient has very severe disease with signs of cor pulmonale, the measurement of *hematocrit, arterial blood gases,* and *pulse oximetry* in the office is likely to be of little value.

PRINCIPLES OF MANAGEMENT

Selection and Initiation of Therapy. Treatment does improve the survival and functional status of patients with obstructive sleep apnea, but a proper matching of disease severity with treatment intensity is critical to achieving the best possible outcome. Unfortunately, few evidence-based criteria are available to guide patient selection and timing of therapy. *Positive findings on polysomnography,* demonstrating more than 20 apneic periods per hour in a symptomatic patient with arterial desaturation during sleep, provides the strongest grounds for initiation of therapy; the risk for complications of obstructive sleep apnea is high in such persons, particularly those with underlying lung disease. A lesser frequency of apneic episodes (<20/h) is a more common finding and necessitates careful consideration of the overall clinical picture before treatment is recommended. At present, no prospective data are available on outcomes in persons with milder disease (<20 episodes per hour) to help in treatment selection. Clinical judgment is required. Patients with preexisting lung disease plus sleep apnea have a worse prognosis than do those with no underlying lung disease, and they should be treated more aggressively. Minimally symptomatic patients with no concurrent pulmonary disease or evidence of impairment might first be prescribed a few potentially useful, noninvasive, simple measures (e.g., weight reduction if obese, changes in sleeping position) and followed expectantly. However, because the consequences of sleep apnea are potentially serious, *empiric therapy* based on clinical suspicion without reference to polysomnography is not recommended because clinical estimates lack the sensitivity and specificity required for a condition in which lifelong therapy may be necessary.

Weight Reduction. A *weight reduction program* should be recommended for patients with mild disease who are obese. Weight reduction is also the centerpiece of the treatment program for those with more symptomatic disease because it can greatly reduce or even cure sleep apnea. The implementation of a comprehensive, personalized program of weight reduction is essential to a successful weight loss effort (see Chapter 233).

Sleep Position. The position one assumes when sleeping can affect airway patency. Lying on one's back increases the risk for apneic episodes; sleeping on one's side reduces the risk. A trial of patient education to change sleeping position is worth a try, but most persons rotate at night during sleep. (One investigator suggested that patients try taping a tennis ball to their back at night to prevent lying in a supine position.)

Continuous Positive Airway Pressure. Nighttime nasal continuous positive airway pressure (CPAP) is becoming an important component of the treatment program for obstructive sleep apnea. A sealed nasal mask is worn at night connected to a blower apparatus that pneumatically sustains sufficient airway pressure to maintain upper airway patency. Patient acceptance is steadily improving, and compliance now exceeds 80% in reported trials (probably closer to 50% in everyday practice), facilitated by advances in apparatus design. CPAP improves survival in persons with more than 20 episodes of apnea per hour. Efficacy in those with less severe disease remains to be established.

Surgery. Surgical approaches are worth considering only if symptoms are severe, more conservative measures have failed, and an obvious obstructing anatomic anomaly is identified. Surgical excision of obstructing tonsils, a nasal mass, or a pharyngeal tumor can be curative. Surgery has also been performed in patients with severe obstructive disease, even in the absence of a single, identifiable obstructing lesion. The procedure used most for this purpose has been the *uvulopalatopharyngoplasty* (UPP). In performing the UPP, the surgeon excises the uvula, part of the soft palate, and any redundant pharyngeal tissue. The problem with recommending such surgery is that only about half of patients obtain a satisfactory result. Moreover, it has not been possible to predict in advance who will benefit from the surgery, and durable results are not always achieved. As a result and with the improvements in CPAP therapy, UPP is becoming a less utilized treatment option.

Oral Appliances. Dental appliances that correct such precipitants as a deep overbite have been tried. Acceptance is variable; long-term efficacy remains to be established. In patients with no such risk factor, but who cannot tolerate CPAP, an oral appliance that keeps tongue from falling back is sometimes tried. Efficacy and compliance are, at best, in the 50% range.

Pharmacologic Approaches. The most important pharmacologic intervention is avoidance of agents that might suppress respiration or neuromuscular function. Patients with sleep apnea should stop using alcohol and drugs with sedative activity. Because apneic episodes are most frequent during REM (rapid eye movement) sleep, the use of nonsedating agents that interfere with the REM phase of sleep, such as the nonsedating tricyclic antidepressant *protriptyline*, has been tried. Another approach is to administer drugs that might stimulate respiration, such as *medroxyprogesterone*. Neither approach has shown much promise and is not recommended. In contrast, treatment of underlying hypothyroidism with *thyroid hormone replacement* is effective in those with documented hypothyroidism as the cause of sleep apnea. *Nocturnal oxygen supplementation* can reduce the desaturation caused by sleep apnea, and some suggest that it be used; however, it can also prolong an apneic episode and should not be administered except in carefully controlled circumstances when an underlying chronic hypoxemia is present (see Chapter 47). Its effect on long-term outcome remains to be established.

INDICATIONS FOR REFERRAL

A patient with daytime tiredness and hypersomnolence should be considered a candidate for referral and consideration of a formal sleep study, especially if the patient's bed companion corroborates a history of loud snoring, disturbed sleep, abnormal respirations, and apneic periods. The presence of marked obesity and difficult-to-control hypertension should further raise the level of suspicion about an obstructive sleep disorder and prompt a consultation. Referral is best made to a pulmonary specialist experienced in the conduct and interpretation of polysomnography; however, it should be made clear that the purpose of the consultation is assessment of the appropriateness of formal sleep testing, and not automatic performance of a polysomnographic study. Consultation with a pulmonary specialist experienced in the treatment of sleep disorders can also be very useful for a patient who fails to improve with weight loss and for whom CPAP and surgical approaches to therapy need to be considered.

PATIENT EDUCATION

Patients brought in by a spouse complaining of their excessive snoring must be given detailed information on the potential seriousness (accidents, cardiovascular morbidity and mortality) of this seemingly harmless condition. Unless they suffer from disabling daytime tiredness and excessive sleepiness, they are unlikely to appreciate the significance of their condition. Patient education is also essential regarding treatment. Because weight loss is so effective in alleviating upper airway soft-tissue obstruction in obese patients, instruction about a comprehensive approach to weight reduction (see Chapter 233) is an essential component of the office encounter. Also important is advice regarding the avoidance of sedatives and alcohol.

A.H.G.

ANNOTATED BIBLIOGRAPHY

Chervin RD, Murman DL, Malow BA, et al. Cost-utility of three approaches to the diagnosis of sleep apnea: polysomnography, home testing, and empirical therapy. Ann Intern Med 1999;130:496. (*A cost–utility analysis demonstrating that polysomnography provided the most quality-adjusted life-years.*)

Fletcher EC, Schaaf JW, Miller J, et al. Long-term cardiopulmonary sequelae in patients with sleep apnea and chronic lung disease. Am Rev Respir Dis 1987;135:525. (*The combination of sleep apnea and chronic lung disease increases the risk for cor pulmonale and worsens the prognosis, but treatment of the apnea improves right ventricular function.*)

Guilleminault C, Stoohs R, Kim Y-D, et al. Upper airway sleep-disordered breathing in women. Ann Intern Med 1995;122:493. (*A retrospective case–control study identifying features of the clinical presentation in women; many were thin and manifested craniofacial anomalies contributing to the obstruction of air flow.*)

He J, Kryger MH, Zorick FJ, et al. Mortality and apnea index in obstructive sleep apnea. Chest 1988;94:9. (*Increased mortality in patients with more than 20 episodes of apnea per hour of sleep; CPAP improved survival.*)

Hla KM, Young T, Bidwell T, et al. Sleep apnea and hypertension: a population-based study. Ann Intern Med 1994;120:382. (*Finds sleep apnea to be an independent risk factor for hypertension.*)

Kramer NR, Cook TE, Carlisle CC, et al. The role of the primary care physician in recognizing obstructive sleep apnea. Arch Intern Med 1999;159:965. (*A retrospective chart audit showing that primary care physicians did recognize severely affected persons but that only a small fraction of patients at risk were identified.*)

Kuna ST, Sant'Ambrogio G. Pathophysiology of upper airway closures during sleep. JAMA 1991;266:1384. (*Excellent review of the mechanisms of upper airway obstruction in sleep apnea.*)

Mooe T, Rabben T, Wiklund U, et al. Sleep-disordered breathing in women: occurrence and association with coronary artery disease. Am J Med 1996;101:251. (*A case–control study finding sleep apnea common in women with coronary artery disease and an independent predictor of coronary artery disease after correction for other risk factors.*)

Pack AI, Gurughagavatula I. Economic implications of the diagnosis of obstructive sleep apnea. Ann Intern Med 1999;130:533. (*An editorial reviewing diagnostic strategies.*)

Roehrs T, Zorick F, Wittig R, et al. Predictors of objective daytime sleepiness in patients with sleep-related breathing disorders. Chest 1989;95:1202. (*Daytime hypersomnolence strongly related to apnea-induced sleep disruption.*)

Schmidt-Nowara WW, Meade TE, Hays MB, et al. Treatment of snoring and obstructive sleep apnea with a dental orthosis. Chest 1991;99:1378. (*A promising but preliminary report of some improvement.*)

Strohl KP, Cherniack NS, Gothe B. Physiologic basis of therapy for sleep apnea. Am Rev Respir Dis 1986;134:791. (*Useful review of pathophysiology and the pathophysiologic basis of available treatment options.*)

Teran-Santos J, Jimenez-Gomez A, Codero-Guevara J, et al. The association between sleep apnea and the risk of traffic accidents. N Engl J Med 1999;340:847. (*Odds ratio of 6.3 in a comparison of persons having more than 10 episodes per hour with normal persons.*)

Viner S, Szalai JP, Hoffstein V. Are history and physical examination a good screening test for sleep apnea? Ann Intern Med 1991;115:356. (*Age, body mass index, male sex, and snoring were predictive of sleep apnea in this logistic regression study, but sensitivity was not much better than that of subjective clinical assessment.*)

Young T, Palta M, Dempsey J, et al. The occurrence of sleep-disordered breathing among middle-aged adults. N Engl J Med 1993;328:1230. (*Prevalence was 24% among men and 9% among women, with sleep apnea among 4% of men and 2% of women—much higher than previously estimated.*)

47
Management of Chronic Obstructive Pulmonary Disease

Chronic obstructive pulmonary disease (COPD), or chronic bronchitis/emphysema, is a major cause of total disability, second only to coronary artery disease, and the fourth leading cause of death. Its prevalence approaches 30/1,000. Although COPD is incurable and often irreversible, improvements in functional status and survival are possible with good care, most of which can be delivered in the outpatient setting by the primary care physician. In many instances, functional impairment can be minimized and exercise tolerance improved. The primary physician needs to know the indications for bronchodilators, corticosteroids, oxygen supplementation, antibiotics, immunizations, and rehabilitative measures in addition to the potential value of surgical approaches. A positive attitude on the part of the physician is an important determinant of patient motivation and success.

PATHOPHYSIOLOGY, CLINICAL PRESENTATION, AND COURSE

Common Mechanisms and Presentations. COPD is a subset of the obstructive pulmonary diseases (which also include asthma, bronchiectasis, and cystic fibrosis). These diverse conditions share a pathophysiologic common denominator: *obstruction* of air flow and a reduction in the expiratory flow rate. This slowing manifests itself as a *reduction in the ratio of forced expiratory volume (FEV$_1$) to forced vital capacity (FVC, VC)*. In COPD, the *small airways* are the site of involvement, with an increase in small-airway resistance being the first detectable manifestation.

Airway *inflammation* plays an important pathophysiologic role in many of the obstructive pulmonary diseases. In stable COPD, the inflammation appears to be predominantly *neutrophilic*. Of the cytokines measured in COPD, those that attract neutrophils (e.g., interleukin-8) are the most markedly elevated. Although lymphocytes are present in increased numbers, they are mainly type 1 helper CD8 T cells. In contrast, the predominant cells in asthma are eosinophils, mast cells, and type 2 helper CD4 T cells. During an acute exacerbation of COPD, the number of eosinophils found in bronchial biopsy specimens is increased 30-fold. These differences in inflammatory cell infiltrates may help to explain the disparate responses to corticosteroids seen in the two conditions and in different phases of COPD (see below).

Despite the differences in inflammatory mechanisms between COPD and asthma, evidence is emerging that the inflammatory pathophysiology of *chronic asthma* might *predispose* patients to COPD, especially smokers. Asthmatic patients who smoke manifest an increased rate of deterioration in FEV$_1$ over time in comparison with nonasthmatic smokers and asthmatic patients who do not smoke. Moreover, bronchial hyperresponsiveness to methacholine challenge is a powerful independent predictor of progression of COPD in smokers. Perhaps the underlying inflammatory process in asthma is an important contributor to the development of COPD in smokers and may account for the steroid responsiveness seen in a subset of COPD patients.

Smoking remains the principal risk factor for the development of COPD; nearly 90% of cases occur in the context of long-term heavy smoking, which increases the risk for COPD 30-fold. Cigarette smoking in excess of 70 pack-years is highly predictive of COPD. The marked increase in COPD prevalence (especially among women) noted since 1980 reflects the heavy smoking habits of the U.S. population in the decades after World War II.

The patient with COPD may present clinically with any combination of *cough*, *sputum production*, *wheezing*, and *shortness of breath*. The presentation is a function of the severity of illness and the relative contributions of chronic bronchitis and emphysema to the clinical picture. Most patients have mixed disease, although one pathophysiology may predominate.

Emphysema is characterized by pathologic enlargement of the air spaces distal to the terminal bronchioles as a consequence of destruction of the alveolar walls and their constituent components. This destructive process remains incompletely understood but appears linked to *excessive alveolar protease activity*. Alveolar tissue contains both proteases and antiproteases, with neutrophil-derived elastase being the most important protease and α_1-antitrypsin being the prime antiprotease. When antitrypsin activity is reduced or elastase levels are increased, alveolar wall destruction is believed to result. Cigarette smoking may contribute to COPD by triggering the influx of elastase-rich neutrophils into the alveoli or by the oxidative inactivation of antitrypsin. Patients who are homozygous for a hereditary deficiency of α_1-*antitrypsin* (<80 mg/L) are at greatly increased risk for the development of emphysema. (They represent fewer than 2% of cases overall but account for many cases among nonsmokers without other environmental risk factors; they present with onset of clinical disease before age 50 and have a positive family history of early-onset emphysema.)

The net result of this pathologic process is fragmentation of the pulmonary elastic tissue, which leads to *destruction of the alveolar architecture* and the *capillary bed* that lies within the alveolar wall. Because both air space and the vascular bed are destroyed, ventilation and perfusion do not become markedly mismatched, and marked hypoxemia does not ensue. Expiratory flow rates decline with loss of the normal elastic recoil of the lung and radial traction on airways; the poorly supported noncartilaginous airways collapse during expiration. In many patients, a *reversible cholinergic component* of airway obstruction is also present that is responsive to muscarinic blockade.

Inspiratory flow rates are normal because airway caliber is normal during inspiration. *Pulmonary compliance* increases with the decline in elasticity. The size of the pulmonary capillary bed is reduced, causing the *carbon monoxide diffusing capacity* (D$_{LCO}$) to drop. The reduction in size of the vascular bed parallels the fall in alveolar surface area. Thus, ventilation still roughly matches perfusion, and significant hypoxemia does not ensue.

The *clinical picture* is dominated by *dyspnea*, particularly on exertion. Cough is only a minor complaint, and sputum production is scant. The patient with advanced disease is *thin* and *tachypneic*, often using accessory muscles of respiration and *pursed-lip breathing*. The latter helps keep noncartilaginous airways from collapsing during expiration. Cyanosis is uncommon because the oxygen tension (P$_{O_2}$) is only minimally reduced—hence the term *"pink puffer."* The neck veins may seem distended, but only during expiration. The *anterior–posterior diameter* of the chest is *increased*, the percussion note is hyperresonant, and the *breath sounds* are *distant*. Usually, no signs of cor pulmonale are present, although the right ventricular impulse may be prominent because of displacement by hyperinflated lungs. As noted, hypoxemia is minimal and little, if any, carbon dioxide retention occurs until the end stages of the disease. Chest radiography demonstrates hyperinflation and hyperlucency, especially at the apices, except in patients with antitrypsin deficiency, whose radiographic changes are greatest at the bases.

Chronic Bronchitis. Inflammation of the cells lining the bronchial wall in conjunction with hyperplasia of the mucous glands and narrowing of the small airways are the predominant pathologic features of chronic bronchitis. Causes of the condition are poorly understood, but chronic infection and airway hyperreactivity are believed to play important roles. Smoking is the major precipitant, along with prolonged exposure to air pollution and other bronchial irritants. However, even after withdrawal of such irritants, the inflammatory process often continues unabated. Airway edema, excess mucous production, and loss of ciliary transport result. Obstruction to air flow occurs with both inspiration and expiration. Widespread bronchial narrowing and mucous plugging produce *hypoxemia* because of mismatching of ventilation and perfusion. *Hypercarbia* results from impeded ventilation. Chronic hypoxia and hypercarbia increase pulmonary arterial resistance and may lead to the development of *pulmonary hypertension* and eventually *cor pulmonale*. Sudden worsening may precipitate acute right-sided heart failure in severe chronic bronchitis. Compared with emphysema, chronic bronchitis causes much less parenchymal damage; diffusing capacity, lung volumes, and compliance are not greatly altered.

Patients with chronic bronchitis are typically *colonized* with *Haemophilus influenzae* and *Streptococcus pneumoniae*; *Moraxella* is also found. However, the role of *infection* in the genesis of acute exacerbations remains unsettled, although evidence from classic double-blind, randomized, placebo-controlled trials demonstrates little difference in outcome between patients given prophylactic tetracycline and those given a placebo. When administered to patients with acute exacerbation of COPD, antibiotic therapy produces a small improvement in outcome in comparison with placebo.

The person with chronic bronchitis is often a *smoker* who presents with a history of chronic, productive cough. By definition, the *cough* must be present for at least *3 months each year during two consecutive years*. At first, the sputum production and cough occur just in the winter months, but soon the patient becomes symptomatic year-round, with a history of frequent exacerbations. By the time dyspnea on exertion sets in, the disease is well advanced. Patients may report having to sit up at night to breathe; at times, this may be a manifestation of congestive heart failure, which is not uncommon, but more careful questioning often reveals that the difficulty is precipitated by cough and relieved by raising sputum. As noted above, cor pulmonale and right-sided heart failure may ensue if chronic hypoxemia and pulmonary hypertension are present.

The chronic bronchitic patient is typically a man in his fifties at the time of presentation, and is often already at a late stage of disease. He may appear *plethoric* and *cyanotic*. The term *"blue bloater"* has been used to describe such patients. Tobacco stains on the fingers and teeth are common, and signs of *cor pulmonale* may be present (distended neck veins, right ventricular heave, right ventricular gallop, and peripheral edema). The lungs sound noisy; *crackles* and *wheezes* are readily evident. The expiratory phase of respiration is prolonged. Because of the mismatching of ventilation and perfusion, *hypoxemia* may be found on measurement of arterial blood gases. The carbon dioxide tension (PCO_2) rises as the ability to move air effectively declines. *Secondary polycythemia* is common, and the chest x-ray film shows increased bronchial vascular markings.

Clinical Course and Estimatation of Prognosis. The clinical course of COPD is generally *progressive*, although some patients seem to reach a plateau clinically—especially if they stop smoking. Early on, before the onset of symptoms, one can often detect an increase in the *closing volume* and a decrease in the *maximum midexpiratory flow rate* (sensitive measures of small-airway disease); measures of large-airway resistance are usually within normal limits during this phase of illness. The presymptomatic, *small-airway stage* of COPD may represent a period of reversible disease; however, early fibrotic changes have been found in airways of such patients. It has not been resolved whether intervention at the time of early small-airway abnormalities will alter the course of disease and improve the prognosis.

Longitudinal studies of symptomatic patients have shown a *steady deterioration* in pulmonary function with time. When the FEV_1 is used as the measure of obstruction, an annual average decrease in flow rate of 50 to 70 mL/s has been noted. By the time the FEV_1 declines to 1 L/s, the mean annual mortality approaches 10%. The rate of decline in FEV_1 can be markedly slowed if the patient stops smoking. The onset of resting tachycardia and signs of cor pulmonale are other indicators of a poor prognosis.

Several parameters are emerging as prognostically useful (Table 47.1). In one important study, significant reductions in 12-year survival were found among patients with a marked reduction in the *ratio of FEV_1 to FVC,* a substantial drop in FEV_1 or FVC, *hypoxemia, hypercarbia,* cor pulmonale, or *decreased diffusing capacity.* The FEV_1 may be a more useful predictor of prognosis in advanced disease than the ratio of FEV_1 to FVC. In late disease, the rate of decline of the FEV_1 often slows and the FVC may fall more rapidly, so that the ratio is preserved even in the setting of clinical deterioration. However, once the FEV_1 falls below 1 L/s, it is a less effective means of distin-

Table 47.1. Predictors of Poor Prognosis in Chronic Obstructive Pulmonary Disease

FEV_1 <40% of predicted, especially <1.0 L/sec
FEV_1/FEV <0.40
Arterial PO_2 <55 mm Hg
Presence of cor pulmonale
Carbon dioxide retention
FVC <80% of predicted
Decreased single-breath diffusing capacity
Decreased mixed venous oxygen concentration

FEV_1, forced expiratory volume in 1 second; FVC, forced vital capacity; PO_2, oxygen tension.

guishing survivors from nonsurvivors. Other predictors of poor prognosis included *heavy smoking* and a more rapid rate of decline of expiratory flow rates over time. Interestingly, the group with the lowest 12-year probability of survival still had a 40% chance of remaining alive.

Differences in patient populations make rigid extrapolation from studies of prognosis to individual patients unwise, but the parameters identified can be of qualitative use clinically. It remains difficult to predict survival in individual patients. Although the prognosis for patients with COPD is not very good, therapy does prolong survival (see below). Cessation of smoking is critical.

WORKUP

Although the selection of treatment modalities is partially empiric, it is still helpful to identify the predominant pathophysiologic defects, their severity and effect on the patient's functional status, and any aggravating or precipitating factors. Clarification of these issues can help focus therapy and serve as a baseline for monitoring efficacy of treatment.

History. One should obtain a careful description of symptoms and limitations of activity experienced in daily life, both at rest and during exercise. A detailed *smoking history* and *environmental* or *work exposures* to pulmonary irritants should be sought and specified. Quasi-quantitative estimates of *exercise capacity* (e.g., number of flights of stairs that can be climbed or distance that can be walked on level ground) are helpful, as is some indication of the progression of symptoms over time. The presence of *leg edema* and worsening exercise tolerance suggest onset of right-sided heart failure in the patient with chronic bronchitis.

Physical Examination. It is important to note any tachypnea, tachycardia, prolongation of the expiratory phase, cyanosis, clubbing, use of accessory respiratory muscles, wheezes, signs of consolidation, diminution of breath sounds, and evidence of cor pulmonale (jugular venous distention, peripheral edema, right ventricular heave, loud pulmonic closure sound, and right ventricular third heart sound).

Laboratory Studies. Testing helps to quantify the degree of the obstructive defect, determine the response to bronchodilators and steroids, and estimate prognosis.

Spirometry is essential to these tasks. The *peak expiratory flow rate,* measured by a hand-held peak flow meter in the office or at home, is a good screening test predictive of obstructive abnormalities on formal spirometry. A measurement of less than 350 L/min is an indication to proceed with formal measurement of lung volumes and flows. The *closing volume* and *maximal midexpiratory flow rate* are useful measures of early small-airways disease; they are most useful in presymptomatic stages of COPD, when other measures of air flow may be normal. Later on, the degree of obstruction in larger airways can be readily assessed by measuring expiratory flow rates with an office spirometer. The most helpful measurement is the *ratio of FEV$_1$ to VC*. Crude estimates of obstruction can be provided by the FEV$_1$ alone. Results are compared with predicted values. Patients with a 50% reduction in FEV$_1$ are often dyspneic and hypoxemic on exertion; by the time the FEV$_1$ falls to 25% of the predicted value, they may note shortness of breath at rest. Determination of the FEV$_1$ *before and after* inhalation of a *bronchodilator* (e.g., albuterol) can provide a quick estimate of the benefit a patient may derive from bronchodilator therapy. The failure to obtain an improvement in flow rate after a few inhalations of a bronchodilator does not rule out the possibility of benefit, but it suggests the likelihood is not great.

Sputum Examination. *Gram's stain* and *culture* of sputum can be helpful when acute pneumonitis is suspected, especially in patients exposed to multiple courses of antibiotics, but one must remember that prior colonization with *S. pneumoniae, H. influenzae,* or *Moraxella* may make interpretation difficult. Preliminary data suggest that examination of an *induced sputum specimen* for *eosinophils* may help predict responsiveness to glucocorticosteroids.

Chest Radiography is helpful, principally to rule out complications of COPD (e.g., pneumonia, pneumothorax) and other forms of chest disease that may present as dyspnea (e.g., heart failure, interstitial lung disease; see Chapter 40). Of the various forms of COPD, only severe emphysema is diagnosed radiologically; the criteria for radiologic diagnosis are the presence of two or more of the following findings: flattening of the diaphragm and blunting of the costophrenic angle on posterior–anterior view, irregularity of lung field lucency, enlargement of the retrosternal space, and flattening or concavity of the diaphragmatic contour on lateral view.

Measurement of Arterial Oxygen Saturation and Blood Gases is worth considering in patients with an FEV$_1$ less than 50% of the predicted value, a point at which hypoxemia is a possibility, especially in persons with chronic bronchitis. *Pulse oximetry* can be used as a screening test; it provides a measure of arterial oxygen saturation (Sao$_2$). If the Sao$_2$ is less than 92%, then measurement of the arterial blood gases is indicated to assess oxygenation and ventilation. Hypoxemia and hypercarbia are indications of severe chronic bronchitis. Blood gas measurement is particularly useful for documenting acute decompensation. In patients with severe chronic bronchitis (FEV$_1$ <35% predicted), baseline and serial studies of blood gasses should be performed, so that measurements of gases obtained at times of marked subjective worsening can be compared with baseline determinations.

Hematocrit and Hemoglobin Concentration provide a rough indication of the severity and chronicity of hypoxemia and the possible need for phlebotomy. Measurement should be undertaken in persons with a Pao$_2$ of less than 50 mm Hg.

Electrocardiogram should be studied for sinus tachycardia, multifocal atrial tachycardia, peaked P waves (P pulmonale), and signs of right ventricular hypertrophy (e.g., tall R wave in lead V$_1$ and deep S wave in lead V$_6$). The electrocardiographic abnormalities that appear in COPD generally reflect the severity of lung disease and the presence of cor pulmonale.

PRINCIPLES OF MANAGEMENT

The prime goals of treatment are improvement of functional status, prolongation of survival, and avoidance of complications. The principal components of management to achieve these goals are elimination of precipitants and risk factors, prevention and treatment of infection, control of bronchospasm, mobilization of secretions, and reversal of chronic hypoxia. The success of treatment is strongly influenced by the physician's interest and the participation of patient and family in the program.

Removal of Precipitants and Prophylaxis against Infection

Smoking Cessation. Regardless of the severity of their disease or the types of deficits present, all patients with COPD *must stop smoking* and should be urged to do so in emphatic terms. As noted earlier, disease progression is accelerated by continued smoking and can be greatly slowed by its cessation. Nonetheless, a surprisingly large number of patients report receiving little or no warning about smoking from their physicians; studies indicate that the physician's urging can be critical to achieving cessation of smoking, especially for those who are symptomatic (see Chapter 54).

A reduction in exposure to other pulmonary irritants should be advised. Readily avoidable pulmonary irritants include aerosol deodorants, hairsprays, paint sprays, and insecticides. An occupational history should be reviewed (see Chapter 39) for important workplace irritants. A change in job or residence (for patients living in areas of severe air pollution) may be necessary but should be urged only when the relationship between exposure and disease is strong; otherwise, the advice might cause more harm than good.

Immunization against Influenza is essential for all patients with COPD. Reductions in outpatient visits, hospitalization, and mortality in elderly persons with COPD have been demonstrated with administration of influenza vaccine. Trivalent influenza vaccine should be given each fall, at least 6 weeks before the onset of the influenza season. Serious reactions are rare unless the patient is allergic to egg protein. Mild fever and myalgias are sometimes noted. Because of ever-changing viral strains, vaccination must be performed yearly (see Chapter 6). Should an outbreak of influenza occur, protection for patients who were not immunized can still be provided (see Chapter 6).

Pneumococcal Vaccine is equally important for patients with COPD. Available preparations incorporate the capsular antigens of 23 species that are responsible for 90% of the cases of pneumococcal pneumonia occurring in the United States. Mild erythema and pain at the injection site are the only common adverse reactions to the vaccine, which is administered as a single IM injection of 0.5 mL. A repeated dose in 5 years may help maximize antibody titers in the elderly (see Chapter 6). The antibody response is not blunted nor is the frequency of adverse reactions increased when the pneumococcal and influenza vaccines are given simultaneously. The only disadvantage is difficulty in determining the cause of hypersensitivity should a reaction occur.

Question of Prophylactic Antibiotics. Evidence regarding the use of prophylactic antibiotics is conflicting. The original studies performed in England suggested a benefit from the prophylactic use of antibiotics during the winter months, with a reduction in the number of exacerbations and days lost from work. Studies in the United States and Canada show a more modest benefit from antibiotic use in general, limited mostly to patients with severe COPD who experience an acute exacerbation of symptoms accompanied by purulent sputum (see below). Long-term antibiotic prophylaxis is not recommended.

Bronchodilation

Bronchodilators remain a mainstay of treatment, providing symptomatic relief of dyspnea in about 50% of patients through reduction of airway resistance. The mechanisms of action are diverse, complex, and less well understood than previously thought. In addition to bronchodilation, positive effects on mucociliary clearance, diaphragmatic action, cardiac contractility, and inflammatory mediator release have been described.

It is not always possible to predict who will respond to bronchodilators on the basis of the response to a single exposure to an inhaled β-agonist. Many patients fail to show a response to a single exposure but demonstrate a significant improvement in symptoms or ventilatory function on repeated testing or after an empiric clinical trial. Those who show considerable improvement in FEV_1 are the best candidates, but all patients with COPD and evidence of a severe obstructive defect should be considered for a trial, even those with air flow obstruction that appears fixed and irreversible (i.e., <15% improvement in FEV_1 after inhalation of a bronchodilator). Although a limited empiric trial is probably reasonable for all patients, bronchodilator therapy should not be continued unless a subjective or objective benefit is clearly shown. No evidence suggests that bronchodilator therapy improves the prognosis.

β**-Agonists** constitute the *first line* of bronchodilator therapy. Their principal role is to provide prompt relief as necessary from acute dyspnea induced by bronchospasm. In patients with mild or moderate disease, β-agonist therapy often suffices. In patients with more severe disease, β-agonists are used in conjunction with longer-acting bronchodilators (see below). The *metered-dose inhaler* (MDI) formulations of the topically active, semiselective *inhaled β_2-agonists* (e.g., *albuterol*, *metaproterenol*) are preferred for their rapid onset of action, minimal systemic side effects (the drugs are relatively bronchoselective), and reasonable duration of action (2 to 4 hours). Oral formulations of these drugs are available but less desirable because they tend to produce a greater number of systemic side effects (especially cardiac effects) without any prolongation in duration of action. At high doses, the relative bronchoselectivity of the inhaled β_2-agonists is lost.

At present, only short-term, as-needed use of these agents is indicated. The advent of long-acting β_2-agonist formulations (e.g., inhaled *salmeterol*) may provide an opportunity for long-term bronchodilation with β_2-agonist therapy, but at present,

data are insufficient to recommend salmeterol over an inhaled muscarinic blocker (see below).

The use of inhaled β-agonists must be accompanied by thorough patient education. Their convenience and rapid onset of action sometimes lead to excessive use, so that development of *tachyphylaxis* is a risk. Conversely, dosing may be inadequate with improper MDI technique (see Chapter 48). The purported advantage of administering β-agonist therapy by means of an *intermittent positive pressure breathing* apparatus has been carefully studied in COPD and found to be lacking in the outpatient setting, even among such potentially relevant subgroups as patients with relatively severe disease, copious sputum, or emphysema. MDI administration is the delivery system of choice in the outpatient setting.

Anticholinergic Agents. Muscarinic blockers provide longer-acting bronchodilation ($\geq$6 hours), which makes them useful as a *second line* of bronchodilator therapy, complementing the shorter-acting β-agonists. An MDI formulation of *ipratropium* (a topically active muscarinic blocker that is poorly absorbed) is the principal means of delivering anticholinergic therapy. The rather slow onset of action of ipratropium, combined with a more sustained effect, makes it best suited for maintenance therapy in persons with persistent bronchospasm-induced dyspnea. It provides more effective bronchodilation than that afforded by round-the-clock use of β-agonists, although patients still benefit from "rescue" doses of a β-agonist when acute worsening occurs. Some patients use ipratropium at bedtime and a β-agonist as needed during the day. MDI application allows convenient delivery with a minimum of systemic side effects. The typical systemic anticholinergic side effects (e.g., blurred vision, urinary outflow obstruction, rapid heart rate) are rarely a problem when the drug is given in proper doses. Sputum volume can be reduced without increasing its viscosity.

Theophylline and its derivatives (e.g., aminophylline) have been relegated to *third-line* bronchodilator status in COPD, reserved for patients in whom β-agonists and ipratropium do not suffice. Although these methylxanthines are inexpensive and symptomatically helpful, they have demonstrated an inconsistent ability to improve objective measures of air flow, a considerable number of cardiovascular side effects, and a narrow therapeutic range. Nonetheless, some patients report subjective benefit, perhaps related to effects other than bronchodilation (e.g., improved diaphragmatic and myocardial function, inhibition of inflammatory mediators). Improvements in respiratory function and dyspnea have been demonstrated in patients with severe COPD, although much of the benefit appears related to enhanced respiratory muscle performance. Patients who experience a worsening of airway hyperreactivity at night despite ipratropium may benefit from the addition of a long-acting, controlled-release theophylline formulation before bed.

The methylxanthines are available for outpatient use in oral and rectal formulations, but only the oral route should be used because rectal administration is associated with erratic absorption and a potential for dangerous sudden rises in serum concentrations. Absorption of an oral dose approaches 90%. Sustained-release preparations can provide therapeutic serum levels (8 to 12 μg/mL) for 12 to 24 hours. The wide variability in levels for a given dose is a consequence of individual differences in clearance, which is predominantly hepatic. Decreased clearance and increased serum levels occur with heart failure, hepatocellular disease, and drugs that inhibit the hepatic cytochrome oxidase system (e.g., cimetidine, macrolide antibiotics); smoking and intake of barbiturates increase clearance.

Serious side effects include *supraventricular* and *ventricular dysrhythmias* and *seizures*. Such adverse effects usually occur only when serum levels rise precipitously, but they can also occur while serum levels are in the "normal" range if concurrent heart failure or hypoxemia develops.

Choice of Agent and Utility of Combination Therapy. The decision to employ bronchodilators and the choice of agent are somewhat empiric; trial and error are usually necessary to arrive at an optimal program. A stepwise program has been recommended by some authorities, in which as-needed use of an inhaled β-agonist is the first line of treatment; the addition of inhaled ipratropium is the second line of bronchodilator therapy, used to maintain control in persons with relatively severe disease. Oral sustained-release theophylline is the third-line of therapy, usually reserved for persons who continue to experience difficulty at night despite administration of first- and second-line therapies. The benefit of reduced-dose combination therapy over full-dose single-agent therapy is not established, but many patients appear to benefit from combination programs.

Corticosteroids

With the growing appreciation for the role of inflammation in COPD has come a renewed interest in glucocorticosteroid therapy. Although steroids have become the mainstay of asthma therapy (see Chapter 48), their usefulness in COPD remains much less well established. In theory, steroid-induced antiinflammatory effects (e.g., suppression of cytokines, inhibition of eosinophils, stabilization of mast cells) have the potential to reduce the acute mucosal edema and bronchoconstriction of COPD flares and the subsequent airway remodeling and progressive loss of lung function of chronic active disease. In reality, well-designed prospective clinical trials have revealed marginal benefit at most. For example, in persons with an acute COPD flare requiring hospitalization, 2 weeks of systemic steroids was found to provide only a modest improvement in rate of treatment failures, length of stay, and pulmonary function. Eight weeks of therapy was no more efficacious than a 2-week course; at 6 months, no improvement in outcomes was demonstrated, and hyperglycemia severe enough to require treatment developed in many patients. In a 3-year trial of smokers with mild, stable COPD, the long-term use of high doses of inhaled steroids failed to reduce progressive loss of lung function. Metaanalytic study finds a modest (10%) chance of a reasonable (20%) improvement in FEV_1 among patients with stable, chronic COPD.

Some speculate that these spotty results and the lesser benefit of steroids in stable COPD than in asthma or COPD flares may be related to the nature of the underlying inflammatory reaction (predominantly neutrophilic in stable COPD and more eosinophilic in acute COPD flares and asthma). That only a small fraction of patients with stable COPD seem to benefit from steroids may reflect the heterogeneity of the COPD population, perhaps made up in part by asthmatic patients who have

progressed to COPD yet remain at least partially steroid-responsive.

The current recommended role for glucocorticosteroids is as a *fourth line* of treatment, reserved for those who are not adequately controlled by the various forms of bronchodilator therapy. An *empiric 2-week trial* of full-dose *systemic steroids* (e.g., 40 mg of prednisone per day) is suggested, with measurement of FEV_1 to document objective improvement (i.e., >20%). Those who demonstrate objective benefit are continued on prednisone, which is tapered to the lowest effective dose, and then switched if possible to a program of *alternate-day prednisone* or an *inhaled nonabsorbable glucocorticosteroid* preparation (see Chapter 48) to limit adverse effects of steroids (see Chapter 105). At 8 weeks, the patient should be retested to confirm that objective benefit continues; otherwise, steroids should be discontinued. For patients with an acute flare necessitating hospitalization, a short course of systemic steroids is worth considering.

Improved means of rapidly identifying patients with steroid-responsive COPD are being sought; use of an induced sputum for the detection of increased numbers of eosinophils is under study.

Oxygen Therapy

Indications. Long-term *continuous oxygen therapy* prolongs survival and reduces the risk for cor pulmonale when administered to patients with COPD who are chronically hypoxemic (Po_2 <55 mm Hg). The more continuous the therapy, the better the effect; round-the-clock oxygen therapy is superior to nocturnal oxygen administration. Maximum benefit requires continuous administration for at least *18 h/d*. Administration for less than 12 h/d is unlikely to be of any help. Although long-term *discontinuous oxygen therapy* at night or during activity is thought to be worthwhile for nonhypoxemic patients with COPD who manifest a drop in PaO_2 during sleep or low-level exertion, such therapy is not of proven benefit with regard to long-term survival or risk for pulmonary hypertension. Nonetheless, both forms of long-term oxygen therapy are reimbursable. (Current clinical criteria are listed in Table 47.2.) Most COPD patients with profound nocturnal hypoxemia also are hypoxic during the day and require continuous administration of oxygen. Concerns about the potential of continuous oxygen therapy to worsen carbon dioxide retention, especially during sleep, when carbon dioxide retention is at its worst, have not been borne out. Administration with nasal prongs usually suffices, and enough oxygen should be delivered to increase the resting Po_2 to 65 mm Hg and the exercise Sao_2 to more than

Table 47.2. Accepted Indications for Reimbursable Long-term Oxygen Therapy

Continuous long-term supplemental oxygen therapy
- Resting Po_2 < 55 mm Hg or
- Resting Sao_2 < 88% or
- Resting Po_2 of 56 to 59 mm Hg with evidence of concurrent right-sided heart failure or secondary polycythemia (hematocrit > 55%)

Noncontinuous long-term supplemental oxygen therapy (no resting hypoxemia)
- Po_2 < 55 mm Hg or Sao_2 < 88% with low-level exertion
- Po_2 < 55 mm Hg or Sao_2 < 88% during sleep, especially with daytime sleepiness, cardiac arrhythmia, or cor pulmonale

90%. Some recommend adding an additional 1 L of flow per minute during sleep and exertion.

The need for *short-term supplemental oxygen* must be considered when *air travel* is planned. Prediction of the need for oxygen and tolerance of the cabin environment can be accomplished by preflight measurement of the arterial Po_2 and FEV_1. A formula has been derived based on these parameters to predict arterial oxygen levels at cruising altitude. Alternatively, one can have the patient inhale a hypoxic gas mixture (17.2% oxygen) that simulates the cabin environment of a jet aircraft at cruising altitude. Although no guidelines have been established for when to administer oxygen supplementation, a drop in Po_2 to below 50 mm Hg or the development of symptoms is a reasonable indication for oxygen supplementation during flights longer than 2 hours. Airlines will provide an oxygen supply if notified at least 48 hours in advance of travel; their units provide flows of 2 to 4 L of 25% or 30% oxygen per minute. Patients are usually not allowed to bring their own oxygen tanks into the cabin of domestic airlines.

Brief administration of oxygen has been touted to *improve exercise tolerance* in COPD patients. In unblinded studies, exercise tolerance improves, but in blinded, placebo-controlled study, little benefit has been demonstrated. Most hypoxemic COPD patients are chronically hypoxic and require continuous oxygen supplementation; brief administration is of no value to them. The small subset of patients who are hypoxemic and markedly dyspneic only with exercise might be candidates for a trial of short-term oxygen supplementation. A convenient means of identifying such patients is to measure their diffusing capacity during routine pulmonary function testing, rather than trying to measure arterial blood gases just after or during exercise. A diffusing capacity above 55% has been shown to be 100% specific in excluding arterial hypoxemia during exercise; sensitivity is 68%. If oxygen is to be tried, it should be limited to those who have a reduced diffusing capacity and demonstrate consistently better performance on oxygen than on air when both are administered in single-blind fashion. Pulse oximetry during exercise is another means of identifying patients who might benefit from oxygen supplementation.

Initiating and Monitoring Therapy. Arterial blood gas measurement is the preferred determination for initiating oxygen therapy and adjusting it, particularly in patients who are at risk for retention of carbon dioxide with application of oxygen. Pulse oximetry is a convenient although slightly less precise substitute for blood gas measurement; it is most useful when therapy is being adjusted, especially if impaired ventilation is not a concern and measurement of the Pco_2 is not necessary.

Control of Secretions

Secretions. Patients bothered by heavy, tenacious sputum may obtain benefit by maintaining good *fluid intake*, ensuring adequate *humidification* of the indoor environment (particularly in centrally heated homes), and practicing *postural drainage* when clearance of secretions is difficult and cough is incapacitating. The simplest method of postural drainage is to have the patient lean over the side of the bed, rest the elbows on a pillow placed on the floor, and cough as a family member or visiting nurse gently pounds on the chest. For hydration, ultrasonic nebulizers are no better than the simple maintenance of good systemic hydration, although the moisture they deliver does reach deep into the tracheobronchial tree. Occasionally, bronchospasm can be triggered by a nebulizer, and its reservoir can become contaminated and serve as a source of airway infection. Nebulized detergents are of no proven use, but *mucolytic agents* such as acetylcysteine are capable of thinning secretions; they are usually reserved for patients on respirators and not commonly used in outpatient practice. Oral *expectorants* are very popular with some bronchitic patients, who report improved ability to raise sputum; however, they are without proven clinical efficacy. These preparations need not be denied to the patient who feels that they are of benefit, but they should not be the mainstay of the therapeutic program. Glyceryl guaiacolate and potassium iodide are the most frequently prescribed expectorants; many are available without a prescription.

Exercise Training and Rehabilitation

The main elements of a pulmonary rehabilitation program are exercise training, breathing retraining, chest physiotherapy, psychosocial support, and patient education. Often, the program is carried out as an intensive intervention at a rehabilitation center for patients with advanced disease who are functionally limited; however, some elements can be initiated at home in earlier phases of the illness (e.g., exercise). The evidence of benefit is strongest for exercise training and psychosocial interventions. The benefit derived from a program of comprehensive pulmonary rehabilitation appears to decline with time after completion of the program, especially after a year; no improvement in survival has been demonstrated.

Exercise Training. Among the simplest and most effective measures for improving exercise tolerance is an *exercise training program*. *Walking* has proved to be the best form of exercise for increasing duration and intensity of activity in COPD patients. Exercises that involve the arms and upper body appear to compromise respiratory mechanics. Three or four sessions per day of walking are recommended, ranging from 5 to 15 minutes each. The pace and duration of activity are matched to the patient's capabilities; most begin the program walking at a half-maximal pace and build gradually through a period of several weeks. At the end of the training period, heart and respiratory rates for a given level of activity are decreased; oxygen consumption also falls. Parameters of ventilatory function are not significantly changed, but increases of 25% are attained in maximum duration and intensity of exercise. Many patients enjoy marked improvement in ability to carry out their daily activities. Although exercise training is often not implemented until patients become severely impaired, there is no reason why a walking program cannot be instituted earlier for most COPD patients.

Breathing Exercises may have some beneficial effect, especially psychologically, in those who readily panic and hyperventilate when dyspneic or show evidence of respiratory fatigue. Teaching the anxious patient to take slow, deep, relaxed breaths and exhale against pursed lips can lessen the work of moving air, provide a sense of control over breathing, and encourage a more relaxed respiratory pattern. Inspiratory muscle training is popular in some centers, with encouraging reports of improvement in exercise performance among patients who experience respiratory muscle fatigue. However, the importance of diaphragmatic dysfunction and the need for exercises continue to be debated.

Psychosocial Support in a comprehensive rehabilitation program entails group and individual meetings with a psychiatrist or other mental health professional in addition to sessions that include families or spouses to help them cope with the depression, anxiety, fear, and family dysfunction that COPD brings upon a household. Behavioral approaches are sometimes taught to patients, such as the breathing relaxation techniques noted above.

Chest Physiotherapy

See above.

Patient Education

See below.

Antibiotics for Acute Exacerbations

The relationship between an acute exacerbation of COPD and infection remains a subject of debate, as does the benefit of antibiotics for COPD flares. Metaanalysis of randomized trials of antibiotics for COPD flares find a positive but modest benefit that is most likely to be of clinical significance in persons with severe disease, especially those who require hospitalization. Because *pneumococci* and *H. influenzae* are the predominant organisms colonizing patients with COPD (*Moraxella* may also be a colonizer), *amoxicillin* or *trimethoprim/ sulfamethoxazole* is a reasonable first choice of antibiotic when evidence of infection (fever, increased sputum production, increased sputum purulence) is present. For patients allergic to penicillin and sulfa drugs, *doxycycline* is a reasonable alternative, although not as effective against pneumococci. More broad-spectrum, penicillinase-resistant antibiotic coverage is worth considering in persons with severe disease who have four or more exacerbations a year or have concurrent heart failure or diabetes. Such patients are at increased risk for infection with gram-negative and resistant organisms. Under such circumstances, amoxicillin/clavulanate, a second- or third-generation cephalosporin, a macrolide, or a fluoroquinolone should be considered. Culturing the sputum can help rationalize antibiotic choice.

Management of Cor Pulmonale

Patients with chronic cor pulmonale can often be made more comfortable by careful attention to their volume status, degree of hypoxemia, and hematocrit. Reduction of excess intravascular volume can reduce edema; *diuretic therapy* (see Chapter 32) is an effective means of volume control. As noted earlier, continuous *low-flow oxygen therapy* is indicated in patients with cor pulmonale who are chronically hypoxic. Survival is improved, although the precise mechanism of improvement is unknown; pulmonary vascular resistance and secondary polycythemia are only modestly decreased. Whether oxygen therapy prevents the development or worsening of cor pulmonale is unsettled.

Focus is shifting to examination of cardiac output as a determinant of survival in patients with cor pulmonale. Augmented cardiac output is a normal response to a fall in Po_2. Many patients with cor pulmonale maintain a high cardiac index. It is suspected that a fall in cardiac output may be a determinant of poor prognosis. If this proves to be the case, then increased efforts at improving cardiac output may be indicated.

Previous attempts at inotropic therapy have produced equivocal results. *Digoxin* seems to help some patients, but not uniformly or predictably. The incidence of digitalis toxicity, which is aggravated by hypoxemia, is high; the clinical response is often equivocal. The drug is worth a try in patients with reduced cardiac output, especially if concurrent left ventricular dysfunction is present (see Chapter 32), but it should be continued only in those who show an objective in addition to a subjective response to therapy. Patients who do appear to improve with digitalis should be given a minimum maintenance dose and should be monitored closely for manifestations of digitalis toxicity (see Chapter 32).

Vasodilators (calcium channel blockers and angiotensin-converting enzyme inhibitors) have proved disappointing, with little improvement in cardiac output or pulmonary artery resistance noted during sustained use in most patients. In some instances, systemic hypotension and even hypoxemia may result.

Phlebotomy is indicated only for urgent treatment when secondary erythrocytosis is severe enough to cause a marked reduction in blood viscosity, significant impairment of oxygen delivery, and exacerbation of cor pulmonale. The risk for such decompensation is greatest when the hematocrit rises above 55%.

Augmentation Therapy for α_1-Antitrypsin Deficiency

The rare patient with emphysema who has significant antitrypsin deficiency (<80 mg/dL) is a possible candidate for augmentation therapy (weekly or monthly infusions of α_1-antitrypsin). Only symptomatic patients with clinical evidence of emphysema and sufficiently low antitrypsin levels are considered appropriate for augmentation therapy because emphysema does not develop in all patients with low concentrations. A history of smoking rules out candidacy.

Surgical Interventions

Bullectomy is worth considering in the rare COPD patient with a few giant bullae unilaterally taking up more than a third of a hemithorax. Additional clinical criteria include being relatively free of severe emphysema and bullae in the contralateral lung, having chest computed tomographic evidence of bullae compressing lung parenchyma, and having an FEV_1 below 50% of the predicted value.

Lung Volume Reduction. This investigational surgical intervention for patients with late-stage nonbullous emphysema entails removing the most severely involved sections of emphysematous lung to improve pulmonary mechanics and gas exchange. Although initial reports are enthusiastic and encouraging, mortality at 1 year can be high (up to 25%). The place of such surgery in the management of emphysema remains to be determined.

Lung Transplant. Although transplant of a single lung has a reasonable 3-year survival rate (up to 70%), most COPD patients are not candidates because of advanced age, continued smoking, or concurrent cardiovascular disease, not to mention the fact that available lungs are in very short supply.

Monitoring Therapy

Functional status and *symptoms* remain among the most important measures of efficacy. Semiquantitative reports from the patient regarding such parameters as number of stairs climbed or distance walked can be useful. Subjective assessment of bronchospasm has been found to correlate surprisingly well with FEV_1 measurement in asthmatic patients, and this probably is valid for COPD patients also. Important aspects of the physical examination to be monitored include ratio of inspiration to expiration, respiratory rate, heart rate, jugular venous pressure, right ventricular impulse, and condition of extremities (edema). In a patient with known carbon dioxide retention, the presence of asterixis is an indication of worsening ventilatory status, further carbon dioxide retention, and encephalopathy. Serial determination of Sao_2, *arterial blood gases*, FEV_1, and *hematocrit* can help in objectively following the course of disease and detecting acute deterioration.

PATIENT EDUCATION

The first priority is to stress the importance of *cessation of smoking*; this should be followed by the design of a specific program (see Chapter 54). Patients should be encouraged to maintain as much activity as possible and be provided with an exercise program if they can be motivated to comply. Patient, family, and physician should be involved in setting reasonable and realistic activity goals. Advice regarding adequate hydration and pulmonary toilet is basic to the care of patients with chronic bronchitis. Patients likely to panic and hyperventilate when they become dyspneic often benefit from being taught how to institute slow, relaxed, deep breathing in such circumstances.

Careful instructions regarding the indications and adverse effects of therapy can help the patient to carry out the prescribed program properly. Complex regimens should be written down and reviewed with both patient and family. It is essential to warn patients with carbon dioxide retention against unauthorized use of tranquilizers and sedatives because of the risk for further suppression of their respiratory drive. Patients for whom inhalers have been prescribed should be thoroughly instructed in their proper use (see Chapter 48); many treatment failures are a consequence of poor technique. Such patients also must be warned that excessive use of β_2-agonists can lead to tachyphylaxis and cardiac side effects; persistent overdoses of inhaled steroids (more than 20 puffs per day) can cause adrenal suppression.

Part of the patient education process should aim to restore a modicum of self-confidence and self-reliance. Instruction in self-adjustment of the medical regimen, in monitoring and reporting functional status, and in implementation of a daily exercise program can have very positive effects on morale. The synergistic interaction of an involved patient and an interested and concerned physician has the potential to enhance the quality, if not the duration, of life for COPD patients.

INDICATIONS FOR ADMISSION AND REFERRAL

The patient with acute respiratory decompensation, especially if accompanied by signs of encephalopathy (e.g., asterixis, lethargy), should be urgently admitted to the hospital; no oxygen should be administered on the way to the hospital for fear of further suppressing the respiratory drive. Those with an acute exacerbation of cough, dyspnea, wheezing, and sputum production that is not immediately responsive to bronchodilator therapy might also require inpatient management and would possibly benefit from a pulmonary consultation. Pulmonary referral is also indicated when the patient remains chronically incapacitated despite a comprehensive program of standard medical therapy. Surgical consultation is not recommended without the prior recommendation of a pulmonary specialist.

THERAPEUTIC RECOMMENDATIONS

Basic Measures for All Patients

- Review the entire treatment program thoroughly with the patient and family; encourage patient participation in setting goals and monitoring functional status.
- Insist on complete *cessation of smoking* and design a comprehensive smoking cessation program (see Chapter 54).
- Advise the patient to reduce exposure to known environmental irritants and allergens (see Chapters 39, 48 and 222).
- Design, with patient participation, an *exercise program*; walking is probably best, although any aerobic exercise will suffice. Begin with an easily achieved level of activity (e.g., half-maximal pace) and increase slowly in small increments. Frequency is three to four times daily, with duration ranging from 5 to 15 minutes.
- Administer trivalent *influenza vaccine* (0.5 mL IM) in the fall of each year, at least 6 weeks before the usual winter onset of the flu season, to all patients with COPD (except those having a known allergy to eggs). Consider administering antiviral therapy to unvaccinated COPD patients during an influenza epidemic (see Chapter 6).
- Administer *pneumococcal vaccine* to all COPD patients. The dose is 0.5 mL IM, and it can be given at the same time as the influenza vaccine. Repeated administration after 5 years may needed in elderly persons (see Chapter 6).
- Advise patients bothered by heavy sputum production to keep well hydrated and to humidify the indoor environment (particularly those living in centrally heated homes). Nebulized detergents and oral expectorants are of no proven benefit. Teach postural drainage techniques to patients bothered by difficulty in raising sputum.
- Perform pulmonary function testing on all patients with a peak flow rate below 350 L/min, obvious bronchospasm, or dyspnea on exertion. Measure FEV_1 before and after inhalation of a rapidly acting bronchodilator (e.g., albuterol) to determine candidacy for bronchodilator therapy.

Stable Disease: Bronchodilator and Antiinflammatory Therapies

- Begin bronchodilator therapy in those who manifest an increase in FEV_1 of more than 200 mL/s or more than 12% in response to bronchodilator inhalation. Also consider an *empiric trial of a bronchodilator* for those who are symptomatically dyspneic or show a substantial reduction in expiratory flow rate (e.g., FEV_1 <1.5 to 2 L/s or FEV_1/FVC <0.50), even if they do not demonstrate a response to a single dose of albuterol (single-dose response does not necessarily predict response to continuous bronchodilator therapy).

- For patients with mild, intermittent symptoms, begin with an MDI formulation of a rapidly acting β_2-agonist (e.g., 1 to 2 puffs of *albuterol* every 4 to 6 hours as needed). Carefully instruct the patient in proper MDI use (see Chapter 48) and warn that the dose is not to exceed 12 puffs in 24 hours. Exert caution in prescribing for patients with heart disease because these agents are relatively cardioselective at low to moderate doses.

- For patients who require or are not adequately controlled by round-the-clock β-agonist therapy, begin an MDI formulation of a topically active, nonabsorbed *anticholinergic* (e.g., 2 to 3 puffs of *ipratropium* four times daily) and supplement as needed with albuterol (1 to 4 puffs as needed for an acute flare or 2 puffs four times daily). Instruct patients to avoid getting ipratropium spray in their eyes, especially if they have narrow-angle glaucoma. The sequencing and timing of combination inhaler therapy do not seem to matter.

- Judge response to bronchodilator therapy on the basis of change in exercise tolerance and expiratory flow rates after about 4 weeks of therapy. Response to a single dose of inhaled bronchodilator does not predict response to continuous treatment. If no response can be demonstrated, then halt inhaled bronchodilator therapy.

- If some bronchodilator response is noted but control of symptoms remains inadequate, especially at nighttime, then consider adding a sustained-release oral *theophylline* preparation before bed (e.g., 200 to 400 mg of generic sustained-release theophylline daily at bedtime). Monitor symptoms closely for a response after about 4 weeks of therapy before deciding to continue therapy longer. Check serum theophylline level and adjust dose to achieve a therapeutic range of 8 to 12 μg/mL. Do not prescribe for patients with cardiac arrhythmias and prescribe with caution for persons with underlying heart disease. Do not use anal suppository preparations.

- Consider initiation of an empiric trial of *glucocorticosteroids* in persons who respond inadequately to bronchodilator therapy and remain symptomatic.

- For patients with stable COPD who fail to achieve adequate control of symptoms with bronchodilators, begin a 2-week trial of oral *prednisone* (40 mg/d) and check FEV_1 for objective improvement (>20%). If a response is noted, try switching to a topically active *inhaled corticosteroid* MDI formulation (e.g., 2 puffs of *beclomethasone* four times daily or 4 puffs twice daily), an alternate-day prednisone program, or the lowest effective dose of daily prednisone.

- After 6 to 8 weeks, evaluate for sustained response; if no symptomatic or objective improvement is noted, then stop inhaled steroid therapy.

Stable Late-stage Disease

- For patients with advanced disease who are functionally limited, consider referral for a comprehensive program of *pulmonary rehabilitation* that includes exercise training, breathing retraining, chest physiotherapy, psychosocial support, and patient education. Emphasis should be on those elements that have proved most beneficial (i.e., exercise training and psychosocial support).

- Teach slow, relaxed, deep breathing to patients likely to hyperventilate when dyspneic; consider targeted inspiratory muscle training in patients with severe COPD; a respiratory therapist may be of help in the teaching effort.

- Be sure the program includes detailed patient and family education to help sustain the benefit of a rehabilitation program once it is completed.

- Begin long-term *continuous oxygen therapy* in patients who are chronically hypoxemic [resting Po_2 <55 mm Hg, or 56 to 59 mm Hg if evidence of concurrent right-sided heart failure or secondary polycythemia (hematocrit >55%) is present].

- Provide continuous administration for at least *18 h/d*. Administration for less time is unlikely to improve long-term outcome and prognosis.

- Consider supplemental *noncontinuous oxygen therapy* during exertion to improve exercise capacity in nonhypoxemic patients only if they exhibit desaturation on pulse oximetry during exercise or a reduced diffusing capacity on routine pulmonary function testing; the patient should demonstrate consistently better performance on oxygen than on air when both are administered in single-blind fashion.

- For patients with cor pulmonale, begin a diuretic program (e.g., 20 to 40 mg of *furosemide* daily) when peripheral edema begins to develop; increase program as needed to control fluid accumulation caused by systemic venous hypertension. Phlebotomize the patient with secondary erythrocytosis (hematocrit >55%) when acute decompensation (worsening of right-sided heart failure or hypoxemia) is present.

- Consider a short-term trial of *cardiac glycoside* therapy (e.g., 0.25 mg of *digoxin* daily) in patients with severe right-sided heart failure; treat for 2 weeks and check for objective signs of improvement (e.g., decreased edema, lower jugular venous pressure, reduced heart size). Use with care in the setting of hypoxemia, and check serum levels regularly. Monitor closely for evidence of digitalis toxicity (see Chapter 32).

- Refer for consideration of *surgical therapies* only severely emphysematous patients with incapacitating disease refractory to a comprehensive program of maximal medical therapy who could tolerate a major thoracic surgical procedure and who have ceased smoking.

Acute Exacerbation

- Initiate intensive MDI bronchodilator therapy with a rapidly acting β-agonist (e.g., 6 to 8 puffs of *albuterol* immediately, then repeated every 30 to 60 minutes). If response is inadequate (e.g., patient still manifests marked dyspnea and severe wheezing) or the drug is poorly tolerated (e.g., palpitations, chest pain), then hospitalize; if response is adequate, add 4 to 8 puffs of *ipratropium* every 6 hours, reduce albuterol to 2 puffs four times daily, and follow closely.

- Consider initiating empiric *antibiotic* therapy, but only for patients with a new onset or marked increase of grossly purulent sputum in conjunction with other signs of infection (e.g., fever, elevated white cell count). Prescribe *amoxicillin* (500 mg three times daily) or *trimethoprim/sulfamethoxazole* (one double-strength tablet twice daily); *doxycycline* (100 mg twice daily) is a reasonable alternative for penicillin-allergic patients.

- Use of a broad-spectrum, penicillinase-resistant antibiotic (e.g., amoxicillin/clavulanate, a later-generation cephalosporin, a second-generation macrolide, or a fluoroquinolone) should be considered only for patients with severe COPD who manifest signs of acute infection plus risk factors for a resistant organism (i.e., more than four exacerbations a year, concurrent heart failure, diabetes). Culturing the sputum in such patients may help rationalize antibiotic choice.
- Consider a 2-week course of *systemic corticosteroids* (e.g., oral *prednisone* starting at 40 mg/d) for those with a severe exacerbation. Taper or if possible switch to alternate-day or high-dose inhaled therapy as soon as possible (see Chapters 48 and 105).

Indications for Consultation

- Obtain pulmonary consultation when the patient remains incapacitated despite a comprehensive, fully implemented program of medical therapy. Surgical consultation is not recommended without the prior recommendation of a pulmonary specialist.
- Refer patients with known α_1-antitrypsin deficiency for consideration of augmentation therapy with α_1-antitrypsin only if they do not smoke, show signs of emphysema, are symptomatic, and have an antitrypsin level below 80 mg/dL.

A.H.G.

ANNOTATED BIBLIOGRAPHY

American Thoracic Society. Standards for the diagnosis and care of patients with chronic obstructive pulmonary disease (COPD) and asthma. Am Rev Respir Dis 1995;152:S77. (*Consensus expert guidelines; second update.*)

American Thoracic Society. Lung volume-reduction surgery. Am J Respir Dis Crit Care Med 1996;154:1151. (*A position paper summarizing the current role of surgery in the care of patients with COPD; emphasizes that data are limited.*)

Anthonisen NR, Connet JE, Kiley JP, et al. Effects of smoking intervention and the use of an inhaled anticholinergic bronchodilator on the rate of decline in FEV₁. JAMA 1994;272:1497. (*Only smoking cessation reduced the rate of decline, and it made a major difference in outcome.*)

Anthonisen NR. Long-term oxygen therapy. Ann Intern Med 1983;99:519. (*Fine review of the recent evidence suggesting improvement in survival with long-term oxygen treatment; 60 references.*)

Anthonisen NR, Wright EC, Intermittent Positive Pressure Breathing Trial Group. Bronchodilator response in chronic obstructive pulmonary disease. Am Rev Respir Dis 1986;133:814. (*Patients with COPD do manifest some bronchodilator responsiveness.*)

Aubier M, DeTroyer A, Sampson M, et al. Aminophylline improves diaphragmatic contractility. N Engl J Med 1981;305:249. (*A finding that may justify a trial of aminophylline despite documented poor bronchodilator effect.*)

Badgett RG, Tanaka DJ, Hunt DK, et al. The clinical evaluation for diagnosing obstructive airway disease in high-risk patients. Chest 1994;106:1427. (*Excellent study showing how useful the history, physical examination, and simple office measures can be.*)

Balter MS, Hyland RH, Low DE, et al. Recommendations on the management of chronic bronchitis: a practical guide for Canadian physicians. Can Med Assoc J 1994;151:1. (*Evidence-based review with especially good discussion of antibiotic use in acute flares.*)

Boushey HA. Glucocorticoid therapy for chronic obstructive pulmonary disease. N Engl J Med 1999;340:1990. (*A very helpful pathophysiologic discussion correlating the observed modest effects of steroids with known and proposed disease mechanisms in COPD.*)

Burrows B, Blood JW, Traver GA, et al. The course and prognosis of different forms of chronic airways obstruction in a sample from the general population. N Engl J Med 1987;317:1309. (*Patients with emphysema had a 10-year mortality of 60%; those with asthmatic bronchitis had a lesser mortality.*)

Callahan CM, Dittus RS, Katz BP. Oral corticosteroid therapy for patients with stable chronic obstructive pulmonary disease. Ann Intern Med 1991;114:216. (*A metaanalysis showing a modest benefit.*)

Celli B, Rassulo J, Make BJ. Dyssynchronous breathing during arm but not leg exercise in patients with chronic airflow obstruction. N Engl J Med 1986;314:1485. (*Leg exercise did not interfere with lung mechanics, but arm exercise did.*)

Dillard TA, Berg BW, Rajagopal KR, et al. Hypoxemia during air travel in patients with chronic obstructive pulmonary disease. Ann Intern Med 1989;111:362. (*Arterial P_{O_2} declined to significantly low levels; oxygen supplementation is urged for patients with severe COPD during air travel.*)

Easton PA, Jadue C, Dhingra S, et al. A comparison of the bronchodilating effects of a beta-2 adrenergic agent (albuterol) and an anticholinergic agent (ipratropium bromide), given by aerosol alone or in sequence. N Engl J Med 1986;315:735. (*Equal efficacy demonstrated; no benefit when a second agent was added to maximum doses of the first.*)

Goldstein RS, Vivekanand R, Bowes G, et al. Effect of supplemental nocturnal oxygen on gas exchange in patients with severe obstructive lung disease. New Engl J Med 1984;310:425. (*Nocturnal oxygen therapy did not induce clinically worrisome increases in P_{CO_2}.*)

Gross NJ. Ipratropium bromide. N Engl J Med 1988;319:486. (*Superb review of inhaled anticholinergic therapy; 110 references.*)

Harver A, Mahler DA, Daubenspeck JA. Targeted inspiratory muscle training improves respiratory muscle function and reduces dyspnea in patients with chronic obstructive pulmonary disease. Ann Intern Med 1989;111:117. (*One of the most careful studies of respiratory muscle training in the treatment of COPD.*)

Himelman RB, Struve SN, Brown JK, et al. Improved recognition of cor pulmonale in patients with severe chronic obstructive pulmonary disease. Am J Med 1988;84:891. (*Echocardiogram proved the most sensitive diagnostic method and was superior to clinical findings and chest radiography.*)

Intermittent Positive Pressure Breathing Trial Group. Intermittent positive pressure breathing therapy of COPD: a clinical trial. Ann Intern Med 1983;99:612. (*Multicenter controlled trial of 985 patients showing that intermittent positive pressure breathing was no better than nebulizer for administration of bronchodilator therapy.*)

Kanner RE, Renzetti AD, Stanish WM, et al. Predictors of survival in subjects with chronic airflow limitation. Am J Med 1983;74:249. (*A 12-year prospective study identifying important determinants of prognosis and confirming findings of earlier studies.*)

Lacasse Y, Guyatt GH, Goldstein RS. The components of a respiratory rehabilitation program: a systematic review. Chest 1997;111:1077. (*The evidence is best for benefit from exercise training and psychosocial support.*)

Lange P, Parner J, Vestbo J, et al. A 15-year follow-up study of ventilatory function in adults with asthma. N Engl J Med 1998;339:1194. (*Marked decline noted in asthmatic patients who continue to smoke, greater than that noted for smokers or other asthmatic patients, which suggests that asthma may predispose to COPD.*)

Matthay RA, Niederman MS, Wiedemann HP. Cardiovascular pulmonary interaction in chronic obstructive pulmonary disease with special reference to pathogenesis and management of cor pulmonale. Med Clin North Am 1990;74:571. (*Detailed review of treatment modalities for cor pulmonale, including vasodilators, oxygen, and phlebotomy.*)

Murciano D, Auclair H-M, Pariente R. A randomized, controlled trial of theophylline in patients with severe chronic obstructive pulmonary disease. N Engl J Med 1989;320:1521. (*Documents improvements in respiratory function and symptoms; attributes them to enhanced respiratory muscle performance.*)

Nichol KL, Baken L, Nelson A. Relation between influenza vaccination and outpatients visits, hospitalizations, and mortality in elderly persons with chronic lung disease. Ann Intern Med 1999;130:397. (*Important evidence for efficacy of influenza vaccination.*)

Niewoehner DE, Erbland ML, Deupree RH, et al. Effect of systemic glucocorticosteroids on exacerbations of chronic obstructive pulmonary disease. N Engl J Med 1999;340:1941. (*Major Veterans Administration study; only modest benefit noted in this multicenter, randomized, placebo-controlled trial.*)

Owens GR, Rogers RM, Pennock BE, et al. The diffusing capacity as a predictor of arterial oxygen desaturation during exercise in patients with COPD. N Engl J Med 1984;310:1218. (*Diffusing capacity measured during routine pulmonary function testing at rest correlated well with degree of hypoxemia during exercise.*)

Paggiaro PL, Dahle RM, Bakran I, et al. Multicentre, randomized, placebo-controlled trial of inhaled fluticasone propionate in patients with chronic obstructive pulmonary disease. Lancet 1998; 351:773. (*Evidence for a modest degree of functional benefit noted.*)

Pauwels RA, Lofdahl C-G, Laitinen LA, et al. Long-term treatment with inhaled budesonide in persons with mild chronic obstructive pulmonary disease who continue smoking. N Engl J Med 1999;340:1948. (*Major European trial failing to find any benefit from inhaled steroid therapy in slowing disease progression.*)

Petty TL. Circadian variations in chronic asthma and chronic obstructive pulmonary disease. Am J Med 1988;85[Suppl 1B]:21. (*Review of the phenomenon and its treatment; 21 references.*)

Pratt PC. Role of conventional chest radiography in diagnosis and exclusion of emphysema. Am J Med 1987;82:998. (*Detailed discussion of use of the chest film in making and excluding the diagnosis of emphysema; very high predictive value when validated criteria are used.*)

Saint S, Bent S, Vittinghoff E, et al. Antibiotics in chronic obstructive pulmonary disease exacerbations: a meta-analysis. JAMA 1995; 273:957. (*A review of randomized trials finding a small but statistically significant improvement in outcome, particularly in persons with severe disease.*)

Shim CS, Williams MH. Bronchodilator response to oral aminophylline and terbutaline versus aerosol albuterol in patients with COPD. Am J Med 1983;75:697. (*Randomized, double-blind crossover study finding the aerosol route to be superior.*)

Silverman EK, Pierce JA, Province MA, et al. Variability of pulmonary function in alpha-1-antitrypsin deficiency: clinical correlates. Ann Intern Med 1989;111:982. (*Finds that many patients with the deficiency do not necessarily have pulmonary impairment attributable to the deficiency.*)

Timms RM, Khaja FU, Williams GW, et al. Hemodynamic response to oxygen therapy in chronic obstructive pulmonary disease. Ann Intern Med 1985;102:29. (*Detailed data showing a modest response; patients with the best response had the best prognosis.*)

Tougaard L, Krone T, Sorknaes A, et al. Economic benefits of teaching patients with chronic obstructive pulmonary disease about their illness. Lancet 1992;339:1517. (*Cost of care reduced.*)

Wewers MD, Casolaro A, Sellers SE, et al. Replacement therapy for alpha-1-antitrypsin deficiency associated with emphysema. N Engl J Med 1987;316:1055. (*Infusions did reverse biochemical abnormalities.*)

48
Management of Asthma

Asthma is a chronic inflammatory disease of airways that affects an estimated 5% to 7% of the population, with prevalence and mortality greatest among inner city residents and increasing. A heightened appreciation for the underlying inflammatory pathophysiology of asthma has markedly altered the approach to therapy in the past decade. Antiinflammatory agents have superseded bronchodilators as the mainstay of treatment.

Although there are no cures for asthma, effective outpatient management is available. Many exacerbations leading to emergency room visits are preventable, so much so that the frequency of emergency room visits for asthma has become a common outcome measure and proxy for quality of primary care. The primary care physician needs to be skilled in asthma management and able to design a practical, cost-effective program that minimizes side effects, maximizes functional status, and reduces the frequency and severity of flares. Because patient involvement in asthma care is essential to a good outcome, the development of a strong patient–doctor relationship

and the provision of detailed patient education are extremely important.

PATHOPHYSIOLOGY, CLINICAL PRESENTATION, AND COURSE

Pathophysiology

Airway inflammation underlies the pathology and pathophysiology of asthma; characteristic features are mast cell degranulation, eosinophilic infiltration, endothelial activation, and recruitment and proliferation of T cells. The normal respiratory epithelium is denuded and replaced by proliferating goblet cells. The resulting edema, inflammatory exudate, and such bronchial hyperresponsiveness lead to airway obstruction. Bronchial hyperresponsiveness is exacerbated by loss of the normal epithelial barrier and can be triggered by exposure to allergens, exercise, cold, and pharmacologic agents. Epidemiologically important allergens leading to *sensitization* include *dust mite* and *cockroach* antigens, which helps to explain the high prevalence of asthma among inner city residents. Air pollutants and occupational exposures sensitize others.

Many precipitants and mediators of the bronchoconstriction, edema, and mucous production that characterize asthma have been identified; however, their precise roles and interrelationships remain to be elucidated. The list of mediators includes *prostaglandin D$_2$, leukotrienes* (slow-reacting substance of anaphylaxis), *eosinophilic chemotactic factor*, and *histamine*. Leukotrienes are emerging as particularly important mediators of inflammation. They increase the migration of eosinophils, production of mucus, airway wall edema, and bronchial hyper-responsiveness. They appear to be important triggers of bronchoconstriction on airway exposure to cold dry air, as in exercise- and cold-induced asthma.

Asthmatic reactions have early and late phases. The *acute bronchoconstrictive phase* involves the rapid development of reversible airway obstruction in response to stimuli that fail to affect normal persons. Stimuli include allergens (e.g., molds, sulfites, animal dander, pollens), aspirin, exercise, emotional stress, viral respiratory infections, and respiratory irritants, such as perfumes and dusts.

In addition to the initial mediator-induced bronchospasm, asthmatic patients experience a second or *late-phase reaction* 6 to 12 hours later. This late-phase reaction is believed to be a manifestation of the inflammatory response that is more refractory to bronchodilator treatment than the initial one. Neutrophil chemotactic factor is believed to play a role. Even some patients with exercise-induced asthma experience a late reaction.

Elements of a *neurogenic pathway* have also been elucidated. Bronchial smooth muscle is responsive to autonomic influences; it has not been determined whether the effect is direct or by way of biochemical mediators. Vagal stimulation and cholinergic drugs cause bronchial constriction; β-adrenergic stimulation appears capable of countering the cholinergic influences. Bronchial irritants and emotional stress are thought to precipitate bronchospasm, in part, by way of triggering vagal reflexes. The nerve endings of asthmatic patients have been found to be devoid of the bronchodilator neuropeptide vasoactive intestinal polypeptide.

Traditionally, asthma has been divided clinically into "extrinsic" and "intrinsic" categories, with extrinsic disease believed to be a manifestation of immunologic reactivity to environmental antigens, and intrinsic disease thought to be unrelated to allergen exposure. However, patients in both groups have demonstrated reactivity related to immunoglobulin E (IgE), which challenges the notion of separate allergen-related and non–allergen-related categories of asthma. Nonetheless, the categories are still used clinically (see following discussion).

It used to be thought that asthma was not associated with any permanent sequelae, but *airway remodeling* has been detected pathologically. The full physiologic significance of this remodeling remains to be determined, but declines in pulmonary function over time have been identified in long-term epidemiologic studies.

Clinical Presentation

Regardless of precipitant, the pathophysiologic final common pathway is airway inflammation, with bronchial edema, smooth-muscle contraction, and excessive mucus production. Clinical manifestations include *wheezing, dyspnea, cough,* and *sputum*. Presentations range from pure bronchospasm, with little cough and sputum production, to a predominance of bronchorrhea and coughing that mimics bronchitis or an upper respiratory tract infection. In fact, cough and sputum production may be the initial symptoms of an asthmatic attack. *Nocturnal exacerbation* of symptoms is common, linked to the diurnal variation in blood levels of catecholamines and vagal tone.

Extrinsic Asthma. Although classifying asthma according to allergen responsiveness may be an oversimplification, the extrinsic and intrinsic categories do describe two relatively distinct clinical presentations. Patients with *extrinsic asthma* typically give a history of atopy, onset of symptoms during childhood or adolescence, predictable seasonal occurrence, and response to environmental stimuli. However, the condition can occur at any age, and attacks may take place seasonally or year-round, precipitated by such common household allergens as dust mites, animal dander, and fungal spores. Anxiety, inhalation of airway irritants, and exposure to perfumes and strong household odors can also precipitate asthmatic episodes in these patients. The course of attacks is usually self-limited, although some patients have severe bouts requiring hospitalization. Prognosis is relatively good, with 70% found to be symptom-free 20 years after onset.

Intrinsic Asthma. Patients with *intrinsic asthma* usually begin having symptoms in the third or fourth decade. Although no identifiable extrinsic allergen is associated with attacks in these patients, they do demonstrate elevations in serum IgE, similar to those of patients with intrinsic disease. Sputum production can be considerable, so that differentiation from chronic bronchitis is sometimes difficult. Minor upper respiratory tract infections often precipitate attacks. Some patients present with exertional dyspnea or cough and no demonstrable wheezing, although expiratory flow rates are clearly reduced. Intrinsic asthma is sometimes more refractory to treatment than is extrinsic disease.

Postexertional Asthma is a form of airway hyperreactivity most common in children and adolescents. The stimulus is believed to be a reduction in the temperature of inhaled air, which leads to mediator release (especially leukotrienes) in susceptible patients. Both initial and late-phase reactions have been identified. Vigorous exercise on a cold, dry day is particularly apt to trigger an attack; airway temperature can become quite low in such circumstances. Although bronchospasm does not occur during exercise, it becomes marked shortly after exercise ends and can last for up to an hour.

Occupational Asthma has gained increasing recognition as an important cause of work-related disability. True occupational asthma involves the development of sensitization through inhalation exposure to an occupationally related allergen. Exposure to irritant or toxic pollutants in the workplace can also trigger bronchospasm, especially in a person with preexisting airway hyperresponsiveness. Cold air, sulfur dioxide in low concentrations, fluorocarbons, and inert dusts are common irritants that stimulate reflex bronchospasm. Toxic gases such as sulfur dioxide in high concentrations, halogens, ammonia, acid fumes, and solvent vapors cause inflammatory bronchoconstriction. Important allergens include animal proteins, enzymes, grain and cereal dusts, seeds, vegetable gums, and legumes. Other substances have pharmacologic activity; histamine-releasing compounds are present in cotton dust, organic acids are found in wood dust, and numerous chemicals have anticholinesterase activity. Some agents provoke asthma through multiple mechanisms; toluene diisocyanate (TDI) has reflex, pharmacologic, β-blocking, and IgE effects.

Patients with occupational asthma caused by toxic or irritant substances characteristically report a direct relation between exposure and onset of symptoms. Those with allergen-induced disease note no symptoms at the time of the first exposure but marked wheezing after even minor repeated contact with the allergen (anamnestic response). Typically, patients with occupational asthma are symptom-free during days off from work, only to have a flare-up on returning (see Chapter 39).

Nasal Polyps and Aspirin Sensitivity comprise a curious but important familial asthma syndrome. The bronchospasm associated with aspirin intake may be marked. The finding of nasal polyps in a person with a history of asthma should lead to consideration of aspirin sensitivity.

Categories of Asthma. For management purposes (see below), four categories of asthma have been defined:

- *Mild intermittent asthma:* symptoms no more than twice weekly and nighttime symptoms no more than twice monthly; lung function [peak flow rate, forced expiratory volume in 1 second (FEV$_1$)] reduced to no less than 80% of predicted; patient asymptomatic between exacerbations and peak expiratory flow rates normal between attacks.
- *Mild persistent asthma:* symptomatic more than two times per week but less than once a day, and nighttime symptoms more than twice monthly; episodes may affect activity; pulmonary function is normal in between episodes and decreases to no less than 80% of normal during episodes.
- *Moderate persistent asthma:* daily symptoms, daily use of β_2-agonists, nocturnal symptoms more than once a week; attacks limit activity; pulmonary function declines to 60% to 80% of normal and may not return to normal after an exacerbation.
- *Severe asthma:* symptoms continuous; frequent acute exacerbations; frequent nocturnal symptoms; activity limited; pulmonary function always abnormal and less than 60% of normal without treatment.

Clinical Course and Natural History

Regardless of the type of asthma, subclinical but significant bronchospasm remains for days to weeks after the wheezing of an acute attack subsides. The continuing bronchial hyperresponsiveness is believed to be related to ongoing inflammation. Often, small airways may remain constricted even after large airways have relaxed. The clinical recurrences that commonly develop shortly after the apparent resolution of an acute attack are most often not new episodes but relapses.

The natural history of asthma and the consequences of airway remodeling that result from chronic airway inflammation remain to be fully established, but in population studies with long-term follow-up, asthmatic patients demonstrate a signifi-cant and steady decline in FEV$_1$ in comparison with those without asthma. This decline is exacerbated by smoking. Overall mortality for all forms of asthma is 0.1% annually; the rate increases markedly to 3.3% for patients with episodes of status asthmaticus. A disturbing increase in asthma mortality has occurred in the past two decades despite the availability of increasingly effective therapy. The cause for this increase is unclear, but much of it is localized to inner city populations in New York and Chicago, which suggests that increased exposure to potent allergens and air pollution may be contributing, in addition to inadequate access to proper health care.

PRINCIPLES OF MANAGEMENT

Strategy

The appreciation of the pivotal role of inflammation in the pathophysiology of asthma has led to a major restructuring of treatment, with *antiinflammatory therapy* emerging as the foundation of treatment for long-term control and *bronchodilators* relegated to a supporting role. The consensus view is that all patients with active disease should be started and maintained on continuous antiinflammatory therapy and that bronchodilators should be used as primary therapy only for those with infrequent, mild exacerbations and to prevent postexertional or cold-induced flares. The previous reliance on long-term bronchodilator therapy as first-line treatment has been largely abandoned because such therapy does not correct the underlying pathophysiology and is associated with poor outcomes (see below). *Patient education* takes on heightened importance because of the need for constant monitoring, compliance, and timely adjustment of the treatment program.

As always, when confronted with an acute attack of bronchospasm and before initiating therapy for asthma, the physician should not forget to consider briefly the other acute causes of wheezing (e.g., pulmonary edema, pulmonary embolization, laryngeal edema, airway obstruction by tumor or foreign body, chronic obstructive lung disease flare; see Chapters 32, 40, 41, and 42).

Practice Guidelines. Recognizing the need to develop and promulgate a new treatment paradigm for asthma, the National Institutes of Health convened expert panels to develop *clinical practice guidelines* for asthma management and published them as the *National Asthma Education Program* (NAEP) (see below). A stepped approach to care is utilized, based on the category of asthma manifested. The regular use of topically active *inhaled corticosteroids* is recommended, supplemented by selective use of *inhaled β_2-agonist* bronchodilators. Oral steroids, other antiinflammatory agents, and other bronchodilators are used in adjunctive fashion. *Patient education* is a central feature of the guidelines because of the importance of compliance to successful management. Underuse of antiinflammatory therapy and failure to monitor peak flows correlate strongly with an increased number of emergency department visits and hospitalizations.

Implementation and Compliance. Like most practice guidelines, many of the NAEP recommendations are supported by the results of randomized, controlled trials (e.g., respective roles for inhaled steroids and bronchodilators), whereas others (e.g., approaches to monitoring and self-care) are based on expert opinion. Primary care physicians may need to customize for individual patients those elements that pertain to patient self-monitoring and self-treatment of an exacerbation. For example, treatment of an exacerbation might need to be stereotyped rather than based on peak flow, and the patient instructed to contact the physician if symptoms do not resolve within a few hours. Surveys indicate that fewer than 50% of asthma patients who should take inhaled steroids daily do so, and fewer than 20% measure their peak flow regularly. Some have suggested that time pressures and staffing limitations in primary care practices may limit the teaching effort and contribute to inadequate outcomes. They propose *disease management* strategies, which emphasize the use of information technology to identify patients, customize the teaching intervention, monitor care, and control costs. The efficacy of the disease management approach is being evaluated.

Treatment Guidelines (Incorporating the National Asthma Education Program Recommendations)

Mild Intermittent Asthma. The treatment of choice is *bronchodilator* therapy as needed with a *short-acting β_2-agonist*, such as albuterol (Table 48.1). As-needed use is preferred to regular use, which is no more effective and may induce tachyphylaxis. *Patient education* includes instruction in proper inhaler use and technique, the role of medication, and avoidance of environmental precipitants. If β_2-agonist therapy is needed more than twice weekly, therapy for mild persistent asthma should be considered.

These agents are also effective as *prophylaxis* for mild episodes of exercise- or cold-induced asthma when taken a few minutes before the inciting activity. If exercise is going to be very prolonged or prolonged protection against unexpected exercise is desired, then one might consider an as-needed dose of a *long-acting β_2-agonist (e.g., salmeterol)*. Regular daily use of a long-acting β_2-agonist is not recommended because of the association of high-dose β-agonist therapy with adverse outcomes (see below). Alternatives for prophylaxis of mild exercise-induced asthma include inhalation of *cromolyn* or *nedocromil* powder before activity and once-daily oral use of *montelukast*.

Mild Persistent Asthma. Antiinflammatory therapy is added to the program to provide long-term control. A *low-dose inhaled glucocorticosteroid* is the treatment of choice (Table 48.1). Alternatives include *cromolyn* or *nedocromil*. Use of a leukotriene-altering agent (e.g., *montelukast*) appears promising as another approach to antiinflammatory therapy for mild disease. Patient education should include initiation of periodic self-monitoring with a *peak flow meter*. Treatment of acute symptoms with as-needed use of a short-acting β_2-agonist continues as for mild intermittent disease; any requirement for daily or increased dosing should lead to consideration of therapy for moderate asthma.

Moderate Asthma. Frequent exacerbations require increasing the dose of *inhaled steroids* to at least *moderate* levels or continuing low doses and *adding an inhaled long-acting β_2-agonist* (e.g., salmeterol) or a bedtime dose of *theophylline*, especially if nocturnal symptoms are present. Although *montelukast*

Table 48.1.   Drugs for Asthma

DRUG	FORMULATION AND AVERAGE DOSAGE	RELATIVE COST
β_2-Agonists—short-acting		
Albuterol-generic;	MDI; 2 puffs prn	1.0
brand (Ventolin, Proventil)	MDI; 2 puffs prn	1.3–1.5
Bitolterol (Tornalate)	MDI; 2 puffs prn	1.5
Pirbuterol (Maxair)	MDI; 2 puffs prn	1.0
(Maxair Autohaler)	Breath-actuated MDI; 2 puffs prn	1.0
Terbutaline	MDI; 2 puffs	0.9
β_2-Agonists—long-acting		
Salmeterol (Serevent)	MDI; 1–2 puffs q12h	3.0
Inhaled corticosteroids		
Beclomethasone		
(Vanceril, Beclovent)	MDI; 4–8 puffs bid	2.4
(Vanceril Double Strength)	MDI; 2–4 puffs bid	2.4
Budesonide (Pulmicort Turbuhaler)	Breath-actuated; 1-2 inhalations bid	1.7
Flunisolide (AeroBid)	MDI; 2–4 puffs bid	3.5
Fluticasone (Flovent)	MDI; 2–4 puffs bid	2.1
(Flovent Rotadisk)	Breath-actuated; 1 inhalation bid	2.1
Triamicinolone (Azmacort)	MDI; 2 puffs tid–qid	1.8
Inhaled nonsteroidal antiinflammatory agents		
Cromolyn (Intal)	MDI; 2–4 puffs tid–qid or prn	3.2
Nedocromil (Tilade)	MDI; 2–4 puffs bid–qid or prn	1.8
Leukotriene modifiers		
Montelukast (Singulair)	Oral 10 mg q am	3.2
Zafirlukast (Accolate)	Oral 20 mg bid	3.0
Zileuton (Zyflo)	Oral 600 mg qid	4.0
Theophylline		
Generic extended-release	300 mg qhs	0.3
(Slo-Bid Gyrocaps)	300 mg qhs	0.7
(Uni-Dur)	200 mg qhs	1.5
(Theo-Dur)	400 mg qhs	0.5

MDI-metered=dose inhaler.

is not as effective for maintenance as are inhaled glucocorticoids, adding this antiinflammatory agent may allow reduction of the steroid dose. Patient education should stress *daily* monitoring of *peak flow* and increasing the dose of inhaled steroid at the first indication of a decline in peak flow. Treatment of acute symptoms with as-needed use of a *short-acting β₂-agonist* is the same as for mild persistent disease; continued requirements for daily or increased dosing should lead to consideration of therapy for severe asthma.

Severe Asthma. The foundation of therapy is *high-dose inhaled steroids*, supplemented during exacerbations by short courses of high-dose *systemic glucocorticosteroids* (e.g., oral prednisone). The prednisone program is rapidly tapered and discontinued after 5 to 10 days. Use of a *long-acting β₂-agonist* or *theophylline* can help control symptoms (particularly nocturnal exacerbations) and may reduce steroid requirements. Daily patient *monitoring of peak flow* and prompt initiation of maximal antiinflammatory therapy (e.g., high-dose prednisone) at the first sign of a marked decline in airway function are critical to avoiding severe exacerbations and emergency department visits. Use of a *short-acting inhaled β₂-agonist*, supplemented if necessary by inhaled *ipratropium*, can help ease the symptoms of a severe bronchospastic attack, but these drugs are no substitute for maximum antiinflammatory therapy. The role of montelukast in severe disease remains to be defined.

Refractory cases require consideration of exacerbating factors, such as exposure to offending allergens, gastroesophageal reflux, sleep apnea, and allergic bronchopulmonary aspergillosis (suggested by an eosinophil count >1,000/mL). *Immunotherapy* is indicated if a responsible allergen is identified, and a trial of proton pump inhibition can be helpful in persons with suspected reflux (see Chapter 61). The most common cause of refractory disease is *poor compliance* with the inhaled corticosteroid program and failure to monitor peak flows, which indicates a need for more patient education and counseling.

Treatment Modalities (In Order of Use in Stepped Care)

β₂-Agonist Bronchodilators. As noted above, bronchodilators have been relegated to a supporting role in the treatment of asthma. The inhaled semiselective β₂-agonists are the bronchodilators of choice; they produce prompt potent bronchodilation and little systemic adrenergic stimulation when used in moderation.

Preparations. Most preparations are available in aerosolized form dispensed from a *metered-dose inhaler* (MDI). A few are breath-actuated, but most require breath–hand coordination. The onset of action is very rapid, and systemic absorption occurs. Some preparations are available as *nebulized solutions*. Nebulized delivery offers few advantages over MDI delivery and costs more, but patients unable to use pressurized aerosols (e.g., the very young, the elderly) may benefit; doses delivered are higher, but the onset of action is slower than with MDIs and the equipment is not portable.

The *short-acting* preparations (e.g., *albuterol, pirbuterol, terbutaline, bitolterol*) have a rapid (2 to 5 minutes) onset of action that lasts 4 to 6 hours. Generic albuterol is well tolerated and among the least expensive. *Levalbuterol*, the L-isomer of albuterol, is available for delivery as a nebulized solution; it offers no particular advantages in safety or efficacy

over racemic albuterol. Some of the short-acting inhaled agents are also available in longer-acting oral formulations; however, these formulations are not recommended because the onset of action is delayed, systemic adrenergic side effects can be considerable, and better-tolerated long-acting formulations are now available.

The inhaled *long-acting β₂-agonists* (e.g., *salmeterol*) provide up to 12 hours of bronchodilation with a minimum of systemic side effects, so that they are well suited for maintenance therapy. Because their onset of action is delayed, they do not obviate the need for a short-acting β₂-agonist when acute bronchospasm arises. At present, they are used only in conjunction with a program of corticosteroid therapy because concern persists (see below) regarding an increase in airway hyperresponsiveness and adverse outcomes when β₂-agonists are used on a regular basis without antiinflammatory therapy. The cost per dose is about two times that of the short-acting preparations.

The modern β₂-agonists have largely replaced the *nonselective β-agonists* (e.g., *isoproterenol, ephedrine, metaproterenol, isoetharine*), which have a very short duration of action and can cause severe adrenergic side effects (palpitations, nervousness, cardiac dysrhythmias).

Adverse Effects. When used in high doses, all semiselective β₂-agents can trigger systemic adrenergic side effects (e.g., *palpitations, tremor, tachycardia*). High doses may also cause *hypokalemia*. A worrisome retrospective report found that overuse of inhaled β₂-agonists was associated with *worsening asthma control* and *increased asthma mortality*, which raises a warning about sole reliance on these agents for asthma management. Explanations for the observed findings range from delay in starting needed antiinflammatory treatment to direct toxic effects, such as exacerbation of *bronchial hyperresponsiveness*. In persons with mild asthma, regular use of inhaled albuterol confers no clinical advantage over as-needed albuterol, but a small significant increase in bronchial hyperresponsiveness results—an increase that could conceivably be injurious to persons with more severe disease. Ongoing prospective study should help clarify the issue. Regular use of both short- and long-acting preparations may lead to *tolerance* to their bronchoprotective effect. Continuous use of salmeterol for prophylaxis shortens the duration of its protective effect.

Recommended Use. The use of *short-acting* inhaled preparations should be limited to providing prophylaxis for exercise- and cold-induced asthma and symptomatic relief of acute symptoms. These agents are to be taken only on an *as-needed basis*. Frequent bronchodilator use is an important sign of disease exacerbation and the need for additional antiinflammatory therapy. The regular use of a *long-acting* preparation may have a role in moderate and severe asthma, but only as an *adjunct* to steroid therapy, helping to sustain control and moderate steroid requirements. Acute attacks still require addition of a short-acting β₂-agonist.

Inhaled Glucocorticosteroids. The *first generation* of inhaled glucocorticoids (e.g., *beclomethasone, triamcinolone, flunisolide*) were developed in an effort to achieve the advantages of long-term steroid therapy without the systemic side effects. With regular use, many of the histologic features of asthma disappear, airway hyperresponsiveness reverts to normal, and the number of exacerbations declines. These agents are topically active, bind to airway cell receptors, and inhibit transcription and translation of cytokines and protein mediators. Airway eosinophilia is reduced, but not entirely eliminated, which suggests that some degree of airway inflammation persists despite their use. The effect on lipoid inflammatory mediators is more variable, with leukotriene synthesis less consistently inhibited.

Systemic absorption of inhaled steroid from the lung is limited, but some of the inhaled dose invariably is swallowed. Effective first-pass hepatic metabolism of drug absorbed from the gastrointestinal tract limits systemic effects, but such effects, including adrenal suppression, can increase with the use of very high doses (see below). *Second-generation* formulations (e.g., *fluticasone, budesonide*) exhibit improved steroid-receptor binding in the lung and enhanced first-pass hepatic metabolism; however, any advantage in clinical outcomes remains to be determined.

Preparations. Most first-generation preparations are dispensed through *MDIs*, which require hand–breath coordination and a chlorofluorocarbon propellant. At equivalent doses, they demonstrate similar efficacy and differ predominantly in dose of steroid delivered per inhalation and cost per canister (Table 48.1). In response to environmental concerns, the halogenated propellants are being phased out. To improve droplet delivery of drug to the lungs and reduce oropharyngeal deposition, a number of preparations come with a built-in *spacer*, which can also be purchased separately. For those who experience difficulty with hand–breath coordination, one of the *inhalation-triggered* dry-powder formulations (e.g., budesonide) may be worth considering (cost is also low). The risk for adverse systemic effects is greatest with preparations delivering the highest dose of inhaled steroid per puff, as fewer puffs are needed to exceed the safe daily limit.

Adverse Effects. When used at moderate doses, the inhaled corticosteroids are well tolerated and produce few adverse systemic effects. The principal localized complaints, *sore throat* and *hoarseness*, are consequences of oropharyngeal deposition of the inhaled steroid and subsequent *oropharyngeal candidiasis* and *vocal cord muscle weakness*. They can be minimized by better inhaler technique (facilitated by use of a spacer, as explained below), rinsing and gargling after MDI use, and use of nystatin mouthwash for established thrush. The risk for adverse systemic effects caused by currently available preparations of inhaled glucocorticoids becomes a concern with sustained use at high doses (750 to 850 μg/d). *Hypothalamic–pituitary–adrenal suppression, decreased bone density, growth retardation in children,* and *glaucoma, cataracts,* and *dermal thinning in the elderly* have all been described. The risks associated with long-term therapy at lower doses remain to be defined.

Use. The topically active, inhaled preparations are preferable to systemic steroids in most instances because systemic adverse effects are limited at the usual doses, so that the risk for systemic steroid–related complications is greatly reduced. Although highly effective, the oral and parenteral preparations of systemic glucocorticoids (e.g., prednisone, methylprednisolone, hydrocortisone) should be reserved for severe exacerbations and refractory disease and used for as short a period as possible (see below).

The original recommendations for inhaled steroids called for administration four times daily, but *twice-daily* regimens are nearly as effective and greatly facilitate compliance with maintenance therapy. Only during exacerbations might dosing four times daily be desirable. The onset of action is usually gradual, and it may take days for the patient to notice improvement—inadequately prepared patients may report that "the drug is not working." Full benefit may not be evident for several weeks. Response is generally dose-related.

The use of *high-dose* inhaled steroids can reduce the need for systemic steroids in many cases of severe asthma, especially when supplemented by β_2-agonists and other drugs. During severe acute exacerbations, a short course of high-dose systemic steroids is indicated because topical steroids may not penetrate obstructed airways, where need is greatest. Patients with extrinsic asthma may benefit from a topically active steroid also applied as a nasal spray during the ragweed season (see Chapter 222).

Oral Glucocorticosteroids. Systemic steroids remain the most effective treatment for asthma, especially the severe, acute exacerbations of this chronic inflammatory disorder. Limiting their use is the set of serious side effects associated with prolonged daily glucocorticosteroid intake (see Chapter 105). *Prednisone* is the most widely prescribed oral preparation; the cost is very low. Its half-life is 12 to 24 hours. Onset of action occurs clinically within 8 to 12 hours of intake.

Use and Adverse Effects. A *short-term course* (5 to 10 days) of high-dose prednisone (40 to 60 mg/d) begun at the earliest signs of an acute exacerbation can control an attack that does not respond promptly to maximum doses of inhaled steroids and bronchodilators. When combined with rapid tapering to full cessation within 5 to 10 days, a short course can obviate the need for emergency department treatment, reduce the risk for acute relapse, and avoid adrenal suppression.

Any *long-term* systemic steroid therapy should be confined to patients with chronic disabling symptoms refractory to maximal doses of all other forms of treatment. The adverse consequences of prolonged daily use of systemic glucocorticoids (osteoporotic fractures, adrenal suppression, skin changes, aseptic necrosis of bone, aggravation of diabetes mellitus) may outweigh the benefits in all but the most severe cases.

In most instances, regular use of high-dose inhaled steroids supplemented by bronchodilator therapy and short courses of systemic steroids can obviate the need for long-term systemic steroid use. If it proves difficult to withdraw oral steroid therapy entirely, one can try an *alternate-day regimen* supplemented by full doses of inhaled steroid; this results in less adrenal suppression and fewer steroid-related adverse effects than does daily systemic therapy (see Chapter 105). Refractory cases require investigation for exacerbating factors (see above).

Although always desirable, a switch from long-term systemic steroids to an inhaled steroid program must be planned carefully to avoid triggering an exacerbation of asthma or precipitating adrenal insufficiency. Slow tapering of the daily dose, use of alternate-day steroid programs, and initiation of full doses of inhaled steroids and adjunctive therapies are essential. Before any long-term program of systemic steroids is discontinued, a Cortrosyn stimulation test (which assays the level of adrenal responsiveness) should be considered to help determine the speed of tapering (see Chapter 105).

Cromolyn Sodium and Nedocromil prevent the degranulation of mast cells, so that they are useful as prophylactic agents for *exercise-* or *allergen-induced asthma* and as substitutes for inhaled steroids in mild persistent disease. They have no direct bronchodilator activity but can decrease airway hyperresponsiveness through their action on mast cells. They are not as effective as inhaled β_2-agonists for immediate use before exercise or exposure to cold air. Their regular use may avert the need for inhaled corticosteroids. A 4-week empiric trial is needed to assess efficacy; there is no way to predict response, and it may take weeks to emerge. Patients who fail a trial should be prescribed inhaled steroids, which are more effective. Because these drugs possess no direct bronchodilator activity, they should not be used to treat attacks.

Preparations and Use. Cromolyn is taken by the *inhaled* route. It is now available in an aqueous solution, so that the frequency of reactions to the often-irritating powdered formulation has been reduced. The dose schedule for patients with chronic asthma is one capsule four times daily. For prophylaxis of exercise-induced asthma, the patient inhales for several minutes before exercise or exposure to a known allergen. (Patients with exercise-induced asthma who cannot tolerate cromolyn can inhale a β_2-adrenergic aerosol a few times before engaging in activity). Cromolyn is expensive but is free of adverse side effects and should be considered a first-line drug in asthma prophylaxis. *Nedocromil* resembles cromolyn in action and effectiveness but is unrelated chemically. Use is similar to that of cromolyn. Side effects are minimal.

Leukotriene Modifiers. Appreciation of the role of inflammation in asthma has stimulated interest in inflammatory mediators and agents that inhibit them. The drugs of this class interfere with leukotriene activity, either by inhibition of synthesis (*zileuton*) or receptor antagonism (*montelukast and zafirlukast*). They are less efficacious than inhaled steroids, but they have proved useful for *prophylaxis* of mild exercise-induced asthma and for *control* of mild to moderate persistent disease. Their role in the treatment of more severe categories of persistent disease, especially in combination with inhaled steroids, remains to be determined; it is hoped they will have a steroid-sparing effect. Predictors of response have not been identified, so that a therapeutic trial is necessary. These drugs are especially effective in the treatment of aspirin-induced asthma. They are costly, and their long-term safety and efficacy, especially in persons with relatively severe disease requiring concurrent use of other drugs, has not been established. A vasculitis-like hypersensitivity reaction has been reported in association with leukotriene modifier therapy when concurrent steroid therapy is cut back.

Preparations. Of the available leukotriene modifiers, *montelukast* is the best tolerated and easiest to use. Its once-daily dosing schedule, reasonable efficacy (effective in two thirds of cases), and few adverse effects (it is the only drug in this class approved by the Food and Drug Administration for use in children under the age of 12) make it a practical though somewhat expensive choice for prophylaxis of exercise-induced asthma. It also shows promise for control of mild to moderate persistent asthma, allowing reductions in steroid and bronchodilator requirements. Drug absorption is not affected by food intake. The other agents in this class are of similar efficacy but more difficult to use. *Zileuton* requires qid dosing and can cause hepatocellular injury, necessitating close monitoring of transaminases. *Zafirlukast* has the disadvantages of reduced bioavailability when taken with food and reduced efficacy when taken with other asthma drugs (e.g.,

theophylline). It also impairs warfarin metabolism, and transaminase monitoring is required.

Theophylline and Its Derivatives. The role of the methylxanthines *theophylline* and *aminophylline* (a derivative salt of theophylline) in asthma care has narrowed with the advent of faster, safer, more effective therapies (see above). Current use is limited to patients with moderate to severe asthma bothered by *nocturnal exacerbations* and to those with refractory, steroid-dependent disease. Although the methylxanthines became popular because they were the first oral active bronchodilators, their current usefulness as an adjunctive therapy may be a function of effects other than bronchodilation. They improve diaphragmatic function, myocardial contractility, and mucociliary transport and demonstrate such antiinflammatory effects as inhibition of anaphylactic mediator release and suppression of mast cell response. Their low cost and the availability of sustained-release preparations facilitate utilization.

Preparations. The preferred oral preparation is *aminophylline*. The half-life of oral theophylline or aminophylline averages 6 hours but can range from 4 to 8 hours; much individual variation is seen because of differences in clearance rates. Clearance occurs predominantly by hepatic biotransformation. Impairment of hepatic microsomal activity raises serum levels and prolongs duration of action. Generic *sustained-release formulations* provide therapeutic serum levels for 12 to 24 hours at low cost and in convenient once- or twice-daily dosing regimens.

A number of formulations previously used for acute bronchodilation are no longer recommended, including *theophylline elixir* (expensive, very short-acting, erratic absorption), aminophylline *suppositories* (erratic absorption, unpredictable serum levels), and *combination preparations* (inability to titrate theophylline dose, irrational combinations of agents).

Adverse Effects are proportional to the serum level. The therapeutic index of these drugs is narrow (10 to 20 μg/mL), and monitoring of serum levels helps to ensure both safety and efficacy. Serum determinations are best obtained from blood drawn 4 to 6 hours after the last dose. The minor gastrointestinal side effects (*nausea, vomiting, reflux, diarrhea*) and the minor neurologic side effects (*agitation, tremor, insomnia*) are largely dose-related but can occur even at subtherapeutic serum levels. The gastrointestinal side effects are not affected by route of administration. Levels above 20 μg/mL are associated with a marked increase in risk for drug toxicity; at levels above 35 μg/mL, life-threatening *ventricular arrhythmias* can occur. *Seizures* refractory to standard anticonvulsant therapy have occurred without warning in patients with serum levels above 40 μg/mL.

Dosage and Use. When used for bronchodilation, methylxanthines were always prescribed in doses sufficient to achieve the "therapeutic range" (i.e., 10 to 20 μg/mL), which bordered on toxicity. Smaller doses of the drug (producing serum levels of 8 to 10 μg/mL) appear sufficient for reducing inhaled steroid requirements and improving nocturnal symptoms. Such supplementary *low-dose programs* are promising and may become the norm, providing a well-tolerated and inexpensive addition to current expensive treatment regimens.

The efficacy and safety of *IV methylxanthine* therapy for acute exacerbations of asthma requiring urgent or room-conducted care remains controversial. Failure in room-conducted studies to demonstrate additional bronchodilation beyond that achieved with β-agonists alone, and the association of such treatment with increased risks for cardiopulmonary toxicity, have blunted enthusiasm for its use. Nonetheless, some have found the need for hospital admission and assisted ventilation to be reduced.

Anticholinergic Therapy: Ipratropium. Ipratropium, a topically active muscarinic blocking agent similar to atropine, is available as an MDI preparation. It is particularly useful in chronic obstructive pulmonary disease, in which its bronchodilator effects rival those of the β-agonists (see Chapter 47). Its efficacy is considerably less in asthma, although it may add some marginal bronchodilation to that provided by β_2-agonist therapy in severe bronchospasm. Compared with β_2-agonists, it is longer-acting but slower to take effect. Unlike atropine, it is poorly absorbed, has little systemic effect, and can be used in patients with glaucoma and prostatism. However, care should be taken to avoid spray contact with the eyes in patients with narrow-angle glaucoma. It is the bronchdilator of choice for β-blocker–induced bronchospasm and appears useful in the elderly. A combination preparation with albuterol is heavily promoted but not approved by the Food and Drug Administration for the treatment of acute bronchospasm.

Other Agents. *Methotrexate* has been studied as a steroid-sparing agent for patients dependent on systemic steroid therapy. Although worth considering in refractory cases, this form of immunosuppressive therapy is not without its own serious toxic side effects (see Chapter 88).

Antibiotics have a limited role in prophylaxis. Although viral upper respiratory infections frequently precipitate attacks—making *influenza vaccination* a must—bacterial infections do not. Heavy sputum production has often been mistakenly attributed to infection when it was actually a manifestation of asthma. However, in cases in which bacterial infection is strongly suggested by sputum Gram's stain, prompt treatment with an appropriate antibiotic (see Chapter 43) is important pending confirmation by culture.

Allergen Avoidance and Immunotherapy. *Allergen identification* is worthwhile, especially in patients with seemingly refractory disease, with incapacitating seasonal disease, or in occupational settings (see Chapter 39). Although history is helpful in suggesting allergens, *skin testing* helps to confirm them and also will identify additional allergens that are likely to be clinically important. Avoidance of exposure and desensitization are too often overlooked as important components of the prophylactic management program.

Desensitization therapy (with intradermal injections of offending allergens; see Chapter 222) has been shown in controlled study to reduce the frequency and severity of asthmatic episodes when a *single offending allergen* can be identified. It can reduce or eliminate the need for systemic steroid therapy. Patients with refractory extrinsic asthma should be considered for allergen testing and desensitization, especially when a single, well-defined, unavoidable seasonal allergen is suspected. Use of immunotherapy for perennial allergic asthma in which the patient is sensitive to multiple allergens has not proved effective.

Avoidance of the offending agent(s) can be an important component of therapy and limit exacerbations even when desensitization is not feasible. Detailed patient education can be very helpful, especially when simple effective measures are recommended (e.g., use of air-conditioning during periods of air pollution, covering mattresses and pillows with impermeable sheets and pillowcases, elimination of wall-to-wall carpets and heavy draperies to limit exposure to dust mite allergen). Unfortunately, avoidance is not always feasible, and pharmacologic methods of prophylaxis may have to be used.

Monoclonal Anti-IgE Antibody. A small proportion of patients with severe asthma and no evidence of atopy often require systemic steroids for control of their disease. Evidence suggests that IgE antibody produced locally in the airway tissue of such patients may be pathophysiologically important. Initial studies of humanized monoclonal anti-IgE antibody to block the action of airway IgE are promising; such therapy may obviate the need for high-dose, long-term systemic corticosteroids.

Monitoring Therapy

Assessment of symptoms, signs, and expiratory flow rates (peak flow and FEV_1) is the basis of monitoring. The patient's subjective perceptions are remarkably accurate and useful for monitoring. *Estimates by patients* of daily changes in airway obstruction and the severity of their condition correlate better with measurements of peak expiratory flow than do the clinical assessments of their physicians.

Certain physical findings, such as the *ratio of inspiration to expiration*, help to judge the degree of bronchospasm semiquantitatively. However, wheezes and related physical findings are not sensitive indicators of airway obstruction. The absence of wheezes does not indicate resolution of bronchospasm (see below). *Pulsus paradoxus* and *sternocleidomastoid retraction* are signs of severe obstruction that suggest an FEV_1 of less than 1 L/s, but these findings are not inevitably present when expiratory flow rates are very low. Moreover, much variation is found between the degree of paradox and the severity of bronchospasm.

Spirometry provides additional sensitivity that helps to identify changes in airway function in the absence of symptoms and to categorize the severity of disease. If possible, the *FEV_1* should be measured by the physician at each office visit and during exacerbations, and the *peak expiratory flow rate* measured by the patient regularly and during exacerbations. The FEV_1 is still prolonged at the time wheezes disappear. Even after the FEV_1 has returned to normal, measures of small-airway obstruction (e.g., *maximum midexpiratory flow rate*) continue to indicate bronchospasm. The clearing of wheezes signifies little more than partial resolution of large-airway bronchospasm; small-airway bronchoconstriction may still be prominent and slower to resolve. Failure to continue therapy beyond the resolution of audible wheezes and acute phase of bronchoconstriction is generally associated with a high rate of relapse.

Self-monitoring is made practical by use of a *hand-held peak expiratory flow meter*. In the NAEP guidelines, monitoring of peak flow both periodically and during exacerbations is central to treatment decisions (see above).

Sputum and *blood eosinophil counts* correlate with the response to therapy in patients treated with steroids for an acute attack. Although blood eosinophilia is not an invariable feature of an acute exacerbation of asthma, it does decline with improvement of expiratory flow rate. The same holds true for sputum eosinophilia. The usefulness of the eosinophil count for predicting relapse and response to therapy is unsettled.

Arterial blood gases provide important information in severe cases, particularly adequacy of ventilation. A carbon dioxide pressure (PCO_2) that is inappropriately high for the respiratory rate indicates ventilatory failure and an urgent need for hospitalization. However, because arterial blood gases are not readily available in most office settings, decisions usually must be made without them. *Chest radiography* rarely provides information of use in decision making.

Thus, some of the most easily obtained parameters (the patient's subjective assessment of severity, ratio of inspiration to expiration, pulsus paradoxus, sternocleidomastoid retraction, peak flow, and FEV_1) are among the more meaningful guides to clinical status and severity of illness.

The Seemingly Refractory Patient

Patient noncompliance is often the cause of "refractoriness." Common shortcomings include *improper inhaler technique*, *underutilization of antiinflammatory medication*, and *overdependence on bronchodilators*. Poor hand–breath coordination, the slow onset of action of inhaled steroids, fear of steroid side effects, and ignorance of the inflammatory nature of the illness contribute to such behavior. Other common patient mistakes include reliance on *nonprescription agents*, such as low-dose adrenergic inhalers, and *alternative medicine remedies* of no proven efficacy (e.g., acupuncture for asthma). Physician *inattention to allergen identification* is another common shortcoming; referral for allergen testing is indicated when the patient appears unresponsive to treatment.

Management of the Pregnant Patient

Fetal morbidity and mortality are increased if asthma is uncontrolled during pregnancy. Most asthma drugs are safe to use during both during pregnancy and breast-feeding, although in some instances data are lacking because of the difficulty in performing controlled studies. Epinephrine increases the risk for fetal malformations, and the safety of the β_2-agonists and cromolyn remains to be established; until safety is proven, they should be avoided if possible. The use of inhaled steroids at moderate doses appears to be without serious consequence, and even systemic steroids can be prescribed if necessary. Theophylline is safe, as is penicillin. Erythromycin is a reasonable alternative in penicillin-allergic patients; tetracycline is contraindicated because it damages fetal liver, bone, and teeth.

PATIENT EDUCATION

Patients need to be made partners in the management of their asthma. Successful outcomes depend on good compliance and proper use of medication. Instruction in *preventive measures* is always appreciated by patients. The bedroom environment deserves particular attention. Covering the mattress and pillows with impermeable materials limits exposure to dust mite allergen, a potential trigger of asthma and its exacerbations. Wall-to-wall carpets are another source of such allergens and should be avoided. Because asthma is a condition characterized by periodic exacerbations, every patient who is capable of understanding and carrying out a medication program should be given instructions for initial self-treatment of an attack, along with strong advice to call the physician promptly if relief does not come quickly. Patients need to know that excessive delay may lead to refractory bronchospasm. Home use of a *handheld flow meter* has helped encourage patient participation in monitoring and adjusting treatment in timely fashion.

Addressing patient concerns and providing written information facilitates *compliance*. Many worry about becoming "dependent" on medication or "immune" to it. These fears need to be addressed openly. A medication booklet that lists prescribing information, side effects, and indications for use alongside a picture of the medication can be helpful to patient and family. Often, patients mistakenly stop the wrong medication or cease therapy altogether because they are fearful or unfamiliar with the side effects of their medications.

Patients in whom bronchospasm is triggered by air pollution, pollens, or exercise need an *activity prescription*. Staying indoors, avoiding physical exertion, and using air-conditioning on particularly bad days are helpful measures. Those with exercise-induced asthma need not restrict themselves so long as prophylactic measures suffice; however, very cold, dry days may be difficult.

Patients with asthma caused by occupational exposure or household factors need careful *counseling* when such difficult alternatives as leaving a job, giving up a favorite pet, or moving to a new location are being considered. Often, less extreme measures are adequate (see above). A number of patients with allergic asthma request advice about desensitization treatment. Allergen testing and consideration of a trial of such therapy are reasonable if episodes are frequent and incapacitating and a single allergen can be identified (see above and Chapter 222).

Patients receiving steroids deserve an extra measure of instruction, particularly when switching over from systemic to aerosol therapy. Writing out the tapering schedule and emphasizing the importance of taking systemic steroids at the time of an exacerbation or major stress will help minimize the risk for adrenal insufficiency.

The *pregnant patient* with asthma will be reluctant to take medication. Detailed counseling about which medications can be used with safety and the importance of asthma control to the health of the fetus is needed to ensure compliance and alleviate concern.

Inhaler Technique. With the growing importance of MDI therapy, proper inhalation technique is essential. The delivery of drug to distal airways is facilitated by *increased duration of breath holding* and by *prolongation and moderation of inspiratory flow*. Rapid inspiration deposits drug in the upper airway; very deep inspiration is no better than moderate inspiration. During periods of respiratory distress, a greater number of inhales may be needed to deliver an adequate dose to the distal airways. Thus, patients need to be instructed to increase the number of inhales during a period of respiratory distress if benefit is not immediately forthcoming; however, they should also be reminded that rapid, deep inhales are neither necessary nor desirable. Extreme care is warranted when the β_2-agonist dose is increased because systemic absorption will occur when drug is deposited in the proximal airway.

Correct MDI use involves hand–breath coordination (i.e., coordinating inspiration with actuation of the MDI), a skill that takes some practice to master. Two recommended approaches are (a) placing the inhaler between closed lips, actuating the inhaler, breathing in, and holding the breath, and (b) holding the mouthpiece 3 to 4 cm from open lips, releasing the medication at the beginning of a full 5-second inspiration, and holding the breath for 10 seconds. The latter technique is a bit more difficult but preferred because less of a jet effect is created to deposit drug on the retropharynx; twice the dose is delivered to the lower respiratory tract if the inspiration is moderate, prolonged, and accompanied by breath holding.

Many patients make the mistake of inhaling first, then actuating the canister, holding their breath for 2 or 3 seconds more, and exhaling before taking the first inhale. Others inhale through the nose. Because many patients cannot perform aerosol inhalation correctly after a demonstration, they need to practice under observation. Moreover, about half forget how to do it when tested on follow-up. Repeated checks of technique are important.

Use of a Spacer. More than 40% of patients cannot master such techniques and need to use an inhalation chamber, often referred to as a "spacer." Commercially available spacers are aerosol-holding chambers that not only eliminate the need for hand–breath coordination but also cut down on oropharyngeal deposition of steroid. They improve delivery substantially, minimize adverse topical effects of inhaled steroids, and improve overall control. They should be considered for persons who cannot master MDI technique and for those who demonstrate inadequate disease control. Their principal disadvantage of most spacers is their bulky size, although some inhalers come with spacers built in.

Breath-actuated Systems. A few β_2-agonists and inhaled steroid preparations are now available in *breath-actuated formulations*. These are triggered by inhalation and do not require as much hand–breath coordination as do MDIs.

INDICATIONS FOR ADMISSION AND REFERRAL

Admission. One of the most difficult determinations is predicting the need for hospitalization at the time of initial presentation. Ability to make such predictions is particularly important for the care of patients with severe attacks who visit the office or emergency department. Some have argued that the response to maximum nonsteroidal therapy is a good predictor of immediate outcome and need for admission. Most studies provide little evidence that any one parameter is predictive, although one group noted that patients who sat bolt upright on admission to the emergency department had a strong likelihood of requiring admission. Another group developed an index of multiple clinical parameters selected by multivariate discriminant analysis to predict the need for hospitalization. A pulse rate of more than 120/min, respiratory rate of more than 30/min, pulsus paradoxus of more than 18 mm Hg, peak expiratory flow rate of less than 120 L/min, moderate to severe dyspnea, accessory muscle use, and wheezing were the presenting clinical parameters used in the index. Although in the investigators' setting the index was capable of distinguishing between those who required admission and those who did not (sensitivity, 95%; specificity, 97%), it did not function nearly as well when applied prospectively by other investigators in their emergency department settings.

Without more definitive means of prediction, clinical status and response to therapy remain the most helpful guidelines for decision making. Consideration of hospital care is indicated for patients with an acute attack who manifest any one of the following:

1. Subjective report of severe difficulty breathing
2. Failure to respond fully and promptly to inhaled β_2-agonist therapy followed promptly by full doses of prednisone
3. Use of accessory muscles of respiration (sternocleidomastoid retraction)
4. Pulsus paradoxus of more than 10 mm Hg
5. FEV_1 of less than 1.0 L/s; peak flow reduced by more than 50% and declining
6. Arterial P_{CO_2} inappropriately high for respiratory rate
7. Underlying cardiac condition
8. Inadequate home situation or a history of poor compliance

Referral. In certain instances, timely referral can be most helpful. Referral for patient *teaching* and *measurement of air flow* is essential if one's practice does not have the time, materials, equipment, or expertise available. *Identification of allergens* and *irritants* is another indication for referral and must be accomplished if the patient is to be advised regarding avoidance of precipitants, even if desensitization is not indicated. *Failure to respond* to treatment, particularly if frequent severe exacerbations necessitate the use of systemic steroids, is yet another indication for referral.

THERAPEUTIC RECOMMENDATIONS

Mild Intermittent Asthma

- Prescribe use as needed of an *inhaled semiselective β_2-agonist* (e.g., 2 to 3 puffs of *albuterol*, repeated in 20 minutes if necessary) for an episode of bronchospasm and for a few minutes before exercise or exposure to cold as prophylaxis for exercise- and cold-induced asthma. Avoid regular use.
- If an alternative to albuterol is desired for prophylaxis, consider a trial of *cromolyn* or *nedocromil* (2 puffs inhaled a few minutes before activity or exposure to cold).
- If exercise is going to be very prolonged or prolonged prophylactic protection against unexpected exercise is desired, prescribe use as needed of a *long-acting β_2-agonist* (e.g., 1 to 3 puffs of *salmeterol* twice daily taken at least half an hour before exercise) or a *leukotriene receptor antagonist* (e.g., 10 mg of *montelukast* every morning). Avoid regular use of salmeterol because it may decrease the duration of protection.
- Teach patient self-management program, including proper inhaler technique, importance of as-needed use only, and avoidance of environmental precipitants.
- Consider advancing to treatment of mild persistent asthma if more than twice-weekly use of β_2-agonist therapy is required.

Mild Persistent Asthma

- Add daily *antiinflammatory* therapy; begin *low-dose* inhaled glucocorticosteroids (e.g., 2 to 4 puffs of *beclomethasone* twice daily); if it is desired to avoid corticosteroids, begin a 4-week trial of a *mast cell stabilizer* (e.g., 2 puffs of *cromolyn* or *nedocromil* two to four times daily) or consider *montelukast* (10 mg every morning).
- Teach the patient how to perform periodic self-monitoring with a *peak flow meter* and how to make a prompt adjustment in the steroid dose with any decline in air flow.

- Continue treatment of acute symptoms with as-needed use of a *short-acting β₂-agonist*. Any requirement for *daily* or *increased* dosing should lead to consideration of therapy for moderate asthma.

Moderate Persistent Asthma

- Advance antiinflammatory program to *intermediate-dose* inhaled *corticosteroids* (e.g., 4 to 8 puffs of *beclomethasone* twice daily).
- If *nocturnal symptoms* are a problem or it is desired to limit steroid exposure, continue low-dose inhaled steroid therapy and add either a *long-acting β₂-agonist* (e.g., 1 to 2 puffs of *salmeterol* every 12 hours) or a methylxanthine (e.g., 300 mg of *extended-release theophylline* daily at bedtime) to the program. Never use a long-acting bronchodilator in the absence of corticosteroid therapy.
- Consider *montelukast* (10 mg every morning) as another alternative for limiting steroid dose in persons with mild to moderate disease.
- Continue treatment of acute symptoms with as-needed use of a *short-acting β₂-agonist*. Any requirement for *daily* or *increased* dosing should lead to consideration of therapy for severe asthma.
- Emphasize the need for *daily* monitoring of *peak flow* and increasing the dose of inhaled steroid at the first sign of a decline in peak flow.
- Continue as-needed use of a *short-acting β₂-agonist* for treatment of acute symptoms; continued requirements for daily or increased dosing should lead to consideration of therapy for severe asthma.

Severe Persistent Asthma

- Advance the antiinflammatory program to *high-dose* inhaled *corticosteroids* (e.g., 4 to 6 puffs of *beclomethasone* four times daily) and supplement with a long-acting β₂-agonist (e.g., 2 puffs of salmeterol every 12 hours) or sustained-release theophylline (300 mg every 12 hours, with regular monitoring of the serum theophylline level).
- For acute severe exacerbations, supplement inhaled steroids with a short course of high-dose *systemic glucocorticosteroids* (e.g., prednisone started at 40 to 60 mg/d and tapered to full cessation within 5 to 10 days).
- Emphasize to the patient the importance of regular daily *monitoring of peak flow* and prompt initiation of high-dose prednisone at the first sign of markedly declining airway function. Have the patient fill a prednisone prescription and keep it for prompt initiation of therapy. Inform the patient that any delay in initiating steroid therapy and overreliance on short-acting bronchodilators can be dangerous.
- Continue as-needed use of a *short-acting β₂-agonist* for treatment of acute symptoms and consider adding a trial of inhaled *ipratropium* (e.g., 2 puffs as needed) if β₂-agonist therapy alone does not suffice for an acute attack. Increase the number of puffs of short-acting bronchdilator and monitor the patient carefully if the exacerbation is marked (e.g., peak flow <60% of predicted). A short course of systemic steroids should be considered and started promptly if improvement is not rapid.
- Consider any persistent requirements for daily or increased dosing of bronchodilator therapy as indications to add daily systemic steroid therapy (e.g., 10 to 20 mg of prednisone every morning).

- Make repeated attempts to taper systemic steroids to the lowest dose sufficient to prevent attacks and, if possible, discontinue systemic steroids; if discontinuation of systemic steroids is not possible, then consider switching to alternate-day therapy (e.g., 10 to 20 mg every other day). To facilitate tapering and maintain control, continue inhaled corticosteroid therapy at full doses in conjunction with long-acting bronchodilator program.
- Taper systemic steroids slowly if the patient has been taking prednisone long enough to cause hypothalamic–pituitary–adrenal suppression (see Chapter 105). At times of stress and severe flares, be sure inhaled steroid therapy is at maximum doses and consider resuming full doses of systemic steroid therapy (e.g., 40 to 60 mg of prednisone per day) until episode passes.
- In *refractory cases*, check for and treat any exacerbating factors, such as exposure to an offending allergen, gastroesophageal reflux, sleep apnea, and allergic bronchopulmonary aspergillosis (suggested by an eosinophil count >1,000/mL). *Immunotherapy* is indicated if a single responsible allergen is identified. Check for *poor compliance* with the inhaled corticosteroid program and failure to monitor peak flows, which indicate the need for more patient education and counseling.

For All Patients

- Before treating for asthma, always briefly consider other causes of bronchospasm and wheezing.
- Identify offending allergens and irritants; consider skin testing, especially if a single allergen is suspected (e.g., seasonal asthma), and desensitization if a single allergen is discovered; design an avoidance program for those with multiple allergens; emphasize smoking cessation for those who continue to smoke.
- Encourage active patient participation in management by providing parameters (such as changes in peak flow or symptoms) for self-initiated adjustments in treatment. Be sure the patient is fully informed about medications, their side effects, and proper use.
- Teach proper use of the *hand-held peak flow meter, MDI*, and *spacer*. Demonstrate and check inhaler and peak flow meter technique. Consider breath-activated inhalers for persons who cannot use MDIs.
- Provide written instructions for carrying out the treatment programs for maintenance and exacerbation, with emphasis on what to do when. Keep it simple and customized to the patient's capacity for compliance. Directly elicit and address any patient concerns.
- Remind patients to avoid overreliance on short-acting bronchodilators for disease control and never to use antianxiety agents or sedatives in the setting of an exacerbation.
- Remember that a severe exacerbation (peak flow <60% of predicted) can occur with any category of asthma and that prompt initiation of a short course of prednisone (40 to 60 mg/d with rapid tapering to cessation in 5 to 10 days) should be considered if a prompt response to bronchodilators and full doses of inhaled steroids does not occur.
- Administer *trivalent influenza vaccine* each fall at least 6 weeks before the start of the flu season. Also administer *pneumococcal vaccine* (see Chapter 6).

- Arrange prompt emergency department care if signs of severe airway obstruction are present (e.g., peak flow reduced by 50%, pulsus paradoxus, $FEV_1 < 1$ L/s, use of accessory muscles of respiration).
- Consider referral for patients who require systemic steroids frequently or persistently.

A.H.G.

ANNOTATED BIBLIOGRAPHY

Adkinson NF, Eggleston PA, Eney D, et al. A controlled trial of immunotherapy for asthma in allergic children. N Engl J Med 1997;336:324. (*One of the few randomized, placebo-controlled trials of immunotherapy showing no benefit for multiple-allergen immunotherapy in children with perennial allergic asthma.*)

Aelony Y. "Noninvasive" oral treatment of asthma in the emergency room. Am J Med 1985;78:929. (*Most patients were fully controlled by nonparenteral means, which would indicate that most emergency department visits are unnecessary.*)

Altman LC, Findlay SR, Lopez M, et al. Adrenal function in adult asthmatics during long-term daily treatment with 800, 1,200, and 1,600 μg of triamcinolone acetonide. Chest 1992;101:1250. (*Inhalation therapy produced no major suppression of adrenal function.*)

Baigelman W, Chodosh S, Pizzuato D, et al. Sputum and blood eosinophils during corticosteroid treatment of acute exacerbations of asthma. Am J Med 1983;75:929. (*Eosinophil counts correlated with objective measures of response.*)

Balon J, Aker PD, Crowther ER, et al. A comparison of active and simulated chiropractic manipulation as adjunctive treatment for childhood asthma. N Engl J Med 1998;339:1013. (*A randomized, controlled trial of an alternative-medicine adjunct to treatment failed to demonstrate any subjective or objective benefit.*)

Burrows B, Lebowitz MD. The beta-agonist dilemma. N Engl J Med 1992;326:560. (*An editorial reassessing the role of β-agonist therapy; argues for a secondary rather than a primary role.*)

Burrows B, Martinez FD, Halonen M, et al. Association of asthma with serum IgE levels and skin-test reactivity to allergens. N Engl J Med 1989;320:271. (*Prevalence closely related to serum IgE levels; patients with both extrinsic and intrinsic asthma had evidence of immunologic hyperreactivity.*)

Busse WW. The precipitation of asthma by upper respiratory infections. Chest 1985;87:44S. (*A review of the mechanisms underlying virus-induced asthma.*)

Chan-Yeung M. Occupational asthma. Am Rev Respir Dis 1986;133:686. (*Useful review of occupations and compounds associated with occupational asthma; guides elimination of environmental precipitants.*)

Dompeling E, van Chayck CP, van Grunsven PM, et al. Slowing the deterioration of asthma and chronic obstructive pulmonary disease observed during bronchodilator therapy by adding inhaled corticosteroids. Ann Intern Med 1993;118:770. (*A prospective, randomized clinical trial showing improvements in flow rate, symptoms, and number of exacerbations.*)

Drazen JM, Israel E, Boushey HA, et al. Comparison of regularly scheduled with as-needed use of albuterol in mild asthma. N Engl J Med 1996;335:841. (*A multicenter, randomized, controlled, double-blinded trial showing no additional benefit from regularly scheduled use of β-agonist therapy in comparison with as-needed use.*)

Ernst P, Spitzer WD, Suisse S, et al. Risk of fatal and near-fatal asthma in relation to inhaled corticosteroid use. JAMA 1992;268:3462. (*Risk markedly reduced by its use.*)

Evans DJ, Taylor DA, Zetterstrom O, et al. A comparison of low-dose inhaled budesonide plus theophylline and high-dose inhaled budesonide for moderate asthma. N Engl J Med 1997;337:1412. (*In this double-blinded, placebo-controlled, randomized trial, modest doses of theophylline reduced steroid requirements.*)

Fiel B, Swartz MA, Glanz K, et al. Efficacy of short-term corticosteroid therapy in outpatient treatment of acute bronchial asthma. Am J Med 1983;75:259. (*A double-blinded, placebo-controlled study showing reductions in symptoms and rate of relapse.*)

Garbe E, Suissa S, LeLorier J. Association of inhaled corticosteroid use with cataract extraction in elderly patients. JAMA 1998;280:539. (*Case–control epidemiologic study finding a three-fold increased risk for cataract extraction with long-term use of high-dose inhaled steroids.*)

Goldstein RA, Paul WM, Metcalfe DD, et al. Asthma: NIH Conference. Ann Intern Med 1994;121:698. (*Excellent basic science review; 78 references.*)

Greenberger PA. Beclomethasone dipropironate for severe asthma during pregnancy. Ann Intern Med 1983;98:478. (*Prevalence of congenital malformations was within the normal range among patients using the drug during pregnancy.*)

Homer CJ. Asthma disease management. N Engl J Med 1997;337:1461. (*A detailed discussion of the possible contributions of disease management techniques in asthma care.*)

Ignacio-Garcia JM, Gonzalez-Santos P. Asthma self-management education program by home monitoring of peak expiratory flow. Am J Respir Crit Care Med 1995;151:353. (*Patient education and self-monitoring found critical to effective control.*)

Lange P, Parner J, Vestbo J, et al. A 15-year follow-up study of ventilatory function in adults with asthma. N Engl J Med 1998;339:1194. (*An important population-based natural history study from Copenhagen showing a clinically and statistically significant decline in FEV_1 over time among asthmatics in comparison with nonasthmatics.*)

Leff JA, Busse WW, Pearlman D, et al. Montelukast, a leukotriene-receptor antagonist, for the treatment of mild asthma and exercise-induced bronchoconstriction. N Engl J Med 1998;339:147. (*A multicenter, randomized, double-blinded study sponsored by the manufacturer of this leukotriene-receptor antagonist found it to be safe and effective in persons with mild, exercise-induced asthma.*)

Legorretta AP, Christian-Herman J, O'Connor RD, et al. Compliance with National Asthma Management Guidelines and Specialty Care. Arch Intern Med 1998;158:457. (*Compliance with preventive guidelines was especially poor among primary care physicians and their patients; compliance was correlated with frequency of emergency room visits and hospitalizations.*)

Malmstrom K, Rodriguez-Gomez G, Guerra J, et al. Oral montelukast, inhaled beclomethasone, and placebo for chronic asthma: a randomized, controlled trial. Ann Intern Med 1999;130:487. (*One of few well-designed comparison studies; oral montelukast found to be more effective than placebo, but not as effective as inhaled beclomethasone.*)

Mathison DA, Stevenson DD, Simon RA. Asthma and the home environment. Ann Intern Med 1982;97:128. (*Editorial describing the allergens associated with house dust, household pets, ubiquitous fungi, and nonallergic irritants.*)

McFadden ER. Methylxanthines in the treatment of asthma: the rise, the fall, and the possible rise again. Ann Intern Med 1991;115:323. (*Editorial reviewing the changing view of methylxanthine use and suggesting a retained role.*)

McFadden ER. Exertional dyspnea and cough as preludes to acute attacks of bronchial asthma. N Engl J Med 1975;292:555. (*Classic article documenting that intermittent episodes of cough and breathlessness represent variants of asthmatic attacks.*)

McFadden ER Jr. Dosages for corticosteroids in asthma. Ann Rev Respir Dis 1993;147:1306. (*Recommendations by a leading authority.*)

McFadden ER, El Sanadi N, Strauss L, et al. The influence of parasympatholytics on the resolution of acute attacks of asthma. Am J Med 1997;102:7. (*A prospective sequential study performed in the emergency department setting showing little additional benefit from addition of ipratropium to the regimen for acute severe flares.*)

Mullarkey MF, Lammert JK, Blumenstein BA. Long-term methotrexate treatment in corticosteroid-dependent asthma. Ann Intern Med 1990;112:577. (*Encouraging report on use of immunosuppressive therapy in place of systemic steroids.*)

National Asthma Education Program. Guidelines for the diagnosis and management of asthma II. Bethesda, MD: National Heart, Lung and Blood Institute, April 1997; US Dept of Health and Human Services publication NIH 92-3091. (*National consensus guidelines, which include an emphasis on prevention and self-monitoring.*)

Nelson JA, Strauss L, Skowronski M, et al. Effect of long-term salmeterol treatment on exercise-induced asthma. N Engl J Med 1998;339:141. (*In a small but well-designed placebo-controlled, random-order, double-blinded crossover trial, long-term administration of salmeterol twice daily continued to provide protection, but the duration of the effect after each dose declined with time.*)

Newhouse MT, Dolovich P. Control of asthma by aerosols. N Engl J Med 1986;315:870. (*Very useful review, with good section on proper technique.*)

Pauwels RA, Lofdahl C-G, Postma DS, et al. Effect of inhaled formoterol and budesonide on exacerbation of asthma. N Engl J Med 1997;337:1405. (*In a randomized trial of asthma patients with exacerbations while on inhaled corticosteroid therapy, the addition of long-acting inhaled β-agonist therapy was superior to high-dose inhaled steroids and without serious adverse effects.*)

Petty TL. Circadian variations in chronic asthma and chronic obstructive pulmonary disease. Am J Med 1988;85[Suppl 1B]:21. (*Documents worsening pulmonary status at night.*)

Picken HA, Greenfield S, Teres D, et al. Effect of local standards on the implementation of national guidelines for asthma. Primary care agreement with national asthma guidelines. J Gen Intern Med 1998;13:659. (*How local physicians respond to national practice guidelines for asthma care; role of customization by primary care physicians.*)

Pope AM. Indoor allergens—assessing and controlling adverse health effects. JAMA 1993;269:2721. (*Brief summary of this increasingly important issue.*)

Rosenstreich DL, Eggleston P, Kattan M, et al. The role of cockroach allergy and exposure to cockroach allergen in causing morbidity among inner-city children with asthma. N Engl J Med 1997;336:1356. (*An important discovery that might explain the high prevalence of asthma among inner city persons.*)

Selner JC. Helping asthmatic patients control their environment. J Respir Dis 1986;8:83. (*Useful practical advice.*)

Shim C, Williams MH Jr. Effects of odors in asthma. Am J Med 1986;80:18. (*Significant decline in FEV$_1$ and worsening of symptoms with exposure to one or more common odors.*)

Simons FER, the Canadian Beclomethasone Dipropionate-Salmeterol Xinafoate Study Group. A comparison of belcomethasone, salmeterol, and placebo in children with asthma. N Engl J Med 1997;337:1659. (*Randomized, placebo-controlled trial; beclomethasone the more effective, but it slowed growth rate in children.*)

Spitzer WO, Siussa S, Ernst P, et al. The use of beta-agonists and the risk of death and near-death from asthma. N Engl J Med 1992;326:501. (*Provocative data; study documents increased risk for treatment refractoriness and death associated with prolonged and excessive β-agonist use.*)

Stephenson BJ, Rowe BH, Haynes RB, et al. Is this patient taking the treatment as prescribed? JAMA 1993;269:2779. (*An excellent piece on compliance with asthma therapy.*)

Weinberger M, Hendeles L. Slow-release theophylline: rationale and basis for product selection. N Engl J Med 1983;308:760. (*Detailed review of these preparations; 35 references.*)

Welsh PW, Reed CE, Conrad E. Timing of once-a-day theophylline dose to match peak blood level with diurnal variation in severity of asthma. Am J Med 1986;80:1098. (*Nocturnal use especially effective.*)

Wrenn K, Slovis CM, Murphy F, et al. Aminophylline therapy for acute bronchospastic disease in the emergency room. Ann Intern Med 1991;115:241. (*Admission rate greatly reduced, even though no additional bronchodilation produced.*)

49

Management of Tuberculosis

BENJAMIN DAVIS
HARVEY B. SIMON

The primary care physician most commonly encounters tuberculosis (TB) as a positive tuberculin skin test result in the absence of active infection. An estimated 7% of the U.S. population may fall into this category. Alternatively, the primary care clinician sees active TB, which is becoming increasingly common among HIV-positive persons and other high-risk populations (see Chapter 38). Through the years, diagnosis and treatment have shifted from the sanitarium and specialist to the community and primary physician.

The rapid diagnosis and treatment of TB are impaired by several factors, including inadequate sensitivity of skin testing and sputum smears, a wide variety of clinical presentations, the several weeks required to obtain confirmatory cultures and antibiotic sensitivities, long treatment regimens (with associated adherence problems), and the emergence of drug-resistant strains. In addition, many clinicians have little experience with the disease and often do not suspect its presence. Even patients admitted to university hospitals may experience a delay in diagnosis, with some cases recognized only at autopsy. In addition, the management of TB has undergone such tremendous changes that studies have demonstrated suboptimal management by many general physicians in the United States. Clearly, the diagnosis and treatment of TB pose major challenges for the primary physician.

PATHOPHYSIOLOGY AND EPIDEMIOLOGY

Virtually all cases are acquired through *person-to-person aerosol* transmission of a nonmotile, acid-fast, gram-positive rod. People with active pulmonary infection shed infected droplets, which are then aerosolized into the environment. Because most infectious patients discharge relatively few organisms, casual contacts are at low risk for infection, and most secondary cases occur among household members, schoolmates, or other close contacts of the index case. TB is more common in immigrants and population groups in which crowding, poverty (especially homelessness), or a high risk for HIV infection is commonplace (see Chapter 38). Among HIV-infected patients, the risk for disease after infection is increased 1,000-fold. Serious outbreaks (with attack rates of 10%) have been reported among patients in hospital wards with a large concentration of AIDS patients.

Most persons harboring the tubercle bacillus mount an immune response sufficient to prevent progression from *primary infection* to clinical illness; they manifest a positive skin test result. About 5% of infected persons fail to contain the primary infection and progress to *active primary disease* within 2 years of initial infection. The proportion of infected persons who progress is much higher among AIDS patients. In the past, primary infection occurred almost entirely in childhood; however, as the epidemiology of tuberculosis has changed (see Chapter 38), primary tuberculosis is now also seen in adults, particularly among elderly nursing home residents and patients on AIDS wards. *Nosocomial tuberculosis* may be developing into an important problem. A worrisome characteristic of some nosocomial outbreaks has been the emergence of organisms *resistant* to one or more antituberculous drugs.

Another 5% of infected patients (again, a higher proportion of AIDS patients) experience *reactivation of latent endogenous infection*, most often within 2 to 4 years of the initial infection or at times of lowered host resistance. However, reactivation can occur many decades after initial infection, as reported among elderly nursing home residents. More than one fifth of patients with reactivated disease have histories of inadequately treated clinical TB. In many instances, a discrete insult to host defenses, such as steroid therapy, alcoholism, malnutrition, neoplastic disease, HIV infection, or gastrectomy, can be implicated, but at times it is impossible to identify the reason for reactivation.

Until the advent of polymerase chain reaction (PCR) technology and development of the techniques of molecular epidemiology, the vast majority of active TB cases in the United States were thought to represent reactivation of latent disease. Several recent studies, however, have suggested that in large metropolitan centers such as San Francisco and New York City, between 35% and 40% of active tuberculosis cases represent *newly acquired infection*. Although the AIDS epidemic accounts for some of this change in epidemiology, it is clear that clinical disease develops shortly after infection in more immunologically "normal" persons than was previously thought.

CLINICAL PRESENTATION AND COURSE

Primary Infection. As noted above, more than 90% of patients are entirely asymptomatic at the time of primary infection and can be identified only through conversion of the tuberculin skin test from negative to positive. The majority of these patients have normal findings on chest radiography. Among the 10% who progress directly to symptomatic disease, four broad syndromes can be identified: (a) *Atypical pneumonia* is the most common, characterized by fever and nonproductive cough. Chest x-ray films may show unilateral lower lobe patchy parenchymal infiltrates or paratracheal or hilar adenopathy. Although such patients should receive full antituberculous chemotherapy when the disease is diagnosed (see below), it usually resolves even without treatment. (b) *Tuberculous pleurisy* and effusion are accompanied by fever, cough, pleuritic chest pain, and occasionally dyspnea. Chest x-ray films reveal unilateral pleural effusions, often without identifiable parenchymal lesions. The tuberculin test result is almost always strongly positive. Diagnosis depends on examination and culture of the pleural fluid or on percutaneous needle biopsy of the pleura because sputum cultures are positive for organisms in only 30% of such cases. (c) *Direct progression* from primary disease to upper lobe involvement is another presentation. (d) Early *systemic dissemination*, which used to be seen exclusively in children, now occurs in HIV-infected patients.

Reactivation (Postprimary) Tuberculosis. Notwithstanding our greater understanding of primary disease, this is still the most common clinical form of TB. Symptoms usually begin insidiously and progress during a period of many weeks or months before diagnosis. Constitutional symptoms are often prominent, including *anorexia*, *weight loss*, and *night sweats*. Most patients have *low-grade fever*, but higher temperatures and even chills may be seen occasionally when the disease progresses more rapidly. In addition, most patients present with pulmonary symptoms, including *cough* and *sputum production*. Dyspnea is relatively uncommon in the absence of underlying chronic lung disease. A frequent complaint is *hemoptysis*, often in the form of bright red streaks of blood caused by bronchial irritation. Although physical examination findings are usually nondiagnostic, chest x-ray films are highly suggestive of the diagnosis. Typical features include *infiltration* in the *posterior apical* pulmonary segments, which may be unilateral or bilateral and progresses to frank *cavitation*. Apical lordotic views and chest tomography may be helpful in documenting cavitary disease. Occasionally, postprimary TB may involve the lower lung fields, and in rare instances the chest radiographic appearance may be normal. The tuberculin skin test result is positive in about 80% of patients with reactivation tuberculosis; patients with advanced disease are often malnourished and thus anergic.

Extrapulmonary Tuberculosis. Approximately 20% of all newly recognized cases of TB in the United States are extrapulmonary. Although the frequency of pulmonary TB is constant, the incidence of extrapulmonary disease is increasing, largely among HIV-positive patients (see below). Although the clinical features of extrapulmonary TB vary widely, certain generalizations are possible. Past history is not a reliable guide to the diagnosis. Only 25% of patients have a past history of TB; of these, virtually all have been inadequately treated. A long latent period between the first episode of infection and the extrapulmonary presentation is typical. Approximately 50% of patients with extrapulmonary disease have entirely normal chest radiographic findings; most of the others have stigmata of old, inactive pulmonary disease, and a minority have coexisting active pulmonary infection. Although extrapulmonary disease can involve all organ systems, either singly or in various combinations, the most commonly affected areas are the genitourinary tract, musculoskeletal system, and lymph nodes.

The most common type of extrapulmonary TB is infection of an individual organ system. The patient is most often afebrile and can be entirely free of constitutional complaints. The illness typically pursues an indolent course characterized by local organ dysfunction and eventual destruction rather than by progressive general decline. In fact, the clinical presentation in these persons more often suggests neoplastic disease than infection. The tuberculin skin test result is almost always positive. Clinical syndromes in this category include genitourinary tuberculosis, tuberculous arthritis and osteomyelitis, tuberculous lymphadenitis, and many others.

HIV-positive patients with TB may experience extrapulmonary disease and dissemination early on. When CD4-cell counts are well preserved (see Chapter 13), tuberculous infection usually causes pulmonary disease that resembles TB in HIV-negative persons. However, in more severely immunocompromised HIV patients, TB is often disseminated at presentation. A high incidence of tuberculous *meningitis* has been reported among HIV-positive patients, often in conjunction with *diffuse lymphadenopathy*. The occurrence of pulmonary or extrapulmonary TB in patients with HIV infection fulfills the criteria for the diagnosis of AIDS.

In HIV-infected patients with disseminated disease, the result of the purified protein derivative (PPD) skin test is often negative. Chest radiographic findings are normal in more than 10% of patients. When infiltrates do occur, they are often nonspecific and involve the lower lobes. Despite these atypical features, the diagnosis can usually be established, if suspected, without much difficulty by visualizing or culturing the causative organism from the sputum or extrapulmonary sites.

Atypical Mycobacterial Infection. Clinical infection with *atypical mycobacteria* is not seen often in primary care practice. Representative syndromes caused by these organisms include cervical adenitis in children (scrofula), pulmonary infection, and cutaneous disease (swimming pool granuloma). Disseminated disease occasionally takes place in immunosuppressed persons. For example, *Mycobacterium avium-intracellulare* has been a major cause of disseminated infection in patients with AIDS. Unlike tuberculous infection in HIV-positive patients, which can be disseminated in the early stages of illness, *M. avium-intracellulare* infection does not cause disseminated disease until late.

DIAGNOSIS

The tuberculin *skin test* is the most sensitive test for the diagnosis of infection with *Mycobacterium tuberculosis* (see Chapter 38); it is far more sensitive than chest radiography. A positive tuberculin test result does not by itself prove the presence of active disease but does indicate that infection has occurred. Negative tuberculin reactions have been documented in 20% of patients with TB, particularly those with overwhelming or advanced disease, malnutrition, and debility. In HIV-positive patients, especially those with low CD4-cell counts, the rate of false-negative skin test results has been as high as 50%. When active pulmonary disease is present, the diagnosis of pulmonary TB can usually be confirmed by examination of the *sputum*, with precautions taken to *avoid spread the of organisms during efforts to obtain sputum*. If patients are not able to produce sputum spontaneously, attempts should be made to *induce sputum* with the aid of hydration, pulmonary physiotherapy, intermittent positive pressure breathing (IPPB), and mucolytic agents.

Bronchoscopy or *bronchoalveolar lavage* may be necessary for obtaining appropriate specimens. Although *cultures* are necessary for a positive diagnosis and are more sensitive than smears, sputum specimens should be examined microscopically either by the traditional *Ziehl-Neelsen (acid-fast) stain*, or by the newer Truant *fluorescent stain*. Sputum or bronchoscopic washings should be examined both directly and after concentration by centrifugation and digestion. Carefully collected individual specimens are preferred to a 24-hour pool of sputum and saliva. Cultures of first morning fasting *gastric aspirates* may also be helpful in children. Because gastric acid is toxic to mycobacteria, the collection bottles should contain a buffer such as sodium bicarbonate. Smears of gastric juice are misleading because of the potential presence of saprophytic mycobacteria, and they should not be performed.

Tissue biopsy is often required for the diagnosis of tuberculous pleurisy or extrapulmonary disease because sputum and gastric samples are usually negative for organisms in these situations.

PRINCIPLES OF TREATMENT

Prophylaxis in Uninfected Persons. In many parts of the world where tuberculosis is common, bacille Calmette-Guérin (BCG) vaccine is used for the prevention of primary infection. It is intended only for prophylaxis and should not be given to patients with positive skin test results (see Chapter 38). Because the incidence of tuberculosis is relatively low in the United States, BCG vaccination is not recommended in this country. All close contacts of patients with active pulmonary tuberculosis should be considered for *isoniazid* (INH) chemoprophylaxis, particularly if they are children, adolescents, or immunocompromised (see Chapter 38).

Prophylaxis in Tuberculin Converters and Persons with Latent Disease. Prevention of active TB can be achieved with INH (see Chapter 38 for detailed guidelines). Patients with a positive skin test result should be evaluated to exclude active infection. One needs to check for cough, fever, sputum production, pleuritic chest pain, lymphadenopathy, meningeal irritation, pleural effusion, pulmonary consolidation, and enlargement of the liver or spleen. Chest radiography is essential, and the results of complete blood cell count, differential, urinalysis, and liver function tests (particularly measurement of alkaline phosphatase) may provide clues of active disease (e.g., "sterile" pyuria or isolated elevation of alkaline phosphatase). If no active infection is identified, the patient should be reassured, and the potential risks and benefits of INH therapy should be explained so the patient can participate in therapeutic decisions.

Treatment of Patients with Active Tuberculosis. Antituberculous drugs are the cornerstone of therapy. Because the patient will not be contagious shortly after starting therapy, most treatment can be administered on an outpatient basis after a brief period in the hospital. The chemotherapy of tuberculosis is different from other antimicrobial programs and proceeds according to a unique set of principles:

- Multidrug regimens and completion of a full course of therapy are necessary to prevent the emergence of drug-resistant organisms.

- Single daily dosing is preferred.
- Prolonged chemotherapy is necessary. Nearly all patients can be cured with regimens lasting 6 months. However, HIV-infected persons may require longer treatment. When INH and rifampin cannot be used simultaneously because of patient intolerance or drug resistance, older, more prolonged regimens of 18 to 24 months are necessary.
- Directly observed therapy (DOT) given twice or thrice weekly should be considered for all new patients.
- No matter what regimen is chosen, it is important to follow patients closely to ensure compliance and monitor for drug efficacy and toxicity.
- Because chemotherapy will control the organisms, surgery is reserved for the treatment of complications, such as restrictive pericardial scarring.
- Elaborate programs of rest and diet have no place in the modern treatment of tuberculosis.
- Prolonged surveillance beyond 1 year after completion of a full course of therapy is generally not necessary because of the efficacy of current chemotherapeutic regimens; however, immunosuppressed patients and those with drug-resistant organisms require more prolonged follow-up.

As little as 2 weeks of multidrug therapy will greatly decrease the infectiousness of patients with tuberculosis, although a few mycobacteria may still be present on sputum smears or cultures. The decision of whether or not to hospitalize patients with newly diagnosed TB should take into account the clinical status of the patient in addition to the health and ages of other people living at home. Certainly, the presence at home of children (especially infants), pregnant women, or persons infected with HIV or having debilitating medical conditions should prompt hospitalization until the index patient can be reliably considered noninfectious. Patients with extrapulmonary tuberculosis are much less infectious and can sometimes be managed entirely as outpatients.

Ensuring Adherence. Poor adherence is the single most important cause of treatment failure and the emergence of multidrug-resistant strains. Conversion to negative cultures takes four times longer in nonadherent patients; their risk for acquiring drug-resistant disease is five times greater, and the treatment time needed to achieve cure is nearly twice as long. However, adherence is a notoriously difficult thing to predict in an individual patient. Probably the most reliable predictors of poor adherence are prior poor adherence, adolescence, and heavy alcohol or IV drug use. Socioeconomic status, race, and ethnicity should not be used to predict adherence.

DOT coupled with a free supply of the necessary drugs appears to be one of the most successful adherence strategies for persons with active tuberculosis. The wide use of DOT has been a cornerstone of public health measures for tuberculosis control in the 1990s and has undeniably contributed to the reversal of the rising incidence in active disease seen in the 1980s. *DOT should be considered initially for all patients with newly diagnosed TB.*

CASE REPORTING AND PATIENT EDUCATION

All cases of tuberculosis should be reported promptly to public health authorities, so that contacts can be investigated and appropriate control measures instituted. However, it must be remembered that, particularly in elderly patients, the diagnosis of tuberculosis still carries a social stigma and dire prognostic implications. Reassurance and education are therefore of great importance. It should be stressed that tuberculosis occurs in all social and economic classes, that modern chemotherapy is truly curative, and that prolonged periods of hospitalization and isolation are no longer necessary.

Patients who are candidates for INH prophylaxis should understand the risks and benefits of INH therapy. If INH therapy is recommended and accepted, the patient should be instructed to discontinue the medication and report to the physician if adverse effects are noted, including skin rash, fever, fatigue, anorexia, abdominal distress, jaundice, and peripheral neuropathic symptoms. The importance of full compliance with the drug regimen, be it for prophylaxis or treatment of active disease, must be stressed.

THERAPEUTIC RECOMMENDATIONS

Prophylaxis

- For more information, see Chapter 38.
- In the decision to use INH for prophylaxis, the risk for drug-induced hepatotoxicity (see next section, Antituberculous Chemotherapeutic Agents) must be weighed against the benefit of preventing active disease. The older the patient, the greater the risk for hepatitis, although the benefit usually outweighs risk, especially in populations with a high incidence of infection and active disease (see Chapter 38 for detailed guidelines).
- Prompt diagnosis and institution of an effective, individualized treatment program are essential to preventing the spread of disease and emergence of resistant organisms. Of particular importance is the early recognition of TB in HIV-infected patients. A high index of suspicion and an awareness of the potentially atypical presentations of TB in these patients (e.g., disseminated disease, meningitis) are essential.

Active Disease

- Patients with active pulmonary or extrapulmonary tuberculosis should be treated for 2 months with INH, rifampin, and pyrazinamide, followed INH and rifampin for 4 months, for a total duration of treatment of 6 months.
- Because nearly all centers in the United States currently report greater than 4% resistance to one of the drugs mentioned above, and because of the now-recognized importance of newly acquired infection, ethambutol (or streptomycin) should be included in the initial regimen until the results of drug susceptibility tests are known, at which time it can be stopped if the presence of a sensitive organism is confirmed.
- The above treatment regimen applies to patients with or without HIV infection. However, because relapse rates are higher in HIV-infected patients, careful clinical follow-up should be the rule. Many authorities advocate continuing INH and rifampin for 6 months following sputum conversion.
- If INH and rifampin cannot be administered simultaneously because of patient intolerance or drug resistance, multiple drug therapy should be continued for 18 to 24 months. Such patients should be referred to an infectious disease specialist or to the local public health authority for optimal management. For patients relapsing after a previous course of antitu-

berculous chemotherapy, or for patients in whom more widespread drug resistance is suspected, the initial therapy may involve six or more drugs and should be coordinated by an infectious disease specialist or public health authority.

- DOT should be considered initially for *all* patients in whom active TB is diagnosed. Twice- and thrice-weekly regimens have established efficacy when given as part of DOT.
- For use in *pregnancy*, INH, rifampin, and ethambutol all appear to be safe.
- After completion of therapy, all patients should be followed for 1 year, with monitoring for evidence of recurrence. Longer follow-up is appropriate for those with drug-resistant organisms, HIV-positivity, or suspected poor compliance.
- *Hospitalization* should be considered in the *initial stages of active pulmonary disease* to minimize the risk for spread. Chemotherapy for 2 weeks usually suffices to render the patient noninfectious.

Antituberculous Chemotherapeutic Agents

Isoniazid. Introduced into clinical use in the early 1950s, INH remains the single most important antituberculous drug. Of importance is the excellent tissue penetration of this small, water-soluble molecule. The distribution of INH includes the central nervous system, tuberculous abscesses, and intracellular sites. The major metabolism of INH is by hepatic acetylation. Although metabolites are excreted by the kidneys, it is not necessary to modify INH doses except in cases of advanced renal failure. INH is available both orally and parenterally. The usual dose is 5 mg/kg of body weight, not to exceed 300 mg/d for an adult.

The major adverse effects of INH include the following:

- *Neurotoxicity*, ranging from peripheral neuropathy (which can be prevented by administration of 50 mg of pyridoxine daily) to much less common manifestations, including encephalopathy, seizures, optic neuritis, and personality changes.
- *Hypersensitivity* reactions, including fever, rash, and rheumatic syndromes with or without the presence of antinuclear antibodies.
- *Hepatocellular injury*, including serious clinical hepatitis in fewer than 2% of cases, but a transient, clinically insignificant rise in transaminase levels in 10% to 20%. The risk for clinically significant hepatitis increases with age.

The U.S. Public Health Service does not recommend routine *transaminase* (aspartate aminotransferase and alanine aminotransferase) determinations in persons who are reliable and able to comply with directions for reporting symptoms of hepatitis. If transaminases are elevated before therapy is begun, however, it is prudent to monitor them at monthly intervals.

In symptomatic patients with an elevated transaminase, INH should be discontinued and liver function should be monitored. In asymptomatic persons with a mild elevation (up to 2.5 times normal), the drug can be continued, but the patient should be monitored weekly. If the transaminase level fails to return to normal in 3 to 4 weeks, it seems prudent to discontinue the INH. On the other hand, even if a patient is asymptomatic, a single, more substantial transaminase elevation may be grounds to discontinue the agent. Again, it must be emphasized that these are "rules of thumb" rather than precise guidelines. INH

treatment may be resumed cautiously in patients for whom it was stopped, with careful monitoring.

Rifampin is a major antituberculous drug and rivals INH in efficacy. Rifampin is a large, fat-soluble molecule that achieves excellent tissue penetration, including the central nervous system. The drug is excreted by the liver; modification of dosage is not required in renal failure but may be necessary in hepatic insufficiency. It is available in both oral and parenteral formulations. The average adult dose is 600 mg/d taken once daily. Patients should be cautioned to expect *orange discoloration of urine, sweat, tears,* and *saliva,* which is of no clinical significance.

Toxicities include *hypersensitivity* reactions (fever, rash, eosinophilia), *hematologic* toxicities (thrombocytopenia, leukopenia, hemolytic anemia), and *hepatitis* (including elevated transaminases in up to 10%). Drug interactions occur; rifampin increases the metabolism of warfarin, quinidine, oral contraceptives, and methadone. Rifampin should never be used in high-dose intermittent therapy because toxic reactions (including hemolytic anemia, thrombocytopenia, and hepatic failure) occur frequently. However, intermittent therapy in doses of 600 mg given twice weekly appears to be well tolerated.

Pyrazinamide, a derivative of nicotinic acid, was introduced in 1952 but was not widely used until its incorporation into short-course regimens in the 1980s. Like INH and rifampin, it is bactericidal, a major asset in short-course therapy. The drug is well absorbed from the gastrointestinal tract and is widely distributed in body tissues and fluids, including the cerebrospinal fluid. It is excreted by mixed hepatic and renal mechanisms. Major toxicities are hepatic dysfunction, hyperuricemia, and hypersensitivity. The usual dose is 15 to 30 mg/kg daily (maximum, 2 g).

Ethambutol was introduced clinically in the United States in 1967 and represented a major advance in antituberculous chemotherapy. Although ethambutol penetrates tissues well—including the central nervous system when the meninges are inflamed—it is not bactericidal; it is only bacteriostatic. The drug is excreted by the kidneys. Dose modification in renal failure should be based on serum ethambutol levels (available through the manufacturer), and patients with renal failure who require the drug should be monitored. The major toxicities of ethambutol include hypersensitivity reactions, such as fever and rash, and optic neuritis, which is dose-related and usually manifested first by a loss of color vision. Less common side effects include neuritis, gastrointestinal intolerance, headache, and hyperuricemia. The usual dose is 15 mg/kg daily; 25 mg/kg may be given daily for the first 2 months. Color vision and visual acuity should be monitored periodically because of a small risk for retinal injury; for this reason, the drug is usually not administered to young children.

Streptomycin, the first effective antituberculous drug, remains useful. Like other aminoglycosides, streptomycin has only a fair tissue distribution, being inactive at an alkaline pH in an anaerobic milieu and penetrating the cerebrospinal fluid very poorly. It must be given parenterally. Streptomycin is excreted by the kidneys, and the dosage should be reduced in patients with renal failure. Major toxicities include hypersensitivity reactions and *toxicity of the eighth nerve,* especially the vestibular division, which results in vertigo. The dose of streptomycin is 15 mg/kg, up to 1 g daily.

"Second-line" Antituberculous Drugs tend to be both less effective and more toxic than the standard agents, but occa-

sionally they are of critical importance in patients with drug-resistant tuberculosis and in those who cannot tolerate the standard therapies. Three of these agents are administered orally, including *paraaminosalicylic acid* (PAS), *ethionamide*, and *cycloserine*. For many years, PAS was considered a first-line drug, but because of its relatively weak tuberculostatic action and the very high incidence of gastrointestinal intolerance associated with its use, it has been relegated to a secondary role. Two other drugs available parenterally, kanamycin and capreomycin, are pharmacologically similar to streptomycin.

Newer Drugs. With the emergence of new multidrug-resistant strains has come an accelerated search for new antituberculous agents. Several fluoroquinolone antibiotics have some activity against *M. tuberculosis*, including *ciprofloxacin*. Their effectiveness has not clearly been demonstrated.

ANNOTATED BIBLIOGRAPHY

American Thoracic Society. Treatment of tuberculosis and tuberculous infection in adults and children. Am Rev Respir Crit Care Med 1994;149:1359. (*Current standards for the treatment of tuberculosis and administration of INH chemoprophylaxis.*)

Berenguer J, Moreno S, Laguna F, et al. Tuberculous meningitis in patients infected with the human immunodeficiency virus. N Engl J Med 1992;326:668. (*HIV-infected patients are at increased risk for TB meningitis.*)

Cohn DL, Catlin BJ, Peterson KL, et al. A 62-dose, 6-month therapy for pulmonary and extrapulmonary tuberculosis: a twice-weekly, directly observed, and cost-effective regimen. Ann Intern Med 1990;112:407. (*Demonstrates efficacy of a strategy for poorly compliant patients.*)

Combs DL, O'Brien RJ, Geiter LJ. USPHS tuberculosis short-course chemotherapy trial 21: effectiveness, toxicity, and acceptability. Ann Intern Med 1990;112:397. (*Outcome measures for a 6-month regimen of INH and rifampin plus pyrazinamide during the first 8 weeks were similar to those for a 9-month regimen of only INH and rifampin.*)

Davidson PT. Treating tuberculosis: what drugs, for how long? Ann Intern Med 1990;112:393. (*Editorial reviewing shorter-course regimens.*)

Dooley SW, Jarvis WR, Martone WJ, et al. Multidrug-resistant tuberculosis. Ann Intern Med 1992;117:3. (*Editorial summing up current knowledge of this serious condition and approaches to coping with it.*)

Edlin BR, Tokars JI, Grieco MH, et al. An outbreak of multidrug-resistant tuberculosis among hospitalized patients with the acquired immunodeficiency syndrome. N Engl J Med 1992;326:1514. (*Documents nosocomial transmission of multidrug-resistant infection among AIDS patients.*)

Frieden TR, Sterling T, Pablos-Mendez A, et al. Emergence of drug-resistant tuberculosis in New York City. N Engl J Med 1993;328:521. (*High prevalence among HIV-positive persons, IV drug abusers, and patients previously treated.*)

Goble M, Iseman MD, Madsen LA, et al. Treatment of 171 patients with pulmonary tuberculosis resistant to isoniazid and rifampin. N Engl J Med 1993;328:527. (*Overall response rate is only about 50%; risk proportional to number of drugs received before current therapy.*)

Horsburgh CR. *Mycobacterium avium* complex infection in the acquired immunodeficiency syndrome. N Engl J Med 1991;324:1332. (*Review of this important opportunistic mycobacterial infection in AIDS patients.*)

Kramer F, Modilevsky T, Waliany AR, et al. Delayed diagnosis of tuberculosis in patients with human immunodeficiency virus infection. Am J Med 1990;89:451. (*Delay in therapy was common among patients with HIV infection; high index of suspicion needed.*)

Pablos-Mendez, Knirsch CA, Barr RG, et al. Nonadherence in tuberculosis: predictors and consequences in New York City. Am J Med 1997;102:164. (*One of the best epidemiologic studies available, in which IV drug abuse and homelessness accounted for about 60% of cases of poor compliance, defined as 2 months or more of failure to take prescribed medications. Nonadherence was associated with a fourfold increase in time required to convert to negative culture, a fivefold increase in risk for drug resistance, nearly a doubling of treatment time required to achieve cure, and twice the likelihood of failure to complete treatment.*)

Small PM, Schecter GF, Goodman PC, et al. Treatment of tuberculosis in patients with advanced human immunodeficiency virus infection. N Engl J Med 1991;324:289. (*Conventional therapy was effective in sterilizing the sputum, improving the chest radiographic pattern, and preventing relapse.*)

Snider DE, Roper WL. The new tuberculosis. N Engl J Med 1992;326:703. (*Editorial addressing the emergence of drug-resistant strains and the rapid transmission of infection among HIV-infected patients.*)

Stead WW. Pathogenesis of the sporadic case of tuberculosis. N Engl J Med 1967;277:1008. (*Lucid and important overview of the "unitary concept" of the pathogenesis of TB. This excellent article clarifies the relationship between primary infection, inactive disease, and reactivated tuberculosis.*)

Stead WW, Kerby GR, Schlueter DP, et al. The clinical spectrum of primary tuberculosis in adults. Ann Intern Med 1968;68:73. (*Classic clinical study of primary TB, which includes an excellent summary of the wide spectrum of events that may occur after initial infection by* M. tuberculosis.)

Stead WW, Lofgren JP, Warren E, et al. Tuberculosis as an endemic and nosocomial infection among the elderly in nursing homes. New Engl J Med 1985;312:1483. (*Exogenous infection can occur in the elderly, and nosocomial TB may be an important problem in nursing homes.*)

Stead WW, To T, Harrison RW, et al. Benefit–risk considerations in preventive treatment for tuberculosis in elderly persons. Ann Intern Med 1987;107:843. (*INH treatment of nursing home patients who had definite skin test conversions was beneficial, and benefits outweighed the risk for hepatitis.*)

Sterling TR, Alwood K, Gachuhi R et al. Relapse rate after short-course (6-month) treatment of tuberculosis in HIV-infected and uninfected persons. AIDS 1999;13:1899. (*Relapse rate of 6.4% in HIV-infected persons, same as that in HIV-seronegative persons.*)

50
Management of the Common Cold
WILLIAM A. KORMOS

The term "common cold" describes a self-limited catarrhal illness caused by a variety of respiratory viruses. It is indeed a common problem, with adults averaging two to four colds per year and almost 7 days lost from work per person per year. Although most patients treat their symptoms at home, physicians are still frequently consulted for upper respiratory infections. The primary task for the physician is to distinguish the common cold from bacterial infections, allergic conditions, and epidemic diseases such as influenza. Once the common cold is diagnosed, reassurance about the self-limited nature of the disease and patient education about its predominantly viral cause is the next step. However, upper respiratory tract infections continue to be a great source of inappropriate use of antibiotics. A recent survey demonstrated that physicians prescribe antibiotics to half of patients labeled with "colds." Instead, physicians should be knowledgeable about symptomatic therapies, including over-the-counter remedies. A targeted treatment plan aimed at the predominant symptoms is not only more effective but also more responsible.

PATHOPHYSIOLOGY AND CLINICAL PRESENTATION

The oropharynx and nasopharynx are lined by a stratified squamous epithelium and are normally teeming with a varied microbial flora. In addition, many potentially pathogenic bacteria can temporarily reside on these epithelial surfaces as "colonizers" without causing true infection. With a few exceptions, such as herpes simplex virus and the Epstein-Barr virus, viruses are not usually long-term members of the normal flora of the respiratory tract.

Numerous host defenses protect the upper airway from infection. The first of these defenses are mechanical; particulate matter is expelled by the cough and sneeze reflexes, entrapped by viscous mucous secretions, and propelled outward by ciliary action. In addition, local immunologic defenses attempt to deal with organisms that have breached the mechanical barriers. These defenses include lymphoid tissue, respiratory secretions that contain immunoglobulin A antibodies, and a rich vasculature capable of rapidly delivering phagocytic leukocytes. Once in the nasal cavity, viruses gain access to the upper airway by binding to ICAM-1 (an intercellular adhesion molecule). Experimental trials are being conducted in which soluble ICAM-1 is used to block this step in the initiation of infection.

Mechanisms of transmission include *airborne transmission* of virus-laden respiratory secretions via small aerosolized particles that remain suspended or large particles that travel only a few feet. However, the most efficient means of transmission is *direct mucous membrane contact* with virus, usually on contaminated hands. Self-inoculation of viruses surviving on the hands is accomplished by touching one's nose or eyes. Children remain an important reservoir of these viruses. The timeless motherly warning that "you'll catch cold if you get wet or damp" has not been borne out by experimental studies, which have demonstrated equal susceptibility in chilled and non-chilled hosts. However, evidence from prospective controlled studies suggests that *psychological stress*, especially chronic life stresses and poor social supports, can increase the risk for infection.

The common cold is caused by viral agents, mostly from five major families of viruses. *Rhinoviruses* are the most common viral agent associated with upper respiratory tract illness. Because there are more than 110 antigenic serotypes, cross-immunity does not exist, and reinfection with another serotype right after a recent cold is common. Coronavirus, parainfluenza virus, coxsackievirus, and respiratory syncytial virus account for the rest of the etiologic agents. *Influenza A* and *influenza B* produce a more severe syndrome that overlaps with the common cold. Influenza infection typically occurs in the winter months (December to March) in the northern hemisphere. The clinical syndrome consists of fever and diffuse myalgia, often accompanied by a nonproductive cough and headache. Lack of fever significantly decreases the probability of influenza. Patients with underlying cardiopulmonary disease and the elderly are at higher risk for development of a secondary bacterial pneumonia following influenza infection.

Incubation periods for viral upper respiratory infections range from 1 to 5 days; virus shedding lasts up to 3 weeks. Typical symptoms include coryza, pharyngitis, laryngitis, headache, malaise, and fever, in various combinations. Experimental evidence suggests that these symptoms are more the results of the body's response to the infection (through mediators like bradykinin, prostaglandin, interleukin, and histamine) than the actual viral infection itself. Ear and sinus discomfort also are often present, frequently caused by mucosal edema that impairs drainage (see Chapters 218 and 219).

Whether known as the common cold, nasopharyngitis, or upper respiratory infection, these problems generally resolve spontaneously. Common viral upper respiratory infections rarely progress to pneumonia; most colds resolve spontaneously within 1 week, although symptoms may linger up to 2 weeks in one fourth of patients.

DIAGNOSIS

The diagnosis of the "common cold" remains a clinical one, based on the typical presentation. Patients should be examined for localized bacterial infection, such as otitis media, sinusitis, or streptococcal pharyngitis (see Chapters 218, 219, and 220). If the patient presents with symptoms typical of influenza, further diagnostic testing can be considered with *rapid testing*, in which antibodies to common influenza antigens are usually used. The sensitivity of these tests appears to be high, and is even higher if nasopharyngeal washings rather than a swab are sent. Although not widely in use at present, these tests may become more important as new treatments for influenza become available (see below). On the other hand, identification of the specific virus causing the "common cold" is neither practical nor important.

PRINCIPLES OF MANAGEMENT

Prevention

The best things one can do to avoid "catching" a cold are to avoid aerosol exposure, wash hands, and keep hands away from mucous membranes (conjunctivae, nasal and oral mucosae). Gargling with "antiseptic" mouthwash is of no benefit. Initial studies on the use of inhaled α_2-interferon have shown promising results for the prevention of rhinovirus infection, but such approaches remain experimental. The enthusiasm surrounding the use of high-dose vitamin C (ascorbic acid) for prophylaxis has waned as controlled studies have failed to demonstrate efficacy. Similarly, zinc lozenges have proved no better than placebo in controlled trials.

Symptomatic Relief

Therapeutic efforts are directed toward relieving nasal congestion, sneezing, rhinorrhea, headache, and grippelike symptoms and preventing complications such as otitis, sinusitis, and lower respiratory tract infection. Targeted therapy aimed at the most bothersome symptoms is preferred to all-inclusive cold remedies, which often contain irrational mixtures or subtherapeutic doses of active ingredients. Sympathomimetics remain the mainstay of decongestant therapy. Data suggesting a cholinergic pathophysiology for rhinorrhea and sneezing have stimulated interest in new forms of anticholinergic therapy.

Decongestants can be helpful, not only for providing symptomatic relief but also for preventing sinus and eustachian tube obstruction that can result in sinusitis and otitis media, respectively.

α-Adrenergic Agents are the most commonly used decongestants. They work by causing generalized vasoconstriction, thereby reducing the formation of secretions. Because they produce systemic vasoconstriction, sympathomimetics may raise blood pressure when used in doses sufficient to alleviate nasal congestion. No oral adrenergic agent provides selective local vasoconstriction; *sympathomimetic nasal sprays* (e.g., Afrin) are more effective for this purpose but may be associated with rebound congestion after as little as 3 days of continuous use, leading to difficulty discontinuing use and an increased risk of chronic abuse. According to most authorities, sympathomimetic nasal sprays are good for very short-term therapy, whereas oral preparations are better when treatment is to continue for longer than 3 to 4 days.

Anticholinergic Agents have been used for years in the treatment of the common cold, mostly in the form of over-the-counter *sedating first-generation antihistamines*, which exert an atropine-like drying effect. It is this effect, not antihistaminic activity, that probably accounts for the symptomatic usefulness of anticholinergics in patients bothered by profuse rhinorrhea and excessive sneezing. However, their marked drying effect can exacerbate symptoms of congestion and cause upper airway obstruction by impairing the flow of mucus. In addition, they cause drowsiness, a side effect that may impair daytime functioning, although it can provide some nighttime rest. These agents can also worsen symptomatic benign prostatic hypertrophy and glaucoma and should be avoided by patients with these conditions. Use of a prescription *second-generation, nonsedating antihistamine* is irrational and has *no place* in management of the common cold because these agents have little anticholinergic activity and cold symptoms have no allergic pathophysiology. Nonetheless, antihistamines continue to be widely consumed for use in colds, both in prescription form (which is extremely expensive and wasteful) and in over-the-counter preparations, usually in combination with a sympathomimetic and other substances (see below).

Ipratropium, a topically active anticholinergic agent now available in a nasal spray preparation, is being heavily promoted for relief of nasal symptoms of the common cold. In a placebo-controlled, double-blind, randomized trial, the nasal spray preparation provided a significant reduction in subjective and objective measures of rhinorrhea and sneezing in comparison with saline placebo spray and with no treatment. Of note, significant benefit was also found with use of the saline control spray in comparison with no treatment. Global ratings by patients for overall effectiveness followed a similar pattern. Observed side effects included increased nasal dryness and blood-tinged mucus in approximately 10% to 15% of subjects. No cases of sinusitis or marked nasal obstruction were reported, which suggests that short-term use of the spray (up to 5 days) might be reasonably well tolerated. The nasal spray is expensive.

Analgesics are useful for relief of the headache, fever, and achiness that often accompany a cold. *Aspirin* and *acetaminophen* have similar analgesic and antipyretic effects and are key ingredients in the combination cold remedies. However, both have been found capable of delaying the immune response to experimental rhinovirus infection, although neither prolongs viral shedding. Nonprescription doses of *ibuprofen* showed similar effects, but prescription doses of *naproxen* did not alter viral shedding or antibody response in one trial. All remain clinically useful for symptomatic relief of the headache, myalgias, and fever that may accompany a cold. Salicylate derivatives such as salicylamide are sometimes used, although they are much less effective than aspirin. Of all the analgesics, plain aspirin is by far the least costly; the other agents can be expensive.

Expectorants and Heated Humidification. Expectorants are included in many preparations in the belief that they stimulate the flow of mucus. There is no evidence to support this view, although these agents are widely prescribed and requested by patients. More important is adequate *hydration*, which helps loosen secretions and prevent upper airway obstruction and the complications that may ensue. *Warm fluids* (including tea and, yes, chicken soup) can increase the rate of mucous flow, providing some symptomatic relief, as can *inhaled steam* (another of grandmother's remedies) or use of a dilute saline nasal spray.

Research suggesting that increasing the nasal mucosal temperature to 37°C could limit viral replication and decrease nasal congestion led to a renewed interest in the inhalation of warm, humidified air. A double-blinded study of steam inhalation through an *active device* showed *no significant benefit* over placebo therapy, although both were associated with considerable subjective improvement. An expensive heated nebulizer device (the Viralizer) has been heavily promoted as a means of promptly and completely relieving cold symptoms. Controlled study has failed to confirm such excessive claims.

Cough Suppressants, including narcotics such as *codeine* and non-narcotic agents such as *dextromethorphan*, are effective and useful symptomatically, especially in allowing the patient to sleep uninterrupted by cough. In many patients, a decongestant is even more effective in suppressing cough because postnasal drip accounts for much of the cough stimulus. These agents are commonly available in combination with expectorants, although they may be prescribed alone, which is more sensible therapy.

Zinc is thought to inhibit viral attachment and replication and improve cellular immune function. Such effects have stimulated interest in its use as a treatment for the common cold. The results of well-designed, controlled studies utilizing zinc gluconate lozenges have been equally divided between showing efficacy and showing no benefit. In the studies with positive findings, adequate blinding has been questioned because zinc lozenges have a distinct taste that may alert study subjects to their allotted treatment. The studies with negative findings have been criticized for subtherapeutic doses or ineffective preparations. One highly publicized study of 100 patients recruited from hospital employees demonstrated a significant reduction (nearly 40%) in the duration of illness, and also in the duration of coughing, nasal drainage and congestion, hoarseness, headache, and sore throat. The lozenges in this study contained 13.3 mg of zinc, and patients were instructed to take them every 2 hours while awake (average of six per day). Side effects included nausea and a bad taste in the mouth, experienced by most of the patients. Patients may be informed of the possible benefit of zinc lozenges but should be forewarned about the likely side effects.

Echinacea. Extracts from plants of the genus *Echinacea* have gained widespread acceptance in Germany as a treatment for the common cold. These plant products are postulated to have immunomodulator activity, such as macrophage activation and interleukin production. Although many randomized trials have suggested a benefit in the reduction of symptoms, the interpretation of results is complicated by the variety of species used (*E. purpurea*, *E. pallida*, and *E. angustifolia*) and the different plant parts (root or herb) and formulations (tablets, liquid extracts, capsules). Further studies based on standardized preparations and validated outcome measures will be needed before recommendations may be made for or against the use of *Echinacea*.

Other Agents and Combination Preparations. Americans spend nearly a billion dollars annually on over-the-counter cold remedies. Most contain a combination of ingredients, including first-generation sedating antihistamines, sympathomimetic amines, and analgesics. Some even contain more than one antihistamine or sympathomimetic. Antitussives, *atropine*, *caffeine*, *vitamin C*, *belladonna alkaloids*, and expectorants are other common additives. *Antacids*, *laxatives*, *quinine*, and *papaverine* are found occasionally. In general, these combination preparations should not be recommended as first-line therapy. As noted above, the vitamin C included has not been shown to have any significant effect, even when given in gram doses.

Management of Influenza

If the diagnosis of influenza is confirmed or highly suspected, several medications may be useful in decreasing the duration of symptoms if administered within the first 48 hours of the illness. *Amantadine* and *rimantadine* are oral antiviral drugs effective against influenza A only. Rimantadine is more expensive but has fewer side effects, notably less central nervous system effects. The dosage for both drugs is 100 mg twice daily except in the elderly, in whom decreased drug clearance allows for once-daily dosing. The drug should be discontinued after 3 to 5 days (or earlier if symptoms resolve) to decrease the opportunity for drug resistance, which may occur in up to one third of treated patients.

Neuraminidase inhibitors, zanamivir and oseltamivir, are newly approved agents for the treatment of influenza. These drugs are sialic acid analogues that inhibit the viral neuraminidase enzyme, essential to replication for both influenza A and influenza B. Early randomized trials of these agents show a decrease in the duration of illness of 1 to 1.5 days if the drug is administered within 48 hours of symptom onset, similar to the effect seen with the older agents. Zanamivir is administered by an inhaler twice daily; oseltamivir is given as a pill (75 mg) twice daily. The advantage of these newer agents is their activity against both influenza A and influenza B; they have not been in use long enough to determine whether viral resistance will be problematic. In addition, because the average cost of these agents is at least 10 times greater than that of influenza vaccine, vaccination is clearly the more cost-effective method to avoid flu symptoms.

PATIENT EDUCATION

Among the most frustrating experiences in primary care practice is the request by patients suffering from a cold for *antibiotics*. Explaining that antibiotics have no role in an uncomplicated viral upper respiratory infection can be time-consuming at best and has the potential to develop into a power struggle. A proactive approach is to send educational materials to patients at the beginning of the upper respiratory infection season. Pamphlets and other informational materials are much appreciated by patients and can help cut down on unnecessary visits and telephone calls. They should include helpful hints at self-care and the indications for seeking medical attention (e.g., high fever; marked pain or tenderness in an ear or sinus; increasingly purulent sputum, dyspnea, pleuritic chest pain). The role of antibiotics in the treatment of viral upper respiratory infection should also be reviewed (i.e., only for complications such as otitis and sinusitis), in addition to the risks of unnecessary antibiotic therapy (e.g., allergic reactions, alteration of bacterial flora, emergence of resistant strains). Unnecessary office visits and telephone calls have been reduced by as much as 30% to 40% through well-designed educational efforts.

THERAPEUTIC RECOMMENDATIONS

Prevention is difficult, but *hand washing,* keeping fingers away from mucous membranes, and avoidance of droplet exposure may help. Relief from cold symptoms and avoidance of complications are facilitated by rest, adequate fluid intake, aspirin, and perhaps inhalation of steam. Taking a *cough suppressant* before bed (e.g., 15 mg of codeine sulfate) and using a *sympathomimetic* nasal decongestant spray for a few days (e.g., phenylephrine; see Chapter 219) may aid in symptomatic management and are superior to expensive combination agents. Symptoms of incapacitating rhinorrhea and sneezing not well controlled by *first-generation antihistamines* may be treated with a short course of *ipratropium* nasal spray (two sprays of a 0.06% solution in each nostril four times daily). Proactive patient education just before the beginning of the cold season may help reduce unnecessary office visits, telephone calls, and requests for antibiotics. Zinc and *Echinacea* remain popular among patients, but their efficacy has not been clearly demonstrated. *Second-generation antihistamines* and antibiotics are of no use in an uncomplicated viral upper respiratory infection.

A.G.M.

ANNOTATED BIBLIOGRAPHY

Barrett B, Vohmann M, Calabrese C. *Echinacea* for upper respiratory infection. J Fam Pract 1999;48:628. (*A review of published trials of* Echinacea *in the prevention and treatment of upper respiratory infections. Although results appear positive, methodologic quality is questioned.*)

Cohen S, Tyrrell DAJ, Smith AP. Psychological stress and susceptibility to the common cold. N Engl J Med 1991;325:606. (*Careful, controlled, prospective study showing a significant, although not particularly strong, relation between stress and risk for getting a cold.*)

Coulehan JL, Eberhard S, Kapner L, et al. Vitamin C and acute illness in Navajo schoolchildren. N Engl J Med 1976;295:973. (*Double-blinded, placebo-controlled trial in 868 schoolchildren, failing to show prophylactic or therapeutic benefit.*)

Douglas RG, Lindgren KM, Couch RB. Exposure to cold environment and rhinovirus common cold. N Engl J Med 1968;279:742. (*Your mother is wrong! Exposure to moisture and cold does not increase susceptibility to upper respiratory infections, at least not in this study of volunteers experimentally infected with rhinovirus.*)

Gaffey MJ, Kaiser DL, Hayden FG. Ineffectiveness of oral terfenadine in natural colds. Pediatr Infect Dis J 1988;7:223. (*No benefit in controlled study; histamine is not a mediator of cold symptoms.*)

Gonzales R, Steiner JF, Sande MA. Antibiotic prescribing for adults with colds, upper respiratory tract infections, and bronchitis by ambulatory care physicians. JAMA 1997;278:901. (*In a national survey of outpatient physicians, antibiotics were prescribed for more than 50% of patients, a disturbing number, to treat conditions that were predominantly viral in origin.*)

Graham NMH, Burrell CJ, Douglas RM, et al. Adverse effects of aspirin, acetaminophen, and ibuprofen on immune function, viral shedding, and clinical status in rhinovirus-infected volunteers. J Infect Dis 1990;162:1277. (*Documents modest reductions in immune function and slight increases in nasal symptoms; no effect on virus shedding.*)

Hayden FG, Diamond L, Wood PB, et al. Effectiveness and safety of intranasal ipratropium bromide in common colds. Ann Intern Med 1996;125:89. (*A randomized, double-blinded, placebo-controlled trial demonstrating significant improvement in rhinorrhea and sneezing, in addition to a global benefit, with use of this anticholinergic nasal spray; well tolerated overall, but nasal dryness and blood-tinged mucus noted in about 15%.*)

Hayden FG, Osterhaus AD, Treanor JJ, et al. Efficacy and safety of the neuraminidase inhibitor zanamivir in the treatment of influenza virus infections. N Engl J Med 1997;337:874. (*Randomized, placebo-controlled trial of 262 patients with confirmed influenza infection showing time to resolution of major symptoms decreased by 1 day in treated patients. In subgroup analysis, no benefit was seen in patients treated 30 hours after onset of symptoms.*)

Jackson JL, Peterson C, Lesho E. A metaanalysis of zinc salts lozenges and the common cold. Arch Intern Med 1997;157:2373. (*Meta-analysis of six trials showing summary odds ratio of 0.50 for persistence of symptoms after 7 days, but no statistical significance.*)

Lane RS, Barsky AJ, Goodson JD. Discomfort and disability in upper respiratory tract infection. J Gen Intern Med 1988;3:540. (*Severity of symptoms was linked in part to the patient's emotional state.*)

Lorber B. The common cold. J Gen Intern Med 1996;11:229. (*A well-written review of the common cold, with discussion of experimental evidence regarding pathogenesis and transmission.*)

Macknin ML, Mathew S, Medendorp SVB. Effect of inhaling heated vapor on symptoms of the common cold. JAMA 1990;264:989. (*No benefit in comparison with control group; both groups showed improvement.*)

Macknin ML, Piedmonte M, Calendine C, et al. Zinc gluconate lozenges for treating the common cold in children: a randomized controlled trial. JAMA 1998;279:1962. (*No difference in time to resolution in this study.*)

Mossad SB, Macknin ML, Medendorp SV, et al. Zinc gluconate lozenges for treating the common cold: a randomized, double-blind, placebo-controlled study. Ann Intern Med 1996;125:81. (*Demonstrated in 100 employees of the Cleveland Clinic a reduction in mean duration of cold symptoms from 7.6 days to 4.4 days; duration of cough, nasal congestion, headache, hoarseness, sore throat, and nasal drainage was significantly shortened; nausea and bad taste were common side effects.*)

Oral cold remedies. Med Lett 1975;17:89. (*Critiques over-the-counter oral cold remedies and warns against high cost, irrational combination of agents, and frequent use of subtherapeutic doses of active ingredients.*)

Simon HB. The immunology of exercise: a brief review. JAMA 1984;252:2735. (*Your mother is wrong again! There is no evidence that exercise lowers "resistance" to respiratory or other infection, nor is it protective.*)

Stergachis A, Newmann WE, Williams KJ, et al. The effect of self-care minimal intervention for colds and flu on the use of medical services. J Gen Intern Med 1990;5:23. (*Simple self-care pamphlet did not affect medical utilization, but article includes an excellent discussion of other such interventions that did.*)

51
Management of Sarcoidosis

Sarcoidosis is a disease characterized by the formation of noncaseating granulomas, particularly in the lungs but also throughout the rest of the body. The precise cause remains unknown, but activation of T-cell lymphocytes in the lung plays an important role in the pathogenesis of granulomas. In the United States, sarcoidosis is 10 times more prevalent in African-Americans than in whites; people of Scandinavian descent also have a high incidence of the disease. Women outnumber men. Onset is most often between the ages of 20 and 45.

Although a large percentage of patients with sarcoidosis are asymptomatic, diverse and clinically important syndromes do result. Granuloma formation in the lung can be especially damaging, as can involvement in a number of other organ systems (e.g., eye, gastrointestinal tract). Once the diagnosis is established, the prime management decision regards the need for corticosteroid therapy. Improved methods of monitoring disease activity have enhanced the clinician's ability to treat sarcoidosis effectively while minimizing the risk for adverse effects from long-term steroids. The primary physician must know the most efficacious means of establishing the diagnosis, determining disease activity, and deciding on whether therapy with systemic steroids is needed, and for how long.

PATHOPHYSIOLOGY, CLINICAL PRESENTATION, AND COURSE

Pathophysiology. The cause of sarcoidosis is unknown. A variety of infectious and exogenous agents have been suggested as inciting factors, but whether one or several agents are involved remains conjectural. It is suspected that the granulomas and inflammatory reactions of sarcoidosis are caused by an abnormal immunologic response to a provocative agent in susceptible hosts.

Although the cause of sarcoidosis is unknown, the pathogenesis of granulomatous inflammation is being clarified. Bronchoalveolar lavage studies reveal that the early stage of pulmonary sarcoid consists of an alveolitis, with an increased number of T lymphocytes. Helper T cells predominate, and "activated" lymphocytes, capable of secreting various soluble mediators or lymphokines that may recruit monocytes and transform them into the macrophages of granulomas, are increased in number. The alveolitis of early disease and subsequent granulomatous inflammation are reversible, either spontaneously or with corticosteroid therapy, but the fibrosis that characterizes advanced chronic sarcoidosis is irreversible.

In contrast to the lungs, in which the numbers and activity of helper T cells are increased, the peripheral blood of patients with sarcoidosis may show a decreased number of T lymphocytes; this may account for the depressed cell-mediated immunity and cutaneous anergy observed in many such patients. However, the blood of patients with sarcoid often reflects increased activity of B lymphocytes, which accounts for the hypergammaglobulinemia and elevated antibody levels and circulating immune complexes that are often observed.

The granulomas of pulmonary sarcoidosis often resolve spontaneously, leaving the lung morphologically unscathed. However, in about 20% of patients, the process is more destructive and is characterized by interstitial fibrosis, obliteration of capillaries, and destruction of the pulmonary architecture. The end stage is characterized by the formation of cystic spaces interspersed with bands of connective tissue.

Clinical Manifestations of sarcoidosis reflect the sites of granulomatous inflammation. The most common presentation, especially in young adults, is *bilateral hilar adenopathy*, which occurs in 50% of patients and is often detected on routine chest radiography. About 25% present with bilateral hilar adenopathy and *pulmonary infiltrates*, and 15% present with infiltrates alone. Disease in the hilum is not associated with invasion or compression of the bronchi or nodal calcification. *Erythema nodosum* or *uveitis* (manifested by red, watery eyes) may accompany hilar adenopathy. Some patients exhibit *cough, shortness of breath, wheezing* or chest discomfort, in addition to constitutional symptoms of *fever, malaise,* and *fatigue.*

Although pulmonary symptoms are the most frequent, sarcoidosis may present with extrathoracic disease, including *hepatomegaly, splenomegaly,* or uveitis. Other presenting manifestations include *fever of unknown origin,* granulomatous *hepatitis,* salivary and lacrimal gland enlargement, *arthritis,* peripheral *adenopathy,* and skin lesions. *Hypercalcemia* as a consequence of increased sensitivity to vitamin D is reported in 10% to 30% but is sustained in only 2% to 3%. Cardiac conduction abnormalities, such as heart block, and neurologic abnormalities, including facial palsies, are each seen in about 5% of cases. In addition, many unusual presentations have been reported.

DIAGNOSIS

The diagnosis of sarcoidosis is sometimes a clinical challenge because the condition may be hard to distinguish from other interstitial lung diseases (see appendix to this Chapter). However, *asymptomatic bilateral hilar adenopathy,* with or without uveitis or erythema nodosum, is likely to be a manifestation of sarcoidosis. In a retrospective series of 100 patients with bilateral hilar adenopathy, conducted before the advent of AIDS, all 30 patients who were asymptomatic had biopsy-proven sarcoidosis. Moreover, 50 of 52 with bilateral hilar adenopathy and negative physical examination findings also had the disease. All 11 patients with neoplasms were symptomatic, and nine had easily identifiable extrathoracic tumor on physical examination. Among symptomatic patients, all with erythema nodosum or uveitis had sarcoid. Thus, in the patient with bilateral hilar adenopathy who is asymptomatic and HIV-negative, and who has negative physical examination findings or erythema nodosum or uveitis, a biopsy is not necessarily required to confirm the diagnosis of sarcoidosis. Nevertheless, some clinicians prefer to obtain a tissue diagnosis in all cases of sarcoidosis, including those with asymptomatic hilar adenopathy.

A decision to perform a *biopsy* must be made by viewing the potential for discovering treatable conditions and balancing this probability against the risks associated with the procedure. For the tissue diagnosis of hilar adenopathy, *mediastinoscopy* is the most direct approach and is usually well tolerated. For the documentation of pulmonary sarcoid, *fiberoptic bronchoscopy* with *transbronchial biopsy* is favored. This procedure has a reported sensitivity of 60% to 80%. In addition, bronchoscopy allows direct visualization of the bronchial tree, so it can be helpful in ruling out tumor and obtaining samples of secretions by *bronchoalveolar* lavage for laboratory study. The major complication of transbronchial lung biopsy is pneumothorax; this is infrequent when the procedure is performed by someone with experience.

In patients with extrathoracic sarcoidosis, accessible sites for biopsy include skin lesions and enlarged peripheral lymph nodes. Biopsy of conjunctivae, salivary glands, and liver may reveal noncaseating granulomas, even if clinical evidence of sarcoid in these tissues is absent. Because of the low morbidity associated with salivary gland and conjunctival biopsies, these may be particularly useful. It must be remembered that the histologic appearance of sarcoid granulomas is not etiologically specific. Therefore, the other known causes of noncaseating granulomas must be ruled out, including tuberculosis, syphilis, berylliosis, brucellosis, Q fever, biliary cirrhosis, Wegener's granulomatosis, drug reactions, and local sarcoid reactions in nodes draining solid tumors. Hodgkin's disease is particularly difficult to exclude with mediastinoscopy in patients presenting with unilateral or asymmetric hilar adenopathy.

The *Kveim test* has also been used in the diagnosis of sarcoidosis. The test requires the intracutaneous injection of heat-sterilized human sarcoid tissue, usually spleen. A positive reaction consists of the development of epithelioid granulomas detected on skin biopsy of the injection site at 4 to 6 weeks. The delay period, variability of the material available for injection, and high incidence of false-positive and false-negative results (resulting from impure batches of antigen) have limited the usefulness of the Kveim reaction. Furthermore, Kveim antigen is not readily available.

Other abnormalities that may be present in patients with sarcoidosis include cutaneous anergy, hyperglobulinemia, abnormal serum liver chemistries, and elevated levels of lysozyme; none of these findings is specific, but together they are supportive of the diagnosis. Similarly, films of the bones of the hands may reveal changes suggestive of sarcoid.

Serum levels of *angiotensin-converting enzyme* (ACE) are elevated in about 70% of patients with active sarcoidosis, but ACE determinations lack both sensitivity and specificity for establishing a diagnosis of sarcoidosis. ACE levels have been studied as markers of disease activity and therapeutic responsiveness, but results have proved disappointing in clinical practice (see below). The same is true of *scanning with gallium 67* (^{67}Ga), although it can help identify extrathoracic disease.

STAGING, NATURAL HISTORY, AND CLINICAL COURSE

Staging. Intrathoracic sarcoidosis can be divided into *four stages*. In *stage 0*, the chest radiographic appearance is normal. In *stage I*, only bilateral hilar adenopathy is present; most pa-

tients are asymptomatic, the lung parenchyma appears normal on chest the film, and pulmonary function tests show normal mechanics, although the carbon monoxide diffusion capacity (D$_{\text{LCO}}$) may be impaired. In *stage II*, both hilar adenopathy and pulmonary infiltrates are present; pulmonary function tests show predominantly restrictive defects. In *stage III* disease, pulmonary infiltrates are present, accompanied by obstructive and restrictive defects; however, hilar adenopathy has resolved. *Stage IV* is marked by advanced fibrosis, bullae, and cysts.

Natural History. Patients with clear lungs and asymptomatic hilar adenopathy have an excellent prognosis. In one large series of untreated cases, complete remission occurred in more than 75% within 5 years. In 50% with untreated pulmonary parenchymal involvement, complete resolution was seen within 2 years. In one third of those in whom clearing did not occur, severe fibrosis developed. Overall, at 5 years, 87% were clinically well, 10% had died of respiratory failure, and 3% were disabled by pulmonary disease.

Most natural history data derive from referral centers. In a report from a nonreferral setting, 86 patients were followed for 10 years in a primary care practice; pulmonary fibrosis developed in only 12, and none experienced respiratory failure or cor pulmonale. This latter study suggests that the course of sarcoid may be more benign than has been reported from referral centers, which are more likely to attract complicated cases.

In general, patients with stage I disease have an 80% chance of spontaneous remission, those with stage II disease have about a 50% remission rate, and those with stage III have about a 20% to 40% chance of spontaneous remission. Stage IV represents irreversible, advanced disease.

Extrathoracic Complications are infrequent. Hepatic granulomas are often present, but the development of clinically symptomatic *granulomatous hepatitis* is much less common; hepatic failure and portal hypertension are rare. Cranial and peripheral neuropathies tend to occur early in the disease and are usually transient; however, in some patients, significant neurologic damage is seen. *Uveitis* affects about 15%, comes on acutely, and often resolves spontaneously. More worrisome is chronic iridocyclitis; it presents as pain and blurring of vision, and cataracts, secondary glaucoma, and blindness may eventually develop. As noted above, *hypercalcemia* persists in about 2% to 3%, although it may be found transiently in up to 30%. Cardiac granulomas are found in 20% of sarcoidosis cases that come to autopsy, but fewer than 5% of patients experience difficulties with conduction or impulse formation. Rarely, infiltration of the myocardium produces pump failure.

The course of patients with sarcoid may occasionally be complicated by *infections* such as tuberculosis, aspergillar fungus balls, candidiasis, and cryptococcosis, attributable in part to the disease and in part to the use of long-term steroid therapy.

PRINCIPLES OF MANAGEMENT, THERAPEUTIC RECOMMENDATIONS, AND MONITORING

The *goals* in the treatment of sarcoid include *relief of symptoms* and *prevention* of significant impairment of organ function. As noted earlier, the natural history of sarcoid is variable, but often favorable. Hence, the indications for therapy are frequently unclear. Patients who present with stage I disease (asymptomatic bilateral hilar adenopathy or erythema no-dosum) usually have a benign course, so that no treatment is indicated unless symptoms develop. Even patients with stage II or III disease may undergo spontaneous remission, and it is not possible to identify whose disease will progress and whose will remit. No evidence is available to indicate that treatment in the early phases of pulmonary sarcoid prevents progression to pulmonary fibrosis.

The view that emerges from available studies is that treatment should be reserved for patients who are symptomatic and have evidence of active pulmonary disease (dyspnea on exertion, abnormal results of pulmonary function studies, infiltrate on chest x-ray films). Gallium scanning and ACE determinations have also been used to provide evidence of disease activity, but in clinical practice they have not proved to be particularly accurate. Additional indications for treatment include important extrathoracic disease, such as uveitis, conduction abnormalities, hypercalcemia, neuropathy, and severe skin involvement (see below).

The principal treatment for sarcoidosis is *systemic corticosteroid therapy*. The great variability in the clinical course of the disease and the previous lack of sensitive indicators of disease activity have made it difficult to document rigorously the efficacy of steroid therapy. Older studies relied on such crude measures as symptoms, radiographic findings, and pulmonary function test values. Recent evaluations examining the effect of corticosteroids on more direct indicators of the disease process (see below) have found marked suppression of the alveolitis, but little influence on anatomic abnormalities present before the initiation of steroid therapy.

Most authorities recommend commencing with large doses of steroids (e.g., 40 to 60 mg prednisone), given on a daily basis for anywhere from 6 weeks to 6 months, then tapering or switching to alternate-day therapy if measures of disease activity indicate response. Improvement is usually evident by 2 to 3 weeks. Steroid therapy is most effective if instituted before the development of pulmonary fibrosis. However, there is no evidence that prophylactic treatment is worth the adverse effects of long-term steroid use (see Chapter 105).

Steroids consistently produce subjective improvement in dyspneic patients with early sarcoidosis and may even reduce pulmonary infiltrates when they are secondary to alveolitis or granulomatous changes. Lung volumes usually improve, but not necessarily the diffusion capacity, which may be permanently altered by destructive changes. Relapses after cessation of therapy are frequent, so that close monitoring is necessary for at least 12 months after discontinuation of treatment. *Alternate-day steroid therapy* (e.g., 15 to 25 mg every other day) has proved successful as a maintenance program in some patients, controlling disease when given after an initial course of daily steroids; this approach minimizes the adverse effects of long-term steroid therapy (see Chapter 105).

Adrenal corticosteroids are also indicated for active ocular disease. Every patient with sarcoid should have an ophthalmologic examination, especially if visual symptoms develop. Topical steroids may be used, but systemic therapy is usually added. Treatment is also indicated in the presence of significant or progressive involvement of any other organ. Onset of hepatitis, facial nerve palsies, meningitis, myocardial conduction defects, hypercalcemia, or persistent constitutional symptoms (fever, fatigue) are all indications for treatment.

In an effort to improve treatment outcomes or to avoid or minimize the toxic effects of prolonged steroid therapy, other approaches have been tried. Inhaled steroids have been used in several randomized trials, either alone or after a course of systemic steroids. At present, the evidence does not support a role for inhaled steroids. Because of its ability to complement systemic steroid therapy in rheumatoid arthritis, methotrexate has been used by some investigators. Case series suggest a modest improvement with a regimen that is well tolerated and able to decrease dependence on steroids, but this has not been documented in a randomized study. A small, randomized trial suggests that chloroquine may be effective. A randomized trial of cyclosporin A does not support its use.

Monitoring. Whenever steroid therapy is undertaken, an objective documentation of the response to treatment is essential. Because the predominant pathologic process in sarcoidosis is an alveolitis leading to granuloma formation, and because corticosteroids work by suppressing the alveolitis, the optimal means of monitoring disease activity and response to therapy would be to follow measures of the alveolitis. It has not been possible to distinguish between the extent of alveolitis and anatomic derangement by means of *chest radiography* and *determination of lung volumes and diffusion capacity*. Although these parameters are certainly useful for assessing the severity of disease, they are relatively insensitive measures of disease activity and suboptimal for judging the adequacy of therapy and the need for continued treatment. Even the sensitivity of the diffusion capacity for measuring disease extent has come under question. In one study, the diffusion capacity was well preserved, whereas lung volumes and measures of oxygenation (e.g., alveolar–arterial oxygen gradient and oxygen saturation) showed declines.

Attempts to improve on such crude measures of disease activity have been discouraging. Parameters generally reflective of inflammation, such as the erythrocyte sedimentation rate and serum globulin levels, have proved inadequate. Initial studies of *determination of ACE levels*, gallium scanning, and serial *bronchoalveolar lymphocyte counts* were encouraging, but a later controlled study found these tests no more sensitive for monitoring and managing steroid therapy than the combination of serial chest radiography and measurement of the diffusion capacity and lung volumes. Some authorities still argue that following the levels of ACE (which is believed to be produced by epithelioid cells within the sarcoid granuloma) can be useful in patients with very high levels before therapy, a situation most common in stage II disease.

Until better tests are devised (an ongoing effort), the best available approach to monitoring appears to be either serial determinations of the diffusion capacity and lung volumes together with chest radiography, or serial determinations of the ACE levels if the initial serum ACE level is markedly elevated.

PATIENT EDUCATION

Serious consequences of sarcoidosis are relatively infrequent. The nature of the disease should be carefully explained, with emphasis on its relatively benign, self-limited nature in the asymptomatic patient. Patients who are treated with steroids should be counseled about side effects and the risks inherent in such treatment (see Chapter 105). Careful follow-up must be emphasized in both the asymptomatic patient (to detect the development of functional abnormalities) and the patient with symptoms (to document objective benefits of treatment). Patients should be instructed about early signs of important complications, such as red eyes, blurred vision, eye pain, and dyspnea on exertion, so that therapy is not unnecessarily delayed.

A.G.M.

ANNOTATED BIBLIOGRAPHY

Baltzan M, Mehta S, Kirkham TH, et al. Randomized trial of prolonged chloroquine therapy in advanced pulmonary sarcoidosis. Am J Respir Crit Care Med 1999;160:192. (*Significant improvement in this small study.*)

Belfer MH, Stevens RW. Sarcoidosis: a primary care review. Am Fam Physician 1998;58:2041. (*Helpful review.*)

Crystal RG, Roberts WC, Hunningham GW, et al. Pulmonary sarcoidosis: a disease characterized and perpetuated by activated lung T-lymphocytes. Ann Intern Med 1981;94:73. (*Comprehensive review of exciting new insights into the pathogenesis and immunology of sarcoidosis; 280 references.*)

Dunn TL, Watters LC, Cherniack, et al. Gas exchange at a given degree of volume restriction is different in sarcoidosis and idiopathic pulmonary fibrosis. Am J Med 1988;85:221. (*Study comparing measures of disease severity; diffusion capacity is a less sensitive measure of disease than are volume change and degree of oxygenation.*)

Gibson GJ, Prescott RJ, Muers MF, et al. British Thoracic Society sarcoidosis study: effects of long-term corticosteroid treatment. Thorax 1996;51:238. (*Improvements in symptoms, respiratory function, and radiographic appearance with long-term steroids.*)

Gottlieb JE, Israel HL, Steiner RM, et al. Outcome in sarcoidosis. The relationship of relapse to corticosteroid therapy. Chest 1997;111:623. (*A 74% relapse rate in the steroid-induced remission group, but only an 8% relapse rate in the spontaneous remission group.*)

Harkleroad LE, Young RL, Savage PJ, et al. Pulmonary sarcoidosis: long-term follow-up of the effects of steroid therapy. Chest 1982;82:84. (*Although only 25 patients were entered into this alternate-case steroid trial, a 15-year follow-up was available; no discernible benefit from early steroid therapy.*)

Israel HL, Fouts DU, Begys RA. A controlled trial of prednisone treatment of sarcoidosis. Am Rev Respir Dis 1973;107:609. (*Prospective study of 90 patients; at 3 months, those on prednisone showed improvement in all parameters measured, but no significant differences noted over the long term.*)

James DG. Kveim revisited, reassessed. N Engl J Med 1975;292:859. (*Reviews the test and its sensitivity and specificity.*)

Johns CJ, Macgregor MI, Zachary JB, et al. Extended experience in the long-term corticosteroid treatment of pulmonary sarcoidosis. Ann N Y Acad Sci 1976;278:722. (*One hundred ninety-two patients with severe disease were treated with prednisone. Clinical improvement resulted from treatment but relapses were frequent when therapy was terminated, so that long-term therapy with 10 to 15 mg of prednisone was necessary, often for years.*)

Kajdasz DK, Judson MA, Mohr LC Jr, et al. Geographic variation in sarcoidosis in South Carolina: its relation to socioeconomic status and health care indicators. Am J Epidemiol 1999;150:271. (*Significant variation was identified, with an increase in sarcoidosis rates in areas near the Atlantic coastline.*)

Koontz CH, Joyner LR, Nelson RA. Transbronchial lung biopsy via the fiberoptic bronchoscope in sarcoidosis. Ann Intern Med 1976;85:64. (*Test sensitivity was 63%, with a higher probability of a positive biopsy result in symptomatic patients.*)

Lawrence EC, Teague RB, Gottlieb MS, et al. Serial changes in markers of disease activity with corticosteroid treatment in sarcoidosis. Am J Med 1983;74:747. (*Initially encouraging data on value of the gallium scan and determination of ACE levels for monitoring response to steroid therapy; see article of Turner-Warwick et al., listed below, for a less sanguine view.*)

Lieberman J, Schleissner LA, Nosal A, et al. Clinical correlations of serum angiotensin-converting enzyme (ACE) in sarcoidosis. A longitudinal study of serum ACE, gallium 67 scans, chest roentgenograms and pulmonary function. Chest 1983;84:522. (*Another enthusiastic early report.*)

Lower EE, Baughman RP. Prolonged use of methotrexate for sarcoidosis. Arch Intern Med 1995;155:846. (*Improvement in two thirds of this series of 50 patients who completed at least 2 years of methotrexate therapy.*)

Lower EE, Broderick JP, Brott TG, et al. Diagnosis and management of neurological sarcoidosis. Arch Intern Med 1997;157:1864. (*Facial nerve paralysis most common but self-limiting; other neurologic signs and symptoms more chronic.*)

Milman N. Oral and inhaled corticosteroids in the treatment of pulmonary sarcoidosis—a critical reappraisal. Sarcoidosis Vasc Diffuse Lung Dis 1998;15:150. (*Concludes that evidence does not support their use.*)

Nagai S, Shigematsu M, Hamada K, et al. Clinical courses and prognosis of pulmonary sarcoidosis. Curr Opin Pulm Med 1999;5:293. (*Functional impairment at time of diagnosis predicts unfavorable prognosis.*)

Peckham DG, Spiteri MA. Sarcoidosis. Postgrad Med J 1996;72:196. (*Useful review.*)

Pietinalho A, Tukiainen P, Haahtela T, et al. Oral prednisolone followed by inhaled budesonide in newly diagnosed pulmonary sarcoidosis: a double-blind, placebo-controlled multicenter study. Finnish Pulmonary Sarcoidosis Study Group. Chest 1999;116:424. (*Early radiographic response not sustained. No change in forced vital capacity.*)

Reich JM, Johnson RE. Course and prognosis of sarcoidosis in a nonreferral setting. Analyses of 86 patients observed for 10 years. Am J Med 1985;78:61. (*Course may be more benign than that reported for referral center populations.*)

Rybicki BA, Maliarik MJ, Major M, et al. Epidemiology, demographics, and genetics of sarcoidosis. Semin Respir Infect 1998;13:166. (*African-Americans and women at greater risk.*)

Siltzbach LE, James DG, Neville E, et al. Course and prognosis of sarcoidosis around the world. Am J Med 1974;57:847. (*Terse summary of clinical findings showing no differences of significance among various races and ethnic groups.*)

Turner-Warwick M, McAllister W, Lawrence R, et al. Corticosteroid treatment and pulmonary sarcoidosis: do serial lavage lymphocyte counts, serum converting enzyme measurements, and gallium 67 scans help management? Thorax 1986;41:903. (*These studies proved no more sensitive than chest radiography and pulmonary function tests.*)

Winterbauer RH, Belic N, Moores KD. Clinical interpretation of bilateral hilar adenopathy. Ann Intern Med 1973;78:65. (*Classic article from the pre-HIV era, providing evidence that asymptomatic patients with only bilateral adenopathy need not undergo biopsy for definitive diagnosis.*)

Wyser CP, van Schalkwyk EM, Alheit B, et al. Treatment of progressive pulmonary sarcoidosis with cyclosporin A. A randomized controlled trial. Am J Respir Crit Care Med 1997;156:1371. (*Higher complication rates not justified by modest improvements in this trial.*)

Appendix: Evaluation of Interstitial Lung Disease

When a chest radiograph shows a diffuse infiltrative pattern that is labeled "interstitial" in appearance, a wide variety of diagnostic possibilities emerge, ranging from sarcoidosis and rheumatoid disease to pneumoconiosis and idiopathic pulmonary fibrosis. With such a large number of diagnostic possibilities at hand, an efficient approach to workup is essential. The primary physician's role is to narrow the differential by careful attention to important elements of the history and physical examination, supplemented by a few well-chosen initial laboratory studies.

PATHOPHYSIOLOGY AND CLINICAL PRESENTATION

Most conditions that cause this diffuse parenchymal radiographic pattern are not truly "interstitial"; in addition to involving the area between the alveolar epithelium and the capillary endothelial basement membrane, they may also affect the gas-exchanging portion of the lung (including the alveolar epithelium, alveolar space, and pulmonary microvasculature).

Most of the interstitial lung diseases begin with parenchymal injury that is followed by an inflammatory response and collagen deposition. It is the widespread nature of the injury and inflammatory response—often compromising the alveolar walls—that accounts for the pathophysiology and clinical presentation. In a few instances, the process is invasive or infiltrative rather than inflammatory; in others, a filling of the alveolar space occurs with an outpouring of material.

The physiologic consequences of such alveolar compromise are the development of a *restrictive defect*; this is manifested by a reduction in forced vital capacity and a *ventilation–perfusion mismatch* that is created when inflammation and fibrosis of the gas-exchanging surfaces cause a reduction in carbon monoxide diffusing capacity and oxygen tension (Po_2). Symptoms may be minimal, although progressive dyspnea is the rule, at times accompanied by a dry cough. The lungs may be clear to auscultation, or basilar crackles may predominate.

DIFFERENTIAL DIAGNOSIS

The conditions responsible for interstitial lung disease can be grouped according to their underlying pathophysiology: drug-induced inflammatory response, connective tissue disease, pneumoconiosis, alveolar filling disease, primary lung disease, and idiopathic disease (Table 51.1).

The most common causes are sarcoidosis and idiopathic pulmonary fibrosis, although in industrial settings the pneumoconioses may predominate.

WORKUP

History should focus on the duration of symptoms, speed of progression, and presence of fever, hemoptysis, pleuritic chest pain, and symptoms of extrathoracic disease (e.g., joint pain, lymphadenopathy, skin changes). Most conditions have a chronic, progressive course, but acute onset with *fever* and a rapidly progressive course suggest a hypersensitivity pneumonitis, usually a consequence of exposure to organic antigens (ranging from cocaine to bird droppings). Fever, bothersome

Table 51.1.   Differential Diagnosis of Interstitial Lung Disease

Pneumoconiosis
Silicosis
Asbestosis
Coal worker's pneumoconiosis
Berylliosis
Organic dusts (pigeons, turkey, duck, chicken, humidifier)

Drugs
Chemotherapeutic agents (busulfan, bleomycin, methotrexate)
Antibiotics (nitrofurantoin, sulfonamides, isoniazid)
Gold
Amiodarone
Penicillamine
Lupuslike reactions (hydralazine, procainamide)
Radiation

Connective Tissue Disease
Systemic lupus erythematosis
Rheumatoid arthritis
Scleroderma
Polymyositis

Primary Lung Disease
Sarcoidosis
Histiocytosis X
Lymphangiomyomatosis
Lymphangiectatic carcinomatosis
Lipoidosis

Alveolar Filling Disease
Diffuse alveolar bleeding (Goodpasture's syndrome, lupus, mitral stenosis, idiopathic pulmonary hemosiderosis)
Alveolar proteinosis
Alveolar cell carcinoma
Eosinophilic pneumonia
Lipoid pneumonia

Other
Idiopathic pulmonary fibrosis
Bronchiolitis obliterans organizing pneumonia
Lymphocytic interstitial pneumonia

Adapted from Schwarz MI. In: Kelley WN. Textbook of Internal Medicine. Philadelphia: JB Lippincott Co, 1989:2060.

dry cough, and a subacute course (2 to 10 weeks) accompanied by a patchy, bilateral air space process characterize bronchiolitis obliterans organizing pneumonia, in which a lymphocytic infiltrate and granulation tissue occupy the distal airways and alveoli. *Productive cough* is rare in interstitial lung disease, but its presence indicates fluid-filled alveoli, as can occur in diffuse alveolar cell carcinoma. *Hemoptysis* suggests conditions that cause diffuse alveolar bleeding (e.g., Goodpasture's syndrome, lupus, severe mitral stenosis, idiopathic pulmonary hemosiderosis). Bleeding that originates from or occurs in the context of upper airway disease is a hallmark of Wegener's granulomatosis. *Pleuritic pain* indicates that the inflammatory process has spread to involve the pleura, which is characteristic of the connective tissue diseases and some drug-induced conditions. Sudden, severe pleuritic pain and acute dyspnea raise the question of a spontaneous pneumothorax, which occurs with many of the primary lung diseases, such as histiocytosis X and lymphangiomyomatosis.

The presence of extrapulmonary symptoms—especially if they predate the development of lung findings—can be diagnostic. *Polyarticular symptoms* and *skin changes* characterize the connective tissue/rheumatoid diseases and sarcoidosis; the latter is often associated with *lymph gland enlargement*. Patients with idiopathic pulmonary fibrosis may have arthralgias, but symptoms of joint inflammation are absent. A history of renal disease, especially *nephritis*, can be a clue for Goodpasture's syndrome and lupus, although in the former, pulmonary disease usually predates renal involvement.

The *drug* and *occupational history* is one of the most important parts of the clinical assessment. Long-term use of such chemotherapeutic agents as methotrexate, busulfan, bleomycin, and cyclophosphamide may result in interstitial lung changes, as may prolonged use of nitrofurantoin, gold, amiodarone, or penicillamine. High-dose procainamide can lead to a lupuslike serositis syndrome. Radiation therapy may trigger a diffuse pneumonitis 6 to 12 weeks after treatment, followed by fibrosis. Occupational exposures, including distant ones, to inorganic dusts such as silicone, asbestos, talc, beryllium, and coal deserve careful review. Patients with a hypersensitivity pneumonitis should be queried about exposure to organic dusts on the job; typically, symptoms are worse at work. They should also be asked about nasal inhalation of cocaine, which has been reported as a cause of hypersensitivity pneumonitis. A *smoking* history is always pertinent. It is uncommon for lung disease to develop in nonsmoking patients with Goodpasture's syndrome.

Physical Examination is particularly useful for signs of extrathoracic disease; the pulmonary findings are usually nonspecific. The skin is checked for signs of connective tissue disease (rheumatoid nodules, malar flush, changes of scleroderma) and sarcoidosis (see above), and the lymph nodes are checked for sarcoid-related enlargement. Patients with hemoptysis should undergo a careful upper airway examination that includes a search for the signs of necrotizing changes in the nasal passages and sinuses that typify Wegener's granulomatosis. The joints are examined for evidence of inflammation (swelling, warmth, redness, effusion), which is indicative of rheumatoid disease but also occurs with sarcoidosis and Wegener's granulomatosis. Enlargement of the liver and spleen are oft-noted features of sarcoidosis and occasional findings in advanced connective tissue disease and histiocytosis X.

As noted earlier, the pulmonary findings are typically nonspecific and may even be grossly normal. Bilateral basilar rales are common in many forms of interstitial lung disease, especially the drug-related, idiopathic, connective tissue, and pneumoconiosis varieties. In those conditions associated with alveolar filling, the rales are likely to be "wet" in quality, whereas those without fluid in the alveoli produce "dry" crackles (sometimes referred to as "Velcro" rales) on end-inspiration. The heart is checked for mitral stenosis if a history of hemoptysis is present, and for signs of cor pulmonale and right-sided failure (right ventricular heave or third heart sound, increased intensity of second heart sound, jugular venous distention, peripheral edema) resulting from chronic hypoxemia-induced pulmonary hypertension.

Chest Radiographic Findings are usually nonspecific but can be helpful. Radiologic adjectives describing the diffuse changes associated with interstitial disease include such terms as "reticular (linear)", "reticulonodular", and "nodular", and "ground glass." The lower lobes tend to be more involved than the upper ones, and a "honeycomb" or cystic appearance to the lung fields develops as fibrous tissue replaces normal alveoli. Exceptions to these generalizations are the upper lobe predilec-

tion and nodular infiltrates of silicosis, berylliosis, chronic hypersensitivity pneumonitis, and histiocytosis X.

Unfortunately, no particular radiographic pattern is diagnostic, although a few emerge as useful. The alveolar filling diseases tend to produce alveolar densities in an ill-defined or "fluffy" nodular pattern; an air bronchogram might ensue as involved alveoli become silhouetted by uninvolved airway. The development of such a pattern in a patient with previously known interstitial disease suggests a superimposed process, such as alveolar cell carcinoma or active inflammation. Frankly nodular infiltrates are seen with sarcoidosis and Wegener's granulomatosis as a result of granuloma formation; nodular infiltrates may even occur with the pneumoconioses and hypersensitivity pneumonitis.

Radiographic findings outside the lung parenchyma are important and worth noting. The concurrent appearance of pleural involvement suggests connective tissue disease, asbestosis, and occasionally sarcoidosis. Bilateral hilar adenopathy can be pathognomonic of sarcoidosis (see above). Diffuse infiltrates, hilar adenopathy, and pneumothorax point to histiocytosis X. A thin rim of calcium in the hilar nodes is characteristic of silicosis.

Pulmonary Function Tests help confirm the interstitial nature of the disease (particularly when radiographic findings are minimal) and provide a baseline with which to judge disease course, although they correlate poorly with degree of pathologic change. As noted earlier, the ratio of *forced expiratory volume* (FEV_1) to *forced vital capacity* (FVC) increases and demonstrates a restrictive pattern secondary to a steady reduction in FVC. Some interstitial conditions (e.g., lymphangiomyomatosis, histiocytosis X) can also cause airway obstruction and may reduce the FEV_1. The diffusion capacity is typically reduced, although it may be preserved until rather late in the course of illness, when mismatching of ventilation and perfusion becomes prominent. *Arterial blood gases* are initially normal, but with disease progression, hypoxemia, hypocarbia, and a respiratory alkalosis ensue. The hypocarbia is a manifestation of tachypnea, triggered predominantly by increased work of breathing as the lung stiffens during progression of the fibrotic process.

Laboratory Studies. Few routine noninvasive laboratory studies are of diagnostic value. A simple yet often overlooked test is *urinalysis*, which can provide important evidence of glomerular injury (red cells, casts, albuminuria), suggestive of connective tissue disease, Wegener's granulomatosis, and Goodpasture's syndrome. Most other tests should be ordered only when the history, physical examination, and chest radiograph indicate a reasonable pretest probability of the condition in question. Unselective testing is associated with a high rate of false-positive results (see Chapter 2). If connective tissue disease is suspected, then *rheumatoid factor*, *antinuclear antibody*, and *DNA binding* studies (see Chapter 146) and a *urinalysis* should be considered. Hypersensitivity pneumonitis, especially if drug-induced, may produce a finding of 10% to 20% eosinophils on the *peripheral smear* examination, but test sensitivity is low (20%). The ACE level is useful for gauging disease activity but lacks sensitivity for the diagnosis of sarcoidosis. Measurement of *precipitating antibodies* is frequently ordered when inhalation of a potentially sensitizing organic dust is suspected, but the test does not distinguish between an etiologic role and exposure. Patients suspected of having Goodpasture's syndrome are usually positive for *antiglomerular basement membrane antibody.* Patients with Wegener's granulomatosis test positive for *antineutrophil cytoplasmic autoantibodies* in only 60% of cases, but specificity is high (<95%).

Fiberoptic bronchoscopy with *bronchoalveolar lavage* provides an opportunity to sample the cellular and fluid contents of the distal airways (counts of total white cells, macrophages, lymphocytes and lymphocyte subsets, neutrophils, and eosinophils; malignant cells; antibodies). Alterations in the normal cellular profile may aid the diagnosis, as can the discovery of malignant cells. However, because of considerable overlap among causes, the findings are usually nonspecific. Lavage data sometimes help stage illness and predict response to therapy.

Except for patients with connective tissue disease, pneumoconiosis, or drug- or radiation-induced disease, most patients with interstitial lung disease usually require a tissue diagnosis. The morbidity of *transbronchial biopsy,* a means of obtaining tissue during bronchoscopy, is low. Unfortunately, however, it rarely establishes a definitive tissue diagnosis. Most forms of interstitial disease that necessitate a tissue diagnosis require more tissue than can be obtained by the transbronchial approach. However, when sarcoidosis, lymphangitic carcinomatosis, or an alveolar filling disease is suspected, a transbronchial biopsy may suffice. In most other instances, an *open lung biopsy* or, when an experienced operator is available, a *video-assisted thoracic lung biopsy* is required.

INDICATIONS FOR REFERRAL AND ADMISSION

Referral to a pulmonary medical specialist is indicated when the diagnosis remains elusive after completion of the noninvasive segment of the evaluation and the need for lavage or a tissue diagnosis is being considered. A thoughtful consultation may save the patient an unnecessary procedure and help select those patients most likely to warrant an invasive evaluation. Hospitalization is indicated when severe ventilation–perfusion mismatching leads to clinically significant hypoxemia (Po_2 <55 mm Hg).

A.H.G./A.G.M.

ANNOTATED BIBLIOGRAPHY

Anonymous. Current world literature. Interstitial lung disease. Curr Opin Pulm Med 1999;5:B109. (*A good place to start for a comprehensive literature review.*)

Cooper JAD, White DA, Matthay RA. Drug-induced pulmonary disease. Part I: cytotoxic drugs. Part II: noncytotoxic drugs. Am Rev Respir Dis 1986;133:321,488. (*Comprehensive, authoritative review.*)

Copper JA Jr. Drug-induced lung disease. Adv Intern Med 1997;42:231. (*Exhaustive review.*)

Crystal RG, Bitterman PB, Rennard SI, et al. Interstitial lung disease of unknown cause. Disorders characterized by chronic inflammation of the lower respiratory tract: parts 1 and 2. N Engl J Med 1984;310:154,235. (*Definitive review and description of these important and difficult diseases, usually referred to as* idiopathic pulmonary fibrosis.)

Ettinger NA, Albin RJ. A review of the respiratory effects of smoking cocaine. Am J Med 1989;87:664. (*Includes description of an acute hypersensitivity interstitial pneumonitis.*)

Ferson PF, Landreneau RJ. Thoracoscopic lung biopsy or open lung biopsy for interstitial lung disease. Chest Surg Clin North Am 1998;8:749. (*Detailed review of advantages and disadvantages of these alternatives for different indications.*)

Gibson PG, Bryant DH, Morgan GW, et al. Radiation-induced lung injury: a hypersensitivity pneumonitis. Ann Intern Med 1988;109:288. (*Interesting data regarding mechanism, and review of clinical presentation.*)

Haupt M, Moore GW, Hutchins GM. The lung in systemic lupus erythematosis. Am J Med 1981;71:791. (*Analysis of pathologic changes in 121 patients.*)

Hunninghake GW, Fauci AS. Pulmonary involvement in the collagen vascular diseases. Am Rev Respir Dis 1979;119:471. (*Classic and comprehensive review.*)

Leatherman JW, Davies SF, Hoidal JR. Alveolar hemorrhage syndromes: diffuse microvascular lung hemorrhage in immune and idiopathic disorders. Medicine 1984;63:343. (*Comprehensive review, including discussion of conditions that also cause renal injury.*)

Nolle B, Specks U, Ludemann J, et al. Anticytoplasmic antibodies: their immunodiagnostic value in Wegener's granulomatosis. Ann Intern Med 1989;111:28. (*Sensitivity averaged 63% during active disease, specificity 95%.*)

Reynolds HY. Bronchoalveolar lavage. Am Rev Respir Dis 1987;135:250. (*Excellent review of the procedure and its findings and diagnostic utility.*)

Reynolds HY. Diagnostic and management strategies for diffuse interstitial lung disease. Chest 1998;113:192. (*Helpful review.*)

52

Approach to the Patient with Acute Bronchitis or Pneumonia in the Ambulatory Setting

WILLIAM A. KORMOS

Although most respiratory tract infections seen in the office setting are limited to the upper airway (see Chapter 50 and Chapters 218 through 220), the differential diagnosis should include lower respiratory tract infection in patients who present with a productive cough, dyspnea, and pleuritic chest pain. In such patients, four questions need to be addressed: (a) Is the process limited to the trachea and bronchi, or is a pneumonia present? (b) Is a diagnostic workup indicated or can empiric treatment be started? (c) Are antibiotics indicated and, if so, which ones? (d) Can the patient be safely treated as an outpatient or is hospital admission necessary? These basic questions are becoming increasingly germane as new strategies emerge for cost-effective management and concerns grow about the rising frequency of antibiotic-resistant organisms. The assessment and decision-making process become considerably more complicated if the patient is HIV-positive (see Chapter 13) or immunosuppressed for other reasons.

PATHOPHYSIOLOGY AND CLINICAL PRESENTATION

Mechanisms

Microorganisms gain access to the lower respiratory tract through inhalation or aspiration. Generally, normal defense mechanisms in the upper and lower respiratory tract protect against infection. Organisms are entrapped by the mucus-producing cells and ciliated epithelium that line the nasal mucosa and oropharynx. Local production of immunoglobulin A in the nasal mucosa prevents bacterial adherence. The cough reflex removes large particles from the lower airways, and ciliated epithelium and mucus in the bronchial tree capture particles too small to be removed by coughing. Alveolar fluid contains complement and immunoglobulin that act as opsonins, and pulmonary macrophages then eliminate bacteria. If the burden is high, macrophages may produce cytokines, including tumor necrosis factor and interleukin-1, to recruit neutrophils to the area.

Infection of the lower respiratory tract occurs when the inoculum or the virulence of a microorganism overwhelms the host defenses. Cigarette smoke interferes with ciliary function and macrophage activity, and alcohol use may increase aspiration (by interfering with the cough reflex) and promote colonization in the upper airway by gram-negative bacteria. Deficiencies in humoral immunity occur in adults with common variable immunodeficiency, hematologic malignancies, or splenectomies. These people are more susceptible to infection with encapsulated organisms such as *Streptococcus pneumoniae* and *Haemophilus influenzae*. Patients with HIV infection have deficiencies in both cell-mediated and humoral immunity, which predisposes them to infection by numerous organisms.

The presentations of bronchitis and pneumonia are similar. Cough may be productive or nonproductive of sputum, and associated symptoms, including fever, chest discomfort, and fatigue, may be present in both entities. Pleurisy or dyspnea tends to suggest more extensive involvement, as seen in pneumonia. "Classic" community-acquired pneumonia presents with a sudden chill followed by fever, pleuritic pain, and productive cough. The "atypical pneumonia" syndrome, associated with *Mycoplasma* or *Chlamydia* infection, often begins with a sore throat and headache followed by a nonproductive cough and dyspnea. Physical examination findings may be misleading, especially in the patient with underlying lung disease. Evidence of consolidation on the lung examination (bronchial breath sounds, egophony) is indicative of pneumonia but is present in few outpatients. The chest x-ray film in acute bronchitis usually reveals no infiltrate or signs of consolidation, in contradistinction to the x-ray film in pneumonia. But even this most clear-cut distinction between bronchitis and pneumonia can be misleading because changes of chronic lung disease can simulate new infiltrates in some patients with bronchitis, whereas dehydration can minimize radiographic abnormalities in patients with pneumonia. The clinical presentations are, in part, a function of the causative organism.

Gram-positive Organisms

Streptococcus pneumoniae is still the most common cause of pneumonia, accounting for 30% to 50% of all cases of bacterial pneumonia. It is especially likely to be the agent infecting healthy young ambulatory patients, but it may affect all age groups. It is also responsible for acute exacerbations in patients with chronic bronchitis, but its role in acute bronchitis in healthy persons is unclear. Classic clinical features of pneumococcal pneumonia include abrupt onset of fever with a single rigor, cough with rusty sputum, and pleuritic chest pain. Radiologic evidence of lobar consolidation is typical, but infiltrates can be patchy, especially in patients with chronic lung disease. The sputum Gram's stain reveals abundant polymorphonuclear leukocytes and gram-positive diplococci (classically lancet-shaped) in pairs or short chains.

The most common complication of pneumococcal pneumonia is bacteremia, which occurs in about one third of patients. Blood-borne distant sepsis (e.g., septic arthritis, peritonitis, meningitis) is much less common. Sterile pleural effusions are common, whereas empyema is less frequent.

Staphylococcus aureus is the etiologic agent in up to 10% of cases of bacterial pneumonia. Except in infancy, when it can be a primary infection, staphylococcal pneumonia most commonly follows a viral respiratory tract infection, particularly *influenza*. It may also occur as a nosocomial infection or as a result of bacteremic seeding of the lungs, especially in patients who have staphylococcal endocarditis or are IV drug abusers. Patients with staphylococcal pneumonia of respiratory or bloodstream origin are usually extremely ill. *S. aureus* produces tissue necrosis, and the distinctive feature of staphylococcal pneumonia is the tendency to produce multiple small lung abscesses. Healing usually leaves some degree of residual fibrosis. Abundant polymorphonuclear leukocytes and gram-positive cocci in pairs, clumps, and clusters are found on the sputum Gram's stain. Local suppurative complications, including lung abscess, empyema, and pneumothorax, are relatively common. Bacteremia with metastatic seeding of distant sites, such as endocardium, bone, joints, liver, and meninges, may occur.

Group A Streptococci are a rather uncommon cause of infection, but this type of pneumonia has occurred in epidemics, especially in closed groups such as military units. Occasionally, streptococcal pneumonia can occur after primary influenza pneumonia. Streptococcal pneumonia usually begins abruptly with fever, cough, and severe debility. Chest pain is prominent in most patients. The distinctive clinical and radiologic feature is rapid spread in the lung, with resultant early empyema formation. Initially, the empyema fluid may be thin, possibly because of the many enzymes elaborated by group A streptococci, but later frank purulence occurs. Other complications, such as lung abscess, bacteremia, metastatic infection, and poststreptococcal glomerulonephritis, are uncommon. In patients with streptococcal pneumonia, the sputum Gram's stain reveals numerous polymorphonuclear leukocytes and gram-positive cocci in pairs and short to long chains.

Gram-negative Organisms

Haemophilus influenzae has long been recognized as a common cause of bronchitis in adults with chronic lung disease; however, recognition of this organism as a cause of frank pneumonias, sometimes with bacteremia, is increasing. Most cases of bronchitis are caused by untypeable strains of *H. influenzae*, but pneumonias are often caused by the more invasive encapsulated strains, especially type b. Radiographically, a bronchopneumonia pattern is typical. Abundant polymorphonuclear leukocytes and small, pleomorphic, gram-negative coccobacillary organisms are the characteristic findings in the sputum of patients with pneumonia or bronchitis cased by *H. influenzae*. Complications of *H. influenzae* pneumonia in adults are uncommon, but in patients with underlying chronic lung disease, the illness may be particularly severe, with development of hypoxia and respiratory failure.

Klebsiella pneumoniae typically produces pulmonary infection in debilitated patients, especially *alcoholics*, and *Klebsiella* pneumonia is one of the few gram-negative bacillary pneumonias seen commonly in ambulatory patients. It usually presents as an acute illness; rarely, it may cause chronic pneumonitis. The organism has a high propensity to produce tissue necrosis, which accounts for the hemoptysis, dense lobar consolidation, and high incidence of abscess formation seen in this illness. Sputum may appear dark red and mucoid ("currant jelly" sputum). Abundant polymorphonuclear leukocytes and large gram-negative bacilli, occasionally with thick capsules, are characteristically seen on sputum Gram's stain. Lung abscess and empyema may occur.

Other Gram-negative Bacillary Pneumonias were once rare but have increased during the past 15 years and now account for up to 20% of cases of bacterial pneumonia. They are principally hospital-acquired infections and remain rare in the ambulatory population. Patients with gram-negative bacillary pneumonia are typically debilitated from other illnesses or elderly and frequently have received antibiotic therapy, during which their normal respiratory flora are replaced with these otherwise unusual pathogens. Abundant polymorphonuclear leukocytes and gram-negative bacilli are seen on sputum Gram's stain. Complications, including lung abscess, empyema, and bacteremia with metastatic spread of infection, may occur.

Moraxella (Branhamella) catarrhalis is a gram-negative coccus that morphologically resembles organisms of the *Neisseria* family but differs in biochemical and DNA characteristics. It is found in the oropharynx of normal hosts and was not considered pathogenic until the 1980s, when it was established as the cause of lower respiratory tract infection in some patients with chronic obstructive pulmonary disease. In more than 80% of *Moraxella catarrhalis* infections, an *underlying pulmonary disease* is present. Diabetes, alcoholism, malignancy, and steroid use are other known risk factors. Cases appear to be concentrated in the *winter* months, perhaps indicating a relation to preceding viral infection. The typical lower respiratory tract infection that ensues is mild and sometimes even self-limited. The organism is readily identified by Gram's stain, and almost all sputum cultures are positive for organisms. Chest radiography shows an interstitial or interstitial–air space infiltrate. Bacteremia is rare, and full recovery with prompt response to antibiotics is the rule, although almost all isolates are positive for β-lactamase.

Bordetella pertussis, a gram-negative pleomorphic bacillus, is a frequently overlooked cause of acute bronchitis. Acquired immunity from childhood wanes after 15 to 20 years, so that young adults are rendered susceptible to pertussis. Several studies have shown that pertussis accounts for up to 25% of patients with acute bronchitis lasting two or more weeks. The disease typically has three phases. The *catarrhal phase* is indistinguishable from an upper respiratory infection, with rhinorrhea, low-grade fever, and mild congestion lasting 1 to 2 weeks. Patients are contagious in this stage and early into the next stage, the *paroxysmal phase*, which lasts for 2 to 4 weeks and is characterized by severe paroxysms of nonproductive coughing, with 10 to 30 coughs in a row. Posttussive syncope and vomiting are not uncommon; the characteristic "whoop" is absent in adults because of their larger airways. Finally, the symptoms gradually resolve during the next 1 to 3 months in the *convalescent phase*. The nasopharyngeal culture, which is used in children to establish the diagnosis, is often negative for organisms by the time adults seek medical attention. A single elevated pertussis serology has been advocated as a rapid means of diagnosing pertussis.

Legionnaires' Disease

First identified in the 1976 Philadelphia hotel outbreak, Legionnaires' disease is now recognized as an important cause of community-acquired pneumonia. *Legionella pneumophila*, an aerobic, fastidious, small, gram-negative bacillus, has been reported as the causative agent in 5% to 10% of all cases of community-acquired pneumonia and in up to 30% of cases of severe community-acquired pneumonia. The organism survives in water and, to a lesser extent, soil; infection is acquired by inhalation of contaminated aerosols or microaspiration of contaminated water. Epidemics have been traced to contaminated cooling systems, whirlpool baths, and potable water; nosocomial infections have occurred through contaminated hospital water supplies. Risk factors for *Legionella* infection include cigarette smoking, chronic lung disease, and immunosuppression. *L. pneumophila* is responsible for more than 90% of all cases; of the 14 serotypes of *L. pneumophila* identified, serogroup 1 is responsible for the majority of these cases. The next most common *Legionella* species is *L. micdadei* (the Pittsburgh pneumonia agent), which can cause cavitary lung disease in immunosuppressed patients.

The spectrum of clinical illness resulting from *Legionella* infection ranges from mild upper respiratory disease (Pontiac fever) and self-limited atypical pneumonia to multifocal pneumonia and respiratory failure. After a short prodrome, the full-blown form of Legionnaires' disease begins acutely with high fever, nonproductive cough, and dyspnea. *Pleuritic chest pain* occurs in about one third of cases. Systemic manifestations such as *diarrhea* or *confusion* are often seen but are not specific to legionellosis.

Relative bradycardia occurs in a few patients, but in most cases the physical examination findings are nonspecific. Chest radiography shows interstitial infiltrates or areas of patchy consolidation with characteristic rapid progression. Extrapulmonary findings are uncommon but include myocarditis, pericarditis, rhabdomyolysis, and renal dysfunction. Sputum is typically absent or scant. The sputum Gram's stain fails to reveal pathogens, but *L. pneumophila* can be cultured on a specialized buffered charcoal yeast extract agar. *Legionella* urinary antigen is very sensitive for disease caused by *L. pneumophila* serogroup 1 (about 70% of all cases) and is easy to obtain.

Mixed Flora

Aspiration pneumonias are usually mixed infections caused by aerobic and anaerobic streptococci, *Bacteroides*, and *Fusobacterium*. These organisms are normal flora of the upper airway that cause pneumonia if they attain a foothold in the lung parenchyma. Predisposing factors include alteration of consciousness (drugs, anesthesia, alcohol, head trauma) and diminution of the gag reflex, which permits aspiration to occur. Patients usually are mildly to moderately ill but can be toxic, especially if lung abscess or empyema occurs. Hospitalized patients, ambulatory patients receiving antibiotics, and edentulous patients have altered respiratory flora and fewer anaerobic organisms, if any. Aspiration of mouth organisms in such persons may result in staphylococcal or gram-negative bacillary pneumonia, as discussed previously, rather than the mixed aerobic–anaerobic infection considered here. The sputum from patients with aspiration pneumonia may be malodorous and characteristically shows abundant polymorphonuclear leukocytes and mixed flora, including gram-positive cocci in pairs and chains and pleomorphic gram-negative rods on Gram's stain. Lung abscess and empyema are fairly common complications of aspiration pneumonia, especially if therapy is delayed.

Nonbacterial Organisms

Mycoplasma pneumoniae is a cell wall–deficient organism that accounts for 10% to 25% of cases of community-acquired pneumonia. It is a leading cause of the *atypical pneumonia syndrome* (fever, dry cough, nonspecific infiltrate on chest film) and also a cause of acute bronchitis in otherwise healthy adults. The organism spreads by way of respiratory droplets and appears to have a long incubation period; onset of illness tends to be insidious. The disease often begins with headache, sore throat, and malaise, then progresses to a nonproductive cough. The physical examination findings are usually unimpressive in comparison with the *patchy peribronchial infiltrates* seen on chest x-ray films. Bullous myringitis has been reported in *Mycoplasma* pneumonia, but it is actually uncommon in clinical practice. Skin examination may show *erythema multiforme*, which is highly correlated with *Mycoplasma* infection in the patient with pneumonia. Laboratory studies reveal a normal white blood cell count and differential in most cases. The sputum is scant, with a predominance of mononuclear cells and no organisms. Sputum culture is not practical because a special medium is required and results do not become available for 2 weeks. Testing for the organism by polymerase chain reaction is a new technique with high sensitivity and specificity, although not widely available. *Cold agglutinins* are present in approximately 50% of cases. *Mycoplasma* pneumonia is usually a mild, self-limited illness, but it can produce severe pneumonia in children with sickle cell anemia, in immunosuppressed hosts, and in the elderly. Uncommon complications include hemolytic anemia, aseptic meningitis, Guillain-Barré syndrome, and myopericarditis.

Chlamydia pneumoniae (TWAR) is an obligate intracellular organism that causes an atypical pneumonia or acute bronchitis. It appears to account for 10% to 20% of cases of community-acquired pneumonia, with higher rates in young adults. *C. pneumoniae* appears to spread from person to person by respiratory droplets. The prodrome resembles that of *Mycoplasma pneumoniae*, with headache and sore throat followed by a dry cough, but the chest radiograph shows less extensive involvement. The diagnosis is difficult because culture requires tissue culture techniques that are not routinely performed. Serology (acute and convalescent titers) has been used to establish the diagnosis, and, as in *Mycoplasma* pneumonia, polymerase chain reaction is an upcoming (but not proven) new technology . The infection is usually self-limited; rare fatalities have been reported in debilitated patients.

Viruses are the most common cause of acute bronchitis, accounting for more than 80% of all cases. Viral pneumonia resembles an atypical pneumonia and is clinically indistinguishable except when it is part of a distinctive systemic viral illness, such as rubeola in children or varicella in adults. Many viruses are capable of producing lower respiratory tract infections, including influenza virus, adenoviruses, respiratory syncytial virus, and parainfluenza virus. Cytomegalovirus is a common cause of viral pneumonia in the immunocompromised host. The most important cause of viral pneumonia is influenza, which can be recognized by its epidemic spread and marked systemic symptoms, such as fever and myalgia. Influenza pneumonia may be mild or a fulminant illness capable of causing lethal respiratory failure. Bacterial pneumonia, especially of the pneumococcal, staphylococcal, or streptococcal variety, is a frequent complication.

Psittacosis is caused by a member of the *Chlamydia* group of obligate intracellular parasites, which are also responsible for lymphogranuloma venereum and trachoma. The disease is transmitted from parrots or other birds (including pigeons and turkeys) to humans. The clinical features of psittacosis are indistinguishable from those of other nonbacterial pneumonias, with prominent headache, nonproductive cough, and fever. Occasionally, a faint macular rash or splenomegaly develops.

Q Fever, caused by *Coxiella burnetii*, is unique among rickettsial infections in that pneumonia is prominent, no rash is associated, and spread is through inhalation of infected dust particles rather than by way of the bite of an insect vector. The organisms reside principally in animals; human contact with cattle, sheep, goats, or infected animal hides or hide products is the most important epidemiologic factor and is often the only clue to diagnosis. The clinical features of Q fever are similar to those of the other nonbacterial pneumonias, except that hepatitis occurs in up to one third of patients.

Fungi and Other Opportunistic Organisms. Immunosuppressed patients (e.g., those taking corticosteroids, HIV-positive patients) are at heightened risk for a community-acquired opportunistic infection (e.g., *Aspergillus*, *Candida*, or *Pneumocystis*; see Chapter 13). HIV-positive patients are also at increased risk for *primary tuberculosis* (see Chapter 49). However, some fungal infections may occur in immunocompetent hosts. For example, exposure to spore-containing dusts may lead to *histoplasmosis* (in the Midwest) or *coccidioidomycosis* (in the Southwest), characterized in the initial phases by a nonproductive cough, flulike illness, liver or splenic enlargement, alveolar infiltrates, and sometimes hilar adenopathy; however, most often the chest radiographic findings are normal.

DIFFERENTIAL DIAGNOSIS

The differential diagnosis of community-acquired pneumonia is listed in Table 52.1. In most epidemiologic studies, *S. pneumoniae* is the most common cause, followed by *H. influenzae*, influenza virus, and *Legionella*.

In addition to the conditions listed in Table 52.1 and detailed above, noninfectious diseases can occasionally mimic infectious processes. Bronchial asthma (see Chapter 48) and hyper-

Table 52.1. Differential Diagnosis of Pneumonia in Ambulatory Patients

Bacterial
Streptococcus pneumoniae
Haemophilus influenzae
Legionella species (most often *L. pneumophila*)
Staphylococcus aureus
Klebsiella pneumoniae (and other *Enterobacteriaceae*)
Moraxella catarrhalis
Streptococcus pyogenes
Mixed aerobic/anaerobic organisms (aspiration)

Nonbacterial
Mycoplasma pneumoniae
Chlamydia pneumoniae
Chlamydia psittaci
Mycobacterium tuberculosis
Coxiella burnetii (Q fever)
Viral (influenza virus, adenovirus)
Pneumocystis carinii
Fungi

sensitivity pneumonitis (see Chapter 51) are common examples. The radiologic findings associated with chronic pulmonary diseases, especially chronic bronchitis (see Chapter 47) and bronchiectasis (see Chapter 41), may be misleading if previous x-ray films are not available. Atelectasis, pulmonary infarction, pulmonary edema (see Chapter 32), and lung tumors may also be confused with pneumonia.

WORKUP

The first task is to differentiate lower respiratory tract infection from the other causes of cough (see Chapters 32, 41, 42, and 51) and from upper respiratory infection (see Chapters 50, 219, and 220). The predominant symptom of a patient presenting with a lower respiratory tract infection is usually cough, either productive or nonproductive of sputum. A predominant symptom of nasal discharge, sore throat, or ear pain can direct the workup away from the lower respiratory tract. Once a lower tract infection is suspected, the focus quickly shifts to the task of diagnosing pneumonia or bronchitis. Unfortunately, the distinction cannot be made reliably on the basis of any single element of the history or physical examination. A search for a specific cause is important if the presentation is unusual, unique exposures are present, or the patient is immunosuppressed.

History. Symptoms of pneumonia were previously classified as "typical" (productive cough, rigors, pleurisy) or "atypical" (nonproductive cough with a prodrome of headache and sore throat). These classifications originally were developed to discriminate pneumococcal pneumonia from pneumonia caused by "atypical" organisms, such as *Mycoplasma* and *Chlamydia*. However, the overlap in symptoms of pneumonia of different causes is substantial, so that this classification is unreliable. As stated above, the type of cough and the presence of dyspnea and fever are also unreliable to differentiate bronchitis from pneumonia.

The history is most useful to determine additional *comorbid conditions* that may influence prognosis or clarify etiology. Advanced age, congestive heart failure, cerebrovascular disease, active malignancy, and renal or liver disease all predict a poorer outcome in patients with pneumonia. In addition, patient characteristics may increase the likelihood of particular organisms. Alcoholics have a higher incidence of infection with gram-negative organisms, especially *K. pneumoniae*, and patients with chronic lung disease are often colonized with *H. influenzae* and *M. catarrhalis*. Nosocomial pathogens, including resistant organisms and *Pseudomonas*, should be considered in nursing home residents. HIV-positive patients are at risk for infection with a number of opportunistic pathogens, such as *Pneumocystis carinii* and *Mycobacterium tuberculosis*.

The history may also be useful in *identifying unusual exposures* or epidemiologic associations to raise the possibility of specific causes. Patients should be assessed for close contact with birds (psittacosis), livestock (Q fever), or rabbits (tularemia). A patient residing in or traveling to the southwestern United States (coccidioidomycosis) or the Midwest (histoplasmosis) may acquire an acute fungal pneumonia, which is usually self-limited without treatment except in immunocompromised hosts. Patients who are at high risk for tuberculosis exposure (immunosuppressed, homeless, exposed to known contact) should be assessed for mycobacterial infection.

Physical Examination. No single physical examination finding can definitively diagnose pneumonia, although the clinician should focus on the vital signs and pulmonary examination to assist diagnosis and prognosis. High fever (>104°F), hypothermia, tachypnea, and tachycardia are all associated with an increased 30-day mortality. Conversely, several studies have demonstrated that the presence of entirely normal vital signs decreases the probability of pneumonia in outpatients to less than 1%. The pulmonary examination in pneumonia often demonstrates crackles, although patients with bronchitis may have similar findings. The classic findings of lung consolidation (dullness to percussion, egophony, bronchial breath sounds) are more specific for pneumonia but are found in fewer than 25% of patients with radiographic evidence of pneumonia. Some physical findings may have etiologic significance. Erythema multiforme is associated with *Mycoplasma* pneumonia, and confusion is seen more often in *Legionella* infection.

Laboratory Studies. In the patient with acute bronchitis, laboratory testing is often unnecessary. However, if pneumonia is suspected, posteroanterior and lateral *chest radiography* is required to confirm the diagnosis. In addition to indicating the extent of disease, the chest x-ray film may also show a pleural effusion, which is associated with a poorer outcome. Unless the pleural effusion is minimal, *thoracentesis* should be performed to assess for the presence of an empyema or complicated parapneumonic effusion. Fluid is sent for Gram's stain, culture, cell count, and determination of glucose, protein, and lactate dehydrogenase levels and pH (see Chapter 43).

The value of routine sputum collection for *Gram's stain* and *culture* remains controversial. In acute bronchitis, the predominance of viral and atypical bacterial organisms makes these tests unlikely to influence treatment decisions. For the patient with pneumonia, the American Thoracic Society has recommended empiric treatment without an aggressive etiologic workup, but more recently the Infectious Disease Society of America has advocated performing sputum Gram's stain and culture in all patients hospitalized with community-acquired pneumonia. This recommendation recognizes the limitations of Gram's stain and culture but also argues for the importance of detecting resistant or atypical organisms and tailoring antibiotic treatment according to culture results. With the increasing presence of resistant organisms, it is reasonable to obtain a specimen for Gram's stain and culture if the patient is producing sputum.

If a sputum sample is obtained, it is essential to ensure that it is adequate. The specimen is obtained from a deep cough, with the use of nebulized saline solution if necessary. For a causative organism to be predicted accurately, the Gram's stain should show fewer than 10 epithelial cells and more than 25 polymorphonuclear cells per low-power field. Interpretation needs to be performed by an experienced observer. Small gram-negative rods may be overlooked by an inexperienced observer, and inadequate decolorization results in misclassification of gram-negative organisms as gram-positive. *Pneumococcal* infections show gram-positive, lancet-shaped diplococci; gram-negative cocci suggest *Moraxella*, and gram-negative coccobacillary forms are indicative of *H. influenzae*. Despite attempts to obtain an adequate specimen, upper respiratory contamination, fastidious pathogens, and delay in transportation all limit the utility of the sputum culture, results of which are negative in about 50% of cases. Ideally, all cultures should be obtained and sent before antibiotics are started, but failure to obtain a sputum specimen should not delay necessary treatment.

In hospitalized patients, additional tests, including a complete blood count, assessment of renal function, and determination of electrolytes, are obtained. Serum liver enzymes are frequently elevated in patients with pneumonia, regardless of the cause. An *arterial blood gas* may be obtained if the patient has an underlying pulmonary disease or the clinical picture warrants the test. *Blood cultures* are positive in about 10% to 15% of patients and may be the only accurate method of identifying the causative organisms. Blood for two sets of cultures should be drawn from different sites before initiation of antibiotic therapy.

Detection of *Legionella urinary antigen* is an accessible and rapid method for diagnosing Legionnaires' disease. The test is very sensitive for *L. pneumophila* serogroup 1, which accounts for more than 70% of cases of pneumonia in humans. The antigen persists in the urine even after antibiotics have been started and may persist for months after infection. A *Legionella* urinary antigen test should be performed in all patients with a clinical picture suggestive of legionellosis. Legionnaires' disease can also be diagnosed in 3 to 5 days by culture of the organism on special media. Serology may also be used to detect infection, but the delay in results makes this a less useful test. A single *antibody titer* of 1:256 is presumptive evidence, but confirmation requires demonstration of a fourfold rise in titer between acute and convalescent specimens.

Additional testing in patients with community-acquired pneumonia is usually unnecessary. Measurement of acute and convalescent serologic titers can confirm infection with *Mycoplasma*, *Chlamydia*, *Coxiella burnetii*, or viral agents. Recognition of influenza is important because contacts can be protected by prophylactic use of amantadine; diagnostic confirmation is worth seeking when influenza is suspected. In the HIV-infected patient with pneumonia, an induced sputum sample or bronchoalveolar lavage is stained for *Pneumocystis* and *M. tuberculosis* (see Chapter 13).

PRINCIPLES OF MANAGEMENT

Many patients with community-acquired lower respiratory tract infections can be managed on an outpatient basis, provided that they are alert, reliable, have help available to them, and have no signs of serious compromise (see Indications for Admission). In the Pneumonia Patient Outcomes Research Trial (PORT), about 50% of patients were identified to be at low risk for complications and appropriate for outpatient treatment. These patients had a 30-day mortality of less than 1%. Therapeutic serum levels can be achieved with oral antibiotic regimens for patients treated at home. The appropriate use of antibiotics is discussed in the next section (see Therapeutic Recommendations).

Patients with bronchitis or pneumonia often ask for medication to relieve the cough that prompted them to seek medical care. Suppression is not encouraged in patients with acute cough because the cough reflex remains an important defense mechanism. Adequate *hydration* is essential to help clear secretions; this can be achieved by fluid intake and local airway humidification. *Expectorants* such as guaifenesin may be helpful to some patients in loosening the sputum, although they have not been proved to make a significant difference in outcome. *Pulmonary physical therapy* may help mobilize secretions, but prospective trials have failed to demonstrate that this time-honored intervention improves outcome (see Chapters 41 and 47).

In some patients, persistent coughing results in severe musculoskeletal chest pain or respiratory fatigue. Nocturnal cough may interfere with sleep and prevent the patient from getting adequate rest. In these cases, several treatments may be offered. In two small trials of patients with acute bronchitis, β_2-agonists, such as albuterol, have decreased the duration of cough. Expiratory flow rates can be decreased in these patients, as in those with reactive airway disease. Because the persistent cough in bronchitis appears to be related to bronchial irritation, not to continuing infection, this treatment makes physiologic sense. However, its use is limited by the lack of large studies, side effects of the medication, and time required to teach inexperienced patients how to use inhalers. *Cough suppressants*, which directly diminish the cough reflex, include dextromethorphan and codeine. These medicines may provide temporary relief, especially when taken before bed (see Chapter 41). Although the tablet form is equally effective, patients may prefer a syrup formulation for cough suppression. Fever, another bothersome symptom, can be controlled with aspirin or acetaminophen (see Chapter 11).

Oxygen therapy may be required in hospitalized patients with pneumonia. In general, treatment should be titrated to the patient's respiratory status and not be focused on a specific oxygen saturation or concentration. Lung consolidation in pneumonia functions as a shunt, and an increase in oxygen may not result in improved arterial oxygenation. In addition, patients with chronic lung disease who retain carbon dioxide may experience respiratory depression with excessive oxygen therapy (see Chapter 47).

Antibiotic therapy should be initiated promptly when appropriate. Because most etiologic testing requires 24 to 48 hours, treatment is usually empiric. Therapy is then modified in response to diagnostic test results and the patient's response to therapy. For most bacterial infections, continued treatment for 10 to 14 days is the standard of care.

THERAPEUTIC RECOMMENDATIONS

Treatment for lower respiratory tract infections is tailored to the clinical syndrome and likely pathogens. Table 52.2 summarizes the empiric antibiotic recommendations for the various clinical syndromes, and Table 52.3 describes the recommendations for specific pathogens.

Table 52.2. Empiric Treatment for Lower Respiratory Tract Infections

CLINICAL SYNDROME	PREFERRED EMPIRIC TREATMENT	ALTERNATIVE TREATMENT
Acute bronchitis	None	Doxycycline, erythromycin
Acute exacerbation of chronic bronchitis	Second-generation cephalosporin	Second-generation macrolide[a], trimethoprim/sulfamethoxazole
Community-acquired penumonia		
Healthy young adults	Macrolide	Doxycycline, newer fluoroquinolone[b]
Elderly (age >60) or comorbid disease	Second- or third-generation cephalosporin	Second-generation macrolide, β-lactam/β-lactamase inhibitor
Hospitalized patient	Third-generation cephalosporin, macrolide, or both	Second-generation macrolide, newer fluoroquinolone

[a]Second-generation macrolides include clarithromycin and azithromycin.
[b]Newer fluoroquinolones are agents with adequate pneumococcal activity, including levofloxacin and sparfloxacin.

Table 52.3. Pathogen-Specific Therapy for Lower Respiratory Tract Infections

ORGANISM	FIRST-LINE AGENT	ALTERNATIVE AGENTS
Streptococcus pneumoniae		
Penicillin-sensitive (MIC <0.1 μg/mL)	Penicillin	Erythromycin
Intermediate penicillin resistance (MIC 0.1–1.0 μg/mL)	Parenteral penicillin	Ceftriaxone
Highly penicillin-resistant (MIC >2.0 μg/mL)	Vancomycin	Newer fluoroquinolone
Legionella pneumoniae	Erythromycin	Second-generation macrolide, newer fluoroquinolone
Haemophilus influenzae	Second-generation cephalosporin	Second-generation macrolide, trimethoprim/sulfamethoxazole
Moraxella catarrhalis		
Chlamydia pneumoniae	Doxycycline or erythromycin	Second-generation macrolide, newer fluoroquinolone
Chlamydia psittaci		
Mycoplasma pneumoniae		
Staphylococcus aureus	Nafcillin	Vancomycin (if methicillin-resistant), cefazolin
Klebsiella pneumoniae	Second- or third-generation cephalosporin	β-lactam/β-lactamase inhibitor, fluoroquinolone
Streptococcus pyogenes	Penicillin	Cephalosporin, erythromycin
Coxiella burnetii (Q fever)	Doxycycline	Chloramphenicol
Mixed anaerobic/aerobic infection (aspiration)	Clindamycin	Penicillin plus metronidazole
Bordetella pertussis	Erythromycin	Second-generation macrolide, trimethoprim/sulfamethoxazole
Influenza A	Amantadine	Rimantadine

MIC, minimum inhibitory concentration.

Acute Bronchitis. At least eight randomized, placebo-controlled trials have failed to show a benefit of empiric antibiotic therapy (doxycycline, trimethoprim/sulfamethoxazole, or erythromycin) in healthy patients with acute bronchitis. In most studies, cough resolved at 1 week regardless of treatment, and persistence of cough for 2 weeks was not unusual. These smaller trials have been combined in two separate systematic reviews that have confirmed the lack of benefit of antibiotics in these patients. Newer antibiotics may have better intracellular penetration and efficacy; however, the lack of placebo-controlled trials, the predominantly viral causes of acute bronchitis, and the preceding data argue against the routine use of antibiotics for acute bronchitis. Despite this evidence, several studies have suggested that physicians prescribe antibiotics for more than 60% of outpatients with acute cough and no underlying lung disease. Epidemiologic studies show that relatively few of these patients actually have pneumonia as the cause of their cough. Healthy patients with acute bronchitis should be treated with conservative measures for cough (see above) and counseled about the natural history of the disease.

The one exception to this approach is the patient with *pertussis*. Early antibiotic therapy with erythromycin can effectively treat *B. pertussis* infection, but most adults who seek medical attention are in the paroxysmal phase, when tracheal damage has already occurred. However, they may still be infectious in the early paroxysmal phase, and treatment can decrease the transmission of *B. pertussis*. Therefore, the patient with documented or suspected pertussis is treated with 500 mg of *erythromycin* four times daily for 7 to 14 days. Prophylactic treatment with the same regimen (adjusted for weight in children) is recommended for household members and close contacts, especially unvaccinated infants. In the patient intolerant of erythromycin, trimethoprim/sulfamethoxazole or a second-generation macrolide (e.g., azithromycin, clarithromycin) may be substituted.

Acute Exacerbation of Chronic Bronchitis. Antibiotics are effective in relieving symptoms and preventing deterioration of lung function in patients with established chronic bronchitis. *S. pneumoniae*, *H. influenzae*, and *M. catarrhalis* are the common pathogens in these patients. A second-generation β-lactam, such as cefuroxime, is the treatment of choice. Alternatives include a second-generation macrolide or trimethoprim/sulfamethoxazole. Additional treatment depends on the patient's condition and underlying lung function (see Chapter 47).

Community-acquired Pneumonia. Antibiotics are clearly indicated for the treatment of community-acquired pneumonia, although no randomized trials have been completed. Evidence consists of the significant decrease in pneumonia mortality since the introduction of antibiotics and the adverse outcomes associated with delayed or inappropriate antibiotic therapy in patients with pneumonia. Increasing drug resistance, notably penicillin-resistance in *S. pneumoniae*, has complicated the empiric selection of antibiotics. The initial treatment is directed at the most common pathogens, and patients are classified by age, comorbidities, and severity of pneumonia.

Healthy Young Adults. In persons less than 60 years old, the most common organisms are *S. pneumoniae*, *Mycoplasma*, *Chlamydia*, and *Legionella*. All these organisms are covered adequately *erythromycin* (500 mg four times daily), which is the first-line treatment. Although macrolide resistance is increasing in *S. pneumoniae*, observational studies have validated this approach as an effective, inexpensive strategy. Penicillins or cephalosporins will not cover the atypical organisms in this age group. Alternative agents include *doxycycline* (100 mg twice daily) or the second-generation macrolides. Newer fluoroquinolones, such as levofloxacin, have adequate activity against the pathogens and are well tolerated. Experience with these agents is limited, however, and indiscriminate use will certainly translate into resistant strains. Older fluoroquinolones (e.g., ciprofloxacin) have less activity against the pneumococcus and are not recommended.

Older Adults and Patients with Comorbidities. S. pneumoniae remains the most common cause of pneumonia, but *H. influenzae*, *M. catarrhalis*, and other gram-negative organisms are alternative possibilities. The atypical organisms such as *Mycoplasma* and *Chlamydia* are unusual in this population. Therefore, the recommended first-line treatment is a *second- or third-generation cephalosporin*. *Cefuroxime* (although not officially approved for pneumonia) is a common choice because it has adequate activity against the common pathogens and is available in twice-daily dosing. Alternatives include β-lactam/β-lactamase inhibitor combinations (e.g., amoxicillin/clavulanate), second-generation macrolides, and fluoroquinolones with adequate pneumococcal coverage.

Patients who are ill enough to be hospitalized for pneumonia often require *parenteral antibiotic therapy*. The causative organisms are similar to those described above, but the potential for worsening respiratory status is higher in these sicker patients. Empiric treatment may be selected based on the patient characteristics described in the first two groups, but therapy is often broadened in sicker patients to cover potentially resistant organisms and a wider spectrum of organisms. For patients with severe pneumonia and an inconclusive Gram's stain, the first-line treatment is a *third-generation cephalosporin* (e.g., 1 g of ceftriaxone daily) *plus a macrolide* in a dose sufficient for *Legionella* infection (e.g., 1 g of erythromycin four times daily). For patients in whom fluid overload is a concern, erythromycin may be equally divided between oral and IV doses. Therapy can then be narrowed after results of diagnostic tests, such as *Legionella* urinary antigen and blood cultures, become available. Focused therapy may also be initiated on presentation when an adequate Gram's stain is highly suggestive of a particular pathogen (see table 52.3). Alternative empiric parenteral treatments include *azithromycin* and several *fluoroquinolones*. These alternatives offer the advantage of single-agent therapy.

Antibiotic Resistance in S. pneumoniae. Previously, S. pneumoniae was almost universally susceptible to penicillin. However, resistance to penicillin, mediated by mutations in penicillin-binding proteins, was first reported in the 1960s in Australia. During the past decade, these resistant organisms have become an increasing concern in the United States. Approximately 25% of pneumococci in the United States have intermediate penicillin resistance (mean inhibitory concentration, or MIC, of 0.1 to 1.0 μmg/mL), and up to 10% are highly penicillin-resistant (MIC >2.0 μmg/mL). These highly resistant organisms are often cross-resistant to multiple antibiotics, including trimethoprim/sulfamethoxazole and erythromycin. Fortunately, parenteral penicillin appears to achieve adequate levels in the tissues for the effective treatment of pneumococci with intermediate resistance. For highly resistant organisms, alternative agents are recommended. Fluoro-quinolone resistance has been very low in *S. pneumoniae*; however, as these agents are used more frequently, resistant strains are being reported. The increasing prevalence of pneumococcal resistance to antibiotics serves to emphasize the need to vaccinate high-risk patients (see below); more than 85% of resistant organisms are serotypes contained in the 23-valent vaccine.

MONITORING THERAPY

Clinical improvement is best indicated by improved vital signs. The Pneumonia PORT validated temperature, respiratory rate, heart rate, and blood pressure as reliable measures of stability. On average, patients achieved "normal" vital signs at a median of 3 days after hospitalization. However, patients were often not completely "afebrile" (temperature < 99°F) until day 6. Once patients reached clinical stability, indicated by normal vital signs along with a normal mental status and an ability to take oral medication, deterioration in clinical status was rare (<1%).

Repeating chest radiography at frequent intervals is wasteful if the patient is progressing well clinically. The clearing of radiologic findings often lags far behind clinical resolution; the continued presence of a slowly resolving infiltrate is neither a sign of poor response to therapy nor indicative of a serious prognosis. This is particularly true of pneumococcal or *Legionella* pneumonia, in which radiography may still show an infiltrate months later. However, when the patient's condition is worsening or fever is not resolving, radiographic examination is important for the detection of complications such as lung abscess and empyema. In addition, the possibility of unusual or resistant organisms should be considered in these patients, and antibiotic therapy appropriately adjusted.

INDICATIONS FOR ADMISSION

As mentioned previously, one of the most important decisions in the care of the patient with a community-acquired lower respiratory infection is selecting the proper setting for care. The decision is obvious in the case of a healthy young patient with an acute bronchitis or a seriously ill patient with overt respiratory compromise. In between are the many patients who are elderly or have underlying cardiopulmonary disease and present in the ambulatory setting with a lower respiratory tract infection; they are a source of concern.

Many studies have examined large numbers of patients with community-acquired pneumonia to determine predictors of poor outcome. Common predictors of worse outcome in these studies include advanced age, comorbidities, and abnormal vital signs. It is important to note that these trials often excluded immunosuppressed patients, who have an overall worse prognosis and are likely to require hospitalization. A useful prediction rule described by Fine et al. has been validated on more than 38,000 inpatients with pneumonia and the more than 2,200 patients of the Pneumonia PORT (Fig. 52.1 and Table 52.4). Patients with none of the comorbidities or vital sign abnormalities indicated in Fig. 52.1 are assigned to class 1 (low risk). Remaining patients are assigned a point score based on the system listed in Table 52.4. Patients with point totals below 90 have a

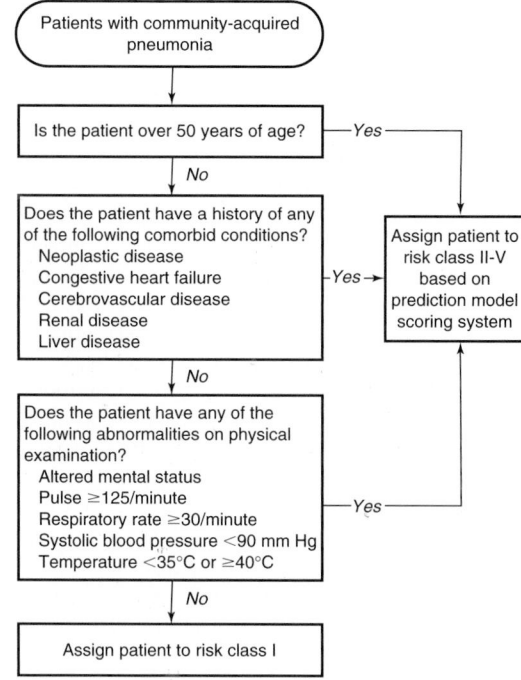

FIG. 52.1. Algorithm for triage in patients with community-acquired pneumonia. (Adapted from Fine MJ, Auble TE, Yealy DM, et al. A prediction to identify low-risk patients with community-acquired pneumonia. N Engl J Med 1997;336:243, with permission.)

low mortality (<1%) and a low risk for deterioration (<6%) and may be considered for outpatient therapy. Of course, any prediction rule does not replace clinical judgment; these rules perform poorly in extreme or unusual circumstances. For example, a 20-year-old man with hypotension, tachycardia, and hypoxia would have a low score but clearly requires hospitalization, if not intensive care.

In addition, the decision for hospitalization will depend on the *quality of the home environment* and the *ability to tolerate oral therapy*. Alternative options, such as home IV therapy and subacute care facilities, have become increasingly practical and cost-effective, especially in the era of managed care.

PATIENT EDUCATION

Patients with lower respiratory tract infections need to be educated about their natural history. As stated above, patients with acute bronchitis often have a persistent cough for 1 to 2 weeks. However, these patients usually show an overall improvement by the end of the first week. In patients with pneu-

Table 52.4. Pneumonia PORT Scoring

PATIENT CHARACTERISTIC	POINTS ASSIGNED[a]
Demographic Factors	
Age: male	age (y)
female	age (y) − 10
Nursing home resident	+10
Comorbid Illnesses	
Neoplastic disease	+30
Liver disease	+20
Congestive heart failure	+10
Cerebrovascular disease	+10
Renal disease	+10
Physical Examination Findings	
Altered mental status	+20
Respiratory rate ≥30/min	+20
Systolic blood pressure	
<90 mm Hg	+20
Temperature <35° C or ≥40°C	+15
Pulse ≥125/min	+10
Laboratory Findings	
pH <7.35	+30
BUN >10.7 mmol/L	+20
Sodium <130 mEq/L	+20
Glucose >13.9 mmol/L	+10
Hematocrit <30%	+10
Po$_2$ <60 mm Hg[b]	+10
Pleural effusion	+10

[a]A risk score (total point score) for a given patient is obtained by summing the patient age in years (age −10 for female) and the points for each applicable patient characteristic.
[b]Oxygen saturation <90% also was considered abnormal.
PORT, Patient Outcomes Research Trial; BUN, blood urea nitrogen.
Adapted from Fine MJ, Auble TE, Yealy DM, et al. A prediction rule to identify low-risk patients with community-acquired pneumonia. N Engl J Med 1997; 336:243, with permission.

monia, the recovery period is much longer. More than 50% of patients with pneumonia continue to report fatigue and cough 1 month after diagnosis. Patients with persistent symptoms often require more outpatient visits during follow-up.

Patients can monitor their own temperature at home if treated in the outpatient setting. Persistent fever, worsening respiratory status, or increasing confusion are reasons to seek medical attention. Patients who smoke should be strongly urged to quit if they have not already done so. In fact, this is an excellent opportunity to encourage patients to quit because many do at this time (see Chapter 54).

Patients who recover from community-acquired pneumonia are eligible to receive pneumococcal and influenza vaccinations. Patients who are elderly (>65 years), have congestive heart failure or obstructive lung disease, are immunosuppressed, or have undergone splenectomy are also candidates for vaccination. The *polyvalent pneumococcal vaccine* (see Chapters 6 and 47) incorporates 23 capsular types of pneumococci, which together account for about 90% of cases of pneumococcal pneumonia in the United States. Revaccination after 5 years is now recommended for immunosuppressed persons, patients with functional asplenia, and elderly persons who received the initial vaccination before age 65. The influenza vaccine, composed of a purified inactivated virus, is modified each year to include prevalent strains of influenza A and influenza B. Hy-

persensitivity to eggs is a contraindication to influenza vaccination. The vaccines may be given at the same time without an increase in side effects or decrease in immunogenicity.

ANNOTATED BIBLIOGRAPHY

Anonymous. Prevention of pneumococcal disease: recommendations of the Advisory Committee on Immunization Practices (ACIP). MMWR Morb Mortal Wkly Rep 1997;46(RR-8):1. (*Guideline for pneumococcal vaccination, with new emphasis on revaccination.*)

Austrian R, Gold J. Pneumococcal bacteremia with special reference to bacteremic pneumococcal pneumonia. Ann Intern Med 1964;60:759. (*Classic study of clinical features and prognostic indicators in bacteremic pneumococcal pneumonia.*)

Bartlett JG, Breiman RF, Mandell LA, et al. Community-acquired pneumonia in adults: guidelines for management. Clin Infect Dis 1998;26:811. (*Guidelines from Infectious Disease Society of America, emphasizing diagnostic workup for patients hospitalized with community-acquired pneumonia.*)

Bent S, Saint S, Vittinghoff E, et al. Antibiotics in acute bronchitis: a metaanalysis. Am J Med 1999;107:62. (*A metaanalysis finding a small benefit, insufficient to justify use.*)

Fahey T, Stocks N, Thomas T. Quantitative systematic review of randomised controlled trials comparing antibiotic with placebo for acute cough in adults. BMJ 1998;316:906. (*Another metaanalysis, examining many of the same studies as in Bent et al.; finds no effect of antibiotics on cough or course of illness.*)

Fang G-D, Fine M, Orloff J, et al. New and emerging etiologies for community-acquired pneumonia with implications for therapy. Medicine (Baltimore) 1990;69:307. (*Despite aggressive diagnostic workup, only 59% of patients with community-acquired pneumonia had an identifiable cause. Legionella was the third most common pathogen.*)

Fine MJ, Auble TE, Yealy DM, et al. A prediction rule to identify low-risk patients with community-acquired pneumonia. N Engl J Med 1997;336:243. (*Prediction rule, prospectively validated on more than 40,000 patients, accurately predicted a low-risk group with 30-day mortality below 1%.*)

Gonzales R, Steiner JF, Sande MA. Antibiotic prescribing for adults with colds, upper respiratory tract infections, and bronchitis by ambulatory care physicians. JAMA 1997;278:901. (*Antibiotics prescribed to 51% of patients with a cold, 52% with upper respiratory infection, and 66% with acute bronchitis. Rates were higher among women and lower among African-Americans.*)

Gonzales R, Steiner JF, Lum A, et al. Decreasing antibiotic use in ambulatory practice: impact of a multidimensional intervention on the treatment of uncomplicated acute bronchitis in adults. JAMA 1999;281:1512. (*Patient education and academic detailing reduced prescription rates from 74% to 48%.*)

Halm EA, Fine MJ, Marrie TJ, et al. Time to clinical stability in patients hospitalized with community-acquired pneumonia: implications for practice guidelines. JAMA 1998;279:1452. (*Most patients reached clinical "stability" by day 3 of hospitalization, and normalized vital signs were a valid basis for a discharge decision.*)

Hoffman J, Cetron MS, Farley MM, et al. The prevalence of drug-resistant *Streptococcus pneumoniae* in Atlanta. New Engl J Med 1995;333:481. (*Centers for Disease Control study showing 25% prevalence of penicillin resistance in invasive streptococcal infections.*)

Hueston WJ. Albuterol delivered by metered-dose inhaler to treat acute bronchitis. J Fam Pract 1994;39:437. (*Small, blinded, placebo-controlled trial showed a significant resolution in cough at 7 days.*)

Jay SJ, Johannson WG, Pierce AK. The radiographic resolution of

Streptococcus pneumoniae pneumonia. N Engl J Med 1975;293:798. (*Classic study showing that delayed resolution of radiographic abnormalities is typical.*)

Kleemola SRM, Karjalainen JE, Raty RKH. Rapid diagnosis of *Mycoplasma pneumoniae* infection: clinical evaluation of a commercial probe test. J Infect Dis 1990;162:70. (*Sensitivity was 95% and specificity 85% when sputum samples were tested with this DNA probe.*)

La Force MA. Community-acquired lower respiratory tract infections: prevention and cost-control strategies. Am J Med 1985;78:52. (*Provocative article examining the utility of diagnostic, preventive, and treatment modalities.*)

Mansel JK, Rosenow EC, Smith TE, et al. *Mycoplasma pneumoniae* pneumonia. Chest 1989;95:639. (*Excellent review of this important cause of atypical pneumonia.*)

Marrie TJ, Grayston JT, Wang S-P, et al. Pneumonia associated with the TWAR strain of *Chlamydia.* Ann Intern Med 1987;106:507. (*Documents that TWAR can cause serious pneumonia in older patients in addition to mild acute respiratory disease in younger ones.*)

Mayer RD. *Legionella* infections: a review of 5 years of research. Rev Infect Dis 1983;5:258. (*Excellent overview of the epidemiology, pathogenesis, diagnosis, and management of this important infection.*)

Metlay JP, Kapoor WN, Fine MJ. Does this patient have community-acquired pneumonia? JAMA 1997;278:1440. (*Discussion of the predictive value of history and physical examination in diagnosing pneumonia.*)

Neiderman MS, Bass JB, Campbell GD, et al. Guidelines for the initial management of adults with community-acquired pneumonia: diagnosis, assessment of severity; and initial antimicrobial therapy. Am Rev Respir Dis 1993;148:1418. (*American Thoracic Society guidelines recommending empiric therapy based on common pathogens in certain patients.*)

Neu HC. New macrolide antibiotics: azithromycin and clarithromycin.

Ann Intern Med 1992;116:517. (*More useful for their expanded spectrum of activity, such as against Lyme disease and atypical mycobacteria, than for their effectiveness against conditions well covered by erythromycin, although more effective against* H. influenzae.)

Plouffe JF, File TM, Breiman RF, et al. Reevaluation of the definition of Legionnaires' disease: use of the urinary antigen assay. Clin Infect Dis 1995;20:1286. (*Urinary antigen was detected in 56% of all cases and was highly specific.*)

Ruiz-Gonzalez, A, Falguera M, Nogues A, et al. Is *Streptococcus pneumoniae* the leading cause of pneumonia of unknown etiology? A microbiologic study of lung aspirates in consecutive patients with community-acquired pneumonia. Am J Med 1999;106:385. (*Accounted for 25% of all cases, and for 33% of cases of otherwise unknown cause.*)

Sarubbi FA, Myers JW, Williams JJ, et al. Respiratory infections caused by *Branhamella catarrhalis*: selected epidemiologic features. Am J Med 1990;88[Suppl 5A]:9S. (*Seasonal pattern; seen in both pediatric and adult populations; many isolates positive for β-lactamase.*)

Sims RV, Steinmann WC, McConville JH, et al. The clinical effectiveness of pneumococcal vaccine in the elderly. Ann Intern Med 1988;108:653. (*Documents 70% efficacy in the elderly.*)

Woodhead MA, MacFarlane JT, McCraqcken JS, et al. Prospective study of the aetiology and outcome of pneumonia in the community. Lancet 1987;1:671. (*A British study;* Pneumococcus *was the most frequent pathogen, identified in 36% of cases;* H. influenzae *accounted for 10%; no cause was identified in 45%; mortality 3%.*)

Wright SW, Edwards KM, Decker MD, et al. Pertussis infection in adults with a persistent cough. JAMA 1995;273:1044. (*Emergency department–based study finding that 21% of patients with cough lasting longer than 2 weeks had evidence of pertussis infection.*)

Wright PW, Wallace RJ, Shepherd JR. A descriptive study of 42 cases of *Branhamella catarrhalis* pneumonia. Am J Med 1990;88[Suppl 5A]:2S. (*Describes a mild clinical illness occurring in many pa-*

53
Approach to the Patient with Lung Cancer

Lung cancer continues to be the leading cause of cancer deaths in the United States and is the second most common cause of cancer death among men and women, trailing prostate and breast cancers, respectively. Cigarette smoking accounts for 95% of lung cancers in men and 85% of those in women (see Chapter 54). Once established, most forms of lung cancer are minimally responsive to therapy, although important exceptions exist. The primary physician needs to be skilled in prevention (see Chapter 54); alert to early signs of lung cancer (see Chapters 41, 42, and 44); capable of conducting the workup, staging, and monitoring of the disease; and knowledgeable about treatment options and their effects on survival and quality of life.

PATHOLOGY, CLINICAL PRESENTATION, AND COURSE

The common types of bronchogenic carcinoma are designated as squamous cell, adenocarcinoma, large-cell, and small-cell. Each has its own epidemiologic and clinical characteris-

tics, although, with the exception of small-cell disease, they share a similar natural history and response to therapy. Consequently, lung cancers are often classified as small-cell (SCLC) and non–small-cell (NSCLC).

Small-cell Lung Cancer (formerly known as oat cell carcinoma) is typically central in location and accounts for 25% of cases. Growth is rapid, with 50% to 75% of patients manifesting evidence of metastatic disease beyond the chest at the time of clinical presentation and initial staging. These tumors derive from endocrine cells of the bronchial mucosa and can produce a variety of paraneoplastic syndromes (see Chapter 92). Untreated, the course of illness is rapid, with a median survival of only a few months. However, these tumors are very responsive to chemotherapy (see below).

Non–Small-Cell Lung Cancer. A fourth to a third of patients with NSCLC present with localized disease (stages I and II).

Table 53.1. Staging and Survival in Non–Small-Cell Lung Cancer

STAGE	TUMOR	NODES	METASTASES	FIVE-YEAR SURVIVAL
I	T1 or T2	N0	M0	50%
II	T1 or T2	N1	M0	30%
IIIa	T1-2 or T3	N1 or N0	M0	15%
IIIb	any T	any N	M0	<5%
IV	any T	any N	M1	0%

Staging for small-cell lung cancer is designed as either "limited disease" (confined to the thorax) or "extensive disease" (metastasis outside the thorax). T1, lesions up to 3 cm in diameter; T2, lesions >3 cm; T3, invasion of mediastinum, diaphragm, or chest wall; T4, invasion of heart, great vessels, or malignant pleural effusion; N0, no nodal involvement; N1, tracheobronchial or hilar node involvement; N2, ipsilateral mediastinal nodes; N3, contralateral or supraclavicular nodes; M0, no metastasis; M1, systemic metastasis. Adapted from Mountain CF. A new international staging system for lung cancer. Chest 1986;89[suppl 4]:225S, with permission.

Another fourth to a third have locally or regionally advanced disease (stages IIIa and b), and a third to a half present with advanced disease and distant metastases (stage IV). Survival is a function of stage at the time of presentation, with nearly 40% of the first group surviving 5 years, 7% of the second group, and fewer than 1% of patients in the last group (Table 53.1).

Squamous cell (epidermoid) carcinoma is the most common lung cancer. It accounts for more than 40% of all cases. Like most other bronchogenic carcinomas, it is strongly associated with smoking. Most of these tumors occur centrally and can produce bronchial obstruction. They tend to ulcerate and may cause bleeding.

Adenocarcinomas account for about 25% of lung cancers and many of those that present peripherally. They sometimes arise in areas of fibrosis secondary to prior pulmonary parenchymal damage. Cancers of this cell type are less closely associated with smoking than others.

Undifferentiated large-cell carcinomas are, in most instances, probably a form of adenocarcinoma. Unlike well-differentiated adenocarcinomas, they are often centrally located and bronchoscopically visible as an endobronchial mass lesion. These cancers tend to metastasize hematogenously relatively early, leading to disease in the bones, liver, and brain.

Clinical Presentation is partially a function of tumor location; *central endobronchial* lesions may produce symptoms *early* in the course of illness. *Hemoptysis, cough, sputum production,* and a *localized wheeze* are among symptoms reported in early phases; however, the frequency with which these symptoms are noted in early disease is low. Hemoptysis occurs as a presenting symptom in only 7% to 10% of patients with lung cancer, although up to 40% will report hemoptysis at some time in their illness. On occasion, a systemic syndrome, such as hypertrophic osteoarthropathy (see Chapter 45), peripheral neuropathy, or inappropriate secretion of antidiuretic hormone, may precede other evidence of disease (see Chapter 92). Symptoms of *advanced disease* include *anorexia, weight loss, nausea* and *vomiting, hoarseness* (recurrent laryngeal nerve involvement), *pleuritic chest pain, bone pain,* and *neurologic deficits.*

In patients who present with metastasis or in whom metastasis later develops, the most frequently involved sites include local or regional *lymph nodes* within the chest (25% to 45%),

liver (30% to 45%), *bone* and *bone marrow* (20% to 40%), and *central nervous system* (20% to 35%).

Clinical Course and Prognosis. Overall 5-year survival remains at a dismal 13%, essentially unchanged in the past three decades. The poor prognosis is related in part to the advanced stage of disease at the time of diagnosis. Unfortunately, local and regional disease is most often asymptomatic. Because the median survival for patients with lung cancer is less than 12 months, late metastasis is rare. Important exceptions to these dim statistics exist, however—in particular, the improved survival for patients with SCLC and those with NSCLC whose tumors are surgically resectable.

As noted above, the clinical course is different for SCLC and NSCLC. For *NSCLC*, clinical course and survival are a function of the surgical pathologic stage. The staging scheme for NSCLC has been revised according to the tumor–node–metastasis (TNM) system (see Table 53.1 and Chapter 86). Survival improves markedly with surgical resectability. For example, those patients whose disease is confined to the lung (stage I) have a 5-year survival approaching 50%. With involvement of the hilar and mediastinal lymph nodes, survival rates decrease significantly, but less so than was previously thought if complete tumor resection is achieved. Unfortunately, only a small minority of patients present with surgically curable disease. Screening efforts have failed to provide satisfactory early detection (see Chapter 37). Preliminary data suggest that monoclonal antibodies directed against some tumor antigens may correlate inversely with prognosis.

SCLC differs substantially from NSCLC in that the prognosis is more independent of anatomic distribution at the time of diagnosis. Before the advent of contemporary chemotherapy, median survival was 1 to 3 months; it has increased several fold to 7 to 16 months, depending on the extent of disease. Five-year survival remains poor (5% to 10%) because of the high probability of metastasis, even among those who present with limited disease.

WORKUP AND STAGING

The basic approach to diagnosis and staging is to begin with noninvasive studies and proceed to increasingly invasive studies only as necessary. Staging is performed to determine prognosis and treatment and, in particular, to assess resectability of the tumor. The advent of computed tomography (CT) has greatly facilitated the noninvasive assessment of hilar and mediastinal node involvement. Invasive studies should be considered only if the results will have a marked effect on treatment plans. Many patients with lung cancer have concurrent chronic lung disease and may be seriously compromised by a complication of an invasive study. The histopathologic diagnosis of lung cancer may be obtained with a variety of procedures, ranging from sputum cytology to thoracotomy (see Chapters 37 and 44).

Diagnosis. *Chest radiography* is the primary diagnostic modality; the appearance of the lesion and its doubling time are helpful in distinguishing benign from malignant disease. Although the detection of lesions as small as 3 mm has been reported, most lesions are not visible until they are at least 5 mm or more in diameter. The finding of a calcified nodule can be helpful, especially if the pattern of calcification is eccentric (see Chapter 44).

Chest CT aids diagnosis by confirming the presence of a suspected lung mass and, if calcium is present, by clarifying its calcification pattern. CT has become critical to staging by determining the presence and extent of hilar and mediastinal node involvement (see below).

Sputum cytology may provide evidence of lung cancer and even cell type. Test sensitivity ranges from 25% to 75%, depending on the site of the tumor. Optimal collection requires obtaining three deep, first morning samples. The presence of pulmonary histiocytes indicates an adequate specimen. A negative cytologic examination result does not rule out cancer, especially in patients with peripheral lesions.

The yield of cytologic testing can be greatly enhanced by the use of *fiberoptic bronchoscopy* complemented by *washings*, *brushings*, or *forceps biopsy*. With centrally located, visualized lesions, washings provide a diagnosis in nearly 80% of instances; for brushings, the yield is 92%, and for forceps biopsy, it is 93%. The yield falls in the case of peripheral lesions; it is 20% to 30% for peripheral lesions less than 3 cm in diameter, and about 40% to 70% for those larger than 3 cm. The complication rate is low in experienced hands, with hypoxemia, hemorrhage, pneumothorax, or laryngospasm occurring in 0.1% to 0.3% of cases. On occasion, *transbronchial biopsy* is deemed the best means of establishing the diagnosis (e.g., in suspected alveolar cell carcinoma; see Chapter 51). The risk for pneumothorax rises to 5%.

With peripheral lesions, *percutaneous transthoracic fine-needle biopsy*—usually guided by CT or chest fluoroscopy—has proved accurate in the diagnosis of lung cancers. Reports on the diagnostic accuracy of these radiologically guided procedures quote sensitivity in excess of 90% and specificity above 95% when they are performed by skilled radiologists using "fine-needle" techniques that allow not only aspiration but also removal of a tiny core of material. However, sensitivity and specificity may be compromised by the occasional inadequacy of the specimen obtained, which is sometimes an aspirate of cytologic material rather than a solid core of tissue; in such instances, the architectural relationships may be obscured or unavailable in cytologic specimens. Pneumothorax ensues in close to 30%, but it is usually small, of little clinical consequence, and resolves spontaneously without the need for a chest tube. Hemorrhage is rare unless a vascular lesion is sampled. For patients with limited pulmonary reserve, who may be unable to tolerate any degree of pneumothorax, a controlled thoracotomy may be preferable to needle aspiration.

Scalene node biopsy is indicated when these peripheral nodes are noted to be enlarged; it can save the patient extensive testing for both diagnosis and staging.

Staging is performed to determine the prognosis and select therapy. The principal challenge is to assess surgical candidacy, which requires an accurate evaluation of hilar and mediastinal lymph nodes. If contralateral involvement of the regional nodes by tumor is noted, the patient is placed in stage IIIb and is not considered for curative surgical therapy; however, ipsilateral disease is no longer de facto grounds for eliminating a patient from surgical candidacy. The challenge is to evaluate the regional nodes accurately.

Chest radiography contributes to staging by providing data on tumor size, and it may show evidence of spread to the chest wall or regional nodes if marked involvement is present, although sensitivity is low.

Chest CT with contrast has been used extensively in the hope of improving the sensitivity of radiologic staging. Although the sensitivity and specificity of CT in the diagnosis of mediastinal disease appear to be reasonable for patients with clinical stage I disease who have a lung lesion larger than 3 cm (T2, N0, M0), results for those with earlier stage I disease (T1, N0, M0; lung nodule <3 cm) have been disappointing. False-positive and false-negative rates of 5% to 10% have been reported for the diagnosis of contralateral mediastinal node involvement in such patients. This has led some authorities to warn against reflexively ordering CT for patients with early stage I disease or depending too heavily on the findings for decision making (e.g., determining surgical candidacy solely on the basis of a result of CT). For patients with a pulmonary lesion larger than 3 cm, CT with contrast continues to be a useful noninvasive step to assess the hilum and mediastinum, but a negative CT result does not rule out microscopic spread from central or late peripheral lesions.

CT is sensitive for the detection of metastasis below the diaphragm (to liver and adrenals); upper abdominal views should be obtained at the time of chest CT. Positive findings, confirmed by needle biopsy, would indicate stage IV disease, for which surgery is inappropriate.

For judging tumor involvement of the chest wall, magnetic resonance imaging (MRI) is superior to CT. MRI is also better for assessing disease in the superior sulcus and defining subcarinal nodal involvement.

Although symptomatic metastasis to head and bone is relatively common, routine use of *head CT* and *bone scanning* is wasteful unless clinical evidence of disease referable to these sites is present (see Chapter 86).

More invasive staging techniques are indicated when the patient's surgical candidacy remains in question after CT. Many thoracic surgeons believe that all patients should undergo *mediastinoscopy* for evaluation of the mediastinum and hilum before thoracotomy because the presence of microscopic tumor in the contralateral mediastinum is a contraindication to resection. Under general anesthesia, a cervical incision is made and mediastinal node biopsy is carried out under direct visualization. They argue that the sensitivity of CT is insufficient, even in the setting of more advanced or central disease, in which the likelihood of microscopic nodal involvement is high. The debate and efforts to improve mediastinal staging continue.

Advances in the techniques of needle biopsy and fiberoptic endoscopy have enhanced the roles of *transthoracic* and *transbronchial needle aspiration biopsy* in the staging of lung cancer. These techniques offer a less morbid alternative to mediastinoscopy for the tissue-based assessment of mediastinal spread. They do not require general anesthesia or a formal surgical procedure and can be performed under CT guidance. Mediastinoscopy can be reserved for those in whom the results of these procedures are inconclusive.

The rest of staging is determined by the tumor cell type. For patients with inoperable *NSCLC*, further staging is of little value because the information will have minimal impact on decision making and estimation of prognosis. Staging is considerably different for patients with *SCLC*. Because the disease usually presents with evidence of bilateral nodal involvement, the issue is extent of disease rather than resectability. The goal is to distinguish between limited and extensive disease (the latter implies spread beyond the hemithorax of origin and regional nodes). Marrow invasion is present in almost 25% of patients, and marrow biopsy is performed routinely. CT of common sites of metastatic disease (e.g., brain) may also be useful if the result will affect plans for therapy (see below).

PRINCIPLES OF MANAGEMENT

Small-Cell Disease

Small-cell disease is biologically unique among bronchogenic cancers in that the cells are extremely sensitive to chemotherapy and radiation, probably in part because of their rapid rate of proliferation. Surgical treatment is usually not possible because 85% of patients have extensive disease at the time of presentation. Irrespective of whether disease is limited to the chest or disseminated, the treatment of choice is *combination chemotherapy*. For patients with limited disease, *radiation* is given as adjunctive therapy. As noted above, survival irrespective of stage has been prolonged fourfold to fivefold by chemotherapy. However, cure rates are very low. Only about 10% of limited-stage patients survive 5 years, and those who survive 2 years have a greater than two-thirds chance of relapse. Essentially all patients with extensive disease die within 2 years.

Chemotherapy. Since the introduction of combination chemotherapy in the 1970s, survival rates have improved modestly, and considerable progress has been made in reducing treatment morbidity, complexity, and duration. The use of a reduced-dose regimen of *etoposide* plus *cisplatin* after a course of three-drug therapy (cyclophosphamide, doxorubicin, vincristine) has improved survival and reduced marrow suppression. Shorter courses of therapy (no more than 4 to 6 months) are standard; longer courses are without additional benefit. In the elderly, single-dose etoposide appears to provide up to 80% of the response without significant compromise of survival.

Radiation. Patients with limited disease show a 90% response rate to irradiation. Survival appears to improve when radiation is used as an adjunct to chemotherapy, although toxicity increases. The optimal means of combining both modalities is under active study, with preliminary data on a synergistic effect noted for concurrent use of cisplatin and radiation. Prophylactic radiation of the cranium decreases the risk for clinical brain metastases, but in the absence of a proven survival benefit, the question of whether the considerable toxicity is justified remains controversial. Cranial irradiation among patients in complete remission has been shown to produce a modest reduction in relative risk for death (0.84) and for recurrence or death (0.75).

Surgery has almost no role in SCLC because of the nearly universal occurrence of occult disease beyond the initial lesion.

Non–Small-Cell Disease

Surgery offers the only possibility for cure. The procedure of choice is a *thoracotomy with resection*. About 35% to 45%

of patients presenting with NSCLC have potentially resectable disease, but only 60% have a successful resection. For the latter group, the 5-year survival or cure rate ranges from 25% to 40%. Thus, at best, fewer than 10% of patients who present with NSCLC can expect a cure. Two concurrent trends dominate the surgical approach to NSCLC: expanding candidacy to patients with stage IIIa disease, and reducing the extent of resection in patients with stage I disease. Patients with a single ipsilateral mediastinal lesion are now considered surgical candidates. Previously, mediastinal nodal involvement was considered incurable, but those with ipsilateral disease that can be grossly removed have shown a 5-year survival ranging from 15% to 30%.

Patients with localized disease are being treated with less radical, more conservative surgery. The goal is to preserve as much functional lung tissue as possible, especially in patients with underlying lung disease. Previously, pneumonectomy was performed in more than 70% of patients and included hilar in addition to mediastinal lymph nodes. A regional excision that employs wedge or segmental resection for stage I peripheral lobe lesions is now preferred. The general surgical dictum is to employ the minimal degree of surgery necessary to remove all macroscopic evidence of tumor.

Surgical excision is particularly indicated for nodules with long doubling times or long disease-free intervals, especially if the nodules are solitary and not associated with extrathoracic disease. The subsequent use of radiation therapy may augment local control, allowing for less extensive surgery.

Radiation Therapy is used for both curative intent and palliation. Preoperative radiation therapy may promote the resectability of tumors and possibly extend survival rates. In patients with tumors of the superior sulcus, preoperative radiation therapy has improved the likelihood of cure despite contiguous extension of such tumors to bone or the chest wall. In general, when surgery is used in combination with prior radiation, the resection must almost always be a pneumonectomy, and in principle, all sites that were diseased before the radiation therapy must be resected.

When radiation is used as sole therapy with a *curative intent*, results have been disappointing. Patients with NSCLC respond poorly to irradiation as a curative therapy, but good intrathoracic control of tumor, even eradication, can be achieved. In a major randomized trial of definitive radiation therapy for patients with unresectable stage III cancer, higher rates of regression and better disease control in the chest were observed with the use of high-dose therapy (60 Gy). However, no improvement in baseline 5-year survival, which remained at 5%, was noted. Although radiation may achieve local control, it does little to prevent relapse, which most often is the result of distant metastases. This has led to attempts to combine chemotherapy with irradiation (see below).

Chemotherapy has a far more limited role in NSCLC than in SCLC. It has been used as adjuvant therapy before surgery in patients with extensive but surgically resectable disease (e.g., stage III), after surgery, and in patients with inoperable disease who are undergoing radiation therapy. The goals are to improve local control and decrease the risk for distant metastasis. Results have been modest at best, but some improvements in survival are being noted. *Cisplatin* in particular has shown promise, although its side effects can be disabling (see Chapter 88). A metaanalysis of trials comparing surgery with surgery plus chemotherapy showed a relative reduction in short-term mortality risk of 13%, which produced an absolute mortality reduction of 5% at 5 years. The same metaanalysis included trials comparing radical radiotherapy with radical radiotherapy plus chemotherapy. Again, the relative reduction in short-term mortality risk was 13%; this produced an absolute mortality reduction of 4% at 2 years. Cisplatin has even produced some improvement in survival for patients with stage IV disease, although the improvement in survival has to be weighed against drug-induced morbidity. Studies indicate that patients who have undergone chemotherapy for NSCLC vary widely in their estimation of the survival benefit that would be necessary to justify toxicity. The majority do not consider the best estimate of median survival benefit (approximately 3 months) sufficient to justify the toxicity. Further refinement of chemotherapy and its use in combined-modality programs offers promise, but much work remains to be done.

Management of Stage III Disease deserves special comment because more than 60% of patients with NSCLC present with inoperable disease. In the majority of patients with stage III bronchogenic carcinoma, distant metastases develop regardless of control of the primary tumor. Survival is a function of the rate and extent of systemic dissemination. Substantial advances in therapy are required before genuine hope can be offered to the patient with this stage of disease. Encouraging developments include the improved survival associated with the surgical treatment of stage IIIa disease, and with the concurrent administration of cisplatin-based chemotherapy and radiotherapy for stage IIIb disease.

MONITORING

Because little can be done for metastatic disease, the monitoring of patients with surgically resectable and potentially curable lung cancer is specifically directed at searching for new primary tumors in this high-risk population. Chest radiography is indicated at regular intervals, ranging from every 3 months during the first 2 years to every 4 to 12 months in later years. Routine monitoring for recurrent disease outside the chest is unnecessary in the absence of specific symptoms suggesting bone, liver, or brain metastasis.

The monitoring of patients with extensive disease is directed at assessing the efficacy of therapy. One needs to select one or more objective measures of tumor burden (see Chapter 86) that can be followed conveniently to gauge response to treatment. Chest radiography, CT, and bronchoscopy are commonly used.

MANAGEMENT OF COMPLICATIONS

Superior Vena Cava Syndrome. Obstruction of the superior vena cava by lung tumor produces the classic clinical syndrome of facial edema, proptosis, suffusion of the conjunctivae, and dilation of the veins of the upper thorax and neck. Asymptomatic neck vein distention is an early manifestation. In late stages, the patient may have relentless headache. In patients with lung cancer, the syndrome is invariably caused by tumor extending into the right side of the mediastinum and compress-

ing the venous system adjacent to the mediastinal lymph nodes. The secondary effects of compression are thrombosis and tumor invasion; without treatment, neurologic function may be compromised. The histopathologic types of lung cancer that lead to the syndrome are variable, but most commonly the culprit is undifferentiated SCLC (see Chapter 92).

The approach to evaluation and therapy has undergone some revision in recent years. Previously, it was believed that emergency radiation therapy was indicated regardless of whether a tissue diagnosis was available; the view was that the risk of an invasive procedure to obtain tissue outweighed the potential contribution to the design of a treatment plan. More recent data indicate that the risk of evaluation in patients lacking a tissue diagnosis is low and that chemotherapy may be superior to radiation in some instances (e.g., SCLC). Because superior vena cava syndrome may be the initial presentation of lung cancer, the issue of need for tissue diagnosis is frequently encountered in this setting. When the result will change the mode of therapy, tissue diagnosis should be attempted, with care taken to minimize risk to the patient.

Even when a tissue diagnosis is not obtained, the response to radiotherapy is rather good; in unselected series, more than 70% of patients demonstrate a response. Although patients with superior vena cava syndrome secondary to lung cancer have an inoperable tumor, their prognosis is no worse than that of other patients with stage III lung cancer.

Malignant Pleural Effusion is another important complication. It occurs in 10% to 15% of patients with carcinoma of the lung and may be secondary to direct pleural implantation or a consequence of mediastinal obstruction to lymphatic drainage of the pleural surface. Only 20% to 30% of pleural effusions that develop as a consequence of bronchogenic carcinoma are cytologically confirmed, and many are transudates. Pleural biopsy is often required for definitive diagnosis.

The median survival for patients in whom a malignant pleural effusion develops is less than 3 months; therefore, the effusion should be monitored and treated only when it causes significant respiratory discomfort. The use of intrapleural chemotherapeutic agents (e.g., bleomycin, fluorouracil) or chemical irritants (e.g., tetracycline, talcum powder, quinacrine) may be effective in 50% to 60% of patients. The specific choice of agent for sealing the pleura is determined by the associated morbidity of the treatment. The chemotherapeutic agents such as bleomycin and fluorouracil are relatively innocuous. On the other hand, nitrogen mustard and the "inert" irritants may result in a major secondary inflammatory response with reactive effusion and fever. Quinacrine (Atabrine) must be instilled repeatedly during a 5- to 7-day period for maximal effect. Radiation therapy to the mediastinum or to the pleura has been of limited effectiveness. Surgical drainage with an intrathoracic tube for 2 to 3 days may result in a secondary inflammatory response adequate to seal the pleural space.

Tumor Humoral Syndromes are associated with SCLC. Because the tumor is derived from endocrine cells of the bronchial mucosa, it is capable of producing adrenocorticotropic hormone, antidiuretic hormone, and even, on occasion, serotonin. The clinical pictures that may result are Cushing's syndrome, inappropriate secretion of antidiuretic hormone, and carcinoid syndrome, respectively. In an autopsy series of 85 patients with

SCLC, it was found that those who manifested a paraneoplastic syndrome tended to have a more benign clinical course and longer survival; in addition, the incidence of metastases to the central nervous system was significantly lower in these patients.

Complications of Surgical Therapy include prolonged air leakage from a bronchopleural fistula and postoperative intrapleural infection with development of empyema. Both are potentially serious and require prompt surgical attention. Pulmonary insufficiency is uncommon as a result of careful preoperative pulmonary evaluation of candidates for resection; however, pneumonia in the remaining lung can lead to respiratory compromise.

Complications of Chemotherapy are related to the use of such agents as cisplatin, cyclophosphamide, doxorubicin (Adriamycin), methotrexate, and nitrosoureas (see Chapter 88). The use of certain chemotherapeutic agents (e.g., nitrosoureas, methotrexate) during the induction phase of radiation therapy in patients with SCLC is suspected of causing some late complications seen in long-term survivors, such as other malignancies.

Complications of Radiation Therapy include radiation pneumonitis, esophageal stricture, pericardial and myocardial fibrosis, rib fractures secondary to radiation-induced osteonecrosis, and radiation fibrosis.

PATIENT EDUCATION

Most lay persons believe that lung cancer is fatal. Although the prognosis and efficacy of treatment are indeed poor in most types of lung cancer, the patient with a newly discovered, suspect pulmonary nodule needs to know that differences in prognosis can be significant, according to tissue type and stage of disease at time of presentation. During the workup and staging, this background information can help sustain patient and family through a worrisome period of uncertainty and provide a rationale for the procedures that need to be carried out.

Once the diagnosis and extent of disease are known, the prognosis and treatment options should be shared with the patient and family. When surgical cure is a genuine possibility and the patient can tolerate the surgery, it should be urged. However, in lung cancer, in which the prognosis is often so poor, the treatment plans should be formulated jointly, and the patient's preferences and willingness to undergo treatment should be elicited and respected. A realistic assessment for the patient and family of prognosis and the pros and cons of treatment are essential for effective decision making. All too often, inappropriately aggressive forms of therapy are rushed into, mostly for the sake of "doing something." Studies have found that socioeconomically advantaged patients tend to undergo more aggressive forms of therapy, although when disease stage is controlled for, no evidence of improved survival is found.

Patients with incurable disease need to know their prognosis, which is best explained at a level of detail consistent with their desire to know. The news of lung cancer in a loved one is very upsetting to family members, who will try to shield the patient from the information. Facilitating communication between family and patient is essential to preserving the patient's quality of life and helping the family to cope (see Chapter 87).

A.H.G./A.G.M.

ANNOTATED BIBLIOGRAPHY

Adjei AA, Marks RS, Bonner JA. Current guidelines for the management of small-cell lung cancer. Mayo Clin Proc 1999;74:809. (*Effective review.*)

Ahmann FR. A reassessment of the clinical implications of the superior vena cava syndrome. J Clin Oncol 1984;2:961. (*Argues that diagnostic workup is safe and useful for proper selection of treatment modality. Based on review of more than 1,800 cases.*)

Auperin A, Arrigada R, Pignon JP, et al. Prophylactic cranial irradiation for patients with small-cell lung cancer in complete remission. Prophylactic Cranial Irradiation Overview Collaborative Group. N Engl J Med 1999;341:476. (*Relative risk for recurrence or death of 0.75 among those in remission when treated with irradiation.*)

Becker GL, Whitlock WL, Schaefer PS, et al. The impact of thoracic computed tomography in clinically staged T1, N0, M0 chest lesions. Arch Intern Med 1990;150:557. (*CT did not prove useful because of an unacceptably high number of false-positive and false-negative results; argues that routine CT is not indicated in such patients.*)

Bunn PA, Licheter AS, Makuch RW, et al. Chemotherapy alone or with chest radiation therapy in limited-stage small-cell lung cancer: a prospective randomized trial. Ann Intern Med 1987;106:655. (*Modest enhancement of benefit from addition of radiation therapy.*)

Bunn PA, Vokes EE, Langer CJ, et al. An update on North American randomized studies in non-small cell lung cancer. Semin Oncol 1998;25:2. (*Effective update.*)

Dillman RO, Seagren SL, Propert KJ, et al. A randomized trial of induction chemotherapy plus high-dose radiation versus radiation alone in stage III non-small cell lung cancer. N Engl J Med 1990;323:940. (*Encouraging results with use of combined-modality therapy.*)

Errett LE, Wison J, Chiu RCJ, et al. Wedge resection as an alternative procedure for peripheral bronchogenic carcinoma in poor-risk patients. J Thorac Cardiovasc Surg 1985;90:656. (*Example of the trend toward less radical surgery in selected patients.*)

Greenberg ER, Chute CG, Stukel T, et al. Social and economic factors in the choice of lung cancer treatment. N Engl J Med 1988;318:612. (*When stage of illness was controlled for, patients of higher socioeconomic status tended to undergo more aggressive therapy without evidence of improved survival.*)

Johnson BE, Grayson J, Makuch RW, et al. Ten-year survival of patients with small-cell lung cancer treated with combination chemotherapy with or without irradiation. J Clin Oncol 1990;8:396. (*Long-term experience of the National Cancer Institute in the treatment of SCLC with chemotherapy.*)

Lin AY, Ihde DC. Recent developments in the treatment of lung cancer. JAMA 1992;267:1661. (*Excellent, authoritative, yet terse review for the general reader; good guide to the plethora of data from clinical trials; 33 references.*)

de la Monte SM, Hutchins GM, Moore GW. Paraneoplastic syndromes and constitutional symptoms in prediction of metastatic behavior of small cell carcinoma of the lung. Am J Med 1984;77:851. (*Autopsy series of 85 patients indicating that patients with paraneoplastic syndromes had a more benign clinical course and less metastasis to the central nervous system.*)

Montazeri A, Gillis CR, McEwan J. Quality of life in patients with lung cancer: a review of literature from 1970 to 1995. Chest 1998;113:467. (*Palliation of symptoms, psychosocial interven-*

tions, and understanding patients' feelings and concerns contribute to improved quality of life.)

Mountain CF. A new international staging system for lung cancer. Chest 1986;89[Suppl 4]:225S. (*Newly adopted and widely used staging system.*)

Non-small Cell Lung Cancer Collaborative Group. Chemotherapy in non-small cell lung cancer: a meta-analysis using updated data on individual patients from 52 randomised clincla trials. BMJ 1995;311:899. (*Addition of chemotherapy to either surgery or radiotherapy afforded a modest benefit, with relative risk for death consistently at 0.87.*)

Perez CA, Pajak TF, Rubin P, et al. Long-term observations of the pattern of failure in patients with unresectable non-oat-cell cancer of the lung treated with definitive radiotherapy: report by the Radiation Oncology Group. Cancer 1987;59:1874. (*Major study showing that disease control was good but survival unaffected because of metastatic disease.*)

Pignon J-P, Arriagada R, Ihde DC, et al. A meta-analysis of thoracic radiotherapy for small-cell lung cancer. N Engl J Med 1992;327:1618. (*Modest improvement in survival among patients with limited disease treated with chemotherapy.*)

Pritchard RS, Anthony SP. Chemotherapy plus radiotherapy compared with radiotherapy alone in the treatment of locally advanced, unresectable, non-small-cell lung cancer. A meta-analysis. Ann Intern Med 1996;125:723. (*Modest reduction in relative mortality risk with chemotherapy added to radiotherapy.*)

Ries LAG, Hankey BF, Miller BA, et al. Cancer Statistics Review 1973–1988. Bethesda, MD: National Cancer Institute, 1991. NIH publication No. 91-2789. (*Little progress in overall 5-year cancer survival, which went from 12% to 13%.*)

Schaake-Konig C, Bogaert WVD, Dalesio Otilla, et al. Effects of concomitant cisplatin and radiotherapy on inoperable non-small-cell lung cancer. N Engl J Med 1992;326:524. (*Significant increase in 3-year survival achieved by combining cisplatin with radiotherapy; local radiation-enhancing effect noted, but 3-year survival still inadequate at 16%.*)

Silvestri G, Pritchard R, Welch G. Preferences for chemotherapy in patients with advanced non-small cell lung cancer: descriptive study based on scripted interviews. BMJ 1998;317:771. (*Overall, 78% of the patients undergoing chemotherapy would opt for supportive care; wide variation in survival benefit perceived as justifying toxicity.*)

Turrisi AT 3rd, Kim K, Blum R, et al. Twice-daily compared with once-daily thoracic radiotherapy in limited small-cell lung cancer treated concurrently with cisplatin and etoposide. N Engl J Med 1999;340:265. (*Twice-daily dosing associated with longer median survival—23 months compared with 19 months.*)

54

Smoking Cessation

NANCY A. RIGOTTI

Cigarette smoking is the major preventable cause of death in the United States. Strong evidence documents benefit from cessation of smoking, even for the elderly and patients in whom chronic tobacco-related disease has already developed. Although the health risks of smoking are widely recognized and the prevalence of smoking has fallen dramatically in the past two decades (from 40% to about 25%), millions of Americans continue to smoke, a substantial fraction more heavily than ever, and adolescents continue to take up the habit in large numbers. Nevertheless, many people are eager to quit and often come to the primary physician for advice. Numerous studies have shown that physicians can change a patient's smoking habits. Extensive evidence indicates that pharmacotherapy increases the likelihood of successful quitting. The primary care physician needs to be expert in motivating patients to quit and in advising them on the best means to accomplish their goal. This requires knowledge about available smoking cessation techniques and an appreciation of how and when to use them.

EPIDEMIOLOGY OF SMOKING AND QUITTING

Since 1964, when the Surgeon General's Report first publicized the health risks of smoking, cigarette smoking by adults in the United States has declined. This decline in the percentage of the population that smokes is averaging about 1.1 percentage points per year, with the percentage of smokers falling to about 25%. This decrease is largely attributable to the increasing number of smokers who have quit, rather than to a fall in the number of smokers taking up the habit. About 30% of smokers report attempting to quit each year. As less addicted smokers quit, the proportion of heavy smokers (>25 cigarettes per day) has increased from about one in four to one in three. Smoking in adolescence—the time when smoking usually begins—has fallen little since its peak in the 1970s. Adolescent girls are smoking in numbers comparable with those in boys; the historical gender difference continues to narrow. This is worrisome because women who smoke during the reproductive years incur special risks with pregnancy and oral contraceptive use. Smoking is increasingly prevalent among populations that are nonwhite, poor, or of low educational status.

Most smokers claim that they are aware of the health hazards of smoking and would like to quit but have difficulty doing so. Although the success rate for any single attempt at quitting is low, smokers who repeatedly try to quit increase their likelihood of success. Lighter smokers are more successful than heavier smokers. Smokers most likely to quit are those who expect their attempt to succeed, have a strong belief in their personal control over events, feel competent and personally secure, and have a good social support system. The smoking habits of the spouse and, in some studies, friends are important; those with nonsmoking spouses are more likely to succeed. Patients with *depression* or a history of depression have a hard time initiating smoking cessation and a poor success rate (40% that of patients who are not depressed) when they try.

More than 90% of former smokers quit on their own without assistance from physicians, groups, patches, gum, hypnosis, acupuncture, or psychological counseling. Those who benefit most from an assisted method are heavy, more addicted smokers. Their chance of successfully quitting is about half that of smokers who quit on their own. Receiving advice from a physician about smoking cessation doubles the chance of a patient making an attempt to quit. Smokers who quit using the "cold turkey" approach are more likely to remain abstinent than those who taper. Reducing cigarette consumption somewhat and switching to a different brand can be part of a smoker's preparation for quitting—being especially helpful in building a sense of confidence and control—but are no substitute for setting a definite date for abrupt and total cessation.

Health concerns are the most common reasons given by former smokers for quitting. However, the risks for lung cancer and heart disease are less often cited than are minor smoking-related ailments such as cough, dyspnea, and sore throat. Minor symptoms may successfully motivate a smoker to quit by making personally salient the more serious health risks of smoking. Illness in one smoker can influence other smokers to quit (e.g., the friend or family member in the intensive care unit), as can personally sustaining a serious smoking-related illness, such as a heart attack. The likelihood that a smoker will quit increases with the severity of the illness. Although fewer than 5% of smokers in the general population quit each year, cessation rates are higher among persons with newly diagnosed coronary heart disease. Many studies report that approximately one third of smokers surviving a myocardial infarction stop smoking permanently. Increased rates of cessation are also reported in smokers with chronic obstructive pulmonary disease. During pregnancy, 20% of women smokers stop smoking, but the majority resume smoking after delivery. Many smokers quit temporarily when they have an acute respiratory illness.

Other reasons for quitting cited by former smokers include a desire to exert self-control over one's life, aesthetic objections to the smoking habit, and fear of setting a bad example for others. The cost of cigarettes exerts little influence among adults.

WHY PEOPLE SMOKE

Smoking is a complex behavior initiated and maintained for different reasons. The influence of peers and parents appears to be most important in the initiation of smoking. Adolescents whose parents and friends smoke are more likely to begin smoking. Once the smoking habit is established, it is sustained by many factors.

Both pharmacologic and psychological models have been proposed to explain what maintains smoking behavior. The *psychological model* regards smoking as a learned behavior that continues because it is rewarding to the smoker. Certain situations, such as finishing a meal, become strongly associated with smoking and trigger the urge to smoke. Smokers also use cigarettes to handle environmental stress and regulate emotions, especially strong negative emotions like anger.

A strong association between *depression* and smoking has been documented. Depressed patients are more likely to be smokers and, as noted above, less likely to attempt quitting or succeed at quitting. It is hypothesized that smoking may represent a form of self-medication for the depressed patient, with nicotine alleviating a dysphoric mood through activation of central neuroreceptors. Such a response would strongly reinforce smoking and might trigger a craving for cigarettes during times of depressed mood. Moreover, withdrawal of nicotine during an attempt at smoking cessation might trigger symptoms of depression, which has been reported in studies of patients with a history of depression who attempt to quit.

The *pharmacologic model* emphasizes physical addiction to nicotine. The evidence for smoking as an addiction is strong, and nicotine has been established as the addicting substance in tobacco smoke. According to this model, the smoker smokes to maintain a constant blood level of nicotine and thereby avert the *withdrawal syndrome*, characterized by falls in heart rate, blood pressure, and basal metabolic rate and changes in electroencephalographic rhythms and rapid-eye-movement (REM) sleep patterns. Craving for nicotine is the most common subjective symptom of withdrawal, but other symptoms include restlessness, irritability, inability to concentrate, daytime drowsiness and fatigue, sleep disturbances, headache, nausea, alteration in bowel habits, and increased appetite. Symptoms begin within hours after cessation of smoking, but their duration and severity are highly variable, representing different degrees of nicotine addiction among smokers. No simple test is available to measure nicotine addiction, but heavily addicted smokers tend to have their first cigarette shortly after arising (i.e., within 30 minutes), smoke more and stronger cigarettes, and have difficulty not smoking for even a few hours.

The pharmacologic model can explain initial difficulties with cessation but cannot explain why smokers have difficulty remaining abstinent after the first few days or weeks. In fact, the majority of smokers who stop temporarily resume smoking within a few months.

TECHNIQUES FOR SMOKING CESSATION

The methods of smoking cessation range from unassisted "cold turkey" to formal treatment programs administered in a group setting, with a host of interventions in between. As noted, the majority of smokers quit in unassisted fashion. As might be expected from the multidimensional nature of the smoking problem, no single method suffices. The most effective approaches address both principal components of the smoking problem: (a) nicotine addiction and (b) behavioral dependency on cigarettes. Combining a number of approaches into a personalized, comprehensive program appears to be the most successful strategy.

Strategies that combine pharmacologic and behavioral techniques appear to be the most effective. Pharmacologic methods are used to relieve symptoms of nicotine withdrawal, freeing the patient to focus on behavioral efforts (Tables 54.1 and 54.2).

Maintaining long-term tobacco abstinence remains the challenge in smoking cessation treatment. Short-term cessation rates of 70% to 80% are common among programs. However, a predictable and rapid return to smoking follows initial cessation. A 1-year cessation rate of 30% to 35% is considered the standard for an effective smoking cessation program.

Pharmacologic Methods

The principal pharmacologic approach is to relieve symptoms of withdrawal by continuing some nicotine exposure, although at reduced and tapered doses. Nicotine delivery is most often achieved transdermally with nicotine patches or through the oral mucosa with nicotine chewing gum. Newer approaches include nicotine nasal spray and nicotine inhalers. Other pharmacologic approaches to minimizing withdrawal symptoms have included the use of clonidine, minor tranquilizers, and drugs that mimic the autonomic effects of nicotine. An alternative pharmacologic approach is the use of antidepressants, especially bupropion, an atypical antidepressant with both dopaminergic and adrenergic effects. Bupropion became available as a prescription drug in 1998 as Zyban, a trade name specific for smoking cessation.

Transdermal Nicotine ("the patch") represents a second-generation form of nicotine reduction therapy, developed after the introduction of nicotine gum more than a decade ago (see below). It provides a convenient means of maintaining nicotine exposure and preventing nicotine withdrawal symptoms while the smoker addresses the behavioral component of the smoking problem. Once the habit is broken, nicotine supplementation is stopped. A smoker on nicotine reduction therapy is already being weaned from nicotine because the pharmacokinetic properties of the patch differ from those of inhaled smoke. The levels of nicotine delivered transdermally are more constant than the peaks and troughs characteristic of smoking.

The *effectiveness* of the patch is related to its ease of administration. In randomized clinical trials of at least 6 months' duration, nicotine patches have been shown to be superior to placebo in helping smokers to stop smoking; the cessation rates of smokers using the nicotine patch were approximately double the rates of smokers receiving placebo patches. In 1996, nicotine patches became available without a prescription. The rationale for this decision of the Food and Drug Administration was to make replacement therapy more accessible because of its proven effectiveness in multiple trials. Since then, several trials have demonstrated the 6-month quit rates obtained with over-the-counter nicotine patches to be 2.5 to 2.8 times those achieved with placebo patches.

Patches are not a panacea, nor are they appropriate for everyone. They should be used only by smokers who (a) want to quit and are willing to set a quitting date; (b) have a signifi-

Table 54.1. Smoking Cessation Strategy for Office Practice

I. Assess smoking habits
  A. Smoking and quitting history
  B. Interest in cessation
  C. Identify potential motivating factors
II. Advise every smoker to stop smoking
III. Motivate the smoker to attempt to quit
  A. Emphasize benefits of cessation
  B. Focus on short-term changes
  C. Tailor to the clinical situation
    1. Asymptomatic smoker
    2. Acute respiratory illness
    3. Chronic cardiopulmonary illness
    4. Pregnancy
IV. Ask for a commitment to quit
V. Help the smoker to quit
  A. Physician counseling/nurse counseling
  B. Self-help materials
  C. Nicotine patch or gum
  D. Referrals to formal smoking withdrawal programs
  E. Anticipate problems
    1. Withdrawal symptoms
    2. Weight gain
VI. Follow-up
  A. Put smoking on the problem list
  B. Follow-up visits with nurse or physician
  C. Continued monitoring at each visit

Table 54.2. Behavioral Program for Smoking Cessation

RATIONALE	SUGGESTIONS FOR THE SMOKER
Preparing to Quit	
1. Increase motivation	Write out a list of reasons to quit.
2. Make a commitment	Set a quit date.
	Sign a contract with family, friends.
3. Develop social supports	Enlist the support of nonsmoking friends, relatives, co-workers.
4. Self-monitoring to identify smoking cues	Keep a record of each cigarette smoked, noting circumstances, time, and how highly desired. Wrap this around cigarette pack with rubber band.
5. Progressive restriction	Eliminate least desired cigarettes; delay smoking first morning cigarette; smoke only at certain times or places.
6. Aversive conditioning	Fill a glass bottle with all your cigarette butts ("butt bottle").
7. Satiation	Oversmoke on the day before quitting.
Initial Cessation	
1. Avoid smoking cues	Eliminate all cigarettes, ashtrays, lighters from home and car.
	Spend the quitting day in places where smoking is not permitted.
2. Positive reinforcement	Reward self with a treat on quitting day.
3. Aversive conditioning	Look at "butt bottle" frequently.
	Wear rubber band on wrist and snap it when urge to smoke occurs.
4. Substitute oral stimuli	Chew on straws, toothpicks, carrot sticks, sugarless candy, or gum.
5. Substitute activities for hands	Rubber bands, paper clips.
Relapse Prevention—Maintaining Nonsmoking	
1. Avoid smoking cues	Spend time in places where smoking is not permitted.
	Substitute situations associated with smoking (coffee, alcohol, end of meal) with other behaviors (tea, soft drink, brushing teeth, or taking a walk at end of meal).
2. Positive reinforcement	Treat self with money saved by not smoking.
3. Aversive conditioning	Wear rubber band on wrist and snap it when urge to smoke occurs.
4. Strategies to cope with urges to smoke	Take slow, deep breaths.
	Relaxation training.
	Incompatible activity (take a shower).
	Contact a nonsmoking friend.

cant amount of nicotine addiction (i.e., smoke more than one pack per day, smoke their first cigarette within 30 minutes of arising, had withdrawal symptoms on prior attempts at quitting); (c) will not smoke while using the patch; and (d) will follow a behavioral program (individual or group) in conjunction with patch use.

Proper use of nicotine patches involves beginning patch application on the day of quitting. The patch is applied to any non-hairy skin site and worn for 16 or 24 hours. Because of possible skin irritation, the patch site should be rotated. Once applied, the patch is impervious to external water (shower, swimming), but it can come loose with perspiration. For this reason, it should put on after exercise. Most patches come in multiple strengths. Most smokers should use the patch for 2 to 3 months and start with the strongest dose (21 mg/d), then gradually taper to lower-dose patches (14 mg/d and 7 mg/d). Those who weigh less than 100 lb are advised to begin with the 14 mg/d strength. A typical program might use the 21 mg/d patch for 4 to 6 weeks, with a switch to the 14 mg/d strength for 2 to 4 weeks and then to the 7 mg/d patch for 2 to 4 weeks. Some argue that patients who smoke less than one pack per day can begin with a 14 mg/d patch, but such patients may not be sufficiently addicted to nicotine to need the patch in the first place.

Side effects are relatively few. The most common is skin irritation, which is usually minor. It is reduced by frequent changes in patch location. Insomnia is also reported, probably caused by the stimulant effect of a constant level of nicotine. The 16-hour patch might be useful for patients bothered by insomnia, or a 24-hour patch can be removed at bedtime. Rash, headache, nausea, vertigo, myalgia, and dyspepsia have been reported, but dependence and abuse have not, although experience is still too limited to rule out the possibility. Isolated cases of myocardial infarction have been reported in patients who continue to smoke while using the patch. In clinical trials, only 5% of patients stopped therapy because of side effects. Because of the vasoconstrictive action of nicotine, patients with recent myocardial infarction, unstable angina, peripheral vascular disease, or serious arrhythmias and women who are pregnant or breast-feeding should avoid patch use.

Patient education is critical. Many patients view the patch as a simple, passive means of quitting, one that requires little effort on their part. Some even continue to smoke while using the patch, under the mistaken belief that it should be used for tapering. Proper patient selection and education are essential to the safe and effective use of the patch. The effectiveness of the patch is enhanced by behavioral smoking cessation therapy.

Nicotine Chewing Gum was the original form of nicotine reduction therapy. It also provides an oral substitute for cigarettes. Nicotine is released from the gum during chewing and absorbed through the oral mucosa, resulting in blood levels lower but more constant than those achieved by smoking. Exposure to the other harmful constituents of cigarette smoke is avoided. In some studies, patients using the gum also gained less weight after cessation of smoking than smokers not using the gum. The preparation initially available contained 2 mg of nicotine. A 4-mg gum was approved for use in 1993 and is probably more effective. Both 2-mg and 4-mg preparations became available without a prescription in late 1995.

Nicotine gum is more effective than placebo when used in conjunction with a behavioral program for self-selected, motivated smokers attending a smoking withdrawal clinic; 1-year cessation rates of 30% to 50% have been reported, representing an advance over rates attained with behavioral treatments alone. The gum, like the patch, may be especially useful in smokers heavily addicted to nicotine. When the gum is used by less motivated patients, cessation rates are lower, and its effectiveness is less certain. Like the patch, the gum is effective only for helping the patient to quit; it is not a substitute for behavioral therapy. Studies of long-term abstinence show little benefit from gum use without a behavioral program.

To use the gum, smokers are instructed to pick a target date when they will stop smoking. After that, they chew the gum whenever they have an urge to smoke, usually consuming a dozen pieces daily at the onset. Gum use should continue for 2 to 3 months. Dependence develops in 5% to 10% of users, who have difficulty stopping. It is important to emphasize to the patient that the best results are obtained when gum use is accompanied by a program that teaches behavioral skills.

Side effects are mostly a consequence of overly vigorous chewing and release of excess nicotine—sore jaw, mouth irritation or ulcers, nervousness, dizziness, nausea, vomiting, hiccups, intestinal distress, headache, and excess salivation. To reduce these symptoms, smokers should chew the gum very slowly, just enough to detect a slight tingling taste in the mouth. Contraindications to use are the same as those for the transdermal patch (see above).

In addition to side effects, factors limiting effectiveness include poor compliance (as many as 35% use the gum for too short a period), improper chewing technique, and adherence to dental appliances and bridgework. Smokers starting the gum need detailed instruction in its proper use. Nicotine absorption may be compromised by the consumption of acidic beverages (e.g., coffee, carbonated drinks). By lowering the pH of saliva, they block nicotine absorption when ingested during or immediately before gum use. Not drinking acid beverages around the time of gum use solves the problem.

Nicotine Nasal Spray was developed to provide more rapid delivery of nicotine and thereby mimic more closely the effect of smoking a cigarette. The delivery device is similar to a nasal antihistamine spray, and one or two doses are taken per hour for a period of about 3 months. As with gum and transdermal patches, the quit rates with the device have proved to be about twice those attained with placebo. Nasal and throat irritation, rhinitis, sneezing, and tearing are common side effects. The role of the nasal spray as an alternative to gum and patches is yet to be defined. It is available only by prescription at the beginning of 2000.

Nicotine Inhalers were introduced as a prescription drug in 1998. The inhaler is a plastic rod with a nicotine plug that delivers nicotine to the buccal mucosa when drawn upon. The pharmacokinetics are similar to those of nicotine gum, as is the effect on quit rates. Its role as an alternative to gum and patches also remains to be defined.

Bupropion, an antidepressant, has proved to be as effective as nicotine replacement therapy, doubling quit rates in comparison with placebo. It is the ideal pharmacologic approach for smokers who prefer not to use nicotine replacement or who have been unable to quit with nicotine replacement. It is equally effective among persons with and without a history of depression. Bupropion is generally started 1 week before the ordained quit date. The usual dosage is 300 mg/d, and treatment is generally continued for 2 to 3 months. Bupropion has been used together with nicotine replacement, and some evidence suggests that the combination is more effective than either approach alone, although results have been conflicting. The most common side effects are dry mouth and insomnia. An increased risk for seizure was an early concern, but that has faded with use of the slow-release preparation at the dosage of 300 mg/d. Nevertheless, alternative treatment is advisable in patients with a history of seizure or other risk factors.

Other Agents. *Clonidine*, the centrally acting adrenergic blocker, has been shown to lessen the symptoms of opiate and alcohol withdrawal and has been tried for smoking cessation. Results of initial studies were encouraging, but randomized, controlled studies with sufficient follow-up found clonidine to be no better than placebo.

Lobeline (Nikoban), a non-nicotine substitute with autonomic effects that mimic those of nicotine, is no more effective than placebo. *Minor tranquilizers* have been prescribed as a means of blunting the anxiety and irritability of nicotine withdrawal, but they are no better than placebo. Furthermore, because daily use of these agents for more than a few days is associated with significant risks for tolerance and dependency (see Chapter 226), they are not appropriate for use in smoking cessation, in which daily use for several weeks is required.

Antidepressant therapy with agents other than bupropion may have a role in the pharmacologic support of smoking cessation. Nortriptyline proved effective in a small, randomized trial, producing a quit rate of 14% at 6 months versus 3% for placebo. Other controlled trials of antidepressant therapy are in progress.

Behavioral Methods

The behavioral model of smoking has inspired a host of techniques to manipulate environmental cues that trigger or reward smoking. These techniques form the core of most smoking cessation programs (Table 54.2).

Strategies for Stimulus Control require smokers to identify and control the environmental stimuli that trigger smoking. Cues are first identified by *self-monitoring*. For example, smokers might be asked to carry a sheet of paper wrapped around their cigarette pack on which they record the circumstances in which each cigarette is smoked. Environmental cues, identified from this daily log, are then progressively avoided or modified so that they no longer trigger smoking. The behavior is separated from the triggers by *progressive restriction* of the situations in which smoking is permitted. At a point in the relearning process, smoking stops altogether.

Controlled studies have not demonstrated impressive long-term cessation with this approach alone. Smokers may decrease their cigarette consumption but are less successful at total cessation, and those who stop have a high relapse rate. By itself, the technique is more effective in preparing the smoker to quit than in achieving long-term cessation.

Aversive Conditioning Techniques pair an unwanted act like smoking with an unpleasant stimulus to make the act less likely to occur. The most effective aversive stimulus is cigarette smoke, which is unpleasant even to a heavy smoker. In the best-known technique, *rapid smoking*, the smoker is required to inhale every 6 seconds until unable to tolerate further smoking because of nausea, headache, or light-headedness. *Smoke holding* is a variation on rapid smoking, believed to produce similar aversive effects with less health risk. A related technique is *satiation*; smokers purposely double or triple their base smoking rate for up to a day before cessation. The safety of rapid smoking and satiation has been a concern because of the smoker's intense exposure to nicotine and carbon monoxide. However, no serious medical complications have been reported with supervised use of rapid smoking among healthy people and even those with mild cardiopulmonary disease, although the technique is not advised for those with more symptomatic heart or lung disease.

Rapid smoking and other aversive techniques are effective for initial abstinence, producing high rates of short-term cessation, but relapse occurs soon unless other techniques are employed.

Hypnosis is of great interest to patients, many of whom hope it offers an effortless way to stop smoking. Most studies evaluating hypnosis have been uncontrolled, with small samples and brief follow-up; they report abstinence rates of 20% to 25% at 1 year, comparable with the standard achieved by behavioral programs. The elements identified as most predictive of success include multiple sessions, supportive therapists, motivated clients, and individualized hypnotic suggestions based on specific motivations for smoking.

Acupuncture, like hypnosis, is widely requested by smokers. Needles are inserted at acupuncture points, often around the ear. Advocates claim the procedure can reduce the urge to smoke and even lead to long-term cessation. Success appears related to belief in the efficacy of acupuncture. Randomized, control trials are few; those that are available found no long-term benefit when acupuncture was used alone. Acupuncture might prove useful for the temporary relief of withdrawal symptoms in addicted patients.

Organized Group Programs. Both nonprofit and commercial organizations offer group programs for smoking cessation. Most programs have a high dropout rate and have not been adequately evaluated. The oldest and best known is the Five-Day Plan, developed in 1963 with the sponsorship of the Seventh Day Adventist Church. Participants meet on five consecutive nights, and the program is low in cost. Techniques used are health education, encouragement to quit, and nonspecific support.

Adding behavior modification techniques to group programs has improved their effectiveness. SmokEnders, a commercial program, consists of weekly meetings run by former smokers. In one long-term study, 70% of participants were not smoking at the end of the program, and 39% remained abstinent 4 years later. However, on repeated analysis, the long-term cessation rate was 24%, equivalent to the standard rates achieved with other behavioral programs. The American Cancer Society and the American Lung Association offer similar group programs at lower cost. More intensive group programs with extended follow-up offered in the medical setting have achieved better results. Patients who appear to benefit most from such programs are women, middle-aged persons, those who are heavy smokers and have made multiple attempts to quit, and persons who are better educated. Overall, however, fewer than 5% of smokers who successfully quit use a group program.

Individual Aids. Booklets, audiovisual aids, telephone services, and nonprescription filters are available to help smokers who wishes to quit on their own. Few have been evaluated. *Self-help manuals* range from booklets with practical tips on how to quit to longer books containing comprehensive programs of behavior modification. Many are available at minimal cost through nonprofit organizations like the American Cancer Society, the American Lung Association, and the National Cancer Institute.

These groups also sponsor *telephone services* that provide education, encouragement, advice, and referrals. Use of the American Lung Association manuals has produced cessation rates of 12% at 1 month and 5% at 1 year.

A series of progressively stronger *filters*, which gradually restrict the delivery of tar and nicotine from a smoker's own cigarettes, has not proved effective.

ROLE OF THE PHYSICIAN

Counseling Smoking Cessation. Because health is the most common reason given by former smokers for quitting, the physician is in a unique position to encourage smoking cessation. The potential importance of the physician's role is underscored by the fact that smokers in whom symptoms of cardiopulmonary disease develop or who become pregnant are more likely to quit. Such patients are particularly motivated to quit and are more responsive to intervention efforts. The chances of making an attempt to quit are doubled by a physician's urging and advice. Providing no more than brief advice to stop smoking to all patients has been shown to be more effective than doing nothing to promote cessation, and it is a cost-effective medical practice. Doing more (i.e., brief, structured smoking cessation counseling) has, in randomized controlled trials, increased patients' efforts to stop smoking and, in some trials, their rates of long-term smoking cessation as well. Surveys indicate that physicians are not taking advantage of their opportunity to alter their patients' smoking habits. Fewer than one half of current smokers recall being told to quit by a physician. In fact, a physician's advice can make a difference. Physicians who devote more time to counseling smokers can expect to be even more effective. In one study, a regularly scheduled follow-up visit for smoking counseling was more effective than one-time advice. The physician can be most effective by advising all smokers to quit and providing additional counseling to susceptible smokers—those with respiratory symptoms or a recently diagnosed serious, smoking-related disease. Physician components identified by the National Cancer Institute as particularly helpful to the cessation effort include making the office a smoke-free site, identifying all smokers in the practice, asking them at each visit about smoking and advising cessation at every appropriate opportunity, helping them set a quit date, providing them with educational and self-help materials, advising nicotine reduction therapy or bupropion when indicated, and arranging follow-up to sustain cessation. A team approach in which a nurse provides more in-depth counseling and follow-up after the physician's introduction to cessation can enhance outcomes and reduce the expenditure of the physician's time (Table 54.1).

Preventing Relapse. *Follow-up* is critical. Studies of physician intervention show that scheduling follow-up visits to discuss smoking increases patients' cessation rates. The importance of continuing to work with the former smoker throughout the first year of cessation cannot be overemphasized, particularly the person with evidence of nicotine addiction. Such patients need to be prepared by the physician to recognize and manage nicotine withdrawal symptoms, prescribed a nicotine reduction program, and followed up within 2 weeks of quitting. Only after a full year of cessation can the patient be considered an ex-smoker. In the interim, repeated visits for reinforcement and support are essential to a successful outcome.

Weight gain must be addressed. Failure to do so risks ignoring a major cause of late relapse. Weight gain may be particularly upsetting to the person who quits out of a desire to improve appearance and personal hygiene. Nicotine increases energy expenditure. After cessation, the loss of such excess expenditure leads to weight gain unless caloric intake is decreased or physical activity is increased. Most smokers gain some weight after they stop smoking, with men averaging 2.8 kg and women 3.8 kg. The risk for large weight gain (>13 kg) is low; it occurs in about 10% of men and 13.5% of women. African-Americans and heavy smokers (>15 cigarettes per day) are also at increased risk. However, weight gain does not cancel the health benefits of smoking cessation. The physician needs to prepare the patient who plans to quit for the risk of weight gain. Prescribing a program of *exercise* (see Chapter 18) can be one of the best complements to the smoking cessation effort, facilitating weight control and providing an enhanced sense of well-being.

Depression also requires attention. Before the patient attempts to quit, the physician should evaluate the patient for an underlying depression (see Chapter 227) because it can be a major cause of smoking and a barrier to successful cessation (see above). If major depression is present, it must be treated before smoking cessation is attempted. As noted above, bupropion has proved to be equally effective at supporting cessation in patients with and without a history of depression, which suggests that its effectiveness in smoking cessation is independent of any beneficial effects on depression. Nevertheless, bupropion may well be the drug of choice in these situations because of the potential for both salutary effects. Patients with a history of depression, but who are not depressed before quitting, are at increased risk for a relapse during the withdrawal period. Depression needs to be watched for and responded to (see Chapter 227).

RECOMMENDATIONS

A smoking cessation strategy for office practice is summarized in Table 54.1.

1. *Assess smoking habits.* Smoking habits should be assessed as a part of every encounter in ambulatory practice. A smoking history should be taken from all smokers to assess the patient's current interest in quitting and anticipate difficulties with cessation, such as a high level of nicotine addiction or lack of social support. The smoker's prior cessation efforts and current medical and social situation can help guide treatment recommendations.
2. *Advise every smoker to stop smoking.* A firm statement to stop smoking should be made to all smokers at every visit. Total cessation is the goal.

3. *Motivate the smoker to attempt to quit.* This is the physician's primary role. The strategy should focus on health concerns, tailored to the individual's clinical situation. The approach should be positive, emphasizing the benefits of cessation and including short-term benefits, such as increased exercise tolerance or improved taste and smell. The contribution of smoking to any of the patient's current symptoms should be emphasized.

The asymptomatic smoker may be the most difficult one to motivate. Most smokers do have minor smoking-related symptoms that would improve with cessation, such as morning cough or limited exercise tolerance. Smokers unable to quit for their own sake may do so for their children's health or to ensure a safe pregnancy.

Smokers with an *acute respiratory illness* commonly stop smoking for a few days on their own. The physician can suggest that the smoker take advantage of the period of reduced desire to stop smoking permanently. For the smoker with a *chronic disease* associated with smoking, the physician should point out the potential for reduced symptoms, improved function, and slowed progression of disease. Radiologic or pulmonary function tests are not recommended for asymptomatic smokers because they do not detect early disease, and normal results may falsely reassure smokers that their health is not being jeopardized.

Smokers reluctant to attempt cessation often harbor a specific concern, such as a fear of failure, weight gain, withdrawal symptoms, or the loss of a pleasurable habit or way to handle life stresses. Helping the smoker to clarify this concern and develop arguments to the contrary can be helpful. If the smoker remains unwilling to consider cessation, the physician should stop with a strong antismoking recommendation but should make a renewed effort at subsequent visits.

4. *Ask for a commitment to quit.* Encourage smokers to set a date on which they will stop smoking, preferably within 4 weeks. Ideal quitting dates are milestones, such as a birthday, anniversary, or New Year's Day, or times when life stresses are minimized, such as the first day of a vacation. The physician should record the date in the medical record, as a reminder to follow the patient's progress.

5. *Help the smoker quit.* The physician should be prepared to offer a personalized and detailed cessation program that will maximize the patient's chances of success and build confidence. Specific behavioral suggestions should be offered (Table 54.2). Smokers concerned about weight gain should be advised to begin a concurrent exercise program and keep low-calorie snacks readily at hand. The addicted heavy smoker should be educated about withdrawal symptoms and considered a candidate for nicotine reduction therapy (transdermal nicotine patch, nicotine gum, or in special circumstances the newer prescription nasal spray or inhaler), especially someone with a history of severe withdrawal or marked weight gain on prior attempts. The patch or gum should be advised in conjunction with a behavioral program; it is not as effective by itself. Total abstinence is a precondition to prescribing reduction therapy, and the patient should be warned of the potential risks of smoking while using nicotine replacement. Smokers in whom cough and sputum production increase immediately after cessation should be reassured that this is temporary and common and represents a return of ciliary clearance activities in the respiratory tract.

Most smokers will initially elect to stop on their own, and an individual attempt should be the physician's initial recommendation. These smokers will benefit from self-help material. For heavy smokers who have failed unassisted quitting attempts, consideration of an assisted program is indicated. Providing information about and referral to such community smoking cessation programs is important.

If an underlying depression is present, it should be treated specifically before cessation is attempted. If depression develops subsequently, it too should be treated directly (see Chapter 227).

6. *Follow-up.* Continued monitoring of the smoking habit is essential. Listing the problem on the patient's medical problem list will remind the physician to manage it as part of the patient's continuing care. One or more return visits for follow-up will increase patients' success rates. The first follow-up should be scheduled shortly after the quit date. At follow-up, smokers who quit should be congratulated but cautioned of the need to maintain vigilance against relapse. Ex-smokers should be monitored carefully during the first year after cessation, which is when most relapses occur. For smokers whose attempts to quit have been unsuccessful, the physician should focus on positive aspects, such as the length of time the smoker was abstinent, and encourage another attempt. Through careful questioning, the physician can help the patient determine what circumstances caused the effort to fail and then encourage the patient to learn from the experience so as to increase the chance of success in the next attempt to quit.

ANNOTATED BIBLIOGRAPHY

Agee LL. Treatment procedures using hypnosis in smoking cessation programs: a review of the literature. J Am Soc Psychosom Dent Med 1983;30:111. (*Identifies components predictive of success with hypnosis.*)

Ahluwalia JS, McNagny SE, Clark WS. Smoking cessation among inner-city African-Americans using the nicotine transdermal patch. J Gen Intern Med 1998;13:1. (*Six-month quit rate was 17%, versus 11% with placebo patch.*)

Anda RF, Williamson DF, Escobedo LG, et al. Depression and the dynamics of smoking. JAMA 1990;264:1541. (*Epidemiologic data showing that smokers who are depressed are 40% less likely to quit than those who are not depressed.*)

Benowitz NL. Pharmacologic aspects of cigarette smoking and nicotine addiction. N Engl J Med 1988;319:1318. (*Comprehensive review of the pharmacokinetics of nicotine and its effects on the cardiovascular, nervous, and endocrine systems; discussion of the regulation of nicotine intake in smokers. Makes the case for smoking as an addiction to nicotine.*)

Benowitz NL, Jacob P, Kozlowski LT, et al. Influence of smoking fewer cigarettes on exposure to tar, nicotine, and carbon monoxide. N Engl J Med 1986;315:1310. (*Patients tended to oversmoke their cigarettes to maintain intake of nicotine, thereby greatly reducing the health benefit of smoking fewer cigarettes.*)

Burt A, Thornley P, Illingworth D, et al. Stopping smoking after myocardial infarction. Lancet 1974;1:305. (*Controlled, prospective study of infarction survivors demonstrating the effectiveness of brief physician advice in the hospital and nurse follow-up after discharge.*)

Cohen SJ, Stookey GK, Katz BP, et al. Encouraging primary care physicians to help smokers quit. Ann Intern Med 1989;110:648. (*Randomized, controlled trial of two practical interventions—use of nicotine gum and labeling of charts; these achieved a twofold to fivefold increase in quitting rate at 12 months.*)

Cummings SR, Coates TJ, Richard RJ, et al. Training physicians in counseling about smoking. Ann Intern Med 1989;110:640. (*Randomized trial; changed the way physicians counseled, but percentage of smokers who achieved long-term cessation increased by only 1% to 2%; useful discussion of reasons for the poor results and implications.*)

Cummings SR, Rubin SM, Oster G. The cost-effectiveness of counseling smokers to quit. JAMA 1989;261:75. (*A careful analysis demonstrating that brief advice during routine office visits is at least as cost-effective as other accepted preventive medical practices.*)

Dale LC, Schroeder DR, Wolter TD, et al. Weight change after smoking cessation using variable doses of transdermal nicotine replacement. J Gen Intern Med 1998;13:9. (*Higher replacement levels of nicotine may at least delay weight gain after cessation.*)

Department of Health and Human Services. The health benefits of smoking cessation: a report of the Surgeon General. Washington, DC: US Government Printing Office, 1990. DHHS publication No. (CDC)90-8416. (*Authoritative and comprehensive update on smoking cessation.*)

Duncan CL, Cummings SR, Hudes ES, et al. Quitting smoking: reasons for quitting and predictors of cessation among medical patients. J Gen Intern Med 1992;7:398. (*Health concerns were the most common reason for quitting, and addiction was the greatest barrier; education, social pressure, provider advice, and formal programs increased chances of quitting.*)

Fielding JE, Phenow KJ. Health effects of involuntary smoking. N Engl J Med 1988;319:1452. (*Comprehensive review of knowledge; increased risk for lung cancer among nonsmokers exposed to passive smoke.*)

Fiore MC, Novotny TE, Pierce JP, et al. Methods used to quit smoking in the United States: do cessation programs help? JAMA 1990;263:2760. (*Important epidemiologic study of smoking cessation methods; among the best available data.*)

Franks P, Harp J, Bell B. Randomized controlled trial of clonidine for smoking cessation in a primary care setting. JAMA 1989;262:3011. (*Clonidine had no effect on withdrawal symptoms or short-term rate of smoking cessation.*)

Fuller JA. Smoking withdrawal and acupuncture. Med J Aust 1982;1:28. (*It helped reduce withdrawal symptoms only.*)

Glantz SA, Parmley WW. Passive smoking and heart disease. Circulation 1992;83:1. (*Reviews evidence supporting increased risk for cardiovascular mortality among persons exposed to passive smoke.*)

Glassman AH, Helzer JE, Covey LS, et al. Smoking, smoking cessation, and major depression. JAMA 1990;264:1546. (*When patients with a history of depression stop smoking, depressive symptoms and even major depression may follow.*)

Greene HL, Goldberg RJ, Ockene JK. Cigarette smoking: the physician's role in cessation and maintenance. J Gen Intern Med 1988;3:75. (*Detailed review of what physicians can do to affect the smoking behavior of their patients; 122 references.*)

Henningfield JE, Radzius A, Cooper TM, et al. Drinking coffee and carbonated beverages blocks absorption of nicotine from nicotine polacrilex gum. JAMA 1990;264:1560. (*Possible reason why some patients fail to benefit from nicotine gum.*)

Hollis JF, Lichtenstein E, Vogt TM, et al. Nurse-assisted counseling for smokers in primary care. Ann Intern Med 1993;118:521. (*Physician burden reduced, and quitting rate enhanced.*)

Howard G, Wagenknecht LE, Burke GL, et al. Cigarette smoking and progression of atherosclerosis. JAMA 1998;279:119. (*Progression, measured by carotid artery intimal–medial thickness, increased by both active and passive smoking.*)

Hughes JR, Goldstein MG, Hurt RD, et al. Recent advances in the pharmacotherapy of smoking. JAMA 1999;281:72. (*Excellent summary of the advances; more than 50 current references.*)

Hurt RD, Sachs DPL, Glover ED, et al. A comparison of sustained-release bupropion and placebo for smoking cessation. N Engl J Med 1997;337:1195. (*One-year quit rate of 23%, compared with 12% for placebo; weight gain also significantly reduced.*)

Iribarren C, Tekawa IS, Stephen S, et al. Effect of cigar smoking on the risk of cardiovascular disease, chronic obstructive pulmonary disease, and cancer in men. N Engl J Med 1999;340:1773. (*Relative risks of 1.27, 1.45, 2.02, and 2.14 for coronary artery disease, chronic obstructive pulmonary disease, aerodigestive tract cancer, and lung cancer, respectively.*)

Jorenby DE, Leischow SJ, Nides MA, et al. A controlled trial of sustained-release bupropion, a nicotine patch, or both for smoking cessation. N Engl J Med 1999;340:685. (*One-year quit rates of 16% in patch-alone and placebo groups, 30% in the bupropion group, and 36% in the patch-plus-bupropion group.*)

Kanner RE, Connett JE, Williams DE, et al. Effects of randomized assignment to a smoking cessation intervention and changes in smoking habits on respiratory symptoms in smokers with early chronic obstructive pulmonary disease: the Lung Health Study. Am J Med 1999;106:410. (*Even with intention-to-treat analysis, smokers randomized to cessation intervention had fewer symptoms 5 years later.*)

Kawachi I, Colditz GA, Stampfer MJ, et al. Smoking cessation in relation to total mortality rates in women: a prospective cohort study. Ann Intern Med 1993;119:992. (*As in men, the risk for mortality among female former smokers declines to approach that of persons who never smoked 10 to 14 years after cessation.*)

Kottke TE, Battista RN, DeFriese GH, et al. Attributes of successful smoking cessation interventions in medical practice: a metaanalysis of 39 controlled trials. JAMA 1988;259:2883. (*Good analysis of available data, although many studies of suboptimal design.*)

LaCroix AZ, Lang J, Scherr P, et al. Smoking and mortality among older men and women in three communities. N Engl J Med 1991;324:1619. (*Finds that mortality risk continues into later life, which makes cessation efforts worthwhile and capable of improving life expectancy in elderly persons.*)

Lam W, Sacks HS, Sze P, et al. Metaanalysis of randomized controlled trials of nicotine chewing gum. Lancet 1987;2:27. (*Metaanalysis demonstrating effectiveness of gum in smoking cessation clinics but not in physician office.*)

Perkins KA, Epstein LH, Marks BL, et al. The effect of nicotine on energy expenditure during light physical activity. N Engl J Med 1989;320:898. (*Nicotine increases energy expenditure markedly during light exercise, a possible mechanism for weight gain during cessation of smoking.*)

Prochazka AV, Weaver MJ, Keller RT, et al. A randomized trial of nortriptyline for smoking cessation. Arch Intern Med 1998;158:2035. (*Six-month quit rate of 14%, versus 3% with placebo.*)

Rigotti NA, Singer DE, Mulley AG, et al. Smoking cessation following admission to a coronary care unit. J Gen Intern Med 1991;6:305. (*Twenty-five percent of smokers admitted to a coronary care unit were not smoking 1 year later. Lighter smokers and those with a new diagnosis of coronary artery disease were most likely to stop smoking.*)

Russell MAH, Wilson C, Taylor C, et al. Effect of general practitioners' advice against smoking. Br Med J 1979;2:231. (*Careful randomized, controlled study in which routine advice to stop smoking resulted in a significant increase in cessation that was sustained during 1 year.*)

Smoking Cessation Clinical Practice Guideline Panel and Staff. The Agency for Health Care Policy and Research clinical practice guideline. JAMA 1996;275:1270. (*Rigorous analysis and synthesis of the evidence.*)

Tonnesen P, Norregaard J, Simonsen K, et al. A double-blind trial of a 16-hour transdermal nicotine patch in smoking cessation. N Engl J Med 1991;325:311. (*Study of patch therapy without a behavioral component; excellent short-term efficacy, but at 1 year only 17% were still off cigarettes; emphasizes need for a combination approach.*)

Williamson DF, Madans J, Anda RF, et al. Smoking cessation and severity of weight gain in a national cohort. N Engl J Med 1991;324:739. (*Average weight gain was 3.8 kg in women and 2.8 kg in men; major weight gain of more than 13 kg in 9.8% of men and 13.4% of women.*)

Wilson D, Wood G, Johnston N, et al. Randomized clinical trial of supportive follow-up for cigarette smokers in a family practice. Can Med Assoc J 1982;126:127. (*Patients scheduled for regular return visits to their family physician for continued smoking counseling were more likely to quit than those receiving one-time advice from their physician.*)

5

Gastrointestinal Problems

55
Screening for Gastric Cancer

Gastric cancer is among the most common malignancies worldwide. It is the leading cause of cancer death in Japan, where population-based screening programs have been sponsored for many years. For unknown reasons, the incidence of gastric cancer in the United States has been decreasing at a rate of 2% to 4% annually for the past several decades. During the 1930s, the death rate for gastric cancer was greater than 30 in 100,000; during the 1970s, the rate was approximately 10 in 100,000. At present, Americans have approximately a 1% chance of acquiring a gastric malignancy during their lifetime. Nevertheless, mortality remains high; approximately 75% of the 25,000 Americans in whom gastric cancer develops each year eventually die of the disease. *Helicobacter pylori* infection has been classified as a carcinogen because of its association with an increased risk for gastric cancer, so that new prevention strategies have become possible by screening for the risk associated with infection.

The usual insidious onset of the disease and the lack of suitable screening tests have heretofore thwarted preventive measures. Advances in endoscopic instrumentation, allowing more complete visualization of the stomach, have raised questions about unmet potential in preventing gastric cancer deaths among high-risk populations. The primary care physician must understand the natural history of gastric cancer and the limitations of diagnostic tools in the detection of early disease.

EPIDEMIOLOGY AND RISK FACTORS

The international variation in the incidence of gastric cancer is marked. Among the countries with the highest incidence are Japan, Chile, Finland, and Iceland. Incidence also varies, predictably, with age and sex. Gastric cancer is twice as likely to develop in men in most countries. More than 60% of cases occur in people over age 65. Fewer than 10% of cases occur in people younger than age 30. The incidence among nonwhites and people in low socioeconomic groups in the United States is twice that among whites and the more well-to-do.

Genetic factors do not play a major role in determining the risk for gastric cancer. It has been documented that migrants from areas of high risk (e.g., Japan) eventually acquire the lower rates of their new home (e.g., the United States). A genetically determined minor risk factor for gastric cancer is blood group; people with type A blood have a 10% increase in risk for the development of gastric cancer.

A number of environmental factors have been suggested as explanations for the geographic variability of gastric cancer incidence. Phenol, present in all smoked foods, and the high salt concentration in salted fish and meat products have been linked to the high incidence of gastric cancer in Finland, Iceland, and Japan. Talc-treated rice has been implicated in Japan and Northern China. Provinces in Chile with high gastric cancer rates are agricultural, with high concentrations of nitrate present in the soil and drinking water. Nitrosamines, derived from nitrates and secondary amines, are suspected causes of gastric cancer in Chile and, to a lesser extent, in the United States, where nitrates and nitrites are used as food additives in meat and fish.

A number of pathologic conditions, including gastric polyps and adenomas, have been associated with an increased risk for stomach cancer. Gastric polyps are relatively infrequent; a prevalence of less than 0.5% has been documented in one autopsy series. The vast majority of polyps are hyperplastic and not associated with an increased cancer risk. People with adenomas, particularly villous adenomas, have the same risk for cancer when the adenomas are found in the stomach as when they are in the colon. Some authorities have argued that peptic ulcer disease predisposes patients to gastric cancer. Carcinoma is found in approximately 3% of surgically resected gastric ulcers. It is likely, however, that ulceration follows carcinoma rather than vice versa. This association is the basis for the clinical practice of taking biopsy specimens from suspected or persistent gastric ulcers, or resecting them.

A number of studies have demonstrated a statistical association between atrophic gastritis and gastric cancer. Achlorhydria and atrophic gastritis are common. Prevalence increases with age. An annual incidence of gastric cancer of 1% among patients with atrophic gastritis has been demonstrated in one study with yearly radiographic examination. The atrophic gastritis associated with pernicious anemia is also a risk factor for gastric cancer. Evidence indicates that patients with pernicious anemia have at least a fourfold increase in risk. Some studies have found even higher rates.

Prior gastric surgery for benign ulcer disease has long been considered a risk factor for subsequent gastric cancer. Increased risk was not evident early after surgery, but several Scandinavian studies suggested that those who lived more than 10 to 15 years after surgery faced a twofold to threefold increase in gastric cancer risk. Recommendations for annual endoscopic examination followed. More recently, a large, population-based study conducted in Olmstead County, Minnesota, found gastric cancer to be no more common among patients with prior gastric surgery than among the population at large.

NATURAL HISTORY OF GASTRIC CANCER AND EFFECTIVENESS OF THERAPY

Gastric cancer typically has an insidious presentation. The most common initial symptom is epigastric discomfort. Later symptoms include early satiety, indigestion, weight loss, and other systemic symptoms. The percentage of patients who survive 5 years has not improved significantly in recent years; it remains at 20% of unselected cases. The patients who are operated on early in the course of their disease have a 60% to 90% 5-year survival rate. Some population-based studies from Japan confirm that 5-year survival rates of 70% can be achieved among patients with gastric cancer detected by screening. Furthermore, follow-up for 15 years suggests that the cancer death hazard rate decreases rapidly for 7 years after detection and treatment of cancer, and then remains very low. Other studies from Japan question the value of screening, especially among people younger than 50 years of age.

Among highly selected patients with "early gastric cancer," defined as gastric cancer confined to the mucosa or submucosa but not extending to the muscularis propria, resection may be curative for as many as 95%. Intensive screening efforts in Japan have increased the proportion of gastric cancers detected in this early stage from approximately 5% to 30%. Efforts have not been as successful elsewhere, where fewer than 10% of cases meet criteria for early gastric cancer. The duration of the asymptomatic detectable period is unknown, but early gastric cancer has been found as long as 3 years after biopsy specimens were originally misread as benign. The natural history of early gastric cancer appears to include protracted cycles of healing and ulceration.

SCREENING AND DIAGNOSTIC TESTS

None of the tests generally used in the United States for the *diagnosis* of gastric carcinoma are suitable for wide screening efforts.

Gastric Cytology. The collection and examination of specimens for gastric cytopathologic analysis, unlike that for cervical cytopathology, is a laborious process. Samples must be obtained either by endoscopic scraping or by gastric lavage. Examination of the resulting slides usually takes 2 to 3 hours rather than the several minutes sufficient for the screening examination of cervical Papanicolaou smears. Many studies have demonstrated the sensitivity of gastric cytopathology studies to be approximately 90%. It is not known how much this figure is influenced by the spectrum of disease—that is, how sensitive

cytology can be for the early, curable cancer. Specificity in a laboratory with experienced personnel should be approximately 97% to 98%. False-positive results are often found in association with healing gastric ulcer and other gastric pathology. Although cytopathology is useful for further diagnosis in documented cases of abnormality of gastric mucosa, it cannot be recommended for indiscriminate screening.

Endoscopy. Similarly, endoscopy must be considered a diagnostic rather than a screening procedure. Its sensitivity in making the diagnosis of gastric cancer is 90%. However, recent evidence suggests that endoscopic visualization is much less sensitive for early cancers, with a visual diagnosis being made in fewer than 50% of cases in some series. Multiple biopsies of any and all suspected lesions can increase the sensitivity to 90%.

Diagnostic Radiology. The sensitivity of contrast studies in the diagnosis of gastric cancer has been reported to be as high as 95%. Obviously, however, it is least sensitive in cases of early disease and is too expensive and time-consuming to be considered a screening test in asymptomatic patients. In Japan, where gastric cancer is the leading cause of cancer death, radiographic techniques have been adapted to mass screening. These modifications in the standard contrast studies have been shown to have a sensitivity and specificity of 90%.

Stool analysis for occult blood (described in detail in Chapter 56) is an appropriate screening procedure for all gastrointestinal malignancies. Yearly guaiac testing has been recommended as part of the general screening for all adult patients. This is especially important for patients with an identified increased risk for gastric cancer, such as those with a history of pernicious anemia or documented atrophic gastritis.

Too little is known about the role of *H. pylori* infection or the effect of its treatment on gastric cancer risk to justify screening asymptomatic persons at this time.

CONCLUSIONS AND RECOMMENDATIONS

- Despite a significant downward trend in incidence, gastric cancer remains a disease of high morbidity and mortality.
- The yearly analysis of stool for occult blood is indicated in all adult patients. This is especially important for those with a history of pernicious anemia, atrophic gastritis, *H. pylori* infection, or other gastric pathology.
- The value of gastric cytology, endoscopy, and contrast studies as routine procedures in high-risk patients is unproven. They are diagnostic procedures and should generally be reserved for symptomatic patients or patients with occult blood demonstrated by stool analysis.

A.G.M.

ANNOTATED BIBLIOGRAPHY

Bedikian AY, Chen TT, Khankhanian N, et al. The natural history of gastric cancer and prognostic factors influencing survival. J Clin Oncol 1984;2:305. (*Useful review of natural history with an emphasis on clinical determinants of survival.*)

Corea P. *Helicobacter pylori* and gastric carcinogenesis. Am J Surg Pathol.1995;19S:S37. (*Describes a multifocal atrophic gastritis associated with* H. pylori *infection in populations at high risk for gastric cancer.*)

Farley DR, Donohue JH. Early gastric cancer. Surg Clin North Am 1992;72:401. (*Review of early gastric cancer and surgical issues.*)

Hitchcock CR, MacLean LD, Sullivan WA. Secretory and clinical aspects of achlorhydria and gastric atrophy as precursors of gastric cancer. J Natl Cancer Inst 1957;18:795. (*Review of data indicating that risk is increased 4.5 and 21.9 times among patients with achlorhydria and pernicious anemia, respectively. Recommends frequent radiographic studies.*)

Kurihara M, Shirakabe H, Yarita T, et al. Diagnosis of small early gastric cancer by x-ray, endoscopy, and biopsy. Cancer Detect Prev 1981;4:377. (*Sensitivity of double-contrast radiography is 75%; that of endoscopy plus biopsy is more than 95%.*)

Logan RFA, Langman MJS. Screening for gastric cancer after gastric surgery. Lancet 1983;2:667. (*Accepts evidence for increased risk but nevertheless does not favor endoscopic screening.*)

Muramaki R, Tsukuma H, Ubukata T, et al. Estimation of validity of mass screening program for gastric cancer in Japan. Cancer 1990; 65:1255. (*Radiographic techniques adapted for mass screening for gastric cancer in Japan achieve sensitivity and specificity of 90%.*)

Parsonnet J, Harris RA, Hack HM, et al. Modeling cost-effectiveness of *Helicobacter pylori* screening to prevent gastric cancer: a mandate for clinical trials. Lancet 1996;348:150. (*Assuming that H. pylori treatment would prevent 30% of attributable gastric cancers, this approach would have a reasonable cost-effectiveness ratio.*)

Schafer LW, Larson DE, Melton LJ, et al. The risk of gastric carcinoma after surgical treatment for benign ulcer disease. N Engl J Med 1983;309:1210. (*No evident increase in the risk for gastric cancer after surgical treatment for benign peptic ulcer disease led the authors to conclude that endoscopic surveillance is not indicated in this population.*)

Yamazaki H, Oshima A, Muramaki R, et al. A long-term follow-up study of patients with gastric cancer detected by mass screening. Cancer 1989;63:613. (*Includes survival curves and hazard rates for more than 1,000 patients with gastric cancer detected by mass screening in Japan.*)

56
Screening for Colorectal Cancer
MICHAEL J. BARRY

Colorectal cancer (CRC) is a common malignancy in both men and women, accounting for about 10% of cancer deaths. Americans face a lifetime risk of CRC of approximately 1 in 17. The majority of CRCs that present with signs or symptoms have already spread beyond the intestinal wall, resulting in a poor 5-year survival rate. However, cancers detected and removed while still localized are associated with a 5-year survival rate in excess of 80%. The long asymptomatic period, the availability of tests that can identify localized disease, and the effectiveness of early therapy suggest that screening for CRC should be a primary care priority. Evidence from multiple randomized trials has now confirmed that such screening can reduce the risk for CRC mortality.

EPIDEMIOLOGY AND RISK FACTORS

The incidence of colorectal cancer is greater in economically developed societies. The high-fat, low-fiber *diet* prevalent in Western societies has been implicated in the etiology of these cancers. Whether intake of dietary fiber among Americans is associated with the risk for CRC has been harder to prove.

Advancing *age* is an important risk factor, with the incidence of CRC rising from about 75 in 100,000 in the sixth decade to 300 in 100,000 in the eighth decade.

Family history is also a risk factor. Having a first-degree relative with CRC raises personal risk twofold to threefold, with risk greatest when cancer has been diagnosed at an early age and when more than one first-degree relative has been affected. Newer evidence suggests that a family history of larger adenomatous polyps also increases the risk for CRC. Autosomal dominant familial adenomatous polyposis confers a risk for CRC of about 50% by age 40, and a number of other familial cancer syndromes also increase risk greatly. Genetic testing is available for one of them, hereditary nonpolyposis colon cancer.

Ulcerative colitis, particularly pancolitis of more than 10 years' duration, increases a patient's risk for CRC fivefold to 10-fold, although isolated left-sided ulcerative proctitis probably confers substantially less or no additional risk. Controversy remains as to whether Crohn's disease is associated with a clinically significant increase in risk for CRC.

In some observational studies, the use of aspirin or NSAIDs has appeared to be associated with a lower risk for CRC. However, among subjects randomized to aspirin in the Physicians Health Study, the incidence of CRC was no lower than the incidence in controls.

Almost all CRCs are believed to arise from *adenomatous polyps*. The prevalence of adenomatous polyps increases with age, occurring in 30% of 50-year-olds (3% >1 cm), 40% of 60-year-olds (4% >1 cm), and 50% of 70-year-olds (5% >1 cm). Once a person has had an adenomatous polyp removed, it has been suggested that their future risk for CRC is higher. However, the magnitude of future risk, if any, is uncertain, especially if the index polyp is small (<1 cm). Because of this association between adenomatous polyps and CRC, it is not surprising that a family history of polyps has also been shown to increase risk for cancer.

Patients with *resected CRCs* have a threefold increase in risk for metachronous cancer in other locations of the colon. Recurrences of index cancers are usually extraluminal and not amenable to detection by endoscopic screening.

The prevalence of *synchronous colonic neoplasia* is high and important to consider in the evaluation of the patient with a positive screening test result. Synchronous adenomas occur in 40% to 50% of patients with an index polyp; 3% to 5% with a carcinoma will harbor a second one.

NATURAL HISTORY OF COLORECTAL CANCER AND EFFECTIVENESS OF THERAPY

Sporadic polyps are common lesions, with the most common being small, hyperplastic outcroppings of the colonic mucosa

Table 56-1. Polypoid Lesions of the Colon and Rectum: Relation of Size to Cancer (1,116 Polypoid Lesions, Massachusetts General Hospital, 1954-1963)

DIAMETER (CM)	PERCENTAGE CANCEROUS
<0.5	0.5
0.5–0.9	1
1.0–1.4	1.8
1.5–1.9	6
2–2.4	10
2.5–3.4	23
≥3.5	29

From Behringer GE. Changing concepts in the histopathologic diagnosis of polypoid lesions of the colon. Dis Colon Rectum 1970;13:1196, with permission.

that do not have a malignant potential. Adenomas are truly neoplastic and may include malignant foci. The risk for malignancy increases with the size of the adenoma, ranging from 0.5% of colonoscopically removed polyps from 0.5 to 0.9 cm in diameter to 25% or more of polyps greater than 3 cm in diameter. Histology also affects cancer risk. Villous adenomas are the polyps with the highest malignant potential, and they tend to be larger and more sessile than tubular or mixed tubulovillous adenomas, which are associated with less risk (Table 56.1). About 10% of polyps have villous histology, tubular adenomas account for 70%, and the remainder have mixed histology. The probability and time frame for the development of a nonmalignant polyp into an invasive cancer are not well defined, although these are important variables in estimating the effectiveness of screening strategies. Interestingly, although the prevalence of polyps increases with age (see above), average polyp size does not, which suggests that most polyps do not progressively enlarge.

Symptoms occur late in the course of CRC growth. The duration of the asymptomatic detectable period is estimated to be several years. When cancers are found after symptomatic presentation, 60% have already disseminated to regional nodes or distant organs. Five-year survival rates vary dramatically with the stage of disease at the time of diagnosis. Patients whose tumors are confined locally to the bowel wall (Dukes stage A) or pericolic fat (Dukes B) have an 80% 5-year survival, whereas those whose tumors exhibit regional lymph node metastases (Dukes C) have a 46% 5-year survival; this drops to 5% with distant metastases (Dukes D).

SCREENING TESTS

Digital Examination

Only about 10% of CRCs are within reach of the examining finger. Although many experts recommend performing this time-honored examination annually among patients who are older than 40 years, there is little evidence to support the practice to screen for CRC.

Fecal Occult Blood Testing

Intermittent occult bleeding occurs with some asymptomatic CRCs and large polyps. Serial sampling of stools for occult blood can be performed to identify this bleeding. Guaiac-impregnated filter paper slides (Hemoccult II and others) are ca-

pable of detecting small amounts of fecal blood, which will be present in some patients with CRC. The fact that colonic tumors selectively enrich the stool surface with blood enhances the sensitivity of guaiac testing of stool samples. Stool sampling is best performed serially because of the intermittent nature of the bleeding (e.g., two samples from a stool on each of 3 days).

Sensitivity, Specificity, and Yield. A six-test guaiac stool sequence has a sensitivity of 30% to 70% for CRC. The lower figure is probably more accurate for early cancers in asymptomatic patients. Sensitivity falls when prepared slides are stored for more than 4 days before being developed. *Rehydration* of the sample before application of developer can increase sensitivity, but at the cost of a loss in specificity. False-positive test results may occur with nonmalignant lesions, aspirin (at doses >325 mg daily) and NSAIDs, rare red meat, or foods with high peroxidase activity. Studies on the ability of iron supplements to cause false-positive guaiac results have been conflicting. A specificity of 97% to 98% can be attained by omitting rare red meat, horseradish, cantaloupe, and uncooked fresh vegetables (especially broccoli, turnip, radish, cauliflower) 2 days before the first sample is collected. High doses of vitamin C increase the false-negative rate. Newer tests and combinations of tests are being evaluated, and clinicians should follow the literature for new developments.

Based on screening results in population studies and randomized trials, the clinician should expect 2% to 4% of persons over the age of 50 to have a positive fecal occult blood test (FOBT) result (Hemoccult II). Of these, about 10% will have CRC and 40% either CRC or polyps. Most of these polyps are too small to cause detectable bleeding but are found serendipitously when follow-up studies are performed after a positive occult blood test result. When rehydration is used, the positivity rate is about 10%. Of these, about 2% will have CRCs and 30% either cancers or adenomas.

A new screening strategy has been proposed that combines a more sensitive guaiac test (HemoccultSENSA) with a more specific immunochemical test (HemeSelect) when the guaiac test result is positive. This strategy may increase the sensitivity of screening for occult blood without as great a loss of specificity as occurs with rehydration of older guaiac cards, but it adds complexity to the testing process.

Individuals with a positive FOBT result require a thorough evaluation for colorectal neoplasia. Smaller polyps produce guaiac positivity only on occasion, but their high prevalence makes them the most common lesions found during the evaluation of patients with occult bleeding. *Colonoscopy* or the combination of *sigmoidoscopy* and *air-contrast barium enema* are acceptable alternatives for follow-up evaluation of the patient with a test positive for occult blood. Colonoscopy offers the advantage of allowing a biopsy or polypectomy to be performed during the same examination and is the more sensitive for detecting smaller polyps. However, given the uncertain natural history of small polyps and the cost of polypectomy (both initially and for any necessary future colonoscopic surveillance), it is not clear whether this higher sensitivity is an advantage or disadvantage.

Outcomes. The best outcome measure of screening efficacy is *reduced CRC mortality*, as judged by prospective, randomized, controlled clinical trials with a long period of follow-up. One such study, The Minnesota Colon Cancer Study, demonstrated a 33% reduction in cumulative CRC mortality (from 8.3 in 1,000 to 5.9 in 1,000 over 13 years) as a result of annual occult blood screening. This trial used a six-sample annual testing protocol, followed by colonoscopy for persons with positive test results. The guaiac cards were rehydrated, which increased the true-positive rate of testing from 81% to 92% but increased the false-positive rate from 2% to 10%. As a result of this decrease in specificity, 38% of screenees underwent colonoscopy during the study. The cumulative incidence of CRC was almost identical in the screened and control groups, which suggests that most of the benefit came from early detection of established cancers rather than from prevention of future cancers by resecting polyps. Compared with the control group, screened patients demonstrated a shift to detection of earlier cancers. Despite the large relative benefit in terms of mortality, the absolute risk that any one man or woman will die of CRC is quite low. As a result, data from this trial indicate that about 300 men would need to be screened annually for 13 years to prevent one CRC death. In a subsequent publication, reporting 18 years of follow-up, the Minnesota investigators reported that even biennial screening reduced CRC mortality by 21%.

As seen from the Minnesota study, rehydration of the guaiac card increases its sensitivity, but it also increases the number of colonoscopies needed, the cost of screening, and the false-positive rate. Two other trials, conducted in Denmark and the United Kingdom, used guaiac cards without hydration and conducted screening biennially rather than annually. Population-based samples of patients were randomized without their knowledge, so it is likely that the persons screened were representative of actual practice. Only 4% of persons screened in the studies underwent colonoscopy. Even under these circumstances, the trials demonstrated 18% and 15% reductions in CRC mortality, respectively.

Sigmoidoscopy

About 25% of colon cancers are within the range of the *rigid sigmoidoscope*, whereas the longer (65 cm) *flexible sigmoidoscope* can potentially detect about 50% of cancers. The risk for a bowel perforation—the major complication of sigmoidoscopy—is low (about 1 to 2 in 10,000 rigid sigmoidoscopic examinations). The risk with flexible scopes has been less well studied. The number of cancers found per 1,000 examinations ranges from 1.5 for the rigid scope to 4 for the 65-cm flexible scope. Adenomatous polyps are found in up to 20% of persons screened. When adenomatous polyps are detected and removed at sigmoidoscopy, the patient then usually undergoes colonoscopy for examination of the rest of the colon.

Sigmoidoscopy can clearly find localized cancers and polyps for removal, but the key question is the effect of the procedure on CRC mortality rates when used for periodic screening. Data from prospective studies are pending, but a retrospective, case–control study of periodic rigid sigmoidoscopy for CRC screening suggested a 60% to 70% reduction in CRC mortality risk. As would be expected, the protective association appeared specific for cancers within reach of the sigmoidoscope; the exposure odds were not reduced for more proximal cancers. The marginal value, in terms of mortality reduction, of adding sigmoidoscopic screening to regular guaiac testing is undefined.

The American Cancer Society recommends annual FOBT and flexible sigmoidoscopy every 5 years, beginning at age 50 for patients at average risk (alternatively, colonoscopy every 10 years or double-contrast barium enema every 5 to 10 years). In light of the mounting evidence from randomized trials, the U.S. Preventive Services Task Force has revised its previous position and now recommends annual FOBT or sigmoidoscopy every 5 years for average-risk persons older than 50 years.

An Overall Screening Strategy

The most commonly recommended approach to screening for CRC is a combination of *annual FOBT* and *flexible sigmoidoscopy every 5 years*, starting at age 50 for average-risk persons. Screening might start at age 40 for those at higher risk (or 10 years before the earliest cancer in a family with a strong history of colorectal cancer). Some experts have suggested as an alternative less frequent examination of the entire colon. In one cost-effectiveness analysis, the combination of annual occult blood tests and an air-contrast barium enema every 5 years was particularly attractive. The high cost of colonoscopy, however, weighs against its periodic use as a screening test for persons of average risk. On the other hand, some experts argue that one or two colonoscopic examinations during a lifetime might be sufficient to reduce mortality from CRC substantially, and reasonably cost-effective because of the small number of studies.

When adenomatous polyps larger than 0.5 cm, multiple lesions, or lesions with villous or tubulovillous histology are found at screening sigmoidoscopy, referral for colonoscopy to search for more proximal synchronous disease is recommended; if it has not already been done, the index polyp should be removed for histologic examination.

CONCLUSIONS AND RECOMMENDATIONS

Conclusions

- The relatively high prevalence of CRC, its slow evolution from adenomatous polyp to cancer, and the accumulating (although not yet definitive) evidence that available screening tests reduce mortality from this disease suggest that an aggressive approach to screening is reasonable and appropriate.

Recommendations: Test Selection and Frequency of Screening

- Most authorities now recommend that all patients, including those at normal risk, be screened with annual FOBT plus periodic sigmoidoscopy or colonoscopy, depending on the estimated risk for CRC.
- To guide screening, annually reassess the patient's CRC risk by reviewing the family history for CRC and larger (>1 cm) adenomas in first-degree relatives, and the past medical history for CRC, larger adenomas, and ulcerative colitis with pancolonic involvement.
- For *high-risk* persons (i.e., those with ulcerative pancolitis for longer than 10 years, familial adenomatous polyposis, or nonpolyposis colon cancer): Refer to a gastroenterologist for surveillance colonoscopy.
- For *intermediate- to high-risk* patients [i.e., those with a personal history of CRC or larger (>1 cm) adenomatous polyps]: Obtain follow-up colonoscopy approximately once every 3 years.

- For *high-intermediate-risk* persons (i.e., those with a strong family history of CRC, larger adenomas in a first-degree relative under 60 years of age, or more than one affected first-degree relative): Begin screening at age 40 with *colonoscopy* approximately once every 5 years.
- For *intermediate-risk persons* [i.e., those with one first-degree relative with CRC or polyps diagnosed after age 60, or with a personal history of a smaller (<1 cm) adenomatous polyp]: Begin screening at age 40 with *annual FOBT and flexible sigmoidoscopy every 5 years.*
- For *average-risk* patients (i.e., those with no risk factors other than age): Begin screening with *annual FOBT* at age 50 and *flexible sigmoidoscopy every 5 years.*
- Because the cost-effectiveness of endoscopic screening remains to be fully determined, the physician can review with the reluctant patient the benefits and risks of available screening strategies and plan an individualized approach.

Recommendations: Test Performance

- Perform *FOBT* by instructing the patient to obtain two samples on each of 3 days, during which dietary peroxidases and rare red meat are restricted.
- Follow any positive FOBT result with colonoscopy or the combination of sigmoidoscopy plus air-contrast barium enema. (This strategy is preferable to repeating any positive test obtained on an undefined diet.)
- Order colonoscopy in any patient with a larger polyp, multiple smaller polyps, or a polyp with tubulovillous or villous histology found on screening sigmoidoscopy.
- Substitute rigid sigmoidoscopy for flexible sigmoidoscopy if the latter is not available (see appendix).

ANNOTATED BIBLIOGRAPHY

Ahlquist DA, McGill DB, Fleming JL, et al. Pattern of occult bleeding in asymptomatic colorectal cancer. Cancer 1989;63:1826. (*Documents the relatively low sensitivity of guaiac tests for asymptomatic cancers.*)

Ahsan H, Neugut AI, Garbowski GC, et al. Family history of colorectal adenomatous polyps and increased risk for colorectal cancer. Ann Intern Med 1998;128:900. (*A reconstituted cohort study showing persons with a first-degree relative who had an adenomatous polyp before age 50 at significantly increased risk for CRC.*)

Allison JE, Feldman R, Tekawa IS. Hemoccult screening in detecting colorectal neoplasm: long-term follow-up in a large group practice setting. Ann Intern Med 1990;112:328. (*Practice-based analysis of the operating characteristics of an FOBT.*)

Allison JE, Tekawa IS, Ransom LJ, et al. A comparison of fecal occult blood tests for colorectal cancer screening. N Engl J Med 1996;334:155. (*Comparison of three different screening tests, and one combination of two tests, suggests that improvement over Hemoccult II sensitivity is possible with only modest loss of specificity.*)

American College of Physicians. Suggested technique for fecal occult blood testing and interpretation in colorectal cancer screening. Ann Intern Med 1997;126:808. (*American College of Physicians guidelines for performing FOBT and following up on suspected results.*)

Byers T, Levin B, Rothenberger D, et al. American Cancer Society guidelines for screening and surveillance for early detection of colorectal polyps and cancer: update 1997. CA Cancer J Clin 1997; 47:154. (*Review of American Cancer Society CRC screening recommendations depending on screenees' risk status: average, moderate, or high.*)

Cannon-Albright LA, Skolnick MH, Bishop DT, et al. Common inheritance of susceptibility to colonic adenomatous polyps and associated colorectal cancers. N Engl J Med 1988;319: 533. (*First-degree relatives have an increased risk for CRC.*)

Eddy DM. Screening for colorectal cancer. Ann Intern Med 1990; 113:373. (*Sophisticated mathematical models examine the cost-effectiveness of CRC screening with a variety of test strategies.*)

Hardcastle JD, Chamberlain JO, Robinson MHE, et al. Randomised trial of faecal-occult-blood screening for colorectal cancer. Lancet 1996;348:1472. (*A population-based trial with a 15% mortality reduction attributable to biennial Haemoccult tests without rehydration.*)

Kronborg O, Fenger C, Olsen J, et al. Randomised study of screening for colorectal cancer with faecal-occult-blood test. Lancet 1996;348:1467. (*In this population-based trial, an 18% mortality reduction was achieved with biennial screening and without rehydration of Hemoccult II tests.*)

Lindsay DC, et al. Should colonoscopy be the first investigation for colonic disease? Br Med J 1988;296:167. (*Randomized trial of colonoscopy versus rigid sigmoidoscopy and air-contrast barium enema in the workup of colonic disease.*)

Mandel JS, Bond JH, Church TR, et al. Reducing mortality from colorectal cancer by screening for fecal occult blood. N Engl J Med 1993;328:1365. (*Randomized, prospective study showing a 33% relative reduction in CRC mortality risk with annual screening for 13 years and use of rehydrated cards.*)

Mandel JS, Church TR, Ederer F, et al. Colorectal cancer mortality: effectiveness of biennial screening for fecal occult blood. J Natl Cancer Inst 1999;91:434. (*In an update of the trial cited above, after 18 years, annual screening reduced CRC mortality 33% and biennial screening reduced CRC mortality 21%.*)

Preventive Services Task Force. Guide to clinical preventive services. Washington, DC: Government Printing Office, 1995. (*Includes revised recommendation for screening with occult blood testing, sigmoidoscopy, or both starting at age 50.*)

Sandler RS. Epidemiology and risk factors for colorectal cancer. Gastroenterol Clin North Am 1996;25:717. (*Comprehensive review of CRC occurrence and risk factors.*)

Ransohoff DF, Lang CA. Small adenomas detected during fecal occult blood test screening for colorectal cancer: the impact of serendipity. JAMA 1990;264:76. (*High predictive value of occult blood tests for polyps is the result of their high prevalence rather than of the fact that they bleed.*)

Ransohoff DF, Lang CA. Screening for colorectal cancer with the fecal occult blood test: a background paper. Ann Intern Med 1997;126:811. (*Background article for the American College of Physicians guideline; presents a detailed review of the methodology and outcomes of FOBT.*)

Rex DK, Lehman GA, Hawes RH, et al. Screening colonoscopy in asymptomatic average-risk persons with negative fecal occult blood tests. Gastroenterology 1991;64:100. (*The negative predictive value of FOBT.*)

St John DJB, McDermott FT, Hopper JL, et al. Cancer risk in relatives of patients with common colorectal cancer. Ann Intern Med 1993;118:785. (*Risk is increased if cancer is present in a first-degree relative, especially if diagnosed at an early age and if other first-degree relatives are affected.*)

St John DJB, Young GP, McHutchison JG, et al. Comparison of the specificity and sensitivity of Hemoccult and HemoQuant in screening for colorectal neoplasia. Ann Intern Med 1992;117:376. (*Cross-sectional study, in which Hemoccult performed better than HemoQuant.*)

Selby JV, Friedman GD, Quesenberry CP, et al. A case–control study of screening sigmoidoscopy and mortality from colorectal cancer. N Engl J Med 1992;326:653. (*Exposure to sigmoidoscopic screening was associated with a substantial reduction in risk of dying of CRC, but only if cancers were within reach of the scope.*)

Selby JV, Friedman GD, Quesenberry CP Jr., et al. Effect of fecal occult blood testing on mortality from colorectal cancer. Ann Intern Med 1993;118:1. (*Retrospective case–control study suggesting that mortality risk might be lowered, but confidence intervals are wide; more data are needed.*)

Towler B, Irwig L, Glasziou P, et al. A systematic review of the effects of screening for colorectal cancer using the faecal occult blood test, Hemoccult. BMJ 1998;317:559. (*In a metaanalysis of randomized trials, guaiac screening reduced CRC mortality by 16%; however, more than 1,000 men would need to be screened biennially for 10 years to prevent one CRC death.*)

Wallace MB, Kemp JA, Trnka YM, et al. Is colonoscopy indicated for small adenomas found by screening flexible sigmoidoscopy? Ann Intern Med 1998;129:273. (*Data from this prospective cohort study suggest the answer is no for a single distal tubular adenoma smaller than 5 mm, but yes for multiple small adenomas or advanced histology.*)

Willett WC, Stampfer MJ, Colditz GA, et al. Relation of meat, fat, and fiber intake to the risk of colon cancer in a prospective study among women. N Engl J Med 1990;323:1664. (*Epidemiologic study suggesting that a high intake of animal fat or red meat increases the risk for colon cancer.*)

Winawer SJ, Zauber AG, O'Brien MJ, et al. Randomized comparison of surveillance intervals after colonoscopic removal of newly diagnosed adenomatous polyps. N Engl J Med 1993;328:901. (*Longer interval just as effective as the shorter one.*)

Winawer SJ, Zauber AG, Gerdes H, et al. Risk of colorectal cancer in the families of patients with adenomatous polyps. N Engl J Med 1996;334:82. (*Siblings and parents of patients with adenomatous polyps are at increased risk for CRC.*)

Appendix: Examination of the Anorectum and Sigmoid Colon with Digital Rectal Examination, Anoscopy, and Sigmoidoscopy

LAWRENCE S. FRIEDMAN

Careful, competent examinations of the anorectal area and distal colon are essential for CRC screening and for evaluation of complaints referable to these structures. The anorectal examination is indicated in all patients who are to undergo sigmoidoscopy and should be incorporated into all complete physical examinations in adults.

ANORECTAL EXAMINATION

Digital Rectal Examination

No bowel preparation is necessary, but the physician must establish rapport with the patient by taking a history and performing other parts of the physical examination first. Apprehension and embarrassment may be minimized by explaining each step, describing the anticipated sensations, and draping the patient to expose only the perineum.

Inspection. The patient may be examined in either the knee–chest or left lateral decubitus (Sims') position. After retraction of the buttocks, the perianal skin and anal orifice are inspected for fecal material (reflecting poor hygiene, painful lesions that make cleansing difficult, or incontinence), drainage, dermatoses, scars, prolapsed hemorrhoids, fistulas, fissures, abscesses, hematomas, condylomata, and carcinomas. Lesions are described anatomically (e.g., anterior, right-sided), not with reference to the face of a clock. Perineal and sacrococcygeal tissues should be palpated with the gloved but unlubricated index finger for tenderness, induration, fluctuance, or masses.

Palpation. Digital examination of the rectum is then performed by placing the gloved, lubricated index finger at the anal orifice and gently inserting as the patient bears down. The small finger may be used in patients with painful or stenotic anal lesions. Anesthetic ointment may be helpful if a tender lesion is present. The anal sphincter tone and strength of contraction are noted, and the finger is swept circumferentially as it is advanced into the rectum. Abnormalities sought include fissures, fistulous tracts, abscesses, sessile and pedunculated polyps, and cancers. Rarely, foreign bodies may be encountered. Internal hemorrhoids are not palpable unless they are thrombosed. In inflammatory bowel disease, the mucosa may feel gritty. Stool in the rectum is deformable, which distinguishes it from other rectal masses. The rectal ampulla should be checked carefully (Fig. 56.1); it is often overlooked and may harbor a neoplasm.

The average effective depth of insertion of the index finger is 7.5 cm. In women, care must be taken not to mistake the cervix for a rectal "tumor" along the anterior rectal wall; the cervix is smooth and symmetric. In men, the prostate and, if possible, the seminal vesicles should be examined. Finally, on withdrawal, the examining finger should be inspected for the character of feces and the presence of blood, pus, or mucus. A test for occult blood should be performed unless gross blood is evident.

Anoscopy

Anoscopy may be a useful adjunct to the anorectal examination, particularly in the evaluation of bright red rectal bleeding, perianal pain, or suspected hemorrhoids. Anoscopes are

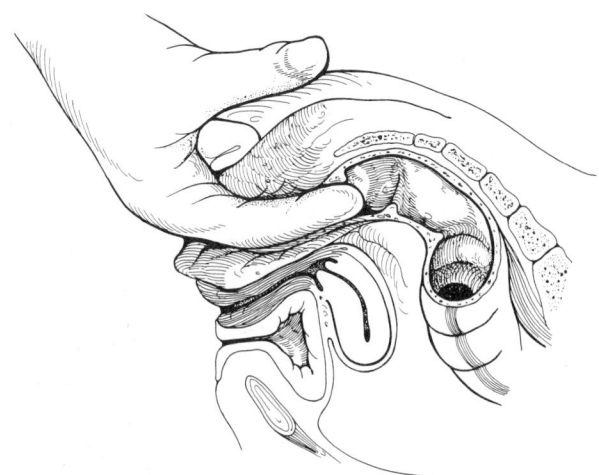

FIG. 56.1. Digital examination.

metal or disposable plastic tubes with a diameter of 2 cm at the tip and a length of 7 cm. A built-in light source may be present or an external light source may be required, depending on the make of anoscope. With the patient in the same position as for the anorectal examination, the lubricated anoscope is held in the right hand with the thumb pressing on the obturator as the instrument is introduced with slow, gentle pressure. The instrument is first directed along the longitudinal axis of the anal canal toward the umbilicus and then pointed more posteriorly at the anorectal angle. It is inserted the full length and held in the left hand so that the flange rests against the anus. The obturator is removed, and the anoscope is slowly withdrawn as the mucosa is examined.

The normal rectal mucosa is pink, with a visible delicate network of submucosal vessels. In patients with proctitis, the vascular pattern is typically obliterated and the mucosa may be friable (i.e., it may bleed easily on gentle swabbing). On withdrawal, the anal mucosa is red. Hemorrhoids appear as purple bulges into the lumen; occasionally, blood may be seen to issue from a hemorrhoid. Fissures may be identified at the anal verge.

SIGMOIDOSCOPY

Indications

Screening for Colorectal Cancer. In asymptomatic persons, sigmoidoscopy can be an important screening procedure for early detection of CRC (see above). About one fourth of CRCs are within reach of the rigid sigmoidoscope, and about 50% are within reach of the flexible sigmoidoscope. Asymptomatic rectal cancers discovered by sigmoidoscopy are less advanced and survival rates are better than in patients with symptomatic cancers. Screening by sigmoidoscopy has been shown to reduce mortality from CRC, and in combination with FOBT, is cost-effective. Moreover, detection of polyps on sigmoidoscopy also leads to reduced mortality from CRC by permitting their removal before they undergo malignant transformation. Polyps that are considered at high risk for malignant transformation and that are markers of additional high-risk polyps in the proximal colon are those larger than 1 cm in diameter or with villous features on histologic examination. The optimal frequency of screening in asymptomatic persons over age 50 and at average risk for CRC appears to be every 5 years. (However, because sigmoidoscopy permits visualization of only the distal colon, sentiment is growing that full colonoscopy, perhaps at age 50 or 60, or both, may prove to be a preferable screening strategy.)

Evaluation of Complaints Referable to the Distal Colon. Sigmoidoscopy permits direct visualization of the colonic mucosa. As such, it is an essential part of the evaluation of patients presenting with a host of complaints or problems referable to the large bowel (Table 56.2). Also, sigmoidoscopy can supplement barium studies by permitting direct observation of abnormalities detected on barium enema, such as polyps and other suspected mass lesions. In patients with known inflammatory bowel disease, sigmoidoscopy is useful for monitoring disease activity and response to therapy.

Rigid Sigmoidoscopy

Preparation. Satisfactory cleansing of the bowel can be achieved in most patients with a single tap water or Fleet

Table 56-2. Indications for Sigmoidoscopy

Symptoms

Rectal pain
Rectal discharge
Bright red bleeding per rectum
Hematochezia
Persistent or recurrent diarrhea
Change in bowel habits
Chronic constipation
Unexplained weight loss

Signs

Rectal mass
Enlarged sentinel lymph node[a]
Positive fecal occult blood test result[a]
Unexplained hepatic nodule or enlargement or other signs of metastatic cancer[a]

Laboratory Abnormalities

Unexplained iron deficiency anemia[a]
Mass or polyp in distal colon on barium enema
Other laboratory manifestation of metastatic disease from unknown primary lesion[a]

Screening

Patients at average risk of colon cancer

[a]Colonoscopy is preferred, but sigmoidoscopy in combination with barium enema is an alternative approach

Phospho-Soda *enema* administered 45 minutes before sigmoidoscopic examination. If the examination has been scheduled in advance, the patient can be instructed to self-administer one or two enemas at home on the morning of examination. After the preparation, the patient should take nothing by mouth. Adequate preparation is particularly advisable in older persons, who often have large amounts of retained stool in the rectal vault.

For patients with diarrhea or suspected inflammatory bowel disease, it is acceptable to forego enema cleansing before sigmoidoscopy. These patients can often achieve adequate preparation by having a *bowel movement* just before the examination. Moreover, because enemas may induce edema and erythema of the mucosa, prior enema administration may make it impossible for the observer to distinguish subtle mucosal changes caused by proctitis from those induced by the enema.

Because of the low risk for endocarditis associated with sigmoidoscopy in patients with valvular heart disease, *antibiotic prophylaxis* is not recommended except for patients with prosthetic valves, a history of endocarditis, or hemodynamically significant right-to-left cardiac shunt; even in these cases, the benefit of antibiotic prophylaxis is uncertain (see Chapter 16). Sedation and analgesia are seldom necessary but may be used in patients with painful anal lesions.

Contraindications to sigmoidoscopy include acute peritonitis, suspected bowel perforation or infarction, a severely uncooperative patient, and refusal of the patient to give consent. Sigmoidoscopy is not contraindicated in pregnancy.

Technique. The patient is examined in the same position as for the rectal and anoscopic examinations. The left lateral decubitus (Sims') position is better tolerated than the knee–chest position by older and debilitated patients and may be less embarrassing to patients in general. However, the knee–chest position permits a greater range of scope motion. If available, a tilt-table designed for sigmoidoscopy minimizes discomfort for the patient and eliminates the rather awkward position required of the examiner when Sims' position is used.

The sigmoidoscope is a rigid metal or disposable plastic tube, 25 cm long and approximately 1.5 cm in diameter. Newer rigid sigmoidoscopes have distal fiberoptic lighting, a proximal magnifying lens, and a connection for air insufflation. Additional standard equipment includes long cotton swabs, suctioning apparatus, and biopsy and grasping forceps. The entire sigmoidoscopic examination should take from 2 to 5 minutes. However, the goal should never be speed, but rather thoroughness and patient comfort.

Insertion. The lubricated instrument is inserted with the right hand holding the obturator firmly in place and with gentle pressure against the anal sphincter as the patient bears down. Alternatively, if the rectal examination is performed with the left index finger, the sigmoidoscope may be guided over the withdrawing examining finger to avoid having to dilate the anal sphincter a second time. The sigmoidoscope is initially directed toward the umbilicus and then posteriorly at the anorectal junction (Fig. 56.2).

Once past the anorectal ring, the obturator is withdrawn, and the sigmoidoscope is advanced with the lumen in view at all times. Unless stool is present, insertion is easy until the rectosigmoid junction is reached at about 12 to 15 cm from the anus. At this point, the lumen bends sharply forward and to the left. The patient may experience painful spasm and should be reassured and instructed to breathe slowly and deeply to ensure relaxation of abdominal muscles as the instrument is slowly advanced. Air insufflation should be kept to a minimum to avoid painful colonic distention. When a tight bend in the lumen is encountered and the direction of the lumen is not obvious, it is best to withdraw the sigmoidoscope slightly until a smooth crescentic band of mucosa appears in the field of view. This band always represents the anterior aspect of the mucosa as it bends behind the band, and the sigmoidoscope can be advanced again just beyond the band and deflected in the same direction, where the lumen should be expected to appear (Fig. 56.3). It is important not to push the sigmoidoscope blindly and to desist when the mucosa blanches or the patient experiences severe pain.

Depth of Insertion. Although it is desirable to pass the sigmoidoscope the entire 25 cm, complete insertion is often not possible. In fact, even in the hands of an experienced sigmoidoscopist, the average depth of insertion is 16 to 20 cm. Furthermore, it is important to note whether the sigmoidoscope is advancing up the lumen or merely pushing the rectal mucosa.

Examination of the Mucosa is conducted on slow withdrawal of the instrument. The tip is swept circumferentially to visualize all areas of the wall, and air is injected in small amounts to flatten out folds and allow adequate inspection. As noted earlier, the normal mucosa is pale pink, with a visible network of submucosal blood vessels. Some blood produced from enema tip trauma may be present. The mucosa should be examined and described; any lesions should be noted, and the distance from the anal verge should be recorded. Occasionally, blood may be found to come from a point above the reach of the instrument; this should be noted.

Biopsy Specimens of suspected lesions and abnormal mucosa may be obtained with angled forceps. Mucosal biopsy specimens should be shallow and taken from the posterior rec-

tal wall, where the risk for perforation is small. Bleeding from biopsy sites usually stops with pressure from a swab or by application of silver nitrate sticks. Because of the risk for perforation, barium enema examination should be avoided for at least 5 days after a sigmoidoscopic biopsy.

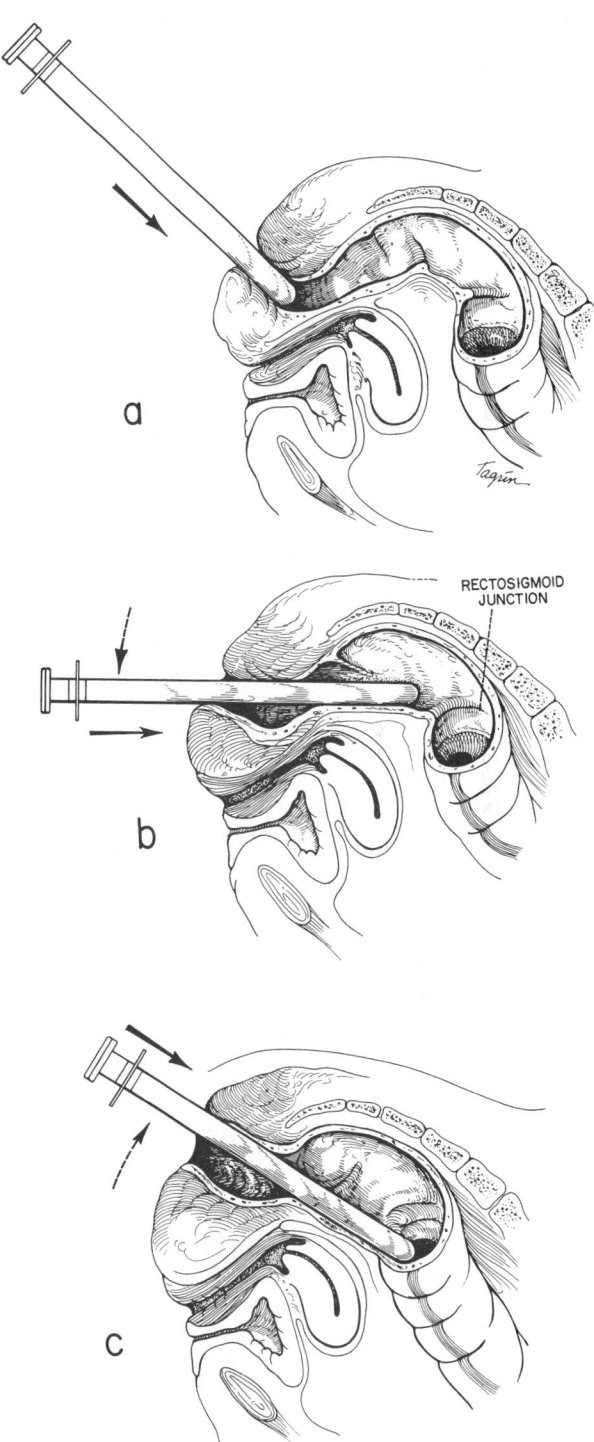

FIG. 56.2. Overview of rigid sigmoidoscopic examination. **A:** Tip of sigmoidoscope is inserted into anal canal in direction of umbilicus. **B:** At anorectal junction (about 3 cm from anus), tip is deflected toward sacrum. **C:** At rectosigmoid junction (about 12 to 15 cm from anus), tip is deflected anteriorly and to the left.

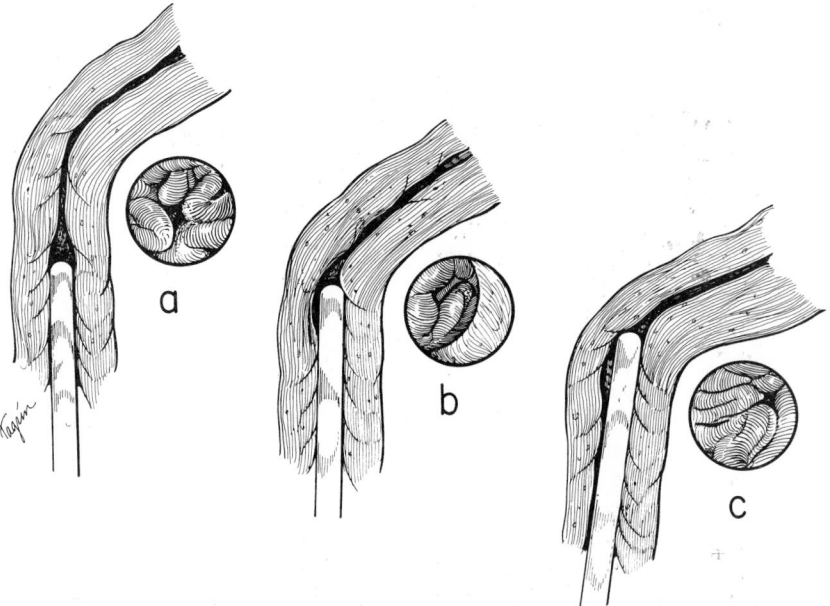

FIG. 56.3. Maneuvering a rigid sigmoidoscope past an angulation in the sigmoid colon. **A:** Advancement of sigmoidoscope through straight portion of colon; view through scope shows concentric lumen with radiating mucosal folds. **B:** As bend in colon is reached, a crescentic band of mucosa is seen in front of the lumen. To maneuver past this angulation, the scope is first withdrawn 1 to 2 cm as the tip is deflected *away* from the lumen. The scope is then readvanced slowly as the tip is deflected back toward the lumen *behind* the crescentic mucosal band. **C:** Lumen reappears as the bend is traversed.

Complications. Perforations are rare, occurring in no more than 1 in 10,000 sigmoidoscopies; they are more likely if the examiner persists in pushing the sigmoidoscope forward in a bowel that is fixed at any point, as by tumor. Bleeding from biopsy sites is infrequent. Arrhythmias have been reported rarely. Informed consent should be obtained before the procedure.

Flexible Sigmoidoscopy

The flexible sigmoidoscopes used most widely in office practice are fiberoptic instruments that are 60 to 65 cm long with large-caliber suction and biopsy channels, full control of tip deflection by two-hand dials, and controls for air insufflation and water instillation. The diameter of the shaft is 11 mm, making the instrument narrower and longer than the rigid sigmoidoscope. The control dials and buttons are managed with the left hand as the examiner views the colon through the eyepiece; advancement of the instrument up the colon is accomplished with the right hand. Acute angulations of the colon are traversed by various combinations of tip deflection, shaft twisting, and repetitive back-and-forth motions; however, even accomplished sigmoidoscopists may encounter difficulty in advancing the instrument through very sharp angles.

Preparation. The procedure can be performed in the office, usually with no sedation or anesthesia and with a preparation of only one or two Fleet Phospho-Soda *enemas.* Some physicians prefer a more rigorous preparation, such as one bottle of *magnesium citrate* taken orally in addition to two Phospho-Soda enemas. In some offices audio or audiovisual stimulation is used to relax the patient during the procedure.

Competency in flexible sigmoidoscopy is usually achieved after performance of about 25 examinations under the supervision of a qualified mentor. Newer video-endoscopes with which the colonic lumen is viewed on a television screen rather than through the eyepiece of the sigmoidoscope are generally used in modern endoscopy suites but are too expensive and impractical for most outpatient primary care practices. The flexible sigmoidoscope has not been widely evaluated in a primary care setting staffed by physicians with no prior experience in flexible endoscopy. Experience to date suggests that nearly any physician as well as nurse practitioners and physician assistants can learn to use the flexible instrument, but only with appropriate supervised instruction.

Comparison with Rigid Sigmoidoscopy. The advantage of the flexible sigmoidoscope over the rigid sigmoidoscope is its ability to examine a longer segment of colon. Whereas the average depth of insertion of the rigid instrument is no more than 20 cm, the average depth of insertion for the flexible instrument in the hands of experienced endoscopists is about 50 cm.

Diagnostic Yield. The yield of flexible sigmoidoscopy is greater than that of rigid sigmoidoscopy. For example, in comparative studies, the flexible instrument identified two to six times more neoplasms and detected some abnormalities, such as diverticula, not generally within reach of the rigid sigmoidoscope. The yield of the flexible sigmoidoscope when used for CRC screening by primary care physicians appears to be acceptable in comparison with the yield obtained with the rigid instrument or by experienced endoscopists. The apparent advantages of flexible sigmoidoscopy must be weighed against the observation that as a screening test, it detects only about half of colorectal polyps and cancers. Moreover, patients undergoing either rigid or flexible sigmoidoscopy for gastrointestinal symptoms may still require additional tests, such as a barium enema or colonoscopy, to complete the evaluation. Thus, the decision to perform flexible rather than rigid sigmoidoscopy in a given instance may be more a matter of physician preference and convenience than of an apparent improvement in diagnostic yield. The clearest advantage of flexible over rigid sigmoidoscopy would appear to be in the screening of asymptomatic patients for CRC, in which case a barium enema or colonoscopy would not be performed unless indicated (see above).

Patient Acceptance, Expense, and Convenience. Patients tolerate the flexible instrument as well as or better than the rigid instrument. However, flexible fiberoptic instruments are much more expensive than disposable plastic rigid sigmoidoscopes and more likely to be damaged, and they require occasional costly repairs. In addition, the flexible instrument must be cleaned thoroughly and disinfected between patients according to rigid protocols, as required by the Occupational Safety and Health Administration (OSHA), and the average duration of examination is at least 10 minutes, so that the time involved in using the instrument per patient is much greater for the flexible than for the rigid instrument. Moreover, cleaning and proper care of the flexible sigmoidoscope require a trained assistant. In a busy clinical practice, use of the flexible sigmoidoscope may be less practical and efficient than use of the rigid instrument. Recently, a flexible fiberoptic sigmoidoscope with a disposable sheath has been introduced; in preliminary studies, it appears to be a reasonable alternative to the standard flexible fiberoptic instrument and obviates the need for rigorous mechanical cleaning and disinfection between cases.

Choice of Procedure

- Rigid sigmoidoscopy is certainly acceptable when a careful examination for rectal pathology is desired, when one is monitoring the activity of ulcerative colitis or evaluating the cause of infectious colitis, and when one wants to avoid contaminating a flexible scope. Although it is not as sensitive a screening test for CRC as is the flexible sigmoidoscope, its use in conjunction with FOBT does decrease CRC mortality in a cost-effective manner.
- Flexible sigmoidoscopy is the more sensitive test for CRC screening and is preferred when determining the source of recurrent rectal bleeding, evaluating a radiologically detected lesion in the sigmoid colon, searching for colitis in a patient with normal rectal mucosa, and evaluating a patient with suspected diverticulitis (see Chapter 75). However, it requires more training to use well and is more expensive to maintain.
- In general, it would seem wise for primary physicians to master the technique of rigid sigmoidoscopy and to consider learning the technique of flexible sigmoidoscopy only if willing to commit sufficient time to develop true proficiency.

Unless expertise has been achieved, the primary care physician should refer patients in need of flexible sigmoidoscopy to a gastroenterologist or surgeon skilled in performing the examination.

ANNOTATED BIBLIOGRAPHY

Ahlquist DA. Triage by flexible sigmoidoscopy: inevitably "short-sighted." Gastroenterology 1998;115:777. (*Editorial discussing the limitations of flexible sigmoidoscopy as a screening tool for CRC because of its inability to detect or predict the presence of proximal colonic neoplasms.*)

Bohlman TW, Katon RM, Lipshutz GR, et al. Fiberoptic pansigmoidoscopy: an evaluation and comparison with rigid sigmoidoscopy. Gastroenterology 1977;72:644. (*In 120 patients, the flexible instrument was inserted nearly three times as far—55 cm versus 20 cm—and identified pathologic lesions three times more often—39% versus 13%.*)

Lehman GA, Buchner DM, Lappas JC. Anatomical extent of fiberoptic sigmoidoscopy. Gastroenterology 1983;84:803. (*A 60-cm examination, achieved in 50% of those examined, viewed the entire sigmoid colon 80% of the time.*)

Lewis JD, Asch DA. Barriers to office-based screening sigmoidoscopy: does reimbursement cover costs? Ann Intern Med 1999;130:525. (*This cost analysis suggests that reimbursement for performing flexible sigmoidoscopy in a primary care practice would be insufficient.*)

Madigan MR, Halls JM. The extent of sigmoidoscopy on radiographs with special reference to the rectosigmoid junction. Gut 1968;9:355. (*Failure to insert the rigid sigmoidoscope to 25 cm in a majority of patients was usually a consequence of the acute angulation of the rectosigmoid junction.*)

McCarthy BD, Moskowitz MA. Screening flexible sigmoidoscopy: patient attitudes and compliance. J Gen Intern Med 1993;8:120. (*Seventy-five percent agreed to the procedure; only 14% said they would not do it again.*)

Nivatvongs S, Fryd DS. How far does the proctosigmoidoscope reach? A prospective study of 1,000 patients. N Engl J Med 1980;303:380. (*Average depth of insertion of the rigid sigmoidoscope was 19.5 cm to 20.3 cm in male and 18.6 cm in female patients.*)

Sardinha TC, Wexner SD, Gilliland J, et al. Efficiency and productivity of a sheathed fiberoptic sigmoidoscope compared with a conventional sigmoidoscope. Dis Colon Rectum 1997;40:1248. (*Because the sterile sheath is disposable, the average reprocessing time for the sheathed sigmoidoscope was only 4.9 minutes, compared with 46.8 minutes for a conventional sigmoidoscope.*)

Schrock TR. Examination and diseases of the anorectum, rigid sigmoidoscopy, and flexible fiberoptic sigmoidoscopy. In: Feldman M, Scharschmidt BF, Sleisenger MH, eds. Sleisenger and Fordtran's gastrointestinal and liver disease: pathophysiology/diagnosis/management, 6th ed. Philadelphia, W.B. Saunders, 1997:1960-1976. (*Comprehensive discussion of indications for and techniques of rigid and flexible sigmoidoscopy, in addition to management of common anorectal disorders.*)

Selby JV, Friedman GD, Quesenberry CP, et al. A case–control study of screening sigmoidoscopy and mortality from colorectal cancer. N Engl J Med 1992;326:653. (*Retrospective study indicating a survival benefit with screening by proctosigmoidoscopy.*)

Wong RCK, Van Dam J. The technique of flexible sigmoidoscopy: a step-by-step guide to the procedure. J Crit Ill 1994;9:797. (*Well-illustrated description of technique and "tricks of the trade," patient preparation, complications, and frequent findings.*)

57
Prevention of Viral Hepatitis
JULES L. DIENSTAG

Viral hepatitis is an infectious disease of the liver estimated to afflict more than 500,000 people in the United States each year. Although the majority of those infected are either asymptomatic or minimally symptomatic, chronic viral hepatitis is associated with substantial morbidity, and fulminant hepatitis, often fatal, may develop in a small proportion of acutely infected patients. Several thousand deaths per year are related to the disease.

Prevention of infection and prophylaxis against clinical disease are prime objectives in the management of viral hepatitis. The primary physician has the major responsibility for these tasks because patients and their contacts often present at a time when infectivity is high. Prevention of viral hepatitis requires a knowledge of the common modes of viral transmission, the periods of maximal communicability, and the efficacy of globulin preparations and vaccines.

EPIDEMIOLOGY AND RISK FACTORS

Viral Types. Five distinct types of viral hepatitis are recognized: A, B, C (formerly labeled non-A, non-B), D, and E (formerly labeled the enteric form of non-A, non-B). Although other types of hepatitis viruses (e.g., "hepatitis G") have been described, none have proved to be true hepatitis viruses or to account for the small proportion of cases that cannot be linked serologically to hepatitis viruses A through E.

Sources of Outbreaks. In general, outbreaks of hepatitis are often traced to a source of hepatitis A virus (HAV) or, in developing countries, to hepatitis E virus (HEV). Occasionally, clusters of hepatitis B follow exposure of several persons to contaminated needles or blood products. Among urban adults presenting to a primary care physician with sporadic cases of hepatitis, hepatitis B accounts for approximately 50% of cases, hepatitis C for 15% to 30%, and hepatitis A for the remainder. More than 95% of transfusion-associated cases were attributable to hepatitis C; however, the frequency of transfusion-related cases has been reduced dramatically to negligible levels by the use of sensitive screening tests for hepatitis C (see below). Hepatitis D is caused by a defective virus that infects only in the presence of infection with hepatitis B virus. Chronic infection with hepatitis B virus (HBV) is prevalent in 0.1% to 0.5% (1 million persons) and chronic infection with hepatitis C virus (HCV) is prevalent in 1.8% (4 million persons) of the U.S. population.

Hepatitis A. HAV is shed in the feces, and transmission occurs predominantly by the *fecal–oral* route (e.g., ingestion of contaminated food, water, shellfish). Prior exposure to hepatitis A is manifested by the presence of antibody to HAV (anti-HAV), which confers lifelong immunity. Many patients over the age of 60 years test positive for anti-HAV, but acute infection is rare in this age group. Because children and adolescents are least likely to have had previous exposure to the virus, they are the most susceptible to infection. Spread of infection is greatest where poor sanitary conditions and crowding exist, with prevalences as high as 75% among low-income people, compared with 20% to 30% for residents in middle- to upper-income neighborhoods. In developed countries, the prevalence of anti-HAV and of immunity to the virus has fallen by approximately 10% per decade since the 1970s. The down side of this declining prevalence of anti-HAV is the growing prevalence of susceptibility to infection in population subgroups that heretofore had been immune. The resulting shift in acute cases from the very young, in whom the disease tends to be subclinical, to adults, in whom the disease tends to be associated with jaundice and relatively severe, has translated into an increased frequency of clinically apparent, severe hepatitis A. There is no carrier state.

Hepatitis B can be transmitted both by *percutaneous* and *nonpercutaneous* modes of spread. The application of sensitive screening methods for the detection of HBV has essentially eliminated posttransfusion hepatitis type B. Reliance on blood obtained from volunteer donors, which is less likely to contain the virus, in addition to blood donor exclusion practices and screening tests to prevent transfusion-transmitted AIDS and hepatitis C, has also contributed to reducing the frequency of hepatitis B after transfusion. Injection drug use remains a common route of exposure. Perinatal transmission from mother to offspring accounts for most HBV infections in developing nations, whereas sexual transmission is an important and efficient mode of spread in the United States and other Western countries. About 0.1% of healthy blood donors are infected; the percentages increase markedly for injection drug users and patients exposed to blood, such as hemophiliacs and those in hemodialysis units. Surgeons, laboratory technicians, oral surgeons, and other medical personnel exposed to blood and body fluids are at increased risk for contracting hepatitis B. Spread of infection from health personnel who are hepatitis B carriers is a rare event.

Hepatitis C, initially labeled "non-A, non-B hepatitis," was first recognized in *transfusion* recipients and found to be the predominant type of hepatitis after transfusion. In the 1970s, it occurred in up to 10% of transfusion recipients, usually within 1 to 3 months after they had received volunteer-donated blood. The frequency of infection fell with the exclusion of blood donors at risk for HIV infection and was further reduced by the use of screening tests for HIV (see Chapter 7), surrogate tests for hepatitis C (e.g., alanine aminotransferase, antibodies to hepatitis B core antigen), and finally direct testing for antibodies to HCV. Currently, the risk for hepatitis C after transfusion is barely measurable. Hepatitis C can be spread by *any percutaneous route*, such as needlestick inoculation (3% to 10% risk of infection) or self-injection among drug users. The risk for hepatitis C resulting from sexual or perinatal transmission is felt to be extraordinarily low, on the order of 5%. In about 40% of patients with acute hepatitis C and in almost all volunteer blood donors with hepatitis C, risk factors are not readily apparent; however, in most such cases, remote or less obvious percutaneous exposures can be identified or inferred. One such route of HCV infection is nasal cocaine inhalation, often associated with mucosal bleeding and practiced with shared inhalation equipment.

Hepatitis D, or Delta Hepatitis, is caused by a defective RNA virus that requires *coinfection with HBV* (a DNA virus) to support its replication. Infection with this agent occurs either simultaneously with acute hepatitis B infection or is superimposed on chronic hepatitis B. Like hepatitis B, hepatitis D is transmitted by *percutaneous inoculation* and *intimate contact.* In nonendemic areas, such as the United States and western Europe, hepatitis D has been confined primarily to populations with frequent percutaneous exposures, such as injection drug users and hemophiliacs. In endemic areas, such as the Mediterranean countries, hepatitis D is transmitted primarily through intimate contact. Hepatitis D remains rare in the United States.

Hepatitis E, prevalent in India, Asia, Central America, and developing countries, is transmitted by the *fecal–oral* route. Rarely encountered in the United States except for imported cases from endemic countries, hepatitis E does not cause chronic infection.

NATURAL HISTORY

Both hepatitis A and E are self-limited and do not lead to chronic liver disease; however, hepatitis B, C, and D can cause chronic hepatitis and cirrhosis; long-standing chronic hepatitis B and C can be complicated by hepatocellular carcinoma.

Hepatitis A has an average incubation period of 30 days (range, 15 to 45 days) from the time of exposure to the onset of symptoms. An early manifestation of disease is elevation of the serum aminotransferase level, which occurs about a week before the onset of flulike symptoms. Fecal shedding of HAV occurs well before the rise in aminotransferase levels and up to 2 weeks before the development of symptoms. HAV can be detected in serum for no more than a few days, and the virus disappears from stool within 2 to 3 weeks, usually at the same time as the onset of jaundice and resolution of prodromal symptoms. A fall in viral titer parallels a rise in the titer of anti-HAV, which persists indefinitely. Initially, the *anti-HAV* is of the *immunoglobulin M (IgM)* class; during convalescence, anti-HAV of the *immunoglobulin G (IgG)* class becomes predominant. Therefore, a diagnosis of acute hepatitis A can be made by demonstrating IgM anti-HAV in a single serum sample. No episodes of chronic hepatitis or a carrier state have been found to result from hepatitis A infection. Fatalities are rare; fewer than 5% of cases of fulminant hepatitis result from HAV infection, but clinically more severe cases are becoming more common (see above).

Hepatitis B is a much more variable disease. The incubation period averages 12 weeks, with a range of 4 weeks to 6 months.

Acute Infection. About 2 to 4 weeks before the onset of symptoms, the viral envelope protein, *hepatitis B surface antigen* (HBsAg), appears in the serum, followed by a rise in aminotransferase levels and symptoms. This antigen usually is cleared from the serum by 4 to 6 months; persistence of anti-

genemia beyond 6 months is considered chronic infection. Symptoms of acute hepatitis B typically last 4 to 6 weeks, but the clinical expression of acute hepatitis B is very variable, ranging from clinically inapparent disease to fulminant hepatitis with hepatocellular failure and death. Determinants of disease severity include age, immunologic competence, undefined host factors, and virulence of the virus.

Chronic Infection. Approximately 1% to 2% of patients with clinically apparent disease acquire *chronic infection* and continue to have circulating HBsAg. A much larger number of cases of chronic hepatitis B do not originate as clinically apparent acute illness, so that the number of chronic cases is much larger than anticipated based on the number of recorded acute cases. Among patients with chronic hepatitis B, some have detectable serologic markers of high-level virus replication and some remain *asymptomatic carriers*. Those with high-level replication tend to have chronic hepatitis that is progressive and of at least moderate severity, whereas asymptomatic carriers lack evidence of high-level virus replication, infectivity, and liver injury (see below). The fatality rate for acute hepatitis B is about 0.1%; however, among those requiring hospitalization, the mortality rate is 1%. Although hepatocellular carcinoma is rare in immunocompetent patients who become chronically infected following adulthood acute infection, this dreaded complication of chronic HBV infection is common among those who become chronically infected after perinatally acquired acute infection. In Asia, where perinatal infection is the most common route of exposure, the lifetime risk for death from cirrhosis and hepatocellular carcinoma may be as high as 40%.

Serology. *Antibody to HBsAg* (anti-HBs) is produced early during infection but becomes detectable with commercially available serologic assays only as HBsAg disappears. More than 95% of patients with self-limited acute hepatitis B acquire detectable levels of anti-HBs, which persist indefinitely.

Antibody to the nucleocapsid core of HBV (anti-HBc) appears in the circulation within a week or so after HBsAg becomes detectable and persists indefinitely. Occasionally, during late acute infection, an interval occurs in which HBsAg has already disappeared and anti-HBs has not yet become detectable. This so-called window period can be identified by the presence of isolated anti-HBc; however, now that tests for HBsAg and anti-HBs are so sensitive, this window period is rarely encountered among patients with acute hepatitis B. Most cases in which anti-HBc occurs in the absence of HBsAg and anti-HBs represent HBV infection in the remote past. In rare instances, isolated anti-HBc represents a false-positive test result, whereas in patients at high risk for blood-borne infections (e.g., injection drug users), isolated anti-HBc may represent low-level HBV infection in which the level of HBsAg does not exceed the detection threshold.

A test for anti-HBc of the IgM class (IgM anti-HBc) can distinguish between acute or relatively recent acute hepatitis B (IgM-positive) and infection in the remote past or current chronic infection (IgM-negative, anti-HBc of the IgG class). In a small proportion of cases of acute hepatitis B, HBsAg does not reach the threshold for detection; in such cases, a diagnosis of acute hepatitis B can be established by detecting IgM anti-HBc.

Hepatitis B early antigen (HBeAg) is a product of the gene that codes for the nucleocapsid core; its presence signifies *high-level virus replication*. As such, patients with HBeAg have a high level of circulating virions and infectivity and substantial liver injury. HBeAg becomes detectable in *all* patients early during acute hepatitis B, and therefore this test has no clinical utility during early acute hepatitis B; however, if circulating HBeAg persists beyond the first 3 months of acute hepatitis, the likelihood of chronic infection is increased.

Testing for HBeAg is more important during chronic infection because the presence of HBeAg denotes a more highly replicative chronic infection, associated with increased infectivity (e.g., 20% to 30% infectivity of a needlestick) and liver injury (chronic hepatitis). When *anti-HBe* can be detected in the absence of HBeAg during chronic infection, the patient can be classified as having a less replicative infection, with *limited infectivity* (e.g., 0.1% infectivity of a needlestick) and liver injury (chronic carrier).

Complicating this simple distinction between highly replicative and relatively nonreplicative chronic hepatitis B are patients with *"pre-core" HBV mutations.* For HBeAg to be produced, the pre-core region of the gene encoding the nucleocapsid core protein must be operative; one of a number of mutations in the pre-core gene precludes elaboration of HBeAg, but this mutation does not prevent production of complete virions or high-level HBV replication. Common in Mediterranean and Asian countries and still rare in the United States but growing in frequency, patients with pre-core mutant HBV have all the virologic (i.e., detectable HBV DNA; see below) and clinical hallmarks of highly replicative HBV infection with the exception of HBeAg.

Quantitative Markers of Hepatitis B Viral Replication. *HBV DNA* is a quantitative marker of HBV replication and is helpful in following patients with chronic disease and in monitoring the success of antiviral therapy (see Chapter 70). Insensitive hybridization assays identify circulating HBV DNA down to a threshold of approximately 105 to 106 virions per milliliter, below which infectivity and liver injury are less common. Clinical assays for HBV DNA are shifting to ultrasensitive amplification techniques such as *polymerase chain reaction*, which can detect HBV DNA in serum down to thresholds of 100 to 1,000 virions per milliliter, well below the level associated with infectivity and liver injury. The presence of a pre-core variant of HBV infection can be inferred in a patient with chronic hepatitis B, high levels of HBV DNA ($>10^5$ or 10^6 virions per milliliter), and anti-HBe in the absence of HBeAg.

Hepatitis C has a mean incubation period of 7 weeks (range, 2 to 15 weeks), with most cases occurring after 5 to 10 weeks of incubation. Only a fourth of patients with acute, transfusion-associated hepatitis C become icteric, compared with two thirds of those with transfusion-induced hepatitis B. However, more than 50% of patients with acute hepatitis C have a chronic elevation of aminotransferase levels, and *chronic infection* (with or without liver injury) occurs in 85% of all acutely infected patients. Contributing to this high rate of chronic infection is the common failure to mount an effective, neutralizing immunologic response.

Progression to Cirrhosis and Hepatocelluar Carcinoma. Among those with chronic hepatitis following acute hepatitis C, 20% may progress to cirrhosis during the first decade of illness, even patients with mild liver disease. On the other hand, morbidity within the first 20 years after acute hepatitis C is limited. Although certain hepatitis C genotypes (e.g., *genotype 1*, occurring in 70% to 80% of U.S. patients) are associated with more severe liver disease, perhaps the best predictor of progression to cirrhosis is *liver histology*. Patients with moderate to severe necrosis, inflammation, or fibrosis almost always progress to cirrhosis during the following 10 to 20 years, whereas those with negligible or mild histologic features usually do not progress to cirrhosis during this interval. After approximately 30 years of infection, patients with chronic hepatitis C have an increased risk for hepatocellular carcinoma. Almost all such patients are already cirrhotic, and the risk for hepatocellular carcinoma in cirrhotic patients with chronic hepatitis C ranges from 1% to 4% annually.

Serology and Markers of Viral Replication. Improved assays for *antibody to hepatitis C (anti-HCV)* yield positive results during acute infection, and results remain positive indefinitely in most patients. They can be used for routine diagnostic purposes during acute hepatitis C. Because of occasional nonspecificity of immunoassays for anti-HCV, a supplemental confirmatory test is needed when a positive result is encountered in a patient at very low risk for blood-borne infection (e.g., the asymptomatic blood donor with no risk factors). In such instances, a *recombinant immunoblot assay (RIBA)* can be performed to identify the viral or nonviral proteins responsible for the positive test result.

Such RIBA tests, still used to supplement anti-HCV–reactive assays among blood donors, are likely to be supplanted by testing for HCV RNA, the most sensitive test for hepatitis C infection. Tests for HCV RNA include a *branched-chain complementary DNA (bDNA)* test, in which the detection molecule is amplified, with a sensitivity threshold of 2×10^5 virion equivalents per milliliter, and a *polymerase chain reaction assay*, with a sensitivity threshold of 100 to 1,000 virion equivalents per milliliter. Both *qualitative* and *quantitative polymerase chain reaction assays* for HCV RNA are available. The qualitative assay is less expensive and can be used to confirm active infection in persons who are antibody-positive.

Hepatitis D (Delta Hepatitis) has an incubation period similar to that for hepatitis B; when both hepatitis B and hepatitis D infections are acquired simultaneously, a single clinically apparent episode of hepatitis may ensue. When the two infections occur simultaneously, the risk for *fulminant hepatitis* is increased slightly, but in general the outcome of simultaneous acute hepatitis B and D is no different from the outcome of hepatitis B alone. In contrast, among patients with chronic hepatitis B infection, superimposed hepatitis D may lead to severe, fulminant hepatitis, convert mild or asymptomatic chronic hepatitis into severe chronic hepatitis, or accelerate the course of chronic hepatitis. A diagnosis of delta hepatitis is made by demonstrating the appearance of *antibody to hepatitis D (anti-HDV)*.

Hepatitis E has a mean incubation period of about 40 days, slightly longer than that for hepatitis A. Its clinical course is similar to that of hepatitis A, except that more patients experience a *cholestatic illness* and the likelihood of fulminant disease is higher (1% to 2%, and 10% to 20% in pregnant women). The disease is *self-limited* and does not progress to chronic infection. The virus is excreted in stool early, and antibodies to HEV become detectable during acute illness. Serologic tests are not available routinely.

PRINCIPLES OF PROPHYLAXIS

The principal means of prophylaxis, *minimizing exposure* to hepatitis viruses and use of *immunoglobulin* preparations (passive immunoprophylaxis) and *vaccines* (active immunoprophylaxis), vary for each of the hepatitis viruses.

Hepatitis A. Precautions against contact with a patient who has hepatitis A are most appropriate during the prodromal stage of illness, when the patient sheds virus most heavily.

Minimizing Exposure. During the early phase of clinical hepatitis, when jaundice first appears, there may still be some shedding of virus; precautions such as avoiding intimate contact and careful washing of hands after contact are probably reasonable for a week or two longer. The patient should not serve food to others and can minimize transmission of virus by using disposable dishes and utensils.

Passive Immunoprophylaxis for hepatitis A can be accomplished by the use of standard *immune globulin* (IG) or formalin-inactivated hepatitis A vaccine. IG preparations contains high titers of anti-HAV and are about 80% effective in preventing clinical disease. IG was thought to protect by passive–active immunization (passively administered antibody acts to minimize clinical illness but does not prevent infection and the durable immunity that follows natural infection). Newer analyses suggest that IG more often prevents infection entirely. IG is currently used exclusively for *postexposure prophylaxis* and must be administered within 1 to 2 weeks of exposure to be most effective. Patients with a prior history of serologically documented hepatitis A need not receive IG because they are already protected by their own anti-HAV. Household contacts and small groups experiencing a common source outbreak should be given IG prophylaxis if the outbreak is identified early enough. Routine immunoprophylaxis is not necessary for casual contacts at work or school.

Active Immunoprophylaxis. For *preexposure prophylaxis*, *hepatitis A vaccine* has supplanted IG. Two "killed" hepatitis A vaccines are available, and both are safe, immunogenic, and highly effective in preventing hepatitis A. Doses of the two vaccines vary slightly, and regimens for the two vaccines vary with age of the vaccinee, but both require at least two injections spaced 6 to 12 months apart. Vaccination is recommended for those who travel to areas of the world where hepatitis A is endemic. (In cases of imminent travel to endemic areas, when inadequate time remains (<4) weeks before travel to achieve vaccine-induced protection, IG should be given along with the first dose of hepatitis A vaccine.) Other candidates for hepatitis A vaccine include military personnel, populations and communities with cyclical outbreaks or high frequencies of hepatitis A, laboratory workers exposed to fecal specimens, day care center employees, primate handlers, patients with chronic hepatitis C, homosexual men, injection drug users, and patients with clotting disorders who require frequent clotting factor concentrates. Vaccine-induced immunity is projected to last 20 years or longer.

Hepatitis B. *Reducing the spread* of hepatitis B has been aided by screening *blood donors* for HBsAg. People discovered to be *asymptomatic carriers* require attention. If such persons are health care workers, they need not be removed from work unless proven to be a source of infection; however, health care workers and professionals with HBeAg who perform "exposure-prone" invasive procedures are advised to have their privileges evaluated by an expert review panel. *Food handlers* have not been implicated in the transmission of hepatitis B, and when HBsAg-positive, they need not be restricted.

Minimizing Exposure is facilitated by having the patient use a separate razor, toothbrush, and other personal items. Avoidance of intimate contact should be recommended, but confinement to home is unnecessary. Ensure that any materials containing HBsAg are handled carefully, particularly blood samples and other body fluids; use of gloves is required. If universal precautions are followed in the handling of clinical materials, additional precautions are unnecessary. Hands should be washed thoroughly after direct contact with the patient or with the patient's blood or body fluids.

Passive Immunoprophylaxis of hepatitis B is achieved by providing the susceptible person with protective antibody, anti-HBs. This can be accomplished by passive immunization with IGs containing anti-HBs. *Hepatitis B immune globulin (HBIG)* is prepared from the plasma of persons with high-titer anti-HBs and contains anti-HBs at titers in the range of 1:100,000 or higher. HBIG, which appears to attenuate clinical illness rather than prevent infection, is recommended in conjunction with vaccine for *postexposure prophylaxis* (see below).

Active Immunization with recombinant *hepatitis B vaccines*, derived from recombinant yeast into which the gene for HBsAg has been inserted, have replaced earlier-generation, plasma-derived vaccines in the United States. Hepatitis B vaccine has been recommended as *preexposure prophylaxis*, primarily for population subgroups considered to be at high risk for exposure to HBV (e.g., health and laboratory workers exposed to blood, hemodialysis staff and patients, residents and staff of custodial institutions, sexually promiscuous persons, injection drug users, patients requiring repeated administration of blood products or clotting factors, and household and sexual contacts of chronic HBsAg carriers).

Universal Vaccination. Although these groups remain targets for vaccination, the attempt to vaccinate them has not been successful in limiting the spread of HBV within the general population of developed countries. Therefore, the U.S. Public Health Service has recommended *universal vaccination in childhood* and also vaccination of adolescents born before universal vaccination was implemented and who were not vaccinated at birth. Three deltoid injections of the vaccine are recommended, the first two given 1 month apart and the third given at 6 months. Doses vary according to age group and vaccine manufacturer.

Postexposure Prophylaxis in susceptible persons is best provided by a combination of *HBIG* and *hepatitis B vaccine*. Babies born to mothers with chronic hepatitis B (or acute hepatitis B during the third trimester of pregnancy), sexual contacts of patients with acute hepatitis B, and those who sustain HBsAg-positive needlesticks should receive HBIG plus hepatitis B vaccine. The HBIG provides immediate, high-level, passively acquired anti-HBs, and the vaccine adds long-lasting immunity and probably attenuation of clinical illness in the postexposure setting. HBIG should be administered as soon as possible after exposure (e.g., no later than 48 hours after a needlestick, in the delivery room for babies). The first dose of vaccine can be given simultaneously or within a few hours in newborns, within a week in those sustaining needlestick exposures, or within 2 weeks in those with sexual exposure. Because early prophylaxis is paramount after an HBsAg needlestick, HBIG should be administered immediately and without a delay to wait for the results of antibody testing. There is no interference between hepatitis B vaccine and HBIG, even when administered simultaneously. Although determination of the HBeAg status of the contact case or inoculum source may provide information about relative infectivity, HBeAg status should not be a criterion for providing prophylaxis to contacts. The delay necessitated by waiting for HBeAg testing may invalidate efforts at prophylaxis, and infectivity can occur in the absence of HBeAg, although the likelihood is reduced. Nonintimate household contacts do not require prophylaxis, nor do casual contacts at work.

Durability of Protection. The duration of protection after hepatitis B vaccination is not definitively known but appears to be at least 10 years. Even after anti-HBs falls below detectable levels, new exposures in nature are likely to be accompanied by an anamnestic immune response, and adequate immunity against clinically apparent infection and chronic infection appear to be maintained. Based on these observations, authorities have not recommended routine booster vaccination in immunocompetent persons. Booster doses are recommended for hemodialysis patients who lose protective levels of anti-HBs after vaccination.

Differentiating between Infection and Immunization. Hepatitis B vaccine consists entirely of HBsAg protein (no core proteins are included); making the distinction between immunization and infection is therefore possible by assaying for the presence of antibody to core protein (anti-HBc).

Hepatitis D (Delta Hepatitis). Prevention of delta hepatitis in persons susceptible to HBV infection can be achieved by administering *hepatitis B vaccine.* Once immune to HBV, a person is immune to hepatitis D also. For those with chronic hepatitis B, immunoprophylaxis against hepatitis D is not available, and prevention of delta hepatitis requires limitation of percutaneous and intimate contacts with patients known to be infected with hepatitis D virus.

Hepatitis C. The incidence of posttransfusion hepatitis C has been dramatically reduced by excluding commercially donated blood and persons highly likely to transmit blood-borne disease, and also by screening prospective donors for anti-HCV. Barrier sexual precautions with latex condoms are recommended for persons with multiple sexual partners or with sexually transmitted diseases; however, no such precautions are recommended for stable, monogamous sexual partners. Persons with hepatitis C, however, should avoid sharing of razors, toothbrushes, and other such implements with sexual partners and family members. Special precautions are not recommended for babies born to mothers with chronic hepatitis C; breast-feeding is not restricted.

Immune globulin and HBIG are of no proven benefit in preventing hepatitis C, and IG is no longer recommended for needlestick, sexual, or perinatal exposure to hepatitis C. There is no vaccine for hepatitis C, and the acquisition of durable immunity after naturally acquired hepatitis C is considered rare. Still, efforts to develop a protective vaccine based on immunization with envelope proteins is being pursued.

Hepatitis E. Immunoprophylaxis for hepatitis E is not available. Whether globulins prepared in developed countries, where hepatitis E is rare, protect against HEV infection in Asia and other parts of the world where hepatitis E is common is not known. Experimental vaccines have been effective in animal models but have yet to be developed for routine use.

RECOMMENDATIONS AND PATIENT EDUCATION

Hepatitis A Precautions (To Be Continued until a Week after Onset of Jaundice)

- Advise the patient to wash hands thoroughly after toilet use.
- The patient need not be confined to home, but intimate contact should be avoided.
- Prohibit the patient from handling and serving food to others.
- Advise others to avoid contact with the patient's fecal material and to wash hands thoroughly if contact is made.

Hepatitis A Prophylaxis

- For postexposure prophylaxis, administer IG to household contacts within 2 weeks of exposure; the dose is 0.02 mL/kg, with an average adult dose of 2 mL IM.
- For preexposure prophylaxis, administer two IM injections of hepatitis A vaccine at least 6 months apart (dose recommendations vary between the two vaccine manufacturers). For imminent travel to endemic areas, when time is too short to achieve vaccine-induced immunization, IG should be administered, at the same dose as for household contacts, along with the first dose of vaccine.

Hepatitis B Precautions (To Be Continued until HBsAg Clears from the Serum)

- All blood donors should be screened for HBsAg.
- Use volunteer blood rather than blood from commercial donors.
- Use disposable syringes and needles.
- Have the patient use a separate razor, toothbrush, and other personal items.
- Have any materials containing HBsAg handled carefully, particularly blood samples and other body fluids; use of gloves is required. Following universal precautions when handling clinical materials makes additional precautions unnecessary.
- Recommend avoidance of intimate contact, but confinement to home is unnecessary.
- Hands should be washed thoroughly after direct contact with the patient or with the patient's blood or body fluids.

Hepatitis B Prophylaxis:

Preexposure.

- Administer three 1-mL IM injections of hepatitis B vaccine at 0, 1, and 6 months to persons in high-risk groups. (Doses for specific age groups may vary according to manufacturer.) High-risk groups include health workers exposed to blood, residents and staff of custodial institutions, household and sexual contacts of chronic HBsAg carriers, promiscuous male homosexuals and promiscuous heterosexuals, patients with hereditary hemoglobinopathies and clotting disorders who require long-term therapy with blood products, and hemodialysis patients.

Postexposure.

- Administer 0.06 mL of HBIG IM per kilogram of body weight (approximately 5 mL) to those who sustain an accidental percutaneous or transmucosal exposure to HBsAg-positive blood or body secretions or needles and instruments contaminated with HBsAg-positive material. This globulin injection should be administered as soon after exposure as possible; although globulin injections are recommended up to 7 days after inoculation, their efficacy is nil beyond 2 days. Passive immunoprophylaxis with HBIG should be followed by a complete, three-injection course of hepatitis B vaccine; these injections can be started at the same time as HBIG or within the first few days to a week after exposure.
- Administer HBIG, at the dose cited above, to sexual contacts of patients with acute hepatitis B as soon after exposure as is practical. Because recognition of hepatitis in a sexual contact is often delayed, early prophylaxis is usually impossible. In one study, prophylaxis within 30 days of recognized exposure was effective, but current recommendations call for prophylaxis within 14 days of exposure. HBIG should be followed by a complete three-injection course of hepatitis B vaccine in all sexual contacts of patients with acute hepatitis B.
- Administer 0.5 mL of HBIG IM to newborns of HBsAg-positive mothers immediately after birth, preferably in the delivery room. This should be followed by a complete three-injection course of hepatitis B vaccine, 0.5 mL per dose, preferably to be started within 7 days of birth (dose may vary according to manufacturer).
- No prophylaxis is necessary for casual contacts or nonintimate household contacts.
- Universal vaccination of all children, in conjunction with routine vaccinations of childhood, is recommended. For children born after the implementation of universal hepatitis B vaccination, vaccination during adolescence is recommended.

Hepatitis D Prophylaxis

- Vaccination against hepatitis B prevents hepatitis D in those susceptible to hepatitis B.
- For those already infected with hepatitis B, prevention of hepatitis D relies on limiting percutaneous and intimate contact with persons known to harbor hepatitis D virus (HDV) infection.

Hepatitis C Precautions and Prophylaxis

- Precautions are the same as those for hepatitis B (i.e., limitation of exposure to the blood and body fluids of infected patients).
- The best means of limiting transfusion-associated hepatitis C is to rely exclusively on volunteer rather than commercial blood donors and to screen donors for anti-HCV.
- IG, which has not been shown to be effective in preventing hepatitis C, is not recommended for those who sustain a needlestick injury, sexual contacts of acute cases of hepatitis C, or babies born to mothers with hepatitis C.
- An effective hepatitis C vaccine has not been developed.

Hepatitis E Prophylaxis

- Approaches to preventing exposure to enteric agents apply to the prevention of hepatitis E (see hepatitis A, above).

- Neither an IG nor a vaccine is available for the prevention of hepatitis E.

ANNOTATED BIBLIOGRAPHY

Alter MJ, Hadler SC, Margolies HS, et al. The changing epidemiology of hepatitis B in the United States: need for alternative vaccination strategies. JAMA 1990;263:1218. (*Argument for a policy of universal hepatitis B vaccination in childhood.*)

Alter MJ, Margolies HS, Krawczynski K, et al. The natural history of community-acquired hepatitis C in the United States. N Engl J Med 1992;327:1899. (*Confirms the high frequency of hepatitis C, even in persons acquiring their acute infections sporadically; persistent asymptomatic viremia was universal, even in those who recovered clinically.*)

Centers for Disease Control and Prevention. Protection against viral hepatitis: recommendations of the Advisory Committee on Immunization Practices (ACIP). MMWR Morb Mortal Wkly Rep 1990;39:1. (*Official recommendations of the U.S. Public Health Service for use of hepatitis B vaccine and HBIG for preexposure and postexposure prophylaxis.*)

Centers for Disease Control and Prevention. Hepatitis B virus: a comprehensive strategy for eliminating transmission in the United States through universal childhood vaccination: recommendations of the Immunization Practices Advisory Committee (ACIP). MMWR Morb Mortal Wkly Rep 1991;40:1. (*Official recommendations of the U.S. Public Health Service for universal hepatitis B vaccination in childhood.*)

Centers for Disease Control and Prevention. Update: recommendations to prevent hepatitis B virus transmission—United States. MMWR Morb Mortal Wkly Rep 1995;44:574. (*This update of hepatitis B vaccine recommendations calls for the vaccination of 11- to 12-year-old children who have not been vaccinated previously. Also included in these revised recommendations for hepatitis B vaccination are unvaccinated children under the age of 11 who are Pacific Islanders or who live in households of first-generation immigrants from countries where hepatitis B infection is endemic.*)

Centers for Disease Control and Prevention. Prevention of hepatitis A through active or passive immunization: recommendations of the Advisory Committee on Immunization Practices (ACIP). MMWR Morb Mortal Wkly Rep 1996;45:1. (*Official recommendations of the U.S. Public Health Service for administration of IG and hepatitis A vaccine to prevent hepatitis A.*)

Centers for Disease Control and Prevention. Recommendations for prevention and control of hepatitis C virus (HCV) infection and HCV-related chronic disease. MMWR Morb Mortal Wkly Rep 1998;47:1. (*Official recommendations of the U.S. Public Health Service for approaches to limiting the spread of hepatitis C virus infection.*)

Chang M-H, Chen C-J, Lai M-S, et al. Universal hepatitis B vaccination in Taiwan and the incidence of hepatocellular carcinoma in children. N Engl J Med 1997;336:1855. (*Hepatitis B vaccination of infants in China has reduced the incidence of hepatocellular carcinoma in children. Thus, hepatitis B vaccine can prevent hepatocellular carcinoma in a population in which hepatitis B is endemic; in essence, hepatitis B vaccine, in addition to preventing acute and chronic hepatitis, is a "cancer vaccine."*)

Conry-Cantilena C, VanRaden M, Gibble J, et al. Routes of infection, viremia, and liver disease in blood donors found to have hepatitis C virus infection. N Engl J Med 1996;334:1691. (*This study of volunteer blood donors found to have antibodies to hepatitis C virus revealed that most did, in fact, have a history of percutaneous exposures or risk factors associated with blood-borne infection. This was the first study to identify nasal cocaine inhalation as a potential risk factor for exposure to hepatitis C.*)

Consensus Statement: EASL International Consensus Conference on Hepatitis C. J Hepatol 1999;30:956. (*A 1999 consensus conference in Paris reviewed contemporary concepts of hepatitis C virology and epidemiology as well as management.*)

Dienstag JL. Non-A, non-B hepatitis. I. Recognition, epidemiology, and clinical features. II. Experimental transmission, putative virus agents and markers, and prevention. Gastroenterology 1983;85:439,743. (*Two-part review compiled before the discovery of hepatitis C; many of the concepts noted in the review were confirmed after hepatitis C virus was identified.*)

Donahue JG, Munoz A, Ness PM, et al. The declining risk of post-transfusion hepatitis C virus infection. N Engl J Med 1992; 327:369. (*Frequency reduced to 0.57% per patient and 0.03% per unit of blood with testing for hepatitis C.*)

Farci P, Alter HJ, Govindarajan S, et al. Lack of protective immunity against reinfection with hepatitis C virus. Science 1992;258:135. (*This report summarizes virologic reassessment of earlier cross-challenge studies in experimentally infected chimpanzees and shows that neither heterologous nor homologous immunity develops after hepatitis C infection.*)

Hadler SC, Francis DP, Maynard JE, et al. Long-term immunogenicity and efficacy of hepatitis B vaccine in homosexual men. N Engl J Med 1986;315:209. (*Detectable anti-HBs persisted for 5 years in 85% of patients, with levels considered protective persisting in 63% of patients; clinically apparent and chronic infection rarely, if ever, occurred.*)

Hoofnagle JH. Type D (delta) hepatitis. JAMA 1989;261:1321. (*Brief but authoritative review that remains current.*)

Houghton M, Weiner A, Han J, et al. Molecular biology of the hepatitis C viruses: implications for diagnosis, development, and control of viral disease. Hepatology 1991;14:381. (*Review by the discoverer of the virus.*)

Hutin YJF, Pool V, Cramer EH, et al. A multistate, foodborne outbreak of hepatitis A. N Engl J Med 1999;340:595. (*Outbreaks of acute hepatitis A continue to occur; this report describes a large outbreak involving persons in many states; the offending contaminated food was frozen strawberries.*)

Katkov WN, Dienstag JL. Prevention and therapy of viral hepatitis. Semin Liver Disease 1991;11:165. (*Review addressing key issues related to hepatitis B vaccine, with brief consideration of hepatitis A vaccine.*)

Koff RS. Hepatitis A. Lancet 1998;341:1643. (*A comprehensive and up-to-date review of hepatitis A.*)

Krawczynski K. Hepatitis E. Hepatology 1993;17:932. (*Authoritative review that remains current.*)

Lemon SM, Thomas DL. Vaccines to prevent viral hepatitis. N Engl J Med 1997;336:196. (*An excellent contemporary review of the development, features, and application of hepatitis B and A vaccines.*)

Major ME, Feinstone SM. The molecular virology of hepatitis C. Hepatology 1997;25:1527. (*A contemporary review of hepatitis C virology, including genotypes, quasi-species diversity.*)

Margolis HS, Coleman PJ, Brown RE, et al. Prevention of hepatitis B virus transmission by immunization: an economic analysis of current recommendations. JAMA 1995;274:1201. (*This analysis indicates that vaccination of infants, and also vaccination of adolescents not vaccinated at birth, is cost-effective.*)

National Institutes of Health Consensus Development Conference. Management of hepatitis C. Hepatology 1997;6[Suppl 1]:1S. (*A comprehensive overview of all aspects of hepatitis C, including excellent sections on diagnosis, diagnostic test methods, epidemiology, and management.*)

Purcell RH. Hepatitis viruses. Changing patterns of human disease. Proc Natl Acad Sci U S A 1994;91:2401. (*A concise but compelling summary of changes in the clinical and epidemiologic expression of hepatitis viruses, some resulting from changes in human behavior and population shifts.*)

Sagliocca L, Amoroso P, Stroffolini T, et al. Efficacy of hepatitis A vaccine in prevention of secondary hepatitis A infection: a randomized trial. Lancet 1999;353:1136. (*Although hepatitis A vaccination cannot always be given in a timely fashion to household contacts of patients with acute hepatitis A, it does prevent secondary cases and should be recommended.*)

Schreiber GB, Busch MP, Kleinman SH, et al. The risk of transfusion-transmitted viral infection. N Engl J Med 1996;334:1685. (*Improvements in blood donor screening, including virus-nonspecific measures and specific viral screening tests, have reduced the frequency of transfusion-associated hepatitis B and C, and HIV infection, to negligible levels.*)

Seeff L, Buskell-Bales Z, Wright EC, et al. Long-term mortality after transfusion-associated non-A, non-B hepatitis. N Engl J Med 1992;327:1906. (*Mortality did not exceed that in control groups of transfused patients in whom hepatitis did not develop.*)

Szmuness W, Stevens CE, Harley EJ, et al. Hepatitis B vaccine: demonstration of efficacy in a controlled clinical trial in a high-risk population in the United States. N Engl J Med 1980;303:833. (*Classic article describing the landmark controlled trial of hepatitis B vaccine in homosexual men, which established the safety and efficacy of the vaccine in preventing clinical and subclinical cases of hepatitis B.*)

Takahashi M, Yamada G, Miyamoto R, et al. Natural history of chronic hepatitis C. Am J Gastroenterol 1993;88:240. (*The likelihood of progression of chronic hepatitis C increases as a function of hepatic histologic classification, with milder forms progressing least and severe forms progressing most.*)

Tong MJ, El-Farra NS, Reikes AR, et al. Clinical outcomes after transfusion-associated hepatitis C. N Engl J Med 1995;332:1463. (*In a tertiary referral center, patients encountered with chronic hepatitis C have progressive disease, including cirrhosis and hepatocellular carcinoma. Progression is more pronounced among those who acquire their disease later in life.*)

Vento S, Garofano T, Renzini C, et al. Fulminant hepatitis associated with hepatitis A virus superinfection in patients with chronic hepatitis C. N Engl J Med 1998;338:286. (*The only report to suggest a high frequency of fulminant hepatitis A in patients with chronic hepatitis C. Although this experience has not been confirmed (actually challenged by other observers), hepatitis A vaccination has been recommended in patients with chronic hepatitis C.*)

Werzberger A, Mensch B, Kuter B, et al. A controlled trial of formalin-inactivated hepatitis vaccine in healthy children. N Engl J Med 1992;327:453. (*The first efficacy trial of a hepatitis A vaccine, which was 100% effective in preventing clinically apparent disease.*)

Wilner IR, Uhl MD, Howard SD, et al. Serious hepatitis A: an analysis of patients hospitalized during an urban epidemic in the United States. Ann Intern Med 1998;128:111. (*This report buttresses the general observation that with a reduction in the frequency of acute hepatitis A in young children, more severe cases are being recognized among adults.*)

58
Evaluation of Abdominal Pain
JAMES M. RICHTER

One of the most challenging problems faced by the primary care physician is the outpatient assessment of the patient with abdominal pain. When the pain is acute in onset, triage decisions have to be made regarding the need for hospital admission and surgical intervention. If the pain is chronic or recurrent, the physician must design a safe, cost-effective plan for workup that will efficiently distinguish among a myriad of possible etiologies. In many instances, the exact cause of pain is not immediately evident, so that a few basic studies are necessary to define the underlying pathophysiology, narrow the differential diagnosis, and effectively guide further assessment and treatment. Also important is the need to decide on the proper speed and extent of evaluation. Etiologies of pelvic pain often overlap with those of abdominal pain (see Chapter 116).

PATHOPHYSIOLOGY AND CLINICAL PRESENTATION

The major mechanisms include obstruction of a hollow viscus, peritoneal irritation, vascular insufficiency, mucosal ulceration, altered bowel motility, capsular distention, metabolic disorder, nerve injury, abdominal wall injury, and referral from an extraabdominal site.

Obstruction. Pain receptors in the bowel, biliary tree, and ureters respond to distention and increased wall tension. The severity of the pain is a function of the speed of onset as well as the degree of distention. Obstruction that develops slowly during weeks to months may be relatively subtle in presentation in comparison with acute obstruction, which produces a more dramatic picture. In acute obstruction, the pain is severe and "colicky" or wavelike in nature; it makes the patient restless.

Small Bowel. The pain of acute *small-bowel* obstruction is greatest when the obstruction is jejunal. The patient is often comfortable between bouts of pain. Severity decreases with time as bowel motility diminishes. Complete strangulation of small bowel is associated with steady pain from secondary vascular insufficiency or peritoneal irritation. Vomiting is common, particularly in proximal obstruction; when the problem is distal, vomiting is less frequent. Flatus and passage of small amounts of stool may occur at the outset, but they soon cease if the obstruction is complete. Diarrhea is noted in some cases of partial obstruction. On examination, the patient appears restless during bouts of pain. The temperature is typically normal or only mildly elevated. The abdomen may be distended, especially when the obstruction is distal. High-pitched, hyperactive bowel sounds are characteristic but not always present. Tenderness to palpation is not impressive unless ischemia or leakage of bowel contents has occurred and caused peritoneal soilage. The stool is usually negative for occult blood.

Large Bowel. Obstruction of the large bowel is, in most instances, less painful and associated with less vomiting than is obstruction of the small intestine. Constipation or a change in bowel habits often precedes complete obstruction. Diarrhea may occur with partial obstruction. Distention is greater than that seen in small-bowel obstruction. Stools are frequently positive for occult blood.

In cases of bowel obstruction, the white blood cell count may be normal, even in association with a strangulating obstruction (i.e., with compromise of the intestinal blood supply in addition to blockage of the lumen). A plain *radiograph of the abdomen* (supine and upright) in patients with small-bowel obstruction often shows distention of loops of small bowel with high air–fluid levels. This, together with an absence of gas in the large bowel (distal to the obstruction), is characteristic of small-bowel obstruction. The radiographic appearance of colonic obstruction varies with the competency (or incompetency) of the ileocecal valve. If the valve is competent, less small-bowel dilation ensues.

Cystic Duct. Sudden obstruction of the cystic duct by a stone produces acute pain, sometimes referred to as *biliary "colic."* Unlike the cramping pain of acute intestinal obstruction, the pain of acute cystic duct obstruction is mostly steady, lasting over an hour after sudden onset. *Acute cholecystitis* is associated with localized peritonitis in addition to obstruction. Pain is typically maximal in the right upper quadrant or epigastrium, radiates to the scapular region, and is accompanied by nausea, vomiting, and fever without jaundice; at times only mild epigastric discomfort is present (see Chapter 69). *Murphy's sign* (inspiratory arrest in response to right upper quadrant palpation) may be seen, and right upper quadrant tenderness to percussion or pressure over the gallbladder is also a suggestive finding. Laboratory investigation usually reveals a leukocytosis and sometimes a modest alkaline phosphatase elevation. In an occasional case, slight hyperbilirubinemia may occur, usually after the initial onset of symptoms. *Gallstones* in the absence of ductal obstruction or gallbladder inflammation produce no characteristic pain (see Chapter 69).

Common Duct. The pain is more likely to be epigastric and less severe than in cystic duct obstruction. Jaundice is noted soon after onset. Emesis may be prominent. Obstruction and dilation that occur gradually are often painless. Physical examination may reveal a tender right upper quadrant, but in comparison with that of acute cholecystitis, tenderness is less focal and deeper. A palpable gallbladder suggests gradual progressive development of ductal obstruction, typically caused by malignancy. Alkaline phosphatase is markedly elevated, as is the serum bilirubin.

Urinary Tract. Obstruction within the urinary tract can present as abdominal pain. Acute ureteral blockade by a stone is extremely uncomfortable. Onset is sudden and the pain is cramping, beginning in the back and flank and radiating into the lower abdomen and groin. If acute pyelonephritis develops, upper abdominal pain, fever, and chills may ensue. Acute bladder outflow obstruction presents as lower abdominal distention and suprapubic pain. Symptoms of prostatism (see Chapter 134) may precede the episode.

Peritoneal Irritation may cause severe pain because of the rich innervation of the parietal peritoneum. Focal injury results in well-localized discomfort that is described as sharp, aching, or burning. Spread of the irritant process leads to more generalized abdominal pain. Severity is related to the nature of the irritant and the speed with which the noxious exposure occurs. Reflex spasm of the overlying abdominal wall musculature can produce involuntary guarding. Rebound tenderness is prominent on physical examination. Most important, the pain is accentuated by pressure changes in the peritoneum; thus, palpation, coughing, or movement may increase the pain, leading the patient to lie still, in contrast to the restlessness of patients with "colicky" pain.

Focal Peritonitis of the retroperitoneum, which is characteristic of *early appendicitis*, may be tested by having the patient lie on the left side and extend the right hip (*psoas sign*). Bowel sounds are often reduced or absent, especially when the irritation is generalized. The origin of the peritoneal irritant need not be intraabdominal.

Familial Mediterranean Fever is an autosomal recessive disorder that causes recurrent, severe attacks of peritoneal irritation. The condition occurs among Armenians and Sephardic Jews and presents in childhood or early adulthood. It is characterized by brief but severe attacks of fever, peritoneal irritation, pleuritis, and synovitis. Patients complain of abdominal swelling and severe pain. Marked elevations in the sedimentation rate and acute-phase reactants accompany attacks. Amyloidosis is a serious consequence, sometimes resulting in renal impairment. Colchicine provides dramatic relief from the pain of an acute attack and also prevents amyloid deposition and renal impairment.

Vascular Disease of the abdomen can result in a host of presentations of abdominal pain, many of which simulate those of other etiologies.

Acute Arterial Insufficiency (resulting from atherosclerosis or embolus) may present with severe abdominal pain, but often the early presentation is more subtle, with mild constant pain the only symptom for several days in the absence of tenderness and rigidity. The diagnosis may not become apparent until signs of peritonitis and shock ensue as a consequence of peritoneal soilage resulting from bowel perforation associated with ischemic necrotic injury.

Chronic Mesenteric Insufficiency characteristically produces dull or cramping postprandial pain ("abdominal angina") localized to the epigastrium or mid-abdomen. Onset is usually within an hour after eating; severity is proportional to the size and fat composition of the meal. Pain is greatest at times of maximal demand for blood supply to the bowel. Symptoms can persist for 2 to 3 hours. The timing, location, and duration reflect meal-triggered ischemia in the territory of the celiac or superior mesenteric artery. Some patients lose considerable amounts of weight because of the fear that eating will induce pain. Symptoms may precede an acute episode of infarction, especially in cases of progressive atherosclerotic disease. Ischemia in the celiac territory may be accompanied by nausea, vomiting, and bloating. In ischemia to the midgut, the predominant complaints are pain and weight loss. Constipation accompanied by occult blood loss characterizes chronic inferior mesenteric artery insufficiency. Abdominal bruits are reported in 20% to 60% of cases. Other signs of vascular insufficiency

(e.g., carotid or femoral bruit) are often detectable. Ischemic abdominal pain also results from vascular occlusive crises of sickle cell anemia.

Aortic Dissection or rupture of an *abdominal aortic aneurysm* produces severe acute abdominal pain that often radiates to the back or genitalia. Before dissection, aneurysms are usually silent, but physical examination may reveal an increase in aortic diameter (>3.0 cm). The greater the increase in aortic diameter on examination, the more likely an aneurysm is present.

Mesenteric Venous Thrombosis is a less common cause of intestinal ischemia than is arterial occlusion. It may present similarly, although it often has a more slowly progressive course. Both aortic dissection and mesenteric thrombosis typically result in pain complaints that are in excess of those elicited by physical examination.

Mucosal Injury. Ulceration or inflammation of the gastrointestinal tract is often accompanied by pain.

Peptic Ulcer Disease. Although the exact mechanism of pain in peptic ulcer disease remains incompletely understood, it is believed that acid plays a major role. This hypothesis is supported by the observation that neutralization of acid often provides immediate relief. The pain pattern of duodenal ulcer disease usually parallels the acid–peptic cycle (see Chapter 68). Unless perforation or penetration into the pancreas is present, the pain is mostly confined to the epigastrium. Patients use such terms as "gnawing," "aching," and "burning" to describe their discomfort. Radiation of pain into the back in patients with duodenal ulcer suggests perforation into the pancreas.

Inflammation of the middle or lower intestine, as seen with acute *gastroenteritis* and acute flares of *inflammatory bowel disease* (see Chapter 73), can disturb motility and absorption. In most instances, the pain is diffuse, but occasionally it is focal and can simulate appendicitis or other surgical conditions. Fever, nausea, and vomiting are often prominent in the early stages of gastroenteritis; bowel sounds are usually hyperactive.

Altered Bowel Motility. This mechanism predominates in functional bowel disturbances, of which irritable bowel syndrome and psychophysiologic disturbances are the best examples.

Irritable Bowel Syndrome. Spasmodic, nonpropulsive, segmental contractions of large bowel result in high intraluminal pressures, manifested by cramping lower abdominal pain and bloating. Constipation alternating with diarrhea and mucous stools are typical findings, as are pain relieved by defecation, more frequent and loose stools with the onset of pain, and a feeling of incomplete evacuation (see Chapter 74). Altered motility and chronically increased intraluminal pressures may lead to *diverticular disease* (see Chapter 75).

Functional Dyspepsia. This condition is characterized by chronic or recurrent upper abdominal discomfort or pain, often in conjunction with food-related dysmotility symptoms (e.g., bloating, fullness, nausea, early satiety). Many patients have concurrent esophageal reflux and irritable bowel syndrome, supporting the concept of "irritable gut syndrome" (see Chapter 74).

Psychiatric Disturbances, especially *anxiety* and *mood disorders*, are common in persons with irritable bowel syndrome who seek medical attention. Symptoms may arise from any area of the intestinal tract—esophagus, stomach, small intestine, and biliary tree as well as the colon. The result is a broad spectrum of presentations that includes nausea, vomiting, dyspepsia, and flatulence in addition to cramping abdominal pain.

Acute Ileus. Causes include *peritonitis* (resulting from a variety of causes), systemic infections, bowel *ischemia*, abdominal *surgery* (a common etiology), abdominal *trauma*, pharmacologic agents (especially *anticholinergics* and *narcotics*), and metabolic disturbances (particularly *hypokalemia*).

Intestinal Pseudoobstruction. Clinical features mimic those of intestinal obstruction. Symptoms may be chronic (recurrent or persistent) or occur acutely (so-called acute ileus). Symptoms can include vomiting and abdominal distention; diarrhea or constipation may also be seen. Plain films of the abdomen demonstrate intestinal dilation, suggestive of partial obstruction. It is noteworthy that the syndrome of chronic pseudoobstruction may precede the recognition of associated systemic diseases by many years (see below). *Chronic intestinal pseudoobstruction* is often idiopathic, although it may occur in the setting of scleroderma, Parkinson's disease, drug use (opiates, phenothiazines, tricyclic antidepressants, or antiparkinso-nian medications), hypercalcemia, diabetes, myxedema, amyloidosis, radiation enteritis, and chronic laxative abuse.

Capsular Distention. Distention of the well-innervated capsule surrounding an organ can be another source of constant, *aching* abdominal pain. *Hepatic* capsular distention may result from hepatic swelling secondary to hepatitis, congestive heart failure, fatty infiltration, or subcapsular hematoma and cause right upper quadrant pain. The pain of *splenic* capsular distention, as may occur secondary to blunt trauma (e.g., in an auto accident), is located in the left upper quadrant. With subdiaphragmatic peritoneal irritation, the patient may experience pain radiating to the ipsilateral shoulder. With splenic trauma, a deceptive period of many hours can pass before peritoneal signs develop if a subcapsular hematoma temporarily retards the spilling of blood into the peritoneum.

Metabolic Disturbances may mimic intraabdominal etiologies or sometimes result from them and exacerbate the clinical presentation.

Ketoacidosis presents with severe abdominal pain in 8% of instances and may be accompanied by emesis and an elevated white blood cell count. Symptoms are caused, at least in part, by accompanying gastroparesis. An acute intraabdominal event such as cholecystitis in a diabetic may be the precipitant.

Porphyria sometimes simulates bowel obstruction because of the cramping abdominal pain and hyperperistalsis that may occur. *Acute intermittent porphyria* presents with moderate to severe colicky abdominal pain, which may be localized or generalized. Abdominal symptoms may be the result of intestinal dysmotility; vomiting and diarrhea are also common complaints. Fever and leukocytosis may be present, but on examination the abdomen is found to be soft. Proximal muscle pain and a range of neuropsychiatric symptoms accompany the abdominal pain. The clinical features of *hereditary coproporphyria* and *variegate porphyria* are similar to those described for acute intermittent porphyria; skin lesions may be prominent.

Lead Poisoning may also present with abdominal pain. Such pain is typically wandering, poorly localized, colicky, and accompanied by a rigid abdomen. Encephalopathy, peripheral neuropathy, and anemia are associated features. The *urine coproporphyrin* test is a more reliable indicator of this entity than is a serum lead level, which can be normal.

Angioneurotic Edema, caused by *C' esterase inhibitor deficiency*, may result in episodic and severe abdominal pain. If this diagnosis is suspected, it is useful to check the serum level of C4, which is low in C' esterase inhibitor deficiency.

Nerve Injury from encroachment or irritation is an important mechanism of abdominal pain. The source of pain may be intraabdominal, as occurs when a pancreatic cancer invades adjacent splanchnic nerves, or it may be extraabdominal, as occurs when a nerve root supplying an abdominal wall dermatome becomes irritated in herpes zoster. Abdominal pain occurs in about 75% of patients with *cancer of the pancreas*; it is usually epigastric and most common in patients with tumor involving the body or tail of the pancreas. Sometimes, the pain radiates to the back or is confined to it. Pancreatic malignancy also causes pain by other mechanisms, including obstruction of the common or pancreatic duct. Nerve root irritation from *herpes zoster* may be mistaken for an intraabdominal process, especially before the rash appears. Often, the patient complains of a severe, lancinating pain resembling that from an intraabdominal source. An associated rectus muscle spasm may simulate peritonitis, but there is no effect on bowel function, as there is with peritoneal irritation, and palpation may actually alleviate the rectus muscle spasm. The pain of herpes infection often precedes the rash by several days and may persist after the skin clears, particularly in the elderly (see Chapter 193).

Abdominal Wall Pathology can also be mistaken for disease inside the abdominal cavity. Traumatic injury to the musculature of the wall produces pain that is constant, aching, and exacerbated by movement or pressure on the abdomen. The muscles may be in spasm, simulating the involuntary guarding of peritonitis. When a generalized myositis is responsible for the muscle pain, discomfort occurs in the limbs as well as in the abdomen. Occasionally, a tender mass in the wall, such as a rectus sheath hematoma, is found to be the source of difficulty.

Referred Pain from a process originating in the chest is sometimes an etiology of abdominal complaints. *Pulmonary infarction* and *pneumonia* of the lower lobes are among the chest problems that may present as pain in the upper abdomen; at times, reflex muscle spasm accompanies the pain. Upper abdominal pain, nausea, and vomiting may be the principal manifestations of an acute *inferior myocardial infarction*. However, most intrathoracic sources of abdominal pain are accompanied by symptoms and signs of cardiac or pulmonary disease.

DIFFERENTIAL DIAGNOSIS

Because the number of possible causes of abdominal pain is large, it is helpful to consider the differential diagnosis in terms of pathophysiologic mechanisms (Table 58.1). Let the nature of the pain suggest a pathophysiology and narrow the differential. Etiologies causing obstruction, peritoneal irritation, and vascular insufficiency are among the most dangerous. In about 70% of cases, mechanical small-bowel obstruction is caused by adhesions or external hernias; 90% of cases

Table 58-1. Principal Mechanisms of Abdominal Pain

Obstruction	**Altered Motility**
Gastric outlet	Gastroenteritis
Small bowel	Inflammatory bowel disease
Large bowel	Irritable bowel syndrome
Biliary tract	Diverticular disease
Urinary tract	
	Metabolic Disturbance
Peritoneal Irritation	Diabetic ketoacidosis
Infection	Porphyria
Chemical irritation (blood,	Lead poisoning
bile, gastric acid)	
Systemic inflammatory	**Nerve Injury**
process	Herpes zoster
Spread from a local	Root compression
inflammatory process	Nerve invasion
Vascular Insufficiency	**Muscle Wall Disease**
Embolization	Trauma
Atherosclerotic narrowing	Myositis
Hypotension	Hematoma
Aortic aneurysm dissection	
	Referred Pain
Mucosal Ulceration	Pneumonia (lower lobes)
Peptic ulcer disease	Inferior myocardial infarction
Gastric cancer	Pulmonary infarction
	Psychopathology
	Depression
	Anxiety
	Neuroses

of large-bowel obstruction are attributable to diverticular disease and carcinoma. Acute arterial insufficiency results most often from systemic embolization secondary to atrial fibrillation, severe atherosclerotic occlusive disease, and hypoperfusional states. Pelvic pathology is a common extraabdominal source of peritoneal irritation.

Other pathophysiologic mechanisms, such as nerve injury, metabolic imbalance, abdominal wall disease, and disordered motility, may produce symptoms that superficially mimic those of a more worrisome etiology; however, conditions associated with these mechanisms are usually more annoying than dangerous (an important exception is diabetic ketoacidosis). Pain referred from an extraabdominal site is more of a problem; significant cardiac disease (e.g., inferior myocardial infarction) or pulmonary pathology (e.g., lower lobe pneumonia) may present as abdominal pain.

WORKUP

The first priority is to determine the likelihood of serious pathophysiology and the pace and extent of workup. Patients with acute pain need to be examined promptly for evidence of obstruction, peritoneal irritation, vascular compromise, and cardiopulmonary disease. The evaluation of chronic pain can be assessed at a more gradual pace, with time allowed to get to know the patient and the problem before extensive testing is undertaken.

History. A complete description of the pain should be obtained, including localization, characterization, area of referral, time course of onset and resolution, and precipitating and alleviating factors. The chronologic sequence of symptom occurrence should be clearly outlined.

Checking for Serious Underlying Pathology. In addition to obtaining a complete description of the patient's pain, one needs to inquire into symptoms and risk factors indicative of pathology requiring urgent attention: prior abdominal surgery; previous episodes of obstruction; known gallbladder or kidney stones; presence and nature of vomitus; presence of rectal bleeding or melanotic stools; passage of flatus; time of last bowel movement; occurrence of diarrhea, constipation, or change in bowel habits; effect of activity on pain; presence of fever and rigors; development of distention; difficulties in urination; presence of atherosclerotic risk factors (especially smoking), any known systemic vascular disease, and any cardiac or pulmonary symptoms. Inquiry into pregnancy and symptoms of pelvic pathology, such as dyspareunia, abnormal vaginal discharge, and irregular menstrual bleeding, should be included in the assessment of every woman with abdominal pain.

Taking into Account Potentially Confounding Variables. The physician must learn to interpret accurately the "true" quality and quantity of the patient's experience, especially in cases of chronic abdominal pain, in which a host of nonmedical factors can alter pain perception and affect daily living. A thorough psychosocial history helps elucidate the psychological and ethnic factors that might contribute. Exploring patient fears, concerns, and expectations is also critical to understanding the patient, designing an effective treatment plan, and communicating a sense of caring and understanding.

Clinical Diagnosis of Functional Disease. The symptoms of functional bowel disease may mimic those of more serious pathology, which makes it necessary first to rule out the latter. Compounding the diagnostic challenge is that the recognition of functional disease relies heavily on the history, as there are no characteristic physical or laboratory findings. Clinical criteria predictive of functional disease have been identified to enable a "positive" diagnosis of functional disease to be made, rather than just an exclusionary one.

Irritable Bowel Syndrome. The widely used *Manning criteria* (visible abdominal distention, pain relief with defecation, more frequent stools with onset of pain, looser stools with onset of pain, passage of mucus per rectum, and feeling of incomplete evacuation) were developed to differentiate irritable bowel syndrome from other gastrointestinal disorders. Predictive value rises with the number of criteria that the patient fulfills and with the exclusion of findings suggestive of underlying bowel pathology. With all six criteria present, the predictive value can be as high as 80% to 90%, although lower in the elderly (70% to 80%) because of the increased risk for colon cancer (which can mimic some of the findings). The *Rome diagnostic criteria* are a refined iteration of the Manning criteria with the following features:

- At least 3 months of continuous or recurrent symptoms of abdominal pain or discomfort associated with any or all of the following:

  a. relief with defecation
  b. change in stool frequency
  c. change in stool consistency
     plus

- Two or more of the following:

  a. altered stool frequency (more than three bowel movements per day or fewer than three per week)
  b. altered stool form (lumpy and hard or loose and watery)

c. altered stool passage (straining, urgency, or incomplete evacuation)

d. passage of mucus

e. bloating or feeling of abdominal distention

Functional Dyspepsia. The *Rome criteria* for this condition identify two forms: ulcer-like and dysmotility-like. For the ulcer-like variant (in which abdominal pain dominates), the principal criterion is 3 months or more of upper abdominal pain with no evidence of organic disease, plus three or more of the following:

- very well-localized pain
- pain relieved by food (>25% of the time)
- pain relieved by antacids or histamine$_2$ blockers
- pain that awakens patient from sleep
- periods of remission and relapse (at least 2 weeks of remission)

Physical Examination. Particular attention ought to be paid to the patient's *general appearance*. The patient who appears reluctant to change position and keeps still is likely to have peritoneal irritation, whereas the patient with obstruction is often restless. It is important to check the *vital signs* for postural changes in the blood pressure or heart rate because obstruction, peritonitis, and bowel infarction can produce large losses of intravascular volume. Any hypotension, atrial fibrillation, or fever should be noted; however, absence of fever does not rule out serious pathology, especially in the elderly or chronically ill patient. The *skin* is examined for jaundice, other stigmata of chronic liver disease, clubbing or spooning of the fingernails, signs of trauma, excoriations, prior surgical scars, and evidence of dehydration, edema, or dermatomal rash. In addition, the sclerae are noted for icterus. The *chest* is checked for splinting, a pleural friction rub, and signs of consolidation (particularly in the lower lobes), and the *heart* is checked for murmurs, chamber enlargement, and signs of heart failure (see Chapter 32).

The *abdominal examination* should be performed with care to avoid unnecessary discomfort. A sharp increase in pain with coughing demonstrates rebound tenderness without the need for palpation and release. Examination of the abdomen includes checking for distention, ascites, altered bowel sounds (increased or absent), hepatic rub, vascular bruit, tenderness, guarding, rebound, hepatosplenomegaly, inguinal hernia, and masses (including a dilated aorta, loops of bowel, stool, distended bladder or uterus). An increased abdominal venous pattern suggests portal hypertension; periumbilical adenopathy suggests pancreatic or ovarian cancer. In a person with risk factors for vascular disease, the abdominal aorta should be palpated to determine its diameter. The index fingers are placed along the lateral margins of the aorta a few centimeters above the umbilicus and the distance between them measured, with the estimated thickness of the skin subtracted. Any diameter larger than 3 to 4 cm raises the possibility of aneurysm and necessitates proceeding to imaging (ultrasonography or computed tomography).

Pelvic and rectal examinations are essential parts of the evaluation, with checks for masses and tenderness. These examinations are certainly more revealing if done gently. The fecal occult blood test is also mandatory.

Examining for *nerve* and *muscle wall* injury is often overlooked in the urgency of searching for more worrisome pathology. Two important signs of nerve involvement are pain in a dermatomal distribution and hyperesthesia. Both occur with nerve injury from herpes zoster or nerve root impingement; however, hyperesthesia is also seen with focal peritoneal irritation. Testing is performed by gentle stroking of the skin overlying the area of pain. The rash of herpes may not appear until the time of the follow-up assessment. Abdominal wall pathology may be discovered by careful palpation of the wall for masses and muscle tenderness and by noting any exacerbation of pain when the muscles are contracted, as occurs with sitting up. Any pain on sitting up should not be confused with that secondary to involuntary muscle spasm associated with peritoneal irritation. The limbs should also be checked for muscle tenderness, which is suggestive of a generalized muscle disorder.

Physical Findings in the Elderly. The usual physical findings of acute peritoneal irritation may be absent in the elderly, especially at the outset. The only manifestations may be unexplained mild fever, tachycardia, reduction in bowel sounds, and vague abdominal discomfort without frank rebound or guarding. A high index of suspicion is required. Acute abdominal pain out of proportion to tenderness on physical examination in a person with known atherosclerotic disease should raise suspicion of vascular compromise.

Suspected Psychogenic Pain. Use of deep palpation while the patient is distracted can provide helpful evidence when a psychogenic etiology or a major degree of psychocultural overlay is suspected. A lack of tenderness is characteristic. A widely used approach is to push down slowly, firmly, and deeply with a stethoscope, distracting the patient by appearing to auscultate. Such a maneuver should be performed only after more serious pathology has been ruled out by history and physical examination.

Laboratory Studies: Initial Office Testing for Serious Acute Etiologies. Relatively few laboratory tests are needed for an initial assessment in the office setting. Studies are aimed at determining the likelihood of obstruction, peritonitis, acute vascular insufficiency, metabolic abnormality, and cardiac or pulmonary disease.

Complete Blood Cell Count and Differential. Although very nonspecific, the complete blood cell count and differential are reasonably sensitive for confirming the presence of an acute inflammatory process. Unfortunately, the complete blood cell count may show little change in the elderly or chronically ill patient, even in an acute intraabdominal emergency. The differential ought to be ordered even if the white cell count is "normal," particularly in the elderly, because a shift to immature forms sometimes occurs without a significant elevation in the white cell count. At times, a relatively benign condition such as viral gastroenteritis may produce an impressive elevation in the white cell count (as high as 20,000 cells per milliliter) accompanied by a marked shift to immature forms, which simulates the peripheral blood picture of a patient with more worrisome disease. The complete blood cell count and differential must be carefully interpreted in the context of the entire clinical picture and not used alone to decide whether to admit the patient. For patients with diarrhea, a microscopic *examination of the stool* for white blood cells is indicated (see Chapter 64).

Pregnancy Testing. Because of the seriousness of an ectopic pregnancy, every woman of reproductive age who presents with lower abdominal pain in the office setting should have pregnancy ruled out early in the assessment and usually before a radiologic study is performed. A *serum human chorionic gonadotropin β-subunit* is the most sensitive test; kit-based urine testing is less sensitive (see Chapter 112).

Plain Films of the Abdomen. Supine and upright films are essential if one suspects bowel obstruction or perforation. Multiple (i.e., 3) air–fluid levels, distention of the small bowel, and absence of gas in the large bowel are characteristic of complete small-bowel obstruction; however, such findings are present in fewer than 50% of cases of bowel strangulation, especially in the early stages of obstruction. Partial mechanical obstruction may produce some loops of bowel with air–fluid levels, but there is also gas in the colon; the same findings are found in patients with adynamic ileus. In colonic obstruction with a competent ileocecal valve, only the large bowel appears distended, but if the valve is not competent, both the large and small bowel demonstrate distention and gas, mimicking the findings of adynamic ileus. Distinguishing partial small-bowel obstruction from ileus requires repeated films or a barium study. Suspected obstruction of the large bowel is an indication for a barium enema and is usually a contraindication to performing an upper gastrointestinal series.

On the plain film, *free air* under the diaphragm indicates perforation of a viscus; *absent psoas shadows* suggest retroperitoneal bleeding, abscess, or mass; and displaced stomach or bowel (determined by gas patterns) may be caused by compression from a tumor. Plain films detect *calcifications*, such as those representing a biliary or renal stone, abdominal aortic disease, or pancreatitis. Calcification of the aortic wall has been found on plain films of the abdomen in more than 60% of abdominal aneurysms; a cross-table lateral view best demonstrates the finding.

Plain films of the abdomen are commonly overused in evaluating abdominal pain. Limiting the study to patients who have moderate to severe tenderness or who are strongly suspected of having bowel obstruction, urinary tract calculi, trauma, ischemia, or gallbladder disease (regardless of degree of tenderness) can reduce utilization by more than 50% without compromising the detection of clinically important pathology. Plain films reveal little unsuspected pathology, especially in patients with mild tenderness on examination. Using plain films to "rule out" serious pathology is possible only with bowel obstruction and perforation, for which the sensitivity of the plain film approaches 100%. Its sensitivity for the detection of other conditions is much lower.

Urinalysis and Chemistries. A *urine specimen* should be checked for pyuria, hematuria, bacteria, sugar, and ketones. Mild to moderate ketonuria is common when the patient has not eaten and is unrelated to diabetes; the diagnosis of ketoacidosis requires urine ketones in large concentrations (see Chapter 102). Red cells in the urine of a patient with flank pain suggest a stone in the ureter (see Chapter 135).

The *blood urea nitrogen, glucose, electrolyte,* and *amylase* levels should be measured. Elevation of the serum amylase occurs not only in pancreatitis but also in intestinal obstruction, perforated ulcer, and biliary tract disease; additional information is needed to identify the source of the elevation (see Chapter 72). Although not especially specific, the serum amylase is sensitive. Serum electrolytes can be helpful in cases of vomiting, diarrhea, or adynamic ileus; tests of renal and liver function should also be performed and blood sugar determined when clinical findings are suggestive.

Chest Film and Electrocardiogram. The initial investigation of acute upper abdominal pain should also include a *chest film* and *electrocardiogram* to look for pleuropulmonary disease in the lower lobes and acute ischemic changes in the inferior myocardium.

Laboratory Studies: Emergent Setting. Patients with evidence of acute obstruction, peritonitis, bowel ischemia, or worrisome metabolic or cardiopulmonary disease need immediate hospitalization and urgent testing. Although testing in the emergency department/urgent care setting is beyond the scope of this book, a few tests in addition to those noted above are worth mentioning for their contributions to initial decision making.

Paracentesis. In the subset of patients with acute pain who have ascites or abdominal trauma, an abdominal paracentesis performed with a small needle inserted into the lower abdomen (where there is less chance of perforating a viscus or a large blood vessel; see Chapter 71) helps to detect peritonitis by providing fluid for detection of blood and white cells. The best sites are nontympanitic areas of the right lower quadrant, left lower quadrant, and linea alba (midline).

Computed Tomography of the Abdomen. Abdominal computed tomography (CT) with Gastrografin oral contrast is the test of choice in patients with suspected *diverticulitis,* especially if there is concern on clinical grounds for abscess formation. CT with IV contrast is indicated for suspected *dissecting aortic aneurysm.* When *appendicitis* is the concern, *helical CT of the appendix* (with Gastrografin contrast) should be performed in the emergency department. This variation of CT technology maximizes diagnostic accuracy (95% to 98%) and, in doing so, shortens time to surgery for those with a positive test result and spares hospitalization and unnecessary surgery in persons with a negative result. The net impact is an improvement in outcomes and a reduction in costs.

Abdominal Ultrasonography. Ultrasonographic examination of the biliary tree is the test of choice for suspected *acute cholecystitis* and *choledocholithiasis.* The test can also detect *aortic aneurysm.* Ultrasonographic examination of the kidneys is needed when *hydronephrosis* from urinary tract obstruction secondary to *ureterolithiasis* is suspected.

Testing for Familial Mediterranean Fever. For Sephardic, Turkish, Arabic, or Armenian patients who present with peritoneal signs and fever, familial Mediterranean fever must be considered before they are subjected to surgery. A high index of suspicion for the diagnosis is warranted in such patients, especially those who have a positive family history or who describe self-limited attacks that may also involve the joints and pleurae. Detecting C5a inhibitor deficiency in serosal or synovial fluid is diagnostic, but not practical. Use of a DNA amplification assay for rapid detection of the responsible genetic mutation is now available in centers where the condition is common.

Laboratory Studies: Subsequent Outpatient Testing. The workup of patients without sufficient evidence of serious acute pathology necessitating immediate hospitalization can be continued on an outpatient basis. Any patient sent home with undiagnosed acute abdominal pain requires careful follow-up and reexamination because several serious etiologies (e.g., bowel ischemia, cholecystitis) may initially present with an indolent picture, particularly in the elderly. Despite the abundance of tests available, a repeated history and physical examination remain among the most productive of diagnostic measures. Additional testing is most productive when directed at working hypotheses suggested by the clinical findings and initial testing. Test selection ought to be judicious and based on the need to confirm or rule out specific diagnoses. Blind searches that involve "running the bowel" in the absence of suggestive clinical evidence are not only wasteful but also potentially misleading and may subject the patient to unnecessary risk. Test selection can be considered in terms of location of pain.

Epigastric Pain that parallels the acid–peptic cycle or responds to food or antacids suggests peptic ulcer disease. If the patient is under the age of 40 and little clinical evidence for malignancy is present (e.g., no dysphagia, weight loss, melena, hematemesis), then *serologic testing* for *Helicobacter pylori* and symptomatic treatment for presumed ulcer disease (see Chapter 68) can be started without first documenting the lesion. However, failure to respond to a 4- to 8-week course of empiric therapy or the development of worrisome symptoms, especially in older patients (who are at increased risk for esophageal and gastric cancers), necessitates direct visualization of the upper gastrointestinal tract by an *upper gastrointestinal series or esophagogastroduodenoscopy* (EGD). Endoscopy provides an opportunity for biopsy and should be considered if there is serious concern for cancer.

Recurrent bouts of epigastric or right upper quadrant pain are an indication for *abdominal ultrasonography*, which provides an important noninvasive approach to the detection of intraabdominal and retroperitoneal conditions presenting as abdominal pain. It is the test of choice for suspected cholecystitis (see Chapter 69) and useful for the detection of biliary and ureteral obstructions (see Chapters 62 and 135, respectively). It can help identify ascites and aortic aneurysm and sometimes localize an intraabdominal abscess. *Duplex scanning* (the combination of *Doppler* with *B-mode ultrasonography*) provides a sensitive, noninvasive approach to screening for mesenteric insufficiency. When performed by skilled operators, sensitivity for celiac and superior mesenteric artery disease is 87% and 96%, respectively. The test deserves consideration when abdominal pain is postprandial in a person with systemic vascular disease or its risk factors (especially smoking).

Periumbilical Pain suggests small-bowel pathology and is an indication for an *upper gastrointestinal series* with *small-bowel follow-through*. A lymphoma or carcinoid tumor may cause an intermittent partial obstruction. When the pain is postprandial, mesenteric ischemia requires consideration; duplex scanning by *Doppler ultrasonography* can provide noninvasive screening (see above).

Lower Abdominal Pain. All patients with lower abdominal pain accompanied by signs of rectal bleeding (be it gross or occult) should be evaluated by *colonoscopy* or the combination of *barium enema* and *sigmoidoscopy* to identify the source (see Chapter 63). However, the young patient (<40 years) with constipation, obvious hemorrhoidal bleeding, and no risk factors for colorectal cancer need undergo only a sigmoidoscopy to rule out associated rectosigmoid pathology, such as that of inflammatory bowel disease. Sigmoidoscopy is ideal for the assessment of suspected rectosigmoid masses or mucosal abnormalities. A full colonoscopy is needed when the source of lower gastrointestinal bleeding is unknown, as in cases of hematochezia or guaiac-positive stools. Barium enema is a reasonable alternative to colonoscopy, although not as sensitive for the detection of some sources of bleeding, such as angiodysplasia. Endoscopic study makes possible not only direct visualization but also biopsy of suspected lesions, polypectomy, and an assessment of the extent of disease in patients with inflammatory bowel disease.

Patients with lower abdominal pain in the absence of bleeding, weight loss, or a change in bowel habits are less likely to benefit from radiologic or endoscopic evaluation unless their symptoms are particularly severe or chronic. At times, the patient insists on having a study for reassurance purposes. The contribution of a normal test result to the patient's peace of mind has to be taken into account in any decision regarding whether or not to test. Carrying out age-appropriate screening for colorectal cancer (see Chapter 56) helps provide appropriate reassurance without excessive testing.

Flank and Adnexal Pains. The patient with flank pain, hematuria, or pyuria may have a renal source of abdominal pain. An *IV pyelogram* may help in detecting disease in the kidneys or ureters or displacement of a ureter by an abdominal or retroperitoneal mass. *Renal ultrasonography* can reveal a stone, tumor, or ureteral dilatation. *Pelvic ultrasonography* is indicated when the patient with adnexal pain has tenderness or a mass noted on bimanual examination.

Suspected Pancreatic Cancer. *Ultrasonography* is the test of choice for screening. Sensitivity ranges from 65% to 85%; specificity is a bit lower but can be greatly enhanced by adding *needle biopsy* of any suspected lesion. A proportion of studies are technically inadequate or indeterminate because of bowel gas or fat, which limits overall sensitivity. Nonetheless, the relatively high sensitivity, low cost, noninvasiveness, and absence of radiation exposure make this the preferred screening test for pancreatic cancer and other forms of pancreatic pathology.

The sensitivity and specificity of *abdominal CT* for the detection of pancreatic cancer parallel those of ultrasonography, but the frequency of indeterminate readings is lower (e.g., 4% vs. 23%). CT is less dependent on the skill of the operator, but it is more expensive and involves radiation exposure, a particularly important consideration in children. In addition to imaging the pancreas, it provides excellent views of the liver, retroperitoneum, and spine. Both ultrasonography and CT visualize the common bile duct, portal vein, and hepatic artery and detect any displacement, encroachment, or encasement of the major intraabdominal vessels and organs.

Endoscopic retrograde cholangiopancreatography (ERCP) is more sensitive and more specific for detecting pancreatic cancer than is ultrasonography, but success is very dependent on the skill of the endoscopist. If ultrasonography is not technically adequate, then CT or ERCP should be ordered. If a mass is found, needle aspiration biopsy is usually needed to confirm a diagnosis of malignancy. Although much progress has been made in identifying pancreatic masses in symptomatic patients, early detection in the asymptomatic period remains an elusive goal.

Suspected Functional Disease. The diagnosis of functional bowel disease is a clinical one, facilitated by careful attention to the history and physical examination. In the absence of history or physical examination evidence (e.g., significant weight loss, positive stool test for occult blood) suggesting a more serious medical condition, the diagnostic screening evaluation can be relatively limited.

For irritable bowel syndrome, the most useful test is *flexible sigmoidoscopy*, because of the considerable overlap between the symptoms of this disease and those of inflammatory bowel disease in younger persons and colorectal cancer in older patients. The routine ordering of chemistry profiles, blood counts, thyroid indices, urinalyses, and tests for ova and parasites appears to add little to the assessment or to decision making in the absence of clinical evidence of the conditions these tests screen for.

For functional dyspepsia, an empiric trial of treatment for peptic ulcer disease is one approach to screening for conditions that may resemble this functional illness. Another is to consider *serologic testing* for *H. pylori* infection, which is etiologic in peptic ulcer disease but not associated with functional dyspepsia. The decision to order upper gastrointestinal endoscopy is more difficult. The rationale is early detection of gastroesophageal malignancy. Because of the expense, discomfort, and potential morbidity associated with the procedure, in addition to a lack of evidence for any significant alteration in outcomes, the controversy regarding the usefulness of upper gastrointestinal endoscopy is considerable. Suggested criteria for its use include onset of symptoms after the age of 40, especially in persons whose symptoms persist without remission for longer than 8 weeks.

Evaluation of Undiagnosed Abdominal Pain. A most vexing problem arises when the cause of abdominal pain remains undetermined despite a careful initial medical evaluation. There may be pressure from patient and family to look still harder for a serious cause and a tendency, from frustration, to order progressively more invasive studies in search of such an etiology. Certainly, further anatomic study is indicated in patients with a strongly positive family history of bowel malignancy (see Chapter 56), significant weight loss, presence of a mass, unexplained iron-deficiency anemia, or a stool test that is positive for occult blood. However, the cause of undiagnosed abdominal pain is often an underlying psychological disturbance or sometimes a condition that can mimic it (e.g., lead poisoning or porphyria) and requires positive identification to facilitate treatment. At other times, no cause can be uncovered, and a plan for observation and follow-up is required.

Identification of Contributory Psychopathology. Abnormal illness behaviors characterize patients with psychosocial problems that present as a bodily complaint such as abdominal pain (see Chapter 230). Such behaviors include an exaggerated presentation with disability out of proportion to the degree of detectable disease, chronic complaints that defy precise diagnosis, persistent attempts to validate suffering, excessive dependence on the physician and others for care, avoidance of health-promoting behaviors, and attempts to maintain the sick role.

Include a history of *multiple bodily complaints*, a *chronic nonprogressive* clinical course that may span many years, *lack of relation* between symptoms and physiologic stimuli, inconsistent or *distractible* physical findings, and presence of the *somatic symptoms of depression* (e.g., early morning awakening, fatigue, decreased libido, altered appetite). Such behaviors and presentations of pain divert attention from the patient's psychosocial suffering and root causes unless they are recognized, understood, and responded to appropriately (see Chapters 226, 227, and 230). In the absence of worrisome objective findings,

one can avoid exhaustive testing of these patients and concentrate more on their underlying psychosocial problems.

The Patient's Perspective. Of particular importance is eliciting the patient's concerns, beliefs, and expectations. Also pertinent are the patient's daily functioning at work and at home, social supports, and psychological state. If elicited early on, these elements can speed recognition of psychosocial distress. The abdominal pain may be only a symptom of psychosocial suffering. Although the patient, family, or friends may be pressing for a medical diagnosis, the real need is for care rather than a diagnostic label. The risk of a missed anatomic diagnosis is less than 3% when the initial evaluation findings are normal and evidence of abnormal illness behavior and clinical features of psychological disturbance are present.

Patients with a clinical picture suggestive of functional disease may also benefit from inquiry into psychosocial issues, such as concurrent stresses, losses, and the effect of the pain on the patient's life and daily activities. However, a suggestion at the outset that the problem is probably psychogenic is inaccurate (about half of patients with functional disease have no etiologic psychopathology), and it also invites resistance and hostility if proclaimed before a careful evaluation is completed.

Avoiding an Adversarial Stance. Care must be taken neither to deny the reality of the patient's pain and suffering nor to emphasize the psychosocial nature of the problem any more than the patient is willing to accept. A detailed and pertinent history and physical examination that address patient concerns along with simple screening laboratory tests should suffice. Any requests for aggressive testing can be postponed as long as a plan for careful longitudinal follow-up is in place and available data show no evidence for dangerous underlying pathology. A caring response and an open-minded attitude help forge a working partnership and avoid triggering an adversarial relationship. In patients with neurotic complaints presenting with irritable bowel syndrome, thorough reassurance that specifically addresses patient concerns can be most effective, especially when delivered in sympathetic and respectful fashion.

Testing for Lead Poisoning and Porphyria. The patient with acute colicky pain but no signs of obstruction or inflammation may have lead poisoning and should have urine samples checked for *coproporphyrin*. Serum lead levels are unreliable. The person with acute intermittent porphyria may also present with colicky pain. Often, such persons are thought to be psychiatrically disturbed because of abnormal behavior during an attack. The diagnosis is suggested by periodic attacks of cramping pain, constipation, nausea and vomiting, and neuromuscular symptoms in conjunction with the altered psychological state. The *Watson-Schwartz test* for *urinary porphobilinogen* is a reliable screening test for acute intermittent porphyria in patients who are symptomatic.

Observation and Follow-up. When the diagnosis remains unclear, close follow-up is essential to proper management.

Acute Pain. If urgent admission does not seem warranted, assiduous, close follow-up is mandatory. Repeated histories and examinations may yield the diagnosis and hence allow proper treatment. Such factors as the degree of distress manifested by the patient, any elevation in temperature or white blood cell count, other laboratory abnormalities, and the ability of the patient to eat and drink all need to be reassessed continually. Judgment also must be made as to whether a patient with undiagnosed abdominal pain should undergo more invasive testing. In general, patients with unexplained abdominal pain in conjunction with recurrent nausea and vomiting, jaundice, fever, weight loss of more than 10% of body weight, or blood in the stool require more extensive evaluation.

Chronic Pain. The patient with chronic or recurrent abdominal pain that defies explanation poses one of the most difficult problems in clinical medicine. In a study of 64 patients with abdominal pain of unknown etiology despite extensive assessment, the younger the age and shorter the duration of the symptoms, the better the chances were for improvement. Older women with pain for more than 3 months were least likely to improve or be given a diagnosis. Of those subjected to *exploratory laparotomy*, a diagnosis was obtained in only 10%; the rate of improvement was the same as for those who did not undergo exploration. In 15% of the total study population, a cause for the patient's abdominal pain was found, but in only 6% did the condition require surgery. Thus, very few patients with abdominal pain of unknown etiology are endangered by continued observation, as long as signs of serious pathophysiology are absent. The morbidity of exploratory laparotomy in such patients greatly exceeds the benefit. Unexplained pain that is present for less than 2 weeks is likely to resolve spontaneously, but such improvement is unlikely when pain has persisted for more than 3 months.

INDICATIONS FOR ADMISSION AND REFERRAL

Admission. Any evidence suggestive of peritoneal irritation, obstruction, or acute vascular compromise is an indication for immediate hospitalization and surgical consultation. Sometimes, further observations made in the hospital can save the patient a surgical procedure, but no patient with the possibility of a condition that might require urgent surgery should be sent home from the office. Elderly patients are especially prone to subtle presentations. The patient with unexplained pain that has defied outpatient diagnostic attempts may benefit from further assessment in the hospital, especially if a need for large amounts of pain medication has developed. Admission provides an opportunity for 24-hour observation, specialty consultation, and assessment of the need for further study.

Referral. Consideration of invasive study is an indication for consultation with the gastroenterologist or surgeon before plans are made to proceed. Conversely, the internist can feel comfortable following the patient who appears well and has an otherwise normal history, physical examination findings, and screening laboratory results. For the overly anxious patient, a session with the gastroenterologist to talk over concerns and review the workup to date can be useful and may obviate need for further testing. Psychiatric consultation is indicated for patients with evidence of serious depression (see Chapter 227) or excessive somatization (see Chapter 230).

SYMPTOMATIC THERAPY

Symptomatic relief may be a high priority in some instances, even before a definitive diagnosis is achieved. Analgesics and therapeutic trials are the principal means utilized, but selective use is essential to ensure patient safety. Behavioral methods can be useful in persons with suspected psychopathology whose symptoms appear refractory.

Analgesics. Although analgesics are inappropriate for most patients with acute abdominal pain of unknown etiology (important diagnostic findings may be obscured), in certain instances their use should not be overlooked. Most important are patients with terminal cancer, for whom the compassionate use of narcotics must not be denied, even if the cause of abdominal pain is not fully defined (see Chapter 90). Patients with undiagnosed chronic pain who request pain medication represent the opposite situation. Many such patients have underlying psychopathology and a strong potential for narcotic abuse. Narcotic analgesics are to be avoided in such instances, even if the request is for "just a few pills."

Therapeutic Trials. Thoughtfully applied empiric therapy can provide relief as well as diagnostically useful information. Patients with suspected *peptic ulcer disease* and no evidence of malignancy are reasonable candidates for a 4-week course of *antacids*, *histamine$_2$ blockers*, or *proton pump inhibitors* (see Chapter 68); they may begin to feel better within days. Those with probable *irritable bowel syndrome* can be tried on a *high-fiber* program, such as a tablespoon of psyllium in 8 oz of water two to three times daily. (Psyllium is preferred to high-fiber cereal because of the need for milk intake with the latter and the associated risk for lactose intolerance in susceptible persons, which can simulate irritable bowel syndrome and confuse the diagnosis; see Chapter 64). As noted earlier, a trial of *antidepressant therapy* (with an agent low in anticholinergic activity) may be useful for patients with abdominal pain who manifest symptoms of major depression (see Chapter 227).

Behavioral Methods. Patients with refractory functional disease linked to underlying psychosocial distress are among the hardest to help, especially when illness behavior is greatly distorted. Although formal psychiatric care may be necessary, the primary physician can help to modify illness behavior by a series of simple actions. One is to provide the patient with techniques to increase control over the illness. Useful approaches include *participating* in treatment decisions, learning relaxation techniques, and beginning an *exercise* program. Even keeping a *symptom diary* can help provide a sense of control.

Equally important for such patients is the reinforcement of positive behaviors and removal of rewards for symptoms. Follow-up should be scheduled at regular intervals rather than as needed for symptoms. However, *setting limits* to time and availability is appropriate, with no more than 20 minutes necessary for a visit and unscheduled visits discouraged. During the visit, the focus should be on *accomplishments* ("What have you been able to do?") rather than on symptoms ("How do you feel?"). Reports of accomplishments are best received with positive reinforcement and requests for elaboration, whereas complaints of suffering and symptoms should be accorded a neutral stance and no request for elaboration unless worrisome new symptoms are reported. Finally, setting *realistic treatment goals* is critical. The emphasis needs to be on improving the quality of life and not on removing symptoms, which may not be possible.

ANNOTATED BIBLIOGRAPHY

Anuras S, Shirazi S. Chronic pseudoobstruction. Am J Gastroenterol 1984;79:525. (*The syndromes of acute and chronic colonic pseudoobstruction are differentiated; 99 references.*)

Council on Scientific Affairs, American Medical Association. Ultrasonic imaging of the abdomen. JAMA 1991;265:1726. (*Expert panel report on its utility; 56 references.*)

Derlet RW, Kinser D, Ray L, et al. Prospective identification and triage of nonemergency patients out of an emergency department: a 5-year study. Ann Emerg Med 1995;25;215. (*Some patients with less dangerous causes of pain can be identified in the emergency department.*)

Donaldson RM, Joyce CM, Feinstein AR. Effect of restraints on diagnostic approaches to abdominal pain and weight loss. Am J Med 1986;81:641. (*Provocative study examining test utilization when quests for economy and "team" approaches to ordering tests are initiated.*)

Drossman DA. Diagnosing and treating patients with refractory functional gastrointestinal disorders. Ann Intern Med 1995;123:688. (*Includes excellent and detailed discussion of approaches to diagnosis of irritable bowel syndrome.*)

Drossman DA, Thompson WG, Talley NJ, et al. Identification of subgroups of functional gastrointestinal disorders. Gastroenterol Int 1990;3:159. (*Consensus panel report on diagnostic guidelines for identification of functional disease and a recommendation that use of diagnostic studies be limited.*)

Eisenberg RL, Heineken P, Hedgcock MW, et al. Evaluation of plain abdominal radiographs in the diagnosis of abdominal pain. Ann Intern Med 1982;97:257. (*Effort to develop criteria for ordering abdominal films in patients with abdominal pain.*)

Eisenberg S, Aksentijeviich I, Deng Z, et al. Diagnosis of familial Mediterranean fever by a molecular genetics methods. Ann Intern Med 1998:129:539. (*Evidence supporting a DNA amplification method for rapid, cost-effective, accurate diagnosis.*)

Friedman G. American College of Gastroenterology Committee on FDA-related Matters. Irritable bowel syndrome I: a practical approach. Am J Gastroenterol 1989;84:803. (*Emphasizes use of fiber and other simple measures.*)

Jorgensen T. Abdominal symptoms and gallstone disease: an epidemiological investigation. Hepatology 1989;9:856. (*No symptoms identifiable as predictive of gallstones in this Danish population study.*)

Lederle FA, Simel DL. Does this patient have abdominal aortic aneurysm? JAMA 1999;281:77. (*A systematic review to determine sensitivity, specificity, and positive predictive value of abdominal palpation, the maneuver of choice for detection by physical examination.*)

Mitchell CM, Drossman DA. The irritable bowel syndrome: understanding and treating a biopsychosocial illness disorder. Ann Behav Med 1987;9:13. (*Comprehensive and multidimensional review of the disorder, with helpful recommendations for management.*)

Moawad J, Gewertz BL. Chronic mesenteric ischemia: clinical presentation and diagnosis. Surg Clin North Am 1997:77:357. (*Useful, terse review; 35 references.*)

Moneta GL, Lee RW, Yeager RA, et al. Mesenteric duplex scanning: a blinded prospective study. J Vasc Surg 1993;17:79. (*Sensitivity study for detection of significant celiac and superior mesenteric artery disease; ranged from 87% to 96%.*)

Rao PM, Rhea JT, Novelline RA, et al. Effect of computed tomography of the appendix on treatment of patients and use of hospital resources. N Engl J Med 1998;338:141. (*A study of CT in 100 consecutive patients with a high index of suspicion for appendicitis; CT findings resulted in a change in management in 58% of cases, reduced rates of unnecessary surgery and hospital days, and saved $447 per patient.*)

Richter JM, Christensen MR, Simeone JH, et al. Chronic cholecystitis: an analysis of diagnostic strategies. Invest Radiol 1987;22:111. (*Analysis of clinical utility of ultrasonography and other studies in the evaluation of abdominal pain.*)

Sarfeh IJ. Abdominal pain of unknown etiology. Am J Surg 1976;132:22. (*An old but still informative study; spontaneous improvement most likely in younger patients with symptoms of less than 2 weeks' duration; laparotomy did not influence the rate of improvement; it established the diagnosis in only 1 of 23 patients explored.*)

Shatila AH, Chamberlain BE, Webb WR, et al. Current status of diagnosis and management of strangulation obstruction of the small bowel. Am J Surg 1976;132:299. (*Still useful for its comparison of presentations of simple obstruction and strangulation; clinical differentiation often not reliable.*)

Silen W. Cope's early diagnosis of the acute abdomen, 18th ed. London: Oxford University Press, 1991. (*Concise, systematic approach to the diagnosis of acute abdominal problems. Emphasis is on history and physical findings; required reading for the primary physician; a classic work.*)

Soll AH. Medical treatment of peptic ulcer disease. JAMA 1996;275;622. (*American College of Gastroenterology guidelines for the treatment of peptic ulcer.*)

Stefansson T, Nyman R, Nilsson S, et al. Diverticulitis of the sigmoid colon: a comparison of CT, colonic enema, and laparoscopy. Acta Radiol 1997;38:313. (*Prospective study finding CT best for detection, especially if abscess is suspected.*)

Tolliver BA, Herrera JL, DiPalma JA. Evaluation of patients who meet clinical criteria for irritable bowel syndrome. Am J Gastroenterol 1994;89:176. (*Prospective study of 196 patients with clinically suspected disease to determine the yield of a wide range of tests.*)

59
Evaluation of Nausea and Vomiting

Nausea and vomiting are extremely common presenting complaints, ranking in one study of primary care practice second only to symptoms of upper respiratory tract infection. Although in most instances the symptoms are caused by self-limited disease, they may be a manifestation of a more serious underlying illness. The primary care physician needs to recognize the more worrisome causes of nausea and vomiting, provide relief from these debilitating symptoms, and correct any important fluid and electrolyte disturbances.

PATHOPHYSIOLOGY AND CLINICAL PRESENTATION

Mechanisms. Two major central nervous system centers are involved in the vomiting reflex—the vomiting center and the chemoreceptor trigger zone. Irritation of vagal and sympathetic afferents in the pharynx, heart, peritoneum, mesentery, bile ducts, stomach, and bowel triggers impulses to the vomiting center in the medullary reticular formation. Gastric irritation, distention of a hollow viscus, myocardial ischemia, increased intracranial pressure, metabolic disturbances, drugs, pharyngeal stimulation, and emotional upset are important noxious stimuli that act through this pathway. Vestibular disturbances, centrally acting drugs, and metabolic derangements stimulate the chemoreceptor trigger zone in the floor of the fourth ventricle, which in turn activates the vomiting center. A cortical pathway to the vomiting center has been postulated to account for some forms of psychogenic vomiting.

Clinical Presentations. The act of vomiting is a stereotyped response that varies little regardless of cause. Even so-called *projectile vomiting* (which is characterized by forceful emesis without prior nausea or retching), supposedly limited to cases of increased intracranial pressure, occurs in other conditions. Moreover, nausea, retching, and nonprojectile vomiting are seen with increased intracranial pressure.

Nausea and vomiting may be only one part of a symptom complex or may dominate the clinical picture (as in psychogenic vomiting, early pregnancy, digitalis toxicity, and metabolic disturbances). Considerable overlap exists among presentations nevertheless. With some causes of nausea and vomiting, symptoms are more likely to occur independently of meals, whereas in others, they are characteristically associated with food intake.

Metabolic Etiologies. Early morning nausea and vomiting are typical of *metabolic causes*. Up to 75% of cases of diabetic ketoacidosis are accompanied by nausea and vomiting. Emesis and nausea are found among as many as 90% of patients in addisonian crisis. Uremia may be heralded by similar symptoms; nausea often improves with correction of any associated hyponatremia, but it can be refractory. *Binge drinkers* experience early morning nausea and dry heaves from excessive alcohol intake.

Early Pregnancy. Early morning nausea and vomiting are characteristic of early pregnancy, occurring in more than 50% of instances. The problem is severe in fewer than 1% of cases but can lead to electrolyte abnormalities, dehydration, and weight loss. Most cases are mild; symptoms begin after the first missed period and terminate by the fourth month. Women with severe cases often have a history of vomiting in response to psychosocial stress. Disturbed motility is also noted in many cases. The diagnosis of pregnancy is sometimes overlooked.

Psychogenic Disease. In contrast to the causes of early morning vomiting, conditions such as psychoneurotic illness, acid or bile reflux, peptic ulcer disease, and gastritis can trigger symptoms shortly after food is ingested. Psychogenic vomiting is characterized by years of recurrent emesis. It can often be traced back to childhood and is more common when a family history of vomiting is present. Patients report that symptoms appear just after intake of food and can be sufficiently controlled voluntarily to avoid vomiting in public. Some patients admit to inducing emesis; most are surprisingly untroubled by the problem. Nausea accompanies almost all episodes. A study of 20 patients with psychogenic vomiting revealed a marked predominance of women engaged in hostile relationships; abdominal pain and depression were uncommon.

Bulimia is a form of psychogenic emesis in which vomiting is self-induced, often after a period of binge eating. A preoccupation with being thin and a poor self-image in a young woman are characteristic. Laxative abuse frequently complicates the clinical picture (see Chapter 234).

Peptic Ulcer Disease and Gastritis. A pyloric channel ulcer or acute gastritis may be associated with marked postprandial emesis. The vomiting in ulcer disease is believed to be in part a consequence of irritation, edema, and spasm of the pyloric sphincter mechanism. Concurrent bleeding can lead to vomiting of "coffee grounds." Patients who undergo surgery for peptic ulcer may be troubled by recurrent *bilious vomiting*, which is believed to be caused by reflux of bile into the stomach or gastric remnant. Patients vomit bile within 15 minutes of eating; little food is present. Nausea and a bad taste in the mouth are present on awakening in the morning.

Gastric Retention results in vomiting of food eaten more than 6 hours previously. A succussion splash is detectable on examination, and food is seen in the stomach on upper gastrointestinal series. In chronic cases, gastric outflow obstruction or atony may be secondary to diabetic neuropathy, anticholinergic use, or gastric malignancy. Transient gastric dilation is a frequent concomitant of pancreatitis, peritonitis, gallbladder disease, and hypokalemia. A *cyclic idiopathic* form of nausea and vomiting has been described with gastric hypomotility demonstrated.

Gastroesophageal Reflux Disease usually does not present with nausea as the predominant symptom (see Chapter 61), but a subset of patients with otherwise unexplained intractable nausea may suffer from reflux. Treatment of their reflux results in resolution of the nausea.

Acute Gastroenteritis. Acute episodes of vomiting accompany a host of conditions that range from the self-limited to life-threatening. The most common is *viral gastroenteritis*. After many years of attributing this illness to viral infection, investigators have finally isolated and identified the responsible viruses. Explosive bouts of nausea and vomiting in conjunction with watery diarrhea, cramping abdominal pain, myalgias, headache, and fever are typical. Recovery is rapid in most instances, but symptoms may linger for 7 to 10 days. Similarly, anorexia, nausea, and vomiting often dominate the prodromal stage of *acute viral hepatitis* (see Chapter 70).

Acute gastroenteritis that results from *food poisoning* secondary to *Salmonella* or *Shigella* infection has a similar clinical presentation and course; onset is 24 to 48 hours after exposure to the contaminated food. Domestic fowl and their eggs represent the largest single reservoir of *Salmonella* infection. Inadequate cooking is often responsible for human infection. Intake of pastries and similar items containing *staphylococcal enterotoxin* causes symptoms indistinguishable from those of viral gastroenteritis, except that onset is within 1 to 6 hours after ingestion of the spoiled food, fever is rare, and complete clearing takes place by 24 to 48 hours. *Clostridial* food poisoning rarely produces prominent nausea and vomiting.

Cholera. Persons who travel to an epidemic area are at risk for contracting *cholera*, especially if they have eaten raw or undercooked seafood or have had drinks chilled with contaminated ice. South America is the latest area to experience an epidemic. High U.S. sanitary standards for the handling of sewage, water, and food have so far prevented outbreaks from spreading to this country. The causative organism is a toxigenic strain of *Vibrio cholerae*, which elaborates an enterotoxin that induces secretion of water and electrolytes from the intestinal mucosa. Mild infection is characterized by a nonspecific diarrheal illness. In 3% to 5% of cases, the disease is much more severe (*cholera gravis*) and presents as profuse watery diarrhea with flecks of whitish mucus ("rice water stools"), vomiting, and dehydration. Vomiting is exacerbated by the acidosis that results from bowel bicarbonate loss. Circulatory collapse, altered consciousness, renal failure, and death are possible outcomes.

Peritoneal Irritation and Acute Obstruction may precipitate acute emesis, usually in the context of severe abdominal pain (see Chapter 58). *Intestinal obstruction*, especially of the proximal small bowel, produces marked nausea and vomiting of bilious material. Distention may be lacking, but intermittent cramping abdominal pain is characteristic. Feculent emesis is found in distal small-bowel obstruction. In *acute pancreatitis*, emesis is seen in 85% of patients; however, upper abdominal pain radiating into the back is the cardinal symptom, occurring in 95% of patients (see Chapter 72). Anorexia, nausea, and vomiting are early symptoms in more than 90% of patients with *acute appendicitis*; usually emesis clears early. As with pancreatitis, pain typically precedes other symptoms. *Acute pyelonephritis* may mimic a gastrointestinal etiology by causing nausea, vomiting, and abdominal pain. *Acute cholecystitis* sometimes triggers acute emesis, but less regularly than does *acute cholangitis* resulting from sudden obstruction of the common duct.

Myocardial Infarction may activate vagal afferents and produce nausea, vomiting, and epigastric discomfort, simulating intraabdominal disease. A prospective series of 62 patients with acute infarction revealed nausea and vomiting at the outset in 69% of those with inferior infarctions and 27% of those with anterior infarctions.

Neurologic Emergencies can provoke severe bouts of acute emesis. In *midline cerebellar hemorrhage*, nausea and vomiting are profuse, in association with severe gait ataxia; meningeal signs and headache are also seen. Within a few hours, the patient may become comatose and die unless the condition is promptly diagnosed and treated (see Chapter 165). One third of patients with *increased intracranial pressure* experience vomiting. When it is sudden, forceful, and not preceded by nausea, it is described as *projectile*, but this presentation is not specific. Concurrent bilateral frontal or occipital headache is the rule. *Migraine headaches* and *vestibular disease* are less worrisome neurologic causes of acute emesis (see Chapters 165 and 166). The former is suggested by photophobia and throbbing unilateral headache, the latter by vertigo.

Drugs. Of the many causes of *drug-induced* vomiting, *digitalis intoxication* is among the most serious. Anorexia is an early sign, followed by nausea and vomiting resulting from stimulation of the chemoreceptor trigger zone. Visual disturbances, such as seeing colored haloes, are suggestive of the diagnosis (see Chapter 32). Hypokalemia and dehydration induced by vomiting may precipitate or worsen digitalis toxicity.

Cancer Chemotherapies and Radiation Therapy produce substantial nausea and vomiting, with cisplatin being among the most problematic of chemotherapy agents. The mechanism of nausea and vomiting is believed to involve drug-induced release of serotonin from enterochromaffin cells, which leads to activation of serotonin receptors on visceral afferent fibers and stimulation of the vomiting center and chemoreceptor trigger zone. Drugs that block such serotonin receptors have proved uniquely effective (see below and Chapter 90).

Drug Withdrawal and Substance Abuse may trigger emesis. Nausea, dry heaves, and retching beginning at about 36 hours

are characteristic features of opiate withdrawal syndrome. Sweats, chills, and restlessness precede other symptoms; the vomiting peaks by 72 hours and then subsides (see Chapter 235).

DIFFERENTIAL DIAGNOSIS

Table 59.1 lists some of the more common and important conditions associated with prominent nausea and vomiting. Causes of simple regurgitation are omitted from the list because they are usually manifestations of esophageal difficulties (see Chapter 61) and unaccompanied by emesis. For convenience, the etiologies are listed according to clinical presentation; however, it is important to keep in mind that overlap and variation in the clinical picture can be considerable. For example, some causes listed as being accompanied by abdominal pain may present with just isolated emesis.

WORKUP

The history and physical examination, supplemented by a few well-chosen laboratory studies, are sufficient for diagnosis in most cases.

Table 59-1.   Some Important Causes of Nausea and Vomiting

Nausea/Vomiting as Predominant or Initial Symptom
Acute
Digitalis toxicity
Ketoacidosis[a]
Opiate use
Cancer chemotherapeutic agents
Early pregnancy
Inferior myocardial infarction[a]
Drug withdrawal
Binge drinking
Hepatitis

Recurrent or chronic
Psychogenic vomiting
Metabolic disturbances (uremia, adrenal insufficiency)
Gastric retention (gastroparesis, outlet obstruction)
Bile reflux after gastric surgery
Pregnancy

Nausea/Vomiting in Association with Abdominal Pain[b]
Viral gastroenteritis
Acute gastritis
Food poisoning
Peptic ulcer disease
Acute pancreatitis
Small bowel obstruction and pseudoobstruction
Acute appendicitis
Acute cholecystitis
Acute cholangitis
Acute pyelonephritis
Inferior myocardial infarction

Nausea/Vomiting in Association with Neurologic Symptoms
Increased intracranial pressure
Midline cerebellar hemorrhage
Vestibular disturbances
Migraine headaches
Autonomic dysfunction

[a]Abdominal pain is sometimes present.
[b]Abdominal pain is sometimes absent.

History should focus on such details as timing of symptoms, their relation to meals, characteristics of the vomitus, and associated complaints.

Timing and Relation to Meals. An early morning onset points to metabolic disturbances, alcoholic binge, and early pregnancy. Emesis precipitated by meals suggests psychogenic vomiting, pyloric channel ulcer, and gastritis. Onset a few hours after eating raises the possibility of obstruction of the gastric outflow tract, gastric atony, or bowel obstruction. Emesis of food that was ingested more than 12 hours earlier strongly suggests gastric stasis and an organic etiology, as does vomiting of large volumes (>1,500 mL daily). However, absence of such features hardly rules out organic disease.

Nature of the Vomitus. Vomiting blood or coffee ground material is indicative of gastritis and ulcer disease. Bilious vomitus means that the pyloric channel is open. When the material vomited is pure gastric juice, peptic ulcer disease and Zollinger-Ellison syndrome are suggested. Lack of acid suggests gastric cancer. Feculent material is a sign of distal small-bowel obstruction and blind-loop syndrome.

Associated Symptoms, Past Medical History, Psychosocial History. The history needs to include inquiry into abdominal pain, fever, jaundice, weight loss, abdominal surgery, external hernias, family history of emesis, symptoms of diabetes, prior renal disease, ischemic heart disease, drug use (e.g., digitalis, narcotics), visual disturbances, headache, ataxia, vertigo, last menstrual period, and concurrent emotional stresses and conflicts. Gentle questioning about self-image, binge eating, and self-induced emesis is indicated when the patient is a young woman suspected of bulimia.

Epidemiologic Data need to be obtained, particularly any exposure to commonly contaminated foods (e.g., raw shellfish, pastries, poultry) or hepatitis and any travel to an area with poor sanitation and outbreaks of cholera. Vomiting in conjunction with diarrhea sufficient to cause severe dehydration in an adult suggests cholera, especially if there are supportive epidemiologic data.

Physical Examination requires a check for *postural hypotension* (indicative of marked volume depletion or circulatory collapse). Other findings to check for include blood pressure elevation, irregularities of rate and rhythm, Kussmaul's respiration, pallor, hyperpigmentation, jaundice, papilledema, retinopathy, nystagmus, stiff neck, abdominal distention, visible peristalsis, abnormal bowel sounds, succussion splash, peritoneal signs, focal tenderness, organomegaly, masses, flank tenderness, muscle weakness, ataxia of gait, and asterixis. If there is a history of vertigo in conjunction with nausea, then Báranáy's maneuver (see Chapter 166) might reproduce symptoms and confirm the diagnosis of a vestibular etiology.

Patients suspected of having a "functional" disorder should be checked carefully for signs of autonomic insufficiency. A finding of postural hypotension, lack of sweat, or blunted pulse and blood pressure responses to Valsalva's maneuver suggests autonomic dysfunction and a bowel motility problem as the underlying etiology of the nausea and vomiting.

Laboratory Studies. Ordering tests is a function of the clinical presentation and is best conducted as a means of testing clinically generated hypotheses, rather than as a routine request for "nausea and vomiting studies."

Acute Emesis with Concurrent Abdominal Pain. In patients with emesis accompanied by acute abdominal pain, the first priority is to rule out an acute surgical cause such as bowel obstruction, peritonitis, or blockage of a hollow viscus. *Plain and upright films of the abdomen* are indicated when such causes are suspected (see Chapter 58). The onset of pancreatitis may be dominated by emesis in addition to abdominal pain, and if pancreatitis is suspected, a serum *amylase* determination is indicated. For suspected acute cholecystitis and choledocholithiasis, liver function studies (e.g., *alkaline phosphatase, aspartate aminotransferase*) and prompt consideration of *abdominal ultrasonography* are required.

Acute Nausea and Vomiting without Associated Abdominal Pain may also be a clue to serious illness. The acute onset of nausea and vomiting in conjunction with ataxia of gait and a stiff neck is very suggestive of a midline cerebellar hemorrhage; emergency *computed tomography* of the posterior fossa is needed (see Chapter 165). If the patient is a known diabetic, ketoacidosis should be suspected and *urine* and *serum ketones* and blood *glucose* should be checked (see Chapter 102). In a patient with risk factors for coronary artery disease, an *electrocardiogram* should be obtained; inferior ischemia may present as gastrointestinal upset (see Chapter 20). Hepatitis may present like acute gastroenteritis, with anorexia, nausea, and vomiting; a *transaminase* determination can be diagnostic. If the patient is taking a medication that potentially causes nausea and vomiting, a *serum drug level* might be informative. If a *digitalis* preparation is being taken, the drug should be withheld, an electrocardiogram obtained, a serum level ordered, and a potassium supplement prescribed if the potassium level is below 4.0 mg/100 mL (see Chapter 32).

Recurrent Vomiting raises the question of a psychogenic cause, but before leaping to such a conclusion, the physician should consider pregnancy, metabolic derangements, and chronic gastroesophageal disease. Metabolic disease and pregnancy are suggested by vomiting that occurs in the early morning. A *urinalysis* and determinations of the serum *blood urea nitrogen, creatinine, electrolytes, glucose*, and, in a woman of childbearing age, *human chorionic gonadotropin β-subunit* ought to be obtained (see Chapter 112).

Gastroesophageal causes are suggested by postprandial symptoms and best investigated by *upper gastrointestinal series* if there is concern about gastric outlet obstruction or retention, and by *endoscopy* if mucosal injury is a possibility (see Chapters 62 and 68).

Psychogenic vomiting is suggested by the characteristic history of chronic emesis, with vomiting around mealtime, partial suppressibility, and a conflict-ridden social situation. The need for additional studies in such cases is best individualized; some patients may insist on further testing, whereas others will be comforted by knowing that extensive studies are not necessary.

Therapeutic Trials. A therapeutic trial may have diagnostic utility and provide symptomatic relief. When a gastroesophageal motility disorder is suspected, a short course of a prokinetic agent such as *metoclopramide* or *cisapride* (e.g., 10 mg half an hour before meals) supplemented by a *proton pump inhibitor* (e.g., 20 mg of omeprazole daily) can be useful. Patients suspected of having an underlying affective disorder sometimes respond to a 4- to 8-week trial of *antidepressant medication*;

an agent with minimal anticholinergic activity (e.g., trazodone, desipramine, or fluoxetine) is preferred to minimize the chances of gastrointestinal side effects.

INDICATIONS FOR REFERRAL AND ADMISSION

Hospital admission for parenteral fluid and electrolyte replacement and additional workup is indicated if postural hypotension is present, especially if the patient is elderly. Prompt hospitalization also is needed for a patient with evidence of bowel obstruction, increased intracranial pressure, or any other gastrointestinal, neurologic, or metabolic emergency.

In the case of a patient whose condition remains undiagnosed after extensive evaluation and is unresponsive to therapeutic trials, and for whom evidence of an underlying psychiatric disturbance is lacking, gastric emptying and motility studies should be considered. These studies are performed at only a few specialty centers; referral should be made in consultation with a gastroenterologist. Patients suspected of psychogenic vomiting require psychiatric consultation because they may be seriously disturbed. Suicidal attempts are not uncommon among bulimic patients and others with psychogenic emesis. Referral to a mental health professional skilled and experienced in the treatment of patients with eating disorders is optimal for those suffering from bulimia (see Chapter 234).

SYMPTOMATIC RELIEF

When a cause has been identified but treatment of the underlying condition does not adequately control the symptoms, antiemetic drug therapy may help provide symptomatic relief. The available agents work by suppressing the vomiting center, the chemoreceptor trigger zone, or peripheral receptors. Symptomatic therapy must not be used in lieu of making a diagnosis.

Phenothiazines and other centrally acting agents are indicated for initial symptomatic treatment of vomiting caused by drugs, metabolic disorders, and gastroenteritis. They suppress the chemoreceptor trigger zone and probably the vomiting center and peripheral receptors also. *Prochlorperazine* (*Compazine*) and *promethazine* (*Phenergan*) are the phenothiazines used most often for vomiting. Prochlorperazine can be given orally in doses of 5 to 10 mg every 6 hours, or rectally in a dose of 25 mg three times daily. The oral dose of promethazine is 12.5 to 25.0 mg every 6-8 hours; the rectal dose is 25 mg three times daily. This class of drugs is not effective for motion sickness or vestibular disease. *Trimethobenzamide* (*Tigan*) is a centrally acting nonphenothiazine antiemetic useful for emesis of central causes. The oral dose is 250 mg three times daily. Rectal suppositories are given three times daily. Like all centrally acting agents, it can cause drowsiness, especially in the elderly. In *hepatitis*, nausea and vomiting may respond to very cautious use of phenothiazines. However, because they are metabolized by the liver and in rare instances can cause cholestasis, they should be used only in limited doses for short periods of time (see Chapter 70).

Antihistamines. For symptomatic relief from the nausea and vomiting of *vestibular disturbances*, the antihistamine *meclizine* (*Antivert*) has proved useful; it acts on the vestibular system and the chemoreceptor trigger zone and helps to control the nausea and vomiting associated with vestibular dysfunction.

Because meclizine can suppress or blunt important clues of vestibular disease, it should not be used unless a diagnosis has been established. Other antihistamines are quite popular for the treatment or prevention of motion sickness because, in comparison with meclizine, they provide either a more rapid onset of action [e.g., *dimenhydrinate* (Dramamine)] or a more prolonged effect (e.g., *transdermal scopolamine*). The average dose of meclizine is 25 mg four times daily for vestibular disease. A single transdermal scopolamine patch applied behind the ear several hours before a trip will provide prophylaxis for up to 3 days. Anticholinergic side effects (constipation, dry mouth, giddiness) are common. Meclizine is teratogenic in animals and is not indicated for vomiting resulting from pregnancy. All antihistamines can cause drowsiness and should not be used before driving or use of machinery.

Prokinetic Agents. For patients with emesis resulting from gastroparesis, the prokinetic agents *metoclopramide* (10 mg after meals and at bedtime) and *cisapride* (10 mg after meals and at bedtime) can help. The latter does not act centrally and thus causes few central nervous system side effects, which makes it more tolerable for long-term use, particularly in the elderly; however, its association with ventricular irritability needs to be taken into account (see Chapter 61).

Antiemetics for Cancer Chemotherapy. The nausea and vomiting associated with *cancer chemotherapy* can be especially uncomfortable and demoralizing. A wide variety of agents have been tried empirically, ranging from phenothiazines to tetrahydrocannabinol (as found in marijuana). Few provide truly satisfactory control, particularly when cisplatin is required. The selective serotonin S_3 receptor antagonist *ondansetron* has proved remarkably effective and safe, probably by virtue of its ability to block the effects of cisplatin-induced serotonin release from enterochromaffin cells. Anticholinergic therapy with high-dose *metoclopramide* has also been used, but cisplatin was superior and better tolerated in double-blinded crossover study (see Chapter 91).

Drugs for Morning Sickness. Morning sickness is best treated with small morning feedings and support; the goal is to try to avoid the use of antiemetics. No antiemetic is approved for use in pregnancy. The more prolonged, severe form of nausea and vomiting in pregnancy (hyperemesis gravidarum) may remit with hypnosis or supportive psychotherapy, but drug therapy is sometimes necessary. *Vitamin B$_6$* (25 mg/d) has proved useful in controlled trials and appears safe. *Metoclopramide* has also been used for years in severe cases without reports of fetal injury. Approval for *Bendectin* has been withdrawn because of concern for teratogenic effects.

Treatment of Psychogenic Vomiting. The best approach involves attention to the conflicts troubling the patient. No controlled studies have been performed of the effectiveness of antiemetics; fortunately, patients often do not request medication for symptomatic relief.

A.H.G.

ANNOTATED BIBLIOGRAPHY

Abell TL, Kim CH, Malagelda JR. Idiopathic cyclic nausea and vomiting—a disorder of gastrointestinal motility? Mayo Clin Proc 1988;63:1169. (*Gastrointestinal motor disturbances found.*)

Ahmed S, Gupta R, Brancato R. Significance of nausea and vomiting during acute myocardial infarction. Am Heart J 1977; 95:671. (*Nausea and vomiting occurred in 69% of patients with inferior infarctions, in comparison with 27% of those with anterior infarctions.*)

Baron TH, Ramirez R, Richter JE. Gastrointestinal motility disorders during pregnancy. Ann Intern Med 1993;118:366. (*Pathophysiology of vomiting in pregnancy.*)

Bothe F, Beardwood J. Evaluation of abdominal symptoms in the diabetic. Ann Surg 1937;105:516. (*Classic study; 75% of patients in ketoacidosis had nausea and vomiting, and 8% had severe abdominal pain and elevated white blood cell counts simulating an acute abdomen; intraabdominal disease can precipitate ketoacidosis.*)

Brzana RJ, Koch KL. Gastroesophageal reflux disease presenting with intractable nausea. Ann Intern Med 1997;126:704. (*A case series of 10 outpatients with intractable nausea demonstrating that all had reflux and that nausea resolved with treatment of the underlying reflux.*)

Cubeddu LX, Hoffman IS, Fuenmayor NT, et al. Efficacy of ondansetron (GR 38032F) and the role of serotonin in cisplatin-induced nausea and vomiting. N Engl J Med 1990;322:810. (*Randomized, placebo-controlled study demonstrating that ondansetron is effective and safe.*)

Hill OW. Psychogenic vomiting. Gut 1968;9:348. (*Classic study; high frequency of hostile living situations and symptoms developing at mealtime.*)

Malagelda JR, Camillieri M. Unexplained vomiting: a diagnostic challenge. Ann Intern Med 1984;101:211. (*Useful review of approaches to this difficult situation. Details neuromuscular disorders that may present as unexplained emesis; 61 references.*)

Richards RD, Valenzuela GA, Davenport KG, et al. Objective and subjective results of a randomized, double-blind, placebo-controlled trial using cisapride to treat gastroparesis. Dig Dis Sci 1993; 38:811. (*Found effective.*)

Rimer D. Gastric retention without mechanical obstruction. Arch Intern Med 1966;117:287. (*Good review of the problem, detailing the causes of this condition; 73 references.*)

Sahakian V, Rouse D, Sipes S, et al. Vitamin B_6 is effective for nausea and vomiting of pregnancy. Obstet Gynecol 1991;78:33. (*A randomized, placebo-controlled, double-blind trial.*)

Swerdlow DL, Ries AA. Cholera in the Americas. JAMA 1992; 267:1495. (*Terse and excellent review of epidemiology, clinical presentation, diagnosis, and treatment; 42 references.*)

60

Evaluation of Dysphagia and Suspected Esophageal Chest Pain

Dysphagia is the unpleasant sensation of difficulty in swallowing as a consequence of neuromuscular or anatomic pathology involving the esophagus (and sometimes the oropharynx). Such pathology may also trigger substernal chest pain and simulate angina (see Chapter 20). *Odynophagia* refers to painful swallowing, which usually results from serious mucosal inflammation. Because esophageal dysfunction and pain may be a manifestation of or mimic important pathology, it deserves to be assessed fully and not dismissed as a trivial problem or glibly invoked to account for symptoms.

PATHOPHYSIOLOGY AND CLINICAL PRESENTATION

Dysphagia implies an abnormality in swallowing and arises from either a loss of coordinated motor activity or mechanical obstruction, be it intrinsic narrowing or extrinsic compression of the esophagus.

Transfer Dysphagia (also referred to as *oropharyngeal dysphagia*) usually occurs as a consequence of neurologic or neuromuscular disease and presents as choking or difficulty in initiating swallowing. In many instances, other neurologic symptoms dominate the clinical picture, but at times, difficulty in swallowing is the major complaint, with aspiration and regurgitation of fluid into the nose. The problem is particularly common among the very old. Cortical and brainstem lesions resulting from stroke, tumor, and degenerative disease are important causes. In addition, medications with central effects (e.g., benzodiazepines, L-dopa, phenothiazines) may blunt the swallowing mechanism. Unlike esophageal disease, oropharyngeal

dysphagia is accurately localized to the suprasternal area. Those with neuromuscular etiologies report more difficulty in swallowing liquids than solids, nasal regurgitation, coughing, and aspiration. Patients with anatomic narrowing and mechanical obstruction of the pharynx or upper esophagus have more difficulty with solids than liquids.

Achalasia, the most common cause of motor dysphagia, is a slowly progressive motility disorder with a chronic course. The pathologic hallmark is a loss of cells in the myenteric ganglia. Lesions in the dorsal vagal nucleus and vagal trunks have also been described. It has been speculated that these changes represent damage caused by a neurotropic virus. As a consequence of a loss of smooth-muscle ganglion cells, the esophagus functions poorly, exhibits episodes of aperistalsis, and demonstrates exquisite sensitivity to gastrin and cholinergic agents. The gastroesophageal sphincter fails to relax properly, leading to functional obstruction at the gastroesophageal junction. In addition, a *loss of peristaltic activity* occurs in the distal esophagus. Dysphagia and substernal chest pain ensue. The resting pressure at the lower esophageal sphincter (LES) rises, and barium study shows an absence of peristalsis and delay in esophageal emptying. Paradoxically, vigorous nonpropulsive (tertiary) esophageal contractions resulting in chest pain may be observed early in the disease in young patients. Swallowing liquids and solids is equally difficult, yet by eating slowly and drinking small amounts, the patient may be able to consume a full meal. Pain is reported by 70% to 80% of patients, especially if they eat or drink rapidly, but pain is not an invariable accompaniment, and only 2% of patients with chest pain caused by esophageal disease have achalasia. Very cold liquids or emotion may provoke symptoms. Patients find that repeated swallowing or performing a rapid Valsalva's maneuver can help pass material into the stomach. Regurgitation is common and can be provoked by changes in position or physical exercise; pulmonary aspiration sometimes results. Patients may have foul breath because of retained esophageal material. Squamous cell carcinoma of the esophagus is sometimes a complication of achalasia; it occurs in 5% to 10% of patients.

Carcinoma-induced achalasia is seen with tumors at the gastroesophageal junction. Adenocarcinoma of the stomach is the most common of these neoplasms. The mechanism by which tumor induces achalasia is unclear, but manometric findings are identical to those of primary achalasia. Patients are typically over the age of 50 and complain of marked weight loss and symptoms of dysphagia of less than a year's duration.

Scleroderma can impair neuromuscular function and result in a decrease in LES tone in addition to a lack of propulsive motor activity. *Reflux* is more of a problem than is dysphagia (helping to distinguish scleroderma from other motility disorders), but as many as 20% of patients may have some difficulty in swallowing. About 75% of patients with scleroderma have esophageal involvement as part of the CREST syndrome (calcinosis, Raynaud's phenomenon, esophageal dysmotility, sclerodactyly, and telangiectasia).

Diffuse Esophageal Spasm is characterized clinically by nonprogressive dysphagia and substernal chest pain that may mimic angina (see below and Chapter 20). Radiologically and manometrically, patients manifest nonpropulsive *simultaneous contractions* (tertiary contractions) throughout the entire esophagus (especially the distal portion) in more than 10% of wet swallows. Such contractions are also observed in normal persons under conditions of emotional stress and dry swallows, which leads some to view this condition as little more than a transient abnormality in motor function induced by stress. However, as noted above, the condition may also be an early manifestation of neuromuscular disease that progresses to achalasia. Unlike achalasia, diffuse esophageal spasm is intermixed with periods of normal peristaltic activity. Dysphagia is noted with both liquids and solids. Diffuse esophageal spasm accounts for about 10% of cases of noncardiac chest pain caused by abnormal esophageal motility. Some asymptomatic patients manifest the radiologic and manometric criteria for esophageal spasm but rarely experience discomfort.

"Nutcracker" Esophagus is a picturesque radiologic description applied to the condition of patients experiencing *very high-amplitude contractions* in the distal esophagus. The resultant pressures exceed the mean by more than two standard deviations. These peristaltic contractions are not only of exceptionally high amplitude but also of long duration. There are no simultaneous contractions, as there are in diffuse esophageal spasm, and only occasionally does impairment of esophageal function lead to dysphagia. The principal symptom is *chest pain* (see below), with nutcracker esophagus accounting for about half of all cases of noncardiac chest pain associated with an esophageal motility disturbance. Occasionally, reflux precipitates the contractile abnormalities. Achalasia develops in about 3% to 5% of patients, and degenerative changes are noted

in ganglia and nerves, suggesting to some a possible link to achalasia. Supersensitivity to gastrin and cholinergic agents can be demonstrated.

Hypertensive Lower Esophageal Sphincter is characterized by increased resting LES pressure but normal relaxation and peristalsis, with no impediment to bolus passage. About half of the patients have high-amplitude contractions, consistent with nutcracker esophagus.

Mechanical Obstruction differs clinically from motor dysfunction in that the patient has more difficulty with solids than with liquids. The duration of symptoms is shorter (<1 year) for patients with malignancy than it is for those with benign causes of obstruction; progression is often rapid. Most patients with tumor are over the age of 50 and report marked weight loss. The location of discomfort does not necessarily correlate with the site of obstruction because the pain may be referred. Spontaneous pain is not a common feature of neoplasm involving the esophagus. Patients with stricture caused by severe esophagitis usually have a long history of reflux.

Inflammatory Lesions of the pharynx or esophagus may cause *odynophagia* (pain on swallowing). Esophageal motility is not disturbed, but swallowing is made difficult by the pain. Even saliva may be irritating. *Radiation therapy*, *tablet ingestion*, and *infection* are important causes of this severe esophageal irritation. Tetracycline, quinidine, potassium tablets, NSAIDs, and iron preparations have been implicated. The elderly are at greatest risk because they are likely to consume more tablets with less water, and saliva production decreases with age. The discomfort is often associated with ingestion of the tablets and generally decreases during a period of a few days.

Infectious esophagitis caused by *Candida*, *herpes simplex virus*, or *cytomegalovirus* is being increasingly recognized in immunocompromised patients, including the growing number with AIDS, and in patients taking broad-spectrum antibiotics on a long-term basis. Onset may be rapid and accompanied by fever, chills, nausea, vomiting, and epigastric pain. Viral or fungal esophagitis rarely occurs in immunologically intact persons; when it does, it is usually short-lived and self-limited.

Esophageal Chest Pain is most often associated with prolonged or severe contractile waves, although distention of stretch receptors and stimulation of chemoreceptors may also contribute. Certain investigators have suggested that some patients subject to attacks of esophageal chest pain may have an esophageal version of irritable bowel syndrome, with motor dysfunction and increased sensitivity to distention and chemical stimuli. They wonder whether there might be an "irritable gut syndrome," with a common pathophysiology extending from the esophagus to the rectosigmoid. They note that many patients with esophageal chest pain also report symptoms of irritable bowel syndrome.

Chest pain is particularly prevalent in patients with nutcracker esophagus. The chest pain associated with esophageal motor disorders can mimic that of angina in terms of location (substernal), quality (tightness), radiation (into the arm or back), and response to nitroglycerine (prompt relief). Adding to the confusion with coronary pain is the fact that esophageal chest pain need not be accompanied by dysphagia, although sometimes heartburn is reported as a preceding symptom. The pain is frequently nocturnal, awakening the patient from sleep. Chest discomfort need not occur in relation to swallowing, but sometimes it is triggered by drinking very hot or very cold liquids.

Conditions Confused with Dysphagia. Sometimes, *globus hystericus*, a condition seen in anxiety disorders, is confused with dysphagia. The patient complains of a constant "lump in the throat" and has a perception of obstruction, although no actual difficulty in swallowing food. An involuntary tightening of the cricopharyngeal muscle has been observed in some patients with this condition and may account for the symptoms. Symptoms are unrelated to swallowing, and esophageal function is normal.

DIFFERENTIAL DIAGNOSIS

The causes of dysphagia can be divided into motor and obstructive categories, and these are often subdivided according to whether they affect the upper or lower esophagus (Table 60.1). Most esophageal cancers are of the squamous cell variety, although half of those in the distal half of the esophagus are adenocarcinomas, which suggests that they arise in the cardia of the stomach. True dysphagia must be distinguished from conditions that may produce esophageal pain without interfering with the mechanics of swallowing, such as most forms of esophagitis and motor disorders with propulsive but high-amplitude contractions (e.g., nutcracker esophagus). The patient with globus hystericus reports a constant sensation of having something in the throat but swallows normally.

No detailed population studies have been performed on the prevalence of dysphagia and the relative frequencies of its causes. However, in a study of 910 patients with noncardiac chest pain, 28% were found to have abnormal esophageal motility. Of these 28%, 48% had nutcracker disease, 36% had nonspecific esophageal motility dysfunction, 10% had diffuse esophageal spasm, and 2% had achalasia.

WORKUP

History

A tentative diagnosis can often be made by history. A British study found that history alone could provide an accurate diagnosis in about 80% of cases. The most important features of the history include the duration and progression of symptoms, relation of symptoms to ingestion of solids and liquids, effect of cold on swallowing, and response to swallowing a bolus. Inquiry into these aspects of the problem help in the important task of differentiating a motor disorder from mechanical obstruction. Motor disease is suggested by gradual onset, slow progression, chronic course, equal difficulty with liquids and solids, aggravation of symptoms on swallowing cold substances, and passage of a bolus by repeated swallowing, forceful drinking, Valsalva's maneuver, or throwing back the head and shoulders. Mechanical obstruction is characterized by more rapid onset and progressive course, more difficulty with solids than with liquids, no aggravation with cold foods, and regurgitation on trying to swallow a bolus. As noted above, the location of discomfort helps to locate the lesion only if it is very high or very low in the esophagus; with a distal lesion, pain may be referred to the neck. Hiccups point to difficulty in the terminal portion of the esophagus. Intermittent dysphagia that occurs only with solid food is indicative of a lower esophageal (Schatzki's) ring.

Other features of the history also have some discriminative value, including the presence of pain, reflux, and neurologic defects. Pain in conjunction with dysphagia suggests spasm or achalasia, although pain may occur in these conditions without concurrent difficulty in swallowing. Pain on swallowing saliva alone is characteristic of mucosal inflammation. A history of heartburn in conjunction with difficulty in swallowing solids argues strongly for a stricture secondary to chronic reflux esophagitis, especially if the problem is chronic. Scleroderma also is suggested when symptoms of reflux occur with dysphagia (together with skin changes and cold extremities). Dysphagia that comes on only after activity and is associated with motor aphasia, diplopia, or dysphonia is indicative of myasthenia. Tremor or difficulty in initiating movement suggests Parkinson's disease (see Chapter 174). Other historical facts to note are recent use of topical upper respiratory or inhaled steroid aerosols or broad-spectrum antibiotics, and concurrent immunodeficiency (e.g., AIDS).

The pace of illness is important to note. Very acute dysphagia suggests infection, irritation, or food impaction. Rapid progression is caused by tumor until proved otherwise, whereas slow progression is most consistent with a motor disorder. Weight loss may occur with any etiology, but in a Mayo Clinic study, it was more predictive of obstruction.

Table 60-1. Differential Diagnosis of Dysphagia

Motor Disease
Pharyngeal (transfer dysphagia)
  Pseudobulbar palsy
  Myasthenia gravis
  Multiple sclerosis
  Amyotrophic lateral sclerosis
  Parkinson's disease
Transesophageal
  Achalasia
  Scleroderma
  Diffuse esophageal spasm
Distal
  "Nutcracker" esophagus
  Hypertensive lower esophageal sphincter

Obstructing Lesions
Upper esophageal
  Tumor
  Zenker's webs (Plummer-Vinson syndrome)
  Goiter
  Enlarged lymph nodes
  Cervical spine osteophytes
Lower esophageal
  Carcinoma
  Stricture (chronic reflux, corrosive agents, intubation)
  Webs and rings
  Foreign bodies
  Food impaction
  Mediastinal tumors
  Aortic aneurysm

Odynophagia
Opportunistic esophageal infection (cytomegalovirus, herpesvirus, *Candida*)
  Tablet-induced irritation
  Severe reflux esophagitis

Physical Examination

The skin is noted for pallor, signs of scleroderma (sclerodactyly, telangiectasia, calcinosis), and hyperkeratotic palms and soles (a rare finding suggestive of esophageal carcinoma). The mouth should be examined carefully for inflammatory lesions, ill-fitting dentures, and pharyngeal masses. The HIV-positive patient with oral candidiasis is at increased risk for esophageal involvement. Lymph nodes are palpated in the neck and elsewhere to detect enlargement suggestive of neoplasm or infection (see Chapter 12), and the thyroid is palpated for a goiter that might extrinsically compress the esophagus. The abdomen is checked for masses, tenderness, and organomegaly, and the stool for occult blood (suggestive of neoplasm and esophagitis). The neurologic examination should be thorough and include testing for motor dysfunction, with a search for tremor, rigidity, and fatigability in addition to cranial nerve deficits, abnormal Babinski's response, and abnormal gag reflex.

Laboratory Studies

The history and physical examination usually provide sufficient evidence to distinguish oropharyngeal from esophageal dysphagia, and a mechanical form of esophageal dysphagia from a neuromuscular one. Making such a determination before laboratory testing helps focus the laboratory workup, interpret the results, and avoid unnecessary studies.

Barium Swallow is usually the first step in the diagnostic evaluation of the dysphagic patient and is especially important if a structural impediment to swallowing is suspected. Its sensitivity is excellent for determining the location and severity of an obstructing mass lesion or stenosis, but it often lacks precision in identifying the nature of the lesion, particularly in distinguishing cancer from postinflammatory scarring and stenosis. For example, some gastric carcinomas may show little more than intrinsic narrowing. Endoscopic biopsy (see below) may be necessary, especially when the history suggests malignancy (e.g., rapid progression, marked weight loss).

By providing fluoroscopic evidence of esophageal function, the barium swallow can sometimes help in documenting motor disorders, although test sensitivity is not high. Early achalasia and esophageal spasm may produce few findings on a routine barium swallow, especially when symptoms are infrequent. The characteristic radiologic features of achalasia include dilation of the distal two thirds of the esophagus, segmental contractions, and termination of the distal esophagus into a narrowed segment (often referred to as a "break"), caused by the tonically contracted LES. When the patient is upright, an air–fluid level may be present on the barium esophagram. If diffuse esophageal spasm occurs during barium examination, it produces multiple tertiary contractions and differs from achalasia in that no break is observed. The functional assessment of dysphagia is facilitated by performing all barium studies with the patient in the supine position to cancel the effect of gravity, and by dipping a piece of bread into barium to trace better the movement of solid food. *Video studies of the oropharyngeal phase* of swallowing are essential in the evaluation of suspected oropharyngeal dysphagia, not only for diagnosis but also to determine the risk for aspiration. Radiologic expertise is required for the interpretation of such films.

Upper Gastrointestinal Endoscopy and Biopsy are needed when an intrinsically obstructing lesion is discovered that may be malignant. As noted above, even stenoses can represent early cancer and should be considered for endoscopy and biopsy if the clinical context is suggestive (e.g., age over 50 years, progressive clinical course). On occasion, even the patient with achalasia may require endoscopy, particularly when contraction of the LES is so persistent that stenosis cannot be ruled out by barium study alone. Stretching of the sphincter can be accomplished at the same time. However, endoscopy for truly radiographically negative dysphagia is generally of low yield.

Acute onset of odynophagia suggests severe esophageal inflammation and, in an immunocompromised host, raises the possibility of an infectious etiology. Endoscopic examination is needed to examine for plaques, vesicles, and pseudomembranes. Brushings and biopsy specimens are obtained as needed and prepared appropriately to detect fungi, giant cells, and intranuclear inclusion bodies. All patients with new-onset odynophagia require endoscopic evaluation.

Manometry. Strong clinical suspicion of motor dysfunction or failure of the barium swallow to reveal a probable etiology raises the question of proceeding to manometry. Although potentially diagnostic, manometry often gives indeterminate data. Many patients suspected of achalasia or esophageal spasm fail to show typical manometric findings at the time of testing. Furthermore, others who are symptom-free may demonstrate abnormalities when tested. Still others end up being placed in a category of nonspecific motility disease. Nevertheless, many authorities insist on manometric data before concluding that a patient has esophageal spasm or a related motor disorder. The diagnosis of nutcracker esophagus is especially dependent on manometric data.

Provocative Testing is most useful and worth serious consideration when the physician is confronted with a patient who complains of *atypical chest pain*. Once cardiac disease is ruled out (see Chapter 20), an esophageal problem is high on the list of possible explanations. Provocative testing provides a ready means in the office of identifying an esophageal origin for an atypical pain, although it does not specify a mechanism and it is of less use in the evaluation of dysphagia. The objective of provocative testing is to reproduce the patient's exact symptoms. Two tests have proved most useful: the Bernstein or acid perfusion test and edrophonium (Tensilon) infusion.

The Bernstein test was initially used to confirm symptoms caused by reflux, but a positive test result has also proved specific for esophageal chest pain, even in the absence of documented reflux. In 7% to 27% of cases, noncardiac chest pain has been associated with a positive Bernstein test result and deemed to be of definite esophageal origin, although evidence of acid reflux may not be found on 24-hour pH monitoring. The test consists of instilling a small amount of acid through a nasogastric tube placed in the esophagus.

Edrophonium testing grew out of a desire to find a safe and well-tolerated means of stimulating esophageal contractions. Ergonovine was originally tried, and although it was successful in reproducing symptoms, its risks of serious cardiac side effects negated its usefulness. Edrophonium (a relatively gentle muscarinic agonist) has proved superior to acid perfusion, bethanechol, and pentagastrin in reproducing atypical chest pain, with 24% to 34% of patients having a positive test result (reproduction of pain during wet swallows). Like the Bernstein test, edrophonium identifies an esophageal origin for the pain but does not specify the mechanism (correlation between response to edrophonium and manometric findings is poor). Side effects of a rapid bolus of IV edrophonium (80 μg/kg of body weight) include mild degrees of light-headedness, nausea, and abdominal cramps, but not the tachycardia, hypertension, or coronary vasoconstriction seen with ergonovine.

Ambulatory Monitoring of both *intraesophageal pH* and *pressures* for 24 hours is becoming increasingly available and may prove useful, especially in cases that defy explanation despite comprehensive testing. Monitoring of esophageal pH during 24 hours has emerged as a useful tool in the evaluation of noncardiac chest pain, as it provides an opportunity to correlate acid reflux with occurrence of symptoms. In a study comparing traditional esophageal tests (manometry, Bernstein test, and edrophonium) with 24-hour pH monitoring, the latter led the field in providing an explanatory correlation in 46% of instances of chest pain, versus 19% for both edrophonium and the Bernstein test, the next-best studies. A single manometric study was of little use. Because no gold standard is available, determinations of sensitivity and specificity are not possible.

As just noted, abnormal motor activity may be difficult to detect at the time of a particular study or may be induced by the study and have little to do with the patient's problem. Round-the-clock pressure monitoring opens up new avenues of evaluation. The precise indications for such testing remain to be defined; studies are ongoing.

SYMPTOMATIC RELIEF AND PATIENT EDUCATION

Motility Disorders. A conservative approach sometimes suffices for patients with mild motor disease. The dysphagic person with achalasia is often able to manage reasonably well by *eating slowly*, *drinking small quantities* at a time, and *avoiding cold foods*. A trial of *sublingual nitrates* or *calcium channel blockers* before eating may sufficiently relax spastic smooth muscle in patients with mild to moderate dysfunction to provide relief.

Patients with *atypical chest pain* caused by esophageal disease benefit greatly from knowing definitively that their pain is not indicative of heart disease. A thorough explanation after a careful evaluation can greatly reduce morbidity and even the frequency of symptoms. Given the presumed relation of atypical chest pain to esophageal spasm, nitrates and calcium channel blockers have been used. The results have been variable, which is not surprising, as the relation of spasm to pain is variable; however, benefit does accrue for some patients, which makes a trial of these agents worthwhile. *Antireflux therapy* (see Chapter 61) can be an important component of the treatment program when the workup suggests acid reflux as a trigger of symptoms. *Antidepressants* with little anticholinergic activity, such as trazodone, have proved effective in patients suspected of having a psychiatric precipitant of esophageal motor dysfunction. *Relaxation techniques* and other *behavioral methods* are worth a try in those with stress-induced esophageal motor dysfunction (see Chapter 226). *Anticholinergic therapy* has been disappointing. When *odynophagia* is present and an inflammatory lesion is suspected as the precipitant, especially

when opportunistic infection might be the cause (e.g., patients with HIV disease), then antifungal or antiviral therapy may be needed (see Chapter 13).

Patients with severe achalasia get little relief from dietary or drug manipulations; *esophageal dilation* or *myotomy* is needed. Myotomy is more effective but requires major surgery and often produces severe reflux that does not respond to antireflux surgery. Consequently, pneumatic esophageal dilation is usually the most effective invasive procedure for treatment of severe motor disease. Dysphagia is relieved immediately, and sufficient LES pressure remains to prevent bothersome reflux.

Obstructing Lesions. Regardless of etiology and pending definitive diagnosis, all patients suspected of having obstruction should be advised to take predominantly liquids or soft solids. The goal is to provide an adequate caloric intake that can be swallowed with a minimum of discomfort. Patients with mechanical obstruction often require dilation or surgery, but there are many exceptions. The best management for a person with a lower esophageal ring is to advise slow intake of small amounts; dilation does not work very well. Restoration of adequate iron intake will reverse the pathologic changes of sideropenic dysphagia unless a carcinoma has developed in the pharynx. Carcinoma of the upper or middle third of the esophagus is often unresectable and best treated by radiation therapy; considerable palliation is sometimes achieved. Oropharyngeal dysphagia caused by obstruction is treated surgically (e.g., removal of a Zenker's diverticulum or large goiter), whereas attention to the underlying neurologic deficit is necessary in cases caused by motor dysfunction, although myotomy may help as well. The patient with globus hystericus can be given thorough reassurance, although symptoms are not likely to resolve easily.

INDICATIONS FOR REFERRAL

Patients with oropharyngeal dysphagia who aspirate more than 10% of a barium test bolus and show barium residue in the oropharynx with subsequent swallows are at great risk for aspiration and should be referred for consideration of a non-oral means of nutrition. In addition, those with evidence of neuromuscular disease severe enough to cause oropharyngeal dysphagia might benefit from a neurologic consultation. The patient with an obstructing lesion requires endoscopic evaluation and referral to a gastroenterologist or surgeon for consideration of endoscopic biopsy. The patient who is referred for further evaluation and therapy should still be followed closely by the primary care physician, especially to monitor nutritional status.

A.H.G./A.G.M.

ANNOTATED BIBLIOGRAPHY

Achem SR, Kotts BE, Wears R, et al. Chest pain associated with nutcracker esophagus: a preliminary study of the role of gastroesophageal reflux. Am J Gastroenterol 1993;88:187. (*Reflux may play a role in up to one third of patients.*)

Bernstein LM, Baker LA. A clinical test for esophagitis. Gastroenterology 1958;34:760. (*Original description of the acid perfusion test.*)

Browning TH. Diagnosis of chest pain of esophageal origin: a guideline of the patient care committee of the American Gastroenterological Association. Dig Dis Sci 1990;35:289. (*Consensus statement offering evaluation guidelines.*)

Clouse RE, Lustman PJ. Psychiatric illness and contraction abnormalities of the esophagus. N Engl J Med 1983;309:1337. (*Documents the association between psychiatric conditions, including depression and anxiety states, and symptomatic esophageal motility disorders, many presenting as chest pain.*)

Cohen S. Esophageal motility disorders and their response to calcium channel antagonists: the sphinx revisited. Gastroenterology 1987;93:201. (*Poor response to these muscle relaxants challenges the view of a simple etiologic association.*)

Cooke RA, Anggiansah A, Chambers JB, et al. A prospective study of oesophageal function in patients with normal coronary angiograms and controls with angina. Gut 1998;42:323. (*The frequency of abnormalities and the correlation of pH events with chest pain was the same among patients with normal coronary angiograms and in controls with angina.*)

Dalton CB, Castell DO, Richter JE. The changing face of the nutcracker esophagus. Am J Gastroenterology 1988;83:358. (*Detailed characterization of the condition in view of accumulating data.*)

Dipalma JA, Prechter GC, Bradie CE. X-ray–negative dysphagia: is endoscopy necessary? J Clin Gastroenterol 1984;6:409. (*Endoscopy in radiographically negative dysphagia is generally of low yield.*)

Domenech E, Kelly J. Swallowing disorders. Med Clin North Am 1999;83:97. (*Useful review.*)

Edwards DAW. Discriminative information in the diagnosis of dysphagia. J R Coll Physicians Lond 1975;9:257. (*Critical discussion of important historical data; diagnostic accuracy by history alone is close to 80%.*)

Goff JS. Infectious causes of esophagitis. Annu Rev Med 1988;39:163. (*Excellent review of these important causes of odynophagia.*)

Hewson EG, Sinclair JW, Dalton CB, et al. Twenty-four-hour esophageal monitoring: the most useful test for evaluating noncardiac chest pain. Am J Med 1991;90:576. (*Test identified an esophageal etiology in 46% of instances.*)

Hurwitz AL, Duranceau A. Upper esophageal sphincter dysfunction: pathogenesis and treatment. Am J Dig Dis 1978;23:275. (*Review of the causes of oropharyngeal dysphagia and a presentation of the results of cricopharyngeal myotomy as a method of relieving symptoms; 48 references.*)

Janssens J, Vantrappen G, Ghillebert G. Twenty-four-hour recording of esophageal pressure and pH in patients with noncardiac chest pain. Gastroenterology 1986;90:1978. (*Correlations between pressure, pH, and chest pain were often variable.*)

Kahrilas PJ. Gastroesophageal reflux disease. JAMA 1996;276:983. (*A systematic review of the management of gastroesophageal reflux disease with esophageal and extraesophageal complications.*)

Katz PO, Dalton CB, Richter JE, et al. Esophageal testing of patients with noncardiac chest pain or dysphagia. Ann Intern Med 1987;106:593. (*Provocative testing proved best in those with chest pain; manometric studies were superior in those with dysphagia.*)

Kilman WJ, Goyal RK. Disorders of pharyngeal and upper esophageal sphincter motor function. Arch Intern Med 1976;136:592. (*Thorough discussion of oropharyngeal motor diseases.*)

Kim CH, Weaver AL, Hsu JJ, et al. Discriminant value of esophageal symptoms. Mayo Clin Proc 1993;68:948. (*Further evidence of the value of a careful history; authors develop a discriminant model, but not one based on a primary care population.*)

Rao SS, Gregersen H, Hayek B, et al. Unexplained chest pain: the hypersensitive, hyperreactive, and poorly compliant esophagus. Ann Intern Med 1996;124:950. (*Lower thresholds for pain and reactive contractions revealed by impedance planimetry after otherwise normal cardiac and esophageal evaluations.*)

Richter JE, Bradley LA, Castell DO. Esophageal chest pain: current controversies in pathogenesis, diagnosis, and therapy. Ann Intern Med 1989;110:66. (*Best review to date, with interesting discussion of the "irritable gut" hypothesis; 119 references.*)

Richter JE, Castell DO. Diffuse esophageal spasm: a reappraisal. Ann Intern Med 1984;100:242. (*Argues for a manometric diagnosis of spasm; critical review of diagnostic criteria.*)

Richter JE, Dalton CB, Bradley LA, et al. Oral nifedipine in the treatment of noncardiac chest pain in patients with the nutcracker esophagus. Gastroenterology 1987;93:21. (*Disappointing results, although these agents show ability to decrease pressure.*)

Rose S, Achkar E, Easley KA. Follow-up of patients with noncardiac chest pain. Value of esophageal testing. Dig Dis Sci 1994;39:2063. (*Many patients continue to blame the esophagus even when tests results are normal.*)

Tavitian A, Raufman JP, Rosenthal L. Oral candidiasis as a marker for esophageal candidiasis in the acquired immunodeficiency syndrome. Ann Intern Med 1986;104:54. (*A useful clinical marker.*)

Ward BW, Wu WC, Richter JE, et al. Long-term follow-up of symptomatic status of patients with noncardiac chest pain: is diagnosis of esophageal etiology helpful? Am J Gastroenterology 1987;82:215. (*The reassurance provided reduced morbidity and even frequency of episodes.*)

Wilcox CM. Esophageal disease in the acquired immunodeficiency syndrome: etiology, diagnosis, and management. Am J Med 1992;92:412. (*Thorough review.*)

Young LD, Richter JE, Anderson KO, et al. Effects of psychological and environmental stressors on peristaltic esophageal contractions in healthy volunteers. Psychology 1987;24:132. (*Data suggesting that stress can induce esophageal motor dysfunction.*)

61

Approach to the Patient with Heartburn and Reflux (Gastroesophageal Reflux Disease)

JAMES M. RICHTER

Heartburn is a nearly universal experience. In one survey of presumably normal hospital staff, 7% reported current daily heartburn and 36% experienced heartburn at least once a month. The term *heartburn* typically refers to retrosternal burning that radiates upward, as a consequence of reflux of gastric acid up into the esophagus. It is characteristically exacerbated by large meals, supine posture, or bending over, and it is alleviated, at least temporarily, by antacids. Heartburn ranges in severity from an occasional episode of postprandial discomfort without sequel to a syndrome of severe esophageal inflammation that can lead to bleeding, stricture, and malignant transformation. Symptoms may be transient or a manifestation of chronic gastroesophageal reflux disease (GERD). Key tasks include deciding who requires endoscopic assessment and selecting the most cost-effective approach to controlling symptoms and preventing serious sequelae.

PATHOPHYSIOLOGY AND CLINICAL PRESENTATION

Normal Esophageal Physiology. The physiologic action of the *lower esophageal sphincter* (LES) is critical to maintaining a pressure barrier between the stomach and the esophagus. The LES is a complicated region of smooth muscle modulated by the interaction of hormonal, neural, and dietary factors. The hormone gastrin increases its resting tone, whereas estrogens, progesterone, glucagon, secretin, and cholecystokinin all decrease sphincter pressure. Vagus nerve input helps maintain resting tone, as does α-adrenergic stimulation. Pharmacologic agents that increase sphincter tone include bethanechol, metoclopramide, pentobarbital, histamine, edrophonium, and antacids. Anticholinergics, theophylline, meperidine, and the calcium channel blockers all decrease the resting tone. Saliva may be an important protective mechanism, inducing peristalsis in addition to aiding in washout, dilution, and neutralization of acid refluxed into the esophagus.

Mechanisms of Reflux. GERD is a multifactorial problem, involving reduction in resting LES tone, transient episodes of inappropriate relaxation of the LES, irritant action of gastric acid and digestive enzymes, decreased secondary peristalsis, and defective mucosal resistance to caustic liquids. Also implicated are impaired esophageal clearance of acid from the esophagus and delayed gastric emptying.

LES pressures vary and overlap enormously between those with and without symptomatic reflux. Normal pressure ranges from 12 to 30 mm Hg. LES pressures below 6 mm Hg are apt to allow reflux, and those above 20 mm Hg usually prevent it. Pressures between 6 and 20 mm Hg are found in both patients and controls. In many patients, reflux occurs as a result of transient episodes of inappropriate sphincter relaxation rather than low basal tone.

Anatomic factors, such as the presence of a *hiatus hernia*, are not as important as they once were believed to be, but patients with hiatus hernia may be modestly predisposed to reflux disease. A certain portion of the esophagus must be situated intraabdominally for optimal esophageal function and sphincter competence; moreover, peristaltic clearing of acid is impaired in patients with a hiatus hernia.

Contributing factors include *tobacco, ethanol, chocolate,* and foods with high concentrations of *fat* or *carbohydrate,* all of which decrease LES pressure and increase heartburn. *Citrus fruits* and fruit juices often exacerbate symptoms; the mechanism by which they cause heartburn is not clear. Although *pregnancy* may cause reflux because of increased intraabdominal pressure, the primary reason for heartburn in pregnancy is reduced sphincter pressure as a consequence of increased circulating levels of progesterone and estrogen. Reflux can be precipitated in normal persons by *exercise*, with jogging after meals the most common cause.

Clinical Features. *Heartburn* predictably accompanies gastroesophageal reflux. The patient characteristically complains of retrosternal ache or burning within 30 to 60 minutes of eat-

ing, especially after large meals. Symptoms are made worse by lying down or bending over; many patients learn to avoid lying down after meals. Reflux may trigger *chest pain* than can mimic cardiac angina, with some patients describing chest heaviness or pressure that, like angina, may radiate to the neck, jaw, or shoulders (see Chapters 20 and 60).

Regurgitation of fluid or food particles may occur, particularly at night. The patient may describe soiling of the pillow with gastric contents or may awake because of coughing or a strangling sensation. *Nocturnal aspiration* is occasionally associated with gastroesophageal reflux and can cause recurrent pneumonias, bronchospasm, and chronic cough. A *reflex salivary hypersecretion* or *"water brash"* is sometimes described by patients with reflux. Water brash is especially common in children, but direct questioning is often required to determine its occurrence. Hoarseness, sore throat, and the feeling of a lump in the throat are other common otolaryngologic manifestations of reflux.

Painful or difficult swallowing (odynophagia, dysphagia) usually suggests long-standing reflux disease with *either* active inflammation, stricture, or both. Solid food may stick in the distal esophagus (with or without stricture formation), although food usually passes into the stomach after repeated swallowing or drinking liquids unless a fairly tight obstruction is present (see Chapter 60). Odynophagia is seen in cases complicated by severe erosion and may be a symptom of malignancy or infection.

Barrett's Esophagus and Adenocarcinoma A strong, dose-related, independent risk for *adenocarcinoma of the esophagus* is conferred by symptomatic reflux. In a substantial number of patients with long-standing severe reflux, a premalignant change develops that is referred to as *Barrett's esophagus*, which denotes metaplastic columnar epithelialization of the distal esophagus. Barrett's esophagus is believed to represent a reparative response to tissue injury from chronic exposure to gastric acid, pepsin, and bile (annual incidence, 0.6% per year; prevalence, 10% among those with reflux lasting longer than 20 years). Histologically, the normal stratified squamous epithelium of the mucosa is replaced by columnar epithelium. Dysplastic transformation may ensue and eventually lead to adenocarcinoma. The risk for the development of adenocarcinoma with onset of Barrett's esophagus is less than 1% annually but rises fivefold with the onset of low-grade dysplasia and 10-fold in persons with high-grade dysplasia. Symptoms are those of reflux and its complications.

Esophageal ulcers, strictures, and hemorrhage may also develop as a consequence of chronic severe esophagitis. *Bleeding* may be slow and chronic, resulting in iron-deficiency anemia, or brisk, resulting in hematemesis.

Dental erosions occur in a substantial proportion of patients with marked reflux as a consequence of the effects of acid and bile on tooth enamel. Patients with teeth erosions of unknown etiology are often found to have reflux on evaluation.

Reflux-induced asthma and laryngitis are among the airway consequences of chronic GERD. Unexplained wheezing, voice change, chronic cough, and lump in the throat are among the symptoms reported; reflux must be considered when such complaints develop in the absence of a known cause.

DIFFERENTIAL DIAGNOSIS

The diagnosis of gastroesophageal reflux disease is secure when the patient describes heartburn and experiences regurgitation of stomach contents. However, many patients report only a dull substernal discomfort or ache, and in such circumstances the physician must consider *myocardial ischemia*, esophageal *spasm* or high-amplitude esophageal peristalsis, *cholelithiasis*, and mediastinal inflammation. Gastroesophageal reflux may accompany *peptic ulcer disease* (particularly in gastric hypersecretory conditions) and *cancer* of the gastroesophageal junction. Esophageal *infections* with opportunistic organisms such as cytomegalovirus, herpesvirus, and *Candida albicans* can cause heartburn in the immunocompromised host. Reflux esophagitis may also accompany intestinal dysmotility syndromes, including idiopathic intestinal pseudoobstruction or secondary pseudoobstruction associated with *scleroderma*. *Diabetic gastroparesis* may predispose a patient to reflux and heartburn because of retarded emptying of gastric contents.

WORKUP

History. The characteristic history of a retrosternal burning sensation radiating upward, associated with large meals and supine posture, is virtually diagnostic of reflux disease. An attempt should be made to identify any aggravating factors, such as intake of fatty foods, concentrated sweets, alcohol, peppermint, coffee, tea, anticholinergics, calcium channel blockers, and theophylline compounds. The use of drugs capable of causing esophageal injury (NSAIDs, quinidine, wax matrix potassium chloride tablets, tetracycline) should also be elicited. Inquiry should be made regarding response to antacids. Surgery near the gastroesophageal junction (e.g., antireflux surgery or vagotomy) may predispose the patient to reflux disease. A history of Raynaud's phenomenon raises the possibility of scleroderma. Consideration of achalasia, malignancy, esophagitis, and stricture is indicated if dysphagia is part of the clinical presentation (see Chapter 60).

Physical Examination. The physical examination is generally unrevealing, but several points are worth special attention. Sclerodactyly, calcinosis, and telangiectasia suggest underlying scleroderma (see Chapter 146). The epigastrium should be carefully examined for the presence of a mass lesion, and the stool should be examined for occult blood.

Laboratory Studies. No single test is accepted as the standard for the diagnosis of reflux disease. Fortunately, a careful history is sufficient to establish the diagnosis in the majority of patients, and laboratory tests are needed only in atypical or severe cases. When a classic reflux story is elicited, initial therapy can be instituted on the basis of history alone for simple heartburn in a young patient.

Esophageal pH monitoring for 24 hours is the most sensitive and specific test for reflux, but it is also very expensive, not universally available, and usually unnecessary. However, it does allow correlation of activity with symptoms and reflux of acid and can be of help in confusing situations, such as atypical chest pain (see Chapter 60).

Barium swallow; esophagoscopy. If dysphagia, painful swallowing, significant weight loss, or occult blood loss is present, the patient should undergo additional study to rule out a neoplasm or a complication of reflux. Suspected damage to the esophageal mucosa from reflux disease is best assessed by *en-doscopy* in conjunction with *biopsy*. The barium swallow may show inflammation, ulceration, or stricture, but findings are normal in most cases of reflux. Although it remains widely used for the diagnosis of reflux, its sensitivity may be as low as 25%, and it is far less accurate than a careful history. Its main utility is in searching for major stricture and tumor in persons with severe or long-standing disease.

In atypical cases, the *Bernstein acid perfusion test* is often employed to see if symptoms are caused by reflux; however, the Bernstein test is rarely needed when the patient gives a classic description of heartburn, and the test requires careful interpretation because false-positives are common. It is of more use in determining whether chest pain is a consequence of acid reflux (see Chapter 60).

SYMPTOMATIC MANAGEMENT

A stepwise approach is recommended by most authorities. Otherwise, healthy patients with a classic history of uncomplicated reflux can be treated empirically, first with simple *nonpharmacologic measures* and then the addition of *pharmacologic intervention* as needed (Table 61.1). In many instances, these measures will suffice. If the patient fails to respond, if heartburn is complicated by dysphagia, weight loss, or anemia, or if a stool test is positive for occult bleeding, then, as noted earlier, a more comprehensive diagnostic investigation is indicated. A detailed evaluation is especially important in older patients, in whom the risk for malignancy is increased.

Table 61-1.   Treatment of Esophageal Reflux

Step 1.
a. Dietary manipulations—avoidance of foods high in fat or carbohydrate (chocolate can be particularly problematic, being high in both)
b. Weight reduction if obese
c. Avoidance of large evening meals near bedtime or before exercise
d. Elevation of the head of the bed with 6-in blocks under the bedposts (pillows are not adequate)
e. Avoidance, if possible, of medications that decrease sphincter tone, including theophylline compounds, calcium channel blockers, meperidine, and anticholinergics
f. Avoidance, if possible, of drugs that may injure the esophageal mucosa (tetracycline, quinidine, wax matrix potassium chloride tablets, NSAIDs)
g. Avoidance of cigarettes, alcohol, coffee
h. Antacids after meals and at bedtime

Step 2. Add:
a. Oral H_2-blocker (bid regimen best, e.g., ranitidine 150 mg, cimetidine 800 mg, famotidine 20 mg)

Step 3. Switch to:
a. Proton pump inhibitor (e.g., omeprazole 20–40 mg/d or lansoprazole 15–30 mg/d), treatment of choice for erosive esophagitis and Barrett's esophagus

Step 4. Add:
a. Metoclopramide (a dopamine antagonist) 10-15 mg qid *or*
b. Cisapride* (a dopamine antagonist) 10-20 mg qid *or*
c. Bethanechol (a cholinergic agent) 25 mg qid) *or*

Step 5. Consider:
a. Antireflux surgery for incapacitating refractory disease

*Use with caution (cardiac side effects—see text).

Nonpharmacologic Measures (Step 1). The first and most important steps are *dietary intervention, life-style modification*, and *antacids* (Table 61.1, step 1, and Tables 68.1 and 68.2). Attention to these measures is essential to a good outcome; they will often suffice. Even if additional therapy is needed, these conservative measures constitute the foundation of all treatment programs and must not be omitted. They represent the most cost-effective approach to therapy for the majority of patients.

Suppression of Gastric Acid Production (Steps 2 and 3). A major objective of symptomatic therapy is a reduction in esophageal exposure to gastric acid. When step 1 measures fail to suffice, pharmacologic measures can be implemented.

Histamine$_2$ blocker (H$_2$-blocker) treatment (Table 61.1, step 2) can be used in place of or in combination with antacid therapy (antacid contributing immediate neutralizing of postprandial acid and H$_2$-blocker providing more sustained acid suppression). Because H$_2$-blocker absorption may by reduced by up to 20% when an H$_2$-blocker is taken with antacids, the two agents should not be taken at the same time. H$_2$-blockers are more convenient to use than a high-dose antacid program and provide better round-the-clock symptom relief and esophageal healing. A twice-daily, full-dose regimen achieves best results (e.g., 800 mg of cimetidine twice daily, 150 mg of ranitidine twice daily, or 20 mg of famotidine twice daily). In milder cases of reflux, a once-daily dose at the time of maximal symptoms often suffices, supplemented when necessary by an antacid for prompt relief of any breakthrough heartburn.

Proton pump inhibitor (PPI) therapy is indicated for patients with symptoms refractory to the full implementation of step 1 and step 2 measures and for those with erosive esophagitis (see Table 61-1, step 3). A single daily dose of a PPI achieves nearly complete suppression of gastric acid production. It has demonstrated efficacy in the healing of erosive lesions and controlling refractory symptoms. However, relapses after completion of therapy are common, so that long-term maintenance therapy must be considered, especially in persons with erosive esophagitis (see below).

The *choice of PPI* should be based on cost and interactions with other medications; side effects are similar (see Chapter 68). At present, lansoprazole is the least expensive PPI, but omeprazole is likely to drop in price as it comes off patent.

Prokinetic Therapy (Step 4). A few patients will report persistent symptoms despite the above measures. In such situations, prokinetic drugs have been used in an attempt to increase LES pressure and halt reflux (Table 61.1, step 4).

Metoclopramide, a dopamine receptor antagonist, is the leading choice for prokinetic therapy. The drug augments gastric emptying and raises LES tone. It is most useful for patients who have reflux without severe heartburn and those with gastroparesis. However, up to a third of patients may not tolerate the drug because of its central nervous system side effects.

Cisapride, a dopamine antagonist that does not cross the blood—brain barrier, represents an advance in prokinetic therapy in that central nervous system side effects are minimal. However, reports of serious cardiac arrhythmias (ven-

tricular tachycardia, ventricular fibrillation, torsades de pointes, and QT prolongation) have emerged, most often in the context of concurrent use of drugs that inhibit hepatic cytochrome P-450 metabolism. These reports have resulted in a warning by the Food and Drug Administration that cisapride is contraindicated when such drugs are being taken. In addition, the agent should not be used in persons with a cardiac rhythm disorder, underlying heart disease, renal failure, electrolyte disturbances, or drugs that may be proarrhythmic. An electrocardiogram should be obtained before cisapride is given and checked for arrhythmias and any prolongation of the QT interval.

Bethanechol, a potent cholinergic agonist, raises LES pressure, increases salivary flow, and improves acid clearance by the esophagus. However, because of its cholinergic side effects, it is not particularly well tolerated. The drug is contraindicated in those with asthma and other conditions in which cholinergic therapy may aggravate symptoms.

Antireflux Surgery (Step 5) includes fundoplication, crural tightening, and return of the esophagogastric junction to below the diaphragm. This represents a more aggressive approach to treatment that is best reserved for patients who experience disablingly refractory symptoms or such complications as stricture, bleeding, Barrett's esophagus, or pulmonary aspiration. Results are best in younger patients and those with preserved function of the esophageal body. A major complication of surgery is difficulty with gastric emptying, which can lead to chronic bloating. Normal gastric emptying should be demonstrated before a patient is subjected to surgery. It appears that a substantial percentage of surgical repairs break down after 5 years, so that reoperation must be considered. Symptoms do not necessarily return.

Long-term Management. Management of gastroesophageal reflux disease can be a challenge because relapse rates are high, so that dietary, postural, behavioral, and even pharmacologic measures must be continued indefinitely. Moreover, severe disease may require long-term pharmacologic intervention.

Treatment of Erosive Esophagitis. Persons with endoscopically documented erosive esophagitis should be considered candidates for long-term maintenance *PPI therapy* (e.g., 15 mg of lansoprazole every morning), but only *after* a symptomatic recurrence has been experienced and only if that recurrence has taken place in the context of full implementation of dietary and other nonpharmacologic measures. Immediate implementation of PPI maintenance therapy *before* a symptomatic recurrence should be reserved for those with a severe erosion (grade 4) and those in whom symptoms cause a reduction in quality of life (>25%). The ability of PPI therapy to reduce the risk for development of Barrett's esophagus remains to be determined.

Initial concerns about the *safety* of long-term PPI therapy (e.g., risk for gastrin-stimulated carcinoid stomach tumors, noted in mice) have not materialized to date, so that most authorities prescribe long-term PPI treatment when necessary. However, the possibility of the development of atrophic gastritis (a risk factor for gastric carcinoma) as a consequence of long-term PPI therapy in persons with concurrent *Helicobacter pylori* infection should be kept in mind, and any *Helicobacter* infection should be eradicated (see Chapter 68).

If prolonged PPI use is a concern, then one can consider a maintenance program of long-term *H₂-blocker* therapy. Sometimes, reduced doses will suffice (e.g., 150 mg of ranitidine daily at bedtime). Although H₂-blockers are not as effective as PPIs in healing and preventing recurrences of erosive esophagitis, they may suffice and can control symptoms. *Antireflux surgery* represents a final option for patients with a serious complication or refractory disease, but durability of the repair is a concern.

Screening for and Management of Barrett's Esophagus. Because of the significant malignant potential associated with chronic GERD, *screening* for Barrett's esophagus is recommended in persons who have had symptomatic GERD for at least 5 years and are sufficiently fit and willing to undergo surgery should severe dysplasia or early cancer be found. The cancer risk appears greatest in older white men with long-standing symptomatic GERD. Endoscopic assessment with biopsy is required because mucosal changes may not be visible. Whether persons who become asymptomatic with therapy and have no evidence of Barrett's esophagus on initial screening benefit from continued screening is unknown.

For those found to have changes of Barrett's esophagus without dysplastic transformation, *surveillance* endoscopy is recommended every 3 years thereafter, based on cost-effectiveness data from retrospective series. The finding of low-grade dysplasia requires more frequent surveillance (e.g., every 6 months); the finding of high-grade dysplasia is an indication for consideration of *surgery*. Improved means for detecting dysplasia are under investigation.

Medical therapy for Barrett's esophagus is similar to that for erosive disease (e.g., long-term *PPI* therapy; see above). The immediate goal is to eliminate symptoms of heartburn and regurgitation. Although Barrett's esophagus is not known to be reversible by medical therapy, it is hoped that long-term PPI therapy will reduce the risk for progression to dysplasia and cancer by minimizing further esophageal injury. The risks associated with long-term PPI treatment are not well known but appear to be modest (see above).

Attempts to reverse the histologic changes associated with Barrett's esophagus are under study and include a variety of ablative approaches based on laser and other techniques in combination with PPI therapy. The hope is that by removing the metaplastic epithelial tissue and providing a reduced acid environment, the esophagus will heal by laying down normal squamous mucosa.

Chronic Cough. In some patients, chronic reflux has resulted in respiratory problems, particularly chronic cough, believed to be caused by nocturnal reflux and subsequent aspiration (see Chapter 41). Pharyngitis, nocturnal coughing and choking spells, and wheezing have also been described. A trial of antireflux therapy is indicated when a patient with chronic pulmonary complaints reports symptoms of reflux. Several weeks of treatment may be needed to allow for airway healing before symptom resolution is noted. Any use of theophylline for pulmonary complaints in patients with reflux should be stopped because it can aggravate the problem by reducing LES pressure (see Chapter 48).

PATIENT EDUCATION AND INDICATIONS FOR REFERRAL

Successful management depends heavily on the patient's compliance with medications, diet, and postural measures. A thorough explanation of the mechanisms of reflux and its aggravating factors helps provide a rational basis for the patient's action. Patients need to realize that no single measure will alleviate the discomfort of reflux, but when all are performed together, relief is extremely likely. The lack of direct connection between hiatus hernia and reflux also deserves mention because this is commonly misunderstood, often leading to a belief that surgery is required for treatment.

The chief indication for referral is consideration of endoscopy, indicated in persons with chronic symptomatic disease of at least 5 years' duration, dysphagia, odynophagia, unexplained weight loss, or iron-deficiency anemia. Surgical referral is worth considering in persons who remain symptomatic despite maximal medical therapy. Modern laparoscopic techniques provide minimally invasive approaches to surgical correction; however, some question remains regarding the durability of such corrections.

ANNOTATED BIBLIOGRAPHY

Achkar E, Carey W. The cost of surveillance for adenocarcinoma complicating Barrett's esophagus. Am J Gastroenterol 1988;83:291. (*Annual incidence is 0.6%; yearly surveillance cost is $62,000, and 78 days of work are lost to find one cancer.*)

Feldman M. Comparison of the effects of over-the-counter famotidine and calcium carbonate antacid on postprandial gastric acid: a randomized controlled trial. JAMA 1996;275:1428. (*Effects on gastric acidity were similar, but the antacid had a rapid onset of action and short duration of action; the H₂-blocker had a delayed onset and long duration.*)

Gaynor EB. Otolaryngologic manifestations of gastroesophageal reflux. Am J Gastroenterol 1991;86:801. (*Voice change, chronic cough, and lump in throat are among the ear, nose, and throat symptoms reported.*)

Harding SM, Richter JE, Guzzo MR, et al. Asthma and gastroesophageal reflux: acid suppressive therapy improves asthma outcome. Am J Med 1996;100:395. (*Evidence for the link between reflux and this suspected respiratory complication.*)

Harris RA, Kupperman M, Richter JE. Prevention of recurrences of erosive reflux esophagitis: a cost-effectiveness analysis of maintenance proton pump inhibition. Am J Med 1997;102:78. (*A decision-analysis study finding that maintenance therapy is cost-effective after a recurrence and at the outset only for those who have grade 4 disease or a marked decline in quality of life.*)

Harvey RF, Hadley N, Gill TR. Effects of sleeping with the bed head raised and of ranitidine in patients with severe peptic oesophagitis. Lancet 1987;2:1200. (*Both were better than either alone; each was equally effective alone.*)

Hillman AL, Bloom BS, Fendrick AM, et al. Cost and quality effects of alternative treatments for persistent gastroesophageal reflux disease. Arch Intern Med 1992;152:1467. (*A decision-analysis study suggests that PPI therapy may be best for patients who fail step 1 therapy.*)

Hinder RA, Perdikis G, Klinger PJ, et al. The surgical option for gastroesophageal reflux disease. Am J Med 1997;103(5A)144S. (*Review of surgical options for treatment.*)

Howden CW, Castell DO, Cohen S, et al. The rationale for continuous maintenance treatment of reflux esophagitis. Arch Intern Med

1995;155;1465. (*A review supporting the long-term prophylactic use of acid neutralization in patients with severe esophagitis.*)

Kitchin LI, Castell DO. Rationale and efficacy of conservative therapy for gastroesophageal reflux disease. Arch Intern Med 1991;151:448. (*Review stressing the importance of dietary, lifestyle, and antacid regimens.*)

Klinkenberg-Knol EC, Festen HPM, Jansen JBMJ, et al. Long-term treatment with omeprazole for refractory reflux esophagitis: efficacy and safety. Ann Intern Med 1994;121:161. (*Treatment of 5 years or more was effective but associated with an increased freqeuency of atrophic gastritis.*)

Kuipers EJ, Lundell L, Klinkenberg-Knol EC, et al. Atrophic gastritis and *Helicobacter pylori* infection in patients with reflux esophagitis treated with omeprazole or fundoplication. N Engl J Med 1996;334:1018. (*Potentially important consequence of this infection and long-term use of PPI therapy.*)

Lagergren J, Bergstrom A, Lindgren A, et al. Symptomatic gastroesophageal reflux as a risk factor for esophageal adenocarcinoma. N Engl J Med 1999;340:825. (*A population study demonstrating a strong, dose-related, independent risk for adenocarcinoma of the esophagus conferred by symptomatic reflux.*)

Mittal RK. Hiatal hernia: myth or reality? Am J Med 1997:103 (5A)33S. (*Good review of the relation of hiatal hernia to GERD.*)

Mittal RK, Balaban DH. The esophagogastric junction. N Engl J Med 1997;336:924. (*Excellent review of pathophysiology; 54 references.*)

Richter JE, Castell DO. Drugs, foods, and other substances in the cause and treatment of reflux esophagitis. Med Clin North Am 1981;65:1223. (*Review of precipitants and importance of attending to them in treatment.*)

Robinson M, Lanza F, Avner D, et al. Effective maintenance treatment of reflux esophagitis with low-dose lansoprazole: a randomized, double-blind, placebo-controlled trial. Ann Intern Med 1996:124:859. (*Low-dose therapy as effective as full-dose program in persons with erosive esophagitis during the course of 1 year.*)

Sabesin SM, Berlin RG, Humphries TJ, et al. Famotidine relieves symptoms of gastroesophageal reflux disease and heals erosions and ulcerations. Results of a multicenter, placebo-controlled, dose-ranging study. Arch Intern Med 1991;151:2394. (*A 20-mg, twice-daily regimen was superior to a single 40-mg dose.*)

Sampliner RE, The Practice Parameters Committee of the American College of Gastroenterology. Practice guidelines on the diagnosis, surveillance and therapy of Barrett's esophagus. Am J Gastroenterol 1998;93;1028. (*Consensus statement on the diagnosis and management of Barrett's esophagus.*)

Sloan S, Rademaker AW, Kahrilas PJ. Determinants of gastroesophageal junction incompetence: hiatal hernia, lower esophageal sphincter, or both. Ann Intern Med 1992;117:977. (*Fresh look at pathophysiologic mechanisms; evidence for both.*)

Spechler SJ. Comparison of medical and surgical therapy for complicated gastroesophageal reflux disease in veterans. N Engl J Med 1992;326:786. (*In men with complicated disease, surgery was better than intensive medical therapy; however, omeprazole was not used.*)

Vigneri S, Termini R, Leandro G, et al. A comparison of five maintenance therapies for reflux esophagitis. N Engl J Med 1995;333;1106. (*PPIs are more effective than H_2-blockers.*)

Winnan GR, Meyer CT, McCallum RW. Interpretation of the Bernstein test. A reappraisal of criteria. Ann Intern Med 1982;96:320. (*Reviews technique and sources of confusion in interpretation of results.*)

Wright TA, Gray MR, Morris AI, et al. Cost-effectiveness of detecting Barrett's esophagus. Gut 1996:39:574. (*Best evidence to date on the cost-effectiveness of surveillance; finds it cost-effective, but study based on retrospective data.*)

62
Evaluation of Jaundice
JAMES M. RICHTER

The onset of jaundice usually prompts the patient or the patient's family to seek medical attention. When associated symptoms are minimal, the patient is likely to present on an ambulatory basis, concerned about hepatitis or cancer. The primary physician needs to distinguish jaundice caused by hepatocellular dysfunction (which can be managed medically) from that caused by biliary tract obstruction (which usually requires an anatomic intervention). More specific determination of etiology is a secondary task that is less important to initial decision making. Effective clinical assessment necessitates familiarity with the mechanisms and clinical presentations of jaundice in addition to the indications for and limitations of the noninvasive diagnostic studies available in the outpatient setting.

PATHOPHYSIOLOGY AND CLINICAL PRESENTATION

The mechanisms responsible for jaundice include excess bilirubin production, decreased hepatic uptake, impaired conjugation, intrahepatic cholestasis, extrahepatic obstruction, and hepatocellular injury. Clinically, jaundice becomes noticeable when the serum bilirubin level reaches 2.0 to 2.5 mg/100 mL.

The yellow hue may be mimicked by carotenemia, but in the latter no scleral icterus is present. Deeply jaundiced patients often demonstrate a greenish tinge resulting from the oxidation of bilirubin to biliverdin.

Excess Bilirubin Production results from accelerated red cell destruction. Occasionally, markedly ineffective erythropoiesis may be responsible. The excessive amounts of hemoglobin and resultant bilirubin released into the bloodstream overwhelm the normal hepatic capacity for uptake, and an unconjugated hyperbilirubinemia ensues. Total bilirubin rises as a result of the increased indirect fraction. The results of all tests of hepatocellular function are normal (as are urine and stool appearances). Symptoms, signs, and laboratory test findings point to hemolysis or ineffective erythropoiesis (see Chapter 79).

Decreased Uptake and Conjugation are other mechanisms of unconjugated hyperbilirubinemia. The only evidence of hepatocellular dysfunction is an increase in unconjugated bilirubin. Frequently, a concurrent acquired illness, such as an infection, cardiac disease, or cancer, is present. Hereditary conditions, such as Gilbert's and Crigler-Najjar syndromes, are often responsible. *Gilbert's syndrome* is the most common cause. This is a benign disorder that produces recurrent, self-limited episodes of mild jaundice. Typically, the unconjugated fraction rises to no more than 1.5 to 3.0 mg/100 mL. In Gilbert's syndrome, fasting and minor illness can precipitate jaundice.

Intrahepatic Cholestasis may occur at a number of levels: intracellularly (e.g., hepatitis), at the canalicular level (when estrogen-induced), at the ductule (phenothiazine exposure), at the septal ducts (primary biliary cirrhosis), and at the intralobular ducts (cholangiocarcinoma). Regardless of site, there are similarities in presentation. Jaundice begins gradually; pruritus is common. The liver is large, smooth, and nontender; it may be firm but not rock-hard. Splenomegaly is unlikely except in primary biliary cirrhosis. Stools are pale, and steatorrhea develops in severe cases. A hyperbilirubinemia is present, predominantly of the conjugated fraction, with marked alkaline phosphatase elevation, mild transaminase rise, and normal serum albumin. Urine is dark and positive for bilirubin. The prothrombin time may be prolonged because of malabsorption, but the prolongation is reversible by vitamin K injection.

Extrahepatic Obstruction occurs when stone, stricture, or tumor block the flow of bile within the extrahepatic biliary tree. A history of gallstones, biliary tract surgery, or prior malignancy may be elicited. The gallbladder is sometimes palpable, especially when obstruction develops gradually, allowing time for painless dilation of the biliary tree. Sudden onset with pain results from passage of a stone that becomes wedged into the common duct; fever and sepsis may follow shortly thereafter, indicating cholangitis. Weight loss is a nonspecific finding, but when it is marked and accompanied by jaundice, it suggests carcinoma of the head of the pancreas or metastatic disease obstructing the common duct. Extrahepatic obstruction and intrahepatic cholestasis may be identical in presentation. The liver is usually enlarged; tenderness is minimal unless cholangitis or rapid distention occurs. A rock-hard mass strongly points to malignancy. As in intrahepatic cholestasis, conjugated bilirubin exhibits the greatest rise in association with a high serum alkaline phosphatase level and a mild to moderate increase in the transaminase level. Any prolongation of the prothrombin time is at least partially reversible with parenteral vitamin K. Urine is dark because of the conjugated bilirubinuria. Stools are pale from absence of bile.

Hepatocellular Disease is typified by hepatitis, with prodromal symptoms of anorexia, nausea, abdominal pain, and malaise preceding jaundice (see Chapters 52 and 70). Hepatic tenderness and some hepatomegaly are common. Ecchymoses may be present. Transaminases may reach dramatic levels, except in cases of hepatitis C and alcoholic hepatitis, in which the rise is no more than five times normal. The alkaline phosphatase rises modestly to two to four times above the baseline. Urine is dark, and stools are pale. There may be evidence of decreased protein synthesis. The prothrombin time is the first measure of synthetic function to become abnormal because the half-lives of the clotting factors made in the liver are less than 7 days. If synthetic function remains de-

Table 62-1.   Differential Diagnosis of Jaundice by Pathophysiologic Mechanisms

Unconjugated Hyperbilirubinemias (urine negative for bilirubin)
Increased bilirubin production
Decreased hepatic uptake of bilirubin
Decreased conjugation
Conjugated Hyperbilirubinemias (urine positive for bilirubin)
Hepatocellular disease
Intrahepatic cholestasis
Extrahepatic obstruction

pressed beyond 2 weeks, the serum albumin begins to fall. Chronic hepatocellular disease may lead to fibrosis and cirrhosis with portal hypertension, peripheral edema, ascites, gynecomastia, testicular atrophy, bleeding, and encephalopathy (see Chapter 71).

DIFFERENTIAL DIAGNOSIS

The causes of jaundice are extensive but can be grouped according to major pathophysiologic mechanisms and type of hyperbilirubinemia (conjugated or unconjugated; Table 62.1). It is important to recognize that more than one mechanism can be operating in a given case. The vast majority of cases are caused by obstruction, intrahepatic cholestasis, or hepatocellular injury. In young patients, hepatitis predominates. In the elderly, stones and tumor are often responsible. Drugs account for many cases of intrahepatic cholestasis, with symptoms often mimicking those of extrahepatic etiologies.

WORKUP

The *history and physical examination* often provide a diagnosis or at least indicate whether the underlying pathophysiology is hepatocellular injury or biliary obstruction. In a study of 61 cases of jaundice documented by liver biopsy, history and physical examination alone correctly identified 70% of viral hepatitis cases, 80% of cirrhosis cases, and 77% of those with obstructive jaundice.

History. Key historical items found useful for discriminating among etiologies include the presence of abdominal pain (indicative of obstruction) and a history of alcoholism, exposure to hepatitis, and flulike onset (all suggestive of a hepatocellular etiology). Of little discriminant value are a history of weight loss, pruritus, nausea, vomiting, and distaste for tobacco. Dark urine and pale stools confirm a conjugated hyperbilirubinemia but do not distinguish between hepatic and obstructive disease. Absence of abdominal pain does not rule out obstruction, especially that which develops slowly from tumor growth or primary biliary cirrhosis. The history should also be checked for other hepatocellular disease risk factors (e.g., previous blood transfusion, travel to an area endemic for hepatitis, consumption of raw shellfish, IV drug abuse, high-risk sexual practices, use of potentially hepatotoxic drugs). A history of gallstones, previous biliary tract surgery, and high fever points toward an obstructive cause. A family history of episodic jaundice in the setting of an intercurrent illness is consistent with Gilbert's disease. Intrahepatic cholestasis is a consideration if the patient reports use of estrogens, phenothiazines, and other drugs that can cause cholestasis.

Physical Examination. Findings that favor a diagnosis of advanced hepatocellular disease include a small liver, signs of portal hypertension (ascites, splenomegaly, prominent abdominal venous pattern), asterixis, peripheral edema (from hypoalbuminemia), spider angiomata, gynecomastia, and palmar erythema. Mild to moderate hepatic enlargement and mild tenderness to punch are also consistent with early or mild hepatocellular disease, especially that caused by acute viral hepatitis. A palpable gallbladder (Courvoisier's sign) suggests malignant obstruction of the common bile duct. Marked hepatic enlargement (6 cm or more below the inferior costal margin) occurs in some instances of extrahepatic obstruction and also in advanced hepatic infiltration, severe passive hepatic congestion, and metastatic cancer to the liver. If obstruction is acute in onset, there may be some associated guarding, rebound tenderness, and fever. The finding of ecchymoses is consistent with both obstructive and hepatocellular mechanisms. The same is true for the detection of pale stools and dark urine.

Laboratory Investigation can be used to identify the predominant pathophysiology and to assess severity, especially when the history and physical examination findings are nondiagnostic. Testing begins with a check of the *urine* for *bilirubin*, a simple, inexpensive, yet often overlooked test that can be performed quickly in the office. Because only conjugated bilirubin appears in the urine, its presence indicates a conjugated hyperbilirubinemia and the possibility of cholestasis, obstruction, or hepatocellular injury; its absence argues for excess bilirubin production, decreased uptake, and impaired conjugation. Determinations of *direct* and *indirect serum bilirubin* levels quantitatively confirm urinary findings and indicate disease severity.

Unconjugated Hyperbilirubinemia. An elevation predominantly of the unconjugated bilirubin fraction and urine negative for bilirubin should initiate a search for hemolysis (see Chapter 79), ineffective erythropoiesis, hereditary causes of jaundice, and concurrent systemic illness. Standard "liver function tests" add little to the assessment of unconjugated hyperbilirubinemia; results are normal or very mildly and nonspecifically elevated.

Conjugated Hyperbilirubinemia: Differentiating Hepatocellular Injury from Intrahepatic and Extrahepatic Cholestasis. The finding of bilirubin in the urine should focus attention on the liver and biliary tree. Testing needs to include determinations of serum *transaminases* [serum glutamic–oxaloacetic transaminase (SGOT), serum glutamic–pyruvic transaminase (SGPT)]; the newer nomenclature refers to them as *aminotransferases* [aspartate aminotransferase (AST), alanine aminotransferase (ALT)]. *Alkaline phosphatase*, *prothrombin time*, and *serum albumin* must also be determined. Mechanical obstruction and intrahepatic cholestasis are characterized by marked rises in *alkaline phosphatase* (four to five times normal) and modest elevations in *transaminases* (two to three times normal). Hepatocellular disease characteristically causes a proportionately far greater rise in serum transaminase levels than in alkaline phosphatase concentrations. As noted earlier, two exceptions are hepatitis C and alcoholic hepatitis, in which transaminases may be only mildly elevated (no more than two to three times the upper limits of normal). SGPT (ALT) elevations are more specific for liver disease; SGOT (AST) also rises with myocardial or skeletal muscle injury.

The differentiation of hepatocellular disease from cholestatic and obstructive conditions can be attempted by studying measures of liver synthetic function and, if need be, their response to vitamin K. A prolonged *prothrombin time* unresponsive to parenteral *vitamin K* (IM or SQ administration is preferred because of reports of anaphylaxis with IV administration) is strongly suggestive of hepatocellular failure. Cholestasis and obstruction may also produce prolongation of the prothrombin time, but it can be reversed by vitamin K. *Serum albumin* levels fall when substantial hepatocellular injury has occurred and synthetic capacity has been suppressed for a few weeks. Interpretation of the albumin level requires consideration of dietary intake and sources of possible protein loss.

Liver biopsy is sometimes needed to determine the cause of hepatocellular injury (see also Chapters 70 and 71), but is unwise in the setting of possible obstructive jaundice because it can lead to bile peritonitis if obstruction is present. Once obstruction is ruled out or relieved, biopsy is an important consideration, especially when evidence of hepatic failure, portal hypertension, or encephalopathy is present, or when jaundice persists longer than 3 months.

Marked Elevation in Alkaline Phosphatase: Differentiating Extrahepatic Obstruction from Intrahepatic Cholestasis. A marked elevation in alkaline phosphatase occurs in the setting of obstructive pathophysiology as well as intrahepatic cholestasis. The latter occasionally occurs in some cases of hepatocellular injury, such as viral, alcoholic, and drug-induced forms of hepatitis. However, a low alkaline phosphatase level (<50 IU/100 mL) is rarely seen in the presence of extrahepatic obstruction. Elevations in alkaline phosphatase also occur in settings of increased bone metabolism. Bony causes can be distinguished from hepatobiliary causes by measuring the *heat-stable fraction* of the enzyme or the *5'-nucleotidase* (these are of hepatobiliary tract origin).

Although hepatocellular disease can usually be distinguished from cholestasis and extrahepatic obstruction on the basis of clinical data and results of liver function tests (including response to vitamin K), cholestasis and obstruction may be indistinguishable without further testing. Clinical evaluation and liver function tests have a sensitivity of 90% for detection of obstruction, but they have a predictive value of only 75%; 25% of patients suspected on clinical grounds of having obstruction turn out to have intrahepatic cholestasis. The distinction is critical to management because mechanical obstruction requires direct surgical, endoscopic, or radiologic intervention to restore bile flow.

Thus, the clinical impression of obstruction must be confirmed by imaging techniques. Only when the clinical likelihood of obstruction is very low is imaging of the biliary tree unnecessary for differentiating intrahepatic cholestasis from extrahepatic obstruction. Available imaging modalities include the following:

Ultrasonography. This is the noninvasive imaging technique of choice to assess the biliary tree in the evaluation of jaundice. Specificity is better than 90%. Sensitivity ranges from 47% to 90%, depending on the duration and degree of bile duct obstruction. Cases of early, acute, or intermittent obstruction may be missed unless ultrasonographic study is repeated after the ducts have had a few days to dilate. False-positive results may occur when ductal dilation persists after cholecystectomy or relief of obstruction. In about half of cases, ultrasonography cannot indicate the level of obstruction, nor is it particularly good at detecting the cause of the obstruction unless it is a mass in the head of the pancreas. Stones in the common duct are frequently missed (sensitivity of 50% if duct not dilated, 75% if duct dilated). Ultrasonographic studies in patients with overlying bowel gas or marked obesity are often of inadequate technical quality, so that a repeated study or computed tomography is required.

Computed Tomography is similar to ultrasonography in sensitivity, specificity, and predictive value for the diagnosis of obstructive jaundice. It has many of the same shortcomings plus greater expense and radiation exposure. As such, it is a second-choice test after ultrasonography. However, results are not obscured by overlying bowel gas or fat, and the ability to detect the level of obstruction is better than with ultrasonography. Moreover, if surgical intervention is being considered, the test is helpful in providing more definitive anatomic information. Nonetheless, cholangiography is usually still necessary.

Other Imaging Modalities: *Percutaneous Transhepatic Cholangiography, Endoscopic Retrograde Cholangiopancreatography, Magnetic Resonance Cholangiopancreatography.* If common duct obstruction is strongly suspected on clinical grounds (even if ultrasonography or computed tomography is nondiagnostic), or if additional anatomic detail is required for planning treatment, then percutaneous trans-hepatic cholangiography or endoscopic retrograde cholangiopancreatography with retrograde cannulation of the common bile duct can be performed. Both procedures are relatively safe, have similar complication rates and rates of visualization, and provide equally diagnostic information. The predictive value of a positive test result is very high, but occasionally stones are missed in dilated ductal systems.

Trans-hepatic cholangiography is technically simple in patients with dilated intrahepatic ducts; however, 3% to 10% of patients experience cholangitis, hemorrhage, or bile leakage.

Endoscopic retrograde cholangiopancreatography (ERCP) is more difficult but allows examination of the ampulla and pancreas and has a slightly lower incidence of serious complications. For patients who may have a retained common duct stone after cholecystectomy, the opportunity to perform an endoscopic papillotomy makes the retrograde cholangiogram advantageous. Techniques have been developed for draining an obstructed biliary tract either endoscopically or trans-hepatically. Overall, both procedures are valuable diagnostically and have therapeutic uses also; final selection is based on the clinical circumstance in addition to local availability and expertise. Selection should be made in consultation with a surgeon, radiologist, or gastroenterologist experienced in evaluating obstructive jaundice.

Magnetic resonance cholangiopancreatography (MRCP) provides a new, noninvasive alternative to these two invasive modalities. Test sensitivity for pathology in the common bile duct, particularly stones, is superior to that of ultrasonography or computed tomography and approaches that of the invasive modalities. The cost is slightly less than that of ERCP, and safety is greater because no dye load or invasive procedure is required. Some have suggested that MRCP be used to screen patients for ERCP candidacy.

Ancillary Testing. Other studies deserve comment, more for their limited usefulness than because they are indicated in evaluation of jaundice. *Plain films* of the abdomen and *upper gastrointestinal series* rarely provide diagnostic information. *Hepatobiliary scintigraphy* is better suited for the diagnosis of cholecystitis; it provides poor anatomic resolution and often cannot aid in distinguishing between intrahepatic cholestasis and extrahepatic obstruction. *Cholescintigraphy* is useful for the diagnosis of acute cholecystitis and cystic duct obstruction (see Chapter 69), but it has no value in the evaluation of jaundice and can be misleading.

INDICATIONS FOR ADMISSION, CONSULTATION, AND REFERRAL

Most patients with jaundice turn out to have acute viral hepatitis and can be managed on an ambulatory basis, unless they are unable to maintain their hydration or begin to show evidence of severe hepatocellular failure (see Chapter 71). Admission is mandatory when jaundice is complicated by fever and peritoneal signs indicative of *cholangitis*. IV antibiotics and prompt surgical consultation are required.

As noted earlier, if extrahepatic obstruction is suspected clinically, consultation with a gastroenterologist, surgeon, or radiologist experienced in the evaluation of jaundice can be very useful, especially when it is difficult to differentiate between intrahepatic cholestasis and extrahepatic obstruction.

When hepatocellular disease is suspected and evidence of hepatic failure, portal hypertension, or encephalopathy is present, or when jaundice persists for longer than 3 months, liver biopsy may be indicated for definitive diagnosis. Consultation should be sought with a gastroenterologist familiar with liver disease and needle biopsy techniques.

SYMPTOMATIC RELIEF

Mild jaundice in itself is innocuous, but more marked elevations in bilirubin may produce considerable pruritus. Presumably, the mechanism involves the deposition of bile salts in the skin, although recent evidence refutes this view. Cholestyramine has been used successfully to treat pruritus and is worth a try in patients who are uncomfortable. One 9-g packet of the powder containing 4 g of cholestyramine resin is mixed in orange juice or apple sauce and taken three times a day. Absorption of fat-soluble vitamins may be impaired by cholestyramine, and oral or parenteral supplements of vitamins A, D, and K can be prescribed. Cholestyramine may also interfere with the absorption of drugs; they should be taken at least 1 hour before cholestyramine. Constipation or diarrhea is a minor common side effect.

ANNOTATED BIBLIOGRAPHY

Barish MA, Yucel EK, Ferrucci JT. Magnetic resonance cholangiopancreatography. N Engl J Med 1999;341:258. (*A review of this new, noninvasive alternative to ERCP for imaging the pancreaticobiliary tree.*)

Chan Y-L, Chan ACW, Lam WWM, et al. Choledocholithiasis: comparison of MR cholangiography and endoscopic retrograde cholangiopancreatography. Radiology 1996;200:85. (*Promising results for magnetic resonance imaging; sensitivity in excess of 90%.*)

Datta D, Sherlock S. Cholestyramine for long-term relief of the pruritus complicating intrahepatic cholestasis. Gastroenterology 1966; 50:323. (*Cholestyramine is effective; 4 to 7 days of therapy is required before relief is obtained.*)

Felsher B, Rickard D, Redeker A. The reciprocal relation between caloric intake and the degree of hyperbilirubinemia in Gilbert's syndrome. N Engl J Med 1970;283:170. (*Increase in unconjugated bilirubin occurred with fasting or very low caloric intake.*)

Frank BB, Members of the Patient Care Committee of the American Gastroenterological Association. Clinical evaluation of jaundice. JAMA 1989;262:3031. (*Comprehensive yet terse overview of the approach to the jaundiced patient.*)

Fregia A, Jensen DM. Evaluation of abnormal liver function tests. Compr Ther 1994;20:50. (*Assessment of abnormal liver function tests from a cost-conscious perspective.*)

Levine R, Klatskin G. Unconjugated hyperbilirubinemia in the absence of overt hemolysis. Am J Med 1964;36:541. (*High proportion traceable to a concurrent illness.*)

Matzen P, Malchow-Moller A, Brun B. Ultrasound, computed tomography, and cholescintigraphy in suspected obstructive jaundice. Gastroenterology 1983;84:1492. (*Presents data on test sensitivity and specificity.*)

Mueller PR, van Sonnenberg E, Simenone JF. Fine needle transhepatic cholangiography. Ann Intern Med 1982;97:567. (*Radiologist's view of this technique and its central role in the evaluation of biliary obstruction.*)

O'Connor KW, Snodgrass PJ, Swonder JE, et al. A blinded prospective study comparing four current noninvasive approaches in the differential diagnosis of medical versus surgical jaundice. Gastroenterology 1983;84:1498. (*Demonstrates the importance and accuracy of clinical evaluation.*)

Richter JM, Silverstein MD, Schapiro RH. Suspected obstructive jaundice: a decision analysis of diagnostic strategies. Ann Intern Med 1983;99:46. (*Comparison of comprehensive diagnostic strategies for the investigation of suspected obstructive jaundice.*)

Saini S. Imaging of the hepatobiliary tract. N Engl J Med 1997; 336:1889. (*Terse, practical review with data on sensitivity and specificity of imaging studies; good guide to test selection.*)

Scharschmidt BF, Goldberg HI, Schmid R. Approach to the patient with cholestatic jaundice. N Engl J Med 1983;308:1515. (*Good review of tests available for workup of obstructive jaundice.*)

Schenker S, Balint J, Schiff L. Differential diagnosis of jaundice: report of a prospective study of 61 proved cases. Am J Dig Dis 1962;7:449. (*Classic study of the merits of clinical features and laboratory tests in the differential diagnosis of jaundice.*)

Sherman KE. Alanine aminotransferase in clinical practice. Arch Intern Med 1991;151:260. (*Review of this increasingly used aminotransferase for detection of hepatocellular injury.*)

Appendix: Evaluation of the Patient with an Incidental Asymptomatic Elevation in Serum Transaminase (Aminotransferase) Levels

An incidental asymptomatic elevation in serum transaminase (aminotransferase) is not infrequently encountered during routine blood testing. Transaminases are often included in standard multiphasic testing packages, so that their determination in the absence of a true clinical indication is rather common. In settings in which the pretest probability of underlying hepatocellular disease is very low, most elevations are likely to represent false-positive results that warrant only a repeated determination in 4 weeks and cessation of intake of alcohol and any potentially offending drugs. However, before the finding is dismissed, it is important to review the history for risk factors for important conditions associated with long-term subclinical hepatocellular injury.

Differential Diagnosis. The causes of such low-grade, subclinical hepatocellular injury include mild, chronic, active *hepatitis C*, *hepatitis B*, and hepatitis associated with *autoimmune* disease (including primary biliary cirrhosis). Chronic occult liver injury may also occur in *hereditary hemochromatosis*, the most common genetic disorder among white Americans. Fatty liver is an important cause, resulting in half of instances from surreptitious *alcohol* abuse; *nonalcoholic steatohepatitis* accounts for the remainder of cases. About half of cases of nonalcoholic statohepatitis are a consequence of *obesity*, *hyperlipidemia*, or *diabetes*, but for another 40% to 50% of cases, no clear precipitant can be found. A rare cause of isolated transaminase elevation is *Wilson's disease*.

Workup. Before a workup is undertaken, the transaminase level should be measured again in 4 weeks, after the patient has refrained from alcohol and any noncritical drugs with potential to cause hepatocellular injury. Once the elevation is confirmed, a focused workup should ensue.

History is reviewed for risk factors for viral hepatitis (see Chapter 57) and alcohol abuse (see Chapter 233), for symptoms of autoimmune disease (see Chapter 146), and for a family history of hemochromatosis or its complications (cirrhosis, heart failure, diabetes, arthritis) not explained by other causes. More commonly, persons with hereditary hemochromatosis may first note fatigue and arthralgias. Medications need to be reviewed in detail. In addition, a review of symptoms pertinent to estimating the severity of hepatocellular injury (fatigue, easy bruising, jaundice) should be included.

Physical Examination should be noted for any etiologic clues, such as hyperpigmentation, arthritis, and liver enlargement. Examining for signs of hepatocellular injury (jaundice, ecchymoses, spider angiomata) is also warranted.

Laboratory Studies can begin with an assessment of the type and severity of hepatocellular injury. Measuring the *alkaline phosphatase* level helps to determine if the problem has a cholestatic component (see above). The *serum albumin* and *prothrombin time* are the best parameters of hepatocellular synthetic function and helpful in determining degree of injury. Potentially useful diagnostic tests should be selected on the basis of clinical suspicion and not simply ordered uncritically as a standard panel for assessment of an isolated SGOT elevation.

If alcohol abuse is suspected, the diagnosis might be supported by a determination of the *SGPT* (ALT) and SGOT (AST); an SGPT-to-SGOT ratio of 2:1 is characteristic of alcoholic liver injury. Risk factors for viral hepatitis are an indication for *hepatitis serology* (e.g., antibodies to hepatitis B virus, hepatitis C virus, and hepatitis B surface antigen; see Chapter 57). Any suspicion of autoimmune disease is an indication for an antinuclear antibody determination (see Chapter 146) in addition to an *antimitochondrial antibody* determination. *Ultrasonography* is helpful to assess suspected fatty liver and the cholestatic pattern on liver function tests (see above).

If the patient has a family history of idiopathic cirrhosis or other features of suggestive of hemochromatosis (fatigue, arthralgias, poor libido, diabetes), the serum *iron, transferrin* (total iron-binding capacity), and *ferritin* should be measured. A transferrin saturation (ratio of serum iron to total iron-binding capacity) above 45% is the screening threshold used by most authorities to diagnose hemochromatosis. The ferritin concentration helps determine the degree of iron overload; treatment is usually indicated when it is above 300 μg/L in men and above 200 μg/L in women. The young patient with concurrent neuropsychiatric disease should be considered for a serum ceruloplasmin determination to check for Wilson's disease.

A key question is the utility of *liver biopsy* in persons who present with incidental transaminase elevation. Biopsy is certainly useful to determine disease extent and severity when a particular condition has been identified before biopsy (e.g., he-

patitis C), but the contribution of biopsy to diagnosis in idiopathic cases is less clear. In a review of biopsies performed in such cases, steatosis was found in the vast majority of cases, and chronic hepatitis plus cirrhosis accounted only for about a fourth. One needs to ask if the result will change management of the patient; if so, then biopsy for diagnosis is worth considering. Given the high frequency of occult steatosis, one might take an alternative approach to biopsy in the obese or diabetic person and recommend exercise, diet, and weight loss followed by a repetition of liver function tests.

A.H.G.

ANNOTATED BIBLIOGRAPHY

Bacon BR, Farahvash MJ, Janney CG, et al. Nonalcoholic steatohepatitis: an expanded clinical entity. Gastroenterology 1994;107: 1103. (*Good review of this increasingly appreciated cause of fatty liver and asymptomatic transaminase elevation.*)

Powell LW, George DK, McDonnell SM, et al. Diagnosis of hemochromatosis. Ann Intern Med 1998;129:925. (*Best review of this important, often missed cause of incidental transaminase elevation; 41 references.*)

63

Evaluation of Gastrointestinal Bleeding

JAMES M. RICHTER

Ambulatory patients frequently report gastrointestinal bleeding to the primary physician. They may complain of *melena* (tarry black stools), *hematochezia* (bright red or maroon blood per rectum), or *hematemesis* (vomiting fresh or changed blood). Sometimes, gastrointestinal bleeding may be evident only as a *positive result on a screening test for fecal occult blood*. Decisions regarding the nature and pace of the evaluation of gastrointestinal bleeding depend on the characteristics, severity, and acuteness of the problem. Proper decision making requires a knowledge of the probability of a serious underlying lesion and of the sensitivity and specificity of contrast studies, endoscopy, and stool guaiac testing.

PATHOPHYSIOLOGY AND CLINICAL PRESENTATION

Hematemesis usually represents bleeding proximal to the ligament of Treitz, although the site of blood loss may on rare occasions be in the jejunum. The absence of hematemesis does not, however, exclude the possibility of active upper gastrointestinal bleeding. *Melena* is usually seen with blood loss proximal to the ileocecal valve, where hemoglobin is converted into hematin, which gives the stool its tarry appearance. Right-sided colonic bleeding may also cause melena when transit is slow. *Hematochezia* most often originates in the left side of the colon or anorectal region, although very brisk movement of blood from the right side of the colon, small bowel, or even stomach can lead to a similar presentation. *Occult gastrointestinal bleeding* may be indicated by a positive result on a test for fecal occult blood or may be suggested by the presence of iron-deficiency anemia without apparent cause. The source of occult bleeding may be anywhere in the gastrointestinal tract.

Manifestations of blood loss are a function of the rate and duration of bleeding. *Postural hypotension* (an orthostatic fall in blood pressure of <10 mm Hg or an increase in heart rate of >10 beats/min on moving from a supine position to standing) in the setting of known bleeding suggests intravascular volume depletion and serious acute hemorrhage. *Fatigue* and *exertional dyspnea* are typical presenting symptoms of anemia resulting from slow, chronic blood loss. Patient descriptions of the volume of bleeding are frequently unreliable.

DIFFERENTIAL DIAGNOSIS

The chief causes of gastrointestinal bleeding can be conveniently grouped by clinical presentation (Table 63.1). Hematemesis prompts consideration of important upper gastroinintestinal etiologies. Melena requires consideration of upper gastrointestinal causes and of small-intestinal and right-sided colonic sources. Hematochezia raises the question of anorectal or colonic disease and, if brisk, a small-bowel or even upper gastrointestinal lesion. The prevalence of specific disorders varies with the population studied, diagnostic methods employed, and time of investigation in relation to bleeding.

Melena or Hematemesis. A British series of 277 patients with melena or hematemesis provides representative prevalence figures in a population composed of both outpatients and patients seen in emergency departments. More than 85% of the patients in this study underwent endoscopy; diagnosis was also made by upper gastrointestinal series or at surgery: 20% had duodenal ulcers, 15% had gastric ulcers, 12% had Mallory-Weiss tears, 11% had esophageal varices, 5% had gastritis, and

Table 63.1. Differential Diagnosis
of Gastrointestinal Bleeding

Hematemesis
Esophageal varices
Esophagitis
Esophageal ulceration
Mallory-Weiss tear
Esophageal cancer
Gastritis or duodenitis
Gastric or duodenal ulcer
Gastric neoplasm (carcinoma, lymphoma, or rarely leiomyoma/
sarcoma)
Telangiectasia
Angiodysplasia, especially in patients with renal failure

Melena
All causes of hematemesis plus:
Meckel's diverticulum
Crohn's disease
Small-bowel neoplasms (rare)

Hematochezia
Hemorrhoid
Anal fissure
Colonic polyp
Colorectal carcinoma
Angiodysplasia
Diverticular disease
Inflammatory bowel disease
Any upper gastrointestinal or small-bowel lesion if bleeding is brisk

1% had gastric cancer. In 21%, no cause was found (half of these patients did not undergo endoscopy), and in 5%, multiple lesions were detected. Patients with chronic renal failure are at increased risk for bleeding, with angiodysplasia and esophagitis being the most common causes.

Hematochezia. In the setting of severe *hematochezia*, age has a major influence on the differential diagnosis. In young adults, Meckel's diverticulum, inflammatory bowel disease, and polyps lead the list of causes. In adults to age 60, diverticulosis, inflammatory bowel disease, and polyps are the predominant etiologies, followed by malignancy and vascular malformations. In persons over the age of 60, vascular ectasia, diverticulosis, malignancy, and polyps are responsible for most cases.

In a study of 311 patients who reported *mild to moderate anorectal bleeding* and were evaluated by careful physical examination, sigmoidoscopy, and barium enema, 79% had lesions of the anal canal, 15% had rectal and colonic disease, and 7% had perianal skin problems. Leading causes were hemorrhoids in 54%, fissure-in-ano in 18%, neoplasm in 6.5%, and inflammatory bowel disease in 5%. In 8%, no cause was found at the time of the examination. The majority of neoplasms were more than 10 cm above the anus, beyond the reach of digital examination.

In a series of 239 patients with *undiagnosed rectal bleeding* who were subjected to colonoscopy, 40% had significant lesions; 16% were found to have polyps, 10% had inflammatory bowel disease, 9% had carcinomas missed by barium enema, and 3% had diverticular disease, hemangiomata, or other causes. In a large percentage of these patients, no cause was found. In a study of anemic competitive runners, an increase in fecal hemoglobin was detected.

Patients with gastrointestinal bleeding while taking *antico-*

agulant medication in a therapeutic range are likely to have an underlying lesion and warrant thorough evaluation. In a study examining 3,800 courses of anticoagulant therapy, gastrointestinal bleeding occurred in 45 patients. In 32 patients, a source was determined; 13 had hemorrhoids, 9 had peptic ulcers, 7 had neoplasms, and 3 had other lesions.

Nosebleeds and *respiratory tract bleeding* must be considered in the differential diagnosis of melena and guaiac-positive stools. A false-positive result on a stool guaiac test can be produced by the use of glycerol guaiacolate (a popular expectorant) or a meal of rare red meat. Black stools may result from bismuth (Pepto-Bismol), iron, charcoal, or spinach intake; red stools can occur after large quantities of beets have been consumed.

WORKUP

The history and physical examination may provide information regarding the location and severity of bleeding, but additional investigations are usually necessary to determine the exact cause. In the previously mentioned series of 311 cases of anorectal bleeding, history and physical examination alone yielded a definite diagnosis in 28%. Nevertheless, history and physical examination have important roles that help in determining the pace of workup and the selection and ordering of tests.

Screening for Major Acute Blood Loss. Whenever active bleeding is suspected in a person presenting to the office, the first priority is to determine the severity and rate of blood loss. The patient should be asked about any *postural light-headedness.* The precise volume lost is not reliably determined by the history, but reports of very large amounts should be taken seriously. When the patient complains of voluminous blood loss or light-headedness, an immediate check of vital signs for *postural hypotension* is indicated. Immediate hospital admission should be considered if the systolic blood pressure falls more than 10 to 15 mm Hg or the heart rate increases by more than 10 to 15 beats/min when the patient stands up from a supine position. The decline in the hematocrit in the acute phase of blood loss may be deceptively small if sufficient time for the reequilibration of intravascular volume has not elapsed.

History. Once it is clear that the degree of blood loss does not pose an immediate hazard, the office evaluation can proceed. Clarifying the nature of the bleeding (melena, hematemesis, or hematochezia) helps not only to assess severity, but also to identify the approximate site of bleeding. Obtaining an accurate description is essential, as is checking for potentially confounding factors. Dark stools must not be mistaken for genuine melena, and one should check for intake of substances that may turn stool black, such as bismuth (Pepto-Bismol), iron, charcoal, or spinach. Red stools can occur after large quantities of beets have been eaten. Factors that can produce a false-positive result on the stool Hemoccult test should be considered (e.g., use of cough syrup containing glycerol guaiacolate, a recent meal of rare red meat), but a positive test result ought not be dismissed lightly.

When hematemesis is reported, sources of esophageal, gastric, and duodenal bleeding must be sought. A history of cirrhosis, chronic liver disease, or alcoholism raises suspicion of esophageal varices. Use of aspirin, alcohol, and antiinflammatory agents suggests bleeding caused by ulceration or gastritis. A history of peptic ulcer or the presence of epigastric pain responsive to antacids or related to food intake raises the possibility of bleeding from a gastric or duodenal ulcer. It is worth noting, however, that another explanation for bleeding may be present in patients with a history typical of ulcer disease, and that more than one potential site of bleeding may be discovered (e.g., esophageal varices).

Even if no hematemesis is noted, the source may still be above the ligament of Treitz; however, small-bowel and colonic lesions become more likely. Diarrhea, urgency, tenesmus, and lower abdominal cramping suggest inflammatory bowel disease (see Chapter 73). With ulcerative colitis, diverticulosis, and other forms of rectosigmoid disease, some frank rectal bleeding is often present. Brisk rectal bleeding in the absence of abdominal pain is particularly common with diverticular disease. Weight loss or change in bowel habits raises suspicion of colonic cancer. A history of diverticular disease may be a clue to the cause of blood loss, but a coincident carcinoma must be ruled out. Many patients with rectal bleeding admit to past or present hemorrhoidal problems, but in almost half of the cases another lesion is found to be the cause of blood loss.

Physical Examination. As noted above, when evidence of acute bleeding is present, the evaluation should begin with a check for *postural signs* and a cardiopulmonary examination to assess the severity of volume loss and the presence of any hemodynamic compromise. Next, the skin is inspected for pallor, ecchymoses, petechiae, telangiectases, and stigmata of chronic liver disease (e.g., jaundice, palmar erythema, spider angiomata). The nose and pharynx are examined for sources of bleeding. Lymph nodes are palpated for enlargement (e.g., left supraclavicular adenopathy suggests an intraabdominal malignancy), and the abdomen is palpated for organomegaly, ascites, and masses. Anorectal lesions are sought on inspection and digital examination; the stool is checked for color and the presence of occult blood (see Chapter 56). Anoscopy is an essential part of the examination for patients who complain of anal symptoms.

If the patient convincingly describes hematemesis, one may assume that the bleeding is from the upper gastrointestinal tract, but if there is evidence of recent significant bleeding of uncertain origin, a nasogastric tube should be passed to aspirate gastric contents and test for the presence of blood. The guaiac test may be insensitive for heme unless the acidic aspirate is neutralized with a few drops of sodium hydroxide.

Laboratory Studies should be performed to determine the chronicity and magnitude of blood loss and the presence of coincident disease. The hemoglobin concentration should be measured in all patients; however, if blood loss is acute, the hemoglobin concentration may not yet accurately reflect the severity of blood loss. A low mean corpuscular volume suggests the possibility of iron deficiency resulting from chronic gastrointestinal blood loss. Studies of coagulation (platelet count, prothrombin time, and partial thromboplastin time) and tests of liver and renal function are useful in checking for factors that may exacerbate bleeding.

Hematochezia. In stable patients, the main concern is the possibility of colon cancer; risk increases with age. Fewer than 5% of such cancers occur in patients under age 40 and fewer than 1% in those under age 30. Thus, if the physical examination or anoscopy reveals a bleeding hemorrhoid or other cause of local anal pathology in a young patient, it may not be necessary to proceed with further tests. The finding on sigmoidoscopy of guaiac-negative stool from above the point of bleeding also provides reassurance. On the other hand, 80% of colorectal malignancies are found in patients over the age of 50. When a person more than 50 years old presents with rectal bleeding, a thorough search for tumor is required, even if a local lesion such as a hemorrhoid is discovered. Twenty-seven percent of patients with carcinoma of the rectum and 10% of those with carcinoma of the sigmoid have been noted to have coincidental hemorrhoids.

Data describing the yields of diagnostic procedures are increasingly available. In the series of 311 patients with bright red rectal bleeding subjected to history, physical examination, sigmoidoscopy, and barium enema, the diagnosis was made by history alone in 5%; physical examination raised the figure to 28%, and the addition of *sigmoidoscopy* provided an explanation in 90%. *Barium enema* raised the yield in this series only another 3%, probably because of the unusually large number of lesions in this study that were within reach of the sigmoidoscope. However, cumulative data suggest that only 30% of colonic malignancies can be viewed by sigmoidoscopy. Consequently, persons with rectal bleeding in the age group at high risk for large-bowel malignancy should undergo additional study. Barium enema has a sensitivity of 70% to 90% for detecting carcinoma and 70% for polyps larger than 5 mm in diameter. Cancers most often missed are in the cecum or rectosigmoid or are obscured by concurrent diverticulosis or ulcerative colitis. Air-contrast techniques improve the results.

Colonoscopy is emerging as the diagnostic procedure of choice for patients with hematochezia who are at risk for colon cancer and whose bleeding is not entirely explained by documented anorectal pathology. About 40% of patients with frank rectal bleeding or occult blood loss in conjunction with normal sigmoidoscopy and barium enema results are found to have previously undetected lesions when studied by colonoscopy. About 10% have cancers, another 10% have polyps, 10% have inflammatory bowel disease, and 5% have telangiectasia. Furthermore, carcinomas and polyps were detected in 20% of patients in whom only diverticula were seen with barium enema. Although the precise role for colonoscopy is not yet entirely settled, most patients over the age of 50 with bleeding are candidates for colonoscopy, either primarily or if barium enema and sigmoidoscopy findings are normal or show only diverticula.

Hematemesis. *Endoscopy* has proved to be diagnostically superior to barium studies and offers the possibility of tissue biopsy for *Helicobacter pylori.* The sensitivity of the upper gastrointestinal series is around 60%, compared with 95% for endoscopy. Esophagitis, Mallory-Weiss tears, and gastritis, which are often undetectable radiologically, are readily seen by endoscopy. Moreover, barium obscures mucosal detail and interferes with endoscopy for 24 to 48 hours. Thus, for suspected acute brisk upper gastrointestinal bleeding, endoscopy is the procedure of first choice, with barium study reserved as a supplementary procedure for patients with inactive bleeding, unexplained chronic blood loss, or suspected small-bowel disease.

The question of whether early endoscopy results in improved outcome for patients with hematemesis remains unresolved. Several studies have failed to demonstrate a significant improvement in outcome among patients who have undergone diagnostic endoscopy. Patients with small bleeds who are hemodynamically stable and do not have liver disease or a significant risk for gastric cancer may be presumed to have peptic ulcer disease and can be treated for *Helicobacter-* or NSAID-induced peptic ulcer (see Chapter 68). Patients at high risk for recurrent bleeding (such as those with evidence of chronic liver disease or an initial bleed that requires a transfusion) and those with persistent bleeding despite medical therapy should undergo endoscopy. In addition, it may be useful to perform upper gastrointestinal endoscopy to exclude esophageal and gastric mucosal features indicative of a high risk for rebleeding (e.g., a "visible vessel" in an ulcer crater).

Melena. Because melena may have an upper or lower gastrointestinal source, one needs to decide which part of the gastrointestinal tract to evaluate first. The decision must be individualized to the patient at hand, although in general, an upper gastrointestinal source of bleeding is more likely.

Occult Bleeding. The evaluation of occult gastrointestinal bleeding is generally aimed at detecting asymptomatic neoplasms at a curable stage. Because colonic adenomas and carcinomas are the most common gastrointestinal neoplasms, evaluation of the colon has greatest utility in this setting. A cost-effectiveness analysis comparing different strategies for evaluating a positive result on testing for fecal occult blood has suggested that colonoscopy would save more lives at lower cost than the combined use of barium enema and flexible sigmoidoscopy. Of seven strategies evaluated, barium enema (without sigmoidoscopy) had the lowest cost-effectiveness ratio but would save fewer lives than colonoscopy. The use of colonoscopy plus barium enema was the only strategy predicted to save more lives than colonoscopy alone, but it does so at significantly higher cost (see Chapter 56).

If no cause of occult bleeding is identified within the colon, evaluation of the upper gastrointestinal tract and small bowel may be considered, although the yield for detection of cancer is likely to be low. In a study of 26 patients followed for 2 to 8 years after a negative result on colonoscopy or barium enema/sigmoidoscopy, only one patient was later found to have a gastric cancer. In five others, a nonmalignant upper gastrointestinal source emerged as the cause of the occult bleeding. A prospective study of patients with iron-deficiency anemia found that site-specific symptoms were predictive of the location of the source of bleeding. Upper gastrointestinal sources were common. Synchronous sources of blood loss were rare, so that further evaluation was unnecessary when an obvious source was found.

PROPHYLACTIC AND SYMPTOMATIC MANAGEMENT

Patients at high risk for upper gastrointestinal bleeding (such as those with varices or a prior history of upper gastrointestinal bleeding, especially if exposed to anticoagulants or high doses of NSAIDs) are candidates for prophylactic measures. Propranolol has been used successfully to prevent a first bleed in patients with known varices (see Chapter 71). *Sclerotherapy* or endoscopic ligation is not indicated for primary prophylaxis because it may actually increase mortality in patients with varices, but these procedures are reasonable in those at high risk for recurrent variceal bleeding. *Histamine$_2$ blockers* and *omeprazole* may be helpful in selected patients with a history of bleeding from an ulcer or gastritis (see Chapter 68). Patients taking steroids do not appear to require such prophylaxis unless an additional risk factor for bleeding is present.

Modest falls in hematocrit that accompany chronic low-grade gastrointestinal blood loss can be treated with oral iron (300 mg of ferrous sulfate three times daily) to make up for the resulting iron deficiency (see Chapter 82). Marked but gradual decreases in hematocrit are usually well tolerated unless the patient has cardiopulmonary disease. Most patients do not need transfusion unless they are symptomatic. Oral iron usually produces a prompt reticulocytosis and at least partial correction of the anemia (see Chapter 82). Patients with presumed anal bleeding can be given fiber supplements or stool softeners to decrease mechanical trauma to the lesion (see Chapter 65).

INDICATIONS FOR ADMISSION AND REFERRAL

The patient with a story of recent or ongoing brisk bleeding, especially if it is accompanied by orthostatic hypotension or other symptoms or signs of hemodynamic compromise, requires emergency department evaluation. Prompt hospitalization is indicated for the person with a profound anemia, even in the absence of evidence for dramatic blood loss. Some patients who are hemodynamically stable may be expeditiously evaluated in a short stay with endoscopy if they have a lesion unlikely to rebleed. Hospitalization should be considered for patients with less severe or perhaps even chronic gastrointestinal blood loss if they have a comorbid condition that might be aggravated by anemia (e.g., ischemic heart disease). For most others, evaluation can proceed safely on an ambulatory basis if the patient does not have serious cardiopulmonary disease and is responsible enough to recognize and promptly report signs of worsening blood loss or volume depletion. Referral to a gastroenterologist should be considered for patients who are potential candidates for endoscopy, and also for patients whose source of bleeding remains elusive after initial evaluation.

ANNOTATED BIBLIOGRAPHY

Barkin JS, Ross BS. Medical therapy of chronic gastrointestinal bleeding of obscure origin. Am J Gastroenterol 1998;93:1250. (*Patients who had chronic occult bleeding, often elderly persons with suspected vascular ectasia, improved with combination estrogen and progesterone therapy.*)

Barry MJ, Mulley AG, Richter JM. Effect of workup strategy on the cost-effectiveness of fecal occult blood screening for colorectal cancer. Gastroenterology 1987;93:301. (*Comparative analysis of seven potential strategies for evaluating the colon in asymptomatic patients with guaiac-positive stool.*)

Boley SJ, Brandt LJ, Frank MS. Severe lower intestinal bleeding. Clin Gastroenterol 1981;10:65. (*Useful enumeration of etiologies by age of patient.*)

Carson JL, Strom BL, Schinnar R, et al. The low risk of upper gastrointestinal bleeding in patients dispensed corticosteroids. Am J Med 1991;91:223. (*Risk was 2.8 cases per 10,000 person-months; argues against prophylactic therapy unless other risk factors are present.*)

Coon U, Willis P. Hemorrhagic complications of anticoagulant therapy. Ann Intern Med 1974;133:386. (*More than half of patients who bled on anticoagulant therapy had an identifiable underlying gastrointestinal lesion.*)

Dooley CP, Larson AW, Stacen H, et al. Double-contrast barium meal and upper gastrointestinal endoscopy. Ann Intern Med 1984;101:538. (*Literature review; endoscopy was substantially more sensitive—92% vs. 5%—and more specific—100% vs. 91%—than double-contrast barium swallow, but no "gold standard."*)

Goulston KJ, et al. Evaluation of rectal bleeding. Lancet 1986;2:261. (*Colorectal malignancies would have been missed on a clinical basis alone.*)

Graham DY. Aspirin and the stomach. Ann Intern Med 1986;104:390. (*Comprehensive review. Notes that degree of mucosal injury seen by endoscopy does not predict risk for or degree of bleeding.*)

Griffiths WJ, Neumann DA, Welsh JD. The visible vessel as an indicator of uncontrolled or recurrent gastrointestinal hemorrhage. N Engl J Med 1979;300:1411. (*Important sign of high risk for a repeated upper gastrointestinal bleed.*)

Knight KK, Fielding JE, Battista RN. Occult blood screening for colorectal cancer. JAMA 1989;261:587. (*General review of the procedure.*)

Laine L, El Newihi HM, Migikovsky B, et al. Endoscopic ligation compared with sclerotherapy for the treatment of bleeding esophageal varices. Ann Intern Med 1993;119:1. (*Endoscopic ligation caused fewer local complications and eradicated varices more rapidly.*)

Layne EA, Mellow MH, Lipman TO. Insensitivity of guaiac slide for detection of blood in gastric juice. Ann Intern Med 1981;94:774. (*Sensitivity of the guaiac test was low, but it was greatly enhanced by neutralizing the acid with a few drops of sodium hydroxide.*)

Lau JYW, Sung JJY, Lam Y-H, et al. Endoscopic retreatment compared with recurrent bleeding after initial endoscopic control of bleeding ulcers. N Engl J Med 1999;340:751. (*Endoscopic retreatment is more cost-effective than emergency surgery.*)

Lindsay DC, et al. Should colonoscopy be the first investigation for colonic disease? Br Med J 1988;296:167. (*Randomized trial of colonoscopy versus rigid sigmoidoscopy and air-contrast barium enema in the workup of colonic disease.*)

Peterson WL, Barnett CC, Smith HJ, et al. Routine early endoscopy in upper gastrointestinal tract bleeding. N Engl J Med 1981;304:925. (*Randomized, controlled trial; no advantage found for early endoscopy, except in those with alcoholic liver disease or continued bleeding.*)

Rockey DC. Occult gastrointestinal bleeding. N Engl J Med 1999;341:38. (*A comprehensive review of testing for occult bleeding and its evaluation.*)

Rockey DC, Cello JP. Evaluation of the gastrointestinal tract in patients with iron-deficiency anemia. N Engl J Med 1993;329:1691. (*Lesions are frequently found; site-specific symptoms help predict location and direct workup.*)

Shapiro RH. The visible vessel: curse or blessing? N Engl J Med 1979;300:1438. (*Editorial reviewing the utility of endoscopy, with emphasis on defining a high-risk group of patients with upper gastrointestinal bleeding.*)

Steer ML, Silen W. Diagnostic procedures in gastrointestinal hemorrhage. N Engl J Med 1983;309:646. (*Concise but very useful review of the operating characteristics of endoscopy, radionuclide imaging, angiography, barium contrast studies, and exploratory surgery.*)

Stewart JG, Ahlquist DA, McGill DB, et al. Gastrointestinal blood loss and anemia in runners. Ann Intern Med 1984;100:843. (*Documents an increase in fecal hemoglobin level associated with competitive running, which may explain anemia and iron deficiency among long-distance runners.*)

Sutton FM. Upper gastrointestinal bleeding in patients with esophageal varices: what is the most common source of bleeding? Am J Med 1987;83:273. (*Varices account for the vast majority of episodes of bleeding, although coexisting sources are not uncommon.*)

Wilcox CM, Truss CD. Gastrointestinal bleeding in patients receiving long-term anticoagulant therapy. Am J Med 1988;84:683. (*Half of episodes were upper gastrointestinal in origin; a lower gastrointestinal origin was noted in 33%. In undiagnosed cases, the risk for a malignancy being encountered later was very low.*)

Zuckerman GR. Upper gastrointestinal bleeding in patients with chronic renal failure. Ann Intern Med 1985;102:588. (*Upper gastrointestinal angiodysplasia was the most common source; esophagitis was also prevalent.*)

64

Evaluation and Management of Diarrhea

JAMES M. RICHTER

Diarrhea is clinically characterized by the frequent passage of unformed stools. Episodes that are brief, self-limited, and well tolerated do not require medical attention, but when diarrhea becomes severe or chronic, a thoughtful evaluation is needed to ensure proper management. The primary care physician needs to know how to conduct an expeditious assessment of acute severe diarrhea and coordinate a cost-effective approach to the evaluation of chronic diarrhea. Diarrhea in the HIV-infected patient requires special attention (see Chapter 13).

PATHOPHYSIOLOGY AND CLINICAL PRESENTATIONS

The pathophysiologic common denominator is increased stool water content, which may be a consequence of increased fluid secretion, decreased water absorption, or altered bowel motility. At times, several mechanisms are operative. *Increased fluid secretion* can be triggered by inflammation, hormones, or enterotoxins. The resulting secretory diarrhea has a stool volume that remains in excess of 500 mL/24 h despite fasting, a low stool osmolality, and a normal stool electrolyte concentration. *Decreased reabsorption of fluid* occurs with abnormalities of the bowel mucosa, loss of reabsorptive surface, or the presence of unabsorbable, osmotically active materials in the bowel lumen, such as lactose in patients with lactase deficiency. Patients with diarrhea resulting from decreased reabsorption typically respond to fasting with a decrease in stool volume to less than 500 mL/24 h; stool osmolality is increased, and its sodium and potassium concentrations are low. *Increased bowel motility* decreases the contact time with the bowel mucosa, limiting fluid reabsorption; it can ensue after vagotomy or may be chemically stimulated, as in hypergastrinemia or with the use of laxatives.

Acute Diarrheas

A diarrhea is categorized as "acute" if its duration is less than 2 weeks. Infectious causes dominate and include viral, bacterial, and parasitic agents. Bacteria may cause diarrhea by producing a toxin in contaminated food or after ingestion, or by invading the bowel mucosa. Some parasites invade the bowel wall, whereas others cling to it and coat the absorptive surface.

Viruses. Viral gastroenteritis has long been the most common cause of acute diarrhea in the United States, although it was not until the late 1970s that the responsible organisms were finally isolated and identified. Epidemics of viral gastroenteritis are particularly common. More than 40% of outbreaks of nonbacterial gastroenteritis investigated by the Centers for Disease Control and Prevention (CDC) during a 5-year period were linked to the *Norwalk virus*. In children, *rotavirus* infection is a common cause. Outbreaks have been found to occur during all seasons and involve water-borne, food-borne, and person-to-person modes of transmission. They last about a week. Vomiting is the prominent symptom in children, diarrhea in adults. After an incubation period of 48 to 72 hours, symptoms usually begin abruptly with diarrhea, nausea, vomiting, headache, low-grade fever, abdominal cramps, and malaise; they resolve spontaneously within 24 to 96 hours. The diarrhea tends to be predominantly secretory in quality. Abdominal examination reveals diffuse tenderness (without guarding) and hyperactive bowel sounds. The white blood cell count is usually normal but may be elevated. Stools are usually free of leukocytes, but occasionally white cells are found, as in an invasive etiology.

Staphylococcus Aureus is a common contaminant of custard-filled pastries and processed meats. The organism produces an enterotoxin that causes nausea, vomiting, abdominal cramps, and diarrhea within 2 to 8 hours after contaminated food has been eaten. Symptoms usually last less than 12 hours. A common-source pattern and lack of fever are typical.

Clostridium Perfringens is another common food contaminant, especially of foods that have been warmed on steam tables. The organism releases an enterotoxin after sporulation in the intestine. Consequently, the incubation period of 8 to 24 hours is a bit longer than that for staphylococcal food poisoning. Symptoms include diarrhea, abdominal cramps, and occasionally some vomiting. It, too, has a common-source epidemiology, and fever is absent.

Escherichia Coli 0157:H7. This pathogen is increasingly recognized as responsible for much food-borne diarrhea. It accounts for up to 2.5% of all cases of acute diarrhea and up to a third of cases of bloody acute diarrhea. Transmission to humans is usually by ingestion of contaminated meat (typically hamburger) that is undercooked. Person-to-person transmission also occurs. Peak incidence is in the summer months. The organism does not directly invade the bowel wall, but the two Shiga-like toxins it produces cause mucosal edema, ulceration, and hemorrhage. The mean incubation period is 3 days (range, 1 to 9 days). Among those who become symptomatic, presentations range from mild, crampy, nonbloody diarrhea to life-threatening hemorrhagic colitis complicated by hemolytic–uremic syndrome or thrombotic thrombocytopenic purpura. The typical presentation starts with crampy abdominal pain followed within hours by watery diarrhea that progresses to grossly bloody stools. Children, the elderly, and compromised hosts are at greatest risk.

Salmonella species cause diarrhea by invading the bowel wall. Achlorhydric patients who lack the antibacterial action of normal gastric acidity are at increased risk. The most common form of *Salmonella* infection is a self-limited diarrheal illness resulting from ingestion of contaminated food (eggs and poultry are the major sources). Children are at greatest risk; late summer and fall are the times of peak incidence. Although most episodes of salmonellosis are mild, debilitated patients are at risk for serious bacteremia. In the typical outpatient case, symptoms begin 12 to 36 hours after ingestion and resolve within 5 days, although diarrhea may persist for up to 2 weeks. The initial presentation is rather nonspecific, although indicative of a small-bowel process: watery diarrhea, cramps, nausea, vomiting, and fever. In addition to colonization, an enterotoxin is released that stimulates the secretory diarrhea. In later stages, invasion spreads to the large bowel, and leukocytes may be noted in the stool. A distinguishing feature of salmonellosis is that the leukocytes are often mononuclear cells. In severe cases, dysentery can develop.

Typhoid fever, a rare but "must-not-miss" form of *Salmonella* disease, is caused by infection with *Salmonella typhi*. About 500 cases occur in the United States each year, mostly among young people. Infections are both water-borne and food-borne. Although diarrhea develops in only a small percentage of patients with typhoid fever, it does occur. The classic and most severe form is a "pea soup" diarrhea developing in the third week of illness. Early symptoms suggestive of the condition are progressive fever, relative bradycardia, evanescent rash on the trunk ("rose spots"), splenomegaly, cough, headache, and right lower quadrant abdominal pain.

Shigella infection produces an invasive diarrheal illness. Transmission is by the fecal–oral route, and stubborn reservoirs include day care centers, Indian reservations, urban ghettos, and rural villages in developing countries. Young children are at greatest risk and often the source of infection within a family. The illness proceeds in two stages. First, colonization takes place in the small bowel, resulting in a watery diarrhea and periumbilical pain, followed in a few days by invasion of the large bowel, associated with frequent small stools, tenesmus, and polymorphonuclear leukocytes on smear. In florid cases, the patient has fever, toxicity, bloody diarrhea, nausea, vomiting, and cramps. Most often, the disease is more subtle and may be difficult to distinguish from other diarrheal illnesses accompanied by fever.

Campylobacter Jejuni infection is responsible for more cases of diarrhea in the United States than is either *Salmonella* or *Shigella*. Infection derives most often from animal sources, such as poultry and household pets; fecal transmission between people also occurs. The incubation period is 2 to 7 days. Clinically, the illness resembles that caused by *Salmonella* or *Shigella*; however, symptoms may persist longer. The relapse rate is as high as 20%, although the illness is usually self-limited and resolves within a week. In half of all cases, a Gram's stain of the stool shows characteristic curved, gram-negative rods arranged in "sea gull wing" fashion. The organism grows best on a special medium incubated at 42°C; it will not grow on plates customarily used for isolation of *Salmonella* and *Shigella*.

Yersinia Enterocolitica also causes an illness that resembles salmonellosis. Patients become infected by eating contaminated meat or dairy products. The incubation period is 12 hours to 3 days. An intense, regional lymphoid reaction may arise in the terminal ileum (the portal of entry for the organism) and result in a clinical picture of fever, right lower quadrant abdominal pain, and diarrhea that can simulate the onset of Crohn's disease. In 10% to 40% of patients, fever, arthralgias, polyarthritis, or erythema nodosum develops. The illness is usually self-limited.

Vibrio Parahaemolyticus and non–toxin-producing *Vibrio cholerae* are pathogenic species that have caused outbreaks of diarrheal disease among people eating raw seafood, particularly oysters and sushi-style red snapper and salmon. The incubation period is measured in hours to several days. The illness that ensues is usually mild and self-limited, although an occasional patient may present with fever, nausea, vomiting, and crampy diarrhea.

Listeria Monocytogenes is another of the food-borne pathogens found increasingly in tainted processed meats and poultry products and also in unpasteurized milk products. Person-to-person transfer does not occur. About 2,000 cases per year occur in the United States. Deaths are common, with mortality rates of 20% to 30% reported. The elderly and the immunocompromised are at greatest risk. Onset of symptoms is typically 1 to 2 days after exposure. Initial symptoms resemble those of a viral gastroenteritis (fever, cramps, myalgias, diarrhea, headache). Days to weeks later, meningitis and bacteremia may ensue, especially in the immunocompromised host.

Vibrio Cholerae causes the prototypical toxin-mediated secretory diarrheal disease that results from drinking water contaminated with the organism. Most outbreaks are pandemic in the Indian subcontinent, Southeast Asia, Africa, and the Middle East. Isolated outbreaks have been reported in Mediterranean countries. In the United States, rare outbreaks sometimes occur along the Gulf coast. The disease ranges in severity from a mild illness to fulminant, life-threatening diarrhea with copious production of gray, watery, mucoid ("rice water") stool. In severe cases, fluid losses may exceed 1 L/h and are accompanied by vomiting, muscle cramps, and severe thirst. Because it is a noninvasive diarrhea involving the small bowel, cholera does not cause tenesmus, and the stool contains no leukocytes. Dehydration, serious volume depletion, and a metabolic acidosis may ensue. In mild cases, the patient reports painless, nonbloody diarrhea of abrupt onset.

Bacillus Cereus is a toxin-producing bacterial contaminant of rice and bean sprouts. One form of toxin-induced illness leads to vomiting but no diarrhea; another is characterized by severe abdominal cramping and diarrhea. The incubation period is 8 to 16 hours after ingestion of contaminated food. The symptoms are self-limited.

Entamoeba Histolytica usually exists in a commensal relationship with its host, and most patients harboring the protozoan are asymptomatic carriers. Occasionally, this relationship breaks down and the ameba invades the colonic wall; an acute bloody diarrhea is the result. The clinical presentation ranges from mild to fulminant illness. Occasionally, the illness is mistaken for inflammatory bowel disease (see Chapter 73) and may have a protracted course with exacerbations and remissions. Asymptomatic carriers such as returning tourists and immigrants are often the source of infection in developed countries. Because the organism does not have a soil phase, amebiasis is not restricted to warmer climates. Well-documented outbreaks

have occurred in the United States and Europe, in addition to those that originate in developing countries. Amebiasis can be spread by sexual contact and is prevalent among promiscuous homosexuals.

Giardia Lamblia ranks as a leading parasitic cause of diarrhea, especially overseas but also in the United States. Infection with the flagellated protozoan is particularly common where water supplies are contaminated by human sewage, but the organism is also endemic to such areas as the Rocky Mountains and St. Petersburg, Russia. The exact means by which *Giardia* causes diarrhea remains unsettled, although heavy infestations can lead to malabsorption by coating large areas of the small bowel, particularly the lower duodenum and upper jejunum. The majority of patients with giardiasis are asymptomatic, but the organism is being recognized more frequently as an important cause of acute, intermittent, and chronic diarrheas in the United States. The ensuing loose stools may be watery or greasy; mucus is often present, but blood is rare. The patient may complain of epigastric or periumbilical discomfort. Mild steatorrhea and malabsorption occur with heavy parasite burdens.

Cryptosporidium, Microsporidia, and Other Protozoans are increasingly recognized as causes of acute watery diarrhea (and sometimes of chronic disease). Point-source outbreaks occur in addition to sporadic cases. Transmission is by person-to-person contact through stool or by water or food contaminated with the spore or oocyst forms of the organism. Intestinal inflammation may develop. Children and immunocompromised adults are at greatest risk for severe and prolonged illness. A profuse, watery diarrhea can develop, with stool volumes that may exceed 3 L daily. Although the illness is usually self-limited, it may persist in immunocompromised hosts. A mild illness develops in otherwise healthy, immunocompetent patients; they may become infected during occupational contact (e.g., animal dung). For them, symptoms resolve spontaneously within 5 to 21 days.

Diarrhea in HIV-infected Patients is a major problem, with a host of possible etiologies (see Chapter 13). In HIV-infected persons who engage in receptive anal intercourse, the presentation may be one of diarrhea, tenesmus, and rectal pain. In this setting, polymicrobial etiologies are not uncommon and may include *Neisseria*, *Giardia*, *E. histolytica*, *Campylobacter*, *Chlamydia*, *Shigella*, *Salmonella*, and protozoans.

Traveler's Diarrheas

Patients traveling from industrialized to developing nations are at considerable risk for the development of diarrhea. Etiologic agents include *E. coli*, *Salmonella*, *Shigella*, *E. histolytica*, *G. lamblia*, *S. typhi*, and *V. cholerae*. Invasive *E. coli* strains can also cause a dysentery syndrome. Although most cases of traveler's diarrhea are associated with travel to developing nations, this is not always true. For example, there is substantial risk of giardiasis with travel to St. Petersburg, Russia, or even to the Rocky Mountains of the United States.

Toxigenic Escherichia coli is responsible for a large proportion of cases labeled as "traveler's diarrhea" or "turista." The agent is transmitted by poor food-handling practices and contaminated water. With enterotoxin production, a watery diarrhea ensues because the toxin promotes fluid secretion in the small bowel.

Drug-induced Diarrheas

Substances associated with diarrhea are listed in Table 64.1.

Acute Diarrhea. Mechanisms of acute diarrhea include excessive fluid secretion (*alcohol, phenolphthalein,* and *castor oil*), reduction of fluid absorption (*magnesium*-containing antacids), and stimulation of bowel motility (*caffeine*-containing beverages and *herbal teas*). An osmotic diarrhea with crampy pain and watery stools may follow oral or parenteral use of *broad-spectrum antibiotics*, which disrupt the salvage of unabsorbed carbohydrate by killing normal colonic flora.

Chronic Diarrhea: Pseudomembranous Colitis. Broad-spectrum antibiotics can cause chronic diarrhea by promoting overgrowth of toxin-producing species such as *Clostridium difficile.* The antibiotics most often responsible are *ampicillin* and *clindamycin,* but other broad-spectrum agents have also been implicated. Immunocompromised patients, the elderly, and those with underlying bowel disease are most susceptible. Pseudomembranous colitis is characterized by fever, abdominal pain, profuse watery stools, and fecal leukocytes. Symptoms may range from mild to severe, usually starting after the initiation of a course of antibiotics, but onset can be delayed for as much as 4 to 8 weeks after cessation of antibiotics. Symptoms may persist for months, mimicking inflammatory bowel disease. The sigmoidoscopic finding of nodular, inflammatory ulcers or yellow-white mucosal plaques is characteristic.

Chronic and Recurrent Diarrheas

Although the number of etiologies is vast, consideration of a few exemplary conditions provides a good sense of the range and types of presentations.

Irritable Bowel Syndrome is the most common of the motility disorders responsible for chronic diarrhea or hyperdefecation (see Chapter 74). It can present as diarrhea alternating with constipation, or as chronic, recurrent diarrhea. Some studies report a high frequency of associated psychiatric disease. In addition to diarrhea and constipation, patients may complain of distention, cramping, and mucus-laden stools. The condition waxes and wanes over many years. Neither fever nor fecal leukocytes are present. Any rectal bleeding that may occur is secondary to anal trauma resulting from straining and passage of hard stool.

Inflammatory Bowel Diseases are typical of the diarrheas that result from inflammatory destruction of the bowel wall (see Chapter 73). Abdominal pain, bloody stools, purulent discharge, and fever are seen in patients with active disease affecting the large bowel. Extraintestinal manifestations may involve the skin, joints, liver, and heart. Microscopic examination of the stool reveals red cells and leukocytes.

Diabetic Enteropathy results from diabetes-induced autonomic neuropathy (see Chapter 102). When the small bowel is involved, the ensuing stasis allows bacterial overgrowth. The bacteria deconjugate bile acids, which leads to fat malabsorption. With involvement of the large bowel, the patient experiences distressing nocturnal diarrhea. Postural hypotension, impotence, and other symptoms and signs of autonomic insufficiency may accompany the diarrhea and suggest the diagnosis.

Dumping Syndrome is another motility disorder, seen most commonly in patients who have undergone vagotomy and gastroenterostomy. Patients complain of sweating, postural light-headedness, tachycardia, and diarrhea following meals. Concentrated carbohydrates are most likely to trigger symptoms. Lying down minimizes symptoms, as does avoidance of concentrated sweets. Onset of the syndrome is shortly after surgery, and symptoms usually subside within 12 months,

Table 64.1. Differential Diagnosis of Diarrhea

ACUTE DIARRHEA	CHRONIC OR RECURRENT DIARRHEA
Viruses	**Protozoa**
Bacterial Toxins	*Giardia lamblia*
Staphylococcus	*Entamoeba histolytica*
Clostridium	*Cryptosporidium*
Bacteria	**Inflammation**
Salmonella	Ulcerative colitis
Shigella	Crohn's disease
Escherichia coli	Ischemic colitis
(including 0157:H7)	Pseudomembranous colitis
Campylobacter	Collagenous colitis
Yersinia	Lymphocytic colitis
Bacillus cereus	
Vibrio parahaemolyticus	**Drugs**
Vibrio cholerae	Laxatives
Listeria	Antibiotics
	Quinidine
Protozoa	Guanethidine; other
Giardia lamblia	antihypertensive agents
Entamoeba histolytica	Caffeine
Cryptosporidium	Digitalis
Microsporidia	
	Functional
Drugs	Irritable bowel syndrome
Laxatives	Diverticulosis
Antibiotics	
Caffeine	**Tumors**
Alcohol	Bowel carcinoma
Antacids	Villous adenoma
	Islet cell tumors
Functional	Carcinoid syndrome
Anxiety	Medullary carcinoma of thyroid
Acute presentations of chronic	
or recurrent diarrhea	**Malabsorption**
(See next column)	Sprue
	Intestinal lymphoma
	Bile salt malabsorption
	Whipple's disease
	Pancreatic insufficiency
	Lactase deficiency
	Other disaccharidase
	deficiencies
	Alpha-beta lipoproteinemia
	Postsurgical
	Postgastrectomy dumping
	syndrome
	Enteroenteric fistulas
	Blind loops
	Parasympathetic denervation
	Short-bowel syndrome
	Bile and diarrhea
	Other
	Cirrhosis
	Diabetes mellitus
	Heavy metal intoxication
	Other neurogenic diarrheas
	Hyperthyroidism
	Addison's disease
	Pellagra
	Scleroderma
	Amyloidosis

although they may persist. Besides dysmotility, osmotic factors may contribute, but their precise role remains unclear.

Villous Adenoma of the rectosigmoid causes a secretory, noninflammatory chronic diarrhea. Watery diarrhea, independent of food and fluid intake, is typical; severe potassium depletion can result. In some patients with this tumor, excessive secretion of mucus occurs, with loss of sufficient protein to produce hypoalbuminemia and a protein-losing enteropathy syndrome.

Malabsorption of Fat or Carbohydrate can lead to an osmotic diarrhea, as occurs in patients with *pancreatic insufficiency*, *sprue*, and *short-bowel* syndrome. Some of the osmotically active substances may also stimulate increased bowel secretion of fluids and electrolytes. Malabsorption of fat characteristically presents as *steatorrhea* (foul, bulky, greasy stools). Patients may note that the stools seem to be "sticky" and difficult to flush down the toilet. Steatorrheic stools "float," not because of their fat content but because of an increase in trapped gas. Associated symptoms are a function of the severity of the caloric and vitamin deficiencies that ensue and may include weight loss, ecchymoses, bone pain, glossitis, muscle tenderness, and peripheral neuropathy. Cramping lower abdominal pain typically precedes bowel movements. Early concerns about severe diarrhea and abdominal pain associated with the regular use of *Olestra*, a nonabsorbable sucrose ester fat substitute used in snack foods, have not been confirmed in randomized, prospective, controlled trials.

Lactase Deficiency (Milk Intolerance) leads to malabsorption of lactose and an osmotic diarrhea. It is particularly common among African-Americans, Indians, Asians, and Jews. Onset is typically in adulthood. A secondary form of the disease may develop in patients with extensive disease of the small bowel. Patients report nausea, bloating, cramps, and diarrhea after ingesting more than their customary intake of milk products. Weight loss and steatorrhea are absent or mild; appetite remains good. Avoidance of milk products (except for yogurt containing live cultures, which provide lactase) terminates symptoms. Diagnosis may be confirmed by a trial of abstinence and by abnormal results on lactose tolerance testing or hydrogen breath testing (which detects excessive hydrogen production resulting from bacterial metabolism of undigested lactose).

Laxative Abuse is an important etiology of chronic diarrhea. Patients with bulimia (see Chapter 234) tend to use laxatives constantly and surreptitiously in a relentless attempt to lose weight. Depending on the type of agent used, either a secretory or osmotic diarrhea may develop. Agents associated with secretory diarrheas include castor oil and phenolphthalein preparations. Osmotic diarrheas occur when the patient takes a preparation that contains magnesium (e.g., milk of magnesia) or another poorly absorbable substance. These substances appear in the stool and can be tested for if laxative abuse is suspected. Patients who abuse laxatives may present with unexplained dehydration, electrolyte depletion, or preoccupation with weight loss.

Lymphocytic Colitis and Collagenous Colitis. These two new conditions associated with refractory chronic diarrhea have recently been recognized. They occur predominantly in women and cause chronic watery diarrhea, often complicated by steatorrhea and malabsorption. The colonic appearance is grossly normal, but biopsy reveals collagenous or lymphocytic infiltrates. The small bowel usually is normal but may show spru-

elike changes in patients with lymphocytic disease, and persons with the condition may present with spruelike malabsorption unresponsive to a gluten-free diet.

Bile Acid Diarrhea is seen after cholecystectomy and ileal reaction. It is an irritant diarrhea caused by the action of excessive bile acids on the bowel and responds to bile acid sequestrants (e.g., cholestyramine).

Incontinence

A number of patients who complain of "diarrhea" actually suffer from incontinence. Typically, their stool volumes are normal (< 2.5 mL/d), although their stools may be soft poor sphincter tone and evidence of stool incontinence are found on physical examination.

DIFFERENTIAL DIAGNOSIS

Acute Diarrhea. The differential diagnosis for acute diarrhea is dominated by infectious agents (Table 64.1). Viruses are the single most important frequent cause. Staphylococcal toxin, clostridial toxin, and ingestion of *Campylobacter*, *Salmonella*, *Shigella*, and enteropathogenic *E. coli* are common bacterial etiologies. Of increasing importance are the potentially life-threatening outbreaks of food-borne disease caused by toxin-producing *E. coli* 0157:H7, *Listeria*, and protozoans such as *Cryptosporidium*. *Giardia* and amebae are less frequent sources of acute diarrhea in the United States. Drug-induced acute disease is associated with the use of antibiotics, laxatives, magnesium-containing antacids, and agents such as quinidine. Alcohol and caffeine-containing beverages should be considered. Most causes of chronic diarrhea are also capable of causing acute presentations.

Traveler's Diarrhea. In more than 50% of acute cases, the cause is exposure to enterotoxigenic *E. coli*. Most of the remainder are accounted for by *Salmonella*, *Shigella*, *Giardia*, or *Campylobacter*.

Chronic Diarrhea. The differential diagnosis is even more extensive (Table 64.1) and includes causes of acute disease that may become chronic (e.g., laxative abuse, pseudomembranous colitis, protozoan infections, amebic infestations) in addition to a host of intrinsic bowel diseases. A *malabsorption* picture may be the consequence of sprue, bile salt deficiency, lactase deficiency, intestinal lymphoma, Whipple's disease, pancreatic insufficiency, or the newly recognized collagenous and lymphocytic forms of colitis. *Postsurgical* diarrhea may reflect postgastrectomy dumping syndrome, fistulas, blind loops, loss of parasympathetic innervation, extensive bowel resection, or excessive bile acid. Diarrhea with *bleeding* may herald neoplasms and inflammatory bowel disease. Diarrhea *alternating with constipation* may be caused by irritable bowel syndrome, Crohn's disease, or diverticular disease of the bowel. A variety of *extraintestinal conditions* may be responsible, including cirrhosis, alcoholism, pellagra, and heavy metal intoxications from lead, mercury, or arsenic. Endocrinopathies also must be considered (e.g., diabetes mellitus, Addison's disease, hyperthyroidism).

Diarrhea of Unknown Etiology. In studies of patients referred for chronic diarrhea of unknown etiology, the vast majority turn out to be abusing laxatives or to have a subtle form of inflammatory bowel disease (including collagenous or lymphocytic varieties) or irritable bowel syndrome. Most of the remainder have a more readily diagnosed condition that was overlooked on initial evaluation.

Diarrhea in the HIV-Infected Patient. The common infectious causes are frequently seen, but such uncommon causes as *Cryptosporidium, Mycobacterium avium–intracellulare,* herpes simplex virus, cytomegalovirus, *Neisseria gonorrhoeae, Giardia,* and *Chlamydia trachomatis* must also be considered (see Chapter 13).

WORKUP

Before embarking on a workup, one needs to confirm that the problem is indeed diarrhea and not simply an occasional loose stool or frequent defecation of formed stools. Stool volume, frequency, and water content should all be increased.

Acute and Traveler's Diarrheas

History. The *nature of the bowel movements* should be determined, including their frequency, consistency, volume, and the presence of gross blood, pus, or mucus (Tables 64.2 and 64.3), and the presence of any *associated symptoms,* such as fever, rash, and abdominal pain, should be noted. Late onset of neurologic deficits or meningeal symptoms should suggest listeriosis.

Epidemiologic Information is critical because the clinical presentation is often nonspecific. Reviews of travel (both international and domestic), personal contacts, and food intake are essential. Among the foods to consider are custard-filled pastries, undercooked processed meats, foods warmed on steam tables, eggs, poultry, raw seafood, unpasteurized milk and fruit juices, rice, and bean sprouts. Important contacts include children who attend day care centers because they may contract rotavirus, *Giardia, Shigella, Cryptosporidium,* or *Campylobacter.* A *sexual history* is indicated if there is concern about polymicrobial infection.

Onset and Associated Symptoms. Diarrhea occurring within hours of ingestion of a potentially contaminated food is suggestive of food poisoning, which is confirmed if others have been similarly affected. Food-borne illness with a short incubation period and no *fever* indicates ingestion of a preformed enterotoxin. Fever and a slightly longer incubation period are characteristic of an infectious etiology (Table 64.3). Some toxin-producing organisms (e.g., *E. coli* 0157:H7) require a few days of incubation.

Drug History. It is particularly important to question about the use of laxatives, magnesium-containing antacids, excess alcohol, caffeine-containing beverages, herbal teas, antibiotics, digitalis, quinidine, loop diuretics (furosemide, ethacrynic acid), antihypertensive agents, and excessive intake of sorbitol-containing "sugar-free" gums and mints.

Physical Examination. Vital signs must be checked. Postural hypotension is a sign of significant volume depletion and an indication for prompt IV repletion. Any elevation in temper-

Table 64.2.   Important Features of Some Acute Diarrheas

ETIOLOGY	NATURE OF DIARRHEA			ASSOCIATED SYMPTOMS AND SIGNS	EPIDEMIOLOGIC DATA	LABORATORY RESULTS
	W/S	OB	GB			
Viral	+/+	−	−	n, v, fever, myalgias, abdominal cramps, HA	Occurs in short-lived epidemics	WBC: nl or elevated Stool: usually no WBC
Staphylococcus aureus	−/+	−	−	n, v, no fever	Custards; incubation: 2-8 h	WBC: nl Stool: no WBC
Clostridium perfringens	+/+	−	−	n, v, no fever	Steam tables; incubation: 8-24 h	WBC nl Stool: no WBC
Bacillus cereus	+/+	−	−	n, v, no fever	Rice, sprouts	WBC: nl Stool: no WBC
Salmonella	+/−	+	+	n, v, fever, in some cases dysentery	Eggs, turtles, poultry	Stool: WBC + culture +
Salmonella typhi	+/+ "Pea soup"	+	−	Rose spots, HA, splenomegaly, bradycardia, fever, toxic	Water, food	Stool: monos, culture +
Shigella	+/− Dysentery	+	−	n, v, fever, toxic in severe cases	Ghettos; day care centers; Indian reservations	Stool: WBC + culture +
Escherichia coli 0157:H7	+/−	+	+	crampy abdominal pain without fever followed by bloody diarrhea, hemolytic uremic syndrome, thrombotic thrombocytopenic purpura	Undercooked contaminated processed meat and poultry	Stool: WBC + culture + toxin +
Campylobacter	+/− Dysentery	+	+	n, v, fever	Poultry, pets	Stool: WBC + culture +
Yersinia	+/+	+	−	Simulates Crohn's disease and appendicitis; joint complaints	Dairy products, meat	Stool: WBC + culture +
Vibrio species	+/+	−	−	n, v, cramps, occasionally fever	Raw seafood; 2-day course	Stool culture +
Cryptosporidium	+/−	−	−	occasionally n, v, cramps, dehydration	AIDS patients, immunosuppressed	Stool for o & p + (spores, oocytes)
Giardia	See Table 64-3					
Entamoeba histolytica	See Table 64-3					

W/S, watery/soft; OB, occult blood; GB, gross blood; n, nausea; v, vomiting; HA, headache; o & p, ova and parasites; +, present; −, absent; nl, normal; WBC, white blood cells.

Table 64.3. Important Features of Traveler's Diarrheas

ETIOLOGY	W/S	OB	GB	NATURE OF DIARRHEA ASSOCIATED SYMPTOMS AND SIGNS	EPIDEMIOLOGIC DATA	LABORATORY RESULTS
Escherichia coli	+/−	−	−	Usually no fever, although occasionally toxicity	Contamination of water, food	Stool: WBC −; can also be +
Entamoeba histolytica	+/+ Dysentery			Can simulate inflammatory bowel disease; asymptomatic carriers	Returning tourists, immigrants	Stool + for o & p; + serology
Giardia	−/+	+/− −	+/− −	Upper abdominal pain	Contamination of water supply	Stool + for o & p
Vibrio cholerae	+/− "Rice water"	−	−	Marked dehydration, cramps, vomiting	Contamination of water supply	Stool: WBC −
Shigella	See Table 64-2					
Salmonella	See Table 64-2					

W/S, watery/soft; OB, occult blood; GB, gross blood; WBC, white blood cells; o & p, ova and parasites.

ature or loss of weight also needs to be noted. The patient who appears markedly dehydrated or toxic is a candidate for hospital admission. The skin is examined for manifestations of sepsis; the macular "rose spot" rash on the trunk is an important clue for typhoid. The lymph nodes are checked for enlargement, and the abdomen for tenderness, guarding, rebound, abnormal bowel sounds, organomegaly, and masses. A rectal examination and fecal occult blood test complete the physical evaluation. When listeriosis is suspected epidemiologically, a careful neurologic examination is in order, with a search for focal deficits and meningeal signs.

Laboratory Studies: Initial Evaluation. The laboratory workup should be individualized. The patient who feels well except for frequent loose stools requires no immediate laboratory testing. On the other hand, the patient who is ill with fever, nausea, abdominal cramps, or other systemic symptoms requires more extensive evaluation, beginning with a stool test for leukocytes, which indicates a potentially serious etiology.

Stool Testing for Leukocytes. A drop of the sample is placed on a microscope slide, mixed thoroughly with two drops of *methylene blue* solution (or Wright's or Gram's stain), and topped with a cover slip for viewing under the microscope. Finding large numbers of white cells suggests an inflammatory or invasive diarrhea, such as occurs with *Shigella*, *Salmonella*, *Campylobacter*, invasive or certain toxigenic *E. coli*, and *Entamoeba*. The presence of mononuclear cells is characteristic of salmonellosis. An occasional white cell is of no pathologic significance. Leukocytes may be absent from the stool in the early phases of shigellosis and pseudomembranous colitis.

Gram's Stain of the Stool will provide etiologic information in selected instances, such as suspected *Campylobacter* infection. In about half of cases, the Gram's stain will demonstrate gram-negative rods arranged in a characteristic sea gull wing configuration.

Stool Cultures. Cultures are usually not necessary in acute diarrhea because most cases are self-limited. However, if the patient appears ill and either occult blood or leukocytes are present in the stool, then *bacterial cultures* should be obtained. Detection of *Campylobacter* or *Yersinia* requires plating on specific medium at 42°; the usual medium for *Salmonella* and

Shigella will not suffice. The laboratory should be notified when *E. coli* 0157:H7 is a consideration because special growth media and other procedures are required to identify the pathogen.

Sigmoidoscopy. Patients with gross blood or large numbers of leukocytes in the stool and severe illness should undergo sigmoidoscopy to examine the appearance of the colonic mucosa; samples of the mucosa and cultures can also be obtained (see following section on the workup for chronic diarrhea for details). Preparatory enemas and cathartics should be avoided so as not to distort the appearance of the bowel wall (see Chapter 56).

Laboratory Studies: Subsequent Evaluation. If the diarrhea persists for 2 weeks or more, a secondary evaluation is indicated. *Stools* should once again be examined for *blood* and *leukocytes*. A second stool should be sent for bacterial *culture*, and a fresh specimen should be examined for ova and parasites.

Stool for Ova and Parasites. Ova and parasite examinations are fraught with limitations that must be kept in mind. If *giardiasis* is a consideration, at least three stool samples are necessary because excretion of the organism is intermittent. Many primary care physicians use a therapeutic trial of metronidazole when they strongly suspect giardiasis. Identifying *E. histolytica* trophozoites by stool examination can be difficult; their visualization is easily impaired by the presence of barium, bismuth, and kaolin compounds. False-negative results of stool examinations also can be caused by the use of preparatory enemas (which lyse the organism) and antibiotics (tetracycline and sulfonamides reduce shedding of trophozoites into the stool).

Other Studies. If symptoms persist and the diagnosis remains uncertain, the patient requires further assessment for a chronic or recurrent diarrheal syndrome (see below). Persons in whom neurologic deficits or meningeal signs develop after a diarrheal illness require culturing of the *blood* and *cerebrospinal fluid* for *Listeria*.

Chronic or Recurrent Diarrhea

History. Diarrhea lasting 4 weeks or more or a pattern of recurrent diarrhea requires an etiologic assessment (Table 64.1).

As in acute diarrhea, *characterization of the diarrhea* and elicitation of any *associated symptoms* are important (Table 64.4).

Suggestive Patterns. A few patterns are suggestive. Frequent passage of *small volumes* of loose stools in association with left lower quadrant crampy abdominal pain or tenesmus points to rectosigmoid pathology. *Large volumes* of loose stools in conjunction with periumbilical or right lower quadrant pain indicate disease of the small bowel, as does diarrhea occurring *shortly after a meal* or ingestion of certain foods. Diarrhea following meals should also lead to a search for malabsorption, an osmotic etiology, the dumping syndrome, or a fistula. The presence of *foul, bulky, greasy* stools further supports the diagnosis of fat malabsorption. *Bloody stools* require investigation for neoplasm, invasive infection, and inflammatory bowel disease. The presence of *fever* has similar diagnostic implications. *Frothy stools* and *excessive flatus* are signs of fermentation of unabsorbed carbohydrates, as occurs in giardiasis. *Alternating diarrhea and constipation* point to irritable bowel syndrome, as does mucus in the stool. The absence of intermittent constipation in a patient with chronic diarrhea does not rule out the diagnosis.

Travel in conjunction with diarrhea that persists for more than 2 weeks raises the possibilities of giardiasis and amebiasis; pseudomembranous colitis is a consideration if the traveler has recently taken antibiotics. The slow resolution of traveler's diarrhea suggests postdysentery lactase deficiency and postdysentery irritable bowel syndrome.

Drugs. A thorough review of drug intake is mandatory; especially important is a check for *antibiotic use*, even if it was a few months before the onset of symptoms. A history of surreptitious *laxative abuse* may be hard to elicit, but inquiring gently and nonjudgmentally about feelings of low self-esteem and a poor body image may provide suggestive information when a young, intense woman presents with chronic diarrhea and wasting.

Prior Surgery. Previous abdominal surgery should be specified, with any procedures that may have produced blind loops and allowed for bacterial overgrowth noted.

Physical Examination. Any fever, dehydration, postural hypotension, or cachexia should be noted. The skin should be inspected for jaundice, pallor, rash, and manifestations of inflammatory bowel disease. The abdomen is examined for distention, ascites, hepatomegaly, tenderness, rebound, and masses. Rectal examination may reveal fecal impaction, perirectal fistula, or a patulous anal sphincter. Stool is tested for occult blood.

Laboratory. Blood tests are helpful but rarely diagnostic. They should include a *complete blood cell count* for evidence of anemia and leukocytosis and determinations of *serum electrolytes* to detect serious losses and imbalances, *amylase* for pancreatic disease, *liver function tests* and *prothrombin time* for hepatobiliary disease, and *serum calcium* and *glucose* for metabolic conditions that can lead to diarrhea. Eosinophil counts are normal in most parasitic infections that cause diarrhea. (The only gastrointestinal parasites that stimulate peripheral eosinophilia are worms.)

Examination of Stool for White and Red Blood Cells. See above. If blood or pus is in the stool, or other evidence of rectosigmoid pathology is present, then one should proceed to sigmoidoscopy (see below).

Other Stool Tests. Additional stool testing can be helpful in selected instances. For suspected laxative abuse, one *alkalinizes the stool*; if it contains phenolphthalein (a common ingredient of many over-the-counter laxatives), it will turn pink. For suspected fat malabsorption, a stool sample is subjected to Sudan stain for *qualitative detection of fat*. Those with a positive result on qualitative study are candidates for a *72-hour*

Table 64.4. Features of Representative Chronic Diarrheas

ETIOLOGY	NATURE OF DIARRHEA			ASSOCIATED SYMPTOMS AND SIGNS	LABORATORY RESULTS
	W/S	OB	GB		
Irritable bowel syndrome	−/+ Mucus prominent	−	−	Bloating, intermittent alternating constipation	Stools: − for WBC/RBC
Ulcerative colitis	+/+	+	+	Fever, abdominal pain, extraintestinal disease, bowel ulcers/inflammation	Stools: + for WBC/RBC Endoscopy: +
Crohn's disease	−/+	+/−	+/−	Abdominal pain, obstruction, skip areas	Proctoscopy +/−; WBC +; o & p −
Pseudomembranous colitis	+/+	+/−	+/−	Simulates inflammatory bowel disease clinically; bowel ulcers/plaques	Stools: + for *Clostridium difficile* toxin/WBC/RBC
Diabetic enteropathy	+/+	−	−	Signs of autonomic insufficiency; occasionally malabsorption	Stools: + for fat (in small-bowel type)
Dumping syndrome	+/+	−	−	Gastric surgery; occurs with meals; sweats, tachycardia	Normal
Malabsorption of fat	−/+ Steatorrhea	−	−	Weight loss, vitamin deficiency, sprue, pancreatic disease	Stools: + for fat
Lactase deficiency	+/+	−	−	Associated with milk products, cramping, bloating	Abnormal lactose tolerance test result
Laxative abuse	+/+	−	−	Wasting, bulimia, dehydration	Stool + for laxatives
Villous adenoma	+/− Secretory, mucus	+	−	Protein wasting, no relation to meats	Hypokalemia, low albumin
Colon cancer	+/+	+	+	Change in bowel habits	Iron deficiency

W/S, watery/soft; OB, occult blood; GB, gross blood; o & p, ova and parasites; WBC, white blood cells; RBC, red blood cells.

quantitative stool fat determination. Normally, stool fat should not exceed 6% of the daily fat intake. Stool fat in excess of 6 g/d while the patient is on a test diet of 100 g of fat per 24 hours indicates fat malabsorption.

Sigmoidoscopy performed without cleansing enemas is a potentially definitive procedure in persons suspected of having inflammatory bowel disease and amebiasis and helps differentiate such conditions from irritable bowel syndrome (see appendix to Chapter 56). The presence of mucosal ulceration, plaques, friability, and bleeding should be noted. The finding of mucus in the absence of evidence of inflammation helps confirm the diagnosis of irritable bowel syndrome, whereas the presence of pus directs the evaluation toward infection and inflammation. Nodular inflammatory ulcers and yellow-white mucosal plaques are characteristic of pseudomembranous colitis. Ulceration is also noted with inflammatory bowel disease and amebic colitis. If Crohn's disease or chronic neoplasia is suspected, *colonoscopy* should be substituted for sigmoidoscopy. Pseudomembranous colitis and amebic disease may produce an endoscopic appearance similar to that of inflammatory bowel disease, so that additional testing is necessary (see below).

Barium Enema and Upper Gastrointestinal Series best demonstrate anatomic abnormalities (blind loops, fistulas, and tumors). A barium enema is an alternative to colonoscopy when inflammatory bowel disease and malignancy are being considered, but the test is not as sensitive and does not allow for biopsy or mucosal sampling. Moreover, amebiasis can simulate inflammatory bowel disease. Because barium obscures the identification of ova and parasites, stool collections must be complete before a barium study is obtained.

Stool for C. difficile Toxin. Patients with recent antibiotic exposure and an inflammatory exudate on sigmoidoscopy require evaluation for pseudomembranous colitis. Up to three stool samples should be assayed for *C. difficile* toxin to maximize sensitivity, although it must be understood that some patients without disease harbor the organism and might show detectable amounts of toxin in the stool.

Mucosal Smears and Stool for Ova and Parasites. If ulceration of the rectosigmoid mucosa is present and *amebic disease* is suspected on the basis of epidemiologic data, fresh mucosal smears should be prepared. Proper technique for the identification of *trophozoites* involves sampling the periphery of the ulcers with a glass rod or metal spatula; cotton swabs are inadequate because the organisms adhere too firmly and do not readily transfer to a slide. Multiple stool examinations for ova and parasites can also be ordered. False-negative results of examinations for trophozoites are common and can be associated with the administration of preparatory enemas, recent exposure to antibiotics, and the concurrent use of barium, bismuth, or kaolin. To detect spore-forming organisms (i.e., *Cryptosporidium*, others), one needs to request that the stool be examined specifically for *spores* and *oocysts.*

Other patients who should have their stools examined for ova and parasites include those who have traveled to areas endemic for *Giardia*, homosexual men, and immunocompromised hosts, including persons with AIDS (who are at risk for harboring a host of pathogens, including *Cryptosporidium*; see below). Fresh loose stools are needed for identification of trophozoites; less fresh specimens can be used for detection of ova. Several stool examinations may be necessary.

Serologic Testing for Amebic Disease. When amebic disease is seriously suspected clinically and epidemiologically, yet results of examinations for ova and parasites are negative, serologic testing is indicated. The standard test is an indirect hemagglutination assay. A positive titer is in excess of 1:128. It takes 2 to 4 weeks for seroconversion to occur. By the time most patients with amebic disease present with diarrhea, they are seropositive. The test is 85% sensitive in the setting of intestinal disease and 95% sensitive with extraintestinal spread. The test works best in nonendemic areas, where most people are seronegative.

Additional Testing for Giardia. Sometimes, *small-bowel aspiration* or even *biopsy* may be necessary to establish the diagnosis of giardiasis or cryptosporidiosis. *Immunologic assay of the stool* based on ELISA (enzyme-linked immunosorbent assay) technology can identify *Giardia* antigen with high sensitivity and specificity (92% and 98%, respectively); the test is rapidly obviating the need for biopsy and aspiration.

Therapeutic Trials sometimes substitute for more elaborate studies. As noted above, cessation of diarrhea in response to *restriction of milk products* strongly supports the diagnosis of lactose intolerance. Other recognized empiric trials include a course of *antibiotic therapy* in patients suspected of blind loop syndrome, and use of *pancreatic enzymes* in patients believed to have pancreatic insufficiency. The once common trial of *metronidazole* for patients with suspected giardiasis is being deferred in favor of sensitive ELISA stool testing for *Giardia* antigen. Some patients are given empiric trials of a gluten-free diet, but bowel biopsy is preferred.

Diarrhea in the AIDS Patient

Often, patients with AIDS experience acute or chronic diarrhea. They especially are susceptible not only to the common pathogens but also to such uncommon ones as *Cryptosporidium*, *M. avium–intracellulare*, herpes simplex virus, cytomegalovirus, *N. gonorrhoeae*, and *C. trachomatis*. Evaluation should focus on finding the pathogen and may require sigmoidoscopic biopsy to obtain tissue for viral or mycobacterial culture (see Chapter 13).

Chronic Diarrhea of Unknown Etiology

The leading possibilities are surreptitious laxative abuse, subtle forms of inflammatory bowel disease, and irritable bowel syndrome. Laxative abuse should be considered in young, professional women who are preoccupied with their weight and have low self-esteem and a poor body image (see Chapter 234). An otherwise unexplained *hypokalemia* is also suggestive. Collagenous and lymphocytic forms of colitis must be considered in women who present with chronic watery diarrhea complicated by steatorrhea and malabsorption, especially those who are thought to have sprue but fail to respond to a gluten-free diet. Irritable bowel syndrome is suggested by the presence of abdominal pain in addition to diarrhea. Although inpatient assessment is often needed, outpatient evaluation can be tried and may obviate the need for hospitalization. Stool analysis and colonoscopy with biopsy are the two most helpful studies.

Stool Analysis. One attempts to characterize the type of diarrhea further by determining *stool volume, osmolality*, and *electrolyte content*. A stool volume of less than 200 mL/d is strongly suggestive of irritable bowel syndrome. Osmotic diarrheas show increased stool osmolality and low sodium and potassium concentrations. The differential diagnosis of osmotic diarrhea includes ingestion of nonabsorbable solutes (magnesium, bran), maldigestion of food, and malabsorption of osmotically active substances (e.g., carbohydrates). Stool volumes in excess of 1 L/d indicate a secretory diarrhea. Occult causes include surreptitious laxative abuse, villous adenoma, carcinoid syndrome, pancreatic cholera (from secretion of vasoactive intestinal peptide), and other rare conditions.

Bowel Biopsy. Because the appearance of the bowel in *collagenous colitis* and *lymphocytic colitis* is grossly normal on endoscopic examination, biopsy is required for diagnosis. Biopsy should be considered in women with unexplained watery diarrhea, especially if complicated by steatorrhea and malabsorption. The small bowel usually is normal but may show spruelike changes in patients with lymphocytic disease.

Inpatient Study. The next step for patients whose condition remains undiagnosed is inpatient evaluation with imposition of a 24- to 72-hour fast and IV hydration. The fast helps to differentiate between osmotic and secretory causes; with the former, diarrhea ceases or is markedly reduced during fasting. Stool analysis is repeated under conditions of fasting and standardized diets.

PRINCIPLES OF MANAGEMENT

Acute Diarrheas

Hydration. The vast majority of cases of acute diarrheal illness should be managed by *maintaining hydration* and waiting for the spontaneous resolution of symptoms. Often, hydration can be maintained with oral fluids, even in cases of profuse diarrhea. Solutions rich in electrolytes and sugar facilitate absorption of water. An 8-oz glass of *fruit juice* to which are added a pinch of table salt and half a teaspoon of honey or a teaspoon of table sugar makes a well-tolerated replacement solution. Nondiet *cola drinks* that have been allowed to stand and lose their carbonation are a reasonable substitute. Either can be taken along with a similarly sized glass of water containing one fourth of a teaspoon of baking soda to replenish losses in stool electrolytes, which in acute infectious diarrhea are sodium (125 mEq/L), potassium (20 mEq/L), bicarbonate (45 mEq/L), and chlorine (90 mEq/L). If adequate hydration cannot be maintained orally, IV therapy is necessary.

Absorbent Preparations are commonly used for symptomatic therapy of simple acute diarrhea. Solutions of *kaolin* and *pectin* have no proven benefit but seem to be harmless; however, they should not be relied on for the treatment of severe diarrhea. Doses of *bismuth subsalicylate (Pepto-Bismol)* in excess of those recommended on the bottle (e.g., 2 to 3 tablespoons every 3 hours) are sometimes effective (see below).

Inhibition of Motility. Opiates such as *diphenoxylate* (dispensed as a combination with small amounts of atropine [Lomotil] to discourage abuse) and *loperamide* (Imodium) are effective in the symptomatic treatment of diarrhea by directly inhibiting the motility of the intestinal smooth muscle. Diphenoxylate and loperamide are derived from meperidine but have less effect on the central nervous system. They should be used cautiously, if at all, in conditions in which toxic megacolon is possible (e.g., inflammatory bowel disease). Their use should also be restricted in certain bacterial diarrheas, such as shigellosis, to avoid prolonging the clinical course. There is also concern for their use in outbreaks of *E. coli* 0157:H7 infection, in which an increased risk for complications has been noted.

The usual dosage of diphenoxylate is 2.5 to 5 mg every 4 hours, up to 20 mg daily. Loperamide is given as 2 or 4 mg every 4 hours, up to 16 mg daily. Lower maintenance doses are often sufficient after initial control has been achieved. Other opiates are potent antidiarrheal agents but carry a higher risk for addiction; they are useful when their coincident analgesic activity is needed. Deodorized tincture of opium (0.5 to 1 mL), paregoric (4 mL), or codeine (30 to 60 mg) can be given orally every 4 hours. *Anticholinergics* are useful only for irritable bowel syndrome (see Chapter 74).

Antibiotics. The *empiric use* of antibiotics is not recommended routinely for acute bacterial diarrheas because most infections are self-limited. Empiric antibiotics have a minimal effect on the course of illness (with the exception of shigellosis outbreaks) and may prolong the asymptomatic bacterial carrier state, especially with *Salmonella* infection. Moreover, one risks triggering an antibiotic-induced diarrhea and inducing antibiotic resistance (e.g., in *Campylobacter*). Antibiotics may also be counterproductive in *E. coli* 0157:H7 infection, in which their use has been associated in some instances with an increased risk for complications.

Antibiotics are best reserved for very ill patients who demonstrate positive stool cultures or other evidence for a specific bacterial etiology (e.g., typhoid fever, salmonellosis, shigellosis, pseudomembranous colitis, *Campylobacter* infection, and *Yersinia* infection).

Salmonella. Elderly patients and others who would be endangered by a *Salmonella* bacteremia (persons with vascular prostheses or sickle cell anemia) should receive a course of antibiotics to limit metastatic infection. *Bacteremia* and *typhoid fever* can be treated with parenteral *ampicillin* or oral *chloramphenicol*; in milder cases, oral *trimethoprim/sulfamethoxazole* (one double-strength tablet of TMS twice daily for 2 weeks) suffices.

Shigella. Patients with severe dysentery caused by shigellosis can be treated with oral *amoxicillin* (500 mg three times daily for 3 to 5 days), but antibiotic sensitivity testing is needed because amoxicillin-resistant strains are common. *TMS* (one double-strength tablet twice daily for 3 to 5 days) is an excellent alternative. Pending stool culture results, a few days of empiric therapy for shigellosis is reasonable if the epidemiologic history is suggestive and the patient is experiencing severe bloody diarrhea. Antiperistaltic drugs are contraindicated.

Campylobacter is sensitive to oral *erythromycin* (500 mg four times daily for 7 days). Most patients with *Yersinia* infection have a self-limited illness, but toxic patients are candidates for oral *chloramphenicol* (50 mg/kg daily in four divided doses for 7 days) or parenteral therapy.

Pseudomembranous Colitis usually resolves without antibiotic treatment, but oral *vancomycin* in a liquid suspension (as little as 125 mg four times daily for 7 to 10 days) and *metronidazole* (250 mg three times daily for 5 to 10 days) have proved equally capable of controlling the disease, although relapses occur in 10% to 20%, so that retreatment is necessary. Metronidazole is preferred for initial use because it is far less expensive. *Cholestyramine* (one packet in water three times daily) is used in conjunction with antibiotics to help bind the enterotoxin; it has proved useful in difficult cases, as have *rifampicin* and *bacitracin*.

Parasitic Infection. Symptomatic patients with diarrhea caused by parasitic infection also benefit from definitive antimicrobial therapy. *E. histolytica* responds to *metronidazole* (750 mg three times daily for 5 to 10 days) for treatment of trophozoites and *diiodohydroxyquin* (650 mg three times daily for 21 days) for elimination of cysts. *Giardiasis* is treated with quinacrine (100 mg three times daily for 7 days) or metronidazole (250 mg three times daily for 7 to 10 days). Retreatment is often necessary.

Traveler's Diarrhea

Prevention. Although much attention has been given to pharmacologic agents for prophylaxis, care in what one eats and drinks remains the single most important means of preventing traveler's diarrhea. Use of local water supplies should be avoided when they are in question. This includes foregoing fresh vegetables, which may have been washed in such water, and even ice cubes. Drinking bottled water is preferable.

Chemoprophylaxis. Because the majority of "turista" cases are caused by enterotoxigenic *E. coli*, chemoprophylaxis has been directed at this organism. *TMS* (one double-strength tablet daily) and *ciprofloxacin* (500 mg daily) can reduce the risk for diarrhea, which ranges from 20% to 30%. For symptomatic relief of acute diarrhea, ciprofloxacin (500 mg twice daily for 3 days) is effective, as is TMS (one double-strength tablet twice daily). Some resistance to TMS is emerging, making ciprofloxacin the preferred agent. *Doxycycline*, a tetracycline derivative, taken on the day of travel (200 mg) and daily (100 mg) while away has also proved useful, although as many as 40% of the toxigenic *E. coli* strains are resistant to the drug, and the drug often causes gastrointestinal upset and photosensitivity. The prophylactic use of antibiotics had been in vogue, but the growing awareness of antibiotic-induced diarrhea, the high frequency of bacterial resistance to some agents, and the efficacy of *bismuth subsalicylate* is leading to less reliance on antimicrobials.

Treatment. Although antibiotics are sometimes used, their disadvantages (see above) suggest the use of other measures first, if possible.

Bismuth Subsalicylate (Pepto-Bismol) has proved effective as both prophylaxis and treatment for traveler's diarrhea when given in large doses (60 mL four times daily). Unlike antibiotics, it has the advantage of not altering the normal bowel flora. Its mechanism of action is believed to involve inhibiting colonization by toxigenic bacterial strains. Bismuth turns the stools black; it is useful to alert patients to this side effect so its occurrence does not cause alarm.

Diphenoxylate or Loperamide is often more convenient for symptomatic relief of traveler's diarrhea than are other measures. In most instances, these agents can be used for brief periods with safety, except when *Shigella* or *Salmonella* infection is a serious consideration (i.e., when fever or rectal bleeding is present). Loperamide has also been a useful adjunct to the antibiotic treatment of symptomatic disease.

Antibiotics are indicated in acute, severe cases. Ciprofloxacin (500 mg twice daily) and TMS (one double-strength tablet twice daily) are both effective, especially when used with loperamide (2 mg after each loose stool, up to 16 mg/d). A 3-day course of antibiotics usually suffices. Giving travelers a 3-day antibiotic supply plus loperamide to carry with them is reasonable and appreciated. Ciprofloxacin is probably preferred because of the emergence of TMS-resistant strains of *E. coli*.

Chronic Diarrhea

Unlike the treatment of acute diarrhea, in which many cases are self-limited and nonspecific measures aimed at symptomatic relief are appropriate, the effective management of chronic diarrhea requires an etiologic diagnosis and specific therapy. Simply suppressing symptoms without identifying a cause may delay identification of a serious underlying condition (e.g., colon cancer or inflammatory bowel disease). Empiric trials are limited to use in diagnosis (see above).

Many causes are treatable. For example, exacerbations of *inflammatory bowel disease* respond to steroids and sulfasalazine; collagenous and lymphocytic forms appear to benefit from a course of bismuth subsalicylate (see Chapter 73). Malabsorption associated with *pancreatic insufficiency* improves with the use of enzyme supplements (see Chapter 72). Steatorrhea caused by *sprue* responds to a gluten-free diet, but not all patients repond to the dietary change because often a concurrent contributing factor is present. *Lactase deficiency* requires limitation of milk products or the use of exogenous lactase. The *dumping syndrome* can be controlled with small feedings. Persistent pseudomembranous colitis is an indication for antibiotic therapy (see above). Cessation of surreptitious *laxative abuse* cures the diarrhea that accompanies it (see Chapter 234). In the setting of *irritable bowel syndrome*, a high-fiber diet is indicated if the clinical picture is predominantly one of constipation interspersed with brief episodes of diarrhea, but if diarrhea predominates, loperamide can be useful for symptomatic relief (see Chapter 74).

Chronic Diarrhea of Unknown Etiology. For patients whose condition remains undiagnosed after an extensive workup yet who appear otherwise well, a trial of therapy for irritable bowel syndrome is reasonable (see Chapter 74). Many such patients with unexplained diarrhea turn out to have a bowel motility disorder and associated psychosocial stresses. Clues to the diagnosis include an absence of weight loss, normal findings on laboratory studies, and a suggestive psychosocial history. Failure to respond after 4 weeks of management should lead to a gastroenterologic consultation. One should not resort to nonspecific antidiarrheal agents to treat patients who have not been given a diagnosis.

INDICATIONS FOR ADMISSION AND REFERRAL

Admission. Most patients with diarrhea can be managed on an outpatient basis. However, for those who are unable to maintain their hydration orally and become significantly volume-depleted (with postural hypotension), hospital admission and parenteral fluid replacement must be seriously considered. Sometimes, several hours of IV fluids given in the emergency department will suffice and obviate an admission. Infants, elderly persons, and persons with chronic or debilitating illnesses such as diabetic renal failure are particularly vulnerable to the complications of volume depletion and warrant close monitoring. Patients with inflammatory diarrhea manifested by bloody, purulent stools and fever are also candidates for admission, as are those with neurologic deficits and meningeal signs following a diarrheal illness, who require assessment for listeriosis. Patients with undiagnosed chronic diarrhea may benefit from the observation and testing possible only during hospitalization.

Referral to a gastroenterologist is indicated for patients who have complicated acute disease (e.g., hemorrhagic diarrhea), poorly controlled inflammatory bowel disease, undiagnosed chronic diarrhea, or who require colonoscopy or intestinal biopsy.

PATIENT EDUCATION

Because most cases of acute diarrhea are self-limited, the patient with no evidence of serious underlying pathology can be reassured and advised to concentrate on maintaining hydration. The sugar and electrolyte preparations described in this Chapter are easy to take and should be encouraged. Many people think that taking fluids will seriously worsen their diarrhea, and they request opiates or antibiotics; the proper role for such agents needs to be reviewed and their unrestricted use should be limited. Many ask if kaolin and pectin preparations are helpful; there is no evidence that they alter symptoms or the course of the illness, but neither are they harmful. Although antibiotics have been in vogue for prophylaxis of traveler's diarrhea, patients should be informed of the emergence of resistant strains, the potential complications of antibiotic use, and the efficacy of bismuth preparations. A few bottles of a bismuth preparation (e.g., Pepto-Bismol), a few tablets of diphenoxylate for "emergencies," and advice to use bottled water and avoid foods likely to be contaminated (e.g., raw vegetables washed with local water) represent reasonable alternatives to antibiotic prophylaxis. Patients with chronic undiagnosed diarrhea need to be prepared for a potentially extensive evaluation. In the meantime, advice on perianal care is much appreciated and ought not to be overlooked while investigation proceeds.

Perianal Hygiene. Much can be done to relieve the perianal discomfort that accompanies severe, unrelenting diarrhea. *Sitz baths* for about 10 minutes two or three times a day can be soothing, followed by gentle drying with absorbent cotton (not toilet paper or towels). Washing with warm water on *absorbent cotton* after each bowel movement is also helpful in lieu of using toilet paper, which can be irritating. Also important is avoidance of soap. Desitin may be effective, and a short course of *hydrocortisone cream* may be useful when considerable anal inflammation is present. Some patients report that cleaning gently with cotton pads soaked in *witch hazel* (Tucks) provides considerable relief. Ointments containing topical anesthetics should be avoided; they can be irritating in themselves.

Recovery Phase. After resolution of diarrhea, it is best to avoid milk and dairy products for approximately another 7 to 10 days because mild lactose intolerance commonly accompanies many cases. The best foods to begin eating are easily digested, high-carbohydrate substances such as bananas, rice, baked potato, and apple sauce. Continued repletion of fluid is important.

ANNOTATED BIBLIOGRAPHY

Afzalpurkar RG, Schiller LR, Little KH, et al. Self-limited nature of chronic idiopathic diarrhea. N Engl J Med 1992;327:1849. (*Clinically useful data on this difficult problem.*)

Bartlett JG. Antibiotic-associated diarrhea. Clin Infect Dis 1992;15:573. (*Authoritative review of pseudomembranous colitis and other forms of diarrhea related to antibiotics.*)

Bayless TM, Rothfeld TM, Massa C, et al. Lactose and milk intolerance: clinical implications. N Engl J Med 1975;292:1156. (*Study of the prevalence, characteristics, and diagnosis of lactose intolerance in adults.*)

Blaser MJ, McDermott KT, Little JR, et al. *Campylobacter* enteritis in the United States: a multicenter study. Ann Intern Med 1983;98:360. (Campylobacter *was more frequently isolated than* Salmonella *and* Shigella *combined.*)

Cann PA, Read NW, Holdsworth CD, et al. Role of loperamide and placebo in the management of irritable bowel syndrome. Dig Dis Sci 1984;29:239. (*Placebo-controlled trial showing reduction in urgency and frequency of bowel movements.*)

Cover TL, Aber RC. *Yersinia* enterocolitica. N Engl J Med 1989;321:16. (*Comprehensive review of this pathogen; 201 references.*)

Dalton C, Austin C, Sobel J, et al. An outbreak of gastroenteritis and fever due to *Listeria monocytogenes* in milk. N Engl J Med 1997;336:100. (*Report of one of a disturbingly more frequent series of outbreaks.*)

Donowitz M, Kokke FT, Saidi R. Evaluation of patients with chronic diarrhea. N Engl J Med 1995;332:725. (*Review plus practical, stepped approach to assessment; 42 references.*)

DuBois R, Lazenby AJ, Yardley JH, et al. Lymphocytic enterocolitis in patients with "refractory sprue." JAMA 1989;262:935. (*Description of this now recognized cause of chronic, watery diarrhea and steatorrhea.*)

Duggan C, Lasche J, McCarty M, et al. Oral rehydration solution for acute diarrhea prevents subsequent unscheduled follow-up visits. Pediatrics 1999;104:29. (*A simple effective therapy.*)

DuPont HL, Ericsson CD. Prevention and treatment of traveler's diarrhea. N Engl J Med 1993;328:1821. (*Excellent review.*)

DuPont HL, Hornick RB. Adverse effect of Lomotil therapy in shigellosis. JAMA 1973;260:1525. (*Lomotil therapy may cause fever and toxicity may be prolonged in patients with shigellosis.*)

DuPont HL, The Practice Parameters Committee of the American College of Gastroenterology. Guidelines on acute infectious diarrhea in adults. Am J Gastroenterol 1997;92:1962. (*Consensus guidelines.*)

Eastham EJ, Douglas AP, Watson AJ. Diagnosis of *Giardia lamblia* infection as a cause of diarrhea. Lancet 1976;2:950. (*Retrospective review of 31 patients found that* Giardia *is not considered often or early enough.*)

Ericsson CD, DuPont HL, Mathewson JJ, et al. Treatment of traveler's diarrhea with sulfamethoxazole and trimethoprim and loperamide. JAMA 1990;263:257. (*Randomized, double-blind study finding combination therapy to be the most effective.*)

Fekety R. Guidelines for the diagnosis and management of *Clostridium difficile*–associated diarrhea and colitis. Am J Gastroenterol 1997;92:739. (*American College of Gastroenterology guidelines.*)

Fine KD, Meyer RL, Lee EL. The prevalence and causes of chronic diarrhea in patients with celiac sprue treated with gluten-free diet.

Gastroenterology 1997;112:1830. (*A host of reasons other than noncompliance detected.*)

Gebhard RL, Gerding DN, Olson MM, et al. Clinical and endoscopic findings in patients early in the course of *Clostridium difficile*–associated pseudomembranous colitis. Am J Med 1985;78:45. (*Useful description of early clinical and sigmoidoscopic appearance of the bowel mucosa.*)

Goodgame RW. Understanding intestinal spore-forming protozoa: *Cryptosporidium, Microsporidia, Isospora,* and *Cyclospora.* Ann Intern Med 1996;124:429. (*Everything you ever wanted to know; 170 references.*)

Goodman LJ, Trenholme GM, Kaplan RL, et al. Empiric antimicrobial therapy of domestically acquired acute diarrhea in urban adults. Arch Intern Med 1990;150:541. (*Randomized, controlled trial; empiric ciprofloxacin was effective for suspected acute bacterial diarrhea; TMS was not.*)

Glynn MK, Bopp C, Dewitt W, et al. Emergence of multidrug-resistant *Salmonella enteritidis* serotype *typhimurium* DT 104 infections in the United States. N Engl J Med 1998;338:1333. (*Documents the widespread nature of this increasingly important pathogen.*)

Gorbach SL, Kean BH, Evans DG, et al. Traveler's diarrhea and toxigenic *Escherichia coli.* N Engl J Med 1975;292:933. (*Classic report documenting that traveler's diarrhea is often caused by enterotoxigenic* E. coli.)

Graham DY, Estes NK, Gentry LO. Double-blind comparison of bismuth subsalicylate and placebo in the prevention and treatment of enterotoxigenic *E. coli*-induced diarrhea in volunteers. Gastroenterology 1983;85:1017. (*Study of 32 volunteers confirming the effectiveness of bismuth subsalicylate in preventing diarrhea.*)

Guerrant RL, Shields DS, Thorson SM, et al. Evaluation and diagnosis of acute infectious diarrhea. Am J Med 1985;78:91. (*Presents a generalizable approach.*)

Harris JC, DuPont HL, Hornick RB. Fecal leukocytes in diarrheal illness. Ann Intern Med 1972;76:697. (*Classic article establishing that fecal leukocytes indicate inflammatory or other tissue-toxic causes of diarrhea, such as shigellosis, salmonellosis, typhoid fever,* E. coli *0157:H7 infection, and inflammatory bowel disease.*)

Kapikian AZ. Viral gastroenteritis. JAMA 1993;269:627. (*A terse discussion of virology, epidemiology, prophylaxis, and treatment.*)

Murphy GS, Bodhidatta L, Echeverria P, et al. Ciprofloxacin and loperamide in the treatment of bacillary dysentery. Ann Intern Med 1993;118:582. (*Found effective.*)

Palmer DL, Koster KT, Islam AF, et al. Comparison of sucrose and glucose in the oral electrolyte therapy of cholera and other severe diarrhea. N Engl J Med 1977;292:1107. (*Discussion of the uses and limitations of oral fluid and electrolyte therapy in severe diarrhea.*)

Palmer KR, Corbett CL, Holdsworth CD. Double-blind, crossover study comparing loperamide, codeine, and diphenoxylate in the treatment of chronic diarrhea. Gastroenterology 1980;79:1272. (*Loperamide was more effective than diphenoxylate and as effective as codeine, and it caused fewer side effects than either agent.*)

Phillips S, Donaldson L, Geisler K, et al. Stool composition in factitious diarrhea: a 6-year experience with stool analysis. Ann Intern Med 1995:123:97. (*Utility of stool analysis documented in cases of chronic diarrhea, with laxative abuse detected.*)

Sandler RS, Zorich NL, Filloon TG, et al. Gastrointestinal symptoms in 3,181 volunteers ingesting snack foods containing Olestra or triglycerides: a 6-week randomized, placbeo-controlled trial. Ann Intern Med 1999;130:253. (*No clinically significant increase in gastrointestinal side effects found.*)

Silva J, Batts DH, Fekety R, et al. Treatment of *Clostridium difficile* colitis and diarrhea with vancomycin. Am J Med 1981;71:815. (*Oral vancomycin proved extremely effective and terminated symptoms within 7 days in all patients tested.*)

Simon D, Brandt LJ. Diarrhea in patients with acquired immunodeficiency syndrome. Gastroenterology 1993;105:1238. (*Comprehensive review of pathogens in cases of AIDS.*)

Slutsker L, Ries AA, Greene KC, et al. *Escherichia coli* 0157:H7 diarrhea in the United States: clinical and epidemiologic features. Ann Intern Med 1997;126:505. (*A population prevalence study that includes clinical features of infection with this increasingly important pathogen.*)

Su C, Brandt LJ. *Escherichia coli* 0157:H7 infection in humans. Ann Intern Med 1995;123:698. (*A systematic review; 217 references.*)

Taylor DN, Sanchez JL, Candler W, et al. Treatment of traveler's diarrhea: ciprofloxacin plus loperamide compared with ciprofloxacin alone. Ann Intern Med 1991;114:731. (*The addition of loperamide was helpful, especially during the first 24 hours.*)

Valdovinos MA, Camilleri M, Zimmerman BR. Chronic diarrhea in diabetes mellitus: mechanisms and approach to diagnosis and treatment. Mayo Clin Proc 1993;68:691. (*Detailed consideration of the consequences of autonomic neuropathy.*)

Weber R, Ledergerber B, Zbinden R, et al. Enteric infections and diarrhea in human inummunodeficiency virus-infected persons. Arch Intern Med 1999;159:1473. (*Data from the Swiss HIV Cohort study on the frequency and causes of acute and chronic diarrhea in this population.*)

Wistrom J, Jertborn M, Ekwall E, et al. Empiric treatment of acute diarrheal disease with norfloxacin: a randomized, placebo-controlled study. Ann Intern Med 1992;117:202. (*Efficacy demonstrated, but benefit limited mostly to the very ill and those with positive cultures.*)

65
Approach to the Patient with Constipation
JAMES M. RICHTER

Constipation is a universal affliction of Western civilization. In the United States, this malady accounts for more than 2.5 million physician visits a year. It is among the most frequent reasons for self-medication and is particularly troublesome in the elderly. More than $500 million are spent annually in the United States on laxatives; a survey of Londoners revealed 30% admitting to recent laxative use.

There is no uniform definition of constipation. To some, it means movements that are too infrequent or stools that are too hard. Others complain of incomplete or difficult evacuation. Among normal people, bowel habits vary widely, and perceptions of what constitutes normal function are diverse. Population studies show that most normal people have more than three bowel movements per week, with men likely to have at least five. Stools of less than 35 g daily are well below the lower limit of normal.

The primary physician must be able to uncover any underlying pathology and provide symptomatic relief to those without a structural lesion. The prevalence of excessive laxative use and inadequate dietary fiber intake make it imperative that the physician be knowledgeable about the actions and adverse effects of available laxative preparations in addition to dietary alternatives to their use.

PATHOPHYSIOLOGY AND CLINICAL PRESENTATION

Normal Physiology. The process of elimination of fecal waste requires two processes: filling of the rectum by colonic transport and reflex defecation of stool. Constipation may arise secondary to interference with either of these processes. The time it takes food to reach the anus is partially a function of the amount of fiber in the diet. Normal people placed on a diet containing 15 g of bran fiber per day have twice the number of movements per week of those on an uncontrolled diet. Patients with constipation solely on the basis of low dietary fiber usually have intermittent complaints that fully resolve with alteration of diet alone. Exercise has an important effect on the propulsion of bowel contents. Colonic transit has been observed to be significantly greater in physically active people than in those who get little exercise.

Inactivity. Previously active persons often become constipated when confined to bed on account of illness. Less dramatic, but probably no less important, is the effect of a sedentary life-style; constipation is common in inactive people.

Metabolic and Endocrine Disturbances can slow colonic transport. Hypokalemia, hypercalcemia, hypothyroidism, and diabetes are the most important of these in terms of frequency or potential reversibility. *Hypokalemia* can produce a generalized ileus and is most often seen in patients who take diuretics. *Chronic laxative abuse* may also produce hypokalemia; surreptitious use of laxatives and diuretics, self-induced vomiting, a pathologic desire to lose weight, and personality disorder are characteristic of such patients, who present with fatigue and electrolyte disturbances. When constipation is caused by *hypothyroidism*, other manifestations of the disease are usually present, although sluggish bowel movements may be the presenting complaint. Constipation is a bothersome problem in some patients with *diabetes*; 20% of those with neuropathy report severe difficulty. Significant *hypercalcemia* (serum calcium level >12 mg/100 mL) can slow bowel motility.

Mechanical Obstruction from tumor, stricture, or volvulus may be responsible for the new onset of constipation. Cramping abdominal pain and distention in conjunction with a marked change in bowel habits are characteristic. Constipation occurs in more than 50% of patients with *colorectal cancers*; it is usually a symptom of advanced disease but may be the presenting complaint. Constipation is a more common presentation of *Crohn's disease* than is diarrhea because transmural involvement predisposes to scarring and obstruction (see Chapter 73).

Motor Dysfunction. Constipation may be the predominant symptom of *irritable bowel syndrome*, a common motility disorder of unknown etiology (see Chapter 74). Patients complain of chronic abdominal discomfort related to alterations in bowel habits and relieved by defecation. They report irregular bowel movements, often diarrhea alternating with constipation (although one may predominate). Passage of mucus, a sense of incomplete evacuation, and bloating or distention add to the clinical picture.

Drug Use may precipitate constipation. *Opiates* and agents with anticholinergic activity such as *antidepressants* are frequently implicated. *Calcium-channel blockers* may slow down bowel motility, and *cholestyramine* may induce constipation by binding bile salts. *Aluminum hydroxide* and *calcium carbonate* antacids are constipating. The habitual use of *laxatives* is associated with impaired motor activity. The typical clinical picture is a long history of chronic constipation or a desire to feel "well cleaned out," followed by increasing laxative dependence, decreasing response, and ultimately a sluggish, poorly contracting bowel. The question of whether a prior underlying motor disorder or actual damage from laxative use is the cause remains unsettled.

Psychiatric Disease and Psychosocial Distress play important roles. An underlying *depression* is often contributory, and bowel complaints may be one of many somatic symptoms (see Chapter 227). Patients with *irritable bowel syndrome* have an increased prevalence of somatization, anxiety, and phobias, which have been linked to triggering disturbances of bowel function. Situational stress appears to play a similar role. The exact mechanisms by which emotional difficulties lead to constipation remain unclear, but their contribution is widely recognized. Disturbances in bowel motility and visceral perception have been documented. Constipation develops in the presence of an excessive degree of nonpropulsive contractions and segmentation of bowel contents. At other times, excessive propulsive activity is noted, typically after meals, resulting in diarrhea.

Neurologic Impairment may present as constipation. *Spinal cord injury* that leads to compression of the cauda equina can halt bowel motility and also cause urinary retention and incontinence. *Multiple sclerosis* may compromise bowel function, as can ganglionic abnormalities. In most instances, other neurologic deficits are present. Disease limited to loss of neurons in the bowel wall typically presents as chronic, refractory constipation; it may date from childhood or, as noted above, be associated with long-standing laxative use. A permanently damaged neuromotor apparatus may also occur as a consequence of *scleroderma*.

Inhibition of the Rectal Defecation Reflex has been documented in cases of painful local anal pathology, neurogenic disease (e.g., Parkinson's disease, multiple sclerosis), long-term use of laxatives, and voluntary suppression. Patients with this problem are found to have stool packed into the rectal ampulla. *Voluntary suppression* of the urge to defecate is usually a concomitant of a hectic daily pace or traveling. The resulting intermittent constipation may lead to excessive use of laxatives and enemas and damage to the reflex emptying mechanism.

Inadequate Fluid Intake may play a role, although this is not well established. Water is known to be an effective means of distending the stomach and stimulating intestinal activity. The consistency of stool is a function of how much water it contains, which is a result, in part, of how much is taken in.

Pelvic Floor Dysfunction accounts for some cases of intractable constipation of unknown etiology. It may be a consequence of inadequate relaxation or inappropriate contraction of the puborectalis and anal sphincter muscles, pelvic floor dyssynergy, or both. Patients complain of the need to strain despite a strong urge to defecate. They may also report a persistent uncomfortable sense of rectal fullness and the need to remove stool digitally from the rectum to obtain relief. With pelvic floor dyssynergy, patients find that supporting the perineum helps during a bowel movement.

DIFFERENTIAL DIAGNOSIS

The causes of constipation can be grouped according to pathophysiology: impaired motility, neurologic disorders, obstruction, and local anorectal pathology (Table 65.1). Many cases remain undiagnosed after initial assessment but respond to empiric therapy. Slow colonic transit and pelvic floor dysfunction often play etiologic roles in such cases, especially in middle-aged and older women with chronic intractable constipation.

WORKUP

History. Evaluation begins with a definition of the size, character, and frequency of bowel movements, followed by a determination of the chronicity of the problem. Acute constipation is more often associated with organic disease than is a long-standing problem. Chronic complaints that wax and wane for months and years point to a functional disturbance, often compounded by habitual laxative use. The patient must be asked about symptoms that suggest an underlying gastrointestinal problem, such as abdominal pain, nausea, cramping, vomiting, weight loss, melena, rectal bleeding, rectal pain, and fever. Anorexia, bloating, belching, flatus, mucus in the stool, headache, depression, and anxiety should also be recorded; these symptoms may be associated with constipation of any etiology but often accompany functional disorders.

Table 65.1.   Important Causes of Constipation

MECHANISM	ETIOLOGY
Impaired Motility	Inadequate dietary fiber
	Inactivity
	Laxative abuse
	Irritable colon syndrome
	Diverticulitis
	Hypothyroidism
	Hypokalemia
	Diabetes
	Hypercalcemia
	Pregnancy
	Scleroderma
	Drugs (opiates, anticholinergics, tricyclic antidepressants, ganglionic blockers, calcium- and aluminum-containing antacids, sucralfate, disopyramide, calcium channel blockers, antihistamines)
Neurologic Dysfunction	Multiple sclerosis
	Spinal cord injury
	Neuroganliomatosis
Psychosocial Dysfunction	Depression
	Situational stress
	Anxiety
	Somatization
	Phobias

It is helpful at the first visit to take a history of working, eating, and bowel habits. Inquiry into dietary fiber intake and physical activity is essential. Use of medications, including nonprescription agents (especially laxatives and antacids), needs to be detailed. The patient's perspective and concerns should be elicited, and a careful psychosocial history obtained, with attention to situational stresses, anxieties, and methods of coping.

Physical Examination. One begins by recording the patient's weight and noting overall nutritional status. Skin is checked for pallor and signs of hypothyroidism (see Chapter 104). The abdomen is examined for masses, distention, tenderness, and high-pitched or absent bowel sounds. Rectal examination includes careful inspection and palpation for masses, fissures, inflammation, and hard stool in the ampulla. The last finding rules out significant obstruction and poor colonic motility and suggests that the problem is inadequate rectal emptying. The stool is noted for color and consistency and tested for occult blood. Anal sensitivity and reflexes are noted. Disordered innervation of the anus is indicated if the anal canal opens wide when the puborectalis muscle is pulled posteriorly. Anoscopy is needed to identify internal hemorrhoids, fissures, tumors, and other local pathology. A neurologic examination should be performed to search for focal deficits and a delayed relaxation phase of the ankle jerks, suggestive of hypothyroidism. A mental status examination includes checking for signs of depression (see Chapter 227), anxiety (see Chapter 226), and somatization (see Chapter 230).

Laboratory Studies. Radiologic investigation is of limited use unless evidence from history and physical examination suggests obstruction or other serious pathology. The acute onset of constipation requires ruling out obstruction and ileus, especially when accompanied by abdominal discomfort. Plain *supine* and *upright films* of the abdomen, plus measurements of serum *potassium* and *calcium* levels, are indicated. More chronic or recurrent forms of constipation should be assessed with a check of the serum glucose level for diabetes (see Chapter 93) and of the serum *thyroid-stimulating hormone* (TSH) for hypothyroidism (see Chapter 104).

If colonic obstruction is suspected (especially if Crohn's disease or cancer is a possibility), *colonoscopy* or *sigmoidoscopy* plus *barium enema* is required. Barium enema is particularly useful and in conjunction with sigmoidoscopy may be preferred to colonoscopy in the assessment of constipation because it is less costly and can demonstrate potentially diagnostic features such as colonic dilation and strictures. Nonetheless, colonoscopy is the test of choice in a case with a positive result on guaiac stool testing, rectal bleeding, anemia, or weight loss in an older patient, all of which suggest the possibility of colorectal cancer (see Chapters 56 and 63). More than 25% of patients with colorectal carcinomas present with constipation.

The elderly person presenting with no evidence of obstruction, anemia, or occult blood loss can probably be followed expectantly for a few weeks, with implementation of an empiric program that includes more dietary fiber, increased exercise, and monitoring with stool guaiac tests, before a decision to subject the patient to colonoscopy or barium enema is made. If symptoms resolve and no other risk factors or findings suggestive of colorectal cancer are present, then the patient can forego bowel visualization at least for the moment. A return visit for repeated assessment of the situation should be scheduled within 4 to 8 weeks. The finding of pigmented colonic mucosa (*melanosis coli*) on direct visualization of the bowel lumen suggests abuse of anthraquinone laxatives such as castor oil or senna.

When the cause of constipation is obscure, it is helpful to stop all nonessential medications. The codeine in a cough suppressant, the calcium in an over-the-counter antacid, or the iron in a multiple vitamin may be responsible for an otherwise puzzling diagnostic problem.

SYMPTOMATIC MANAGEMENT AND PATIENT EDUCATION

Empiric symptomatic management is appropriate for the patient with a suspected functional etiology, but only after obstruction and other forms of serious organic pathology have been ruled out.

Basic First Steps. The first intervention after a careful workup is to reassure the patient that no evidence for a serious underlying illness has been found. Cancer is a common fear, especially in elderly patients with new onset of constipation. Careful *patient education* about diet, exercise, and use of laxatives is the next priority. Explanation is needed to reassure the patient that a daily bowel movement is not essential to good health and that comfortable patterns of elimination depend on good living and eating habits. *Daily exercise* should be prescribed, based on the patient's physical capacity (see Chapter 18). Adequate fluid intake (1.5 to 2 L daily; 6 to 8 glasses of water) is also essential, especially if a high-fiber diet is prescribed.

The patient should *stop taking laxatives, enemas, and nonessential drugs* that may suppress colonic motility. Trying to establish a convenient, uninterrupted *time for defecation* each day may be useful; 15 to 20 minutes after breakfast provides a good opportunity because spontaneous colonic motility is greatest during that period. Continuing this routine each day regardless of travel or situational stress ought to be encouraged. Although no controlled studies are available to prove the efficacy of this approach, it seems to help some people, although days or weeks can pass before success is noted.

In general, these first steps can relieve constipation, but in chronic cases, it may take weeks to months for more satisfactory bowel function to return. Often, immediate results are expected; when they do not appear, the patient becomes despondent, stops the program, and returns to laxative and enema use.

Dietary Fiber and Fiber Supplements. The use of fiber and bulk laxatives can help alleviate symptoms by softening stools and reducing abdominal discomfort. Most clinicians prefer to start with fiber before resorting to bulk laxatives; data on relative efficacy and safety are limited. One begins to increase the fiber content of the diet by adding bran, fruits, green vegetables, and whole-grain cereals and breads. Most studies show that 15 g of fiber per day is needed for the best effects, but the amount can be individualized. A large breakfast including bran cereal, juice, milk or coffee, and whole-grain bread is helpful.

Some patients refuse to eat bran because it makes them feel bloated and gassy. The patient can be reassured that these side effects usually resolve within a month of continued use. If dietary and exercise efforts fail or the patient insists on medication, a *nondigestible fiber residue* such as ground *psyllium* seed (Metamucil), *methylcellulose* (Citrucel), or *polycarbophil* can be beneficial. It acts to increase bulk by means of its hydrophilic properties, but it must be taken with plenty of fluids to prevent formation of an obstructing bolus; the usual dose is one teaspoon in 8 oz of liquid three times a day. Placebo-controlled studies show significant improvement in symptoms with use, but the placebo groups also show improvement, which suggests that explanation, reassurance, and increased attention are also important to improved bowel function.

Laxatives of First Choice. The constipation of some elderly patients will remain refractory to the above measures, and they will press for prescription of a laxative. A few classes are relatively safe and worth considering when simpler measures have failed. Efficacy in controlled trials is similar to that of fiber.

Nonabsorbable Saccharide/Bulk Laxatives (e.g. lactulose, sorbitol) have been shown to be safe and effective when used on a long-term basis in the elderly. These agents induce a potent osmotic effect, retaining fluid in the bowel lumen and softening the stool. The cost of sorbitol (30 to 60 mL daily at bedtime) is about a tenth that of lactulose, and sorbitol has been shown in double-blind crossover studies to be equal in effect and slightly better tolerated. Side effects include excessive flatulence, bloating, and cramping.

Magnesium-containing Laxatives (e.g., milk of magnesia, magnesium citrate) are also osmotically active, but they should be used more cautiously because they may induce magnesium and sodium overload in older persons with renal dysfunction. They are less expensive than sorbitol.

Surfactant Laxatives such as docusate soften stool by promoting the mixing of water and fat. They are worth a try in patients reporting hard stools, but evidence supporting their efficacy is limited (see below) and their cost is high.

Other Laxative Preparations. Most other laxatives are probably worth avoiding for regular use because of the potential for adverse effects (although definitive data documenting adverse effects are limited).

Stimulant/Irritant Laxatives include the derivatives of diphenylmethane (*bisacodyl*), anthraquinone (*senna*), and cascara. These irritants trigger colonic contraction acutely; long-term use is associated with an increased risk for bowel refractoriness and worsening constipation (*laxative abuse syndrome*).

Prokinetic Agents. *Cisapride* is a prokinetic agent producing dopaminergic stimulation. Experience is still limited regarding its use in chronic constipation; however, when used in esophageal reflux, it is associated with an increased risk for ventricular dysrhythmias, which limits its appropriateness in the elderly.

Enemas. When *fecal impaction* is present, a *hypertonic enema* (e.g., Fleet) will often relieve the situation. *Soapsuds enemas* should be avoided because colitis has been reported with their use. The patient with impaction who is taking an enema can be instructed to squat over the toilet by standing on a chair in front of the bowl, which provides a more favorable position for evacuating the rectum. Only rarely does one need to resort to disimpaction.

Prevention of constipation during an illness that requires bed rest can be achieved with a high-fiber diet, bulk agents, and use of a commode in preference to a bedpan. Correction of any coincident hypokalemia is important (see Chapter 32). There is no evidence that prophylactic use of laxatives or stool softeners is effective. A randomized, controlled study of dioctyl sodium sulfosuccinate (Colace), a popular and expensive stool softener, failed to demonstrate any effect on the quality or frequency of stools. Use of minor tranquilizers in overly anxious patients has little direct effect on constipation. When severe depression requires use of antidepressants, the least constipating agent should be selected (i.e., one with minimal anticholinergic activity). All tricyclic antidepressants have at least some anticholinergic activity, but desipramine, nortriptyline, and trazodone seem to have the least. Alternatively, a nontricyclic antidepressant such as sertraline might be a reasonable choice (see Chapter 227).

The Patient–Doctor Relationship. The importance of establishing a trusting, therapeutic patient–doctor relationship cannot be overemphasized, especially when the probability of underlying psychosocial distress is high. One facilitates the establishment of trust by eliciting concerns and perspective and taking time to explain and answer questions. A patient who has used a particular agent for decades needs to be told why it is being removed from the program; otherwise, chances of compliance are small. Long-term laxative users should be warned that it may take 4 to 6 weeks before spontaneous bowel movements return. Patience and sympathetic support can be rewarding, but expectations of quick results must not be raised (see also Chapter 74).

ANNOTATED BIBLIOGRAPHY

Almy TP. Management of the irritable bowel syndrome. Ann Intern Med 1992;116:1027. (*Editorial perspective on this difficult problem.*)

Baron TH, Ramirez B, Richter JE. Gastrointestinal motility disorders in pregnancy. Ann Intern Med 1993;118:366. (*Constipation is common; mechanisms reviewed.*)

Burkitt D, Walker A, Paintner N. Effect of dietary fibre on stools and transit times and its role in causation of disease. Lancet 1972;2:1408. (*Classic article on fiber and its link to constipation and other bowel problems.*)

Camileri M, Thompson WG, Fleshman JW, et al. Clinical management of intractable constipation. Ann Intern Med 1994;121:520. (*A review of both the basic approach and the tertiary center's protocol for patients who fail standard therapy.*)

Camilleri M, Prather CM. The irritable bowel syndrome: mechanisms and a practical approach to management. Ann Intern Med 1992;116:1001. (*Excellent review and a balanced, pathophysiologic approach to therapy; 78 references.*)

Cann PA, Read NW, Holdsworth CD. What is the benefit of coarse wheat bran in patients with irritable bowel syndrome? Gut 1984;25:168. (*Double-blind, placebo-controlled study demonstrating efficacy.*)

Connell A, Hilton C, Irvine R, et al. Variation of bowel habits in two population samples. Br Med J 1965;2:1095. (*Population study helping to define the range of normal for bowel activity and the prevalence of constipation.*)

Darlington RC. Over-the-counter laxatives. J Am Pharm Assoc 1966;6:470. (*Data on spending for over-the-counter preparations; dated but enlightening and still valid.*)

Drossman DA, Thompson WG. The irritable bowel syndrome: review and a graduated multicomponent treatment approach. Ann Intern Med 1992;116:1009. (*Emphasizes the biopsychosocial model and the importance of the patient–doctor relationship to a successful outcome.*)

Goodman J, Pang J, Bessman A. Dioctyl sodium sulfosuccinate: an ineffective prophylactic laxative. J Chronic Dis 1976;29:59. (*Randomized, prospective study of patients admitted to the hospital. The drug made no difference in quality or frequency of stools.*)

Graham DY, Moser SE, Estes MK. The effect of bran on bowel function and constipation. Am J Gastroenterol 1982;77:599. (*Twenty grams of wheat or corn bran reduced transit time by 50% and improved constipation clinically in 6 of 10 constipated women.*)

Holdstock D, Misiewicz JJ, Smith T, et al. Propulsion in the human colon and its relationship to meals and somatic activity. Gut 1970;11:91. (*Physical activity was found to stimulate mass movements, and inactivity reduced them.*)

Hull C, Greco RS, Brooks DL. Alleviation of constipation in the elderly by dietary fiber supplementation. J Am Geriatr Soc 1980;28:410. (*In an institutional geriatric population, adding bran prevented constipation and reduced laxative use.*)

Katz L, Spiro H. Gastrointestinal manifestations of diabetes. N Engl J Med 1966;275:1350. (*A classic review; constipation is a frequent gastrointestinal complaint of diabetics.*)

Kirwn WO, Smith AN. Colonic propulsion in diverticular disease, idiopathic constipation and the irritable bowel syndrome. Scand J Gastroenterol 1974;12:331. (*Transit time is prolonged in all three diseases and can be significantly reduced by bran.*)

Lederle FA, Busch DL, Mattox BS, et al. Cost-effective treatment of constipation in the elderly: a randomized double-blind comparison of sorbitol and lactulose. Am J Med 1990;89:597. (*Demonstrates efficacy and comparability; useful in elderly patients with refractory functional disease.*)

Longstreth GF, Fox DD, Youkeles MS, et al. Psyllium in irritable bowel syndrome: a double-blind study. Ann Intern Med 1981;95:53. (*Both treatment and control groups showed equally impressive degrees of improvement, which suggests that other factors are also operative.*)

Matthews DA, Suchman AL, Branch WT Jr. Making "connections": enhancing the therapeutic potential of patient–clinician relationships. Ann Intern Med 1993;118:973. (*Useful piece with important insights into the treatment of patients with functional bowel disease.*)

Oster JR, Materson BJ, Rogers AI. Laxative abuse syndrome. Am J Gastroenterol 1980;74:451. (*Review article outlining this important cause of chronic constipation.*)

Roth HP, Fein SB, Shurman JF. The mechanisms responsible for the urge to defecate. Gastroenterology 1957;32:717. (*Describes normal process of defecation and provides physiologic basis for understanding disease states.*)

Sonnenberg A, Koch TR. Epidemiology of constipation in the United States. Dis Colon Rectum 1989;32:1. (*Accounts for more than 2.5 million physician visits per year.*)

Tramonte SM, Brand MB, Mulrow CD, et al. The treatment of chronic constipation in adults: a systematic review. J Gen Intern Med 1997;12:15. (*A look at the evidence from randomized trials; finds that both fiber and laxatives help, but few data on which treatment is best.*)

66
Approach to the Patient
with Anorectal Complaints

Anorectal complaints often go incompletely evaluated. Although they are usually a result of minor conditions such as hemorrhoids or fissures, causes range beyond the trivial to inflammatory bowel disease, cancer, and infection. In addition, anorectal problems generate a substantial amount of worry and discomfort. As a result, they deserve careful consideration by the primary care physician. An increasingly frequent diagnostic challenge is the evaluation of anorectal problems in male homosexuals.

PATHOPHYSIOLOGY AND CLINICAL PRESENTATION

Anorectal complaints result from traumatic, vascular, infectious, inflammatory, neurologic, and malignant causes. Symptoms include pain, discharge, itching, mass, and fecal incontinence. *Pain* is most often a manifestation of anal pathology; anal and perianal skin are richly innervated with pain-sensitive nerve fibers; rectal tissue is relatively insensitive to pain. A fissure, distention by abscess or hemorrhoid, invasion by tumor, or marked inflammation can lead to considerable discomfort. Secondary anal sphincter spasm may ensue, prolonging and intensifying the pain. *Discharge* results from inflammation of the rectal mucosa or drainage of an abscess. Cancer, abscess, and thrombosed hemorrhoids can produce an anorectal *mass*; condylomata acuminata may also cause anal skin nodularity. *Itching* represents a minor form of skin irritation that occurs with a variety of mechanical and inflammatory lesions; it is intensified by moisture in the perianal area. Chronic itching leads to excoriation, edema, thickening, fissuring, and lichenification of the perianal skin. *Bleeding* is a common and important manifestation of anorectal pathology; its causes range from hemorrhoids and fissures to carcinoma and inflammatory bowel disease (see Chapter 63).

Hemorrhoids. The most common of all anorectal problems, hemorrhoids affect about half of patients over the age of 50. They represent dilations of the anorectal vascular network. Epidemiologically, they are associated with diets high in fat and low in fiber. Theories explaining the development of hemorrhoids invoke a number of mechanisms, including increased venous pressure secondary to upright posture and straining at stool, arteriovenous communications in rectal tissue, and prolapsed cushions of tissue secondary to loss of support. Clinically, hemorrhoids are associated with pregnancy, portal hypertension, and constipation. The relative absence of hemorrhoids in African populations that have high-residue diets has led to the suggestion that an increase in dietary fiber might prevent the development of hemorrhoids.

Although the traditional view is that hemorrhoids are venous varicosities resulting from straining at stool, they do not always present in a fashion consistent with this postulate. For example, hemorrhoids appear in early pregnancy in many young women, long before the development of significant intraabdominal pressure from a large fetus. Moreover, hemorrhoidal blood is characteristically arterial in quality (bright red) rather than the dark variety that would be expected from a strictly venous source. Nonetheless, many patients with hemorrhoids have been found to have increased resting anal sphincter pressures, which supports the hypothesis that increased anal pressure causes straining at stool. The straining stresses and compromises the supporting fibrous tissue of the rectal mucosa, allowing the now poorly supported mucosa to slide down and become entrapped by the sphincter. Venous engorgement is a consequence of the entrapment.

Classification. Hemorrhoids may be classified by presentation as *first-degree* when they merely bleed, *second-degree* if they prolapse on high pressure but return spontaneously, and *third-degree* when the anal suspensory ligament is stretched to the point of permanent prolapse. Hemorrhoids are considered to be *internal* when derived from the superior hemorrhoidal plexus above the dentate line, and *external* when located below the dentate line and covered by squamous epithelium. External hemorrhoids are covered by pain-sensitive anal skin and arise from the inferior hemorrhoidal plexus. Internal hemorrhoids are covered by the much less pain-sensitive rectal mucosa and represent dilations of the superior hemorrhoidal plexus.

Clinical Presentation. Pain, incomplete defecation, constipation, excessive moisture, rectal itching, bleeding, or a prolapsed mass are the common presentations. Clinical presentation depends in part on the location of the hemorrhoid and the presence of complications. External hemorrhoids that have thrombosed present as tender, bluish swellings. Internal hemorrhoids often bleed, but only when they prolapse do they present as a mass; when irreducible, they are subject to thrombosis. Recurrent bleeding may be seen with either type; sudden rupture may cause rather dramatic, although relatively harmless, bright red bleeding. Hemorrhoids are regularly encountered as incidental findings on physical examination. Skin tags are evidence of previous hemorrhoids that have thrombosed, leaving connective tissue. The most bothersome complications of hemorrhoids include bleeding, prolapse, and thrombosis.

Fistula-in-ano is a communication between the anal canal and the perianal skin. It is usually nontender. The external opening may be single or multiple, with a granulation tissue bud and chronic seropurulent drainage. Occasionally, an indurated cord of tissue may be palpable, extending from the external fistulous opening toward the anal canal. The fistula may result from rupture or surgical drainage of a perirectal abscess; other causes include Crohn's disease, carcinoma, tuberculosis, radiation therapy, lymphogranuloma venereum, and anal fissure. Patients complain of persistent and irritating drainage of blood, pus, or mucus.

Perirectal Abscess and fistula-in-ano are two stages of the same disease process, beginning as an infection in the anal glands that empty into the anal crypts at the mucocutaneous junction, and subsequently spreading into the adjacent tissue. The abscess thus formed often drains through the perianal skin. Symptoms and signs are a function of the size and location of the abscess. The first manifestation is rectal pain, which may occur before any mass becomes palpable. Patients characteristically complain of constant, throbbing pain in the perianal region or in the rectum. A mass may be identified externally on examination of the anus or internally during palpation the rectum. The formation of perirectal abscesses is a particularly important problem in patients with Crohn's disease, immunodeficiency states, and hematologic disorders.

Infected Pilonidal Cyst or Sinus is most common in boys and young men between the ages of 16 and 30. These are midline, in the area of the natal cleft. Multiple sinuses may be present. Recurrent secondary infections are frequent.

Carcinoma of the Anus. Carcinoma involving the perianal skin or anorectal tract typically does not cause pain until relatively late in its clinical course, often in the setting of a large, ulcerated, bleeding lesion. Earlier lesions present as painless nodules or plaques. Pruritus, mucoid drainage, and changes in bowel habits are more subtle manifestations that sometimes occur.

Proctalgia Fugax, as the term implies, is fleeting but severe rectal pain believed to be related to spasm of the levator ani and coccygeal muscles. Although usually brief, symptoms can last for more than 30 minutes. Suspected precipitants include chronic trauma from poor posture; psychogenic factors may also be operative. No associated physical findings are present, except for muscle tenderness on digital examination.

Proctitis, inflammatory disease of the rectum, is associated with a wide variety of conditions, ranging from infection and trauma to radiation and inflammatory bowel disease. Regardless of the cause, the presentation is usually one of mucopurulent discharge, rectal bleeding, and, in severe cases, rectal pain and tenesmus. Patients with *ulcerative proctitis* demonstrate on sigmoidoscopy an inflamed rectal mucosa and a clearly demarcated upper border, above which the mucosa is normal. Systemic symptoms and extraintestinal manifestations are rare when the disease is limited to the rectum. The risk for carcinoma is small, and diffuse colitis develops in fewer than 10% to 15% of patients.

Infectious Proctitis occurs mostly among promiscuous *male homosexuals* who engage in frequent rectal intercourse with multiple partners. Gonorrhea, amebic disease, chlamydial infection, and herpes simplex infection are prominent in this population (see below). *Gonococcal proctitis* is especially common. The rate of asymptomatic carriage of gonorrhea among promiscuous male homosexuals is reportedly as high as 60% to 70%. Symptomatic gonococcal proctitis presents with discharge and rectal discomfort (see below). Diarrhea is the hallmark of symptomatic *amebic infection*, *shigellosis*, and *Campylobacter* infection (see Chapter 64). *Herpes sim-*

plex proctitis can be a very painful condition, accompanied by tenesmus, constipation, rectal ulceration, and discharge. Involvement of the sacral nerve roots can lead to bladder and erectile difficulties, paresthesias, and pain in the thighs and buttocks.

Solitary Rectal Ulcer is a rare condition of unknown cause associated with rectal discharge, bleeding, and, occasionally, dull pain. The characteristic finding on sigmoidoscopy is a single shallow ulcer 7 to 10 cm from the anus; its borders may be heaped or nodular. Chronicity is the rule; complications are rare. These lesions must be distinguished from cancer and lymphogranuloma venereum by biopsy.

Pruritus Ani (chronic perianal itching) is not a diagnosis but rather a syndrome that results from a variety of mechanical and inflammatory lesions. Anatomic lesions that produce chronic discharge (such as *fistulas*, *fissures*, and *hemorrhoids* with intermittent mucosal eversion) can result in pruritus ani. Infectious causes are numerous. *Anogenital warts (condylomata acuminata)* are viral in origin and generally transmitted by sexual contact. They may be confined to the perianal region or also involve the penis, vulva, and anal canal. Multiple, soft, filiform excrescences characterize these lesions, which may enlarge, become confluent, and even bleed. *Gonococcal proctitis* can lead to anal soreness, burning, and purulent discharge. Infestations with *pinworm (Enterobius vermicularis)* typically cause nocturnal anal itchiness, especially among children, but sometimes spread to involve adult family members. Nocturnal symptoms are caused by the daily evening migration of the female pinworm downward to deposit eggs on the perianal skin. Anal involvement is characteristic of some systemic dermatologic diseases, such as *psoriasis* and scabies. *Contact dermatitis* or *eczema* resulting from use of a topical agent is common and can complicate the diagnosis of the original cause of pruritus. Applied initially as a remedy for itching, the agent may only aggravate the problem by causing skin sensitization. Itching is intensified by moisture in the perianal area and often aggravated by the use of topical agents applied in an attempt to quell symptoms. The passage of *alkaline stools* (as occurs in severe diarrhea) can have an irritant effect on the anal skin. Persistent anal itching may be a form of *neurodermatitis*; such patients characteristically present with multiple excoriations. *Candida infection* is found among diabetics, homosexuals, and those recently taking broad-spectrum antibiotics; perianal erythema and itching are presenting manifestations.

Fecal Impaction ranks as one of the major sources of anorectal discomfort among the elderly and bedridden. Chronic incomplete evacuation leads to formation of an obstructing bolus of desiccated hard stool in the rectum. Symptoms of anal discomfort and constipation are typical, but anorexia, malaise, or nonspecific lower abdominal fullness may be all that is reported. Paradoxically, diarrhea rather than constipation is sometimes the only complaint; this is caused by the collection of liquid stool that distends the proximal colon and passes around the obstructing bolus. Unless this problem is corrected by disimpaction, complications such as intestinal obstruction, rectal prolapse, and even bowel perforation may ensue.

Table 66.1. Differential Diagnosis of Anorectal Problems

PROBLEM	DIFFERENTIAL DIAGNOSIS
Anal discomfort	Hemorrhoids Fissure-in-ano (hard bowel movement, cancer, venereal disease) Fistula-in-ano (perirectal abscess, Crohn's disease, carcinoma, radiation, TB, lymphogranuloma venereum) Perirectal abscess (Crohn's disease, immunodeficiency, hematologic disorders) Infected pilonidal cyst Carcinoma of the anal epidermis Infections (syphilis, candidiasis, condylomata acuminata)
Rectal discomfort	Proctitis (ulcerative, gonococcal, amebic, herpetic), often accompanied by discharge and bleeding Perirectal abscess Impaction Proctalgia fugax Solitary rectal ulcer
Pruritus ani	Excess moisture (poor hygiene), pinworms, eczema, scabies, diabetes, liver failure, irritants (topical agents, alkaline stools), fissure, early cancer, neurodermatitis, and infections (see above)
Incontinence	Rectal surgery, neurologic disease, perianal disease

Fecal Incontinence follows damage to the normal anal sphincter mechanism. Perianal disease, anal surgery, and neurologic disease can have devastating psychosocial consequences when the anal sphincter becomes compromised. Some patients lose the ability to sense rectal distention and to constrict the external sphincter. In others, with only a weakened sphincter, the prognosis is less grim; biofeedback methods can be employed to help them regain continence.

Anorectal Problems in Homosexuals and others engaging in receptive anal intercourse can be complex in etiology and presentation. In a major study, more than 80% of homosexual men presenting to a venereal disease clinic with anorectal or intestinal symptoms were infected with one or more sexually transmissible anorectal or enteric pathogens. Three principal syndromes were noted: a *proctitis* characterized by anorectal pain, lesions, and discharge, but no evidence of disease above the rectum; a *proctocolitis* that, in addition to manifestations of proctitis, included diarrhea, tenesmus, and inflammation extending into the sigmoid mucosa; and an *enteritis* (see Chapter 64) that consisted of diarrhea and abdominal pain, but no anorectal symptoms or signs.

As noted above, gonococcal, herpetic, chlamydial, and syphilitic forms of proctitis occur with increased frequency among these patients. *Gonorrhea* occurs in about a third of patients; *herpes simplex type 2 virus* is cultured from about one fifth, who also manifest rectal mucosal ulcerations. About 3% of symptomatic persons have anal syphilitic chancres, and another 3% show evidence of secondary anorectal syphilitic disease (erythematous nodular or indurated rectal mucosal lesions from which biopsy specimens test positive).

A clinical and sigmoidoscopic picture of *proctocolitis* occurs in about 15% of cases. Such patients complain of anorectal discomfort, tenesmus, diarrhea, constipation, and abdominal cramps. On sigmoidoscopy, inflammatory changes start at the rectum and extend beyond 15 cm into the sigmoid colon. *Campylobacter*, *Entamoeba histolytica*, *Chlamydia*, and *Clostridium difficile* are significantly correlated with the enterocolitis; often, more than one organism is recovered. Polymicrobial infection is commonplace among symptomatic male homosexuals with many sexual partners.

Although much of the proctitis in this population is infectious in origin, *culture-negative proctitis* occurs with some frequency and has been linked to exposure to the *coloring agents* and scents found in some of the lubricants used for anal intercourse. Manifestations of several causes may present simultaneously. The patient complaining of hemorrhoidal pain may actually have concurrent gonorrhea, allergic proctitis, and chlamydial infection. Traumatic complications of rectal intercourse include prolapsed hemorrhoids, anal fistulas and fissures, perirectal abscesses, rectal ulcers, and anal tears. Foreign bodies are sometimes recovered.

DIFFERENTIAL DIAGNOSIS

The differential diagnosis of anorectal problems can best be considered in anatomic terms, depending on whether symptoms and signs are predominantly anal, anorectal, or rectocolonic (Table 66.1). This is particularly true when the causes of anorectal disease in male homosexuals are considered (Table 66.2).

WORKUP

History. Although a careful physical examination is the single most important part of the evaluation, the history can provide important epidemiologic and etiologic information. Determining whether the condition is predominantly anal (local pain only), anorectal (local anal pain plus rectal discomfort, tenesmus, rectal discharge, constipation), or rectocolonic (rectal discomfort, tenesmus, and rectal discharge plus diarrhea, abdominal pain, bloating, nausea) helps to focus the evaluation.

Patients with anal complaints ought to be questioned about masses, nodules, focal tenderness, history of hemorrhoids, psoriasis, passage of hard stool, bleeding, discharge, generalized itching, nocturnal pattern, and recent trauma. Detailed inquiry into the use of topical medications (many of which are sensitizing), involvement of other household members or sexual partners, and hygienic practices should also be made.

Table 66.2. Differential Diagnosis of Anorectal Problems in Male Homosexuals

SYNDROME	ETIOLOGY
Proctitis	*Neisseria gonorrhoeae* Herpes simplex *Chlamydia* (nonlymphogranuloma strains) Syphilis Condylomata acuminata Trauma Chemical irritants
Proctocolitis	*Campylobacter* *Shigella* *Entamoeba histolytica* *Chlamydia* (lymphogranuloma strains)
Enteritis	*Giardia lamblia*

For patients with anorectal involvement, the physician should check into symptoms of inflammatory bowel disease (see Chapter 73), obtain a careful and detailed sexual history focusing on the number of partners and practice of receptive rectal intercourse, and note any reports of inguinal adenopathy (seen with herpes and lymphogranuloma), sacral root paresthesias, and difficulty with micturition (other telltale symptoms of herpes simplex infection). Those with rectocolonic symptoms are likely to have either inflammatory bowel disease or a polymicrobial infection from rectal intercourse; consideration of associated symptoms and risk factors is indicated.

Physical Examination. Thorough and gentle inspection of the anus and perianal region is the *sine qua non* for a successful diagnosis of anorectal problems. One examines the anal skin for erythema, eczema, psoriatic patches, ulcerations, vesicles, fistulas, fissures, condylomata, nodules, hemorrhoids, and inflammatory changes. The presence of perianal or rectal ulcers in association with proctitis in a male homosexual is indicative of syphilis or herpes simplex. If the lesions appear as scaling plaques, a look at the skin of the extensor surfaces of the extremities might provide additional evidence for a diagnosis of psoriasis. In a very anxious patient with multiple excoriations over other parts of the body, neurodermatitis should be suspected as the cause of pruritus ani. If an inflamed anorectal mucosa is encountered, gonorrhea needs to be considered and inquiry into rectal intercourse needs to be pursued.

Stretching the perianal skin will reveal fissures, which come into view at the anal verge, most often in the posterior midline but occasionally in the anterior midline. With chronic fissures, scarring and induration are seen in addition to an associated hypertrophied anal papilla at the pectinate line; a skin tag marks the external limit. Crohn's disease is likely in those with multiple fissures, recurrent fistulas, or perirectal abscesses. A painless hard nodule or plaque in the anal region may represent carcinoma. When the lesion is ulcerated, the diagnosis is more obvious and the disease is more advanced.

Digital rectal examination is almost always an essential component of the examination. However, in the presence of a painful fissure, this can be an extremely painful procedure that is likely to alienate the patient and cause such pain as to make adequate examination impossible. The same applies to the use of anoscopy in such patients. On the other hand, rectal examination should never be deferred in patients who are not acutely and severely uncomfortable.

One needs to check for masses (both fluctuant and firm), discharges, ulcerations, and other mucosal changes and also to test the stool for occult blood. Ascribing anorectal symptoms to hemorrhoids without performing as complete an examination as possible is a common reason for delay in the diagnosis of carcinoma.

Palpation for enlarged lymph nodes should not be overlooked. Prominent inguinal adenopathy is characteristic of herpetic and chlamydial infections (lymphogranuloma venereum species).

Diagnostic Studies. Unless the patient has a very painful lesion, *anoscopy* needs to be performed (see appendix, Chapter 56) to visualize the canal and mucosa adequately and obtain samples of any discharge. One inspects for mucosal inflammation, fissure, fistula, mass, plaque, ulcer, and discharge. Patients with rectal inflammation, fistula formation, nonhealing fissures, bleeding, or diarrhea are candidates for *sigmoidoscopy*. Involvement of the sigmoid mucosa suggests inflammatory bowel disease (see Chapter 73) and infectious forms of colitis (see Chapter 64). Patients with atypical fissures (especially those that fail to heal), painless hard anorectal nodules, and mucosal ulcerations are candidates for *biopsy* to rule out malignancy, inflammatory bowel disease, and chronic infection (syphilis, tuberculosis). Children with nocturnal pruritus ani can be evaluated for pinworm infestation by taking a cellophane tape impression of the anus and microscopically examining it under low power for the characteristic eggs.

Male homosexuals engaging in receptive anal intercourse with many sexual partners should undergo anoscopy to determine the nature of rectal involvement and to obtain samples of mucus for *Gram's stain* and culture on *Thayer-Martin plates*. A positive smear with Gram's stain is excellent presumptive evidence of gonorrhea, although a negative smear does not rule out the diagnosis. Any chancrelike lesions should be subjected to *dark-field* examination for spirochetes. A *serologic test for syphilis* is also obtained.

Homosexual patients with evidence of rectal pathology on anoscopy require *sigmoidoscopy*; establishing the extent of mucosal involvement helps narrow the list of possible causes. Those with a *proctocolitis* picture of mucosal involvement extending above 15 cm or symptoms of colitis (diarrhea, nausea, abdominal cramping) should have specimens *cultured for Campylobacter*, *Chlamydia* (lymphogranuloma strains), and *Shigella* and have their stools examined for the *ova* and *trophozoites* of *Entamoeba histolytica*. Those with *proctitis* only (no mucosal disease above 15 cm) are more likely to have gonorrhea, herpes simplex, or chlamydial infection (nonlymphogranuloma strains), and specimens can be cultured accordingly. Viral cultures are not necessary because the diagnosis of herpes simplex proctitis can usually be made on the basis of its characteristic clinical presentation (severe anorectal pain, multiple perianal ulcers, rectal ulceration, inguinal adenopathy, difficult micturition, impotence, and paresthesias in the S-4 and S-5 distributions).

SYMPTOMATIC MANAGEMENT AND INDICATIONS FOR REFERRAL

Acute Anal Fissure. Patients with anal pain caused by fissure should initially be treated symptomatically. Lubricants, such as mineral oil, and agents providing a soft, bulky stool, such as methylcellulose, will decrease trauma and counteract the attendant sphincter spasm. Frequent warm sitz baths provide intermittent relief of pain and spasm. Topical analgesics are of limited use and may result in skin sensitization. Systemic analgesics are sometimes necessary, but if narcotics are used, constipation may be aggravated.

Chronic Anal Fissure. If the pain has not improved with conservative measures in several days to weeks, the patient should be referred for consideration of surgical treatment, which has a high success rate. In general, chronic or recurrent fissures will require surgery more often than acute or superficial fissures. In patients in whom the pain of fissure precludes digital or instrumental examination at the first visit, these may be performed at the time of surgical treatment under adequate anesthesia. *Sphincterotomy* is used to counter the internal sphincter spasm that maintains the tear, but because the procedure permanently weakens the sphincter, it may be followed by incontinence. Up to 30% of patients undergoing sphincterotomy may be so affected. Less invasive alternatives include one to two injections of *botulinum toxin* into the internal anal sphincter (95% healing rate) and daily application of *topical nitroglycerine* ointment for 2 to 6 weeks (60% healing rate). Botulinum toxin injection appears to heal fissures with a frequency equal to that of surgery without inducing long-term incontinence.

Perirectal Abscess will not resolve on antibiotics alone; the proper treatment is surgical drainage. Antibiotic therapy should be reserved for patients with extensive cellulitis, signs of systemic infection, immunosuppression, valvular heart disease, or intravascular prostheses. Incision and drainage of a perirectal abscess usually requires anesthesia and is not often an office procedure. Similarly, the treatment for an infected pilonidal sinus is surgical drainage, which is accomplished satisfactorily under local anesthesia.

Fistula-in-ano. The only successful treatment is surgical. However, patients with inflammatory bowel disease should not undergo surgery for fistula because this will usually fail as long as any active proximal disease is present. Surgery is reserved for palliation of the complications of fistula (i.e., drainage of recurrent perirectal abscess).

Suspected Carcinoma and the need for biopsy require surgical consultation, as does the patient with severe recurrent discomfort from *hemorrhoids* (see appendix).

Pruritus Ani. Specific therapy is related to identification of a specific cause (e.g., diabetes in the patient with candidiasis). Identification of the cause may be a challenging exercise to the primary physician. Pruritus resulting from anatomic lesions generally remits after correction of the underlying problem. *Anogenital warts* are effectively treated with topical application of 25% podophyllin in tincture of benzoin repeated every 1 to 2 weeks. The patient is instructed to bathe between 6 and 12 hours after the application. Care should be taken to avoid applying the compound to intact skin. If anoscopy reveals intraanal warts at the initial examination, curettage and electrocoagulation under anesthesia will be necessary.

Pinworms. All family members should be treated simultaneously. Pyrantel pamoate (Antiminth) is the drug of choice; a one-time oral dose of 11 mg/kg of body weight usually suffices. Preventive measures are difficult to enforce, except for hand washing before meals and after bowel movements. The best prevention is simultaneous treatment of all members of the household.

Idiopathic. No specific cause is found. Pruritus appears to be a form of neurodermatitis affecting the perianal skin. However, the symptoms are often relieved by careful attention to *perianal hygiene* after bowel movements; the perianal skin is kept dry with the application of witch hazel, and topical steroid ointments (0.25% hydrocortisone ointment) are used for several weeks to break the cycle of itching and skin changes caused by scratching. When contact dermatitis is thought to be caused by topical agents, the offending medication should be discontinued.

Gonorrheal Proctitis. See Chapter 137.

Proctitis in Homosexuals. Pending the results of cultures, those with a nonspecific *proctitis* (inflammation limited to the lower 15 cm of the bowel and no ulcers) should be treated empirically by covering for gonorrhea and *Chlamydia* (see Chapters 136 and 137). Both infections may be present simultaneously. The presence of ulceration suggests syphilis and herpes simplex but does not rule out concurrent gonorrhea and chlamydial infection; polymicrobial infection is found in about 25% of patients.

Fecal Incontinence. Patients have achieved some benefit from *biofeedback* technique. However, only those who retain some degree of rectal sensation are candidates for biofeedback. The technique requires responding to the feeling of rectal fullness. Manometry is sometimes helpful to retrain the anal sphincter response to rectal distention.

PATIENT EDUCATION

When poor or excessive personal hygiene, application of irritating agents, or neurotic behavior is responsible for symptoms, the relationship between rectal discomfort and precipitants should be explained so that the patient can take appropriate corrective action. Patients who obtain temporary relief of symptoms by applying a topical sensitizing agent may be reluctant to halt their medication if no other therapy is advised. Daily sitz baths can be prescribed in its place. Prevention through counseling is an important component of therapy in male homosexuals. Patients need to know that receptive anal sex with multiple partners carries a very high risk for intestinal infection and that they should certainly refrain from sexual activity if they become symptomatic.

A.H.G.

ANNOTATED BIBLIOGRAPHY

Alexander-Williams J. Causes and managements of anal irritation. Br Med J 1983;287:1528. (*Good review with the British clinical approach.*)

Brisinda G, Maria G, Bentivoglio AR, et al. A comparison of injections of botulinum toxin and topical nitroglycerin ointment for the treatment of chronic anal fissure. N Engl J Med 1999;341:65. (*Botulinum toxin superior to nitroglycerine ointment in this randomized trial of nonsurgical therapies.*)

Goodell SE, Quinn TC, Mkrtichian PA, et al. Herpes simplex virus proctitis in homosexual men. N Engl J Med 1983;308:868. (*Documents the high frequency and distinctive clinical presentation of this infection.*)

Jensen SL, et al. Management of acute anal fissure. Br Med J 1986;292:1167. (*Sitz baths and bran worked best.*)

Lebedeff DA, Hochman EB. Rectal gonorrhea in men: diagnosis and treatment. Ann Intern Med 1980;92:463. (*Prospective study of 1,200 men detailing the clinical presentation, utility of Gram's stain and culture, and response to therapy.*)

Lieberman DA. Common anorectal disorders. Ann Intern Med 1984;101:837. (*Superb review; 107 references.*)

Maria G, Cassetta E, Gui D, et al. A comparison of botulinum toxin and saline for the treatment of chronic anal fissure. N Engl J Med 1998;338:217. (*Double-blind, placebo-controlled trial demonstrating efficacy for healing chronic fissures.*)

Owen WF. Sexually transmitted disease and traumatic problems in homosexual men. Ann Intern Med 1980;92:805. (*Good review of the multitude of problems faced by homosexual men practicing receptive anal intercourse; 60 references.*)

Quinn TC, Goodell SE, Fennell C, et al. Infections with *Campylobacter jejuni* and *Campylobacter*-like organisms in homosexual men. Ann Intern Med 1984;101:187. (*Describes the clinical presentation of infection with this class of organisms; about 25% of symptomatic patients were infected with the organism.*)

Quinn TC, Goodell SE, Mkrtichian E. *Chlamydia trachomatis* proctitis. N Engl J Med 1981;305:195. (Chlamydia trachomatis *of LGV immunotypes is associated with severe acute proctitis that mimics Crohn's disease.*)

Quinn TC, Stamm WE, Goodell SE, et al. The polymicrobial origin of intestinal infections in homosexual men. N Engl J Med 1983;309:576. (*Important article documenting the polymicrobial nature of intestinal infection in this population.*)

Ramanujmps PRA, Sad ML, Abcarian H, et al. Perianal abscesses and fistulas: a study of 10,023 patients. Dis Colon Rectum 1984;27:595. (*One of the largest series.*)

Smith LE, Henrich SD, McCullah RD. Etiology and treatment of pruritus ani. Dis Colon Rectum 1982;25:358. (*Practical article on mundane but important issue.*)

Wald A. Biofeedback therapy for fecal incontinence. Ann Intern Med 1981;95:146. (*Technique proved helpful in those who retain some degree of rectal sensation.*)

Appendix: Management of Hemorrhoids

Hemorrhoids are a source of much misery, although they are of no consequence unless they become thrombosed, prolapse, or bleed. Therapy is directed toward relief of symptoms and should be accomplished with a minimum of discomfort, cost, and time lost from work. Simple approaches to pain relief and sensible modification in bowel habits to prevent progression constitute the essentials of medical therapy. The primary physician must be certain that symptoms are attributable to hemorrhoids, alleviate any anxiety about neoplasm, provide conservative medical therapy, and decide on the need for and timing of surgery.

PRINCIPLES OF MANAGEMENT

In most cases, it is not necessary to remove hemorrhoids to treat them effectively. Symptomatic relief and a halt to progression can usually be achieved by use of simple local measures and minor changes in diet. For a painful attack, a *cold pack* applied for the first few hours offers considerable relief. Hot *sitz baths* (with a little salt added to the water to make it a more isotonic solution) are soothing and effective when used at least once or twice daily for about 20 to 30 minutes. Softening the stool helps minimize straining and can be accomplished by increasing *dietary fiber* and making short-term use of *stool softeners* (e.g., dioctyl sodium sulfosuccinate). Irritant laxatives should be avoided. Patients should set aside a regular time each day to have an unhurried bowel movement and avoid vigorous wiping. Stubborn itching and inflammation respond well to *topical corticosteroids*; *hydrocortisone cream* and suppositories are adequate and relatively inexpensive. Topical hydrocortisone cream (1%), which can be purchased without a prescription, provides good relief from itching caused by mild inflammation

of anal tissue. It has been added to many of the popular over-the-counter preparations, although generic hydrocortisone is the least expensive formulation.

A host of *over-the-counter preparations* are heavily promoted. Many contain a topical anesthetic, such as benzocaine or pramoxine. *Benzocaine* may produce some temporary pain relief, but it is quite sensitizing; the resultant allergic response may actually worsen symptoms. *Pramoxine* is another topical anesthetic found in popular over-the-counter preparations (Anusol, Tronolane Cream, and so forth). It is similar in efficacy to benzocaine but is less sensitizing; it acts within 3 to 5 minutes of application, and effects lasts several hours. However, the cream formulation can still be irritating because of the presence of paraben preservatives. *Preparation H* is among the best-selling and most widely advertised over-the-counter hemorrhoidal therapies. It contains shark liver oil, live yeast cell derivatives, and phenyl mercuric nitrate; none of these agents, singly or in combination, has been shown to have any beneficial effect on hemorrhoids, although they are promoted as being able to shrink hemorrhoids and reduce inflammation.

Hemorrhoids that bleed repeatedly, prolapse, produce intractable pain, or become thrombosed deserve surgical evaluation. Internal hemorrhoids that have been bleeding persistently or have prolapsed can be removed in the surgeon's office with the use of *rubber band ligation*. A rubber band is placed at the base of the hemorrhoid; within a week the lesion sloughs. Multiple attempts are sometimes necessary. *Injection of sclerosing agents* (e.g., 5% phenol in oil) into the upper pole of internal hemorrhoids is another means of dealing with them; the procedure has fallen out of favor because of its association with scarring of the anal canal. *Cryosurgery* is relatively painless and does not require anesthesia, but a foul-smelling discharge is produced for about a week after the procedure, and stricture is occasionally a late occurrence. Excruciatingly painful external hemorrhoids that have become thrombosed can be excised under local anesthesia and the *clot removed*. Excellent nonsurgical results have been reported with the use of heat delivered through an infrared *photocoagulation probe* to treat first- and second-degree hemorrhoids. The heat is directed to the root of the hemorrhoid to interrupt its vascular supply, which causes it to contract.

Definitive *hemorrhoidectomy* is the treatment of last resort. In contrast with the other surgical therapies mentioned, it requires hospitalization, and the recovery period can last several weeks. Moreover, there is a risk for compromising the competence of the anal sphincter. Nevertheless, it does represent a serious treatment option for patients with disabling, refractory disease.

THERAPEUTIC RECOMMENDATIONS

- Advise frequent hot sitz baths for relief of pain. At the initial recognition of pain, the patient can apply a cold pack for the first few hours, then take hot baths three or four times a day.
- If inflammation and itching are present, prescribe a suppository preparation containing a steroid (e.g., hydrocortisone). If symptoms are predominantly external, prescribe 1% or 2.5% hydrocortisone cream.
- Topical anesthetics may be useful for the acute relief of severe pain. If this form of therapy is to be used, an agent that is minimally sensitizing (e.g., pramoxine) should be chosen.

- Treat constipation by having the patient increase dietary fiber and use a stool softener, such as 100 mg of dioctyl sodium sulfosuccinate three times daily. After resolution of acute symptoms, the high-fiber diet should be continued.
- For thrombosed hemorrhoids, the following measures may be helpful:
  1. Instruct the patient to lie prone with ice applied to the thrombosed hemorrhoid.
  2. Prescribe oral analgesics; codeine may be required.
  3. Prescribe stool softeners.
  4. Conservative therapy should be successful in 3 to 5 days; otherwise, refer the patient for surgical removal of the clot, which will relieve the pain promptly.
- Intractable symptoms require surgical therapy. The specific method chosen depends on the surgical expertise available in the community.

PATIENT EDUCATION AND PREVENTION

Instruction concerning proper diet and bowel habits is extremely helpful.

- Advise the patient to increase the intake of dietary fiber; suggest bran, carrots, green vegetables, and fruits with skin. Consider use of a psyllium preparation. Some people find foods such as chili, onions, and alcohol irritating. If this applies to your patient, suggest that they be avoided.
- Emphasize the importance of providing a regular time to have bowel movements. After bowel movements, the patient should avoid vigorous wiping; patting ought to suffice, and it minimizes irritation.

- Instruct the patient not to linger on the toilet or strain at stool. Long periods of standing should be avoided.
- Caution the patient against the use of irritant laxatives.
- At the first sign of recurrent symptoms, institute frequent hot sitz baths.
- Instruct the patient to pat dry rather than wipe or rub.

ANNOTATED BIBLIOGRAPHY

FDA Advisory Review Panel on OTC Hemorrhoidal Drug Products. Federal Register 1980;45:35576. (*Concludes it is unclear whether topical anesthetics are effective for the treatment of hemorrhoids.*)

Johnson JF, et al. The prevalence of hemorrhoids and chronic constipation. Gastroenterology 1990;98:380. (*Best data, with divergent patterns noted.*)

Lieberman DA. Common anorectal disorders. Ann Intern Med 1984;101:837. (*Extensive review of the anatomy and physiology of the anus and rectum, with special attention to hemorrhoids, fissure-in-ano, pruritus ani, and fecal incontinence; required reading for all primary physicians.*)

Murie JA, Sim AJ, MacKenzie I. Rubber band ligation versus haemorrhoidectomy for prolapsing haemorrhoids. Br J Surg 1982;69:536. (*Long-term prospective clinical trial showing that ligation is effective, except for permanently prolapsed painful lesions.*)

Prasad GC, et al. Studies on etiopathogenesis of hemorrhoids. Am J Proctol 1976;27:33. (*Excellent review of the pathogenesis of hemorrhoids.*)

Stern H, McLeod R, Cohen Z, et al. Ambulatory procedures in anorectal surgery. Adv Surg 1987;20:217. (*Includes discussion of hemorrhoid treatments offered by the surgeon in the office setting.*)

To tie; to stab; to stretch, perchance to freeze [Editorial]. Lancet 1975;2:645. (*Concludes that hemorrhoidectomy should be reserved for failure of other methods.*)

67
Approach to the Patient with an External Hernia

Abdominal hernias are exceedingly common, often causing occupational disabilities and posing the risk for incarceration and strangulation of bowel. Fortunately, adequate evaluation can usually be performed in the office by means of history and physical examination. The primary physician must distinguish between patients who require surgical referral and those who may be managed expectantly.

PATHOPHYSIOLOGY AND CLINICAL PRESENTATION

Pathophysiology. A hernia is a defect in the normal musculofascial continuity of the abdominal wall that permits the egress of structures not normally passing through the parietes. In general, the significant feature of hernia is not the size of the protrusion or the sac, but the size and rigidity of the defect in the abdominal wall. Fixation and rigidity of the hernial ring are the features that lead to incarceration and strangulation. The distinction between congenital and acquired hernia is not often clear because many hernias that appear after trauma or straining represent a congenital predisposition, such as indirect in-

guinal hernia in the adult. This distinction has little bearing on management, although it can make a considerable difference to the patient, who may be compensated if the hernia can be attributed to trauma at work. Some of these hernias are incidental to, and antedate, the perceived injury.

Disorders resulting in increased intraabdominal pressure may contribute to the appearance of a hernia and affect the postoperative management also. For example, chronic cough resulting from cigarette smoking or bronchitis can precipitate or worsen herniation; the same is true of symptomatic prostatism.

Clinical Presentations

Reducible Hernia. The symptoms of an uncomplicated or reducible external hernia are related not to its size but to the degree of pressure on its contents. Patients with large scrotal hernias containing much intestine may have few symptoms other than a dragging sensation. A mass appears on standing, which reduces when the patient is supine. Pain may be intermittent, disappearing when the hernia is reduced. Patients with small hernias containing an entrapped knuckle of bowel may have rather severe pain and nausea. Many patients with femoral, umbilical, or epigastric hernias may be entirely unaware of their existence.

Irreducible or Incarcerated Hernia is one in which the contents cannot be replaced into the abdomen. Here, the mass remains palpable with the patient relaxed and in the supine position. A *strangulated hernia* is an irreducible hernia in which the blood supply to the entrapped bowel loop has been compromised, resulting in small-bowel obstruction and infarction. These patients complain of colicky abdominal pain, nausea, and vomiting and show signs of small-bowel obstruction with distention, tympany, and hyperperistalsis. In addition, careful examination demonstrates a tender, irreducible groin or ventral hernia.

Inguinal Hernias. *Indirect inguinal hernias*, which account for one half of all hernias in adults, pass through the internal abdominal inguinal ring along the spermatic cord through the inguinal canal and exit through the external inguinal ring. In male patients, these can descend into the scrotum. *Direct inguinal hernias* pass through the posterior inguinal wall medial to the inferior epigastric vessels, through Hesselbach's triangle. *Femoral hernias* pass through the femoral canal inferior to the inguinal ligament and become subcutaneous in the fossa ovalis. It is often difficult to distinguish between these three forms, especially when incarceration is present and the sac is large.

Indirect inguinal hernias are eight to ten times more common in men than in women, whereas femoral hernias are three to five times more common in women than in men. Nevertheless, the most common hernia in women is the indirect inguinal type. The diagnosis is less often made in women because physical examination of the external inguinal ring is more difficult. Direct hernias increase in incidence with advancing age and are the least likely of the external hernias to become incarcerated or strangulated.

Strangulation is common in femoral hernias. The majority of patients with strangulated inguinal hernias are aware of the hernia before strangulation. In contrast, nearly half of those with strangulated femoral hernias are unaware of the hernia before strangulation. In addition, groin pain and tenderness are absent in a significant percentage of cases of strangulated femoral hernia.

Ventral Hernias. The commonly encountered ventral hernias include umbilical, epigastric, and incisional varieties. Ventral hernias are often more obvious when the patient is standing. *Umbilical hernias* pass through the umbilical ring and represent failure of the ring to be obliterated after birth. In the infant, these often close spontaneously within the first 2 years of life. In the adult, they are more common in women and are associated with obesity, multiparity, and cirrhosis with ascites. Umbilical hernias are often missed because they are obscured by subcutaneous fat. They are associated with a high risk for incarceration and strangulation, and mortality rates are higher than with inguinal hernias because large bowel is frequently entrapped.

Incisional Hernias are those that develop in the scar of a previous laparotomy or in a drain site. They are associated with a previous postoperative wound infection, dehiscence, malnutrition, obesity, and smoking. They are more common in vertical than in transverse scars. Incisional hernias often have mul-

tiple defects and several rings. They are frequently irreducible or only partially reducible because of adhesions within the sac. Patients with very large incisional hernias may be remarkably free of symptoms of intestinal obstruction, although incarceration is common; strangulation is relatively uncommon because of the usually large size of the defects.

Epigastric Hernias occur through the linea alba between the xiphoid process and the umbilicus. They may be difficult to detect in the obese patient and must be looked for in patients with epigastric pain. Incarcerated epigastric hernia may produce symptoms that mimic those of peptic ulcer disease or biliary colic.

DIFFERENTIAL DIAGNOSIS

Recognizing a hernia usually presents little difficulty, although distinguishing one type of inguinal hernia from another can sometimes be complicated. The differential diagnosis of an entrapped femoral hernia includes not only inguinal hernia but femoral lymphadenopathy, saphenous varix, psoas abscess, and hydrocele. On occasion, it is impossible to differentiate an incarcerated femoral hernia from a single enlarged femoral lymph node (the lymph node of Cloquet). Other causes of groin pain or swelling include muscle strain, hip arthritis, inguinal adenopathy, and undescended testicle.

WORKUP

The diagnosis and evaluation of external hernias require no more than a brief history and careful physical examination; laboratory and radiologic studies are unnecessary unless major complications have resulted.

History. The patient is questioned about groin pain, swelling, ability to reduce the hernia, circumstances of onset, and aggravating and alleviating factors, such as exacerbation on standing, straining, or coughing. Acute onset of colicky abdominal pain, nausea, and vomiting suggest entrapment and strangulation in a patient with a known hernia.

Physical Examination is directed toward differentiating herniation from other causes of inguinal swelling or pain and distinguishing among (a) hernias that are uncomplicated and require no therapy, (b) those that can be repaired electively, and (c) those in which emergency surgery is the safest course. The physical examination is also important in distinguishing the anatomic type of hernia; the prognosis and likelihood of incarceration and strangulation differ among the various types.

Inspection. Patient should be examined in both the supine and standing positions. Inspection is often as important as palpation for detection. Examination should include Valsalva's maneuver to increase intraabdominal pressure. In male patients, small inguinal hernias are looked for by invaginating the scrotal skin while the patient is standing. To detect ventral hernias, patients should be supine and then asked to lift their head from the examining table and bear down to tense the abdominal wall.

Palpation. Palpation follows and is best performed with the patient standing. In male patients, one inserts the index finger into the *inguinal canal* by following the spermatic cord. Distinguishing a direct from an indirect hernia can be difficult. An indirect hernia projects more inferiorly, and protrusion into the scrotum is almost always a sign. To detect a femoral hernia, one palpates the *fossa ovalis*, inferior to the inguinal canal. If a groin hernia is detected, one should gently attempt reduction of the hernia while the patient relaxes the abdominal muscles.

Examination of the Irreducible Hernia. If a hernia is irreducible, the physician should look for local tenderness, discoloration, edema, fever, and signs of small-bowel obstruction. It is often difficult to distinguish a simple incarceration from early strangulation; for this reason, these two lesions are managed identically by immediate referral to a surgeon. Surgical exploration is the only way to be certain that no compromised bowel is trapped in the hernia sac. Conversely, when signs of small-bowel obstruction are present, it is essential to examine thoroughly for a strangulated femoral hernia because groin pain and tenderness may be absent.

Additional Groin Examination. The groin area also is checked for *lymphadenopathy* and other masses that do not change with position or Valsalva's maneuver. If groin pain is present but no mass, then a musculoskeletal cause is suggested and a careful examination of *hip* movement is indicated.

Checking for Associated Conditions. A few conditions are believed to have more than a chance association with hernias, and some argue that they should be screened for. Whether the adult patient with a recent hernia is more likely to have an occult *carcinoma of the colon* remains a source of controversy. It has been suggested that patients undergo screening for colorectal cancer (see Chapter 56). However, if the patient reports no change in bowel habits and the stools are repeatedly negative for blood on guaiac testing, it is unnecessary to submit the patient to more extensive investigation for occult malignancy. Symptoms and signs of prostatism are frequently present in elderly men with hernia and may require relief before herniorrhaphy. The entire abdomen ought to be examined for masses, hepatomegaly, and ascites, which are sometimes associated with hernia formation.

PRINCIPLES OF MANAGEMENT AND INDICATIONS FOR REFERRAL

Conservative Therapy versus Surgery. The key determination is the need for surgery, which can be based on the findings at physical examination.

Reducible Inguinal Hernia. Patients with an *asymptomatic*, easily reducible inguinal hernia can be managed expectantly without resorting to surgery. Surgery is elective but should probably be carried out if the patient is young. Should pain ensue or signs of incarceration develop, then surgery may be indicated. Patients with a *symptomatic* reducible inguinal hernia should undergo elective repair for relief of symptoms and prevention of strangulation. Reduction by means of a *truss* may be unsatisfactory, even in patients with relative medical contraindications to surgery. Moreover, surgical repair can be performed under local anesthesia in the high-risk patient, and newer laparoscopic techniques (see below) make for less perioperative morbidity.

Nontender Incarcerated Inguinal Hernia. If the hernia is of recent onset and signs of inflammation or bowel obstruction are absent, it may be safe to attempt *gentle reduction* (*"taxis"*). This is best accomplished with the patient supine and the hips and knees flexed. If gentle pressure over the hernial sac fails to reduce the mass further, efforts should be abandoned and the patient should be referred for surgery forthwith. Often, patients have more experience in reducing their own hernia than does the physician. Patients with evidence of strangulated groin hernias should be subjected to immediate operation regardless of medical contraindications; if they are not treated, death will result from bowel necrosis.

Reducible Femoral Hernias should undergo prompt elective repair because of the high incidence of strangulation. Whenever there is a question of an incarcerated femoral hernia, it is safest to proceed immediately with surgical exploration.

Umbilical Hernias. Surgery is unnecessary if physical examination reveals a small, asymptomatic fascial defect without protrusion. When herniation is detected, however, umbilical defects should be repaired because the risk for incarceration and strangulation is high. The danger of strangulation is compounded by the greater likelihood of colonic entrapment, which is associated with a higher mortality rate than is strangulation of small intestine. Therefore, all incarcerated umbilical hernias should be managed as if they were strangulated. Elective umbilical herniorrhaphy should be avoided in patients with ascites; instead, efforts should be directed toward reducing the ascites (see Chapter 71). The problem in patients with cirrhosis and ascites is made more difficult when the skin overlying the sac thins out and poses the risk of rupture.

Small-neck Incisional Hernias or Tender Incarceration should undergo repair on an urgent basis. Patients who have trophic changes or ulceration in the skin overlying incisional hernias are also candidates for urgent surgery. In some instances, cellulitis of the skin overlying the hernia sac develops and is difficult to distinguish from strangulation of the contents of the sac. Management of large incarcerated incisional hernias that occur in the abdomen in very obese patients is a particular problem. Major efforts should be directed toward weight reduction before repair if it is possible to procrastinate. If, however, the presence of intestinal obstruction is a possibility or the viability of the contents of the sac is doubtful, the advice of a surgeon should be sought promptly.

Treatment of Contributing Factors. Factors contributing to hernia formation should be corrected if possible. *Prostatism* that leads to straining at urination needs attention, be it medical or surgical (see Chapter 138). Patients with *chronic cough* secondary to chronic obstructive pulmonary disease, cigarette smoking, asthma, or esophageal reflux should have the underlying condition addressed promptly (see Chapter 41) to diminish symptoms caused by the hernia and to decrease the possibility of postoperative complications.

Conventional versus Laparoscopic Hernia Repair. The effective application of laparoscopic techniques to the repair of inguinal hernias provides an alternative surgical approach for patients. In the largest multicenter, randomized prospective study to date, laparoscopic repair proved superior to open repair in terms of time required for recovery from surgery (1 week vs. 2 weeks), return to work (2 weeks vs. 3 weeks), and resumption of athletic activities (3 weeks vs. 5 weeks). In addition, the risk for recurrence was reduced by 50%, and fewer wound infections were noted. Most recurrences that did follow laparoscopic surgery were traceable to errors in surgical technique. The duration of surgery was similar for both procedures. The time to discharge was less, as was the degree of postoperative pain, with laparoscopic surgery. Disadvantages include the higher cost of surgery, need for general anesthesia, and additional surgical skill required. (A clear and prolonged learning curve is associated with laparoscopic surgery, with the potential for inexperienced operators causing serious complications, such as viscus perforation, when unsupervised.) If the requisite surgical skill is available, then patients capable of undergoing general anesthesia and desiring a more rapid return to activity can be offered laparoscopic repair.

PATIENT EDUCATION

Patients who are to be managed conservatively must be taught to watch for signs of complications. It is the responsibility of the physician to instruct the patient in the symptoms of incarceration and strangulation and in the urgency of seeking help should they occur. If the patient is deemed incompetent to make such observations and to obtain help promptly, a strong case can be made for proceeding with surgery. Patients scheduled for elective surgery also require instruction because incarceration occasionally occurs before the planned operation.

Many patients with asymptomatic or mildly symptomatic reducible hernias will be reluctant to undergo surgery because their symptoms are minimal. If they fall into the high-risk group (e.g., femoral or small-neck incisional hernias), they should be informed of the strong likelihood of strangulation and the minuscule morbidity and mortality associated with surgery.

Patients who are advised to have surgery appreciate estimates of time to walking (same day for local anesthesia and general anesthesia in the morning), time to return to physically undemanding work (2 to 3 weeks), time to resumption of unlimited activity (3 to 6 weeks), risk for recurrence (10%), and effect on sexual function (none). A discussion of the advantages and disadvantages of open versus laparoscopic repair is also worthwhile in the context of a review of the patient's surgical candidacy.

ANNOTATED BIBLIOGRAPHY

Barry MK, Donohue JH, Harmsen WS, et al. Transabdominal preperitoneal laparoscopic inguinal herniorrhaphy: assessment of initial experience. Mayo Clin Proc 1998;73:717. (*The Mayo Clinic initial experience; useful article in that it shows the importance of the learning curve in achieving optimal outcomes.*)

Flanagan L Jr., Bascom JV. Repair of the groin hernia: outpatient approach with local anesthesia. Surg Clin North Am 1984;64:257. (*An increasingly common approach that reduces cost considerably.*)

Gilbert AI. An anatomic and functional classification for the diagnosis and treatment of inguinal hernia. Am J Surg 1989;157:331. (*Useful, terse summary.*)

Liem MSL, van der Graaf Y, van Steensel CJ, et al. Comparison of conventional anterior surgery and laparoscopic surgery for inguinal hernia repair. N Engl J Med 1997;336:1541. (*Multicenter, randomized, prospective study showing significant advantages for laparoscopic surgery.*)

68
Management of Peptic Ulcer Disease

Peptic ulcer disease continues to be a major source of morbidity, affecting up to 2.0% of the U.S. population at any one time. Men outnumber women by two to one. The peak prevalence for duodenal ulcer (which accounts for 80% of cases) is between ages 45 and 54; gastric ulcer peaks between the ages of 55 and 64.

Advances in understanding peptic ulcer pathogenesis have revolutionized treatment and markedly improved outcomes. The primary care physician must be capable of designing and implementing a cost-effective program that alleviates pain, promotes healing, limits complications, and prevents recurrences. Other tasks include the timely identification of patients who require endoscopy or consideration of surgery. The management of non-ulcer dyspepsia, which may mimic peptic ulcer disease, shares aspects of peptic ulcer treatment (see Chapter 74).

PATHOPHYSIOLOGY AND CLINICAL PRESENTATION

Peptic ulcers arise principally in the stomach and duodenum, areas exposed to gastric acid and pepsin. Although the precise mechanisms of ulcer formation remain incompletely understood, the process appears to involve the interplay of acid production, pepsin secretion, *Helicobacter pylori* infection, and mucosal defense mechanisms.

Gastric Acid Production, Pepsin Secretion, and Mucosal Defenses

Acid Production and Pepsin Secretion. Excess acid production is the hallmark of duodenal ulcer disease, with significant increases noted in basal and peak acid outputs, parietal and chief cell masses, and responses to food and hormonal stimulation. Zollinger-Ellison syndrome (with its associated hypergastrinemia and parietal cell overproduction) is the prototypical acid hypersecretory condition resulting in ulcer formation. Some patients with duodenal ulcer demonstrate *rapid gastric emptying*, which raises the acid exposure of the proximal duodenum. *Pepsin* secretion is also elevated in duodenal ulcer disease. Gastric acid production is relatively normal in patients with gastric ulcers.

Mucosal Defense. An appreciation for the importance of mucosal defense mechanisms is emerging. Major determinants of mucosal integrity include secretion of mucus, production of bicarbonate, mucosal blood flow, and cellular repair mechanisms. *The mucous barrier may become compromised* by an increased degradation of mucus, decreased secretion, or production of defective mucus. Bile acids, pepsin, pancreatic enzymes, and mechanical forces contribute to the degradation of mucus. *Gastric prostaglandin production* appears important to sustaining production of mucus, secretion of bicarbonate, and mucosal repair. By helping to maintain a neutral pH and aqueous environment at the surface of the gastric epithelium, mucus and bicarbonate protect the mucosa from acid, pepsin, and other potentially injurious agents (see below).

Role of Aspirin and Other Nonsteroidal Antiinflammatory Drugs

Mechanisms. The relation of aspirin and nonaspirin NSAIDs to ulcer disease largely involves their potent *inhibition of gastric mucosal prostaglandin synthesis*. With long-term use, all NSAIDs (including enteric-coated and non-aspirin salicylates and NSAID prodrugs) are capable of producing solitary deep *gastric ulcers*. The risk for clinically important ulceration is estimated by the U.S. Food and Drug Administration to be 2% per patient-year of NSAID use. No major differences are found among NSAID preparations in regard to ulcer risk (despite highly advertised claims to the contrary). About 15% of long-term NSAID users demonstrate gastric ulceration at endoscopy. Risk generally increases with dose and duration of therapy, but up to one fourth of complications have been observed within the first month of therapy. The elderly are at greatest risk (reported relative risk of about 4.0).

In addition to inhibiting prostaglandin synthesis, many NSAID preparations produce acute diffuse mucosal injury by means of a *direct erosive effect*. Endoscopic study has shown significant mucosal injury to result from both plain and tablet forms of buffered aspirin, although not with enteric-coated aspirin preparations, unless gastric emptying is delayed. Similar acute erosions occur with uncoated NSAIDs, but not with enteric-coated preparations or prodrug formulations. Such diffuse acute injury is rarely associated with symptoms or clinically significant ulceration, although minor occult bleeding may ensue. Smoking, alcohol use, alcohol-related disease, and preexisting peptic ulcer disease greatly increase the risk for ulcer and ulcer complications in NSAID-treated patients. Concurrent *H. pylori* infection also may predispose the patient to NSAID-related injury.

Gastric versus Duodenal Disease. NSAID use is associated primarily with gastric ulceration, not with new *duodenal ulceration*, but preexisting duodenal ulceration may be exacerbated and complicated by NSAID use. It is estimated that more than half of ulcer complications associated with NSAID use occur in patients with preexisting duodenal ulcers. Much of the ulcer morbidity associated with NSAID use may be related to preexisting, subclinical disease.

Role of *Helicobacter pylori* Infection

Infection with *H. pylori* has emerged as a major, if not the major, precipitant of peptic ulcer disease; it is associated with 95% to 99% of cases of *duodenal ulcer* and ulcer recurrence and with more than 90% of *gastric ulcers* unrelated to NSAID use. *Helicobacter* infection also is strongly associated with antral *gastritis* and is a risk factor for *gastric carcinoma* and *MALT lymphoma* (mucosa-associated lymphoid tissue) of the stomach; its eradication results in remission of the latter. Cancer risk appears to increase when *H. pylori* is present in the setting of atrophic gastritis.

Cure of *Helicobacter* infection can speed ulcer healing and greatly reduce rates of recurrence. The organism does not appear to cause ulcers *per se*, but rather seems to enhance mucosal susceptibility to the injurious actions of acid and pepsin. Acid hypersecretors may be particularly vulnerable to ulcer formation in the context of *Helicobacter* infection and subject to slow healing and a high rate of recurrence. The prevalence of *H. pylori* infection increases with age, approaching 90% in ulcer patients over age 65. The mode of transmission is unclear, although person-to-person fecal-oral spread is suspected because clusters occur in families.

Other Precipitants

A host of psychological, dietary, pharmacologic, and hereditary factors have been implicated in the cause or aggravation of ulcer disease.

Stress has long been considered a key precipitant, a view supported by a higher incidence of chronic stress in ulcer patients than in controls, increased acid production in response to stress, and a more prolonged course and poorer prognosis in those with chronic severe anxiety. Patients in whom ulcers develop view life stresses more negatively than do controls. Acid hypersecretion and ulcer formation have been observed in small-scale studies of patients undergoing severe emotional stress; with subsidence of stress, acid secretion falls and ulcers heal. Confirmation of these small-scale observations will strengthen the association between stress and ulcer disease.

Smoking is an important risk factor, identified by epidemiologic studies. For example, ulcers are twice as likely to develop in cigarette smokers as in nonsmokers. The risk for gastric ulcer correlates with the number of cigarettes smoked, and those with ulcers have increased rates of smoking. The rates of recurrence are dramatically increased in those who smoke, and healing is markedly slowed. Impaired prostaglandin production has been demonstrated in the gastric mucosa of smokers.

Alcohol and Coffee have also been implicated. Coffee, including decaffeinated forms, stimulates acid secretion, as do other caffeine-containing beverages, but evidence proving ulcer causation is lacking. *Ethanol* can compromise the mucosal barrier and cause gastritis, and beer is almost as potent a stimulant of acid secretion as is gastrin. Nonetheless, data on the link between alcohol use and ulcer disease are conflicting. However, patients with alcohol-related cirrhosis are at increased risk for ulcer formation and complications.

Glucocorticosteroids. Their contribution has been debated ever since these agents first became available, with randomized controlled trials and metaanalyses producing conflicting results. Discrepancies are related in part to failure to control for concurrent NSAID use. The risk appears to be nil if the patient is not taking NSAIDs concurrently and the dose is less than 30 mg daily. However, high-dose steroid therapy (>30 mg/d) may confer an increment of risk, as might the underlying disease for which the prednisone is being taken. In the absence of concurrent NSAID use, overall risk appears to be very modest.

Heredity plays some role. The incidence of ulcer in the parents, siblings, and children of ulcer patients is increased, and studies of twins show greater concordance (e.g., both twins affected) among identical than among fraternal twins. Increased meal-stimulated gastrin release and pepsin secretion have been found to be hereditary traits among ulcer patients and their families.

Clinical Presentation

Peptic ulcers usually occur at or near mucosal transition zones, areas thought to be particularly vulnerable to the effects of acid, pepsin, bile, and pancreatic enzymes. Gastric ulcers are found in the *antrum* at the *lesser curvature*, near the junction of the acid-secreting parietal cells and the antral mucosa. Duodenal ulcers arise mostly at the *junction* of the *antrum* and *duodenum*.

The clinical presentations of gastric and duodenal peptic ulcers often overlap and may be nonspecific. Patients can present with pain, bleeding, or obstruction, or they may be symptom-free. Epigastric pain, relieved by antacids and occurring as clusters of daily symptoms for a few weeks separated by pain-free periods of months, is characteristic of peptic disease. Duodenal ulcer pain is classically relieved by food, absent before breakfast, and responsible for awakening the patient at night; it starts 2 to 3 hours after a meal. However, careful studies of patients with documented duodenal ulcers have shown that in some of them pain is often worsened by meals, present before breakfast, and continuous rather than periodic. Gastric ulcer pain is more likely to be precipitated by food and often radiates from the epigastrium to the back or substernal region. It too can awaken the patient and be relieved by food. In both conditions, the pain may be dull, aching, gnawing, or burning in quality, consistent with its visceral quality.

Symptoms may be absent and dissociated from mucosal changes. Silent disease is particularly common among the elderly and those using NSAIDs. A complication is the first clinical manifestation of ulcer disease in about 25% of persons with ulcer disease unrelated to NSAID use; the figure is considerably higher in the setting of NSAID use.

Natural History and Clinical Course

Natural History and Clinical Course without *Helicobacter* Eradication. Because most patients receive some form of treatment, available data reflect the clinical course more than the true natural history. Studies performed before the advent of aggressive use of antacids or histamine$_2$ (H$_2$)-receptor antagonists showed that a large majority of ulcers heal completely by 4 weeks, although large ones in the stomach can take up to 12 weeks. The majority of patients in such studies became pain-free within the first 4 weeks; however, little correlation was noted between the cessation of pain and healing of the ulcer. Recurrences were frequent. The 5-year recurrence rates ranged from 30% to 90%. Although it was rare for a patient to have more than two or three recurrent gastric ulcers, multiple recurrences were not unusual for those with duodenal ulcers. No correlation was found between recurrence rate and ulcer size, duration of symptoms, or location. Recurrent ulcers healed just as rapidly and completely as original lesions. The rate of development of a major complication, such as hemorrhage, perforation, or obstruction, was less than 1% annually. Bleeding was slightly more common from duodenal than from gastric ulcers and two to three times more common than perforation.

Clinical Course with *Helicobacter* Eradication. With eradication of *H. pylori* infection and the use of potent agents to suppress acid production, the clinical course of peptic ulcer disease has improved markedly. Complete *healing* is now achieved in up to 95% of cases within 4 to 6 weeks of initiation of treatment with antibiotics to eradicate *H. pylori* and proton pump inhibitors (PPIs) to suppress acid production maximally (see below). The 1-year risk for relapse is about 5% with eradication of *Helicobacter*, but more than 50% when acid suppression is the only form of initial therapy.

Surgical therapy has also affected the clinical course. Antrectomy lowers the recurrence rates for duodenal ulcer to 5% annually; selective proximal gastric vagotomy also substantially lowers recurrences, although to a lesser extent (see below).

WORKUP

A presumptive diagnosis of acid-peptic disease can often be made on clinical grounds alone (see Chapter 58). Aside from the testing of all patients for *H. pylori* infection (see below), the initial workup of uncomplicated peptic ulcer disease need not include confirmation by barium study or endoscopy. Cost-effectiveness studies demonstrate that commencement of empiric therapy is superior to prior confirmation of the diagnosis by endoscopy or upper gastrointestinal series. The only time confirmatory studies are needed initially is when clinical findings suggest a complication of peptic ulcer disease or gastric cancer (e.g., weight loss, dysphagia, recurrent nausea and vomiting, iron-deficiency anemia, and stool test positive for occult blood, especially in a person over 40 years of age).

Testing for Helicobacter infection. There is no "gold standard," but the reference method remains endoscopic antral mucosal *biopsy* with *special staining* [Warthin-Starry (silver) stain, with a sensitivity of 90% and a specificity of 100%]. The CLO test provides a more rapid means of endoscopic diagnosis (sensitivity 90%, specificity 96%). Noninvasive testing is possible with the ^{13}C-urea breath test (sensitivity 91%, specificity 91%) and by *serologic testing*, which measures immunoglobulin G and immunoglobulin A antibodies to *Helicobacter* (sensitivity 71%, specificity 85%). Because no statistically significant difference between these test performances has been found in head-to-head study, noninvasive testing is preferred in persons who do not need to undergo initial endoscopy.

Role of Serologic Testing. Serologic testing is used by many primary care physicians in lieu of endoscopic examination or breath testing because it is readily available, convenient, reasonably sensitive and specific, and inexpensive. This approach has proved cost-effective for the detection of infection in persons who have never been treated, but it cannot be used to determine cure or recurrence of infection because the test result often remains positive for years after eradication of the organism. Positivity means only prior exposure to the organism.

Role of Breath Testing. Breath testing takes advantage of the urease production of the organism and, unlike serology, provides direct evidence of active infection. Consequently, breath testing is considered the preferred nonivasive method for *determining the eradication of infection*, which becomes important in the settings of relapse, recurrence, and disease complicated by bleeding. Utilizing carbon dioxide labeled with ^{13}C or ^{14}C, this technology provides diagnostic sensitivity and specificity approaching that of endoscopic measures. The test is still not widely available, and its cost is currently greater than that for serology, so that it is relegated to a secondary role for initial testing.

Role of Endoscopy and Upper Gastrointestinal Series. At the time of *initial presentation*, patients over 40 years of age who have any clinical findings that raise concern about gastric cancer or complicated ulcer disease (see above) should promptly undergo visualization of the stomach and duodenum. The most cost-effective approach to initial testing remains a subject of debate. Endoscopists correctly argue that gastroscopy is superior to barium study for the detection of gastric ulcer, malignancy, and *H. pylori* because brushings, biopsy, CLO test, and cultures can be performed at the same time. However, radiologists aver that with the use of air-contrast techniques, the sensitivity of endoscopy to detect malignancy can be approached with a procedure that entails one-third the cost and is safer and more comfortable for the patient. The debate continues; test selection should be individualized.

Later in the course of illness, the patient with refractory or recurrent disease in the absence of evidence for persistent *H. pylori* infection should undergo endoscopy to check for gastric malignancy, as should the person with an ulcer that appears suspect on barium study.

Evaluation of the Benign-appearing Ulcer on Barium Study. About 4% of all gastric ulcers prove to be malignant. The sensitivity of barium study for the detection of gastric malignancy is in the range of 80% to 85%, compared with 95% for endoscopy with biopsy and brushing. Most malignant ulcers manifest radiologic signs of cancer, including irregular shape, nodular base, absence of radiating gastric folds, folds that are blunted or stop before the ulcer, and rigidity of adjacent stomach. Ulcers in the fundus are more likely to be malignant; those within 1 cm of the pylorus are almost always benign. Ulcers that appear malignant by any of these criteria require biopsy.

Subjecting all patients with benign-appearing ulcers on barium study to endoscopy is likely to be of low yield and add little to survival. For persons presenting with an ulcerated gastric carcinoma, the 5-year survival is only 25% to 35%. A more productive alternative might be to refer for endoscopy and biopsy only those patients with a radiologically suspect gastric ulcer and those with an ulcer that fails to heal fully despite documented eradication of *Helicobacter* infection (see below). The literature should be followed for further cost–benefit studies.

PRINCIPLES OF THERAPY

Treatment Objectives and Therapeutic Options: Overview

The major objectives of therapy are to speed healing, reduce pain, and prevent complications and recurrences while minimizing the costs and side effects of therapy. Although peptic ulcer disease represents a heterogeneous set of disorders, the overall approach to medical therapy is similar and centers on eradicating any *Helicobacter* infection, reducing gastric acidity, and protecting the mucosal barrier.

Antibiotics that eradicate *Helicobacter* infection are critical to effective treatment of peptic ulcer disease (except in cases related to NSAID use). Their use promotes effective ulcer healing and prevents relapse. Combination programs are required because of the high frequency of antibiotic resistance to single agents.

Antacids, Histamine₂ Blockers, and Proton Pump Inhibitors all speed ulcer healing by reducing gastric acidity, but unless they are used on a long-term basis, they do not prevent recurrence. *Antacids* provide a low-cost, safe means of neutralizing gastric acid but require frequent dosing. *H₂-receptor antagonists* and *PPIs* block acid secretion; they are well tolerated and convenient to use but very expensive when taken for prolonged periods.

Sucralfate acts locally, forming a cytoprotective coating over the injured mucosa, perhaps also absorbing pepsin and inactivating bile acids. Its principal use is to facilitate ulcer healing. It must be taken frequently, is costly, and can cause gastrointestinal upset.

Misoprostol, a prostaglandin analogue, counters the prostaglandin inhibition associated with NSAID use. The drug reduces the risk for ulcer formation associated with NSAID therapy and prevents the recurrence of NSAID-induced gastric ulceration and bleeding. Its cost is high and gastrointestinal side effects are common.

Avoidance of substances and activities potentially injurious to the gastric mucosa (aspirin, NSAIDs, smoking, stress) complement the therapeutic effort.

Surgery remains an option for the treatment of refractory disease and its complications.

Combination Programs are often utilized, particularly in instances of *Helicobacter*-induced disease. Antibiotics are prescribed to treat the underlying infection, and acid suppression is given to speed ulcer healing and promote relief of symptoms. Misoprostol plus acid suppression with a PPI is an effective combination in ulcers related to NSAID use.

Nonpharmacologic Therapies

Avoidance of Agents Injurious to the Mucosal Barrier. Any program to speed healing, limit recurrences, and prevent complications must address both short-term and prolonged use of agents injurious to the mucosal barrier. *Aspirin* and most *NSAIDs* should be avoided, if possible, because they greatly increase risk and refractoriness to therapy. Using *enteric-coated* and *prodrug* NSAID formulations and taking them with meals might mitigate superficial erosive injury but do little to prevent the deep ulcers that ensue with long-term use of these potent prostaglandin inhibitors. Consequently, if NSAID therapy must be continued, other means must be found to ensure their safe use (see below).

Although not an independent risk factor, *alcohol* should probably be restricted because it may impair healing and cause complications. Although *glucocorticosteroids* may exacerbate the chance of an ulcer developing in the context of NSAID therapy, they pose little direct risk, and a concurrent prophylactic regimen is not required unless other risk factors are present or large doses (e.g., >30 mg of prednisone daily) are going to be used for prolonged periods.

Alleviating Emotional Stress. Persons with difficult home or work situations may benefit from counseling. Treatment begins with a careful history eliciting pertinent psychosocial information. The very act of discussing these issues and the opportunity to ventilate one's feelings to a supportive listener may lessen tension and help point the way to solutions. A brief course of minor tranquilizer therapy is sometimes helpful to augment supportive psychotherapy and enable the patient to cope with the combination of stress and illness (see Chapter 226). Before the days of cost containment, very stressed patients were hospitalized to facilitate ulcer healing; however, only stays in excess of 4 weeks were shown to be effective.

Smoking Cessation. Smoking impedes the healing of peptic ulcers and may interfere with the action of H_2-receptor antagonists (gastric ulcer patients who continue to smoke have blunted responses to cimetidine therapy). Cessation should be urged during recovery from an ulcer. Although the role of smoking as a causative factor in ulcer disease is less well established, there is ample medical justification to advise its discontinuation (see Chapter 54).

Diet. Contrary to common belief, evidence is lacking that any particular dietary manipulation promotes healing or reduces acidity. The one exception is that not eating before bedtime probably reduces nocturnal gastric acid levels because the postprandial stimulus to acid secretion is avoided. Otherwise, bland diets, frequent feedings, small feedings, and avoidance of spices, fruit juices, and acidic foods have never been shown to affect the course of ulcer disease. Milk is also without specific benefit; in fact, its high content of protein and calcium stimulates gastric acid secretion. Some patients claim that certain foods "disagree" with them; these can be avoided, but not for the sake of altering acid production. Intake of *coffee* (including decaffeinated forms) and other caffeinated beverages ought to be limited but need not be eliminated entirely; their link with ulcer disease is not especially strong.

Pharmacologic Therapies

Antibiotics. The eradication of *H. pylori* infection is emerging as the principal treatment objective for peptic ulcer disease (except in cases related to NSAID use). The efficacy of such treatment in preventing relapses, resolving refractory disease, and eliminating the need for expensive, long-term acid suppression/inhibition therapy is becoming increasingly evident. One to two weeks of antibiotic therapy reduces the relapse rate at 1 year from 50% to as little as 5% to 10%. As effective as antibiotic therapy is, empiric use is not recommended because of the emerging risk for *Helicobacter* drug resistance in the community. However, selective empiric use may be reasonable when the clinical probability of infection is very high (e.g., objectively documented duodenal ulcer in a person not taking NSAIDs).

Cost-effectiveness. The efficacy, safety, and low cost of antibiotic therapy have made eradication of *Helicobacter* infection the mainstay of cost-effective management for peptic ulcer disease; antibiotic therapy usually obviates the need for long-term or recurrent use of expensive acid suppression therapy. Even with the cost of endoscopy figured in, antibiotic treatment for *Helicobacter* is a far more cost-effective approach to peptic ulcer disease than is maintenance acid suppression. Cost-effectiveness data strongly favor the treatment of *Helicobacter* over traditional acid suppression therapy. Once infection is eradicated, the rate of recurrence falls not only dramatically but often permanently.

Available Agents. Multidrug regimens are required because of the high frequency of resistance to single agents. Agents with anti-*Helicobacter* activity include *tetracycline, amoxicillin, bismuth subsalicylate, metronidazole,* and *clarithromycin,* in addition to the *PPIs.* Antibiotic resistance has been reported, particularly for metronidazole (in 10% to 50%) and more recently for clarithromycin. Persons with prior exposure to these antibiotics should be treated with other agents. Acid suppression therapy (with H_2-blockers or PPIs) is often added to speed ulcer healing and provide more rapid symptomatic relief, but prevention of relapse depends primarily on the eradication of *Helicobacter.*

Standard Triple Therapy. The standard regimen is so-called *triple therapy* with *metronidazole, tetracycline* (or *amoxicillin* for those patients allergic to tetracycline), and *bismuth subsalicylate* given four times daily for *2 weeks.* Rates of eradication are in excess of 90% under study conditions but are probably lower in everyday practice. A lack of compliance and antibiotic-induced diarrhea are common problems with triple therapy, especially when 2 weeks of therapy are prescribed. A *1-week program* that adds a *PPI* (omeprazole or lansoprazole) to the regimen achieves similar eradication results while shortening the length of treatment.

Dual Regimens. Because triple antibiotic therapy poses problems related to compliance and side effects, simpler, better-tolerated programs have been explored. *Clarithromycin*-based regimens, which combine the antibiotic (taken three times daily for 2 weeks) with either *omeprazole* or *ranitidine/bismuth citrate* (taken twice daily for a month), improve compliance and are better tolerated; however, eradication rates are not quite as good as with triple therapy (70% to 85%), and cost increases substantially (an order of magnitude more expensive than triple therapy)! Substituting amoxicillin for clarithromycin in a dual regimen markedly reduces eradication rates and is not recommended.

Two Antibiotics Plus Proton Pump Inhibitor. Treatment programs that enhance compliance and minimize side effects without compromising efficacy or affordability continue to be tested. A particularly promising program involves two antibiotics (*clarithromycin* plus *metronidazole* or *amoxicillin*) in combination with a *PPI* (omeprazole or lansoprazole). The principal advantages include twice-daily dosing and few side effects. The cost is considerably greater than with standard triple therapy, but eradication rates are in excess of 90%. Comparative cost-effectiveness data are not yet available.

Antacids. Because they are effective, inexpensive, and safe, antacids remain a mainstay of therapy. The preferred preparations are those containing magnesium hydroxide, aluminum hydroxide, or a combination of the two. Those containing calcium carbonate (e.g., Tums, Rolaids) have considerable acid-neutralizing capacity and are inexpensive, convenient, and well tolerated, but laboratory studies have demonstrated rebound acid hypersecretion with the use of calcium-containing antacids. Nonetheless, no clinical evidence suggests that acid rebound is clinically important, but more study of the issue is needed. In persons with renal disease, antacid use can cause hypercalcemia and systemic alkalosis.

Effectiveness. When taken in four-times-daily regimens, antacids have been shown endoscopically to be more effective than placebo, and comparable with H_2-blockers and sucralfate in promoting the healing of duodenal ulcers. Their effectiveness in gastric ulcer disease and in preventing recurrences of gastric and duodenal ulcers is less well established. These agents are no more effective than placebo for the relief of pain from duodenal ulcer, although they are better than placebo for symptoms attributable to gastric ulcer. This effect on gastric ulcer pain and the recently demonstrated efficacy of frequent but non-neutralizing antacid doses has stimulated speculation, especially in regard to aluminum-containing antacids, about mechanisms of action beyond simple acid neutralization (e.g., protective coating, inactivation of irritant bile acids, stimulation of prostaglandin synthesis).

Buffering Capacities of liquid antacid preparations vary considerably, ranging from 6 to 128 mEq/15 mL. Liquids are superior to tablets in buffering capacity. Calcium carbonate preparations are among the most potent in neutralizing capacity but can cause acid rebound of unclear significance. The most effective liquid antacids contain magnesium and aluminum hydroxides. When the aluminum hydroxide mixes with acid, nonabsorbable aluminum salts are formed, which are constipating. The magnesium salts formed are also poorly absorbed but frequently cause diarrhea, an effect that may not be completely canceled by the constipating action of the aluminum. If diarrhea becomes a problem, one can alternately use an antacid containing only aluminum hydroxide. Many of the liquid antacids contain considerable amounts of sodium. A low-sodium preparation is sometimes needed to avoid sodium excess in patients who must restrict salt intake.

Dosage. Substantial doses of antacids are needed in the treatment of duodenal ulcer; however, as little as 120 mEq daily has proved effective in healing gastric ulcers. Previous failures to demonstrate the effectiveness of antacids may have been a consequence of inadequate doses. About 140 mEq at a time is necessary to bring the gastric pH into the range of 3.5 to 5.0. Typical 30-mL doses of many popular antacids provide only 60 mEq. Although the contents listed on labels of weak and strong antacid preparations are similar, the relative amounts and solubilities of ingredients do vary, which accounts for differences in potency.

Timing of the antacid dose affects the degree of acid neutralization. If given with a meal, the antacid is wasted because food is a perfectly adequate buffer. When an antacid is given 1 hour after eating, gastric acidity is minimized for another 1 to 2 hours, countering the food-induced stimulation of acid secretion. A second dose 3 hours after a meal provides another hour of acid neutralization and tides the patient over to the next meal.

Side Effects are relatively few but important to recognize. *Diarrhea* is common as a result of the cathartic effect of insoluble magnesium salts. Alternating with an antacid containing only aluminum hydroxide can help. Antacids enhance the absorption of dicumarol and L-dopa and decrease the absorption of H_2-blockers, phenothiazines, sulfonamides, isoniazid, and penicillin. Potent antacids can cause the premature release of aspirin from enteric-coated tablets when both are taken simultaneously. *Phosphate depletion* is possible in patients using an aluminum-containing antacid; insoluble aluminum phosphate forms. In renal failure, excess aluminum may accumulate and cause central nervous system toxicity. There is also concern, although no proof, about the relation of dementia to serum aluminum excess in the elderly (see Chapter 169). Excess sodium absorption has already been mentioned. Magnesium-containing antacids should be avoided in renal failure because of the risk for *hypermagnesemia*; the small amounts of magnesium absorbed cannot be eliminated. Calcium can be absorbed and precipitate *hypercalcemia* if renal function is depressed. As noted, calcium also triggers *rebound acid secretion*, raising at least a theoretical concern about overall efficacy.

Cost-effective Prescribing for duodenal ulceration employs an agent with a high degree of neutralizing capacity and a low cost per therapeutic dose. Several liquid preparations have such qualities and stand out as the best buys; moreover, they have low sodium levels (Tables 68.1 and 68.2). Compared with tablets, they are less expensive but not as convenient; tablets are particularly well suited for patients who must take medication while at work. Although antacids are safe and effective, their cost and inconvenience can mount when they must be taken seven times a day. Trying to achieve adequate acid neutralization with antacid tablets alone can become difficult; at least eight tablets must be taken just to obtain 140 mEq of acid-neutralizing capacity. For the treatment of gastric ulcer,

Table 68.1. Characteristics of Major Liquid Antacids

PREPARATION	NEUTRALIZING CAPACITY (MEQ/5ML)	VOLUME FOR 140 MEQ (OZ)	SODIUM CONTENT (MG/5 ML)	RELATIVE COST[a]	BUFFERS
Maalox TC	27	0.86	<1.0	1.7	Al/MgOH$_2$
Titralac Plus	11	2.12	<1.0	1.9	CaCO$_3$
Mylanta Double Strength	25	0.93	1.0	1.2	Al/MgOH$_2$
Gaviscon	3	8.0		14.5	Al/MgCO$_2$
Riopan Plus	15	1.56	<1.0	1.7	Magaldrate
Riopan Plus Double Strength	30	0.78	<1.0	1.3	Magaldrate
Mylanta	12	1.94	<1.0	1.8	Al/MgOH$_2$
AlternaGEL	16	1.46	2.0	2.7	AlOH$_2$
Maalox	13	1.74	1.0	1.6	Al/MgOH$_2$
Maalox Extra Strength	29	0.88	1.0	1.0	Al/MgOH$_2$
Riopan Double Strength	30	0.78	<1.0	1.3	Al/MgOH$_2$
Amphojel	10	2.33	7.0	4.4	AlOH$_2$

[a]Reference cost is that of a 140-mEq dose of Maalox Extra Strength liquid. (Personal communication, Harold S. Delmonaco, Massachusetts General Hospital Pharmacy.)

Table 68.2.   Characteristics of Major Antacid Tablets

PREPARATION	NEUTRALIZING CAPACITY (MEQ/TABLET)	DOSE FOR 140 MEQ (TABLETS)	SODIUM CONTENT (MG/TABLET)	RELATIVE COST[a]	BUFFERS
Gaviscon	0.5	280	19.0	36.9	$Al/MgOH_2$
Mylanta II	23	6	1.3	1.0	$Al/MgOH_2$
Mylanta	21	12	0.8	1.4	$Al/MgOH_2$
Tums	10.5	14	2.0	0.8	$CaCO_3$
Riopan Plus	13.5	10	0.1	1.4	$Al/MgOH_2$
Titralac	7.5	19	0.3	2.1	$CaCO_3$
Gelusil II	11	13	0.8	2.1	$Al/MgOH_2$
Rolaids	7.3	19	53.0	1.2	$Ca/MgOH_2$
Maalox Plus	11.4	12	0.8	5.9	$Al/MgOH_2$
Maalox Extra Strength	25.4	6	1.4	1.0	$Al/MgOH_2$
Maalox	9.7	14	0.7	2.2	$Al/MgOH_2$
Amphojel	8	18	1.8	3.1	$AlOH_2$

[a]Reference cost is that of a 140-mEq dose of Maalox Extra Strength Tablets. (Personal communication, Harold S. Delmonaco, Massachusetts General Hospital Pharmacy.)

acid neutralization is less of an issue, and much smaller doses may suffice (e.g., two to three extra-strength tablets of an aluminum-containing antacid, such as Mylanta Double Strength or Extra Strength Maalox Antacid Plus taken four times daily). The cost of antacid regimens is about one-fourth that of H_2-blocker therapy or sucralfate.

Histamine$_2$-Receptor Antagonists. These drugs block the H_2-receptors of parietal cells, which results in a 50% to 80% reduction in basal, postprandial, and vagally stimulated acid production. The available preparations include cimetidine, ranitidine, famotidine, and nizatidine. Despite advertising claims of major differences among these agents, they are remarkably similar in efficacy. No clinically significant differences have been found in rates of ulcer healing or prevention of relapse. About 75% of duodenal ulcers are healed by 4 weeks, and 84% to 97% by 8 weeks; 55% to 65% of gastric ulcers are healed by 4 weeks, and 80% to 90% by 8 weeks. Recurrence rates after completion of therapy range from 45% to 70% at 3 months to 75% to 90% at 1 year and are no different from those noted with other treatments. Rarely is maintenance therapy necessary if *Helicobacter* infection has been eradicated.

Cimetidine was the first H_2-blocker and is available in generic formulation, so that it is the least expensive of the drugs in its class. It is also available without prescription in half-strength doses.

Pharmacokinetics. Absorption is rapid and complete after oral administration. Peak blood levels occur 45 to 90 minutes after a 300-mg dose. Originally thrice-daily or four-times-daily dosing was recommended, but equivalent results have been achieved with a single 800-mg dose at bedtime or 400 mg twice daily. A low-dose maintenance program (400 mg daily at bedtime) has been shown to reduce the recurrence rate substantially to 15% to 25% yearly. Absorption is reduced 10% to 20% by concurrent intake of magnesium- or aluminum-containing antacids; a 2-hour staggering of doses helps maximize benefit, although it is not essential. Absorption is not affected by meals. Most of the drug is excreted unchanged in the urine; 15% is metabolized by the liver. Patients in renal failure require less frequent administration (e.g., every 12 hours when the serum creatinine rises above 3.0 mg/dL). The drug crosses the placental barrier.

Side Effects and Adverse Reactions are relatively minor and occur infrequently (<5% of patients). In controlled studies, the frequency of side effects was indistinguishable from that for placebo; however, in long-term studies, the frequency of adverse reactions exceeds that for placebo. The most commonly experienced adverse reactions include *diarrhea, nausea, vomiting, rash, dizziness, and headache.* The incidence of each is less than 1%. The drug crosses the blood-brain barrier in humans and can cause *lethargy, confusion, slurred speech, agitation, and visual hallucinations,* particularly in the elderly, the very young, patients with renal or liver disease, and those receiving high doses. *Gynecomastia* and *sexual dysfunction* rank among the most troubling of side effects and are especially prevalent among patients taking the drug at high doses (2,400 mg daily) for the treatment of Zollinger-Ellison syndrome. The mechanism is believed to involve the ability of the drug to impair estradiol metabolism and bind to androgenic receptors, which also results in a slightly reduced sperm count.

Isolated cases of *bone marrow suppression* have been reported in the setting of severe underlying illness and use of multiple drugs. Small, clinically insignificant decreases in *creatinine clearance* are sometimes noted. The effect is dose-related and more common when daily doses exceed 2,000 mg. On occasion, the creatine clearance might fall by as much as 25%, but no permanent renal injury results. Frank *hep-atotoxicity* is rare, but transient twofold to threefold increases in aminotransferase (transaminase) levels sometimes ensue; however, these usually disappear, even with continuation of therapy.

Drug–Drug Interactions. Cimetidine slows hepatic drug metabolism by *inhibiting microsomal enzymes.* These effects are dose-related but occur with as little as 800 mg daily. Clearance is reduced by 20% to 30%, so that serum half-lives are increased. Although such impairment is usually not clinically significant, it can be important when hepatically metabolized drugs with a narrow therapeutic range are taken concurrently (e.g., *warfarin, benzodiazepines, phenytoin, procainamide, and theophylline compounds*). Cimetidine also reduces the hepatic metabolism of *propranolol* and *carbamazepine* by about 20%. The net effect is a potentiation of drug effect. Dose reductions are essential, as is monitoring of serum levels. The effect of cimetidine on hepatic microsomal enzymes lasts for about 2 weeks after the drug is stopped. *Ketoconazole* absorption is reduced by up to 65% when the drug is taken within 2 hours after a cimetidine dose, so that it must be administered at least 2 hours before intake of an H_2-blocker.

Ranitidine, Famotidine, and Nizatidine were developed after cimetidine and are more potent on a weight basis. Their single-dose ability to inhibit acid secretion is equal or superior to that of cimetidine, and the effect of a single dose lasts 12 to 24 hours. They can promote healing in a proportion of patients with refractory gastric ulcer, duodenal ulcer, or Zollinger-Ellison syndrome who have not responded to cimetidine. A single dose at night has been found to be as effective as cimetidine in preventing recurrence of duodenal ulcer; recurrence rates are reduced to less than 25%.

Pharmacokinetics. Absorption after oral administration ranges from 45% for famotidine to 100% for nizatidine, a difference that is not clinically important. Concurrent intake of food does not reduce absorption, but the use of aluminum or magnesium antacids does, by 10% to 20%. About 30% of each of these agents is metabolized by the liver. Metabolites plus unmetabolized drug are excreted by the kidneys. Drug half-life is prolonged in renal failure. Like cimetidine, ranitidine is excreted in breast milk.

Side Effects are similar and only slightly different from those of cimetidine (which can be attributed at least in part to less clinical experience with the newer agents). *Headache* occurs in about 5% of patients taking famotidine and in 3% of those taking ranitidine; migraine may be exacerbated. *Confusion* is slightly less common with these agents than with cimetidine but still may occur, especially in elderly patients taking large doses. Gynecomastia has not been reported, but *impotence* has been encountered among a few patients taking extremely high doses. The only reported cases of bone marrow suppression are a few isolated instances of thrombocytopenia in patients taking famotidine. Renal function is unimpaired, but hepatoxicity has been noted in a few instances. These drugs interfere less with *microsomal enzyme* function than does cimetidine, but interference may occur with ranitidine, although usually only at high doses. The clearance rates of warfarin, theophylline, benzodiazepines, phenytoin, and procainamide appear normal, but the metabolism of propranolol may be slowed, as may absorption of ketoconazole.

Choice of Histamine₂ Blocker. When prescribed in therapeutic doses, these agents are similar in efficacy and side effects. Drug–drug interactions are slightly more common with cimetidine because inhibition of hepatic microsomal enzymes occurs at lower doses. Most other adverse effects are typically minor and usually of concern only when these drugs are used in the elderly or when very large doses are prescribed (as in treatment of hypersecretory states). The predominant difference among H₂-blockers is cost, with generic cimetidine being the least expensive (at about half the daily cost of the other agents). In the past, when it was recommended that cimetidine be taken three or four times daily, the once- or twice-daily dosing of the newer H₂-blockers offered a considerable compliance advantage. However, now that twice-daily dosing of cimetidine has been shown to be effective, this advantage is less important, although the newer H₂-blockers may have a slight advantage in efficacy. With ranitidine becoming available generically, it too may offer a reduced-cost option. Billions of dollars per year are spent on H₂-blocker therapy, so that a cost-conscious approach to their use is necessary.

Proton Pump Inhibitors. The gastric H⁺/K⁺-ATPase ("proton pump") inhibitors are the most potent of the acid-inhibiting drugs, reducing 24-hour acid production by more than 90% with a single daily dose of 20 to 30 mg. In comparison, acid production is reduced 50% to 80% with standard doses of H₂-blockers. With higher PPI doses, acid production is almost completely stopped.

Effectiveness. The speed of ulcer healing and pain reduction (40% to 80% at 2 weeks and 80% to 95% at 4 weeks) are greater with these agents than with standard doses of H₂-blockers. Ulcers refractory to high doses of H₂-blockers can be healed by 20 to 40 mg of a PPI daily, a principal indication for their use. However, rates of relapse are similar to those with other forms of acid suppression therapy, so that treatment directed against *H. pylori* infection must be considered (see below). Interestingly, these agents appear to have some antibacterial effect on *Helicobacter* and are useful in regimens to eradicate *Helicbacter* infection (see above). The PPIs are the drugs of choice for *Zollinger-Ellison syndrome.*

Adverse Effects. These agents are well tolerated. Some patients experience mild gastrointestinal upset. Important adverse effects include drug–drug interactions and an increase in serum gastrin levels. *Drug–drug interactions* are a consequence of the metabolism of PPIs by *hepatic microsomal enzymes.* Omeprazole displaces such microsomally metabolized drugs as benzodiazepines, phenytoin, and warfarin (but not theophylline and propranolol), so that serum levels of these agents are increased. It also increases absorption of digoxin and decreases prednisone efficacy. Lansoprazole increases clearance of theophylline.

Risk for Gastric Carcinoid. One consequence of potent inhibition of gastric acid production is hypergastrinemia. Most patients experience a twofold to fourfold increase above baseline (still within normal limits). About 10% exhibit a 10-fold increase (>500 ng/L), which is associated with an increased rate of argyrophil cell hyperplasia and atrophic gastritis (but not of dysplasia or cancer). Prolonged hypergastrinemia has been associated with hyperplasia of enterochromaffin cells and development of *carcinoid tumors* in rats given high doses of omeprazole—presumably a consequence of the trophic effects of *hypergastrinemia* on enterochromaffin cells. No such tumors have been reported with prolonged omeprazole use in humans (see Chapter 61).

Atrophic Gastritis. Although PPI therapy by itself might not increase cancer risk, there is concern about its contribution in the setting of *Helicobacter* infection. *Atrophic gastritis* (a precancerous change) seen in the context of high-dose, long-term PPI therapy may exacerbate the gastric cancer risk associated with *H. pylori* infection (see above). Lack of gastric acid may contribute to bacterial overgrowth and the elaboration of bacterial carcinogens. Any person requiring long-term, high-dose PPI therapy ought to be tested and treated for *H. pylori* infection.

Vitamin B₁₂ Deficiency. Patients with Zollinger-Ellison syndrome requiring long-term PPI therapy to suppress gastric acid overproduction demonstrate significant (30%) reductions in vitamin B₁₂ levels, especially when achlorhydria is achieved. Whether this effect pertains to other persons taking long-term, high-dose PPI therapy remains to be established, but periodic monitoring of serum B₁₂ levels might be reasonable, especially in the elderly.

Prostaglandin Analogues (Misoprostol). NSAID-induced cases of peptic ulcer disease are related to prostaglandin inhibition. Misoprostol is a prostaglandin analogue used for the treatment and prophylaxis of NSAID-induced peptic ulcer disease.

Efficacy and Cost-effectiveness in NSAID-induced Ulcer Disease. Although more effective than placebo, misoprostol is less effective than H₂-blockers or PPIs for the treatment of non–NSAID-induced peptic ulcers. However, the prostaglandin analogue is very effective in the treatment of *NSAID-induced* peptic ulcers, with resolution achieved in more than 70% of cases at 8 weeks, about the same rate achieved with H_2-blockers but somewhat less than that achieved with PPI therapy. Misoprostol is the only drug approved by the Food and Drug Administration for the *primary prevention of NSAID-induced* peptic ulcers; it is effective when taken in full doses at least two to three times per day concurrently with NSAID therapy. (No prospective comparisons with PPI therapy for primary prevention have been undertaken.)

For treatment and prophylaxis in persons with a history of NSAID-induced ulceration who require continued NSAID use (*secondary prevention*), misoprostol is less effective than PPI therapy for sustaining a remission, although both agents are effective for healing the initial ulcer and superior to H_2-blockers.

Misoprostol has also been examined for ability to prevent the complications of NSAID-induced ulcer disease, such as gastrointestinal bleeding. Because of its high cost, misoprostol has not proved cost-effective in the *primary prevention* of NSAID-induced *upper gastrointestinal bleeding*, but its use for *secondary prevention* does appear more reasonable from a cost-effectiveness perspective. NSAID-induced primary duodenal ulceration is infrequent, but complications are common, and misoprostol is thought to help reduce their frequency (as might PPI therapy).

Side Effects. Dose-related *diarrhea* is common (20% with 100-μg doses four times daily, 40% with 200-μg doses four times daily) and an important form of intolerance to the drug that results in its discontinuation by patients. A reduced dose is often tried, but efficacy is reduced. Maintaining full doses but reducing dosing frequency to twice or three times daily appears to be a more productive strategy for sustaining a prophylactic program; much of the benefit is preserved while gastrointestinal side effects are substantially reduced. Taking the drug with meals also helps to reduce the severity of diarrhea. The drug is an *abortifacient*; it is contraindicated in women who are pregnant or who may be pregnant and should be prescribed for sexually active women of childbearing age only with proper warning and detailed patient education. Those considering taking misoprostol should be capable of reliable use of birth control. Consideration of an alternative to misoprostol is probably a safer approach in such women.

Sucralfate is a complex of aluminum hydroxide and sulfated sucrose; it is believed to act by forming a barrier on the ulcer base, inhibiting pepsin activity, and binding bile salts. It has no acid-neutralizing activity and little is absorbed, although aluminum salts are released and some aluminum is absorbed. Its principal role in outpatient management of peptic ulcer disease is as an alternative to acid suppression therapy in persons who cannot tolerate antacids, H_2-blockers, or PPI therapy.

Efficacy. The drug is comparable to cimetidine and ranitidine for healing of *duodenal ulcers*. Maintenance therapy (1 g twice daily) to prevent recurrences appears slightly less effective than that with H_2-blockers. Available data suggest some benefit for treatment of *gastric ulcer*; however, more data are needed, and the Food and Drug Administration has not yet approved sucralfate treatment for this condition. Although some clinicians add sucralfate to H_2-receptor antagonist therapy to promote healing of gastric ulcers, evidence to support this approach is lacking. The claim that sucralfate preferentially heals ulcers in smokers has not been substantiated. Sucralfate is most effective when taken 1 hour before meals and at bedtime, although twice-daily administration of double-strength doses has proved adequate for treatment of duodenal ulcer.

Side Effects. The main side effect is constipation. The drug binds phosphate and has been reported to cause *hypophosphatemia* and *aluminum toxicity* in patients with chronic renal failure. Sucralfate may interfere with the *gastrointestinal absorption* of tetracycline, fluoroquinolone antibiotics (e.g., ciprofloxacin, norfloxacin), digoxin, phenytoin, and, to a clinically insignificant degree, H_2-blockers. No data are available regarding safety in patients who are pregnant, nursing, or of advanced age. The cost of daily sucralfate therapy is intermediate between that of cimetidine and other H_2-blockers.

Anticholinergic Agents can suppress the parasympathetic muscarinic activity that triggers gastric acid secretion, especially the nocturnal surge. These agents are not nearly as potent as H_2-receptor antagonists in suppressing acid production. The frequency and severity of anticholinergic side effects make therapy intolerable for many patients. Because agents that are more effective and better tolerated are available, anticholinergics are rarely prescribed anymore.

Follow-up

Monitoring Response: Gastric Ulcer. If a *gastric* lesion has been detected initially by radiography and has all the hallmarks of a benign lesion (see above), if symptoms resolve fully, and if no clinical findings suggestive of cancer or complicated disease are present (see above), then follow-up barium study or endoscopy can probably be foregone. Although some authorities advocate routine endoscopic or radiologic *documentation of healing*, no studies show this to be cost-effective in uncomplicated cases in which symptoms resolve within 4 to 6 weeks and do not recur. However, if a refractory gastric ulcer is suspected (e.g., persistent pain after 8 weeks despite a full medical regimen), then *endoscopic examination* and *biopsy* are needed, especially in patients over age 40, who are at increased risk for gastric cancer. Barium study is not sufficient because even malignant ulcers may shrink in size in response to therapy. Earlier endoscopic evaluation is indicated if evidence of bleeding or obstruction or another reason for concerned about gastric carcinoma is present (see above).

Monitoring Response: Duodenal Ulcer. In the case of a *duodenal* ulcer (where cancer risk is nil), follow-up radiologic or endoscopic evaluation should be restricted to patients with persistence or recurrence of pain, symptoms of gastric outlet obstruction, or evidence of bleeding. Periodic repetition of studies is unnecessary and expensive, even when typical symptoms recur, unless a different course of therapy, such as surgery, is contemplated. Following results of stool guaiac tests and blood cell counts can help detect bleeding, as can careful questioning of the patient.

Duration of Therapy. The standard duration for an initial acid suppression regimen is 4 weeks to achieve full healing in 90% of patients. Up to 12 weeks of such treatment may be necessary for very large benign ulcers. However, without eradication of *Helicobacter* infection, the risk for ulcer recurrence within 1 year is greater than 50%, so that long-term acid suppression therapy is often implemented. As noted earlier, 1 to 2 weeks of combination antibiotic therapy eradicates more than 90% of *Helicobacter* infections, reduces 1-year recurrence rates by 90%, and eliminates the need for most courses of long-term acid suppression therapy. Resolution of pain cannot be used as a therapeutic end point because cessation of pain correlates poorly with completion of healing or eradication of infection. Unfortunately, patients commonly terminate treatment when their symptoms resolve, which increases their risk for relapse.

Maintenance Therapy for Secondary Prevention. The need for maintenance acid suppression to prevent *recurrence* has declined markedly with the eradication of *Helicobacter* infection. One-year recurrence rates for non–NSAID-related ulcers are about 5% when initial therapy is aimed at elimination of *Helicobacter* and in excess of 50% without use of antibiotics. Before the advent of treatment for *Helicobacter* infection, maintenance acid suppression was commonly prescribed to prevent recurrences. Although prevention of ulcer recurrence has been demonstrated with the long-term use of H_2-receptor antagonists and PPIs, the risk returns to its previous level once such acid suppression therapy has been discontinued. Even with continuation of adequate maintenance therapy, silent breakthrough ulceration can be demonstrated by repeated endoscopy in up to 50% of patients, although most is usually of little clinical consequence. Just a single course of antibiotic therapy that eradicates *H. pylori* infection reduces the risk for recurrence to less than 5%. Medical therapy that cures *H. pylori* infection also markedly reduces the risks for *hemorrhage, perforation, and obstruction* but shows little advantage over placebo for pain relief, in part because of a very strong placebo effect.

Indications. Maintenance suppression of gastric acid production is currently recommended only for those with a history of *upper gastrointestinal bleeding*, concurrent *oral anticoagulation* and recent peptic ulcer (see Chapter 83), an *ulcer recurrence* within 1 year that fails to respond to *Helicobacter* therapy, or a history of *NSAID-induced peptic ulcer* that requires continued NSAID therapy.

Efficacy. Effective long-term suppression of gastric acid production is provided by a maintenance program of PPI therapy (e.g., 20 mg of omeprazole daily), which reduces 24-hour acid production by more than 90% with a single daily dose. This compares with a 50% to 80% reduction in acid production with standard doses of H_2-blockers. Almost complete cessation of acid production is achieved with higher PPI doses. As noted earlier, PPI therapy can markedly reduce the risk for ulcer recurrence and complications in the settings for which maintenance therapy is recommended. H_2-blocker maintenance is signficantly less effective.

Dosing. Daily dosing is required to achieve the best outcomes. Concern about the effects of long-term suppression of acid production (see below) have prompted some to suggest an every-other-day or every-3-days PPI maintenance program; the impact on efficacy is not known, nor is the benefit. The rationale for less frequent dosing is to allow some acid production to occur, which reduces hypergastrinemia and its possible adverse consequences (see below). Another alternative to daily maintenance therapy is empiric treatment of pain recurrences, a common self-treatment approach. Its safety and efficacy are unknown but likely to be problematic, given the poor correlation between symptoms and risk for complications of ulcer disease.

Cost. Long-term PPI therapy is very expensive, but the cost is likely to decrease markedly as these drugs come off patent and become available generically. The least expensive preparation should be sought. *H_2-blockers* are less effective and not much less expensive. *Misoprostol* (200 μg twice daily) is a reasonable alternative for prophylaxis in persons who need long-term NSAID therapy, but expense is high and gastrointestinal side effects can be troublesome. Antacids are much less costly, but their efficacy as maintenance therapy is unknown.

Duration. Although most authorities recommend continuing maintenance treatment for 1 year or for the duration of the indication (e.g., NSAID or anticoagulation use), the optimal duration of such therapy remains unknown; the consequences of prolonged suppression of gastric acid production are also unknown (see below). The relapse rate for medical maintenance therapy is 10 times that for surgical therapy, but most patients can be spared an operation, particularly if attention is paid to *Helicobacter* infection as a major cause of relapsing disease.

Concerns Regarding Long-term Acid Suppression. Debate continues about the safety of shutting down gastric acid production on a long-term basis, as is possible with prolonged PPI therapy. Concerns include a risk for carcinoid tumors, gastric cancer, and vitamin B_{12} deficiency (see above). The best means of avoiding these potential adverse consequences is to minimize the need for prolonged PPI therapy, which is best achieved by eradicating *Helicobacter* infection and minimizing the use of NSAIDs. The literature should be followed closely for more data on the consequences of prolonged suppression of gastric acid production.

Refractory or Recurrent Disease

Persistence of pain 4 weeks after the initiation of proper therapy suggests an unhealed ulcer. If endoscopic evaluation was carried out initially to rule out a malignant lesion and a large ulcer was found, then acid suppression therapy can be continued, with high-dose PPI therapy utilized to speed healing. Eight to 12 weeks of treatment may be necessary. If *H. pylori* infection was not tested for and treated initially, then it should be at this time. If compliance with the anti-*Helicobacter* treatment regimen has been complete, then testing for the eradication of infection can help guide further action. If, despite eradication of *Helicobacter* infection, symptoms persist beyond 4 to 8 weeks, then endoscopic evaluation is needed (if not performed initially) to rule out malignancy or complicated disease. Recurrent disease raises the question of persistent *Helicobacter* infection, repeated NSAID exposure, Zollinger-Ellison syndrome, and malignancy.

Testing for Active *Helicobacter* Infection. The potential contribution of *Helicobacter* infection to persistent or recurrent disease necessitates testing for active infection. *Serologic testing* is appropriate for the initial identification of *H. pylori* infection; eradication may be documented by repeated serologic testing, but test sensitivity for detecting cure of infection is wanting. Much more sensitive is ^{14}C or ^{13}C *breath testing* (see above). If this is unavailable, repeated quantitative serologic testing may suggest eradication if antibody has cleared from the serum or titers are significantly reduced from initial levels. If persistent infection is found, it should be fully treated with a different multidrug antibiotic regimen to counter any possible antibiotic resistance (see above).

Checking for Noncompliance and Aggravating Factors. In addition to checking for *Helicobacter*, it is crucial to check for noncompliance and aggravating factors such as *smoking* and *stress*. Many instances of refractory disease and recurrence are closely linked to continued smoking, severe stress, and failure to follow a prescribed medical regimen. Concurrent *NSAID use* may also contribute to refractoriness.

Switching to Another Agent is worth consideration when an ulcer is slow to heal. Patients genuinely failing H$_2$-blocker treatment may achieve a more rapid and complete response with *PPI* therapy, but more important is eradicating *Helicobacter* infection (see above) and checking for malignancy and Zollinger-Ellison syndrome (see below).

Assessing for Malignancy and Zollinger-Ellison Syndrome. Truly refractory cases (i.e., those in which *Helicobacter* infection, aggravating factors, and noncompliance have been addressed) ought to be evaluated endoscopically for malignancy and studied biochemically for *Zollinger-Ellison syndrome*, especially if multiple ulcers, occurrences in unusual places, marked abdominal pain, or a secretory diarrhea (resulting from hypergastrinemia) is present. Patients with Zollinger-Ellison syndrome often manifest evidence of multiple endocrine adenomatosis (e.g., concurrent hyperparathyroidism and pituitary adenomas). A fasting serum gastrin level in excess of 500 pg/mL in the presence of acid hypersecretion is diagnostic.

Consideration of Prophylactic Therapy. If an NSAID must be continued (e.g., because of disabling rheumatoid disease), then prophylactic treatment with *misoprostol* or a *PPI* may be required (see above). Sometimes, *increasing the dosage* of a prophylactic agent may help. If the patient has been on low-dose maintenance therapy when a recurrence develops, full-dose therapy should be initiated. Those taking an H$_2$-blocker may benefit from doubling the dose or *switching* to a PPI, which provides better prophylaxis. Convincing evidence is lacking that the addition of a second agent (e.g., H$_2$-blocker plus sucralfate) achieves better results in the treatment of refractory disease than does the administration of full doses of a single agent.

Surgery. Surgery for peptic ulcer disease is becoming increasingly uncommon with the advent of effective medical therapy. The most compelling *indications for surgery* include brisk bleeding of 6 to 8 U of blood in 24 hours (see Chapter 63), recurrent episodes of bleeding, perforation, gastric outlet obstruction refractory to medical therapy, and failure of a benign gastric ulcer to heal after 15 weeks. Operations are most often performed on patients who fail to respond to medical therapy and have disabling symptoms.

The *proximal gastric vagotomy* effectively limits recurrences without producing the disabling side effects associated with earlier forms of surgery for duodenal ulcer disease. The operation involves selective severing of the nerve supply to the acid-secreting fundus; the nerves to the antrum are left intact, so that control of gastric emptying is preserved. The incidence of ulcer recurrences is slightly higher (10%) than with vagotomy and antrectomy (5%) but similar to that with vagotomy and pyloroplasty (12%). Surgical mortality is lower, and such potentially disabling postsurgical side effects as the dumping syndrome and diarrhea are much less common. The operation is technically demanding and should be considered only by sur-

geons specifically trained to perform it. The procedure should not be carried out in patients with delayed gastric emptying. Distal gastrectomy with excision of the ulcer remains the procedure of choice for gastric ulcer.

PATIENT EDUCATION

Enlisting the patient's active involvement and overcoming much of the mythology surrounding ulcer disease are prime objectives of the patient education effort.

Advice. Patients appreciate dietary instruction, such as knowing what foods they can eat and what substances to avoid. Many ulcer patients unnecessarily put themselves on a "bland diet" and increase their intake of milk products, hoping these actions will help their ulcers to heal. Others take aspirin or over-the-counter NSAIDs for relief of ulcer pain. Use of coffee, alcohol, and tobacco also needs to be reviewed. Many physicians insist that coffee drinking be stopped, although this may cause more difficulty than is warranted by its role in pathogenesis. Switching to decaffeinated coffee offers little advantage. On the other hand, cessation of smoking is essential and detailed cessation counseling is critical (see Chapter 54) because continuation of the habit greatly impedes healing. Alcohol intake should also be discouraged

Maximizing Compliance. Even when an effective medical program has been designed, inadequate compliance can be a problem. Full compliance with the multidrug antibiotic regimens used to treat *Helicobacter* infection can be especially problematic, particularly when a 2-week thrice-daily or four-times-daily dosing regimen is required. The more expensive twice-daily regimens may be worth the extra initial expense for patients whose ability to comply fully is questionable. Alternatively, a 1-week thrice-daily program can be considered, which is almost as effective.

Other common compliance errors that need to be addressed include stopping medication as soon as symptoms disappear, taking antacids with meals (which wastes the antacid), and taking cimetidine at the same time as antacids (which partially impairs cimetidine absorption).

Counseling the patient with situational stress is often beneficial, but any suggestion to change jobs or family situations because an ulcer has developed is probably unwarranted and potentially counterproductive. There is no evidence that such extreme solutions contribute to healing, and they may actually heighten stress. One useful supplement to counseling is teaching simple *relaxation techniques*; these are especially useful for patients bothered by multiple somatic manifestations of stress (see Chapter 226).

Self-Monitoring. The patient needs to be taught to watch for complications of ulcer disease. In particular, the manifestations of gastrointestinal bleeding (see Chapter 63) should be well understood so that the patient does not delay in seeking help.

Shared Decision Making. If the question of elective surgery arises, the patient should be made a full partner in the decision because few definite guidelines for operation are available. A value judgment is necessary, and the costs and benefits of surgery versus continued medical therapy need to be discussed.

INDICATIONS FOR REFERRAL AND ADMISSION

Refractoriness to therapy is an indication for referral to a gastroenterologist for review of the program and consideration of endoscopy. Admission is mandatory when symptoms of *hemorrhage, peritoneal irritation, or gastric outlet obstruction* are present; both surgeon and gastroenterologist need to be consulted.

A most difficult issue is when and whom to select for *elective surgery*. Much has to do with the patient's preferences; gross generalizations are meaningless. Clearly, those with recurrent major bleeds, gastric outlet obstruction, or evidence of malignancy need to be seen by the surgeon. Seventy-five percent of patients with intractable pain obtain relief when treated surgically, but subgroups with alcohol abuse, character disorders, or severe neuroses do poorly after surgery. The decision to resort to elective surgery for recurrent disease should be made in conjunction with the patient, and the small risk for operative mortality and the morbidity of postgastrectomy syndrome should be weighed against the morbidity and cost of recurrent pain, time lost from work, and the need for long-term drug therapy.

THERAPEUTIC RECOMMENDATIONS

Nonpharmacologic Interventions and Initial Testing

- Avoid, or at least limit to the extent medically possible, the use of agents potentially injurious to the mucosa, including aspirin, excess alcohol, NSAIDs, and perhaps long-term, high-dose glucocorticosteroids.
- Insist on total *cessation of smoking* (see Chapter 54).
- Suggest a decreased intake of coffee (including decaffeinated forms) and other caffeine-containing beverages; however, complete cessation of intake is unnecessary.
- Do not restrict any foods or insist on a bland or milk-laden diet. Frequent small feedings are unnecessary, and a bedtime snack may stimulate nocturnal acid secretion. The patient should avoid only foods that cause discomfort.
- Attend to stress-related issues, but avoid recommending a major job or geographic change.
- Test for *Helicobacter* infection. For initial noninvasive testing, obtain quantitative serology and use a reference laboratory. Alternatively, perform a ^{14}C or ^{13}C breath test for noninvasive detection. If endoscopy is required (see below), have a rapid urease test (e.g., CLO test) performed at the same time.
- Order upper gastrointestinal endoscopy or barium study before initiating therapy if clinical findings suggest malignancy or complicated disease (e.g., patient manifests weight loss, gastrointestinal bleeding, or persistent nausea and vomiting).

Initial Pharmacologic Therapy

- For ulcer patients who test positive for *Helicobacter*, begin a multidrug antibiotic program.
  1. When cost is a major consideration but compliance is not, prescribe 250 mg of *metronidazole* four times daily, 500 mg of *tetracycline* four times daily (or 500 mg of *amoxicillin* four times daily if the patient is unable to tolerate tetracycline), and two tablets (525 mg) of *bismuth subsalicylate* (e.g., Pepto-Bismol) four times daily; continue for 2 weeks or limit to 1 week by adding a concurrent course of *PPI* therapy (e.g., 20 mg of omeprazole daily or 30 mg of lansoprazole daily).
  2. When side effects and compliance with a four-times-daily regimen are major concerns but cost is not, consider a 2-week program consisting of 500 mg of *clarithromycin* and 20 mg of *omeprazole* twice daily plus 500 mg of *metronidazole* or 500 mg of *amoxicillin* twice daily.
  3. Acid suppression therapy is *not required* in patients with *Helicobacter* infection, but it speeds healing and attainment of symptomatic relief.
- For all patients, begin an *acid suppression* program consisting of either antacids [e.g., 30 mL of a high-potency magnesium hydroxide–aluminum hydroxide liquid antacid after meals and at bedtime (Table 68.1)], an H_2-receptor antagonist (e.g., 400 mg of cimetidine twice daily), or a PPI (e.g., 20 mg of omeprazole twice daily or 30 mg of lansoprazole daily). Base selection on affordability, severity of disease, capacity for compliance, and potential for interaction with other medications.
- For patients with an active NSAID-induced ulcer, begin treatment with either a *PPI* (e.g., 20 mg of omeprazole twice daily) or *misoprostol* (200 mg with each meal and before bed); continue for 4 to 8 weeks depending on severity at time of presentation. There is no need to test for or treat *Helicobacter* infection because its eradication does not improve outcome in NSAID-induced disease.
- For patients with a prior history of NSAID-induced peptic ulceration or of upper gastrointestinal bleeding who absolutely require continuous NSAID therapy for maintenance of function, initiate prophylaxis with a *PPI* (e.g., 20 mg of omeprazole daily); consider *misoprostol* (200 mg with breakfast and supper) as a slightly less effective alternative for secondary prevention of NSAID-induced diseease, but as a reasonable (although not very cost-effective) first choice for primary prevention.
- Thoroughly instruct the patient on how to carry out the therapeutic program and review common misconceptions to maximize compliance.

Refractory or Recurrent Disease

- Check for failure to eradicate *H. pylori* infection, preferrably by *breath test* (if available); alternatively, repeat quantitative serology and compare pretreatment titers with current titers (seroconversion from positive to negative is highly specific but not sensitive).
- Reemphasize the importance of compliance, smoking cessation, and avoidance of NSAIDs.
- Institute PPI therapy, but limit its duration if possible; if not, be sure to eradicate any concurrent *H. pylori* infection so as to avoid development of atrophic gastritis. Institute long-term PPI therapy for treatment of Zollinger-Ellison syndrome.
- If *Helicobacter* infection persists, retreat with a new antibiotic regimen rather than repeating the original program.
- For persistent or recurrent disease unresponsive to treatment, refer for endoscopic examination and biopsy to rule out malignancy and complicated disease, especially if endoscopy was not performed initially.
- Refer the patient with refractory multiple ulcers, frequent recurrences, or associated secretory diarrhea for consideration of Zollinger-Ellison syndrome when symptoms are accompanied by marked hypergastrinemia in the context of acid hypersecretion.
- Admit patients with evidence of bleeding, gastric outlet obstruction, or perforation and obtain surgical consultation.

A.H.G.

ANNOTATED BIBLIOGRAPHY

Anda RF, Williamson DF, Escobedo LG, et al. Smoking and the risk of peptic ulcer disease among women in the U.S. Arch Intern Med 1990;150:1437. (*First National Health and Nutrition Examination Survey; relative risk 1.8 overall and increased with amount smoked; estimates 20% of all ulcers in women are a consequence of smoking.*)

Buchman E, Kaung DT, Dolank D, et al. Unrestricted diet in treatment of duodenal ulcer. Gastroenterology 1969;56:1016. (*Dietary restrictions made little or no difference.*)

Cantu TG, Korek JS. Central nervous system reactions to histamine$_2$-receptor blockers. Ann Intern Med 1991;114:1027. (*All H$_2$-blockers are capable of causing central nervous system effects, not just cimetidine.*)

Conn Ho, Blitzer BL. Nonassociation of adrenocorticosteroid therapy and peptic ulcer. N Engl J Med 1976;294:473. (*The first of two studies examining pooled data; concludes there is little association between steroids and risk for ulcer.*)

Cutler AF, Prasad VM, Santogade P. Four-year trends in *Helicobacter pylori* IgG serology following successful eradication. Am J Med 1998;105:18. (*Even with full eradication of infection, antibody titers plateau and persist in more than 70%.*)

Cutler AF, Havstad S, Ma CK, et al. Accuracy of invasive and noninvasive tests to diagnose *Helicobacter pylori* infection. Gastroenterology 1995;109:136. (*^{13}C-urea breath test and serology are as accurate as biopsy and CLO test for diagnosis.*)

Curatolo PW, Robertson D. The health consequences of caffeine. Ann Intern Med 1983;98:641. (*Thorough review; examines the evidence linking caffeine with ulcer disease and acid secretion; 281 references.*)

Dooley CP, Larson AW, Stace NH, et al. Double-contrast barium meal and upper gastrointestinal endoscopy. Ann Intern Med 1984;101:538. (*A randomized study indicating superior sensitivity and specificity for endoscopy but admitting that cost–benefit relationship is not established.*)

Drake D, Hollander D. Neutralizing capacity and cost-effectiveness of antacids. Ann Intern Med 1981;94:215. (*Excellent reference data on comparative characteristics of available antacids.*)

Feldman M, Cryer B, Lee E, et al. Role of seroconversion in confirming cure of *Helicobacter pylori* infection. JAMA 1998;280:363. (*Seroconversion had a sensitivity of 60% and a specificity of 100%, which suggests possible usefulness as an initial test for cure, but many with cure still had detectable antibody.*)

Fendick AM, Chernew ME, Hirth RA, et al. Alternative management strategies for patients with suspected peptic ulcer disease. Ann Intern Med 1995;123:260. (*Noninvasive management strategies were more cost-effective than immediate endoscopy.*)

Friedman DG, Siegelaub AB, Seltzer C. Cigarettes, alcohol, coffee and peptic ulcer. N Engl J Med 1974;290:469. (*Increased prevalence of ulcer disease in smokers. Coffee consumption and alcohol were not independent predictors of ulcer disease.*)

Gabriel SE, Jaakkimainen L, Bombardier C. Risk for serious gastrointestinal complications related to use of nonsteroidal antiinflammatory drugs. Ann Intern Med 1991;115:787. (*Relative risk increased about three times; other risk factors include age over 60, concomitant NSAID use, and prior ulcer disease.*)

Graham DY, Lew GM, Klein PD, et al. Effect of treatment of *Helicobacter pylori* infection on the long-term recurrence of gastric and duodenal ulcer. Ann Intern Med 1992;116:705. (*Randomized, controlled trial showing that eradication of the organism can lead to cure.*)

Graham DY, Smith JL. Aspirin and the stomach. Ann Intern Med 1986;104:390. (*Excellent review emphasizing the differences between acute and chronic effects; 98 references.*)

Graham DY, White RH, Moreland LW, et al. Duodenal and gastric ulcer prevention with misoprostol in arthritis patients taking NSAIDs. Ann Intern Med 1993;119:257. (*Randomized, controlled clinical trial showing reduction by misoprostol of rate of ulcer development.*)

Griffin MR, Piper JM, Daugherty JR, et al. Nonsteroidal antiinflammatory drug use and increased risk for peptic ulcer disease in elderly persons. Ann Intern Med 1991;114:257. (*Risk substantial and increases with dose and recency of use.*)

Hade JE, Spiro HM. Calcium and acid rebound: a reappraisal. J Clin Gastroenterol 1992;15:37. (*A critical review of the literature finding no evidence that the original laboratory findings of acid rebound are clinically significant; argues for reconsideration of the role of calcium carbonate antacids in treatment of peptic ulcer disease.*)

Hansson L-E, Nyren O, Hsing AW, et al. The risk of stomach cancer in patients with gastric or duodenal ulcer disease. N Engl J Med 1996;335:242. (*A Swedish population study; incidence ratio 1.8 for gastric ulcer, 0.6 for duodenal ulcer.*)

Hawkey CJ, Karrasch JA, Szczepanski L, et al., for the OMNIUM Study Group. Omeprazole compared with misoprostol for ulcers associated with nonsteroidal antiinflammatory drugs. N Engl J Med 1998;338:727. (*A two-part prospective, double-blind, randomized study showing both agents effective for healing NSAID-induced injury, but omeprazole better tolerated and superior for maintenance therapy.*)

Hentschel E, Brandstatter G, Dragosics B, et al. Effect of ranitidine and amoxicillin plus metronidazole on the eradication of *Helicobacter pylori* and the recurrence of duodenal ulcer. N Engl J Med 1993;328:308. (*Randomized, controlled study showing that eradication of* Helicobacter pylori *infection significantly speeds healing and prevents recurrences.*)

Ippolitto A, Elashoff J, Valenzuela J, et al. Recurrent ulcer after successful treatment with cimetidine or antacid. Gastroenterology 1983;85:875. (*Recurrence rates after antacid therapy were 29% at 3 months and 56% at 6 months, compared with 36% and 55% after cimetidine.*)

Isenberg JI, Peterson WL, Elashoff JD, et al. Healing of benign gastric ulcer with low-dose antacid or cimetidine. N Engl J Med 1983;308:1319. (*Demonstrates efficacy for both cimetidine and low-dose antacids, although cimetidine was superior.*)

Kim JG, Graham DY. *Helicobacter pylori* infection and development of gastric or duodenal ulcer in arthritis patients receiving chronic NSAID therapy. Am J Gastroenterol 1994;89:203. (*No increased risk for ulceration with* Helicobacter *infection.*)

Kuipers EJ, Lundell L, Klinkinberg-Knol EC, et al. Atrophic gastritis and *Helicobacter pylori* infection in patients with reflux esophagitis treated with omeprazole or fundoplication. N Engl J Med 1996;334:1018. (*Increased risk for this premalignant gastric change in persons with complete acid suppression and concurrent* Helicobacter *infection.*)

Levant JA, Walsh JH, Isenberg J. Stimulation of gastric secretion and gastrin release by single oral doses of calcium carbonate. N Engl J Med 1973;289:555. (*Calcium carbonate causes rebound acid hypersecretion, although it is a good neutralizing agent.*)

Lipsy RJ, Fennerty B, Fagan TC. Clinical review of histamine$_2$-receptor antagonists. Arch Intern Med 1990;150:745. (*Compares cimetidine, ranitidine, famotidine, and nizatidine; differences are more subtle than previously thought; 99 references.*)

Mahl GF. Anxiety, HCl secretion and peptic ulcer etiology. Psychosom Med 1950;12:158. (*Classic study showing that acute anxiety raises acid secretion.*)

Maton PN. Omeprazole. N Engl J Med 1991;324;965. (*Comprehensive review; 181 references.*)

Maton PN, Vinayek R, Frucht H, et al. Long-term efficacy and safety of omeprazole in patients with Zollinger-Ellison syndrome: prospective study. Gastroenterology 1989;97:827. (*Safety and efficacy demonstrated.*)

McCarthy DM. Sucralfate. N Engl J Med 1991;325:1017. (*Best review; 159 references.*)

Messer J, Reitman D, Sacks HS, et al. Association of adrenocorticosteroid therapy and peptic ulcer disease. N Engl J Med 1983;309:21. (*Second analysis of pooled data; finds an increased risk for ulcer disease, although the absolute risk is small.*)

Peterson WL, Cook DJ. Antisecretory therapy for bleeding peptic ulcer. JAMA 1998;280:877. (*Critical review of evidence concluding that PPI therapy is worthwhile.*)

Peterson WL. *Helicobacter pylori* and peptic ulcer disease. N Engl J Med 1991;324:1043. (*Excellent, terse review of the data; 97 references.*)

Peterson WL, Sturdevant RA, Frankl HD, et al. Healing of duodenal ulcer with an antacid regimen. N Engl J Med 1977;297:341. (*Classic placebo-controlled study; documents the efficacy of high-dose therapy at 1,000 mEq daily, surprisingly high rate of pain relief by placebo, and delayed healing in cigarette smokers.*)

Piper JM, Ray WA, Daugherty MS, et al. Corticosteroid use and peptic ulcer disease: role of nonsteroidal antiinflammatory drugs. Ann Intern Med 1991;114:735. (*Corticosteroid use was associated with an increased risk for ulcer only in the context of concurrent NSAID use.*)

Pounder R. Silent peptic ulceration: deadly silence or golden silence? Gastroenterology 1988;96[Suppl]:626. (*Symptoms and ulceration are frequently dissociated.*)

Raskin JB, White RH, Jackson JE, et al. Misoprostol dosage in the prevention of nonsteroidal anti-inflammatory drug-induced gastric and duodenal ulcers: a comparison of three regimens. Ann Intern Med 1995;123:344. (*Multicenter, randomized, placebo-controlled trial finding that twice-daily and three-times-daily regimens are better tolerated than four-times-daily programs and yet retain efficacy and reduce cost.*)

Rutter M. Psychological factors in short-term prognosis of physical disease. 1. Peptic ulcer. J Psychosom Res 1963;7:45. (*Another classic; severe anxiety prolongs recovery and makes relapse more likely.*)

Sogtag S, Graham DY, Belisto A, et al. Cimetidine, cigarette smoking, and recurrence of duodenal ulcer. N Engl J Med 1984;311:689. (*Smoking is a major factor in the recurrence of duodenal ulcer.*)

Soll AH, for the Practice Parameters Committee of the American College of Gastroenterology. Medical treatment of peptic ulcer disease: practice guidelines. JAMA 1996;275:622. (*Consensus view emphasizing the importance of eradicating H. pylori infection and eliminating NSAID use.*)

Sonnenbberg A, Townsend WF. Costs of duodenal ulcer therapy with antibiotics. Arch Intern Med 1995;155:922. (*A cost-effectiveness analysis comparing antibiotic therapy plus short-term acid suppression with long-term acid suppression alone, vagotomy, and intermittent acid suppression; finds antibiotics plus short-term acid suppression the most cost-effective by a wide margin.*)

Spiro HM. Is the steroid ulcer a myth? N Engl J Med 1983;309:45. (*Editorial that examines the contradictory data on this topic.*)

Steinberg WM, Lewis JH, Katz DM. Antacids inhibit absorption of cimetidine. N Engl J Med 1982;307:400. (*Original U.S. report of this interaction; degree of inhibition modest at 10% to 20%.*)

Sung SJY, Chung SCS, Ling TKW, et al. Antibacterial treatment of gastric ulcers associated with *Helicobacter pylori*. N Engl J Med 1995;332:139. (*One hundred patients randomized to 1 week of triple antibiotic therapy or 4 weeks of omeprazole; recurrence rate at 1 year was 52.3% with omeprazole alone, 4.5% with antibiotics.*)

Termanini B, Gibril F, Sutliff VE, et al. Effect of long-term gastric acid suppressive therapy on serum vitamin B_{12} levels in patients with Zollinger-Ellison syndrome. Am J Med 1998:104;422. (*Thirty percent reduction in serum B_{12} found in persons on long-term, high-dose omeprazole therapy.*)

Thompson JC. The role of surgery in peptic ulcer disease. N Engl J Med 1982;307:550. (*Editorial that nicely summarizes the indications for surgery.*)

Walan A, Bader JP, Classen M, et al. Effect of omeprazole and ranitidine on ulcer healing and relapse rates in patients with benign gastric ulcer. N Engl J Med 1989;320:69. (*Major European study showing omeprazole superior to H₂-blocker therapy.*)

Wolfe MM, Lichtenstein DR, Singh G. Gastrointestinal toxicity of nonsteroidal antiinflammatory drugs. N Engl J Med 1999;340:1888. (*Comprehensive review; 113 references.*)

Wolfe MM. Diagnosis of gastrinoma: much ado about nothing? Ann Intern Med 1989;111:697. (*Editorial suggesting that a screening serum gastrin level might be warranted in patients with duodenal ulcer.*)

Yeomans ND, Tulassay Z, Juhasz L, et al., for the ASTRONAUT Study Group. A comparison of omeprazole with ranitidine for ulcers associated with nonsteroidal antiinflammatory drugs. N Engl J Med 1998;338:719. (*A randomized, prospective, international trial of 541 patients showing omeprazole to be superior to ranitidine for healing and prophylaxis.*)

69
Management of Asymptomatic and Symptomatic Gallstones

Gallbladder disease afflicts over 20 million Americans, with more than 500,000 undergoing cholecystectomy each year. Prevalence is particularly high among middle-aged obese women. Most patients with gallstones are asymptomatic, whereas a few suffer from recurrent bouts of abdominal discomfort. Occasionally, a complication such as acute cholecystitis, pancreatitis, or choledocholithiasis may ensue. The primary physician needs to know when treatment is necessary and how to help the patient choose between elective surgery, medical therapy, and expectant management.

PATHOPHYSIOLOGY, CLINICAL PRESENTATION, AND COURSE

Pathophysiology and Risk Factors. Most gallstones are cholesterol laden, developing as a consequence of bile becoming supersaturated with cholesterol. Hereditary factors play a strong role, as do female gender and obesity, due to the lithogenic effects of estrogen and the increased risk associated with even moderate degrees of weight gain and caloric excess (relative risk, 2 to 3). Rapid weight loss is also an important risk factor. In men, regular exercise protects against developing symptomatic disease (the effect is unknown in women).

Presentation. Gallbladder disease may be asymptomatic or manifested by recurrent pain. Characteristically, *biliary colic* is rather sudden in onset, builds to a maximum within 1 hour, is steady, localized to the right upper quadrant or epigastrium, lasts 2 to 4 hours, and occasionally radiates to the left or right scapula. There is often nausea and vomiting. *Dyspeptic symptoms*, fatty food intolerance, belching, and bloating have also been attributed to chronic gallbladder disease, but the association has never been proven. Prospective studies have shown that such symptoms are just as common in middle-aged women without gallstones as in those with them. When patients with these symptoms are operated on, the dyspepsia often persists after cholecystectomy. Reflux of bile into the stomach has been noted in such individuals.

The clinical presentation of choledocholithiasis may be highly variable, ranging from acute nausea, vomiting, fever, upper abdominal pain, and jaundice to mild recurrent episodes of biliary colic. In many instances the patient may be asymptomatic for years before an attack develops, occurring when a stone blocks the distal end of the common duct.

The rare patient with true biliary colic but a normal gallbladder study on ultrasound may have *acalculous gallbladder disease* (an uncommon condition) or multiple small stones undetectable by conventional methods. These subtle forms of gallbladder disease may be discovered by observing delayed gallbladder emptying in response to a fatty meal or cholecystokinin.

Clinical Course. The clinical course of untreated gallbladder disease depends whether the patient has been asymptomatic or not. Two prospective studies, totaling 1,300 symptomatic patients who had at least one bout of pain, showed that over a follow-up period of 5 to 20 years, 30% had *recurrent pain* and 20% experienced *complications* such as jaundice, cholangitis, or pancreatitis; half remained asymptomatic. Because all patients in these studies had pain requiring a hospital admission, this patient population probably represents a group with a greater likelihood of complications than one with a predominance of *asymptomatic* stones. In a more representative retrospective cohort study of 123 people with silent gallstones, there was no mortality from the condition and a 15-year accumulative probability of biliary pain of only 18%.

Although there is no certainty that the onset of complications will be preceded by episodes of biliary pain, a study of 600 patients found that more than 90% of patients who suffered a complication of gallbladder disease had prior warning symptoms of biliary colic, although these were often mild and ignored. Most patients with pain on presentation had similar patterns of pain on follow-up. When 112 patients with asymptomatic stones were followed without surgery for 10 to 20 years, 27% eventually complained of dyspepsia, 19% had biliary colic, and 4.5% experienced transient jaundice. No deaths resulted from delay of surgery. In a separate study of symptomatic patients, those with small stones (diameter less than 5 mm) demonstrated a fourfold increase in risk of pancreatitis. In men, increased physical activity correlates inversely with risk of symptomatic disease.

Overall, asymptomatic patients appear to have a relatively favorable prognosis, but symptomatic individuals with episodes of true biliary colic have twice the rate of complications. Increased risk in asymptomatic patients is associated with very large stones (greater than 2.5 cm), age over 60, and diabetes. In symptomatic patients, small stones (less than 0.5 cm) may increase the risk of gallstone pancreatitis.

Some authorities believe there is a cause-and-effect relationship between gallstones and *carcinoma of the gallbladder*. The cancer occurs mostly in older women. The initial association with stone formation was based on circumstantial autopsy data. Community-based study has shown a much weaker association, pertaining only to men.

DIAGNOSIS

Asymptomatic Gallstones. Asymptomatic disease is usually detected as an incidental finding during radiologic or ultrasound investigation that encompasses the upper abdomen for a reason other than suspected gallbladder disease. With the advent and widespread application of ultrasound and computed tomography (CT) techniques, the frequency of detection of asymptomatic disease has been on the increase.

Acute Cholecystitis. The occurrence of classic biliary colic provides strong presumptive evidence for the diagnosis of cholecystitis; dyspepsia and fatty food intolerance do not. Real-time *ultrasound* of the gallbladder and biliary tree is the test of choice for evaluation of symptomatic patients with suspected acute cholecystitis. The only preparation necessary is 6 hours or more of fasting. The test takes about 15 minutes. Adequate images are obtained in about 98% of instances, although obesity can reduce visualization. Ultrasound can be performed rapidly, provides anatomic information, is low in cost, and allows examination of other potentially causative abdominal structures. Major criteria for a positive study are presence of stones or nonvisualization of the gallbladder (no fluid-filled lumen). Minor criteria include tenderness of the gallbladder during ultrasound examination, thickening of the gallbladder wall, and a rounded shape. Sensitivity and specificity are in excess of 95%.

Patients with a nondiagnostic ultrasound, but still strongly suspected of having acute cholecystitis (e.g., presence of biliary colic, mild elevations in liver function tests), should have the test repeated. The stone may have passed from the gallbladder into the common bile duct (see below). Besides presence of stone, other findings correlate with presence of cholecystitis, including localized tenderness over the gallbladder ("*sonographic Murphy's sign*") and gallbladder wall thickening.

An alternative to ultrasound for detection of acute cholecystitis is *scintigraphy* with the radionuclide *HIDA*. The isotope is taken up by the liver and excreted into the bile. Images are obtained after 1 hour. The patient needs to be fasting (but no longer than 2 to 4 hours) and free of underlying hepatocellular disease and alcoholism (which cause false-positive tests). The gallbladder, cystic duct, common bile duct, and duodenum are visualized by 60 minutes in the normal person. Nonvisualization of the gallbladder after 1 hour is characteristic of acute cholecystitis (the common bile duct and duodenum remain visualized). Sensitivity and specificity approach that of ultrasound, but cost is greater and the test takes more time. Scintigraphy can help determine patency of the cystic duct.

Ultrasound has largely replaced the *oral cholecystogram* for the diagnosis of acute cholecystitis, because it is more sensitive, equally specific, and provides results much faster and with none of the gastrointestinal upset and allergic reactions associated with oral cholecystography. *CT* of the gallbladder is not sufficiently sensitive to warrant its use for detection of stones; gallstones and bile can have the same density.

Choledocholithiasis. Symptomatic patients with recurrent pain plus persistent mild elevations in liver function tests, a dilated common bile duct, jaundice, or signs of acute pancreatitis require further evaluation for a stone in the common bile duct. As noted, ultrasound may be nondiagnostic because the sensitivity of a single study for detecting stones in the duct is only 50% when there is no ductal dilatation and 75% when ductal dilatation is present. Overlying bowel gas can obscure visualization of a common duct stone. If clinical suspicion remains high, a repeat ultrasound study is indicated. *CT* has about the same sensitivity (75%) as ultrasound for detection of a common duct stone. If noninvasive testing is nondiagnostic in the setting of suspected common duct stone, then *endoscopic retrograde cholangiopancreatography* (ERCP) deserves consideration. Sensitivity exceeds 90%, and therapeutic sphincterotomy can be performed at the same time. *Magnetic resonance imaging* of the biliary tree appears promising; initial reports of test sensitivity are in excess of 90% and no contrast or invasive procedure is required. Magnetic resonance imaging cholangiography has the potential to obviate the need for diagnostic ERCP and improve selection of candidates for a therapeutic ERCP.

Chronic Cholecystitis. *Ultrasound* is the diagnostic test of choice in patients with recurrent episodes of biliary colic. The *oral cholecystogram* has come back into use in patients who are being considered for lithotripsy or gallstone dissolution, because the test can provide information on gallbladder function and stone composition (see below).

PRINCIPLES OF MANAGEMENT

Given the rather benign natural history of asymptomatic stone disease, watchful waiting usually suffices in most patients, but one still needs to identify high-risk patients who require closer follow-up and possible consideration of elective cholecystectomy. Symptomatic patients want advice on treatment options, which include open cholecystectomy, laparoscopic cholecystectomy, and gallstone dissolution, both chemical and physical. There have yet to be randomized controlled clinical trials comparing treatment options, necessitating extrapolation from available data on natural history of disease and on the risks and outcomes of interventions.

Asymptomatic Gallstones

There is no evidence that the vast numbers of patients with asymptomatic gallstones would benefit from surgery or stone dissolution. Although surgical mortality is only 0.5%, only 20% of asymptomatic patients will ever develop biliary colic and acute cholecystitis, and only a small fraction of these people will experience a complication such as pancreatitis. In most patients, the risks of conservative management are not much different from those of surgery and involve far less expense, morbidity, and time lost from work. A substantial fraction of the 500,000 cholecystectomies done each year for asymptomatic gallstones and stones accompanied by dyspeptic symptoms (but not true biliary colic) could probably be avoided. Many such patients continue to have symptoms after surgery. Similarly, there is no evidence that stone dissolution therapy improves outcomes in patients with asymptomatic stones, although data on this issue are sparse. Patients at high risk for gallbladder cancer might be reasonable candidates for prophylactic cholecystectomy, but few risk factors have been identified (other than calcified gallbladder and stones more than 3 cm in diameter).

Acute Cholecystitis

Patients presenting with symptoms of acute cholecystitis require hospitalization for prompt diagnosis, intravenous fluids, and surgical consultation. The elderly, diabetics, and other debilitated persons are at particularly high risk of a complication from cholecystitis. Although *immediate surgery* may not be necessary, inpatient care for assessment and initial supportive care is warranted. There is considerable debate among surgeons as to whether urgent surgery is indicated. Available analyses suggest little risk to delaying surgery until the acute inflammatory phase of the illness has receded, provided there are no acute complications such as choledocholithiasis or pancreatitis. Performing nonelective open cholecystectomy raises the mortality risk fourfold (i.e., up to 10% in the elderly). Long-term outcomes are similar for *open* and *laparoscopic cholecystectomy* (see below). In general, laparoscopic surgery shortens length of hospital stay and time required for return to work but also increases risks of injury to the common bile duct and retained stones.

Symptomatic Gallstones

Symptomatic patients with recurrent attacks of biliary colic and confirmed gallstones should be advised to undergo *elective cholecystectomy*, provided they are reasonable surgical candidates. Before the advent of laparoscopic surgery, it was unclear which form of therapy was best for such patients, and several analytic studies found little difference between medical versus traditional surgical approaches. However, with development of minimally invasive laparoscopic surgical techniques, the decision has shifted in favor of gallbladder removal by laparoscopic cholecystectomy (see below). Here, the risk of complications from gallbladder disease (although relatively low) exceeds the risk of surgery.

Patients unwilling or too frail to undergo general anesthesia and surgery are candidates for medical therapy, which aims at stone dissolution by use of bile acids, lithotripsy, ether instillation, or a combination of modalities. Some patients will refuse all forms of treatment, preferring to "see how it goes." Such patients subject themselves to a small increase in mortality risk, but recent studies suggest the risk is actually modest and that the real issue is the patient's willingness to risk future attacks of pain and possible morbid complications (e.g., pancreatitis). Patients with only a single episode of biliary colic and no risk factors for complications of gallstone disease (i.e., diabetes, age more than 60, stones more than 2.5 cm or less than 0.5 cm) are probably the best symptomatic candidates for an expectant approach to treatment, having a reasonable chance of remaining symptom free into the future.

Surgery is the most definitive means of effecting a long-term cure. *Conventional open cholecystectomy* remains one of the most commonly performed of all surgical procedures, although laparoscopic cholecystectomy has become very popular and has replaced the traditional cholecystectomy in many settings (see below). Mortality rates for conventional open cholecystectomy range from 0.3% to 0.5% in patients under the age of 50 and rise to 1.4% to 2.7% in those over age 70. The complication rate from traditional elective surgery is 5% and doubles for nonelective surgery. Conventional surgery is successful; only about 4% experience chronic postoperative pain, with a retained stone often the cause. Surgery is sometimes undertaken to relieve dyspeptic symptoms, although results are inconsistent and usually disappointing. This is not surprising given the poor correlation between stones and dyspepsia.

Laparoscopic cholecystectomy provides the opportunity for a much less invasive procedure, with length of hospital stay reduced from an average of 6 days to 1.2 days. Over three fourths of patients return to work within 10 days, compared with a month for conventional gallbladder surgery. The procedure takes about 30 minutes longer to perform than an open cholecystectomy. The reported complication rate among surgeons experienced in the technique is 5%, similar to that for open surgery in such patients, but the proportion of serious complications is reduced. The overall rate of bile duct injury is slightly higher (0.5% versus 0.2%) but in a major study fell to 0.1% after a 2.2% rate for the initial 13 cases. Only one case of trocar-induced bowel perforation occurred in over 1,500 procedures, and no deaths were attributable to surgery or a postoperative complication. The most common problem was superficial infection at the site of the insertion of the umbilical trocar. About 5% of cases had to be converted to open procedures, mostly due to poor visualization of the gallbladder.

The laparoscopic approach represents an excellent option in patients with uncomplicated symptomatic gallstone disease. Suspicion of common duct stone necessitates consideration of an open procedure; however, common duct exploration is possible with laparoscopic surgery. If a common duct stone is found, the procedure needs to be converted to an open cholecystectomy or followed postoperatively by ERCP to achieve stone removal. With increasing availability and surgical skill, this procedure is likely to become the treatment of choice for uncomplicated symptomatic gallbladder disease. Although cost per patient has declined markedly with the advent of laparoscopic surgery, total costs have not fallen because more patients are undergoing surgery.

Medical Therapy is an option for patients who are poor surgical candidates or reluctant to undergo elective cholecystectomy. The objective is stone dissolution by biochemical or physical means.

Bile Acids. Up to 80% of gallstones have cholesterol as the major constituent, making them potentially dissolvable in the presence of increased bile acid. Only the naturally occurring bile acid *ursodeoxycholic acid (ursodiol)* has proven both effective in dissolving stones and free of the serious gastrointestinal side effects that accompanied trials of other bile acids (e.g., *chenodiol*, which causes liver injury, diarrhea, and low-density-lipoprotein cholesterol elevations). Ursodiol is safe for long-term use. The agent not only dissolves stones directly but also desaturates the cholesterol content of the bile by suppressing hepatic cholesterol synthesis and biliary cholesterol secretion. It is the only bile acid approved by the U.S. Food and Drug Administration for stone dissolution, replacing chenodiol.

Gallstone dissolution is achievable in patients with small (2 cm) *cholesterol stones*, especially if there is a *functioning gallbladder* (as determined by oral cholecystogram). The overall stone dissolution rate is just under 50% and higher for those with pure cholesterol stones (as determined by the oral cholecystogram findings of floating radiolucent stones in a functioning gallbladder). Results are best in those with a few small stones. Many patients become pain free even before full stone dissolution is achieved, and 40% become stone free after 2 years of continuous bile acid therapy. Patients with larger (more than 10 mm) or calcified stones fail to achieve complete stone dissolution.

The effects of therapy can be well documented by periodic oral cholecystogram or gallbladder ultrasound. Therapy is contraindicated in patients with inflammatory bowel disease or peptic ulcer, because the drug increases bile acids, which may be harmful to colonic and gastric mucosa. Stones recur at the rate of 15% per year. This high recurrence rate suggests a role for chronic suppressive therapy. Continued symptoms despite dissolution occur in about 4%.

Ursodiol is expensive, costing upward of $2 to $3 per day. However, a major cost-to-benefit analysis showed that ursodiol treatment is a reasonable alternative to surgery in patients deemed poor surgical risks (although comparisons with laparoscopic surgery have not been performed). Some authorities have even advocated using ursodiol initially in all symptomatic patients and operating only on those who fail medical therapy. However, the excellent results reported with laparoscopic surgery, particularly the marked reductions in recovery time and perioperative morbidity, have probably tilted the equation back in favor of surgery for most patients who can tolerate general anesthesia.

Bile salt treatment has an adjuvant role in patients treated with lithotripsy or methyl-*tert*-butyl ether (see below). Stone fragments that remain after initial therapy are subjected to a course of ursodiol in an attempt to dissolve them. Bile salt treatment is also prescribed to prevent new stone formation in high-risk persons such as morbidly obese persons attempting rapid weight reduction.

Extracorporeal Shock-Wave Lithotripsy is worth considering in the 10% of symptomatic gallstone patients who have a small number of *calcium-containing stones* (with the calcium deposited in the core or along the rim) and a *functioning gallbladder*. Lithotripsy will effectively shatter such stones in over 95% of instances. Results are not as good with more than three stones or if greater than 3 cm in diameter. After the stone is shattered, follow-up therapy with ursodiol is required to achieve full dissolution or at least painless stone passage. The procedure is contraindicated in patients with acute cholecystitis or a coagulation deficit and can cause such adverse effects as cardiac arrhythmias, pain, bacteremia, hematuria, cutaneous abdominal wall petechiae, and transient liver injury. About 10% suffer stone-related symptoms after the procedure due to passage of stone fragments. Although transiently popular as a nonsurgical means of gallstone removal, lithotripsy has been supplanted by laparoscopic surgery . However, for patients with calcium-containing stones who are not surgical candidates, it remains a treatment option available at a few centers. The availability of lithotripsy has been limited by very high equipment costs and concerns about cost effectiveness.

Methyl-Tert-Butyl Ether dissolves cholesterol stones and has been used in a few centers to treat highly selected populations of patients with multiple or large cholesterol stones. Instilled directly into the gallbladder by way of a percutaneous catheter, the ether can dissolve stones in less than 3 days of continuous application. However, catheter placement and ether installation are difficult and potentially dangerous, necessitating an experienced team to perform the procedure. Stones reform in about 15%, and another 20% report biliary colic after treatment, probably due to a retained small insoluble nidus. Ursodiol is often used as an adjunct.

In summary, medical therapy represents an alternative for symptomatic patients with cholesterol gallstones who are too sick or unwilling to undergo elective cholecystectomy. Definition of stone composition, size, and number is required, as is willingness to take bile acid medication for a prolonged period of time.

Choledocholithiasis

Stones in the common duct are associated with increased risks of complications and death. Consequently, they need to be removed. Endoscopic sphincterotomy and retrieval of stones by balloon catheter or basket can performed during ERCP. Stones too large to be extracted can be performed broken up by lithotripsy or dissolved by use of ursodiol.

Prevention

Diet and Exercise. Although obesity and caloric excess are major risk factors for gallstone formation in women, there is no evidence that a low-fat low-cholesterol diet per se alters the course of gallbladder disease. Some gallstone patients with dyspeptic symptoms feel better if they avoid fatty foods; however, the relationship between stones and fatty food intolerance is tenuous at best (see Chapter 74). Multivariate analysis shows that it is the number of calories consumed rather than the proportion of calories coming from saturated fat or cholesterol intake that seems to correlate best with risk. One case-control epidemiologic study did find a reduction in risk associated with increased consumption of vegetable protein and vegetable fat, but this finding needs to be confirmed. Although obesity and caloric excess can lead to stone formation, rapid weight loss through fasting and starvation diets are contraindicated because they cause bile to become very lithogenic. Perhaps modest weight reduction achieved in gradual fashion might be of some prophylactic value in high-risk patients such as obese women.

Prospective study of dietary factors is sorely needed. Exercise appears to be protective of symptomatic disease in men; it has not been studied in women.

Alcohol and Tobacco. Daily consumption of small amounts of alcohol (about 1 oz per day) has been found in retrospective studies of women to correlate with a 20% reduction in risk of symptomatic gallstone disease. This closely parallels the 20% lower bile cholesterol saturation found among modest drinkers compared with control subjects. Smoking also appears to reduce risk in women, probably by its adverse effects on estrogen production and degradation.

Avoidance of Lithogenic Medications. Risk of gallstone formation rises markedly with use of *estrogen* and *clofibrate*. Patients with known gallstones should not take them, and those taking such drugs should be monitored for gallstone formation, particularly if there is a strongly positive family history of stone disease. *Thiazide* use is associated with a modest increase in relative risk of gallstones (relative risk, 2.0 to 2.9).

PATIENT EDUCATION

The truly asymptomatic gallstone patient can be reassured of the low probability of becoming symptomatic or suffering a complication. Such patients can be followed expectantly and should not be pushed into surgery, medical therapy, or unnecessary dietary restriction. Previously, asymptomatic patients with large stones, diabetes, or advanced age were considered candidates for prophylactic stone removal because they had an increased mortality risk from a complication. However, improvements in medical and surgical therapy of symptomatic patients have greatly reduced risk for such patients, making prophylactic surgical or stone-dissolution therapy unnecessary.

Because symptomatic patients have a slightly increased mortality risk and a modest chance of a complication, they need to be informed of the available therapeutic options so that patient preferences and treatment modality can be matched. The principal therapeutic benefit is a reduction in frequency of symptoms and in risk of complications; mortality benefit is small and almost clinically insignificant. The wish to refuse therapy can be respected, so long as the patient understands the risks of choosing expectant therapy. However, the short hospital stay, low morbidity, and speedy recovery afforded by laparoscopic cholecystectomy may be particularly appealing to previously reluctant symptomatic patients. Ursodiol is also well tolerated and may be an attractive option for qualifying patients fearful of any surgery.

Any dyspepsia should be clearly differentiated from biliary colic. Patients need to know that the link between dyspepsia and gallstones is not well founded and that the presence of dyspeptic symptoms is not an indication for surgery, lithotripsy, or medical therapy, although other measures might help (see Chapter 74).

INDICATIONS FOR REFERRAL AND ADMISSION

Patients with evidence of acute cholecystitis should be admitted to the hospital for evaluation, surgical consultation, and supportive measures. Consultation with a surgeon regarding elective cholecystectomy is also indicated for patients with recurrent biliary colic. Referral for consideration of laparoscopic cholecystectomy should be made exclusively to a surgeon skilled and experienced in performing the procedure. High levels of morbidity (e.g., bile duct injury, perforation) and mortality have resulted from inadequately trained personnel performing the procedure. A gastroenterologic referral may be useful for symptomatic patients who are deemed too frail to undergo elective surgery as well those with a suspected common duct stone who may require ERCP.

THERAPEUTIC RECOMMENDATIONS

- Patients with asymptomatic cholelithiasis can be managed expectantly, because the risk of developing symptomatic disease or a complication is only 1% per year.
- Patients with a single episode of biliary colic are also reasonable candidates for expectant management, as long as they continue free of recurrent pain.
- Patients with documented gallstones and recurrent biliary colic or a history of a complication of gallstone disease (cholecystitis, pancreatitis) should be advised to undergo elective cholecystectomy, provided they can tolerate general anesthesia and surgery. *Laparoscopic cholecystectomy* has become the surgical procedure of choice, reducing perioperative morbidity and shortening the recovery period when performed by a surgeon skilled in the procedure.
- Symptomatic nonsurgical patients with a functioning gallbladder and radiolucent (i.e., cholesterol) gallstones can be given a trial of bile acid therapy with *ursodiol* (10 to 15 mg/kg/d). Therapy is continued for at least 12 months and often for 24. Results are best in those with stones that are less than 2 cm in diameter and three in number. Presence of calcification rules out bile acid therapy. The effects of therapy should be monitored with a gallbladder ultrasound every 6 months. Risk of recurrence is high after bile acid therapy is stopped.
- *Lithotripsy* is worth consideration in symptomatic nonsurgical patients with calcium-containing stones. Results are best in those whose stones are less than 3 cm in diameter and less than four in number. Patients require referral to a center with expertise in the procedure.
- Estrogen preparations, clofibrate, and other drugs that may trigger stone formation should be stopped or dosages should be decreased in persons with gallstones or high risk of developing them.
- Restricting *fat* and *cholesterol* is of little or no benefit in altering the clinical course of gallstone disease. However, obesity and caloric excess are major risk factors, and gradual weight reduction through modest caloric restriction might be helpful. Fasting and starvation diets are to be avoided because they make the bile even more lithogenic. Modest *alcohol* consumption (less than 1 oz per day) is not harmful. *Exercise* can be recommended as a preventive measure.
- Dyspeptic symptoms should not be considered grounds for medical or surgical treatment because their relation to gallstone disease is tenuous at best. Dyspeptic symptoms are likely to respond better to other measures (see Chapter 74).

A.H.G.

ANNOTATED BIBLIOGRAPHY

American College of Physicians. Guidelines for the treatment of gallstones. Ann Intern Med 1993;119:620. (*Consensus recommendations.*)

Barkun AG, Ponchon T. Extracorporeal biliary lithotripsy. Ann Intern Med 1990;112:126. (*Review of experimental studies and clinical results; 71 references.*)

Bates T, Mercer JC, Harrison M. Symptomatic gallstone disease: before and after cholecystectomy. Gut 1984;25:579. (*One year after surgery nearly half of patients complain of digestive symptoms.*)

Broomfield PH, Chopra R, Sheinbaum RC, et al. Effects of ursodeoxycholic acid and aspirin on the formation of lithogenic bile and gallstones during loss of weight. N Engl J Med 1988;319:1567. (*Ursodiol prevented lithogenic changes in bile.*)

Carveth SW, Priestley JT, Gage R. Size and number of gallstones in acute and chronic cholecystitis. Mayo Clin Proc 1959;34:371. (*Stones larger than 2.5 cm are more likely to precipitate attacks of cholecystitis than are smaller stones.*)

Chan Y-L, Chan ACW, Lam WWM, et al. Choledocholithiasis: comparison of MR cholangiography and endoscopic retrograde cholangiopancreatography. Radiology 1996;200:85. (*Promising results for magnetic resonance imaging; sensitivity in excess of 90%.*)

Cooperberg PL, Burhenne HJ. Real time ultrasonography in calculus gallbladder disease. N Engl J Med 302:1277;1980. (*One of the original studies establishing ultrasound as the test of choice; sensitivity 98%, specificity 95%; comparison with oral cholecystography in a subsample showed greater sensitivity and similar specificity.*)

Dolgin SM, Schwartz JS, Kressel HY, et al. Identification of patients with cholesterol or pigment gallstones by discriminant analysis of radiographic features. N Engl J Med 1981;304:808. (*Describes oral cholecystogram findings that help identify patients with cholesterol stones; buoyancy was highly predictive of cholesterol composition.*)

Fullearton GM, Bell G, and the West of Scotland Laparoscopic Cholecystectomy Audit Group. Prospective audit of the introduction of laparoscopic cholecystectomy in the west of Scotland. Gut 1994;35:1121. (*Total costs did not go down because more patients chose to have surgery.*)

Gracie WA, Ransohoff R. The natural history of silent gallstones. N Engl J Med 1982;307:798. (*Retrospective cohort study of 123 people identified no mortality associated with asymptomatic gallstones and a 15-year accumulative probability of biliary pain of only 18%.*)

Health and Policy Committee, American College of Physicians. How to study the gallbladder. Ann Intern Med 1988;109:752. (*Consensus statement on recommended approaches to imaging the gallbladder.*)

Leitzmann MF, Giovannucci EL, Rimm EB, et al. The relation of physical activity to risk for symptomatic gallstone disease in men. Ann Intern Med 1998;128:417. (*A major prospective cohort study of male health professionals; physical activity inversely correlated with risk of symptomatic gallstone disease.*)

Maclure KM, Hayes KC, Colditz GA, et al. Weight, diet, and the risk of symptomatic gallstones in middle-aged women. N Engl J Med 1989;321:563. (*Prospective data confirming the strong association between obesity and symptomatic gallstones; moderate overweight increases risk; alcohol decreases it.*)

Maringhini A, Moreau JA, Melton J, et al. Gallstones, gallbladder cancer, and other gastrointestinal malignancies. Ann Intern Med 1987;107:30. (*Community study showing only a minor increase in risk and much less risk than previously reported from autopsy studies.*)

McSherry CK, Ferstenberg H, Calhoun WF, et al. The natural history of diagnosed gallstone disease in symptomatic and asymptomatic patients. Ann Surg 1985;202:59. (Documents very favorable prognosis in 691 patients followed for an average of 5 years.)

Mulley AG. Shock-wave lithotripsy. N Engl J Med 1986;314:845. (Editorial suggesting caution regarding applicability of lithotripsy to therapy of gallstones.)

NIH Consensus Development Panel on Gallstones and Laparoscopic Cholecystectomy. Gallstones and laparoscopic cholecystectomy. JAMA 1993;269:1018. (Recent consensus view on the indications for laparoscopic gallbladder surgery.)

Pastides H, Tzonou A, Trichopoulos D, et al. A case-control study of the relationship between smoking, diet, and gallbladder disease. Arch Intern Med 1990;150:1409. (One of the few studies examining the relationship of these factors to symptomatic gallbladder disease.)

Pickleman J, Gonzalez RP. The improving results with cholecystectomy. Arch Surg 1986;121:930. (Review of outcomes in 389 consecutive cases; finds rates of mortality lower than previously reported and lower complication rates for the elderly and diabetics.)

Price WH. Gallbladder dyspepsia. Br Med J 1963;3:138. (Frequency and severity of dyspeptic complaints are unrelated to presence or absence of gallstones.)

Ransohoff DF, Gracie WM. Management of patients with symptomatic gallstones: a quantitative analysis. Am J Med 1990;88:154. (Decision analysis study indicating that survival benefit from surgery or medical therapy is modest at best and that management decisions should be based on considerations other than mortality.)

Ransohoff DF, Gracie WA. Treatment of gallstones. Ann Intern Med 1993;119:606. (Authoritative review of risks and benefits of available treatment strategies; 92 references.)

Ransohoff DF, Gracie WA, Wolfenson LB, et al. Prophylactic cholecystectomy or expectant management for silent gallstones. Ann Intern Med 1983;99:199. (Decision analysis suggesting a very small survival benefit for prophylactic cholecystectomy that may well be offset by monetary costs, morbidity, and time preferences.)

Rosenberg L, Shapiro S, Slone D. Thiazides in acute cholecystitis. N Engl J Med 1980;303:546. (Relative risk of acute cholecystitis among patients who used thiazide during the month before hospital admission was 2; for those who used thiazides for 5 or more years, the relative risk was 2.9.)

Rubin RA, Kowalskin TE, Khandelwal M, et al. Ursodiol for hepatobiliary disorders. Ann Intern Med 1994;121:207. (Best review of bile acid therapy; 142 references.)

Sackmann M, Delius M, Sauerbruch T, et al. Shock-wave lithotripsy of gallbladder stones. N Engl J Med 1988;318:393. (Report of the first 175 cases, finding that results were best when combined with bile acid therapy.)

Saini S. Imaging of the hepatobiliary tract. N Engl J Med 1997;336:1889. (Terse practical review with data on sensitivity and specificity of imaging studies.)

Salen G, Tint GS. Nonsurgical treatment of gallstones. N Engl J Med 1989;320:665. (Excellent editorial tersely reviewing the methods, indications, and results from nonsurgical therapies for gallstones.)

Schein CJ. Acute cholecystitis in the diabetic. Am J Gastroenterol 1969;51:511. (Cholecystitis can be a lethal disease in the diabetic; documents increased risk in this subpopulation, although later studies have shown the risk to be lower than the one reported here.)

Thistle JL, Cleary PA, Lachin JM, et al. The natural history of cholelithiasis: the National Cooperative Gallstone Study. Ann Intern Med 1984;101:171. (Among 305 patients receiving placebo therapy, the most important predictor of biliary tract pain was a history of pain; only 4% required elective cholecystectomy in 2 years of follow-up.)

Thistle JL, May RR, Bender CD, et al. Dissolution of cholesterol gallbladder stones by methyl-tert-butyl ether administered by percutaneous transhepatic catheter. N Engl J Med 1989;320:633. (Report of successful application of this treatment modality.)

Weinstein MC, Coley CM, Richter JM. Medical management of gallstones: a cost-effectiveness analysis. J Gen Intern Med 1990;5:277. (Finds medical therapy with ursodiol to be a cost-effective alternative to conventional surgery, especially in the elderly.)

70
Management of Hepatitis
JULES L. DIENSTAG

Viral and nonviral forms of hepatitis are more common than generally thought. More than 50,000 cases of viral hepatitis in the United States are reported to the Centers for Disease Control and Prevention each year, although the actual number is estimated to be 10 times as high. Hepatitis B accounts for 30% to 35% of cases of acute viral hepatitis, hepatitis A for 45% to 50%, and hepatitis C for 15% to 20%; a few percent cannot be attributed to any known hepatitis virus. In addition, a proportion of patients with acute types B, C, and D progress to chronic infection. Some become asymptomatic carriers; others have chronic hepatitis, which is associated with an increased risk of cirrhosis and death. Approximately 25% to 40% of chronic liver disease in the United States and Europe derives from chronic hepatitis C infection and 10% to 15% from hepatitis B. Other important causes include chronic alcohol abuse, hemochromatosis, and autoimmune hepatitis. In about 15% to 20% of cases, the cause is unknown ("cryptogenic").

The primary physician needs to be skilled in the management of both viral and nonviral forms of hepatitis, because these are illnesses usually encountered in the outpatient setting. Effective outpatient management requires knowledge of diagnosis (see Chapters 57 and 62), natural history, and treatment options. Immunosuppressive therapy for nonviral disease, interferon and nucleoside analogues for viral disease, and transplantation for end-stage forms have widened the therapeutic options greatly. Although many treatment decisions require subspecialty consultation, the primary physician retains responsibility for long-term management and follow-up. This requires knowing the indications and contraindications for the various treatment options and the best means of monitoring clinical course and therapeutic interventions.

CLINICAL PRESENTATION AND NATURAL HISTORY

Acute Viral Hepatitis

In most instances, acute viral hepatitis is a self-limited illness; on the order of 85% of hospitalized patients and over 95% of outpatients recover completely and uneventfully within 3 months (except in hepatitis C; see below). Most persons with acute viral hepatitis never become jaundiced; their illness is mistakenly labeled as a nonspecific viral syndrome unless liver biochemical tests, such as aminotransferase levels, are ordered. A large proportion of patients remain asymptomatic, especially children. In elderly or immunologically compromised patients, the prognosis is more guarded, with an increased risk of severe and protracted disease.

Prodromal symptoms occur after an *incubation period* of 2 to 4 (rarely 6) weeks for hepatitis A, 4 to 24 weeks for hepatitis B (with or without simultaneous acute delta hepatitis infection), and 3 to 15 weeks (80% within 5 to 10 weeks) for hepatitis C. Characteristically, *prodromal symptoms* consist of 1 to 2 weeks of malaise, anorexia, nausea, vomiting, change in senses of taste and smell, low-grade fever, right upper quadrant or midepigastric abdominal discomfort, and fatigue. Aminotransferase elevations may precede or coincide with the onset of prodromal symptoms.

If jaundice develops, it usually does so as prodromal complaints begin to subside, although persistence of prodromal symptoms is observed in more severe cases. By the time 6 to 8 weeks have elapsed, most patients are well on their way to full recovery. Occasionally, an isolated mild aminotransferase elevation persists after clinical recovery. If it resolves within 3 to 6 months, the mild elevation has no prognostic significance.

Fulminant Acute Disease. This is the most ominous form of acute disease, characterized by overwhelming liver cell necrosis and signs of liver failure—encephalopathy, ascites, and coagulopathy. This complication is seen more often in cases of hepatitis B (especially with simultaneous delta hepatitis infection) than in those of hepatitis A or C, although, as noted earlier, the frequency is particularly high among pregnant women with hepatitis E. Before the availability of liver transplantation, the mortality of fulminant hepatitis approached 80%, despite the best intensive medical care.

Other Variants of Acute Hepatitis. In 5% to 10% of cases of acute type B hepatitis, the prodromal phase of illness may be characterized as a *serum sickness–like syndrome*, with urticaria, arthralgias, fever, and polyarticular arthritis. Some patients with acute viral hepatitis, especially those with hepatitis A or E, have a *cholestatic* illness, with marked jaundice, elevation of serum alkaline phosphatase activity, and pruritus lasting 1 month to several months.

Approximately 5% to 10% of patients with viral hepatitis appear to suffer mild *relapses* during convalescence. Such clinical and biochemical relapses are now well recognized in patients with acute hepatitis; in patients with acute hepatitis B, what appears clinically as a relapse may represent the clinical expression of simultaneous delta hepatitis infection. Episodic swings in aminotransferase levels are common during acute and chronic hepatitis C. In some instances, these recurrent elevations are accompanied by clinical "relapses."

Progression to Chronic Hepatitis. The risk of progression varies among the several types of viral hepatitis. Although an occasional case of hepatitis A may be slow to resolve and last more than 6 months, no cases of chronic hepatitis have been linked to hepatitis A infection. Similarly, hepatitis E does not progress to chronic infection. There are no reliable early pre-dictors of chronicity. In patients with hepatitis B, persistence of *hepatitis B surface antigen (HBsAg) and hepatitis Be antigen (HBeAg)* increases the risk of chronic hepatitis, although early presence of either has no predictive value. Similarly, no reliable predictors of chronicity have been identified in patients with acute hepatitis C. Clinical manifestations of progression to chronic viral hepatitis may be subtle, with little more than persistence of mild symptoms and biochemical abnormalities for 6 or more months. Many patients remain asymptomatic and almost all remain anicteric.

Hepatitis B can progress to chronic hepatitis, but usually at a very low rate (1% to 2%) among immunocompetent adults. When accompanied by high levels of hepatitis B virus (HBV) replication, patients with chronic hepatitis B tend to have chronic liver injury categorized as mild, moderate, or severe chronic hepatitis. Those with negligible virus replication become asymptomatic carriers of HBsAg.

The likelihood of chronic HBV infection is higher, approaching 90%, when acute infection occurs at birth or in *early childhood* or when acute infection occurs in an *immunocompromised host*. Most patients who present with chronic hepatitis B have no history of having experienced an acute hepatitis-like clinical illness, acquiring their infection subclinically. In patients with simultaneous acute *hepatitis B and D* (delta hepatitis), the likelihood of *chronicity* is not increased, but *severity* of acute and chronic hepatitis is increased.

Although most HBsAg carriers are asymptomatic and have a nonprogressive course, a small proportion may actually have subtle and insidious progression to chronic liver disease. Rarely, acute hepatitis-like exacerbations can occur. Such events may represent superimposed infection with another hepatitis virus (A, C, D) or reactivation of hepatitis B. Occasionally, an acute hepatitis-like elevation of aminotransferase activity represents a successful spontaneous seroconversion from highly replicative, HBeAg-positive, high-level HBV DNA infection to relatively nonreplicative, anti-HBe–positive, low-level HBV DNA infection; when such seroconversions occur, chronic liver injury gives way to an asymptomatic carrier state. With early-generation clinical assays for HBV DNA, the level of HBV DNA in "nonreplicative" carriers fell below the detection threshold, but with exquisitely sensitive amplification techniques, HBV DNA can be detected in carriers, albeit at a threshold below 10^5 to 10^6 virions per milliliter.

More recently, another category of chronic hepatitis B has been recognized, *"pre-core" mutant hepatitis B*. The C gene, which codes for the nucleocapsid core protein (HBcAg), also codes for HBeAg protein; HBeAg production requires an intact pre-core gene sequence. When one of several mutations in the pre-core region prevents elaboration of HBeAg, HBcAg and intact virus particles can still be synthesized, leading to highly replicative hepatitis B, despite the absence of HbeAg. Patients with such pre-core mutations can have high levels of HBV DNA and substantial liver injury despite the absence of HBeAg, the conventional marker for high-level HBV replication and infectivity. Often, these variants emerge after many years of HBeAg-reactive chronic hepatitis B. Pre-core–mutant chronic hepatitis B appears to be relatively refractory to antiviral therapy.

Patients with chronic hepatitis B, especially those with infection acquired early in life, are at markedly increased risk of progression to *cirrhosis* and *hepatocellular carcinoma*.

Hepatitis C. In hepatitis C, 50% to 60% of patients experience elevations in aminotransferase that persist for more than a year after acute infection, and almost all of these go on to have long-standing chronic hepatitis. Moreover, even among patients in whom aminotransferase elevations resolve within the first 6 months, chronic viremia persists in almost all. Between the 50% and 60% with chronic hepatitis after acute hepatitis C virus (HCV) infection and the remainder with *chronic viremia*, chronicity of HCV infection occurs in more than 85% of acutely infected persons. What is more, patients with chronic viremia remain at risk for the development of chronic hepatitis.

Among patients with chronic hepatitis C, *cirrhosis* develops in 20% of cases within 10 years after onset of acute infection. Most have little impact of their disease for many decades, but in patients with moderate to severe chronic hepatitis on liver biopsy, the risk of progression to cirrhosis over 10 to 20 years remains high. Among those with cirrhosis, 10-year survival is very good, approximately 80%; in compensated cirrhotics with chronic hepatitis C, hepatic *decompensation* occurs in approximately 4% to 5% per year; the risk of *hepatocellular carcinoma* (rare during the first three decades of infection) increases at a rate of 1% to 3% per year.

Toxic and Drug-induced Hepatitis

Drugs can trigger hepatocellular injury through a direct toxic effect or by means of an idiosyncratic reaction. Some agents are associated with a cholestatic reaction, either as part of an idiosyncratic process or independent of it.

Direct Toxins. Directly toxic reactions are dose-related and predictable. The latency period is short, and there are no manifestations suggestive of a hypersensitivity reaction. *Acetaminophen* is the most commonly used drug that is directly hepatotoxic, though only when taken in massive doses.

Idiosyncratic Reactions. These were once thought to be immunologically mediated but actually result from the hepatotoxic effects of drug metabolites. They are less predictable than direct toxins. Latency is variable, and there is little relationship to dose. In about 25% of patients, extrahepatic manifestations suggestive of a hypersensitivity reaction (e.g., fever, rash, arthralgias, eosinophilia) occur. Hepatitis resulting from *halothane, isoniazide, methyl dopa, valproic acid,* and *trimethoprim-sulfamethoxazole* has a strong idiosyncratic component.

Cholestatic Reactions. There are two types of cholestatic reactions, *bland cholestasis,* with little evidence of hepatitis and *inflammatory cholestasis.* As is the case for other types of drug hepatotoxicity, some categories of cholestatic drug injury appear to represent predictable, dose-dependent, direct toxicity and others unpredictable, non–dose-dependent, idiosyncratic reactions. Oral contraceptives cause bland cholestasis, and the reaction is dose dependent and variable in onset. *Erythromycin* (especially the estolate preparation but also other forms) and *chlorpromazine* are capable of causing idiosyncratic cholestasis with hepatitis, as are other phenothiazines, amoxicillin-clavulanic acid, and oxacillin. *Anabolic steroids* (17α-substituted androgens) also can cause cholestasis, often accompanied by a mild degree of hepatocellular injury. Other drugs cause a clinical picture reminiscent of sclerosing cholangitis, with inflammatory destruction of intrahepatic bile ducts (e.g., the chemotherapeutic agent FUDR), whereas others (e.g., carbamazepine, chlorpromazine, tricyclic antidepressant agents) can result in disappearance of bile ducts, "ductopenic" cholestasis, reminiscent of chronic rejection after liver transplantation.

Drug-induced Steatosis. Macrovesicular or microvesicular steatosis or fatty infiltration with accompanying hepatitis (steatohepatitis) complicates therapy with several drugs. Among patients treated with antiretroviral infection for HIV infection, severe steatohepatitis, a reflection of mitochondrial toxicity, has been observed in association with reverse transcriptase inhibitors such as *zidovudine* and *didanosine* and with *protease inhibitors* such as indinavir and ritonavir.

Clinical Course. Severity of drug-induced hepatitis can range from an asymptomatic increase in liver enzymes to life-threatening illness. Prompt cessation of the drug is essential to limiting further hepatic injury; rechallenge may lead to an exaggerated reaction. Most cases are self-limited, provided that severe injury has not already occurred.

Chronic Hepatitis

Classification by Grade and Stage. The distinctions between what used to be labeled "chronic persistent" and "chronic active" hepatitis are no longer recognized as valid and are being phased out of clinical use. Chronic persistent hepatitis, which now is called *minimal* or *mild chronic hepatitis*, referred to more indolent disease, whereas chronic active hepatitis was the designation for more progressive disease that is now labeled *as moderate to severe chronic hepatitis*. The obsolete distinctions have been replaced by assessments of relative inflammatory activity (grade) and fibrosis (stage). In clinical trials of chronic hepatitis, especially of chronic viral hepatitis, a numerical histologic index is used to assess severity (grade) and progression (stage). The *histologic activity index* includes numeric scores for periportal necrosis (including piecemeal and bridging necrosis; range, 0 to 10), intralobular necrosis (range, 0 to 4), portal inflammation (range, 0 to 4), and fibrosis (range, 0 to 4).

Mild Chronic Hepatitis has mononuclear-cell inflammation confined to the portal tract, the limiting plate of periportal hepatocytes is not eroded, hepatocellular necrosis and inflammation do not extend into the lobule, and fibrosis is absent or very limited. This mild category of chronic hepatitis was believed in the past to be predictive of a good prognosis and limited progression; however, although the benignity of mild chronic hepatitis tends to persist, the prognostic value of this designation is now recognized to be more limited and does not preclude progression to more severe chronic hepatitis or even cirrhosis.

Moderate to Severe Chronic Hepatitis is characterized histologically by a mononuclear-cell portal infiltrate that not only expands portal zones but also extends beyond the portal tract into the adjacent periportal lobular area with erosion of the limiting plate of periportal hepatocytes (*"piecemeal necrosis" or "interface hepatitis"*). Fibrous septae extending into the lobule are also characteristic, fibrosis can range from mild to severe, and a proportion of such patients may have cirrhosis on their initial liver biopsies. A more severe form of this lesion includes *"bridging necrosis,"* in which confluent necrosis and cell dropout span lobules (portal–portal and portal–central bridges).

Chronic Viral Hepatitis. In the chronic forms of viral hepatitis, the *level of virus replication* appears to be the most important determinant of progression, even more so than histologic pattern. Nonetheless, *histologic appearance*, especially as a reflection of the degree of virus replication, may also serve as a determinant of prognosis. In patients with chronic hepatitis B, one fourth of patients with mild chronic hepatitis B can still become cirrhotic. Similarly, in patients with histologically mild chronic hepatitis C, 20% can progress to cirrhosis over one to two decades. Superinfection with *hepatitis D* can cause progression to more severe liver disease among persons with chronic mild hepatitis B.

Hepatitis B. The 15-year survival of histologically mild chronic hepatitis B is in excess of 95%, that of more severe chronic hepatitis B about 85%, and of the more histologically severe forms of chronic hepatitis B *with* cirrhosis about 40%. Progression to cirrhosis has been noted in 13% of those with mild chronic hepatitis B, in 16% of patients with moderate chronic hepatitis B (without bridging necrosis), and in 88% of those with severe chronic hepatitis B (with bridging necrosis).

The determinant of prognosis that underlies histology in chronic hepatitis B is virus replication. *Level of virus replication* (as measured by serum concentration of HBV DNA and presence of HBeAg) is probably the most important determinant of progression to cirrhosis in patients with chronic hepatitis B. For example, in one study, cirrhosis developed in 53% of those with persistent HBV DNA but in none of those able to clear HBV DNA. In patients with chronic hepatitis B, *conversion from HBeAg to anti-HBe* may signal an improvement in liver histology, whereas superinfection with the *delta agent* is usually associated with a deterioration in histology in up to one third of patients and an acceleration of the disease process.

In sum, although histologic appearance is important, liver biopsy provides only a measure of disease at one point in time. Degree of virus replication activity may be the best predictor of prognosis. *Life-long infection* with HBV, such as occurs primarily among those infected at or shortly after birth, is associated with an increased risk of *hepatocellular carcinoma*, whether cirrhosis is present or not.

Hepatitis C. Episodic bursts of inflammatory activity often punctuate the clinical course of patients whose liver biopsies show mild chronic hepatitis C. Like hepatitis B, histologic features of chronic hepatitis C can change, and even patients with clinically and histologically mild chronic hepatitis C can progress insidiously and slowly to cirrhosis. Chronic hepatitis C is commonly associated with erosion of the limiting plate of periportal hepatocytes (piecemeal necrosis) but rarely with clinical or histologic criteria for severe chronic hepatitis (10-fold elevation of aminotransferase activity, disabling symptoms, multilobular collapse). Still, despite this apparent relative benignity, chronic hepatitis C may progress insidiously, even in the absence of symptoms or marked elevations in aminotransferase activity, and may lead to cirrhosis in 20% within 10 years. Although a wide range of frequencies of progression to cirrhosis have been reported and although most patients with chronic hepatitis C do very well with limited clinical conse-

quences over several decades, patients with long-standing chronic infection often demonstrate histologic progression. Although a correlation exists between HBV replication and disease progression, a similar correlation between HCV replication and disease progression cannot be demonstrated invariably. Among the several variables associated with progression in chronic hepatitis C, duration of infection is probably the most important. The best clinical predictor of progression may be histologic stage and grade. Mild inflammation and necrosis and mild fibrosis characterize a cohort of patients with an excellent prognosis and limited progression to cirrhosis over time, whereas moderate to severe necrosis/inflammation and/or fibrosis portend progression to cirrhosis almost invariably over one to two decades.

Nonviral (Autoimmune, Idiopathic) Chronic Hepatitis. An autoimmune mechanism is believed to account for many cases of nonviral chronic hepatitis. The sensitivity of histologic change may have a degree of prognastic value. Although in autoimmune hepatitis histologic severity may have a degree of prognostic value. Like other autoimmune diseases, the condition predominates in women between ages 20 and 40. An acute form with severe fatigue, jaundice, fever, amenorrhea, and anorexia sometimes occurs, but some present asymptomatically. There is a high incidence of extrahepatic manifestations, including arthritis, rash, thyroiditis, glomerulonephritis, and pleuropericarditis. Asymptomatic patients are typically discovered when an incidental modest elevation in aminotransferase is noted on routine testing. Marked elevation in *gamma globulin* (more than two times normal) is characteristic, as are high titers of *antinuclear antibody* and *antibody to smooth muscle*. Enzyme immunoassays for antibody to hepatitis C may yield false-positive readings in such patients; therefore, in patients with what appears to be autoimmune hepatitis, if screening tests for anti-HCV are reactive, a confirmatory test, such as a test for HCV RNA, should be done. The bilirubin may be higher than in viral hepatitis. Histology and disease activity are more important determinants of prognosis for nonviral disease.

Untreated severe autoimmune hepatitis (defined by disabling symptoms, sustained aminotransferase elevations more than 10 times normal, gamma globulin levels twice normal, bridging or multilobular collapse on biopsy) may progress to cirrhosis and eventual death. The 6-month fatality rate is 40% in patients with these findings. Bridging or multilobular necrosis on biopsy specimen is associated with cirrhosis in 40% and death in 20% after 5 years. In contrast, patients with less severe disease (piecemeal necrosis alone, minimal symptoms) are usually not at risk for death, and progression to cirrhosis is rare (3% to 10%).

Mild autoimmune chronic hepatitis has a good prognosis in most cases but is not uniformly benign. This lesion has been documented to deteriorate to more severe chronic hepatitis and to progress to cirrhosis in certain patients, such as those with an initial histologic diagnosis of severe hepatitis whose liver biopsies improve with therapy and in immunosuppressed patients with a histologic diagnosis of mild chronic hepatitis.

PRINCIPLES OF MANAGEMENT

Acute Viral Hepatitis

Being a generally benign and self-limited illness, acute viral hepatitis can be managed in most cases on an outpatient basis. Hospitalization should be reserved for high-risk patients (e.g., elderly, immunocompromised, difficult-to-manage underlying chronic diseases) and those with signs of severe hepatocellular injury (e.g., marked prothrombin time prolongation, encephalopathy, ascites and edema, inability to maintain oral intake, hypoglycemia, or hypoalbuminemia). Other than specific antiviral therapy (see below), there is no specific therapy for acute viral hepatitis that will accelerate convalescence or prevent sequelae. The usual goals of care are to maintain *adequate nutrition* and *patient comfort*, to *avoid* additional *hepatocellular insults* from hepatotoxic medications and alcohol, and to *prevent the spread* of infection to others.

Neither *specific dietary manipulations, corticosteroids, nor* strict *bedrest* has any beneficial effect on the course or prognosis of acute uncomplicated or acute severe viral hepatitis. *Oral contraceptives* do not necessarily need to be stopped, but *alcohol* intake should be omitted, and use of other drugs known to cause liver injury should be discontinued or monitored carefully. *Exercise* does not interfere with recovery; patients should be encouraged to engage in as much physical activity as they can tolerate without discomfort or undue fatigue.

Symptoms may be incapacitating. Nausea and vomiting can be controlled by cautious use of antiemetics; however, because phenothiazines cause cholestatic hepatitis in approximately 1% of patients, *nonphenothiazine antiemetics*, such as *trimethobenzamine*, should be used. Small *frequent feedings*, especially in the morning when nausea is at a low ebb, can ensure adequate calorie intake. No specific foods need be restricted. In patients with cholestasis and pruritus, *cholestyramine* usually provides relief. Certainly, the identification of a patient with acute viral hepatitis should prompt consideration of prophylactic measures to limit the spread of infection to contacts (see Chapter 57).

Hepatitis B. Because patients with clinically apparent acute hepatitis B almost always recover, specific antiviral therapy is not indicated. For the unfortunate 1% to 2% who remain chronically infected, antiviral therapy can be instituted once chronicity is documented.

Hepatitis C. For patients encountered with acute hepatitis C, antiviral therapy during early acute hepatitis has been shown to reduce the frequency of chronicity and is recommended (see below). In clinical practice, such acute cases are being recognized in growing frequency among health workers who sustain accidental needle sticks or other percutaneous exposures.

Monitoring and Follow-up. The patient is monitored clinically by observing symptoms and checking hepatocellular function. An *aminotransferase* level obtained weekly at the outset and then monthly is useful to judge the presence of ongoing disease, although the absolute level is not a particularly sensitive determinant of disease severity in the acute phase of illness. *Prothrombin time* is a good measure of hepatocellular synthetic function and should be checked when the patient first presents and when there is suspicion of worsening. *Serum bilirubin*, a marker of hepatic excretory function, also correlates with severity. A fall in *serum albumin* indicates reduced hepatocellular synthetic function, but because its half-life is 28 days, this change does not become apparent until late in the acute illness. In patients with acute hepatitis C, early antiviral therapy with a standard course (see above) of interferon and ribavirin should be initiated.

An office visit 1 to 2 weeks after the first presentation is often helpful to be sure there is no worsening and that the patient is managing satisfactorily. Thereafter, follow-up depends on how well the patient feels. At 3 months, a repeat aminotransferase, bilirubin, albumin, prothrombin time, and, in cases of hepatitis B, an *HBsAg* determination should be performed to ascertain disease activity, severity, and antigen status.

If symptoms and laboratory evidence of activity persist after 3 months, repeat evaluations at monthly intervals are indicated. *Liver biopsy* is not indicated in patients with acute viral hepatitis unless clinical suspicion of chronic hepatitis is present.

Fulminant Acute Hepatitis. Neither corticosteroids nor any other specific medical therapy has proven effective. The best approach involves meticulous attention to details of the multisystem dysfunction that accompanies acute liver failure. Such patients should be admitted to an intensive care unit and considered for early referral to a transplantation center. *Liver transplantation* is the only intervention that has truly life-saving potential. With timely transplantation, survival rates of 50% to 60% are possible. Recurrent viral hepatitis may occur in the new liver, but not invariably, and antiviral therapy for hepatitis B and C can be used after transplantation to reduce the impact of reinfection. Experimental trials are underway to assess a variety of hepatic assist devices, but none have yet been proven effective. Reversal of acute fulminant hepatitis B has been observed anecdotally with early administration of the nucleoside analogue lamivudine (see below).

Drug-induced Hepatitis

Treatment is largely supportive. All possible offending agents should be stopped. Immunosuppressive and anti-inflammatory drugs are of no benefit.

Chronic Viral Hepatitis

Treatment of viral chronic hepatitis depends on the etiology and severity of disease. Therapy focuses on termination of viral replication, the principal determinant of prognosis. Immunosuppression, which is useful in nonviral hepatitis (see below), has no place and may even be detrimental, resulting as it does in an increase in viral replication. Therapeutic decisions may be made independently of histologic severity, but *liver biopsy* is indicated to establish the presence of necroinflammatory liver disease, to assess the stage and grade of the disease, and to exclude other causes for abnormal liver chemistry tests (e.g., infiltration with fat or iron). In patients considered for antiviral therapy, a brief period of observation before instituting treatment is helpful to ensure that the patient is not in the process of spontaneous improvement.

Hepatitis B. Antiviral therapy is the cornerstone of treatment, using the interferon alfa or the inhibitor of viral replication, lamivudine.

Interferon alfa was the first antiviral drug to be approved for treatment of chronic hepatitis B. When given to patients with *compensated replicative chronic hepatitis B* (i.e., with circulating HBV DNA and HBeAg), approximately 30% experience seroconversion to nonreplicative infection (loss of HBeAg and HBV DNA detectable by conventional hybridization assays). Treatment consists of a 16-week course of either daily subcutaneous injections of 5 million units or thrice weekly injections of 10 million units. About one fourth of responders in early trials also lost detectable HBsAg. Improvements in serum aminotransferase activity and liver histology occur as well in those with sustained reductions in viral replication.

Interferon is effective in patients with modest levels of HBV replication and with elevated aminotransferase activity but ineffective in those with very high levels of HBV replication and in those with normal or near-normal aminotransferase activity. Among patients who respond (as manifested by disappearance of circulating HBV DNA and HBeAg), there is improvement in the natural history of the disease (80% clearing of HBsAg over the decade after therapy), improved survival without decompensation, and reduced risk of hepatocellular carcinoma. Those not responding well to interferon include immunosuppressed patients, those infected in early childhood, and patients with pre-core hepatitis B mutations (see above). In *decompensated patients*, the acute hepatitis-like exacerbation that accompanies successful interferon therapy may precipitate liver failure, making them poor candidates for routine interferon treatment.

Adverse Effects. Major adverse effects of interferon include *flulike symptoms, marrow suppression, irritability* (sometimes depression), and autoimmune *thyroiditis* (rarely, other autoimmune disorders). Successful interferon therapy is often accompanied by a transient, acute, hepatitis-like elevation in aminotransferase activity, believed to represent an enhancement of cell-mediated immune cytolysis of HBV-infected hepatocytes.

Lamivudine, a potent inhibitor of HBV and HIV reverse transcriptase, has been approved for routine use in patients with chronic "replicative" hepatitis B. For hepatitis B, lamivudine therapy is rapidly supplanting interferon as first-line therapy, because lamivudine does not require injections, has no appreciable side effects, and is at least if not more effective than interferon. Patients with decompensated chronic hepatitis B are not good candidates for interferon therapy but may respond to lamivudine, sometimes with reversal of clinical signs of decompensation.

Efficacy. Daily doses of 100 mg/d (a third of the dose for HIV infection) suppress HBV DNA by four orders of magnitude. A 12-month course of therapy results in HBeAg loss in approximately 30%, seroconversion from HBeAg to anti-HBe in approximately 16% to 20%, normalization of alanine aminotransferase in more than 40%, and histologic improvement in more than 50%. Among the histologic changes are a reduction in necroinflammatory activity in 60% and a halting of progression to fibrosis in 20%. Among those with HBeAg responses (loss or seroconversion), the antiviral response is durable in approximately 80%; an HBeAg response can be used as a landmark for discontinuing therapy. In the absence of an HBeAg response, however, continued therapy may be required.

Although lamivudine suppresses HBV replication substantially in almost all patients, a sustained response is less likely in patients with normal aminotransferase activity and in patients with pre-core HBV variants who nevertheless do benefit histologically and biochemically. Side effects are negligible, and transient elevations in aminotransferase activity occur in about one fourth of patients but no more frequently than in placebo recipients. After discontinuation of therapy, however, in the absence of an HBeAg response, aminotransferase elevations (acute hepatitis-like flares) occur in 20% to 30% of patients, but these flares are transient and clinically mild in most cases. Close posttreatment monitoring is essential to identify and re-

treat severe posttreatment exacerbations. Losses of HBsAg are uncommon during lamivudine therapy but are observed after therapy in those with HBeAg loss.

Resistance. The frequency of HBeAg responses increases with each year of lamivudine therapy, but the downside of long-term therapy is the emergence of viral *resistance*. In 15% to 30% of patients treated for a year and in 50% of those treated for 3 years, a viral variant emerges (e.g., YMDD), reflecting a *mutation* in HBV DNA polymerase. Although YMDD variants are less responsive to lamivudine than wild-type HBV, measures of disease activity remain well below baseline levels, perhaps because variants replicate less effectively than wild-type HBV. Withdrawal of lamivudine results invariably in a return of wild-type HBV and more severe liver injury. Consequently, continued therapy even after the emergence of YMDD variants is recommended, at least until other antivirals are developed. In the future, multidrug regimens will be introduced and will reduce the likelihood of viral resistance. Overall, many authorities rely on lamivudine as first-line therapy for chronic hepatitis B.

Adverse Effects. Lamivudine has no recognized side effects or impact on nonhepatic laboratory values.

Famciclovir and ganciclovir, nucleoside analogues with antiviral activity, have limited activity against HBV.

Monitoring and Followup. *Aminotransferase* levels are *monitored* once a month during therapy. For patients being treated with interferon or lamivudine, monitoring of *HBV DNA* is indicated at intervals of 1 to 3 months; *HBeAg* is checked, at a minimum, at the end of therapy, but an interval HBeAg testing during therapy is helpful. For patients treated with interferon, monitoring of *white blood cell* and *platelet* counts is indicated at weeks 1, 2, and 4 and then monthly to detect any marrow suppression. Aminotransferases are monitored monthly, and bilirubin and albumin are checked periodically. Periodic monitoring of thyroid function (*thyroid-stimulating hormone*) at 1- to 3-month intervals identifies patients with thyroiditis who are candidates for reduction or cessation of interferon or initiation of thyroid hormone-replacement therapy.

Liver Transplantation. Decompensated patients who are refractory to antiviral therapy may be candidates for *liver transplantation* or investigative protocols. The success of liver transplantation for chronic hepatitis B is approximately 75% now that antiviral regimens are offered routinely. The most common approach is a combination of high-dose hepatitis B immune globulin plus lamivudine.

Hepatitis D. *Interferon* achieves reductions in hepatitis D virus RNA and a fall in aminotransferase, but cessation of therapy is followed almost invariably by a return of these markers to pretreatment levels. Long-term high-dose interferon therapy continued for a full year may produce more durable results, and multiyear therapy may be required to control the disease. The benefit of antiviral therapy remains to be demonstrated; corticosteroid therapy is ineffective. Lamivudine is not effective for hepatitis D. *Liver transplantation* has been successful in patients with end-stage disease, with an outcome better than that for hepatitis B alone.

Hepatitis C. Major advances in the treatment of chronic hepatitis C have been made possible with the advent of interferon alfa and ribavirin. Candidates for antiviral therapy include those with compensated chronic hepatitis C and moderate-to-severe chronic hepatitis on liver biopsy. No consensus exists on treatment of patients with asymptomatic or histologically mild disease; such patients tend to do well without therapy, and therapy has not been shown to have a beneficial impact in this cohort. Decompensated patients are unlikely to respond. Cirrhosis per se is not a contraindication to antiviral therapy, but reports of primarily retrospective studies suggesting that interferon therapy in cirrhotics prevents hepatocellular carcinoma may represent a selection bias favoring treatment in patients with less advanced disease, not a true treatment effect. The role of interferon in preventing complications of cirrhosis and hepatocellular carcinoma needs to be tested in prospective trials. Corticosteroids have never proven useful in treatment of chronic viral hepatitis. *HCV genotype* and quantitative testing for *HCV RNA* ("*viral load*") should be determined before therapy to help determine the duration of treatment (6 months for patients with low viral loads and genotypes other than 1; 12 months for patients with high viral loads and genotype 1).

Interferon Alfa is U.S. Food and Drug Administration approved for treatment of chronic hepatitis C. After receiving a dose of 3 million units three times a week for 24 weeks, 50% of patients with chronic hepatitis C experience a normalization of aminotransferase levels (biochemical response) and approximately 30% have a loss of detectable HCV RNA (virologic response). Histologic improvement occurs in as many as three fourths of patients assessed at the end of therapy. The relapse rate after cessation of therapy is high, yielding a sustained response rate (usually measured at least 6 months after completion of therapy) after 6 months of therapy of only 10%. The frequency of sustained responses can be increased to approximately 20% by increasing the duration of interferon monotherapy from 6 to 12 months; dose escalation has a negligible effect, and switching from one interferon preparation to another is also of limited benefit.

Induction therapy with initial high-dose intensive regimens has been advocated, but they have not improved ultimate sustained response rates. Sustained response rates have been improved with long-acting interferons bound to polyethylene glycol. Pegylated interferons have longer half-lives and are eliminated more slowly, allowing once-a-week administration and achieving a prolonged concentration plateau. In preliminary trials, sustained responses have been observed in more than 30% of patients treated for a year. The likelihood of a response to interferon is increased in patients with low-level HCV RNA (less than 2 million copies/mL) and in those with HCV genotypes other than 1.

Ribavirin. combination interferon–ribavirin therapy is the treatment of choice. Initial responses during therapy and sustained responses after therapy are achieved most frequently by *combining* interferon with the nucleoside analogue ribavirin (1,000 mg by mouth once a day for patients weighing less than 75 kg and 1,200 mg/d for patients weighing 75 or more kg). Although ribavirin monotherapy is ineffective, the combination administered for a year can yield sustained response rates of 40%. Sustained responses are even more likely for patients with low viral loads and HCV genotypes other than 1; in fact, in this subgroup, 6 months of therapy is just as effective as a year and need not be extended for the full year. Therefore, in the absence

of contraindications (coronary artery disease, cerebrovascular disease, anemia, pregnancy, etc.; see below), combination interferon–ribavirin represents first-line therapy for chronic hepatitis C.

Interferon–ribavirin combination therapy is also effective in patients who relapsed after a course of interferon monotherapy, achieving a sustained response rate in 50%. Combination therapy, however, has been disappointing in nonresponders to interferon therapy.

Side effects of combination interferon–ribavirin therapy are similar to those for interferon alone (see above), but ribavirin can cause *hemolysis*, mild in most cases but severe and brisk in an unpredictable proportion of patients. Therefore, combination therapy is contraindicated in patients who cannot tolerate anemia, including patients who are already anemic and those with, or with risk factors for, coronary artery disease or cerebrovascular disease, in whom anemia can result in a life-threatening ischemic event. Because ribavirin is renally excreted and teratogenic, the drug is *contraindicated* in patients with *renal insufficiency* and during *pregnancy* (birth control should be used in fertile patients who take ribavirin).

Monitoring and Follow-up. In patients taking ribavirin, monitoring for hemolysis is carried out by attention to the *complete blood count*, supplemented when suspicion is high by the *reticulocyte count*. During treatment, quantitative HCV RNA should be checked periodically; an undetectable level at 1 month may portend an ultimate sustained response, but most treating physicians will test HCV RNA at 3 months for patients undergoing a 6-month course and at 6 months for patients undergoing a 12-month course. If HCV RNA remains detectable at these landmarks, the likelihood of achieving a response during treatment is low. Whether to continue treatment under these circumstances is still debated. Finally, HCV RNA should be repeated at the end of therapy to document a complete end-treatment response, and in those with an end-treatment response, HCV RNA testing should be repeated intermittently over the next 6 months to document a sustained response. The need for and value of *repeat liver biopsies* at regular follow-up intervals are controversial. After the initial biopsy, which is necessary to initiate therapy, many authorities make subsequent decisions about duration and direction of therapy based on clinical and biochemical responses without reliance on liver histology.

Liver Transplantation is indicated for those with end-stage decompensated chronic hepatitis C. Although reinfection of the allograft is universal, its clinical impact on the new liver is negligible in most cases over the early years after transplantation, and antiviral therapy with interferon and ribavirin has the potential to limit the impact of reinfection considerably.

Nonviral (Autoimmune or Idiopathic) Chronic Hepatitis. Approaches to therapy of nonviral and viral types of chronic hepatitis are distinctly different. In nonviral disease, histology plays a predominant role in determining prognosis, and immunosuppression is an important treatment modality in severe cases.

In *mild asymptomatic* autoimmune and idiopathic forms of chronic hepatitis, the prognosis is excellent. *No treatment*, beyond simple symptomatic relief, is indicated. Long-term high-dose immunosuppressive therapy (e.g., with prednisone) is not indicated because the high probability of adverse effects (see

Chapter 105) outweighs any potential benefit. More randomized controlled trials are needed to better define the efficacy of other forms of immunosuppressive therapy in such patients.

Moderate-to-severe chronic nonviral hepatitis tends to be a more serious and progressive disease. *Severe cases* have been shown to respond to *immunosuppressive–anti-inflammatory* therapy (*prednisone/azathioprine*). However, only 15% to 20% of patients with autoimmune or idiopathic chronic hepatitis fulfill criteria for severe disease. The need for and efficacy of immunosuppressive therapy in symptomatic patients with less severe disease remains unknown.

Prednisone/Azathioprine. Immunosuppressive–antiinflammatory therapy using *high-dose prednisone* alone or the combination of *reduced-dose prednisone* plus *azathioprine* produces clinical, biochemical, and histologic resolution in 80% of persons with severe disease and significantly reduces mortality. Histologic remission to mild hepatitis or to normal occurs within 6 to 36 months. In the prednisone-only regimen, treatment begins at 60 mg/d, and the dose is reduced over the course of a month to a maintenance level of 20 mg/d. Promising results have been obtained with lower dose corticosteroid-only regimens in which the high-dose phase is omitted, but confirmation is needed. The combination regimen is initiated with 30 mg/d prednisone combined with 50 mg/d azathioprine. The azathioprine dose remains constant, whereas the prednisone dose is reduced over the course of the first month to a maintenance level of 10 mg. Neither azathioprine alone nor alternate-day prednisone therapy has been found to be effective as alternative regimens.

Adverse Effects. About two thirds of patients treated with high-dose steroids alone experience severe steroid complications (see Chapter 105), compared with fewer than 20% of those treated with prednisone plus azathioprine. Azathioprine-induced *bone marrow suppression* may occur in patients receiving the combination-therapy regimen, necessitating close monitoring. Occasionally, unacceptable drug toxicity, intolerable gastrointestinal upset, compression fractures, or failure to respond necessitates premature cessation of therapy.

Duration of Therapy. Therapy is continued until there is objective evidence of remission (i.e., a fall in *aminotransferase activity* to a level under twice normal and improvement in *morphologic features* of chronic hepatitis). Although aminotransferase levels do not always reflect histologic activity absolutely faithfully, such biochemical monitoring has been documented to be valuable and a satisfactory substitute for repeat invasive biopsies. In responsive cases, symptoms improve within 6 months, aminotransferase levels within 12 months, and histology within 24 months. Rarely, more than 36 months are necessary to achieve remission. After 4 years, the likelihood of drug-induced complications becomes greater than the likelihood of beneficial drug effect. Nevertheless, some patients cannot be weaned from maintenance treatment and require indefinite continuation of therapy.

Once remission is achieved, therapy is discontinued by gradual tapering of prednisone over 6 weeks. Patients are monitored closely for signs of relapse, which occur in 50% of patients. Relapse is especially common in patients with cirrhosis, often necessitating prolonged therapy for many years or multiple courses of treatment. Approximately 20% of patients fail to respond to conventional doses but may respond to higher doses. Relapses usually occur early. If remission lasts more

than 6 months after cessation of therapy, relapse is less likely. Most cases of relapse are accompanied by symptoms and biochemical abnormalities, but in 10% of cases, the only sign of relapse is a change in histology. After relapse, 80% of patients respond again to reinitiation of therapy. After cessation of therapy, again, the relapse rate is 50%. The likelihood of relapse after combination prednisone-azathioprine therapy may be reduced by maintenance azathioprine monotherapy after steroid withdrawal.

Monitoring and Follow-up. In nonviral disease, patients with *mild* chronic hepatitis may be followed casually, but those who are symptomatic deserve careful monitoring and periodic reassessment to be sure there are no signs of progression. When *severe* chronic disease has been identified, very close follow-up monitoring is vital. If prednisone and azathioprine are used, weekly and later monthly *platelet and white blood cell counts* are required. *Aminotransferase, bilirubin,* and *gamma globulin* levels ought to be obtained at 2 weeks and then every 1 to 3 months to monitor response and to identify treatment failure. Patients with mild-to-moderate chronic disease who do not receive therapy should be monitored in similar fashion and biopsied again if symptoms or biochemical tests worsen.

Transplantation. For patients with end-stage disease who have sustained a life-threatening complication, referral to a liver transplantation center is an appropriate consideration (see below).

INDICATIONS FOR REFERRAL AND ADMISSION

Referral

Prompt consultation is indicated in most patients with fulminant or severe forms of hepatitis, whether viral or nonviral, because treatment decisions are difficult and increasingly effective antiviral and immunosuppressive therapies are becoming available.

Viral Hepatitis. Referral is indicated for consideration of liver biopsy when prognostic information or confirmation of disease severity is needed. Examples include patients with acute viral hepatitis B or C who fail to show signs of recovery within 6 months and who were not treated at the time of initial diagnosis and those with progressive or severe cases of chronic hepatitis B or C who might be candidates for antiviral therapy. It is particularly important to obtain help from a hepatologist, gastroenterologist, or pathologist experienced in interpreting biopsy material obtained from patients with chronic hepatitis; diagnosis depends on histologic appearance and can be difficult.

Autoimmune and Idiopathic Chronic Hepatitis. Referral for biopsy to confirm the diagnosis is indicated for patients with suspected autoimmune or idiopathic chronic hepatitis (e.g., hyperglobulinemia, autoantibodies).

Admission

Admission to the hospital is indicated for *worsening mental status, bleeding, refractory ascites,* or *poor home environment.* When decompensation does not respond readily to medical therapy, then referral to a *liver transplantation center* is indicated. Spontaneous or recurrent hepatic encephalopathy, wasting, refractory ascites, variceal bleeding, and spontaneous bacterial peritonitis are among the indications for transplantation in patients with chronic liver disease. Given the long waiting time for a donor liver, patients should be referred as early as possible for transplantation candidacy evaluation.

PATIENT EDUCATION

Hepatitis often affects previously vigorous people accustomed to full activity. The prolonged course and magnitude of malaise commonly precipitate a reactive depression. Thorough explanation of the disease's course, design of a sensible treatment program that actively involves the patient and family, and close follow-up can maximize compliance and minimize depression.

Instruction concerning diet and activity is central to a comprehensive treatment program. In particular, it is important to prevent unnecessary restriction of activity and to ensure adequate nutrition. Patients can be told to do as much as they feel like doing, as long as they avoid overtiring themselves. Small frequent meals, especially in the morning, are tolerated best. Foods do not need to be restricted, but carbohydrates seem to be the best-tolerated food when nausea is pronounced. Alcohol should be proscribed. Today, many patients with hepatitis take "alternative" therapies of no proven benefit. Most of these preparations are harmless, but some can actually injure the liver. Although patients should be discouraged from taking these substances, such warnings often fall on deaf ears.

Patients and household members have many questions regarding transmissibility of viral hepatitis. Explicit instructions regarding preventive measures are greatly appreciated (see Chapter 57). Of particular concern is sexual activity, especially for young persons who might want to have children. In hepatitis B, the risk of transmission by sexual intercourse is high, but prophylaxis with hepatitis B immune globulin and vaccine reduces the risk in the patient's sexual partner. In hepatitis C, the risk of sexual transmission is negligible, especially between monogamous stable sexual partners, making it possible to allow unprotected intercourse for purposes of conception.

THERAPEUTIC RECOMMENDATIONS
(SEE CHAPTER 57 FOR PROPHYLACTIC MEASURES)

Acute Viral Hepatitis

- Maintain adequate caloric intake and a balanced diet. Small feedings are tolerated best, especially in the morning. No foods need to be restricted.
- Ensure adequate rest, but activity does not need to be unduly restricted if the patient feels capable of it.
- Omit potentially hepatotoxic agents, especially alcohol.
- Treat severe pruritus with cholestyramine.
- Treat severe nausea and vomiting with a nonphenothiazine antiemetic, such as trimethobenzamide (Tigan) suppositories.
- Admit the patient to the hospital if signs of marked worsening of hepatocellular function occur (e.g., encephalopathy, bleeding, prolongation of prothrombin time). Also consider admission for maintaining adequate caloric and fluid intake when symptoms are severe or for managing complicated underlying diseases.
- Refer patients with fulminant hepatitis for consideration of liver transplantation. In cases of hepatitis B, a trial of lamivu-

dine may be considered but should not interfere with evaluation for transplantation.
- For patients with acute hepatitis C, therapy with interferon plus ribavirin should be initiated as soon as possible.
- Check aminotransferase, prothrombin time, bilirubin, albumin/globulin, and HBsAg at onset and at 12 weeks; aminotransferase levels should be monitored at 1- to 4-week intervals during acute illness. Retest any patient with evidence of persistent symptoms or laboratory abnormalities every 4 weeks. Refer for liver biopsy those with a combination of failure to resolve infection and inflammation by 6 to 12 months and persistence of disabling symptoms.

Drug-induced Hepatitis

- Stop all drugs that might be responsible and institute supportive measures.
- Avoid rechallenging the patient with the same agent.

Nonviral Chronic Hepatitis

- Follow patients with *mild* chronic hepatitis at regular intervals and rebiopsy if there are signs of marked worsening. Otherwise treat symptomatically. Steroids are not indicated.
- For patients with *severe* chronic hepatitis (multilobular or bridging necrosis, disabling symptoms, and marked aminotransferase and globulin elevations), begin high-dose *prednisone* (60 mg/d) or combination prednisone (30 mg/d) plus *azathioprine* (50 mg/d). Combination therapy is preferred for the elderly, diabetics, and others who cannot tolerate long-term high-dose steroids. Because of the impact of azathioprine on fertility, this drug should be avoided, if possible, in young adults who are planning to raise families.
- Taper prednisone by 5 to 10 mg at a time over the course of a month until a maintenance dose of 10 mg/d (with 50 mg/d azathioprine) or 20 mg/d is established.
- Monitor aminotransferase, bilirubin, and globulins at 2 weeks and then every 1 to 3 months. If the patient is taking azathioprine, obtain platelet and white cell counts at weeks 1 and 2 and then monthly thereafter.
- Continue maintenance therapy for at least 24 to 36 months and then consider attempting discontinuation of therapy with a 6-week period of tapering medication.
- Obtain a consultation if there is failure to achieve clinical improvement within 2 to 8 months of initiating therapy; high-dose treatment may be indicated.
- Treat relapses in the same manner as new cases.

Chronic Viral Hepatitis

- Avoid immunosuppressive therapy in patients with chronic viral hepatitis.
- Consider *interferon alfa* in patients with compensated chronic hepatitis B who demonstrate sustained presence of HBV DNA and HBeAg. If deemed appropriate by a consultant, begin a 16-week course of 5 million units administered subcutaneously daily or 10 million units every other day.
- Most authorities would choose, instead of interferon, to consider lamivudine therapy for chronic "replicative" hepatitis B. Treatment consists of 100 mg daily by mouth for 12 months.

Therapy can be stopped in patients who lose HBeAg; in those who retain HBeAg, therapy may need to be prolonged.

- Treat patients with compensated chronic *hepatitis C* who manifest sustained elevations of aminotransferase and detectable HCV RNA with *interferon* at a dose of 3 million units subcutaneously three times a week plus oral ribavirin at a daily dose of 1,000 mg (for those weighing less 75 kg) or 1,200 mg (for those weighing 75 or more kg) for a full year. In patients with genotypes other than 1 and with a low viral load (less than 2 million viral copies), a 6-month course of therapy may suffice. For patients who relapse whenever therapy is stopped and for nonresponder patients, long-term maintenance therapy is a consideration, currently being evaluated in clinical trials.
- Consider *interferon alfa* for patients with *hepatitis D*. Long-term high-dose therapy (as much as 9 million units three times a week for a year) is required. Some patients may benefit from indefinite maintenance therapy.
- Monitor patients receiving interferon by checking leukocyte, granulocyte, and platelet counts at weeks 1, 2, and 4 and monthly thereafter. Check aminotransferase levels monthly and thyroid-stimulating hormone every 1 to 3 months. In patients with hepatitis B treated with interferon or with lamivudine, monitor HBV DNA monthly to every few months and measure HBeAg periodically and at the end of therapy. In patients being treated for hepatitis C, monitor HCV RNA at approximate intervals of 3 months. Those receiving ribavirin need close monitoring of hematocrit/hemoglobin.
- Admit the patient to the hospital when there is evidence of marked worsening of hepatocellular function. Consider liver transplantation for patients with hepatic decompensation.

ANNOTATED BIBLIOGRAPHY

Bizollon T, Palazzo U, Ducer FC, et al. Pilot study of the combination of interferon alfa and ribavirin as therapy of recurrent hepatitis C after liver transplantation. Hepatology 1997;26:500. (*Preliminary trial; suggests that combination therapy may help prevent recurrence.*)

Consensus Statement. EASL international consensus conference on hepatitis C. J Hepatol 1999;30:956. (*Succinct contemporary assessment of the clinical-epidemiologic features; recommendations for antiviral therapy, updated to include combination interferon-ribavirin therapy.*)

Czaja AJ. Chronic active hepatitis: the challenge for a new nomenclature. Ann Intern Med 1993;119:510. (*A review of viral agents and other causes, pathophysiology, and nomenclature, which can be confusing.*)

Czaja AJ. Autoimmune hepatitis: evolving concepts and treatment strategies. Digest Dis Sci 1995;40:435. (*An updated overview of autoimmune hepatitis and its management.*)

Czaja AJ, Wolf AM, Baggenstoss A. Laboratory assessment of severe chronic active liver disease during and after corticosteroid therapy: correlation of serum transaminase and gamma globulin levels with histologic features. Gastroenterology 1981;80:687. (*These blood tests are reliable indicators, making most follow-up biopsies unnecessary.*)

Davis GL, Esteban-Mur R, Rustgi V, et al. Interferon alfa-2b alone or in combination with ribavirin for the treatment of relapse of chronic hepatitis C. N Engl J Med 1998;339:1493. (*Multicenter, prospective, randomized trial; interferon/ribavirin resulted in a 50% sustained response rate in patients who relapsed after an initial course of interferon monotherapy.*)

Davis GL, Balart LA, Schiff ER, et al. Treatment of chronic hepatitis C with recombinant interferon alfa: a multicenter randomized controlled trial. N Engl J Med 1989;321:1501. (*The study that established the efficacy of interferon for chronic hepatitis C.*)

Desmet VJ, Gerber M, Hoofnagle JH, et al. Classification of chronic hepatitis: diagnosis, grading, and staging. Hepatology 1994; 19:1513. (*An authoritative overview of how chronic hepatitis is classified based on cause, severity [grade], and progression [stage].*)

Di Bisceglie AM. Hepatitis C. Lancet 1998;351:351. (*A concise but thorough description of the diagnosis, epidemiology, clinical features including natural history, and contemporary management of hepatitis C.*)

Di Bisceglie AM (guest editor). Treatment advances in chronic hepatitis C. Semin Liver Dis 1999;19[Suppl 1]:1. (*An entire issue devoted to, and covering every aspect of, antiviral therapy for chronic hepatitis C; useful for a more in-depth understanding of the approach to and practical issues involved in treating patients.*)

Dienstag JL. Non-A, non-B hepatitis. I. Recognition, epidemiology, and clinical features. II. Experimental transmission, putative virus agents and markers, and prevention. Gastroenterology 1983;85: 439. (*Although written before identification of hepatitis C virus, its discussion of clinical features and outcome remains a useful resource.*)

Dienstag JL, Schiff ER, Wright TL, et al. Lamivudine as initial treatment for chronic hepatitis B in the United States. N Engl J Med 1999;341:1256. (*Randomized, placebo-controlled trial finding lamivudine to be safe and effective.*)

Farci P, Mandas A, Coriana A, et al. Treatment of hepatitis D with interferon alfa-2a. N Engl J Med 1994;330:88. (*Response found in half of patients, but relapse common after treatment stopped; a randomized controlled trial.*)

Fattovich G, Brollo L, Alberti A, et al. Chronic persistent hepatitis type B can be a progressive disease when associated with sustained virus replication. J Hepatol 1990;11:29. (*Important natural history study; progression in one third of those positive for HBV DNA.*)

Fattovich G, Brollo L, Giustina G, et al. Natural history and prognostic factors for chronic hepatitis type B. Gut 1991;32:294. (*Progression to cirrhosis predicted by histologic findings and persistence of HBV DNA.*)

Fattovich G, Giustina G, Degos F, et al. Morbidity and mortality in compensated cirrhosis type C: a retrospective follow-up study of 384 patients. Gastroenterology 1997;112:463. (*A European retrospective natural history study; 80% 10-year survival; annual mortality 1.9%; annual decompensation 3.9%; annual rate of hepatocellular carcinoma 1.4%.*)

Gane EJ, Portman BC, Naoumov NV, et al. Long-term outcome of hepatitis C infection after liver transplantation. N Engl J Med 1996;334:815. (*Although reinfection of the new liver is universal after liver transplantation for end-stage chronic hepatitis C, the clinical impact is limited.*)

Hoofnagle JH, di Bisceglie AM, et al. The treatment of chronic viral hepatitis. N Engl J Med 1997;336:347. (*A brief authoritative review of antiviral therapy for hepatitis B, C, and D.*)

Ishak K, Baptista A, Bianchi L, et al. Histologic grading and staging of chronic hepatitis. J Hepatol 1995;22:696. (*An update of histologic grading and staging by the original investigators.*)

Krawitt EL. Autoimmune hepatitis. N Engl J Med 1996;334:897. (*A concise, contemporary, authoritative review.*)

Lai CL, Chien RN, Leung NW, et al. A one-year trial of lamivudine for chronic hepatitis B. N Engl J Med 1998;339:61. (*A randomized, placebo-controlled, multicenter trial in Asian patients; the 100-mg dose was more effective, resulting in HBeAg-to-anti-HBe seroconversion in 14% and histologic improvement in 52%.*)

Lau DTY, Everhart J, Kleiner DE, et al. Long-term follow up of patients with chronic hepatitis B treated with interferon alfa. Gastroenterology 1997;113:1660. (*Loss of detectable HBeAg during interferon therapy is associated with an 80% chance of losing HBsAg and normalizing alanine aminotransferase over the ensuing decade.*)

Lin SM, Sheen IS, Chien RN, et al. Long-term beneficial effect of interferon therapy in patients with chronic hepatitis B virus infection. Hepatology 1999;29:971. (*Interferon treatment in Asian patients with chronic hepatitis B improved the natural history of the disease and reduced the risk of hepatocellular carcinoma.*)

Markowitz JS, Martin P, Conrad AJ, et al. Prophylaxis against hepatitis B recurrence following liver transplantation using combination lamivudine and hepatitis B immune globulin. Hepatology 1998;28:585. (*Preliminary trial; the combination of hepatitis B immune globulin infusions plus oral lamivudine was effective in preventing hepatitis B reinfection after liver transplantation.*)

McHutchison JG, Gordon SC, Schiff ER, et al. Interferon alfa-2b alone or in combination with ribavirin as initial treatment for chronic hepatitis C. N Engl J Med 1998;339:1485. (*Large, randomized, controlled trial; combination therapy for 12 months had the best outcome, with a sustained response just under 40%.*)

National Digestive Diseases Information Clearinghouse. Chronic hepatitis C: current disease management. NIH Publication No. 99-4230, 1999. (http://www.niddk.nih.gov/health/digest/pubs/chrnhepc.htm) (*This comprehensive overview of hepatitis C—virology, diagnosis, clinical and epidemiologic features, antiviral therapy, etc.—is updated periodically and appears on the web site of the National Institutes of Health.*)

National Institutes of Health Consensus Development Conference. Management of hepatitis C. Hepatology 1997;26[Suppl 1]:1S. (*NIH consensus guidelines on every aspect of hepatitis C evaluation and management; all recommendations are evidence based.*)

Niederau C, Heintges T, Lange S, et al. Long-term follow-up of HBeAg-positive patients treated with interferon alfa for chronic hepatitis B. N Engl J Med 1996;334:1422. (*Natural history study; patients who responded experienced a marked improvement in survival and survival without hepatic decompensation.*)

Perrillo RP, Schiff ER, Davis GL, et al. A randomized, controlled trial of interferon alfa-2b alone and after prednisone withdrawal for the treatment of chronic hepatitis B. N Engl J Med 1990;323:295. (*The study establishing efficacy of interferon for chronic hepatitis B. Pre-interferon prednisone withdrawal did not improve the response to interferon.*)

Perrillo RP, Rakela R, Rakela J, et al. Multicenter study of lamivudine therapy for hepatitis B after liver transplantation. Hepatology 1999;29:1581. (*An open-label multicenter trial supporting the benefit of lamivudine as therapy for recurrent hepatitis B after liver transplantation.*)

Poynard T, Marcellin P, Lee SS, et al. Randomized trial of interferon α2b plus ribavirin for 48 weeks or for 24 weeks versus interferon α2b plus placebo for 48 weeks for treatment of chronic infection with hepatitis C virus. Lancet 1998;352:1426. (*A large, European, randomized, controlled trial; combination therapy for 12 months had the best outcome, with a sustained response rate of 40%.*)

Rosenberg PM, et al. Therapy with nucleoside analogues for hepatitis B virus infection. Clin Liver Dis 1999;3:349. (*A contemporary overview of current and experimental nucleoside analogue therapy for chronic hepatitis B.*)

Samuel D, Muller R, Alexander G, et al. Liver transplantation in European patients with the hepatitis B surface antigen. N Engl J Med 1993;329:1842. (*Retrospective European analysis; marked improvement provided by long-term hepatitis B immune globulin infusions after liver transplantation.*)

Sorrell MF, Shaw BWJ. A primer of liver transplantation for the referring physician. Semin Liver Dis 1989;9:159. (*Excellent reading for the nontransplantation physician.*)

Starzl TE, Demetris AJ, Van Thiel D. Liver transplantation. N Engl J Med 1989;321:1014. (*Two-part review by the pioneers in the field.*)

Summerskill WHJ, Korman MG, Ammon HV, et al. Prednisone for chronic active liver disease: dose titration, standard dose, and combination with azathioprine compared. Gut 1975;16:876. (*Important double-blind randomized trial showing that prednisone or prednisone plus azathioprine was superior to placebo and azathioprine alone in nonviral hepatitis.*)

Weissberg JI, Andres LL, Smith CT, et al. Survival in chronic hepatitis B: an analysis of 379 patients. Ann Intern Med 1984;101:613. (*Five-year survival rates were a function of histologic severity at presentation; age more than 40, bilirubin elevation, ascites, and spider nevi also associated with poor prognosis and high risk of death; follow-up extended to 15 years.*)

Wright EC, Seeff LB, Bark PD, et al. Treatment of chronic active hepatitis: an analysis of 3 controlled trials. Gastroenterology 1977;73:1422. (*Critical review; finds that reduction in cirrhosis and mortality is achieved by steroids in patients with severe nonviral chronic hepatitis.*)

Yano M, Kumada H, Kage M, et al. The long-term pathological evolution of chronic hepatitis C. Hepatology 1996;23:1334. (*Unique Japanese study; serial liver biopsies over 20 years; severity of histologic grade and stage at baseline predictive of clinical course.*)

71

Management of Cirrhosis and Chronic Liver Failure

Cirrhosis represents an irreversible state of chronic liver injury. The best treatment is *prevention*, detecting and addressing conditions that can lead to it, including *chronic hepatitis, chronic alcohol abuse, hemochromatosis, and primary biliary cirrhosis* (see Chapters 57, 70, and 228). Even after its onset, the patient can be kept comfortable, active, and independent if precipitants of further hepatocellular injury are eliminated and complications are prevented or treated promptly. Although consultative help from specialists is often necessary, responsibility for long-term management usually rests with the primary care physician. One needs to be capable of treating etiologies and dealing with such complications as ascites, peripheral edema, encephalopathy, infection, bleeding, renal dysfunction, and electrolyte imbalances.

CLINICAL PRESENTATION AND COURSE

Clinical Presentation. Onset may be rather dramatic if the initial presentation is a late-stage complication such as brisk *variceal bleeding* or *encephalopathy*. In the office setting, the patient may present more subtly with complaints of *fatigue,* easy *bruising,* mild abdominal *swelling,* or new onset of bilateral *ankle edema.* In the setting of portal hypertension, *splenomegaly,* abdominal distention with *shifting dullness,* and a prominent *abdominal venous pattern* may become significant. Additional signs of chronic hepatic dysfunction include *palmar erythema, Dupuytren's contractures, spider angiomata, parotid and lacrimal gland hypertrophy, gynecomastia, testicular atrophy,* loss of *axillary* and *pubic hair,* and *clubbing.* Although nonspecific abnormalities in routine liver function tests are common, the best measures of hepatocellular synthetic impairment are prolongation of the *prothrombin time* (PT) and decline in the *serum albumin.* PT prolongation occurs first, because of the short serum half-lives of the hepatically synthesized clotting factors (e.g., 7 days) that determine it. The decline in serum albumin follows later because of the longer serum half-life of albumin (28 days).

Most presentations of cirrhosis and chronic hepatic failure are nonspecific, but the initial manifestations of a few treatable etiologies are worth noting because of the potential benefit of early recognition and treatment.

Hemochromatosis. *Primary hemochromatosis* is among the most common of autosomal hereditary conditions, having an estimated prevalence of 1:250 among whites. The mutation causes excessive iron absorption, resulting in iron overload. Decades of chronic iron deposition in parenchymal cells of the liver, heart, pancreas, and gonads eventually produce organ failure as cells suffer peroxidative damage; fibrosis ensues. Initially, the patient may be asymptomatic or incidentally noted to have a mild elevation in serum transaminase level. Mild *fatigue* or *arthralgias* might be the first symptoms. By the fifth or sixth decade, organ failure begins to appear, heralded by *dyspnea, glucose intolerance, arthritis,* and *gonadal dysfunction* and by manifestations of *cirrhosis* and chronic hepatocellular dysfunction. The skin might appear slate gray or *bronzelike* from the chronic iron deposition. Early diagnosis of the homozygous state is achieved by finding a *transferrin saturation* (serum iron/total iron binding capacity) more than 60% in men and more than 50% in women. A *ferritin* level more than twice normal for age and gender (e.g., more than 300 μg/L in men, more than 200 μg/L in women) indicates iron overload. At this stage, liver biopsy is indicated to determine the extent of iron deposition, degree of hepatic fibrosis, and need for initiation of therapy.

Primary Biliary Cirrhosis. The condition predominates in women aged 30 to 65 years. Autoimmune injury of the intrahepatic biliary tree leads to chronic *cholestasis* and culminates in fibrosis, *cirrhosis, portal hypertension,* and *severe pruritus.* Other autoimmune diseases may coexist with the condition (e.g., *Sjögren's syndrome, Hashimoto's thyroiditis). Fatigue* and *itching* are often the initial complaints. *Hepatomegaly* may be the first physical finding, and a markedly *elevated alkaline phosphatase* is the the principal laboratory abnormality before onset of manifestations associated with cirrhosis. *Hyperlipidemia* is common. *Jaundice* with skin excoriations accounts for the initial presentation in about one fourth of patients. The sedimentation rate is markedly elevated; liver function tests reveal a cholestatic pattern. *Steatorrhea* may ensue, compromising absorption of fat-soluble vitamins. *Antimitochondrial antibody* is

found in about 90% of cases, and *IgM antibody titers* are elevated. Diagnosis is made by *liver biopsy* with staining for copper that reveals characteristic interlobular ductal inflammation and fibrosis.

Alcoholic Liver Disease. Early hepatic injury may be manifested by mild elevations in aminotransferase levels. A ratio of 2:1 for alanine aminotransferase/aspartate aminotransferase is characteristic of alcoholic liver injury. A palpable liver from *fatty infiltration* is another early presentation. Risk factors for development of cirrhosis include prolonged consumption of *excess alcohol* (e.g., more than 16 oz/d for 10 years or more), *female sex,* and concurrent *viral hepatitis C* infection. Simultaneous use of *acetaminophen* (even at normal doses) and excess alcohol increases the risk of liver injury, especially when the patient is fasting. *Gastritis* and *upper gastrointestinal (GI) bleeding* are common consequences of alcohol excess and may be presenting manifestations.

Chronic Hepatitis (see Chapter 70)

Clinical Sequelae. *Portal hypertension, fluid retention,* and *encephalopathy* are the major sequelae of cirrhosis; they lead to *varices, ascites, hypersplenism, peripheral edema,* and *altered mental status.* Variceal bleeding occurs in 20% to 30% of all cirrhotic patients: one third may die during the initial hospitalization, one third rebleed within 6 weeks, and one third survive 1 year or more. The principal causes of death in patients with cirrhosis are variceal bleeding, encephalopathy, and infection. In addition, patients with cirrhosis, especially those with chronic hepatitis B infection, are at increased risk for hepatocellular carcinoma.

Prognosis is determined by the nature, severity, and activity of the underlying illness. The traditional prognostic indicator, the Pugh modification of the *Child-Turcotte prognostic classification,* is widely used to semiquantitatively estimate risk of invasive interventions (Table 71.1). A newer approach to predicting survival uses a discriminant function (DF) based on the serum bilirubin and PT (DF = 4.6 [PT − control] + bilirubin [mg/100 mL]). An ADF greater than 32 indicates a short-term mortality risk of 35%.

Prognosis in a few common causes of cirrhosis is illustrative of the basic determinants of cirrhosis and survival. Continued alcohol consumption in the context of alcoholic hepatitis is associated with an 80% chance of developing cirrhosis, whereas complete abstinence lowers the risk to 15%. Even after *alco-*

Table 71.1. Child-Pugh Classification of Hepatic Decompensation

CLINICAL FEATURE	CLASS		
	1	2	3
Encephalopathy grade	0	1–2	3
Ascites	None	Slight	Moderate
Bilirubin (mg/dL)	1–2	2–3	>3
Albumin (g/dL)	>3.5	2.8–3.5	<2.8
Prothrombin time prolongation (s)	1–4	5–6	>6

Adapted from Pugh RN, Murrary-Lyon IM, et al. Transection of the oesophagus for bleeding oesophageal varices. Br J Surg 1973;60:646-649, with permission.

holic cirrhosis has developed, survival continues to be affected by alcohol ingestion. Five-year survival is 60% to 85% in those who abstain, compared with 40% to 60% for those who continue to drink. Onset of jaundice or ascites further decreases 5-year survival (to 30% in drinkers). In symptomatic *primary biliary cirrhosis*, the average length of survival from the onset of symptoms is about 12 years, whereas the survival of asymptomatic patients did not differ from that of a control population matched for age and sex. The prognosis of patients with *postnecrotic cirrhosis* is difficult to assess because it is hard to date its onset; the cirrhosis develops insidiously over years from subclinical chronic active hepatitis.

Irrespective of etiology, development of ascites, encephalopathy, hyperbilirubinemia, variceal bleeding, hypergammaglobulinemia (from bypass of the hepatic reticuloendothelial system), and hypoalbuminemia are poor prognostic signs, as is decreased liver size. Onset of ascites is associated with a 50% 2-year mortality rate, and variceal bleeding has a 35% short-term mortality rate. The 2-year mortality for worsening renal function is 33%.

PRINCIPLES OF MANAGEMENT

Treatment of the underlying etiology and the manifestations and complications of cirrhosis and chronic hepatic failure constitute the basic elements of management. Outcomes can be improved when all elements are addressed in the treatment program.

Treatment of the Underlying Etiology

Alcoholic Cirrhosis requires complete *abstinence* from further alcohol intake (see Chapter 228), because prognosis is markedly worsened by continued drinking (see above). Attention to good nutrition, daily multiple vitamin supplements (including 1 mg of folic acid), and correction of any iron deficiency or electrolyte deficits are important supportive measures. The search continues for agents that might halt hepatic fibrosis and promote hepatocyte regeneration. Glucocorticosteroids and portacaval shunting have failed to demonstrate an improvement in survival, although cortico-steroids do improve short-term survival in patients with acute alcoholic hepatitis. A randomized, placebo-controlled, long-term study of *colchicine* revealed a doubling of 5- and 10-year survival. The drug is an inhibitor of collagen deposition. However, confirmatory data are needed before it or other drugs found experimentally to improve survival (e.g., *propylthiouracil*) can be recommended. *Liver transplantation* is sometimes considered in patients who have become totally and permanently abstinent.

Primary Biliary Cirrhosis used to be thought of as a relentlessly progressive autoimmune disease leading to liver transplantation or death. Medical therapy now appears capable of altering this dismal prognosis. *Ursodiol*, which is well tolerated, may stabilize the disease and even improve survival. *Colchicine* provides some biochemical improvement, but the survival benefit is unclear. *Methotrexate* appears very promising in persons unresponsive to ursodiol or colchicine alone, achieving histologic, biochemical, and clinical remissions when added to the treatment program in selected patients. Corticosteroids and penicillamine do not improve survival and cause serious ad-

verse side effects. *Liver transplantation* has proven to be a viable option.

Severe pruritus associated with this condition can be relieved by *cholestyramine* in a dose of 4 g orally with meals. Refractory pruritus responds to opiate antagonists. Because of decreased fat absorption from low intestinal bile-salt concentrations, these patients are particularly prone to develop deficiencies of the *fat-soluble vitamins*. They may require supplemental vitamin K (10 mg SC every 4 weeks), vitamin D (50,000 U orally two to three times a week or 100,000 U intramuscularly every 4 weeks) with oral calcium (1 g daily), and vitamin A (25,000 U orally per day). Night blindness unresponsive to vitamin A may be due to zinc deficiency, which is treated with oral *zinc sulfate* (220 mg/d). For patients with steatorrhea, *medium-chain triglyceride* preparations often help.

Secondary Biliary Cirrhosis can be halted by relieving or bypassing the obstruction to bile flow (see Chapter 62).

Hemochromatosis is treated with weekly *phlebotomies* of 500 mL until the serum iron and ferritin levels fall to normal; then, phlebotomies are performed as needed based on serum ferritin levels. Early recognition and timely initiation of treatment are essential to minimizing the chance of developing cirrhosis. Repeated studies have shown that iron removal by phlebotomy improves survival and decreases morbidity and may lead to normal life expectancy if started before onset of cirrhosis or diabetes. Unfortunately, delay in diagnosis and treatment are common, underscoring the importance of early recognition (see above).

Chronic Hepatitis of the nonviral variety may benefit from *corticosteroid/azathioprine* therapy; viral hepatitis responds to *interferon alfa* plus *ribavirin* (see Chapter 70).

Wilson's Disease responds to *d-penicillamine* therapy, which should be administered in conjunction with a hepatologist experienced in using the drug, because of its potential for serious side effects.

Treatment of Complications

Ascites and Edema result from increased portal pressure, hypoalbuminemia, secondary hyperaldosteronism, and impaired free water clearance. Its presence is strongly suggested by the clinical findings of a *fluid wave, shifting dullness*, and *peripheral edema*. Abdominal *ultrasound* can be used for confirmation and to rule out venoocclusive disease involving the hepatic veins or the hepatic region of the inferior vena cava (Budd-Chiari syndrome). Although ascites is not a hazard, gross ascites can cause abdominal discomfort and respiratory compromise; under such circumstances, it should be treated.

Diagnostic Paracentesis is indicated before treatment is initiated in patients with new onset of ascites, worsening hepatic function, fever, or increasing encephalopathy to exclude infection and malignancy. Although it was once believed that differentiating exudative from transudative ascitic fluid could aid in identifying infection and malignancy, such a differentiation has proven insufficiently sensitive and specific to be reliable. Fluid protein concentrations in excess of 2.5 g/dL are seen not only in conditions causing exudates but also in patients with transudative processes subjected to diuresis. Moreover, the ascitic fluid protein concentration of patients with spontaneous bacterial peritonitis is typically less than 1 g/dL. However, the *serum-to-ascites albumin gradient* (serum albumin concentration minus the ascites albumin concentration) can help differentiate portal hypertension from other causes of ascites, especially when the ascitic protein concentration is high. A gradient of greater than 1.1 mg/dL is indicative of portal hypertension; ascites in the presence of a gradient less than 1.1 suggests a mechanism other than portal hypertension. Ascitic fluid should also be sent for cytologic examination, cell count, and culture. A leukocyte count in excess of 2,500/mL is strongly suggestive of spontaneous bacterial peritonitis in the patient with abdominal pain and fever. Culture is positive in over 80% of cases when 10-mL aliquots are injected into three blood culture bottles; Gram stain is usually negative.

Salt and Fluid Restrictions. A reduction in daily sodium intake is the first priority in treating ascites due to portal hypertension. One begins with a *2-g sodium diet*, a reasonable compromise between maximizing sodium restriction and dietary palatability. Adequate nutrition is critical. In the absence of encephalopathy, a daily protein intake of at least 50 g is recommended. Excessive water intake should be prohibited, and *free water* should be restricted to 1,500 mL/d if hyponatremia ensues. An effective program of salt and water restriction requires a cooperative patient and a conscientious family. A dietitian can provide invaluable assistance. The patient should be instructed to check weight daily. Measuring abdominal girth is an unreliable index of fluid loss because of variations due to gaseous distention of the GI tract. About 15% of patients will respond to sodium and fluid restrictions alone. Bedrest is of no added benefit.

Diuretic Therapy is indicated if a diuresis has not occurred spontaneously after a full week of salt restriction. *Spironolactone* is the agent of first choice, because it inhibits the hyperaldosteronism of portal hypertension. Being a specific aldosterone antagonist, it counters the hypokalemic alkalosis commonly seen in cirrhotic patients with ascites. Its diuretic action is mild and unlikely to cause rapid intravascular volume depletion. The initial dosage of spironolactone is 100 mg/d orally in divided doses. If diuresis does not follow within 1 week, the daily dosage may be increased by 100 mg every 4 or 5 days to a maximum of 400 mg daily (higher doses may cause hyperkalemic acidosis). It is useful to monitor urinary electrolyte concentrations, because diuresis should follow a significant rise in urinary sodium and a fall in urinary potassium. If natriuresis and diuresis do not occur on a maximal dosage of spironolactone, a loop diuretic such as *furosemide* (starting at 20 to 40 mg/d) may be added. *Bumetanide or metolazone* may be added to the diuretic program, but such potent diuretics must be used with extreme care to avoid precipitating renal failure, hypokalemia, and encephalopathy.

Monitoring blood urea nitrogen, creatinine, and electrolytes is critical during treatment of ascites. However, some cirrhotic patients with renal impairment do not manifest an elevated serum creatinine (believed related to reduced creatine synthesis by the liver). This reduces the sensitivity of the serum creatinine in some cirrhotic patients and can complicate monitoring of their renal status. Other measures of renal function may be required.

The maximum amount of ascitic fluid that can be mobilized in 24 hours is about 700 to 900 mL, although peripheral edema can be mobilized at a faster rate. This translates to a daily weight loss of 0.5 kg in patients with ascites alone and of 1 kg in those with both ascites and peripheral edema. Daily weight loss in excess of these amounts suggests overdiuresis, with its attendant risk of intravascular volume depletion leading to hepatorenal syndrome and encephalopathy. A falling urine output accompanied by orthostatic signs (rise in pulse and fall in blood pressure on change from supine to standing) suggests inadequate intravascular volume. An oral fluid challenge of several hundred milliliters of isotonic fluid can confirm the presence of hypovolemia by inducing a temporary increase in urine output.

Refractory Ascites. Some patients with incapacitating ascites are *truly refractory* to sodium restriction and diuretics. For them, *large-volume paracentesis* and *peritoneovenous (LeVeen) shunting* become therapeutic considerations. Removal of more than 1 to 2 L of ascitic fluid at a time by paracentesis was once considered to be unwise, because of the risk of precipitating serious intravascular volume depletion from the shift of intravascular fluid into the emptied peritoneal cavity. Moreover, protein depletion and increase in renin activity and aldosterone secretion might ensue. By infusing *albumin* intravenously (6 to 8 g/L of ascitic fluid removed) at the time of paracentesis, large volumes (5 to 6 L) of ascitic fluid can be removed without precipitating adverse reactions. Results are comparable with those achieved by shunting procedures, although admissions for reaccumulation of fluid are more frequent (every 10 to 30 days). The best candidates are those with peripheral edema and relatively well-preserved renal function.

Before the development of large-volume paracentesis, peritoneovenous (LeVeen) shunting was the principal means of dealing with refractory ascites. Although effective in treating ascites, shunt placement does not improve survival. Moreover, insertion can precipitate disseminated intravascular coagulation. Infection and shunt obstruction are common complications. Compared with large-volume paracentesis, LeVeen shunting requires fewer readmissions for treatment of ascites but an overall similar number of hospitalizations due to shunt occlusions. Its potentially serious complications and the advent of large-volume paracentesis has led to a decline in use of LeVeen shunts. Refractory ascites has also been treated with placement of a *transjugular intrahepatic portosystemic shunt (TIPS)*. Although helpful in some persons and successful in decreasing portal pressure, the procedure increases the risk of encephalopathy and carries its own procedural morbidity and mortality (see below).

Spontaneous Bacterial Peritonitis develops in about 10% of ascitic patients per year. Risk is especially great if the total protein concentration of the ascitic fluid falls below 1.0 g/dL. Under such circumstances, primary antibiotic prophylaxis (e.g., *trimethoprim-sulfamethoxazole*, one double-strength tablet every 5 of 7 days/wk) is worth considering. Secondary prophylaxis is indicated in those with a prior episode.

Hepatic Encephalopathy is thought to be produced by one or more intestinally derived toxic substances that escape hepatic detoxification as a result of portasystemic shunting and hepatocellular dysfunction. Candidates include ammonia, benzodiazepine-like substances, mercaptans, phenol, neuroinhibitors, false neurotransmitters, and short-chain fatty acids. Elevations of arterial and venous *ammonia levels* usually, but not always, correlate with the presence of hepatic encephalopathy. Venous levels may be falsely elevated when a tourniquet is left on too long at the time of blood drawing. Ammonia levels are useful in following the clinical state of individual patients. Mild encephalopathy may be managed on an ambulatory basis.

Patients should also be monitored with routine mental status examinations that include five-point star and signature testing and examination for asterixis.

Treating Precipitants. The first goal of treatment is to address the major precipitants. Important precipitating factors include GI bleeding; excessive dietary protein intake; hypokalemic alkalosis; infection; constipation; use of sedative, opiate, or hypnotic drugs; surgical procedures; and volume depletion resulting from diuresis or paracentesis. Precipitants are identified in about 50% of patients; the prognosis is usually better in those with an identifiable contributory factor than in those in whom the onset of encephalopathy is associated only with worsening hepatocellular function.

Reducing Ammonia Production. The mainstay of therapy is *restriction of dietary protein* intake to 30 to 40 g/d while maintaining a daily caloric intake of 1,500 kcal. Controlled trials support dietary protein restriction and substitution of animal protein with vegetable sources; their metabolism produces less ammonia. Sometimes, oral *amino acid supplements* (high in branched-chain varieties and low in aromatic amines) are added to prevent negative nitrogen balance and to reduce production of false neurotransmitters. Their efficacy in treatment of encephalopathy appears to be transient. Simple gut cleansing with enemas or cathartics is effective when bleeding, constipation, or a large dietary protein intake has led to encephalopathy. *Lactulose* (a synthetic nonabsorbable disaccharide metabolized to organic acids by enteric bacteria) causes an osmotic catharsis and also suppresses the growth of ammonia-forming urease-producing bacteria in favor of lactose-fermenting organisms. The initial dosage for patients with mild encephalopathy is 15 to 30 mL orally every 4 to 6 hours, with adjustments thereafter to produce two to three loose stools a day. Side effects of oral lactulose include diarrhea and abdominal distress, which usually resolve after a reduction in dosage.

Use of poorly absorbed antibiotics to decrease the intestinal concentration of ammonia-forming bacteria is a proven approach to treating encephalopathy. *Neomycin*, a poorly absorbed broad-spectrum aminoglycoside antibiotic, is about as effective as lactulose, but prolonged use of doses in excess of 4 g/d (especially in patients with renal insufficiency) may lead to ototoxicity and nephrotoxicity. The recommended maximum oral dose is 1 g twice daily. The drug also causes malabsorption. In patients who fail to respond to either lactulose or neomycin, the two may be given together; in some patients, the effect appears to be additive. *Metronidazole* (800 mg/d for 1 week) may be used instead of neomycin; when used for short periods, it is less toxic. Eradication of *Helicobacter pylori* is meeting with some initial success in uncontrolled studies, presumably because of its contribution to ammonia production (being a urea-splitter). Repopulating the colon with nonurease-producing organisms, such as *Lactobacillus acidophilus*, has been tried with variable success; *Enterococcus faecium* use has been more promising.

Improving Ammonia Metabolism. Dietary supplements of *ornithine aspartate, benzoate, and phenylacetate* are thought to increase ammonia metabolism, and available studies are encouraging, with benefits approaching those seen with lactulose in persons with mild encephalopathy. *Zinc*, a required cofactor of several enzymes of the urea cycle, is often deficient in cirrhotics. Treatment of zinc deficiency with 600 mg/d of zinc supplement has been helpful in some but not all controlled trials of this element.

Reducing False Transmitters. The restriction of aromatic amino acids and use of preparations rich in branched-chain amino acids is based on the hypothesis that such an approach reduces production of false neurotransmitters. Results of controlled trials are equivocal at best. Nitrogen balance may improve, but improvement in encephalopathy may be hard to come by.

Inhibition of GABA-Benzodiazepine Receptors. Although binding of ligands to this receptor is believed to be pathophysiologically important in hepatic encephalopathy, receptor antagonist therapy with flumazemil has not produced significant benefit.

Variceal Bleeding. Primary and secondary prophylaxis against bleeding are the principal concerns of the primary care physician. In patients with known varices, risk of bleeding is high. Independent risk factors include marked hepatocellular dysfunction, ascites, encephalopathy, large varices, and presence of dilated venules on the varices. Risk of a first bleed is as high as 65% in the first year. Because clinical and endoscopic risk factors are independent and therefore not predictive of one another, some authorities recommend endoscopic assessment of all cirrhotic patients to determine risk and candidacy for treatment.

Beta-blockers are useful in patients at high risk for variceal bleeding. When prescribed in dosages that produce beta-blockade (a reduction in heart rate of about 25%), these agents can lower portal venous pressure and decrease the risk of variceal bleeding by about 50%. The rate of death from hemorrhage is also reduced, but all-cause mortality is not. Although disappointing for secondary prophylaxis, beta-blockers have demonstrated efficacy for prevention of a first variceal bleed and should be considered for use in high-risk patients (large varices). Other agents are being investigated for their ability to further reduce portal pressure.

Endoscopic Injection Sclerotherapy is used to control acute variceal bleeding and, when repeated several times over 2 to 3 months, to prevent recurrences. Controlled trials have shown it to be superior to placebo in preventing repeat variceal hemorrhage but having little impact on the risk of all-cause upper GI bleeding, which remains at close to 40%. The procedure is not effective in preventing a first bleed. Addition of *octreotide* infusion to sclerotherapy reduces the short-term risk of rebleeding and transfusion requirements. The procedure has a high complication rate (up to 20%) and a mortality risk of nearly 5%. Like portasystemic shunt surgery (see below), sclerotherapy may only substitute one form of morbidity and mortality for another. Sclerotherapy largely replaced portasystemic shunt surgery, which is reserved for those who bleed despite repeated sclerotherapies and other approaches to treating varices.

Endoscopic Band Ligation of varices has been used to improve upon injection sclerotherapy. It requires fewer treatments than sclerotherapy and causes fewer complications. Outcomes are about the same; consequently, it is replacing sclerotherapy.

TIPS involves angiographic placement of a stent from a branch of the hepatic vein through the liver parenchyma and into a branch of the portal vein. It represents an increasingly effective option in persons who fail endoscopic therapy. TIPS decompresses the portal system and reduces the risk of bleeding. Stent failure occurs in up to 50% of cases and represents the principal cause of rebleeding. Improvements in stent design are lowering the failure rate. The procedure has a 5% mortality risk, similar to that for sclerotherapy. In a randomized controlled trial comparing TIPS with endoscopic sclerotherapy, TIPS produced a dramatic decrease in portal pressure and was superior in preventing rebleeding; however, there was no difference in survival, although a positive trend toward improved survival was noted. The major drawback to stent placement is encephalopathy or its worsening, which can be especially problematic if present before the procedure.

Portasystemic shunt surgery remains the final treatment option for patients with recurrent variceal hemorrhage due to portal hypertension. Although reducing the risk of hemorrhage, shunt surgery increases the risk of encephalopathy. The likelihood of recurrent variceal bleeding is significantly reduced after portasystemic shunting, but long-term survival is not. Reasons for lack of improvement in survival include high operative mortality rates and no benefit to hepatic function, the principal determinant of survival. Consequently, portasystemic shunt surgery is not indicated in patients with varices who have never bled. Selective shunt procedures were developed to reduce the risk of encephalopathy, a common consequence of shunt surgery. For example, the selective *distal splenorenal shunt* attempts to preserve portal blood flow in patients with demonstrable preoperative portal perfusion. Its incidence of postoperative encephalopathy is lower than with conventional portacaval shunting, but long-term benefit is reduced as collateral channels develop. *Side-to-side portacaval or proximal splenorenal shunts* are the most effective operations for decompressing hepatic sinusoids and reducing ascites, but they still risk precipitating encephalopathy. For patients awaiting liver transplantation, TIPS can be used to bide time.

Coagulopathy results from reductions in vitamin K–dependent clotting factors (II, VII, IX, and X) secondary to decreased hepatic protein synthesis and increased plasma proteolytic activity. In addition, bile-salt deficiency, neomycin therapy, and malnutrition may contribute to malabsorption of vitamin K, and hypersplenism may account for thrombocytopenia. If a patient with cirrhosis is discovered to have a prolonged PT, a trial of *vitamin K*, 10 mg subcutaneously daily for 3 days, will correct hypoprothrombinemia caused by bile-salt deficiency, neomycin, or malnutrition but not hypoprothrombinemia related only to hepatocellular disease. In the absence of bleeding, measures to correct abnormal coagulation parameters are generally not indicated.

Role of Liver Transplantation. In the face of terminal hepatocellular failure, liver transplantation becomes a consideration. In properly selected patients, 5-year survival may be as high as 85%. The best candidates are those who are highly motivated, emotionally stable, and willing to comply with a medical program. Postnecrotic cirrhosis, primary biliary cirrhosis, and primary sclerosing cholangitis are among the primary indications. Alcohol-induced liver disease associated with continued drinking is a strong relative contraindication, as is hepatitis B liver disease, hepatocellular carcinoma, and renal failure. Absolute contraindications are AIDS, extrahepatic sepsis, metastatic cancer, and severe cardiopulmonary disease. Advanced age is not a poor prognostic factor, nor is alcoholic liver disease in a person who abstains from drinking for 6 months before transplantation.

THERAPEUTIC RECOMMENDATIONS AND MONITORING

General Measures

- The patient should maintain a caloric intake of at least 2,000 to 3,000 kcal/d.
- Use of alcohol or other hepatotoxic agents must be prohibited.
- The patient should avoid tranquilizers and sedatives.
- Monitor PT, serum albumin, and bilirubin to assess the severity and progression of hepatocellular dysfunction.
- Have the patient keep a record of daily weights.
- Check stools at each visit for evidence of occult bleeding.
- Check for asterixis and other signs of encephalopathy at each visit.
- Check the abdomen for evidence of ascites (shifting dullness, fluid wave, bulging flanks). Ultrasound examination is useful to confirm the presence of ascites and rule out venoocclusive disease.

Management of Ascites

- Perform a diagnostic paracentesis in patients with the new onset of ascites or clinical deterioration in the setting of pre-existing ascites. The fluid should be sent for cell count and differential, total protein and albumin concentrations, culture, and cytologic examination.
- Instruct patients with ascites to restrict daily sodium intake to no more than 2 g and to consume at least 50 g protein/d. Consult with a dietitian and provide patient and family with specific menus and food lists.
- Restrict fluid intake to 1,500 mL when there is marked hyponatremia (serum sodium concentration less than 125 mEq/L).
- If salt restriction does not result in diuresis, begin spironolactone 100 mg daily in divided doses. If natriuresis and diuresis do not occur after 1 week, increase the daily dose of spironolactone by 100 mg every 4 to 5 days to a maximum of 400 mg/d.
- If spironolactone alone is ineffective in causing diuresis, add furosemide 20 to 40 mg/d to the regimen and cautiously increase dosage as necessary.
- Adjust diuretic dose so that no more than 0.5 kg of fluid (approximately 1 lb) is lost per day in patients with ascites alone, and no more than 1 kg/d (2 lb) in those with both ascites and peripheral edema. Halt diuretics at the first sign of intravascular volume depletion.
- Consider daily potassium supplementation (20 to 40 mEq KCl elixir) in patients receiving furosemide; administer cautiously, if at all, to patients concurrently taking a potassium-sparing diuretic such as spironolactone.
- Monitor serum potassium, blood urea nitrogen, creatinine, daily weight, and postural signs to avoid inducing intravascular volume depletion, renal failure, hypokalemia, and encephalopathy. Be aware that in some patients the serum creatinine may be falsely normal and remain within normal limits despite worsening renal function.
- Consider large-volume paracentesis (5 to 6 L) with concurrent intravenous albumin infusion (6 to 8 g/L of fluid removed) for patients with refractory ascites that is disabling. Admit for the procedure.

Encephalopathy

- At the first sign of encephalopathy, restrict dietary protein intake to 20 to 30 g/d. Obtain dietary consultation to construct a diet emphasizing plant protein over animal protein. Consider use of an oral supplement rich in branched-chain amino acids if protein intake is insufficient.
- Monitor mental status and check for asterixis; use five-point star or signature testing. Monitoring venous ammonia levels is less useful; in drawing blood for a determination, avoid prolonged tourniquet application.
- When protein restriction fails to control encephalopathy, begin oral lactulose, 15 to 30 mL every 4 to 6 hours, with subsequent adjustments in the dosage to allow two to three soft stools a day. Add oral *neomycin* 1 g twice daily or *metronidazole* 250 mg three times a day if lactulose alone does not suffice. Metronidazole is probably the better tolerated for short-term use.
- Consider dietary supplementation with *ornithine aspartate, benzoate,* or *phenylacetate* in patients with mild encephalopathy.

Prevention of Variceal Bleeding and Bleeding Due to Clotting Factor Deficiency

- Begin a beta-blocker (e.g., propranolol 80 mg/day) for primary prevention in patients with risk factors for variceal bleeding (marked hepatocellular dysfunction, ascites, encephalopathy, large varices, and presence of dilated venules on the varices).
- Consider endoscopic sclerotherapy, endoscopic variceal banding, and shunt procedures (e.g., TIPS) for prevention of recurrent variceal bleeding.
- Monitor PT and platelet count. Administer vitamin K (10 mg SC daily for 3 days) if there is prolongation of PT due to drug-induced bile-salt malabsorption, neomycin, or malnutrition. Platelet transfusions are unwarranted unless there is active bleeding in the context of a very low platelet count (see Chapter 81).

INDICATIONS FOR REFERRAL AND ADMISSION

Prompt hospitalization is required for patients with GI bleeding, worsening encephalopathy, increasing azotemia, signs of peritoneal irritation, or unexplained fever. Intractable ascites may respond to elective admission for large-volume paracentesis. Decisions about the management of refractory ascites, encephalopathy, variceal bleeding, and uncommon etiologies of cirrhosis (e.g., primary biliary cirrhosis, Wilson's disease, hemochromatosis) are best made in consultation with a gastroenterologist skilled in treating liver disease. The same pertains to candidacy for liver transplantation. When urine output falls in the absence of a clearcut explanation, a nephrologic consultation may be of considerable help, especially because creatinine level may not adequately reflect renal function.

PATIENT EDUCATION AND SUPPORT

It should be emphasized to the patient and family that prognosis can often be greatly improved and symptoms lessened by careful adherence to the prescribed medical program. In particular, dietary discipline and omission of alcohol are central to a successful outcome and should be stressed. Many of these patients are chronic alcoholics with low self-esteem. A nonjudgmental sympathetic physician can be instrumental in providing support, raising self-esteem, and improving the chances of compliance (see Chapter 228). Depression is a frequent accompaniment of the later stages of chronic liver disease and is manifested by failure to comply with the medical regimen and outright expressions of wanting to die. Treatment is very difficult. Antidepressant drugs may cause oversedation and thus are risky. There are no simple measures, but the physician's concern and support can help enormously (see Chapter 227).

A.H.G.

ANNOTATED BIBLIOGRAPHY

Black M, Friedman AC. Ultrasound examination in the patient with ascites. Ann Intern Med 1989;110:253. (*Editorial urging its routine use in patients with new onset of ascites, both for its confirmation and to rule out a venoocclusive etiology.*)

Borowsky SA, Strome S, Lott E. Continued heavy drinking and survival in alcoholic cirrhotics. Gastroenterology 1981;80:1405. (*80% of those who continued to drink heavily died an average of 7.2 months after discharge; 95% of abstainers were still alive at 14 months.*)

Campra JL, Reynolds TB. Effectiveness of high-dose spironolactone therapy in patients with chronic liver disease and relatively refractory ascites. Dig Dis Sci 1978;23:1025. (*Doses as high as 600 mg per day found effective in patients with ascites presumed to be "refractory."*)

Cello JP, Ring EJ, Olcott EW, et al. Endoscopic sclerotherapy compared with percutaneous transjugular intrahepatic portosystemic shunts after initial sclerotherapy in patients with acute variceal hemorrhage. A randomized controlled trial. Ann Intern Med 1997;126:858. (*TIPS was associated with a lower rate of rebleeding, but an increased risk of encephalopathy.*)

Conn HO, Levy CM, Vlahcevic ZR, et al. Comparison of lactulose and neomycin in the treatment of chronic portal systemic encephalopathy; a double-blind controlled trial. Gastroenterology 1977;72:573. (*Found to be equally effective and free of significant toxicity at the doses used.*)

Epstein M. Treatment of refractory ascites. N Engl J Med 1989;321:1675. (*Editorial summarizing data on LeVeen shunting and large volume paracentesis; argues that paracentesis may be preferable.*)

Gines P, Arroyo V, Vargas V, et al. Paracentesis with intravenous infusion of albumin as compared with peritoneovenous shunting in cirrhosis with refractory ascites. N Engl J Med 1991;325:829. (*Randomized comparison showing equal effectiveness and similar total hospital days.*)

Graham DY, Smith JL. The course of patients after variceal hemorrhage. Gastroenterology 1981;80:800. (*One third died in the initial hospitalization, one third rebleed within 6 weeks, and one third survived at least 1 year. Long-term survival after the initial 2 weeks no different from that of unselected cirrhotics without bleeding.*)

Kaplan MM, DeLellis RA, Wolfe HJ. Sustained biochemical and histologic remission of primary biliary cirrhosis in response to medical treatment. Ann Intern Med 1997;126:682. (*Very promising results in persons treated with methotrexate in combination with ursodiol or colchicine.*)

Kershenobich D, Vargas F, Garcia-Tsao G, et al. Colchicine in the treatment of cirrhosis of the liver. N Engl J Med 1988;318:1709. (*Randomized, placebo-controlled study; 14 years of follow-up; survival doubled.*)

Lucey MR, Carr K, Beresford TP, et al. Alcoholic liver disease is not a contraindication to liver transplantation. Hepatology 1997;25:1223. (*Prognosis is good; up to 2/3 who abstain for 6 months prior to transplantation never drink again.*)

McDonnell SM, Preston BL, Jewell SA, et al. A survey of 2,851 patients with hemochromatosis: symptoms and response to treatment. Am J Med 1999;106:619. (*Diagnosis and treatment are often delayed, but treatment is effective in improving many symptoms.*)

Niederau C, Fischer R, Purschel A, et al. Long-term survival in patients with hereditary hemochromatosis. Gastroenterology 1996;110:1107. (*Iron removal by phlebotomy improves survival and decreases morbidity, and may lead to normal life expectancy if started before onset of cirrhosis or diabetes.*)

North Italian Endoscopic Club. Prediction of the first variceal hemorrhage in patients with cirrhosis of the liver and esophageal varices. N Engl J Med 1988;319:983. (*Multivariate analysis identifying risk factors predictive of bleeding.*)

Ochs A, Rossle M, Haag K, et al. The transjugular intrahepatic portosystemic stent-shunt procedure for refractory ascites. N Engl J Med 1005:332:1192. (*An uncontrolled prospective study showing symptomatic benefit, but high levels of morbidity and mortality.*)

Pagliaro L, D'Amico G, Sorensen TIA, et al. Prevention of first bleeding in cirrhosis: A meta-analysis of randomized trials of nonsurgical treatment. Ann Intern Med 1992;117:59. (*Beta-blockers prevent first bleeding in high-risk patients; sclerotherapy is of unproven efficacy for primary prophylaxis.*)

Papadakis MA, Arieff AI. Unpredictability of clinical evaluation of renal function in cirrhosis. Am J Med 1987;82:945. (*Some cirrhotics with reduced glomerular filtration have normal serum creatinine levels, which may remain within normal limits despite worsening of renal function.*)

Powell LW, George K, McDonnell SM, et al. Diagnosis of hemochromatosis. Ann Intern Med 1998;129:925. (*Useful review of screening and workup; 41 references.*)

Powell WJ Jr., Klatskin G. Duration of survival in patients with Laennec's cirrhosis. Am J Med 1968;44:406. (*Classic paper showing improved survival in cirrhotic patients who abstained from alcohol compared with those who continued to drink heavily.*)

Poynard T, Cales P, Pasta L, et al. Beta-adrenergic antagonist drugs in the prevention of gastrointestinal bleeding in patients with cirrhosis and esophageal varices. N Engl J Med 1991;324:1532. (*Analysis of pooled data showing reduction in risk of first bleeding and mortality from hemorrhage.*)

Rector WG Jr., Reynolds TB. Superiority of serum ascites albumin differences in "exudative" ascites. Am J Med 1984;77:83. (*Better than total protein for differential diagnosis.*)

Riordan SM, Williams R. Treatment of hepatic encephalopathy. N Engl J Med 1997;337:473. (*A very useful pathophysiologic approach to treatment adopted for this Chapter.*)

Shear L, Ching S, Gabuzda GJ. Compartmentalization of ascites and edema in patients with hepatic cirrhosis. N Engl J Med 1970;282:1391. (*Classic elegant study; maximum rate at which ascites can be absorbed was 930 mL per 24 hours; concludes that the therapeutic aim in patients with ascites should be weight loss of no more than 0.5 kg daily.*)

Stanley MM, Ochi S, Lee KK, et al. Peritoneovenous shunting as compared with medical treatment in patients with alcoholic cirrhosis and massive ascites. N Engl J Med 1989;321:1632. (*Ascites alleviated, but survival unchanged.*)

Williams JW, Simel DL. Does this patient have ascites? How to divine fluid in the abdomen. JAMA 1992;267:2645. (*Best review of the diagnostic utility of history and physical examination methods.*)

72
Management of Pancreatitis
JAMES M. RICHTER

The primary physician encounters pancreatitis in three forms that lend themselves to ambulatory management: 1) recovery phase of acute pancreatitis; 2) chronic mild relapsing pancreatitis presenting as recurrent abdominal pain; and 3) pancreatic insufficiency, with steatorrhea and weight loss.

In the United States, most cases of pancreatitis are a result of excess ethanol ingestion or biliary tract disease, chiefly among middle-aged alcoholic men and elderly women with gallstones, respectively. A penetrating duodenal ulcer, trauma, hypercalcemia, hypertriglyceridemia, vascular insufficiency, tumor, heredity, ampullary stenosis, and drugs such as thiazide diuretics, glucocorticosteroids, azathioprine, and sulfasalazine are also associated with pancreatitis. In patients with AIDS, the risk of acute pancreatitis increases by 35 to 500 times, due in part to some of the drugs used to treat the condition and to increased risk of infection. In some cases of acute pancreatitis, no etiology is found. The course, response to therapy, and prognosis are largely functions of the etiology.

The primary physician must be able to distinguish acute pancreatitis from other causes of acute upper abdominal pain (see Chapter 58), pancreatic insufficiency from other causes of steatorrhea (see Chapter 64), and chronic abdominal pain due to pancreatitis from that due to pancreatic carcinoma and other important etiologies (see Chapters 58 and 76). Objectives of management include relief of pain, removal of precipitants, and assurance of adequate nutrition.

DIAGNOSIS, CLINICAL PRESENTATION, AND COURSE

Acute Pancreatitis

The manifestations of acute pancreatic disease are produced by inflammatory breakdown of pancreatic architecture, with release of digestive enzymes into the interstitium of the gland, leading to autolysis. Typically, acute pancreatitis produces constant epigastric, periumbilical, or left or right upper abdominal pain radiating to the back, often increased by food and decreased by upright posture. Vomiting can be persistent. Examination reveals abdominal tenderness and may include decreased bowel sounds, distention, and fever. The clinical presentation in HIV-infected patients is similar to that in immunocompetent patients but often obscured by other concurrent illnesses.

Diagnosis. The diagnosis of acute pancreatitis is supported by increases in the serum amylase and serum lipase. The *serum amylase* is elevated principally in pancreatic disease but may also be high in renal insufficiency, salivary gland disease, biliary tract obstruction, aortic dissection, and such other intraabdominal conditions as perforated peptic ulcer, mesenteric infarction, and small bowel obstruction without detectable pancreatitis. Patients with AIDS may have hyperamylasemia from salivary gland pathology or macroamylasemia. Macroamylasemia is also seen in connective tissue diseases, lymphoma, and liver disease. The *serum lipase* is more specific but less sensitive; it is a good confirmatory test. Assays of *amylase isoenzymes* have also been developed as confirmatory tests, especially useful when nonpancreatic sources of hyperamylasemia need to be ruled out (e.g., as in AIDS). An *amylase-creatinine clearance ratio* greater than 5 was thought to convey added specificity, but further study found it to be merely a nonspecific consequence of decreased renal amylase clearance that can occur in the setting of any severe acute stress, including diabetic ketoacidosis and cutaneous burns.

Improved rapid screening methods for diagnosis acute pancreatitis continue to be sought. *Trypsinogen-2 dipstick testing* of the urine is being studied as a means of quickly ruling out acute pancreatitis in the urgent care/emergency room setting. The qualitative version of the test has a sensitivity of 94% and a specificity of 95% for acute pancreatitis. When applied to patients with acute abdominal pain, a negative result effectively rules out acute pancreatitis; a positive result needs confirmation because the test has a 5% false-positive rate.

At present, the serum amylase remains the best initial diagnostic study. At times *ultrasonography* can be used for diagnostic purposes; it shows edema of the gland and any biliary tract pathology. Contrast-enhanced *computed tomography (CT)* of the abdomen can also be used to detect such findings and to provide an estimate of severity. Intraglandular necrosis, surrounding edema, and fluid collections can also be detected. The test is considered the gold standard for severe cases of acute pancreatitis but is less sensitive for mild disease. The disadvantages of CT include high cost and need for potentially injurious contrast agents.

Clinical Course. The course of acute pancreatitis depends on the severity of the disease and the underlying etiology. Patients with HIV infection or frank AIDS have particularly poor prognoses. In a patient recovering from acute pancreatitis, symptoms are reliable indicators of disease activity. Elevated enzymes in an otherwise asymptomatic patient are usually of no significance. The serum amylase routinely falls to normal within several days but may remain elevated for weeks after an uncomplicated illness. In other instances, persistently elevated enzymes in an asymptomatic person may be a clue to the presence of a silent pseudocyst. If a mass is palpable or pain recurs, a *pseudocyst* should be ruled out by ultrasonography of the upper abdomen. Pseudocysts arise in about half of patients with severe pancreatitis, mostly in those with alcohol-induced disease or AIDS. Spontaneous resolution occurs over 3 months in about 50% of patients; those with persistent lesions over 5 cm usually require surgical drainage.

Chronic Pancreatitis characteristically presents and proceeds as bouts of mild to severe recurrent epigastric pain, often occurring in *alcoholic patients* after years of excessive drinking. Sometimes chronic pancreatitis is heralded by a severe attack of acute pancreatitis. At other times, there may be mild pain or simply the painless insidious onset of exocrine insuffi-

ciency and diabetes. The pain of chronic pancreatitis is not entirely constant and often varies in intensity over days to weeks. There may be exacerbations of pain, nausea, and vomiting after eating or drinking alcohol. Elevated serum *amylase* and *lipase* levels are helpful, but the sensitivity of these tests is lower than in acute pancreatitis.

Diagnosis. Individuals who present with chronic recurrent abdominal pain and a history of relapsing pancreatitis usually do not present difficult diagnostic problems, but the patient without such a history requires more extensive assessment. A *plain film of the abdomen* may reveal *pancreatic calcification*, a late finding in alcoholic pancreatitis. *Ultrasonography* may demonstrate a diffusely enlarged gland, local mass, or pseudocyst. If ultrasound evaluation is normal and pancreatic disease is strongly suspected on clinical grounds, *CT* of the upper abdomen should be performed. If a solitary mass is found, *needle biopsy* should be performed to help diagnose cancer. If uncertainty about cancer or chronic pancreatitis persists, *endoscopic retrograde pancreatography* may prove diagnostically useful. *Abdominal angiography* can be substituted for retrograde pancreatography, if the latter is unavailable or fails.

Clinical Course. The clinical course of chronic pancreatitis is variable and depends on elimination of precipitating factors. Gallstones, particularly common bile duct stones, should be promptly removed, either surgically or endoscopically. Successful and early removal greatly reduces the risk of recurrent or chronic pancreatitis. With recurrent disease, *pancreatic insufficiency* may gradually develop over years, manifested by weight loss and steatorrhea. Although mild glucose intolerance may occur early in the disease process, the onset of clinical *diabetes* is a late complication and a sign of advanced disease. There appears to be an increased risk of pancreatic cancer.

Pancreatic Insufficiency. Patients with pancreatic exocrine insufficiency complain of *weight loss* and frequent greasy bowel movements (i.e., steatorrhea). Weight loss is often striking but nonspecific in this population, which tends to substitute alcohol for other forms of nourishment. Steatorrhea is a late development, not seen until more than 80% of pancreatic exocrine function has been lost. Objective evidence of maldigestion may be obtained by a *qualitative examination for stool fat* with Sudan stain. Where this is not available, a 72-hour *quantitative stool fat analysis* can also be used to establish the presence of steatorrhea and a *d-xylose test* to exclude small bowel mucosal disease. The *bentiromide test* is a simple outpatient study for detecting pancreatic exocrine insufficiency. When bentiromide (500 mg) is given orally, it normally is acted on by pancreatic chymotrypsin to produce para-aminobenzoic acid, which is absorbed by the small bowel and excreted in the urine. In normal persons, greater than 50% is excreted in 6 hours. This test appears to have a sensitivity of 80% and a specificity of 90% for exocrine insufficiency. A trial of pancreatic enzyme replacement may be valuable diagnostically.

When significant uncertainty persists, direct pancreatic function tests, such as secretin stimulation, may be needed to demonstrate exocrine insufficiency objectively. A small group of patients with pancreatic insufficiency who do not give a history of alcoholism or recurrent abdominal pain should be evaluated for hemochromatosis and cystic fibrosis.

PRINCIPLES OF MANAGEMENT

Acute Pancreatitis. About 50% of patients have mild self-limited disease and will recover spontaneously. Such patients with mild pain and no vomiting may be treated on an ambulatory basis with restriction of fat and protein and careful monitoring. Patients with more severe disease who require hospitalization generally tolerate a full diet before discharge from the hospital, although a *diet moderately restricted in fat* is often recommended to lessen the degree of pancreatic stimulation. *H2-receptor antagonists, antacids,* and *anticholinergics* are frequently given with the hope of reducing the stimulus to pancreatic secretion but are of no proven benefit. A patient who returns with severe pain and vomiting should be readmitted.

Identification and treatment or removal of precipitants, such as alcohol abuse, hypercalcemia, gallstones, and hypertriglyceridemia, are essential to successful therapy. Of the conditions associated with pancreatitis, alcoholism is the most difficult to deal with. Even the pain of pancreatitis often does not dissuade the dedicated drinker from abusing alcohol. Nevertheless, the *treatment of alcoholism* should be undertaken with considerable effort (see Chapter 228), because there is much to gain by the cessation of drinking. A check for drugs associated with pancreatitis is indicated (thiazides, corticosteroids, estrogens, azathioprine). In the *HIV-infected patient,* treatment of potentially etiologic opportunistic infections (e.g., toxoplasmosis, cytomegalovirus) and elimination of inciting medications (e.g., didanosine, pentamidine, sulfonamides, corticosteroids) are priorities in addition to the standard approaches to treatment.

All patients should undergo evaluation of the biliary tract by *ultrasonography* to rule out gallstone disease, a treatable cause of pancreatitis. However, in acute pancreatitis, early stone removal by *endoscopy retrograde cholangiopancreatography* in the absence of obstructive jaundice is no better than conservative therapy and fraught with more serious complications. After an acute episode, the serum calcium should be repeated, because *hypercalcemia* can be masked by the decrease in calcium that may result from an attack. Repeatedly marked elevations in *fasting triglyceride* concentration suggest the diagnosis of hypertriglyceridemia, which responds to gemfibrozil (see Chapter 27).

Chronic Pancreatitis. Patients with chronic pancreatitis may develop recurrent bouts of pain and vomiting indistinguishable from acute pancreatitis. Those with severe pain and inability to maintain hydration orally should be admitted. Others with less severe exacerbations may be managed on an outpatient basis. Many are bothered by chronic pain.

Initial treatment consists of eliminating causative factors (see above) and attempting to control the often disabling *pain.* Pancreatic enzymes and low-fat diets may decrease pancreatic secretion but do not reliably lessen the pain. Nonnarcotic analgesics (aspirin, ibuprofen, acetaminophen) should be tried but are usually inadequate, necessitating use of more potent agents. *Methadone* and *sustained-release morphine* are the narcotics best suited for long-term outpatient use. Sometimes, *tricyclic antidepressants* are useful adjuncts for pain control (see Chapter 227). The establishment of a *supportive doctor–patient relationship* complements pharmacologic pain control efforts.

Numerous *surgical procedures* have been designed to alleviate the pain of chronic pancreatitis; none is totally effective. Patients with persistent pain in the absence of gallbladder disease or alcoholism should have an endoscopic *retrograde pancreatogram* to search for a surgically treatable anatomic abnormality, such as pancreas divisum. If a markedly dilated duct is found, a modified *Puestow sphincteroplasty procedure* can be performed to improve drainage of pancreatic juices into the small bowel. The operation may provide reasonable pain relief without removal of pancreatic tissue. Large persistent pseudocysts should be drained internally; however, reduction in pain is not consistently achieved. Sometimes partial or even subtotal pancreatectomies are attempted for control of pain; at best, results are equivocal.

In patients with severe active disease, the pancreas is progressively destroyed, and eventually the pain subsides as the disease "burns" itself out. Then the management priority shifts to treatment of pancreatic insufficiency.

Pancreatic Insufficiency. Management of pancreatic insufficiency begins with a therapeutic trial of oral pancreatic enzymes to judge efficacy of therapy. The patient who benefits from use of exogenous enzymes will tolerate the unpleasant taste and mild discomfort they cause. *Pancreatin* contains trypsin, amylase, and some lipase, whereas *pancrealipase* contains trypsin, amylase, and extra amounts of lipase. The usual dose is 0.5 to 2.5 g with each meal. Because enzyme preparations are partially inactivated by gastric acid or require increased alkalinity in the duodenum, they may work better when given with antacids, bicarbonate, or H2-receptor antagonists. *Medium-chain triglycerides* are often helpful because they can be absorbed in the absence of lipase. Therapy can be assessed by monitoring symptoms, weight, and qualitative stool fat determinations. Clinically significant fat-soluble vitamin deficiencies are uncommon, perhaps because intact bile secretion prevents complete fat malabsorption.

Most patients with chronic pancreatitis have abnormal glucose tolerance tests. Mild glucose intolerance can be watched, but insulin dependence may occur. Hypoglycemia may be a problem, because loss of glucagon secretion leads to a "brittle" diabetic state, but ketoacidosis is rare. The vascular complications of diabetes are infrequent but eventually occur if severe pancreatic insufficiency persists.

PATIENT EDUCATION

Most patients know little about the pancreas and its role in digestion. Moreover, few are aware of the connection between alcohol abuse and pancreatitis. Patient cooperation regarding diet, alcohol intake, and use of enzyme extracts may be facilitated by a better understanding of the function of the pancreas and the nature of pancreatitis. Also, patients with acute pancreatitis who are making good recoveries can be comforted by the fact that recurrence is not common when the underlying cause is treated.

The patient with intractable pain and narcotic dependence poses one of the most difficult problems encountered in clinical medicine. A major pitfall is the development of an adversarial relationship between patient and physician concerning the need for narcotics. Although there are no simple solutions, it is essential to elicit, understand, and respond to patient concerns, fears, and needs at the outset. A well-informed patient who has confidence in the physician and in him- or herself requires less pain medication than one who is scared, feels abandoned, and is in conflict with the physician.

INDICATIONS FOR ADMISSION AND REFERRAL

Some patients present with rather mild symptoms but later develop a fulminant illness. Patients over age 55 are at risk for a serious progression, as are those who manifest fever, tachycardia, hyperglycemia, serum calcium below 8.0 mg/dL, or amylase over 1,000 mg/dL at the time of initial presentation. Such individuals deserve admission for careful monitoring, even if they do not appear seriously ill at the outset. Patients who cannot maintain oral hydration also require admission. Patients with refractory pain might benefit from evaluation by a gastroenterologist skilled in endoscopic retrograde pancreatography. Surgical consultation is indicated if an anatomic abnormality, pseudocyst, or obstructive lesion is detected on workup of the pancreas and biliary tract. Patients with chronic refractory pain may benefit from a psychiatric or pain management assessment, supplemented by tricyclic antidepressant therapy.

MANAGEMENT RECOMMENDATIONS

Recovery Phase of Acute Pancreatitis

- Begin feedings with foods rich in carbohydrates and low in protein and fat. Gradually increase the amount of protein in the diet as tolerated, followed by slow resumption of fat intake.
- Check for and treat any underlying alcohol abuse (see Chapter 228), hypertriglyceridemia (see Chapter 27), or hypercalcemia (see Chapter 96).
- Eliminate, if possible, use of drugs associated with pancreatitis (azathioprine, estrogens, thiazides, corticosteroids). In the HIV-infected patient, check for and treat any toxoplasmosis or cytomegalovirus infection and eliminate any potentially inciting medication (e.g., didanosine, pentamidine, sulfonamides, corticosteroids).
- Obtain ultrasound examination of the gallbladder and biliary tract; refer the patient for consideration of surgery if stones are found. There is no benefit to early endoscopic retrograde cholangiopancreatography and stone removal in persons with biliary pancreatitis who are not jaundiced.

Chronic Pancreatitis

- Check for and treat any inciting cause, such as alcoholism, biliary tract disease, hypercalcemia, or hyperlipidemia (see above).
- Readmit the patient if severe recurrent acute pancreatitis develops.
- Temporarily limit fat intake during flare-ups.
- Begin with mild analgesics for pain control, such as aspirin or acetaminophen 600 mg every 4 hours.
- Pain unrelieved by mild analgesia is an indication for a course of narcotic analgesics, such as methadone 5 or 10 mg every 6 or 8 hours.
- Further evaluation is needed to rule out carcinoma, pseudocyst, and biliary tract disease. Begin with ultrasonography and proceed to CT if ultrasonography is technically unsatisfactory.
- Refer the patient for surgery if a treatable lesion is found.
- Aggressive surgical procedures other than sphincteroplasty aimed at relieving ductal obstruction do not reliably relieve pain.

- Consider a trial of tricyclic antidepressant therapy (see Chapter 227) for patients with refractory pain. Psychiatric or pain management consultation may also help.

Pancreatic Insufficiency

- Give oral pancreatic extract with each feeding in doses of 0.5 to 2.5 g (two to eight tablets) with full meals and 0.5 g with snacks. Lack of effect may require addition of an antacid (e.g., 60 mL of Mylanta with each meal) or H_2-receptor antagonist (e.g., ranitidine, 150 mg twice daily) to neutralize gastric acid and prevent enzymes from becoming inactivated.
- Provide a high-calorie diet rich in carbohydrate and protein.
- Supplement the diet with a medium-chain triglyceride preparation. Restrict fat in symptomatic steatorrhea.
- Monitor glucose tolerance and treat clinical diabetes, if present, with insulin, cautiously; these patients often exhibit brittle disease.

ANNOTATED BIBLIOGRAPHY

Agarwal N, Pitchumoni CS, Sivaprasad AV. Evaluating tests for acute pancreatitis. Am J Gastroenterol 1990;85:356. (*Current analysis of serologic and imaging studies.*)

Ammann RW, Akobintz A, Largiader F, et al. Course and outcome of chronic pancreatitis: a longitudinal study of a mixed medical-surgical series of 245 patients. Gastroenterology 1984;86:820. (*Excellent clinical course/natural history study.*)

Bank S, Marks IN, Vinik AI. Clinical and hormonal aspects of pancreatic diabetes. Am J Gastroenterol 1975;64:13. (*Classic clinical description of pancreatic diabetes, its therapy, and its distinctive properties.*)

Baron TH, Morgan DE. The diagnosis and management of fluid collections associated with pancreatitis. Am J Med 1997;102:555. (*A discussion of the management of pseudocysts and peripancreatic fluid collections.*)

Dassopoulos T, Ehrenpreis ED. Acute pancreatitis in human immunodeficiency virus-infected patients: A review. Am J Med 1999;107:78. (*Excellent review for the generalist reader; 102 references.*)

Folsch UR, Nitsche R, Ludtke R, et al. Early ERCP and papillototomy compared with conservative treatment for acute biliary pancreatitis. N Engl J Med 1997;336:237. (*In those without obstructive jaundice, early ERCP and papillotomy was fraught with more severe complications and no improvement in outcomes compared with conservative therapy.*)

Gress F, Schmitt C, Sherman S, et al. A prospective randomized comparison of endoscopic ultrasound- and computed tomography–guided celiac plexus block for managing chronic pancreatitis pain. Am J Gastroenterol 1999;94:900. (*Celiac block can be helpful in some patients with severe chronic pain.*)

Karasawa E, Goldberg HI, Moss AA, et al. CT pancreatogram in carcinoma of the pancreas and chronic pancreatitis. Radiology 1983;148:489. (*Irregular calcified ducts are characteristic of chronic pancreatitis, whereas in pancreatic cancer, smooth or beaded dilatation is the most frequent finding.*)

Kemppainen EA, Hedstrom JI, Puolakkainen PA, et al. Rapid measurement of urinary trypsinogen-2 as a screening test for acute pancreatitis. N Engl J Med 1997;336:1788. (*A negative test had a high negative-predictive value; a positive test required further confirmation.*)

Lowenfels AB, Maisonneuve D, Cavallini G, et al. Pancreatitis and the risk of pancreatic cancer. N Engl J Med 1993;328:1433. *(An association found.)*

Lowenfels AB, Maisonneuve P, Cavallini G, et al. Prognosis of chronic pancreatitis: an international multicenter study. Am J Gastroenterol 1994;89:1467. *(Age at diagnosis, smoking, and continued drinking were the key prognostic factors.)*

Mallory A, Kern F Jr. Drug-induced pancreatitis: a critical review. Gastroenterology 1980;78:813. *(Useful paper that includes how to separate the presumptive from the definite.)*

Moosa AR. Surgical treatment of chronic pancreatitis: an overview. Br J Surg 1987;74:661. *(Excellent review of the data on surgical approaches to the problem.)*

Niederau C, Grendell JH. Diagnosis of chronic pancreatitis. Gastroenterology 1985;88:1973. *(This remains an excellent comprehensive review of biochemical and imaging approaches to the diagnosis of chronic pancreatitis; 247 references.)*

Pitchumoni CS, Agarwal N, Jain NK. Systemic complications of acute pancreatitis. Am J Gastroenterol 1988;83:597. *(Best available review.)*

Richter JM, Schapiro RH, Mulley AG, et al. Association of pancreatitis and its treatment by sphincteroplasty of the accessory ampulla. Gastroenterology 1981;81:1104. *(Patients with pancreas divisum develop recurrent acute pancreatitis more frequently than people with normal anatomy.)*

Sachdeva CK, Bank S, Greenberg R, et al. Fluctuations in serum amylase in patients with macroamylasemia. Am J Gastroenterol 1995;90:800. *(An important cause of hyperamylasemia in the absence of pancreatitis.)*

Steer ML, Waxman I, Freedman S. Chronic pancreatitis. N Engl J Med 1995;332:1482. *(Comprehensive review.)*

Steinberg W, Tenner S. Acute pancreatitis. N Engl J Med 1995;332:1198. *(Best current review.)*

Steinberg WM, Goldstein SS, Davis SS, et al. Diagnostic assays in acute pancreatitis. Ann Intern Med 1985;102:576. *(Compares sensitivity and specificity of amylase, lipase, trypsinogen, and amylase isoenzymes; recommends use of amylase as the initial study.)*

Toskes P. Bentiromide as a test of exocrine function in adults with pancreatic exocrine insufficiency. Determination of appropriate dose of urinary collection interval. Gastroenterology 1983;85:565. *(Standardization of the bentiromide test as a simple outpatient test for pancreatic insufficiency.)*

Twersky Y, Bank S. Nutritional deficiencies in chronic pancreatitis. Gastroenterol Clin North Am 1989;18:543. *(Thorough and useful discussion of the problem and its management.)*

Van Dyke JA, Stanley RJ, Berland LL. Pancreatic imaging. Ann Intern Med 1985;102:212. *(Critical review of CT, ultrasound, and other imaging techniques; considers CT the best initial study, because ultrasonography often compromised by overlying bowel gas; 50 references.)*

Warshaw AL, Banks PA, Fernandez-Del Castillo, C. AGA technical review: treatment of pain in chronic pancreatitis. Gastroenterology 1998;115;765. *(A current review of the medical and surgical management of chronic pancreatitis.)*

73

Management of Inflammatory Bowel Disease

JAMES M. RICHTER

Ulcerative colitis and Crohn's disease account for most inflammatory bowel disease seen in primary care practice. Abdominal pain, diarrhea, and bleeding are among the presenting manifestations. The first priority is to distinguish inflammatory bowel disease from other causes of diarrhea (see Chapter 64). The chronicity, potentially disabling symptoms, risk of malignancy (in the case of ulcerative colitis), and occasional refractoriness to medical therapy make management a major challenge. The primary care physician needs to know how to treat exacerbations, maintain remissions, and psychologically sustain these patients through difficult times. Competent care is based on a thorough understanding of the roles for medical and surgical therapy and skill in providing psychological support. Although patients with severe or refractory disease may need to be referred to the gastroenterologist, most others can be well managed by the primary care physician.

PATHOPHYSIOLOGY, CLINICAL PRESENTATION, AND COURSE

Ulcerative Colitis

Ulcerative colitis is an idiopathic diffuse inflammatory disease of the *bowel mucosa*. Although pathogenesis remains poorly understood, there is growing evidence of a primary immune mechanism (e.g., high prevalence of antibodies to intestinal epithelial antigens in asymptomatic relatives of patients and in patients themselves). The disease typically begins in adolescence or young adulthood but may occur at almost any age. Whites are affected more often than African-Americans. Prevalence is highest among Jews of Eastern European descent, and there is a 10-fold increase in risk for having the disease among first-degree relatives of patients.

Clinical Presentation. The cardinal symptoms are *bloody diarrhea* and *abdominal pain*; in severe cases, *fever, anorexia,* and *weight loss* are present as well. The variability of presentations is remarkable, ranging from malaise and no symptoms referable to the colon, to fever, prostration, abdominal distention, and passage of large volumes of liquid stool. The disease need not be confined to the bowel; extracolonic manifestations include *arthritis, uveitis, jaundice,* and *skin lesions*. The course is characteristically chronic, recurrent, and unpredictable. An insidious presentation does not predict a benign course, and a fulminant onset may be followed by long relatively asymptomatic periods.

Ulcerative colitis almost always involves the *distal colon* and *rectum*, making diagnosis possible by sigmoidoscopy. The mucosa becomes edematous, obscuring the fine network of submucosal vessels. The moist glistening mucosal surface is lost, and a *granular* appearance develops. The bowel wall is friable, bleeding spontaneously or when touched with a swab.

In advanced cases, *pseudopolyps* and discrete *ulcers* may be seen. Smears of mucus from the bowel wall show polymorphonuclear leukocytes. Barium enema documents the extent of disease. Radiologic findings range from mucosal denudation to frank ulceration, with loss of haustral markings and a tubular appearance. There are *no skip areas*. Liver involvement occurs in the form of *pericholangitis* and *fatty infiltration*; these are common histologic findings in ulcerative colitis but are seldom symptomatic. Much less frequently, *chronic active hepatitis, cirrhosis,* or sclerosing *cholangitis* is seen. A migratory *monoarticular arthritis* affecting the large joints develops in 10% of patients. This arthritis often coincides with an exacerbation of colitis and resolves with control of the underlying disease. *Ankylosing spondylitis* also occurs but runs a course independent of the colitis. Uveitis or episcleritis may be seen at any time during the course of the disease. *Erythema nodosum, pyoderma gangrenosum,* or *oral aphthous ulcerations* are found in about 5% of patients, usually during active colitis.

Course. The prognosis for patients with ulcerative colitis seen in the primary care setting is far better than that for patients studied in referral centers who are likely to have more severe disease. Long-term community-based studies find that nearly 90% go into complete remission after the first attack and less than 10% develop chronic persistent disease. Among those with chronic disease, nearly three fourths have disease limited to the distal bowel (rectum or rectosigmoid). Overall mortality in community-based populations of ulcerative colitis patients is no different from that of the general population, although it is increased in patients with severe first attacks or extensive disease.

There is an increased *risk of cancer* that correlates with the extent and duration of disease and age at diagnosis. Risk begins to increase substantially after 8 years of illness. Absolute risk of colon cancer in the setting of pancolitis has been found to be 30% after 35 years from time of diagnosis. Those with pancolitis diagnosed before the age of 15 manifest an absolute risk of 40%. These figures are slightly lower than traditional risk estimates of 1% to 2% per year derived from referral center cohorts.

Ulcerative Proctitis

Typically, the patient with ulcerative proctitis is a young adult who presents with rectal bleeding and tenesmus. The bleeding is usually not severe; it is sometimes mistakenly attributed to hemorrhoids. Diarrhea or constipation may accompany the bleeding, but often there are only small frequent bowel movements associated with a small amount of mucus. On sigmoidoscopy, an edematous friable rectal mucosa is observed; the bowel above the rectosigmoid is uninvolved. On barium enema or colonoscopy, the remainder of the large bowel is normal. The clinical presentation of ulcerative proctitis is not pathognomonic; the condition must be distinguished from infectious forms of proctocolitis, including AIDS-related etiologies (see Chapters 13 and 66).

Ulcerative proctitis is a variant of ulcerative colitis, distinguished by the limited extent of inflammation, its good prognosis, and paucity of serious complications. However, relapses are common. Fewer than 15% progress to generalized ulcerative colitis. The distant complications of ulcerative colitis are rare, and carcinoma of the rectum develops no more often than in unaffected individuals.

Crohn's Disease

Pathophysiology. Crohn's disease is a chronic relapsing inflammatory disorder of the alimentary tract that appears to have an autoimmune pathophysiology. There are high levels of selected T-cell populations and high prevalence of antibodies to intestinal epithelial antigens in patients and in their asymptomatic relatives. Of therapeutic interest is the role of inflammatory mediators. T helper cells in the bowel mucosa of patients with Crohn's disease appear to produce increased amounts of tumor necrosis factor-α. Infusion of monoclonal antibodies directed against these cytokines can produce remission of otherwise refractory disease (see below). Other potentially important cytokines include interleukin-12 and interferon-γ. There may also be inadequate production of counter-regulatory substances. Pathologically, the distribution of bowel inflammation is *discontinuous*, with diseased segments of bowel separated by normal areas. Because the granulomatous inflammatory process may extend through *all layers* of the bowel wall, it has a tendency to cause *strictures, fistulas,* and *abscesses*.

Clinical Presentation. Peak incidence is in the second and third decades. The condition often affects the distal ileum and right colon, but frequently it involves only the small bowel or colon. It may occur in any portion of the alimentary tract, from the buccal mucosa to the anus. Extraintestinal involvement occurs in 15% to 20% of cases, with *arthritis, ankylosing spondylitis, uveitis, erythema nodosum, aphthous oral ulcers,* and *pyoderma gangrenosum* being the predominant manifestations of disease outside the bowel. In addition, *cholelithiasis* and *nephrolithiasis* have a higher incidence in these patients than in the general population.

Symptoms vary, depending on the location and extent of disease. *Diarrhea* and *abdominal pain* (particularly in the right lower quadrant) are cardinal symptoms, occurring in almost 80% of patients. *Weight loss, vomiting, fever, perianal discomfort,* and *bleeding* are also common complaints. *Constipation* may be an early manifestation of obstruction. Symptoms can develop subtly or can present in fulminant fashion with the patient systemically toxic.

Physical examination may reveal a discrete abdominal mass, especially in the right lower quadrant, but usually a normal abdomen or doughy loops of bowel are found. Abdominal or perianal fistulous tracts are noted on examination in up to 10% of patients. Extraintestinal findings include inflamed joints, spinal deformities, erythema nodosum, pyoderma, uveitis, and aphthous ulcers.

Sigmoidoscopy is abnormal in fewer than 20% of cases; fistulous tracts and discrete inflammatory ulcers are sometimes encountered in the rectosigmoid. *Barium enema and upper gastrointestinal series* often show segmental involvement of large and small bowel, often with strictures, fistulas, and ulcers. The primary abnormality in Crohn's disease is submucosal, causing radiologic studies to sometimes appear normal. In such cases, *colonoscopy* aids diagnosis by demonstrating segmental disease and ulceration that may be missed on barium enema.

Prognosis. Although it is difficult to extrapolate from referral center data to patients seen in primary care settings, a pattern emerges of disease activity that waxes and wanes over many years. Disease-free intervals may last as long as several years or even decades, but recurrences are the rule. Several years of relief from symptoms may be afforded by surgical resection, but there is no evidence that any medical and surgical therapy alters the ultimate course of the illness. In referral center series, as many as 70% of patients ultimately require surgical resection.

WORKUP

Proper management requires confirming the diagnosis and determining the extent of disease. One proviso should be kept in mind: Because these illnesses often occur in women of childbearing age, attempts should be made to minimize their x-ray exposure and carefully select only the most necessary radiologic studies.

Ulcerative Colitis

Diagnosis. The diagnosis is usually based on the clinical presentation, sigmoidoscopic demonstration of inflammation, and the exclusion of bacterial and parasitic infections by culture and examination for ova and parasites (see Chapter 64). Because the disease almost invariably affects the distal colon and rectum, *sigmoidoscopy* is an essential component of the workup. The procedure is best performed without cleansing preparations, so as not to distort the appearance of the bowel mucosa (see Appendix in Chapter 56). In acute phases of the illness, the mucosa appears *friable* and inflamed; there is loss of the normal vascular pattern. As the disease progresses, a *purulent exudate* and discrete small *ulcers* may form. With severe colitis, there may be pus and spontaneous bleeding and large ulcers. Chronic phases of the disease are characterized by a granular mucosa and inflammatory *pseudopolyps* (tags of damaged mucosa and granulation tissue).

When the sigmoidoscopic picture is nonspecific, one should *culture* and examine the stool for *Clostridium difficile, Entamoeba histolytica, Campylobacter, Shigella, Salmonella,* and *Neisseria gonorrhea* (see Chapters 64 and 66). Rectal biopsy is indicated when one needs to confirm the diagnosis and exclude conditions such as Crohn's disease of the rectosigmoid, amoebic colitis, pseudomembranous colitis, cytomegalovirus infection, and herpetic pancolitis. *Barium enema* or *colonoscopy* can be used to provide supportive evidence when the diagnosis is in doubt and helps document the extent of disease. However, they should not be performed during a flare-up because there is a small risk of perforation when the procedure is performed on an acutely inflamed bowel.

Estimating Disease Activity and Severity. The appearance of the bowel mucosa on *colonoscopy* remains the mainstay of assessment of disease activity. Scoring systems based on clinical parameters are sometimes used in research settings but have little utility in clinical practice. A host of radionuclide imaging methods has been tried, but they lack specificity. Disease severity is defined more clinically. *Mild disease* is defined as less than four bowel movements a day and no signs of toxicity (i.e., no fever, tachycardia, anemia, or elevation of sedimentation rate). *Moderate disease* is characterized by four or more bowel movements a day plus minimal toxicity. *Severe disease* is manifested by six or more bowel movements a day and/or signs of toxicity.

Crohn's Disease

Diagnosis. Crohn's disease of the colon may mimic ulcerative colitis clinically. Differentiating features include *skip areas* in the colon, significant *small bowel* involvement, *fistulas*, and *granulomas* on biopsy. The diagnosis is suggested by a history of recurrent postprandial lower abdominal pain and altered bowel habits in a young person; it is reinforced by finding on physical examination a mass or tenderness in the right lower quadrant. Radiologic contrast studies are needed for a more definitive assessment. The small bowel phase of an upper gastrointestinal series shows *segmental narrowing*, areas with loss of the normal mucosal pattern interspersed with areas of normal mucosa, fistula formation, and the *"string sign"* (a narrow band of barium flowing through an inflamed or scarred area) in the terminal ileum.

Colonic disease may be documented by *air contrast barium enema*, with asymmetric segmental changes distinguishing Crohn's disease of the large bowel from ulcerative colitis. Disease of the terminal ileum can often be detected on barium enema; however, radiologic involvement of the terminal ileum is not unique to Crohn's disease. Some ulcerative colitis patients also demonstrate inflammatory changes in the terminal ileum ("backwash ileitis"), but they lack the skip pattern characteristic of Crohn's disease.

Sigmoidoscopy demonstrates rectosigmoid inflammation in the 20% to 50% of patients with disease in this area; however, the findings are often nonspecific (mild erythema). *Colonoscopy* is needed in difficult cases and helps in judging the extent and severity of disease. *Biopsy* can be diagnostic but is usually unnecessary unless the diagnosis remains unsubstantiated; it should be avoided when acute inflammation is present.

Estimating Disease Activity and Severity. Disease activity in the colon is best assessed by *colonoscopy* and in the small bowel by *barium contrast study*. Disease severity is categorized clinically. *Mild-to-moderate disease* is defined as having symptoms but functioning adequately on an ambulatory basis, maintaining oral intake of food and fluids, and showing no signs of toxicity or complications. In *moderate-to-severe disease*, symptoms are more severe, sometimes interfering with daily activity and not responding fully to treatment. In *severe disease*, there may be toxicity, complications, and failure to respond to full doses of oral corticosteroids.

PRINCIPLES OF MANAGEMENT

The inflammatory bowel diseases are chronic illnesses that require long-term comprehensive management. Such management entails attention to the patient's medical, psychological, and nutritional needs and support for the family. For the most part, treatment is empirical and directed at providing symptomatic relief; however advances in the understanding of inflammatory bowel disease pathophysiology are leading to a host of new treatments that have the potential to improve treatment outcomes.

Ulcerative Colitis

Because the disease typically follows a relapsing course with acute exacerbations and intervals of remission, the approach to treatment depends on the patient's current clinical status. During remission, treatment is prophylactic; during flare-ups, the goal is control of the inflammatory process. Surgery is a consideration for those with refractory disease, especially when it is widespread.

Dietary and Nutritional Measures. No specific diet improves or exacerbates ulcerative colitis. However, reduction in dietary *fiber* may be of some benefit during periods of active disease. In patients with inactive disease, 1 or 2 teaspoons of *psyllium* hydrophilic colloid (Metamucil) in water daily often helps to bind the stool. There is an increased incidence of lactase deficiency in these patients; an empirical trial of a *milk-free diet* is reasonable when diarrhea persists despite other evidence of clinical remission. Those who are anemic from blood loss need oral or parenteral *iron* supplementation (see Chapter 82). Oral iron may be poorly tolerated, necessitating parenteral administration. Anemia may also be due to folic acid deficiency. *Folic acid* supplementation is indicated when intake of leafy vegetables and fresh fruits is poor or when sulfasalazine is being taken (see below). Anemia may also be due to chronic disease and may not respond to dietary and nutritional measures.

Sulfasalazine. The drug is recommended as initial treatment for mild to moderate disease and for prevention of relapses. After oral administration, about 70% reaches the colon, where it is metabolized by intestinal bacteria, resulting in the local release of sulfapyridine and the salicylate analogue *5-aminosalicylate (5-ASA)*, which is believed to be the active moiety. Sulfasalazine's precise mechanism of action remains speculative. Hypotheses include effects on prostaglandin synthesis (particularly arachidonic acid metabolism) and inhibition of migration of polymorphonuclear leukocytes.

Efficacy. Randomized controlled studies have shown the drug to be effective as *initial treatment* for patients with mild to moderate symptoms when given in doses of 4 g/d for 2 to 4 weeks. About 80% of patients respond. Because sulfasalazine is less effective than corticosteroid therapy, it is reserved for relatively mild cases; however, combined use with steroids has been suggested for early treatment of severe disease.

Controlled studies have also documented the drug's efficacy for *prophylaxis* and maintaining remissions. In one major study, more than 65% of patients given maintenance doses of 2 g/d remained symptom-free for at least 1 year compared with 25% of patients given placebo. The prophylactic effect of maintenance therapy persists when the drug is continued beyond 1 year. The optimum dose is 2 g/d (4 g/d provides even better protection, but the frequency of side effects is markedly increased).

Adverse Effects. Sulfasalazine is usually well tolerated (being safe enough to use during pregnancy and when breastfeeding), but up to 20% experience adverse effects, mostly due to the sulfapyridine moiety. These range from common forms of dose-related gastrointestinal upset (*nausea, vomiting, anorexia, heartburn*) and mild *hypersensitivity* reactions (*rash, fever*) to uncommon but potentially serious idiosyncratic reactions such as *agranulocytosis, hepatocellular injury, and lupuslike phenomena*. Patients unable to tolerate full doses of sulfasalazine because of gastrointestinal upset often do better when reintro-

duced to the drug more gradually. Taking it with meals also helps. Other potential hematopoietic effects include *anemia* (from folic acid deficiency, hemolysis, or marrow suppression), *granulocytopenia*, and *thrombocytopenia*. *Low sperm counts* and qualitative sperm abnormalities have been noted in men taking the drug, usually after about 2 months of therapy; these conditions reverse when the medication is stopped. *Desensitization* (starting with fractions of a tablet and slowly advancing over 2 to 4 weeks to therapeutic doses) can overcome minor allergic reactions (rash, fever), but most often sulfa-intolerant patients are now switched to a sulfa-free 5-ASA preparation (see below).

Drug interactions associated with sulfasalazine include inhibition of *folic acid* absorption (usually not clinically significant) and a 25% reduction in *digoxin* bioavailability. Sulfasalazine's metabolism is slowed when *cholestyramine* or *broad-spectrum antibiotics* are used concurrently, an effect of uncertain clinical significance. *Ferrous sulfate* appears to have a similar effect on sulfasalazine, although iron absorption is not appreciably hindered; these drugs should not be taken at the same time. Because of the risk of neutropenia, any concurrent use with azathioprine or 6-mercaptopurine (6-MP) requires extreme caution and close monitoring.

Sulfapyridine-free 5-Aminosalicylate Agents. These agents were developed to provide a sulfapyridine-free means of delivering 5-ASA to affect bowel and in doing so eliminate most the adverse effects seen with sulfasalazine. The first developed was *olsalazine*, which is just two 5-ASA molecules bound by an azo bond that is cleaved by bacteria in the colon, releasing the active 5-ASA moiety. It is useful for achieving control of mild-to-moderate disease and for maintaining remissions. Diarrhea is the most common side effect, is dose related, and is diminished by increasing dose gradually and by giving the drug with meals.

Mesalamine is 5-ASA specially coated to produce delayed release. The oral tablet formulation (Asacol) dissolves at a pH of 7, the lumenal pH of the terminal ileum and colon. The methylcellulose capsule formulation (Pentasa) releases 5-ASA into the small bowel and the colon. In controlled trials, oral 5-ASA agents perform at least as well as sulfasalazine in the treatment of active mild-to-moderate ulcerative colitis and in maintaining remissions. Benefit appears to be dose related. Side effects are nil, but 5-ASA–related interstitial nephritis (seen in animal studies and case reports) is a concern with long-term high-dose use. Idiosyncratic reactions include pleuropericarditis, pancreatitis, and nephrotic syndrome. Those with very active disease should probably take mesalamine with meals if they note that the coated tablet is being passed undissolved, because taking the pill with food can slow transit and allow more time for dissolution.

Although these oral 5-ASA agents appear better tolerated than sulfasalazine, they are considerably more expensive. Nonetheless, patients who do not tolerate sulfasalazine deserve a trial of a sulfapyridine-free agent.

Topical 5-ASA enemas were also developed as an alternative to sulfasalazine and represent a reasonable option in patients with distal colitis. At maximum dose, they are more effective than hydrocortisone enemas and useful for persons with mild-to-moderate disease limited to the distal large bowel. Relapse is common with cessation of enema therapy; however, unlike hydrocortisone enemas, a maintenance program (alternate-day dosing) of topical 5-ASA therapy helps to maintain remission. The safety profile is excellent; adverse effects are nil other than idiosyncratic reactions, and the only common side effects are local itching and mild rectal irritation. Cost is considerably higher than that of a hydrocortisone enema. However, unlike steroid enemas, there is no concern about systemic steroid absorption.

Glucocorticosteroids. Steroids suppress the inflammatory process of ulcerative colitis and have important roles both as systemic agents in severe disease and as topical agents in disease confined to the rectosigmoid. When uveitis and colitis flare simultaneously, oral steroids are often effective for both. (In the absence of active colitis, the uveitis may be treated with topical steroids and mydriatics.) The best means of treating other systemic manifestations (erythema nodosum, pyoderma gangrenosum, oral aphthous ulcerations) is to control the underlying disease with systemic steroids. Patients with severe disease requiring daily steroids should receive calcium and vitamin D supplementation, because absorption may be impaired.

Systemic preparations are used in moderate-to-severe and severe disease, especially in markedly symptomatic patients with extensive bowel involvement. Those without systemic toxicity can be treated on an outpatient basis starting with the equivalent of 60 mg/d of *prednisone*. Patients too ill for oral therapy (i.e., those with vomiting, high fever, or signs of bowel distention) should be admitted to the hospital. Once symptoms lessen, steroids are gradually tapered over 4 to 8 weeks to the lowest dose that maintains control. Whenever possible, every effort should be made to taper and terminate systemic steroid therapy, both because only some ulcerative colitis patients benefit from chronic steroid use and because the adverse effects of chronic steroid therapy can be disabling (see Chapter 105). *Alternate-day* steroid administration often suffices after a flare-up has been brought under control and poses much less risk of steroid side effects. Newer corticosteroids with fewer systemic effects are under development. The best studied is a slow-release oral preparation of *budesonide*, which provides release in the colon with minimal systemic side effects.

Topical preparations are useful for disease confined to the rectosigmoid area. *Hydrocortisone* enemas as widely prescribed and effective, but prolonged high-dose use can lead to systemic steroid side effects (some hydrocortisone does get absorbed). The topically active steroid *beclomethasone* has been found equally efficacious to topical hydrocortisone but with less systemic absorption and no effect on serum cortisol levels; however, cost is greater.

Immunosuppressive Agents. Patients who require chronic high-dose steroid therapy might benefit from a trial of steroid-sparing immunosuppressive therapy with *6-MP* or *azathioprine*. Because onset of action can be slow (up to 6 months), concurrent therapy with a second agent is necessary until the drug's effect sets it. Side effects are less frequent than with systemic steroids, but these can be serious (see below). Intravenous administration of *cyclosporine* is sometimes used in very ill patients not responding to intravenous steroids. Results from controlled trials are variable and risk of toxicity is high.

Opiates are useful for providing symptomatic relief of diarrhea during acute phases of illness and chronic active colitis.

They must be used with caution in acutely ill patients because of the risk of precipitating *toxic dilatation*. Diphenoxylate, codeine, tincture of opium, paregoric, and loperamide all limit the number of bowel movements. They are given before meals and at bedtime. *Loperamide* is among the most effective and least addicting but is considerably more expensive. *Codeine* is excellent for short-term use and superior to diphenoxylate in efficacy. *Tincture of belladonna* and other anticholinergics help to control cramps.

Psychological Support. Although psychological disturbances are more prevalent in patients with inflammatory bowel disease than in control subjects, there is little evidence that psychiatric disease is etiologically linked to the development of ulcerative colitis. However, recent data suggest a correlation between stress, immunologic dysfunction, and onset of symptoms. Formal psychotherapy directed at uncovering intrapsychic conflict has not proven useful, but a close, supportive, and empathetic patient–doctor relationship is invaluable to psychologically sustaining the patient through this illness (see below). Fears and worries about debility, surgery, colostomy, and body image contribute markedly to the psychosocial impairment and disability associated with this illness.

Surgery. Total colectomy offers the potential for complete cure of bowel disease and remission of most peripheral manifestations. As such, it represents an important therapeutic consideration, albeit a difficult one. Indications include *high-grade dysplasia, suspected cancer*, and *unresponsiveness* of bowel or systemic symptoms to maximal medical management. Patients with severe persistent disease requiring continuous *high-dose corticosteroids* that cannot be tapered after 6 to 12 months also warrant serious consideration for surgery, as do those with frequent severe *relapses* or *complications* from prolonged exposure to systemic steroids.

The traditional procedure is *proctocolectomy with Brooke ileostomy*. It has the advantage of being the fastest and safest procedure. The disadvantages of an ileostomy include incontinence, need to frequently empty an external ileostomy appliance, skin excoriations, and potential need for stomal revision (in about 10% to 20%). *Total proctocolectomy with continent ileostomy* (Koch pouch) creates a continent ileostomy that does not require wearing an appliance; it is best suited for those who desire control of stomal output. *Park's procedure* (total colectomy, rectal mucosectomy, ileal reservoir, and ileoanal anastomosis) provides the opportunity to retain continence and avoid a stoma. Although there is likely to be some incontinence initially, this usually passes. About four to eight bowel movements per day are common, helped by chronic use of low-dose antidiarrheal therapy (e.g., loperamide). Potential complications include pelvic infection, strictures, small bowel obstruction, and "pouchitis." Although complications occur in up to 30%, most patients are pleased with the procedure and its outcomes.

Regardless of the surgical procedure chosen, the morbidity of active disease and the threat of cancer must be weighed against the risks of major surgery. The mortality of elective colectomy is 1% to 3%, with most patients having no postoperative complications. Stoma revision is necessary in 10% to 20% of cases.

Screening for Cancer.
All patients with clinical or radiologic evidence of *pancolitis of 7 or more years* should be considered for colon cancer

screening. At this point, cancer risk begins to rise substantially. Because the bowel cancer is often multicentric, the best method of screening is *colonoscopy* with multiple biopsies. Cancer screening should begin at 7 years with 3-year intervals until 20 years, when it should become more frequent. Worrisome findings include *stricture* and *dysplasia*. Mild dysplasia is an indication for repeat study in 3 months. Severe dysplasia and stricture formation require consideration of colectomy; the risk of cancer is very high in the presence of such findings.

Crohn's Disease

Most patients can be treated on an outpatient basis by judicious use of medications and careful follow-up. A strong working alliance between the patient and primary physician is essential, because the disease is chronic, relapsing, and incurable.

Diet. Adequate nutrition is critical to the promotion of healing. Sufficient protein and calories must be provided but in a manner that limits the stress put on an inflamed and often strictured bowel. Patients with cramps and diarrhea should have the *fiber* content of their diet *reduced*; those with steatorrhea will benefit from a *decrease in fat intake* to less than 80 g/d. An empiric trial of *restricting milk products* may terminate diarrhea due to lactase deficiency, which often accompanies the illness. More severely ill patients require partial *bowel rest*, which removes the stimulus that food has on bowel motility and secretion. *Elemental diet preparations* (e.g., Magnacal, Ensure, Sustacal, Isocal) have been found to induce remission, improve symptoms, and decrease disease activity in patients with acute disease. They are convenient and usually well tolerated sources of the extra nutrition needed during exacerbations. *Total parenteral nutrition* should be used in patients whose oral intake is not adequate or in whom surgery is indicated.

Vitamin and mineral deficiencies are common and must be corrected for proper healing and avoidance of such complications as anemia and bone disease. *Folic acid* supplementation is particularly important in patients taking sulfasalazine, which impairs its absorption. Patients who have had ileal surgery may need extra *vitamin B12*. *Vitamin D* levels are likely to be low when intake is poor or steatorrhea is a problem. An oral supplement of 4,000 IU or more usually suffices. Most vitamin and mineral deficiencies can be overcome by taking a multiple vitamin containing about five times the normal daily vitamin requirements and such minerals as iron, calcium, magnesium, and zinc.

Antidiarrheal Agents. The use of these agents in Crohn's disease is similar to that in ulcerative colitis (see above). The risks include addiction and exacerbation of obstructive symptoms.

Sulfasalazine and Other 5-Aminosalicylate Preparations. The National Cooperative Crohn's Disease Study demonstrated modest efficacy of sulfasalazine in patients with disease of the colon and no benefit in those with disease limited to the small bowel. Doses of 2 to 4 g/d are used to treat acute exacerbations of abdominal pain and diarrhea in patients with colonic involvement. Improvement typically occurs within 4 to 8 weeks. Patients who respond to sulfasalazine but experience an adverse

effect attributable to the sulfa moiety are candidates for a *sulfa-free 5-ASA* preparation (e.g., *mesalamine* or *olsalazine*). Olsalazine delivers 5-ASA exclusively to the colon, making it useful only for those with disease confined to the large bowel. Mesalamine tablets (Asacol) are formulated to deliver 5-ASA to the cecum and large bowel; mesalamine capsules (Pentasa) release 5-ASA to the entire small bowel and colon. Because they are costly, the 5-ASA preparations should not be used before sulfasalazine for treatment of active disease. Sulfasalazine does not sustain remissions, but meta-analytic data and subsequent controlled trials suggest that mesalamine may reduce risk of recurrence by up to 40%, with benefit most notable for disease of the small bowel and for sustaining remission and after surgery. Nonetheless, the safety and efficacy of routine long-term prophylactic use of mesalamine in Crohn's disease is not established. Combination of sulfasalazine with corticosteroids has not been shown to have a steroid-sparing effect or allow more rapid tapering of steroids once a remission has been induced.

Adverse Effects (see above, under Ulcerative Colitis)

Metronidazole, in doses of approximately 10 to 20 mg/kg/d (e.g., 250 to 500 mg three times a day), is effective in the treatment of patients with Crohn's ileocolitis or colitis and is a reasonable next step in patients who fail to respond adequately to a 5-ASA agent. In addition, uncontrolled studies have demonstrated healing of rectovaginal fistulas, abscesses, and proctocolectomy wounds. It appears that *maintenance* therapy at a lower dose can minimize recurrence of perineal disease. Patient acceptability is sometimes limited by gastrointestinal upset, metallic taste, and paresthesias (a manifestation of peripheral neuropathy associated with chronic use). There is a small risk (1% to 2%) of an *Antabuse-like reaction* occurring with concurrent alcohol use. Persons on long-term therapy who would like to have an occasional drink can conduct a trial of modest alcohol intake at home (where any vomiting will not be embarrassing) to see if they are at risk.

Other Antibiotics. The fluoroquinolone antibiotics (e.g., ciprofloxacin) have also demonstrated efficacy in very ill patients with fistulas and abscesses.

Glucocorticosteroids. If a patient is acutely ill or has moderate-to-severe disease not responding to 5-ASA therapy, then systemic steroids are indicated. Patients with small bowel involvement are especially responsive. *High doses* (e.g., the equivalent of 60 mg prednisone/d) should be used initially. Steroids plus sulfasalazine are more effective than sulfasalazine alone in bringing an acute flare-up under control, but, like sulfasalazine, they are ineffective in preventing a relapse. Sulfasalazine has no steroid-sparing effect.

As acute disease activity subsides, the steroid dose is empirically tapered to the minimum necessary to control symptoms. Sometimes, *alternate-day regimens* will suffice to control disease activity; they have the advantage of minimizing the steroid side effects (see Chapter 105). As long as 4 months of steroid therapy may be necessary to treat an exacerbation.

Newer oral steroid preparations are being developed, such as controlled-release *budesonide*, which is topically active in the terminal ileum and proximal small bowel yet much less likely to cause systemic side effects because it is 90% inactivated after the first pass through the liver. It has proven more effective than mesalamine in persons with active mild to moderate disease yet relatively free of adverse systemic effects. Its full role in treatment of Crohn's disease (including use as maintenance therapy) is being actively explored; it should soon be available in the United States.

Although steroids occupy a central place in the treatment of Crohn's disease, they are *ineffective for maintaining remissions* or preventing exacerbations. Prophylactic steroids are not indicated in Crohn's disease. Moreover, some extraintestinal manifestations and perianal disease do not respond well to glucocorticoids. An important goal of treatment is discontinuation of steroids, necessitating consideration of maintenance mesalamine, metronidazole, immunosuppressive therapy, and the newly developed monoclonal antibody preparations.

6-Mercaptopurine, Azathioprine. These closely related *immunomodulators* are especially useful for their steroid-sparing effects, providing an option for maintenance therapy that is considerably less toxic than chronic steroids. In controlled studies, these agents achieve or maintain control and allow a reduction or discontinuation of steroids in two thirds to three fourths of patients. Treatment is initiated at low doses and increased if no response is noted. There can be a delay in onset of effect of weeks to months, necessitating continuation of concurrent therapy until the effect sets in. Treatment is typically continued for about 12 months and then cessation is attempted. Unlike other forms of medical treatment for Crohn's disease, chronic immunosuppressive therapy has been shown to be capable of maintaining remission, especially in patients with fistulas or frequent relapses.

Limitations to immunosuppressive therapy include slow onset of action and potentially serious side effects. Onset of action may take as long as 3 to 6 months in some patients, necessitating a 6-month trial that includes a doubling of the starting dose. In addition, immunosuppressive therapy may induce infection, pancreatitis, bone marrow suppression, or drug-induced hepatitis. Monitoring of blood counts is essential. Despite the potential for such adverse effects, 6-MP and azathioprine have a good safety profile, especially if the dose is 50 mg/d or less. A total dose of 1.5 to 2.0 mg/kg/d should not be exceeded. Initiation of immunosuppressive therapy should not done without first consulting a gastroenterologist familiar with use of these agents.

Other Immunomodulating/Anti-inflammatory Agents. A host of other agents have been examined for use as steroid-sparing therapy. They should used only in consultation with a gastroenterologist familiar with their use in inflammatory bowel disease.

Methotrexate, the folic acid antagonist with anti-inflammatory effects, has been found in a double-blind placebo-controlled trial of Crohn's disease patients requiring chronic steroid therapy to reduce steroid needs and improve disease control. However, elevations in transaminases and nausea caused nearly a fifth of patients to withdraw from therapy. More study is needed to fully determine the role of methotrexate in Crohn's disease and to develop guidelines for its safe use. Some speculate that its efficacy in achieving short-term control may make it useful as a complement to azathioprine or 6-MP.

Monoclonal Antibody cA2 (infliximab) directed against *tumor necrosis factor-α* has demonstrated efficacy and minimal toxicity in well-designed short-term trials in patients with moderate-to-severe disease resistant to other forms of therapy. Patients with refractory fistulas treated with one to three intravenous infusions over 6 weeks achieve a marked clinical response, with some fistulas healing completely. However, relapse is common, and safety and efficacy of maintenance infusions remains to be established. Serum sickness–like reactions have occurred with repeat infusions and some lymphomas, and antinuclear antibody positivity has been noted in patients receiving cA2 therapy. Cost is very high (in the thousands of dollars) for a single infusion. Whether these impressive short-term results will hold up in long-term study remains to be determined. Consultation is required for cA2 use.

Omega-3 Fatty Acids, found in fish oil and believed to suppress inflammatory mediators such as the leukotrienes and prostaglandins, have produced modest improvements in acute disease and in maintenance of remission.

Cyclosporine A, an immunomodulator with a faster onset of action than that of azathioprine and 6-MP, has produced promising results in uncontrolled studies but unimpressive findings in placebo-controlled trials. Risk of toxicity is high.

Surgery. Unlike ulcerative colitis, surgery in Crohn's disease does not cure the patient. It is therefore best reserved for patients who have intractable disease, perforation, obstruction, or severe bleeding. It has been estimated that the probability of surgery is 78% at 20 years and 90% at 30 years from the onset of Crohn's disease symptoms. The objective of surgery is to remove grossly involved bowel and spare as much normal-appearing bowel as possible. Postoperative recurrence rates have been estimated to be 30% to 50% per decade and are inversely related to preoperative disease duration. The most common operation is removal of a diseased portion of the terminal ileum with an end-to-end ileocolonic anastomosis. For patients with colonic involvement, colectomy with an internal anastomosis connecting the ileum to the sigmoid or total proctocolectomy with Brooke ileostomy is the procedure of choice. Ileostomy is necessary in patients with marked rectosigmoid disease. Twenty percent to 40% of ileostomies need revision within 5 years because of disease in the stomal area.

Surgical treatment is undertaken with reluctance and only in the setting of severely disabling disease or serious complications. The patient presenting with obstruction may respond sufficiently to bowel rest, nasogastric suction, steroids, and other conservative measures, avoiding the need for immediate surgery, unless the obstruction persists or recurs quickly. In patients with multiple surgeries and much bowel already resected, stricturoplasty might be considered in lieu of yet another resection of bowel. All attempts should be made to use a conservative surgical approach to preserve functional bowel. Loss of bowel, especially right colon, can lead to disabling postsurgical diarrhea.

Management of the Pregnant or Nursing Patient with Inflammatory Bowel Disease

For patients with a flare-up of inflammatory bowel disease during nursing or pregnancy, both sulfasalazine and steroids are safe and effective. To maintain remission throughout pregnancy in ulcerative colitis, sulfasalazine should be continued in conjunction with folic acid supplementation. Metronidazole and immunosuppressive agents may be injurious to the fetus or nursing child and should be avoided. Women with ulcerative colitis are prone to suffer new attacks or exacerbations during the first trimester of pregnancy and have a spontaneous abortion rate of about 10%. Pregnancy seems to inhibit relapses during later trimesters. Women with active ulcerative colitis should be counseled to postpone getting pregnant until they have been in remission for about a year.

PATIENT EDUCATION

The education and support of the patient and the family are essential. Fears abound when patients are told they have ulcerative colitis or Crohn's disease. These diagnoses conjure up images of colostomy, recurrent hospitalizations, invalidism, and social isolation. It is important to emphasize that the vast majority of patients lead fully functional lives and many obtain satisfactory control of their disease through medical therapy.

Because these are chronic diseases that affect young adults, the questions of *conception, pregnancy, and childbearing* will arise. Although there is some familial pattern to the occurrences of the inflammatory bowel diseases, transmission is not purely genetic, and there is ample evidence that when the disease is in remission, fertility is essentially normal, and healthy full-term infants can be delivered. However, conception might be a problem when the male patient is taking sulfasalazine (see above).

The issue of *cancer risk* in patients with long-standing and extensive ulcerative colitis can be addressed directly and clearly, reassuring those with minimal disease that their risk is no greater than that of the general population. Even those with extensive disease appreciate knowing the magnitude of the risk.

The primary physician can do much to prepare the patient who requires *colectomy* and subsequent *ileostomy*. Thorough patient education combined with a caring approach that includes a willingness to listen to concerns and fears is invaluable and greatly appreciated. Many patients have fears and anxieties that they will not discuss unless they are broached by the physician. Also helpful in preparation for ileostomy is to have an ileostomy patient of the same age and sex discuss the procedure and its consequences with the surgical candidate. Seeing that one can go on to lead a fully active life is comforting. Where available, a local association of ostomates is a valuable resource. Finally, the more widespread use of ileoanal anastomosis in carefully selected patients may increase the acceptability of surgery.

Many patients can be taught to *adjust their medication* within a prearranged set of guidelines and limits. Dosages of sulfasalazine to be used for mild exacerbations can be specified and extra supplies of medication can be provided, allowing the patient to play an active role in his or her care and ensuring prompt treatment of a flare-up. Antidiarrheal agents can also be provided for as-needed use but only to reliable patients who are not likely to abuse them. Patients should be *instructed to call* if fever develops, diarrhea worsens, bleeding occurs, or abdominal pain becomes marked.

The need for a steady exchange of information with the patient, including careful explanation of procedures and therapies, and the importance of close follow-up and availability cannot be overemphasized. Attentiveness and responsiveness alleviate much of the fear and worry that accompany inflammatory bowel disease and support the development of an effective therapeutic alliance. Additional information and support is available to the patient from the local Chapter of the National Ileitis and Colitis Foundation.

INDICATIONS FOR REFERRAL AND ADMISSION

Referral for gastroenterologic consultation is indicated when full dosages of sulfasalazine in combination with oral corticosteroids ($\pm$ metronidazole in patients with Crohn's disease) fail to control symptoms. In addition, Crohn's disease patients who require high doses of chronic daily steroid therapy should be referred for consideration of immunosuppressive therapy. Ulcerative colitis patients with disabling, chronic, refractory disease ought to have a surgical consultation. The pancolitis patient with long-standing disease who is at increased risk for cancer needs referral for periodic colonoscopy and biopsy. Patients with extraintestinal disease should undergo an ophthalmologic consultation that includes a slit-lamp examination to check for uveitis.

Prompt hospitalization for parenteral management is indicated for patients who are toxic, bleeding heavily, in severe pain, or too sick to obtain adequate nutrition orally. Bowel rest, nasogastric feeding of elemental diets, and parenteral steroids are prescribed, and surgical consultation is obtained, especially if there is severe bleeding, toxicity, distention, or evidence of peritoneal irritation. Home nasoenteric feeding has been demonstrated for carefully selected patients with malabsorption and weight loss refractory to conventional outpatient therapy. Nocturnal tube feedings of a low-fat elemental diet can correct such nutritional problems, but the program requires patients who can insert their own feeding tubes at night.

MANAGEMENT RECOMMENDATIONS

Ulcerative Colitis

General Measures

- Document mucosal inflammation with sigmoidoscopy.
- Reduce dietary fiber during an exacerbation.
- Advise adequate rest and sleep.
- Prescribe a *folic acid* supplement (1 mg/d) when leafy vegetables are restricted or sulfasalazine is being used.
- Add oral *iron* supplementation (300 mg ferrous sulfate three times daily) when there is considerable rectal bleeding and documented iron-deficiency anemia.
- Schedule visits frequently in the early phases of the illness to provide psychological support and close monitoring. Phone checks are helpful.
- Prescribe a short course of opiate therapy (e.g., *loperamide* 2 to 4 mg or codeine 15 mg before meals and at bedtime) for temporary symptomatic control of troublesome diarrhea in patients with mild to moderate disease; avoid prolonged use and use in patients with severe disease (high risk of toxic dilatation).
- If mild diarrhea persists during remissions, initiate a trial of psyllium hydrophilic colloid (1 teaspoon in 8 oz of water once or twice daily); if this is still unsuccessful, try restricting milk products.

- Refer for consideration of periodic colonoscopy and biopsy those patients who have pancolitis lasting more than 8 years.

Mild to Moderate Disease

- Begin *sulfasalazine*, 500 mg four times a day with meals, and increase the dosage as tolerated over several days to 4 g/d. Continue this dosage for 2 to 4 weeks until symptoms abate, and then decrease it to the smallest dosage that maintains control of symptoms (usually 2 g/d, although sometimes 4 g/d are required).
- Substitute a nonsulfa 5-ASA preparation (e.g., *olsalazine*, 500 mg twice a day; *mesalamine*, 1 g four times a day) in patients who are sulfa allergic, cannot tolerate sulfasalazine, or experience a suboptimal response from sulfasalazine.
- If sulfasalazine or another 5-ASA preparation fails to achieve control within a few weeks, begin oral *prednisone*, starting with a dose of 40 mg/d. Initially give in divided doses for patients who are having symptoms round the clock but change to an every-morning program as soon as possible to limit the degree of adrenal suppression. Continue this dosage for 7 to 10 days.
- If control is achieved, begin tapering prednisone by 5 to 10 mg every 2 weeks to the lowest dosage necessary to suppress disease activity. An alternate-day program (using the same total weekly dose that maintains control) may be tried to minimize chronic steroid therapy side effects (see Chapter 105).
- Once steroids are tapered off and disease activity ceases, decrease sulfasalazine to a maintenance dose of 2 g/d and continue for at least 1 year to maintain remission. If olsalazine is being used, prescribe 1 g/d for maintenance.

Moderate to Severe Disease

- Start with *prednisone*, 60 mg/d in divided doses, and *sulfasalazine* at 4 g/d. Once the symptoms come under control, give the entire prednisone dose in the morning and begin tapering empirically by 5 mg/wk. Continue the sulfasalazine at 1 g four times a day indefinitely.
- If food intake is inadequate over time because of nausea or abdominal pain, consider supplementing the diet with a nutritionally balanced *low-residue liquid dietary preparation* (e.g., Magnacal, Ensure, Sustacal, Isocal).
- Monitor carefully for marked blood loss, volume depletion, severe abdominal pain, distention, and peritoneal signs; any of these is an indication for prompt hospital admission, parenteral therapy, and urgent surgical consultation.
- Refer for consideration of steroid-sparing immunosuppressive therapy (6-MP or azathioprine) patients requiring persistently high doses of steroids.
- Refer for consideration of elective surgery, patients refractory to maximal medical therapy, those requiring daily steroids for prolonged periods (more than 6 months), and those found on cancer screening to have a stricture or dysplasia.

Ulcerative Proctocolitis

- If disease is limited to the rectosigmoid, begin treatment with oral sulfasalazine (as noted above) or a topical agent. Enemas of *hydrocortisone or 5-ASA* are both effective topically. Hydrocortisone can be administered rectally using a 100-mg *retention enema* taken once nightly, a 25-mg *suppository* once or twice daily, or a 90-mg *foam* preparation once or twice

daily. Selection of preparation can be based on patient preference and empirical results. Use a 5-ASA enema if there is concern about steroid absorption and systemic side effects. Dose is 2 to 4 g/d for acute symptoms and 1 g/d for maintenance. Continue therapy until symptoms clear; continue sulfasalazine or isoleucine for prophylaxis.

Crohn's Disease

General Measures

- Document the extent of disease by barium studies or colonoscopy. Postpone barium enema and colonoscopy until disease activity subsides.
- Limit the fiber content of the diet in patients with cramps and diarrhea.
- Decrease the fat intake to less than 80 mg/d when there is steatorrhea.
- Conduct a trial of restricting milk products from the diet of patients with diarrhea; if the diarrhea promptly improves, continue with a lactose-restricted diet.
- Supplement the diet with a multivitamin preparation that contains five times the normal daily vitamin requirements plus iron, calcium, magnesium, and zinc.
- Consider short-course opiate therapy (e.g., *loperamide* 2 to 4 g or codeine 15 mg with meals and before bed) for symptomatic relief of diarrhea; use caution, obstruction may be aggravated, and prolonged use can lead to narcotic dependence.
- Advise partial bowel rest and use of elemental low-residue dietary preparations when cramps and diarrhea are severe.
- Admit for refractory disease, severe bleeding, toxicity, abdominal pain, abscess formation, or evidence of obstruction. Such patients need surgical consultation.

Colonic Disease

- Begin *sulfasalazine* (500 mg four times a day) and quickly increase the dosage to 1 g four times a day over several days; continue for 4 to 8 weeks. Use *olsalazine* (500 mg twice a day) or *mesalamine* (up to 4.8 g/d) for the sulfa-intolerant patient or the patient unresponsive to sulfasalazine.
- If there is a response to sulfasalazine, continue for 4 to 6 months and then stop if symptoms have ceased. Maintenance sulfasalazine and olsalazine do not prevent recurrences, but there is a prophylactic benefit associated with mesalamine use. For maintenance, prescribe mesalamine at the lowest dose that sustains a remission (usually 2.4 to 3.6 g/day).
- If there is no response to 5-ASA agents, *switch to metronidazole* in doses of 10 to 20 mg/kg/d (e.g., 250 to 500 mg three times a day) and continue for a 4-week trial. If there is a satisfactory response, continue for 4 to 6 months, then stop if symptoms have ceased.
- If there is inadequate response to metronidazole, switch to *prednisone* 60 mg/d; four times a day dosages may be required at the outset for round-the-clock control.
- As disease activity subsides, give the entire dosage in the morning and begin tapering it to the lowest dosage that controls the symptoms (often as little as 5 mg/d). Continue this dosage until all evidence of disease activity ceases (and then at least for 1 year); an alternate-day schedule may suffice.
- For refractory disease or patients requiring chronic steroid therapy, refer for consideration of immunosuppressive therapy with *6-MP, azathioprine* (both 50 mg/d), or one of the

newer anti-inflammatory/immunomodulator therapies (e.g., *methotrexate, infliximab*).

Perianal Disease

- Prescribe *metronidazole* (750 to 2,000 mg/d) for refractory perianal disease; a prolonged course of treatment may be necessary.

Ileal Disease

- The effectiveness of sulfasalazine for ileal disease is not well established, although some patients with mild disease may benefit. *Olsalazine* (500 mg twice a day) or *mesalamine* capsules (up to 4.8 g/day) may provide better results and is worth a 4- to 6-week trial.
- If there is no response or if ileal symptoms are severe, then prescribe *prednisone* (60 mg/d) and use in the same fashion as for colonic involvement (see above).
- Consider use of *6-MP or azathioprine* (50 mg/d) for patients with fistulas, refractory symptoms, or persistent requirements for very high steroid dosages. A 6-month trial is often necessary. Treatment is continued for 12 months and then cessation is attempted, although long-term therapy is sometimes necessary and successful in maintaining remission. Because immunosuppressive therapy can cause marrow suppression and carcinogenesis, gastroenterologic consultation is essential if it is to be used.

ANNOTATED BIBLIOGRAPHY

Belluzzi A, Brignola C, Campieri M, et al. Effect of an enteric-coated fish-oil preparation on relapse in Crohn's disease. N Engl J Med 1996;334:1557. (*Decreased rate of relapse.*)

Bernstein LH, Frank MS, Brandt LJ, et al. Healing of perineal Crohn's disease with metronidazole. Gastroenterology 1980;79:375. (*Documents the drug's usefulness in therapy of chronic perianal abscesses and fistulas.*)

Collins RH Jr., Feldman M, Fordtran JS. Colon cancer, dysplasia, and surveillance in patients with ulcerative colitis. N Engl J Med 1987;316:1654. (*Provocative paper critical of routine surveillance in patients with ulcerative colitis.*)

Disanayake AS, Truelove SC. A controlled therapeutic trial of long-term maintenance treatment of ulcerative colitis with sulfasalazine. Gut 1973;14:923. (*The original data documenting efficacy of sulfasalazine for prophylaxis; recurrence rate one fourth that of the control group.*)

Donaldson RM. Management of medical problems in pregnancy: inflammatory bowel disease. N Engl J Med 1985;312:1616. (*Practical approach to this important management issue.*)

Drossman DA. Psychosocial aspects of inflammatory bowel disease. Stress Med 1986;2:119. (*Good review of psychological and psychosocial dimensions.*)

Dworken HJ. Ulcerative colitis. A clearer picture. Ann Intern Med 1983;99:717. (*Reviews data on prognosis derived from community-based studies and argues for a more optimistic view of the illness.*)

Ekbom A, Helmick C, Zack H, et al. Ulcerative colitis and colorectal cancer: a population-based study. N Engl J Med 1990;323;1228. (*Best available data for estimation of risk for colorectal cancer.*)

Farmer RG, Whelan G, Fazio VW. Long-term follow up of patients with Crohn's disease. Gastroenterology 1985;88:818. (*Relationship between clinical pattern and prognosis.*)

Feagan BG, Rochon J, Fedorak RN, et al. Methotrexate for the treatment of Crohn's disease. N Engl J Med 1995;332:292. (*Multicenter placebo-controlled trial in patients with chronically active disease finding the drug superior to placebo in improving symptoms and reducing steroid requirements.*)

Fiocchi C, Roche JK, Michener WM. High prevalence of antibodies to intestinal epithelial antigen in patients with inflammatory bowel disease and their relatives. Ann Intern Med 1989;110:786. (*Evidence suggesting that immune sensitization is a primary phenomenon.*)

Garrett, JW, Drossman DA. Health status in inflammatory bowel disease; review of biologic and behavioral considerations. Gastroenterology 1990;99:90. (*Outcomes appear to be a function of both disease and quality of life factors.*)

Gendry JP, Mary JY, Florent C, et al. Oral mesalamine (Pentasa) as maintenance treatment in Crohn's disease. A multicenter placebo-controlled study. Gastroenterology 1993;104:435. (*Relapse rate significantly reduced.*)

Glotzer DJ, Gardner RC, Goldman H, et al. Comparative features and course of ulcerative and granulomatous colitis. N Engl J Med 1970;282:582. (*Classic review comparing and contrasting the two conditions.*)

Greenberg GR, Feagan BG, Martin F, et al. Oral budesonide as maintenance treatment for Crohn's disease: a placebo-controlled dose-ranging study. Gastroenterology 1996;110:45. (*Achieved a more prolonged remission but not sustainable beyond 1 year.*)

Klotz UK, Maier K, Fischer C, et al. Therapeutic efficacy of sulfasalazine and its metabolites in patients with ulcerative colitis and Crohn's disease. N Engl J Med 1980;303:1499. (*Classic paper that establishes that 5-aminosalicylate is the active moiety of sulfasalazine.*)

Kornbluth A, Sachar DB. Ulcerative colitis practice guidelines in adults. American Gollege of Gastroenterology Practice Parameters Committee. Am J Gastroenterol 1997;92:204. (*Current consensus practice guidelines.*)

McLeod RS, Wolff BG, Steinhart AH, et al. Prophylactic mesalamine treatment decreases postoperative recurrence of Crohn's disease. Gastroenterology 1995;109;404. (*Effective prophylactically when used following surgery.*)

National Cooperative Crohn's Disease Study. Gastroenterology 1979;77:825. (*Multicenter prospective controlled trial demonstrating efficacy of sulfasalazine in acute disease of the colon. No improvement observed in patients with disease confined to the small bowel.*)

Pearson DC, May GR, Fick GH, et al. Azathioprine and 6-mercaptopurine in Crohn disease: a meta-analysis. Ann Intern Med 1995;122:132. (*The analysis found these agents effective in treating active disease and in maintaining remission; however, adverse effects requiring withdrawal are common.*)

Peppercorn MA. Advances in drug therapy for inflammatory bowel disease. Ann Intern Med 1990;112;50. (*Especially useful is the discussion of the 5-ASA drugs, but also covers other aspects of medical therapy.*)

Peppercorn MA. Sulfasalazine: pharmacology, clinical use, toxicity and related new drug development. Ann Intern Med 1984;101:377. (*All you ever wanted to know; 140 references.*)

Present DH, Korelitz BI, Wisch N, et al. Treatment of Crohn's disease with 6-mercaptopurine. N Engl J Med 1980;302:981. (*Long-term, randomized, double-blind study showing that 6-MP is effective in the management of refractory Crohn's disease. The accompanying editorial by Sleisenger puts the study's results into context.*)

Present DH, Meltzer SJ, Krumholz MD, et al. 6-Mercaptopurine in the management of inflammatory bowel disease: short- and long-term toxicity. Ann Intern Med 1989;111:641. (*Reports an 18-year experience.*)

Present DH, Rutgeerts P, Targan S, et al. Infliximab for the treatment of fistulas in patients with Crohn's disease. N Engl J Med 1999;

340;1398. (*Infliximab is established as an effective medical therapy for fistulous Crohn's disease.*)

Provenzale D, Kowdley KV, Arora S, et al. Prophylactic colectomy or surveillance for chronic ulcerative colitis? A decision analysis. Gastroenterology 1995;109:1188. (*Both increase life expectancy.*)

Rijk MC, van Hogezand RA, van Lier HJ, et al. Sulfasalazine and prednisone compared with sulfasalazine for treating active Crohn disease. Ann Intern Med 1991;114:445. (*Double-blind, randomized, multicenter trial showing that prednisone helped only in speeding initial improvement.*)

Robertson DAF, Ray J, Diamond I, et al. Personality profile and affective states of patients with inflammatory bowel disease. Gut 1989;30:623. (*Personality disturbances were frequent and correlated with duration of disease; many reported stress preceding onset of symptoms.*)

Steinhart AH, Hemphill D, Greenberg GR. Sulfasalazine and mesalamine for the maintenance therapy of Crohn's disease: a meta-analysis. Am J Gastroenterol 1994;89:2116. (*A meta-analysis of the efficacy of sulfasalazine and mesalamine in Crohn's disease.*)

Targan SR, Hanauer SB, van Deventer SJH, et al. A short-term study of chimeric monoclonal antibody cA2 to tumor necrosis factor alpha for Crohn's disease. N Engl J Med 1997;337:1029. (*A double-blind placebo-controlled trial in persons with moderate-to-severe treatment-resistant disease showing significant reduction in symptoms over 12 weeks.*)

Thomsen OO, Cortot A, Jewell D, et al. A comparison of budesonide and mesalamine for active Crohn's disease. N Engl J Med 1998;339:370. (*A double-blind multicenter trial in persons with active mild-to-moderate Crohn's disease showing budesonide to be superior to slow-release mesalamine and not suppressing adrenal function.*)

Tremaine WJ, Sandborn WJ. Practice guidelines for inflammatory bowel disease: an instrument for assessment. Mayo Clin Proc 1999;74;495. (*Guidelines for inflammatory bowel disease management and suggestions for their assessment.*)

Ursing B, Almy T, Barney F, et al. A comparative study of metronidazole and sulfasalazine for active Crohn's disease. A Cooperative Crohn's Disease Study in Sweden. II. Results. Gastroenterology 1982;83:550. (*Metronidazole produced results comparable with those of sulfasalazine; moreover, the drug worked in some patients who failed to respond to sulfasalazine.*)

Whelan G, Farmer RG, Fazio VW. Recurrence after surgery in Crohn's disease, relationship to location and disease. Clinical pattern and surgical indication. Gastroenterology 1985;88:1826. (*Six hundred fifteen patients followed by the Cleveland Clinic from 1966 to the present show a high index of recurrence after operation.*)

74

Approach to the Patient with Functional Gastrointestinal Disease

Functional gastrointestinal (GI) disease accounts for a large proportion of the GI complaints seen in office practice, not only in the primary care setting but also in the referral practices of gastroenterologists. The international working group consensus definition of functional GI disease is "a variable combination of chronic or recurrent GI symptoms not explained by structural or biochemical abnormalities. They include symptoms attributed to the pharynx, esophagus, stomach, biliary tree, small and large intestine or anorectum." Included under the rubric of functional GI disease are two common often troubling syndromes: *irritable bowel syndrome (IBS) and nonulcer dyspepsia*. The former is associated with large bowel discomfort or pain, disturbed defecation, and distention, often predominated by constipation, diarrhea, or gaseousness. The latter is characterized by upper abdominal discomfort, bloating, distension, and nausea, which is often but not necessarily exacerbated or triggered by eating. Another increasingly appreciated functional malady is *irritable esophagus* (sometimes referred to as esophageal spasm; see Chapter 61). In many cases of functional disease, there is a strong interplay between biopsychosocial factors and gut physiology.

The primary care physician needs to become expert in the recognition and management of these conditions, not only because they can mimic more serious disease (sometimes leading to unnecessary testing and treatment), but also because they are the source of much worry, functional impairment, and substantial health care expenditures.

IRRITABLE BOWEL SYNDROME

IBS is a functional disturbance of intestinal motility and visceral perception, strongly influenced by emotional factors. It accounts for about half of GI complaints seen by physicians. Epidemiologic studies suggest that nearly 20% of adults suffer from some form of the condition, although only a fraction actually seek medical attention. "Spastic bowel," "mucous colitis," and "spastic colitis" are less accurate terms sometimes used to connote the syndrome. When mistaken for organic disease, it can result in unnecessary testing or frustrating attempts at therapy. Careful diagnosis and a comprehensive approach to management (including a strong patient–doctor relationship) are essential to optimizing patient outcomes.

Pathophysiology and Clinical Presentation

The Emerging Pathophysiologic View of IBS is one of functional disturbances in motor activity and visceral perception, triggered or exacerbated by psychological distress and luminal irritants. *Abnormal motor function* is a hallmark of this syndrome, capable of producing both *diarrhea* and *constipation*. Both may occur in alternating fashion or one may predominate. Nonpropulsive colonic contractions and slow-wave myoelectric patterns at two to three cycles per minute constitute about 40% of electrical and contractile activity at rest in patients with IBS, compared with 10% in healthy patients. When excessive, these contractions may impede propulsion of stool, prolong transit time, and cause constipation. Diarrhea occurs when the increase in contractility is localized to the small bowel and proximal colon. A pressure gradient develops, causing accelerated movement of intestinal contents. Meals normally cause an increase in colonic contractions, but controlled study has shown that patients with irritable colon syndrome have a significantly exaggerated increase in motor response to food. Patients with diarrhea-predominant disease have more jejunal, fast, and high-amplitude contractions postprandially than do healthy individuals, resulting in reduced colonic transit time.

Abnormalities in motor function may help explain the constipation and diarrhea but do not adequately account for the *abdominal pain* and *anorectal discomfort* experienced. Recent balloon manometry studies of patients with IBS show *excessive sensitivity* to balloon distention in the ileum, rectosigmoid, and anorectum. In patients with a predominance of diarrhea, there are reduced thresholds for initiation of reflex motor activity and discomfort; urgency is precipitated at abnormally small volumes of balloon distention. In patients with constipation, the threshold for reflex motor activity is abnormally high, and emptying is delayed. Fecal material collects and hardens, and the bowel becomes distended. Pain ensues.

The combination of abnormal motor and sensory functioning has the potential to cause the patient much discomfort. For example, increased sensitivity can trigger excessive reflex motor activity, leading to a cycle of anorectal discomfort or pain before a bowel movement, a sense of incomplete evacuation after one, and increased frequency of movements. Data also suggest that patients with IBS experience alterations in flow of visceral sensory afferent data and abnormalities in its central processing, perhaps as a result of learned behavior or underlying psychopathology.

Situational stress has long been considered an important contributing factor. Hypermotility in response to stress has been documented in both healthy persons and patients with IBS, but the latter show a significantly higher frequency of life stress.

In addition, a high prevalence of *psychopathology* has been uncovered in patients with IBS presenting for care. Somatization, personality disturbances, anxiety, and depression are among the conditions frequently identified. Although it is well recognized that psychological stress may alter bowel function, careful study of IBS reveals psychopathology to be more a *predictor of illness behavior* than a direct cause of the bowel disease. Psychiatric symptoms and poor coping skills usually predate bowel complaints. Disturbances in bowel function can be especially troubling to patients with preexisting psychopathology and more likely to precipitate medical encounters than might similar symptoms in otherwise well-adjusted persons. This finding has been invoked to explain why only a fraction of patients with IBS ever present for medical care. Patients with IBS who do not consult physicians have been found to be psychologically similar to control subjects.

What seems to characterize the patient persistently bothered by symptoms is the greater prevalence of serious situational stresses, psychopathology, and perhaps learned visceral responses to bowel discomfort and threatening situations. Such factors may modify the underlying pathophysiology and illness behavior, determining severity of symptoms, frequency of episodes, and thresholds for seeking and continuing with medical care.

Recently, a greater appreciation has emerged for *intraluminal factors* that might alter bowel motor function and cause it to behave in an "irritable" manner, such as selective *malabsorption* of certain sugars, like *lactose* (the common dairy product sugar), fructose (the common citrus fruit sugar), and *sorbitol* (often found in "sugar-free" candy). Sorbitol is a common sweetener in candies and chewing gum and is capable of causing bloating and diarrhea if taken in large amounts, as are milk products in patients with lactose intolerance. One study suggests that *food allergies* may play a role in some patients. *Bile acid* malabsorption has been detected in up to 10% of patients with diarrhea-predominant IBS. The resulting large quantities of fatty acids descending on the colon can trigger painful rapid contractions, leading to marked discomfort and diarrhea.

Clinical Presentation is illustrated by a series of 50 patients treated in an outpatient unit. Most patients (62%) experienced onset of symptoms before age 40; 50% were under 30 at time of onset; and one fourth were under 20. *Chronicity* was the rule, with little change in symptoms over time, except for waxing and waning. Duration was in years. *Abdominal pain* was present in 90%, *mucous* stools in 36%, *pelletlike stools* in 38%, *diarrhea* alone in 10%, and *excessive flatus* in 36%. Fifty percent considered their symptoms related to stress, 34% denied this, and 66% manifested symptoms of anxiety or depression. Abdominal pain was most often in the left lower quadrant or lower abdomen (62%), but in 28% there were multiple sites of pain. Upper abdominal involvement occurred in 38%. The pain was typically achy rather than crampy, often relieved by a bowel movement or passage of flatus. It was unusual for the pain to awaken the patient. Radiation was variable and even extended into the left chest and arm when gas was trapped in the splenic flexure.

Small, hard, infrequent stools and an empty rectal ampulla characterize constipation. Prolonged retention of stool allows full absorption of intestinal water content. The diarrhea is typically small in volume, associated with visible amounts of mucus, and may follow a hard movement by a few hours. There may be urgency. Dyspepsia and excessive gaseousness are also reported (see above). Weight loss is rare; symptoms usually parallel situational stresses. Rectal bleeding is absent unless there is coincident hemorrhoidal disease.

Clinical Course

IBS is a chronic relapsing condition with no evidence of significant morbidity or mortality. A prospective British study providing follow-up at 2-month intervals over 3 years found that severity waxed and waned but the constellation of symptoms remained remarkably constant. At 1 year, 50% were unchanged, 36% improved, 12% were symptom free, and 20% were worse. The symptom-free period was usually less than a few months. One third of employed patients lost time from work. There was no correlation between time lost and number of visits to the doctor; 40% made five or fewer visits and 46% made none at all. At 2 years, a similar pattern was found. Only one patient remained symptom free from the first year.

Studies on clinical course identified groups of patients with different prognoses. The group with symptoms triggered by a major life stress enjoyed long symptom-free periods after the acute problem abated, whereas those with continuous intestinal complaints in response to daily living rarely became asymptomatic.

Diagnosis and Initial Evaluation

Clinical criteria for diagnosis of IBS were specified by *Manning* and colleagues in the late 1970s. Although not derived quantitatively (e.g., by multiple regression analysis), these symptom-based criteria have been largely validated and are widely used for suggesting the diagnosis of IBS:

- Continuous or recurrent symptoms during several months of abdominal pain or discomfort relieved with defecation or associated with a change in frequency or consistency of stool, and/or
- An irregular or varying pattern of disturbed defecation at least 25% of the time, consisting of two or more of the following: altered frequency; altered consistency; straining, urgency, or feeling of incomplete evacuation; passage with mucus; and bloating or feeling of distention.

Although the sensitivity and specificity of the Manning criteria have, for the most part, been confirmed, there are some questions regarding the discriminant value of individual items. Moreover, some clinical situations require ruling out organic pathology that might resemble and be mistaken for IBS (see below). A combination of detailed history taking and careful physical examination, combined with selective parsimonious testing and a few diagnostic trials of therapeutic measures, will usually provide the best combination of completeness and cost efficacy.

The *Rome criteria* are another commonly used set of diagnostic criteria, very similar to the Manning criteria and often used for patient selection in clinical studies.

Overall Approach to Workup. Because many patients with IBS harbor fears of serious underlying disease, they commonly pressure physicians into ordering a plethora of diagnostic studies. Such cost-ineffective testing can be minimized by conducting a detailed history and careful physical examination that specifically elicits and addresses patient concerns, concluding the initial visit with a thorough review of key findings and their meaning (see below), and using the clinical presentation to determine the need for any further diagnostic testing. Often, the diagnosis of IBS can be made exclusively on clinical grounds. When a careful initial assessment is conducted, there is little risk of missing organic illness. Prospective studies with up to 30 years of follow-up have shown only a 1% rate of missed diagnoses of organic disease in patients carefully assessed at the outset.

When constipation predominates, it may be necessary to rule out a malignancy, particularly in patients over the age of 40 who have weight loss or a family history of colon cancer. In such patients, one needs to consider *flexible sigmoidoscopy with or without barium enema* or *colonoscopy* (see Chapter 65). In most others, a *stool test for occult blood* and a *complete blood count* (for microcytic anemia) should suffice. The absence of evidence for GI blood loss helps exclude organic disease. A clinical trial of *increased dietary fiber, stool softeners* (dioctyl sodium sulfosuccinate), or an *osmotic laxative* (psyllium) complements the diagnostic assessment. Patients taking diuretics should have a serum *potassium* checked, because hypokalemia may reduce bowel contractility and produce an ileus.

When diarrhea predominates, dietary review is essential for clues of intolerance to lactose or sorbitol. A check of *blood sugar* is needed to rule out diabetes mellitus (which may present as diarrhea due to diabetic gastroenteropathy; see Chapter 102), as is a check of the *stool for ova and parasites.* A diagnostic trial of eliminating sorbitol-containing candies and restricting lactose-containing milk products (yogurt containing live cultures are relatively lactose free) helps rule out contributions from intraluminal factors. A *lactose-hydrogen breath test* is an alternative means of testing for lactose intolerance. A trial of the bile acid-binding resin *cholestyramine* serves as a simple test for bile acid malabsorption. If diarrhea persists undiagnosed, a *sigmoidoscopy with or without mucosal biopsy* might be reasonable to exclude inflammatory bowel disease and collagenous and lymphocytic forms of colitis (see Chapter 64).

Abdominal pain and bloating necessitate ruling out obstruction. During an episode of pain, a timely *plain film of the abdomen* should suffice. Such bloating and discomfort may also occur with lactose, fructose, or sorbitol intolerance, which can be tested for as detailed above.

Psychological Assessment. Because the prevalence of underlying psychopathology is very high in patients with IBS, definitive therapy often requires identifying and addressing the patient's psychological difficulties. In the context of conducting a thorough workup, the clinician needs to sensitively elicit details of the patient's life situation, aspirations, accomplishments, frustrations, and losses. Concerns, fears, expectations, and responses to previous life stresses can also be very informative, as can the mental status of the patient on examination. *Anxiety disorders* are commonly identified (see Chapter 226), but *depression* (see Chapter 227) and *somatization* (see Chapter 230) often go unrecognized.

Principles of Management

Establishing a strong patient–doctor relationship, treating important underlying psychopathology, modifying diet, and supplementing these efforts with judicious use of medication constitute the basic approaches to management of the patient with IBS. No single treatment modality has proven successful in randomized placebo-controlled studies, but patient confidence in the diagnosis and a strong patient–doctor relationship are central to effective management. Such a relationship helps to minimize unnecessary repetition of diagnostic evaluations, dependence on drugs for provision of symptomatic relief, and excessive use of ambulatory medical services.

Establishing a Strong Patient–Doctor Relationship. The first rule in the care of patients with IBS is to *take their symptoms seriously* and not dismiss them as inconsequential. Such an approach communicates a sense of caring and is essential to the formation of an effective patient–doctor relationship, the *sine qua non* of IBS management. As noted earlier, it begins with a careful history and physical examination that addresses potentially serious etiologies, especially those of concern to the patient (e.g., cancer, inflammatory bowel disease). One cannot overemphasize the therapeutic importance of such an initial evaluation.

Once IBS has been identified (usually by the end of the initial or second office visit), the physician needs to *review the di-*

agnosis with the patient. Anxious emotionally troubled patients, such as those who present with IBS, often believe there is something seriously awry and will not accept a simplistic "there's nothing wrong with your bowels." They appreciate knowing the basis for their diagnosis and how more worrisome conditions were ruled out. In this way, the patient does not leave frustrated, feeling the "doctor cannot find what is wrong."

The establishment of a supportive *doctor–patient relationship* in conjunction with providing reassurance, explanation, and advice can have an important impact on outcome. When such care was given to patients in the prospective British study cited earlier, most reported feeling better, less concerned about their bowels, and more able to cope with their symptoms and the stresses of daily life. Although relapses were frequent, these seemed to be less important when they occurred in the context of close medical support. The failure of many physicians to provide adequate support is suggested by the 20% rate of self-referral to alternative medicine practitioners noted in patients with IBS. Developing a positive doctor–patient relationship has been found to be a key determinant in reducing use of ambulatory health services by IBS patients.

Management of Underlying Psychopathology. A distinguishing characteristic of patients who present to physicians with IBS is their high probability of underlying psychopathology. Often this is manifested by an exaggerated emotional response to bowel symptoms. Sometimes, the best intervention is withdrawing all previously prescribed medications and simply listening empathically to the patient's problems, helping them cope with their life situation. When specific underlying psychopathology is identified, treatment should be directed toward it. Success rates are high in such circumstances. When bowel symptoms are not due to a well-defined psychiatric illness, use of psychotropic agents is less effective and not recommended. Casual use of popular combination preparations such as a benzodiazepine/antispasmodic formulation should be avoided. A double-blind controlled study of 52 patients manifesting nonspecific anxiety showed that *diazepam* had no effect on bowel complaints compared with placebo.

Depression. Patients with IBS who manifest evidence of depression and receive antidepressant therapy have a high rate of improvement. Both *amitriptyline* and *desipramine* in low doses (50 to 100 mg qhs) have been found to be particularly effective in depressed IBS patients with diarrhea, due in part to their anticholinergic activity reducing bowel hyperactivity (see below). In patients with constipation, a tricyclic with strong anticholinergic effects may actually worsen symptoms. An antidepressant with minimal anticholinergic activity might be a better choice (e.g., a *selective serotonin receptor inhibitor* [SSRI] such as *sertraline* or a *tricyclic antidepressant* with minimal anticholinergic activity [*nortriptyline*]).

Chronic Anxiety. Many patients with IBS suffer from chronic anxiety, but one must be careful not to prescribe anxiolytics chronically because of their strong potential for inducing addiction and causing withdrawal syndromes (see Chapter 226). An *antidepressant with anxiolytic properties* may be a reasonable substitute (e.g., *doxepin, nortriptyline, trazodone, or an SSRI*; see Chapter 227).

Somatization Disorder. Treatment of patients with somatization disorders first requires withdrawing the vast array of medications prescribed by the multitude of physicians they have visited over the years and then setting up regularly scheduled visits for them to talk about their symptoms and personal problems. Such supportive therapy by the primary physician often suffices to alleviate much of their complaining and need for medication (see Chapter 230).

Behavioral methods are worth considering in highly motivated patients. The emphasis is on changing behavior rather than on gaining insight. They provide a sense of control and enhance health-promoting behaviors. *Relaxation techniques* help those with exaggerated sympathetic responses to stress. Patients are taught how to blunt such responses and relax skeletal muscles. *Biofeedback* is used predominantly for treatment of fecal incontinence, aiming for improved control over internal sphincter activity. The method is expensive, but promising. *Hypnosis* has been used successfully to reduce pain perception.

Psychotherapy represents an important treatment option for patients who seek to deal with their illness through better understanding. To be successful, the therapy has to be viewed as personally relevant. The goal is learning to understand and cope with psychosocial stresses. Controlled studies have found psychotherapy plus medication to be superior to medication alone in reducing bowel symptoms. Methods range from traditional insight-focused therapy to cognitive-behavioral approaches, where the emphasis is on identifying stressors and thoughts that precipitate symptoms.

A *multifaceted approach* seems to be the best strategy. In a study of combined therapy that included medication, psychotherapy, and relaxation techniques, results were best when the treatment program used a combination of approaches. Predictors of a good response included presence of overt anxiety or depression, short duration of bowel symptoms, and absence of constant or diffuse pain.

Dietary Measures. Although a major part of the therapeutic effort in IBS involves redirecting the patient's attention away from his or her bowels, it is often necessary to provide patients with symptomatic relief before they are willing to turn their attention to the factors precipitating their symptoms. Dietary manipulations are sometimes helpful in this regard.

Foods that might exacerbate IBS should be avoided, including caffeinated beverages, alcohol, sorbitol-containing candies and gums, citrus fruits in those with fructose intolerance, and milk products in those who prove lactose intolerant. Reducing intake of such poorly digestible carbohydrates as beans and cabbage may help patients suffering from bloating, gas, and abdominal pain.

Many IBS patients insist they have *food allergies* as the cause of their symptoms. Although recent study suggests an increased incidence of food allergies in IBS, true food allergies are rare and typically cause acute hypersensitivity reactions, not chronic GI complaints. No changes in colonic motor activity have been found to occur in such patients on intake of the offending food. However, food intolerance (as noted above) is often noted in patients with IBS, and it may be worthwhile trying to avoid foods that seem poorly tolerated. Some food intolerance is mislabeled as IBS. For example, patients with gluten intolerance (adult celiac disease, nontropical sprue) may present with abdominal discomfort and diarrhea. Persistent diarrhea, bloating, cramping, and excessive flatus may be manifestations of underlying lactose intolerance. A 1- to 2-week trial of restricting a suspected offending food or substance is reasonable when clinical suspicion is high. On the other hand, patients who present having already restricted an unnecessarily large number of foods can have them added back. Rechallenging them with the purported offending agent rebuilds their confidence and avoids nutritional deficiency.

Increasing dietary fiber can help restore propulsive colonic motor activity. However, clinical studies examining bran and high-fiber diets have produced variable results, often no better than control diets due, in part, to a large placebo effect. In a double-blind trial of 50 patients eating a standardized bran biscuit or placebo, both groups reported subjective improvement in more than 50% of the subjects. A more recent controlled but unblinded British study of 26 patients showed significant improvement in symptoms and colonic motor activity in the bran-fed group compared with control subjects. Certainly there is no harm in prescribing a high-fiber diet, and it may have other health benefits such as reducing the risk of colon cancer (see Chapter 76). However, some patients report worsening of bloating and gaseousness with initiation of a high-fiber diet due to bacterial metabolism of nondigestible fiber, although this subsides with time. It is best to start with the equivalent of about 1 tablespoon of bran daily and build up to 3 tablespoons per day as tolerated.

An alternative is to use *bulking agents*, such as the hydrophilic colloid *psyllium* (Metamucil). A total daily dose of 15 to 25 g/d is necessary to achieve benefit and most helpful in IBS patients bothered predominantly by constipation. *Low-residue diets* have been tried. There is no evidence that they are of any use.

Drug Therapy. Pharmacologic intervention should proceed only in the context of a balanced program that includes patient education and support. Precipitously or prematurely resorting to pharmacologic measures in a hasty attempt to suppress symptoms completely can lead to frustration and excessive, even dangerous, escalations of drug intake. In fact, at the outset of therapy, it is often useful to *stop all nonessential medicines* that may affect bowel function, especially irritant laxatives. Nevertheless, there is a role for carefully selected short-term applications of medication when some symptomatic relief is deemed necessary.

Diarrhea. Patients suffering from disabling diarrhea may benefit from use of an opiate derivative. Transit time is prolonged, water and ion absorption is enhanced, and anal sphincter tone is strengthened. These effects result in less diarrhea, rectal urgency, and fecal soiling. *Loperamide* (in doses of 2 to 4 mg four times a day) is the preferred opiate derivative, being less habit forming and less likely to exert central nervous system effects than other derivatives, such as *tincture of opium* or *diphenoxylate*. Patients with diarrhea due to bile acid malabsorption experience improvement with *cholestyramine*. As noted earlier, those with an underlying depression may benefit from use of a tricyclic antidepressant with anticholinergic activity (e.g., *amitriptyline* 50 to 100 mg/d).

Constipation. No drugs have been proven safe and effective for use in IBS patients suffering from constipation. The prokinetic agent *cisapride* is under investigation and may soon be available. It facilitates acetylcholine release from the myenteric plexus. Although transiently helpful in patients with constipation, the drug appears best for dyspeptic symptoms. *Metoclopramide* does not act on the lower bowel and is not recommended for use in IBS. Drugs with anticholinergic activity should be avoided, because they are likely to worsen constipation. As noted above, if antidepressants are needed, it is best to select a preparation without anticholinergic activity (e.g., trazodone, fluoxetine).

Abdominal Pain and Distention. Patients suffering from postprandial pain and distention often request symptomatic relief. *Anticholinergic agents* have been used in such circumstances. The rationale is to reduce the cholinergic stimulation of colonic activity that occurs in response to a meal. The anticholinergic *dicyclomine* (10 to 20 mg before a meal) is the preparation most often recommended in this context. Although such agents have been shown to inhibit the postprandial increase in nonpropulsive colonic contractions, their clinical effectiveness is unproven. However, the consensus is that they are worth a try in cases in which nonpharmacologic measures have failed. They are best prescribed for short-term use. Chronic use should be avoided, because of the risk of worsening constipation and pain. *Combination preparations* containing a tranquilizer (e.g., a benzodiazepine or a barbiturate) and an anticholinergic are promoted as *"bowel relaxants"* or *"antispasmodics."* They are heavily advertised yet of no proven benefit and best avoided because of their habituation potential and poor efficacy. Whether the newer anxiolytics, which are nonsedating and free of habituation potential (e.g., *buspirone* 15 to 30 mg/d), will prove beneficial remains to be proven. Studies are ongoing on the use of opioids, enkephalins, and other agents that have potential for blocking or modulating gut pain receptors.

Herbal Therapy. Herbal therapies have become very popular among patients who suffer from chronic functional conditions that resist a simple approach to cure. Most herbal therapies have not been subjected to scientific study. Chinese herbal medicine is a centuries-old remedy for GI symptoms. In the only randomized, double-blind, placebo-controlled trial to date using standardized preparations of Chinese herbal medicine in patients fulfilling standard diagnostic criteria for IBS, patients treated with the herbal preparation for 16 weeks showed significant improvements in scores for bowel symptoms and global state and in patient scores for daily functioning. Such intriguing preliminary findings need to be confirmed and more importantly need to prove durable over time, because symptoms returned rapidly in the above study after cessation of herbal therapy.

Patient Education

Because IBS is a condition characterized by an exaggerated response to symptoms, patient education is central to effective management. As noted earlier, the basic elements of the patient education effort include addressing patient fears, providing a specific diagnosis, and explaining the pathophysiologic basis of symptoms. In patients with symptoms triggered by psychosocial stress, an explanation (perhaps aided by diagrams) of how such stress can lead to functional alterations in bowel motility helps patients to better understand their condition and cope with it.

When important situational stress or psychopathology is uncovered, it needs to be discussed openly so that the patient can begin to focus on the underlying issues rather than on bowel symptoms. Sometimes, having the patient keep a diary of symptoms, stresses, and feelings can help reveal connections that have otherwise eluded the patient. The major lesson to be mastered by patients with IBS is the relationship between their psychological state and symptoms, a message that often takes patience, sensitivity, and skill to communicate effectively. It is important not to push discussion and treatment of psychological issues beyond what the patient is prepared to accept. Patients initially unwilling to consider such issues should be respected, but once a supportive relationship is established, they often begin to cope better and spend less time obsessing about their bowels and more on the underlying issues triggering their "disease."

Patients not psychologically minded can still be helped greatly by changing the focus of their care from cure of symptoms to improvement in functional status. At each office visit, instead of asking for an in-depth recitation of bowel complaints, the physician spends more time inquiring into how the patient is dealing with the demands of daily life and helping the patient to cope with them. The visit agenda shifts from eliminating symptoms to solving problems. Such a shift is often remarkably refreshing and revealing; it helps improve functional capacity and reduces the intensity of bodily complaints.

Indications for Referral and Admission

This is a condition in which a continuous relationship is essential, and any perceived need for referral should be acted on only after thorough discussion with the patient. In general, referral is helpful when there are refractory disabling symptoms, such as uncontrollable diarrhea, or when serious psychopathology is encountered. Less disturbed patients may also benefit from psychiatric referral, but only if the patient is accepting of a psychological dimension to the illness and is motivated to delve into it. A hospital admission may, in rare circumstances, be appropriate and very beneficial in helping the patient to learn new means of coping with stress and providing a respite from an intolerable living situation.

Management Recommendations

- Take the patient's bowel complaints seriously; do not minimize their importance or deny their "reality."
- Elicit a full psychosocial database and a complete history of the patient's bodily symptoms.
- Conduct a thorough workup that includes a detailed investigation of all possible etiologies, both organic and psychological.
- Provide a thorough explanation of the diagnosis and directly address the patient's concerns and fears.
- Establish a supportive relationship and begin supportive psychotherapy for patients with underlying situational or psychosocial stresses.
- Identify, discuss, and treat specifically any underlying depression (see Chapter 227), anxiety disorder (see Chapter 226), somatization (see Chapter 230), or other psychiatric condition.
- When treating a depressed patient with antidepressant medication, consider its degree of anticholinergic activity and match it appropriately to bowel symptoms (e.g., amitriptyline 50 to 100 mg qhs is helpful for the patient with diarrhea; an SSRI [e.g., sertraline 25 mg/d] is a better choice in the patient

with IBS bothered by constipation; see Chapter 227).
- Stop all nonessential medicines that may affect bowel function, especially irritant laxatives.
- For the patient bothered predominantly by constipation, increase dietary fiber and recommend regular exercise. Add a bulking agent such as psyllium (Metamucil), 1 rounded teaspoon in 8 oz of water three times a day if constipation is still troublesome. A stool softener (e.g., dioctyl sodium sulfosuccinate) is sometimes helpful.
- If the patient finds abdominal pain and distention intolerable, resort to a trial of anticholinergic therapy (e.g., dicyclomine 20 mg four times a day), but only if other measures have failed. It may also be useful for diarrhea. Use only for a short period of time. Tricyclic antidepressants with anticholinergic activity may also be worth a trial (e.g., amitriptyline 50 to 100 mg qhs), but avoid these if constipation is bothersome.
- For the patient with diarrhea, evaluate first for underlying bowel pathology (e.g., parasitic disease, colitis; see Chapter 64) and then limit intake of potentially contributing substances such as caffeine, sorbitol-containing candies and chewing gums, alcohol, and dairy products (except for yogurt preparations). When short-term symptomatic relief is essential, prescribe a 2- to 5-day supply of loperamide, 1 tablet twice a day as needed. Exercise caution with opiate use because of its addiction potential in this chronic condition.
- For patients with refractory diarrhea, consider a diagnostic trial of cholestyramine (4 g three or four times a day), which will counter any concurrent bile acid malabsorption.
- Major dietary restrictions are usually unnecessary. However, if there is a strongly suggestive history of intolerance to a food or substance, consider a 1- or 2-week trial of omitting its intake. Sorbitol and lactose are the most common offenders.
- Despite the presence of chronic anxiety, avoid use of sedatives, tranquilizers, and combination preparations containing benzodiazepines or barbiturates. The risks of habituation and withdrawal outweigh any benefit. Antidepressants with anxiolytic activity (e.g., amitriptyline, trazodone, doxepin) are reasonable alternatives, as might be the nonaddicting azapirone anxiolytics (e.g., buspirone).
- Help redirect the patient's attention away from bowel symptoms and endless searches for cure and toward better coping with daily stresses; focus on accomplishments rather than symptoms, on taking control through exercise, good eating habits, and behavioral changes rather than on repeated recitation of symptoms.
- For motivated patients with well-identified psychosocial stressors, consider referral for a combination of behavioral techniques and psychotherapy.
- At this time there is insufficient evidence to recommend a trial of Chinese herbal medicine.
- See patient at regular intervals and be available for help at times of increased stress.

NONULCER DYSPEPSIA

Nonulcer dyspepsia is a poorly defined condition characterized by recurrent upper abdominal pain and discomfort that frequently, but not exclusively, occurs with eating. The discomfort may encompass bloating, nausea, distention, early satiety, and anorexia. The term *dyspepsia* literally means "bad digestion," although it is not meant to be synonymous with or inclusive of other symptoms of "indigestion" (such as heartburn, eructation, or regurgitation). Rather, the emphasis is on the abdominal pain, which may resemble the discomfort of peptic ulcer disease, thus the term "nonulcer." Older terms for this condition also alluded to its ulcer-negative status, including "x-ray–negative dyspepsia" and "functional dyspepsia."

Nonulcer dyspepsia is twice as prevalent as ulcer-related dyspeptic disease and one of several GI conditions that can cause upper abdominal pain in the absence of an ulcer (see Chapter 58). Billions of dollars are spent annually on its evaluation and treatment, yet remarkably little is known about its pathogenesis. However, new data are emerging, and the primary care physician needs to understand the relative importance of diet, smoking, acid secretion, gastric motility, stress, and *Helicobacter* infection to fashion a rational and cost-effective treatment plan.

Pathophysiology, Clinical Presentation, and Course

Mechanisms. The pathophysiology of nonulcer dyspepsia remains largely unknown. A number of factors have been proposed, and as in many other functional disorders, the etiology is probably multifactorial.

Dysmotility. Among the most consistent abnormalities is disordered upper GI motility. Gastric emptying is delayed, and gas transit is slowed in about half of dyspeptic patients. Distention and bloating are common and thought to be manifestations of this slowing.

Altered Nociception (visceral perception) is suggested by the increase in pain reported by about half of dyspeptic patients to intragastric balloon inflation at volumes that do not cause pain in normal persons.

Psychological Factors. Patients who present with dyspepsia have higher frequencies of anxiety, depression, and neuroticism, and exacerbations of symptoms often coincide with increases in situational stress. However, investigators cannot tell if this pattern is because of the role of psychological factors in dyspepsia or because of the role of such factors in health-seeking behavior. It is noteworthy that persons with dyspepsia report greater stress in their lives.

Excessive Acid Production. Although excess acid production may play some role in nonulcer dyspepsia (especially patients who go on to develop a peptic ulcer), it does not appear to be the predominant pathogenic factor. Patients and control subjects show little difference in gastric acid secretion. H_2-blocker therapy and antacids are little better than placebo in providing relief, but combination therapy and use of proton-pump inhibitors does provide relief for some patients, probably those with an underlying ulcer "diathesis" or concurrent esophageal reflux.

Helicobacter Infection. Of great interest has been the contribution of *Helicobacter pylori* infection because it can cause gastritis. *H. pylori* infection is present in about 60% of cases of nonulcer dyspepsia, but this high frequency is not much greater than that for the population at large. Large-scale, randomized, placebo-controlled studies of eradicating *Helicobacter* infection have shown only modest benefit (e.g., 25% long-term cure rates compared with rates of 7% to 21% in omeprazole-treated control subjects). These results indicate that although *Helicobacter* infection may be important in a small subset of patients, it is not the major causative that was hypothesized.

Maldigestion/Malabsorption of Carbohydrates. Dyspeptic symptoms are common in persons with lactase deficiency and those who take in large amounts of nonabsorbable sugars through heavy use of chewing gum, diet foods, and related products with sorbitol, fructose, or mannitol.

Other Factors. A number of other potential precipitants have been examined. *Smoking, alcohol, coffee, and tea* were not found to have any relation to nonulcer dyspepsia. Although *fatty food intolerance* is a common complaint in dyspeptic patients, controlled studies using disguised meals fail to confirm fatty foods as precipitants. *Bile reflux* has been proposed and when found can cause dyspepsia-like symptoms, but no increase in bile concentrations have been found in dyspeptic patients who have not undergone prior surgery. *NSAIDs* and *aspirin* are well-recognized gastric irritants, but in case-controlled studies no relation was found between their use and nonulcer dyspepsia.

Clinical Presentation. Recurrent upper abdominal pain and discomfort are the hallmarks. In about half of instances, symptoms are associated with meals. Bloating and gaseous distention may accompany the pain. Acid reflux, biliary colic, painful or altered defecation, and chronic pain are not considered part of its presentation but rather features of other forms of nonulcer upper abdominal pain; however, they often coexist with dyspepsia (e.g., 25% of dyspeptic patients also report reflux symptoms).

Clinical course is benign, with little evidence that the condition ultimately leads to peptic ulceration or other forms of upper GI pathology. Previously, nonulcer dyspepsia was seen as part of a continuum that progressed to duodenitis and frank peptic ulceration, but this suspicion has not been confirmed (although a small subset of patients go on to develop a peptic ulcer). Typically, the condition is chronic. Although it may wax and wane, it usually does not worsen substantially.

Workup

Because the symptoms of nonulcer dyspepsia are nonspecific and may mimic more serious pathology, the diagnostic task is to rule out the must-not-miss etiologies. At the top of the list are gastric carcinoma, complicated peptic ulcer disease, and erosive esophagitis and low-grade chronic pancreatitis, biliary tract disease, and IBS. Upper GI endoscopy can readily identify and distinguish among many of these conditions—particularly gastric cancer, peptic ulcer, and esophagitis—but the high frequency and harmlessness of nonulcer dyspepsia and the high cost of endoscopy necessitate some risk stratification.

Upper Endoscopy. Selectivity is necessary for cost-effective workup. If everyone was studied endoscopically at the time of initial presentation, the yield would be extremely low and the testing would be wasteful, because most will have nonulcer dyspepsia and a normal study. Most authorities recommend a workup strategy based on risk stratification for the serious pathology noted above. Consensus criteria cite age older than 45 years (or any other demographic risk factor for gastric cancer) and unexplained weight loss, persistent nausea and vomiting, dysphagia, odynophagia, jaundice, iron deficiency anemia, or a positive guaiac stool test as indicative of increased risk of serious underlying pathology. Although a relatively low threshold is set for endoscopy by using a cutoff age of 45 years (some use older than 50 years, others older than 55 years), the cost of endoscopy can be quickly surpassed by indefinite unnecessary use of commonly used empiric therapies (e.g., acid suppression, prokinetic agents), not to mention the cost of delay in diagnosis of a more serious potentially treatable condition and the persistent worry about cancer by the patient.

These recommendations are based on cost-effectiveness analyses; they need to be validated by prospective study. Nonetheless, those who are deemed low risk can skip endoscopy and proceed to consideration of Helicobacter testing (see below). Subsequent endoscopic investigation of low-risk patients deserves consideration in those who fail to respond to a trial of empiric therapy or later develop any of the manifestations suggestive of more serious disease.

Testing for *H. pylori* Infection. Low-risk patients benefit from testing for *Helicobacter* infection, because eradication cures symptoms in the 20% of *Helicobacter*-positive dyspeptics who prove to have a peptic ulcer or a peptic ulcer "diathesis" and the 20% of *Helicobacter*-positive dyspeptics with nonulcer dyspepsia who respond to eradication of the infection. Serologic study for *Helicobacter* antibodies (see Chapter 68) usually suffices for this purpose.

Other Studies. The clinical presentation can also determine the need for other investigations. Patients with heartburn are likely to have gastroesophageal reflux and should be worked up accordingly (see Chapter 61). Patients reporting paroxysmal attacks of constant epigastric or right upper quadrant pain lasting a few hours and radiating into the back require consideration of biliary tract disease and *abdominal ultrasound* and *liver function testing* (see Chapter 69). Unrelenting upper abdominal pain radiating into the back, especially if alcohol related, suggests chronic pancreatitis. Serum *amylase* and abdominal ultrasound are indicated (see Chapter 72). Altered bowel habits in conjunction with upper abdominal pain argue for IBS involving the transverse colon; colitis and bowel cancer may need to be ruled out by *colonoscopy or barium enema* (see above).

Principles of Management

Given the poor understanding of the precise pathophysiology of nonulcer dyspepsia, its likely multifactorial nature, and the lack of tight correlation between clinical presentation and response to treatment, it should not be surprising that there is little consensus on how best to treat the condition. Options include eradication of *Helicobacter* infection, chronic acid suppression, prokinetic therapy, dietary manipulations, and psychotherapy.

Eradication of *Helicobacter* Infection. Those who are *Helicobacter*-positive are reasonable candidates for eradication of the *H. pylori* infection (see Chapter 68), even though most test-positive nonulcer dyspeptics are unlikely to respond. Because there are other benefits to *Helicobacter* eradication beside cure of dyspeptic symptoms (see Chapter 68), treatment is not without merit even if there is no response clinically.

Acid Suppression. Contrary to common belief, there is little evidence that acid-inhibiting or acid-neutralizing treatment significantly improves symptoms in patients with documented nonulcer dyspepsia. Much of the confusion about the efficacy of such antiulcer therapy seems to result from a substantial placebo effect, the heterogeneous nature of patients with dyspepsia, and poor characterization of patients in many studies. Randomized controlled trials have failed to demonstrate consistent benefit from use of antiulcer therapy in patients with carefully documented nonulcer dyspepsia. This correlates with data showing little excess acid production in most of these patients. Those who respond to empiric therapy may be the subset with an underlying peptic ulcer diathesis. Some interpret response to empiric proton-pump inhibition as a sign of underlying gastroesophageal reflux or peptic ulcer disease. More and better data are required to clarify the use of these very expensive drugs in dyspepsia. In the meantime, physicians are likely to continue prescribing acid-suppression antiulcer therapy empirically because there is little else to offer patients. If such therapy is to be offered, it should be given for a limited time and not continued if symptoms fail to resolve.

Enhancing Gastric Motility. If indeed nonulcer dyspepsia is a disease of altered upper GI motility, then drugs that facilitate such motility would be expected to be beneficial. *Metoclopramide*, the original dopaminergic blocking agent available for stimulating gastric motility, provides some benefit as short-term therapy. Unfortunately, long-term administration of the drug is associated with risk of tardive dyskinesia, making it inappropriate for prolonged use. *Cisapride* is the first of another class of prokinetic agents that release acetylcholine at the myenteric plexus to stimulate upper GI motility. It appears better tolerated than metoclopramide, but data on its efficacy and long-term safety are still pending. A proarrhythmic effect has been noted and caution is indicated when used with other agents (see Chapter 61).

Diet, Alcohol, Smoking, and Stress. No data indicate that a low-fat diet, restriction of alcohol, cessation of smoking, or reduction of stress have any consistently positive effect on nonulcer dyspepsia. The lack of effect may be as much a function of the heterogeneous nature of the dyspeptic population as it is an indication of true absence of benefit. Most authorities recommend taking a careful history to identify any precipitants and responding to them. In otherwise refractory cases where there is a clearcut association between dyspepsia and psychosocial factors, the latter should be addressed thoroughly (see Chapters 226, 227, and 230).

Patient Education and Indications for Referral

Patients who present with recurrent upper abdominal pain are fearful of cancer and other serious forms of GI pathology. For many, the first priority is knowing that they do not have a life-threatening illness. As with any disorder that can mimic more worrisome illness, the patient's concerns should be taken seriously and addressed directly (see the Reassurance section on IBS above; the same principles and approach apply here).

Referral to a gastroenterologist is indicated when endoscopy is considered. The most appropriate candidates are those at increased risk of gastric malignancy and other serious upper GI pathology (see above). At times, a consultation with the gastroenterologist will help reassure the low-risk but overly concerned patient, although the need for such referrals can be kept to a minimum by thorough patient education and support.

A.H.G.

ANNOTATED BIBLIOGRAPHY

Irritable Bowel Syndrome

Almy T. Experimental studies on the irritable colon. Am J Med 1951;10:60. (*Classic paper on relation of stress to bowel activity.*)

Bensoussan A, Talley NJ, Hing M, et al. Treatment of irritable bowel syndrome with Chinese herbal medicine. JAMA 1998;280:1585. (*The only randomized, double-blind, placebo-controlled trial to date; improvements noted in symptom score and quality of life; benefit ceased with cessation of therapy except in those given a customized program.*)

Camilleri M, Prather CM. The irritable bowel syndrome: mechanisms and a practical approach to management. Ann Intern Med 1992;116:1001. (*Best review of pathophysiology and a very useful mechanistic approach to treatment; 78 references.*)

Cann PA, Read NW, Holdsworth CD. What is the benefit of coarse wheat bran in patients with irritable bowel syndrome. Gut 1984;25:168. (*Bran did help pain, constipation, diarrhea, and urgency, as did placebo, except for constipation, which responded better with bran.*)

Cann PA, Read NW, Holdsworth CD, et al. Role of loperamide and placebo in management of irritable bowel syndrome. Dig Dis Sci 1984;29:239. (*Proved superior to placebo in patients with diarrhea, urgency, and incontinence.*)

Deutsch E. Relief of anxiety and related emotions in patients with gastrointestinal disorders. Am J Dig Dis 1971;16:1091. (*Diazepam relieved anxiety but did not improve bowel symptoms any better than did placebo.*)

Drossman DA, McKee DC, Sandler RS, et al. Psychosocial factors in the irritable bowel syndrome. A multivariate study of patients and nonpatients with irritable bowel syndrome. Gastroenterology 1988;95:701. (*Underlying psychopathology is a major predictor of becoming a patient.*)

Drossman DA, Thompson WG. The irritable bowel syndrome: review and a graduated multicomponent treatment approach. Ann Intern Med 1992;116:1009. (*An outstanding review and the best on psychosocial factors and their management; 117 references.*)

Esler M, Goulston K. Levels of anxiety in colonic disorders. N Engl J Med 1973;288:16. (*Patients with predominant diarrhea were significantly more anxious and more neurotic by psychometric testing than normal persons or those with constipation and pain.*)

Greenbaum, Mayle JE, Vanegeren LE, et al. Effects of desipramine on irritable bowel syndrome compared with atropine and placebo. Dig Dis Sci 1987;32:257. (*The antidepressant was best in patients with diarrhea.*)

Guthrie E, Creed F, Dawson D, et al. A controlled trial of psychological treatment for the irritable bowel syndrome. Gastroenterology 1991;100:450. (*Useful data on efficacy and patient selection.*)

Hislop I. Psychological significance of the irritable colon syndrome. Gut 1971;12:452. (*Fifty-six of 67 patients with irritable colon syndrome were treated with tricyclic antidepressants. More than 80% reported significant improvement.*)

Jones AV, McLaughlan P, Shorthouse M, et al. Food intolerance: a major factor in the pathogenesis of the irritable bowel syndrome. Lancet 1982;2:115. (*The evidence for intolerance to wheat, corn, dairy products, coffee, tea, and citrus fruits.*)

Klein KB. Controlled treatment trials in the irritable bowel syndrome: A critique. Gastroenterology 1988;95:232. (*Important article on methodologic shortcomings of most studies; essential reading before reviewing the literature.*)

Kruis W, Thieme C, Weinzierl M, et al. A diagnostic score for the irritable bowel syndrome, its value in the exclusion of organic disease. Gastroenterology 1984;87:1. (*Elaborate regression study providing a weighted score with high specificity and sensitivity; blood in the stool rules out the diagnosis.*)

Longstreth GF, Fox DD, Youkeles MS, et al. Psyllium therapy in the irritable bowel syndrome. Ann Intern Med 1981;95:53. (*Randomized, double-blind, controlled study; both treatment and controlled groups improved significantly, suggesting strong psychological overlay of symptoms and efficacy of supportive measures.*)

Manning AP, Thompson WG, Heaton KW, et al. Towards positive diagnosis of the irritable bowel syndrome. Br Med J 1978;2:653. (*Most widely accepted criteria for diagnosis.*)

Merrick MV, Eastwood MA, Ford MJ. Is bile acid malabsorption underdiagnosed? An evaluation of accuracy of diagnosis by measurement of SeHCAT retention. Br Med J 1985;290:665. (*Diagnosis and the role for bile acid malabsorption.*)

Mertz H, Fullerton S, Naliboff B, et al. Symptoms and visceral perception in severe functional and organic dyspepsia. Gut 1998;42:814. (*Half of dyspeptic patients have pain on intragastric balloon inflation at volumes too low to cause pain in normals.*)

Nanda R, James R, Smith H, et al. Food intolerance and the irritable bowel syndrome. Gut 1989;30:1099. (*Reviews the evidence for the role of food intolerance.*)

Newcomer AD, McGill DB. Clinical importance of lactose deficiency. N Engl J Med 1984;310:42. (*Editorial summarizing the data on lactose deficiency in clinical syndromes, including its role in IBS.*)

Owens DM, Nelson DK, Talley NJ. The irritable bowel syndrome: long-term prognosis and the physician-patient interaction. Ann Intern Med 1995;122:107. (*The Olmstead county experience: prognosis is good; the initial diagnosis is unlikely to change; and use of ambulatory health services is reduced by development of a strong patient–doctor relationship.*)

Prior A, Colgan SM, Whorwell PJ. Changes in rectal sensitivity after hypnotherapy in patients with irritable bowel syndrome. Gut 1990;31:896. (*Pain threshold raised, suggesting a mechanism and role for hypnotherapy in IBS.*)

Rumessen JJ, Gudmand-Hoyer E. Functional bowel disease: malabsorption and abdominal distress after ingestion of fructose, sorbitol, and fructose-sorbitol mixtures. Gastroenterology 1988;95:694. (*Evidence for their role in some cases of IBS.*)

Schwarz SP, Taylor AE, Scharff L, et al. Behaviorally treated irritable bowel syndrome patients: A four-year follow-up. Behav Res Ther 1990;28:331. (*Lasting response demonstrated.*)

Smart HL, Mayberry JF, Atkinson M. Alternative medicine consultations and remedies in patients with irritable bowel syndrome. Gut 1986;27:826. (*Up to 20% make use of alternative treatment; suggests needs are not being met by their physicians.*)

Smith RC, Greenbaum DS, Vancouver JB, et al. Psychosocial factors are associated with health care seeking rather than diagnosis in irritable bowel syndrome. Gastroenterology 1990;98:293. (*The title says it all.*)

Sullivan M, Cohen S, Snape W. Colonic myoelectric activity in irritable bowel syndrome. N Engl J Med 1978;298:878. (*Patients with IBS and abnormally prolonged increase in postprandial motor activity, which was reduced by an anticholinergic agent.*)

Svendsen JH, Munck LK, Andersen JR. Irritable bowel syndrome—prognosis and diagnostic safety. Scand J Gastroenterol 1985;20:415. (*Disease waxes and wanes; only rarely [0 to 3% of cases] is there a missed diagnosis of organic disease, even after 5 years of follow-up.*)

Talley NJ, Thieme C, Weinzierl M, et al. Diagnostic value of the Manning criteria in irritable bowel syndrome. Gut 1990;31:77. (*Best critique of these diagnostic criteria.*)

Treacher DF, et al. Irritable bowel syndrome: is barium enema necessary? Clin Radiol 1986;37:87. (*Retrospective analysis of 114 patients; barium enema rarely revealed useful information in patients who had normal hematologic and biochemical screening, especially in those under age 50.*)

Van Outryve M, Milo R, Toussant J, et al. Prokinetic treatment of constipation–predominant irritable bowel syndrome: a placebo controlled study of cisapride. J Clin Gastroenterol 1991;13:49. (*Benefit demonstrated.*)

Whitehead WE, Holtkotter B, Enck P, et al. Tolerance for rectosigmoid distention in irritable bowel syndrome. Gastroenterology 1990; 98:1187. (*Sensation thresholds are altered.*)

Young S, Alper D, Norland C, et al. Psychiatric illness and the irritable bowel syndrome. Gastroenterology 1970;70:162. (*Seventy-two percent of patients with IBS in a general group practice have an underlying psychiatric illness; only 28% were properly recognized and diagnosed.*)

Zwetchkenbaum JF, Burakoff R. Food allergy and the irritable bowel syndrome. Am J Gastroenterol 1988;83:901. (*Disputes the role of food allergy; see also Nanda et al. above.*)

Nonulcer Dyspepsia

Blum AL, Talley NJ, O'Morain C, et al. Lack of effect of treating Helicobacter pylori infection in patients with nonulcer dyspepsia. N Engl J Med 1998;339:1875. (*A well-designed, randomized, placebo-controlled study showing no difference in symptoms at 12 months despite documented eradication of infection.*)

Fisher RS, Parkman HP. Management of nonulcer dyspepsia. N Engl J Med 1998;339:1376. (*A useful review of management, most notably for its excellent discussion of theories of pathogenesis; 59 references.*)

Friedman LS. *Helicobacter pylori* and nonulcer dyspepsia. N Engl J Med 1998;339:1928. (*An editorial summarizing the best evidence available and proposing very reasonable recommendations.*)

Health and Public Policy Committee, American College of Physicians. Endoscopy in the evaluation of dyspepsia. Ann Intern Med 1986;102:266. (*Recommends a 6- to 8-week course of empiric antiulcer therapy in low-risk patients before considering endoscopic evaluation.*)

Johannessen T, Petersen H, Kristensen P, et al. Cimetidine for symptomatic relief of dyspepsia. Scand J Gastroenterol 1992;27:189. (*Evidence for benefit with H_2-blocker therapy.*)

Johnson AF. Controlled trial of metoclopramide in the treatment of flatulent dyspepsia. Br Med J 1971;2:25. (*Nausea and pain were relieved.*)

McColl K, Murray L, El-Omar E, et al. Symptomatic benefit from eradicating Helicobacter pylori infection in patients with nonulcer dyspepsia. N Engl J Med 1998;339:1869. (*A randomized placebo-controlled study showing a modest long-term benefit [21% vs. 7%] from antibiotic therapy in patients positive for H. pylori.*)

Nyren O, Adami HO, Bates S, et al. Absence of therapeutic benefit from antacids or cimetidine in nonulcer dyspepsia. N Engl J Med 1986;314:339. (*Evidence against benefit from antiulcer therapy.*)

Ofman JJ, Etchason J, Fullerton S, et al. Management strategies for Helicobacter pylori–seropositive patients with dyspepsia: clinical and economic consequences. Ann Intern Med 1997;126:280. (*A decision-analysis study supporting the cost effectiveness of serologic testing and treatment for Helicobacter infection.*)

Rosch W. Cisapride in nonulcer dyspepsia. Results of a placebo-controlled trial. Scand J Gastroenterol 1987;22:161. (*Promising results with this prokinetic agent.*)

Strauss RM, Wang TC, Kelsey PB. Association of Helicobacter pylori infection with dyspeptic symptoms in patients undergoing gastroduodenoscopy. Am J Med 1990;89:464. (*Prevalence of infection was greater in those with dyspepsia.*)

Talley NJ, Boyce P, Jones M. Dyspepsia and health care seeking in a community: how important are psychological factors? Dig Dis Sci 1998;43:1016. (*Increased incidence of psychological factors found among patients; a pathophysiologic mechanism or a cause of health seeking?*)

Talley NJ, McNeil D, Piper DW. Environmental factors and chronic unexplained dyspepsia: Association with acetaminophen but not other analgesics, alcohol, coffee, tea, or smoking. Dig Dis Sci 1989;33. (*Surprising but well-documented findings.*)

Talley NJ, Phillips SF. Nonulcer dyspepsia: potential causes and pathophysiology. Ann Intern Med 1988;108:865. (*Exhaustive, slightly dated, but still useful review with excellent discussions of disease mechanisms, possible precipitants, and workup, all with practical implications; 268 references.*)

Talley NJ, Silverstein MD, Agreus L, et al. AGA technical review: evaluation of dyspepsia. Gastroenterology 1998;114:582. (*A consensus guideline.*)

Zell SC, Budhraja M. An approach to dyspepsia in the ambulatory care setting: evaluation based on risk stratification. J Gen Intern Med 1989;4:144. (*Argues for a diagnostic approach that assigns low-risk patients to empiric antiulcer treatment rather than endoscopic study.*)

75

Management of Diverticular Disease

Diverticula, abnormal herniations of colonic mucosa through the muscularis, are extremely common and increase with age. Autopsy studies estimate their presence in 20% of people over 40 and in 70% of those over 70. About 15% of people with the condition develop attacks of *diverticulitis*, in which the diverticula become plugged and inflamed. It is possible that the recent emphasis on increasing the fiber content of the diet will reduce the incidences of diverticula and their complications in Western countries. The primary physician encounters many elderly patients with gastrointestinal (GI) complaints referable to diverticular disease. The physician must effectively and economically recognize and treat mild manifestations of disease, reduce the chances of complications, and decide when admission and surgical intervention are necessary.

PATHOPHYSIOLOGY, CLINICAL PRESENTATION, AND COMPLICATIONS

Pathophysiology. Increased intracolonic pressure causes herniation of colonic mucosa. Consequently, diverticula occur most frequently in the sigmoid colon, where the colon is narrowest and pressure is greatest; however, diverticula can occur anywhere within the colon, including the ascending portion, which makes for atypical clinical presentations. Diverticula show a predilection for points of relative weakness in the muscularis, especially where branches of the marginal artery penetrate the colonic wall. The possibility of muscular degeneration has been suggested but remains unproven. Current research indicates that the *low fiber content* of modern diets has an important causal role, producing less bulky stool and increased intracolonic pressure. *Irritable bowel syndrome*, with its abnormal colonic motor activity and segmentation, might contribute to diverticular formation by way of increased intraluminal pressures.

The diverticular sac that ensues is a thin purely mucosal structure. Obstruction of the sack's neck by undigested food residues or a fecalith leads to distention and *microabscess* formation as mucous secretions accumulate and bacteria proliferate. If the blood supply to the sac becomes mechanically compromised, the sac may perforate. *Microperforations* commonly occur, producing peridiverticular and pericolonic inflammation and abscess formation. Walling off is the rule because these perforations typically occur adjacent to mesocolon. The bowel lumen is typically uninvolved. Even if a peridiverticular abscess ruptures into the peritoneal cavity, gross peritonitis from fecal soilage usually does not occur because the diverticular neck is sealed by obstructing material.

A less common but potentially catastrophic complication of diverticular disease is *free colonic perforation*, which occurs from rupture of an uninflamed diverticulum. Fecal soilage follows, because there is no plug in the diverticular neck to prevent leakage of bowel contents. Frank peritonitis is the consequence.

Clinical Presentation and Course. *Diverticulosis* is usually asymptomatic and often discovered incidentally on barium enema. However, colonic motor activity is sometimes disturbed, and intermittent left lower quadrant pain may result. Constipation is common, as is constipation alternating with diarrhea, and occasionally there is tenderness.

Diverticulitis is characterized by left lower quadrant pain, tenderness, fever, and leukocytosis in a patient with known diverticulosis. Frequently a tender mass is noted. Right-sided presentations are possible, especially in Asian populations, and may mimic appendicitis or Crohn's disease. The diagnosis is made clinically during an acute attack and confirmed later by barium enema, once the risk of perforation subsides. At times, the radiologic findings resemble those of cancer or Crohn's disease, and colonoscopy is needed for more definitive evaluation. In rare instances, there are extraintestinal manifestations (arthritis, pyoderma gangrenosum) that may simulate those of Crohn's disease and lead to misdiagnosis. Bladder symptoms (dysuria, urgency, frequency) may occur if the process occurs adjacent to the bladder or bladder nerves.

The major *complications* of diverticular disease are perforation, obstruction, and bleeding. *Perforations* may lead to abscess formation. The abscesses may spontaneously drain into the bowel or erode into an adjacent organ, such as the ureter, bladder, or vagina, forming *fistulas*. Perforations that fail to become walled off may cause peritonitis. Those that enter the vagina result in vaginal gas or feces; those that erode into the urinary tract lead to dysuria or pneumaturia. Chronic inflammation can thicken the bowel wall and cause *obstruction*. Erosion into a blood vessel may result in brisk rectal *hemorrhage*. Diverticular disease is one of the most common causes of lower GI hemorrhage and a leading consideration in patients who present with brisk rectal bleeding (see Chapter 63). In a 15-year study from the Lahey Clinic, the incidence of hemorrhage, obstruction, or perforation from diverticular disease was 15%.

DIAGNOSIS

Diverticulosis. As noted earlier, diverticulosis is usually an incidental finding in a patient undergoing a *barium enema or colonoscopy* for another reason. However, the diagnosis should also be considered in a patient presenting with relatively painless but brisk rectal bleeding. If the bleeding is not too severe, *proctosigmoidoscopy* can be performed to confirm the diagnosis and site of blood loss.

Diverticulitis. The diagnosis of acute diverticulitis should be suspected in an older patient who presents with new onset of left lower quadrant abdominal pain, low-grade fever, focal tenderness with or without guarding, and an elevated white blood cell count. In rare instances, the pain may be suprapubic or localized to the right lower quadrant if there is a redundant sigmoid or a right-sided diverticulum. Nausea, vomiting, and diarrhea or constipation may accompany the bowel complaints and simulate gastroenteritis. Absence of bowel sounds suggests peritoneal inflammation. In situations of diagnostic uncertainty, confirmatory testing can be obtained.

Computed tomography (CT) of the abdomen has become the test of choice for immediate confirmation of acute diverticulitis, supplanting barium enema. Although more expensive than barium enema, CT has proven more cost effective. Diagnostic findings include inflammation of pericolic fat, peridiverticular abscess, thickening of bowel wall more than 4 mm, and presence of diverticula. The test can be used to differentiate cancer from diverticulitis and provides the opportunity for guiding needle aspiration and drainage of large abscesses (greater than 5 cm). Although CT is the current diagnostic test of choice, it is not without its shortcomings. The false-negative rate can be as high as 20%, due in part to inability to detect small abscesses and to differentiate tumor from diverticulitis when there is marked bowel wall thickening.

Proctosigmoidoscopy performed with a flexible sigmoidoscope can be done comfortably, safely, and with a minimum of bowel preparation when it is essential to rule out other causes of serious colonic pathology, such as inflammatory bowel disease and cancer. Inability to pass the flexible sigmoidoscope beyond the rectosigmoid junction due to acute bowel inflammation is strongly suggestive of acute diverticulitis.

Barium enema can demonstrate diverticulitis; the finding of contrast outside the bowel lumen is an important diagnostic feature. However, many clinicians are reluctant to order a barium enema during the acute phase of illness, because of concern that the air insufflation used to perform the test might sufficiently increase intraluminal pressure to dislodge the obstructing diverticular plug and cause bowel perforation and fecal soilage. Although this concern is disputed, it is common practice to delay performing a barium contrast study until after inflammation quiets down. The diagnostic accuracy of barium study has been questioned by some investigators, especially its ability to differentiate between diverticular disease and malignancy, which is better detected by endoscopic study.

Differentiating Diverticulitis from Colon Cancer. One of the most important diagnostic tasks in the assessment of suspected diverticulitis is differentiation from colon cancer. Both produce similar clinical presentations and similar radiologic findings on barium enema. CT at the time of initial diagnosis sometimes can help make the distinction, but sensitivity falls in the setting of marked bowel wall thickening. Lower GI *endoscopy* is the more definitive test, allowing for direct visualization and biopsy if tumor is present. The test is usually done after acute symptoms have quieted down.

PRINCIPLES OF MANAGEMENT

Diverticulosis. The goals of therapy are prevention of symptoms, relief of pain, and avoidance of complications. Because diverticular disease is believed to be, in part, a manifestation of a low-fiber diet, *bran* has been tried in therapy. Prospective British studies of bran use have shown reversal of abnormal bowel physiology and reduction in symptoms in over 90% of cases. The average amount of bran needed to achieve an effect is 15 g/d. Some individuals are bothered by flatulence and bloating during the first 2 to 3 weeks of bran use, but this usually resolves with continued bran intake.

Patients unable to tolerate bran may be treated with bulk agents such as *psyllium* (Metamucil). Irritant laxatives should be avoided. The efficacy of *anticholinergics* is controversial; painful spasm may be lessened, but the risk of constipation is increased, raising the likelihood of inspissation of fecal material. Indigestible materials (e.g., seeds) that may block the mouth of a diverticulum should be omitted from the diet.

Acute Diverticulitis. This can be treated at home when symptoms are mild and there is no evidence of widespread peritoneal inflammation. A key requirement is ability to maintain good oral intake of fluids. One aim of therapy is to markedly reduce bowel activity and thus lessen the chance of perforation. *Rest* and *clear liquids* usually suffice. Strong analgesics and antipyretics should not be prescribed because they may mask signs of worsening inflammation. A course of broad-spectrum oral *antibiotics* is commonly prescribed (e.g., *trimethoprim-sulfamethoxazole* or *ciprofloxacin*, plus *metronidazole* for anaerobic coverage), especially when there is fever, although its efficacy is unproven. Antibiotic treatment is continued for 3 to 5 days beyond resolution of fever.

An important decision in the therapy of diverticulitis is whether to treat the patient medically or opt for *elective surgical resection* of the involved bowel after initial resolution of symptoms. Proponents of surgical therapy argue that the frequency of complications warrants prophylactic operation once a patient experiences an attack of diverticulitis. The courses of 132 patients at Yale–New Haven Hospital with documented uncomplicated diverticulitis were analyzed. Of the 99 treated medically and 33 treated surgically, the rates of recurrence were almost identical. Moreover, three fourths of the patients never had more than one attack. The increased length of hospitalization and postoperative morbidity were not balanced by any marked reduction in rate of recurrence or

complications. However, the presence of abscess, perforation, or obstruction is an indication for *immediate surgery*. Although controlled data are lacking, most authorities recommend treatment with a high-fiber diet after acute symptoms have ceased.

INDICATIONS FOR ADMISSION AND REFERRAL

The development of a temperature greater than 101°F on antibiotic therapy, inability to take fluids orally, or worsening or persistence of pain or peritoneal signs indicate need for admission. Sometimes, a markedly elevated white blood cell count may be the only clue to a deteriorating situation; many patients with diverticulitis are elderly and may not demonstrate much fever, abdominal pain, or peritoneal signs. The management of a patient with bleeding, abscess, or perforation requires surgical consultation; operative intervention may be urgent.

THERAPEUTIC RECOMMENDATIONS AND PATIENT EDUCATION

Diverticulosis. For the patient with known diverticula and occasional pain or constipation, the following recommendations should be observed:

- Increase the fiber content of the diet. The best sources are bran, root vegetables (particularly raw carrots), and fruits with skin. Bulk laxatives such as psyllium hydrophilic mucilloid (Metamucil) can be used in patients who cannot tolerate bran, but these are relatively expensive.
- Inform patients that any bloating or flatulence due to bran intake usually resolves with continued use.
- Advise patients to avoid foods with seeds or indigestible material that may block the neck of a diverticulum, such as nuts, corn, popcorn, cucumbers, tomatoes, figs, strawberries, and caraway seeds.
- Have patients avoid laxatives, enemas, and opiates because they are potent constipating agents.
- Anticholinergics are worth considering in patients with recurrent cramping pain, but they may increase constipation and the risk of inspissation of fecal material.
- Instruct patients to report fever, tenderness, or bleeding without delay.

Diverticulitis. For patients with mild diverticulitis (temperature less than 101°F, white cell count below 13,000 to 15,000), the following recommendations should be observed:

- Prescribe bedrest and a clear liquid diet.
- Use mild nonopiate analgesics for pain.
- Monitor temperature, pain, abdominal examination for signs of peritonitis, and white blood cell count for elevation.
- If the patient is febrile, consider a broad-spectrum antibiotic program (e.g., trimethoprim-sulfamethoxazole DS 1 tablet twice a day or ciprofloxacin 500 mg twice a day, plus metronidazole 500 mg four times a day) and continue until patient is afebrile for 3 to 5 days.
- Arrange for prompt hospitalization if temperature goes above 101°F despite antibiotics, pain worsens markedly, peritoneal signs develop, or white cell count continues to rise.

A.H.G.

ANNOTATED BIBLIOGRAPHY

Almy T, Howell DA. Diverticular disease of the colon. N Engl J Med 1980;302:324. (Classic review; 119 references.)

Boles R, Jordan S. Clinical significance of diverticulosis. Gastroenterology 1958;35:579. (Classic natural history study; mean duration of follow-up 15 years. Frequency of hemorrhage, obstruction, or perforation was 15%.)

Boulos PB, Karamanolis DG, Salmon PR, et al. Is colonoscopy necessary in diverticular disease? Lancet 1984;1:95. (Authors argue that air-contrast barium enemas yield inaccurate results in one third of cases; colonoscopy detected neoplasms in 31% of patients with diverticulosis.)

Ferzoco LB, Raptopoulos V, Silen W. Acute diverticulitis. N Engl J Med 1998;338:1521. (Terse thoughtful review; 51 references.)

Horner JL. Natural history of diverticulosis of the colon. Am J Dig Dis 1958;3:343. (Study of 503 patients followed in the ambulatory setting for a mean of 8 years; incidence of diverticulitis was 15%.)

Klein S, Mayer L, Present DH, et al. Extraintestinal manifestations in patients with diverticulitis. Ann Intern Med 1988;108:700. (Report of three cases of pyoderma gangrenosum and arthritis in patients with carefully documented diverticulitis.)

Larson D, Masters S, Spiro H. Medical and surgical therapy in diverticular disease. Gastroenterology 1976;71:734. (Patients followed for a mean of 9.8 years; no difference in outcome, and in about 75% of instances, no further problems occurred among those in either group.)

Markham NI, Li KC. Diverticulitis of the right colon—experience from Hong Kong. Gut 1992;33:547. (Good description of this uncommon but important variant.)

Munson KD, Hensien MA, Jacob LN, et al. Diverticulitis: a comprehensive follow-up. Dis Colon Rectum 1996;39:318. (Modern data on risk of recurrence, including that after surgery.)

Nicholas GG, Miller WT, Fitts WT, et al. Diagnosis of diverticulitis of the colon: role of barium enema in defining pericolic inflammation. Ann Surg 1972;176:205. (Argues that the risk of the study is small, even in the setting of acute inflammation.)

Painter N, Almeida A, Colebourne K. Unprocessed bran in treatment of diverticular disease of the colon. Br Med J 1972;2:137. (Seventy patients treated with bran in a prospective but uncontrolled study. More than 90% showed marked improvement in symptoms.)

Siewert B, Raptopoulos V. CT of the acute abdomen: findings and impact on diagnosis and treatment. AJR Am J Roentgenol 1994;163:1317. (Documents utility of CT for diagnosis of acute diverticulitis.)

Taylor I, Duthie H. Bran tablets and diverticular disease. Br Med J 1976;2:988. (Crossover trial of bran tablets, high roughage diet, and a bulk agent plus an antispasmodic; each improved bowel function, but bran was the most effective in relieving symptoms and normalizing colonic motor activity.)

76
Management of Gastrointestinal Cancers

Gastrointestinal malignancies are among the most common tumors found in adults. The treatment of local disease is the province of the surgeon, but management of advanced disease is a responsibility often shared by the primary physician in close conjunction with oncologic colleagues. It is important for the primary physician to know the indications, limitations, efficacy, and side effects of available treatment modalities to help counsel the cancer patient and make best use of therapies offered by the surgeon, radiation therapist, and oncologist.

Recent developments in combining chemotherapy and radiation therapy with surgery for treatment of gastrointestinal cancer have added substantially to palliation and potential for cure, although mortality is still high (50% to 80%). Moreover, improvements in management of the gastrointestinal complications of cancer, such as obstruction, ascites, and cachexia, have improved the quality of life for these patients (see Chapter 91).

ESOPHAGEAL CANCER

Carcinoma of the esophagus is difficult to diagnose and treat because symptoms usually do not occur until late in the course of illness. As a result, by the time symptoms develop, palliation is often the only therapeutic option. Of the 12,000 new cases of esophageal cancer diagnosed annually, less than 10% survive 5 years. Consequently, emphasis is on early detection and prevention. There are two histologic types: epidermoid (squamous cell) and adenocarcinoma; they currently occur with about equal frequency, but adenocarcinoma is increasing in frequency more rapidly than any other cancer in the United States.

Risk Factors. Precipitants of epidermoid carcinoma include heavy smoking, excessive alcohol use, achalasia, and distant lye ingestion. The risk factors for adenocarcinoma are less well established, but chronic severe gastroesophageal reflux is a principal etiologic factor; both duration and severity contribute to risk.

Clinical Presentation. Adenocarcinoma often appears in the setting of Barrett's esophagus, a premalignant metaplastic change that is the consequence of prolonged severe acid reflux disease. Barrett's esophagus has a significant potential for dysplastic transformation leading to malignancy (see Chapter 61). Aside from heartburn, such patients are usually asymptomatic at the time of malignant transformation.

The first symptoms of esophageal cancer may go unnoticed because they can be nonspecific (e.g., a mild burning discomfort associated with swallowing, sometimes referred to as odynophagia). More typically, the symptoms at time of presentation include dysphagia and progressive inanition, manifestations of late disease. Dysphagia indicates a markedly narrowed esophageal lumen and a substantial tumor burden.

Although these tumors begin as superficial mucosal lesions, they tend to spread silently under the mucosa and extend readily into the mediastinum, because the esophagus has no serosal surface barrier. Tumor may extend regionally into the trachea and regional lymph nodes and vertically up and down the esophageal mucosa and submucosa. Distant metastases occur in the liver and intraabdominal node-bearing areas. At the time of diagnosis, less than one third of patients have cancer confined to the esophageal wall, the stage in which cure is possible with surgical resection.

Diagnosis. Early diagnosis is among the best means of improving outcome and requires a high index of suspicion. Patients with a long-standing history of severe heartburn should be considered for *endoscopy* and *biopsy*, because they have an increased risk of Barrett's esophagus and adenocarcinoma. Those found to have metaplastic change indicative of Barrett's esophagus are candidates for a program of regular surveillance endoscopy and biopsy (see Chapter 61). Those who show dysplastic change need referral for possible surgical resection. New onset of odynophagia in a heavy smoker or drinker should also trigger consideration of endoscopy. Although the presence of small nodules, minor erosions, thickened folds, or mucosal depressions is suggestive of early cancer, mucosal biopsy is required for definitive diagnosis.

Staging. Besides biopsy to determine depth of tumor penetration (the primary determinant of staging), there are a number noninvasive means useful to the staging evaluation. Physical examination should include a check for supraclavicular adenopathy and hepatomegaly. *Computed tomography (CT)* of the chest and upper abdomen should be performed to check for mediastinal invasion. CT provides about the same degree of sensitivity for detection of invasion as does *magnetic resonance imaging (MRI)*, which can also be used for this purpose, although it is more expensive than CT. *Endoscopic ultrasound* is proving useful in determining depth of invasion and appears superior to CT for this purpose.

T1 and T2 disease refers to tumor confined to the esophageal wall, T3 refers to invasion through the wall, and T4 indicates metastatic disease. Nearly 80% who present with dysphagia have at least T3 disease.

Principles of Management. The few controlled studies available find surgery the modality of choice for primary therapy, which includes attempt at cure. However, only some patients have potentially curable disease at the time of detection. Moreover, treatment with curative intent is fraught with high rates of local recurrence and distant metastasis. Combination programs are being explored to reduce the risk of recurrence. In most instances, therapy remains palliative.

Nutrition is one of the first priorities. The morbidity of esophageal carcinoma is due largely to the severe dysphagia, odynophagia, and inanition that characterizes advanced disease. Many patients are unable to swallow their own saliva. Even partial obstruction leads to weight loss and cachexia. A more than 10% weight loss at the time of presentation is a poor prognostic sign. Good nutrition helps sustain immunologic competence and ability to tolerate the stresses of treatment. Blenderized diets and liquid diet supplements are helpful, and hyperalimentation is used as a temporary means in patients with the potential for meaningful survival.

Surgery currently is the modality of choice for *primary therapy*. It provides the potential for cure for the 10% of cases found to have disease confined to the mucosa and for those with

severe dysplasia or carcinoma in situ found during surveillance biopsy of Barrett's esophagus (see Chapter 61). The type of *esophagectomy* performed is determined by the location of the tumor. Achieving tumor-free margins of at least 2 cm is required. Except for very early disease picked up by surveillance (which might allow for a more localized resection), most cases usually require resection of at least a substantial portion of the esophagus, necessitating a major thoracoabdominal procedure. Perioperative morbidity and mortality are high in such surgeries, with death rates of nearly 10% and major nonfatal complications in up to 30%. Median survival for patients undergoing surgery for cure is about 2 years, although considerably higher for those with very early disease confined to a small area of mucosa. Three-year survival in the largest of randomized surgical series is in the range of 25%. Preoperative irradiation does not appear to add much benefit, but when combined with preoperative chemotherapy, the results are more promising (see below).

Most authorities also consider surgery the *palliative treatment* of choice, performed to reestablish the ability to swallow. Palliative surgical resection is most successful in patients with disease confined to the distal esophagus. However, even partial esophagectomy is a major procedure, with high risk of major postoperative complications and surgical mortality. The best results reported for palliative surgery include an 85% rate of symptomatic improvement, 17-month mean survival, and 20% 5-year survival.

Radiation Therapy is a consideration in persons with locally advanced disease not amenable to surgical resection. Such therapy has theoretic appeal because many of these cancers are squamous cell tumors, which tend to be very radiosensitive; however, their central intrathoracic location adjacent to the such key structures as the heart, lungs, and spinal cord makes delivery of curative doses difficult without causing radiation injury. A program of chemotherapy (see below) added to radiation enables use of lower radiation doses and provides superior survival (25% at 5 years) compared with radiation alone (6%) in patients with localized disease, be it adenocarcinoma or squamous cell cancer. Local-regional persistence of disease is the principal cause of treatment failure, suggesting to some that surgery after chemoradiation might be worthwhile (see below).

Chemotherapy. The high risk of distant and local failures with surgery and radiation has prompted trials of chemotherapeutic regimens for use in *combination* with curative-intent surgery or radiation. The addition of *cisplatin* and *fluorouracil* improves outcomes in patients treated with radiation therapy but not in those undergoing surgical resection. Better chemotherapeutic regimens are being sought. Initial results with *paclitaxel* show it to be highly active against esophageal cancers.

Multimodality Therapy. The combination of all three modalities appears promising, particularly when chemoradiation is applied before surgery. In the best randomized trial to date of such multimodal therapy, mean survival was 16 months versus 11 months for surgery alone, and 3-year survival was 32% versus 6%. More data are needed on long-term survival to judge the benefit.

Laser Therapy is available for palliation in patients too ill to undergo surgery or radiation. Results are encouraging, adverse effects are few, and therapy can be performed on an outpatient basis after an initial 2- to 3-day hospitalization. Relief is achieved, but there is no change in survival rate.

Stenting and Dilatation. For dysphagic patients too ill for surgery, palliation can be provided by endoscopic placement of a polyvinyl *stent.* Esophageal *dilatation* is useful for temporary relief. Gastrostomy may be of help for nutrition but provides no symptomatic relief from disabling dysphagia.

Prevention remains the most effective means of dealing with this devastating cancer. Efforts to achieve cessation of *smoking and alcohol abuse* (see Chapters 54 and 228) are essential to reduce the risk of epidermoid cancers. Surveillance *endoscopy* plus biopsy of high-risk patients (e.g., those with Barrett's esophagus) offers the potential to identify dysplastic transformation and early adenocarcinoma, hopefully leading to marked improvements in survival. The optimal approach to surveillance remains to be determined (see Chapter 61). Similarly, the identification of chronic symptomatic reflux as a risk factor for adenocarcinoma raises the possibility that acid-suppression therapy (e.g., by proton-pump inhibition) might reduce the chances of malignant transformation of esophageal mucosa (see Chapter 61). Prospective randomized study is needed.

GASTRIC CANCER

There are approximately 20,000 new cases of gastric cancer in the United States each year and 14,000 deaths attributable to it annually; however, the incidence has been decreasing markedly in the United States, although this cancer remains one of the most common worldwide. Mortality remains relatively unchanged. Overall 5-year survival is about 10%. Onset is rare before the age of 45 years, but incidence increases markedly thereafter. Improvement in outcome has been linked to advances in early diagnosis. Patients with early gastric carcinoma (disease confined to the mucosa and submucosa) have a 5-year survival in excess of 90%. Unfortunately, extension occurs rather early.

About 95% of gastric malignancies are *adenocarcinomas,* with those that are well differentiated and circumscribed having a much better prognosis than those that are poorly differentiated and infiltrative. Lymphomas account for most of the remaining 10%.

Risk Factors. Throughout the world, dietary factors appear to play a major role, linked at least in part by the contribution of *Helicobacter pylori* infection to pathogenesis. Large-scale epidemiologic studies find a strong independent association between *Helicobacter* infection and risk of gastric carcinoma. *H. pylori* infection is most prevalent among populations with inadequate means of food preservation and high risk of food spoilage, populations with the highest prevalences of gastric cancer. The unexplained decline in gastric cancer in the United States over the last half century may be related to improvements in food handling. Infection of the gastric mucosa by the organism leads to chronic inflammation and development of atrophic gastritis, a recognized premalignant change. Infection during childhood is believed to be especially harmful. It is estimated that up to 70% of cases are causally related to *Helicobacter* infection, but only a small number of persons with the infection develop gastric carcinoma, suggesting additional causative factors.

In countries where risk is high, research suggests that dietary *nitrate* sources are important risk factors. Foods associated with increased risk of gastric cancer include dried salted fish, which are rich in *nitrates.* The nitrates may be converted to carcinogenic nitrites and nitroso compounds by bacteria found in unrefrigerated partially decomposed food. This may account for the high rates of gastric cancer among lower socioeconomic groups. (Well-refrigerated and carefully handled raw fish popular in Japan and more recently in the United States as served in sushi bars does not appear to carry a nitrite risk). In the United States, nitrate sources include hot dogs and other processed meats such as cold cuts.

Other identified risk factors include *previous gastric surgery* (usually Billroth II anastomosis) and *achlorhydria.* Increased prevalences also occur among Native Americans, Asians, Hispanics, and Scandinavians.

Clinical Presentation. Clinical presentation can be subtle, making early diagnosis difficult. Unexplained iron deficiency *anemia* or asymptomatic *guaiac stool test positivity* may be the only manifestation. Nonspecific abdominal pain, gastric ulceration with or without bleeding, weight loss, and obstruction are the major patterns of clinical presentation, but most are manifestations of advanced disease. About 75% of patients with early disease have *epigastric pain* as the initial complaint; it may be subtle and resemble *dyspepsia.* Most are free of the nausea, vomiting, anorexia, and weight loss that characterize more advanced disease. *Gastric ulcer* is an important presentation, characterized by a suspicious appearance on barium study or endoscopy or a more benign-appearing radiologic defect that fails to heal completely or quickly recurs after 6 weeks of ulcer therapy (see Chapter 68). The disease often progresses silently until signs of metastatic disease, such as enlargement of the *left supraclavicular lymph nodes or ascites,* become evident and cause the patient to seek medical attention.

Diagnosis. A high index of suspicion is warranted; early diagnosis provides the best chance for survival. Patients over the age of 45 years presenting with any of the manifestations noted above should undergo testing as early as possible. *Endoscopy* with *brushings* and *biopsy* is the preferred method for definitive diagnosis. In the absence of an ulcer, all atypical areas of mucosa should be biopsied. Endoscopy has largely replaced upper gastrointestinal series for diagnosis, in part because it permits the obtaining of biopsy specimens.

Course. Spread occurs by direct extension and by seeding of the lymphatics, blood vessels, and peritoneal surface. Metastases develop locally and at distant sites, most frequently the *liver* (40%), *lung* (15%), and *bone* (15%). Among patients who come to surgery, approximately 80% are found to have *lymph node* metastases, whereas 40% have *peritoneal involvement* and 35% show spread to the liver or lung.

Principles of Management. Surgery is the treatment of choice, but the ability to achieve cure is limited by the finding of metastatic disease at surgery in 80%. Adjuvant chemotherapy is being used to reduce the high risk of metastasis, but the overall survival rate has not changed in the past two decades. Prevention and early detection are the best hopes at present in improving outcomes.

Surgery is the primary mode of treatment, both for cure and palliation. Median survival for patients managed by complete surgical resection is in excess of 3 years. The 5-year survival rate varies according to location of the tumor: it is 25% in patients with distal lesions and 10% for those with proximal ones. When lymph node involvement is found, survival falls by 50%. The surgical loss of the stomach's food reservoir function necessitates small frequent feedings. Without careful patient education and use of high-calorie supplements, total gastrectomy can lead to malnutrition. Subtotal or total gastrectomy is optimal for management of bleeding or obstruction related to tumors at the gastroesophageal junction. *Linitis plastica* or total wall involvement of the stomach is incurable and not manageable by surgery.

Chemotherapy (using such agents as 5-fluorouracil [5-FU]) as the sole mode of treatment in patients with metastatic disease produces responses in almost 40% of patients. The average duration of response is 9 months, but there is no improvement in survival. Complete responses are rare. Reports of efficacy for *adjuvant chemotherapy* after surgical resection are encouraging but require confirmation. Unlike adenocarcinoma, gastric *lymphomas* are responsive to chemotherapy after gastrectomy (see Chapter 84), with 5-year survival approaching 40%. Combination chemotherapy is being considered for patients with primary gastric lymphoma that is unresectable.

Radiation. Adenocarcinomas of the stomach are not radiosensitive at tolerable doses. Neither radiation used alone nor as part of an adjuvant program with chemotherapy has improved survival. Likewise, postoperative radiation does not seem to be of much benefit in patients with gastric lymphoma.

Patient Monitoring should be guided by symptoms and not by routine testing for potential metastatic sites, because only palliative therapeutic options exist for patients with advanced disease.

Prevention and Early Detection. Although the relationship between *Helicobacter* infection and gastric carcinoma is becoming increasingly well established, it remains to be proven that eradication or prevention of *Helicobacter* infection will reduce risk (see Chapter 68). Nonetheless, improvement in food handling and preservation and assuring that young children are not exposed to spoiled food seem like reasonable public health measures at this time. Early detection through endoscopic or radiologic screening has been carried out in populations where risk is very high (e.g., Japan). Such measures would not be cost effective in the United States, where disease prevalence is relatively low and declining.

PANCREATIC CANCER

Carcinoma of the pancreas is the fourth leading cause of cancer death in the United States. Mortality is high (close to 99% at 5 years); fewer than 20% survive 1 year. High death rates are due partially to difficulties in early detection, which stem from the tumor's retroperitoneal location. For decades, pancreatic cancer had been increasing in frequency, but incidence has plateaued since 1973. There are about 25,000 new cases annually. The disease is rare before age 45, but incidence rises rapidly thereafter. There is a slight male predominance.

Hypotheses regarding pathogenesis include concentration and excretion of carcinogens by acinar cells inducing neoplastic transformation among ductal cells. Established risk factors include heavy *alcohol consumption* and heavy *smoking*. Diabetes mellitus, chronic pancreatitis, and exposures to dry-cleaning chemicals and gasoline are also suspected contributing factors. The validity of a statistical association with coffee consumption has been disproved.

Clinical Presentation. In most instances, the tumor remains silent until late in the course of disease, with presentation determined largely by the tumor's location. In about two thirds of cases, the cancer begins in the head of the pancreas; in the remainder, it occurs in the body or tail. Disease that originates in the pancreatic head near the pancreaticobiliary junction may extend locally to obstruct bile flow and cause *painless jaundice*—one of the few potentially early symptomatic presentations of pancreatic cancer. Jaundice, with or without pain, is an eventual manifestation in about 50% of patients, although in many it is due to metastasis or late extension.

More often than not, symptoms are late in onset and nonspecific. Disease of the body or tail may present with vague upper abdominal or back *pain* or *discomfort*, unexplained *weight loss*, unexplained *depression*, or even migratory *thrombophlebitis*. Carcinomas of the tail may not cause symptoms until they metastasize. Pancreatic cancer is also an important cause of ectopic hormone production (insulin, glucagon, corticotropin) and unexplained onset of *diabetes* or *pancreatitis*. Persistent *nausea and vomiting* suggest invasion and obstruction of the upper gastrointestinal tract.

The clinical course of pancreatic carcinoma is dominated by regional extension into the retroperitoneum and liver. The tumor tends to spread perineurally and lymphatically. Median survival for patients with extrapancreatic tumor is 12 weeks from time of presentation and 19 to 42 weeks for those with tumor confined to the pancreas.

Diagnosis no longer requires laparotomy, but tissue may still be needed because symptoms and signs may be nonspecific and there are no definitive blood tests. The workup begins with abdominal *ultrasonography or CT*. Both have the capacity to detect lesions as small as 2 cm and to image the biliary tree and pancreatic ducts. In many cases, both are ordered. Ultrasound is usually the initial study in patients with jaundice, because the test is readily available and provides a quick and inexpensive means of diagnosing common bile duct obstruction. It also can detect tumor before it distorts the pancreatic contour, an advantage it has over CT. CT provides better definition of the tumor and adjacent structures, helping to determine anatomy and detect metastasis to the liver and draining lymph nodes. MRI techniques offer no advantages over CT, although advances in MRI may eventually prove useful. Pancreatic radionuclide scanning is not used due to poor diagnostic accuracy.

When a distinct pancreatic mass is identified, *fine-needle aspiration biopsy* can be performed percutaneously, guided by direct ultrasound or CT visualization. Limiting the yield from needle biopsy is the large zone of fibrosis and inflammation that typically surrounds the tumor. The procedure is the confirmatory test of choice in patients with disease believed to be metastatic or unresectable. Drawbacks include a substantial false-negative rate and the risk of seeding along the needle tract.

Patients with a mass at the pancreaticobiliary junction are excellent candidates for *endoscopic retrograde cholangiopancreatography (ERCP)*. Early ampullary lesions causing jaundice can be visualized and biopsied directly, leading to prompt diagnosis, definitive treatment, and improved 5-year survival (as high as 50%). A pancreatogram is taken during ERCP, with ductal narrowing, obstruction, and extravasation of dye comprising additional signs of malignancy (although they also can occur in chronic pancreatitis). An irregular stricture longer than 10 mm is characteristic of cancer. Cytologic sampling, especially that obtained by brushing, has a reported sensitivity approaching 85%, although results vary.

Serum tumor markers have always been appealing, although of limited use in diagnosis. *CA 19-9*, a tumor marker developed with monoclonal antibody technology, has been tested for its utility in detecting and monitoring pancreatic cancer. Although sensitive in the setting of advanced disease, the test is often normal in early stages. In addition, specificity has been disappointing; high levels have been reported in other gastrointestinal cancers (bile duct, colon). It is not recommended for screening but can be useful in differentiating chronic pancreatitis from pancreatic cancer and in follow-up surveillance (provided levels were high before surgery and fall immediately after). Other serum tumor markers examined include carcinoembryonic antigen (CEA) and the ratio of testosterone to dihydrotestosterone. None has proven sufficiently sensitive or specific to warrant use in routine diagnosis.

Principles of Management. The chance for cure is limited because it depends on surgically removing the entire tumor, which is usually well advanced by the time it is detected. Careful staging is critical. One needs to distinguish between tumors that are localized and resectable, localized and not resectable, and metastatic. In addition, patients with duodenal obstruction need to be identified because they require operation.

Staging. CT with contrast is the staging procedure of choice for visualizing the tumor and detecting liver and large lymph node metastases. Such metastases rule out resectability. Microscopic nodal disease is not visible by CT, but neither is it considered a contraindication to surgery (although palliation rather than cure may be the objective). Many surgeons view data from *angiography* as useful—major vascular involvement indicates inoperability. The utility of a staging *laparoscopy* for patients being considered for surgery has become evident. Upward of 40% of such patients are found at laparoscopy to have previously undetected peritoneal or omental metastases, which rule out resectability. These three tests are complementary and greatly increase the determination of surgical candidacy. They can save many patients from undergoing unnecessary laparotomy. If any one test is positive, only 5% will have a resectable tumor at laparotomy, but if all three are negative, the rate increases to 78%. *Endoscopic ultrasound with transendoscopic fine-needle aspiration* is a new technology that allows determination of spread beyond the pancreatic capsule and determination of local nodal involvement.

Surgery. Only patients with relatively small lesions confined to the head of the pancreas are candidates for *curative surgery*. This accounts for no more than 5% to 22% of patients who present with the disease. The risks of surgery are great, the operations formidable, and postoperative complications serious. Operative mortality frequently approaches or even exceeds the 5-year survival rate. The decision to subject a patient with pancreatic cancer to a major operation with a high degree of operative mortality and only modest chances for substantially improved survival must be made individually.

The operation of choice is the *Whipple procedure* (pancreatoduodenectomy), which requires a surgical tour de force and should be attempted only by surgeons able to perform it with less than 5% mortality. Five-year survival rates are best in patients with a small (2 cm or less) tumor, approaching 30% at centers with surgical expertise in performing the operation. Survival increases to 57% if lymph nodes prove to be negative (unfortunately, an uncommon occurrence). Overall 5-year survival had been 5%, but reports of 15% to 25% are now appearing in conjunction with advances in staging, case selection, and operative technique. Regional pancreatectomy or total pancreatectomy provides no survival benefit.

Surgery is also recommended for *palliation*. Patients with biliary obstruction are candidates for biliary bypass or endoscopic stent placement, which can relieve jaundice and lower the risk of cholangitis. Surgical or percutaneous ablation of the celiac ganglion can provide relief from intractable pain.

Radiation Therapy is applied to patients with localized but unresectable disease. However, only when used in conjunction with 5-FU therapy does it prolong survival. Intraoperative radiation is also being promoted, but survival benefit remains to be defined. Preoperative courses of radiation and chemotherapy are being studied. Radiation therapy has also been used for control of intractable retroperitoneal pain; 4 to 6 months of relief have been reported.

Chemotherapy has traditionally offered little to persons with unresectable disease. The standard chemotherapeutic agent, *5-FU*, has a poor response rate (about 20%) and no proven ability to prolong survival. *Gemcitabine*, a recently developed nucleoside analogue, appears to be more effective than 5-FU, able to reduce pain, improve functional status, and slightly improve survival. This agent is now U.S. Food and Drug Administration approved for use as first-line therapy in persons with locally advanced or metastatic disease and in those previously treated with 5-FU.

Supportive Measures are essential, not only to patients who are dying of their disease (see Chapter 87) but also to those who have undergone pancreatectomy. In the latter group, insulin therapy and pancreatic enzyme preparations are needed. Insulin requirements are in the range of 20 to 30 units per day.

COLORECTAL CANCER

Colorectal cancer is one of the most common malignancies and, although one of the more potentially curable cancers, results in 50,000 deaths annually. Over 150,000 new cases develop each year.

Risk Factors. Among the suspected etiologic factors is an increased exposure to chemical carcinogens present within the bowel lumen. High-risk patients are those with a *first-degree relative* with colorectal cancer (especially if cancer developed at an early age), long-standing *pancolitis, familial polyposis,* or *Gardner's syndrome* (polyps, osteomas, epidermoid cysts, soft tissue tumors). Loss of the tumor suppressor gene p53 has been found in colorectal cancer patients. High-fiber diets may lessen risk, but recent large-scale epidemiologic data in women cast some doubt on earlier positive findings. Epidemiologic evidence does suggest that regular use of aspirin may reduce the risk of fatal colon cancer. Calcium supplementation moderately reduces the risk of recurrent adenomatous polyp formation. Early diagnosis through screening is a high priority in the approach to this condition, offering the best chance of reducing mortality (see Chapter 56).

Adenomatous polyps, villoglandular polyps, and *villous adenomas* represent premalignant lesions that may also harbor early cancers. Most colon cancers derive from these lesions, making their timely detection and removal essential. Hyperplastic "polyps" are not premalignant lesions (see below and Chapter 56).

Clinical Presentation. The clinical presentation of colorectal cancer is related to the site of the tumor. Tumors of the ascending colon may be asymptomatic until late stages, producing little more than mild *iron deficiency anemia* or intermittently *guaiac-positive stools*. Tumors of the descending colon and rectosigmoid can cause symptoms earlier in the course of illness, presenting as rectal *bleeding or change in bowel habits* (diarrhea and constipation). At the time of surgery, 50% to 75% of patients demonstrate tumor that has penetrated the bowel wall; 60% of these show regional metastases.

Rectal cancers commonly present with occult or frank rectal bleeding, with or without an alteration in bowel habits. *Tenesmus* is usually a late symptom representing extension of the tumor beyond the bowel wall. Rectal or perianal pain is a consequence of the invasion of the pararectal structures in the sacral plexus. Tumor often arises on the posterior wall, making it particularly important to examine the rectal ampulla on routine rectal examination.

Prognosis and Clinical Course. Prognosis depends on extent of penetration and local spread. A modification of the standard *Dukes' classification* serves as a useful system for staging (Table 76.1). Stage A patients have tumor limited to the submucosa and a 5-year survival in excess of 90%. Those with stage B disease have a 5-year survival ranging from 70% to 85%. Once the serosal surface and lymph nodes are involved, stage C, survival falls to 30% to 65%. Prognosis is also adversely affected by presence of polyploidy and mucin production in the tumor and by preoperative elevation of serum CEA level (more than 5 ng/mL).

The most common sites of metastasis are the *liver* (60% overall and 30% of solitary metastases) due to portal blood flow draining the intestines, the *peritoneal surface* (30%), and the *lung* (20%). Brain, skin, and local recurrences occur in less than 5%. Rectal cancers tend to invade locally and to recur in the pelvis alone or in association with distant metastases to the liver or lung, bypassing the intraabdominal cavity.

Diagnosis in a patient suspected of colorectal cancer (e.g., because of guaiac-positive stools, rectal bleeding, unexplained iron-deficiency anemia, or change in bowel habits) is best accomplished by *colonoscopy* that extends to the cecum. The combination of flexible *sigmoidoscopy plus barium enema* is a second choice where colonoscopy is not available, but barium study does not allow for biopsy and the false-negative rate can be as high as 40% for single-contrast studies. Sensitivity is improved with use of air-contrast techniques, but elderly patients find such barium studies uncomfortable.

For patients in whom a cancer is detected in the rectosigmoid, a preoperative examination of the entire colon all the way to the cecum is required, either by colonoscopy or air-contrast barium enema, because *synchronous tumors* are present in up to 5% of patients. Similarly, colonoscopy is needed when a benign adenomatous polyp is found on examination of the rectosigmoid.

Staging for colon cancer is based predominantly on findings at surgery and pathologic examination (Table 76.1). Liver scanning and CT are not usually performed preoperatively because the results do not affect the decision to remove the tumor. However, *CT or MRI* of the pelvis can help determine extent of a rectal cancer and candidacy for surgery. A preoperative CEA level provides a baseline for postoperative monitoring of colorectal cancer and helps assess prognosis. Detailed examination of draining lymph nodes is especially important in patients with stage B (stage II) disease. Histopathologically, negative nodes may still contain tumor, necessitating molecular testing to uncover micrometastasis that is associated with a much worse prognosis and a need for stage C treatment.

Treatment. Patients with disease detected in the early stages have an excellent prognosis, emphasizing the important of early diagnosis and treatment, including removal of polyps that represent premalignant disease (see Chapter 56).

Surgery is the primary modality of therapy, both for cure and for palliation (e.g., to prevent or relieve bowel obstruction). For colon cancer, *colectomy* is the procedure of choice. Because the tumor spreads lymphatically, adequate amounts of bowel on both sides of the lesion must be removed to avoid cutting into intramural lymphatics that may contain cancerous cells. Patients presenting with obstruction may benefit from a temporary diverting colostomy followed at a later date by reanastomosis. *Salvage surgery*, often with curative intent for a single resectable recurrence of tumor (e.g., in the abdomen, lung, or liver), is being increasingly offered by surgeons, encouraged by the low perioperative mortality risk and the roughly 25% 5-year disease-free survival rate.

Surgical management of *rectal cancer* consists of *abdominoperineal resection*, aided by adjuvant radiation therapy. When possible, an effort is made to preserve the anal sphincter. Tumors of the upper two thirds of the rectum can usually be resected in conjunction with construction of an anastomosis; those of the lower third require an abdominoperineal resection with a permanent sigmoid colostomy. Sometimes unwise attempts are made to limit the resection to preserve the sphincter; inadequate surgical margins are taken, leading to local recurrence and death. Alternatives to abdominoperineal resection include local excision, fulguration, and intrarectal radiation ther-

76.1. Staging for Colorectal Cancer

STAGE	DESCRIPTION	5-YEAR SURVIVAL (%)
A	Lesion confined to submucosa; nodes negative	>90%
B1[a]	Muscularis involved but not serosa; nodes negative	80–85
B2[a]	Lesion extends through serosa; nodes negative	70–75
C1[a]	Lesion extends into muscularis only; nodes positive	70–75
C1[a]	Lesion extends through serosa; 1–4 nodes positive	60–65
C2[a]	Lesion extends through serosa; >4 nodes positive	30–40

[a]Gastrointestinal Tumor Study Group modification of Dukes' staging system. Adapted from Steel G, et al. *Cancer manual*, 8th ed. Massachusetts Division, Boston: American Cancer Society. 1990:244, with permission.

apy. Only patients with small exophytic tumors in the lower third of the rectum should be considered for such alternative therapy.

The appreciation that adenomatous polyps, villoglandular polyps, and villous adenomas may harbor cancers or be premalignant has led to the recommendation of *polypectomy* when detected, aided greatly by fiberoptic colonoscopy and sigmoidoscopy. Cancer confined to the polyp is considered carcinoma *in situ*; detectable invasion of the stalk or muscularis necessitates *colectomy*.

Radiation therapy has no established role in colon cancer, in contrast to its important place in the treatment of rectal cancer. The tendency of rectal cancers that have penetrated the bowel wall to recur locally is high (30% to 50%). Adjunctive use of radiation therapy in such patients significantly reduces the risk of local recurrence and improves survival. Patients with extensive local disease are irradiated preoperatively. This reduces tumor size and allows for subsequent resection. Postoperative radiotherapy is reserved for those whose findings at surgery suggest high risk of recurrence (i.e., those with stage B2 or C). In addition, the application of adjuvant radiation therapy postoperatively has permitted an anterior resection with primary anastomosis in many patients who would otherwise require a colostomy.

Chemotherapy, consisting of postoperative application of *levamisole and 5-FU*, can significantly reduce the risk of recurrence in patients with resected stage C colon cancers. In the largest prospective randomized clinical trial of this adjuvant program, the recurrence rate decreased by 40% and the death rate by 33%. Levamisole alone had minimal effect on outcomes. Typically, treatment is begun as soon as possible after surgery.

For patients with advanced nonresectable disease, 5-FU remains the only option. None of the other drugs or drug combinations has proven superior to 5-FU alone. The response rate is about 20%, but there is little chance of a meaningful prolongation of survival. The addition of *leukovorin* to 5-FU increases the response rate modestly to 30% to 35% but does not enhance survival and has side effects of its own.

Other Modalities. have been asserted. At one point, claims were made for high-dose *vitamin C*. Randomized, double-blind, control study has shown that such therapy is no better than placebo. No benefit has been found with *immunotherapy*.

Monitoring. Attentive follow-up is essential because of the risk of a second bowel cancer (occurring in up to 5% of patients) and appearance of new polyps. Moreover, a new primary in the bowel or a single metastasis to the lung or liver is amenable to curative resection with a 25% chance of disease-free survival at 5 years. Regularly scheduled *colonoscopy* should begin 6 months after surgery and take place every 24 to 36 months if no polyps are found and every 6 months if they are. Any encountered polyps are removed. If colonoscopy is unavailable or cannot reach the cecum, air-contrast *barium enema* is an adequate substitute in conjunction with sigmoidoscopy.

Early detection of potentially resectable recurrent or metastatic disease in the abdomen or lung requires additional monitoring. Periodic *chest x-ray* every 6 months for the first 12 to 48 months has been suggested as a low-cost approach to screening for lung metastasis. The *CEA* is a marker that correlates with tumor burden in colorectal cancer. It has proven useful in detection of disease recurrence and is used in monitoring after initial resection. The recommended interval for CEA determinations is every 6 months for the first 2 years, provided that the CEA was elevated before surgery and fell to low levels within 2 to 4 weeks after it. If the CEA rises by 30% or more per month from its postoperative level, then a search for curable recurrent disease should be undertaken. However, sensitivity and specificity have been found wanting, especially for early detection of liver metastases, causing some investigators to suggest periodic abdominal *ultrasound* or *CT* for this purpose. Evidence that CEA surveillance is cost effective and saves a significant number of lives remains to be obtained. Careful patient selection is warranted. *MRI* does not appear to offer any advantages over CT and costs considerably more to perform. The most cost-effective approach to monitoring remains to be established.

As noted earlier, one should also monitor symptoms (weight loss, fatigue, change in bowel habits), the physical examination (especially chest and abdomen), and *alkaline phosphatase* (rises with infiltration of the liver) to help detect recurrent but curable disease.

Supportive Therapy. Patients who have undergone abdominoperineal resection with permanent or temporary colostomy need careful counseling pre- and postoperatively to help them adapt to their situation. Becoming comfortable with the details of ostomy care and having an opportunity to discuss their fears and concerns (sexual function, odor, appearance, bag changes, recurrence of cancer) are essential components of the rehabilitation effort. Ostomy groups and stoma nurses are important resources for the patient, but there is no substitute for a supportive understanding patient–doctor relationship.

Patients presenting with nonresectable disease benefit from a comprehensive review of prognosis, available treatment modalities, and patient and family preferences. A meeting set up by the primary care physician to include the patient and family can be most helpful in facilitating communication, addressing the obvious but difficult questions regarding prognosis and treatment, and formulating a personalized plan that aims to maximize the patient's quality of life, comfort, and dignity. It helps assure the patient and family of close follow-up and a program of support that makes sense to all. Such a meeting may also be an opportune time to address the elements necessary to complete an advance directive (see Chapter 1).

Prevention. A host of approaches are available, ranging from endoscopic screening to genetic testing to lifestyle modifications.

Screening. The best approach to prevention is a screening program that includes fecal occult-blood testing and sigmoidoscopy, complemented by colonoscopy or barium enema in high-risk patients (see Chapter 56). All polyps detected need to be removed and subjected to pathologic examination.

Genetic Testing. The contribution of genetic testing to prevention is just beginning to be explored as genetic risk factors are identified in familial forms of colorectal cancer. In *hereditary nonpolyposis colorectal cancer* (the most common of the familial colorectal cancer syndromes), upward of 25% of family members are found under study conditions to have deleterious mutations in the *hMSH2* or *hMLH1* gene, mutations that confer a significantly increased risk of cancer and warrant heightened surveillance and preventive measures. Such high frequencies of important prognostic information suggest routine genetic testing as a future management recommendation for hereditary forms of colon cancer, especially for hereditary nonpolyposis. New colorectal cancer patients who should be suspected for hereditary nonpolyposis include those with a family history of a first-degree relative with colorectal or endometrial cancer, age less than 50 years at time of diagnosis of colorectal cancer, or a history of multiple cancers. Some authorities suggest molecular screening of such patients and the subsequent testing of the families of those who manifest important gene mutations.

Diet, Vitamins, and Exercise. A number of dietary preventive measures have been touted with varying degrees of supporting evidence. Ever since Burkett's observation of very little colorectal cancer in African societies taking a high-fiber diet, *dietary fiber* has been viewed as useful in prevention of colorectal cancer. Numerous case-control studies support this view, but the well-designed prospective Nurses Health Study failed to find any benefit from increased fiber intake, at least in women. In the same Nurses Health Study, long-term (more than 15 years) use of multivitamins, particularly *folic acid*, was associated with significantly reduced cancer risk. A high *calcium* intake is associated with a moderate reduction in risk of polyp recurrence. *Physical activity* in men appears beneficial (truncal obesity is detrimental).

Hormones and Medications. *Hormone replacement therapy* in postmenopausal women has been shown in some studies to decrease risk of colorectal cancer and large adenomas by nearly 35%, but the association is not well established by prospective study and the benefit disappears quickly with cessation of hormone therapy. The use of *aspirin* and other NSAIDs initially appeared to be beneficial, but subsequent large-scale study failed to confirm the association between NSAID use and reduced risk.

Management of Colorectal Polyps (see also Chapter 56)

The finding of a sporadic polyp on screening sigmoidoscopy is a common event. Most are not true polyps but just small *hyperplastic* mucosal outcroppings that have no malignant potential. Polyps representing true neoplasia with the potential for malignant transformation include *villous adenomas, tubular adenomas, and mixed tubulovillous adenomas.* Villous adenomas have the highest malignant potential and tend to be larger and more sessile than tubular or mixed tubulovillous adenomas (see Chapter 56, Table 56.1). With adenomatous polyps, the risk of malignancy increases with polyp diameter. Lesions less than 1 cm have a 0.5% chance of harboring malignancy; for polyps greater than 3.0 cm, the risk increases to over 15%. Small tubular adenomas account for nearly 70% of the polyps found. Polypectomy reduces the risk of new colon cancers by 70% to 90%.

All polypoid lesions found should be excised and sent for histologic categorization. Those that prove to be hyperplastic require no additional action, but truly neoplastic lesions are an indication for colonoscopy, because of the increased risk of synchronous premalignant polyps or even cancer-containing lesions proximal to the reach of the sigmoidoscope. However, the magnitude of this risk and thus the need for colonoscopy is uncertain in the large group of patients found to have only a single small (less than 0.5 cm) tubular adenoma on sigmoidoscopy. Of the two best prospective cohort studies performed in primary care settings in persons with diminutive tubular adenomas, one found the risk of proximal disease to be nil, whereas the other noted a 5% risk of concurrent cancer and a 30% risk of another polyp. Subsequent cross-sectional analysis of data from a large health maintenance population population found that tubulovillous or villous histology in the distal lesion was the most powerful predictor of proximal pathology; also predictive were age greater than 65 years, more than one distal adenoma, and positive family history of colorectal cancer. Pending additional data to help settle the controversy, one can use these risk factors to help select for colonoscopy patients most likely to have an important proximal lesion.

The optimal frequency for repeat colonoscopy is unsettled. The best determinant of frequency is individual risk. Current consensus guidelines recommend performing the first follow-up study in 3 years, followed by one every 5 years if the first study is normal (see Chapter 56). Patients with familial adenomatous polyposis are at very high risk of developing colorectal cancer (approximately 50% by age 40). Prophylactic colectomy is often recommended for such persons. Colonoscopic surveillance is an effective alternative to prophylactic colectomy in persons with hereditary nonpolyposis colorectal cancer mutations discovered through genetic screening.

A.H.G.

ANNOTATED BIBLIOGRAPHY

Esophageal Cancer

Cello JP, Gerstenberger PD, Wright T, et al. Endoscopic neodymium-YAG laser palliation of nonresectable esophageal malignancy. Ann Intern Med 1985;102:610. (*Laser use to alleviate luminal obstruction; a promising therapy for patients with inoperable disease.*)

Cooper JS, Guo MD, MacDonald JS, et al. Chemoradiotherapy of locally advanced esophageal cancer: long-term follow-up of a prospective randomized trial (RTOG 85-01). JAMA 1999;281:1623. (*Results found to be durable; 5-year survival 26%.*)

Kelsen DP, Ginsberg TF, Pajak TF, et al. Chemotherapy followed by surgery compared with surgery alone for localized esophageal cancer. N Engl J Med 1998;339:1979. (*Preoperative chemotherapy with cisplatin and 5-FU did not provide any survival benefit.*)

Lagergren J, Bergstrom A, Lindgren A, et al. Symptomatic gastroesophageal reflux as a risk factor for esophageal adenocarcinoma. N Engl J Med 1999;340:825. (*A population study demonstrating a strong, dose-related, independent risk of adenocarcinoma of the esophagus conferred by symptomatic reflux.*)

Lehr L, Rupp N, Siewert JR. Assessment of resectability of esophageal cancer by computed tomography and magnetic resonance imaging. Surgery 1988;103:344. (*Roughly equivalent results with each; still some difficulty in detecting penetration into the mediastinum.*)

Sampliner RE, The Practice Parameters Committee of the American College of Gastroenterology. Practice guidelines on the diagnosis, surveillance and therapy of Barrett's esophagus. Am J Gastroenterol 1998;93:1028. (*Consensus statement on the diagnosis and management of Barrett's esophagus.*)

Schattenkerk ME, Obertop H, Mud HJ, et al. Survival after resection for carcinoma of the oesophagus. Br J Surg 1987;74:165. (*Useful outcome statistics for surgical therapy.*)

Tio TL, Coene LO, Luiken HM, et al. Endosonography in the clinical staging of esophagogastric cancer. Gastrointest Endosc 1990;35:S2. *(Overall accuracy [89%] much better than that available from CT; overstaging 6%, understaging 5%.)*

Walsh TN, Noonan N, Hollywood D, et al. A comparison of multimodal therapy and surgery for esophageal adenocarcinoma. N Engl J Med 1996;335:462. *(Promising early results for combination of radiation and chemotherapy followed by surgery.)*

Wright TA, Gray MR, Morris AI, et al. Cost effectiveness of detecting Barrett's esophagus. Gut 1996:39:574. *(Best evidence to date on the cost effectiveness of surveillance; finds it cost effective, but based on retrospective data.)*

Gastric Cancer

Cutler AF, Havstad S, Ma CK, et al. Accuracy of invasive and noninvasive tests to diagnose *Helicobacter pylori* infection. Gastroenterology 1995;109:136. *(^{13}C-urea breath test and serology as accurate as biopsy and CLO test for diagnosis.)*

Eckardt VF, Giebler W, Kanzler G, et al. Clinical and morphological characteristics of early gastric cancer. Gastroenterology 1990;98:708. *(Very useful data on the presentation, diagnosis, clinical course, and outcome of early gastric cancer in the community setting.)*

Haber DA, Mayer RJ. Primary gastrointestinal lymphoma. Semin Oncol 1988;15:154. *(Useful review of this important gastric malignancy.)*

Hansson L-E, Nyren O, Hsing AW, et al. The risk of stomach cancer in patients with gastric or duodenal ulcer disease. N Engl J Med 1996;335:242. *(A Swedish population study; incidence ratio 1.8 for gastric ulcer and 0.6 for duodenal ulcer.)*

Parsonnet J, Friedman GD, Wandersteen DP, et al. *Helicobacter pylori* infection and the risk of gastric carcinoma. N Engl J Med 1991;325:1127. *(Important case-control study providing strong epidemiologic evidence for a link between the two conditions.)*

Pancreatic Cancer

Cameron JL, Crist DW, Sitzmann JV, et al. Factors influencing survival after pancreaticoduodenectomy for pancreatic cancer. Am J Surg 1991;161:120. *(Small tumor size, negative nodes, and lack of vessel involvement predict good results.)*

Gordis L. Consumption of methylxanthine-containing beverages and risk of pancreatic cancer. Cancer Lett 1990;52:1. *(Critical and detailed review of all published data; concludes no increased risk.)*

Kalser MH, Barkin J, MacIntyre JM. Pancreatic cancer: assessment of prognosis by clinical presentation. Cancer 1985;56:397. *(Onset of symptoms is usually a sign of advanced disease, although jaundice may be an early manifestation in some.)*

Lowenfels AB, Maisonneuve P, Cavallini G, et al. Pancreatitis and the risk of pancreatic cancer. N Engl J Med 1993;328:1433. *(Positive association found.)*

MacMahon B, Trichopoulos D, Warren K, et al. Coffee and cancer of the pancreas. N Engl J Med 1981;304:630. *(Study that started the controversy.)*

Gemcitabine for treatment of pancreatic cancer. Med Lett Drugs Ther 1996;38:102. *(Terse summary of evidence for efficacy and safety.)*

Muller MF, Meyenberger C, Bertschinger P, et al. Pancreatic tumors: evaluation with endoscopic, ultrasound, CT and MRI imaging. Radiology 1994:190:745. *(Good comprehensive comparative review of imaging modalities.)*

Parsons L, Palmer CH. How accurate is fine-needle biopsy in malignant neoplasia of the pancreas? Arch Surg 1989;124:681. *(Sensi-

tivity 57% to 94%, few false positives but many false negatives due to sampling errors and fibrosis and inflammation surrounding the tumor.)*

Steinberg W. The clinical utility of the CA 19-9 tumor-associated antigen. Am J Gastroenterol 1990;85:350. *(Useful for monitoring but not for screening or early diagnosis.)*

Venu RP, Geenen JE, Kini M, et al. Endoscopic retrograde brush cytology: a new technique. Gastroenterology 1990;99:1475. *(Greatly enhances the diagnostic yield from ERCP.)*

Warshaw AL, Fernandez del Castillo C. Pancreatic carcinoma. N Engl J Med 1992;326:455. *(Definitive review, including excellent discussion of surgical therapy; 186 references.)*

Colorectal Cancer and Polyps

Atkin WS, Morson BC, Cuzick J. Long-term risk of colorectal cancer after excision of rectosigmoid adenomas. N Engl J Med 1992;326:658. *(Risk increased only in patients with villous, tubulovillous, or large adenomas.)*

Baron JA, Beach M, Mandel JS, et al. Calcium supplements for the prevention of colorectal adenomas. N Engl J Med 1999;340:101. *(A randomized controlled trial in persons who had a previous adenoma, finding a significant but only moderate reduction in rate of recurrence.)*

Bond JH, for the Practice Parameters Committee of the American College of Gastroenterology. Polyp guideline: diagnosis, treatment, and surveillance for patients with nonfamilial colorectal polyps. Ann Intern Med 1993;119:836. *(Recommends first surveillance after polypectomy at 3 years, then every 5 years.)*

Bresalier RS, Kim YS. Diet and colon cancer. N Engl J Med 1985;313:1413. *(Summarizes the data linking dietary factors and colon cancer.)*

Creagan ET, Moertel CG, O'Fallon JR, et al. Failure of high-dose vitamin C therapy to benefit patients with advanced cancer. N Engl J Med 1979;301:1189. *(Despite anecdotal claims to the contrary, this careful study conclusively demonstrates that high-dose vitamin C is no more effective than placebo.)*

Fletcher RH. Carcinoembryonic antigen. Ann Intern Med 1986;104:66. *(Thoughtful review indicating that surveillance by CEA can detect recurrences, but few lives actually saved.)*

Fuchs CS, Giovannucci EL, Colditz GA, et al. Dietary fiber and the risk of colorectal cancer and adenoma in women. N Engl J Med 1999;340:169. *(Data from the Nurses Health Study failing to confirm a protective effect for dietary fiber.)*

Giardiello FM. Treatment of colonic and rectal adenomas with sulindac in familial adenomatous polyposis. N Engl J Med 1993;328:1313. *(Some benefit suggested.)*

Giovannucci E, Ascherio A, Rimm EB, et al. Physical activity, obesity, and risk for colon cancer and adenoma in men. Ann Intern Med 1995;122:327. *(Prospective cohort study; physical activity was associated with reduced risk, abdominal adiposity with increased risk.)*

Giovannucci E, Stampfer MJ, Colditz GA, et al. Multivitamin use, folate, and colon cancer in women in the Nurses Health Study. Ann Intern Med 1998;129:524. *(Prospective cohort study showing long-term use, especially for folate, associated with reduced risk.)*

Goldberg RM, Fleming TR, Tangen CM, et al. Surgery for recurrent colon cancer: strategies for identifying resectable recurrence and success rates after resection. Ann Intern Med 1998;129:27. *(Evidence suggesting that monitoring for and removing surgically resectable recurrences improves outcomes.)*

Goldstein F, Martinez E, Platz EA, et al. Postmenopausal hormone use and risk for colorectal cancer and adenoma. Ann Intern Med

1998;128:705. *(Prospective cohort study; benefit found while taking replacement therapy, but it persisted only if treatment continued.)*

Ivanovich JL, Read TE, Ciske DJ, et al. A practical approach to familial and hereditary colorectal cancer. Am J Med 1999;107:68. *(A review that stresses the importance of a detailed family history followed by more intensified screening, cancer risk assessment, genetic testing, and consideration of prophylactic surgery.)*

Levin TR. Predicting advanced proximal colonic neoplasia with screening sigmoidoscopy. JAMA 1999;281:1611. *(A cross-sectional study from an HMO identifying risk factors predictive of finding an advanced lesion on colonoscopy.)*

Liefers G-J, Cleton-Jansen A-M, de Velde CJH, et al. Micrometastases and survival in stage II colorectal cancer. N Engl J Med 1998; 339:223. *(Molecular methods uncovered micrometastases with an adverse prognosis.)*

Moertel CG, Fleming TR, MacDonald JS, et al. Fluorouracil plus levamisole as effective adjuvant therapy after resection of stage III colon carcinoma: a final report. Ann Intern Med 1995;122:321. *(After a mean follow-up of 6.5 years, this randomized controlled trial demonstrated a 40% reduction in recurrence and a 33% reduction in mortality for patients with advanced disease.)*

Read TE, Read JD, Butterly LF. Importance of adenomas of 5 mm or less in diameter that are detected by sigmoidoscopy. N Engl J Med 1997;336:8. *(Found a high risk for proximal pathology and argues that colonoscopy be performed.)*

Selby JV, Friedman GD, Quesenberry CP, et al. A case-control study of screening sigmoidoscopy and mortality from colorectal cancer. N Engl J Med 1992;326:653. *(Mortality from cancer of the distal colon and rectum reduced.)*

Sturmer T, Glynn RJ, Lee I-M, et al. Aspirin use and colorectal cancer: post-trial follow-up data from the Physicians' Health Study. Ann Intern Med 1998;128:713. *(No benefit found.)*

Swedish Rectal Cancer Trial. Improved survival with preoperative radiotherapy in resectable rectal cancer. N Engl J Med 1997;336:980. *(Randomized controlled trial; long-term survival improved by 15%.)*

Syngal S, Fox EA, Li C, et al. Interpretation of genetic test results for hereditary nonpolyposis colorectal cancer. JAMA 1999;282:247. *(Deleterious mutations useful to management were found in 25% of families examined.)*

Syngal S, Weeks JC, Schrag D, et al. Benefits of colonoscopic surveillance and prophylactic colectomy in patients with hereditary nonpolyposis colorectal cancer mutations. Ann Intern Me 1998;129: 787. *(A decision-analysis study of the options for patients with high genetic risk of malignancy.)*

Wallace MB, Kemp JA, Trnka YM, et al. Is colonoscopy indicated for small adenomas found by screening flexible sigmoidoscopy? Ann Intern Med 1998;129:273. *(Disagrees with Read et al.; finds risk of proximal disease is nil.)*

Winawer SJ. Randomized comparison of surveillance intervals after colonoscopic removal of newly diagnosed adenomatous polyps. N Engl J Med 1993;328:901. *(Suggests that the interval need not be as short as previously thought.)*

Winawer SJ, Zauber AG, Ho MN, et al. Prevention of colorectal cancer by colonoscopic polypectomy. N Engl J Med 1993;321:1977. *(Risk of cancer reduced by 70% to 90%; best prospective study.)*

6

Hematologic and Oncologic Problems

77
Screening for Anemia

Anemia is a sign of illness rather than a diagnosis in itself. The incidental finding of a low hematocrit or hemoglobin level suggests a host of underlying conditions that range from the trivial to the life-threatening. Patients with fatigue or other subjective symptoms often ask about their "blood count." The absence of anemia in such instances is reassuring. But is the patient who is otherwise well likely to benefit from either the identification or the treatment of asymptomatic anemia? The answer to this question depends on the prevalence and nature of the conditions most likely to cause asymptomatic anemia, and on the relationship between the hemoglobin level and those symptoms attributed to its reduction.

EPIDEMIOLOGY AND RISK FACTORS

By far the most common cause of asymptomatic anemia is *iron deficiency* resulting from the inadequate dietary replacement of iron lost from the body. Daily iron requirements for men and postmenopausal women are between 0.5 and 1 mg. Because additional iron is needed by menstruating and pregnant women, their daily requirements are 2 mg and 2.5 mg, respectively. Because only 5% to 10% of the 10 to 20 mg of the iron contained in the average adult diet is absorbed, it is not surprising that iron deficiency is common in women of childbearing age. Population studies have found 10% to 20% of menstruating women to have abnormally low concentrations of hemoglobin (usually <12 g/100 mL). Between 20% and 60% of pregnant women have hemoglobin levels below 11 g/100 mL. Anemia is less likely to occur in women taking birth control pills and more likely to occur in women with intrauterine devices. Iron deficiency is rare in male adults; if present, it is a clear indication for diligent investigation of the gastrointestinal tract. Absorption of iron may be decreased after gastrectomy or in the presence of achlorhydria.

Sideroblastic and megaloblastic anemias are much less common. The prevalence of *pernicious anemia*, the most common form of vitamin B_{12} deficiency, is 0.1% in persons of Northern European extraction. Pernicious anemia is much less common among other ethnic and racial groups. *Folate deficiency* is common during pregnancy and in patients with alcoholic liver disease, in whom it is often accompanied by sider-

oblastic anemia. Anticonvulsant drugs, including phenytoin, primidone, and phenobarbital, may interfere with folate absorption, so that megaloblastic anemia results. *Thalassemia* minor is a common cause of mild anemia in patients of Mediterranean or Far Eastern extraction. *Sickle cell disease* and trait, by far the most common forms of hemoglobinopathy, are discussed separately (see Chapter 78).

NATURAL HISTORY OF ANEMIA AND EFFECTIVENESS OF THERAPY

Obviously, the natural history of anemia depends on the underlying cause. What symptoms can mild or moderate anemia be expected to produce? The hyperkinetic symptoms that follow compensatory increases in cardiac stroke volume and heart rate are rarely present before hemoglobin levels have fallen to 7.5 g/100 mL. Other highly subjective symptoms, including irritability, fatigue, and headache, have been attributed to milder degrees of anemia. A British survey, however, found no relationship between the frequency of such symptoms and the level of hemoglobin (ranging from 8 to 12 g/100 mL) among women found to have iron-deficiency anemia during a screening program. Indirect evidence showed that levels under 8 g/100 mL were associated with symptoms severe enough to prompt presentation to a physician. Among the asymptomatic women identified by screening, no benefits of treatment were detected. It has been noted by some investigators that symptoms associated with vitamin B_{12} deficiency may predate the onset of anemia (see Chapters 79 and 82).

Most studies of screening for anemia have been conducted in the preoperative or inpatient setting. The few that have been performed on outpatients have shown little benefit. In a Swiss study of the utility of the complete blood cell count in 595 outpatients attending a university-based clinic, 34 (5.8%) had a low hemoglobin level, and a new diagnosis (iron deficiency without serious underlying pathology) was made in only three of them (0.5%). Another report from Britain demonstrated a 10% prevalence of anemia among screened women. The absence of treatable underlying conditions other than iron deficiency was noteworthy, and, again, no benefits of treatment could be demonstrated.

Iron-deficiency anemia is not uncommon among pregnant women and has been associated with a twofold to threefold increased risk for low birth weight, preterm delivery, and perinatal mortality. Screening for anemia is generally recommended as part of the first prenatal evaluation. The results of randomized trials of iron supplementation for pregnant women without anemia or with mild anemia have been mixed. When iron supplementation is prescribed for women who already have children, they should be reminded of the risk of overdose among toddlers; 30% of fatal pediatric overdoses can be attributed to iron supplements.

SCREENING AND DIAGNOSTIC TESTS

The laboratory measurements of *hematocrit* and *hemoglobin concentration* are straightforward. Automated methods are reliable and reproducible when specimens are properly handled. The mean hematocrit for adult men at sea level is 46%, with a range of 41% to 51%; for women, the mean is 42% and the range is 37% to 47%. Slight differences may be noted when automated techniques are used to measure the hematocrit. The normal mean hemoglobin concentration is approximately 16 g/100 mL for men, with a range of 14 to 18 g/100 mL; for women, the mean is 14 g/100 mL and the range is 12 to 16 g/100 mL. In men over 65, the mean falls to 13.5 g/100 mL, and in women over 65, it falls to 13.1 g/100 mL. It must be remembered, as with all continuous laboratory variables, that the choice of a reference value for defining normality is arbitrary. This is particularly true in light of the unclear relationship between significant symptoms and mild "anemia."

CONCLUSIONS AND RECOMMENDATIONS

- Anemia is a common condition. It may be secondary to serious underlying disease or a simple dietary deficiency. Determination of the hemoglobin concentration or hematocrit is recommended as an important part of the evaluation of a variety of presenting complaints, including fatigue, weight loss, abdominal pain, and gastrointestinal bleeding (see Chapters 8, 9, 58, and 63).
- Although determination of the complete blood cell count may provide clues in asymptomatic patients to the presence of early treatable disease, such as gastrointestinal malignancy, more sensitive and more specific screening methods are available and preferred (e.g., stool guaiac testing and sig-

moidoscopy for early detection of colorectal cancer; see Chapter 56).
- No clear relationship has been found between mild to moderate degrees of anemia and significant symptoms. No clearly measurable benefits after the treatment of mild anemia have been identified in screening studies.
- Thus, routine screening for anemia in nonpregnant, asymptomatic patients is not recommended.
- Iron-deficiency anemia is common among pregnant women and is associated with poorer outcomes of pregnancy. Screening for anemia at the time of the first prenatal visit is recommended.

A.G.M./A.H.G.

ANNOTATED BIBLIOGRAPHY

Elwood PC, Shinton NK, Wilson IL, et al. Haemoglobin, vitamin B_{12} and folate levels in the elderly. Br J Haematol 1971;21:557. (*In 10% of elderly men, hemoglobin levels are below 13 g/100 mL; in 10% of elderly women, they are below 12.5 g/100 mL. No megaloblastic anemia found.*)

Elwood PC, Waters WE, Greene WJW, et al. Symptoms and circulating haemoglobin level. J Chron Dis 1969;21:615. (*Symptoms not correlated with hemoglobin level in those found anemic on screening.*)

Elwood PC, Waters WE, Greene WJ, et al. Evaluation of a screening survey for anemia in adult nonpregnant women. Br Med J 1967;4:714. (*Not very extensive follow-up, but no serious underlying disease detected among anemic women.*)

Institute of Medicine. Iron-deficiency anemia: recommended guidelines for the prevention, detection, and management among U.S. children and women of childbearing age. Washington, DC: National Academy Press, 1993. (*Authoritative review and recommendations.*)

Murphy JF, O'Riordan J, Newcombe RG, et al. Relation of haemoglobin levels in first and second trimester to outcome of pregnancy. Lancet 1986;1:992. (*Association with increased risk for low birth weight, preterm delivery, and perinatal mortality.*)

Ruttman S, Clemencon D, Dubach UC. Usefulness of complete blood counts as a case-finding tool in medical outpatients. Ann Intern Med 1992;116:44. (*One of the few studies performed in the outpatient setting; yield of 5.8%, but no significant pathology found in this middle-aged population.*)

U.S. Preventive Services Task Force. Guide to clinical preventive services, 2nd ed. Baltimore: Williams & Wilkins, 1996. (*Screening for anemia recommended for pregnant women at their first prenatal visit and for high-risk infants.*)

78

Screening for Sickle Cell Disease and Sickle Cell Trait

Sickle cell disease is the most common of the clinically significant hemoglobinopathies. In the United States, the disease and trait occur almost exclusively among African-Americans. Sickle cell disease afflicts 1 in 375 African-Americans and 1 in 60,000 whites. During the late 1960s and early 1970s, sickle cell disease received a great deal of attention in the medical and

lay press. The importance of screening for the disease and trait was stressed. Some states legislated mandatory screening programs.

Sickle cell disease (the hemoglobin SS homozygous state) is usually identified during childhood. Patients in whom anemia is not identified by screening are often given the diagnosis after they present with impaired growth, increased susceptibility to infection, or painful crisis. Screening of adults is aimed at the identification of asymptomatic carriers of sickle cell trait (the hemoglobin AS heterozygous state). The principal objective is to reduce the prevalence of the homozygous condition by means of genetic counseling. Whether or not screening benefits the people screened has been debated. Screening performed without subsequent education and counseling can be harmful. An understanding of the natural history of sickle cell trait and disease, sensitivity to the concerns of affected patients, and selective use of available screening tests are all necessary if such harmful effects are to be avoided.

EPIDEMIOLOGY AND RISK FACTORS

Sickle cell disease has a prevalence of less than 0.35% among African-American children in the United States. Double heterozygotes, including those with hemoglobin SC or S-β-thalassemia, are even less common. The prevalence of sickling disease is lower among adults because the life span of SS homozygotes and double heterozygotes is decreased.

Screening surveys have documented a prevalence of sickle trait of 7.4% among African-American veterans and 8.7% in the African-American community of San Francisco. Some studies have shown regional differences in prevalence. Prevalence does not decrease with age. Sickle cell trait is present with a low frequency in Southern Italy and with a higher frequency in parts of Greece. It remains a rare finding in Americans of Mediterranean extraction.

NATURAL HISTORY OF SICKLE CELL DISEASE AND EFFECTIVENESS OF THERAPY

The natural history of *sickle cell disease* is variable. Most children exhibit failure to thrive and have frequent infections. Anemia is usually moderate but can become severe, often as a result of infection or folate deficiency. The course is punctuated by painful crises precipitated by infection, dehydration, or hypoxia. Organ infarction, congestive heart failure, cholelithiasis, and skin ulcers are some of the complications of chronic disease. Because supportive care has improved, the life expectancy of patients with sickle cell disease has increased; however, it still remains significantly shortened, by 25 to 30 years in comparison with that of African-Americans who do not have sickle cell disease.

In contrast, life expectancy is not affected by *sickle cell trait*. AS red blood cells sickle at a much lower oxygen tension than do SS cells. The only clinical abnormality that occurs with any frequency among patients with sickle cell trait is painless hematuria, presumably the result of small infarcts of the renal medulla, where red cells are particularly susceptible to sickling.

Concern about a risk for sudden death during extreme physical exertion in patients with sickle trait has been raised by case reports and population studies of military recruits. Indeed, the presence of sickle trait was associated with an increased risk for otherwise unexplained sudden death among military recruits who were engaged in extreme exertion during basic training. This led to a suggestion that African-American recruits and athletes be screened for sickle trait. However, although the relative risk for sudden death may be elevated, the absolute risk still appears to be very small (about 1 in 3,000 in the Army recruit study) and practically nil for physically well-conditioned persons during exercise (no episodes of sudden death attributable to sickle trait among Olympic or professional athletes, even when they performed at high elevations).

Thus, for untrained persons with sickle trait, a small increase in risk may indeed exist, especially at extremes of exertion and altitude, but under most other circumstances, sickle trait appears to be a benign condition. Some data even suggest that the reason for an occasional sudden death in patients with what appears to be ordinary sickle trait is the undetected presence of an electrophoretically silent hemoglobin variant migrating like hemoglobin A but causing significant sickling in patients heterozygous for hemoglobin S.

If sickle trait is a generally benign condition, then the principal reason for screening adults is to provide genetic counseling. It is important to consider the effectiveness of such counseling. Evidence suggests that the identification and counseling of heterozygotes do not alter marriage and parenthood decisions. The person who does not wish to make such decisions on the basis of carrier status is not likely to benefit from screening. Some families have been traumatized by questions of paternity raised by indiscriminate screening. Because of the confusion among patients and physicians about differences between sickle cell disease and trait, unnecessary anxiety may be the most common result. Surveys have demonstrated that many internists and general practitioners do not sufficiently understand the implications of screening test results to be able to counsel patients properly.

SCREENING AND DIAGNOSTIC TESTS

Screening tests for sickle cell trait are inexpensive and reproducible. Results of tests for sickling, including the use of 2% metabisulfite solution and the more expensive commercial methods, are positive in the presence of hemoglobin S, but the tests do not distinguish between homozygotes, heterozygotes, and double heterozygotes (hemoglobin S combined with thalassemia or hemoglobin C). Hemoglobin electrophoresis can also be performed inexpensively; however, it is not a substitute for a test of sickling because some nonsickling hemoglobin variants travel in the same electrophoretic band as hemoglobin S (e.g., hemoglobin Lepore). Examining a peripheral blood smear and checking a reticulocyte count provide supportive data for diagnosis of sickle cell disease (see Chapter 79).

A number of techniques have been developed to diagnose sickle cell disease during early gestation of fetuses at risk. Chorionic biopsy has been used successfully to identify sickle cell disease during the first 6 to 8 weeks of pregnancy. The availability of prenatal diagnosis should be explained before screening. Careful counseling must also precede the responsible application of any prenatal diagnostic method. Risks of the procedure to mother and fetus, risks of false-positive and false-negative test results, and the acceptability of therapeutic abortion should be discussed.

CONCLUSIONS AND RECOMMENDATIONS

- Sickle cell disease is a serious health hazard that usually presents during early childhood. Screening of newborn infants permits appropriate prophylaxis and immunization and is recommended.

- Sickle cell trait is generally a benign condition. Although there is some question of an increased relative risk for sudden death in untrained persons required to exert extreme physical effort at very high altitude, the absolute risk is extremely low and nil in trained persons.
- Thus, the principal reason for screening adults for the presence of sickle trait is to facilitate genetic counseling. Screening of high-risk pregnant women at their first prenatal visit should be preceded by counseling about the subsequent need for paternal testing and the availability of prenatal diagnosis. Indiscriminate screening followed by inadequate counseling may be harmful and is not likely to provide benefits to those persons who will not revise marriage and parenthood decisions on the basis of test results.
- Screening for sickle trait should be offered to African-American adults in reproductive age groups. The implications of test results should be fully explained before testing is performed.

A.G.M./A.H.G.

ANNOTATED BIBLIOGRAPHY

Agency for Health Care Policy and Research. Sickle cell disease: screening, diagnosis, management and counseling in newborns and infants. Clinical practice guideline No 6. AHCPR Publication No 93-0562. Rockville, MD: Agency for Health Care Policy and Research, US Department of Health and Human Services, Public Health Service, 1993. (*Guidelines based on critical synthesis of the evidence.*)

Charache S. Sudden death in sickle trait. Am J Med 1988;84:459. (*Editorial summarizing the evidence; concludes risk is very small and clinically unimportant under most circumstances.*)

Farfel MR, Holtzman NA. Education, consent, and counseling in sickle cell screening programs: report of a survey. Am J Public Health 1984;74:373. (*Of 52,000 persons screened in Maryland during a 1-year period, 25% were screened without informed consent.*)

Goossens M, Dumez Y, Kaplan L, et al. Prenatal diagnosis of sickle-cell anemia in the first trimester of pregnancy. N Engl J Med 1983;309:831. (*Earlier diagnosis of sickle cell disease is possible through chorionic biopsy techniques.*)

Kark JA, Posey DM, Schumacher HR, et al. Sickle-cell trait as a risk factor for sudden death in physical training. N Engl J Med 1987;317:781. (*Increased risk for sudden death found among recruits with sickle cell trait.*)

Kellon DB, Beutler E. Physician attitudes about sickle cell disease and sickle cell trait. JAMA 1974;227:71. (*Finds many primary care practitioners misunderstand the implications of sickle cell screening.*)

Martin TW, Weisman IM, Zeballos RJ, et al. Exercise and hypoxia increase sickling in venous blood from an exercising limb in individuals with sickle cell trait. Am J Med 1989;87:48. (*At 4,000 m, sickling increased significantly in venous blood, but not in arterial blood; oxygen consumption and exercise performance same as for controls.*)

Motulsky AG. Frequency of sickling disorders in U.S. blacks. N Engl J Med 1973;288:31. [*Estimates prevalence of double heterozygosity and of SS disease in newborns (1 in 625 with SS, 1 in 833 with SC, and 1 in 1,667 with S-β-thalassemia) and in the population.*]

Murphy JR. Sickle cell hemoglobin in black football players. JAMA 1973;225:981. (*Rate of hemoglobin AS among African-American football players in the National Football League was 6.7%.*)

Petrakis NL, Wiesenfeld SL, Sams BJ, et al. Prevalence of sickle-cell trait and glucose-6-PD deficiency. N Engl J Med 1970;282:767. (*An 8.7% prevalence of sickle trait among more than 4,000 African-Americans in San Francisco.*)

Platt OS, Brambilla DJ, Rosse WF, et al. Mortality in sickle cell disease: life expectancy and risk factors for early death. N Engl J Med 1994;330:1639. (*The life expectancy of African-Americans with sickle cell disease is on average 25 to 30 years shorter than that of other African-Americans.*)

Sears DA. The morbidity of sickle cell trait. Am J Med 1978;64:1021. (*Extensive review. Although certain abnormalities do occur with increased frequency in sickle cell trait, survival is not impaired; 296 references.*)

79
Evaluation of Anemia

In most instances, the office presentation of anemia is incidental, with no obvious cause and no hemodynamic compromise. Because anemia is not a diagnosis, its appearance necessitates identification of the underlying cause, especially in men, women who are neither menstruating nor pregnant, and the elderly; in all these groups, the probability of disease is high. In more than 50% of cases, a clinically important cause is discovered. The task for the primary physician is to design a cost-effective assessment that concentrates on testing for causes of prognostic significance.

DEFINITION, PATHOPHYSIOLOGY, AND CLINICAL PRESENTATION

Definition. Anemia is defined as a reduction in the hematocrit or hemoglobin concentration. The widely accepted World Health Organization definition is expressed in terms of hemoglobin concentration: for male adults, below 13 g/dL; for nonpregnant women, below 12 g/dL; for pregnant women, below 11 g/dL. Although the cutoff points are somewhat arbitrary, derived statistically from population data, these numbers can have meaning for individual patients, as they tend to correlate with health status and prognosis, particularly in the elderly. Although the mean hemoglobin concentration tends to decline with age, the significance of anemia does not, and consequently the diagnostic criteria are not adjusted downward for age. Because anemia is defined in terms of red cell mass and hemoglobin concentration, a spurious diagnosis of anemia may be made when the plasma volume is expanded. Similarly, if the plasma volume is contracted, a true anemia may be masked.

Pathophysiology. Anemia may result from *bleeding, inadequate red cell production,* or *excessive red cell destruction;* often, two or more mechanisms are operating simultaneously.

Production is decreased when defects in stem cell proliferation or differentiation, DNA synthesis, or hemoglobin synthesis, or a combination of these deficiencies, is present. Excessive destruction can result from membrane disorders, abnormal hemoglobins, enzyme deficiencies, and a host of extrinsic problems, such as mechanical disruption or antibody-mediated injury.

The development of symptoms and signs depends on the abruptness and severity of onset, age of the patient, and ability of the cardiopulmonary system to compensate for the decrease in blood volume and oxygen-carrying capacity. When onset is gradual, symptoms may be minimal because there is adequate time for compensatory adjustments to occur. Important responses include an increase in 2,3-diphosphoglycerate, which facilitates oxygen delivery to tissues, and expansion of the plasma volume.

Clinical Presentation. Symptoms are a function of the severity and speed of onset of the anemia. Patients experiencing a rapid onset of anemia, with little time for compensatory mechanisms to act, are likely to have the most symptoms. Those who have a hematocrit above 30% and a gradual onset and are otherwise in good health rarely note symptoms. However, if the hematocrit falls further, *exertional dyspnea* and *fatigue* may begin to appear after strenuous activity. Greater reductions in the hematocrit result in cardiopulmonary symptoms that come with less activity. Age and cardiopulmonary reserve are also important determinants of symptoms. A potpourri of nonspecific complaints frequently accompanies anemia, including headache, tinnitus, poor concentration, palpitations, vague abdominal discomfort, anorexia, nausea, and diarrhea or constipation. *Tachycardia* and diminished peripheral resistance occur as the hemoglobin falls below 7.5 g/100 mL; a *systolic flow murmur* resulting from high output is common. *Pallor* is an obvious finding, best seen in the conjunctiva, but it is of little help as an indicator of severity. More specific clinical findings depend on the underlying cause, which can best be classified on the basis of red cell morphology (determined by appearance on a Wright-stained peripheral smear, mean corpuscular volume calculated by an autoanalyzer, and degree of anisocytosis).

Microcytic Anemias

Iron Deficiency. *Inadequate dietary intake, inadequate absorption,* and excessive *blood loss* may result in iron-deficiency anemia. Most patients with mild disease are asymptomatic, manifesting only a low-grade microcytic anemia. In otherwise healthy menstruating women, iron deficiency is often blamed for a host of symptoms, including *fatigue, headache, paresthesias,* and *irritability.* Although fatigue may certainly be a manifestation of severe anemia, the correlation between these symptoms and hemoglobin concentration has been poor in women with mild anemia. In placebo-controlled double-blinded studies, they fail to show consistent symptomatic benefit with iron therapy. *Menorrhagia* is attributed by some investigators to instances of iron deficiency, but this is disputed by others. *Pica* and *dysphagia* (caused by an esophageal web) are classic, although rare, features today.

The physical findings that occur in iron deficiency are a bit more specific. *Atrophic glossitis* is commonly found, as is *cheilitis*; koilonychia, with spooning, ridging, and thinning, is

rare. Other physical findings and symptoms are manifestations of the underlying cause. The earliest laboratory changes are depletion of marrow iron stores and a corresponding *fall in serum ferritin*. These are followed by a *decrease in serum iron* and an *increase in transferrin*, which produce in many cases a reduction in the *transferrin saturation* to *less than 16%*. The first change in the peripheral blood is a drop in the *hematocrit* and *hemoglobin concentration*. An *anisocytosis* develops, manifested by an elevation in the *red cell distribution width* (RDW). Later, with increasing severity of anemia (hemoglobin concentration <9 g/dL), red cells become *microcytic* and eventually *hypochromic*.

Anemia of Chronic Disease. A common accompaniment of chronic inflammatory diseases and malignancy, the anemia of chronic disease is believed to involve trapping of iron by activated macrophages, which renders the iron unavailable for erythropoiesis. In addition, some suppression of erythropoiesis by humoral substances (interleukins, tumor necrosis factor, prostaglandins), elaborated in the course of the underlying chronic disease process, often occurs. Interestingly, erythropoietin is inappropriately low in almost all cases. The anemia is usually moderate, with hemoglobin levels in the range of 7 to 11 g/dL. Both serum iron and iron-binding capacity are reduced. The smear is most often *normocytic* but can be *hypochromic* and even *microcytic*, mimicking iron deficiency. The *serum iron falls* before anemia sets in; *transferrin saturation* may be below 16%, again simulating iron deficiency. However, marrow iron stores and *ferritin* levels are *normal* or increased.

Another important anemia of chronic disease is that associated with *HIV infection*, which affects the bone marrow. Myelofibrosis occurs. Anemia is seen in about 15% of asymptomatic HIV-positive persons, 45% with AIDS-related complex, and 75% of those with untreated AIDS. For unknown reasons, *erythropoietin* is inappropriately *low*. The smear in most cases is *normochromic–normocytic*. *Rouleaux* formation resulting from circulating immune complexes sometimes develops, but hemolysis is uncommon. The anemia can be exacerbated by *medications* used in the treatment of HIV infection (zidovudine, pentamidine, trimethoprim, sulfonamides). Zidovudine is especially toxic to marrow, causing anemia in about 30% of instances. *Neutropenia* and *thrombocytopenia* occur to a lesser extent. Patients most susceptible to the adverse hematologic effects of zidovudine are those with a low CD4-cell count, pre-existing anemia, concurrent vitamin B_{12} deficiency, or neutropenia.

Thalassemia Minor (Thalassemia Trait). This condition is typically detected in asymptomatic patients undergoing an evaluation for a microcytic hypochromic anemia that does not respond to iron. A gene defect leads to impaired red cell maturation by causing an excess of either α- or β-chains of hemoglobin to accumulate. The most prevalent form is β-thalassemia trait, common among persons of Mediterranean ancestry. It is associated with an increase in *hemoglobin A_2*. There are no characteristic physical findings. The red cell count is elevated, and the smear may reveal *target cells, basophilic stippling, polychromatophilia, poikilocytosis,* and *anisocytosis* in addition to microcytosis. α-Thalassemia trait is seen among

African-Americans. The hemoglobin A_2 level is normal, but a mild anemia, hypochromia, and microcytosis are present.

Sideroblastic Anemias are a heterogeneous set of disorders that include a *primary* type, which may be a preleukemic state; a *congenital* pyridoxine-responsive variant; and *secondary* variants associated with rheumatoid arthritis, polyarteritis, malabsorption, chronic alcoholism, cancer, porphyria, lead poisoning, and true pyridoxine deficiency. These, too, are conditions of abnormal red cell maturation. They can lead to significant anemia requiring repeated transfusion of red cells. Their hallmark is the accumulation of nonheme iron within the mitochondria of red cells. When stained for iron, immature red cells demonstrate a ring of stain around the nucleus (*ringed sideroblasts*). In the primary type, patients are typically over the of age 60 and may have *primary myelodysplasia*, a proliferative disease of the bone marrow in which a clone of stem cells suppresses production of other cell lines. A *secondary myelodysplastic syndrome* occurs as a consequence of cancer chemotherapy. The spleen is usually not enlarged, as it is in myeloproliferative disorders. The smear is classically microcytic but may be macrocytic or dimorphic, especially in acquired forms. Cells can be hypochromic, which leads to confusion with iron deficiency. Anisocytosis and poikilocytosis are pronounced. *Serum iron* is *elevated*, as is *transferrin saturation*. Marrow iron stains show many abnormal ringed sideroblasts. The anemia may be refractory, sometimes followed by marrow failure and acute myeloid leukemia.

Macrocytic Anemias

Vitamin B_{12} Deficiency. A classic cause is reduced gastric production of intrinsic factor, as occurs in *pernicious anemia* and after subtotal *gastrectomy*. The association of pernicious anemia with *Hashimoto's thyroiditis* and *vitiligo* suggest an autoimmune mechanism, confirmed by the identification of autoantibodies to intrinsic factor and parietal cells. Dietary lack is rare because vitamin B_{12} is available in everyday foods, and body stores can hold up to a 3-year reserve. However, patients with achlorhydria or hypochlorhydria resulting from atrophic gastritis or gastric surgery may fail to split cobalamin from food, resulting in so-called *food-cobalamin malabsorption*, which is thought to be responsible for much of the B_{12} deficiency seen in the elderly and those with prior gastric surgery. Population studies find a prevalence of vitamin B_{12} deficiency of 1.9% in persons over the age of 60 years. *Blind-loop syndrome* and *terminal ileal disease* are other causes.

Onset is gradual. In pernicious anemia, symptoms usually become evident in the sixth decade. Gastrointestinal problems such as *anorexia* and *diarrhea* may predominate. *Sore tongue* resulting from *atrophic glossitis* is a classic presentation, as is *numbness* and *tingling* in the extremities associated with peripheral neuropathy. The neurologic deficits result from defects in the maintenance of myelin integrity. Besides peripheral neuropathy, injury to the posterior columns and corticospinal tracts of the spinal cord (i.e., *subacute combined degeneration*) may be present, manifested by disturbances of *position* and *vibratory sense* and *incoordination*, *spasticity*, and *upturned toes*. Cerebral dysfunction may also ensue, leading to *memory loss*, *depression*, and *irritability*. If vitamin B_{12} deficiency is uncor-

rected, demyelination can progress to axonal degeneration and irreversible neuronal death. Nerve damage can occur in the absence of anemia.

By the time the anemia is discovered, it may be severe. *Hypersegmented polymorphonuclear leukocytes* are an early finding on peripheral blood smears that is specific for the megaloblastic anemias. *Oval macrocytes* are also characteristic, although poikilocytosis is considerable. Classically, the mean corpuscular volume rises above 100 μm^3 and the serum vitamin B_{12} level falls below 100 pg/mL, but in up to a third of cases macrocytosis may be absent or the vitamin B_{12} level may be greater than 100 pg/mL. The serum concentration of *holotranscobalamin II* (the vitamin B_{12} carrier protein) begins to decline before the vitamin B_{12} level does. Macrocytosis may be absent if concurrent iron deficiency is present, but the hypersegmented polymorphonuclear leukocytes persist. In pernicious anemia, *achlorhydria* is found on stimulation testing. Serum *homocysteine* levels frequently become elevated, which may predispose to vascular disease (see Chapter 31); levels of the *methylmalonic acid* increase.

Folate Deficiency. Inadequate dietary intake is the usual cause, as body stores are limited to a 3-month reserve. Chronic alcohol abuse is the classic cause. Increased demand sometimes occurs, as in pregnancy, hemolysis, malignancy, or severe psoriasis. Decreased uptake resulting from malabsorption or drugs (e.g., phenytoin, other anticonvulsants) also can trigger the anemia. The same is true for folate antagonists such as methotrexate, trimethoprim, and triamterene. Hematologic features resemble those of vitamin B_{12} deficiency; no neurologic deficits are present. Folate deficiency is an important cause of *hyperhomocysteinemia*, which is associated with increased risk for arterial and venous thrombosis (see Chapter 31).

Liver Disease. Hepatocellular disease is responsible for a host of anemias, especially when accompanied by alcoholism and poor diet. It accounts for many cases of macrocytic anemia. Folate deficiency, marrow suppression, hypersplenism, bleeding, and bile salt alteration of the red cell membrane all contribute. The smear shows considerable poikilocytosis with *spiculated red cells* and some *macrocytes*; if folate deficiency occurs, a megaloblastic picture is superimposed.

Sideroblastic Anemia. See above.

Normochromic–Normocytic Anemias

Hemolytic Anemias are a diverse group. Inherited forms are caused by intrinsic red cell defects; acquired types depend primarily on extrinsic mechanisms, such as immunologic or mechanical injury. Clinical presentations vary according to rate of destruction, compensatory adaptations, and underlying cause. Jaundice sets in when the capacity of the liver to conjugate excess bilirubin from hemoglobin breakdown is exceeded; the serum level of unconjugated bilirubin climbs. *Splenomegaly* evolves as trapping of damaged red cells progresses. Sudden fever, chills, headache, back and abdominal pain, and *hemoglobinuria* characterize severe acute hemolysis.

The reticulocyte count is elevated unless an accompanying marrow defect is present. The peripheral smear usually appears normochromic–normocytic but may be macrocytic because of the release of immature forms during rapid red cell destruction and regeneration. Polychromatophilia is common, and *nucleated red cells*, *stippling*, *schistocytes*, and *Howell-Jolly bodies* may be noted. *Spherocytes* occur in *hereditary spherocytosis*, a condition of reduced cell membrane area resulting from a defect in synthesis of the membrane protein spectrin. *Spherocytosis* is also seen in *immune hemolytic anemia* as a consequence of membrane loss.

Sickle Cell Disease is the most prevalent hemolytic condition in the African-American population. *Sickle cell trait* is asymptomatic and anemia is absent, although mild hematuria caused by sickling in the hypertonic renal medulla sometimes occurs. The peripheral smear is normal except for an occasional *target cell*. Hemoglobin electrophoresis reveals less than 50% of total hemoglobin to be of the S variety. Patients homozygous for the sickle cell gene have *sickle cell anemia*, a much more serious condition in which painful crises are precipitated by stress (especially infection). Intravascular sickling ensues, the red cells become rigid, and vascular occlusion may result, leading to arterial desaturation, hemolysis, and organ damage. *Leg ulcers*, *hepatomegaly*, *hematuria*, *renal concentrating defects*, and mild *jaundice* commonly occur. Patients report acute, severe *pain* in the lower extremities, back, or abdomen. *Fever* and *leukocytosis* may also be present. Attacks typically last from a few hours to a few days, then resolve spontaneously. Aplastic crises develop when a concurrent illness suppresses erythropoiesis. The smear is normochromic; *sickled cells* may be noted in addition to target forms. Hemoglobin electrophoresis reveals a predominance of *hemoglobin S*. Addition of a reducing agent, such as metabisulfite, to a drop of blood causes the cells to sickle within a few minutes and confirms the diagnosis.

Glucose-6-phosphate Dehydrogenase Deficiency is a sex-linked red cell defect compromising the enzyme that maintains hemoglobin in an unoxidized state. In its episodic form, seen in African-Americans, the condition causes hemolysis after exposure to oxidant compounds (sulfonamides, antimalarials) or infection. A chronic variety occurs in persons of Mediterranean ancestry.

Drug-induced Hemolytic Anemias usually manifest an immune mechanism, such as adsorption to the red cell of drug–antibody complexes (quinidine); adsorption to the red cell of drug to form a hapten, followed by binding of antidrug antibody (high-dose penicillin); or induction of a red cell "autoantibody" (long-term methyldopa). The hallmark of most drug-related hemolytic episodes is a positive *direct Coombs' test* result. Withdrawal of the offending agent ends the process.

Autoimmune Hemolytic Anemias result when patients produce antibodies against their own red cells. They are classified according to the type of antibody produced (immunoglobulin G or immunoglobulin M). Those of the *IgG class* are directed against the Rh antigen. Most are *"warm" autoantibodies*; although many are idiopathic, about 50% occur in the context of lymphoma, lupus, ulcerative colitis, or chronic lymphocytic leukemia. The diagnosis is made by detecting IgG and C3d proteins on the red cell surface. Macrophages that can detect these proteins bind the involved red cells. Hemolysis is mostly extravascular. The red cells are cleared by the spleen. The *IgM* form of autoimmune hemolytic anemia is a *cold hemagglutinin* condition. These antibodies are seen in mycoplasmal, Epstein-Barr virus, or cytomegalovirus infection and in lymphoprolifer-

ative conditions. *Cold agglutinin* titers are markedly elevated in the setting of hemolysis (>1:$1,000$).

Aplastic Anemias are usually idiopathic but may be linked to a marrow toxin (cytotoxic drugs, radiation), an idiosyncratic drug reaction (chloramphenicol, gold, sulfur compounds, carbamazepine), or a viral infection (hepatitis B virus, hepatitis C virus, cytomegalovirus, HIV, parvovirus). Onset is gradual, with fatigue and bleeding noted first; infection is a later problem. No organomegaly occurs. The smear appears normochromic–normocytic, but the number of platelets is diminished. There are no signs of increased red cell production. The reticulocyte count is zero, and a pancytopenia is present.

Renal Failure. The anemia of chronic renal failure is caused by a reduction in both production and survival of red cells. Lack of erythropoietin and metabolic injury to erythrocytes are postulated mechanisms. The severity of the anemia parallels the degree of azotemia. The smear is normochromic–normocytic; burr cells are sometimes prominent.

Hypothyroidism is associated with a number of anemic states. The most common is a mild normochromic–normocytic anemia. Iron deficiency may occur secondary to heavy menstrual bleeding. Also, a macrocytic picture that clears after administration of exogenous thyroid hormone is sometimes encountered. A true megaloblastic anemia caused by vitamin B_{12} deficiency occurs in about 10% of hypothyroid patients with a macrocytic smear; the relation between hypothyroidism and pernicious anemia is unresolved, but an autoimmune mechanism is postulated.

Anemia of Chronic Disease. See above.

DIFFERENTIAL DIAGNOSIS

A practical method for organizing the many causes of anemia is to group them according to (a) the appearance of the Wright-stained smear of the peripheral blood and (b) the electronically determined red cell indices. This method allows causes to be classified into normochromic–normocytic, hypochromic–microcytic, and macrocytic categories (Table 79.1) and facilitates workup.

Iron deficiency accounts for most of the anemias seen in the office setting. In community-based primary care practices, iron deficiency is the underlying cause in 95% of anemic women and 50% of anemic men. In male patients and the elderly, the source is typically occult bleeding from an underlying gastrointestinal lesion, which is identified in about half of cases. The prevalence of iron deficiency anemia among premenopausal women is conservatively estimated to be 15%, rising to well over 30% during pregnancy. Even in menstruating women with iron deficiency, an underlying gastrointestinal lesion is not uncommon. Iron deficiency resulting from malabsorption may be the initial presentation of adult celiac disease. Among immigrants from impoverished countries, hookworm infestation is a leading malabsorptive cause of iron deficiency.

Other common causes of anemia include vitamin B_{12} deficiency (nearly 10% of cases) and chronic disease (at least 5% of cases). Among the elderly, vitamin deficiencies are common,

Table 79.1.   Differential Diagnosis of Anemia
(Representative Etiologies)

Microcytic (MCV <80)
1. Iron deficiency
2. Anemia of chronic disease
3. Thalassemia trait
4. Sideroblastic anemia

Normocytic (MCV 80–100)
1. Hemolysis
   a. Drug-induced
   b. Autoimmune (idiopathic, collagen disease, lymphoma)
   c. Cold agglutinin–induced (viral infection, lymphoma)
   d. Hemoglobinopathy (sickle cell disease, G-6-PD deficiency)
   e. Hereditary spherocytosis
   f. Microangiopathy (heart valve, jogging, vasculitis, DIC)
2. Chronic disease, including HIV infection
3. Renal failure
4. Hypothyroidism
5. Myelofibrosis
6. Early stage or iron deficiency
7. Sideroblastic anemia
8. Mixed anemia (e.g., iron and vitamin B_{12} deficiencies)

Macrocytic (MCV >100)
1. Vitamin B_{12} deficiency
2. Folate deficiency
3. Aplastic anemia
4. Acute hemolysis or hemorrhage with brisk reticulocytosis
5. Chronic liver disease
6. Myelodysplastic syndromes
7. Hypothyroidism, severe

MCV, mean corpuscular volume; G-6-PD, glucose-6-phosphate dehydrogenase; DIC, dissented intra vascular coagulation.

Table 79.2.   Classification of Anemias by Use of Data from Automated Cytometry

MCV <80 MICROCYTOSIS	MCV 80–100 NORMOCYTOSIS	MCV >100 MACROCYTOSIS
Low RDW		
Anemia of chronic disease	Hypoproliferation (e.g., renal failure)	Aplastic anemias
Most thalassemias	Hereditary spherocytosis	Myelodysplastic syndromes
	Anemia of chronic disease	
High RDW		
Iron deficiency	Sickle cell disease	Megaloblastic anemias
Sideroblastic anemia	Early iron deficiency	Acute hemolysis or hemorrhage
Hemoglobin H	Marrow infiltration Chronic hemolysis	Liver disease

MCV, mean corpuscular volume; RDW, red cell distribution width.

with folate deficiency accounting for about 15% of cases and vitamin B_{12} deficiency for about 10%.

WORKUP

Diagnosis and Morphologic Categorization of Anemia

The diagnosis of anemia is based on measurement of the *hematocrit* or *hemoglobin concentration* of venous blood. Any abnormal test result needs to be repeated for confirmation before further evaluation is undertaken. Proper interpretation requires consideration of the patient's *intravascular volume status*. An overly expanded plasma volume will dilute the red cell mass and lead to a false-positive diagnosis. Conversely, dehydration can mask an underlying anemia.

Morphologic categorization helps focus the subsequent evaluation, which proceeds according to whether the anemia is microcytic, macrocytic, or normocytic. Examination of the Wright-stained *peripheral blood smear* and determination of the *red cell indices* (mean corpuscular volume, or MCV, and mean corpuscular hemoglobin concentration, or MCHC) with an autoanalyzer are the time-tested means of classifying anemias morphologically. Recent advances in flow cytometry have made possible an automated means of determining the degree of variability in size of a patient's red cells. This measure of anisocytosis is referred to as the *red cell distribution width* (RDW). Technically, the RDW is the coefficient of variation of cell volume; it serves as a means of detecting red cell heterogeneity, which could previously be done only by examination of the peripheral smear. Although examination of the Wright-stained smear still provides morphologic information unattain-

able from other sources, the combined use of the MCV and RDW for the initial classification of anemias markedly enhances interpretation (Table 79.2).

The peripheral smear and red cell indices should be analyzed together; they provide complementary information. Overdependence on machine-generated indices can lead to errors in diagnosis. For example, anemia resulting from deficiencies of both iron and vitamin B_{12} often produces a dimorphic population of microcytic and macrocytic red cells readily observed on peripheral smear, yet the electronically determined MCV will calculate the average size and erroneously suggest a normocytic type of anemia. Moreover, some vitamin B_{12}–deficient patients with normal ferritin levels have normocytic indices.

The Wright-stained smear can also mislead when used alone, and it often lacks sensitivity. Cells that are easily flattened out (as in liver disease) may appear larger on smear than they actually are; the MCV will give a more correct determination of size. The sensitivity of the smear in the detection of iron deficiency has been found to be as low as 49%.

Determination of red cell size on the peripheral smear is facilitated by using the nucleus of the mature small lymphocyte as a good reference standard for normal red cell diameter. One can also prepare a control smear of known blood to help judge abnormalities. Use of the MCV and appearance on peripheral smear serves to classify the anemia morphologically and facilitate evaluation.

Not all automatically determined cell indices have proved valuable. Careful studies suggest that the MCHC and the mean corpuscular hemoglobin (MCH) add little to the evaluation of anemia, although the MCHC is still used as a means of quantifying the degree of hypochromia.

Workup by Morphologic Category: Microcytic Anemia

Initial Assessment. The basis for the classification of microcytosis is the presence of small red blood cells on smear and an *MCV of less than 82* fL. A prime consideration should be iron deficiency and the important underlying conditions that might precipitate it, but thalassemia and anemia of chronic disease are also important to consider, and sometimes sideroblastic anemias.

History should focus on any abnormal blood loss, change in bowel habits, melena, heavy use of aspirin or NSAIDs, family history of anemia (especially in those of Mediterranean descent), concurrent malignancy, HIV infection, symptoms of other chronic infections or chronic inflammatory disorders, number of pregnancies, pica, dysphagia, history of lead exposure, dietary iron intake, quantity of menstrual blood loss, gastric resection, changes in nails, and soreness of the tongue.

Physical Examination includes checking for glossitis, cheilitis, koilonychia, lymphadenopathy, hepatosplenomegaly, rectal mass, stool positive for occult blood, pelvic mass, and other signs of chronic infectious, inflammatory, and neoplastic disorders.

Laboratory Studies usually allow one to differentiate iron-deficiency anemia, thalassemia, sideroblastic anemia, and anemia of chronic disease, although some overlap does occur and may cause confusion and wasteful expenditures if tests are not thoughtfully selected.

Testing for Iron Deficiency. The test of choice for screening and diagnosis of iron deficiency is determination of the level of serum *ferritin*, the storage protein for iron, which correlates best with marrow iron stores. Levels are somewhat higher in men than in women and increase gradually with advancing age. The test is highly sensitive and specific for the diagnosis of iron deficiency. For example, a serum concentration below 15 μg/L has a predictive value for iron deficiency of more than 90% when the pretest probability is only 50%. A level above 100 μg/L virtually rules out the diagnosis. Ferritin is also an acute-phase reactant that rises in response to inflammatory disease or hepatocellular dysfunction, which potentially limits the sensitivity of this test in such settings. However, when the serum ferritin level is below 50 μg/L in the setting of inflammatory or liver disease, the test retains much of its predictive value for iron deficiency. Levels between 50 and 100 μg/L constitute a diagnostic "gray zone," in which case careful attention to other clinical and laboratory data is required to obtain an accurate diagnosis.

Measurements of the *serum iron* level and *total iron-binding capacity* (TIBC) and of the *transferrin saturation* [calculated as a percentage: (Fe/TIBC) × 100] have been traditional components of the workup for iron deficiency, but under most circumstances, they add little information beyond that obtained from the ferritin determination and they lack its sensitivity or specificity. These tests need not be ordered routinely in patients with microcytic anemia. Nonetheless, a transferrin saturation below 16% has been used as a criterion for iron deficiency. However, the specificity of the figure is limited because some patients with the anemia of chronic disease manifest similar reductions in transferrin saturation. Nonetheless, the more typical pattern for the anemia of chronic disease is a low iron level and low TIBC, in contrast to the low iron level and increased TIBC characteristic of iron deficiency. The *RDW* is almost always increased.

Bone marrow aspiration and examination of a sample stained for *iron stores* comprise the "gold standard" for the diagnosis of iron deficiency, but up to 20% of aspirates are unsatisfactory, yielding insufficient marrow stroma. Ferritin testing has all but eliminated the need for marrow aspiration in the diagnosis of iron deficiency, but the test is sometimes necessary in confusing cases. A *therapeutic trial* of oral iron therapy can also be used in uncomplicated cases as a simple alternative to determination of the ferritin level or examination of the marrow. The reticulocyte count is monitored during a 7- to 10-day period. A significant rise in the reticulocyte count is strong evidence for the diagnosis of iron deficiency.

When the cause of the iron deficiency is not evident, a *workup for gastrointestinal blood loss* is indicated. Idiopathic iron-deficiency anemia is associated with a gastrointestinal tract lesion in about one half to two thirds of cases. The most common upper gastrointestinal lesion is peptic ulcer; colon cancer is the leading colonic lesion in this setting. Site-specific symptoms are predictive of the location of the lesion. Concomitant lesions are present in fewer than 1% of cases, so that it is unnecessary to study both the upper and lower gastrointestinal tract if a likely source is found on the first examination. *Endoscopy* is the test methodology of choice (see Chapter 63). Barium studies are considerably less sensitive, and their yield is nil in the setting of a negative endoscopic evaluation. The vast majority of patients with no detectable lesion on upper and lower gastrointestinal endoscopy have a favorable prognosis; most respond to iron therapy. Those who do not are likely to have an underlying medical illness. Menstruating women require workup just as do other patients; screening for occult gastrointestinal blood loss is particularly important. A positive fecal occult blood test result, hemoglobin below 10 g/dL, and abdominal symptoms are predictive of the endoscopic finding of a gastrointestinal lesion in an anemic menstruating woman.

When iron *malabsorption* is suspected clinically, consideration should be given to testing for adult celiac disease (*antiendomysial IgA antibodies, small-bowel biopsy*); if the patient is from an undeveloped country, checking the *stool* for evidence of hookworm *ova* and *parasites* is in order.

Testing for Thalassemia. Once iron deficiency has been ruled out as the cause of microcytic anemia, the focus shifts to differentiating between anemia of chronic disease, thalassemia, and sideroblastic anemia. History is very important in this regard. A person of Mediterranean extraction without underlying chronic illness is likely to have thalassemia trait, which necessitates a look at the *peripheral smear* for abnormalities of red cell morphology (e.g., *target cells, poikilocytosis*) and a check of the *red cell indices* for *reduced MCHC* and *increased red cell count*. Determination of the *hemoglobin A$_2$* level can confirm the diagnosis, but it may not be elevated if concurrent iron deficiency is present. A *hemoglobin electrophoresis* may be needed when thalassemia trait is suspected in an African-American patient because hemoglobin A$_2$ is not increased in α-disease.

Differentiating Anemia of Chronic Disease from Sideroblastic Anemia. Once iron deficiency and thalassemia trait are deemed to be of low probability, then the task shifts to differentiating anemia of chronic disease from sideroblastic anemia. Here, the *serum iron* level and *TIBC* may be of help. In the anemia of chronic disease, the serum iron level and *transferrin saturation* are likely to be below normal or reduced; in sideroblastic anemia, both are often increased, as is the serum *ferritin*.

Such an increase in the absence of another reason for iron overload suggests a sideroblastic state and the need for a bone marrow aspirate to search for ringed sideroblasts.

Workup by Morphologic Category: Macrocytic Anemia

Initial Assessment. The criteria for inclusion in this group are an MCV above 95 fL, a normal MCHC, and macrocytes on smear. Often, the latter are hard to detect in mild cases. Marked macrocytosis (MCV >115 fL) identified electronically is associated with a high probability of folate or vitamin B_{12} deficiency, liver disease, or alcoholism accompanied by liver disease.

Megaloblastic versus Nonmegaloblastic. The first objective is to distinguish megaloblastic from nonmegaloblastic causes. The *peripheral smear* is the single most helpful test. The presence of *hypersegmented polymorphonuclear leukocytes* (having nuclei with five or more lobes) is among the earliest and most specific signs of a megaloblastic anemia, seen in more than 65% of cases. *Oval macrocytes* are also an early and characteristic finding but may be absent in the setting of concurrent iron deficiency. An increase in hypersegmented polymorphonuclear leukocytes can be screened for by counting the number of neutrophils with five or more lobes in a routine 100-cell differential. Finding three neutrophils with five lobes or even one with six is strong presumptive evidence for megaloblastic anemia.

Bone marrow aspiration may be needed in confusing situations (such as differentiating a sideroblastic anemia from a truly megaloblastic type, or searching for megaloblastic changes in a patient with a low-normal vitamin B_{12} level), but a peripheral smear suffices in most instances. It must be remembered that megaloblastic marrow changes can revert to normal within 12 to 24 hours of therapy, and thus treatment should be delayed if marrow examination is anticipated. However, neutrophil hypersegmentation may persist for up to 2 weeks after initiation of vitamin replacement.

Folate versus Vitamin B_{12} Deficiency. Once a megaloblastic anemia has been identified, the focus shifts to folate versus vitamin B_{12} deficiency. History and physical examination can give important clues. A history of gastric surgery, inflammatory bowel disease, Hashimoto's thyroiditis, vitiligo, or raw fish intake (fish tapeworm) may provide the substrate for vitamin B_{12} deficiency. Neuropsychiatric symptoms and signs in addition to those of subacute combined system disease further suggest vitamin B_{12} deficiency, as do the findings of glossitis and diarrhea. Alcoholism, poor nutrition, pregnancy, blood dyscrasias, sprue, severe psoriasis, and anticonvulsant intake suggest folate lack. Antimetabolite therapy with folate antagonists such as methotrexate can cause a megaloblastic picture with normal serum folate levels.

Serum folate and *vitamin B_{12}* determinations are helpful, but a number of pitfalls are encountered in interpreting the results. The bioassay for vitamin B_{12} is affected by recent antibiotic intake. Assays in which radioactive cobalt or immunologic techniques are used are not affected. However, up to a third of patients with documented pernicious anemia will have vitamin B_{12} levels above 100 ng/L (the often-cited cutoff for diagnosis). Persistence in pursuing the diagnosis is necessary when clinical suspicion is high. Vitamin B_{12} levels may be artificially low in patients with folate deficiency alone; folate and vitamin B_{12} levels must always be measured together. Recent intake of green vegetables can cause a false rise in the serum folate level. Concomitant measurement of serum and red cell folate is needed to establish the diagnosis of a true folate deficiency.

Serum measurements of *methylmalonic acid* and *total homocysteine* enhance sensitivity of diagnostic testing and are helpful in cases in which the serum vitamin B_{12} or folate result is confusing. Both folate and vitamin B_{12} are needed for the conversion of homocysteine to methionine. In both folate and vitamin B_{12} deficiency, homocysteine is increased, but only in B_{12} deficiency is methylmalonate increased.

An empiric means of determining vitamin B_{12} or folate deficiency is to conduct a *therapeutic trial* of replacement therapy. Such a trial is appropriate when serum assays are unavailable or the results are equivocal. The hematocrit and reticulocyte counts are measured twice before administration, then followed every few days for up to 10 days after a small but effective dose of vitamin B_{12} (e.g., 100 μg IM) or folate (1 mg IM) has been given. The trial result is positive if a significant rise in reticulocyte count occurs within 10 days. It is important to use only small folate doses in such trials. Large folate doses can transiently and nonspecifically improve the hematologic picture in a patient with vitamin B_{12} deficiency and lead to its progression by obscuring the diagnosis.

Determining the Cause of Vitamin B_{12} Deficiency. To distinguish vitamin B_{12} deficiency caused by malabsorption from that caused by lack of intrinsic factor, an *oral Schilling test* with and without intrinsic factor is used. An unlabeled IM dose of 1,000 μg of vitamin B_{12} is given to saturate binding sites. Then an oral dose of radioactive vitamin B_{12} without intrinsic factor is given, and both urine and plasma samples are taken to determine the amount of vitamin B_{12} absorbed. The test is repeated with the addition of intrinsic factor. In malabsorptive states, no improvement will occur with intrinsic factor, whereas it will in pernicious anemia. One difficulty with the test is that vitamin B_{12} deficiency can cause malabsorption, which confuses test interpretation. Thus, the test should be postponed until the deficiency is corrected. In addition, sensitivity is not very high; false-negative results occur in up to 40% of cases. The commonly used double isotope method of performing the Schilling test (labeled free cobalamin and labeled cobalamin bound to intrinsic factor are administered at the same time) often produces false-negative results. The Schilling test is not helpful for detecting food-cobalamin malabsorption. Such patients have a normal test result because the test uses free cobalamin and does not assay the ability to split cobalamin from food.

Two other tests can improve the diagnostic accuracy and yield in cases of suspected pernicious anemia. Testing for *anti–intrinsic factor antibody* provides a highly specific approach to diagnosis. The test helps confirm the presence of pernicious anemia; specificity is high so long as no vitamin B_{12} is injected within 48 hours of testing; sensitivity is only modest (60% to 70%). Determination of the *serum gastrin* level may also be helpful because it is elevated in more than 80% of cases. *Antiparietal cell antibodies* are present in more than 90% of cases, but the false-positive rate can be as high as 10% to 30%.

If pernicious anemia is found, *endoscopic examination* of the stomach is indicated because of the increased risk for gastric cancer and carcinoid tumors; thyroid function needs to be assayed by determination of the thyroid-stimulating hormone level.

Nonmegaloblastic Macrocytic Anemias. These can be divided into subgroups according to whether marrow activity is increased, normal, or decreased. To make this determination, a *reticulocyte count* is obtained. (A normal value is 0.8% to 2.5% in male patients and 0.8% to 4.1% in female patients; correction for anemia is made by multiplying the reticulocyte count by the hematocrit and dividing the result by 0.45.) Reticulocytes are increased by hemorrhage or hemolysis; in the absence of overt bleeding, a workup for hemolysis is indicated (see below). Low-normal or decreased counts occur in myxedema and chronic liver disease and are indications for performing thyroid and liver function studies (see Chapters 71 and 104). Marked reductions may occur in myelophthisic states and sideroblastic anemia. The patient should be questioned and examined carefully for symptoms of any of these conditions, and the smear should be studied again for teardrop and fragmented forms and for sideroblasts, respectively. A *bone marrow biopsy* is indicated when a sideroblastic anemia or a myelophthisic process is a concern; aspiration of the marrow may yield only a dry tap and is insufficient.

Workup by Morphologic Category: Normochromic–Normocytic Anemia

This category encompasses a diverse group of conditions that can be classified according to the marrow response, manifested by the *reticulocyte count.*

Elevated Reticulocyte Count: Workup for Hemolysis. If no evidence of recent brisk bleeding is present, then hemolysis and its precipitants require consideration. The history is reviewed thoroughly for medications (e.g., penicillins, cephalosporins, macrolides, tetracyclines, sulfa drugs, quinidine, methyldopa); symptoms of sickle cell disease (e.g., fever and attacks of chest, musculoskeletal, and abdominal pain); a family history of anemia; symptoms of a viral infection (mononucleosis, cytomegalovirus infection, viral hepatitis); lymphoproliferative disease; and systemic lupus. During the physical examination, the patient is checked for splenomegaly and signs of an underlying viral, lymphoproliferative, or connective tissue disease (see Chapters 12, 84, and 146).

The laboratory assessment includes a check of hemolytic indices: *bilirubin, haptoglobin,* and *lactic dehydrogenase.* Haptoglobin is the most sensitive but least specific because it is an acute-phase reactant. Lactic dehydrogenase and unconjugated bilirubin are less sensitive but more specific for significant hemolysis. In a patient taking a potentially offending drug, a *direct Coombs' test* should be undertaken to assess the possibility of drug-related hemolysis. A drug-related or infection-related episode in an African-American patient should also raise the question of glucose-6-phosphatase deficiency, especially when the drug is a sulfonamide or an antimalarial. An African-American patient presenting with painful episodes of hemolysis should have a smear examined and a *hemoglobin electrophoresis* obtained, and a *metabisulfite test* for sickling of red cells should be performed. If an underlying lymphoproliferative disorder or connective tissue disease is detected, then consideration of an immune hemolytic anemia is appropriate and a sampling of the blood for *IgG autoantibodies* is indicated. Concurrent viral infection or lymphoproliferative disease raises the question of an IgM-based hemolytic process and the need to check *cold hemagglutinin* levels. Bone marrow examination in cases of suspected hemolysis is unnecessary.

Reticulocyte Count Not Appropriately Elevated: Workup for Metabolic Disease. A metabolic basis of marrow suppression is suggested by this presentation. Causes that require consideration include renal failure, myxedema, Addison's disease, and alcoholic liver disease. Even early forms of vitamin B_{12} deficiency and iron deficiency may present with relatively normal red cell indices, as can the anemia of chronic disease, so that they also must be checked for (see above).

Reticulocyte Count Nil: Workup for Aplastic Anemia. A very low or absent reticulocyte count is suggestive of an aplastic anemia, especially if accompanied by evidence of pancytopenia on the peripheral smear and cell counts. A history of drug use (e.g., chloramphenicol, phenylbutazone, antimetabolites, gold, zidovudine, pentamidine), toxin exposure (benzene, insecticides), or recent viral illness may provide a clue to the cause. In the majority of instances, the history is unrevealing. Bone marrow biopsy is indicated if the condition persists after all drugs are halted.

SYMPTOMATIC THERAPY

Few patients who present with an anemia of gradual onset require immediate correction of the anemia. The one exception is the patient with significant cardiopulmonary disease, who may be compromised by a decrease in oxygen-carrying capacity (i.e., hematocrit <30%). In almost all other instances, evaluation should proceed in an orderly manner, and therapy should be withheld until a specific diagnosis can be made and a specific therapy can be implemented (see Chapter 82). The exception to this rule is the use of therapy as a diagnostic trial (e.g., vitamin B_{12} replacement). All too common is the practice of simultaneously prescribing multiple hematinics, which obscure important findings and the detection of serious underlying disease. The elderly and others with limited cardiopulmonary reserve should be admitted for inpatient evaluation and consideration of transfusion therapy when they are experiencing dyspnea, angina, or marked fatigue because of their anemia.

PATIENT EDUCATION

Many patients think anemia is caused by a vitamin deficiency or iron deficiency and consequently attempt self-treatment before seeing a physician. Others request vitamin therapy. A common error among both patients and physicians is to attribute symptoms of depression, such as fatigue and listlessness, to an underlying anemia. Unless the hematocrit is well below 30%, or the patient has very little cardiopulmonary reserve, this attribution is unjustified (see Chapter 8). Finally, the patient needs to be told to what extent the anemia accounts for symptoms, what the possible causes are, and what the appropriate workup will be.

RECOMMENDATIONS

All Cases

- Classify the anemia and conduct the workup on the basis of peripheral smear and MCV: microcytic if MCV is below 82 fL and red cells are small, macrocytic if MCV is above 95 fL and red cells are large, and normocytic if MCV is between 82 and 95 fL and red cells are normal in size.

Microcytic Anemia

- Test first for iron deficiency. Obtain a serum ferritin, the test of choice for iron deficiency. One need not order a serum iron or TIBC for a diagnosis of iron deficiency unless there is reason to suspect that the ferritin may be elevated as a consequence of acute inflammation. If iron deficiency is found but its cause is not evident, begin a search of the gastrointestinal tract for a source of occult blood loss (see Chapter 63).
- If iron deficiency is ruled out, assess for thalassemia. Check for Mediterranean extraction and family history of anemia or thalassemia. Examine the peripheral smear and red cell indices for characteristic manifestations (e.g., target cells, teardrops, increased red cell count, reduced MCHC), and consider testing for hemoglobin A_2 level.
- If iron deficiency and thalassemia have been ruled out, obtain a transferrin saturation and ferritin level to help differentiate anemia of chronic disease from sideroblastic anemia. If both are elevated, then consider a bone marrow aspirate to check for ringed sideroblasts.

Macrocytic Anemia

- Examine the peripheral smear for hypersegmented polymorphonuclear leukocytes and oval macrocytes. If they are present, obtain serum vitamin B_{12} and folate levels.
- If the serum vitamin levels are not diagnostic, obtain serum homocysteine and methylmalonate levels enhance diagnostic sensitivity or alternatively, perform a diagnostic trial with a small dose of vitamin B_{12} or folate, monitoring reticulocyte count.
- If vitamin B_{12} deficiency is detected, consider a Schilling test to differentiate lack of intrinsic factor from malabsorption.
- If the macrocytic anemia is nonmegaloblastic, obtain a reticulocyte count and examine the peripheral smear to determine if marrow activity is increased, normal, or decreased.
- If the reticulocyte count is high in the absence of hemorrhage, check for hemolysis; if it is normal or slightly reduced, consider hepatic and thyroid dysfunction; if markedly reduced, review peripheral smear for teardrops and ringed sideroblasts and consider bone marrow biopsy.

Normocytic Anemia

- Check the reticulocyte count and determine if it is elevated, inappropriately normal, or low.
- If the count is elevated, evaluate for evidence of recent hemorrhage; if none, confirm hemolysis with haptoglobin, bilirubin, and lactate dehydrogenase determinations.
- If hemolysis is confirmed, check for a drug-induced cause (direct Coombs' test), an autoimmune type (IgG or cold agglutinins), or a hemoglobinopathy (sickle cell disease, glucose-6-phosphatase deficiency).
- If the reticulocyte count is not elevated, search for underlying hepatocellular, endocrine, and renal failure (see Chapters 71, 104, and 142, respectively) and for early iron-deficiency anemia and anemia of chronic disease (see above).
- If the reticulocyte count is nil, the peripheral blood count and smear show pancytopenia, teardrop forms and fragmented cells, and halting all potentially offending medications does not result in prompt restoration of marrow function, then order a bone marrow biopsy.

A.H.G.

ANNOTATED BIBLIOGRAPHY

Beutler E. Glucose-6-phosphate dehydrogenase deficiency. N Engl J Med 1991;324:169. (*Authoritative review; 85 references.*)

Bini EJ, Micale PL, Weinshel EH. Evaluation of the gastrointestinal tract in premenopausal women with iron deficiency anemia. Am J Med 1998;105:281. (*A positive fecal occult blood test result, a hemoglobin level below 10 g/dL, and the presence of abdominal symptoms were predictive of finding a gastrointestinal lesion endoscopically.*)

Bunn HF. Pathogenesis and treatment of sickle cell disease. N Engl J Med 1997;337:762. (*One in a series of excellent reviews of basic mechanisms and the implications for treatment.*)

Carmel R. Prevalence of undiagnosed pernicious anemia in the elderly. Arch Intern Med 1996;156:1097. (*Prevalence found to be nearly 3% in the diverse sample studied.*)

Carmel R. Pernicious anemia. The expected findings of very low serum cobalamin levels, anemia, and macrocytosis are often lacking. Arch Intern Med 1988;148:1712. (*The title says it all.*)

Cash JM, Sears DA. The anemia of chronic disease: spectrum of associated diseases in a series of unselected hospitalized patients. Am J Med 1989;87:638. (*Although based on an inpatient sample, the spectrum may be wider than previously suspected.*)

Committee on Iron Deficiency. Iron deficiency in the United States. JAMA 1968;203:407. (*Article on natural history and epidemiology that is still useful.*)

Corazza GR, Valentini RA, Andreani ML, et al. Subclinical coeliac disease is a frequent cause of iron-deficiency anemia. Scand J Gastroenterol 1995;30:153. (*Found in 5% of patients in this population presenting with iron deficiency; makes the point that this may be the presenting manifestation.*)

Crosby WH. Reticulocyte count. Arch Intern Med 1981;141:1747. (*Detailed discussion of this important test and its clinical significance.*)

Edwin E. The segmentation of polymorphonuclear neutrophils in hypovitaminosis B_{12}. Acta Med Scand 1967;182:401. (*Classic article; 64% of patients exhibited hypersegmentation on smear. Good discussion of errors in counting lobes.*)

Forman SJ. Myelodysplastic syndrome. Curr Opin Hematol 1996;3:297. (*Useful review of classification and diagnosis.*)

Gulati FL, Hyun BH. The automated CBC. A current perspective. Hematol Oncol Clin North Am 1994;8:593. (*A review of the technical and performance characteristics of these measurements, with implications for their clinical use.*)

Guyatt GH, Oxman AD, Ali M, et al. Laboratory diagnosis of iron-deficiency anemia. J Gen Intern Med 1992;7:145. (*Detailed literature review; ferritin is the test of choice; 73 references.*)

Izaks GJ, Westendorp RGJ, Knook DL. The definition of anemia in older persons. JAMA 1999;281:1714. (*A community-based study finding that a reduced hemoglobin concentration is predictive of underlying illness.*)

Kis AM, Carnes M. Detecting iron deficiency in anemic patients with concomitant medical problems. J Gen Intern Med 1998;13:455. (*Finds a ferritin level below 100 μg/L is best for detection in the context of inflammation, infection, or malignancy.*)

Olivieri NF. The beta-thalassemias. N Engl J Med 1999;341:99. (*Definitive review; 120 references*)

Rockey DC, Cello JP. Evaluation of the gastrointestinal tract in patients with iron-deficiency anemia. N Engl J Med 1993;320:1691. (*High prevalence of gastrointestinal lesions; site-specific symptoms predictive of location; concomitant lesions rare; prospective study.*)

Scadden DT, Zon LI, Groopman JE, et al. Pathophysiology and management of HIV-associated hematologic disorders. Blood 1989;74:1455. (*Excellent review of this increasingly important cause of anemia.*)

Serjeant GR, Ceulaer CD, Lethbridge R, et al. The painful crisis of homozygous sickle cell disease: clinical features. Br J Haematol 1994;87:568. (*One of the best systematic studies of the condition; skin cooling a perceived precipitant; low-grade fever common.*)

Stabler SP, Marcell PD, Podell ER, et al. Elevation of total homocysteine in the serum of patients with cobalamin or folate deficiency detected by chromatography–mass spectrometry. J Clin Invest 1988;81:466. (*Utility of measuring homocysteine levels.*)

Thompson WG, Babitz L, Cassino C, et al. Evaluation of current criteria used to measure vitamin B_{12} levels. Am J Med 1987;82:291. (*Use of an MCV above 95 fL or a vitamin B_{12} level below 100 pg/mL may lead to false-negative results.*)

Toh B-H, van Driel IR, Gleeson PA. Pernicious anemia. N Engl J Med 1997;337:1441. (*An authoritative review of pathophysiology.*)

Tudhope G, Wilson G. Anemia in hypothyroidism. Q J Med 1960;29:513. (*Classic study of 116 cases of hypothyroidism, revealing anemia in more than 30%; pernicious anemia occurred in 7%.*)

Van der Weyden M, Rother M, Firkin B. Metabolic significance of reduced B_{12} in folate deficiency. Blood 1972;40:23. (*Classic report. Low B_{12} levels found in folate deficiency; level is moderately reduced and improves with folate replacement, which can mask B_{12} deficiency.*)

Wilcox CM, Alexander LN, Clark WS. Prospective evaluation of the gastrointestinal tract in patients with iron deficiency and no systemic or gastrointestinal symptoms or signs. Am J Med 1997;103:405. (*Half found to have an underlying lesion; prognosis good if none found.*)

Wood M, Elwood P. Symptoms of iron deficiency anemia: a community survey. Br J Prev Soc Med 1966;20:117. (*In 295 patients studied, little correlation was found between symptoms and serum hemoglobin concentration.*)

Young NS, Maciejewski J. The pathophysiology of acquired aplastic anemia. N Engl J Med 1997;1365. (*Excellent review of mechanisms.*)

Zauber NP, Zauber AG. Hematologic data on healthy very old people. JAMA 1987;257:2181. (*Increasing age alone does not cause anemia.*)

80
Evaluation of Erythrocytosis (Polycythemia)

When an elevated red cell count, hemoglobin concentration, or hematocrit occurs unexpectedly, it raises the question of *polycythemia*, a term used to denote an absolute increase in circulating red cell mass (some use the term *erythrocytosis* for all increases in red cell mass except those with an autonomous etiology). The upper limit of normal for a hematocrit is 52% for men and 47% for women. In the context of marked dehydration or severe chronic lung disease, the elevation may come as no surprise. In the absence of obvious concurrent disease, a search for an important underlying illness (e.g., polycythemia vera, occult malignancy, right-to-left shunt, hemoglobinopathy) is warranted. The finding may even be spurious because of volume contraction. In most instances, the primary physician should be able to distinguish among the variety of causes on clinical grounds, aided by a few simple laboratory studies.

PATHOPHYSIOLOGY AND CLINICAL PRESENTATION

An absolute increase in red cell mass may represent abnormal stem cell proliferation (as in polycythemia vera), a response to chronic hypoxemia (as in chronic lung disease), or a manifestation of renal disease or extrarenal malignancy.

Polycythemia Vera is a *myeloproliferative* disorder affecting all marrow elements; it results from clonal proliferation of a multipotent hematopoietic stem cell. Not only is red cell mass increased, but so are leukocyte and platelet counts. Other consequences include *extramedullary hematopoiesis, splenomegaly, hyperuricemia*, a hypercellular bone marrow, and often myeloid metaplasia and *myelofibrosis*. The condition is uncommon, with an incidence in the United States of four to five cases per million per year, or about 1,000 new cases annually. However, the prevalence is higher because survival is prolonged in the majority of patients. The peak age at onset is 50 to 60 years. Some patients have a relatively benign course, with red cell volume controlled by occasional phlebotomy, but others experience a much more malignant illness characterized by recurrent thrombosis and evolution toward myeloid metaplasia, myelofibrosis, and acute leukemia. Prior exposure to myelosuppressive therapy is a risk factor for malignant transformation.

It is not surprising that the presence of true polycythemia is often unsuspected because symptoms develop gradually and are frequently vague and rather nonspecific. In early stages, the patient may be entirely asymptomatic, with an elevated hematocrit as the only manifestation. As the disease progresses, the white blood cell (WBC) and platelet counts also rise, and symptoms and signs ensue as the red cell volume expands. Most symptoms are attributable to *hyperviscosity, hypervolemia,* and the resultant sluggish blood flow, which develop when the hematocrit rises above 55%. Disturbed hemostasis ensues, exacerbated by defective platelet function. Patients may present with either *thrombosis* (often in uncommon sites, such as hepatic, mesenteric, or retinal veins) or *bleeding* in the form of epistaxis, menorrhagia, easy bruisability, or oozing from the gums. The patient with advancing disease has a deep red appearance; peripheral cyanosis and ecchymoses may be noted. Blood pressure is usually normal, but *neurologic symptoms* are common (e.g., headache, dizziness, vertigo, tinnitus, "fullness" of the head, and blurred vision). Patients may complain of angina pectoris or claudication when coexisting atherosclerotic disease is present. Generalized *weakness*, fatigue, sweating, and lassitude are frequently reported. Gastrointestinal complaints may predominate (e.g., fullness, belching, epigastric or left upper quadrant discomfort); hepatomegaly is present in 40% and *splenomegaly* in 70%. A classic symptom is *pruritus* after bathing, believed to be caused by abnormal histamine release. Also, gouty joint symptoms occur in the context of marked secondary hyperuricemia caused by increased cell turnover.

Typically, the serum hemoglobin concentration is above 18.5 g/dL in men and above 16.5 g/dL in women, or an unexplained increase in hemoglobin concentration of 2 g/dL is present. In about 60% to 70% of cases, the WBC count rises above 12,000/mm^3. More than half of patients experience an increased platelet count. The red cells appear normochromic and normocytic unless iron deficiency develops, in which case the red cells may appear microcytic and hypochromic. The erythrocyte sedimentation rate is frequently very low. *Erythropoietin* levels are never elevated (in contrast to erythropoietin levels in other forms of polycythemia) and are often low. Leukocyte alkaline phosphatase concentrations are increased in 80%, as are vitamin B_{12} levels, a consequence of an increase in vitamin B_{12}–binding proteins.

Reactive Erythrocytosis (Secondary Polycythemia). Chronic hypoxemia triggers *erythropoietin* production, which in turn stimulates marrow production of red cells. The increase is usually an appropriate physiologic response to tissue hypoxia and occurs when the arterial oxygen tension (Pao_2) continually falls below 55 mm Hg or, more precisely, when the arterial oxygen saturation (Sao_2) drops below 92%. Residence at a *high altitude* and *severe pulmonary disease* are common causes of chronic hypoxemia. Other etiologies include *cyanotic heart disease* with right-to-left shunt, heavy cigarette *smoking* (associated with excessive levels of carboxyhemoglobin), and a *hemoglobin variant* that poorly releases oxygen to tissues.

Pathologic Secondary Erythrocytosis. When *erythropoietin* production is increased in the absence of tissue hypoxemia, then pathologic secondary polycythemia may ensue. Renal disease and a host of extrarenal malignancies have been implicated. Such instances of inappropriate erythropoietin production are unusual, but their occurrence can be an early clue of underlying disease. In about 1% to 3% of renal cell carcinomas, erythrocytosis is a manifestation, occurring at a time when cure

is possible. Focal glomerulonephritis, hydronephrosis, renal artery stenosis, and polycystic kidney diseases are occasionally associated with elevations in erythropoietin and erythrocytosis. The mechanism is thought to involve a reduction in blood flow to renal tissue involved in erythropoietin production. Huge uterine myomas, cerebellar hemangiomas, and hepatomas are also causes, although the mechanisms are unclear; up to 10% of patients with hepatoma in one series had erythrocytosis. In rare instances, an increase in circulating androgens is associated with polycythemia.

Relative (Spurious) Erythrocytosis. This term denotes a heterogeneous set of conditions, characterized by an increase in hematocrit without an increase in red cell mass. The most common and usually self-evident cause is *dehydration*. More controversial is a group of patients who appear to have a normal to increased erythrocyte mass and a low to normal plasma volume (also referred to as *Gaisböck's syndrome* or *stress erythrocytosis*). There is some debate as to the actual existence of such a state, but it has been reported in obese, smoking, middle-aged, hypertensive men. Such men manifest an increased risk for thromboembolization.

DIFFERENTIAL DIAGNOSIS

Patients with erythrocytosis can be separated on the basis of their underlying pathophysiology into three diagnostic categories: (a) polycythemia vera; (b) secondary erythrocytosis; and (c) relative (spurious) erythrocytosis. Secondary erythrocytosis can be subdivided into physiologic and pathologic varieties (Table 80.1).

WORKUP

The cause of erythrocytosis can usually be identified clinically, with the aid of a few well-selected laboratory tests. The

Table 80.1. Differential Diagnosis of Polycythemia

Polycythemia Vera

Secondary polycythemia
1. Physiologic (systemic hypoxia)
   a. High altitude
   b. Right-to-left shunt
   c. Heavy smoking
   d. Severe pulmonary disease
   e. Abnormal hemoglobin with high O_2 affinity
2. Pathologic (no systemic hypoxia)
   a. Renal cell carcinoma
   b. Uterine myoma
   c. Cerebellar hemangioma
   d. Hepatoma
   e. Hydronephrosis
   f. Cystic kidney disease
   g. Renal artery stenosis

Relative Polycythemia
1. Marked volume depletion
   a. Protracted vomiting
   b. Persistent diarrhea
   c. Excessive diuretic use
   d. Renal
2. High-to-normal erythrocyte mass, low-to-normal volume: hypertensive, obese, middle-aged, male smoker

first task is to rule out decreased plasma volume and then to determine if the true increase in hematocrit is a physiologic response or a pathologic process.

History. The history should first be checked for risk factors for volume depletion (e.g., diuretic use, vomiting, diarrhea) and for precipitants of chronic hypoxemia (e.g., residence at a high altitude, known cyanotic heart disease, smoking more than two packs per day, chronic lung disease). Inquiry into familial occurrence of polycythemia helps identify an abnormal hemoglobin, and a history of renal disease is also useful for recognition of pathologic secondary erythrocytosis. Important clues for polycythemia vera are easy bruising, bleeding, and thrombosis, especially if the clotting involves an unusual site (e.g., retina, hepatic or portal vein, mesenteric vasculature). Symptoms of hyperviscosity should be reviewed, although most are nonspecific (e.g., lassitude, headache, sweating). It is common to ask about pruritus worsened by bathing, a classic symptom of polycythemia vera. Any report of abdominal discomfort should be noted, as it might be a manifestation of the organomegaly associated with polycythemia vera.

Physical Examination. Postural signs should be checked for evidence of volume depletion (see Chapter 24). The integument is noted for plethora, cyanosis, clubbing, and ecchymoses. A comprehensive cardiopulmonary examination is essential and should include a search for signs of chronic lung disease (see Chapter 40), structural heart disease with a right-to-left shunt (see Chapter 21), hepatic enlargement, splenomegaly, and abdominal and pelvic masses. Splenomegaly can be an important clue for polycythemia vera because it is not found in most other forms of erythrocytosis; however, its absence does not rule out the diagnosis, particularly in the early phases of the disease.

Laboratory Evaluation. Testing should begin with a *complete blood cell count, platelet count,* and *peripheral blood smear examination* because two thirds of patients with polycythemia vera have an elevated WBC count (usually to 12,000 to 25,000/mm³, and occasionally 50,000 to 100,000/mm³), with increased numbers of immature forms and basophils; moreover, half have elevated platelet counts in the range of 450,000 to 1 million per cubic millimeter. Large, bizarre platelets and megakaryocytic fragments may be seen on the blood smear. In polycythemia vera, cell morphology becomes abnormal with progression of disease. For example, in the setting of myeloid metaplasia, anisocytosis and poikilocytosis with tear drop forms, ovalocytes, elliptocytes, and nucleated red blood cells may be seen. A microcytic, hypochromic smear may be noted if concurrent iron deficiency is present (found in about 10% of cases and sometimes obscuring the diagnosis). In secondary and spurious forms of erythrocytosis, the WBC count, platelet count, and blood smear are normal, which helps to differentiate these conditions from polycythemia vera.

Distinguishing Polycythemia Vera from Pathologic Secondary Erythrocytosis. Because no single test is pathognomonic for polycythemia vera, testing for the condition should be limited to patients with a reasonable pretest probability of having the disease. Patients should manifest at least one or two of the characteristic features in addition to an elevated hematocrit, such as generalized pruritus after bathing, splenomegaly, persistent leukocytosis, persistent thrombocytosis, or atypical

thrombosis. Proper patient selection, in conjunction with utilization of newer testing modalities, is markedly improving laboratory confirmation of polycythemia vera.

Traditionally, either direct measurement of *red cell mass* or an estimation based on *red cell volume* was considered necessary for diagnosis; however, this measurement is expensive and often not readily available, and it does not distinguish between polycythemia vera and pathologic secondary erythrocytosis, the most important differentiation that needs to be made. Increasingly, determinations of serum *erythropoietin* levels and assays of *in vitro growth of erythroid colonies* are being used to make this important distinction. A high erythropoietin level virtually rules out polycythemia vera and suggests secondary erythrocytosis, as erythropoietin production should be suppressed in polycythemia vera. A low erythropoietin level strongly supports the diagnosis of polycythemia vera while ruling out pathologic secondary erythrocytosis (which is driven by excess erythropoietin production). If the erythropoietin level is normal (which can occur in mild disease, after phlebotomy, and with secondary disease), then erythroid stem cells are obtained for *in vitro* testing. In polycythemia vera, erythroid stem cells manifest colony growth in the absence of exogenous erythropoietin, a characteristic unique to this form of erythrocytosis.

Measurement of erythropoietin levels and erythroid colony assays are replacing the *traditional consensus diagnostic criteria* for polycythemia vera: (a) an elevated total red cell volume, a normal arterial oxygen saturation, and splenomegaly; or (b) in the absence of splenomegaly, an elevation in at least two of the following: *platelet count* (>400,000/mm³), *WBC count* (>12,000/mm³), *leukocyte alkaline phosphatase level, serum B_{12} level,* or unbound B_{12}-*binding capacity.*

Testing for Secondary Polycythemia (Reactive Erythrocytosis). Although history and physical examination will often suffice, an *arterial blood gas* or *arterial oxygen saturation* determination can be important in the assessment of less obvious cases. A PaO_2 below 55 mm Hg and an SaO_2 below 92% indicate significant hypoxemia. The SaO_2 should be measured directly rather than calculated from the PaO_2 because false-negatives occur in smokers. When a strong family history of polycythemia is present, one should obtain a *hemoglobin electrophoresis* in search of a mutant hemoglobin with an abnormally high oxygen affinity. *Cardiac ultrasonography with Doppler* (and bubble study if available) is indicated when structural heart disease with right-to-left shunt is suspected.

Testing for Causes of Pathologic Secondary Erythrocytosis. One should look for signs and symptoms of renal lesions and tumors, especially renal cell carcinoma. *Renal ultrasonography* or *IV pyelography* with nephrotomograms is a reasonable screening test for such lesions; a positive study result is followed by contrast-enhanced *computed tomography* of the abdomen. *Abdominal ultrasonography* is a useful screening test for hepatoma, and *pelvic ultrasonography* can help confirm a large uterine myoma when one is suspected on physical examination.

Testing for Relative Erythrocytosis. A postural decline in blood pressure and rise in pulse usually suffice for a diagnosis of dehydration, but a ratio of *blood urea nitrogen* to *creatinine* above 20 can provide supporting evidence if desired. Only when the clinical evidence is insufficient to distinguish relative erythrocytosis from other forms should a *determination of red cell mass* be ordered. The calculation of red cell mass is rather elaborate and requires a laboratory experienced in the test. A radioisotope label (chromium 51) is administered to tag the red cells so that the mass can be calculated. The patient's body habitus needs to be taken into account when the result is interpreted. Tall, muscular persons will have a greater red cell mass than short, fat persons because blood volume is greater in muscle than in fat. A normal red cell mass is diagnostic of relative erythrocytosis.

SYMPTOMATIC THERAPY

When possible, treatment should be directed at the underlying cause (e.g., correction of a right-to-left shunt, removal of a erythropoietin-secreting tumor). *Cessation of cigarette smoking* (see Chapter 54) is an important goal; in patients with relative erythrocytosis or reactive polycythemia resulting from heavy smoking and high carboxyhemoglobin levels, the hematocrit will begin to fall within a week and return to normal 3 to 4 months after smoking is terminated. For selected patients with severe chronic obstructive pulmonary disease, *long-term oxygen therapy* may help normalize the arterial oxygen saturation (see Chapter 47).

The risks associated with erythrocytosis (hyperviscosity, thrombosis, impaired hemostasis) begin to rise substantially as the hematocrit moves into the 55% to 60% range. When the condition cannot be treated etiologically in prompt fashion, *phlebotomy* should be performed. Phlebotomy improves oxygen delivery, relieves hyperviscosity symptoms, and prevents the thromboembolic and hemorrhagic complications of polycythemia. The target hematocrit is in the low to middle 40s, the level at which tissue oxygenation is optimal in normovolemic patients. Phlebotomy is especially useful in patients with polycythemia vera and pathologic secondary erythrocytosis. Even in cases in which the rise in red cell mass represents a physiologic accommodation to chronic hypoxemia, phlebotomy may be indicated if the erythrocytosis becomes excessive (hematocrit >60%) and threatens oxygen delivery. Reducing the hematocrit below 55% improves exercise tolerance in patients with severe chronic obstructive pulmonary disease.

Phlebotomy is conducted by removing up to 500 mL of blood as often as every 2 to 3 days to achieve a hematocrit below 55%. For patients who cannot tolerate such large losses of volume (e.g., the elderly), phlebotomy is limited to removal of no more than 250 mL once or twice a week. Iron deficiency may ensue but should not be corrected in cases of polycythemia vera or pathologic secondary erythrocytosis because such treatment may stimulate a fulminant recurrence of red cell production. In patients with cardiopulmonary disease, a modest amount of iron replacement to correct microcytosis is probably beneficial because microcytic erythrocytes increase blood viscosity and decrease oxygen delivery. The severely erythrocytic patient who is to undergo surgery requires phlebotomy to prevent compromised hemostasis. Preoperative phlebotomy should be followed by administration of a volume expander to correct volume depletion.

Treatment of Polycythemia Vera. Control of polycythemia vera with phlebotomy alone is usually possible in cases in which the platelet count and WBC count remain relatively normal. Phlebotomy has been shown to increase median survival from 2 to 12 years by reducing the risk for thrombosis. The frequency of treatments is a function of the hematocrit and symptoms. Most symptoms can be alleviated by reducing the hematocrit to around 50%; however, continued frequent phlebotomy is recommended until a normal hematocrit is achieved (middle 40s in men, low 40s in women). A maintenance schedule can then be set up based on monthly monitoring.

Bothersome *pruritus* can be controlled by the use of histamine blockers. The combination of a histamine$_1$ blocker (e.g., 60 mg of *fexofenadine* every morning; 4 mg of *chlorpheniramine* daily at bedtime) and a histamine$_2$ blocker (e.g., 400 mg of *cimetidine* three times daily) will often suffice. Secondary *hyperuricemia* occurs in this disease and can lead to acute gout; *allopurinol* (300 mg administered once daily) prevents gouty attacks and should be considered when the uric acid level rises above 9 to 10 mg/dL.

Myelosuppressive therapy deserves consideration when phlebotomy proves inadequate, thrombocytosis develops, or extramedullary hematopoiesis ensues. The optimal treatment is yet to be identified; a longitudinal investigation by the Polycythemia Vera Study Group has compared P 32, alkylating agents, and hydroxyurea. Although P 32 and *alkylating agents* (e.g., chlorambucil) are effective, they are also leukemogenic over time; as such, they are reserved for elderly patients. *Hydroxyurea* appears to be preferred, as it is less likely to cause malignant transformation but can suppress the disease. Its disadvantages include the need for frequent administration and the ingestion of a large number of pills, and remissions are far less sustained than with P 32. Patients who fail hydroxyurea therapy can be given a treatment of P 32, especially if they are elderly; it will induce a 6- to 24-month remission and is less leukemogenic than alkylating agents.

Thrombosis and bleeding are the most important complications of polycythemia vera. Prophylactic therapy with *aspirin* and other antiplatelet agents has failed to halt thrombosis. The most effective approach to limiting such risk appears to be phlebotomy with volume expansion. Development of thrombosis is an indication for *oral anticoagulation*, but the risk for bleeding is increased in patients with polycythemia vera who are taking warfarin.

In the later stages of the illness, painful splenic infarction or congestive splenomegaly may necessitate splenectomy. Transition to leukemia is associated with a lack of responsiveness to chemotherapy and a very poor prognosis.

PATIENT EDUCATION AND INDICATIONS FOR REFERRAL

Patient education is essential to encourage smokers to give up cigarettes (see Chapter 54) and patients with chronic obstructive lung disease to follow a maximal program for improving oxygenation (see Chapter 47). The patient's understanding of the basis of the disease and its prognosis should help in achieving compliance (see Chapter 1). When polycythemia vera is a strong diagnostic consideration, the patient should be referred to a hematologist for confirmatory testing and design of a treatment program. Referral is also appropriate when the diagnosis is difficult and measurement of red cell mass or bone marrow biopsy is being considered.

A.H.G.

ANNOTATED BIBLIOGRAPHY

Balcerzak SP, Bromberg PA. Secondary polycythemia. Semin Hematol 1975;12:353. (*Excellent review of the pulmonary physiology related to tissue hypoxia-induced polycythemia and other classes of secondary polycythemia.*)

Berk PD, Goldberg JD, Donovan PD, et al. Therapeutic recommendations in polycythemia vera based on Polycythemia Vera Study Group protocols. Semin Hematol 1986;23:132. (*Still valid and based on the best trials.*)

Berk PD, Goldberg JD, Silverstein MN, et al. Increased incidence of acute leukemia in polycythemia vera associated with chlorambucil therapy. N Engl J Med 1981;304:441. (*Incidence of acute leukemia was 13 times that of patients treated with phlebotomy and 2.3 times that of patients given P 32.*)

Berlin NI. Diagnosis and classification of the polycythemias. Semin Hematol 1975;12:339. (*Traditional consensus criteria.*)

Birgegard G, Wide L. Serum erythropoietin in the diagnosis of polycythemia vera and after phlebotomy treatment. Br J Haematol 1992;81:603. (*Useful, but phlebotomy can induce false-negative results.*).

Brown SM. Spurious (relative) polycythemia: a nonexistent disease. Am J Med 1971;50:200. (*Patients with this condition were men with high-normal red cell masses and low-normal plasma volumes.*)

Chetty KG, Brown SE, Light RW. Improved exercise tolerance of the polycythemic lung patient following phlebotomy. Am J Med 1983;74:415. (*The exercise tolerance of patients with chronic obstructive pulmonary disease improves when the hematocrit is lowered by phlebotomy to under 55%.*)

Editorial. Polycythemia due to hypoxemia: advantage or disadvantage? Lancet 1989;2:20. (*Fresh look at the pathophysiology.*)

Fairbanks VF, Klee GG, Wiseman GA, et al. Measurement of blood volume and red cell mass: re-examination of ^{51}Cr and ^{125}I methods. Blood Cells Mol Dis 1996;22:169. (*Critical look at the utility of testing for red cell mass and plasma volume.*)

Golde DW, Hocking WG, Koeffler HP, et al. Polycythemia: mechanisms and management. Ann Intern Med 1981;95:71. (*Comprehensive review of pathophysiology, evaluation, and therapy.*)

Gruppo Italiano Studio Policitemia. Polycythemia vera: the natural history of 1,213 patients followed for 20 years. Ann Intern Med 1995;123:656. (*Prognosis is poorer in those treated with myelosuppressive therapy.*)

Kaplan ME, Mack K, Goldberg JD, et al. Long-term management of polycythemia vera with hydroxyurea. Semin Hematol 1986; 23:167. (*Found moderately effective and quite safe.*)

Lamy T, Devillers A, Bernard M, et al. Inapparent polycythemia vera: an unrecognized diagnosis. Am J Med 1997;102:14. (*Emphasizes the importance of clinical features for diagnosis.*)

Lederle FA. Relative erythrocytosis: an approach to the patient. J Gen Intern Med 1987;2:128. (*Useful review; 31 references.*)

Milligan DW, MacNamee R, Roberts BE, et al. The influence of iron-deficient indices on whole blood viscosity in polycythemia. Br J Haematol 1982;50:467. (*Iron deficiency increases viscosity; replacement may be necessary in selected patients.*)

Perloff JK, Rosove MH, Child JS. Adults with cyanotic congenital heart disease: hematologic management. Ann Intern Med 1988;109:406. (*Very useful article about an often-overlooked issue.*)

Smith JR, Landaw SA. Smokers' polycythemia. N Engl J Med 1978;298:6. (*Occurs in heavy smokers and resolves when smoking is stopped.*)

Tefferi A. Diagnosing polycythemia vera: a paradigm shift. Mayo Clin Proc 1999;74:159. (*An algorithm in which clinical features plus serum erythropoetin levels and endogenous erythroid colony growth are used in lieu of red cell mass for the diagnosis of polycythemia vera.*)

Weinberg RS. *In vitro* erythropoiesis in polycythemia vera and other myeloproliferative disorders. Semin Hematol 1997;34:64. (*Use of in vitro growth of stem cells as a diagnostic test for polycythemia vera.*)

81

Evaluation of Bleeding Problems and Abnormal Bleeding Studies

The problems of bleeding encountered in the office setting range from abnormal results on screening studies to easy bruising, petechial rashes, and recurrent episodes of unexplained frank blood loss. Sometimes, the only manifestation is a low platelet count, prolonged prothrombin time (PT), or a delay in the bleeding time. When the volume of blood loss is small, rate of bleeding is slow, and risk for serious hemorrhage is low, evaluation may take place in the outpatient setting. The workup involves examination of the intrinsic and extrinsic clotting systems in addition to an evaluation of blood vessels, platelet function, and platelet quantity to identify which part of the hemostatic apparatus is at fault. Often, a careful history and physical examination, supplemented by a few simple laboratory studies, can yield a clinically meaningful answer and guide therapy. An important objective is to determine if the problem is inherited or acquired. At times, an anatomic lesion coexists with a bleeding diathesis; the clinician always needs to address this possibility, especially when the bleeding originates from the lung, gastrointestinal tract, vagina, or urinary tract (see Chapters 42, 63, 111, and 129, respectively).

PATHOPHYSIOLOGY AND CLINICAL PRESENTATION

Hemostasis is achieved by the interplay of the coagulation cascade, platelets, and vessel wall. The platelets provide the initial primary hemostatic plug in response to vascular injury, followed secondarily by generation of fibrin at the site of damage. Blood coagulation is a carefully controlled process, limited by endogenous anticoagulants. Normal hemostasis represents a delicate balance between coagulant and anticoagulant factors. Any upset in this system of checks and balances may result in bleeding or thrombosis.

Disorders of primary hemostasis involve the platelets or vessel wall and present as spontaneous bleeding or bleeding into superficial tissues (skin and mucous membranes, including the lining of the bowel and genitourinary tract). The appearance of petechiae and slow oozing after trauma, rather than brisk bleeding, are typical. Menorrhagia or epistaxis may be a presenting complaint.

Disorders of secondary hemostasis involve the clotting factors or the fibrinolytic system and lead to bleeding that is characteristically deep and visceral, causing such problems as hemarthrosis, retroperitoneal hemorrhage, and deep hematomas.

Qualitative Platelet Disorders

Platelet function defects can be classified according to the step in platelet activity that is affected: adhesion, aggregation, activation, secretion, or acceleration of coagulation. Patients with isolated qualitative platelet defects have a prolonged bleeding time in conjunction with normal-appearing platelets that are adequate in number.

Defective Adhesion. The most important condition of impaired adhesion is *von Willebrand's disease*, which is inherited in an autosomal dominant pattern and associated with decreased secretion or abnormal synthesis of a glycoprotein polymer (von Willebrand's factor) needed for platelet adherence to a site of vascular endothelial injury. The release of von Willebrand's factor in the classic form of the disease can be stimulated by desmopressin (DDAVP). Rarer forms of the disease are not corrected by DDAVP. Cryoprecipitate can also correct the problem. In addition, because of a deficiency of factor VIII procoagulant, the partial thromboplastin time (PTT) is prolonged. Platelet agglutination fails to occur in the presence of the antibiotic ristocetin, a laboratory characteristic of this disease that is useful for its detection. Mucous membrane bleeding is a frequent manifestation. The severity of bleeding is variable and most severe among homozygous persons, who may bleed from the gastrointestinal tract; hemarthrosis is rare. Acquired forms of the disease also exist, which occur in the context of lymphoma, other malignancies, and connective tissue disease.

An acquired adhesion defect occurs when high doses of *semisynthetic penicillins* or *cephalosporins* are taken; these agents can coat the platelet surface and reduce binding to glycoprotein.

Defective Activation and Secretion. Patients with activation problems have impaired production or an impaired response to prostaglandin-dependent activators such as thromboxane A_2, which attracts platelets and constricts vessels. *NSAIDs* affect platelet activation and secretion by inhibiting cyclooxygenase, which helps convert arachidonic acid to thromboxane. In addition, NSAIDs inhibit the release of adenosine diphosphate, which is needed for platelet aggregation. Irreversible inhibition of cyclooxygenase occurs with even small, single doses of aspirin and persists for the life span of the platelet (7 days). Reversible inhibition is seen with the use of other NSAIDs and omega-3 fatty acids (found in oily fish). Severe bleeding does not result, but an underlying bleeding diathesis may be aggravated. In patients with *storage pool disease*, the adenosine diphosphate and serotonin contents of platelet granules are reduced or released prematurely,

as occurs in patients who have undergone *cardiopulmonary bypass*. Bleeding is typically mild, and the bleeding time is only mildly prolonged.

Defective Aggregation. Patients with a rare hereditary defect in platelet aggregation, *Glanzmann's thrombasthenia*, are missing a bridging protein called glycoprotein IIb/IIIa. The platelets of such persons cannot bind to fibrinogen and thus fail to aggregate by way of fibrinogen cross-links. *Clot retraction is abnormal*; the bleeding time is markedly prolonged. Serious bleeding can occur. Patients taking high doses of *semisynthetic penicillins* or *cephalosporins* also demonstrate reduced binding to fibrinogen.

Defective Acceleration of Coagulation. When platelets bind factors V and X on their surface, the rate of prothrombin conversion is greatly accelerated. Patients whose platelets cannot bind these clotting factors have a mildly prolonged PT, normal bleeding time, and normal platelet aggregation.

Mixed or Unknown Defects in Function. A number of conditions are associated with poorly defined but potentially important qualitative defects in platelet function. *Uremia* is the most important and is believed to be related to a dialyzable toxin. In addition to dialysis, correction of anemia and administration of DDAVP, conjugated estrogens, and cryoprecipitate can reduce the prolongation in bleeding time. *Dysproteinemias* and *myeloproliferative diseases* also produce complex defects in platelet function, as can high parenteral doses of β-lactam *antibiotics*.

Quantitative Platelet Defects

A normal platelet count ranges from 150,000 to 300,000/mm^3. *Thrombocytosis* (by definition, counts >400,000) may lead to impairment of platelet function, occasionally causing mucous membrane bleeding or hemorrhage following trauma or surgery. Bleeding from thrombocytosis most often occurs in the setting of myeloproliferative disease. *Thrombocytopenia*, defined as a platelet count below 100,000, is associated with a prolonged bleeding time. The diagnosis requires confirmation with a peripheral smear because spurious forms occur caused by *in vitro* clumping of platelets in response to citrate or small amounts of circulating cold agglutinin.

The risk for serious bleeding from true thrombocytopenia does not occur until the platelet count falls well below 50,000. Easy bruising is seen with counts of 30,000 to 50,000; spontaneous bruising, menorrhagia, and prolonged bleeding with trauma arise as the count drops below 20,000. Below 10,000, spontaneous epistaxis, gastrointestinal and genitourinary bleeding, and an increased risk for central nervous system hemorrhage occur. A petechial rash of the lower legs may be an initial manifestation. The lesions differ from those of vasculitis in that they are painless, flat, nonpruritic, and without an erythematous blush. Hemorrhagic bullae in the buccal mucosa are another characteristic finding. Bleeding may begin from the gastrointestinal or urinary tract. Thrombocytopenia develops when platelet destruction is increased (trauma, immune injury, disseminated intravascular coagulation, thrombotic thrombocytopenic purpura), production is decreased (marrow failure), or abnormal pooling occurs (hypersplenism).

Increased Destruction is the most common cause of thrombocytopenia. The primary mechanism is immunologic, occurring in association with drugs, viruses, lymphoproliferative disorders, and connective tissue diseases as well as idiopathically.

Idiopathic Thrombocytopenic Purpura ranks among the major causes of platelet destruction. Although a platelet-bound immunoglobulin G (IgG) antibody has been detected in 80% of cases and found useful for diagnostic purposes, its pathophysiologic significance remains to be determined. Free antibody in the serum is less common and highly variable. The condition is most common in young adults, children, and women. In adults, the condition is more chronic, being characterized by a waxing and waning course with few spontaneous remissions. It may present as bleeding in the context of aspirin or NSAID use, as an incidental finding on routine blood count, or as menorrhagia, epistaxis, or purpuric rash following a viral infection. The physical examination findings are otherwise normal, and the spleen usually is not palpable, although it may be slightly enlarged. No lymphadenopathy, hepatomegaly, or sternal tenderness is present, which helps to distinguish it from immune thrombocytopenia of other causes (HIV infection, connective tissue disease, lymphoproliferative disease). Mild fever is sometimes noted.

Immune Thrombocytopenias associated with *chronic lymphocytic leukemia* and *systemic lupus erythematosus* follow clinical patterns similar to that of idiopathic thrombocytopenic purpura. In addition, lymphadenopathy and splenomegaly are found in the majority of patients with chronic lymphocytic leukemia, and 25% have hepatomegaly also. In systemic lupus erythematosus, arthritis and arthralgias are reported in 90%, skin rash in 70%, lymphadenopathy in 60%, and renal disease in 50%. Platelet counts below 100,000 are not frequent, being reported in about 15% of cases. *HIV infection* is also associated with an immune thrombocytopenia, affecting 10% of asymptomatic carriers and 30% of patients with AIDS.

Drug-induced Thrombocytopenia that results in increased destruction is idiosyncratic and immune-mediated. *Heparin* (less likely with the low-molecular-weight preparations), histamine$_2$ blockers, *quinidine, sulfonamides,* and *penicillins* are common precipitants, although *any* drug may be responsible. A rapid fall in the platelet count to levels below 10,000 can occur, and acute hemorrhage may ensue. A prompt return of the count to safe levels is typical as soon as the responsible drug is withheld.

Thrombotic Thrombocytopenic Purpura causes platelet consumption, rather than outright destruction, as hyaline–platelet complexes form in small vessels, trapping platelets. No consumption of clotting factors or fibrin deposition is seen, as it is in disseminated intravascular coagulation. The cause is unknown. Ironically, use of the platelet aggregation inhibitor *ticlopidine* has been associated with thrombotic thrombocytopenic purpura. In most instances, an immune mechanism is postulated. Microangiopathic hemolytic anemia ensues, fever develops, and microvascular damage to the kidneys and central nervous systems may become manifest. The lactic dehydrogenase level can rise markedly. The combination of *anemia*, a peripheral smear showing *schistocytes*, and *thrombocytopenia* in conjunction with fever, *neurologic symptoms,* and *renal dysfunction* comprises the clinical syndrome. Patients with the acute fulminant form of the disease are unlikely to present in the outpatient setting, but those with the chronic relapsing form may do so.

Decreased Production. The bone marrow may be suppressed by drugs, depressed after a viral infection, or replaced by tumor. Thrombocytopenias associated with conditions causing *marrow failure* or a *myelophthisic process* usually occur in the context of a generalized pancytopenia (see Chapter 80). On occasion, individual *drugs* cause selective *inhibition of platelet production.* Chlorothiazide, tolbutamide, and ethanol are among the best documented. Megakaryocyte production is reduced in *megaloblastic anemia,* and quick recovery is noted with replacement therapy. Transient thrombocytopenia may follow influenza, hepatitis, rubella, and other viral diseases. The thrombocytopenia of HIV disease involves viral invasion of megakaryocytes in addition to increased peripheral destruction.

Increased Pooling can be seen in disorders associated with an abnormally enlarged spleen. Splenomegaly results in excessive trapping and a fall in the number of circulating platelets.

Defects of the Intrinsic Pathway

These conditions prolong the *PTT* (the PT remains normal) by impairing the synthesis or functioning of intrinsic pathway clotting factors. Detection may be difficult because the PTT will not become prolonged until the reduction in the concentration of a functioning intrinsic clotting factor exceeds 75%. Fortunately, many clotting factor deficiencies do not cause serious bleeding, but the most common ones, the hemophilias, do.

Deficiencies of Factor VIII and IX. *Hemophilias A* and *B* represent deficiencies of factors VIII and IX, respectively. They account for more than 80% of patients with an inherited bleeding diathesis and, because they are X-linked, affect only males. The risk for bleeding depends on the degree of factor deficiency. Patients with concentrations as low as 5% of normal experience little bleeding, except after surgery or major trauma; those with concentrations 1% to 5% of normal may bleed after minor trauma; those with concentrations below 1% of normal undergo spontaneous hemorrhage, typically into muscle and weight-bearing joints. Bleeding can also occur into the central nervous system, genitourinary tract, and retroperitoneum. As noted, detection may be difficult if factor levels are in excess of 25% of normal because the PTT will be normal. Chromosomal mapping is being developed to help detect female carriers. Relatively early prenatal detection is available by DNA analysis of chorionic villi tissue, provided tissue is also available from other affected family members. Fetal blood may be sampled for the determination of antihemophilic factor levels later in pregnancy by ultrasonographically guided aspiration.

Factor XI Deficiency occurs mostly among Ashkenazi Jews, inherited as an autosomal recessive disorder. A severe insult such as major trauma or surgery is needed to precipitate bleeding.

Other Deficiencies of intrinsic pathway factors may cause a prolongation of the PTT but do not lead to clinical bleeding, even in the setting of major surgery or serious trauma.

Inhibitors. The *lupus anticoagulant* is an IgG antibody elicited in the setting of connective tissue disease and phenothiazine use. Bleeding complications are rare, but a hypercoagulable state is sometimes seen in patients with this anticoagulant that leads to an increased risk for venous thrombosis and spontaneous abortion (see Chapter 22). Both the PTT and PT are prolonged because the antibody is directed against phospholipids used in both assays. Hemophiliacs who have had multiple transfusions of antihemophilic factor have close to a 15% risk for the development of antihemophilic factor inhibitors, IgG antibodies against the replaced factors. Such antibodies are also noted in patients with connective tissue or lymphoproliferative disease, those who are pregnant, and persons of advanced age.

Defects of the Extrinsic Pathway

The major clotting factors of the extrinsic pathway (II, VII, X) depend for their synthesis and modification on a healthy liver and an adequate dietary intake of vitamin K. Some vitamin K also derives from bacterial production by gut flora. Hereditary deficiencies of extrinsic pathway factors are rare. Most bleeding traced to the extrinsic pathway is the consequence of impaired vitamin K production or liver disease. Causes include *hepatocellular insufficiency, cholestasis* (which impairs absorption of lipid-soluble vitamin K), *poor dietary intake,* and use of *broad-spectrum antibiotics* that kill normal gut flora. The characteristic laboratory finding is a prolongation of the PT. Prolongation of the PT also occurs with warfarin anticoagulant therapy. *Warfarin* inhibits the vitamin K–dependent postsynthetic modification of factors II, VII, IX, and X; this prevents them from being able to bind calcium and achieve biologic activity (see Chapter 83).

Vascular Defects

Vascular defects are characterized by *purpuric bleeding* into the skin and mucous membranes in the absence of a detectable clotting factor or platelet abnormality. Ecchymoses and petechiae are the predominant manifestations. The most common form occurs as a result of aging, so-called *senile purpura.* Atrophy of connective and fatty tissues makes the vessels fragile and subject to ecchymotic bleeding, especially in areas of constant sun exposure (face, neck, dorsum of hands, forearms). The skin fragility and easy bruising seen with *Cushing's syndrome* are believed to have a similar basis, the catabolic effects of prolonged corticosteroid excess. *Scurvy* causes defective collagen synthesis; affected patients may present with gingival bleeding or hemorrhage into subcutaneous tissue and muscle. Perifollicular bleeding is characteristic. *Purpura simplex* is a mild condition seen in otherwise healthy women; they experience ecchymoses mostly in the lower extremities (sometimes colorfully referred to as "devil's pinches"), especially during menstrual periods. Most cases are believed to be acquired, and some have been linked to the use of NSAIDs.

Hereditary Disorders of connective tissue (e.g., *Marfan syndrome, Ehlers-Danlos syndrome*) produce structural defects in supporting connective tissue and major vessels. Bleeding ranges from easy bruising to serious hemorrhage. In *Rendu-Weber-Osler disease,* the developmental anomaly is *telangiectasis* formation because of a lack of vessel support and contractility. Bleeding from these thin, convoluted networks of venules and capillaries can result from minor trauma or occur spontaneously. The telangiectatic lesions are violaceous, flat, and usually no larger than a few millimeters, and they range in shape from pinpoint to spidery. They occur on the mucous membranes, face, trunk, and palmar and plantar surfaces. Lesions also arise in major viscera, which leads to a risk for serious hemorrhage. The clinical course is often one of repeated hemorrhagic episodes.

Pharmacologic Agents can induce purpuric bleeding in the absence of demonstrable platelet or clotting factor abnormalities. *Drug-induced vascular purpura* is thought to have an autoimmune mechanism, with antibodies directed at the endothelial surface, although the responsible antibodies have yet to be identified. Drugs in this category include *procaine penicillin, thiazides, quinine, iodides, sulfa drugs,* and *coumarins.* The bleeding ceases when the drug is withdrawn.

Immune Complex Formation can result in minor purpuric bleeding, as sometimes occurs with *systemic lupus, rheumatoid arthritis,* and *Sjögren's syndrome.* In *amyloidosis,* deposition of amyloid protein in the skin and subcutaneous tissue leads to vascular fragility, especially about the orbits and upper torso. The "raccoon eyes" appearance of such patients is characteristic.

Mixed Defects

A number of conditions impair the hemostatic apparatus at multiple levels. Chronic renal failure, dysproteinemias, chronic liver disease, and consumption coagulopathies are the most important examples.

Uremia interferes with platelet function and causes deficiencies in the production of clotting factors. Prolonged oozing from arterial and venipuncture sites is common. Dialysis and correction of the anemia help reduce the bleeding tendency, which ranges from purpura and mucous membrane bleeding to gastrointestinal hemorrhage.

Dysproteinemias, including cryoglobulinemia, macroglobulinemia, and myeloma, can lead to damage of the endothelial surface as immune complexes and paraproteins precipitate from the serum. The sludging and hyperviscosity commonly associated with these conditions also result in capillary anoxia. Impaired clotting factor and platelet activity and endothelial damage cause a multifactorial bleeding diathesis.

Chronic Liver Disease precipitates bleeding by a number of routes. Patients with severe hepatocellular failure can no longer make adequate amounts of vitamin K–dependent clotting factors, even with the administration of vitamin K. In addition, fibrinogen production suffers, and the fibrinogen that is made is defective. Patients with portal hypertension may become thrombocytopenic from platelet sequestration in the spleen, although in itself this rarely causes bleeding. However, varices are common in such patients, which increase the risk for gastrointestinal hemorrhage (see Chapter 63).

Disseminated Intravascular Coagulation occurs in the setting of illness that causes exposure of blood to tissue thromboplastin (e.g., snake bite, extensive burn, serious infection, cancer). Activation of the extrinsic pathway in the microcirculation consumes clotting factors and platelets; it leads to bleeding that ranges from minor petechiae to hemorrhage. The condition is rarely encountered in the office setting.

DIFFERENTIAL DIAGNOSIS

The causes of a bleeding diathesis can be organized according to the subdivisions of the hemostatic apparatus: platelet function, platelet number, intrinsic pathway, extrinsic pathway, and vessels (Table 81.1). Differential diagnosis proceeds by identifying which segment of the clotting system is at fault.

WORKUP

When a patient presents with easy bruising or bleeding, the clinician needs to ascertain the likelihood of an underlying defect in hemostasis. Bleeding from multiple sites, easy bruising, spontaneous bleeding, ecchymoses greater than 3 cm in diameter, or prolonged bleeding after a surgical or dental procedure strongly suggest a bleeding diathesis. Before embarking on a detailed evaluation in the office, one should be sure that no serious hemorrhage or major volume depletion is present. Inquiry is required into dyspnea, light-headedness, marked postural fatigue, and observed quantity of blood loss. A quick check of postural signs, skin color, and skin temperature will provide

added objective evidence of intravascular volume status and degree of anemia. Once the presence of or risk for severe hemorrhage has been ruled out, the outpatient evaluation can commence.

The next task is to ascertain which segment(s) of the hemostatic system are at fault. This determination, along with an assessment of whether the condition is acquired or hereditary, can greatly help focus the evaluation (Table 81.2).

History

One needs a detailed history of the bleeding problem, including its onset, precipitants, location, clinical course, prior history, associated family history, and drug history. Inquiry into past surgery, childbirth, menstruation, nosebleed (both nostrils), dental extraction, trauma, laceration, and injection can provide important information. Especially important is the history of a transfusion requirement after minor trauma or surgery when such transfusion would ordinarily not be required.

On the other hand, not all patients with a history of easy bruising have a bleeding diathesis. Easy bruising is common and often occurs in otherwise normal patients. Bruises that occur on the limbs and are less than 3 cm in diameter are likely to be harmless and caused by inapparent trauma in the absence of

Table 81.1. Differential Diagnosis of Bleeding by Mechanism

Qualitative Platelet Disorders	
Defective adhesion	Von Willebrand's disease: high doses of semisynthetic penicillins and cephalosporins
Defective aggregation	Glanzmann's thrombasthenia; high doses of semisynthetic penicillins and cephalosporins
Defective activation	NSAIDs; dipyridamole; cardiopulmonary bypass
Defective acceleration	Factor V deficiency
Quantitative Platelet Disorders	
Thrombocytosis	Myeloproliferative disease
Thrombocytopenia	
Decreased production	Thiazides, alcohol, viral infection, marrow failure, megaloblastic anemia, myelophthisic process
Increased destruction	Quinidine, methyldopa, sulfa, phenytoin, barbiturates, lupus, infection, idiopathic thrombocytopenic purpura, chronic lymphocytic leukemia
Increased sequestration	Hypersplenism
Intrinsic Pathway Defects	
Factor VIII deficiency	Hemophilia A
Factor IX deficiency	Hemophilia B
Factor XI deficiency	Ashkenazi Jews
Extrinsic Pathway Defects	
Vitamin K–dependent factor deficiency	Poor diet, cholestasis, hepatocellular failure, coumarin, broad-spectrum antibiotics
Vascular Defects	
Connective tissue fragility	Age, Cushing's syndrome, scurvy, purpura simplex
Hereditary defect	Marfan syndrome, Rendu-Weber-Osler disease
Drug-induced	Procaine penicillin, sulfa, thiazides, quinine, iodides, coumarin
Paraproteinemia	Myeloma, macroglobulinemia, cryoglobulinemia
Connective tissue disease	Lupus, rheumatoid arthritis, Sjögren's synrome
Multiple Defects	
Uremia	
Chronic hepatocellular failure	
Disseminated intravascular coagulation	
HIV infection	

Table 81.2. Differentiating Platelet, Coagulation, and Vascular Disorders

CLINICAL FEATURES	PLATELET	COAGULATION	VASCULAR
Onset	Immediate	Delayed	Immediate
Duration	Short	Prolonged	Variable
Precipitant	Trauma	Often spontaneous	Variable
Site	Skin, mucous membranes, GI tract	Joints, muscle, viscera	Skin, GI tract
Family history	Absent	Usually present	Usually absent
Drug-related	Often	Rarely	Sometimes
Sex predominance	Often female	Usually male	Usually female
Response to focal pressure	Usually effective	Ineffective	Effective
Platelet count	Normal, low, or excessive	Normal	Normal
Prothrombin time	Normal	Abnormal in cases of factor II, VII, IX, and X deficiency	Normal
Partial thromboplastin time	Normal	Abnormal with factor VIII or IX deficiency	Normal

GI = gastrointestinal.

recalled injury. Likewise, minor bleeding up to 2 days after a molar extraction is within normal limits. However, ecchymoses occurring spontaneously on the trunk or measuring greater than 3 cm in diameter on the limbs are more worrisome.

As noted earlier, bleeding that is transient, superficial (confined to the skin and mucous membranes), and spontaneous or immediately posttraumatic suggests a platelet problem or vascular fragility. In contrast, patients with serious clotting factor problems characteristically report bleeding that is deep (into tissues or viscera), delayed, and prolonged. A past medical history or family history of abnormal bleeding is strong presumptive evidence of a hereditary disorder, but its absence does not rule it out. For example, 30% of hemophiliacs give no family history of bleeding. In a patient with a suspected hereditary cause, gender should be noted because many hereditary bleeding disorders are sex-linked, especially those involving clotting factors.

A thorough review of *medications* is essential. The use of medications capable of interfering with platelet function (aspirin, NSAIDs, semisynthetic penicillins, cephalosporins, dipyridamole), platelet number (thiazides, alcohol, quinidine, methyldopa, sulfa, phenytoin, barbiturates), or coagulation factor synthesis (warfarin) should be noted.

The presence of a recent or *concurrent illness* that might affect hemostasis ought to be given particular attention, including chronic liver disease, uremia, viral infection, connective tissue disease, myeloproliferative states, and paraproteinemias.

Physical Examination

After taking the vital signs and checking for significant volume depletion, one can proceed with a systematic examination. The general appearance is noted for cushingoid habitus and marfanoid appearance. On examination of the skin, the size, number, and location of any *purpuric lesions* should be recorded, and note should be made of whether they are *petechial* (<3 mm) or *ecchymotic* (>3 mm). Purpura represents bleeding into the skin, usually the result of vessel breakage or leakage. Petechial lesions occur with thrombocytopenia, quali-

tative platelet disorders, and vascular defects. Petechial rashes are also a hallmark of vasculitis, but the lesions in vasculitic cases are characteristically palpable, tender, and pruritic, and are surrounded by an erythematous flush. One can readily distinguish petechiae from nonpurpuric erythematous skin lesions by noting their failure to blanch when compressed with a glass slide. *Blanching* lesions must not be dismissed too hastily because they may be *telangiectases*, which are an important clue to Rendu-Weber-Osler syndrome. Ecchymoses occurring in areas subject to trauma are a common finding in normal people; however, ecchymotic lesions greater than 6 cm in the absence of major trauma are likely to represent an underlying bleeding abnormality. The skin is also noted for signs of chronic liver disease (spider angiomas, jaundice).

The mucous membranes are examined for bleeding, the lymph nodes for enlargement, the abdomen for hepatosplenomegaly, and the joints and muscles for hematomas and hemarthroses. Rectal and pelvic examinations are conducted for evidence of bleeding. In a patient with thrombocytopenia, careful examination for splenomegaly is important because it may be the only clue of sequestration. Percussion of the Traube space (the area of resonance over the stomach) for dullness, combined with splenic palpation with the patient in the right lateral decubitus position, is the best means of detecting splenomegaly by physical examination (sensitivity of 46%, specificity of 97%).

Laboratory Studies

Although the history and physical examination often provide important clues regarding etiology, laboratory investigation helps to classify the cause of the bleeding more definitively. Primary hemostasis is assessed by *platelet count* and *bleeding time*. The *PT* best assays the extrinsic clotting system, and the PTT, the intrinsic one.

Platelet Count is usually performed by an automated particle-counting machine on a sample of blood collected into a tube containing the anticoagulant ethylenediaminetetraacetic acid

(EDTA). Falsely low counts occur when platelets clump on exposure to EDTA, a common phenomenon when blood is processed at low temperatures. It can be prevented by warming the blood slightly before processing, using another anticoagulant, or performing a finger-stick platelet count. The presence of a cold agglutinin in the blood will also cause clumping and a falsely low level, as will antibody that produces rosettes of platelets about white cells. A confirmatory look at the peripheral smear is always helpful. Finding platelets on examination of a peripheral smear is good presumptive evidence of adequate quantity.

Bleeding Time is a sensitive but nonspecific test of qualitative platelet function; values are also abnormal in thrombocytopenia, uremia, von Willebrand's disease, and afibrinogenemia. Even anemia may produce a prolonged bleeding time, correctable by transfusion of red cells alone. The test often gives false-positive readings, demonstrated by the high rate of normal findings on follow-up platelet aggregation studies.

The Ivy method is the standard technique for performance of the test. A cut is made in a relatively avascular area of the forearm, with use of a template to ensure an incision of 1 cm in length and 1 mm in depth, while venous return is obstructed with a blood pressure cuff inflated to 40 mm Hg. Blotting paper is applied to the edge of the incision; a normal result is cessation of blotter-detected oozing by 9 minutes. Recent aspirin or current NSAID use will produce a modest prolongation in the bleeding time, although this usually does not represent a significant risk for bleeding unless a preexisting bleeding diathesis is present.

Prothrombin Time and Partial Thromboplastin Time assay the extrinsic and intrinsic clotting factor cascades, respectively, in addition to the common pathway. The PT assesses factor VII and common pathway factors X, V, prothrombin, and fibrinogen. The PTT reflects levels of kininogen, prekallikrein, and factors VIII, IX, XI, and XII, in addition to those of the common pathway. Its sensitivity is limited; clotting factor deficiency in excess of 75% is needed to prolong the PTT. The PT is slightly more sensitive, becoming prolonged when factor VII falls by 55% to 65%. However, bleeding is rare in the absence of such reductions. PTT prolongations not associated with bleeding include those caused by deficiencies of factor XII, kininogen, or prekallikrein, and the presence of an inhibitor.

Screening for an inhibitor is carried out by mixing equal volumes of the patient's plasma and normal donor plasma. If the prolongation in PT or PTT is corrected, then no inhibitor is present and the workup proceeds to determine the missing clotting factor. If it is not corrected, then this is strong suggestive evidence of the presence of an inhibitor, and identifying it is the next step. The PT and PTT do not assess the final factor XIII-dependent cross-linking of fibrin; urea clot solubility testing is required. Testing for fibrinolysis also must be performed separately.

Testing for a Qualitative Platelet Defect. In the setting of bleeding consistent with defective initial hemostasis (see above) and a normal platelet count, normal PT, and normal PTT, one should consider determining the bleeding time, provided that no explanation is readily evident (e.g., recent aspirin or NSAID use, uremia, and so forth). An abnormal study is followed by *in vitro* testing of platelet function. *Aggregation testing* is conducted by adding an aggregating substance such as adenosine diphosphate, epinephrine, collagen, or thrombin to a platelet-rich plasma sample. If the bleeding time and the PTT are prolonged, then *ristocetin-induced agglutination* of platelets can be performed to check for von Willebrand's disease. Aggregation is normal in von Willebrand's disease, but the platelets fail to agglutinate. Aggregation and ristocetin studies are best ordered in consultation with a hematologist.

Testing for the Cause of Thrombocytopenia. First, pseudo-thrombocytopenia must be ruled out. Then the task turns to differentiating increased destruction from decreased production and sequestration. Examination of the *peripheral blood smear* is helpful in this regard. A pancytopenia strongly suggests marrow failure. The presence of large immature platelets on the peripheral smear in a patient with an isolated thrombocytopenia points to increased destruction. Isolated thrombocytopenia is almost always caused by increased destruction. If uncertainty persists, a *bone marrow examination* can provide further clarification of the mechanism. A hypocellular marrow in the setting of pancytopenia indicates marrow failure; an increase in megakaryocytes argues for increased destruction. Sequestration is best determined by examining for an enlarged spleen.

Increased destruction may be immune or nonimmune. Immune destruction is by far the more common, but before ordering elaborate tests for antibodies, one should consider a few preliminary investigations that may obviate the need for more sophisticated studies. For example, simply withdrawing all potentially offending drugs (especially those most likely to be responsible, such as quinidine, gold, trimethoprim/sulfamethoxazole) and monitoring the platelet count may suffice for the diagnosis of a medication-induced condition. Testing for the presence of HIV infection (enzyme-linked immunosorbent assay and Western blot), connective tissue disease (antinuclear antibody), or mononucleosis (heterophile) is indicated when clinical evidence is suggestive. In the absence of such common precipitants and in the setting of an otherwise normal complete blood cell count (mild lymphocytosis included), one should consider idiopathic thrombocytopenic purpura. Whole blood is tested for the presence of *platelet-bound IgG autoantibodies* (serum may contain little of the antibody). Detection is complex, and controversies abound concerning the meaning of findings.

To check for consumption of platelets, a peripheral smear (with an examination for red cell schistocytes) is useful. Their presence suggests a microangiopathic condition, such as occurs with thrombotic thrombocytopenic purpura and disseminated intravascular coagulation. The PTT is normal in the former and abnormal in the latter.

Preoperative Screening for a Bleeding Disorder

The most important component of preoperative screening is the history. The absence of abnormal bleeding during a previous surgical procedure or trauma is strong evidence of normal hemostasis. Current medication use also needs to be carefully reviewed, especially NSAIDs, salicylates, and drugs known to precipitate thrombocytopenia. Although the platelet count, PT,

PTT, and bleeding time are frequently determined, the yield is low in patients with unsuspected deficits. In particular, little if any correlation is found between bleeding time and risk for surgical bleeding. Routinely obtaining a preoperative bleeding time in a patient with no known or suspected bleeding abnormality is of no proven value.

The PTT, PT, and platelet count continue to be ordered routinely, but their value in the absence of a condition known to compromise hemostasis remains unproven. In a study of 829 consecutive and otherwise healthy patients undergoing PT and PTT screening before orthopedic surgery, unexpected abnormalities were found in about 8%. None had an impact on patient management.

SYMPTOMATIC MANAGEMENT AND PATIENT EDUCATION

Patients with a clinically insignificant laboratory abnormality deserve detailed reassurance that their hemostasis is adequate. For example, the patient with a minor prolongation of bleeding time on preoperative testing yet no prior history of abnormal bleeding is unlikely to have anything more serious than recent salicylate exposure. Functional hemostasis will usually be preserved and no special precautions or further action (other than repeating the bleeding time) need be taken. However, the patient with a clinically important bleeding diathesis requires some basic advice, even as evaluation proceeds. The nature of the advice depends on the type of bleeding abnormality at hand.

Vascular Defects. Patients with purpura simplex and senile purpura can be reassured. Occasionally, these patients take large doses of vitamins C and K in the hope of lessening their easy bruising; such self-treatment measures are without proven efficacy and only add unnecessary expense. NSAIDs may exacerbate the cosmetic problem and can be withheld if the easy bruising disturbs the patient, but they ought not to be avoided if the case of an important indication for their use. Patients with recurrent bleeding from more serious vascular disease (e.g., hereditary hemorrhagic telangiectasia) should be advised to avoid any agent that might compromise hemostasis. Episodes of bleeding respond to compression if the rest of the hemostatic system is kept intact. Patients with vascular defects often have an iron deficiency from recurrent bleeding; the resulting anemia responds well to oral iron (see Chapter 82).

Platelet Disorders. Patients with a known qualitative platelet disorder and a history of bleeding should be counseled to avoid salicylates and NSAIDs. Patients with no history of abnormal bleeding before NSAID use can probably continue on the agent, provided the bleeding is clinically unimportant and the indication for drug use is compelling. However, the drug should be stopped in anticipation of a major surgical procedure.

Patients with platelet counts below 50,000 are at risk for posttraumatic bleeding and should be advised to put off surgery, dental extraction, and contact sports until the problem is corrected. The use of stool softeners and a soft toothbrush is recommended. Those with counts below 20,000 are at risk for serious spontaneous bleeding and require hospitalization. While workup is in progress to identify a cause, all but the most essential medications should be halted, with substance exposures (solvents, insecticides, alcohol) limited and NSAIDs and salicylates prohibited.

In most instances, treatment of thrombocytopenia should be etiologic and carried out in consultation with a hematologist. A few exceptions are worth noting: Thrombocytopenia associated with HIV infection is an indication for prompt initiation of *antiretroviral therapy* (see Chapter 13). Idiopathic thrombocytopenic purpura is an indication for immediately starting *high-dose steroid therapy* (e.g., 1 mg of prednisone per kilogram per day), especially if the patient is symptomatic. Prednisone can be tapered after 1 to 2 weeks if the platelet count normalizes; if it does not, then splenectomy may be needed. In both instances, hematologic consultation is still warranted, but it should not delay the implementation of initial therapy.

Clotting Factor Problems. Most patients on warfarin who exhibit bleeding from excessive anticoagulation need to hold their dose for only a few days to allow the PT to drift back into a safe therapeutic range (see Chapter 83). Large doses of vitamin K should not be used to correct the PT unless anticoagulation is no longer desired because it is difficult to resume anticoagulation quickly in a patient who has recently received large doses; smaller doses are less problematic. An urgent need to correct the PT without impairing future anticoagulation efforts can be met by administering fresh-frozen plasma.

Patients with a poor intake or malabsorption of vitamin K can be given oral vitamin K supplements (2.5 to 10 mg/d) or parenteral doses (10 to 25 mg IM); in addition, the underlying cause of the malabsorption should be treated (see Chapter 64). Patients with severe hepatocellular failure will not respond to vitamin K because synthetic function has been compromised (see Chapter 71).

Hemophilia. The patient with hemophilia and the patient's family face lifelong problems. A detailed discussion of the management of such patients is beyond the scope of this chapter, but basic management includes specifying guidelines for permissible physical activity and teaching proper first aid. If the degree of bleeding has been only mild to moderate, then one can encourage participation in noncontact sports and other activities that entail little risk for injury. The goal is to allow as much normal activity as possible. First aid treatment of an acute hemarthrosis should be learned by the family. One immobilizes the joint and applies ice packs to reduce pain and swelling. Splinting and elastic bandages can help ensure that a position of good joint function is maintained.

Pain control is important. Aspirin and related nonsteroidal agents must be avoided. Acetaminophen and codeine work well when given in adequate doses for short periods of time. The primary physician should not try to aspirate a hemarthrosis; the risk for causing further bleeding and introducing infection is high.

Administration of *factor VIII concentrate* has been the mainstay of therapy, used for episodes of acute bleeding and before surgery and dental work. Carefully obtained and elaborately treated concentrate preparations have greatly reduced the risk for transfusion-related HIV infection, and *recombinant preparations* are now available, although more expensive. *DDAVP* is being used in place of factor VIII to treat patients with mild to moderate hemophilia or von Willebrand's disease and is proving effective for both episodes of acute bleeding and prophylaxis. If future studies support these encouraging results, desmopressin should offer hemophiliacs an alternate means of acute treatment.

Genetic counseling is an important component of hemophiliac care. Definitive identification of women who are carriers of the hemophilia gene has been difficult, but DNA analysis techniques offer hope of improved identification to facilitate genetic counseling. Early prenatal diagnosis is also available (see above).

INDICATIONS FOR ADMISSION AND REFERRAL

Bleeding problems carry the potential for serious harm and bear very careful evaluation and monitoring. If the severity of the condition is in doubt, prompt hospital admission should be considered. Patients who manifest volume depletion, gross bleeding, bleeding from multiple sites, or a change in mental status require emergency admission. The person who otherwise appears well but has a dangerously low platelet count (<20,000), an absence of platelets on smear, or a markedly prolonged bleeding time is best evaluated and monitored in the hospital. Hemophiliacs with acute bleeding require emergency transfusion of factor VIII.

Referral or consultation with a hematologist can be helpful when a patient with clinical bleeding is suspected of having a qualitative platelet disorder. Proper test selection and interpretation will be facilitated. Referral is also indicated for patients with unexplained, clinically significant clotting factor deficiencies, severe thrombocytopenia, or suspected hemophilia or von Willebrand's disease.

A.H.G.

ANNOTATED BIBLIOGRAPHY

Antonarakis SE, Waber PG, Kittur SD, et al. Hemophilia A: detection of molecular defects and of carriers by DNA analysis. N Engl J Med 1985;313:842. (*An accurate method of detecting carriers, which had previously been problematic.*)

Ballem PJ, Belzberg A, Devine DV, et al. Kinetic studies of the mechanism of thrombocytopenia in patients with HIV infection. N Engl J Med 1992;327:1779. (*Increased destruction, but also decreased production as a consequence of viral infection of megakaryocytes.*)

Barber A, Green D, Galluzzo T, et al. The bleeding time as a preoperative screening test. Am J Med 1985;78:761. (*Not found to be of value for routine use.*)

Barkun AN, Camus M, Green L, et al. Bedside assessment of splenic enlargement. Am J Med 1991;91:512. (*Percussion of Traube space followed by palpation recommended.*)

Bennett Cl, Weinberg PD, Rozenberg-Ben-Dor K, et al. Thrombotic thrombocytopenic purpura associated with ticlopidine: a review of 60 cases. Ann Intern Med 1998;128:541. (*Thrombotic thrombocytopenic purpura ironically found as a complication of using this inhibitor of platelet aggregation.*)

Bushick JB, Eisenberg JM, Kinman J, et al. Pursuit of abnormal coagulation screening tests generates modest hidden preoperative costs. J Gen Intern Med 1989;4:493. (*Routine PT and PTT added little additional cost, but impact of abnormal results was nil.*)

Cohen AJ, Kessler CM. Treatment of inherited coagulation disorders. Am J Med 1995;99:675. (*Best review for the generalist reader, especially the section on von Willebrand's disease.*)

de la Fuente B, Kasper C, Rickles FR, et al. Response of patients with mild and moderate hemophilia A and von Willebrand's disease to treatment with desmopressin. Ann Intern Med 1985;103:6. (*Vasopressin analogue both effective and safe in treatment and prevention.*)

Furie B, Furie BC. Molecular and cellular biology of blood coagulation. N Engl J Med 1992;326:800. (*Excellent short review of basis mechanisms.*)

George JN, Raskob GE, Shah SR, et al. Drug-induced thrombocytopenia: a systematic review of published case reports. Ann Intern Med 1998;129:886. (*Critical look at the evidence, finding many instances in which a causal relationship is lacking.*)

Gernsheimer T, Stratton J, Ballem PJ, et al. Mechanisms of response to treatment in autoimmune thrombocytopenic purpura. N Engl J Med 1989;320:974. (*Prednisone stimulated platelet production; splenectomy prolonged survival.*)

Kitchens CS. The anatomic basis of purpura. Prog Hemost Thromb 1980;5:21. (*Interesting discussion of purpura from the perspective of blood vessel structure and function.*)

Lind SE. The bleeding time does not predict surgical bleeding. Blood 1991;77:2547. (*Review of available data; finds little predictive value.*)

Lusher JM, Arkin S, Abildgaard CF, et al. Recombinant factor VIII for the treatment of previously untreated patients with hemophilia A. N Engl J Med 1993;328:453. (*Major multicenter report of its safety and efficacy, and the development of inhibitors.*)

Mannucci PM. Hemostatic drugs. N Engl J Med 1998;339:245. (*Terse, general overview.*)

McMillan R. Therapy for adults with refractory chronic immune thrombocytopenic purpura. Ann Intern Med 1997;126:307. (*Includes excellent summary of first-line therapy that can be administered by the primary physician, in addition to indications for referral.*)

Rodgers RPC, Levin J. A critical appraisal of the bleeding time. Semin Thromb Hemost 1990;16:1. (*Detailed review of its utility and shortcomings.*)

Suchman AL, Griner PF. Diagnostic uses of the activated partial thromboplastin time and prothrombin time. Ann Intern Med 1986; 104:810. (*Screening with the PT and PTT adds little in the absence of a history of bleeding. Normal PT and PTT values rule out a clotting factor abnormality in the patient with a bleeding problem.*)

Warkentin TE, Levine MN, Hirsh J, et al. Heparin-induced thrombocytopenia in patients treated with low-molecular-weight heparin or unfractionated heparin. N Engl J Med 1995;332:1330. (*Risks for thrombocytopenia, thrombotic events significantly less with low-molecular-weight heparin.*)

White GC, Shoemaker CB. Factor VIII gene and hemophilia A. Blood 1989;73:1. (*Excellent discussion of detection and genetic and prenatal counseling.*)

82
Management of Common Anemias

Most of the anemias encountered in the outpatient setting are sufficiently mild or chronic to allow time for the careful design of a cost-effective treatment program. The ease with which a number of anemias (e.g., deficiencies of iron, folate, and vitamin B_{12}) can be corrected sometimes leads to empiric therapy or self-treatment without adequate workup for the underlying cause. The skillful application of appropriate treatment is based on a thorough etiologic evaluation (see Chapter 79). Once the cause is understood, attention can be turned to treatment modalities. Increasingly prominent among treatment options is erythropoietin therapy, with an expanding list of indications, so that an understanding by the primary care physician of evidence-based applications is necessary. Those caring for patients with sickle cell anemia who are subject to painful crises need to be familiar with the first line of treatment so as to prevent such disabling episodes.

IRON-DEFICIENCY ANEMIA

Iron-deficiency anemia is extremely common, occurring in about 10% to 15% of premenopausal women; it may also be a manifestation of gastrointestinal blood loss. Proper management necessitates identifying the underlying cause (see Chapter 79). Ascribing the anemia to a trivial cause (e.g., menstruation, hemorrhoids) and treating it empirically without a thorough workup for more serious disease (e.g., bowel malignancy) can seriously compromise outcome. A response to iron replacement should not be taken as a sign of a benign cause. The physician must determine whether inadequate intake, poor absorption, increased loss, or a combination of factors is responsible for the anemia. Knowing the most economical, effective, and best-tolerated forms of supplemental iron facilitates design of an optimal replacement therapy program.

Clinical Presentation and Course

In menstruating women, the balance between dietary iron intake (1 mg/d) and loss (15 mg/mo) is precarious. Low-grade anemia, especially when losses from pregnancy (approximately 500 mg) are not made up, is common. However, the many vague symptoms in otherwise healthy menstruating women that are attributed to "low iron" have not been found to correlate with degree of anemia or respond to correction of anemia in controlled studies (see Chapter 79).

Iron-deficiency anemia is usually slow in onset, so that compensatory changes such as increases in 2,3-diphosphoglycerate and cardiac output minimize symptoms. When blood loss has been rapid or the anemia severe (hemoglobin level below 7 g/dL), patients are likely to become symptomatic, especially if cardiopulmonary reserve is limited. Replacement therapy is required in such cases, regardless of underlying cause. The degree of anemia does not correlate with the seriousness of the cause.

Pica (defined as a craving for ice, starch, clay, or any other substance) is particularly common in patients with severe iron deficiency, but often goes unreported. Up to 50% of iron-deficient patients may exhibit pica, with pagophagia (the craving for ice) accounting for the vast majority of cases. No correlation has been found between the presence of pica and the cause of iron deficiency. Symptoms resolve with treatment.

The occasional patient with severe iron deficiency who presents with glossitis, angular stomatitis, koilonychia, or esophageal web improves after correction of the deficiency. Whether the *menorrhagia* sometimes seen with iron deficiency is corrected by iron is a subject of debate. Patients who have undergone *subtotal gastrectomy* and gastrojejunostomy have up to a 60% chance of incurring iron deficit because of a loss of acid-secreting capacity, rapid gastric emptying, and bypass of the duodenum. *Pregnancy* is almost certain to produce iron deficiency because a net loss of more than 500 mg of iron occurs. Iron deficiency from chronic gastrointestinal blood loss has been documented in *long-distance runners*.

Unless the cause of the iron deficiency is removed, recurrence rates are high, even when treatment is prescribed. In a series of 100 cases, 29 relapses were noted: In 24 instances, inadequate iron was being taken; in 12, blood loss continued in excess of iron therapy; and in four patients, malabsorption was documented.

Principles of Management

As noted above, the importance of identifying and treating the underlying cause cannot be overemphasized, especially when the anemia is found in male patients or the elderly. Even in menstruating women, the probability of finding silent but important gastrointestinal disease is substantial. Correcting iron deficiency without attending to the underlying cause can mask an important clue to treatable disease and compromise timely treatment.

Indications. Symptoms are often minimal and the morbidity from a mild anemia is low, so that treatment in such situations is less important than discovery of the underlying cause. Moreover, as noted previously, correction of the iron deficit is not certain to alleviate the host of vague symptoms often attributed to it. Nevertheless, replacement therapy makes sense when (a) the patient is symptomatic and has a limited cardiopulmonary reserve; (b) the anemia has become moderately severe (hemoglobin level of 8 to 9 g/dL); (c) the patient is pregnant; (d) the patient has undergone a subtotal gastrectomy and gastrojejunostomy; (e) continued heavy blood loss is anticipated; or (f) the patient is recovering from megaloblastic anemia.

Absorption occurs best under conditions of low pH in the proximal small bowel, such as 1 to 2 hours before a meal or at bedtime. Antacid use reduces absorption, as does food intake; the phytates and phosphates in food bind iron. When iron tablets are taken with meals, absorption drops by more than 50%. Absorption also varies according to the severity of the deficit. About 20% of an oral dose is taken up initially, but absorption falls to 5% after 1 month of replacement therapy, even though the anemia remains incompletely corrected. Ascorbic acid improves absorption in achlorhydric patients.

Side Effects. Upper and lower gastrointestinal symptoms are the principal side effects of oral iron therapy; they can be severe enough to interfere with treatment. The upper gastrointestinal effects are especially troublesome and include *nausea, vomiting, epigastric cramping,* and *acid reflux.* Onset is usually within an hour of iron intake. Upper gastrointestinal symptoms are proportional to the amount of ionized iron delivered to the stomach and proximal small bowel, and they decrease with a reduction in dose. Many patients mistakenly attribute their symptoms to the type of iron preparation used and switch to another; however, most often it is the amount of iron released in the upper digestive tract that accounts for symptoms. Dose reduction is all that is required. The lower gastrointestinal side effects of *constipation* and *diarrhea* are reported by about 25% of users, but these are less a function of the amount of iron available for absorption than are upper gastrointestinal side effects. Constipation usually responds to dietary fiber or a stool softener.

The IM administration of iron has been associated with the development of *sarcomas* at injection sites and should be avoided. Fatal *anaphylactic reactions* and *asthma* have been associated with all parenteral forms of iron administration. If parenteral iron must be given, it should be administered by the IV route, first a very small test dose and then a slow drip; a syringe with epinephrine should be drawn up at the same time and kept on hand.

Preparations. Ferrous iron is required for oral use; ferric iron is poorly absorbed. The most cost-effective approach to oral iron replacement is use of generic *ferrous sulfate.* It is the least expensive (as little as 10% of the cost of other preparations) and provides the most elemental iron. All commonly used ferrous salts (i.e., sulfate, *gluconate, citrate*) have equivalent rates of absorption, differing principally in the amount of elemental iron released. Choice is a matter of cost and side effects. The severity of gastrointestinal upset is predominantly a function of the amount of iron released rather than the type of ferrous salt used. This is the reason for the increased frequency of gastrointestinal upset associated with the use of ferrous sulfate, which releases the most elemental iron. Some preparations contain ascorbic acid to facilitate absorption, but ferrous sulfate provides sufficient iron to make absorption-enhancing measures unnecessary in most instances. *Slow-release* and *enteric-coated* preparations have been touted as producing fewer side effects and requiring only once-daily administration. However, they dissolve slowly and can bypass the proximal small bowel (where most absorption takes place) before dissolving to a significant degree. There is *no* evidence they are worth the extra cost, which can be several times that of unadulterated ferrous sulfate. An ingenious but expensive ferrous sulfate formulation utilizes a *gastric delivery system* that is activated by stomach secretions; as a result, the capsule floats and remains within the stomach for a few hours after food has passed. The capsule slowly releases iron during this period, so that iron absorption

is enhanced by two to three times, gastrointestinal upset is minimized, and the necessary frequency of dosing is reduced.

Parenteral iron has a very limited role. It should be used only in patients who have had an adequate trial of oral iron and have shown a genuine intolerance to all available preparations. Patients with inflammatory bowel disease may require parenteral iron because of the irritant effect of oral iron and the need to take large doses to keep up with blood loss. Parenteral iron has also been suggested for patients with malabsorption, but most are able to absorb a sufficient amount of oral iron. Parenteral iron is best given by the *IV* route (see above).

Dosing. The *recommended oral dose* for iron deficiency is 300 mg of ferrous sulfate three times daily. As noted, absorption is maximized by dosing 1 to 2 hours before a meal or at bedtime. Although taking iron with a meal reduces absorption, it also lessens disagreeable gastrointestinal symptoms, such as nausea and epigastric discomfort. For alleviation of gastrointestinal side effects, reducing frequency of dosing is less effective than reducing the dose taken.

Drug–Drug Interactions. The *effect of iron on absorption* of other drugs needs to be kept in mind. When iron is ingested simultaneously, the absorption of *levodopa, methyldopa, tetracycline,* and *fluoroquinolone antibiotics* is reduced by up to 90%. A similar but more variable effect on thyroxine has been noted. Iron intake should be delayed for several hours after intake of these other medications, and monitoring of their efficacy should be stepped up during iron therapy.

Drugs that neutralize or inhibit acid secretion (e.g., *antacids, histamine$_2$ blockers, proton pump inhibitors*) may reduce iron absorption because a low pH is required in the proximal small bowel for optimal uptake. Taking iron with orange juice (rich in ascorbic acid) or using an ascorbic acid–containing preparation can help in situations in which suppression of gastric acid is needed.

Duration of Therapy. The response to iron is apparent within 10 days of initiatiation of therapy; a reticulocytosis is first noted, followed by a rise in the hemoglobin concentration of 0.1 to 0.2 g/dL daily. Therapy for several weeks is required to bring the hemoglobin level back up to normal, and replenishing iron stores may take months. However, speed is not an issue unless blood loss is rapid, in which case blood transfusion rather than iron therapy is the treatment of choice. The response to parenteral iron therapy is no more rapid than that seen with oral preparations.

Patient Education and Prevention of Iron Deficiency

To maximize compliance, patients need to be instructed about the best means of minimizing gastrointestinal side effects. Starting with a small dose of ferrous sulfate (e.g., 300 mg/d) and building to 900 mg/d avoids initial intolerance. Taking iron just after eating may also help. It needs to be made clear that therapy has to be continued on a regular basis for weeks and often months.

The prevention of iron deficiency is most important in those with increased needs (i.e., pregnant women and young children). The average American diet contains 12 mg of iron per 2,000 calories. Twenty percent is absorbed by markedly iron-deficient patients and 5% to 10% by others; thus, about 0.6 to 1.2 mg is taken up under normal circumstances each day. The daily requirement for men and postmenopausal women is 0.5 to 1.0 mg, so that dietary intake should suffice. However, the requirement for menstruating women is 1.5 mg/d, and that for pregnant women is 2.5 mg/d. Iron-rich foods can be added to the diet to avoid the need for iron supplements. Liver, oysters, and heavily iron-enriched cereals (containing >45% of the recommended daily iron allowance) are the best dietary sources, providing more than 5 mg of iron per serving. Lean beef, veal, moderately iron-fortified cereals (containing >25% of the daily allowance), and beans are good sources, providing 3 to 5 mg of iron per serving. Fish, chicken, egg yolks, raisins, and fortified breads and pasta are fair sources, providing 1 to 3 mg per serving. Green vegetables are rich in iron, but the iron is less readily available for absorption because it is bound to the phosphates and phytates present in these foods.

When diet alone seems inadequate and needs are very high, as in pregnancy, a once-daily dose of 150 to 300 mg of ferrous sulfate is recommended to avoid significant iron deficiency. It must be emphasized that most people who eat a balanced diet do not require iron supplements. Taking widely promoted supplements that contain iron, vitamins, and minerals is expensive and unnecessary in most instances. Excessive iron is associated with increased risks for malignancy and atherosclerotic disease. Those taking expensive vitamin preparations should be advised that much simpler, less costly, yet equally efficacious preparations are available.

VITAMIN B$_{12}$ DEFICIENCY

Vitamin B$_{12}$ deficiency can result from inadequate intake, impaired absorption, increased requirements, or faulty utilization. Poor intake is distinctly rare, occurring mostly in ultrastrict vegetarians who refrain from eating eggs and dairy products as well as meat. Many cases of vitamin B$_{12}$ deficiency are secondary to pernicious anemia; the lack of intrinsic factor compromises absorption. Absorption can also be impaired by achlorhydria, disease of the terminal ileum, bacterial overgrowth resulting from stasis, and gastrectomy. Faulty utilization is uncommon; it occurs with genetic defects in the synthesis of transcobalamin, the plasma protein that transports vitamin B$_{12}$.

Clinical Presentation and Course

Irrespective of cause, vitamin B$_{12}$ deficiency may lead to slowly evolving *megaloblastic anemia*, *glossitis*, and *neuropathy*. Macrocytosis is usually the first hematologic manifestation and can precede anemia by as much as 1 to 2 years. Hypersegmentation of neutrophils is another early hematologic finding. Because of the body's large vitamin B$_{12}$ storage capacity, the onset of clinical manifestations may take months to years. Although megaloblastic anemia and glossitis also occur with folic acid deficiency, the neuropathy is distinctive. Traditionally, neurologic symptoms were thought to be a late development, associated with a vitamin B$_{12}$ level below 100 pg/mL. However, careful studies have documented vitamin B$_{12}$–responsive neuropsychiatric deficits in the absence of such marked vitamin B$_{12}$ deficiency, anemia, or machine-determined macrocytosis (although hypersegmentation and macrocytosis were often noted on examination of the peripheral smear).

Classically, the neurologic syndromes include those of peripheral neuropathy and subacute combined degeneration (symmetric paresthesias in the hands and feet, and progression to ataxia resulting from loss of vibratory and position sense as the posterior columns of the spinal cord become involved). However, cortical involvement is also prevalent and may present as memory loss (simulating dementia), disorientation, depression, hallucinations, agitation, personality change, perversions of taste and smell, irritability, or central visual scotomas. If left untreated, many neurologic deficits can become permanent.

In pernicious anemia, coincident thyroid disease, rheumatoid arthritis, vitiligo, or gastric cancer may be present. *Achlorhydria* after histamine stimulation is characteristic. The diagnosis is usually made by the Schilling test, with the use of exogenous intrinsic factor to help document its absence (see Chapter 79).

Principles of Management

Prompt recognition and treatment are essential to minimize the risk for permanent neurologic damage. Early disease produces reversible demyelination; if uncorrected, it progresses to nerve death and permanent neurologic dysfunction. Thus, in a patient with neurologic symptoms suggestive of vitamin B$_{12}$ deficiency, prompt diagnosis (see Chapters 79, 167, and 169) and treatment are paramount. Parenteral therapy is preferred (except in the rare patient with poor intake) because most vitamin B$_{12}$ deficiency is secondary to impaired absorption. However, the use of large oral doses (>100 μg/d) may result in sufficient absorption of vitamin B$_{12}$ in some cases. *Cyanocobalamin* is the most commonly used parenteral formulation, although *hydroxycobalamin* is better bound to serum proteins and less rapidly excreted, so that less frequent administration is possible. In practice, either form of vitamin B$_{12}$ suffices.

Replacement Regimens. A host of initial replacement regimens are available, all of which are adequate. For example, in a program commonly used for pernicious anemia, a patient is initially treated with 100 to 1000 μg of IM cyanocobalamin or hydroxycobalamin daily for 1 to 2 weeks, after which the same dose is given twice weekly for another month, and then once a month for the remainder of the patient's life. If neurologic symptoms are present, a twice-monthly follow-up dose is recommended for 6 months.

Some argue that 1,000-μg doses are unnecessary because only 100 μg can be effectively metabolized at one time, with the remainder promptly excreted in the urine. However, because of their low cost and safety, maintenance doses of 1,000 μg are often given. Others note that monthly injections after initial replacement are unnecessary, finding that an injection once every 3 to 4 months suffices for many patients. The optimal program can be individualized, although it is probably best to continue with a monthly regimen in patients with neurologic sequelae. More important than the interval of therapy is its indefinite continuation, which must be ensured. Relapse of symptoms is common in the absence of continued therapy. Compliance with a monthly injection program is often poor; having the visiting nurse or family member give the injection is helpful and far less inconvenient than a monthly office visit.

Vitamin B$_{12}$ deficiency can be prevented in the elderly, in whom gastric atrophy, hypochlorhydria, and food-cobalamin malabsorption (see Chapter 79) are frequent findings, with a daily oral intake of 25 to 1,000 μg of cyanocobalamin. About 1% is absorbed.

Response to Treatment can be dramatic, with marked reticulocytosis noted within 72 hours and a rapid improvement in neurologic deficits, especially those that are mild or of short duration. However, neurologic problems that have been present longer may take 6 to 12 months to improve, and deficits that persist after 12 to 18 months of therapy are probably permanent, which underscores the importance of a timely diagnosis for successful therapy.

During recovery, serious *hypokalemia* can develop in patients who have had a severe depletion of vitamin B_{12} as potassium is taken up by new red cells. The serum potassium level should be monitored, and supplements should be provided if it falls below normal. Concurrent folic acid supplementation is not needed. In fact, the inappropriate use of a large pharmacologic dose of oral folate (e.g., 5 mg) alone may partially and nonspecifically correct the anemia and mask an underlying vitamin B_{12} deficiency, which puts the patient at risk for an acute, marked deterioration of neurologic function if vitamin B_{12} is not given. There is no harm in having the patient take folate in addition to vitamin B_{12}, but this is rarely necessary unless the diet is extremely poor.

Other Treatment Modalities. Patients with a vitamin B_{12} deficiency caused by bacterial overgrowth or disease of the terminal ileum require treatment directed at the underlying bowel problem. Oral *antibiotic therapy* with tetracycline or amoxicillin provides temporary relief from bacterial overgrowth. More definitive treatment of inflammatory bowel disease may be indicated (see Chapter 73).

Unnecessary Vitamin B_{12} Therapy. Many well-intentioned physicians have used parenteral vitamin B_{12} as a nonspecific therapy for patients bothered by fatigue or other vague symptoms. In one study of a rural health clinic, 10% of all patients attending the clinic were found to be receiving such treatment regularly, 6% in the absence of appropriate indications for its use. Many persons without a vitamin B_{12} deficiency report symptomatic benefit from monthly injections, probably as a consequence of a strong placebo effect. Even after being told that it is unnecessary, a large proportion remain reluctant to halt such therapy or stop temporarily, only to seek out a physician willing to restart it. Although giving vitamin B_{12} entails little direct risk, its use can be misleading and should be abandoned in favor of a more comprehensive and etiologic approach to the patient's underlying problems, be they those of anxiety, depression, somatization, or an underlying medical problem (see Chapters 8, 226, 227, and 230). Patients taking vitamin B_{12} injections unnecessarily should be counseled on the need to explore the underlying cause of their symptoms.

FOLIC ACID DEFICIENCY

Causes. Most folic acid deficiency results from inadequate intake, although occasionally increased need or impairment of absorption or utilization is encountered. *Dietary deficiency* is in part a consequence of the limited capacity to store folate; within 3 months of initiation of an inadequate diet, mega-

loblastic changes and anemia can develop. Foods rich in folate include green vegetables (asparagus, lettuce, spinach, broccoli), liver, yeast, and mushrooms. Excessive boiling of vegetables in water can remove a substantial amount of available folic acid. *Alcoholism* is responsible for many cases of inadequate intake.

Impaired absorption is seen in the context of ileal disease (e.g., tropical and nontropical sprue, heavy infestation with *Giardia*), short-bowel syndrome, and phenytoin use. *Increased demand* takes place in the setting of pregnancy, severe hyperthyroidism, hemolytic anemia, malignancy, and florid psoriasis. *Utilization* is *hindered* by the use of methotrexate; triamterene and trimethoprim have similar although less marked effects on dihydrofolate reductase. Patients undergoing hemodialysis experience substantial folic acid *loss*, so that replacement therapy is necessary.

Clinical Presentation. Folate deficiency is one of the megaloblastic anemias. It is sometimes accompanied by glossitis. Anemia occurs within 3 to 4 months of the onset of deficiency. Diagnostic features include a low serum folate level (<15 ng/mL) and a marked reticulocytosis in response to physiologic doses (200 μg per) of folic acid. The response to treatment with folic acid is prompt. No neurologic deficits are associated with folic acid deficiency, but elevations in serum homocysteine occur, which are associated with premature arterial occlusive disease and a heightened risk for venous thrombosis (see Chapters 31 and 35).

Treatment for most patients involves orally administered pharmacologic doses of folic acid (1 to 2 mg/d). Most forms of folic acid deficiency, even malabsorptive types, can be overcome by oral therapy. Four to five weeks of treatment usually reverse the anemia and replenish body stores. When the underlying cause persists (e.g., malabsorption, malignancy, psoriasis, hemodialysis), long-term therapy is indicated. Patients taking methotrexate can be given folinic acid, which bypasses inhibition of dihydrofolate reductase. As noted above, the nonspecific use of folic acid to treat a megaloblastic anemia is ill-advised because it may mask an underlying vitamin B_{12} deficiency and precipitate neurologic symptoms. If alcoholism is the basis of the folate deficiency, then the drinking problem requires careful attention in its own right (see Chapter 228). Patients with folate deficiency will benefit from dietary counseling and perhaps a referral to the nutritionist.

ERYTHROPOIETIN DEFICIENCY STATES AND PREOPERATIVE ANEMIA

Erythropoietin Deficiency States. Anemias secondary to erythropoietin deficiency states (e.g., end-stage renal disease) have been among the most refractory to treatment. Erythropoietin replacement therapy, made possible by the advent of recombinant human erythropoietin, represents a major advance in the management of such anemias. Randomized, controlled trials have established the cost-effective application of such treatment in a number of settings. In dialysis patients with regular transfusion requirements, an almost universal elimination of such requirements, a normalization of the hematocrit, and an improved quality of life with thrice-weekly IV injections of recombinant erythropoietin (150 U/kg) have been demonstrated. Side effects are few but include increases in blood pressure and iron deficiency. Concurrent iron supplementation is often necessary. Erythropoietin has also proved cost-effective in other situations associated with severe anemia and reduced serum erythropoietin levels (e.g., HIV infection, malignancy, cancer chemotherapy). Erythropoietin has made more aggressive therapy possible and has markedly reduced transfusion requirements.

Preoperative Anemia. A reduced requirement for allogeneic transfusions has become a major objective for patients undergoing elective surgery. The donation of autologous blood has become a standard practice in many settings. The presence of anemia before surgery is a major predictor of the need for intraoperative or postoperative transfusion. The increasing desire to reduce exposure to allogeneic blood has stimulated a demand for autologous transfusion and an interest in the contribution of erythropoietin therapy. Weekly preoperative erythropoietin therapy can limit transfusion requirements (and so the need for allogeneic blood) and facilitate the donation of autologous blood. A preoperative program of two to four weekly SQ doses of erythropoietin (averaging 300 to 600 U/kg) plus autologous blood donation appears to limit the risk for exposure to allogeneic blood significantly. The best candidates for such preoperative measures appear to be patients with a preoperative hematocrit in the range of 33% to 39% who are to undergo surgery entailing an expected blood loss of 1 to 3 L. Once-weekly erythropoietin administration is the most cost-effective mode of administration in this setting. Work is ongoing (including better methods for procurement of autologous blood) to bring the costs of this approach down to the range of that for allogeneic transfusion.

SICKLE CELL DISEASE

The need to treat sickle cell disease is especially pressing in patients with painful crises. Vascular occlusion may result from hemolytic episodes induced by sickling; this leads in turn to the chest pain syndrome and stroke, which can be life-threatening, and to asplenia. Transfusion requirements can be high. Theoretically, the ideal approach to therapy would be to block sickling (hemoglobin S polymerization), reduce the intracellular hemoglobin concentration, and induce the formation of hemoglobin F.

Direct Inhibition of Sickling and Reduction of Intracellular Hemoglobin Concentration. To date, no sufficiently safe and effective drugs are available that directly inhibit sickling. Reducing the intracellular hemoglobin concentration is a less direct means of inhibiting sickling; the rate of sickling is proportional to the concentration of hemoglobin S. To achieve a lower intracellular concentration, efforts have focused on increasing intracellular water. This is accomplished through the inhibition of potassium loss with low-dose *clotrimazole* therapy, which blocks one set of potassium channels. The results of initial studies are promising, but confirmation and safety of long-term use remain to be demonstrated. *Magnesium* supplements have been shown to block other modes of potassium egress from red cells and are being studied in sickle cell disease.

Increasing Hemoglobin F. Hemoglobin F inhibits the polymerization and sickling of hemoglobin S. Efforts to encourage the synthesis of hemoglobin F have led to use of the myelosuppressive drug *hydroxyurea* in the treatment of sickle cell disease. Although the mechanism by which hydroxyurea increases hemoglobin S synthesis remains unknown, it has proved effective in national prospective, randomized trials in reducing hemolysis, which necessitates transfusion, and the number and severity of painful crises and episodes of chest pain syndrome. Paradoxically, the increase in hemoglobin F is only short-lived, yet the effect of the drug persists, which correlates with its suppression of neutrophil and reticulocyte counts. The major concern with the long-term use of hydroxyurea is that it is associated with induction of malignancy. This concern has stimulated searches for alternatives. Results with erythropoietin are mixed; butyric acid and its analogues are also being studied for their effects on hemoglobin F synthesis. Gene therapy is likely to be applied in the future to manage this classic genetic disease.

A.H.G.

ANNOTATED BIBLIOGRAPHY

Boggs DR. Fate of a ferrous sulfate prescription. Am J Med 1987;82:124. (*Most patients received a more expensive, less effective enteric-coated or slow-release form, even when not ordered.*)

Brise H, Hallberg L. Influence of meals on iron absorption in oral iron therapy. Acta Med Scand Suppl 1962;171:376. (*Absorption fell 40% when oral iron was taken with meals.*)

Bunn HF. Pathogenesis and treatment of sickle cell disease. N Engl J Med 1997;337:762. (*Excellent review of basic mechanisms and implications for treatment.*)

Campbell NR, Hasinoff BB. Iron supplements: a common cause of drug interactions. Br J Clin Pharmacol 1991;31:251. (*Good summary of these important interactions; most occur when tablets are taken simultaneously.*)

Campbell NR, Hasinoff BB, Stalts H, et al. Ferrous sulfate reduces thyroxine efficacy in patients with hypothyroidism. Ann Intern Med 1992;117:1010. (*Taking both at the same time reduces thyroxine efficacy; binding to iron suspected.*)

Charache S, Terrin ML, Moore RD, et al. Effect of hydroxyurea on the frequency of painful crises in sickle cell anemia. N Engl J Med 1995;332:1317. (*Major national randomized trial demonstrating efficacy.*)

Crosby W. Who needs iron? N Engl J Med 1977;297:543. (*Terse and still pertinent review of iron requirements and the need for supplementation.*)

Elwood P, Williams G. A comparative trial of slow-release and conventional iron preparations. Practitioner 1970;204:812. (*No therapeutic advantage found for slow-release preparations.*)

Erslev AJ. Erythropoietin. N Engl J Med 1991;324:1339. (*Excellent review; 54 references.*)

Fry J. Clinical patterns and course of anemias in general practice. Br Med J 1961;2:1732. (*Recurrence rate of iron deficiency was 30% after treatment if the underlying cause was not corrected.*)

Goodnough LT, Monk TG, Andriole GL. Erythropoietin therapy. N Engl J Med 1997;337:933. (*Evidence for perioperative use to reduce requirements for allogeneic transfusion.*)

Hallberg L, Ryttinger L, Solvell L. Side effects of oral iron therapy. Acta Med Scand 1966;459[Suppl]:3. (*Blinded controlled trial found only 7% had to stop therapy because of gastrointestinal intolerance.*)

Lawhorne L, Ringdahl D. Cyanocobalamin injections for patients without documented deficiency: reasons for administration and patient responses to proposed discontinuation. JAMA 1989;261:1920. (*Well-documented example of unwarranted empiric use.*)

Lindenbaum J, Healton EB, Savage DG, et al. Neuropsychiatric disorders caused by cobalamin deficiency in the absence of anemia or macrocytosis. N Engl J Med 1988;318:1720. (*Emphasizes need for high index of suspicion and early treatment.*)

Rector WG. Pica—its frequency and significance in patients with iron-deficiency anemia due to chronic gastrointestinal blood loss. J Gen Intern Med 1989;4:512. (*Found to be frequent and resolved with therapy; no relation to etiology.*)

Savage D, Lindenbaum J. Relapses after interruption of cyanocobalamin therapy in patients with pernicious anemia. Am J Med 1983;74:765. (*Emphasizes importance of ensuring indefinite provision of therapy.*)

Stevens RG, Jones DY, Micozzi MS, et al. Body iron stores and the risk of cancer. N Engl J Med 1988;319:1047. (*Just an epidemiologic reminder that too much iron can be harmful.*)

Toh B-H, van Driel IR, Gleeson PA. Pernicious anemia. N Engl J Med 1997;337:1441. (*An authoritative review of pathophysiology, diagnosis, and treatment.*)

Wood M, Elwood P. Symptoms of iron-deficiency anemia: a community survey. Br J Prev Soc Med 1966;20:117. (*Classic study; the correlation between hemoglobin concentration and symptoms was poor. Iron therapy produced no statistically significant reduction in symptoms.*)

83

Outpatient Oral Anticoagulant Therapy

ELAINE M. HYLEK
ROBERT A. HUGHES

Oral anticoagulant therapy with coumarin derivatives effectively prevents thromboembolism in a variety of conditions, ranging from venous thrombosis to atrial fibrillation to transient ischemic attacks. Oral platelet inhibitors help prevent thrombosis and restenosis of coronary arteries. This expanded range of applications for oral anticoagulants makes their proper use an important responsibility of the primary care physician. To optimize patient care, physicians must know (a) the indications for warfarin and antiplatelet therapy, (b) how to initiate and maintain patients on oral anticoagulants in the outpatient setting, (c) common complications, and (d) the drugs and conditions that interfere with or potentiate the anticoagulant effect. This chapter focuses primarily on coumarin derivatives and aspirin (see Chapter 30 for a discussion of the use of other antiplatelet agents).

WARFARIN

Mechanism of Action

Warfarin and other coumarin derivatives act by inhibiting the action of vitamin K in the γ-carboxylation of glutamic acid residues on coagulation factors II, VII, IX, and X. Without γ-carboxylation, these proteins cannot participate in coagulation. The warfarin-induced decline in active, carboxylated coagulation factors is a function of the half-life of each factor, which varies from 5 hours for factor VII to 72 hours for factor II. The prothrombin time (PT) may be prolonged after only 2 to 3 days of therapy, but this represents primarily depression of factor VII. The full antithrombotic effect of warfarin is achieved only after 5 to 7 days, with depletion of factor II.

Indications

Therapy is indicated in conditions associated with a high risk for thrombus formation and subsequent embolization. These include the following:

- Atrial fibrillation (see Chapters 28 and 33)
- Valvular heart disease and prosthetic heart valves (see Chapter 33)

- Systemic embolization (see Chapter 171)
- Deep venous thrombosis (see Chapter 35)
- Pulmonary embolization (see Chapter 35)
- Dilated cardiomyopathy and left ventricular thrombus (see Chapter 32)
- Following myocardial infarction in selected patients (see Chapter 31)

Atrial Fibrillation is highly prevalent, found in 5% of people over 60 and nearly 10% of people over 80. It increases the risk for stroke more than fivefold; the patient in atrial fibrillation has a 5% average annual risk for stroke. Patients with atrial fibrillation secondary to valvular heart disease are at even greater risk.

Prosthetic Heart Valves increase the risk for systemic emboli, especially stroke. The risk is higher with caged-ball and tilting-disk valves, and with valves in the mitral rather than aortic position. Anticoagulation is continued indefinitely. Patients with bioprosthetic valves need only short-term (e.g., for 3 months) anticoagulation unless another indication, such as atrial fibrillation or a history of systemic embolism, is present.

Deep Venous Thrombosis and Pulmonary Embolism are indications for anticoagulation. A 3- to 6-month course may suffice when risk factors are reversible or time-limited, such as surgery, temporary immobilization, or estrogen use. Patients with a first event who are found to be heterozygous for activated protein C resistance (factor V Leiden) but no other risk factors should also receive a 3- to 6-month course of treatment. Patients with a first episode of idiopathic deep venous thrombosis should be treated for at least 6 months. In patients with recurrent deep venous thrombosis or pulmonary embolism, a known hypercoagulable state, or homozygosity for factor V Leiden, anticoagulation should be continued indefinitely.

Dilated Cardiomyopathy puts patients at risk for embolization. When this condition was accompanied by atrial fibrillation, the annual risk for embolic events in the absence of anticoagulation exceeded 15% in one cohort study. Without atrial fibrillation, the risk is in the 1% to 5% range. The absence of randomized trials demonstrating risk reduction with anticoagulation precludes definitive recommendations. Potential benefits and risks must be weighed for individual patients.

Myocardial Infarction. Some patients may benefit from anticoagulation following myocardial infarction. *Anterior Q-wave infarction*, particularly with evidence of *mural thrombosis*, or atrial fibrillation warrants anticoagulation. Otherwise, there is no evident advantage for warfarin over aspirin in chronic stable angina or in the secondary prevention of myocardial infarction.

Contraindications

Contraindications to the use of oral anticoagulants need to be considered in the context of urgency of anticoagulation, risk and seriousness of potential complications, and duration of therapy (see Table 83.1). Patients with *previous central nervous system bleeding*, recent *neurosurgery*, or *frank bleeding* should not receive warfarin. Important relative contraindications include *active peptic ulcer disease*, *chronic alcoholism*, *blindness* (unless in supervised situations), *bleeding diathesis*, and *severe hypertension*. When taken in *early pregnancy*, coumarins may cause birth defects; when they are used at *delivery*, fetal hemorrhage can occur. Heparin should be used in place of warfarin during early pregnancy and childbirth. Embarking on oral anticoagulant therapy is unwise when follow-up cannot be readily maintained, when laboratory facilities for accurately measuring the PT are inadequate, or when the patient is unreliable.

Initiating and Monitoring Therapy

Initiation. Patients with *acute pulmonary embolization* or acute systemic embolization should be admitted to the hospital for immediate administration of *IV heparin* to halt clot propagation. Warfarin should be started on the first day of heparin therapy and overlapped with heparin for at least 4 days to ensure adequate reduction in prothrombin levels. Heparin can then be discontinued once the *international normalized ratio* (INR; see below) exceeds 2.0 on two consecutive days. Warfarin treatment should be initiated with sequential 5-mg doses and daily measurement of the INR. Studies have shown that such initial 5-mg doses (in comparison with initial 10-mg doses) are less likely to induce excessive anticoagulation and are equally effective in lowering levels of prothrombin.

Table 83.1. Contraindications to Anticoagulant Therapy with Warfarin

Absolute Contraindications
 Previous central nervous system bleeding
 Recent neurosurgery
 Active frank bleeding
 Early pregnancy and delivery

Relative Contraindications
 Active peptic ulcer disease
 Chronic alcoholicm
 Bleeding diathesis
 Severe hypertension

For patients with *deep venous thrombosis*, SQ administration of *low-molecular-weight heparin* is an effective alternative to IV administration of unfractionated heparin for initial anticoagulation (see Chapter 35). It allows for a shortened hospital stay or an entirely at-home anticoagulant treatment program, which reduces costs. Warfarin therapy is instituted in the same fashion as IV heparin therapy.

Patients who are in less urgent need of immediate full anticoagulation (e.g., *stable atrial fibrillation*) can be safely started on warfarin alone as outpatients. A generally accepted approach to initiating outpatient warfarin therapy is to give 5 mg daily, measure the INR at 5 to 7 days, and adjust the dose accordingly. The starting dose should be set at 2.5 mg daily in patients who weigh less than 110 lb, are older than 75 years, or are at increased risk for bleeding. Warfarin is best taken on an empty stomach at a specific time each day. Administration at bedtime allows for changes to be made in the dosage on the same day the INR is measured. The Food and Drug Administration has approved several generic warfarins; the same generic or brand formulation should be used consistantly to avoid patient confusion and INR fluctuaion.

Monitoring. The intensity of anticoagulation is measured with the *PT test* and expressed as the *prothrombin time ratio* (PTR), which is the ratio of the patient's PT to the control PT of the laboratory. Standardization of the PTR across laboratories is necessary to account for the different sensitivities of the various thromboplastin reagents used in the assay. The *INR* has replaced the PTR as the universally accepted measurement of anticoagulation intensity. To calculate the INR, the PTR is raised to the power of the international sensitivity index (ISI) of the specific reagent used (i.e., PTR^{ISI}).

It can take up to 3 months to achieve a stable warfarin dosage. Once stabilized, the INR can be checked every 3 to 4 weeks. The variability in the warfarin dose response mandates frequent monitoring. Changes in the warfarin requirement may be precipitated by a change in diet, particularly the intake of foods with a high content of vitamin K (e.g., most leafy vegetables), or by medications that interfere with the hepatic clearance of warfarin. Many commonly used drugs potentiate the anticoagulant effect of warfarin and should prompt close monitoring (see below). In about 75% of patients, dosage adjustments over time are unnecessary.

Patients with *lupus anticoagulants* (one of the *antiphospholipid antibodies* that can cause hypercoagulability and thromboembolization; see Chapter 35) pose a particular problem in monitoring because these antibodies can interfere with the PT assay. Both overestimation and underestimation of the degree of anticoagulation can result. Consultation with a hematologist is needed to design the anticoagulation monitoring program for such a patient.

Recommended Intensity of Therapy. After initiation of therapy, dosage should be adjusted to maintain the therapeutic range. Extensive study supports the use of lower ranges of anticoagulation intensity (INR target range of 2.0 to 3.0) for most groups of patients. Efficacy is maintained while the risk for hemorrhagic complications is reduced. Only those patients at highest risk for thromboembolism (e.g., mechanical prosthetic heart valves) should receive anticoagulation in an INR range of 2.5 to 3.5.

Adjustment of Dose. The dose can be adjusted in numerous ways when the INR is out of range. One method designed to maximize safety and avoid wide swings in the INR is based on 10% changes in the weekly dose unless the INR is grossly out of range. For example, if the patient is taking 7.5 mg/d, the weekly dose is 52.5 mg. If the INR is too low, the weekly dose is increased by 10%, so that on 2 days of the week the patient takes 10 mg, and 7.5 mg on the other 5 days. The INR is then measured weekly for the next 2 weeks, with continued adjustment in dose if necessary.

Outpatient anticoagulation requires facilities for accurate INR measurement and reliable collection of blood samples, and the ability to contact patients promptly. Careful monitoring and follow-up are essential for a safe and successful outpatient anticoagulation program. At the beginning of therapy, patients should attend an educational session with a nurse who can instruct them in the use of warfarin, answer questions, test their understanding, and provide informative booklets for them to take home. Patients who fail to keep an appointment for an INR test should be contacted immediately. A computer system can provide reminders so that no patient is lost to follow-up. Commercial laboratory services are sometimes employed to draw samples at home for patients who have difficulty coming to the office. Home monitoring devices are under development.

Duration. In the absence of hemorrhagic complications, anticoagulation should be continued indefinitely in patients with atrial fibrillation, valvular heart disease, systemic embolization, or mechanical prosthetic heart valves. Patients with recurrent deep venous thrombosis, recurrent pulmonary embolism, or a known hypercoagulable state should also receive anticoagulants indefinitely. Those with a single episode of deep venous thrombosis caused by a self-limited risk factor and no known hypercoagulable state can stop their warfarin after 3 to 6 months (see Chapter 35).

Complications

Reports of the incidence of *hemorrhagic complications* in patients on long-term anticoagulant therapy have varied widely, depending on the definition of bleeding used and the INR target under study. Several series have demonstrated that hemorrhage severe enough to require hospitalization or transfusion should occur in fewer than 5% of patients who are carefully monitored. The rate of intracranial hemorrhage among patients managed in a structured setting was 0.6% annually. *Risk factors* for hemorrhagic complications include an *INR higher than 4.0, recent initiation of anticoagulation*, and *wide fluctuation in the INR*. A *history of gastrointestinal bleeding* is a risk factor; peptic ulcer disease *per se* is not. Older patients generally experience a higher incidence of complications, but this may be mediated through other risk factors more common among the elderly.

Patients experiencing urinary, gastrointestinal, or gynecologic bleeding while on anticoagulant therapy should undergo a diagnostic evaluation to identify any underlying pathologic lesion. In several series, a lesion responsible for the bleeding was detected in more than 50% of patients.

Hemorrhagic necrosis of the skin (more common among women) and *cyanotic toes* (more common among men) occur rarely, even with INRs in the therapeutic range. The mechanism may be a transient inhibition of endothelial vitamin K–dependent antithrombotic proteins (proteins S and C) in patients congenitally deficient in such factors.

Effects of Drugs and Concurrent Illnesses

Potentiation. Drugs that potentiate the effect of warfarin may do so by preventing the synthesis or absorption of vitamin K, displacing warfarin from binding sites, inhibiting microsomal degradative enzyme activity, increasing catabolism of clotting factors, or impairing platelet function (Table 83.2). The risk for bleeding is particularly high with concurrent use of NSAIDs. In the elderly, a 13-fold increase in hemorrhagic peptic ulcer disease results from taking NSAIDs plus warfarin. Substitution of daily *acetaminophen* for NSAIDs reduces the risk for bleeding from gastric injury, but it raises the risk for excessive anticoagulation by potentiating the effects of warfarin; close INR monitoring and warfarin dose adjustment are critical with daily use of acetaminophen.

Hepatocellular failure results in impaired synthesis of clotting factors and albumin; cholestasis makes for less efficient absorption of vitamin K. Both conditions are capable of prolonging the INR and potentiating the effects of warfarin.

Inhibition. Anticoagulant effects are decreased by agents that induce microsomal enzymes, decrease the absorption of warfarin, or increase the synthesis of clotting factors or binding proteins (see Table 83.2). Moreover, coumarins cause a decrease in the metabolism of tolbutamide and phenytoin by competing for the same degradative enzymes. The INR should be measured when any change in a drug program is made, and it should be followed closely thereafter.

Reversal of Anticoagulation and Elective Interruptions in Therapy

Rapid Reversal. Serious bleeding, a dangerously high INR (>20), or a need for urgent surgery are among the circumstances in which rapid reversal of oral anticoagulation is indicated. Administration of *fresh-frozen plasma* provides rapid correction of the INR but involves exposure to blood products and a large colloid load. Alternatively, administration of *vitamin K* (which stimulates hepatic synthesis of the clotting factors inhibited by warfarin) is also effective but somewhat slower, taking 12 to 48 hours to reduce the INR to a safe level. IV, SQ, and oral preparations are available. The *high-dose IV preparation of vitamin K* (1 to 10 mg) is the most potent and most rapidly acting of the various formulations, but it is also the most likely to overshoot, impair repeated anticoagulation, and subject the patient to the risk for an acute anaphylactic reaction (a rare but serious complication). *Low-dose IV vitamin K* (0.1 to 0.5 mg) appears only slightly less effective and is less likely to overshoot. The same holds for *sc vitamin K* (1 to 3 mg), but systemic absorption can be erratic, leading to treatment failure. *Oral vitamin K* (2.5 mg) can reverse INRs of less than 10 but may require slightly more time to work than parenteral forms.

Interruptions. The decision to discontinue anticoagulant therapy in the context of nonemergent bleeding or elective surgery needs to be individualized. The risk for embolization must be balanced against the risk for hemorrhage. The risk for

Table 83.2.   Common Drugs That Interact with Oral Anticoagulants

Effect	Mechanism	Drug
Prolongation of PT	Inhibits clearance	Metronidazole
		Trimethoprim sulfamethoxazole
		Cimetidine[a]
		Omeprazole[a]
		Sulfinpyrazone[a]
		Disulfiram
		Anabolic steroids
	Inhibits vitamin K	Cephalosporins, 2nd, 3rd generation
	Increases metabolism of clotting factors	L-Thyroxine
	Unknown	Erythromycin
		? Tamoxifen
		? Phenytoin
		? Isoniazid
		? Ketoconazole
		? Piroxicam
Reduction of PT	Increases warfarin clearance	Barbiturates
		Carbamazepine
		Rifampin
	Reduces warfarin absorption	Cholestyramine
	Increases synthesis of clotting factors	Estrogens
	Unknown	Penicillins

[a]Causes only minimal prologation of prothrombin time (PT).
Adapted from Hirsh J. Oral anticoagulant drugs. N Engl J Med 1991:324:1865, with permission.

embolization is substantial and greatest for persons with acute deep venous thrombosis or acute arterial embolization who have been taking warfarin for less than 1 month. A somewhat lesser risk is associated with recurrent deep venous thrombosis, nonvalvular atrial fibrillation with previous arterial embolization, placement of a mechanical heart valve, and deep venous thrombosis after more than 1 month of warfarin. The risk for postoperative bleeding can be minimized by withholding anticoagulation for about 4 days before elective surgery to allow the INR to drift below 1.5, the level at which most surgery can be carried out with little risk for hemorrhage.

When patients are at high risk for thromboembolization, *perioperative heparin* must be considered. A 2-day preoperative course is of low risk when stopped 6 hours before surgery. Postoperative heparinization, begun 12 hours after surgery (without a loading bolus), is associated with a 3% daily risk for major hemorrhage and should be reserved for those patients at highest thromboembolic risk whose risk for postoperative bleeding is acceptable. If the risk for bleeding is unacceptably high in such persons, then a *vena cava filter* should be considered preoperatively.

Patient Education

Before initiation of outpatient therapy, the patient and designated family member(s) need to (a) understand the risks and benefits of warfarin; (b) become familiar with the requirements for taking warfarin responsibly (e.g., avoidance of NSAIDs and excessive amounts of alcohol); (c) be able to recognize signs of abnormal bleeding (e.g., melena); and (d) be versed in the triage protocol for hemorrhagic complications. Instruction of the patient by a nurse trained in anticoagulation management, supplemented by an information booklet appropriate to the patient's educational level, constitute the essentials of the patient education effort. Any patient who is incapable of understanding the instructions or is deemed unreliable should not be placed on therapy because the risks for hemorrhage probably outweigh any possible benefits. The one exception is the patient who can be closely supervised by family members or health care professionals.

The physician should know the tablet color coding of the warfarin brand the patient is using. This helps ensure that proper doses are being taken. Constancy of brand should be advised, both to minimize dosing errors and to ensure consistency of anticoagulant effect.

ANTIPLATELET THERAPY

Aspirin inhibits platelet aggregation by irreversibly acetylating and inactivating platelet prostaglandin H synthase and its cyclooxygenase activity. The major side effect of aspirin is gastrointestinal hemorrhage. Newer platelet-active drugs, *ticlopidine* and *clopidogrel*, inhibit adenosine diphosphate–induced platelet aggregation and do not interfere with the prostaglandin protective effect on the gastric mucosa. The cost of ticlopidine and its association with agranulocytosis has reduced its use as an alternative to aspirin. Clinical studies of clopidogrel are ongoing.

Indications

Aspirin has been shown to be effective in the treatment and prevention of atherothrombosis.

Current indications for aspirin therapy include the following:

- Primary and secondary prevention of myocardial infarction (see Chapters 18 and 31)
- Chronic stable angina (see Chapter 30)

- Unstable angina (see Chapter 20)
- Acute myocardial infarction
- Transient cerebral ischemia and ischemic stroke (see Chapter 171)
- Acute ischemic stroke
- Coronary stent implantation (combined with clopidogrel or ticlopidine for at least 14 days; see Chapter 30)

The minimum effective dose of aspirin for these indications ranges from 80 to 160 mg/d.

Aspirin as an Adjunct or Alternative to Warfarin

As Adjunct. Patients with mechanical prosthetic heart valves, specifically those with caged-ball or caged-disk valves, or others with additional risk factors for thromboembolism can optimally be managed by adding aspirin therapy (80 to 100 mg/d) to warfarin, with an INR target range of 2.5 to 3.5.

As Alternative. For most conditions in which anticoagulation is indicated, aspirin has been found to be either ineffective or equivocally effective. Among patients with atrial fibrillation, only those deemed to be at low risk for stroke or for whom warfarin is contraindicated are appropriate candidates for aspirin therapy (see Chapters 28 and 33).

CONCLUSIONS AND RECOMMENDATIONS

Warfarin

- Warfarin is highly effective in preventing thromboembolism. The recommended intensity of anticoagulation for most indications is an INR of 2.0 to 3.0. Patients with metallic prosthetic heart valves should be given aspirin in addition to warfarin, with a target INR of 2.5 to 3.5.
- Only patients felt to be at low risk for stroke or those in whom anticoagulant therapy is contraindicated should be treated with aspirin for prophylaxis against stroke in atrial fibrillation.
- Patients with temporal risk factor–related deep venous thrombosis or pulmonary embolism should be treated with warfarin for 3 to 6 months. Patients with idiopathic deep venous thrombosis or pulmonary embolism should be treated for at least 6 months. Patients with recurrent thrombosis or an ongoing hypercoagulable state or who are homozygous for activated protein C resistance should be treated indefinitely with warfarin.
- Rapid reversal of anticoagulation therapy is indicated for severe bleeding, an INR above 20, and urgent surgery. Administration of fresh-frozen plasma achieves reversal within hours. Vitamin K accomplishes the same in 6 to 48 hours, depending on dose and route of administration.
- The decision to discontinue anticoagulant therapy in the context of nonemergent bleeding or elective surgery needs to be individualized. The risk for embolization must be balanced against the risk for hemorrhage.
- Reversal of oral anticoagulation for elective surgery can be accomplished simply by withholding warfarin for 4 days or until the INR is below 1.5, the level at which the risk for hemorrhage becomes minimal in most forms of surgery. For high-risk patients, perioperative heparinization must be considered.

- Anticoagulant therapy mandates frequent monitoring, lifestyle changes, and commitment by the patient and health care team to optimize its safety and efficacy.

Aspirin

- Aspirin should be used by all persons at risk for atherothrombosis. Aspirin can reduce the risk for vascular events, including myocardial infarction, stroke, and transient ischemic attack.
- Aspirin combined with clopidogrel or ticlopidine should be used for at least 14 days after coronary stent implantation.

ANNOTATED BIBLIOGRAPHY

Ansell JE, Hughes R. Evolving models of warfarin management: anticoagulation clinics, patient self-monitoring, and patient self-management. Am Heart J 1996;132:1095. (*Reviews benefits of anticoagulation clinics and feasibility of patient self-monitoring.*)

Ansell JE, Patel N, Ostrovsky D, et al. Long-term patient self-management of oral anticoagulation. Arch Intern Med 1995;155:2185. (*Patients are able to adjust warfarin doses successfully on the basis of fingerstick determination of PT performed at home.*)

Azar AJ, Cannegieter SC, Deckers JW, et al. Optimal intensity of oral anticoagulant therapy after myocardial infarction. J Am Coll Cardiol 1996;27:1349. (*Assuming equal harm of thrombotic and hemorrhagic complications, an INR of 2.0 to 4.0 is considered optimal.*)

Boston Area Anticoagulation Trial for Atrial Fibrillation Investigators. The effect of low-dose warfarin on the risk of stroke in patients with nonrheumatic atrial fibrillation. N Engl J Med 1990;323:1505. (*One of several randomized trials demonstrating benefit in patients with chronic or paroxysmal atrial fibrillation; also shows efficacy of low-intensity therapy.*)

Cannegieter SC, Rosendaal FR, Wintzen AR, et al. Optimal oral anticoagulant therapy in patients with mechanical heart valves. N Engl J Med 1995;333:11. (*Recommends a target INR of 3.0 to 4.0.*)

Dutch TIA Trial Study Group. Comparison of two doses of aspirin (30 mg versus 383 mg per day) in patients after a transient ischemic attack or minor ischemic stroke. N Engl J Med 1991;325:1261. (*Low-dose aspirin was as effective as higher doses in preventing stroke recurrence.*)

European Atrial Fibrillation Trial Study Group. Optimal oral anticoagulant therapy in patients with nonrheumatic atrial fibrillation and recent cerebral ischemia. N Engl J Med 1995;333:5. (*Recommends target INR of 3.0.*)

Ezekowitz MD, Bridgers SL, James KE, et al. Warfarin in the prevention of stroke associated with nonrheumatic atrial fibrillation. N Engl J Med 1992;327:1406. (*Veterans Administration study further confirming that low-intensity therapy reduces risk in patients older than 70 years.*)

Feder W, Auerback R. Purple toes: an uncommon sequela of oral coumarin drug therapy. Ann Intern Med 1961;55:911. (*Original report of complication seen in 1% of patients, now known to be caused by congenital deficiency of factor S or C worsened by warfarin therapy.*)

Fihn SD, McDonell M, Martin D, et al. Risk factors for complications of chronic anticoagulation. Ann Intern Med 1993;118:511. (*High-intensity anticoagulation, wide fluctuations in PT, recent initiation of therapy, and poor patient selection were major risk factors.*)

Gurwitz JH, Avorn J, Ross-Degnan D, et al. Aging and the anticoagulant response to warfarin therapy. Ann Intern Med 1992;116:901.

(Response increases with age, so that close monitoring becomes particularly important in the elderly.)

Harrison L, Johnston M, Massicotte MP, et al. Comparison of 5-mg and 10-mg loading doses in initiation of warfarin therapy. Ann Intern Med 1997;126:133. (*The 5-mg dose takes effect nearly as fast, but with less risk of complications.*)

Hass WK, Easton JD, Adams HP Jr, et al. Randomized trial comparing ticlopidine with aspirin for the prevention of stroke in high-risk patients. N Engl J Med 1989;521:501. (*Double-blind, randomized trial of more than 3,000 patients with transient ischemic attack or minor stroke showing a significant reduction, approximately 10%, in risk of complications.*)

Hirsh J. Oral anticoagulant drugs. N Engl J Med 1991;324:1865. (*Exhaustive but clinically useful review; 132 references.*)

Hirsh J, Levin MN. The optimal intensity of oral anticoagulant therapy. JAMA 1987;258:2723. (*Argues that low-intensity therapy is best for most indications.*)

Hylek EM, Heiman H, Skates SJ, et al. Acetaminophen and other risk factors for excessive warfarin anticoagulation. JAMA 1998; 279:657. (*Case–control study; acetaminophen was independently associated with excessive anticoagulation.*)

Hylek EM, Singer DE. Risk factors for intracranial hemorrhage in outpatients taking warfarin. Ann Intern Med 1994;120:897. (*The odds of hemorrhage increase sharply as PTR exceeds 2.0 or INR exceeds 3.7 to 4.3.*)

Hylek EM, Skates SJ, Sheehan MA, et al. An analysis of the lowest effective intensity of prophylactic anticoagulation for patients with nonrheumatic atrial fibrillation. N Engl J Med 1996;335:540. (*The odds of stroke rise sharply as the INR falls below 2.0.*)

Kearon C, Hirsh J. Management of anticoagulation before and after elective surgery. N Engl J Med 1997;336:1506. (*A critical review that provides practical recommendations.*)

Koopman MMW, Prandoni P, Piovella F, et al. Treatment of venous thrombosis with intravenous unfractionated heparin administered in the hospital as compared with subcutaneous low-molecular-weight heparin administered at home. N Engl J Med 1996;334:682. (*Safety and ethicasy as good if not better for LMWH.*)

Lancaster TR, Singer DE, Sheehan MA, et al. The impact of long-term warfarin therapy on quality of life. Arch Intern Med 1991;151:1944. (*Quality of life well preserved.*)

Landefeld CS, Goldman L. Major bleeding in outpatients treated with warfarin: incidence and prediction by factors known at the start of outpatient therapy. Am J Med 1989;87:144. (*Age over 65 years, history of stroke or gastrointestinal bleeding, serious comorbid condition, and atrial fibrillation were predictors of risk.*)

Landefeld CS, Rosenblatt MW, Goldman L. Bleeding in outpatients treated with warfarin: relation to the prothrombin time and important remediable lesions. Am J Med 1989;87:153. (*Companion study confirming that risk for bleeding increases with intensity of anticoagulation; confirms value of checking for underlying lesions.*)

Levine M, Gent M, Hirsh J, et al. A comparison of low molecular weight heparin administered primarily at home with unfractionated heparin administered in the hospital for proximal deep vein thrombosis. N Engl J Med 1996;334:677. (*Randomized trial; evidence for ethicasy and safety of LMWH.*)

Meltzer RS, Visser CA, Fuster V. Intracardiac thrombi and systemic embolization. Ann Intern Med 1986;104:689. (*Excellent review of data justifying oral anticoagulation.*)

Moll S, Ortel TL. Monitoring warfarin therapy in patients with lupus anticoagulants. Ann Intern Med 1997;127:177. (*Prospective case series demonstrating overestimation and underestimation of anticoagulation by PT assay in such persons.*)

Petty GW, Brown RD Jr, Whisnant JP, et al. Frequency of major complications of aspirin, warfarin, and intravenous heparin for secondary stroke prevention: a population-based study. Ann Intern Med 1999;130:14. (*Provides rates from "real world" practice.*)

Raj G, Kumar R, McKinney WP. Safety of intramuscular influenza immunization among patients receiving long-term warfarin anticoagulation therapy. Arch Intern Med 1995;155:1529. (*Small study found no effect on PT and no local hemorrhagic complications.*)

Shorr RI, Ray WA, Dougherty JR, et al. Concurrent use of nonsteroidal antiinflammatory drugs and oral anticoagulants places elderly persons at high risk of hemorrhagic peptic ulcer. Arch Intern Med 1993;153:1665. (*Risk increases 13-fold.*)

Smith P, Arneson H, Holme I. The effect of warfarin on mortality and reinfarction after myocardial infarction. N Engl J Med 1990;323:147. (*Intriguing data from Europe suggesting that warfarin may reduce rate of reinfarction.*)

Stafford RS, Singer DE. National patterns of warfarin use in atrial fibrillation. Arch Intern Med 1996;156:2537. (*Documents dramatic differences in the rates at which patients in atrial fibrillation are given anticoagulants by different specialists and in different regions of the country.*)

Stroke Prevention in Atrial Fibrillation Investigators. Predictors of thromboembolism in atrial fibrillation. Ann Intern Med 1992;116:1,6. (*Two-part study; recent congestive heart failure, hypertension, previous embolism, left ventricular dysfunction, and left atrial enlargement were independent predictors of stroke risk.*)

Whitling AM, Bussey HI, Lyons RM. Compairing different routes and doses of phytonadione for reversing excessive anticoagulation. Arch Intern Med 1998;158:2136. (*A retrospective study, but provides useful data on efficacy and safety of various vitamin K preparations.*)

84

Approach to the Patient with Lymphoma

The lymphomas are a diverse group of malignancies, with non-Hodgkin's lymphoma about twice as common as Hodgkin's disease and increasing at a rate of 4% annually. Together, they account for more than 60,000 new cases of cancer per year in the United States, having doubled in incidence during the past 20 years. Multiple subtypes are found, each with specific immunologic and pathologic characteristics and a distinctive clinical presentation and therapeutic response. Non-Hodgkin's lymphoma strikes much later than Hodgkin's disease; peak incidence is in the fifth decade, compared with the second decade for Hodgkin's disease (although a second peak occurs in the fifth decade). The prognosis for non-Hodgkin's lymphoma is less favorable in terms of long-term cure, although survival and responsiveness to therapy are substantial. Cure is possible for many patients with Hodgkin's disease.

Although the treatment of these conditions is the province of the oncologist, the primary physician has an important role in diagnosing and staging the disease, coordinating plans for management, and delivering follow-up care on an outpatient basis. Because they are likely to conduct the initial evaluation, it is essential that primary physicians be prepared to discuss with patients and their families the meaning of findings. Even after referral, the primary physician often encounters requests for advice, being the physician the patient knows best. Consequently, a serious working knowledge of the clinical presentation, prognosis, staging methods, and treatment options is important for the primary physician if the patient is to be served well.

HODGKIN'S DISEASE

Pathology, Clinical Presentation, and Course

The histology of Hodgkin's disease incorporates four categories: lymphocyte predominance, nodular sclerosis, mixed cellularity, and lymphocyte depletion. *Lymphocyte predominance* occurs in 10% to 15% of patients, *nodular sclerosis* in 20% to 50%, *mixed cellularity* in 20% to 40%, and *lymphocyte depletion* in 5% to 15%. In about 15% of cases, classification is difficult and requires expert interpretation of the histology. In all instances, the *sine qua non* of diagnosis is the pathognomonic *Reed-Sternberg cell*.

The condition originates in the lymph nodes. Conceptually, Hodgkin's disease is *unicentric* in origin and progresses by contiguous extension along lymphatic pathways. Consequently, the adenopathy tends to be asymmetric. This pattern of evolution is in contrast to that of non-Hodgkin's lymphomas, which are multicentric and generally at more advanced stages at initial presentation. Most patients present with disease above the clavicle. Fewer than 15% present with disease originating below the diaphragm, although any node may be involved (including those of the mediastinum, axilla, or groin). Typically, the nodes are firm and nontender; although often matted, they may be discrete and even freely movable. Subsequent spread to the spleen is a regular occurrence and is the first manifestation of disease below the diaphragm, followed by involvement of the liver and bone marrow. Fever, weight loss, night sweats, or alcohol-induced pain may develop and almost always represents advanced disease.

The differential diagnosis of Hodgkin's disease includes infectious mononucleosis, HIV infection, and other nonbacterial adenopathies in the young (see Chapter 12). In the elderly, other malignancies are a common diagnostic consideration; they are particularly suspect in the presence of a fever of unknown origin. Excisional biopsy rather than needle aspiration is needed for diagnosis.

Classification by Stage. Because prognosis and treatment are so dependent on the extent of disease, classification by stage plays a central role in Hodgkin's disease. The *Ann Arbor staging system* of classification is the one most widely referred to. In it, *stage I* is defined as disease confined to a single node-bearing area or localized involvement of a single extranodal site. *Stage II* involves two or more contiguous node-bearing areas on the same side of the diaphragm or more than one nodal region in conjunction with localized involvement of an extra-

lymphatic organ on the same side of the diaphragm. *Stage III* is nodal involvement on both sides of the diaphragm, with or without involvement of the spleen or a local extranodal organ or site. Additional subcategories have been developed for patients with intraabdominal disease. *Stage III1* represents disease confined to the upper abdomen; it is generally microscopic. *Stage III2* designates disease extending into the pelvis with grossly involved nodes or bulky retroperitoneal tumor. *Stage IV* represents diffuse visceral disease (liver, lung parenchyma, bone marrow).

The special category designated *E* (for extranodal) was created because of data indicating that involvement of an organ contiguous with a lymph node–bearing area is associated with a distinctly better prognosis than is hematogenous visceral involvement. Nonetheless, the prognosis is not as good as it would be without any organ involvement. *S* denotes disease in the spleen.

Approximately 20% of patients have *fever, night sweats*, or *significant weight loss* (>10%). These systemic symptoms are incorporated into the staging system because they are important determinants of prognosis. When absent, the designation is *A*; when any of the three is present, the designation is *B*. Patients with pruritus only are no longer included in the B group. Early (I and II) and advanced (III and IV) stages of Hodgkin's disease are relatively equally distributed in terms of frequency. More sophisticated staging by pathologic and clinical procedures generally tends to advance the stage of disease.

The *prognosis* of Hodgkin's disease has improved dramatically with the advent of careful staging and improved radiation technology and chemotherapy programs. Overall 5-year survival is 80%; when all stages of disease are combined, 65% experience 5-year relapse-free survival (Table 84.1). The principal determinants of outcome are stage, patient age, presence or absence of symptoms, and tumor bulk. Histology is also a factor, although not as important as the others.

Staging

Staging (Table 84.2) is critical to the design of a therapeutic program and an estimation of prognosis. *Clinical staging* involves an assessment of the history and the findings on physical examination and radiology. The history should ascertain the presence of fever, night sweats, or weight loss. Careful palpation of all lymph nodes and assessment of liver and spleen size are important, although enlargement discovered by physical examination does not necessarily indicate involvement by the disease. One half of patients with a palpable spleen do not have histologic splenic involvement, and one fourth with normal-sized spleens do.

About 90% of patients are thought to have stage I or II disease at the time of initial clinical staging. However, most treatment decisions require *pathologic staging* (which includes biopsy) because up to two thirds of patients who present with clinical stage I or II disease are found to have disease below the diaphragm on pathologic staging. About half of patients with B symptoms will manifest disease below the diaphragm at laparotomy, compared with 25% of patients with A symptoms. The principal staging procedures include chest radiography, computed tomography (CT), lymphangiography, and bone marrow biopsy. Staging laparotomy is indicated in selected instances.

Table 84.1. Hodgkin's Disease: Stages, Relative Incidences, and Prognosis

STAGE	DEFINITION	RELATIVE INCIDENCE (%)	THERAPY	CURE (%)
I	Confined to single node-bearing area	30	Radiation	70–90
II	Confined to two contiguous node-bearing areas on one side of diaphragm	25	Radiation	
III	In nodal areas on both side of diaphragm	25	Radiation and chemotherapy	50–60
IV	Visceral lesions (liver, lung) *not* in contiguity with nodes	20	Chemotherapy	
Special categories				
E	Visceral extranodal disease in continuity with nodes (e.g., lung mass extending out from hilum)		Radiation +/– chemotherapy	
B	Symptoms of fever, weight loss, or sweats		Chemotherapy +/– radiation	

Adapted from DeVita VT Jr, Hellman S, Jaffee ES. Hodgkin's disease. In: DeVita VT Jr, Hellman S, Rosenberg SA, eds. Cancer: principles and practice of oncology, 5th ed. Philadelphia: JB Lippincott Williams and Wilkins, 1997:2250, with permission.

Chest Radiography and Computed Tomography. All patients should undergo *chest radiography* because some of the most common forms of Hodgkin's disease involve the mediastinum. Even if the chest radiographic findings are abnormal, *CT of the chest* is indicated because it provides enhanced sensitivity for detection and definition of mediastinal, hilar, and paravertebral adenopathy. The need for chest CT in a patient with totally normal findings on the chest x-ray film depends on whether the result will alter therapy or prognosis. CT is more sensitive than chest radiography for the detection of disease in the mediastinum and adjacent structures.

Complementary information about disease below the diaphragm is provided by *CT of the abdomen* and lymphangiography. CT is best for demonstrating the number and size of nodes in the retroperitoneum and pelvis. It also may show evidence of hepatic or splenic involvement, although no radiologic test (including *magnetic resonance imaging* and *radionuclide scanning*) is sensitive enough to rule out splenic involvement. Abdominal CT provides anatomic information about nodes in areas not well visualized by lymphangiography (mesenteric, subhepatic, perisplenic, celiac, and periaortic regions). CT cannot detect microscopic disease and gives less information than the lymphangiogram about nodal architecture. Magnetic resonance imaging offers no advantage over CT.

Lymphangiography can provide complementary information about the structure of retroperitoneal nodes and is capable of detecting disease in nodes that are not enlarged. The sensitivity of lymphangiography by itself is low, with a false-negative rate of 20%. However, when strict radiologic criteria for nodal involvement are used, the specificity reaches 95%, with a false-positive rate below 5% noted. Thus, a positive study result is helpful, but negative findings on the lymphangiogram do not rule out disease below the diaphragm. Moreover, even with a positive result, the test does not detect involvement of the liver or spleen, which is an important determinant of therapy. The test is important to perform in patients with clinical stage I or II disease without B symptoms, particularly those patients in whom laparotomy is scheduled, to identify the lymph nodes to be removed. About 25% of patients classified clinically are reclassified on the basis of lymphangiogram results. The dye load associated with lymphangiography carries a small risk for pulmonary insufficiency related to extravasation of dye into the lung parenchyma, and it should not be performed in persons with severe lung disease.

Table 84.2. Staging Procedures for Hodgkin's Disease

STUDY	INDICATION
Radiographic Studies	
Chest roentgenogram	All patients; CT if mediastinal or hilar disease
Chest CT	If x-ray findings abnormal or if results would change therapy
Lymphangiogram	*Only if* (a) no clinical evidence of infradiaphragmatic disease, (b) no mass or lung disease, or (c) no advanced stage signs or B symptoms
Abdominal CT	Complements lymphangiogram; same indications
Surgical Studies	
Laparoscopy	Preferable to laparotomy in presence of B symptoms; to identify liver pathology
Laparotomy	Stage I or II disease and no symptoms
Hematologic Studies	
Bone marrow biopsy	Only if clinical stage IIB or more

CT = computed tomography.

Bone Marrow Biopsy. Biopsy of the marrow is a useful staging procedure in patients with systemic symptoms or disease beyond stage II; results are positive in up to 20% of such patients. Because disease in the marrow is often focal, multiple biopsies are necessary to avoid sampling error. Marrow aspiration is never useful. A positive result on a marrow study classifies the disease as stage IV and makes laparotomy unnecessary. Patients with clinical stage I or IIA disease have never been reported to have positive findings on marrow biopsy, but stage IIB is associated with marrow involvement in 9% of patients.

Staging Laparotomy and Laparoscopy. Removal of the spleen is reserved for patients in whom the result will change the approach to therapy (e.g., asymptomatic patients with clinical stage I or II disease who are being considered for radiotherapy alone). The procedure has the advantage of allowing a more precise definition of the extent of disease and frequently results in reclassification and implementation of a different treatment program. It includes wedge biopsy of the liver, splenectomy, and examination of the lymph nodes in contiguous chains, exclusive of mesenteric nodes. The surgery is associated with a low mortality rate (0.5% to 1.0%) and negligible early morbidity. However, patients who receive radiation and chemotherapy after splenectomy are at increased risk (up to 28% in the first 6 years) for fulminant sepsis, with its attendant 50% mortality. Those who undergo splenectomy but do not receive chemotherapy appear to be much less vulnerable to serious infection. Because of the risk for infection, only those who will have their treatment program altered by the results of laparotomy should undergo the operation. Immunizations for pneumococcal disease and other potentially life-threatening infections should be conducted before splenectomy.

Laparoscopy has been advocated as a less invasive means of identifying liver involvement in patients with a high probability of disease below the diaphragm (e.g., those with B symptoms). Liver biopsy specimens are taken from suspected areas under direct visualization. Laparoscopy is superior to percutaneous liver biopsy (20% yield vs. 5%), but its yield does not match that of open biopsy performed during staging laparotomy. Few patients with hepatic involvement are free of systemic complaints; on the other hand, neither hepatomegaly detected by physical examination or scan nor elevated alkaline phosphatase levels identify patients likely to have positive findings on biopsy.

Radionuclide Scanning. Conventional liver/spleen and bone scans lack sufficient sensitivity or specificity to warrant their routine use in staging. Results of *gallium 67 scanning* may be positive in areas of disease involvement, and occasionally previously unknown disease is discovered. Its main use is to detect residual disease in the mediastinum after treatment of bulky mediastinal disease.

Overall Approach. The history is reviewed for characteristic systemic symptoms; the physical examination focuses on lymph node–bearing areas. Chest radiography and CT are performed, as is lymphangiography and abdominal CT in patients who are clinically in stage I or II. If the patient is clinically in stage I or II and would be treated by radiation alone, a staging laparotomy should be performed to identify occult disease below the diaphragm. Until it becomes possible to predict more accurately who is likely to have occult disease in the abdomen, one must rely on the laparotomy. When systemic symptoms are present, a laparoscopy and bone marrow biopsy can be performed as preliminary studies; if either result is positive, the need for laparotomy is obviated. Lymphangiography produces too many false-negative results to be relied on without intraabdominal evaluation, and even if the result is positive, it fails to provide information about the liver and spleen, which is necessary for selecting radiation therapy, chemotherapy, or both.

Prognostic Scoring

Although staging is the single most important determinant of prognosis, staging has not been sufficient to predict fully the outcome of treatment, especially in persons presenting with advanced (i.e., stage III and IV) disease. Clinical, biologic, and demographic data have been examined by regression analysis to identify independent predictors of prognosis. Partially validated scoring systems have emerged from such analyses. One of them, derived from the International Prognostic Factors Project, is based on a serum level of *albumin* below 4.0 g/dL, a *hemoglobin* concentration below 10.5 g/dL, *male sex*, *age* older than 45 years, *stage IV* disease, *white cell count* above 15,000/mm³, and *lymphocytopenia* (<600 cells per milliliter or <8% of white cells). Patients with two features have a nearly 20% greater chance of being free of progression of disease than do patients with three features. Separate work on biologic factors of possible prognostic value find potential for *CD30* levels, number of *activated cytotoxic T cells*, presence of *CD15* in biopsy specimens, and presence of *interleukin-16*.

To be maximally useful in choice of therapy, prognostic systems will have to become better at identifying patients at greatest and least risk. Although effective, therapy for Hodgkin's disease can have morbid consequences. Carefully matching disease prognosis with aggressiveness of therapy is essential to maximize outcomes and minimize the risks of treatment.

Treatment

Although selection of a treatment regimen is the responsibility of the oncologist, it is important for the primary physician to be cognizant of the major treatment regimens and their outcomes. Treatment is a function of disease stage, not of cell type. Therapy for Hodgkin's disease achieves a substantial cure rate in all stages (Table 84.1).

Stages I and II. *Radiation therapy* is the treatment of choice. For patients with stage IA or IIA disease, *local* and *extended-field radiotherapy* to contiguous node-bearing areas and adjacent regions has resulted in an 85% to 90% cure rate. *Total nodal radiation therapy* has been used in stages IB and IIB, delivered at a dose of 3,500 to 4,500 rads during a 3- to 4-week period through a portal referred to as the "mantle" for chest radiation and the "inverted Y" for intraabdominal lymph nodes. Patients with stage IB and IIB disease have a 70% to 75% chance of cure with such radiation therapy. However, to be curative, radiation therapy must be performed with great precision, and the extent of disease must be well documented. One study found that 37% of treatment portals did not cover the entire extent of disease. *Side effects* of radiation therapy include dental problems and increased risks for *thyroid cancer* (20-year latency), *hypothyroidism* (50%), radiation *pneumonitis* (6% to 20%), accelerated *coronary artery disease* and *myocardial infarction*, and a *second solid tumor* (incidence approximately 1% annually). The risk for *leukemia* is also increased in patients receiving high doses of radiation to the bone marrow.

Chemotherapy is added to radiation when a large mediastinal mass (exceeding one-third the diameter of the chest) is present, and is substituted for radiation if the patient fails to respond or relapses. Some have argued that because success rates with chemotherapy are so great, all patients with early-stage disease should receive it. The debate continues, but radiation therapy remains the treatment of choice.

Stages III and IV. *Combination chemotherapy* is the cornerstone of treatment. The Mustargen, Oncovin, prednisone, procarbazine (*MOPP*) program was the prototype. Doxorubicin (Adriamycin), bleomycin, vinblastine, dacarbazine (*ABVD*) is currently in wide use. Combination regimens are designed to address issues of tumor resistance and drug toxicity. Hybrids and alternation of combinations have also proved effective. All are based on the identification of agents with individually distinctive mechanisms of antitumor activity. Their side effects are nonadditive, which helps to limit the amount of drug-related morbidity. Response rates for stage III and IV disease are in the 80% range, and complete remission of disease is the rule. For patients with advanced disease who experience remission, the chance of cure is 50%. By manipulation of dosages and schedules of drugs, most such chemotherapy can be delivered conveniently on an outpatient basis. In most instances, chemotherapy is administered for 6 months, at which time restaging is carried out; in the absence of residual disease, therapy is discontinued. No benefit is derived from a "maintenance program."

Choice of program remains a subject of much debate among oncologists. Of particular concern is the 20% rate of failure to respond, which has led to the use of seven-drug and alternating four-drug regimens. Problems occur with both, especially the need to prolong therapy beyond 6 months, which greatly increases the risk for toxicity. Some authorities argue that the real cause of failure to respond is the inability to administer adequate doses. In the absence of a definitive means of identifying the very high-risk patient (see above), balancing response rates with treatment-related adverse effects remains an art form that requires an oncologist experienced in the treatment of Hodgkin's disease.

Adverse effects of combination chemotherapy include sterility, secondary malignancy, and increased susceptibility to infection, in addition to those associated with individual drugs (see Chapter 88). MOPP produces *sterility* in almost all male patients. Sperm banking is indicated before initiation of therapy. Close to 90% of women over age 26 become infertile, but most younger women are able to have children; however, premature menopause is common. The incidence of sterility is significantly lower with ABVD. The risk for *leukemia* is increased for up to 10 years after chemotherapy (peak is at 5 years), especially when the program includes an alkylating agent (as in MOPP). In a comprehensive analysis of leukemia in treated Hodgkin's disease, the relative risk was 9.0 over that for radiation therapy and did not increase with concomitant radiation. Risk did increase with dose and duration of chemotherapy, stage of disease, age, and splenectomy. Leukemia risk is thought to be lower with ABVD. Despite the risk for leukemia, the gain in survival afforded by combination chemotherapy greatly outweighs its adverse effects.

Other chemotherapy-related side effects include severe *emesis*, *bone marrow suppression*, and *neuropathy* (see Chapter 88). The risk for overwhelming *pneumococcal sepsis* associated with splenectomy can be lessened by the use of polyvalent *pneumococcal vaccine*. The vaccine is often given before splenectomy but can be administered after surgery; antibody response is just as adequate after splenectomy. However, antibody production is blunted if chemotherapy is begun within 10 days of vaccination. As noted above, the risk for overwhelming sepsis approaches 30%, with a 50% fatality rate.

Radiation is sometimes employed for stage III patients. Those with stage III1A disease appear to do equally well with radiation or chemotherapy. When patients with stage IIIA disease have a large mass of mediastinal tumor, radiation is often added to their program.

Treating Relapses. Relapse occurs in 20% to 35% of patients. The probability of responding to repeated treatment ("salvage" therapy) is a function of the length of the initial remission and approaches 95%, even if the original chemotherapeutic regimen is used. A non–cross-resistant regimen, such as ABVD, can be used either in place of the original program or in some form of combination with it. Relapse-free survival of 45% at 10 years has been noted for patients retreated after an initial remission of more than 12 months; however, overall survival falls to 24% because of complications of retreatment (e.g., second malignancy). For those with an initial remission of less than 12 months, the survival after retreatment is about 10% at 10 years. The use of *autologous bone marrow transplantation* in drug-resistant patients has provided new options. Retreatment after transplantation produces remission in 50% and extended disease-free periods in a fourth to a half of those who respond.

Monitoring Therapy

Periodic examination of involved nodes is the simplest means of judging response to therapy. Many laboratory parameters have been developed but offer little advantage over physical examination and chest radiography. The need for periodic restaging is a judgment to be made in consultation with the oncologist. Patients receiving MOPP require close surveillance (see Chapter 88). Patients being treated with radiation should be watched for bone marrow suppression and, when lung fields are involved, radiation pneumonitis and thyroid dysfunction.

The likelihood of *late relapse* (36 months or more after completion of therapy) is small, but large enough to warrant continued monitoring. The risk for late relapse is low, but patients with stage I disease show the highest rates, perhaps because of failure to irradiate all involved nodes. Also at risk for recurrence are patients presenting with a large mediastinal tumor; local recurrence is typical. Gallium scanning has proved useful in such cases, although biopsy confirmation is necessary because false-positives do occur. Most relapses are detected by history, physical examination, or chest radiography; abdominal CT may also help detect late disease. Careful late follow-up is warranted, even after 3 years, because response to retreatment is good.

Patient Education and Indications for Consultation and Referral

Many patients will greet the diagnosis of Hodgkin's disease with dread, equating it with a fatal outcome. Without raising false hopes, the physician can point to the excellent 5-year survival rates and the high percentage of patients who are disease-free after 10 years. Patients who have undergone splenectomy should be advised to undergo vaccination with polyvalent pneumococcal vaccine before starting chemotherapy or radiation.

Because chemotherapy can cause permanent sterility, it is important to review this prospect with the patient before treatment is begun. Pretherapy sperm storage has been advocated. Young women (under age 26) can be counseled in encouraging terms because they have been found capable of bearing phenotypically normal children.

Once the diagnosis is confirmed and clinical staging is completed, referral to the oncologist for a discussion of pathologic staging and design of a treatment program is indicated. During the period of initial treatment, the patient will be followed closely by the oncologist, but the primary physician can and should serve to coordinate care and provide support to the patient and family.

NON-HODGKIN'S LYMPHOMAS

The non-Hodgkin's lymphomas represent a diverse group of malignancies originating from lymphocytes. About 85% arise from B cells, with the remainder deriving from T cells. The wide range of histologic appearances that characterize the non-Hodgkin's lymphomas is believed to represent arrest of maturation at different stages of cellular development. The etiology remains unknown, but risk factors include viral infection, mutation of oncogenes, connective tissue disease, prior Hodgkin's disease, and immunodeficiency states.

Classification, Prognosis, and Clinical Presentation

Classification and Prognosis. In contrast to the histopathologic characteristics of Hodgkin's disease, those of the non-Hodgkin lymphomas are major determinants of prognosis and response to therapy, whereas stage at the time of presentation is of less importance. A host of histologic classification schemes have been put forward. The most widely accepted is the one referred to as the *Working Formulation* (Table 84.3). It relates histology to prognosis, with nodal architecture, degree of differentiation, and cell type being the important determinants.

Three *histopathologic categories* emerge: *low-grade* (indolent), *intermediate-grade* (aggressive), and *high-grade* (highly aggressive). Survival for patients with untreated low-grade disease extends for years; for those with intermediate-grade disease, it declines to several months; and for high-grade disease,

it is measured in weeks. However, the response to therapy often follows an inverse pattern, with some of the many aggressive tumors responding readily to therapy and exhibiting a potential for cure, whereas most low-grade lymphomas prove stubborn and typically relapse.

Clinical Presentation. Unlike Hodgkin's disease, non-Hodgkin's lymphomas are multicentric in origin and can appear in discontinuous lymph node chains. *Localized* and *regional* lymphomas (stages I and II, respectively; see below) account for fewer than 10% of cases. Most of the remainder present with *disseminated* disease (stage III or IV). Non-Hodgkin's lymphomas can occur in nodal sites, viscera, or both. Mediastinal disease is found in 20%. *Extranodal disease* is often solitary and likely to be confined to the organ of origin. Waldeyer's ring, the upper gastrointestinal tract, testes, and bone are the most commonly involved extranodal sites, accounting for up to 15% of cases. Extranodal disease can have a favorable prognosis, particularly in the absence of nodal involvement. Five-year survival rates are as high as 30% to 50% irrespective of pathologic type. A unique site of extranodal disease is the central nervous system, especially the epidural space, leptomeninges, and cerebral hemispheres. This form of lymphoma has a high association with HIV infection. The propensity for the development of central nervous system lymphoma is also related to histologic type (lymphoblastic), distribution (marrow spread), and age (younger patients).

Presentation is affected by tumor grade. Patients with high-grade disease are likely to present with a rapidly growing, symptomatic mass confined to a single nodal or extranodal site. Low-grade disease typically manifests as slowing enlarging nodes at multiple sites. Fever, night sweats, and weight loss are more common in non-Hodgkin's lymphoma than they are in Hodgkin's disease.

Anemia is a common consequence of lymphoma. Mechanisms include immune hemolysis, hypersplenism, and marrow infiltration. In some patients, the lymphoma cells circulating in the blood may be sufficiently numerous to appear on a peripheral blood smear. In others, a *leukemic phase* may develop and account for the appearance of malignant cells on peripheral smear.

Immune dysfunction occurs in many patients, which should not be surprising given that most lymphomas are B-cell disor-

Table 84.3. Working Formulation of Non-Hodgkin's Lymphomas

GRADE AND CELL TYPE	FREQUENCY (%)	SURVIVAL (Y)
I. Low-Grade Lymphoma	39% total	5–7 years
A. Small lymphocytic	4	
B. Follicular, small cleaved cell	26	
C. Follicular, mixed, small cleaved cell	9	
II. Intermediate-Grade Lymphoma	41% total	2–5 years
D. Follicular, predominantly large cell	4	
E. Diffuse small cleaved cell	8	
F. Diffuse mixed, small, large cell	7	
G. Diffuse large cell, cleaved/noncleaved	22	
III. High-Grade Lymphoma	20% total	0.5–2 years
H. Diffuse large cell; immunoblastic	9	
I. Lymphoblastic	6	
J. Small noncleaved cell (Burkitt's, non-Burkitt's	5	

Adapted from Rosenberg SA. National Cancer Institute–sponsored study of classifications of non-Hodgkin lymphomas: summary and description of a working formulation for clinical usuage. Cancer 1980;45:2188, with permission.

ders. Humoral immunity is particularly impaired, leading to hypogammaglobulinemia, monoclonal gammopathies, hemolytic anemias, and immune destruction of platelets.

Staging

The staging system for lymphoma is identical to that used for Hodgkin's disease, with the exception that there are no categories for symptoms or designations for contiguous visceral involvement or splenic disease. As noted above, stage is less a determinant of prognosis and treatment selection than it is for Hodgkin's disease, but it still plays some role in the selection and intensity of treatment. Pending a better staging system, the Ann Arbor scheme (Table 84.4) continues to be used for non-Hodgkin's lymphoma, although distinctions between stages have less meaning. For patients with low-grade disease, the main issue therapeutically is whether their disease is localized or disseminated. For more aggressive forms of disease, extent of disease is less important.

Although the approach to staging is in part determined by tumor histology (see below), some generalizations are appropriate. A thorough *physical examination* of all node-bearing areas is essential, including such sites as the epitrochlear nodes, Waldeyer's ring, and the preauricular area. The liver and spleen are commonly enlarged when involved and should be carefully checked. Radiologic investigations are especially important in patients thought to have local or regional disease. *Chest radiography* and *CT* of the *chest, abdomen,* and *pelvis* are obtained. In many centers, CT of the abdomen and pelvis has replaced *lymphangiography* for nodal survey and has the added advantage of providing information about liver and spleen size. However, lymphangiography is a reasonable alternative where CT is unavailable. CT is considerably better at detecting disease in the pelvis and retroperitoneum.

Hematologic assessment is critical and includes examination of the *peripheral smear* and *bone marrow* (aspirate plus biopsy specimen). Bilateral or multiple bone marrow biopsies can identify occult stage IV disease. In a series of 131 patients, 27% had positive biopsy findings when more than one marrow site was sampled. Aspiration is inadequate because the false-negative rate is 30%; a solid bone marrow specimen is essential.

Much of the staging workup depends on clinical or histopathologic findings. For example, patients with intermediate-grade disease found in the area of Waldeyer's ring are at increased risk for gastrointestinal involvement and need to undergo endoscopy if the clinical picture is suggestive. Patients with a high-grade histologic pattern are almost certain to have advanced disease at the time of presentation and need not undergo extensive study. *Lumbar puncture* should be considered in patients at risk for central nervous system spread (i.e., those with marrow involvement, lymphoblastic histology, young age, or HIV infection).

Several staging procedures are unnecessary. *Laparotomy* is *not* indicated because the yields from CT and bone marrow biopsy are so high that rarely do the findings from laparotomy influence clinical decision making. *Gallium scanning* is also not very helpful.

Therapy

Chemotherapy is the predominant mode of treatment for non-Hodgkin's lymphoma (Table 84.4) because most patients already have widespread disease at the time of initial clinical presentation. It may be administered as a single agent or as a complex multidrug regimen. Radiation plays a role in the management of localized disease. As noted, histology and stage are, respectively, the primary and secondary determinants of response to therapy. Absence of bulky disease, minimal extranodal disease, absence of B symptoms, young age, and female gender are other predictors of response to therapy and prolonged survival.

Low-grade (Indolent) Disease. The curability of low-grade disease remains a subject of controversy. Most forms of therapy produce responses and remissions, but relapses are the rule. The rare patient with true early-stage disease is typically treated with *radiation*. For patients with more advanced indolent disease, treatment is controversial. Most histopathologic types appear to respond with complete remission to *combination*

Table 84.4. Treatment of Non-Hodgkin's Lymphomas

GRADE AND STAGE	TREATMENT	LONG-TERM REMISSION (1%)[a]
Low-Grade		Unknown
Early stage	Radiation	
Late stage	Controversial (single or multiagent chemotherapy interferon,[b] radiation,[b] watchful waiting[b])	
Intermediate-Grade		
Early stage	Multiagent chemotherapy +/− radiation	85–95
Late stage	Multiagent chemotherapy	60–80
High-Grade		
All stages	High-dose multiagent chemotherapy, autologous marrow transplantation[b]	20–40

[a]Long-term remission is *not* synonymous with cure; cure rates actually increase with advancing grade of disease.
[b]Investigational method.
Adapted from Longo DL, DeVita VT Jr, Jaffee ES, et al. Lymphocytic lymphomas. In: DeVita VT Jr, Hellman S, Rosenberg SA, eds. Cancer: principles and practice of oncology, 5th ed. Philadelphia: JB Lippincott Williams and Wilkins, 1997:2250, with permission.

chemotherapy, high-dose single-agent therapy, radiation, or *combined-modality therapy*, but relapse is common after 2 years. Remission after retreatment is common, but cure has never been reported (except for those with the follicular mixed cell type), and the benefit of aggressive chemotherapy versus watchful waiting remains to be demonstrated. Overall, median survival is about 10 years, regardless of type of therapy used. Some centers use aggressive chemotherapy plus radiation, followed by *autologous bone marrow transplantation* in selected patients who relapse. The approach must still be considered investigational until long-term results are available, but they appear to be encouraging. Another approach is the use of *interferon alfa* plus combination chemotherapy, which appears to give better results than chemotherapy alone. *Isotope-labeled monoclonal antibodies* are also under investigation.

Intermediate-grade (Aggressive) Disease. Among patients with *localized disease*, *combination chemotherapy* [e.g., with CHOP (cyclophosphamde, hydroxydaunomycin, Oncovin, prednisone)] with or without *local radiation* to the involved area provides 5-year disease-free results in as many as 85% to 95%. Besides histopathology and stage, outcome is adversely affected by advancing age, B symptoms, marrow involvement, elevations in lactate dehydrogenase, a large abdominal mass, and multiple extranodal sites. In patients who fail to respond or who relapse after an initial response, secondary therapy is employed, consisting of non–cross-resistant drugs such as bleomycin and doxorubicin.

Advanced-stage disease has been treated with more *aggressive combination chemotherapy*, which provides complete remissions in 80% and long-term survival in up to 70% of patients who can tolerate full therapy. However, drug-related toxicity and serious complications are far more frequent with the more aggressive programs, so that dose reductions are often necessary that compromise outcomes and result in long-term survival rates of only 30%. High-level expression of the *BCL-2* oncogene is associated with a poor prognosis. The survival of patients who relapse is improved with *high-dose chemotherapy* and *autologous bone marrow transplantation*.

High-grade (Highly Aggressive) Disease. *Intensive chemotherapy* utilizing multidrug regimens is indicated for patients with symptomatic or rapidly progressive disease. For localized disease, the addition of *radiation* therapy improves absolute rates of survival by more than 13 percentage points. Tumor burden, lactate dehydrogenase levels, *p53* gene mutations, and interleukin-6 levels correlate with prognosis. High-dose chemotherapy in combination with *autologous bone marrow transplantation* has proved superior to standard-dose therapy in persons with diffuse large-cell disease. Lymphoblastic and some Burkitt's lymphomas are treated with regimens similar to those for acute leukemia. Response rates with multidrug therapy approach 95%, with a median survival in excess of 2 years. For some subgroups, combination chemotherapy may result in cure for 20% to 40% of patients.

Investigational Therapies include the use of monoclonal antibodies, autologous bone marrow transplantation, and interferon. Because most lymphomas are of B-cell origin, identification of a specific antigen allows a *monoclonal antibody* against the tumor cell to be developed. Monoclonal antibodies have induced remissions but are associated with the development of immune responses against the immunoglobulin in some patients. Another approach is to perform *autologous bone marrow transplantation*, sometimes after treating the marrow with monoclonal antibodies to purge it of tumor cells. The best candidates for transplantation appear to be those who are responsive to chemotherapy and are in a second remission. Five-year disease-free results have been reported in 30% to 60% of carefully selected patients, but risk is high, with up to 10% of patients dying of complications associated with the procedure. Clinical trials with *interferon* are under way; partial remissions have been achieved.

Monitoring Therapy

Monitoring patients on chemotherapy requires close surveillance (see Chapter 88). Bone marrow suppression is the leading complication. Relapse or recurrence generally develops in the areas of previous disease (in contrast to Hodgkin's disease, in which relapse is extranodal or visceral). Relapse typically occurs within 12 to 18 months of initiation of treatment. Watching for the development of neurologic symptoms is particularly important in those with a predisposition to central nervous system spread (see above).

Patient Education

The encouraging results of chemotherapy, particularly in patients with aggressive advanced disease, provide new hope. As with Hodgkin's disease, the patient can be given a fairly accurate assessment of the prognosis after careful histologic study and staging have been carried out. Often, the prognosis is far better than the patient's fearful expectations and can be shared profitably. Even elderly patients are candidates for treatment of life-threatening disease.

A detailed review of possible adverse effects of therapy (e.g., sterility, infection; see Chapter 88) must be reviewed, as must the experimental nature of those therapies for which data on long-term outcomes are lacking. A key question remaining is what constitutes the best approach to advanced stages of indolent disease.

Indications for Referral

These malignancies are potentially curable. Referral to the oncologist should be made early, when the diagnosis is first suspected. Management of the patient with Hodgkin's disease or lymphoma needs to be a cooperative venture from the start, with the primary physician working closely with the oncologist experienced in lymphoma. Selection of a treatment modality requires the judgment of an oncologist who is knowledgeable about available protocols, which are constantly undergoing revision. The primary physician monitors response and adverse effects, maintains continuity, and provides psychological support.

A.H.G.

ANNOTATED BIBLIOGRAPHY

Hodgkin's Disease

Aisenberg A. The staging and treatment of Hodgkin's disease. N Engl J Med 1978;299:1288. (*Classic article establishing the utility of staging laparotomy.*)

Bookman MA, Longo DL. Concomitant illness in patients treated for Hodgkin's disease. Cancer Treat Rev 1986;13:77. (*Exhaustive review of medical problems associated with the illness and its treatments.*)

Brice P. Prognostic factors in advanced Hodgkin's disease—can they guide therapeutic decisions? N Engl J Med 1998;33:1547. (*A critical look at predictors; concludes that they are getting better and can help in some decisions, but not yet in the most important ones.*)

Devita VT Jr, Hubbard SM. Hodgkin's disease. N Engl J Med 1993;328:580. (*Authoritative review of chemotherapy, including a discussion of treatment according to stage, program selection, and salvage therapy; 63 references.*)

Hasenclever D, Diehl V. A prognostic score for advanced Hodgkin's disease. N Engl J Med 1998;339:1506. (*A partially validated means of determining prognosis by using readily available patient and clinical data.*)

Hoppe RT, Coleman CN, Cox RS, et al. The management of stage I–II Hodgkin's disease with irradiation alone or combined-modality therapy: the Stanford experience. Blood 1982;59:455. (*Radiotherapy curative for early-stage disease.*)

Horning SJ, Hoppe RT, Kaplan HS, et al. Female reproductive potential after treatment for Hodgkin's disease. N Engl J Med 1981;304:1377. (*Women under the age of 26 successfully treated for Hodgkin's disease became pregnant and delivered phenotypically normal children.*)

Kaldor JM, Day NE, Clarke EA, et al. Leukemia following Hodgkin's disease. N Engl J Med 1990;322:7. (*Case–control study of international cancer registries; risk for leukemia greatly increased by chemotherapy, but not by radiation.*)

Phillips GL, Wolff SN, Herzig RH, et al. Treatment of progressive Hodgkin's disease with intensive chemoradiotherapy and autologous bone marrow transplantation in refractory Hodgkin's disease. Blood 1989;73:2086. (*Improved response achieved.*)

Rosenberg SA, Kaplan HS. The evolution and summary results of the Stanford randomized clinical trials of the management of Hodgkin's disease: 1962–1984. Int J Radiat Oncol Biol Phys 1985;11:5. (*Summary report focusing on radiation therapy from a leading center.*)

Seymour JF, Talpaz M, Hagemeister FB, et al. Clinical correlates of elevated serum levels of interleukin-6 in patients with untreated Hodgkin's disease. Am J Med 1997;102:21. (*Levels correlated with severity, activity, and response to treatment.*)

Siber GR, Gorham C, Martin P, et al. Antibody response to pretreatment immunization and post-treatment boosting with bacterial polysaccharide vaccines in patients with Hodgkin's disease. Ann Intern Med 1986;104:467. (*Antibody response was not affected by the timing of immunization relative to splenectomy, but was blunted if chemotherapy was begun within 10 days of immunization.*)

Somers R, Carde P, Henry-Amar M, et al. A randomized study in stages IIIB and IV Hodgkin's disease comparing eight courses of MOPP versus an alternation of MOPP with ABVD. J Clini Oncol 1994;12:279. (*A major multicenter European trial; the alternating program improved response and failure-free survival, but not overall survival.*)

Non-Hodgkin's Lymphoma

Aisenberg AC. Cell lineage in lymphoproliferative disease. Am J Med 1983;74:679. (*Still one of the most lucid discussions on designating lymphomas on the basis of T- or B-cell origin.*)

Anderson T, Chabner BA, Young RC, et al. Malignant lymphoma. Histology and staging of 473 patients at the National Cancer Institute. Cancer 1982;50:2699. (*Review of histology and staging in a retrospective series, with emphasis on relationship to prognosis and response to therapy.*)

Armitage JO. Treatment of non-Hodgkin's lymphoma. N Engl J Med 1993;328:1023. (*Detailed but very useful review for the generalist reader.*)

Brunning R, Bloomfield C, McKenna R, et al. Bilateral trephine bone marrow biopsies in lymphoma and other neoplastic diseases. Ann Intern Med 1975;82:365. (*Reports a 37% yield from bilateral sampling, compared with a 20% yield from unilateral sampling.*)

Gianni AM, Bregni M, Siena S, et al. High-dose chemotherapy and autologous bone marrow transplantation compared with MACOP-B in aggressive B-cell lymphoma. N Engl J Med 1997;336:1290. (*Randomized trial; high-dose therapy plus transplantation proved best.*)

Gordon LI, Harrington D, Andersen J, et al. Comparison of a second-generation combination chemotherapeutic regimen (m-BACOD) with a standard regimen (CHOP) for advanced diffuse non-Hodgkin's lymphoma. N Engl J Med 1992;327:1342. (*Less aggressive program provided equivalent remission and survival results, with lower rates of adverse effects.*)

Ichiwawa A, Kinoshita T, Watanabe T, et al. Mutations of the p53 gene as a prognostic factor in aggressive B-cell lymphoma. N Engl J Med 1997;337:529. (*Mutations associated with poor prognosis.*)

Miller TP, Dahlberg S, Cassady JR, et al. Chemotherapy alone compared with chemotherapy plus radiotherapy for localized intermediate- and high-grade non-Hodgkin's lymphoma. N Engl J Med 1998;339:21. (*Multicenter prospective, randomized trial; combined-modality therapy was superior.*)

National Cancer Institute. Classification of non-Hodgkin's lymphomas: summary and description of a working formulation for clinical usage. Cancer 1982;49:2112. (*International effort to construct a working classification scheme.*)

Phillip T, Guglielmi C, Hagenbeek A, et al. Autologous bone marrow transplantation compared with salvage chemotherapy in relapses of chemotherapy-sensitive non-Hodgkin's lymphoma. N Engl J Med 1995;333:1540. (*Improved response rate and event-free and overall survival.*)

Preti HA, Cabanillas F, Talpaz M, et al. Prognostic value of serum interleukin-6 in diffuse large-cell lymphoma. Ann Intern Med 1997;127:186. (*A retrospective cohort analysis; serum levels of interleukin-6 found to be an independent prognostic factor.*)

Simon R, Durrleman S, Hoppe RT, et al. The non-Hodgkin lymphoma pathologic classification project. Ann Intern Med 1988;109:939. (*Outcome predominantly a function of histology and stage.*)

Smalley RV, Andersen JW, Hawkins MJ, et al. Interferon alfa combined with cytotoxic chemotherapy for patients with non-Hodgkin's lymphoma. N Engl J Med 1992;327:1336. (*Interferon improved outcome in patients with low- to intermediate-grade tumors.*)

Straus DJ, Gaynor JJ, Leiberman PH, et al. Non-Hodgkin's lymphomas: characteristics of long-term survivors following conservative treatment. Am J Med 1987;82:247. (*Good histology, little bulk, age below 60, no B symptoms, early-stage disease correlated with good outcome.*)

Vose JM, Armitage JO, Weisenburger DD, et al. The importance of age in survival of patients treated with chemotherapy for aggressive non-Hodgkin's lymphoma. J Clin Oncol 1988;6:1838. (*Although advancing age may reduce the response rate, it does not obviate the benefit of treatment.*)

Young RC, Longo DL, Dlatstein E, et al. The treatment of indolent lymphomas: watchful waiting vs. aggressive combined-modality treatment. Semin Hematol 1988;25[Suppl 2]:11. (*Addresses one of the key questions; interim data.*)

85
Approach to the Patient with Metastatic Tumor of Unknown Origin

A malignancy is designated as a tumor of unknown origin (TUO) after meeting several criteria: (a) the tissue is histologically confirmed to be malignant and a primary tumor of the organ is ruled out; (b) routine screening fails to identify the primary source; and (c) a very late metastasis (as occurs in breast cancer, melanoma, and renal cell carcinoma) is also ruled out.

A TUO poses several problems, ranging from the utility of pursuing further workup to the efficacy of empiric therapy for disease that is already widely metastatic. Any decision to conduct a more extensive evaluation or treat empirically must include a consideration of the low probability that a treatable cancer is present. Moreover, the evaluation of a TUO can prove expensive and uncomfortable. However, within this very heterogeneous group are a few very responsive malignancies that can be effectively treated if recognized.

Guided by the principle of looking only for treatable disease, the primary physician should be able to conduct the major part of an effective workup in the outpatient setting and work closely with the oncologist in presenting thoughtful treatment options to the patient.

CLINICAL PRESENTATION AND NATURAL HISTORY OF DISEASE

Clinical Presentation. Common sites of metastatic presentation are the lung, mediastinum, liver, bone, and lymph nodes. Others include the bone marrow, brain, spinal cord, peritoneum, and retroperitoneum. In the *lung*, a TUO may present as a solitary nodule, multiple nodules, or recurrent pleural effusion (see Chapters 43 and 44). When a TUO presents in the mediastinum, it often does so as a catastrophic secondary complication, such as dysphagia, stridor or respiratory difficulty, or superior vena cava syndrome. In *bone*, a TUO may appear as a lytic or blastic lesion of the axial skeleton, long bones, or skull. Sometimes, the patient reports bone pain or has a pathologic fracture. Often, a TUO is discovered as an incidental radiographic finding. *Bone marrow* invasion may be heralded by pancytopenia or a myelophthisic picture.

An isolated hard *lymph node* is another important presentation of a TUO. Asymmetric cervical, axillary, or inguinal disease is characteristic. Axillary nodes that histologically manifest adenocarcinoma are most commonly associated with ipsilateral breast cancer, even in the presence of normal findings on a breast examination and mammogram. The presence of carcinoma in an inguinal node may represent local spread from carcinoma of the vulva, prostate, perineum, endometrium, or ovary, or it may represent systemic involvement by lymphoma. Metastasis from testicular cancer usually does not present as inguinal adenopathy except in cases of previous pelvic and retroperitoneal node dissection.

Liver involvement is usually discovered when results of liver function tests are abnormal (e.g., isolated elevation of alkaline phosphatase), a hepatic nodule is detected on physical examination, or a focal defect is noted on abdominal ultrasonography or liver scan. When a primary is discovered, the most frequent sites of origin prove to be the pancreas, liver, bowel, and stomach. Tumor that has spread to the *peritoneum* can lead to malignant ascites. Involvement of the *retroperitoneum* is usually a silent consequence of spread by lymphomas and genital cancers. *Brain* metastasis may be asymptomatic, but the new onset of a focal deficit or headache is suggestive. *Spinal cord* involvement may present urgently with symptoms of cord compression (see Chapter 167).

A number of newly appreciated treatment-responsive tumors that often present as TUOs have been defined. Most manifest a poorly differentiated or undifferentiated histologic appearance. For example, *poorly differentiated carcinoma* of *neuroendocrine origin* (determined by electron microscopy) is quite responsive to treatment (60% response rate) and typically involves the mediastinum, peripheral lymph nodes, and retroperitoneum. *Extragonadal germ cell cancers* are another subset of poorly differentiated carcinomas that respond to treatment. They too manifest as disease of the mediastinum, retroperitoneum, or lymph nodes. Other features are patient age of less than 50 years and elevations in serum human chorionic gonadotropin (HCG) or α-fetoprotein (AFP) levels. *Adenocarcinoma of the peritoneum* causing malignant ascites in a woman with no known primary responds to treatment for ovarian carcinoma, even when no ovarian disease can be found; median survival increases to 23 months. Atypical presentations of *prostate cancer* may include a poorly differentiated or undifferentiated histology and little clinical evidence of a primary lesion.

Natural History and Clinical Course. Because a TUO represents metastatic disease, it should not be surprising that overall median survival is usually no more than 3 to 4 months; about 25% survive 1 year, and fewer than 10% are alive after 5 years. Overall survival is not improved by treatment when all TUO patients are considered as a group, although outcomes for responsive clinical and histopathologic subgroups can be improved considerably with treatment (see below).

DIFFERENTIAL DIAGNOSIS

Based on data from autopsy studies, pancreatic carcinoma leads the list of causes of cancer of unknown origin, accounting for about 25% of cases. Cancers of the lung, kidney, colorectum, and prostate cancer together account for another 30%. From the perspective of workup and management, a consideration of potentially treatable cancers is most important (Table 85.1); this is aided by a differential diagnosis according to region of presentation (Table 85.2). In older men, the most common treatable malignancy is prostate cancer; in younger men, it

Table 85.1. Treatable Malignancies That May Present as a Tumor of Unknown Origin

Potentially curable, even when metastatic
Gestational trophoblastic tumors
Germ cell cancer, gonadal (e.g., testicular carcinoma)
Hodgkin's disease
Non-Hodgkin's lymphoma
Squamous cell carcinoma of the oropharynx
? Poorly differentiated carcinoma of neuroendocrine type[a]
? Poorly differentiated carcinoma of extragonadal germ cell origin[a]

Very responsive to treatment, although not curable when metastatic
Prostate cancer
Breast cancer
Small-cell carcinoma of the lung
Ovarian carcinoma
Endometrial cancer
Thyroid cancer
Poorly differentiated carcinoma of neuroendocrine type[a]
Poorly differentiated carcinoma of extragonadal germ cell origin[a]
Peritoneal carcinomatosis[a]

[a]Presents as tumor of unknown origin with poorly differentiated or undifferentiated histology.

is testicular carcinoma. In women, breast and ovarian cancers lead the list. Other important causes are cancers of the nasopharynx, oropharynx, and lung (small-cell type). As noted, even patients with a poorly differentiated or undifferentiated histology may have a treatable cancer, such as lymphoma, neuroendocrine carcinoma, extragonadal germ cell cancer, peritoneal carcinomatosis, or carcinoma of the prostate. Although a number of other subtly presenting tumors (e.g., pancreatic carcinoma, melanoma) are probably responsible for many TUO presentations, they are not sufficiently responsive to treatment to warrant listing.

WORKUP

Searching for Treatable Disease

When faced with a TUO, the priority is to search for treatable disease. Conducting the workup on the basis of probability rather than on responsiveness to therapy (Table 85.3) may lead to searches that have little impact on outcome. The expense and discomfort incurred by the many diagnostic studies ordered in search of likely but poorly responsive disease can be avoided if the physician adopts the discipline of searching for malignancies that respond to treatment (Tables 85.1 through 85.4). In similar fashion, once a metastatic lesion has been identified, it is *not necessary to stage* the patient for other sites of metastases because the incurable nature of the tumor has already been revealed. Thus, the patient who presents with a pulmonary nodule and is found to have breast cancer as a primary source does not require a liver scan to document the presence of liver disease. Treatment in patients with cancer is determined first and foremost by stage of disease, but once metastases have been identified, the tumor is sufficiently staged.

Histologic Diagnosis

The importance of *biopsy* and histologic diagnosis cannot be overstated. Before other investigations are initiated in search of a treatable cancer, a thorough *histologic assessment* of tissue from the metastatic site should be conducted. Because im-

Table 85.2. Treatable Causes of Metastic Disease by Site of Presentation

SITE OF PRESENTATION	SOURCE OF PRIMARY
Lung and mediastinum	Lung (small cell)
	Breast
	Hodgkin's disease
	Estragonadal germ cell
	Neuroendocrine
	Germ cell (testicular)
Bone	
Osteoblastic lesions	Prostate
	Lung (small-cell)
	Hodgkin's disease
Osteolytic or mixed lesions	Breast
Liver	Breast
	Lung (small-cell)
Brain	Breast
	Lung (small-cell)
	Lymphoma
Bone marrow	Breast
	Lung (small-cell)
	Prostate
Lymph nodes	
High cervical	Squamous cell cancer
	Hodgkin's disease, lymphoma
	Neuroendocrine
Axillary	Breast (ipsilateral)
	Lymphoma
	Lung (small-cell)
Inguinal	Prostate
	Ovary
	Endometrium
	Lymphoma
Retroperitonal	Lymphoma
	Hodgkin's disease
	Testes
	Prostate
	Ovarian
	Neuroendocrine
	Extragonadal germ cell

Table 85.3. Common Cancers and Their Responsiveness to Therapy

TUMOR	RESPONSE RATE (%)
Responsive	
Breast	40–60
Ovary	60–70
Prostate	60–70
Head, neck	50–70
Testicular	80–100
Lymphoma	80
Lung (small-cell)	80
Marginally Responsive	
Neurosecretory	30–50
Sarcoma	30
Colon, other GI tumors	10–15
Melanoma	10–15
Hepatoma	20
Unresponsive	
Renal	
Lung (non-small-cell)	
Brain	

GI, gastrointestinal.

Table 85.4. Diagnosis of Some Treatable Cancers Presenting as Tumor of Unknown Origin

MALIGNANCY	DIAGNOSTIC FEATURES OR STUDIES
Squamous cell, nasopharynx oropharynx	PE (nodule, plaque), CT or MRI, blind biopsy
Lymphoma	PE (adenopathy) immunohistochemical stains
Ovarian cancer	PE (ascites or mass), pelvic CT or MRI, AFP, HCG, peritoneal implants
Prostate cancer	PE (nodule), PSA, prostate ultrasonography, immunohistochemical stains
Breast cancer	PE (breast nodule), receptor studies
Testicular cancer	PE (testicular nodule), ultrasonography, serum AFP, HCG
Extragonadal germ cell cancer	PE (adenopathy), CT (lung nodules, mediastinal mass, retroperitoneal mass), immunohistochemical studies, serum AFP, HCG
Neuroendocrine carcinoma	PE (adenopathy), CT (retroperitoneal nodes, mediastinal nodes), EM

PE, physical examination; CT, computed tomography; MRI, magnetic resonance imaging; AFP, α-fetoprotein; HCG, human chorionic gonadotropin; PSA, prostate-specific antigen; EM, electron microscopy.

munohistochemical, electron microscopic, and receptor studies may need to be performed on the sample, adequate tissue must be obtained and processed properly. One portion is quick-frozen for immunohistologic study, another placed in formalin for hematoxylin and eosin staining, and a third placed in glutaraldehyde for electron microscopy. Cytologic sampling is usually insufficient because it does not provide architectural information, which can be critical for diagnosis. Moreover, cytologic preparation may misrepresent nuclear and cytoplasmic abnormalities, which can be induced by inflammation or drugs. Therefore, in patients with serositis and pleural or peritoneal effusions, the cytologic diagnosis should be confirmed by tissue diagnosis.

The histologic assessment begins with diagnosis of the tumor by cell type (adenocarcinoma, lymphoma, small-cell carcinoma of the lung, sarcoma, squamous cell carcinoma, melanoma, undifferentiated). *Special stains*, such as the one for *mucin* (found in cancers of the prostate and kidney), may be utilized. The histologic designation of *adenocarcinoma* does not definitively establish the primary source of the tumor. A glandular malignancy can develop in any organ. The histologic distinction between adenocarcinoma of the ovary, stomach, lung, or breast is sometimes possible by pathology laboratory methods, but other approaches may be needed, including clinical assessment (see below).

The histologic designation of *undifferentiated carcinoma* presumes a level of anaplasia that precludes reliable identification of the origin of the malignancy. If this is encountered, *immunohistochemical staining* is used to search for diagnostically important intracellular substances, such as prostate-specific antigen (PSA) and prostatic acid phosphatase for prostate cancer, and AFP and HCG for germ cell tumors. The technique may also detect substances useful in differentiating a carcinoma

from a lymphoma, melanoma, or germ cell tumor. Immunohistochemical analysis has become the ancillary test of choice in the workup of undifferentiated carcinoma.

Electron microscopy can be useful when immunohistochemistry is inconclusive. Subcellular structures are examined for evidence of differentiation from which one can infer the cell line of origin (i.e., its histogenesis). Such a review of ultrastructure can help classify a cell as epithelial, mesenchymal, mesothelial, or melanocytic in origin, and subclassify within each category according to characteristic ultrastructural features (e.g., melanosomes, membrane-bound secretory granules, elongated microvilli, lysosomes, large bundles of tonofilaments, membrane-bound mucin vacuoles). However, because of problems with sampling and cell preservation, the sensitivity and specificity of electron microscopy are not high. The sample must be cut into very small cubes (which makes for sampling errors) and preserved in glutaraldehyde promptly (any delay in processing or use of a fixative other than glutaraldehyde can distort cell architecture).

Other studies include testing for the presence of *estrogen* and *progesterone receptors*, which helps to identify breast cancer, although these receptors are also found in ovarian and endometrial cancers. *Cytogenetic studies* are a promising diagnostic technique and likely to enhance tumor identification as the methodology matures. Among the growing list of molecular diagnostic methodologies is *polymerase chain reaction* technology, which allows specific nucleic acid sequences to be detected.

Clinical Assessment

All patients should undergo a careful *physical examination* that concentrates on the detection of treatable malignant disease (i.e., cancer of the breast, uterus, or ovaries in women; cancer of the prostate or testicles in men; lymphoma in all patients). Depending on the site of metastasis, other elements of the physical examination may also prove useful (see below and Table 85.4).

Similarly, *laboratory studies* are guided by the same principle of looking for treatable cancer rather than conducting an extensive workup for all possible primary tumors. An unfocused search can lead to the ordering of many unnecessary, uncomfortable, or expensive tests. Studies should be directed at the detection of treatable cancer [e.g., *mammography* for breast cancer, *ultrasonography* for a testicular or prostatic cancer, *computed tomography* (CT) for ovarian disease]. The clinical presentation (see Table 85.2 and below) in conjunction with pathologic data can help guide the workup. Most routine blood chemistries are not helpful, although a few *serologic markers* (e.g., prostate-specific antigen, AFP, β-HCG subunit) can aid in searching for treatable disease (Table 85.4).

Pulmonary Nodules, Pleural Effusions, and Mediastinal Masses. An *open biopsy* procedure is generally necessary to obtain sufficient tissue for detailed histopathologic study and definitive diagnosis. A needle aspiration rarely suffices. Of particular importance is the identification of small-cell, neuroendocrine, and extragonadal germ cell cancers and lymphoma, which are among the more treatable malignancies that present as mediastinal or rapidly growing pulmonary mass lesions. In most other instances, identification of the primary does not affect outcome. Detailed study by the pathologist can be very useful. *Electron microscopy* and *immunohistochemical studies* are essential, complemented by *serologic testing* for *AFP* and β-HCG subunit.

Pleural effusions caused by malignancy can be identified cytologically, but a *pleural biopsy* in conjunction with aspiration is more informative (see Chapter 43). A diagnosis of adenocarcinoma in cytologic fluids does not identify the primary source; one must look specifically for the source by immunohistochemical, receptor, and mammographic studies.

Mediastinal disease that produces symptoms of dysphagia, respiratory difficulty, or superior vena cava syndrome is almost invariably a consequence of primary lung cancer, metastatic breast cancer, or lymphoma. All can be rather well managed by local radiation therapy; thus, extensive evaluation and a search for the primary tumor are usually unwarranted. Clinically more silent mediastinal disease may be caused by neuroendocrine or extragonadal germ cell cancer, which can be identified by the methods noted earlier.

Osseous Metastases. The identification of an isolated bony lesion that is radiographically characteristic of neoplasia should be followed by a biopsy if tissue is not obtainable elsewhere. The appearance of the lesion on *plain film* should be noted to determine whether it is lytic, blastic, or mixed, which can help limit the differential diagnosis (Table 85.2) and focus the evaluation. If the bony lesion is difficult to sample, a *bone marrow biopsy* at the iliac crest represents a reasonable alternative. The vast majority of patients with bony metastases have multiple lesions that often invade the bone marrow. Should this not prove diagnostic, one can obtain a *bone scan* to identify other sites of tumor that may be more easily accessible to biopsy. Having established a histologic diagnosis of malignancy in the bone, the search for the primary should, as always, be confined to treatable disease. Tumors of the lung and kidney (usually not very treatable) prove to be the most common sources of skeletal metastases of unknown cause.

Liver Metastases are usually diagnosed by ultrasonography or *CT-guided needle biopsy*. Most are adenocarcinomas with gastrointestinal sources, although breast and lung are other important origins. Once a metastatic adenocarcinoma has been identified in the liver, further testing to identify the primary is usually unwarranted because few are sufficiently responsive to justify the workup. Symptomatic patients with hepatic metastases have a life expectancy of less than 6 months, but asymptomatic persons have a significantly longer survival.

Ascites. Malignant ascites is most likely to derive from metastatic cancer of the pancreas, stomach, or colon involving the peritoneal surface. However, a search for such cancers is of little value because little can be done to alter prognosis. However, in women, an important treatable cause of malignant ascites is diffuse peritoneal involvement by ovarian cancer. *Pelvic ultrasonography*, CT, or magnetic resonance imaging (MRI) and testing for the tumor marker serum *CA-125* are indicated, although peritoneal implants have been noted in patients without detectable ovarian disease. Serologic studies (HCG, AFP) and immunohistochemical study of the tumor may suggest this responsive lesion.

High Cervical Lymphadenopathy. Because enlargement of a high cervical node may result from a contiguous primary tumor in the nasopharynx or oropharynx or a lymphoma (two treatable cancers), intensive assessment is warranted. A careful examination of the nasopharynx, oral cavity (including base of the tongue), and larynx is essential, as is detailed examination of all lymph nodes. *CT* or *MRI* is helpful in the examination of the deeper submucosal and neck structures. If node biopsy reveals squamous cell or epidermoid histology but no primary is evident, then *blind biopsies* of areas likely to harbor nasopharyngeal tumor (base of the tongue, nasopharynx) are conducted. If the histopathology is adenocarcinoma, then sinuses or the salivary glands may be the primary source. Again, careful physical examination supplemented by CT or MRI may help reveal the primary. If histologic studies indicate a lymphoma or Hodgkin's disease, then the evaluation shifts to staging activities (see Chapter 84).

Axillary Adenopathy necessitates a careful breast examination and mammography. The diagnosis of breast cancer may be assisted by performing *estrogen* and *progesterone receptor assays* on nodal tissue obtained from the axilla. *Immunohistochemical study* for markers of lymphoma is also indicated. *Chest CT* may be warranted if small-cell histology is suggested.

Inguinal Adenopathy is approached diagnostically in much the same manner as cervical adenopathy, with an emphasis on local disease and lymphoma, because they are quite responsive to treatment (Table 85.3). Detailed pathologic study is essential and should include *immunohistochemical* and *receptor studies* of the tissue obtained at biopsy. Careful pelvic and anorectal examinations are performed, complemented by ultrasonographic study of the pelvis. If inguinal node biopsy identifies a lymphoma, then workup proceeds for staging (see Chapter 84).

Retroperitoneal Mass. An incidentally discovered retroperitoneal mass is likely to represent advanced-stage lymphoma or metastatic prostate, germ cell, or ovarian cancer. All are responsive to therapy and thus important to identify. Because it is difficult to obtain samples from this site, a search for a more accessible site is indicated. Careful physical examination of the peripheral nodes, prostate and testicles in men and pelvic organs in women is indicated. Ultrasonographic examination may help detect a small prostatic or testicular lesion. Ultrasonography may also help identify an ovarian tumor. Serum marker studies (AFP, β-HCG subunit, and prostate-specific antigen) aid the diagnostic effort.

Brain. The search focuses on breast, small-cell, and lymphomatous disease (see above). Consideration of brain biopsy is usually unnecessary unless no tissue is available peripherally. If a brain biopsy is performed, detailed immunohistochemical and receptor studies should be conducted.

Bone Marrow Invasion. When pancytopenia or a myelophthisic picture with leukoerythroblastic changes is encountered, marrow invasion should be considered and confirmed by *bone marrow biopsy* (see Chapter 79). The marrow examination includes a search for clusters of malignant cells, which may help in identification. Once their presence is confirmed, a search for the several treatable tumors can commence (Table 85.1).

TREATMENT

As emphasized above, the workup focuses intensively on identification of treatable cancers (Tables 85.1 and 85.3). However, when the primary remains unknown (as in a substantial proportion of cases), the options for treatment become more problematic, with the choices being between empiric treatment and watchful waiting. Data on the efficacy and cost-to-benefit ratio of both approaches are limited. Interpretation of published outcomes data is often hindered by the absence of careful, detailed characterization of patients and their tumors. Only a few prospective, randomized, controlled trials have been performed, and although responses have been documented, median survival seems to improve little, if at all. Many optimistic reports suffer from selection biases. Consequently, any discussion with the patient and family must address the uncertain benefit of empiric treatment and its likely adverse effects. When patients with germ cell and neuroendocrine TUOs are excluded, response rates are in the range of 25% to 30%. With certain exceptions, only those who are symptomatic ought to be considered for treatment because the response is likely to be brief, side effects prominent, and chances of long-term benefit small.

Empiric Therapy. Of the two basic approaches to *empiric therapy*, one is to use *"broad-spectrum" chemotherapy* (e.g., Adriamycin and mitomycin C). These are potent agents with a high potential for toxicity. Monitoring for marrow suppression is necessary. Treatment is halted if no response is noted after two courses. The other empiric approach is to treat based on a prudent estimate of the *most likely treatable tumor*, judged by cell type, age, sex, site, and so on (Tables 85.1, 85.2, and 85.4). If the pathologic type is undifferentiated, treatment is directed toward the most responsive tumors in this class—namely, lymphoma and germ cell neoplasms. Metastatic adenocarcinoma in men can be treated as metastatic prostate cancer, and in women as metastatic ovarian or breast cancer, as these are the most treatable malignancies. Metastatic prostate cancer shows a very high response rate to hormonal therapy. Carcinoma of the breast shows a similar response rate to therapy; modalities include hormonal treatment for some patients and chemotherapy for others (see Chapter 122).

One of the more effective empiric therapies for TUO is *radiation* with or without node dissection in patients who have high cervical adenopathy and epidermoid or squamous cell histology. Treatment is conducted on the ipsilateral site, with cure rates of 20% to 35% reported. Adenocarcinoma of an inguinal node without a known primary may be treated by local radiation therapy bilaterally if no evidence of an anal or prostatic lesion is found on blind biopsy. Radiation may also provide reasonable *palliation* for patients with localized symptomatic disease, especially that which involves bone, mediastinum, or lymph nodes. Bony metastases are generally not treated systemically. When symptomatic, they are treated palliatively with local radiation therapy and, if necessary, stabilized orthopedically. In the absence of symptoms, a bony metastasis may be monitored unless a definitively responsive tumor, such as prostate or breast cancer, can be identified.

PATIENT EDUCATION AND INDICATIONS FOR REFERRAL

The finding of metastatic cancer is always very upsetting news, and even more perplexing when a source is hard to identify. However, an intelligently designed, selective search for treatable disease can provide considerable reassurance and hope. Such a diagnostic strategy should be shared with patient and family, both to provide hope and a sense of control over a difficult situation and to reduce irrational pressure to "find the cause" at all costs.

A search that proves unrevealing poses the issue of empiric therapy. Here, a thoughtful and frank consultation with the oncologist is indicated to review the options. The lack of adequate data on cost and benefit often make counseling difficult, but an experienced and wise oncologist can be of great help to the patient and family. The patient suspected of having a metastatic lesion of the spinal cord requires urgent hospital admission and prompt referral to the radiation oncologist.

A.H.G.

ANNOTATED BIBLIOGRAPHY

Abbruzzese JL, Abbruzzese MC, Lenzi R, et al. Analysis of a diagnostic strategy for patients with suspected tumors of unknown origin. J Clin Oncol 1995;13:2094. (*A predefined limited diagnostic study was evaluated in an attempt to define a cost-effective approach to workup.*)

Bataini JP, Rodriquez J, Jaulerry C, et al. Treatment of metastatic neck nodes secondary to an occult epidermoid carcinoma of the head and neck. Laryngoscope 1987;97:1080. (*Very high rates of response and some cures.*)

Copeland EM, McBride CM. Axillary metastases from unknown primary sites. Ann Surg 1972;178:25. (*The breast is the most common primary source in women with an undifferentiated axillary lesion.*)

Gatter KC, Heryet A, Alcock C, et al. Clinical importance of analyzing malignant tumors of uncertain origin with immunohistological techniques. Lancet 1985;1:1302. (*Terse discussion of these important methods.*)

Gentile PS, Carloss HW, Huang T-Y, et al. Disseminated prostatic carcinoma simulating primary lung cancer. Cancer 1988;62:711. (*The presentation of this very treatable malignancy may be quite atypical.*)

Greco FA, Vaughn WK, Hainsworth JD. Advanced poorly differentiated carcinoma of unknown primary site: recognition of a treatable syndrome. Ann Intern Med 1986;104:547. (*Patients with poorly differentiated histology and tumor in the mediastinum, retroperitoneum, and lymph nodes responded well to cisplatin-based chemotherapy.*)

Hainsworth JD, Greco FA. Treatment of patients with cancer of an unknown primary site. N Engl J Med 1993;329:257. (*Among the best reviews of the subject.*)

Hainsworth JD, Johnson DH, Greco FA. Poorly differentiated neuroendocrine carcinoma of unknown primary site. Ann Intern Med 1988;1090:364. (*Identification of a very treatable subgroup; electron microscopy useful.*)

Kirsten F, Chi CH, Leary JA, et al. Metastatic adeno or undifferentiated carcinoma from an unknown primary site. Q J Med 1987;62:143. (*A detailed discussion of the natural history and approach to workup.*)

Le Chevalier TL, Cvitkovic E, Caille P, et al. Early metastatic cancer of unknown primary origin at presentation. Arch Intern Med

1988;148:2035. (*In an autopsy study, pancreas, lung, kidney, and colon were the most common primary sites; authors recommend a workup strategy.*)

Levine MN, Drummond MF, LaBelle RJ. Cost-effectiveness in the diagnosis and treatment of carcinoma of unknown primary origin. Can Med Assoc J 1985;133:977. (*Argues that much diagnostic work is wasteful and treatment ineffective.*)

McMillan JH, Levine E, Stephens RH. Computed tomography in the evaluation of metastatic adenocarcinoma from an unknown primary site. Radiology 1982;143:143. (*A retrospective series comparing CT with other radiologic modalities finds CT superior.*)

Miettinen M. Immunohistochemistry in tumor diagnosis. Ann Med 1993;25:221. (*A terse review.*)

Nystrom JS, Weiner JM, Wolf RM, et al. Identifying the primary site in metastatic cancer of unknown origin: inadequacy of roentgenographic procedures. JAMA 1979;241:381. (*Standard radiographic studies proved insensitive.*)

Schapira DV, Jarrett AR. The need to consider survival, outcome, and expense when evaluating and treating patients with unknown primary carcinoma. Arch Intern Med 1995;155:2050. (*A retrospective look revealing high costs, very low yield, and poor survival when these issues are not taken into account in planning the workup and treatment.*)

Sporn JR, Greenberg BR. Empiric chemotherapy in patients with carcinoma of unknown primary site. Am J Med 1990;88:49. (*Outstanding review of the entire issue, including identification of patients with responsive disease; 43 references.*)

86
Approach to Staging and Monitoring

Staging and monitoring are essential components of cancer management. Staging is performed to assess the extent of disease, and it is used to help determine prognosis and choice of therapy. Monitoring serves to detect the reappearance or progression of cancer and contributes importantly to updating prognosis and revising treatment plans. Staging and monitoring strategies are determined by tumor type, natural history, response to therapy, and characteristic pattern of spread. The frequency and duration of monitoring depend on the rate of disease recurrence.

The primary physician is in an ideal position to conduct much of the noninvasive staging and monitoring needed in the care of the cancer patient. To do so effectively requires an understanding of the limitations of the many available laboratory tests and radiologic procedures, so that important decisions about test and procedure selection can be made effectively and unnecessary expense and discomfort can be avoided.

TERMINOLOGY, PRINCIPLES, AND PROCEDURES OF STAGING

Cancer stage is defined by the anatomic distribution of disease. The task of staging is to identify the amount and distribution of tumor. Several staging systems are used to express the extent of disease. At times, there appear to be almost as many staging schemes as there are malignancies. Some are so tumor-specific and idiosyncratic that they make for considerable confusion. However, most incorporate designations for *local disease* (confined to a visceral site), *regional extension* (with or without involvement of contiguous lymph nodes), and *distant metastasis*.

The TNM System

To standardize staging, the *TNM system* has been proposed and used with increasing frequency. The *T* refers to *tumor*, the *N* to *nodes*, and the *M* to *metastases*. Numbers are added to des-

ignate subcategories, reflecting the size of the tumor (T1 to T5), the degree of nodal involvement (N0 to N3), and the absence or presence of distant metastases (M0 or M1).

Although varying slightly among tumors, the various subcategory designations have specific meaning. For the T categories, *Tis* indicates carcinoma *in situ*; *T1*, the smallest measurable tumor mass or tumor confined to mucosa or submucosa; *T2*, larger tumor mass or tumor extending directly to adjacent structures; *T3*, very large tumor or still further direct extension; *T4*, tumor of any size with very profound local tissue invasion and marked direct extension; and *T5*, extension beyond adjacent organs. As regards N categories, *N0* designates no nodal metastasis; *N1*, ipsilateral or regional involvement or movable regional nodes; *N2*, more extensive regional disease or fixed, matted nodes; *N3*, contralateral or distant nodal metastasis.

The TNM staging classification is increasingly preferred because of its consistency, comparability, and precision. Other staging systems commonly used for particular cancers have direct correlates to the TNM system and can be expressed in its terms (Table 86.1).

Staging Principles and Procedures

A well-designed staging evaluation reflects the characteristic pattern of a malignancy and the speed of local and metastatic spread. Staging is performed both *clinically* (by means of history, physical examination, imaging procedures, and serum markers) and *pathologically* (by direct sampling of tissue). The two are complementary.

History and Physical Examination. Although much emphasis is placed on laboratory and radiologic procedures in clinical staging, the history and physical examination continue to play central roles in the determination of tumor mass, local spread, and metastasis. In almost every cancer workup, historical and physical data are required for intelligent staging and determination of the need for additional study. The failure to conduct a

Table 86.1.   TNM Staging and Correlation with Conventional Staging Systems for
Cancers of the Lung, Breast, and Colon

TUMOR	CONVENTIONAL STAGE/ TNM DESIGNATION		COMMENTS
Lung	0	Tis, N0, M0	Carcinoma *in situ*
	1	T1–2, N0, M0	Local tumor ± visceral pleura involved
	2	T1–2, N1, M0	Ipsilateral hilar, peribronchial nodes
	3a	T3, N0–1, M0	Extension to chest wall, diaphragm
	3b	T1–3, N2, M0	Ipsilateral mediastinal nodes involved
	4	Any T, any N, M1	
Breast	0	Tis, N0, M0	Paget's of nipple, no palpable tumor, carcinoma *in situ*
	1	T1, N0–1a, M0	Tumor <2 cm, nodes feel normal
	2	T0 or T1, N1b, M0	Nodes feel diseased
	3	T2, N1a or b, M0	Tumor 2–5 cm in diameter
	3	T3, N1–2, M0	Tumor >5 cm in diameter
	4	T4, any N, any M	Direct involvement of chest wall and skin
		Any T, N3, any M	Supraclavicular nodes
		Any T, any N, M1	
Colon	0	Tis, N0, M0	
	A	T1, N0, M0	Confined to mucosa, submucosa
	B1	T2, N0, M0	Transmural disease, no extension
	B2	T3–5, N0, M0	Transmural disease plus extension
	C1	T1–2, N1, M0	Regional nodes, no direct extension
	C2	T3–4, N1, M0	Regional nodes plus extension
	D	Any T, any N, M1	

American Joint Committee on Cancer. Manual for Staging of Cancer, 2nd ed. Philadelphia: JB Lippincott, 1983.

careful history and physical examination risks subjecting the patient to unnecessary or misguided studies.

Imaging Procedures. If, after a detailed history has been taken and a physical examination performed, it is deemed necessary to obtain further information noninvasively regarding the anatomic extent of disease, then one usually considers imaging studies. Among the most frequently ordered are computed tomography (CT), magnetic resonance imaging (MRI), ultrasonography, and radionuclide scanning (particularly the bone scan). Even the plain film of the chest or bone can sometimes provide diagnostic information. Limitations include lack of specificity and inability to detect very early lesions.

Computed Tomography and Magnetic Resonance Imaging represent important advances over older contrast and radionuclide studies. They provide not only improved detection of tumor but also better quantification of tumor burden. CT is the less expensive and more readily available of the two technologies, but MRI provides enhanced resolution in some areas, particularly the central nervous system. *Chest CT* has proved superior to conventional full-lung tomography for the detection of pleural, mediastinal, and parenchymal lesions. The test is particularly useful for staging patients with lung cancer and those with sarcomas and testicular cancers, malignancies with high rates of metastasis to the lung and mediastinum. *CT of the abdomen* enhances evaluation of the retroperitoneum by identifying enlarged lymph nodes that were previously difficult to detect noninvasively. A positive scan result can obviate the need for surgical exploration. CT has also improved the detection, sampling, and quantification of tumor in the pancreas, liver, adrenal gland, and kidney. Results of pelvic CT for the detection and staging of early ovarian and prostate cancers have been variable; the test often lacks sensitivity in the detection of early disease or early spread to pelvic nodes. *CT of the head* has virtually eliminated invasive and radionuclide staging studies of

the central nervous system. Conducting the study with iodinated contrast further improves sensitivity.

Particularly in the central nervous system, *MRI* has contributed to the staging and monitoring of cancer. Compared with CT, it is more sensitive and offers a better assessment of the posterior fossa and spinal cord. Its increased cost is justified when enhanced sensitivity is required. In addition, MRI is being investigated as a means of staging of pelvic malignancies. Although early results have been disappointing, methodologic advances in imaging ovarian and prostate cancers may improve sensitivity. Sensitivities have been reported in the range of 40% to 50% for early disease and 60% to 70% for more advanced disease. It is too soon to recommend MRI for routine use in staging pelvic malignancies, but the literature should be followed closely.

Radionuclide Scanning remains the most sensitive means of detecting metastasis to *bone*. It is far superior to plain films, except in cases of myeloma. However, bone scan results can be nonspecific, so that confirmation by other means is sometimes necessary. In cancers with a high propensity for spread to bone (prostate, breast, small-cell cancers), the bone scan has become an integral part of the initial evaluation. In other instances, it is used late in the course of disease to evaluate bone pain. *Liver* scans are still frequently ordered to stage gastrointestinal cancers, but they rarely detect disease that is not predicted on the basis of abnormal serum liver chemistries (e.g., elevated alkaline phosphatase) or clinical hepatomegaly. Furthermore, a large percentage of abnormal findings on hepatic scans represent secondary drug effects or incidental inflammatory disease. True-positive liver scans are found in fewer than 1% of patients with otherwise operable primary breast or colon cancer; routine liver scanning for metastases is unwarranted in these conditions. As noted, CT and MRI have largely ended the use of radionuclide *brain* scanning for the detection of central nervous system disease. The sensitivity and specificity of gallium scanning are inadequate because the radionuclide also readily enters inflamed tissue. Nevertheless, the test is recommended by some for staging melanoma and lymphoma. Because of the discomfort of the study, which requires frequent enemas, and its high false-negative rate, it has been relegated to infrequent use.

Ultrasonography has proved extremely useful for assessment of the prostate, ovaries, testes, liver, pancreas, kidneys, and thyroid. Ultrasonography accurately distinguishes solid from cystic masses, an important advantage in the evaluation of pelvic, testicular, renal, and thyroid masses. It can also help guide needle biopsy. Resolution for transabdominal studies wanes for lesions less than 1 cm in diameter. The results of about 20% of such studies are inadequate because of overlying bowel gas. Transrectal ultrasonographic techniques have improved the detection and staging of early prostate cancer. Ultrasonography appears to provide results comparable to those of MRI for the staging of early prostate disease, but at much lower cost.

Standard Radiographs, such as the *metastatic series*, have a high false-negative rate and are relatively insensitive, although false-positive rates are relatively low. *Contrast studies*, such as IV pyelography, venography, and angiography, are infrequently applied to staging, although they may aid in planning surgery. Conventional chest tomography has been supplanted by chest CT (see above), which has a lower false-negative rate.

Lymphangiography was developed primarily for the evaluation of retroperitoneal lymph nodes in the staging of Hodgkin's disease, but it has been similarly employed for lymphoma. The usefulness of the test for staging has declined because treatment no longer depends heavily on its findings (see Chapter 84). In lymphoma, the test has been replaced by abdominal CT, but it is still used for staging in Hodgkin's disease.

Serum Chemistries and Markers. An isolated elevation in *alkaline phosphatase* (liver fraction) indicates hepatic infiltration; it may be an early sign of metastasis to liver and often precedes a radiologically detectable lesion. Marked elevations in *prostate-specific antigen* suggest a large tumor burden and the likelihood of extracapsular spread of prostate cancer.

Surgical Staging is indicated when the results will alter therapeutic decision making. Clinical staging may underestimate the extent of disease by virtue of its limited ability to detect microscopic spread. However, invasive study should be conducted only when the choice of therapy will be affected; otherwise, the morbidity and risks incurred may not be justifiable.

Lymph Node Dissection was initially undertaken in patients with breast cancer, prostate carcinoma, and malignant melanoma in the hope of eliminating contiguous sites of disease. However, it has been demonstrated that lymphadenectomy at the time of surgery for the primary lesion does not extend survival, although it does serve as a prognostic and therapeutic determinant in cancers of the prostate and breast. Lymph node evaluation of distant disease has become a recognized staging procedure in some tumors. For example, scalene or retroperitoneal node biopsy is sometimes performed in patients with testicular cancer. *Sentinel node biopsy* with the use of radionuclide markers for nodal identification is being applied in malignant melanoma and breast cancer as an alternative to standard node dissections. This approach involves performing intraoperative lymph node mapping to allow selective lymphadenectomy.

Laparotomy to detect intraabdominal disease that will affect choice of therapy is central to the staging of colon cancer, helpful in selected patients with Hodgkin's disease, and useful in ovarian cancer. *Mediastinoscopy* helps to determine operability for patients with lung cancer; the more invasive *Chamberlain procedure* is sometimes necessary. *Bone marrow biopsy* provides an efficient means of pathologic staging in cancers that frequently metastasize to bone marrow (e.g., lymphoma, small-cell carcinoma, prostate cancer).

PRINCIPLES AND PROCEDURES OF MONITORING DISEASE

Monitoring for disease recurrence is appropriate for asymptomatic patients who have undergone curative cancer therapy.

Monitoring usually adds little to the care of patients with incurable disease except when it is desired to document tumor response to palliative treatment objectively. Monitoring activities that can affect decision making and improve outcomes are the only ones that should be undertaken. All others just add expense and may even cause harm in the case of a false-positive result. The cost-effectiveness of many routine programs of monitoring has been called into question by some. Although a host of increasingly sophisticated tests are available, few have demonstrated an ability to affect outcomes. The history and physical examination supplemented by a few simple laboratory studies remain among the most cost-effective of measures.

Monitoring Techniques

Many of the techniques useful for staging are pertinent to monitoring. Checking for residual disease or a new primary is the objective when curative therapy is employed; monitoring for reduction in tumor burden is the goal when palliation is undertaken. The frequency and duration of monitoring depend on the rate of disease recurrence. Tumor type, response to therapy, stage of disease, and pattern of metastasis also influence the selection of monitoring activities. Test sensitivity and specificity are important considerations. As noted, the emphasis should be on monitoring activities that will affect decision making and outcomes. Aggressive routine follow-up is pointless when the findings will not influence management or improve results.

Tumor Markers have been sought with the hope of obtaining a means of tumor detection more sensitive than those provided by other clinical methods. Although initially developed to aid in early diagnosis, most markers have actually proved better suited for monitoring of disease recurrence or progression after curative or palliative therapy. Baseline and posttreatment levels are obtained and follow-up readings repeated at regular intervals.

Carcinoembryonic Antigen is present in both normal and malignant tissue; serum levels in excess of 2.5 ng/mL are suggestive of tumor, but the test is too nonspecific for screening. Its most useful application is in early the detection of recurrence, especially for cancers of the colon and rectum, breast, and lung. The consensus is that serial determinations of carcinoembryonic antigen are the best currently available noninvasive means for identifying recurrent colorectal cancer after surgery.

α-Fetoprotein has been found in high serum concentrations in association with hepatomas, testicular carcinomas, and extragonadal germ cell tumors. Although lacking sufficient specificity for diagnostic purposes, repeated determinations of the α-fetoprotein level can be used to monitor for disease recurrence and assess adequacy of treatment.

β-Human Chorionic Gonadotropin Subunit is another useful tumor marker for germ cell tumors of the testes and ovaries. Monitoring of the β-human chorionic gonadotropin subunit provides information similar to that obtained from the α-fetoprotein level.

Prostate-specific Antigen is unique to prostate tissue and is found in both malignant and normal cells. A concentration in excess of 10 ng/mL is strongly suggestive of cancer and is found in fewer than 2% of patients with benign prostatic hypertrophy. Levels increase with the tumor burden and rise briefly after needle biopsy or with prostatitis, but not after a prostate examination. False-negatives occur with the use of finasteride.

Levels of CA-125, produced by 80% of epithelial ovarian cancers, correlate with the clinical course and are useful for monitoring. The specificity is high. This marker is the first of what promises to be a host of tumor-specific markers detected by monoclonal antibody methods.

Many other markers are under development (e.g., CA19-9) and are being applied experimentally in monitoring such cancers as those of the breast and pancreas.

Monitoring Local or Regional Disease. Patients with local or regional disease subjected to curative therapy may be monitored by history and physical examination supplemented by more detailed study of the disease site at routine intervals or as clinically indicated. The periodic evaluation of patients with regional disease who have undergone curative primary therapy should be directed less at detecting the presence of asymptomatic metastases and more at *finding new primary tumors* in the involved organ. *Endoscopy* for colorectal cancer and *mammography* for breast cancer are prime examples of this approach.

In the absence of symptoms or signs of recurrence, monitoring is conducted at 3-month intervals for the first year following operation, and at 4-month intervals for the second year. Thereafter, follow-up may be accomplished at 6-month intervals for a minimum of 5 years. In general, most tumors recur at a maximum rate during the first 2 years following the initial operation—if in fact they are destined to recur. Three malignancies are notorious for late recurrence: breast carcinoma, melanoma, and renal cell carcinoma. In some patients with these tumors, the lag period before the development of detectable metastases may extend beyond 10 years after initial diagnosis.

Monitoring Metastatic Disease. Follow-up examinations for patients with metastatic disease who receive systemic therapy should be performed at intervals determined by the time expected for an objective clinical response. For hormonal therapy of breast cancer, clinical evidence of response may take as long as 3 months to appear. The effects of cytotoxic chemotherapy may be seen rapidly—for example, within two courses of treatment or 4 to 6 weeks. This is particularly true for exquisitely responsive tumors such as breast, testicular, ovarian, and oat cell carcinomas.

Patients with metastatic disease receiving palliative systemic therapy should be examined for evidence of new disease. Unnecessary chemotherapy-induced morbidity can be avoided if ineffective palliative systemic therapy is discontinued at the first signs of new disease. Response to therapy may be objectively demonstrated after a predictable interval, but new growth or spread may be noted on earlier examination.

An important corollary to the monitoring of patients with metastatic disease on systemic therapeutic regimens is to define the most objective site of disease to be followed and to avoid additional staging procedures if they do not alter the therapeutic plan. For example, a patient with hepatic metastases from a primary breast cancer need not undergo a bone scan unless bone pain or a fracture occurs. The tumor is already established as being incurable, and therapy is determined by the presence of liver metastases. Alternatively, the patient with bony metastases that are difficult to monitor may undergo selective staging to identify a more measurable marker of metastatic disease, such as plasma carcinoembryonic antigen. Identification of asymptomatic metastases by radionuclide scanning is of little use because the early detection and treatment of asymptomatic metastatic disease does not necessarily improve survival.

A.H.G.

ANNOTATED BIBLIOGRAPHY

American Joint Committee on Cancer. Manual for staging of cancer, 2nd ed. Philadelphia: JB Lippincott, 1983. (*Basic outline of TNM staging scheme.*)

American Society of Clinical Oncology. Clinical practice guidelines for the use of tumor markers in breast and colorectal cancer. J Clin Oncol 1996;14:2843. (*Evidence-based expert panel recommendations.*)

American Society of Clinical Oncology. Recommended breast cancer surveillance guidelines. J Clin Oncol 1997;15:2149. (*An example of evidence-based consensus guidelines for follow-up.*)

Bast RC Jr, Klug TL, St John E, et al. Radioimmunoassay using a monoclonal antibody to monitor the course of epithelial ovarian cancer. N Engl J Med 1983;309:883. (*The development of the CA-125.*)

Beard DB, Haskell CM. Carcinoembryonic antigen in breast cancer. Am J Med 1986;80:241. (*A review of the role of carcinoembryonic antigen in breast cancer; especially useful in patients with advanced disease.*)

Edelman MJ, Meyers FJ, Siegel D. The utility of follow-up testing after curative cancer therapy. A critical review and economic analysis. J Gen Intern Med 1997;12:318. (*Reviews most follow-up strategies for common treatable malignancies and finds aggressive routine follow-up to be of questionable value in most cancers.*)

Fletcher RH. Carcinoembryonic antigen. Ann Intern Med 1986;104:66. (*A critical review pointing out the limitations of its usefulness.*)

Friedman MA, Resser KJ, Marcus FS, et al. How accurate are computed tomographic scans in assessment of changes in tumor size? Am J Med 1983;75:193. (*Documents the sensitivity of CT for determining changes in size; authors argue the test is the best means available.*)

Harris MN, Shapiro RL, Roses DF. Malignant melanoma: primary surgical management (excision and node dissection) based on pathology and staging. Cancer 1995;75:715. (*A review of the role of lymph node dissection and of intraoperative lymph node mapping to allow selective lymphadenectomy.*)

Rifkin MD, Zerhouni EA, Gatsonis CA, et al. Comparison of magnetic resonance imaging and ultrasonography in staging early prostate cancer. N Engl J Med 1990;323:621. (*No difference; both found wanting in early disease, better for more advanced disease. This study was performed before the advent of the rectal probe; sensitivities are in the range of 40% to 50% for early disease, 60% to 70% for more advanced disease.*)

Smalley RV, Malmud LS, Ritchie WGM. Preoperative scanning: evaluation for metastatic disease in carcinoma of the breast, lung, colon, bladder, and prostate. Semin Oncol 1980;7:358. (*A critical analysis of radionuclide scanning, ultrasonography, and CT.*)

Stamy TA, Yang N, Hay AR, et al. Prostate-specific antigen as a serum marker for adenocarcinoma of the prostate. N Engl J Med 1987;317:909. (*The original report. More sensitive than acid phosphatase; both elevated in benign prostatic hypertrophy.*)

Van Dyke JA, Stanley RJ, Berland LL. Pancreatic imaging. Ann Intern Med 1985;102:212. (*A detailed review that discusses the use of abdominal CT in documenting the presence and extent of tumor.*)

87

Comprehensive Care of the Cancer Patient

The treatment of cancer is multifaceted, involving the interdigitation of physician support and treatment with surgery, radiation, cytotoxic agents, and, most recently, biologic response modifiers. Comprehensive care requires a team approach, in which the primary physician plays a central role in coordinating the effort. To succeed in this role, the primary physician needs to understand the major issues of cancer management and be capable of interacting effectively with cancer specialists. The patient and family are likely to request the opinion of the primary physician, so that an ability to explain and assess management recommendations is necessary. Most cancer patients can remain at home with their families and receive optimal therapy on an outpatient basis when a primary physician is able to work closely with a cancer center or a local specialist in cancer management.

Curative treatment that focuses on the primary tumor site has traditionally been the province of surgery, with radiation and chemotherapy relegated to palliative roles. More recently, radiation and chemotherapy have been employed as adjuvants in the treatment of local disease, enhancing the capability of surgery to cure. Advances in radiation therapy have effected cures of some cancers in early stages. Biologic response modifiers hold promise for achieving further improvements in outcome.

Effective care of the cancer patient begins with communicating the diagnosis and strengthening the relationship between patient and physician. It also requires the establishment of a close working partnership with the cancer specialist, whose job will be to design and implement the treatment program. The primary physician can and should maintain a central role in the care of the cancer patient, but to do so requires a thorough understanding of the natural history of the tumor, its staging and monitoring (see Chapter 86), and its responsiveness to treatment. In addition, the patient will call on the primary physician for relief from symptoms related to the tumor or its treatment. This necessitates a thorough knowledge of measures to control pain (see Chapter 90), emesis (see Chapter 91), and related side effects of cancer therapy (see Chapters 88 and 89).

SUPPORTING THE PATIENT AND FAMILY THROUGH DIAGNOSIS AND TREATMENT

For most patients, the diagnosis of cancer evokes images of pain, suffering, mutilation, and certain death. These basic fears are so intertwined with the word "cancer" that confirmation of the diagnosis places extreme emotional stress on both patient and family. It is in managing this anguish that the primary physician plays a most important role as the person to whom the patient and family can turn. One must be not only the source of scientific and medical expertise but also the provider of emotional support and understanding.

Giving Bad News

It is always difficult to give bad news. Physicians sometimes avoid telling the patient the diagnosis in accurate and specific terms at the outset, resorting to such euphemisms as "lump," "mass," and "lesion." Further inhibiting communication may be the ill-advised, although well-intentioned, insistence of family members that the diagnosis be kept from the patient out of fear of precipitating a severe depression. Such concerns are usually ill-conceived. It is rare that ignorance of the diagnosis or prognosis is helpful for the patient or family. Quite the contrary. Patients and their families deal better with cancer when they are well informed.

The *goal* in communicating the diagnosis and prognosis is to be accurate without destroying all hope. First and foremost, the words "cancer" and "malignant tumor" should be used at the outset of the interview and not avoided, although constant repetition of the terms is usually unnecessary. The term "fatal" ought to be omitted in discussions of the prognosis because it implies little hope of control. When informed of an incurable malignancy, the patient and family want to know, "How much time is left?" A rough estimate may be necessary when patients must arrange their affairs, but if possible, the physician should avoid indicating a specific period of time because it is apt to be inaccurate. Preferably, the physician should direct the patient toward realistic therapeutic approaches and reinforce the role of living instead of dying.

The *candor* expressed by telling the diagnosis "as it is" facilitates the development of trust among patient, family, and medical staff and breaks down the barrier that often isolates cancer patients from their families. Being well informed also helps alleviate the sense of hopelessness and loss of control that can be one of the most frightening aspects of living with a malignant disease. Families are especially grateful for full and frequent reports of the patient's status and prognosis.

The *consequences* of not fully informing the patient and family can be considerable. The patient who is unaware of the diagnosis and prognosis may fail to put affairs in order and continue to have unrealistic plans or uncomfortable relationships with other members of the family, which might otherwise be resolved if all were to understand the prognosis. Similarly, the uninformed family is unable to grieve gradually over time, and death may appear to be sudden. The resulting unresolved grief may profoundly affect the surviving family members (see Chapter 227). Both patient and family may need to grieve and resolve their own fears and anxieties. By virtue of having a long-standing relationship with the patient and family, the primary physician is in an ideal position to provide effective support and guidance.

The Patient's Response

Cancer patients have been observed to pass through a series of emotional states. These include periods of denial, hostility, anger, hope, depression, and finally acceptance. The physician can help alleviate the more dysfunctional reactions and facilitate the patient's coping. The reactions of patients at the time of presentation of the diagnosis depend on preconceived ideas about cancer and what the specter of cancer suggests to them. Common misconceptions include the certainty of death, intractable pain, and erosive, disfiguring disease. To avoid needless worry, it is essential at the outset to address these common concerns directly, even if the patient does not express them. Nonetheless, a good number of patients will respond with denial, hostility, rejection of loved ones, regression, or even withdrawal. It is important to recognize such reactions as psychological defense mechanisms and respond to them in an understanding and patient manner.

Denial of the diagnosis is generally a transient reaction. When denial is mild, physicians may need only to reinforce their remarks with a repeated presentation of the facts or a provision of objective and tangible evidence. However, in some patients, denial is extreme and functions as a crude psychological defense mechanism, necessary for sustaining the psyche. A constant onslaught of evidence and reinforcement of the diagnosis or prognosis may be counterproductive and is not justified.

Hostility is occasionally an early reaction to the diagnosis. Anger may be directed against the medical team for the delayed diagnosis or for inadequate attention, and also toward family members, who may be viewed as not particularly upset and happy to finally "get their way." This phase is generally transient, receding as the patient comes to recognize the reality of the situation and the need for family and physician. Hostility is difficult for both patient and doctor and may be intense enough to lead the physician and family to reject the patient emotion-

ally. If recognized, this reaction should be allowed to run a natural course without withdrawal of support.

Regression is an accentuated response commonly occurring in the patient with a dependent personality who may have appeared overly independent before illness. If it is more than transient, the regression may turn infantile and must be mitigated by providing a parental figure who will be, on the one hand, supportive and, on the other hand, stern and demanding. Infantile regression places an inordinate burden on the family, who are called on to provide extraordinary amounts of support.

Withdrawal is an extreme form of regression, often tinged with elements of hostility. Direct confrontation is essential for the patient who withdraws; constant encouragement and the setting up of goals to be achieved (e.g., ambulation, planning trips, visiting friends) are critical.

Family Reactions to the Diagnosis

Reactions of the family are critical to the patient's well-being and to aiding the health care team in providing maximum support. Thus, the physician must be concerned with the family's responses to the patient and the diagnosis. The physician is frequently obliged to deal with many members of the family, often with differing levels of need for information and support. Not uncommonly, complete families—wives, husbands, and children—may be alienated by the patient, who disallows them the opportunity to resolve their confusion. Such alienation, which may approach pathologic proportions, can be understood with the help of the physician. A frequent family reaction is to provide smothering protection in compensation for guilt over previous misunderstandings with the patient and the need to resolve such differences. Again, the physician can help alleviate such pathologic reactions.

Psychological Reactions to Cancer Treatment

The patient who enters treatment for cancer is subjected to a reinforcement of the diagnosis and a rekindling of the fears regarding threats to self-esteem and self-image. The latter may be particularly demoralizing if the cancer treatment involves bodily disfigurement or a physical limitation that is either cosmetically mutilating or functionally disabling. Thus, the patient who requires a mastectomy, jaw resection, amputation, or colostomy faces a significant and frightening change in self-image. The distortions that are incorporated into the patient's unconscious, perhaps as a result of real or imagined experiences with friends, are potentially devastating. Often, these distortions are unrealistic and unsubstantiated, but more importantly, they may not be expressed. The physician must inquire into the patient's concerns and offer a realistic appraisal to minimize unnecessary anguish (see Chapter 1).

Patient education is a most important component of the approach to dealing with the stress of therapy. It additionally serves to cushion the stress by allowing the patient to intellectualize about the disease and its treatment. In this "demythologizing process," patient fears are identified and dealt with openly. Often, the result is a more acceptable view of one's illness and treatment. Educational materials available from the American Cancer Society and the National Cancer Institute can complement the educational effort by addressing common questions that patients have about cancer therapy. Detailed explanation of the therapy in terms of its effect on the tumor and its potential side effects allows the patient to approach treatment realistically. The use of support groups and meditation techniques can facilitate the patient's coping with the stresses of cancer therapy.

Such supportive efforts are designed to strengthen the patient psychologically and improve quality of life. Whether they affect survival or immune function is uncertain, but they certainly can help morale and coping with illness.

APPROACHES TO TREATMENT

The approach to treatment is determined by tumor type and stage (see Chapter 86). In the earliest stages of disease, the malignancy is localized and cure is possible through locally or regionally applied therapy. Regional spread reflects more advanced disease, and the chances of cure are lessened, but not eliminated. More systemic forms of therapy are added to local measures. With important exceptions (e.g., testicular cancer), distant metastasis indicates that cure is unlikely, and the goal is palliation through the use of systemic therapies.

Local Tumor Control: Surgery and Radiation

Surgery has traditionally played the dominant role in the management of localized cancer. The diagnosis is established and confirmed by surgical biopsy, and cure may be effected by operation. Nonetheless, the emphasis has shifted recently toward minimizing surgical procedures, particularly when the prognosis is determined by factors such as distant metastases and when salvage by secondary local modalities can be accomplished. For example, lymph node dissection for malignant melanoma, limb amputation for osteogenic sarcoma, ostomy and abdominoperineal resection for rectal cancer, and radical mastectomy for breast cancer have been scaled down in many cases to lesser procedures, so that morbidity is reduced without a compromise in survival. The surgical approach to these lesions may be modified by the addition of local therapy (e.g., radiation) or systemic therapy (e.g., cytotoxic agents).

Radiation Therapy has become more effective through the development of high-energy linear accelerators and technical improvements in delivery, which have lowered rates of morbidity and increased rates of survival and local control. For example, radiation has become the therapy of choice for early stages of Hodgkin's disease (see Chapter 84). Radiation in conjunction with surgery may be curative in some tumors when administered preoperatively or postoperatively. In other malignancies, the combined application of radiation and either surgery or chemotherapy may promote palliation and chances for long-term survival, although it rarely achieves cure (see Chapter 89).

Regional Cancer: Surgery Plus Adjuvant or Combined Therapy

Adjuvant therapy involves the addition of chemotherapy or radiation to surgical procedures. The rationale for adding radiation therapy is primarily to promote the local control of presumed residual microscopic tumor. In theory, chemotherapy functions as an adjuvant modality because of the possibility that tumor cells are released into the circulation at the time of surgery. In addition, adjuvant chemotherapy may be effective because it affects existing micrometastases at a time when they are rapidly proliferating and likely to be quite drug-sensitive.

Adjuvant therapy has been proposed or is part of ongoing trials of treatments for a number of regional cancers and is a proven and established therapy for others. For example, in breast cancer, premenopausal women with positive lymph nodes and pathologic stage II disease have benefited from the addition of chemotherapy. It has reduced the incidence of recurrence and prolonged disease-free survival. In patients with rectal cancer extending beyond the bowel wall (so-called Duke's stage B2 or C lesions), the use of radiation therapy has reduced local recurrence rates and possibly increased survival time. The role of preoperative radiation therapy in comparison with postoperative radiation therapy has not been definitely established.

With the vast majority of tumors, regional disease is incurable despite the use of adjuvant modalities, and some have a particularly poor prognosis. Long-term survival is seen in fewer than 5% of patients with lung, renal cell, or pancreatic cancers that are regionally advanced. Thus, multimodality therapy is generally not employed for patients with these tumors unless it is being used investigationally. Because of the high frequency of selection bias in many trials, it is critical to refer to results from randomized studies for a determination of efficacy. For some tumors (testicular cancer, osteogenic sarcoma, Hodgkin's disease), the role of ancillary modalities is important in extending survival time and limiting the morbidity of regional disease.

The advent of a host of advances in treatment (e.g., more effective cytotoxic drugs, *dose-intensified* therapy, *marrow transplantation*, hematologic *growth factors*, *biologic response modifiers*, local *radiation* for site sterilization; see Chapters 88 and 89) should improve approaches to local, regional, and even advanced cancers and become an increasing part of standard management. The optimal application of such forms of therapy will require reference to data from well-designed randomized trials.

Metastatic Cancer: Cytotoxic Drugs, Biologic Response Modifiers

The management of advanced disease is largely palliative and involves systemic therapy provided by cytotoxic drugs. Biologic response modifiers may begin to play an increasingly active role as research into their efficacy advances.

Chemotherapeutic Regimens have become increasingly sophisticated and complex, but they are also more effective because of the development of new agents and multiple-drug regimens (see Chapter 88). Decisions concerning the use and timing of cytotoxic therapy in advanced disease are difficult because of the potential morbidity associated with such therapy and the frequent lack of established benefit in promoting cure or even in prolonging survival. The decision to use chemotherapy in advanced disease is often a philosophical and psychological one, based on the feelings of patient, family, and physician.

Any decision to employ chemotherapy should involve an analysis of host tolerance in addition to potential tumor responsiveness. Most important, the use of chemotherapy must be preceded by informed consent of the patient, who should be aware of the side effects as well as the potential for response. A common misconception is that the drugs invariably create morbidity and prolong life only at the cost of agonizing discomfort. In fact, when effective, chemotherapy can improve the quality of life as well as prolong it, and when it is ineffective, it will not necessarily induce more than transient morbidity. Some of the newer chemotherapy regimens for this phase of illness utilize weekly administrations of drugs that are well tolerated at modest doses (e.g., paclitaxel, gemcitabine).

In addition to these considerations, the primary indications for the use of chemotherapy in advanced disease include the following:

1. A probability of tumor responsiveness to chemotherapy of more than 30% for a partial response and more than 5% for a complete response
2. Progressive tumor growth during a period of observation (e.g., pulmonary nodules doubling in fewer than 30 days)
3. Symptomatic metastatic disease (e.g., pleural effusion)

Within these guidelines, cytotoxic therapy can be administered with a reasonable risk–benefit balance.

The use of *experimental drug therapy* should be reserved for the following:

1. Patients who have failed with known effective drugs (i.e., drugs with a response rate >30% and an established ability to prolong survival)
2. Patients who wish to have or insist on a new form of treatment
3. Patients who have a measurable parameter that can be monitored to judge the effectiveness of therapy

Biologic Response Modifiers, such as the *interleukins* and *interferons*, are new forms of systemic treatment, designed to promote a generalized response that can affect tumors at any site. Although in most instances their use remains highly experimental, some have been approved for application in patients with cancer (e.g., interferon alfa for hairy cell leukemia and Kaposi's sarcoma; levamisole for Duke's stage C colon cancer). They offer considerable promise as an adjunct to cytotoxic chemotherapy. The literature should be followed closely (see also Chapter 89).

Management of the Preterminal Phase

(See also Chapter 90.)

"Terminal cancer" is an expression commonly employed by both patients and physicians, but with distinctly different definitions. Strictly defined, "terminal cancer" means that death will ensue within a 4-week period. The physician should avoid using the term "terminal" in talking with the patient or family. Not infrequently, patients may absorb the label and yet live for months or even years. The term imposes on both family and patient a tremendous stress that often results in withdrawal.

The physician's role in the terminal phase is a crucial one. It is essential to remain sensitive to all the patient's needs and, specifically, to the patient's need to know that the physician is always available. If the patient is at home, frequent home visits may be enormously appreciated. It may be helpful to allow the patient to come to the office once or twice a week, even though no specific medications are to be administered.

It is not incumbent on the physician to reinforce the inevitability of death to patients who have entered a preterminal or terminal state and are sustaining hope for a reversal of the tumor. More importantly, however, the family must be apprised precisely during this period to allow them to pass through the grieving process successfully.

The best approach to the management of the preterminal patient is to initiate *hospice care,* a comprehensive program of physical and psychological comfort measures delivered by skilled health care professionals either at home or in an inpatient facility. Hospital routines, laboratory studies, and life-sustaining therapies are omitted in favor of psychological and symptomatic support. Priorities include relief of pain (see Chapter 90) and psychological support of the patient and the family.

Psychotropic Drugs

Antidepressant therapy (e.g., use of an selective serotonin reuptake inhibitor, such as sertraline, at a dosage of 25 to 50 mg each morning) can help with the somatic symptoms of depression, such as marked fatigue and awakening in the early morning (see Chapter 227). Pain control may also be enhanced. Unless a contraindication is present, tricyclics should not be withheld on the basis of the common clinical misconception that "the patient is appropriately depressed, considering the diagnosis and prognosis." Checking for suicidal ideation is important because tricyclic overdose can be fatal. Asking about suicide does not suggest the act to the patient; rather, it conveys an understanding of how profoundly the patient is suffering. *Benzodiazepines* (e.g., 2 mg of diazepam daily at bedtime) given for short periods can facilitate coping with particularly stressful situations and the resultant difficulty in falling asleep. Patients with panic disorder may require more prolonged therapy with anxiolytics (see Chapter 226).

Nutrition and Pain Control

(See Chapters 90 and 91.)

Alternative or Complementary Approaches to Care

So-called "alternative" or "complementary" approaches to standard modern oncologic care are frequently sought by patients and their families, more as "natural" or "holistic" supplements to standard care than as substitutes. Subsumed under the rubric of "alternative medicine" are *meditation, relaxation* techniques, *mental imagery, massage, herbal remedies, megavitamins, chiropractic manipulation,* and *acupuncture.* To date, few data from randomized, controlled trials are available on which to base their use (although this is likely to change as U.S. government support for such trials emerges). Most claims of efficacy are based on anecdotal reports at best. Many patients view these measures as "natural" and therefore harmless and thus worth a try. Sociodemographic factors correlating with the use of alternative therapies include upper levels of income, younger age, and higher levels of education. Other triggers of use identified in cohort studies of cancer patients include depression, fear of recurrence of cancer, and psychosocial distress.

The primary care physician needs to be cognizant of the highly frequent use of alternative medicine among cancer patients and of the increased likelihood of underlying fear and psychosocial distress that may be driving the patient to seek such therapy. Eliciting and effectively addressing such fear and distress may be one of the most therapeutic responses one can make to the patient's use of or request for alternative medicine. Valuing informed medical opinions, patients hope their physicians will be knowledgeable about the safety and efficacy of such practices. The scientific literature should be followed closely and patients provided with the best of available information when it is desired. In this manner, patient safety and satisfaction can be maximized and unnecessary expense avoided.

APPROACH TO THE CARE OF CANCER SURVIVORS

Patients who survive cancer are increasing in number and are more commonly encountered than ever before in primary care practice. They present challenges in management that reflect both the psychological and physiologic consequences of the disease and its therapy. An expanding appreciation of their needs is essential to helping them return to full and productive lives.

Psychological Consequences. Although surviving cancer may be expected to be a cause for joy, studies show that considerable anxiety persists. Having had cancer appears to produce a heightened *sense of vulnerability* and fear of death and a decreased feeling of control and mastery over one's life. Fear of death wanes as the duration of survival increases, but *anxiety about recurrence* may persist and result in hypochondriasis or avoidance of follow-up health care. Contact with patients having active disease can be very stressful, rekindling feelings of fear and vulnerability. Conversely, some demonstrate marked anxiety over the loss of close contact with the health care team that characterized the active phase of their illness. Frank *separation anxiety* has been reported. Others begin to express feelings of *anger* over perceived shortcomings in diagnosis and care.

Physical disabilities resulting from cancer or its treatment can have a profound psychological impact, with *depression* being the most common and important. If not appreciated, it may present as fatigue or other physical complaints that generate concern in both patient and physician. Preoccupation with bodily sensations is another common manifestation of depression (see Chapter 227) that might be encountered in the surviving cancer patient. When not appreciated, symptoms of depression can be mistaken for more serious disease.

Interpersonal and Social Consequences. The psychosocial effects of having had cancer are equally important to keep in mind in helping the patient to adjust to survivorship. Some will miss the privileges that the *sick role* provided and may have difficulty in returning to the responsibilities of normal life. Family members and work colleagues may find it awkward to relate, not knowing whether to treat the survivor as still partially incapacitated or back to normal. A return to sexual activity may be a source of concern for the patient. Most patients with a close supportive marital relationship and no permanent loss of sexual capacity appear to do reasonably well, but preexisting marital problems or the absence of a close relationship can lead to considerable *sexual dysfunction*. Such dysfunction may result in

depression. Sexual dysfunction may also be a symptom of an underlying depression unrelated to sexual issues. Of course, patients who have sustained gonadal injury or bodily mutilation are prime candidates for sexual dysfunction and its interpersonal consequences. Overall, psychological distress appears to be highest in patients lacking a close, supportive relationship. Single patients are most vulnerable.

Elements of *interpersonal isolation* have been reported, especially among those who are single and reluctant to share information about their cancerous past with a potential mate. Feelings of isolation may also be triggered by difficulty in discussing the cancer experience with friends, family, or co-workers. *Work difficulties* are often encountered. Survivors have fears, real or imagined, of losing their job. Prolonged absence and a perceived inability to perform may compromise their previous position and lead to long-term job insecurity. With job insecurity comes concern about maintaining adequate and affordable *health insurance*, especially in light of a past history of major illness and the tendency of insurance companies to "cherry pick" those whom it will insure. It is hoped that insurance reform with community rating will alleviate this major worry of surviving cancer patients.

Physiologic Consequences. (See Chapters 88 and 89 and the chapters on specific cancers for a detailed discussion of physiologic consequences.)

Supportive Therapy and Preparing the Patient. An understanding of the difficulties that cancer survivors may encounter helps the physician prepare the patient for life after cancer therapy. Counseling the patient and family about the challenges and potential difficulties likely to be experienced can go a long way toward ensuring an effective return to daily life. The counseling is carried out in the same honest, open, and supportive manner that characterized discussions in earlier phases of the illness. The issues can be every bit as difficult for the patient and require that physician support continue unabated. Regularly scheduled office visits for a check of symptoms, physical findings, and progress in returning to normal life are greatly appreciated and extremely therapeutic. Studies suggest that it takes as long as 3 years after the time of successful treatment for survivors to regain the confidence and social functioning that was lost as a result of having had cancer. Many survivors also exhibit a wisdom and sense of value and proportion that comes from having faced death, an appreciation of life that benefits all whom they encounter.

A.H.G.

ANNOTATED BIBLIOGRAPHY

American Society of Clinical Oncology. Recommendations for the use of hematopoietic colony-stimulating factors: evidence-based clinical practice guidelines. J Clin Oncol 1997;15;3288. (*Recent update of guidelines for use; example of evidence-based approach to effective implementation of new approaches to therapy.*)

Anderson BL. Sexual functioning morbidity among cancer survivors. Cancer 1985;55:1835. (*Differentiates between dysfunction secondary to physiologic and psychological factors.*)

Burstein HJ, Gelber S, Guadagnoli E, et al. Use of alternative medicine by women with early-stage breast cancer. N Engl J Med 1999;340:1733. (*A cohort study finding that the use of alternative medicine is a marker for psychosocial stress and poor quality of life.*)

Cassileth BE, Zupkis RV, Sutton-Smith K, et al. Information and participation preferences among cancer patients. Ann Intern Med 1980;92:832. (*Most patients prefer maximum amounts of information; those who are more hopeful want to participate in treatment decisions.*)

Cassileth BE, Walsh WP, Lusk EJ. Psychosocial correlates of cancer survival. J Clin Oncol 1988;6:1753. (*A long-term study with practical implications.*)

Christakis NA, Escarge JJ. Survival of Medicare patients after enrollment in hospice programs. N Engl J Med 1996;335:172. (*Outcomes-based study of hospice care; some selection bias, but one of the best studies of benefits and limitations.*)

Fauci AS, Rosenberg SA, Sherwin SA, et al. Immunomodulators in clinical medicine. Ann Intern Med 1987;106:421. (*A basic science and clinical review of biologic response modulators.*)

Garcia-Carbonero R, Hidalgo H, Pax-Ares L, et al. Patient selection in high-dose chemotherapy trials: relevance in high-risk breast cancer. J Clin Oncol 1997;15:178. (*Documents a great deal of selection bias, which can compromise results in nonrandomized trials.*)

Goldie JH, Goldman AJ, Gudauskas GA. Rationale for the use of alternating non–cross-resistant chemotherapy. Cancer Treat Rep 1982;66:439. (*The theoretical basis for modern multiple-drug regimens.*)

Hartmann O, Le Corroller AG, Blaise D, et al. Peripheral blood stem cell and bone marrow transplantation for solid tumors and lymphomas: hematologic recovery and costs. A randomized trial. Ann Intern Med 1997;126:600. (*An example of recent advances in hematologic support of aggressive chemotherapy; use of peripheral blood stem cells was associated with more rapid recovery at lower cost.*)

Lieberman M. The role of self-help groups for helping patients and families cope with cancer. CA Cancer J Clin 1988;38:162. (*The many pluses and some minuses reviewed.*)

Lynn J, Teno JM, Phillips RS, et al. Perceptions by family members of the dying experience of older and seriously ill patients. Ann Intern Med 1997;126:97. (*A prospective cohort study finding that although families often think the goal is comfort, life-sustaining measures are often used.*)

Papper S. Care of patients with incurable, chronic neoplasm: one patient's perspective. Am J Med 1985;78:271. (*A deeply moving essay written by a leading clinician while dying of myeloma.*)

Reiser SJ. Words as scalpels: transmitting evidence in the clinical dialogue. Ann Intern Med 1980;92:837. (*A very thoughtful article on communicating the diagnosis, with an interesting historical perspective.*)

Rose PG, Bundy BN, Watkins EB, et al. Concurrent cisplatin-based radiotherapy and chemotherapy for locally advanced cervical cancer. N Engl J Med 1999;340:1144. (*An important example of combined-modality therapy prolonging survival in locally advanced disease.*)

Silberfarb PS. Psychiatric treatment of the patient during cancer therapy. CA Cancer J Clin 1988;38:133. (*Very practical advice.*)

Spiegel D, Bloom JR, Yalom I. Group support for patients with metastatic cancer. Arch Gen Psychiatry 1981;38:527. (*Documents benefits of support group interactions.*)

Thomas LR. Does bone marrow transplantation confer a normal life span? N Engl J Med 1999;341:50. (*An editorial that considers benefits and risks.*)

Weeks JC, Cook EF, O'Day SJ, et al. Relationship between cancer patients' predictions of prognosis and their treatment preferences. JAMA 1998;279:1709. (*Overestimation of prognosis found to drive desire for life-extending therapy.*)

Welch-McCaffrey D, Hoffman B, Leigh SA, et al. Surviving adult cancers. Part 2: psychosocial implications. Ann Intern Med 1989;111:517. (*Best review to date on the subject, with an excellent review of the literature and a useful discussion of key issues; 58 references.*)

88
Principles of Cancer Drug Therapy

Chemotherapy and, more recently, biologic agents represent important components of cancer management. However, such agents are potent and can be relatively unselective, with adverse effects that can offset their beneficial antitumor qualities. A well-constructed program attempts to strike an effective balance between beneficial and adverse effects and requires the expertise of the oncologist. The primary care physician has an important supportive role, which is increasing as more cancer chemotherapy is conducted on an outpatient basis and away from cancer centers. While maintaining a close working relationship with the oncologist, the primary physician may be called on to monitor the effects of therapy closely and provide initial care for the wide range of medical and emotional problems that may arise (see Chapter 87). These responsibilities necessitate a knowledge of the general indications for chemotherapy and biologic agents, and an awareness of the major toxic and adverse side effects of commonly employed agents. The primary care physician must also know how to evaluate the response to treatment and alleviate side effects.

PRINCIPLES OF THERAPY

Types of Regimens and Their Indications

Chemotherapy may be given as preoperative (neoadjuvant) therapy, as postoperative (adjuvant) therapy, or as palliative (occasionally curative) therapy for advanced disease.

Neoadjuvant Chemotherapy is used for the preoperative treatment of *locally invasive tumors* that are moderately sensitive and responsive to drugs (e.g., stage III non–small-cell *lung* cancer and stage III *breast* cancer; see Chapters 53 and 122, respectively). The goal is to decrease tumor bulk and make possible a more conservative surgical approach, and also to reduce the risk for systemic disease via micrometastasis. For patients with locally invasive disease, an early consultation with the medical oncologist may be helpful and even precede the surgical referral.

Postoperative Adjuvant Therapy has now been established as a standard form of treatment for several cancers, including stages I and II *breast* cancer (see Chapter 122) and Duke's stage C *colon* cancer (see Chapter 76). The rationale behind giving chemotherapy to patients who have undergone what appears to be curative surgery is the frequency of distant micrometastases and local recurrences. Chemotherapy applied just after surgery has been more successful in prolonging survival than therapy delayed until clinical evidence arises of recurrence or spread.

Chemotherapy of Advanced Disease has evolved from a strictly palliative modality to a *curative* one in some instances (e.g., *lymphoma* and *testicular cancer*; see Chapters 84 and 143, respectively). This change has resulted from the discovery of increasingly effective chemotherapeutic agents and the development of *multiple-drug regimens* that have increased not only response rates but also the duration of response and the rates of complete clinical remission and cure. Nonetheless, much of chemotherapy in advanced disease remains *palliative*, designed to reduce morbidity and prolong survival without placing too heavy a burden on the patient. This is not always possible, and it takes good judgment to decide what and when to offer and when to withhold palliative therapy. When patients fail to demonstrate a clinically meaningful response, their chemotherapy regimen should be stopped or at least changed to an alternative program.

Basic Chemotherapy Strategies

Designing combination programs and applying dose-intensified therapy through the use of marrow transplantation and marrow growth factors are important chemotherapy strategies that maximize outcomes while helping to minimize risk.

Combination Chemotherapy. The use of regimens comprising agents with different modes of cellular action increases the effectiveness of therapy without greatly increasing toxicity. The best choices are drugs with nonadditive side effects. Synergistic effects are achieved while adverse effects are minimized. A meaningful response to cytotoxic chemotherapy is usually expected within two courses of treatment.

Dose Intensification. Using the highest possible doses is essential to ensuring effectiveness of therapy, especially when treating with curative intent. The use of too small a dose produces inferior outcomes. When cure is being attempted, it is best to try to maintain maximal doses and treat drug side effects by means other than dose reduction. Reductions in dose are among the most common causes of drug failure. Dose intensity and consequent long-term survival can be increased substantially by complementing chemotherapy with marrow-supportive efforts that include bone marrow transplantation and the use of hematopoietic growth factors.

Bone Marrow Transplantation. Efficacy is best established for its use in the treatment of lymphomas, myelomas, and leukemias. The role of bone marrow transplantation in breast cancer remains controversial and requires additional study. For the leukemias, the *allogeneic transplantation* of HLA-matched donor marrow cells has produced the best outcomes once cancerous marrow cells are eliminated by dose-intensified chemotherapy. In some instances, *autologous transplantation* and the use of *peripheral stem cells* has also produced meaningful results, especially in patients with solid tumors, extending the use of high-dose chemotherapy and reducing the costs and risks of marrow reconstitution. Risks are substantial; the most serious of these are life-threatening infection and acute graft-versus-host reactions in the short term, lymphomas and hematopoietic disorders within the first several years (a consequence of compromised immune function and Epstein-Barr virus infection), and solid tumors later in life (especially in patients also receiving radiation). Chronic graft-versus-host disease may also compromise outcomes. Such risks underscore the importance of careful patient selection, follow-up, and attending to cancer risk factors such as smoking. Although risk–reward ratios often favor proceeding to transplantation, the decision to proceed should be informed by data from well-designed randomized, controlled trials with long-term follow-up.

Growth Factors. *Granulocyte colony-stimulating factor* (G-CSF), *granulocyte–macrophage colony-stimulating factor* (GM-CSF), and *interleukin-1* (IL-1) can provide support to specific marrow cell lines and lessen the risks for infection that can result from intensive chemotherapy. These agents are expensive but are cost-effective when used prophylactically in situations in which febrile neutropenia is highly likely. They are not used routinely to treat episodes of neutropenia, but they do have a role in supporting allogeneic and autologous marrow transplantation and the use of peripheral stem cells. Recombinant *IL-11*, a cytokine that stimulates marrow, has been approved by the Food and Drug Administration to treat severe thrombocytopenia resulting from chemotherapy for nonmyeloid cancers. Under study is the use of *erythropoietin* and *thombopoietin*. For the former, the principal issue is cost-effectiveness; for the latter, the principal concerns involve long-term safety (i.e., risks for thrombosis, myelofibrosis, and stimulation of abnormal cells).

Follow-up. Only rarely does continued treatment in the absence of initial response result in an increased response; usually, more therapy is unwarranted. Follow-up assessment for response and determination of further chemotherapy is usually conducted within 2 months of initiation of the treatment program.

Cytotoxic Chemotherapeutic Agents

Cytotoxic drugs have been grouped into categories based on their mechanism of action or the chemical derivation of the drug (Table 88.1).

Alkylating Agents. In general, the alkylating agents have a broad spectrum of antitumor activity, chemically interacting directly with DNA. As just noted, secondary malignancy is a concern associated with their use. The most commonly used drugs in this class are *cyclophosphamide* and *nitrogen mustard*. *Ifosfamide* is a newer alkylating agent that has shown promise in treating cancers of the testicle, lung, and cervix.

Table 88.1.   Cytotoxic Chemotherapeutic Agents

CLASS/AGENTS	DOSE FREQUENCY	ACUTE TOXICITY			OTHER TOXICITY	ELIMINATION	PLASMA HALF-LIFE (hours)
		Leukocyte	Platelet	Nausea/vomiting			
Plant Derivatives							
Paclitaxol	q 3 wk	Moderate	Moderate	Mild	Anaphylactoid response, sensory neuropathy, alopecia	M	6–8
Vincristine	qwk	Mild	Mild	Mild	Distal neuropathy, inappropriate ADH	M	2.6
Vinblastine	qwk	Marked	Marked	Mild	Mucositis	M	3.1
VP-16 (etoposide)	qd x 5	Moderate	Mild	Mild	Distal neuropathy	M, R	6
Antibiotics							
Dactinomycin	qd x 5	Marked	Marked	Moderate	Alopecia, mucositis	M, R	?
Doxorubicin	q 3 wk	Marked	Marked	Moderate	Alopecia, cardiomyopathy	M	3–25
Daunorubicin	3 d, q 3 wk	Marked	Marked	Moderate	Alopecia, cardiomyopathy	M	3–?
Mitomycin C	qd x 3, q 3 wk	Marked	Marked	Moderate	Renal, pulmonary	M	?
Bleomycin	qwk	Rare	Rare	Mild	Skin, pulmonary, fibrosis, fever, allergic reactions	R	0.4–2
Antimetabolites							
Methotrexate (high-dose with leucovorin	q 3 wk q6h x 7 doses	Mild	Mild	Moderate	Hepatic dysfunction, renal failure	R M	2–8
Methotrexate	Twice weekly	Moderate-marked	Moderate-marked	Mild	Stomatitis	R	2–8
5-Fluorouracil	qwk or qd x 5, q 4 wk	Moderate-marked	Moderate-marked	Mild	Cerebellar, conjunctivitis	M	0.3
5-Fluorouracil with leucovorin	qwk x 6, qd x 5 q 4 wk	Marked	Marked	Mild	Diarrhea, stomatitis	M	0.3
6-Mercaptopurine	qd x 5	Moderate-marked	Moderate-marked	Mild	Cholestasis	M	0.3–0.6
Cytarabine (cytosine arabinoside)	q12h x 5–10 d	Marked	Marked	Moderate	Cholestasis, mucositis	R, M	0.15
Hydroxyurea	qd x 5	Marked	Moderate	Moderate	None	R, M	1.7
Fludarabine	qd x 5	Moderate	Mild	Mild	Pneumonitis, neurotoxicity	R, M	9.3
Alkylating Agents							
Cyclophosphamide	qd x 5	Marked	Mild	Moderate	Cystitis, water retention, alopecia	M	1–4
Ifosfamide	qd x 5	Moderate	Moderate	Mild	Neurotoxicity, urothelial neurotoxicity	M	5–6
and mesna	qd x 5.5	None	None	None	None	M	?
Melphalan	qd	Moderate	Moderate	Mild	Leukemia	M	2
Busulfan	qd	Marked	Marked	Mild	Pulmonary fibrosis	M	?
CCNU (lomustine)	q 6 wk	Marked	Marked	Moderate	Leukemia, pulmonary fibrosis, renal failure	M	?
BCNU (carmustine)	q 6 wk	Marked	Marked	Marked	Leukemia, pulmonary fibrosis, renal failure	M	1.0
Streptozocin	qd x 5 q 3–4 wk	Mild	Mild	Moderate-marked	Renal failure, hyperglycemia, hepatic enzyme elevation	R	0.25

Table 88.1. Cytotoxic Chemotherapeutic Agents—*cont'd*

CLASS/AGENT	DOSE FREQUENCY	ACUTE TOXICITY			OTHER TOXICITY	ELIMINATION	PLASMA HALF-LIFE (hours)
		Leukocyte	Platelet	Nausea/vomiting			
Chlorambucil (*cis*-diaminedi-chloroplatinum)	qd q 3–4 wk	Moderate Moderate	Moderate Moderate	Mild Severe	Leukemia Renal failure, Mg²⁺ wasting, peripheral neuropathy, ototoxicity	M R, M	1.5 0.3
Carboplatin	q 3–4 wk	Marked	Marked	Mild		R	
Miscellaneous							
DTIC (dacarbazine)	qd x 5	Mild	Mild	Marked	Flulike syndrome, venoocclusion	M	0.65
Procarbazine	qd x 10–14 d	Moderate	Moderate	Mlld	Sensitivity to amines	M	?
Mitoxantrone	q 3 wk	Moderate	Moderate	Mild	Cholestasis, cardiac	M	0.25–37

ADH, antidiuretic hormone; M, Metabolized Heliver exasperated; R, Renally.

Adapted from Chabner BA. Anticancer drugs. In: DeVita VT, Hellman S, Rosenberg SA, eds. Cancer: principles and practice of oncology, 4th ed. Philadelphia; JB Lippincott Co, 1993:325, with permission.

Antimetabolites. These drugs interfere with the synthesis of DNA by blocking the action of important metabolic precursors and cofactors. Their greatest effect is on rapidly growing cells. The most commonly used agents in this class are *fluorouracil* and *methotrexate*. The antimetabolites are rapidly metabolized and excreted in the urine. Methotrexate is distributed throughout total body water, so that pleural effusions and ascitic fluid are potential reservoirs of the drug. Newer antimetabolites include *gemcitabine* (for pancreatic, bladder and lung cancers) and *fludarabine*, *DCF*, and *2-CDA* (for chronic lymphocytic leukemia and hairy cell leukemia, respectively).

Topoisomerase Inhibitors. *Etoposide* and the anthracycline antibiotics (*doxorubicin* and *bleomycin*) impair the action of the reversible nucleases that create nicks in the DNA strands needed for DNA replication. The spectrum of activity of doxorubicin is comparable to that of the alkylating drugs. In combination with the alkylating drugs, doxorubicin appears to have a synergistic antitumor effect.

Mitotic Spindle Inhibitors. These agents inhibit mitosis. *Paclitaxel*, *vincristine*, and *vinblastine* are the best-known examples. Paclitaxel has the unique property of interfering with microtubular function. Much excitement accompanied the demonstration of its efficacy in the treatment of advanced ovarian cancer.

Miscellaneous or Mixed-mechanism Agents include two important drugs: the *nitrosoureas* and *cisplatin*. The *nitrosoureas* are alkylating drugs that cross the blood–brain barrier. *Cisplatin* is effective in the treatment of testicular and ovarian cancers.

Adverse Effects of Chemotherapeutic Agents

The principal factor limiting the usefulness of chemotherapeutic agents is their relative *lack of selectivity* for the tumor cell (Table 88.2). Cytotoxic drugs adversely affect normal cells, especially those populations with a rapid turnover (bone marrow, hair follicles, gastrointestinal mucosa). This leads to the development of *bone marrow suppression*, *alopecia*, and *gastroenteritis* shortly after the initiation of chemotherapy.

Typically, *acute marrow suppression* begins 7 to 10 days after the administration of chemotherapy and may last about 1 week. Continuous cytotoxic therapy may cause a more lasting *cumulative suppression of the bone marrow*. However, most forms of adjuvant chemotherapy are usually not associated with persistent marrow suppression, although a transient fall in cellular constituents may occur.

The most serious risks of chemotherapy are *leukopenia*, leading to overwhelming sepsis, and *thrombocytopenia*, resulting in hemorrhage. In most instances, leukopenia and thrombocytopenia are dose-related and may be prevented or lessened by dose adjustment in patients with marginal marrow reserve because of marrow invasion, advanced age, or prior therapy. Nonetheless, the goal of most chemotherapeutic regimens is to induce some degree of leukopenia, which can serve as a measure of the cytotoxic effect and a guideline to dosage.

The *gastrointestinal toxicity* of chemotherapy can be debilitating. It includes nausea, vomiting, mucosal injury (stomatitis), and diarrhea. Although not as life-threatening as leukopenia and thrombocytopenia, gastrointestinal side effects can significantly compromise quality of life, morale, and willingness to undergo further chemotherapy.

Alopecia is a consequence of most forms of chemotherapy. It is usually partial, but with doxorubicin the hair loss is generally total. It begins approximately 2 weeks after the initiation of treatment and becomes complete by 4 to 6 weeks. Hair loss is almost always transient, and often some hair grows during the course of treatment; however, total restitution does not take place until chemotherapy is stopped. When hair growth returns, darker, finer, more curly hair is usually produced, but with time, the normal texture and color return.

Of concern for younger patients, especially those undergoing curative-intent therapy for leukemia or a lymphoma, is the significant risk for a *secondary malignancy*. Acute leukemia may arise a decade or two after treatment for lymphoma; lymphoma is seen in some leukemic patients years after chemotherapy, especially when alkylating agents have been used. Although the evidence for risk is compelling, the benefits of treatment continue to outweigh the risks.

Table 88.2.   Side Effects of Some Commonly Used and Important New
Chemotherapeutic Agents

CLASS AND AGENT	SIDE EFFECTS
Alkylating Agents	
Cyclophosphamide	Early: n/v, facial burning, metallic taste, blurred vision, hypersensitivity Delayed: bone marrow depression, alopecia, hemorrhagic cystitis, bladder cancer, pulmonary infiltrates and fibrosis, SIADH, leukemia
Ifosfamide	Early: n/v, confusion, nephrotoxicity, metabolic acidosis, cardiotoxicity Delayed: bone marrow depression, hemorrhagic cystitis, alopecia, SIADH, renal failure, neurotoxicity
Antimetabolites	
Methotrexate	Early: n/v, diarrhea, hepatic injury, hypersensitivity Delayed: oral and GI ulceration with possible perforation, bone marrow depression, hepatotoxicity with cirrhosis late; renal toxicity; pulmonary infiltrates and fibrosis, osteoporosis, alopecia, conjunctivitis, depigmentation, menstrual dysfunction, infertility, encephalopathy, lymphoma
5-Fluorouracil	Early: n/v, diarrhea, hypersensitivity rarely Delayed: oral and GI ulcers, bone marrow depression; diarrhea, cerebellar nerologic defects, arrhythmias, angina, alopecia, hyperpigmentation, conjunctivitis, palmar–plantar dysesthesias, heart failure, seizures
6-Mercaptopurine	Early: n/v, diarrhea Delayed: bone marrow depression, cholestasis, oral and intestinal ulcers, pancreatitis
Cytarabine	Early: n/v, diarrhea, anaphylaxis, acute respiratory distress (high doses) Delayed: bone marrow depression, conjunctivitis, megaloblastic anemia, oral ulceration, liver injury, fever, pulmonary edema, neuropathy (high doses), rhabdomyolysis, pancreatitis, rash
Gemcitabine	Early: fatigue, n/v Delayed: bone marrow depression, edema, pulmonary toxicity, anal pruritis
Fludarabine	Early: n/v, diarrhea, hypersensitivity Delayed: bone marrow depression, immunosuppression, CNS effects, visual disturbances, renal injury at high doses, pulmonary infiltrates
Topoisomerase Inhibitors	
Etopside	Early: n/v, diarrhea, fever, hypotension, local phlebitis, hypersensitivity Delayed: bone marrow depression, alopecia, rash, peripheral neuropathy, leukemia, mucositis and liver injury with high doses.
Doxorubicin	Early: n/v, red urine, local tissue damage, diarrhea, fever, ECG changes, ventricular irritability, anaphylaxis Delayed: bone marrow depression, cardiotoxicity (very late), alopecia, stomatitis, anorexia, conjunctivitis, acral pigmentation, dermatitis, acral erythrodysesthesia, hyperuricemia
Bleomycin	Early: n/v, rarely diarrhea Delayed: bone marrow depression, pulmonary infiltrates and fibrosis, alopecia, gynecomastia, ovarian failure, hyperpigmentation, azoospermia, leukemia, cataracts, hepatitis, seizures, secondary malignancy with prolonged use
Irinotecan	Early: n/v, diarrhea, fever Delayed: diarrhea, anorexia, stomatitis, bone marrow depression, asthenia, alopecia, abdominal cramping and pain
Topotecan	Early: n/v, diarrhea, headache, flulike illness Delayed: bone marrow depression, asthenia, stomatitis, alopecia, abdominal pain
Mitotic Spindle Inhibitors	
Vinblastine	Early: n/v, local tissue injury from extravasation Delayed: bone marrow depression, alopecia, peripheral neuropathy, stomatitis, jaw pain, paralytic ileus
Vincristine	Early: local tissue injury from extravasation Delayed: peripheral neuropathy, alopecia, mild bone marrow depression, constipation, ileus, jaw pain, SIADH, optic atrophy
Paclitaxel	Early: hypersensitivity reactions Delayed: bone marrow depression, peripheral neuropathy, alopecia, myalgias, cardiac toxicity, mucositis

n/v, nausea and vomiting; SIADH, syndrome of inappropriate secretion of antidiuretic hormone; GI, gastrointestinal; CNS, central nervous system; ECG, electrocardiographic.

Adapted from Drugs of choice, revised ed. New Rochelle, NY: The Medical Letter, 1999:39.

New Cytotoxic Therapies: The Biologic Agents

Interleukins. Naturally occurring cytokines such as the interleukins are produced by activated T cells and demonstrate immunostimulatory and antineoplastic effects. IL-2 triggers peripheral mononuclear cells to release a host of biologically active cytokines that in turn modulate the activity of natural killer cells, B cells, and suppressor cells, with eventual lysis of cancer cells. The best antitumor effects have been observed in patients with metastatic renal cell carcinoma, for which IL-2 treatment is approved by the Food and Drug Administration. Adverse effects are caused by the release of tumor necrosis factor and IL-1 and include fever, chills, lethargy, diarrhea, thrombocytopenia, liver dysfunction, and myocarditis. Vascular leakage is a major side effect. Adverse effects are dose-related and rapidly reversible.

Interferons are biologic response modifiers—proteins with antiproliferative and immunomodulatory properties. *Interferon alfa*, an interferon with antitumor activity, is produced by leukocytes, often in response to viral infection. It induces lymphocyte activation and has demonstrated antitumor effects clinically, most notably in chronic myelogenous leukemia, hairy cell leukemia, and, to a lesser extent, Kaposi's sarcoma. Interferon alfa is also moderately useful as adjuvant therapy in melanoma, renal cell carcinoma, and multiple myeloma. Although interferon alfa can exert antitumor effects when used as monotherapy, it often produces better outcomes in combination with chemotherapeutic agents (e.g., with cytarabine in chronic myelogenous leukemia). Adverse effects are dose-dependent and can be troublesome, frequently causing therapy to be stopped. The most common is a flulike syndrome of fevers, sweats, fatigue, and myalgias, experienced by most patients during the first several weeks of therapy. The flulike symptoms are often transient and likely to resolve unless the dose is increased, but a host of even more disabling symptoms may follow. These include marked anorexia, depression, anxiety, emotional lability, hair loss, tinnitus, reversible hearing loss, and thyroid dysfunction. An increased susceptibility to bacterial infection and cardiotoxicity may also develop.

Monoclonal Antibodies. Although treatment with monoclonal antibodies is still experimental for cancer, the efficacy of these agents in the treatment of Crohn's disease and rheumatoid arthritis has already been demonstrated. The use of antibodies is also being intensively studied as a means of enhancing the specificity of chemotherapeutic agents. The promise of these approaches is considerable and likely to result in major advances. The reader is urged to follow the literature closely for data on efficacy, safety, and indications for use.

PRACTICAL ISSUES

Administration of Chemotherapy. Sometimes, the administration of chemotherapy is assigned to the primary physician, particularly when the services of the oncologist are not locally available. Under such circumstances, it is particularly important to be aware of the potential hazard of *extravasation* associated with certain IV agents [e.g., doxorubicin, vincristine, vinblastine, dacarbazine (DTIC), carmustine (BCNU), nitrogen mustard]. The best treatment is prevention, with proper venous access being the most important element. When extravasation does occur, it results in tissue irritation and secondary inflammation that leads to ulceration and necrosis. Surgical grafting and debridement are sometimes necessary. In the event of extravasation, the infusions should be stopped immediately and *ice* applied. Any accumulation of drug should be removed by aspiration. The actual inflammation and necrosis may not occur for 3 to 10 days following injection, although pain is generally present early on. Corticosteroids have been used, but definitive evidence of efficacy has not been demonstrated.

Even without extravasation, the repeated use of irritating IV chemotherapy drugs can lead to sclerosis and endothelial deterioration, particularly when small-caliber veins are used for infusion. Large-diameter veins in the antecubital fossa or higher are preferred. Devices for venous access facilitate administration.

Suppression of Nausea and Vomiting. The drugs most likely to induce severe nausea and vomiting include cisplatin, dacarbazine, doxorubicin, nitrogen mustard, and high doses of cyclophosphamide. Some agents cause vomiting that begins approximately 30 to 45 minutes following injection; with others, particularly cyclophosphamide and doxorubicin, the vomiting begins 4 to 5 hours after injection. Recent advances in understanding the mechanisms of chemotherapy-induced nausea and vomiting have led to the development of effective multifaceted programs (see Chapter 91).

Management of Bone Marrow Suppression. Generalized marrow suppression is common. The pattern of suppression is a function of the type of drug, dose, and schedule of administration (Table 88.3). Standard approaches to this problem include adjustments in dose and timing of chemotherapy. Dose adjustments for subsequent courses of therapy are based on the nadir levels observed. In monitoring patients on chemothera-

Table 88.3. Chronologic Patterns of Marrow Suppression Secondary to Chemotherapy

AGENT	NADIR DAY	OPERATION
Nonsuppressive Drugs		
Bleomycin		
Vincristine		
Streptozotocin		
Corticosteroids		
Dacarbazine (DTIC)		
Marrow-Suppressive Drugs		
Alkylating drugs		
Cyclophosphamide		
Nitrogen mustard	5–8	Variable
Mitomycin C	Delayed	Cumulative
Antibiotics		
Doxorubicin	12–14	5 d
Dactinomycin		
Antimetabolites		
5-Fluorouracil	5–10	<5 d
Cytosine arabinoside		
Methotrexate		
Natural products		
Vinblastine	8–12	3 d
Others		
Nitrosoureas	14–28	Cumulative
Hydroxyurea	Variable	
Procarbazine	Variable	

peutic regimens, the anticipated nadir days for blood counts are the most crucial times to obtain follow-up complete blood cell counts. For patients in whom leukopenia develops, the observation period should be intensified, depending on the level of the count and the presence of associated fever or sepsis. Emerging data suggest that *prophylactic oral antibiotics* (e.g., 500 mg of levofloxacin daily) reduce the number of hospitalizations in patients whose absolute neutrophil count falls below 1,000/mm³. The advent of marrow growth factors (see above) has enhanced our ability to administer the optimal doses of chemotherapy, which ordinarily might be limited by the onset of marrow suppression. Growth factors work best when given prophylactically, rather than after marrow suppression has set in. They are expensive but can prevent hospitalizations and limit complications.

EVALUATION OF RESPONSE TO THERAPY

Patients on chemotherapeutic regimens are monitored for adverse effects at the same time that the effectiveness of treatment is evaluated (see also Chapter 87). Objective tumor measurements are often difficult to define, but generally the oncologist depends on them to gauge the response to therapy (Table 88.4).

The criteria of response are often difficult to evaluate because partial responses may be influenced by nontumor factors. In addition, some forms of metastatic disease simply cannot be measured, such as osseous metastases and, particularly, osteoblastic lesions. Criteria for some metastatic patterns have been established, such as hepatomegaly, in which the criterion for response is a 30% decrease in the sum of measurements made below the costal margin at the midclavicular and midxiphoid lines. Peritoneal masses, pleural effusions, and skin ulcerations are not considered amenable to evaluation. *Ultra-sonography* and *computed tomography* have helped quantify lesions in the retroperitoneum.

Tumor markers (see Chapter 86) have facilitated gauging the response to therapy objectively. Serum levels of markers, monitored sequentially, correlate well with tumor mass and often predict recurrence before it becomes clinically evident. For example, measurement of levels of human chorionic gonadotropin has proved useful in the management of testicular cancer, and determination of carcinoembryonic antigen in colorectal cancer. Markers derived from monoclonal antibody techniques are increasingly important, including CA19-9 for pancreatic cancer, prostate-specific antigen for prostate cancer, CA15-3 for breast cancer, and CA-125 for ovarian cancer. Other biochemical parameters, such as levels of alkaline phosphatase and the various hepatic enzymes, have proved uniformly inadequate in the evaluation of the effectiveness of treatment.

PATIENT EDUCATION

The ability to tolerate chemotherapy is enhanced by a strong and trusting patient–doctor relationship. Fully educating patients and families about diagnosis, prognosis, and the rationale and side effects of planned treatment can greatly facilitate the development of trust and confidence (see Chapter 88). Concerns about alopecia, sterility, gastrointestinal upset, and other side effects should be elicited and directly addressed. The probability of response also deserves review. A comprehensive educational effort appropriate for the patient's level of understanding allows the patient to participate meaningfully in decision making and encourages a sense of partnership in the undertaking, an attitude that can help sustain the patient through this often difficult time.

INDICATIONS FOR ADMISSION AND REFERRAL

The onset of febrile neutropenia (absolute neutrophil counts <1,000/mm³) requires immediate hospitalization. The development of bleeding in the setting of thrombocytopenia is an indication for urgent hospitalization and consideration of platelet transfusion. The asymptomatic patient with severe thrombocytopenia (platelet count <20,000/mm³) also deserves consideration for admission and platelet transfusion. Counts of 20,000 to 50,000 are an indication for close observation and warning the patient to avoid trauma.

Chemotherapy programs are in a constant state of revision as new combinations are tried and new agents developed. Each patient's treatment program must be designed in conjunction with an oncologist. When such expertise is not locally available, patients may have to travel to a regional center for therapy. Computer-based chemotherapy protocol advisory systems are now available to help provide expert input where it may not otherwise be obtainable.

A.H.G.

Table 88.4.   Criteria of Response to Therapy

Survival

Measured from time of diagnosis, metastasis, or initiation of treatment in days, weeks, or months, to be compared by median (as opposed to mean) with a randomized control or historical control not receiving treatment or receiving alternative treatment. Survival as a measurement of time may also be supplemented by a time measurement of diagnosis to point of recurrence and is translated as disease-free survival.

Objective Reduction in Tumor

Partial Response

Equals a 50% reduction in the product of the maximum perpendicular diameters of the most easily measurable lesion without increase in other lesions and with a minimum duration of 4 weeks.

Complete Response

Equals a 100% reduction in all evidence of tumor for minimum of 4 weeks without appearance of new lesions.

Stable Disease

Equals a less than 25% decrease in measurable disease without development of other lesions.

No Response (Progressive Disease)

Equals a more than 25% increase in the size of the lesion or the development of new lesions.

Improvement

Equals a 25%–50% reduction in the product of maximum perpendicular diameters lasting at least 4 weeks.

ANNOTATED BIBLIOGRAPHY

Curtis RE, Rowlings PA, Deeg HJ, et al. Solid cancers after bone marrow transplantation. N Engl J Med 1997;336:897. (*Long-term cohort study finding increased risk for new solid cancers years after transplantation.*)

Duell T, van Lint MT, Ljungman P, et al. Health and functional status of long-term survivors of bone marrow transplantation. Ann Intern

Med 1997;126:184. (*Retrospective multicenter study finding most patients in good health after 5 years, but late cancers and chronic graft-versus-host disease are problematic for some.*)

Fojo AT, Ueda K, Slamon DJ, et al. Expression of a multidrug-resistant gene in human tumors and tissues. Proc Natl Acad Sci U S A 1987;84:265. (*Mechanism of multiple-drug resistance reported.*)

Garcia-Carbonero R, Hidalgo M, Paz-Ares L, et al. Patient selection in high-dose chemotherapy trials: relevance in high-risk breast cancer. J Clin Oncol 1997;15:3178. (*Study inclusion criteria actually found to be an independent predictor of good outcome, which underscores the importance of reading studies carefully for sources of bias.*)

Goldie JH, Goldman AJ, Gudauskas GA. Rationale for the use of alternating non–cross-resistant chemotherapy. Cancer Treat Rep 1982;66:439. (*The theoretical basis for combination chemotherapy.*)

Guilhot F, Chastang C, Michallet M, et al. Interferon alfa-2b combined with cytarabine versus interferon alone in chronic myelogenous leukemia. N Engl J Med 1997;337:223. (*Major study providing an example of interferon efficacy, especially when combined with conventional chemotherapy.*)

Hartmann O, Le Corroller AG, Blaise D, et al. Peripheral blood stem cell and bone marrow transplantation for solid tumors and lymphomas: hematologic recovery and cost. A randomized, controlled trial. Ann Intern Med 1997;126:600. (*Use of peripheral blood stem cells produced more rapid marrow recovery at lower cost.*)

Hryniuk W. Is more better? J Clin Oncol 1986;4:621. (*An editorial reviewing the issue of dose intensity.*)

Pui C-H, Boyett JM, Hughes WT, et al. Human granulocyte colony-stimulating factor after induction chemotherapy in children with acute lymphoblastic leukemia. N Engl J Med 1997;336:1781. (*Example of application of G-CSF in setting of intensive chemotherapy.*)

Rowinsky EK, Donehower RC. Paclitaxel (Taxol). N Engl J Med 1995;332:1004. (*Excellent review of this increasingly important chemotherapeutic agent.*)

Singal PK, Iliskovic N. Doxorubicin-induced cardiomyopathy. N Engl J Med 1998;339:900. (*Reviews major dose-related complication of this commonly used chemotherapeutic agent.*)

Vadhan-Raj S, Murray LJ, Bueso-Ramos C, et al. Stimulation of megakaryocyte and platelet production by a single dose of recombinant thrombopoietin in patients with cancer. Ann Intern Med 1997;126:673. (*A phase I and phase II clinical cohort study.*)

89

Principles of Radiation Therapy

THOMAS DELANEY

Modern radiation therapy represents an important means of achieving local and regional control of malignancy in addition to providing palliation. When given with the intent of controlling disease and attempting cure, it is termed *radical*; when given for symptomatic relief, it is designated *palliative*. Although the design and implementation of such therapy is the responsibility of the radiation oncologist, the primary physician shares in the decision to use the modality, monitors and supports the patient while it is being administered, and watches for and treats late complications. The primary care physician needs to be familiar with basic aspects of radiation therapy, its applications, and its side effects.

PRINCIPLES OF MANAGEMENT

Response to Irradiation

Determinants of Radiosensitivity. Exponential killing of both tumor and normal cells occurs after an initial, sublethal accumulation of radiation damage. The ability of cells to accumulate some radiation damage before cell death is manifested is believed to be linked to *repair capacity*. The general shapes of the radiation response curves of cells in culture are remarkably similar, with most of the difference in *"radiosensitivity"* a consequence of subtle differences in the ability of cells to accumulate and repair radiation damage. Cells in the S phase of the cell cycle (when DNA synthesis is taking place, but no mitosis) are the least sensitive to radiation, probably because of the enhanced capacity for repair in this phase. In response to radiation injury, normal cells initially stop proliferating because of "checkpoints" in the cell cycle designed to allow the cell to repair DNA damage before cell division is attempted. Malignant cells often have mutations in these critical cell cycle regulatory genes (such as *p53*) that perturb the checkpoint function, so that progress through the cell cycle is uninterrupted despite the presence of radiation-damaged DNA; as a consequence, cell death occurs during mitosis.

The response to irradiation is also affected by the *volume* of the tumor. Except for uniquely radiosensitive tumors (lymphomas and seminomas), larger tumors are more difficult to eradicate with any given dose of irradiation. This is in part related to the larger number of tumor cells that must be killed. Another part of the reason for this resistance, however, is *tissue hypoxia*. Oxygen facilitates the cytotoxic effect of x-rays, which is mediated in part by oxygen free radicals. Hypoxic cells are about three times more refractory to irradiation than are cells treated in the presence of oxygen. Interior areas of large tumors can become hypoxic and relatively refractory to radiation. However, as the tumor shrinks, the access of its hypoxic cells to oxygen increases, and they become more susceptible to radiation if doses are given in sequential fractionated fashion (see below). Nevertheless, the presence of anemia (hemoglobin levels <10 to 12.5 g/dL) has been shown to have a negative impact on radiotherapy treatment outcome in multiple anatomic sites, which has led to the clinical practice of administering red cell transfusions or erythropoietin to maintain hemoglobin levels during a course of radiotherapy.

Strategies to Improve Response. Effective approaches include the use of *particle beams*, concurrent *chemotherapy*, and compounds that *sensitize hypoxic tumor cells*. Particle beams such as neutrons are less dependent on oxygen for their cytotoxic action than are x-rays and represent another means of treating large, poorly vascularized tumors. Other particles, such as protons, have significantly better dose distribution properties than conventional x-rays do, so that the dose to the tumor can be increased substantially while adjacent normal tissue is spared. Many chemotherapy compounds, such as *cis*-platinum, 5-fluorouracil, and paclitaxel, enhance radiation cytotoxicity, which results in simultaneous improvement in local and distant control of tumor. Compounds that sensitize hypoxic tumor cells and improve their response to radiation therapy are under investigation.

The *dose* of irradiation that can be safely directed at a malignancy is limited by the tolerance of the organs surrounding it. Although the energy (i.e., voltage) of the radiation determines its ability to penetrate tissue, it is the amount of radiation actually absorbed that determines the biologic effects. *High-energy* megavoltage beams spare the skin, with better cosmetic results. Focusing beams on a tumor from multiple directions concentrates the dose in the tumor and avoids excessive irradiation of critical adjacent normal structures. Damage can be particularly injurious when radiation is absorbed by cells of the heart, liver, brain, intestines, bone marrow, kidneys, or lung (see below). These structures have defined radiation tolerances that are related to the volume irradiated and the dose received. Usually, trade-offs must be made between therapeutic benefits and adverse effects.

Minimizing Adverse Effects. The probability of radiation-induced complications depends on how narrow the difference is between the dose needed for control of the tumor and the dose that causes injury to normal tissue. (The ratio of the two doses is termed the *therapeutic ratio*.) The greater the difference in doses, the better the result. Dose fractionation, shielding of normal tissue, and use of imaging techniques to define tumor volume and location precisely have helped limit the adverse effects of radiation therapy.

Fractionating the dose helps to widen the margin of safety and improve the selective killing of tumor cells. Normal cells repair sublethal radiation damage more effectively than do tumor cells. Traditional fractionation programs provide about 200 centigray (cGy) or rads per treatment, applied five times per week. Newer fractionation schemes hyperfractionate radiation with two to three treatments per day to exploit differences in radiation repair capacity between tumor and normal tissue maximally and accelerate the treatment to overcome the repopulation of tumor cells that occurs during the conventional treatment of some tumors.

Shielding helps protect vital organs adjacent to the portal from radiation exposure. Often, custom-fabricated lead shields or analogous, automated blocking devices in the head of the treatment machine (multileaf collimators) are used to prevent the irradiation of normal tissue abutting the tumor.

Computed tomography (CT) and *magnetic resonance imaging* (MRI) have improved the delineation of tumor volume and the surrounding anatomic structures so that the target can be more precisely defined. *Simulation* reproduces the geometry of the actual radiation portal and helps to ensure that only the desired tissue is irradiated. CT-based simulation is increasingly used for this purpose; patients are scanned in the treatment position with markers on the skin or other structures to allow the

tumor to be referenced to a reproducible, spatial coordinate system. The CT data set is transferred electronically to a three-dimensional treatment system that allows the tumor, normal tissues, and doses to be displayed in three dimensions. This technology permits the radiation dose to the tumor to be escalated, so that the tumor control rate is increased, while normal tissue is simultaneously protected; as a result, fewer side effects to normal tissue are produced. Specific applications of this technology include *stereotactic radiosurgery* for the treatment of intracranial tumors. In this technique, the patient is rigidly immobilized in a head frame for CT and radiation treatment. In addition, amifostine is the first compound to be shown to be a clinically useful and preferential protector of normal tissue from radiation damage.

Clinical Applications

Three basic *delivery modes* are currently used. External sources (teletherapy or external beam) are the most frequently applied. Brachytherapy, in which encapsulated sources are placed directly into the body at tumor sites, has selective advantages in the treatment of very localized disease. Improvements in imaging and radiation treatment planning have resulted in a resurgence of interest in brachytherapy at such sites as the prostate, where the therapeutic ratio for this technique is high. Systemic delivery via radionuclides is the third mode. Investigational forms entail IV administration of radionuclide-labeled monoclonal antibodies designed to attack a target cancer selectively. The theoretical attractiveness of the latter two methods is closer proximity to the tumor and the limited exposure of normal tissue to radiotherapy.

Radiation is applied for to achieve cure and control in addition to palliation. It may be the sole treatment or an alternative therapy, or it may be combined with other modalities (Table 89.1).

As Sole or Alternative Therapy. Like surgery, radiation therapy is primarily a method of treating local or regional disease. The goal is to "sterilize" both the primary site and likely areas of local and regional spread. In some instances, such as stage I *Hodgkin's disease* or early low-grade *non-Hodgkin's lymphoma* (see Chapter 84), radiation therapy is the treatment of choice. When preservation of function and appearance can be achieved with comparable survival outcome, radiation may be preferred by some patients over surgery (as in localized *breast cancer*, localized *prostate cancer*, or early *head* and *neck cancers*). When surgery and radiation provide similar rates of cure and control, the choice depends largely on the impact of treatment on the patient.

As Combination Therapy. Several characteristics of radiation therapy make it a good complement to *surgery*. Surgery is the more effective of the two modalities in the management of bulky disease, whereas radiation appears to be more effective in the treatment of small-volume, locally invasive disease, which is the basis for the sequence of surgery for local disease followed by radiation as adjunctive therapy. Radiation can also reduce tumor bulk and destroy microscopic disease, thereby facilitating surgical removal and local control. By allowing the use of lower doses of radiation and less radical surgery, combination therapy minimizes side effects and has become the cor-

Table 89.1. Applications of Radiotherapy

TUMOR	COMMENTS
Radiation Therapy Alone Curative	
Hodgkin's disease	Stage IA–IIA; 90% 10-year survival
Lymphoma (indolent)	Stage I–II; 50% 10-year survival
Cervical cancer	Curative for early-stage disease; stage IB–IIA 85% 5-year disease-free survival
Testicular cancer	Seminomas; cure rates for early-stage disease >95%
Head and neck cancer	Early-stage disease (T1, T2); results comparable with those of surgery with less functional and cosmetic loss
Prostate cancer	External beam or brachytherapy excellent alternatives to surgery for organ-confined disease; external beam and hormonal therapy for locally advanced disease
Radiation Combined With Another Modality Potentially Curative	
Uterine cancer	With surgery, good results for stages I, II, and III; 60–90% 5-year survival
Head and neck cancer	With surgery and/or chemotherapy in locally advanced cases
Soft-tissue sarcomas	In combination with surgery, often function- or limb-sparing
Breast cancer	In combination with surgery and chemotherapy/hormonal therapy, breast preservation with survival equivalent to that of mastectomy possible for tumors ≤ 5 cm
Esophagus	Chemoradiation cures 25% of patients with localized disease
Lung	Chemoradiation cures 15% of patients with locally advanced non–small-cell and 20–25% of patients with limited small-cell carcinoma
Bladder	Chemoradiation is an organ-sparing option with similar treatment outcome as cystectomy
Rectum	Addition of chemoradiation to radical surgery improves outcome in patients with node-positive or transmural tumors
Anus	Chemoradiation has replaced surgery as the primary treatment, curing 75% of patients
Radiation Therapy Palliative	
Bony metastases	For pain not controlled by analgesics, chemotherapy, or hormonal therapy
Brain metastases	Stereotactic radiosurgery an alternative to craniotomy for patients with 1 to 2 lesions
Spinal cord compression	Treat emergently with steroids especially when there is a single focal obstructing lesion; patients with myeloma, lymphoma, and small-cell cancers respond especially well to radiation.

nerstone of the organ-preservation treatments for cancer. Such combination therapy often also includes chemotherapy (see below).

With Surgery. Whether to administer radiation before, during, or after surgery depends on several practical and theoretical issues. Favoring *preoperative treatment* are the need to reduce tumor size for easier resection and the desirability of sterilizing tumor cells that might be spread during surgery. Moreover, *postoperative irradiation* may be less effective if the vascular bed is surgically reduced and oxygen delivery impaired. Factors favoring postoperative treatment include prompt performance of surgery, ability to determine the need for radiotherapy based on a pathologic review of the resected specimen, avoidance of radiation effects on wound healing, and destruction of any remaining microscopic disease. *Intraoperative treatment* allows one to displace normal abdominal organs (which are quite intolerant of the high radiation doses necessary to sterilize gross tumor) and target diseased tissue more precisely.

With Chemotherapy. The application of radiation in combination with chemotherapy to achieve cure is established for advanced stages of *Hodgkin's disease*, and the combination has been demonstrated in the last decade to result in improved outcome in locally advanced cancers of the *head* and *neck, lung, esophagus, rectum, anus,* and uterine *cervix* in comparison with radiotherapy alone. The rationale is to treat local disease with radiation and administer chemotherapeutic agents that both in-

crease the efficacy of radiation against the primary tumor and target occult systemic metastases. Radiation can also be used to treat areas not readily accessible to chemotherapy, such as the brain in patients with small-cell lung cancer. Although improved survival has been demonstrated, acute and late toxicities can be additive. Marrow suppression can be the limiting problem. Other instances of additive adverse effects include the following: Cyclyphosphamde (Cytoxan) and radiation produce acute hemorrhagic cystitis; 5-fluorouracil and radiotherapy cause acute mucositis of the oral cavity and acute radiation enteritis; *cis*-platinum, etoposide, and taxanes combined with thoracic radiotherapy produce acute esophagitis, and combination chemotherapy with radiation increases the risk for leukemia. Some drugs enhance radiation reactions in normal tissues, even when given up to a year after radiotherapy. Adriamycin is the most prominent example of a drug producing this *"recall phenomenon."*

At present, the optimal strategies for the application of combined-modality therapy are continuing to evolve. The literature should be followed for the results of studies now ongoing.

As Palliative Therapy. Radiation serves an important function in providing symptomatic relief to some patients with incurable disease. For those tumors that respond to chemotherapy or hormonal therapy, radiation should be held in reserve. However, if localized tumor is not sensitive to other modalities, palliative radiation may be an effective means of providing symptomatic relief. In most instances, the treatment of asymptomatic lesions yields little benefit, although prophylactic brain irradiation appears useful in patients with small-cell lung cancer. One of the best examples of palliative therapy is for painful *bony metastases* from such tumors as those of breast and prostate. Within 2 to 3 weeks of the start of a relatively short course of radiotherapy (2 weeks), many patients experience relief from bone pain. Radiation to bony metastases has also been used to stabilize a weight-bearing bone, but if cortical involvement is present, then surgical stabilization of the bone may be necessary. Radiation plays an important role in the urgent treatment of certain oncologic emergencies, including *spinal cord compression* and *superior vena cava syndrome* (see Chapter 92).

Adverse Effects

As noted previously, many normal cells tolerate radiation better than do malignant cells. However, the degree of tolerance varies greatly (Table 89.2). Tissues with high rates of turnover and large stem cell populations are among the most vulnerable. Even organs with almost no proliferative capacity are at risk by virtue of the vulnerability of their vascular endothelium. Much radiation-induced injury is vascular in nature. Toxicity may be acute or chronic. Acute toxicity is noted in tissues with the highest rates of turnover (e.g., marrow, skin, gastrointestinal mucosa). *Acute radiation toxicity* is often defined as that appearing within 90 days after the start of radiotherapy. It usually resolves with supportive care in the majority of patients without significant late consequences. *Toxicity appearing later*, however, is usually more serious and clinically significant, as it may involve irreversible injury to the involved normal tissue.

Tolerance to radiotherapy decreases as the dose is increased. The *dose limit* for a tissue can be expressed as the cumulative dose that produces a 5% incidence of toxicity when radiation is delivered in 200-cGy fractions for 5 days a week. Beyond the dose limit, the incidence of toxicity rises quickly.

Bone Marrow Suppression. The bone marrow is the most radiosensitive tissue, with marrow suppression developing when exposure exceeds 250 cGy. Suppression is usually transient and reversible, unless large marrow volumes are irradiated. Skin, gastrointestinal mucosa, and lung are of intermediate sensitivity.

Radiation Pneumonitis starts to appear when the dose to a large volume of the lung surpasses 2,000 cGy; the incidence reaches 100% at doses of 4,000 cGy. The onset, usually within 6 to 12 weeks, is characterized by dyspnea, cough, low-grade fever, hypoxemia, and a "ground glass" appearance on chest x-ray films. CT may show straight lines that match the radiotherapy field. Restrictive defects and chronic hypoxemia follow if fibrosis sets in, which typically takes place during the ensuing 6 to 24 months. Treatment is mainly supportive. High-dose steroids (1 mg of prednisone per kilogram initially with gradual taper as tolerated) and oxygen can alleviate symptoms during the acute phase; once fibrosis occurs, no treatment is available. The best approach is prevention through careful limitation of the radiation portal.

Other Radiation-induced Organ Injury. *Nephrosclerosis* is the renal response to doses in excess of 2,000 cGy. *Hepatitis* is a consequence of doses to the liver above 3,000 cGy. Gastrointestinal *ulceration* followed by perforation or fibrosis are complications of bowel doses exceeding 4,500 cGy. *Pericarditis* and *spinal cord infarction* are risks of 4,500-cGy doses to the heart and spinal cord, respectively. With mediastinal irradiation, pericarditis can become constrictive, and valvular injury has also been noted.

Although acute reactions are common, the skin can tolerate as much as 5,500 cGy given over time; *dermatitis* becomes a problem at higher doses. The brain (except the brainstem) can withstand up to 6,000 cGy before the risk for *necrosis* begins to rise. Radiation can also induce cataracts and retinal damage and can lead to blindness. Gonadal radiation is likely to induce permanent *sterility*, and pelvic irradiation during the first trimester of pregnancy is teratogenic.

Risk for Secondary Malignancy. A genuine risk for secondary malignancy in the field of treatment exists; it is usually small, approximately 0.2% at 10 years, but in some instances can be considerably higher. In children with bilateral retinoblastoma and mutations of the tumor suppressor gene, this risk may approach 1% each year.

Minor and Temporary Side Effects can be quite disabling unless anticipated and dealt with. *Nausea* occurs with abdominal irradiation; onset can be as soon as 1 to 2 hours after treatment. Prior administration of prochlorperazine, ondansetron, or granisetron helps to lessen gastrointestinal upset. Small, frequent feedings are better tolerated than large ones. If nausea and vomiting become problems, the daily radiation dose can be scaled back or treatment temporarily halted. Head and neck irradiation may cause dryness in the mouth and *difficulty* with *mastication* and *swallowing*. Initiation of pilocarpine (Salagen)

Table 89.2. Serious Adverse Effects of Radiotherapy

TISSUE	ADVERSE EFFECT	DOSE LIMIT [cGy (rads); ≤5% TOXICITY]
Bone marrow	Marrow suppression	250
Kidney	Nephrosclerosis	2,000
Lungs	Pneumonitis	2,000
Liver	Hepatitis	3,000
Heart	Pericarditis	4,500
Spinal cord	Myelitis	4,500
Small intestine	Ulceration, fibrosis	4,500
Skin	Dermatitis, sclerosis	5,500
Brain	Necrosis	6,000

Modified from Chabner BA. Principles of cancer therapy. In: Wyngaarden JB, Smith LH, eds. Cecil's textbook of medicine, 16th ed. Philadelphia: WB Saunders, 1982:1034, with permission.

treatment with the start of radiotherapy can help to maintain salivary function. The use of blenderized meals or liquid dietary supplements can help to maintain adequate caloric intake. *Diarrhea* resulting from bowel radiation responds to diphenoxylate (Lomotil) and loperamide. *Skin care* can sometimes be overlooked. Although the use of megavoltage machines has reduced skin exposure to 30% of the total dose delivered, avoidance of heat and excessive sun exposure helps preserve the integrity of irradiated skin.

PATIENT EDUCATION

Patients undergoing radiation therapy need plenty of emotional support. The fears associated with cancer are compounded by the awesome machinery and concerns about exposure to radiation. Patients who are well informed tolerate therapy better than those who are not. Answering questions and addressing concerns about the rationale for radiation therapy, the side effects to be expected, and how they will be controlled are essential to the successful conduct of a radiation therapy program. Printed information about radiation treatment can be very useful for the patient. In particular, one needs to review the risk for sterility with patients of reproductive age and the chances of a second malignancy in patients considering curative radiotherapy. Such cost–benefit discussions are critical to helping the patient make an informed choice. Knowing that treatment can be adjusted to one's tolerance to therapy is also reassuring.

COORDINATION OF CARE

Conducting a radiotherapy program is the province of the radiation oncologist, carried out in the context of an overall treatment plan developed by the surgeon, medical oncologist, and radiation oncologist in consultation with the primary care physician. The primary physician can ensure that the therapeutic program is well suited to the patient's needs and carefully monitored. A multidisciplinary team approach works best when one member has been designated as the person to whom the patient can always turn for advice and help; in many instances, this important role can be best carried out by the primary care physician.

ANNOTATED BIBLIOGRAPHY

Auchter RM, Lamond JP, Alexander E, et al. A multiinstitutional outcome and prognostic factor analysis of radiosurgery for resectable single brain metastasis. Int J Radiat Oncol Biol Phys 1996;35:27. (*Results of radiosurgery similar to those of resection for single brain metastases.*)

Fletcher GH. The evolution of the basic concepts underlying the practice of radiotherapy. Radiology 1978;127:3. (*The development of combination therapy with radiation as one component.*)

Gunderson LL, Willett CG, Harrison L, et al. Intraoperative irradiation: current and future status. Semin Oncol 1997;24:715. (*Details rationale and results.*)

Lichter AS, Lawrence TS. Recent advances in radiation oncology. N Engl J Med 1995;332:371. (*A review emphasizing recent technical advances and treatment results, in addition to providing an overview of the basic principles of radiation therapy; 115 references.*)

Morris AD, Morris RD, Wilson JF, et al. Breast-conserving therapy vs. mastectomy in early-stage breast cancer: a meta-analysis of 10-years. Cancer J Sci Am 1997;3:6. (*An example of curative radiotherapy.*)

Press OW, Eary JF, Appelbaum FR, et al. Phase II trial of ^{131}I-B1 (anti-CD20) antibody therapy with autologous stem cell transplantation for relapsed B-cell lymphomas. Lancet 1995;346:336. (*A promising report of systemic radiotherapy in which a radionuclide is coupled to a monoclonal antibody.*)

Ragde H, Blasko JC, Grimm PD, et al. Interstitial iodine 125 radiation without adjuvant therapy in the treatment of clinically localized prostate carcinoma. Cancer 1997;80:442. (*Template-guided brachytherapy under real-time ultrasonographic visualization yields excellent treatment results at 7 years.*)

Shipley WU, Winter KA, Kaufman DS, et al. Phase III trial of neoadjuvant chemotherapy in patients with invasive bladder cancer treated with selective bladder preservation by combined radiation therapy and chemotherapy: initial results of Radiation Therapy Oncology Group 89-03. J Clin Oncol 1998;16:3576. (*Excellent example of the use of conservative surgery, chemotherapy, and radiotherapy as a paradigm for organ-preserving approaches to cancer treatment.*)

Stewart JR, Fajardo LF, Gillette SM, et al. Radiation injury to the heart. Int J Radiat Oncol Biol Phys 1995;31:1205. (*Constrictive pericarditis, valvular thickening, and infarction may occur.*)

Taghian A, de Vathaire F, Terrier P, et al. Long-term risk of sarcoma following radiation treatment for breast cancer. Int J Radiat Oncol Biol Phys 1991;21:361. (*Cumulative incidence of sarcoma was 0.2% at 10 years.*)

Tannock IF. Treatment of cancer with radiation and drugs. J Clin Oncol 1996;14:3156. (*Critical review of the status of combined chemotherapy and radiation.*)

Thames HD, Ang KK. Altered fractionation: radiobiological principles, clinical results, and potential for dose escalation. Cancer Treat Res 1998;93:101. (*A discussion of fractionation.*)

Tucker MA, Coleman CN, Cox RS, et al. Risk of second cancers after treatment for Hodgkin's disease. N Engl J Med 1988;318:76. (*Found to be 1% annually for patients undergoing curative therapy.*)

Zelefsky MJ, Leibel SA, Gaudin PB, et al. Dose escalation with three-dimensional conformal radiation therapy affects the outcome in prostate cancer. Int J Radiat Oncol Biol Phys 1998;41:491. (*Technical innovations allow escalation of radiation dose and improve outcome.*)

90
Management of Chronic Cancer Pain and Palliative Care

Part 1: Management of Chronic Cancer Pain
LINDA A. KING and J. ANDREW BILLINGS

Relief of pain is an essential objective in the treatment of the cancer patient at all phases of the illness. Unrelieved pain interferes with a patient's ability to work, enjoy life, and function maximally in family and society. Effective amelioration of pain can almost always be achieved with proper use of analgesics. Unfortunately, undertreatment of pain is frequent. Common barriers to effective pain management reflect problems with health care professionals, patients, and the health care system, and they need to be explored actively and addressed (Table 90.1).

Fear of unrelieved cancer pain is widespread. The primary care physician must know the appropriate treatments and their limitations, and must also be able to support the cancer patient and minimize the emotional suffering that is invariably intertwined with the perception of pain.

PATHOPHYSIOLOGY AND CLINICAL PRESENTATION

Pain in cancer patients may result from direct effects of the tumor (e.g., infiltration into bone, viscera, nerves), from treatments directed at the cancer (e.g., chemotherapy, radiation, surgery), or from causes unrelated to the cancer (e.g., arthritis, migraines). Three broad physiologic categories describe the underlying pathophysiology: somatic, visceral, and neuropathic.

Table 90.1. Barriers to Cancer Pain Management

Problems Related to Health Care Professionals
Inadequate knowledge of pain management
Poor assessment of pain
Concern about regulation of controlled substances
Fear of patient addiction
Concern about side effects of analgesics
Concern about patients becoming tolerant to analgesics

Problems Related to Patients
Reluctance to report pain
    Concern about distracting physician from treatment of underlying disease
    Fear that pain means disease is worse
    Concern about not being a "good patient"
Reluctance to take pain medications
    Fear of addiction or of being thought of as an addict
    Worries about unmanageable side effects
    Concern about becoming tolerant to pain medications

Problems Related to the Health Care System
Low priority given to cancer pain treatment
Inadequate reimbursement and prohibitive costs
Restrictive regulation of controlled substances
Problems of availability of treatment or access to it

From Jacox A, Carr DB, Payne R, et al. Management of cancer pain. Clinical practice guideline No.9, AHCPR Publication No. 94-0592. Rockville, MD: Agency for Health Care Policy and Research, U.S. Department of Health and Human Services, Public Health Service, March 1994.

Multiple pain complaints caused by multiple mechanisms are the rule.

Somatic pain arises from the activation of nociceptors in cutaneous or deep musculoskeletal tissues. This pain is usually well localized and often described as dull or aching. Examples of somatic pain include that from bone metastases, surgical incision, and radiation burns.

Visceral pain results from infiltration, compression, or distention of thoracic or abdominal viscera. Visceral pain is usually poorly localized and often described as deep, squeezing, or as if caused by pressure. Referral of the pain to overlying or distant cutaneous sites is common. Causes of visceral pain include liver metastases that distend the capsule and obstruct the biliary tree, bowel, or urinary tract.

Neuropathic pain results from direct injury to peripheral or central nervous system structures. Pain from nerve injury may be described as constant, aching, or as if caused by a vise; paroxysms of sharp, burning, or shocklike pain are superimposed. The pain may follow a nerve distribution and can be associated with sensory or motor (including sphincter) disturbances. Causes of neuropathic pain include spinal nerve root compression, radiation-induced plexopathy, and chemotherapy-associated neuropathy.

Common Pain Syndromes

In cancer patients, a number of pain syndromes occur frequently; some involve a single mechanism, and others operate through multiple mechanisms.

Osseous Pain. Metastases to the bony skeleton may cause pathologic fractures; the development of pain in a bony site is invariably secondary to interruption of the cortex, which may or may not be observed radiographically. Common sites are vertebrae, long bones, pelvis, and skull. Another form of osseous metastasis involves the bone marrow or medullary cavity. Intramedullary tumor is characteristic of leukemia but may also be observed in some solid tumors. These produce a pain syndrome characterized by diffuse bone sensitivity in the presence of normal radiographic findings.

Thoracic Pain. Pain associated with thoracic disease is generally a consequence of local invasion of the intercostal nerves. Pleuritic pain may develop if the malignancy spreads to involve the pleura. Direct invasion of a contiguous bony structure may result in local or referred pain.

Abdominal Pain may develop as a consequence of intestinal obstruction; cramping pain is characteristic (see Chapter 58). Ascites can be uncomfortable as a consequence of abdominal distention. Hepatic metastases may cause pain by distending the liver capsule or irritating the peritoneal surface secondary to tumor necrosis. The latter is often associated with a friction rub.

Nerve Root Compression. Pain originating in the back and radiating down an extremity is characteristic of root compression. When an associated neurologic deficit is present, it suggests the possibility of evolving cord compression. The tumor most commonly extends either from the retroperitoneal space or from a contiguous involved bony structure. Bone scans or radiographs often demonstrate lytic or blastic lesions. Compression syndromes may also occur as a consequence of vertebral body collapse secondary to tumor without direct tumor compression of the nerve.

Peripheral Nerve Compression. The relatively uncommon nerve compression syndromes result in pain in the shoulder or arm (brachial plexus), buttocks and perineum (sacral plexus), lumbar area (paraspinal nerves), and mouth or face (trigeminal nerve). All are secondary to nerve entrapment and, occasionally, to nerve invasion by tumor growth.

Special Pain Syndromes. The *phantom limb syndrome* characteristically develops following amputation in patients with osteogenic sarcoma, especially when the tumor has been present for a long period. Persistence of phantom limb pain may lead to narcotic dependence. It is only after a protracted period of time that the reverberating neural circuit is eventually exhausted.

Herpes zoster (shingles) occurs in patients with hematologic malignancies, particularly Hodgkin's disease, the non-Hodgkin's lymphomas, and chronic lymphocytic leukemia. Post-herpetic pain may persist in the absence of typical skin lesions; herpes zoster should be suspected in patients who have pain in a dermatomal distribution (see Chapter 193).

Hypertrophic pulmonary osteoarthropathy produces a periarticular pain syndrome in patients with primary or metastatic tumors of the lung and with mesotheliomas. The mechanism of periarticular pain is unclear.

WORKUP

Prompt, careful assessment of the cancer patient's pain is essential to the timely design and implementation of a rational treatment plan. Assessment should be carried out at the time of the initial report of pain, at regular intervals thereafter, and with any treatment changes. As noted above, cancer patients commonly report multiple types of pain. Each complaint should be individually assessed and prioritized. Because pain is a subjective phenomenon, the patient's report of pain must be taken seriously. The focus of the workup includes an assessment of the underlying mechanism(s) of pain in addition to their impact on the patient's quality of life and ability to carry out the activities of daily living.

History. A careful pain history includes the intensity, duration, location, and quality of the pain, in addition to aggravating and alleviating factors and associated symptoms. It is worth noting whether the pain is well localized, which suggests a somatic mechanism; more diffuse, which is indicative of visceral pain; or in the distribution of a nerve, which points to a neuro-

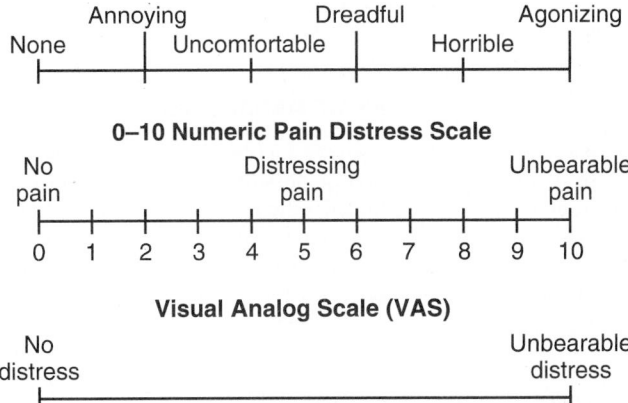

FIG. 90.1. Pain Assessment Intensity Scales.*

*From Jacox A, Carr DB, Payne R, et al. Management of cancer pain. Clinical practice guideline No. 9. AHCPR Publication No. 94-0592. Rockville, MD: Agency for Health Care Policy and Research, US Department of Health and Human Services, Public Health Service, March 1994.

pathic cause. If the pain is somatic in quality, is there a history of bony metastases, surgical incisions, or radiation burns? If the pain is more diffuse and visceral in quality, one needs to consider capsular distention and also obstruction of a viscus, be it bowel, biliary tree, or urinary tract, depending on the location of the pain. If the pain appears neuropathic in distribution, one needs to ask about sensory and motor disturbances (including those involving sphincters).

Another important component of the history is elucidating the impact of the pain on the patient's psychosocial state and on activities of daily living (sleeping, dressing, eating, moving around). A numeric rating scale (Fig. 90.1) helps to quantify pain intensity and follow it over time. Exploring the past use of analgesic therapies, their effectiveness, and their side effects helps in the design of the treatment program. Identifying how the patient interprets the meaning of the pain provides an opportunity to understand and ease the worry contributing to the pain.

Physical Examination. A focused physical examination can provide essential corroborating evidence for the underlying mechanism(s) and site(s) of pain suggested by the history. For example, if the patient's story suggests neuropathic pain, then a careful neurologic examination confirming the neuronal distribution of the pain and examining for motor and sensory deficits and sphincter incompetence is critical. Similarly, somatic pain should be confirmed by the finding of focal tenderness. If the pain is poorly localized, then checking for an obstructed viscus or distended organ capsule is in order.

Laboratory Studies. Imaging studies and other laboratory means of confirming the cause of pain are especially important to management when a surgical, chemotherapeutic, or radiotherapeutic approach to pain control is being considered. Determining the specific cause of the pain (e.g., bone metastases, bowel obstruction, spinal cord compression) allows appropriate, disease-specific therapy to be instituted. Patients with advanced disease who are not candidates for such aggressive therapeutic measures need not undergo extensive testing unless the results will affect clinical decision making. In such patients, the decision to initiate or escalate an analgesic program may require little more than a good clinical assessment. While the workup is proceeding, troublesome pain should be treated empirically.

PRINCIPLES OF MANAGEMENT

After a thorough assessment has been completed and the cause of the pain identified, if possible, an appropriate treatment regimen can be instituted. Often, a multifaceted approach is necessary. Analgesics, psychological support, control of tumor, neurosurgical procedures, and behavioral methods are among the important modalities for the treatment of cancer-related pain.

Pharmacologic Measures

General Principles. Selection of the appropriate analgesic therapy must be individualized for each patient. The *World Health Organization analgesic ladder* (Fig. 90.2) provides a standard initial approach to drug selection for cancer pain based on pain severity and previous analgesic use. The ladder begins with the use of acetaminophen, aspirin, or NSAIDs for *mild to moderate pain.* When pain *persists* or *increases*, a weak opioid or a stronger opioid at a low dosage is added. Pain that is *moderate to severe* at presentation or more persistent should be treated with opioids at higher dosages or a stronger opioid preparation. The simplest route and dosage schedule and the least invasive pain management measures are preferred for initial use. *Chronic cancer pain* requires around-the-clock (*not as-needed*) dosing, supplemented by as-needed ("rescue") doses for breakthrough pain.

Acetaminophen, Aspirin, and Nonsteroidal Antiinflammatory Drugs. These non-opioid drugs comprise the analgesics useful as initial therapy for mild pain (Table 90.2). Except for acetaminophen (which has no antiinflammatory effects), they have analgesic, antipyretic, and antiinflammatory effects. Adding aspirin or acetaminophen to an oral opioid regimen can boost the analgesic effect, which allows lower doses of opioids to be used and also limits side effects. Unlike opioids, none of these drugs produces tolerance or physical dependence. There is a ceiling to their analgesic effects, beyond which no additional analgesia is achieved. Long-term use of oral NSAIDs for pain control in cancer has not been well studied, but available

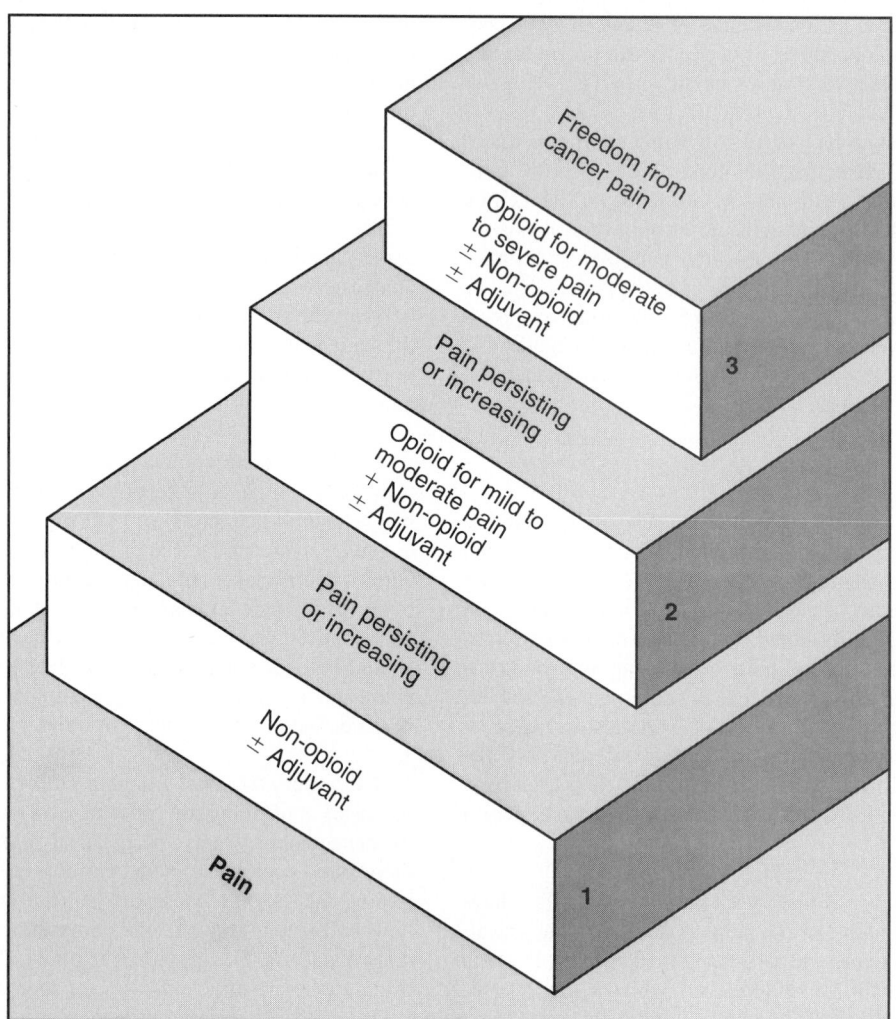

FIG. 90.2. The WHO three-step analgesic ladder.

Table 90.2. Non-opioid Analgesics

DRUG	USUAL ADULT DOSE
Acetaminophen	650 mg q4h
	975 mg q6h
Aspirin	650 mg q4h
	975 mg q6h
Choline magnesium	
trisalicylate (Trilisate)	750–1500 mg tid
Salsalate (Disalcid)	750–1500 mg tid
Ibuprofen (Motrin, Advil)	600 mg q6h
Naproxen (Naprosyn, Aleve)	250–500 mg bid
Ketorolac (Toradol)	10 PO mg q6h
	30 mg IM q6h (up to 5 days)
Celecoxib (Celebrex)	100–200 mg bid
Rofecoxib (Bioxx)	12.5–25 mg per day

Adapted from Jacox A, Carr DB, Payne R, et al. Management of cancer pain. Clinical practice guideline No. 9 AHCPR Publication No. 94-0592. Rockville, MD: Agency for Health Care Policy and Research, U.S. Department of Health and Human Services, Public Health Service, March 1994.

evidence suggests reasonable efficacy, especially for bone pain or pain with an inflammatory component.

The analgesia provided by NSAIDs is equivalent to that of aspirin, acetaminophen, and opioids at low dosages. NSAIDs are available in various oral formulations, including tablets, capsules, and liquids. Ketorolac, the only parenteral NSAID preparation, is recommended for short-term (<5 days) use only. Because responses to individual NSAIDs vary, titration of the dose and trials of different preparations are often necessary to achieve the best response. (For a discussion of adverse effects, see Chapters 68 and 156).

Cyclooxygenase-2 Inhibitors. The selective cyclooxygenase-2 (Cox-2) inhibitors (e.g., *celecoxib*) block both isoforms of cyclooxygenase to inhibit prostaglandin synthesis. The Cox-1 isoform is found in abundance in platelets, and its inhibition by NSAIDs is responsible for many of the side effects of these drugs. Cox-2 inhibitors are believed to cause fewer gastrointestinal and platelet side effects than do the traditional NSAIDs, but these drugs are expensive and may not have comparable analgesic efficacy.

Opioids are the preferred analgesics for the management of *moderate to severe* cancer pain. They are highly effective, easily titrated, and generally well tolerated.

Titration and Dosing. Opioid doses are *titrated* in each patient to maximize pain relief promptly and minimize side effects. Dosage requirements vary greatly among patients and with time, so that careful and ongoing titration is necessary to achieve and maintain adequate analgesia. The degree of analgesia that can be provided by increasing the dose of opioids is not limited, as it is with non-opioid analgesics. To provide optimal pain control, opioids should be prescribed on a *regularly scheduled* (around-the-clock) basis, rather than on an as-needed basis. This regimen actually minimizes the total daily amount of opioid required to control pain.

Dose titration is best accomplished by using a *short-acting preparation* and rapidly increasing the dose until pain resolves. At the end of every dosing interval, the dose is increased by at least 25% if pain persists; 50% increases are appropriate for severe pain. The goal is rapid implementation of effective pain control, accomplished by going "fast and high." Once the nec-

essary daily opioid dose is established, a *long-acting oral preparation* that is taken twice daily can be substituted for the shorter-acting preparation. The shorter-acting oral opioids should be kept on hand for episodes of *breakthrough pain*. Breakthrough doses should be approximately 10% to 20% of the total 24-hour dose of the long-acting preparation and should be used every 2 to 4 hours as needed.

Routes of Administration. The *oral* route of opioid administration (Table 90.3) is ideal for patient convenience, but other routes (Table 90.4) are available for patients who cannot take their medication by mouth. The *IV* route allows for continuous administration of opioids, in addition to intermittent boluses as needed, although at a greater cost than that of other routes. *IM* dosing should be avoided because of the discomfort associated with injection and the availability of other equally effective routes of delivery. Equi-analgesic dosage guidelines and the duration of action must be understood when opioids or routes of administration are switched. In general, the same opioid dosages are required for oral, sublingual, buccal, and rectal administration. Likewise, roughly the same dosages are required for IM, IV, and SQ administration.

Side Effects. The most common side effects of opioids include *constipation* and *sedation*; less commonly, these agents produce *nausea* and *vomiting*, *pruritus*, *myoclonus*, *dry mouth*, and *urinary retention*. Significant *respiratory depression*, a dreaded side effect in the treatment of acute pain, is extremely rare and not a concern in carefully conducted management of

Table 90.3. Oral Opioid Preparations

DRUG	OPIOID DOSE (mg)
Morphine	
MSIR tablets or capsules	15, 30
MSIR "soluble" tablets	10, 15, 30
Roxanol (elixir)	10/5 mL, 20/5 mL, 100/5 mL
MS Contin	15, 30, 60, 100, 200
Oramorph SR	15, 30, 60, 100
Hydromorphone	
Dilaudid, generic	2, 4, 8
Codeine	
Codeine sulfate tablets	15, 30, 60
Codeine with acetaminophen	
Tylenol No. 2, No. 3, No. 4	15, 30, 60, respectively
Codeine with aspirin	
Empirin No. 3, No. 4	30, 60, respectively
Hydrocodone with acetaminophen	
Lortab	2.5, 5, 7.5, 10
Lorcet	5, 7.5, 10
Vicodin	5, 7.5
Oxycodone	
Roxicodone	5
OxyContin	10, 20, 40, 80
Oxycodone with acetaminophen	
Percocet, Roxicet, Tylox, generic	5
Oxycodone with aspirin	
Percodan	5
Levorphanol	
Levo-Dromoran, generic	2
Methadone	
Dolophine, generic	5, 10

Adapted from Weissman DE, Dahl JL, Dinndorf PA. Handbook of cancer pain management. Madison, Wisconsin Cancer Pain Initiative. 1996, with permission.

Table 90.4.   Approximate Equianalgesic Doses of Short Acting Opioids
for Chronic Pain[a,b]

ORAL DOSE (mg)	USUAL ORAL DOSING INTERVAL	ANALGESIC	PARENTERAL DOSE (mg)	USUAL PARENTERAL DOSING INTERVAL
200	q3–4h	Codeine	130	q3–4h
30	q3–4h	Hydrocodone (Vicodin, Zydone)		
20–30		Oxycodone (Percodan, Percocet, Tylox, Roxicet, Roxicodone, Roxiprin)[c,d]		
30	q4h	Morphine[c,e,f]	10	q3–4h
20	q4–6h	Methadone (Dolophine)[g]	10	q4–6h
7.5	q3–4h	Hydromorphone (Dilaudid)[e]	1.5	q3–4h
4	q4–6h	Levorphanol (Levo-Dromoran)	2	q4–6h

Fentanyl (Duragesic) patch or other long-acting opioids should be considered for patients with a relatively stable basal opioid dosage and relatively well controlled pain. According to the manufacturer, a 10-mg IM [or SC/IV] or 60 mg oral dose of morphine every 4 hrs. for 24 hrs. (total 60 mg/day [2.5 mg/hr SC/IC] or 360 mg/day oral) is approximately equivalent to transdermal fentanyl 100 µg/hr. Palliative care clinicians generally divide the 24-hour oral morphine dosage by 3.8 to get the roughly equivalent hourly dosage/hr of fentanyl. Patches should be replaced every 48-72 hrs.

[a]All dosages and intervals are approximate, and should be adjusted according to the patient's response. When a patient has been on a particular opioid for weeks or months, conversion to a relatively lower dosage of another opioid is often adequate, especially with methadone, which has occasionally been reported as 10-20 times as potent as predicted by this kind of table when used after prolonged or high-dose treatment with other opioids.

[b]This table does not include meperidine (Demerol) or pentazocine (Talwin), which generally should not be used for chronic cancer pain.

[c]Oxycodone is available as a long-acting preparation, (Oxycontin). Morphine is also available in long-acting preparations. MS Contin, Oramorph SR, lasting 8-12 hours or Kadian, lasting 24 hours. Sustained-action tablets should not be crushed or chewed.

[d]Some oxycodone preparations are compounded with acetaminophen or aspirin. Do not exceed 4,000 mg/day acetaminophen for prolonged periods.

[e]Morphine and hydromorphone (Dilaudid) are available as suppositories. Rectal dosage and intervals are generally the same as with oral administration.

[f]Liquid morphine preparations can be administered by the sublingual or buccal route. Dosage and intervals are similar to those for oral administration.

[g]Methadone's long half-life may be associated with accumulation of opioid and delayed development of toxicity, and may allow for longer dosing intervals.

chronic pain. One monitors for side effects and treats constipation prophylactically. Tolerance to many of the side effects, including nausea, sedation, and respiratory depression, occurs quickly. Constipation persists and should be managed with regularly scheduled laxative regimens (see Chapter 91).

Tolerance. Opioid tolerance is defined as the need for an increasing amount of drug to achieve the same analgesic effect. Tolerance develops with regular opioid use and is manifested by a *shortened duration of pain control* and an overall increase in perception of pain. *Concurrent use* of a *non-opioid analgesic* (see above) or an *adjuvant drug* (see below) can delay the onset of tolerance by allowing the use of lower opioid doses and less frequent dosing. The simplest means of overcoming tolerance is to increase the dose or dose frequency. *Cross-tolerance* is common but not complete after prolonged opioid administration, so that it is possible to boost analgesia by *switching* to another opioid, starting at as low as one tenth and usually at about one half of the equi-analgesic dose.

Dependence. *Physiologic dependence* presents as the development of opioid *withdrawal* symptoms if opioids are abruptly discontinued or if opioid antagonists are administered. A withdrawal syndrome, although usually mild in patients with cancer pain, can be easily avoided by tapering the opioid dose by roughly 25% to 50% a day within a few days to a week. *Psychological dependence* (addiction) is an abnormal behavior pattern in which a person becomes overwhelmingly involved in the acquisition and use of a drug. Addiction remains very uncommon in cancer patients who take opioids for pain relief. Patients and their families should be counseled about the rarity of addiction when opioids are prescribed for cancer pain, as misconceptions often result in avoidance of pain medications or underreporting of pain. Similarly, health care professionals often inappropriately withhold opioids from patients who could benefit from these analgesics.

Pseudo-addiction describes the development of behaviors resembling psychological dependence. This state arises as a result of inadequate and inappropriate pain regimens, such as "only-as-needed" dosing for continuous pain, dosing intervals exceeding the duration of action of the medication, or inadequate doses. The "drug-seeking" behaviors observed are eliminated if an appropriate analgesic regimen is prescribed.

Choice of Opioid Agent. Choice should coincide with the patient's needs. For patients with mild to moderate pain that is becoming persistent, a low-potency opioid such as *codeine* is a reasonable choice. It is the least potent opioid; starting doses (15 to 30 mg) provide pain control comparable to that achieved with full analgesic doses of aspirin, acetaminophen, or an NSAID. Codeine in combination with acetaminophen provides effective analgesia at low cost for patients with mild to moderate pain. The related compounds *oxycodone* and *hydrocodone* are eight times more potent than codeine and are similar in potency to morphine. These opioids are also available in combination with aspirin and acetaminophen. The toxicities of the non-opioids in these formulations limit the overall dose of opioid that can be administered daily. Oxycodone is available in a long-acting, slow-release formulation (OxyContin) with an effect lasting up to 12 hours.

Morphine is the prototype opioid analgesic for severe cancer pain. It is effective both orally and parenterally and has a duration of action of approximately 3 to 4 hours. The use of sustained-release preparations (e.g., MS Contin, Oramorph SR) provides prolonged analgesia (8 to 12 hours) with less frequent dosing, but the cost can be substantial. These long-acting formulations cannot be crushed or chewed.

Hydromorphone (Dilaudid) is more potent than morphine and also more costly. Its duration of action and strength are reduced considerably when it is given orally rather than parenterally. Because hydromorphone is more potent and more soluble than morphine, a smaller injected volume can be used in patients requiring parenteral opioid infusions.

Methadone and *levorphanol* also have proved useful because of their longer duration of action. The cost of methadone is low, which makes it an attractive alternative to long-acting morphine preparations. With repeated dosing, excessive sedation and central nervous system depression can result because of the sustained half-life of these agents. Careful dose titration is required for proper use.

Although *meperidine* (Demerol) is commonly prescribed and available for both oral and parenteral use, it is not recommended for chronic cancer pain because of the rapid inactivation of an oral dose and overall short duration of action. In addition, its metabolite, normeperidine, causes dysphoria, tremors, and irritability, especially in patients with impaired renal function. In patients taking monoamine oxidase (MAO) inhibitors, meperidine can cause serious and sometimes lethal side effects.

Fentanyl, a potent opioid, is available as a transdermal preparation that provides 3 days of continuous analgesia. The fentanyl patch is generally more expensive than oral opioids and requires careful titration to avoid excessive sedation. The starting dose should be based on the patient's previous morphine requirement or determined empirically by starting with the patch of the lowest strength, which provides 25 μg of fentanyl per hour (the equivalent of about 90 mg of oral morphine per day or 30 mg of parenteral morphine per day).

Some synthetic opioids have antagonist in addition to agonist activity. *Pentazocine* (Talwin) and *butorphanol tartrate* (Stadol) are opioid agonists–antagonists available orally and as a nasal spray, respectively. The opioid antagonist qualities of these drugs can precipitate withdrawal in a patient already taking an opioid agonist; therefore, they are not optimal drugs for cancer patients with long-standing opioid requirements.

Adjuvant Agents. Various agents can be used to enhance the effectiveness of the analgesics discussed above (Table 90.5). The *tricyclic antidepressants* (see Chapter 227) are effective for neuropathic pain, concurrent depression, and sleep disturbance related to ongoing pain. The analgesic effects may occur at lower doses and may develop more quickly than the antidepressant effects. Starting doses of desipramine (Norpramin) or

amitriptyline (Elavil) as low as 10 to 25 mg at bedtime can reduce pain, with upward dose adjustment as necessary. Anticholinergic side effects and sedation may limit titration, especially in the elderly.

Anticonvulsants including *gabapentin* (Neurontin), *carbamazepine* (Tegretol), and *phenytoin* (Dilantin) are also helpful in relieving neuropathic pain. Again, doses should be started low and titrated to effect. Local anesthetics such as IV *lidocaine* and oral *mexiletine* have also been used effectively for neuropathic pain.

Stimulants, such as *dextroamphetamine* (Dexedrine) and *methylphenidate* (Ritalin), are sometimes used to counter the somnolence associated with opioid use. They can also have the beneficial effects of increasing energy and appetite. *Glucocorticoids* may lessen the pain associated with tumor-associated inflammation or infiltration while providing a stimulant effect in addition to an improved appetite and sense of well-being. The anticipated side effects of ongoing corticosteroid use (hyperglycemia, edema, infection, gastrointestinal bleeding) may limit their long-term use. *Benzodiazepines* are helpful on an intermittent basis if a patient reports situational stress or anxiety or increased pain with resultant difficulty in falling asleep. However, agitation caused by depression should be treated with an antidepressant and not a benzodiazepine.

Patients with pain caused by bone metastases may benefit from therapy with *bisphosphonates* or *calcitonin*, which both inhibit osteoclast activity and reduce bone pain. Monthly pamidronate therapy has been shown to reduce bone pain and the incidence of pathologic fractures in certain cancers.

Nonpharmacologic Measures: Physical and Psychological Modalities

These interventions represent an important component of a multifaceted approach to pain management. Such interventions should be used with, not instead of, appropriate analgesic regimens.

Physical Modalities. *Cutaneous stimulation* by the application of *cold* or *hot* packs or by the use of *massage, vibration, transcutaneous electrical stimulation* (TENS), or *acupuncture* helps to manage pain when employed in conjunction with appropriate analgesics. These modalities are easy to use and relatively inexpensive, and they cause minimal morbidity.

Psychosocial Interventions. *Relaxation* techniques (focused-breathing exercises, meditation, music therapy), *guided imagery, biofeedback*, and *hypnosis* can be very helpful, especially for episodic pain and pain related to specific activities. These easily learned techniques enable patients to gain a sense of control over the pain. Belief in the validity of the underlying method strongly correlates with a positive outcome.

Psychological Support. The importance of psychological support from both physician and family cannot be overemphasized. The active involvement of the primary physician is vital to the successful control of pain. The understanding and concern expressed, with attention to the patient's worry in addition to the pain itself, are as central to effective pain relief as are tumor control and proper use of analgesics (see Chapter 87).

Table 90.5. Adjuvant Analgesics

DRUG	USUAL ADULT DOSE RANGE
Antidepressants	
Amitriptyline (Elavil)	10–150 mg qhs
Nortriptyline (Pamelor)	10–150 mg qhs
Anticonvulsants	
Gabapentin (Neurontin)	100–400 mg tid
Carbamazepine (Tegretol)	100–800 mg bid
Phenytoin (Dilantin)	300–500 mg qd
Psychostimulants	
Dextroamphetamine (Dexedrine)	5–10 mg qd–bid
Methylphenidate (Ritalin)	2.5–15 mg qd–bid
Glucocorticoids	
Dexamethasone (Decadron)	4–96 mg bid–qid
Prednisone	10–100 mg qd–bid

Adapted from Jacox A, Carr DB, Payne R, et al. Management of cancer pain. Clinical practice guideline No. 9. AHCPR Publication No. 94-0592. Rockville, MD: Agency for Health Care Policy and Research, U.S. Department of Health and Human Services, Public Health Service, March 1994.

Nonpharmacologic Measures: Invasive Modalities

Anesthetic Procedures. Patients in whom adequate pain control is not achieved with application of all the above measures or who experience intolerable side effects may be candidates for invasive anesthetic or neurosurgical procedures. Before such an invasive measure is utilized, a multidisciplinary team including oncologists, pain specialists, and neurosurgeons should review the situation to ensure appropriate patient selection. It is important to characterize the pain as precisely as possible to target the planned interventions appropriately. A number of approaches are available.

Epidural or *intrathecal injection* of opioids and local anesthetics can be used for either short-term or long-term control of intractable pain in the lower part of the body. Operator expertise is essential to ensure proper catheter placement and manage potential complications, including respiratory depression, hypotension, and infection.

Nerve blocks utilize the application of a local anesthetic, corticosteroid, or neurolytic to control intractable pain related to an identifiable nerve structure. Application of a short-acting local anesthetic provides useful diagnostic and management information by confirming the specific source of pain and predicting likely side effects. Once an appropriate site has been identified by diagnostic block, a neurolytic agent such as ethanol or phenol is injected to destroy the involved nerve and provide long-term pain relief. Neurolytic blocks can relieve pain related to tumor infiltration of the upper abdominal organs (celiac block), pelvic organs (hypogastric block), head and neck (stellate ganglion block), and legs (lumbar sympathetic block). Precise technique is required for the successful implementation of a nerve block and to prevent damage to surrounding tissue and other nerves.

Neurosurgical Procedures for pain control are now used less frequently because of the development of more advanced, radiologically guided techniques for anesthetic blocks. Pituitary ablation (hypophysectomy) has been used successfully in rare patients with refractory disseminated pain.

INDICATIONS FOR REFERRAL AND ADMISSION

Successful management of cancer pain requires a team approach. The primary physician plays a major role in the design and implementation of an effective analgesic program and in monitoring the patient for painful complications of the malignancy. When such complications arise, prompt consultation with the oncologist, radiation therapist, or surgeon is often indicated because of the potential need for further systemic treatment or additional local measures. Patients with *refractory pain* in the absence of evident, focally approachable disease may benefit from consultation with a specialist in the treatment of chronic pain. The patient with new onset of pain suggestive of *spinal cord compression* or *pathologic fracture* requires prompt consultation and hospital admission.

PATIENT AND FAMILY EDUCATION

Patients endure their condition much better when they know that maximum pain relief is available. The educational effort should take into account any cultural or language barriers that might contribute to undertreatment, a phenomenon noted with increased frequency among minority patients with cancer. To avoid underdosing, all family and health care team members need to be informed of the patient's analgesic needs and the low risk for true addiction. The issues of drug tolerance and physiologic dependence should be reviewed and their significance discussed. Few patients should have to endure disabling pain, given the array of effective treatment modalities available. Many patients do best when they maintain an active role in their care. Enlisting their help in the design, implementation, and monitoring of the pain management program can be of considerable psychological benefit. Effective pain control is central to sustaining a reasonable quality of life and is one of the most basic requests of cancer patients.

RECOMMENDATIONS

- Carefully assess each complaint of pain. Patients may have multiple pains with multiple origins and mechanisms.
- Attempt to diagnose each underlying cause because specific causes respond best to specific treatments. In particular, be alert for bone pain, neuropathic pain, and cord compression.
- Treat the worry in addition to the discomfort. Psychological support contributes greatly to effective pain control.
- Utilize the stepped approach for analgesic use as outlined by the World Health Organization analgesic ladder, while recognizing that analgesic therapy must be individualized for each patient.
  - For *mild to moderate* pain, begin with acetaminophen, aspirin, or NSAIDs.
  - When pain *persists* or *increases*, add a weak opioid or a stronger opioid at a low dosage.
  - For pain that is *moderate to severe*, treat with higher dosages of opioids or a stronger opioid preparation.
  - Treat *chronic cancer pain* with around-the-clock (*not as-needed*) dosing, supplemented by as-needed ("rescue") doses for breakthrough pain.
- Initiate opioid therapy by quickly establishing the necessary opioid dose. Do this by titrating with a short-acting preparation, increasing each dose by 25% to 50% until satisfactory pain control is achieved. Once the effective dose is established, switch to a long-acting preparation (e.g., MS Contin, OxyContin, Oramorph SR, Duragesic patch). Use as high a dose of opioid as is necessary to achieve effective pain relief.
- Treat *"breakthrough"* pain with doses of a short-acting opioid equal to 10% to 20% of the total 24-hour opioid dose and give every 2 to 4 hours as needed.
- Use the simplest route of administration, the most convenient dosage schedule, and the least invasive pain management measures. Oral therapy is preferred.
- Address common misunderstandings about addiction to minimize underdosing.
- Consider adding simple nonpharmacologic modalities, such as application of heat or cold, massage, relaxation techniques, and guided imagery, which can complement appropriate analgesic regimens.
- If *tolerance* to one opioid seems to be developing, consider switching to another opioid. Use equi-analgesic doses when switching between different opioids and routes.

- To help control severe *neuropathic* or *bone pain*, consider an adjuvant agent (e.g., tricyclic antidepressant or anticonvulsant for neuropathic pain, bisphosphonate for bone pain).
- Minimize adverse effects of opioid use by periodically retitrating and prescribing such measures as laxatives to prevent severe constipation.
- For *pain caused by severe localized disease*, consider tumor-specific therapy (e.g., radiation, surgery, chemotherapy).
- For *poorly controlled pain* or problematic side effects, consider referral for nerve block or placement of an epidural catheter.
- Reassess frequently and at regular intervals, especially when pain worsens and after medication changes have been made.
- When pain is not responding well to treatment, reevaluate the role of psychosocial factors, consider whether pain is neuropathic, and seek help from pain specialists.

ANNOTATED BIBLIOGRAPHY

American Pain Society. Principles of analgesic use, 4th ed. Skokie, IL: American Pain Society, 1999. (*Excellent resource on pain medications and their proper use.*)

American Pain Society. Quality improvement guidelines for the treatment of acute and cancer pain. JAMA 1995;274:1874. (*Describes five key elements to improve pain management practices.*)

Bernabei R, Gabmassi G, Lapane K, et al. Management of pain in elderly patients with cancer. JAMA 1998;279:1877. (*Highlights populations at particular risk for inadequate pain management.*)

Cleeland CS, Gonin R, Baez L, et al. Pain and treatment of pain in minority patients with cancer. The Eastern Minority Outpatient Pain Study. Ann Intern Med 1997;127:813. (*A prospective study; increased rate of inadequate pain control among minority patients, especially Hispanic patients.*)

Drugs for pain. Med Lett Drugs Ther 1998;40[Issue 1033]:79-84. (*Terse overview; very useful comparisons of drugs.*)

Edwards M. Barriers to effective pain/symptom control. Am J Hospice Palliative Care 1998;15:107. (*A thoughtful review of common barriers to symptom control.*)

Jacox A, Carr DB, Payne R, et al. Management of cancer pain. Clinical practice guideline No 9. AHCPR Publication No 94-0592. Rockville, MD: Agency for Health Care Policy and Research, US Department of Health and Human Services, Public Health Service, March 1994. (*The most complete guideline for clinical practice; includes an accompanying clinician quick reference guide and patient guide.*)

Levy MH. Pharmacologic treatment of cancer pain. N Engl J Med 1996;335:1124. (*A practical, succinct, and up-to-date review.*)

Liss AL, Portenoy RK. Strategies for limiting the side effects of cancer pain therapy. Semin Oncol 1997;24[Suppl 16]:S16. (*Details common opioid side effects in addition to the concepts of tolerance and addiction.*)

Pereira J, Mancini I, Walker P. The role of bisphosphonates in malignant bone pain: a review. J Palliative Care 1998;14:25. (*A review of pharmacology, use, and toxicities of bisphosphonates and their growing role in treating cancer pain.*)

Rowlingson JC. Interventional cancer pain management. Anesth Analg 1998; [Suppl]:106. (*A review of nerve blocks and other anesthetic modalities for treating cancer pain.*)

Weissman DE, Dahl JL, Dinndorf PA. Handbook of cancer pain management. Madison Wisconsin Cancer Pain Initiative, 1996. (*A pocket-sized, spiral-bound guide full of practical information and clinical examples.*)

Part 2: Palliative Care
ERIC L. KRAKAUER

Palliative care is comprehensive care focused on alleviating suffering and promoting the quality of life of patients living with a life-threatening or terminal illness. Major concerns are pain and symptom management, information sharing and advance care planning, psychosocial and spiritual support of both patient and family, and coordination of care, including arranging for services in the community. The orchestration and provision of palliative care is part of the purview of any primary physician who cares for a dying patient. It may be provided in an acute care hospital, a skilled nursing facility, an inpatient hospice, or the home. Community hospice organizations and visiting nurse associations can assist in arranging palliative care outside the hospital.

PRINCIPLES OF PALLIATIVE CARE

Transition to Palliative Care. Although attention to palliation and comfort should be part of the care plan for all patients, including those receiving curative or life-sustaining treatments, many patients reach a point at which they want the primary focus of care to shift to comfort and achievement of the best possible quality of life. Helping patients and surrogates to determine the timing of this shift requires (1) an assessment of their understanding of the diagnosis and prognosis, (2) the communication of information about the illness—what is wrong, the likely outcomes, the potential benefits and burdens of each treatment option, (including no treatment); and (3) an understanding of patients' goals and values. Previously executed advance directives such as a living will or health care proxy form can be useful in these discussions. Factors that may impede a patient's ability to make treatment decisions, such as delirium, dementia, or denial, should be taken into account. When the patient's capacity to understand medical information is questionable, a psychiatric consultation may be useful. Efforts should be made to discern and respect cultural and familial factors that may inform a patient's decisions.

Non-abandonment. As the goal of care shifts from cure or life support to comfort, it is important to reassure patients, surrogates, and families through words and deeds that they will not be ignored or abandoned and that attentive palliative care will be provided. A decision to forego "aggressive" interventions, or to request a "Do Not Resuscitate" or "Comfort Care Only" order, should never lead to a diminution of attention to the patient's well-being. Phoning to "check in" or a home visit can be very comforting.

Proportionality. When deliberating with patients or surrogates about specific treatments, it is important to weigh the potential benefits against the potential or certain burdens. If a treatment seems likely to be more burdensome than beneficial, the physician should suggest that it not be used.

Withholding and Withdrawing Treatments. It sometimes can be emotionally more difficult for surrogates and families to withdraw life-sustaining treatments that have been initiated than to withhold them. However, no medically, ethically, or legally relevant distinction can be made between withdrawing and withholding such treatments if the patient would not want them or if their burdens to the patient would outweigh the benefits. When discussing with surrogates or families the withdrawing or withholding of artificial nutrition and artificial hydration, it may be helpful to allay the common misconception that lack of nutrition or dehydration is inevitably uncomfortable and thus inhumane (see sections below on the management of anorexia and dry mouth).

Comprehensive Care. Palliative care is best provided by a team, directed by the physician, that may include nurses, a social worker, a chaplain, hospice workers, health aides, and specialists in oncology, radiation therapy, psychiatry, or palliative care. Regular case review with team members is necessary to ensure coordinated, high-quality care. Although the patient is the focus of care, the family's emotional, social, and spiritual needs also require attention, both for their own well-being and for the patient's. After the patient's death, grieving families may benefit from bereavement care.

Maximizing Dignity and a Sense of Control. Patients may fear the loss of dignity and control as much as any physical symptom. The care plan should be developed so as to maximize the patient's personal sense of dignity and to give the patient as great a sense of control as possible.

Double Effect. It is important to make clear to patients, surrogates, families, and clinicians that palliative care or a shift of focus to comfort is not euthanasia or physician-assisted suicide. Rather, palliative care is standard, appropriate medical care when curative or life-sustaining treatment is no longer beneficial or desired. It is particularly important to make this clear when control of the patient's symptoms may require the administration of opioids, benzodiazepines, or other medications in doses high enough to cause serious side effects. In this situation, the principle of double effect, a centuries-old tenet of the Catholic Church, is critical to the physician.

The principle of double effect states that "an action with two possible effects, one good and one bad, is morally permitted if the action (a) is not in itself immoral; (b) is undertaken only with the *intention* of achieving the possible good effect, without *intending* the possible bad effect even though it may be *foreseen*; (c) does not bring about the possible good effect by means of the possible bad effect; and (d) is undertaken for a proportionately grave reason." For example, a patient with advanced metastatic lung cancer and intractable pain may be given opioids even at the risk of side effects including sedation, hypotension, respiratory depression, respiratory arrest, and death as long as the action (giving opioids to relieve pain) (a) is not in itself immoral (giving opioids for pain is not); (b) is intended only to relieve pain and suffering and to ensure comfort; (c) does not intend to achieve relief and comfort by means of the possible side effect (death); and (d) is undertaken for the purpose of relieving the pain and suffering of a gravely ill patient.

Patients who wish to be made comfortable, their families, and other caregivers should be assured that the intention of treatment is to use the minimum doses of medications necessary for comfort, no more but also no less. When it is anticipated that adequate symptom control may unintentionally hasten the patient's death, the patient or surrogate should be advised of this and reassured that this is medically appropriate and ethically legitimate as well as compassionate.

PALLIATIVE CARE ASSESSMENT

A thorough palliative care assessment includes a comprehensive history and physical examination. It should address not just the medical issues of the patient but also the psychosocial and spiritual issues, and the needs of the family and significant others. Certain aspects of the palliative care assessment require particular attention.

Review of Symptoms. The palliative care assessment replaces the standard review of systems with a review of *symptoms* that is designed to explore typical causes of suffering at the end of life. It generally should cover pain, shortness of breath, nausea, vomiting, constipation, anorexia, dry mouth, odynophagia, insomnia, anxiety, and depression. Further review of symptoms should be tailored to the patient's illness.

Functional Status. The patient's performance status currently and during the past 2 weeks should be assessed. Categories might include the following: fully active, restricted strenuous activities, ambulatory/not able to work, limited self-care, confined to bed or chair/no self-care.

Awareness of Illness and Preferences for Care. The patient's and family's understanding of the diagnosis and prognosis should be explored. Patients should be asked whether they would like to receive all diagnostic and prognostic information and make all necessary decisions. Some patients may prefer instead that a surrogate receive this information and make these decisions, or that decisions be made by the physician. The existence of any advance directive such as a living will or health care proxy form (durable power of attorney) should be established. The physician particularly needs to know whom the patient wishes to serve as surrogate in case of decisional incapacity. The patient's hopes and goals for care should be explored and discussed. Helpful questions include the following: "Are there important tasks that would require your immediate attention if you were unable to function well in the future?" "If time were limited, what would be your priorities?" "Are there any upcoming events, such as births, weddings, or graduations, that are especially meaningful to you?" The patient's preferred location of care—home or hospital—should be explored. If possible without upsetting the patient, the preferred location of death also should be explored. Finally, any wishes to forego specific life-sustaining treatments, such as cardiopulmonary resuscitation, endotracheal intubation and mechanical ventilation, artificial nutrition, and artificial hydration, should be explored if the patient is ready to do so.

Social History. The social history should probe for sources of social suffering and identify psychosocial supports for both the patient and family. It should include the patient's living situation, names of all immediate and close family members and friends, work history, religion and degree of participation in organized religion, major sources of joy, major losses and disappointments, including deaths in the family, and the patient's and family's history of coping with these losses.

Medications. When the focus of care is shifted to palliation, the medication list should be reviewed and irrelevant medications such as cholesterol-lowering drugs discontinued.

Physical Examination should focus on evaluating current symptoms and anticipating future symptoms. Care should be taken to minimize the discomfort of the examination itself.

Laboratory and Imaging Studies. Diagnostic tests not needed for comfort care should not be performed. Occasionally, additional studies are indicated to help determine the prognosis, plan optimal palliative care, or maximize the patient's quality of life.

Impression. This should include a determination of prognosis and a list of actual and potential causes of discomfort. A differential diagnosis of an uncomfortable symptom should be performed whenever the cause is not obvious.

Plan. The treatment plan should be organized primarily by *symptom* rather than by organ system or disease. The list of symptoms should be exhaustive and should include anticipated symptoms. For example, three actual or potential symptoms—chest pain, hemoptysis, and acute respiratory distress—may be caused by the same underlying disease, but each symptom requires separate management. The preferred location of care should be identified and contingency plans made for major changes in the patient's condition. Psychosocial and spiritual supports (family, friends, social worker, clergy, visiting nurses, home health aides, hospice volunteers) should be identified. If relevant, financial or insurance problems should be addressed. Plans should be made to facilitate communication between the physician and the primary caregiver, nurses, and other physicians involved in the patient's care. If the patient wishes to forego resuscitation in the event of cardiac arrest or respiratory failure, a plan should be made to protect the patient from unwanted resuscitation in the event 911 is called. Many states have established protocols for this purpose.

MANAGEMENT OF MAJOR SYMPTOMS IN PALLIATIVE CARE

Dyspnea is a common symptom among terminally ill patients with primary or secondary lung neoplasms, pneumonias, cardiogenic or noncardiogenic pulmonary edema, chronic obstructive pulmonary disease, pulmonary embolism, and other conditions frequently seen at the end of life. The cause (or causes) of dyspnea should be identified and treated as aggressively as is compatible with the overall goal of comfort. Chest radiography, computed tomography, antibiotics for pneumonia, or thoracentesis, chest tubes, and pleurodesis for large pleural effusions may or may not be appropriate, depending on the pa-

tient's wishes and the plan of care. Occasional patients are maintained at home on positive inotropic agents for end-stage congestive heart failure. The workup for pulmonary embolism is rarely indicated for a patient whose care is focused on comfort.

When air hunger persists despite maximal appropriate treatment of the underlying condition, palliative treatment with *morphine* is indicated. Mild symptoms can be treated with 5 to 10 mg PO every 4 hours as needed (or around the clock if the symptoms are constant), and the dose can be titrated upward (e.g., to 15, 20, 30 mg) to achieve the desired effect. The regimen for patients who persistently require frequent doses should be changed to a long-acting opioid (e.g., MS Contin) at the equi-analgesic dose, with a short-acting dose available as needed for breakthrough dyspnea (see Part 1 of this chapter). For sudden, severe, or rapidly progressing dyspnea that is typical of massive pulmonary embolism, septic shock, or intrapulmonary lymphangitic spread of tumor, SQ or IV morphine often is necessary. Even at home, a constant SQ or IV infusion can be administered by means of a small infusion device and titrated to comfort. The starting dose will depend on the previous dose of opioids and the severity of symptoms. When a change is made from oral to parenteral morphine, the total daily parenteral dose should equal one third of the total daily oral dose. An opioid-naive patient can be started on an infusion of 1 to 2 mg/h. Bolus doses of 2 to 10 mg can be given for worsening symptoms and when the infusion rate is titrated upward. In the setting of severe respiratory distress, opioid doses necessary to achieve comfort may have the unintended but foreseeable side effect of hastening death (see preceding discussion of the principle of double effect).

Dyspnea frequently is associated with anxiety. *Benzodiazepines* can be helpful adjuncts to opioids when anxiety is prominent. Troublesome respiratory secretions causing choking, coughing, or respiratory distress can be treated with *scopolamine* transdermal patches (most patients need at least 1 mg/d) or glycopyrrolate via a nebulizer (0.8 mg every 6 hours), orally (1 to 2 mg three times daily), or parenterally (0.1 to 0.2 mg IV or SQ every 6 hours). Secretions are often reduced or absent in patients whose artificial nutrition and artificial hydration is discontinued before the terminal phase. Oxygen sometimes relieves dyspnea even in patients who are not hypoxic, as does a cool breeze from a fan.

Anorexia can be the consequence of any of the causes of chronic nausea. It also can be caused by factors elaborated by tumors (e.g., tumor necrosis factor), a massive tumor burden, chronic infection (e.g., viral hepatitis, AIDS), an increased basal metabolic rate (as in cancer, AIDS, end-stage congestive heart failure), gastroparesis, bowel surgery (e.g., short-bowel syndrome, dumping syndrome), and depression. Treatable underlying causes should be addressed. Medications that enhance the appetite for some patients include *megestrol acetate* (Megace; 160 to 800 mg PO daily), low doses of a corticosteroid (2 to 4 mg of *dexamethasone* PO twice daily), or *dronabinol* (Marinol; 2.5 to 5 mg PO twice daily before meals). Artificial nutrition by means of nasogastric, gastrostomy, or jejunostomy tubes or parenteral nutrition often is not appropriate in patients for whom the goal of care is comfort; these interventions may be more burdensome than beneficial by prolonging the dying process and worsening terminal respiratory distress.

Dry Mouth. Xerostomia, a very common symptom among dying patients, may be caused by dehydration, mouth breathing, or opioids and other medications with anticholinergic side effects, or it may follow head and neck surgery or radiation. Patients may take sips or ice chips if they wish. In severe cases, or when patients are unable to sip fluids, a saliva substitute (several commercial brands) should be applied every 4 hours around the clock and as needed. Petroleum jelly may be applied to the lips three times a day. Patients and families worried about discontinuing artificial hydration for fear of discomfort from dehydration may be assured that dry mouth is usually the only uncomfortable symptom of dehydration and that careful oral care is effective in preventing it.

Thrush. Candidal infection of the oropharynx and esophagus is common in patients who are immunosuppressed because of cancer, cancer therapy, AIDS, or the use of immunosuppressive medications such as corticosteroids. Mild cases may be treated with *nystatin* (5-mL Swish and Swallow four times daily) or *clotrimazole* (10-mg troche five times daily for 14 days). More severe cases require *fluconazole* (200 mg PO or IV on the first day, followed by 100 mg PO or IV for 2 weeks or until symptoms are resolved). Suppressive therapy with *fluconazole* is 100 mg PO weekly.

Constipation. This very common symptom can cause serious distress in terminally ill patients, who are typically immobile, somewhat dehydrated, and taking constipating medications such as opioids. Opioid regimens should virtually always be accompanied by a bowel regimen. Patients should be advised to make sure they move their bowels at least every 2 to 3 days. A typical starting regimen is senna (Senokot, 1 to 2 tablets PO twice daily; hold as needed in case of loose stools) and lactulose (30 mL PO at bedtime as needed if no bowel movement in 1 to 2 days) (see also Chapter 65).

Bowel Obstruction causing abdominal pain or vomiting, even when proximal, can sometimes be managed medically with a combination of IV morphine, scopolamine, and haloperidol. *Octreotide* IV or SQ often is useful to reduce gastrointestinal secretions and vomiting. *Dexamethasone* may help reduce the obstruction from complete to partial. When vomiting is refractory, *decompression* is required with a nasogastric tube. If the obstruction persists and the patient's prognosis is longer than a few days, permanent decompression with a gastrostomy tube may be considered.

Delirium and Agitation. The myriad possible causes of delirium and agitation in dying patients include side effects of medications, metabolic derangements (e.g., electrolyte abnormalities, uremia, liver failure), pain, infection, and central nervous system lesions. Underlying causes should be addressed if this can be done with minimum discomfort. Among medications, common offenders are opioids and the very drugs used to treat agitation, such as benzodiazepines and neuroleptics. When an opioid is felt to be the offending agent, an alternate opioid can tried. Because of incomplete cross-tolerance to opioids,

pain relief is often adequate with no more than one half of the equi-analgesic dose of the alternate agent. Because of the risk for delirium and paradoxical agitation, *benzodiazepines* such as *lorazepam* (Ativan) and neuroleptics such as *haloperidol* should be used cautiously in elderly or debilitated patients. Often, haloperidol (0.5 mg PO at bedtime or two or three times daily) is all that is needed to induce sleep or relieve agitation.

Depression. For rapid treatment of depression in a patient with a short prognosis, psychostimulants such as *dextroamphetamine* (Dexedrine) or *methylphenidate* (Ritalin) are the treatments of choice. The dosage for either is 2.5 to 5 mg PO each morning, titrated upward to 5 to 10 mg PO twice daily, at 8 a.m. and noon (see also Chapter 227.)

Sedation is a common side effect of opioids and other medications used frequently in palliative care. It can be treated with dextroamphetamine or methylphenidate (see also Chapter 226).

Myoclonus is a common side effect of opioid analgesics, particularly when given in high doses. Its appearance is idiosyncratic and may resolve with a switch to an alternate opioid. Again, adequate analgesia often can be maintained with less than the equi-analgesic dose of the alternate agent because of incomplete cross-tolerance. Mild myoclonus may cause no discomfort. If myoclonus is severe or clearly uncomfortable and not controlled by switching to an alternate opioid, lorazepam (Ativan; started at 0.5 to 1 mg PO or IV every 6 hours) or diazepam (Valium; started at 2 to 5 mg PO or IV every 8 hours) may be effective.

Hemorrhage. Sudden massive hemorrhage can be very distressing to the patient and family members. However, some highly motivated patients and families may remain at home during hemorrhage if they are properly prepared by the primary care physician and if adequate home nursing is available to ensure comfort. If massive hemorrhage is a likely scenario, the physician should explore the patient's desire to remain at home and the family's willingness to do whatever is necessary to keep the patient at home. The physician should reconfirm that the goal of care is comfort, that no resuscitation is to be performed, and that no blood products are to be given. The physician also should ascertain that a hospice or visiting nurse is available around the clock and able to get to the home in less than 1 hour. The physician should discuss the possibility of massive hemorrhage with the primary nurse and review the management plan. The physician then should explain to the patient and family what might happen, what the patient might feel, and exactly what measures would be taken to ensure comfort.

When hemorrhaging occurs, several simple steps are appropriate. First, the patient and family should be calmed and reassured that the situation can be handled. The nurse or other clinician on the scene should cover the blood or melena and remove it frequently. Morphine or a benzodiazepine such as lorazepam should be given IV or SQ to calm the patient. A constant IV or SQ infusion of morphine should be started and titrated to comfort. As the patient exsanguinates, additional symptoms may arise, such as shortness of breath, chest pain from ischemia, light-headedness, and anxiety. Additional morphine (and sometimes also benzodiazepine) in IV or SQ bolus doses should be given to control these symptoms quickly.

Pain. (See Part 1 of this chapter.)

Ascites. (See Chapters 71, 91, and 92.)

Hiccups. (See Chapter 221.)

Nausea and Vomiting. (See Chapters 59 and 91.)

Dysphagia, Odynophagia. (See Chapter 60.)

Insomnia. (See Chapter 232.)

Seizure. (See Chapter 170.)

Pressure Ulcers. (See Chapter 197.)

Pruritus. (See Chapter 178.)

Terminal Distress. (See section above on dyspnea.)

OTHER ISSUES AND INDICATIONS FOR ADMISSION

Hospice and Home Services. Hospice services are available in inpatient hospices, in some nursing homes, and at home through home hospice organizations or visiting nurse associations. The primary care physician may choose to remain in charge of the patient's care in all settings. Most hospices accept patients only when the patient and family are aware of the terminal diagnosis and prognosis and accept care focused purely on comfort.

Psychosocial and Spiritual Support. Emotional and spiritual support and counseling can be extremely important for dying patients and their loved ones. All accredited hospice organizations have a social worker, chaplain, and volunteers available. They can assist with the search for meaning in the dying process, religious and spiritual issues, anticipatory grieving, life review, preparation of a legacy, and financial issues.

Bereavement. Hospices also make available some form of support for bereaved family members and loved ones. A note of condolence from the physician with an offer to be available by phone to answer any lingering questions can be very comforting. The physician also might call the family to provide support, answer questions, and assess the need for a referral for formal bereavement counseling.

Indications for Admission. In some situations, it is necessary to admit a patient to the hospital to protect the patient from end-of-life suffering. For example, a patient with severe or refractory pain, dyspnea, or seizures may require treatments not available at home. In other cases, adequate home nursing care may not be available or the family may be overwhelmed. Patients who are near death may be admitted for terminal care. Others are admitted just long enough to control symptoms and arrange appropriate end-of-life care in a skilled nursing facility, inpatient hospice, or the home.

CONCLUSIONS AND RECOMMENDATIONS

- Patients with chronic life-threatening illnesses and their families need reassurance that attentive comfort care can be provided if desired in lieu of aggressive, life-sustaining treatment.
- The benefits and burdens of all diagnostic and therapeutic measures should be weighed and the physician should suggest that more burdensome measures not be used.
- No medical, ethical, or legal distinction is made between withdrawing and withholding a treatment that is more burdensome than beneficial or not desired by the patient.
- Artificial nutrition and hydration are medical treatments that may be provided or not provided, like any other intervention, depending on the benefit-to-burden ratio and the patient's or surrogate's wishes.
- Treatments intended only to relieve serious refractory symptoms in a terminally ill patient often may be provided even at the risk of unintended but foreseeable side effects, including a hastening of death.
- Sources of physical and social suffering should be thoroughly explored, along with the patient's awareness of the diagnosis and prognosis and preferences for end-of-life care.
- A differential diagnosis of uncomfortable symptoms should be performed and the underlying cause treated to the fullest extent consistent with the goal of comfort.
- Anticipate sources of terminal distress and make treatment plans in advance.
- Treat dyspnea with morphine administered orally, sublingually, or rectally. If the dyspnea is severe, morphine can be administered IV or SQ.
- Troublesome respiratory secretions can be treated with anticholinergics such as scopolamine or glycopyrrolate.
- Treat xerostomia with a saliva substitute around the clock, particularly in dehydrated patients.
- Inpatient and outpatient hospice services are available to help manage symptoms and psychosocial problems under the direction of the physician. Hospice teams include nurses, social workers, chaplains, health aides, and volunteers.
- Dying patients sometimes must be admitted to the hospital to control refractory symptoms.

ANNOTATED BIBLIOGRAPHY

Block SD. Assessing and managing depression in the terminally ill patient. Ann Intern Med 2000;132:209. (*A superb review of grief and clinical depression in the terminally ill patient, with an overview of treatment recommendations.*)

Block SD, Billings JA. Patient requests to hasten death: evaluation and management in terminal care. Arch Intern Med 1994;154:2039. (*An excellent discussion of ways to understand and manage patients' requests to hasten death.*)

Bruera E, MacEachern T, Ripamonti C, et al. Subcutaneous morphine for dyspnea in cancer patients. Ann Intern Med 1993;119:906. (*A crossover, placebo-controlled trial demonstrating the beneficial effect of morphine on dyspnea in terminally ill cancer patients.*)

Covinsky KE, Goldman L, Cook EF, et al. The impact of serious illness on patients' families. JAMA 1994;272:1839. (*A good analysis of the often severe social and economic burdens on family members of terminally ill patients.*)

Dunn PM, Levinson W. Discussing futility with patients and families. J Gen Intern Med 1996;11:689. (*A nice analysis of pitfalls encountered in discussing end-of-life care with patients and families.*)

Finucane TE, Christmas C, Travis K. Tube feeding in patients with advanced dementia: a review of the evidence. JAMA 1999;282:1365. (*A thorough review of the literature revealed that tube feeding for patients with advanced dementia provides little or no benefit and risks substantial burdens.*)

Khoo D, Hall E, Motson R, et al. Palliation of malignant intestinal obstruction using octreotide. Eur J Cancer 1994;30A:28. (*A study demonstrating the usefulness of octreotide to control vomiting in the setting of malignant bowel obstruction.*)

Koenig BA, Gates-Williams J. Understanding cultural difference in caring for dying patients. West J Med 1995;163:244. (*The importance of culture and religious belief in determining attitudes toward death and dying; includes guidelines for sensitively assessing these attitudes.*)

Krakauer EL, Penson RT, Truog RD, et al. Sedation for intractable distress of a dying patient: acute palliative care and the principle of double effect. Oncologist 2000;5:53. (*A discussion of medical and ethical issues involved in sedating dying patients with intractable distress.*)

Landry FJ, Parker JM, Phillips YY. Outcome of cardiopulmonary resuscitation in the intensive care unit. Arch Intern Med 1992;152:2305. (*One of the best studies of cardiopulmonary resuscitation outcomes in patients with various underlying diseases.*)

McCann RM. Comfort care for terminally ill patients: the appropriate use of nutrition and hydration. JAMA 1994;272:1263. (*A study demonstrating that artificial nutrition and hydration are usually not beneficial and may be burdensome to terminally ill patients.*)

Sulmasy DP, Pellegrino ED. The rule of double effect. Arch Intern Med 1999;159:545. (*A good overview of the principle of double effect and its critical importance to palliative care.*)

SUPPORT Investigators. A controlled trial to improve care for seriously ill hospitalized patients. JAMA 1995;274:1591. (*A summary of the most comprehensive study to date of end-of-life care.*)

Ventafridda V, Ripamonti C, Caraceni A, et al. The management of inoperable gastrointestinal obstruction in terminal cancer patients. Tumori 1990;76:389. (*A study of a technique for managing malignant bowel obstruction without nasogastric suction that can be used in the home.*)

Wanzer SH, Federman DD, et al. The physician's responsibility toward hopelessly ill patients. N Engl J Med 1989;320:844. (*An eloquent statement of the importance of high-quality palliative care.*)

Weil JV, McCullough RE, Kline JS, et al. Diminished ventilatory response to hypoxia and hypercapnia after morphine in normal man. N Engl J Med 1975;292:1103. (*A classic study demonstrating a physiologic reason for the effectiveness of morphine in treating air hunger resulting from hypoxia or hypercapnia.*)

91
Managing the Gastrointestinal Complications of Cancer and Cancer Treatment

The gastrointestinal symptoms that accompany cancer and cancer therapy are among the most difficult for the patient to bear, often compromising nutritional status and quality of life. Problems may arise from primary disease, metastases, side effects of therapy, or metabolic disturbances. Successful primary care of the cancer patient necessitates attending to the anorexia, nausea, vomiting, weight loss, abdominal pain, ascites, and related gastrointestinal problems that often worsen their lives.

NAUSEA AND VOMITING

Cancer therapies are far and away the leading cause of nausea and vomiting in patients with malignancy. Treatments often have to be stopped or limited by the onset of emesis. This makes the control of nausea and vomiting important, not only for restoring patient comfort but also for ensuring completion of a full course of treatment. The presentation of emesis may precede, acutely follow, or follow after a short delay the application of cancer therapy; it may also become persistent.

Pathophysiology and Clinical Presentation

Current models postulate both peripheral and central components of therapy-induced nausea and vomiting. The peripheral pathway involves acute injury to the rapidly dividing cells of the gastric mucosa. The resultant cellular damage and accompanying inflammation cause the release of serotonin from gastric enterochromaffin cells into the gastric lumen, with subsequent activation of *serotonin S_3-receptors* in the gut wall and centrally in the brainstem vomiting center. Central stimulation of the vomiting center is also believed to occur when chemotherapy drugs directly stimulate the chemoreceptor trigger zone. A number of central receptors effecting emesis have been identified, including those responsive to *dopamine, endorphin, serotonin,* and *substance P.*

Most treatments produce *acute,* self-limited emesis that lasts only a few hours; however, the experience can be very uncomfortable, exhausting, and demoralizing. A milder, *delayed* emesis that can occur 1 to 5 days after therapy is most commonly seen with cisplatin therapy and is believed to be related to the development of gastritis and the persistence of active drug metabolites. Although less severe, it is discouraging and can impede nutrition. *Anticipatory* vomiting is a psychogenic behavioral phenomenon, derived from the association of severe emesis with the administration of cancer treatment. Nausea and vomiting can be brought on just by the anticipation of chemotherapy. *Refractory emesis* suggests a metabolic or anatomic complication of cancer or cancer therapy (see below).

Antiemetic Agents

Serotonin S₃-receptor Blockers (Ondansetron, Granisetron, Dolasetron) have proved effective in the prevention of both acute and delayed chemotherapy-induced nausea and vomiting. When the drugs are used alone, complete prevention of acute nausea and vomiting is achieved in about 40% to 50% of patients; more than 70% have no vomiting, but some nausea. When they are combined with a program of acute glucocorticoid therapy (e.g., *dexamethasone*), their prophylactic efficacy rises to 90% for prevention of emesis and to 70% for prevention of both nausea and vomiting. All three available serotonin blockers are similar in regard to efficacy and side effects, which include mild headache, mild dizziness, and a transient, clinically insignificant prolongation of electrocardiographic intervals. These drugs can be administered IV or orally. Ondansetron is the least expensive of the oral preparations (two 8-mg doses are administered orally); dolasetron is the least expensive IV agent.

Glucocorticoids have proved effective, especially in the prevention of delayed nausea and vomiting (perhaps because of their antiinflammatory effects). In controlled trials, they have outperformed phenothiazines in the prevention of acute emesis and have provided protection similar to that afforded by the serotonin-receptor blockers. They are superior to the latter in preventing delayed nausea and vomiting (50% rates of complete prevention vs. 30%) and provide enhanced control when used in combination with them. A typical program is a 4-mg oral dose of dexamethasone given just before chemotherapy, followed by three more doses given every 6 hours.

Metoclopramide blocks both dopaminergic and serotonin receptors, which accounts for its antiemetic action and its side effects. Given parenterally in high doses just before chemotherapy, it too can suppress emesis, but to a considerably lesser degree than the serotonin-receptor blockers (42% complete suppression vs. 75%). It is frequently used in combination with other agents, especially to prevent delayed emesis. Its dopaminergic blocking effect promotes gastric emptying and gastroesophageal sphincter closure but also leads to dystonia in young patients and mental confusion in older patients. It too is administered IV in a loading dose (1 to 3 mg/kg) 30 minutes before chemotherapy. It can be continued as a slow IV infusion, given as another dose 90 minutes after the first dose, or continued orally.

Substance P Blockade (Neurokinin-1-receptor Antagonists). The identification of substance P receptors in the central sites triggering emesis has led to the investigation of agents that block such receptors and inhibit substance P–mediated effects. Although such therapy is still investigational, initial trials of substance P blockers in combination with granisetron and dexamethasone show significant additional benefit, especially in the prevention of delayed emesis. More data on efficacy and safety should be forthcoming. If initial results are confirmed, then improved prevention of delayed emesis may soon be available.

Benzodiazepines potentiate the activities of the central inhibitory neurotransmitter γ-aminobutyric acid (GABA) and can enhance the antiemetic effects of other agents. They also cause a desirable degree of mild amnesia. A short-acting preparation such as *lorazepam* is commonly given before chemotherapy. It too is best used as part of a combination program. Some prescribe an *antihistamine* (e.g., diphenhydramine) in place of a benzodiazepine. *Psychogenic vomiting* that occurs in anticipation of chemotherapy responds to IV lorazepam or oral alprazolam in conjunction with behavioral *desensitization* therapy; however, the best treatment is prevention of emesis at the outset of chemotherapy.

Phenothiazines, such as *prochlorperazine* (Compazine), are well established as a treatment for mild nausea and vomiting associated with other conditions, but they are less effective in chemotherapy if used alone. However, when combined with other antiemetic agents, they may help provide additional prophylaxis. Phenothiazines act centrally, blocking serotonin and dopamine receptors in the chemoreceptor trigger zone. Sedation accompanies their use and is often desired, but extrapyramidal symptoms may also ensue. They are available in oral, suppository, and parenteral forms. The route of administration has little influence on effectiveness. On the day of treatment, a prochlorperazine capsule or suppository is given 4 to 8 hours before the administration of chemotherapy and again on a regularly scheduled basis for the next 24 hours. The main drawback to phenothiazine therapy is the precipitation of extrapyramidal symptoms, which are most likely to occur when daily doses exceed 50 mg. Their onset necessitates discontinuation of therapy. Under such circumstances, the mild antiemetic *trimethobenzamide* (Tigan) is worth a try, although it is less effective than prochlorperazine. *Haloperidol*, a major tranquilizer that is not a phenothiazine, is similar to prochlorperazine in antiemetic and extrapyramidal effects. It blocks dopaminergic receptors. Side effects are similar to those of metoclopramide.

Cannabinoids and Marijuana were transiently popular, but they were found to be little better than phenothiazines and have been supplanted by more effective regimens with fewer side effects. Evidence suggests some antinausea and appetite-stimulant effects with the use of purified tetrahydrocannabinol, but no evidence that smoking crude marijuana is required to achieve these effects has been found.

Design of a Comprehensive Prophylactic Program

The optimal goal of antiemetic therapy is to prevent the nausea and vomiting associated with cancer therapy. This eliminates the dread of undergoing therapy and prevents any behaviorally triggered emesis. To design an effective prophylactic program, the physician must be familiar with the propensity of various agents to cause emesis (Table 91.1) and the mechanisms and synergistic effects of available antiemetic drugs (Table 91.2).

A combination strategy takes advantage of the mechanistic synergistic effects afforded by administering effective drugs with different modes of action. More complete and extended prophylaxis, the use of lower doses of individual agents, and therefore a reduction in side effects become possible. For example, to treat a patient with anticipatory, acute, and delayed forms of emesis, an effective program might include a benzodi-

Table 91.1.   Chemotherapeutic Agents and Their Emetic Potential

AGENT	EMETIC POTENTIAL	AGENT	EMETIC POTENTIAL	AGENT	EMETIC POTENTIAL
Cisplatin	High	5-Fluorouracil	Low	Lomustine	Moderate
Dacarbazine	High	Methotrexate	Low	Doxorubicin	Moderate
Dactinomycin	High	Vincristine	Low	Procarbazine	Moderate
Mechlorethamine	High	Vinblastine	Low	Daunorubicin	Moderate
Cyclophosphamide	High	Chlorambucil	Low	Cytosine arabinoside	Moderate
		Etoposide	Low	Carmustine	Moderate
		Bleomycin	Low		
		Mitomycin C	Low		

Adapted from Gralla RJ. In: DeVita VT, Hellman S, Rosenberg SA, eds. Cancer: principles and practice of oncology, 3rd ed. Philadelphia: JB Lippincott Co, 1989:2138, with permission.

Table 91.2.   Combination Approach to Prophylaxis of Chemotherapy-Induced Emesis

Select

1. Neurotransmitter Blocking Agent
   a. Ondansetron (blocks serotonin S$_3$-receptors, peripheral and central)
   b. Metoclopramide (blocks dopamine $\pm$ serotonin receptors)
   c. Phenothiazine (blocks central dopamine $\pm$ receptors)

Plus

2. Benzodiazepine or Antihistamine
   a. Lorazepam (increases central inhibitory transmission; mild amnesia)
   b. Diphenhydramine (sedates)

Plus

3. Corticosteroid
   a. Dexamethasone (mechanism unknown; ? antiinflammatory role)
   b. Methylprednisolone (same)

azepine (lorazepam), a serotonin-receptor blocker (e.g., ondansetron), and a corticosteroid (dexamethasone). Normal food intake before chemotherapy is encouraged because it minimizes retching on an empty stomach, which produces muscle cramps and pain. The chemotherapy schedule should comprise no more than two to three applications per month.

Refractory Emesis. A few treatable causes need to be considered when a patient presents with refractory emesis. Persistent vomiting can be a manifestation of *bowel obstruction* or severe *ileus*, which respond to decompression by *nasogastric suctioning*. *Hypercalcemia* and *hypokalemia* may be causes as well as consequences of vomiting; monitoring of electrolytes and correction of any imbalances can help lessen the anorexia, nausea, and vomiting that sometimes accompany them.

ANOREXIA AND WEIGHT LOSS

The cachexia of cancer is one of its hallmark manifestations, characterized by anorexia, early satiety, profound weight loss, and inanition. Maintaining adequate nutrition becomes very difficult in this situation.

Pathophysiology

Although multifactorial, *cachexia* has been strongly linked to elaboration of the macrophage-derived protein *cachectin* (also referred to as *tumor necrosis factor*), which is capable of inducing a wasting syndrome in animals and mediating adverse metabolic changes in human malignancy. Increased gluconeogenesis, excessive catabolism of body protein (especially muscle), abnormal fat metabolism, and abnormal substrate use have all been observed. In addition to cachectin, tumor-induced tissue breakdown, caloric wasting, and sequestration of protein-rich ascitic fluid in the abdomen may also contribute. Further aggravating the situation are disorders of digestion and absorption that are associated with malnutrition, obstructive lesions, and surgical therapies such as gastrectomy or intestinal bypass procedures. Abnormal caloric utilization is a consequence of tumor-related changes of metabolism, with food intake and lean body mass being channeled to support the caloric demands of the tumor.

The mechanisms behind *anorexia* remains incompletely understood. A paraneoplastic syndrome has been postulated, linked to a tumor-induced polypeptide that can affect the satiety center in the brain. Additionally, radiation and chemotherapeutic agents may contribute by distorting taste, causing stomatitis, and injuring the gastrointestinal mucosa and liver.

Management

The single most effective means of overcoming anorexia and cachexia is to achieve control of the underlying malignancy. In the interim, patients need practical suggestions that can be put to immediate use.

Dietary Measures. *Small, frequent feedings* (about six per day) of foods high in protein and calories should be advised. *Liquid dietary supplements* in the form of milk shakes and commercial preparations are excellent if tolerated. If nausea is prominent, the patient should be advised to try foods that are *salty*, beverages that are *cool* and *clear*, and desserts such as *gelatin* and *popsicles*. Dry foods such as *toast* and *crackers* also help. Dietitians recommend that the food be served in a *relaxed* family or group setting, *attractively prepared* and readily available. When *altered taste* makes food unpalatable, meat should be avoided and dairy products substituted as the main source of protein. *Acidic foods* may stimulate the appetite when taste acuity seems to wane, as may *extra seasoning* and spicy foods. The use of *zinc* to treat dysgeusia has been reported, but results are not very impressive. Foods best to *avoid* when nausea is prominent include those that are overly *sweet*, *greasy*, or *high in fat*.

Medications. *Tricyclic antidepressants* (e.g., amitriptyline) have a nonspecific appetite-stimulating effect that is sometimes helpful and often independent of the antidepressant effect. *Corticosteroids* have sometimes been used to stimulate appetite, but their effect is transient and not worth the major side effects associated with the high doses and prolonged administration needed to achieve a sustained increase in appetite. *Megasterol* has been administered as an anabolic steroid with some success.

Treatment of Stomatitis. Stomatitis is an often overlooked cause of poor intake and weight loss. The management of chemotherapy-induced stomatitis includes avoidance of smoking, alcohol, and foods that are very hot, cold, spicy, or salty. A mixture of *Benadryl elixir* and *Kaopectate* used as a mouth wash is often helpful and well tolerated. *Chlorhexidine gluconate* is an antimicrobial oral rinse that can be used as a preventative, but a non–alcohol-based mouthwash is better once sores occur. *Viscous Xylocaine* preparations are not very helpful because they wash away quickly and thus provide only very transient relief; paste preparations last considerably longer. Unfortunately, taste can be distorted as a consequence of the topical anesthetic effect.

When radiation therapy to the head and neck results in *xerostomia* and *mucositis*, the dryness and thick secretions can be lessened by chewing gum or sucking on hard candy, which helps stimulate salivation. The use of gravies and avoidance of dry foods helps deglutition in patients whose salivary glands are damaged by radiation. In refractory situations, artificial saliva preparations can be used.

MALNUTRITION

One of the most serious consequences of nausea, vomiting, and cachexia is malnutrition. A self-perpetuating and debilitating cycle of food rejection and malnutrition weakens host immune defenses and permits further tumor growth. Moreover, host tolerance to radiation and chemotherapy is compromised, so that the ability to tolerate therapeutic doses of either form of treatment is restricted. The goals and methods of nutritional therapy vary according to the patient's clinical situation. In most instances in which gastrointestinal function remains intact, minor dietary alterations and oral dietary supplements are sufficient. More elaborate means of nutritional support are sometimes necessary and appropriate on a temporary basis to tide the patient over a difficult period. Such therapy is rarely indicated in the very late stages of cancer.

Detection. Recognition of mild to moderate malnutrition is important. Manifestations include a 10% weight loss, serum albumin level below 3.5 g/dL, total lymphocyte count of less than 1,500/mm³, and serum creatinine level that is low for the patient's size. More severe malnutrition is characterized by fur-

ther weight loss, a serum albumin level below 3.0 g/dL, and a lymphocyte count of less than 1,000/mm³.

Use of Supplements. For patients who have upper alimentary discomfort but can still swallow liquids, a *nutritionally complete liquid preparation* may offer a more comfortable and palatable means of keeping well nourished. These preparations are available commercially and are reasonably well tolerated. Most contain all the necessary vitamins and minerals. Lactose-free formulations are available for those who may have acquired lactose intolerance. Blenderized meals are another alternative.

Hyperalimentation. More intensive temporary nutritional support is worth considering during difficult phases of cancer therapy, although evidence of cost-effectiveness is often wanting and indiscriminate use can be counterproductive and increase morbidity. Most controlled studies of hyperalimentation and other nutritional therapies have failed to demonstrate any significant improvement in response to chemotherapy or radiation, lessening of side effects of these treatment modalities, prolongation of survival, or improved tolerance to higher doses or longer periods of treatment. However, the selective use of hyperalimentation may be of benefit in some instances.

Enteral hyperalimentation is utilized for the nutritional support of malnourished patients with an obstructed or injured upper alimentary tract, provided the remainder of the gastrointestinal tract is intact. Such hyperalimentation is particularly well suited to patients recovering from radiation or surgery in the upper alimentary tract. A feeding tube is either passed or surgically placed beyond the point of obstruction or injury. An enteral hyperalimentation program can then commence. The use of long (43-in), flexible silicon nasal feeding tubes makes it possible to administer feedings directly into the distal duodenum or proximal jejunum, so that the risks for aspiration and reflux that occur with gastrostomy feedings are avoided. When a feeding tube cannot be passed nasally, feedings can be administered through a jejunostomy.

Enteral hyperalimentation utilizes milk-based and soy-based formulas, in addition to less viscous formulations, although sometimes a pump is needed. The formulas are quite hypertonic and must be started at less than full strength (usually at half-strength) and increased during several days, as tolerated. Cramps, symptoms of dumping syndrome (flushing, tachycardia, sweating), and diarrhea are the major manifestations of intolerance. The goal is a daily intake of 2,000 to 3,000 calories.

Total parenteral nutrition is an alternative form of nutritional support reserved for short-term use in persons whose oral or enteral intake is likely to be inadequate for more than 10 to 14 days. The best evidence for its efficacy is in severely malnourished cancer patients about to undergo surgery; morbidity and mortality are reduced with preoperative administration of total parenteral nutrition. It can be carried out *at home* so long as the patient and family are capable of mastering the procedures necessary to ensure the sterility of the line and integrity of the infusion apparatus. Visits by a hyperalimentation nurse are also helpful. The access site can be maintained as a heparin lock, which allows the patient to disconnect easily from the infusion. About 12 to 14 hours are needed for infusions daily, which are administered as solutions containing 4.2% or 5.2% amino acids and 20% to 25% glucose. The infusion schedule provides the patient with 10 to 12 hours of independence each day and an opportunity to ambulate. Careful monitoring of metabolic parameters, including glucose, calcium, phosphate, magnesium, blood urea nitrogen, and creatinine levels, is essential, as is close coordination with a hyperalimentation consultant.

DIARRHEA AND CONSTIPATION

Diarrhea is another gastrointestinal nemesis familiar to cancer patients. When it ensues from radiation- or chemotherapy-induced enteritis, the problem is usually self-limited, resolving within the 1 to 2 weeks needed for the mucosal surface to reconstitute itself. If it is persistent or troublesome, low doses of *diphenoxylate* (Lomotil) or nonprescription *loperamide* (Imodium) can be prescribed for symptomatic relief (see Chapter 64). *Steatorrhea* is experienced by patients who have undergone pancreatectomy or who have pancreatic insufficiency; intake of several *pancreatic enzyme* tablets with each meal (see Chapter 72) usually alleviates the problem. The postgastrectomy patient is at risk for the symptoms of the *dumping syndrome*. Avoidance of *sweets* and large *fluid volumes* (especially those rich in sugar) helps prevent attacks, as does lying down after a meal (see Chapter 64).

Constipation can be a very troublesome and often unavoidable consequence of *narcotic use* for pain control. However, prophylactic institution of some simple measures can help prevent disabling symptoms and fecal impaction. These include a *high-fiber diet*, good *fluid intake* (at least 2 L/d), use of *stool softeners* (e.g., dioctyl sodium sulfosuccinate), and, if necessary, administration of a gentle *laxative* before bed (e.g., 15 mL of milk of magnesia). Constipation may also be a sign of *obstruction* in the lower intestinal tract or ileus, conditions that need to be ruled out before laxative therapy is escalated. *Hypokalemia* and *hypercalcemia* are two other important causes that deserve attention.

MALIGNANT ASCITES

Ascites may occur as a complication of diffuse peritoneal implantation or the combination of portal venous hypertension and hypoalbuminemia. When it is caused by peritoneal implants and the primary is unknown, one should consider treatable malignancies such as ovarian cancer. Occasionally, the ascites will cause disabling symptoms such as marked abdominal distention and pain. Only in debilitating circumstances should it be treated. The most direct means is *therapeutic paracentesis*. Recent experience with large-volume paracentesis suggests that it can be performed with safety so long as care is taken to preserve intravascular volume. About 4 to 6 L of ascitic fluid is removed slowly during 60 to 90 minutes. (An infusion of albumin is administered simultaneously in severely hypoalbuminemic patients.)

Large-volume therapeutic paracentesis has reduced the need for *peritoneal venous shunting*, which is associated with a high rate of complications, including encephalopathy, disseminated intravascular coagulation, peritonitis, sepsis, and superior vena cava syndrome (see Chapter 71). Shunting should be considered only in the most refractory and disabling

of cases. The use of surgical drainage for ascites is not as effective as it is for effusions of the pleural space. Similarly, intraabdominal instillation of chemotherapeutic agents and radioisotopes has been relatively ineffective. Sclerosing drugs and irritants to seal the peritoneal space are not recommended because an irritant effect on the bowel may result in necrosis, perforation, or secondary fibrosis and adhesions leading to obstruction.

PERITONEAL IMPLANTS, BOWEL OBSTRUCTION, AND FISTULAS

Peritoneal implants within the abdominal cavity may develop in a diffuse miliary pattern or coalesce into large mass lesions capable of causing obstruction. A surgical *bypass* procedure or regional surgical resection (*"debulking"*) is indicated under such circumstances for palliation when there is some hope of prolonging meaningful survival. For patients with an indolent malignancy, particularly those with a localized point of obstruction, an aggressive surgical approach is worthy of consideration. When implants are centered in the pelvic area, fistulas communicating with the bladder or skin may form; local *surgical excision* or *radiation therapy* can help control the problem.

OBSTRUCTIVE JAUNDICE

Surgery used to be the traditional treatment, but it is often not feasible in patients with extensive disease of the porta hepatis extending into the liver. More recently, endoscopic or percutaneous *placement of a stent* has provided a less invasive alternative. The procedure should be attempted only by persons skilled in placement of such stents. Major complications do occur, particularly recurrent cholangitis. The procedure can be uncomfortable, and the stents tend to become dislodged. However, if the procedure is successful, significant palliation and an improved quality of life can result for the patient willing to undergo stent placement.

Radiation therapy has also been used to treat obstructive jaundice caused by tumor in the porta hepatis. It is particularly useful in patients with radiosensitive neoplasms (e.g., breast cancer, lymphoma).

A.H.G.

ANNOTATED BIBLIOGRAPHY

Beck TM, Ciociola A, Jones SE, et al. Efficacy of oral ondansetron in the prevention of emesis in outpatients receiving cyclophosphamide-based chemotherapy. Ann Intern Med 1993;118:407. (*Demonstrated safe and effective, with 66% experiencing no emetic episodes.*)

Cubeddu LX, Hoffmann IS, Fuenmayor NT, et al. Efficacy of ondansetron (GR 38032F) and the role of serotonin in cisplatin-induced nausea and vomiting. N Engl J Med 1990;322:810. (*Major initial evidence of efficacy and the importance of serotonin S₃-receptors.*)

Epstein M. Refractory ascites. N Engl J Med 1989;321:1675. (*Editorial summarizing methods of treatment.*)

Gralla RJ, Itri LM, Pisko SE, et al. Antiemetic efficacy of high-dose metoclopramide. N Engl J Med 1981;305:905. (*A randomized, controlled study establishing efficacy in cisplatin-induced vomiting.*)

Klein S, Koretz RL. Nutritional support in patients with cancer: what do the data really show? Nutr Clin Pract 1994;9:91. (*A good review of the evidence.*)

Kris MG, Gralla RJ, Clark RA, et al. Consecutive dose-finding trials: adding lorazepam to the combination of metoclopramide plus dexamethasone. Cancer Treat Rep 1985;69:1257. (*Evidence for the efficacy of multiple-drug, multiple-mechanism therapy.*)

Kris MG, Gralla RJ, Clark RA, et al. Incidence, course, and severity of delayed nausea and vomiting following the administration of high-dose cisplatin. J Clin Oncol 1985;3:1379. (*Cisplatin is the major cause.*)

Marty M, Pouillart P, Scholl S, et al. Comparison of the 5-hydroxytryptamine (serotonin) antagonist ondansetron (GR38032) with high-dose metoclopramide in the control of cisplatin-induced emesis. N Engl J Med 1990;322:816. (*Ondansetron proved far superior.*)

Morrow GR, Morrell C. Behavioral treatment for the anticipatory nausea and vomiting induced by cancer chemotherapy. N Engl J Med 1982;307:1476. (*Describes the phenomenon and details behavioral approaches to treatment.*)

Navari RM, Reinhardt RR, Gralla RJ, et al. Reduction of cisplatin-induced emesis by a selective neurokinin-1-receptor antagonist. N Engl J Med 1999;340:190. (*Randomized, placebo-controlled trial of a new class of antiemetic; found to enhance control of delayed emesis markedly and add some prevention of acute emesis to that provided by dexamethasone and granisetron.*)

Rivadeneira DE, Evoy E, Fahey TJ III, et al. Nutritional support of the cancer patient. CA Cancer J Clin 1998;48:69. (*Very practical, fully documented discussion of the best approaches to nutritional support and supporting evidence.*)

The Italian Group for Antiemetic Research. Dexamethasone, granisetron, or both for the prevention of nausea and vomiting during chemotherapy for cancer. N Engl J Med 1995;332:1. (*The combination program provided the best results.*)

Voth EA, Schwartz RH. Medical applications of delta-9-tetrahydrocannabinol and marijuana. Ann Intern Med 1997;126:791. (*Literature review concluding that a modest benefit may be derived from the use of pure tetrahydrocannabinol for chemotherapy-induced nausea and anorexia, but that the use of crude marijuana adds no value and entails many disadvantages.*)

92
Complications of Cancer: Oncologic Emergencies and Paraneoplastic Syndromes

The complications of cancer are great in number and variable in degree of urgency. They range from commonly experienced gastrointestinal difficulties and pain syndromes (see Chapters 90 and 91) to true emergencies, stubborn malignant effusions, and the uncommon, but important, paraneoplastic phenomena. Most oncologic emergencies and malignant effusions are consequences of anatomic spread. Paraneoplastic syndromes result from hormonal and immunologic disturbances. The primary care physician's important role in monitoring the cancer patient requires familiarity with the early presentations of these complications, many of which are amenable to intervention. In most instances, hospital admission for inpatient treatment will be necessary, so the emphasis is on early detection.

ONCOLOGIC EMERGENCIES AND URGENCIES

The anatomic spread of tumor is capable of causing emergent complications, including spinal cord compression, cardiac tamponade, and hypercoagulability with acute bleeding or clotting. Urgent adversities associated with malignancy ensue from a combination of tumor invasion and metabolic/immunologic effects (e.g., superior vena cava syndrome, hypercalcemia, fever, infection).

Spinal Cord Compression

Extradural or epidural cord compression occurs in approximately 5% of patients with cancer. It is a *true emergency*, with early diagnosis and treatment essential to preventing serious, permanent neurologic damage. The majority of cases of epidural compression result from bony metastases in the vertebral bodies extending into the epidural space. Less frequently, metastatic tumor reaches the epidural space hematogenously or by direct extension through the intervertebral foramina. Malignancies with a propensity to spread to bone (e.g., myeloma, lymphoma, melanoma, renal cell carcinoma, and tumors of lung, breast, and prostate) are associated with the greatest risk for cord compression. Lymphoma may metastasize directly to the epidural space and not produce any bony changes. In more than 90% of cases, the initial symptom is *back pain*, often radicular in nature. The course is progressive; weakness and sensory deficits in the extremities follow. Sphincter incontinence is a late development, unless the cauda equina is the initial site of compression.

Diagnosis. *Plain films* of the spine should be obtained in all cancer patients with back pain. If the radiographic findings are normal in the area of pain, the patient does not have lymphoma, and no neurologic deficits are present, no further workup need be carried out immediately, but the patient should be followed closely. If the radiographic findings are abnormal or if neurologic deficits are noted, then immediate hospital admission and prompt neurologic and oncologic consultations are needed.

Magnetic resonance imaging (MRI) is the diagnostic procedure of choice, being the most sensitive and least invasive of the imaging procedures, especially when gadolinium enhancement is used. It allows identification of all affected areas without the need for injection of contrast into the spinal canal. If MRI is not available, imaging of the spinal cord can also be performed by standard *myelography* with iodinated contrast or by *computed tomography* (CT) with water-soluble contrast. The use of a non-resorbable iodinated dye for the myelogram allows follow-up films to be obtained conveniently without the need for repeated injections of dye, but the thick dye does not always pass an obstructing lesion, so that multiple procedures are sometimes necessary to assess different sites. Use of a water-soluble dye (metrizamide) plus CT may provide better definition of an obstructing lesion. If myelography is performed, a sample of cerebrospinal fluid should be obtained at the time of lumbar puncture and sent for cytology, cell count, and determination of protein and glucose levels.

Treatment. *High-dose corticosteroids* (e.g., 4 mg of dexamethasone every 6 hours) and *radiation therapy* are the mainstays of treatment, with *surgical decompression* indicated when neurologic function deteriorates rapidly. Patients with myeloma, lymphoma, or small-cell cancers respond well to irradiation. Chemotherapy is worth considering in those with multifocal obstructing disease. The prognosis depends on the extent of neurologic damage at the time of presentation. Patients who are ambulatory have a 60% to 80% chance of leaving the hospital able to walk; those with paraplegia have less than a 20% chance of regaining their ability to walk.

Meningeal Carcinomatosis. Diffuse seeding of the meninges with malignant cells is a serious complication of a number of solid tumors (lymphoma, melanoma, cancers of breast, lung, and stomach) and leukemias. Even if true cord compression is not present, the entire neuraxis may become involved, with the development of meningeal, cranial nerve, and root symptoms. The diagnosis is confirmed by lumbar puncture, which typically reveals malignant cells in the cerebrospinal fluid. Corticosteroids, irradiation, and intrathecal administration of cytotoxic agents are the treatment modalities of choice.

Cardiac Tamponade

Life-threatening tamponade may arise as a complication of malignancy, either indolently or rapidly, depending on the progression of the underlying tumor. Compression may be caused by tumorous encasement, malignant effusion, or scarring from radiation-induced pericarditis. Cancers associated with tamponade include tumors of the breast and lung, lymphoma, leukemia, and melanoma. In some instances, symptoms and signs of pericarditis (see Chapter 20) precede those of tamponade. The presence of *pulsus paradoxus* strongly suggests significant tamponade. Unexplained elevation of neck veins, narrowed pulse pressure, inspiratory distention of neck veins, and a pericardial friction rub should raise suspicion. Unfortunately, a pericardial friction rub is often absent in cases of tamponade caused by a malignant pericardial effusion. The usual accompanying symptoms (dyspnea, weakness, chest discomfort, cough) are nonspecific. More definitive diagnosis is best made by *cardiac ultrasonography*, the most sensitive and specific noninvasive test for documenting the problem and its physiologic significance.

A strong clinical suspicion of tamponade necessitates urgent hospitalization for prompt sonography and cardiac consultation. Sometimes a right-sided heart catheterization is performed when the degree of tamponade is unclear or the diagnosis is still questionable. *Pericardiocentesis* is the treatment of choice for urgent tamponade and may also yield positive cytology.

Hypercoagulability

A number of the natural inhibitors of clotting, many of which are endothelial in origin (protein C, protein S, tissue plasminogen factor, antithrombin III), are disrupted directly by tumor invasion or indirectly by substances elaborated by cancers. Patients with adenocarcinomas appear particularly susceptible to recurrent or migratory *thrombophlebitis* or even thrombotic arterial occlusions. A more disseminated consumption coagulopathy (*disseminated intravascular coagulation*, or DIC) sometimes develops and can present acutely as a generalized bleeding diathesis. Acute DIC is a true medical emergency. Suggestive laboratory findings include prolongations in the prothrombin time, partial thromboplastin time, and thrombin time, a low platelet count, and elevated concentrations of fibrin split products. The peripheral smear shows a microangiopathic picture (schistocytes). Chronic DIC is more subtle in presentation, with thrombotic end-organ damage and thrombosis being the principal manifestations. Acute DIC requires immediate hospitalization to stop the bleeding. Platelet and plasma transfusions are given to replace those blood elements that have been consumed. More definitive therapy requires treatment of the underlying malignancy.

Superior Vena Cava Syndrome

Obstruction of the superior vena cava is usually caused by extrinsic compression. The majority of cases are associated with bronchogenic carcinoma (especially small-cell carcinoma), lymphoma, and metastatic disease. The earliest manifestation is asymptomatic, unexplained *distention of the neck veins*. Late signs include swelling of the face, neck, and upper extremities, plethora, shortness of breath, and persistent headache. Although the condition is rarely fatal, increased intracranial pressure and thrombosis leading to neurologic deficits may ensue. The clinical diagnosis is reinforced by the finding of a mass on chest radiography in the right superior mediastinum or hilar area. Venography and other flow studies are unnecessary in most instances.

At one time, it was considered essential to treat the mass immediately with emergency *radiotherapy*. Now, the view is one of *urgency* rather than emergency. The first task is to consider whether a *tissue diagnosis* should be obtained before radiotherapy is instituted (see Chapter 44), as a host of tumors with different degrees of radiosensitivity may be responsible for the condition. Although many malignancies respond within 1 week to radiation, some may respond better to chemotherapy, and occasionally a nonmalignant process that would not benefit from radiation is the cause (e.g., tuberculous adenopathy, substernal goiter). When a tissue diagnosis will alter therapy, invasive study to obtain tissue should proceed. If a small-cell carcinoma or lymphoma is found, *chemotherapy* might be placed ahead of radiation as the treatment of choice (see Chapters 53 and 84).

Optimal therapy depends on the underlying diagnosis, prior treatment, and overall clinical status of the patient. Diuretics and corticosteroids can occasionally diminish local symptoms, but the effect is transient, and these agents are no substitute for more definitive therapy. The use of heparin provides no benefit. The occurrence of superior vena cava syndrome does not worsen the prognosis (if adjusted for stage of disease), particularly in cases of small-cell lung cancer.

Hypercalcemia

Hypercalcemia is a accompaniment of advanced carcinomas with extensive *lytic bony involvement* (breast cancer, myeloma, hematologic malignancies) and also a complication of epidermoid cancers (renal cell, ovarian, bladder, head and neck, and epidermoid and squamous cell lung cancers) with little or no bony metastasis. In the latter case, hypercalcemia has been linked to tumor elaboration of a protein with some parathyroid hormone–like activity (*parathyroid hormone–related protein*, or PTHRP). Cancers that invade bone and trigger a blastic response (e.g., prostate, oat cell cancers) are rarely associated with hypercalcemia.

Monitoring the serum calcium level provides the simplest means of early detection. Initially, the patient is asymptomatic. Later, such nonspecific symptoms as weakness, fatigue, lethargy, nausea, and constipation ensue. If the hypercalcemia progresses, it leads to an osmotic diuresis manifested by thirst and polyuria. The electrocardiogram may undergo change, with prolongation of the PR interval, shortening of the QT interval, and widening of the T wave. Dysrhythmias become a risk at very high calcium levels. Calcium potentiates the effects of digitalis and can trigger digitalis toxicity.

Hospitalization is needed if one decides to treat the hypercalcemia. (When it occurs in the setting of terminal illness, therapy may not be indicated.) One begins vigorous rehydration with *IV saline solution*, followed by *furosemide* to accelerate saline diuresis. *Calcitonin* also rapidly reduces serum calcium levels, but daily injections are required, and tachyphylaxis may be induced. *Corticosteroids* are useful for acute–subacute management, especially in cases of myeloma, lymphoma, and metastatic breast cancer. Long-term control can be achieved with the use of *bisphosphonates*; second-generation agents (e.g., *pamidronate*) are more effective than first-generation drugs (e.g., *etidronate*). Treatment of the underlying tumor remains the most definitive measure. Even with control of hypercalcemia and relief of symptoms, prognosis is poor and life expectancy limited.

Fever in the Setting of Neutropenia

Infection ranks as the leading cause of death in patients with leukemia and the cause of death in half of those with lymphoma and solid tumors.

Malnutrition, immune dysfunction, mechanical compromise, and a lowered neutrophil count (mostly caused by cytotoxic therapy) all contribute to the high risk of mortality from infection. Neutropenia is defined in cancer patients as granulocyte counts of less than 500/mL, the minimum needed to counter infection. Prophylactic therapy with *granulocyte colony-stimulating factor* (G-CSF) is being used to prevent neutropenia and lower the attendant risk of infection, but G-CSF is not effective as a treatment for febrile neutropenia.

Patients in whom fever develops during periods of neutropenia should be considered infected until proven otherwise. The majority of neutropenic cancer patients with fever will have a bacterial infection (often caused by a gram-negative organism). The possibility of viral, fungal, or parasitic infection is increased in patients who have leukemia or who are on long-term steroid therapy or prolonged broad-spectrum antibiotic coverage.

Often, neutropenic patients lack the usual signs of inflammation, which makes it hard to determine the site of infection at the time of presentation. Bacteremia without an identifiable primary site and pneumonitis lead the list of presentations. Onset of fever in the neutropenic patient is an indication for *prompt hospitalization*, regardless of whether or not any additional signs of infection are present. The mortality in such patients ranges from 18% to 40% within the first 48 hours. Outpatient management is not appropriate.

Once the patient is admitted, cultures of urine, sputum, and blood samples will be needed, as will samples of material from any suspected site (e.g., cerebrospinal fluid). In the absence of an identified pathogen, broad-spectrum antibiotic therapy is initiated, often with a *third-generation cephalosporin* (e.g., *ceftazidime*) or a *semisynthetic penicillin* (e.g., *imipenem*); an *aminoglycoside* is added when *Pseudomonas* infection is a concern. The short-term prognosis for patients treated early and aggressively is good. With the aggressive use of antibiotics, 60% to 90% of neutropenic, febrile cancer patients will recover from their infection.

Malignant Effusions

Some malignant effusions can be life-threatening (e.g., those in the pericardium; see above). Others are an important source of discomfort and disability.

Malignant ascites can lead to marked abdominal distention and respiratory compromise; treatment is supportive in most instances because the finding is a sign of end-stage disease. No randomized trials have compared treatment options, which range from peritoneal–venous shunt to intermittent drainage to medical management. Also largely unknown is the benefit of intracavitary versus systemic antitumor therapy. A wide range of agents have been tried intraperitoneally, but results are modest at best. Although peritoneal–venous shunting was at first applied with enthusiasm, an increased recognition of its risks (infection, DIC, venous thrombosis) and disappointing performance (frequent shunt clogging and failure) have limited its application. Only a small subset of patients (life expectancy longer than 3 months; nonloculated, nonbloody, viscous ascitic fluid; uncomfortably rapid reaccumulation of fluid despite repeated paracentesis and medical therapy) should be considered for shunting (see Chapter 91).

Malignant pleural effusions resulting from pleural implants or lymphatic obstruction can impair respiration. Lung, breast, and ovarian cancers are important causes of pleural implants; lymphomas lead to lymphatic obstruction. The optimal therapy is systemic treatment of the underlying malignancy. Repeated thoracentesis is ineffective and associated with considerable morbidity. Definitive local therapy requires placement of an indwelling chest tube for several days to allow thorough drainage and closure of the third space. Instillation of a sclerosing agent (e.g., tetracycline) after drainage promotes the scarring process and helps to limit reaccumulation of exudate.

Thrombocytopenia and Bleeding

(See Chapter 81.)

PARANEOPLASTIC SYNDROMES

Ectopic Hormone Syndromes

Small-cell (oat cell) carcinoma of the lung is the archetypal tumor capable of ectopic hormone production. A variety of other tumors may behave in similar fashion. One or more polypeptides may issue forth from the tumor and lead to such complications as Cushing's syndrome and inappropriate secretion of antidiuretic hormone (ADH).

Cushing's Syndrome develops in approximately 5% of patients with small-cell carcinoma of the lung because of the ectopic production of *adrenocorticotropic hormone* (ACTH), although some degree of ectopic ACTH synthesis may take place in as many as 80% of patients with the tumor. The clinical syndrome can be subtle and is usually not manifested by the typical cushingoid appearance; rather, it is characterized by *increased pigmentation* and metabolic and immunosuppressive effects, such as severe, recalcitrant *hypokalemia* and *impaired resistance* to infection. The hypokalemia requires extraordinary doses of supplemental potassium and the use of spironolactone. Serum and urinary ketosteroids are especially abundant, with some patients demonstrating virilization. Metabolic inhibitors of adrenal hormone synthesis (metyrapone, mitotane, amino-glutethimide) have been tried; success has been variable. The prognosis is very poor; median survival is less than 2 months.

Syndrome of Inappropriate Secretion of Antidiuretic Hormone is not unique to cancers, but small-cell carcinomas (about 10% of cases) and a host of other cancers are capable of elaborating a polypeptide with ADH activity. The earliest manifestations are *hyponatremia* and renal sodium wasting. *Urine osmolality is inappropriately elevated.* If the serum sodium falls to very low levels, confusion and disorientation may ensue. Treatment includes the use of *lithium carbonate* or *demeclocycline*, two agents that counter the action of ADH. A *restricted intake of free water* also helps to restore the serum sodium level. Infusions of hypertonic saline solution are to be avoided because these patients, although not edematous, tend to be volume-overloaded. However, diuretics are contraindicated because of sodium depletion. Inappropriate secretion of ADH is rapidly reversible with effective *treatment of the underlying tumor*.

Hypercalcemia associated with epidermoid cancers is, as noted above, caused by the ectopic production of PTHRP, a protein with *parathyroid hormone–like activity*. Unlike the hypercalcemia of osteolytic disease, the hypercalcemia associated with epidermoid cancers is characterized by elevations in urinary cyclic adenosine monophosphate and serum PTHRP. Because symptoms may not develop until the serum calcium becomes markedly elevated, routine monitoring of the serum calcium is the best means of early detection and is worthwhile in patients with tumors that frequently lead to this complication (squamous cell cancers of the head, neck, and lung; ovarian cancer; bladder cancer; hypernephroma). The diagnosis requires a high index of suspicion and direct testing for PTHRP; the protein is too different structurally from parathyroid hormone (PTH) to be detected by standard assays for PTH. Symptomatic relief can be achieved acutely by lowering the serum calcium (see above and Chapter 96). Treatment of the underlying cancer is more definitive.

Hyperthyroidism and Acute Thyrotoxicosis have resulted from ectopic production of chorionic gonadotropin (which functions like thyroid-stimulating hormone). Choriocarcinomas are the main source of the overproduction. Patients can present with all the typical hypermetabolic manifestations of thyrotoxicosis. *β*-Blockers are only modestly effective; primary treatment must be directed at the tumor.

Others. The ectopic production of *human chorionic gonadotropin* by testicular and lung cancers is sometimes sufficient to cause *gynecomastia*. *Fasting hypoglycemia* is a classic manifestation of insulinoma and a rare complication of sarcoma.

Immunologically Mediated Paraneoplastic Syndromes

A series of syndromes, mostly neurologic in nature, have been linked to aberrations in immune function. The precise identification of the mediator or immune complex has not been possible in all instances; at times, the link to an immune mechanism is merely speculative.

Myasthenic (Eaton-Lambert) Syndrome occurs most commonly in patients with small-cell carcinoma of the lung and characteristically results in *proximal muscle weakness* of the limbs. Its electromyographic pattern is distinct from that of true myasthenia, being characterized by facilitation and an increasing evoked muscle potential. Clinical management includes the administration of *guanidine*; the anticholinesterases used to treat myasthenia do not work.

Subacute Cerebellar Degeneration is another remote neurologic syndrome, characterized by injury to the Purkinje cells of the cerebellum. Ataxia, dysarthria, dysphagia, and even dementia may comprise the clinical picture. It has been associated most commonly with small-cell carcinoma of the lung and with ovarian and breast cancers.

Peripheral Neuropathy is the most common form of neurologic deficit in cancer. The mechanism(s) are poorly defined but likely to be multifactorial. The most typical is a symmetric sensory neuropathy seen in patients with advanced malignant disease. Motor and mixed sensory and motor neuropathies have also been described.

Paraneoplastic Syndromes of Unknown Etiology

A host of other purportedly paraneoplastic syndromes have been described, linked to malignancy by the fact that symptoms recede with effective treatment of the underlying tumor. A tumor secretory product or other mechanism has not yet been identified.

Hypertrophic Pulmonary Osteoarthropathy presents with the findings of digital clubbing and tenderness along the distal long bones. Most commonly, the syndrome occurs in the setting of primary or metastatic lung tumors. Radiography of the long bones shows an elevated periosteum, and radionuclide scanning demonstrates a distinctive pattern of increased uptake along the cortical margins. The exquisite pain accompanying these changes is relieved by removal of the tumor. The mechanism of the syndrome remains unknown.

Hyperpyrexia and Tumor-related Fever have been observed in patients with hepatic metastases, typically from colon cancer, and also as a manifestation of the "B" syndrome associated with Hodgkin's disease. The release of pyrogens from tumor has been proposed as the cause of fever, but other possibilities include the inability to detoxify endogenous endotoxin and an alteration in the metabolism of fever-producing steroids. The fever can be controlled with the administration of *NSAIDs*, which can also serve as a diagnostic test for the condition.

Nephrotic Syndrome. In some patients with Hodgkin's disease, massive edema with proteinuria and hypoalbuminemia develops. The renal lesion appears as an accumulation of immune complexes along the basement membrane. The nature of the antigen is unknown. The problem does not respond to steroid therapy but does regress with control of the malignancy.

Cachexia. (See Chapter 91.)

Cutaneous Paraneoplastic Syndromes

Cutaneous paraneoplastic syndromes are quite rare, but they are important to recognize as clues to the presence of internal malignancy. They may be a consequence of hormone secretion, such as the hyperpigmentation or *melanosis* associated with ACTH-producing tumors or the *necrotizing erythema* seen with glucagon-secreting malignancies of the pancreas. The proliferation of *seborrheic keratoses* can be a sign of internal malignancy; *acanthosis nigricans* or freckling and hyperpigmentation in the axillary folds suggest neurofibromatosis and intestinal cancer. *Acquired ichthyosis* is associated with lymphomas and several other tumors.

A.H.G.

ANNOTATED BIBLIOGRAPHY

Abrahm JL. Management of pain and spinal cord compression in patients with advanced cancer. Ann Intern Med 1999;131:37. (*A thoughtful, case-based discussion.*)

Ahmann FR. A reassessment of the clinical implications of the superior vena cava syndrome. J Clin Oncol 1984;2:961. (*Argues that taking the time and effort to make a tissue diagnosis helps to select treatment properly.*)

Baker WF Jr. Clinical aspects of disseminated intravascular coagulation. Semin Thromb Hemost 1989;15:1. (*A comprehensive review that includes a discussion of DIC in cancer.*)

Burtis WJ, Brady TG, Orloff JJ, et al. Immunochemical characterization of circulating parathyroid hormone–related protein in patients with humoral hypercalcemia of cancer. N Engl J Med 1990;322:1106. (*Identifies PTHRP and links it convincingly to humoral hypercalcemia.*)

Byrne TN. Spinal cord compression from epidural metastases. N Engl J Med 1992;327:614. (*One of the best reviews of the subject.*)

Callahan JA, Seward JB, Nishimura RA, et al. Two-dimensional echocardiographically guided pericardiocentesis. Am J Cardiol 1985;55:476. (*Ultrasonographic technique useful for diagnosis and treatment.*)

Chang JC, Gross HM. Utility of naproxen in the differential diagnosis of fever of undetermined origin in patients with cancer. Am J Med 1984;76:597. (*Found to be remarkably distinguishing, although size of sample very small.*)

Gucalp R, Ritch P, Wiernik PH, et al. Comparative study of pamidronate disodium and etidronate disodium in the treatment of cancer-related hypercalcemia. J Clin Oncol 1992;10:134. (*The second-generation bisphosphonate pamidronate was superior.*)

Hainsworth JD, Workman R, Greco A. Management of the syndrome of inappropriate antidiuretic hormone secretion in small-cell lung cancer. Cancer 1983;51:161. (*Antitumor chemotherapy resulted in resolution of the syndrome of inappropriate secretion of ADH.*)

Martinez-Lavin M, Matucci-Cerinic M, Jajic I, et al. Hypertrophic osteoarthropathy: consensus conference on its definition, classification, assessment, and diagnostic criteria. J Rheumatol 1993; 20:1386. (*Comprehensive consideration of the condition.*)

Nussbaum SR, Younger J, VanderPol CJ, et al. Single-dose intravenous therapy with pamidronate for the treatment of hypercalcemia of malignancy. Am J Med 1993;95:297. (*Evidence for efficacy of second-generation bisphosphonates.*)

Portenoy RK, Lipton RB, Foley KM. Back pain in the cancer patient: an algorithm for evaluation and management. Neurology 1987;37:134. (*Emphasizes the importance of a high index of suspicion for spinal metastasis and cord compression.*)

Posner PB. Paraneoplastic syndromes. Neurol Clin 1991;9:919. (*Excellent review by a leading authority.*)

Ralston SH, Gallacher SJ, Patel U, et al. Cancer-associated hypercalcemia: morbidity and mortality. Ann Intern Med 1990;112:499. (*Prognosis poor even if corrected, but morbidity can be reduced.*)

Sarpel S, Sarpel C, Yu E, et al. Early diagnosis of spinal-epidural metastasis by magnetic resonance imaging. Cancer 1987; 59:1112. (*Enhanced capacity for detection of early lesions.*)

Wilkes JB, Fidios P, Vaickur L, et al. Malignancy-related pericardial effusion: 127 cases from Roswell Park Cancer Institute. Cancer 1995;76:1377. (*Large series providing details of presentation, clinical course, and treatment.*)

Worschmidt F, Bunemann H, Geilmann HP, et al. Small-cell lung cancer with and without superior vena cava syndrome: a multivariate analysis of prognostic factors in 408 cases. Int J Radiol Oncol Biol Phys 1995;33:77. (*Superior vena cava syndrome actually associated with a favorable prognosis.*)

Wysolmerski JJ, Broadus AE. Hypercalemia of malignancy: the central role of parathyroid hormone–related protein. Annu Rev Med 1994;45:189. (*Review of the causes of hypercalemia and the important role of PTHRPs.*)

7

Endocrinologic Problems

93
Screening for Diabetes Mellitus

Diabetes is, after obesity and thyroid disease, the most common metabolic disorder seen by the primary care physician. Patients' concerns about the possible need for insulin injections and about such well-known complications as blindness, kidney disease, premature vascular disease, and impotence make diabetes one of the most feared diagnoses. Detection campaigns and advertising have further heightened public awareness. Diabetes screening is commonly requested by patients, even in the absence of symptoms or risk factors. There is no question that treatment effectively reduces symptoms associated with the metabolic derangements induced by diabetes. Results of the Diabetes Control and Complications Trial (DCCT) have definitively answered long-standing questions about the reduction in complication rates that can be achieved with intensive efforts to control glucose level, at least for type 1 disease. Less definitive but consistent results are also available for type 2 disease from the U.K. Prospective Diabetes Study Group. Nevertheless, the benefits of treatment initiated in the asymptomatic phase have not been demonstrated. Furthermore, labeling a patient "diabetic" on the basis of results of a nonspecific screening test may be harmful. Although some advise screening for high-risk groups, uncertainty about the natural history of diabetes and its complications precludes making definitive recommendations.

EPIDEMIOLOGY AND RISK FACTORS

Diabetes mellitus is heterogeneous. The destruction of β-cells in the islets of Langerhans through a number of pathophysiologic mechanisms is responsible for the clinical syndrome of type 1 mellitus, previously referred to as *insulin-dependent diabetes* (IDDM). The etiology and pathogenesis of type 2 diabetes, previously called *non–insulin-dependent diabetes mellitus* (NIDDM), may be even more heterogeneous; multiple lesions include a blunted β-cell response to glucose, a defect at the insulin receptor, and a defect in hepatic uptake of glucose that contributes to glucose intolerance. Depending on the diagnostic criteria used, the prevalence of all types of diabetes in the United States is between 3% and 7%; type 2 diabetes is nearly 10 times more common than type 1 diabetes.

Type 1 Diabetes is generally manifested in childhood or early adulthood. Only 20% of patients with type 1 diabetes have a first-degree relative with diabetes. However, a predisposition to type 1 diabetes, apparently mediated through the immune system, is inherited. This pathologic predisposition to autoimmune destruction of the β-cells has been linked to the presence of certain HLA antigens, some of which are also associated with other autoimmune diseases, including Hashimoto's thyroiditis and Addison's disease. Conversely, other HLA antigens seem to be associated with protection against diabetes. Overall, the risk for eventual development of diabetes in a sibling of a patient with type 1 disease is between 3% and 6%. However, the risk for siblings can be defined by comparing HLA antigens with those of the index case. Although siblings who are HLA-identical to the diabetic patient face a risk for diabetes that is 25 times greater than that of the general population, the relative risk for those who share no antigens or are haplo-identical is only two or three times greater. The role of autoimmune destruction of β-cells in many patients with type 1 diabetes is attested to by the presence of islet cell antibodies in a large proportion of newly diagnosed cases. Islet cell antibodies can also be detected in nondiabetic relatives of patients with type 1 disease.

At least in some cases, islet cell destruction is the result of viral infection, which perhaps initiates the autoimmune response. coxsackieviruses, particularly coxsackievirus B4, have been most strongly implicated. Mumps virus, cytomegalovirus, Epstein-Barr virus, and hepatitis viruses have also been associated with type 1 diabetes. The role of viral infection has been linked to a seasonal variation in the incidence of type 1 disease and has raised questions about a relationship between socioeconomic status and risk for type 1 diabetes, but the evidence is equivocal.

Type 2 Diabetes has a much stronger *genetic component* than does type 1 diabetes; concordance in identical twins is greater than 90%. The genetic link is not related to HLA antigens, and islet cell antigens are no more prevalent than in the general population.

The overwhelming risk factor for type 2 diabetes is overnutrition and resulting *obesity*. Eighty percent of diabetic adults are obese or have a history of obesity. Among adults who are at least 25% over their ideal body weight, one of every five has elevated fasting blood sugar levels, and three of every five have abnormal results on glucose tolerance tests. Obesity increases insulin levels and decreases the concentration of insulin receptors in tissue, including skeletal muscle and fat. The relationship between the concentration of insulin receptors and glucose tolerance is modified, however, by intracellular sequences following insulin binding that are poorly understood. Exercise increases the concentration of insulin receptors, and a *sedentary life-style* is associated with glucose intolerance. Regular exercise has been shown to be associated with a decreased incidence of type 2 diabetes after adjustments for body mass index.

Steroids reduce receptor affinity for insulin, as do uremia and hepatic failure. Other drugs can impair glucose tolerance by further diminishing the sluggish response of β-cells to glucose. These include *thiazide* diuretics, β-adrenergic blockers, α-adrenergic stimulants, and phenytoin. Prostaglandin inhibitors, including indomethacin and salicylate, may increase β-cell release of insulin.

Persons with *impaired glucose tolerance* are also at greater risk for frank type 2 diabetes (see below). Although long-term follow-up studies indicate that as many as half of those with impaired glucose tolerance will have normal glucose tolerance test results 5 to 10 years later, somewhere between 1% and 5% of these patients become diabetic each year.

In approximately 3% of previously euglycemic women, glucose intolerance develops during pregnancy. The fetal hyperglycemia and hyperinsulinemia that accompany maternal diabetes result in increased neonatal morbidity and mortality and the increased birth weight common in infants of diabetic mothers. *Gestational diabetes* in the mother resolves after delivery in 90% of cases, but type 2 diabetes eventually develops in more than half of these women.

NATURAL HISTORY OF DIABETES AND EFFECTIVENESS OF THERAPY

The natural history of diabetes mellitus has been difficult to define because the condition is so heterogeneous. This problem has historically been confounded by studies that have defined diabetes according to varying degrees of glucose intolerance.

The natural history of asymptomatic impaired glucose intolerance is variable; only 15% to 30% of these patients progress to frank diabetes during 10 to 15 years. Patients with impaired glucose tolerance are at increased risk for the development of the macrovascular complications that result from accelerated atherogenesis. However, unless glucose intolerance progresses to frank diabetes, characteristic diabetic microangiopathy does not develop in these patients.

The *asymptomatic detectable period* seems to be much shorter for type 1 diabetes than it is for type 2 diabetes. Despite some evidence for a longer asymptomatic period than was previously estimated, the markedly lower prevalence of asymptomatic type 1 diabetes, in comparison with type 2 disease, makes such patients a very small target for screening efforts.

The incidence of *vascular* and *neurologic complications* clearly tends to increase with the duration of clinical diabetes. However, some long-term studies of patients followed for as long as 40 years have indicated that clinical evidence of mi-crovascular disease, atherosclerosis, or neuropathy may occur in only 20% to 40% of type 1 patients.

The increased risk for vascular and neurologic complications is reflected in the relative mortality rates of diabetics. The relative risk for death of diabetic patients, in comparison with that of age-matched nondiabetic persons, increases with the duration of known disease. In one study of patients followed for up to 25 years, the increase in mortality risk with increased duration was greater after age 40 and among women. *Coronary artery disease* is the most common cause of death among diabetics. Autopsy studies indicate that coronary disease is two to three times more common among diabetics than in nondiabetics. Peripheral vascular disease is also very common among diabetics; clinical studies have indicated a prevalence of about 60%. Diabetics in the Framingham study were shown to be four to five times more likely to have *intermittent claudication* and two to three times more likely to suffer the morbid consequences of stroke than were nondiabetics. On the other hand, the presence of peripheral vascular disease in a nondiabetic person increases the risk for eventual development of NIDDM.

Retinopathy is the most common specific complication of diabetes. In general, the incidence of retinopathy increases with the duration of diabetes, regardless of age at onset. Prevalence ranges of 40% to 80% have been reported among patients with known diabetes lasting 20 to 30 years. In one study of patients whose diabetes began before age 30, nearly all had retinopathy 25 to 30 years later and about 50% had proliferative changes. Retinopathy was less prevalent among those whose diabetes began later in life and those not receiving insulin. Laser photocoagulation has been shown to decrease the progression of diabetic retinopathy. However, this does not provide a basis for recommending screening for diabetes; retinopathy that warrants treatment is very rare early in the course of disease. (Once diabetes is diagnosed, screening for retinopathy is indicated.)

Renal disease has been reported in 15% to 80% of diabetic patients at autopsy. Renal failure is the cause of death in 6% to 12% of diabetic patients. Prevalence estimates vary widely from study to study, but it is clear that the risk for glomerulosclerosis with clinically evident functional impairment increases dramatically with the duration of disease.

Although the *duration of glucose intolerance* and associated metabolic abnormalities can be related to many of the complications of diabetes, the variability of the natural history must be kept in mind. It has been argued that all complications, including specific microangiopathic changes, have been identified in patients without evident glucose intolerance. Whether or not the morbidity and mortality associated with the complications can be influenced by therapy is a matter of long-standing debate (see Chapter 102). The DCCT provided compelling evidence that rates of microvascular complications and other consequences of diabetes could be reduced with intensive efforts to control glucose levels among patients with type 1 diabetes. Intensive therapy was associated with an increased frequency of hypoglycemic episodes and considerable inconvenience and cost. Questions remain about whether these findings apply to patients with type 2 diabetes and about whether treatment during the asymptomatic period would improve outcomes.

Gestational diabetes is a special case. As noted, it occurs in 3% of pregnancies, although considerable variation is noted in different populations. It is associated with perinatal morbidity, including macrosomia and the associated increased risk for serious birth trauma and cesarean section. Evidence from observational studies and randomized trials supports the contention that identification of gestational diabetes, followed by management with diet, insulin, or both, can reduce the incidence of macrosomia and perhaps improve birth outcomes.

SCREENING AND DIAGNOSTIC TESTS

In 1979, the National Diabetes Data Group (NDDG) published criteria for the diagnosis of diabetes. In 1997, these criteria were updated by a committee of the American Diabetes Association. According to these revised criteria, at least one of the following conditions must be met to establish the diagnosis of diabetes in the nonpregnant adult:

1. Symptoms of diabetes plus a *casual glucose* concentration of 200 mg/dL (11.1 mmol/L) or more. Casual is defined as any time of day without regard to time since last meal. The classic symptoms of diabetes include polyuria, polydipsia, and unexplained weight loss.
2. A *fasting plasma glucose* concentration of 126 mg/dL (7.0 mmol/L) or more (fasting defined as no caloric intake for at least 8 hours).
3. A 2-hour postprandial level of 200 mg/dL or more during an oral glucose tolerance test, performed as described by the World Health Organization (glucose load equivalent to 75 g of anhydrous glucose dissolved in water).

To confirm a diagnosis of diabetes, any one of the criteria must also be met on a subsequent day. It is worth noting that capillary blood glucose levels are lower than plasma levels by approximately 10 mg/dL during fasting, but are equal to or higher than plasma levels after a glucose load.

In addition to defining these diagnostic criteria, which have since been widely accepted in the United States, the group suggested new designations for persons with glucose intolerance who do not meet the criteria for frank diabetes. The term impaired glucose tolerance is reserved for patients with a glucose tolerance between normal and that of frank diabetes (e.g., fasting plasma glucose from 110 to 125 mg/dL).

It should be remembered that any criteria for the diagnosis of diabetes based on glucose levels are, by necessity, arbitrary. The sensitivity and specificity of the tests will depend on the arbitrary levels chosen. At the time of their publication, the principal effect of the NDDG criteria, which require higher levels than were commonly used previously, was to increase the specificity of the criteria at the expense of sensitivity. This trade-off reflected the judgment that little benefit can be expected from aggressive identification and treatment of early or mild degrees of glucose intolerance, and that the label diabetes can engender substantial anxiety and morbidity. The recommendations made in 1997 increase sensitivity at the expense of specificity, reflecting an implicit judgment that more benefit than harm will result from identifying and labeling patients with less severe levels of glucose intolerance as diabetic.

Despite the widespread acceptance of these diagnostic tests, the indications for performing oral glucose tolerance tests and any blood glucose measurements to screen asymptomatic persons remain controversial. The American Diabetes Association advocates use of a fasting glucose level to screen for diabetes among people over age 45. They recommend earlier screening for those at higher risk for diabetes because of racial background, family history, obesity, or prior evidence of impaired glucose tolerance. However, no evidence from a prospective, randomized trial is available to support such recommendations. The U.S. Preventative Services Task Force has concluded that sufficient evidence for or against routine screening for diabetes in asymptomatic adults is lacking.

The detection of autoantibodies as predictors of type 1 diabetes among asymptomatic persons with a strong family history of type 1 disease has also received considerable attention. However, because no interventions have been proved to slow or prevent onset of disease, this approach is not recommended in the general population.

Screening for gestational diabetes is generally accomplished between 24 and 28 weeks of gestation by administering 50 g of glucose orally and measuring the glucose level 1 hour later. A level above 140 mg/dL would prompt further evaluation with an oral glucose tolerance test (see Chapter 102). This generally accepted policy is not supported by conclusive evidence from randomized trials; both the U.S. Preventative Services Task Force and the Canadian Task Force on the Periodic Health Examination have recommended neither for or against this practice. Recently, selective screening on the basis of age (over 35), body mass index, and race has been advocated.

Some have advocated the use of hemoglobin A_{1c} measurements to screen for and diagnose diabetes. However, in population-based studies, fasting glucose levels have been found to be more sensitive and more specific.

CONCLUSIONS AND RECOMMENDATIONS

- Diabetes mellitus is a common but heterogeneous condition. The most important risk factor for type 1 diabetes is a family history of diabetes in a twin, sibling, or parent. Family history is even more predictive for type 2 diabetes, but the most important risk factor is obesity. Persons with a history of gestational diabetes or with impaired glucose tolerance also are at risk for the development of frank diabetes.
- The natural history of diabetes and the incidence of complications is highly variable. The incidence of diabetic complications increases with duration of disease. Close control of glucose levels in patients with type 1 diabetes has been shown to reduce the incidence of microvascular diabetic complications, at the expense of increased rates of hypoglycemia and substantial inconvenience and cost. Consistent but less conclusive evidence exists for type 2 diabetes, but no effect on the macrovascular complications that confer much higher burdens of morbidity and mortality was noted. No evidence is available to indicate that therapy of asymptomatic, nonpregnant patients with diabetes or impaired glucose tolerance offers any benefit.
- Therefore, the routine measurement of blood glucose levels to screen asymptomatic, nonpregnant adults for diabetes is not recommended.

A.G.M.

ANNOTATED BIBLIOGRAPHY

Diabetes Control and Complications Trial Research Group. The effect of intensive treatment of diabetes on the development and progression of long-term complications in insulin-dependent diabetes mellitus. N Engl J Med 1993;329:977. (*Intensive therapy reduced retinopathy, proteinuria, and neuropathy in symptomatic patients.*)

Ellenberg M. Diabetic complications without manifest diabetes. JAMA 1963;183:926. (*Early review. Virtually any of the common "complications" can precede detectable abnormalities in carbohydrate metabolism.*)

Expert Committee on the Diagnosis and Classification of Diabetes Mellitus. Report of the Expert Committee on the Diagnosis and Classification of Diabetes Mellitus. Diabetes Care 1997;20:1183. (*Recommends revised criteria for diagnosis and screening.*)

Garcia MJ, McNamara PM, Gordan T, et al. Morbidity and mortality in diabetics in the Framingham populations. Diabetes 1974;23:105. (*Insulin-treated diabetic women have the greatest relative mortality. Increased mortality among diabetics is not entirely explained by associated obesity, hypertension, and hyperlipidemia.*)

Genuth SM, Houser HB, Carter JR, et al. Observations on the value of mass indiscriminate screening for diabetes mellitus based on a 5-year follow-up. Diabetes 1978;27:377. (*About 3 of nearly 2,000 patients with abnormal oral glucose tolerance test results had normal results 5 years later.*)

Harris MI, Hadden WC, Knowler WC, et al. Prevalence of diabetes and impaired glucose tolerance and plasma glucose levels in U.S. population ages 20 to 74 years. Diabetes 1987;36:523. (*Extrapolation of survey results provides a prevalence estimate of 6.6%—3.4% previously diagnosed and 3.2% undiagnosed.*)

Manson JE, Nathan DM, Krolewski AS, et al. A prospective study of exercise and incidence of diabetes among U.S. male physicians. JAMA 1992;268:63. (*Relative risk was 0.77 for those who exercised once a week and 0.58 for those who exercised five or more times weekly.*)

Nathan DM, Singer DE, Godine JE, et al. Retinopathy in older type II diabetics: association with glucose control. Diabetes 1986;35:797. (*Duration of diabetes and hemoglobin A_{1C} were major predictors of retinopathy among 185 patients with type 2 diabetes ages 55 to 75.*)

Naylor CD, Sermer M, Chen E, et al. Selective screening for gestational diabetes mellitus. N Engl J Med 1997;337:1591. (*Selecting women for screening based on age, race, and body mass index can reduce the number of screening tests by one third without a loss in sensitivity.*)

O'Sullivan JB, Mahan CM. Prospective study of 352 young patients with chemical diabetes. N Engl J Med 1968;278:1038. (*Only 32% of those with chemical diabetes by Fajans and Conn criteria progressed to overt diabetes within 10 years.*)

Paz-Guevara AT, Hsu T-H, White P. Juvenile diabetes mellitus after 40 years. Diabetes 1975;24:559. (*Insulin-induced hypoglycemia was the most common complication. The prevalence of complications was significant: visual impairment in 50%, nephropathy in 59%, neuropathy in 50%, peripheral vascular disease in 40%, and major cardiac complications in 20%.*)

Singer DE, Nathan DM, Fogel HA, et al. Screening for diabetic retinopathy. Ann Intern Med 1992;116:660. (*Reviews natural history of diabetic retinopathy and makes the case for screening among patients with diagnosed diabetes.*)

Singer DE, Samet JH, Coley CM, et al. Screening for diabetes mellitus. Ann Intern Med 1988;109:639. (*Well-reasoned analysis of the issues, with emphasis on evidence that supports screening for gestational diabetes.*)

University Group Diabetes Program. Effects of hypoglycemic agents on vascular complications in patients with adult-onset diabetes. VIII. Evaluation of insulin therapy: final report. Diabetes 1982;31[Suppl 5]:1. (*Only 15% of patients taking variable doses of insulin had poor control, compared with 34% and 45% of those treated with fixed doses and diet, respectively. However, complications were rare, and no significant differences were detected.*)

UK Prospective Diabetes Study Group. Intensive blood glucose control with sulphonylureas or insulin compared with conventional treatment and risk of complications in patients with type 2 diabetes. Lancet 1998;352:837. (*Intensive therapy reduced risk for microvascular complications by 25%, but no evident effect on macrovascular disease was noted.*)

94
Screening for Thyroid Cancer

Cancer of the thyroid is a relatively rare disease with a low mortality rate. Approximately 14,000 cases are diagnosed each year in the United States; the number of deaths caused by the tumor is about 1,000 annually—only 0.2% of cancer deaths. Nevertheless, this disease is of major significance for the primary physician because of its iatrogenic relationship to childhood irradiation of the head and neck. A high prevalence of thyroid cancer, diagnosed after a long latent or asymptomatic period, has repeatedly been documented among patients exposed to such irradiation. The appropriate approach to the evaluation and management of radiation-exposed patients remains a subject of debate.

EPIDEMIOLOGY AND RISK FACTORS

Generally, the incidence of thyroid cancer increases with age. This is particularly true of tumors with an anaplastic or follicular histopathologic pattern and of the medullary carcinomas derived from the parafollicular cells. The most common tumors, with a papillary histopathologic pattern, have a bimodal, age-specific incidence, peaking in the thirties and late in life. Thyroid tumors occur more than twice as frequently in women. In the United States, African-Americans seem to be at lower risk than others. Wide variations in thyroid cancer prevalence at autopsy have been reported internationally, from 3% to more than 10% in nonirradiated thyroids, with the highest rates reported in Japan. Approximately 20% of the rare medullary carcinomas, which comprise fewer than 10% of thyroid cancers, are familial.

The major identifiable risk factor for the development of thyroid cancer is a history of *external irradiation of the head and neck*. External irradiation was used as early as 1907 to shrink an enlarged thymus in infancy. During the 1920s and subsequently until the 1950s, it was used extensively to treat enlarged tonsils and adenoids, cervical adenitis, mastoiditis, sinusitis, hemangiomas, tinea capitis, and acne. Concern about ill effects began to mount in 1950 when a history of neck irradiation was noted in 9 of 28 cases of childhood thyroid cancer with a latency period of 5 or more years. Further documentation followed, and radiation to the neck was discontinued. In 1973, attention focused on the issue again when 40% of a series of adults with thyroid cancer were found to have a history of irradiation. Clearly, the latent period between exposure and the diagnosis of cancer could be measured in decades. It was also clear that the exposed population at risk was substantial—estimates ranged from 1 million to 2 million persons—and largely unidentifiable.

Successive reports focused on the risk among exposed persons. Large studies indicated that more than 25% had detectable thyroid abnormalities; the prevalence of cancer was estimated at 7% to 9%. These figures must, however, be considered in the light of information available regarding the prevalence of thyroid abnormalities, including carcinoma, in the general population.

At least one investigation has questioned the value of thyroid screening in persons with a history of radiation exposure based on the legitimate questions that can be raised about the effects of sampling bias and observer bias on the results of most studies. In a small, retrospective cohort study comparing irradiated persons with siblings or patient-selected controls, the investigators found no difference in the prevalence of malignant and nonmalignant thyroid abnormalities. This study has in turn been challenged, however, because of its own potential biases and limited power.

Preliminary evidence suggests that some radiation-exposed persons may be at greater risk than others. Radiation during infancy may be most carcinogenic, with cancer risk decreasing as age at the time of radiation increases. Although the threshold dose for cancer risk appears to be low, risk may be greatly increased for persons who received multiple treatments.

NATURAL HISTORY OF THYROID CANCER AND EFFECTIVENESS OF THERAPY

The prevalence of occult carcinoma of the thyroid is not well defined. Autopsy studies have indicated that the prevalence ranges from 5% to 13%. An often-quoted study showing an overall prevalence of 5.7% found the highest age-specific rates in the fifth and sixth decades.

A high prevalence of asymptomatic thyroid cancer is not surprising considering the benign clinical course of most thyroid tumors after diagnosis. Follow-up studies have determined that the probability of survival depends on the tissue type and age of the patient. For localized papillary carcinoma, survival approximates that of age-matched controls; in one large study, no deaths occurred among patients younger than 40 years of age during 10 to 15 years of follow-up. The course of follicular cancer is only slightly more aggressive. Anaplastic tumors, on the other hand, run a rapid clinical course to death.

The relatively high prevalence of occult thyroid cancer presumed to be present in general raises a number of questions about the significance of tumors found during the evaluation of patients with radiation exposure. It is worth noting that in the largest study, conducted at Michael Reese Hospital in Chicago, 47% of the tumors were incidental findings identified after surgery was recommended because of palpable or scan abnormalities. That is, 29 of 60 cancers were not found in or near the benign nodule that prompted surgery. No evidence indicates that tumors found in patients with past radiation exposure are more likely to result in morbidity or mortality than are occult tumors found in the general population. However, they do have a high frequency of recurrence.

SCREENING AND DIAGNOSTIC TESTS

The sensitivity of *history taking* in identifying persons at risk is not known. Many who were irradiated during early childhood may be unaware of their exposure. *Physical examination* of the thyroid gland is often difficult, and the palpable nodule is a nonspecific finding that can be found in 4% to 7% of the adult population. *Thyroid scan* is more sensitive in detecting thyroid abnormalities, but because it fails to distinguish between benign and malignant disease, it is even less specific. A number of studies indicate that physical examination itself becomes more sensitive after scanning has been performed and the physician is aware of scan results.

Large studies utilizing both multiple examinations and technetium (^{99m}Tc) scanning indicate that 60% of thyroid abnormalities (identified by either or both modalities) will be identified by palpation alone. Scanning alone will be more than 95% sensitive. However, palpable abnormalities appear to be more specific for cancer. In one study of patients with palpable nodules who ultimately underwent thyroidectomy, the prevalence of cancer was 34%; it was 19% among patients who went to surgery on the basis of scan abnormalities alone. Physical examination was nearly 80% sensitive in identifying thyroid glands containing cancers. Cancers found in glands with scan abnormalities alone were often incidental, unrelated to the scan abnormality.

The availability of high-resolution *ultrasonography* has increased our capacity to identify small thyroid nodules. Ultrasonography has been shown to be better than physical examination, isotope scanning, magnetic resonance imaging, and computed tomography in detecting nodules. However, no specific sonographic criteria distinguish between benign and malignant nodules. In one study, 14% of cystic thyroid lesions were cancers, compared with 23% of solid lesions.

Attempts to use measurements of serum thyroglobulin as a screening test for thyroid cancer have not been successful. Despite poor specificity, thyroglobulin abnormalities are disappointingly insensitive.

When abnormalities are detected on examination or on scan, additional diagnostic steps are indicated. The refinement of *fine-needle aspiration biopsy* with *cytologic examination* has made this the first-line diagnostic test in many centers (see Chapter 95).

In cases of questionable physical examination or scan findings, some physicians have suppressed the thyroid for 3 to 6 months in an effort to shrink normal thyroid tissue and thereby increase the sensitivity of the examination for autonomous nodules. Although this remains a reasonable approach when cancer risk is low, it must be kept in mind that regression following thyroid hormone suppression is neither perfectly sensitive nor highly specific for thyroid cancer. Cases have been reported of confirmed carcinomas that apparently responded to suppression therapy; only a minority of nodules that do not respond prove to be malignant.

On the basis of animal experiments, long-term thyroid suppression as prophylaxis for thyroid cancer has also been advocated for all patients with a history of exposure or, more selectively, those with questionable scan findings.

Patients with a familial risk for medullary thyroid cancer may be tested for an exaggerated increase in serum calcitonin levels in response to calcium or pentagastrin stimulation. Such a response is reasonably sensitive, but it is not specific for medullary thyroid cancer. High-resolution ultrasonography may play a role in the screening of these rather rare patients.

CONCLUSIONS AND RECOMMENDATIONS

- Childhood irradiation is an important risk factor for thyroid carcinoma, which may be diagnosed as long as 35 years after exposure.
- The prevalence of thyroid abnormalities among the estimated 1 to 2 million patients with a history of exposure is about 25%. The prevalence of thyroid cancer has been estimated to be 7% to 9%.
- The significance of occult thyroid cancer in exposed patients is not known. The prevalence of occult tumors in the general population appears to be a high.
- Identification of patients at risk is an important part of history taking.
- Patients at risk should be carefully examined yearly, or at least every 2 years.
- Needle biopsy may be preferred in cases in which a single nodule has been identified. Multiple examinations by experienced examiners may be necessary. Thyroid suppression may increase the sensitivity of thyroid palpation. The examination of patients with normal examination but abnormal scan findings should be repeated yearly.

A.G.M.

ANNOTATED BIBLIOGRAPHY

Davis NL, Gordon M, German E, et al. Clinical parameters predictive of malignancy of thyroid follicular neoplasms. Am J Surg 1991;161:567. (*Age above 50 years, nodule size larger than 3 cm, and history of neck irradiation were associated with a surgical diagnosis of cancer when needle aspiration biopsy findings were consistent with follicular neoplasm.*)

De los Santos ET, Keyhani-Rofagha S, Cunningham JJ, et al. Cystic thyroid nodules. The dilemma of malignant lesions. Arch Intern Med 1990;150:1422. (*Of 71 cystic lesions, 14% were malignant, compared with 23% of 150 solid lesions. Sensitivity and specificity of fine-needle aspiration cytology were 88% and 52%, respectively, for cystic lesions, and 100% and 55%, respectively, for solid lesions.*)

Friedman M, Toriumi DM, Mafee MF. Diagnostic imaging techniques in thyroid cancer. Am J Surg 1988;155:215. (*Argues that refinement of fine-needle aspiration cytology has made radionuclide scanning and other imaging studies second-line diagnostic tools for thyroid cancer.*)

Gagel RF, Tashjian AH, Cummings T, et al. The clinical outcome of prospective screening for multiple endocrine neoplasia type 2a. N Engl J Med 1988;318:478. (*Reports 86% disease-free survival in 22 patients followed for a mean of 11 years after being given a screening diagnosis of medullary thyroid carcinoma.*)

Gharib H, Goeller JR. Fine-needle aspiration biopsy of the thyroid: an appraisal. Ann Intern Med 1993;118:282. (*Advocates fine-needle aspiration as the first step in diagnosis.*)

Gonzalez-Villalpando C, Frohman LA, Bekerman C, et al. Scintigraphic thyroid abnormalities after radiation. Ann Intern Med 1982;97:55. (*Palpable and nonpalpable thyroid nodules were much more common among patients with prior radiation exposure than among controls.*)

McTiernan AM, Weiss NS, Daling JR. Incidence of thyroid cancer in women in relation to previous exposure to radiation therapy and history of thyroid disease. J Natl Cancer Inst 1984;73:575. (*Relative risk for exposed women was 16.5.*)

McTiernan AM, Weiss NS, Daling JR. Incidence of thyroid cancer in women in relation to reproductive and hormonal factors. Am J Epidemiol 1984;120:423. (*Despite the impact on the production of thyroid-stimulating hormone, pregnancy and use of exogenous estrogens had little or no effect on the risk for thyroid carcinoma in this case–control study.*)

Miki H, Inoue H, Komaki K, et al. Value of mass screening for thyroid cancer. World J Surg 1998;22:99. (*Only 36 cancers found among 18,619 screenees in Japan.*)

Negri E, Ron E, DalMaso L, et al. A pooled analysis of case–control studies of thyroid cancer. Cancer Causes Control 1999;10:143. (*Any associations between thyroid cancer and menstrual or reproductive factors are weak.*)

Refetoff S, Lever EG. The value of serum thyroglobulin measurement in clinical practice. JAMA 1983;250:2352. (*A review. No value in cancer screening.*)

Sampson RJ, Woolner LB, Bahn RC, et al. Occult thyroid carcinoma in Olmstead County, Minnesota: prevalence of autopsy compared with that in Hiroshima and Nagasaki, Japan. Cancer 1974;34:2072. (*Prevalence of 5.6% among 157 autopsies of patients with clinically occult thyroid cancer. Highest age-specific prevalence between 40 and 60 years.*)

Schneider AB, Favus MJ, Stachura ME. Plasma thyroglobulin in detecting thyroid carcinoma after childhood head and neck irradiation. Ann Intern Med 1977;86:29. (*Thyroglobulin levels not found to be very useful.*)

Schneider AB, Recant W, Pinsky SM. Radiation-induced thyroid carcinoma. Ann Intern Med 1986;105:405. (*Describes the clinical course of Michael Reese cohort at mean follow-up of 10 years; a high frequency of recurrent disease noted. Small nodules managed conservatively.*)

VanHerle AJ, Rich P, Ljung BE, et al. The thyroid nodule. Ann Intern Med 1982;96:221. (*An extensive review of the diagnostic value of fine-needle aspiration, thyroid scanning, and ultrasonography, including an analysis of alternative sequencing strategies; fine-needle aspiration followed by scan in patients with cytologically suspect lesions is recommended.*)

Woolner LB, Beahrs OH, Black BM, et al. Classification and prognosis of thyroid carcinoma: a study of 885 cases observed in a 30-year period. Am J Surg 1961;102:354. (*Noninvasive disease without significant morbidity or mortality.*)

95
Evaluation of Thyroid Nodules

Thyroid nodules are an extremely common phenomenon clinically, radiographically, and histologically. A palpable thyroid nodule can be detected in 4% to 7% of the adult population (10 to 20 million people in the United States alone). The prevalence of nodules in autopsy series approaches 50%, a figure that is approximated by patients undergoing modern high-resolution, real-time ultrasonography of the thyroid. The incidence of thyroid nodules increases with age and neck irradiation; it is six to nine times more common in women than in men.

The principal objective in evaluating thyroid nodules is to differentiate malignant from benign lesions. About 70% of nodules subjected to fine-needle biopsy prove to be benign, and 4% malignant; in the remainder, the cytologic findings are either inadequate or indeterminate. Additional tasks are to determine the functional status of a nodule and assess any adverse effect on neighboring structures.

Because of the high frequency and potential importance of thyroid nodules, the primary care physician must be able to coordinate a cost-effective evaluation; to that end, familiarity with the indications for and utilities of scanning, ultrasonography, and fine-needle aspiration is necessary. In addition, an understanding of the respective roles of surgery, suppressive therapy, and watchful waiting facilitate the formulation of an appropriate program of symptomatic management.

PATHOPHYSIOLOGY AND CLINICAL PRESENTATION

Thyroid nodules may be single or multiple, with or without underlying disturbances of hormonal homeostasis. A solitary nodule is usually more worrisome because it may represent a malignancy, although on occasion a multinodular gland may harbor a cancer. Benign and malignant thyroid nodules are usually asymptomatic and discovered incidentally by the patient or examining physician. Large nodules may cause a cosmetic problem or compress an adjacent structure. The nodules are usually painless unless rapid growth, inflammation, or hemorrhage occurs and produces significant discomfort.

Solitary Nodule

Solitary thyroid nodules represent benign adenomas, carcinomas, or multinodular conditions in which only a single nodule is palpable.

Benign Adenomas account for most nonmalignant truly solitary nodules. The majority are designated as *follicular* and have a true capsule; the remainder are labeled *colloid* or *adenomatous nodules* and are not well encapsulated. Both behave similarly. Growth is typically slow, extending over many years. Follicular adenomas rarely become large enough to encroach on the trachea or esophagus. Thyroid-stimulating hormone (TSH) receptors are present in most, making them hormonally responsive. Most do not produce much thyroid hormone, and their limited radioiodine uptake on scan sometimes gives the appearance of a "cold" nodule. Benign adenomas that outgrow their blood supply may undergo necrosis, degenerate, become filled with fluid, and appear on ultrasonography as nodules with solid and cystic elements. Adenomas make up a significant proportion of such "cystic" lesions. A few follicular adenomas produce such large quantities of thyroid hormone that the patient presents with thyrotoxicosis (see Chapter 103). This is particularly true of so-called *"toxic" adenomas* exceeding 3 cm in diameter. They function autonomously, suppress TSH (which renders the rest of the gland atrophic), and appear as *"hot" nodules* on thyroid scan. Patients with a smaller hot nodule may remain euthyroid, although enough thyroid hormone is produced to suppress the rest of the gland and render it atrophic.

Thyroid Carcinomas are uncommon; the current incidence is 2.5/100,000 persons annually, although it is higher in areas with radiation exposure. They are more frequent in women than in men. A major risk factor is prior head or neck irradiation. On radioiodine scan, most thyroid carcinomas present as *"cold" nodules*, failing to take up iodine, although on technetium scan a rare malignant nodule will take up the radionuclide. On ultrasonography, most cancers are solid, although a mixed cystic–solid appearance is encountered in about 20%, and even a purely cystic-appearing lesion may occasionally be malignant.

Papillary and *mixed papillary–follicular* carcinomas are the most common and account for 60% to 70% of all thyroid malignancies. The lesions tend to be very slow-growing, spreading locally to adjacent lymph nodes but not metastasizing distantly until very late. Consequently, the prognosis is good even after local spread has occurred. Although most are solid, some may present as mixed cystic–solid lesions because of necrosis and liquefaction.

Follicular carcinomas, which make up another 15% to 20% of thyroid cancers, are also slow-growing. Local spread to regional nodes may occur without invasion of the thyroid capsule, but this does not alter the prognosis. Hematogenous spread can develop early, and the initial presentation is often a metastasis to lung or bone.

Anaplastic carcinomas comprise another 10% to 12% of cases; these are very invasive, usually inoperable, and fatal within 1 year.

Medullary carcinomas, derived from the parafollicular cells of the thyroid, represent 10% of thyroid cancers. Sporadic and familial forms of the disease are seen; among the latter are familial medullary cancers unaccompanied by other conditions and *multiple endocrine neoplasia* types II and III (which occur in conjunction with pheochromocytoma and hyperparathyroidism). The malignancy often presents as a nodule located in the upper half of the thyroid gland. It can be multicentric, especially in the familial forms. At least 50% of medullary carcinomas of the thyroid occur sporadically. *Calcitonin*, produced by the parafollicular or "C" cells, is a unique tumor marker for medullary carcinoma.

Lymphoma may sometimes develop as a primary lesion within the thyroid of a patient with chronic lymphocytic thyroiditis. Its clinical course is a function of tissue type and stage at time of presentation (see Chapter 84). Spread to local nodes is common and prominent.

Multiple Nodules

Hashimoto's Thyroiditis, an autoimmune condition, is the leading cause of multinodular goiter in the United States. Evidence of the condition can be found in about 4% of the general population and up to 15% of women over the age of 65. Women patients outnumber men by a ratio of 3:1. Pathologically, a chronic inflammatory cell infiltrate, formation of germinal centers, fibrosis, and Hürthle cell changes are seen to involve follicular epithelial cells. Although not unique to this condition, *antimicrosomal antibodies* are found in 70% to 95% of patients. About one third of patients manifest a multinodular goiter, although euthyroid goiter is actually the most common presentation. The immunologically mediated injury impairs thyroxine synthesis and increases leakage of hormone into the circulation. A third of patients experience progressive loss of glandular function and eventually become hypothyroid. Hyperthyroidism in uncommon but can occur in patients with a prominent lymphocytic infiltrate.

Multinodular Goiter is the second most common cause of a multinodular gland in adults. It represents an advanced stage of focal autonomous hyperplasia, which initially presents as a diffusely enlarged gland but then progresses to multinodularity as areas of focal hyperplasia undergo degenerative changes. Nodules may also develop when colloid accumulates in hyperplastic cells (*colloid cysts*). Uptake of radioiodine on scan is heterogeneous; some areas may not take up iodine and appear "cold." The thyroid gland feels less firm than it does in Hashimoto's disease. The TSH level may be slightly reduced, reflecting the autonomous nature of the thyroxine output of the gland, but free thyroxine levels are usually within normal limits.

Cancers may arise in a multinodular gland, although this is very uncommon. Thyroid cancer and lymphoma are the leading causes. Cervical adenopathy, hoarseness (resulting from recurrent laryngeal nerve compression), and the continued enlargement of a "cold" nodule on thyroid scan are distinguishing features of the clinical presentation. A history of neck irradiation or family history of thyroid cancer (suggestive of hereditary disease) are risk factors. The nodule may be tender if the tumor is rapidly growing (as with lymphoma), a finding atypical of other multinodular goiters.

Incidentalomas

This term is used to refer to nonpalpable thyroid lesions detected incidentally in the course of imaging of the neck area by ultrasonography or other sensitive diagnostic modalities. The risk for malignancy is low when the diameter of the lesion is less than 1.5 cm. Even if some incidentalomas represent early papillary cancers, the rate of growth is likely to be very slow for lesions smaller than 1.5 cm.

DIFFERENTIAL DIAGNOSIS

The vast majority of solitary nodules are benign, even those that fail to take up radionuclide on thyroid scan (see below). In the United States, Hashimoto's thyroiditis accounts for the majority of cases of multinodular goiter. Cancers account for about 10% to 20% of solitary thyroid nodules; the prevalence is lower in patients with multinodular glands (Table 95.1.)

WORKUP

As noted earlier, the main objective is to differentiate a carcinoma from benign causes of nodularity. Although a definitive assessment cannot be made by history and physical examination alone, these elements provide important information regarding risk and need for biopsy or excision. Other tasks include identification of autonomous function and compression of adjacent structures.

History

The history is reviewed not only for the clinical presentation of the nodule and associated symptoms but also for important cancer risk factors, such as a history of neck irradiation in

Table 95.1. Differential Diagnosis of Thyroid Nodularity

CAUSE	DISTINGUISHING CHARACTERISTICS
Solitary Nodule	
Benign adenoma	Solid or mixed cystic and solid; most euthyroid and responsive to TSH; those >3 cm may become autonomous and present as a "hot" nodule on scan
Cancer	
Papillary or mixed	Single hard nodule; local adenopathy; "cold" on scan; slow-growing; metastasizes very late
Follicular	Same, although metastasizes earlier; some cystic
Medullary	May be familial; multiple endocrine neoplasia; calcitonin elevated; "cold" nodule
Lymphoma	Primary cancer arises in patients with chronic lymphocytic thyroiditis; prominent regional nodes
Multinodular	
Hashimoto's thyroiditis	Multinodular, rubbery gland; antithyroid antibodies; one third hypothyroid; heterogeneous uptake; TSH-responsive
Multinodular goiter	Multiple nodules, enlarged gland; heterogeneous uptake on scan with some areas of decreased or absent uptake; clinically euthyroid, although some with mild decrease in TSH; autonomous gland
Cancer	
Thyroid	Same as above
Lymphoma	May arise in a Hashimoto's gland

TSH, thyroid-stimulating hormone.

childhood, exposure to excessive environmental radiation, and a positive family history of thyroid cancer. Age and sex are also relevant. Patients younger than 40 years and male patients are at increased risk for a malignant thyroid nodule. Symptoms suggestive of local compression or invasion (e.g., *hoarseness, dysphagia,* and *tracheal wheezing*) should be noted, as should the new appearance of a nodule or rapid growth of an existing one. However, bleeding into a benign cyst or subacute thyroiditis may cause a similarly abrupt change and new onset of symptoms. Conversely, many thyroid cancers are slow-growing and may have been present for years; duration is not particularly useful for distinguishing benign from malignant disease. Such factors as residence in an iodine-deficient area, presence of goiter, or intake of goitrogens (e.g., lithium, turnips, beets) favor a benign thyroid lesion, as does a family history of goiter (as opposed to thyroid cancer). Symptoms of hypothyroidism or hyperthyroidism argue against malignancy.

Physical Examination

The physical examination focuses on the gland and adjacent lymph nodes. The gland is noted for its overall size, consistency, and number and size of nodules. A solitary hard nodule that is irregular and fixed (fails to move with swallowing) is suggestive of malignancy. However, finding a soft nodule does not rule out the diagnosis of cancer because a papillary carcinoma that has undergone cystic degeneration can be soft to the touch. Finding a single nodule increases the chances of cancer; few multinodular goiters harbor a cancer.

The adjacent lymph nodes, especially those on the same side as the nodule, require detailed examination. A thyroid nodule with associated cervical adenopathy should be viewed with marked suspicion. A single node may represent metastasis from the thyroid, whereas multiple nodes in a young person with a thyroid nodule raise the possibility of lymphoma. The vocal cords should be viewed in patients with hoarseness.

Laboratory Studies

Fine-needle Aspiration Biopsy has become the test of choice for the initial evaluation of most euthyroid patients with a thyroid nodule, having supplanted the radionuclide thyroid scan and ultrasonography in determining who needs surgical excision. The fine ("skinny") needle is inserted into the nodule and its contents are aspirated for cytologic examination. In skilled hands, the sensitivity of fine-needle biopsy exceeds 95%. Although radionuclide scanning and ultrasonography also provide high sensitivity, their specificity is poor. The specificity of fine-needle biopsy ranges from 70% when patients with "suspicious" readings are included in the group in need of surgery to more than 90% when they are not. In comparison with ultrasonography and radionuclide scan, fine-needle biopsy has reduced by half the number of patients who undergo operations needlessly, doubled the incidence of malignancy in surgically excised nodules, and reduced costs by more than 25%. The procedure is safe, inexpensive, and readily performed in the office setting. A skilled physician is needed to perform the procedure and an experienced pathologist to interpret the results so that errors in sampling and interpretation are minimized. Failure to drain a cystic lesion completely and obtain samples from the residual mass is an important source of false-negative results. With cytologic information provided by aspiration biopsy only, it can be difficult for even experienced pathologists to differentiate benign Hürthle cell and follicular adenomas from their malignant counterparts. Patients with lesions labeled "suspicious" or "indeterminate" usually must undergo surgical excision of the nodule, although sometimes malignancy can be ruled out by radionuclide scanning.

Radionuclide Scanning. As noted above, radionuclide scanning has been supplanted by fine-needle aspiration biopsy as the initial test of choice in patients with a euthyroid nodule. Although it is true that most malignant disease has the appearance of a "cold" nodule on scan, only 15% to 20% of all "cold" nodules are malignant. Moreover, uptake in a nodule ("warm" nodule) does not entirely rule out malignancy. Thus, radionuclide scanning is best relegated to a supplemental role, performed after fine-needle biopsy in patients with "suspicious" cytologic findings. A "hot" nodule on the scan of such patients indicates an autonomously hyperfunctioning nodule, which is associated with a very low risk for cancer. A "suspicious" nodule that is "warm" or "cold" on scan is more likely to be cancerous, so that surgical excision must be considered. A radionuclide scan can also be of help in detecting multinodularity, although thyroid ultrasonography is even more sensitive.

Thyroid Ultrasonography has an excellent sensitivity in the detection of nodules (down to 1 mm) and a unique ability to differentiate solid from cystic lesions, and it plays a role in helping to localize a lesion for biopsy. However, even with the development of new, high-resolution ultrasonographic technology to detect ever-smaller lesions, the test still lacks diagnostic specificity because no clearly defined architectural criteria are available for differentiating benign from malignant lesions. Recently compiled combined data show that 21% of solid lesions, 12% of mixed lesions, and 7% of purely cystic lesions are malignant. Now that "cystic" is no longer considered synonymous with "benign," the test has fallen into disuse as a means of determining risk for malignancy. It is excellent for determining multinodularity, but the meaning of such multinodularity is unclear because up to 40% of all patients with a solitary nodule clinically are found by modern ultrasonography to have multiple nodules.

Ancillary Laboratory Studies. Most are usually of little direct help in deciding who should undergo biopsy, but they occasionally provide supportive information. An abnormal *TSH level* is uncommon in malignant disease, as are high titers of *antimicrosomal antibodies* (useful in suspected cases of Hashimoto's and subacute lymphocytic thyroiditis). Routine use of plain films is not cost-effective. A very high *erythrocyte sedimentation rate* in the setting of an acutely tender gland is very suggestive of subacute granulomatous thyroiditis. A serum *calcitonin* determination is indicated when the patient has a strong family history of thyroid cancer. No other markers are known at present for thyroid cancers. *Thyroglobulin* elevations do occur with cancer, but also with benign nodular thyroid disease. The response to *TSH suppression* (by administration of thyroid hormone) is not reliable for differentiating cancer from benign disease because both may either shrink or not in response to exogenous hormone. In rare instances, a plain film of the chest may incidentally reveal punctate calcifications characteristic of the psammoma bodies of papillary carcinoma or the shell-like calcification characteristic of a benign lesion, but routinely obtaining such films is of low diagnostic yield.

Testing Sequence. The most cost-effective testing sequence for the euthyroid patient with a single thyroid nodule on physical examination is to begin with *fine-needle aspiration biopsy*. If the cytology is "malignant," then surgery is indicated. If the reading is "benign," then observation for 1 year and *follow-up ultrasonography* are reasonable. If the reading is "suspicious," then *radionuclide scan* for determination of nodule uptake is indicated. A "hot" nodule indicates a very low risk for cancer and requires only clinical follow-up with or without treatment, depending on whether the patient is euthyroid or thyrotoxic. A "warm" or "cold" nodule in a patient with "suspicious" cytology raises the question of cancer and necessitates surgical excision.

If after 1 year of observation the follow-up thyroid ultrasonography indicates an increase in nodule size, then repeated biopsy is indicated. An enlarging nodule that continues to appear benign on repeated biopsy can be treated with levothyroxine suppressive therapy (see below) and restudied by ultrasonography in another year's time. If the nodule has stopped enlarging on suppressive therapy, then suppressive therapy can be continued and the patient reassessed annually. If size is increasing, then surgical removal is undertaken. Malignant or suspect pathologic findings are always an indication for surgery.

Patients with Multinodular Glands. Biopsy is usually not required unless the concern for cancer is increased because of neck irradiation, cervical adenopathy, rapid growth of a single nodule in an otherwise stable gland, or onset of recurrent laryngeal nerve palsy. Most cases represent Hashimoto's thyroiditis, and a diagnosis can be made by obtaining antithyroid antibody determinations. High titers of *antimicrosomal antibodies* correlate best with biopsy-proven disease. Antithyroglobulin titers are less useful. The risk for *lymphoma* of the thyroid is increased in patients with Hashimoto's disease, so that *needle biopsy* of the gland is mandated in the presence of an enlarging tender goiter, cervical adenopathy, or a goiter markedly enlarging on thyroid hormone suppressive therapy (which should cause the nodule size to decrease in Hashimoto's disease).

Further Evaluation of the Benign Adenoma. When a lesion is found to be a benign adenoma, the question arises of whether it is functioning autonomously and thus posing a risk for toxicity. Adenomas smaller than 2 cm rarely change much in size or function and can be followed. Those larger than 3 cm are at risk for progressing to toxicity within a few years. Autonomous function is determined by performing *serial radionuclide scans* and demonstrating little change in uptake in a comparison of scans taken before and after *stimulation by thyrotropin-releasing hormone* (TRH) or *suppression by thyroid hormone*. Observation rather than ablation is now preferred for the smaller, low-risk lesions. Annual determination of the nodular size and hormonal output usually suffices. Every 5 years, scanning can be repeated to see if suppression of extranodular tissue function is increasing, a sign of impending toxicity. Other signs include size greater than 3 cm, a rise in serum triiodothyronine (T_3) to the upper limits of normal, and decreasing responsiveness to stimulation or suppression.

Incidentalomas. A stance of watchful waiting is reasonable as long as the patient has no risk factors for thyroid cancer and the lesion is smaller than 1.5 cm in diameter. Biopsy is not necessary under such circumstances, but careful follow-up with repeated examination is essential. Patients with lesions larger than 1.5 cm, prior head or neck irradiation, a strongly positive family history of thyroid cancer, or ultrasonographic findings suggestive of malignancy do require biopsy at the outset.

SYMPTOMATIC THERAPY

Euthyroid Patients with a Benign Solitary Nodule. The best approach to management remains unclear because no definitive data from prospective, randomized studies are available. *Low-dose suppressive therapy* (sufficient to reduce the TSH level to low but not indetectable levels) with *levothyroxine* is advocated by some as a relatively safe means of reducing the risk for nodule growth and decreasing the nodule size. In approximately 10% to 30% of patients with a nontoxic solitary nodule, the nodule size will decrease when doses of levothyroxine sufficient to suppress TSH are given, although such treatment does not appear to work in patients with colloid nodules. The rationale for suppressive therapy is that reducing TSH stimulation should diminish the size of lesions that are TSH-responsive (e.g., follicular adenomas, Hashimoto's thyroiditis). The required dosage of levothyroxine is in the range of 0.1 to 0.15 mg daily, with small doses (e.g., 0.05 mg/d) given first and increased gradually until the TSH level declines to about 0.3 mU/L. Further suppression markedly increases the risk for thyroxine-induced osteoporosis (see Chapter 104). The therapy is relatively contraindicated in the elderly and those with underlying coronary disease (see Chapter 103). It is not known whether therapy prevents an increase in nodule size in patients in whom it fails to effect a decrease.

Others counter that the risk for nodule growth is small and the ability of suppressive therapy to reduce nodule size is modest at best. Moreover, even partially suppressive doses of levothyroxine are associated with a risk for osteoporosis, especially in postmenopausal women, who comprise the majority of patients. Pending better data, one suggested approach is to observe the nodule for a year after the initial biopsy, recheck its size by ultrasonography, perform another biopsy on any nodule that appears to be enlarging, and, if the nodule is benign, institute modest suppressive therapy in an attempt to halt enlargement and achieve some reduction in size. If the nodule continues to enlarge, then *surgical removal* is recommended; otherwise levothyroxine is continued and the nodule size is checked at regular intervals.

Nontoxic Multinodular Goiter. Such nodular glands often do not shrink much because they are composed of a great deal of fibrous tissue. Dominant nodules caused by bothersome *large cysts* may require *surgical removal*, but smaller ones can be *aspirated* as necessary, both to rule out malignancy (incidence about 1%) and to increase comfort and improve appearance. Hormone therapy has no effect on the recurrence of thyroid cysts after aspiration or on nodular disease because glandular function typically becomes increasingly autonomous with age. *Radioiodine* is sometimes used, but high doses are required, which increases the chances of precipitating Graves' disease (5%) and possibly late malignancy.

Toxic Nodules and Autonomously Functioning Solitary Adenomas. Patients with these lesions are at high risk for thyrotoxicosis, especially if the nodule is larger than 3 cm in diameter, the serum triiodothyronine level is at the upper limit of normal, and the nodule is increasingly unresponsive to thyroxine suppression. Such patients should be considered for *ablative therapy*. Ablation is mandatory for those with autonomous nodules that have already become toxic. One needs to choose between surgery and radioiodine. *Surgery* represents a definitive approach with low risk if performed by a skilled thyroid surgeon. Young patients are the best candidates. *Radioiodine* is simpler and usually the treatment of choice in the elderly. The theoretical risk of inducing cancer in the remaining thyroid tissue makes radioiodine a less attractive option for young people, although no increase in the incidence of malignancy has been reported. A palpable nodule often remains after irradiation; it is of no consequence except for the cosmetic effect. The patient needs to be monitored for the development of posttreatment hypothyroidism (see Chapter 103).

Incidentalomas. As noted earlier, a stance of watchful waiting is reasonable as long as the patient has no risk factors for thyroid cancer and the lesion is smaller than 1.5 cm. Careful follow-up is critical.

PATIENT EDUCATION

The primary care physician should counsel and closely follow patients who have undergone previous head or neck radiation (see Chapter 94). Regular follow-up is important for any patient with a nodule, and the patient should be instructed to call if a change in size, development of lymphadenopathy, pain, dysphagia, or hoarseness is noted.

The patient with an autonomous nodule or a multinodular goiter should be advised to avoid substances containing high concentrations of iodine (medications, kelp, radiographic contrast media) because they may precipitate thyrotoxicosis. If a contrast study is necessary, the patient should be started on a β-blocking agent 10 days before the study.

INDICATIONS FOR REFERRAL

Detection of a solitary thyroid nodule in a clinically euthyroid patient should prompt a referral to a consultant skilled in performing fine-needle biopsy of the thyroid. Finding a worrisome nodule (see above) in a patient with a multinodular gland represents another indication for consideration of biopsy. Patients with a toxic or large (>3 cm) autonomously functioning adenoma require consultation for discussion of ablative therapy. Those with goiters that are unresponsive to thyroid hormone and are causing obstruction or unpleasant cosmetic effects may be surgical candidates.

A.H.G.

ANNOTATED BIBLIOGRAPHY

Asp AA, Georgitis W, Waldron EJ, et al. Fine needle aspiration of the thyroid: use in an average health care facility. Am J Med 1987;83:489. (*Excellent sensitivity and specificity demonstrated, which indicates that the procedure can be performed in the community setting provided the physician and pathologist are well trained.*)

Baker BA, Gharib H. Correlation of thyroid antibodies and cytologic features in suspected autoimmune thyroid disease. Am J Med 1983;74:941. (*Establishes that antimicrosomal antibodies are the antibody test of choice for Hashimoto's disease.*)

Belfiori A, La Rosa GL, La Porta GA, et al. Cancer risk in patients with cold nodules: relevance of iodine intake, sex, age and multinodularity. Am J Med 1992;93:363. (*Male sex and age below 30 or over 60 years were predictors of cancer, but multinodularity was not.*)

De los Santos ET, Keyhani-Rofagha S, Cunningham JJ, et al. Cystic thyroid nodules: the dilemma of malignant lesions. Arch Intern Med 1990;150:1422. (*A retrospective study; 20% of cystic lesions were malignancies.*)

Fogelfeld L, Wiviott MBT, Shore-Freedman E, et al. Recurrence of thyroid nodules after surgical removal in patients irradiated in childhood for benign conditions. N Engl J Med 1989;320:835. (*A study of the utility of treatment with exogenous thyroid hormone; rate of recurrence reduced, but not risk for cancer.*)

Gharib H, Goellner JR, Zinsmeister AR, et al. Fine-needle aspiration biopsy of the thyroid. Ann Intern Med 1984;101:25. (*Addresses the difficult issue of what to do with the "suspicious" finding.*)

Gharib H, James EM, Charboneau JW, et al. Suppressive therapy with levothyroxine for solitary thyroid nodules. N Engl J Med 1987;317:70. (*A double-blinded, randomized study of patients with colloid nodules; no benefit.*)

Gharib H, Mazzaferri EL. Thyroxine suppressive therapy in patients with nodular thyroid disease. Ann Intern Med 1998;128:386. (*A review of published evidence; concludes that most patients with benign findings on cytology are best followed without suppressive therapy because most nodules do not continue to enlarge.*)

Hamburger JI. The autonomously functioning thyroid adenoma. N Engl J Med 1983;309:1512. (*An editorial summarizing diagnosis and treatment.*)

Hamburger JI. Lymphoma of the thyroid. Ann Intern Med 1983;99:685. (*A clinical review drawing attention to the relation between the condition and Hashimoto's thyroiditis; provides indications for biopsy.*)

Hamburger JI. The various presentations of thyroiditis. Ann Intern Med 1986;104:219. (*Authoritative review with detailed discussions of Hashimoto's and subacute thyroiditis; 51 references.*)

Hermus AR, Huysmans DA. Treatment of benign nodular thyroid disease. N Engl J Med 1998;338:1438. (*Excellent general review; 77 references.*)

Mandel SJ, Brent GA, Larsen PR. Levothyroxine therapy in patients with thyroid disease. Ann Intern Med 1993;119:429. (*Includes discussion of use of thyroxine to reduce size of solitary nodules.*)

McCowen KD, Reed JW, Fariss BL. The role of thyroid therapy in patients with thyroid cysts. Am J Med 1980;68:853. (*Treatment with hormone did not prevent recurrence of cysts after aspiration.*)

Rallison ML, Dobyns BM, Meikle AW, et al. Natural history of thyroid abnormalities: prevalence, incidence, and regression of thyroid diseases in adolescents and young adults. Am J Med 1991;91:363. (*Data from a population exposed to high levels of environmental radiation; emphasizes the dynamic nature of these conditions.*)

Ridgway EC. Medical treatment of benign thyroid nodules: have we defined a benefit? Ann Intern Med 1998;128:403. (*This editorial on the management of benign thyroid nodules proposes, in the absence of definitive data, a reasonable and practical algorithm for follow-up and the selective use of suppressive therapy; the algorithm is incorporated into the assessment and follow-up strategy presented in this chapter.*)

Rojeski MT, Gharib H. Nodular thyroid disease. N Engl J Med 1985;313:428. (*Useful review, especially of evaluation methods; 115 references.*)

Ross DS, Ridgway EC, Daniels GH. Successful treatment of solitary toxic thyroid nodules with relatively low-dose iodine 131, with low prevalence of hypothyroidism. Ann Intern Med 1984;101:488. (*Reports excellent results with no induction of hypothyroidism.*)

Simpson WJ, McKinney SE, Carruthers JS, et al. Papillary and follicular thyroid cancer. Am J Med 1987;83:479. (*Extrathyroidal extension, poor differentiation, and older age were most predictive of reduced survival.*)

Tan GH, Gharib H. Thyroid incidentalomas: management approaches to nonpalpable nodules discovered incidentally on thyroid imaging.

Ann Intern Med 1997;126:226. (*A literature review finding the prognosis good for patients with a nodule diameter smaller than 1.5 cm and no thyroid cancer risk factors; close follow-up is critical, but biopsy not necessary initially.*)

Zelmanowitz F, Genro S, Gross JL, et al. Suppressive therapy with levothyroxine for solitary thyroid nodules: a double-blind controlled clinical study and cumulative meta-analysis. J Clin Endocrinol Metab 1998;83:3881. (*Evidence in support of suppressive therapy; degree of benefit clinically modest but statistically significant.*)

96
Approach to the Patient with Hypercalcemia
SAMUEL R. NUSSBAUM

The advent of automated laboratory screening has led to an increased recognition of asymptomatic persons with hypercalcemia, with the annual incidence rising from 7.8/100,000 to 51/100,000. In addition, outpatients with nonspecific complaints, such as fatigue, weakness, abdominal discomfort, or constipation, may have hypercalcemia discovered during biochemical testing. Mild hyperparathyroidism is usually the explanation for these often inadvertently recognized elevations in calcium levels. Hypercalcemia may also herald other important underlying diseases, such as malignancy or sarcoidosis. Asymptomatic hyperparathyroidism is not necessarily a benign condition. The effect of excessive levels of parathyroid hormone for prolonged periods on target organs, such as bone and kidney, may lead to skeletal loss and impaired renal function.

The primary physician must be able to interpret an abnormal calcium value and diagnose its cause. If hyperparathyroidism is present, one must decide between surgery and medical therapy. The treatment of hypercalcemia resulting from malignancy can improve the quality of life and deserves consideration.

PATHOPHYSIOLOGY AND CLINICAL PRESENTATION

The serum calcium concentration is maintained within narrow limits by parathyroid hormone. Precise calcium homeostasis is necessary because of the vital role of calcium in membrane function, hormonal secretion and action, and neuromuscular function. The free or ionized portion of serum calcium is responsible for its physiologic actions. Slightly less than 50% of serum calcium is in the form of free calcium ions; the remainder is bound to plasma proteins, mostly albumin. Globulins can also bind serum calcium. Calcium binding by serum proteins is pH-dependent. Increased binding at alkaline pH explains the common symptom of paresthesias that occur in conjunction with hyperventilation. The normal range for serum calcium is 8.5 to 10.4 mg/dL, or 2.12 to 2.59 mmol/L. The normal range for ionized serum calcium is 1.16 to 1.34 mmol/L. True hypercalcemia requires an increase in the ionized fraction of serum calcium. A convenient correction factor to apply to the total serum calcium is the subtraction or addition of 1 mg/dL to the calcium concentration for every 1.0 g/100 mL of serum albumin above or below 4.0 g/100 mL.

Hyperparathyroidism. The hypercalcemia of hyperparathyroidism is caused by an increase in osteoclastic bone resorption, mediated by the binding of excess parathyroid hormone (PTH) to receptors on osteoblasts, in addition to an increase in gut calcium absorption. PTH also increases renal tubular reabsorption of calcium, which results in phosphate wasting. Pathologically, approximately 80% of patients are found to have a single parathyroid adenoma, whereas 20% have four-gland hyperplasia. Parathyroid cancer accounts for approximately 1% of all cases of hypercalcemia attributed to excess parathyroid hormone secretion.

The incidence of hyperparathyroidism increases with age, peaking in the fourth through sixth decades of life, and hyperparathyroidism occurs more commonly in women than men, by approximately a 2:1 ratio. It is not certain whether the increased recognition of the disease relates to multiphasic biochemical screening or whether the number of cases of the disease has increased, possibly as a result of head and neck irradiation in infancy or other environmental factors that affect parathyroid cell proliferation.

The majority of patients with hyperparathyroidism do not have symptoms. The "classic" presentation of "stones, bones, abdominal groans, and psychic moans" has been replaced by a more subtle and nonspecific presentation. *Fatigue, weakness,* mild gastrointestinal symptoms (*constipation, abdominal pain*), changes in intellectual performance, and depression may all be manifestations of hypercalcemia or excessive PTH. Often, such nonspecific symptoms are recognized only after successful parathyroid surgery has been performed, when the patient describes an improved sense of well-being.

The resultant hypercalcemia of hyperparathyroidism can lead to a renal concentrating defect and *increased urination.* Hyperparathyroidism is also associated with an increase in *calcium oxalate stones,* particularly in patients with elevated levels of 1,25-dihydroxyvitamin D_3 and urinary calcium excretion in excess of 300 to 350 mg/24 h. Bone pain results from skeletal fracture and osteitis fibrosa cystica. A possible but somewhat controversial increase in peptic ulcer disease and pancreatitis has been noted, and a spectrum of psychiatric disease. In persons with mild disease, survival appears to be unaffected.

Hyperparathyroidism may be observed in familial settings, such as the autosomal dominant syndromes of *multiple endocrine neoplasia* (MEN) types 1 and 2. In MEN 1, parathyroid hyperplasia occurs in conjunction with adenomas of the pituitary and pancreas. In MEN 2, parathyroid hyperplasia may occur with medullary cancer of the thyroid and bilateral adrenal pheochromocytoma.

Patients with *"normocalcemic hyperparathyroidism"* often have serum calcium levels at the upper limit of normal, which on repeated determinations fluctuate into the frankly elevated range. *Thiazide diuretics* may transiently elevate serum calcium by reducing urinary calcium excretion. More sustained elevations suggest mild underlying hyperparathyroidism that is unmasked by thiazide therapy.

Familial Hypocalciuric Hypercalcemia may cause hypercalcemia as often as MEN type 1. This condition is associated with an abnormality of calcium sensing by the parathyroid, which leads to parathyroid gland hyperplasia. Serum PTH is not elevated. Urinary calcium excretion is often less than 100 mg/24 h.

Malignancy is the second most frequent cause of hypercalcemia and more common among hospitalized patients than outpatients. Cancers of the *breast*, *lung*, and *kidney* lead the list of malignant causes, accounting for 50% to 60% of such cases. The incidence of hypercalcemia during the course of breast cancer ranges from 18% to 42%, and in lung cancer, from 6% to 16%. Other malignancies associated with hypercalcemia include *multiple myeloma* (incidence of 30% to 100%), squamous cell carcinomas of the head and neck (2%), lymphoma and leukemia (1%), and genitourinary cancer (1%).

Several *mechanisms* for the hypercalcemia of malignancy have been identified, with a common theme being increased osteoclastic bone resorption. Such resorption and resultant hypercalcemia can occur with or without bony metastasis, and many tumors that commonly metastasize to bone do not cause hypercalcemia. Squamous cell cancers produce a parathyroid hormone–related protein (PTHRP), a *PTH-like peptide* with an amino terminal structure similar to that of PTH and a nearly identical effect on mineral ion homeostasis. Myeloma cells produce *interleukin-1β* and *interleukin-6*, which stimulate osteoclast-mediated bone resorption. In some patients with lymphoma and leukemia, an increase in *1,25-dihydroxyvitamin D_3* is implicated.

Hypercalcemia is rarely the sole presenting manifestation of an underlying malignancy. The presence of hypercalcemia in association with malignancy indicates a grim prognosis, as the median survival is approximately 2 months. Very high levels of serum calcium (>14 mg/dL) are most often associated with malignancy, but levels up to 20 mg/dL may be seen in acute primary hyperparathyroidism caused by large parathyroid adenomas.

Other Causes. In *sarcoidosis*, enhanced conversion of inactive vitamin D to its active 1,25-dihydroxy form by granulomatous tissue increases absorption of calcium from the gut and resorption of bone. *Vitamin D intoxication* and *milk–alkali syndrome* are being seen increasingly with the popularization of calcium and vitamin D supplements to avert osteoporosis. Hypercalcemia may occur when an excess of 50,000 U of vitamin D and an excess of 3 to 5 g of calcium are consumed daily.

The *thiazide diuretics* cause a transient, mild increase in serum calcium, generally within the normal range. As noted earlier, a sustained increase in serum calcium beyond 10 days implies underlying metabolic bone disease, usually hyperparathyroidism. Some investigators have used thiazides as a provocative test for hyperparathyroidism in patients with borderline hypercalcemia. *Theophylline* excess is another pharmacologic cause of hypercalcemia.

Hyperthyroidism is associated with mild elevations in serum calcium in approximately 20% of patients because of increased skeletal turnover. *Immobilization* in young persons who have not completed skeletal growth and in patients with Paget's disease may cause severe hypercalcemia. *Lithium* therapy for manic–depressive illness is sometimes associated with hypercalcemia. Persons taking lithium may have an altered calcium set point for PTH secretion. *Addison's disease* and severe *liver disease* may cause hypercalcemia; mechanism(s) remain unknown.

DIFFERENTIAL DIAGNOSIS

Hyperparathyroidism is overwhelmingly the most likely cause of hypercalcemia in the medically well, asymptomatic patient. In a Swedish population survey that yielded 95 persons with hypercalcemia, hyperparathyroidism was suspected in 88 patients and confirmed surgically in 57 of the 59 who underwent neck exploration for cure of hyperparathyroidism. Primary hyperparathyroidism accounts for more than 60% of hypercalcemic patients and is extremely likely to be the explanation for hypercalcemia in patients with an elevation of serum calcium dating back several years. *Malignancy, granulomatous disease, hyperthyroidism, Addison's disease,* and *excess ingestion* of *vitamin D* and *calcium* are the causes of most other cases. Occasionally, an underlying *MEN syndrome* or *hypocalciuric hypercalcemia* is present.

WORKUP

Because a more extensive laboratory evaluation is undertaken, a *repeated calcium determination* is indicated to confirm the elevation. Measuring serum albumin and globulin levels helps to confirm that the calcium elevation is not an artifactual result of elevated protein binding of calcium. Hypercalcemia that appears ephemeral may be spurious, caused by prolonged application of the tourniquet at the time of blood drawing. Should hypercalcemia be confirmed, then evaluation can proceed.

History. In the "asymptomatic" patient, subtle manifestations of hyperparathyroidism, such as fatigue, weakness, lethargy, arthralgias, nonspecific gastrointestinal complaints, impairment of intellectual performance, and depression, should be specifically sought. Associated conditions such as hypertension, gout, pseudogout, and nephrolithiasis should be recognized. A history of increased urination may indicate calcium-related defects in urine-concentrating ability. Symptoms of underlying malignancy, particularly of breast, lung, and hematologic origin, should be pursued. Review of intake of antacids, food additives, and health food store preparations may uncover excessive ingestion of vitamin D or calcium. Symptoms of hyperthyroidism (see Chapter 103) also need to be considered.

Physical Examination in the totally asymptomatic patient is generally unrevealing. However, a careful search for signs of malignancy (breast mass, lymphadenopathy, bone tenderness) and sarcoidosis (lymph node enlargement, abnormalities on lung examination) should be undertaken. Signs of hyperparathyroidism are not readily apparent; band keratopathy is rarely visible without the slit lamp.

Laboratory Studies. After confirmation of hypercalcemia and in the absence of an obvious cause, one should obtain a *serum PTH* determination. Improvements in the sensitivity and specificity of immunoradiometric assays for the intact PTH molecule have proved to be a great advance in differentiating patients with hyperparathyroidism from those with other causes of hypercalcemia. In virtually all patients with hyperparathyroidism, PTH 1-84 is either frankly elevated, in 90%, or at the upper limit of the normal range (10 to 60 pg/mL), in 10%. In hypercalcemia associated with malignancy, PTH is either undetectable or below normal in most patients. Therefore, a single laboratory test confirms the diagnosis of hyperparathyroidism.

When hyperparathyroidism is under consideration, serum *electrolytes* and *phosphate* concentrations can provide indirect evidence of the diagnosis. Fasting hypophosphatemia, hyperchloremia, and mild metabolic acidosis suggests the diagnosis. This is because PTH induces renal phosphate and bicarbonate wasting. A normal serum phosphate level does not exclude the diagnosis of hyperparathyroidism, and hypophosphatemia can be observed in malignancy. Furthermore, phosphate must be measured in the fasting state, as intake of food causes phosphate to shift into cells as glucose is phosphorylated. *Alkaline phosphatase* elevation implies increased osteoblastic activity and can be seen in malignancy, hyperparathyroidism with PTH bone disease, and Paget's disease.

Although *anemia* and an *elevated erythrocyte sedimentation rate* can be seen in severe hyperparathyroidism with osteitis fibrosa cystica, these laboratory findings are more suggestive of multiple myeloma, the diagnosis of which requires a serum *immunoelectrophoresis* or, occasionally, a urine immunoelectrophoresis for light-chain excretion. *Chest radiographic findings* of hilar adenopathy or pulmonary parenchymal abnormalities, in conjunction with an elevated *angiotensinconverting enzyme*, is indicative of sarcoidosis. The hypercalcemia of sarcoidosis may be more severe following an interval of sun exposure, so that more sophisticated diagnostic studies may be required, including diffusing capacity, a hydrocortisone suppression study in which orally administered hydrocortisone (40 mg three times daily for 10 days) normalizes the hypercalcemia of sarcoidosis, and even bronchoscopy or mediastinoscopy with biopsy for histologic confirmation (see Chapter 48).

A *bone scan* will detect the skeletal metastases of breast cancer. *Skeletal radiography* may show lytic or metastatic lesions. Radiographic findings are frequently normal in hyperparathyroidism, but the finding of *subperiosteal bone resorption* is specific for and diagnostic of hyperparathyroidism. Cortical bone is lost preferentially in hyperparathyroidism. Therefore, it is important that noninvasive measurements of

skeletal mass include cortical bone, which predominates at sites such as the wrist (in contrast to trabecular bone, which predominates in the spine and is lost earliest following the menopause).

Familial hypocalciuric hypercalcemia can be considered and excluded in patients without frankly elevated serum PTH by the finding of a 24-hour *urinary calcium excretion* of 80 to 100 mg. *Thyroid hormone* determinations (see Chapter 103), particularly total triiodothyronine by radioimmunoassay, and measurements of serum cortisol following administration of Cortrosyn should be performed if the patient has a history suggestive of hyperthyroidism or Addison's disease, respectively. A *1,25-dihydroxyvitamin D₃* assay will unequivocally allay concerns of excessive vitamin D intake.

Despite the occasional usefulness of such determinations to exclude the myriad causes of hypercalcemia, the most direct approach to the workup is to measure the PTH level with the sensitive, specific PTH immunoradiometric assay that is now available. In principle, an elevated PTH concentration or an inappropriately "normal" level in the setting of hypercalcemia should indicate hyperparathyroidism. Older carboxyl terminal and midregion radioimmunoassays for PTH recognized PTH-like factors present in the serum in some patients with hypercalcemia of malignancy. The elevation noted by such PTH assays was minimal for the degree of hypercalcemia present. These assays do not test for PTHRP.

MANAGEMENT OF HYPERPARATHYROIDISM

A basic decision in the management of hyperparathyroidism is whether to treat definitively with surgery or follow expectantly and consider medical modalities. The decision must take into account the degree of symptomatology and the natural history of the disease. Prospective studies have attempted to ascertain the natural history of disease in asymptomatic patients. Only in rare instances does recurrent nephrolithiasis, pancreatitis, or hypercalcemic crisis develop. The major consequence of untreated disease appears to be a decrease in skeletal mass, which may predispose to fracture. There is no way to predict who will suffer these effects; monitoring is required. Routine skeletal radiography and alkaline phosphatase measurements are insufficient for long-term follow-up of bone demineralization. *Bone densitometry* is required (see Chapter 164). Because cortical bone loss is most prominent, measurements are made in the proximal wrist. Marked elevation of *urinary calcium* may predict the development of nephrolithiasis.

Candidacy for Surgical Cure. Most authorities agree that the *symptomatic patient* with recurrent kidney stones or parathyroid bone disease or a serum calcium level higher than 12.5 to 13.0 mg/dL is a candidate for surgery. Less clear are the indications for surgery in *asymptomatic* or minimally or nonspecifically symptomatic patients with mild hypercalcemia. A 1990 National Institutes of Health consensus conference to establish guidelines for the management of hyperparathyroidism in asymptomatic persons formulated a set of criteria for surgical intervention (Table 96.1). Surgical cure is warranted for all persons younger than age 40, for those who have a cortical bone density that is two standard deviations below normal, and perhaps for patients with a urinary calcium excretion greater than 350 to 400 mg in 24 hours, which implies, on a restricted cal-

Table 96.1.   Indications for Surgical Treatment of Hyperparathyroidism

Marked elevation of serum calcium, usually >12.5 mg/dL

History of an episode of life-threatening hypercalcemia

Reduced creatinine clearance

Presence of kidney stones detected by abdominal radiography

Markedly elevated 24-hour urine calcium excretion

Substantially reduced bone mass determined by direct measurement

Medical surveillance neither desirable nor suitable:
    Patient is young (<50 years old).
    Patient requests surgery.
    Consistent follow-up is unlikely.
    Coexistent illness complicates management.

Adapted from Proceedings of the NIH Consensus Development Conference on Diagnosis and Management of Asymptomatic Primary Hyperparathyroidism. J Bone Miner Res 1991;6[Suppl 1–2]:S1.

cium intake, that a negative calcium balance is occurring. Cure rates for the initial neck exploration in experienced surgical centers are better than 90%.

As just noted, curative surgical treatment should be a serious consideration for persons with asymptomatic hyperparathyroidism who are young or middle-aged because of the likelihood of progression of skeletal disease, particularly in women, who must anticipate the synergistic effects of menopausal bone loss. The cost of medical surveillance, which includes yearly or biannual assessment of renal function and skeletal mass, may surpass the cost of surgical cure after 5 to 10 years of follow-up studies. Some now recommend parathyroidectomy for nearly all patients. Long-term follow-up study finds that surgery results in normalization of biochemical abnormalities and an increase in bone density. However, three fourths of asymptomatic patients who do not undergo surgery experience no progression of their disease within 10 years, which suggests that for truly asymptomatic patients, an alternative to surgery is close follow-up. For such patients, biannual serum calcium determinations and annual measurements of urinary calcium excretion and bone mineral density allow timely recognition of the need for operative cure. Nonetheless, asymptomatic patients at high risk for disease progression, especially women as they enter menopause, should be advised about a surgical option.

Before surgery, localization of the parathyroid adenoma may be helpful, even to the skilled surgeon. Ultrasonography and technetium Tc 99m sestamibi scanning with computer programs that subtract thyroidal uptake of technetium have localized parathyroid adenomas in approximately 70% of patients preoperatively. Anatomic localization by selective angiography or, less commonly, by venous sampling is generally reserved for patients in whom neck exploration by an experienced parathyroid surgeon fails to cure the disease.

Medical Therapy. For patients who do not undergo surgical cure for hyperparathyroidism, several medical alternatives exist. These alternatives may help limit nonspecific symptoms of hypercalcemic hyperparathyroidism and, more importantly, may prevent skeletal loss.

Estrogen and progestogen therapy given to postmenopausal women may lower or even normalize serum calcium, reduce bone resorption, and increase skeletal mass. It represents a reasonable therapeutic option in older women without any contraindications for estrogen therapy (see Chapter 164). In women with a family or personal history of breast cancer, *tamoxifen* treatment has a beneficial effect on the skeleton and may be of therapeutic value.

Oral phosphate therapy, particularly for patients with moderate hypophosphatemia, may lessen fatigue and weakness and reduce urinary calcium excretion, thereby reducing the likelihood of renal stones. Serum calcium is lowered by the oral administration of phosphate, given as 250 mg to 500 mg of neutral phosphate four times daily. The most common side effect of this therapy is dose-related frequent bowel movements, which are often preferred to the constipation of hyperparathyroidism. Phosphate should be very cautiously administered in cases of renal insufficiency because the calcium phosphate solubility product of 65 might be exceeded and calcium be deposited in skeletal and extraskeletal sites. Phosphate therapy has a potential drawback: it increases PTH secretion and, theoretically, can accelerate bone resorption.

Diuretics, such as *furosemide* or *bumetanide*, increase renal calcium excretion. *Thiazides* may actually decrease PTH secretion and urinary calcium excretion. However, the risk for dehydration requires caution in the use of diuretic agents.

Calcitonin and *bisphosphonates* have *not* proved useful on a long-term basis in hyperparathyroidism. Tachyphylaxis develops with calcitonin therapy, and bisphosphonates result in only transient decreases in osteoclastic bone resorption and serum calcium levels.

Most physicians limit *dietary calcium* in patients with hyperparathyroidism. However, this restriction of dietary calcium may result in accelerated bone resorption as the body responds by maintaining the "set point" elevation of serum calcium with increased PTH secretion. It is prudent to increase the dietary calcium intake to 1 to 1.5 g daily in patients with hyperparathyroidism but no associated nephrolithiasis or increased levels of 1,25-dihydroxyvitamin D_3.

Patients who are taking phosphate or estrogen therapy or are being followed expectantly for hypercalcemia and the development of skeletal or renal disease should be instructed to maintain a *fluid intake* of at least 2 L daily and report any illness that might lead to dehydration and worsening hypercalcemia.

MANAGEMENT OF HYPERCALCEMIA OF MALIGNANCY

(See Chapter 92.)

INDICATIONS FOR REFERRAL AND HOSPITALIZATION

Because one cannot predict in which patients with asymptomatic hyperparathyroidism the progressive complications of disease will develop, recommendations for who should be referred for surgical cure cannot be rigidly applied. The decision to refer for surgery should take into account the patient's preferences and willingness to cooperate with the demands of long-term surveillance, and the availability of skilled surgical care. As noted above, the patients who should be urged to consider surgery are those who are younger than age 40, have a cortical bone density two standard deviations below normal, or have a urinary calcium excretion greater than 350 to 400 mg/24 h (which, on a restricted calcium intake, implies a negative calcium balance). Patients for whom surgical cure is being planned should be referred to surgeons experienced in the complexities of parathyroid surgery, not only for cure of potential hyperplasia and discovery of a parathyroid adenoma in an unusual location, but also for prevention of the complications of recurrent laryngeal nerve injury and hypoparathyroidism.

Hospitalization is necessary for patients with severe hypercalcemia. Hydration and bisphosphonates such as pamidronate that limit osteoclastic resorption of bone are helpful.

PATIENT EDUCATION

Several recommendations will prevent the likelihood of more severe hypercalcemia in patients with mild hyperparathyroidism. Adequacy of fluid intake and prevention of dehydration that might occur during an acute gastrointestinal illness should be encouraged. Although the administration of thiazide diuretics and calcium has been discouraged, thiazides may actually limit hypercalciuria and renal stone disease, and dietary calcium may decrease PTH secretion and limit negative calcium balance. Patients should be encouraged to remain active and avoid immobilization. The necessity of surveillance for PTH-induced skeletal disease and the delineation of symptoms that might represent manifestations of hyperparathyroidism (e.g., symptoms of nephrolithiasis and pancreatitis) should be carefully reviewed.

Sharing with patients information on the clinical course of hyperparathyroidism helps them choose among treatment options. The truly asymptomatic patient with mild disease needs to know that without surgery there is only a 25% chance of disease progression. Symptomatic patients are at greater risk.

ANNOTATED BIBLIOGRAPHY

Bilezikian JP. Management of acute hypercalcemia. N Engl J Med 1992;326:1196. (*A current review of treatment options.*)

Broadus AD, Horst RL, Lang R, et al. The importance of circulating 1,25-dihydroxyvitamin D in the pathogenesis of hypercalciuria and renal stone formation in primary hyperparathyroidism. N Engl J Med 1980;302:421. (*In a subgroup of patients with hyperparathyroidism, renal stones are likely to form because of elevated 1,25-dihydroxyvitamin D_3 levels, which increase gut absorption of calcium and produce marked hypercalciuria.*)

Christensson T, Hellstrom K, Wengle B, et al. Prevalence of hypercalcemia in a health screening in Stockholm. Acta Med Scand 1976;200:131. (*In a population of more than 15,000, hypercalcemia was confirmed in 95 patients, with probable hyperparathyroidism in 88.*)

Gartenberg F, Silverberg SJ, Bilezikian JP. Optimal dietary calcium intake in primary hyperparathyroidism. Am J Med 1997;102:543. (*Intake can be liberalized as long as 1,25-dihydroxyvitamin D_3 levels are not elevated.*)

Heath H III, Hodgson SF, Kennedy MA. Primary hyperparathyroidism: incidence, morbidity, and potential economic impact in a community. N Engl J Med 1980;302:189. (*Increased case finding with the advent of multiphasic biochemical screening and the increasing recognition of the disease in older women.*)

Insogna KL, Mitnick ME, Stewart AF, et al. Sensitivity of the parathyroid hormone–1,25-dihydroxyvitamin D axis to variations in calcium intake in patients with primary hyperparathyroidism. N Engl J Med 1985;313:1126. (*Parathyroid function may be suppressed by dietary calcium in some patients with hyperparathyroidism. Perhaps we should be encouraging an increased calcium intake in nonhypercalciuric patients.*)

Marcus R, Madvig P, Crim M, et al. Conjugated estrogens in the treatment of post-menopausal women with hyperparathyroidism. Ann Intern Med 1984;100:633. (*Estrogen therapy normalized serum calcium and decreased bone turnover in 10 women with hyperparathyroidism for up to 2 years.*)

Marx SJ, Attie MF, Levine M, et al. The hypocalciuric or benign variant of familial hypercalcemia: clinical and biochemical features in 15 kindreds. Medicine (Baltimore) 1981;60:397. (*A genetic, clinical, and physiologic review of familial hypocalciuric hypercalcemia.*)

McPherson ML, Prince SR, Atamer ER, et al. Theophylline-induced hypercalcemia. Ann Intern Med 1986;105:52. (*Documents elevations in the settings of both excess and therapeutic theophylline levels.*)

NIH Consensus Development Conference on Diagnosis and Management of Asymptomatic Primary Hyperparathyroidism. Proceedings of the Conference. J Bone Miner Res 1991;Suppl[1-2]:S1. (*A scholarly compendium of the clinical spectrum and treatment options for hyperparathyroidism, especially asymptomatic disease.*)

Nussbaum SR. Pathophysiology and management of severe hypercalcemia. Endocrinol Metab Clin North Am 1993;22:343. (*A review of mechanisms of hypercalcemia, with an emphasis on the newer inhibitors of osteoclastic bone resorption, especially bisphosphonates.*)

Nussbaum SR, Zahradnik R, Lavigne J. Highly sensitive two-site immunoradiometric assay for parathyrin and its clinical utility in evaluating patients with hypercalcemia. Clin Chem 1987;33:1364. (*Immunoradiometric assay for intact PTH can distinguish hypercalcemic patients with hyperparathyroidism from those with malignancy, providing an advantage over earlier, region-specific assays.*)

Palmer M, Adami HO, Bergstrom R. Survival and renal function in persons with untreated hypercalcemia: a population-based cohort study with 13 years of follow-up. Lancet 1987;1:59. (*Decreased survival among 176 hypercalcemic patients was largely explained by cardiovascular deaths. Are some long-term consequences of hyperparathyroidism not currently recognized?*)

Parisien M, Silverberg SJ, Shane E, et al. The histomorphometry of bone in primary hyperparathyroidism: preservation of cancellous bone structure. J Clin Endocrinol Metab 1990;70:930. (*Disproportionate loss of cortical bone in hyperparathyroidism; skeletal study must assess cortical bone.*)

Rao DS, Wilson RJ, Kleerekoper M, et al. Lack of biochemical progression or continuation of accelerated bone loss in mild asymptomatic primary hyperparathyroidism: evidence for biphasic disease course. J Clin Endocrinol Metab 1988;67:1294. (*Longitudinal follow-up demonstrated unchanged calcium and PTH levels and other biochemical parameters, and a low risk for renal or skeletal disease; larger numbers of African-Americans in the study population, with greater bone mass than whites, may explain the skeletal findings.*)

Silverberg SJ, Shane E, Jacobs TP, et al. A 10-year prospective study of primary hyperparathyroidism with or without parathyroid surgery. N Engl J Med 1999;341:1249. (*A long-term follow-up study demonstrating the risks and benefits of curing the condition in asymptomatic persons.*)

Simeone JF, Mueller PR, Ferucci JT, et al. High-resolution real-time sonography of the parathyroid. Radiology 1981;141:745. (*Ultrasonography may demonstrate the location of a parathyroid adenoma in 70% to 80% of patients.*)

Stewart AF, Horst R, Deftos LJ, et al. Biochemical evaluation of patients with cancer-associated hypercalcemia. Evidence for humoral and non-humoral groups. N Engl J Med 1980;303:1377. (*The "classic" study segregating cancer patients with humoral hypercalcemia, often without bone metastases, from patients with metastatic disease.*)

Strewler GJ. The physiology of parathyroid hormone–related protein. N Engl J Med 2000;342:177. (*Basic science review of this protein, which mediates the hypercalcemia of cancer.*)

Taillefer R, Boucher Y, Potvin C, et al. Detection and localization of parathyroid adenomas in patients with hyperparathyroidism using a single radionuclide imaging procedure with technetium 99-sestamibi (double-phase study). J Nucl Med 1992;33:1801. (*This technique reliably detects parathyroid adenomas and greatly simplifies surgery.*)

Utiger RD. Treatment of primary hyperparathyroidism. N Engl J Med 1999;341:1301. (*An editorial recommending surgery for nearly all patients, arguing that almost everyone is symptomatic.*)

Wermers RA, Kholsa S, Atkinson EJ, et al. Survival after the diagnosis of hyperparathyroidism: a population-based study. Am J Med 1998;104:115. (*Survival is normal in persons with mild disease.*)

Wysolmerski JJ, Broadus AE. Hypercalcemia of malignancy: the central role of parathyroid hormone–related protein. Annu Rev Med 1994;45:189. (*Detailed review of the evidence for the role of PTHRP in cancer.*)

97

Evaluation of Hypoglycemia

Except in cases of diabetes, the workup for hypoglycemia is most often an exercise in ruling out underlying pathology, triggered by nonspecific symptoms (e.g., irritability, fatigue, sweats, confusion, palpitations, tremulousness) that are attributed to a "low blood sugar." At other times, the assessment is precipitated by the chance finding of a low blood glucose level. In the setting of diabetes, tight glucose control leading to hypoglycemic episodes is common and readily confirmed (see Chapter 102). In patients who do not have diabetes, confirmation may be more problematic, made difficult by a lack of glucose measurements taken during symptomatic periods and the nonspecific nature of the hypoglycemic symptoms. Compounding the diagnostic problem are unaddressed manifestations of psychopathology, which the patient may prefer to attribute to "hypoglycemia." Although true hypoglycemia in the absence of diabetes is rarely encountered in the office setting, its causes include serious, treatable conditions that must not be missed. These factors make the workup of hypoglycemia challenging. The primary care physician needs to know how to differentiate suspected from true hypoglycemia, and, in the nondiabetic patient, how to identify the rare case that requires an in-depth search for serious underlying disease. A cost-efficient strategy for assessment is needed because the question of hypoglycemia comes up all the time.

PATHOPHYSIOLOGY AND CLINICAL PRESENTATION

Mechanisms. Hypoglycemia can result from increased insulin secretion, enhanced glucose utilization, or inadequate functioning of one or more compensatory regulatory mechanisms. When hypoglycemia occurs, the liver responds with increased glycogenolysis and gluconeogenesis, stimulated by glucagon and epinephrine, which activate hepatic phosphorylase. In addition, the pituitary secretes growth hormone, which inhibits the utilization of glucose by muscle and enhances lipolysis, and adrenocorticotropic hormone (ACTH), which promotes cortisol production. The increased cortisol acts to stimulate gluconeogenesis and diminish muscle uptake of glucose.

No single threshold of glucose concentration invariably triggers hypoglycemic symptoms or characterizes patients with a disorder of glucose homeostasis. Glucose levels lower than 45

mg/dL (2.5 mmol/L) have been documented in metabolically normal men during prolonged exercise and in healthy asymptomatic women. More than 20% of normal patients demonstrate serum sugar levels below 50 mg/dL during glucose tolerance testing. Conversely, hypoglycemic thresholds may rise in poorly controlled diabetes, in which levels as high as 75 mg/dL (4.3 mmol/L) may trigger symptoms. This has led to the view that the onset of hypoglycemic symptoms is related to the robustness of counterregulatory responses in addition to the rate of fall in serum glucose and the absolute serum glucose concentration. In patients with intensively controlled insulin-dependent diabetes, the catecholamine response is blunted, and they may exhibit few symptoms until their glucose concentration falls to a very low level.

Clinical Manifestations of Hypoglycemia. Hypoglycemic symptoms are typically categorized as *neuroglycopenic* (confusion, lethargy, visual disturbances, behavioral changes, impaired performance of routine tasks) or *catecholamine-mediated* (anxiety, tremulousness, headache, palpitations, sweats). Adrenergic symptoms characteristically accompany acute, rapid falls in blood sugar, especially if levels drop to concentrations below 40 mg/dL. Neuroglycopenic symptoms can develop in the absence of premonitory adrenergic complaints.

In the outpatient setting, most cases of true hypoglycemia occur among persons who look well. Their condition is a consequence of insulin excess, and they may have no apparent symptoms indicative of the underlying cause. Those cases resulting from a failure of counterregulatory mechanisms usually occur in very ill patients, who are typically hospitalized with end-stage disease.

Exogenous Insulin or Oral Hypoglycemic Agents account for most of the cases of spontaneous hypoglycemia seen in clinical practice, which develops in persons attempting tight control of their diabetes. Although the hypoglycemia associated with diabetic therapy may occur at any time in relation to meals, it tends to be most severe in the fasting state. The hypoglycemia associated with the use of potent, long-acting oral agents can be particularly severe and prolonged (see Chapter 102). *Surreptitious administration* is seen among self-destructive persons, typically nurses with access to diabetic medications and syringes. Patients injecting insulin secretly may have high levels of immunoreactive insulin but very low serum levels of C-reactive protein or proinsulin because they produce little endogenous insulin. However, those taking excessive doses of oral hypoglycemic agents have high levels of insulin and C-reactive protein because the drugs stimulate endogenous insulin secretion. The diagnosis requires finding excessive amounts of oral agent and oral agent metabolites in the urine.

Early Adult-onset Diabetes. Postprandial hypoglycemia may occur 3 to 5 hours after meals as a consequence of delayed insulin release, a characteristic feature of type 2 diabetes. Insulin levels may be inappropriately high for the level of serum glucose at hand. In most type 2 diabetic patients, the mismatching of insulin and serum glucose levels is not sufficient to cause true symptomatic hypoglycemia, but on occasion it may be noted.

Insulinomas, a rare but important cause of uncontrolled insulin production, account for the large majority of patients with endogenous hyperinsulinemia. More than 85% of insulinomas are benign islet cell tumors. Many occur in the setting of multiple endocrine neoplasia type 1, which also includes parathyroid hyperplasia and pituitary adenoma. The clinical presentation of insulinomas can be confusing and highly variable in timing and severity. The only valid generalizations are that fasting and exercise may precipitate symptoms, and that profound degrees of hypoglycemia may ensue (leading to seizures in 10%). Levels of serum glucose are not always low after an overnight fast. In a series of 39 patients with proven islet cell tumors, about half still had glucose levels above 60 mg/dL after 10 hours of fasting. Another series found symptoms to occur with equal frequency early in the morning, late in the afternoon, and several hours after a meal. Nonetheless, evidence of hyperinsulinism is evident in more than 75% of patients after 24 hours of fasting, and 80% report a combination of neuroglycopenic and adrenergic symptoms. Serum levels of insulin and C-peptide (split from proinsulin) are high.

Non–Islet Cell Tumors. Some large mesenchymal tumors, hepatomas, gastric cancers, and adrenocortical carcinomas synthesize and release large amounts of the prohormone form of *insulin-like growth factor II* ("big" IGF-II). IGF-II inhibits the uptake of glucose by the liver and increases glucose uptake by the tumor itself and by insulin-responsive tissues (e.g., muscle and fat); hypoglycemia is the result. Insulin secretion is suppressed, so that levels of immunoreactive insulin in the serum become very low. The presentation is that of hypoglycemia in the setting of a known malignancy. Rarely, the tumor may be silent, but usually its presence dominates the clinical picture. Serum insulin and C-peptide levels are low. IGF-II may be detected in the serum in elevated quantities. Reduction in tumor bulk alleviates the hypoglycemia.

Defects in Glycogenolysis or Gluconeogenesis are uncommon in the office setting; they are seen predominantly among very sick and often hospitalized patients with advanced pituitary or adrenal insufficiency, end-stage liver or renal disease, or severe HIV infection. The common pathophysiologic denominator is failure of glucose counterregulatory mechanisms to maintain glucose homeostasis. Symptoms may be exacerbated by poor nutritional intake. On occasion, symptomatic hypoglycemia may be noted after severe binge drinking in the absence of food intake. Ill patients are particularly sensitive to the hypoglycemic effects of drugs, including pentamidine when given for *Pneumocystis* pneumonia, trimethoprim/sulfamethoxazole in the setting of renal failure, quinine or quinidine in the setting of malaria, and propoxyphene in renal failure.

True Reactive Hypoglycemia (after Gastric Surgery). Onset of true hypoglycemia 1 to 2 hours after eating characterizes the reactive hypoglycemia of patients who have undergone gastric surgery. About 5% to 10% of such patients experience a reactive hypoglycemia, believed related to pyloric sphincter incompetence and the excessively rapid entry of concentrated carbohydrates into the small bowel. Unidentified gut factors are stimulated, causing the release of excessive insulin. Symptoms should not be confused with those of the dumping syndrome (see Chapter 64), which consist of nausea, fullness, and weakness developing within an hour after eating. An occasional patient with a functional defect in gastric emptying may present in similar fashion.

Functional Reactive "Hypoglycemia" designates a common postprandial syndrome in which autonomic hypoglycemia-like symptoms occur within 2 to 4 hours after a meal and may be relieved by eating a snack. Patients may report that symptoms are especially likely to occur with the intake of concentrated sweets. Some authorities argue that the designation of "functional reactive hypoglycemia" is inappropriate because the serum glucose is usually normal at the time symptoms occur, so that the criteria of Whipple's triad are not met. Insulin secretion is normal, and no relation between glucose levels and symptoms can be demonstrated. The pathophysiology of this alimentary variant is unknown, but it may respond to a high-protein, low-carbohydrate diet. The "functional reactive hypoglycemia" label is also sometimes applied inappropriately to asymptomatic patients who manifest a low serum glucose during a 5-hour glucose tolerance test, a normal occurrence in 10% to 20% of healthy persons.

DIFFERENTIAL DIAGNOSIS

The traditional classification of fasting versus reactive hypoglycemia is fading from use as it becomes increasingly appreciated that reactive hypoglycemia is not a diagnosis except in patients who have undergone gastric surgery. Proposed new classification schemes categorize causes of hypoglycemia according to "healthy versus ill-appearing patient" and "insulin-related versus non–insulin-related." For the purposes of office-based differential diagnosis by the primary care physician, the main diagnostic issue is less one of determining the cause of hypoglycemia than of confirming its presence. Nonetheless, categorizations can be helpful (Table 97.1).

Two important groups of nonhypoglycemic patients must be differentiated from patients who manifest genuine falls in glucose in conjunction with symptoms. One group comprises persons with *anxiety* or *depression* who have multiple bodily complaints of a functional or psychophysiologic nature (see Chapters 226, 227, and 230). The most common symptoms include fatigue, headache, spasms, palpitations, numbness,

Table 97.1.   Some Important Causes of True Hypoglycemia Seen in the Office Setting

Patient Looks Healthy/Insulin-Related
Excessively tight diabetic control with insulin or sulfonylurea therapy
Factious hypoglycemia induced by surreptitious insulin administration
Sulfonylurea overdose
Insulinoma
Intense exercise
Prior gastric surgery
Early type 2 diabetes

Patient Looks Ill/Non–Insulin-Related
End-stage renal disease
End-stage liver disease
HIV infection, severe
Pituitary failure
Alcohol binge, severe, with little food intake
Hepatic dysfunction secondary to severe congestive heart failure, sepsis, infiltrative disease
Insulin-like growth factor II production by malignancy (most patients are ill)

Patient Looks Ill/Drug-Related
Pentamidine for *Pneumocystis* pneumonia
Salicylates in renal failure
Propoxyphene in renal failure
Trimethoprim/sulfamethoxazole in renal failure
Quinine in cerebral malaria

---

sweating, and mental dullness. These patients attribute their symptoms to "hypoglycemia" to explain their difficulties and avoid the psychosocial issues at hand. Requests for glucose tolerance testing are frequent. A second group is bothered by postprandial symptoms very similar to those experienced by patients with reactive hypoglycemia, but in the context of normal serum sugar levels.

WORKUP

The first task is to confirm that the patient with low blood glucose or "hypoglycemic" symptoms actually has true hypoglycemia. Complicating the evaluation is the difficulty of documenting the relationship between symptoms and blood glucose level. Once the criteria of Whipple's triad have been met, then the focus shifts to detecting important treatable disease, which may sometimes be obvious; however, in other cases, a search for occult disease or surreptitious patient behavior may be necessary.

Identifying True Hypoglycemia

Diagnostic Criteria (Whipple's Triad). The diagnostic criteria include (a) symptoms consistent with neuroglycopenia (blurred or double vision, confusion, odd behavior, lethargy) or adrenergic stimulation (anxiety, tremulousness, headache, palpitations, sweats); (b) a low serum glucose concentration (<50 mg/dL, 2.8 mmol/L) at the time of symptoms; and (c) relief of symptoms when the glucose level returns to normal. These criteria are sometimes referred to as *Whipple's triad,* named for the physician who first suggested them as a means of distinguishing normal persons from those with underlying disease. Simply having adrenergic symptoms or a low serum glucose level in the absence of symptoms does not suffice because many healthy persons may have an isolated glucose level below 50

mg/dL. The objective is to document the correlation between symptoms and a low serum glucose concentration. Without such documentation, one cannot make a diagnosis of physiologically significant hypoglycemia. The occurrence of symptoms in the presence of a normal blood glucose level rules out true hypoglycemia.

Testing and Confirming True Hypoglycemia. Determination of the *serum glucose at the time of symptoms* is essential for diagnosis and helps eliminate from consideration the large number of cases with symptoms that are not caused by hypoglycemia. In a study of patients referred with a presumptive diagnosis of reactive hypoglycemia, fewer than 20% actually had a serum glucose level below 50 mg/dL during symptoms—a finding that emphasizes the importance of a blood sugar determination at the time of symptoms. If the blood glucose level is above 50 mg/dL at the time of symptoms, then true hypoglycemia is ruled out. The traditional 5-hour oral *glucose tolerance test* is not indicated because it provides no useful information. Even if a low blood glucose level is detected during glucose tolerance testing (which occurs in up to 20% of normal persons), the number is meaningless in the absence of a correlation with symptoms. Thus, the glucose tolerance test can be skipped. More important is a determination of the glucose level at the time of symptoms.

Finger-stick methods have improved the ability to sample blood sugar at the time of symptoms, although reagent strip techniques may be inaccurate at low glucose concentrations and self-testing poorly performed when patients are symptomatic. Venipuncture is more accurate but less convenient. However, a sample is worth obtaining as long as symptoms are present because the serum glucose level is usually low in the presence of symptoms.

Patients not fulfilling criteria for hypoglycemia should be evaluated for other conditions. It is essential that one avoid mislabeling them as hypoglycemic, even if symptoms follow meals. In a study of 28 patients with suspected postprandial hypoglycemia, only 20% had abnormal glucose levels at the time of symptoms. Patients with no correlation between their symptoms and serum glucose levels are unlikely to have an underlying disturbance in glucose homeostasis. For them, an alternative explanation for symptoms should be sought. Symptoms of *anxiety* disorders, *depression,* and *hyperthyroidism* may mimic those of hypoglycemia. A story of early morning awakening, chronic fatigue, and disturbed appetite and libido in conjunction with a history of personally significant losses provides strong presumptive evidence for depression (see Chapter 227). Paroxysms of anxiety, palpitations, difficulty in breathing, and chest tightness unrelated to meals suggest a panic attack disorder (see Chapter 226). The presence of heat intolerance, weight loss despite normal food intake, constant nervousness unrelated to meals, and skin and hair changes point to hyperthyroidism (see Chapter 103).

Evaluating True Hypoglycemia

History. Once hypoglycemia has been established, the evaluation proceeds to determine whether the condition is insulin-related or not. In diabetics, the use of *insulin* and *sulfonylurea agents* needs to be reviewed (biguanides and thiazolidinediones do not in themselves confer a risk for hypoglycemia; see Chapter 102). As noted earlier, intensive insulin therapy may reduce the counterregulatory responses to hypoglycemia and lower the glucose level at which symptoms occur, so that a high index of suspicion is necessary. A person using such drugs surreptitiously is likely to deny any intake, but a *vocational history* of medical or paramedical work should raise one's index of suspicion. If *postprandial* symptoms develop, then one should check for a history of *type 2 diabetes* or *gastric surgery*. In a patient with a history of gastric surgery, onset within 1 to 2 hours after eating is very strong evidence for rapid emptying as the underlying pathophysiology. Symptoms beginning 3 to 5 hours after eating in a patient with a family history of diabetes or recent development of polyuria/polydipsia argues for early type 2 diabetes.

The physician checks for non–insulin-related causes by inquiring into recent *binge drinking* in the absence of food intake, end-stage *liver* or *kidney disease*, *adrenal insufficiency*, marked *hypopituitarism*, and a history of *malignancy*. Such persons are ill and the cause is usually evident, with symptoms of the underlying condition dominating the clinical presentation (see Chapters 71, 101, and 142).

Patients with *insulinomas* report few symptoms other than those related to their hypoglycemia, which typically worsen *after exercise* or in the *absence of food intake* (e.g., just before breakfast or late in the afternoon, especially with exercise). The occurrence of neuroglycopenic symptoms (blurred vision, diplopia, sweats, confusion, poor memory) during these periods should raise suspicion of the diagnosis. Because insulinomas often develop in the context of multiple endocrine neoplasia type 1, symptoms of hypercalcemia may be evident (see Chapter 96).

Physical Examination. In most cases of reactive hypoglycemia, few etiologically suggestive physical findings are noted. The exception is the upper abdominal surgical scar in a patient who has undergone gastric surgery. Patients with fasting hypoglycemia should be checked for postural hypotension, alcohol on the breath, needle marks at common insulin injection sites, jaundice, ecchymoses, hyperpigmentation, visual field defects, abdominal mass, ascites, and other signs of hepatocellular failure (see Chapter 71). A careful neurologic examination is essential to rule out focal neurologic injury, which would indicate a cause of symptoms other than hypoglycemia.

Laboratory Studies can help in the differentiation between insulin-related and non–insulin-related causes. Concurrent measurements of serum *insulin*, *C-peptide* (formed as proinsulin and split during endogenous synthesis), and *glucose* at the time of symptoms are key to the differentiation. Often, an *overnight fast* is sufficient to elicit hypoglycemia and make possible these simultaneous determinations. Because exercise promotes a fall in serum glucose, it may be used in conjunction with fasting to elicit hypoglycemia and precipitate symptoms. In two thirds of patients with insulinomas, hypoglycemia develops within 24 hours; fewer than 5% have to fast for 72 hours (which requires an inpatient admission).

Inappropriately high levels of insulin in the presence of a low glucose level suggest an insulin-related cause; low or normal insulin levels are indicative of a cause other than insulin. An insulin-to-glucose ratio in excess of 0.3 is consistent with insulinoma and characteristically increases as fasting progresses. An insulin level above 6 to 10 μg/mL and a C-peptide level above 0.2 to 0.4 nmol/ml strongly suggest insulinoma but may also occur with surreptitious sulfonlyurea use, which can be identified by testing a urine or serum sample for the presence of *sulfonylurea*. A high insulin level in the setting of a low C-peptide level indicates an exogenous insulin source. When insulinoma is a concern and more laboratory evidence is desired, a *C-peptide suppression test* can be performed. Insulin is infused during 1 hour, and C-peptide levels are monitored. Failure to suppress C-peptide formation strongly suggests insulinoma.

Testing to locate an insulinoma can be difficult. In most settings, preoperative assessment by *ultrasonography* or *computed tomography* is adequate for lesions larger than 1.5 cm in diameter but insufficient for smaller lesions. A host of modalities for improved preoperative localization are being developed, but palpation by the surgeon with the aid of intraoperative ultrasonography remains the best means of localization at present.

The need for additional studies in patients with non–insulin-dependent hypoglycemia depends on the clinical context. *Cortisol* and *ACTH* determinations are indicated if hypopituitarism or adrenal insufficiency is suspected (see Chapter 101). Extensive liver function testing may be superfluous if the patient is floridly jaundiced and ecchymotic, but the prothrombin time and serum albumin remain the best measures of hepatocellular synthetic function (see Chapter 71). When tumor-induced hypoglycemia is suspected, an *IGF-II* determination can be considered; usually, the tumor has been identified earlier.

SYMPTOMATIC MANAGEMENT

Hypoglycemia is best treated by attending to the underlying cause (e.g., removing the insulinoma, debulking a tumor producing IGF-II, arranging for psychotherapy for self-destructive behavior, adjusting the diabetes treatment regimen; see Chapter 102). Those with postprandial hypoglycemia (e.g., *after gastric surgery*) may respond to dietary interventions, such as *frequent feedings* (six per day) and diets *high in protein* and *low in concentrated carbohydrate*. In addition, treatment with anticholinergic agents (e.g., 7.5 mg of propantheline before meals) delays gastric emptying; results are fair at best. Other approaches include administration a β-blocking agent before meals (e.g., 10 mg of propranolol), reversal of a 10-cm segment of the jejunum, and administration of pectin.

Patients who have postprandial symptoms without hypoglycemia (i.e., those previously labeled as having *functional reactive hypoglycemia*) may benefit from similar dietary measures, although no controlled studies have established the efficacy of any of these dietary manipulations. Some patients note that avoidance of concentrated sweets is helpful, but the mechanisms of symptom production and reduction remain unclear.

PATIENT EDUCATION

The patient who seeks medical attention because of a fear of hypoglycemia should be taken seriously, but once the diagnosis has been ruled out, reassurance and refocusing attention to other possible causes of symptoms should follow. Patients with underlying psychopathology may initially refuse to accept the fact that hypoglycemia is not responsible for their symptoms because the attribution serves as a psychologically comfortable explanation. One needs to explore their concerns sympathetically while redirecting further evaluation to an exploration of anxiety, depression, and somatization disorders (see Chapters 226, 227, and 230). The patient with "functional reactive hypoglycemia" whose glucose levels are normal during the occurrence of symptoms can be reassured that although the symptoms are "real," they are not related to low blood glucose or disturbances in glucose homeostasis, and that simple dietary recommendations (see above) may be helpful. Requests for glucose tolerance testing are common, but they are readily withdrawn when the lack of specificity of the test is explained. Patients with a suspected insulinoma appreciate being told that almost all cases are benign, and that removal of the tumor cures their condition, with little risk for relapse or recurrence.

INDICATIONS FOR ADMISSION AND REFERRAL

Patients with suspected insulinoma are at risk for a profound fall in serum glucose and should be referred promptly to an endocrinologist and surgeon familiar with the management of this rare condition. Those with severe symptoms (seizure, mental confusion) should be admitted immediately to the hospital for glucose infusion and detailed evaluation. Routine referral of patients with postprandial symptoms for glucose tolerance testing is no longer considered appropriate.

A.H.G.

ANNOTATED BIBLIOGRAPHY

Boyle PJ, Schwartz NS, Shah SD, et al. Plasma glucose concentrations at the outset of hypoglycemic symptoms in patients with poorly controlled diabetes and in nondiabetics. N Engl J Med 1988;318:1487. (*Symptoms occur at higher glucose levels when the diabetes is poorly controlled.*)

Charles MA, Hofeldt F, Shackelford A, et al. Comparison of oral glucose tolerance tests and mixed meals in patients with apparent idiopathic postabsorptive hypoglycemia. Diabetes 1981;30:465. (*Mixed meals did not cause hypoglycemia, but a glucose load did; provides a rationale for treatment.*)

Cryer PE, Binder C, Bolli GB, et al. Hypoglycemia in IDDM. Diabetes 1989;38:1193. (*Excellent review of the problem.*)

Fajans SS, Floyd JC. Fasting hypoglycemia in adults. N Engl J Med 1976;294:766. (*A physiologically oriented review of fasting hypoglycemia, with a table of causes organized around pathophysiologic mechanisms.*)

Felig P, Cherif A, Minagawa A, et al. Hypoglycemia during prolonged exercise in normal men. N Engl J Med 1982;306:895. (*A normal event during maximal exertion.*)

Gastineau CF. Is reactive hypoglycemia a clinical entity? Mayo Clin Proc 1983;58:545. (*An example of the debate surrounding the issue.*)

Kioschinsky T, Dannehl K, Gries FA. New approach to technical and clinical evaluation of devices for self-monitoring of blood glucose. Diabetes Care 1988;11:619. (*Useful critique of self-monitoring techniques.*)

LeRoith D. Insulin-like growth factors. N Engl J Med 1997;338:633. (*Detailed summary for the generalist reader, including mechanisms of hypoglycemia in patients with tumors.*)

Lev-Ran A, Anderson RW. The diagnosis of postprandial hypoglycemia. Diabetes 1981;30:996. (*Data indicating a diagnosis of reactive hypoglycemia, with a discussion focusing on what constitutes a "low" glucose level.*)

Merimee TJ, Tyson JE. Stabilization of plasma glucose during fasting—normal variations in two separate studies. N Engl J Med 1974;291:1275. (*Fasting blood sugar levels in normal women may be as low as 40 mg/dL.*)

Oberg K, Skogseid B, Eriksson B. Multiple endocrine neoplasia type I: clinical, biochemical, and genetic investigations. Acta Oncol 1989;28:383. (*Comprehensive review of this syndrome, which can include insulinoma.*)

Palardy J, Havrankova J, LePage R, et al. Blood glucose measurements during symptomatic episodes in patients with suspected postprandial hypoglycemia. N Engl J Med 1989;321:1421. (*Study of a referral population indicating that postprandial hypoglycemia is infrequent and that glucose tolerance testing is of little diagnostic utility.*)

Ritholz MD, Jacobson AM. Living with hypoglycemia. J Gen Intern Med 1998;13:799. (*Qualitative study underscoring the experiential dimension of the problem.*)

Scarlett JA, Mako ME, Rubenstein AH, et al. Factitious hypoglycemia: diagnosis by measurement of serum C-peptide and insulin-binding antibodies. N Engl J Med 1977;297:1029. (*Documents the usefulness of these measures in patients who self-administer insulin surreptitiously.*)

Service FJ. Hypoglycemic disorders. N Engl J Med 1995;332:1144. (*Iconoclastic review by one of the leading authorities in the field, who proposes a new classification; 113 references.*)

Service FJ. Hypoglycemia and the postprandial syndrome. N Engl J Med 1989;321:1472. (*An editorial emphasizing that most patients with postprandial syndrome do not have hypoglycemia.*)

Service FJ, Horwitz DL, Rubenstein AH, et al. C-peptide suppression test for insulinoma. J Lab Clin Med 1977;13:571. (*Initial description of the test.*)

Simonson DC, Tamborlane WV, DeFronzo RA, et al. Intensive insulin therapy reduces counterregulatory hormone responses to hypoglycemia in patients with type I diabetes. Ann Intern Med 1985;103:184. (*Documents risk for profound hypoglycemia in such patients.*)

Yeager J, Young RT. Nonhypoglycemia as an epidemic condition. N Engl J Med 1974;291:907. (*A succinct discussion of how to manage patients with self-diagnosed "hypoglycemia."*)

98
Evaluation of Hirsutism
SAMUEL R. NUSSBAUM

Hirsutism in women is caused by increased androgenic activity and is characterized by the excessive growth of hormone-dependent pubic, axillary, abdominal, chest, and facial hair. Women are likely to present for evaluation when such hair growth is viewed as exceeding that of others in their societal, geographic, or racial environment. For a woman living in a society preoccupied with stereotyped perceptions of beauty, hirsutism may be extremely upsetting and connote loss of femininity and sexuality. For the primary physician, hirsutism raises the question of an underlying endocrinopathy, ranging in severity from minor changes in androgen metabolism to the development of a hormonally active neoplasm.

When confronted with women with excessive hair growth, the primary care physician must decide whom to begin evaluating for endocrine disease and whom to reassure or treat symptomatically. Women with signs of virilization, progressive hair growth beginning after age 25, or concurrent amenorrhea should undergo endocrine evaluation (see below).

PATHOPHYSIOLOGY AND CLINICAL PRESENTATION

Pathophysiology. Hirsutism is a manifestation of excessive androgenic effect. The hormonal stimulus for hair growth is *5-α-dihydrotestosterone,* a potent testosterone metabolite derived from the peripheral conversion at the hair follicle of testosterone by 5-α-reductase. *δ-4-Androstenedione* and *dehydroepiandrosterone* (DHEA), produced by the ovaries and adrenal glands, are the *precursors* for 50% to 70% of circulating testosterone in women; the remainder of the testosterone is secreted directly by the ovaries or occasionally by the adrenals.

Hirsute women generally have *increased production rates of DHEA* and δ-4-androstenedione, which are relatively weak androgens, or of *testosterone,* a more potent androgen. Serum measurements of the total concentrations of androgens reflect the binding of sex steroid hormones to sex hormone–binding globulin; however, only the free fraction, which in the case of testosterone is 1% of total testosterone, is biologically active. The source of enhanced androgen production may be the *ovary,* the *adrenal gland,* or both. *Hyperinsulinism* resulting from insulin resistance has been noted to trigger excess ovarian androgen production, providing a possible link between *obesity* and hirsutism, a common association. In addition, obesity leads to a reduction in the concentration of sex hormone–binding globulin.

Virilization (temporal hair recession, acne, deepening voice, increased muscle mass, and clitoromegaly) develops when autonomous androgen production originating in an adrenal or ovarian neoplasm results in extremely high levels of circulating androgens.

Clinical Presentation. Hair follicles are located over the entire body except for the palms and soles. Hair growth is of two types; lanugo (neonatal) or vellus hair is soft, unpigmented, and rarely more than 2 cm long, whereas terminal hair is coarse and pigmented and grows in excess of 2 cm. A survey of college women revealed that one fourth had easily noticeable facial hair, one third reported hair extending along the linea alba from the pubic area (male escutcheon), and 17% had periareolar hair. Three fourths of women over age 60 have a measurable growth of facial hair. Hirsutism has familial, ethnic, and racial patterns. Eastern European women are more hirsute than Scandinavian women; white women are more hirsute than black women, who have more body hair than Asian women. The *Ferriman-Gallwey scale* is used to define and grade hirsutism. Hair growth in each of nine androgen-dependent areas of the body is graded from 0 (no hair growth) to 4 (frankly virile growth). A score of 8 or more is generally accepted as indicative of hirsutism.

Ovarian Sources. The majority of women with nonvirilizing hirsutism in conjunction with oligomenorrhea or amenorrhea have *polycystic ovary disease.* Gonadotropin dynamics are abnormal, with a loss of pulsatile secretion of luteinizing hormone (LH), an increased ratio of LH to follicle-stimulating hormone (FSH), and elevated levels of LH. Concurrent obesity and insulin resistance are noted in many patients, which contribute to androgen excess. Both LH and insulin stimulate excessive secretion of ovarian testosterone and androstenedione. Large numbers of small ovarian follicles form, but follicular growth is abnormal and no preovulatory follicles develop. Menstrual abnormalities and infertility are the consequence (see Chapter 112). The ovaries may be of normal size or enlarged, and they characteristically contain multiple follicular cysts.

Ovarian hyperthecosis, which may be seen in association with the syndrome of acanthosis nigricans and insulin resistance, and *ovarian tumors,* including arrhenoblastomas and hilar cell tumors, are capable of causing *virilization* through an excess production of testosterone. The virilized patient often has testosterone levels exceeding 200 ng/dL.

Adrenal Sources. *Late-onset congenital adrenal hyperplasia* designates a heterogeneous group of mild disorders of cortisol biosynthesis (most commonly partial deficiency of 21-hydroxylase or 3-δ-hydroxydehydrogenase) that are increasingly recognized as an important cause of adult-onset hirsutism. The enzyme deficiencies lead to the production of abnormal amounts of adrenal androgen. These conditions are inherited as an autosomal recessive trait closely linked to the HLA gene. Menstrual abnormalities are noted in conjunction with hirsutism, but clinically significant glucocorticoid deficiency does not occur.

Cushing's syndrome, especially if the underlying cause is an *adrenocortical carcinoma,* may produce virilization. Other causes of Cushing's syndrome are more likely to produce excess hair growth and typical cushingoid features without true virilization.

Androgen excess may accompany *hyperprolactinemia* because prolactin stimulates androgen production, particularly DHEA. Characteristic features are amenorrhea and galactorrhea (see Chapter 113).

Other Causes. Hirsutism in women with normal periods and normal plasma androgens is often labeled *idiopathic.* Although initially believed to be a consequence of overproduction of testosterone, idiopathic disease is now viewed as a condition of enhanced peripheral conversion of testosterone to dihydrotestosterone by increased 5-α-reductase activity in hair follicles and skin.

Drugs are another important cause of hirsutism. Most potent are the *anabolic steroids* (methyltestosterone, oxandrolone), used surreptitiously by some women engaged in competitive body building or athletics. The sex steroid precursor *androstenedione* is available without prescription and is very popular among adolescents; it is estimated that 2.5% of all adolescent girls take the drug regularly, especially those engaged in competitive athletics. When used in doses of 300 mg/d by young men, it results in increased levels of testosterone and estradiol. Similar increases in sex hormones are likely in young women, although they are not yet documented. Danazol, used to treat endometriosis, may also bring on hirsutism. In an occasional patient, oral contraceptives containing androgenic progestogens may stimulate hair growth (see Chapter 119), although this is not a frequent side effect. Phenytoin, glucocorticoids, cyclosporine, diazoxide, and minoxidil stimulate hair growth by poorly understood, nonandrogenic mechanisms.

DIFFERENTIAL DIAGNOSIS

The causes of hirsutism can be divided into those that do and do not cause virilization and categorized according to adrenal and ovarian sources of androgen excess (Table 98.1). In a series of 100 outpatients presenting to an endocrine unit for evaluation of true hirsutism, about 75% had polycystic ovary

Table 98.1. Differential Diagnosis of Hirsutism

CAUSE	MECHANISM
Hirsutism without Virilization	
Idiopathic	Increased peripheral conversion of androgens
Late-onset congenital adrenal hyperplasia	Adrenal androgen overproduction
Cushing's syndrome (ACTH-induced)	Adrenal androgen overproduction
Polycystic ovary disease	Ovarian androgen overproduction
Insulin resistance/obesity	Ovarian androgen overproduction
Drugs: anabolic steroids, danazol, minoxidil, phenytoin, diazoxide, glucocorticoids	Varies, ranging from direct androgenic activity to nonandrogenic effects
Hirsutism with Virilization	
Ovarian hyperthecosis	Autonomous ovarian androgen production
Ovarian neoplasms	Autonomous ovarian androgen production
Adrenal neoplasms, especially adrenal carcinoma	Autonomous adrenal androgen production

ACTH, adrenocorticotropic hormone.

disease, 15% were labeled idiopathic, and 3% had late-onset congenital adrenal hyperplasia. In the remainder of the cases, Cushing's disease, ovarian tumor, prolactinoma, or drug use was identified as the cause. In addition, some patients with anorexia nervosa report an increase in body hair (see Chapter 234), and excessive tweezing (hypertrichosis) may traumatize the hair follicle and cause coarse hair to grow at the site of repeated injury.

WORKUP

The paramount objective in the evaluation of hirsutism is to identify the women who are likely to have important underlying endocrine disease.

History

Features suggestive of serious endocrine disease include *virilization* (voice change, temporal hair recession, increased muscle mass, acne); *rapid progression*, particularly a sudden increase in hair growth after age 25; *amenorrhea* or menstrual changes; and *galactorrhea*. The new onset of *hypertension* in the setting of hirsutism should also raise suspicion. A peripubertal onset of hirsutism is generally reassuring. A detailed *drug history* (anabolic steroids, oral contraceptives, danazol, phenytoin, corticosteroids, minoxidil, cyclosporine, diazoxide) is essential. Inquiry into any daily or regular use of nonprescription sex hormone precursors, such as *androstenedione*, is essential because the substance is popular among adolescent competitive athletes who take it to enhance their performance (estimated prevalence of regular use among adolescent women is 2.5%). *Southern European* or *Mediterranean ancestry* in conjunction with hirsutism of a similar degree in a mother, grandmothers, aunts, and sisters reduces the probability of serious disease. However, a positive family history may also be found in some patients with polycystic ovary disease and partial congenital adrenal hyperplasia.

Physical Examination

Terminal hair on the face, about the areolae, and on the lower abdomen is normal, but new growth, especially on the upper abdomen, sternum, upper back, and shoulders, suggests androgen excess and hirsutism. Virilization is indicated by temporal and vertical scalp hair loss, a deep voice, acne, an increase in muscle mass, and clitoromegaly. Cushing's syndrome should be suspected when centripetal obesity, muscle wasting with myopathy, and violaceous striae are encountered. Patients with oligomenorrhea require a pelvic examination to detect bilaterally enlarged cystic ovaries; however, a significant number of women with polycystic ovary physiology do not have palpable ovarian abnormalities. Women with virilization and amenorrhea should be examined carefully for a palpable adrenal or ovarian neoplasm. Most of these tumors are inefficient producers of androgens and do not result in high levels of circulating androgens until they become quite large.

Laboratory Studies

An abundance of costly endocrinologic hormonal assays may be performed in the evaluation of hirsutism. To avoid the expense of unnecessary testing, it is important to define the likely diagnostic considerations and the goals of therapy for hirsutism so that appropriate hormonal evaluation may be obtained, rather than the indiscriminate measurement of all ovarian and androgen sex steroids and pituitary hormones. On the basis of the history and physical examination findings, patients can be categorized as likely to have idiopathic or familial, oligomenorrheic/amenorrheic, cushingoid, or virilizing forms of disease.

Idiopathic and Familial Forms of Hirsutism. A young woman with a minor increase in facial hair beginning in the peripubertal period but with perfectly regular ovulatory menses is most likely free of serious underlying disease and need not undergo detailed testing. The same pertains to the normally menstruating woman of southern European ancestry whose female relatives have similar amounts of facial and body hair.

Oligomenorrheic/Amenorrheic Disease. When amenorrhea or oligomenorrhea, obesity, and hirsutism occur, especially in the context of infertility, polycystic ovary disease needs to be considered. Because pelvic examination may not reveal bilaterally enlarged cystic ovaries, *pelvic ultrasonography* and laboratory testing can help to confirm the clinical suspicions. Testosterone, particularly *unbound testosterone*, and *ratios of LH to FSH* are increased. Because an increase in androgens suppresses sex hormone–binding globulin, measurement of the unbound or *free serum testosterone* is more valuable than measurement of the total testosterone. Free testosterone correlates best with testosterone production rates. Because testosterone secretion is episodic, *three serum samples* taken 15 minutes apart may be pooled for immunoassay.

Patients with menstrual irregularities but no evidence of polycystic disease should be evaluated for a late-onset congenital adrenal hyperplasia (most often 21-hydroxylase deficiency). This condition can be identified by performing an *ACTH stimulation test* and measuring the *plasma 17-hydroxyprogesterone* 30 to 60 minutes after the IV administration of one ampule (25 μg) of cosyntropin (synthetic ACTH). A pretest level of 17-hydroxyprogesterone above 300 ng/dL is suggestive, but many patients have normal levels, so that ACTH stimulation testing is necessary. A posttest level above 1,200 ng/dL at 30 minutes is diagnostic. Although these patients represent a minority of hirsute women, no distinguishing clinical features of this entity set it apart from the more common polycystic ovary syndromes. *Prolactin* should be measured in women with oligomenorrhea or amenorrhea, especially if galactorrhea is also present.

Cushingoid Appearance. Patients with clinical features of Cushing's syndrome should be screened with either a *24-hour urinary free cortisol determination* or an *overnight dexamethasone suppression test*. The 24-hour urinary free cortisol determination, which is the more specific study, is above 100 μg in Cushing's syndrome. *Urinary 17-ketosteroids* are elevated in adrenocortical carcinoma. For overnight dexamethasone suppression, the patient is given 1 mg of dexamethasone at midnight, and the plasma cortisol is measured at approximately 8:00 a.m. the next day. Cortisol should be suppressed to below 5 μg/dL. If the 24-hour urinary free cortisol is elevated, or an elevated cortisol is not suppressed by dexamethasone, more extensive dexamethasone testing to determine the likelihood and cause of Cushing's syndrome needs to be pursued.

Virilization. When virilization is present, *serum testosterone* and *urinary 17-ketosteroids* should be measured. The serum testosterone level will be above 200 ng/dL in women with masculinizing ovarian or adrenal neoplasms. Measurement of 17-ketosteroids detects elevated adrenal androgens, such as androstenedione and DHEA in adrenal cortical carcinoma. Although both the adrenals and ovaries can synthesize all the androgenic steroids, adrenal hormonal production is best assessed by measuring *DHEA sulfate*, as more than 90% is formed in the adrenal gland. A serum DHEA level above 800 μg/dL strongly suggests an adrenal tumor. Androstenedione is synthesized equally by the adrenal and ovary glands. When the presence of a tumor is suspected in one of these glands, *ultrasonography* or *computed tomography* is required. Before a search for tumor is begun, the history should again be checked for the regular use of exogenous androstenedione, as in competitive athletes, especially adolescent girls, for body building.

SYMPTOMATIC MANAGEMENT AND PATIENT EDUCATION

Alternative approaches to the management of hirsutism are based on the underlying pathophysiology. They include (a) supportive reassurance that no important underlying endocrine disease is present; (b) cosmetic manipulations, such as bleaching, waxing, use of depilatories, and electrolysis; (c) medical therapy with estrogens or glucocorticoids directed at suppressing ovarian and adrenal hormone overproduction; (d) medical therapy directed at antagonizing the action of androgens at the receptor level; and (e) definitive curative therapy of underlying diseases such as Cushing's syndrome or masculinizing ovarian neoplasms.

Supportive Measures and Cosmetic Manipulations. Patients free of significant endocrine disease can be effectively managed with *reassurance* that hirsutism does not impair sexuality or fertility. Adolescents taking exogenous sex hormone precursors such as androstenedione to enhance their athletic performance will benefit from a nonjudgmental review of the cosmetic and developmental consequences of taking these "natural" supplements.

If a woman is concerned about her appearance, cosmetic manipulation or medical therapy is appropriate. Hair may be bleached with a *6% hydrogen peroxide* solution or commercially available cream bleaches. Shaving removes unwanted hair; however, because hair grows at the rate of 1 mm/d, "stubble" appears within several days. *Epilation* with tweezers or hot wax may retard hair growth for several months but may cause low-grade folliculitis. *Chemical depilation* may require the use of low-concentration hydrocortisone topically to prevent irritation. *Electrolysis*, the only permanent method of hair removal, involves electrocoagulation and destruction of the hair root. It is a costly and time-consuming process and should be performed only by a licensed electrologist.

Suppression of Ovarian and Adrenal Androgen Overproduction. *Oral contraceptives* containing estrogen and progestin suppress ovarian and adrenal androgen production by decreasing levels of FSH and LH. In addition, the estrogen increases sex hormone–binding globulin levels, competes with the cytosolic receptor for dihydrotestosterone, and limits (along with progestogens) endometrial hyperplasia in hyperandrogenic patients with *polycystic ovaries*. Oral contraceptives also work well for patients with *idiopathic disease* by reducing the amount of available androgenic substrate. Preparations containing at least 35 μg of ethinyl estradiol or 50 μg of mestranol are needed to reduce androgen levels; those with lower amounts of estrogen are less effective. The least androgenic progestins, such as norethindrone (1 mg) or ethynodiol acetate in combination with mestranol and ethinyl estradiol, are preferred. If the hormonal and clinical responses to these therapies, determined at 3 months, are inadequate, an oral contraceptive containing larger amounts of estrogen should be used. Side effects of these drugs, including an increased risk for thromboembolism in smokers (see Chapter 119), must be reviewed. A decrease in hirsutism is usually not evident for 3 to 6 months; a decrease in the rate of hair growth is noted initially, followed by a transformation to lighter, finer hair.

Glucocorticoids may reduce hirsutism and induce ovulation in partial *congenital adrenal hyperplasia*, in which the androgens are of adrenal origin. Adrenal suppression with a concomitant decrease in androgens can best be accomplished by administering 1 mg of dexamethasone at bedtime. Potential concerns with this form of therapy are suppression of the hypothalamic–pituitary–adrenal axis and induction of a cushingoid appearance. Alternate-day corticosteroid therapy may suffice and reduce the risk for such adverse effects. Following the changes in the 17-hydroxyprogesterone concentration is an effective means of monitoring therapy.

Weight reduction should be part of any program for the obese hirsute woman. Normalization of weight limits the peripheral conversion of androstenedione to testosterone by fatty tissue and reduces the hyperinsulinism that may contribute to ovarian production of androgens. Impressive results can be achieved.

Antagonizing Testosterone at the Target Tissue. *Spironolactone*, an antihypertensive diuretic, decreases androgen levels by decreasing testosterone biosynthesis and antagonizing peripheral action on the hair follicle. Dosages as high as 100 mg twice daily have been shown to diminish hirsutism during a 3-month observation interval but may cause menstrual disturbances. One might begin therapy with 50 mg twice daily taken from day 4 through day 22 of each menstrual cycle. The drug is teratogenic and should not be used in large doses by women of childbearing age. It is often given as an adjunct to oral contraceptives in patients with severe polycystic ovary disease.

Cimetidine, a histamine$_2$-receptor antagonist, competes with androgens for target tissue binding; it appears to be less effective than spironolactone.

Flutamide, a selective androgen receptor antagonist, and *finasteride*, a 5-α-reductase inhibitor, offer improved blockade of testosterone action at the target tissue. Studies are ongoing.

INDICATIONS FOR REFERRAL

Patients with virilization and elevated testosterone levels require evaluation by an endocrinologist and a gynecologist because a virilizing tumor may be present. If polycystic ovary syndrome is present and if infertility is an issue, referral for clomiphene therapy and evaluation for endometrial hyperplasia with endometrial biopsy is appropriate. Hyperprolactinemia necessitates coronal computed tomography or magnetic resonance imaging to recognize a prolactinoma or pathologic process interrupting the dopaminergic inhibition of prolactin. Patients with Cushing's syndrome should be referred for endocrinologic evaluation of a pituitary, adrenal, or ectopic origin.

ANNOTATED BIBLIOGRAPHY

Barnes R, Rosenfield RL. The polycystic ovary syndrome: pathogenesis and treatment. Ann Intern Med 1989;110:386. (*Comprehensive review of disease mechanisms, including loss of LH pulsatility, and treatment modalities based on them.*)

Cumming D, Yang JC, Rebar RW, et al. Treatment of hirsutism with spironolactone. JAMA 1984;247:1295. (*A study of 39 patients; responses observed as early as 2 months, and side effects limited.*)

Ehrmann DA, Rosenfield RL. Hirsutism—beyond the steroidogenic block. N Engl J Med 1990;323:909. (*An editorial summarizing current knowledge and focusing on late-onset congenital adrenal hyperplasia.*)

Eldar-Geva T, Hurwitz A, Vecsei P, et al. Secondary biosynthetic defects in women with late-onset congenital adrenal hyperplasia. N Engl J Med 1990;323:855. (*High incidence of the condition found among Israeli women with hirsutism, menstrual disorders, and unexplained infertility; mechanisms examined.*)

Leder BZ, Longcope C, Catlin DH, et al. Oral androstenedione administration and serum testosterone in young men. JAMA 2000;283:779. (*In an open-label, 7-day randomized trial in young men, increases in both testosterone and estradiol were found when androstenedione was taken at a dosage of 300 mg/d. The study was too brief and limited to male patients, but sex hormone levels were often above normal, which indicates that prolonged use can cause hirsutism and even virilization.*)

Rittmaster RS, Loriaux DL. Hirsutism. Ann Intern Med 1987;106:95. (*Very useful review, with a detailed discussion of idiopathic disease; exhaustively referenced with 246 citations.*)

Siegel SF, Finegold DN, Lanes R, et al. ACTH stimulation tests and plasma dehydroepiandrosterone sulfate levels in women with hirsutism. N Engl J Med 1990;323:849. (*Basal levels were unrevealing, but levels measured after ACTH stimulation differed between normal subjects and many of those with hirsutism.*)

Vigersky RA, Hehlman I, Glass AR, et al. Treatment of hirsute women with cimetidine. N Engl J Med 1980;303:1042. (*Cimetidine produced a decrease in rate of hair growth without a decrease in serum androgen.*)

Wagner RF Jr. Physical methods for the management of hirsutism. Cutis 1990;45:319. (*Useful information to give patients.*)

Yesalis CE, Barsukiewicz CK, Kopstien AN, et al. Trends in anabolic–androgenic steroid use among adolescents. Arch Pediatr Adolesc Med 1997;151:1197. (*Use among female adolescents estimated to be 2.5%.*)

99
Evaluation of Gynecomastia

Gynecomastia is defined as enlargement of the male breast as the result of an increase in glandular tissue, which distinguishes it from simple obesity. Some patients present out of fear of loss of masculinity or onset of breast cancer. Others may not have recognized the change and come to the physician at the suggestion of friends or family. Gynecomastia is a normal transient physiologic event in 70% of pubertal boys; its prevalence in adults is less than 1%. The primary physician must be able to recognize gynecomastia and initiate an evaluation to rule out such important potential causes as adrenal and testicular cancers, cirrhosis, and hyperthyroidism. In most instances, the cause is more benign and the tasks are to allay fears and help the patient decide about treatment.

PATHOPHYSIOLOGY AND CLINICAL PRESENTATION

Pathophysiology

Estradiol is the growth hormone of the breast. Gynecomastia represents a phenomenon of relative estradiol excess leading to the proliferation of breast tissue. Under normal circumstances, most estradiol in men is derived from the peripheral conversion of testosterone and adrenal estrone. The basic mechanisms of gynecomastia are a decrease in androgen production, an absolute increase in estrogen production, and an increased availability of estrogen precursors for peripheral conversion to estradiol. Blocking of androgen receptors and increased binding of androgen are additional modes of reduced androgen effect.

Reduced Androgen Production accounts for many cases seen in older men or men with testicular endocrine failure, as after bilateral orchiectomy and other forms of cancer therapy. Ketoconazole inhibits testosterone production in a dose-related manner. *Androgen availability is reduced* in both hyperthyroidism and cirrhosis because of an increase in the serum concentration of sex hormone–binding globulin. *Blockade of androgen receptors* accounts for the gynecomastia associated with use of spironolactone, cimetidine, flutamide, and perhaps marijuana.

Increased Estrogen Production may be seen with Klinefelter's syndrome, adrenal carcinomas, tumors producing ectopic human chorionic gonadotropin (hCG), and Leydigs cell tumors of the testes. Tumors that produce hCG stimulate the testicular production of estradiol. Teratomas of the testes and carcinomas of the lung, pancreas, and colon are known sources of ectopic hCG. The transient gynecomastia of puberty represents a brief physiologic increase in testicular estrogen secretion and lasts 1 to 2 years before receding.

Increased Estrogen Precursor Availability is the mechanism of gynecomastia in patients who have androgen-secreting tumors or congestive heart failure, or who use *exogenous androgen*, which leads to an increased conversion of testosterone and androstenedione to estradiol and estrone. This effect has been documented with the use of *androstenedione*, the popular "natural" sex hormone precursor supplement taken by body builders and adolescents. Hyperthyroidism causes an *increased peripheral conversion*. Much of the conversion takes place in fatty tissue. An *exogenous estrogen effect* is seen with the use of digitalis and synthetic estrogens. Ketoconazole and spironolactone cause a *release of free estrogen* by displacement from sex hormone–binding globulin.

Clinical Presentations

The most noticeable feature is an increase in breast tissue, unilateral in a third of cases. Tenderness may also be noted in a third of patients, but actual pain is less frequent. Enlargement is usually central and symmetric, although it is occasionally eccentric. Idiopathic and drug-induced gynecomastia is usually unilateral, whereas in pubertal and hormonal cases, the changes are often bilateral. It may be that asymmetry is a more accurate description than unilateral enlargement, based on the prevalence of bilaterally histologic but not clinically evident gynecomastia in autopsy series.

A few distinctive clinical presentations are noted. In *Klinefelter's syndrome*, gynecomastia develops around puberty in a patient with long limbs, small and firm testes, infertility, and normal or deficient secondary sex features. In cirrhosis, patients present with loss of libido, loss of body hair, and testicular atrophy (see Chapter 71).

Recovery from *malnutrition* or *serious chronic illnesses* (severe heart failure, renal failure, liver failure) leads to a picture resembling a second puberty, with development of transient gynecomastia.

Carcinoma of the male breast is distinct from gynecomastia; it is characterized by a unilateral, eccentrically located firm mass that may be fixed. Male breast cancer is rare; it is generally not more frequent in patients with gynecomastia, although the incidence in patients with Klinefelter's syndrome is higher.

DIFFERENTIAL DIAGNOSIS

In healthy pubertal boys, transient physiologic gynecomastia is the most likely explanation (Table 99.1). Testicular or adrenal tumors are rare in this age group, but Klinefelter's syndrome may account for a number of cases.

The two most common causes of gynecomastia in adults are drugs and alcohol-related liver disease. Estrogens, androgens, androstenedione, spironolactone, digitalis preparations, flutamide, ketoconazole, cimetidine, and marijuana have all been associated with gynecomastia. The association also exists but is more tenuous with use of phenothiazines, amphetamines, reserpine, methyldopa, isoniazid, imipramine, phenytoin, and heroin. In one series, 22% of patients had a history of taking a drug associated with gynecomastia, and 26% had alcoholic liver disease.

Table 99.1.   Differential Diagnosis of Gynecomastia

Inhibition of Androgen Effect
Spironolactone (at high doses only)
Cimetidine (common at high doses)
Flutamide

Decreased androgen availability secondary to increased binding or conversion
Cirrhosis (very common)
Hyperthyroidism (uncommon, except with thyrotoxicosis)

Decreased Androgen Synthesis
Testicular failure, primary (Klinefelter's syndrome) or secondary (orchiectomy, cancer drugs, ketoconazole)

Increased estrogen synthesis or estrogen effect
Estrogen-secreting tumor of the testis or adrenal gland (very rare)
Klinefelter's syndrome (about 15% of pubertal cases)
Ectopic hCG-secreting tumor of testis, lung, colon, pancreas (rare)
Digitalis (uncommon)
Exogenous estrogen (dose-related)

Increased Availability of Estrogen Substrate
Androgen-producing tumor (rare)
Exogenous androgen (common)
Congestive heart failure (common)

Physiologic
Puberty
Recovery from chronic illness or starvation
Old age

hCG, human chorionic gonadotropin.

Less common causes include recovery from malnutrition or a serious chronic illness. Much rarer forms are tumor-related ectopic hCG production and feminizing adrenal, testicular, and pituitary tumors. In just under 10% of cases, a probable cause is not identified. Gynecomastia must be distinguished from carcinoma of the male breast.

WORKUP

History. The onset, location, duration, and course deserve note. The most important aspect is a detailed inquiry into drug use, including chronic alcoholism and the use of cimetidine, spironolactone, flutamide, digitalis, ketoconazole, or exogenous estrogens or androgens. The use of androstenedione by adolescents and body builders is common and needs to be checked. Any symptoms of hyperthyroidism (see Chapter 103), heart failure (see Chapter 32), or hepatocellular failure (see Chapter 71) should be noted, as should the resolution of a chronic illness and any changes in libido, skin, voice, testicles, and hair quality and distribution. Weight loss, chronic cough, hemoptysis, change in bowel habits, headaches, or visual field disturbances can be important etiologic clues.

Physical Examination. Onset at puberty should trigger an examination for features of Klinefelter's syndrome (arm span greater than height, small and firm testes, absence of secondary sex characteristics). In adults, one needs to look at the skin for signs of hepatocellular failure (jaundice, spider angiomas, ecchymoses, pallor, palmar erythema) and hyperthyroidism (warm, sweaty skin and fine hair). The eyes are checked for exophthalmos, and the neck palpated for goiter.

During the breast examination, the glandular texture of true gynecomastia must be distinguished from the fatty consistency of breast enlargement related to obesity and the nodularity of a carcinoma. Asymmetry and nodules deserve special note, and careful palpation of the axillary nodes is necessary. The question of malignancy in the breast tissue must always be considered in gynecomastia. If the enlargement is unilateral and eccentric, the breast is particularly firm or nodular, or axillary adenopathy is present, then a biopsy should be performed.

On cardiopulmonary examination, one checks for signs of heart failure (see Chapter 32), and on abdominal examination for signs of cirrhosis (see Chapter 71). The abdomen must be palpated for masses and the stool tested for occult blood. The testicles are examined for atrophy and nodules. The presence of a testicular nodule requires workup for a carcinoma (see Chapter 131).

Laboratory Studies. Gynecomastia not associated with puberty, drugs, hyperthyroidism, hepatocellular failure, or another obvious cause requires further evaluation. Laboratory testing should begin with measurement of *serum gonadotropins* (*luteinizing hormone* and *follicle-stimulating hormone*).

High concentrations are consistent with testicular failure, Klinefelter's syndrome, and hCG-secreting tumors. Ectopic hCG production can be identified by finding elevated *serum β-hCG subunit* levels. This should trigger a search for the source of ectopic gonadotropin production (see Chapter 92). To check for Klinefelter's syndrome, a buccal smear is obtained and examined for chromatin positivity (Barr bodies). If the smear is negative, the diagnosis is most likely primary testicular failure or a chromatin-negative variant of Klinefelter's syndrome.

Low gonadotropin concentrations are more worrisome because they raise the question of autonomous androgen or estrogen production (in addition to exogenous sex steroid use). Repeated questioning of the patient regarding exogenous steroid use, including regular use of popular precursor preparations such as *androstenedione*, is critical. If the patient's responses are convincingly negative, then levels of *free testosterone* and *estradiol* should be measured, but with full cognizance of the pitfalls involved in interpreting the results. For example, total testosterone may be affected by the concentration of sex hormone–binding protein and not reflect the free testosterone concentration. Consequently, free testosterone must be measured. However, testosterone secretion can fluctuate greatly, so that three samples obtained during 15 minutes should be pooled for best results. The estradiol concentration measured may correlate poorly with the rate of estrogen production because of vagaries in peripheral uptake. Thus, normal levels do not necessarily rule out an estrogen-secreting tumor, although marked elevations are very suggestive, provided exogenous use has been ruled out. If serum estrogens are elevated, then adrenal cancer and Leydigs cell tumor of the testes should be ruled out.

Normal gonadotropin and *sex hormone levels* make serious underlying endocrinopathy unlikely and can be followed expectantly with periodic reevaluation. It is important to keep in mind that gynecomastia may resolve after the condition that caused it resolves. The search for an underlying cause may yield few clues if the cause was transient and self-limited.

SYMPTOMATIC MANAGEMENT, PATIENT EDUCATION, AND INDICATIONS FOR REFERRAL

Removal of the offending drug usually produces regression of breast enlargement within a month or two. Counseling adolescents who are using androstenedione on a daily basis for body building is especially important because it may help prevent adverse developmental consequences (see Chapter 238). The gynecomastia that accompanies puberty or refeeding after starvation is a transient phenomenon that can be managed by providing reassurance. Resolution of gynecomastia usually follows treatment of hyperthyroidism. Gynecomastia attributable to alcoholic liver disease or Klinefelter's syndrome is not likely to respond to any treatment. When hCG-secreting tumors are discovered, resection of the tumor is indicated if possible.

The persistence of gynecomastia may produce cosmetic problems. Patients who are considerably bothered by breast enlargement may elect to undergo *mastectomy*, but this should be performed only after the underlying cause has been elucidated. Experimental use of the antiestrogen tamoxifen has been useful in reducing breast size in patients with painful gynecomastia.

When a benign condition such as drug-induced gynecomastia is discovered, the patient can be reassured that the condition is not a reflection of loss of maleness or a carcinomatous process. It must be remembered that some conditions that produce gynecomastia may reduce potency; this situation must be confronted and discussed with the patient. No evidence of carcinomatous degeneration in gynecomastia has been found except in Klinefelter's syndrome. Pain, irritation, or social problems that may arise should be dealt with symptomatically and sympathetically.

Consultation with an endocrinologist is essential when a case of Klinefelter's syndrome is suspected, and also when ectopic hCG production is a concern or autonomous sex hormone production is under consideration (low gonadotropin levels). Referral is also indicated when treatment of gynecomastia is being considered, be it medical therapy or surgery.

A.H.G.

ANNOTATED BIBLIOGRAPHY

Bannagan GA, Hajdu SI. Gynecomastia: clinicopathologic study of 351 cases. Am J Clin Pathol 1972;57:431. (*Idiopathic and drug-induced cases of gynecomastia are usually discrete and unilateral, whereas endocrine and pubertal cases are bilateral.*)

Braunstein GD. Gynecomastia. N Engl J Med 1993;328:490. (*Comprehensive review of pathogenesis and clinical issues.*)

Braunstein GD, Vaitukaitis JL, Carbone PP, et al. Ectopic production of human chorionic gonadotropin by neoplasms. Ann Intern Med 1973;78:39. (*One of the original reports of ectopic production of hCG.*)

Cavanaugh J, Niewoehner CB, Nutall FQ. Gynecomastia and cirrhosis of the liver. Arch Intern Med 1990;150:563. (*Factors other than ratio of estrogen to testosterone are operative.*)

Courtiss EH. Gynecomastia: analysis of 159 patients and current recommendations for treatment. Plast Reconstr Surg 1987;79:740. (*The plastic surgeon's perspective.*)

Feldman D. Ketoconazole and other imidazole derivatives as inhibitors of steroidogenesis. Endocr Rev 1986;7:409. (*Detailed discussion of the effects of this important class of drugs on testosterone production.*)

Jensen RT, Collen MJ, Pandol HD. Cimetidine-induced impotence and breast changes in patients with gastric hypersecretory states. N Engl J Med 1983;308:883. (*A side effect of high-dose, long-term therapy; resolves with cessation of cimetidine therapy.*)

Leder BZ, Longcope C, Catlin DH, et al. Oral androstenedione administration and serum testosterone in young men. JAMA 2000;283:779. (*In an open-label, 7-day randomized trial, increases in both testosterone and estradiol were found when androstenedione was taken at a dosage of 300 mg/d; the study was too short to document long-term effects, but sex hormone levels were often above normal.*)

Parker LN, Gray DR, Lai MK, et al. Treatment of gynecomastia with tamoxifen: a double-blind, crossover study. Metabolism 1986;35:705. (*Medical therapy with an antiestrogen proved beneficial for patients with painful gynecomastia.*)

Wilson JD. Gynecomastia: a continuing diagnostic dilemma. N Engl J Med 1991;324:334. (*An editorial emphasizing the difficulties encountered in evaluating this condition.*)

Yesalis CE, Barsukiewicz CK, Kopstien AN, et al. Trends in anabolic–androgenic steroid use among adolescents. Arch Pediatr Adolesc Med 1997;151:1197. (*Rate of use among male adolescents estimated to be 4.9%.*)

100
Evaluating Galactorrhea and Hyperprolactinemia

PATHOPHYSIOLOGY AND CLINICAL PRESENTATION

Discharge of milk or colostrum from the breast in the absence of nursing is referred to as *galactorrhea*. When it is accompanied by disturbed menses or infertility, it suggests the possibility of hyperprolactinemia and the associated risk for pituitary neoplasm. When a patient presents with galactorrhea, underlying pituitary disease must be carefully considered.

Galactorrhea. Normal milk production involves the interplay of prolactin and breast tissue primed by estrogen and progestin. Prolactin secretion is under hypothalamic control, mediated by inhibitory dopaminergic transmission. Other hormones (e.g., thyroxine, insulin) are thought to play supporting roles in facilitating lactation. Galactorrhea can occur in the setting of a normal or elevated serum prolactin level. The normal range for serum prolactin is 1 to 20 ng/mL.

Normoprolactinemic Galactorrhea is believed to be a consequence of local breast stimulation or irritation in women with hormonally primed breast tissue. It is hypothesized that stimulation of the breast may cause a mild, transient elevation in prolactin secretion, although this is not sustained. Many cases are associated with a distant pregnancy or the use of oral contraceptives. Gonadal function is preserved, with menses and fertility remaining normal. Galactorrhea in the absence of sustained hyperprolactinemia is usually noted as an isolated symptom or an incidental finding on breast examination.

Hyperprolactinemic Galactorrhea develops as a consequence of excessive prolactin production, caused either by a loss of hypothalamic inhibition of lactotrophs in the anterior pituitary or by the development of an autonomously functioning pituitary adenoma. In rare instances, hyperprolactinemia results from a decreased clearance of prolactin (as in renal failure). Even in the context of high prolactin levels, galactorrhea does not occur unless the breast is primed by estrogen, which accounts for the rarity of the condition in men. Amenorrhea is a common accompaniment, which develops when high prolactin levels suppress the secretion of hypothalamic gonadotropin-releasing hormone (GnRH).

Hyperprolactinemia. Very high serum concentrations of prolactin are associated with autonomously functioning *prolactinomas*, derived from lactotrophs in the anterior pituitary. The degree of hyperprolactinemia tends to correlate with tumor size. Prolactinomas larger than 10 mm in diameter ("macroadenomas") are associated with extremely high prolactin levels (>1,000 ng/mL). Except in pregnancy, serum prolactin in excess of 300 ng/mL is almost always the result of a prolactinoma. Microadenomas (<10 mm in diameter) may produce less impressive elevations. They typically have a benign course and undergo little additional enlargement.

Moderate degrees of hyperprolactinemia are characteristic of conditions that interfere with hypothalamic control of the anterior pituitary. In nonpregnant patients with galactorrhea, only slightly more than half of those with prolactin levels above 100 ng/mL had a functioning pituitary tumor; the remainder had a problem that compromised hypothalamic inhibition. Interruption of hypothalamic inhibition can occur with use of a centrally active *dopaminergic blocking agent* (e.g., a phenothiazine), with *anatomic interference* by a sellar or suprasellar mass, and in *hypothyroidism*, in which thyrotropin-releasing hormone (TRH) stimulates lactotrophs in the anterior pituitary. Transient prolactin elevations have been observed in patients undergoing emotional stress, physical trauma, and nipple stimulation.

Because patients with hyperprolactinemia are at risk for hypogonadism, they may experience, in addition to galactorrhea, disturbed menses, *amenorrhea*, *infertility*, and *osteoporosis*. In hyperprolactinemic men, galactorrhea is rare, but *impotence* is common. Those with a substantially enlarging sellar mass may complain of *headache* or a *visual field cut*.

DIFFERENTIAL DIAGNOSIS

The differential diagnosis of galactorrhea can be organized according to whether prolactin is elevated or not, and according

Table 100.1.   Differential Diagnosis of Galactorrhea

Normoprolactinemic Galactorrhea
 Local breast stimulation/irritation (suckling, trauma, inflammation)
 Oral contraceptive use
 Recent pregnancy
 Idiopathic (? transient elevation in prolactin from stress, breast stimulation)

Hyperprolactinemic Galactorrhea
 Impairment of hypothalamic pituitary inhibition
  Drugs (phenothiazines, metoclopramide, heroin, reserpine, methyldopa, haloperidol)
  Lesions of the pituitary stalk (nonfunctioning sellar tumors, infarction)
  Hypothalamic disease (craniopharyngioma, infiltrative disease, infarction)
 Overproduction by a pituitary adenoma
  Prolactinoma
  Hypothyroidism (simulates adenoma by TRH stimulation of lactotrope cells)
 Idiopathic
  ? Microadenoma not detectable by neuroimaging
  ? Stress, trauma, breast stimulation

TRH, thyrotropin-releasing hormone.

to whether an elevation in prolactin is the result of a decrease in hypothalamic inhibition or overproduction by a functioning adenoma (Table 100.1). Only 20% of patients with galactorrhea have hyperprolactinemia. In patients with galactorrhea, amenorrhea, and hyperprolactinemia, prolactinoma is a leading cause. Other causes originating in the region of the pituitary include empty sella syndrome, craniopharyngioma, pinealoma, and parasellar sarcoidosis. Nonprolactinomic disease about and within the pituitary accounts for about one third of cases of galactorrhea and amenorrhea. Persistent galactorrhea after childbirth accounts for just under 10% of cases. Drugs associated with galactorrhea include oral contraceptives and agents with central dopaminergic-blocking activity (phenothiazines, haloperidol, metoclopramide) and, less commonly, reserpine, methyldopa, isoniazid, and imipramine.

WORKUP

History and Physical Examination. The workup for galactorrhea should include careful questioning about menstrual pattern, recent pregnancy, infertility, medications, change in libido, symptoms of hypothyroidism (see Chapter 104), breast stimulation, chest trauma, and the presence of headache or visual complaints. A careful review of drug use, particularly oral contraceptives and drugs that block central dopaminergic transmission (see above), needs to be pursued. The physical examination should include a detailed examination of the breasts to be sure the discharge is indeed milky and not caused by local breast disease, although no increased risk for breast cancer has been found in patients with true galactorrhea. Confrontation testing of the visual fields and funduscopic examination are important, although the findings are usually normal. Any signs of hypothyroidism (see Chapter 104) should be noted and then confirmed by measuring the thyroid-stimulating hormone (TSH) level.

Laboratory Testing. The development of accurate prolactin assays and the association of galactorrhea with high prolactin levels and pituitary tumors have made determination of the *serum prolactin concentration* an essential part of the diagnostic evaluation. However, caution is warranted in obtaining and interpreting a prolactin level. The prolactin concentration may be transiently elevated by stress, time of day, sleep, meals, or breast stimulation. Accuracy is enhanced by placing a catheter in the patient's vein and having the patient rest in a recumbent position for an hour before the sample is drawn. The morning is the best time. The patient with galactorrhea and amenorrhea is at increased risk for a pituitary neoplasm, and her prolactin concentration must be measured unless the explanation for both is apparent (e.g., recent pregnancy, medication).

Patients with galactorrhea, menstrual irregularities, and an otherwise unexplained elevation in serum prolactin should undergo neuroimaging of the sellar region. *Magnetic resonance imaging* (MRI) *with gadolinium enhancement* is the procedure of choice, although *computed tomography* (CT) is a reasonable alternative if MRI is unavailable. Gadolinium enhancement of MRI of the sellar structures is based on differences in vascularity between normal pituitary tissue and adenomas. Nonetheless, microadenomas can be difficult to detect, although the absence of a visible lesion rules out an anatomically threatening neoplasm. Even patients with modest unexplained elevations of prolactin (<200 ng/mL) should undergo neuroimaging of the pituitary region because another type of sellar or parasellar mass can be responsible for the mild elevation. Finding a lesion in excess of 10 mm in a patient with a modest rise in prolactin necessitates consideration of other types of pituitary tumors. The prolactin rise is likely to represent compression of the pituitary stalk.

Formal visual field testing should be performed in all patients with a sellar mass or visual symptoms.

From a practical standpoint, regular menses and a normal prolactin level in a patient with galactorrhea make the likelihood of a clinically important pituitary tumor remote. Patients in whom the likelihood of tumor is low can be followed carefully with periodic determinations of prolactin, usually at 1-year intervals; if prolactin levels become elevated, neuroimaging of the sella can be pursued.

SYMPTOMATIC MANAGEMENT

No Evidence of a Mass Lesion. Patients with normal periods and normal prolactin levels need no treatment. They can be reassured and followed. For patients with galactorrhea secondary to the use of a dopaminergic-blocking agent, a reduced dose of the drug can be tried, although full cessation may be necessary to terminate symptoms. If hypothyroidism is the contributing factor, it should be corrected (see Chapter 104). Symptomatic patients with *idiopathic disease* (galactorrhea, abnormal periods, elevated prolactin, normal MRI findings, no other evident disease) who want relief from their symptoms can be treated as if they have a microadenoma (see below).

Prolactinoma. The treatment approach depends on the size of the lesion and its natural history. *Microadenomas* (<10 mm in diameter) have an excellent prognosis. Long-term studies of untreated patients demonstrate that in 80% to 90% of cases, the size of a microadenoma remains the same, or the tumor regresses with time; only 10% to 20% continue to grow. Prolactin levels follow a similar pattern. However, with microadenomas that grow, the correlation between tumor size and prolactin

level may not be close, so that close monitoring of both parameters is necessary.

Despite the favorable prognosis, many patients with stable microadenomas may be bothered by menstrual irregularities, severe galactorrhea, and infertility. As noted earlier, osteoporosis is also a risk. The treatment of choice for such symptomatic patients is the dopaminergic agonist *bromocriptine*. The drug inhibits prolactin synthesis, secretion, and cellular proliferation. In many instances, prolactin levels return to normal, galactorrhea ceases, tumor size decreases, menses resume as gonadal function returns, and osteoporosis recedes. For control of symptoms, continuous bromocriptine administration is required, although in some patients the tumor undergoes spontaneous regression. A 2-year course of treatment followed by a trial of cessation is a common approach to bromocriptine therapy for patients with a symptomatic microadenoma. The doses needed to control symptoms range from 2.5 to 10 mg/d, although smaller doses often suffice for maintenance. Dopaminergic agonists with fewer side effects are under development. An alternative to bromocriptine therapy when pregnancy is not desired is the use of *oral contraceptives*, the benefits of which include regular periods, birth control, and the prevention of osteoporosis.

Macroadenomas are also treated initially with *bromocriptine*. In many instances, the drug suffices to control symptoms and shrink the adenoma. The doses needed to establish control range from 5 to 20 mg/d. Tumor size and prolactin concentration decline substantially. Lower doses (0.625 to 10 mg/d) are effective for maintenance. Indefinite treatment is the rule because spontaneous regression is rare. *Surgery* is reserved for patients with rapidly progressing visual loss or symptoms refractory to bromocriptine therapy. Because the recurrence rate after surgery is high, its use is limited. *Radiation therapy* is sometimes considered.

PATIENT EDUCATION AND INDICATIONS FOR REFERRAL

Patients with pituitary adenomas understandably worry about further tumor growth. Concern can be lessened by explaining the very favorable prognosis for the vast majority of microadenomas and the excellent response of most prolactinomas to bromocriptine. The patient with galactorrhea and amenorrhea should be informed that numerous options for induction of fertility are available and that these may be pursued according to the patient's wishes. By providing accurate information, moral support, and close follow-up, the primary physician can spare the patient a great deal of unnecessary concern.

Although the basic evaluation of galactorrhea and hyperprolactinemia can be effectively carried out by the primary physician, a consultation with the endocrinologist is indicated in a number of situations (e.g., macroadenoma, suspected pituitary neoplasm other than prolactinoma, failure to respond to bromocriptine, visual loss, desire to become pregnant).

A.H.G.

ANNOTATED BIBLIOGRAPHY

Dalkin AC, Marshall JC. Medical therapy of hyperprolactinemia. Endocrinol Metab Clin North Am 1989;18:259. (*Comprehensive review, with particularly detailed and useful section on the use of bromocriptine.*)

Fish LH, Mariash CN. Hyperprolactinemia, infertility, and hypothyroidism. A case report and review of the literature. Arch Intern Med 1988;148:709. (*Makes the important observation that hypothyroidism may mimic prolactinoma.*)

Hooper JH, Welsh VC, Shackleford RT. Abnormal lactation associated with tranquilizing drug therapy. JAMA 1961;178:506. (*Abnormal lactation occurred in 26 of 100 women receiving major tranquilizers; the effect was dose-dependent.*)

Kleinberg DL, Noel GL, Frantz AA. Galactorrhea: a study of 235 cases, including 48 pituitary tumors. N Engl J Med 1977;296:589. (*In one of the largest reported series, 34% had concurrent amenorrhea, and 32% had idiopathic galactorrhea without amenorrhea.*)

Klibanski A, Biller BMK, Rosenthal DI, et al. Effects of prolactin and estrogen deficiency in amenorrheic bone loss. J Clin Endocrinol Metab 1988:67:124. (*Bone loss results from prolactin-induced hypogonadism.*)

Koppelman MC, Jaffe MJ, Rieth KG, et al. Hyperprolactinemia, amenorrhea and galactorrhea. Ann Intern Med 1984;100:115. (*Most untreated patients experienced either no growth or spontaneous regression, with resumption of menses in some.*)

Liuzzi A, Dallabonzana D, Oppizzi G, et al. Low doses of dopamine agonists in the long-term treatment of macroprolactinomas. N Engl J Med 1985;313:656. (*Efficacy of low maintenance doses demonstrated, but therapy could not be halted.*)

Molitch ME. Pathologic hyperprolactinemia. Endocrinol Metab Clin North Am 1995;24:549. (*Thorough review of diagnosis and treatment.*)

Newton DR, Dillon WP, Norman D, et al. Gd-DTPA-enhanced MR imaging of pituitary adenoma. Am J Neuroradiol 1989;10:949. (*Data on the efficacy of gadolinium-enhanced MRI of pituitary adenomas.*)

Pellegrini I, Rasolonjanahary R, Gunz G, et al. Resistance to bromocriptine in prolactinoma. J Clin Endocrinol Metab 1989;69:500. (*Mechanisms of resistance reviewed, and need to monitor therapy carefully emphasized.*)

Schlechte J, Dolan K, Sherman B, et al. The natural history of untreated hyperprolactinemia: a prospective analysis. J Clin Endocrinol Metab 1989;68:412. (*Resumption of normal periods, normal prolactin levels, and resolution of the prolactinoma noted in 6 of 30 patients.*)

101
Evaluation of Suspected Diabetes Insipidus

When a patient presents with polyuria and polydipsia, the primary care physician needs to include diabetes insipidus (DI) in the differential diagnosis. DI is characterized clinically by the excretion of large volumes of inappropriately dilute urine. Although uncommon, DI may be a manifestation of important hypothalamic–pituitary disease or renal tubular dysfunction. The primary care physician needs to know how to screen for DI in a patient with polyuria and polydipsia and how to proceed with the basic elements of the diagnostic investigation.

PATHOPHYSIOLOGY AND CLINICAL PRESENTATION

Plasma osmolality is carefully regulated to maintain a level of 285 to 290 mOsm/kg. Any increase to much above 290 mOsm/kg stimulates hypothalamic osmoreceptors, following which *antidiuretic hormone* (ADH), also called *vasopressin*, is released from the posterior pituitary. ADH increases renal distal tubular permeability to water, so that water resorption is enhanced. Osmoreceptor stimulation also triggers *central thirst mechanisms*. These actions serve to reestablish normal serum osmolality. A lesion in any portion of this osmoregulatory system can result in DI and its attendant water diuresis. Dehydration and hypertonicity may ensue unless the thirst mechanism remains intact and access to water is adequate.

Clinically, DI is characterized by the excretion of large volumes of dilute urine in conjunction with thirst and polydipsia. A true polyuria occurs, defined as the excretion of more than 3 L/24 h. Craving for ice water is common (especially with central DI). The urine is almost always colorless, even in the morning, because of its dilute nature. Urine osmolality is inappropriately low (<250 mOsm/kg). Nocturia is common. Serum osmolality may be increased, especially if the thirst mechanism is impaired.

Central or Neurogenic Diabetes Insipidus is the most common form of DI, occurring in the context of an injury to the hypothalamus or posterior pituitary. Mechanisms of central DI include idiopathic degeneration of vasopressin-secreting neurons, destruction by malignant or granulomatous disease, vascular insult, and pituitary surgery. Because the thirst center is situated near the hypothalamic osmoreceptors, it too may be involved, although in many cases the thirst mechanism is preserved and dehydration avoided. Anterior pituitary adenomas usually do not cause DI unless they extend posteriorly or beyond the sella.

Nephrogenic Diabetes Insipidus results from conditions or medications that damage renal tubulointerstitial function and concentrating ability (e.g., hypercalcemia, hypokalemia, sickle cell disease, lithium, obstruction, pyelonephritis). ADH levels are appropriate, but the renal response is impaired.

Primary Polydipsia also produces polyuria, but unlike DI, this condition appears to originate with an altered perception of thirst. It is particularly prevalent among patients with chronic psychiatric disturbances (especially schizophrenia) but is also seen with organic brain disease (e.g., multiple sclerosis). Detailed study of such patients has revealed multiple defects in the regulation of osmolality, including problems with urinary dilution, regulation of water intake, and ADH secretion. Increased thirst and fluid intake are followed by polyuria, although some patients may hide this behavior. A fall in serum osmolality (<285 mOsm/kg) may be accompanied by hyponatremia. Symptoms tend to be episodic.

Table 101.1. Differential Diagnosis of Polyuria/Polydipsia in the Outpatient Setting

Solute Diuresis
  Diabetes mellitus
  Diuretics

Water Diuresis
  Diabetes insipidus
    Central
      Idiopathic
      Trauma
      Tumor (local or metastatic to the sellar region)
      Granulomatous disease (sarcoidosis, tuberculosis)
      Postsurgical (removal of pituitary adenoma)
      Vascular (Sheehan's syndrome, old stroke)
    Nephrogenic
      Drugs (lithium, demeclocycline, amphotericin)
      Tubulointerstitial disease (pyelonephritis, polycystic kidney
        disease, sickle cell disease, obstructive uropathy)
      Metabolic (hypercalcemia, hypokalemia)
    Primary polydipsias
      Psychogenic (schizophrenia)
      Central nervous system disease (multiple sclerosis)
      Idiopathic

DIFFERENTIAL DIAGNOSIS

The differential diagnosis for patients with polyuria and polydipsia in the outpatient setting includes *diabetes mellitus* (see Chapter 102), *diuretic use*, *DI*, and *primary polydipsia*. The differential can be organized as follows: (a) whether the diuresis is related to water or solute; (b) if related to water, whether it is a manifestation of DI or primary polydipsia; and (c) if DI, whether it is central or nephrogenic (Table 101.1). Other causes of urinary frequency unaccompanied by polydipsia (e.g., *urinary tract infection, bladder dysfunction*) need to be ruled out (see Chapters 133, 134, and 140).

WORKUP

The initial diagnostic evaluation of the patient with polyuria can proceed logically and efficiently by addressing a set of basic questions:

Is This True Polyuria or Just Urinary Frequency? A history of frequently voiding large volumes of dilute (colorless or pale) urine, both day and night, suggests true polyuria, whereas frequent voiding of small volumes of concentrated urine is indicative of bladder dysfunction caused by infection or other local disease. A *24-hour urine collection* provides objective confirmation of true polyuria when the volume exceeds 3 L.

If True Polyuria, Is This a Water Diuresis or a Solute Diuresis? Measurement of the *urine osmolality* is very helpful. Patients with a concentrated urine (>350 mOsm/L) have a condition causing a solute diuresis. Those with a dilute urine (<250 mOsm/L) have a water diuresis. Patients with a urine osmolality between these levels may have either. To differentiate, one calculates the *total solute excretion* (urine volume per day multiplied by the average urine concentration). If it is less than 1,200 mOsm/d, then a water diuresis is likely. If a solute diuresis is suspected, checking the urine for glucose and electrolytes can be confirmatory.

If a Water Diuresis, Is This Diabetes Insipidus or Primary Polydipsia? Measurement of the *serum osmolality* can be helpful. A clearly elevated serum osmolality (>290 mOsm/L) in the context of inappropriately dilute urine (*osmolality <275 mOsm/L*) suggests DI, although many patients with DI and an intact thirst mechanism and access to water have a serum osmolality close to normal. A low serum osmolality suggests primary polydipsia. Direct measurement of the *serum vasopressin* (ADH) would help to clarify the situation, but reliable assays are not widely available. Very low levels would occur with central DI; very high levels would indicate renal DI; inappropriately elevated levels would suggest primary polydipsia.

The clinical context may help suggest the cause of the water diuresis. When it occurs in the setting of known renal tubulointerstitial disease or drug use, nephrogenic DI is likely. A central mechanism is suggested when the patient presents with other manifestations of pituitary disease or has a condition that may damage the central nervous system (e.g., cancer, granulomatous disease). Onset in a patient with mental illness raises the probability of primary polydipsia.

Desmovasopressin Testing. When the cause remains uncertain and in the absence of a reliable measure of ADH, it may be necessary to admit the patient for a *trial of desmovasopressin* (DDAVP), an ADH analogue. The response to DDAVP helps clarify the underlying mechanism of the water diuresis. A 50% decrease in urine volume, an increase in urine osmolality, and a return of serum osmolality toward normal confirm central DI. Lack of response identifies renal DI. DDAVP also causes a decrease in polyuria and an increase in urine osmolality in patients with primary polydipsia, but the serum osmolality will decrease to subnormal levels and hyponatremia may ensue. Because of such risks and the need to monitor fluid intake and excretion closely, inpatient testing is usually recommended for a DDAVP trial.

Pituitary–Hypothalamic Imaging. Biochemical evidence of central DI is an indication for neuroimaging to determine if a mass lesion or other disease is compromising the integrity of the pituitary. *Magnetic resonance imaging* (MRI) with *gadolinium* enhancement is the procedure of choice, although *computed tomography* (CT) is a reasonable alternative if MRI is unavailable or cost is a major issue. Gadolinium enhancement of MRI of the sellar structures is based on differences in vascularity between normal and abnormal tissues.

Is This Definitely Primary Polydipsia? When primary polydipsia is suspected (low–normal or low serum osmolality, polyuria, low urine osmolality, concurrent psychiatric disease), an inpatient *water restriction test* can be confirmatory; all parameters will return to normal when water is restricted. Because such dehydration testing can be very dangerous for patients with other causes of a water diuresis, it is necessary to conduct this test in a carefully supervised inpatient setting. Supervised water restriction is also necessary because patients with primary polydipsia tend to be psychotic and drink surreptitiously.

SYMPTOMATIC RELIEF

The advent of *DDAVP* as a *nasal spray* has greatly facilitated the treatment of central DI. The intranasal vasopressin is taken before bed to eliminate nocturnal polyuria. The dose is adjusted to allow normal amounts of daytime urination. Excessive doses can lead to a DDAVP-induced syndrome of inappropriate secretion of ADH.

Drugs that enhance ADH secretion (clofibrate, chlorpropamide, carbamazepine) are also helpful. Somewhat paradoxically, *thiazide diuretics* relieve the symptoms of DI. By inducing a mild sodium diuresis, they enhance the proximal resorption of sodium and water, so that the amount of water that reaches the distal tubule is reduced. *NSAIDs* are sometimes helpful in nephrogenic DI. By inhibiting renal prostaglandins (which are active in settings of renal disease), they reduce water delivery to the distal tubule. Treatment of the underlying psychiatric disturbance is the only treatment at present for primary polydipsia.

INDICATIONS FOR ADMISSION AND REFERRAL

As noted above, patients requiring DDAVP testing or a trial of water restriction need to be admitted. An endocrinologic consultation can be helpful in further planning the diagnostic evaluation and in interpreting its results. Patients in whom central DI is suspected are candidates for neuroimaging of the sella region (MRI is best) and endocrinologic consultation for further testing of the hypothalamic–pituitary axis. Renal DI suggests extensive renal tubulointerstitial disease and the need for further investigation and consultation. The patient with primary polydipsia should undergo a careful psychiatric workup to search for an underlying thought disorder.

A.H.G.

ANNOTATED BIBLIOGRAPHY

Berl T. Psychosis and water balance. N Engl J Med 1988;318:441. (*An editorial summarizing disturbances of regulation of osmolality in psychotic persons.*)

Goldman MB, Luchins DJ, Robertson GL. Mechanisms of altered water metabolism in psychotic patients with polydipsia and hyponatremia. N Engl J Med 1988;318:397. (*Defects in regulation of osmolality and secretion of ADH found.*)

Halperin M, Skorecki KL. Interpretation of the urine electrolytes and osmolality in the regulation of body fluid tonicity. Am J Nephrol 1986;6:241. (*Written for the subspecialist, but some very useful sections for the generalist reader.*)

Robertson GL. Diabetes insipidus. Endocrinol Metab Clin North Am 1995;24:549. (*Authoritative review.*)

Robertson GL. Differential diagnosis of polyuria. Annu Rev Med 1988;39:425. (*Comprehensive treatment of causes and workup.*)

Tetiker T, Sert M, Kocak M. Efficacy of indapamide in central diabetes insipidus. Arch Intern Med 1999;159:2085. (*Example of the efficacy of a thiazide-like diuretic; 40% reduction in urinary volume.*)

Zeerbe RL, Robertson GL. A comparison of plasma vasopressin measurements with a standard indirect test in the differential diagnosis of polyuria. N Engl J Med 1981;305:1539. (*Use of the assay improves the workup for polyuria.*)

Vokes TJ, Robertson GL. Disorders of antidiuretic hormone. Endocrinol Metab Clin North Am 1988;17:281. (*Authoritative review, with good section on inadequate production.*)

102
Approach to the Patient with Diabetes Mellitus

Diabetes mellitus, the most prevalent endocrinologic problem encountered in primary care practice, is characterized by hyperglycemia, a relative or absolute deficiency of insulin, insulin resistance, and a propensity to the development of long-term microvascular and macrovascular complications. If recent trends showing a dramatic increase in prevalence (believed to be a consequence of a decline in physical activity and excessive caloric intake) continue, then the condition will soon affect nearly 20 million people in the United States. The primary physician is in the unique position to provide comprehensive care to the diabetic patient. The ultimate goals of therapy are the prevention of microvascular and macrovascular complications, consequences of diabetes that make the condition a major risk factor for cardiovascular disease, stroke, visual impairment, renal failure, impotence, peripheral neuropathy, limb loss, and death.

Effective management requires care that is thoughtful and meticulous, incorporating intensive patient education. Euglycemic control, with the level of hemoglobin A_{1c} (HbA_{1c}) kept below 7.0 mmol/L, has emerged as a major treatment objective because of its association with a marked reduction in the risk for microvascular complications. The challenge for the primary care physician is to design a therapeutic program that is safe, practical, and acceptable to the patient. Important decisions include determining when to initiate pharmacologic therapy, selecting among available agents, and setting an achievable goal for glycemic control. Practical tasks include creation of an effective means for diabetic surveillance and provision of education and encouragement that enable the patient to become a partner in management.

PATHOPHYSIOLOGY, CLINICAL PRESENTATION, AND COURSE

Diagnostic Criteria. The increasing appreciation of the pathologic significance of hyperglycemia and the importance of early diagnosis has resulted in a revision of diagnostic criteria by the Expert Committee on the Diagnosis and Classification of Diabetes Mellitus. The threshold for diagnosis based on the *fasting blood glucose level* has been revised downward from 140 mg/dL to *126 mg/dL*) to increase the sensitivity of this determination. The 2-hour-postprandial glucose determination conducted as part of a glucose tolerance test is more sensitive for the diagnosis of diabetes than the fasting glucose level is, but it is less convenient to perform, especially in the evaluation of populations. Thus, for populations, the fasting glucose level with a reduced threshold is now deemed the preferred measurement. For individuals, the diagnosis can be made based on the presence of any one of three glucose abnormalities found on two separate days:

1. Fasting plasma glucose >126 mg/dL
2. Random plasma glucose >200 mg/dL in a person with diabetic symptoms, or
3. Two-hour-postprandial plasma glucose level >200 mg/dL after administration of the equivalent of a 75-g glucose load

If the fasting blood glucose is between 100 mg/dL and 126 mg/dL, the diagnosis can be made on the basis of a 75-g oral glucose tolerance test showing a *2-hour-postprandial plasma glucose and one other value between 0 and 2 hours above 200 mg/dL.*

Classification. The major forms of diabetes may be classified pathophysiologically. The use of the terms *insulin-dependent* and *non–insulin-dependent* is now discouraged because exogenous insulin may be needed to treat either form of the disease, so that the terms are meaningless. The major classifications of diabetes are as follows:

Type 1 Diabetes is characterized by an absolute deficiency of insulin. Patients are *ketosis-prone* and require insulin to live. Onset is typically in youth but may occur at any age.

Type 2 Diabetes. Insulin is present, but in amounts insufficient to meet metabolic needs in a timely fashion. Because they have some insulin, these patients are *not ketosis-prone* (except under severe stress of infections or surgery). They exhibit *impaired insulin secretion* at any plasma glucose concentration and *"insulin resistance"* (impaired insulin action at the level of the insulin receptor or signal transudation). *Obesity*, which is present in 60% to 80% of patients with type 2 diabetes, is believed to play a major role in insulin resistance.

Impaired Glucose Tolerance. Patients are identified on the basis of a *fasting glucose* between *110 mg/dL* and *126 mg/dL* or a *2-hour-postprandial glucose* between *140 mg/dL* and *200 mg/dL.* The risk for the development of overt type 2 diabetes is increased (1% to 5% annually), as is the risk for cardiovascular disease. Microvascular complications do not develop in those who do not progress to diabetes.

Gestational Diabetes. In pregnancy, even minor degrees of glucose intolerance can be important (see below). Screening for the condition is conducted at 24 to 28 weeks of gestation by testing for a plasma *glucose above 140 mg/dL at 1 hour after oral administration of a 50-g glucose load.*

Pathogenesis. The basic pathogenesis of diabetes remains incompletely understood; genetic and acquired factors have been identified. The principal lesion in type 1 disease is pancreatic β-*cell failure*, which leads to a loss of insulin production. Type 2 disease is characterized by defects in both the production and peripheral action of insulin; *impaired insulin secretion, decreased muscle glucose uptake*, and *inappropriate hepatic glucose production* are the pathophysiologic hallmarks. The latter two features are sometimes characterized as manifestations of *insulin resistance* because they occur despite the secretion of insulin. Insulin resistance is an important component of the broader metabolic perturbations that are features of diabetes, including weight gain, dyslipidemia, hypertension,

and a strongly increased risk for macrovascular atherosclerotic disease. Coronary risk is two to four times greater in diabetic than in nondiabetic persons.

Weight gain is an important contributor to type 2 disease, exacerbating insulin resistance. Glucose intolerance in diabetic patients may also be worsened by infection, stress, thiazides, glucocorticoids, and pregnancy. Excess secretion of growth hormone, cortisol, catecholamines, or glucagon may contribute to glucose intolerance, as can diseases that destroy a substantial portion of the pancreas (e.g., chronic pancreatitis, hemochromatosis, cystic fibrosis).

Clinical Presentation and Course. Type 2 diabetes is often discovered as an incidental finding on screening urinalysis or blood sugar measurement. Occasionally, the diagnosis is made during an evaluation for cardiovascular, renal, neurologic, or infectious disease. A complication such as myocardial ischemia, stroke, intermittent claudication, impotence, peripheral neuropathy, proteinuria, or retinopathy may be the initial manifestation. Sometimes, fatigue is the predominant symptom. In patients with more significant hyperglycemia, polyuria, polydipsia, and polyphagia with weight loss are encountered. The natural history of both type 1 and type 2 diabetes is characterized by the relentless progression of β-cell failure with time, even in the setting of tight glycemic control. The most important determinant of daily glycemia is the fasting glucose level, so that efforts to normalize it are given top priority. A reduction is also important, but the postprandial glucose level is a lesser determinant of overall control.

Complications of diabetes occur with a very high frequency. Most correlate with the magnitude and duration of hyperglycemia; there does not appear to be any glycemic threshold for the development of such complications. The major complications of diabetes can be categorized as vascular, neurologic, ocular, and infectious. Diabetic vascular disease includes both *large-vessel* atherosclerotic disease and *microangiopathic* occlusive changes.

Macrovascular Disease. As noted, the increase in the risk for coronary events is marked and similar to that of a nondiabetic patient who has had a previous myocardial infarction. Premature atherosclerosis may develop in large and medium vessels, leading to coronary ischemia, stroke, and peripheral arterial insufficiency. The effects of smoking, hypertension, and other risk factors for vascular disease appear to be synergistic with those of hyperglycemia. The pathophysiology remains poorly understood. Current hypotheses include hyperglycemic alteration of lipid deposits to make them more atherogenic. In addition, it has been suggested that the insulin resistance of type 2 disease leads to a state of *hyperinsulinism*, with its associated adverse cardiovascular effects of *increased blood pressure, reduced levels of high-density lipoprotein (HDL) cholesterol*, and *increased levels of very low-density lipoprotein (VLDL) cholesterol*—an atherogenic phenotype termed *syndrome X*. It is suspected but remains to be proved that tight control reduces the risk for large-vessel atherosclerosis. However, major reductions in the risk for coronary events and stroke can be achieved by correcting other major cardiovascular risk factors, such as smoking, hypertension, and hyperlipidemia. Effective treatment of such risk factors appears more important than normalization of glucose *per se* in the prevention and limitation of cardiovascular complications.

Microvascular Disease accounts for much of the morbidity of diabetes, causing nephropathy, retinopathy, and neuropathy. The risk for these microvascular complications can be markedly reduced by achieving tight glucose control (see below).

Diabetic Nephropathy is one of the leading causes of end-stage renal failure in adults, accounting for 25% of cases (see Chapter 142). Characteristic renal changes include glomerular basement membrane thickening and mesangial proliferation. Mesangial proliferation correlates strongly with the onset of proteinuria and hypertension. Subclinical and histologic findings for diabetic nephropathy are present long before the stage of clinical proteinuria. An elevated glomerular filtration rate (hyperfiltration), genetic determinants, and hypertension contribute to the progression of renal impairment. With persistent proteinuria, hypertension becomes established and glomerular filtration begins to decline at the rate of 1 mL/min per month.

The risk for the development of nephropathy correlates with the duration of disease and the degree of hyperglycemia. Renal failure eventually develops in 30% to 50% of type 1 diabetics and 6% to 9% of type 2 patients. Tight control of the blood glucose can reduce the risk for renal failure, particularly if instituted early. It can reverse mild proteinuria in insulin-dependent diabetics who do not yet have renal insufficiency. In the presence of significant proteinuria (>500 mg/d), near-normalization of the plasma glucose may not slow the rate of renal deterioration. Bladder dysfunction and resultant urinary tract infections can also contribute to renal impairment in patients with diabetic neuropathy.

Retinopathy. The risk for retinopathic changes (see Chapter 209) is related to the duration and degree of hyperglycemia. After 20 years of diabetes, all age groups show a 75% to 80% prevalence of retinopathy. The cumulative incidence of retinopathy can be reduced by more than 50% with intensive insulin therapy. Reversible changes in the lens configuration occur with wide fluctuations in plasma glucose and may cause transiently blurred vision. In addition, cataracts and glaucoma occur with increased frequency (see Chapters 207 and 208).

Neuropathy may lead to a peripheral sensory deficit, autonomic dysfunction, or a mononeuritis. Mechanisms include *myoinositol depletion* in nerve cell membranes (which prolongs conduction time) and hyperglycemia-induced *sorbitol accumulation* in nerve tissues that have a polyol pathway for glucose metabolism (e.g., Schwann cells). *Microangiopathic changes* that decrease the blood supply to the myelin sheaths are believed responsible for the mononeuropathy. The *peripheral neuropathy* is predominantly sensory; sensation is reduced in the lower extremities, and the condition may progress to cause pain and dysesthesias. *Autonomic neuropathy* most commonly presents as impotence. Gastrointestinal motility disturbances, orthostatic hypotension, and urinary retention are other potential manifestations. Autonomic neuropathy is almost always seen in association with distal polyneuropathy. Its presence is an important predictor of foot and other infections. Diabetic *mononeuropathy* involves discrete cranial or peripheral nerves, singly or as a mononeuritis multiplex. Cranial nerves III and VI are most commonly affected. In contrast to other diabetic neuropathies, mononeuropathies resolve almost completely within 1 year of onset.

Increased Susceptibility to Infection in diabetics appears to result from impaired leukocyte function, compromised vascular supply, and neuropathy. Cellulitis and candidiasis occur, with infections of ischemic foot lesions especially serious because they may lead to osteomyelitis, which requires amputation. Overall, the occurrence of perioperative infections correlates with end-organ involvement by diabetes and marked degrees of hyperglycemia. Recent studies show a sixfold increase in all perioperative complications (stroke, infection, and renal insufficiency) in patients with end-organ disease. Urinary tract infections are common in patients with an autonomic bladder (see Chapter 134).

PRINCIPLES OF MANAGEMENT

Treatment Goals and Strategy

Treatment Goals. The goals of therapy in diabetes are *normalization of blood glucose* and prevention of multisystem complications that may result from hyperglycemia. The Diabetes Control and Complication Trial (DCCT) and the U.K. Prospective Diabetes Study (UKPDS), landmark prospective clinical trials comparing standard with tight-control regimens in types 1 and 2 disease, respectively, convincingly demonstrated that maintaining blood glucose concentrations close to the normal range (e.g., HbA_{1c} <7.0%) delays the onset and limits the progression of the long-term microvascular complications of diabetes—retinopathy, nephropathy, and neuropathy. In addition, a strong trend was noted in the UKPDS toward a reduction in coronary events.

Based on these data, the *American Diabetes Association* recommends a *treatment goal of HbA_{1c} < 7.0%*. Although tight glucose control can markedly decrease the morbidity associated with small-vessel disease, it remains to be proved whether it can reduce the serious large-vessel consequences of diabetes (which cause death in the majority of patients with type 2 diabetes). Nonetheless, normalization of carbohydrate metabolism stands as a major treatment objective for all diabetics. The challenge is how to accomplish normalization and reduce risk, given the still imperfect treatment modalities and monitoring methods currently available. Strong patient motivation and close support are essential. Advances in treatment promise to facilitate achievement of control.

Normalization of blood sugars to nondiabetic postprandial and fasting levels is an ideal objective that is not without risk. The risk for hypoglycemia with intensive insulin therapy is a serious concern; it can be especially dangerous in patients who have underlying coronary or cerebrovascular disease. However, the goal of safe and convenient glucose normalization is becoming easier to achieve. Until implantable glucose sensors and insulin delivery systems automate the control process, the maintenance of normoglycemia still requires attention to the details of diet, exercise, weight control, and the many facets of medical therapy to achieve the best possible outcome.

Treatment Strategy. The strategy is pathophysiologically based, with a focus on the importance of establishing euglycemia as quickly as possible, as diabetic complications are mostly a function of the degree and duration of hyperglycemia. Because the fasting glucose level is the most important determinant of daily glycemia, efforts to normalize it are given top priority. A reduction in postprandial glucose is also important, but the postprandial glucose level is a lesser determinant of overall control. For type 1 disease, the emphasis is on intensive insulin therapy to make up for the loss of insulin production. In type 2 disease, the treatment strategy is multidimensional; impaired insulin secretion is countered by the therapy with sulfonylurea, repaglinide, or insulin; decreased muscle glucose uptake and inappropriate hepatic glucose production are treated with diet, weight reduction, exercise, and biguanides or thiazolidinediones. Combination programs are often necessary to attain the treatment goals of a fasting glucose level below 140 mg/dL and an HbA_{1c} level $<$ below 7.0%, especially as the disease advances.

Diet and Exercise

The cornerstone of therapy for all overweight patients with type 2 diabetes is *weight reduction* through calorie restriction and exercise. Achieving ideal body weight is the single most important goal for the physician to encourage and advance to achieve metabolic control. Weight loss has been shown to enhance the sensitivity of peripheral insulin receptors to endogenous insulin and reduce the requirements for administered insulin. It is not possible to predict the exact improvement in glucose control from each pound lost, but a reduction of body weight may lead to an improvement in glucose tolerance.

The hyperglycemia of most type 2 diabetics can be controlled by achieving an ideal body weight; however, such weight reduction is often difficult to maintain, as a permanent restriction in caloric intake is required. An effective *exercise program* (see Chapter 18) enhances weight loss because caloric consumption is increased. Exercise can help obese persons, who may require fewer calories to maintain their body weight, to lose weight. Rigidly developed and prescribed diets should be avoided in favor of diets adapted to the patient's lifestyle. The goal is gradual, sustained weight reduction of approximately 1 to 2 lb each week (see Chapter 233).

Diet Composition for type 2 diabetics is less critical than achieving an ideal body weight. At present, the American Diabetes Association recommends diets high in carbohydrate, up to 60%, with a significant amount of polyunsaturated fats. In mild glucose intolerance, isocaloric increases in carbohydrate, up to 80%, may improve glucose tolerance, particularly when complex carbohydrate, high-fiber diets are consumed. Hypertriglyceridemia secondary to the increase in carbohydrates has not been a problem, and in several studies, triglycerides and cholesterol levels have fallen substantially. Recent studies in type 2 diabetics, however, show unchanged or worsened glycemic control with high-carbohydrate diets and increases in VLDL triglyceride and cholesterol. All carbohydrates are not similar; some, such as those from potato, cause greater increases in blood glucose than do those from beans or wheat. Even the inclusion of sucrose or ice cream in mixed meals does not necessarily adversely affect glucose control. Preliminary data suggest that *vitamin E* and *β-carotene* supplements may decrease the oxidation of polyunsaturated fatty acids and help prevent the accelerated atherogenesis of diabetes (see Appendix, Chapter 27.)

High-fiber diets, generally associated with a higher intake of complex carbohydrates and a decreased intake of refined carbohydrates and animal fats, are associated with a low prevalence of diabetes mellitus. *Increasing dietary fiber content* with unprocessed natural foods that include cereals, grains, fruits, and vegetables results in improved glucose tolerance in type 2 diabetics and decreased insulin requirements in type 1 diabetics. The likely mechanism for this improvement in glycemic control is delayed absorption.

Exercise has important effects on glucose control in diabetes. It increases glucose consumption and reduces insulin resistance. All forms of exercise, even walking and other forms of nonvigorous activity, improve insulin sensitivity. A few precautions are worth noting in those who may engage in more vigorous activity. The increased absorption of insulin in an exercising limb may precipitate hypoglycemia in patients on insulin; therefore, the abdomen should be used as the site for insulin injection. Because of the possibility of underlying ischemic heart disease, an exercise electrocardiogram (ECG) should be considered before a rigorous exercise program is undertaken by a sedentary person with longstanding diabetes or other atherosclerotic risk factors (see Chapters 18 and 36).

Special Considerations for Patients on Insulin. For type 1 *insulin-requiring diabetics* who are at ideal body weight, the essential aspect of dietary therapy is the *regularity of caloric intake* and the spacing of meals. Three meals, supplemented by snacks midmorning, midafternoon, and before bed, are needed to provide a source of glucose during the sustained presence of exogenously administered insulin. The commonly used American Diabetic Association diets recommend 2/9 of calories at breakfast, 2/9 at lunch, 4/9 at dinner, and 1/9 as snacks. The timing of meals must match peak insulin effects and activity schedules; increased activity requires increased food intake or a decrease in insulin dosage to prevent hypoglycemia. Simple sugars are generally restricted because they worsen postprandial hyperglycemia; however, patients should carry a source of simple sugar, such as fruit juice or sugar candy, to limit an insulin reaction. Patients who are not taking insulin do not require elaborate exchange systems, careful timing of meals, or other special dietary accommodations.

Drug Therapy: Oral Agents

If diet, exercise, and weight reduction to an ideal body weight fail to control of blood sugar reasonably well (i.e., fasting glucose $>$140 mg/dL, postprandial glucose $>$160 mg/dL, or HbA_{1c} $>$7.0%), relieve symptoms, or prevent ketosis, then drug therapy is indicated. Drug therapy is also indicated if it is unlikely that the patient can lose weight or if the patient is pregnant. Insulin remains the agent of first choice in persons with severe hyperglycemia (fasting glucose $>$240 mg/dL), whether from type 1 or type 2 disease. Oral agents—the sulfonylureas, biguanides (e.g., metformin), thiazolidinediones (e.g., the glitazones), and glucosidase inhibitors (e.g., acarbose)—are effective in type 2 disease with moderate hyperglycemia (fasting glucose between 140 and 240 mg/dL). The recommended American Diabetes Association glycemic goals of drug treatment based on the DCCT and UKPDS data are a *fasting glucose level below 140 mg/dL* and an *HbA_{1c} level below 7.0%*.

Sulfonylureas. With the advent of potent, long-acting, second-generation preparations and increasing evidence of their efficacy and safety, the sulfonylureas have become a mainstay of treatment for *mild to moderately severe type 2 disease (fasting glucose between 140 and 240 mg/dL)*. An absolute average reduction in HbA$_{1c}$ of 1.5 to 2.0 percentage points, along with a reduction in fasting glucose of 60 to 70 mg/dL, is achieved in most cases.

Mechanism of Action. The sulfonylureas acutely increase the sensitivity of β-cells to glucose and stimulate endogenous insulin release. This action can lead to hypoglycemia—hence the term *oral hypoglycemic agents*. These agents are effective in persons who require additional insulin secretion and have an adequate β-cell reserve. Enhancement of basal insulin secretion inhibits basal hepatic glucose production and improves the fasting glucose level. Efficacy declines with time as β-cell function deteriorates, so that glycemic control worsens despite the use of maximum doses. Although these agents also increase insulin receptor binding and enhance tissue sensitivity to insulin, such effects are minor compared with the stimulation of insulin release and are insufficient to sustain glycemic control when insulin release declines.

Preparations. The *first-generation sulfonylureas* (e.g., chlorpropamide, tolbutamide, tolazamide) have given way to *second-generation agents*, such as *glyburide* (Micronase, DiaBeta), *glipizide* (Glucotrol), and *glimepiride* (Amaryl), in the treatment of type 2 diabetes. Second-generation drugs are more potent and longer-acting. All are of equal efficacy. Although they cost 5 to 10 times more than first-generation drugs, they remain the least costly of the oral agents; all are similarly priced. These drugs are non-ionically bound to plasma proteins and are less variable in their bioavailability than the earlier oral agents. They are inactivated by the liver and consequently should be used with caution in reduced dosages in patients with liver disease. Glyburide is excreted in bile and urine, which is a potential advantage in patients with renal insufficiency. Glipizide releases insulin slightly more rapidly than the others, but this feature provides no special long-term advantage. In contrast to chlorpropamide, the second-generation agents do not cause inappropriate secretion of antidiuretic hormone, and only rarely cause disulfiram (Antabuse)-like effects. Like those of their predecessors, the effects of these agents may be potentiated by sulfonamides, salicylates, and clofibrate, or inhibited by warfarin.

Dosing Schedules for these agents are convenient because the duration of action is 12 to 24 hours. A sustained-release glipizide preparation allows for once-daily dosing, which is a marginal convenience benefit but a means of reducing the cost of therapy if used in place of a twice-daily program. The duration of action of glimepiride is slightly longer than that of other preparations (16 to 24 hours), so that once-a-day dosing is also possible. A lower-dose formulation is available for glimepiride than for sustained-release glipizide, which facilitates its use in the elderly and those with mild hyperglycemia. The starting doses of the second-generation agents are 2.5 mg for glyburide, 5.0 mg for glipizide, and 1 mg for glimepiride, taken once daily in the morning. Treatment is started at low doses and increased every 1 to 2 weeks, with monitoring of fasting and postprandial sugars. Failure to demonstrate any reduction in glucose early on suggests that oral agent therapy will probably fail, even at increased doses. The maximum daily dose is 15 to 20 mg/d for glipizide and glyburide, usually given on a twice-daily schedule for optimal effectiveness. For

glimepiride, the maximum dose is 8 mg, given once daily. Monitoring of blood sugars and HbA$_{1c}$ is required (see below).

Efficacy. In about 25% of patients, treatment goals are achieved with sulfonylurea therapy alone. In another 50% to 60% of patients, the initial response is good, but an additional agent is required over time to achieve treatment goals. The 15% who fail to exhibit a primary response probably have more advanced disease or slowly progressive type 1 diabetes. Predictors of a good response include newly diagnosed diabetes, mild to moderate disease, good β-cell function (high levels of C-peptide), and no history of prior insulin therapy or presence of islet cell antibodies. In the UKPDS, when the goals of intensive therapy were reached, reductions in long-term microvascular complications could be demonstrated, although no decreases in the risk for macrovascular disease were noted.

In careful side-by-side comparisons, second-generation sulfonylureas can achieve results comparable with those of single-dose NPH (neutral protamine Hagedorn) insulin in lowering HbA$_{1c}$. However, as β-cell function declines with time, pharmacologic coaxing of further insulin output is less likely to succeed. In the UKPDS, only 24% of patients on sulfonylurea monotherapy had adequate control 9 years after diagnosis. Addition of a second agent is usually necessary, either one that reduces peripheral resistance to endogenous insulin (e.g., metformin) or one that provides exogenous hormone (see below).

Adverse Effects. The principal risk of sulfonylurea use is *hypoglycemia* (a result of increased insulin release). Hypoglycemia (which tends to be prolonged) occurs at a frequency of 4% with the use of glyburide and 2% to 4% with glipizide. Occasionally, patients whose diabetes has become refractory to a first-generation sulfonylurea may benefit from substitution with a second-generation agent. Doses in excess of 15 to 20 mg/d provide little additional control. The risk for hypoglycemia is greatest with potent, long-acting sulfonylureas, which can cause sustained, severe hypoglycemia. Under study conditions, about 5% of patients experience hypoglycemia with sulfonylurea use. Outside study settings, the risk is likely to be higher.

Concern about an increase in *cardiovascular risk* was suggested by data from the University Group Diabetes Project (UGDP), which revealed a small but significant increase in the rate of cardiovascular death in patients on long-term tolbutamide therapy. Questions about the UGDP study design and the veracity of the finding triggered an extensive controversy. Oral agent use declined for several years because of concern about this observation, and a new generation of sulfonylureas was developed. The controversy appears to have been put to rest by new long-term data from the UKPDS, which found, after 10 years of follow-up, no increase in the incidence of coronary events associated with the prolonged use of oral agents.

The effect on cardiovascular risk factors is important to note. *Weight gain* is an important consequence of the enhanced insulin secretion stimulated by oral agent therapy. Weight gain may be on the order of 5 to 10 lb with most agents, although there is some suggestion that it may be less with long-acting glipizide. *Triglycerides* decrease modestly, but overall effects on *lipids* are minimal.

Patient Selection. These agents are commonly prescribed as initial pharmacologic therapy for patients who remain moderately hyperglycemic (fasting glucose between 140 and 240 mg/dL) despite dietary and exercise measures. The insulin requirements of such patients may be increased, especially if they are obese, and they initially benefit from the increased release of endogenous insulin. The best results are achieved in patients who are not obese. The sulfonylurea drugs are a first choice for oral agent therapy and the least costly. Their convenience of use in comparison with insulin and their minimal side effects make them a popular choice for patients with type 2 diabetes. In the very elderly, they should be prescribed with care because of the increased vulnerability of these patients to the adverse consequences of hypoglycemia.

Biguanides (e.g., Metformin). These agents, also referred to as *oral antihyperglycemics*, differ from the oral hypoglycemics in that they do not stimulate endogenous insulin secretion; rather, they enhance tissue responsiveness to insulin. Consequently, they are less likely to induce hypoglycemia and are effective in the treatment of patients with tissue resistance to insulin, such as obese persons.

Mechanism of Action. These drugs facilitate insulin uptake by peripheral tissue, especially muscle, and decrease hepatic gluconeogenesis and basal glucose output, thereby helping to lower fasting glucose levels. Glucose utilization also improves in adipose and intestinal tissues. The net result is an improvement in fasting and postprandial hyperglycemia. Insulin demand declines as glucose utilization improves. Serum lipid abnormalities also improve.

Preparations. Metformin is the only biguanide currently approved in the United States for the treatment of type 2 diabetes. The drug is well absorbed and excreted unchanged by the kidneys. Impaired renal function (creatinine >1.5 mg/dL in men and >1.4 mg/dL in women) is a contraindication for use. The drug is not metabolized by the liver. Its cost is about two to three times that of the oral hypoglycemics. The original biguanide, *phenformin*, is no longer marketed because of its associated risk for lactic acidosis (see below).

Dosing. The starting dose of metformin is 500 mg twice daily, given with the two largest meals of the day to minimize gastrointestinal upset. The dose is increased by 500 mg every 2 weeks until treatment goals are met or the maximum dosage of 2,000 to 2,500 mg/d is reached.

Efficacy. The efficacy of metformin is about the same as that of a second-generation sulfonylurea used as monotherapy in an obese person with moderate glucose intolerance; it lowers fasting glucose and glycosylated hemoglobin levels to the same degree (see above). Metformin has a synergistic effect when combined with sulfonylurea therapy in patients who do not respond well to monotherapy. Unlike the sulfonylureas, metformin is effective even in severe fasting hyperglycemia (>300 mg/dL), indicative of poor β-cell responsiveness. In the UKPDS, obese diabetics who attained tight control with metformin treatment exhibited a reduction in *microvascular disease*, and they were also the only group to show a reduced risk for *macrovascular* complications (i.e., myocardial infarction, stroke and cardiovascular death). Plasma triglycerides and LDL cholesterol levels were decreased.

Adverse Effects. The most common side effect of biguanide therapy is dose-related *gastrointestinal upset* (nausea, diarrhea, abdominal discomfort). The risk for serious prolonged *hypoglycemia* is minimal. *Lactic acidosis* represents the most potentially serious adverse effect. One of the original biguanides, *phenformin*, was taken off the market by the Food and Drug Administration in 1977 because of its association with fatal episodes of lactic acidosis. The risk for lactic acidosis associated with metformin is 5% that of phenformin (three cases per 100,000 patient-years of use). The risk is greatest in the setting of hypoxemia and in renal insufficiency (creatinine >1.5 mg/dL). Accumulation of the drug secondary to reduced excretion results in impaired hepatic metabolism of lactate. Other risk factors include binge drinking, use of IV radiologic contrast agents, hepatic failure (lactate is metabolized by the liver), and serious underlying illness, particularly heart failure. Long-term data on safety have yet to be accumulated. Because insulin secretion is not increased with metformin use, weight gain does not occur; some patients may even lose weight.

Patient Selection. Obese patients are particularly good candidates for metformin therapy because the drug helps reverse their insulin resistance. Peripheral responsiveness to insulin improves and insulin needs decrease, so that hyerinsulinism and its adverse effects, including weight gain, are minimized. The typical candidate is a *moderately obese person with type 2 diabetes* who has persistent moderate hyperglycemia (fasting glucose between 140 mg/dL and 240 mg/dL, glycosylated hemoglobin >7.0%) despite a full program of diet and exercise. Other candidates for metformin include obese patients who do not achieve tight control while taking a sulfonylurea at maximal doses. In this setting, metformin is *added to the oral hypoglycemic program* to improve control through its complementary mode of action. The sulfonylurea dose is reduced to lessen the risk for hypoglycemia. Combination therapy is most effective when initiated before the onset of symptomatic hyperglycemia (fasting glucose >250 mg/dL). If delayed, combination programs offer little benefit in altering disease progression or delaying the need for exogenous insulin. Patients who become unresponsive to maximal doses of a sulfonylurea may have exhausted their β-cell reserve and can be *switched to metformin* or considered for exogenous insulin therapy (sometimes in conjunction with metformin). The same pertains to the severely hyperglycemic obese patient (fasting glucose >300 mg/dL). Some diabetologists use metformin to *supplement an insulin program* in obese type 2 diabetics who require large insulin doses and have difficulty losing weight. The combined program helps to reduce insulin requirements and the appetite stimulation and weight gain that accompany hyperinsulinism. Caution and careful patient monitoring are required when a patient already taking exogenous insulin is started on metformin; the insulin requirement may drop considerably, putting the patient at risk for hypoglycemia.

Thiazolidinediones, (e.g. troglitazone, pioglitazone, rosiglitazone) are a new class of oral agents for treatment of type 2 diabetes. They appear to work predominantly by reducing insulin resistance in peripheral tissues, including fat and muscle, affording an additional opportunity to counter insulin resistance. They have become very popular because they are generally well-tolerated, do not cause hypoglycemia, and can enhance glycemic control when used in conjunction with other oral agents or insulin. The major concern surrounding their use has been idiosyncratic hepatocellular injury, occurring in such high frequency with troglitazone use that the drug has been withdrawn from the market.

Mechanism of Action. The main sites of action are muscle and fat, with improved sensitivity to insulin. Compared to metformin, there is less of an effect on hepatic responsiveness, which might account for the reduced efficacy. Adipocytes proliferate, possibly accounting for the observed increase in weight.

Efficacy. These drugs have about half the effectiveness of sulfonylureas and metformin in terms of lowering the fasting glucose and glycosylated hemoglobin. Onset of action may be evident by 7 days, manifested by a drop in fasting blood sugar, but full effect may take 4-6 weeks. About 25 percent of patients manifest no benefit; most have a low fasting C-peptide level. All thiazolidinediones have about the same degree of efficacy; 15-20 percent reductions in serum glucose levels can be expected. Modestly favorable improvements in triglyceride and HDL cholesterol levels occur, but LDL cholesterol may also increase, offsetting any improvement in lipid profile.

Adverse Effects. Because both short-term and long-term use of troglitazone is associated with rapid onset of *idiopathic hepatocellular injury* severe enough to result in death or require liver transplantation, the manufacturer has withdrawn the drug from the market. So far, the newer drugs in this class have not demonstrated this degree of hepatocellular risk, but experience with them is still limited. Careful, regular monitoring of hepatocellular enzymes is recommended at this time until there is sufficient experience with their use to better determine overall risk of liver injury. Any increase in ALT level beyond 1.5 to 2.0 times the upper limit of normal is an indication for weekly ALT monitoring and considering cessation of therapy. *Weight gain* occurs, especially when used in combination with sulfonylureas.

Preparations, Dosing, and Patient Selection. With troglitazone removed from the market, the two newer drugs in this class remain available for use. *Pioglitazone* is begun at 15 mg/day and *rosiglitazone* at 2 mg/day. Treatment is advanced on a monthlyl basis until maximum doses are reached (45 mg/d for pioglitazone and 8 mg/d for rosiglitazone). With the exception of troglitazone, these agents are approved for use both as *monotherapy* and in *combination* with either insulin or the sulfonylureas. Until more experience with them accumulates and hepatocellular safety is more firmly established, they should be used cautiously and only in patients without underlying liver disease who are willing to have their liver function monitored regularly.

Acarbose is a poorly absorbed complex oligosaccharide of bacterial origin. When taken at the beginning of a meal, it interferes with the pancreatic enzymatic hydrolysis of dietary carbohydrates (particularly disaccharide and complex carbohydrates), thereby slowing absorption. Glucose uptake from the bowel occurs more slowly and more distally, so that absorption can be better matched with insulin release in type 2 disease. Less than 1% of the drug is absorbed. Significant additional reductions in levels of postprandial glucose and glycosylated hemoglobin have been noted when acarbose is used in conjunction with diet, oral agents, or insulin. Its efficacy is about midway between that of diet alone and that of oral agents. Few data are available regarding its use in type 1 disease.

The principal side effects are gastrointestinal (abdominal cramping, distention, flatulence, and diarrhea) and are caused by the fermentation of unabsorbed carbohydrate by colonic bacteria. The effect is dose-related and seems to decrease with time. Occasional impairment of iron absorption may lead to microcytic anemia. Use with oral hypoglycemics or insulin may increase the risk for hypoglycemia, which must be treated with glucose because the drug interferes with the absorption of sucrose and other sugars. Concurrent use with metformin is problematic because acarbose potentiates the bioavailability of metformin and exacerbates its gastrointestinal side effects. The drug does not cause significant weight loss. The starting dosage is 25 mg three times daily, taken at the beginning of meals. The maximum dosage is 50 to 100 mg three times daily, depending on weight. The cost is about two to three times that of the oral hypoglycemics and similar to that of metformin.

Although acarbose can improve glycemic control in persons with type 2 disease and complement other forms of therapy, its gastrointestinal side effects limit its clinical acceptability for long-term use. Nonetheless, it represents an additional treatment option that can be useful in selected cases.

Repaglinide (Prandin). This agent, like the sulfonylureas, increases β-cell secretion of insulin; it is not yet known whether its effects are additive with those of the sulfonylureas, but its efficacy is similar. The onset of action is rapid and the duration short, so that use just before a meal is possible. The starting dosage is 0.5 mg three times daily; doses are taken 15 minutes before meals. The main adverse effect is hypoglycemia, which tends to be slightly less frequent and severe than in sulfonylurea therapy. Weight gain is noted; effects on lipids are minimal. The cost is 2.5 times that of brand name sulfonylureas.

Drug Therapy: Insulin

Insulin is the drug therapy of choice for diabetics in whom ketosis develops, for patients with symptomatic type 2 diabetes whose disease cannot be controlled by diet alone or a program of oral agent therapy, and for diabetics in whom near-normalization of blood sugar is a goal of therapy.

Preparations. In 1980, *highly purified* insulins prepared by high-performance liquid chromatography and containing less than 1 ppm of proinsulin were introduced. In 1982, *human recombinant insulin* was approved by the U.S. Food and Drug Administration. The increased use of human recombinant insulin and highly purified insulins has led to a decline in the incidence of local reactions, insulin allergy, immune resistance, and lipoatrophy. In some patients, human insulin may be absorbed more rapidly than animal insulins and have a shorter duration of action. Although antibody formation is less pronounced against human insulin than against insulin from animal species, a measurable increase in anti-insulin antibodies in a minority of patients treated with the recombinant preparation has been noted. More favorable pricing has made the cost of recombinant insulin similar to that of animal insulins, so insulin therapy should be initiated with human insulin.

Standard Preparations. Insulin is available in short-, intermediate-, and long-acting preparations. Intermediate types of insulin, *NPH* and *Lente*, with a peak action at 6 to 12 hours and an effect lasting 24-hours, are the most commonly used. The short-acting insulins, *regular (crystalline zinc insulin,* or CZI) and *Semilente,* have an earlier onset of action that peaks at 2 to 4 hours and lasts for a shorter time (5 hours). Long-acting insulins, *protamine-zinc* insulin and *Ultralente* insulin, may be most useful when given in intensive insulin therapy programs to provide a basal release of insulin in conjunction with multiple injections of short-acting insulin. Intermediate-acting Lente insulin contains crystalline structures that have absorption characteristics similar to those of NPH insulin, which makes it possible to avoid the use of a foreign protein that delays the absorption of NPH insulin.

Insulin Lispro, a newly synthesized preparation, has a faster onset and shorter duration of action. The positions of lysine and proline are switched in the B-chain of the molecule, which makes it less likely to polymerize; it is therefore more readily absorbed into the systemic circulation after SQ injection. The net result is a faster-acting insulin (45 to 60 minutes to peak) with a shorter duration of action (3 hours). Dosing is more convenient and compliance probably improved because insulin can be administered 10 to 15 minutes before a meal (in comparison with 30 to 45 minutes for regular insulin). In addition, the frequency of hypoglycemic episodes is modestly reduced (10% to 15%) in patients with type 1 disease because of a better match in the timing of insulin administration and food intake (no reduction in frequency of hypoglycemia noted with use in type 2 patients). Overall glycemic control and fasting glucose levels are significantly improved because the drug has no effect on basal insulin levels. Insulin lispro must be taken in combination with a longer-acting basal insulin program. Reasonable candidates are persons with type 1 disease who have achieved tight control with intensive insulin therapy but are at high risk for hypoglycemia. Such patients, especially those with a very active life-style and unpredictable schedule, appreciate the convenience and freedom of action afforded by insulin lispro. Patients with poor control and little risk for hypoglycemia are not candidates. Other potential users include those with a recent onset of type 1 disease who retain some basal insulin secretion. Fetal safety is not established, so that insulin lispro must be avoided by women of childbearing age unless they are utilizing birth control. The cost is considerably more than that of regular insulin.

Insulin Programs. Insulin is the treatment of choice for type 1 disease, an option as initial therapy for type 2 diabetes, and an essential component for the later stages of type 2 disease (Table 102.1). Because of the increasingly recognized value of tight glycemic control, traditional insulin regimens have been reexamined and new programs developed that provide better control. The goal is to enhance control of blood glucose without increasing the frequency and severity of hypoglycemic episodes. Both basal and prandial components of the insulin regimen must be considered.

Basal Insulin. The basal program is essential because it influences the fasting glucose level, the principal determinant of overall glycemic control. Typically, *twice-daily* (*"split"*) doses of an *intermediate-acting insulin* (NPH or Lente) or a *single dose* of a *long-acting insulin* (Ultralente) is administered to maintain normoglycemia during the fasting state.

A principal problem with such basal regimens is that increasing the dose to improve control increases the risk for *hypoglycemia* because the action of these insulin preparations often peaks at times of fasting rather than at times of food intake. A typical twice-daily split-dose program of NPH insulin taken before breakfast or dinner will produce peak insulin effects be-

Table 102.1. Common Insulin Regimens

STANDARD REGIMENS: RESPONSE TO INSULIN	REGIMEN
Early (type A)	Two-thirds dose intermediate insulin before breakfast One-third dose intermediate insulin before dinner
Normal (type B)	Full dose of intermediate insulin before breakfast
Late (type C)	Reduced dose of intermediate insulin plus a short-acting insulin before breakfast Small dose of short-acting insulin before dinner if postprandial evening hyperglycemia occurs

MORE INTENSIVE INSULIN REGIMENS: DEGREE OF CONTROL	REGIMEN
Tight	Divide total daily intermediate insulin dose into injections before breakfast and before dinner Add to each of the intermediate insulin doses a small dose of short-acting insulin
Very tight[a]	Long-acting insulin at night Short-acting insulins before each meal or more frequently based on self-monitored glucose measurements to achieve preprandial glucose between 70 and 120 mg/dL, postprandial glucose of <180 mg/dL, and normal HbA$_{1C}$ of <6.05% Pump therapy

[a]Intensive insulin therapy used in the Diabetes Control and Complication Trial.

tween 4 to 10 hours after injection, depending on whether the patient is an early (type A), normal (type B) or late (type C) reactor to insulin. The time of peak action with such basal regimens can be the very time when food intake is least likely (e.g., afternoon, early morning). Unless the timing of dosing or food intake is changed (e.g., moving the evening dose to before bed or having a good lunch and/or a late afternoon snack), the likelihood of hypoglycemia increases as control is tightened. Paradoxically, fasting *hyperglycemia* may be noted as a consequence of rebound glucose production (i.e., the *Somogyi effect*). Hyperglycemia may also ensue if the insulin effect peaks too early (e.g., when the dose is taken with dinner) or if the dose is insufficient to suppress morning hepatic glucose production ("dawn phenomenon").

If twice-daily intermediate insulin proves inadequate, the current alternative is to try Ultralente insulin. Its use is sometimes made problematic by an uneven absorption pattern. Safe basal control requires achieving a constant basal insulin level. The increasing desire to achieve tight control has led to interest in the development of ultralong-acting insulin preparations that provide a more constant rate of release and of novel delivery systems, such as inhaled preparations, pumps, and implants.

Prandial Insulin. In traditional single- or split-dose programs, *regular insulin* (CZI) is often used in conjunction with a basal insulin program to provide better postprandial glycemic control. In many instances, regular insulin is mixed with a longer-acting preparation and administered as a single injection to minimize the number of daily injections. The addition of regular insulin makes it necessary to administer the *mixed insulin regimen* at least 30 to 45 minutes before breakfast and dinner to ensure that the peak action of CZI is properly timed and not too late. The CZI timing requirement can be awkward for persons whose mealtimes are irregular or unpredictable; poor compliance and postprandial hyperglycemia or hypoglycemia are often the result. Also because of the CZI timing requirement, administration of the longer-acting insulin preparation can be timed poorly (as noted above). The net result is a wide daily fluctuation in blood sugar with periods of hypoglycemia and hyperglycemia and suboptimal overall control.

Intensive Insulin Therapy attempts to overcome the limitations of basal and prandial control associated with typical mixed and split insulin regimens. An intensive regimen is based on frequent home glucose monitoring, multiple daily injections of short-acting insulin before meals to provide better prandial control, and use of a long-acting insulin preparation for basal control. Regular insulin has typically been used for the prandial component, but its required lead time of 30 to 45 minutes before a meal is inconvenient and compromises compliance; moreover, its 4- to 6-hour duration of action increases the risk for hypoglycemia. The development of fast-acting, short-duration insulins (e.g., insulin lispro) and the pending arrival of more constantly absorbed long-acting preparations hold considerable promise for facilitating the achievement of safe, effective glycemic control through intensive insulin therapy.

In a typical intensive insulin program, *Ultralente* insulin is administered at 6 p.m. and *Semilente* insulin or *CZI* before meals. As noted earlier, *insulin lispro* can be used as the short-acting insulin for patients who achieve tight control but experience frequent hypoglycemic episodes, and for those who would benefit from its convenient schedule of administration. However, adequate basal insulin therapy is all the more important with lispro; because of its short duration of action, lispro contributes minimally to basal insulin levels. Intensive therapy requires careful self-monitoring of glucose to adjust dose and schedule. A 3 a.m. blood glucose determination is occasionally added to ensure that nocturnal hypoglycemia is not occurring. The major complication of intensive insulin therapy remains frequent and relatively severe *hypoglycemia.*

Intensive therapy is indicated in pregnancy because of the proven benefit of glucose control in limiting fetal morbidity and mortality and the potential for preventing congenital malformations, which are increased in children of diabetic mothers. Type 1 diabetics and younger, sophisticated, motivated patients without established complications may also be considered for intensive therapy. The expansion of intensive insulin therapies and the resources needed to apply intensive therapies across the entire diabetic population will increasingly involve discussions and decisions regarding broad health care and public policy.

Open-loop Pump Therapy. Pump therapy represents an attempt to duplicate the normal physiologic pattern of insulin release. Insulin infusion devices (worn externally and connected to an indwelling catheter) and multiple daily injections are being widely applied in gestational diabetes and in patients with type 1 diabetes that is difficult to control. This therapeutic approach requires patient motivation and sophistication, close monitoring, and careful supervision to be safe and effective. Comparable control of glycemia can be achieved by insulin pump and conventional intensive therapy. The major advantage of insulin pumps is that they facilitate frequent insulin administration. Complications include catheter infection, inadvertent catheter displacement from the skin, and cost.

Combined Oral Agent and Insulin Programs. In type 2 disease, with its multiple mechanisms of glucose intolerance, combination programs are a logical consideration when maximal doses of insulin or oral agents prove insufficient. In patients with type 2 disease who require very large insulin doses and experience unacceptable weight gain, the addition of *metformin* can improve glycemic control and reduce insulin requirements by countering insulin resistance in liver and muscle. Weight gain and other adverse effects of hyperinsulinism can be minimized. Likewise, a patient whose oral agent program is ineffective may benefit substantially from supplementation with a single modest dose of *NPH insulin* administered before bed. The small amount of insulin suppresses early morning hepatic glucose production (the dawn phenomenon), thereby reducing morning hyperglycemia without inducing hypoglycemia; overall glycemic control improves significantly.

Initiation of Therapy. Insulin therapy can be started safely on an ambulatory basis as long as the patient is reliable, nonketotic, and not severely hyperglycemic with intercurrent illness. Treatment should be initiated with 10 to 15 U of an intermediate-acting insulin and increased by approximately 2 U each day, depending on the results of urine or, preferably, blood sugar monitoring performed by the patient. Double-voided urine glucose determinations, commonly used in the past, have limitations (see below).

Technique and Storage. Insulin is injected SQ and is absorbed directly into the circulation. The abdomen and limbs are convenient injection sites; rotation among sites minimizes discomfort and, rarely, lipoatrophy. Rotation among multiple abdominal *injection sites* is preferable to limb injections in athletically active diabetic patients because of the possibility of more rapid insulin absorption from an exercising limb. Insulin, best *stored* in the refrigerator, may be left at room temperature for up to 12 hours without loss of biopotency.

Degree of Control. As noted earlier, the large-scale, long-term, randomized, controlled DCCT (for type 1 disease) and UKPDS (for type 2 diabetes) have firmly established that normalization of glycemia (HbA$_{1c}$ <7.0%) significantly reduces the risks for microvascular complications. Very tight control (HbA$_{1c}$ between 6.0% and 7.0%) is the objective of intensive insulin regimens. Whether and under what conditions such control can also reduce the risk for macrovascular complications remains to be determined. So far, only obese patients achieving tight glycemic control with metformin have experienced significant reductions in cardiovascular and stroke risk. That the weight gain seen with intensive insulin therapy might be a manifestation of the insulin resistance syndrome, which includes hypertension and an increased coronary risk, is a concern. Efforts to counter such insulin resistance may be necessary to achieve a reduction in coronary risk. More study is needed.

The practical issue is whether such tight control can be accomplished safely in a given patient and whether the means of therapy currently available are compatible with patients' lifestyles and personal choices for therapy. In type 1 disease, an in-

Table 102.2.   Important Causes of Worsening Hyperglycemia During Insulin Therapy

Inadequate dose
Increased caloric intake
Failure to take insulin properly
Occult infection (especially urinary tract)
Coronary ischemia
Severe emotional stress
Use of corticosteroids
Somogyi phenomenon
Insulin resistance
Growth hormone surge in early morning

telligent, well-motivated, reliable person can be taught to regulate daily insulin doses, but less capable patients risk hypoglycemic reactions when tight control is attempted. In type 2 diabetes, the advent of well-tolerated agents that turn off hepatic gluconeogenesis and peripheral insulin resistance has made it possible to improve control with a lesser risk for hypoglycemia.

Worsening Hyperglycemia during Insulin Therapy. In a patient taking a previously adequate dose of insulin, hyperglycemia requires prompt attention (Table 102.2). Although important changes in caloric intake or failure to take insulin properly may be the explanation for worsening hyperglycemia, occult infection (especially in the urinary tract), coronary ischemia, severe emotional stress, and Somogyi phenomenon (rebound hyperglycemia) must be investigated. A recently recognized phenomenon, worsening hyperglycemia in the early morning hours, is caused by the surges in growth hormone levels that occur during sleep. An intermediate-acting insulin given at bedtime can provide excellent coverage for such early morning hyperglycemia.

The Somogyi Phenomenon, in which rebound hyperglycemia and possibly ketosis occur after insulin-induced hypoglycemia, may be mistaken for inadequate control. The hypoglycemia usually goes unnoticed because it occurs at night or in a patient with severe autonomic neuropathy. Hypoglycemia is followed by several days of poor control. Clues to recognizing nocturnal hypoglycemia include night sweats, poor sleep, nightmares, and morning headaches. Urinary monitoring reveals negative urinary glucose and ketones in the evening followed by trace urinary sugar and large ketones in the morning. The best way to recognize the Somogyi effect is to be cognizant of its potential existence and to measure blood glucose at a time of suspected hypoglycemia. Appropriate therapy, which involves slowly decreasing the dosage of insulin, may be commenced after hypoglycemia has been documented. If detection is impractical, a diagnostic trial of reduced insulin may be used to confirm the clinical suspicion. Doses of insulin should be decreased slowly each day rather than precipitously because a dramatic decrease in insulin dosage will cause hyperglycemia to worsen.

Insulin Resistance is occasionally the cause of poor control. It is arbitrarily defined as the requirement for *more than 200 U of insulin daily.* Most cases of insulin resistance result from obesity; restoring normal weight is the best treatment. As noted earlier, the hepatic and muscle refractoriness to insulin seen in type 2 disease may respond to therapy with metformin or a thiazolidinedione. More classic insulin resistance is immunologically mediated by antibodies directed at bovine or porcine insulin, or against protamine or protamine-insulin complexes. There appears to be no increased frequency of antibody production against insulin lispro.

For patients with immunologic insulin resistance, switching therapy to a Lente insulin preparation or to human recombinant insulin may be advantageous. At times, high-dose glucocorticoids (80 to 100 mg of prednisone daily) may be necessary. Most patients respond, and steroid therapy can often be rapidly tapered. Immunologic insulin resistance is commonly seen in patients who have been receiving insulin in intermittent treatment programs. In patients who receive insulin for limited intervals only (e.g., during myocardial infarction or weight reduction for obesity), human insulin represents the best choice of therapy to limit antibody development.

Hypoglycemia and Insulin Reactions. When food intake is delayed or diminished, physical activity is increased, or the insulin dose is excessive, hypoglycemia may ensue. Symptoms include those of increased sympathomimetic activity: sweating, palpitations, tremor, and weakness. In addition, *neuroglycopenic symptoms* (fatigue and changes in mentation) may be seen with a less precipitous decline in blood sugar. Profound hypoglycemia may lead to loss of consciousness. If autonomic neuropathy is present, or if a patient is taking a β-adrenergic blocker, many hypoglycemic symptoms will be masked and mental confusion may be the paramount symptom. Patient and family education and the availability of a syringe containing glucagon are important (see below). In patients who experience frequent hypoglycemic episodes, an apparent decline in the blood glucose level that occurs with time triggers an autonomic response, so that careful home glucose monitoring is necessary when patients engage in a program of intensive insulin therapy.

Insulin Allergy, manifested as cutaneous reactions to insulin, occurs in approximately 5% of patients. Urticaria, angioedema, or anaphylaxis is rare. Insulin allergy may be treated by a change to human insulin administered with antihistamines. Desensitization may be necessary if systemic allergic manifestations have occurred. Lispro insulin has not been associated with an increased risk for insulin allergy.

Insulin and Surgery. In the management of the diabetic patient during surgery, modest hyperglycemia is allowed and hypoglycemia and ketosis are assiduously avoided. The preoperative medical evaluation is critical because most perioperative complications relate not to hyperglycemia or hypoglycemia, but rather to coexisting cardiac or renal disease. Importantly, the potential for infection must be considered carefully and sources of fever, such as pulmonary, skin, and urinary tract infection, need to be investigated. Many insulin programs for operative management have been advanced. In general, the dose of insulin should be reduced by approximately one third to one half on the morning of surgery and carbohydrate supplied as IV 5% dextrose at the rate of 150 mL/h. Surgery should, if possible, be performed early in the day, with postoperative monitoring of blood sugar and renal function. An ECG should be obtained because of the higher incidence of silent myocardial ischemia and infarction in diabetics. Until the patient resumes eating, the insulin dosage may need to be decreased unless an increased secretion of counterregulatory hormones (e.g., growth hormone, cortisol, catecholamines) worsens hyperglycemia and an increased dose is necessary. A risk for infection has been found in patients whose HbA_{1c} is 11.5%, an indication of marked hyperglycemia in the preoperative interval.

Control of Associated Cardiovascular Risk Factors

As noted earlier, control of hyperglycemia prevents or limits the microvascular, neurologic, and renal complications of diabetes. Except in obese patients with type 2 diabetes who achieve tight control with metformin, it has not yet been proved that the risk for macrovascular disease is similarly reduced by tight control. Consequently, it is most important that all associated risk factors for the development of coronary artery disease be meticulously controlled. Diabetes confers a degree of coronary risk similar to that associated with prior myocardial infarction. In diabetics, aggressive efforts to control hypertension, reduce hypercholesterolemia, and cease smoking (see Chapters 26, 27, and 54) result in marked reductions in the risk for coronary events and stroke and in all-cause mortality. With 75% of deaths in diabetic patients caused by cardiovascular problems, the importance of reducing atherosclerotic risk factors cannot be overemphasized. These efforts are even more productive than attempts at tight control of blood sugar and must not be overlooked.

Hypertension. The treatment of hypertension in diabetics requires attention not only to the degree of control achieved but also to its effects on metabolic control, recognition of hypoglycemia, and "renal hyperfiltration." The drugs of choice are the *angiotensin-converting enzyme* (ACE) *inhibitors*. They appear to limit hyperfiltration and preserve renal function (see below). Patients must be monitored for hyperkalemia. The *thiazide* diuretics may modestly compromise glucose intolerance, which makes them less desirable than the ACE inhibitors as first-line agents, especially in full doses. In smaller doses, they have few adverse effects on blood glucose and may facilitate blood pressure control. *β-Blockers* are effective but can mask the sympathomimetic warning symptoms of hypoglycemia. They should be used with care in patients undergoing intensive insulin therapy. Impotence and postural hypotension are features of diabetes that may affect the choice of antihypertensive therapy (see Chapter 26).

Lipid Disorders. Lipid abnormalities are a consequence of diabetes and sometimes also of treatments for diabetes. HDL cholesterol is often low, and VLDL and LDL cholesterols and triglycerides increased. Effective control of hyperglycemia often improves the lipid profile by reducing triglycerides and raising HDL cholesterol, but intensive insulin therapy that causes weight gain may actually increase LDL cholesterol and lower HDL cholesterol. Metformin use is associated with reductions in triglycerides and LDL cholesterol and slight increases in HDL cholesterol. The thiazolidindiones decrease triglycerides and raise HDL cholesterol, but they also increase LDL cholesterol. The sulfonylureas and acarbose have no effects on lipids. The drugs used to treat lipid disorders are usually well tolerated in diabetes; the statins can very effectively lower LDL cholesterol and modestly raise HDL cholesterol; the fibrates are effective for reducing triglycerides and raising HDL cholesterol (see Chapter 27), but they should not be used with statins.

Niacin is effective for raising low HDL cholesterol but can exacerbate glucose intolerance (see Chapter 27).

Management of Complications

Renal Failure. *ACE inhibitors* reduce proteinuria and significantly slow the progression of azotemia. The beneficial effect on nephropathy occurs even in normotensive patients and is independent of reduction in blood pressure. It is believed related to afferent arteriolar dilation and reduced hyperfiltration. Control of hypertension still remains important, particularly as renal function declines (see Chapter 26). Studies suggest that treating all diabetic patients prophylactically with an ACE inhibitor may be cost-effective, irrespective of renal sediment findings. *Protein restriction* (0.5 mg/kg) may also reduce hyperfiltration in early nephropathy, but ACE inhibitor therapy is likely to be more acceptable. The progression to renal failure may be inexorable once heavy proteinuria (>3 g/d) develops. However, the primary care physician may still be able to prevent some forms of late renal insufficiency, such as that associated with bladder dysfunction, pyelonephritis, and acute papillary necrosis, and the contrast-induced acute renal failure that occurs in diabetics with moderate to advanced renal insufficiency. Prompt and aggressive *treatment of urinary tract infections* (see Chapters 133 and 140), therapy to *limit urinary retention*, which increases the risk for infection (see Chapter 134), and avoidance of unnecessary contrast studies all help to prevent renal insults. If *dye studies* are necessary, *hydration must be maintained*, as small a dye load as possible used, and mannitol administered after the study. Nephrotoxic antibiotics and *NSAIDs* (which can inhibit renal prostaglandin activity) should be avoided. *Metformin* use needs to be restricted in the setting of renal insufficiency (creatinine >1.5 mg/dL in men, >1.4 mg/dL in women) because it is excreted by the kidneys and high doses increase the risk for lactic acidosis.

During the past decade, the outlook for the diabetic patient undergoing hemodialysis or renal transplantation has improved, although the mortality rate for diabetics on these treatment modalities remains higher than that of nondiabetics. Continuous ambulatory *peritoneal dialysis* has been offered to diabetic patients because of concerns that the heparin used in hemodialysis may worsen diabetic retinopathy. However, early information suggests that infection rates are higher in diabetic patients on continuous peritoneal dialysis.

Peripheral Vascular Disease. The microvascular and macrovascular complications of diabetes are readily evident in the limbs. Ischemic skin ulcers, claudication, and limb loss are common complications. Amputation of a lower extremity is often the consequence of peripheral vascular disease and neuropathy in patients with diabetes. In comparison with a control diabetic population, diabetic amputees had more severe neuropathy and vascular impairment and lower HDL cholesterol levels, and they had received less outpatient diabetic education. Management includes tightening glycemic control, reducing atherosclerotic risk factors, exercising, quitting smoking, and maintaining meticulous foot care (see Chapter 34).

Foot Problems. Because of vascular insufficiency and neuropathy, diabetic patients have unique foot care problems. Early detection of diminished sensation is facilitated by testing with a standardized monofilament, which is superior to the conventional physical examination for detecting protective foot sensation. Meticulous foot care is essential to prevent cellulitis, osteomyelitis, and the need for amputation. Feet must be kept clean, interdigital spaces dry, calluses pared down, and toenails carefully trimmed. Frequent inspection for skin breakdown and cellulitis by the patient needs to be stressed, as does the importance of wearing properly fitting shoes. Before bathing, diabetic patients should use their hands to test the water temperature, so that scalding injuries that may occur because of a loss of temperature sensation in the lower extremities can be prevented. Regular podiatric care is a well-considered preventive measure for all diabetics, especially those who are elderly or have poor eyesight, a history of foot infection, or a significant loss of sensation.

Neuropathy. Neuropathic *pain* has been treated with phenytoin, carbamazepine, tricyclic antidepressants, and phenothiazines, but no singularly effective treatment program has emerged. The tricyclic *amitriptyline* is the standard treatment. Initial data from placebo-controlled studies of *gabapentin* are very encouraging; comparative study is required to assess its relative benefit. *Phenytoin* seems to cause the least toxicity and should be tried first. The *postural hypotension*, impotence, and urinary retention associated with autonomic neuropathy are usually permanent. Postural hypotension may respond to the synthetic mineralocorticoid *Florinef. Impotence* is a reasonable indication for consideration of *sildenafil* (Viagra), which can be moderately effective in diabetic men (see Chapter 132). Anxiety and depression, which are often superimposed on neurologic dysfunction, must be excluded (see Chapters 132 and 229).

Enteropathy. Gastrointestinal motility problems, which include *gastroparesis* and *diabetic diarrhea*, can be difficult to treat. Small, frequent feedings and cholinergic drugs such as *cisapride* may lessen the symptoms of gastroparesis. Patients with diarrhea caused by bacterial overgrowth of the bowel can be treated with a trial of a broad-spectrum antibiotic (e.g., *neomycin*). *Cholestyramine* has been found to be of benefit in controlling the diarrhea of diabetic autonomic neuropathy. Fortunately, refractory nocturnal diarrhea often resolves spontaneously.

Regular dental examinations are a necessity because of the higher incidence in diabetic patients of *pyorrhea* and abscesses, which may also reduce diabetic control.

Ophthalmopathy. Diabetic *retinopathy* is the most important systemic disease causing blindness. Proliferative retinopathy accounts for the majority of cases of blindness among type 1 diabetics, whereas *macular edema* resulting from nonproliferative retinopathy accounts for most cases of blindness in type 2 diabetes. Prevention is the best treatment, achieved by a reduction in hyperglycemia. Even partial normalization of glucose levels is helpful. Photocoagulation with laser therapy can retard visual loss by 50% (see Chapter 209). Cataracts and glaucoma are also important complications (see Chapters 207 and 208 for a discussion of management).

Glucose Intolerance and Pregnancy

Fetal hyperglycemia contributes to excessive fetal growth, which increases the risks for birth trauma, asphyxia, neonatal respiratory distress syndrome, and death *in utero*. In addition, the need for cesarean section is increased. Maintenance of blood sugars in the physiologic range (60 to 120 mg/dL) takes on added importance during pregnancy because the complications of fetal hyperglycemia can be prevented and perinatal mortality reduced to the rate seen in nondiabetics. Even in nondiabetic pregnant women in whom an otherwise insignificant degree of hyperglycemia (2-hour-postprandial blood sugars in the range of 140 to 160 mg/dL) develops, the risk for macrosomia and its complications is increased. Women with postprandial readings in excess of 165 mg/dL have an increased incidence of diabetes in later life.

The importance of glucose intolerance during pregnancy has led to the recommendation by the American Diabetic Association that all pregnant women be screened for glucose intolerance by the 24th to 28th week of gestation. Data from the Nurses' Health Study have shown an advanced maternal age, family history, nonwhite ethnicity, higher body mass index, weight gain in early adulthood, and cigarette smoking identified to be independent risk factors. Screening is conducted with a 50-g oral glucose load, which can be given at any time of day. Patients with a 1-hour serum glucose level in excess of 140 mg/dL should be given a 100-g glucose tolerance test and treated if the level is above 165 mg/dL at 2 hours. Some argue, on the basis of studies showing an increased fetal risk associated with levels of glucose intolerance previously considered "normal" (120 to 160 mg/dL), that even more modest elevations are grounds for therapy, at least with dietary measures.

All patients with glucose intolerance should be treated with diets that limit simple sugars and total calories (35 to 38 calories per kilogram of ideal weight before pregnancy) and tested for elevation of blood sugar every 1 to 2 weeks until delivery is indicated. Patients showing fasting sugars in excess of 105 mg/dL or postprandial levels above 120 mg/dL should be considered for insulin therapy; consultation with a diabetologist is indicated.

For diabetic patients already on insulin, adjustments in dose may be necessary. During the first trimester, the insulin dose of a patient with type 1 diabetes should be reduced because insulin requirements decrease and the risk for hypoglycemia is increased. In the second trimester, the type 1 diabetic requires more insulin as the diabetes becomes more labile and the chances for the development of ketoacidosis (with its associated risk for fetal death) rise. Third-trimester dose requirements usually do not change, but the increase in the glomerular filtration rate can lower the tubular threshold for glucose and make urine testing unreliable. Within a few hours of delivery, insulin requirements fall considerably, returning completely to prepregnancy levels within 1 to 2 weeks. Optimal control is facilitated by the use of home glucose monitoring (see below).

Monitoring

Monitoring must address three parameters: glycemic control, diabetic complications, and adverse drug effects.

For Control of Glycemia. The traditional means of monitoring was the double-voided urine test for glucose and ketones, usually performed before breakfast and before the evening meal by patients taking insulin. The technique requires voiding fully, then voiding again an hour later and testing the urine sample by means of tape or tablets; a colorimetric response indicates the urine glucose and ketone concentrations. At best, the correlation between urine and serum glucose concentrations is approximate. It varies from patient to patient and from time to time in the same patient because of differences and changes in the renal tubular threshold for glucose, renal blood flow, and urine volume. Moreover, the test result is compromised in patients with bladder dysfunction who have a postvoid residual.

Home Glucose Monitoring. The finger-stick method represents a marked improvement in monitoring. The patient obtains a finger-stick sample of capillary blood, which is tested for glucose concentration by colorimetric reading of a reagent strip to which a drop of blood is applied. More sophisticated meters and color charts are now available for the glucose determination. Insurance companies are increasingly covering the costs. Measurements are most useful for patients on insulin therapy; hour-to-hour and day-to-day adjustments can be made based on the results of blood sugar monitoring. Frequent measurements, both in the fasting state and at several intervals postprandially, are valuable when an insulin program is being started or adjusted and also during periods of illness or worsening control. Most patients can be taught the method. Numerous devices automatically perform the finger-stick. Once a stable insulin dose has been achieved, a single measurement need be taken only once every several days, typically before breakfast. Patients who are capable of adjusting their own insulin doses can use home monitoring to keep their sugars in the mid-100 range after a meal. Home monitoring does not obviate the need to inform the patient carefully about symptoms of hyperglycemia and hypoglycemia (see below).

Hemoglobin A_{1c} is the glycosylated form of hemoglobin in the red cell. The degree of glycosylation reflects the glucose concentration in the red cell environment during the life span of the cell. Measurement of the HbA_{1c} concentration allows an assessment of overall glycemic control for the preceding 2 to 3 months. It correlates well with the results of frequent blood glucose determinations. Levels of less than 8.0% indicate blood sugar levels of less than 200 mg/dL; values of 11% to 12% correlate with glucose levels in excess of 300 mg/dL and indicate poor carbohydrate control. This test has superseded the *random blood sugar* determination as the best means of assessing control over time. For the patient with mild non–insulin-dependent diabetes, a periodic HbA_{1c} determination suffices for monitoring glycemia control. Patients taking insulin require both short- and long-term measurements of blood sugar.

Checking for Complications. Patients with diabetes should undergo at least an annual office evaluation that includes a check of the blood pressure for elevation; the skin for infection; the eyes for background retinopathy (see Chapter 209); the cardiovascular system for evidence of carotid, coronary, and peripheral vascular disease; and the feet for ischemic lesions. The evaluation should conclude with a careful neurologic examination for signs of neuropathy. Of particular importance is the need to test for and vigorously treat other risk factors for vascular disease, such as hypertension (see Chapter 14), hypercholesterolemia (see Chapter 15), and smoking (see Chapter 54). More frequent office visits are usually necessary for patients on insulin therapy and with complications of diabetes. Laboratory monitoring should include a urinalysis to check for proteinuria

and sediment and a determination of blood urea nitrogen and creatinine to estimate renal function. A diabetic summary sheet placed in the patient's record makes it possible to note quickly the extent, severity, and progression of the disease and its complications. Teaching the patient to watch for skin, eye, neurologic, and cardiovascular changes is an important part of the monitoring effort (see below).

Monitoring for Adverse Effects of Drug Therapy. Patients prescribed *troglitazone* and other thiazolidinediones require regular monitoring of *serum liver enzymes* (e.g., ALT; see above). Testing should be conducted biweekly at the start of troglitazone therapy and continued monthly for the first year. Any ALT elevations in excess of three times the upper limit of normal are an indication for immediate cessation of therapy, and cessation should also be considered if any sustained increases are noted. The *renal* and *hepatic* function of patients on *metformin* must be monitored. The onset of renal or hepatic insufficiency necessitates that metformin therapy be discontinued because of the increased risk for lactic acidosis.

PATIENT EDUCATION

The success of a program for metabolic control depends on patient compliance. Because *weight reduction* to ideal body weight is the most important therapy that can be offered to patients with type 2 diabetes, instruction about *diet* and choosing healthful foods should take place in a setting that includes both patient and family. Sample diets can be obtained from the American Diabetic Association. The emphasis on diet therapy for the type 2 diabetic should focus more on caloric restriction than on actual percentages of carbohydrate or simple sugars.

The patient receiving insulin requires continuous education and encouragement, particularly as more intensive insulin treatment programs are applied to patients with type 2 diabetes to limit the end-organ consequences of hyperglycemia. In many hospital-based practices and several office practices, a nurse specializing in diabetes education offers patients careful instruction in drawing up insulin into syringes (particularly if the patient is visually impaired), insulin injection techniques, and the complications of excess insulin administration, and is readily available for telephone communication with patients. Some physicians consider deliberately creating mild insulin reactions in their patients so that they are able to recognize their own unique warning symptoms of hypoglycemia. A *syringe with glucagon* for IM injection is given to each patient in the event that the patient becomes profoundly hypoglycemic. Oral administration of juices to an unconscious and obtunded patient may lead to pulmonary aspiration.

The importance of skin and foot care must be emphasized (see Chapter 34). Referral of elderly diabetic patients with vision loss to podiatrists for regular foot care is indicated.

INDICATIONS FOR ADMISSION AND REFERRAL

Patient care programs that encourage communication between patients and health care professionals reduce the need for hospitalization for dehydration, marked hyperglycemia, ketoacidosis, and infection. Making diabetes management a collaborative process involving the complementary efforts of teams including nurses or physician assistants also helps in this regard; controlled trials have demonstrated improved glycemic control.

Acute hospitalization for IV administration of fluids is necessary for diabetic patients with protracted nausea and vomiting who are becoming dehydrated and hyperglycemic. Often, cellulitis of the foot requires IV antibiotic therapy, as does acute pyelonephritis. In general, elderly diabetic patients with pneumonia or urinary tract infections benefit from brief hospitalizations. Referral to an endocrinologist is indicated for the diabetic patient who is subject to marked fluctuations in blood sugar, with frequent episodes of hypoglycemia and hyperglycemia. When proteinuria is in the nephrotic syndrome range and the creatinine level begins to rise above 2.5 mg/dL, referral to a nephrologist for consideration of dialysis or transplantation is necessary. Indications for coronary artery bypass grafting are not different for the diabetic patient. Because of the potential severity of cholecystitis and ascending cholangitis, cholecystectomy for cholelithiasis may be a reasonable clinical choice, although more recent experience favors watchful waiting for asymptomatic cholelithiasis (see Chapter 69). Ophthalmologic referral is indicated when background diabetic retinopathy first becomes evident.

THERAPEUTIC RECOMMENDATIONS

All Diabetic Patients

- Attempt to normalize hyperglycemia; the goal is an HbA_{1c} concentration below 7.0% and a fasting glucose level below 126 mg/dL.
- Emphasize the importance of maintaining ideal body weight. For those who are obese, institute caloric restriction without compromising the regularity of meal timing.
- Prescribe exercise and healthful diet.
- Pay assiduous attention to the diagnosis and treatment of all additional atherosclerotic risk factors, such as hypertension, hyperlipidemia, and smoking (see Chapters 26, 27, and 54).
- Teach all diabetic patients, especially those on insulin therapy, how to monitor glycemic control daily with *home blood glucose determinations.*
- Assess long-term glucose control with *HbA_{1c} measurements* three or four times yearly.
- Carefully investigate the causes of worsening hyperglycemia (Table 102.2).
- Perform a comprehensive history, physical examination, and selected laboratory studies (blood urea nitrogen, creatinine, HbA_{1c}, cholesterol, urinalysis) at least annually. Search for evidence of coronary artery disease, cerebrovascular disease, peripheral vascular disease, diabetic neuropathy, renal insufficiency, proteinuria, and retinopathy.
- Carefully monitor *renal function* for azotemia and check the *urinary sediment* for proteinuria and microscopic hematuria. Promptly institute tighter control of hyperglycemia and prescribe an *ACE inhibitor* at the first sign of nephropathy. Even for patients with no sign of nephropathy, consider instituting ACE inhibitor therapy if they are middle-aged to reduce the risk for development of nephropathy. When the serum creatinine level reaches 3 mg/dL, obtain a nephrology consultation regarding candidacy for dialysis or transplantation.
- Exercise caution in the use of *iodinated contrast agents*, especially in the setting of renal impairment.
- Refer diabetic patients who have background retinopathy or who have had diabetes for 5 to 10 years to an ophthalmolo-

gist for prompt *indirect ophthalmoscopy* and, if necessary, fluorescein angiography. Arrange for an annual ophthalmic diabetic eye examination for all others (see Chapter 209).
- Emphasize *foot care* to diabetic patients with neuropathy or vascular insufficiency. Arrange regular podiatric care for such patients.
- Perform a careful perioperative assessment of diabetic patients undergoing surgery. Pay particular attention to worsening hyperglycemia and diligently observe for infection and occult coronary artery disease, particularly in those with evidence of microvascular disease.
- Consider including a well-trained nurse, nurse practitioner, or physician assistant in the long-term management program to complement and support physician efforts at achieving glycemic control.

Patients with Type 1 Disease

- Consider early institution of *intensive insulin therapy* to achieve very tight control (HbA_{1c} 6.0% to 7.0%), especially for highly motivated patients willing to perform multiple glucose determinations each day and self-administer insulin according to the results of each test. Consider less intensive insulin therapy or infusion pump technology for those unable to carry out an intensive insulin regimen.

For those attempting intensive insulin therapy:
- Start with a modest dose of long-acting insulin, such as Ultralente or one of the new long-acting preparations as they become available, administered once daily in the evening; start with a dose of 15 U and increase in increments of 2 U, based on fasting glucose determinations.
- Also begin a program of short-acting insulin, such as regular (CZI) or Semilente, started at 5 U administered 30 to 45 minutes before each meal and adjusted according to the results of postprandial home glucose measurements.
- Prescribe human recombinant insulin for newly treated diabetics to minimize risks for insulin allergy, insulin resistance, and antibody development.
- Consider prescribing insulin lispro (or another fast-onset, very short-acting insulin), administered 10 to 15 minutes before each meal, to patients achieving tight control but bothered by frequent hypoglycemic episodes or the inconvenience of a standard regimen of regular insulin.

For those unable to carry out an intensive insulin program:
- Begin a twice-daily insulin regimen with an intermediate-acting insulin (e.g., NPH or Lente), administered before breakfast and before the evening meal for basal coverage, mixed with a short-acting insulin (e.g., CZI, Semilente) for prandial control.
- Adjust doses according to fasting and 4 p.m. glucose determinations.
- Teach the importance of regular caloric intake and regular spacing of meals to match peak insulin effects and activity schedules.

Patients with Type 2 Disease

- Emphasize *weight reduction* to ideal body weight as the cornerstone of therapy for type 2 diabetes. The composition of the diet *per se* is less important, but the diet should have a high ratio of polyunsaturated to saturated fat and contain cholesterol and complex carbohydrates. Diets low in protein may be beneficial in averting diabetic nephropathy (see Chapter 132).

- Prescribe a practical program of regular exercise that fits the patient's life-style (see Chapter 18).

If after 4 to 8 weeks of diet and exercise the treatment goals have not been achieved and the patient shows *mild to moderate glucose* intolerance (fasting glucose <240 mg/dL), then:

- Begin oral agent therapy with either a *second-generation sulfonylurea* (e.g., 2.5 mg of *glyburide*, 5 mg of *glipizide*, or 1 mg of *glimepiride*) or a *biguanide* (e.g., 500 mg of *metformin* twice daily, with breakfast and the evening meal). Choose metformin if the patient is obese.
- Increase the oral agent dose every 1 to 2 weeks as needed. Consider twice-daily dosing for glyburide and glipizide to maximize control or once-daily dosing of a sustained-release glipizide. Advance until glycemic goals are achieved or maximum dose is reached (20 mg/d for glyburide and glipizide, 8 mg/d for glimepiride).
- If after 4 to 8 weeks of monotherapy glycemic goals have not been achieved, then add a second oral agent from a different class (e.g., metformin if a sulfonylurea was given first and vice versa) or add a small dose of an intermediate-acting insulin taken before bedtime (e.g., 10 U of NPH). If the sulfonylurea was the starting drug, reduce the sulfonylurea dose to avoid the risk for prolonged hypoglycemia.
- If after 4 to 8 weeks of two-drug oral agent therapy control has not been achieved, then consider adding either a dose of *intermediate insulin* before bed (e.g., 10 U of NPH) or a third oral agent (e.g., a thiazolidinedione or acarbose).
- If adding a *thiazolidinedione* (e.g., *pioglitazone, rosiglitazone*) start with a low dose (for pioglitazone, 15 mg/day, and for rosiglitazone, 2 mg/day, and monitor liver function (ALT) montly for at least the first several months, halting therapy at the first sign of persistent elevation. Until proven hepatically safe, consider thiazolidinediones only if all other attempts to date have failed to achieve reasonable glycemic control and the patient is reliable, free of underlying liver disease, and willing to have close monitoring of liver function tests.
- If a program of insulin supplementation is considered, be aware that initially supplementing oral agent therapy with a small bedtime dose of insulin may suffice but usually latter stages of type 2 disease require insulin as the mainstay of the treatment program, supplemented by a thizolindinedione (eg. pioglitazone, rosiglitazone) or metformin to reduce insulin resistance and keep the insulin dose manageable.

If after 4 to 8 weeks of diet and exercise treatment goals have not been achieved and the patient is very symptomatic or manifests *moderate to severe glucose intolerance* (fasting glucose >240 mg/dL), then:

- Begin *insulin* therapy with an intermediate-acting insulin preparation (Lente or NPH) at a modest once-daily dose (e.g., 10 U before breakfast).
- Specify human recombinant insulin for newly treated diabetic patients to minimize the risks for insulin allergy, insulin resistance, and antibody development.
- Advance the insulin program according to glucose monitoring results with reference to target levels.
- If high doses of insulin, poor control, and weight gain become problems, consider adding metformin to the insulin

program to improve tissue responsiveness and reduce insulin requirements and weight gain. A thiazolidinedione can also improve insulin responsiveness and control, but does not halt weight gain.

A.H.G.

ANNOTATED BIBLIOGRAPHY

Arky R. Current principles of dietary therapy of diabetes mellitus. Med Clin North Am 1978;62:655. (*A classic review of dietary methods of controlling diabetes.*)

Aviles-Santa L, Sinding J, Raskin P. Effects of metformin in patients with poorly controlled insulin-treated type 2 diabetes mellitus: a randomized, double-blind, placebo-controlled trial. Ann Intern Med 1999;131:182. (*Strong evidence for the effectiveness of adding metformin to an insulin program.*)

Aubert RE, Herman WH, Waters J, et al. Nurse case management to improve glycemic control in diabetic patients in a health maintenance organization: a randomized, controlled trial. Ann Intern Med 1998;129:605. (*Glycemic control improved in this collaborative effort between physicians and nurse practitioners.*)

Backonja M, Beydoun A, Edwards KR, et al. Gabapentin for the symptomatic treatment of painful neuropathy in patients with diabetes mellitus: a randomized controlled trial. JAMA 1998;280:1831. (*A placebo-controlled study finding significantly reduced pain and improved quality of life; however, no comparison with other agents.*)

Bailey CJ, Turner RC. Metformin. N Engl J Med 1996;334:574. (*Detailed review of this important treatment modality; 66 references.*)

Campbell PJ, Bolli G, Cryer P, et al. Pathogenesis of the dawn phenomenon in patients with insulin-dependent diabetes mellitus. N Engl J Med 1985;312:1473. (*Physiologic studies implicating growth hormone, not catecholamines, in the preawakening rise in glucose.*)

Chiasson JL, Josse RG, Hunt JA, et al. The efficacy of acarbose in the treatment of patients with non–insulin-dependent diabetes mellitus: a multicenter controlled clinical trial. Ann Intern Med 1994;121:928. (*Provides moderate benefit when used as monotherapy or when added to an existing program.*)

Colditz GA, Willett WC, Rotnitzky A, et al. Weight gain as a risk factor for clinical diabetes mellitus in women. Ann Intern Med 1995;122:481. (*Even a modest weight gain, to 5 kg above weight at age 18, in women ages 35 to 50 years correlated with a significant increase in risk for type 2 diabetes.*)

DeFronzo RA. Pharmacologic therapy for type 2 diabetes mellitus. Ann Intern Med 1999;131:281. (*Outstanding review of evidence for the use of oral agents, including a discussion of treatment strategies; 175 references.*)

DeFronzo RA, Goodman AM, and the Multicenter Metformin Study Group. Efficacy of metformin in patients with non–insulin-dependent diabetes mellitus. N Engl J Med 1995;333:541. (*A randomized, controlled trial comparing metformin, glyburide, combination therapy, and placebo in obese patients with type 2 diabetes not adequately controlled by diet or sulfonylurea therapy. Metformin was well tolerated and proved capable of improving diabetic control in these patients.*)

DeFronzo RA, Bonadonna RC, Ferrannini E. Pathogenesis of NIDDM. A balanced overview. Diabetes Care 1992;15:315. (*A comprehensive review of hyperinsulinemia and insulin resistance in the pathogenesis of type 2 diabetes.*)

Diabetes Control and Complications Trial Research Group. Effect of intensive therapy on residual β-cell function in patients with type 1 diabetes in the Diabetes Control and Complications Trial: a randomized, controlled trial. Ann Intern Med 1998;128:517. (*Early onset of intensive therapy helped preserve β-cell function, which facilitated control and reduced risk for hypoglycemia.*)

Diabetes Control and Complications Trial Research Group. The effect of intensive treatment of diabetes on the development and progression of long-term complications in insulin-dependent diabetes mellitus. N Engl J Med 1993;329:977. (*This landmark prospective multicenter trial of 1,441 patients randomized to intensive or conventional insulin therapy, which demonstrated dramatic reductions in retinopathy, proteinuria, and clinical neuropathy, has confirmed the value of tight glycemic control in patients with type 1 disease.*)

Diabetes Control and Complications Trial Research Group. The effect of intensive diabetes therapy on the development and progression of neuropathy. Ann Intern Med 1995;122:561. (*Risks for development of neuropathy and progression of existing neuropathy were significantly reduced with tight glycemic control.*)

Gabbe SG. Gestational diabetes. N Engl J Med 1986;315:1025. (*An editorial reviewing the condition. Data suggest development of complications, even with modest degrees of hyperglycemia.*)

Golan L, Birkenmeyer JD, Welch HG. The cost-effectiveness of treating all patients with type 2 diabetes with angiotension-converting enzyme inhibitors. Ann Intern Med 1999;131:660. (*Finds that treating all middle-aged diabetic patients can be cost-effective.*)

Haffner SM, Lehto S, Ronnemaa T, et al. Mortality from coronary heart disease in subjects with type 2 diabetes and in nondiabetic subjects with and without prior myocardial infarction. N Engl J Med 1998;339:229. (*Diabetes confers a degree of risk similar to that associated with prior myocardial infarction.*)

Haffner SM, Miettinen H. Insulin resistance implications for type II diabetes mellitus and coronary heart disease. Am J Med 1997;103:152. (*A review of the literature on the relation of diabetes and insulin resistance to coronary risk, with a discussion of implications for therapy; 106 references.*)

Holleman F, Hoekstra JBL. Insulin lispro. N Engl J Med 1997;337:176. (*A review of the evidence for this new form of insulin. The authors conclude that its principal benefits are a decreased risk for hypoglycemia and convenience, which make it most useful for patients who achieve tight control while taking multiple doses of insulin but have frequent insulin reactions; 84 references.*)

Jenkins DJA, Thomas DM, Wolever MS, et al. Glycemic index of foods: a physiological basis for carbohydrate exchange. Am J Clin Nutr 1981;34:362. (*An analysis of the glycemic effects of various carbohydrates; beans cause less hyperglycemia than do potatoes or corn.*)

Jovanovic-Peterson L, Peterson CM. Pregnancy in the diabetic woman. Endocrinol Metab Clin North Am 1992;21:433. (*Comprehensive review of evidence supporting the benefits of normalization of blood sugar and the management necessary to achieve tight control of diabetes in pregnancy.*)

Lewis EJ, Hunsicker LG, Bain RP, et al. Effect of angiotensin-converting enzyme inhibition on diabetic nephropathy. N Engl J Med 1993;329:1456. (*Marked reduction in proteinuria and progression to renal failure; important advance.*)

MacKenzie CR, Charlson ME. Assessment of perioperative risk in the patient with diabetes mellitus. Surg Gynecol Obstet 1988;167:293. (*End-organ consequences of diabetes, rather than hyperglycemia per se, predict infectious and renal complications of surgery.*)

Maggs DG, Buchanan TA, Burant CF, et al. Metabolic effects of troglitazone monotherapy in type 2 diabetes mellitus. Ann Intern Med 1998;128:176. (*A randomized, double-blinded study demonstrating a decrease in fasting and postprandial serum glucose concentrations, achieved by augmentation of glucose disposal.*)

Mayer-Davis EJ, D'Agostino R, Karter AJ, et al. Intensity and amount of physical activity in relation to insulin sensitivity: the Insulin Resistance Atherosclerosis Study. JAMA 1998;279:669. (*All forms of exercise improved insulin sensitivity.*)

Miller LV, Goldstein J. More efficient care of diabetic patients in a community hospital setting. N Engl J Med 1972;286:1388. (*Demonstrates the importance of communication between patient and health care provider in reducing acute hospitalization for diabetes.*)

Nathan DM, Singer DE, Hurxthal K, et al. The clinical information value of the glycosylated hemoglobin assay. N Engl J Med 1984;310:341. (*Original report establishing the value of the HbA_{1C} assay.*)

Ohkubo Y, Kishikawa H, Araki E, et al. Intensive insulin therapy prevents the progression of diabetic microvascular complications in Japanese patients with non–insulin-dependent diabetes mellitus: a randomized, prospective, 6-year study. Diabetes Res Clin Pract 1995;28:103. (*The first study confirming that tight control has the same effect on microvascular complications in type 2 diabetes as it does in type 1 disease.*)

Purnell JQ, Hokanson JE, Marcovina SM, et al. Effect of excessive weight gain with intensive therapy of type 1 diabetes on lipid levels and blood pressure: results from the DCCT. JAMA 1998;280:140. (*Intensive therapy found to induce weight gain, which was associated with elevations in blood pressure and lipids.*)

Reaven GM, Laws A. Insulin resistance, compensatory hyperinsulinemia and coronary heart disease. Diabetologia 1994;37:948. (*A review of syndrome X, an atherogenic phenotype. The theory is that hyperinsulinemia causes hypertension, low HDL cholesterol, and high VLDL cholesterol and triglyceride.*)

Reiber GE, Pecoraro RE, Koepsell TD. Risk factors for amputation in patients with diabetes mellitus. A case–control study. Ann Intern Med 1992;117:97. (*Impaired circulation in the lower extremity was the most powerful predictor, along with neuropathy and low HDL cholesterol levels.*)

Report of the Expert Committee on the Diagnosis and Classification of Diabetes Mellitus. Diabetes Care 1997;20:1183. (*The first update of diagnostic criteria and classification in almost 20 years; does away with some categories and provides new recommendations for diagnosis.*)

Saudek CD, Duckworth WC, Giobbie-Hurder A, et al. Implantable insulin pump vs. multiple-dose insulin for non–insulin-dependent diabetes mellitus: a randomized clinical trial. JAMA 1996;276:1996. (*Good comparison study revealing relative risks and benefits.*)

Schwartz S, Raskin P, Fonseca V, et al. Effect of troglitazone in insulin-treated patients with type II diabetes mellitus. N Engl J Med 1998;338:861. (*A randomized, placebo-controlled trial of this agent in patients with poorly controlled disease requiring at least 30 U of insulin daily; glycemic control significantly improved by addition of troglitazone.*)

Smieja M, Hunt DL, Edelman D, et al. Clinical examination for the detection of protective sensation in the feet of diabetic patients. J Gen Intern Med 1999;14:418. (*Evidence for efficacy of monofilament testing.*)

Solomon CG, Willet WC, Carey VJ, et al. A prospective study of pregravid determinants of gestational diabetes. JAMA 1997;278:1078. (*Data from the Nurses' Health Study; advanced maternal age, family history, nonwhite ethnicity, higher body mass index, weight gain in early adulthood, and cigarette smoking identified as risk factors.*)

Stenmans S, Melander A, Groop PH, et al. What is the benefit of increasing the sulfonylurea dose? Ann Intern Med 1993;118:169. (*Little benefit above the equivalent of 15 mg of glyburide per day.*)

Taguma Y, Kitamoto Y, Futaki G, et al. Effect of captopril on heavy proteinuria in azotemic diabetics. N Engl J Med 1985;313:1617. (*The original report of a reduction in proteinuria in diabetic nephropathy associated with ACE inhibitor therapy.*)

Tallarigo L, Giampietro O, Penno G, et al. Relation of glucose tolerance to complications of pregnancy in nondiabetic women. N Engl J Med 1986;315:989. (*Even limited degrees of glucose intolerance during pregnancy were associated with increased risks for macrosomia and its attendant complications.*)

Turner RC, Cull CA, Frighi V, et al. Glycemic control diet, sulfonylurea, metformin, or insulin in patients with type 2 diabetes mellitus: progressive requirement for multiple therapies (UKPDS 49). JAMA 1999;281:2005. (*Control declined markedly by 9 years after diagnosis in this report from the 20-year prospective, randomized UKPDS.*)

United Kingdom Prospective Diabetes Study Group. Tight blood pressure control reduced diabetes mellitus–related deaths and complications and was cost-effective in type 2 diabetes (UKPDS 38). BMJ 1998;317:703. (*Evidence for the importance of aggressive treatment of cardiovascular risk factors in diabetes.*)

United Kingdom Prospective Diabetes Study Group. Intensive blood glucose control with sulphonylureas or insulin compared with conventional treatment and risk of complications in patients with type 2 diabetes (UKPDS 33). Lancet 1998;352:837. (*Landmark 20-year prospective, randomized, controlled trial of diet, sulfonylureas, insulin, and later metformin in patients with type 2 disease. The study confirms that, as in type 1 disease, the risk for microvascular com-plications is reduced by tight control; HbA$_{1c}$ below 7.0% was identified as being necessary to minimize microvascular risk.*)

United Kingdom Prospective Diabetes Study Group. Effect of intensive blood-glucose control with metformin on complications in overweight patients with type 2 diabetes (UKPDS 34). Lancet 1998;352:54. (*First documented reduction in macrovascular complications with intensive therapy.*)

United Kingdom Prospective Diabetes Study Group. A 6-year randomized, controlled trial comparing sulfonylurea, insulin, and metformin therapy in patients with newly diagnosed type 2 diabetes that could not be controlled with diet therapy (UKPDS 24). Ann Intern Med 1998;128:165. (*Therapy with an oral agent proved just as effective as insulin and caused less weight gain and fewer hypoglycemic episodes.*)

Wilson RM, Clark P, Barkes H, et al. Starting insulin treatment as an outpatient. JAMA 1986;256:877. (*Data indicate that this is both safe and cost-effective.*)

Yki-Jarvinen H, Ryysy S, Nikkila K, et al. Comparison of bedtime insulin regimens in patients with type 2 diabetes mellitus: a randomized, controlled trial. Ann Intern Med 1999;130:389. (*Evidence for the effectiveness of combining metformin with bedtime insulin; the program provided the best results with regard to control and prevention of weight loss.*)

103

Approach to the Patient with Hyperthyroidism

Hyperthyroidism is the clinical expression of a heterogeneous group of disorders that produce elevations of free thyroxine (T_4), triiodothyronine (T_3), or both. Well-recognized causes of hyperthyroidism include diffuse toxic goiter (Graves' disease), toxic multinodular goiter, toxic single nodular goiter (toxic nodule), and excessive doses of levothyroxine. Transient hyperthyroidism has been noted in the settings of chronic lymphocytic (Hashimoto's) thyroiditis and subacute (granulomatous) thyroiditis.

Hyperthyroidism is relatively common and much more likely to occur in women than in men. Community-based studies have found a prevalence of 1.9% in women and 0.16% in men. Approximately 15% of recognized cases occur in persons over the age of 60. The clinical presentation of hyperthyroidism in the elderly is often atypical. The primary physician should be able to recognize hyperthyroidism, identify its cause, and design a therapeutic program appropriate to the patient's underlying pathophysiology, age, clinical condition, and personal preferences. The indications and limitations of surgery, radioiodine therapy, and antithyroid agents must be understood.

PATHOPHYSIOLOGY, CLINICAL PRESENTATION, AND COURSE

The pathophysiologic common denominator of hyperthyroidism is an excess of circulating thyroid hormone. The mechanisms responsible for this excess include increased production of thyroid-stimulating hormone (TSH), stimulation of thyroid TSH receptors by immunoglobulins, autonomous thyroid hormone production, increased release of thyroid hormone without increased production, and intake of exogenous hormone.

Thyroid hormone stimulates calorigenesis and catabolism and enhances sensitivity to catecholamines. Excessive amounts of the hormone lead to the classic picture of heat intolerance, nervousness, tremor, increased appetite, weight loss, excessive sweating, lid lag, stare, and muscle weakness. Diarrhea or, more precisely, frequent defecation may also ensue.

In the elderly thyrotoxic patient, the characteristic manifestations of hyperthyroidism may be absent and the clinical picture dominated instead by apathy, weight loss, and otherwise unexplained atrial fibrillation. This *apathetic hyperthyroidism of the elderly* has been mistaken for depression and occult malignancy.

Elevations in alkaline phosphatase and angiotensin-converting enzyme may accompany thyrotoxicosis and persist even after treatment. The pathophysiologic significance of these elevations remains unclear, but the findings might suggest thyroid disease and save extensive workup when other explanations for their occurrence are lacking.

Graves' Disease is an autoimmune condition in which an apparent deficiency of thyroid-specific suppressor T-cell lymphocytes allows a *thyroid-stimulating immunoglobulin G antibody* (TSab) to form. TSab binds to TSH receptors on the surface of thyroid cells and triggers the synthesis of excess thyroid hormone. Graves' disease is the most common disorder causing hyperthyroidism and accounts for about 90% of cases seen in persons younger than age 40.

Ophthalmopathy can be a troubling accompaniment of Graves' disease, affecting about 40% of patients. It is a consequence of antibody-mediated inflammation and infiltration. TSab does not appear to be directly involved, although the onset of ophthalmopathy generally parallels that of the hyperthyroidism. Antibodies to extraocular muscle and orbital fibroblasts capable of inducing *in vitro* the pathologic changes found *in vivo* have been detected. The inflammatory infiltrate causes the extraocular muscles to enlarge; they in turn cause proptosis by displacing the eye forward and orbital edema by compressing orbital veins. In general, the eye problems develop concurrently with the onset of hyperthyroidism and change little once established, although up to 20% of patients may experience a gradual worsening with treatment (see below). Manifestations range from mild periorbital edema and conjunctival inflammation to extraocular muscle dysfunction, corneal injury, and optic nerve damage. The lid lag and stare of hyperthyroidism may make the ophthalmopathy look worse than it actually is. Other associated ocular symptoms include pain, diplopia, proptosis, and blurred vision. The cosmetic changes may be among the most disturbing. The proptosis is a true one, differentiated from the stare, lid lag, and apparent proptosis that may accompany other forms of hyperthyroidism.

Pretibial myxedema is a less common immune-mediated infiltrative process that affects an occasional patient with Graves' disease. The onset typically occurs years after treatment for hyperthyroidism, usually in patients with a history of ophthalmopathy. The condition is characterized by the appearance of erythematous, mildly scaly plaques limited to the skin of the ankles and pretibial area. The plaques are indurated but not tender. They usually resolve spontaneously.

The thyroid gland in Graves' disease is diffusely enlarged, and a bruit may be heard in severe cases. The classic symptoms and signs of thyrotoxicosis are common. The skin is velvety and the hair silky. Onycholysis, vitiligo, and gynecomastia are found in some cases and may suggest the diagnosis. Cardiac complications are infrequent because of the relative youth of the patient population, but a reversible cardiomyopathy has been identified, manifested by a fall in the ejection fraction with exercise. Heart failure is rare, but impaired exercise tolerance is often reported, perhaps caused by the decreased ejection fraction.

The clinical course of Graves' disease waxes and wanes, with exacerbations and remissions of unpredictable duration. After many years, mild hypothyroidism may ensue, especially in patients with small goiters and mild hyperthyroidism at the time of onset.

Toxic Multinodular Goiter (Plummer's Disease) accounts for an increasing proportion of cases of hyperthyroidism in middle-aged and elderly persons. The condition is often associated with a long-standing simple goiter. The gland is clinically and pathologically indistinguishable from the gland of patients with nontoxic multinodular goiters. Cardiovascular symptoms may dominate the clinical presentation; new onset of heart failure, atrial fibrillation, or angina is not uncommon and reflects the high prevalence of coexisting organic heart disease in this older population. In a series of 85 hyperthyroid patients between ages 60 and 82, two thirds experienced heart failure and 20% reported angina. Only a minority evidenced the more typical symptoms of hyperthyroidism; for example, fewer than 11% had polyphagia. On the other hand, 33% had anorexia, and constipation was as prevalent as diarrhea. Lid lag may be noted on occasion, but exophthalmos does not occur. Sometimes, apathy and weight loss are the most prominent clinical features and can be so profound as to suggest occult malignancy or severe depression.

An increased risk for the development of thyrotoxicosis on exposure to iodides (including iodinated contrast agents) has been demonstrated in elderly patients with large, nontoxic nodular goiters. The problem is most prevalent among patients who come from areas where iodine intake is low (e.g., Europe) but can also occur in nonendemic cases of multinodular goiter and thyroid adenoma. The mechanism involves an increased release of stored hormone. The clinical course is self-limited. Laboratory findings include a low uptake of radioactive iodine and an absence of antithyroid antibodies.

Single Toxic Nodule ("Hot" Nodule). The autonomously functioning toxic nodule presents clinically much like the toxic multinodular goiter. The principal difference is the finding of a "hot" nodule surrounded by suppressed gland on radioiodine thyroid scan. The larger the nodule, the greater its propensity to cause thyrotoxicosis, with the risk quite high once the nodule reaches 3 cm in diameter. Often, the onset of toxicity is first manifested by an isolated increase in serum T_3 levels; later, T_4 levels rise. Sometimes, hemorrhagic infarction terminates the overproduction of hormone and limits the progression to thyrotoxicosis.

Triiodothyronine Toxicosis is an important entity to consider when patients with clinically apparent hyperthyroidism have normal T_4 levels. The condition has been reported in association with both diffuse and nodular goiters. The clinical presentation is no different from that of hyperthyroidism caused by elevations in T_4. Isolated elevations in T_3 concentration may also occur in euthyroid patients who have no underlying thyroid disease (see below).

Transient Hyperthyroidism may occur in association with subacute (granulomatous) or chronic (lymphocytic) thyroiditis. As noted above, the mechanism appears to be uncontrolled release of hormone from an inflamed gland. Iodine uptake is reduced during the period of hyperthyroidism. The clinical manifestations of hyperthyroidism are usually mild. The course is self-limited, and hypothyroidism often follows as intrathyroidal stores of the hormone are depleted.

Subacute Thyroiditis typically follows a viral illness, producing a tender, multinodular gland. The occasional case associated with hyperthyroidism has an abrupt onset characterized by thyrotoxic symptoms. The erythrocyte sedimentation rate is high, and a thyroid scan characteristically shows little or no uptake of radioiodine.

Lymphocytic Thyroiditis resulting in hyperthyroidism is thought to be an uncommon variant of Hashimoto's disease. In some cases, it may be caused by coexisting Graves' disease. High titers of antibodies to microsomes and thyroglobulin are present. The prevalence is highest in middle-aged women and among the elderly, in whom it may go unrecognized. The gland feels rubbery and is enlarged, sometimes asymmetrically. Hypothyroidism eventually develops in a substantial number of cases.

Postpartum (Subacute Lymphocytic) Thyroiditis, a previously unappreciated but surprisingly frequent problem (incidence as high as 5% in one series) can precipitate transient mild hyperthyroidism. The onset is within 3 to 6 months of delivery, and the condition often is mistaken for anxiety associated with the stress of caring for a new baby. The gland is nontender and may resemble that of Hashimoto's thyroiditis. A low uptake of radioactive iodine and the detection of antithyroid antibodies suggest an immunologic mechanism. The condition may persist for months before eventually resolving. A period of hypothyroidism may occur before the condition abates. It tends to recur with subsequent pregnancies.

Overproduction of Thyroid-stimulating Hormone. A small number of *pituitary adenomas* produce excessive TSH. The result is a diffusely enlarged gland simulating that of Graves' disease, but ophthalmopathy does not occur. A similar clinical picture may be caused by a tumor producing human chorionic gonadotropin (hCG), such as a *hydatidiform mole* or a *choriocarcinoma.* The thyroid-stimulating activity of hCG is weak, but when it is produced in massive quantities, it can cause hyperthyroidism.

Ectopic Thyroxine Production and Intake of Exogenous Hormone. When the source of excess thyroid hormone is extrathyroidal, the thyroid gland will appear small because of the absence of TSH stimulation. A dermoid tumor of the ovary, *struma ovarii,* with elements of thyroidlike tissue, is the only neoplasm regularly capable of synthesizing excessive amounts of thyroid hormone. (Rarely, thyroid cancers can cause hyperthyroidism, but only in the context of a massive tumor burden.) The intake of thyroid hormone in excess of daily requirements (>200 μg of levothyroxine per day) will make a person hyperthyroid. Sometimes, the intake is surreptitious. The gland is small, and TSH is absent.

Subclinical Hyperthyroidism is characterized by low or undetectable levels of TSH in the setting of normal levels of free T_4 and T_3. The most common cause is suppressive thyroid hormone therapy. Other causes include an autonomously functioning goiter and mild Graves' disease. Progression to thyrotoxicosis is rare. The risks associated with this state are a moderately increased frequency of atrial fibrillation in the elderly and osteoporosis in postmenopausal women.

DIFFERENTIAL DIAGNOSIS

The differential diagnosis of hyperthyroidism can be organized according to pathophysiology (Table 103.1). The most common cause is Graves' disease, followed by multinodular goiter, toxic adenoma, thyroiditis, and exogenous thyroid hormone. Pituitary adenoma, struma ovarii, and chorionic cancers are very rare causes.

WORKUP

Diagnosis of Hyperthyroidism. Clinical recognition of hyperthyroidism can sometimes be difficult, especially when symptoms are mild or when the condition occurs in an elderly or pregnant patient. Moreover, the correlation between symptoms and thyroid hormone levels is often poor, so that careful

Table 103.1.   Causes of Hyperthyroidism

PATHOPHYSIOLOGY	CAUSE
Autonomous hormone production	Toxic multinodular goiter Toxic adenoma
Increased hormone release	Subacute thyroiditis Lymphocytic (Hashimoto's) thyroiditis Iodide exposure
Increased glandular stimulation	Graves' disease (TSab) Functioning pituitary adenoma (TSH) Choriocarcinoma (hCG)
Exogenous hormone intake	Intake of >20 μg of levothyroxine per day
Extraglandular production	Struma ovarii Metastatic thyroid cancer

TSab, thyroid=stimulating antibody; TSH, thyroid= timulating hormone; hCG, human chorionic gonadotropin.

laboratory confirmation of the diagnosis and the severity of the condition are necessary.

Thyroid-stimulating Hormone Assay. The *serum TSH* determination has become the test of choice for screening patients for hyperthyroidism. A marked improvement in the sensitivity of the TSH assay through the use of radioimmunologic techniques now makes it possible to diagnose hyperthyroidism solely on the basis of an absence of detectable TSH. As long as the hypothalamic–pituitary axis is intact, an absence of TSH represents the appropriate response to too much circulating thyroid hormone. A normal TSH level by radioimmunoassay virtually rules out hyperthyroidism unless a functioning pituitary adenoma is present. A low TSH level (<0.1 mIU/L) suggests subclinical hyperthyroidism resulting from suppressive thyroxine therapy or an autonomously functioning gland (e.g., thyroid adenoma, subclinical Graves' disease). It may also be seen in older persons without hyperthyroidism. Undetectable TSH by second- or third-generation assay is diagnostic of hyperthyroidism.

Thyroid Hormone Levels. The sensitivity of second- and third-generation TSH assays has markedly reduced the need for thyroid hormone determinations in screening for hyperthyroidism. They can, however, help to confirm the diagnosis and determine the severity of disease and should be obtained when the TSH level is low or undetectable. The *free T_4* or *free T_4 index* (an excellent proxy for the free T_4, calculated by multiplying the serum T_4 by the T_3 resin uptake) is the most useful and consequently the preferred determination of circulating thyroid hormone. Measurement of the serum *total T_3* is usually not necessary unless the patient is clinically thyrotoxic in the setting of normal or only slightly elevated levels of free T_4. Routinely measuring the serum T_3 is probably wasteful because T_3 toxicosis is uncommon.

As useful as thyroid hormone levels are for diagnosis, overreliance on them and failure to use the TSH assay can be misleading. *Euthyroid hyperthyroxemia* occurs when an increase in thyroid-binding globulin (e.g., pregnancy, estrogen use, liver disease) produces an increase in total T_4, while the free T_4 remains normal. More confusing are euthyroid states with increases in both free and total T_4. Patients with autoantibodies against thyroid hormones may manifest surprisingly high levels of free hormone because of interference by these immunoglobulins with the standard radioimmune assays for thyroid hormones. Acute medical, surgical, and psychiatric illnesses, in addition to intake of high doses of propranolol, amiodarone, and gallbladder dyes, can impair the peripheral conversion of T_4 to active T_3 and lead to a rise in free T_4 concentration in conjunction with a reduction in T_3 and an increase in reverse T_3. An unexpectedly normal or low T_3 level in a patient who is clinically euthyroid but has elevated T_4 and free T_4 levels should suggest the possibility of euthyroid hyperthyroxemia. The T_3 concentration helps in the differentiation.

Thyrotropin-releasing Hormone stimulation testing is sometimes used when hyperthyroidism is suspected but serum thyroxine levels are equivocal. In patients with genuine hyperthyroidism, the TSH response to thyrotropin-releasing hormone (TRH) is minimal or absent. This reflects suppression of the pituitary by elevated levels of thyroid hormone. However, cortisol hypersecretion can also suppress the TSH response to TRH, simulating the pattern seen with hyperthyroidism. With the advent of a very sensitive TSH assay, TRH stimulation testing is rarely necessary, but it remains among the most sensitive of tests for the detection of hyperthyroidism.

Identifying the Underlying Cause. Etiologic assessment should proceed once the diagnosis of hyperthyroidism has been confirmed because treatment based on such an assessment is usually the most successful.

History. Inquiry should be made into goiter, thyroid nodule, use of iodides or thyroid hormone, eye changes, recent pregnancy or viral illness, and known ovarian, pituitary, or thyroid neoplasm. A review of systems should include a search for symptoms of a pituitary tumor (see Chapters 100 and 101).

Physical Examination focuses on the *thyroid gland*, with a check for overall size and nodularity. A diffusely enlarged, nontender gland suggests Graves' disease; in rare instances, a TSH-secreting tumor may be responsible for such diffuse glandular stimulation. A bruit may accompany the diffusely enlarged gland of Graves' disease. An exquisitely tender, diffusely enlarged gland occurring in the context of a viral illness points to subacute thyroiditis. The gland in lymphocytic thyroiditis is nontender and diffusely, but only modestly, enlarged. A small gland indicates an extrathyroidal source of hormone. Multinodularity is consistent with a toxic multinodular goiter and also occurs in patients with Hashimoto's thyroiditis. An otherwise atrophic gland with a single nodule, especially if larger than 3 cm in diameter, strongly suggests toxic adenoma.

Extrathyroidal findings may be of diagnostic significance and should be noted. *True proptosis* (eye protrusion of >20 mm from the orbital bone) is a hallmark of Graves' disease, as is *pretibial myxedema*. Lid lag and stare are nonspecific consequences of hyperthyroidism and may simulate proptosis. The neck nodes should be checked for adenopathy. Painless cervical lymphadenopathy raises the question of a thyroid malignancy. A pelvic examination and visual field testing are important to check for ovarian and pituitary sources.

Laboratory Studies. The *thyroid scan* can help differentiate among possible causes when the clinical picture remains uncertain. A toxic adenoma will be identified as a "hot" nodule, with little uptake by the rest of the gland. Uptake will be low in patients with thyroiditis, exogenous hormone intake, extraglandular hormone production, and iodide exposure. Uptake will be diffusely increased in patients with Graves' disease or a functioning pituitary adenoma.

Antithyroid antibodies (including those directed against microsomal peroxidase) are increased in both Graves' disease and lymphocytic (Hashimoto's) thyroiditis, so that their diagnostic utility is limited. *Serum thyroglobulin* determination serves as an elegant yet simple means of detecting a patient who is surreptitiously taking thyroid hormone. Exogenous hormone use results in the suppression of thyroglobulin synthesis. *Whole-body scanning* will identify the rare cases of extrathyroidal hormone synthesis, such as occurs in a struma ovarii or a metastasis from a thyroid malignancy.

A host of nonspecific hematologic and serum chemistry abnormalities accompany hyperthyroidism, but they are of little etiologic significance. They include a mild degree of anemia, granulocytosis, lymphocytosis, hypercalcemia, transaminase elevation, and alkaline phosphatase elevation.

Screening for Osteoporosis. Excessive amounts of thyroid hormone are associated with an increased risk for osteoporosis, especially in cortical bone, because of increased bone turnover. The risk for thyroid-induced osteoporosis and hip fracture is greatest in postmenopausal women with a history of hyperthyroidism or thyroid suppressive therapy. Such women should have a screening bone density examination of the hip or wrist (sites with a predominance of cortical bone).

PRINCIPLES OF THERAPY

The goals of therapy are to correct the hypermetabolic state with a minimum of side effects and the smallest possible incidence of hypothyroidism. For definitive therapy, one must choose among antithyroid drugs, radioiodine, and thyroidectomy. β-Blocking agents are useful for prompt, temporary control of hyperadrenergic symptoms. Hyperthyroidism should not go untreated, particularly in the elderly, who are at risk for cardiovascular complications. Moreover, not only are symptoms uncomfortable, but thyrotoxic crisis may ensue if the untreated patient unexpectedly encounters a severe stress, such as emergency surgery or acute sepsis.

Therapeutic Modalities

β-Blocking agents inhibit the adrenergic effects of excess thyroid hormone. As such, they provide excellent, prompt, symptomatic relief from many of the catecholamine-mediated manifestations of hyperthyroidism (e.g., tremor, palpitations, heat intolerance, nervousness). However, β-blockers have no intrinsic antithyroid activity, except perhaps at very high doses (which may slow the peripheral conversion of T_4 to T_3). Control of symptoms can often be achieved within a few days, so that these agents are an excellent choice for first-line therapy and preoperative treatment. β-Blockers may suffice for the treatment of transient hyperthyroidism, but they must be used in conjunction with other treatment modalities for the definitive control of persistent disease.

β-Blockers are particularly valuable for minimizing the major cardiac complications of hyperthyroidism (e.g., atrial fibrillation and angina; see Chapters 28 and 30). Patients with rate-related heart failure will also benefit from β-blockade, but the condition of those with heart failure resulting from myocardial pathology will worsen with such therapy. Consequently, β-blockade must be administered with care in elderly patients and those with preexisting heart disease (see Chapter 32).

Of the β-blockers, propranolol remains the most widely used for control of hyperthyroidism, but other agents in this class (e.g., atenolol, metoprolol, nadolol) demonstrate comparable efficacy. Those with a more sustained half-life (e.g., atenolol) are particularly useful for patients who are to undergo surgery. Adequacy of the dose is determined by monitoring the resting and exercise heart rates and the degree of symptomatic relief.

One important benefit of β-blockade is that it becomes possible to proceed safely with thyroid surgery within 1 to 2 weeks. With antithyroid drugs (see below), 6 to 8 weeks of preoperative treatment is required. The addition of *potassium iodide* to β-blocker therapy produces more rapid and greater preoperative control in patients with Graves' disease who are to undergo thyroidectomy; it is especially useful in those whose condition is not adequately controlled on β-blockers alone (control being defined as a resting pulse of <90 beats/min and a blunting of exercise-induced tachycardia).

Antithyroid Drugs. *Methimazole* and *propylthiouracil* (PTU) are the most important antithyroid agents. PTU acts by interfering with the synthesis of T_4 and blocking the peripheral conversion of T_4 to T_3, although at conventional doses, this latter effect does not appear to be clinically important. Methimazole does not have any peripheral effect but is more potent. Both drugs suppress thyroid autoimmunity and decrease circulating TSab. A biochemical response to the antithyroid drugs is detectable within 1 to 2 weeks; the clinical response typically takes 4 to 8 weeks.

These antithyroid agents are widely used in *young* and *middle-aged patients*, particularly for the long-term control of *Graves' disease*. They are also used for preoperative control and in many instances for therapy before and after radioiodine ablation. The average initial dosage of PTU is 300 mg/d (100 mg every 8 hours). For methimazole, the starting dosage is 15 mg/d, which can be given as a single dose because its half-life is much longer. Therapy is adjusted as needed to attain clinical and biochemical control. Once control is achieved, the dose can be tapered to the lowest amount needed to maintain a euthyroid state. Usually, treatment is continued for 12 to 24 months and then halted to see if relapse occurs.

The chance for long-term remission in Graves' disease is enhanced by 1 to 2 years of antithyroid drug therapy. PTU induces a remission in approximately 50% of patients with Graves' disease who are treated for 1 to 2 years, but one third to one half of those who respond eventually relapse. Reports of a remission rate of 40% after only 3 to 5 months of antithyroid therapy initially raised hopes that a shorter course of treatment might suffice, but longer-term follow-up revealed increased rates of relapse. Combination programs in which higher doses of antithyroid medication are given in conjunction with thyroxine have not proved advantageous, and they increase the risk for adverse effects of antithyroid drugs. The risk for inducing hypothyroidism is low. For patients who relapse or fail to achieve remission, radioiodine or surgical therapy must be considered.

Common adverse effects include skin rash, fever, and arthralgias; these are usually not of major clinical significance. However, the rare (0.3% to 0.6% of patients) but potentially fa-

tal complication of *agranulocytosis* necessitates careful patient selection and close monitoring of therapy. The risk for agranulocytosis increases with age (beginning at about age 40) and is independent of the dose for PTU but dose-dependent for methimazole. Onset is usually within 2 months, rarely beyond 4 months. The development of agranulocytosis has not been reported in any patients taking less than 30 mg of methimazole per day, so this drug is the safer of the two.

Because the drop in granulocyte count is precipitous, it is not clear that close monitoring of blood counts is beneficial, but many clinicians consider it advisable during the first 4 months of therapy. Mild leukopenia is common, occurring in up to 10% of patients, and does not require cessation of treatment. If the leukocyte count falls below 1,500/mm³, therapy should be withheld.

Choice of antithyroid agent has been a subject of debate. With proper monitoring, either antithyroid drug is a reasonable choice. Although PTU is more widely prescribed, *methimazole* appears *preferable* in terms of cost, hematologic side effects, and ease of administration. It also has no adverse effect on the response to radioiodine therapy when used before ablative therapy, an effect sometimes seen with PTU. At doses up to 30 mg/d, methimazole is about 30% lower in cost than a comparable dose of PTU, is much less likely to induce agranulocytosis, and needs to be taken only once daily. PTU is preferable during pregnancy and breast-feeding (see below).

Ablation with Radioactive Iodine (Iodine 131), an important form of therapy, was first introduced in 1942 and is widely used today, especially for older hyperthyroid patients, in whom the long-term effects of radiation exposure are not a major concern. It is indicated for patients with Graves' disease when antithyroid drugs do not suffice, when they are elderly or noncompliant or have a solitary toxic nodule, and when surgery is contraindicated or the patient is reluctant to undergo surgery. Advantages include established efficacy, relative safety, and ease of administration. Disadvantages are delayed control of symptoms and a high incidence of hypothyroidism following therapy.

Among the *side effects* of radioactive iodine therapy, the most common complication is *hypothyroidism*. High-dose radioiodine provides predictable relief but is associated with a high incidence of early hypothyroidism (70% in the first year). The early risk for hypothyroidism is lower with low-dose regimens (15% in the first year), but they provide less control of the disease (50% of patients still hyperthyroid at 1 year). Long-term follow-up studies of patients given low-dose treatment indicate a steady increase in the cumulative incidence of hypothyroidism (75% at 11 years), suggesting that its early advantages fade with time. Regardless of the dose used, the risk for eventual hypothyroidism requires that patients be regularly reevaluated, typically at 6-month intervals.

Worsening ophthalmopathy is a concern and is more common with radioiodine therapy than with other forms of antithyroid treatment for Graves' disease. Risk is exacerbated by *cigarette smoking*. As noted earlier, up to 20% of patients with Graves' disease and eye involvement predating treatment for hyperthyroidism experience an exacerbation after treatment for hyperthyroidism. Correction of hyperthyroidism does not appear to cause ophthalmopathy *de novo*, but treatment-induced hypothyroidism (which is common in patients treated with radioiodine) appears to increase the risk for worsening eye problems. The mechanism is unclear; a treatment-induced outpouring of antibody-stimulating antigen is hypothesized.

Prophylactic treatment with oral *prednisone* for 3 months (started at 40 mg/d a few days after radioiodine therapy and continued for 1 month before taper to full cessation over 8 weeks) prevents ophthalmopathy in persons with little or none before treatment. Although steroids are tapered after the first month, the incidence of steroid side effects (see Chapter 105) is high. Cyclosporine has also been tried. It is less effective than prednisone but has proved helpful in combination for refractory cases. At present, avoidance of hypothyroidism appears to be the best mode of prevention. The mode of therapy may also be germane (see also Chapter 204).

Risks for cancer and *birth defects* have been long-standing concerns. The gonadal radiation dose from iodine 131 therapy is small, the equivalent of that from a barium enema or an IV pyelogram. To address the question of cancer risk, cohort studies have followed tens of thousands of patients for decades. Recent analyses indicate that the risk for overall cancer mortality is not increased, but the rate of thyroid cancer deaths is increased fourfold in comparison with that of patients who received other forms of therapy. Although this increase in relative risk is statistically significant, the absolute risk remains very small. Interestingly, more than a year after treatment, a slight increase in total cancer mortality risk was noted for patients treated with antithyroid medications. More study is needed to define these comparative risks. Radioiodine therapy is also associated with increased risks for cardiovascular disease, stroke, and osteoporotic fracture. Whether this is a consequence of the therapy or the underlying thyroid status of these patients remains to be clarified.

Surgery represents the most direct ablative approach to hyperthyroidism. The objective is to reduce the thyroid mass sufficiently to cure the hypermetabolic state without inducing a hypothyroid condition. Unfortunately, the incidence of permanent hypothyroidism is substantial, and smaller but perceptible risks for hypoparathyroidism and laryngeal paralysis exist. Moreover, hyperthyroidism may recur despite subtotal thyroidectomy in Graves' disease. Prior preparation of the patient with antithyroid drugs is required to avoid precipitating thyroid storm. Surgery is particularly useful for relieving esophageal obstruction; cosmesis and pregnancy are other indications. It is also a choice when antithyroid drugs fail or produce complications, or when patients are noncompliant or refuse radioiodine. Young patients with moderate to severe disease do particularly well. However, treatment with iodine 131 has largely replaced surgery because it is less expensive and associated with less morbidity.

Iodides are sometimes useful as supplemental agents because they can block peripheral conversion of T_4 to T_3 and inhibit hormone release. *Potassium iodide* was the earliest of the iodides to be employed. The *organic iodide radiographic contrast agents* (e.g., ipodate, iopanoate) have supplanted the inorganic iodides. However, control is sometimes problematic. Paradoxical increases in hormone release can occur. Thus, iodides are best utilized for preoperative control in patients who require a second drug to counter the hyperthyroidism and in those for whom β-blockers and other antithyroid medications are contraindicated.

Treatment of Osteoporosis. Bone-preserving therapy should be considered for hyperthyroid women found to be osteoporotic, especially if they are menopausal (see Chapter 164).

Choice of Therapy

Graves' Disease. There is little consensus among thyroidologists regarding the best treatment for Graves' disease, except in the case of *elderly patients*, for whom *radioactive iodine* is considered the treatment of choice. Surveys of opinion regarding the treatment of *middle-aged* and *younger patients* reveals marked diversity of opinion, split between antithyroid drugs and radioiodine, with surgery deemed best reserved for those who are not candidates for either. An initial trial of *antithyroid drug* therapy represents a reasonable starting point for treatment, supplemented by β-blocker therapy to help establish a euthyroid state and control adrenergic symptoms. When such therapy fails to achieve control, or the patient is unable to tolerate it or experiences a relapse after it has been completed, radioiodine can be considered. Despite the absence of evidence for long-term genetic risk, concern persists about giving radioiodine to patients in their reproductive years.

Contributing to the diversity of opinion is dissatisfaction with available therapies. None appears capable of definitively halting the underlying immunopathologic process, which remains poorly understood. Adding *thyroid replacement therapy* to antithyroid drug therapy decreases the frequency of recurrence of Graves' disease and reduces the production of antibodies to TSH receptors.

Treatment of ophthalmopathy also remains a challenge. Etiologic therapy awaits a better understanding of the underlying disease mechanisms. Although ophthalmopathy may worsen with treatment of the hyperthyroidism, especially if hypothyroidism is induced, no evidence has been found that scaling back treatment prevents an exacerbation. However, radioiodine appears to be the modality most likely to worsen ophthalmopathy, perhaps because it is the most likely to induce hypothyroidism. This has led some to recommend thyroxine supplementation to prevent hypothyroidism. Moderately high doses of glucocorticoids given at the time of antithyroid treatment can reduce the risk for ophthalmopathy, but such prophylactic therapy is not recommended for routine use because of the high incidence of adverse side effects, the inability to predict who will experience an exacerbation, and the low incidence (7%) of severe ophthalmopathy. However, patients with moderate to marked preexisting ophthalmopathy may be reasonable candidates for such prophylactic treatment. Good eye care is also a priority.

With a host of alternative therapies available, each with its own advantages and disadvantages, it is important to individualize treatment according to the patient's needs, capabilities, and clinical status. For now, one must settle for treating the hyperthyroidism; etiologic therapy is awaited.

Toxic Nodule. Radioiodine is the treatment of choice for elderly patients with this condition. Because the rest of the gland is suppressed by the hyperfunctioning nodule, the incidence of posttreatment hypothyroidism is far less than that seen with treatment of Graves' disease. The optimal radioiodine dose remains a subject of debate. A relatively low dose of iodine 131 (5 to 15 mCi) appears to provide excellent results with minimal adverse effects (75% of patients euthyroid by 2 months, >90% within 6 months, posttreatment hypothyroidism very rare). Surgical removal may be preferable in young patients.

Hyperthyroidism in Pregnant and Nursing Patients. The choice is between antithyroid drugs and surgery; radioiodine is contraindicated because it crosses the placenta and concentrates in the fetal thyroid. Antithyroid drug therapy is considered safer than surgery, with surgery reserved for refractory cases and patients who refuse to take their medication. Among the *antithyroid agents*, *PTU* is preferred; methimazole has been associated with aplasia cutis in the fetus. The risk that drug will cross the placenta and induce hypothyroidism in the fetus is small and not strictly dose-related, but precipitation of hypothyroidism in the mother can compromise the fetus and should be avoided. Pregnant women with Graves' disease may transfer large amounts of TSab to the fetus and induce fetal thyrotoxicosis, even after thyroid ablation. Testing the newborn for thyrotoxicosis is essential in this setting. Evidence that treatment of pregnant thyrotoxic patients leads to impaired intellectual development in the offspring has not been found. The optimal antithyroid drug regimen for the fetal thyroid status appears to be one that maintains maternal levels of free T$_4$ near the upper limit of normal.

Breast-feeding mothers can transfer antithyroid medication in milk, but the amount is small, especially of PTU, and not likely to induce significant hypothyroidism. However, a discussion of potential risks and the need for careful monitoring is important.

The short-term use of *β-blocking agents*, *iodides*, or both provides prompt, effective, and safe control of thyrotoxic symptoms. Symptoms improve within 2 to 7 days. Longer-term use of these agents is more problematic. *β*-Blocking drugs have been linked to retarded intrauterine growth, small placenta, and postnatal bradycardia and hypoglycemia. Nevertheless, the complication rate is low, and use during pregnancy is generally safe. Extended use of iodides is riskier, with large, obstructing fetal goiters reported.

Surgery is usually reserved for the patient who has failed or is a poor candidate for medical treatment. Operative mortality, although low, still exceeds that associated with drug therapy. Before subtotal thyroidectomy, preoperative medical therapy is indicated to attain control and prevent thyroid storm.

Thyroiditis. As noted above, hyperthyroidism associated with thyroiditis can be managed symptomatically with *β-blocking agents* because spontaneous resolution is the rule. Aspirin and occasionally corticosteroids are indicated in subacute thyroiditis to control inflammatory symptoms.

Monitoring Therapy

Monitoring treatment requires attention to the clinical status and indices of thyroid function. Clinical status is assessed by taking note of any changes in weight, degree of heat intolerance, tremulousness, anxiousness, appetite, level of energy, resting heart rate, ophthalmopathy, skin texture, or skin temperature. The *TSH* level provides the best measure of the treatment end point (normalization of TSH) and the earliest evidence of overtreatment and development of hypothyroidism. The amount of circulating thyroid hormone can be assessed by

monitoring changes in the serum concentration of *free T$_4$* (or total T$_3$ in the case of T$_3$ toxicosis), but assessment is needed only when the TSH level is abnormal.

In patients with Graves' disease, monitoring the serum level of *antibodies to TSH receptors* also helps predict the clinical course. Relapse is a strong possibility if TSab remains elevated and is less likely, although not ruled out, when it is reduced or absent.

For patients taking antithyroid drugs, routine monitoring of the *leukocyte count* should be considered, especially for those taking PTU or more than 30 mg of methimazole per day. Risk is greatest during the first 4 months of therapy.

PATIENT EDUCATION

Patients with hyperthyroidism are often relieved to know that their "nervousness" is caused by an underlying medical illness rather than an emotional problem and that it will improve with therapy. Patients who are taking antithyroid agents need to be instructed about prompt reporting of symptoms suggestive of agranulocytosis (e.g., fever, chills), especially during the first 4 months of therapy. Those with prominent exophthalmos should be warned to see the physician at the first sign of diplopia or visual impairment. Hyperthyroid mothers taking antithyroid drugs and eager to breast-feed their infants need not be prohibited from breast-feeding so long as one takes the time to explain the potential risks and the importance of careful monitoring. Patients treated with radioiodine should be told to watch for symptoms of hypothyroidism.

INDICATIONS FOR REFERRAL AND ADMISSION

Patients who are candidates for therapy with iodine 131 should undergo a thyroid scan and be seen by the endocrinologist or radiation therapist for calculation of the dose of iodine 131 to be administered. Consultation with an endocrinologist is also indicated in the management of the pregnant or lactating hyperthyroid patient and the patient with severe ophthalmopathy of Graves' disease. Visual impairment caused by severe ophthalmopathy may require hospital admission for very high-dose systemic steroid therapy or surgical decompression. Referral for consideration of surgical therapy is also indicated when the patient's swallowing is obstructed and when the patient is pregnant, desires cosmetic improvement, or fails antithyroid drug therapy. Prompt hospital admission is needed if heart failure, rapid atrial fibrillation, or angina develops.

THERAPEUTIC RECOMMENDATIONS

- For prompt control of adrenergic symptoms of hyperthyroidism, regardless of underlying cause, start treatment immediately with a *β-blocking agent* (e.g., 80 mg of propranolol per day, 50 mg of atenolol per day). Increase dose daily until symptoms are controlled. Use with extreme caution in patients who have preexisting heart failure unrelated to thyroid disease.
- For *nonpregnant young* and *middle-aged* patients with *Graves' disease*, start *methimazole* (20 to 30 mg/d) in addition to the *β*-blocker program. Continue both methimazole and *β*-blockade for 4 to 8 weeks, and then taper the *β*-blocker as the antithyroid agent takes effect. Adjust the antithyroid

drug dose according to the clinical status and thyroid indices (TSH, free T_4). Use the lowest possible dose that maintains biochemical and biologic control. Monitor closely to avoid precipitating hypothyroidism. Monitor leukocyte count if more than 30 mg of methimazole is being taken per day or if the patient is elderly.

- If a response is obtained, continue antithyroid therapy for 12 to 24 months. One can measure TSab at 12 months. If TSab is absent and the patient appears to be in remission clinically and biochemically, then try discontinuing therapy. If relapse occurs, then consider resumption of antithyroid therapy for 12 more months or radioiodine therapy.

- For the *pregnant patient* with *Graves' disease*, consider antithyroid drug therapy, but obtain endocrinologic consultation before initiating treatment. *PTU* is preferred (starting dose is 100 mg three times daily) and can also be given to the patient who is eager to breast-feed. Risks of such therapy should be fully explained and understood by the patient. Careful monitoring of thyroid status in both mother and baby is essential. Maintain the pregnant patient's free T_4 levels near the upper limit of normal; monitor TSH closely.

- For all patients taking antithyroid medication, consider *monitoring* the *leukocyte count* every 2 to 4 weeks during the first 4 months of therapy, then every 4 to 6 months. Stop therapy if the neutrophil count falls below 1,500/mL. The risk for agranulocytosis and the need for close monitoring are greatest in elderly patients and those taking PTU or more than 30 mg of methimazole per day.

- For patients with Graves' disease who have severe symptomatic ophthalmopathy, obtain a prompt endocrinologic consultation. Options include very high-dose systemic glucocorticoids (120 to 150 mg of prednisone per day), local steroid injection, surgical decompression, and radiation therapy.

- For patients with Graves' disease who have mild to moderate ophthalmopathy, minimize the risk for worsening eye disease by avoiding posttreatment hypothyroidism. The routine use of systemic daily steroid therapy for prophylaxis of posttreatment exacerbation is not recommended but may be considered for patients who begin radioiodine treatment with moderately severe eye changes already established (20 to 40 mg of prednisone per day for the first month, followed by taper to full cessation during the next 8 weeks). For periorbital edema, advise elevating the head of the bed and prescribe a mild diuretic (e.g., 50 mg of hydrochlorothiazide per day). Prescribe methylcellulose drops to prevent corneal drying (see also Chapter 204).

- Consider *therapy with iodine 131* for patients with a *solitary toxic nodule, elderly patients with Graves' disease*, and other patients with Graves' disease who fail or cannot be maintained on therapy with antithyroid drugs (relapse, agranulocytosis). Continue β-blockade for the 2- to 3-month period that it takes for the radioiodine to exert its full effect on the gland. Between 3 and 6 months after onset of treatment and at 3- to 6-month intervals thereafter, monitor TSH for evidence of hypothyroidism; correct promptly by starting thyroid replacement therapy before hypothyroidism develops.

- Refer for consideration of *surgery* any patient who has a *neck obstruction* or a *cosmetic concern* or who is *poorly compliant* in taking medication. Surgery should also be considered when antithyroid drug therapy has failed or is contraindicated. Young patients do particularly well. If surgery is con-

templated, continue antithyroid or β-blocking therapy up to the moment of surgery. Monitor for postoperative hyperthyroidism.

- Treat patients with *transient hyperthyroidism* associated with thyroiditis symptomatically with *β-blockade* until the condition resolves on its own.

- Screen and treat hyperthyroid women for *osteoporosis* (see Chapters 144 and 164); they are at increased risk for hip fracture.

A.H.G.

ANNOTATED BIBLIOGRAPHY

Bartalena l, Marocci C, Bogazzi F, et al. Relation between therapy for hyperthyroidism and the course of Graves' ophthalmopathy. N Engl J Med 1998;338:1998. (*Radioiodine therapy is more likely than methimazole to cause or worsen ophthalmopathy; the problem is often transient and can be prevented by treatment with prednisone.*)

Bartalena L, Marcocci C, Tanda ML, et al. Cigarette smoking and treatment outcomes in Graves' ophthalmopathy. Ann Intern Med 1998;129:632. (*Smoking increases the risk and decreases the efficacy of corticosteroids and orbital irradiation.*)

Borst GC, Eil C, Burman KD. Euthyroid hyperthyroxemia. Ann Intern Med 1983;98:366. (*A detailed review of the mechanisms and syndromes of hyperthyroxemia in clinically euthyroid patients; 229 references.*)

Burch HB, Solomon BL, Watofsky L, et al. Discontinuing antithyroid drug therapy before ablation with radioiodine in Graves' disease. Ann Intern Med 1994;121:553. (*Suggests that antithyroid therapy before ablation has little effect on short-term course after radioiodine therapy.*)

Burrow GN. The management of thyrotoxicosis in pregnancy. N Engl J Med 1984;313:562. (*A terse but clinically useful review; 49 references.*)

Cantalamessa L, Baldini M, Orsatti A, et al. Thyroid nodules in Graves' disease and the risk of thyroid carcinoma. Arch Intern Med 1999;159:1705. (*Risk for thyroid cancer in nodules detected with ultrasonography was low.*)

Chopra IJ, Hershman JM, Pardridge WM, et al. Thyroid function in nonthyroidal illnesses. Ann Intern Med 1983;98:946. (*Discusses the changes in thyroid hormone levels and their consequences in nonthyroidal illness.*)

Cooper DS. Which antithyroid drug? Am J Med 1986;80:1165. (*Favors methimazole over PTU for most cases.*)

Cooper DS, Goldminz D, Levin AA, et al. Agranulocytosis associated with antithyroid drugs. Ann Intern Med 1983;98:26. (*Increasing age and dose of methimazole were associated with increased risk; the risk with PTU was independent of dose.*)

Forar JC, Muir AL, Sawers SA, et al. Abnormal left ventricular function in hyperthyroidism. N Engl J Med 1982;307:1165. (*Provides evidence for a reversible cardiomyopathic state directly related to excess thyroid hormone.*)

Franklin JA, Maisonneuve P, Sheppard MC, et al. Mortality after the treatment of hyperthyroidism with radioactive iodine. N Engl J Med 1998;338:1998. (*Increased mortality found in all-cause, cardiovascular, and cerebrovascular categories.*)

Graham GD, Burman KD. Radioiodine treatment of Graves' disease. Ann Intern Med 1986;105:900. (*Comprehensive review of potential risks; 72 references.*)

Greenspan SL, Greenspan FS. The effect of thyroid hormone on skeletal integrity. Ann Intern Med 1999;130:750. (*In a systematic review, hyperthyroidism and the use of hyroxine to supress TSH were found to be associated with an increased risk for osteoporosis, particularly in cortical bone; a bone density examination of the hip or forearm is recommended for women with a history of either.*)

Hashizume K, Ichikawa K, Sakurai A, et al. Administration of thyroxine in treated Graves' disease—effects on the level of antibodies to thyroid-stimulating hormone receptors and on the risk of recurrence of hyperthyroidism. N Engl J Med 1991;324:947. (*An intriguing approach in which adding thyroxine reduces TSab levels and the risk for recurrence.*)

Helfand M, Redfern CC. Screening for thyroid disease: an update. Ann Intern Med 1998;129:144. (*Thoughtful review of the evidence for screening; includes good discussion of the value of detecting subclinical hyperthyroidism.*).

Hermus AR, Duysmans DA. Treatment of benign nodular thyroid disease. N Engl J Med 1998;338:1438. (*A review that includes a discussion of the management of toxic nodular goiter.*)

Klein I, Becker DV, Levey GS. Treatment of hyperthyroid disease. Ann Intern Med 1994;121:281. (*A useful review.*)

Mariotti S, Martino E, Cupini C, et al. Low serum thyroglobulin as a clue to the diagnosis of thyrotoxicosis factitia. N Engl J Med 1982;307:410. (*An excellent way to detect surreptitious use.*)

Masters PA, Simons RJ. Clinical use of sensitive assays for thyroid-stimulating hormone. J Gen Intern Med 1996;11:115. (*Review that includes a discussion of use of the assay to detect hyperthyroidism.*)

Momotani N, Noh J, Oyanagi H, et al. Antithyroid drug therapy for Graves' disease during pregnancy. N Engl J Med 1986;315:24. (*The optimal antithyroid regimen for the fetus appears to be one that maintains maternal free T_4 in the mildly hyperthyroid range.*)

Rittmaster RS, Abbott EC, Douglas R, et al. Effect of methimazole, with or without L-thyroxine, on remission rates in Graves' disease. J Clin Endocrinol Metab 1998;83:814. (*No benefit from combined therapy, and increased risk for adverse drug effects from the higher doses used.*)

Ron E, Doody MM, Becker DV, et al. Cancer mortality following treatment of adult hyperthyroidism. JAMA 1998;280:347. (*No increase in overall cancer mortality with use of radioiodine, but a fourfold increase in thyroid cancer deaths in this cohort of more than 35,000 patients followed for a mean of 21 years.*)

Ross DS, Ardisson LJ, Meskell MJ. Measurement of thyrotropin in clinical and subclinical hyperthyroidism using a new chemiluminescent assay. J Clin Endocrinol Metab 1989;69:684. (*Original report establishing the enhanced sensitivity of the assay and its use in determining TSH levels to diagnose hyperthyroidism.*)

Ross DS, Ridgeway EC, Daniels GH. Successful treatment of solitary toxic thyroid nodules with relatively low-dose iodine 131, with a low prevalence of hypothyroidism. Ann Intern Med 1984;101:488. (*Reports excellent efficacy and safety; argues that high doses are unnecessary.*)

Singer PA, Cooper DS, Levy EG, et al. Treatment guidelines for patients with hyperthyroidism and hypothyroidism. Standards of Care Committee, American Thyroid Association. JAMA 1995; 273:808. (*Consensus clinical guidelines.*)

Sundbeck G, Jagenburg R, Johansson PM, et al. Clinical significance of low serum thyrotropin concentration by chemiluminometric assay in 85-year-old women and men. Arch Intern Med 1991;151:549. (*Elderly persons may have a low TSH level but remain euthyroid.*)

Surks MI, Sievert R. Drugs and thyroid function. N Engl J Med 1995;333:1688. (*Best review of drugs causing hyperthyroidism.*)

Surks MI, Chopra IJ, Mariash CN, et al. American Thyroid Association guidelines for use of laboratory tests in thyroid disorders. JAMA 1990;263:1529. (*Recommends TSH measurement supplemented by free T_4 measurement as the principal tests.*)

Tajiri J, Noguchi S, Murakami T, et al. Antithyroid drug–induced agranulocytosis—the usefulness of routine leukocyte count monitoring. Arch Intern Med 1990;150:621. (*Evidence for regular monitoring.*)

Tallstedt L, Lundell G, Torring O, et al. Occurrence of ophthalmopathy after treatment for Graves' hyperthyroidism. N Engl J Med 1992;326:1733. (*A randomized, controlled trial; iodine 131 therapy was more likely to be followed by worsening ophthalmopathy than were other therapies, especially in older patients.*)

Utiger RD. β-Adrenergic antagonist therapy for hyperthyroid Graves' disease. N Engl J Med 1984;310:1597. (*An editorial summarizing the use of β-blockade and other modalities in the treatment of Graves' disease.*)

Utiger RD. Pathogenesis of Graves' ophthalmopathy. N Engl J Med 1992;326:1772. (*Mechanisms reviewed, particularly in relation to mode of antithyroid therapy.*)

104
Approach to the Patient with Hypothyroidism

The development of accurate and relatively inexpensive diagnostic techniques and the availability of low-cost, high-quality levothyroxine preparations have greatly facilitated the diagnosis and management of hypothyroidism. Hashimoto's thyroiditis accounts for most of the cases of hypothyroidism seen in the United States. Other causes of thyroid injury include idiopathic thyroid atrophy, previous radioactive iodine (iodine 131) therapy, and subtotal thyroidectomy. Women are more frequently affected than men. The prevalence of hypothyroidism increases with age. As much as 5% of the elderly population manifests evidence of hypothyroidism, most of it resulting from thyroiditis. Less common causes include neck irradiation, iodide administration, and the use of lithium or paraaminosalicylic acid. Pituitary insufficiency can result in secondary hypothyroidism. Rarely, hypothalamic disease is the source of difficulty. Assessment for hypothyroidism includes an evaluation of the patient taking long-term thyroid hormone replacement therapy for unclear reasons. The primary physician should be able to determine when replacement therapy is indicated and to prescribe it with safety and precision.

PATHOPHYSIOLOGY, CLINICAL PRESENTATION, AND COURSE

Pathophysiology

The basic mechanisms of hypothyroidism can be divided into those that impair thyroid function (primary hypothyroidism) and those that principally involve hypothalamic–pituitary function (secondary hypothyroidism). In primary disease, the hypothalamus responds with an increased output of thyrotropin-releasing hormone (TRH), which triggers pituitary thyrotropin (TSH) secretion. This in turn stimulates thyroid gland enlargement, goiter formation, and the preferential synthesis of triiodothyronine (T_3) over thyroxine (T_4). In secondary hypothyroidism, the TSH response is inadequate, the gland is normal or reduced in size, and both T_4 synthesis and T_3 synthesis are equally reduced.

Primary Hypothyroidism may occur as a result of blockade of thyroid TSH receptors, impairment of thyroxine production, or inhibition of thyroxine release. In *Hashimoto's thyroiditis*, the most common form of hypothyroidism, *immune-mediated injury* may damage all three components of glandular function. The precipitants of excessive antibody production remain ill-defined, but TSH receptors and microsomal enzymes (e.g., peroxidase) are among the targeted antigens. In fact, antimicrosomal antibodies serve as a convenient laboratory marker for the condition (see below). Pathologically, a lymphocytic infiltrate and glandular enlargement are noted; frank nodularity may develop (see Chapter 95). Antibodies directed against glandular antigens can impair the response to TSH and the synthesis and release of hormone. Although most patients with Hashimoto's thyroiditis remain euthyroid, a fraction experience transient hyperthyroidism because of the premature release of thyroid hormone (see Chapter 103). If hormone synthesis is sufficiently compromised, hypothyroidism may ensue and can be permanent. Most patients with Hashimoto's thyroiditis have mild disease and remain euthyroid, although a modest goiter may develop.

Postpartum thyroiditis is believed to be a common variant of Hashimoto's thyroiditis (see Chapter 103), affecting up to 5% of women postpartum. Antibody production peaks 3 to 4 months after delivery and then declines. A period of transient hyperthyroidism may be followed by hypothyroidism, but most patients return to euthyroid status. The symptoms of mild hyperthyroidism may be mistakenly attributed to "tension" and are followed by fatigue and depression resulting from the onset of hypothyroidism. The symptoms resolve spontaneously within 2 to 3 months but tend to recur with subsequent pregnancies.

Radiation-induced hypothyroidism is another leading cause of thyroid injury in the United States. It is a common and permanent consequence of iodine 131 therapy and also of external neck irradiation that exceeds 2,500 rads (used to treat lymphoma and head and neck cancers). Onset is within 3 to 6 months of treatment.

Subacute thyroiditis following a viral upper respiratory infection is a more transient form of thyroid injury. In this condition, the gland is very tender and enlarged, sometimes asymmetrically. A brief period of hyperthyroidism may precede glandular hypofunction, but spontaneous remission and restoration of normal thyroid function are the rule. Pathologically, a granulomatous giant cell infiltrate and a marked reduction in iodine uptake characterize the condition. The clinical course ranges from weeks to a few months.

Subtotal thyroidectomy produces transient hypothyroidism in most patients and permanent hypothyroidism in about half within the first year after surgery. *Drugs* with antithyroid activity, such as *lithium*, can induce some evidence of hypothyroidism in about a fifth of cases, but only 5% become clinically hypothyroid. *Iodide excess* impairs thyroxine synthesis and release, especially in patients with preexisting thyroid disease; *iodide deficiency* inhibits hormone synthesis. Drugs that have an antithyroid effect produce a rapid but reversible form of hypothyroidism.

Secondary Hypothyroidism occurs most commonly as a result of injury to thyrotropes by a functioning or nonfunctioning pituitary adenoma. Many other forms of sellar or suprasellar disease can produce the same net result, which is inadequate production of TSH leading to an atrophic thyroid gland and hypothyroidism. Other hormone-producing cells of the pituitary may also be involved and cause a host of associated endocrinopathies (see Chapters 100 and 101). Primary hypothyroidism can sometimes mimic secondary disease by causing the pituitary to enlarge; however, the pituitary shrinks in response to exogenous thyroid hormone in primary disease, but not in secondary disease.

Clinical Presentation

Subclinical Hypothyroidism. Along with the ability to detect early disease (see below) comes the designation of subclinical hypothyroidism, defined as an asymptomatic elevation in serum TSH concentration (ranging from 6 to 14 mU/L, depending on the specificity desired) accompanied by thyroid hormone levels within normal limits. The general population prevalence averages 7% for women and 2.5% for men. In about 20% of patients with a TSH concentration above 6 mU/L, clinically symptomatic hypothyroidism develops within a period of 5 years; the incidence of clinical disease rises to almost 100% for those with a TSH level above 14 mU/L. Patients with high titers of antithyroid antibodies are at greatest risk for becoming overtly hypothyroid, which suggests that Hashimoto's thyroiditis plays an important role. The meaning of an isolated TSH between 6 and 10 mU/L remains unclear, although some evidence has been found of an increased risk for coronary artery disease resulting from lipid abnormalities.

Clinical Hypothyroidism. The overt symptomatic manifestations of hypothyroidism reflect the decreases in metabolic rate and sensitivity to catecholamines that result from insufficient circulating thyroid hormone. Early symptoms are gradual in onset and may occur before serum free thyroxine levels fall below normal limits, although the TSH level rises as soon as circulating levels of thyroid hormone are sensed to be inappropriately low. The patient typically complains of *fatigue*, moderately *dry skin*, *heavy menstrual periods*, a slight *weight gain*, or *cold intolerance*. These symptoms are followed during the next few months by the development of very dry skin, coarse hair, hoarseness, continued weight gain (although appetite is minimal), and slightly *impaired mental activity* (e.g., minor diminution in psychomotor activity, visual–perceptual skills, or memory). Later, depression may become evident.

In late stages, hydrophilic mucopolysaccharide accumulates subcutaneously, producing the *myxedematous changes* that characterize the severe form of the disease. The skin becomes doughy, the face puffy, the tongue large, the expression dull, and mentation slow, even lethargic. *Muscle weakness*, *arthralgias*, *diminished hearing*, and *carpal tunnel syndrome* are also found. Daytime sleepiness in severely myxedematous patients suggests that obstructive sleep apnea may be occurring. *Dementia* may ensue and be only partially responsive to thyroid replacement therapy.

On examination, a *goiter* may be evident. If Hashimoto's disease is the cause, the goitrous gland may feel rubbery, nontender, and even nodular. In the case of subacute thyroiditis, it will be very tender and enlarged, although not always symmetrically. Diffuse enlargement also occurs with hereditary defects in thyroxine synthesis or the use of iodides, paraaminosalicylic acid, or lithium. An atrophic gland is characteristic of secondary hypothyroidism. The heart may show signs of dilatation or an effusion. Bowel sounds are diminished, and the relaxation phase of the deep tendon *reflexes* is slowed or *"hung up."*

In *secondary hypothyroidism*, signs of accompanying ovarian and adrenal insufficiency (e.g., loss of axillary and pubic hair, amenorrhea, postural hypotension) may be seen as a consequence of concurrent loss of luteinizing hormone (LH), follicle-stimulating hormone (FSH), and adrenocorticotropic hormone (ACTH) production. Myxedematous changes tend to be less marked than with primary hypothyroidism, and the gland is smaller.

Laboratory Manifestations

As noted earlier, in primary hypothyroidism, *TSH elevation* may precede clinical manifestations. The earliest development is an increase in TRH, followed by the TSH response. At this stage, thyroid hormone levels may still be reported as "within normal limits," although in reality, they are reduced from baseline. Only later does free thyroxine fall to overtly abnormal levels. *Hypercholesterolemia*—an increase in low-density lipoprotein (LDL) cholesterol and a reduction in high-density lipoprotein (HDL) cholesterol—is often noted. Hypothyroidism is associated with a number of *anemic states*. The most common is a mild normochromic normocytic anemia. In addition, a microcytic anemia may ensue from iron deficiency secondary to heavy menstrual bleeding. Also, a macrocytic picture that clears on administration of exogenous thyroid hormone is sometimes encountered. A true megaloblastic anemia resulting from *vitamin B$_{12}$* deficiency occurs in about 10% of hypothyroid patients with a macrocytic smear; the relation between hypothyroidism and pernicious anemia is unresolved, but an autoimmune mechanism is postulated.

In severe cases of myxedema, dilutional hyponatremia occurs as a result of inadequate renal blood flow. A warning of impending myxedema coma is a rise in arterial carbon dioxide tension (Paco$_2$), which takes place as the respiratory drive weakens.

DIFFERENTIAL DIAGNOSIS

The causes of hypothyroidism can be categorized according to whether they impair the thyroid gland (primary hypothyroidism) or the hypothalamic–pituitary axis (secondary hy-

Table 104.1. Differential Diagnosis of Hypothyroidism

Primary Hypothyroidism
Hashimoto's thyroiditis
Postpartum disease (transient)
Postirradiation disease
Subtotal thyroidectomy
Subacute thyroiditis (transient)
Antithyroid drugs (lithium, PAS, PTU, methimazole, iodide excess)
Iodide deficiency
Infiltrative disease (hemochromatosis, amyloidosis, scleroderma)
Biosynthetic defect, hereditary

Secondary Hypothyroidism
Pituitary macroadenoma
Empty sella syndrome
Infarction
Infiltrative disease (e.g., sarcoidosis)
Surgery or radiation-induced injury

PAS, para-aminosalicylic acid; PTU, propylthiouracil.

pothyroidism) (Table 104.1). Primary disease is far more prevalent than secondary disease. Hashimoto's thyroiditis and postirradiation disease are the leading causes in the United States.

WORKUP

Screening for Hypothyroidism

The test of choice to screen for hypothyroidism is a *serum TSH determination*, the most sensitive and cost-effective of available tests. Modern TSH assays provide a very sensitive means of detecting hypothyroidism, often long before the patient becomes overtly symptomatic. Measurement of *thyroid hormone levels* is indicated if the TSH is elevated, but not for screening, because the test sensitivity is lower and the cost is no less.

Despite the ease and effectiveness of detection, considerable controversy remains regarding the value of adding a TSH determination to the periodic health examination. The frequency of hypothyroidism is low in men, and the impact of treatment on asymptomatic patients is unclear. Although screening for hypothyroidism has been calculated to be as cost-effective as many other generally accepted preventive medical practices ($9,000 to $23,000 per quality-adjusted life-year), such calculations are based on benefits noted in observational studies of symptomatic patients; no randomized trials have evaluated the treatment of asymptomatic patients detected by screening. Nonetheless, patients in subgroups with an increased prevalence of hypothyroidism might be reasonable candidates for screening, and for them a TSH determination should at least be considered. These include women over the age of 50 years (especially if hyperlipidemic) and patients with goiter, Hashimoto's thyroiditis (presence of antithyroid antibodies), recent radioiodine or external neck irradiation, or recent thyroid surgery. In addition, the prevalence of hypothyroidism is high among patients with mental dysfunction admitted to geriatric units and among women older than age 40 with such nonspecific complaints as fatigue.

Diagnosis of Hypothyroidism

Although the history (cold intolerance, skin changes, unexplained weight gain, hoarseness, fatigue, heavy periods) and physical findings (dry skin, coarse hair, goiter, "hung-up" reflexes) often suggest the diagnosis, confirmation and the detection of early disease require laboratory study.

The diagnosis of *primary hypothyroidism* is readily achieved by demonstrating an *increased TSH level* and a *low free T_4 level* (or *free T_4 index*). The TSH is the more sensitive indicator of primary hypothyroidism and the test of choice. The designation of *"subclinical hypothyroidism"* is given to the asymptomatic patient with a modest elevation in TSH (6 to 10 mU/L) and a free T_4 index remaining within normal limits. However, the range of normal for the free T_4 index is wide. A single free T_4 determination may not detect the patient who has a modest yet physiologically important decline in hormone level because the serum concentrations may remain within normal limits. Moreover, antithyroid antibodies can interfere with the commonly used immunoassays and produce falsely high or low readings, depending on the type of assay used. Nevertheless, the free thyroxine level is a better measure of thyroid function than the *total T_4*, which is affected by changes in thyroid-binding globulin that are independent of thyroid function.

Often, measurement of *total T_3* is routinely ordered as part of a battery of thyroid function tests. The assay is expensive to perform, and the results correlate poorly with thyroid status, affected by such events as a fall in peripheral conversion of T_4 to T_3, which is common in the elderly and in nonthyroidal illness. Determinations of serum *cholesterol* and *thyroglobulin* and of *radioactive iodine uptake* are also insensitive tests that contribute little to the diagnostic evaluation.

Secondary hypothyroidism should be suspected when the TSH level is inappropriately low in the setting of overt hypothyroidism. Concurrent amenorrhea, galactorrhea, postural hypotension, or visual field deficits also suggest pituitary–hypothalamic disease. Imaging of the sellar region is indicated. *Computed tomography* (CT) is best for detecting small lesions within the sella; *magnetic resonance imaging* (MRI) is best for imaging the suprasellar region (see Chapter 100). *TRH stimulation* is sometimes used to confirm secondary hypothyroidism, but the test often fails to distinguish among its causes.

Patients who are taking a thyroid preparation but in whom hypothyroidism has not been documented can be evaluated by stopping replacement therapy. Abrupt cessation of exogenous thyroid hormone therapy is not dangerous so long as the patient has no prior history of severe hypothyroidism. Prompt and adequate (although submaximal) responses of the pituitary and thyroid gland occur when hormone intake is halted. However, because it takes about 5 weeks for full functioning of the hypothalamic—pituitary–thyroid axis to return, testing for hypothyroidism should be delayed until then to avoid a false-positive diagnosis of hypothyroidism.

Identifying the Underlying Cause

History should be checked for possible etiologic factors, such as exposure to iodine 131, neck irradiation, recent viral infection, use of medications with antithyroid activity (lithium, excess iodide), residence in an area of iodide deficiency, subtotal thyroidectomy, pituitary surgery or irradiation, and recent pregnancy.

Physical Examination should include a careful look at the thyroid gland for size, consistency, and nodularity. An exquis-

itely tender gland suggests subacute thyroiditis. A nontender, diffusely enlarged gland is seen in early Hashimoto's disease, iodide deficiency, and congenital biosynthetic defects, and after childbirth. A rubbery, multinodular goiter suggests more advanced Hashimoto's thyroiditis. When secondary hypothyroidism is suspected clinically, the blood pressure should be checked for postural hypotension and the visual fields for deficits.

Laboratory Investigation is relatively limited. The *TSH* level (to differentiate primary from secondary disease) and *antimicrosomal antibody* titer (presence of antibodies strongly suggestive of Hashimoto's thyroiditis) are the most useful. In patients with a sellar mass lesion, determination of the serum levels of LH, FSH, ACTH, and prolactin may be indicated (see Chapters 100 and 101). A *lipid profile* (see Chapter 15) should be obtained in all hypothyroid patients because it is likely to be abnormal and require attention. Those with suspected Hashimoto's disease should also have a *complete blood cell count* and a serum *vitamin B_{12}* determination.

PRINCIPLES OF MANAGEMENT

The availability of high-quality, inexpensive preparations of levothyroxine make restoration of the euthyroid state readily achievable. The issues are when to initiate therapy, how best to do so, how best to monitor the patient, and how long to continue treatment.

Subclinical Hypothyroidism

The need for replacement therapy in subclinical hypothyroidism is a matter of debate. Favoring therapy is the opportunity to correct secondary lipid abnormalities (elevated LDL cholesterol, reduced HDLs) and decrease the size of the gland if it is enlarged. Also, some persons are actually symptomatic, although the relation of symptoms to thyroid disease is not appreciated until treatment is instituted and the patient reports feeling considerably better. This is especially true for patients with neuropsychiatric symptoms. Against treatment is the lack of evidence from prospective, controlled trials that treatment is beneficial, safe, and cost-effective. No evidence has been found that early treatment affects the natural history of the underlying cause. Lipid and symptom responses to replacement therapy in patients with only modest elevations in TSH (e.g., <10 mU/L) appear modest at best. Moreover, osteoporosis or atrial fibrillation can be induced with excessive treatment, which can easily occur in patients with minimally elevated TSH levels.

Given these present uncertainties, a reasonable approach would be to follow expectantly truly asymptomatic persons with mild elevations in TSH (<10m U/L) and to consider treating those with more substantial increases in TSH (i.e., >10 mU/L). Those who are to be managed expectantly should undergo an annual assessment that includes a TSH determination, and they should be treated if they are becoming symptomatic or the TSH increases substantially.

Clinical Hypothyroidism

For patients who are clinically hypothyroid, replacement therapy is indicated. Treatment of mild to moderate disease is best instituted gradually because hypothyroid patients are very sensitive to the effects of thyroid hormone. (An excessive rate of replacement may cause tremor, nervousness, and palpitations.) Adequate replacement should result in resolution of fatigue, loss of excess weight, and reversal of autonomic symptoms. The first signs of response are a modest loss of weight, increase in the pulse rate, and resolution of constipation. Myxedematous skin changes, pleural and pericardial effusions, and elevated creatine phosphokinase levels also normalize, but this requires more time. Most patients feel better within 2 weeks, and clinical resolution is usually complete by 3 months. Therapy for primary hypothyroidism is continued indefinitely, except in patients with transient disease, such as those with postpartum or subacute thyroiditis.

Replacement Program. Levothyroxine remains the preparation of choice for most patients (see below). A replacement dose of 100 to 125 μg/d usually suffices. The elderly tend to have a 20% lower daily requirement because of decreased T_4 clearance. Current levothyroxine replacement doses are lower than those previously cited because contemporary levothyroxine preparations are more potent.

The *starting dose* and rate of adjustment depend on age, height, weight, presence of chronic disease (especially coronary artery disease), severity and duration of symptoms, and pretreatment TSH level. Young, otherwise healthy patients can be started on a nearly full dose of levothyroxine (100 μg/d). The dose can be adjusted in 25- to 50-μg increments until a euthyroid state is achieved. In patients older than age 50 (who are at increased risk for silent coronary disease) and those with known heart disease, more cautious replacement is indicated to avoid precipitating angina, arrhythmias (atrial fibrillation, sinus tachycardia), and even heart failure. In this setting, it is best to initiate therapy with 25 to 50 μg/d and increase it in 25-μg steps. If angina or other cardiac symptoms occur, the dosage of thyroid hormone should be reduced. Some advocate the concurrent administration of a *β-blocking agent* (e.g., propranolol) to protect the heart from the increase in myocardial oxygen demand associated with thyroxine therapy.

The onset of effect is usually gradual, becoming evident in 2 to 4 weeks. One should allow 4 to 6 weeks between dose adjustments because it can take that long for a given dose to become fully effective.

Preoperative management has been a subject of concern. Coronary patients found to be mildly to moderately hypothyroid can safely undergo urgent surgery (including bypass procedures) without prior replacement. The rate of complications is no greater than that for nonhypothyroid patients, and the cardiac risks are less than when replacement therapy is initiated preoperatively. However, careful preoperative planning of anesthesia is essential because the clearance of anesthetics is reduced.

Replacement Preparations. The replacement preparation of choice for most patients continues to be *levothyroxine* (L-T_4), based on uniform bioavailability, cost, safety, and ease of monitoring therapy (see below). The half-life is about 24 hours, which allows for convenient once-daily administration. Some of the drug is converted peripherally to T_3, so that it is usually unnecessary to use the more expensive preparations containing mixtures of T_4 and T_3. Patients who continue to be bothered by *neuropsychiatric symptoms* clearly referable to their hypothyroidism may benefit from a trial of *mixed therapy*, in which

12.5 μg of *triiodothyronine* is substituted for 50 μg of levothyroxine. However, *antidepressant therapy* (see Chapter 227) should be considered for patients with major depression if thyroid hormone replacement is not helping. The exclusive use of exogenous T_3 is considered inadvisable for replacement purposes, especially in older patients, because it causes rapid increases in metabolic rate and oxygen demand and can precipitate angina. Moreover, its short half-life produces wide swings in T_3 levels and makes frequent administration necessary. For these reasons, it is best to switch patients from desiccated thyroid hormone or T_3 preparations to levothyroxine.

Levothyroxine has its own shortcomings. In the early 1980s, variations in the biologic activity and hormonal content of some commercial preparations were reported. Quality control efforts mandated by the Food and Drug Administration have eliminated most of this variability. Although pharmacokinetic differences are found between different preparations, those that have been thoroughly tested appear relatively interchangeable. Nonetheless, it is probably best, if possible, to stay with a particular levothyroxine preparation as long as it appears to provide adequate replacement and a consistent performance. Using a brand name preparation has no particular advantage. The absorption of levothyroxine is impaired by simultaneous ingestion of ferrous sulfate, which binds to it. Because T_3 is the pertinent feedback hormone and derives from conversion of T_4, the amount of thyroxine necessary to normalize the TSH level may produce serum free thyroxine levels in the high-normal to slightly elevated range.

Monitoring and Adjusting Replacement Therapy is best accomplished by measuring the serum *TSH* with the sensitive TSH assay, the results of which closely correlate with physiologic measures of thyroid hormone effect. However, reliance on the TSH determination can lead to erroneous conclusions during the initial 6 to 12 months of therapy because it can take that long for the TSH level to normalize despite adequate replacement doses. *Free T_4* levels may also correlate poorly with the physiologic status during this initial period of therapy. For these reasons, objective monitoring is difficult during the start-up phase of treatment, so that reliance on symptoms and signs is necessary.

The role of *symptoms* and *signs* in monitoring therapy is the subject of debate. Most studies suggest that the correlation between test results and clinical findings is poor, but more data are needed. For now, TSH testing appears to be the preferred method of monitoring, supplemented by correlation with the clinical state during periods when the TSH changes may lag behind the changes in the physiologic state (e.g., during initiation of therapy). Thus, if the patient becomes clinically euthyroid during the early phase of replacement therapy but the TSH level is still elevated, it is best to leave the dose unchanged and repeat the TSH determination in 4 to 8 weeks. If the TSH falls but remains elevated and the patient continues to be clinically hypothyroid, then an increase in the thyroxine dosage is warranted. If the TSH level of the hypothyroid patient shows no change, then poor compliance is the most likely explanation and no dose adjustment is warranted. If TSH is undetectable, then the replacement dose is excessive.

When an excessive dose is suggested by a very low or absent TSH, measurement of the *free T_4* (or *free T_4 index*, which is an excellent proxy for the free T_4) can help determine just how excessive the current dose is.

Once a stable replacement dosage has been achieved, twice-yearly TSH determinations are probably sufficient. Any upward adjustments in dosage should be made in small increments and followed by repeated TSH testing in 6 to 8 weeks.

Secondary Hypothyroidism

Treatment and monitoring must take into account the lack of TSH response and any coexisting adrenal or ovarian hypofunction. Because thyroid replacement and the resultant rise in metabolic rate can precipitate an addisonian crisis, adrenal function should be assessed with an ACTH stimulation test before replacement therapy is prescribed in any patient suspected of having secondary hypothyroidism. Patients with an inadequate ACTH response would be candidates for treatment with cortisone acetate before levothyroxine replacement.

MANAGEMENT RECOMMENDATIONS

Screening and Diagnosis

- Consider TSH screening for women over the age of 50 years (especially if hyperlipidemic or with complaints of fatigue); persons with Hashimoto's thyroiditis, recent radioiodine or external neck irradiation, or recent thyroid surgery; and patients with mental dysfunction admitted to geriatric units.
- Stop any exogenous thyroid or antithyroid medication if the reason for its use is unclear; recheck the TSH level 4 to 6 weeks after treatment is stopped.
- Confirm the diagnosis of hypothyroidism with TSH and free T_4 or free T_4 index determinations.
- If the patient appears clinically and biochemically hypothyroid but the TSH is not appropriately elevated, test for pituitary insufficiency.

Primary Hypothyroidism

- If possible, stop all drugs with a potential antithyroid effect (e.g., iodides, para-aminosalicylic acid, lithium).
- Begin replacement with a once-daily morning dose of levothyroxine. Initiate therapy with 50 to 100 μg/d in young, otherwise healthy patients and with 25 to 50 μg/d in older patients; the size of the dose is a function of patient age and weight, severity and duration of hypothyroidism, and the presence of underlying heart disease. Particular caution is indicated in the presence of underlying coronary disease; small starting doses are required for these patients.
- Monitor initial therapy by TSH determination and clinical state. The goal is normalization of the TSH, but be aware that the TSH level may initially require several months to normalize despite adequate thyroid hormone replacement. If the patient is clinically euthyroid but the TSH is still elevated, continue the same dose and repeat the TSH determination in 4 to 8 weeks. A check of the free T_4 (or free T_4 index) may be of use if TSH is low or absent. Also monitor for side effects (e.g., tremor, angina, arrhythmias).
- Increase the dose in increments of 25 to 50 μg; the lower increment is appropriate for elderly patients and those with heart disease.
- Allow 4 to 6 weeks for a new dose to take full effect before considering another increase in dose.
- Patients who continue to be bothered by *neuropsychiatric symptoms* clearly referable to their hypothyroidism may ben-

efit from a trial of *mixed therapy*, in which 12.5 μg of *triiodothyronine* is substituted for 50 μg of levothyroxine. However, patients with major depression should be considered for *antidepressant* therapy (see Chapter 227) if thyroid hormone replacement is not helping.
- The average levothyroxine replacement dose for most adults is 100 to 125 μg/d; for the elderly, the average dose is 20% less.
- Avoid excessive doses of replacement therapy (TSH <0.5 mU/L) because of the risk for inducing osteoporosis.
- Once the proper dose has been achieved, monitor therapy every 6 to 12 months with a TSH determination.
- Levothyroxine is the thyroid replacement preparation of choice; select and stay with a particular manufacturer's preparation. The use of desiccated thyroid and the sole use of T_3 preparations is not recommended.
- Patients with mild to moderate hypothyroidism and underlying coronary disease need not receive replacement therapy before urgent surgery. However, careful planning of anesthesia is necessary.

Secondary Hypothyroidism

- Perform an ACTH stimulation test to assess adrenal reserve. If it is low, give cortisone acetate *before* prescribing thyroid replacement.
- Replace thyroid hormone as for primary hypothyroidism.
- Monitor therapy by following clinical signs and free T_4.

PATIENT EDUCATION

Euthyroid patients who are inappropriately placed on exogenous thyroid hormone for the treatment of fatigue or obesity are often reluctant to give up the medication. Documenting that their thyroid status is perfectly normal is an essential first step in taking them off the medication successfully. Often, they will agree to a request from the physician to halt thyroid hormone for 5 weeks and have their TSH and free T_4 measured. Usually, patients note little change in how they feel, and this helps to convince them that exogenous hormone is unnecessary.

Hypothyroid patients need to be warned of the danger of increasing their medication too rapidly or taking more than is prescribed. Unfortunately, some patients adjust their dosages on the basis of other symptoms that they mistakenly attribute to hypothyroidism, such as symptoms of depression. All patients should be instructed to measure and record their weight regularly and report any unexplained change of 5 lb or more.

It is imperative that the patient and family be instructed about the signs of worsening hypothyroidism. Hypothyroid patients have been known to stop taking their thyroid medication. The importance of continuing therapy indefinitely must be emphasized to patients and the persons close to them.

A.H.G.

ANNOTATED BIBLIOGRAPHY

Amino N, Mori H, Iwatani Y, et al. High prevalence of transient postpartum thyrotoxicosis and hypothyroidism. N Engl J Med 1982;306:849. (*The initial report of this phenomenon, which was attributed to an autoimmune thyroiditis; incidence was 5%.*)

Bauer DC, Ettinger B, Browner WS. Thyroid function and serum lipids in older women: a population-based study. Am J Med

1998;104:546. (*Elevated TSH levels associated with increased LDL cholesterol and reduced HDL cholesterol; women with multiple lipid abnormalities twice as likely to have an elevated TSH level.*)

Bunevicius R, Kazanavicius G, Salinkevicius R, et al. Effects of thyroxine as compared with thyroxine plus triiodothyronine in patients with hypothyroidism. N Engl J Med 1999;340:424. (*A crossover study of 33 patients treated with each approach for 5 weeks; in the group given mixed treatment, relative improvements in mood and neuropsychological functioning were noted.*)

Danese MD, Powe NR, Sawin CT, et al. Screening for mild thyroid failure at the periodic health examination: a decision and cost-effectiveness analysis. JAMA 1996;276:285. (*Screening for subclinical hypothyroidism found cost-effective, especially in elderly women.*)

Dong BJ, Hauck WW, Gambertoglio JG, et al. Bioequivalence of generic and brand-name levothyroxine products in the treatment of hypothyroidism. JAMA 1997;277;1205. (*A pharmacokinetic study of four generic and one brand name product concluded that they differ but are bioequivalent and interchangeable for most patients.*)

Dugbartey AT. Neurocognitive aspects of hypothyroidism. Arch Intern Med 1998;158:1413. (*Reviews the data relating neurocognitive symptoms to thyroid disease and their responsiveness or lack thereof to thyroid replacement therapy.*)

Fish LH, Schwartz HL, Cavanaugh J, et al. Replacement dose, metabolism, and bioavailability of levothyroxine in the treatment of hypothyroidism. N Engl J Med 1987;316:764. (*Detailed study of pharmacokinetics; mean replacement dose was 112 μg/d.*)

Greenspan SL, Greenspan FS. The effect of thyroid hormone on skeletal integrity. Ann Intern Med 1999;130:750. (*Hyperthyroidism and the use of thyroxine to suppress TSH are associated with an increased risk for osteoporosis, particularly in cortical bone; bone density examination of the hip or forearm is recommended for women with a history of either.*)

Greenspan SL, Greenspan FS, Resnick NM, et al. Skeletal integrity in premenopausal and postmenopausal women receiving long-term L-thyroxine therapy. Am J Med 1991;91:5. (*Bone loss is minimal at most when replacement therapy is carefully administered.*)

Helfand M, Redfern CC. Screening for thyroid disease: an update. Ann Intern Med 1998;129:144. (*Thoughtful review of the evidence for screening; includes detailed discussion of the value of screening for subclinical hypothyroidism.*).

Helfand M, Crapo LM. Screening for thyroid disease. Ann Intern Med 1990;112:840. (*Whole-population screening found to be of little value, although it may be of benefit in groups with a high prevalence of hypothyroidism.*)

Krugman L, Hershman J, Chopra I, et al. Patterns of recovery of the hypothalamic–pituitary–thyroid axis in patients taken off chronic thyroid therapy. J Clin Endocrinol Metab 1975;41:70. (*Full recovery of pituitary and thyroid responsiveness to TRH occurred in euthyroid patients 5 weeks after withdrawal of long-term thyroid hormone therapy.*)

Levine HD. Compromise therapy in the patient with angina pectoris and hypothyroidism. Am J Med 1980;69:411. (*Details the difficulties of adequately controlling angina while fully correcting hypothyroidism.*)

Mandel SJ, Brent GA, Larsen PR. Levothyroxine therapy in patients with thyroid disease. Ann Intern Med 1993;119:492. (*Includes detailed discussion of replacement therapy for hypothyroidism.*)

Nordyke RA, Reppun T, Madanay LD, et al. Alternative sequences of thyrotropin and free thyroxine assays for routine thyroid function testing: quality and cost. Arch Intern Med 1998;158:266. (*A literature review of cost-effectiveness; obtaining the TSH level first found to be the most cost-effective approach to testing.*)

Robuschi G, Safran M, Braverman LE, et al. Hypothyroidism in the elderly. Endocr Rev 1987;8:142. (*Comprehensive review of pathophysiology, clinical presentation, and treatment.*)

Ross DS. Monitoring L-thyroxine therapy: lessons from the effects of L-thyroxine on bone density. Am J Med 1991;91:1. (*Outlines an approach to replacement therapy that minimizes the risk for osteoporosis by carefully titrating dose and TSH response.*)

Sawin CT, Geller A, Hershman JM, et al. The aging thyroid—the use of thyroid hormone in older persons. JAMA 1990;261:2653. (*Epidemiologic data showing 10% prevalence of use in the elderly; in 10% of these patients, use was inappropriate and treatment could be discontinued.*)

Schectman JM, Pawlson LG. The cost-effectiveness of three thyroid function testing strategies for suspicion of hypothyroidism in a primary care setting. J Gen Intern Med 1990;5:9. (*A TSH-first strategy proved best.*)

Singer PA, Cooper DS, Levy EG, et al. Treatment guidelines for patients with hyperthyroidism and hypothyroidism. Standards of Care Committee, American Thyroid Association. JAMA 1995;273:808. (*Consensus clinical guidelines.*)

Staub JJ, Althaus BU, Engler H, et al. Spectrum of subclinical and overt hypothyroidism. Am J Med 1992;92:631. (*One of the most detailed studies of subclinical hypothyroidism to date.*)

Surks MI, Sievert R. Drugs and thyroid function. N Engl J Med 1995;333:1688. (*Best review of drugs causing hypothyroidism.*)

105
Glucocorticoid Therapy

The therapeutic potency of glucocorticoids has led to their widespread use. Although benefits can be substantial, adverse effects are numerous, including serious metabolic derangements and suppression of the hypothalamic–pituitary–adrenal (HPA) axis. To maximize the therapeutic response and minimize the risks, a number of questions must be addressed before steroid therapy is initiated: (a) Is the underlying disorder of such severity that the benefits of therapy outweigh the risks? (b) Will prolonged treatment be required, or will a brief, limited course suffice? (c) Have alternative, less morbid therapies been maximally utilized? (d) Does the patient have any underlying condition that will worsen on steroid therapy or predispose to drug-induced complications? (e) Can a less suppressive regimen (e.g., alternate-day therapy) be utilized?

The primary physician must decide when and how to institute steroid therapy, whether to use daily or alternate-day treatment, and how to withdraw long-term glucocorticoid treatment safely.

ADVERSE EFFECTS

Most adverse effects of glucocorticoids are a function of degree of systemic absorption, dosage, and duration of use. A few are irreversible; fortunately, most resolve within several months of termination of therapy.

Suppression of the Hypothalamic–Pituitary–Adrenal Axis. Suppression compromises the physiologic response to major stress (e.g., surgery, injury), putting the patient at risk for hypotension and hypoglycemia. Symptoms and signs include *light-headedness*, *nausea*, *postural hypotension*, and *hypoglycemia*. Risk correlates with *dose* and *duration* of therapy, but it is hard to predict HPA responsiveness accurately on the basis of dose and duration alone. Other factors are believed to be operative also. Even the so-called "physiologic dose" of 7.5 mg of prednisone that supposedly corresponds to daily endogenous glucocorticoid synthesis is suppressive in some patients. Moreover, individual patients vary widely. Some experience clinically important HPA suppression with the use of as little as 5 mg of prednisone taken daily for a few weeks, whereas others manifest no measurable HPA suppression despite the use of much higher daily doses.

Scheduling of the *dose* has some effect on the degree of HPA suppression. *Daily* physiologic doses of glucocorticoids (e.g., 5 to 7.5 mg of prednisone) given in the morning do not cause suppression of any consequence, but if the same doses are given at night, normal diurnal cortisol secretion is inhibited. Doses just above the physiologic range are suppressive after about a month of use. *Alternate-day* therapy, in which short- or intermediate-acting preparations are taken at 8 a.m. every other day, does not induce clinically significant HPA suppression, nor does a *cyclic* program of 5 days of daily therapy followed by 2 to 4 weeks off therapy. However, cycles of 2 weeks on and 2 weeks off do lead to HPA suppression. A single daily pharmacologic dose of glucocorticoid produces less HPA suppression than does the same dose divided and taken at intervals during the course of the day.

Recovery from HPA suppression can take up to 12 months. Hypothalamic–pituitary function returns first, reappearing 2 to 5 months after cessation of suppressive therapy, and is manifested by appropriate plasma adrenocorticotropic hormone (ACTH) levels that demonstrate a normal diurnal pattern. Signs of adrenal recovery become evident at 6 to 9 months, with a return of the baseline serum cortisol level to normal. Maximal adrenal response to ACTH may not reappear until 9 to 12 months after cessation of therapy. There is no proven method for accelerating the restoration of normal HPA function once it has been inhibited. The administration of ACTH does not seem to speed adrenal recovery.

Like predicting the onset of HPA suppression, estimating how long clinically important hyporesponsiveness will persist is also difficult. Again, individual variation is great, and the degree of suppression cannot be reliably estimated by the basal serum cortisol concentration. In the setting of such uncertainty, *testing of the HPA axis* becomes an important adjunct to clinical decision making. Of the available stimulation tests (insulin-induced hypoglycemia, corticotropin, metyrapone, corticotropin-releasing hormone), the *corticotropin (ACTH) test* is the most widely used; results correlate well with cortisol levels measured during the stress of surgery. A blood sample is drawn to measure the serum cortisol, after which a one-ampule (250-μg) bolus of synthetic ACTH (*cosyntropin*) is injected IV. Additional samples of blood are drawn at 30 and 60 minutes for cortisol determinations. The test produces a few false-positive results in comparison with insulin-induced hypoglycemia (the "gold standard" for testing HPA function), but it is safer and more convenient to perform. False-negatives may occur if cen-

tral suppression, but not yet adrenal suppression, has developed. A low-dose (1 μg) cosyntropin test may be helpful in identifying central suppression when a standard-dose test result is suspected to be a false-negative. Some argue that the corticotropin-releasing hormone (CRH) test combines the sensitivity and specificity of insulin-induced hypoglycemia with the convenience of corticotropin testing, but few direct comparisons have been made. The test can be performed in the outpatient setting, but CRH is very expensive. The basal cortisol level has shown little correlation with the results of stimulation testing and is not a substitute for such testing.

Although HPA suppression is important to detect, it is not the only factor determining the ability of corticosteroid-exposed patients to respond appropriately to stress. Some patients manifest a hypotensive response to stress despite a normally responding HPA axis, and patients with a blunted HPA response may manifest no signs of clinical adrenal insufficiency. More work is needed to elucidate the mechanisms governing stress response in steroid-treated patients.

Metabolic and Endocrinologic Side Effects. A *negative nitrogen balance* (the result of inhibition of protein synthesis and enhancement of protein catabolism) is believed to be partially responsible for reduced muscle mass, weakness, thinning of the skin, and striae formation. *Fat redistribution* accounts for the characteristic truncal obesity and cushingoid appearance. Both fat redistribution and negative nitrogen balance are minimized by using alternate-day therapy or giving no more than a physiologic dose each morning, but not by using ACTH or daily pharmacologic glucocorticoid doses. Acne is seen, more often with ACTH than with glucocorticoid use, because of stimulation of adrenal androgen production.

Glucose intolerance is common. Mechanisms include increases in peripheral insulin resistance, gluconeogenesis, glucagon secretion, and substrate availability. Usually, the glucose intolerance is mild, does not lead to ketosis, and resolves when therapy is stopped. When carbohydrate intolerance develops, the effect appears to be dose-related.

Hypertension and *fluid retention* with peripheral edema are more common when agents with mineralocorticoid effects are used, and they are not dependent on any prior elevation of blood pressure (Table 105.1). Again, dosage and duration of therapy are important factors. *Electrolyte derangements* are common, especially hypokalemia.

Enhanced Susceptibility to Infection results from the antiinflammatory and immunosuppressive actions of corticosteroids. Bacterial infections are common. Candidiasis and aspergillosis sometimes develop. Herpes zoster, varicella, vaccinia, and cytomegalovirus infection are the principal viral infections encountered in patients on steroids. Reactivation of tuberculosis is a well-recognized risk (see Chapter 49).

Osteoporosis develops when steroids are used for prolonged periods. The exact incidence of clinically significant loss is unknown, but estimates are in the 50% range, making this underappreciated consequence one of major importance. The precise relation between dosage, duration of use, and risk for osteoporosis remains unclear, although some evidence suggests that alternate-day therapy minimizes the chance of serious osteoporosis. Even as little as 5 mg of prednisone per day over

Table 105.1.   Commonly Used Glucocorticoids

DURATION OF ACTION	GLUCOCORTICOID POTENCY[a]	EQUIVALENT GLUCOCORTICOID DOSE (mg)	MINERALOCORTICOID ACTIVITY
Short-Acting			
Cortisol (hydrocortisone)	1	20	Yes[b]
Cortisone	0.8	25	Yes[b]
Prednisone	4	5	No
Prednisolone	4	5	No
Methylprednisolone	5	4	No
Intermediate-Acting			
Triamcinolone	5	4	No
Long-Acting			
Betamethasone	25	0.60	No
Dexamethasone	30	0.75	No

[a]The values given for glucocorticoid potency are relative. Cortisol is arbitrarily assigned a value of 1.

[b]Mineralocorticoid effects are dose-related. At dosages close to or within the basal physiologic range for glucocorticoid activity, no such effect may be detectable.

Adapted from Axelrod L. Glucocorticoid therapy. Medicine (Baltimore) 1976;55:39, with permission.

time can result in bone loss. Patients with a predisposition to osteoporosis, such as menopausal women and immobilized persons, appear to be among the most susceptible. The *axial skeleton* is affected more than the limbs, and vertebral compression fractures may result. *Aseptic necrosis of the femoral head* and other bones is a well-recognized and serious, but relatively rare, skeletal complication. Sometimes it may be a manifestation of the underlying illness for which corticosteroids are being given, such as rheumatoid arthritis or systemic lupus. However, the risk is markedly increased with an increase in steroid dose and prolonged therapy.

Gastrointestinal Effects. Gastritis, peptic ulceration, and gastrointestinal bleeding have all been attributed to steroid use. Multiple randomized, controlled trials have produced conflicting results, as have major metaanalyses examining pooled data from such trials (see Chapter 68). Hotly debated is the degree to which ulcer risk is a function of dosage and duration of exposure. The risk appears small until dosages in excess of the equivalent of 30 mg of prednisone per day are reached and continued for more than a month. Even then, the increase in rate of peptic ulceration is in the range of only 1% to 2%. Most peptic ulceration is caused by the concurrent use of nonsteroidal antiinflammatory agents. Antacids and food do not interfere with absorption of oral steroid preparations.

Acute pancreatitis is noted with increased frequency in patients taking corticosteroids. *Panniculitis* is unique to iatrogenic Cushing's syndrome.

Myopathy may result from the prolonged intake of large doses. Proximal muscle wasting and weakness of the lower extremities are characteristic. Patients have difficulty climbing stairs. The average time of onset is 5 months into treatment. Muscle enzymes are normal. The complication is reversible, and exercise may help minimize it.

Psychological and Behavioral Changes are particularly common in the elderly. The reported incidence ranges from 25% to 40%, mostly among patients receiving high doses. Increased appetite, mild euphoria, and changes in sleep patterns are rather common at the beginning of treatment. Psychoses,

which are not predictably related to dosage or duration of therapy, can occur; they slowly respond to reduction or cessation of steroid use. Some clinicians argue that the patient's premorbid personality plays a role; others deny this. Steroid therapy can exacerbate previous psychiatric disease.

Cataracts of the posterior subcapsular type are reported in 10% to 35% of cases and are predominantly dose- and duration-dependent. A few require removal; most do not.

Adverse Effects of Inhaled Glucocorticoids. The inhaled topically active steroid preparations used for asthma are usually well tolerated and not associated with significant adverse effects, even when used daily for months at a time. However, the growing appreciation of the need for long-term therapy with inhaled steroids and the development of increasingly potent preparations (e.g., fluticasone) have raised concerns about the potential for systemic effects. Metaanalytic study finds that the risk for HPA suppression is greatest when the dosage of most inhaled steroids exceeds 1.5 mg/d (>0.75 mg/d for fluticasone). Fluticasone demonstrates greater biologic activity and confers a greater risk on a milligram per milligram basis in comparison with beclomethasone, budesonide, and triamcinolone. Similar relationships and dose thresholds have been noted in regard to the risks for osteoporosis and posterior subcapsular cataracts. A lesser risk for ocular hypertension and glaucoma has been observed, but no evidence of permanent growth retardation in children. Skin bruising parallels HPA suppression.

PRINCIPLES OF THERAPY

The challenge of glucocorticoid use is to obtain maximal therapeutic benefit with a minimum of adverse effects. In most instances, steroids do not cure disease or alter its natural history; rather, they suppress or alter the inflammatory and immunologic responses and, in doing so, reduce symptoms. Therefore, one must carefully weigh the perceived therapeutic benefit against the potential risks. The risk is negligible for a short-term course of therapy (7 to 14 days), even with high doses, which can be very effective in selected situations (e.g., acute asthma, contact dermatitis). Appetite stimulation and restlessness are the principal side effects. No long-term consequences have been noted. The decision to initiate more prolonged steroid therapy requires additional consideration of the risks involved (see above).

Selection of Agent. Corticosteroid preparations differ principally in duration of action and degree of mineralocorticoid activity (Table 105.1). *Short-acting agents* are less likely to cause HPA suppression, especially when prescribed for morning use in low doses as part of an alternate-day program (see below). Long-acting agents are preferred for situations in which a high-dose steroid effect must be sustained (e.g., increased intracranial pressure). Mineralocorticoid activity is desirable in adrenal insufficiency but not in situations of excessive inflammation or immunoreactivity. Regardless of the agent selected, it is essential to continue maximal nonsteroidal therapy, insofar as it reduces steroid requirements.

Prednisone is the most widely prescribed of the glucocorticoids. Its short half-life, low cost, and negligible mineralocorticoid effect make it useful for most immunosuppressive and antiinflammatory indications. *Prednisolone* is the active hepatic metabolite of prednisone and is useful in the setting of liver failure. *Dexamethasone* is the long-acting glucocorticoid of choice, being about seven times more potent on a weight basis than prednisone and having a half-life of 24 hours. This potency makes the agent useful for suppressive testing of the HPA axis. *Hydrocortisone* (cortisol) is the naturally occurring glucocorticoid. It has one fourth the glucocorticoid potency of prednisone but exerts some mineralocorticoid effect when used in pharmacologic doses, which makes it useful for parenteral supplementation in a patient believed to have adrenal suppression. *Florinef* (9-α-fluorohydrocortisone), a potent mineralocorticoid with virtually no glucocorticoid effect, is used primarily for replacement in adrenal cortical insufficiency.

Theoretically, the use of *ACTH* would appear attractive because it might avoid adrenal suppression, but it also induces undesirable mineralocorticoid and androgenic responses. Moreover, it must be given parenterally, and there is no way to know how much glucocorticoid effect is obtained from a given dose. These disadvantages limit its usefulness, although it is given preferentially by many neurologists for exacerbations of multiple sclerosis (see Chapter 172).

Selection of Dosing Schedule: Alternate-day versus Daily. Most conditions that require prolonged corticosteroid treatment, such as asthma (see Chapter 48), sarcoidosis (see Chapter 51), inflammatory bowel disease (see Chapter 73), and nephrotic syndrome (see Chapter 142), can be well controlled with *alternate-day therapy*, although it is often necessary to begin with a program of daily steroids when the disease is very active and symptoms are severe. Important advantages of alternate-day treatment are avoidance of significant HPA suppression and minimization of cushingoid side effects without a substantial loss of antiinflammatory activity. It appears that the antiinflammatory effects of glucocorticoids persist longer (up to 3 days) than the undesirable metabolic effects. Other adverse effects that are reduced or eliminated by an alternate-day schedule include inhibition of delayed hypersensitivity, susceptibility to infection, negative nitrogen balance, fluid retention, hypertension, and psychological and behavioral disturbances.

Alternate-day therapy by itself will not prevent HPA suppression if a long-acting steroid preparation is used (e.g., dexamethasone). Moreover, therapy must really be given on alternate days, with the total dose taken first thing in the morning every other day. Intermittent therapy or doses taken throughout the day every other day do not preserve HPA responsiveness.

Daily steroid therapy is indicated during acute exacerbations of disease and in the limited number of conditions that are controlled only by daily glucocorticoid administration, such as temporal arteritis (see Chapter 161) and pemphigus vulgaris. When daily therapy is necessary, HPA suppression can be minimized by having the patient take the entire daily dose first thing in the morning and by prescribing a short-acting glucocorticoid at the lowest possible dose. Daily single-dose regimens may be as effective or nearly as effective as divided-dose regimens in controlling underlying illness. However, manifestations of Cushing's syndrome are not prevented, as they are with alternate-day therapy.

Switching from a Daily to an Alternate-day Schedule. Most patients who experience a remission on daily therapy are candidates for a trial of alternate-day steroids (see above for exceptions). Switching makes it possible for the patient to transfer to a less morbid program without a diminution in disease control. In switching, the *same total steroid dose* is continued, whereas in tapering, it is gradually reduced. Switching is carried out by gradually increasing the dose on the first day and decreasing it on the second day until a double dose is taken every other day, with no drug taken on the in-between days.

How fast the changeover can be made varies, depending on the activity of the underlying disease, duration of therapy, degree of HPA suppression, and cooperativeness of the patient. A rough guideline for switching to alternate-day therapy is to make changes in increments of 10 mg of prednisone (or its equivalent) when the daily prednisone dose is greater than 40 mg, and in 5-mg increments when the daily dose is between 20 and 40 mg. For daily doses smaller than 20 mg, the changes should be made in increments of 2.5 mg. The interval between changes ranges from 1 day to several weeks and is determined empirically, based on the clinical response. It is important to keep in mind that most patients who have been on a daily steroid program for more than 2 to 4 weeks probably have some degree of HPA suppression.

Tapering and Withdrawing Therapy. The abrupt withdrawal of steroid therapy after a patient has been on daily doses of prednisone greater than 20 to 30 mg for more than a month can precipitate adrenal insufficiency, a flare-up of the underlying illness, or a withdrawal syndrome. There is no way to speed HPA recovery, nor are specific schedules available for reducing the daily dose. One must monitor disease activity and decrease the dose empirically by small amounts, watching for flare-up of disease or signs of adrenal insufficiency, such as postural hypotension, weakness, and gastrointestinal distress.

One empirical approach to reducing the dose toward physiologic levels is to make changes in decrements of 10 mg of prednisone or its equivalent every 1 to 3 weeks, so long as the daily dose is above 40 mg. Below 40 mg, the decrement is 5 mg. Once a physiologic dose of prednisone is reached (5 to 7.5 mg/d), the patient can be switched to 1-mg prednisone tablets or the equivalent dose of hydrocortisone, so that further reductions in dose can be made in smaller steps than is possible when 5-mg prednisone tablets are used. Weekly or biweekly reductions can then be carried out in steps of 1 mg of prednisone at a time, as permitted by disease activity.

During the tapering process, a *steroid withdrawal syndrome* develops in some patients, characterized by depression, myalgias, arthralgias, anorexia, headaches, nausea, and lethargy. Studies have failed to show a relationship between these symptoms and low cortisol or 17-hydroxycorticosteroid levels. In most instances, symptoms are reported when levels are normal, or even elevated, but falling rapidly. HPA responsiveness has also been found to be normal in many of these patients. The mechanisms responsible for this syndrome are unknown but seem to be linked to the rapidity with which the dose is tapered.

Identification and Treatment of Steroid-induced Adrenal Suppression. At times of anticipated stress (e.g., impending surgery), it is important to know how responsive the HPA axis is and whether or not supplementary steroid therapy will be needed. As noted earlier, it is very difficult to predict the onset and duration of HPA suppression, so that testing of the HPA axis is a useful adjunct for deciding who will need supplementation. In the office setting, the administration of *cosyntropin* (250 μg of synthetic ACTH) is a convenient, safe, and effective means of testing for suppression (see above). If the serum cortisol level at 60 minutes is above 18 μg/dL or an increase from baseline of at least 10 μg/dL is noted, then adrenal responsiveness is sufficient to sustain the patient through a stress equivalent to general anesthesia. Testing can be carried out in similar fashion by administering 100 μg of *CRH* as an IV bolus; CRH testing is more expensive, but it is more sensitive and helpful when pituitary dysfunction is a concern. Alternatively, a low-dose ACTH test (with 1 μg of synthetic ACTH) may help detect central disease.

If the patient cannot mount an adequate cortisol response, or testing is impractical because of urgency or unavailability of agents or assays, corticosteroid supplementation should be administered for acute stress. *Hydrocortisone* is usually prescribed because it provides both glucocorticoid and mineralocorticoid effects. Depending on the severity of the stress, one administers 100 to 400 mg of hydrocortisone per day in divided doses. The lower end of the dose range is appropriate for the stress of gastroenteritis, influenza, or dental extraction. During major stress, such as trauma or surgery, the patient should be given 100 mg of hydrocortisone parenterally every 6 to 8 hours. A prepackaged syringe containing 4 mg of *dexamethasone* phosphate can be prescribed for the patient or family to carry for parenteral use in an emergency should medical care be unavailable and the patient become unconscious or so ill that steroids cannot be taken by mouth. The need to continue supplementation is based on the duration of the stress and the underlying state of the HPA axis.

Prophylaxis and Treatment of Osteoporosis. Patients requiring long-term daily steroid therapy are at high risk for osteoporotic fracture, and prophylaxis and treatment should be considered for them. Even modest doses of prednisone (e.g., 7.5 mg/d) are associated with a risk for significant bone loss when used on a daily basis for a prolonged period. Vertebral compression fractures are of particular concern, as trabecular bone seems most affected. Bone density should be measured (see

Chapter 144), especially if the patient is menopausal. If osteoporosis is not particularly severe and the woman is menopausal, then standard *estrogen* replacement therapy should be considered in conjunction with *vitamin D* and *calcium* supplementation (see Chapter 164). If the patient has severe osteoporosis, is at high risk (e.g., prolonged high-dose therapy, inactivity), or has a history of vertebral compression fracture, then the bisphosphonate *alendronate* appears to offer the best prophylaxis. For most patients, a 5-mg dose of alendronate taken once daily with a large glass of water on arising in the morning is safe and effective. Postmenopausal patients not taking estrogen replacement therapy obtain better protection with 10 mg of alendronate per day. Careful instruction on the proper administration of alendronate is essential to its safe use (see Chapter 164).

Minimizing Risk of Inhaled Corticosteroids. The single most important means of reducing the risk for systemic effects is to keep the daily dose as low as possible (i.e., <1.5 mg/d for beclomethasone, flunisolide, budesonide, triamcinolone; <0.8 mg/d for fluticasone). The ways to accomplish this without compromising asthma control include concurrent use of a long-acting β-agonist (e.g., salmeterol) or leukotriene inhibitor (e.g., montelukast), and immunotherapy (see Chapter 48).

PATIENT EDUCATION

Steroids should be given with caution to patients whose reliability or intelligence is in question because of the risk of HPA suppression and adrenocortical insufficiency. Patients on alternate-day therapy must be instructed about the importance of keeping to the alternate-day schedule and taking their medication around 8 a.m. so as to minimize the risk for suppression. Patients on a suppressive dose of steroid should be informed about the need for steroid supplementation when stress or illness occurs and should wear an identification bracelet stating that they take a corticosteroid. Patients must understand the need to contact the physician and increase the steroid dose when they are subjected to physiologic stress.

Many patients are reluctant to discontinue long-term steroid therapy because they fear recrudescence of the underlying illness or experience malaise as the drug is tapered. A detailed review of the side effects of prolonged therapy is necessary so that the rationale for reducing the dose and the desirability of eventually discontinuing corticosteroid therapy are understood and appreciated. Any change in dosage and schedule should be written out. When prolonged daily high-dose therapy is required, the psychological impact of adverse effects (e.g., cushingoid features) can be lessened by informing the patient that they are likely to occur but are at least partially reversible.

THERAPEUTIC RECOMMENDATIONS

- Prescribe glucocorticoids only when maximal doses of other forms of therapy have proved insufficient and when the risks of steroid use are outweighed by the therapeutic benefit expected.
- To minimize the steroid dose required, always try to *add steroid therapy* to the ongoing treatment program rather than replace it.
- In the setting of active *autoimmune* or *inflammatory* disease, initiate a full-strength program of daily glucocorticoid ther-

apy with *prednisone* (40 to 60 mg/d, or prednisolone in cases of hepatocellular failure). When replacement therapy for adrenal cortical insufficiency is needed, use *hydrocortisone* (see below). The long-acting *dexamethasone* is reserved for testing the HPA axis and for the rare situation in which very high-dose, sustained-action therapy is required (e.g., increased intracranial pressure). All glucocorticoids can be taken with food; absorption is not impaired.

- To *minimize the risk for HPA suppression*, avoid prescribing long-acting preparations, give the entire glucocorticoid dose in the morning or, better yet, on alternate days, and continue for the shortest possible time.

- Try initiating therapy on an *alternate-day* basis when symptoms are not severe and the condition is not one with an absolute requirement for daily treatment (i.e., temporal arteritis, pemphigus vulgaris, severe inflammatory bowel disease).

- Once control is achieved, *taper* to the lowest dose that maintains control and terminate if possible. Tapering is carried out empirically; the patient is monitored for disease activity and evidence of adrenal insufficiency (postural hypotension, gastrointestinal upset, fatigue, muscle weakness, hypoglycemia).

- For very brief courses of corticosteroid therapy (<7 to 14 days), taper rapidly over 7 to 10 days to full cessation provided that disease activity remains quiescent. When longer courses of therapy are required, taper more slowly, reducing the dose in 10-mg decrements when the daily dose is above 40 mg and in 5-mg steps when it is below 40 mg. The *rate of tapering* is determined by disease activity and the appearance of symptoms of steroid withdrawal or adrenal insufficiency. Once the dosage has been reduced to 5 mg of prednisone every other day, therapy can be stopped or switched to 5-mg hydrocortisone or 1-mg prednisone tablets and reduced in decrements of 2.5 mg of hydrocortisone or 1 mg of prednisone.

- If tapering is unsuccessful or prolonged therapy is deemed necessary, then ascertain and maintain the lowest effective dose and try *switching to an alternate-day regimen* if it is not already being utilized.

- When switching to alternate-day therapy, begin by modestly reducing the second day's dose and adding that amount to the first day's dose. In this manner, the same total dose is maintained. If the daily dose is above 40 mg, reduce the dose on the alternate day by the equivalent of 10 mg of prednisone, and by 5 mg if the daily dose is below 40 mg. Below 20 mg, the increment is 2.5 mg. The interval between changes in dose is determined empirically, based on the clinical status of the patient. The end point of switching is attained when the previous entire 2-day dose is being given once every other day.

- If withdrawal symptoms are a problem on alternate-day therapy, a small morning dose of hydrocortisone (10 to 20 mg) given on the off day may help alleviate symptoms without prolonging HPA suppression.

- When HPA responsiveness is in question, perform a *cosyntropin stimulation test*. Administer 250 μg parenterally and measure serum cortisol immediately before and 30 and 60 minutes after administration.

- Because 9 to 12 months of HPA suppression may begin after as little as 2 to 4 weeks of 20 to 30 mg of prednisone daily, advise patients taking daily pharmacologic doses to supplement their steroid intake when under stress or experiencing an acute illness. In the setting of injury, surgery, or an inability to take oral medication, prescribe parenteral hydrocortisone or its equivalent. The total daily stress dose is 100 to 400 mg of hydrocortisone, given in divided doses every 6 to 8 hours. Provide a prepackaged syringe containing 4 mg of dexamethasone for IM emergency use.

- To prevent or treat *steroid-induced osteoporosis*, begin by measuring the vertebral bone density. If the patient is markedly osteoporotic, prescribe 5 mg of *alendronate* per day; if the patient is postmenopausal, prescribe a dose of 10 mg/d. Instruct the patient regarding the proper intake of alendronate to the minimize risk for esophageal irritation (see Chapter 164). Alternatively, consider estrogen replacement therapy in conjunction with calcium and vitamin D supplementation for menopausal women taking corticosteroids if the degree of osteoporosis is not severe and the risk for steroid-induced disease is not great (see Chapter 164).

A.H.G.

ANNOTATED BIBLIOGRAPHY

Aagaard EM, Lin P, Modin GW, et al. Prevention of glucocorticoid-induced osteoporosis: provider practice at an urban county hospital. Am J Med 1999;107:456. (*Documentation of relative lack of awareness and suggestions for improvement.*)

Abdu TA, Elhadd TA, Nearly R, et al. Comparison of the low-dose short synacthen test (1 μg), the conventional-dose short synacthen test (250 μg), and the insulin tolerance test for assessment of the hypothalamo–pituitary–adrenal axis in patients with pituitary disease. J Clin Endocrinol Metab 1999;84:838. (*Evidence that the low-dose test may be more sensitive than the conventional test and may obviate the need for insulin tolerance testing.*)

Anatruda TT Jr, Hurst MM, D'Esposo ND. Certain endocrine and metabolic facets of the steroid withdrawal syndrome. J Clin Endocrinol Metab 1965;25:1207. (*A classic study showing that the steroid withdrawal syndrome is not a consequence of inadequate serum levels of steroid.*)

Axelrod L. Glucocorticoid therapy. Medicine (Baltimore) 1976;55:39. (*A superb and comprehensive review that is slightly dated but still well worth reading; 188 references.*)

Boumpas DT, Chrousos GP, Wilder RL, et al. Glucocorticoid therapy for immune-mediated diseases: basic and clinical correlates. Ann Intern Med 1993;119:1198. (*Excellent National Institutes of Health conference on the topic; 98 references.*)

Byyny RL. Withdrawal from glucocorticoid therapy. N Engl J Med 1976;295:30. (*Still a very practical approach.*)

Carella MJ, Srivastava LS, Gossain VV, et al. Hypothalamic–pituitary–adrenal function 1 week after a short burst of steroid therapy. J Clin Endocrinol Metab 1993;76:1188. (*Finds that clinically evident adrenal insufficiency is rare after a 1-week course of steroid therapy.*)

Christy NP. Pituitary–adrenal function during corticosteroid therapy: learning to live with uncertainty. N Engl J Med 1992;326:266. (*An editorial reviewing the tests for HPA suppression and the difficulty of predicting it.*)

Dale DC, Fauci AS, Wolff SM. Alternate-day prednisone, leukocyte kinetics and susceptibility to infections. N Engl J Med 1974;29:1154. (*Classic article; alternate-day steroid therapy does not reduce leukocyte count, inflammatory response, or neutrophil half-life.*)

Graeber AL, Ney RL, Nicholson WE, et al. Natural history of pituitary–adrenal recovery following long-term suppression with corticosteroids. J Clin Endocrinol Metab 1965;25:11. (*In most patients taking glucocorticoids for 1 to 10 years, full restoration of function was noted within 1 year; hypothalamic–pituitary function returned in the first 2 to 5 months; 17-hydroxycorticosteroid levels normalized during months 6 to 9.*)

Krasner AS. Glucocorticoid-induced adrenal insufficiency. JAMA 1999;282:671. (*A useful case-based discussion; 34 pertinent references.*)

Laan RF, van Riel PL, van de Putte LB, et al. Low-dose prednisone induces rapid, reversible axial bone loss in patients with rheumatoid arthritis: a randomized, controlled study. Ann Intern Med 1993; 119:963. (*Evidence that even low doses can produce bone loss.*)

Liworth BJ. Systemic adverse effects of inhaled corticosteroid therapy: a systematic review and metaanalysis. Arch Intern Med 1999; 159:941. (*Finds increased risk for adrenal suppression, cataracts, and ocular hypertension, but not osteoporosis, with high-potency formulations.*)

Meikle AW, Tyler FH. Potency and duration of action of glucocorticoids. Effects of hydrocortisone, prednisone, and dexamethasone on human pituitary–adrenal function. Am J Med 1977;63:200. (*The intrinsic potency and relative rate of disappearance from plasma are the two most important factors determining the relative potency of orally administered glucocorticoids.*)

Messer J, Reithman D, Sacks HS, et al. Association of adrenocorticosteroid therapy and peptic ulcer disease. N Engl J Med 1983;309:21. (*Metaanalysis showing that high-dose corticosteroids do increase the risk for peptic ulcer and gastrointestinal hemorrhage. However, although the relative risk was 2, the absolute risk was quite small— 2% vs. 1% in controls.*)

Papanicolaou DA, Tsigos C, Oldfield EH, et al. Acute glucocorticoid deficiency is associated with plasma elevations of interleukin-6: does the latter participate in the symptomatology of the steroid withdrawal syndrome? J Clin Endocrinol Metab 1996;81:2303. (*Evidence suggesting that this cytokine is an important factor.*)

Piper JM, Ray WA, Daugherty JR, et al. Corticosteroid use and peptic ulcer disease: role of nonsteroidal antiinflammatory drugs. Ann Intern Med 1991;114:735. (*The increased risk was caused by concurrent NSAID use.*)

Saag KG, Schnitzer TJ, Brown JP, et al. Alendronate for the prevention and treatment of glucocorticoid-induced osteoporosis. N Engl J Med 1998;339:292. (*A 48-week randomized, placebo-controlled trial of 477 patients requiring long-term daily steroid therapy; significant improvement in bone density was achieved regardless of baseline bone density, steroid dose, or duration of steroid therapy.*)

Schlagkecke R, Kornely E, Santen RT, et al. The effect of long-term glucocorticoid therapy on pituitary–adrenal responses to exogenous corticotropin-releasing hormone. N Engl J Med 1992; 326:226. (*HPA responsiveness could not be reliably predicted from dose or duration of steroid therapy or from basal plasma cortisol level; CRH testing was nearly as accurate as insulin-induced hypoglycemia for determining HPA suppression.*)

Streeten DH, Anderson GH Jr, Bonaventrua MM. The potential for serious consequences of misinterpreting normal responses to the rapid adrenocorticotropin test. J Clin Endocrinol Metab 1996; 81:285. (*Excellent discussion of pitfalls.*)

Streeten DH. Shortcomings of low-dose (1 μg) ACTH test for the diagnosis of ACTH deficiency states. J Clin Endocrinol Metab 1999;84:835. (*A critique of this new approach to identifying central dysfunction of the axis.*)

8

Gynecologic Problems

106
Screening for Breast Cancer

Breast cancer is among the most feared illnesses that afflict women, especially in North America and northern Europe where incidence rates are five to six times higher than in Asia and Africa. More than 150,000 women develop breast cancer each year in the United States, accounting for more than one in four cancer diagnoses among women. Of these, 50,000 eventually die of the disease, accounting for one in five female cancer deaths. The lifetime probability that an American woman will develop breast cancer is approximately 12%. The morbidity and mortality associated with this disease, coupled with the importance of the breasts to many women's self-image, make breast cancer a topic of intense interest.

Breast cancer is one of only a few conditions for which benefits of screening have been well documented in randomized controlled trials, but there is controversy about which women should be screened and how often. Advances in molecular biology, including identification of breast cancer susceptibility genes, have improved our ability to estimate risk and predict behavior of breast cancer for some women, but the clinical introduction of these techniques poses new challenges. These and other controversies and advances are heralded by the media, increasing public awareness and expectations. The primary care provider deals with breast cancer screening and diagnosis or associated fears on a daily basis. Knowledge of various recommendations is insufficient. Primary care providers must understand the benefits and harms of breast cancer screening and other modes of prevention and communicate these effectively to patients.

EPIDEMIOLOGY AND RISK FACTORS

The epidemiology of breast cancer has been studied extensively. Furthermore, analysis of familial patterns and identification of breast cancer susceptibility genes have refined our understanding of risk associated with age and family history.

Age. Risk of breast cancer increases with age. The median age at the time of diagnosis is about 55 years; 45% of cases occur after age 65. However, breast cancer is not uncommon in women younger than 40 in whom approximately 20% of cases occur. When breast cancer does occur earlier in life, it is more likely to be associated with a susceptibility gene. For example,

before age 40, about 5% of non-Jewish women with breast cancer and about 25% of Jewish women with breast cancer can be expected to have *BRCA1* mutations.

Family History. Overall, a family history of breast cancer, whether among maternal or paternal relatives, increases the risk approximately two- to threefold. For women who have a family history, specific risk depends heavily on the age at onset of cancer for combinations of first-degree and second-degree relatives. For example, if one first-degree or second-degree relative had cancer diagnosed at or after age 50, the cumulative breast cancer risk by age 80 is approximately 10%, not significantly different than risk for the general population. If a first-degree relative had cancer before age 50, cumulative risk may be as high as 20%. With a history of early onset in two first-degree relatives, the probability that the family is affected by a dominant breast cancer susceptibility gene is substantial, and cumulative cancer risk by age 80 approaches 50%.

Susceptibility genes account for about 5% to 10% of all breast cancers. In addition to family clustering and early age at onset of disease, family history of bilateral or multifocal breast cancer and ovarian cancer suggest inherited cancer predisposition. *BRCA1*, which accounts for about half of all inherited breast cancer, confers a cumulative breast cancer risk of approximately 85% and an ovarian cancer risk of 50%. Women with *BRCA2* mutations face approximately the same risk of breast cancer but a significantly lower (10% to 20%) risk of ovarian cancer. Many members of families affected by breast cancer susceptibility genes have indicated a preference not to be tested. Also, the response to learning about susceptibility is varied. Some women choose to have prophylactic surgery (bilateral mastectomies and/or oophorectomies); others do not. Prophylactic surgery reduces risk by about 90%.

Reproductive History. Generally, there is an inverse relationship between breast cancer risk and parity, but maternal age at the time of first full-term pregnancy may be the most important factor related to reproductive history. In a woman with high parity, whose first birth occurs before the age of 20, the risk of breast cancer is half that of a nulliparous woman and one third that of the woman with one or two births after the age of 30. It has been suggested that childbirth transiently increases risk of breast cancer but reduces risk in later years. Either spontaneous or induced abortion may increase risk slightly, but the association is weak and could be due to reporting bias. Lactation appears to reduce slightly the risk of premenopausal cancer.

Menstrual History. Both late menarche and early natural menopause reduce breast cancer risk. Women who experienced menarche after age 16 have half the risk of those who experienced it earlier. Women in whom menopause occurred before age 45 have half the risk of those in whom menopause occurred after age 55. Women with early surgical menopause seem to be similarly protected.

History of Benign Breast Disease. The relative risk of breast cancer is two- to threefold greater in women who have a history of benign breast disease. Some have estimated higher relative risks and others have questioned whether or not benign breast disease confers any additional risk. Most women with benign breast disease worrisome enough to prompt biopsy have nonproliferative changes and are not at increased risk for eventual breast malignancy. Risk is concentrated among those women who have proliferative changes, especially those with atypical hyperplasia, on biopsy. Women with proliferative disease without atypical hyperplasia account for one in four breast biopsies and have a twofold increase in risk. Those with atypical hyperplasia have a fivefold increase in risk but account for only 1 in 25 biopsies.

History of Previous Malignancy. Approximately 10% of women who survive 10 years after the diagnosis of breast cancer will have a second primary malignancy, usually in the contralateral breast. Increasing popularity of breast-sparing surgery for minimal breast cancer will increase the incidence of second breast cancers; about 10% to 20% of women who choose breast-sparing surgery followed by radiation experience ipsilateral in-breast recurrences during the 10-year period after treatment of the initial tumor. Women with a history of endometrial carcinoma have slightly increased risk of breast cancer.

Diet, Drugs, and Other Factors. Breast cancer incidence varies fivefold among different countries and is positively associated with national dietary intake of fat. Diets high in fat have produced increased rates of mammary tumors in laboratory animals. Data from case-control studies have suggested a positive association, but prospective studies, including a recent overview of studies involving more than 300,000 women and nearly 5,000 cases, have found no evidence of a positive association between dietary fat and breast cancer. Low levels of vitamin A have also been linked to increases in risk. Obesity has been associated with minor increases in risk.

The role of drugs is controversial. Evidence for increased risk after oral contraceptive use is equivocal; risk may be slightly increased (relative risks in the range of 1.1 to 1.2) for younger women and for long-time users. Breast cancer risk from postmenopausal estrogen and combined estrogen-progestin hormone replacement therapy is also uncertain. A recent case-control study found no association, but a 16-year cohort analysis of the Nurses' Health Study found increased relative risk among women currently using hormones (1.32 for estrogen alone and 1.41 for estrogen plus progestin), as compared with postmenopausal women who had never used hor-

mones. Women who were former but not current users had no greater risk than women who never used hormones.

Several studies have demonstrated an association between daily moderate alcohol consumption and modest increase in breast cancer risk.

A study suggesting that women who had undergone breast augmentation had lower cancer risk received substantial media attention. However, the analysis was found to be faulty, and a subsequent analysis showed no difference in risk after breast implants.

NATURAL HISTORY OF BREAST CANCER AND EFFECTIVENESS OF EARLY THERAPY

Little can be said with certainty about the natural history of breast cancer. The few observational studies of untreated invasive breast cancer have shown widely variable tumor doubling times ranging from less than a week to more than 6 months.

Younger women tend to have faster growing tumors than older women. The average time for development of an invasive tumor that can be detected by mammography for women aged 35 to 49 is 15 months. The average time that a tumor is detectable by mammography before a clinical diagnosis is made is thought to be approximately 3 years. Again, however, progression is likely to be faster among younger women.

There is even greater uncertainty about the natural history of noninvasive breast cancer. Dramatic increases in the incidence of ductal carcinoma *in situ* (DCIS) in recent years are attributable to mammographic screening. DCIS incidence rates increased approximately 4% annually during the decade ending in 1983 and approximately 18% annually for the subsequent decade. More than 25,000 new cases of DCIS are now diagnosed among American women each year. Many of these lesions appear to be slow growing, and evidence suggests that 50% or more of untreated women with DCIS would not develop invasive disease.

Therapy for early-stage breast cancer is highly effective (see Chapter 122). DCIS does not affect survival during the first 1 to 9 years after diagnosis and treatment. Women with small invasive cancers (e.g., 1 cm) and negative axillary nodes can expect a disease-free survival of 90% to 95% during the 5 to 10 years after either mastectomy or breast-conserving surgery followed by radiation. Cumulative recurrence risk rises sharply with increase in tumor size and/or metastasis to axillary lymph nodes.

Attention to breast cancer screening has dramatically increased the proportion of breast cancers that are in earlier stages of development at the time of diagnosis. Alone, this stage shift is inadequate evidence for screening benefit (see Chapter 3). But breast cancer screening, particularly mammographic screening, has been shown to decrease breast cancer morbidity and mortality for some women. Controversy remains about which women should be screened and how often.

SCREENING METHODS

Mammography

Mammography has become the cornerstone of breast cancer screening programs. Clinical trials have demonstrated that screening mammography can reduce breast cancer mortality by 25% to 30% for women aged 50 years or older. These same trials have reported no statistically significant reduction in breast cancer mortality in women aged 40 to 49 after 7 to 10 years of follow-up. The few studies that have longer follow-up for women in this age group do show a nonsignificant trend toward mortality reduction. An overview of nine randomized trials and four case-control studies estimated the relative risk for breast cancer mortality for women aged 50 to 74 to be 0.74 (95% confidence interval, 0.66 to 0.83). For women aged 40 to 49, the relative risk estimate was 0.93, but the 95% confidence interval (0.76 to 1.13) included 1.

The sensitivity of initial screening mammography increases with age as fat replaces more dense and radiopaque breast tissue. After age 50, the sensitivity approaches 95%. For women aged 30 to 39 and 40 to 49, sensitivity is approximately 75% and 85%, respectively. Specificity is approximately 95% and does not vary significantly with age. However, false-positive results, including interpretations that request follow-up examination of some kind, are not at all uncommon and are a source of considerable anxiety. In one large retrospective cohort study, false-positive results, defined broadly, occurred in 6.5% of mammograms; cumulative incidence after 10 mammograms was estimated to be 50%. Cumulative incidence of false-positive mammograms leading to biopsy approached 20%.

It is important to note that as many as 50% of breast cancers detected after abnormal mammography in women under age 50 are DCIS; in older women, DCIS accounts for only one in five cancers detected by mammography.

Physical Examination

A physical examination by the patient's clinician can detect cancers that are not detected by mammography. Much of the benefit evident in the Health Insurance Plan study was derived from the physical examination rather than from mammography; only 44% of cancers in women aged 50 to 59 and 19% of those in women aged 40 to 49 were found on mammography alone. In the younger age group, 58% of cancers were found by physical examination alone. In the Canadian trial, in which women aged 50 to 59 were randomized to clinical examination and mammography or clinical examination alone, clinical examination alone was as effective as the combination. However, in a recent meta-analysis of trials and case-control studies, no difference was found in mortality reduction between studies that offered both examination and mammography and those that offered mammography alone. Nevertheless, physical examination and mammography should be viewed as complementary procedures; a substantial proportion of cancers, particularly among younger women, will be missed by physicians who rely too heavily on mammography and thereby neglect careful systematic inspection and palpation of the breasts.

Breast Self-Examination

Breast self-examination has both supporters and detractors. Surveys have disclosed that many women perform breast self-examination but that most do not perform the procedure monthly and do not spend sufficient time to do it correctly. Age, education, marital status, having been instructed by a health professional, regular professional breast examinations, and a family history of breast cancer have all been shown to influence breast self-examination behavior.

Some question the effectiveness of self-examination in the early detection of disease and point to the psychological morbidity related to the fear, dread, and burden of responsibility that self-examination engenders in some women. All agree that effectiveness depends on breast size, shape, and the density of breast tissue. Small or poorly supported pendulous breasts are most suitable. Examination of large well-supported breasts is difficult for both patients and physicians. Repeated episodes of brief instruction have been shown to be highly effective in increasing self-examination proficiency and frequency. Seven to 10 days after menses is the best time for premenopausal women who choose to practice self-examination; postmenopausal women can pick a regular calendar date, such as the first of each month.

PATIENT EDUCATION

Many women are frightened by what they learn about breast cancer from the popular media. This is especially true for women with a family history of breast cancer, whose fears may have been heightened by the identification of breast cancer susceptibility genes. With regard to screening and prevention, fear is more an obstacle than a motivator for many patients. The primary care provider now has greater responsibility to provide accurate information about genetic predisposition and other risk factors.

One reason that breast cancer fears may be exaggerated is frequent reference to lifetime cumulative incidence rates such as the often-cited one in eight or one in nine figures for the general population. Often, younger women do not appreciate the effect of age on breast cancer incidence and dramatically overestimate their chances of being diagnosed or dying of breast cancer in the near future. For example, a 30-year-old woman may have a 12% chance of developing breast cancer during the remainder of her lifetime, but the probability that she will develop cancer in the next 10 years is less than 5 in 1,000 and the probability that she will die of breast cancer in the same period is 1 in 1,000. For a 40-year-old woman, the comparable 10-year incidence and mortality figures are 15 in 1,000 and 2 in 1,000, respectively.

The debate about which women should receive routine mammography can best be summarized for patients by asking them to consider the likely outcomes of initial screening mammograms for women younger than 50 years and those 50 and older, as presented in Table 106.1.

Table 106.1. Estimated Outcomes of First-Screening Mammography Stratified by Age

	≤ 50 YEARS OLD	≥ 50 YEARS OLD
No. women screened	1,000	1,000
No. abnormal reports	53	71
No. diagnostic procedures	102	132
No. biopsies	13	25
No. invasive cancers	1	7.5
No. dectal carcinoma *in situ*	1	2.5

Modified from Kerlikowske K, Grady D, Barclay J, et al. Positive predictive value of screening mammography by age and family history of breast cancer. JAMA, 1993;270:2444-2450, with permission.

Alternatively, the discussion can focus on the mortality reduction benefits of mammography. For example, the probability of dying in the next 15 to 20 years of breast cancer that develops in the next 10 years is reduced approximately from 0.8% to 0.7% for the 40-year-old woman, from 1.3% to 1.1% for the 50-year-old woman, from 2.0% to 1.4% for the 60-year-old woman, and from 2.5% to 1.7% for the woman who is 70 years or older.

CONCLUSIONS AND RECOMMENDATIONS

- Breast cancer is common. Although risk factors allow identification of subgroups at particularly high risk, women without risk factors are nonetheless at substantial risk and should be educated about breast cancer and the benefits and harms of screening.
- Testing and counseling related to breast cancer susceptibility genes and family history must be conducted with utmost care. The implications of inherited breast cancer, including limitations of available prevention strategies, should be discussed before referral for testing.
- Breast cancer mortality is reduced 25% to 30% by mammographic screening among women aged 50 to 74; regular mammograms should be performed in this age group at 1- to 2-year intervals.
- Among women younger than 50 years, a modest benefit (approximately 10% mortality reduction) seems likely based on trial results, but mammography has not been proven to be beneficial. Furthermore, younger women face a higher likelihood of mammographic detection of DCIS and the subsequent difficult therapeutic decisions leading to potentially unnecessary surgery. Women in this age group should be engaged in a dialogue about their wishes regarding mammography. Ideally, this should include quantitative estimates of the benefits and harms of screening. When regular mammography is performed for women younger than 50 years, a shorter screening interval (e.g., every year) may be more appropriate.

A.G.M.

ANNOTATED BIBLIOGRAPHY

Alexander FE, Anderson TJ, et al. Fourteen years of follow-up from the Edinburgh randomised trial of breast-cancer screening. Lancet 1999;353:1903. *(13% reduction in breast cancer mortality increased to 21% after adjustment for demographics. No benefit for women whose cancers were diagnosed before age 50.)*

Bains CJ, To T. Changes in breast self-examination behavior achieved by 89,835 participants in the Canadian National Breast Screening Study. Cancer 1990;66:570. *(Competence and frequency of breast self-examination increased dramatically after brief episodes of instruction.)*

Bryant H, Brasher P. Breast implants and breast cancer. N Engl J Med 1995;332:1536. *(The incidence of breast cancer is no different after breast augmentation.)*

Burman ML, Taplin SH, Herta DF, et al. Interval breast cancer screening in a health maintenance organization. Ann Intern Med 1999;131:1. *(False-positive results did not decrease adherence to subsequent mammogram at recommended interval.)*

Chu KC, Smart CR, Tarone RE. Analysis of breast cancer mortality and stage distribution by age for the Health Insurance Plan clinical trial. J Natl Cancer Inst 1988;80:1125. *(Analysis of late follow-up of the Health Insurance Plan study that finds evidence to support screening women in their forties.)*

Collins FS. *BRCA1*—lots of mutations, lots of dilemmas. N Engl J Med 1996;334:186. *(Summary of prevalence of BRCA1 mutations in young women with breast cancer.)*

Elmore JG, Barton MB, Moceri VM, et al. Ten-year risk of false-positive screening mammograms and clinical breast examinations. N Engl J Med 1998;338:1089. *(Retrospective cohort study suggests cumulative risk for false-positive result for women who undergo 10 mammograms is 50% or more; risk for biopsy after 10 mammograms approximates 20%.)*

Ernster VL, Barclay J, Kerlikowske K, et al. Incidence of and treatment for ductal carcinoma in situ of the breast. JAMA 1996; 275:913. *(Mammography has produced an "epidemic" of DCIS; treatment patterns may vary substantially in different geographic regions.)*

Feig SA. Strategies for improving sensitivity of screening mammography for women aged 40 to 49 years. JAMA 1996;276:73. *(Addresses the questions about what to do about the 35,000 American women each year in this age group who are diagnosed with breast cancer.)*

FitzGerald MG, MacDonald DJ, Krainer M et al. Germ-line BRCA1 mutations in Jewish and non-Jewish women with early-onset breast cancer. N Engl J Med 1996;334:143. *(The specific BRCA1 mutation 185delAG is strongly associated with breast cancer before age 40 in Jewish women.)*

Gammon MD, Bertin JE, Terry MB. Abortion and the risk of breast cancer. JAMA 1996;275:321. *(Discusses potential for ascertainment bias as explanation for occasional association.)*

Garber JE, Schrag D. Testing for inherited cancer susceptibility. JAMA 1996;275:1928. *(Cites the challenges associated with identifying and counseling patients with cancer susceptibility genes.)*

Harris R, Leininger L. Clinical strategies for breast cancer screening: Weighing and using the evidence. Ann Intern Med 1995;122:539. *(Describes a practical patient-centered approach to presenting the benefits and harms of screening mammography.)*

Hartmann LC, Schaid DJ, Woods JE, et al. Efficacy of bilateral prophylactic mastectomy in women with a family history of breast cancer. N Engl J Med 1999;340:77. *(Bilateral prophylactic mastectomy reduces cancer risk by 90%.)*

Hoskins KF, Stopfer JE, Calzone KA, et al. Assessment and counseling for women with a family history of breast cancer. JAMA 1995;273:577. *(Detailed discussion of practical approach to risk assessment and counseling.)*

Hunter DJ, Spiegelman D, Adami H, et al. Cohort studies of fat intake and the risk of breast cancer—a pooled analysis. N Engl J Med 1996;334:356. *(A meta-analysis of seven studies finding no association between total dietary fat intake and breast cancer.)*

Kelsey JL. Lactation and the risk of breast cancer. N Engl J Med 1994;330:136. *(Editorial discusses implications of modest reduction in risk.)*

Kerlikowske K, Grady D, Barclay J, et al. Positive predictive value of screening mammography by age and family history of breast cancer. JAMA 1993;270:2444. *(After mammography, women 15 and older undergo about 15 diagnostic procedures for each cancer detected; women younger than 50 undergo 50 procedures for each cancer detected.)*

Kerlikowske K, Grady D, Barclay J, et al. Effect of age, breast density, and family history on the sensitivity of first screening mammography. JAMA 1996;276:33. *(Sensitivity is lower in younger women and particularly low with longer screening intervals.)*

Kerlikowske K, Grady D, Barclay J, et al . Likelihood ratios for modern screening mammography. JAMA 1996;276:39. *(Estimates likelihood ratios for different mammographic interpretations.)*

Kerlikowske K, Grady D, Rubin SM, et al. Efficacy of screening mammography. JAMA 1995;273:149. *(Meta-analysis combining results of 13 studies with conclusion that screening mammography may be effective in reducing mortality in women age 40 to 49 after 10 to 12 years, but that the same benefit could likely be achieved by starting at age 50.)*

Lambe M, Hsieh C, Trichopoulos D, et al. Transient increase in the risk of breast cancer after giving birth. N Engl J Med 1994;331:5. *(Evidence to support the hypothesis that pregnancy has a dual cancer risk: increasing it in the short-term, then decreasing risk.)*

Langston, AA, Malone KE, Thompson JD, et al. BRCA1 mutations in a population-based sample of young women with breast cancer. N Engl J Med 1996;334:137. *(BRCA1 mutations were found in 10% of women with breast cancer onset before age 35.)*

Lerman C, Narod S, Schulman K, et al. BRCA1 testing in families with hereditary breast-ovarian cancer. JAMA 1996;275:1885. *(Among family members affected by BRCA1-linked hereditary breast-ovarian cancer, 40% did not want to be tested.)*

Lerman C, Trock B, Rimer BK, Boyce A, et al. Psychological and behavioral implications of abnormal mammograms. Ann Intern Med 1991;114:657. *(Documents threefold greater prevalence of mood affected by worry among women who had an abnormal mammogram 3 months earlier.)*

Lindfors KK, Rosenquist J. The cost-effectiveness of mammographic screening strategies. JAMA 1995;274:881. *(A Markov model analysis suggesting that annual mammography for ages 40 to 49 and biennial mammography for ages 50 to 79 is more cost effective than annual mammography for the older age group.)*

Miller AB, Baines CJ, To T, et al. Canadian National Breast Screening Study. 1. Breast cancer detection and death rates among women aged 40 to 49 years. Can Med Assoc J. 1992;147:1459. *(After 7 years of follow-up among women age 40 to 49, the risk for dying of breast cancer was higher among the women randomized to the screening intervention, which included annual physical examination and mammography.)*

Miller AB, Baines CJ, To T, et al. Canadian National Breast Screening Study. 2. Breast cancer detection and death rates among women aged 50 to 59 years. Can Med Assoc J 1992;147:1477. *(Clinical examination alone performed as well as clinical examination and mammography.)*

National Institutes of Health Consensus Development Panel. Breast cancer screening for women ages 40–49, January 21–23, 1997. J Natl Cancer Inst 1997;336:1243. *(Conclusion that the available evidence did not support a universal recommendation for mammography for all women in their forties proved highly controversial.)*

Newcomb PA, Storer BE, Longnecker MP, et al. Lactation and reduced risk of premenopausal breast cancer. N Engl J Med 1994;330:81. *(A reduction in risk of approximately 20% is restricted to premenopausal women.)*

Newcomb PA, Storer BE, Longnecker MP, et al. Pregnancy termination in relation to risk of breast cancer. JAMA 1996;275:283. *(A relative risk of 1.12 is reported.)*

Page DL, Jensen RA. Ductal carcinoma in situ of the breast. JAMA 1996;275:948. *(Describes the current treatment options and lack of evidence for an informed choice.)*

Shapiro S, Goldberg JD, Hutchinson GB. Lead time in breast cancer detection and implications for periodicity of screening. Am J Epidemiol 1974;100:357. *(Average duration of preclinical disease previously estimated to be 20 months. Lead time estimated to be 19 months at the initial examination and 11 to 13 months at subsequent screenings.)*

Shattuck-Eidens D, McClure M, Simard J, et al. A collaborative survey of 80 mutations in the BRCA1 breast and ovarian cancer susceptibility gene. JAMA 1995;273:535. *(Reports on BRCA1 testing from nine laboratories.)*

Sox H. Screening mammography in women younger than 50 years of age. Ann Intern Med 1995:122:550. *(A clear articulation of a clinical approach for the primary care provider.)*

Taber L, Fagerberg G, Duffy SW, et al. Update of the Swedish Two-County Program of mammographic screening for breast cancer. Radiol Clin North Am 1992;30:187. *(After 11 years of follow-up, no detectable benefit of screening for women in their forties.)*

Weber B. Breast cancer susceptibility genes: current challenges and future promises. Ann Intern Med 1996;124:1088. *(Editorial that provides estimates of the probability of BRCA1 mutation based on family history.)*

107

Screening for Cervical Cancer

In the United States, the annual incidence of invasive cervical cancer exceeds 15,000 cases and annual mortality is approximately 5,000. For an American woman, the lifetime probability of developing invasive cervical cancer is about 0.7%. The incidence of carcinoma in situ is more than three times that of invasive disease. There is a very long asymptomatic period during which cytologic detection of cervical neoplasia is possible. Early therapy is often curative. Appropriately, the Papanicolaou (Pap) smear is one of the most widely used cancer screening tests.

EPIDEMIOLOGY AND RISK FACTORS

Age and sexual activity are the principal risk factors for cervical cancer. The age-specific prevalence rates for carcinoma in situ follow a bimodal distribution with the dominant first peak of about 6 per 1,000 women occurring in the 30-to-45 age group. A second peak of about 5 per 1,000 occurs among women older than age 60. The highest carcinoma *in situ* incidence rates are in the 25-to-29 age group. The prevalence of invasive carcinoma is highest in older age groups, rising precipitously after age 50. A breakdown in host barriers at the time of menopause has been proposed as an explanation for the decreased *in situ* and increased invasive prevalence rates observed in these patients.

Many factors have been associated with cervical neoplasia. Most are related to sexual activity. First intercourse at a *young age* (i.e., before age 18) and *multiple sexual partners* (four or more) are the factors most consistently associated with high risk. Increasing parity, poor personal hygiene, a history of venereal disease, an uncircumcised partner, and a high number of sexual partners of the husband or regular sexual partner have also been linked to cervical cancer. The extremely low risk of cervical neoplasia in women who have never had intercourse and the consistent association with variables that define sexual exposure has sparked several hypotheses about cervical cancer as a venereal disease. An association between herpes simplex type 2 virus and cervical cancer has been described, but more recent findings do not suggest a causal link. The strongest evidence points to *human papillomavirus* (HPV), particularly types 16 and 18, as potential venereally transmitted oncogenic agents. It is now thought that the combination of exposure to such agents and the presence of susceptible cervical epithelium leads to cervical neoplasia. Observations that normal immature squamous epithelium in the transformation zone of the cervix is particularly sensitive to viral infections may explain some of the long-observed epidemiologic correlates of cervical cancer. Immature squamous cells are present in the developing transformation zone after menarche and during remodeling of the transformation zone after pregnancy. Women who are sexually active early in life and who have multiple pregnancies may be more likely to come in contact with oncogenic agents when their cervical epithelium is susceptible to infection. This theory would also explain the two- to fourfold increase in risk of dysplasia and carcinoma *in situ* in women exposed *in utero* to diethylstilbestrol. Persistent susceptibility to oncogenic agents may stem from immature metaplastic squamous cells that arise in the areas of cervical and vaginal adenosis frequently found in women exposed to diethylstilbestrol (see Chapter 110).

Other factors have been associated with cervical neoplasia, but it is difficult to control for sexual exposure. The incidence of cervical cancer is decreased in Jewish women and increased in African-Americans, native Americans, and Hispanics. *Socioeconomic status* may be the most important predictor, inasmuch as the racial and ethnic disparities are reduced or eliminated when socioeconomic factors are controlled. Smoking has been identified as a potentially important independent risk factor for cervical cancer in a number of studies that controlled for both sexual activity and socioeconomic status. Although the issue remains controversial, the weight of current evidence supports the association. One theory holds that smoking may make women more susceptible to the oncogenic effects of viruses. Evidence suggests that use of oral contraceptives confers a modest increase in cervical cancer risk. Women infected with HIV are at increased risk of HPV infection, and the prevalence of cervical dysplasia ranges from 10% to 60% depending on the severity of immunosuppression.

The most compelling risk information comes from the Pap smear itself, in that the risk of carcinoma is 100 times greater in women with dysplasia than in those with a normal cervix.

NATURAL HISTORY OF CERVICAL CANCER AND EFFECTIVENESS OF THERAPY

Cervical cancer classically presents with *intermenstrual bleeding* prompted by coitus or douching. Symptoms invariably occur late in the course of the disease. Epidemiologic evidence indicates that the natural history of cervical neoplasia should be viewed as a progression from mild dysplasia, through carcinoma *in situ*, to invasive carcinoma. Only some mildly dysplastic lesions progress to carcinoma. It is not clear that carcinoma *in situ* invariably becomes invasive, but epidemiologic data suggest that progression occurs in most cases. Both of these premalignant lesions, which are referred to together as cervical intraepithelial neoplasia, are reliably detected by cytologic techniques.

The mean duration of the detectable asymptomatic period, as estimated from incidence and prevalence rates, is very long. The mean duration of carcinoma *in situ* varies with age but averages about 10 years. The duration of asymptomatic invasive carcinoma is 5 years for all age groups. It should be emphasized that these are estimated means; the proportion of cervical cancers that become invasive early in their development is not known.

There is no doubt that the earlier the clinical stage of the tumor when detected and treated the better the prognosis. Survival for carcinoma *in situ* treated with hysterectomy is essentially 100%. However, the uncertainty about the natural course of carcinoma *in situ* must be kept in mind. Relative 5-year survival rates for localized and regional invasive carcinoma are about 80% and 40%, respectively. The 5-year experience of one screening program demonstrated that 86% of cases detected by cytologic screening were limited to regional invasion, whereas only 44% of those presenting symptomatically were in this early stage.

SCREENING METHODS AND DIAGNOSTIC TESTS

There are three techniques of cell collection for Pap staining and cytologic screening of the cervix. The easiest and least effective is aspiration from the vaginal pool. More sensitive, but requiring visualization of the cervix with a vaginal speculum, are *endocervical swabbing and cervical scraping*. The sensitivity of the vaginal aspirate technique has been reported in a range from 62% to 92% in the presence of invasive carcinoma and from 31% to 70% in the presence of carcinoma *in situ*. The range of reported sensitivities for swabbing is 82% to 92% and that for scraping, 86% to 100%. There is no consistent difference in detection rates between invasive carcinoma and carcinoma *in situ* with the swabbing and scraping techniques. Current recommendations suggest that two cell smears should be taken for each test: one from the endocervical canal, with either a saline-moistened cotton swab or a cytologic brush designed specifically for the purpose, and one scraped with a spatula from the os of the cervix, which contains the squamous-columnar junction or transformation zone. Smears should be interpreted by an experienced cytopathologist. Use of the endocervical brush is more likely to collect endocervical cells than use of a cotton swab, but it is not known whether this increases the detection rate for abnormal smears or affects clinical outcomes.

Recent reports indicate that sensitivity in actual practice may be substantially lower because of poor cell collection technique or faulty interpretation. To roughly estimate the practical false-negative rate resulting from the combination of these potential errors, investigators have defined a smear as falsely negative if a woman subsequently developed a confirmed lesion within a defined follow-up period. In one such study, 17% of women developed such lesions within 2 years of a negative smear. These findings have prompted recommendations that the screening interval should be kept short between the first and second smear for women regularly screened. There have also been developments in automated interpretation of smears, both to enrich samples for rescreening and as a strategy to improve the efficiency of screening without a loss in sensitivity.

The *specificity* of cytologic diagnosis is very high. In a 2-year period, 151 of 25,000 cytologic examinations of the cervix performed at the Massachusetts General Hospital were read as positive. Eighty percent of these women had cervical cancer. Clearly, more than 99% without disease had negative smears. This high specificity limits the costs associated with false-positive results.

The *frequency* of cervical cancer screening has been controversial. Because of the usually long duration of the asymptomatic detectable period of cervical intraepithelial neoplasia, which is easily controlled and cured when detected, the American Cancer Society and others have moved away from earlier recommendations of annual Pap smears. Generally, smears are now recommended every 3 years after two successive negative smears 1 year apart at ages 20 and 21 or younger if the patient is sexually active. The purpose of the short first interval is to improve sensitivity of the first screening effort. Though women who are at high risk because of early age at first intercourse, multiple sexual partners, or other risk factors may be tested more frequently, the clinician should be mindful that the decision about test frequency depends more on the duration of the asymptomatic detectable disease rather than a woman's individual risk.

Some recommendations for more frequent screening among young women reflect concern about evidence that a greater proportion of carcinoma *in situ* among younger women may be rapidly progressive. For example, in 1982 the Canadian Task Force recommended that women who have had sexual intercourse should be screened annually between ages 18 and 35. Pap smears every 5 years are recommended for women ages 35 to 60. Screening is not recommended for women who have never had intercourse. Subsequent findings, however, do not support the hypothesis that there is an increased frequency of lesions that move rapidly from carcinoma *in situ* to invasion.

Screening is recommended until age 65. Screening after age 65 is not cost effective in women who have been undergoing regular screening and have had normal smears. However, those who have not been screened previously should be (cervical cancer screening is now a Medicare benefit).

Cytologic smears are not read as simply positive or negative. The original Papanicolaou system included five classes ranging from normal (class I) to suggestive of invasive cancer (class V). Subsequently, a World Health Organization committee recommended classifying specimens as "normal," "atypical," "dysplasia" (mild, moderate, or severe), "carcinoma *in situ*," "invasive cervical cancer," and "adenocarcinoma." In 1988, a committee of the National Cancer Institute recommended the Bethesda System, which replaces the older class II "atypical" category with the designation "reactive and reparative change." This term is used to describe cellular changes in response to inflammation and other nonneoplastic processes. The Bethesda System also introduced the term "squamous intraepithelial lesion," which includes two grades. Low-grade squamous intraepithelial lesions are consistent with HPV infection and mild dysplasia and correspond to the old class III mild dysplasia category. High-grade lesions include the moderate and severe dysplasia and carcinoma *in situ* designations. Women whose smears show high-grade squamous intraepithelial lesions (i.e., moderate to severe dysplasia) or carcinoma *in situ a*nd those with smears suggestive of invasive cancer

should be referred to a gynecologist experienced in the use of the colposcope. Colposcopic examination will allow the gynecologist to select sites for biopsy and determine the limits of the lesion. This will allow informed choice between conservative measures such as electrocautery and cryotherapy, which are used increasingly frequently, and more traditional measures such as conization and hysterectomy. Such decisions will be based not only on the size, location, and histology of the lesion but also on the patient's age, parity, and reliability for follow-up.

Because of the association between HPV infection and cervical cancer, some have advocated HPV testing as primary screening for cervical cancer. However, there is wide variation in prevalence rates of HPV positivity in different populations. Among younger women, where reactivity is often transient, it appears to be more a marker for sexual activity than for cancer risk. Among older less sexually active women, the persistence of HPV is an indication of increased risk. Results of screening studies, most of which have been conducted among high-risk women, have been mixed. Current evidence does not support HPV testing for primary screening.

CONCLUSIONS AND RECOMMENDATIONS

- The high prevalence, long mean duration of asymptomatic detectable disease, and availability of a highly specific screening test make cervical cancer screening an important task for all primary care providers.
- Known risk factors, including early sexual activity and high number of sexual partners, allow selection of high-risk patients and populations.
- Because of the long duration of preinvasive detectable disease in women of reproductive age, annual screening in the absence of specific risk factors may be unnecessary. Two screens with a short interval (e.g., 1 year) may be used to reduce the number of false-negative prevalence cases. The interval between subsequent screens can be lengthened for low-risk individuals. The presence of a risk factor, particularly in the menopausal or postmenopausal patient, may be an indication for more frequent (i.e., yearly) screening.
- Annual Pap smears after two negative smears 6 months apart is the recommended strategy for women who are infected with HIV. However, benefits for women with only 1 to 2 years of life expectancy due to late-stage HIV infection are modest.
- A cytologic smear positive for cancer or a high-grade squamous intraepithelial lesion is an indication for referral to a gynecologist for further evaluation, including appropriate biopsies.
- A smear suggestive of reactive or reparative changes or mild dysplasia can be further evaluated by the nongynecologist. If a concurrent infection is evident, the smear should be repeated after specific treatment of the infection. If no infection is present, the smear may be repeated after a 3- to 6-month interval. Women with repeatedly abnormal smears should be referred for colposcopy or biopsy.
- Screening can cease after age 65 in women with a history of regularly obtained negative smears but should be performed if not done regularly before age 65 or if smear has been abnormal.

A.G.M.

ANNOTATED BIBLIOGRAPHY

Brinton LA, Fraumeni FJ Jr. Epidemiology of uterine cervical cancer. J Chronic Dis 1986;39:1051. (*Good review of epidemiology and risk factors.*)

Canadian Task Force on Cervical Cancer Screening Programs. Cervical cancer screening programs: summary of the 1982 Canadian Task Force report. Can Med Assoc J 1982;127:581. (*Recommendations for more frequent screening among younger women.*)

Crum CP, Ikenberg H, Richart RM, et al. Human papillomavirus type 16 in early cervical neoplasia. N Engl J Med 1984;310:880. (*HPV 16 virus was isolated from condylomata of the uterine cervix that contained abnormal mitotic figures and appeared to be precursors of invasive cancer of the cervix.*)

Cuzick J, Szarewski A, Terry G, et al. Human papilloma virus testing in primary cervical screening. Lancet 1995;345:1533. (*Predictive value positive 42% in this study.*)

Devesa SS. Descriptive epidemiology of cancer of the uterine cervix. Obstet Gynecol 1984;63:605. (*Documents a decline in cervical cancer mortality in all age groups accompanied by a sharp rise in incidence of diagnosis of carcinoma in situ.*)

Eddy DM. Screening for cervical cancer. Ann Intern Med 1990;113:214. (*An excellent review of the literature and in-depth analysis that provides estimates of the benefits and harms of alternative screening strategies.*)

Fahs MC, Mandelblatt J, Schecter C, et al. Cost-effectiveness of cervical cancer screening for the elderly. Ann Intern Med 1992;117:520. (*Not cost effective after age 65 if done regularly before 65 and normal smears found.*)

Goldie SJ, Weinstein MC, Kuntz KM, et al. The costs, clinical benefits, and cost-effectiveness of screening for cervical cancer in HIV-infected women. Ann Intern Med 1999;130:97. (*This analysis confirms the reasonableness of the Centers for Disease Control and Prevention recommendation for annual screening after two negative screens 6 months apart.*)

International Agency for Research on Cancer Working Group on Evaluation of Cervical Cancer Screening Programmes. Screening for squamous cervical cancer: duration of low risk after negative results of cervical cytology and its implications for screening policies. BMJ 1986;293:659. (*Documents diminishing returns when screening interval is reduced below 3 years.*)

Kashgarian M, Dunn JE. The duration of intraepithelial and preclinical squamous cell carcinoma of the uterine cervix. Am J Epidemiol 1970;92:211. (*Detailed analysis of incidence and prevalence data from Memphis study providing estimates of preclinical duration of disease.*)

Massachusetts Department of Public Health. Papanicolaou testing—are we screening the wrong women? N Engl J Med 1976;294:223. (*Points out high frequency of screening of young women with low risk.*)

Miller AB. The cost-effectiveness of cervical cancer screening. Ann Intern Med 1992;117:529. (*An editorial supporting cessation of Pap testing after age 65 in women previously tested on a regular basis.*)

Mitchell H, Drake M, Medley G. Prospective evaluation of risk of cervical cancer after cytological evidence of human papilloma virus infection. Lancet 1986;1:573. (*Among 846 women with cytologic evidence of HPV infection followed for 6 years, 30 developed carcinoma in situ, leading to a 15.6 estimate of the relative risk.*)

National Institutes of Health. Consensus Development Conference. Statement on cervical cancer. Gynecol Oncol 1997;66:351. (*Authoritative consensus statement includes observation that half of American women with newly diagnosed invasive cervical cancer have never had a Pap smear.*)

Spitzer M. Cervical screening adjuncts: recent advances. Am J Obstet Gynecol 1998;179:544. (*Comprehensive review of automated screening devices and HPV screening and newer approaches to visualization of the cervix.*)

Trevathan E, Layde P, Webster LA. Cigarette smoking and dysplasia and carcinoma in situ of the uterine cervix. JAMA 1983;250:499. (*A case-control study suggesting substantially increased risk of cervical cancer among young women who smoke cigarettes.*)

Van der Graaf Y, Vooijs GP. False negative rate in cervical cytology. J Clin Pathol 1987;40:438. (*Among women followed for 2 years after negative smears, 17% developed significant lesions.*)

108
Screening for Ovarian Cancer

Ovarian cancer is less common than breast cancer and other gynecologic malignancies; the lifetime probability is approximately 1 in 70. However, it has a high case fatality rate. Each year in the United States, more than 20,000 new cases are diagnosed and more than 12,000 women die from the disease. Ovarian cancer deaths among prominent public figures, the recent availability of new diagnostic tests, and the general trend toward increased interest in disease prevention among women has focused attention on screening for ovarian cancer. The primary care provider needs to understand the epidemiology and risk factors for this disease, as well as the value and limitations of available tests, to respond appropriately to patients' questions and, when appropriate, recommend a screening intervention.

EPIDEMIOLOGY AND RISK FACTORS

Increasing age and family history are risk factors for ovarian cancer. The annual incidence is 20 per 100,000 among women aged 30 to 50 and increases to 40 per 100,000 among women aged 50 to 75. The incidence among older women is even higher when one restricts the denominator to women who have not had their ovaries surgically removed.

A family history of ovarian cancer is present in about 10% of women with the disease. Most of these women have a family history of sporadic ovarian cancer. Some of these women are members of families with inherited predisposition to cancer, including those with *BRCA1* and *BRCA2* mutations. For some subsets of patients with inherited predisposition, cumulative lifetime risk of ovarian cancer may be as high as 85%. But for most women with *BRCA1 mutation*, the cumulative risk by age 70 years is closer to 25%. For women with *BRCA2 mutation*, the cumulative risk is lower—approximately 10% by age 70 years.

A family history of the more common sporadic ovarian cancer also confers risk. The best estimate is that ovarian cancer in one first- or second-degree relative increases risk threefold. When two relatives have had the disease, risk is increased fivefold.

Use of the oral contraceptive pill and parity are associated with reduced risk of ovarian cancer in unselected women. Any use of oral contraceptives appears to reduce risk by 35%, and use for 5 or more years by 50%. A recent case-control study indicates similar protection afforded to women with known mutations in either the *BRCA1* or *BRCA2* gene. Any pregnancy reduces risk by about 50%; increasing number of pregnancies is associated with decreasing risk. Other factors, including age at first pregnancy, infertility, menstrual history, hormone replacement therapy, and dietary factors, may modify risk of ovarian cancer, but evidence is inconclusive. Tubal ligation and possibly hysterectomy appear protective.

NATURAL HISTORY OF OVARIAN CANCER AND EFFECTIVENESS OF THERAPY

Mortality rates for ovarian cancer have changed little over the past three decades. When ovarian cancer is diagnosed after clinical presentation with signs or symptoms, three of four cases have already spread beyond the ovary. Under these circumstances, the 5-year survival rate is less than 20%. In contrast, 5-year survival rates of patients with tumor confined to the ovary has been greater than 70% in older studies and greater than 90% in recent case series. It is not surprising that there is great enthusiasm for using newer diagnostic modalities to advance the time of diagnosis and thereby reduce the burden of morbidity and mortality associated with ovarian cancer. It must be remembered, however, that we know little about the preclinical course of ovarian cancer, including variability in its biologic behavior. Any current estimates of screening benefit will be confounded by lead time and time-linked sampling biases. Until randomized trials of screening demonstrate reduction in population mortality rates, estimates of the benefits of screening will remain tentative.

DIAGNOSTIC TESTS

There has been little formal evaluation of the pelvic examination as a screening test for ovarian cancer among asymptomatic women. Evaluations that have been conducted comparing the physical examination with other diagnostic modalities have produced mixed results. In two studies, pelvic examination failed to detect three stage I tumors that were detected by transvaginal or abdominal ultrasound. However, in other studies, pelvic examination was able to detect early tumors. There is a general consensus that pelvic examination alone is insufficiently sensitive to be of value as a screening test.

Although early use of ultrasonography to diagnose ovarian cancer used the transabdominal approach, more recent work has focused on *transvaginal ultrasonography,* with the addition of color-flow Doppler techniques to improve specificity. The sensitivity of ultrasound has been estimated in studies of women with known ovarian cancer and in screening studies. In the former case, estimates of sensitivity range from 80% to 100%. Estimates are higher in the screening studies, but this may reflect failure to diagnose cancer among screened-negative study subjects. Estimates of specificity derived from screening studies range from about 75% to 97%. A recent analytic review provided summary estimates of sensitivity and specificity of 83% and 93%, respectively. Some studies have shown improvements in specificity of transvaginal ultrasound with addition of color-flow Doppler techniques, which can detect tumor neovascularization. Ultrasound is a safe diagnostic modality. Interpretations can be highly variable and depend on the skill of the operator. Timing the study to avoid ovulation may improve specificity. Cost, personnel, and patient inconvenience limit its use as a primary screening test. Furthermore, the limited specificity of the test results in low predictive values in the screening situation.

There is a great deal of interest in the use of *CA-125* to screen for ovarian cancer. CA-125 is an antigenic determinant on a glycoprotein that is present in the serum at elevated levels in 80% of women with epithelial ovarian cancers. CA-125 levels are also elevated in late-stage endometrial cancers and in about 60% of pancreatic cancers. Levels may also be elevated in patients with benign ovarian cysts, uterine leiomyoma, pregnancy, endometriosis, and pelvic inflammatory disease. Estimates of sensitivity derived from women with known ovarian cancer, using a reference level of 35 U/mL, range from 61% to 96%. In the screening situation, sensitivity has been estimated at 67% to 100%. However, reported sensitivities for stage I disease have ranged from 25% to 75%. The specificity of CA-125 in large screening studies, with the reference level of 35 U/mL, has been approximately 99%. Specificity is much lower in premenopausal women, because CA-125 levels fluctuate with the menstrual cycle and because of a higher prevalence of the benign gynecologic conditions that are associated with elevated levels.

Given the sensitivity and specificity of CA-125 and the prevalence of ovarian cancer in the population of women older than age 50, the expected positive predictive value of a CA-125 level greater than 35 U/mL in that population would be 3%. If screening were restricted to women with ovarian cancer in one first-degree relative or in two or more relatives, the positive predictive values with the same reference level would be 9% and 15%, respectively. These predictive values indicate that many screened women would have false-positive results that would require invasive diagnostic evaluation, often including laparotomy.

Evidence from a pilot randomized trial combining CA-125 and ultrasound suggests that screening may be possible with a moderate number of negative biopsies. Among nearly 11,000 women screened, 468 had levels of 30 U/mL or higher. Of these, only 29 had ovarian volume estimated 8.8 mL or greater on ultrasonography and were referred for biopsy; 6 had cancers.

CONCLUSIONS AND RECOMMENDATIONS

- Women from families with genetic predisposition to ovarian cancer are at high risk and should be screened annually with CA-125 and ultrasound beginning at approximately age 35. Women known to be *BRCA1* mutation carriers are at higher risk than those with *BRCA2* mutations. Screening beginning at an earlier age (e.g., 25 years) on a semiannual basis may be advisable.

- Women with a family history of sporadic ovarian cancer may benefit from screening with CA-125, but because of the low predictive value and the morbidity associated with further diagnostic evaluation, *routine* screening is not recommended. However, women should be advised of the potential benefits and harms of screening. Similarly, *routine* screening is not recommended for pre- and postmenopausal women without a family history of ovarian cancer.
- Women in their childbearing years should be advised of the ovarian cancer risk reduction afforded by oral contraceptive use. This may be especially important for women with a family history or with known genetic predisposition. Women should be apprised of the potential slight increase in breast cancer risk associated with current use of oral contraceptives, but it is likely that the benefit of ovarian cancer risk reduction outweighs this potential harm.

A. G. M.

ANNOTATED BIBLIOGRAPHY

Andolf E, Jorgensen C, Astedt B. Ultrasound examination for detection of ovarian carcinoma in risk groups. Obstet Gynecol 1990;75:106. *(Pelvic examination did not detect the ovarian cancer detected by ultrasound.)*

Bell R, Pettigrew M, Sheldon T. The performance of screening tests for ovarian cancer: results of a systematic review. Br J Obstet Gynaecol 1998;105:1136. *(Estimates that between 3 and 60 women would undergo surgery for every cancer detected.)*

Bourne TH, Whitehead MI, Campbell S, et al. Ultrasound screening for familial ovarian cancer. Gynecol Oncol 1991;43:92. *(Women with a family history of ovarian cancer have a higher prevalence of benign ovarian abnormalities.)*

Burke W, Daly M, Garber J, et al. Recommendations for follow-up care of individuals with an inherited predisposition to cancer. II. BRCA1 and BRCA2. JAMA 1997;277:997. *(Recommends annual or semiannual screening starting at age 25 to 35.)*

Einhorn N, Sjovall K, Knapp RC, et al. Prospective evaluation of serum CA 125 levels for the early detection of ovarian cancer. Obstet Gynecol 1992;80:14. *(Prospective cohort study of 5,550 women yielding estimates of sensitivity and specificity of 67% to 100% and 99.4%, respectively.)*

Hankinson SE, Colditz GA, Hunter DJ, et al. A quantitative assessment of oral contraceptive use and risk of ovarian cancer. Obstet Gynecol 1992;80:708. *(Relative risk of ovarian cancer among ever-users of oral contraceptives pills was 0.65.)*

Hankinson SE, Hunter DJ, Colditz GA, et al. Tubal ligation, hysterectomy, and risk of ovarian cancer: a prospective study. JAMA 1993;270:2813. *(Tubal ligation and possibly hysterectomy may reduce risk.)*

Hartge P, Schiffman MH, Hoover R, et al. A case-control study of epithelial ovarian cancer. Am J Obstet Gynecol 1989;161:10. *(One of many case-control studies which collectively provide highly variable estimates of relative risks.)*

Jacobs IJ, Skates SJ, MacDonald N, et al. Screening for ovarian cancer: a pilot randomized trial. Lancet 1999;353:1207. *(In this randomized trial including 10,958 screened women, 468 had elevated CA-125 and 29 were referred for biopsy after ultrasound disclosed an enlarged ovary. There were six cancers.)*

Kerlikowske K, Brown JS, Grady DG. Should women with familial ovarian cancer undergo prophylactic oophorectomy? Obstet Gynecol 1992;80:700. *(Weighs the risks and benefits of prophylactic surgery.)*

Koch M, Gaedke H, Jenkins H. Family history of ovarian cancer patients: a case-control study. Int J Epidemiol 1989;18:782. *(One of many case-control studies that collectively provide highly variable estimates of relative risks.)*

Menon UA, Talaat A, Jeyarajah AR, et al. Ultrasound assessment of ovarian cancer risk in postmenopausal women with CA-125 elevation. Br J Cancer 1999;80:1644. *(Among women with elevated CA-125, ultrasound distinguished between those with baseline risk and those with relative risk greater than 300.)*

Narod SA, Risch H, Moslehi R, et al. Oral contraceptives and risk of hereditary ovarian cancer. N Engl J Med 1998;339:424. *(Risk reduced by 50% for those with any past use, 60% for those with six or more years of use.)*

Pittaway DE, Fayez JA. Serum CA-125 antigen levels increase during menses. Am J Obstet Gynecol 1987;156:75. *(Documents cyclic variation which could have a profound effect on sensitivity and specificity among premenopausal women.)*

Schapira MM, Matchar DB, Young MJ. The effectiveness of ovarian cancer screening: a decision analysis model. Ann Intern Med 1993;118:838. *(Found limited effect on life expectancy and not recommended for routine use.)*

Skates SJ, Singer DE. Quantifying the potential benefit of CA 125 screening for ovarian cancer. J Clin Epidemiol 1991;44:365. *(Presents a sophisticated mathematical model for estimating effects of CA-125 screening.)*

Sparks JM, Varner RE. Ovarian cancer screening. Obstet Gynecol 1992;77:787. *(A good summary of the issues.)*

Van Nagell JR, DePriest PD, Puls LE, et al. Ovarian cancer screening in asymptomatic postmenopausal women by transvaginal sonography. Cancer 1991;68:458. *(Reports a sensitivity of 100% including all stage I cancers.)*

109
Screening for Endometrial Cancer

More than 95% of the cancers of the uterine corpus are adenocarcinomas arising from the endometrium. In the United States, endometrial cancer is nearly three times more common than invasive cervical cancer. There are approximately 30,000 cases and 6,000 endometrial cancer deaths among American women each year. The lifetime probability of developing endometrial carcinoma is 3%. Most cases occur in women in whom risk factors are well defined. The tumors often present symptomatically at a time when cure is still possible. Diagnostic tests suitable for indiscriminate screening are not available.

It is the responsibility of the primary care provider to be aware of the risk factors and limitations of diagnostic tests, to elicit the pertinent history, and to respond to worrisome symptoms.

EPIDEMIOLOGY AND RISK FACTORS

Advancing age is an important risk factor for endometrial cancer. Most tumors occur during the sixth and seventh decades; fewer than 5% occur before age 40. The risk is increased among first-degree relatives of patients with endometrial cancer. Epidemiologic studies have also shown an association with cancer of the breast and cancer of the colon. Case-control studies have also demonstrated a surprisingly high prevalence of obesity and glucose intolerance among patients with endometrial cancer. Many studies have documented an association between obesity and endometrial cancer with relative risks ranging as high as 20 in some studies. The wide range depends in part on varying definitions of obesity, but most studies have estimated relative risks above 2.0. Up to 40% of patients with endometrial cancer in some studies have diabetes mellitus, but the strength of this association independent of obesity is unclear.

There is strong evidence that *estrogens*, either endogenous or exogenous, play a principal role in the etiology of endometrial carcinoma. The histologic precursor of endometrial cancer is atypical endometrial hyperplasia. Retrospective studies have indicated a progression from cystic hyperplasia through adenomatous hyperplasia to atypical hyperplasia, associated with unopposed estrogen effects. Prospective studies have demonstrated a cumulative incidence of carcinoma of 10% to 30% among patients with atypical endometrial hyperplasia.

A number of clinical syndromes that include ovarian estrogen excess have been associated with the increased risk of endometrial cancer. Postmenopausal women with estrogen-secreting tumors have been reported to have a 10% to 24% incidence of endometrial cancer. There is also a high incidence of cancer in patients with *polycystic ovary disease*; 19% to 25% of young women with endometrial carcinoma have underlying Stein-Leventhal syndrome. It is likely that less well-defined abnormalities of estrogen control explain the association of endometrial cancer with menstrual abnormalities and infertility. Approximately half of all women with endometrial carcinoma and 20% to 30% of married women with endometrial carcinoma are nulliparous.

The principal estrogen in postmenopausal women is estrone, which is peripherally converted from androstenedione produced in the adrenal glands. Peripheral conversion of androstenedione to estrone has been shown to be increased in patients with endometrial cancer, and estrone to estradiol ratios are higher. Peripheral conversion by adipose cells may be the explanatory link between obesity and endometrial cancer.

A number of retrospective case-control studies indicate that the use of *estrogens postmenopausally* substantially increases the risk of endometrial cancer. Rates of endometrial cancer among estrogen users ranged from 4 to 14 times those among control patients. Several studies demonstrated a dose–response relationship in that use of estrogen for longer periods of time was associated with greater risk. It has been argued that the association between estrogens and endometrial cancer can be explained in part by a greater likelihood of detection of preexisting tumors in women for whom estrogens are prescribed. Implications of this link between exogenous estrogens and endometrial cancer for treatment of menopausal symptoms are discussed in Chapter 118. Case-control data suggest a 50% decrease in risk among women who have used combination birth control pills for a minimum of 12 months, with the protective effect lasting from 8 to 15 years. A program of estrogen plus progesterone for postmenopausal hormone replacement therapy is not associated with an increased risk of endometrial carcinoma.

NATURAL HISTORY OF ENDOMETRIAL CANCER AND EFFECTIVENESS OF THERAPY

Postmenopausal bleeding, by far the most common symptom associated with endometrial cancer, must always be pursued aggressively. Clinical studies have indicated that, depending on patient selection, cancer is the explanation from 10% to 70% of women who present with postmenopausal bleeding. In one review of more than 400 presentations of bleeding at least 2 years after menopause, 16% of patients had endometrial cancer. The likelihood of malignancy increased with the span of years since menopause.

In a series of more than 500 patients with endometrial cancer from the Mayo Clinic, nearly all presented with postmenopausal bleeding or similar symptoms; only 3% of the tumors were detected in asymptomatic women. In this series, there was little if any correlation between the duration of symptoms and the clinical stage of the tumor at the time of diagnosis. The prognosis for endometrial cancer is generally favorable. In the Mayo series, a 5-year survival rate of 75% was reported.

DIAGNOSTIC TESTS

Available data suggest that endometrial cancer presents with symptoms early in its natural history. There is little evidence that cytopathologic screening can appreciably advance the time of diagnosis in most patients. The diagnosis of endometrial cancer can be made on the basis of a *Papanicolaou (Pap) smear* of cells aspirated from the *vaginal pool* or scraped from the *cervical os*. However, a number of studies have indicated that the sensitivity of the Pap smear in the diagnosis of endometrial cancer is only 70% to 80%. A retrospective review of patients with endometrial cancer who had Pap smears during the year before diagnosis found that only 18% had smears that were suggestive of cancer.

Jet wash and aspiration techniques have been used for sampling cells from the uterine cavity. These techniques proved to be less painful and effective substitutes for dilation and curettage in some diagnostic situations. However, the value of using these techniques to screen asymptomatic women for premalignant and malignant lesions has not been demonstrated.

Transvaginal ultrasound has proven to be an effective means of assessing endometrial thickness related to the probability of finding significant pathology with subsequent curettage in postmenopausal women. This approach has been advocated to monitor women at high risk of endometrial cancer, including those at iatrogenic risk due to unopposed estrogen treatment for menopause (rarely advised for women with intact uteri) or tamoxifen treatment for breast cancer. Estimation of endometrial thickness has also been advocated as a means to avoid diagnostic curettage in postmenopausal women who experience abnormal bleeding. Its value in screening asymptomatic women has not been defined.

SUMMARY AND CONCLUSIONS

Endometrial carcinoma is a source of substantial morbidity and mortality and has well-defined risk factors. Evidence indicates that endogenous and exogenous estrogen stimulation play an etiologic role. Although Pap smears potentially advance the diagnosis of cervical cancer, there are no tests as suitable for endometrial cancer screening. A prompt diagnostic workup, with transvaginal ultrasound perhaps preceding endometrial biopsy, must be initiated by the primary care provider in patients presenting with postmenopausal bleeding. Ultrasound followed by endometrial sampling and other diagnostic interventions should be considered for women at risk because of hormonal therapy. Risk associated with postmenopausal estrogen therapy can be reduced by adding progesterone to the hormone replacement program (see Chapter 118).

A.G.M.

ANNOTATED BIBLIOGRAPHY

Antunes CMF, Stolley PD, Rosenshein NB, et al. Endometrial cancer and estrogen use. N Engl J Med 1979;300:9. *(Overall sixfold increased risk in estrogen users. Increased risk with dosage and duration. Stage 0 and 1 tumors are more common in estrogen users.)*

Beral V, Hannaford P, Kay C. Oral contraceptive use and malignancies of the genital tract. Results from the Royal College of General Practitioners' oral contraception study. Lancet 1988;2:1331. *(Found an 80% reduction in risk.)*

Burke JR, Lehman HF, Wolf FS. Inadequacy of Papanicolaou smears in the detection of endometrial cancer. N Engl J Med 1974; 291:191. *(Only 18% of Pap smears taken within a year of presentation with endometrial cancer were suggestive of malignancy.)*

The Cancer and Steroid Hormone Study of the Centers for Disease Control and the National Institute of Child Health and Human Development. Combination oral contraceptive use and risk of endometrial cancer. JAMA 1987;257:796. *(Risk reduction of 40% after 1 year's use that lasted up to 15 years.)*

Centers for Disease Control Cancer and Steroid Hormone Study. Oral contraceptive use and the risk of endometrial cancer. JAMA 1983;249:1600. *(Combination pill use for more than 1 year showed a protective effect in this case-control study, particularly among nulliparous women.)*

Horwitz RI, Feinstein AR. Alternative analytic methods for case-control studies of estrogen and endometrial cancer. N Engl J Med 1978;299:1089. *(Points out the potential of bias in case finding but does not refute increased risk.)*

Koss LG, Schreiber K, Oberlander SG, et al. Detection of endometrial carcinoma and its hyperplasia in asymptomatic women. Obstet Gynecol 1984;64:1. *(Vaginal pool and endometrial sampling were used to screen 2,586 women; 17 endometrial cancers were diagnosed.)*

Malkasian GD, McDonald TW, Pratt JH. Carcinoma of the endometrium. Mayo Clin Proc 1977;52:175. *(Detailed review of 523 cases with 74% 5-year survival rate.)*

Pachecho JC, Kempers RD. Etiology of postmenopausal bleeding. Obstet Gynecol 1968;32:40. *(Sixteen percent of 401 women with postmenopausal bleeding had endometrial cancer.)*

Pritchard KI. Screening for endometrial cancer: is it effective? Ann Intern Med 1989;110:177. *(Reviews the basis for the Canadian Task Force recommendation against screening.)*

Smith DC, Prentice R, Thompson DJ, et al. Association of exogenous estrogen and endometrial carcinoma. N Engl J Med 1975;293: 1164. *(Case-control study showing 4.5 times greater risk among exposed women.)*

110
Vaginal Cancer and Other Effects of Diethylstilbestrol Exposure

Vaginal cancer is a rare disease, accounting for approximately 1% of gynecologic malignancies. More than 90% of vaginal cancers are squamous cell tumors. Elderly women are at greatest risk, and because of the extensive lymphatic drainage of the vagina, the 5-year survival rate is only 20% to 25%.

Of greater concern to the primary care provider is adenocarcinoma, or clear cell carcinoma of the vagina, which occurs in young women who were exposed to diethylstilbestrol (DES) or other synthetic estrogens *in utero*. Although these tumors are quite rare, the population at risk is large. The anxiety among DES-exposed persons is substantial. In addition to the association with vaginal cancer, other abnormalities of the genital tract, including some that may affect reproductive function, have been reported. The primary physician should understand the risks that follow DES exposure and the natural history of the associated conditions to counsel and evaluate these patients appropriately.

DIETHYLSTILBESTROL AND ABNORMALITIES OF THE GENITAL TRACT

DES is a synthetic estrogen first produced in 1938. After early studies indicated it was helpful in preventing spontaneous abortion, it and other synthetic estrogens were used extensively from the 1940s until 1971 in pregnant women at risk for miscarriage. It has been estimated that between 100,000 and 160,000 women born between 1960 and 1970 were exposed to DES or similar drugs *in utero*. Because these agents were used more extensively in the 1940s and 1950s, well over 1 million women are estimated to have been exposed.

In 1970, a cluster of cases of the then very rare adenocarcinoma of the vagina, occurring in daughters who had been exposed to DES *in utero,* was reported from Massachusetts General Hospital. Since that time, the association has been confirmed, and several hundred cases of clear cell carcinoma have been recorded and investigated. A history of DES exposure has been elicited in approximately two thirds of all cases of malignancy.

Subsequent prospective studies of exposed women identified the abnormalities of the cervix and vagina that can be found in women at risk, in addition to clear cell carcinoma. Vaginal adenosis, the presence of glandular epithelium in the vagina, occurred in 35% of exposed women but in only 1% of matched control subjects. Cervical erosion was present in more than 75% of exposed women and in only one third of control subjects. Gross structural abnormalities of the cervix were found in more than 20% of exposed women but were not found among control subjects. The cumulative incidence of carcinoma in exposed daughters is estimated to be 1.5 per 1,000 women. The relative risk of vaginal clear cell adenocarcinoma conferred by DES exposure has been estimated to be approximately 40. The embryonic development of the female genital tract begins as early as the 4th week of gestation and is completed by the end of the 18th week. Patients exposed early during this period (i.e., weeks 4 to 18) are most likely to have the epithelial changes and structural abnormalities.

Although tumors have been identified in pre-teenaged patients as young as age 7, more than 90% of tumors have been found in daughters age 14 or older. The peak incidence of tumors occurs between the ages of 14 and 20, suggesting that the period of greatest risk occurs when the abnormal vaginal or cervical epithelium is stimulated by ovarian hormones with the onset of puberty. Incident cases after age 29 years are rare, but incident vaginal adenocarcinoma has been reported in exposed women in their forties.

Findings from the National Collaborative Diethylstilbestrol Adenosis (DESAD) Project indicate that women exposed to the drug *in utero* have a twofold increase in risk of *cervical* intraepithelial neoplasia over nonexposed control subjects. But there is no increase in risk of invasive cervical cancer.

Questions have also been raised about the ability of DES-exposed offspring to conceive. A high prevalence of uterine and fallopian tube abnormalities has been described in case series of exposed women who have undergone hysterosalpingography. A controlled cohort study from the DESAD Project, however, found no difference in fertility between exposed and control subjects. Subsequent studies have suggested a modest increase in risk of primary *infertility* in association with the higher prevalence of abnormal hysterosalpingograms among exposed daughters. DES-exposed women who become pregnant have been shown to be more likely to have an *unfavorable outcome* of pregnancy. It has been estimated that DES-exposed women are approximately eight times more likely to have an ectopic pregnancy, twice as likely to have a miscarriage, and five times as likely to deliver prematurely. Nevertheless, more than 80% of such women had at least one full-term live birth during the course of the DESAD study.

A large cohort study with an average follow-up of 16 years found no increased risk of cancer other than clear cell adenocarcinoma of the vagina. Because of the relatively young age of the cohort, definitive conclusions await further study. Mothers exposed to DES during their pregnancy face a modest increase in breast cancer risk, with a relative risk of 1.35.

Genital abnormalities and infertility have also been described in male offspring of mothers who took DES early in pregnancy. It is likely that these findings were influenced by selection and ascertainment biases; the only controlled study addressing this question found no differences in rates of genitourinary abnormalities, infertility, or testicular cancer in exposed and nonexposed men.

SYMPTOMS AND NATURAL HISTORY OF VAGINAL CANCER AND EFFECTIVENESS OF THERAPY

The natural history of clear cell carcinoma is uncertain. Cases can present with *abnormal vaginal bleeding or discharge*, but because of increasing public and professional awareness, a substantial percentage of cases are detected in the asymptomatic stage. Adenosis has been found in proximity to adenocarcinoma in more than 95% of cases, and it is therefore considered a malignant precursor by some. Transitions from adenosis to carcinoma have not, however, been clearly documented.

Limited follow-up information indicates that clear cell carcinoma is an aggressive tumor. Metastases have been found at the time of surgery in 17% of cases of stage I disease and in most cases of stage II disease. Short-term follow-up of registry cases of clear cell carcinoma has indicated that recurrence, death, or both occur in approximately 25% of patients.

It is too early to know whether cervical dysplasia and carcinoma *in situ* in DES-exposed young women have the same natural history as nonexposed women (see Chapter 107). However, it seems prudent to follow such patients with vigilance and yearly Papanicolaou (Pap) smears.

DIAGNOSTIC TESTS

Although the discovery of abnormal cytology has led to the detection of some cases of clear cell carcinoma, the *Pap smear* has been shown to have a relatively low sensitivity (80%) for detecting this lesion. This may be explained by the relatively high degree of differentiation of the neoplastic cells, which may resemble endocervical cells. The cells may also be obscured by a heavy polymorphonuclear infiltration. The initial examination of a woman exposed *in utero* to DES or similar drugs must therefore include, in addition to direct inspection of the vagina and cervix and cytologic sampling, careful *Schiller's iodine staining and biopsies* of areas that appear red or fail to stain with the iodine solution. *Colposcopy* is a complementary procedure, particularly useful in patients with abnormal iodine staining or cytology. Colposcopy should be performed by an experienced gynecologist.

Despite the poor sensitivity of the Pap smear for clear cell cancer, Pap smears should be done yearly in all women with an exposure history. This is especially important in light of the increased risk of cervical intraepithelial neoplasia, particularly among women with evidence for human papillomavirus infection or other risk factors related to sexual activity.

CONCLUSIONS AND RECOMMENDATIONS

- As many as 1 million women are at risk for abnormalities of the genital tract, including clear cell adenocarcinoma, because of *in utero* exposure to DES or other synthetic estrogens.
- Risk of malignancy among exposed women is low. Nevertheless, because of the significant morbidity and mortality associated with these tumors, careful case finding and evaluation are indicated. Because routine screening procedures such as

the Pap smear are inadequate, patients at risk must be identified by careful history taking if they are to receive proper evaluation and counseling.

- It is recommended that exposed daughters with symptoms such as vaginal discharge or bleeding are examined promptly regardless of age. Asymptomatic daughters with a history of exposure should have an initial evaluation at age 14 with subsequent yearly examinations.
- More frequent examinations are advised when extensive epithelial changes are present. When possible, such examinations should be performed by a gynecologist experienced in the use of the colposcope.

A.G.M.

ANNOTATED BIBLIOGRAPHY

Barnes AB, Colton T, Gunderson J, et al. Fertility and outcome in pregnancy in women exposed in utero to diethylstilbestrol. N Engl J Med 1980;302:609. *(Fertility was not affected by DES exposure; there was, however, an increased risk of unfavorable outcome of pregnancy associated with DES exposure—the relative risk was 1.69.)*

Calle EE, Mervis CA, Thun MJ, et al. Diethylstilbestrol and risk of fatal breast cancer in a prospective cohort of U.S. women. Am J Epidemiol 1996;144:645. *(Confirms the earlier Colton study with relative risk of 1.34.)*

Colton T, Greenberg ER, Noller K, et al. Breast cancer in mothers prescribed diethylstilbestrol in pregnancy. JAMA 1993;269:2096. *(The relative risk of breast cancer in mothers exposed during pregnancy was 1.35.)*

Hatch EE, Palmer JR, Titus-Ernstoff L, et al. Cancer risk in women exposed to diethylstilbestrol in utero. JAMA 1998;280:630. *(No increased cancer risk except for clear cell carcinoma of the vagina in a cohort of 4,536 women followed for an average of 16 years.)*

Heinonen OP. Diethylstilbestrol in pregnancy: frequency of exposure and usage pattern. Cancer 1973;31:573. *(Drug utilization data for 1960s indicated that 100,000 to 160,000 women born in the United States during that decade were exposed in utero.)*

Herbst AL, Poskanzer DC, Robboy SJ, et al. Prenatal exposure to stilbestrol: a prospective comparison of exposed female offspring with unexposed controls. N Engl J Med 1975;292:332. *(Prospective examination of 110 exposed and 82 unexposed females. No cancers were found, but adenosis and other abnormalities were common among exposed individuals.)*

Leary FJ, Resseguie LJ, Kurland LT, et al. Males exposed in utero to diethylstilbestrol. JAMA 1984;252:2984. *(Careful urologic and fertility evaluation of exposed and unexposed subjects showed no increased risk of abnormalities.)*

Melnick S, Cole P, Anderson D, Herbst A. Rates and risks of diethylstilbestrol-related clear cell adenocarcinoma of the vagina and cervix. N Engl J Med 1987;316:514. *(Risk of vaginal cancer from birth through age 34 is about 1 in 1,000.)*

Robboy SJ, Noller KL, O'Brien P, et al. Increased incidence of cervical and vaginal dysplasia in 3980 diethylstilbestrol-exposed young women. JAMA 1984;252:2979. *(The incidence of dysplasia and carcinoma in situ was 15.7 versus 7.9 per 1,000 person-years in exposed and nonexposed women, respectively.)*

Senekjian EK, Potkul RK, Frey K, et al. Infertility among daughters either exposed or not exposed to diethylstilbestrol. Am J Obstet Gynecol 1988;158:493. *(Primary infertility in 33% of exposed and 14% of unexposed, with high prevalence of abnormal hysterosalpingograms among the exposed.)*

Sharp GB, Cole P. Vaginal bleeding and diethylstilbestrol exposure during pregnancy: relationship to genital tract clear cell adenocarcinoma and vaginal adenosis in daughters. Am J Obstet Gynecol 1990;162:994. *(The relative risks of vaginal clear cell adenocarcinoma for in utero exposure were 3.66 and 4.59 when vaginal bleeding did and did not occur during the index pregnancy.)*

Wingard DL, Cohn BA, Helmrich SP, et al. DES awareness and exposure: the 1994 California Behavioral Risk Factor Survey. Am J Prevent Med 1996;12:437. *(Among respondents in the age group exposed, one in five men and two in five women had ever heard of DES.)*

111

Approach to the Woman with Abnormal Vaginal Bleeding

Abnormal vaginal bleeding is bleeding that occurs at an inappropriate time (less than 21 or more than 36 days after last period) or in an excessive amount (clots lasting more than 7 days). About one half of all women presenting with this problem are over age 40 years. In these peri- and postmenopausal patients, uterine malignancy must be ruled out. Pelvic pathology is also a possibility in younger women, but disturbances of the hypothalamic-pituitary-ovarian axis are more common precipitants of abnormal bleeding. This is especially true among adolescent and immediately postadolescent women who constitute about 20% of those presenting with abnormal bleeding. When bleeding is anovulatory and occurs in the absence of an anatomic lesion, it is sometimes referred to as "dysfunctional." The terms "anovulatory" and "dysfunctional" are used interchangeably by clinicians. The former is more explanatory and is less likely to have negative connotations for the patient.

The differentiation of anovulatory bleeding from bleeding due to anatomic pathology in the presence of normal ovulation is the goal of the primary physician's initial evaluation and an important determinant of therapy. Anovulatory bleeding is common for young women just beginning to ovulate and may last 1 to 2 years before menses become regular. It is also common as ovarian function declines in the perimenopausal woman where it presents a particular challenge, because this is also a time for increased risk of endometrial cancer.

PATHOPHYSIOLOGY AND CLINICAL PRESENTATION

Normal Menstrual Bleeding

Normally, in the absence of implantation of a fertilized ovum, the ovarian corpus luteum undergoes regression within 9 to 11 days of ovulation. Estrogen and progesterone production fall and menstruation ensues. The normal menstrual cycle ranges from 23 to 39 days (mean, 29 days). Cycle length shortens as menopause approaches. The menstrual period usually lasts 2 to 7 days, with most blood lost during the first few days. Presence of clots or duration of bleeding in excess of 1 week indicates excessive blood loss. Abnormal bleeding may occur in the context of normal ovulation or in its absence.

Abnormal Bleeding in the Setting of Normal Ovulatory Cycles

In normally ovulating women, abnormal vaginal bleeding may present as *menorrhagia* (bleeding that is normal in timing but excessive in amount and duration) or *intermenstrual bleeding*. Most often the cause is an *endometrial or cervical lesion* (Table 111.1). However, it sometimes is the presenting symptom of a *bleeding diathesis*, most often the consequence of thrombocytopenia or a qualitative platelet disorder (see Chapter 81).

Normal ovulation may be accompanied by a small amount of midcycle vaginal staining and pelvic pain (especially on the right side). It is sometimes referred to as "*mittelschmerz*," which occurs in the context of ovarian follicle rupture and release.

Uterine Fibroids or leiomyomas are the most common cause and account for about one third of cases. Fibroids occur in 20% to 25% of women before age 40 and in up to half of all women

Table 111.1. Differential Diagnosis of Abnormal Vaginal Bleeding

Ovulatory Bleeding
1. Normal variant
   a. "Mittelschmerz"
2. Anatomic lesion
   a. Uterine fibroids
   b. Cervical disease (inflammation, polyp, cancer)
   c. Endometrial carcinoma
   d. Pelvic inflammatory disease
   e. Intrauterine device
3. Concurrent disease
   a. Bleeding diathesis
   b. Foreign body

Anovulatory Bleeding
1. Hypothalamic dysfunction
   a. Puberty
   b. Perimenopausal state
   c. Situational stress, excessive exercise, weight loss
   d. Excess androgen, prolactin, cortisol; hypothyroidism
   e. Polycystic ovary syndrome
2. Oral contraceptive use
   a. Inadequate estrogen dose

Postmenopausal Bleeding
1. Endometrial pathology
   a. Fibroid
   b. Cancer
   c. Polyp
2. Cervical pathology
   a. Cancer
   b. Polyp
   c. Erosion
3. Vaginal pathology
   a. Atrophic vaginitis

Pregnancy
1. Ectopic pregnancy
2. Postabortion (retained products of gestation)
3. Failing pregnancy

overall. However, only those fibroids that are submucosal in location and involve the uterine cavity cause bleeding. Location is more important than size. Because they are so common, they may coexist with another cause of abnormal vaginal bleeding. Periods are often very heavy.

Carcinoma of the Cervix is among the more serious sources of abnormal bleeding in ovulating patients, although it accounts for only about 3% of cases. *Postcoital bleeding* and slight intermenstrual spotting are characteristic when there is surface ulceration, which may occur in early stages of the disease (see Chapter 123).

Endometrial Carcinoma is more typically a disease of abnormal vaginal bleeding in postmenopausal women (see below), but 20% have the disease while still menstruating (although almost all are over the age of 40). Heavier than normal periods are noted as well as an intermenstrual watery discharge containing small amounts of blood early on.

Polyps, Erosions, and Infection. *Cervical polyps, cervical erosions, and vaginal lesions* present similarly, with slight spotting noted intermenstrually, especially after coitus. *Pelvic inflammatory disease*, with its fever, pelvic pain, and discharge, may lead to postcoital, intermenstrual, or heavy menstrual bleeding by causing cervicitis, endometritis, or salpingitis.

Foreign Bodies. *Intrauterine devices* also alter the endometrial surface and can be similarly responsible for heavy menstrual bleeding or intermenstrual bleeding. Vaginal wall irritation from *tampon* use may lead to minor vaginal bleeding.

Anovulatory Bleeding

This type of bleeding is usually a manifestation of a disturbance within the hypothalamic-pituitary-ovarian axis. *Metrorrhagia*—prolonged bleeding occurring at irregular intervals—is characteristic.

Hypothalamic Dysfunction. The pathophysiologic common denominator is *inadequate progesterone* production, most often due to lack of a *luteinizing hormone (LH) surge* at midcycle, a consequence of an alteration in the normal pattern of gonadotropin-releasing hormone (GnRH) release from the hypothalamus. This pattern is typical of patients with mild hypothalamic dysfunction who may experience irregular menses in the context of moderate *situational stress, weight loss, or exercise training*. However, oligomenorrhea and amenorrhea may follow if the functional disturbance is more severe, impairing follicle-stimulating hormone (FSH) secretion and estrogen production (see Chapter 112). Those who bleed have an estrogen-withdrawal type of bleeding. The severity of the bleeding is a function of the amount of estrogen produced. The bleeding that occurs from mild hypothalamic dysfunction is sometimes referred to as "dysfunctional." *Hyperprolactinemia, hypothyroidism*, and excess production of *androgen* and *cortisol* can also disturb hypothalamic rhythmicity. Even *iron deficiency anemia* has been found to inhibit ovulation.

Histoanatomically, unruptured ovarian follicles persist, and functioning corpora lutea are absent. The endometrium shows hyperplasia resulting from unopposed estrogen effect. There is little if any secretory pattern because of the lack of progesterone. Ovulation does not occur, and anovulatory bleeding results when progesterone production returns or excessive proliferation causes sloughing of the overstimulated endometrium. There is irregularity of the menstrual interval, periods of amenorrhea, and episodes of very heavy and prolonged bleeding if there has been sufficient estrogen-induced buildup of the endometrium.

Polycystic Ovary Syndrome. This incompletely understood condition affects about 5% of reproductive-age women and represents a leading cause of chronic anovulatory bleeding. In addition to a life-long history of irregular periods, patients may report infertility, hirsutism, obesity, and amenorrhea. Disordered hypothalamic rhythmicity is believed to cause excessive LH production without a midcycle surge, leading to ovarian overproduction of *testosterone* and *androstenedione*. Some of this androgen is converted to *estrone*, which can stimulate endometrial proliferation that ends in irregular episodes of bleeding. Serum concentrations of both estrogen and testosterone rise. *Insulin resistance* with hyperinsulinism are common and believed to be linked to ovarian androgen overproduction. The consequences of androgen excess range from hirsutism to frank virilization (see Chapter 98), although the latter is uncommon. Chronic unopposed endometrial estrogen stimulation can lead to adenomatous hyperplasia, cellular atypicality, and even endometrial carcinoma. Risk of cancer is increased threefold.

Puberty. The anovulatory bleeding of puberty is a consequence of immaturity of the positive-feedback mechanism responsible for the LH surge that triggers progesterone secretion. In the absence of adequate progesterone production, estrogen-withdrawal bleeding takes place. The pattern of anovulatory bleeding is irregular and may occur anytime between 22 and 45 days.

Perimenopausal Bleeding. The irregular menstrual bleeding that characterizes the perimenopausal period is also an anovulatory estrogen-withdrawal phenomenon. As the number of functioning ovarian follicles declines, insufficient estrogen is produced to cause an LH surge and ovulation. In the absence of progesterone production, an estrogen-withdrawal type of irregular bleeding occurs. Such perimenopausal bleeding can continue for months to years, but it eventually stops when estrogen production ceases.

Postmenopausal, Pregnancy-related, and Breakthrough Types of Bleeding

Postmenopause. Here the major concern is cancer, although *uterine fibroids* still account for most cases. Women who have had chronic unopposed estrogen stimulation are at increased risk of *endometrial carcinoma*. Early on, bleeding may be subtle and little more than minor vaginal staining (see Chapter 123). Postmenopausal women with marked *atrophic vaginitis, cervical polyp, or cervicitis* from a prolapsed uterus may also experience some blood-stained vaginal discharge or minor spotting. Cervical carcinoma is uncommon after age 55 in women who have had Papanicolaou (Pap) smears regularly but may be the cause of bleeding in the early postmenopausal period.

Pregnancy. One of the most serious causes of acute abnormal vaginal bleeding in women of reproductive age is *ectopic pregnancy*, which is characterized by delay of the regular period followed by vaginal blood spotting, often in conjunction with unilateral pelvic pain. Intraperitoneal hemorrhage can ensue if tubal rupture occurs, but this happens in fewer than 5% of cases. A *failing pregnancy* may be heralded by onset of bleeding. *Retained products of gestation* represents a very common cause of abnormal uterine bleeding after abortion; blood loss is often heavy.

Oral Contraceptives. If an oral contraceptive contains insufficient estrogen or if compliance is inadequate, then abnormal vaginal bleeding may occur. The characteristic pattern is one of "*breakthrough bleeding*" or staining that occurs intermenstrually (see Chapter 119).

DIFFERENTIAL DIAGNOSIS

The differential diagnosis can be divided into ovulatory, anovulatory, postmenopausal, and pregnancy-related etiologies (Table 111.1). Among postmenopausal women, endometrial cancer accounts for up to 25% of cases of bleeding, although most are due to submucosal uterine fibroids. In women of reproductive age, the etiology is often an anovulatory disturbance, although cancer remains a concern. As noted, girls going through puberty and perimenopausal women who complain of irregular menses are most likely to have anovulatory bleeding.

WORKUP

Among women of reproductive age who complain of abnormal vaginal bleeding, the initial tasks are to rule out pregnancy and determine if the bleeding is ovulatory or anovulatory. Postmenopausal bleeding has its own workup, which focuses on identifying the anatomic site of bleeding.

History

A careful and detailed menstrual history is essential. Most important is information on the patient's normal menstrual cycle (duration, frequency, intensity) and how the current bleeding pattern compares with it. If the patient is of childbearing age, then inquiry should be made into unprotected intercourse and symptoms of pregnancy (breast engorgement, morning sickness, cessation of normal menses). If menstrual regularity persists despite an increase in intensity or duration of flow or onset of intermenstrual staining, then an ovulatory etiology is likely. This is further supported by presence of premenstrual symptoms, such as breast engorgement, pelvic cramping, fluid retention, and mood swings. Anovulatory bleeding is suggested by the absence of such symptoms plus complete irregularity of menstrual periods, especially if accompanied by months of amenorrhea. Although intensity of the bleeding (e.g., by number of pads or tampons used) is more useful for management than for diagnosis, the new onset of clots or duration of more than 7 days argues for abnormal bleeding.

Ovulatory Bleeding. History should include query into symptoms of a bleeding diathesis and medicines that inhibit normal clotting (see Chapter 81). Equally important is checking for dyspareunia, postcoital bleeding, vaginal discharge, pelvic pain, fever, trauma, and intrauterine device use. Risk factors for endometrial carcinoma should be reviewed (see Chapter 123).

Anovulatory Bleeding. One should ask about important precipitants, such as emotional stress, weight loss, exercise, and chronic illness. If the patient is an adolescent girl, one should check for a history of irregular periods since the onset of menarche and the common precipitants just noted. Review of medications for use of oral contraceptives is essential, with attention to the estrogen dose and history of breakthrough bleeding. For the perimenopausal woman, menstrual irregularity and the skipping of periods suggest a functional etiology but do not rule out cancer. Androgen excess is suggested by symptoms of hirsutism and virilization (see Chapter 98) and a history of infertility. Rapid onset of hirsutism and virilization raises the possibility of a functioning adrenal or ovarian tumor-making androgens. A life-long history of irregular menses, hirsutism, infertility, and obesity suggests polycystic ovary syndrome. Inquiry into galactorrhea and development of cushingoid appearance check for prolactin and cortisol excess, respectively. Any symptoms of hypothyroidism (see Chapter 104) and iron deficiency (see Chapter 79) should be noted.

Postmenopausal Bleeding. Any history of bleeding, even if just minor staining, should be taken as evidence of a possible malignancy. However, inquiry into symptomatic atrophic vaginitis and uterine prolapse may provide useful clues.

Physical Examination

Regardless of presumed etiology, all patients should be checked for *postural signs* indicative of significant intravascular volume depletion. In addition, careful *speculum and bimanual pelvic examinations* are essential, with particular care taken to note any vaginal or cervical erosions, uterine or adnexal masses, focal tenderness, or purulent or bloody discharge. Signs of pregnancy (engorged breasts, pigmented areolae, bluish cervix, enlarged uterus) should be sought in women of reproductive age.

Suspected ovulatory bleeding necessitates concentrating on the pelvic examination, but one should also check for signs of a bleeding diathesis (petechiae, ecchymoses, splenic enlargement). The patient with *suspected anovulatory bleeding* should be carefully examined for hirsutism, virilization, cushingoid appearance, milky nipple discharge, goiter, dry skin, coarse hair, and "hungup" reflexes. Visual field testing is indicated if there is suspicion of a large pituitary adenoma. Presence of hirsutism or virilization necessitates thorough pelvic and abdominal examinations for an ovarian or adrenal mass.

On examination of the *postmenopausal woman*, particular note should be taken of the friability of the vaginal mucosa and cervix and the presence of any uterine or adnexal masses.

Laboratory Studies

All patients of reproductive age with abnormal vaginal bleeding should be tested for pregnancy (a *serum human chorionic gonadotropin β subunit* is the most sensitive; see Chapter 112). A *complete blood count* is always useful. The *hematocrit* will help assess the severity of chronic blood loss (although not of acute hemorrhage; see Chapter 79) and a mean *red cell volume* may reveal the microcytosis of iron deficiency.

Ovulatory Bleeding. Here the goal is identification of pelvic pathology after ruling out concurrent disease that may predispose to heavy bleeding. Determinations of *blood urea nitrogen, creatinine, and platelet count* should be obtained when there is concern about a bleeding diathesis. Otherwise, one should proceed directly to *pelvic ultrasound* examination, with transvaginal study being the most sensitive noninvasive means of searching for uterine and adnexal pathology; it is superior to the standard transabdominal approach.

A *Pap smear* is indicated if the cervix appears abnormal. In women over age 40, *vaginal cytologic sampling* from the posterior cervical fornix may detect abnormal endometrial cells shed into this accessible area. Acetic acid can be added to cytology preservative if the smear sample is bloody. A *cervical culture* for gonorrhea and for other pathogenic organisms is needed in the patient with pain on motion of the cervix and adnexal tenderness (see Chapter 117); an elevated *sedimentation rate* suggests pelvic inflammation.

Endometrial sampling is central to the evaluation of ovulatory bleeding when noninvasive evaluation is unrevealing. It is contraindicated in the presence of cervical stenosis, infection, or pregnancy. Transvaginal ultrasound or hysteroscopy should generally precede diagnostic dilation and curettage.

Anovulatory Bleeding. No additional studies are necessary when the etiology is evident (e.g., situational stress, puberty, chronic illness, marked weight loss). If perimenopausal bleeding is suspected, an *FSH* can be confirmatory; if more than 40 IU/mL, then ovarian failure is imminent. An LH-to-FSH ratio of greater than 2:1 is characteristic of polycystic ovary syndrome. When hirsutism or virilization is noted, a serum *testosterone* is the best test. If the onset of such changes is rapid or the serum testosterone is greater than 600 nmol/L (190 ng/mL), then a functioning adrenal or ovarian neoplasm may be the source and a *17-hydroxyprogesterone* can facilitate the diagnosis. A *fasting serum insulin* level is also indicated in patients with elevated testosterone (more than 350 nmol/L, 100 ng/mL). A *fasting insulin* level in excess of 180 pmol/L is suggestive of insulin resistance.

Postmenopausal Bleeding. Noninvasive study for pelvic pathology is conducted as noted above. Because concern about endometrial cancer is high in this age group, endometrial sampling or diagnostic dilation and curettage is appropriate, even when noninvasive study is unrevealing.

SYMPTOMATIC MANAGEMENT AND PATIENT EDUCATION

Acute anovulatory bleeding that is not severe can often be managed by the primary care physician in the office setting. To stop the abnormal bleeding, one can administer a course of oral *medroxyprogesterone* (Provera; 10 mg/d for 10 days) or a single intramuscular injection of *progesterone* (100 mg). These will convert a proliferative endometrium to a secretory one. Bleeding should stop within 24 to 48 hours of initiating progestin therapy, and menstrual flow should occur on its completion. If this so-called medical dilation and curettage does not stop acute bleeding, then referral for dilation and curettage and hysteroscopy is indicated.

Chronic Anovulatory Bleeding can be treated symptomatically by monthly administration of progesterone therapy. By causing regular endometrial shedding, it protects against adenomatous changes and lowers the risk of endometrial cancer associated with long-term unopposed estrogen stimulation. A course of *medroxyprogesterone* given for the last 10 to 12 days of each month will usually suffice. Cessation of further abnormal bleeding episodes argues strongly against a structural lesion, but resumption of such bleeding on progestin therapy necessitates referral for dilation and curettage.

Ovulation may resume on this program, particularly in the young person, and periodically the treatment should be halted for a month or two to observe for the return of normal cycles. If abnormal bleeding recurs despite correction of all possible precipitating factors, then maintenance hormonal therapy may be used. In patients who do not desire pregnancy, an *estrogen-progestin* oral contraceptive preparation may be used in place of the medroxyprogesterone (see Chapter 119). Oral contraceptive therapy has the advantage of improving the hyperandrogenism that accompanies some causes of chronic anovulatory bleeding. The patient with anovulatory bleeding who desires pregnancy should be referred for consideration of clomiphene therapy. Any iron deficiency (see Chapter 82) or pelvic infection should be treated (see Chapter 117).

Nonsteroidal anti-inflammatory agents may decrease bleeding by as much as 50%. They may also provide relief for any associated dysmenorrhea. They may be used along with oral contraceptives. Danazol may also be effective but has some undesirable androgenic side effects. GnRH analogues produce a menopausal state in women of reproductive age. They are used primarily for preoperative management of uterine fibroids and for endometrial preparation before ablation procedures.

When anovulatory bleeding is diagnosed, it is important for the patient to know that reproductive capacity is not lost, that some causes are self-limited, and that the possibility of malignancy is very low under age 30. Addressing any contributing factors (e.g., situational stress, dieting, excessive exercise, hypothyroidism [see Chapter 104], hyperprolactinemia [see Chapter 100], polycystic ovary syndrome [see Chapter 112]) is essential to successful therapy.

Perimenopausal Bleeding may be the result of anovulatory periods, but an irregular pattern may also represent intrauterine disease. When discussed openly, the concerns that most patients already harbor can be addressed and often lessened, because most cases are not likely to be cancerous. Once a structural lesion has been ruled out, symptomatic therapy with monthly *medroxyprogesterone* (10 mg/d for 10 to 12 days) can commence. It will correct the irregular bleeding. Therapy is continued monthly until withdrawal bleeding stops, indicating arrival of ovarian failure and menopause. Until menopause, some ovulatory periods may still take place and cause bleeding independent of progesterone therapy. In such instances, an oral contraceptive can be used as an alternative to progesterone, provided the patient is a nonsmoker, normotensive, and not hyperlipidemic.

Breakthrough Bleeding. Patients experiencing breakthrough bleeding on low-dosage estrogen oral contraceptives need to be sure they are adhering carefully to their regimen. If they are taking the medication on schedule, switching to a preparation with a higher estrogen dose is indicated.

INDICATIONS FOR ADMISSION AND REFERRAL

Immediate hospital admission is essential for any woman who is bleeding heavily and manifests signs of intravascular volume depletion. Immediate hospital admission and gynecologic consultation are particularly important if ectopic pregnancy is a possibility, because life-threatening hemorrhage is a real, albeit slight, risk. The same applies to cases of recent abortion, because placental tissue may be retained. Bleeding in pregnancy is a definite indication for an emergency obstetric consultation.

Any patient with abnormal vaginal bleeding who has a mass lesion detected on pelvic examination, an abnormal appearing cervix, an abnormal Pap test, or risk factors for carcinoma of the cervix or endometrium (see Chapters 107 and 109) should be referred to the gynecologist. The consultation is essential for any perimenopausal or postmenopausal woman who experiences the new onset of staining or abnormal bleeding, because the risk of malignancy is greatly increased. In one retrospective series, 23% of women with postmenopausal bleeding were found to have endometrial carcinoma. Dilation and curettage, generally after transvaginal ultrasound or hysteroscopy, is usually required. Patients under age 30 with an otherwise normal examination are at very low risk and need not be referred. However, risk of cancer begins to increase over age 30, necessitating consideration of referral for invasive evaluation, especially in the ovulating patient with abnormal bleeding.

When medical therapy fails to adequately control chronic bleeding, there are surgical options. By this time, most women will already have been referred to a gynecologist for invasive evaluation. They may be offered endometrial ablation or hysterectomy. The primary care provider should maintain a supportive role in the decision making, ensuring that the patient is adequately informed about the harms and benefits of surgical intervention. It is especially important that women approaching menopause appreciate that their symptoms will diminish over time with "watchful waiting" and symptomatic therapy.

A.G.M./A.H.G.

ANNOTATED BIBLIOGRAPHY

Archer DF, Lobo RA, Land HF, et al. A comparative study of transvaginal uterine ultrasound and endometrial biopsy for evaluating the endometrium of postmenopausal women taking hormone replacement therapy. Menopause 1999;6:201. (*Found endometrial thickness to be inconclusive among women taking hormone replacement therapy.*)

Barnes R, Rosenfield RL. Polycystic ovary syndrome: pathogenesis and treatment. Ann Intern Med 1989;110:386. (*Excellent review of pathophysiology; 169 references.*)

Bayer SR, DeCherney AH. Clinical manifestations and treatment of dysfunctional uterine bleeding. JAMA 1993;269:1823. (*Helpful approach to workup and symptomatic management.*)

Berga SL, Mortola JF, Girton L, et al. Neuroendocrine aberrations in women with functional hypothalamic amenorrhea. J Clin Endocrinol Metab 1989;68:301. (*The normal pattern of GnRH release is disturbed.*)

Brenner PF. Differential diagnosis of abnormal uterine bleeding. Am J Obstet Gynecol 1996;175:766. *(Well-organized review with emphasis on systemic disease as a contributor to abnormal uterine bleeding.)*

Carlson KJ, Miller BA, Fowler FJ. The Maine Women's Health Study. II. Outcomes of nonsurgical management of leiomyomas, abnormal uterine bleeding and chronic pelvic pain. Obstet Gynecol 1994;83:566. *(More than 300 women followed with nonsurgical therapy with most improving.)*

Fraser IS, McCarron G, Markham R. A preliminary study of factors influencing perception of menstrual blood loss volume. Am J Obstet Gynecol 1984;149:788. *(Finds patient reports of amount of blood loss are inaccurate.)*

Goldfarb JM, Little AB. Abnormal vaginal bleeding. N Engl J Med 1980;302:666. *(Reviews pathophysiology, diagnosis, and treatment of anovulatory bleeding.)*

Isaacs JH, Ross FH. Cytologic evaluation of the endometrium in women with postmenopausal bleeding. Am J Obstet Gynecol 1978;131:410. *(A retrospective series of 143 women with postmenopausal bleeding found endometrial carcinoma in 23%.)*

Jennings JC. Abnormal uterine bleeding. Med Clin North Am 1995; 79:1357. *(Cogent summary.)*

Shangold M, Rebar RW, Wentz AC, et al. Evaluation and management of menstrual dysfunction in athletes. JAMA 1990;263:1665. *(Useful discussion with very practical recommendations; 36 references.)*

Smith-Bindman R, Kerlikowske K, Feldstein VA, et al. Endovaginal ultrasound to exclude endometrial cancer and other abnormalities. JAMA 1998;280:1510. *(A sensitivity for cancer of 96% using a 5-mm endometrial thickness as a threshold.)*

Spencer CP, Cooper AJ, Whitehead MI. Management of abnormal uterine bleeding in women receiving hormone replacement therapy. BMJ 1997;315:37. *(Good treatment of this common dilemma including description of normal and abnormal bleeding patterns with sequential and combined regimens.)*

Weissberg SM, Dodson MG. Recurrent vaginal and cervical ulcers associated with tampon use. JAMA 1983;250:1430. *(Case reports plus review of the literature of what may be a frequent cause of minor abnormal vaginal bleeding.)*

112
Evaluation of Secondary Amenorrhea

Secondary amenorrhea is defined as cessation of menses for 3 or more months in a woman with previously normal cycles. The incidence of secondary amenorrhea is about 3% in unselected populations. The primary physician is frequently consulted by women who have missed one or more menstrual periods. Concerns about pregnancy and menopause are prominent. Knowing how to initiate an efficient workup for functional or structural abnormalities of the hypothalamic-pituitary-ovarian axis and knowing when to refer are important com-ponents of the primary care of women with this problem.

PATHOPHYSIOLOGY AND CLINICAL PRESENTATION

Amenorrhea reflects an interruption in the mechanisms of normal menstruation and may result from a disturbance at the level of the hypothalamus, pituitary, ovaries, or uterus.

Hypothalamic Amenorrhea most often results from a *functional disorder of gonadotropin-releasing hormone (GnRH) release* causing *loss of a luteinizing hormone (LH) surge* and failure to ovulate. The most profound disturbances of GnRH release may occur in the context of *marked weight loss* (less than 70% ideal, as in anorexia nervosa and other eating disorders; see Chapter 233), *severe emotional upset, or excessive exercise* (competitive athletes). Up to half of women who are competitive long distance runners experience secondary amenorrhea, believed linked to endorphin-mediated inhibition of normal GnRH release. Some weight-stable nonathletic women with functional hypothalamic amenorrhea exhibit evidence of subclinical eating disorders characterized by severe restriction of dietary fat. In patients with severe functional impairment of GnRH release, follicle-stimulating hormone (FSH) release and estrogen levels can fall so far below normal that the patient is at risk for osteopenia; *osteoporosis* may ensue if the condition goes untreated for a prolonged period of time. In addition, there is little or no endometrial proliferation, so that withdrawal bleeding does not occur upon uterine exposure to progesterone. Persons with severe functional hypothalamic amenorrhea can achieve a return of GnRH release and restoration of normal periods with correction of the underlying problem. However, the bone loss may be permanent.

Milder functional forms of impaired GnRH release are seen in the settings of *situational stress* and *mild weight loss*. In mild functional hypothalamic disease, FSH secretion continues at a low-normal level, allowing estrogen production that results in endometrial proliferation. Withdrawal bleeding occurs upon exposure to progesterone, be it endogenous or exogenous.

A host of endocrinopathies may cause amenorrhea by interfering with normal GnRH release. Excess production of *cortisol, androgens,* and *prolactin* have been linked to impairment of GnRH release. *Hypothyroidism* may present as amenorrhea by its ability to trigger prolactin secretion.

Drugs are sometimes responsible, including oral contraceptives and agents with dopaminergic activity (e.g., phenothiazines). Menses usually return within 2 months of stopping oral contraceptives, although "post-pill amenorrhea" can last up to 6 months. More prolonged amenorrhea suggests underlying pathology unrelated to oral contraceptive use.

Pituitary Pathology. Most *pituitary neoplasms* are relatively infrequent causes of amenorrhea, but *prolactinomas* are responsible for up to one fourth of cases. Excess prolactin production *inhibits normal GnRH release* and impairs gonadotropin production. The characteristic clinical picture is one of *galactorrhea, infertility,* and *amenorrhea* (see Chapter 100). As prolactin levels rise, plasma concentrations of gonadotropins and estradiol begin to fall. Early on, estrogen levels may still be sufficient to produce withdrawal bleeding upon exposure to progesterone, but eventually this ceases. Most prolactinomas are small (less than 10 mm in diameter) and designated as "*microadenomas*." Patients with microadenomas usually have otherwise normal pituitary function, whereas those with "*macroadenomas*" (more than 10 mm) may experience reduced secretion of other pituitary trophic hormones. In cases where high levels of prolactin are produced that markedly impair gonadotropin secretion, *estrogen deficiency* may ensue and put the patient at risk for *osteoporosis*. If large enough, the tumor can displace pain-sensitive neurologic structures and cause headache; impinging on the optic chiasm may result in a visual field defect. Over time, most patients with microadenomas experience a decrease in prolactin production and a return of ovulation; however, among those who become pregnant, there is approximately a 10% chance of the neoplasm enlarging. Overall, only some patients with prolactinomas suffer an increase in tumor size.

Less common pituitary lesions include *sellar tumors, postpartum pituitary necrosis* (Sheehan's syndrome)*, empty sella, and granulomatous disease* (e.g., sarcoidosis). These destructive lesions can impair functioning pituitary tissue. Growth hormone production is usually the first to suffer but usually without causing symptoms, followed by *reduced FSH and LH synthesis*, leading to amenorrhea, which may be the presenting complaint. Headache and visual field defects may follow later, as might manifestations of panhypopituitarism. In empty sella syndrome, there appears to be herniation of the arachnoid down into the sella, compressing its contents and producing a ballooning of the bony sella on x-ray. The typical patient is female, obese, multiparous, and complaining of headache. Mild hyperprolactinemia may result from loss of normal inhibition of prolactin secretion and may lead to amenorrhea.

The dopamine blocking effects of antipsychotics, notably risperidone, can increase prolactin to levels associated with amenorrhea.

Ovarian Dysfunction leading to amenorrhea is characterized by marked *elevations in LH and FSH* and *low levels of estrogen and progesterone*. In all types of ovarian failure, estrogen deficiency is marked and osteoporosis may ensue.

Normal Menopause results from depletion of ovarian follicles. As estrogen production declines, gonadotropins increase, reaching extreme levels as the serum estradiol concentration drops to less than 5% of normal (about 5 pg/mL). Early manifestations include hot flashes, anovulatory bleeding, and missed periods, followed by total cessation of periods (see Chapter 118). *Premature menopause* presents in a similar fashion, except that the patient is under the age of 40. There are no associated endocrinopathies or systemic illnesses in this *idiopathic* form of premature ovarian failure. There are no ovarian follicles on biopsy.

Polycystic Ovary Syndrome (formerly Stein-Leventhal syndrome) is an important ovarian cause of amenorrhea, characterized clinically by *hirsutism, anovulation, and oligomenorrhea or amenorrhea*. Many patients are obese and have bilaterally enlarged polycystic ovaries. Biochemical features include *elevations in free and total testosterone, reduced sex hormone-binding globulins, elevated LH levels* (without a midcycle surge), and *hyperinsulinemia*. In addition, many of these patients are *obese* and manifest *insulin resistance*, although frank diabetes mellitus is not the rule. *Infertility* occurs in about 75% of cases, hirsutism in 70%, and amenorrhea in 50%. Characteristically, both ovaries are enlarged and polycystic, although not invariably, and not all women with cystic ovaries have the hormonal syndrome. The precise pathophysiology appears to be multifactorial and remains poorly understood, but hyperinsulinemia appears to play an important role in some persons. Treatment to correct hyperinsulinemia can cause many of the biochemical features of the disease to revert toward normal and periods to resume. It is postulated that in genetically susceptible persons, hyperinsulinemia may trigger excessive ovarian production of testosterone and high levels of LH production.

Autoimmune Polyglandular Failure is associated with about one half of cases of premature ovarian failure. It may present as adrenal insufficiency and progress to ovarian, thyroid, and pancreatic endocrine dysfunction. Myasthenia gravis or pernicious anemia sometimes accompanies the condition, which is hereditary and transmitted in an autosomally recessive fashion. Cancer treatment may cause direct irreversible ovarian injury when *radiation therapy* is used (see Chapter 89) and reversible suppression in the setting of *alkylating agent chemotherapy* (see Chapter 88). Premature ovarian failure also occurs without evidence of autoimmune disease or known precipitants. Extensive *endometriosis* may compromise ovarian function, as might mumps-related *oophoritis*. *Ovarian resistance to FSH* is a rare condition, with premature ovarian follicles present on biopsy but no response to FSH. *Ovarian tumors* rarely destroy enough ovarian tissue to cause amenorrhea, but granulosa-cell tumors, which produce excess estrogen, and arrhenoblastomas, which synthesize excess androgen, may be responsible for amenorrhea.

Uterine Pathology. Endometrial scarring may occur as a consequence of radiation therapy, septic abortion, or overly vigorous curettage. Adhesions can obliterate the uterine cavity (Asherman's syndrome). Similarly, cervical trauma can result in scarring.

DIFFERENTIAL DIAGNOSIS

Table 112.1 lists the causes of secondary amenorrhea, distinguishing among hypothalamic, pituitary, ovarian, and uterine etiologies. In one representative series of patients with secondary amenorrhea, hypothalamic dysfunction accounted for 30% of cases, polycystic ovary syndrome for 30%, pituitary disease (mostly prolactinomas) for 15%, ovarian failure for 12%, and uterine problems for about 5%.

WORKUP

The first priority is to *rule out pregnancy*. History is reviewed for recent unprotected intercourse and symptoms of early pregnancy (e.g., morning sickness). Any possibility of pregnancy should lead directly to a *serum human chorionic gonadotropin (hCG) β subunit* determination. The test is the most sensitive and specific test for pregnancy, capable of providing a definitive answer rapidly and at a much earlier stage of pregnancy than is possible with urine testing for human chorionic gonadotropin. However, the *urine human chorionic gonadotropin-precipitation slide test* is more convenient and can be performed at home on a first-morning voided urine. It can achieve 90% sensitivity about 6 weeks after the last menstrual period under ideal conditions. But actual sensitivity when the urine testing is performed by patients is closer to 75%. A negative urine test requires retesting in a week or proceeding directly to serum testing. Once the question of pregnancy is settled, eval-

Table 112.1.   Important Causes of Amenorrhea

1. Hypothalamic dysfunction
   a. Mild
      1. Situational stress
      2. Dieting
      3. Concurrent illness
      4. Increased exercise
      5. Drugs (phenothiazines, oral contraceptives)
      6. Idiopathic
   b. Marked
      1. Anorexia nervosa with severe weight loss
      2. Serious emotional stress or psychopathology
      3. Serious concurrent illness
      4. Competitive long-distance running
      5. Excess androgen, prolactin, or cortisol
      6. Idiopathic
2. Pituitary disease
   a. Prolactinoma
   b. Other pituitary neoplasm
   c. Empty sella syndrome
   d. Pituitary infarction (Sheehan's syndrome)
   e. Granulomatous disease (sarcoidosis)
3. Ovarian
   a. Menopause
   b. Polycystic ovary syndrome (may have hypothalamic etiology)
   c. Premature ovarian failure (idiopathic, autoimmune disease, radiation therapy, chemotherapy, endometriosis, oophoritis)
   d. FSH resistance
4. Uterine
   a. Obliteration of uterine cavity by intrauterine scarring and synechiae formation—Asherman's syndrome (overly vigorous curettage, septic abortion, radiation)
   b. Cervical scarring with resultant os closure
5. Endocrinopathies
   a. Thyroid disease
   b. Cushing's syndrome
   c. Hyperandrogenism
6. Pregnancy

FSH; follicle-stimulating hormone.

uation for other etiologies can proceed in logical systematic fashion.

History and Physical Examination

History should begin with a detailed menstrual history and the circumstances of the amenorrhea. Age of menarche, character of normal cycles, timing of missed periods, and any prior pregnancies or abortions should be ascertained. A detailed psychosocial history may provide evidence for hypothalamic amenorrhea and should include inquiry into situational stresses (job, school, family, friends), emotional problems, excessive dieting, bulimia, marked weight loss, and heavy physical training. Nutritional imbalance including severe dietary fat restriction may be relevant. Oral contraceptive use and intake of other medications such as antipsychotics needs to be carefully reviewed.

Review of systems needs to include a check for hot flashes, skin changes of hypothyroidism (see Chapter 104), development of hirsutism, headache, visual disturbances, thyroid enlargement, breast changes or lactescent nipple discharge, increase or decrease in libido, and change in muscle mass or body habitus.

Several patterns are suggestive. Amenorrhea in the context of marked weight loss suggests anorexia nervosa (see Chapter 234). If periods were very irregular before onset of amenorrhea,

then anovulatory bleeding was probably occurring and one of its etiologies is likely (see Chapter 111). Amenorrhea accompanied by galactorrhea is strongly suggestive of hyperprolactinemia, which may be due to a prolactinoma, a destructive lesion of the sella, or hypothyroidism (see Chapter 100). A history of irregular periods since menarche in conjunction with obesity and hirsutism raises the probability of polycystic ovary syndrome. Rapid onset of amenorrhea, hirsutism, and frank virilization suggests an androgen-producing neoplasm, usually of adrenal or ovarian origin.

Physical Examination starts by taking specific note of the patient's general appearance, especially for manifestations of low body weight, marked obesity, hirsutism, virilization (see Chapter 98), and Cushing's syndrome. The integument is examined for signs of hypothyroidism (see Chapter 104) and adrenal disease. Vision is checked for visual field defects and the breasts for a lactescent nipple discharge. On pelvic examination, note should be made of any clitoromegaly, atrophy of the vaginal mucosa, scarring of the cervical os, ovarian or adnexal masses, and uterine enlargement or masses.

Laboratory Studies

When history and physical examination are unremarkable and pregnancy has been ruled out, one needs to decide whether further evaluation is indicated. An otherwise healthy-appearing young woman undergoing situational stress can be followed expectantly if only one or two periods have been missed and pregnancy has been ruled out. In patients with more prolonged amenorrhea or clinical evidence suggestive of more serious underlying pathology, an algorithmic approach is sometimes helpful (Fig. 112.1) but is best used in the context of clinical findings rather than carried out in ritualistic fashion. For example, a woman with amenorrhea and galactorrhea should proceed directly to prolactin testing rather than be subjected first to earlier steps in the algorithm.

Short Course of Progesterone. Administration of either a single 100-mg dose of *progesterone* or 5 days of oral *medroxyprogesterone* (10 mg/d), is typically the first test performed after pregnancy has been ruled out. Onset of *withdrawal bleeding* after progestin administration indicates adequacy of FSH secretion, estrogen synthesis, and uterine responsiveness but inadequate progesterone synthesis. Another way to make the same assessment is to note the pattern made by cervical mucus on a glass slide: the mucus from a patient with adequate estrogen secretion forms a fernlike pattern.

Patients with Withdrawal Bleeding in response to a progestin trial have a problem with proper LH release from the pituitary. It may be due to *mild hypothalamic dysfunction* disrupting normal GnRH release, which impairs the LH secretion necessary to trigger ovulation and ensure a functioning corpus luteum. Alternatively, the patient who exhibits withdrawal bleeding may be suffering from too much LH secretion, as seen in *polycystic ovary syndrome*. In both, there is no LH surge, but the former is characterized by too little circulating LH and the latter by too much. Serial serum *LH determinations* can help differentiate. Persistently high or high-normal levels without a midcycle surge are characteristic of polycystic disease. Low or low-normal levels that lack a midcycle surge are consistent with mild hypothalamic dysfunction.

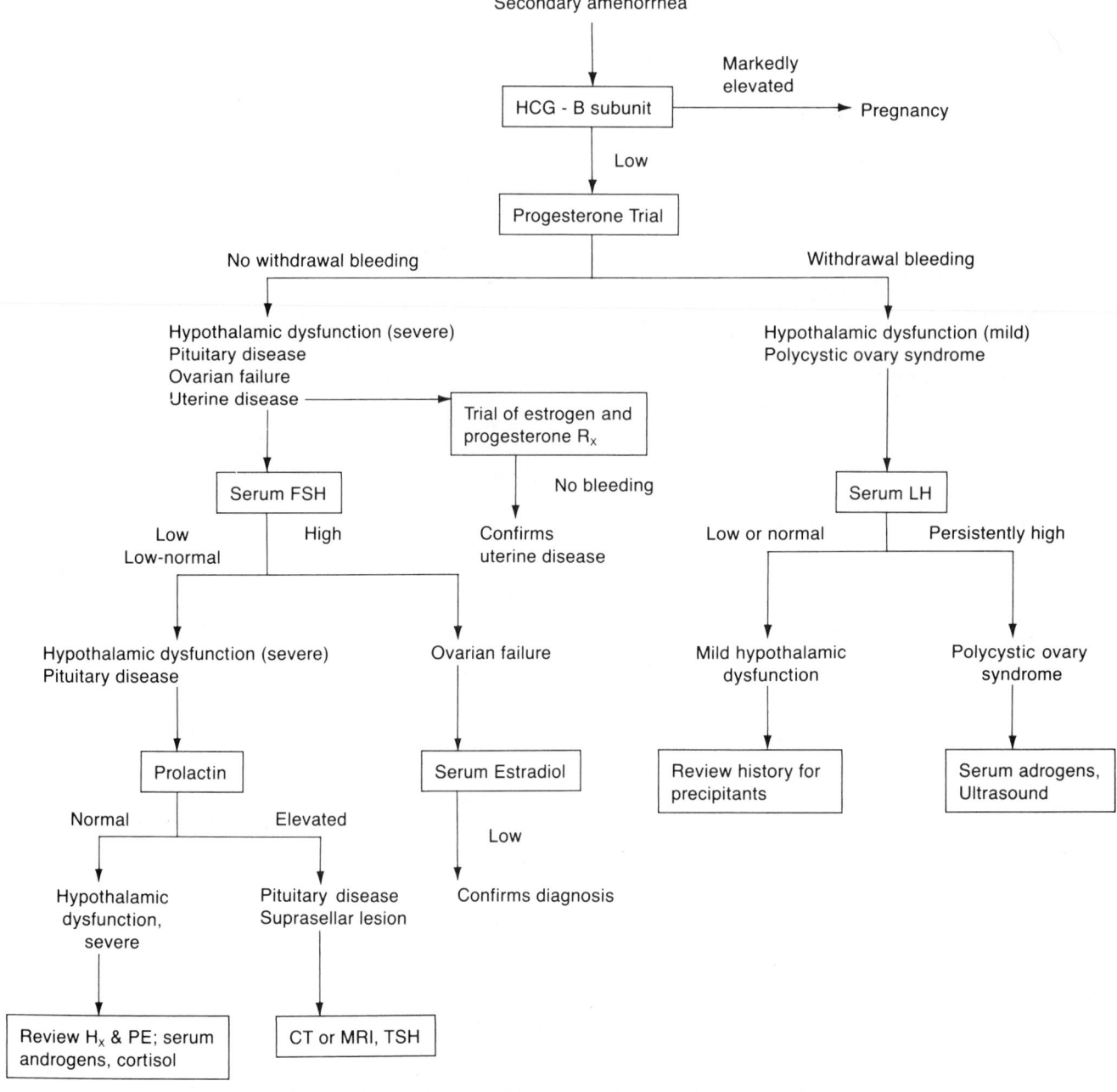

Fig. 112.1.   Initial testing of the patient with secondary amenorrhea.

The patient with withdrawal bleeding, a life-long history of menstrual irregularities, infertility, hirsutism, and an elevated LH has a high probability of polycystic ovary syndrome and is a candidate for further testing. Serum levels of *estrone, androstenedione,* and *total testosterone* may be elevated and support the diagnosis, but sometimes only the *free testosterone* level is abnormally high. The latter is a rather expensive test but may provide the only biochemical evidence of androgen excess. *Ultrasonography* for detection of enlarged polycystic ovaries can be performed for anatomic evidence of the condition, although the finding is nonspecific and its absence does not rule out the diagnosis. *Laparoscopy* and biopsy are reserved for difficult cases.

Patients Without Withdrawal Bleeding are likely to have more serious hypothalamic dysfunction, pituitary disease, or

ovarian failure. In rare instances, the cause is uterine. If uterine disease is not a serious consideration, then one can proceed directly to an *FSH determination* to differentiate ovarian from pituitary and hypothalamic etiologies. The FSH is more sensitive than the LH for this purpose.

Low or Low-Normal FSH is consistent with both severe hypothalamic dysfunction and pituitary disease. Most hypothalamic etiologies are functional and suggested by the history (e.g., competitive athletics, marked weight loss, psychiatric disturbance, anorexia nervosa). Those due to excessive production of androgen, prolactin, or cortisol are usually shown by the clinical presentation (e.g., hirsutism/virilization, galactorrhea, cushingoid appearance, respectively) and can be confirmed by serum determination of the suspected hormone (*testosterone,* *prolactin, or cortisol*). Rapid onset of hirsutism suggests a functioning ovarian or adrenal tumor, especially if accompanied by virilization and a serum testosterone in excess of 2.0 ng/mL. An overnight 1-mg dexamethasone suppression test with 8 a.m. serum cortisol remains the best screening test for Cushing's syndrome. A markedly elevated prolactin level suggests a pituitary prolactinoma.

Some authorities recommend that all amenorrheic patients should have a prolactin level obtained because of the frequency with which hyperprolactinemia is responsible for amenorrhea, even in the absence of galactorrhea. To avoid making a false-positive diagnosis of a hyperprolactinemic condition, the prolactin determination should be done with the patient off all medications known to stimulate prolactin secretion, including estrogens, phenothiazines, and reserpine. L-Dopa, nicotine, and ergotamine reduce prolactin output and may mask or blunt an elevation.

If prolactin is found elevated, then a search for pituitary and suprasellar pathology is indicated. *Computed tomography of the sella* is the most sensitive test for detection of small pituitary tumors (resolution is measured in a few millimeters). *Magnetic resonance imaging* is best for imaging larger pituitary tumors and suprasellar pathology (see Chapter 100). If an adenoma is found, it should be monitored closely if the patient becomes pregnant, because a small percentage of prolactinomas will grow.

A check for primary hypothyroidism by thyroid-stimulating hormone (TSH) determination is also indicated, because the thyrotropin-releasing hormone elevation that develops in this condition can stimulate prolactin secretion (see Chapters 100 and 104).

Elevated FSH is a strong indicator of ovarian failure, especially in the context of a four- to fivefold increase. Confirmation can be obtained by a serum *estradiol* determination. In the absence of a readily evident cause for ovarian failure (e.g., radiation therapy, chemotherapy), one should consider autoimmune disease, which is likely to involve the adrenals, thyroid, and the ovaries. Appropriate testing of these glands (*Cortrosyn stimulation* testing [see Chapter 104] and *TSH* determination in conjunction with serum *free thyroxine* [see Chapter 104]) is indicated.

Patients with No Withdrawal Bleeding but Normal FSH and Normal Estradiol are likely to have uterine pathology. History should be very suggestive (e.g., previous endometritis from abortion or delivery, vigorous curettage). Failure of a course of conjugated estrogens (1.25 mg/d for 21 days) followed by progestin (medroxyprogesterone 10 mg/d for 5 days) to induce withdrawal bleeding is strongly supportive of the diagnosis of uterine disease and necessitates gynecologic referral for further evaluation.

SYMPTOMATIC THERAPY

Mild Hypothalamic Dysfunction: Patients with Withdrawal Bleeding. Usually, patients with *mild hypothalamic amenorrhea* need only advice and reassurance (see below). Their periods are likely to return quickly once the precipitant is withdrawn (be it situational stress, dieting, or exercise). There is no immediate medical need to reestablish menstrual cycles unless the patient is uncomfortable living with the uncertainty of waiting for menstrual flow to resume or the condition is

chronic and associated with prolonged unopposed estrogen stimulation of the endometrium (a possible risk factor for endometrial cancer). In such instances, a periodic 5-day course of *medroxyprogesterone* (10 mg/d) will usually cause shedding of the proliferative endometrium and bring on withdrawal bleeding; the process can be repeated as needed on a monthly or bimonthly basis. The bimonthly program allows for detection of spontaneous remission.

Severe Hypothalamic Dysfunction. When the cause is anorexia nervosa, menses will not resume until *weight* is *restored* to 90% or more of normal. Treatment can be difficult (see Chapter 234). However, if weight begins to return to normal, GnRH secretion will revert from a prepubertal pattern to a pubertal one. Competitive athletes may have to cut down on their training program to achieve restoration of menses. They sometimes exhibit excessive weight loss and eating disorders, which may also contribute to the problem and deserve attention. Those with marked hypothalamic dysfunction due to chronic illness will have to await the resolution of their underlying illness before normal menses will resume.

When severe hypothalamic amenorrhea results in inadequate secretion of both estrogen and progesterone (as seen by absence of withdrawal bleeding after progestin administration), then *hormonal replacement therapy* should be considered to prevent osteoporosis. A typical replacement program includes *conjugated estrogens* (0.625 to 1.25 mg/d) on days 1 to 25 plus *medroxyprogesterone* (10 mg/d) starting on day 15 and continuing for 12 days. The progesterone is added to induce adequate shedding of endometrial tissue. Some authorities recommend withholding such therapy periodically (e.g., every 6 months) to see if menses have returned.

Pituitary Disease. Patients with *hyperprolactinemia* can often achieve restoration of normal GnRH release, ovulation, and menstruation with use of the dopamine agonist *bromocriptine*, which blocks excessive prolactin secretion in up to 95% of cases (see Chapter 100). More invasive treatment is reserved for patients with a pituitary tumor that threatens adjacent structures (e.g., other areas of the pituitary or the optic chiasm).

Patients with destructive pituitary lesions (Sheehan's syndrome, tumor, granulomatous disease) may require *replacement therapy*. The program should be tailored to the deficiencies detected. Estrogen and progesterone are usually necessary; thyroid hormone and adrenal steroids are less commonly required.

Ovarian Etiologies. Patients with ovarian failure should receive *estrogen/progesterone* replacement therapy. Because some forms may be reversible, a 1- to 2-month pause every year is recommended to see if there is a return of ovarian function. Premature ovarian failure and drug-induced disease are among the reversible forms.

Polycystic Ovary Syndrome. Not all women who suffer from infertility, hirsutism, or glucose intolerance require treatment. To restore ovulation and fertility, bilateral *wedge resection* of the ovaries remains a traditional approach, although benefit is usually short term only. *Clomiphene* administration and preparations of *GnRH, GnRH analogues,* and *gonadotropins* are used by fertility specialists to achieve ovulation. *Oral contraceptives* will inhibit gonadotropin release and ovarian androgen overproduction. Alternatively, *spironolactone* (50 to 150 mg/d for days 1 to 25) can be used for its ability to antagonize androgen effect without causing glandular suppression. Both finasteride and flutamide have also been used, most often to reduce hirsutism. Flutamide is more effective in this regard. Glucose intolerance and hyperinsulinism are best treated by a program of weight loss and exercise, supplemented, if necessary, by oral hypoglycemics (see Chapter 102). *Metformin*, effective for treatment of insulin resistance and hyperinsulinemia in obese diabetics, is being studied as a possible therapy for polycystic ovary syndrome. Initial studies show ability to normalize the hyperinsulinemia and most other biochemical abnormalities associated with the condition.

Uterine Disease. When the cause is granulomatous disease, treatment of the underlying disease offers the best hope for restoration of menses (see Chapters 49 and 51). Asherman's syndrome may respond to a combination of *recurettage* that severs bridging synechiae, which obliterate the uterine cavity, and *glucocorticosteroids*, which inhibit formation of new scar tissue.

PATIENT EDUCATION

Patient education occupies a central role in the management of amenorrhea. Little could be of more concern to a woman than her reproductive capacity and endocrinologic health. For the person with mild hypothalamic dysfunction, addressing fears such as pregnancy, infertility, and premature menopause and reviewing how situational stresses can lead to the amenorrhea comprise the principal means of treatment. Simple advice regarding proper degrees of exercise and dieting and how to cope with situational stresses ensure a good outcome. The competitive marathon runner with more severe hypothalamic dysfunction may care little about menses and fertility at this stage of her life, but she needs to be informed about the risk of osteoporosis and the need for hormonal replacement therapy.

Patients whose amenorrhea followed use of oral contraceptives can be reassured that they have not been rendered infertile and that normal ovulatory periods resume in more than 99% of patients by 6 months. If conception is not desired, the need for mechanical contraception should be stressed, because the incidence of spontaneous ovulation is high in functional amenorrhea.

Women in their late 30s and early 40s who become amenorrheic fear premature menopause and its consequences. Usually, such concerns are best met by prompt assessment for ovarian failure (see above) and communication of results rather than by adopting a wait-and-see approach.

Patient education is no less important when the suspected etiology is more serious (e.g., pituitary tumor, polycystic ovary syndrome, anorexia nervosa). Sometimes, such patients may rationalize their amenorrhea, ascribing it to a benign etiology, and delay proper evaluation and treatment.

INDICATIONS FOR REFERRAL

A very significant proportion of the initial amenorrhea evaluation can be effectively carried out by the primary physician. However, referral for more intensive study and treatment is indicated when there is evidence of serious anatomic disruption (e.g., uterine synechiae), neoplasm (e.g., pituitary tumor), premature ovarian failure, or marked hypothalamic dysfunction. A gynecologic endocrine consultation can be very helpful, especially in the setting of severe functional disease, hyperprolactinemia, or premature ovarian failure. Such referral is of particular importance to the woman who desires to become pregnant, because a number of therapeutic options are available. Rapid onset of hirsutism, especially if accompanied by virilization and elevations in serum androgens, suggests a functioning ovarian or adrenal tumor and necessitates prompt endocrinologic consultation. Management of a large pituitary neoplasm that threatens adjacent structures requires the advice of the endocrinologist and neurosurgeon. Patients with idiopathic hyperprolactinemia or a microadenoma (especially those desiring to become pregnant) will appreciate a gynecologic endocrine consultation for confirmation of the diagnosis, counseling, and consideration of bromocriptine therapy.

A.H.G./A.G.M.

ANNOTATED BIBLIOGRAPHY

Barnes R, Rosenfield RL. Polycystic ovary syndrome: pathogenesis and treatment. Ann Intern Med 1989;110:386. *(Excellent review of pathophysiology; 169 references.)*

Bastian LA, Nanda K, Hasselblad V, et al. Diagnostic efficiency of home pregnancy test kits. A meta-analysis. Arch Family Med 1998;7:465. *(The discriminating ability is greatly affected by the user; sensitivity falls from 0.91 to 0.75 when test is performed by actual patients.)*

Berga SL, Mortola JF, Girton L, et al. Neuroendocrine aberrations in women with functional hypothalamic amenorrhea. J Clin Endocrinol Metab 1989;68:301. *(The normal pattern of GnRH release is disturbed.)*

Biller BMK, Klibanski A. Amenorrhea and osteoporosis. Endocrinologist 1991;1:294. *(Estrogen production is reduced and bony changes may ensue in women with severe hypothalamic amenorrhea.)*

Conn PM, Crowley WF. Gonadotropin-releasing hormone and its analogues. N Engl J Med 1991;324:93. *(Useful basic science review with good clinical correlations; 180 references.)*

Davis PC, Hoffman JC Jr, Spencer T, et al. MR imaging of pituitary adenoma: CT, clinical, and surgical correlation. AJR Am J Roentgenol 1987;148:797. *(A series of 25 patients, in which MR was best for imaging large adenomas and computed tomography for detection of microadenomas.)*

Falsetti L, Gambera A, Legrenzi L, et al. Comparison of finasteride versus flutamide in the treatment of hirsutism. Eur J Endocrinol 1999;141:361. *(Both effective in women with polycystic ovary disease and idiopathic hirsutism, but flutamide is more effective.)*

Falsetti L, Scalchi S, Villani MT, et al. Premature ovarian failure. Gynecol Endocrinol 1999;13:189. *(Of 40 women studied extensively, 18 had immunologic failure and 21 were idiopathic.)*

Fries H, Nillius SJ, Pettersson F, et al. Epidemiology of secondary amenorrhea. II. A retrospective evaluation of etiology with special regard to psychogenic factors and weight loss. Am J Obstet Gynecol 1974;118:473. *(Documents relation of secondary amenorrhea to weight loss and stressful life events.)*

Kiningham RB, Apgar BS, Schwenk TL. Evaluation of amenorrhea. Am Fam Physician 1996;53:1185. *(General review.)*

Kleinberg DL, Davis JM, de Coster R, et al. Prolactin levels and adverse events in patients treated with risperidone. J Clin Psychopharmacol 1999;19:57. *(Both haloperidol and risperidone produce dose-related increases in plasma prolactin level among men and women.)*

Koppelman MC, Jaffe MJ, Rieth KG, et al. Hyperprolactinemia, amenorrhea and galactorrhea. Ann Intern Med 1984;100:115. *(Important data on the natural history of hyperprolactinemic conditions.)*

Laufer MR, Floor AE, Parsons KE, et al. Hormone testing in women with adult onset amenorrhea. Gynecol Obstet Invest 1995;40:200. *(In this series, 10% had abnormal FSH levels, 7.5% abnormal prolactin levels, and 4.2% abnormal TSH levels.)*

Loucks AB, Mortola JF, Girton L, et al. Alterations in the hypothalamic-pituitary and the hypothalamic-pituitary-adrenal axes in athletic women. J Clin Endocrinol Metab 1989;68:402. *(Heavy exercise programs can disrupt these axes and lead to amenorrhea.)*

McIver B, Romanski SA, Nippoldt TB. Evaluation and management of amenorrhea. Mayo Clin Proc 1997;72:1161. *(General review.)*

McKenna TJ. Pathogenesis and treatment of polycystic ovary syndrome. N Engl J Med 1988;318:558. *(Terse but very useful review; 54 references.)*

Melmed S, Braunstein GD, Chang RJ, et al. Pituitary tumors secreting growth hormone and prolactin. Ann Intern Med 1986;105:238. *(Comprehensive discussion of pathophysiology, diagnosis, and treatment; 167 references.)*

Nestler JE, Jakubowicz DA. Decreases in ovarian cytochrome P450c17alpha activity and serum free testosterone after reduction of insulin secretion in polycystic ovary syndrome. N Engl J Med 1996;335:617. *(By correcting hyperinsulinemia, metformin reduced ovarian cytochrome testosterone synthesis and many of the other biochemical abnormalities of polycystic disease.)*

Reindollar RH, Novak M, Tho SPT, et al. Adult onset of amenorrhea. Am J Obstet Gynecol 1986;155:531. *(A series of 262 patients, providing a useful breakdown of etiologies.)*

113
Evaluation of Breast Masses and Nipple Discharges

A solitary or dominant breast mass or an abnormal nipple discharge may be a harbinger of breast cancer, the most common malignancy among women. Because such a finding, whether discovered by the patient or by her physician, will raise legitimate fears, the primary physician must be able to proceed with deliberate speed in reaching a diagnosis that excludes carcinoma.

PATHOPHYSIOLOGY AND CLINICAL PRESENTATION

Breast Mass

Pathophysiology. A breast mass may represent proliferative changes in epithelial or mesenchymal tissue or fluid-filled cysts. The breast is a complex organ composed of epithelium that forms acini and ducts, fibrous tissue that provides support, and fat. It is exquisitely sensitive to its hormonal milieu. Estradiol stimulates proliferation of epithelial cells and accompanying increases in periductal vascularity. Progesterone induces the development of acini and opposes the mesenchymal actions of estrogens.

With each menstrual cycle, the breast exhibits its own cycle of proliferation and desquamation of duct lining. But the response of epithelium, fibrous tissue, and fat to the same hormonal stimulation is variable. Certain areas of the breast may overshoot in the monthly preparation for pregnancy, causing thickening of the breasts and lumpiness. The overgrowth may involve proliferation of fibrous tissue alone or also involve epithelial cells of the ducts and glands, leading to *fibroadenomas* or *ductal dysplasia*. Lumps can also be caused by the collection of fluids, essentially colostrum or dissolved cellular debris, which form microcysts or macrocysts.

These physiologic events may combine to produce a breast that is *fibrocystic* in quality (hence the advice by experts to drop the term *fibrocystic disease*). Fibrocystic changes can be found clinically in approximately 50% of women during their reproductive years and histologically in 90%. Most investigators believe that benign breast disease, including neoplasms such as fibroadenomas and intraductal papillomas and fibrocystic change, represents a spectrum of responses to normal hormonal stimulation rather than distinct diseases.

Although the variable response of breast tissue to physiologic proliferative and involutional hormonal stimuli is responsible for most benign masses, there are other causes. *Infection*, usually associated with duct obstruction, can result in an inflammatory mass. Redness, warmth, and tenderness are prominent features. *Mammary duct ectasia* can result in infection and yet may simulate cancer, because it can produce nipple discharge, nipple inversion, and a mass. Periareolar infection may ensue. Blunt trauma can lead to hematoma formation.

The proportion of solitary or dominant breast masses that prove to be cancers varies from 5% to 20%. It depends on the age of patients and on where in the clinical process the case series is assembled. Masses noted by either patients or primary care clinicians are often not confirmed on surgical examination. The proportion of confirmed masses that prove to be cancer is higher than the proportion of all masses brought to their attention.

Breast cancers derive from ductal or epithelium cells. They may invade immediately or grow *in situ*. Breast cancer in younger women tends to be *lobular* in pathologic appearance and multicentric but not calcifying or rapidly invading. *Ductal carcinomas* are prominent in older women. They are typically unicentric, readily calcified (producing the characteristic microcalcifications helpful in radiologic detection), and much more rapidly invasive than lobular lesions.

Growth is often associated with increasingly malignant behavior, characterized by loss of estrogen and progesterone receptors, metastasis, and more aggressive local invasion. Although metastasis can occur early, it is not an invariably early event and usually does not occur in lesions less than 1 cm in diameter (unless lymphatics have been invaded). Local growth may extend to the skin or chest wall. Axillary nodes are typically the first clinical site of spread beyond the breast.

Clinical Presentation. Cancer in the breast typically presents as a painless discrete mass. Pain is a presenting symptom in fewer than 7% of cases and is almost always accompanied by a mass. Early on, the mass may be movable; later, it can become fixed. Nipple retraction or inversion of new onset may also herald an underlying cancer. Signs of more advanced disease include skin retraction, change in breast contour, thickening or dimpling of the skin, and fixation of the mass to the chest wall. A ductal carcinoma may present as an isolated serosanguinous nipple discharge (see below).

Benign lesions may be present in a manner clinically indistinguishable from that of cancers, but a few patterns are characteristic. In *fibrocystic change*, the breasts are diffusely lumpy and fibrous in quality. One breast may be more involved than the other. An isolated cyst may also be a presentation of benign disease, but those that yield blood on aspiration or recur after aspiration may be related to a malignant process.

Nipple Discharge

A nipple discharge that is unilateral, spontaneous, and localized to one duct should be considered pathologic. Nonlactescent unilateral breast discharges may reflect local inflammatory or neoplastic lesions, most of which are benign. Benign etiologies include chronic cystic mastopathy and intraductal papilloma. Many papillomas are not palpable. Approximately 5% of women with a breast discharge have cancer. The most worrisome nipple discharge is a bloody one, which occurs in 70% to 85% of cancers that present with a nipple discharge. However, only 25% of bloody discharges prove to be due to cancer. The discharge may predate onset of a clinically detectable mass. The chance of a nipple discharge being associated with cancer increases with age. Onset of a lactescent nipple discharge (galactorrhea) in a woman who is not nursing may be a sign of a prolactinoma (see Chapter 100).

DIFFERENTIAL DIAGNOSIS

The differential diagnosis of a breast mass is confusing because of lack of agreement or standardization in clinical and pathologic terminology. The category of "fibrocystic disease" has been dropped because it does not represent a pathologic state. Among lesions that come to biopsy, the most common discretely palpable solid mass is the fibroadenoma. As many as 20% of solitary or dominant breast masses are cancers.

A serous or bloody discharge may occur with intraductal papillomas, ductal ectasia, and ductal carcinoma. In one reported series, 44% had papilloma or papillomatosis, 23% had ductal ectasia, 16% had fibrocystic changes, and only 11% had cancer.

WORKUP

Breast Mass

Physical Examination. The key finding is a *dominant nodule*. Most glandular tissue is found in the upper outer quadrant of the breast and changes with the menstrual cycle. Dominant masses are characterized by their unchanging and persistent nature throughout the cycle. Breast tenderness to examination in the absence of a dominant mass is of no pathologic significance.

Much is made of the clinical characteristics of breast masses in estimating the probability of malignant disease. Easy mobility within the breast, regular borders, and a soft or cystic feel on palpation all suggest a benign process. However, these signs are not reliable; 60% of cancers are freely movable, 40% have regular borders, and 40% feel soft or cystic. A "benign" physical finding reduces the probability of cancer no further than to approximately 10%.

The young woman with multiple nodules and diffuse thickening consistent with fibrocystic change has difficult breasts to evaluate. Reexamination at different times in the menstrual cycle is often informative and reassuring when no dominant nodule emerges. A persistent solitary or dominant nodule requires biopsy.

Examination of the lymph nodes is required in all patients with a breast lump, because it may provide important supporting evidence for a malignancy, especially if otherwise unexplained adenopathy is found in the ipsilateral axilla.

Breast Imaging. *Mammography* can be a valuable diagnostic test, especially in the woman over 30 with breast symptoms, but it must be emphasized that a negative mammogram does not obviate the need for biopsy of a clinically suspicious breast mass. Studies in which the most advanced techniques were used by the most experienced clinicians have repeatedly indicated that mammography has a false-negative rate of 8% to 10%. A mammogram should be obtained before biopsy and preoperatively for any woman undergoing breast surgery. The preoperative study can also help to delineate the mass and identify any occult lesions in the ipsilateral or contralateral breast. Mammography is used to guide needle biopsy of small lesions.

Ultrasonography can be used to differentiate a cystic from a solid palpable mass, especially in women under 30, and help guide needle aspiration. A host of improved imaging techniques are under development.

Biopsy. *Needle aspiration biopsy* of solid and cystic lesions, with cytologic examination of the material obtained, is sometimes a means to avoid open biopsy. It can be performed in the office or in the radiologic suite under the guidance of imaging techniques. Adequate specimens are obtained in about 60% to 85% of instances. Among adequate samples, sensitivity is in excess of 80% and specificity is over 99%. Negative cytology from a solid lesion does not rule out cancer. However, a cystic lesion that is successfully aspirated, cytologically negative, and nonrecurring requires only follow-up breast examination and mammography. Solid lesions that have negative or suspicious cytology and cystic lesions containing serosanguineous fluid require *excisional* biopsy. The procedure is usually done as an outpatient procedure.

Nipple Discharge

The patient should undergo a careful *breast examination* that includes careful palpation and noting if the discharge is unilateral or bilateral, spontaneous or expressible, and localized to one or many ducts. If unilateral and expressed only from a single duct, one should note the quadrant of the breast from which it seems to be coming. Guaiac testing helps to detect occult blood, and cytologic examination may sometimes reveal abnormal cells, although sensitivity is low. These measures are followed by *mammography*, looking for dilated ducts or occult masses. Patients with nipple discharge that remains unexplained (especially if bloody) requires referral to a surgeon experienced in evaluating breast disease. The risk of cancer in such patients remains real, and *ductal exploration* may be the only means of detecting an early ductal malignancy.

SYMPTOMATIC MANAGEMENT AND PATIENT EDUCATION

The woman with painful breasts associated with fibrocystic change can be reassured that the discomfort is not a sign of cancer and that symptoms usually improve with the cyclical decrease in hormonal stimulation. Moreover, it is important to emphasize that the finding is not a risk factor for breast cancer. The physiologic nature of fibrocystic changes, their extremely high prevalence, and their favorable natural history can be reviewed. Oral contraceptives provide no benefit in treatment or prevention of the condition. Commonly recommended measures include use of a support bra, Vitamin E supplements plus avoidance of chocolate and caffeinated beverages. Efficacy is variable.

The woman with a dominant breast mass or bloody discharge is more concerned with the possibility of breast cancer than with symptoms. Explaining that the likelihood of a benign etiology is still greater than that of cancer can provide a modicum of reassurance and perspective while more definitive diagnostic measures are undertaken. A prompt efficient diagnostic evaluation is the best medicine. Reassurance can be given to the patient who fears spread of cancer from breast compression (as occurs with mammography) or needle biopsy.

A.H.G./A.G.M.

ANNOTATED BIBLIOGRAPHY

Atkins H, Wolff B. Discharges from the nipple. Br J Surg 1964;51:602. *(A review of 203 cases from the Breast Clinic at Guys Hospital.)*

Beitler AL, Hurd TC, Edge SB, et al. The evaluation of palpable breast masses: common pitfalls and management guidelines. Surg Oncol 1997;6:227. *(A surgical perspective on errors of omission and commission in the early evaluation of breast masses.)*

Ernster VL. The epidemiology of benign breast disease. Epidemiol Rev 1981;3:184. *(A thoughtful review emphasizing the problem of case definition and reviewing evidence for its precipitants.)*

Evans WP. Breast masses. Appropriate evaluation. Radiol Clin North Am 1995;33:1085. *(Comprehensive review from the radiologist's perspective.)*

Gulay H, Bora S, Kilicturgay S, et al. Management of nipple discharge. J Am Coll Surg 1994;178:41. *(Extensive case series with 448 cases of nipple discharge of whom 140 proceeded to biopsy. Nearly 48% of these had intraductal papillomas; 14% had cancers.)*

London RS, Sundaram GS, Goldstein PJ. Medical management of mammary dysplasia. Obstet Gynecol 1982;59:519. *(Reviews hormonal therapy, vitamin E, and avoidance of methylxanthines.)*

Love SM, Gelman RS, Silen W. Fibrocystic "disease" of the breast—a nondisease? N Engl J Med 1982;307:1010. *(A critical review of clinical and histologic definitions of fibrocystic disease in a careful exploration of its role as a risk factor for breast cancer.)*

Morrow M, Wong S, Venta L. The evaluation of breast masses in women younger than forty years of age. Surgery 1998;124:634. *(Masses were confirmed by surgeon examination in about 30% of women referred because of a mass detected by themselves or their physicians. Carcinoma was present in 5% of each group.)*

Murad TM, Contesso G, Mouriesse H. Nipple discharge from the breast. Ann Surg 1982;195:259. *(Provides data on etiologies, prevalences, and presentations.)*

Mushlin AI. Diagnostic tests in breast cancer. Ann Intern Med 1985;103:79. *(A superb review, logical and carefully reasoned, of test characteristics with recommendations based on diagnostic probabilities. Accompanies a position statement of the American College of Physicians in the same issue.)*

Okazaki A, Hirata K, Okazaki M, et al. Nipple discharge disorders: current diagnostic management and the role of fiber-ductoscopy. Eur Radiol 1999;9:583. *(Describes both low-tech and high-tech diagnostic approaches.)*

Preece P, Baum M, Mansel R. The importance of mastalgia in operable breast cancer. Br Med J 1982;284:1299. *(Pain was the presentation in only 7% of cancers and in the absence of a mass not associated with cancer.)*

Rongione AJ, Evans BD, King KM, et al. Ductography is a useful technique in evaluation of abnormal nipple discharge. Am Surg 1996;10:785. *(Ductal abnormalities were identified in 73% of cases, most of which were explained by benign findings rather than cancer.)*

114
Evaluation of Vulvar Pruritus

Vulvar itching can be a very annoying symptom for the patient. In the genital area, only the vulvar and perineal skin have sensory receptors that trigger the sensation of itching. However, vulvar pruritus may be secondary to a vaginal infection and a vulvar dermatitis or primary skin disease. In older women, it is likely to be related to declining estrogen levels and, in rare cases, may be a manifestation of a malignancy. The primary care physician should be familiar with the appearance of inflammatory, infectious, and malignant conditions of the vulva to tailor appropriate therapy and avoid delays in the detection of carcinoma.

PATHOPHYSIOLOGY AND CLINICAL PRESENTATIONS

The most common causes of vulvar pruritus are listed in Table 114.1. Patients with vaginitis often complain of itching. In *candidal vulvovaginitis*, the vulva is erythematous, often with a sharp scalloped border demarcating the area of involvement. "Satellite" lesions are characteristic, as is the cheesy discharge of the associated vaginitis (see Chapter 117). Primary cutaneous candidiasis of the vulva can also occur without evidence of vaginitis or discharge. It is more commonly seen in women with diabetes or those who are pregnant or obese. In-

Table 114.1.   Causes of Vulvar Pruritus

Infections
 Candida
 Trichomonas
 Bacterial vaginosis
 Hidradenitis suppurativa
 Herpes simplex
 Human papillomavirus
 Dermatophytes
 Scabies

Dermatoses
 Lichen sclerosis
 Lichen simplex chronicus
 Lichen planus (erosive vaginitis)
 Psoriasis
 Seborrheic dermatitis

Low Estrogen States: Atrophic Vaginitis
 Postpartum
 Postmenopausal

Premalignant/Malignant Conditions
 Vulvar intraepithelial neoplasia
 Squamous cell carcinoma
 Adenocarcinoma

Irritants
 Contact dermatitis

tense vulvar inflammation also occurs with *trichomonal infection*, and, rarely, bacterial vaginosis may present with itching. *Hidradenitis suppurativa*, which is caused by inflammation or infection of the apocrine sweat glands in the vulva, can cause itching or burning and progress to fistula formation.

Lesions of *herpes genitalis* are caused in most cases by herpes simplex virus type 2. The lesions, which begin as vesicles and progress to ulcers, cause burning, itching, and often pain and tenderness of the vulva. Vulvar lesions caused by *human papillomavirus* (HPV), also called condyloma acuminata, are generally multifocal and appear on the labia or fourchette, causing itching and often vaginal discharge. The umbilicated lesions of *molluscum contagiosum* may also be pruritic. This infection, which is generally self-limited, is also sexually transmitted. Dermatophyte lesions (tinea cruris) are a rare cause of itching in women.

Infestation with mites or lice can cause intense pruritus. Scabies produces papular lesions and itching, which may occur in several areas on the body, including wrists, finger webs, elbows, axillae, genitals, and buttocks. *Pediculosis* is confined to areas covered by hair, because eggs are deposited on the hair shafts (see Chapter 195).

The term vulvar dystrophy has been replaced by the term *vulvar dermatoses* to describe the large group of nonneoplastic papulosquamous lesions that occur on the vulva. All of these may cause pruritus in addition to other symptoms. Any of the lesions may appear white, because they are hyperkeratotic, but less than 5% are premalignant. *Lichen sclerosis* presents as a symmetric "keyhole" pattern of pale atrophic epidermis with fine wrinkling or scaling on a whitened dermis. Chronic contact or *irritant reactions* can cause persistent scratching and lichenification (lichen simplex chronicus), which leaves the vulva thickened and furrowed. *Lichen planus*, a chronic erosive vaginitis, occurs with pruritic purple polygonal papules and

plaques ("the five Ps"). *Psoriasis* may appear as moist red plaques with a silvery scale on the labia majora. *Seborrheic dermatitis* of the vulva presents with scaling erythematous lesions of the vulva.

Atrophic vaginitis occurs in low estrogen states, including postmenopause (natural and surgical) and postpartum (see Chapter 117). The mucosa is red and thin; sometimes a mild discharge is present.

Malignancy may develop in association with dermatoses such as lichen sclerosis or with infections; vulvar intraepithelial neoplasia in association with HPV is an example. Paget's disease of the vulva, which appears as a diffuse scaling process often involving the anal region as well, is associated in 5% of cases with an underlying adenocarcinoma.

Squamous carcinoma of the vulva is the most ominous cause of vulvar pruritus, occurring primarily in older women: 70% of cases appear in women older than age 60. Delay in presentation is common; often the patient gives a history of unsuccessful trials of topical agents for symptomatic relief from itching. Squamous cell carcinoma of the vulva may present with single or multiple papules or macules, which can be confluent or discrete, usually on the labia majora or minora. The lesions can be red, white, or pigmented and may be in multiple locations on the labia. They typically arise on the vulvar skin in areas already long involved with premalignant change. Spread is to inguinal and deep pelvic nodes. Occasionally, a patient with carcinoma complains of a lump or an ulcerated lesion. Itching may be intense, sometimes in conjunction with a slightly bloody discharge.

Vulvar intraepithelial neoplasia, which occurs in younger women (mean age, 39), is akin to cervical intraepithelial neoplasia in its relationship to previous HPV infection. A certain percentage of women who have one will have the other, necessitating a full evaluation with colposcopy. However, vulvar intraepithelial neoplasia progresses to malignancy at a much slower rate than cervical intraepithelial neoplasia.

Vulvar irritation caused by scratching, maceration, and chemical agents is common. Deodorants, soaps, douching agents, bubble baths, and contraceptive foams may incite allergic reactions or chemical irritations, leading to itching. The vulva may appear erythematous, and edema or secondary excoriations may be present. The precipitant may be inadequate or overly aggressive genital hygiene. A warm moist environment, which promotes infection, can occur in patients who are obese or who wear tight-fitting pants or nylon underwear. Chafing fosters maceration of the mucosa in conjunction with the itching and scratching. Elderly women, who experience urinary incontinence, may be forced to wear pads, which can cause irritation. Younger women who shave their pubic hair are often bothered by pruritus from a secondary folliculitis.

DIFFERENTIAL DIAGNOSIS

In young women, vaginitis, pediculosis, scabies, chemical irritants, and allergic reactions are the major causes of vaginal itching. The same etiologies apply to older women, but atrophic vaginitis, dermatoses, and vulvar carcinoma also become major considerations. In any woman with a persistently pruritic vulva, the possibility of a primary dermatosis should be considered.

WORKUP

It is important to inquire about vaginal discharge, any skin rashes, urinary incontinence, vulvar lesions, and other sites of itching. Possible irritants and allergies need to be identified, such as creams, soaps, bubble baths, vaginal deodorants, douches, and contraceptive foams. The sexual history or presence of genital itching in partners or roommates may suggest infection or infestation. Information related to the duration of the problem and responses to prior treatments can be useful. Presence of an ulceration or nodule that has persisted or grown should be ascertained. Any history of HPV or herpes simplex virus–associated lesions or abnormal Papanicolaou smears should be obtained.

The vulva and perineal skin is inspected for macules, papules, scaling, erythema, ulcerations, pigmented lesions, hypopigmentation, excoriation, rash, lice, and mites. A close look at the hair shaft may reveal lice eggs (nits), which are pathognomonic of the infestation (see Chapter 195). A speculum examination helps to identify any vaginitis or discharge (see Chapter 117). Inguinal nodes should be palpated. A smear of the discharge for identification of an organism and a urinalysis for glycosuria are the major laboratory studies needed. Any suspicious lesions should be referred for biopsy.

SYMPTOMATIC MANAGEMENT, PATIENT EDUCATION, AND INDICATIONS FOR REFERRAL

The management of vulvar pruritus is most likely to be successful when a specific etiology can be identified. Self-treatments and use of potentially irritating soaps or creams should be stopped. Atrophic vaginitis responds well to a topical estrogen cream (see Chapter 118). Occasionally, an antihistamine may be used at night to relieve itching and break the itch/scratch cycle. In some cases, where the etiology is known, the short-term use of steroid creams may be beneficial to reduce inflammation. Any persistent suspicious vulvar lesions should be referred to the dermatologist or gynecologist for biopsy.

Patients should be educated about factors that contribute to persistent vulvar irritation, including excessive hygiene or moisture (secondary to tight-fitting jeans, panty hose, nylon underwear, or exercise clothes). Women should be encouraged to perform regular vulvar self-examination. They should be taught to use a hand mirror to inspect the vulva, looking for moles, changes in pigmentation, warts, ulcers, and sores.

A.G.M.

ANNOTATED BIBLIOGRAPHY

Abramov YU, Elchalel U, Abramov D, et al. Surgical treatment of vulvar lichen sclerosis: a review. Obstet Gynecol Surv 1996;51:193. *(Reviews indications for vulvectomy, cryosurgery, and laser ablation.)*

Apgar BS, Cox JT. Differentiating normal and abnormal findings of the vulva. Am Fam Physician 1996;53:1171. *(Emphasizes tendency to overdiagnose micropapillae of the inner labia or acetowhite changes of the vulva secondary to human papilloma virus infection.)*

Fischer G, Spurett B, Fischer A. The chronically symptomatic vulva: aetiology and management. Br J Obstet Gynaecol 1995;102:773. *(The most common cause was dermatitis, which occurred alone in 55% and together with evidence of HPV infection in another 9%.)*

Hatch KD. Vulvovaginal human papillomavirus infections: clinical implications and management. Am J Obstet Gynecol 1991;165:1183. *(Good review of the subject.)*

Heller DS, Randolph P, Young A, et al. A five-year experience of the Columbia Presbyterian Medical Center Cutaneous-Vulvar Service. Dermatology 1997;195:26. *(The most common presenting condition was vulvar vestibulitis at 36% followed by lichen sclerosis and vaginitis, at 19% and 15%, respectively.)*

McKay M. Vulvitis and vulvovaginitis: cutaneous considerations. Am J Obstet Gynecol 1991;165:1176. *(Good descriptive review of vulvar dermatoses and other vulvar lesions.)*

115

Medical Evaluation of Female Sexual Dysfunction

Sexual dysfunction is highly prevalent. Community-based surveys conducted in the United States and the United Kingdom indicate that the prevalence among women is greater than 40%. The problem focus may be one of the sexual pain disorders, including dyspareunia and vaginismus. Alternatively, problems may relate to the woman's level of interest in and desire for sexual activity, her physiologic and subjective level of arousal in response to sexual stimuli, or the frequency with which she achieves orgasm. These disorders of desire, arousal, and orgasm may either cause or result from difficulties in the relationship with a spouse or partner. Most women do not discuss sexual problems with their physicians. The primary care physician is often in the best position to open the dialogue, begin the evaluation, and facilitate definitive treatment of these conditions that can have a significant negative impact on quality of life when left unaddressed.

PATHOPHYSIOLOGY AND CLINICAL PRESENTATION

Dyspareunia may be the form of female sexual dysfunction most likely to be brought to the attention of the primary care clinician. Several mechanisms may be responsible for painful intercourse (Table 115.1), depending on whether the symptoms occur with initial insertion of the penis or deep penetration. Pain is experienced in the former case because of failure of lubrication or inadequate stimulation, vaginal or vulvar irritation, and structural impediments secondary to surgery, inflammation, or anatomic variants. Deep pain can arise from friction against inflamed tissue or by jarring of inflamed parametrial structures. The psychological mechanisms of dyspareunia reflect a variety of issues.

Pain on Insertion can also be caused by irritation of the vulva, which in turn is caused by multiple factors, including vulvovaginal infections (see Chapters 114 and 117). A *cyst of the Bartholin's gland duct* occurs when mechanical irritation and

Table 115-1.   Important Causes of Dyspareunia

Pain greatest on insertion	Pain greatest on deep penetration
Inadequate lubrication	Pelvic inflammatory disease
Vaginitis	Ovarian cyst
Incompletely ruptured hymen	Endometriosis
Bartholin's gland cyst	Pelvic adhesions
Stricture	Relaxation of pelvic support
Inadequate episiotomy	Uterine fibroids
Vulvovaginal atrophy	
Vulvar vestibulitis	
Pudendal neuralgia	
Vaginismus	

the attendant inflammatory reaction obstruct the ductal lumen. Thin vulvar surface and vaginal mucosa are less resilient and more susceptible to *trauma*. These vaginal changes take place in women who are anorexic, breastfeeding, or menopausal or who have had pelvic irradiation.

In premenopausal women, *inadequate lubrication*, because of insufficient foreplay, is among the most frequent causes of dyspareunia. Women who are postpartum may also experience short-term vaginal dryness and resultant dyspareunia, which can continue while they are breastfeeding. In postmenopausal patients, vaginal atrophy is the most important cause of inadequate lubrication. Finally, scant production of vaginal secretions may reflect fears about sexual intercourse or risk of infection, misunderstandings, or conflicts with a sexual partner.

Chronic vulvar vestibulitis, an uncommon cause of introital dyspareunia, is defined as pain of the vestibule on vaginal entry, associated with erythema of the vulva. The syndrome may be associated with subclinical human papillomavirus infection, recurrent candidiasis, or bacterial vaginosis and an elevated vaginal pH. A biopsy shows only chronic inflammatory changes.

Pudendal neuralgia is another cause of vulvar burning; patients with this symptom may complain of superficial burning or deep aching pain, but few have physical findings. *Vaginismus* is defined as involuntary spasm of the perineal muscles induced by an attempt at physical penetration. It is an important and treatable, though uncommon, cause of dyspareunia usually with a large psychogenic component.

Deep Dyspareunia may occur with endometriosis, ovarian cysts, adhesions, and pelvic inflammatory disease. Penile thrusting moves the entire uterus, with resultant pulling on the peritoneum. Acute or defervescing *pelvic inflammatory disease or endometritis* will produce pain even on gentle motion.

Inhibited or *hypoactive sexual desire* and *difficulty achieving orgasm* are more common than the various forms of painful intercourse. In each case, it is important to determine whether the dysfunction is primary or secondary. The physician is most likely to encounter patients with secondary dysfunction from a variety of causes. Psychological etiologies, including relationship difficulties, predominate. Systemic illnesses when present is often a major contributor.

Drug-induced decrease in sexual desire may be caused by many medications, especially antihypertensive agents and antidepressants. Selective serotonin reuptake inhibitors are associated with sexual dysfunction in 40% to 80% of men and women taking them. Problems with desire and arousal and/or orgasmic dysfunction predominate among women. Libido is a very sensitive indicator of general physical health, and any intercurrent illness (acute or chronic) will blunt it. There is no evidence that estrogen deficiency alone has an impact on libido, but androgen deficiency does; several studies suggest that small doses of testosterone may be helpful for postmenopausal women who experience loss of libido (see Chapter 118).

Secondary orgasmic dysfunction from medical causes is seen in patients who previously functioned normally. As with desire and excitement phase problems, any illness can interfere with this part of sexual activity. For example, in one study, loss of orgasmic capacity occurred in 35% of diabetic women and severity correlated with duration of the diabetes.

DIFFERENTIAL DIAGNOSIS

All the causes of dyspareunia, listed in Table 115.1, should be considered according to the age of the patient and whether there is pain on insertion or on deep penetration. Causes of problems with desire, excitement phase, and orgasm are listed in Table 115.2.

WORKUP

In the history, one needs to determine whether dyspareunia was noticed with the first experience of sexual intercourse or has developed recently, secondary to organic change or a situational problem. The patient should be asked whether pain occurs before penetration, on penetration, or only after deep penetration. It is important to establish whether the patient can insert a tampon without pain; if she can, mechanical obstruction is unlikely. A history of recent infection, previous surgery, or pelvic pathology may suggest the etiology. The clinician should take a complete history, including current and previous sexual experiences. Recent studies underscore a new awareness of the prevalence of sexual abuse, including incest, rape (including date rape), and domestic violence. It is not surprising that the patient may not be forthcoming with these experiences. Any history of sexual fears should be explored. An understanding of the patient's current sexual experience (circumstances, time spent on foreplay, etc.) and feelings toward the partner should be sensitively obtained (see Chapter 229). Sexual prob-

Table 115-2.   Secondary Causes of Sexual Dysfunction

Medical	Psychiatric
Cushing's disease	Bipolar disorder
Addison's disease	Anxiety disorder
Diabetes mellitus	Major depression
Hypopituitarism	Panic disorder
Hyperprolactinemia	Somatization disorder
Degenerative joint disease	Somatiform pain disorder
Hypothyroidism	
Multiple sclerosis	
Temporal lobe lesions	
Coronary heart disease	

lems cluster with self-reported psychological and social problems among women. Interviewing the husband or sexual partner is part of a complete evaluation and is appropriate in many cases.

The most important part of the workup is the pelvic examination. The physician inspects for signs of vulvovaginitis, atrophic vaginitis, narrowed introitus, cervicitis, and congenital abnormalities. Palpation may identify a uterine mass, a retroverted uterus, or tenderness. The cervix should be manipulated to see if pain is produced. Examination for loss of pelvic support, rectocele, or cystocele is needed. A smear should be obtained for cervical cytology to detect underlying malignancy.

A complete blood count, sedimentation rate, and cervical culture are indicated if there is evidence on physical examination suggesting pelvic inflammatory disease (see Chapter 116). Pelvic ultrasonography may be indicated to help define a suspected pelvic mass. Referral to a gynecologist for laparoscopy is indicated if endometriosis, adhesions, or an adnexal mass is under consideration.

Vaginal anatomy, measured by introital caliber, length, and vulvovaginal atrophy, does not correlate well with sexual function, including symptoms of dyspareunia and vaginal dryness. Studies of the biopsychosocial profiles of women with dyspareunia indicate that pain with intercourse is greatest among those with evident pathology on examination, including for instance vulvar vestibulitis. Psychological symptoms are no more prominent among these women than among women without dyspareunia. Women with dyspareunia who do not have evident pathologic findings are more likely to have psychological symptoms and/or relationship maladjustment.

SYMPTOMATIC MANAGEMENT, PATIENT EDUCATION, AND INDICATIONS FOR REFERRAL

The patient without organic pathology who is troubled by inadequate lubrication should be reassured and offered advice about the benefits of more prolonged foreplay or the use of a water-soluble lubricant jelly. Contraceptive creams should not be used for lubrication, because they often cause dehydration and may worsen soreness. A variety of lubricant products are available over the counter. Oral-genital foreplay, trying different positions for coitus, and guiding the man's penis for insertion are other suggestions that can be made. The postmenopausal woman with an atrophic vaginal mucosa can be given estrogen cream to use topically on an intermittent basis (see Chapter 118).

If there is an underlying vaginal or pelvic infection, it should be treated and the patient advised to refrain temporarily from intercourse (see Chapters 116 and 117). A cyst of the Bartholin's gland duct may spontaneously drain after frequent warm soaks in the bathtub, which sometimes relieves the obstruction; marsupialization by a gynecologist may be required to provide adequate drainage if the cyst is badly inflamed and infected. Patients troubled by pain from herpes simplex infection can obtain relief with use of acyclovir (see Chapter 193). Retained suture material in episiotomy scars, vulvar islands of adenosis (ectopic columnar epithelium), or nerve endings previously damaged by herpetic infection may require local excision for relief of pain.

As noted, there is little correlation between vaginal introitus caliber or other measures of vaginal anatomy and dyspareunia.

Nonetheless, the patient with an unusually narrow introitus might be referred to a gynecologist for consideration of a trial of vaginal dilators. Vaginismus may be managed by education, relaxation, and Kegel exercises, all of which are usually best accomplished by an experienced therapist or sex therapy clinic. Patients bothered by pain on deep penetration may be more comfortable lying on one side during coitus so that deep penetration is limited.

Initial failure to identify or relieve dyspareunia should prompt referral. This should be done only after a thorough evaluation has been performed, the sexual history has been elicited, any infection has been treated, advice on sexual technique has been provided, and lubricants have been tried. If there is still uncertainty about an anatomic etiology, referral to a gynecologist would be appropriate. Otherwise, referral to a psychologist or sex therapist, involving both the patient and her sexual partner, might be considered (see Chapter 229).

In a few cases where the problem focus is related primarily to desire, excitement, or orgasm, the cause may be easily identified in the primary care setting. Changes in antihypertensive or antidepressant regimens may be enough to solve the problem. When selective serotonin-reuptake inhibitors are implicated but clearly indicated, the addition of buspirone has been shown to be effective in alleviating symptoms. But for many cases, referral to a sex therapist for the patient and her partner will be indicated when medical causes have been ruled out. Small doses of testosterone has been used to increase desire in postmenopausal women. Sildenafil is being studied to assess its effects on vaginal lubrication, clitoral sensation, and orgasm. Ephedrine and oral phentolamine have also been used to treat female sexual arousal disorder. Because of the preliminary nature of this evidence and the strong interplay with psychological and relationship issues, referral is the prudent course for the primary care clinician who has not developed special expertise in this area. It is important to be aware of well-trained resources in the community. Recognition of underlying psychopathology and psychosocial distress is also essential (see Chapter 229).

A.G.M

ANNOTATED BIBLIOGRAPHY

Anonymous. Drugs that cause sexual dysfunction: an update. Med Lett Drugs Ther 1992;34:73. *(The list continues to expand.)*

Bergeron S, Binik YM, Khalife S, et al. Vulvar vestibulitis syndrome: a critical review. Clin J Pain 1997;13:27. *(Systematic literature review of the entity that is the most common cause of dyspareunia in some series of premenopausal women.)*

Dunn KM, Croft PR, Hackett GI. Sexual problems: a study of the prevalence and the need for health care in the general population. Fam Pract 1998;15:519. *(Current sexual dysfunction reported by 41% of women.)*

Dunn KM, Croft PR, Hackett GI. Association of sexual problems with social, psychological, and physical problems in men and women: a cross-sectional population survey. J Epidemiol Community Health 1999;53:144. *(Sexual problems cluster with physical problems among men and with psychological and social problems among women.)*

Glatt AE, Zinner SH, McCormack WM. The prevalence of dyspareunia. Obstet Gynecol 1990;75:433. *(Among college graduates with 10 to 20 years of sexual activity, more than 60% had dyspareunia at some time and a third had at least episodic pain chronically.)*

Kaplan SA, Reis RB, Kohn IJ, et al. Safety and efficacy of sildenafil in postmenopausal women with sexual dysfunction. Urology 1999;

53:481. (*Improvements in lubrication and clitoral sensitivity but not overall subjective response.*)

Landon M, Eriksson E, Agren H, et al. Effect of buspirone on sexual dysfunction in depressed patients treated with selective serotonin reuptake inhibitors. J Clin Psychopharmacol 1999;19:268. (*Improvement for 58% on buspirone compared with 30% on placebo.*)

Laumann EO, Paik A, Rosen RC. Sexual dysfunction in the United States: prevalence and predictors. JAMA 1999;281:1174. (*More prevalent in women at 43% than men at 31%.*)

Leiblum SR. Definition and classification of female sexual disorders. Int J Impot Res 1998;10:S104. (*Hypoactive sexual desire disorder is the most common disorder followed by orgasmic disorder, but women's dissatisfaction often stems from aspects of affection, communication, nongenital touching, and issues of attraction and passion.*)

Marinoff SC, Turner MLC. Vulvar vestibulitis syndrome: an overview. Am J Obstet Gynecol 1991;165:1228. (*Reviews evidence regarding etiology of syndrome involving pain on contact with the vestibule or on vaginal entry.*)

Meston CM, Heiman JR. Ephedrine-activated physiological sexual arousal in women. Arch Gen Psychiatry 1998;55:652. (*Significantly increased physiologic response to erotic stimuli.*)

Read S, King M, Watson J. Sexual dysfunction in primary medical care: prevalence, characteristics and detection by the general practitioner. J Public Health Med 1997;19:387. (*Prevalence among women was 42%.*)

Rosen RC, Phillips NA, Gendrano NC, et al. Oral phentolamine and female sexual arousal disorder. J Sex Marital Ther 1999;25:137. (*Mild positive effect across all measures of arousal in this pilot study.*)

116

Approach to the Patient with Menstrual or Pelvic Pain

Pelvic pain is a major source of concern and morbidity for many women. Dysmenorrhea, or painful periods, affects approximately half of menstruating women at some time, and an estimated 10% of women are significantly impaired by the problem. Acute episodes of pelvic pain are also common and may represent potentially serious pathology. The primary care physician should be able to distinguish pain of a functional nature from that due to infection or an anatomic lesion and know when referral to a gynecologist or urgent hospital admission is indicated. The generalist should also be able to initiate treatment and educate patients about the most common causes of pelvic pain.

PATHOPHYSIOLOGY AND CLINICAL PRESENTATION

The causes of pelvic pain can be organized into acute, chronic, and recurrent categories, with the latter group subdivided based on the relationship of the pain to the menstrual period (Table 116.1).

Acute Pain

Pelvic pain of acute onset may result from pelvic inflammatory disease, ectopic pregnancy, torsion of the fallopian tube or ovary, rupture of an ovarian cyst, or extrapelvic pathology such as acute appendicitis or ureteral stones.

Pelvic Inflammatory Disease (PID) usually causes little pain until the infection has spread from the cervix through the lymphatics into the parametria and fallopian tubes. This process may not occur until weeks or even months after initial exposure to an infected partner. The consequent acute salpingitis is characteristically bilateral, although one side may be more involved than the other. Peritoneal signs may occur if infected discharge escapes from the fallopian tube and soils the overlying peritoneum. Mixed microbial infection is common. Organisms commonly implicated include α streptococci, *Chlamydia trachomatis*, *Escherichia coli*, *Neisseria gonorrhea*, *Mycoplasma*, and anaerobic organisms such as *Bacteroides*.

Although epidemiologic reports of sexually transmitted diseases suggest that *N. gonorrhea* infections are decreasing in incidence, antibiotic resistance appears to be increasing. All cases of PID should be treated presumptively for penicillin-resistant *N. gonorrhea*, pending cultures. The PID associated with chlamydia appears to be less acute in onset (higher likelihood of asymptomatic cases) than that due to gonorrhea, but it is more likely to result in tubal damage and subsequent ectopic pregnancy and infertility. Because of the high prevalence of mixed infections, treatment regimens should always include coverage for *C. trachomatis* and *N. gonorrhea* (see Chapter 117).

Sequelae of PID include recurrent PID, ectopic pregnancy, infertility, and chronic pelvic or back pain. Twenty-five percent of patients with PID will have a subsequent pelvic infection. A prior episode of PID increases the risk of ectopic pregnancies 7- to 10-fold. Recurrent pelvic infections also increase the risk of infertility: one episode is associated with a 12% risk of infertility, two episodes with 35% risk, and three episodes with a risk of 75%. Pelvic infection may also result in chronic pelvic pain.

Physical examination in patients with PID is notable for purulent cervical discharge, friability of the cervix, cervical motion tenderness, or adnexal tenderness. Occasionally, there may be peritoneal signs.

Ectopic Pregnancy is a much-feared cause of acute pelvic pain because catastrophic hemorrhage can result from tubal rupture. The incidence of ectopic pregnancies in the United States from 1970 to 1987 increased from 4.5 to 16.8 per 1,000 pregnancies. The case-fatality rate, however, decreased dramatically, from 35.5 per 10,000 to 3.4 per 10,000 ectopic pregnancies. The drop in fatality rates was probably caused by improved diagnosis resulting from the sensitive radioimmunoassay for human chorionic gonadotropin (hCG), high-resolution ultrasonography, and the frequent use of laparoscopy. In most cases of ectopic pregnancy, the menses is delayed by 1 to 2 weeks, followed by recurrent spotting. Pain is generally unilateral. Severe

Table 116.1.   Important Causes of Pelvic Pain

Acute Pain
  Pelvic inflammatory disease
  Ectopic pregnancy with rupture
  Torsion of the fallopian tube, ovary, or ovarian cyst
  Ruptured ovarian cyst
  Extrapelvic disease (e.g., appendicitis)

Recurrent Pain with Menstruation
  Primary dysmenorrhea
  Secondary dysmenorrhea
    Endometriosis
    Adenomyosis
    Chronic pelvic inflammatory disease
    Intrauterine devices

Recurrent Pain Unrelated to Menstruation
  Mittelschmerz (midcycle pain)
  Leaking ovarian cysts
  Nongynecologic pathology: adhesions, IBD, functional bowel

Chronic Pain
  Benign neoplasms
  Malignancy
  Enigmatic or psychogenic pain

IBD; inflammatory bowel disease.

hemorrhage occurs in fewer than 5% of cases, causing sudden extreme pain and hypotension.

Patients with a prior history of PID, prior ectopic pregnancies, tubal surgery to enhance fertility, use of intrauterine devices, or ovulation-inducing drugs (which alter steroid hormone levels and affect tubal motility) may be predisposed to subsequent ectopic pregnancies.

Torsion of the fallopian tube with or without ovarian involvement is seen most commonly in women of reproductive age. The adnexae may be normal except for the resulting ischemia, although most cases have cysts of the ovaries. Severe, acute, unilateral pain and distension are found without an elevation of white blood cell count, fever, or increased sedimentation rate, unless complicated by ischemic necrosis. Most patients will have an adnexal mass on ultrasound.

Ovarian Cysts may spontaneously rupture or twist on their pedicles. Rupture can be associated with rapid blood loss, similar to a ruptured ectopic pregnancy. More commonly, only small amounts of fluid or blood are released, resulting in unilateral and often recurrent discomfort. Torsion of the pedicle of the cyst can cause ischemia and lead to extreme pain with acute peritoneal signs, fever, and leukocytosis.

Extrapelvic Pathology that can cause acute pelvic pain includes appendicitis, kidney stones, urinary tract infections, bleeding from a Meckel's diverticulum, intestinal obstructions, and intestinal abscesses.

Chronic or Recurrent Pain

Conditions that result in recurrent or chronic pelvic pain are generally less urgent than those responsible for acute pain. Common etiologies include primary dysmenorrhea; secondary dysmenorrhea caused by endometriosis, adenomyosis, chronic PID, and intrauterine devices (IUDs); uterine fibroids; ovarian cysts; nongynecologic pathology such as adhesions, inflamma-

tory bowel disease, or irritable bowel syndrome; and psychogenic pain.

Primary Dysmenorrhea. *Dysmenorrhea* represents the major source of recurrent pelvic pain. It is classified as "primary" when there is no pelvic pathology and "secondary" when it occurs in the setting of an underlying gynecologic problem, such as endometriosis, PID, or IUD use. Primary dysmenorrhea affects as many as 50% of postpubertal women. It occurs in ovulatory cycles, therefore beginning at the time of menarche or soon after when the cycles become regular. The pain occurs at the onset menstrual blood flow and generally lasts for 48 to 72 hours. It is generally cramping in nature and can be located in the suprapubic region, the low back, or the inner aspect of the thighs. Dysmenorrhea, which begins several years after menarche, is usually secondary to gynecologic pathology.

Menstrual pain occurs because of increased prostaglandin production and release by the endometrium, which leads to abnormal uterine muscle activity. Several studies have showed increased menstrual fluid prostaglandin levels (primarily PGF_{2a}) and increased circulating leukotriene and vasopressin levels in women with primary dysmenorrhea. High levels of these hormones lead to increased uterine tone and dysrhythmic contractions followed by reduction in uterine blood flow and ischemia. The pain may be either from the abnormal contractions, uterine ischemia, or stimulation of sensory pain fibers by the prostaglandins and bradykinin. NSAIDs, which reduce prostaglandin synthesis, are extremely effective at reducing menstrual pain.

Premenstrual Syndrome. Many physiologic changes occur during the menstrual cycle. Women who suffer from premenstrual syndrome (PMS) appear to have an *abnormal response* to the *normal hormonal changes* associated with the menstrual cycle, particularly those changes that precede the midluteal phase. The precise mechanisms by which normal hormonal changes result in symptoms are poorly understood, but their effects on *serotonergic and γ-aminobutyric acid receptors* appear to be important. For example, serotonergic activity decreases in some women with PMS during the luteal phase. Personality testing done during symptomatic periods does reveal abnormalities, but retesting at other stages of the menstrual cycle shows resolution of the changes, suggesting that psychologic factors may be a manifestation rather than a cause of the problem. PMS is thought to be pathophysiologically distinct from dysmenorrhea, unrelated to prostaglandins, and unresponsive to nonsteroidals.

Symptoms, which may seriously disrupt daily activities and impair life-style, include pelvic pain, irritability, fatigue, bloating, food cravings, headache, inability to concentrate, breast tenderness, anxiety, and depression. Onset is typically 7 to 10 days before menses commence, continues through 4 days of blood flow, and is recurrent with each cycle. The diagnosis of PMS is based on the history of symptoms and their correlation with the menstrual cycle. It is helpful to have patients keep a daily chart of their symptoms and their menses for 2 or more months to assess the pattern.

Endometriosis is presumed to be a common cause of secondary dysmenorrhea. Endometriosis is caused by the presence of functioning ectopic endometrial tissue, located in such places as the ovaries, uterosacral ligaments, cul de sac, and peritoneum. It occurs in 1% to 5% of reproductive women and approximately 30% of infertile women between ages 30 and 40. Pain from this condition can begin days or even a week before menstruation. It tends to subside with the onset of bleeding. It is usually bilateral and may radiate to the rectum or perineal region. There is frequently a history of infertility, dyspareunia, or menorrhagia. Symptoms of endometriosis depend on actively functioning endometrial tissue, with resolution at menopause. The frequency of dysmenorrhea has been found to be no different in patients with endometriosis compared with normal control subjects; however, patients with extensive endometriosis (stage III or IV by laparoscopy) were more likely to have acyclic pain. Diagnosis of endometriosis can only be made by laparoscopy or laparotomy.

Adenomyosis is caused by the presence of functioning ectopic endometrial tissue in the myometrium. It appears to be most common in women aged 41 to 50. The condition can cause menorrhagia, dysmenorrhea, and an enlarged sometimes tender uterus. Pain may be referred to the back and rectum. There is a slightly increased rate of endometrial carcinoma in patients with adenomyosis.

Chronic PID is another source of secondary dysmenorrhea. A history of previous sexually transmitted disease, dyspareunia, menstrual irregularity, backache, rectal pressure, or pelvic pain with fever is often obtained. The physical examination typically reveals tender thickened adnexae. Bilateral involvement is characteristic, although one side may predominate.

IUD are an important source of secondary dysmenorrhea. The rate of removal because of pain and bleeding ranges from 4% to 15%. Crampy menstrual pain may occur in a woman with a newly placed IUD who has never experienced dysmenorrhea. It is important to rule out concomitant PID in women with abdominal pain and an IUD.

Ovarian Cysts are usually painless unless complicated by torsion or rupture, which produces severe abdominal pain. Chronic intermittent discomfort that is worse at the time of ovulation or in the latter half of the cycle may be seen secondary to leakage of irritant contents.

Uterine Fibroids (Leiomyomas) may produce a constant chronic ache in the pelvis or back. They may also cause urinary symptoms (increased frequency and incontinence) and bleeding, particularly when they are submucosal. Significant pain and/or obstruction of the ureters is noted usually when the uterus is larger than 12 weeks gestation. Severe pelvic pain and fever, in a woman with a history of fibroids, can suggest necrosis of the tumor.

Nongynecologic Pathology may also cause chronic pelvic pain; this would include adhesions, inflammatory bowel disease, and irritable bowel syndrome. Of note, symptoms from irritable bowel syndrome such as pain, cramping, and change in bowel habits may also worsen in the second half of the menstrual cycle secondary to the effect of progestins on gastrointestinal motility.

Mittelschmerz or intermenstrual pain is not a form of dysmenorrhea, because it occurs in midcycle at the time of ovulation. It is more common on the right side than the left and may be accompanied by bleeding. There is some evidence that the ovary is the source of the blood loss. The pain, believed due to distention of the ovarian capsule, is harmless but annoying and a source of concern.

Enigmatic or Psychogenic Pain. The terms *enigmatic pain* and *psychogenic pain* are applied to chronic pelvic pain lasting more than 6 months without clear organic pathology. Approximately one third of laparoscopies performed for long-standing symptoms fail to reveal any pathology. Even when pathology is found, it is unclear whether or not it is the cause of the pain. Studies have found, for instance, that endometriosis and adhesions are as common in women without pain as in those with pain.

Numerous theories for the pain have been proposed, including pelvic vascular congestion, retrodisplacement of the uterus, and rotation of the fundus on the cervix as a universal joint (this was believed to be secondary to lacerations of the broad and cardinal ligaments from prior obstetric procedures and to cause pain because of the hypermobility of the cervix with relation to the fundus in all directions). Surgical treatments have included antefixation of a retroverted uterus, hysterectomy with or without salpingo-oophorectomy, and presacral neurectomy. Although initial reports demonstrated some success with each of these techniques, most patients continued to have pain. Studies have also reported continued symptoms in patients even with total exenteration of pelvic organs.

Because of lack of improvement with current surgical and medical regimens and the low incidence of demonstrable pathology, attention has turned to psychogenic etiologies and treatments for patients with chronic pelvic pain. Recent reports have demonstrated a significant association between a childhood history of sexual abuse and chronic pelvic pain. Women with chronic pelvic pain have also been found to have higher rates of alcohol and drug dependency, although it is unclear whether this is in response to their chronic pain.

WORKUP

In the patient with acute pain, it is important to determine the need for immediate hospitalization. Vital signs, including a rectal temperature, and postural changes in blood pressure and pulse are essential. Physical examination should determine whether there are signs of peritoneal irritation (rigidity, percussion tenderness, rebound), presence of bowel sounds, cervical motion tenderness, or abnormal masses. Laboratory evaluation should include a complete blood count, differential, sedimentation rate, urinalysis, and serum β-hCG subunit pregnancy test. Urine hCG testing is less sensitive; a negative urine hCG test within the first 6 weeks after the last menstrual period does not rule out an ectopic pregnancy. The serum hCG radioimmunoassay, on the other hand, can be positive as soon as 1 week postovulation.

Any patient with a high fever, orthostatic hypotension or tachycardia, or an acute abdomen should be sent immediately to the hospital, even before laboratory studies are available. However, even if the situation is urgent, a few historical facts can help establish the diagnosis. Important questions would include any delay in the menstrual period, dyspareunia, IUD use, shaking chills, abnormal vaginal discharge or bleeding, recent abortion, and the location and radiation of the pain. Development of generalized severe pain is a worrisome symptom, indicating possible peritoneal involvement, especially in conjunction with a rigid abdomen and absent bowel sounds. Unilateral pain suggests a local tubal or ovarian problem, whereas bilateral involvement is more indicative of PID or diffuse pelvic irritation. Symptoms of constipation, nausea, vomiting, diarrhea, flank pain, and dysuria need to be elicited to rule out nongynecologic etiologies such as appendicitis, acute pyelonephritis, or urethral stone.

If the pain is chronic or recurrent, a more detailed history should be obtained during the office visit, including the relationship of the pain to the menstrual cycle and a complete menstrual and obstetric history. Onset of pain, quality and radiation of pain, and any exacerbating or ameliorating factors should be noted. Pain due to cervical, uterine, or vaginal pathology is often referred to the low back or buttock, whereas that due to tubal or ovarian problems is generally localized to one side and referred to the medial aspect of the thigh. A detailed pelvic and rectal examination should be done to look for adnexal thickening, cervical discharge, uterine masses, fixation of any structures, ovarian masses, and focal tenderness.

Laboratory testing should include a serum hCG, complete blood count, sedimentation rate, urinalysis, and culture of the cervix and rectum for gonorrhea and chlamydia. If a mass is felt, ultrasonography (possibly with transvaginal probe) is indicated to confirm the finding, better localize the mass, and distinguish a solid from a cystic lesion. Laparoscopy or dilation and curettage may be necessary to establish the diagnosis.

TREATMENT

Acute Pelvic Pain. PID may be treated on an outpatient basis if the patient is nontoxic and reliable. Antimicrobial regimens should include coverage for *N. gonorrhea* and *C. trachomatis* (see Chapter 117). Patients and their partners should be educated about safe sexual practices and the sequelae of PID to prevent subsequent infections.

Other etiologies of severe acute pelvic pain, such as ectopic pregnancy, torsion of the fallopian tube or ovary, and ruptured ovarian cysts, are best managed by a specialist and should be referred immediately to a gynecologist.

Recurrent Pelvic Pain. *Primary dysmenorrhea* can be managed symptomatically with *NSAIDs.* Lower dose over-the-counter formulations are frequently effective. Treatment is started up to a week before expected onset of menses and continued several days into it. Oral contraceptive pills are also helpful in decreasing dysmenorrhea because they suppress ovulation. Progestins also inhibit ovulation but do not appear to be as effective at reducing pain. This may be related to their effects on prostaglandin synthesis. Patient education about the mechanism of pain during menstruation may be helpful in alleviating symptoms.

PMS is related to normal hormonal events during the menstrual cycle; therefore, there is no benefit to hormonal manipulations such as estrogen and/or progesterone supplementation. In controlled study, such supplements have not proven useful and might even worsen symptoms. However, complete ovarian hormonal suppression by use of a *gonadotropin releasing-hormone agonist* (GnRH) such as *leuprolide* will terminate symptoms in many PMS sufferers. Alternatives proven effective in randomized controlled trials and shown to dramatically reduce both the physical and psychological symptoms of PMS include the *semiselective serotonin reuptake inhibitors (SSRIs) and alprazolam (Xanax),* which act on GABA receptors. SSRIs have a more rapid onset of action than when used for depression; therapy can be limited to the luteal phase. In fact, some studies suggest that such intermittent therapy is more effective than therapy that continues through the follicular phase. There appears to be more benefit for behavioral symptoms (75% reduction) than for the physical symptoms (40% reduction). Vitamin B6 in doses up to 100 mg/d may well reduce symptoms. Though conclusions are limited by poor quality of most studies, a systematic review of randomized trials of vitamin B6 suggests an odds ratio relative to placebo of overall symptom improvement of 2.32. A randomized trial of calcium supplementation at 1,200 mg/d showed a smaller but significant effect. Symptoms were reduced by 48% compared with 30% with placebo. *Life-style changes* such as participating in regular aerobic exercise and eliminating xanthines, alcohol, and salt from the diet offer only limited improvement. PMS, unlike primary dysmenorrhea, is unresponsive to NSAID therapy.

Endometriosis will most likely be managed by specialists, because the diagnosis is made only by laparoscopy or laparotomy. However, it is important to be aware of the medications used to treat endometriosis because they can have some significant side effects. Oral contraceptive pills may be used continuously to achieve a "pseudo-pregnancy" effect on the endometrial tissue. Cessation of menstrual periods may decrease the painful symptoms. Danazol and GnRH agonists both inhibit gonadal function, leading to a pharmacologic menopause. Danazol is associated with androgenic side effects such as hirsutism, acne, and weight gain, whereas GnRH agonists typically have more hypoestrogenic side effects, such as hot flashes, osteoporosis, and vaginal dryness.

Other causes of recurrent pelvic pain, such as IUDs, uterine fibroids, and ovarian cysts, are best managed by a gynecologist. Indications for hysterectomy for uterine fibroids are substantial bleeding, significant pelvic pain or obstruction, or anemia refractory to iron replacement.

Chronic Pelvic Pain. This is best managed by a combination of psychological, behavioral, and medical treatments. Primary care physicians are in a unique position to coordinate this type of therapy. Patients with chronic pain need reassurance that further diagnostic testing is unnecessary, that the physician is not abandoning them, and that there is treatment for their suffering. Psychological therapy can help pinpoint triggers for their pain and address previous sexual trauma (if any). Behavioral therapy can help decrease pain through relaxation techniques. Self-hypnosis may also be beneficial. Because of the frequency of concomitant depression and the known beneficial effects of the tricylic antidepressant amitriptyline in patients with chronic pain, it may be useful to consider an antidepressant medication in some cases.

INDICATIONS FOR REFERRAL

Patients with pelvic pain and an acute abdomen should be sent immediately to the hospital with referral to a gynecologic surgeon. Women with a pelvic mass detected by physical examination should be referred, although it may be helpful to obtain an ultrasound before the patient's initial visit with the gynecologist. Suspicion of chronic PID, endometriosis, adenomyosis, ovarian cyst, or other condition best assessed by laparoscopy should prompt consultation with a gynecologist.

A.G.M.

ANNOTATED BIBLIOGRAPHY

ACOG. Technical bulletin. Chronic pelvic pain. Int J Gynaecol Obstet 1996;54:59. *(Comprehensive summary.)*

Bider D, Mishiach S, Dulitzky M, et al. Clinical, surgical, and pathologic findings of adnexal torsion in pregnant and nonpregnant women. Surg Gynecol Obstet 1991;173:363. *(Case series of women with adnexal torsion at laparotomy.)*

Carlson KJ, Nichols DH, Schiff I, et al. Indications for hysterectomy. N Engl J Med 1993;328:856. *(Discussion of the indications for hysterectomy including uterine leiomyomas, endometriosis, and chronic pelvic pain.)*

Coc AS. Primary dysmenorrhea. Am Fam Physician 1999;60:489. *(Reviews prevalence, quality-of-life impact, diagnosis and treatment.)*

Deuster PA, Adera T, South-Paul J. Biological, social, and behavioral factors associated with premenstrual syndrome. Arch Fam Med 1999;8:122. *(Prevalence in this community-based survey of women aged 18 to 44 was 8%; associations with exercise and perceived stress and alcohol consumption.)*

Dingfelder JR. Prostaglandin inhibitors: new treatment for an old nemesis. N Engl J Med 1982;307:746. *(An editorial examining the pathophysiology and treatment of primary dysmenorrhea, with emphasis on prostaglandins.)*

Freeman E, Rickels K, Sondheimer SJ, et al. Ineffectiveness of progesterone suppository treatment of premenstrual syndrome: a placebo-controlled, randomized, double-blind cross-over study. JAMA 1990;264:349. *(No benefit found.)*

McCormack WM. Pelvic inflammatory disease. N Engl J Med 1994;330:115. *(Excellent review of clinical characteristics, pathogenesis, and treatment.)*

Mortola JF. Premenstrual syndrome–pathophysiologic considerations. N Engl J Med 1998;338:256. *(An editorial summarizing current pathophysiologic understanding of PMS.)*

Muse KN, Cetel NS, Futterman LA, et al. The premenstrual syndrome: effects of "medical ovariectomy." N Engl J Med 1984;311:1345. *(An intriguing double-blind placebo-controlled study showing that use of an experimental GnRH agonist is effective in providing symptomatic relief.)*

Ory SJ. New options for diagnosis and treatment of ectopic pregnancy. JAMA 1992;267:534. *(Information on diagnosis and treatment options.)*

Peters AAW, et al. A randomized clinical trial to compare two different approaches in women with chronic pelvic pain. Obstet Gynecol 1991;77:740. *(Study showing the efficacy of an integrated approach to patients with chronic pelvic pain by addressing psychological, dietary, and environmental factors in addition to somatic complaints.)*

Reiter RC. Evidence-based management of chronic pelvic pain. Clin Obstet Gynecol 1998;41:422. *(Superb review.)*

Schmidt PJ, Nieman LK, Danaceau MA, et al. Differential behavioral effects of gonadal steroids in women with and in those without premenstrual syndrome. N Engl J Med 1998;338:209. *(A very clever study using GnRH agonist therapy to shut down hormonal activity and then testing the effects of shutdown and replacement therapy on symptoms. Shows that suppression of activity is the only beneficial approach.)*

Thys-Jacobs S, Starkey P, Bernstein D, et al. Calcium carbonate and the premenstrual syndrome: effects on premenstrual and menstrual symptoms. Am J Obstet Gynecol 1998;179:444. *(Calcium in a dose of 1,200 mg/day reduced symptoms by 48%; placebo reduced symptoms by 30%.)*

Trobough GE. Pelvic pain and the IUD. J Reprod Med 1977;20:167. *(A thorough review of the role of IUDs in producing pelvic pain; 36 references.)*

Walker E, et al. Relationship of chronic pelvic pain to psychiatric diagnoses and childhood sexual abuse. Am J Psychiatry 1988;145:75. *(Comparison study of women with chronic pelvic pain and women undergoing laparoscopy for infertility or tubal ligation for rates of sexual abuse, depression, alcohol, and drug use.)*

Wood SH, et al. Treatment of premenstrual syndrome with fluoxetine: a double-blind, placebo-controlled, crossover study. Obstet Gynecol 1992;80:339. *(A well-controlled study demonstrating significant reduction [62%] in both physical and psychological symptoms with fluoxetine.)*

Wyatt KM, Dimmock PW, Jones PW, et al. Efficacy of vitamin B6 in the treatment of premenstrual syndrome: systematic review. BMJ 1999;318:1375. *(Overall symptoms and depressive symptoms showed improvement.)*

Young SA, Hurt PH, Benedek DM, et al. Treatment of premenstrual dysphoric disorder with sertraline during the luteal phase: a randomized, double-blind, placebo-controlled crossover trial. J Clin Psychiatry 1998;59:76. *(Demonstrated SSRI effectiveness when limited to luteal phase.)*

117

Approach to the Patient with a Vaginal Discharge

Vaginal discharge is one of the most common reasons that women consult physicians in office practice in the United States. Vaginal infections not only are extremely prevalent but also result in considerable discomfort for symptomatic patients. Some vaginal infections put women at risk for upper genital tract disease and complications of a concurrent pregnancy. A history; a systematic examination of the vulva, vagina, and cervix; and a microscopic examination of the discharge will enable one to identify the cause in most cases and choose the appropriate therapy. Patient education can help to allay fears, encourage compliance, and reduce recurrences.

PATHOPHYSIOLOGY AND CLINICAL PRESENTATION

Normal vaginal discharge contains desquamated vaginal epithelial cells, secretions from cervical glands and from the uterus, and bacteria and bacterial products, including lactic acid. Under the microscope, the vaginal microflora of healthy asymptomatic women appear as moderate numbers of unclumped rodlike organisms. These consist of a wide variety of anaerobic and aerobic bacterial genera and species dominated by *Lactobacillus*. The pH of a normal vagina is between 3.5 and 4.1. The vaginal environment, which is in a delicate balance, is easily altered by numerous internal and external influences. The

Table 117.1.   Common Causes of Vaginal Discharge

Infectious
Bacterial vaginosis
Vulvovaginal candidiasis
Trichomonas vaginitis
Mucopurulent cervicitis (*C. trachomatis*)
Gonorrhea
Condyloma acuminata
Herpes virus type 2
Cytolytic vaginosis

Normal Discharge Secondary to Hormonal Changes
Physiologic leukorrhea (midcycle cervical mucus/postintercourse)
Atrophic vaginitis

Other
Chemical/allergic vaginitis, foreign body
Desquamative inflammatory vaginitis (erosive lichen planus)
Chronic cervicitis
Cervical ectropion
Cervical polyps
Cervical and endometrial cancer
Collagen vascular diseases

amount or quality of vaginal discharge can be affected by normal changes in the body's hormonal milieu, such as midcycle mucus production with ovulation, menstruation, or the atrophic mucosal changes that occur after menopause.

The most common cause of an abnormal discharge is infection with bacteria, yeast, or parasites (Table 117.1). Infections with organisms such as *Trichomonas vaginalis* and *Candida albicans* generally induce an inflammatory response in the vaginal wall, which is accompanied by an increased number of leukocytes in the vaginal fluid, so-called "vaginitis." The most common infection causing vaginal discharge is *bacterial vaginosis*, a condition of bacterial overgrowth in which inflammation is not a feature. Bacterial vaginosis is responsible for 40% to 50% of vaginal infection, followed closely by vulvovaginal candidiasis (20% to 25%) and finally trichomoniasis, which occurs less frequently (15% to 20%). The clinical presentation, including type, amount, and odor of discharge, depends in part on the underlying etiologic agent.

Trichomoniasis occurs in approximately 3 million women annually. Contrary to previous belief, *Trichomonas vaginalis*, a small mobile protozoan, is not part of normal vaginal flora. It is sexually transmitted and frequently occurs in the presence of other infections. It occurs in 13% to 25% of women attending gynecologic clinics and 7% to 35% of women attending clinics for sexually transmitted diseases. Sexual contact may not be the only mode of transmission. *T. vaginalis* can survive in hot tubs, tap water, and chlorinated swimming pools. The belief that *T. vaginalis* is sexually transmitted is also supported by the high prevalence (30% to 70%) in male partners of infected women and the improved cure rates of infected women whose partners are also treated. Fewer than 20% of men with *T. vaginalis* in their urine are symptomatic. A substantial percentage of women with trichomoniasis (10% to 50%) are also asymptomatic, but one third of asymptomatic infected women become symptomatic within 6 months.

Symptoms include vaginal discharge, pruritus, dyspareunia (caused by vulvar edema), dysuria, increased frequency of micturition, and abdominal pain. Physical examination generally reveals vulvar erythema and edema and, occasionally, characteristic petechial hemorrhages of the external genitalia and cervix (strawberry cervix is seen by the naked eye in only 1%

to 2% of patients). Vaginal discharge may be minimal or abundant, frothy, and foul smelling. Signs and symptoms alone are not sufficiently helpful to make the definitive diagnosis.

Candidiasis is very common in the vagina. Yeast is often recovered as a commensal organism in the vagina. In one private practice study, the incidence of candidiasis was 8.5%, and of these individuals, 25% were asymptomatic. In women with symptoms, complaints include vulvar pruritus and burning associated with a discharge. Symptoms are usually rather rapid in onset, occurring shortly before menstruation when the pH of the vagina falls. On physical examination, erythema, edema, and excoriation of the vulva are often prominent; sometimes there are pustules apparent on the skin. The discharge is typically thick, white, and adherent, often described as resembling cottage cheese.

Bacterial Vaginosis, previously referred to as gardnerella vaginitis or "nonspecific vaginitis," can be asymptomatic in up to 50% of women. The clinical picture tends to be one of mild discomfort, although in 10% to 20% of cases the vaginal burning and itching are more pronounced. Sometimes patients note a disagreeable odor. The discharge ranges from grayish to occasionally a yellow-green color. Wet mount of the discharge shows short motile rods and characteristic "*clue cells*" (vaginal epithelial cells with a stippled appearance due to the adherence of bacilli on their surfaces). The diagnosis of bacterial vaginosis is made by the presence of three of the four following criteria: vaginal pH greater than 4.5; thin, white, homogenous discharge; positive amine test; and clue cells on saline wet prep.

Several other infectious etiologies need to be considered in the differential diagnosis of a vaginal discharge. *Gonorrhea* (also covered in Chapter 137) can produce a thick, purulent, irritating discharge involving the cervix, vagina, and urethra. In *type 2 herpes virus* (discussed in Chapter 192), the infection can extend to the cervix in 75% of cases, producing ulceration, friability, and a grayish exudate in conjunction with a profuse watery discharge. *Condyloma acuminata*, genital warts caused by papillomavirus, can cause in severe cases a profuse irritating vaginal discharge (see Chapter 141). *Mucopurulent cervicitis* caused by *Chlamydia trachomatis* is characterized by a thick yellow-white discharge coming from the cervical os in conjunction with 10 or more leukocytes per microscopic field (high-power oil immersion) on Gram's stain examination. Erythema, friability, and ectocervical ulceration may occur.

Cytolytic Vaginosis is a condition thought to be caused by an overgrowth of lactobacilli and possibly other bacteria, which causes cytolysis of vaginal epithelium and a frothy white discharge. Symptoms, which usually increase during the second half of the menstrual cycle, include dyspareunia, vulvar pruritus, and dysuria. Physical examination is remarkable for the presence of white frothy discharge and a pH level between 3.5 and 4.5. The four diagnostic criteria observed on wet mount are absence of *Trichomonas*, bacterial vaginosis, and *Candida*; few leukocytes; increased lactobacilli; and cytolysis of vaginal epithelial cell. Patients with cytolytic vaginosis are frequently misdiagnosed as having chronic yeast infections and treated unsuccessfully with various antifungal medications, especially when the health care provider relies on the patient's symptoms and not on a thorough examination of the wet mount.

Atrophic Vaginitis is the most common cause of vaginal discharge in older postmenopausal women. Among postmenopausal women attending a vaginitis clinic in one study, a defined diagnosis of *T. vaginalis, C. albicans*, or bacterial vaginosis could be made in only one third. Estrogen deficiency leads to thinning of the vaginal epithelium with a decrease in the superficial layer. The vaginal pH increases to 7.0, and the potential pathogens change from those listed above to streptococci, coliform bacteria, and gut anaerobes. Symptoms include vaginal and vulvar burning and soreness, occasional bleeding or itching, and dyspareunia. External burning on urination is sometimes noted, resulting from localized irritation of raw and inflamed mucosa rather than from infection of the urinary tract. Examination of the vaginal mucosa reveals a thin erythematous surface and scant watery discharge.

Other Causes. A variety of other processes cause vaginal discharge less frequently. *Lichen planus* is an idiopathic inflammatory mucocutaneous disease that causes a desquamative vaginitis. Certain *collagen vascular diseases* can also produce a type of vaginal inflammation and discharge. *Chronic cervicitis* can result from extensive chronic cervical inflammation and has been implicated in the pathogenesis of cervical eversion, squamous metaplasia, basal cell hyperplasia, leukoplakia, polyps, and carcinoma. The discharge is thick, tenacious, and yellowish white and may be streaked with blood. Cervical inspection reveals edematous, grossly inflamed, and friable tissue. *Cervical ectropion* is found in 15% to 20% of healthy young women. It represents columnar epithelium that is found farther out on the exocervix, causing the cervix to appear granular and red. An increase in a nonirritating vaginal discharge consisting of mucus can be seen with a large ectropion.

DIFFERENTIAL DIAGNOSIS

The most common cause of an abnormal vaginal discharge in women of childbearing age is infection. If an infectious etiology is not identified, other causes must be considered, including hormonal changes, allergens, and foreign bodies. The most common irritants are intrauterine devices; condoms; spermicidal foams, jellies, and creams; deodorants; sprays; soaps; and any chemical douches. Foreign bodies include forgotten tampons, condoms, diaphragms, and intrauterine devices. Some vaginal discharge is expected after conization or cauterization. Cervical polyps and uterine fibroids and neoplasms of the vulva, vagina, uterus, ovaries, or fallopian tubes may produce abnormal discharge (Table 117.1).

WORKUP

History should include the onset of the discharge, its appearance, amount, odor (if any), and any associated symptoms. The relation of the discharge to phase of menstrual cycle, coitus, and use of medication (especially antibiotics) should be noted. Details about associated symptoms such as dysuria, pruritus, pain, dyspareunia, and skin rash provide additional information. Use of a pad or tampon can be a precipitating factor or a sign of excessive discharge. Asking the patient for a detailed sexual history will aid in understanding whether she is at particular risk for any infections. Questions should be asked about possible exposure to sexually transmitted diseases and whether the patient's partner has a complaint of penile discharge or le-

sion. Known allergies need to be reviewed in conjunction with use of spermicidal preparations and douches. Patients should be asked about use of foreign bodies and bubble baths, soaps, or genital deodorants. A history of a previous vaginal infection, diabetes, or the recent use of antibiotics or corticosteroids needs to be considered in a search for alterations in vaginal flora or host defenses. Any self-treatment should be carefully inquired about, because antifungal medication is now readily available over the counter. Women with chronic or recurrent discharge also turn to a wide range of alternative treatments, including oral and vaginal acidophilus pills, oral and vaginal yogurt, and douches with vinegar and boric acid. These self-remedies may complicate diagnosis and management.

Physical Examination begins with careful inspection of the vulva and vaginal canal for evidence of lesions, discharge, erythema, atrophy, or prolapse. During the speculum examination, the surface of the cervix should be examined carefully, looking for any lesions, erosion, erythema, or friability. The color, consistency, pH, and odor of the discharge can provide useful clues to the etiology. On bimanual examination, the provider should check for tenderness on cervical motion and for adnexal and uterine masses.

Laboratory Studies. A wet-mount examination of the discharge is simple and potentially diagnostic. A fresh sample is placed on a microscopic slide to which a drop or two of normal saline is added, and a cover slip is placed over the suspension. The pH should be tested and the slide examined before the sample dries. Although the sensitivity of the wet mount for the detection of the motile, ovoid, trichomonads is low (25%), the finding is very specific and permits immediate diagnosis. The sample pH for *Trichomonas* is usually greater than 5.0. Although Gram's and Giemsa stains show no advantage to wet mount, cultures (which have been anaerobically incubated) have a sensitivity of up to 95% for the presence of trichomonads.

Saline wet mount of patients with bacterial vaginosis characteristically show few polymorphonuclear neutrophils and many (more than 20%) clue cells. Two additional diagnostic criteria for bacterial vaginosis are a sample pH higher than 4.5 and a positive amine test (the presence of a "fishy odor" after adding potassium hydroxide [KOH] to a sample).

Adding a drop of 10% KOH to a sample of the discharge also aids in the recognition of *Candida*. The KOH dissolves most cellular material except for the filamentous hyphae and budding forms of *Candida*; the sensitivity of the test ranges from 40% to 80%. Gram's stain has an even higher sensitivity for detection of *Candida*. The vaginal pH with a candidal infection is closer to normal. Vaginal cultures for *Candida* are not routinely used but can be done on Nickerson's medium if microscopy is negative and presentation is highly suggestive of *Candida*. A wet smear of a patient's discharge that is suspected to have cytolytic vaginosis should show few leukocytes; no *Trichomonas*, clue cells, or filamentous hyphae; and an increased number of lactobacilli with evidence of epithelial cytolysis and a pH close to normal.

When other causes of vaginal discharge, such as gonorrhea and chlamydia, are being considered, a Gram's stain of the discharge can yield additional information (see Chapters 125 and 137). A Gram's stain is useful in identifying mucopurulent cer-

Table 117.2.   Treatment for Common Vaginal Infections[a]

Infection	Medication	Dose	Relative Cost
Candida	Butoconazole (Femstat)	Suppository or cream for 3–7 days	3.0 (28 g cream)
	Clotrimazole (Mycelex)		2.4 (vag. supp.)
	Miconazole (Monistat)		2.4 (vag. supp.)
	Terconazole (Terazol)		3.6 (vag. supp.)
	Nystatin	Suppository or cream for 7–14 days	1.2 (vag. supp.)
	Ketoconazole	100 mg qd up to 6 mo (for recurrent infections and pending FDA approval for acute infection)	8.0 (#20 tablets)
Bacterial vaginosis	Metronidazole	2 g PO single dose or	1.0
		500 mg PO bid for 7 days	1.6
	Metronidazole gel	Suppository bid for 5 days	3.1
	Clindamycin	300 mg PO bid for 7 days or	4.8
		2% cream bid for 7 days	4.6
Trichomonas	Metronidazole	2 g PO single dose or	1.0
		500 mg PO bid × 7 days	1.6

[a]Includes treatment of initial episodes only. For recurrent infections, see text.

FDA; Food and Drug Administration.

vicitis due to chlamydial infection, because the presence of more than 10 leukocytes per oil-immersion field distinguishes it from other types of cervicitis. Further suspicion of *chlamydia* infection can be followed up with direct immunofluorescent staining or culture.

A few other laboratory studies may be helpful. A complete blood count is indicated if pelvic pain or dysuria is present. Urinalysis should be obtained to check for pyuria and bacteriuria, especially if there is concurrent dysuria or flank pain. Women with poorly controlled and, occasionally, new-onset diabetes mellitus can present with persistent or recurrent yeast infections, and a fasting blood sugar may be useful. A Papanicolaou (Pap) smear should be done, recognizing that it may be abnormal in the presence of inflammation (see Chapter 107). In some patients with obvious infection, it may be reasonable to defer the Pap test until the vaginitis or cervicitis has been treated. However, with chronic inflammation of the cervix, Pap testing and probably colposcopy are indicated.

MANAGEMENT

Trichomonal Vaginitis. *Metronidazole* is the treatment of choice for trichomoniasis (Table 117.2). This drug is probably most effective if administered orally in a dosage of 500 mg twice daily for 7 days, with cure rates up to 95%. A one-time oral dose of 2.0 g is less effective (80% to 88%) but has better compliance rates. Efficacy for single-dose therapy is increased if the male partner is also treated. Some authorities advocate simultaneous treatment of male sexual partners in all cases; others treat the male only if the female relapses. Recommended therapy for recurrent *T. vaginalis* infections is an additional 1-week treatment with metronidazole (500 mg twice a day) and, if symptoms persist, 2 g every day for 3 to 5 days. Patients should be instructed to avoid alcohol intake while taking the drug because of its disulfiram-like effects. Other side effects include nausea and transient neutropenia. Meta-analyses have not found an association between metronidazole exposure during pregnancy and birth defects. The one-time oral dose of 2.0 g is generally recommended. For patients allergic to metronidazole, alternative but less-effective therapies include topical clotrimazole or Betadine jelly. Vinegar douches may be palliative.

Candidal Vaginitis. In considering treatment for candidal vaginitis, precipitants such as the use of broad-spectrum antibiotics, oral contraceptives, or corticosteroids or the presence of diabetes need to be addressed. First-line treatment for candidiasis for women with infrequent episodes is the use of over-the-counter preparations of topical miconazole and clotrimazole, generally for 7 days. Miconazole is also available in a more concentrated form for 3-day regimens. These agents often provide symptomatic relief within 2 days, although patients should be encouraged to complete their treatment course (3 to 7 days). The lower dose miconazole in the form of 100-mg suppositories for 7 days is usually recommended during pregnancy. Symptomatic relief of vulvar irritation can be obtained by using witch hazel compresses or cool water and recovery hastened by application of nystatin or a synthetic imidazole cream directly to the vulva.

Prescription regimens can generally be reserved for women who do not improve with the over-the-counter regimens. Terconazole (as a 0.4% cream for 7 days, a 0.8% for 3 days, or an 80-mg suppository for 3 days) may be more effective against *Candida glabrata*. One-day oral regimens include fluconazole 150 mg or itraconazole 200 mg. They are as effective as longer topical regimens, but as many as 15% of women suffer gastrointestinal side effects.

For recurrent vulvovaginal candidiasis, prophylactic treatment has been achieved with 100 mg ketoconazole each day for 6 months, but the drug is very expensive, and hepatotoxicity is a concern with such prolonged use. Fluconazole, 150 mg weekly or monthly, is an alternative with less hepatotoxicity. When infection is related to menstruation, 100-mg clotrimazole vaginal suppositories nightly for several days preceding menstruation may be effective. An alternative is 200 mg ketoconazole orally twice a day for 5 to 7 days beginning before menstruation. Because *Candida* is normally found in the gastrointestinal tract, perianal contamination is thought to be a possible cause of recurrent infections. Therefore, educating the patient about proper hygiene is important (see patient information section). Treatment of male partners is not usually recommended.

Bacterial Vaginosis. The best results for treatment of bacterial vaginosis have occurred with *metronidazole* therapy with a usual oral dose of 500 mg twice daily for 7 days. A single dose of 2 g metronidazole is also effective and is generally recommended for treatment during pregnancy. Single-dose therapy is less likely to lead to secondary yeast infections and is just as effective with initial cure rates of 80% to 90% but may be associated with higher recurrence rates than 7-day regimens. Metronidazole intravaginal *gel* 0.75% for a 5-day twice-daily treatment is equally effective with fewer systemic side effects but is more expensive than oral metronidazole regimens. This disadvantage may be mitigated by recent evidence that once-daily dosing with the gel for 5 days is as effective as twice-daily dosing. If there are contraindications or side effects to metronidazole use, oral (300 mg twice daily for 7 days) or topical (2% cream vaginally for 7 nights) *clindamycin* is an alternate. Only limited success in treatment has occurred with use of ampicillin or amoxicillin, because of β-lactamase produced by vaginal flora. Treatment of the sexual partner is not indicated.

Mucopurulent Cervicitis. This condition results from *chlamydia* and responds to *doxycycline* (100 mg twice a day for 7 days) or *erythromycin* (500 mg four times a day for 7 days), with treatment of the partner and follow-up culture 1 week after completed treatment. Ofloxacin and azithromycin are also effective but more expensive.

Cytolytic Vaginosis. This is treated with *sodium bicarbonate douches* two to three times a week and then once or twice a week as needed to increase the pH of the vagina and decrease the amount of lactobacilli. The recommended douching solution should include 30 to 60 g of sodium bicarbonate to 1 L of warm water. Commercially prepared sodium bicarbonate douches are also available.

Atrophic Vaginitis. *Estrogen cream* applied vaginally works to restore mucosal layers of squamous epithelium. Treatment is best achieved by topical use of estrogen cream for 1 to 2 weeks, followed with treatment for 1 to 2 days for occasional symptom control. Although they are less effective, oral conjugated estrogens can be prescribed (see Chapter 118).

PATIENT EDUCATION AND INDICATIONS FOR REFERRAL

Patient education is important whether the vaginal discharge is caused by normal physiologic changes, an infection, or a noninfectious process. All women should be educated about hormonal changes and their effect on the presence and appearance of normal physiologic vaginal discharge. Most infectious causes of vaginal discharge, except for bacterial vaginosis, candidiasis, and cytolytic vaginosis, are known to be sexually transmitted. Patients with discharge caused by *Trichomonas* or *Chlamydia* should be given information about the need for examination and concurrent treatment of partners and the role of barrier methods of contraception. In the prevention of these infections, women with recurrent yeast infections should be advised to avoid nylon underwear, panty hose, wet bathing suits, and tight jeans.

All patients with vaginitis, especially allergic vaginitis, should be advised to avoid douches, irritant soaps, bubble baths, and genital deodorants. Patient education about personal hygiene, including wiping from front to back after urination, is

important. Often the patient's vulvar and vaginal discomfort is relieved after a few days of treatment, yet the patient should be encouraged to complete the treatment course and to abstain from intercourse during treatment to prevent recurrence or further irritation.

Referral is needed for any patient with suspicious cervical or vaginal lesions, especially if there are erosions and ulcerations that fail to clear with treatment of a known pathogen. Colposcopy and biopsy are indicated.

A.G.M.

ANNOTATED BIBLIOGRAPHY

Caro-Paton T, Carvajal A, Martin de Diego I, et al. Is metronidazole teratogenic? A meta-analysis. Br J Clin Pharmacol 1997;44:179. *(Did not find a relationship between first-trimester exposure and birth defects.)*

Carr PL, Felsenstein D, Friedman RH. Evaluation and management of vaginitis. J Gen Intern Med 1998;13:335. *(Excellent comprehensive review with 119 references.)*

Cibley L, Cibley L. Cytolytic vaginosis. Am J Obstet Gynecol 1991; 165:1245. *(Review of a relatively unknown type of vaginosis.)*

Faro S. Bacterial vaginosis. Clin Obstet Gynecol 1991;34:582. *(Bacterial vaginosis has a significant impact on the number of office visits per year, a woman's psychosocial well-being, and the development of subsequent obstetric/gynecologic infections.)*

Hillier SL, Nugent RP, Eschenbach DA, et al. Association between bacterial vaginosis and preterm delivery of a low-birth-weight infant. N Engl J Med 1995;333:1737. *(Bacterial vaginosis confers twofold risk of first-trimester abortion. No evident effect on conception rates.)*

Horowitz B. Mycotic vulvovaginitis: a broad overview. Am J Obstet Gynecol 1991;165:1188. *(Mycotic vulvovaginitis is on the rise, especially due to varied species.)*

Kent H. Epidemiology of vaginitis. Am J Obstet Gynecol 1991; 165:1168. *(Epidemiology of candidiasis, bacterial vaginosis, and trichomoniasis in the United States and Scandinavia.)*

Krieger JN, Tam MR, Stevens CE, et al. Diagnosis of trichomoniasis. JAMA 1988;259:1223. *(Includes data on sensitivity and specificity of wet mount, cytologic study, and antibody testing.)*

Lago-Miro V, Green M, Mazur L. Comparison of different metronidazole therapeutic regimens for bacterial vaginosis. JAMA 1992;268:92. *(The 2-g oral dose as effective as any program.)*

Livengood CH, Soper DE, Sheehan KL, et al. Comparison of once-daily and twice-daily dosing of 0.75% metronidazole gel in the treatment of bacterial vaginosis. Sex Transm Dis 1999;26:137. *(Once-daily equally effective in this randomized trial.)*

McCormack WM. Pelvic inflammatory disease. N Engl J Med 1994;330:115. *(Excellent review of pathogenesis, clinical presentation, and treatment.)*

Nyirjesy P, Weitz MV, Grody MH, et al. Over-the-counter and alternative medicines in the treatment of chronic vaginal symptoms. Obstet Gynecol 1997;90:50. *(Use is common, often when specifically treatable etiologies are present and often without the physician's knowledge.)*

Ralph SG, Rutherford AJ, Wilson JD. Influence of bacterial vaginosis on conception and miscarriage in the first trimester: a cohort study. BMJ 1999;319:220. *(Infection does not decrease rate of conception but does increase first-trimester miscarriage risk.)*

Redondo-Lopez V, et al. Emerging role of lactobacilli in the control and maintenance of the vaginal bacterial microflora. Rev Infect Dis 1990;12:856. *(Interaction between Lactobacilli and other bacterial species and the maintenance of normal vaginal flora.)*

Schaaf VM, Cook RL, Sobel JD, et al. The limited value of symptoms and signs in the diagnosis of vaginal infections. Arch Intern Med 1990;150:1929. (*Discusses the limitations of signs, symptoms, and microbiologic diagnosis.*)

Sobel JD. Vaginal infections in adult women. Med Clin North Am 1990;74:1573. (*Excellent comprehensive review concentrating on bacterial vaginosis, vulvovaginal candidiasis, and trichomoniasis.*)

Spinillo A, Bernuzzi AM, Cevini C, et al. The relationship of bacterial vaginosis, *Candida* and *Trichomonas* infection to symptomatic vaginitis in postmenopausal women attending a vaginitis clinic. Maturitas 1997;27:253. (*The three common infectious etiologies were responsible for symptoms in only one third.*)

118
Approach to the Menopausal Woman

Using the generally accepted definition of menopause as a full year without menstrual flow in a previously menstruating woman, the incidence of menopause is 10% by age 38, 20% by age 43, 50% by age 48, 90% by age 54, and 100% by age 58. In addition, the prevalence of surgically induced menopause is estimated to be 25% to 30% of women in their mid-fifties. Despite its inevitability for the woman who lives through her sixth decade, menopause can be difficult in a society that ostensibly celebrates youthfulness. Although many of the emotional and physical changes blamed on menopause are not related to decreased estrogen levels, the cessation of menstruation has major symbolic significance, and, as a result, many symptoms and complaints are attributed to it. Hormone replacement therapy (HRT) is very effective in dealing with the specific symptoms of estrogen deficiency and confers disease-prevention benefits, particularly for prophylaxis of osteoporosis and cardiovascular disease. But HRT also involves potential harm, including an increased risk of cancer in some women. The primary care physician can do a great deal to help women cope with menopause and make informed choices regarding options for symptom relief and disease prevention.

PHYSIOLOGY AND CLINICAL PRESENTATION

The essential cause of menopause is decreased estrogen due to decreased responsiveness to follicle-stimulating hormone in aging ovaries. This results in cessation of menses and increase in gonadotropins. Some estrogen production continues, but its source is primarily peripheral conversion of androstenedione. The diagnosis of menopause is confirmed by a marked increase in the gonadotropins; maximum levels of follicle-stimulating hormone and luteinizing hormone occur within 1 to 2 years of onset and remain high for 10 to 15 years. The physiologic events are similar in surgically induced menopause, but the time course is shorter, with follicle-stimulating hormone and luteinizing hormone rising to high levels within 20 to 30 days. Approximately 25% of women do not experience any symptoms, perhaps because of nonovarian sources of estrogen production.

Hot Flashes, associated with the rate of estrogen withdrawal and resultant vasomotor instability, are among the most specific of menopausal symptoms. An uncomfortably warm sensation radiates upward from the chest to neck and face and lasts seconds to a few minutes before subsiding. Skin temperature generally increases by about 2.5°C. The response is thought to be triggered by a hypothalamic mechanism related to catecholamine metabolism. Eating, exertion, emotional upset, and alcohol are known precipitants. As many as 20 episodes per day may occur; in most patients, the condition lasts for 2 to 3 years, but it may continue for 6 years or more. Prevalence of severe disabling hot flashes ranges from 10% to 35% of menopausal women. No link between emotional makeup and symptoms has been shown, though it is clear that the flashes can be the cause of considerable morbidity.

Atrophy of the Vaginal and Vulvar Epithelium with Associated Sexual Dysfunction is another important manifestation of estrogen decline. The vagina becomes smaller and less compliant; lubrication decreases. Women may present with complaints of itching, discharge, bleeding, or painful intercourse. The uterus becomes smaller, but this causes no symptoms. Of interest is the finding that sexually active women show less vaginal atrophy. Whether this is a cause or effect is unclear. Some women experience a decrease in libido and/or increased difficulty in achieving orgasm after menopause. Again the relationship to estrogen decline is unclear. The little evidence that is available suggests that estrogen replacement is not effective but that addition of low doses of androgens may be helpful. The atrophic effects of estrogen decline extend to the urethra and perineal bacteria colonize the area, increasing the risk of urethritis and dysuria.

Sleep Disturbances occur in many menopausal women. Some are associated with nocturnal hot flashes. In addition, abnormalities in the sleep pattern, with decrease in rapid-eye-movement sleep, have been documented independent of hot flashes.

Cardiovascular Disease is the leading cause of mortality among postmenopausal women. Among other cardiovascular effects, the loss of estrogen causes an unfavorable change in lipoprotein profile. Estrogens increase high-density-lipoprotein cholesterol and decrease low-density-lipoprotein cholesterol. For women, the increase in heart disease risk with age is mediated in part by decreasing estrogen levels at menopause. The risk of heart disease increases substantially in the postmenopausal years.

Osteoporosis represents an important consequence of estrogen decline; decreased activity, inadequate nutrition, and the aging process also contribute, to varying degrees. Although irreversible by HRT, osteoporosis can be prevented by prophylactic administration of estrogen at the onset of menopause (see below and Chapter 164). Risk factors for postmenopausal osteoporotic fractures include thin body build, premature surgical menopause, cigarette smoking, and heavy alcohol use. Prolonged bedrest is a potent stimulus of osteoporosis. Long-acting benzodiazepines, anticonvulsants, caffeine, and impaired visual function are other risk factors for hip fracture.

Other Symptoms, such as *headache, nervousness, and depression,* which frequently occur during the climacteric, are more a reflection of the emotional stress that may be associated with this stage of life rather than a result of a change in hormonal milieu. Some women report feeling better emotionally on estrogen therapy, but this may represent a placebo effect. No specific psychiatric problems have been found to be linked specifically to menopause. Women who experience a prolonged symptomatic perimenopausal phase may exhibit some depressive symptoms, but depression is not a consequence of the menopause itself.

Cosmetic Changes associated with aging have been attributed by some to a decrease in estrogens, but clinical evidence is to the contrary. Breast atrophy, loss of skin turgor, and redistribution of fat to the abdomen and thighs have not been shown to be influenced by estrogen therapy and most likely are part of the more general process of aging.

PRINCIPLES OF MANAGEMENT

Short-term objectives are to alleviate any bothersome symptoms that result from estrogen deficiency and to provide support for any emotional and functional problems that may accompany this phase of life. The use of HRT to prevent disease and thereby extend and improve the quality of life is also an important consideration. Relatively short-term therapy suffices for symptom relief. A minimum of 10 to 20 years of HRT is often necessary when prevention is the goal. In either case, benefit and harm will vary for different women and must be assessed with attention to the individual's risk factors and personal preferences. Nonhormonal approaches also exist and provide women with a choice of options for dealing with menopausal changes.

Hormone Replacement Therapy

Because much of the medical morbidity of menopause, including symptoms such as hot flashes and vaginal dryness, relate to estrogen deficiency, the clinician and patient are faced with the difficult decision of when to use HRT. This necessitates careful consideration of benefits and risks.

Benefits of Hormone Replacement Therapy. The benefits range from symptom relief to prevention of major causes of morbidity and mortality.

Resolution of Hot Flashes. Hot flashes severe enough to be a serious bother to the patient are an important indication for estrogen replacement. In most instances, the symptoms are self-limited, but relief during the year or two that symptoms are most severe can mean much and is one of the principal benefits of treatment for symptomatic women. HRT is effective in the vast majority of cases, although it may take several weeks to achieve relief.

Reversal of Atrophic Vaginitis. Atrophic vaginitis responds well to both topical and oral administration of estrogen. Even when vaginal creams are used, systemic estrogen absorption does take place and risks of adverse estrogen effects must still

be considered a possibility, though probably to a lesser degree than with the use of systemic therapy. Milder symptoms (e.g., mild dryness with intercourse) may respond well to use of a water-soluble vaginal lubricant and obviate the need for estrogen in the woman who wants to avoid its use. Resolution of atrophic vaginitis decreases frequency of urinary tract infections as the mucosal barrier is reestablished.

Improvement of Sleep Disorders. Sleep disorders may improve with estrogen replacement. Increases in the rate of rapid-eye-movement sleep have been documented, regardless of whether or not hot flashes have been experienced.

Prevention of Postmenopausal Osteoporosis. Osteoporosis can be prevented by long-term prophylactic estrogen therapy. Controlled studies have shown that rates of vertebral, wrist, and hip fractures can be reduced very significantly by estrogen replacement and that this protective effect is not impaired by addition of progestin. The risk of hip fracture is reduced by 25% in women who have used estrogen in the past and to an even greater extent among current and recent users.

Because the rate of bone loss is greatest in the early postmenopausal years, it has been argued that prophylactic therapy should start no later than 5 years after onset of menopause and ideally in the perimenopausal period. However, there is also evidence that the benefit of HRT in reducing risk of fractures is lost at some point after cessation of therapy. Because baseline risk of fracture increases with age, those who choose to limit duration of HRT to minimize any increased risk of breast cancer (see below) might reasonably start therapy later rather than sooner.

For women willing to accept the increased risk of breast cancer and other possible risks associated with very prolonged HRT use (see below), the combination of estrogen therapy in conjunction with exercise and dietary calcium supplementation offers one of the best options for prevention of postmenopausal osteoporosis (see Chapter 164). Women who are reluctant to take HRT should be strongly encouraged to engage in regular weight-bearing exercise and maintain adequate calcium intake (see below). These measures can slow osteoporotic changes but not as effectively as estrogen. Women who are reluctant to take HRT and who are at particular risk for osteoporosis should be encouraged to consider additional approaches to prevention of osteoporosis such as alendronate or raloxifene (see Chapter 164).

Reduction in Risk of Cardiovascular Disease. Observational studies indicate that morbidity and mortality are markedly reduced by HRT. Relative risk of cardiovascular mortality among women who are current users of HRT compared with those who have never used HRT ranges from 0.50 to 0.89. Benefit is greatest for women with multiple cardiovascular risk factors. A randomized trial among women with established cardiovascular disease suggests that HRT may increase coronary events during the first year, after which there seems to be a reduction in the rate of new events. It has been hypothesized that the early increased risk can be explained by the thrombogenic effect of estrogen (see below) in women with established coronary disease and that the later reduction in risk is a result of reduced progression of atherosclerosis. Compared with control subjects, women taking HRT in the Postmenopausal Estrogen/Progestin Intervention (PEPI) trial had an early increase in concentration of inflammation-sensitive proteins, suggesting another explanatory hypothesis for early adverse events. A 10% to 50% reduction in mortality would be extremely important on a population basis because coronary heart disease is the leading cause of death among postmenopausal women. Studies designed to reduce our uncertainty about HRT effects in primary prevention of cardiovascular disease are currently in progress.

Other Benefits of Hormone Replacement Therapy. Accumulating evidence suggests that HRT reduces risk of colorectal cancer. In the Nurses' Health Study, the relative risk of colorectal cancer among current hormone users was 0.65 (95% confidence interval, 0.50 to 0.83). A meta-analysis confirms this finding and suggests a relative risk of 0.80 for women who have ever used HRT. There is also suggestive evidence that women who use estrogens are also at lower risk of Alzheimer's disease, with a risk reduction of as much as 50% in some groups. Finally, hormone replacement may prevent the decrease in wound healing that occurs in postmenopausal women.

Risks of Hormone Replacement Therapy. Although relief of symptoms and disease prevention benefits have been clearly documented, so have risks of HRT.

Endometrial Cancer. This is the major risk associated with use of unopposed systemic estrogen. More than 35 epidemiologic studies have evaluated the association between estrogen replacement therapy and endometrial cancer, and the vast majority have found a significant and substantial increase in risk. Relative risk of endometrial cancer among estrogen users has been estimated to be as low as 2 and as high as 15. Risk increases with dosage and duration of estrogen use. Pooled relative risk estimates range from 2.31 for women who have ever used exogenous estrogens to 8.22 for those taking them for 8 or more years, including some who were using doses higher than those used today. For women taking 0.625 mg for at least 5 years, risk is increased fourfold.

Estrogens cause cystic hyperplasia of the endometrium, a premalignant condition. Prolonged continuous use causes excessive stimulation, leading to malignant change. Fortunately, the tumors induced by estrogen therapy in postmenopausal women tend to be of low grade and in early stages when detected. Progestins prevent the development of endometrial hyperplasia that is otherwise associated with unopposed estrogen use. The incidence of atypical or adenomatous endometrial hyperplasia decreases from 35% to 1% with progestin use. At least five studies have examined the effect of estrogen plus progestin therapy on endometrial cancer risk, and none found a significant increase.

Breast Cancer. After considerable uncertainty, it now seems that risk of developing breast cancer increases significantly with duration of exposure to estrogen replacement therapy. The addition of progestin confers no protective effect. Previous analytic studies found a history of any estrogen use produced little increase in relative risk (estimate, 1.01). However, as confirmed in the Nurses' Health Study, the relative risk of developing breast cancer is a function of duration of treatment and ranged from 1.09 to 1.46. There was a 43% increase in deaths from breast cancer in patients who took HRT for more than 10 years. Pooled estimates of relative risk for women who have used estrogen for 8 to 15 years have been in the 1.25 to 1.30 range. Duration of therapy less than 5 years does not appear to cause a significant increase in breast cancer risk. It has

been suggested that HRT increases risk of breast cancers that have more favorable prognoses.

Other Adverse Effects. Other effects of exogenous estrogen include *fluid retention, blood pressure elevation, gallstones* (due to a change in bile cholesterol content), *glucose intolerance,* and *headaches.* Often there is *recurrent uterine bleeding,* especially with cyclic progesterone use (see below). This bleeding can complicate clinical recognition of endometrial cancer and cause inconvenience and concern. There appears to be a threefold increased risk of thromboembolism among menopausal women on estrogen replacement, but the absolute risk remains very low for women who are otherwise healthy and active. A history of thromboembolism is a relative contraindication to estrogen use. In the Nurses' Health Study, estrogen replacement has been associated with a twofold increase in risk of *systemic lupus erythematosus*, but the absolute risk is very low.

Specific Treatment Regimens. HRT regimens have evolved over the years to reduce risks, side effects, and inconvenience without compromising efficacy. Progestin use has nullified the endometrial cancer risk and can eliminate cyclic bleeding without any apparent loss in benefit from estrogen replacement or increase in other risks. Because clinical benefits and adverse effects of HRT are a function of dose and duration of therapy, it is important to pay considerable attention to design of the treatment regimen.

Dosing. The established dose of conjugated estrogens (Premarin) necessary to prevent osteoporosis and capable of reducing cardiovascular risk is 0.625 mg daily. Lower doses (e.g., 0.3 mg or the equivalent) often suffice to control hot flashes, but as much as 2.5 mg/d may be necessary. Symptomatic atrophic vaginitis may be treated with vaginal estrogen cream, 1 g every 2 to 3 days, but this is not effective for osteoporosis prophylaxis. Progestin doses of 2.5 to 10.0 mg/d of medroxyprogesterone (Provera) are required to induce either endometrial atrophy when used continuously or endometrial shedding when used cyclically.

Oral Regimens. Three approaches to oral hormone replacement are commonly used.

1. *Continuous estrogen with cyclic progesterone* was the first estrogen/progesterone replacement program designed for postmenopausal women with an intact uterus. The rationale for cyclic progesterone is to produce endometrial shedding so as to avoid continuous endometrial proliferative stimulation. A typical program is 0.625 mg conjugated estrogens (Premarin) daily with 10 mg of medroxyprogesterone acetate (Provera) for 10 to 14 consecutive days each month. Lower doses of Provera (5 mg) may be substituted. In the PEPI trial, cyclic micronized progesterone (200 mg daily for 12 days each month) had a more favorable impact on high-density-lipoprotein cholesterol than cyclic Provera. Disadvantages of this regimen include periodic bleeding and the difficulty in telling if the bleeding is a sign of underlying endometrial pathology.

2. *Continuous estrogen with continuous progesterone* has surpassed the cyclic progesterone program in popularity among women with an intact uterus because it does not result in cyclic bleeding. The advantage of this regimen

is induction of endometrial atrophy and eventual cessation of uterine bleeding. Long-term safety is yet to be established but appears similar to the cyclic progesterone regimen. A standard daily regimen consists of 0.625 mg of conjugated estrogen daily plus 2.5 to 5.0 mg of medroxyprogesterone. The proper progesterone dose is that which results in full cessation of vaginal bleeding. This is program is taken continuously.

3. *Continuous unopposed estrogen* is best reserved for postmenopausal women without a uterus. Unopposed estrogen (i.e., 0.625 mg of conjugated estrogens) is taken daily. The practice of interrupting estrogen dosing for 5 to 7 days confers no additional advantages. Moreover, cyclic estrogen therapy does not reduce rates of endometrial hyperplasia or endometrial cancer in women with an intact uterus. Consequently, unopposed estrogen is not recommended for women with a uterus. Moreover, its use in such women necessitates special monitoring for development of endometrial cancer (see below).

Transdermal Estrogen is also an option. A 50-mg patch applied twice each week produces estradiol levels similar to those resulting from oral doses of 0.625 mg of Premarin daily. This approach might make most sense for the woman without a uterus who has no need for progestins. Cost is increased and beneficial effect on lipoproteins may be less than with oral therapy.

Topical Estrogen is effective for atrophic vaginitis causing dysuria or dyspareunia. Symptoms will respond to topically applied estrogen cream used as seldom as once or twice a week. Systemic absorption occurs, and there is concern about localized endometrial stimulation with prolonged daily use, but limited use on a short-term basis is probably safe.

Duration of Therapy. At present, there is much uncertainty about the optimal duration of HRT. Programs for symptomatic relief are usually short term (1 to 2 years) and self-limited. However, to achieve durable prophylactic benefits requires prolonged use, which may increase cancer risk. Significant reductions in risk of osteoporotic disease might require initiation of HRT therapy at the onset of menopause and continuation indefinitely. After several years of cessation, there is little demonstrable benefit to having taken HRT (see Chapter 164). The same holds true for prophylaxis of cardiovascular disease. However, as the Nurses' Health Study points out, mortality risk from breast cancer increases markedly with prolonged continuous use (more than 10 years). Treatment duration of less than 5 years does not seem to significantly increase breast cancer risk.

Perhaps a mixed approach to prophylaxis will prove the safest, using both HRT and non-HRT modalities in sequential manner during the decades of postmenopausal life to maximize benefit and minimize adverse effects. And HRT is increasingly being delayed for as long as 10 years after menopause because osteoporosis and heart disease occur later in life and protection is greatest for current users. The literature should be watched closely for more data to guide clinicians on duration and timing of therapy.

Patient Selection. For the purpose of prolonging life, the best candidates for HRT are postmenopausal women with many cardiovascular risk factors and little added risk of breast cancer. The marked cardiovascular survival benefit associated with long-term HRT found in the Nurses' Health Study greatly overshadows the moderately increased risk of breast cancer. Survival is least improved by HRT for women with little cardiovascular risk and multiple risk factors for breast cancer. Women who fall between both ends of the breast cancer/heart disease spectrum require a more customized approach that takes into account their preferences and concerns and includes consideration of alternative approaches.

In regards to HRT for prevention of osteoporotic fractures, patient selection requires assessment of osteoporotic risk (see Chapter 164). Women with increased risk of osteoporosis and hip fracture are likely to benefit most from hormone replacement. A single measurement of bone mineral density may be useful if the decision to treat would be influenced by the three-fold increase in risk associated with low bone density. Because of the increased risk of breast cancer with prolonged estrogen exposure, women concerned about breast cancer risk might best be offered alternative treatment for osteoporosis (e.g., exercise, calcium supplementation, vitamin D, bisphosphonates; see Chapter 164).

Given the potentially serious adverse effects of HRT and the fact that some are still poorly defined, the primary physician must exert care and judgment in selecting patients for HRT. The decision to use such therapy needs to be made with full consideration of the patient's willingness to undertake the risks in exchange for specified benefits. One woman may be willing to accept the risk of breast cancer in return for prevention of disabling osteoporosis and decreased risk of cardiovascular disease; another might not. The addition of progestin to the hormone replacement program can reduce the risk of endometrial cancer but not breast cancer, and other long-term effects remain to be defined.

Monitoring. Current evidence does not support definitive recommendations for monitoring women taking HRT. However, because of the increased risk of breast cancer with increasing duration of HRT, it is recommended that clinical breast examination and mammography are performed yearly in women on long-term therapy, especially those taking HRT for more than 10 years. Women taking progestins, as well as estrogens, do not need either baseline or subsequent routine endometrial evaluations.

For the occasional case of a women with an intact uterus who desires to take unopposed estrogens, a baseline pelvic examination with endometrial sampling and a baseline mammogram may be well advised. An alternative to endometrial sampling is screening with transvaginal ultrasound, with sampling reserved for women with a thickened endometrium. Any vaginal bleeding should be reported by the woman taking unopposed estrogens, and the report should prompt endometrial evaluation. In the absence of bleeding, screening with transvaginal ultrasound and/or endometrial sampling should be performed yearly.

Other Treatment Modalities

Advances in the prevention and treatment of osteoporosis (see Chapter 164) and cardiovascular disease provide menopausal women a host of preventive and therapeutic options for conditions related to menopause. HRT is not the only effective modality available. For example, a *diet* low in fat, high in calcium, combined with regular weight-bearing aerobic *exercise* can do much to reduce cardiovascular and osteoporotic risks. Even patients at high risk for osteoporotic disease have nonhormonal options, such as *bisphosphonates* (see Chapter 164).

Diet and exercise can slow osteoporotic changes but not as effectively as estrogen. Nevertheless, the addition of 1.0 to 1.5 g of dietary calcium carbonate per day will compensate for the intestinal malabsorption of calcium that results from estrogen deficiency and will retard bone loss, especially when combined with regular exercise. *Vitamin D* treatment is not beneficial unless serum levels of 25-OH vitamin D_3 are low. Small doses (400 U/d) are helpful in preventing vitamin D deficiency in elderly women; large doses are unnecessary. Bisphosphonate therapy (e.g., alendronate) can reduce vertebral compression fractures by close to 50%.

Patients with worrisome lipid profiles have multiple lipid-lowering options (see Chapter 27) to supplement dietary measures. Vaginal dryness that interferes with intercourse can be treated nonhormonally with a *water-soluble lubricant*, if there is a reason to avoid any estrogen exposure. Decrease in libido and/or orgasmic dysfunction that was clearly associated with the onset of menopause but persists with estrogen replacement might justify consideration of androgen therapy (see Chapter 115).

Overly medicalizing menopause by emphasizing HRT runs the risk of turning a normal phase of life into a disease state and unintentionally triggering depression. A more constructive approach is to advise the menopausal women about her options, emphasizing the range of possibilities and providing a sense of empowerment rather than one of hopelessness.

PATIENT EDUCATION

Because the emphasis in our society is on youth and vitality, the physician has an important supportive role to play in helping the menopausal woman adjust psychologically and maintain her sense of self-worth and well-being. Discussion of the physiologic consequences of menopause and their clinical manifestations can give the patient a rational basis for understanding her own symptoms and properly attributing them. This might save many anxious phone calls and office visits. One can take advantage of this milestone to interest the patient in a program of regular exercise, attainment of ideal weight, and cessation of self-destructive habits, such as smoking. The patient needs to know that any incapacitating symptoms caused by lack of estrogen can be controlled and that many are self-limited. During the perimenopausal period, women should be reminded to use contraception because ovulation and unwanted pregnancy may occur. Reassurance that capacity for normal sexual activity will continue after menopause is often tremendously comforting. Lack of need for special vitamin supplements should be pointed out because the lay press heavily encourages their use, and this unnecessary expense can be considerable.

If estrogen therapy is being considered, the patient must share in the decision with full awareness of the potential risks and benefits. Patients with intact uteri on unopposed estrogen therapy must be reminded about the need for regular endometrial evaluation. The need for regular follow-up and prompt reporting of any abnormal vaginal bleeding, breast masses, leg swelling, and so forth must be emphasized.

INDICATIONS FOR REFERRAL

Women with an intact uterus who are taking HRT and who experience irregular vaginal bleeding that does not clear with adjustment of progesterone dose require gynecologic evaluation to rule out important endometrial pathology. The postmenopausal patient who develops major depression and does not respond to first-line antidepressant therapy and counseling should be considered for psychiatric consultation.

THERAPEUTIC RECOMMENDATIONS

- **Review Risks and Benefits.** Decisions about treatment of postmenopausal changes require careful weighing and thorough discussion of risks and benefits. The postmenopausal woman's preferences and concerns should be elicited and addressed in the design of any program.

- **For Hot Flashes.** For symptomatic relief of incapacitating hot flashes, consider *oral estrogen* at the lowest dose necessary (often as little as 0.3 mg/day of conjugated estrogens). The need for continued treatment should be reevaluated regularly. If the patient has an intact uterus and requires treatment indefinitely, then consider adding a *progestin* to the program (see below).

- **For Atrophic Vaginitis** with severe dysuria or unacceptable dyspareunia, prescribe a *topical estrogen preparation* (e.g., conjugated estrogen cream) applied as seldom as once or twice a week. Systemic absorption occurs, but its effect is uncertain. However, avoid prolonged daily use because of the risk of endometrial stimulation. In instances of painful coitus only, advise trying a *water-soluble lubricant*, especially if there is a desire to avoid estrogen exposure.

- **For Depression.** Treat specifically for depression with supportive psychotherapy and/or a standard antidepressant drug regimen (see Chapter 227); HRT is not a substitute.

- **For Prophylaxis of Osteoporosis.** Explain the need for long-term therapy and its attendant risks. For those at increased risk of osteoporosis and willing to undergo indefinite treatment, initiate oral HRT (see below) at the onset of menopause. Continue for a minimum of 10 years and indefinitely if possible. Incorporate a 1.5 g/d *calcium* intake, consider vitamin D supplementation in the elderly, and prescribe a weight-bearing aerobic exercise program. Consider bisphosphonate therapy as an alternative to indefinite hormone supplementation, particularly in a patient with a prior vertebral compression fracture (see Chapter 164). HRT cannot replace lost bone; it is *not* a therapy for reversing established osteoporosis. However, for women without increased risk of osteoporosis, HRT may reasonably be delayed until age 60.

- **For Prophylaxis of Cardiovascular Disease.** Initiate oral HRT (see below) for those with multiple cardiovascular risk factors who are willing to accept long-term treatment and the associated increase in risk of breast cancer. Women with established coronary disease may also incur increased early risk. Also incorporate appropriate diet, exercise, and pharmacologic measures pertinent to the patient's major risk factors (see Chapters 18, 26, 27, and 30).

- **Oral Hormone Replacement Regimens.** For women with an intact uterus, treat with either continuous daily estrogen combined with daily low-dose progestin (e.g., 0.625 mg conjugated estrogens plus 2.5 to 5.0 mg/d of medroxyprogesterone acetate or equivalent) or continuous daily estrogen plus cyclic progestin (e.g., 0.625 mg conjugated estrogens plus 5 to 10 mg of medroxyprogesterone acetate added on 10 to 14 consecutive days of the month). Choice should be based on desirability and acceptability of periodic vaginal bleeding.

- For women who have had a hysterectomy, treat with continuous daily estrogen therapy (e.g., 0.625 mg/d of conjugated estrogens). There is no benefit to adding a progestin.

A.G.M./A.H.G.

ANNOTATED BIBLIOGRAPHY

Avis NE, Brambilla D, McKinlay S, et al. A longitudinal analysis of the association between menopause and depression: results from the Massachusetts Women's Health Study. Ann Epidemiol 1994; 4:12. (*Depression associated with a long symptomatic perimenopause rather than the menopause itself.*)

Barrett-Connor E. Hormone replacement therapy. BMJ 1998;317:457. (*A superb focused review of the harms and benefits as understood in 1998.*)

Barrett-Conner E. Postmenopausal estrogen therapy and selected (less-often-considered) disease outcomes. Menopause 1999;6:14. (*Provides 10-year literature review addressing evidence for positive associations with multiple conditions, including arthritis, systemic lupus erythematosus, pancreatitis, asthma, and diabetes.*)

Bergkvist L, Adami HO, Persson I, et al. The risk of breast cancer after estrogen and estrogen-progestin replacement. N Engl J Med 1989;321:293. (*The relative risk for women who have ever used unopposed estrogen was 1.1; for women with 9 or more years of unopposed estrogen use, relative risk was statistically significant at 1.8. For women with 6 to 9 years of estrogen and progestin use, relative risk was 1.4.*)

Cauley JA, Seeley DG, Ensrud K, et al. Estrogen replacement therapy and fractures in older women. Ann Intern Med 1995;122:9. (*A prospective cohort study of nearly 10,000 women demonstrating risk reduction with HRT for wrist fractures and all nonspinal fractures; initiation soon after menopause was important.*)

Colditz GA, Hankinson SE, Hunter DJ, et al. The use of estrogen and progestins and the risk of breast cancer in postmenopausal women. N Engl J Med 1995;332:1589. (*Extended follow-up from the Nurses' Health Study indicating a relative risk of 1.32 for women using estrogen alone and 1.41 for women using estrogen plus progesterone.*)

Collaborative Group on Hormonal Factors in Breast Cancer. Breast cancer and hormone replacement therapy: collaborative reanalysis of data from 51 epidemiological studies of 52 705 women with breast cancer and 108 411 women without breast cancer. Lancet 1997;350:1047. (*The risk of breast cancer in women using HRT increases with increasing duration of use reaching 1.35 after 5 years. This effect is reduced after HRT cessation and has largely disappeared after about 5 years.*)

Cummings SR, Browner WS, Grady D, et al. Should prescription of postmenopausal hormone therapy be based on the results of bone densitometry? Ann Intern Med 1990;113:565. (*Advocates single measurement of bone density if risk for osteoporosis would influence the hormone replacement decision.*)

Cushman M, Legault C, Barrett-Connor E, et al. Effect of postmenopausal hormones on inflammation-sensitive proteins: the Postmenopausal Estrogen/Progestin Intervention (PEPI) Study. Circulation 1999;100:717. (*HRT rapidly increased concentration of the inflammation factor C-reactive protein suggesting an explanatory hypothesis for adverse early effects.*)

Davidson NE. Hormone-replacement therapy—breast versus heart versus bone. N Engl J Med 1995;332:1638. (*Discusses trade-offs required by HRT.*)

Ditkoff EC, Crary WG, Cristo M, et al. Estrogen improves psychological function in asymptomatic postmenopausal women. Obstet Gynecol 1991;78:991. (*Estrogen therapy may improve mood and mental function, even in asymptomatic postmenopausal women.*)

Falkeborn M, Persson I, Terent A, et al. Hormone replacement therapy and risk of stroke. Arch Intern Med 1993;153:1201. (*Population study from Sweden; risk reduced 30%.*)

Felson DT, Zhang Y, Hannan MT, et al. The effect of postmenopausal estrogen therapy on bone density in elderly women. N Engl J Med 1993;329:1141. (*Very long-term therapy required to produce clinically meaningful benefit to women older than 75 years.*)

Ganz PA, Greendale GA, Kahn B, et al. Are older breast carcinoma survivors willing to take hormone replacement therapy? Cancer 1999;86:814. (*More so to relieve symptoms than for prevention.*)

Gatspur SM, Morrow M, Sellars TA. Hormone replacement therapy and risk of breast cancer with a favorable histology: results of the Iowa Women's Health Study. JAMA 1999;281:2091. (*In this study, increased risk was for invasive breast cancers with a favorable prognosis.*)

Grady D, Hulley SB, et al. Venous thromboembolic events associated with hormone replacement therapy. JAMA 1997;278:477. (*The increased risk of thromboembolic events confirmed in an RCT.*)

Grady D, Rubin SM, Petitti DB, et al. Hormone therapy to prevent disease and prolong life in postmenopausal women. Ann Intern Med 1992;117:1016. (*A comprehensive and scholarly analytic review of the literature, accompanied by practical recommendations; 265 references.*)

Greendale GA, Lee NP, Arriola ER. The menopause. Lancet 1999; 353:571. (*Well-organized and referenced review.*)

Grodstein F, Newcomb PA, Stampfer MJ. Postmenopausal hormone therapy and the risk of colorectal cancer: a review and meta-analysis. Am J Med 1999;106:574. (*Relative risk of 0.80 among ever users and 0.66 among current users.*)

Grodstein F, Martinez E, Platz EA, et al. Postmenopausal hormone use and risk of colorectal cancer and adenoma. Ann Intern Med 1998;128:705. (*Current use of hormones reduced risk of colorectal cancer by 35% in the Nurses' Health Study.*)

Grodstein F, Stampfer MJ, Colditz GA, et al. Postmenopausal hormone therapy and mortality. N Engl J Med 1997;336:1769. (*Best available epidemiologic investigation, based on data from the Nurses' Health Study; mortality is lower among users than nonusers; survival benefit decreases with duration of use and is considerably diminished in those with a low cardiovascular risk.*)

Hulley S, Grady D, Bush T, et al. Randomized trial of estrogen plus progestin for secondary prevention of coronary heart disease in postmenopausal women. Heart and Estrogen/progestin Replacement Study (HERS) Research Group. JAMA 1998;280:605. (*Key study.*)

Jick H, Derby LE, Myers MW, et al. Risk of hospital admission for idiopathic venous thromboembolism among users of postmenopausal oestrogens. Lancet 1996;348:981. (*Relative risk of 3.6 among current users in this case-control study.*)

Keating NL, Cleary PD, Rossi AS, et al. Use of hormone replacement therapy by postmenopausal women in the United States. Ann Intern Med 1999;130:545. (*Best data on use.*)

Kritz-Silverstein D, Barrett-Conner E. Long-term postmenopausal hormone use, obesity, and fat distribution in older women. JAMA 1996;275:46. (*HRT is not associated with the weight gain and central obesity commonly seen in postmenopausal women.*)

Leiblum S, Bachmann G, Kemmann E, et al. Vaginal atrophy in the postmenopausal woman. JAMA 1983;249:2195. (*Less vaginal atrophy was apparent in sexually active women compared with sexually inactive women; women with less vaginal atrophy had higher levels of estrogens and gonadotropins.*)

McNagny SE, Wenger NK, Frank E, et al. Personal use of postmenopausal hormone replacement therapy by women physicians in the United States. Ann Intern Med 1997;127:1093. (*Women physicians have a higher rate of HRT use than that reported in cross-sectional U.S. surveys.*)

Myers LS, Dixen J, Morrissette D, et al. Effects of estrogen, androgen, and progestin on sexual psychophysiology and behavior in postmenopausal women. J Clin Endocrinol Metab 1990;70:1124. (*In this study, there was no improvement in libido and sexual enjoyment among estrogen-treated women.*)

Naessen T, Persson I, Adami HO, et al. Hormone replacement therapy and the risk for hip fracture. A prospective, population-based cohort study. Ann Intern Med 1990;113:95. (*Cohort study showing relative risk of 0.8 for women who had ever used unopposed estrogens.*)

Pedersen AT, Lidegaard O, Kreiner S, et al. Hormone replacement therapy and risk of non-fatal stroke. Lancet 1997;350:1277. (*No apparent effect of HRT on risk in this study.*)

The PEPI Writing Group. Effects of estrogen or estrogen/progestin regimens on heart disease risk factors in postmenopausal women. JAMA 1995;273:199. (*Associated with increased high-density-lipoprotein cholesterol, decreased low-density-lipoprotein cholesterol, and other favorable changes in cardiovascular risk factors.*)

The PEPI Writing Group. Effects of hormone replacement therapy on endometrial histology in postmenopausal women. JAMA 1996; 275:370. (*Unopposed estrogen produced marked hyperplasia in 34% compared with 1% in those also taking a progestin.*)

Sarrel PM. Psychosexual effects of menopause: role of androgens. Am J Obstet Gynecol 1999;180:319. (*Review of available clinical evidence concluding that the addition of androgens to HRT provides greater improvement in psychologic and sexual symptoms.*)

Schneider DL, Barrett-Connor EL, Morton DJ. Timing of postmenopausal estrogen for optimal bone mineral density. The Rancho Bernardo study. JAMA 1997;277:543. (*HRT effective when delayed until age 60.*)

Stampfer MJ, Colditz GA, Willett WC, et al. Postmenopausal estrogen therapy and cardiovascular disease. Ten-year follow-up from the Nurses' Health Study. N Engl J Med 1991;325:756. (*Relative risk for women who have ever-used estrogen therapy was 0.6.*)

Steinberg KK, Thacker SB, Smith SJ, et al. A meta-analysis of the effect of estrogen replacement therapy on the risk of breast cancer. JAMA 1991;265:1985. (*Analytic review finding no increased risk for women who have ever used estrogen and relative risk of 1.3 for women who had used estrogens for at least 15 years.*)

Tang MX, Jacobs D, Stern Y, et al. Effect of estrogen during menopause on risk and age at onset of Alzheimer's disease. Lancet 1996;348:429. (*Data suggesting significant preventive effect for estrogen replacement.*)

Utian WH, Boggs PP. The North American Menopause Society 1998 Menopause Survey. Part I. Postmenopausal women's perceptions about menopause and midlife. Menopause 1999;6:122. (*The majority of respondents were happiest and most fulfilled between the ages of 50 and 65 years.*)

Yaffe K, Sawaya G, et al. Estrogen therapy in postmenopausal women: effects on cognitive function and dementia. JAMA 1998;279:688. (*Reviews 10 observational studies and four trials concluding that evidence is too poor to have confidence in modest risk reductions that have generally been reported.*)

119

Approach to Fertility Control

NANCY J. GAGLIANO
SUSAN OLIVERIO

The ideal contraceptive is perfectly safe, effective, inexpensive, acceptable, and available. None exists. The efficacy of individual contraceptive agents is expressed in several ways. *Theoretic effectiveness* refers to the ability of the medication, device, or procedure to prevent pregnancy if applied under ideal conditions. *Use effectiveness* combines theoretic effectiveness with inherent patient-related lapses in application. *Extended use effectiveness* adds the dimension of time. All are important aspects of evaluation of approaches to fertility control.

The primary physician should be knowledgeable about the effectiveness, difficulties, and adverse effects of available contraceptive methods to help the patient or couple intelligently select the one that suits them best.

NATURAL METHODS

Natural methods of birth control do not meet the demands of most sexually active individuals in industrialized societies. Faithfully practiced *rhythm*, with daily basal body temperature recording, usually results in one pregnancy every 2 years or at least one more child than planned by the couple by their late thirties. Rhythm practiced by abstinence according to menstrual dates is less effective. Rhythm controlled by following the cervical mucus cycle is confounded by infections, dietary changes, douching habits, oral medications, patient understanding of her anatomy, and availability of testing materials. One needs to understand reproductive anatomy and physiology and to have privacy to conduct such tests. These ingredients are unavailable to many Americans. The *amenorrhea of lactation* is useful, but the duration of ovarian inactivity in an individual is hard to predict or follow. *Withdrawal* is probably the most commonly used natural contraceptive technique. Unfortunately, sperm migration from the female perineum can occur, due to discharge of semen before ejaculation.

BARRIER CONTRACEPTIVES

Condoms have moderate extended use effectiveness. Pregnancies may occur in up to 15 per 100 couples per year using condoms. When properly used, this method is 85% to 95% effective. For a few cents more than the cheapest devices, high-quality thin condoms are available, use of which is accompanied by very little loss of sensation. When used in conjunction with a spermicidal foam or jelly, its effectiveness may rise to 96%. The condom is inexpensive and widely available. It requires no medical intervention or prescription. Failure by means of rupture is rare but easily recognized. The condom has received more attention recently due to its protective effects against infectious agents such as the HIV, *Chlamydia*, gonococci, herpes simplex virus, and possibly the human papillomavirus. This effect appears to be dependent on the use of nonoxynol-9, a spermicide found in most condoms.

Diaphragms are synthetic latex barriers mounted on covered rims that deny access of sperm and penis to the anterior vaginal wall and cervical os. The largest diaphragm that will cover the cervix and anterior vagina from the pubis symphysis to the posterior fornix should be selected. The diaphragm should be comfortable so that the woman barely notices its presence. It should not stretch the rest of the vagina or put undue pressure on the urethra. Only significant weight changes of 25% or more of body weight require diaphragm refitting. Refitting should be performed 6 weeks or more postpartum as well. When used properly, diaphragms with a small amount of spermicidal cream or jelly are up to 96% effective. Four pregnancies per 100 fertile women per year would be expected. The cream facilitates insertion but need not be used in the large amounts recommended by the manufacturers, as it is unpleasantly messy. Additional spermicidal cream needs to be applied intravaginally for repeated intercourse. The diaphragm is worn for 6 hours after the last coital event, because this is the length of time during which sperm motility persists. It may be worn for longer periods of time, but like all vaginal contraceptives, it will then become associated with an unpleasant odor. It may also be worn while the patient is swimming or during menstruation.

The two most frequent complaints regarding the diaphragm are latex allergy and increased frequency of urinary tract infections. The Wide Seal diaphragm may be prescribed to women with urinary tract infections. The wider band around the rim puts less direct pressure on the urethra and may reduce the frequency of urinary tract infections. The woman should also be advised to void after intercourse and use adequate lubrication. The Wide Seal diaphragm is often not stocked by pharmacies, and the practitioner who frequently prescribes diaphragms may wish to stock this item.

A physician, nurse, or trained technician must fit the diaphragm to the individual woman. The cost of the diaphragm is reasonable, but manufacturers advocate massive use of creams, which adds to the expense. The patient must have some understanding of her anatomy and not be concerned about exploring her reproductive organs. Some adolescents reject the diaphragm because they are uncomfortable with touching themselves. Its use represents premeditated sexual intercourse, which they find less acceptable than spontaneous events. Women in their twenties seldom voice such a complaint. Some women cannot be fitted adequately with a diaphragm for anatomic reasons. The cervix may not protrude into the vagina adequately (absent pars vaginalis). The cervix may be displaced posteriorly by retroversion or extreme anteversion.

Cervical Caps fit snugly over the cervix and are slightly more difficult to insert and remove. Their use requires significant physician or nurse teaching, and they are more costly than diaphragms. Currently, four sizes are manufactured, and some women cannot be fit. For these reasons, they are less popular than the diaphragm. For women who have recurrent urinary tract infections, however, they are particularly useful because they do not press on the urethra. Additionally, they can be worn for 48 hours, during which time intercourse may be repeated without the addition of spermicidal cream. There is evidence of a 4% increased incidence of abnormal Papanicolaou (Pap) tests; therefore, it is recommended that a Pap test is performed 3 months after initiating use of the cap. If the Pap smear is normal, then the woman can proceed with yearly Pap tests.

Female Condoms are approved by the U.S. Food and Drug Administration (FDA). The condom is a lubricated polyurethane pouch that lines the vagina. One outer ring lies outside the body and a smaller inner ring is pushed up toward the cervix to hold the condom in place. It gives a woman an additional choice and freedom to protect herself from sexually transmitted diseases and pregnancy. Because it is made from polyurethane, the female condom can be used by latex allergic individuals. Female condoms appear to have failure rates similar to those of the male condom. Unfortunately, they currently cost about twice as much as the male condom.

Spermicidal Creams and Jellies may have a high theoretic effectiveness, but they have lesser use effectiveness. Most contain nonoxynol-9 as the spermicidal agent. The physical nature of the creams and jellies and difficulty in their application often result in inadequately smearing the cervical os, so that sperm invasion is not prevented. Both men and women complain of the dehydrating effect of spermicidal agents and may report burning sensations. Nonoxynol-9 has the added advantage of being toxic *in vitro* to HIV, gonococci, *Chlamydia*, and other genital pathogens; some clinical evidence suggests an *in vivo* effect as well. *Foams* have better physical properties, allowing more adequate smearing of the cervical os; however, foams are effective for short periods of time only, and reapplications are necessary. This increases their cost. They also contain nonoxynol-9 and may cause irritation. Failure rates up to 25% are reported. When used in conjunction with the condom, excellent pregnancy protection has been demonstrated, reaching 96% effectiveness. Foams have the advantage of being readily accessible in both supermarkets and drugstores, and they do not require medical instruction or prescription.

INTRAUTERINE DEVICES

The idea of inserting materials into the uterine cavity to prevent nidation is ancient. Nevertheless, the precise mechanism of intrauterine device (IUD) action remains unknown. What appears to be important is the area of surface contact. Copper enhances effectiveness. The 1% to 5% first-year pregnancy rates with IUD use are among the lowest attainable form of birth control method and are comparable with those of oral contraceptives. The lack of constant compliance greatly enhances efficacy. Another advantage is the lack of systemic effects, a major problem with oral contraceptives (see below). A major limitation to efficacy is expulsion, which is particularly frequent in nulliparous women. The overall expulsion rate is 19 per 100 women per year, lower with copper devices. Occasionally, it is necessary to remove an IUD because of bleeding or pain, which occurs at a rate of about 11% per year. Copper devices are better tolerated by nulliparous women.

The confirmation of a markedly increased risk of tubal infertility associated with IUD use has greatly discouraged IUD placement as a means of safe birth control, especially among nulliparous women. In 1986, sale of all IUDs, except Progestasert, was discontinued. In 1988, Paragard, a new copper IUD, was approved by the FDA. Clinical or subclinical pelvic inflammatory disease is believed to account for the tubal infertility. Risk of pelvic inflammatory disease in nulliparous sexually active women with an IUD has been found to be seven times that for similar women not using an IUD; for parous women, the risk is three times greater. In view of the infertility risk, IUD use is best confined to multiparous women and nulliparous women with a single sexual partner. The nulliparous woman considering an IUD as a means of birth control should be fully informed of the risk of tubal infertility before any decision is made regarding its use.

ORAL CONTRACEPTIVES

Combinations of synthetic estrogen and progesterone have been found to have use effectiveness rates that exceed most estimates of effectiveness of barrier methods, spermicides, and IUDs. Although some report failure rates as high as 5% to 10%, most report only one failure per 100 users per year. The combination pill appears to prevent cyclic release of follicle-stimulating hormone (FSH) and luteinizing hormone, which are required for ovulation; alter the cervical mucus, thereby decreasing sperm motility; and alter the endometrial lining to inhibit implantation. At the present time, combination pills consist of an estrogen (ethinyl estradiol or mestranol) and a progestin (norethindrone, norethynodrel, norgestrel, levo-norgestrel, ethynodiol diacetate, desogestrel, gestodene, and norgestimate). Pill cycles are 28 days long. Pill packets contain 21 or 28 pills depending on the brand. Twenty-eight–day packets contain placebo pills for part or all of the last week of the pill pack. Patients are instructed to start on the first Sunday of the menstrual cycle or the first day of bleeding.

Preparations. More than two dozen combination preparations are available in the United States. In general, it is most useful to renew any prescription with which a patient is satisfied, as long as the patient has no new symptoms or habits that warrant discontinuation of any oral contraceptive.

Cardiovascular risks have been a significant concern when prescribing the pill. Because of the concern that these risks might increase with estrogen dosage and progestin potency, emphasis in recent years has been on use of preparations that have the *lowest effective estrogen dose* (20 to 35 μg ethinyl estradiol) and the least progestin potency. Fortunately, efficacy of 30 to 35 μg of estrogen for prevention of pregnancy is about the same as that of the older 50-μg estrogen pill.

It is best to begin with a pill containing 30 to 35 μg of ethinyl estradiol. The *lowest possible progestin dosage* helps minimize bothersome side effects such as increased appetite, steady weight gain, acne, and depression. Many newer and more expensive oral contraceptives are heavily marketed. They may offer some theoretic benefits and perhaps fewer actual ones. Currently, a line of generic birth control pills offer a range of options at a much lower cost to the patient or insurer. It is prudent to reserve the high-cost oral contraceptive pills for patients who have a medical need for a specialized contraceptive

Table 119.1. Effects of Synthetic Progestins[a]

ESTROGENIC	ANDROGENIC
Norethynodrel	Norgestrel
Ethynodiol	Norethindrone
All others have none	Norethindrone acetate
	Ethynodiol
	Norethynodrel (has none)

[a]In order of decreasing potency.

pill. A good basic pill to start with contains 1 mg norethindrone and 35 μg ethinyl estradiol (generic Necon 1/35 = Ortho Novum 1/35).

Patients who have a history of symptoms suggesting hyperresponsiveness to endogenous estrogens (premenstrual breast engorgement and soreness, cyclic weight gain, heavy periods) may benefit from a preparation containing a low estrogen and a *progestin with minimal estrogenic effect* (e.g., Necon 0.5/35, a generic preparation; norethindrone 0.5 mg/ethinyl estradiol 35 μg; or Ovcon with ethinyl estradiol 35 μg and norethindrone 0.4 mg). Similarly, a patient bothered by acne or hirsutism should be given a preparation with low androgenic progestin such as desogestrel or norgestimate (Table 119.1). Other side effects such as nausea seem related to estrogen content.

The *disadvantages* of using lower dose agents are higher rates of spotting, breakthrough bleeding, and amenorrhea. Moreover, women who use oral contraceptives containing less than 30 μg of estrogen may experience a greater chance of pregnancy. To counteract this reduced efficacy, newer pills with 20 μg of ethinyl estradiol have lengthened the hormone cycle with as few as 2 days of hormone-free placebo in the 28-day cycle. In an attempt to improve rates of breakthrough bleeding and pregnancy associated with low-estrogen/weak-progestin formulations, manufacturers have developed *biphasic* (e.g., Ortho-Novum 10/11) and *triphasic* (e.g., Ortho-Novum 7/7/7, Tri-Norinyl, Triphasil) formulations. The rationale is to more closely mimic normal ovarian patterns. Efficacy is similar to that obtained with other low-estrogen/weak-progestin preparations; no controlled evidence to date suggests that they are superior in terms of breakthrough bleeding. There is evidence that the monophasics are superior to triphasic pills in suppressing ovarian function and should be the pill of choice in women with a history of large ovarian cysts. All low-dose preparations need to be taken religiously to be maximally effective and to minimize the chances of breakthrough bleeding.

Progesterone-only pills—"the minipill"—are available and prescribed for women who should not take estrogens. Lactating women, women with complex migraine headaches, women over age 35 who smoke, and women with thromboembolic disease may be given this preparation.

It is helpful to become familiar with four or five pills and their minor differences rather than using the most recently marketed combinations. Providing the patient with full understandable information at the initiation of therapy will ward off many anxious phone calls. In particular, if one pill is missed, it can be made up by doubling the next dose. If two pills are missed, the patient should double the dose for the next 2 days, but barrier contraception is recommended for the remainder of the cycle. If three or more consecutive pills are missed, the pills should be stopped altogether, allowing withdrawal bleeding to occur. A new pill pack should be started 1 week after the last pill was taken. Recurrent failure to take oral contraceptives regularly is an indication for trying another form of birth control.

Because contraceptive pills are often prescribed until menopause, knowing just when to stop or switch to post-menopausal estrogen replacement can give the patient and physician pause. One approach is to check an FSH near the age of 50. The FSH should be checked on day 7 of the placebo or pill-free week. If the FSH is significantly elevated (close to 100), then it would be appropriate to stop or switch to estrogen replacement therapy. If the FSH is normal or midrange, then continuing the pill and rechecking the FSH in another year would be prudent.

Breakthrough bleeding is a common side effect of the pill. If it occurs late in the cycle or in the first few months of initiation of the pill, it is usually caused by too little progesterone. If it occurs early in the cycle or after years of use, it may be caused by inadequate estrogen. This problem may be temporarily resolved by having the patient take two pills a day for 3 days. The additional pills should be obtained from a separate package of pills.

If the problem recurs repeatedly after the first 3 months, then changing the pill to a stronger estrogenic or progestinal pill would be appropriate. The physician should always rule out other causes of irregular bleeding, such as infection and pregnancy.

Another common complaint is that of *morning nausea*. It may be improved by having the patient take the pill with her evening meal and then consume a light breakfast daily. If the symptoms persist, switching to a lower estrogen pill or a progesterone-only pill (e.g., Micronor) may be indicated.

Patients require follow-up care 6 to 12 weeks after initiation of the birth control pill to check for hypertension, review proper use, and discuss side effects. The patients should then be seen yearly, checking for headaches, hypertension, breast masses, cervical abnormalities, phlebitis, and signs of cardiovascular or cerebrovascular disease.

Physicians are generally unaware of the high discontinuation rate among oral contraceptive users. Factors involved include the patient's perceptions of need and attitudes about taking medications that affect the sex organs. Oral contraceptives are expensive and require a medical prescription, important barriers for adolescents. Despite these factors and known side effects, birth control pills continue to be the most used safest birth control method for most nonsmokers. The pill's relative safety is most apparent in countries where the risk of dying in childbirth is high.

Adverse Effects. The major hazards of oral contraceptives are cardiovascular. The relative risks of cardiovascular events in users compared with nonusers had been reported to be 4 to 11 times greater for *thromboembolism*, 4 to 9.5 times greater for *thrombotic stroke*, 2 times greater for *hemorrhagic stroke*, and 2 to 12 times greater for *myocardial infarction*. These earlier studies, which demonstrated a slight increase in risk, were done on women taking 50-μg doses of estrogen. Currently, it is thought that any increased risk is due to embolic events. The Nurses' Health Study demonstrated no significant differences in the rates of various cardiovascular diseases between never-users and past users of oral contraceptives. The studies consis-

tently showed increased risks *in smokers*. Mortality from myocardial infarction rises sixfold in women older than age 40 who are smokers. The overall excess death rate annually has been estimated to be 20 per 100,000, with risk concentrated in women older than 35, especially if they smoke cigarettes and have used oral contraceptives for 5 years or longer. Division of data at age 35 is arbitrary, and it would be prudent to assume that risk gradually increases with age. Cardiovascular risk is much lower with 35-μg estrogen pills.

Progestin potency may also be associated with increased cardiovascular risk, probably because of its ability to raise low-density-lipoprotein (LDL) cholesterol and lower high-density-lipoprotein (HDL) cholesterol (see Chapter 15). Initial concern that the newer progestins such as desogestrel may be related to an increase in thromboembolic disease and deep vein thrombosis *(DVT)* has not been borne out in further studies.

Any population of women provided with oral contraception will show a rise in mean blood pressure in about 3 months. Prospective studies have found that the incidence of *hypertension* increases two- to sixfold in users compared with nonusers. It is wise to check blood pressure before renewing a patient's prescription. The progesterone in the birth control pill, like the progesterone in the secretory phase of the menstrual cycle, increases aldosterone secretion, and estrogen increases renin substrate.

There is a twofold increase in the risk of *gallbladder disease* in users compared with nonusers, because of increased cholesterol saturation of bile. The frequency of gallstones appears to rise after 2 years' usage and to reach a plateau after 4 to 5 years' usage. This risk must be balanced against the increased risk of gallbladder disease associated with multiparity. Another hepatobiliary problem is the rare development of highly vascular *hepatic adenomas*, which can rupture spontaneously, resulting in serious hemorrhage. Isolated cases have appeared in the literature; in most cases, patients had been using the pill longer than 5 years. The actual risk is unknown. Finally, estrogen use has been associated with *cholestatic jaundice*, but oral contraceptive use does not worsen cases of mild viral hepatitis and need not be discontinued unless cholestasis or hepatocellular injury is severe.

Studies concerning risk of breast cancer associated with the use of oral contraceptives remain conflicting and controversial. Although there may be a small increased risk in premenopausal *breast cancer,* there is no consensus as to which subgroups of women might be at increased risk. Data from several recent studies are inconsistent. Estrogens may stimulate the growth of certain cancers; these include carcinoma of the breast (see Chapter 122), cervix, and endometrium (see Chapter 123). Most studies have shown diminished incidences of fibroadenomas, ovarian and endometrial cancers, and benign fibrocystic disease of the breast in pill users.

Metabolic and endocrinologic effects are numerous. Thyroid-binding globin levels increase, which in turn raises the serum thyroxine level. Glucose tolerance falls as circulating growth hormone rises and peripheral resistance to insulin occurs. Triglyceride levels increase, sometimes dramatically, with the concurrent boost in lipoprotein production. The estrogen component tends to result in a rise in HDL cholesterol, whereas the progestin may result in a rise in LDL cholesterol. There is no evidence to suggest that the oral contraceptive pill should not be prescribed in women with hypercholesterolemia. However, it may be prudent to use a pill shown to have minimal lipid-worsening effect. Such pills are those with low doses of norethindrone (e.g., Necon 0.5/35 or Ovcon) or those with newer progestins (e.g., Desogen).

A few miscellaneous effects are noteworthy. Birth control pills may increase the frequency of *migraine headache* in patients with prior migraine attacks. However, they are only contraindicated in the woman with neurologic symptoms associated with her migraine headache. Anecdotal reports of *exacerbation of lupus erythematosus* appear in the obstetric literature. Sensitivity to sunlight and chloasma (mask of pregnancy) are seen in some users and fade with discontinuation.

Certain medications such as antibiotics and seizure medications have been found to affect the efficacy of the oral contraceptive pill. Anticonvulsants such as Dilantin induce hepatic metabolism and therefore effect the circulating level of hormone. Gabapentin is not metabolized and therefore unlikely to effect contraceptive hormone levels. It is prudent to advise women who are prescribed oral antibiotics to use back-up contraception for that month. However, the data to support this practice are limited.

A number of gynecologic conditions are affected by use of these agents; effects may be beneficial or detrimental. Patients with menstrual irregularities before oral contraceptive use will have regular pill-induced periods while taking the medication. Patients should have a full evaluation of the etiology of their irregular menses before initiation of the oral contraceptive pill. On discontinuation of the pills, some will revert to their previous irregularity. Rarely, *amenorrhea* due to ovarian suppression will persist for several months, even a year after pill cessation (see Chapter 112). Usually, menses return promptly, and fertility rates in the first 3 months of discontinuation are increased. Occasionally, a patient will notice nipple discharge (nonpuerperal lactation) with use of oral contraceptives. The mechanism is not clear. No increased incidence of pituitary prolactinomas has been observed.

Many patients with *dysmenorrhea* find marked relief with oral contraceptives (see Chapter 116). If the dysmenorrhea is associated with endometriosis, the response is variable, with many patients complaining of exacerbation of symptoms rather than relief.

With these side effects in mind, absolute and relative contraindications can be listed (Table 119.2). Patients exposed to diethylstilbestrol have used birth control pills with no evidence to date of either beneficial or deleterious effects.

Postcoital (Emergency) Contraception. Several regimens provide 97% to 99% effective emergency contraception if started within 12 to 24 hours of unprotected intercourse: 1) *estrogen/progestin* (ethinyl estradiol 100 μg plus levonorgestrel 1.0 mg – eg, 2 Ovral tablets) repeated in 12 hours; 2) *high-dose estrogen* (ethinyl estradiol 0.5 mg) bid for 5 days; 3) *progestin only* (levonorgestrel 0.75 mg) repeated in 12 hours; or 4) *mifespristone* (600 mg, single dose; FDA approval pending). Nausea and vomiting occur with estrogen-based programs The only contraindication is pregnancy. If emesis occurs within one hour of taking an estrogen containing pill then the dose can be repeated.

SUBDERMAL AND INTRAMUSCULAR PROGESTINS

Norplant is a method of contraception using six slender Silastic tubes surgically implanted subdermally. Levonorgestrel, a progestin, is released continuously at a very low

Table 119.2. Contraindications of Oral Contraceptives

Absolute Contraindications
Thromboembolic disorders, cardiovascular disease, thrombophlebitis, or a past history of these conditions or other conditions that predispose to them
Markedly impaired liver function from severe hepatitis, alcoholism, etc.
Known or suspected estrogen-dependent neoplasm (cancers of the breast, endometrium, etc.)
Undiagnosed genital bleeding
Known or suspected pregnancy

Relative Contraindications
Migraine headache
Hypertension
Familial hyperlipidemia
Epilepsy
Uterine leiomyoma
History of idiopathic obstructive jaundice of pregnancy
Smoking one-half pack or more per day
Diabetes mellitus
Severe heart disease
Patient unreliability
Age >35 yr

level for 5 years and appears to suppress ovulation. Cumulative pregnancy rates over the 5 years are 0.6% to 4% and are highest among women who have regular menstrual cycles while using Norplant. The advantages are 5 years of continuous contraception and very low hormone levels, resulting in no clinically significant metabolic effects. The disadvantages are irregular bleeding (in 66%) lasting many months and a cost of hundreds of dollars.

Depo-Provera has also been FDA-approved for use as a contraceptive. Medroxyprogesterone acetate 150 mg is administered intramuscularly every 3 months. Care should be taken to ensure that the woman is not pregnant initially, and it is recommended that the drug be administered during the first 5 days of the cycle. If a patient waits longer than 14 weeks between injections, a pregnancy test should be performed before her next injection. The pregnancy rate is 1% if used correctly. Disadvantages include irregular bleeding and the displeasure of patients receiving injections.

ABORTION (see Chapter 121)

Studies by Planned Parenthood have not found that a substantial number of American women rely on abortion as the sole method of birth control or has any trend to such a reliance been noted. Rather, abortion is used as a backup when other methods fail. Frequently, the necessity for an abortion initiates effective contraceptive use, particularly in those younger than age 20. No adverse affect of first-trimester induced abortion on future childbearing has been demonstrated. The effect of second-trimester abortions in rupturing cervical tissue is controversial. Rarely, an anomalous cervix may become incompetent, requiring cerclage if the patient wishes to carry future pregnancies to term. Morbidity and mortality in teenagers from induced abortion is lower than in older women.

Since 1988, mifepristone (RU-486), an antiprogesterone, has been successfully used in Europe for medical termination of early pregnancy. It is given as an oral dose in combination with a self-administered vaginal prostaglandin analogue. It has been found to be safe, highly effective, and acceptable to women. In addition, it is being studied for other clinical uses, including the treatment of leiomyomata, endometriosis, breast cancer, and potential estrogen-free contraceptive. To date, it has yet to gain FDA approval for use in the United States, likely due to social issues surrounding the abortion debate.

OVERALL RISKS

Used alone by women younger than 30, condoms, diaphragms, IUDs, birth control pills, and first-trimester abortion have a mortality risk of 1 to 2 per 100,000, significantly lower than the 12 per 100,000 delivery-related risk rate. After age 30, the risk of birth control pills rises, especially in smokers, but it is still less than the morbidity and complications of childbearing without fertility control. The birth control pill may be prescribed to women until menopause, but it is contraindicated in a smoker past the age of 35. The lowest level of mortality is achieved by a combination of contraception with access to early abortion.

STERILIZATION

In 1965, one third of the married couples in the United States used oral contraception, sterilization, or IUDs. By 1975, almost three fourths used one of these methods. Sterilization is now the most frequently used method of contraception among couples married for a decade or longer and among couples who have had all the children they want.

Vasectomy is the simplest and safest means of sterilization. Only a few surgical instruments and local anesthesia are required. The procedure may be done in a clinic, doctor's office, ambulatory surgical day care unit, or hospital. The procedure does not lead to impotence; rather, men with problems associated with impotence may blame vasectomy. It takes about 90 days of average ejaculatory activity to completely empty the spermatic cord and accessory glands of residual sperm. Thus, the vasectomy subject should have a postoperative semen analysis before he is considered sterile. Alternative methods of birth control should be used in the interim. Circulating antibodies to sperm may be induced by foreign proteins and by sperm. The effect of elevated sperm antibodies on a man's health is not clear but has been the subject of much concern. Retrospective cohort study of more than 10,000 vasectomized men fails to support such concerns; no serious immunopathologic consequences of vasectomy were noted. Further evidence of safety emerges from use-control and cohort studies showing no relation between vasectomy and cardiovascular disease. The only adverse effects are an increased risk of epididymitis, orchitis, and testicular changes leading to infertility (see below). Vasectomy still appears safe and effective, and it is the least expensive form of permanent sterilization. Recanalization when ends of the vas are tied too closely together may account for failures. Reanastomosis may be carried out with microsurgical techniques; however, only about one third of patients undergoing reanastomosis father live-born children. The causes of diminished fertility are multifactorial and include damage to nerves adjacent to the vas, the development of interstitial fibrosis within the testicle, and age.

Procedures on the Fallopian Tubes (Tubal Sterilization). Tubal sterilization is currently the leading form of contracep-

tion in the United States, with over 10 million women having undergone the procedure and 1 million being performed annually. The procedure is not foolproof; the pregnancy rate is 1% to 2%, depending on the type of tubal procedure performed. Of the pregnancies that do occur after tubal sterilization, a substantial proportion (0.15 to 0.65) are ectopic.

Postpartum Surgical Division of the Fallopian Tubes shortly after delivery is easily accomplished, either with normal vaginal delivery or with cesarean section. The procedure adds 1 to 2 days to the patient's hospitalization. Procedures that leave the two ends of the fallopian tubes in close proximity (Pomeroy technique, in which a suture ties a knuckle of tube and the apex of the knuckle is excised) may have a failure rate of 2%. Other methods that leave the two severed ends well separated have failure rates of less than 1%. When there is concern for the survival of the newborn, postpartum sterilization is contraindicated.

Vaginal tubal ligation is usually not done postpartum through the vagina because of the increased vascularity and the risk of sepsis. A skilled obstetrician-gynecologist can do interval sterilizations under local anesthesia, usually in a day care or hospital facility. However, leiomyoma, endometriosis, or previous infection may obstruct the approach to the tube.

The *minilaparotomy* involves a small abdominal incision of 1 to 2 inches done under local anesthesia through the peritoneum. Each fallopian tube is identified, ligated, and divided. The incision is closed with resorbable sutures, and a bandage is applied. The patient is able to go home within a few hours.

These methods have the advantage of simplicity and require commonly used instruments. They have been taught to surgical technicians in Third World countries. Such procedures may be unsuitable in an obese or anxious patient. In fact, other methods are more commonly used in the United States.

Laparoscopy requires expensive special instrumentation and an experienced gynecologist or surgeon. Although it can be done under local anesthesia, general endotracheal anesthesia is more commonly used. A fiberoptic endoscope is inserted through a subumbilical incision, and a second instrument accompanies the endoscope or is inserted through the pelvic incision. The tubes are cauterized or both cauterized and divided. Alternatively, plastic rings or clips are used to occlude them. Cauterization has the lowest failure rate; however, clips are advocated as being less likely to cause damage to bowel. In fact, complications and failures with clips are often remedied by cauterization. Furthermore, the half-life of the plastic materials used for occlusion has not been clearly defined, and very little 5-year data are available.

In experienced hands, laparoscopy is highly effective with minimal risk in a healthy woman. Laparoscopy may be accomplished on a 1-day basis or in day care facilities. The patient may be expected to continue her normal menstrual life and menopause. Anastomosis of severed fallopian tubes can be accomplished by careful surgical procedures with or without optical magnification. However, as with vasectomy, the rate of achieving patency is higher than that of live births. Motivating factors, patient age, concurrent disease, or attitudes of the partner and surgical technical details account for the low fertility rate.

In general, tubal sterilization should be considered irreversible. The procedure is indicated when the patient requests it. Many requests for anastomosis of divided tubes come when the procedure is initially advocated by a physician or partner. A woman of 23 with three children may be firm in her desire for sterilization, whereas a woman of 34 with five children may be unwilling to consider it. On the average, women are aged 28 to 30 at the time of tubal sterilization; 88% are married, 6% have never been married. Of note, risk of ovarian cancer appears to be reduced by tubal sterilization procedures; the mechanism is unknown.

The federal government will not reimburse for sterilization done at the time of abortion, because the combined procedure has been found to be more hazardous than either done separately. The rare instance in which this does not hold true is the patient in whom the risk of anesthesia is unduly high, such as a woman with myasthenia gravis. There is no federal reimbursement for sterilization of minors or mentally incompetent patients. Though awkward in individual cases, on the whole such regulations have been necessary to prevent widespread abuse of easily accomplished low-risk surgical procedures done without due respect for the patient's understanding or desires. In addition, the government will not pay for hysterectomies done solely for the purpose of sterilization.

CHOICE OF METHOD

The choice of birth control is best viewed in terms of the patient's age and family expectations. *Unmarried adolescents and women in their early twenties* may use oral contraceptives with a high degree of safety and acceptability. Contraindications are infrequent in this age group, and the cost, in general, is not beyond their reach. Diaphragms may be as effective but often are less acceptable. Condoms and foam are an excellent choice given their effectiveness and protection from sexually transmitted diseases. Their use depends on motivation, which can be lacking at times. Though less effective and not usually recommended by physicians as a sole means of contraception, the sponge is convenient and, as such, more likely to be used by young women. IUDs are effective, but the risk of pelvic sepsis that may affect future childbearing is a concern.

For sexually active *26 to 35 year olds*, birth control pills, diaphragms, and condoms may be equally effective, and choice is simply a matter of preference. IUDs may be a reasonable choice for parous women aware of the small risk of pelvic inflammatory disease and willing to seek help promptly at the first sign of infection. The smoker should be asked to stop tobacco use if she wants to use oral contraceptives. Many patients in this age group have completed their families and request sterilization. Nulliparous women in this age group who desire sterilization present a problem to many health care providers. If the patient is not well known to the clinic or physician, one can suggest she practice contraception for a year, then undergo sterilization if she still wants to. When such advice is given, perhaps half the patients return for the procedure. The others go elsewhere or change their minds.

For *women older than age 35*, the birth control pill may be prescribed as long as she is a nonsmoker. Diaphragms, condoms, sterilization, and more recently the pill are commonly chosen by *women older than age 40.*

PATIENT EDUCATION

There are few areas in primary care in which patient education is so important to decision making. Diagrammatic and written materials are available from most commercial distributors of contraceptive products, Planned Parenthood, many women's advocacy organizations, the American College of Obstetrics and Gynecology, and the American Medical Association. It is most important that information is clearly written in the patient's native language and that the patient is given an opportunity to ask questions and demonstrates her understanding.

The need to offer sympathetic and nonjudgmental counseling cannot be overemphasized. Regardless of the physician's personal views on abortion and birth control, the patient should be able to obtain factual information from her primary care physician or should be referred to someone who is willing to provide the information and care desired.

INDICATIONS FOR REFERRAL

Patients may need or request referral for counseling on emotional responses to sexual activity and contraceptive techniques. Referral to a social worker, sex therapist, or psychiatrist with an interest in the area may be useful, but thorough discussion between the primary physician and patient usually suffices.

When a surgical procedure is being considered, the patient should meet with the gynecologist to discuss the issue in more detail. Referrals of medically uncomplicated patients may be made by phone. For patients with known medical problems, a careful history and physical examination and written referral to the specialist are helpful, so that the risks of the various procedures may be carefully discussed and therapy individualized. Patients who seem unable to use any form of birth control offered may also be referred to any of the above-named specialists, in the hope that an alternative approach will enhance motivation.

ANNOTATED BIBLIOGRAPHY

Beral V, Hermon C, Kay C, et al. Mortality associated with oral contraceptive use: 25 year follow up of cohort of 46 000 women from Royal College of General Practitioners' oral contraceptive study. BMJ 1999;318:96. *(Current and recent users with relative risk of 0.2 for ovarian cancer, 1.9 for cerebrovascular disease.)*

Berenson AB, Weimann CM, Rickerr VI, et al. Contraceptive outcomes among adolescents prescribed Norplant implants versus oral contraceptives after one year of use. Am J Obstet Gynecol 1997; 176:586. *(A case-control study demonstrates better contraception protection but higher side effect rate with Norplant when compared with oral contraceptives.)*

Burkman RT. Lipid metabolism effects with desogestrel-containing oral contraceptives. Am J Obstet Gynecol 1993;168:1033. *(A review of the studies suggests that desogestrel has minimal effect on lipoprotein metabolism.)*

Chang CL, Donaghy M, Poulter N. Migraine and stroke in young women: case control study. BMJ 1999;318:13. *(Oral contraceptives increase risk of stroke associated with migraine.)*

Chasan-Taber L, Stampfer MJ. Epidemiology of oral contraceptives and cardiovascular disease. Ann Intern Med 1998;128:467. *(Extensive review of literature reveals that cardiovascular risk is lower with any of the current new preparations as compared with prior high estrogen dose pills. Cardiovascular risk is significant in smokers.)*

Collins D. Selectivity information on desogestrel. Am J Obstet Gynecol 1993;168:1010. *(Review of desogestrel's progestational effect reveals that it is weakly androgenic while retaining strong progestational activity.)*

Coukell AJ, Balfour JA. Levonorgestrel subdermal implants. A review of contraceptive efficacy and acceptability. Drug 1998 55:861. *(A review of Norplant reveals that despite a high incidence of menstrual irregularity, levonorgestrel subdermal implants are a good choice of contraceptive method in women who are looking for an alternative to an oral regimen.)*

Dardano KL, Burkman RT. The intrauterine contraceptive device: an often-forgotten and maligned method of contraception. Am J Obstet Gynecol 1999;181:1. *(Despite many advantages for some women, used by fewer than 1% of American women who use contraception.)*

Delbanco SF, Stewart FH, Koenig JD, et al. Are we making progress with emergency contraception? Recent findings on American adults and health professionals. J Am Womens Med Assoc 1998;53:242. *(Only 11% of women knew enough about emergency contraception to use it.)*

Eldon MA, Undwerwood, BA, Randinitis EJ, et al. Gabapentin does not interact with a contraceptive regimen of norethindrone acetate and ethinyl estradiol. Neurology 1998;50:1146. *(Gabapentin may be a good choice anticonvulsant for women on oral contraceptives.)*

Farmer RD, Lawrenson RA, Thompson CR, et al. Population-based study of risk of venous thromboembolism associated with various oral contraceptives. Lancet 1997;349:83. *(A large-scale record review found no significant increase in rate of thromboembolic disease in users of newer progestins.)*

Gaspard UJ, Lefebvre PJ. Clinical aspects of the relationship between oral contraceptives, abnormalities in carbohydrate metabolism, and the development of cardiovascular disease. Am J Obstet Gynecol 1990;163:334. *(Low-dose oral contraceptives with reduced progestogen content have the least effect on glucose tolerance.)*

Hankinson SE, Colditz GA, Manson JE, et al. A prospective study on oral contraceptive use and risk of breast cancer (Nurses' Health Study, United States). Cancer Causes Control 1997;8:65. *(Cohort study of women found no increase in breast cancer risk in women over 40 years of age.)*

Hannon PR, Duggan AK, Serwint JR, et al. The influence of medroxyprogesterone on the duration of breast-feeding in mothers in an urban community. Arch Pediatr Adolesc Med 1997;151:490. *(Prospective cohort study revealed no detrimental effect on lactation from medroxyprogesterone.)*

Henkinson SE, Hunter DJ, Colditz GA, et al. Tubal ligation, hysterectomy, and risk of ovarian cancer. JAMA 1993;270:2813. *(Risk is reduced significantly by tubal ligation.)*

Lobo RA, Skinner JB, Lippman JS, et al. Plasma lipids and desogestrel and ethinyl estradiol: a meta-analysis. Fertil Steril 1996;65:1100. *(Meta-analysis reveals that desogestrel-ethinyl estradiol combination results in increased HDL and lower LDL cholesterol when compared with baseline.)*

Maharani DK, London SN. Mifepristone (RU 486). Fertil Steril. 1997;68:967. *(A review of the literature concerning mechanism of action, pharmacodynamics and potential new uses of RU-486.)*

Mant J, Painter R, Vessey M. Risk of myocardial infarction, angina and stroke in users of oral contraceptives: an updated analysis of a cohort study. Br J Obstet Gynaecol 1998;105:890. *(A cohort study of 17,032 revealed a slight increase risk of ischemic stroke [relative risk, 2.9] in all users and myocardial infarction only in smokers.)*

Narod SA, Risch H, Moslehi R, et al. Oral contraceptives and the risk of hereditary ovarian cancer. N Engl J Med 1998;339:424. *(A case-control study of 386 women revealed reduced risk of ovarian cancer in women with the BRCA1 or BRCA2 gene in oral contraceptive users.)*

Peterson HB, Xia Z, Hughes JM, et al. The risk of ectopic pregnancy after tubal sterilization. N Engl J Med 1997;336:762. *(A multicenter cohort study of over 10,000 women followed for 8 to 14 years after tubal sterilization; cumulative rate of ectopic pregnancy was 7.3 per 1,000 procedures, with the bipolar technique 27 times more likely to cause ectopic pregnancy that partial salpingectomy.)*

Rabe T, Nitsche DC, Runnebaum B. The effects of monophasic and triphasic oral contraceptives on ovarian function and endometrial thickness. Eur J Contracept Reprod Health Care 1997;2:39. *(Monophasic pills are superior to triphasics in reducing ovarian function.)*

Rosenberg L, Palmer JR, Rao RS, et al. Case-control study of oral contraceptive use and risk of breast cancer. Am J Epidemiol 1996; 143:25. *(Case-control study revealed an increase in relative risk in women aged 25 to 34.)*

Rossing MA, Standford JL, Weiss NS, et al. Oral contraceptive use and risk of breast cancer in middle-aged women. Am J Epidemiol 1996;144:161. *(Case-control study supports absence of any strong association between oral contraceptive use and breast cancer risk.)*

Rushton L, Jones DR. Oral contraceptive use and breast cancer risk: a meta-analysis of variations with age at diagnosis, parity and total duration of oral contraceptive use. Br J Obstet Gynaecol 1992;99:239. *(A meta-analysis revealing a relative risk of breast cancer with oral contraceptive use of 1.16 in younger women, 1.21 in nulliparous women, and 1.27 for duration greater than 8 years.)*

Schaff EA, Stadalius LS, Eisinger SH, et al. Vaginal misoprostol administered at home after mifepristone (RU486) for abortion. J Fam Practice 1997;44:353. *(A prospective trial with women up to 8 weeks pregnant wanting an abortion. Misoprostol was found to be safe, highly effective, and acceptable to women).*

Schwartz SM, Siscovick DS, Longstreth WT Jr, et al. Use of low-dose oral contraceptives and stroke in young women. Ann Intern Med 1997;127:596. *(Population-based case-control study reveals no increase risk in oral contraceptive users for stroke. Question of possible increased risk in users of norgestel-containing oral contraceptive was raised.)*

Shoupe D, Mishell DR, Bopp BL, et al. The significance of bleeding patterns in Norplant implant users. Obstet Gynecol 1991;77:256. *(Cohort study of 234 Norplant users revealing 66.3% of women with irregular bleeding during the first year of use and 37.5% with irregular bleeding by the fifth year.)*

Spitz IM, Bardin CW. Mifepristone (RU-486)—a modulator of progestin and glucocorticoid action. N Engl J Med 1993;329:404. *(Authoritative review of this potent abortifacient.)*

Spitzer WO. Bias versus causality: interpreting recent evidence of oral contraceptive studies. Am J Obstet Gynecol 1998;179:S43. *(Review of methodology of earlier studies reveals that bias rather than causality demonstrated increase DVT rates in newer progestins. Difference in cardiovascular event rates of new progestin-containing oral contraceptives are trivial and not clinically significant.)*

Spona J, Elstein M, Feichtinger W, et al. Shorter pill-free interval in combined oral contraceptives decreases follicular development. Contraception 1996;54:71. *(Reducing hormone-free days to 5 in a 28-day cycle appears to improve contraceptive safety margin in very low estrogen pills.)*

Stampfer MJ, Willet WC, Colditz GA, et al. Past use of oral contraceptives and cardiovascular disease: a meta-analysis in the context of the Nurses' Health Study. Am J Obstet Gynecol 1990;163:285. *(Large cohort study that prospectively looked at cardiovascular events and found no difference among past users as compared with never-users of the oral contraceptive.)*

Task Force on Postovulatory Methods of Fertility Regulation. Randomised controlled trial of levonorgestrel versus the Yuzpe regimen of combined oral contraceptives for emergency contraception. Lancet 1998;352:428. *(Levonorgestrel regimen better tolerated and more effective.)*

Task Force on Postovulatory Methods of Fertility Regulation. Comparison of three single doses of mifepristone as emergency contraception: a randomised trial. Lancet 1999;353:697. *(A dose as low as 10 mg as effective as 600 mg.)*

Thomas DB. Oral contraceptives and breast cancer: review of the epidemiologic literature. Contraception 1991;43:597. *(In-depth review of studies reveals little or no overall increase in the risk of breast cancer. There may be a slight increase risk in very young women or women who use the pill for a long duration.)*

Van Os WA, Edelman DA, Rhemrev PE, et al. Oral contraceptives and breast cancer risk. Adv Contracept 1997;13:63. *(A review of the medical literature supports the view that oral contraceptive use is associated with small increased risks of premenopausal breast cancer, but there is no consensus on which subgroups of women might be at increased risk.)*

120
Approach to the Infertile Couple

A couple that has been engaging in regular sexual intercourse without contraception for at least a year without conceiving is considered infertile. Ten percent to 20% of American couples in their childbearing years are infertile. New technologies and rising expectations have produced significant increases in the numbers of couples seeking help, more than doubling in the past decade and now exceeding three million. The primary physician is often the first to be consulted and is responsible for initiating a medical evaluation of the couple. Although the usual request is to find or rule out a medical cause for the problem, there is also a need to identify any psychological or socioeconomic barriers to conception. Treatment is frequently carried out by individuals specializing in infertility, but the primary care physician should become proficient in performing the initial assessment and knowing when referral is indicated. Principal tasks include providing accurate advice and uncovering treatable etiologies.

PATHOPHYSIOLOGY AND CLINICAL PRESENTATION

Any disorder involving the male or female reproductive system may interfere with function to a degree sufficient to cause infertility.

Men

Infertility in the male can be classified in terms of gonadal, gonadotropic, obstructive, and functional etiologies and considered according to whether they present with azoospermia, oligospermia, or normal sperm counts.

Azoospermic Etiologies. Patients with primary hypogonadism affecting both spermatogenesis and testosterone synthesis have azoospermia, a low testosterone, and elevations of luteinizing hormone (LH) and follicle-stimulating hormone (FSH). *Klinefelter's syndrome* is the archetype example, characterized by two X chromosomes and one Y chromosome. The extra chromatin is visible as the Barr body seen on examination of buccal mucosa cells.

Men with predominantly germinal compartment failure are also azoospermic but manifest relatively normal testosterone and normal LH and elevated FSH. *Sertoli cell–only syndrome*, adult *mumps* orchitis, and *cancer therapy* are among the more common congenital and acquired varieties, respectively. In a study comparing childhood and adolescent cancer survivors to sibling control subjects, overall relative fertility was 85%, with radiation therapy below the diaphragm reducing it by 25% and alkylating therapy alone causing a 40% reduction.

Hypogonadotropic hypogonadism also causes azoospermia. It too may be congenital or acquired (Table 120.1). Patients present with azoospermia and low levels of FSH, LH, and serum testosterone. Congenital disease is often associated with anosmia (*Kallmann's syndrome*). Pituitary tumors account for much of the acquired disease; a *prolactinoma* may be responsible. Large sellar tumors can lead to panhypopituitarism, with features of hypothyroidism and adrenal insufficiency dominating the clinical picture. *Drugs* (including alcohol and marijuana) can interfere with hypothalamic-pituitary function.

Azoospermia in association with normal levels of LH, FSH, and testosterone characterize *retrograde ejaculation* (due to diabetes or drugs) and *obstruction* of the ejaculatory system. There may be *congenital obstruction* of the epididymis and vas deferens or the vas may be absent. Most other types of obstruction are more proximal, giving normal testicular size and normal semen fructose.

Oligospermic Etiologies. Patients with a large *varicocele* may present with the typical "bag of worms" appearance to the testicle, but at times the only manifestation is a faint pulsation along the spermatic vein on Valsalva or coughing. The varicocele may be unilateral (usually on the left) or bilateral. There is no correlation between size of the varicocele and degree of infertility. Testicular size may be reduced, even though the scrotal contents appear enlarged. The mechanism by which varicocele results in infertility remains undetermined; some even question the association, but repair of the varicocele by spermatic vein ligation often restores normal sperm quantity and function. Effects on fertility are less clear.

Another large group of oligospermic patients with normal LH and testosterone have no detectable pathology and are labeled *idiopathic*. The condition results in a quantitative abnormality of spermatogenesis without any identifiable anatomic or endocrinologic precipitant. FSH is normal unless the sperm count falls below 20 million/mL, in which case it may begin to rise. At times, the acquired forms of selective tubular damage (*chemotherapy, irradiation, adult mumps*) may leave the patient

Table 120.1.   Important Causes of Male Infertility

Hypothalamic/pituitary
   Prolactinoma
   Idiopathic
   Drugs (e.g., alcohol, marijuana)

Testicular
   Klinefelter's syndrome
   Sertoli cell–only syndrome
   Irradiation
   Adult mumps
   Alkylating agents

Anatomic/functional
   Obstruction of epididymis or vas
   Impotence
   Retrograde ejaculation
   Infection
   Antisperm antibodies
   Idiopathic defects in sperm quantity or quality

oligospermic rather than azoospermic. Testosterone and LH are normal, but thyroid-stimulating hormone is elevated.

In milder forms of acquired *hypothalamic-pituitary dysfunction*, some spermatogenesis may be preserved. FSH and LH are low to low normal and testosterone is low. Prolactin may be elevated due to a *microadenoma*. In *partial androgen resistance,* testosterone and LH are elevated, whereas FSH remains normal. Gynecomastia develops as a result of excess estradiol production by the testicle and peripheral conversion of testosterone.

Etiologies with Normal Sperm Counts. Most patients demonstrate abnormal sperm morphology or motility and suffer from many of the same conditions as those with oligospermia (e.g., varicocele). In addition, *genitourinary tract infection* may cause such qualitative sperm changes; leukocytes sometimes appear in the semen. *Antisperm antibodies* are noted in some patients, and an autoimmune mechanism may be operative in some instances, although the relationship between antibodies and infertility remains to be fully established.

Impotence or erectile dysfunction ranks as a leading, although frequently overlooked, etiology. Hormone concentrations and sperm parameters are usually normal in "functional" types (although depression and situational stress can transiently reduce sperm counts). In organic etiologies of impotence, these parameters reflect the underlying pathology (see Chapters 132 and 229). Anatomic anomalies, such as proximal location of the urinary meatus, may lead to infertility because of deposition of sperm and semen too far from the cervical os.

Women

Disorders of Ovulation are among the most frequent causes of failure to conceive, comprising 20% to 40% of cases in which a female factor is responsible for the infertility. Anovulatory bleeding (irregular menses), amenorrhea, or infertility may be the presenting complaint. *Polycystic ovary syndrome* and other forms of *hypothalamic dysfunction* account for most cases (see Chapters 111 and 112). Pathophysiologically, the normal pattern of gonadotropin-releasing hormone (GnRH) release is disrupted, impairing the normal midcycle surge in LH. The result is failure to ovulate and inadequate corpus luteum formation. Treatment can restore fertility.

Premature ovarian failure may be autoimmune or idiopathic, but an important acquired source is *cancer therapy* in children and adolescents (see above). In the study noted above comparing survivors of childhood and adolescent cancers with their siblings, overall relative fertility for women was 85%, with radiation therapy below the diaphragm reducing it by 25% but alkylating therapy having relatively little effect.

Tubal Disorders account for about 25% of cases. *Pelvic inflammatory disease* (particularly indolent nongonococcal forms such as that due to *Chlamydia trachomatis*; see Chapters 116 and 117) is the leading cause of tubal damage. In a prospective study, 12% of those with a single episode of salpingitis had tubal occlusion; 35% of those with two infections had occlusion; and 75% of those with three or more had occlusion. Other pelvic and abdominal infections (such as a *ruptured appendix* in childhood) may lead to tubal adhesions. Infections associated with intrauterine devices are a problem. *Postpartum infection* has an unusually frequent association with tubal occlusion. Infections after induced abortion, particularly if inadequately treated (e.g., with inappropriately low doses of antibiotics), unrecognized, or not brought to medical attention, may lead to infertility.

Oil-based dyes used for uterotubograms (hysterosalpingograms) in some countries have also been associated with adhesions. Uncommon causes include *pelvic trauma* from vehicular accidents, *inflammatory bowel disease*, tuberculosis, and schistosomiasis. In general, processes that cause adhesions rather than tubal epithelial damage seem to have a better prognosis. *Endometriosis*, found in 8% to 15% of fertility clinic populations, may cause tubal obstruction and uterine disturbances.

Uterine Pathology represents about 5% of cases. *Congenital anomalies*, such as absence or duplication of the uterine fundus, often present as repeated pregnancy wastage. Complete duplication of cervix and uterus tends to diminish fertility but less so than anomalies causing distortion of a single uterine cavity. Septate and deeply arcuate uteri may be more useful after hysteroscopic or operative repair. Urinary tract anomalies are estimated to occur with 25% of congenitally abnormal uteri. They are found more frequently in the completely duplicated situation or when one side of the müllerian duct is missing.

Uterine Fibroids and Endometriosis may distort or obstruct the uterine cavity. Resection and reresection of fibroids have been surprisingly successful. The *forgotten intrauterine device* is occasionally a cause of infertility. The role of uterine glycosaminoglycan in stimulating conversion of sperm proacrosin to acrosin, a step necessary for sperm penetration of the zona pellucida, is an area of ongoing investigation.

Cervical Factors are increasingly appreciated sources of infertility. *Cervical incompetence* may lead to repeated abortion or later trimester pregnancy losses. The incompetence can result from inadequate innervation, disturbances in synthesis or breakdown of prostaglandin, or defects in muscle and collagen fibers. Incompetence of the cervix may also compromise its role in resisting the entry of infectious agents into the sterile uterine cavity.

The precise role of *cervical mucus* is still not well understood, but normal viscosity and ferning are essential to conception and represent evidence of adequate estrogen stimulation and response. The importance of cervical mucus *antibodies* and proteins as a cause of infertility continues to be a focus of much research.

Vaginal Factors are occasionally implicated. An intact or nearly *intact hymen*, a septum, or a constricting ring in the upper vagina can limit access to the cervix. Total absence of the vagina is only rarely associated with sufficient development of the cervix and uterus to allow fertility at all. As a site of *infection*, the vagina may prove to be an important cause of pregnancy wastage. *Trichomonas, Candida albicans, Chlamydia, Mycoplasma, Gardnerella*, streptococci, and gonococci are all associated with cervical and vaginal discharge (see Chapter 117). Their role in vaginally related obstructions to conception is not clear, although their role in pregnancy wastage is established. When these organisms lead to pelvic inflammatory disease, they become more clearly accountable for infertility.

Viral Infections of the Vulva and Labia, particularly herpes vaginalis and condyloma accuminata, are usually only temporary impediments to fertility (see Chapter 192). Vulvar surgery per se need not cause infertility. Similarly, paralysis or hemipelvectomy may or may not be blamed for infertility; much of the impediment derives from the social and emotional impact of these conditions.

Both Partners

Interpersonal problems (see Chapter 229) are an important etiologic factor, because they may lead to sexual dysfunction. The desire for children may not be shared equally by both partners. This may be overt, with one partner seeking medical assistance to persuade the other. More often, it is covert. There may be anxiety over how family responsibilities will interfere with career development, or one partner may not want to lose the economic and social freedom of a childless couple. Sometimes one partner may be concerned about sharing the other's affection with a child. Some may feel inadequate or unwilling to assume parental duties. Such concerns can lead to sexual inactivity. Transient situational problems arise. The young professional person may be under considerable job pressure; travel may interfere with optimal timing of intercourse for conception or lead to hypothalamic dysfunction. Acknowledged or unrecognized homosexual preference may also interfere with fertility.

Controversy surrounds the role of *genital* Mycoplasma *infection* in the genesis of infertility. In one study, if the husband was culture positive, treatment of the infertile couple for *Mycoplasma* led to a 60% pregnancy rate if the infection was eradicated versus a 5% rate when it was not. Other studies fail to show any association between the *Mycoplasma* infection and infertility.

DIFFERENTIAL DIAGNOSIS

In about a third of instances, a male factor is the predominant etiology. In another third, a female factor predominates. In the remainder, either the cause resides with both partners or the etiology is unknown. In most cases attributed to a male factor, there is either a quantitative or qualitative sperm defect of unknown etiology. Among female factors, ovulatory disturbances account for up to 40%, tubal disorders for 10% to 30%, cervical factors for 20%, and uterine factors for about 5%. Tables 120.1 and 120.2 list some of the most important etiologies.

Table 120.2. Important Causes of Female Infertility

Hypothalamic/pituitary
  Hypothalamic dysfunction
  Polycystic ovary syndrome
  Prolactinoma

Ovarian
  Primary failure (e.g., premature menopause)
  Irradiation

Tubal
  Pelvic inflammatory disease
  Endometriosis
  Adhesions

Uterine
  Fibroids
  Scarring (Asherman's syndrome)
  Anatomic abnormalities

Cervical
  Poor mucus quality
  Infection
  Anatomic abnormalities

WORKUP

Initial Evaluation

The prognosis even for untreated couples is favorable (see below). An extensive "infertility workup" need not be undertaken on first visit, unless the couple is older (mid to late 30s and upward), has been unable to conceive despite trying seriously for over a year, or has a similar good reason to hasten the pace of evaluation. Otherwise, a reasonable approach to the first visit is to limit the assessment to a careful general history and physical examination, checking for such important causes as endocrinopathy, tumor, genitourinary tract infection, anatomic disorder, and interpersonal problems.

In the Male. *History* should include inquiry into drug and medication use (marijuana, alcohol, antihypertensive agents), urethral discharge, headache and other symptoms of a pituitary tumor (see Chapter 100), past history of radiation therapy or cancer chemotherapy, mumps, toxin exposure, and systemic illnesses (especially diabetes with associated retrograde ejaculation). A sexual history that reviews the marital relationship, sexual techniques, erectile function, and frequency of intercourse is also important.

Physical examination begins with noting general appearance and any signs of diminished androgenization (decreased body hair, gynecomastia, eunuchoid proportions). The scrotum is examined for testicular size, presence of a varicocele, hypospadias, and absent vas deferens. Soft small testes (less than 4 cm in longest diameter) are consistent with primary testicular failure and pituitary-hypothalamic insufficiency. A Valsalva maneuver performed while the patient is standing will help reveal a small varicocele. The urethra is observed for discharge, and the prostate and seminal vesicles are observed for tenderness and other signs of infection. If a pituitary condition is suspected, visual field testing by confrontation might reveal an important field defect; a normal study does not rule out a mass lesion. Testing deep tendon reflexes may uncover delay in relaxation suggestive of hypothyroidism (see Chapter 104).

In the Female. *History* focuses on the menstrual and reproductive history, including any abortions, complicated deliveries, curettages, menstrual irregularities, or episodes of amenorrhea. A life-long history of menstrual irregularities is suggestive of polycystic ovary syndrome, especially if accompanied by hirsutism and obesity. Any situational or emotional stress, marked weight loss, or excess exercise should be noted, because it can lead to hypothalamic dysfunction and impairment of ovulation (see Chapters 111 and 112). Similarly, checking for symptoms of hypothyroidism (see Chapter 104), hyperprolactinemia (see Chapter 100), Cushing's syndrome (see Chapter 100), and androgen excess (see Chapter 98) may yield clues of conditions that can impair hypothalamic function. Inquiry into headaches, visual field disturbances, galactorrhea, symptoms of pituitary insufficiency (see Chapter 100), and a history of postpartum hemorrhage helps to screen for a sella tursica esion. Checking for a history or symptoms of pelvic inflammatory disease (vaginal discharge, pelvic pain, fever, dyspareunia) is also essential. Any malignant disease history is important to note, especially if treatment included irradiation or alkylating agents. One should also obtain a detailed psychosocial history that reviews pertinent details of the marital relationship and sexual activity. Loss of libido may signify psychosocial or hormonal dysfunction.

Physical examination focuses on checking for obesity, excessive weight loss, hirsutism, cushingoid appearance, stigmata of hypothyroidism (see Chapter 104), visual field disturbances, and goiter. Most important is a careful pelvic examination, taking special note of any ovarian, uterine, or adnexal masses, thickening, or tenderness. Examination of the cervix should include checking for erosions, discharge, polyps, masses, scarring, and pain on cervical motion. The hirsute patient is examined for clitoromegaly.

Both Partners. An empathic, supportive, nonjudgmental exploration of the marital relationship is essential; it is often best done by interviewing the couple together (to observe their interactions) and each partner separately.

Further Evaluation

Couples with no evidence of serious pathology on initial evaluation can be reassured and informed that more than half of such couples go on to conceive without the aid of treatment. Those who have been trying to conceive for less than 1 year can be advised to delay further evaluation until 12 months have passed, provided they are willing to do so and have no compelling reason for proceeding directly to more extensive testing. Couples who have failed to conceive after continuously trying for 12 months or who insist on further workup at the time of initial visit can undergo a set of basic laboratory studies to more fully define the problem and guide further evaluation and treatment.

In the Male. The first test to perform is a *semen analysis*, collecting two to three specimens over a 4- to 6-week period. Quantitative analysis includes number of sperm per milliliter of semen (counts more than 20 million/mL are normal) and semen volume (less than 1.5 mL may be inadequate to buffer vaginal acidity). Patients with normal counts should have qualitative studies of the sperm performed (motility, morphology, cervical mucus interaction), although these studies are often more useful for identifying the infertile individual than for defining a specific course of therapy (see below). In normal persons, the counts for motile forms and spermatozoa with oval heads are in excess of 50%.

Patients with azoospermia or oligospermia are candidates for serum gonadotropin (*LH and FSH*) and *testosterone* determinations, because of the possibility of an underlying disorder within the hypothalamic-pituitary-testicular axis. Proper sampling technique is important to avoid misleading results. One draws three serum samples 20 minutes apart and pools them. High concentrations of gonadotropins and low or low-normal testosterone suggest a primary gonadal problem. Both gonadotropins and testosterone being low characterize a pituitary-hypothalamic etiology. Normal FSH, testosterone, and testicular size in a patient with azoospermia suggests obstruction. Normal hormone and gonadotropin concentrations in the setting of oligospermia are characteristic of patients with varicocele or idiopathic disease. Small testes, gynecomastia, an elevated FSH, and a reduced testosterone suggest Klinefelter's syndrome. The diagnosis is confirmed by a *buccal smear* that shows the extra chromatin of a Barr body.

The patient with suspected pituitary disease needs a *prolactin level* and *computed tomography* (CT) of the sella turcica to search for a tumor. An elevated prolactin in the setting of a normal CT may be due to a drug-induced problem, but CT should be repeated in 6 months to be sure that an early tumor has not been missed.

The utility of more elaborate studies (e.g., antisperm antibodies, sperm-cervical mucus interaction, penetration testing) is best determined by the infertility specialist.

In the Female. The first task is to establish that ovulation is taking place. The time-tested approach is to use a *temperature chart*. Ovulation is accompanied by a rise in progesterone secretion, which leads to a 0.3° rise in basal body temperature after ovulation. Temperature is measured orally each morning before rising from bed. One uses a special thermometer graduated in tenths of degrees Fahrenheit. Absence of a rise indicates failure to ovulate. Alternatively, one can measure the *serum progesterone* on days 21 to 23 of the cycle. A level greater than 10 ng/mL indicates ovulation and a functioning corpus luteum. Endometrial biopsy may also be useful but is more expensive, more painful, and may remove the long-awaited pregnancy. If the patient is deemed anovulatory, further testing proceeds with measurement of *serum prolactin, FSH, and LH* (see Chapters 111 and 112).

A *postcoital examination* is used to assess cervical mucus function and the competency of the partner. An appointment is scheduled just before the time of ovulation, and the woman is asked to come within 2 to 12 hours of coitus. A specimen of cervical mucus is obtained from the endocervical canal. Five or more motile sperm found in the specimen confirms her partner's competence. Mucus is also examined for viscosity (stretching to 6 cm is normal) and "ferning," manifestations of estrogen effect.

If after the initial history, physical examination, postcoital test, and serum progesterone, it appears that tubal or uterine disease may be responsible for infertility, then *hysterosalpingography* and *laparoscopy* deserve consideration. Choice of test should be made by the gynecologist experienced in evaluation of infertility. Hysterosalpingoscopy involves injection of a contrast agent into the uterus by way of a cervical catheter. Pretreatment doxycycline antibiotic coverage is provided. Films reveal uterine and tubal anatomy. Laparoscopy requires general anesthesia but can detect adhesions, endometriosis, an unpalpable fibroid, and polycystic ovaries. Tubal patency and position may also be confirmed, often more accurately than by radiologic investigation. Not to be forgotten is the importance of negative findings.

PRINCIPLES OF MANAGEMENT AND INDICATIONS FOR REFERRAL

Studies from infertility clinics have shown that many couples go on to conceive without treatment (e.g., 44% of those with ovulation deficiency; 61% of those with endometriosis, tubal defects, or seminal deficiencies; and 96% of those with cervical factors or idiopathic infertility). A conservative approach of watchful waiting is reasonable in such cases, provided there is no evidence of tumor, infection, anatomic defect, or serious endocrinopathy. Counseling can be a very important adjunct (see below).

When the workup suggests causative organic pathology, an appropriate referral for confirmatory testing and design of a treatment program is indicated. The participation of the primary physician in the care of the couple should continue, but the subtleties of specialized care that some types of infertility treatment require argue for referral rather than for treatment by the primary physician. Successful referral depends to a large extent on proper patient selection.

Men. A neurologic or anatomic cause of *impotence*, a suspected acquired *obstructive defect*, and *varicocele* are indications for urologic consultation. Surgical ligation of a varicocele is commonly performed, but results are often disappointing even though sperm counts may rise. Treatment of obstruction requires a urologist skilled in microsurgical techniques, as does vasectomy reversal.

Hypothalamic-pituitary disorders have a high rate of success with treatment by the reproductive endocrinologist. Those with idiopathic hypogonadotropic disease often respond successfully to gonadotropin or GnRH administration. When prolactin levels are elevated and CT reveals a microadenoma, bromocriptine can often restore fertility. Larger pituitary adenomas may require neurosurgical intervention.

Idiopathic oligospermia (no evidence of a varicocele; normal LH, FSH, and testosterone) has no proven therapy. Clomiphene and other antiestrogens, GnRH factor, gonadotropins, and low doses of androgen have been tried but without confirmed long-term benefit. There is no evidence that vitamins (A, E, C), zinc, thyroid hormone, or a host of home remedies are at all useful in men with normospermia or oligospermia. Such patients should be referred to the reproductive endocrinologist for consultation.

Men who have quantitatively and qualitatively *normal sperm* and *normal LH, FSH,* and *testosterone* pose a challenge. When *antisperm antibodies* are found in high titers in the semen, their levels can be lowered with a course of high-dose corticosteroids. However, the efficacy of this therapy is controversial. Careful patient selection by referral to the re-

productive specialist is essential. In vitro fertilization is an alternative.

Artificial insemination and other assisted reproductive technologies are available for patients with otherwise *refractory qualitative sperm defects*. Patients with retrograde ejaculation might also effect pregnancy with artificial insemination, using semen recovered in the urine.

Subclinical infection, especially with *Mycoplasma*, has been suggested as a cause of infertility. Culturing both partners and treating the couple if one partner is culture positive has produced inconsistent results. There are no known treatments for patients with gonadal failure or androgen insensitivity.

Women. Women with *hypothalamic dysfunction* have a good prognosis. Those with mild dysfunction are likely to resume ovulating without therapy and need only counseling at the time of initial evaluation. Those with moderate dysfunction often respond well to treatment, especially when FSH, thyroid function, and prolactin remain normal. Such persons have a 50% chance of conceiving with use of clomiphene, which is given for 3 to 5 days followed by a month of waiting for either pregnancy or an ovulatory period. Patients suffering from more severe hypothalamic dysfunction may fail clomiphene, but respond to synthetic GnRH therapy. GnRH is administered by parenteral pulse infusions, mimicking normal GnRH secretion. Careful dose adjustments are necessary to avoid multiple pregnancies. Only an experienced reproductive endocrinologist should prescribe such therapy. Those with a prolactin-secreting microadenoma require endocrinologic consultation. Bromocriptine may help restore fertility (see Chapter 100).

Gynecologic referral is indicated for patients with suspected *tubal scarring*. Microsurgical tubal reconstruction is required for successful repair, which leads to pregnancy in 10% to 60% of cases. In making the referral for tubal repair, it is important to select a gynecologist skilled in microsurgical techniques. Success rates vary considerably.

Women with *abnormal postcoital testing* may be candidates for intrauterine insemination if they are ovulating and the semen analysis is normal. Couples who have *failed other methods* may still be candidates for in vitro fertilization or gamete intrafallopian tube transfer. These are elaborate technologies that require the consultative and technical services of a specialized reproductive center. One must have adequate sperm, ovarian follicles, and a competent uterus to qualify for in vitro fertilization. These plus fallopian tube patency and accessibility are the minimum determinants for gamete intrafallopian tube transfer.

Couples. Infertility resulting from a *psychosocial problem* (e.g., lack of privacy, work exhaustion, marital discord) needs to be approached with careful and understanding explanation. Some individuals may attempt to view the situation as a medical problem when there is unlikely to be a strictly medical solution. Attention needs to be directed to the home environment, work situation, and marital relationship. When *sexual dysfunction* is detected, treatment is best directed toward it (see Chapter 229). However, artificial insemination is sometimes used when there is a strong desire to have a child as soon as possible.

The infertility evaluation may lead to reconsideration and redesign of treatment regimens for *underlying medical conditions* such as cancer and hypertension (see Chapters 26, 88, and 89).

PATIENT EDUCATION

Couples are eager for information about their chances of conceiving. At one end of the spectrum are men and women with permanent gonadal failure who have no chance of conceiving. At the other end are those with a transient functional deficit who are likely to conceive without any treatment other than reassurance and time. The couple that remains unsuccessful after a year of trying can be given some reassurance as they begin to undergo evaluation. Up to one fourth of such couples achieves pregnancy within 3 months. Published findings from infertility clinics show that, overall, 25% to 35% of couples achieve conception within 1 to 2 years of registration. The percentages continue to rise over the next 4 to 5 years.

There is a slight decrease in fecundity after 30 and a marked decrease after age 35. There appears to be little or no difference in prognosis between infertile couples who have conceived in the past and those who have never conceived. The prognosis for women who experience recurrent spontaneous abortions is better than the approximately 20% live-birth rate previously estimated. Patients with ovulatory problems do reasonably well; those with tubal problems have more difficulty. As noted earlier, rates for live births after tubal repair range from 10% to 60%, depending on the severity and site of the scarring, quality of semen, age of the women, and a host of other factors. Couples whose infertility involves multiple factors do less well than those in whom only one factor is identified.

Whenever an evaluation is normal, it is important to reassure patients about their normality, particularly if one harbors guilt or fear about an episode of infidelity, a previous abortion, an out-of-wedlock pregnancy, or some other potentially adverse event.

The investigation of infertility provides an opportunity to educate patients about normal human reproduction and prevention of sexually transmitted disease. Education for both partners about the menstrual cycles, the best time to attempt conception, and the frequency of coitus needed to achieve pregnancy can be very helpful, sometimes even curative. The importance of using a condom to prevent spread of sexually transmitted diseases that might lead to tubal scarring cannot be overemphasized to teenagers and other patients with multiple partners. Screening such persons for chlamydial infection and treating when present may help prevent tubal infertility (see Chapter 117). A review of sexual attitudes and concerns may also be of benefit. At times, the infertility evaluation encourages couples to take better care of themselves.

A.H.G./A.G.M.

ANNOTATED BIBLIOGRAPHY

Agarwal SK, Haney AF. Does recommending timed intercourse really help the infertile couple? Obstet Gynecol 1994;84:307. *(Evidence suggests that peak fertility is often missed if coitus is timed with menstrual calendar, basal body temperature, or LH kit.)*

Byrne J, Mulvihill JJ, Myers MH, et al. Effects of treatment on fertility in long-term survivors of childhood or adolescent cancer. N Engl J Med 1987;317:1315. *(A retrospective cohort study; fertility rates varied by sex, site of therapy, and type.)*

Collins JA, Wrixon W, Janes LB, et al. Treatment-independent pregnancy among infertile couples. N Engl J Med 1983;309:1201. *(A retrospective review indicating that the potential for a spontaneous cure is high.)*

Collins JA, Ying SO, Wilson EH, et al. The postcoital test as a predictor of pregnancy among 355 infertile couples. Fertil Steril 1984;41:703. *(Predictive value was good.)*

Gleicher N, Vanderlaan B, Pratt D, et al. Background pregnancy rates in an infertile population. Hum Reprod 1996;11:1011. *(Spontaneous annual pregnancy rate in this infertile population was 20%.)*

Himmel W, Ittner E, et al. Management of involuntary childlessness. Br J Gen Pract 1997;47:111. *(A review for the primary care provider.)*

Hull MG, Cahill DJ. Female infertility. Endocrinol Metab Clin North Am 1998;27:851. *(Reviews basic investigations and summarizes cumulative pregnancy rates for alternative interventions.)*

Kaufman DG, Nagler HM. Significance and pathophysiology of the varicocele: current concepts. Semin Reprod Endocrinol 1988;6:349. *(A review of the debate.)*

Magid MS, Cash KL, Goldstein M. The testicular biopsy in the evaluation of infertility. Semin Urol 1990;8:51. *(Especially useful in the assessment of men with normal endocrine function and suspected ductal obstruction.)*

Moran C, Garcia-Hernandez E, et al. Prognosis for fertility analyzing different variables in men and women. Arch Androl 1996;36:197. *(Women older that 32 had a cumulative pregnancy rate at 30 months of 31% compared with 65% among younger women and couples with primary infertility had a rate of 45% compared with 88% for those with a previous pregnancy.)*

Morell V. Basic infertility assessment. Prim Care 1997;24:195. *(Describes the role of the primary care provider in diagnosis, treatment, and support.)*

Mueller BA, Daling JR, Moore DE, et al. Appendectomy and the risk of tubal infertility. N Engl J Med 1986;315:1506. *(Risk increased only in cases of ruptured appendix.)*

Schwartz D, Mayaux MJ. Female fecundity as a function of age. N Engl J Med 1982;306:404. *(A slight but significant decrease after age 30; more marked after age 35.)*

Swerdloff RS, Overstreet JW, Sokol RZ, et al. Infertility in the male. Ann Intern Med 1985;103:906. *(A comprehensive yet practical review of the pathogenesis, evaluation, and treatment; 132 references.)*

Van Balen F, Trimbos-Kemper TC. Factors influencing the well-being of long-term infertile couples. J Psychosom Obstet Gynaecol 1994;15:157. *(Secrecy with regard to infertility was associated with a lower sense of well-being.)*

121
Approach to the Woman with an Unplanned Pregnancy

More than half of the pregnancies that occur in the United States are unintended. An equal proportion of unintended pregnancies end in abortion and in birth. The woman who suspects an unplanned or unwanted pregnancy often calls on her primary care provider to confirm a diagnosis and formulate a care plan. To provide support and assistance, the physician first must accurately diagnose the pregnancy. He or she can then inform the patient about community services available for prenatal care, abortion, and adoption. If the physician feels his or her beliefs interfere with objective counseling, then referral to another provider is necessary. Awareness of the patient's social and cultural environment is essential to lending appropriate support.

CLINICAL PRESENTATIONS

Women presenting with unplanned pregnancies have highly variable experiences. Responses to the diagnosis, coping mechanisms, and capacity to take responsibility for decision making may differ greatly from woman to woman.

A pregnancy may be untimely or unwanted because of the severe hardship a child would create. A limited single or dual income may be insufficient to support either a first or additional child. A pregnancy may hinder opportunities for education and career advancement. These factors may conflict with the woman's desire for motherhood, creating great ambivalence. For many women, fear that an abortion will hinder future reproductive function adds to the concern. Some women who desire children may have a partner opposed to parenting or may need family or social support to raise a child alone. They may feel pressured to terminate the pregnancy yet be unwilling to do so.

The woman who desires pregnancy but suffers from a chronic or life-threatening illness such as diabetes, systemic lupus erythematosus, or cancer endures unique stress when she faces an unplanned pregnancy. The pregnancy may jeopardize her health and her ability to care for her family, and she may face conflicting opinions regarding termination. Additionally, the impact of pregnancy on certain disease processes is not well understood.

Many women of childbearing age are infected with HIV. The rate of transmission of the HIV to the fetus is estimated to be 25% to 50%. This raises concerns for the primary care physician who must consider the welfare of both the mother and the unborn child. It is unclear whether pregnancy adversely affects the HIV disease process in the mother. Additionally, the difficult dilemma of whether to carry a potentially infected fetus to term poses many ethical questions.

Substance abuse among pregnant women continues to rise. The most significant increase is seen with cocaine, but use of heroin, methadone, and amphetamines has also grown. Cocaine use has been associated with lower birth weight and preterm labor. Heroin use during pregnancy can lead to a withdrawal syndrome in the infant. In addition to toxic drug effects, poor pregnancy outcomes may result from transmission of disease from "dirty needles," hazardous behavior to support a drug habit, malnutrition, and poor prenatal care. Often there is evidence of polysubstance abuse with additive effects. Additionally, alcohol remains a significant problem during pregnancy. The fetal alcohol syndrome, manifested by intrauterine growth retardation, microcephaly, and developmental abnormalities, occurs in approximately 1 in 2,000 live births. Some substance abusers may respond to pregnancy with denial or indifference.

A woman with a severe poorly controlled psychiatric illness presents many concerns. Some evidence suggests that pregnant patients with psychiatric disorders may have worsening of their mental health during pregnancy. In addition, some studies indicate that patients with severe disorders may have increased birth complications resulting from poor prenatal care, concurrent substance abuse, increased incidence of homelessness, use of psychiatric medications during pregnancy, and unrecognized physical illness. The primary care physician may be asked to provide counseling and to act as a liaison between obstetric and psychiatric providers.

Some patients undergoing amniocentesis or chorionic villus sampling to identify genetic abnormalities do so on the assumption that they will consider an induced abortion. A patient may look to her primary care provider for guidance with this difficult decision-making process.

Almost 1 million adolescents in the United States become pregnant yearly. Consequences for the future of these teenagers may be immense. Pregnancy may lead to dropping out of school, limited job opportunities, and dependence on the welfare system. Adolescents may intentionally or unintentionally become pregnant for various reasons. They may exhibit risk-taking behavior in response to peer pressure, to experiment, or to test parental limits. Failure to properly use contraception may result from lack of adequate information or stem from the belief that "it will never happen to me." Some adolescents who feel deprived of love and security from parents or partners may see a child as a companion who will provide them with unconditional love. Often, teenagers present at a later gestational age because of denial or unawareness of how to get help. This delay may result in significant negative consequences with increased morbidity and mortality from the pregnancy or termination.

A number of presentations are particularly important because of their psychosocial circumstances. In both rural and urban areas, sexual abuse (including rape) persists to a greater extent than most professional people assume. It may occur between father and daughter, but frequently it involves another adult male in the household, such as uncle, older brother, or boyfriend. The victim may be repulsed at the thought of a baby inside her from such a traumatic experience and may not present for care until later in the pregnancy. In some states, the physician is mandated to report sexual abuse involving minors.

PRINCIPLES OF MANAGEMENT
AND PATIENT EDUCATION

Diagnosis. Immunologic tests, including home pregnancy kits or office slide kits that measure human chorionic gonadotropin (hCG), are commonly used for first diagnosis of pregnancy. These use urine or serum, are accurate 4 to 14 days from a missed period, and can give false-positive results because of luteinizing hormone cross-reactivity. More sensitive and specific tests include the ELISA, using serum or urine, and serum radioimmunoassay tests. These detect lower hCG levels and appear positive earlier (12 days and 7 days postconception, respectively). They are specific for the β-hCG subunit and are not affected by luteinizing hormone cross-reactivity. The availability of monoclonal antibodies to the subunit has improved test accuracy. The half-life of hCG after delivery is 1.5 days, so failure to normalize after pregnancy termination indicates remaining tissue, as with incomplete abortion or gestational trophoblastic disease.

Counseling. Once a diagnosis of pregnancy is confirmed, a nonjudgmental supportive examination of the patient's feelings is needed. A thorough psychosocial history should be gathered so her options can be fully explored. Special attention to issues of rape and incest are necessary if this history is elicited or appears to be a possibility. Formal counseling is indicated in this instance. Community support groups may also be helpful.

Surgical Therapeutic Abortion. Abortion is one of the most common gynecologic procedures performed in the United States. Data regarding the use of abortion have remained fairly stable in recent decades. In 1990, the national abortion ratio (number of legal abortions per 1,000 live births) was 344 and the abortion rate (number of legal abortions per 1,000 women aged 15 to 44 years) was 24. In that year, about 55% of women undergoing pregnancy termination were younger than age 25, 79% were unmarried, and approximately 64% were white. Approximately 88% of abortions occur within the first 12 weeks of gestation, with half occurring within 8 weeks of gestation.

When performed appropriately, surgical pregnancy termination is safe, with less than one death per 100,000 procedures. In developed countries, legal first-trimester terminations result in lower death rates than those from pregnancy across all age groups. Termination is safest when performed earlier in gestation. Risk increases with gestational age, maternal age, and higher parity. With legalization of abortion in the United States, morbidity has decreased. There is increased physician training and expertise; increased use of the safer suction curettage procedure rather than sharp curettage, uterine instillation, and surgical procedures; and improved access, allowing earlier procedures. Service availability and practices regarding waiting periods, parental consent, and abortion funding all have an impact on a woman's obtaining services. Additional barriers to services include cost (earlier and nonhospital procedures are cheaper than second-trimester hospital procedures), harassment of patients at abortion facilities, and vandalism of facilities.

Preprocedure assessment includes determining any underlying medical problems that would necessitate an inpatient rather than outpatient procedure. Usual laboratory evaluation includes pregnancy testing, urinalysis, complete blood count, blood type and Rh factor determination, syphilis serologies, gonorrhea and chlamydia testing, and Papanicolaou smear. Additional studies such as HIV testing and sonography can be considered. Contraception may also be addressed at this time, because oral contraceptives can be initiated the day after termination and intrauterine device placement can occur with the procedure. This addresses the concern about frequent no-show rates for follow-up appointments. Rh immune globulin should be given after the procedure to Rh-negative unsensitized individuals. Postabortion instructions include no intercourse, douching, or tampons for 1 to 2 weeks.

Local anesthesia is used for first-trimester procedures. Paracervical block using lidocaine, with or without epinephrine, and preoperative analgesics or sedatives are generally safe and inexpensive. General anesthesia is most often used for procedures done later in pregnancy.

First-trimester abortions are performed at 12 weeks gestation or sooner, and most in the United States are performed by suction curettage. Menstrual regulation, the least invasive procedure, is performed up to 2 weeks after a first missed period in an outpatient facility, without anesthesia. A flexible plastic catheter is inserted with no more difficulty than performing endometrial biopsy or intrauterine device placement, and suction is applied. Because the procedure is done so early in pregnancy, failure to aspirate all the tissue may occur, manifested by a persistent positive pregnancy test and absent postoperative bleeding. This may require a repeat procedure. Later first-trimester terminations involve suction curettage, commonly requiring cervical dilation. Intravaginal or oral administration of misoprostol has been shown to be effective in facilitating cervical dilation, especially in nulliparous women. Suction using a cannula removes the pregnancy. The complication rate is 2 per 1,000 procedures. A small percentage (3%) of pregnancy terminations use sharp curettage (the traditional dilation and curettage). These are most often later first-trimester procedures (10 to 12 weeks) or earlier second-trimester procedures.

Second-trimester terminations are mostly dilation and evacuation procedures involving placement of an osmotic dilator 6 to 12 hours before the procedure, which is either suction or sharp curettage. The complication rate for dilation and curettage is 7 per 1,000 procedures. From 16 weeks' gestation, induction terminations may be performed using intrauterine instillation of agents inducing labor. A small amount of amniotic fluid is removed and urea, prostaglandins, or rarely saline is introduced, resulting in labor and delivery over the next 12 to 24 hours. Intramuscular and vaginally-placed prostaglandin preparations are also used to induce labor. This is a hospital-based procedure, with a higher complication rate (up to 20% at some institutions) than earlier procedures and may take several days to complete. Complications from hypertonic saline inductions include disseminated intravascular coagulation, hypernatremia, and hemorrhage from retained tissue. Prostaglandins have side effects of nausea, vomiting, diarrhea, and fever.

Hysterotomy and *hysterectomy* are rarely performed second-trimester procedures (accounting for less than 0.05% of reported procedures). These have higher morbidity and mortality. Tubal sterilization can be done at the same time as hysterotomy. Hysterectomy is generally performed for an existing condition requiring hysterectomy with a coexisting pregnancy.

Nonsurgical Therapeutic Abortion. Extensive experience from other countries with mifepristone indicates that it provides a safe and effective alternative to surgical therapeutic abortion for women who are no more than 7 weeks pregnant. Mifepristone, formerly known as RU-486, is a synthetic steroid that binds progesterone receptors, blocking normal activity and preventing implantation or inducing menstruation after implantation. Mifepristone is generally followed by progesterone administration. Effectiveness of this approach exceeds 95%. An alternative approach to medical abortion is the use of methotrexate, generally followed by misoprostol administered vaginally.

Abortion-related *complications* are affected by time of gestation, method of procedure, and coexisting complicating illnesses. Major complications of surgical abortion, including uterine perforation, hemorrhage, and infection, occur at a rate of 1 case per 1,000 procedures. The termination needs to be repeated 2.3 times per 1,000 abortions. Presentations suggestive of these complications include bleeding, fever, abdominal pain or cramping, and uterine tenderness. Minor complications, including infection, cervical stenosis, cervical tear, and bleeding or incomplete abortion requiring resuctioning, occur in 8 per 1,000 procedures. Complication rates increase with gestational age and are estimated as follows: at 8 weeks gestation, 2 per 1,000; at 14 weeks, 6 per 1,000; at more than 20 weeks, 15 per 1,000. Complications of medical abortions include bleeding and pain and gastrointestinal side effects.

A number of studies have examined women's preferences for either medical or surgical abortion. In one trial conducted in Scotland among women in the first 9 weeks of gestation, 20% of women preferred medical abortion, 26% preferred surgical evacuation, and 56% were sufficiently indifferent to permit randomization. Women in the eighth and ninth week were more likely to prefer the surgical approach. Short-term and long-term outcomes, including satisfaction, were comparable, highlighting the importance of the individual woman's preferences.

There are no conclusive data showing that serious emotional problems result after pregnancy termination in the United States. Existing data indicate that women generally experience relief and reduced anxiety and distress after pregnancy termination. Negative emotional reactions are more common among women with prior psychiatric illnesses, second-trimester terminations, terminations for medical or genetic reasons, or with significant ambivalence about the decision.

Women who have undergone a single first-trimester vacuum aspiration procedure are at no significant increased risk for infertility, miscarriage, ectopic pregnancy, stillbirth, or major pregnancy or delivery-associated complication. The effect of multiple abortions on future childbearing is uncertain; some evidence suggests a subsequent two- to threefold increased risk of pregnancy loss after two or more abortions. Second-trimester dilation and evacuation procedures are believed to be associated with development of an incompetent cervix, which can lead to spontaneous abortion, premature delivery, and low birth weight.

Illegal abortions occur rarely today. Reasons for this choice have included financial limitations, secrecy, geographic location, and knowledge deficits regarding legal termination or choosing an ethnically familiar provider. Complication rates are unknown but are thought to be higher than those of legal procedures. In 1989, 2 of 20 reported abortion-related deaths followed illegal procedures. Patients may present to hospital emergency rooms with hemorrhage and sepsis.

Adoption. Placing a child for adoption is an alternative for a woman who believes it is impossible to raise a child and who would prefer not to undergo an abortion. Women choosing this option often do so with the belief that their child will have a better upbringing than they can provide. Additionally, placement may allow a woman to defer or delay parenthood, complete her education, establish economic security, or pursue goals. Adoptions, however, have declined significantly over the past decades. Fewer than 3% of never-married women in recent years relinquished their infants. Societal acceptance of single motherhood, legalization of abortion, and establishment of programs offering financial assistance all contribute to this trend. If a woman decides to place her child for adoption, she may enlist a state-run or private agency. She should be encouraged to investigate an agency carefully to ensure that she is not pressured and that she agrees with its policies. Open adoption, where there is some future contact with the child, is becoming more common.

Keeping the Child. Keeping the child may emerge as a realistic option if a problematic social situation is amenable to change. Identification of social supports include extended family. Community agencies may facilitate this process. Adolescents need special counseling because teenage pregnancy is a serious problem resulting in poverty and child neglect.

Birth Control. Whether a patient chooses to proceed with or terminate a pregnancy, a discussion of future contraceptive options is essential (see Chapter 119).

Providing care to the woman faced with an unplanned and/or unwanted pregnancy is a challenge to the primary care provider. The provider must explore the patient's beliefs, fears, support network, and psychosocial history. Options must be explained thoroughly and without judgment. Only then can one formulate an appropriate care plan that incorporates the woman's personal circumstances and preferences.

A.G.M.

ANNOTATED BIBLIOGRAPHY

Adler NE, David HP, Major BN, et al. Psychological responses after abortion. Science 1990;248:41. (*Brief review of U.S. studies examining women after legal terminations.*)

Blendon RJ, Benson JM, Donelan K. Public controversy over abortion. JAMA 1993;270:2871. (*Survey data on public attitudes about abortion.*)

Centers for Disease Control and Prevention. Abortion surveillance, 1990. MMWR Morb Mortal Wkly Rep 1992;41:936. (*Updated review of current information.*)

Council on Scientific Affairs, American Medical Association. Induced termination of pregnancy before and after Roe v Wade, trends in the mortality and morbidity of women. JAMA 1992;268:3231. (*Good review article.*)

Edwards J, Carson SA. New technologies permit safe abortion at less than six weeks gestation and provide timely detection of ectopic gestation. Am J Obstet Gynecol 1997;176:1101. (*Case series of more than 1,500 procedures at less than 6 weeks with no serious complications.*)

Forrest JD. Epidemiology of unintended pregnancy and contraceptive use. Am J Obstet Gynecol 1994;170:1485. (*More than half of pregnancies in the United States are unintended; of these, equal proportions end in birth and abortion.*)

Grimes DA, Schulz KF, Cates W, et al. Mid-trimester abortion by dilatation and evacuation: a safe and practical alternative. N Engl J Med 1977;296:1141. (*Compared more than 6,000 evacuation procedures with nearly 9,000 saline abortions and found greater effectiveness and fewer complications for the latter.*)

Hakin-Elahi E, Tovell HMM, Burnhill MS. Complications of first-trimester abortion: a report of 170,000 cases. Obstet Gynecol 1990;76:129. (*Retrospective review of New York City Planned Parenthood cases. Letter in response in Obstet Gynecol 1990;76:1145.*)

Henshaw RC, Naji SA, Russell IT, et al. Comparison of medical abortion with surgical vacuum aspiration: women's preferences and acceptability of treatment. BMJ 1993;307:714. (*In this preference trial, 20% preferred medial abortion, 26% preferred aspiration, and 54% were willing to be randomized.*)

Howie FL, Henshaw RC, Naji SA, et al. Medical abortion or vacuum aspiration? Two year follow-up of a patient preference trial. Br J Obstet Gynaecol 1997;104:829. (*No differences in outcome.*)

Levin AA, Schoenbaum SC, Monson RR, et al. Association of induced abortion with subsequent pregnancy loss. JAMA 1980;243:2495. (*Found two- to threefold increased risk of pregnancy loss up to 28 weeks among women with two or more prior abortions.*)

Paul M. Office management of early induced abortion. Clin Obstet Gynecol 1999;42:290. (*Good review including procedural advances.*)

Penney GC, Thomson M, Norman J, et al. A randomised comparison of strategies for reducing infective complications of induced abortion. Br J Obstet Gynaecol 1998;105:599. (*Routine antibiotic prophylaxis proved more effective and less costly than a screen-and-treat strategy in this trial.*)

Skjeldestad FE, Atrash HK. Evaluation of induced abortion as a risk factor for ectopic pregnancy. Acta Obstet Gynaecol Scand 1997;76:151. (*No association in this case-control study.*)

Sperling RS, Stratton P. Treatment options for human immunodeficiency virus–infected pregnant women. Obstetric Gynecologic Working Group of the AIDS Clinical Trials Group of the National Institute of Allergy and Infectious Diseases. Obstet Gynecol 1992;79:443. (*Review of HIV in pregnancy, including demographics and therapeutics.*)

Spitz IM, Bardin CW. Mifepristone (RU-486)—a modulator of progestin and glucocorticoid action. N Engl J Med 1993;329:404. (*Authoritative review of this potent abortifacient.*)

Sunderland MA, Handte J, Moroso G, et al. The impact of human immunodeficiency virus serostatus on reproductive decisions of women. Obstet Gynecol 1992;79:1027. (*Discusses the impact of HIV status on deciding to carry or terminate a pregnancy.*)

122

Management of Breast Cancer

Breast cancer is one of the most common malignancies in the United States. About 12% of American women will develop breast cancer during their lifetime, more than 170,000 cases per year. Unfortunately, despite the expanded therapeutic armamentarium for breast cancer, approximately 30% of women who develop the disease die from it.

Women with newly diagnosed breast cancer face a difficult and complex series of treatment decisions at a time when they may be least able to think rationally or bear the burden of decision-making responsibility. The breast cancer diagnosis evokes anger, a sense of isolation, irrational guilt, and, most of all, vulnerability. Clearly, this mix of emotions makes it difficult for the communication tasks necessary for the patient to be involved in decision making. Yet the most important determinants of the "right" decision for each patient are her attitudes toward the possible treatment outcomes and risks. New information about the relative effectiveness of alternative approaches to primary therapy and adjuvant therapy has added to the complexity of these decisions. The primary care physician can be a critically important source of empathy, support, and information about treatment options. After primary treatment, with or without subsequent adjuvant therapy, the primary care provider may be principally responsible for monitoring the patient's psychosocial adjustment to breast cancer and its treatment and for evidence of disease recurrence. Finally, the primary care role is critically important in decision making about treatment for the woman with advanced breast cancer.

CLINICAL PRESENTATION AND COURSE

The term *"early-stage breast cancer"* is generally applied to stage I and stage II tumors. *Stage I* disease is defined as a primary tumor of less than 2 cm in diameter with no axillary lymph node involvement (Table 122.1). Approximately 55% of patients with primary breast cancer now present with stage I disease, in part because of improved screening methods. *Stage II* disease is still considered a localized disease, but it does include involvement of axillary lymph nodes. About 25% of patients with *clinical* stage I disease turn out to have pathologic stage II disease on sampling of the axillary nodes. Interestingly, a similar percentage of patients with clinical stage II disease (palpable axillary lymph nodes) turn out to have no tumor in the nodes on pathologic examination. In *stage III* disease, there is extensive tumor (more than 5 cm) at the primary site, and lymph nodes are larger than 2 cm with or without fixation. In *stage IV* disease, there are distant metastases.

Because of greater use of mammographic screening, cases are increasingly identified with small lesions, including those without evidence of invasion. *Noninvasive cancer,* or *carcinoma in situ* (CIS), is characterized as ductal or lobular based on histology and location, cytologic features, and growth patterns. These two lesions behave very differently. With ductal CIS (DCIS), mastectomy results in cure for 98% to 99% of women. Similar rates can be achieved with lumpectomy without subsequent radiation if the surgical margins are adequate.

Table 122.1. Curability of Breast Cancer by Stage

Stage	Tumor extent	10-Year disease-free survival (%)
I	Confined to breast	70–80
II	Involves the axillary nodes	20–40
III	Tumor >5 cm; nodes >2 cm; with or without fixation	<5
	Inflammatory	0

Table 122.2. Patterns of Recurrence and Survival in Breast Cancer

Pattern	Incidence (%)	Median time (mos) Relapse	Median time (mos) Survival
Multiple metastases	19	9	4
Pulmonary	12	36	18
Bone	26	15	29+
Effusions[a]	16	39	44
Skin and subcutaneous[b]	26	15	27+

[a] + Minor skin nodules.

[b] + Minor bone metastases.

One reason for the very good prognosis after therapy is the indolent course for many cases of DCIS. Much remains uncertain about the natural history, but there is evidence that many women with DCIS lesions would not progress to invasive disease if left untreated. DCIS now accounts for 12% of all newly diagnosed breast cancers in the United States and 30% of cancers detected by mammography. With more than 10,000 mastectomies performed each year for DCIS, it is obvious that more information and education about the clinical significance of DCIS are needed. Lobular CIS has very different treatment implications. It is not clear whether it is indeed a premalignant lesion or simply a marker for increased risk of invasive disease elsewhere in the breast(s). The incidence of invasive cancer in women with lobular CIS is about 1% per year.

Prognosis. For women with early-stage breast cancer, the prognosis is largely determined by the size of the tumor and the number of positive nodes. For women with negative nodes, 5-year cumulative recurrence rates for women with tumors smaller than 1 cm, 1 to 2 cm, and 2 to 5 cm in diameter are 10%, 20%, and 30%, respectively. Among women with one to three positive nodes, 40% have a recurrence within 5 years. For women with 4 to 10 nodes positive, the 5-year recurrence rate is 60% to 70%. For women with more than 10 nodes positive, or with stage III disease, long-term survival is less than 5%. Inflammatory breast cancer has a worse prognosis than noninflammatory lesions.

In addition to the stage of tumor and tumor size, *estrogen receptor* and *progesterone receptor* status affect the prognosis. Patients with stage I or stage II disease whose tumors have estrogen or progesterone receptors, or both, have a better prognosis than those with the same stage of disease whose tumors are receptor negative.

Breast cancer may metastasize to almost any site in the body, but five general categories have been distinguished by Smalley et al., which are correlated with predictable response to therapy and prognosis (Table 122.2). It is evident that even in patients with metastatic disease, median survival may exceed 3 years, and there does not have to be significant change in quality of life when palliative radiation and chemotherapy or hormonal therapy are used throughout that period (see below). Today, more than 50% of patients with metastatic breast cancer may respond to therapy, but only a small portion (perhaps fewer than 10%) show complete regression. The median duration of response is approximately 12 to 18 months.

The clinical course of breast cancer is unique in that metastatic lesions may develop after a long period of freedom from disease, even after as long as 20 years. Thus, 5 years without evidence of metastatic spread does not indicate cure.

PRINCIPLES OF MANAGEMENT

The therapeutic options for women diagnosed by an incisional or excisional biopsy have expanded in recent years, accompanied by greater patient participation in choice of therapy. It is no longer justified to perform a biopsy and immediate mastectomy under the same anesthesia. Patients should be fully informed of the diagnosis, promptly staged, and advised of the therapeutic options.

Primary Treatment of Early-stage Breast Cancer. Most women with early-stage breast cancer have a choice of surgical treatments. Multiple randomized trials have demonstrated that survival is the same with either *mastectomy* or *breast-conserving surgery* ("lumpectomy" or "quadrantectomy") *followed by radiation*. There are some relative contraindications to breast-conserving surgery, including tumors that are large relative to breast size, cancer that is near or involves the nipple, and tumors with extensive intraductal components within or adjacent to the primary tumor. Also, women with large breasts may fare worse cosmetically with radiation therapy. Chemotherapy has been used before surgery to reduce tumor size and make breast conserving an option for more women with large tumors relative to their breast size. Termed *neoadjuvant chemotherapy*, this approach has been used increasingly in recent years. Radiation therapy after the breast-conserving option is essential. Without it, there is a 40% rate of ipsilateral breast recurrence after breast-conserving surgery. Even with radiation therapy, ipsilateral recurrences do occur, at a rate of 1% to 2% per year. These can usually be treated with mastectomy and, as noted, do not result in decreased survival for women who opt for the breast-conserving approach.

Mastectomy is preferred by some women who do not want to live with the anxiety associated with the possibility of having to deal with an ipsilateral recurrence in the breast that they chose to keep. Others prefer mastectomy simply because it does not usually involve subsequent radiation and it thereby lets them put primary therapy behind them more quickly. However, some recent studies suggest that women who are at high risk of recurrence because of a tumor larger than 4 cm or the presence of more than four positive nodes benefit from radiation therapy after mastectomy. After mastectomy, some women opt for breast reconstruction, whereas other feel no need for surgery for cosmetic purposes.

Adjuvant Therapy of Breast Cancer. Adjuvant therapy is administered to decrease the likelihood of, or delay, cancer recurrence and death. The most commonly used regimens are cyclophosphamide, methotrexate, and fluorouracil and other regimens that include adriamycin. Recent studies indicate that newer agents provide additional benefit. The antiestrogen tamoxifen has become the standard hormonal therapy.

The effectiveness of adjuvant therapy in decreasing rates of recurrence and breast cancer death among node-positive women has been proven for some time. More recent evidence indicates that adjuvant therapy is as effective in node-negative women. That is, the relative risk reduction afforded by either chemotherapy or hormonal therapy is the same in node-positive and node-negative women. However, the absolute risk difference is much smaller for node-negative women because their baseline risk is lower. For example, women with two positive nodes and women with negative nodes and tumors less than 1 cm might receive the same 30% risk-reduction benefit from adjuvant chemotherapy or hormonal therapy. For the former, that means a reduction from 40% to 28% or an increase in disease-free survival from 60% to 72%. For the node-negative woman, the same proportional benefit means a reduction from 10% to 7% or an increase in disease-free survival from 90% to 93%. The significant morbidity associated with adjuvant therapy may or may not be justified, depending on the absolute benefit and the woman's attitudes toward the alliterative outcomes.

Adjuvant chemotherapy has been the standard of care for premenopausal women with positive nodes, regardless of hormone receptor status, and tamoxifen has been the standard for postmenopausal women with positive nodes, particularly those with positive hormone receptor levels. Ongoing analysis by the Early Breast Cancer Trialists' Collaborating Group of individual patient experiences for tens of thousands of women who have participated in scores of randomized trials continues to refine our understanding of adjuvant therapy effects. Tamoxifen is effective regardless of age or menopausal status in women who are estrogen-receptor or progesterone-receptor positive. The effects of chemotherapy and tamoxifen are greater than either intervention alone for these women. The relatively nontoxic response has led to increasing use of tamoxifen among node-negative women who are receptor positive. Treatment of node-negative women who are receptor negative is more controversial. The source of the controversy is the question of whether the risk-reduction benefits are sufficiently great to justify the significant morbidity associated with adjuvant chemotherapy. Women who choose this option should have a clear understanding of the benefits and realistic expectations of side effects, including nausea and vomiting, alopecia, and premature menopause.

The inclusion of a *bisphosphonate* in the adjuvant regimen has recently gained favor. The antiosteolytic effect of bisphosphonates has been shown to significantly reduce the incidence of bone pain, pathologic fractures, and hypercalcemia in women with breast cancer and bone metastases. And recently, the adjuvant use of the bisphosphonate clodronate in women at high risk for distant metastases has been shown to reduce the incidence of bony and visceral metastases by 50%.

Monitoring. After primary therapy, women with breast cancer should be seen at regular intervals. Psychosocial adjustments and clinical status need careful attention. A mammogram should be obtained annually. Follow-up examination of the bones should be undertaken only in patients who develop symptoms of bone pain. The crucial concern in monitoring patients with breast cancer is the increased risk of a second primary tumor, which may also be curable. The identification of early metastatic disease is less consequential, because systemic therapy should be used only for patients with either rapidly growing tumor or symptomatic disease.

Treatment of Advanced Disease. Stage III breast cancer is an inoperable local disease confined to the skin, breast, or lymph nodes. It may be treated either with systemic therapy (either hormonal or chemotherapy) to determine the effectiveness of the systemic treatment and to reduce the bulk of tumor or with local therapy, which may be either mastectomy followed by radiation therapy or radiation therapy alone. The median length of survival after effective treatment is 18 to 24 months.

The management of stage IV (metastatic) breast cancer is determined in part by sites of metastases, menopausal status, and hormone receptor status. The decision to treat and the timing of therapy depend on the presence or absence of symptoms and the growth rate of the tumor. There are three categories of systemic therapy for advanced breast cancer: hormone therapy, chemotherapy, and combination therapy. Radiation therapy is also very effective for palliation, and, as noted, bisphosphonate therapy reduces the incidence of complications associated with bony metastases.

Hormone therapy can be very effective for tumors that have high concentration of estrogen receptor protein in the cytoplasm. Tumors with progesterone receptors are also more likely to be hormonally responsive. The sites of disease most often responsive to hormones are pulmonary nodules, pleural effusions, and osseous lesions. There is a much lower likelihood of response to hormonal manipulation for patients with hepatic metastases, lymphangitic pulmonary involvement, brain metastases, or skin lesions. Hormone management also depends on menopausal status. The least responsive group is perimenopausal. After an initial response to hormonal therapy, a relapse usually occurs, but a subsequent secondary response to an alternative hormonal manipulation is not uncommon. For the most part, such secondary responses are short lived and are not of the quality of the initial response. It is important to recognize that the effect of hormonal therapy on tumor bulk may not be observed for 1 or 2 months, even though the agent may begin working immediately. Relief of bone pain is much more rapidly achieved.

Hormonal therapy occasionally results in exacerbation of bone pain or tumor growth. The mechanism is not known. In a small percentage of these patients, the opposite hormonal maneuver (i.e., ablation or supplementation) may induce an antitumor effect. In some institutions, patients are monitored in the hospital for a 10-day period to determine whether or not tumor stimulation and serious hypercalcemia occur.

The development of drugs for use in place of adrenalectomy has eased the burden of treatment for patients with advanced disease. *Tamoxifen,* a competitive inhibitor of endogenous estrogen, binds to estrogen receptors and achieves an antitumor effect by an unknown mechanism. The drug has a low rate of toxicity and a response rate comparable with that of other forms of hormone therapy. As a result, tamoxifen is the usual first-line hormonal therapy.

Chemotherapy should be considered for patients with advanced disease after hormonal manipulations have failed or when they are deemed inappropriate (e.g., in receptor-negative patients). However, the likelihood of response is reduced when the tumor has proven resistant to other forms of treatment. The chemotherapeutic regimens most commonly used to manage advanced disease include the same regimens commonly used for adjuvant therapy. As with adjuvant therapy, combinations of hormonal manipulations and multidrug programs have been advocated on the basis of a possible synergistic interaction.

Breast cancer is particularly sensitive to *radiation therapy.* Metastatic bony lesions are present in more than 60% of patients with breast cancer, and lytic lesions are often associated with pain. Local radiation therapy at the relatively low doses of 2,000 to 3,500 rads may relieve pain, although persistent structural defects as a consequence of cortical bony erosion may necessitate orthopedic support and even internal fixation for weight-bearing bone structures. Another important role for radiation therapy is in palliation of patients who develop metastatic brain lesions, which occur in more than 10% of patients.

Autologous bone marrow transplantation in conjunction with high-dose chemotherapy has been used extensively in the United States among women deemed at high risk of distant metastases and death, usually because of extensive lymph node involvement. However, it should be thought of as an investigative approach because of unproven benefits. A recent trial with median follow-up of more than 4 years did not show a survival benefit for the high-dose approach.

PATIENT EDUCATION

Whether or not a woman has had a role in decision making about breast cancer treatment can be an important determinant of her psychosocial adjustment. The primary care provider is well positioned to provide empathetic support and vital information about the benefit and harm of alternative treatment options.

A.G.M.

ANNOTATED BIBLIOGRAPHY

Al-Ghazal SK, Fallowfield L, Blamey RW, et al. Patient evaluation of cosmetic outcome after conserving surgery for treatment of primary breast cancer. Eur J Surg Oncol 1999;24:344. *(More than 90% of women in this series were satisfied.)*

Cox C, Pendas S, Cox J, et al. Guidelines for sentinel node biopsy and lymphatic mapping of patients with breast cancer. Ann Surg 1998;227:645. *(Describes the rationale for the sentinel node technique and findings for nearly 500 patients with different size tumors.)*

Diel IJ, Solomayer E-F, Costa SD, et al. Reduction in new metastases in breast cancer with adjuvant clodronate treatment. N Engl J Med 1998;339:357. *(Demonstrates 50% reduction in both bony and visceral metastases over a median follow-up of 3 years.)*

Early Breast Cancer Trialists' Collaborating Group. Systemic treatment of early breast cancer by hormonal, cytotoxic, or immune therapy. Lancet 1992;339:71. *(Landmark overview and analysis of worldwide randomized trial experience with treatment of early breast cancer.)*

Early Breast Cancer Trialists' Collaborating Group. Effects of radiotherapy and surgery in early breast cancer: an overview of the randomized trials. N Engl J Med 1995;333:1444. *(Further results from the landmark meta-analysis.)*

Early Breast Cancer Trialists' Collaborative Group. Tamoxifen for early breast cancer: an overview of the randomised trials. Lancet 1998;351:1451. *(Overview of trial experience of 37,000 women who received tamoxifen for 1, 2, or approximately 5 years with or without adjuvant chemotherapy: some years of tamoxifen therapy substantially improves 10-year survival for women with estrogen receptor-positive tumors.)*

Farrow DC, Hunt WC, Samet JM. Geographic variation in the treatment of localized breast cancer. N Engl J Med 1992;326:1097. *(Wide variations in the rates of breast-conserving surgery in different regions.)*

Fisher B. Highlights from recent National Surgical Adjuvant Breast and Bowel Project studies in the treatment and prevention of breast cancer. CA Cancer J Clin 1999;49:159. *(Very effective review of recent and ongoing trials.)*

Fisher B, Anderson S, Fisher ER, et al. Significance of ipsilateral breast tumor recurrence after lumpectomy. Lancet 1991;338:327. *(Ipsilateral in-breast recurrences occurred at a rate of 1.4% per year despite radiation after lumpectomy.)*

Fisher B, Dignam J, Wolmark N, et al. Tamoxifen in treatment of intraductal breast cancer: National Surgical Adjuvant Breast and Bowel Project B-24 randomised controlled trial. Lancet 1999;353:1993. *(Addition of tamoxifen reduced cancer events over 5 years from 13.4% to 8.2%.)*

Fisher B, Redmond C, Poisson R, et al. Eight-year results of a randomized clinical trial comparing total mastectomy and lumpectomy with or without irradiation in the treatment of breast cancer. N Engl J Med 1989;320:822. *(Further evidence for the equivalence of the two primary treatment options in terms of distant recurrence and survival.)*

Gail MH, Costantino JP, Bryant J, et al. Weighing the risks and benefits of tamoxifen treatment for treating breast cancer. J Natl Cancer Inst 1999;91:1829. *(Benefits are greatest for younger women at higher risk of breast cancer.)*

Harris JR, Lippman ME, Veronesi U, et al. Breast cancer. N Engl J Med 1992;327:319. *(Extensive review, first of three parts.)*

Hojris I, Overgaard M, Christensen JJ, et al. Morbidity and mortality of ischaemic heart disease in high-risk breast cancer patients after adjuvant postmastectomy systemic treatment with or without radiotherapy. Lancet 1999;354:1425. *(Postmastectomy radiation does not increase ischemic heart disease risk over 12 years.)*

Hortobagyi GH, Theriault RL, Porter L, et al. Efficacy of pamidronate in reducing skeletal complications in patients with breast cancer and lytic bone metastases. N Engl J Med 1996;335:1785. *(Monthly infusions of this bisphosphonate reduced the incidence of bony complications in women with stage IV breast cancer.)*

Loprinzi CL, Kugler JW, Sloan JA, et al. Lack of effect of coumarin in women with lymphedema after treatment for breast cancer. N Engl J Med 1999;340:346. *(No effect in this randomized trial.)*

McGuire WL, Clark GM. Prognostic factors and treatment decisions in axillary-node-negative breast cancer. N Engl J Med 1992; 326:1756. *(Excellent review of prognostic variables among node-negative women.)*

Rodenhuis S, Richel DJ, van der Wall E, et al. Randomised trial of high-dose chemotherapy and haemopoietic progenitor-cell support in operable breast cancer with extensive axillary lymph-node involvement. Lancet 1998;352:515. *(Randomized trial of 97 women with extensive axillary node metastases randomized to conventional or high-dose chemotherapy after neoadjuvant chemotherapy and primary therapy: no difference in survival was seen with a mean follow-up of 49 months.)*

Schover LR. The impact of breast cancer on sexuality, body image, and intimate relationships. CA Cancer J Clin 1991;41:112. *(Conflicting evidence about comparative effects of mastectomy and breast-conserving surgery. Impact of adjuvant therapy may be underappreciated.)*

Silverstein MJ, Lagios MD, Groshen S, et al. The influence of margin width on local control of ductal carcinoma in situ of the breast. N Engl J Med 1999;340:1455. *(Very low rates of recurrence in women with lumpectomy and margins of 1 cm or more with no benefit from radiation.)*

123

Management of the Woman with Genital Tract Cancer

Cancers of the genital tract account for about 20% of cancers in women and 10% of cancer deaths. They range from the readily detectable and curable carcinoma of the cervix to the very problematic ovarian carcinoma, with its tendency to remain inconspicuous until very late. Endometrial carcinoma has come to be one of the most common genital cancers of the postmenopausal years. Cervical cancer is now predominantly a disease of younger women.

Treatment of the woman with genital tract cancer is usually the province of the oncologist and gynecologist, but the primary physician remains an important part of the collaborative effort. Patient counseling, monitoring, and management of ongoing medical problems are among the important responsibilities.

CARCINOMA OF THE CERVIX

The incidence of invasive cervical carcinoma peaks between the ages of 48 and 55. The peak for carcinoma in situ is between ages 25 and 40. Most women with the disease present in their twenties and thirties thanks to early detection from use of the Papanicolaou (Pap) smear (see Chapter 107). Among proven risk factors are early sexual intercourse, multiple sexual partners, and infection with human papillomavirus (particularly types 16 and 18).

Principles of Management

Diagnosis. Postcoital bleeding should raise suspicion for the diagnosis. In most cases of early disease, the patient is asymptomatic and, as noted above, detection is by screening *Pap test* (see Chapter 107). Diagnosis requires biopsy confirmation of a sufficiently abnormal Pap test or a grossly suspicious-looking lesion. Patients with only mild atypia on the Pap smear (also referred to as reactive or reparative change) can be followed without biopsy but require repeat Pap testing (usually in 3 to 6 months) to be sure there is no progression to the more serious dysplasia. If there is ongoing infection, it should be treated before the Pap smear is repeated. Patients with dysplasia seen on Pap smear are at greater risk and should be referred to the gynecologist for *colposcopy* and *biopsy*. If colposcopic examination fails to identify the area for biopsy, cervical conization is required.

Staging. Clinical staging is based on findings from biopsy, physical examination, and radiologic study. An estimate of extent of local disease can be made by *pelvic examination*, carefully palpating to see if there is lateral extension to the vagina or pelvic wall. Palpating lymph nodes may detect a distant nodal metastasis, but clinical staging for involvement of pelvic nodes and the more distant paraaortic ones requires *lymphangiography* and/or *computed tomography* (CT). The latter has been especially helpful in assessment of paraaortic nodes. Stud-

ies of *magnetic resonance imaging* suggest some usefulness in delineating local extension.

Stage of disease is designated by the TMN system (Table 123.1). Prognosis worsens with advancing stage of local disease, development of regional and distant nodal metastases (especially paraaortic nodes), and histologic grade. Risk of nodal metastasis rises with growth of tumor to greater than 4 cm, lymphovascular invasion, invasion deep into the cervical stroma, and histologic grade.

Treatment and Prognosis. Early stages of carcinoma of the cervix are curable. Patients sometimes ask the opinion of their primary physician regarding the choices of therapy for early stage disease. Consequently, these choices are worth reviewing here.

For *stage 0 disease*, the treatment of choice has been *conization*. In instances where the lesion is readily visible by colposcopy and the patient can be counted on to come for regular follow-up, outpatient *cryotherapy* or *laser ablation* can serve as an alternative to conization. *Hysterectomy* is reserved for those who have intraepithelial neoplasia at the margins of the cone biopsy and do not care for future childbearing. Cure is in excess of 99%.

Stage IA1 is treated with *vaginal hysterectomy* when childbearing is not an issue. When it is desired, *conization* and close follow-up are the alternative if the cone margins are free of tumor. Five-year survival is over 90%. There is debate regarding the best approach to *stage IA2* disease. If invasion is greater than 3 mm or there is lymphovascular invasion, then these patients are usually treated like stage IB. If invasion is less than 3 mm and there is no lymphovascular involvement, then they are treated like IA1. *Intracavitary irradiation* is another curative option.

Stages IB and IIA are treated by *radical hysterectomy* plus *pelvic lymphadenectomy* or by definitive *irradiation*. Surgery is preferred in young women, because the ovarian function can be spared and the vagina is more pliable than after irradiation. Also, radiation effects on bowel and other adjacent structures are avoided. Radiation therapy spares the need for an extensive surgical procedure and its attendant complications. With either procedure, 5-year survival is equally good, with rates averaging about 85% for patients with no pelvic node disease. If there is involvement of pelvic nodes, 5-year survival falls to about 50%.

Stages IIB and beyond are treated with *irradiation*. Five-year survival averages about 60% for patients with IIB disease and falls to about 35% for stage IIIB and to 20% for stage IV.

The high likelihood of nodal metastasis associated with advancing stages of local disease markedly lowers the chances of cure. Clinically inapparent involvement of paraaortic nodes is a particularly difficult problem, leading some to advocate surgical sampling. Prophylactic radiation to the area does not seem to improve survival.

Table 123.1.   Staging of Cervical Cancer

Primary Tumor			
0			Carcinoma *in situ*
I			Confined to uterus
	A		Preclinical invasive disease
		A1	Minimal stromal invasion
		A2	Invasion $\leq$ 5 mm
	B		Invasion $\geq$ 5 mm
II			Invasion beyond uterus but not to pelvic wall or lower third of vagina
	A		Without parametrial invasion
	B		With parametrial invasion
III			Invasion to pelvic wall, lower third of vagina, or causes hydronephrosis
	A		Only invasive to lower third of vagina
	B		Invasive to pelvic wall or hydronephrosis
IV			Invasion of bladder, rectum, or beyond true pelvis
Regional lymph nodes			
N0			No regional node metastasis
N1			Regional node metastasis
Distant metastasis (includes paraaortic nodes)			
M0			No distant metastasis
M1			Distant metastasis

Adapted from Beahrs OH, Henson DE, Hutter RVP, et al., eds. Manual for staging of cancer, 3rd ed., Philadelphia; J.B. Lippincott, 1988:151, with permission.

Patient Education

Young patients need to know that carcinoma of the cervix is potentially curable and that early disease can be successfully treated without compromising childbearing capacity. Such knowledge ensures that the young woman with carcinoma in situ or severe dysplasia will not refuse timely treatment out of fear. Older patients presenting with more invasive disease can still obtain some comfort from knowing the prognosis remains very favorable for most stages of this disease.

CARCINOMA OF ENDOMETRIUM

This disease continues to be the most common female genital cancer, accounting for about half of all new cases (about 33,000 per year). It predominantly strikes postmenopausal women. Peak incidence is between ages 55 and 60. Only 5% of cases occur in women under the age of 40. Risk factors include obesity, nulliparity, late menopause, and prolonged unopposed estrogen stimulation of the uterus (either from replacement therapy or polycystic ovary syndrome; see Chapter 111). Uninterrupted estrogen stimulation in the absence of progestin risks induction of cystic and adenomatous hyperplasia, which are considered premalignant changes. Obesity may contribute by the ability of adipose tissue to convert circulating androstenedione into estrogen. Postmenopausal bleeding (defined as uterine bleeding occurring 6 months after the onset of menopause) may be the only early clue to the development of this tumor. Occasionally, a mass is felt on routine pelvic examination.

Principles of Management

Diagnosis. Suspicion of the diagnosis mandates gynecologic referral for *fractional curettage*. When there is confusion as to whether a pelvic mass is ovarian or uterine, ordering a *pelvic ultrasound* examination can help make the distinction noninvasively, but the test is insufficient for definitive diagnosis of an intrauterine lesion. Biopsy by way of curettage is required.

Staging and Prognosis. Prognosis is a function of the extent of disease and of histologic type. The gynecologist will attempt to determine if the problem is confined to the uterine corpus or extends into the cervix and beyond. A careful *pelvic examination, CT, and chest x-ray* comprise the clinical staging process. Surgical staging is based on findings at the time of hysterectomy. Histologic grade, depth of myometrial penetration, and lymph node metastases influence prognosis in patients with early-stage disease. Overall survival is about 80% for those with stage I disease (confined to the corpus), 50% for stage II (involves corpus and the cervix), 27% for stage III (spread beyond the uterus but within the pelvis), and 9% for stage IV (invades bladder or rectum, extends beyond the pelvis).

Treatment. Patients with the *premalignant* change of adenomatous hyperplasia are usually advised to undergo *hysterectomy* because of the risk of developing cancer. However, a second option is *progestin therapy* followed by repeat curettage. Patients with *stage I or stage II* disease are curable when treated with *hysterectomy/bilateral salpingo-oophorectomy plus irradiation*. The addition of radiation therapy is especially useful in stage II disease. The precise type of radiation therapy depends on histologic type and degree of spread. Intracavitary and external beam treatments are considered. The treatment of *stage III* disease is individualized, determined by findings on laparotomy. Patients with more advanced disease are inoperable and treated with radiation, progestins, or chemotherapy for palliation.

Patient Education

Patients who are considering estrogen therapy for treatment of postmenopausal osteoporosis need to consider the risk of developing endometrial cancer. Although patients who do develop cancer from estrogen therapy are often detected early at a curable phase of illness, the disease still represents a serious consequence of an elective form of therapy. Adding a progestin to the estrogen program helps prevent unopposed endometrial proliferation and development of cystic hyperplasia (see Chapters 117 and 158).

OVARIAN CARCINOMA

Ovarian cancer ranks fourth in cancer deaths among women and leads all gynecologic cancers. Incidence increases with age, beginning shortly after menarche and continuing through the eighth decade. Risk heightens among women in their 40s, especially among those who are nulliparous. Up to 10% of cases are *familial*, with many of these demonstrating germ-line mutations of the *BRCA1* gene on chromosome 17 and to lesser degree mutations in the related *BRCA2* gene. It is believed that these genes function as tumor suppressor genes and that mutations at this site account for the greatly increased risk of ovarian cancer in the hereditary form of the disease. Mutations in these genes have also been identified in families with increased risk of breast cancer.

Women in families with a history of ovarian cancer have a lifetime risk of the malignancy that ranges from 20% to 40%. BRCA mutations are rare in the sporadic form of the disease, and risk is minuscule in family members with sporadic disease compared with that of women with a positive family history. Although risk of developing the disease is greatly increased in hereditary ovarian carcinoma, the prognosis appears much more favorable. Among patients with advanced disease (the most common stage at presentation), those with the hereditary form that includes mutation of BRCA1 survive nearly three times as long as those with sporadic disease, making mutation at BRCA1 the single most important determinant of prognosis.

Screening remains inadequate, despite the advent of transvaginal ultrasound for detection of ovarian masses and monoclonal antibody techniques for detection of the tumor-associated antigen CA-125 (see Chapter 108). *Genetic testing* for BRCA mutations holds considerable promise, but the implications for management must be more fully defined before meaningful guidelines can be constructed. Possible uses might include testing of women from families with a strongly positive history of ovarian cancer if they are contemplating prophylactic removal of both ovaries or other forms of prophylactic therapy. Study results could help inform the decision.

Clinical Presentation is typically late, because the disease is usually silent in its early stages. Over 80% of ovarian tumors derive from the epithelial surface of the ovary, disseminating silently by surface shedding or lymph node invasion. Initial symptoms when they do occur may be extremely vague, such as nonspecific gastrointestinal complaints that seem to persist in the absence of objective evidence for bowel disease. In later stages, the disease may be manifested by an abdominal or pelvic mass or development of ascites. Almost 70% of patients have already reached advanced-stage disease at the time of initial presentation.

Diagnosis

Because the disease is so silent or nonspecific in its presentation, a high index of suspicion is required. Family history

should be checked carefully for ovarian cancer. Peri- and postmenopausal women with unexplained pelvic or abdominal complaints should have a thorough *pelvic examination* with emphasis on careful palpation of the adnexae for a mass. Ability to palpate the ovary in a postmenopausal woman is suspicious of pathologic enlargement, because the ovary normally involutes to less than 2 cm in size.

A *transvaginal ultrasound* can help confirm the presence of an ovarian mass and is superior to transabdominal study. The finding of a simple cyst less than 4 cm is unlikely to represent cancer but warrants further observation, especially in postmenopausal women who do not have functioning ovarian cysts. In women of reproductive age, ovarian enlargement is common and usually due to functioning follicular or corpus luteum cysts. These typically regress within one to three menstrual cycles. Finding a complex cyst increases the risk of malignancy to about 10% and necessitates *surgical exploration*, as does discovery of a solid mass. Spread to the opposite ovary occurs in up to 15% of cases, so the finding of bilateral disease should increase rather than decrease suspicion. *CT* delineates pelvic and abdominal masses, liver and pulmonary metastasis, and retroperitoneal node involvement. It can be used to assess the ovary when pelvic ultrasound study is obscured by bowel gas.

As just noted, suspicious cases require surgical exploration. Laparoscopy is not a substitute, because laparoscopically guided needle aspiration or biopsy risks spilling malignant cells into the peritoneum and washings are of insufficient sensitivity.

Use of the tumor marker *CA-125* to achieve earlier detection of ovarian cancer has proven disappointing, perhaps because only 50% of women with clinically detectable disease have elevated levels of the marker. In addition, many women with positive studies prove to already have advanced disease, because the frequency of marker elevation increases with tumor stage and bulk. Nonetheless, a markedly elevated CA-125 in a patient with a suspicious adnexal mass only increases the importance of proceeding with surgical exploration. A negative study does not obviate the need to refer for consideration of exploration. Combining CA-125 with transvaginal ultrasound appears to have little impact on survival when used as a screening technique in the general population. Its efficacy in persons with hereditary disease may be better, but the effect on survival remains unknown (see Chapter 108).

Principles of Management

Prophylaxis. Because ovarian carcinoma is hard to detect in its early stages, much attention has been directed toward prophylactic approaches to disease. The prime candidates for consideration of prophylaxis are women at very high risk (i.e., those with a family history of hereditary disease and mutation of the BRCA genes). Options include *regular screening* by CA-125 and ultrasound (see above), *prophylactic oophorectomy*, and *oral contraceptive therapy*. Because data on efficacy and relative benefit are sparse (no randomized trials), the options need to be reviewed with each woman at high risk to help her reach a personally acceptable decision.

Prophylactic Oophorectomy can be accomplished laparoscopically as an ambulatory surgical procedure with minimal adverse effects. It is a reasonable consideration for women with a family history of hereditary disease and BRCA mutations who have completed childbearing. Such persons have a 20% to

40% chance of getting the disease and might be willing to undergo surgery. However, there is still a small risk (1% to 2%) of the tumor arising from a primary peritoneal site in high-risk persons with hereditary disease. Hormone replacement therapy would usually be prescribed after surgery to obviate the consequences of a surgical menopause; however, such therapy increases the relative risk of breast cancer by about 20%—a concern in this population already at increased risk for breast cancer by virtue of the *BRCA1* mutation.

Oral Contraceptive Therapy. Epidemiologic observations demonstrate that the risk of ovarian cancer in unselected populations of women is reduced by approximately 50% when there is a history of long-term oral contraceptive use. A retrospective analysis of women with the BRCA mutations and a positive family history shows a similar reduction in risk with 6 or more years of oral contraceptive use. However, women with BRCA mutations are also at increased risk of breast cancer, and estrogen therapy does modestly increase the relative risk of breast cancer in unselected populations. There are no data on breast cancer risk when oral contraceptive therapy is used as prophylaxis for hereditary ovarian cancer. Many women with known hereditary predisposition may well be inclined to opt for the risk-reduction benefits afforded by oral contraceptive use during their childbearing years, after which prophylactic oophorectomy may become an acceptable strategy for some women. Those opting for estrogen therapy will require close monitoring and regular mammographic screening for breast cancer.

Staging and Monitoring. Staging is performed predominantly by surgical exploration. Precise staging necessitates a meticulous *laparotomy* to assess the diaphragmatic surface and the omentum and other intraabdominal sites to which spread is common. Disease limited to the ovaries is considered stage I; if confined to the pelvis, it is considered stage II. Stage III designates involvement of regional nodes or disseminated peritoneal seeding with spread to the upper abdomen. Stage IV signifies distant or visceral metastasis. Ascites and bulky peritoneal tumor are frequent manifestations of advanced-stage disease. About 75% of patients present with stage III or IV disease. In the near future, staging is likely to include genetic testing for BRCA1 status, because of its important contribution to prognosis. BRCA1 status could become extremely important if it is found to predict responses to treatment modalities.

The disease most commonly recurs within the abdominal cavity. Monitoring techniques include *CA-125 levels, laparoscopic examination, ultrasonography, and second-look surgery*. Miliary implants on the serosal surface may go undetected by imaging studies. Elevations in CA-125 are associated with residual tumor at the time of second-look surgery.

Treatment Modalities. Although the tumor is responsive to cancer treatment measures, its bulk and spread limit the results. Cure is still limited. In advanced stages of the disease, prognosis correlates with amount of residual disease after initial surgery. Those with less than 2 cm of residual disease do better than those with greater amounts of tumor remaining. Consequently, treatment often begins with "*debulking*" or tumor removal. *Omentectomy* and *total abdominal hysterectomy* and *bilateral salpingo-oophorectomy* are performed, in addition to the reduction of tumor masses throughout the abdominal cavity.

This is believed to lessen the host-tumor burden and increase the effectiveness of ancillary or adjunctive therapeutic modalities, such as radiation or chemotherapy.

A major advance in *chemotherapy* has been achieved with the *combination regimen of cisplatin and paclitaxel*. Complete clinical response has been achieved in over 70% of persons with advanced stage disease (stage III or IV with residual tumor after surgery). Median survival in responding patients has increased to 38 months, a marked improvement from the 12 to 24 months achieved with older regimens. In patients appearing to respond to chemotherapy, a *second-look operation* is performed to remove residual disease, check response, and, at times, place intraperitoneal catheters for *intraperitoneal infusion* therapy with cisplatin. The regression of disease, confirmed by second-look operations, suggests that multidrug therapies should be the standard approach to ovarian cancer.

Radiation therapy to the pelvis or to the abdomen (for patients with disease that extends beyond the pelvis) has been advocated as a routine adjunct to surgery in patients with advanced stage disease, although impact on survival appears minimal. The rationale for abdominal and pelvic irradiation is based on the fact that ovarian tumors frequently cause recurrent ascites and bowel obstruction, leading to progressive inanition.

Survival. As noted above, median survival has increased dramatically. More than two thirds of patients used to die within a year. Now over two thirds of women who present with advanced disease can expect a complete clinical response to combination chemotherapy and a median survival of 38 months. Prognosis correlates with amount of residual tumor after initial surgery, stage of disease, tumor grade, age, histologic type, and BRCA1 gene status. Those with stage I or II disease, less than 2 cm of residual disease, grade I tumor, and mucinous histology have the best chance of achieving complete remission and long-term survival from postoperative therapy. Relatively young age at time of diagnosis and mutation of the BRCA1 gene are among the most powerful determinants of favorable prognosis. Median survival of those who have a mutation of BRCA1 is over 6 years.

Patient Education

Patients with ovarian cancer have a long and difficult clinical course. Mortality rates are high, and tumor bulk leads to considerable morbidity. Women with this disease and their families need all the support, interest, and comprehensive care that one can muster (see Chapter 87). With the advent of improved chemotherapy regimens, some hope for prolongation of survival can now be offered to those with advanced disease. Careful counseling, perhaps in conjunction with genetic testing for BRCA1 status, is essential for women with a family history of ovarian carcinoma.

CARCINOMA OF THE VULVA

Being a disease of a readily visible area, carcinoma of the vulva lends itself to early detection and treatment. Associations between the disease and low socioeconomic class and infection with herpes simplex virus and human papillomavirus have been observed. The median age for initial presentation of carcinoma in situ is 44; for invasive disease it is 61, suggesting a slowly progressive course. Presentations include a mass or growth, vulvar pruritus, and bleeding. About 20% are asymptomatic. Lesions may be flat and raised or verrucal. Coloration ranges from white (leukoplakia) to brown (hyperpigmentation) to red. The term *Bowen's disease* refers to the hyperpigmented variety, and Paget's disease refers to the leukoplakial form. The best means of early diagnosis is a high index of suspicion. Surgical excision is the treatment of choice. More conservative approaches are now being used to decrease short- and long-term morbidity without sacrificing chance for cure. Cure rates in excess of 90% are achievable for localized disease less than 2 cm in greatest dimension. Radiation therapy is used for nonresectable disease.

CARCINOMA OF THE VAGINA

This is a relatively rare disease. Cancer found in the vagina is more likely to represent spread of disease from the cervix. Primary vaginal carcinomas are mostly squamous cell lesions, although those related to diethylstilbestrol exposure are of the clear cell variety. Prior irradiation may be a predisposing factor. Most lesions appear on the posterior wall and in the upper third of the vaginal vault. The tumor spreads directly and by lymphatic channels. It may present as an ulcerated lesion or as an exophytic mass extending into the vaginal vault. Preinvasive disease is asymptomatic. Invasive disease may present as postmenopausal or postcoital bleeding. Careful inspection of the posterior and distal aspects of the vagina is important in locating the lesion. Diagnosis is made by biopsy. Carcinoma *in situ* can be treated with local excision. Laser techniques are popular. Invasive disease is treated with radiation.

A.H.G./A.G.M.

ANNOTATED BIBLIOGRAPHY

Gusberg SB. The changing nature of endometrial cancer. N Engl J Med 1980;302:729. *(Examines the increased incidence, clinical course, and treatment.)*

Koutsky L. Epidemiology of genital human papillomavirus infection. Am J Med 1997;102:3. *(Prevalence among sexually active adults is 15%.)*

Lee YN, Wang KL, Lin MH, et al. Radical hysterectomy with pelvic lymph node dissection for treatment of cervical cancer. Gynecol Oncol 1989;32:135. *(Excellent results for treatment of stages IB and IIA.)*

Lovecchio JL, Averette HE, Donato D, et al. 5-Year survival of patients with periaortic nodal metastases in clinical stage IB and IIA cervical carcinoma. Gynecol Oncol 1989;34:43. *(Survival falls from 85% to about 50% with positive nodes.)*

Mangioni C, Bolis G, Pecorelli S, et al. Randomized trial in advanced ovarian cancer comparing cisplatin and carboplatin. J Natl Cancer Inst 1989;81:1464. *(Establishes the role of platinum agents in treatment of this disease.)*

McGuire WP, Hoskins WJ, Brady MF, et al. Cyclophosphamide and cisplatin compared with paclitaxel and cisplatin in patients with stage III and stage IV ovarian cancer. N Engl J Med 1996;334:1. *(A randomized prospective trial establishing that combination of paclitaxel and cisplatin is the treatment of choice, producing significant improvements in progression-free survival and overall survival.)*

Narod SA, Risch H, Moslehi R, et al. Oral contraceptives and the risk of hereditary ovarian cancer. N Engl J Med 1998;339:424. *(A retrospective case-control study showing a 50% to 60% reduction in risk associated with long-term oral contraceptive therapy.)*

National Cancer Institute. The Bethesda System for reporting cervical/vaginal cytologic diagnoses. JAMA 1989;262:931. *(An improved system that is increasingly used for designating Pap smear results.)*

Omura GA, Brady MF, Homesley HD, et al. Long-term follow-up and prognostic factor analysis in advanced ovarian carcinoma. J Clin Oncol 1991;9:1138. *(Tumor bulk, stage, and histology were among the key determinants.)*

Oriel KA, Hartenbach EM, Remington PL, et al. Trends in United States ovarian cancer mortality, 1979–1995. Obstet Gynecol 1999;93:30. *(Mortality rates have changed little overall but are increasing among older women and decreasing among younger women.)*

Rodriguez MH, Platt LD, Medearis AL, et al. The use of transvaginal sonography for evaluation of postmenopausal ovarian size and morphology. Am J Obstet Gynecol 1988;159:810. *(Documents its utility and enhanced sensitivity for disease detection.)*

Rubin SC, Benjamin I, Behbakht K, et al. Clinical and pathological features of ovarian cancer in women with germ-line mutations of BRCA1. N Engl J Med 1996;335:1413. *(A retrospective study, but the first evidence that mutation of BRCA1 gene is strongly associated with a more favorable clinical course.)*

Rubin SC, Hoskins WJ, Hakes TB, et al. Serum CA 125 levels in surgical findings in patients undergoing secondary operations for epithelial ovarian cancer. Am J Obstet Gynecol 1989;160:677. *(Level correlates with amount of tumor found.)*

Rustin GJ, Jennings JN, Nelstrob AE, et al. Use of CA 125 to predict survival of patients with ovarian cancer. J Clin Oncol 1989;7:1667. *(Those with high levels had a worse prognosis.)*

Schapira MM, Matchar DB, Young MJ. The effectiveness of ovarian cancer screening: a decision analysis model. Ann Intern Med 1993;118:838. *(Limited effect on survival predicted by this decision-analysis study.)*

Whittemore AS, Haris R, Itnyre J, et al. Characteristics relating to ovarian cancer risk: collaborative analysis of 12 US case-control studies. Am J Epidemiol 1992;136:1184. *(A meta-analysis demonstrating a 50% reduction in risk of ovarian cancer associated with oral contraceptive use in a general population.)*

9

Genitourinary Problems

124
Screening for Syphilis
BENJAMIN DAVIS
HARVEY B. SIMON

The prevalence of syphilis in the United States began to decline with the introduction of penicillin therapy in the 1940s, falling to about 7,000 cases in 1956. Since then, reported cases of syphilis have increased. In the 1970s, much of the increase was a consequence of infection in homosexual men. The AIDS epidemic produced changes in sexual behavior that have reduced the incidence of syphilis in homosexual men; however, syphilis has increased dramatically in African-Americans, Hispanics, and inner-city residents. This trend peaked in 1990, when more than 50,000 cases of primary and secondary syphilis were reported, representing a 9% increase in just 1 year. Since then, the reported cases of syphilis have declined to a new low in 1997.

If a patient is not identified and treated during the primary or secondary stages of the disease, the infection becomes latent and is identifiable only by means of laboratory tests until late, often irreversible, clinical manifestations appear. The prevention of destructive cardiovascular and neurologic lesions by means of appropriate screening for latent syphilis is an important task for the primary physician. Because false-positive results are common and are potentially traumatic for the patient, it is critical that the sensitivity and specificity of the various serologic tests be understood.

EPIDEMIOLOGY AND RISK FACTORS

With the exception of infection in utero or, rarely, by means of blood transfusion, syphilis is transmitted exclusively by *direct sexual contact* with infectious lesions. It follows that risk increases with sexual activity. Because syphilis is readily treated with antibiotics, it is less common in populations with access to medical care. The reported incidence of syphilis in nonwhites in the United States is much higher than in whites. Rates are highest in urban areas. It must be remembered, however, when incidence rates in different populations are compared, that case reporting has been shown to be more complete in public clinics than among private practitioners.

The age-specific incidence rates parallel those of gonorrhea, with the peak incidence for both diseases occurring between ages 20 and 25. A diagnosis of gonorrhea, nongonorrheal urethritis, HIV infection, or another sexually transmitted disease should be considered a risk factor for syphilis. Drug abuse has become an important risk factor. Male homosexuals are also at high risk.

The importance of an accurate sexual history in determining the risk for syphilis is obvious. Patients with early syphilis report an average of three recent sexual contacts. The probability that syphilis will develop in a known contact following a single exposure has been shown to be approximately 30%.

NATURAL HISTORY OF SYPHILIS AND EFFECTIVENESS OF THERAPY

Treponema pallidum enters the bloodstream within a few hours after inoculation through intact mucous membranes or abraded skin. A primary lesion occurs at the site of the inoculation between 10 and 90 days after contact. The incubation period depends on the size of the inoculum but is usually less than 3 weeks. The painless chancre usually resolves within 4 to 6 weeks, ending the *primary stage*. The *secondary stage* is usually heralded by a maculopapular rash that appears approximately 6 weeks after the primary lesion has healed. When the rash subsides, after 2 to 6 weeks, untreated syphilis enters the *latent stage* (arbitrarily divided into *early latent* for the first year and *late latent* thereafter). If untreated, patients with secondary syphilis may relapse clinically during early latency.

Because anorectal or vaginal chancres are not likely to be brought to medical attention, primary syphilis is often not diagnosed among homosexual men or among women. Whereas more than 40% of syphilis cases are detected in the primary stage among male heterosexuals, only 23% and 11%, respectively, are detected in the primary stage among male homosexuals and among females.

Natural history studies from Oslo and Tuskegee indicate that clinically manifest tertiary disease develops in approximately one third of persons with untreated syphilis, and that evidence of cardiovascular syphilis can be found in more than half at autopsy. In the retrospective Oslo study, 10% of patients had clinically evident cardiovascular syphilis, 7% had neurosyphilis, and 16% had gummatous disease. The incidence of cardiovascular syphilis was higher and that of neurosyphilis was lower in the prospective Tuskegee study.

Factors that influence the progression to clinical tertiary disease are incompletely understood. Congenital syphilis or disease contracted before age 15 does not predispose to cardiovascular tertiary disease. In general, late complications seem more likely to occur among untreated men than among untreated women.

The antibiotic regimens recommended in Chapter 141 are highly effective in eradicating early syphilis. If the response to therapy is appropriately monitored by following the quantitative VDRL or RPR titer, the risk for late complications is virtually eliminated. Antibiotic treatment of late syphilis has less predictable results. Improvement among patients with general paresis has been reported in 40% to 80% of cases. Not surprisingly, structural cardiovascular changes caused by syphilis are not reversed by antibiotic treatment.

SCREENING AND DIAGNOSTIC TESTS

Two groups of serologic tests can be used to diagnose syphilis: nontreponemal tests and treponemal tests.

Nontreponemal Tests, first introduced by Wasserman in 1906, use *cardiolipin* antigens extracted from mammalian tissues. These tests depend on cross-reactivity with antibodies against *T. pallidum*. The *rapid plasma reagin* (RPR) test, *Venereal Disease Research Laboratory* (VDRL) test, and *automated reagin test* (ART) are among the most widely used. Their advantages include low cost, simplicity, and automated processing for mass screening. Many of the results can be quantified to allow serologic monitoring of response to therapy.

Nontreponemal tests are well suited for *screening* because they are highly sensitive. Virtually all patients with secondary syphilis are seropositive. Most with primary disease become seropositive within a week of the appearance of symptoms, but in a minority, detectable antibodies fail to develop in early infection. Patients with concomitant HIV and *T. pallidum* infection usually have positive findings on serologic testing for syphilis (titers are often high). Even without treatment, 25% of patients with syphilis become seronegative in late latent disease.

A disadvantage of nontreponemal tests is that their specificity is only about 70%. *Acute false-positive reactions*, which spontaneously revert to negative within 6 months, may follow many bacterial and viral infections. *Chronic false-positive reactions* occur in patients with elevated serum globulins. Such reactions are particularly common in IV drug abusers (about 25%), patients with systemic lupus (15%), and healthy elderly persons (10%). Chronic false-positive tests also occur in patients with chronic liver disease, other connective tissue diseases, myeloma, and other advanced malignancies.

Treponemal Tests. All patients with positive nontreponemal test results should be retested with specific treponemal antigens. Although these tests are more sensitive and specific than the nontreponemal tests, they are better suited for diagnostic confirmation than for screening. The *microhemagglutination–T. pallidum test* (MHA–TP) is now the most widely used. Others include the *fluorescent treponemal antibody–absorbed test* (FTA-ABS), the *hemagglutination treponemal test* for syphilis (HATTS), and the now rarely performed *T. pallidum immobilization test* (TPI).

In general, the results of treponemal tests become positive earlier than do the results of nontreponemal tests, and they tend to remain positive throughout life. However, it has been noted that in about 13% of patients receiving prompt treatment for primary syphilis, MHATP test results become negative within 3 years of therapy.

CONCLUSIONS AND RECOMMENDATIONS

- After decades of decline, syphilis is becoming more common, especially among IV drug abusers, the urban poor, and HIV-infected persons.
- Screening for latent disease is simple, and the late manifestations of syphilis are entirely preventable if treatment is instituted early.
- Many patients have been screened routinely at the time of marriage, during prenatal care, before giving blood, or on hospital admission. Frequent screening is unnecessary, but the nonreactivity of sexually active persons, particularly those with multiple sex partners, should be documented at approximately 5-year intervals.
- Special indications for screening include exposure to or infection with other sexually transmitted diseases, pregnancy, IV drug abuse, and HIV infection.
- All patients with syphilis should be counseled about HIV infection and advised to accept HIV testing.
- Nontreponemal tests such as the RPR or VDRL are appropriate for screening because of their sensitivity and simplicity. MHATP or other treponemal tests should be reserved for confirming a diagnosis suspected on the basis of clinical presentation or positive nontreponemal test results.

ANNOTATED BIBLIOGRAPHY

Andrus JK, Fleming DW, Harger DR, et al. Partner notification: can it control syphilis? Ann Intern Med 1990;112:539. (*The answer is no because of too many anonymous sexual contacts.*)

Centers for Disease Control and Prevention. Primary, secondary syphilis—United States, 1981–1990. JAMA 1991;265:2940. (*Details of the changing epidemiology of the disease.*)

Clark EG, Danbold N. The Oslo study of the natural course of untreated syphilis. Med Clin North Am 1964;48:613. (*A restudy of case material of untreated syphilis collected from 1891 to 1910.*)

Hart G. Syphilis tests in diagnostic and therapeutic decision making. Ann Intern Med 1986;104:368. (*An evaluation of available tests, with consideration of their sensitivity and specificity.*)

Hutchinson CM, Hook EW. Syphilis in adults. Med Clin North Am 1990;74:1389. (*Excellent review of syphilis in adults, including serologies and treatment.*)

Rockwell DH, Yobs AR, Moore MB Jr. The Tuskegee study of untreated syphilis. Arch Intern Med 1964;114:792. (*A prospective 30-year study of untreated syphilis in 412 male blacks; notable for the ethical questions raised in addition to the natural history of syphilis.*)

Waring GW. False-positive tests for syphilis revisited. The intersection of Bayes' theorem and Wassermann's test. JAMA 1980;243:2321. (*A reminder that as the incidence of a disease declines, so does the specificity of its screening test. The overall sensitivity of a positive result on a serologic test for syphilis was calculated at 85%.*)

125
Screening for Chlamydial Infection
BENJAMIN DAVIS

Chlamydia trachomatis is responsible for close to 4 million cases of genitourinary tract infection each year in the United States. Transmission is by sexual contact. Because symptoms may be absent, mild, or nonspecific, treatment is often delayed or missed. Undetected or untreated infection can lead to pelvic inflammatory disease, with such consequences as tubal scarring, infertility, and ectopic pregnancy. More than 50,000 women are left sterile each year. The estimated direct and indirect costs of such adverse outcomes is in excess of $2.4 billion per year. Screening for chlamydial infection should be a consideration in the provision of routine primary care to women. Key issues are who should be screened and with what method(s).

EPIDEMIOLOGY AND RISK FACTORS

Chlamydial infection is a sexually transmitted disease (STD) present in epidemic proportions. Its prevalence varies by clinical setting. Among women seen in primary care practice, the prevalence is 3% to 5%. In family planning clinics, the prevalence increases to 9%; in STD clinics, the rate rises to 17% to 28%. Prevalence is very high among adolescents (18%), and one study of college campus women found 50% to be infected. Among female military recruits, the prevalence of chlamydial infection was 9%; the rate for the youngest recruits, 17 years of age, was 12%. Between 1987 and 1995, the reported rates of chlamydial infection increased by 281%. Although much of this rise is accounted for by increased screening, chlamydial infection is still very prevalent in the United States.

Women are at greater risk for contracting *C. trachomatis* infection than are men, and they also suffer more serious consequences. The risk in a single act of unprotected intercourse with an infected partner is 40% for women and 20% for men. The increased risk for women reflects the fact that they receive an ejaculate of infected secretions from their partner's genital tract. Men do not receive such a large inoculum unless they have an intact foreskin, which can serve as a reservoir for the woman's infected cervical secretions.

Among women with documented urogenital infection, the cervix is infected in 75% and the urethra in 50%. Endometritis can be demonstrated in about 33%; it is often clinically silent, but infection may spread to the tubes. In studies of salpingitis, *Chlamydiae* is recovered from the tubes in up to 50% of subjects. Vaginal infection is rare.

Chlamydiae may also colonize the pharynx and rectum in women engaging in oral and anal sex, respectively. Among those attending an STD clinic, the rate for oral recovery of organisms was 3.2%; the rectal colonization rate was 5.2%. Rectal involvement has been noted even in the absence of rectal intercourse.

In men, the urethra is the predominant site of infection, with more than 82% having a symptomatic or visible urethral discharge. In 1% to 2% of infected men, the infection ascends to the epididymis to produce acute scrotal pain and discomfort. Homosexual men demonstrate even higher rates of oral and anal recovery of organisms. Lymphogranuloma strains are often present.

Age is a powerful predictor of infection. Women *younger than 21 years* are at the greatest risk. Other important risk factors include having had a *new partner* in the last 2 months, *more than one partner* in the last 6 months, or a *partner known to have other partners*. Nonetheless, even among women who are monogamous or who have been sexually inactive in the last 2 months, prevalence can be as high as 7% to 10%.

Other significant predictors of chlamydial infection identified by multivariate analysis include *African-American race, low level of education, unprotected intercourse, mucopurulent cervical discharge*, and *induced mucosal bleeding* on swabbing of the cervix. Among patients with *gonococcal infection*, 30% to 50% have concurrent chlamydial disease.

SCREENING

Screening women at risk for the disease is essential because infection is so frequently asymptomatic despite being associated with extensive inflammation of the female genital tract. The rising rate of chlamydial infection in the past decade surely reflects, in part, wider acceptance and implementation of screening programs. However, when family planning clinics (where chlamydial screening is universal) are analyzed, the rate of chlamydial infection has actually *declined* from 9% to 3% in the past decade. This very likely reflects the impact that screening programs have had on the incidence of untreated disease, and quite possibly a reduction in infertility caused by chlamydial infection. In fact, a randomized controlled trial of screening of asymptomatic women enrolled in a health maintenance Organization demonstrated a 50% reduction in subsequent pelvic inflammatory disease.

DIAGNOSIS
Clinical Recognition

In women, clinical recognition can be difficult because most patients are asymptomatic or have only minor symptoms. Although vaginal discharge, bleeding, lower abdominal discomfort, and dysuria may accompany infection, these symptoms are nonspecific and require a detailed workup in their own right (see Chapters 111, 116, 117, and 133). The only features of the history that reliably suggest the problem are the risk factors identified above.

In the absence of definitive symptoms, physical findings take on additional importance. *Mucopurulent discharge, cervical ectopy, edema* in the area of ectopy, and easily *induced mucosal bleeding* have proved predictive of *C. trachomatis* infection, as has the presence of more than 10 neutrophils per high-power field. *Uterine* or *adnexal tenderness* in a patient with a mucopurulent cervical discharge is suggestive of chlamydial pelvic inflammatory disease (see Chapters 116 and 117).

In men, nongonococcal *urethritis* is the most common presentation, with dysuria, penile discharge, and the presence of more than five neutrophils per high-power field (see Chapter 136). About a third of men with chlamydial urethritis have no symptoms or signs, although pyuria may be noted. A small number experience acute testicular pain from an ascending epididymitis (see Chapter 131).

Diagnostic Tests

Culture is the gold standard for identification. However, because *chlamydiae* are obligate intracellular organisms, cell culture techniques similar to those used for viruses are required to isolate and identify them. Such cultures are technically difficult and expensive, take up to a week, and require refrigeration of the specimen and transport to the laboratory within 24 hours.

Modifications in traditional cell culture techniques have simplified isolation of the organism. Cell monolayers set up in microtiter plates are helpful in settings where titers are likely to be high (e.g., STD clinics). Fluorescein-conjugated monoclonal antibodies are useful for identifying chlamydial inclusions in infected monolayers. Combining both advances provides a 14% increase in diagnostic yield and sensitivity, makes second-pass testing unnecessary, and shortens test time to 3 days.

Antigen Detection techniques were developed to overcome the difficulties and limitations posed by culture. *Direct immunofluorescence* staining of smears, with the use of monoclonal antibodies, and *enzyme-linked immunosorbent assay* (ELISA) of antigen eluted from swabs are commercially available. When culture is used as the gold standard, the sensitivity of the direct immunofluorescent technique in women ranges from 77% in intermediate-prevalence populations to 90% in high-prevalence ones. Specificity is above 95% in both. The ELISA has a sensitivity of 85% to 89% and a specificity in excess of 95%. Cost-effectiveness studies indicate that screening for *Chlamydia* with antigen detection techniques becomes cost-effective when the pretest probability of disease exceeds 7%. Prescreening the urine for white blood cells can facilitate identifying asymptomatic men for testing.

DNA Detection techniques represent a further advance in diagnosis and have made detection possible by sampling of urine in addition to the traditional urethral or cervical swab. When a polymerase chain reaction or ligase chain reaction is used to detect minute quantities of chlamydial DNA, sensitivity rises into the 90% range and specificity approaches 100%. The convenience of an accurate urine test for *Chlamydia* makes the polymerase chain reaction and ligase chain reaction ideal for screening high-risk, asymptomatic patients.

EFFECTIVENESS OF TREATMENT

Several effective treatment regimens are available for chlamydial urogenital tract infection (see Chapters 117, 135, and 141). For urethritis and cervicitis without evidence of pelvic inflammatory disease, the treatment of choice is a *single 1-g oral dose of azithromycin*. The cost is comparable to that of 1 week of *doxycycline* (100 mg twice daily) or *tetracycline* (500 mg four times daily), and ensured compliance is a major benefit. If the patient is pregnant or unable to take tetracycline or azithromycin, then 500 mg of *erythromycin* base four times daily for 7 days is recommended.

CONCLUSIONS AND RECOMMENDATIONS

- Screening for chlamydial genitourinary infection is definitely worthwhile, but universal screening is not recommended in most primary care practices because the prevalence of asymptomatic infection in this setting is likely to be below the threshold that makes universal screening cost-effective.
- In settings where prevalence is very high (e.g., >10%), universal screening deserves consideration.
- Antigen testing becomes cost-effective among patients whose pretest risk is above 7%. Culturing becomes cost-effective among patients whose pretest risk is above 14%. DNA-based testing with polymerase chain reaction amplification lowers the prevalence threshold for cost-effective screening.
- A policy of selective screening is recommended based on a clinical estimate of the risk for chlamydial infection.
- Because the prevalence of chlamydial infection among sexually active girls and women *under the age of 21* is high and because the risk for sterility resulting from subclinical infection is also very high, annual screening of patients with or without symptoms has been recommended.
- The Centers for Disease Control and Prevention has recommended annual screening for women *ages 20 to 24 years* if either of the major risk factors for chlamydial infection is present: *lack of barrier contraception, or new or multiple partners in the preceding 3 months*. Women *older than 24 years* who have both these risk factors should also be screened.
- All men presenting with a urethral discharge and all women with mucopurulent cervicitis should be screened for chlamydial infection.
- Partner notification and treatment, either by patient referral or provider referral, is a critical step in interrupting the cycle of reinfection by asymptomatic partners.
- Although antigen testing of a cervical or urethral swab is the least expensive screening method, DNA-based polymerase chain reaction technology is recommended as the testing method of choice, especially in settings of lower prevalence, because its sensitivity is superior and it allows testing of urine in addition to cervical specimens, which lowers the prevalence threshold at which screening is cost-effective.
- All young women coming for routine gynecologic care who do not desire pregnancy should be urged to insist on condom use during intercourse.

ANNOTATED BIBLIOGRAPHY

Aronson MD, Phillips RS. Screening young men for chlamydial infection. JAMA 1993;270:2097. (*An editorial review of the data on screening young men.*)

Brunham RC, Paavonen J, Sevens CE, et al. Mucopurulent cervicitis—the ignored counterpart in women of urethritis in men. N Engl J Med 1984;311:1. (*The presence of cervical mucopus and more than 10 polymorphonuclear leukocytes per high-power field is predictive of* C. trachomatis *infection.*)

Centers for Disease Control and Prevention. *Chlamydia trachomatis* genital infections—United States, 1995. MMWR Morb Mortal Wkly Rep 1995;46(09);193. (*epidologic data.*)

Centers for Disease Control and Prevention. Recommendations for the prevention and management of *Chlamydia trachomatis* infections, 1993. MMWR Morb Mortal Wkly Rep 1993;42(RR-12). (*Guidelines for screening and treating* Chlamydia *infection in men and women.*)

Chow JM, Yonekura ML, Richwald GA, et al. The association between *Chlamydia trachomatis* and ectopic infection. JAMA 1990; 263:3164. (*A case–control study finding an odds ratio of 3.0 and a relative risk of 2.4; suggests that douching may increase risk.*)

Gaydos CA, Howell MR, Pare B, et al. *Chlamydia trachomatis* infections in female military recruits. N Engl J Med 1998;339:739. (*Population-based prevalence data of asymptomatic* Chlamydia *infection. Offers a rationale for screening all women below age 25.*)

Howell MR, Quinn TC, Gaydos CA. Screening for *Chlamydia trachomatis* in asymptomatic women attending family planning clinics: a cost-effectiveness analysis of three strategies. Ann Intern Med 1998;128:277. (*Analysis of cohort data from two family planning clinics; finds that age-based screening provides the greatest cost savings but that universal screening may be useful when prevalence of infection is very high.*)

Johnson BA, Poses RM, Fortner CA, et al. Derivation and validation of a clinical diagnostic model for chlamydial cervical infection in university women. JAMA 1990;264:3161. (*Identifies risk factors for chlamydial infection as a means of determining who should be screened.*)

Marrazzo JM, White CL, Krekeler B, et al. Community-based urine screening for *Chlamydia trachomatis* with a ligase chain reaction assay. Ann Intern Med 1997;127:796. (*Among adolescents, 9% of girls and 5% of boys infected.*)

Martin DH, Mrockowski TF, Dalu ZA, et al. Controlled trial of a single dose of azithromycin for the treatment of chlamydial urethritis and cervicitis. N Engl J Med 1992;327:921. (*Found to be as effective as standard therapy.*)

Phillips RS, Aronson MD, Taylor WC, et al. Should tests for *Chlamydia trachomatis* cervical infection be done during routine gynecologic visits? Ann Intern Med 1987;107:188. (*A cost-effectiveness study indicating that if prevalence is greater than 7%, antigen testing is worth performing.*)

Phillips RS, Hanff PA, Holmes MD, et al. *Chlamydia trachomatis* cervical infection in women seeking routine gynecologic care: criteria for selective testing. Am J Med 1989;86:515. (*Multivariate study; identifies low level of education, partner with other partners, and sex with other partners as predictors of infection and indications for screening.*)

Scholes D, Stergachis A, Heidrich FE, et al. Prevention of pelvic inflammatory disease by screening for cervical *Chlamydia* infection. N Engl J Med 1996;334:1362. (*Screening asymptomatic women for* Chlamydia *results in a 50% decline in subsequent pelvic inflammatory disease.*)

Sellor JW, Picard L, Gafni A, et al. Effectiveness and efficiency of selective vs. universal screening for chlamydial infection in sexually active young women. Arch Intern Med 1992;152:1837. (*Two selection rules were developed by regression analysis and tested; selective testing is preferred in low-prevalence settings.*)

Shafer M-A, Schachter J, Moncada J, et al. Evaluation of urine-based screening strategies to detect *Chlamydia trachomatis* among sexually active asymptomatic young males. JAMA 1993;270:2065. (*Prescreening the urine for white blood cells followed by antibody testing of persons with urine positive for white cells was most cost-effective.*)

Stamm WE. Diagnosis of *Chlamydia trachomatis* genitourinary infections. Ann Intern Med 1988;108:710. (*Excellent review, with very useful discussion of clinical findings, culture, and antigen methods; 93 references.*)

Vogels WHM, van Vooster-Vader PC, Schroder FP. *Chlamydia trachomatis* infection in a high-risk population: comparison of polymerase chain reaction and cell culture for diagnosis and follow-up. J Clin Microbiol 1993;31:1103. (*Test characteristics of the new DNA-based methods.*)

Workanski KA, Lampe MF, Wong KG, et al. Long-term eradication of *Chlamydia trachomatis* genital infection after antimicrobial therapy. JAMA 1993;270:2071. (*Treatment completely eradicates the organism.*)

126

Screening for Prostate Cancer

MICHAEL J. BARRY
JOHN D. GOODSON

Prostate cancer is a common cause of morbidity and mortality among older men in the United States. The lifetime probability of a man having clinical prostate cancer diagnosed in the "PSA era" is between 10% and 20%, but the probability of death from prostate cancer is stable, at approximately 3%. This ratio of cumulative incidence to mortality indicates that most patients in whom prostate cancer is diagnosed die of something else.

Patients and clinicians face a great deal of uncertainty in making clinical decisions about the early detection and treatment of prostate cancer. These tumors are exceedingly common and have the potential to cause significant morbidity and mortality. They also have a variable, often indolent course and a higher prevalence in elderly men whose health is often more limited by other diseases. The clinician should be aware of the unpredictable natural history of the disease and the limitations of current knowledge about the benefits of therapy when considering the use of screening tests for prostate cancer.

EPIDEMIOLOGY AND RISK FACTORS

The incidence of prostate cancer increases with age. Age-specific prevalence rates derived from autopsy studies are about 15% for men in their sixth decade, 25% for those in their seventh, and 40% or higher for men older than 70. The incidence of prostate cancer rose dramatically in the United States with increasing use of the prostate-specific antigen (PSA) test after about 1990, and it is now falling. Mortality from prostate cancer, however, has been relatively stable (Fig. 126.1). African-Americans have a twofold to threefold higher incidence of

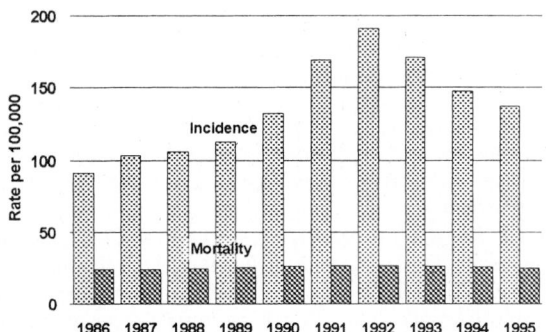

FIG. 126.1. Mortality and incidence of prostate cancer.

prostate cancer. A brother or father with prostate cancer increases risk twofold. A diet high in fat (particularly red meat) may also be a risk factor, and there is some suggestion that selenium, vitamin E, and tomato products (lycopenes) are protective. Evidence linking prostate cancer with prior vasectomy has been equivocal. No strong evidence has linked prostatitis or benign prostatic hyperplasia (BPH) to the development of prostate cancer.

NATURAL HISTORY OF DISEASE AND EFFECTIVENESS OF THERAPY

Clinical Presentation and Course. The biologic behavior of prostate cancer can vary, making individual cases unpredictable. Early prostate cancers are asymptomatic; older men not infrequently have concurrent lower urinary tract symptoms caused by BPH. Early prostate cancers may be discovered through screening activities or diagnosed incidentally when men undergo prostatectomy for BPH. Advanced cancers may present with obstructive symptoms, bleeding, and pelvic or bone pain.

The prognosis of prostate cancer depends as much on the degree of histologic differentiation of the tumor as on the extent of the disease, at least before detectable metastases are evident. Histologically, prostate cancers are often heterogeneous. Pathologists commonly assign a *Gleason score* of 1 to 5 to the most common and next most common histologic patterns, and add the two scores to obtain a Gleason sum ranging from 2 to

10. Cancers with Gleason sums of 2 to 4 are considered well differentiated, 5 to 7 moderately differentiated, and 8 to 10 poorly differentiated (although cancers with sums of 7 in fact behave in an intermediate fashion between moderate and poorly differentiated cancers). Most cancers discovered by screening are Gleason 5 to 7.

Clinically localized prostate cancers generally have doubling times measured in years. The prognosis of prostate cancers depends on tumor factors such as grade, and patient factors such as age. Table 126.1 provides estimates of the 15-year probability of being alive, dying of other causes, or dying of prostate cancer for different combinations of these factors in the absence of initial attempts at curative therapy with surgery or radiation. These data were generated from men in whom cancer was diagnosed in the pre-PSA era. Men with cancer diagnosed in the PSA era will generally do even better because the lead time afforded by early detection through PSA measurement appears to be at least 5 years, on average.

Effectiveness of Therapy. The variability in the natural history of this disease complicates an assessment of therapeutic efficacy. Some have argued that early and aggressive intervention [surgical extirpation of involved tissue (radical prostatectomy), radiation therapy (either external beam radiotherapy or implantation of radioactive seeds, also called interstitial radiotherapy or brachytherapy), or both] may improve survival for patients in whom the tumor appears to be localized to the gland. However, no form of intervention has yet been shown to improve survival in randomized clinical trials. In very old patients, many specialists withhold treatment until symptoms appear. A recent trend has developed toward more aggressive therapy in younger patients and older patients without coincident disease. This strategy may eventually prove beneficial, but it presents a higher immediate risk to the patient. Others argue that smaller, well-differentiated or moderately differentiated cancers are unlikely to need treatment because of their good prognosis, whereas larger, more poorly differentiated tumors are unlikely to benefit from curative treatment. These questions are being addressed in clinical trials, but it will likely be at least a decade before definitive answers become available. In the meantime, nonexperimental comparisons of treatment outcome from the pre-PSA era suggest a small advantage for more aggressive

Table 126.1. Estimated Percentage of Patients with Putatively Localized Prostate Cancer Managed Conservatively, by Age and Gleason Score at Diagnosis, with Each Outcome after 15 Years

	AGE AT DIAGNOSIS											
	% 55–59 YR			% 60–64 YR			% 65–69 YR			% 70–74 YR		
GLEASON SCORE	ALIVE	DECEASED FROM OTHER DISEASE	DECEASED FROM PCA	ALIVE	DECEASED FROM OTHER DISEASE	DECEASED FROM PCA	ALIVE	DECEASED FROM OTHER DISEASE	DECEASED FROM PCA	ALIVE	DECEASED FROM OTHER DISEASE	DECEASED FROM PCA
2–4	69	27	4	55	40	5	38	56	6	20	73	7
5	67	27	6	53	39	8	35	55	10	18	71	11
6	57	25	18	41	36	23	25	48	27	11	59	30
7	15	15	70	14	24	62	11	36	53	7	51	42
8–10	3	10	87	3	16	81	3	25	72	2	38	60

PCA, prostate cancer.

From Albertsen PC, Hanley JA, Gleason DF, et al. Competing risk analysis of men aged 55 to 74 years at diagnosis managed conservatively for clinically localized prostate cancer. JAMA 1998;280:975, with permission.

Table 126.2. Ten-year Disease-specific Survival in Patients with Clinically Localized Prostate Cancer by Intention to Treat

| | TEN-YEAR CANCER-SPECIFIC SURVIVAL | |
	NO.	PERCENTAGE (95% CI)
Grade 1		
Prostatectomy	3,854	94 (91–95)
Radiotherapy	4,065	90 (87–92)
Conservative	9,804	93 (91–94)
Grade 2		
Prostatectomy	14,287	87 (85–89)
Radiotherapy	7,939	76 (72–79)
Conservative	6,198	77 (74–80)
Grade 3		
Prostatectomy	5,133	67 (62–71)
Radiotherapy	2,596	53 (47–58)
Conservative	2,236	45 (40–51)

CI, confidence interval.
From Lu-Yao GL, Yao S. Population-based study of long-term survival in patients with clinically localised prostate cancer. Lancet 1997;349:906, with permission.

treatment of moderate and poorly differentiated cancers (Table 126.2), although these advantages may simply represent biases resulting from case selection. The side effects of these treatments are considerable and include a small but finite risk of mortality, in addition to problems of incontinence and sexual dysfunction.

SCREENING AND DIAGNOSTIC TESTS

Digital Rectal Examination (DRE) for evidence of either prostate or rectal cancer is a time-honored screening maneuver. Many clinicians believe a curled lateral decubitus position, with the legs drawn to the chest, and a standing position, with toes together and heels apart and the patient leaning over an examination table, to be the two best. Symmetric enlargement and firmness may be seen with BPH. Asymmetric areas of firmness or frank nodules are suggestive, and a stony hard, asymmetric prostate is highly suggestive, of malignancy. Fixation to adjacent tissue and a loss of the lateral prostate sulcus suggest local spread. Interobserver agreement regarding suggestive DRE findings is poor, even among urologists.

Test Characteristics of the DRE are poor for the earliest stages of prostate cancer. Compared with a multimodal screening battery including both transrectal ultrasonography (TRUS) and PSA determination, DRE has an estimated *sensitivity* of 60% to 70%. The *positive predictive value* (see Chapter 2) for a suspected abnormality detected on DRE is between 20% and 40%; however, cancer is often found by random biopsies in areas separate from the palpable abnormality. As many as 60% to 70% of the cancers detected initially by rectal examination are later found to have spread beyond the capsule of the gland. It has been estimated that abnormal findings on DRE double the odds of intracapsular cancer but increase the odds of extracapsular disease threefold to ninefold. Two case–control studies have evaluated whether DRE is associated with reduced mortality from prostate cancer, with conflicting results.

Prostate-Specific Antigen is a unique glycoprotein produced by both benign and malignant prostate epithelial tissue.

Measurement of PSA can clearly find more cancers than DRE alone. Because a number of assays are commercially available, physicians should know which assay is used by their local laboratory. Elevations can be seen after cystoscopy, acute urinary retention, or prostate trauma (such as a needle biopsy or prostatectomy), or with infection (especially prostatitis). DRE does not raise the PSA level; however, ejaculation may cause minor increases for a day or two. BPH can also produce modest PSA elevations, and separating BPH from early prostate cancer is a major clinical problem with PSA screening.

Test Characteristics. The true *sensitivity* and *specificity* of PSA measurement are unknown, as generally only men with suggestive results undergo biopsy. Gann and colleagues indirectly estimated the sensitivity of PSA to detect cancers ultimately destined to present clinically at 50% to 75%, with a specificity of about 90%; specificity deteriorates among older men or men with symptoms suggesting BPH. The predictive value of an elevated PSA level (above 4 ng/mL) for prostate cancer is about 30%, regardless of age (rising prevalence cancels the effect of decreasing specificity with age).

Prostate-specific Antigen Derivatives such as an *age-specific biopsy threshold* and *PSA rates of change over time* (i.e., the *"PSA velocity"*) have been proposed to separate men with early prostate cancer from those with BPH more effectively. Some aggressive urologists have begun to perform biopsies in all men with PSA levels above 2.5 ng/mL, finding cancer in 10% to 20% of men with levels of 2.6 to 4.0 ng/mL. Increases in PSA of more than 0.75 ng/mL yearly suggest cancer, but these must be based on at least three annual samples. Most recently, measurements of circulating *free PSA* (not bound to macromolecules) have been suggested for the same reason; men with higher ratios of free to total PSA are less likely to have prostate cancer. Some experts have suggested that in men with mildly elevated PSA levels (in the range of 4.0 to 10.0 ng/mL), biopsies need not be performed if free PSA comprises more than 25% of total PSA. However, the probability of prostate cancer in men with these ratios still appears to be about 10%. Given the lack of evidence regarding the benefit of screening with total PSA, no one of these modifications can be recommended over another. Similarly, recommendations for annual PSA screening are arbitrary.

Outcomes. No randomized trials have documented a *mortality* reduction from PSA screening. A recently published trial revealed no reduction in prostate cancer mortality among residents of Montreal randomized to screening; however, only a small percentage of men accepted the screening invitation. Among these men, mortality was lower, but self-selection for testing may have been an important source of bias. Advocates of PSA screening point out that there is also *no* convincing evidence that early detection programs do not reduce prostate cancer mortality. As a result, groups like the American College of Physicians recommend presenting the potential benefits and known risks of PSA screening to patients, and helping them reach an informed decision about whether or not to undergo PSA testing. At minimum, patients undergoing PSA screening should be informed that false-positive and false-negative PSA test and biopsy results can occur, and that no one knows whether regular PSA screening will reduce the risk of death from prostate cancer. However, even advocates of early detection and aggressive treatment doubt its value, at least in terms of reducing mortality, in men who have less than a 10-year life expectancy, or who are about age 75 or older with average comorbidity.

Transrectal Ultrasonography of the prostate is no longer widely promoted as a primary screening test because of poor sensitivity and specificity. It is, however, used to evaluate abnormalities found on DRE and PSA screening and to guide transrectal biopsy by identifying suspect hypoechoic areas. The yield from biopsy depends on the number of samples obtained. When the results of a rectal examination and PSA measurement are both negative, the positive predictive value of ultrasonography drops to 5% or less. Because of the limited sensitivity of TRUS, urologists usually systematically obtain six or more biopsy specimens from men with an elevated PSA level when no hypoechoic areas are seen.

CONCLUSIONS AND RECOMMENDATIONS

- Evidence regarding DRE screening for prostate cancer is conflicting. Many clinicians, however, simply consider the DRE an extension of a thorough physical examination of older male patients.
- If a prostatic abnormality on DRE is identified in a younger patient or an older patient without significant comorbid disease who would be eligible for curative treatment, a urologic referral for biopsy should be made. A normal PSA result does not exclude cancer in the presence of a palpable abnormality.
- PSA measurement can be considered at the age of 50 (and perhaps at age 40 among men at higher-than-average risk, such as those with a positive family history). However, because there is no evidence that such screening reduces long-term mortality, screening is optional. Patients should understand the pros and cons of screening before undergoing the test.
- When to proceed to biopsy is controversial; a PSA threshold of 4.0 ng/mL is commonly used.
- Screening periodicity has not been established, but repeating the PSA measurement at 1- to 2-year intervals is probably reasonable (the longer interval should be used when the initial PSA level is lower). Early detection efforts are not indicated for men with a life expectancy of less than 10 years.
- Routine TRUS is no longer recommended as a primary screening test; its main role is in the evaluation of abnormalities found on DRE or PSA measurement.

ANNOTATED BIBLIOGRAPHY

Albertsen PC, Hanley JA, Gleason DF, et al. Competing risk analysis of men aged 55 to 74 years at diagnosis managed conservatively for clinically localized prostate cancer. JAMA 1998;280;975. (*Provides 15-year outcomes for men of different ages with tumors of different histologic types managed conservatively.*)

Catalona WJ, Smith DS, Ratliff TL, et al. Measurement of prostate-specific antigen in serum as a screening test for prostate cancer. N Engl J Med 1991;324:1156. (*Reports outcome of a screening program involving 1,653 healthy male patients. About a third of the cancers found in this study would not have been detected by DRE alone. Many believe this article marked the start of the "PSA era."*)

Catalona WJ, Smith DS, Wolfert RL, et al. Evaluation of percentage of free serum prostate-specific antigen to improve specificity of prostate cancer screening. JAMA 1995;274:1214. (*Free PSA can stratify cancer risk to some degree, but it appears to add little to help in decision making regarding biopsy at this point in time.*)

Catalona WJ, Smith DS, Ornstein DK. Prostate cancer detection in men with serum PSA concentrations of 2.6 to 4.0 ng/mL and benign prostate examination. JAMA 1997;277;1452. (*These investigators obtained biopsy specimens from volunteers with PSA levels in the range of 2.6 to 4.0 ng/mL and normal findings on DRE, below the traditional biopsy threshold, and found cancer in 22%.*)

Chan ECY, Sulmasy DP. What should men know about prostate-specific antigen screening before giving informed consent? Am J Med 1998;105:266. (*Used focus groups of physicians and patients to attempt to define what patients should be told before undergoing PSA testing.*)

Chybowski FM, Bergstahl EJ, Oesterling JE. The effect of digital rectal examination on the serum prostate-specific antigen concentration. J Urol 1992;148:83. (*No effect noted; can order test on same day that DRE is performed.*)

Coley CM, Barry MJ, Fleming C, et al. Early detection of prostate cancer. Part I: prior probability and effectiveness of tests. Ann Intern Med 1997;126:394. (*Comprehensive review focusing on the performance of DRE and PSA measurement as screening tests.*)

Coley CM, Barry MJ, Fleming C, et al. Early detection of prostate cancer. Part II: estimating the risks, benefits, and costs. Ann Intern Med 1997;126;468. (*Second part of review focusing on outcomes of screening.*)

Flood AB, Wennberg JE, Nease RF, et al. The importance of patient preference in the decision to screen for prostate cancer. J Gen Intern Med 1996;11:342 (*Men who were well informed were evenly divided on the screening decision.*)

Friedman GD, Hiatt RA, Quesenberry CP Jr, et al. Case–control study of screening for prostate cancer by digital rectal examinations. Lancet 1991;337:1526. (*A case–control study showing that the relative risk for metastatic cancer was no lower among men who had undergone one or more rectal examinations in the preceding 10 years.*)

Gann PH, Hennekens CH, Stampfer MJ. A prospective evaluation of plasma prostate-specific antigen for detection of prostate cancer. JAMA 1995;273:289. (*PSA measurement had a sensitivity of 73% in detecting cancers diagnosed within 4 years of the time test serum was obtained in the Physicians' Health Study.*)

Jacobsen SJ, Katusic SK, Bergstrahl EJ, et al. Incidence of prostate cancer diagnosis in the eras before and after serum prostate-specific antigen testing. JAMA 1995;274:1445. (*Largely because of PSA testing, the age-adjusted incidence of prostate cancer increased from 64/100,000 person-years in 1983 to 215/100,000 in 1992.*)

Jacobsen SJ, Bergstrahl EJ, Katusic SK, et al. Screening digital rectal examination and prostate cancer mortality: a population-based case–control study. Urology 1998;52:173. (*In contrast to the Friedman study cited above, this study found fatal prostate cancer to be associated with a 50% lower probability of having undergone a DRE in the 10 previous years.*)

Labrie F, Candas B, Dupont A, et al. Screening decreases prostate cancer death: first analysis of the 1988 Quebec prospective randomized trial. Prostate 1999;38:83. (*Despite the title, men randomized to PSA screening did not have a lower death rate from prostate cancer; only the small subset who accepted screening had lower mortality, which may represent the effect of selection bias.*)

Litwin MS, Hays RD, Fink A, et al. Quality-of-life outcomes in men treated for localized prostate cancer. JAMA 1995;273:129. (*Treatment for prostate cancer produces a temporary decrease in measures of sexual and urinary function and quality of life.*)

Lu-Yao GL, Yao S. Population-based study of long-term survival in patients with clinically localised prostate cancer. Lancet 1997; 349:906. (*Provides statistics on 10-year survival for almost 60,000 men treated for prostate cancer with conservative management, radiation, or surgery.*)

Pienta KJ, Esper PS. Risk factors for prostate cancer. Ann Intern Med 1993;118:793. (*Comprehensive review; 178 references.*)

Potosky AL, Miller BA, Albertsen PC, et al. The role of increasing detection in the rising incidence of prostate cancer. JAMA 1995;273:548.

(*The age-adjusted incidence of prostate cancer among men more than 65 years old in four SEER (Surveillance, Epidemiology, and End Results) Program regions was 20% in 1990 and 19% in 1991.*)

Richie JR, Catalona WJ, Ahmann FR, et al. Effect of patient age on early detection of prostate cancer with serum prostate-specific antigen and digital rectal examination. Urology 1993;42;365. (*This six-center screening study involving more than 6,000 men provides predictive values of DRE and PSA measurement in prostate cancer for men of different ages.*)

127

Screening for Asymptomatic Bacteriuria and Urinary Tract Infection

Efforts to detect and treat asymptomatic bacteriuria are based on the assumption that treatment reduces the likelihood of subsequent morbidity from symptomatic infection, sepsis, or chronic renal disease. The risk for such complications depends on the clinical situation, including the age and sex of the patient. For some, risk is well defined and treatment is indicated; for most, however, the most significant morbidity may be related to the side effects of inappropriate treatment. It is therefore critical that the physician appreciate the implications of bacteriuria in different settings.

EPIDEMIOLOGY AND RISK FACTORS

The prevalence of bacteriuria depends on age and sex. Among neonates, positive cultures are found in about 1% of both boys and girls. During school age, the prevalence among boys is as low as 0.03%, in comparison with 1% to 2% among girls. The prevalence among women increases by 1% of the population per decade; throughout the childbearing years, the prevalence is 2% to 4%, and by age 50, it has reached 5% to 10%. Elderly men are almost as likely to have bacteriuria as women because of the high incidence of prostate and other urologic disease and subsequent instrumentation in this group. Prevalence in these older age groups reaches 15%.

The greater susceptibility of younger women and girls can be explained anatomically in that a short urethra allows easier access to the bladder, so that colonization by perineal organisms is facilitated. Risk increases with local trauma associated with sexual activity and relaxation of the pelvic supporting structures with age. Anatomic changes may also explain the higher prevalence of bacteriuria (4% to 7%) among pregnant women. Alternatively, because users of birth control pills also have an increased risk, the higher prevalence may also reflect estrogen-mediated dilation of the urethra.

The prevalence of bacteriuria is even higher in diabetic women. The relative risk for bacteriuria among women with diabetes, in comparison with nondiabetic women, is approximately 3. The risk among diabetic men is not increased.

It must be kept in mind that prevalence figures indicate the extent of bacteriuria at a single point in time. Because risk factors are shared by many and bacteriuria frequently resolves spontaneously as well as after therapy, the cumulative prevalence of bacteriuria is higher. By age 30, approximately 25% of women have experienced symptoms consistent with urinary tract infection.

Structural abnormalities (including obstruction of the urethra or ureters), significant vesicourethral reflux, neurologic lesions, and the presence of foreign bodies are important additional risk factors for bacteriuria.

NATURAL HISTORY OF ASYMPTOMATIC BACTERIURIA AND EFFECTIVENESS OF THERAPY

Asymptomatic and symptomatic urinary tract infections have the same epidemiologic correlates. Asymptomatic infections can become symptomatic; bacteriuria can persist after symptoms have resolved. Ninety percent of women with bacteriuria have had symptoms some time in the past, nearly 70% within the preceding year. Although both asymptomatic and symptomatic infections can resolve spontaneously, the urine is more likely to become sterile after treatment. Approximately 80% of women with bacteriuria have sterile urine after appropriate antibiotic treatment. However, follow-up studies indicate that only 55% of those treated will have sterile urine at the end of 1 year. Sterile urine developed spontaneously in fully 36% of untreated bacteriuric women during the same period. Significantly, women who had recurrences of infection after treatment were more likely to have associated symptoms than those who had persistent or relapsing bacteriuria. Symptomatic infection recurs within 3 years in 40% of women.

The importance of chronic or recurrent bacteriuria as a cause of chronic renal failure has been deemphasized as diverse noninfectious etiologies for the pathologic findings of interstitial nephritis have been recognized. Patients with bacteriuria are more likely to be hypertensive. They are also more likely to have identifiable abnormalities on intravenous pyelogram, including small kidneys, delayed excretion, caliceal dilation and blunting, ureteral reflux, stones, and other obstructive lesions. However, chronic renal failure rarely occurs as a complication of urinary tract infection in the absence of structural abnormalities. Evidence indicates that such abnormalities predispose patients to both chronic renal failure and recurrent infection. Definitive studies that address this important question have not yet been performed.

In addition to symptomatic urinary tract infection and chronic renal disease, the clinician must also be concerned with the possibility that chronic asymptomatic infection is a potential source of disseminated infection, such as endocarditis. This danger is particularly likely in the male patient with prostate disease and infection who requires instrumentation. Bacteremia has been documented in as many as 50% of male patients whose urine is infected at the time of the procedure; it is relatively rare when the urine is sterile. In elderly populations, asymptomatic bacteriuria has been associated with increased mortality. Obviously, such increased rates may be a consequence of either bacteriuria or other factors that increase the risk for both bacteriuria and death. Recent evidence suggests the latter; studies among among elderly women and men have found no difference between patients with and without bacteriuria when comorbidity such as cancer was controlled.

Special risks are associated with bacteriuria during pregnancy. Asymptomatic bacteriuria, defined by repeated recovery of more than 10^5 colony-forming units per milliliter in voided urine or suprapubic aspirates positive for bacteria, occurs in approximately 5% of pregnancies. In one study, the risk for onset of bacteriuria was greatest between weeks 9 and 17 of gestation. Among women with bacteriuria identified early in pregnancy, the incidence of acute pyelonephritis without prophylactic treatment is 40%. Women with bacteriuria are nearly twice as likely to deliver low-birth-weight infants, and the relative risk for perinatal mortality in their infants has been estimated at 1.6. Randomized trials of treatment of asymptomatic bacteriuria during pregnancy have demonstrated efficacy in reducing the incidence of pyelonephritis and delivery of low-birth-weight infants.

SCREENING AND DIAGNOSTIC TESTS

Asymptomatic bacteriuria is a laboratory diagnosis that requires careful definition. Because voided urine is easily contaminated by urethral and (in women) perineal flora during micturition, clean voided urine must be cultured quantitatively. The probability of infection when a specimen contains 10^5 colony-forming units per milliliter is nearly 100% for male patients but only 80% for female patients. The finding of two such positive cultures in a female patient increases the probability of infection to 95%. False-negative findings are more likely if the patient is undergoing vigorous diuresis, if the urine is unusually acidic (pH 5.5), or if the specimen has inadvertently been contaminated with antibacterial detergents. Spurious positive cultures are more common because of unclean collection technique, contaminated collection equipment, or failure to culture the urine promptly.

Collection of a single urine specimen with 10^5 colony-forming units per milliliter during urethral catheterization has a predictive value of infection of 95%. Catheterization should be limited to patients requiring relief of obstruction or those who absolutely cannot cooperate with collection techniques. The risk of introducing infection during catheterization may be as high as 5%. The risk of inducing bacteremia in men with an infected urinary tract approaches 50%. When suprapubic percutaneous bladder aspiration is performed, either in young children or in adults with confusing problems that must be resolved, infection can be presumed if growth of any bacteria other than skin contaminants occurs.

Nonquantitative approaches to diagnosis include microscopic examination for bacteria and clinical tests of bacterial activity, such as the reduction of nitrate to nitrite. Dipstick ni-

trite testing for bacteriuria has been shown to have a sensitivity of better than 90%, but specificity is limited and variable, ranging from 35% to 85% in different studies. This variation may be explained by differences in the prevalence of bacteria that do not reduce nitrates and variation in the time interval between collection and testing of urine. Dipstick tests for leukocyte esterase activity as a marker of pyuria are more sensitive but less specific. Reported sensitivity of the leukocyte esterase dipstick test for bacteriuria ranges from 72% to 97%; the reported range for specificity is 64% to 82%. Dipstick tests have been shown to be less sensitive when the prior probability of infection is low based on clinical findings. These and other nonspecific signs of urinary tract inflammation, such as the presence of microscopic pyuria or hematuria and the presence of proteinuria, may be helpful in making a presumptive diagnosis in the symptomatic patient. They may also indicate the need for urine culture when incidental abnormalities are detected in the asymptomatic patient. Confirmation of infection with quantitative culture technology should precede a therapeutic decision in the absence of symptoms.

CONCLUSIONS AND RECOMMENDATIONS

- Bacteriuria, both symptomatic and asymptomatic, is a common phenomenon with well-defined risk factors.
- Treatment is moderately effective in the short run, but because of high rates of spontaneous recurrence and resolution, the likelihood that bacteriuria will be noted with longer follow-up is not significantly influenced by short-term therapy.
- Symptomatic infections are generally not prevented by the treatment of asymptomatic bacteriuria in nonpregnant women.
- Although an association exists between bacteriuria and renal abnormalities, there is no evidence that this is an etiologic relationship. Furthermore, there is no evidence that treatment of infection in the absence of urinary tract abnormalities prevents progressive renal disease.
- Screening for asymptomatic bacteriuria is recommended only in selected high-risk populations, including (a) pregnant women; (b) elderly men with clinical prostatism or other urologic abnormalities, before and after required instrumentation; (c) all patients recently catheterized; and (d) patients with known renal calculi or other structural abnormalities of the urinary tract.
- Screening with reagent strips is not sufficiently sensitive to be used among patients who are at high risk and likely to benefit from detection and treatment. Screening of pregnant women should include urine culture.

A.G.M.

ANNOTATED BIBLIOGRAPHY

Abrutyn E, Mossey J, Berlin JA, et al. Does asymptomatic bacteriuria predict mortality and does antimicrobial treatment reduce mortality in elderly ambulatory women? Ann Intern Med 1994;120:827. (*Treatment reduces bacteriuria, no association with mortality has been found.*)

Asscher AW, Sussman M, Waters WE, et al. The clinical significance of asymptomatic bacteriuria in the nonpregnant woman. J Infect Dis 1969;120:17. (*Controlled trial of treatment of asymptomatic bacteriuria. Concludes that screening for bacteriuria in nonpregnant women is unlikely to be of value.*)

Kass EH, Zinner SH. Bacteriuria and renal disease. J Infect Dis 1969; 120:27. (*Exhaustive review of the links between bacteriuria and renal disease. Authors conclude that a causal relationship has been demonstrated in cases of pyelonephritis in pregnancy and bacteremia after catheterization but not in progressive renal disease among adults.*)

Kunin CM, Polyak F, Postel E. Periurethral bacterial flora in women. JAMA 1980;243:134. (*Intensively monitored small cohort of women with and without history of urinary tract infection. The most notable finding is a high frequency of asymptomatic bacteriuria, with spontaneous resolution in both groups.*)

Lachs MS, Nachamkin I, Edelstein PH, et al. Spectrum bias in the evaluation of diagnostic tests: lessons from the rapid dipstick test for urinary infection. Ann Intern Med 1992;117:135. (*Sensitivity for documented bacteriuria is much lower, approximately 50%, when the prior probability of infection is deemed to be low on clinical grounds.*)

Nicole LE, Mayhew WJ, Bryan L. Prospective randomized comparison of therapy and no therapy for asymptomatic bacteriuria in institutionalized elderly women. Am J Med 1987;83:27. (*No differences were noted in genitourinary morbidity or mortality; antimicrobial therapy was associated with adverse effects and a higher reinfection rate.*)

Nicole LE. Urinary infections in the elderly: symptomatic or asymptomatic. Int J Antimicrob Agents 1999;11:265. (*Neither urine culture nor symptomatic presentation allows a diagnosis to be made with confidence.*)

Nordenstam GR, Brandberg CA, Oden AS, et al. Bacteriuria and mortality in an elderly population. N Engl J Med 1986;314:1152. (*Nine-year cohort study found no difference in mortality among women with and without bacteriuria, and also no difference among men when those with cancer were excluded.*)

Pels RJ, Bor DH, Woolhandler S, et al. Dipstick urinalysis screening of asymptomatic adults for urinary tract disorders. II. Bacteriuria. JAMA 1989;262:1220. (*A careful review of the literature offering estimates of sensitivity and specificity plus recommendations.*)

Romero R, Oyarzun E, Mazor M, et al. Metaanalysis of the relationship between asymptomatic bacteriuria and preterm delivery/low birth weight. Obstet Gynecol 1989;73:576. (*Metaanalysis of eight trials.*)

Schieve LA, Handler A, Hershow R, et al. Urinary tract infection during pregnancy: its association with maternal morbidity and perinatal outcome. Am J Public Health 1994;84:405.(*Risk for preterm delivery and low birth weight increased 1.5- to 2-fold.*)

Stamm WE. Prevention of urinary tract infections. Am J Med 1984;76:148. (*Thoughtful review of risk factors and preventive approaches; recommends screening only for pregnant women.*)

Stenquist K, Dahlen-Nilsson I, Lidin-Janson G, et al. Bacteriuria in pregnancy. Frequency and risk of acquisition. Am J Epidemiol 1989;129:372. (*In a study of more than 3,000 pregnancies, the risk for onset of bacteriuria was greatest between weeks 9 and 17 of gestation.*)

Takahashi M, Loveland DB. Bacteriuria and oral contraceptives. JAMA 1974;227:762. (*Prevalence 50% higher among oral contraceptive users.*)

Tincello DG, Richmond DH. Evaluation of reagent strips in detecting asymptomatic bacteriuria in early pregnancy: prospective case series. BMJ 1998;316:435. (*Sensitivity too low for use in pregnant women.*)

128
Screening for Cancers of the Lower Urinary Tract

Lower urinary tract cancers include tumors of the renal pelves, ureters, bladder, and urethra. These lesions can logically be considered together because of their similar cell types—more than 95% consist of transitional cells, squamous cells, or a combination of the two—and because of common epidemiologic correlates.

Cancer of the lower urinary tract is viewed by many primary physicians as a relatively benign tumor that principally affects the elderly. Nevertheless, more than 50,000 new cases occur each year in the United States, and 11,000 deaths per year can be attributed to bladder cancer. The lifetime probability of incurring cancer of the bladder is approximately 3% for white men and 1% for white women. The probability of dying of bladder cancer, however, is approximately 1% and 0.3% for white men and white women, respectively.

Risk factors, including a strong association with occupational exposure, have been well defined. A weaker association with tobacco use has more recently been demonstrated. A prospective study of fluid intake and development of bladder cancer during 10 years suggests that a high intake of fluids decreases risk. Screening tests are available. Although the natural history of bladder cancer is still insufficiently understood to allow specific screening recommendations, the physician should understand the epidemiology of these tumors and the potential costs and benefits of various screening practices.

EPIDEMIOLOGY AND RISK FACTORS

Cancer of the lower urinary tract is a tumor of older age groups; in the United States, the mean age at the time of diagnosis is 68 years. The incidence increases at a constant rate during adult life, varying from 1 in 100,000 per year at age 20 to 200 in 100,000 per year at age 80 for white men. Women have approximately one-third the risk of men. In the United States, whites are twice as likely to have bladder tumors as nonwhites. Urban dwellers, too, have consistently been shown to have a higher incidence of lower urinary tract tumors than do people who live in rural or suburban areas.

The most notable risk factor for the development of lower urinary tract cancers is *occupational exposure* to aromatic amines, first noted in England in 1895. Subsequently, dyestuff workers were shown to have a 10- to 50-fold increased risk for bladder carcinoma. Compounds most closely associated with bladder carcinogenesis include 2-naphthylamine and benzidine. Recent case–control studies indicate excess risk among men who work with dyestuffs, rubber, leather, paints, and organic chemicals. It has been estimated that these occupational exposures are responsible for 18% of bladder cancer cases. As little as 2 years' exposure may be sufficient to increase the risk, but the time between exposure and subsequent cancer may be as long as 45 years.

Smoking has been implicated as a risk factor for bladder cancer in many studies, most of which indicate that smokers have a twofold increase in risk in comparison with nonsmokers. Other suggested risk factors include pelvic irradiation, which was used in the past for dysfunctional bleeding, and abuse of phenacetin-containing analgesics. Early case–control studies suggested an association with coffee consumption, but the weight of evidence does not support a significant increase in risk.

Because direct contact of the bladder urothelium with carcinogens excreted in the urine may contribute to bladder cancer, it has been hypothesized that a high consumption of fluids could reduce risk by diluting the urine or reducing contact time. Evidence has been inconsistent, but the largest prospective study suggests that men in the highest quintile of fluid consumption face about half the risk of those in the lowest quintile. Case–control and cohort studies also suggest that long-term use of diuretics may increase the risk for bladder cancer by as much as twofold.

NATURAL HISTORY OF LOWER URINARY TRACT CANCERS AND EFFECTIVENESS OF THERAPY

The natural history of lower urinary tract tumors is not well defined. The prognosis at the time of diagnosis depends on both clinical stage, defined by depth of penetration and extent of metastases, and histologic grade of the tumor. Depth of penetration and histologic grade are often closely correlated. Urothelial tumors are grossly subdivided into papilloma, papillary carcinoma, and transitional cell carcinoma. These gross morphologic distinctions have histologic counterparts that are highly predictive of 5-year survival. Grade 1 papillary carcinoma (papilloma) has a 5-year cure or clinical control rate of approximately 95%. Grade 2 papillary carcinoma (papillary carcinoma) has a 5-year survival rate of only 25%. The outlook for grade 3 papillary and infiltrating carcinoma (transitional cell carcinoma) is worse. The prognosis for patients with squamous carcinoma is also very poor unless the tumor is well differentiated. Clinical staging systems that distinguish between levels of tumor penetration of the bladder have also been shown to have good prognostic value. Overall, about 50% of patients with treated bladder cancer survive for 5 years. However, multiple synchronous and asynchronous tumors are the rule in lower urinary tract cancer and contribute to morbidity and eventual mortality.

Hematuria is the most common presentation of lower urinary tract cancer. Other symptoms suggestive of cystitis may also occur. Although it has been claimed that 75% of tumors promptly diagnosed after a first episode of hematuria are localized, few data on this subject are available. The likelihood that screening tests, including urinalysis and urinary cytology, would significantly advance the time of diagnosis is likewise unproven. A progression from urothelial atypia to sessile carcinoma in situ or papilloma to higher-grade malignancy has been postulated. Studies of the natural history of urothelial carcinoma in situ indicate that the majority of lesions progress to more malignant forms. Although early lesions are much less likely to be detected cytologically, 3.7% of detected tumors were *in situ* in one study. The usual synchronous and asynchronous multiplicity of such tumors makes it difficult to assess the benefits of early detection.

SCREENING TESTS

Efforts to screen for asymptomatic bladder cancer have focused on the detection of asymptomatic hematuria with urine dipsticks and urine cytology. Studies of dipstick urinalysis have been conducted in older men at increased risk for bladder cancer. Daily screening for 2 weeks or 10 serial screens conducted on a daily or weekly basis have produced at least one positive screen result in about 205 men. The predictive values positive for any urologic malignancy (bladder, prostate, or renal) in these two studies were 6% and 8%. One-time screening in general outpatient populations has a significantly lower yield and predictive value. In one such study, dipstick screening of more than 20,000 patients disclosed only one bladder cancer and two cancers of the prostate. In a second study, only 2% of patients with a positive screen result had any significant urologic disease. The predictive value for urologic cancer diagnosed anytime in the ensuing 3 years was 0.5%.

Urinary cytology is less sensitive but more specific than hematuria on dipstick as a screening test for lower urinary tract cancers. Reported rates of the sensitivity of cytology in detecting bladder carcinoma vary from 50% to 90%. Studies have consistently demonstrated that sensitivity increases with the grade of malignancy. Although invasive transitional cell carcinoma can regularly be detected with a sensitivity of 90% or greater, sensitivity rates for papillomas and papillary carcinomas range from zero to 50%.

Studies of cytologic screening of high-risk populations have been conducted. In one such study, screening of 285 exposed workers produced positive results in 31, 10 of whom had the diagnosis of cancer confirmed at cystoscopy. Within 4 years, 11 additional tumors developed among the 21 cytology-positive, cystoscopy-negative patients. Cystoscopy was also performed in the 254 workers with negative cytologic findings; only one case of bladder cancer was diagnosed on that examination. In general, the specificity of urinary cytology depends on the skill of the cytologist. False-positive rates as low as 1% and as high as 20% have been reported.

The value of other urinary sediment abnormalities, particularly hematuria, has not been well defined. In one study of cytologic detection, hematuria was absent in 50% of true-positive cytologic diagnoses.

Cystoscopy and radiographic procedures cannot be considered screening tools. They should be reserved for patients who present with symptoms suggestive of urinary cancer or who have positive findings on cytology. Frequent follow-up cystoscopy is also part of the postoperative care of the patient with bladder cancer.

CONCLUSIONS AND RECOMMENDATIONS

- Lower urinary tract cancer is associated with significant morbidity and mortality.
- Risks of occupational exposure to dyestuffs, rubber, leather and leather products, paint, and organic chemicals have been

well defined. Smoking is also associated with a significant increase in risk.

- High levels of fluid intake may reduce the risk for bladder cancer.
- Urinary cytology is an imperfect but useful screening test for high-risk groups.
- There is no evidence that screening significantly advances the time of diagnosis in an individual case or that early treatment influences the outcome. Nevertheless, because of the relatively high specificity and lack of morbidity associated with cytologic screening, identification of patients at high risk because of occupational exposure, with subsequent yearly cytologic screening, may be indicated in the occupational health setting. Screening of asymptomatic smokers without risk of occupational exposure is not recommended.

A.G.M.

ANNOTATED BIBLIOGRAPHY

Britton JP, Dowell AC, Whelan P, et al. A community study of bladder cancer screening by the detection of occult urinary bleeding. J Urol 1992;148:788. (*Among the 20% of men with one positive result in 10 screens, the predictive value for urologic malignancy was 6%.*)

Cole P, Hoover R, Friedell GH. Occupation and cancer of the lower urinary tract. Cancer 1972;29:1250. (*Case–control study identifying excess risk among five occupation categories: dyestuffs, rubber, leather and leather products, paint, and organic chemicals. No risk could be identified in those who worked with nonorganic chemicals, petroleum, or printing products.*)

Cole P, Monson RR, Haning H, et al. Smoking and cancer of the lower urinary tract. N Engl J Med 1971;284:129. (*Case–control data indicating that smokers have a twofold greater risk for the development of bladder cancer.*)

Foot NC, Papanicolaou GN, Holmquist ND, et al. Exfoliative cytology of urinary sediments (a review of 2,829 cases). Cancer 1958; 11:127. (*Sensitivity of 62% in detecting tumors of renal pelves,*

bladder, or ureters, 8% in renal tumors, 15% in prostatic tumors; high specificity.)

Grossman E, Messerli FH, Goldbourt U. Does diuretic therapy increase the risk of renal cell carcinoma? Am J Cardiol 1999;83: 1090. (*Systematic review of case–control and cohort studies suggesting that long-term use of diuretics increases risk for bladder cancer, with an odds ratio or risk ratio of 1.5 to 2.0.*)

Heney NM, Ahmed SW, Flanagan MJ, et al. Superficial bladder cancer: progression and recurrence. J Urol 1983;30:1083. (*Useful description of the natural history of the disease.*)

Matanoski GM, Elliott EA. Bladder cancer epidemiology. Epidemiol Rev 1981;3:203. (*Extensive review of descriptive epidemiology and risk factors, including smoking, coffee drinking, use of sugar substitutes, and occupational exposures.*)

Messing EM, Young TB, Hunt VB, et al. Home screening for hematuria: results of a multi-clinic study. J Urol 1992;148:289. (*Among 21% with a positive result on one screen, the predictive value positive was 8%.*)

Messing EM, Young TB, Hunt VB, et al. Comparison of bladder cancer outcome in men undergoing hematuria home screening versus those with standard clinical presentations. Urology 1995;45:387. (*Mortality during 2 years was lower among screenees.*)

Michaud DS, Spiegelman D, Clinton SK, et al. Fluid intake and the risk of bladder cancer in men. N Engl J Med 1999;340:1390. (*Men in the highest quintile for fluid intake had half the risk of men in the lowest quintile.*)

Mohr DN, Offord KP, Owen RA, et al. Asymptomatic microhematuria and urologic disease. JAMA 1986;256:224. (*Prevalence of hematuria was 13%, but only 2% of these had urologic disease.*)

Morrison AS, Buring JE. Artificial sweeteners and cancer of the lower urinary tract. N Engl J Med 1980;302:537. (*A case–control study that did not detect a significant association between the use of artificial sweeteners and excess risk of lower urinary tract cancer.*)

van der Meijden APM. Bladder cancer. BMJ 1998;317:1366. (*Review of diagnosis and treatment.*)

Viscoli CM, Lachs MS, Horwitz RI. Bladder cancer and coffee drinking: a summary of case–control research. Lancet 1993;341:1432. (*No significant association.*)

129
Evaluation of the Patient with Hematuria
LESLIE S.-T. FANG

Virtually every disease of the genitourinary tract can produce hematuria. The primary physician may encounter a patient with gross hematuria or may find microscopic hematuria on routine examination of the urine. Sometimes, the cause is a harmless condition, especially when asymptomatic microscopic hematuria occurs in an otherwise healthy, young patient. At other times, hematuria may be the only symptom of genitourinary neoplasia. Its presence demands careful consideration and often a thorough investigation to ascertain the underlying cause. One needs to be able to initiate an effective workup and decide how comprehensive and invasive it ought to be; this includes deciding when referral for urologic evaluation or renal biopsy is necessary.

PATHOPHYSIOLOGY AND CLINICAL PRESENTATION

Normally, fewer than 1,000 red blood cells are excreted in the urine each minute. Microscopic hematuria ensues if the rate

of excretion rises to 3,000 to 4,000 red blood cells per minute; two to three red blood cell per high-power field will appear on microscopic examination of the urine. If the excretion rate exceeds 1 million red blood cells per minute, macroscopic or gross hematuria will result. Definitions of clinically significant hematuria are somewhat arbitrary; however, more than eight red blood cells per high-power field is considered a reasonable cutoff for separating the likelihood of a benign cause from that of potentially serious disease.

Any intrinsic lesion within the genitourinary tract involving the kidneys, ureter, bladder, prostate, or urethra can produce hematuria. Hematuria may also result from periurethral problems in the pelvis or colon, systemic diseases, bleeding diatheses, and the use of certain drugs (e.g., cyclophosphamide).

Symptoms associated with hematuria may provide important clues to etiology. The flank pain of renal colic is usually secondary to renal calculi but may occasionally be associated

Table 129.1. Diagnosis in 1,000 Referred Cases of Gross Hematuria

DIAGNOSIS	PATIENTS (%)
Kidneys	15.0
Tumor	3.5
Infection	3.0
Calculus	2.7
Trauma	2.0
Obstruction	1.5
Others	2.3
Ureters	6.5
Calculus	5.3
Tumor	0.7
Others	0.5
Bladder	39.5
Infection	22.0
Tumor	14.9
Others	2.6
Prostate	23.6
Benign hyperplasia	12.5
Infection	9.0
Tumor	2.1
Urethra	4.3
Stricture	1.7
Calculus	1.3
Others	1.3
Essential hematuria	8.5

From Lee LW, Davis E, et al. Gross urinary hemorrhage: a symptom, not a disease. JAMA 1953;153:782, with permission.

with the passage of clots. Frequency, dysuria, urgency, and suprapubic pain occur with inflammatory lesions of the lower urinary tract. Dull flank pain with fever and chills may accompany pyelonephritis (see Chapter 133).

Occasionally, complaints such as fever, rash, or joint pains may indicate an underlying systemic disease. Uncommonly, hematuria occurs without any associated symptoms, although the majority of cases have a definable cause. When a thorough workup fails to reveal one, the patient is said to have "essential hematuria." Renal biopsy of such patients often shows minimal glomerular or interstitial disease. The long-term prognosis of these patients is excellent.

DIFFERENTIAL DIAGNOSIS

Intrinsic genitourinary lesions involving the kidneys, ureters, bladder, prostate, and urethra can all produce hematuria (Tables 129.1 and 129.2). Gross hematuria is most commonly associated with infections and neoplasms. Microscopic hematuria is most commonly associated with infection and benign prostatic hypertrophy. The prevalence of serious underlying disease (e.g., cancer, polycystic disease) in community-based study of asymptomatic microscopic hematuria is 0.1%, in comparison with 10% in referred populations. Even among high-risk groups (e.g., older men), the prevalence in community-based study is only 5%.

Rarely, periureteral inflammatory lesions in the appendix, colon, or pelvic structures produce microscopic hematuria. On occasion, a systemic illness such as lupus erythematosus, bacterial endocarditis, or rheumatic fever is the source of hematuria. Blood dyscrasias (e.g., hemophilia, sickle cell disease,

polycythemia vera, and leukemia) and hemorrhagic disorders (e.g., thrombocytopenic purpura and various coagulation defects) can be responsible for red cells in the urine.

Drugs such as anticoagulants, salicylates, methenamine preparations, and sulfonamides have been known to cause hematuria. Cyclophosphamide can induce hemorrhagic cystitis or microscopic hematuria (see Chapter 88). Hematuria in a patient on anticoagulants requires evaluation because an underlying urologic lesion is often found (see Chapter 83).

Fever, strenuous exercise, and long-distance running are among the harmless causes of microscopic hematuria in otherwise healthy patients.

Conditions occasionally mistaken for hematuria include menstrual bleeding and the intake of substances that can darken the urine, such as beets, rhubarb, and the drugs phenazopyridine (Pyridium) and rifampin.

WORKUP

The appropriate workup depends on whether the patient has macroscopic hematuria or asymptomatic microscopic hematuria, on the age and sex of the patient, and on the mode of clinical presentation. As indicated in the previous section, the likelihood of finding a significant genitourinary tract disease is higher in patients with macroscopic hematuria, particularly in older men. Asymptomatic microscopic hematuria in young adults, on the other hand, carries a much lower risk. Evidence from five population-based studies indicates that 1% to 5% of children and adults will show evidence of microhematuria on routine urinalysis and that fewer than 2% of these patients will have a serious and treatable urinary tract disease. However, the incidence of urinary tract cancers rises dramatically with age and is more than twice as high in men as in women. An investigation of microscopic hematuria in the older male patient should therefore be pursued.

Table 129.2. Diagnosis in 500 Referred Cases of Asymptomatic Microscopic Hematuria

DIAGNOSIS	PATIENTS (%)
Kidneys	6.2
Calculus	3.4
Cyst	1.2
Hydronephrosis	0.6
Tumor	0.4
Others	0.6
Ureters	0.8
Calculus	0.4
Ureterocele	0.4
Bladder	8.6
Infection	6.6
Tumor	1.8
Others	0.2
Prostate	23.6
Benign hyperplasia	23.6
Urethra	23.4
Infection	21.2
Calculus	1.8
Others	0.4
Essential hematuria	44.0

From Greene LF, O'Shaughnessy EJ Jr, Hendricks ED. Study of 500 patients with asymptomatic microhematuria. JAMA 1956;161:610, with permission.

History is of paramount importance in narrowing the scope of the workup. A history of trauma ought to direct attention to possible renal, ureteral, or urethral injury. Massive hematuria is usually associated with bladder neoplasm, benign prostatic hyperplasia, or trauma. The passage of large, bulky clots implicates the bladder as the source, whereas long, shoestring-shaped clots suggest a ureteral origin. A past history of analgesic excess makes analgesic nephropathy a possibility. A prior history of nephritis requires consideration of chronic nephritis as the basis of the hematuria. A family history of renal diseases may suggest polycystic kidney disease or hereditary nephritis. Benign familial hematuria has been described and is inherited in a pattern consistent with autosomal dominant transmission; checking for hematuria in relatives may avoid an extensive workup in otherwise healthy-appearing patients. Harmless, self-limited forms of microscopic hematuria are suggested by a recent history of strenuous exercise, long-distance running, or a minor febrile illness.

Physical Examination should include observation of any fever, hypertension, rash, purpura, petechiae, friction rub, heart murmur, or joint swelling. The presence of hypertension suggests renal parenchymal disease. The abdomen has to be examined carefully for enlargement of one or both kidneys, liver, or spleen. Thorough examination of the prostate in the male patient and the pelvis in the female patient is essential.

Laboratory Testing. A repeated urinalysis is worthwhile in patients suspected of having a self-limited or trivial cause for their hematuria, such as low-grade infection, a menstrual period, or vigorous exercise. An entirely normal result of a repeated study in a healthy young person requires no further investigation other than a follow-up urinalysis in a month or two. However, in an older patient, whose risk for malignancy is much greater, an abnormal number of red blood cells on urinalysis should be taken seriously, even if a second urine specimen is clear. A urinary tract malignancy may present in just this manner. The urine sediment should be carefully examined. The presence of white cells and bacteria favors a diagnosis of cystitis; casts of white cells imply the presence of pyelonephritis or interstitial nephritis. Red cell casts strongly suggest glomerulonephritis. The presence of dysmorphic red cells under phase contrast microscopy is also highly suggestive of a glomerular origin of the red cells. A urine specimen should be sent for routine culture when pyuria is noted (see Chapter 133). Culture for urine acid-fast bacillus needs to be obtained if sterile pyuria and hematuria persist.

The need for further workup is determined by the probability of important underlying pathology. For example, a patient over age 50 is at increased risk for urinary tract cancer; it must be ruled out. On the other hand, an otherwise healthy young patient with an unremarkable history, normal findings on physical examination, and an otherwise benign urinary sediment need not undergo invasive testing because the likelihood of malignancy or other serious pathology is low. In a major population study, the frequency of clinically significant microscopic hematuria was 2.3%, with only 0.5% of patients having bladder or renal cell carcinoma; malignant lesions were found almost exclusively in patients over age 50.

The *three-glass test* (see Chapter 139) can be performed to attempt to identify the site of the bleeding. Initial hematuria is usually associated with anterior urethral lesions, such as stenosis and urethritis. Terminal hematuria usually arises from a lesion in the posterior urethra, bladder neck, or trigone. Total hematuria is associated with lesions at the level of the bladder or above.

Renal function is checked when renal parenchymal disease is suspected. In patients with proteinuria, a *24-hour urine collection for creatinine and protein determinations* should be performed to assess renal function and assess the degree of proteinuria quantitatively. Heavy proteinuria (>3 g/24 h) is usually associated with glomerular lesions (see Chapter 130). In the presence of renal colic, the urine should be strained to detect calculi or papillae. Three first-void morning urine specimens are sent for *cytology* in patients over the age of 40 with hematuria because they are at increased risk for a neoplasm. Normal findings on cytology do not rule out a malignancy (see Chapter 128); cystoscopy is indicated if suspicion remains. *Flat plate and upright films* of the abdomen are obtained and carefully examined to ascertain renal size and detect the presence of calcification.

If these tests fail to define the origin of the hematuria, an *intravenous pyelogram with tomograms* should be performed. Renal and ureteral abnormalities can be defined accurately. A *postvoid film* should be obtained to assess the amount of postvoid residual urine, which can be used to estimate the degree of bladder neck obstruction. *Ultrasonography*, *computed tomography* of the body, and *magnetic resonance imaging* are useful to differentiate a solid mass from a cystic lesion if the differentiation cannot be made on nephrotomograms. *Renal angiography* is reserved for evaluation of possible renal trauma, suspected renal masses, and possible arteriovenous malformations.

If clinical evidence of glomerular disease (red cell casts, dysmorphic red cells, heavy proteinuria) is present, *immunologic studies* should be performed and a renal biopsy should be considered. The immunologic tests of diagnostic use include the following: antinuclear antibody (ANA), anti-DNA antibody, and complement levels [C3, C4, and CH50 (hemolytic complement)] for the diagnosis of systemic lupus erythematosus (see Chapter 130); antistreptolysin-O (ASLO) titer and antihyaluronidase, antistreptokinase, and complement levels for the diagnosis of poststreptococcal glomerulonephritis; serum and urine immunoelectrophoresis for the diagnosis of multiple myeloma; serum immunoglobulin A level for patients suspected of having Berger's disease (IgA nephropathy) or Henoch-Schönlein purpura; serum antiglomerular basement membrane antibody levels for patients suspected of having Goodpasture's syndrome; and antineutrophil cytoplasmic antibody (ANCA) levels for pauciimmune glomerulonephritis.

INDICATIONS FOR REFERRAL

In a patient over age 50, if a distinct lesion is still not defined or a bladder lesion is suspected, it is necessary to proceed to *cystoscopy* (see Chapter 128). The procedure is particularly useful during periods of active bleeding. Careful examination of the ureteral orifices for bleeding and biopsy of suspected lesions are essential.

Patients with evidence of glomerulonephritis should be referred to a nephrologist for consideration of *renal biopsy*, which is indicated only to establish a diagnosis that will affect the selection of therapy (see Chapter 130) and should be reserved for patients with clinical evidence of glomerular disease. Rarely, renal biopsy may be indicated if the preceding studies have not led to a diagnosis.

PATIENT EDUCATION

It is essential to impress on the older patient the necessity of a complete evaluation of hematuria. The high incidence of potentially curable neoplasms in patients over age 50 (see Chapter 143) makes thorough investigation in this group mandatory.

ANNOTATED BIBLIOGRAPHY

Bard RH. The significance of asymptomatic microscopic hematuria in women and its economic implications. Arch Intern Med 1988;148:2629. (*No bladder lesions found in 10 years; suggests cystoscopy might be unnecessary in such persons, although study population small.*)

Blumenthal SS, Fritsche C, Lemann J. Establishing the diagnosis of benign familial hematuria. The importance of examining the urine sediment of family members. JAMA 1988;259:2263. (*Suggests checking for hematuria in relatives before launching extensive investigation.*)

Cespedes RD, Peretsman SJ, Blatt SP. The significance of hematuria in patients infected with the human immunodeficiency virus. J Urol 1995;154:1455. (*No occult tumors found among 331 young HIV-infected patients, but full evaluations were performed in only 20%.*)

Corwin HL, Silverstein MD. Microscopic hematuria. Clin Lab Med 1988;8:601. (*Review of methods for detection of hematuria, prevalence, causes, and diagnostic strategies in patients with microscopic hematuria.*)

Culclasure TF, Bray VJ, Hasbargen JA. The significance of hematuria in the anticoagulated patient. Arch Intern Med 1994;154:649. (*Anticoagulation is not associated with increased incidence or prevalence of hematuria.*)

Grossfeld GD, Carroll PR. Evaluation of asymptomatic microscopic hematuria. Urol Clin North Am 1998;25:661. (*The urologist's perspective.*)

Miller MI, Puchner PJ. Effects of finasteride on hematuria associated with benign prostatic hyperplasia: long-term follow-up. Urology 1998;51:237. (*Finasteride reduced hematuria associated with benign prostatic hypertrophy in this small study.*)

Mohr DN, Offord KP, Owen RA, et al. Asymptomatic microhematuria and urologic disease: a population-based study. JAMA 1986;256:224. (*Community-based prevalences of underlying disease.*)

Thaller TR, Wang LP. Evaluation of asymptomatic microscopic hematuria in adults. Am Fam Physician 1999;60:1143. (*Helpful review.*)

Van Savage JG, Fried FA. Anticoagulant-associated hematuria: a prospective study. J Urol 1995;153:1594. (*Of 24 patients with gross hematuria, two had bladder cancer.*)

Woolhandler S, Pels RJ, Bor DH, et al. Dipstick urinalysis screening of asymptomatic adults for urinary tract disorders. JAMA 1988;262:1215. (*In a review of five population-based studies, fewer than 2% of patients with a positive result on heme dipstick testing had a serious and treatable urinary tract disease.*)

Yamagata K, Yamagata Y, Kobayashi M, et al. A long-term follow-up study of asymptomatic hematuria and/or proteinuria in adults. Clin Nephrol 1996;45:281. (*Of patients with asymptomatic hematuria, proteinuria developed in 11% during follow-up with a mean duration of 6 years.*)

130

Evaluation of the Patient with Proteinuria

LESLIE S.-T. FANG

Normal persons excrete less than 150 mg of urinary protein each day; the mean is 40 to 50 mg. Excretion in excess of 150 mg/24 h is classified as clinically significant proteinuria. Causes range from benign conditions, such as exercise and orthostatic proteinuria, to glomerulonephritis with rapidly deteriorating renal function. Office evaluation is frequently prompted by an incidental finding of proteinuria on routine urinalysis. The objective of the outpatient workup is to establish the presence of significant proteinuria, search noninvasively for treatable underlying conditions, and select patients who require referral for renal biopsy.

PATHOPHYSIOLOGY AND CLINICAL PRESENTATION

Small amounts of protein (2 to 8 mg/100 mL) are normally found in the urine of healthy persons, but at a concentration below that detectable by routine methods. Two thirds of this protein is low-molecular-weight globulin of serum origin; the remainder is albumin and nonserum protein.

Significant proteinuria can occur through a number of mechanisms:

1. Increased glomerular permeability
2. Increased production of abnormal proteins small enough to pass freely through the glomerulus (e.g., Bence Jones protein)
3. Decreased tubular reabsorption (e.g., because of interstitial nephritis)
4. Lower urinary tract disease, including infection
5. Fever, heavy exertion, congestive heart failure, postural changes, and surgical trauma—all believed to affect renal blood flow

Clinical Presentations

Proteinuria can present as an isolated asymptomatic finding on urinalysis, as edema of unknown cause, or as part of the clinical picture in a patient with known renal or systemic disease.

Isolated Proteinuria. Asymptomatic patients excreting less than 1 g of protein daily and appearing otherwise healthy, with no other evidence of renal dysfunction or systemic disease, are considered to have isolated proteinuria. The urine sediment is normal. Two varieties have been described: benign, transient proteinuria and persistent, isolated proteinuria.

Benign forms are characterized by their transient nature. A *functional* variety has been observed in the context of emotional or physical stress, an acute illness, or even a bout of congestive heart failure. The proteinuria is believed to reflect physiologic changes in renal hemodynamics. Although all forms of proteinuria worsen with standing, some persons experience proteinuria only on standing; it is absent when they are recumbent. The condition is common in persons under the age of 30 (especially males) and is labeled *orthostatic proteinuria*. In many persons, the postural proteinuria resolves after a few years; in others, it remains. Long-term (20-year) follow-up studies show no development of progressive renal impairment.

Other forms of benign disease in young people include *idiopathic transient proteinuria*, characterized by an occasional positive result on dipstick testing that is unrelated to posture or stress, and *intermittent proteinuria*, in which about half of dipstick test results are positive for albumin. The former is considered a physiologic variant of normal. The latter is sometimes associated with minor abnormalities on renal biopsy, but progressive disease is rare and the condition is usually self-limited. Intermittent proteinuria in older persons carries a slightly higher risk for renal impairment.

Persistent isolated proteinuria carries a worse prognosis, although the urine sediment and renal function are entirely normal. The condition is most common in healthy young men. Mild forms of glomerular and tubular injury have been found among these patients. Long-term follow-up studies of patients with persistent isolated proteinuria reveal a 40% chance for the development of renal insufficiency, usually secondary to glomerular disease. In some instances, nephrotic syndrome may ensue. However, even when persistent and accompanied by minor glomerular changes on biopsy, the condition has an excellent prognosis provided no associated abnormalities of the urine sediment are present.

Proteinuria in the Setting of Renal or Systemic Disease. Albuminuria in excess of 1 g/24 h suggests significant renal impairment. When it exceeds 3 g/24 h, underlying *glomerular disease* is likely; lesser amounts are consistent with either glomerular or tubular dysfunction. Early in the course of glomerular injury, *microalbuminuria* (urine albumin concentration >20 mg/dL) appears. *Obstruction* and *reflux* are important treatable causes of tubular protein leakage. Glomerular injury may be caused by intrinsic renal disease or a systemic process (e.g., diabetes, systemic lupus).

Nephrotic syndrome is said to be present when more than 3.5 g of protein is excreted in 24 h and the serum albumin falls to less than 3.0 g/dL. Such heavy proteinuria usually indicates significant glomerular disease (either primary or secondary to systemic illness), but it may occur with severe tubular injury. If the serum albumin concentration drops to less than 2 g/dL, then plasma oncotic pressure may fall sufficiently to cause *edema*, typically beginning in the medial aspect of the ankles; on occasion, however, periorbital puffiness may be the principal manifestation. *Hypercholesterolemia* is a common accompaniment

reflecting increased hepatic synthesis of low-density lipoprotein (LDL) and very low-density lipoprotein (VLDL) cholesterol. *Lipiduria* is a diagnostic feature of the urine sediment. A *hypercoagulable* state may ensue, believed linked to reductions in protein S (an inhibitor of thrombosis). Venous thromboembolism occurs in about 20% of cases. The source of embolization may be a clinically silent *renal vein thrombosis*. The risk for *bacterial infection* is increased in those with marked urinary loss of immunoglobulins. Excessive urinary loss of vitamin D may develop, causing *hypocalcemia* and secondary hyperparathyroidism. Other presenting symptoms reflect associated renal dysfunction or underlying systemic diseases.

DIFFERENTIAL DIAGNOSIS

Asymptomatic Proteinuria. Proteinuria without other abnormalities in an asymptomatic patient can be transient or persistent (Table 130.1). *Transient* forms include functional, orthostatic, idiopathic, and intermittent varieties. *Persistent isolated proteinuria* suggests underlying glomerular or tubular disease.

Symptomatic Proteinuria. As noted above, heavy proteinuria resulting in nephrotic syndrome is usually the result of either intrinsic or secondary glomerular disease (Table 130.2), but occasionally severe tubular injury is responsible (Table 130.3). About 50% to 75% of cases are associated with intrinsic glomerular disease; the remainder are associated with systemic illnesses that cause glomerular injury (e.g., long-standing diabetes mellitus, systemic lupus, amyloidosis). In adults, *membranous nephropathy* is the most common histologic abnormality seen on the biopsy specimens of patients with nephrotic syndrome. It may be idiopathic or secondary to systemic lupus, hepatitis B, cancer (breast, lung, colon), or medication (gold, penicillamine, captopril). It accounts for close to 50% of patients with idiopathic disease. *Minimal-change disease* is the glomerulopathy most common in children but is also seen in patients with Hodgkin's disease and hypersensitivity reactions to drugs such as NSAIDs. *Focal and segmental glomerulosclerosis* is the pathologic picture in about 25% of cases of intrinsic renal disease but is also a feature of HIV infection and IV heroin abuse. *Membranoproliferative glomerulonephritis* accounts for about 15% of patients with idiopathic disease and also occurs in the setting of infection, non-Hodgkin's lymphoma, cryoglobulinemia, and some forms of systemic lupus.

Table 130.1.   Differential Diagnosis of Proteinuria

Asymptomatic–Transient
    Exercise
    Upright posture
    Lower urinary tract disease (e.g. infection)
    Fever (occasionally)
    Congestive heart failure (occasionally)

Asympotomatic–Persistent
    Idiopathic
    Fixed postural type
    Mild glomerular injury
    Mild tubular injury

Symptomatic
    Glomerular disease
    Severe tubular disease (see Table 130.3)

Table 130.2.   Important Glomerular Causes of Nephrotic Syndrome

CAUSE	PATHOLOGIC FEATURES	PROGNOSIS
Idiopathic Glomerular Injury		
Membranous nephropathy	Basement membrane thickening, granular deposits of IgG and C3	Fair–good
Minimal-change disease	Normal light microscopy; no immune deposits	Excellent
Focal and segmental glomerulosclerosis	Segmental sclerosis, tubular atrophy	Fair–poor
Membranoproliferative glomerulonephritis	Hypercellular glomeruli and duplicate basement membrane; immune deposits	Poor
Secondary Glomerular Injury		
Diabetetes mellitus	Nodular sclerosing	Fair–poor
Light-chain disease	Nodular sclerosing	Poor
Amyloidosis	Nodular sclerosing	Fair–poor
Systemic lupus	Membranoproliferative or membranous	Poor–good
Infection (endocarditis, malaria, syphilis, hepatitis B)	Membranoproliferative	Fair–poor
Non-Hodgkin's lymphoma	Membranoproliferative	Poor
Hodgkin's disease	Minimal change	Fair
Drug hypersensitivity	Minimal change	Good
Hepatitis B	Membranous	Fair–good
Cancer (lung, colon, breast)	Membranous	Fair
Nephrotoxins (gold, other heavy metals, high-dose captopril, penicillamine)	Membranous	Poor–good
Heroin	Focal glomerulosclerosis	Poor–fair
HIV infection	Focal glomerulosclerosis	Poor
Mechanical (renal vein thrombosis, IVC obstruction)		Fair–poor
Pregnancy (preeclampsia)		Good

IVC, inferior vena cava; IgG, immunoglobulin G; C3, complement component 3.

Table 130.3.   Tubular Disorders Associated with Proteinuria

Analgesic abuse

Pyelonephritis

Fanconi's syndrome

Cadmium and mercury poisoning

Balkan nephropathy

Lowe syndrome

Hepatolenticular degeneration

WORKUP

Confirming Proteinuria and Its Significance

Repeat *urinalysis* that includes examination of the *urine sediment* should be the initial step when proteinuria is detected by *dipstick* in a routine random urine sample. The dipstick test is specific for albumin and can detect concentrations in excess of 30 mg/dL. A single negative test result does not rule out significant proteinuria because protein excretion may be intermittent (e.g., orthostatic proteinuria), or a protein other than albumin (e.g., light chains in myeloma) can be excreted. Orthostatic proteinuria can be differentiated from more serious types by collecting a urine sample from the patient on arising and another after the patient has been continuously upright for 2 hours. False-positive dipstick reactions can be seen in patients who are dehydrated, have gross hematuria, or are receiving large doses of nafcillin or a cephalosporin. The specific gravity should be noted along with the test results.

Detection of microalbuminuria (urine albumin concentration >20 mg/dL) is becoming increasingly important in the management of diabetes (see Chapter 102) and other conditions in which early treatment of glomerular impairment can reduce the risk for progression to renal failure. *Radioimmunoassay* is the most sensitive and specific mode of detecting microalbuminuria, but the procedure is costly and not widely available. Combined testing with a *dipstick* (e.g., Chemstrip) plus *sulfosalicylic acid* provides a high degree of sensitivity (95%) and can function well as a low-cost *screening* procedure. However, specificity is low (64%), and false-positives occur frequently with such testing. When the result will affect management, samples that test positive by screening methods can be subjected to radioimmunoassay.

Sediment examination is critical and should be performed on a freshly collected specimen. Red cell casts indicate glomerulonephritis (although the absence of erythrocytes on one sample does not rule out glomerulonephritis). White cell casts are found in pyelonephritis and interstitial nephritis. Oval fat bodies are a consequence of lipiduria in patients with nephrotic syndrome.

A confirmed urinalysis for protein should be followed by a *24-hour urine collection* to quantify the proteinuria. In addition to the urinary *albumin*, the urine *creatinine* should also be noted. The latter determination enables assessment of adequacy of collection. Depending on muscle mass, the total 24-hour urine creatinine level should be 15 to 24 mg/kg. In conjunction with a serum creatinine measurement, the urine creatinine determination can also be used to calculate the *creatinine clearance*. Recent reports indicate some progress in developing quantitative estimates of heavy proteinuria with use of a spot urine sample. For now, 24-hour collection remains necessary.

Once significant proteinuria has been established, the evaluation turns to determining whether the patient is asymptomatic or symptomatic and, if asymptomatic, whether the proteinuria is transient or persistent. If the patient is asymptomatic, several urinalyses are performed (as described above). If the proteinuria is found to be transient (especially if orthostatic or exercise-induced), then it is likely to be benign, usually occurring in young adults with no underlying renal disease. Invasive procedures and extensive workup are unnecessary. On the other hand, persistent asymptomatic proteinuria is associated with a high incidence of renal disease and warrants the same investigation as that performed in patients with symptomatic proteinuria. For such patients, a careful history and physical examination are required, followed by selected laboratory testing.

History and Physical Examination

History should begin by focusing on risk factors for glomerular disease. These include long-standing diabetes, systemic lupus, paraproteinemia, infectious disease (HIV infection, malaria, syphilis, endocarditis), medications (gold, penicillamine, NSAIDs, antibiotics, high-dose angiotensin-converting enzyme inhibitors), hepatitis B, toxin exposure (heavy metals, heroin), allergen exposure (bee sting, serum sickness), and malignancy (lymphoma, Hodgkin's disease, cancer of breast, lung, or colon). Risk factors for tubular disorders also should be sought, including analgesic abuse (especially with phenacetin-containing compounds), heavy metal exposure, family history of proteinuria, and history of pyelonephritis.

Physical Examination begins with a careful blood pressure determination.

Hypertension is a poor prognostic sign, raising the specter of significant renal impairment. The patient is also checked for vasculitic skin changes, other rashes, retinopathy, lymphadenopathy, signs of right-sided heart failure and constrictive physiology, abdominal masses, organomegaly, stool positive for occult blood on guaiac testing, prostatic enlargement, peripheral edema, and joint inflammation.

Laboratory Studies

Several laboratory studies are helpful regardless of etiology:

- The *creatinine clearance* is the best determination of renal function, as it approximates the glomerular filtration rate. A serum creatinine and a 24-hour urine collection for urinary creatinine levels are simultaneously obtained. Random measurements of *blood urea nitrogen* or serum *creatinine* are less accurate than a clearance determination but are useful for following the patient once the creatinine clearance is known.
- The *complete blood cell count* will identify any anemia resulting from severe subacute or chronic renal insufficiency. Anemia is also present at some point in all cases of myeloma.
- The *serum albumin level* is worth monitoring because it correlates inversely with the severity of proteinuria.
- The *protein selectivity index* is useful for diagnosis and therapy in patients with nephrotic syndrome. Proteinuria is considered selective when the urine contains large amounts of proteins of low molecular weight. A high degree of selectiv-

ity in patients with nephrotic syndrome suggests minimal-change disease, which is responsive to corticosteroids (see below).

- Radiographic examination of the *kidneys, ureters, and bladder* can be used to judge kidney size, which may help to elucidate etiology (e.g., small, shrunken kidneys suggest significant chronic bilateral disease). *Renal ultrasonography* may be more accurate and informative, as it can detect cystic disease, mass lesions, and obstruction. *IV pyelography* is indicated when chronic pyelonephritis is under consideration. It also provides an estimate of individual kidney function, based on how well each concentrates and excretes the contrast material. However, when creatinine clearance is reduced by more than 75%, the kidneys may not concentrate the contrast medium sufficiently for visualization. Contrast-induced acute renal failure is a risk in patients with preexisting renal disease, especially those with diabetes or multiple myeloma.

Additional studies may prove useful when based on clinical findings, although they are not always necessary. The patient with long-standing diabetes mellitus accompanied by retinopathy, significant proteinuria, and azotemia is almost certain to have diabetic glomerulosclerosis and requires little additional workup other than exclusion of concurrent urinary tract infection or obstruction. On the other hand, in a young woman with polyarthritis, red cell casts, and heavy proteinuria, the ANA, anti-ds (double-stranded) DNA, and serum C3 and C4 complement levels should be determined. Hepatitis serology and cryoprotein determinations are useful in the patient with a history of jaundice, hepatitis B, or its risk factors. Serum and urine electrophoresis is indicated when myeloma is under consideration (elderly patient with elevated globulins, unexplained anemia). Although occult malignancy is occasionally a possible cause, a search beyond careful breast, lymph node, abdominal, and rectal examination, chest radiography, mammogram, and stool guaiac testing has not been shown to be of sufficient yield to warrant more extensive testing. Extensive testing for all possible causes of proteinuria is unlikely to be of much diagnostic value when the pretest probabilities of the conditions being tested for are low. Such indiscriminate testing is more likely to yield false-positive results (see Chapter 2).

Kidney biopsy deserves consideration when treatable disease remains a possibility but the cause continues to be elusive despite careful and thorough clinical and laboratory evaluations (see below).

INDICATIONS FOR REFERRAL

A referral for consideration of renal biopsy is indicated if the result will have important therapeutic or prognostic implications. Most causes of glomerulonephritis do not respond to therapy; thus, biopsy is of academic interest only. However, at times, it will be clinically impossible to rule out a treatable form of glomerulonephritis, and either a biopsy or an empiric course of therapy may be indicated. The advice of an experienced nephrologist is essential.

Referral is also indicated when a cause (e.g., membranous disease) potentially responsive to immunosuppressive therapy is suspected clinically. Because the morbidity associated with therapy can be high, consultation is indicated for optimal design of the treatment regimen.

PRINCIPLES OF MANAGEMENT
AND PATIENT EDUCATION

Asymptomatic Proteinuria. *Transient proteinuria* is, by and large, benign. Patients should be reassured; therapy is not warranted. Patients with idiopathic and fixed orthostatic forms of proteinuria that occur as isolated findings without other associated abnormalities have been found to have an excellent prognosis in prospective studies with 5 to 20 years of follow-up.

Asymptomatic patients with *persistent isolated proteinuria* can also be followed expectantly. However, they are at greater risk for eventual development of renal impairment and should be carefully followed with annual checks of blood pressure, urine, blood urea nitrogen, and creatinine. Referral to a nephrologist for consideration of renal biopsy and treatment is indicated if the urine sediment becomes abnormal or the blood pressure begins to rise.

Symptomatic Proteinuria/Nephrotic Syndrome. Marked proteinuria associated with systemic diseases such as multiple myeloma, diabetes, or systemic lupus erythematosus is best countered by treating the underlying disease. In addition, *angiotensin-converting enzyme inhibitors* (see Chapter 26) help reduce albumin loss and preserve renal function, presumably by limiting hyperfiltration. The edema of nephrotic syndrome is aggravated by sodium retention, which can be countered by *sodium restriction* and the judicious use of loop and distally acting diuretics. Modest *dietary protein restriction* (approximately 1.0 g/kg daily) may be of benefit in slowing the course of patients with progressive renal disease. Patients for whom protein restriction is prescribed require close nutritional follow-up to ensure adequate nitrogen balance. Onset of hypercholesterolemia is initially treated with a *diet low in saturated fat and cholesterol*, but use of a lipid-lowering agent (e.g., a statin) may be necessary. If severe hypocalcemia or renal failure develops, *1,25-dihydroxyvitamin D* plus *calcium* supplementation can limit onset of secondary hyperparathyroidism (see Chapter 142). Because of an increased risk for infection, all nephrotic patients should receive the *pneumococcal* and *influenza vaccines*.

In idiopathic nephrotic syndrome, therapy also depends on the renal pathology defined by biopsy. Minimal-change disease responds to *corticosteroids* and *immunosuppressive agents*, which can enhance the already favorable rate of remission. Most patients with focal and segmental glomerulosclerosis are resistant to steroid therapy and experience renal insufficiency within 5 years of diagnosis. Some patients with idiopathic membranous nephropathy respond to high-dose, alternate-day corticosteroids with partial or complete remission of proteinuria. However, 40% undergo spontaneous remission, and steroid treatment overall confers no additional improvement in long-term renal survival. Adding an alkylating agent to the steroid regimen does little to improve outcome. Membranoproliferative disease is progressive, ending in renal failure in about 50% of cases. Treatment appears to have little impact on renal survival.

ANNOTATED BIBLIOGRAPHY

Abuelo JG. Proteinuria: diagnostic principles and procedures. Ann Intern Med 1983;98:186. (*A terse review including a detailed discussion of patients with isolated proteinuria.*)

Ahmed Z, Lee J. Asymptomatic urinary abnormalities. Hematuria and proteinuria. Med Clin North Am 1997;81:641. (*Helpful review.*)

Bernard DB. Extrarenal complications of the nephrotic syndrome. Kidney Int 1988;33:1184. (*These include edema, hyperlipidemia, hypercoagulable state, hypocalcemia, and increased susceptibility to infection.*)

Carbone L, D'Agati VD, Cheng J-T, et al. Course and prognosis of human immunodeficiency virus-associated nephropathy. Am J Med 1989;87:389. (*More common in African-Americans and IV drug abusers; rapidly progressive.*)

Cirillo M, Senigalliesi L, Laurenzi M, et al. Microalbuminuria in nondiabetic patients. Relation of blood pressure, body mass index, plasma cholesterol levels, and smoking: the Gubbio Population Study. Arch Intern Med 1998;158:1933. (*These cardiovascular risk factors were associated with microalbuminuria.*)

Falk RJ, Hogan SL, Muller KE, et al. Treatment of progressive membranous glomerulopathy. Ann Intern Med 1992;116:438. (*A randomized trial comparing cyclophosphamide and corticosteroids with corticosteroids alone; no difference found.*)

Ginsberg JM, Chang BS, Matarese RA, et al. Use of single voided samples to estimate quantitative proteinuria. N Engl J Med 1983;309:1543. (*An attempt to identify significant proteinuria from a spot urine sample; those with a protein-to-creatinine ratio above 3.5 were likely to have significant proteinuria.*)

Glassock RJ. Postural (orthostatic) proteinuria: no cause for concern. N Engl J Med 1981;305:639. (*An editorial summarizing the condition and arguing that reassurance and monitoring are all that is necessary.*)

Johnson RJ, Couser WG. Hepatitis B infection and renal disease. Kidney Int 1990;37:663. (*A very useful review of this increasingly appreciated association.*)

Levey AS, Lan S-P, Corwin HL, et al. Progression and remission of renal disease in the Lupus Nephritis Collaborative Study. Ann Intern Med 1992;116:114. (*Prognosis is a function of the initial creatinine level and response to initial therapy.*)

Levey AS, Lau J, Pauker SG, et al. Idiopathic nephrotic syndrome: puncturing the biopsy myth. Ann Intern Med 1987;107:697. (*An alternative strategy suggested—empiric trial of alternate-day steroid therapy in lieu of biopsy.*)

Madaio MP, Harrington JT. The diagnosis of acute glomerulonephritis. N Engl J Med 1983;309:299. (*A useful guide to further evaluation once glomerulonephritis is suspected; role of complement levels addressed.*)

Pegoraro A, Singh A, Bakir AA, et al. Simplified screening for microalbuminuria. Ann Intern Med 1997;127:817. (*A cross-sectional study finding that the combination of sulfosalicylic acid and Chemstrip testing provides a sensitive, low-cost approach to the detection of microalbuminuria.*)

Robinson RR. Orthostatic proteinuria: definition and prognosis. Kidney 1971;4:1. (*Review of pathogenesis and prognosis of orthostatic proteinuria.*)

Robinson RR. Idiopathic proteinuria. Ann Intern Med 1969;71:1019. (*Short review of idiopathic benign proteinuria.*)

Springberg PD, Garrett LE, Thompson AL Jr, et al. Fixed and reproducible orthostatic proteinuria: results of a 20-year follow-up study. Ann Intern Med 1982;97:516. (*Prognosis was excellent, with no renal impairment developing in the vast majority.*)

Yamagata K, Yamagata Y, Kobayashi M, et al. A long-term follow-up study of asymptomatic hematuria and/or proteinuria in adults. Clin Nephrol 1996;45:281. (*Among patients with asymptomatic hematuria, proteinuria developed in 11% during follow-up with a mean duration of 6 years.*)

131
Evaluation of Scrotal Pain, Masses, and Swelling

A mass, generalized enlargement, or acute pain involving the scrotum may be noted by the patient or discovered incidentally on physical examination. Patients with scrotal complaints are often concerned about loss of sexual function and the possibility of cancer. The primary physician needs to be able to recognize torsion and epididymitis promptly and to differentiate benign masses from those suggestive of testicular malignancy, which require referral for urologic evaluation.

PATHOPHYSIOLOGY AND CLINICAL PRESENTATION

Testicular Cancer. Almost all testicular neoplasms are malignant and of germ cell origin. Fortunately, these tumors are uncommon, accounting for fewer than 1% of all deaths from neoplasms in men. However, testicular cancers are the most common malignancy in male patients ages 15 to 35, with an estimated incidence of 3 in 100,000. Incidence is increased in those with an undescended testicle and remains high even if orchiopexy is performed or the testicle is removed; the risk seems to be genetically determined. Peak incidence occurs between ages 20 and 40. In patients over age 60, testicular lymphoma is the most common testicular malignancy.

Typically, the tumor presents as a hard, heavy, firm, nontender testicular mass that does not transilluminate, but sometimes it is smooth or even resilient in nature, so that it is mistaken for a benign lesion even though it blocks transmission of light. Although these lesions are usually painless, about 20% cause some discomfort in the scrotum, and frank pain may be reported and tenderness noted, especially if hemorrhage into the tumor is present. Metastasis to the retroperitoneum may cause vague pain in the back or abdomen. Spread to the chest can lead to dyspnea, cough, or hemoptysis. A palpable left supraclavicular node or epigastric mass may be noted. On occasion, extensive metastasis occurs with little evidence of the primary tumor. The metastatic lesion may be histologically different from the primary lesion. A few of these malignancies produce chorionic gonadotropin or estrogen and are associated with gynecomastia (see Chapter 99).

Nonmalignant Testicular Disease. *Testicular torsion* presents with acute pain and a firm tender mass in a young patient. The intense pain may be associated with nausea and vomiting and may be confused with an abdominal process. The condition is mostly one of adolescent boys and young men. A history of recurrent episodes of testicular pain is often present. The testicle dangles within an abnormally enlarged tunica, likened to the clapper of a bell. An attack can come on during sleep; there need not be a history of antecedent trauma. *Testicular trauma* produces acute testicular pain and swelling similar to that associated with torsion or infection. It does not predispose to cancer. *Mumps orchitis* is usually seen 7 to 10 days after parotitis; most often, it is unilateral and accompanied by fever, swelling, pain, and tenderness. On occasion, parotitis is absent. The condition is more common in adults than in children.

Cystic and Vascular Scrotal Masses. Cystic masses containing fluid or sperm often develop spontaneously. They are slow-growing and usually painless, and they may be large and fluctuant. *Hydroceles* are cystic accumulations of clear or straw-colored fluid within the tunica vaginalis or processus vaginalis. *Epididymal cysts* are common and benign. *Spermatoceles* are intrascrotal cysts containing sperm that derive from the small tubules of the epididymis. The space between the testicle and tunica vaginalis may also fill with fluid secondary to impaired drainage or inflammation.

Varicoceles arise from incompetent venous valves. They occur on the left in 97% of cases because the left spermatic vein empties directly into the renal vein and considerable hydrostatic pressure is transmitted into the scrotum when the valves are incompetent and the patient stands. A right-sided varicocele may occur in the context of venous obstruction or renal carcinoma. Varicoceles have a "bag of worms" appearance and are usually nontender; they decrease in size when the patient is recumbent.

Epididymitis. In men under age 35, epididymitis may occur as a consequence of gonococcal or chlamydial infection. *Ureaplasma* infection has also been implicated. Being a sexually transmitted disease, it may be accompanied by symptoms of urethritis (dysuria, discharge). In older men, the cause is more likely to be prostatitis, recent urinary instrumentation, or a structural lesion. Epididymitis can occur with carcinoma of the testes. Initially, tenderness and swelling are confined to the epididymis, but as the condition progresses, the inflammation may spread to the adjacent testicle, making for a large, ill-defined, tender scrotal mass.

Nontesticular Intrascrotal Malignancies are rare and usually firm, and they do not transilluminate, which differentiates them from benign extratesticular scrotal pathology.

Inguinal Herniation can lead to scrotal enlargement and discomfort as bowel tracks through the inguinal canal and pushes down into the scrotum.

Referred Pain. Extrascrotal sources can cause scrotal pain by stimulating one of the nerves (genitofemoral, iliofemoral, or posterior scrotal) supplying the scrotum. Scrotal examination is unremarkable.

DIFFERENTIAL DIAGNOSIS

The differential diagnosis can be considered in terms of the clinical presentation. A clearly extratesticular, soft scrotal mass that transilluminates may be represent a hydrocele, spermatocele, epididymal cyst, or even generalized edema. A "bag of worms" presentation is characteristic of a varicocele. A tender, inflamed extratesticular mass is likely early epididymitis. Acutely painful testicular swelling may represent epididymitis, orchitis, torsion of the spermatic cord, trauma, or hemorrhage into a testicular cancer. A firm, nontender, testicular nodule that does not transilluminate represents carcinoma until proven otherwise. A malignancy also has to be considered in the setting of a nontransilluminating extratesticular nodule, although benign etiologies are more common.

An extrascrotal source is suggested by pain in the absence of scrotal pathology. Causes include abdominal aortic aneurysm, ureteral colic, retrocecal appendix, retroperitoneal cancer, and prostatitis.

WORKUP

Because testicular cancer and testicular torsion are serious but potentially curable diseases, they are prime, must-not-miss considerations in young men who present with a complaint referable to the scrotum or testicles. Epididymitis is similarly curable and important to recognize because it may represent sexually transmitted disease.

History should include inquiry into the acuteness of symptoms, duration, clinical course, tenderness, recent trauma, urethral discharge, dysuria, fever, inguinal herniation, and concurrent infection (e.g., mumps, gonorrhea, prostatitis). A complaint of scrotal heaviness is common but nonspecific, found in conditions ranging from tumor to hydrocele and epididymitis. The patient's age is worth noting because testicular cancer is a disease of men under the age of 40 and torsion is most common among adolescents and young men. A history of an undescended testicle raises the possibility of testicular cancer. Vague abdominal, back, or chest complaints should not be dismissed because they may herald the onset of metastatic testicular cancer. Recurrent episodes in a young person suggest torsion (see below). Concurrent flank pain, abdominal pain, prostatitis, or known extratesticular cancer suggests an extrascrotal source, especially in the absence of scrotal pathology on physical examination.

Physical Examination. The key elements of the examination are careful palpation of the scrotal contents and transillumination of any palpated mass. One should try to assess whether a lesion is cystic or solid, testicular or nontesticular. During inspection, the examiner should note any erythema, masses, hernias, or varices. To palpate the scrotal contents properly, one stands to the side and uses both hands, one to support the testicle and the other to feel and identify each structure, beginning with the uninvolved side. The head of the epididymis is usually situated above the testis; the body and tail run posteriorly. All are separately palpable from the testis. The normal testicle is freely movable and uniform in consistency. It is checked for abnormalities that may provide clues to disease on the involved side, such as horizontally oriented "bell clapper" mobility in a person at risk for torsion. The scrotal structures are identified and examined for tenderness, warmth, swelling, and nodularity. If a mass or nodule is found, one attempts to determine if it is testicular or extratesticular

and if it feels solid or cystic. The inguinal canal is examined for a hernia.

Transillumination with a penlight in a darkened room is necessary to help determine whether the lesion is cystic or solid. Cystic lesions allow transmission of light in most instances, although a bloody exudate may not. A mass that appears extratesticular and cystic is most likely benign and either a spermatocele, a cyst of the epididymis, or hydrocele. If it is hard, does not transilluminate, or is reported to be steadily growing, tumor must be considered, and urologic evaluation is necessary even if the mass appears to be extratesticular.

In patients suspected of having a testicular tumor, a careful check of the supraclavicular lymph nodes, chest, and abdomen is needed because more than 50% present with metastatic disease. In addition, the breasts are examined for gynecomastia. (Inguinal adenopathy does not suggest testicular cancer because the testicular lymphatics drain into the paraaortic nodes. Scrotal nontesticular lymphatics drain into the inguinal nodes.)

A tender scrotum in the absence of a mass, redness, increased warmth, or swelling should trigger a look for extrascrotal pathology. Careful examination of the abdomen for signs of appendicitis, aneurysm, and inguinal hernia is warranted, as is a check of the prostate and flanks for tenderness.

Laboratory Studies. When a mass is noted or uncertainty persists, *testicular ultrasonography* is helpful in determining whether the lesion is testicular or extratesticular, solid or cystic. Measurement of human chorionic gonadotropin and α-fetoprotein levels is more useful for monitoring testicular cancer than for diagnosis (see Chapter 143), but a marked elevation in either is suggestive. Unfortunately, sensitivity is low; a negative study does not rule out cancer. If metastatic disease is suspected, *chest radiography* and *abdominal computed tomography* are performed as part of the staging process.

A *urinalysis* is helpful for detection of pyuria or bacteriuria in cases suggestive of an infectious process. Semen analysis should be performed only when infertility is a concurrent complaint. A right-sided varicocele or suddenly appearing left-sided varicocele requires further evaluation because of the possibility of venous obstruction or renal carcinoma. In such cases, an *IV pyelogram* or *renal ultrasonography* is indicated.

When extrascrotal pathology is suspected, appropriate direction of the workup is required (see Chapters 58 and 139).

Approach to the Patient with Acute Pain and Swelling. An acutely painful, swollen testicle requires urgent assessment because if torsion of the testes is present, permanent damage may occur if treatment is not initiated within 4 hours of onset. Acute epididymitis and torsion are the two dominant considerations. Hemorrhage into a testicular cancer is a third. In an older man with concurrent prostatitis or a younger one with urethritis (see Chapter 136), epididymitis is the more likely cause of the problem. The presence of a urethral discharge, tender prostate, pyuria, or bacteriuria further supports the diagnosis of epididymitis. A firm, tender mass of acute onset in an afebrile young man with a history of prior episodes must be considered to represent torsion until proven otherwise. The diagnosis is further supported by finding a testicle with a horizontal lie on the uninvolved side. Urgent urologic consultation is necessary to determine whether the scrotum should be explored. Sometimes, it can be difficult to distinguish torsion from acute epididymitis on clinical grounds, and urgent surgical exploration is mandatory.

PATIENT EDUCATION AND INDICATIONS FOR REFERRAL

It has been suggested that teaching testicular self-examination might help shorten or eliminate the delay in presentation common in patients with testicular carcinoma. The patient with a clearly extratesticular, transilluminating scrotal lesion can be reassured that cancer is virtually ruled out and that no further evaluation for cancer is necessary other than a periodic follow-up examination. On the other hand, the person with a solid testicular mass needs prompt referral to the urologist, regardless of whether the mass is tender. Testicular cancer confined to the testicle is almost 100% curable by orchiectomy alone (see Chapter 143).

As noted above, referral to a urologist should be swift in cases of suspected torsion because surgical exploration must not be delayed if a viable testicle is to be preserved. Patients in whom testicular cancer is strongly suspected are also likely to require surgical evaluation, although whenever a testicular malignancy is suspected, exploration should be conducted through an inguinal incision. Transscrotal biopsy may cause spillage of tumor into the scrotum and areas of lymphatic drainage. Any mass that cannot be confidently defined as cystic and separate from the testicle should be subjected to a urologist's examination.

A patient with varicocele should be referred if it does not deflate when he lies down, is painful, or is associated with infertility, although conception is often not achieved after correction of the varicocele (see Chapter 120). Referral to a general surgeon is needed for the patient with a poorly reducible hernia.

Most hydroceles and cystic lesions do not require surgical therapy, but the patient should be instructed to return if the enlargement becomes uncomfortable or interferes with intercourse. The patient should understand that surgery is an option that will not threaten virility or fertility. Patients may want a hydrocele removed for cosmetic reasons or for relief of discomfort. Aspiration of a hydrocele is to be avoided. Patients with inguinal hernias that are at risk of causing bowel strangulation should be advised to have them repaired (see Chapter 67).

A.G.M./A.H.G.

ANNOTATED BIBLIOGRAPHY

Davis BE, Noble MJ, Weigel IW, et al. Analysis and management of chronic testicular pain. J Urol 1990;143:936. (*Very useful discussion.*)

Dilworth JP, Farrow GM, Oesterling JE. Testicular tumors of nongerm cell origin. J Urol 1991;37:399. (*Comprehensive review; 126 references.*)

Doll DC, Weiss B. Malignant lymphoma of the testis. Am J Med 1986;81:515. (*The most common cause of testicular malignancy in men over age 60.*)

Hainsworth JD, Greco FA. Testicular germ cell neoplasms. Am J Med 1983;75:817. (*A comprehensive review of evaluation and therapy; 121 references.*)

Haynes BE, Bessen HA, Haynes VE. The diagnosis of testicular torsion. JAMA 1983;249:2522. (*Emphasizes the importance of early diagnosis.*)

McGee SR. Referred scrotal pain. J Gen Intern Med 1993;8:693. (*Case reports and a review; more common than appreciated.*)

Junnila J, Lassen P. Testicular masses. Am Fam Physician 1998; 57:685. (*Emphasizes "must-not-miss" diagnoses: torsion, epididymitis, acute orchitis, strangulated hernia, and testicular cancer.*)

Krone KD, Carroll BA. Scrotal ultrasound. Radiol Clin North Am 1985;23:121. (*Comprehensive review.*)

Richie JP, Birnholz J, Garnick MB. Ultrasound as a diagnostic adjunct for the evaluation of masses in the scrotum. Surg Gynecol Obstet 1982;154:695. (*Found to be a very useful test in indeterminate cases.*)

Scott RF, Bayliss AP, Calder JF, et al. Indications for ultrasound in the evaluation of the pathological scrotum. Br J Urol 1986;58:178. (*Documents value of ultrasonography in a series of 156 men.*)

Williamson RCN. Death in the scrotum: testicular torsion. N Engl J Med 1977;296;338. (*A succinct discussion of the problem and its clinical diagnosis.*)

Witherington R, Jarrell T. Torsion of the spermatic cord in adults. J Urol 1990;143:62. (*Presentation is usually earlier in life, but adult onset does occur.*)

Zornow DH, Landes RR. Scrotal palpation. Am Fam Physician 1981;23:150. (*Detailed review of the physical examination.*)

132

Medical Evaluation and Management of Erectile Dysfunction

Most normal men have occasional episodes of erectile failure, especially at times of stress, fatigue, or distraction. Only when the rate of failure approaches 25% is it proper to invoke the clinical diagnosis of impotence or erectile dysfunction, defined as the repeated inability to achieve or sustain an erection sufficient to engage in sexual intercourse. The condition is estimated to affect up to 10% of men at any given point in time; prevalence increases among older men. Other forms of male sexual dysfunction, including premature ejaculation, which is more common among younger men, are addressed in Chapter 229.

In recent years, the primary physician has taken a more active role in the evaluation and management of sexual problems, helped by a better understanding of sexual pathophysiology and more open discussions of sexual problems. Men with erectile dysfunction who suspect their problem may have an organic basis (e.g., diabetics, those taking medications, and the elderly) are especially insistent on a medical evaluation before they are willing to consider psychological issues. It is estimated that up to 50% of erectile dysfunction is organic in origin, a number that is bound to increase as the mean age of the population rises. Nonetheless, the workup of erectile dysfunction requires thorough investigation from both medical and psychological perspectives (see Chapter 229), and it often begins with a visit to the primary physician.

Many treatments require subspecialty consultation and intervention, but a substantial number of patients appreciate an opportunity to review possible treatments with their primary physician, which necessitates an understanding of the advantages and limitations of available therapeutic options.

NORMAL AND PATHOLOGIC PHYSIOLOGY AND CLINICAL PRESENTATIONS

A working knowledge of both normal and abnormal erectile function is essential to conducting a proper evaluation.

Normal Physiology

Erection is predominantly a hemodynamic process, mediated by neurogenic, endothelial, endocrinologic, and cortical (psychogenic) influences. It begins when blood flow increases into the large, vascular corpora cavernosa, which comprise much of the penile shaft. Flow varies according to the contractile state of smooth muscle lining the corporal arterioles and sinusoids. In the flaccid state, corporal smooth-muscle tone is high, and arterial flow into the penis is minimal. In addition, venous outflow is facilitated by copious arteriovenous shunts. On sexual stimulation, the smooth muscle relaxes, arterioles dilate, and blood flows in, engorging the corporal sinusoidal spaces. This engorgement and its restriction by the bandlike tunica albuginea compress the venous plexuses and arteriovenous shunts, impairing venous outflow. The net effect is a strong erection in which systemic arterial pressure may be approached. Detumescence occurs when smooth-muscle tone returns, blocking arterial inflow and opening venous channels. *Cyclic guanosine monophosphate (GMP)* is essential to achieving smooth-muscle relaxation in the corpus cavernosum.

Mediators. In the flaccid state, penile vascular smooth-muscle contraction is maintained by sympathetic *α-adrenergic* tone, which results in *norepinephrine* release. The vasodilation of erection can be triggered by *parasympathetic* stimulation, which releases *acetylcholine*, and by *nonautonomic* neurotransmission, which is believed to involve vasoactive intestinal peptide. Vascular endothelial cells contribute to relaxation by releasing *endothelium-derived relaxing factor*, a locally active vasodilator. *Prostaglandins* produced by corporal tissue are also capable of inducing both contraction and relaxation of smooth muscle and may play a regulatory role. *Nitric oxide* is released by cavernous nerves and endothelial cells in response to sexual stimulation. Nitric oxide, in turn, stimulates the formation of *cyclic GMP*, which causes cavernosal smooth-muscle relaxation. Although *androgens* have a clear effect on sexual development, behavior, and libido, their influence on erectile capacity is less well defined. Erection can occur with visual stimuli, even if circulating testosterone levels fall to castration levels. However, nocturnal erections are lost.

Control Centers. Erections may be triggered by psychic (cortical) stimulation or reflexively by tactile stimulation of the genitals. In most instances, both are operable and synergistic. A host of erotic stimuli can elicit cortical and subcortical responses, which are transmitted to the medial anterior hypothalamus, integrated, and projected down into the spinal reflex centers. There they modulate sympathetic and parasympathetic outflow to corporal smooth muscle.

There are two spinal reflex centers. The *sympathetic* reflex center is situated in the *thoracolumbar* region. It controls adrenergic tone and sustains the vasoconstriction of the flaccid state. The *parasympathetic* reflex center occupies the *midsacral* region and effects vasodilation. Tactile stimulation of the genitals produces afferent impulses carried by the internal pudendal nerve, which has synapses in the reflex erectile center (sacral cord segments 2 through 4). From there, efferent impulses pass over the pelvic nerves (nervi erigentes) to the parasympathetic plexuses innervating the corpora cavernosa.

Pathophysiology and Clinical Presentations

Impairment of any element of the erectile apparatus or its control can lead to erectile dysfunction. Included among the major organic causes are injury to the reflex centers in the spinal cord, severance of cortical input, injury to peripheral nerves, diabetes-induced autonomic and endothelial dysfunction, and medication-induced disruption of autonomic function.

Spinal Cord Injury. The location of the injury and its severity determine the degree of sexual dysfunction. Even if the cord is functionally severed, some erectile capacity is likely to be maintained if the thoracic and sacral reflex centers are left intact. Also, less severe injury is associated with a greater likelihood of erection remaining possible. About 60% of paraplegics regain the capacity for penile erection 1 to 24 months after injury. The percentage of erections is higher if the injury is above T-11, lower if below. More than 75% of all persons with cord injuries demonstrate some erectile capacity, but only 25% are able to engage successfully in intercourse. The erection is reflexive in nature, requiring constant penile stimulation to be maintained. Erections are totally abolished when local destruction of spinal segments S-2 to S-4 or their roots is complete. Again, the higher the location of the lesion, the better the chances of a good erection.

Ejaculation is rare when the lower thoracic and upper lumbar segments (approximately to L-3) of the cord are so extensively damaged that the nearby sympathetic components are destroyed. Sexual sensation is abolished with transection anywhere above the sacral level. After tactile stimulation, a paraplegic must look to confirm that reflex erection has occurred. Ejaculation can be documented only by feeling wetness with the fingers. Orgasm can be recognized only by feeling for perineal muscle contractions.

Herniated intervertebral disks and metastatic cancer of the vertebral column, especially between T-10 and L-5, which cause local swelling and destruction of spinal cord tissue, may produce a similar clinical picture.

Surgical Procedures. Erectile dysfunction results from transection of autonomic fibers. In simple prostatectomy, whether transurethral, suprapubic, or retropubic, erectile dysfunction is only occasional and is a function of age, prior potency, extent of surgical dissection, and psychological expectations. However, in up to 80% of patients undergoing simple prostatectomy, regardless of the type of procedure performed, some degree of retrograde ejaculation will develop as a result of surgical destruction of the internal sphincter mechanism at the bladder neck. The surgically destroyed or neurologically incompetent internal sphincter allows retrograde flow of seminal fluid into the bladder, producing a dry emission. Normal ejaculation will not occur under these circumstances because the external sphincter tightens to retain urine. Simple perineal prostatectomy is associated with a much higher incidence of erectile dysfunction because of unavoidable direct dissection of parasympathetic fibers along the posterior capsule.

Open *perineal biopsy* and posterior urethral reconstruction can result in erectile dysfunction; transperineal or transrectal needle biopsy of the prostate does not. *Radical prostate, bladder*, or *colorectal surgery* can produce erectile dysfunction as a result of surgical damage to the pelvic autonomic nerves, notably the nervi erigentes as they course through the perirectal retroperitoneal tissues. Improved understanding of the course of these autonomic fibers has led to revised surgical techniques that spare them and lower the risk for erectile dysfunction. Good results have been achieved in younger patients undergoing radical prostatectomy. After radical *retroperitoneal lymph node dissection* for testicular tumors, ejaculatory failure may develop in young men as a result of bilateral resection of the paraaortic sympathetic ganglia, but erectile dysfunction rarely develops. *Bilateral sympathectomy* of lumbar ganglia at L-1 will inhibit ejaculatory capacity, but not orgasmic sensation, in more than half of cases.

Diabetes Mellitus. Erectile dysfunction may be the presenting symptom and is reported in up to 50% of men with the disease. Parasympathetically mediated smooth-muscle relaxation becomes defective, although sympathetic tone remains normal. Cholinergic transmission in corporal smooth muscle declines because of decreased synthesis of acetylcholine. In addition, endothelium-derived relaxing factor becomes deficient. Occlusive disease of larger vessels plays a much less important role than was previously thought, although the presence of hemodynamically significant atheromatous plaques may slow the onset of erection.

The risk for erectile dysfunction appears to parallel the duration and severity of diabetes. With conventional means of achieving glucose control, the majority of diabetic men experience some degree of erectile dysfunction, with fewer than 10% achieving restoration of normal function. Aggressive control of type I diabetes has effected a marked reduction in the risk for development of autonomic neuropathy. Whether initiating tight control in an already impotent diabetic will restore erectile capacity remains to be determined. The forerunner of erectile dysfunction in the diabetic is most often retrograde ejaculation. The presence of dry orgasm or milky postcoital urine augurs a loss of erectile function within a year.

Other Endocrine Disease. The common denominator of most other endocrinopathies causing erectile dysfunction is decreased libido and a decline in serum testosterone. *Hypogonadism*, whether a result of chromosomal, pituitary, or testicular disorders, involves nondevelopment or regression of the secondary male sex characteristics, along with feeble libido and waning potency. When the cause is testicular failure, gonadotropin levels will be very high; when a pituitary or hypothalamic cause is present, gonadotropin levels will be low. *Hyperprolactinemia* is an important source of pituitary-derived erectile dysfunction. Serum testosterone levels fall as gonadotropins decline, although erectile dysfunction seems more closely related to the degree of prolactin elevation. Reduction in prolactin restores erectile function. Hyperprolactinemia may be idiopathic, the result of a functioning pituitary adenoma, or a consequence of *hypothyroidism* (stimulated by high levels of thyroid-stimulating hormone; see Chapter 100).

Addison's disease tends to lead to loss of libido and erectile dysfunction. *Cushing's syndrome*, except when associated with adrenal carcinoma, impairs libido and potency after an initial period (weeks or months) of marked increase. *Acromegaly* leads to early impairment of potency and premature extinction of function. The decline in function is frequently preceded by a hyperlibidinal period.

Drugs. Although it is a common observation that drugs can interfere with sexual functioning, the precise mechanisms remain incompletely understood. Drug effects are often unpredictable and may vary from patient to patient and with dosage and duration. Most are reversible by reducing or discontinuing the medication.

Antihypertensives are frequently to blame (see Chapter 26), with methyldopa, clonidine, β-blockers, reserpine, and diuretics leading the list. Most of these are centrally acting agents, which are believed to interfere with neurotransmitter activity. Erectile dysfunction has also been observed in patients taking antihypertensives with peripheral activity (e.g., hydralazine, thiazides, prazosin). On theoretical grounds, one might expect peripheral vasodilators and α-blockers to facilitate trabecular smooth-muscle relaxation, but clinically these antihypertensives are more likely to be the cause rather than the cure. However, agents with peripheral α-agonist activity (e.g., clonidine) can worsen erectile dysfunction by increasing trabecular smooth-muscle tone. In patients with underlying vascular insufficiency, antihypertensives may contribute to erectile dysfunction by lowering perfusion pressure. Ganglionic blockers may inhibit parasympathetic activity from the sacral segments of the cord or sympathetic activity from the sympathetic chain. Although most antihypertensives have been implicated, the calcium channel blockers and angiotensin-converting enzyme inhibitors appear to interfere least with sexual function.

Psychotropic agents may also be responsible for unpredictable forms of sexual dysfunction. The *phenothiazines* suppress central sympathetic activity. They are capable of producing such side effects as decreased libido, impaired ejaculation, erectile dysfunction, and retrograde ejaculation. The anticholinergic effects of *tricyclic antidepressants* may interfere with erection, although sexual function often improves after drug treatment of depression (see Chapter 227). The serotonin reuptake inhibitors *fluoxetine* and *sertraline* have also been found to impair sexual functioning. Large doses of alcohol can acutely depress the sexual reflexes to the point of abolishing them. Chronic alcoholism leads to nerve damage, liver failure, and high levels of circulating estrogens (see Chapter 71). *Exogenous estrogen* therapy may have a similar effect of diminishing the libido.

Drug abuse involving barbiturates, heroin, morphine, or methadone can result in major disturbances of sexual potency. Most cases are reversible. Marijuana, amyl nitrite, hashish, and lysergic acid diethylamide may heighten the perception of the sexual experience but do not specifically increase or decrease potency. Amphetamines, in moderate users, may increase libido and delay orgasm, thus prolonging the sexual act; however, erectile dysfunction often occurs with long-term, heavy use. Cocaine increases both male and female sexual excitability, but side reactions, including a flight of ideas, may interfere with sustained sexual performance. Episodes of painful priapism may develop in chronic abusers.

Prostatic Disease. Erectile dysfunction may be the first symptom of *prostate cancer*. Advancing centrifugal growth of neoplastic tissue in the posterior lobe of the prostate may induce local swelling and destruction of the parasympathetic fibers that run along the posterolateral aspect of the prostate. *Prostatitis* may cause painful ejaculations and even hematospermia. Premature ejaculation and postcoital fatigue occur, but erectile dysfunction is not characteristic. *Benign prostatic hypertrophy* does not interfere with sexual functioning.

Compulsive vesiculoprostatitis represents a chronic congestive syndrome. It occurs in the context of habitual self-inhibited masturbation, lifelong limitation of sexual activities, chronic coitus interruptus with a sexually inert partner, or habitually hastened intercourse fraught with anxiety related to threatened interruptions. The onset is gradual and progressive weakening of erectile strength may occur, although complete erectile dysfunction is not a primary feature. Other symptoms of this psychosomatic syndrome may include sacroiliac ache, irritating sensations in the glans penis, urinary urgency and frequency, minor weakness of the urinary stream, overflow prostatorrhea (especially after straining), and sometimes hematospermia.

Injury to the Penis or Urethra. *Pelvic fracture*, resulting from a crash injury in which the posterior urethra is ruptured, causes erectile dysfunction in 25% to 30% of cases. Nonperformance may result from painful intromission associated with *Peyronie's disease, balanitis,* acute *gonorrhea, herpes genitalis,* or *phimosis.* Hypospadias with a chordee of the shaft can preclude intercourse. With *priapism,* erection may be only partial and insufficient for intercourse because irreversible fibrosis of the corpora cavernosa has occurred. A large hernia or hydrocele may mechanically interfere with coitus, although potency should remain intact.

Vascular Disease. *Arterial insufficiency* is usually listed as a leading cause of erectile dysfunction in older men. Unexplained, progressive slowing of erection followed by decreased rigidity can be among the first symptoms of aortoiliac vascular disease when plaque obstructs the iliac arteries immediately distal to the aortic bifurcation. Erectile dysfunction develops in almost 40% of men with stenosis and nearly 75% of those with occlusion. Symptoms of claudication in association with erec-

tile dysfunction, aortic or femoral bruits, and diminished peripheral pulses describe Leriche's syndrome. In some cases, the patient has the ability to initiate an erection but cannot maintain it. Patients with hypertension, diabetes, and hypercholesterolemia, or who smoke, are at increased risk for compromise of penile perfusion by atheromatous disease. Radiation therapy and pelvic trauma are other risk factors for vascular injury.

Venous dysfunction can be equally important and result from age- or lipid-induced loss of venous fibroelastic compressibility. Several authorities argue that venous dysfunction may be more important than previously suspected.

Psychogenic Conditions. Anxiety and depression are potent precipitants of erectile dysfunction. The marked sympathetic outflow that accompanies anxiety increases α-adrenergic tone and impedes trabecular smooth-muscle relaxation. In addition, cortical influences may inhibit sacral cord reflexes that would normally trigger erection by way of parasympathetic stimulation (see Chapter 229).

Zinc Deficiency has been touted in the lay literature as a possible cause of erectile dysfunction, with health food stores promoting zinc preparations. Although zinc replacement has benefited dialysis patients with erectile dysfunction, the frequency of such severe zinc deficiency in most other patients is probably very low. More study of the issue is needed, especially in patients taking diuretics, which may lower zinc concentrations.

DIFFERENTIAL DIAGNOSIS

In a review of 165 men with sexual dysfunction seen at the Cleveland Clinic, 51% were found to have functional disorders, 47% had organic disorders, and 2% had incomplete evaluations. The incidence of sexual dysfunction peaked between the ages of 50 and 59. Among patients with organic sexual dysfunction, diabetes mellitus accounted for 41.5% of cases. In 16.8%, sexual dysfunction was caused by vascular insufficiency. Those with Peyronie's disease (15.5%) could not penetrate because of marked chordee or an inability to achieve sufficient erection. In 12.9%, hypogonadism, resulting from low levels of serum testosterone, was a factor. In 10.3%, erectile dysfunction followed a variety of surgical procedures. Sexual dysfunction secondary to various neurologic diseases occurred in 9%.

The Cleveland Clinic data represent the experience of a referral practice. Reports from primary care practices reveal a higher frequency of medications and alcohol as causes of sexual dysfunction, but not a substantially greater prevalence of psychological disease.

The widespread use of drugs affecting the autonomic nervous system makes pharmacologic agents an epidemiologically important source of erectile dysfunction and ejaculatory disturbances. Table 132.1 provides a listing of some of the more important causes of secondary erectile dysfunction and ejaculatory disturbances.

In many patients, especially the elderly, sexual dysfunction is multifactorial in origin. Both psychological and organic factors are often present, and in many instances, more than one medical condition is involved.

Table 132.1. Important Organic Causes of Secondary Sexual Dysfunction

CAUSE	EFFECT		
	DECREASED LIBIDO	IMPOTENCE	EJACULATORY FAILURE
Drugs			
Alcohol	+	+	+
Amphetamines		+	
Antidepressants		+	
Antihypertensive agents (methyldopa, clonidine, β-blockers, diuretics, reserpine)		+	
Barbiturates		+	
Cocaine		Priapism with chronic abuse	
Guanethidine	+		+ (Retrograde)
H₂-blockers (cimetidine)	+	+	
Methadone		+	
Phenothiazines	+	+	+
Cord Lesions			
Well above T-11	Sensation abolished		+/−
Below T-11	Sensation abolished	+	+
Peripheral Autonomic Neuropathy			
Diabetes		+	+ (Retrograde)
Surgical Procedure			
Simple prostatectomy (all approaches)		Occasional	+ (Retrograde)
Perineal prostatectomy		+	
Open perineal biopsy		+	
Radical prostatectomy, bladder or rectal surgery		+	
Radical retroperitoneal node dissection			+
Bilateral sympathectomy			+
Prostatic Disease			
Benign prostatic hypertrophy		No effect on function	
Cancer of the prostate		+	
Vesiculoprostatitis		+/−	
Prostatitis			Painful
Penile and Urethral Lesions			
Pelvic fractures		+	+
Hypospadias			+
Priapism			+
Phimosis, herpes, balanitis		Painful intromission	
Peyronie's disease		Painful intromission	
Hernia or hydrocele		Interferes with coitus	
Endocrine–Metabolic Disease			
Addison's disease	+	+	
Cushing's syndrome	+	+	
Hypothyroidism	+	+/−	
Acromegaly		+	
Hypogonadism	+	+	
Hyperprolactinemia		+	
Zinc deficiency (severe, in dialysis patients)		+	
Vascular Disease			
Aortoiliac insufficiency		+	
Venous disease		+	

H₂, histamine₂.

WORKUP

Advances in the pathophysiologic understanding of erectile dysfunction have yielded an array of new diagnostic methods, many of which require referral to a specialized laboratory to be performed properly. Nonetheless, history and physical examination remain an integral part of proper diagnosis. Obtaining a description of what the patient means by "impotence" is the first task and is best carried out by taking a detailed sexual history. It is essential to establish that erectile function is significantly compromised before an extensive workup is undertaken. Once the presence of erectile dysfunction has been confirmed, the evaluation shifts to differentiating psychogenic from organic disease. If psychogenic disease is deemed likely, the evaluation concentrates on underlying causes (see Chapter 229).

If organic disease is more probable, then the search begins for historical and physical findings suggestive of an underlying precipitant.

History

Differentiating Organic from Psychogenic Disease. The onset of the condition, its clinical course, and its effect on morning erections help differentiate psychogenic from organic mechanisms. A sudden onset and the preservation of erections on awakening or masturbation are characteristic features of psychogenic disease. A gradual onset and the progressive loss in duration and strength of morning erections and erections associated with masturbation and coitus suggest organic disease. These distinctions are not absolute. For example, depression may be associated with a temporary loss of morning erections, mimicking organic disease. Inquiry into libido is also important. A decrease in the context of erectile dysfunction raises the possibility of endocrinopathy in addition to psychogenic disease.

Because an intact nervous system, blood supply, and sexual apparatus are necessary to achieve an erection, any occurrence of erection and ejaculation, even if rare, suggests that the problem may be emotional rather than organic. However, it is important to recognize that in the early phases of organically determined erectile dysfunction, many patients retain some erectile function and are more likely to report a decrease in number of erections, rapid detumescence after penetration, or inability to obtain a sufficiently hard erection for intercourse. Further confusing the issue, early organic disease almost always triggers performance anxiety. Finally, the absence of an erection does not rule out a psychogenic cause, but usually one is able to elicit from patients with a psychogenic etiology a story of an occasional erection (particularly on awakening from sleep).

Inquiry into Medical Etiologies. Of primary importance is checking for symptoms of diabetes (see Chapter 102), alcohol abuse (see Chapter 228), and aortoiliac disease (see Chapter 23). As noted above, unexplained, progressive slowing of erection followed by decreased rigidity may be the presenting manifestation of aortoiliac insufficiency. Atherosclerotic risk factors (hypertension, smoking, diabetes, hyperlipidemia) should be noted. All medications are reviewed, especially antihypertensives, major tranquilizers, antidepressants, other drugs with anticholinergic activity, and histamine₂ blockers with antiandrogenic effects (e.g., cimetidine). Careful inquiry into substance abuse is also indicated (see Chapter 235). If libido is reduced, it is worth checking for symptoms of thyroid disease (see Chapters 103 and 104), hyperprolactinemia (see Chapter 100), hypogonadism (see Chapter 120), and adrenal disease. Past medical history is reviewed for radical prostate or pelvic surgery, pelvic irradiation, spinal cord injury, multiple sclerosis, cancer, and pelvic fracture.

Physical Examination

The vital signs are checked for postural fall in blood pressure (indicative of autonomic or adrenal insufficiency), the general appearance for loss of secondary sexual characteristics, and the skin for spider angiomata, palmar erythema, excessive dryness, hyperpigmentation, and other dermatologic signs of endocrinopathy. The neck is noted for goiter.

The flaccid penis ought to be inspected for tumor, inflammation, discharge, phimosis of the foreskin, and the hard plaques of Peyronie's disease along the dorsolateral aspect of the shaft. If possible, assessment of the erect penis should be attempted, especially if disease of the shaft is suspected, so that precise information on the degree of chordee or erectile weakness can be obtained. Testicles and prostate are checked for size, masses, nodules, and tenderness. Small, soft testes suggest hypogonadism. Intrascrotal pathology such as varicocele, hydrocele, or inguinal hernia may mechanically interfere with performance and can be readily detected by a careful examination (see Chapter 131).

The aorta and femoral arteries need to be palpated and auscultated for bruits and other signs of occlusive disease, especially if the patient has a history of claudication (see Chapter 23). Any femoral bruits are noted. The spine is checked for focal tenderness and evidence of cord compression (see Chapter 147). Neurologic assessment includes testing for pain sensation in the genital and perianal areas and checking the bulbocavernosus reflex to determine the integrity of second, third, and fourth sacral segments of the spinal cord. This reflex is achieved when the anal sphincter contracts around the examining finger as the glans is squeezed. A positive response indicates that S-2, S-3, and S-4 are intact. Other aspects of neurologic function also deserve thorough testing. Evidence of a cortical, brainstem, spinal cord, or peripheral deficit may be an important clue to etiology.

Laboratory Studies

Ordering a routine battery of "impotence" tests is rarely cost-effective. Moreover, no single test or set of tests "rules out" organic disease. The best approach is to tailor the laboratory workup to match the patient's clinical presentation.

Chemistries. A 2-hour postprandial serum *glucose* determination is indicated when diabetes is suspected (see Chapter 93). Hypothyroidism is best confirmed by an elevated *thyroid-stimulating hormone* level. Measurement of serum total *testosterone* and *luteinizing hormone* is indicated when reduced libido accompanies erectile dysfunction. Pooled samples of each (obtained 30 to 60 minutes apart) are necessary to avoid a sampling error from the large oscillations in serum concentration that can occur every few hours. A consistently low testosterone level confirms hypogonadism. Luteinizing hormone and *prolactin* levels help differentiate pituitary etiologies from primary gonadal failure (see Chapter 120). Abnormally high concentrations of total testosterone are seen with hyperthyroidism and represent an indication for testing of thyroid-stimulating hormone. If evidence of peripheral vascular disease is present, a *cholesterol* profile can help guide therapy (see Chapter 27). The usefulness of a serum *zinc* determination is still unproven, except perhaps in dialysis patients. The literature should be followed to see if more widespread measurement has physiologic meaning and therapeutic implications.

Study of Nocturnal Penile Tumescence. Tumescence study serves to confirm loss of erectile function in the patient who reports a total absence of erections, including those normally experienced on awakening from sleep. The physiologic basis for testing at night is the observation that 80% to 95% of young men experience erections during rapid eye movement (REM) sleep. Although the percentage falls with age, nocturnal monitoring represents the most sensitive available means of testing for intactness of the erectile apparatus. The absence of nocturnal tumescence indicates advanced organic disease and remains the "gold standard" for detecting organic erectile dysfunction. However, in early organic disease, some erectile function and morning episodes may persist. Thus, demonstration of tumescence does not negate the need for further medical evaluation.

Formal tumescence study is very expensive and is performed overnight in a special sleep laboratory that monitors the electroencephalogram and eye movements in addition to measures of penile tumescence. The *"postage stamp test"* is a much simpler, inexpensive method of screening for nocturnal tumescence. The patient is instructed to wrap a ring of postage stamps snugly around the flaccid penis at night before going to bed, and to moisten the overlapping stamps to seal the ring. A positive test result is breakage along the perforations on awakening in the morning. Because sleep is not monitored, a single negative test result does not rule out the capacity for nocturnal tumescence. Continued failure on repeated testing is more suggestive. Other devices for home monitoring have been developed, including plastic wires that break at different tensile strengths and a tumescence scanning device (Rigiscan) that entails wearing two rings for three nights.

Other Studies. Most other studies are the province of the specialist in male erectile dysfunction and should be ordered only on the basis of a consultation. A few are worth mentioning because of their popularity. The vascular apparatus can be assessed by *Doppler ultrasonography*, both in the flaccid state and, more meaningfully, after an *intracavernosal injection* of a vascular smooth-muscle relaxant. Color flow technology provides excellent images. Papaverine alone or in combination with the α-blocker phentolamine can be used for the intracavernosal injection. Inability to achieve a full erection within 5 to 10 minutes of injection or an erection that is only partial or lasts less than 1 hour strongly suggests vascular disease. However, the very anxious patient with a normal vasculature may have a false-positive result. One study suggests an increased specificity with a second injection because the patient is less anxious about the diagnostic procedure itself.

Patients in whom sacral neurologic injury is suspected clinically can be objectively tested by measuring the *sacral nerve reflex latency time*. One applies an electrical stimulus to the penile shaft and measures the time it takes for the bulbocavernosal muscles to contract. A time in excess of 35 ms is strongly suggestive of pathology in the nerves comprising the sacral reflex arc.

SYMPTOMATIC MANAGEMENT AND PATIENT EDUCATION

Psychological Support. The deeply upsetting nature of erectile dysfunction necessitates an empathic, understanding, and thorough approach to the problem. Education is essential to help the patient comprehend and cope with the condition. Reviewing the mechanism of erection and how it is impaired can be very useful in providing a rational basis for diagnosis, prognosis, and treatment. These informational and supportive needs are no less intense for the elderly, many of whom derive considerable self-esteem from maintaining their ability to engage in intercourse. The loss can be very demoralizing.

Most patients with organic etiologies acquire performance anxieties when their ability to engage in sexual intercourse becomes impaired. The onset of anxiety can result in full loss of function in a patient who is only partially compromised physiologically. In such instances, patient and partner should come in for supportive counseling, both to remove blame and inappropriately exclusive psychological attributions and to educate about prognosis and available therapy. Fortunately, many options for treatment are available.

Adjustment of Medication Program. Patients taking an antihypertensive medication implicated in erectile dysfunction might benefit from a trial of dose reduction, or from switching to an angiotensin-converting enzyme inhibitor (e.g., captopril), a calcium channel blocker (e.g., nifedipine), or a relatively selective β-blocking agent (e.g., atenolol) (see Chapter 26). The patient experiencing erectile dysfunction and loss of libido with use of cimetidine can be switched to ranitidine, which is similar in efficacy but has no antiandrogen effect. The depressed patient whose erectile dysfunction is clearly related to drug therapy can be tried on a tricyclic antidepressant with less anticholinergic activity (e.g., nortriptyline, desipramine), but switching to a serotonin reuptake inhibitor (e.g., sertraline, fluoxetine) may not help because they too can impair sexual functioning. The psychotic patient with sexual dysfunction believed linked to the medication program should be referred to the psychiatrist for adjustment of the drug regimen.

Sildenafil (Viagra). Effective oral therapy for erectile dysfunction of most causes is now available with the advent of sildenafil (Viagra). The drug selectively inhibits the enzyme that metabolizes cyclic GMP, a mediator of smooth-muscle relaxation in the corpus cavernosum. So long as some sexual arousal occurs that results in nitric oxide-induced production of cyclic GMP, erectile function will improve with sildenafil use. In the absence of arousal, sildenafil will not induce or sustain an erection, nor is it effective when marked vascular insufficiency limits the inflow of blood or when cavernosal fibrosis is present. Preliminary data also indicate that sildenafil is not effective among men who have undergone radical prostatectomy for prostate cancer unless bilateral sparing of the neurovascular bundles has been possible. However, for almost all other forms of erectile dysfunction, including those of psychogenic and mixed causes, it can be helpful. At maximum doses, a 100% improvement in erectile function is noted among responders in comparison with baseline, with successful sexual intercourse achieved in more than two thirds of attempts. Although the drug has no effect on sexual desire, some improvement in orgasmic function occurs. Sildenafil is taken 1 hour before planned intercourse, the time to maximum serum levels. The minimum dose is 25 mg, and the maximum is 100 mg. No more than one dose per day is recommended.

The cost is very high, averaging well over $10 per dose.

It is important to inform patients that the drug has no effect on sexual desire and that it works only in the context of sexual arousal. Although sildenafil works for a wide range of etiologies, a thorough work-up for the cause of erectile dysfunction should always be conducted to identify serious underlying organic and/or psychogenic illness that requires attention in its own right.

Adverse effects are transient and include *flushing, headache, visual disturbances* (alterations in hue or brightness)*, and dyspepsia.* Priapism has not been reported. The drug does cause some vasodilation, and several reported deaths of men taking sildenafil have been associated with significant *hypotension,* which occurs when the drug is given concomitantly with agents that lower blood pressure, especially nitrates used in the treatment of ischemic heart disease. Sildenafil should not be prescribed for patients taking nitrates because of the risk for nitrate potentiation resulting in severe hypotension. Subgroup analyses of men with erectile dysfunction and ischemic heart disease who are not taking nitrates suggest that sildenafil is effective and safe. However, the ability to engage in sexual intercourse safely and a lack of hypotension during exercise and drug use should be established before the drug is prescribed. The lowest dose (25 mg) should always be prescribed initially.

Intracavernosal Injection Therapy. Local intracavernosal injection of smooth-muscle relaxants and α-adrenergic blockers has been effective in a wide variety of patients. Diabetics, patients with neurologic injury, those with psychogenic erectile dysfunction, and even some with vascular insufficiency have regained their ability to engage in successful sexual intercourse with intracavernosal injection therapy, a substantial advance for many patients. Follow-up of men introduced to penile injection therapy indicate that more than 70% are sufficiently satisfied to continue treatment. Of those who stop, most do so because of cost; fewer than one in seven who stop do so because of ineffectiveness.

Among the agents used for intracavernosal therapy are *papaverine*, which directly relaxes trabecular smooth muscle; *phentolamine*, a short-acting, α-adrenergic blocker that increases arterial inflow; and most recently, *alprostadil* (an aqueous preparation of prostaglandin E_1) that both relaxes smooth muscle and causes vasodilation. Within 10 to 15 minutes of injection in responding patients, an erection develops and lasts for up to 1 hour. Patients with neurologic disease and psychogenic erectile dysfunction respond most readily and require the smallest doses of medication. Underlying vascular disease is less responsive and necessitates larger doses.

Alprostadil, the only agent approved by the Food and Drug Administration for the intracavernosal treatment of erectile dysfunction, is highly effective. Ninety-four percent of men in mixed populations achieved erections in 87% of attempts, with a good average duration of erection (64 minutes). Furthermore, the risk for priapism (0.4% to 1.0%) or fibrosis (2% to 3%) is smaller than with papaverine (see below). Long-term safety remains to be determined, but the risk for fibrosis is small with continuous use of up to 6 months. The most common side effect of alprostadil is pain at the injection site in 20% to 50%, but this is problematic only in about 11% and depends on the preparation used. Combining a modest dose of alprostadil with papaverine provides better results and less pain than papaverine plus phentolamine or larger doses of alprostadil alone. The recommended frequency of use is no more than three times per week and no more than once in 24 hours. Dosage determination requires titration in the office, started at 1.25 to 2.50 μg and increased by 2.5- to 5.0-μg increments.

Patients with psychogenic or neurogenic forms of erectile dysfunction may require as little as 2 μg to achieve an adequate erection. The goal is to identify the least amount of alprostadil necessary to sustain an effective erection for 1 hour. After undergoing titration of dose, patients are set up for self-administration of the therapy at home. Cost is moderate.

Papaverine, used either alone or with phentolamine, achieves response rates of about 50% in mixed populations of impotent men. Duration of erection averages 50 minutes. Adverse effects include pain at the site of injection and a risk for hepatocellular enzyme elevation, priapism, and painless fibrotic nodules. Ischemic injury and scarring of the corporeal tissue may result when erections last longer than 4 hours. Such injury can lead to permanent damage of corporeal tissue and must be treated promptly by intracavernosal injection of an α-agonist (epinephrine, phenylephrine). Penile fibrosis occurs in up to 60% of patients after 1 year of treatment, with some men experiencing sufficient corporeal fibrosis to distort the penile shaft. Alprostadil has replaced papaverine as the drug of first choice for intracavernosal injection, but papaverine appears to be useful as an adjunct in some instances (see above).

Insulin syringes with a very fine (27- to 30-gauge) needle are used for the intracavernosal injection, which is usually placed into the proximal third of the penis in the dorsolateral area of the corpus cavernosum. Unilateral injection suffices because the vessels from each side interconnect. Sides are alternated. Erection usually ensues within 10 minutes of injection and lasts 30 to 60 minutes. Side effects are most common during the titration period, when excessive duration of erection and hypotension occur from doses that are too large. Patients with cardiovascular compromise may be suboptimal candidates for this therapy.

The optimal candidate for intracavernosal injection is one with an intact vascular apparatus and the intelligence and dexterity to self-inject properly. However, even those with concurrent vascular disease may benefit, although higher doses may be required, which increases the risk for side effects and complications. Diabetics have especially benefited because the treatment directly addresses their underlying pathophysiology.

Penile Implants and Other Mechanical Devices. More than 30,000 prostheses are implanted annually in the United States. A prosthesis is a consideration for the patient with refractory erectile dysfunction who expresses a serious need to regain his capacity to engage in coitus. Of the three types of prostheses available, the simpler ones (the semirigid and adjustable malleable types) have proved the most satisfactory. They are least likely to fail and have the fewest complications associated with their implantation and use. Although they might seem the most "natural," the inflatable prostheses have much higher breakdown and complication rates, so that surgical revision is often necessary. Reoperation rates range as high as 44%. The reservoir tends to leak, and infection is a risk on the order of 1% to 10%.

Overall, patient and partner satisfaction with prostheses is in the range of 80% to 90%, with little difference reported among users of the various types. Careful counseling is required before implant surgery is elected. If the cause of erectile dysfunction is a poor interpersonal relationship, then a prosthesis is going to have little effect.

A *vacuum suction device* has been advocated, especially in the elderly. A plastic cylinder is placed over the flaccid penis and connected to a hand-operated vacuum pump. The negative pressure in the cylinder facilitates passive blood flow into the penis. A band is placed at the base of the penis to retard venous outflow, and the cylinder is removed. The device works best in patients who respond to penile injection therapy and is an alternative to such therapy. Pain, ecchymoses, and difficulty ejaculating are experienced by about 10%. Coitus is successfully achieved in about 80% after 3 months of use.

Vascular Surgery. Patients with vascular insufficiency have yet to achieve consistently successful results after reconstructive surgery. Correction of aortoiliac disease often meets with disappointing results because of the high frequency of coexisting disease in distal vessels. Microsurgical techniques have been employed to correct vascular disease within the penis. Success rates range from 20% to 80%. The best results are obtained in young men with traumatic vascular injury; the worst results are in older men with diffuse atherosclerotic involvement of the cavernosal artery.

Hormone Therapy. *Testosterone* therapy should be reserved for patients with hypogonadism, manifested by a low serum testosterone level, and testosterone should not be used as an all-purpose sexual stimulant. It has little effect in impotent patients with normal testosterone concentrations (although it may add to frustration by increasing their libido). In such patients, particularly the elderly, the use of testosterone is associated with a high incidence of adverse effects, including sodium retention, prostatic enlargement, gynecomastia (from peripheral conversion to estrogens), and polycythemia. Patients with concurrent adenocarcinoma of the prostate may experience a serious flare of their testosterone-responsive disease.

Treatment is given every 3 to 4 weeks by IM injection of a long-acting preparation. A period of trial and error to find the optimal dose requires patience on the part of both physician and patient. Oral preparations are rapidly inactivated. A transdermal delivery system is under development.

Patients with hyperprolactinemia-induced hypogonadism may not respond to testosterone replacement therapy because of the androgen-antagonizing effect of prolactin. Consequently, treatment of the underlying hyperprolactinemia is necessary to restore potency.

Yohimbine is an α-blocker touted as a medical treatment for erectile dysfunction. In a double-blind, randomized study of the drug in patients with organic erectile dysfunction, it was found ineffective. However, it did prove helpful in a similarly designed study of patients with psychological erectile dysfunction, probably because of their high level of anxiety and sympathetic tone.

Treatment of Underlying Urologic Disease. At least temporary relief from the acute discomfort of prostatosis ensues from repeated prostatic massage (see Chapter 138). Selected patients with Peyronie's disease are candidates for plaque resection and replacement with a dermal skin graft. The ability to perform sexually may return after removal of a large hydrocele or repair of an inguinal hernia. Patients recovering from routine simple prostatectomy (either transurethral or suprapubic) can be reassured that potency and ability to engage in coitus are likely to return within 4 to 8 weeks after surgery.

INDICATIONS FOR REFERRAL

Patients with urologic disease should have a urologic consultation to see if they are candidates for surgical correction. Diabetics and impotent patients with otherwise refractory disease who have a relatively well-preserved penile vascular apparatus are reasonable candidates for referral to consider intracavernous injection therapy if they have failed sildenafil. Even those with a degree of vascular insufficiency may be candidates. The risks and benefits of prosthetic surgery can also be reviewed at the same time. Referral is best made to a urologist experienced in the treatment of erectile dysfunction. Patients found to have symptomatic aortoiliac disease require evaluation by a vascular surgeon (see Chapter 34). Endocrinologic advice is indicated for patients with elevated prolactin levels, primary hypogonadism (low levels of testosterone, high levels of luteinizing hormone), or evidence of pituitary–hypothalamic disease (low concentrations of luteinizing hormone). Patients suspected of harboring a cord lesion need urgent neurologic consultation.

Psychiatric referral is essential when depression, anxiety disorder, or interpersonal conflict appears to be an etiologic factor in a case of erectile dysfunction. However, premature referral to a psychiatrist before an appropriate medical evaluation has been completed should be avoided because of the risk for inappropriately labeling the condition as purely psychological and alienating the patient. Referral may also be useful when the patient with organic disease fails to respond to supportive psychotherapy offered by the primary physician (see Chapter 229).

A.G.M./A.H.G.

ANNOTATED BIBLIOGRAPHY

Broderick GA, Allen GA, McClure RD. Vacuum tumescence devices: the role of papaverine in the selection of patients. J Urol 1990;145:284. (*A 94% positive predictive value.*)

Cappeleri JC, Rosen RC, Smith MD, et al. Diagnostic evaluation of the erectile function domain of the International Index of Erectile Function. Urology 1999;54:346. (*This index appears to be useful in the clinical setting and for research.*)

Carter JN, Tyson JE, Tolis G, et al. Prolactin-secreting tumors and hypogonadism in 22 men. N Engl J Med 1978;299:847. (*An important report on the association of hyperprolactinemia and erectile dysfunction.*)

Conti CR, Pepine CJ, Sweeney M. Efficacy and safety of sildenafil in the treatment of erectile dysfunction in patients with ischemic heart disease. Am J Cardiol 1999;83:29C. (*Effective and safe in patients with erectile dysfunction and ischemic heart disease who are not taking nitrate therapy.*)

Fischer C, Gross J, Zuch J. Cycle of penile erection synchronous with dreaming (REM) sleep. Arch Gen Psychiatry 1965;12:29. (*The classic report describing the association between rapid eye movement [REM] sleep and nocturnal erections.*)

Frosch WA. Psychogenic causes of impotence. Med Asp Hum Sex 1978;12:57. (*Differentiates psychogenic from organic causes by history.*)

Goldstein I, Lue TF, Padma-Nathan H, et al. Oral sildenafil in the treatment of erectile dysfunction. N Engl J Med 1998;338:1397. (*A placebo-controlled, dose–response study of 329 men who had erectile dysfunction with a wide variety of causes; a 100% improvement in function was found with the highest dose, and side effects were minimal during 32 weeks of use.*)

Jarow JP, Burnett AL, Geringer AM. Clinical efficacy of sildenafil citrate based on etiology and response to prior treatment. J Urol

1999;162:722. (*Best predictors of satisfaction were baseline function and etiology.*)

Kedia S, Zippe CD, Agarwal A, et al. Treatment of erectile dysfunction with sildenafil citrate after radiation therapy for prostate cancer. Urology 1999;54:308. (*Positive response for 71%.*)

Kessler WO. Nocturnal penile tumescence. Urol Clin North Am 1988;15:1. (*A discussion of available tests.*)

Krane RJ, Goldstein I, Saenz de Tejada I. Impotence. N Engl J Med 1989;321:1648. (*Excellent review, with emphasis on pathophysiology; 150 references.*)

Linet OI, Ogrinc FG, for the Alprostadil Study Group. Efficacy and safety of intracavernosal alprostadil in men with erectile dysfunction. N Engl J Med 1996;334:873.

Mahajan SK, Abbasi AA, Prasil AS, et al. Effect of oral zinc therapy on gonadal function in hemodialysis patients. Ann Intern Med 1982;63:357. (*One of the few well-documented instances of zinc therapy proving effective.*)

Merrick GS, Butler WM, Lief JH, et al. Efficacy of sildenafil citrate in prostate brachytherapy patients with erectile dysfunction. Urology 1999;53:1112. (*Favorable response in 80%.*)

Morales A, Condra MS, Owen JA, et al. Is yohimbine effective in the treatment of organic impotence? Results of a controlled trial. J Urol 1987;137:1168. (*The answer is no for organic disease but yes for psychogenic disease.*)

Mulhall JP, Jahoda AE, Cairney M, et al. The causes of patient dropout from penile self-injection therapy for impotence. J Urol 1999; 162:1291. (*Attrition rate was 31%; the most common reason was cost, and only one in seven who quit did so because of lack of effectiveness.*)

Mulligan T, Katz PG. Erectile failure in the aged: evaluation and treatment. J Am Geriatr Soc 1988;36:837. (*Causes examined; use of vacuum pump suggested.*)

NIH Consensus Conference. NIH Consensus Development Panel on Impotence. JAMA 1993;270:83. (*Addresses impact, diagnosis, treatment modalities, and education.*)

Rendell MS, Rajfer J, Wicker PA, et al. Sildenafil for treatment of erectile dysfunction in men with diabetes: a randomized controlled trial. JAMA 1999;281:421. (*At 12 weeks, 56% of sildenafil patients had improved, in comparison with 10% of those on placebo.*)

Saenz de Tejada I, Goldstein I, Asadzoi K, et al. Impaired neurogenic and endothelium-mediated relaxation of penile smooth muscle from diabetic men with impotence. N Engl J Med 1989;320:1025. (*Mechanisms of diabetic erectile dysfunction delineated; provides basis for use of intracavernosal smooth-muscle relaxant.*)

Zelefsy MJ, McKee AB, Lee H, et al. Efficacy of oral sildenafil in patients with erectile dysfunction after radiotherapy for carcinoma of the prostate. Urology 1999;53:775. (*Significant improvement in 74%.*)

Zippe CD, Kedia AW, Kedia K, et al. Treatment of erectile dysfunction after radical prostatectomy with sildenafil citrate. Urology 1999;52:963. (*Of those who had undergone bilateral nerve-sparing procedures, 80% responded. Those who had undergone unilateral or non–nerve-sparing procedures did not respond.*)

133
Approach to Dysuria and Urinary Tract Infections in Women

LESLIE S.-T. FANG

Among adult women, urinary tract infection (UTI) is the most common of all bacterial infections. Between 20% and 30% of women have a UTI in their lifetime, and 40% of women with one infection have a recurrence. Thus, UTIs represent a significant source of morbidity among women. Evaluation by the primary physician should be directed at the detection of any anatomic abnormalities that may predispose the patient to recurrent infections. Therapy should be aimed at the eradication of infection to minimize morbidity.

PATHOPHYSIOLOGY AND CLINICAL PRESENTATION

Current evidence suggests that most episodes of UTI in adult women are secondary to *ascending infection*. Bacteria reach the bladder through the urethra and may then ascend to the kidneys through the ureters. Hematogenous spread has rarely been implicated in the pathogenesis of UTIs.

Bacteria that commonly cause UTI are found in the periurethral area in up to 20% of adult women. This *colonization* of the *vaginal introitus* has been shown to be the essential first step in the production of bacteriuria and plays an important role in recurrent UTIs. Colonization with *Enterobacteriaceae* occurs in postmenopausal women and is believed to account for much of the increase in susceptibility to UTI seen in this age group. Entry of bacteria into the bladder through the relatively short female urethra can occur spontaneously. In addition, *sexual intercourse* and use of a *diaphragm* correlate with risk for infection. The use of spermicide with a diaphragm or on a condom predisposes specifically to infection with *Staphylococcus saprophyticus*. Significant increases in bacteriuria follow 30% of intercourse episodes. The use of tampons and wiping from back to front are not risk factors for UTI.

The establishment of a bladder infection also depends on the virulence of the bacteria introduced, the number of organisms introduced, and, most importantly, a lapse in normal host defense mechanisms. A number of *host defense mechanisms* normally act together to decrease the likelihood of infection. Normal voiding eliminates some organisms. Certain chemical properties of the urine are antibacterial; urine with a high concentration of urea, low pH, and high osmolarity supports bacterial growth poorly. The most important host defense mechanism is phagocytosis of bacteria that come into contact with the bladder mucosal surface. Vaginal epithelial cell characteristics also contribute. Susceptibility to UTI correlates with increases in cellular bacterial adhesiveness. Abnormalities in these host defense mechanisms result in recurrent and complicated UTIs. Inability to express blood group antigens is a risk factor.

In approximately 30% of cases of sustained bladder infection, the infection extends further through the ureters into the kidneys. The presence of *reflux* increases the chance that infection will ascend. Once infected urine gains access to the renal pelvis, it can enter the renal parenchyma through the ducts of Bellini at the papillary tips and then spread outward along the collecting ducts to cause parenchymal infection.

Clinical Syndromes

Urinary tract infections are associated with a number of clinical syndromes, ranging from acute urethral syndrome to pyelonephritis. Most are accompanied by dysuria, frequency, urgency, and suprapubic or flank discomfort. Other features are unique to each syndrome.

Acute Urethral Syndrome (Symptomatic Abacteriuria) occurs in about 10% to 15% of women who present with symptoms suggestive of UTI. Patients in this category have fewer than 10^5 organisms per milliliter on urine culture. In addition, urinalysis findings are usually unimpressive—few white blood cells (WBCs) and no bacteria. These patients can be subdivided into two groups. Approximately 70% have some degree of pyuria (>2 to 5 WBCs per high-power field in a centrifuged sample) and true infection, either with bacterial counts of fewer than 10^5 organisms or with *Chlamydia trachomatis*. Those with bacterial counts in the range of 10^2 to 10^4 may have early UTI with infection not yet established in the bladder. The remaining 30% have no pyuria and no infection. The cause of their dysuria is unknown. Only those without pyuria have proved to be truly abacteriuric. A subset of truly abacteriuric women with urinary frequency report chronic pelvic pain relieved by voiding, suprapubic tenderness, and dyspareunia. They have normal findings on urinalysis. Cystoscopic dilation reveals submucosal hemorrhages. The term *interstitial cystitis* has been used to designate their condition. The cause is unknown, and the course is chronic. Tricyclic antidepressants are sometimes helpful.

Asymptomatic Bacteriuria. (See Chapter 126 for a discussion of this entity.)

Symptomatic Bacteriuria, in the form of cystitis or pyelonephritis, is the most common of the clinical syndromes. *Cystitis* has traditionally been thought to present primarily as frequency, urgency, dysuria, and bacteriuria. *Pyelonephritis*, on the other hand, is generally believed to be associated with fever, flank pain, and systemic symptoms such as nausea and vomiting. Unfortunately, numerous investigations have shown that the ability to differentiate between bladder and kidney infection on clinical grounds alone is limited. Studies using bilateral ureteral catheterization to localize directly the site of infection have demonstrated that many patients with upper tract infection present with symptoms supposedly characteristic of lower tract infection. Moreover, patients whose infection is limited to the bladder may occasionally have fever, flank pain, and systemic symptoms usually associated with pyelonephritis. Thus, the traditional clinical clues are at best imprecise for identifying the site of infection.

Recurrent Infections are characteristic of some patients. Two basic patterns of recurrence are recognized: (a) *relapse*, in which the original organism is suppressed by antimicrobial therapy and then reappears when the antibiotic is stopped, and (b) *reinfection*, in which the original organism is eradicated by antimicrobial therapy and the recurrent infection is caused by a new bacterial strain. Approximately 80% of recurrences represent reinfection. Ureteral catheterization studies have demonstrated that most reinfections occur in patients in whom infec-

tion is restricted to the bladder, whereas most relapses occur in patients with renal parenchymal infection.

Groups frequently bothered by recurrent infections include (a) sexually active women, who report a temporal relationship of urinary symptoms to intercourse; (b) patients with host defenses compromised by underlying systemic illness or residual urine in the bladder; (c) patients with upper tract infections; and (d) pregnant women.

The consequences of recurrent uncomplicated infections are, for the most part, minimal and rarely result in progressive renal impairment. However, patients with infections in the setting of vesicoureteral reflux, pregnancy, or diabetes are at greater risk. *Vesicoureteral reflux* is associated with residual urine in the bladder, ascending infection, chronic pyelonephritis, and a high risk for renal scarring, which leads to focal glomerulosclerosis, proteinuria, and progressive renal failure. Patients most likely to have vesicoureteral reflux are those who report a long history of UTIs beginning in childhood. UTI during pregnancy has been linked to increased rates of fetal complications and prematurity, especially when the infection occurs within 2 weeks of delivery. The mother has an enhanced risk for pyelonephritis. Patients with diabetes show an increased susceptibility to upper tract infection.

DIFFERENTIAL DIAGNOSIS

Dysuria. The differential diagnosis of dysuria includes *UTI*, *vaginitis*, and *urethritis*. Patients with vaginitis may occasionally be mistakenly thought to have UTI. Vaginal discharge, "external" discomfort (from urinary irritation of inflamed labial tissue), absence of frequency or urgency, and urine cultures negative for bacteria distinguish vaginitis from UTI. *Trichomonas vaginalis* and *Candida albicans* are the most commonly responsible organisms. Women with dysuria and an absence of bacterial growth on routine urine culture may have *urethritis* caused by *Neisseria gonorrhoeae* or *herpes simplex virus*, although, as previously noted, most cases will be caused by *Chlamydia trachomatis* (see Chapter 125). The onset is usually gradual, dysuria is mild, and vaginal discharge may be present. Pelvic pain and vaginal or cervical discharge suggest spread of infection into the cervix and fallopian tubes, a serious development (see Chapters 116 and 117).

Pyuria typically accompanies gonococcal and trichomonal infection as well as chlamydial infection. Patients with acute urethral syndrome and no pyuria may have dysuria on the basis of *local trauma* or *irritation* rather than infection, problems that occur in postmenopausal women secondary to desiccation of vaginal and urethral tissue.

Flank Pain. Patients with *renal calculi* or *embolic infarction* may present with flank pain and hematuria, mimicking *pyelonephritis*. However, urine cultures are sterile and no bacteria are seen on Gram's stain, as they are in UTI.

WORKUP

The pace, extensiveness, and order of the evaluation are largely dictated by the patient's clinical presentation. Candidates for outpatient evaluation include dysuric patients with no evidence of systemic toxicity or obstruction.

Acutely Ill Patients

Those presenting with fever, flank pain, and systemic symptoms require prompt evaluation for the possibility of urinary tract *obstruction* and superimposed infection. Such patients should be questioned about a history of diabetes, sickle cell anemia, and excessive analgesic use; patients with these problems are at higher risk for renal papillary necrosis and subsequent obstruction by sloughed papillae. Likewise, a history of renal calculi is cause for concern in this setting. The patient with any of these risk factors who appears toxic (high temperature, prostration) and restless on examination and who has marked tenderness in the costovertebral angle requires immediate urologic evaluation to rule out obstruction. Infection behind an obstruction constitutes a medical and urologic emergency necessitating urgent therapeutic intervention.

Dysuric Patients

History. The acutely dysuric woman ought to be questioned about vaginal discharge, external irritation on urination, and pain on intercourse to differentiate vaginal causes of dysuria from those referable to the urinary tract. Also helpful is a sexual history to identify risk factors for chlamydial urethritis, including new sexual partners, a partner with a penile discharge or recent urethritis, mucoid vaginal discharge, or gradual onset of symptoms. A recent history of gonorrhea or exposure to gonorrhea should be elicited.

Physical Examination. One begins with a temperature determination, followed by percussion of the costovertebral angle to test for tenderness and palpation of the suprapubic region to detect discomfort and distention. The pelvic examination is essential; any urethral discharge, vaginal erythema, discharge, or atrophy, and cervical discharge, erosion, vesicles, or tenderness on motion must be noted.

Laboratory Studies.

Urinalysis and Gram's Stain of the unspun urine are often diagnostic. Proper collection of the urine specimen is essential. The *clean-voided technique* has withstood the test of time and minimizes contamination from vaginal and labial sources. The female patient is told to straddle or squat over the toilet and to spread the labia with the nondominant hand. This position is maintained throughout collection. With the other hand, the vulva is swabbed front to back with three sterile gauze pads soaked in sterile water or with a sponge soaked in a mild non-hexachlorophene soap. A small amount of urine is then passed. This is a urethral specimen and can be saved if bacterial or protozoan urethritis is suspected. More urine is voided and collected in a sterile cup. Alternatively, the patient can be told to slide the cup into a freely flowing stream to collect a true midstream specimen. The adequacy of collection can be confirmed by examining for epithelial cells; their presence indicates vulvar or urethral contamination.

With an elderly patient, the assistance of a family member or a nurse may be needed. When repeated contamination is suspected, *straight catheterization* of the bladder can be performed with relatively little risk.

Examining the urine promptly minimizes artifactual findings. The finding of *pyuria* (>25 WBCs per high-power field

on examination of a spun sediment) is indicative of UTI and predictive of a response to antibiotic therapy. The absence of pyuria suggests a vaginal cause for the dysuria or a noninfectious variant of the acute urethral syndrome. The presence of one organism on high-power field examination of a Gram's-stained unspun urine sample represents clinically significant bacteriuria ($>10^5$ organisms per milliliter).

Culture. The traditional criterion for infection has been a colony count of more than 10^5 organisms per milliliter; it provides high specificity but poor sensitivity. Studies using suprapubic aspirates find that half of dysuric women with "negative" urine cultures by the traditional criterion are truly infected, although the colony counts were in the range of 10^2 to 10^5. Colony counts of more than 10^2 obtained on clean-voided specimens from acutely dysuric women are diagnostic of true coliform infection. Many such women who previously were labeled as having symptomatic abacteriuria fall into this category. As noted earlier, the presence of pyuria identifies those who are infected and will respond to antibiotics.

The need to obtain a urine culture for every acutely dysuric woman with mild to moderate symptoms has been challenged. The vast majority of organisms that cause infection in this group are sensitive to the antibiotic regimens commonly prescribed (see below). Even when disk-sensitivity testing designates an organism as "resistant" to an antibiotic, the resistance is only relative and the organism is usually susceptible to the much higher antibiotic concentrations found in the urine. Many authorities now recommend basing the decision to treat with antibiotics and the selection of an agent on the results of urine sediment examination and Gram's stain, with urine culture reserved for patients with a recurrence or a report of several UTIs within the past year. Empiric therapy has also been advised. A compromise is patient-initiated antibiotic therapy after a dip-slide urine culture has been performed.

At the other extreme are patients who present acutely with severe symptoms and risk for urosepsis. They require not only urine sediment examination, Gram's stain, and culture, but also at least two sets of *blood cultures* before antibiotics are initiated.

When the urine culture is obtained, familiarity with important urinary pathogens facilitates interpretation of culture results. The most common urinary pathogen in community-acquired UTI is *Escherichia coli*. Occasionally, the other gram-negative rods are responsible. Of the gram-positive organisms involved in UTI, enterococci, *Staphylococcus aureus*, and group B streptococci are common isolates. Less appreciated as a urinary pathogen is *S. saprophyticus*, a coagulase-negative organism frequently found to cause UTIs in female outpatients. Diphtheroids, lactobacilli, and α-hemolytic streptococci represent contaminants.

Intravenous Pyelography and Other Urinary Tract Investigations. Recurrent infection raises the specter of a structural lesion. However, as already noted, the vast majority of recurrences represent reinfection in the absence of upper tract disease or other pathology. IV pyelography, excretory urography, and cystoscopy in women with recurrent infection are of very low yield and are not recommended. Such radiographic and urologic evaluations should be reserved for those in whom anatomic abnormalities are suspected (e.g., onset of UTIs in childhood) or in whom obstruction is likely or renal insufficiency is developing. If evidence of reflux is suggested by IV pyelography, a voiding cystourethrogram should be performed to document the degree of reflux. Urologic evaluation is indicated when urethral meatal stenosis is strongly suspected (see Chapter 134).

PRINCIPLES OF THERAPY

The intensity and duration of therapy should match the patient's clinical presentation and risk for complications. In general, patients who are sick require consideration for hospitalization and parenteral antibiotics, especially if they are metabolically or immunologically compromised or have an anatomic or functional defect of the urinary tract.

Acutely Ill Patients: Pyelonephritis, Urosepsis. Those presenting with high fever, chills, flank pain, costovertebral angle tenderness, nausea, and vomiting may have upper tract or even bloodstream infection and should be hospitalized, especially if elderly. They require fluids, thorough evaluation for treatable precipitants (see above), and prompt initiation of parenteral antibiotics. The choice of initial antibiotic program should be consistent with the findings on urine Gram's stain, although Enterobacteriaceae account for more than 90% of cases.

Often, broad-spectrum coverage is selected in this setting because of concern for *Pseudomonas* species and other multiply resistant gram-negative rods. In addition, coverage for enterococci is usually included, although the pathogen is more common in men. *Ampicillin* plus *gentamicin* is the time-honored choice for serious UTI, providing effective coverage at low cost. Expensive alternatives for initial treatment include imipenem/cilastatin, ciprofloxacin, and ceftriaxone. When culture and sensitivity results become available, the regimen can be revised to provide more focused coverage. Urosepsis requires 2 to 3 weeks of IV antibiotics. Pyelonephritis without bloodstream invasion can be treated parenterally until fever resolves, then with oral antibiotics to complete a 14-day course.

Outpatient Treatment of Pyelonephritis. Otherwise healthy patients with less severe but still acutely incapacitating symptoms often have *uncomplicated* pyelonephritis; this can be treated entirely on an outpatient basis with 10 to 14 days of oral antibiotics provided that the patient is reliable, can take fluids, is not seriously immunocompromised, and has no obstruction. The choice of initial therapy is based on Gram's stain findings. For infection with gram-negative rods, *trimethoprim/ sulfamethoxazole* (TMS) or a fluoroquinolone (e.g., *ciprofloxacin, norfloxacin*) is a reasonable choice. Up to 30% of community-acquired *E. coli* infections are now ampicillin-resistant, so that this antibiotic less effective for initial outpatient treatment of pyelonephritis, although the combination preparation of *amoxicillin/clavulanic acid* (Augmentin) produces cure in more than 90% of cases. TMS resistance is also becoming more common, approaching 15% in some areas. With increasing TMS and ampicillin resistance among community-acquired *Enterobacteriaceae,* fluoroquinolone therapy may emerge as the preferred selection for outpatient treatment of pyelonephritis, with amoxicillin/clavulanic acid also assuming an increasingly important role. Gram-positive cocci seen on urine Gram's stain suggest enterococci and *S. saprophyticus,* both of which are best treated with *amoxicillin.*

Repeated culturing 2 to 4 days after completion of therapy is essential. Failure to respond to an appropriate antibiotic program suggests an anatomic or functional abnormality and the

need for radiologic evaluation and urologic consultation (see above).

Mild to Moderate Symptoms: Uncomplicated Urinary Tract Infection. Most patients with mild to moderate symptoms have cystitis and respond well to a short course of oral antibiotics. The choice of agent is again based on urine Gram's stain. With *gram-negative rods*, TMS or *amoxicillin* should suffice for most cases of lower UTI, even those caused by "resistant" strains, because of the very high bladder antibiotic concentrations achieved. For patients allergic to both sulfa drugs and penicillin, a fluoroquinolone (e.g., *ciprofloxacin*) is an effective alternative. For *gram-positive cocci, amoxicillin* is the drug of choice.

The optimal duration of therapy for uncomplicated UTI has been a subject of much interest ever since it was found that *single-dose regimens* could provide nearly the same results as conventional 7- to 10-day programs while significantly reducing cost and risk for vaginal candidiasis, rash, diarrhea, poor compliance, and emergence of resistant organisms. Single-dose amoxicillin (3 g orally) and TMS (two double-strength tablets) have been used successfully, with better results reported for TMS. Ciprofloxacin (1 g) is also effective. The oral cephalosporins—cephaloridine, cefadroxil, and cefaclor—have been disappointing. A *3-day course* of antibiotics achieves a slightly higher rate of cure than does a 1-day program yet retains most of the advantages of single-dose therapy. Suboptimal candidates for short-course therapy include patients with diabetes, a history of relapses, more than three UTIs in the past year, and immunocompromise. Such patients are best treated with a more conventional course of antibiotics (up to 2 weeks).

Failure to Respond. Failure to respond to short-course therapy has proved to be a reliable clinical criterion for upper tract disease, correlating well with results of formal localization tests. Patients may report no relief of symptoms or a relapse within days of treatment. Such patients are likely to have subclinical uncomplicated pyelonephritis and should be treated accordingly (see above).

Acute Urethral Syndrome. Patients with *pyuria*, no bacteria on Gram's stain, and no clinical evidence for chlamydial, gonococcal, or other venereal forms of urethritis can be treated with *single-dose antibiotic therapy* in the same manner as any patient with lower tract infection. Alternatively, they can be treated with *TMS* (one single-strength tablet twice daily for 10 days) or *doxycycline* (100 mg twice daily for 10 days). Doxycycline is effective against *Chlamydia* and gonococci and also most common urinary pathogens (see Chapters 125 and 137). Recurrences are common in patients with acute urethral syndrome.

Patients *without pyuria* do not respond to antibiotics. Symptomatic therapy with fluids and urinary analgesics such as phenazopyridine (Pyridium) are usually prescribed.

Recurrent Infection. Patients bothered by frequent symptomatic recurrences are potential candidates for prophylactic measures. Recurrent infection should be confirmed at least once by repeated culture. The clinical setting helps determine the appropriate approach to therapy. As noted earlier, recurrences in *sexually active women* are most often reinfections. Prophylaxis at the time of intercourse with *single-tablet* ther-

Table 133.1. Antibiotic Regimens for Urinary Tract Infections in Women

CLINICAL SITUATION	REGIMEN
Acutely ill and toxic patient	Hospitalization; parenteral antibiotics; ampicillin plus gentamicin if urosepsis suspected; otherwise, ciprofloxacin if Gram's stain shows GNR; ampicillin if it shows GPC
Uncomplicated pyelonephritis	Oral TMS (1 double-strength tablet) bid for 2 wks or ciprofloxacin 500 mg bid for 2 wks
Uncomplicated lower UTI	Single-dose TMS (2 double-strength tablets), ciprofloxacin (1 g) or amoxicillin (3 g) if Gram's stain shows GNR; amoxicillin if it shows GPC; 3-day course if more symptomatic with TMS (1 double-strength tablet) bid, ciprofloxacin 500 mg bid, amoxicillin 500 mg tid; 7- to 10-day course if diabetes, recurrent UTI, age >65
Relapse	Same drug as for uncomplicated UTI, but continued for at least 2 weeks
Acute urethral syndrome with pyuria	TMS as for uncomplicated UTI, or doxycycline 100 mg bid for 10 days if *Chlamydia* infection suspected
Acute urethral syndrome without pyuria	No antibiotics
Recurrent infection	
Sexually active	Prophylaxis with nocturnal single-tablet dose of ampicillin, TMS, or ciprofloxacin
Elderly patient with large postvoid residual	Prophylaxis with nightly dose of TMS (half of a single-strength tablet) or ciprofloxacin (250 mg)
Pregnancy	Ampicillin, amoxicillin, and oral cephalosporins have proved safe; nitrofurantoin safe for the fetus, but potentially toxic for the mother; fluoroquinolones should be avoided

TMS, trimethoprim/sulfamethoxazole; GNR, gram-negative rod; GPC, gram-positive cocci; UTI, urinary tract infection.

apy has proved effective in minimizing their frequency and severity. In reliable patients with fewer than three UTIs per year, a patient-initiated *1- or 3-day course* of standard antibiotic therapy for uncomplicated UTI at the first sign of symptomatic infection has proved effective. In *postmenopausal* women, a course of topical *vaginal estrogens* can prevent recurrent infection, presumably by returning the vaginal flora to its premenopausal composition with few *Enterobacteriaceae*. For *very elderly patients* with bladder distention, postvoid residual urine, and recurrent reinfection, *continuous prophylaxis* with nightly TMS (one half of a single-strength tablet daily at bedtime) usually suffices and works better than regimens of sulfisoxazole or methenamine mandelate (Mandelamine) and ascorbic acid. Once prophylaxis is stopped, there is no residual benefit. In patients with defined anatomic abnormalities, such as significant reflux or nephrolithiasis, surgical correction to decrease the severity and frequency of recurrences should be considered.

Treatment of the Pregnant Patient. Treatment of symptomatic UTI in pregnancy is recommended because of an increased risk for upper tract infection in the mother and potential injury to the fetus (low birth weight, prematurity). Antibiotics proved safe for use in pregnancy include ampicillin, amoxicillin, and oral cephalosporins. The combination preparation of amoxicillin/clavulanic acid (Augmentin) is recommended for use against organisms demonstrating resistance to multiple drugs. Nitrofurantoin has also been used without evidence of fetal toxicity; however, its associated risk of inducing peripheral neuropathy, pulmonary fibrosis, and hepatic injury in adults makes it a less preferable choice. The fluoroquinolones should be avoided in pregnant patients.

Treatment of Asymptomatic Bacteriuria in the Elderly. Because the risk for urosepsis, renal failure, or mortality is not increased, the need for antibiotics is not urgent. The risk for asymptomatic infection is increased, but the benefit of treat-

ment is unclear. Antibiotics are indicated if obstruction is present or the patient is to undergo a genitourinary procedure.

THERAPEUTIC RECOMMENDATIONS

Table 133.1 summarizes the therapeutic recommendations for UTIs.

INDICATIONS FOR REFERRAL OR ADMISSION

Hospitalization is indicated in patients with severe symptoms such as rigors, high fever, flank pain, nausea, and vomiting. Patients with suspected obstruction and those unable to maintain oral intake also require hospitalization. Referral to a urologist is indicated if a surgically correctable anatomic abnormality is detected or suspected.

PATIENT EDUCATION

Certain general measures are important in minimizing the possibility of recurrent infection. The patient should be instructed about increasing fluid intake during symptomatic periods and maintaining urine flow around the clock. Patients with UTIs temporally related to sexual intercourse would probably benefit from voiding after intercourse. The importance of compliance with antibiotic regimens and follow-up for repeated urinalysis and culture must be impressed on patients with serious infections and relapses.

ANNOTATED BIBLIOGRAPHY

American College of Physicians. Common uses of intravenous pyelography in adults. Ann Intern Med 1989;111:83. (*A position paper recommending against routine use in women with UTI.*)

Boscid JA, Abrutyn E, Kaye D. Asymptomatic bacteriuria in elderly persons: to treat or not to treat? Ann Intern Med 1987;106:764. (*In most instances, no treatment is needed.*)

Dolan JG, Bordley DR, Polito R. Initial management of serious urinary tract infection: epidemiologic guidelines. J Gen Intern Med 1989;4:190. (*A retrospective study; TMS was effective for young women; older women had a higher likelihood of a TMS-resistant organism; men required coverage for* Pseudomonas.)

Echols RM, Tosiello RL, Haverstock DC, et al. Demographic, clinical, and treatment parameters influencing the outcome of acute cystitis. Clin Infect Dis 1999;29:113. (*A metaanalysis of six trials including more than 3,000 women with acute cystitis treated with 11 different regimens. Not using a diaphragm was associated with a successful bacteriologic outcome.*)

Fang LST, Tolkoff-Rubin NE, Rubin RH. Efficacy of single-dose and conventional amoxicillin therapy in urinary tract infection localized by the antibody-coated bacteria technique. N Engl J Med 1978;298:413. (*Efficacy of single-dose therapy for lower UTI demonstrated.*)

Fihn SD, Boyko EJ, Chi-Ling C, et al. Use of spermicide-coated condoms and other risk factors for urinary tract infection caused by *Staphylococcus saprophyticus*. Arch Intern Med 1998;158:281. (*Nonoxynol 9 increased the risk for infection with this organism.*)

Fihn SD, Johnson C, Roberts PL, et al. Trimethoprim-sulfamethoxazole for acute dysuria in women: a single-dose or 10-day course. A double-blind, randomized trial. Ann Intern Med 1988;108:350. (*Risk for failure at 6 weeks no different.*)

Fowler JE, Pulaski ET. Excretory urography, cystography and cystoscopy in the evaluation of women with urinary tract infection. N Engl J Med 1981;304:462. (*Very low yield, even in women with two or more recent UTIs.*)

Gupta K, Scholes D, Stamm WE. Increasing prevalence of antimicrobial resistance among uropathogens causing acute uncomplicated cystitis in women. JAMA 1999;281:736. (*Documents increasing resistance to ampicillin, cephalothin, trimethoprim, and TMS.*)

Hooton TM, Running K, Stamm WE. Single-dose therapy for cystitis in women. A comparison of trimethoprim-sulfamethoxazole, amoxicillin, and cyclacillin. JAMA 1985;253:387. (*TMS was effective, but the trial was stopped because one in every three receiving the other drugs failed treatment.*)

Hooton TM, Stamm WE. Management of acute uncomplicated urinary tract infection in adults. Med Clin North Am 1991;75:339. (*Authoritative review that remains very helpful nearly a decade after publication.*)

Hooton TM, Winter C, Tiu F, et al. Randomized comparative trial and cost analysis of 3-day antimicrobial regimens for treatment of acute cystitis in women. JAMA 1995;273:41. (*TMS was the most effective.*)

Huang X, Hartzema AG, Raasch RH, et al. Economic assessment of three antimicrobial therapies for uncomplicated urinary tract infection in women. Clin Ther 1999;21:1578. (*TMS was the most effective.*)

Komaroff AL. Diagnostic decision: urinalysis and urine culture in women with dysuria. Ann Intern Med 1986;104:212. (*Urinalysis was the most reliable indicator of treatable infection; urine culture was of limited value except in cases of suspected upper UTI.*)

Komaroff AL. Acute dysuria in women. N Engl J Med 1984;310:368. (*A review emphasizing the importance of pyuria as a sign of UTI and predictor of response to therapy; good discussion of the acute urethral syndrome; 106 references.*)

Kremery S, Hromec J, Tvrdikova M, et al. Newer quinolones in the long-term prophylaxis of recurrent urinary tract infections. Drugs 1999;58:99. (*Daily dosing effective during a 12-month period in four of every five premenopausal women with a history of recurrent infection.*)

Kunin CM, White LV, Hua TH. A reassessment of the importance of "low-count" bacteriuria in young women with acute urinary symptoms. Ann Intern Med 1993;119:454. (*Likely to represent an early phase of UTI.*)

Latham RH, Running K, Stamm WE. Urinary tract infections in young adult women caused by *Staphylococcus saprophyticus*. JAMA 1983;250:3063. (S. saprophyticus *was the second most common cause of UTIs, accounting for 11%.*)

McCarty JM, Richard G, Huck W, et al. A randomized trial of short-course ciprofloxacin, ofloxacin, or trimethoprim/sulfamethoxazole for the treatment of acute urinary tract infection in women. Ciprofloxacin Urinary Tract Infection Group. Am J Med 1999;106:292. (*These three drugs were equally effective.*)

Mushlin AI, Thornbury JR. Intravenous pyelography: the case against its routine use. Ann Intern Med 1989;111:58. (*Little justification for its routine use found in women with UTI.*)

National Institutes of Arthritis, Diabetes, and Digestive and Kidney Diseases. Workshop on Interstitial Cystitis. J Urol 1988;140:203. (*A brief summary of this often overlooked condition.*)

Norrby SR. Short-term treatment of uncomplicated urinary tract infections in women. Rev Infect Dis 1990;12:458. (*A metaanalysis suggesting that 3-day regimens are generally more effective than 1-day programs.*)

Pinson AG, Philbriack JT, Lindbeck GH, et al. Oral antibiotic therapy for acute pyelonephritis: a methodologic review of the literature. J Gen Intern Med 1992;7:544. (*Critical look at available studies.*)

Raz R, Stamm WE. A controlled trial of intravaginal estriol in postmenopausal women with recurrent urinary tract infections. N Engl J Med 1993;329:753. (*Prevents recurrent UTI.*)

Safrin S, Siegel D, Black D. Pyelonephritis in adult women: inpatient versus outpatient therapy. Am J Med 1988;85:793. (*Results are comparable; cost is greatly reduced by outpatient management.*)

Schaeffer AJ, Stuppy BA. Efficacy and safety of self-start therapy in women with recurrent urinary tract infections. J Urol 1999:161:207. (*Patient initiation of norfloxacin after a dip-slide urine culture was effective in this small trial.*)

Stamm WE, Counts GW, Running KR, et al. Diagnosis of coliform infection in acutely dysuric women. N Engl J Med 1982;307:463. (*A criterion of 10^5 organisms per milliliter is too insensitive for infection in this setting.*)

Stamm WE, Counts GW, Wagner KF, et al. Antimicrobial prophylaxis of recurrent urinary tract infections. Ann Intern Med 1980;92:770. (*All regimens proved effective and were well tolerated; no emergence of resistant strains.*)

Stamm WE, Hooton TM. Management of urinary tract infections in adults. N Engl J Med 1993;329:1328. (*Terse review of the major clinical questions; 60 references.*)

Stamm WE, McKevitt M, Counts GW. Acute renal infection in women: treatment with trimethoprim-sulfamethoxazole or ampicillin for two or six weeks. Ann Intern Med 1987;106:341. (*Treatment for 2 weeks sufficed; TMS was better.*)

Stamm WE, McKevitt M, Counts GW. Is antimicrobial prophylaxis of urinary tract infections cost-effective? Ann Intern Med 1981;94:251. (*Prophylaxis became cost-effective when women had three infections per year.*)

Stamm WE, Wagner KF, Cimsel R, et al. Causes of the acute urethral syndrome in women. N Engl J Med 1980;303:409. (*Patients with pyuria had infection with coliform bacteria,* S. saprophyticus, *or C.* trachomatis; *those without pyuria had no organism isolated.*)

Strom BL, Collins M, West SL, et al. Sexual activity, contraceptive use, and other risk factors for symptomatic and asymptomatic bacteriuria. Ann Intern Med 1987;107:816. (*Intercourse, diaphragm use, and past history of UTI were the only independent risk factors; tampon use and wiping improperly were not.*)

Wong ES, McKevsitt M, Running K, et al. Management of recurrent urinary tract infections with patient-administered single-dose therapy. Ann Intern Med 1985;102:302. (*A safe, effective, convenient, and inexpensive approach.*)

134
Approach to Incontinence and Other Forms of Lower Urinary Tract Dysfunction
JOHN D. GOODSON

Patients with lower urinary tract dysfunction may present with incontinence, hesitancy, dribbling, loss of stream volume or force, frequency, or urgency. Such complaints are particularly prevalent among the elderly and a common problem in primary care practice. An efficient and parsimonious evaluation strategy is essential, given the large number of possible causes and available studies.

Incontinence can have a major impact on one's life and family. At the least, it is an embarrassment and an inconvenience. Constant incontinence can predispose to local skin breakdown, serious infection, and social isolation. In many instances, it is the culminating event that leads to nursing home placement. The primary physician must be attuned to the nature of the problem and the needs of the patient and family to design and implement an effective treatment program. Substantial progress has been made in the management of incontinence, and one should be familiar with available treatment strategies and their indications.

PATHOPHYSIOLOGY AND CLINICAL PRESENTATION

Normal Bladder Function and Continence. The *detrusor muscle* of the bladder is normally under simultaneous *sympathetic* and *parasympathetic* control. During the filling phase, sympathetic tone predominates, whereas parasympathetic tone is inhibited. The internal bladder sphincter tightens under *α-adrenergic* influence, and the detrusor relaxes under *β-adrenergic* influence. During voluntary emptying, parasympathetic stimulation produces detrusor contraction; at the same time, sympathetic tone decreases, the external sphincter of the pelvic floor relaxes, and abdominal muscles tighten. Normally, the urethra is oriented to the bladder so as to facilitate continence. With the initiation of voluntary voiding, the *urethrovesicular angle* changes so as to permit full drainage. Complete bladder emptying depends on unimpeded flow.

The process of voiding usually begins with a sensation of bladder fullness mediated by proprioceptive fibers in the detrusor. A reflex arc between the detrusor and the brainstem initiates and amplifies bladder contraction by parasympathetic stimulation. This arc is under cortical inhibition. Voiding occurs with the release of inhibition and voluntary relaxation of the pelvic external sphincter.

Incontinence. The pathophysiology and clinical presentations of incontinence can be divided on clinical and mechanistic grounds into categories of detrusor instability (urge incontinence), sphincter or pelvic incompetence (stress incontinence), reflex incontinence, overflow incontinence, and functional incontinence. Clinically, two or more processes frequently coexist to varying degrees in the same patient.

Detrusor Instability (Urge Incontinence) is characterized by reduced bladder capacity resulting from excessive and inappropriate detrusor contraction. For many, the condition appears to arise as a concomitant of *aging*, although the mechanism is unclear. In some, it seems to be the result of *decreased cortical inhibition* of detrusor contraction. Loss of cortical input can ensue from such conditions as cerebral infarction, Alzheimer's disease, brain tumor, and Parkinson's disease. For others, the detrusor overactivity is linked to *bladder irritation* from such causes as trigonitis (a common accompaniment of cystitis), chronic interstitial cystitis, postradiation fibrosis, and detrusor hypertrophy from outflow tract obstruction. Patients note a few moments of warning, frequent episodes of urgency, moderate to large volumes, and nocturnal wetting. In roughly half of patients, detrusor instability is associated with poor detrusor function. For these patients, voiding is frequent and incomplete.

Sphincter or Pelvic Incompetence (Stress Incontinence) is Usually a Consequence of Pelvic Floor Laxity and is the most common form of urinary incontinence in women. Less frequently, it develops from *partial denervation* that reduces sphincter tone. Pelvic laxity is seen as a concomitant of normal aging and of difficult or multiple vaginal deliveries or direct perineal injury. In some cases, a cystocele forms and further impedes control. Estrogen deficiency in women reduces the competency of the internal sphincter and can also cause urethral symptoms (dysuria and frequency). In men, pelvic incompetence may result from prostatic surgery, although in most cases the abnormality resolves within 6 months if innervation remains largely intact. Patients complain of incontinence, which occurs predominantly at times of straining (coughing, laughing, sneezing, lifting). There is loss of small to moderate volumes of urine, very infrequent nighttime leakage, and little postvoid residual.

Reflex Incontinence derives mostly from *spinal cord damage* above the sacral level. Interference with sensation and coordination of detrusor and sphincter activity secondary to inhibited or absent central control leads to *detrusor spasticity* and *functional outlet obstruction*. The patient is unable to sense the need to void. Spinal cord injury is the most common cause. Diabetes, multiple sclerosis, tabes dorsalis, and intrinsic or extrinsic cord compression from tumor or disk herniation are also important causes. Reflex incontinence takes place day and night with equal frequency and without warning or precipitating stress. Volumes are moderate, and voiding is frequent. Voluntary sphincter control and perineal sensation are reduced; sacral reflexes remain intact.

Detrusor Hypotonia (Overflow Incontinence) results from either long-standing *outlet obstruction, detrusor insufficiency,* or *impaired sensation.* The bladder becomes hypotonic, flaccid, and distended. Voiding consists primarily of overflow spillage. In outflow tract obstruction (most often from long-standing prostatic hypertrophy), the detrusor is constantly overstretched and gradually becomes incapable of generating sufficient pressure to ensure bladder emptying. Retrograde flow of urine and increased ureteral pressures can compromise renal function if the condition is left uncorrected. Often, detrusor insufficiency is a consequence of lower motor neuron damage, as occurs with injury to the sacral cord or the development of peripheral neuropathy. Importantly, numerous medications (e.g., anticholinergics, tricyclic antidepressants) can reduce detrusor tone. Distinguishing clinical characteristics include a palpably *distended bladder* and a *large postvoid residual*. Patients void frequently, especially after fluid loads and diuretics. A history of incomplete emptying, slow or interrupted flow, hesitancy, and the need to strain are reported. Injury either to peripheral nerves (as in diabetes or vitamin B_{12} deficiency) or to the spinal cord may be accompanied by losses of perineal sensation and sacral reflexes.

Functional Incontinence refers to situations in which physical or mental disability makes it impossible to void independently, even though the urinary tract may be intact. Patients with disabling illness or simply an acute change to a bedridden state may be unable to maintain sufficient control over lower urinary function to avoid incontinence. Sedating drugs in such situations may only exacerbate the problem. Patients who are aware of their condition will describe their unsuccessful attempts to maintain continence. Patients with frontal lobe dysfunction secondary to cortical degenerative disease or normopressure hydrocephalus may be unaware of their own voiding and, therefore, functionally incontinent. Rarely, a severely disturbed patient is deliberately incontinent.

Urinary Frequency in Conjunction with Dysuria. Frequency accompanied by dysuria is a common presentation of lower *urinary tract infection*. Inflammation of the bladder trigone and urethra are responsible for most acute symptoms. *Chronic interstitial cystitis, acute urethral syndrome*, and *prostatosis* have been implicated as causes in cases without identifiable infection, although some of these may have inapparent infection with *Chlamydia* (see Chapters 125, 133, 136, and 139). *Carcinoma* of the bladder trigone or urethra is a rare but important cause of dysuria, frequency, and symptoms of outflow tract obstruction.

Urinary Frequency in Conjunction with Difficulty Voiding. When associated with slow stream, hesitancy, and a sense of incomplete emptying, frequency is likely to be a manifestation of *outflow tract obstruction* (extrinsic or intrinsic). At first, the patient may notice only minor slowness of stream. If the obstruction persists, bladder instability may ensue and cause frequent voiding of small volumes, followed later by chronic distention and overflow incontinence (see above). Strictures, tumor (especially prostatic enlargement), and occasionally stones are responsible for most cases of obstruction. In the setting of severe constipation, the rectal vault can become sufficiently impacted that it actually blocks the urethra and prevents bladder emptying. *α-Adrenergic* agents and *β-blockers* can increase sphincter tone and impair voiding acutely, especially in patients with preexisting lower urinary tract dysfunction. *Anticholinergic drugs* may interfere with bladder contraction.

Urinary Frequency and Polydipsia. When frequency presents in association with increased thirst, it suggests a diabetic condition leading to increased urine volume and the resultant polyuria. *Diabetes mellitus* is distinguished by significant glycosuria (see Chapter 102). *Neurogenic (idiopathic central) diabetes insipidus* is manifested by sudden onset, craving for huge volumes of cold water, and prodigious urine outputs (5 to 10 L/d). Inability to concentrate the urine after overnight fluid deprivation and response to parenteral antidiuretic hormone (ADH), with formation of a concentrated urine, characterize the condition. Patients with *nephrogenic diabetes insipidus* differ from those with the neurogenic variety in that their kidneys do not respond to intrinsic or parenteral ADH. Hypercalcemia, lithium therapy, and pregnancy are precipitants of the acquired variety. Patients with *psychogenic polydipsia* may be hard to distinguish from those with nephrogenic diabetes insipidus because they have washed out their renal concentrating system and also do not adequately respond to parenteral ADH. They do respond normally to fluid deprivation, a diagnostically useful finding, although some patients with neurogenic disease respond in a similar fashion (see Chapter 101).

Isolated Urinary Frequency. Isolated frequency may be a manifestation of reduced bladder capacity, or a presentation of mild diabetes mellitus, mild diabetes insipidus, minor urinary tract infection, or bladder irritation. A large *extrinsic* or *intrinsic mass* impinging on the bladder can reduce its capacity and produce frequent urination, usually of small volumes, which distinguish it from other forms of polyuria. Pelvic surgery, chronic interstitial cystitis, or irradiation can have a similar effect by reducing bladder capacity. Patients who surreptitiously abuse *diuretics* rarely complain of frequency, but those who take them for therapeutic purposes are often bothered by the side effect. Nocturnal urinary frequency and occasional incontinence can represent the *mobilization of fluid* in patients with dependent edema associated with congestive heart failure or intake of certain medications, such as some of the calcium channel blockers.

DIFFERENTIAL DIAGNOSIS

The differential diagnosis of incontinence can be classified according to clinical presentation and mechanism (Table 134.1). The differential diagnosis of dysuria and frequency is that of urinary tract infection and its related syndromes (see Chapters 133 and 140). Most of those with difficulty voiding are men with prostatic enlargement (see Chapter 138). Among other causes of difficult voiding are drugs (anticholinergics, β-blockers, sedatives), urethral stricture, congenital valves, stone, tumor, pelvic abscess, and fecal impaction. Causes of urinary frequency in the absence of other urinary tract symptoms include diabetes mellitus, diabetes insipidus, psychogenic polydipsia, diuretics, and bladder compression.

WORKUP

The evaluation of incontinence and other lower urinary tract symptoms requires assessment of the major neuromuscular and anatomic elements involved in maintaining urinary continence and flow. Much can be gleaned from the history and physical examination, which provide important clues to the underlying pathophysiology and precipitants.

Table 134.1.   Important Causes of Incontinence

TYPE	MECHANISM	CHARACTERISTICS
Detrusor Instability Bladder infection Chronic cystitis CNS disease (dementia, stroke) Detrusor hyperreflexia Detrusor hypertrophy Irradiation	Unstable detrusor	Warning; frequent episodes; nocturnal wetting; small postvoid residual, intact reflexes; normal sensation
Stress Incontinence Aging Autonomic neuropathy Estrogen deficiency Pelvic laxity Perineal injury Urologic surgery	Inadequate sphincter	Upon straining; small to moderate volumes; rarely at night; small postvoid volume

Reflex Incontinence
Disk herniation
Multiple sclerosis
Spinal cord disease
Tumor
	Upper neurologic tract disease (autonomous bladder)
	    Spinal cord injury
	    Severe cortical disease
		No warning or precipitants; severe neurologic disease; episodes can occur day and night; frequent; moderate volumes; loss of control and sensation; reflexes intact

Overflow Incontinence Diabetes Medications Outflow obstruction Peripheral neuropathy Sacral cord lesion Tabes dorsalis Vitamin B_{12} deficiency	Bladder outlet obstruction, lower motor neuron injury, or impaired sensation; toxic impairment of detrusor contraction	Distended bladder; history of obstructive symptoms; frequent loss of small volumes; loss of reflexes and sensation if caused by neurologic injury; large postvoid residual
Functional Incontinence Acute illness Medications Psychiatric disease	Inability to reach toilet in time	Functionally impaired patient

History. For the assessment of incontinence, one cannot overemphasize the importance of a detailed history, with emphasis on the circumstances, precipitants, timing, frequency, and volume of urine loss, the presence of warning symptoms, and the intactness of perineal and bladder sensation. When the history is sketchy, asking the patient or family to keep a *diary* of events and contributing factors can be of considerable help. This diary should include the following: time of urination; an estimate of the volume; the symptoms associated with each void, such as leakage; and any precipitating events, such as laughing or coughing.

Several clinical pictures are indicative of mechanism. Incontinence triggered only by *straining* indicates stress incontinence, although an occasional patient with overflow incontinence will report leakage under similar circumstances. Patients with overflow differ in that they also experience frequent loss of *small volumes* without warning or straining and are bothered by nocturnal episodes. A history of long-standing obstructive symptoms, such as difficulty with stream initiation or weakened urine flow, suggests an etiology for the overflow physiology.

In contrast to those with overflow disease, patients who have frequent episodes of *urgency*, lose small amounts of urine, yet retain perineal sensation are likely to have detrusor instability. Although there may be a few moments of warning, they too report nocturnal incontinence. When this is accompanied by dysuria, a search for urinary tract infection is indicated (see Chapters 133 and 140). Frequent voiding of small volumes and

urgency are also consistent with a small bladder resulting from extrinsic compression.

Reflex incontinence is suggested by a history of spinal cord injury, diabetes, multiple sclerosis, or dementia with neurologic deficits. Severe loss of cortical function is also a precipitant of detrusor instability. Furthermore, recent physical disability and confinement to bed may produce functional incontinence.

Regardless of the history and type of underlying pathology, the patient and family should be carefully questioned about *medications*, especially those with anticholinergic, α-adrenergic, β-adrenergic blocking, tranquilizing, or diuretic effects (e.g., tricyclic antidepressants, major and minor tranquilizers, decongestants, and antihypertensives). Any excessive use of coffee, tea, or alcohol should be noted.

Patients with isolated urinary frequency need to be asked about *increased thirst*, a feature consistent with diabetes mellitus and diabetes insipidus. Compulsive water drinkers with psychogenic polydipsia may deny their intake of water but do not report nocturia, a feature of both diabetes mellitus and diabetes insipidus. The sudden onset of intense thirst for ice-cold water is very suggestive of diabetes insipidus.

Those with symptoms of slow stream and hesitancy are likely to have outflow obstruction and should be checked for prostatism, stricture, stone, tumor, and fecal impaction.

Physical Examination. For the patient with incontinence, the examination begins by noting general appearance and any lack of attention to personal hygiene. A careful urogenital examination is essential and includes suprapubic palpation and percussion of the bladder after voiding to detect distention and masses. When appropriate, the *rectum* should be checked for impaction or *prostatic enlargement*. Absence of palpable prostatic enlargement does not rule out obstruction, especially in a patient with obstructive symptoms; median lobe encroachment on the urethra is often not palpable. Likewise, a large prostate does not predict severe obstruction.

Woman with stress incontinence should be examined in the lithotomy position. *Pelvic motion* and continence should be noted during cough or Valsalva's maneuver. Testing for stress incontinence is best done with the bladder full, unless the problem is severe and requires little provocation. Check the *vaginal mucosa* for atrophic changes (red, thin mucosa with a watery discharge) indicative of inadequate estrogen. A *bimanual examination* completes the evaluation, with note taken of any uterine or adnexal masses.

Neurologic control of voiding needs to be assessed to determine the presence of any deficits above, within, or distal to the autonomic reflex arc. Checking the *bulbocavernosus reflex* tests the integrity of the arc. Normally, squeezing the clitoris or glans penis will cause anal sphincter contraction. Lack of response suggests interruption. Another means of testing the arc is to note *anal sphincter tone*. Because control of the anal sphincter is similar to that of the bladder, the examiner can indirectly estimate its competence by checking the anal tone on rectal examination and by noting the patient's ability to contract the sphincter voluntarily. Loss of sphincter tone in a patient who retains sensation suggests a motor neuron lesion within the arc.

Perineal sensation is also tested; if it is lacking, yet sacral reflexes are preserved, reflex incontinence from a lesion above the arc is suggested, such as one caused by diabetes, multiple sclerosis, or spinal cord injury. Patients with loss of both sensation and reflexes are likely to have overflow incontinence because of neurologic injury to the reflex arc. Incontinent patients who retain their reflexes and sensation have detrusor instability, stress incontinence, overflow incontinence, or a functional problem.

A mental status examination is usually not necessary to detect underlying dementia in the patient with incontinence; in most cases, the condition is apparent by the time incontinence occurs.

Laboratory Studies. Often, a careful history and examination are sufficient to arrive at a working diagnosis for the patient with lower urinary tract symptomatology. A *urinalysis* and a few simple chemistry studies (*blood urea nitrogen, creatinine,* and *glucose*) are appropriate for most patients. Consider a *serologic test for syphilis* in patients with overflow incontinence. All patients should have a *urinalysis* and possible *culture* to exclude concurrent infection. *Pelvic ultrasonography* offers a noninvasive method of assessing postvoid residual and is especially useful when outflow obstruction or detrusor failure is suspected. *Straight catheterization* after voiding is a simple office technique for determining residual volume, a useful measure when overflow incontinence is in question. A volume over 50 mL is abnormal.

The *cystometrogram* is rarely needed but can help to sort out complicated mixed conditions. Normal persons sense bladder filling between 100 and 200 mL, have a nonurgent desire to void at 250 to 350 mL, and experience detrusor contraction at 400 to 550 mL (Fig. 134.1A). A spastic bladder will demonstrate a small capacity and recurrent uninhibited contraction (Fig. 134.1B). An atonic bladder will show a large volume and little contractile force (Fig. 134.1C).

Measurement of *urine flow* rates provides information on outflow obstruction and aids in monitoring the progression of obstruction. Normal flow rates are 10 mL/sec with more than 200 mL in the bladder. The normal curve (Fig. 134.2A) shows an early peak flow rate, whereas the curve of the obstructed bladder manifests a delayed and reduced flow rate (Fig. 134.2B).

Patients with polyuria should be checked for glycosuria, hypercalcemia, and hypokalemia. Those with normal levels should have their urine-concentrating ability tested; this is accomplished by measuring *urine osmolality* after 8 hours of *fluid restriction* (usually overnight). Normal persons and those with psychogenic polydipsia should be able to concentrate their urine to more than 700 mOsm/L after 8 hours of fluid restriction. Inability to concentrate requires further testing, including measurement of serum osmolality before and after water restriction and parenteral administration of ADH. Direct measurement of ADH may be helpful (see Chapter 101).

MANAGEMENT OF INCONTINENCE

General Measures. Management is best guided by the mechanism(s) responsible for the incontinence, the patient's overall medical and mental status, and the capabilities of the family or caretakers (Table 134.2). However, some general measures apply to all incontinent patients:

- Restrict fluid loads, coffee, tea, and alcohol.
- Limit the use of diuretics, and, if necessary, give them in the morning.
- Anticholinergic drugs for nonurologic purposes should be given with care and in the lowest possible dosages.
- Avoid use of indwelling catheters because of the risk for infection, exacerbation of detrusor instability, and leakage.
- Avoid use of condom catheters, except for short, well-supervised periods.

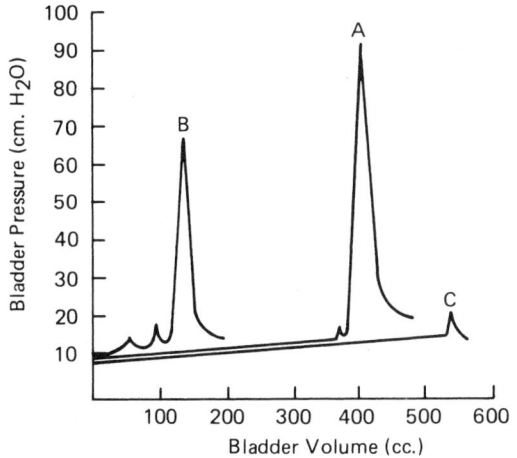

FIG. 134.1. Cystometrogram findings. **A:** Normal pressure–volume relationship. **B:** Uninhibited neurogenic bladder. **C:** Atonic bladder.

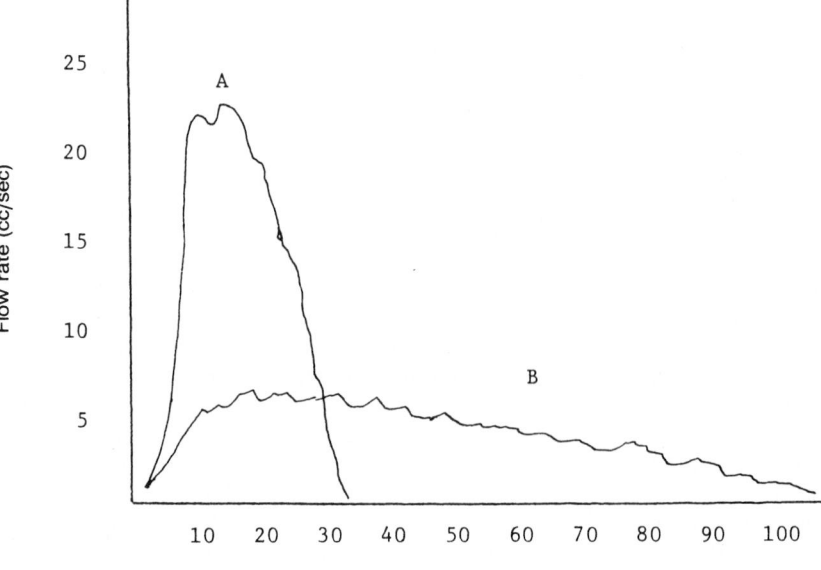

FIG. 134.2. Urinary flow studies. **A:** Normal voiding. **B:** Obstructed voiding. The area under each curve represents the volume voided.

Table 134.2. Drugs Used to Treat Incontinence

DRUGS	DOSAGE RANGE	ACTION	SIDE EFFECTS	POSSIBLE CONTRAINDICATIONS
Detrusor Instability				
Imipramine hydrochloride (Tofranil)	10–25 mg qd to qid	Decreases detrusor and increases internal sphincter tone	Dry mouth, blurred vision, constipation, postural hypotension, palpitations	Anatomic obstruction, cardiac arrhythmias, hyperthyroidism, glaucoma, hepatic or renal disease, pregnancy
Oxybutynin chloride (Ditropan)	2.5–5 mg qd to qid	Decrease detrusor tone	Same	Same
Tolterodine (Detrol)	1–2 mg bid	Selectively decreases detrusor tone	Same	Same
Detrusor Atony				
Bethanechol chloride (Urecholine)	5–25 mg bid to qid	Increases detrusor tone	Salivation, flushing, abdominal cramps, diarrhea, sweating	Anatomic obstruction, asthma, guanethidine peptic ulcer, hyperthyroidism, age
Prazosin (Minipress)	1–5 mg bid to qid	Decreases internal sphincter tone	Light-headedness	Postural hypotension
Doxazosin (Cardura)	2–8 mg qd	Same	Same	Same
Terasozin (Hytrin)	1–2 mg qd	Decreases internal sphincter tone	Same	Same
Tamsulosin (Flomax)	0.4 mg qd to bid	Selectively decreases internal spinchter tone	Same	Possible postural hypotension
Sphincter Incompetency				
Imipramine hydrochloride (Tofranil)	10–25 mg qd to qid	Decreases detrusor and increases internal sphincter tone	See above	See above
Estrogen cream (in women) (Premarin)	qd initially then biw, tiw	Increases internal sphincter tone	Uterine cancer, possibly breast cancer, hypertension, cholelithiasis, glucose intolerance, thromboembolic disease	Uterine or breast malignancy, uterine fibroid tumors
Phenylpropanolamine	25 mg qd to qid	Increases internal sphincter tone	Abdominal distress, insomnia, palpitations, anxiety	Hypertension, hyperthyroidism, glaucoma
Reflex Incontinence				
Prazosin (Minipress)	1–5 mg bid to qid	Decreases internal sphincter tone	See above	See above
Doxazosin (Cardura)	2–8 mg qd	Same	Same	Same
Terazosin (Hytrin)	1–10 mg qd	Same	Same	Same
Tamsulosin (Flomax)	0.4 mg qd to bid	Selectively decreases internal spinchter tone	Same	Possible postural hypotension

- Advise use of an adsorbent pad for patients with refractory symptoms and recommend that it be changed frequently to prevent skin breakdown.
- If long-term indwelling catheterization is unavoidable, the catheter should be inserted only by trained personnel under aseptic conditions, drained with the bag always below the patient's bladder, manipulated as little as possible, irrigated only if flow is reduced, changed if blocked, and removed if upper tract infection is suspected. Antibiotic prophylaxis is not recommended.

Detrusor Instability (Urge Incontinence). Before symptomatic therapy is initiated, one should attend to treatable etiologic factors, such as outflow obstruction or chronic bladder irritation. In most instances, the cause cannot be identified or is not amenable to definitive treatment, so that symptomatic relief becomes the major objective. Much can be done.

- Teach the patient to void at regular, frequent intervals. Patients can learn to suppress the urge to void by contracting pelvic muscles and then relaxing them slowly or by engaging in distracting activities (such as mathematical calculations or conversations). Over time, the intervals can be increased. Sometimes, merely keeping a voiding diary improves urinary control.
- Provide a bedside commode or urinal for the patient.
- Initiate a trial of a tricyclic agent, such as imipramine (10 to 100 mg/d in divided doses).
- Initiate a trial of an agent with both smooth-muscle relaxant and anticholinergic properties, such as oxybutynin (2.5 to 5 mg three times daily). Lower doses can be effective in the elderly, and untoward central nervous system side effects and intolerable dry mouth are thereby avoided. The selective bladder smooth-muscle relaxant tolterodine (1 to 2 mg twice daily) has fewer side effects than oxybutynin and may be better tolerated.

Detrusor Atony (Overflow Incontinence). The first priority is definitive treatment of any mechanical obstruction or reversible neurologic deficit (e.g., herniated disk, vitamin B_{12} deficiency), followed by efforts to reduce the postvoid residual and prevent infection. If a fixed obstruction is present, relief may be sufficient to allow detrusor function to return.

- For both acute and chronic obstruction, place an indwelling catheter or repeatedly catheterize the patient to decompress the bladder.
- If this does not restore bladder function, then teach the patient to void while performing a Credé's maneuver (suprapubic external compression) or Valsalva's maneuver.
- Add an α-blocker such as prazosin (2 to 20 mg/d in divided doses), doxazosin (2 to 8 mg/d), terazosin (1 to 10 mg/d), or tamsulosin (0.4 to 0.8 mg/d) to reduce sphincter resistance.
- Add bethanechol (25 to 125 mg/d in divided doses) to augment bladder contraction.
- Monitor the effects of these agents by checking postvoid residuals; patients with a residual in excess of 300 mL require repeated sterile catheterization on an intermittent basis (three to four times per day).

Sphincter Incompetence (Stress Incontinence). The condition responds well to simple measures, beginning with exercises to strengthen the perineal muscles that terminate the urinary stream. For postmenopausal women, estrogen cream can also help. Surgical approaches are reserved for patients with persistently incapacitating difficulty.

- Instruct the male patient to exercise by voluntarily contracting the anal sphincter slowly 15 times once or twice a day.
- Instruct the female patient in the Kegel exercises.
- For a female patient with evidence of atrophic vaginitis, prescribe a topical estrogen cream (Table 134.2). It should be applied daily for the first 3 weeks and then once or twice weekly thereafter to maintain sufficient estrogen to restore internal sphincter and uretheral tone in postmenopausal women. Continuous use may increase the risk for uterine cancer in women with an intact uterus. This risk can be eliminated with the concurrent use of a progestin (see Chapter 118).
- Prescribe the α-adrenergic agonist phenylpropanolamine (50 to 100 mg/d in divided doses) for patients who need more than exercises. This agent is especially useful in the presence of weakened pelvic muscles and after surgical instrumentation of the urethra. It can be found in most over-the-counter cold remedies but should not be given to patients with hypertension.
- Try a course of imipramine (10 to 100 mg/d in divided doses) for those with symptoms of both bladder irritability and stress incontinence.
- Pessaries come in a variety of shapes and can be successfully fitted to improve continence. They must be changed and cleaned regularly.
- A penile clamp may be necessary in men who do not respond to other measures. Careful monitoring and a competent patient are necessary.

Reflex Incontinence. A major problem is a dyssynergy between bladder contraction and sphincter relaxation that results in ureteral reflux and the potential for hydronephrosis. The bladder needs to be decompressed. An α-adrenergic blocking agent or mechanical maneuvers may help. For frequent urination, the mechanical measures and behavioral techniques are similar to those for detrusor instability.

- In a patient with bladder–sphincter dyssynergy, try pharmacologically decompressing the bladder by giving prazosin (2 to 20 mg/d in divided doses), doxazosin (2 to 8 mg/d), terazosin (1 to 10 mg/d), or tamsulosin (0.4 to 0.8 mg/d).
- Consider an agent used for detrusor instability (see above). A sphincterotomy may be required to ensure bladder emptying.

Functional Incontinence. The prime effort is to ease the patient's access to a urinal, bed pan, or commode. Bedside placement is the obvious solution. For more disabled patients, regular use of absorbent diapers, frequent straight catheterization, or rarely condom or indwelling catheterization can be considered.

PATIENT EDUCATION

Incontinence is hard for both patient and family. The primary care physician must ensure that all understand the problem and its cause so that no one blames the patient for being incontinent. The need to provide palliative relief early in the course of the evaluation makes it important to teach symptomatic measures even before the workup is completed. The use of adult diapers, pads, and scheduled voiding times, plus elimination of xanthine-containing beverages and alcohol and rescheduling of medication intake, can do much to lessen symptoms and the stress on patient, family, and caretakers.

INDICATIONS FOR REFERRAL

The incontinent patient with a suspected cord lesion or other form of neurologic injury should be promptly referred for neurologic consultation. Urologic referral is needed in cases of outflow tract obstruction, especially those severe enough to cause a hypotonic bladder and a large postvoid residual (>100 mL). The risk for ureteral reflux and the development of hydronephrosis makes definitive therapy essential. Women with refractory stress incontinence are candidates for reconstructive surgical efforts; referral should be made to a surgeon experienced with correcting pelvic incompetence. Those with stubborn detrusor instability or hypotonia are potential candidates for biofeedback therapies. Patients with severe sphincter dyssynergy and reflex incontinence may require a sphincterotomy if all else fails.

ANNOTATED BIBLIOGRAPHY

Abrams P, Freeman R, Anderstrom C, et al. Tolterodine, a new antimuscarinic agent: as effective but better tolerated than oxybutynin in patients with an overactive bladder. Br J Urol 1998;81:801. (*Prospective, randomized, controlled trial of 293 men and women with urgency or urge incontinence. Oxybutynin and tolterodine were equally effective, although oxybutynin caused more side effects, mostly dry mouth.*)

Brechtelsbauer DA. Care with an indwelling catheter. Postgrad Med 1992;92:127. (*Addresses the key issues of catheter use in a terse, well-referenced review.*)

Burgio KL, Whitehead WE, Engel BT. Urinary incontinence in the elderly. Bladder–sphincter biofeedback and toilet training skills. Ann Intern Med 1985;104:507. (*A report of encouraging results obtained with behavioral methods.*)

Burgio KL, Locher JL, Goode PS, et al. Behavioral vs. drug treatment for urge urinary incontinence in older women. JAMA 1998;280:1995. (*Behavioral therapy produced an 80.7% reduction in incontinence episodes, in comparison with a 68.5% reduction for drug therapy and a 39.4% reduction for placebo in this randomized, controlled trial.*)

DuBeau CE. Interpreting the effects of common medical conditions on voiding dysfunction in the elderly. Urol Clin North Am 1996;23:11. (*Reviews mechanisms by which common medical conditions affect urinary continence.*)

Fantl JA, Wyman JF, McClish DK, et al. Efficacy of bladder training in older women with urinary incontinence. JAMA 1991;265:609. (*Reduced incontinent episodes by 57% in those with sphincter or detrusor instability.*)

Fantl JA, Cardoza L, McClish DK, and the Hormone and Urogenital Therapy Committee. Obstet Gynecol 1994;83:12. (*Metaanalysis of 166 studies. All forms of estrogen subjectively improve urinary incontinence in women.*)

Hu TW, Igou JF, Kaltreider L, et al. A clinical trial of a behavioral therapy to reduce urinary incontinence in nursing homes. JAMA 1989;261:2656. (*Behavioral methods can be very helpful.*)

Kozoil JA, Clark DC, Gittes RF, et al. The natural history of interstitial cystitis: a survey of 374 patients. J Urol 1993;149:465. (*Symptoms exacerbated by acidic, alcoholic, or carbonated beverages or by tea or coffee in 50%. More than 80% had to restrict their activities.*)

Messing EM, Stamey TA. Interstitial cystitis. Urology 1978;12:381. (*The diagnosis should be considered in women with persistent lower urinary tract symptoms and negative findings on cultures and workup.*)

Ouslander JG, Schnelle JF. Incontinence in the nursing home. Ann Intern Med 1995;122:438. (*Prompted voiding and reminders by caregivers every 2 hours reduce daytime incontinence in up to one third of nursing home patients.*)

Resnick NM, Valla SV, Laurino E. The pathophysiology of urinary incontinence among institutionalized elderly persons. N Engl J Med 1989;320:1. (*Sixty-one percent had detrusor overactivity; 50% had impaired contractility.*)

Resnick NM, Valla SV. Management of urinary incontinence in the elderly. N Engl J Med 1985;313:800. (*Terse, clinically useful review; 71 references.*)

Stern P, Valtin H. Verney was right, but . . . N Engl J Med 1981;305:1581. (*An editorial on the approach to the workup of diabetes insipidus; underscores the pitfalls and problems.*)

Zeitlin MP, Lebherz TB. Pessaries in the geriatric patient. J Am Geriatr Soc 1992;40:635. (*Pessaries are indicated for the control of symptomatic uterine prolapse and should be assessed frequently.*)

135
Approach to the Patient With Nephrolithiasis
LESLIE S.-T. FANG

Nephrolithiasis is a significant medical problem incurring substantial morbidity and cost. One autopsy series estimated the prevalence as 1.12%. In most industrialized countries, 1% to 3% of the population may be expected to have a calculus at some time, and the likelihood that stone disease will develop in a white man by age 70 is about 1 in 8. The annual frequency of hospitalization for nephrolithiasis is estimated at 1 in 1,000 population. The recurrence rate without treatment for calcium oxalate renal stones is about 10% at 1 year, 33% at 5 years, and 50% at 10 years. In the outpatient setting, the primary physician may encounter patients with a history of renal calculi, asymptomatic nephrolithiasis, or acute colic. Others may present with hematuria or urinary tract infection. One needs to identify the nature of the stone and any precipitating factors, prevent further stone formation, and know when referral for surgical intervention or lithotripsy is needed.

PATHOPHYSIOLOGY AND CLINICAL PRESENTATION

Two major groups of factors are important in the pathogenesis of stones: (a) changes that increase the urinary concentration of stone constituents; and (b) physicochemical changes.

Increase in concentration can occur with reductions in urinary volume or increases in the excretion of calcium, oxalate, uric acid, cystine, or xanthine.

Calcium-containing Stones. The majority of calcium-containing stones contain calcium oxalate; hypercalciuric and hyperoxaluric states promote stone formation. In some instances, hyperuricemia also contributes to calcium stone formation.

Hypercalciuric states can be categorized into three groups according to cause: increased gut absorption of dietary calcium, increased resorption of calcium from bone, and the presence of a renal calcium leak. Combinations of these factors can be at play in certain clinical settings. About 50% of patients with calcium stones are found to be hypercalciuric.

Hyperoxaluria is less common than hypercalciuria, but recent studies indicate that up to 30% of patients with calcium oxalate stones are hyperoxaluric. Hyperoxaluria may result from increased absorption of dietary oxalate, as occurs in patients with small-bowel disease; from increased endogenous production of oxalate, as occurs in patients with a genetic deficiency of enzymes in the glyoxalate pathway or of pyridoxine (an important cofactor in glyoxalate metabolism); or, rarely, from markedly increased ingestion of oxalate or one of its precursors.

Some patients with calcium-containing stones may be hyperuricosuric. It is believed that adsorption of glutamic acid onto a uric acid nidus allows for the growth of calcium oxalate crystals.

Magnesium Ammonium Phosphate Stones (Struvite). Struvite formation occurs in an alkaline environment and is almost invariably associated with urinary tract infection produced by a urea-splitting organism.

Uric Acid Stones. Most patients with uric acid stones have persistently acid urine, which decreases the solubility of uric acid. Some patients may be hyperuricosuric. Hyperuricosuric states are seen in patients with a high dietary intake of protein and with primary and secondary gout. In patients who have myeloproliferative disorders or are undergoing chemotherapy, significant hyperuricosuria can occur, and uric acid stones can form if adequate urine flow and alkalinization are not maintained.

Cystine Stones. Cystine stones are found exclusively in patients with cystinuria. These patients have an inherited disorder in which renal and gastrointestinal transport of cystine, ornithine, lysine, and arginine is abnormal.

Xanthine Stones. These occur in the setting of xanthinuria, an extremely rare genetic disorder of purine metabolism associated with a deficiency of xanthine oxidase. Rarely, xanthine stones may be seen in patients taking xanthine oxidase inhibitors for the treatment of uric acid disorders.

Physicochemical factors that have been identified as important in stone formation include changes in urinary pH and urinary concentrations of potential inhibitors of stone formation, such as magnesium, citrate, sulfate, organic matrix, and pyrophosphate. As noted earlier, an alkaline pH facilitates struvite formation, and an acidic pH facilitates the formation of uric acid and xanthine stones.

Magnesium, citrate, pyrophosphate, and certain anions in high urinary concentrations are potent inhibitors of stone formation. Deficiencies in one or more of the inhibitors have been identified in some patients with recurrent stones.

Three major theories have been advanced to explain stone formation and growth. The *matrix nucleation* theory suggests that some matrix substances (e.g., uric acid) form an initial nucleus for subsequent stone growth by precipitation. The *precipitation–crystallization* theory suggests that when the urinary crystalloids are present in a supersaturated state, precipitation and subsequent growth occur. The *inhibitor absence* theory postulates that the deficiency of one or more of numerous agents known to retard stone formation leads to nephrolithiasis. Evidence for and against each of these theories has been advanced; multiple factors may be involved in any patient.

Clinical presentation is one of pain, bleeding, or silent obstruction. *Renal "colic"* is typically a constant unilateral pain, abrupt in onset, localized to the flank when a stone sits in the upper tract and radiating into the groin when a stone lodges in the lower portion of the ureter. The presentation may be mistaken for pyelonephritis and occasionally for abdominal and pelvic processes, but the initial workup should rapidly lead to the correct diagnosis.

Any *obstruction* that occurs is usually transient and of no lasting significance; however, in some instances, it persists and may be silent and progressive. Occasionally, asymptomatic calcareous calculi are detected on abdominal x-rays films taken for other reasons. Calculi extending from one renal calix to another ("staghorn" calculi) can result in significant renal parenchymal damage, particularly in association with infection.

Natural history of stone formation is still a matter of some controversy. The likelihood of *recurrence* of calcium stones with time was examined prospectively in one study of patients in whom single stones formed. An exceedingly high incidence of recurrence was found, with a mean time to recurrence of 6.78 years. With time, the incidence of cumulative recurrence approached 100%. Recurrence appeared early in half of the patients but took up to 20 years in others.

Other studies have found a more benign course. In one, a group of 101 patients was followed for an extended period (mean, 7 years); additional stone formation was observed in only a third of the patients. These differences in recurrence rates undoubtedly reflect heterogeneity among patients in the respective referral groups. In any case, the incidence of recurrence is high enough to justify evaluation and consideration of preventive treatment.

Most kidney stones pass spontaneously; however, 10% to 30% do not and may cause continuing pain, infection, or obstruction.

DIFFERENTIAL DIAGNOSIS

In the United States, about two thirds of all renal calculi are composed of either calcium oxalate or calcium oxalate mixed with calcium phosphate (Table 135.1). Stones of pure uric acid account for about 10%. Struvite or magnesium ammonium phosphate stones occur almost exclusively in patients with urinary tract infections caused by urea-splitting organisms, and they constitute about 9% of all stones analyzed. Other stones occur infrequently and are composed of cystine, xanthine, and silicates.

Table 135.1.   Types of Renal Calculi

Calcium oxalate	58.8%
Calcium phosphate	8.9%
Mixed calcium oxalate and phosphate	11.4%
Uric acid	10.1%
Struvite (magnesium ammonium phosphate)	9.3%
Cystine	0.7%
Miscellaneous	0.8%

The disease states associated with nephrolithiasis are best categorized according to the type of stones formed. In many instances, stone formation is a manifestation of systemic disease (Table 135.2).

WORKUP

In the evaluation of the patient with recurrent nephrolithiasis, knowledge of the stone composition is essential to rational management. Obtaining the stone for analysis is the single most important study; therefore, urine should be strained for stones when renal colic is present. Ideally, studies of the stone should include quantitative chemical analysis in addition to crystallographic examination.

History. When no stone is available for analysis, certain aspects of the clinical history can be helpful in the evaluation. The *age* of the patient at the onset of nephrolithiasis should be obtained because metabolic disorders such as hyperoxaluria, cystinuria, xanthinuria, and renal tubular acidosis are often associated with stones at an early age; idiopathic calcareous nephrolithiasis and primary hyperparathyroidism commonly develop after age 30. The *sex* of the patient can also be helpful; idiopathic nephrolithiasis is common in males, whereas primary hyperparathyroidism is more common in females. A *past history* of stones is invaluable if their composition has been previously determined. Any prior history of systemic illness (e.g., sarcoidosis or cancer) and any prior urinary tract infection should be noted. A *family history* of nephrolithiasis increases the risk for stone disease and may suggest a hereditary metabolic disorder. A careful *dietary history* should also be taken to rule out excessive protein, oxalate, or calcium intake. Consumption of apple juice and grapefruit juice has been associated with an increased risk for stone formation. Consumption of alcoholic beverages is associated with a decreased risk. It is important to check for the use of *drugs* that promote stone formation. Medications that result in an increased risk for stone formation include vitamins A, C, and D, loop diuretics, acetazolamide, ammonium chloride, calcium-containing medications, alkali, and antacids. Medications may increase urinary concentrations of calcium (vitamin D, loop diuretics, calcium-containing medications, ammonium chloride), alter urinary pH (acetazolamide, ammonium chloride, and alkali), or decrease urinary concentrations of inhibitors (ammonium chloride, absorbable antacids, and alkali can decrease urinary citrate concentration).

Physical Examination is not particularly revealing in most cases, but the patient should be checked for evidence of a systemic disease, such as sarcoidosis (lymphadenopathy, organomegaly) or cancer (adenopathy, breast mass, and so forth).

Laboratory Evaluation should include *urinalysis* for determination of pH and an examination of urinary sediment for crystals. An alkaline pH suggests infection with urea-splitting organisms and struvite formation. *Urine culture* is needed. Inability to acidify the urine pH below 5.3 despite systemic acidosis suggests renal tubular acidosis. Serum should be obtained for determination of calcium, uric acid, blood urea nitrogen, and creatinine levels, and a *24-hour urine* should be collected for creatinine, calcium, uric acid, and oxalate.

Repeated determinations of *fasting serum calcium* and *phosphorus* are necessary if primary hyperparathyroidism is suspected. The serum albumin should be determined at the same time because 40% to 45% of the serum calcium is protein-bound. If the serum calcium is elevated and hyperparathyroidism is suspected clinically, the diagnosis can be confirmed by obtaining a simultaneous *parathyroid hormone* determination, which should reveal an inappropriately elevated level (see Chapter 96). If the clinical presentation suggests a rare cause of nephrolithiasis, such as cystinuria or xanthinuria, special 24-hour collections of urine should be sent for study.

Roentgenographic evaluation includes a plain film of the *kidneys, ureter, and bladder* (KUB), and an *IV pyelogram*. The flat-plate radiograph of the abdomen can provide an estimate of renal size and is important in detecting the presence of small, radiopaque stones. Staghorn calculi usually denote magnesium

Table 135.2.   Important Conditions Associated with Nephrolithiasis

Calcium Stones
Increased gastrointestinal calcium absorption
    Primary hyperparathyroidism
    Sarcoidosis
    Vitamin D excess
    Milk–alkali syndrome
    Idiopathic nephrolithiasis

Increased bone calcium resorption
    Primary hyperparathyroidism
    Neoplastic disorders
    Immobilization
    Distal renal tubular acidosis

Renal calcium leak
    Idiopathic hypercalciuria

Hyperoxaluria
    Small-bowel disease
    Enzymatic deficiency
    Pyridoxine deficiency
    Increased ingestion

Magnesium Ammonium Phosphate Stones
Alkaline environment
    Urinary tract infection caused by urea-splitting organism

Uric Acid Stones
Increased uric acid production
    Primary gout
    Secondary gout (myeloproliferative disorder, chemotherapy)

Cystine Stones
Inherited disorder for amino acid transport

Xanthine Stones
Xanthine oxidase deficiency
Use of xanthine oxidase inhibitor

ammonium phosphate or cystine stones. The latter usually have a more laminated appearance. The *IV pyelogram* provides better details of any renal abnormalities that may be present, in addition to the level of the obstruction caused by the renal calculus. *Renal ultrasonography* is useful for detecting hydronephrosis but is not a substitute for the IV pyelogram in the initial workup of urolithiasis.

The laboratory evaluation permits the identification of stones and hyperexcretory states and therefore allows rational therapy.

PRINCIPLES OF MANAGEMENT

Because of the high incidence of stone formation and its attendant morbidity, preventive therapy is indicated in all patients with nephrolithiasis.

In general, maintenance of dilute urine by means of *vigorous fluid therapy* around the clock is beneficial in *all forms of nephrolithiasis*. A number of studies have indicated that the relative probability of a kidney stone forming decreases with urinary volume. Enough fluid to maintain an output of 2 to 3 L of urine needs to be taken daily. In general, 250 mL of fluid should be taken every 4 hours, and 250 mL of fluid should be taken with meals. A high fluid intake has been associated with a 40% reduction in recurrence risk. Specific therapy should be tailored to the type of stones involved.

Calcium-containing Stones. During the past decade, a considerable amount of information has become available to suggest that dietary manipulation is helpful in the management of calcium-containing stones. Increasing evidence has accumulated to indicate that *restriction of dietary protein* is helpful in preventing the formation of calcium-containing stones. Population studies indicate a clear correlation between increased dietary protein and an increased incidence of stone formation. Protein loading in patients results in an increase in urinary excretion of both calcium and uric acid. A high dietary intake of protein also decreases urinary concentrations of inhibitors such as citrate. These metabolic abnormalities are corrected with restriction of dietary protein. *Sodium intake should also be restricted.* Restriction of dietary sodium predictably results in a decrease in urinary calcium excretion. Oxalate is a metabolic end product of glycine, and the bulk of the urinary oxalate is derived from metabolic pathways. However, in some patients, dietary excesses of oxalate can result in hyperoxaluria. These patients would benefit from a *restriction of dietary oxalate. Evidence does not support dietary restriction of calcium.* Calcium restriction results in an increased intestinal absorption of oxalate, which leads to hyperoxaluria in addition to mobilization of calcium from the bone because of a negative calcium balance. Cohort studies have demonstrated an inverse relationship between dietary calcium intake and stone formation. In other words, a high dietary intake of calcium decreases the risk for symptomatic stone disease. However, supplemental calcium intake has been associated with a modest increase (relative risk, 1.20) in stone formation.

Dietary manipulations have been shown to prevent further stone formation. In one series, in which patients with first-time stones were placed on a dietary program, only a 27% recurrence of stones was noted during a 5-year follow-up.

For patients with recurrent stone formation despite dietary therapy, every effort should be made to rule out underlying systemic conditions (Table 135.2) before *drug therapy* is initiated. Patients with underlying primary hyperparathyroidism should be treated surgically when feasible. Drugs that can promote calcium stone formation should be stopped. Patients with sarcoidosis may benefit from steroid therapy.

Thiazides decrease urinary calcium excretion, and hydrochlorothiazide (50 mg once a day) has been found to be effective in *reducing recurrent stone formation*. Primary hyperparathyroidism has to be ruled out before thiazides are given to avoid hypercalcemia.

Patients with *hyperoxaluria* should have their dietary intake of oxalates limited. Tea, rhubarb, and many leafy green vegetables should be avoided. Dietary calcium, on the other hand, should not be severely restricted because severe calcium restriction has been shown to cause increases in the urinary excretion of oxalate. In the rare patient with pyridoxine deficiency, replacement would improve the hyperoxaluric state.

Patients with *hyperuricosuria* benefit from protein restriction and *allopurinol*. Reduction of the urinary uric acid concentration minimizes the likelihood of calcium oxalate crystal growth around acid adsorbed to uric acid. Two randomized trials have shown that stone recurrence rates are lower with allopurinol treatment.

Studies in patients with *no identifiable metabolic disorder* have demonstrated a drastic reduction in new stone formation when patients are given a *thiazide* and *allopurinol*. In one study, six stones formed in 30 such patients, compared with a predicted 31.8 stones, during a 1- to 7-year follow-up period.

In addition to the therapeutic interventions outlined, several other, less well-evaluated modes of therapy have been advocated. Administration of *magnesium oxide* may improve the solubility of urinary oxalate. In patients with documented hypocitraturia, *potassium citrate* may be useful in inhibiting new stone formation. These forms of therapy have not been evaluated with rigorous controlled trials.

Magnesium Ammonium Phosphate Stones. These are often very large and may have to be removed surgically. Acidification of the urine with ascorbic acid, along with a prolonged (often at least 2 months) course of appropriate *antibiotic treatment* to eradicate any *Proteus* urinary tract infection, is essential to prevent recurrences of struvite stones.

Uric Acid Stones. *Hydration* to maintain copious urine flow, *allopurinol* therapy, and *alkalinization* of the urine are the mainstays of therapy. The solubility of uric acid is 100 times higher at pH 7 than at pH 4.5, and every attempt should be made to maintain alkaline urine by giving 100 to 150 mEq of *sodium bicarbonate* every 24 hours in divided doses. In patients with myeloproliferative disorders who are undergoing chemotherapy, the prophylactic use of allopurinol, saline diuresis, and alkalinization should eliminate the incidence of uric acid stone formation.

Cystine Stones. A copious urine flow and urinary pH maintained above 7.5 are important in preventing and dissolving cystine stones. D-Penicillamine has also been shown to be effective, but significant side effects may be encountered.

Xanthine Stones. Limitation of dietary purines, maintenance of urine flow, and maintenance of very high urine pH

(>7.6) minimize difficulties. Prophylactic alkalinization and forced diuresis should be employed in patients with myeloproliferative disorders who are taking xanthine oxidase inhibitors.

INDICATIONS FOR ADMISSION AND REFERRAL

In a patient with renal colic, the need for hospitalization and other interventions is dictated by the clinical presentation. Patients with mild to moderate pain can be managed as outpatients with oral analgesics and instructed to maintain a high fluid intake and urine output around the clock. These patients should be told to strain the urine to retrieve calculi for stone analysis.

Patients with severe pain, nausea, and vomiting require hospitalization for IV hydration and pain control. In these patients, KUB and IV pyelogram are indicated to localize and determine the extent of the obstruction. In the majority of cases, stones will pass spontaneously. Patients with severe symptoms and persistent obstruction beyond 3 to 4 days should be referred for urologic evaluation.

Patients presenting with fever, chills, and symptoms of renal colic require hospitalization and prompt intervention. If the presence of an infection behind an obstructed ureter is indeed confirmed, antibiotic coverage (see Chapter 133) and surgical decompression are mandatory.

Surgical intervention for nephrolithiasis has changed dramatically with the introduction of a number of new techniques; *lithotripsy* and *ureteroscopic interventions* have largely obviated the need for lithotomy in most patients. In lithotripsy, the stone is shattered by subjecting it to focused ultrasonic shock waves, delivered either percutaneously through a nephrostomy or extracorporeally. *Extracorporeal shock wave lithotripsy* is an excellent choice for fragmentation and removal of simple stones in the kidneys and upper ureters. Its very low complication rate and high degree of efficacy are rapidly eliminating the need for surgical lithotomy in the centers where the lithotriptor is available. Because the equipment needed to perform the procedure is expensive and not widely available, *percutaneous ultrasonic lithotripsy* represents an acceptable alternative and may be the preferred initial therapy for upper tract stones lodged in the ureter for more than 4 to 6 weeks. The procedure is also indicated for larger (>2.5 cm) stones. *Ureteroscopic* approaches have allowed basketing of stones that have lodged in the ureters, obviating the need to resort to open lithotomy.

The expense and operator skill required for these technologies limit their availability to regional centers. Patients with documented stones, especially those that are located in the upper tracts and kidney or that cause continuous pain, infection, or obstruction, should be referred to such centers for intervention.

PATIENT EDUCATION

Meticulous care must be taken in giving dietary instructions. Patients should also be instructed regarding how to divide their fluid intake evenly to maintain a dilute urine at all times. As noted previously, a daily fluid intake of 2 to 3 L is needed to help minimize stone formation. Consumption of apple and grapefruit juice has been associated with increased risk, and alcoholic beverages appear to decrease risk. Because there is some evidence that soft drinks acidified solely with phosphoric acid may contribute to stone recurrence, patients might be advised to avoid them. However, most soft drinks also contain citric acid, and the combination appears to have no effect on stone recurrence. Patients who need to alkalinize their urine should be instructed in how to measure urinary pH with litmus test tapes. Long periods of immobilization should be avoided, and appropriate fluid intake should be prescribed if such situations are anticipated.

ANNOTATED BIBLIOGRAPHY

Curhan GC, Willett WC, Rimm EB, et al. Body size and risk of kidney stones. J Am Soc Nephrol 1998;9:1645. (*Body size is associated with risk for stone formation, and the magnitude of risk varies by sex.*)

Curhan GC, Willett WC, Speizer FE, et al. Comparison of dietary calcium with supplemental calcium and other nutrients as factors affecting the risk for kidney stones in women. Ann Intern Med 1997;126:497. (*Intake of dietary calcium was inversely associated with risk for kidney stones, and intake of supplemental calcium was positively associated with risk.*)

Curhan GC, Willett WC, Rimm EB, et al. Prospective study of beverage use and the risk of kidney stones. Am J Epidemiol 1996;143:240. (*Risk decreased with consumption of coffee and alcoholic beverages and increased with consumption of apple juice and grapefruit juice.*)

Curhan GC, Willett WC, Rimm EB, et al. A prospective study of dietary calcium and other nutrients and the risk of symptomatic kidney stones. New Engl J Med 1993;328:833. (*High dietary intake of calcium decreases risk for symptomatic kidney stones.*)

Curhan GC, Willett WC, Rimm EB, et al. Family history and risk of kidney stones. J Am Soc Nephrol 1997;8:1568. (*A family history of kidney stones substantially increases the risk for stone formation.*)

Curhan GC, Rimm EB, Willett WC, et al. Regional variation in nephrolithiasis incidence and prevalence among United States men. J Urol 1994;151:838. (*Those in the Southeast have a moderately greater risk.*)

Curhan GC, Willett WC, Speizer FE, et al. Beverage use and risk for kidney stones in women. Ann Intern Med 1998;128:534. (*Risk is decreased 59% by wine consumption and increased 44% by consumption of grapefruit juice.*)

Goldfarb S. The role of diet in the pathogenesis and therapy of nephrolithiasis. Endocrinol Metab Clin North Am 1990;19:805. (*Excellent review of the various aspects of diet that are important to consider in the patient with nephrolithiasis, including intake of fluid, protein, calcium, oxalate, and sodium.*)

Lingeman JE, Woods J, Toth PD, et al. The role of lithotripsy and its side effects. J Urol 1989;141:793. (*Critical examination of the technology.*)

Madore F, Stampfer MJ, Rimm EB, et al. Nephrolithiasis and risk of hypertension. Am J Hypertens 1998;11:46. (*Prior occurrence of nephrolithiasis increases the risk for subsequent hypertension in men.*)

Madore F, Stampfer MJ, Willett WC, et al. Nephrolithiasis and risk of hypertension in women. Am J Kidney Dis 1998;32:802. (*A history of nephrolithiasis is also associated with an increased risk for subsequent hypertension in women.*)

Menon M, Koul H. Clinical review: calcium oxalate nephrolithiasis. J Clin Endocrinol Metab 1993;74:703. (*An excellent review of the pathogenesis of calcium oxalate stones and management options.*)

Pak CY. Medical prevention of renal stone disease. Nephron 1999;81:60. (*Reviews indications for and effectiveness of medical treatment.*)

Riese RJ, Sakhaee K. Uric acid nephrolithiasis: pathogenesis and treatment. J Urol 1992;148:765. (*A review of the pathogenesis of uric acid stones and an examination of various treatment options, including allopurinol and potassium citrate therapy.*)

Shuster J, Jenkins A, Logan C, et al. Soft drink consumption and urinary stone recurrence: a randomized prevention trial. J Clin Epidemiol 1992;45:911. (*Reduction in consumption of soft drinks reduced risk for stone recurrence.*)

Smith LH. The pathophysiology and medical treatment of urolithiasis. Semin Nephrol 1990;10:31. (*Review of the pathogenesis of stone formation, with emphasis on the medical treatment of stone disease.*)

Wilson DM. Clinical and laboratory evaluation of renal stone patients. Endocrinol Metab Clin North Am 1990;19:773. (*An in-depth review of the available tools for evaluation of the patient with renal stone.*)

136
Approach to the Male Patient with Urethritis
JOHN D. GOODSON

A penile discharge or urethral discomfort may be the presenting manifestation of a sexually transmitted disease (STD) and, as such, requires prompt attention. Nongonococcal urethritis (NGU) has surpassed gonorrhea as the principal cause of urethral symptoms in men and has reached epidemic proportions in sexually active adolescents and college-age persons. It can occur as an isolated infection or in conjunction with gonorrhea or other STDs. Because NGU is fast becoming the most common STD among heterosexuals in the United States and a potential source of female infertility and infant morbidity, the primary physician needs to be especially cognizant of its clinical manifestations, epidemiologic importance, and antibiotic treatment.

PATHOPHYSIOLOGY, CLINICAL PRESENTATION, AND CLINICAL COURSE

Most penile discharges are a consequence of urethral infection or inflammation. Numerous bacterial and nonbacterial organisms can invade its mucosal lining. Organisms causing NGU are characterized by their low levels of tissue invasiveness. In older men, a discharge may result from an inflamed prostate gland or, in rare instances, a tumor.

Gonococcal Urethritis. The typical presentation of symptomatic gonococcal disease is a 2- to 4-day history of dysuria and a thick and purulent penile discharge. The Gram's stain reveals polymorphonuclear leukocytes and gram-negative intracellular diplococci. Systemic gonococcemia develops in approximately 3% of patients, manifested by rash, fever, and polyarthritis (see Chapter 137). *Mixed infections*, involving both gonococci and chlamydiae, occur in up to 20% of patients presenting with gonococcal urethritis. Such patients complain of persistence of symptoms after being effectively treated only for gonorrhea.

Gonococcal urethritis responds well to proper antibiotic therapy, with resolution of symptoms and no sequelae. In men, even untreated disease may resolve spontaneously within a few weeks. An asymptomatic carrier state may ensue, or a chronic low-grade discharge may remain. Stricture is a possible consequence of untreated disease.

Nongonococcal Urethritis. Regardless of etiology, the clinical presentation of NGU is rather stereotypical. Compared with gonococcal urethritis, NGU tends to be an indolent illness of longer duration (e.g., 3 to 4 weeks). Dysuria, if present, is not as severe, and the discharge is less purulent, mucoid, sometimes scanty, or even absent. The urethral Gram's stain shows some neutrophils (by definition >4 cells per high-power field) and, at most, a few mixed extracellular pleomorphic organisms, features that help to distinguish NGU from gonococcal infection. Only 20% of ambiguous Gram's stains (rare extracellular gram-negative diplococci) are shown by subsequent culture to represent gonococcal infection. The absence of neutrophils (<10 cells per high-power field) on analysis of the first 15 to 30 cm^3 of urine or a urine dipstick test negative for leukocyte esterase is highly specific for urethritis (i.e., a negative test result makes infection highly unlikely).

Chlamydia trachomatis infection of the urogenital tract has reached epidemic proportions, with 20% to 50% penetration of some populations. Prevalence is greatest among sexually active adolescents and young adults, especially those under the age of 20 with multiple partners. The condition is also concentrated among poor, inner-city African-Americans. In heterosexual men, urethritis with penile discharge, dysuria, or both is the most common symptomatic clinical presentation, but 25% to 50% may manifest neither symptoms nor leukocytes on urethral swab. Proctitis can develop in homosexual men engaging in receptive anal intercourse.

In untreated cases, symptoms may wax and wane during several weeks. Spontaneous resolution can occur. Complications are rare. Prostatitis and epididymitis have been reported in untreated or poorly treated cases. Epididymitis may also be part of the initial clinical presentation. Chlamydial infection accounts for about half of the cases of epididymitis in the United States.

Female counterparts of chlamydial NGU have been identified, including mucopurulent cervicitis and urethritis (see Chapters 117, 125, and 133). The prevalence of chlamydial infection among female partners of men with chlamydial NGU is very high (almost 70%; see Chapter 125).

Ureaplasma urealyticum has finally been established as a cause of NGU after decades of debate. It accounts for 10% to 40% of NGU cases and is sexually transmitted.

Mycoplasma genitalium invades epithelial cells and has emerged as a common cause of NGU, especially in male homosexual partners. The urethritis is indistinguishable from NGU of other causes. Persistence of symptomatic urethritis after appropriate antibiotic treatment of NGU has been linked to tetracycline-resistant strains. However, most recurrent NGU represents reinfection by an untreated sexual partner rather than infection with a resistant organism.

Trichomonas vaginalis infection is a common cause of vaginitis in women and also an important source of urethritis in men. A 22% urethral prevalence was found among male partners of women with known trichomonal infection and a 6% prevalence among heterosexuals attending a clinic for STD. About 50% of patients are symptomatic and have a discharge on examination. Others have symptoms but no visible discharge. The odds ratio for trichomonal infection in patients with nongonococcal, nonchlamydial urethritis has been found to be 3.8. The condition should be suspected in patients with symptoms but little or no discharge on physical examination.

Reiter's Syndrome The finding of genetic overlap between the histocompatibility antigen HLA-B27 (found in up to 96% of patients vs. 10% of controls) and certain *Klebsiella* and *C. trachomatis* antigens suggests infection in susceptible persons may play a role in the pathogenesis of Reiter's syndrome. It usually presents as urethritis in conjunction with a host of other mucocutaneous and musculoskeletal symptoms. Various combinations of conjunctivitis, iritis, fever, acute asymmetric polyarthritis (see Chapter 146), nonarticular bony pain (e.g., of the heel), circinate balanitis, keratoderma blennorrhagicum, and mucosal ulcerations may be present at any one time. The most characteristic presentation is onset of mild dysuria and a mucopurulent urethral discharge about 2 to 4 weeks after a diarrheal illness or sexual contact. Many patients present first with the urethritis, although involvement of other organ systems is frequently present in subclinical form or develops within a few weeks. Most patients with Reiter's syndrome experience a self-limited illness of 6 to 12 months' duration, although a minority progress to chronic or recurrent symptoms in conjunction with bouts of arthritis.

In older men, prostatic hyperplasia predisposes to obstruction and infection. *Prostatitis* may also represent infectious spread to the prostate. Minor penile discharge may be noted, exacerbated by prostatic massage. Symptoms of urinary outflow obstruction and perineal discomfort may dominate the clinical picture (see Chapters 138 and 139).

DIFFERENTIAL DIAGNOSIS

The differential diagnosis of a penile discharge is traditionally divided into gonococcal and nongonococcal etiologies, with NGU accounting for the majority of cases. Among the causes of NGU are chlamydial, *Ureaplasma,* and trichomonal infections of the urethra, Reiter's syndrome, prostatitis, and urethral malignancy. Chlamydial disease is responsible for about half of cases of NGU. In up to a third of NGU cases, no pathogen is identified. Occasionally, urethral infection with herpes simplex virus or human papillomavirus may be responsible for the problem.

WORKUP

History and Physical Examination

History. The duration and character of the discharge can be informative. Acute onset of a profuse purulent discharge usually suggests gonococcal infection. Several weeks of a more indolent, less profuse, mucoid discharge point toward a nongono-

coccal etiology. However, presentations overlap to some degree, and the history is not sufficient for diagnosis. A blood-tinged discharge raises the question of prostatitis or urethral tumor. Inquiry should be made concerning the number of sexual partners during the past few months and the use or nonuse of barrier contraception (important considerations in assessing risk for chlamydial infection and other STDs). The history is also checked for symptoms of prostatitis (slow stream, perineal discomfort), localized or systemic gonorrheal infection (pharyngitis, proctitis, arthritis, punctate skin lesions, sepsis), and Reiter's syndrome (polyarthritis, dermatitis, conjunctivitis, bony pain). Any history of penile warts or herpes simplex viral infection should be noted, as should sexual contact with a partner known to have had trichomonal infection.

Physical Examination. The temperature is taken and the integument carefully examined for signs of gonococcemia (fever; punctate, centrally hemorrhagic, necrotic skin lesions; tenosynovitis; polyarthritis). Similarly, manifestations of Reiter's syndrome are sought, including conjunctivitis, iritis, oral or meatal mucosal ulcerations, circinate balanitis (ulceration and erythema on the penile glans), keratoderma blennorrhagicum (pustular or hyperkeratotic lesions on the soles of the feet), inflamed joints (knees, ankles, sacroiliac joints), and nonarticular bone pain (especially of the heel). The urethral meatus is examined for herpetic lesions and warts, the epididymis is palpated for tenderness and swelling, and the prostate for enlargement, bogginess, and tenderness. An acutely inflamed prostate should be examined very gingerly because abscess is a possible concomitant.

Laboratory Studies

Gram's Stain of the urethral discharge should be the first study performed because it helps to distinguish gonococcal from nongonococcal disease. Even if no visible discharge is present, a swab is gently inserted into the urethral meatus and a sample obtained. A first morning sample before urination or one several hours after urination offers the best yield. Some of the sample is plated onto Thayer-Martin medium for culture of *Neisseria gonorrhoeae* (see Chapter 137), and the remainder is placed on a glass slide and Gram's-stained. The finding of polymorphonuclear leukocytes with gram-negative intracellular diplococci is highly predictive of gonococcal urethritis. The sensitivity and specificity of the Gram's stain exceed 95%. Four or more polymorphonuclear leukocytes per high-power field and mixed gram-negative and gram-positive pleomorphic extracellular organisms or leukocytes with no visible organisms are indicative of NGU. If no definite gram-negative intracellular diplococci are seen on Gram's stain, then a tentative diagnosis of NGU is appropriate. The diagnosis is confirmed by a negative gonococcal culture. Alternative testing for *N. gonorrhoeae* urethral infection is available with DNA probes or DNA amplification techniques (see Chapter 137); the latter has been approved for urine testing. Both techniques are useful for diagnosing pharyngeal or rectal infection.

Chlamydial Testing. It is not practical to culture for *Chlamydia* or *Ureaplasma* because of the expense, technical difficulty, and 2 to 3 days required to obtain results. However, antigen detection methods provide more rapid, less expensive detection of chlamydial infection. At the time an intraurethral swab is obtained for Gram's stain, a second swabbing should also be performed and the specimen saved for chlamydial testing. Such testing can be valuable, even if the patient is going to be treated presumptively for chlamydial infection, because the information thus obtained often helps to improve compliance, facilitate counseling, and guide care if symptoms persist. Patients with a presumptive diagnosis of gonorrhea may also benefit from chlamydial testing because both infections can exist concurrently.

Direct fluorescent antibody staining of urethral smears and *enzyme immunoassay* of secretions are the antigen detection methods most widely available. The former is more sensitive and specific; the latter is cheaper and better suited for laboratories that process large numbers of specimens. They are the preferred chlamydial testing methods for men with symptomatic urethritis. Sensitivity exceeds 70% and specificity approaches 99% in symptomatic men. Sensitivity is enhanced by obtaining a specimen several hours after the last urination. Enzyme immunoassay may give a false-positive result if lower urinary tract infection is present, which makes the test less useful in older men with prostatic disease. Test results are available within 36 to 72 hours. If posttreatment testing is desired, it should not be performed until 3 weeks after completion of treatment—sufficient time for clearing of antigen. *Rapid chlamydial testing* kits are packaged for office use and provide results within 30 minutes. They too make use of antigen detection methods and are subject to the same false-positive results. In addition, quality control problems arise because of the relatively unskilled persons performing the test.

DNA amplification tests based on ligase or polymerase chain reactions have proved reliable and predictive. These tests are 15% to 35% more sensitive then other nonculture urethral testing techniques and have better than 99% specificity.

Other Studies. When routine cultures and Gram's stains are not diagnostic and an empiric trial of treatment for NGU is unsuccessful (see below), then reevaluation and consideration of culturing for *Ureaplasma* or *trichomonads* may be appropriate. When Reiter's syndrome is suspected clinically, the patient can be checked for the presence of the *HLA-B27* histocompatibility antigen. However, its presence is not diagnostic of Reiter's syndrome, nor does its absence rule out the condition. Bloody discharge warrants referral to the urologist for consideration of *cystoscopy*.

MANAGEMENT OF NONGONOCOCCAL URETHRITIS

Because chlamydial infection accounts for 50% of NGU cases, ranks as the most common STD among heterosexuals in the United States, and represents a potential source of morbidity to female partners and their infants, all patients with NGU should be treated, regardless of whether definite identification of *Chlamydia* has been achieved. Female partners of NGU patients should be tested; if testing is not available, they too should be treated for presumptive chlamydial infection. Male homosexual partners should be tested. Empiric treatment of asymptomatic male homosexual partners is not recommended because of the reduced incidence of *Chlamydia* infection in this population.

Initial Treatment. The Centers for Disease Control and Prevention recommendation for the treatment of NGU is *doxycy-* *cline* (100 mg twice daily for 7 days) or *azithromycin* (1 g orally in a single dose). Although expensive, azithromycin provides greatly enhanced ease of use and compliance. Pregnant patients and others who should not take doxycycline or azithromycin can be treated with *erythromycin base* (500 mg four times daily for 7 days; erythromycin estolate is contraindicated in pregnancy). These antibiotic regimens are usually also effective against *Ureaplasma*. *Ofloxacin* (300 mg twice daily for 7 days) is also effective for the treatment of NGU, with excellent activity against both *Chlamydia* and *Ureaplasma*. It is superior to other fluoroquinolone antibiotics for the treatment of NGU and has also proved effective against *N. gonorrhoeae* (see Chapter 137). Cost is high. *Minocycline*, a once-a-day tetracycline, appears as effective as doxycycline. At a dose of 100 mg/d, vestibular toxicity is uncommon.

Management of Recurrent Nongonococcal Urethritis. Although most patients with NGU experience resolution of symptoms with onset of therapy, up to 30% relapse. Some relapses have been attributed to tetracycline-resistant strains of *Ureaplasma* and others to poor compliance with medication, reinfection, or the presence of prostatitis. Because *erythromycin* is effective against tetracycline-resistant strains of *Ureaplasma* and penetrates the prostate well, it has been used as a 3-week treatment program (500 mg four times daily) for recurrent disease. Such a regimen is particularly useful for patients with NGU caused by prostatitis. However, one should confirm the presence of prostatitis (see Chapter 139) and also evaluate for reinfection before resorting to empiric antibiotics. *Chlamydia* and *Trichomonas* are often found in patients with recurrent disease. If the latter is found, treatment with *metronidazole* (2.0 g as a single dose or 250 mg three times daily for 1 week) may prove useful. Endoscopic urethral examination in search of intrinsic urethral pathology is of low yield and not recommended in patients with recurrent NGU.

Treatment of Reiter's Syndrome. Treatment for *Chlamydia* may shorten the duration of illness and prevent recurrences in patients who appear to have the illness on the basis of sexually transmitted chlamydial infection.

Treatment of Gonococcal Urethritis. See Chapter 137.

PATIENT EDUCATION

The most important message to patients is the importance of prevention through the use of condoms. In addition, successful treatment of the disease requires contacting and treating recent sexual partners. The asymptomatic sexual partner is an important reservoir for reinfection. Treated male patients should be told to return for follow-up evaluation if symptoms return. Female partners should undergo retesting after 3 weeks to ensure eradication of chlamydial infection. No firm data are available concerning abstinence from unprotected intercourse during the treatment period, but it seems reasonable to suggest at least 7 days of treatment before sexual activity is resumed.

RECOMMENDATIONS

- Inquire into the number of sexual partners during the past few months and use or nonuse of barrier contraception.
- Check for symptoms of prostatitis, gonorrheal infection, and

Reiter's syndrome and for reports of penile warts, herpes simplex viral infection, and sexual contact with a partner known to have had trichomonal infection.

- Measure the temperature and examine for signs of gonococcemia and Reiter's syndrome. Also check the urethral meatus for herpetic lesions and warts and the testes and prostate for signs of epididymitis and prostatitis, respectively.
- Obtain a urethral swab for Gram's stain and for plating onto Thayer-Martin medium for culture of *Neisseria gonorrhoeae*.
- Obtain a second swabbing for chlamydial antigen detection, either by *direct fluorescent antibody* staining or *enzyme immunoassay*.
- Alternatively, send the second swab for *DNA amplification testing*, which is more sensitive and specific.
- Test female partners of NGU patients; if testing is not available, treat them empirically for presumptive chlamydial infection. Male homosexual partners should also be tested but not treated empirically.
- When routine cultures and Gram's stains are not diagnostic and an empiric trial of treatment for NGU is unsuccessful (see below), then reevaluate and consider culturing for *Ureaplasma* or *trichomonads*.
- Treat all patients with NGU for chlamydial infection, regardless of whether definite identification of *Chlamydia* has been achieved. Test nonetheless because the information often helps to improve compliance, facilitate counseling, and guide care if symptoms persist.
- Treat NGU initially with *doxycycline* (100 mg twice daily for 7 days) or *azithromycin* (1 g orally in a single dose).
- Treat documented NGU recurrences with *erythromycin* (500 mg four times daily for 3 weeks).

ANNOTATED BIBLIOGRAPHY

Centers for Disease Control and Prevention. 1998 Guidelines for treatment of sexually transmitted diseases. MMWR Morb Mortal Wkly Rep 1998;47:1. (*Excellent review of diagnostic methods and authoritative guidelines for treatment; essential reading.*)

Hooton TM, Wong ES, Barnes RC, et al. Erythromycin for persistent or recurrent nongonococcal urethritis. Ann Intern Med 1990; 113:21. (*A 3-week course of treatment proved beneficial, especially in those with prostatitis.*)

Jacobs NJ, Kraus SJ. Gonococcal and nongonococcal urethritis in men. Ann Intern Med 1975;82:7. (*Sensitivity of Gram's stain was 97%, and specificity was 98% for diagnosis of gonococcal urethritis; 21% of specimens that were equivocal on staining were positive for gonococci on culture.*)

Krieger JN, Jenny C, Verdon M, et al. Clinical manifestations of trichomoniasis in men. Ann Intern Med 1993;118:844. (*Found to be a cause of urethritis and sexually transmitted.*)

Marrazzo JM, White CL, Krekeler B, et al. Community-based urine screening for *Chlamydia trachomatis* with a ligase chain reaction assay. Ann Intern Med 1997;127:796. (*Risk factors for male chlamydial infection: being nonwhite, having had two or more sexual partners in previous two months, not using a condom. The positive predictive value of urinary leukocyte esterase testing was 38.4%; the negative predictive value was 97.7%.*)

Martin DH, Pollack S, Kuo CC. *Chlamydia trachomatis* infections in men with Reiter's syndrome. Ann Intern Med 1984;100:207. (*Documents infection and an exaggerated immune response in some patients in whom Reiter's syndrome later develops.*)

Schwartz MA, Hooton TM. Etiology of nongonococcal nonchlamydial urethritis. Sex Transm Dis 1998;16:72. (*Most nonspecific urethritis is caused by organisms other than* Chlamydia, *such as* Ureaplasma urealyticum, Mycoplasma genitalium, *and* Trichomonas vaginalis.)

Stamm WE. Diagnosis of *Chlamydia trachomatis* genitourinary infections. Ann Intern Med 1988;108:710. (*Excellent review, with very useful discussion of clinical findings, culture, and antigen methods; 93 references.*)

Stamm WE, Hicks CB, Martin DH, et al. Azithromycin for empiric treatment of the nongonococcal urethritis syndrome in men. JAMA 1995;274:545. (*Cure rates for* Chlamydia *infection were 83% for single-dose azithromycin and 90% for 7 days of doxycycline.* Ureaplasma *cure rates were 45% and 47%, respectively.*)

Stamm WE, Koutsky LA, Benedetti JK, et al. *Chlamydia trachomatis* urethral infections in men. Ann Intern Med 1984;100:47. (*Details prevalence, risk factors, and clinical manifestations.*)

Taylor-Robinson D, McCormack WM. The genital mycoplasmas. N Engl J Med 1980;302:1003. (*A comprehensive two-part review detailing the role of* Ureaplasma *infection in nongonococcal urethritis and other genital infections.*)

Wong ES, Hooton TM, Hill CC, et al. Clinical and microbiological features of persistent or recurrent nongonococcal urethritis in men. J Infect Dis 1988;158:1098. (*Noncompliance and reinfection were the main causes;* Chlamydia *and* Trichomonas *were often found.*)

137

Approach to the Patient with Gonorrhea

BENJAMIN DAVIS
HARVEY B. SIMON

Like other sexually transmitted diseases, gonorrhea remains a major public health problem in the United States. Although penicillinase-producing strains have become increasingly prevalent, antibiotic resistance cannot be blamed for the failure to control gonorrhea. In fact, excellent alternative drugs are available. Rather, the continued spread of gonorrhea represents the failure of "safe sex" programs to influence human behavior. Theoretically, primary prevention could control this age-old infection, but 1 million cases of gonorrhea are reported each year in the United States. Because of underreporting, it can be safely estimated that at least 3 million cases occur annually. Gonorrhea is most prevalent among teenagers and young adults, especially those belonging to minority groups and dwelling in the inner city; however, the infection crosses all age and socioeconomic barriers.

The great majority of patients with venereal disease present to an ambulatory care facility and should be diagnosed and treated in this setting. At the same time, the physician must be alert to serious systemic complications requiring hospitalization. In addition, patient education is critical to prevent inadequate treatment and recurrent infections. Finally, the responsibility of the physician must extend beyond the diagnosis and treatment of an individual patient to the identification and treatment of sexual contacts who may otherwise harbor and further disseminate these infections.

PATHOPHYSIOLOGY AND CLINICAL PRESENTATION

Gonococcal infection invariably begins with the direct infection of a mucosal surface during sexual activity. Organisms may then gain access to the bloodstream to produce bacteremia and systemic spread of infection. This is most common in women, especially at the time of menstruation, but it occurs in men also. The clinical features of gonorrhea differ greatly between the sexes. Moreover, symptoms of the primary gonococcal infection may be absent or mistaken for those of another condition, making the diagnosis more difficult.

In men, clinical symptoms usually follow within 2 to 10 days of sexual exposure. The risk that a man will acquire gonorrhea after a single exposure to an infected partner is approximately 35%. Absence of symptoms does not indicate absence of infection. Indeed, up to 10% of infected men are asymptomatic carriers of the gonococcus and are fully capable of transmitting the disease. In men, gonorrhea is principally an infection of the anterior urethra, and hence the major symptom is purulent *urethral discharge*, often accompanied by urinary frequency and dysuria. Although spread of infection to the *prostate* or *epididymis* is uncommon in the antibiotic era, gonococci occasionally gain entry into the *bloodstream* to produce disseminated infection.

In women, the *cervix* is the favored site of gonococcal infection. However, up to 25% of women with gonococcal infection are asymptomatic and must be identified through epidemiologic case finding. When symptoms do occur, cervical discharge is most common. Although the vagina is usually spared, the gonococcal infection may spread downward from the cervix to produce *urethritis*, which presents as dysuria and frequency. Infection of *Bartholin's glands* presents as labial swelling and pain, and rectal infection presents as anorectal discomfort. If, on the other hand, gonococcal infection spreads upward from the cervix, more serious processes may develop. Such upward spread is particularly likely at the time of menstruation and can produce a variety of syndromes. Gonococcal *endometritis* can cause pelvic pain and abnormal vaginal bleeding, whereas *salpingitis* characteristically leads to fever, chills, leukocytosis, and a tender adnexal mass. Both systemic and pelvic signs and symptoms are even more pronounced in frank *pelvic peritonitis*, and further intraperitoneal spread may produce gonococcal *perihepatitis* with right upper quadrant pain and tenderness.

Primary extragenital infections are being encountered more frequently as a result of changing sexual practices. Gonococcal infection of the pharynx is usually asymptomatic but can present as an acute *exudative pharyngitis*, with fever and cervical lymphadenopathy. Gonococcal *proctitis* is also most often asymptomatic but can present as proctitis with anorectal discomfort, tenesmus, or rectal bleeding and discharge.

Gonococcal bacteremia is manifested by the *"dermatitis–arthritis" syndrome*. Patients have fever, chills, and other constitutional symptoms. Skin lesions are an important clue to diagnosis; these are typically pustular, hemorrhagic, or papular, are few in number, and tend to be most common on the distal extremities. *Tenosynovitis*, especially involving the extensor surfaces of the hands and feet, and *migratory polyarthritis* are typically seen. During the early stage of systemic infection, blood cultures are often positive, but joint cultures are characteristically negative. Later in the course of untreated disease, however, gonococci can produce frank *septic arthritis*. Such patients have less fever, no skin lesions, and negative blood cultures but more impressive joint swelling and pain, often with purulent synovial fluid in which gonococci can be demonstrated by Gram's stain or culture. In rare instances, gonococci can produce *osteomyelitis* or even life-threatening bacterial *meningitis* or *endocarditis*.

DIFFERENTIAL DIAGNOSIS

The organisms besides *Neisseria gonorrhoeae* capable of producing female genital infections include *Chlamydia, Gardnerella, Trichomonas,* and *Candida* (see Chapter 117). The differential diagnosis of gonococcal salpingitis and peritonitis mainly encompasses the causes of nongonococcal pelvic inflammatory disease (see Chapter 116), but other conditions, such as appendicitis, ectopic pregnancy, hemorrhagic ovarian cysts, and endometriosis, can produce similar clinical findings and often require urgent therapy very different from that of pelvic inflammatory disease. In the male patient, the causes of nongonococcal urethritis enter the differential diagnosis (see Chapter 136). Gonococcal infection also needs to be considered among the causes of pharyngitis (see Chapter 220) and proctitis (see Chapter 66).

WORKUP

History and Physical Examination. The diagnosis of gonorrhea requires a high index of suspicion and a careful *sexual history*. Physical examination findings in men with urethritis are usually normal except for purulent *urethral discharge*. In asymptomatic women, the physical examination findings are normal, but *cervicitis* may produce cervical inflammation, discharge, and marked cervical tenderness. *Adnexal tenderness* and fullness are signs of salpingitis and may be unilateral or bilateral in women with gonorrhea. Tubal abscesses may be suspected because of a palpable mass, and rebound tenderness is a sign of pelvic peritonitis.

Pelvic inflammatory disease caused by organisms other than the gonococcus may present similarly. Clinical features favoring the gonococcus include purulent cervical discharge, onset early in the menstrual cycle, no previous history of pelvic inflammatory disease, and exposure to a male partner with urethritis.

Laboratory Studies. A properly performed *Gram's stain* of the urethral discharge can be a highly reliable diagnostic tool. A Gram's stain is considered "positive" when biscuit-shaped gram-negative diplococci are seen within polymorphonuclear leukocytes, "equivocal" if diplococci are only extracellular or if intracellular organisms are morphologically atypical, and "negative" if no diplococci are found. Sensitivity of the Gram's stain is more than 95% in symptomatic men but declines to 50% to 60% in those with asymptomatic urethral infection. Gram's stains are much less reliable in cervical, rectal, and pharyngeal infections.

Cultures confirming the diagnosis of gonorrhea are mandatory in both sexes. *N. gonorrhoeae* is a fragile and fastidious organism that requires special handling in the laboratory. The gonococcus is readily killed by drying, so all cultures must be plated promptly. Ideally, this should be done by the physician at the time of examination by streaking the swab across the surface of the culture medium in a *Z*-shaped pattern. Special culture media must be used. Although chocolate agar has been the traditional medium used, a modified *Thayer-Martin medium* is preferred for specimens obtained from genital, anal, or pharyngeal sites because the addition of antibiotics to this medium suppresses the growth of nonpathogenic *Neisseria* species and other bacteria. The culture medium should be at room temperature at the time of inoculation. Because the gonococcus requires a high carbon dioxide concentration to grow, cultures should be promptly incubated in a candle jar or carbon dioxide incubator. When this is not possible, the cultures should be planted on modified Thayer-Martin medium in bottles with a 10% carbon dioxide atmosphere. These bottles should be kept capped until the moment of inoculation and should be held in an upright position when open to prevent the loss of carbon dioxide, which is heavier than air.

In the male patient, cultures of the anterior *urethra suffice* unless homosexual contacts are suspected, in which case cultures of the anal canal and pharynx are also indicated. In the female patient, the *endocervix* should be cultured by inserting a swab into the cervical os through a speculum that has been lubricated only with water. In all women, *rectal* cultures are indicated because rectal infection can result simply through direct spread from the genital tract. When pharyngitis is suspected, *throat* culture is mandatory. When acute arthritis is present, *joint fluid* should be obtained by arthrocentesis and should be evaluated with cell counts, Gram's stain, and culture. *Blood* cultures are indicated in patients with fever, skin lesions, and tenosynovitis or arthritis.

PRINCIPLES OF MANAGEMENT AND THERAPEUTIC RECOMMENDATIONS

Overcoming Penicillin Resistance. The therapy of gonorrhea has undergone dramatic changes during the past 40 years. Penicillin has been used for decades, but during this time penicillin resistance has increased steadily. The recommended dosages of penicillin are 30 times greater than those initially used with success in 1943. Until recently, penicillin resistance was just a matter of degree because it was based on chromosomal mutations that decreased the permeability of the cell wall to penicillin and other antibiotics. Simply increasing the dosage of penicillin sufficed.

Another form of penicillin resistance was recognized in 1975, when gonococcal strains were isolated that resisted the effects of even massive doses of penicillin by producing penicillinase. These strains were found to contain plasmids that produce β-lactamase. In the United States, infections with plasmid-containing strains were initially sporadic, but the number of such infections has increased dramatically and is no longer limited to a few groups of patients. More recently, very high-level, chromosomally mediated penicillin resistance has emerged. In all, about 5% of gonococcal strains are penicillin-resistant. A significant number of clinical isolates are also tetracycline-resistant, and heavy use of spectinomycin has led to emergence of strains resistant to that agent.

Unless the isolate is proven to be penicillin-sensitive, a regimen effective for resistant strains should be used. When possible, drugs that are also effective against syphilis are preferred. Because of problems with patient compliance, single-dose regimens are recommended. The parenterally administered *ceftriaxone* and the orally administered *cefixime* presently meet these requirements.

Concurrent Infection. In addition to the problem of antibiotic resistance, the management of gonorrhea is complicated by the need to treat coexisting sexually transmitted infections. Chlamydial disease is of greatest concern, coexisting with gonococcal infection in up to 20% of men and 50% of women with sexually transmitted disease. As a result, all patients with gonorrhea should also be treated for chlamydial infection. Although much less common than chlamydial infection, incubating syphilis can be a more serious problem, and patients should be screened for syphilis (see Chapters 124 and 117). Confidential testing for HIV infection may be of benefit not only for case identification, but also for promotion of safer sexual practices (see below).

THERAPEUTIC RECOMMENDATIONS

Uncomplicated Gonorrhea (Including Urethral, Cervical, and Rectal Infection)

- Prescribe ceftriaxone (125 mg IM once), cefixime (400 mg PO once), ciprofloxacin (500 mg PO once), or ofloxacin (400 mg PO once) *plus* azithromycin (1 g PO once) or doxycycline (100 mg twice daily for 7 days).
- Prescribe spectinomycin (2 g IM once) for patients who are allergic to β-lactam antibiotics (i.e., cephalosporins and penicillins) or who cannot take fluoroquinolones (e.g., pregnant women).
- Prescribe erythromycin base (500 mg four times daily for 7 days) for patients who cannot take doxycycline (e.g., pregnant women and those allergic to the drug).

Disseminated Gonococcal Infection

- Hospitalize initially and begin *ceftriaxone* (1 g IV or IM every 24 hours for 7 days).
- Treat with higher doses for a more prolonged period if meningitis, endocarditis, or osteomyelitis is present.
- Treat with *spectinomycin* (2 g IM every 12 hours for 7 days) those persons who are allergic to β-lactam antibiotics.
- Discharge those who respond well to the initial 1 to 2 days of parenteral therapy, provided they return daily for IM ceftriaxone or complete a week of oral therapy with *ciprofloxacin* (500 mg twice daily).
- Treat also for chlamydial infection, as in uncomplicated disease.

Monitoring

Because treatment failures with ceftriaxone–doxycycline are rare, immediate *follow-up cultures* are not mandatory. It may be more cost-effective to delay repeated evaluation with cultures until 1 to 2 months have passed. This allows detection of reinfection and treatment failures and reinforcement of patient education. Patients treated with regimens other than ceftriaxone–doxycycline do require follow-up cultures 4 to 7 days after therapy has been completed.

All patients with gonorrhea should undergo *serologic testing for syphilis*. Seronegative patients treated with ceftriaxone do not require follow-up serologies because this regimen is effective for incubating syphilis. However, patients receiving other antibiotic regimens do require repeated serologic testing in 3 months. All patients with gonorrhea should be offered confidential *testing for HIV* infection. All gonorrhea cases should be reported to the appropriate local health department. Because many patients are asymptomatic, vigorous case finding represents the only present means of controlling this epidemic.

PATIENT EDUCATION AND PREVENTION

Health education about the prevention of sexually transmitted disease is extremely important. Properly used barrier methods of contraception are effective means of preventing gonorrhea. *Condoms* do not permit transmission of the gonococcus or *Chlamydia*. The diaphragm or contraceptive sponge may also offer some protection against gonorrhea and chlamydial infection, especially when used with a *vaginal spermicide* containing nonoxynol 9, the active ingredient in many preparations. However, diaphragms and sponges *do not reduce the risk for HIV transmission*.

Preventive measures also include attention to *partner notification*. Patients should be encouraged to notify their sexual partners of their exposure and encourage them to seek medical care. This is *patient referral*. If patients are unwilling or unable to notify their partners, then the assistance of state and local departments of public health can be enlisted. This is *provider referral*.

INDICATIONS FOR ADMISSION

Patients with disseminated disease who are febrile, who are unreliable, or who have evidence of osteomyelitis, endocarditis, or meningitis must be hospitalized. The same is true of the woman with pelvic inflammatory disease who appears toxic, pregnant, or unlikely to comply, or who has pelvic pain of unclear etiology in association with peritoneal signs.

ANNOTATED BIBLIOGRAPHY

Allen S, Serufilira A, Bogaerts J, et al. Confidential HIV testing and condom promotion in Africa: impact on HIV and gonorrhea rates. JAMA 1992;268:3338. (*Condom use went up 300%, and the prevalence of gonorrhea fell by more than half.*)

Centers for Disease Control and Prevention. Sexually transmitted diseases treatment guidelines. MMWR Morb Mortal Wkly Rep 1989;38[Suppl 8]:1. (*Expert committee consensus recommendations.*)

Faro S, Martens MG, Maccato M, et al. Effectiveness of ofloxacin in the treatment of *Chlamydia trachomatis* and *Neisseria gonorrhoeae* cervical infection. Am J Obstet Gynecol 1991;164:1380. (*Proved effective for both organisms.*)

Handsfield HH, Lipman TO, Harnisch JP, et al. Asymptomatic gonorrhea in men. N Engl J Med 1974;290:117. (*Asymptomatic men may be an important reservoir of infection; all sexual contacts should be cultured, whether male or female and whether symptomatic or not.*)

Handsfield HH, McCormack WM, Hook EW, et al. A comparison of single-dose cefixime with ceftriaxone as treatment for uncomplicated gonorrhea. N Engl J Med 1991;325:1337. (*Oral cefixime produced results equivalent to those obtained with parenterally administered ceftriaxone.*)

Hook EW, Holmes KK. Gonococcal infections. Ann Intern Med 1985;102:229. (*Highly recommended authoritative review; 157 references.*)

Hutt DM, Judson FN. Epidemiology and treatment of oropharyngeal gonorrhea. Ann Intern Med 1986;104:655. (*Not to be forgotten as a cause of severe pharyngitis.*)

Jick H, Hannan MT, Stergachis A, et al. Vaginal spermicides and gonorrhea. JAMA 1982;248:1619. (*Suggests a protective effect against gonorrhea.*)

Judson FN. Management of antibiotic-resistant *Neisseria gonorrhoeae*. Ann Intern Med 1989;110:5. (*An editorial that succinctly reviews the options.*)

Kelaghan J, Rubin GL, Ory HW, et al. Barrier-method contraceptives and pelvic inflammatory disease. JAMA 1982;248:184. (*A relative risk of 0.6 for women using barrier methods.*)

Klein EJ, Fisher LS, Chow AW, et al. Anorectal gonococcal infection. Ann Intern Med 1977;86:340. (*A clinical review of such infections in women and male homosexuals.*)

Kreiss J, Ngugi E, Holmes K, et al. Efficacy of nonoxynol 9 contraceptive sponge use in preventing heterosexual acquisition of HIV in Nairobi prostitutes. JAMA 1992;268:447. (*Rate of gonococcal infection was reduced by 60%, although risk for HIV infection increased by 60%.*)

O'Brien JP, Goldenberg DL, Rice PA. Disseminated gonococcal infection: a prospective analysis of 49 patients and a review of pathophysiology and immune mechanisms. Medicine 1983;62:395. (*A comprehensive study of 49 patients and review of the literature.*)

Phillips RS, Safran C, Aronson M, et al. Should women be tested for gonococcal infection of the cervix during routine gynecologic visits? An economic appraisal. Am J Med 1989;86:297. (*This decision-analysis study suggests the answer is yes in high-risk persons.*)

Platt R, Rice PA, McCormack WM. Risk of acquiring gonorrhea and prevalence of abnormal adnexal findings among women recently exposed to gonorrhea. JAMA 1983;250:3205. (*Risk was 50%, 86%, and 100% for one, two, and more than two exposures, respectively; spread in the upper genital tract was a common early complication.*)

Schwarcz SK, Zenilman JM, Schnell D. National surveillance of antimicrobial resistance in *Neisseria gonorrhoeae*. JAMA 1990;264:1413. (*Twenty-one percent found resistant to penicillin, tetracycline, cefoxitin, or spectinomycin; all sensitive to ceftriaxone.*)

138

Approach to Benign Prostatic Hyperplasia

MICHAEL J. BARRY
JOHN D. GOODSON

Benign prostatic hyperplasia (BPH) is a common condition among older men, causing morbidity primarily through lower urinary tract symptoms. The primary physician should attempt to distinguish BPH from the other causes of such symptoms, objectively determine symptom severity, and, when the symptoms are bothersome enough, design a therapeutic approach that offers symptomatic improvement. For patients who elect a course of "watchful waiting" or medical therapy, a strategy of regular follow-up visits should be instituted to monitor for symptom changes or BPH complications. The treatment of BPH has changed substantially in recent years, with increasing emphasis on nonsurgical approaches. The result is an expanded role for primary care providers in BPH management.

PATHOPHYSIOLOGY AND CLINICAL PRESENTATION

Pathophysiology. BPH arises from *nodular hyperplasia* of prostatic stromal and glandular elements. Growth begins in the *periurethral* glandular tissue. As these nodules expand and coalesce over years, the true prostatic tissue is compressed outward and forms a "surgical capsule" around the adenomatous hyperplasia. The etiology of age-related prostatic hyperplasia is still unknown, although it is reasonably well established that androgenic stimulation at the cellular level has a major influence. A better understanding of these influences on prostatic hyperplasia is beginning to help define hormonal manipulations that may affect the natural history of the disease.

As the gland enlarges, urethral resistance to urine flow increases and *bladder muscle hypertrophy* ensues. *Bladder instability* may develop, and emptying may become incomplete. The resulting *residual urine* predisposes to infection, which in turn may produce further bladder irritation. *Bladder herniations* can form between the thickened, overlapping muscular bands that comprise the detrusor. These diverticula are incompletely emptied with voiding, which further predisposes to infection.

A large fluid load, impairment of the contractile function of the bladder by anticholinergics, or increased outflow resistance resulting from sympathomimetic drugs may lead to *acute urinary retention*. Some proportion of acute retention may be precipitated by painless infarction in the enlarged gland. The hyperplastic prostate is highly vascular and predisposed to *bleeding*; painless hematuria can occur.

The late-stage complications of chronic retention caused by BPH include *hydroureter*, *hydronephrosis*, and *renal failure*. Fortunately, these complications are rare.

Clinical Presentation and Course. BPH manifests clinically through lower urinary tract symptoms. Although BPH is the most common cause of such symptoms among older men, other diseases can cause them also. The old term "prostatism" implies a diagnostic specificity to these symptoms that does not in fact exist; as a result, this term should be avoided. Simplistically, "voiding" (or "obstructive") symptoms (such as a weak stream, straining, hesitancy, and intermittency) have been attributed to mechanical bladder outlet obstruction, whereas "filling" (or "irritative") symptoms (such as frequency, nocturia, and urgency) have been attributed to secondary detrusor instability. In reality, the situation is much more complex; the way that the histologic process of BPH eventually leads to symptoms is in fact poorly understood. The severity of lower urinary tract symptoms correlates poorly with prostate size and urodynamic measurements of the severity of bladder outlet obstruction, and some treatments (such as microwave thermotherapy) can reduce symptoms considerably without having much effect on these parameters.

It is quite common for patients to have a waxing and waning symptomatic course, with very gradual deterioration through many years. Sometimes, urinary tract infection is the first indication of bladder outlet obstruction secondary to BPH. Hematuria may be an early symptom of BPH, but neoplasm must be considered as an alternative diagnosis.

In the elderly, BPH can have protean manifestations. It may occasionally cause a lower abdominal mass because of bladder enlargement with a paucity of symptoms. Confusion, anorexia, a palpable kidney, anemia, and a bleeding diathesis secondary to hydronephrosis and uremia constitute a rare presentation of advanced disease. Other symptoms include sleep disturbance and incontinence related to detrusor instability or overflow.

DIAGNOSIS

The digital rectal examination of the prostate provides a rough estimate of overall gland volume but is of little help in assessing the degree of mechanical obstruction. Severity can be assessed by symptoms and a few basic laboratory studies (see below). Clinicians tend to underestimate prostate size, but the inability to palpate the distal margins of the gland generally indicates massive enlargement (more than three times normal size).

Assessing Severity of Symptoms. In older men presenting with lower urinary tract symptoms thought likely to be caused by BPH, the clinician should first objectively document symptom severity. The seven-item *American Urological Association (AUA) Symptom Index* is a quick, self-administered questionnaire that is widely used for this purpose (Fig. 138.1). Scores on individual questions can be summed to yield an *AUA symptom score* ranging from 0 to 35. Scores of 0 to 7 represent mild symptoms, 8 to 19 moderate symptoms, and 20 to 35 severe symptoms. Importantly, clinicians should determine the extent to which the patient is bothered by his symptoms.

A *creatinine* determination and a *urinalysis* should be obtained for all patients to assess renal function and check for in-

	not at all	less than 1 time in 5	less than half the time	about half the time	more than half the time	almost always
1. Over the past month or so, how often have you had a sensation of not emptying your bladder completely after you finished urinating?	0 ☐1	1 ☐2	2 ☐3	3 ☐4	4 ☐5	5 ☐6
2. Over the past month or so, how often have you had to urinate again less than two hours after you finished urinating?	0 ☐7	1 ☐8	2 ☐9	3 ☐10	4 ☐11	5 ☐12
3. Over the past month or so, how often have you found you stopped and started again several times when you urinated?	0 ☐13	1 ☐14	2 ☐15	3 ☐16	4 ☐17	5 ☐18
4. Over the past month or so, how often have you found it difficult to postpone urination?	0 ☐19	1 ☐20	2 ☐21	3 ☐22	4 ☐23	5 ☐24
5. Over the past month or so, how often have you had a weak urinary stream?	0 ☐25	1 ☐26	2 ☐27	3 ☐28	4 ☐29	5 ☐30
6. Over the past month or so, how often have you had to push or strain to begin urination?	0 ☐31	1 ☐32	2 ☐33	3 ☐34	4 ☐35	5 ☐36

	None	1 time	2 times	3 times	4 times	5 or more times
7. Over the last month, how many times did you most typically get up to urinate from the time you went to bed at night until the time you got up in the morning?	0 ☐37	1 ☐38	2 ☐39	3 ☐40	4 ☐41	5 ☐42

Score = sum of questions 1-7 = ___ ___

FIG. 138.1. American Urological Association symptom index for benign prostatic hypertrophy.

fection or hematuria. Measurements of *postvoid residual urine* can be made by catheterization (>50 to 100 mL of residual urine is abnormal) or, less invasively, by transabdominal ultrasonography. However, these measurements are poorly reproducible in individual patients and probably helpful only if persistently and grossly increased (>350 mL).

Urinary flow studies have become widely available. These tests do not require catheterization and are particularly useful in assessing patients whose presentations are atypical (e.g., younger patients or men with dominantly filling symptoms). A normal peak flow rate (>15 mL/s) in the setting of lower urinary tract symptoms should prompt further evaluation for alternative explanations. However, men with true bladder outlet obstruction may sometimes maintain normal flow rates by generating high bladder pressures. Similarly, men with hypotonic bladders may have low flow rates without physiologic obstruction. A low voided volume <150 mL may produce a falsely low peak flow rate.

Imaging studies are not routinely necessary in typical cases of BPH. Radiographic assessment of the bladder and upper urinary tract is not recommended unless an elevated creatinine level, hematuria, or another specific indication is present. If necessary, transabdominal *ultrasonography* can be used to exclude hydronephrosis and assess the postvoid residual volume without an *IV pyelogram*, which entails the risk for a contrast reaction. Similarly, cystourethroscopy should be performed only when specifically indicated (e.g., prior genitourinary instrumentation, hematuria). More sophisticated *urodynamic studies* (cystometrics and pressure–flow studies) are best reserved for patients with conflicting results on simple tests (e.g., severe symptoms

but a normal flow rate), neurologic disease, or prior unsuccessful prostatectomy.

Assessing Significance of Symptoms. For some, frequency and nocturia significantly interfere with a restful night of sleep, whereas for others, they are a minor inconvenience. It is generally best to monitor the patient for 3 to 6 months, often while he attempts some life-style changes (discussed below), to determine the stability or progression of symptoms before making any major therapeutic decisions. It is essential that the physician understand the *importance of symptoms* to the patient and their impact on his quality of life because the individual patient may be willing to accept a given level of symptomatology and a small risk for future BPH complications to avoid surgery.

Checking for Prostate Cancer. When the digital rectal examination findings are not suggestive of prostate cancer, a test for serum *prostate-specific antigen* (PSA) is optional for men with symptomatic BPH. The sensitivity of PSA in this setting is 60% to 70%, and specificity is only 50% to 70%. Moreover, the "prior probability" of subclinical cancer does not seem to be appreciably elevated in the presence of lower urinary tract symptoms. No trials have documented that early detection of prostate cancer improves patient outcomes (although, in fairness, trials have not ruled out such a benefit either). Even advocates of PSA screening do not advise the test for men with less than a 10-year life expectancy (ages 75 and older for men with average comorbidity), given its dubious impact on mortality among these men. Nevertheless, men of any age with BPH should understand that they run a 10% to 15% risk for harboring coincidental prostate cancer and that further tests are available if the patient and his physician wish to screen for prostate cancer (see Chapter 126).

PRINCIPLES OF MANAGEMENT

General Measures. Most patients with urinary symptoms arising from BPH that are not particularly bothersome should simply be followed (*"watchful waiting"*). The decision to proceed to prostatectomy should rarely be made quickly. Complicating and exacerbating factors, such as infections, should be treated, and medications that impair lower urinary tract function should be eliminated if possible. In particular, *diuretics* should be stopped if possible or taken early in the day to avoid nocturnal bladder distention. Drugs that can exacerbate the symptoms of bladder outflow obstruction (e.g., *anticholinergics, tricyclic antidepressants, disopyramide*) should be used only with great care. Patients should be warned about over-the-counter *decongestants* and cough-and-cold preparations. The patient should be told to *void frequently*, take extra time to void completely, and to avoid *beverages* that are likely to produce a diuresis (coffee, tea, alcohol), particularly before bed.

α-Blockers. The efficacy of these agents in reducing symptoms in men with BPH has been documented in clinical trials of up to a year's duration. They probably work mainly by relaxing the bladder neck and prostatic smooth-muscle tone, thereby relieving some of the "dynamic" component of obstruction. Selective α_1-blockers (*prazosin, doxazosin, terazosin*) have fewer side effects than nonselective α-blockers (phenoxybenzamine), and doxazosin and terazosin can be given just once a day. These drugs can induce orthostatic hypotension, particularly in the frail elderly, and can cause fatigue and dizziness unrelated to blood pressure changes. Doses need to be escalated carefully, with monitoring of supine and standing blood pressure. *Tamsulosin* is a new α-blocker developed to reduce prostatic rather than vascular smooth-muscle tone; this agent does not appear to affect blood pressure. Whether tamsulosin has fewer side effects than doxazosin or terazosin (most of which are not blood pressure-related) has not been tested in head-to-head clinical trials.

Many physicians give α-blockers at night to reduce side effects (particularly the first dose at a particular strength), but whether the strategy accomplishes this aim is poorly documented. Doses should be increased (unless side effects ensue) until the patient is satisfied with the result; underdosing is a common reason for treatment failure. Typical dose escalations are from 1 to 2 mg up to 4 to 8 mg daily for doxazosin, or 1 to 2 mg up to 5 to 10 mg for terazosin. Tamsulosin is started at 0.4 mg daily and can be increased to 0.8 mg. About 70% of patients report symptomatic improvement on α-blockers. Whether α-blockers reduce the rates of BPH complications (such as acute urinary retention or progression to surgery) is not well documented.

Inhibition of 5-α-Reductase. *Finasteride* blocks the conversion of testosterone to its metabolite dihydrotestosterone, a potent intraprostatic androgen. The drug reduces prostate size by about 20% during a year of treatment. Mild improvements in symptoms and urinary flow rates relative to placebo have been demonstrated in some trials but not others. The efficacy of the drug appears restricted to men who have large prostates. A Veterans Administration randomized trial comparing finasteride alone, terazosin alone, finasteride and terazosin, and placebo demonstrated efficacy for terazosin but not finasteride; the addi-

tion of finasteride to terazosin produced no additional benefit in terms of symptom relief. On the other hand, long-term trials have demonstrated that finasteride use significantly reduces the risk for acute urinary retention or progression to prostatectomy. Because the absolute risks of these events are low, about 16 men would have to take the drug for 4 years to prevent one event (acute retention or surgery). However, this "number needed to treat" is more favorable among men with higher prostate volumes, or higher baseline levels of PSA (>3.2 ng/mL), the latter probably serving as a practical proxy for prostate volume.

Sexual dysfunction in the form of decreased libido, impotence, or ejaculatory difficulties occurs in about 5% of men taking finasteride. Finasteride is given at a dose of 5 mg daily and does not require dose titration. It can take 6 to 12 months of continuous use before benefit is noted. The drug reduces serum PSA levels by an average of 50%, which means PSA results need to be interpreted differently among men on this drug. One common strategy is simply to double the PSA value in a man on finasteride and then interpret the results in the same way as for a man not on the drug.

Phytotherapy, or treatment with plant extracts, is widely prescribed for men with BPH by clinicians in Europe and is being used more commonly by men in the United States. The best studied of these medications are extracts of the *saw palmetto plant (Seranoa repens)*. In a recent meta-analysis of trials of saw palmetto extracts, this therapy was found to reduce symptoms somewhat more than placebo, and was roughly equivalent to finasteride. Side effects were few. Given the marginal efficacy of finasteride in reducing symptoms, however, this impact is not impressive. Whether saw palmetto extracts share the ability of finasteride to prevent future BPH complications is unknown. A problem with this treatment is that many products are available, without standardization of dose.

Surgical Approaches. Prostatectomy is indicated in patients who have acute retention without a predisposing cause, hydronephrosis, repeated urinary tract infections, recurrent or refractory gross hematuria, or an elevated creatinine level that responds to a period of bladder decompression with catheter drainage. More commonly, refractory, bothersome symptoms are an indication to consider surgery. The primary care physician must integrate the patient's report of his symptoms with an assessment of how bothered the patient is by these complaints. Surgery does provide excellent symptomatic relief in most cases, but any procedure entails risks and costs that some patients may not be willing to undertake. Furthermore, there are patients for whom surgery might not provide much benefit, particularly if concurrent detrusor abnormalities are present.

Transurethral prostatectomy (TURP) is the most common surgical procedure for BPH, with a dominant track record of effectiveness at reducing both symptoms and the risk for BPH complications. The degree of symptom reduction is, on average, much greater than that achieved with any of the medical therapies. A *retropubic* or a *suprapubic ("open") prostatectomy* may be required if the gland is substantially enlarged. The mortality rate for all these operations is low (<1% for TURP). TURP has classically been said to be associated with potential complications such as incontinence and erectile dysfunction, but a Veterans Administration trial that randomized men to immediate TURP versus a strategy of watchful waiting found that the risk for these problems was no higher after TURP. On the other hand, retrograde ejaculation and resulting infertility are common complications of prostatectomy and should be discussed with the patient before operation. A *transurethral incision* of the prostate (TUIP) may be a good choice for younger men with small prostate glands. TUIP has been shown to be nearly as effective as TURP in providing symptom relief and carries a lower risk for retrograde ejaculation and other complications. More recently, urologists have been using *laser* energy or *electrical vaporization* to destroy prostate tissue, still via a transurethral approach. These procedures seem to cause less bleeding than TURP does and can often be performed as "day surgery," but results of comparative trials with long-term follow-up are not available.

Operations for BPH leave a substantial amount of prostatic tissue in place. The postoperative risk for future malignancy is the same. Because residual prostatic tissue may continue to grow, symptoms may recur after surgery. Patients undergo reoperation at a rate of about 1% per year.

Device Therapies. *Balloon dilation* has lost favor because of frequent relapse of symptoms. Two newer therapies for BPH are *transurethral microwave thermotherapy* (TUMT) and *transurethral needle ablation* (TUNA). In both, a device generates heat to coagulate prostate tissue. In the former, a microwave antenna is placed in the urethra surrounded by a cooling jacket (to protect the urethra), and in the latter, radiofrequency energy is delivered directly to the prostate via intraprostatic needles. Both procedures can be performed in a single outpatient session and may be complicated by urinary retention requiring catheter drainage. In general, studies have suggested short-term symptom relief somewhat less than that obtained with TURP but greater than obtained with medical therapy. The mechanism of symptom relief with these treatments is unclear, as the coagulated intraprostatic tissue is not removed. Long-term trials comparing the results of TUMT and TUNA with TURP or medical therapy are not yet available.

INDICATIONS FOR REFERRAL

A urologist should be consulted when a patient presents with absolute indications for surgery, as discussed previously. In addition, consultation can be helpful when the diagnosis is unclear, particularly when evidence of an alternative cause of a patient's lower urinary tract symptoms is present. Most commonly, a consultation will be called for when a patient still has bothersome symptoms despite maximal medical therapy and would like to consider a surgical intervention.

PATIENT EDUCATION

One cannot overestimate the value of patient education in the effective management of BPH. When patients are provided with information about the waxing and waning natural history of symptoms and the advantages and risks of the full range of treatment options, they are likely to choose differently than when exposed only to a surgical opinion. Reviewing such information enables the primary physician and the patient to make a joint management decision. A joint management strategy ensures a therapeutic approach best suited to the patient's preferences. Watchful waiting is a reasonable choice for patients without absolute indications for surgery, provided both patient and physician share a commitment to periodic review and reassessment.

TREATMENT RECOMMENDATIONS

- The primary care physician should objectively assess the severity of lower urinary tract symptoms and determine their effect on the patient's quality of life.
- All patients with symptoms likely caused by BPH should have a baseline creatinine determination and urinalysis.
- Routine urinary tract imaging is not necessary. Upper tract imaging, preferably by ultrasonography, is indicated if hydronephrosis is a concern (a large postvoid residual urine volume or an elevated creatinine level).
- A urine flow rate measurement may be useful when symptomatology is confusing or ambiguous; it helps to identify patients who have symptoms but little evidence of obstruction (peak flow rates >15 mL/s).
- Patients should be made aware of the possible coexistence of prostate cancer and BPH and the availability of further evaluation, including PSA screening. However, the impact of early detection of prostate cancer on prostate cancer mortality is doubtful in men with a life expectancy of less than 10 years.
- Most patients can be followed expectantly unless evidence of hydronephrosis, recurrent or persistent infection, or deterioration in renal function is present. Such complications warrant prompt surgical attention. Nighttime fluids and drugs that affect lower urinary tract function should be avoided.
- Selective α_1-blocker therapy (*doxazosin, prazosin, terazosin, tamsulosin*) can provide symptomatic relief for some patients.
- The 5-α-reductase inhibitor *finasteride* may be worth considering in persons with larger prostate glands (reflected by baseline PSA levels >3.2 ng/mL), primarily to reduce the future risk for acute retention or surgery. It is less effective than α-blocker therapy in reducing lower urinary tract symptoms in the short run.
- Elective urologic consultation is indicated when the diagnosis is confusing or when, despite medical therapy, the quality of life is sufficiently compromised to warrant consideration of an operation to achieve symptomatic relief.
- Less invasive treatments for BPH will provide an increased array of treatment options in the coming years, but *prostatectomy* remains the standard for long-term symptom relief.

ANNOTATED BIBLIOGRAPHY

Barry MJ, Fowler FJ, O'Leary MP, et al. The American Urological Association Symptom Index for benign prostatic hyperplasia. J Urol 1992;148:1549. (*Validation of seven-item questionnaire to assess symptom severity in men with BPH.*)

Boyle P, Gould L, Roehrborn CG. Prostate volume predicts outcome of treatment of benign prostatic hyperplasia with finasteride: meta-analysis of randomized clinical trials. Urology 1996;48:398. (*The efficacy of finasteride is best for men with a prostate weighing more than 40 g.*)

Bruskewitz RC, Christensen MM. Critical evaluation of transurethral resection and incision of the prostate. Prostate 1990;3[Suppl]:27. (*TUIP is an option for younger patients with small glands.*)

Christensen MM, Bruskewitz RC. Clinical manifestations of benign prostatic hyperplasia and indications for therapeutic intervention. Urol Clin North Am 1990;17:509. (*The urologist's perspective; few noncontroversial indications for surgical intervention in patients with BPH.*)

De La Rosette JJMCH, D'Ancona FCH, Debruyne FMJ. Current status of thermotherapy of the prostate. J Urol 1997;157:430. (*Review of some studies of transurethral microwave thermotherapy; a generic problem is lack of long-term follow-up.*)

Eri LM, Tveter KJ. Alpha-blockade in the treatment of symptomatic benign prostatic hyperplasia. J Urol 1995;154:923. (*An overview of 29 α-blocker trials showing improvement in symptom scores, flow rates, and residual urine volume.*)

Gormley GJ, Stoner E, Bruskewitz RC, et al. The effect of finasteride in men with benign prostatic hyperplasia. N Engl J Med 1992; 327:1185. (*Symptoms improved, flow increased; slight increase in risk for sexual dysfunction.*)

Lepor H, Auerbach S, Puras-Baez A, et al. A randomized, placebo-controlled multicenter study of the efficacy and safety of terazosin in the treatment of benign prostatic hyperplasia. J Urol 1992; 148:1467. (*A key trial documenting the short-term outcomes of α-blocker treatment.*)

Lepor H, Williford WO, Barry MJ, et al, for the Veterans Affairs Cooperative Studies Benign Prostatic Hyperplasia Study Group. The efficacy of terazosin, finasteride and the combination in benign prostatic hyperplasia. N Engl J Med 1996;334:533. (*Terazosin but not finasteride was effective, and the combination was no more effective than terazosin alone.*)

McConnell JD, Barry MJ, Bruskewitz RC, et al. Benign prostatic hyperplasia: diagnosis and treatment. Clinical practice guidelines, No. 8. AHCPR publication No. 940582. Rockville, MD: Agency for Health Care Policy and Research, Public Health Service, U.S. Department of Health and Human Services, February 1994. (*Practical guidelines for clinicians and their BPH patients. A guide designed for BPH patients is available from the same source as publication No. 940584.*)

Narayan P, Tewari A. Overview of alpha-blocker therapy for benign prostatic hyperplasia. Urology 1998;51[Suppl 4A]:38. (*Comprehensive review of the therapeutic and adverse effects of the α-blockers, including tamsulosin.*)

Naslund MJ. Transurethral needle ablation of the prostate. Urology 1997; 50:167. (*Review of the technique and results of this new technology.*)

Neal DE, Ramsden PD, Sharples L, et al. Outcome of elective prostatectomy. Br Med J 1989;299:762. (*In a nonrandomized cohort study of men undergoing elective prostatectomy, 79% had a satisfactory subjective response to surgery; an unsatisfactory response to surgery could not be predicted.*)

Oesterling JE. Benign prostatic hyperplasia. Medical and minimally invasive treatment. N Engl J Med 1995;332:99. (*Extensive review of BPH, medical therapy, microwave therapy, and laser prostatectomy.*)

Roehrborn CG, McConnell JD, Lieber M, et al. Serum prostate-specific antigen concentration is a powerful predictor of acute urinary retention and need for surgery in men with benign prostatic hyperplasia. Urology 1999;53:473. (*In this subgroup analysis of a 4-year placebo-controlled trial, men with a baseline serum PSA level above 3.2 ng/mL had the greatest absolute benefit in terms of reduced risk for prostatectomy and acute retention.*)

Wasson JH, Reda DJ, Bruskewitz RC, et al. A comparison of transurethral surgery with watchful waiting for moderate symptoms of benign prostatic hyperplasia. N Engl J Med 1995;332:75. (*This randomized trial documented superior symptom improvement and fewer treatment failures with surgery. However, the men managed expectantly also had relatively good outcomes.*)

Wilt TJ, Ishani A, Stark G, et al. Saw palmetto extracts for treatment of benign prostatic hyperplasia: a systematic review. JAMA 1998;280:1604. (*Extracts of the saw palmetto plant reduced lower urinary tract symptoms more than placebo and as much as finasteride, with fewer side effects.*)

139

Management of Acute and Chronic Prostatitis

JOHN D. GOODSON

Prostatitis is the most important cause of urinary tract infection in men. Chronic prostatitis is a common infection that can cause persistent and annoying symptoms, whereas acute prostatitis is less common but potentially much more serious. Both conditions require accurate recognition and treatment by the primary physician. Prompt initiation of therapy is especially important for acute prostatitis. Pain in the male perineum can arise from both infectious and noninfectious inflammation and can represent pain referred from retroperitoneal structures and low sacral nerve roots. Further complicating management is the ongoing controversy about the role of low-level commensal microorganisms that can be cultured from symptomatic patients. Experts continue to disagree about the value of extended antibiotic treatment and empiric therapy. A consensus panel has addressed some of this confusion by proposing a scheme for classifying prostatitis syndromes (Table 139.1).

CLINICAL PRESENTATION, PATHOPHYSIOLOGY, AND COURSE

Bacterial prostatitis may ensue from ascending urethral infection, reflux of infected urine, extension of rectal infection, or hematogenous spread. Gram-negative bacilli (predominantly *Escherichia coli*, *Proteus*, *Klebsiella*, and *Pseudomonas*) and *enterococci* account for most of the single isolates obtained from culture. Occasionally, *Chlamydia*, *Ureaplasma*, a virus, or *Trichomonas* may be the etiologic agent. In the immune-compromised patient, infection with fungi, such as *Aspergillus*, should be considered.

Small numbers of bacterial isolates from prostatic fluids are very difficult to interpret, especially when the organisms identified are not usually thought of as urinary tract pathogens (e.g., gram-positive organisms such as *Staphylococcus epidermidis* or *Corynebacterium* species). When bacterial growth is associated with evidence of prostate inflammation (defined below), then antibiotic treatment is warranted. When no evidence of inflammation is present, then treatment may be warranted, but neither physician nor patient should anticipate success.

Acute Prostatitis. The condition is readily identified by the onset of diminished urine flow, perineal pain, dysuria, and fever. On gentle rectal examination, the gland is enlarged, exquisitely tender, and boggy. Abdominal examination occasionally reveals striking bladder distention. Some patients may appear toxic at the time of presentation.

Chronic Prostatitis. In older men, the symptoms are generally those of bladder outflow obstruction. Patients complain of frequency, dribbling, loss of stream volume and force, double voiding, hesitancy, and urgency. Younger men more often complain of dysuria and dribbling, intermittent discomfort in the perineum, low back, or testicles. Some patients present initially with hematuria, hematospermia, or painful ejaculations. Rectal examination usually reveals an enlarged prostate with a variable amount of asymmetry, bogginess, and tenderness. Untreated or incompletely treated chronic prostatitis is characterized by recurrent symptomatic exacerbations, although these may be separated by long asymptomatic intervals.

Both acute and chronic prostatitis can cause urinary tract and systemic complications. The acutely infected gland may lead to renal parenchymal infection or bacteremia. Rarely, acute infection will progress to a well-defined abscess of the gland. Chronic infection can produce small prostatic stones, which may serve as a nidus for further inflammation and recurrent symptomatic bouts of infection.

Prostatodynia. Patients with prostatodynia complain primarily of persistent *pelvic* and *perineal* pain, but no bacterial pathogen can be identified and no evidence of prostatic inflammation can be documented. Sometimes, the pain may be associated with urinary symptoms such as frequency, urgency, decreased stream flow, and decreased bladder capacity. As noted, some of these patients will be found on extensive culturing to have small numbers of commensal gram-positive organisms in their prostate secretions, and for this reason, low-level infection with bacterial or nonbacterial agents has been argued as the cause of this syndrome. However, a sizable number of patients have negative cultures, and this group remains a management challenge. Some of these patients may have nonperitoneal causes of peritoneal pain, such as pain referred from other pelvic structures or sacral nerve root irritation.

DIFFERENTIAL DIAGNOSIS

Acute prostatitis is readily evident by the clinical presentation and exquisitely tender prostate found on rectal examination. However, chronic prostatitis presents a more difficult diagnostic problem, often resembling, in clinical presentation, other common forms of urinary outflow tract obstruction, such as benign prostatic hypertrophy (see Chapter 138), prostatic carcinoma (see Chapter 143), and urethral stricture (see Chapter 134). The lower urinary tract irritative symptoms associated

Table 139.1. Classification and Definition of Prostatitis

Category I	Acute bacterial prostatitis	Acute infection
Category II	Chronic bacterial prostatitis	Persistent infection
Category III	Chronic abacterial prostatitis	No infection
IIIA	Inflammatory	WBCs in EPS or VB$_3$ (postmassage urine)
IIIB	Non-inflammatory	WBCs in EPS or VB$_3$ (postmassage urine)
Category IV	Asymptomatic inflammatory prostatitis	WBCs in EPS or VB$_3$ (postmassage urine) or on biopsy specimen, but no symptoms

WBC, white blood cell; EPS, expressed prostatic secretion, VB, voided bladder. After Nickel JC. Prostatitis: myths and realities. Urology 1998;51:363, with permission

with chronic prostatitis may be seen with urethritis (see Chapter 136), bladder carcinoma (see Chapter 143), sphincter dyssynergy, and neurogenic bladder (see Chapter 134).

WORKUP

History and Physical Examination. The pertinent history and physical examination depend on the clinical presentation. For suspected *acute prostatitis*, check for acute onset of fever, perineal pain, dysuria, and diminished urine flow. A urethral discharge is sometimes reported. On rectal examination, the prostate is exquisitely tender. Examination should proceed cautiously to avoid precipitating bacteremia. If symptoms of urinary outflow obstruction are present, then the abdomen should be checked for bladder distention. For *chronic prostatitis*, inquire into recurrent perineal, back, or testicular discomfort, dribbling, slow stream, dysuria, and hematospermia. The prostate is enlarged, boggy, and sometimes tender on examination.

Laboratory Studies. Because the documentation of prostate inflammation and the identification of infecting organisms are essential to categorizing prostatitis, and because prostatic infection can be recurrent and elusive, it is well worth the effort to obtain *prostatic fluid* and *urine* for analysis.

Prostatic Fluid. The most rigorous approach is to obtain a series of specimens before and after *prostate massage*. Specimens representing urethral, bladder, and post-massage urine are collected and labeled VB$_1$, VB$_2$, and VB$_3$ (voided bladder; see appendix), in addition to any expressed prostatic secretions (EPS) that can be obtained as a result of massage. Vigorous massage should be avoided in patients with severe acute prostatitis because of the risk for inducing bacteremia. Gram's stain of the EPS or the spun VB$_3$ will sometimes demonstrate organisms or white blood cells (>10 cells per high-power field is abnormal). Fewer than 10 white blood cells per high-power field on EPS examination excludes prostatic infection with a specificity of 88%. Cultures of the EPS and VB$_3$ should show significant growth (>5,000 colony-forming units per milliliter), whereas the VB$_1$ and VB$_2$ should be sterile or have a colony count that is smaller by one order of magnitude.

Urine. On a more practical level, when urethritis is not suspected clinically and no prostatic secretions can be obtained, then urine specimens can be collected before and after prostate massage (*pre-massage/post-massage test*). If leukocytes are present in the urine after massage when none were present before, then prostatic inflammation can be inferred. Occasionally, the *urine culture* after massage will show a single organism or mixed organisms when none were present before massage. Even low levels of bacterial growth (<100,000 colony-forming units per milliliter) should be identified and sensitivities determined. Some laboratories require notification to do this. When no bacterial growth is identified on the EPS, VB$_3$, or post-massage urine despite the presence of leukocytes in any of the three, then bacterial infection has been missed, a nonbacterial infectious agent such as *Chlamydia* is present, or a noninfectious inflammation is present. Unfortunately, these patients cannot reliably be further differentiated. Older men who are without evidence of infection yet are bothered by lower urinary tract irritative symptoms should undergo *urine cytology* to help exclude a bladder malignancy. A bladder carcinoma located in the trigonal region can mimic chronic prostatitis.

Other Studies. Cystoscopy may be indicated when the diagnosis is not confirmed by urine culture data. *Blood urea ni-*

trogen and *creatinine* levels should be determined at the initial visit and periodically thereafter depending on the chronicity and severity of symptoms. An *IV pyelogram* or *spiral computed tomography* is indicated when evidence of renal deterioration or symptoms of persistent outflow obstruction are present. *Abdominal* and *pelvic computed tomography* may be indicated to exclude a retroperitoneal process, and occasionally *lumbosacral magnetic resonance imaging* is indicated to exclude sacral nerve entrapment or impingement.

PRINCIPLES OF MANAGEMENT

Acute Prostatitis. When accompanied by severe pain, high fever, rigors, and marked leukocytosis, acute prostatitis requires *hospitalization* for *IV antibiotic therapy*. Such patients should be examined gently for the presence of a fluctuant prostatic mass suggestive of an abscess, which may necessitate surgical drainage. Less toxic patients can be treated as outpatients with an oral antibiotic program. *Trimethoprim/sulfamethoxazole* (TMS), a fluoroquinolone such as *ciprofloxacin* or *levofloxacin*, and *doxycycline* all work well. Extended therapy, 4 to 6 weeks, is recommended to prevent acute infection from becoming established. Most other antibiotics effective against gram-negative rods (e.g., *amoxicillin*) penetrate the acutely inflamed prostate well and work satisfactorily in the acute phase of illness, but not so well in subacute and chronic states.

Local measures can help reduce discomfort. Sitz baths two to three times a day for 20 minutes can relieve perineal pain. Stool softeners, antipyretics, analgesics, and bed rest are all helpful.

Chronic Prostatitis. This condition is more difficult to eradicate, partly because of poor penetration by oral antibiotics into the prostate. Curative antibiotic therapy requires elimination of bacteria from prostatic fluid. Because the prostatic secretions are normally acidic (pH 6.5 to 7.4), the most efficacious drugs are those that readily penetrate membranes (lipid-soluble) and become ionically trapped (high pH). *TMS*, the *fluoroquinolones*, and *erythromycin* have these characteristics, with good prostatic fluid levels demonstrated. Because *TMS* and *ciprofloxacin* are more effective than *erythromycin* against gram-negative bacteria, they are preferred. However, *TMS* is not effective against enterococci. *Carbenicillin* and *doxycycline* also penetrate the prostate reasonably well. The latter is especially active against *Chlamydia* and some *Ureaplasma* organisms.

With chronic infection, the prostatic fluid becomes increasingly alkaline, which tends to reduce antibiotic penetration. As a result, prolonged treatment may be necessary. Some patients may not achieve cure even after 8 to 12 weeks of antibiotics. Cure rates with TMS range from 30% to 70%; slightly higher rates have been reported with 2 to 4 weeks of ciprofloxacin. To demonstrate cure, the EPS or VB$_3$ (post-massage urine) should be inspected and cultured after the treatment period. Because causative organisms are hard to identify and treatment is frequently empiric, analysis of the prostate fluid after treatment is valuable. If evidence of infection is still present (>10 white cells per high-power field in the EPS or pus in the urine after massage), then a longer course of antibiotics is indicated. After 12 weeks of antibiotic therapy, cure is unlikely; 6 to 12 months of treatment is not unreasonable.

Peripheral *α-adrenergic blockers,* such as doxazosin, tamsulosin, or terazosin, should be used in conjunction with antibiotic therapy for both acute and chronic prostatitis to reduce symp-

toms. Some data suggest that these drugs also help facilitate cure.

The relatively low cure rate achieved with antibiotics in chronic prostatitis requires that therapeutic goals be adjusted to the patient's age. In most cases, α-adrenergic blockade can be used to control symptoms. If infection relapses, one *TMS* tablet daily appears to be an effective *suppressive regimen*. *Transurethral prostatic resection* (TURP), *transurethral thermotherapy*, and *total prostatectomy* provide alternatives when repeated courses of antibiotics fail. Such procedures are associated with significant morbidity, including possible impotence or sterility, and should be reserved for carefully selected patients. Recurrent infection associated with prostatic stones is an indication for removal of the gland.

Local measures can help reduce symptoms in patients with chronic prostatitis. The patient with obstructive symptoms can try voiding while in a warm water bath with the pelvic muscles relaxed. The value of prostatic massage is a subject of debate. Many claim that *prostatic massage* relieves gland congestion in chronic cases and should be repeated every 1 to 2 weeks. (Massage of the acutely infected gland is contraindicated.) The patient should avoid alcohol, coffee, tea, or other beverages that might produce rapid bladder expansion. The physician should discontinue or reduce the dosage, if possible, of anticholinergics, sedatives, and antidepressants, all of which can impair bladder function (see Chapter 134). Ejaculation is not contraindicated.

Prostatodynia or Chronic Perineal and Pelvic Pain. Patients with pain and urinary symptoms and no evidence of infection should be watched for the emergence of infection. A limited (4 to 6 weeks) course of antibiotics may be worthwhile; antibiotics can then be continued for an extended course (3 to 4 months) if a clinical response is noted. α-Adrenergic blockade has been used with some success in these patients.

PATIENT EDUCATION

Patients should be advised of the chronic and relapsing nature of the disease and alerted to the early signs of infection in the upper urinary tract. They can also be reassured that isolated prostatitis does not cause infertility or impotence. Local measures that can be suggested for symptomatic relief include sitz baths and voiding into a warm water bath. The importance of compliance with the prolonged antibiotic course and physician monitoring of the response to treatment needs to be stressed.

THERAPEUTIC RECOMMENDATIONS

Acute Prostatitis

- Obtain Gram's stain and culture of the EPS or VB$_3$ (post-massage urine) and treat immediately.
- For the nontoxic patient, oral antibiotic therapy is sufficient. Prescribe either double-strength *TMS* (160 mg trimethoprim, 800 mg sulfamethoxazole twice daily), *ciprofloxacin* (500 mg twice daily), or *levofloxacin* (500 mg daily) for 4 weeks. *Amoxicillin* (500 mg three times daily), *doxycycline* (100 mg twice daily), and *carbenicillin* indanyl sodium (1 g four times daily) are reasonable alternatives, all given for 4 weeks.

Chronic Prostatitis

- Document an infectious organism and the presence of prostatic inflammation, either with sequential urinary culturing and EPS examination or with the pre-massage/post-massage test.

- Treat with a prolonged course of antibiotics, such as double-strength TMS (twice daily for 8 to 12 weeks), or *ciprofloxacin* (500 mg twice daily) or *levofloxacin* (500 mg daily) for 4 weeks. The latter two are considerably more expensive.
- After treatment, follow closely for return of infection. A second course of antibiotics with the same or an alternative drug for up to 12 weeks may be necessary in partially responsive infections. For patients who fail to respond initially, prescribe a 12-week course of *doxycycline* (100 mg twice daily), *erythromycin* (500 mg four times daily), or *carbenicillin* indanyl sodium (1 g four times daily).
- Schedule a return 1 to 2 weeks after the completion of treatment to assess the effects of therapy by checking the EPS or VB$_3$ (post-massage urine specimen).
- Prescribe a peripheral α-adrenergic blocker such as *doxazosin* (2 to 8 mg daily), *terazosin* (2 to 10 mg daily), or *tamsulosin* (0.4 to 0.8 mg daily) with the initiation of antibiotic therapy. Continue as long as the patient derives benefit.

Prostatodynia or Chronic Pelvic and Perineal Pain

- Prescribe a trial of a peripheral α-adrenergic blocker, as above.

INDICATIONS FOR ADMISSION AND REFERRAL

Patients with high fever, leukocytosis, and severe perineal pain require IV antibiotics, antipyretics, and analgesics; hospitalization is indicated. In the presence of marked outflow obstruction, suprapubic bladder decompression may be necessary. A fluctuant prostatic mass suggestive of an abscess may require surgical drainage. Until culture and sensitivity data are available, treatment of the toxic patient is directed toward gram-negative bacteria and enterococci, with parenteral administration of ampicillin and gentamicin or levofloxacin.

Patients with outflow tract obstruction or refractory chronic infection should have a urologic consultation. Patients with prostatodynia or an unexplained chronic pelvic and perineal pain syndrome should be referred to a urologist with expertise in this area.

ANNOTATED BIBLIOGRAPHY

Barbalias GA. Prostatodynia or painful male prostate syndrome? Urology 1990;36:146. (*A discussion of pathogenesis and possible mechanisms.*)

Barbalias GA, Nikiforidis G, Liatskos EN. α-Blockers for the treatment of chronic prostatitis in combinations with antibiotics. J Urol 1998;159:883. (*Concurrent use of an α-blocker and antibiotics was associated with a reduction in recurrence rate and improved symptom relief.*)

Brunner H, Weidner W, Schiefer HG. Studies on the role of *Ureaplasma urealyticum* and *Mycoplasma hominis* in prostatitis. J Infect Dis 1983;147:807. (*Thirteen percent had documented Ureaplasma infection; more than 80% responded to tetracycline.*)

Drach GW, Nolan PE. Chronic bacterial prostatitis: problems in diagnosis and therapy. Urology 1986;27[Suppl]:26. (*When strict criteria were used, only 20% of patients referred for evaluation of prostatitis had definitely positive results on cultures.*)

Lowentritt JE, Kawahara K, Human LG, et al. Bacterial infections in prostatodynia. J Urol 1995;154:1378. (*Of 22 patients with prostatodynia, 9 had very low levels of infection documented, mostly with commensal organisms. Of 7 patients treated, 5 became culture-negative and improved.*)

Meares EM Jr. Long-term therapy of chronic bacterial prostatitis with trimethoprim-sulfamethoxazole. Can Med Assoc J 1975;112:225. (*Twelve weeks produced an initially good response in 74%, but only 31% remained cured for a 30-month follow-up period.*)

Meares EM Jr. Infected stones of the prostate gland. Urology 1974;4:560. (*Found in 13.8% of men; most are asymptomatic, but when recurrent infection is demonstrated, the gland and stones must be removed.*)

Nickel JC. Effective office management of chronic prostatitis. Urol Clin North Am 1998;25:677. (*Describes and advocates the more practical pre-massage/post-massage test for screening purposes. Test sensitivity and specificity cannot be determined in the absence of any diagnostic "gold standard."*)

Nickel JC, Sorenson R. Transurethral microwave thermotherapy for nonbacterial prostatitis: a randomized double-blind sham controlled study using new prostatitis-specific assessment questionnaires. J Urol 1996;155:150. (*More than a 50% improvement in symptoms was noted in 7 of 10 treated patients, in comparison with 1 of 10 sham patients. This study was small but well done and offers some hope for this group of patients.*)

Roberts RO, Lieber MM, Bostwick DG, et al. A review of clinical and pathological prostate syndromes. Urology 1997;49:809. (*The Mayo Clinic experience. The authors advocate 4 to 6 weeks of treatment for acute prostatitis and 3 to 4 months of treatment for chronic prostatitis.*)

Thin RN, Simmons PD. Chronic bacterial and nonbacterial prostatitis. Br J Urol 1983;55:513. (*The EPS leukocyte counts for bacterial and nonbacterial prostatitis were similar; the test is highly specific but poorly sensitive.*)

Appendix: Urine and Prostatic Fluid Collections in Men

Standard Clean-voided Specimen. Specimen collection in *male patients* varies with the clinical situation. When cystitis is suspected, the patient is traditionally instructed to retract the foreskin and clean the glans penis with three moist gauze pads or soap sponges. A small amount of urine is voided into the toilet and then a midstream specimen is collected. Cleansing and retraction of foreskin make no difference if a midstream specimen is obtained. However, omitting these steps does lead to contamination of initial specimens. When urethritis or prostatitis is suspected, voided bladder specimens are indicated.

Voided Bladder Specimens. The patient retracts the foreskin and cleans the glans penis. The first 10 mL is collected and labeled VB$_1$ (Fig. 139.1). This represents a urethral specimen,

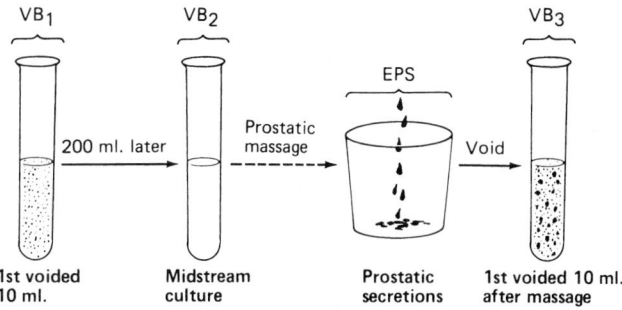

FIG. 139.1. Segmented culture of the lower urinary tract in male patients. (Adapted from Meares EM, Stamey T. Bacteriologic localization patterns in bacterial prostatitis and urethritis. Invest Urol 1968;5:492, with permission.)

which is also useful in cases of suspected urethritis (see Chapters 125 and 136). A midstream specimen is collected in the standard fashion. This is labeled VB_2. The bladder must not be completely emptied. The physician then massages the prostate with continuous strokes. The resulting prostatic fluid, which either comes from the meatus or is milked from the penis by the patient, is collected in a sterile container labeled EPS; this can be used for culture and Gram's stain or acid-fast stain. If no fluid can be collected, the patient is told to void another 10 mL into a sterile container. This specimen, labeled VB_3, represents roughly a 100:1 dilution of prostatic fluid and can be cultured or spun and stained. Vigorous prostatic massage can produce a transient bacteremia and should be avoided if acute prostatitis is suspected. If the patient has chronic prostatitis and known valvular heart disease, endocarditis prophylaxis may be necessary (see Chapter 16).

The EPS and VB_3 can be inspected under the microscope for the presence of fat globules, leukocytes, and organisms. If fewer than 10 leukocytes are seen per high-power field, bacterial prostatic infection is unlikely. A Gram's stain may aid in identifying the responsible organism. With bacterial prostatitis, growth will occur in VB_3 and EPS, but not in VB_1 and VB_2.

When bacterial growth is noted in both VB_2 and VB_3 samples, a prostatic infection may be masked by a bladder infection. In this situation, antibiotics that sterilize the bladder contents but do not penetrate the prostate [e.g., 500 mg of penicillin G four times a day orally, or 100 mg of nitrofurantoin (Macrodantin) three times a day orally] may be given for 2 to 3 days before specimen collection. With bacterial prostatic infection, the EPS will still grow organisms.

Urethral catheterization of male patients is rarely required for culture and should be reserved for the symptomatic relief of marked outflow obstruction.

ANNOTATED BIBLIOGRAPHY

Lipsky BA, Inui TS, Plorde JJ, et al. Is the clean-catch midstream void procedure necessary for obtaining routine urine culture specimens from men? Am J Med 1984;76:257. (*Data suggest the answer is no.*)

Meares EM, Stamey T. Bacteriologic localization patterns in bacterial prostatitis and urethritis. Invest Urol 1968;5:492. (*Detailed description of the methodology and rationale for voided bladder specimens.*)

140
Management of Urinary Tract Infection in Men

Urinary tract infection (UTI) is rare in young men, but the incidence begins to increase with age, particularly after the age of 50. By age 65, it equals that of women. In elderly debilitated patients confined to nursing homes, the prevalence may reach as high as 20% to 50%. The primary physician needs to know the clinical significance of UTI in men, what type of workup is indicated, and what modes of therapy are most cost-effective.

PATHOPHYSIOLOGY, CLINICAL PRESENTATION, AND COURSE

Young Men. UTI in young men usually represents *urethritis* or introduction of bacteria through *instrumentation* (e.g., bladder catheterization for surgery). At times, a *congenital anomaly* of the urinary tract is responsible, although usually the presentation is at an earlier age. Dysuria, frequency, and urgency accompany most forms, with urethral discharge characteristic of urethritis. Most cases of urethritis are venereal in origin and respond well to treatment (see Chapter 136). The condition of patients with an anatomic defect does not improve unless the structural problem is alleviated. Patients who respond fully to a 7-day course of antibiotics are unlikely to have any serious underlying pathology.

In some young men, uncomplicated *cystitis* may develop because of exposure to uropathogenic strains of *Escherichia coli*. The exposure is seen among homosexual men engaging in anal intercourse and in heterosexual men having vaginal intercourse with a colonized partner. Lack of circumcision is a risk factor, as is HIV infection with a CD4-lymphocyte count below $200/mm^3$.

Middle-aged Men. The increase in rate of UTI that occurs in men ages 50 to 65 parallels the increase in prostate size that occurs with hyperplasia of the gland. The enlargement leads to bladder outflow tract obstruction, and a postvoid residual begins to develop in the bladder. The reduced antibacterial activity of prostatic secretions among men in this age group may also contribute to infection risk. Infection of the prostate may serve as a nidus for recurrent UTI.

Elderly Men. With further prostatic enlargement, the *postvoid residual* and consequently the risk for infection continue to rise. Use of condom or urethral *catheters*, urinary incontinence, and history of a previous UTI are other risk factors for UTI in this age group. Asymptomatic bacteriuria may occur, especially among nursing home residents. Additional contributing factors include neurogenic bladder dysfunction (see Chapter 134) and *concomitant illness* (pneumonia is a common precipitant of UTI).

Despite the high prevalence of infection with pathogenic organisms, the vast majority of infected elderly men remain asymptomatic and seem to be at low risk for serious complications. However, the usual manifestations of serious, symptomatic UTI may be absent, replaced by such vague findings as "failure to thrive" or worsening mental status. Gram-negative sepsis from a urinary tract source can be life-threatening. Debate continues as to whether bacteriuria per se increases mortality; studies controlling for comorbid conditions show no increase.

Bacteriology. In patients with infection caused by a single organism, *E. coli* accounts for about 25% of cases, other gram-negative rods (*Proteus, Pseudomonas, Providencia*) for another 50%, and *enterococci* and *coagulase-negative staphylococci* for the remaining 25%. Patients with indwelling catheters and those with recurrent infections and multiple antibiotic exposures are likely to have unusual organisms with resistance to multiple antibiotics. Multiple organisms are found in as many as a third of infected nursing home patients.

WORKUP

History and Physical Examination

In men, complaints of dysuria, frequency, and urgency have a predictive value of about 75% for UTI. Acute onset of hesitancy, nocturia, slow stream, and dribbling have a predictive value for UTI of about 33%. No symptoms differentiate upper from lower tract infection, with the possible exception of fever (which is rare in men with lower tract disease).

The temperature should be taken and a careful genitourinary tract examination performed. The urethral meatus is examined for erythema and discharge, the testes and epididymides for tenderness and swelling, and the prostate for enlargement, nodularity, and pain on palpation. In the patient with suspected acute prostatitis, palpation should be very gentle to avoid causing a bacteremia. The abdomen is checked for suprapubic distention and tenderness in the costovertebral angles.

Laboratory Studies

Urine Culture and Microscopic Examination. Unlike women, men require a urine culture because of the wider range of causative agents and their less predictable drug sensitivities. A diagnosis of UTI is justified on isolation of a pure culture of 10^3 colony-forming units (CFU) per milliliter of urine. A culture that grows fewer than 10^3 CFU/mL or three or more organisms (without one being predominant) is suggestive of contamination. A midstream urine sample or even an initial void sample without prior cleansing of the glans suffices for most clinical situations, even if the patient is uncircumcised. Sensitivity and specificity are in excess of 97%. Initial and midstream urine samples correlate very well with bladder specimens ($r = .96$).

Both spun and unspun urine specimens should be examined. The spun sediment is examined for the presence of white blood cell casts (indicative of pyelonephritis) and pus, and a Gram's stain is performed to identify a predominant organism, if present. Gram's stain of the unspun urine is also performed. The finding of a single organism or white blood cell per high-power field on Gram's stain of the unspun urine has a sensitivity of 85% for UTI and a specificity of 60%, about the same as those of other rapid diagnostic methods.

Culturing the Incontinent Patient. Specimens from patients with an indwelling catheter can be obtained for culture by first cleansing the side port of the catheter with a povidone–iodine

solution and then drawing up urine through a needle attached to a sterile syringe. A culture of urine drawn from an indwelling catheter is positive for organisms when 100 or more CFU/mL are present. Most patients with indwelling catheters have positive cultures.

A specimen from an *incontinent patient* can be obtained for culture without resorting to catheterization by cleansing the glans penis with povidone–iodine solution, applying a fresh *condom catheter* and drainage system, and collecting the first voided specimen in the drainage bag within 2 hours. The criterion for a positive study is the presence of more than 10^5 CFU/mL; lesser growth is considered to represent contamination.

Straight catheterization and direct bladder aspiration are alternative methods of obtaining urine for culture in incontinent patients. The former carries a slight risk of inducing a bacteremia (see Chapter 16); skill is required to perform the latter procedure.

Measurement of Renal Function. Some UTIs or their causes may compromise renal function. Blood urea nitrogen and creatinine are reasonable determinations. A white cell count usually contributes little to the diagnosis but may provide confirmatory evidence in the patient who appears toxic.

Intravenous Pyelography. The dictum that all UTIs in men are complicated (i.e., caused by an anatomic or functional disruption of the urinary tract) has led many to obtain an IV pyelogram routinely when a UTI is detected in a male patient. In the absence of suspected obstruction or refractory infection, there is little evidence to support such a practice in male adults. (In bacteriuric infants and boys, the situation is different.) Although it is true that the prevalence of abnormalities on IV pyelogram is high in men with UTI, the contribution of these findings to management is often minimal. Pending better data regarding who benefits most from IV pyelography, many authorities recommend reserving the test for those with recurrent infection, suspected upper tract obstruction, or pyelonephritis. The IV pyelogram also provides an estimate of the postvoid residual. Renal ultrasonography offers a dye-free means of checking for obstruction.

Determination of Residual Volume. In the elderly patient with recurrent UTI, assessment is often directed at identifying risk factors for recurrence. Residual volume is among the most prominent. Straight catheterization after voiding is a simple technique to determine residual volume. It entails a very low risk for infection if performed after the urine is sterilized. A volume of more than 50 mL is abnormal. The IV pyelogram also provides an estimate of residual volume. Whether reduction in residual volume by treatment of bladder outlet obstruction reduces the risks and morbidity of UTI remains to be determined.

Testing for Prostate Involvement. In the setting of recurrent or relapsing UTI, there is usually some concern that the prostate may be harboring organisms. A *three-glass test*, which includes culture and Gram's stain of the expressed prostatic secretions (see Chapter 139), may provide objective evidence for prostatic infection. However, the test is expensive (several cultures are required), and its interpretation remains uncertain (no "gold standard" test is available to provide a basis for comparison). Under most clinical circumstances of recurrent UTI, it is assumed that the prostate is involved to some degree, and treatment is initiated empirically without the need for such testing (see below). However, when the results of testing for prostate infection would alter clinical decision making (e.g., as in planning prostate surgery), then the test may prove worthwhile.

Localization Studies. Differentiating upper from lower tract infection is helpful because of the implications for clinical course and treatment. Clinical findings are usually nonspecific. Instrumentation (ureteral catheterization, bladder washout) is the only proven method for making such a determination. *Antibody coating* is useful as a research technique but not in clinical practice because false-positives occur in patients with prostatic involvement. The best available test has been the response to an initial course of antibiotics.

Testing for Sexually Transmitted Disease in Young Patients. Sexually transmitted diseases may present with urethral symptoms and mimic UTI. Young patients with acute urethral symptoms, even if unaccompanied by discharge, need to be tested for chlamydial infection, which has reached epidemic proportions among adolescents and young adults. Urethral swabbing is carried out (see Chapters 125 and 136). Methods that can identify chlamydial infection from a urine sample are under development. In addition, any urethral discharge should be Gram's-stained, examined for gonococci and leukocytes, and plated promptly on Thayer-Martin medium (see Chapter 137).

PRINCIPLES OF MANAGEMENT

Symptomatic Infection

Initial Infection. Acute onset of a symptomatic UTI in a male patient should be treated. In the absence of evidence for serious renal parenchymal disease or marked obstruction, one can immediately start a course of oral antibiotics. The initial choice of agent is based on Gram's stain findings, pending culture results. If gram-negative rods are found, then one double-strength tablet of *trimethoprim/sulfamethoxazole* (TMS) twice daily usually suffices. If the organisms are gram-positive cocci, then *amoxicillin* (500 mg three times daily) represents a better choice. The initial program can be revised, if need be, after urine culture results and antibiotic sensitivities become available. As noted above, urine culturing is important in men because of the wide range of organisms and drug sensitivities.

Unlike women, who respond well to single-dose and 3-day treatment regimens, men are customarily treated with a *7- to 10-day* course of antibiotics, based on the view that all male UTIs are at least partially "complicated." Hardly any data are available on abbreviated antibiotic regimens in men. If symptoms clear, no further evaluation or repeated culturing is necessary.

Refractory or Recurrent Infection. Failure to clear symptoms or quick relapse suggests persistence of the original infection. Prostatic involvement (about half of instances), obstruction, anatomic anomaly, or functional disease may be responsible, necessitating repeated urine culture and consideration of IV pyelogram, three-glass testing, and a prolonged course of therapy (6 to 12 weeks) with an antibiotic that both penetrates the prostate and is active against resistant organisms. Many authorities recommend the fluoroquinolone antibiotics in this setting (e.g., 400 mg of *norfloxacin* twice daily). Although a third more effective than *TMS* (which is also prescribed in this setting), the fluoroquinolones are several times more expensive.

Overall, about 65% to 90% of men are cured by a prolonged course of antibiotics. The variability in results depends on the frequency and severity of important underlying pathology. A patient with prostatitis and no postvoid residual has a reasonable chance for cure, but the person with a large postvoid residual is unlikely to derive lasting benefit until the underlying cause has been addressed. Looking for and correcting any treatable precipitants of infection (obstruction, bladder dysfunction, anatomic anomaly) is likely to be more productive than depending solely on repeated or prolonged courses of increasingly potent antibiotics.

Long-term antibiotic prophylaxis against symptomatic recurrences is sometimes prescribed (e.g., double-strength tablet of TMS daily at bedtime). However, concerns about selecting for resistant strains, drug toxicity, and cost have limited this practice to a very small number of patients (those with frequent incapacitating episodes and those at high risk for a serious complication of infection). Because even the frail elderly have low rates of UTI complications, very few patients are treated with long-term antibiotics.

Asymptomatic Infection

Debate continues on the need to treat the debilitated elderly nursing home patient who has asymptomatic bacteriuria. The issue will remain moot so long as it continues to be virtually impossible to eradicate infection in many such patients, especially those who become incontinent and require indwelling or condom catheterization on a long-term basis. In those with an indwelling catheter for more than 30 days, infection becomes a near certainty. Antibiotics may temporarily clear the infection, but relapse within 4 weeks is the rule. Only those who become symptomatic derive benefit from a course of antibiotics. More important are regularly scheduled catheter changes, which reduce the risks of encrustation and obstruction. Although the incidence of bacteriuria is lower with use of a condom catheter, it still approaches 40%. A daily change of the collecting system apparatus helps to cut the rate of infection.

The role of antibiotic therapy is different for men with asymptomatic bacteriuria who are scheduled to undergo surgery and will require short-term urinary tract instrumentation. Preoperative urine testing and treatment are essential to avoid introduction of bacteria into the upper urinary tract and bloodstream. This is especially important for patients scheduled to undergo urologic surgery or surgery in which a foreign body is to be introduced. A fluoroquinolone antibiotic is a reasonable choice for antibiotic therapy under these conditions, but culture and sensitivity results are the best determinants of antibiotic choice.

INDICATIONS FOR REFERRAL AND ADMISSION

Any UTI patient who appears toxic or obstructed requires immediate hospitalization. Urosepsis is a potentially life-threatening complication of UTI that necessitates high-dose parenteral antibiotics and prompt evaluation and treatment of the underlying precipitant. Symptoms of pyelonephritis and urosepsis in elderly patients may be vague (change in mental status, new onset of "failure to thrive"), so a high index of suspicion is warranted. The patient with recurrent symptomatic UTI who promptly relapses after a 6-week course of fluoroquinolone therapy should be considered for urologic evaluation, as should the person with UTI in the context of declining renal function. An infectious disease consultant can also be helpful in these difficult situations.

A.G.M./A.H.G

ANNOTATED BIBLIOGRAPHY

Baldassarre JS, Kaye D. Special problems of urinary tract infection in the elderly. Med Clin North Am 1991;75:375. (*Includes the question of treating asymptomatic bacteriuria.*)

Barnes RC, Daifuku R, Roddy RE, et al. Urinary tract infection in sexually active homosexual men. Lancet 1986;1:171. (*Anal intercourse is a risk factor for cystitis.*)

Berger RE, Alexander ER, Monda GD, et al. *Chlamydia trachomatis* as a cause of acute idiopathic epididymitis. N Engl J Med 1978; 298:301. (*Eight of 13 men under age 35 had* C. trachomatis *infection; 8 of 10 over 35 had coliform infections.*)

Boscia JA, Abrutyn E, Kaye D. Asymptomatic bacteriuria in elderly persons: treat or do not treat? Ann Intern Med 1987;106;764. (*The evidence favors not treating.*)

Collins MM, Stafford RS, et al. Distinguishing chronic prostatitis and benign prostatic hyperplasia symptoms: results of a national survey of physician visits. Urology 1999;53:921. (*Pain is the distinguishing feature.*)

Krieger JN, Ross SO, Simonsen JM. Urinary tract infections in healthy university men. J Urol 1993;149:1046. (*Mean incidence of 5 in 10,000 men annually.*)

Lipsky BA. Urinary tract infections in men: epidemiology, pathophysiology, diagnosis, and treatment. Ann Intern Med 1989;110:138. (*The best review; 107 references.*)

Lipsky BA. Prostatitis and urinary tract infection in men: what's new; what's true. Am J Med 1999;106:327. (*Authoritative review.*)

Lipsky BA, Ireton RC, Fihn SD, et al. Diagnosis of bacteriuria in men: specimen collection and culture interpretation. J Infect Dis 1987; 155:1341. (*The best study of the question. Initial and midstream specimens are equally valid; meatal cleansing is unnecessary.*)

Litwin MS, McNaughton-Collins M, et al. The National Institutes of Health chronic prostatitis symptom index: development and validation of a new outcome measure. J Urol 1999;162:369. (*Presents a validated nine-item index to help gather and interpret more evidence about this difficult condition.*)

Nordenstam GR, Brandberg CA, Oden AS, et al. Bacteriuria and mortality in an elderly population. N Engl J Med 1986;314:1152. (*No lowering of survival with bacteriuria when cancer is excluded.*)

Ouslander JG, Greengold BA, Silverblatt FJ, et al. An accurate method to obtain urine from culture in men with external catheters. Arch Intern Med 1987;147:286. (*A useful method in incontinent persons that avoids catheterization.*)

Saffaj, Hoagland VL, Cook T. Norfloxacin versus cotrimoxazole in the treatment of recurring urinary tract infections in men. Scand J Infect Dis 1986;48[Suppl]:48. (*Norfloxacin was about one-third more effective.*)

Saint S, Lipsky BA. Preventing catheter-related bacteriuria: should we? Can we? How? Arch Intern Med 1999;159:800. (*Evidence-based review concludes that infection can be delayed but not prevented during long periods of catheterization.*)

Smith JW, Jones SR, Reed WP, et al. Recurrent urinary tract infections in men. Ann Intern Med 1979;91:544. (*Half had underlying prostate infection, more than 70% grew* E. coli; *most failed to respond to a standard 10-day course of therapy, whether they were symptomatic or not.*)

Spach DH, Stapleton AE, Stamm WE, et al. Lack of circumcision increases the risk of urinary tract infection in young men. JAMA 1992;267:679. (*An important risk factor for cystitis in young men.*)

Stamm WE, Hooton TM. Management of urinary tract infections in adults. N Engl J Med 1993;329:1328. (*Includes excellent discussion of UTI in the elderly; 60 references.*)

141

Management of Syphilis and Other Sexually Transmitted Diseases

BENJAMIN DAVIS
HARVEY B. SIMON

SYPHILIS

In 1943, the dramatic efficacy of penicillin treatment was established, and for the next 15 years the incidence of new cases of syphilis declined steadily to a low of about 6,500 in 1956. Although *Treponema pallidum*, the spirochete that causes syphilis, has not developed resistance to penicillin, the incidence of syphilis has increased progressively in the last 25 years, largely because of a change in sexual mores, with many new cases occurring in adolescents, young adults, and homosexuals. An accelerating resurgence had been noted among inner-city residents, IV drug abusers, and HIV-infected persons, which peaked in 1991. Since then, the rates have declined steadily to an all-time low since reporting began.

Pathophysiology, Clinical Presentation, and Course

Humans are the only natural reservoir of *T. pallidum*. Except for cases of transplacental transmission, virtually all cases are acquired by sexual contact with persons having active infectious lesions. *T. pallidum* readily penetrates abraded skin and intact mucous membranes to multiply locally and disseminate through the lymphatics and bloodstream.

The course of syphilis can be divided into primary, secondary, latent, and tertiary phases.

Primary Syphilis. The lesion of primary syphilis is the chancre, which occurs at the site of inoculation about 3 weeks after exposure. The chancre is usually located on the genitalia, but, depending on sexual practices, it can occur in the anal canal, on oral mucosa, on the hands, and in other locations. The lesion begins as a small papule that enlarges and undergoes superficial necrosis to produce an ulcer with a clean base and sharp margins. The chancre is typically painless, and patients are free of constitutional symptoms, although regional nodes may be enlarged. The chancre is teeming with spirochetes and is highly infectious. Even without therapy, the chancre heals completely in 2 to 6 weeks.

Secondary Syphilis. About 2 months after the primary infection, the features of secondary syphilis may appear. Secondary syphilis is a systemic disease. A flulike syndrome is common, as is generalized lymphadenopathy. The most characteristic feature of secondary syphilis is a generalized skin eruption. Lesions may be macular, papular, or papulosquamous but tend to be symmetric and uniform in size; typically, the palms and soles are involved. Patches and split papules often occur on the mucous membranes. Secondary syphilis can involve many other organs; clinical manifestations may include aseptic meningitis, hepatitis, nephritis, or uveitis. Patients with secondary syphilis are contagious. As in primary syphilis, the manifestations of secondary syphilis resolve spontaneously even without therapy, although up to 25% of patients exhibit a brief relapse of secondary lesions.

Latent and Tertiary Syphilis. Untreated patients without active lesions are considered to have latent syphilis. About two thirds of these people remain entirely asymptomatic, but in the remaining third, the lesions of tertiary syphilis develop, usually 10 to 40 years after primary infection. The major forms of tertiary syphilis include (a) *cardiovascular syphilis*, characterized by aneurysmal dilation of the ascending aorta and aortic insufficiency; (b) *neurosyphilis*, which may be asymptomatic; alternatively, it may present as general paresis with disorders of intellect and personality, or as tabes dorsalis, with ataxic gait, impaired pain and temperature sensation, autonomic dysfunction, and hypoactive reflexes; and (c) *gummas*, which are isolated, slowly progressive, destructive granulomatous lesions of skin, bone, liver, or other organs.

Infection of the Central Nervous System infection may occur at any point in the natural history of untreated syphilis and may be more likely in HIV-positive patients. Even in the absence of neurologic symptoms, about 25% of patients with primary, secondary, or latent infection have cerebrospinal fluid abnormalities (pleocytosis, elevated protein, serologies positive for syphilis). Although it is not clear how many of these patients will ultimately be affected by symptomatic neurosyphilis, concern is warranted. Organisms have been detected from the central nervous system in 30% of patients with untreated primary and secondary disease.

Syphilis and HIV Disease. Patients with syphilis are at increased risk for other sexually transmitted diseases, including HIV infection. Moreover, those with HIV infection are at increased risk for syphilis. Some studies find that HIV-infected patients have unusually high titers in their syphilis serology, whereas others find that seroconversion can be delayed or blunted by concomitant HIV infection, particularly in patients with symptomatic AIDS. In addition to being more common in HIV-infected persons, syphilis in these patients may be clinically atypical, unusually severe, or more difficult to treat successfully. Central nervous system syphilis is also more likely in HIV-positive patients.

Congenital Syphilis occurs as a result of transplacental transmission of spirochetes during the second or third trimester of pregnancy. Fetal loss is about 60%, and up to half of surviving infants have stigmata, which can result in serious permanent handicaps. Congenital syphilis can be prevented by prompt treatment of maternal infection.

Diagnosis

Treponema pallidum cannot be cultured in vitro, but the diagnosis of syphilis can be made by direct visualization of treponemas from the chancre. This is a specialized technique that requires *dark-field* or *fluorescent microscopy* and very experienced observers. As a result, the diagnosis usually depends on clinical features and serologic testing.

The most widely used serologic tests for syphilis employ a nontreponemal antigen (lipoidal extract of mammalian tissues). Examples include the *Venereal Disease Research Laboratory* (VDRL), *Hinton*, and *rapid plasma reagin* (RPR) tests. These are excellent screening tests, but the false-positive rate is as high as 30%, often as the result of unrelated infections or inflammatory diseases that produce hyperglobulinemia. More specific serologic tests employ treponemal antigens and can distinguish true-positive from false-positive results. The most frequently used treponemal test is the *microhemagglutination–T. pallidum* (MHA-TP) test (see Chapter 124).

Some patients with primary syphilis manifest false-negative nontreponemal and treponemal test results. False-negatives are most likely to occur in patients with infections of less than 30 days' duration. For persons with a suspect primary lesion, dark-field examination should be performed and serologic studies repeated in 10 to 14 days. For *HIV-infected* patients with suspect skin lesions and negative serology, skin biopsy may be necessary to rule out syphilis. The Warthin-Starry stain can be used to visualize organisms in biopsy specimens.

Principles of Management and Therapeutic Recommendations

The results of treatment of early syphilis are excellent. *T. pallidum* is very sensitive to *penicillin*. Because the organism multiplies slowly, the goal is to attain long-lasting antibiotic levels. Present recommendations include the following:

- For early syphilis (primary, secondary, early latent stages), treat with 2.4 million units of *benzathine penicillin* IM at a single session. Penicillin-allergic patients should receive 500 mg of oral *tetracycline* four times daily for 14 days or 100 mg of *doxycycline* twice daily for 14 days. Doxycycline and tetracycline are contraindicated in pregnancy.
- For syphilis of more than 1 year's duration (latent, tertiary, or unknown duration), treat with 2.4 million units of *benzathine penicillin* IM weekly for 3 weeks consecutively. Penicillin-allergic patients should receive 500 mg of oral *tetracycline* four times daily for 28 days or 100 mg of *doxycycline* twice daily for 28 days.
- Neurosyphilis should be treated with 18 to 24 million units of *aqueous penicillin G* IV, divided every 4 hours, for 14 days. Some experts recommend a single dose of 2.4 million units of *benzathine penicillin* IM at the end of IV therapy. After

therapy, the cerebrospinal fluid should be reexamined every 6 months until findings are normal.

- HIV infection may increase the risk for neurosyphilis, but cerebrospinal fluid abnormalities are common in HIV-infected patients, and their presence is of uncertain significance. Lumbar puncture should be considered. There are no data to suggest that the treatment regimens prescribed for HIV-negative patients will be less effective in HIV-positive patients. HIV-infected patients should be monitored closely after therapy.
- Syphilis in pregnancy and neurosyphilis should always be treated with penicillin. Patients allergic to penicillin should be desensitized if necessary.
- A febrile reaction (the Jarisch-Herxheimer reaction), often with headache and myalgia, may occur within the first 24 hours after treatment of syphilis, especially early syphilis. Patients should be warned of this possibility, but treatment should not be delayed.

Immunity to syphilis is incomplete and reinfection may occur, especially in patients treated with penicillin within a year of infection. Follow-up of patients is essential. Quantitative nontreponemal serologies at 3, 6, and 12 months after treatment help determine adequacy of therapy. HIV-infected patients should be followed more closely. Failure to sustain a fourfold decline in titers with therapy suggests treatment failure or reinfection, and examination of the cerebrospinal fluid should be considered. If lumbar puncture is not possible, retreatment with a regimen used for syphilis of more than 1 year's duration should be considered.

All cases of syphilis should be reported to the appropriate public health authorities so that appropriate case finding can be performed. Like all patients with sexually transmitted diseases, syphilis patients need to be screened for other venereal infections, including HIV infection, chlamydial infection, and gonorrhea (see Chapters 7, 125, and 137), and counseled about HIV infection and safe sex practices.

CHANCROID AND GRANULOMA INGUINALE

Chancroid, which is endemic in some areas of the United States, is caused by the gram-negative bacillus *Haemophilus ducreyi*. It typically produces painful genital ulcers that are often accompanied by regional adenopathy. Azithromycin (1 g PO) or ceftriaxone (250 mg IM), both given as a single dose, are the treatments of choice.

Painless, slowly progressive genital ulcers are characteristic of *granuloma inguinale*, caused by the gram-negative bacterium *Donovania granulomatis*. Double-strength *trimethoprim/sulfamethoxazole* twice daily or 100 mg of *doxycycline* twice daily, both for 21 days, are the treatments of choice. Both chancroid and granuloma inguinale are rare in temperate climates.

LYMPHOGRANULOMA VENEREUM

A microorganism belonging to the *Chlamydia* group of obligate intracellular parasites is the cause of lymphogranuloma venereum. In this disease, the primary genital lesion is a small, painless papule that heals spontaneously and often escapes no-tice. The major impact of the disease is on the regional lymphatics. Inguinal nodes enlarge and may suppurate to produce chronic draining sinuses. Scarring and lymphatic obstruction may result. Women and homosexual men may have proctocolitis, which can lead to rectal fibrosis, strictures, and fistulas. A 21-day course of doxycycline (100 mg twice daily) is the treatment of choice. An alternative is a 21-day course of erythromycin (500 mg four times daily).

OTHER SEXUALLY TRANSMITTED DISEASES

Gonorrhea. See Chapter 137.

Chlamydial Infection. See Chapters 125 and 136.

HIV Infection. See Chapters 7 and 13.

Genital Herpes. See Chapter 192.

Condylomata Acuminata. See Chapter 194.

Pubic Lice. See Chapter 195.

ANNOTATED BIBLIOGRAPHY

Centers for Disease Control and Prevention. 1998 Guidelines for treatment of sexually transmitted diseases. MMWR Morb Mortal Wkly Rep 1998;47(RR-1):1. (*An authoritative and comprehensive reference.*)

Centers for Disease Control and Prevention. Primary, secondary syphilis—U.S. 1981–1990. MMWR Morb Mortal Wkly Rep 1991;40:314. (*The changing epidemiology of syphilis.*)

Gourevitch MC, Selwyn PA, Davenny K, et al. Effects of HIV infection on the serologic manifestations and response to treatment of syphilis in intravenous drug users. Ann Intern Med 1993;118:350. (*HIV infection did not alter the clinical presentation or course of syphilis in this cohort.*)

Hart G. Syphilis tests in diagnostic and therapeutic decision making. Ann Intern Med 1986;104:368. (*A critical look at available diagnostic tests.*)

Hook EW 3rd, Stephens J, Ennis DM. Azithromycin compared with penicillin G benzathine for treatment of incubating syphilis. Ann Intern Med 1999;131:434. (*Azithromycin in a single 1.0-g dose seemed effective.*)

Jackman JD. Cardiovascular syphilis. Am J Med 1989;87:425. (*A review of cardiovascular manifestations of tertiary disease.*)

Musher DM. Syphilis, neurosyphilis, penicillin, and AIDS. J Infect Dis 1991;163:1201. (*Excellent review of the need for intensive therapy in HIV-infected patients.*)

Musher DM, Hamill RJ, Baughn RE. Effect of human immunodeficiency virus (HIV) infection on the course of syphilis and on the response to treatment. Ann Intern Med 1990;113:872. (*Intensive therapy and follow-up are recommended.*)

Romanowski B, Sutherland R, Fick GH, et al. Serologic response to treatment of infectious syphilis. Ann Intern Med 1991;114:1005. (*Therapeutic response must be based on illness episode and pretreatment RPR titer; seroconversion can occur after 36 months.*)

Woodward C, Fisher MA. Drug treatment of common STDs. Am Fam Physician 1999;60:1387. (*First of two-part series that succinctly reviews changes in the 1998 Centers for Disease Control recommendations.*)

142

Management of the Patient with Chronic Renal Failure

LESLIE S-T. FANG

Although many diseases can lead to chronic renal failure, the resulting clinical manifestations and functional derangements are remarkably constant. The primary physician is often responsible for initial conservative management, including interventions that have been shown to delay progression of disease. Additional objectives are to prevent or minimize the complications of uremia, monitor disease progression, and judge when referral to the nephrologist is indicated for consideration of dialysis or transplantation.

PATHOPHYSIOLOGY, CLINICAL PRESENTATION, AND COURSE

Pathophysiology

Chronic renal failure can result from glomerular, vascular, or tubular disease. Congenital anomalies, infection, metabolic diseases, obstructive uropathy, and collagen vascular disease can all lead to renal insufficiency. Irrespective of underlying disease, the major clinical manifestations of chronic renal failure result from disturbances in electrolyte and fluid balance, elimination of metabolic wastes and toxins, erythropoietin production, and blood pressure control. The role of urea and other toxins in the production of symptoms remains controversial.

Fluid and Electrolyte Problems. These include hyperkalemia, volume overload, hypocalcemia, hyperphosphatemia, and metabolic acidosis. With moderate renal insufficiency, the *urinary concentrating ability* is impaired, so that to handle the same solute load, patients have to drink and excrete more water than normal. This results in polydipsia, polyuria, and nocturia. The ability to dilute urine is compromised with further renal impairment, producing isosthenuria and obligate fluid intake. As renal function continues to decline, oliguria supervenes. The situation is similar with sodium; moderate renal failure produces mild *salt wasting*. In the later stages, sodium excretion becomes limited, *salt retention* develops, and edema supervenes.

Potassium excretion is usually preserved until late in the course, when *potassium retention* occurs as oliguria develops and the ability of the distal tubules to secrete potassium is compromised.

Decreased renal function produces *phosphate retention*, *secondary hypocalcemia*, and, consequently, *secondary hyperparathyroidism*. Decreased intestinal calcium absorption secondary to impaired hydroxylation of vitamin D also contributes to hypocalcemia.

Acidosis results from an inability to excrete urinary ammonium and, with further impairment, titratable acid. Loss of bicarbonate exacerbates the problem. *Uric acid* levels increase as urate excretion falls.

Endocrine Problems. Impairment of renal endocrine function contributes to anemia, hypertension, and congestive failure, which may further compromise renal function. *Decreased erythropoietin* production results in a mild to moderate normochromic normocytic anemia. Anemia also develops as a consequence of increased hemolysis and bleeding, aggravated by impaired platelet adhesiveness. *Increased renin* levels sometimes occur, causing modest hypertension and fluid retention. In addition to renal osteodystrophy, *secondary hyperparathyroidism* may lead to alterations in central nervous system calcium, which have been implicated in some of the neurologic manifestations of renal failure.

Hematologic Problems. Anemia in the patient with chronic renal failure develops as renal production of erythropoietin declines. The anemia may be severe enough to cause symptoms, which usually occur when the creatinine level rises above 4 mg/dL and the hematocrit falls to less than 25%.

Clinical Presentation and Course

Early in renal failure, anorexia, lassitude, fatigability, and weakness are prominent symptoms. As renal failure worsens, the patient may complain of pruritus, nausea, vomiting, constipation, or diarrhea. Shortness of breath may occur secondary to cardiomyopathy and fluid overload. Edema, hypertension, and pericarditis are common late in the course. Neurologic manifestations include drowsiness, lethargy, peripheral myopathy, seizures, and, terminally, coma.

The course of renal failure is punctuated by periods of rapid deterioration, often precipitated by dehydration or infection. The rate of progression depends, in part, on the underlying renal disease, being more rapid in patients with diabetic nephropathy or severe hypertension and slower in patients with polycystic kidneys. However, in patients with advanced renal failure (creatinine level >10 mg/dL), mean survival without intervention is 100 to 150 days.

PRINCIPLES OF MANAGEMENT

Conservative management of renal failure can prolong survival and preserve quality of life by compensating for the excretory, regulatory, and endocrine functions of the kidney. The goals of therapy are to reduce symptoms, slow progression, and avoid preventable complications.

Drug Therapy to Slow Progression to End-stage Renal Failure. Early initiation of therapy with *angiotensin converting-enzyme inhibitors* (ACE inhibitors) reduces the risk for progression to end-stage renal disease. This effect was first established in diabetic renal disease (both normotensive and hypertensive), but it also pertains to cases with nondiabetic causes.

Protein Intake. The excretory function of the kidneys involves the removal of nitrogenous waste. Reduction of dietary protein intake has long been the cornerstone of therapy for uremia. Early in the course of renal disease, reduction of protein intake helps reduce the rate of progression, but the degree of benefit is actually quite modest. Late in the course of renal disease, reduction of protein intake is useful in preventing azotemia from worsening.

Restricting the daily intake of protein to 0.5 g/kg usually allows sufficient amounts for daily requirements while slowing the progression of renal failure. Foods rich in *essential amino acids* are the most effectively utilized source of nitrogen.

Blood Pressure Control. Hypertension is a common complication of renal disease. Rigid control of blood pressure is the most important of factors influencing the rate of disease progression. Blood pressure control is beneficial regardless of the antihypertensive agent or agents employed. However, the best results are associated with the use of *ACE inhibitors*, particularly if they are administered early. ACE inhibitors are thought to slow the rate of injury by decreasing glomerular hyperfiltration. Renal function should be monitored carefully during ACE inhibitor therapy because acute deterioration in renal function may be seen in some patients, particularly those with bilateral renal vascular disease. Calcium channel blockers have also been shown to delay the onset of nephropathy in patients with type I diabetes. Alternative antihypertensive agents include α- and β-blockers, diuretics, and vasodilators. Patients with pronounced proteinuria respond best to aggressive reduction in blood pressure.

Fluids and Electrolytes. Judicious fluid and electrolyte management is exceedingly important because patients with chronic renal failure have difficulty adjusting to variations of either excessive intake or rigid restriction of salt and fluids.

Sodium. In the early and middle stages of renal failure, salt and fluid intake must be adequate to match the excess losses that occur as tubular functions begin to deteriorate. Restriction of intake can actually accelerate renal damage by causing decreased extracellular volume and reduced renal perfusion. The concentrating ability can be measured by determining the specific gravity of a first morning urine specimen, and sodium requirements can be estimated by testing a 24-hour urine collection for sodium excretion. In later stages, as excretion of sodium and water becomes limited, cautious sodium and fluid restriction becomes necessary.

Potassium. Because potassium excretion is preserved until late in the course of renal failure, there is usually no need to restrict its intake until oliguria sets in. However, it is prudent to *avoid* or at least use with caution *drugs* that predispose to potassium retention, such as potassium-sparing diuretics, potassium supplements, β-adrenergic blockers, and NSAIDs. Because acidosis worsens hyperkalemia, it should be corrected promptly. On the other hand, severe protracted hypokalemia can itself cause tubular damage; therefore, serum potassium should be monitored regularly and low levels corrected.

Calcium. Hypocalcemia and secondary hyperparathyroidism are best countered by reducing the elevations in serum phosphate that result from decreased renal excretion of the anion. The principle of therapy is to lower serum phosphate by reducing dietary sources, inhibiting absorption, and maintaining adequate calcium levels with pharmacologic doses of *vitamin D* and exogenous *calcium*. In patients with hypocalcemia and hyperphosphatemia, calcium citrate can be used to help with phosphate binding. It should be administered either shortly before or shortly after a meal to maximize phosphate binding. Aluminum hydroxide antacids are now used infrequently because of concern that excessive ingestion may lead to aluminum-induced osteomalacia and neuropathy.

In advanced disease, renal hydroxylation of 25-hydroxyvitamin D is impaired, so that the use of 1,25-dihydroxyvitamin D_3 becomes necessary. This reduces the prevalence of secondary hyperparathyroidism and the ensuing metabolic bone disease. In patients with severe hyperparathyroidism, partial parathyroidectomy should be considered.

Hyperuricemia. Urate reduction is necessary only if gouty attacks develop (see Chapter 158).

Acidosis. Correction of acidosis becomes desirable when the serum bicarbonate level falls below 15 mEq/L. Any external acid loads, such as aspirin, vitamin C, or excess protein intake, should be removed. *Sodium bicarbonate* is given as long as the sodium load can be tolerated. The goal is to titrate the serum bicarbonate level to 16 to 20 mEq/L.

Hematologic Problems. The advent of *recombinant erythropoietin* has greatly enhanced the management of the anemia of chronic renal failure. After patients become symptomatic (usually when the hematocrit falls below 25%), erythropoietin therapy can be started, administered either SQ or IV three times per week in doses of 1,000 to 6,000 units. Patients require close monitoring of hemoglobin, reticulocyte count, and ferritin. Iron supplementation must be provided to patients who are iron-deficient to maximize the efficacy of erythropoietin therapy. Most patients with symptomatic anemia respond well, with improvement in quality of life in addition to hematologic parameters. Judicious use of erythropoietin can usually raise the hematocrit to the 30% level and avoid the need for repeated transfusions.

Transfusion therapy is sometimes used, but repeated transfusions carry the risk for hepatitis (see Chapter 70) and sensitization to leukocyte HLA antigens, which can complicate finding a compatible cadaver donor for renal transplantation.

Patients with chronic renal failure should be cautioned to avoid antiplatelet drugs. Abnormalities in platelet function can be aggravated by drugs such as aspirin and other NSAIDs (see Chapter 81). The abnormalities can be corrected by dialysis or the administration of cryoprecipitates, DDAVP (deamino-8-D-arginine vasopressin), or estrogens. Uremia-induced megaloblastic changes are unresponsive to folate or vitamin B_{12}.

Cardiovascular Complications. The onset of congestive heart failure poses a very difficult problem, especially late in the course of the disease, when the ability to excrete sodium may be very limited. *Salt restriction* and a trial of a *loop diuretic* (e.g., furosemide) may be tried, but these measures are often insufficient. *Metolazone* can be added to a loop diuretic regimen; it often augments the diuretic effect. Renal function and the electrolyte profile should be carefully monitored. Digitalization must be carried out with care, as the renal excretion of digoxin is compromised (see Chapter 32). *Dialysis* may be the only recourse in patients with refractory fluid overload.

Uremic pericarditis is another late cardiovascular complication. Patients may have symptoms of atypical chest pain and progress to pericardial tamponade. The development of pericarditis is an indication to proceed with dialysis.

Neuromuscular Difficulties. Lethargy, an inability to concentrate, and asterixis improve with *protein* restriction. However, peripheral neuropathies often progress despite comprehensive conservation therapy. Muscle cramping and tetany respond to correction of hypocalcemia.

Itching, Hiccups, and Nausea. These symptoms are not life-threatening but certainly contribute to the patient's misery and require attention. Pruritus can be quite stubborn but responds to topical measures (see Chapter 178). *Prochlorperazine* is effective in lessening hiccups and nausea.

Adjustment of Medications and Avoidance of Nephrotoxic Agents. Doses of drugs and other substances that are excreted renally or are potentially nephrotoxic must be adjusted. This is one of the most crucial aspects in the management of chronic renal failure. *Digoxin* (see Chapter 32), *aminoglycoside* antibiotics, radiographic *contrast media*, *ACE inhibitors*, and *NSAIDs* are important examples of agents to be used with extreme care in uremic patients. Elderly azotemic patients, who are likely to have some degree of renal vascular impairment, are particularly susceptible to agents that affect the renin–angiotensin system (e.g., ACE inhibitors) or inhibit renal prostaglandin production (e.g., NSAIDs). Diabetics with underlying renal disease may experience acute deterioration in renal function from a dye load, such as may be administered for angiography or even pyelography.

Not all drugs that cause an elevation in serum creatinine are necessarily nephrotoxic. Cimetidine and trimethoprim compete with creatinine for tubular excretion; elevations in serum creatinine may ensue, especially in patients who are azotemic. Methyldopa and cefoxitin interfere with some autoanalyzer measurements of creatinine and can give falsely elevated readings.

Aggravating Conditions. Of chief importance is early detection and correction of any condition that may further compromise renal function. Urinary tract infection, dehydration, gastrointestinal bleeding, and congestive heart failure can cause acute decompensation.

PATIENT EDUCATION AND SUPPORT

Successful therapy and good morale depend strongly on a well-developed doctor–patient relationship. The patient must be educated about chronic renal failure and the rationale behind therapy because compliance is central to successful conservative management, especially if the treatment requires dietary restrictions. Renal failure is a serious chronic disease that often precipitates depression, denial, anger, and noncompliance. The physician's patience, understanding, support, and interest are powerful but sometimes underutilized elements of the treatment program.

Keeping the patient well informed enhances a sense of control and facilitates compliance. Treatment alternatives must be presented honestly and completely. Discussions about diet, medications, prognosis, and therapeutic options should include the family. Psychosocial management should aim at minimizing dependence and social isolation.

INDICATIONS FOR REFERRAL AND ADMISSION

Patients can generally be managed as outpatients, but referral to a nephrologist should be made if clinical deterioration continues despite maximal supportive therapy. As the serum creatinine level approaches 10 mg/dL, mean survival drops to between 100 and 150 days, so that consideration of dialysis or transplantation is warranted. Moreover, vascular access for hemodialysis needs to be constructed with 2 to 3 months of lead time to permit maturation of the fistula and revisions. Decisions regarding dialysis and transplantation require a comprehensive evaluation of the patient's medical, psychological, and social situation, which necessitates a close working relationship between the patient, family, primary physician, and nephrologist.

Continuous ambulatory peritoneal dialysis (CAPD) and *continuous cycling peritoneal dialysis* (CCPD) are outpatient options that provide a high degree of independence for the patient and the physiologic advantage of a slow, continuous dialysis process. Dialysate administrations are conducted through an indwelling abdominal catheter three to five times per day. Results are comparable with those of hemodialysis. The main disadvantage is a substantial risk for peritonitis; fortunately, most cases are mild and can be managed on an outpatient basis by self-administration of antibiotics through the catheter.

Hospitalization may be required for control of fluid overload, hypertension, hyperkalemia, or infection. In general, the multiplicity of possible metabolic disturbances in the patient with chronic renal insufficiency demands careful follow-up and constant adjustments of the treatment program.

MANAGEMENT RECOMMENDATIONS

Angiotensin-converting Enzyme Inhibitors to Slow Progression to End-stage Renal Failure

- Consider initiation of ACE inhibitor therapy (e.g., 25 mg of captopril two to three times daily) early in the course of renal failure, especially in patients with diabetes, but also in persons with nondiabetic renal disease. Hypertension is not a prerequisite for such treatment. Exert caution with ACE inhibitor use in the setting of acute dehydration. Monitor blood pressure, renal function, and serum potassium regularly. Omit in persons with bilateral renal artery stenosis.

Protein and Calories

- Restrict protein intake to 0.5 g of high-quality protein per kilogram daily if the patient is symptomatic or acidotic, and to 0.5 to 0.75 g/kg daily if the blood urea nitrogen level is above 75 mg/dL but the patient is asymptomatic.
- Maintain calorie intake at 40 to 50 cal/kg daily.

Fluids

- With mild to moderate renal insufficiency, fluid restriction is not necessary unless concomitant hypertension or congestive heart failure is present.
- Restrict fluids only in the presence of oliguria. Intake should equal urine output and insensible losses.

Hypertension

- ACE inhibitors are the treatment of choice, especially in diabetics and those with marked proteinuria, but also in those with nondiabetic renal disease. Calcium channel blockers have also been shown to delay onset of nephropathy in patients with type I diabetes. The choice of agent can be on the basis of cost and convenience (e.g., 25 mg of captopril three times daily); monitor renal function. Alternatives include α- and β-blockers and vasodilators (see Chapter 26).
- Attempt to achieve the lowest blood pressure possible in patients with marked proteinuria.

Sodium

- With mild to moderate renal insufficiency, salt restriction is not necessary.
- In patients with hypertension or congestive heart failure, salt restriction to 2 g of sodium daily may be necessary.
- Restrict sodium in the presence of oliguria or congestive heart failure.

Potassium

- For hypokalemic patients, administer potassium supplements in low doses and check levels frequently. Do not maintain potassium supplementation indefinitely.
- Avoid potassium-sparing diuretics in patients with moderate renal insufficiency.
- Monitor potassium frequently in oliguric patients. Treat levels above 6 mEq/L and admit if electrocardiographic changes accompany levels above 6.5 mEq/L. Mild chronic hyperkalemia is best treated with exchange resins such as sodium polystyrene sulfonate (Kayexalate), given by mouth or instilled as an enema in sorbitol. Kayexalate exchanges sodium ion for potassium ion; therefore, be alert to possible sodium and volume overload.

Calcium and Phosphate

- Correct hyperphosphatemia with calcium citrate (667 mg three times daily before meals).
- Symptomatic or severe hypocalcemia despite normalization of serum phosphate requires calcium supplements (e.g., 600 mg of calcium carbonate twice daily), vitamin D in pharmacologic doses (e.g., calcitriol 0.25 mg daily), or both.

Acidosis and Hyperuricemia

- Treat if serum bicarbonate concentration is less than 15 mEq/L.
- Remove external acid load.

- Treat acidosis with 600 mg of sodium bicarbonate twice daily initially, and titrate bicarbonate to the range of 16 to 20 mEq/L. Follow serum potassium and calcium levels during the treatment of acidosis because both may fall.
- Treat hyperuricemia only if symptomatic gout develops; use allopurinol (see Chapter 158).

Anemia

- Treat with 1,000 to 6,000 units of erythropoietin SQ three times per week; monitor hemoglobin, hematocrit, reticulocyte count, and serum ferritin.
- Avoid antiplatelet drugs.
- Give 325 mg of oral ferrous sulfate per day to patients with iron deficiency.
- Transfuse for high-output failure or angina. Avoid unnecessary blood work and injections.

Congestive Heart Failure

- Treat with restriction of salt.
- Add furosemide if congestive failure persists.
- Add metolazone (2.5 to 5 mg) if refractory fluid overload is present; monitor renal function and electrolytes closely.
- Consider use of an ACE inhibitor (e.g., start with 12.5 to 25 mg of captopril two to three times daily); monitor renal function closely.
- Digoxin can be used, but frequent monitoring of digoxin levels is needed.

Itching, Hiccups, and Nausea

- Minimize symptoms by reducing dietary protein intake.
- Prescribe 5 to 10 mg of prochlorperazine orally four times daily for nausea.
- Treat itching topically with menthol or phenol lotion or a trial of capsaicin cream; cholestyramine and ultraviolet light have also been used successfully (see Chapter 178).

Dialysis and Transplantation

- The conservative management outlined is directed toward prolongation of the symptom-free period. If dietary therapy becomes intolerable or is no longer effective, dialysis or transplantation must be considered. Referral to a nephrologist is necessary at this point. The primary physician should continue to participate in the important decisions about dialysis and transplantation.

ANNOTATED BIBLIOGRAPHY

Ayanian JZ, Cleary PD, Weissman JS, et al. The effect of patients' preferences on racial differences in access to renal transplantation. N Engl J Med 1999;341:1661. (*Preferences differ, but not enough to explain the substantial racial differences in access to transplantation.*)

Abuelo JG. Diagnosing vascular causes of renal failure. Ann Intern Med 1995;123:601. (*Excellent review emphasizing helpful clinical clues and laboratory confirmation.*)

Aradhye S. Clinical management of early progressive renal failure. Dis Mon 1998;44:178. (*Good basic review for the generalist.*)

Bennett WM, Aronoff GR, Morrison G, et al. Drug prescribing in renal failure. Am J Kidney Dis 1983;3:155. (*Extensive tables and discussion of dosing guidelines for adults with renal failure, including those on dialysis.*)

Eschback JW. The anemia of chronic renal failure. Kidney Int 1989;35:134. (*Pathophysiology and the effects of recombinant erythropoietin.*)

Evans RW, Rader B, Manninen DL, et al. The quality of life of hemodialysis recipients treated with recombinant human erythropoietin. JAMA 1990;263:825. (*Both quality of life and hematocrit improved.*)

Fraser CL, Arieff AI. Nervous system complications of uremia. Ann Intern Med 1988;109:143. (*Intellectual dysfunction, dialysis dementia, peripheral neuropathy, and disequilibrium syndrome reviewed; 119 references.*)

Giatras I, Lau J, Levey AS, et al. Effect of angiotensin-converting enzyme inhibitors on the progression of nondiabetic renal disease: a meta-analysis of randomized trials. Ann Intern Med 1997;127:337. (*This analysis of randomized, controlled studies found ACE inhibitors to be more effective than other antihypertensives in reducing the risk for worsening renal failure.*)

Harris LE, Luft FC, Rudy DW, et al. Effects of multidisciplinary case management in patients with chronic renal insufficiency. Am J Med 1998;105:464. (*Intensive, multidisciplinary case management of no measurable benefit among patients with modest degrees of renal failure.*)

Herzog CA, Ma JZ, Collins AJ. Poor long-term survival after acute myocardial infarction among patients on long-term dialysis. N Engl J Med 1998;339:799. (*Mortality of 59%, 73%, and 90% at 1, 2, and 3 years, respectively, after myocardial infarction among patients on dialysis.*)

Hirth RA, Turenne MN, Woods JD, et al. Predictors of type of vascular access in hemodialysis patients. JAMA 1996;276:1303. (*Large variations in relative use of fistulas and grafts, with a disconcerting trend away from fistula use.*)

Hsu C. Are we mismanaging calcium and phosphate metabolism in renal failure? Am J Kidney Dis 1997;4:641. (*Argues that phosphate control is the most important means to prevent secondary hyperparathyroidism.*)

Ifudu O. Care of patients undergoing hemodialysis. N Engl J Med 1998;339:1054. (*Excellent comprehensive review.*)

Ihle BU, Whitworth JA, Shahinafar S, et al. Angiotensin-converting enzyme inhibition in nondiabetic progressive renal insufficiency: a controlled double-blind trial. Am J Kidney Dis 1996;27:489. (*Decrease in rate of progression is in addition to that afforded by decrease in blood pressure.*)

Kaufman JS, Reda DJ, Fye CL, et al. Subcutaneous compared with intravenous epoetin in patients receiving hemodialysis. N Engl J Med 1998;339:578. (*Less epoetin necessary to maintain hematocrit in hemodialysis patients when it is administered SQ rather than IV.*)

Kimmel PL, Thamer M, Richard CM, et al. Psychiatric illness in patients with end-stage renal disease. Am J Med 1998;105:214. (*Nearly 9% of dialysis patients in this cohort were admitted for psychiatric illness during 1993; psychiatric illness was more likely to develop among patients who were male, younger, or African-American.*)

Klahr S, Levey AS, Beck G, et al. The effects of dietary protein restriction and blood pressure control on the progression of chronic renal disease. N Engl J Med 1994;330:877. (*A small but significant benefit was noted with a diet low in protein; low blood pressure was helpful in patients with pronounced proteinuria.*)

Lewis EJ, Hunsicker LG, Bain RP, et al. The effect of angiotensin-converting enzyme inhibition on diabetic nephropathy. N Engl J Med 1993;329:1456. (*ACE inhibitor therapy slows the progression of renal failure in type I diabetics; benefit found to be independent of effect on blood pressure.*)

Mackenzie HS, Brenner BM. Current strategies for retarding progression of renal disease. Am J Kidney Dis 1998;31:161. (*Emphasis on evidence for ACE inhibitors, protein restriction, and blood pressure control.*)

Mailloux LU, Bellucci AG, Mossey RT, et al. Predictors of survival in patients undergoing dialysis. Am J Med 1988;84:855. (*Advancing age and diabetes described the highest-risk group, yet these patients still benefited.*)

Mailloux LU, Haley WE. Hypertension in the ESRD patient: pathophysiology, therapy, outcomes, and future directions. Am J Kidney Dis 1998;32:705. (*In-depth review of the literature that points out the limitations of evidence.*)

Malluche HM, Faugere M-C. Renal osteodystrophy. N Engl J Med 1989;321:317. (*A terse summary of its etiology and treatment.*)

Mooradian AD, Morley JE. Endocrine dysfunction in chronic renal failure. Arch Intern Med 1984;144:351. (*A short but useful summary of the effects of chronic renal failure on endocrine function, including a discussion of workup and therapy.*)

Moore MA, Epstein M, Agodoa L, et al. Current strategies for management of hypertensive renal disease. Arch Intern Med 1999;159:23. (*Recommends that blood pressure be reduced to 130/85 mm Hg, and to 120/75 mm Hg in African-Americans.*)

Moscone L, Ruggenenti P, Perna A, et al. Nitrendipine and enalapril improve albuminuria and glomerular filtration rate in non–insulin-dependent diabetes. Kidney Int 1996;49:S91. (*A small study showing improvement equivalent to that achieved with ACE inhibitors.*)

Nolph KD, Lindblad AS, Novak JW. Continuous ambulatory peritoneal dialysis. N Engl J Med 1988;318:1595. (*Terse but authoritative discussion for the general reader; includes clinical indications and complications.*)

Pastan S, Bailey J. Dialysis therapy. N Engl J Med 1998;338:1428. (*Effective review of technical aspects of dialysis procedures and prognostic information, which is valuable to patients if communicated effectively.*)

Pedrini MT, Levey AS, Lau J, et al. The effect of dietary protein restriction on the progression of diabetic and nondiabetic renal diseases: a metaanalysis. Ann Intern Med 1996;124:627. (*Relative risk for renal failure or death is reduced 33% and 44% for nondiabetic and diabetic renal disease, respectively.*)

Rahman M, Smith MC. A diagnostic and therapeutic approach. Arch Intern Med 1998;158:1743. (*Well-referenced review with summary of evidence supporting clinical recommendations.*)

Rahman M, Smith MC. Chronic renal insufficiency: a diagnostic and therapeutic approach. Arch Intern Med 1998;158:1743. (*Excellent review of recent studies and their implications for practice.*)

Ravid M, Savin H, Jutrin I, et al. Long-term stabilizing effect of angiotensin-converting enzyme inhibition on plasma creatinine and on proteinuria in normotensive type II diabetic patients. Ann Intern Med 1993;118:577. (*Benefit found in type II diabetics.*)

Ritz E, Orth SR. Primary care: nephropathy in patients with type 2 diabetes mellitus. N Engl J Med 1999;341:1127. (*Effective clinical review.*)

Sherrard DJ, Andress DL. Aluminum-related osteodystrophy. Ann Intern Med 1989;39:307. (*Review of aluminum toxicity and its consequences.*)

Walser M. Assessing renal function from creatinine measurements in adults with chronic renal failure. Am J Kidney Dis 1998;32:23. (*Reviews methods for assessing renal function, including determination of creatinine clearance after oral administration of cimetidine, which blocks tubular secretion of creatinine.*)

Whelton A, Stout RL, Spilman PS, et al. Renal effects of ibuprofen, piroxicam, and sulindac in patients with asymptomatic renal failure. Ann Intern Med 1990;112:568. (*Prospective study of NSAID effects; some worsening noted, especially with ibuprofen use.*)

143
Management of Genitourinary Cancers in Men

Cancers of the genitourinary tract in men are often localized, and, if so, they can be managed by surgery or radiation. Unfortunately, advanced disease is common and requires a team approach involving the surgeon, oncologist, radiotherapist, and primary physician. The responsibilities of the primary physician include prevention, screening for early disease (see Chapter 126), counseling, support, and monitoring of patients with advanced disease. A more active role in therapy has been created by the advent of hormonally active therapy for advanced prostate cancer.

CARCINOMA OF THE PROSTATE

Epidemiology and Risk Factors

Carcinoma of the prostate has become the leading cancer in men, with an estimated 200,000 new cases annually. Incidence rose during the years before 1992 but has since leveled off, in part because of advances in the detection of prevalence cases, but perhaps also because of increases in dietary, environmental, and genetic precipitants. Evidence is mounting for possible pathogenetic roles for monounsaturated fats, heavy metals, and certain oncogenes. Some familial clustering has been observed, and risk doubles among first-degree relatives. These factors may account for some of the differences in prevalence encountered across geographic and racial boundaries. Testosterone is likely to play a major role, evoked as the cause of the high prevalence of this disease among African-American men and its absence among those who have been castrated. No association with benign prostatic hypertrophy or sexual activity has been found. However, age is a major determinant, with incidence and mortality rising sharply after age 50. By the ninth decade, more than 70% of men have at least microscopic evidence of prostate carcinoma at autopsy.

Although prostate cancer may be a common affliction of older men, it is far from being harmless. Approximately 30,000 die annually from the disease, making it the second leading cause of cancer death among men in the United States. Lifetime risk for a 50-year-old man developing clinical cancer is estimated to be 10%; lifetime risk of dying from the cancer is 3%.

Pathophysiology, Clinical Presentation, and Course

Most of the prostate cancers found at autopsy are *incidental* and have no clinical import. They are small in volume, well differentiated, diploid, and noninvasive, and they originate from the transition zone; prostate-specific antigen (PSA) levels are often normal. *Clinically important* lesions are larger, less well differentiated, invasive, and nondiploid, and they originate from the peripheral zone; PSA is often elevated. What converts microscopic pathology to clinically evident disease remains unknown. It is also unclear what percentage of all prostate cancers become clinically important.

In 85% of cases, clinically evident tumor arises in the *periphery* of the gland (posterior lobe or lamella), so that detection by digital examination is possible in many instances. However, only 30% of new cases are discovered by this means. Many patients now present with nonpalpable, asymptomatic lesions, detected by PSA screening followed by prostate ultrasonography (see Chapter 126). Others present with nonspecific symptoms of urethral obstruction (see Chapter 134). Renal insufficiency resulting from prolonged urinary tract obstruction ensues in a small but important fraction. About 15% of patients have bone pain or other manifestations of metastatic disease as the presenting complaint. Osteoblastic metastases predominate; they can be painful and are the major cause of morbidity. Metastasis to regional lymph nodes is common and usually asymptomatic. It may occur even when disease appears clinically to be confined to the gland and before spread to bone.

Prognosis is a function of disease stage at the time of diagnosis, histologic grade of the tumor, and level of PSA. Because of the advanced age of this patient population, many men die of other conditions.

Staging

Staging is essential to formulating a prognosis and selecting therapy. However, clinical staging continues to underestimate the extent of disease. Metastases to regional lymph nodes often go undetected. The inadequacy of clinical staging accounts in part for the often-noted poor correlation between clinical stage and response to therapy. It is also the reason for the conflicting reports of treatment results that pervade the prostate cancer literature. Attempts to compensate for the shortcomings of clinical staging and to estimate better the likelihood of metastatic disease include the designation of subcategories within each stage and consideration of the histologic pattern (patients with histology of a higher grade are more likely to harbor lymph node metastases).

Determining Extent of Local Disease. The clinical assessment begins with careful *palpation* of the prostate to establish the extent of local tumor. Emphasis is on establishing tumor size and any spread into the surrounding soft tissue. However, digital examination understages about one third of patients thought to have disease limited to the prostate. The *PSA* concentration correlates with tumor volume. Levels in excess of 15 ng/mL (Hybritech assay) suggest extension through the capsule or into the seminal vesicles. Transrectal *ultrasonography* and *magnetic resonance imaging* (MRI) are often used to stage local disease, but the accuracy of such imaging studies has been disappointing (range, 58% to 69%), so that biopsy confirmation of any positive findings is necessary. MRI adapted for transrectal use is being studied and may prove better. Computed tomography (CT) is not useful.

Determining Metastatic Involvement. Physical examination initiates the search, with careful palpation of all nodes, bones, and the abdomen. PSA determination has become increasingly useful. If the PSA concentration exceeds 20 ng/mL (Hybritech assay), distant metastasis to bone is likely and a *bone scan* should be ordered. If the result of the bone scan is positive, more elaborate imaging studies are unnecessary because the disease is already stage D2 (see below). A PSA level below 20 ng/mL greatly reduces the likelihood of bony involvement (<1%) and obviates the need for bone scan, but regional metastasis still needs to be considered. *CT* of the pelvis and abdomen is often ordered to assess pelvic and retroperitoneal lymph node involvement noninvasively, but results have been disappointing in predicting outcome. Sensitivity is especially poor. Biopsy confirmation of a positive finding is required. *Lymphangiography* has also proved inadequate because of poor visualization of obturator–hypogastric nodes, which are the only site of nodal disease in up to one third of patients. Pelvic lymphadenectomy is the only definitive means of establishing nodal disease, but its morbidity is substantial. It is typically performed when radical prostatectomy is being considered for cure.

Staging Categories and Prognosis. A typical A, B, C, and D staging system is used, based on TMN categories. In *stage A*, palpable evidence of tumor is absent. Disease at this stage consists of malignancy found incidentally during prostatectomy for treatment of benign prostatic hyperplasia. *Stage A1* represents disease with a microscopic focus of well-differentiated malignant cells occupying less than 5% of tissue examined. Risk for progression is low (12% to 18%), with little effect on survival of older men. *Stage A2* denotes multiple foci or more poorly differentiated disease, with a markedly increased risk for mortality if the tumor is left untreated. Pathologically, as many as 25% of these patients already have lymph node metastases.

In *stage B*, a palpable prostatic nodule is noted on rectal examination. If the lesion is less than 1.5 cm in diameter and confined to one lobe, it is designated *stage B1*. Clinical B1 disease usually proves to be confined to the gland and has a very good prognosis with treatment. If the palpable lesion is larger than 1.5 cm or extends beyond one lobe, it is considered *stage B2*. Patients with clinical stage B2 have a 15% to 45% chance of having occult metastases to lymph nodes at the time of presentation. Consequently, their prognosis is less favorable.

In clinical *stage C*, rectal examination reveals local extension beyond the prostate to the pelvic wall, seminal vesicles, or bladder neck. In C1 disease, tumor is not fixed to the pelvic wall; in C2 disease, it is. Bone scan findings are normal, suggesting localized disease, but 40% to 80% of patients at this clinical stage have lymph node metastases. Thus, many people with clinical stage C disease already have metastases and a poor prognosis.

Stage D designates metastatic disease. *D1* denotes spread to pelvic lymph nodes. *D2* indicates distant metastasis, usually to bone. Palliation is the most that can be expected.

Histologic Grading

Histologic grading helps to overcome some of the prognostic shortcomings of clinical staging. Adenocarcinomas are scored according to the *Gleason system* on a *scale of 2 to 10*. The more disrupted and undifferentiated the normal glandular architecture, the higher the grade of tumor and the poorer the prognosis.

Retrospective cohort studies indicate that men who have a Gleason score in the *range of 2 to 4* rarely die of prostate cancer in the ensuing 15 years regardless of age at diagnosis. For men with a Gleason score in the *range of 8 to 10*, the prognosis is much worse, with 15-year case fatality rates of 80% or more except for the oldest men, who face a higher risk for death from other causes because of their age. Cancers with a Gleason score of 5 confer a prognosis similar to that for cancers with a Gleason score of 2 to 4. Gleason 7 scores are similar to Gleason 8 to 10. The prognosis for men with a Gleason 6 score is intermediate.

Principles of Management

For lack of a better method, the selection of a treatment modality is determined largely by clinical stage, with some adjustment according to histologic grade (especially in stage A disease).

Stage A1. Elderly patients with stage A1 disease and low-grade histology *need not be treated* because survival is unaffected by the disease. Such patients do require regular follow-up that includes monitoring the PSA, checking the prostate, and inquiring about symptoms. Patients with 10 or more years of life expectancy have a definite risk for disease progression and should undergo curative therapy (see below).

Stages A2 and B. These patients are candidates for curative therapy, either with radical prostatectomy or radiation. The 10-year disease-specific survival rates for these patients are similar for both treatment modalities and approach 90%. *External beam radiation* is a relatively low-morbidity procedure and the radiation therapy procedure of choice. It rarely causes incontinence, and potency is preserved in well over 50% of patients. Proper technique spares permanent rectal injury, although temporary diarrhea, tenesmus, and rectal bleeding may occur. The problem of *residual tumor* after radiation therapy remains unresolved. PSA often remains detectable, and biopsy sometimes reveals residual tumor. Its importance and the need for further treatment are subjects of ongoing study. The frequency of the problem is estimated to be as high as 35% in patients treated by radiation therapy and is an argument against the use of radiation, especially in younger persons who have many years of life expectancy. The use of ultrasonographically guided interstitial implant therapy, or *brachytherapy*, has received a great deal of attention, but evidence to date is insufficient for valid comparisons to be made with external beam radiation. Although the approach has real appeal for men who want to avoid the complications of other treatment options, all men considering brachytherapy should understand the limited evidence for this approach, especially men at intermediate or high risk.

Radical prostatectomy used to cause permanent impotence in almost all patients and was shunned by many for that reason. Advances in surgical technique have made the preservation of erectile function possible, but so-called *nerve-sparing* procedures are not always possible and not always successful when they are possible. When impotence does occur, the vascular apparatus and capacity for erection via injection therapy or sildenafil may remain intact (see Chapter 132). Although postoperative incontinence occurs in most patients, it clears by 5 weeks in more than 50%. It remains a long-term problem in approximately 30%. Bilateral pelvic lymphadenectomy is usually performed before removal of the prostate. The frozen-section findings determine whether proceeding with curative surgery is appropriate. Node dissection and prostatectomy increase the risk for thrombophlebitis and lymphocele. Postoperatively, PSA becomes undetectable when all tumor is removed. Factors favorable to radical prostatectomy are a small stage B lesion.

Stage C. Treatment remains unsatisfactory, with the optimal approach yet to be defined. Radiation is useful for local control of tumor but fails to sterilize pelvic nodes, which are highly likely to be involved by tumor. Surgery fails for similar reasons. *Antiandrogen therapy* (see below) may represent the most effective approach. Studies are in progress.

Stage D. The mainstay of treatment for symptomatic metastatic disease is hormonal manipulation. Prostate cancers contain both hormone-dependent and hormone-sensitive cells and hormone-independent cells. Hormone-dependent cells die a programmed death in the absence of testosterone. Hormone-sensitive cells stop dividing, but hormone-independent cells continue to grow. As a result, although prostate cancer can be halted by antiandrogen therapy, such treatment does not effect a permanent cure.

Orchiectomy. Castration is the time-honored hormonal manipulation. Bilateral removal of the testes can be performed at low cost on an outpatient basis. This reduces by 95% the total body production of androgen. A small amount of adrenal androgen synthesis persists. Psychologically, orchiectomy is difficult for many patients, including the elderly. Prostheses can be placed to lessen the psychological impact.

Luteinizing Hormone-releasing Hormone Agonists. Many patients want a biochemical alternative to castration. Synthetic peptides that act as *luteinizing hormone-releasing hormone* (LH-RH) *agonists* have been developed. *Leuprolide* was the first to be commercially available, packaged as a 7-mg depot preparation given IM once a month. These agents prevent the pulsatile release of luteinizing hormone necessary for testosterone secretion and effect castration levels of testicular androgens after causing an initial stimulative effect. The LH-RH agonists are convenient to use, effective, and well tolerated, but they are very expensive, costing several thousand dollars per year. Hot flashes are the main side effect. Because of the initial stimulative effect, this therapy should be given in conjunction with an antiandrogen at the outset. Some studies suggest that combination use with an antiandrogen improves survival (see below).

Estrogen Therapy. The estrogen *diethylstilbestrol* has been used for decades to achieve a "chemical castration." It inhibits LH secretion and competitively blocks circulating androgens. Doses of 3 mg daily halt testosterone production but are associated with an increased risk for thromboembolic disease. The thromboembolic risk is reduced with lower doses (e.g., 1 mg daily) and aspirin therapy, but lower doses do not suppress testosterone secretion as well. Gynecomastia is another side effect, which can be prevented by prophylactic low-dose irradiation of breast tissue. The effect is comparable to that of orchiectomy in inducing tumor regression. The combination of orchiectomy plus estrogen is no better than each used alone.

Moreover, patients failing to respond to orchiectomy are unlikely to benefit from estrogen.

Antiandrogens. These agents block the effects of testosterone at the receptor level, which makes them useful for countering adrenal androgen secretion and the surge that accompanies early LH-RH agonist therapy. They may be steroidal (e.g., megestrol acetate) or nonsteroidal (e.g., *flutamide, bicalutamide*). These drugs cannot be used as monotherapy because they induce an increase in LH release that eventually stimulates sufficient testosterone secretion to overcome their blocking effect. Side effects include gynecomastia and diarrhea; a chemical hepatitis sometimes develops. Although they do not induce a hypercoagulable state or gynecomastia, they do cause impotence.

Combination Therapy. Although monotherapy with a hormonally active agent appears to provide some symptomatic relief (tumor shrinks, bony pain lessens), there is little evidence that it prolongs life in patients with metastatic disease. Consequently, such therapy is reserved for the onset of symptoms. About 10 years ago, evidence of a survival advantage emerged with the use of combination programs that provide *total blockade* of both testicular and adrenal sources of androgen. Total androgen blockade is a conceptually attractive option for the treatment of a testosterone-responsive tumor like prostate cancer. The most widely studied is the combination of *leuprolide plus flutamide*. A significant benefit (2-year increase in survival) was observed in patients with asymptomatic bony metastasis and excellent functional status. Such findings suggest that total androgen blockade be considered early in patients with metastatic disease. The cost could be lowered by substituting orchiectomy for LH-RH agonist therapy. Combination therapy is little better than monotherapy in patients with advanced, symptomatic, metastatic disease. It is best reserved for nonpalliative use.

New evidence emerging from the group that initially showed a survival benefit with long-term combination therapy now challenges that finding, raising doubt about the validity of the initial findings and the need for indefinite antiandrogen therapy in persons subjected to castration. The addition of long-term flutamide in persons treated with castration did not confer an additional survival advantage. However, data are available only for patients undergoing surgical castration; whether the findings also pertain to "biochemical castration" with an LH-RH agonist remains to be determined.

Secondary Hormonal Therapy. When initial hormonal monotherapy fails, flutamide is sometimes considered. Responses average 6 months and occur in only about 20% of patients. Hydrocortisone, aminoglutethimide, and ketoconazole have all been used to suppress adrenal androgen production. Under investigation are the *5-α-reductase inhibitors* (e.g., finasteride), which block the peripheral conversion of testosterone to its more active metabolite dihydroxytestosterone.

Much can be done to make the patient with advanced disease comfortable. In addition to the palliative measures mentioned above, the use of adequate analgesia (see Chapter 91) should not be overlooked.

Radiation and Chemotherapy. External beam radiation is an effective means of palliation for patients with bone pain. It can prevent fracture and is used in cases of impending spinal cord compression (see Chapter 92). Chemotherapy has been disappointing, with no agent altering survival. Response rates are somewhat less than 20%.

Monitoring Therapy. The serum *PSA* determination is the best means of monitoring response to therapy. The 48-hour half-life of PSA allows it to reflect changes in tumor activity and mass quickly. The serum concentration directly correlates with tumor burden. Although prostatic procedures may transiently elevate the PSA level, it quickly returns to baseline so that interpretation is usually unaffected by recent examinations or procedures.

Although the *bone scan* is sensitive for detection of bony involvement, its findings are not specific. Areas of increased uptake may reflect repair as much as damage. Thus, the test may provide confusing information when used to monitor response to therapy. It is best reserved for the initial evaluation or when bone pain of unclear significance arises.

For the asymptomatic patient not currently receiving therapy, regular inquiry into the development of *symptoms* has proved an economical yet effective means of monitoring. The routine repetition of blood tests and radiographic studies can become expensive and should be considered only when the result will substantively alter clinical decision making.

Patient Education and Indications for Referral and Admission

The primary physician plays a central role in helping the patient choose among a variety of options that he is likely to face. For the patient with curable disease, the choice will be between radiation and radical prostatectomy. Risks of impotence, incontinence, and recurrence need to be reviewed. For the person with early metastatic disease, the issue of initiating total androgen blockade and the decision of whether to undergo orchiectomy or commit to a program of leuprolide therapy will need to be faced. Patients are surprised and comforted to realize that they will not become feminized after removal of the testes.

These difficult decisions require consultative help, but the patient will often return to the primary physician for discussion, which requires one to keep abreast of the options in the treatment of prostate cancer. Because the patient knows the primary physician best, the patient is likely to ask his primary care doctor to select the option that would best meet his needs. Phone calls to one's consultants may be helpful in this situation.

Referral to the urologist is indicated at the time a prostate cancer is first suspected. Careful planning of the evaluation is necessary, and a tissue sample will be needed (see Chapter 126). Although most staging of the tumor can be performed by the primary physician, the limitations of imaging techniques must be kept in mind. When curable disease is suspected, referrals to the urologist and radiation oncologist are indicated to help in choosing the optimal approach. When metastatic disease is encountered, an oncology consultation may facilitate design of antiandrogen therapy. Urgent hospital admission is indicated if spinal cord compression is deemed imminent (see Chapter 92).

TESTICULAR CANCER

Testicular cancer is the most common malignancy in men between the ages of 15 and 35 and is a major cause of death in this age group. Its seriousness and curability, both in early stages and, more recently, in advanced stages, make it an important disease for the primary physician. One needs to encourage self-examination, screen young men during routine checkups (see Chapter 131), and help guide the patient with advanced disease through his illness.

Pathophysiology, Clinical Presentation, and Course

Known predisposing factors are testicular atrophy (secondary to an undescended testicle) and Klinefelter's syndrome. Suspected risk factors include natural exposure to intrapartum estrogens, exposure to insecticides, and prior history of a testicular tumor. Trauma is not a known precipitant.

Almost all testicular cancers are germ cell tumors. *Seminomas* account for 40% to 50%. Most are confined to the testicle at the time of presentation. The remainder are termed *nonseminomatous germ cell tumors* (NSGCTs). These include *teratomas*, *choriocarcinomas*, *embryonal cell carcinomas*, and *endodermal sinus tumors*. Many are of mixed cell type. Their metastases may be less differentiated than the primary.

Both groups commonly present as solid, painless, nontransilluminating testicular masses in young men (see Chapter 131). Some patients describe "heaviness" in the scrotum. Pain is less common. These tumors grow rapidly and spread by the lymphatics and blood. Local extension to the epididymis occurs in 10%. Occasionally, the tumor is occult at the primary site, with metastases already established. If chorionic gonadotropin is secreted (as may occur with several of the NSGCTs), gynecomastia may be an initial complaint. Disease already established in the lung may present with cough or hemoptysis.

Diagnosis and Staging

Any solid, nontransilluminating, painless testicular mass in a young man should be presumed to represent a primary testicular cancer until proven otherwise. *Testicular ultrasonography* should be performed to obtain a more definitive determination of the location of the lesion. If testicular, prompt urologic consultation is required for consideration of surgical removal of the involved testicle. Testicles with suspect lesions are subjected to *orchiectomy* through an inguinal canal approach to minimize the risk for seeding the scrotum, as might occur with a transscrotal operative procedure. If the lesion is extratesticular, urologic consultation is less urgent but still advisable. Surgical removal is less likely.

Staging Procedures and Surveillance. Staging begins with *orchiectomy* findings and proceeds to *chest radiography* and *chest CT* for metastatic disease of the chest, and to *abdominal CT* for assessment of retroperitoneal lymph nodes. Circulating *tumor markers* also provide a means to detect occult disease. The *β-subunit of human chorionic gonadotropin* (HCG) is always elevated in choriocarcinoma and in about half of the other NSGCTs (it is rarely elevated in pure seminoma, but a number of seminomatous cases have mixed disease and elevated HCG). *α-Fetoprotein* is produced by about 80% of patients with embryonal cell cancer. Both markers also provide an excellent means of monitoring response to therapy (see below). *Lactic dehydrogenase* is sometimes elevated in germ cell tumors.

False-positive rates are low for abdominal CT, but false-negative rates are as high as 30%, with the poorest results in thin persons. Previously, if no evidence of metastatic disease was found by staging studies, then an ipsilateral complete *lymphadenectomy* and a contralateral partial lymphadenectomy to the level of the aortic bifurcation were considered mandatory, especially for NSGCT, because of the high incidence of microscopic nodal involvement. However, lymphadenectomy is now being used less often because advances in chemotherapy have made it possible to achieve high rates of cure even if the diagnosis of metastasis is delayed. Moreover, lymph node dissection involves extensive surgery, with an attendant risk for ejaculatory failure (a risk that has been reduced by improvements in surgical technique). Finally, retroperitoneal lymph node dissection is unnecessary if the primary cancer is a seminoma and a course of radiation therapy to the nodes (which is highly curative) is being planned. *Lymphangiography* is sometimes useful in patients with seminomatous tumors whose CT results are negative. Abnormal paraaortic nodes are detected in 13% to 22%.

The decision of whether to proceed with nodal dissection or opt for close surveillance with measurement of tumor markers and repeated CT remains a judgment call. Factors associated with an increased risk for relapse and thus favoring node dissection include a high percentage of embryonal cell carcinoma in the primary tumor, a marked degree of local disease, and the presence of vascular or lymphatic invasion. If surveillance is elected after orchiectomy, it must be done rigorously, with monthly monitoring of tumor markers, repeat CT scanning every 2 to 3 months, and periodic physical examination. Noninvasive staging may be followed by chemotherapy, with secondary surgical exploration to evaluate the retroperitoneum after treatment.

Clinical Stages. A host of staging systems are used, with one set for seminomatous disease and another for nonseminomatous disease. Common designations are stage I or stage A for disease confined to the testis, stage II or stage B for spread to regional nodes, and stage III or stage C for spread beyond retroperitoneal nodes. Within each stage are subcategories denoting the degree of tumor burden.

Management

Treatment decisions are based on stage, histology, and levels of tumor markers.

Seminomatous Tumors. *Stage I* disease is treated with inguinal *orchiectomy*, which is followed by adjuvant retroperitoneal node *irradiation* in most centers, although surveillance is now considered an option by some. The cure rate is close to 100%. Patients who relapse are candidates for combination chemotherapy, which is extremely effective (see below). Patients with *stage IIA* disease are also treated with retroperitoneal radiation, but they no longer undergo prophylactic mediastinal irradiation because of its associated morbidity and the success of chemotherapy in treating relapses. Cure rates are still close to 100% at this stage. Patients with stage *IIB* and stage *III* disease are treated with *cisplatin-based chemotherapy*. Cure rates exceed 90%.

Nonseminomatous Tumors. *Stages I and IIA* NSGCT disease is treated with *surgery only*. Surgical cure rates average

95% when lymph node dissection shows no regional disease. Even when retroperitoneal disease is detected, lymphadenectomy is likely to suffice for treatment as long as nodes are less than 3 cm in diameter. Patients with stage IIB disease have a high probability of relapse and thus are candidates for chemotherapy, as are patients with stage III disease.

Cisplatin-based Chemotherapy. Multiple-agent chemotherapy based on cisplatin represented an important breakthrough in treatment of testicular cancer. Even patients with distant metastatic disease now have a high probability of cure. The need for maintenance therapy has been eliminated. Even the severe nausea and vomiting associated with the use of cisplatin have become much less problematic with the advent of *ondansetron*, a serotonin receptor-blocking agent capable of reducing cisplatin-induced emesis. Cisplatin-induced renal toxicity is preventable with good hydration.

Monitoring. Close monitoring of the response to therapy is essential. *HCG* and *α-fetoprotein* levels are used to detect subclinical relapse and failure to respond to treatment. An elevated serum marker level failing to decline with therapy suggests resistance to therapy. Its rise during follow-up indicates relapse. Patients having isolated elevations in tumor markers as the sole manifestation of relapse have nearly a 100% chance of cure when treated promptly with chemotherapy. In patients with advanced disease, a decline in HCG after initial chemotherapy is an excellent predictor of response to treatment. *Periodic physical examination* to check for the development of palpable adenopathy or an abdominal mass and chest and abdominal CT are additional components of the monitoring and surveillance processes (see above).

Patient Education

Although most of the details of care are related by the oncologist, the primary physician is often consulted by the patient and needs to be familiar with some of the basic questions regarding prognosis, treatment options, and side effects. Patients are greatly relieved to know the favorable prognosis for testicular cancer, especially those with metastatic disease. Nonetheless, treatment is not without its adverse effects. Lymph node exploration is an extensive procedure and thus not without considerable morbidity. Retrograde ejaculation and subsequent infertility are still associated risks, although they have been reduced to about 12%. The ability to achieve an erection is only rarely compromised. Radiation therapy is associated with a risk for decreased spermatogenesis in the remaining normal testicle, although shielding methods have reduced the radiation exposure and, consequently, the period of infertility associated with low sperm counts. The fear of chemotherapy can be lessened by reassurance that there are effective means of minimizing its adverse effects. If the risk of infertility is greater than 5%, sperm banking should be considered before treatment. A pretreatment sperm count may be helpful in decision making.

CARCINOMA OF THE BLADDER

Bladder cancer strikes about 45,000 patients annually in the United States, causing about 10,000 deaths per year. Prevalence is greatest among persons ages 60 to 70. Risk factors include smoking, exposure to naphthalene or aromatic amine antioxidants, use of cyclophosphamide, and schistosomiasis.

Clinical Presentation and Course

Tumors of the bladder are usually detected when gross or microscopic hematuria is noted. In most instances, the hematuria is otherwise asymptomatic, but, in elderly men especially, dysuria, urgency, frequency, or voiding of small volumes of uninfected urine may be noted. Such symptoms of vesicle irritation suggest carcinoma in situ. Because urothelial tissue extends up into the ureters and renal pelvis and down into the proximal urethra, cancer of the urothelium can present in any of these areas.

More than 90% of bladder cancers are transitional cell carcinomas; squamous cell tumors account for most of the others. A few are undifferentiated. Multiple tumors may arise simultaneously. About 80% are superficial and remain so; the remainder are invasive from the outset. Depth of invasion is the most important predictor of survival, although histologic grade is also a factor. Five-year survival with appropriate treatment is 95% for patients with carcinoma in situ, 60% for disease that invades the subepithelial connective tissue, 35% for superficial muscle invasion, 15% for deep-muscle invasion, and nil for extension to the pelvis. Spread to the lymph nodes is common in patients with deep-muscle invasion.

Diagnosis and Staging

Cystoscopy and *biopsy* of multiple sites are required for diagnosis. Urine cytology is not sensitive enough to obviate the need for invasive study, although a positive result may provide the only means of detecting an otherwise occult carcinoma in situ. *IV pyelography* is performed to detect evidence of an infiltrated bladder wall, a filling defect, or a bladder diverticulum.

Staging is performed by *cystoscopy with biopsy and bimanual rectal–abdominal examination* under anesthesia to determine the depth of tumor penetration and infiltration into the bladder wall. Although the tumors of almost half of patients with infiltration into deep muscle have spread to the lymph nodes (which carries a poor prognosis), such spread is hard to detect without resorting to pelvic lymphadenectomy. Early spread involves the hypogastric and obturator nodes. *Abdominal CT* is obtained to evaluate them. Chest radiography, determination of the alkaline phosphatase level, and a bone scan are commonly ordered to check for distant metastases.

The *prognosis* has also been linked to the presence of blood group antigens on the surface of bladder cancer cells. Patients with tumors that elaborate A, B, or H antigens have a better prognosis than those with tumors that do not. A separate T antigen correlates with invasiveness.

Treatment

Noninvasive stages of disease are often curable with local measures. *Excision* at the time of cystoscopy in conjunction with fulguration represents a most effective form of therapy for early disease. In the setting of multiple tumors, a cytotoxic agent can be instilled. *Thiotepa* has been widely used. *Bacille Calmette-Guérin* (BCG) has emerged as a superior treatment for carcinoma in situ in patients with superficial transitional cell

disease. It decreases the risk for progression to invasive disease and improves survival in comparison with resection alone. Irradiation of the bladder can effect tumor regression, but the recurrence rate is high. Rapid recurrence of multiple lesions is an indication for combined *cystectomy and prostatectomy*. Diffuse carcinoma in situ with persistently positive washings despite treatment has a poor prognosis and may necessitate early cystectomy.

Infiltrative disease carries a poor prognosis because of the substantial likelihood of lymph node metastases (see above). Options include *partial bladder resection*, *cystectomy* with urinary diversion via an *ileal loop*, radical radiation, and combination therapy. Although partial cystectomy has the attraction of preserving some of the bladder, only a few patients are suitable candidates. *Combination therapy* consisting of *preoperative irradiation plus cystectomy* is often used. Complications include a surgical mortality rate of 5%, postoperative problems necessitating a prolonged hospitalization in about 25%, and the possibility of a need for revision of the ileal loop. Hyperchloremic metabolic acidosis sometimes occurs in these patients.

Those with *deeply invasive disease* are not candidates for surgery. External beam *megavoltage irradiation* provides a reasonable chance (50%) for local control and a small chance (no more than 25%) for cure. The rate of bowel and bladder complications is 10% to 15%. About half of these patients maintain sexual potency. In patients with *distant metastases*, *cisplatin* in conjunction with *cyclophosphamide* and *doxorubicin* has achieved substantial, but not lasting, regression. Intravesicle cisplatin is associated with anaphylaxis.

Because many patients with bladder cancer present with advanced disease, the focus of treatment is often palliative. If not previously used, radiation can provide relief from pelvic and bone pain. The onset of ureteral obstruction and subsequent uremia presents a relatively comfortable means of dying to patients with advanced disease; relief of the obstruction is rarely indicated.

Monitoring. Monitoring patients treated for early disease is essential. Surveillance cystoscopy and washings are conducted every 3 months during the first year and then at less frequent intervals. Monoclonal antibody staining of washings has enhanced the detection of tumor cells, as has the use of hematoporphyrin derivatives, which stain malignant urothelium and make them more visible at cystoscopy.

Patient Education

The best treatment for bladder cancer is prevention. Risk factors such as smoking and occupational exposure should be addressed. Patients who are to undergo cystectomy need prior counseling about management of the ileal loop. Most adjust reasonably well to managing the stoma and bag. Stoma groups and instruction by a stoma nurse can be helpful.

RENAL CELL CARCINOMA (HYPERNEPHROMA)

Renal cancer is uncommon, accounting for fewer than 2% of all cancers. However, it is a potentially curable disease if detected before it penetrates through the capsule. There is no systemic treatment.

Clinical Presentation and Course

The disease is notorious for its protean presentations. *Painless hematuria* is the most common, found in 50% to 75% of cases. Aching flank pain and a palpable mass are other classic, although far less frequent, manifestations and represent advanced disease. Unexplained weight loss, nausea and vomiting, fever of unknown origin, and a markedly elevated erythrocyte sedimentation rate (ESR) are sometimes systemic clues of early disease, occurring in up to a third of patients. Paraneoplastic syndromes are associated with this disease, including polycythemia and hypercalcemia secondary to production of a parathyroid hormone–like substance.

The natural history of the tumor is unique, with occasional spontaneous regression and long intervals before the appearance of metastases. Nevertheless, in a major proportion of patients with hypernephroma, metastases are found at presentation or develop later.

Diagnosis

A high index of suspicion is needed to make an early diagnosis of this disease. Hematuria in the setting of a normochromic, normocytic anemia and a markedly elevated ESR are suggestive, as is the triad of fever, elevated ESR, and increased α_1-globulin.

If suspicion remains high, radiologic evaluation should begin with *IV pyelography*. If a mass is found on IV pyelography, it must be determined whether it is cystic (and therefore most likely benign) or solid. Renal *ultrasonography* plus *CT* or *MRI* helps to determine the local extent of disease, including perinephric involvement, renal vein obstruction, and spread to the retroperitoneal nodes. MRI has the advantage of detecting vessel invasion and caval thrombosis. Needle aspiration biopsy can be performed under imaging guidance if cytologic confirmation is desired.

Management

Tumor confined to the kidney is curable. When it extends beyond Gerota's capsule, the prognosis is poor. Some authorities suggest that removal of the primary tumor may trigger the regression of metastases, although the only evidence derives from case reports. Large series have failed to demonstrate such an effect or an improvement in survival. Most argue that the primary tumor in patients with metastatic disease should be removed only for control of local pain or bleeding. Metastases to lung, bone, and brain are treated with chemotherapy or irradiation.

Effective chemotherapeutic regimens are lacking for this disease. Hormonal therapies (progesterone and androgens) have produced responses in some patients, but without prolonging survival. A minority of patients have partial or complete responses to interferon, interleukin-2, or both, but the response is rarely durable. Studies are ongoing.

A.G.M./A.H.G.

ANNOTATED BIBLIOGRAPHY

Prostate Cancer

Adolfsson J, Steineck G, Whitmore WF Jr. Recent results of management of palpable, clinically localized prostatic cancer. Cancer 1993;72:310. (*Risk for death reduced by 50% with treatment.*)

Albertsen PC, Hanley JA, Gleason DF, et al. Competing risk analysis of men aged 55 to 74 years at diagnosis managed conservatively for clinically localized prostate cancer. JAMA 1998;280:975. (*Men with a low Gleason score are unlikely to die of prostate cancer, regardless of their age at onset.*)

Bolla M, Gonzalez D, Warde P, et al. Improved survival in patients with locally advanced prostate cancer treated with radiotherapy and goserelin. N Engl J Med 1997;337:295. (*Five-year overall survival of 79% with goserelin, 62% without.*)

Chodak GW, Thisted RA, Gerber GS, et al. Results of conservative management of clinically localized prostate cancer. N Engl J Med 1994;330:242. (*A pooled analysis of data from more than 800 cases favoring initial conservative therapy in older patients with low-grade histology.*)

Chybowski FM, Keller JJ, Bergstraih EJ, et al. Predicting radionuclide bone scan findings in patients with newly diagnosed untreated prostate cancer. J Urol 1991;145:313. (*PSA level was found to be superior to other clinical parameters.*)

Crawford ED, Eisenberger MA, McLeod DG, et al. A controlled trial of leuprolide with and without flutamide in prostatic carcinoma. N Engl J Med 1989;321:419. (*Combination therapy was superior to monotherapy in patients with advanced disease.*)

D'Amico AV, Whittington R, Malkowicz B, et al. Biochemical outcome after radical prostatectomy, external beam radiation therapy, or interstitial radiation therapy for localized prostate cancer. JAMA 1998;280:969. (*No difference in PSA failure during 5 years for low-risk patients, but implant patients did not do as well as others if risk was moderate or high.*)

Eisenberger MA, Blumenstein BA, Crawford ED, et al. Bilateral orchiectomy with or without flutamide for metastatic prostate cancer. N Engl J Med 1998;339:1036. (*From the same group that initially showed a benefit from long-term combination therapy, in the form of flutamide plus leuprolide, come these findings, which show no additional benefit from long-term administration of flutamide.*)

Garnick MB, Fair WR. Prostate cancer: emerging concepts. Ann Intern Med 1996;125:118,205. (*Comprehensive two-part review.*)

Gerber GS, Thisted RA, Scardino PT, et al. Results of radical prostatectomy in men with clinically localized prostate cancer. Multi-institutional pooled analysis. JAMA 1996;276:615. (*Ten-year disease-specific survival rates were 94%, 80%, and 77% for grades 1, 2, and 3 tumors, respectively.*)

Gittes RF. Carcinoma of the prostate. N Engl J Med 1991;34:236. (*Comprehensive review with especially helpful discussions of staging and treatment; 150 references.*)

Hanks GE, Krall JM, Pilepich MV. Comparison of pathologic and clinical evaluation of lymph nodes in prostate cancer. Int J Radiat Oncol Biol Phys 1991;21:1099. (*Results of CT were not predictive of response to therapy; results of lymphadenectomy were.*)

Johansson JE, Adami HO, Andersson SO, et al. High 10-year survival rate in patients with early, untreated prostatic cancer. JAMA 1992;267:2191. (*Watchful waiting is appropriate for those with stage A1 who are elderly.*)

Johansson JE, Holmberg L, Johansson S, et al. Fifteen-year survival in prostate cancer: a prospective, population-based study in Sweden. JAMA 1997;277:467. (*Of 642 conservatively treated men with well, moderately, and poorly differentiated disease, 6%, 17%, and 56%, respectively, died of prostate cancer during 15 years.*)

Lange PH. Controversies in management of apparently localized cancer of the prostate. Urology 1989;34[Suppl 4]:13. (*Radiation and radical prostatectomy provide similar 10-year survival rates.*)

Kattan MW, Cowen ME, Miles BJ. A decision analysis for treatment of clinically localized prostate cancer. J Gen Intern Med 1997;12:299. (*Concludes that benefit is likely for younger men and harm is likely for older men.*)

Lee HHK, Warde P, Jewett MA, et al. Neoadjuvant hormonal therapy in carcinoma of the prostate. Br J Urol 1999;4:438. (*Good review of what remains inadequate evidence.*)

Litwin MS, Flanders SC, Pasta DJ, et al. Sexual function and bother after radical prostatectomy or radiation for prostate cancer: multivariate quality-of-life analysis CaPSURE. Urology 1999;54:503. (*Sexual function improved somewhat during the first year following either therapy.*)

McCammon KA, Kolm P, Main B, et al. Comparative quality-of-life analysis after radical prostatectomy or external beam radiation for localized prostate cancer. Urology 1999;54:509. (*Physicians' estimates of urinary incontinence more favorable than patients'.*)

Rifkin MD, Zerhouni EA, Gatsonis CA, et al. Comparison of magnetic resonance imaging and ultrasonography in staging early prostate cancer. N Engl J Med 1990;323:621. (*Accuracy is poor for both; positive test results require biopsy confirmation.*)

Thompson IM, Middleton RG, Optenberg SA, et al. Have complication rates decreased after treatment for localized prostate cancer? J Urol 1999;162:107. (*Yes, but they remain high.*)

Testicular Cancer

Bosl GJ, Motzer RJ. Testicular germ-cell cancer. N Engl J Med 1997;337:242. (*Excellent comprehensive review.*)

Cubeddu LX, Hoffmann IS, Fuenmayor NT, et al. Efficacy of ondansetron (GR 38032F) and the role of serotonin in cisplatin-induced nausea and vomiting. N Engl J Med 1990;322:810. (*Helps considerably.*)

Donohue JP, Foster RS, Rowland RG, et al. Nerve-sparing retroperitoneal lymphadenectomy with preservation of ejaculation. J Urol 1990;144:287. (*Advances in technique have reduced the risk for infertility.*)

Dunphy CH, Ayala AG, Swanson DA, et al. Clinical stage I nonseminomatous mixed germ-cell tumors of the testis: a clinicopathologic study of 93 patients on a surveillance protocol after orchiectomy alone. Lancet 1988;62:1202. (*The use of surveillance as an alternative to lymph node dissection.*)

Einhorn LH, Donohue J. Cis-diaminedichloroplatinum, vinblastine, and bleomycin combination chemotherapy in disseminated testicular cancer. Ann Intern Med 1977;87:293. (*The original report on this most important advance in the treatment of testicular cancer.*)

Lange PH, McIntire R, Waldmann TA, et al. Serum alpha-fetoprotein and human chorionic gonadotropin in the diagnosis and management of nonseminomatous germ-cell testicular cancer. N Engl J Med 1976;295:1237. (*The original report of the utility of these tumor markers in staging and monitoring.*)

Marks LB, Walker TG, Shipley WU, et al. The role of lymphangiography in staging testicular seminoma. Urology 1991;38: 264. (*Yield is about 15% in patients with negative findings on CT.*)

McLeod DG, Weiss RB, Stablein DM, et al. Staging relationships and outcome in early-stage testicular cancer. J Urol 1991;146:1178. (*Excellent outcomes achieved; 5-year survival in excess of 90%.*)

Nichols CR. Testicular cancer. Curr Probl Cancer 1998;22:187. (*Detailed, comprehensive review of all aspects.*)

Picozzi VJ, Freiha FS, Hannigan JF, et al. Prognostic significance of a decline in serum human chorionic gonadotropin levels after initial chemotherapy for advanced germ-cell carcinoma. Ann Intern Med 1984;100:183. (*A fall in level was very predictive of an excellent long-term response to therapy.*)

Warde P, Jewett MA. Surveillance for stage I testicular seminoma. Is it a good option? Urol Clin North Am 1998;25:425. (*Pros and cons of alternative approaches.*)

Williams SD, Stablein DM, Einhorn LH, et al. Immediate adjuvant chemotherapy versus observation with treatment at relapse in pathological stage II testicular cancer. N Engl J Med 1987; 317:1433. (*Equivalent cure rate achieved.*)

Bladder Cancer

Cookson MS, Herr HW, Zhang ZF, et al. The treated natural history of high-risk superficial bladder cancer: 15-year outcome. J Urol 1997;158:62. (*At 15 years, 34% were dead of bladder cancer, 27% were dead of other causes, and 37% were alive, including 27% with functioning bladders.*)

Droller MJ. Bladder cancer: state-of-the-art care. CA Cancer J Clin 1998;48:269. (*Excellent review.*)

Herr W, Laudone VP, Badalament RA, et al. Bacillus Calmette-Guérin therapy alters the progression of superficial bladder cancer. J Clin Oncol 1988;6:1450. (*An important advance in the treatment of early superficial disease.*)

International Collaboration of Trialists. Neoadjuvant cisplatin, methotrexate, and vinblastine chemotherapy for muscle-invasive bladder cancer: a randomised, controlled trial. Lancet 1999; 354:533. (*Not effective.*)

Lamm DL, Torti FM. Bladder cancer. CA Cancer J Clin 1996;46:93. (*Clinical review.*)

Raghavan D, Shipley WM, Garnick MB, et al. Biology and management of bladder cancer. N Engl J Med 1990;322:1129. (*Review of new developments; 155 references.*)

Renal Cell Carcinoma

Figlin RA, Abi-Aad AS, Belldegrum A, et al. The role of interferon and interleukin-2 in the immunotherapeutic approach to renal cell carcinoma. Semin Oncol 1991;18:102. (*Promising results.*)

Lokich JJ, Harrison JH. Renal cell carcinoma: natural history and chemotherapeutic experience. J Urol 1975;114:371. (*Still useful descriptions of its myriad presentations and unusual clinical course.*)

Motzer RJ, Russo P, Nanus DM, et al. Renal cell carcinoma. Curr Probl Cancer 1997;21:185. (*Exhaustive review.*)

Richie JP, Garnick MB, Seltzer S, et al. Computed tomography for diagnosis and staging of renal cell carcinoma. J Urol 1983;129:1114. (*CT provides important information.*)

Vogelzang NJ, Stadler WM. Kidney cancer. Lancet 1998;352:1691. (*Succinct review of natural history and therapy.*)

10
Musculoskeletal Problems

144
Screening for Osteoporosis

One of the major concerns of postmenopausal women is the development of osteoporosis. Osteoporotic fractures in aging women represent a major health problem in industrialized nations. In the United States, approximately 150,000 hip fractures occur annually in women over the age of 65, with 15% to 25% of these women experiencing excess mortality or needing long-term nursing home care. Current expenditures for osteoporotic fractures and their consequences are well in excess of $15 billion annually and rising with the aging of the population. The pathophysiologic mechanisms for postmenopausal osteoporosis are imperfectly understood, but the means to ensure maximal skeletal growth and strength, prevent loss of bone mass, and noninvasively evaluate bone mass are now available (see Chapter 164).

The frequency and clinical significance of osteoporosis, combined with the capabilities to detect and treat it effectively so as to prevent fractures, argue strongly for screening. Many now recommend that osteoporosis screening become an essential part of the health maintenance program for women; however, data from prospective, long-term, randomized studies identifying those who are best served by screening are yet to emerge, so that clinical judgment is necessary in selecting candidates for osteoporosis screening. Effectively advising the perimenopausal woman requires a knowledge of the epidemiology of osteoporosis, and of the risk factors, screening tests, and treatment modalities for this disease.

EPIDEMIOLOGY AND RISK FACTORS

Epidemiology. As the life expectancy of women reaches the mid-80s, osteoporosis takes on epidemic proportions, especially among Caucasian women in industrialized societies. In the United States, the prevalence of low bone density in older adults approaches 50%; a woman's risk for an osteoporotic fracture by age 80 is approximately 40% (several times greater than the risk for breast cancer). The risk for death after a hip fracture is nearly 25%. The disability and expense attributable to the consequences of osteoporosis are enormous and growing.

Risk Factors. Epidemiologic studies have identified *major risk factors*:

- Family history of osteoporosis in a first-degree relative
- Body mass index below the 25th percentile (<22 kg/m^2)
- History of fracture during adulthood
- Current cigarette smoking

In addition, a number of *contributing risk factors* have emerged. These include *lifelong inadequate intake of calcium, Caucasian race, inadequate physical activity, early menopause* (onset before the age of 45), and *excessive intake of alcohol.* All may predispose a woman to a lower bone mass and osteoporotic fractures with aging. Women in whom osteoporosis does not develop may have a larger skeletal mass, which can be increased through physical activity and calcium supplementation.

Medical conditions that are *secondary causes* of osteoporosis include *Cushing's syndrome,* exogenous *glucocorticoid* administration, prolonged heparin therapy, thyrotoxicosis (including excessive replacement therapy), *hypogonadism, hyperprolactinemia, anorexia nervosa,* and *hyperparathyroidism.* However, these diseases account for only a small percentage of cases of osteoporosis.

NATURAL HISTORY AND EFFECTIVENESS OF THERAPY

Natural History. The resorption and formation of bone are a continuous process throughout life. Under physiologic circumstances, the rates of these processes are equal and coupled. Skeletal mass is usually maximal by age 35 and declines in women after age 40 and in men after age 50, when the rate of new bone formation no longer equals the rate of bone resorption. The rate of decline in skeletal mass is most rapid in women within 2 years of menopause and averages 2% to 4% a year during the first 7 years after menopause. Bone mineral content may decline by 25% to 33% during this period. Afterward, loss continues, but at a slower rate (1% to 2% a year). The areas of greatest loss include the femoral neck and lumbar vertebrae, sites rich in *trabecular bone* and subject to future fracture. *Cortical bone*, comprising 80% of skeletal bone, is lost less rapidly.

The progressive decline in skeletal mass becomes clinically manifest when fractures are sustained spontaneously or after minimal trauma. A loss of height and developing kyphosis generally indicates vertebral compression fracture. Fractures most commonly occur in the sacral and lumbar vertebrae, hip, humerus, and wrist. The clinical course and frequency of fractures in individual patients are hard to predict.

Effectiveness of Therapy. (See also Chapter 164.) *Estrogen replacement* can prevent bone loss and even lead to skeletal accretion. Observational studies have consistently noted a 35% to 50% reduction in hip, wrist, and vertebral fractures in women who have used estrogen for at least 5 years after menopause. After 10 years of estrogen use, the risk for fracture decreases 75%. However, if estrogen is discontinued, bone loss rapidly ensues, and it is difficult to reverse the significant bone loss that occurs in the first few years of menopause. Beyond age 75, the effect of as many as 7 to 10 years of estrogen therapy started at the time of menopause is barely appreciable, which indicates that very prolonged estrogen therapy or restarting it in later years may be necessary. The bisphosphonate *alendronate* prevents bone loss and increases bone density at least as well as estrogen replacement. Fracture risk in osteoporotic patients is reduced by up to 50%. The selective estrogen receptor modulator *raloxifene* also halts bone resorption and modestly increases bone mineral density. *Calcium supplementation* with *vitamin D* helps preserve cortical bone mass but does not prevent bone loss to the degree that estrogen therapy does. The combination of calcium supplementation and *weight-bearing exercise* is more effective at stemming bone loss.

Utility of Bone Densitometry for Osteoporosis Screening. The chances for the development of significant osteoporosis and subsequent fracture cannot be adequately predicted by a review of clinical and epidemiologic risk factors. Measurement of bone mineral density is also required. Bone mineral density strongly correlates with the risk for osteoporotic fracture. The test of choice to measure bone mineral density is *dual energy x-ray absorptiometry* (DEXA), which provides rapid, accurate screening with minimal radiation exposure. Because the bone mineral density can vary at different sites of the body, dual energy x-ray absorptiometry should optimally include separate determinations at the hip and spine. The bone density at the wrist is also predictive of fracture, providing a reasonable approximation of body bone mineral density; the study is less expensive and of interest as an economical alternative for mass screening. Nonetheless, direct assessment of bone mineral density at the hip and spine maximizes test sensitivity and is the most accurate assessment of osteoporotic risk.

Bone mineral density measurement is expressed as the number of standard deviations from the mean for normal young adults of the same sex (*T-score*) and as the number of standard deviations from the mean for persons of the same sex and age (*Z-score*). The World Health Organization diagnostic criterion for *osteoporosis* is a *T-score of less than -2.5*. *Osteopenia* is defined as a *T-score between -1.0 and -2.5*. A *Z-score of less than -1.5* suggests a *secondary cause* of osteoporosis. The risk for osteoporotic fracture increases twofold to fourfold for every standard deviation of reduction in bone mineral density.

Cost-effectiveness analysis suggests that up to age 65, bone mineral density screening should be reserved for persons with one or more of the major risk factors for osteoporosis. In those with no risk factors at this age, the bone mineral density measurement is discretionary. After age 65, bone mineral density screening appears cost-effective for all women. Bone mineral density screening is also appropriate at any age for patients with an underlying medical condition that might cause osteoporosis (see above). Although many decision-analysis and cost-effectiveness studies of screening for osteoporosis have been performed, no data from long-term, prospective, randomized trials are yet available to confirm the value of screening. Clinical judgment and individualized decision making continue to be essential. If bone density measurement will affect clinical decision making, then screening makes sense for the individual patient. If it will not, then another compelling reason should exist.

CONCLUSIONS AND RECOMMENDATIONS

- Osteoporosis is a common affliction of postmenopausal women that results in important morbidity. Irreversible bone loss is most rapid in the early phases of menopause but continues indefinitely.
- Effective means to prevent postmenopausal bone loss are available; therapy with estrogen replacement, bisphosphonates, and possibly selective estrogen receptor modulators can halt bone loss and even stimulate modest amounts of remineralization.
- Clinical and epidemiologic parameters are limited in predicting low bone mass.
- Advances in the measurement of bone density have improved test accuracy and predictive value in the assessment of risk for osteoporotic fracture.
- Dual energy x-ray absorptiometry involving bone mineral density measurement of the spine and femur is the screening test of choice for the detection of osteoporosis; study of the forearm only provides a low-cost alternative but is not as sensitive.
- Criteria for optimal patient selection remain to be defined, but the best available data and cost-effectiveness studies suggest that biannual screening begin at menopause for women with a major risk factor for osteoporosis and after age 65 for those with no risk factors.
- Screening is not recommended when the results will have no effect on decision making (e.g., persons already taking medication for osteoporosis prevention, refusing it, or unable to take it).
- Definitive benefit from screening plus prophylactic therapy remains to be demonstrated by large-scale, randomized, controlled trials.

A.H.G.

ANNOTATED BIBLIOGRAPHY

Bauer DC, Browner WS, Cauley JA, et al. Factors associated with appendicular bone mass in older women. Ann Intern Med 1993;118:657. (*Age, weight, muscle strength, and estrogen use were the major factors.*)

Black DM, Cummings SR, Karpf DB, et al. Randomised trial of effect of alendronate on risk of fracture in women with existing vertebral fractures: Fracture Intervention Trial Research Group. Lancet 1996;348:1535. (*Major study finding a 47% reduction in rate of new fractures in comparison with placebo group.*)

Cauley JA, Seeley DG, Esrud K, et al. Estrogen replacement therapy and fractures in older women: Study of Osteoporotic Fractures Research Group. Ann Intern Med 1995;122:9. (*Relative risk for nonspinal fracture reduced by 34%.*)

Cummings SR, Black DM, Thompson DE, et al. Effect of alendronate on risk of fracture in women with low bone density but without vertebral fractures: results from the Fracture Intervention Trial. JAMA 1998;280:2077. (*Significantly reduced risk for hip fracture.*)

Cummings SR, Nevitt MC, Browner WS, et al. Risk factors for hip fracture in white women. N Engl J Med 1995;332:767. (*Finds family history of osteoporosis, low body mass index, history of bone fracture as adult, and current smoking to be the major risk factors.*)

Cummings SR, Black D. Bone mass measurement and risk of fracture in Caucasian women: a review of findings from prospective studies. Am J Med 1995;98:245. (*Strong correlation between bone mass and incidence of fractures; evidence supporting bone density measurement.*)

Cummings SR, Black DM, Nevitt MC, et al. Appendicular bone density and age predict hip fracture in women. JAMA 1990;263;665. (*Reduction in bone density found to correlate with risk for hip fracture.*)

Eastell R. Treatment of postmenopausal osteoporosis. N Engl J Med 1998;338:736. (*A review that focuses on the evidence for efficacy of therapy.*)

Eddy DM, Johnston CC Jr, Cummings SR, et al. Osteoporosis: review of the evidence for prevention, diagnosis, and treatment and cost-effectiveness analysis. Osteoporos Int 1998;8[Suppl 4]:S1. (*Extensive review of the evidence; concludes that screening appears to be cost-effective, especially for women with major risk factors.*)

Grady D, Rubin SM, Petitti DB, et al. Hormone therapy to prevent disease and prolong life in postmenopausal women. Ann Intern Med 1992;117:1016. (*Includes comprehensive review of the data on costs and benefits of estrogen replacement to prevent osteoporosis.*)

Hui SL, Slemenda CW, Johnston CC Jr. Baseline measurement of bone mass predicts fracture in white women. Ann Intern Med 1989;111:355. (*Predictive value of wrist bone density measurement demonstrated.*)

Kanis JA, Melton LJ III, Christiansen C, et al. The diagnosis of osteoporosis. J Bone Miner Res 1994;9:1137. (*World Health Organization consensus criteria for the diagnosis of osteoporosis; emphasizes importance of bone mineral density determination.*)

Kellie SE, AMA Council on Scientific Affairs. Measurement of bone density with dual energy x-ray absorptiometry (DEXA). JAMA 1992;267:286. (*The test of choice for screening.*)

Liberman UA, Weiss SR, Broll J, et al. Effects of oral alendronate on bone mineral density and the incidence of fractures in postmenopausal osteoporosis. N Engl J Med 1995;333:1437. (*Large, randomized, controlled trial revealing 9% increase in bone mineral density of spine and 6% increase at hip; 50% reduction in vertebral spine fracture.*)

Looker AC, Orwoll ES, Johnston CC Jr, et al. Prevalence of low femoral bone density in older U.S. adults from NHANES III. J Bone Miner Res 1997;12:1761. (*High prevalence found in this major epidemiologic study.*)

Rizzoli R, Slosman D, Bonjour JP. The role of dual energy x-ray absorptiometry of lumbar spine and proximal femur in the diagnosis and follow-up of osteoporosis. Am J Med 1995;33S. (*Good summary of test utility and shortcomings.*)

145
Evaluation of Acute Monoarticular Arthritis

Acute monoarticular arthritis calls for a prompt diagnostic evaluation because of the possibility of bacterial infection, which can lead to rapid joint destruction and septic sequelae. In certain noninfectious forms of inflammation, notably crystal-induced arthropathy, quick diagnosis and treatment are also beneficial. Most patients present for care on an outpatient basis, so that the diagnosis of monoarticular arthritis is an important responsibility of the primary physician.

PATHOPHYSIOLOGY AND CLINICAL PRESENTATION

The principal mechanisms of monoarticular arthritis can be broadly categorized as inflammatory and noninflammatory, with the inflammatory mechanisms subdivided into infectious and noninfectious.

Inflammatory Disease

Septic Arthritis. The arthritis of sepsis derives predominantly from hematogenous seeding of the synovium. Occasionally, it is caused by direct extension from a site of trauma or by osteomyelitis.

Disseminated Gonorrhea. Among previously healthy, sexually active patients, disseminated gonorrhea is the most frequent cause of joint infection. Women account for two thirds of cases. Pregnancy and menstruation appear to the increase risk for dissemination, which occurs in about 1% to 3% of persons with gonorrhea (see Chapter 137). An initial bacteremic stage is characterized by fever, polyarthralgias, transient scattered tendinitis, minimal joint effusion, necrotic skin lesions, blood cultures positive for organisms, and sterile joint fluid. This phase of the illness may be followed in several days by a septic joint stage, with monoarticular or occasionally polyarticular pain, marked joint swelling, and effusion. During the septic joint stage, gonococci can be recovered from the joint in about 50% of patients.

Nongonococcal Septic Arthritis. More than 80% of cases are monoarticular, with gram-positive organisms, especially *Staphylococcus aureus*, predominating (60% of infectious cases, most of them methicillin-resistant). *Streptococcus* species account for about 18%. *Gram-negative Enterobacteriaceae* also cause septic arthritis, particularly in IV drug abusers, immunocompromised persons, and the chronically ill. Joint sepsis is more likely in patients with altered host defenses (diabetes, cirrhosis, immunodeficiency), previously damaged joints (rheumatoid arthritis), or prosthetic joints. Fever, chills, and joint inflammation are usually prominent, but the presentation may be devoid of systemic symptoms, especially if the patient is debilitated or immunosuppressed. A larger joint, such as a knee or hip, is most likely to be involved. Sternoclavicular joint infection is characteristic of IV drug abusers. Articular destruction can be rapid. Within 10 days of nongonococcal infection, radiographic evidence of cartilaginous and bony damage may appear. Joint injury from gonococcal arthritis is less precipitous, so that more time is available for treatment. Permanent damage is uncommon in patients who are treated.

Lyme Disease. An acute oligoarthritis can develop months after the initial infection in untreated persons, with about 60% experiencing the problem (see Chapter 160). Large joints are typically involved, especially the knees. Intermittent attacks of acute arthritis lasting weeks to months are sometimes seen, as is chronic erosive arthritis. Swelling may be more prominent than pain.

Mycobacterial Infection. HIV-infected patients are at increased risk for mycobacterial joint infection, as are persons who have had repeated glucocorticoid injections into a joint. Often, periarticular bony disease develops in addition to joint inflammation. A chronic picture remains more common than acute inflammation.

HIV Infection. An acute monoarticular or oligoarticular arthritis may be part of a syndrome accompanying the onset of HIV infection. The lower extremities are the usual site of involvement (see Chapter 13).

Noninfectious Inflammatory Disease. The underlying mechanism is usually crystal-induced inflammation, but occasionally one of the immunologically mediated diseases may present as monoarticular disease.

Acute Gout. Gout is a common cause of acute monoarticular arthritis. Sodium urate crystals in the synovium incite a brisk inflammatory response after they are ingested by polymorphonuclear leukocytes. The condition is found most commonly among middle-aged and older men. Onset is rapid, peaking within 12 to 24 hours. The metatarsophalangeal joint of the great toe is the classic site, but the midfoot, ankles, knees, wrists, and olecranon bursae are other important locations. Sodium urate crystals are found in the joint fluid. They are needlelike and negatively birefringent under the polarizing microscope. Although the likelihood of a gouty attack increases with serum uric acid levels, uric acid levels are not diagnostically helpful except if extremely high. Alcoholic binges or the new use of thiazide diuretics may precipitate gouty attacks. A mild fever may even be present. Rapid response to colchicine helps differentiate crystal-induced arthritis from infection (see Chapter 158).

Pseudogout. Pseudogout results when crystals of calcium pyrophosphate induce joint inflammation, and it resembles gout pathophysiologically, although clinical features differ. Knees and wrists are the sites most commonly affected. Under the polarizing microscope, weakly positively birefringent rhomboid forms of calcium pyrophosphate are revealed in the synovial fluid. Chondrocalcinosis is usually present on radiography. Pseudogout tends to occur in older patients and seems to be associated with hyperparathyroidism, hemochromatosis, and severe degenerative joint disease.

Immunologic Disease. Immunologically mediated conditions typically cause polyarthritis but may present initially as a monoarthritis. These include rheumatoid arthritis, Reiter's syndrome, ankylosing spondylitis, psoriatic arthritis, the arthritis of inflammatory bowel disease, and the arthritis of sarcoidosis (see Chapter 146).

Noninflammatory Disease

Acute traumatic causes include juxtaarticular ligament or meniscus *injury*, frank bone *fracture* extending through to the joint space, or minor trauma in patients with impaired coagulation that results in *hemarthrosis*. A variety of mechanical disorders, collectively referred to as "internal derangements" of the knee, may produce chronic recurrent pain and noninflammatory effusion. *Osteoarthritis*, characterized by the degeneration of articular cartilage with adjacent bony sclerosis and proliferation, often produces chronic, gradually increasing joint symptoms but may present as an acutely painful joint with a noninflammatory or mildly inflammatory effusion.

DIFFERENTIAL DIAGNOSIS

The most immediately important entities in the differential diagnosis of acute monoarthritis are infection, crystal-induced arthropathy, and trauma. The gonococcus is the leading infectious agent, followed in frequency by gram-positive organisms (staphylococci, streptococci) and in compromised hosts by gram-negative coliforms. Gout and pseudogout are the important crystal-induced arthropathies.

As noted earlier, several polyarticular diseases may initially present with one acutely inflamed joint or with symptoms that are most pronounced in a single joint. These monoarticular presentations of polyarticular disease are seen in rheumatoid arthritis, Reiter's syndrome, ankylosing spondylitis, psoriatic arthritis, the arthritis of inflammatory bowel disease, and sarcoidosis.

Despite the wide range of diagnostic possibilities, it should be appreciated that recent series of monoarthritis have revealed that the most prevalent diagnoses are osteoarthritis, septic arthritis, gout, and pseudogout.

WORKUP

The first objective is to establish whether the joint is infected. Although examination of the joint fluid is the single most important diagnostic test, history and physical examination may provide useful information regarding the likelihood of infection and also its source.

History

Onset, associated symptoms, location, risk factors, and concurrent illness are essential items to check. Abrupt onset in conjunction with fever and chills points to a septic cause, as does a history of skin lesions, vaginal or urethral discharge, exposure to gonorrhea, tick bites, diabetes, concurrent rheumatoid arthritis, joint prosthesis, immunosuppression, HIV infection, IV drug abuse, and previous trauma. Acute trauma increases the probability of periarticular injury, internal derangement, and hemarthrosis. Prior attacks are indicative of gout and pseudogout. Alcohol abuse predisposes to gout, trauma, and infection.

Inflammation in the first metatarsophalangeal joint points to gout, especially in an elderly male patient; however, in patients with diabetes, extension of osteomyelitis into the joint must be ruled out. Associated back pain and stiffness raise the possibility of one of the spondyloarthropathies. Age can be a helpful clue. Pseudogout is most common in older patients. Disseminated gonococcal infection, Reiter's syndrome, and ankylosing spondylitis are diseases of young people.

Physical Examination

All joints are carefully examined to ascertain the location and nature of the problem. Signs of inflammation are sought (increased warmth, swelling, redness, effusion). One needs to differentiate inflammation of the joint space from a periarticular process such as tendinitis, bursitis, or cellulitis, which can be mistaken for it. Sometimes this distinction is impossible to make, but preservation of range of motion despite pain in the area reduces the likelihood of true joint involvement. The probability of a periarticular process is increased by the finding of localized tenderness that does not encompass the entire joint space. Although painful limitation of motion suggests articular disease, tendinitis and cellulitis can also cause discomfort with movement.

Once it is suspected that joint inflammation is present, the focus shifts quickly to differentiating between infectious and noninfectious causes. The patient's temperature should be taken. Almost all patients with septic arthritis are febrile. Low-grade fever may also be noted in gout and rheumatoid arthritis, but a high fever suggests infection. The integument is noted for necrotic lesions on the extremities (indicative of gonococcemia), the splinter hemorrhages of endocarditis, manifestations of HIV disease (see Chapter 13), needle tracks, tophi, rheumatoid nodules, pitting of the nails and other psoriatic manifestations, erythema nodosum (seen with sarcoidosis and inflammatory bowel disease), and the keratoderma blennorrhagicum and circinate balanitis of Reiter's syndrome. The eyes are examined for conjunctivitis and iritis, the fundi for signs of endocarditis, the mouth for mucosal ulceration, and the heart for murmurs. The genitalia need to be checked for signs of gonococcal urethritis and cervicitis (see Chapters 136 and 137). The spine should be examined carefully for restriction of motion and tenderness, indicative of spondylitis.

Laboratory Studies

No "standard" laboratory workup exists for acute monoarticular disease. Appropriate test selection should be based on the clinical presentation; only conditions suggested by the history and physical are worth investigating further. Running a standard battery of "arthritis tests" is both wasteful and potentially misleading. A few guidelines for initial test selection have been suggested by the American College of Rheumatology:
- If trauma or focal bone pain is present, then the first study should be radiography of the area.
- If an effusion or other signs of inflammation are noted, then the test of first choice is joint aspiration with fluid cell count and differential to confirm the presence of inflammation.
- If no effusion or trauma is present, then testing for trigger points and tender points (see Chapter 159) is indicated to assess for tendinitis and fibromyalgia, respectively.

Examination of Joint Fluid. Aspirating and examining the joint fluid is the single most important diagnostic procedure in the evaluation of acute monoarticular arthritis when evidence of inflammation is found. Taking note of the appearance of the joint fluid may be of help in determining the cause of arthropathy. A turbid appearance to the fluid points to inflammation; blood suggests trauma, coagulopathy, pseudogout, or neoplasm; a clear, straw-colored fluid is seen with degenerative disease and minor trauma. With sepsis, one may aspirate frank pus.

The fluid should be sent promptly for *cell count* and *differential* while it is fresh, and separate samples should be put aside briefly to be sent quickly for microscopic examination for *crystals* and *organisms* and for culture if the initial fluid examination shows evidence of inflammation. A white blood cell count above *2,000/mm³* is suggestive of an *inflammatory process*. A predominance of *neutrophils (>75%)* confirms an inflammatory process. In gout and septic joints, the white blood cell count often exceeds 50,000/mm³. Crystal examination under a polarizing lens provides the most rapid and sure method of diagnosing gout and pseudogout. However, urate crystals can often be seen under the microscope with normal light; the crystals of pseudogout are harder to identify in this manner. The *glucose* concentration is often measured; it may be suggestively low in infection and rheumatoid disease.

The fluid in a case of suspected infection should be sent for *Gram's stain* in addition to culture. Gram-positive bacteria are seen in about 80% of the cases in which they are the responsible agent. *Enterobacteriaceae* show up on Gram's stain less frequently. *Neisseria gonorrhoeae* is rarely seen. It is most important to *culture* the joint fluid immediately onto proper media (including Thayer-Martin plates for detection of gonococci). Smears of the joint fluid may show organisms in the absence of a culture positive for organisms if antibiotics have already been taken. A repeated tap of the joint will improve the diagnostic yield of Gram's stain and culture if results of the first arthrocentesis are negative.

Other Testing. When joint fluid cannot be obtained, the *complete blood cell count* and *erythrocyte sedimentation rate* are moderately helpful in distinguishing inflammatory from noninflammatory disease, but clearly the initial results of the synovial fluid examination are the most helpful to guide further testing. If inflammatory joint fluid is sterile, a workup for connective tissue disease (see Chapter 146), Lyme disease (see Chapter 160), and sarcoidosis (see Chapter 51) must be considered. Reviewing the history and physical examination findings for pertinent clinical clues can help determine to what extent testing for each of these conditions should be performed. If the fluid is frankly bloody, then determination of the prothrombin time, partial thromboplastin time, and platelet count is in order. The finding of characteristic crystals obviates the need for *serum uric acid* or *calcium* determinations; values are often normal despite an acute attack of crystal-induced disease. The serum uric acid level is useful only if markedly elevated. *Blood cultures* are indicated when sepsis is suspected. Culturing other possible foci of infection, such as skin lesions, urethral discharge, and the cervix, should be considered if infection is a possibility. Testing the joint fluid by polymerase chain reaction analysis for evidence of *Borrelia burgdorferi* can be diagnostic when Lyme disease is a real concern, but test availability may be limited.

Serologic Studies. A host of serologic studies are routinely offered for the assessment of arthritis. However, they are rarely diagnostic of the cause of an acute monoarticular arthritis, and false-positives are common in the setting of acute inflammation. Nonetheless, they can be helpful when used carefully. Testing for *HIV antibodies* is indicated when evidence of immune compromise or high-risk sexual behavior is found (see Chapter 13). Testing for *antinuclear antibodies* (ANA) and *rheumatoid factor* can help in the diagnosis of connective tissue disease, but false-positives are very common, especially in the elderly and persons with other inflammatory conditions (see Chapter 146), so they should be ordered only when clinical suspicion is substantial. *Lyme antibody titers* add little to the diagnosis except in cases with strongly supporting clinical and epidemiologic evidence for *Borrelia* infection (see Chapter 160).

Radiography. *Plain films* are most useful when evidence of trauma or focal bone pain is present. Plain films may also reveal fracture, neoplasm, osteomyelitis, and chondrocalcinosis. A diagnosis of osteoarthritis cannot be based solely on the presence of osteoarthritic changes, but their absence makes osteoarthritis unlikely. Radiography in patients with an acute inflammatory arthropathy often shows little more than soft-tissue swelling, especially in early phases of the disease. Films are of little use unless a baseline study for later comparison is desired. *Magnetic resonance imaging* is overused, but the technology is worth considering when traumatic internal knee derangement is suspected and confirmation is required (see Chapter 152). *Bone scan* or magnetic resonance imaging is indicated if osteomyelitis is suspected.

Despite optimal efforts, many cases of acute monoarthritis elude diagnosis. In one study, one third of cases were never satisfactorily diagnosed. Fortunately, however, the majority of these patients improved, or at least did not get worse. If infection, trauma, and, less importantly, crystal-induced arthritis are ruled out, the evaluation can be approached less hurriedly.

SYMPTOMATIC MANAGEMENT

Until a diagnosis is established, the patient may feel better resting, immobilizing the joint, and administering ice packs. Antiinflammatory agents should be postponed for at least 12 to 24 hours so that cultures can grow and arthrocentesis can be repeated if the first result is nondiagnostic. If pain is unbearable and a diagnosis is not yet established, an analgesic without antiinflammatory effects (e.g., acetaminophen or codeine) may be used. After a second negative result of arthrocentesis, it is reasonable to institute antiinflammatory therapy even in the absence of a specific diagnosis provided all cultures are negative for organisms and the patient is deemed to be at very low risk for infection. More definitive therapy of acute monoarticular arthritis must be based on the underlying cause (see Chapters 137, 156, 158, and 160).

INDICATIONS FOR REFERRAL AND ADMISSION

A patient with septic arthritis requires hospital admission, treatment with IV antibiotics, and consultation with an infectious disease specialist. When a case of acute monoarticular arthritis remains undiagnosed but the white blood cell count is high, infection is a possibility and an infectious disease spe-cialist should be consulted to consider an empiric course of IV antibiotics. The more chronic case that eludes diagnosis may benefit from a rheumatologic consultation. Closed synovial biopsy or arthroscopy may be needed.

A.H.G.

ANNOTATED BIBLIOGRAPHY

American College of Rheumatology Ad Hoc Committee on Clinical Guidelines. Guidelines for the initial evaluation of the adult patient with acute musculoskeletal symptoms. Arthritis Rheum 1996;39:1. (*Evidence-based consensus guidelines.*)

Baker DG, Schumacher HR. Acute monoarthritis. N Engl J Med 1993;329:1013. (*Clinically useful review, with excellent section on analysis of the joint fluid; 60 references.*)

Brown SL, Hansen SL, Linguine JJ. Role of serology in the diagnosis of Lyme disease. JAMA 1999;282:62. (*A review of the test performance of commercially available serologic kits. Finds great variability among tests, low reproducibility, and disappointing sensitivity and specificity under many circumstances; recommends that serologic testing be limited to those with an intermediate pretest probability of disease and that a two-step approach to testing be used.*)

Edeiken J. Arthritis: the roles of the primary care physician and the radiologist. JAMA 1975;232:1364. (*Differentiates conditions with mainly clinical findings from those with specific radiographic manifestations.*)

Freed JF, Nies KM, Boyer RS, et al. Acute monoarticular arthritis: a diagnostic approach. JAMA 1980;243:2314. (*Discusses the prevalence of various diagnoses and which tests were useful; one third of cases were never diagnosed.*)

Fries JF, Mitchell DM. Joint pain or arthritis. JAMA 1976;235:199. (*Still relevant for its emphasis on clinical diagnosis and judicious use of the laboratory.*)

Gatter RA, Schumacher HR Jr. Joint aspiration: indications and technique. In: Gatter RA, Schumacher HR Jr, eds. A practical handbook of synovial fluid analysis. Philadelphia: Lea & Febiger, 1991:14. (*Best guide to joint aspiration.*)

Goldenberg DL. Infectious arthritis complicating rheumatoid arthritis and other chronic rheumatic diseases. Arthritis Rheum 1989;32:496. (*Increased risk for infection; comprehensive review of the issue.*)

Goldenberg DL, Reed JI. Bacterial arthritis. N Engl J Med 1985;312:764. (*Reviews pathophysiology, risk factors, diagnosis, and therapy; emphasizes importance of early recognition and treatment.*)

Holmes K, Counts G, Beaty H. Disseminated gonococcal infection. Ann Intern Med 1971;74:979. (*Arthritis occurred in almost 90% with disseminated disease. Classic article describing the syndrome; 141 references.*)

Juby AF, Davis P, McElhaney JE, et al. Prevalence of selected autoantibodies in different elderly subpopulations. Br J Rheumatol 1994;33:1121. (*Increased prevalence with age; many with positive test results show no signs of disease.*)

Pascual E, Tovar J, Ruiz MT. The ordinary light microscope: an appropriate tool for provisional detection and identification of crystals in synovial fluid. Ann Rheum Dis 1989;48:983. (*One does not need a polarizing microscope to identify urate crystals.*)

Rowe IF, Forster SM, Seifert MH, et al. Rheumatic manifestations of human immunodeficiency virus infection. Am J Med 1988;85:59. (*Best description of joint involvement in HIV disease.*)

Shmerling RH, Delbanco T. How useful is the rheumatoid factor? Analysis of sensitivity, specificity, and predictive value. Arch Intern Med 1992;152:2417. (*The answer is that it is not too useful when ordered in low-probability situations; high rate of false-positives and false-negatives.*)

Shmerling RH, Delbanco T, Tosteson ANA, et al. Synovial fluid tests: what should be ordered? JAMA 1990;264:1009. (*Good discussion of the contribution of synovial fluid studies to diagnosis.*)

Slater CA, Davis RB, Shmerling RH. Antinuclear antibody testing. A study in clinical utility. Arch Intern Med 1996;156:1421. (*Test of-ten ordered in low-probability situations; positive predictive value very low in the setting of a low clinical probability for lupus.*)

Steere AC, Schoen RT, Taylor E. The clinical evolution of Lyme arthritis. Ann Intern Med 1987;107:725. (*The multiple presentations of Lyme arthritis.*)

Weissman BN, Hussain S. Magnetic resonance imaging of the knee. Rheum Dis Clin North Am 1991;17:637. (*Good review of indications for its use.*)

146
Evaluation of Polyarticular Complaints

Polyarticular complaints are among the most frequent in primary care practice and are often associated with considerable loss of function. Although osteoarthritis accounts for many of the more obvious cases (particularly in the elderly), the differential diagnosis can encompass a bewildering array of conditions, both articular and nonarticular, inflammatory and noninflammatory (Table 146.1). Careful attention to the history and physical examination findings helps chart a logical course to minimize diagnostic error and cost and maximize patient benefit. In most instances, the workup can proceed in deliberate, sequential fashion, but its pace is best matched to that of the underlying illness. The initial evaluation should focus on answering the following basic questions:

1. Are the patient's symptoms truly articular or nonarticular?
2. Is the arthritis inflammatory or degenerative?
3. Is the problem local or systemic?
4. How sick is the patient?

PATHOPHYSIOLOGY AND CLINICAL PRESENTATION

Pathophysiology

Polyarthritis can result from a degenerative, relatively noninflammatory process or from an inflammatory one. *Noninflammatory* forms of arthritis are, in most cases, the result of breakdown in joint cartilage and secondary mechanical disruption of the joint. This can be a primary process, or it can be associated with an underlying disease, such as hemochromatosis. Signs of inflammation are minimal, although occasionally a small joint effusion may be present. Other mechanisms of noninflammatory joint injury include synovial infiltration (amyloidosis), periosteal proliferation at the ends of long bones (hypertrophic osteoarthropathy), and ischemic injury (sickle cell disease).

Inflammatory arthritis develops as a consequence of the aggregation of inflammatory cells and their products in the joint space and synovium. Infection, gout, pseudogout, and the immunologically mediated diseases—rheumatoid arthritis, lupus, the spondyloarthropathies—all produce an inflammatory type of arthritis, characterized by joint swelling, warmth, redness, effusion, and tenderness. Joint constituents may be the targets of immunologic attack or may be caught up in a more generalized inflammatory process.

Periarticular disease involving muscles and tendons may also present as pain referable to joints, although it is not a true arthritis. Mechanisms range from autoimmune inflammatory processes to purported vasomotor instability.

Clinical Presentation: Inflammatory Polyarthritides

The hallmark of these conditions is synovitis, with manifestations of inflammation (erythema, warmth, swelling) encompassing the entire joint.

Rheumatoid Arthritis typically presents in subacute fashion with symmetric polyarthritis, although atypical forms include

Table 146.1. Differential Diagnosis of Polyarticular Pain

Inflammatory Joint Disease
Rheumatoid arthritis
Systemic lupus erythematosus
Scleroderma
Psoriatic arthritis
Reiter's syndrome
Ankylosing spondylitis
Polyarticular gout
Pseudogout
Sarcoidosis
Lyme disease
Disseminated gonococcemia
Rheumatic fever
Hepatitis B
Subacute bacterial endocarditis
Vasculitis

Noninflammatory Joint Disease
Osteoarthritis
Hypertrophic pulmonary osteoarthropathy
Myxedema
Amyloidosis
Sickle cell disease

Inflammatory Periarticular Disease
Polymyalgia rheumatica
Dermatomyositis, polymyositis
Eosinophilia–myalgia syndrome

Noninflammatory Periarticular Disease
Fibromyalgia syndrome
Reflex sympathetic dystrophy

Adapted from Mainardi CL. Approach to the patient with pain in more than one joint. In: Kelley WN, ed. Textbook of internal medicine, 2nd ed. Philadelphia: JB Lippincott Co, 1993:1002, with permission.

Table 146.2.   Diagnostic Criteria for Rheumatoid Arthritis[a]

1. Morning stiffness for more than 6 weeks
2. Arthritis involving three or more joint areas for more than 6 weeks
3. Arthritis of hand joints for more than 6 weeks
4. Symmetric arthritis for more than 6 weeks
5. Rheumatoid nodules
6. Serum rheumatoid factor in elevated titers
7. Radiologic changes (bony erosion in or adjacent to involved hand or wrist joints)

[a]Presence of any four or more criteria is necessary for a diagnosis of definite rheumatoid arthritis.
Adapted from Arnett FC, Edworthy SM, Block DA, et al. The American Rheumatism Association 1987 revised criteria for the classification of rheumatoid arthritis. Arthritis Rheum 1988;31:315, with permission.

Table 146.3.   Criteria for Diagnosis of Systemic Lupus Erythematosus[a]

1. Malar rash
2. Discoid rash
3. Photosensitivity
4. Oral or nasopharyngeal ulceration
5. Nonerosive arthritis
6. Pleuritis or pericarditis
7. Persistent proteinuria or casts
8. Seizures or psychosis
9. Hemolytic anemia, leukopenia, or thromboyctopenia
10. Antinuclear antibody
11. Anti-DNA antibody, anti-Sm antibody, or false-positive serologic test for syphilis

[a]Presence of any four or more criteria is necessary for a diagnosis of definite SLE, although many authorities accept fewer criteria in clinical practice, particularly if an antibody test result is positive.
Sm, Smith antigen.
Adapted from Tan EM, Cohen AS, Fries JF, et al. The 1982 revised criteria for the classification of systemic lupus erythematosus. Arthritis Rheum 1982;25:1271, with permission.

monoarticular and asymmetric disease. The most common sites are the wrists, proximal interphalangeal (PIP) joints, and metacarpophalangeal (MCP) joints, but elbows, neck, hips, knees, ankles, and feet may also be involved. Extraarticular manifestations include vasculitis, pulmonary nodules or interstitial fibrosis, mononeuritis multiplex, Sjögren's syndrome, and Felty's syndrome (splenomegaly, anemia, thrombocytopenia). Fatigue may dominate the early clinical presentation and precede the onset of joint symptoms. Other systemic symptoms (fever, weight loss) are prominent in severe cases. Women are more often affected than men. Morning stiffness is almost universal, with Raynaud's phenomenon a common accompaniment. Rheumatoid factor (RF) is found in approximately 75% of cases and is associated with skin nodules and more aggressive articular and extraarticular disease. Tendinous inflammation and joint destruction may ensue, producing characteristic changes (subluxation, swan neck deformities of the fingers, ulnar deviation of the wrists). Because no single clinical feature or test finding is definitive, the diagnosis requires the presence of a constellation of findings (Table 146.2). Current criteria are believed to have a sensitivity and specificity of approximately 90%.

Systemic Lupus Erythematosus usually occurs in young women, with a high prevalence in blacks. Malar rash, symmetric polyarthralgias, and nondeforming arthritis are characteristic, as is multisystem involvement, but morning stiffness and joint destruction are not as prominent as in rheumatoid arthritis (RA). Both large- and small-vessel vasculitis may occur. Oral ulcers are common. Serositis leading to pleuritis, effusion, or pericarditis develops in about a third of patients with systemic lupus erythematosus (SLE). Hematologic manifestations include leukopenia, immune thrombocytopenia, and hemolytic anemia. The most serious complications are glomerulonephritis and cerebritis. Results of testing for *antinuclear antibody* (ANA) by indirect immunofluorescence are positive in 95% to 99% of cases. *Antibody to native double-stranded DNA (antidsDNA)* is specific for lupus and is found in more than 70% of cases, especially those with renal involvement. *Antibody to the Smith antigen (anti-Sm)* is present in 30% and is also specific for SLE. Results of cardiolipin-based serologic tests for syphilis are false-positive. As with RA, no single finding or test is diagnostic for SLE; the presence of several characteristic features is necessary to confirm the diagnosis (Table 146.3).

Systemic Sclerosis (Scleroderma) initially presents as either hand arthralgias, mild inflammatory hand arthritis, or

Raynaud's phenomenon. Florid joint inflammation is uncommon. Skin thickening, a hallmark of the condition, follows several months later. Two clinical variants are described. One is a very slowly progressive form in which visceral involvement does not become significant until after decades of activity. It is manifested by the CREST syndrome: subcutaneous calcinosis of the digits, Raynaud's phenomenon, esophageal dysmotility, sclerodactyly, and telangiectasia. In the more aggressive form, skin thickening progresses rapidly to extend to the proximal limbs and trunk (hence the term *scleroderma*), and the onset of visceral involvement is accelerated (i.e., kidneys, lung, heart, and gastrointestinal tract). The results of ANA testing are positive in most patients with diffuse organ system disease, and a speckled pattern is characteristic and disease-specific when it corresponds to *antibody* to the nuclear enzyme *topoisomerase (anti-Scl-70)*.

Vasculitis may be a consequence of rheumatoid disease (e.g., RA, SLE) or an idiopathic necrotizing process that can lead to multisystem injury. Typically, vasculitis comes to attention after the appearance of palpable purpura, livedo reticularis, or skin ulceration, consequences of inflammatory injury to small dermal blood vessels (see Chapter 179). Multisystem involvement is characteristic, heralded by neurologic deficits, hematuria and proteinuria, abdominal pain, or asymmetric polyarthritis. The diagnosis is usually made by biopsy of an affected organ; skin is the most convenient.

Mixed Connective Tissue Disease is a term sometimes used to describe an indistinct clinical syndrome that contains features of systemic sclerosis, lupus, and Sjögren's syndrome. With time, the presentation usually evolves into one of these three conditions, so that some investigators have concluded that this is not a unique condition but rather an early, nonspecific clinical presentation.

Psoriatic Arthritis has both peripheral and axial forms. The peripheral form is asymmetric, oligoarticular, and often erosive. The distal interphalangeal (DIP) joints are most often affected, and the nails are pitted. Sausage-shaped digits and a "pencil-in-cup" radiologic appearance of the affected joints caused by erosion are found in advanced disease. Psoriatic skin changes (see

Chapter 187) usually predate the onset of arthritis, often by months to years, but they can be subtle. The spondylitic form of the disease (associated with HLA-B27 positivity) may resemble ankylosing spondylitis, but the extent of spinal involvement is less.

Reiter's Syndrome is primarily a disease of young men. Oligoarthritis, nongonococcal urethritis, and ocular inflammation (i.e., conjunctivitis, iritis) are the defining features. The latter two features may be fleeting and nonconcurrent. Dermatologic features include circinate balanitis (shallow, painless ulcers of the glans penis) and keratoderma blennorrhagicum (a hyperkeratosis of the feet). Onset sometimes follows a recent bacillary dysentery or chlamydial urethritis, which has led to speculation that the condition represents an immunologic cross-response in genetically predisposed hosts. HLA-B27 positivity is common and is believed to be related to the pathogenesis (i.e., shared antigenicity with the infectious agents). Joint involvement is asymmetric and affects the lower extremities. Heel pain with plantar fasciitis and calcaneal periostitis is distinctive. Mild spondylitis is common. ANA is absent.

Ankylosing Spondylitis begins insidiously and affects young men most severely, producing inflammation of the spinal joints and connective tissue with subsequent calcification and ossification. Characteristic radiographic findings include sacroiliitis and a diffuse proliferation of syndesmophytes leading to spinal fusion. Peripheral arthritis does occur, more often in women. In men, it tends to develop only after spinal disease has become evident. Large proximal joints such as the hips or knees are the predominant peripheral sites. Uveitis and HLA-B27 positivity are found, but their presence is not necessary for the diagnosis to be made. The arthritis of inflammatory bowel disease has many of the same features (see also Chapter 147).

Polyarticular Gout of an acute nature almost always occurs in patients with a prior history of monoarticular or oligoarticular gouty attacks, although hyperuricemia is not always present. The acute arthritis may be migratory but usually is confined to the lower extremities. The diagnosis is made by the finding of urate crystals in synovial fluid (see Chapter 145). A chronic arthritis occurs in patients with tophaceous disease. Acute attacks may be superimposed (see Chapter 158).

Pseudogout, like gout, is mostly an acute monoarticular disease but is on occasion polyarticular. Patients are usually elderly, with degenerative disease of the knees. The finding of calcium pyrophosphate crystals in the synovial fluid is diagnostic, although cartilage calcification can be seen on radiography. A subacute form, referred to as "pseudorheumatoid" arthritis, has been described, characterized by morning stiffness, synovial thickening, an elevated erythrocyte sedimentation rate (ESR), and low titers of RF.

Gonococcal Arthritis is the bacterial arthritis most likely to present in polyarticular fashion. Fever is usually present, and a papulovesicular rash indicative of disseminated disease develops in about two thirds of cases. Initially, the patient may have diffuse polyarticular symptoms, and signs of tenosynovitis may be found in the wrists, fingers, ankles, and toes. These manifestations are followed by a purulent arthritis in a limited number of joints, usually confined to the wrists, knees, or ankles (see Chapter 137).

Acute Rheumatic Fever causes an acute migratory polyarthritis if streptococcal infection is not treated. Abrupt onset of arthritis and fever are the predominant manifestations in adults. Both synovitis and periarticular inflammation occur, especially in the knees and ankles. Erythema of the overlying skin may be noted. Anti-DNAase B titers are elevated.

Lyme Disease may begin with migratory polyarthralgias and progress to attacks of asymmetric oligoarthritis in large joints (especially the knees) beginning about 6 months after infection in untreated patients. Later, a chronic monoarticular or oligoarticular arthritis may follow. The knees are a common site of chronic involvement. *Erythema chronica migrans*, the diagnostic annular red lesion at the site of the tick bite, occurs in 50% to 80% of cases during the early phase of illness. The diagnosis of late disease can be difficult because serologic testing is imprecise (see below and also Chapter 160).

Acute Viral Hepatitis B and other viral infections may present with an immune polyarthritis, often in conjunction with urticaria. The condition is symmetric, affecting the proximal joints of the hands. Onset in hepatitis B is during the preicteric phase. The condition clears spontaneously (see also Chapter 70).

Subacute Bacterial Endocarditis also causes an immune-mediated polyarthritis similar to that noted with hepatitis B. Fever, petechiae, splinter hemorrhages, heart murmur, and hematuria may be seen.

Sarcoidosis can cause an acute arthritis of the knees, wrists, PIP joints, and ankles that is accompanied by fever and simulates arthritis with an infectious cause. Erythema nodosum, hilar adenopathy, and periarticular involvement help to differentiate the condition from those with other causes. A destructive arthritis develops in a few persons; it is asymmetric and relapsing.

Clinical Presentation: Noninflammatory Arthritides

These conditions produce joint pain with few of the manifestations of inflammation, although sometimes a small effusion or mild synovial thickening may be noted.

Osteoarthritis typically presents as deep, aching joint pain that is aggravated by motion and weight bearing and by periods of inactivity. The involved joint can be enlarged as a result of osteophyte formation, but swelling is usually inconsequential, as soft-tissue involvement and inflammation are minimal. In later stages, pain occurs on motion and at rest in conjunction with stiffness. Nocturnal pain after vigorous activity is common. Patients with advanced disease have pain on weight bearing and joint instability. Examination often reveals crepitus and discomfort on movement of the joint. Occasionally, slight warmth is noted in severely affected weight-bearing joints, but erythema and marked warmth are absent. Limitation of motion, malalignment, and bony protuberances from spurs are frequent findings. The joints most commonly affected include the DIP joints of the hands (with formation of Heberden's nodes), MPC joint at the base of the thumb, hips, knees, and cervical and lumbosacral vertebral joints.

Hypertrophic Pulmonary Osteoarthropathy may lead to diffuse bony pain in the lower extremities that is worsened by dependency. New bone formation and periostosis are the source of discomfort. Articular and periarticular symptoms may be encountered. Clubbing is a hallmark, although it is not readily evident in about 25% of cases. Intrapulmonary disease is an important precipitant (see Chapter 45).

Hypothyroidism severe enough to cause myxedema is associated with symmetric peripheral joint swelling that can mimic RA. The white blood cell count in the joint fluid is low, and no clinical signs of inflammation are present. Nonarticular neuromuscular symptoms include myalgias and hand pain related to carpal tunnel syndrome.

Amyloidosis can cause swelling of large joints secondary to synovial infiltration. Because of the symmetric distribution and gradual onset, an immunologic cause of arthropathy may be suspected, but the joint fluid shows no signs of inflammation or immune hyperreactivity. Concurrent involvement of the skin, heart, liver, and peripheral nerves is characteristic. Carpal tunnel syndrome may be present.

Sickle Cell Disease sometimes produces a 2- to 3-week noninflammatory arthropathy affecting large joints that is characterized by swelling, tenderness, and effusion. The synovial fluid is noninflammatory.

Clinical Presentation: Nonarticular Disease

Polymyalgia Rheumatica develops gradually during weeks or months. Pain and stiffness of periarticular structures of the neck and shoulders is the presentation in two thirds of cases, with hip and thigh involvement accounting for the other third. Many patients have both shoulder and thigh involvement. Morning stiffness and pain with movement are highly characteristic; muscle strength is unimpaired. Synovitis has been documented histologically; muscle biopsy specimens are usually normal or show minor inflammatory infiltrates. Sometimes, low-grade fever, weight loss, and fatigue precede the onset of musculoskeletal symptoms. The condition is usually symmetric, but if asymmetric it may be mistaken for shoulder bursitis or hip arthritis. Most patients are elderly. The association with cranial arteritis makes this an important condition to recognize. Marked elevation of the ESR is characteristic. No serologic abnormalities are found (see also Chapter 161).

Myositis of any type may present as musculoskeletal pain and be confused with polyarthritis, although weakness is typically more prominent than pain. *Polymyositis* is the prototypical inflammatory muscle disease, characterized by proximal muscle weakness, soreness, and elevated levels of muscle enzymes. It may present as *dermatomyositis* in the elderly. *Eosinophilia–myalgia* syndrome is a serious myositis observed in association with ingestion of L-tryptophan preparations. Marked peripheral eosinophilia, muscle weakness and pain, and serum aldolase elevations comprise the initial presentation.

Skin induration, pulmonary infiltrates, cardiac rhythm disturbances, and peripheral neuropathy may ensue.

Fibromyalgia Syndrome (Fibrositis, Fibromyositis) occurs predominantly in women. An inflammatory mechanism has been suspected (hence the "itis" designation) but never demonstrated. Characteristic manifestations include morning stiffness worsened by changes in the weather and heavy exercise, fatigue caused by disordered sleep, and tenderness at multiple symmetric *trigger points* concentrated in the upper back and neck. The musculoskeletal discomfort is typically diffuse and poorly localized, but exacerbations caused by extremes of joint motion may produce pain referable to the joints. All hematologic and serologic parameters are normal (see also Chapter 159).

Reflex Sympathetic Dystrophy Syndrome causes diffuse musculoskeletal discomfort, swelling, weakness, and limitation of motion. A single limb is affected, usually an arm. The limb is swollen and the skin shiny, often dusky in appearance and cool to the touch. Pain can be severe and burning. Periarticular structures are especially tender. Preceding trauma accounts for 50% of cases. A vasomotor mechanism is postulated.

DIFFERENTIAL DIAGNOSIS

The causes of polyarticular complaints can be divided into articular and nonarticular categories, and these can be subdivided into inflammatory and noninflammatory conditions (Table 146.1).

WORKUP

Overall Strategy

The initial assessment of the patient who presents with multiple joint symptoms is facilitated by addressing the following questions:

1. Is the underlying disease process inflammatory or noninflammatory?
2. Is the problem systemic or focal?
3. Is it truly articular or periarticular?
4. Is vital organ function or joint integrity endangered?

In the vast majority of cases, the answers to these questions can be provided by a careful history and physical examination, supplemented by a few basic blood tests or a radiographic study suggested by the clinical picture. Synovial fluid analysis is sometimes helpful if an accessible effusion is present. The laboratory workup is best used to modify one's initial clinical impression. Routinely ordering an "arthritis panel" of blood tests is wasteful, and it also risks the generation of false-positive results, which can have devastating consequences.

It is important to note that official criteria for the diagnosis of RA and SLE are designed more to ensure uniformity in epidemiologic and therapeutic studies than to diagnose disease in individual patients. The American Rheumatism Association criteria for RA emphasize chronicity and symmetry of polyarthritis, so they are less sensitive for use in early disease. The diagnosis of SLE by official criteria poses similar problems. For the individual patient, a diagnosis of one of these conditions should be considered if some, but not necessarily all, of the characteristic clinical features of the disease are present.

History

Differentiating Articular from Nonarticular Disease. Patients complain of pain, stiffness, and loss of function and often confuse neuropathic pain, bone pain, or myalgias with arthritis. The physician should attempt to identify the anatomic basis of the symptoms by asking the patient to specify exactly where the pain is located, what aggravates it, and what functional loss has occurred. For the most part, the symptoms of joint disease are well localized to the joint and bear a logical relation to its use. Nonarticular disease rarely has a specifically articular location and does not produce loss of articular function, although range of motion may be affected to some degree. After the location of the process has been established, the underlying disease mechanism should be elucidated.

Differentiating Inflammatory from Noninflammatory Disease. One inquires into the characteristic hallmarks of inflammation: redness, warmth, soft-tissue swelling, and tenderness. If such symptoms are localized to and encompass an entire joint, one has excellent presumptive evidence for synovitis and an inflammatory process. It is important not to mistake tenderness in a segment of the joint or a small effusion as evidence of inflammation. The response to antiinflammatory agents is sometimes useful for differentiation, although most nonprescription agents, such as aspirin and other NSAIDs, also have analgesic activity that may provide nonspecific relief. Patients with RA reach for their aspirin as soon as they awaken and clearly feel worse if they miss a dose. The response in patients with osteoarthritis is much less dramatic.

Elucidation of a Specific Cause. The basic determinations of site and disease process help narrow the differential diagnosis and enable a more focused consideration. Attention to other elements of the history, such as distribution of involved joints, associated symptoms (including those suggesting systemic disease), and age and sex, facilitate identification of the cause.

Distribution and Temporal Pattern are of considerable diagnostic value, so that careful inquiry about all the joints affected and the sequence of involvement is necessary. Problems that at first appear monoarticular or asymmetric may turn out to be polyarticular or symmetric on further questioning. Several patterns are quite suggestive. Symmetric noninflammatory involvement of the PIP and DIP joints, without MCP or wrist involvement and without morning stiffness, argues for osteoarthritis. Asymmetric inflammatory disease of these joints points to psoriatic arthritis. Symmetric inflammatory involvement of the MCP, PIP, carpal, or metatarsophalangeal (MTP) joints supports a diagnosis of rheumatoid disease. Bilateral heel pain suggests Reiter's syndrome and the other spondyloarthropathies, as does back pain. Hip and shoulder girdle symptoms in an elderly patient with noninflammatory, nonarticular disease provide strong presumptive evidence for polymyalgia, whereas a vague distribution in conjunction with the presence of trigger points supports a diagnosis of fibromyalgia.

The temporal pattern deserves attention. A chronic, subacute, additive process is consistent with rheumatoid disease. The sudden, explosive onset of symmetric polyarthritis suggests an acute hypersensitivity reaction, such as that seen with early hepatitis B infection or penicillin allergy. A migratory pattern raises the possibilities of rheumatic fever, disseminated gonococcemia, Reiter's syndrome, and Lyme disease, among others.

Associated Symptoms aid in the diagnosis and may provide evidence for systemic involvement. A careful review of systems is essential. *Morning stiffness* is very suggestive of rheumatoid disease, which produces maximal stiffness after inactivity. In contrast, osteoarthritis is characterized by maximal symptoms with use. If some stiffness occurs with rest in osteoarthritis, it passes quickly with activity. Acute onset of fever points to an infectious origin or a marked hypersensitivity reaction, whereas low-grade fever may herald the onset of rheumatoid disease. The development of a *rash* may be diagnostic for such conditions as SLE, gonococcemia, Lyme disease, and vasculitis (see later discussion). New onset of *Raynaud's phenomenon* raises the possibility of scleroderma, SLE, or RA. A history of chronic or bloody *diarrhea* suggests inflammatory bowel disease. Symptoms of *urethritis* and *conjunctivitis* are suggestive of Reiter's syndrome. *Sleep disorder* and *chronic fatigue* point to fibromyalgia. Chronically *dry mouth* and *dry eyes* suggest Sjögren's syndrome, a common accompaniment of RA. Systemic involvement with SLE is evidenced by reports of nasopharyngeal ulcers, pleuritic chest pain, or mental status changes.

Age and Sex. Patients with SLE and RA are predominantly female, whereas those with Reiter's syndrome are predominantly male. The onset of rheumatic fever or ankylosing spondylitis nearly always occurs before age 40. The peak incidence for SLE is in the premenopausal period, although later onset is not rare. The incidence of RA is less dependent on age, with new onset occurring in elderly as well as young persons. Gout in women is mainly a postmenopausal disease; in men, it occurs at all adult ages. SLE is particularly common among black women.

Severity and effect on daily activity help assess the functional significance in addition to underlying cause. Joint pain awakening the patient at night indicates severe arthritis; alternatively, it may signify a bony or neuropathic process. Marked daily fatigue, the need for afternoon naps, weight loss, and fever all suggest active systemic illness. The assessment of the functional impact must take into account not only the severity of the condition but also the patient's premorbid level of activity and attitudes toward work and pain.

Past Medical History and Family History. Recurrent attacks and a genetic propensity are characteristic of many conditions. Gout may present as polyarthritis, but more often one uncovers a prior history of podagra or another form of acute monoarthritis in a lower extremity. A history of travel or residence in an area endemic for Lyme disease, in addition to a history of recent tick bite, should be elicited. The spondyloarthropathies, gout, and the Heberden's nodes of osteoarthritis all have a familial preponderance, which should be explored.

Physical Examination

The physical examination is basically a continuation of the same approach, with documentation of the pattern and type of joint involvement and the nature of any extraarticular disease. The myriad extraarticular manifestations of the arthritic diseases makes a detailed general physical examination mandatory. Certain aspects deserve emphasis.

Skin and Integument. Important dermal clues to underlying cause include the malar rash of SLE, annular erythema chronica migrans of Lyme disease, papulovesicular lesions with a necrotic center of disseminated gonococcemia, nail pitting and scaling of psoriasis, urticarial lesions of hepatitis B infection, and palpable purpura, ulceration, or livedo reticularis of vasculitis. In a patient with suspected Reiter's syndrome, the glans penis should be checked for the ulcers of circinate balanitis and the heels for the hypertrophic changes of keratoderma blennorrhagicum. One should carefully palpate around the elbows, Achilles tendons, and pinnae and search for rheumatoid nodules and tophi, which are specific indicators of RA and gout, respectively. The nails should be examined for pitting and clubbing. Nail pitting adjacent to erosive DIP arthritis can justify a diagnosis of psoriatic arthritis in the absence of any skin psoriasis. Fingertip atrophy with healed or active ulcers suggests severe Raynaud's phenomenon and should prompt a search for the calcinosis, subungual telangiectases, and skin tightening of scleroderma. The presence of the red, tender, subcutaneous lesions of erythema nodosum raises the possibilities of sarcoidosis and inflammatory bowel disease. Dry, doughy skin and loss of the outer third of the eyebrows are signs of hypothyroidism.

Head, Ears, Nose, Throat, Neck, Lungs, Heart. The anterior eye should be checked for conjunctivitis and iritis, which are suggestive of Reiter's syndrome and spondylitis (see Chapter 199), and the posterior eye for retinal hemorrhages, exudates, and ischemic lesions, which are consistent with systemic lupus and vasculitis. "Cotton-wool" exudates are the most common eye lesion in SLE. The oral and nasal mucosa should be examined for ulcers, which if painful suggest SLE and if painless suggest Reiter's syndrome. Thyroid evaluation may reveal a goiter. The chest is examined for signs of effusion, pleuritis, and pericarditis. Pleural and pericardial rubs are found in RA and SLE. Heart murmurs characterize rheumatic fever and SLE, mitral valve murmurs sometimes occur in SLE, and aortic regurgitant murmurs occur in the spondyloarthropathies. The abdominal examination includes checking for splenomegaly, which is found in a variety of rheumatic diseases, including RA and SLE.

Musculoskeletal Examination. One checks for signs of serositis, noninflammatory articular disease, and periarticular disease. As emphasized earlier, inflammatory joint disease involves the entire joint; tenderness, warmth, redness, soft-tissue swelling, and often an effusion are present. In contrast, noninflammatory disease is usually associated with only focal tenderness and few, if any, signs of inflammation, although a small noninflammatory effusion may be present. The distribution of disease is noted, as are any mechanical abnormalities, such as limitation of motion, instability, subluxation, or tendon injury.

A careful look at the periarticular tissues (tendons, bursae, muscles) is also indicated. Bursitis and tendinitis commonly mimic arthritis. Subacromial bursitis and bicipital tendinitis can be confused with shoulder joint disease (see Chapter 150), lateral epicondylitis (tennis elbow) and olecranon bursitis with elbow joint disease (see Chapter 153), trochanteric bursitis with hip disease (see Chapter 151), and anserine bursitis with knee disease (see Chapter 152). Muscle soreness and proximal muscle weakness raise the question of a myositis. Checking for pressure points in the upper back and neck is indicated in patients with suspected fibromyalgia syndrome.

Another important type of periarticular disease is that manifested by "frozen" joints and flexion contractures. Severe limitation of motion may occur in an intrinsically normal joint. Disuse because of neurologic disease or periarticular pain may lead to tightening of periarticular fibrous tissue and secondary contractures. The clinical presentation can be mistaken for that of arthritis, but normal radiographic findings in a joint and a lack of indicators of inflammatory arthritis, plus an awareness of a predisposing illness, lead to the correct diagnosis.

If a patient has hand stiffness or pain, a valuable screening test for finger joint and tendinous disease is *"curling."* The patient is asked to extend the MCP joints and then maximally flex the PIP and DIP joints, but not to make a fist. Curling is normal if a patient can bring the fingertips into apposition with the palm. Any disease of the PIP or DIP joints interferes with curling, as does any inflammation along the dorsal extensor tendons.

For patients with a suspected spondyloarthropathy, *Schober's test* provides a useful assessment of lumbar mobility. Two marks are made on the patient's back while the patient is standing: one at the level of the posterior iliac spine and the other exactly 10 cm above the first. When the patient bends forward maximally, the two marks should be at least 15 cm apart. An abnormal Schober's test result is nonspecific, but if an abnormal result is combined with other evidence for a spondyloarthropathy, it can advance the diagnosis.

Neurologic Examination. Evidence of peripheral neuropathy is sought by assessing motor and sensory function in the extremities, and the mental status is carefully evaluated in patients with suspected SLE and HIV infection (central nervous system involvement is a sign of serious disease).

Laboratory Studies

Approach to Testing. A large number of laboratory tests, both simple and esoteric, are routinely used in the evaluation of polyarthritic symptoms. Panels of tests are sometimes offered by laboratories as a means of "screening" for arthritic conditions. They range from a set of basic studies (e.g., ANA and RF titers, uric acid level, ESR) to elaborate panels that may include testing for anti-dsDNA, anti-Ro, anti-La, anti-Scl-70, anti-Sm, and anti-ribonucleoprotein. All such batteries of tests have been found to be wasteful, of little use diagnostically when ordered in the absence of clinical evidence, and a source of potentially misleading false-positive results. Nonetheless, test panels continue to be popular, even when the pretest probability of disease is so low that a positive test result will have almost no positive predictive value (see Chapter 2). Perhaps it is the desire to "rule out" disease that drives such testing (negative predictive value is high, but it is usually already very high before testing). Repeated studies demonstrate and expert panels reaffirm that the best means of diagnosing or ruling out "must-not-miss" conditions is a careful history and physical examination, complemented by thoughtfully selected tests that specifically address conditions for which at least some clinical evidence is present. Diagnostic confusion that persists at the end of the physical examination is rarely resolved by "pan-scanning" for arthritic disease. Careful test selection and interpretation are especially important in the elderly because the frequency of abnormal test results in the absence of disease increases with age, especially with the most commonly ordered studies (e.g., ESR, uric acid level, ANA and RF titers); the false-positive rate can be as high as 90%. Test selection is guided by whether the clinical assessment suggests inflammatory or noninflammatory disease.

Suspected Inflammatory Articular Disease. In this setting, a determination of the *ESR* provides useful but nonspecific confirmation of inflammatory disease activity and can be followed as a measure of disease activity. A markedly elevated reading (e.g., >60 mm/h) suggests considerable inflammatory activity. A normal ESR in the setting of active joint symptoms reduces the probability of active inflammatory pathophysiology. However, the ESR is a relatively poor test for the detection of inflammatory disease that is in remission. A *complete blood cell count* can be obtained at the same time to check for hematologic involvement by the underlying disease process.

If symptoms are acute and new in onset, then tests for infectious causes should be considered. *Blood cultures* are essential if endocarditis or disseminated gonococcemia is suspected. Currently available *Lyme antibody* assays lack specificity, so their results are difficult to interpret (see Chapter 160) and less useful than a careful clinical assessment. DNA-based assays with polymerase chain reaction technology are not yet widely available and very expensive. Liver function testing (e.g., measurement of aminotransferases) may help confirm suspected viral hepatitis; hepatitis serology should follow if serum liver chemistries are abnormal.

If the duration of symptoms is more than 6 weeks, then the possibility of rheumatoid disease and other chronic forms of inflammatory joint disease need to be explored further, especially if the patient has systemic symptoms.

Rheumatoid factor is helpful if the pretest probability of RA is intermediate and further supporting evidence is sought. In general, 70% to 80% of all patients meeting strict criteria for RA are RF-positive. The higher the RF titer, the more likely the diagnosis of RA. RF negativity does not rule out RA; 25% of patients with RA are RF-negative. On the other hand, RF positivity does not rule in RA; it also occurs in other inflammatory conditions (e.g., SLE, subacute bacterial endocarditis, vasculitis, and even viral infection). Moreover, 5% to 15% of "normal" persons (the percentage increases with age) are RF-positive.

Antinuclear Antibody testing is very sensitive (99%) for the diagnosis of SLE, but specificity is lacking (50% to 85%). The test result can also be positive in other forms of connective tissue disease (sensitivity of about 50% for RA, and considerably higher for Sjögren's syndrome and progressive systemic sclerosis), in chronic hepatitis, and in elderly persons without any connective tissue disease. The higher the ANA titer, the more likely the diagnosis of lupus. A titer of 1:40 is usually listed as the criterion for a positive test result, but such a cutoff produces a 35% false-positive rate in a general medical setting. An ANA titer criterion of 1:160 reduces the false-positive rate to 5% while reducing sensitivity only minimally (to 95%). Titers of ANA fluctuate with time but do not necessarily parallel disease activity. The test is most useful in the setting of inflammatory polyarthritis and systemic symptoms. ANA negativity rules out SLE; however, the test is not specific enough for a positive result to rule in the condition, but it would justify further testing.

Follow-up Tests for Patients with a Positive Antinuclear Antibody Test Result. Because ANA positivity is a nonspecific finding, additional testing is required for patients with a positive test result. The specific nuclear constituents represented by the ANA titer function as convenient autoantigens. Testing for antibodies against these antigens often provides the desired specificity but should not be performed in the absence of characteristic clinical features (i.e., a reasonable pretest probability is required); otherwise, poor likelihood ratios (ratio of true-positives to false-positives) are likely to result. *Antibody to native dsDNA* occurs in up to 70% of patients with SLE and is specific for the condition and also predictive of an increased risk for nephritis. Testing for anti-dsDNA is used to confirm the diagnosis of SLE in patients with suspected disease and ANA positivity. *Antibody to Smith antigen* is similarly specific but is found in only 30% of patients with SLE. *Antibody to Scl-70* (a nuclear topoisomerase) is highly specific for *systemic sclerosis*, but its sensitivity is low (20%). In *Sjögren's syndrome*, anti-Ro and anti-La antibodies provide 60% to 70% sensitivity and more than 90% specificity. *Lip biopsy* is the definitive test, but it is often not necessary in the context of characteristic clinical and serologic findings.

Synovial Fluid Analysis is useful and indicated if a joint effusion is present and the diagnosis remains undetermined. One seeks to differentiate between inflammatory and noninflammatory disease (see Chapter 145), and also to check for crystal-induced arthropathy and investigate any suspected infection (see Chapter 145). A white blood cell count above 2,000/mm³ with more than 75% polymorphonuclear leukocytes supports the presence of inflammation; a cell count below 1,000/mm³ indicates noninflammatory disease. A count between 1,000 and 2,000/mm³ is ambiguous. Often, one obtains a synovial fluid white blood cell count of 5,000 to 20,000/mm³ without crystals, bacteria, or other distinctive attributes, which allows for little more than a designation of inflammatory arthritis, type unspecified.

Serum Uric Acid levels are obtained unnecessarily in most arthritis patients and too often serve as the primary basis for a diagnosis of gout. The definitive diagnosis is best made by observing urate crystals in the synovial fluid. A normal serum uric acid level does not rule out the diagnosis of gout, nor does an elevated level rule it in.

Radiography is usually of minimal diagnostic value in the early stages of inflammatory polyarthritis, showing little more than soft-tissue swelling. Films obtained during later stages may manifest more characteristic bony changes, but usually a diagnosis has already been established. However, early *sacroiliac films* are of value in suspected spondyloarthropathy because they may reveal sacroiliitis, a diagnostic finding. Another early radiologic change in spondyloarthropathy is squaring of the superior and inferior margins of the vertebral bodies. Only later do prominent syndesmophytes appear.

HLA-B27 Testing has not proved diagnostically useful. Although the prevalence of HLA-B27 antigen positivity in the seronegative spondyloarthropathies is high (≥90%), the fact that positivity for HLA-B27 is seen in 6% to 8% of normal persons negates the utility of HLA-B27 testing in the diagnosis of this uncommon condition.

Urinalysis and Routine Chemistries. Urinalysis is essential to screen for glomerular injury in rheumatoid disease. Routine serum chemistries are less rewarding, although assessment of renal function by measurement of *blood urea nitrogen* and *creatinine* levels is indicated in patients with proteinuria or hematuria.

Suspected Noninflammatory Polyarticular Disease. In os-teoarthritis, *joint radiographic findings* are abnormal by the time the patient becomes symptomatic and can confirm the diagnosis. However, degenerative changes are commonly found in asymptomatic joints also. Films of long bones can be obtained to confirm hypertrophic osteoarthropathy, but the diagnosis can usually be made clinically by the presence of clubbing. Suspected hypothyroidism can be confirmed by a *thyrotropin* (TSH) determination.

Suspected Inflammatory Nonarticular Disease. The *ESR* should be measured in patients with clinical evidence for polymyalgia rheumatica. A high rate supports the diagnosis; a low one reduces the probability. If headache, jaw claudication, visual disturbance, or a tender cranial artery is noted, then evaluation for cranial arteritis should proceed promptly (see Chapter 161). A *complete blood cell count* and *differential* are indicated in patients with suspected eosinophilia–myalgia; referral for skin and muscle biopsy is then appropriate if florid peripheral eosinophilia is noted. Suspected polymyositis is evaluated by measuring serum *creatine kinase* levels and, if they are markedly elevated, proceeding to consideration of *muscle biopsy*.

Suspected Noninflammatory Nonarticular Disease. The diagnosis of fibromyalgia is a clinical one. No associated laboratory abnormalities are found (see Chapter 159). Similarly, the diagnosis of reflex sympathetic dystrophy is predominantly clinical. Plain films of the hand may show a nonspecific but suggestive patchy osteopenia.

INDICATIONS FOR ADMISSION AND REFERRAL

The diagnosis of polyarticular arthritis may remain uncertain for a long period. For the most part, the underlying condition is not immediately life-threatening, and the workup can take place in the outpatient setting during several visits. Short-term risk to the patient is posed primarily by extraarticular disease and infection. If any evidence of bloodstream infection, vasculitis, or involvement of the eyes, lungs, heart, kidneys, or nervous system is found, hospitalization and consultation should be promptly considered. The same recommendation pertains to persons with severe constitutional symptoms (e.g., disabling fatigue, fever, weight loss). Rheumatologic consultation is also appropriate if a patient with less serious illness remains without a diagnosis after the initial evaluation has been completed. A timely referral for consultation with a well-trained rheumatologist is likely to be far more productive than exhaustive serologic testing, with its attendant risks of false-positive results.

SYMPTOMATIC THERAPY

Treatment should be etiologic (see Chapters 155 through 163), but the definitive diagnosis of an inflammatory polyarthritis may take time. Pending results, and provided infection has been ruled out, the patient bothered by symptoms of joint inflammation may be given either high-dose aspirin (up to twelve 325-mg tablets daily) or a generic NSAID preparation (e.g., 400 to 800 mg of ibuprofen four times daily).

A.H.G.

ANNOTATED BIBLIOGRAPHY

American College of Rheumatology Ad Hoc Committee on Clinical Guidelines. Guidelines for the initial evaluation of the adult patient with acute musculoskeletal symptoms. Arthritis Rheum 1996;39:1. (*Evidence-based consensus guidelines.*)

Arnett FC, Edworthy SM, Bloch DA, et al. The American Rheumatism Association 1987 revised criteria for the classification of rheumatoid arthritis. Arthritis Rheum 1988;31:315. (*A collaborative study showing a sensitivity and specificity for the official criteria of approximately 90%.*)

Brown SL, Hansen SL, Linguine JJ. Role of serology in the diagnosis of Lyme disease. JAMA 1999;282:62. (*A review of the test performance of commercially available serologic kits. Finds great variability among tests, low reproducibility, and disappointing sensitivity and specificity under many circumstances; recommends that serologic testing be limited to those with an intermediate pretest probability of disease and that a two-step approach to testing be used.*)

Goldenberg DL. Fibromyalgia syndrome: an emerging but controversial condition. JAMA 1987;257:2782. (*Thoughtful description of the condition and how to recognize it.*)

Harler NM, Franck WA, Bress NM, et al. Acute polyarticular gout. Am J Med 1974;56:715. (*A study of this uncommon presentation of a very common disease.*)

Homburger HA. Cascade testing for autoantibodies in connective tissue diseases. Mayo Clin Proc 1995;70:183. (*The argument against unselective testing.*)

Juby AF, Davis P, McElhaney JE, et al. Prevalence of selected autoantibodies in different elderly subpopulations. Br J Rheumatol 1994;33:1121. (*Increased prevalence with age; many with positive test results show no signs of disease.*)

Juby AF, Johnston C, Davis P. Specificity, sensitivity, and diagnostic predictive value of selected laboratory-generated autoantibody profiles in patients with connective tissue diseases. J Rheumatol 1991;18:354. (*Data on test performance characteristics.*)

Kahn MA, Kahn MK. Diagnostic value of HLA-B27 testing in ankylosing spondylitis and Reiter's syndrome. Ann Intern Med 1982;96:70. (*The test is usually unnecessary.*)

Keat A. Reiter's syndrome and reactive arthritis in perspective. N Engl J Med 1983;309:1606. (*An extensive review, including a discussion of joint manifestations.*)

Kozin F. Reflex sympathetic dystrophy. Bull Rheum Dis 1986;36:1. (*Good summary of pathophysiologic hypotheses and clinical manifestations.*)

Lichtenstein MJ, Pincus T. How useful are combinations of blood tests in "rheumatic panels" in diagnosis of rheumatic diseases? J Gen Intern Med 1987;3:435. (*Positive predictive value of only 34% leads to many false-positive results.*)

Mainardi CL. Approach to the patient with pain in more than one joint. In: Kelley WN. Textbook of internal medicine, 2nd ed. Philadelphia: JB Lippincott Co, 1993:1000. (*Provides a useful categorization of the differential diagnosis, adapted for use in this chapter.*)

Medsger TA. Tryptophan-induced eosinophilia–myalgia syndrome. N Engl J Med 1990;322:926. (*An editorial summarizing current understanding.*)

Plotz PH, Dalakas M, Leff RL, et al. Current concepts in idiopathic inflammatory myopathies. Ann Intern Med 1989;111:143. (*Comprehensive review that includes useful discussions of polymyositis and dermatomyositis.*)

Rahn DW, Malawista SE. Lyme disease: recommendations for diagnosis and treatment. Ann Intern Med 1991;114:472. (*Still useful for its discussion of clinical manifestations and the shortcomings of antibody testing.*)

Slater CA, Davis RB, Shmerling RH. Antinuclear antibody testing. A study in clinical utility. Arch Intern Med 1996;156:1421. (*Test frequently ordered in low-probability situations; positive predictive value very low in the setting of a low clinical probability for lupus.*)

Stere AC, Schoen RT, Taylor E. The clinical evolution of Lyme arthritis. Ann Intern Med 1987;107:725. (*Attacks of asymmetric oligoarthritis begin in large joints, especially the knees, about 6 months after infection in untreated patients.*)

Tan Em, Feltkamp TE, Smolen JS, et al. Range of antinuclear antibodies in "healthy" individuals. Arthritis Rheum 1997;40:1601. (*Many normal persons have an elevated ANA titer; increasing the cutoff for a positive result to 1:160 markedly reduces the false-positive rate without significantly compromising sensitivity.*)

Tan EM, Chan EK, Sullivan KF, et al. Antinuclear antibodies (ANAs). Clin Immunol Immunopathol 1988;47:121. (*Most comprehensive review of their diagnostic meaning and pathophysiologic significance.*)

Tan EM, Cohen AS, Fries JF, et al. The 1982 revised criteria for the classification of systemic lupus erythematosus. Arthritis Rheum 1982;25:1271. (*The official criteria, although more stringent than those used in practice.*)

147
Evaluation of Back Pain

Back pain is a common complaint in primary care practice and one of the leading causes of disability. Most back pain is caused by musculoligamentous strain, degenerative disk disease, or facet arthritis and responds to symptomatic treatment. Disk disease is often responsible for recurring mild discomfort of the low back and episodes of severe back pain with sciatica. Occasionally, back pain may result from problems originating outside the spinal axis. Serious underlying problems such as tumor, infection, or vertebral compression fracture must be kept in mind. The prevalence of back pain requires that the primary physician be skilled in its assessment and conservative management and knowledgeable about the indications for referral and surgery.

PATHOPHYSIOLOGY AND CLINICAL PRESENTATION

Musculoligamentous Strain. Muscle fibers or distal ligamentous attachments of the paraspinal muscles may tear, usually at the iliac crest or lower lumbar/upper sacral region. Resultant bleeding and spasm cause local swelling and marked tenderness at the site of injury. The patient typically presents after a specific episode of bending, twisting, or lifting. The strain is usually severe and is associated with a feeling of something giving way in the lower back. The onset of pain in the lower lumbar area is immediate. Pain radiates across the low back, often to the buttock and upper thigh posteriorly. Radiation of pain into the lower leg is rare because usually no injury to the nerve roots has occurred.

Lumbar Disk Disease. The pathophysiology of disk disease remains incompletely understood but involves degenerative changes in the disk. It is thought that degeneration and attritional changes in the lower lumbar disks are caused by the concentration of stress at the lumbosacral level. Stresses resulting from the enormous longitudinal and sheer forces that are a consequence of upright posture are aggravated by bending strain. Injury, inflammation, and weakening of the disk annulus may occur and lead to localized back pain. Pain receptors in the longitudinal ligaments probably mediate the recurring attacks of local back pain. Eventually, the disk may become so weakened that it bulges circumferentially beyond the disk interspace. Less often, a focal or asymmetric extension beyond the interspace, termed a disk *protrusion*, develops. Extreme extension of the disk beyond the interspace has been called *extrusion*. Historically, the term *herniation* has been used to describe all these phenomena. It has been suggested that use of the more specific terms will sharpen our understanding of the relationship between disk disease and pain syndromes. Regardless of the vocabulary, compression and irritation of a lower lumbar or upper sacral nerve root may result, and the radicular symptoms of *sciatica* develop.

Sciatica is the symptomatic hallmark of nerve root irritation. Disk protrusion or extrusion is present in 95% of cases. It presents as sharp or burning pain radiating down the posterior or lateral aspect of the leg to the ankle or foot (depending on the specific nerve root involved). The pain may be worsened by cough, Valsalva's maneuver, or sneezing and is often accompanied by paresthesias and numbness. Weakness may also develop in the areas supplied by the irritated nerve root.

More than 95% of disk protrusions and extrusions occur at the L4-5 or L5-S1 level, with the L-5 and S-1 nerve roots affected, respectively. With S-1 root irritation, pain, numbness, and paresthesias involve the buttock, posterior thigh, calf, lateral aspect of the ankle and foot, and lateral toes. Calf atrophy can occur, the ankle jerk can be diminished or absent, and plantar flexion weakness may be noted. With L-5 root compression, pain radiates to the dorsum of the foot and great toe, and the only neurologic deficits may be extensor weakness of the great toe and numbness of the L-5 area on the dorsum of the foot at the base of the great toe (Fig. 147.1). In the rarer instance of high lumbar disk disease, pain radiates to the anterior thigh, and the knee jerk may be diminished or absent. Quadriceps atrophy and weakness may be found.

With lower lumbar disk disease, especially disk extrusion, lumbar paraspinal muscle spasm often occurs and limits lumbar motions. A list away from the side of the disk extrusion, so-called sciatic scoliosis, may develop, and often tenderness of the lower lumbar spine and sciatic notch is present. *Straight leg raising (SLR)* on the affected side is limited by back and leg pain that increases on ankle dorsiflexion at the extreme of SLR. With upper lumbar disk disease, reverse SLR often reproduces the back and anterior thigh pain (see later discussion).

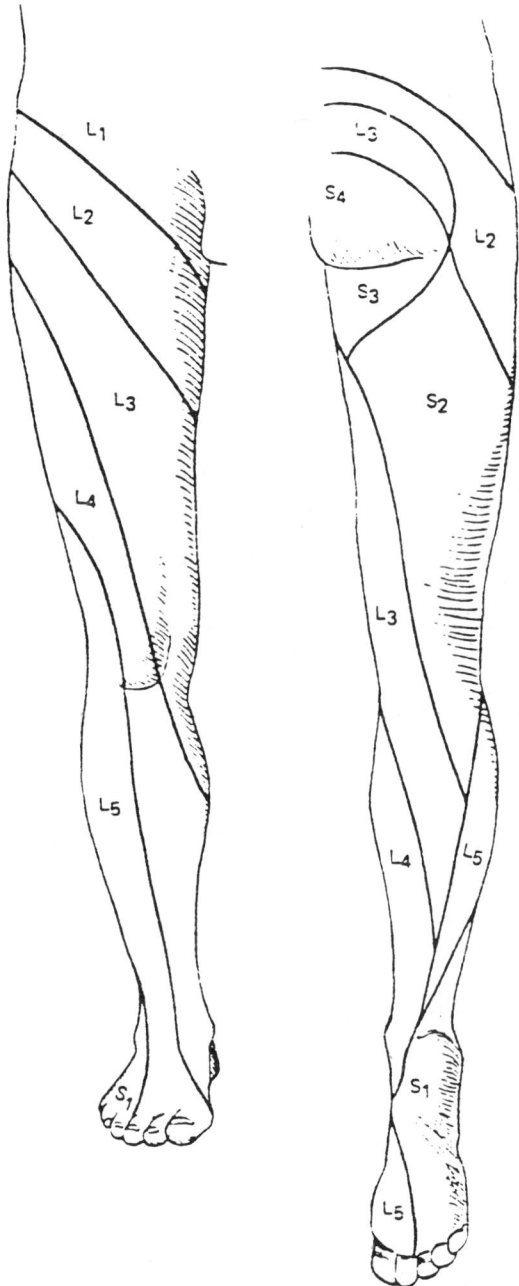

FIG. 147.1. Dermatomes of the lower extremity. (From Finneson BE. Low back pain. Philadelphia: JB Lippincott Co, 1973, with permission.)

The clinical course may begin with a several-year history of recurring mild mid-low back pain related to minor back strain, with symptoms clearing spontaneously within a few days. Attacks typically increase in frequency and severity at intervals of several months to several years. Finally, an episode of persistent pain accompanied by sciatica develops, often triggered by a seemingly trivial stress (e.g., bending over in the shower to pick up the soap).

Spinal Stenosis has become better appreciated as an important cause of chronic low back and lower extremity complaints. It occurs predominantly in elderly individuals with os-teoarthritic spurring, chronic disk degeneration, and facet joint arthritis. Spinal stenosis is also found in young people who have a congenitally narrowed lumbar spinal canal. In either case, the changes narrow the canal and the neuroforamina, leading to root impingement and pain.

The characteristic symptom is pain that is worsened by standing, walking, or other activities that cause spinal extension and is relieved by rest, especially by sitting or lying down and flexing the spine and hips. Patients report pain in the low back, gluteal region, or lower extremities; often, it is bilateral. Numbness or weakness may accompany the pain in the legs. Because symptoms are often worsened by walking and relieved by sitting down and resting, they can mimic vascular insufficiency and are sometimes referred to as *pseudoclaudication.*

On examination, the spine demonstrates good range of motion and little focal tenderness. SLR is usually normal. Minor neurologic deficits (e.g., a diminished ankle jerk) may be present, but no pattern is characteristic.

Spondylolisthesis denotes forward subluxation of a vertebral body. In adults, the condition results from degenerative changes and arthritis of the facet joints, usually at L4-5 or L5-S1, with forward slippage of 10% to 20% of the diameter of the vertebral body. About 70% of patients with spondylolisthesis have chronic low back pain; sciatica is infrequent. The pain is caused by strain imposed on the ligaments and intervertebral joints.

Vertebral Compression Fracture. In normal bone, this fracture requires severe flexion–compression force. It is acutely painful. Spontaneous vertebral body collapse, or pathologic fracture, is most commonly seen in elderly persons with severe osteoporosis (see Chapter 164), in patients taking long-term glucocorticoids (see Chapter 105), and in cancer patients with lytic bony metastases. Usually, the history is one of sudden back pain brought on by a minor stress. The discomfort is noted at the level of fracture, with local radiation across the back and around the trunk, but rarely into the lower extremities. The fracture is more likely to occur in the middle or lower levels of the dorsal spine, which helps differentiate the problem from lumbar disk herniations, 95% of which occur at the level of the L-4 or L-5 disk.

Neoplasms. The most common spinal tumor is *metastatic carcinoma,* which often presents with waist-level or midback pain of insidious onset, gradually increasing in severity and aggravated by activity. About 80% of patients are older than 50 years of age. Although only 30% give a history of previous cancer, in those that do, the probability of spinal metastasis is high. Approximately 90% report night pain and pain unrelieved by lying down or bed rest. A history of prior malignancy and insidious increase in midback pain that is not relieved by lying down is highly predictive of metastatic tumor.

Breast, lung, prostate, gastrointestinal, and genitourinary neoplasms often metastasize to the spine. Purely lytic lesions, which are often caused by renal or thyroid carcinoma, are seen occasionally. The disk spaces are spared. Disk space height is usually maintained, although collapse of the vertebral body as a result of destruction and weakening of bone is common. *Myeloma* is the most common primary bone tumor involving the spine. Early in its course, the tumor may be difficult to differentiate from compression fracture if osteoporosis is present.

Intraspinal tumors may present in the same manner as herniated disks. However, marked progression of neurologic deficits despite adequate conservative therapy is a clue to the existence of a tumor inside the spinal canal. *Extraspinal tumors* may eventually cause root impingement and simulate diskogenic sciatica. Tumors of the retroperitoneum, pelvis, and large bowel may extend to the roots. This is a very late development; metastases may occur earlier.

Infection. Back pain resulting from infection is rare but important to detect. An identifiable source is found in 40% of cases; possibilities include urinary tract infection, skin abscess, indwelling catheter, and IV drug abuse. *Vertebral osteomyelitis* is usually hematogenous in origin but may occasionally result from a spinal procedure, such as lumbar puncture, myelography, diskography, or disk surgery. It extends into the disk space in addition to affecting the vertebral bodies. Dull, continuous back pain is the usual presentation, often in conjunction with low-grade fever and spasm over the paraspinous muscles. Tenderness to percussion over the involved vertebrae is common, but fever is absent in up to half of cases. A compression fracture or an epidural abscess may ensue.

Epidural abscess develops in the context of bacteremia or osteomyelitis. The infection presents as back pain, focal tenderness, and fever. Fever and spinal tenderness are present in about 85% of cases. If the condition is not promptly treated, it may extend to compromise the local blood supply to the spinal cord and rapidly progress from spinal ache to major motor and sensory deficits within hours to a few days.

Ankylosing Spondylitis. This seronegative spondyloarthropathy has both peripheral and axial skeleton manifestations (see also Chapter 146). Spinal involvement is most prominent in young men. Morning spinal stiffness, symptomatic improvement with exercise, gradual onset, and persistence of pain for more than 3 months are characteristic but relatively nonspecific features. The mechanism of disease is unknown, but the incidence of HLA-B27 positivity is high, suggesting an immune pathophysiology. Some patients have a history of inflammatory bowel disease. Early clinical findings include morning back stiffness and diminished chest expansion. Spinal radiographic findings are often unremarkable in the early phases, but films of the sacroiliac joints may show narrowing of the joint space and reactive sclerosis ("sacroiliitis"). Eventually, the sacroiliac joint space becomes obliterated, and fusion follows. Squaring of the vertebral bodies is the first spinal radiologic manifestation, followed by the development of syndesmophytes. Similar although less florid changes may occur in the other seronegative spondyloarthropathies (see Chapter 146).

Psychogenic Disease. Patients with *depression* may present complaining of chronic low back pain. Often, they have a history of previous back problems or onset at the time of a minor injury, with the depression amplifying the presentation and prolonging the clinical course. Mild muscle spasm may be noted on physical examination. Characteristically, the intensity of the symptoms and degree of disability are much greater than the minor limitations found on examination would suggest. Multiple somatic symptoms are common (see Chapter 227).

Other patients may have an underlying *somatization* disorder. Many of these patients appear refractory to therapy and are often unwilling to take an active role in their own treatment. Some even seem to derive a sense of legitimacy and self-worth from their suffering (see Chapter 230).

Malingering implies conscious deception for the sake of obtaining gain from being ill. Inconsistencies among symptoms and physical findings typify the malingerer. These often can be brought out by distracting the patient.

Cauda Equina Syndrome. Although the spinal cord ends at the L-1 level, the collection of nerve roots that make up the cauda equina are subject to injury by any process that compromises the spinal canal below the L-1 level. Massive midline disk herniation is the most common cause of cauda compression and a serious, although very infrequent, event that requires prompt attention. In contrast to the clinical presentation of simple root impingement, the presentation in cauda equina syndrome includes urinary retention in almost 90% of cases. Another characteristic feature is "saddle anesthesia" (reduction in sensation over the buttocks, upper posterior thighs, and perineum), reported by about 75% of patients. Both of these clinical findings are a consequence of sacral root compression, as is a decrease in anal sphincter tone, noted in about two thirds of cases. Sciatica and lower extremity motor and sensory deficits are prominent and often bilateral. Patients may report falling.

DIFFERENTIAL DIAGNOSIS

The differential diagnosis of back pain can be considered in terms of whether or not root pain is present (Table 147.1).

In primary care practice, about 85% of patients with back pain have musculoligamentous injury or degenerative change. Up to 5% have symptomatic disk protrusion or extrusion, with about half of these coming to surgery; 4% have compression fracture, 3% have spondylolisthesis, and another 1.5% have either tumor, infection, or ankylosing spondylitis. The prevalence of spinal stenosis remains unknown. Bulging disks at at least one level have been found on magnetic resonance imaging in half, and disk protrusions in 30%, of asymptomatic persons. Disk extrusions are much less common, occurring in only 1%.

Table 147.1. Important Causes of Back Pain

Conditions Commonly Presenting with Sciatica
Disk herniation
Spinal stenosis
Compression fracture
Epidural abscess
Vertebral osteomyelitis (late)
Compression fracture
Intraspinal tumor
Spinal metastasis
Spondylolisthesis (occasionally)

Conditions Usually Presenting without Sciatica
Musculoligamentous strain
Ankylosing spondylitis
Spondylolisthesis
Depression
Vertebral osteomyelitis (early)
Epidural abscess (very early)
Retroperitoneal neoplasm

WORKUP

Even with the advent of sophisticated spinal imaging techniques, the history and physical examination remain critical to the effective evaluation and management of back pain. The findings elicited are often diagnostic, and even if they are not, they can help guide test selection and ensure timely referral. Overreliance on imaging studies often results in false-positive diagnoses.

History

In elucidating the basic features of back pain (i.e., quality, location, onset, radiation), one should also inquire specifically into symptoms potentially indicative of serious underlying disease (e.g., fever, progressive neurologic deficits, bilateral deficits, bladder dysfunction, saddle anesthesia, persistent pain unresponsive to bed rest). A history of recent injury and a prior history of cancer are other critical elements to be noted, as are previous therapy for back problems, recent lumbar puncture, concurrent infection, and prolonged use of high-dose corticosteroids.

The presence of sciatica helps narrow the differential diagnosis (Table 147.1).

Aggravating and alleviating factors may have diagnostic meaning. Morning stiffness in the back that is relieved by activity suggests ankylosing spondylitis or other inflammatory conditions. Worsening or onset of symptoms with standing or walking and relief with bending or sitting is characteristic of spinal stenosis, whereas worsening with sitting, driving, or lifting points to lumbar disk herniation.

The patient should be asked to describe the impact of the back pain on daily activities. Emotional and social stressors are sought if severity and duration of the symptoms appear disproportionate for the amount of organic disease present. Under such circumstances, it is important to check for depression (see Chapter 227) and manifestations of somatization disorder (see Chapter 230).

Physical Examination

Before examining the back, one should check the abdomen, rectum, groin, pelvis, and peripheral pulses for conditions that might mimic the symptoms of spinal disease. In addition, one looks for fever, skin abscess, breast mass, pleural effusion, prostate nodule, lymphadenopathy, joint inflammation, and other signs of systemic or malignant disease that may affect the spine. Thigh and calf circumferences are measured to detect evidence of atrophy, and joint motions of the lower extremities are tested.

Back Examination begins with the patient standing and the back uncovered. One checks for any abnormalities in symmetry, muscle bulk, posture, and spinal curvature. Flexibility is assessed, with any muscle spasm or spinal segments that do not move freely noted. A description of what limits back motion is more important than an estimation of degrees of motion, which is imprecise at best. The spine is palpated for focal tenderness suggestive of tumor, infection, fracture, or disk herniation. Sensitivity of the lower lumbar spine and sciatic notch is usually found with lower lumbar disk problems. Sacroiliac tenderness to deep palpation is sometimes present in ankylosing spondylitis, but the finding is nonspecific.

Straight Leg Raising (SLR) Test is an important component of the assessment for disk disease. The maneuver serves as a sensitive indicator of lower lumbar disk herniation, particularly in patients with sciatica. SLR testing is based on the observation that an L-5 or S-1 nerve root tethered by a herniated disk causes radicular pain if stretched. In the presence of a severely herniated disk, the additional root stretching causes impingement and pain, especially with an L5-S1 disk injury.

Straight leg raising is performed in the supine position with passive lifting of the patient's leg at the heel while the knee is kept fully extended. The test is performed both on the side of the reported sciatica (*"ipsilateral" SLR testing*) and on the opposite side (*"contralateral"* or *"crossed" SLR testing*). A test result is positive if the sciatica is reproduced as the leg is elevated between 30 and 70 degrees. Reproduction of the sciatica should not be confused with hamstring muscle tightness, which can also cause discomfort on SLR, especially as elevation approaches 90 degrees. (Elevation beyond 80 degrees exerts little additional stretch on the nerve root and is not of much meaning.) If severe pain is reported on elevation and resistance occurs, yet the leg can be raised another 20 or 30 degrees when the patient is distracted, the test result is "negative" and other causes of the pain should be sought, such as hamstring muscle tightness. Dorsiflexion of the ankle at the extreme of SLR may exacerbate the pain of disk herniation on SLR testing and is particularly useful if the SLR test result is equivocal.

The earlier the onset of pain during the test, the more specific the result and the greater the degree of disk herniation. Test sensitivity averages 80% for ipsilateral SLR; specificity is low (about 40%). The specificity of a positive contralateral SLR test result is considerably higher (75%), but the sensitivity is only 25%. A large disk herniation with an extruded fragment is an important cause of a positive contralateral SLR result.

Much less L-4 and minimal L-2 or L-3 movement occurs during SLR testing, so that it is less useful to detect disk herniation above L4-5. Femoral nerve sensitivity is usually present with higher lumbar (L-2, L-3, or L-4) root irritation. Flexing the knee with the patient lying in a prone position may reproduce the back and anterior thigh pain of upper lumbar disk herniation.

Neurologic Examination is most efficiently performed by concentrating on the areas of compromise suggested by the history. The patient with sciatica is most likely to have deficits in the territory of the L-5 and S-1 roots and should be tested accordingly. The person with back pain radiating to the anterior thigh and associated quadriceps weakness should be tested for L-4 function. A history of urinary retention requires a check of sacral root motor and sensory function.

Tests for *S-1 root* function (L5-S1 disk) include tiptoe walking, plantar flexion against resistance, ankle deep tendon reflexes, and lateral foot sensation. Loss of plantar flexion occurs only with severe disk herniation (low sensitivity, high specificity). Tests for *L-5 root* function (L4-L5 disk) include heel walking (an imprecise test), dorsiflexion of the ankle and big toe against resistance, and sensation on the anterior medial dorsal foot (Fig. 147.1). For a suspected upper lumbar disk lesion (*L-4 root*), one notes the knee deep tendon reflexes, quadriceps strength, and sensation about the medial ankle.

The sensitivity of any single neurologic test for the diagnosis of lumbar disk protrusion or extrusion is no greater than 50%, but it can be enhanced to almost 90% when clusters of findings are considered. The most accurate assessment of sensory function is attained by pinprick testing, most efficiently performed by limiting the examination to a few key distal dermatomal areas in the feet (Fig. 147.1) and noting any asymmetry of response. Responses in patients with psychological stress to neurologic testing and spinal examination may appear neuroanatomically inappropriate, but often they are diagnostically meaningful. Disturbances in strength or sensation that do not correspond to nerve root innervation patterns, inconsistency of responses to maneuvers, overreaction to palpation or passive movement, superficial or widespread tenderness, and pain on sham testing of spinal rotation (arms kept at sides while hips are rotated) are among the characteristic responses. The presence of three or more of these responses suggests considerable psychological overlay to the patient's back pain.

Laboratory Studies

For the majority of patients with low back pain, a careful history and physical examination usually suffice for diagnosis at the time of the initial office visit. The utility of imaging studies is limited to a few specific situations, many of which are also indications for referral or consultation (see later discussion).

Lumbosacral Spine Films. In most instances, the routine ordering of plain lumbosacral spine films in patients presenting with back pain is low in yield and neither cost-effective nor useful for decision making. The finding of normal disk spaces does not rule out disk herniation, and the finding of a narrowed disk space does not distinguish between disk rupture and asymptomatic degeneration. The presence of osteophytes extending from the vertebral bodies indicates little more than long-existing disk degeneration and attempts at repair.

Nonetheless, early radiography of the back is indicated in some situations, as when the physician suspects (a) malignancy (patient older than 50 years, focal persistent bone pain unrelieved by bed rest, history of malignancy); (b) compression fracture (prolonged corticosteroid therapy, postmenopausal woman, severe trauma, focal tenderness); (c) ankylosing spondylitis (young male patient, limited spinal motion, sacroiliac pain); (d) chronic osteomyelitis (low-grade fever, high sedimentation rate, focal tenderness); (e) major trauma; and (f) major neurologic deficits. Back pain localized to the high lumbar or thoracic region is also an indication for prompt spinal radiography because compression fracture and metastatic tumor are common in these areas. Plain films may be needed for patients seeking compensation for back pain and for those who desire reassurance, but they are of little use in early osteomyelitis (in which bony changes take 10 to 14 days to appear).

Computed Tomography and Magnetic Resonance Imaging. If severe symptoms persist for several weeks despite conservative therapy and disk herniation or other surgically correctable disease is suspected, then computed tomography (CT) or magnetic resonance imaging (MRI) may be useful. These are both very sensitive tests for the detection of lumbar disk disease or spinal stenosis and can provide anatomic detail of some surgical value. The cost of CT of the lumbosacral spine is less than the cost of MRI, but CT involves radiation exposure and does not provide the visualization of the entire spine or upper vertebrae that MRI does (desirable features if the differential diagnosis includes intraspinal tumor and disk herniation at an upper level). Besides being costly, MRI often triggers a claustrophobic response, but no radiation exposure is involved. MRI is the best available test to detect early osteomyelitis and is also the noninvasive test of choice for spinal cord tumors, epidural abscess, and cord compression. In many instances, it obviates the need for myelography. CT provides excellent bony detail and shows changes in vertebral bodies caused by tumor and infection. MRI may reveal such pathologic findings even earlier than CT because it can detect marrow changes, which precede bony changes.

MRI and CT should be limited to patients who are either sufficiently symptomatic that surgical intervention must be considered or are suspected of having serious systemic disease. The high sensitivity of these tests for disk disease can produce misleading results unless the patient and clinician are aware that disk bulges and protrusions are extremely common (50% and 30%, respectively) in asymptomatic people.

Myelography has been largely replaced by MRI. It is best performed in conjunction with CT on patients with progressive neurologic deficits, especially those with findings suggestive of injury to the spinal cord (e.g., loss of sphincter control, bilateral numbness and weakness). The temptation to perform myelography in the patient with chronic refractory pain is strong, but the test should be reserved for patients with objective findings that are amenable to surgery or radiation therapy.

Radionuclide Scanning. The moderately high sensitivity of the technetium bone scan for osteomyelitis and metastatic disease and its wide availability make it a reasonable consideration for the patient presenting with any combination of fever, weight loss, persistent back pain, history of malignancy, concurrent infection, and markedly elevated sedimentation rate. Gallium scanning is sometimes useful in defining soft-tissue involvement by infection or abscess formation.

Immunoelectrophoresis of serum and urine samples diagnoses most cases of myeloma; crude screening with a complete blood cell count and determination of the erythrocyte sedimentation rate and serum globulin level is probably sufficient if clinical suspicion is not high. A diagnosis of myeloma must be suspected if back pain in an older person is accompanied by unexplained anemia and a very high sedimentation rate. However, such findings are quite nonspecific and may also be caused by a chronic inflammatory process.

Electromyography may be needed to document peripheral nerve deficits and help select patients who require myelography.

SYMPTOMATIC MANAGEMENT AND PATIENT EDUCATION

Acute Back Pain

Acute musculoligamentous strain, degenerative disk disease, and lumbar disk disease with or without sciatica are best managed conservatively. Bed rest was formerly a mainstay of treatment, but randomized trials have demonstrated that recovery is more rapid in patients who continue their ordinary activities within the limits permitted by pain than in those who go to bed.

Some patients are severely incapacitated by pain at rest as well as with movement. The acute discomfort usually persists for at least several days. Symptomatic measures consist of local application of heat or warm baths and the use of mild analgesics. Antiinflammatory agents have been shown to be effective in randomized trials and are preferred over narcotics for all but the first night or two of symptoms. Most so-called muscle relaxants are actually minor tranquilizers; they have little direct effect on muscles but can be of help to the patient who cannot sleep. The patient in pain should be advised to experiment to find the most comfortable position in bed. Lying supine with pillows behind the knees and a low pillow for the head usually suffices. Lying on one's side with the hips and knees flexed is sometimes quite comfortable; lying prone is usually not.

Even for patients with continuing pain and evidence of disk protrusion or extrusion, there is little evidence to support prolonged bed rest. Deconditioning with bed rest can contribute to physical and psychological morbidity.

Activity Prescription. For patients with disk protrusion or extrusion, a major goal is to avoid prolonged inactivity and the deconditioning that accompanies it. A reasonable activity program during the first week consists of walking for about 20 minutes three times a day, interspersed with several hours of bed rest. After the spine has healed sufficiently to allow sitting without pain, the patient can ease into a program of endurance exercises that may help prevent future back problems (see later discussion).

A reasonable program of back care should be discussed after recovery from acute symptoms allows gradual mobilization and resumption of normal activities. The patient must understand that pain is a normal protective response to injury or inflammation. Discomfort should be used as a guideline to determine the pace at which to increase activity. However, minor discomfort, stiffness, soreness, or mild aching should not interfere with progressive mobilization.

If symptoms recur or marked pain develops in relation to a specific activity or level of activity, the patient should temporarily limit activity for several days. If the patient undertakes a new or higher level of activity and pain increases within 24 hours, the activity should be halved each day until a tolerable level is reached and then gradually increased. The patient should be encouraged to progress as rapidly as symptoms permit.

Exercises and Back Care. Proper back care should become a way of life for the patient, even though acute symptoms subside with rest. The patient is advised to avoid activities that cause pain, and also potentially injurious actions such as repetitive bending, heavy lifting, and shoveling snow. Increasing evidence suggests that physical therapy programs designed to improve muscle strength and flexibility are effective, helping to maintain good posture and reduce the chances of recurrent injury. Instruction sheets are often useful to supplement instruction in the office (Figs. 147.2 and 147.3). Controlled trials have failed to confirm any benefit from the use of traction or braces in patients with disk herniation. In fact, it is of concern that re-

striction of movement may promote muscle weakness. A program of mild daily exercise with more vigorous endurance exercise two to three times a week is also encouraged and appears more useful than traditional isometric exercises. Brisk walking for 20 minutes once or twice a day, supplemented by swimming twice weekly for up to 30 minutes, fulfills such an exercise requirement. Stationary bicycling or jogging can be substituted for swimming.

Spinal Manipulation by chiropractors and osteopaths may be the most common treatment for back pain. Overviews of trials suggest that such treatment may be some benefit in acute back pain. The safety of spinal manipulation in the setting of root compression, either by disk protrusion or extrusion or spinal stenosis, is not established. Most physicians advise patients with evidence of disk root impingement to avoid spinal manipulation therapy. A randomized trial comparing physical therapy, chiropractic manipulation, and an educational booklet for patients with acute back pain found no clinically significant differences in relief of back pain. Patients seen by either a physical therapist or chiropractor were more satisfied with their care. There is no evidence to suggest that manipulation is effective in the treatment of chronic back pain.

Persistent Pain or Worsening Neurologic Deficits

Patients with evidence of lumbar disk herniation who experience (a) persistent disabling root pain despite 4 to 6 weeks of comprehensive conservative therapy, (b) progressive neurologic deficits in the lower extremities, or (c) disruption of bowel or bladder control are strong candidates for surgery. *Disk excision (diskectomy)* by open surgery is mandatory and urgent for patients with massive disk herniation causing a cauda equina syndrome. It is also indicated in cases of major progressive neurologic deficit, calcified disk, extruded disk fragments that are not in continuity with the disk space, or pain caused primarily by bony abnormalities rather than by disk herniation. Relative indications for surgery include chronic disabling low back pain that persists after resolution of more acute symptoms, and frequent acute recurrences of severe back pain that the patient cannot prevent by following a careful program of back care.

Chymopapain disk injection is an option for patients who do not require an open procedure, although it is not indicated for backache alone. This naturally occurring enzyme acts to solubilize the nucleus pulposus, and in doing so, it decreases nerve root pressure with an effect very much like that of surgical disk excision. Hazards include possible nerve damage from the technique of lateral needle placement, diskitis, infection, and, in 1% to 2% of cases, an anaphylactic response. The incidence of complications is very low, and the drug is thought to be quite safe overall. However, many patients still experience back spasm and pain for several weeks after the treatment, so that the recovery period is about the same as that for surgery. Although enthusiasm for the procedure has waned, in experienced hands it still represents a less invasive means of treating disablingly painful disk herniation.

Some patients seek treatment from chiropractors, acupuncturists, and other paramedical practitioners. In a double-blinded, controlled study, *acupuncture* proved no better than placebo for the treatment of chronic back pain. No controlled studies of *chiropractic manipulation* for chronic back pain have

How to get along with your back

Sitting: Use a hard chair and put your spine up against it; try and keep one or both knees higher than your hips. A small stool is helpful here. For short rest periods, a contour chair offers excellent support.

Standing: Try to stand with your lower back flat. When you work standing up, use a footrest to help relieve swayback. Never lean forward without bending your knees. Ladies take note: shoes with moderate heels strain the back less than those with high heels. Avoid platform shoes.

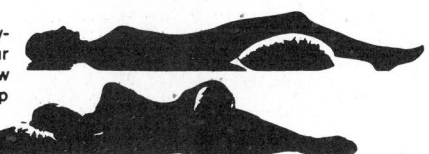

Sleeping: Sleep on a firm mattress; put a bedboard (³/₄″ plywood) under a soft mattress. Do not sleep on your stomach. If you sleep on your back, put a pillow under your knees. If you sleep on your side keep your legs bent at the knees and at the hips.

Driving: Get a hard seat for your automobile and sit close enough to the wheel while driving so that your legs are not fully extended when you work the pedals.

Lifting: Make sure you lift properly. Bend your knees and use your leg muscles to lift. Avoid sudden movements. Keep the load close to your body, and try not to lift anything heavy higher than your waist.

Working: Don't overwork yourself. If you can, change from one job to another before you feel fatigued. If you work at a desk all day, get up and move around whenever you get the chance.

Exercise: Get regular exercise (walking, swimming, etc.) once your backache is gone. But start slowly to give your muscles a chance to warm up and loosen before attempting anything strenuous.

See your doctor: If your back acts up, see your doctor; don't wait until your condition gets severe.

FIG. 147.2. Sample instruction sheet describing care of the back. (Courtesy of McNeil Laboratories, Fort Washington, PA.)

been performed. *Injection of facet joints* with corticosteroids has been used in some patients with chronic back pain, under the presumption that a component of facet joint arthritis might be contributing to the pain. Controlled trials have shown it to be no better than placebo. The findings are similar for epidural injection to treat sciatica caused by a herniated nucleus pulposus. Despite initially enthusiastic reports, a controlled study also found *transcutaneous electrical nerve stimulation* (TENS) to be ineffective.

Chronic Refractory Back Pain in the Absence of Anatomic Deficits

Patients with chronic refractory back pain and no clear anatomic deficits pose one of the most difficult long-term man-

agement problems encountered in primary care practice. Persistence of symptoms may be encouraged by social factors such as *pending litigation* or *application for disability*. At other times, the patient's amplification of symptoms and refractoriness to treatment may be manifestations of an underlying *depression* or *somatization disorder* (see Chapters 227 and 230).

There are no simple solutions to the management of these patients. Many patients do not take an active role in their own treatment and frustrate the well-intentioned efforts of physicians while they continue to complain of discomfort. However, some important objectives can be achieved: identification and treatment of underlying psychopathology; avoidance of inappropriate tests, addictive medications, ineffective therapies, and unnecessary surgery; and preservation of the patient's capacity to function independently.

Exercises for low back pain

General Information:

Don't overdo exercising, especially in the beginning. Start by trying the movements slowly and carefully. Don't be alarmed if the exercises cause some mild discomfort which lasts a few minutes. But if pain is more than mild and lasts more than 15 or 20 minutes, *stop* and do no further exercises until you see your doctor.

Do the exercises on a hard surface covered with a thin mat or heavy blanket. Put a pillow under your neck if it makes you more comfortable. Always start your exercises slowly— and in the order marked—to allow muscles to loosen up gradually. Heat treatments just before you start can help relax tight muscles. Follow the instructions carefully; it will be well worth the effort.

Do exercises marked (X)

in numerical order

for _____ minutes

_____ times a day.

Take the medication

prescribed for you

_____ times daily

for_____ .

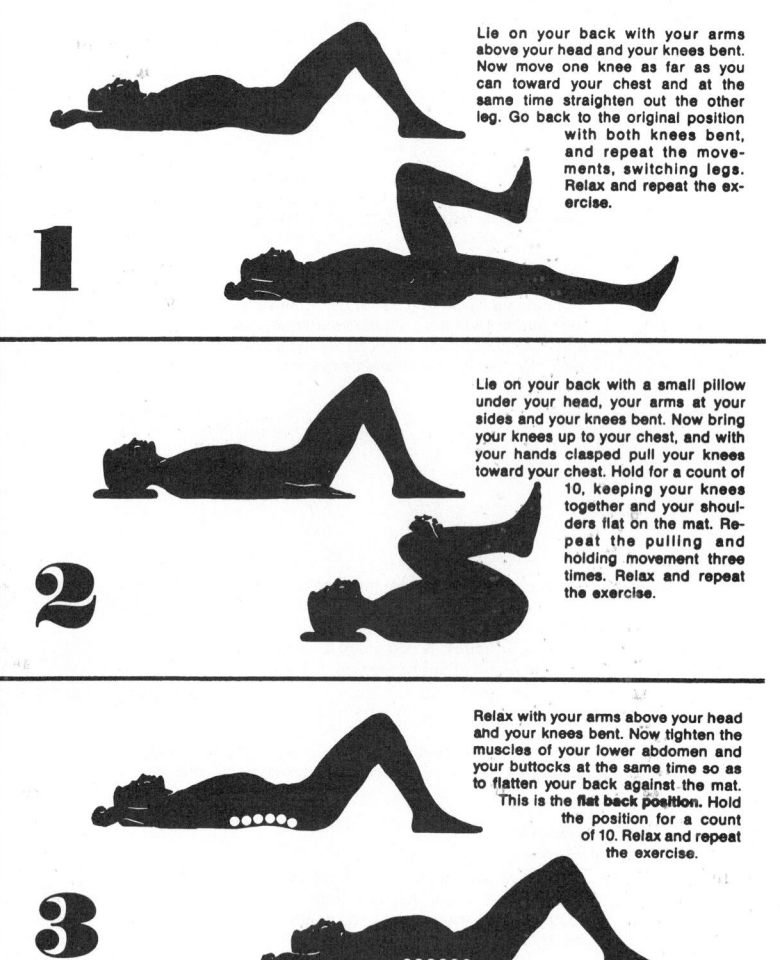

1 Lie on your back with your arms above your head and your knees bent. Now move one knee as far as you can toward your chest and at the same time straighten out the other leg. Go back to the original position with both knees bent, and repeat the movements, switching legs. Relax and repeat the exercise.

2 Lie on your back with a small pillow under your head, your arms at your sides and your knees bent. Now bring your knees up to your chest, and with your hands clasped pull your knees toward your chest. Hold for a count of 10, keeping your knees together and your shoulders flat on the mat. Repeat the pulling and holding movement three times. Relax and repeat the exercise.

3 Relax with your arms above your head and your knees bent. Now tighten the muscles of your lower abdomen and your buttocks at the same time so as to flatten your back against the mat. This is the flat back position. Hold the position for a count of 10. Relax and repeat the exercise.

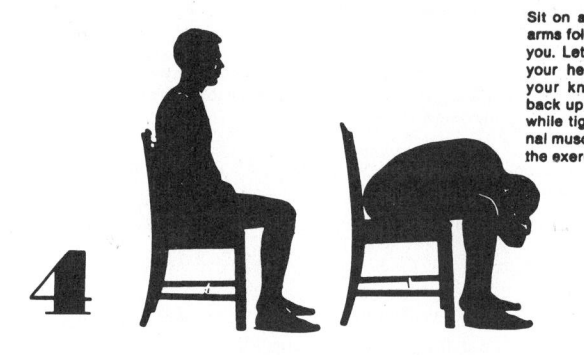

4 Sit on a hard chair with your arms folded loosely in front of you. Let your body drop until your head is down between your knees. Pull your body back up into a sitting position while tightening your abdominal muscles. Relax and repeat the exercise.

FIG. 147.3. Sample instruction sheet describing exercises for low back pain. (Courtesy of McNeil Laboratories, Fort Washington, PA.)

Addressing Underlying Psychopathology and Social Factors. If depression is encountered, it should be treated (see Chapter 227) regardless of whether it is the cause or result of the patient's condition. For the person with a suspected somatization disorder, therapeutic efforts are best directed at helping the patient to find ways other than suffering to achieve a sense of self-worth. Attempts to "cure" such persons physically actually remove their one source (albeit maladaptive) of personal value. Such efforts are bound to be sabotaged by patients unless they find something to replace their back pain (see Chapter 230). Patients with pending legal matters should be strongly encouraged to settle them as quickly as possible. If a disability determination is needed, it should be expedited. Arranging an independent evaluation may be best. This avoids jeopardizing the patient–doctor relationship, particularly if the physician does not feel comfortable certifying that the patient is physically disabled.

Protecting the Patient from Unnecessary Procedures and Narcotics. Patients with chronic refractory back pain are at considerable risk for invasive testing (e.g., myelography) and surgery, even though they may lack symptoms and signs that are considered proper indications for such procedures. The primary physician needs to protect such patients from unnecessary and potentially harmful interventions. One way to accomplish this objective is to arrange a consultation for the patient with an orthopedic surgeon or a neurosurgeon experienced in back problems, so that the patient does not feel the need to "shop around" for a willing surgeon.

Avoiding prolonged or repeated reliance on narcotics for pain control is a key management priority. A patient may repeatedly demand strong analgesic agents, but unless an acute and reversible cause of the pain is found, the use of narcotics should be avoided if at all possible. An assessment for substance abuse should be considered when a patient with back pain persistently requests narcotics (see Chapter 235).

Preserving Capacity to Function Independently. Establishing a strong doctor–patient alliance (see Chapter 1) and attending to underlying psychosocial issues are prerequisites to engaging the patient in a program of self-help. The caring, concern, and responsiveness that characterize a strong relationship help foster patient confidence and receptiveness. Even though symptoms may not disappear, it is often possible to keep the patient functioning independently through cultivation of the relationship and promulgation of a program of activity and exercise. Arranging regularly scheduled visits at intervals meaningful to the patient facilitates the sense of support and can forestall many anxious phone calls and unannounced office appearances.

PATIENT EDUCATION

The importance of patient education cannot be overemphasized for the person with back pain. Surveys of patients with back pain find that a lack of information is the greatest source of dissatisfaction with care. Patients suffering from a condition that suddenly disables them are extremely anxious and in need of detailed information about what has happened, what can be done, and what lies ahead. Even if the diagnosis has not been established, a review of the working differential helps one deal with the uncertainty of the situation. The use of a model of the spine greatly simplifies explanation and helps many patients better understand their condition. Patients with disk herniation can be reassured that the natural history of their condition is generally favorable, with most responding well to conservative therapy and very few suffering prolonged physical disability. Active patients are greatly relieved to know that jogging, stationary cycling, and swimming are not only possible but often desirable, and that reemergence of mild to moderate discomfort with resumption of activity is to be expected and is not a worrisome prognostic sign. At the same time, it is important to review with the patient the symptoms of serious neurologic injury that would necessitate prompt reporting and hospital admission. The rationale and anatomic basis for back hygiene measures and exercises also need to be reviewed to ensure compliance and proper implementation. A good outcome is greatly facilitated by keeping the patient well informed.

INDICATIONS FOR ADMISSION AND REFERRAL

Patients with rapidly progressive neurologic deficits require prompt neurologic and surgical consultations. Urgent admission and referral are indicated if symptoms suggestive of cauda equina syndrome or cord compression develop (e.g., new bilateral neurologic deficits, urinary retention, sphincter incontinence, saddle anesthesia). The same is true for patients with acute vertebral collapse because spinal stability may be compromised by the fracture. Suspicion of osteomyelitis or epidural abscess is an indication for immediate hospitalization and infectious disease consultation. Particularly in patients with epidural abscess, treatment must be initiated early to be effective.

If back pain remains severe and intractable after 4 to 6 weeks of conservative therapy, or if an important neurologic deficit develops (e.g., foot drop, gastrocnemius–soleus or quadriceps weakness), then further evaluation and consideration of surgery are indicated and referral to an orthopedist or neurosurgeon with a particular interest in back problems can be helpful. Even if the patient does not have sciatica or neurologic deficits and is therefore not a candidate for surgery, the referral can serve to reassure the patient that a surgically correctable lesion is not being overlooked and that the efforts of the primary physician are appropriate.

A.G.M.

ANNOTATED BIBLIOGRAPHY

Atlas SJ, Deyo RA, Keller RB, et al. The Maine Lumbar Spine Study, Part II. One-year outcome of surgical and nonsurgical management of sciatica. Spine 1996;21:1777. (*Definite improvement in dominant symptoms in 71% of surgical patients and 43% of nonsurgical patients.*)

Atlas SJ, Deyo RA, Keller RB, et al. The Maine Lumbar Spine Study, Part III. One-year outcome of surgical and nonsurgical management of lumbar spinal stenosis. Spine 1996;21:1787. (*Definite improvement in dominant symptoms in 55% of surgical patients and 21% of nonsurgical patients.*)

Baker AS, Ojemann RG, Swartz MN, et al. Spinal epidural abscess. N Engl J Med 1975;293:463. (*An important condition to recognize. The typical progression was from spinal ache to root pain, followed by weakness and paralysis within a few days. Osteomyelitis was the cause of 38% of the abscesses and bacteremia of 26%.*)

Bates DW, Reuler JB. Back pain and epidural spinal cord compression. J Gen Intern Med 1988;3:191. (*Detailed review of this spinal presentation of metastatic disease; 52 references.*)

Carette S, Marcoux S, Truchon R, et al. A controlled trial of corticosteroid injections into facet joints for chronic low back pain. N Engl J Med 1991;325:1002. (*No evidence of benefit found.*)

Carette S, Leclaire R, Marcoux S, et al. Epidural corticosteroid injection for sciatica due to herniated nucleus pulposus. N Engl J Med 1997;336:1634. (*No evidence for significant clinical benefit in this study.*)

Carey TS, Garrett J, Jackman A, et al. The North Carolina Back Pain Project. The outcomes and costs of care for acute low back pain among patients seen by primary care practitioners, chiropractors, and orthopedic surgeons. N Engl J Med 1995;333:913. (*Symptoms diminished rapidly, with fewer than 20% of patients having persistent functional impairment lasting 25 days after the initial visit.*)

Cherkin DC, Deyo RA, Battie M, et al. A comparison of physical therapy, chiropractic manipulation, and provision of an educational booklet for the treatment of patients with low back pain. N Engl J

Med 1998;339:1021. (*No clinically significant differences in outcome among the three groups. However, those seen by either a physical therapist or chiropractor were more satisfied with their care.*)

Deyo RA. Conservative therapy for low back pain. JAMA 1983; 250:1057. (*Reviews 59 therapeutic trials; also useful for its critique of study designs.*)

Deyo RA, Diehl AK, Rosenthal M. How many days of bed rest for acute low back pain? N Engl J Med 1986;315:1064. (*A randomized clinical trial showing that for patients without neuromotor deficits, 2 days of bed rest was as effective as 7 days.*)

Deyo RA, Loeser JD, Bigos SJ. Herniated lumbar intervertebral disk. Ann Intern Med 1990;112:598. (*Terse, critical look at diagnostic and therapeutic modalities; 41 references.*)

Deyo RA, Rainville J, Kent DL. What can the history and physical examination tell us about low back pain? JAMA 1992;268:760. (*Required reading. Article summarizes available data on the diagnostic utility of historical and physical findings; many of its observations and conclusions are cited in this chapter.*)

Deyo RA, Walsh N, Martin D, et al. A controlled trial of transcutaneous electrical nerve stimulation (TENS) and exercise for chronic low back pain. N Engl J Med 1990;322:1627. (*TENS was no better than the control intervention.*)

Edelman RR, Warach S. Magnetic resonance imaging. N Engl J Med 1993;328:708. (*A major review with a useful section on spinal imaging.*)

Hadler NM. Regional back pain. N Engl J Med 1986;315:1090. (*An editorial that provides an overview of the problem and suggests that patients may be the best judge of how long to rest in bed.*)

Hall S, Bartleson JD, Onofrio BM, et al. Lumbar spinal stenosis. Ann Intern Med 1985;103:271. (*Excellent review of this often overlooked cause.*)

Hoffman RH, Wheeler KJ, Deyo RA. Surgery for herniated discs. A literature review. J Gen Intern Med 1993;8:487. (*Finds many shortcomings in study design, but overall impression is that properly selected patients derive some benefit from diskectomy.*)

Javid MJ, Nordby EJ, Ford LT, et al. Safety and efficacy of chymopapain (Chymodiactin) in herniated nucleus pulposus with sciatica. JAMA 1983;249:2489. (*Useful data that help to put the procedure in perspective.*)

Jensen MC, Brant-Zawadzki MN, Obuchowski N, et al. Magnetic resonance imaging of the lumbar spine in people without back pain. N Engl J Med 1994;331:69. (*Among asymptomatic people, 52% had bulges, 27% protrusions, and 1% extrusions.*)

Kostuik JP, Harrington I, Alexander D, et al. Cauda equina syndrome and lumbar disc herniation. J Bone Joint Surg Am 1986;68:386. (*Clinical features of this important syndrome are delineated.*)

Lahad A, Malter AD, Berg AO, et al. The effectiveness of four interventions for the prevention of low back pain. JAMA 1994;272:1286. (*Limited evidence to recommend exercise; insufficient evidence to recommend risk factor modification, mechanical supports, or education.*)

Liang M, Komaroff AL. Roentgenograms in primary-care patients with acute low back pain: a cost-effectiveness study. Arch Intern Med 1982;142:1108. (*Cost is high, yield low if films are ordered on a first visit.*)

Malmivaara A, Hakkinen U, Aro T, et al. The treatment of acute low back pain—bed rest, exercises, or ordinary activity? N Engl J Med 1995;332:351. (*More rapid recovery among those who continued activity than in those treated with bed rest or exercise programs.*)

Mendelson G, Selwood T, Kranz H, et al. Acupuncture treatment of chronic back pain. Am J Med 1983;74:49. (*A double-blinded, placebo-controlled study showing no difference in results.*)

Moffett JK, Torgerson D, Bell-Syer S, et al. Randomised controlled trial of exercise for low back pain: clinical outcomes, costs and preferences. BMJ 1999;319:279. (*Patients with subacute pain who participated in an eight-session exercise program did significantly better, with improvements on the Roland Disability Scale.*)

Shekelle PG, Adamas AH, Chassin MP, et al. Spinal manipulation for low-back pain. Ann Intern Med 1992;117:590. (*A metaanalysis finding short-term value in patients with uncomplicated acute back pain; data insufficient for determining utility in chronic back pain.*)

Volinn E. Between the idea and the reality: research on bed rest for uncomplicated acute low back pain and implications for clinical practice patterns. Clin J Pain 1996;12:166. (*Good review of evidence for shift away from recommending bed rest.*)

Von Korff M, Barlow W, Cherkin D, et al. Effects of practice style in managing back pain. Ann Intern Med 1994;121:187. (*Practice styles consistent with self-care for back pain yielded similar long-term pain and functional outcomes at lower cost.*)

Waddell G, McCulloch JA, Kummel E, et al. Nonorganic physical signs in low back pain. Spine 1980;5:117. (*Describes physical findings, noted in this chapter, suggestive of persons with psychological distress.*)

Weber H. Lumbar disc herniation: a controlled prospective study with 10 years of observation. Spine 1983;8:131. (*The only randomized trial comparing medical and surgical therapy; earlier relief achieved with surgery, but no difference in outcomes after 3 to 4 years.*)

148
Evaluation of Neck Pain

The primary physician is often faced with the patient who complains of a stiff neck; most of the time, the problem is musculoskeletal in origin. Although the majority of musculoskeletal causes are not serious, they can result in considerable discomfort. One should be able to provide symptomatic relief to the person with a minor neck problem and to identify the patient with a serious complication of cervical spine disease, such as root compression or cord injury, that requires surgical attention.

PATHOPHYSIOLOGY AND CLINICAL PRESENTATION

Neck Strain. The most common form of neck pain is caused by *cervical paraspinal muscle spasm*, usually secondary to minor strain or prolonged, unconscious muscle contraction associated with emotional stress. The problem is usually self-limited. Neck pain caused by minor muscle ligament strain is usually self-limited if aggravating activities are avoided. A relapsing clinical course is not uncommon. Muscle spasm also occurs with cervical degenerative disease (see below).

Severe neck strain is seen in *cervical hyperextension* (*"whiplash"*) *injury*, typically sustained in an automobile accident. Sudden hyperextension of the neck followed by flexion results in musculoligamentous strain. Tearing of muscle fibers leads to bleeding, swelling, severe muscle spasm, and pain. Symptoms increase gradually during several hours, often becoming most severe the day following the acute event. The anterior or posterior ligaments of the cervical spine may be disrupted. Neurologic deficits are rare unless a cervical spine fracture is present that leads to root or cord compression. Refractory pain lasting more than 6 months may represent injury to a zygapophyseal joint, although other causes include the psychological stress of ongoing litigation and pending legal proceedings.

Degenerative Disease. Trauma or degenerative changes in the intervertebral disks or joint facets can be a source of neck pain and result in ankylosis or subluxation of the cervical spine, termed *cervical spondylosis*. Immobility and consolidation of the joint may ensue. Usually, the process is localized to the lower cervical levels, such as C4-5, C5-6, or C6-7. Degenerative changes and spurring at the cervical disk spaces are prominent. The condition presents as recurring neck stiffness and mild aching discomfort, with progressive limitation of neck motion over months to years. Lateral rotation and lateral flexion of the neck toward the painful side are limited; pain is precipitated or increased by such motions.

Cervical disk degeneration can lead to narrowing of the neural foramina that causes *root impingement* and pain. Pain radiates in the distribution of the affected nerve root, and paresthesias, numbness, and weakness may be associated. The C-5, C-6, and C-7 nerve roots are most often affected. C-5 root compression results in the development of pain, paresthesias, and numbness in the anterosuperior shoulder and anterolateral aspect of the upper arm and forearm; a decreased biceps jerk and weakness of elbow flexion are found on examination. Compression of the C-6 nerve root produces symptoms in the dorsoradial aspect of the forearm and thumb, whereas C-7 impingement is denoted by altered sensation in the middle of the hand. The brachioradialis tendon reflex is affected by conditions altering C-5 and C-6, and the triceps jerk by injury to the C-7 and C-8 roots.

Inflammatory Disease. *Rheumatoid* disease can produce neck pain; it is typically worse in the morning. Concurrent symmetric polyarthropathy and subluxation at C1-2 (identifiable on plain films of the neck in flexion and extension) are characteristic. In the *spondyloarthropathies*, neck pain occurs in the context of diffuse back and sacroiliac discomfort. The earliest radiologic signs are those of sacroiliitis visible on sacroiliac joint films; advanced disease produces syndesmophytes. In *polymyalgia rheumatica*, neck pain may accompany the aching discomfort and stiffness of the shoulders and hip girdle that predominate in this condition. Polymyalgia complicated by *giant cell arteritis* with carotid artery involvement can produce focal neck tenderness along one or both carotid arteries, sometimes referred to as *carotodynia*.

Malignancy. Tumor may infiltrate the spinal cord or the vertebral bodies and produce pain that is worse at night or while lying down. Cord involvement may be heralded by neurologic deficits in addition to the nocturnal pain.

Referred Pain. Neck pain radiating to the jaw is characteristic of *coronary ischemia*, which is usually precipitated or worsened by physical activity. Concurrent arm pain may simulate a cervical radiculopathy. *Esophageal* disease may produce pain referable to the neck; if a cancer of the esophagus extends into the prevertebral space, posterior pain may develop.

DIFFERENTIAL DIAGNOSIS

The musculoskeletal causes of neck pain include muscle strain, muscle spasm, cervical spondylosis, and cervical root compression. Lymphadenopathy, thyroiditis (see Chapter 104), angina pectoris (see Chapter 20), and meningitis are important causes of cervical pain that may be mistaken for a musculoskeletal problem.

WORKUP

History. Inquiry should focus on elucidating precipitating events, aggravating and alleviating factors (particularly specific neck movements), area of maximal tenderness, radiation of pain, presence of numbness or weakness in the extremities, course, past history of similar problems, and previous therapeutic efforts. One also should consider symptoms suggestive of coronary artery disease (see Chapter 30) or meningeal irritation.

Physical Examination must include full visualization of the neck, thorax, and upper extremities. Neck motions are assessed, including flexion–extension, left and right lateral flexion, and left and right rotation. The neck must be carefully palpated to identify the point of local tenderness, which gives the best indication of the structure involved. Careful examination of the upper extremities is also required and should include an evaluation of tendon reflexes, strength, sensation, range of motion, and pulses. Every patient with fever and neck pain should be tested for meningeal signs.

Laboratory Studies. In cases of nontraumatic neck strain, no studies are necessary. The only finding may be a loss of the normal lordotic curve. In cases of traumatic neck strain caused by a hyperextension injury, *cervical spine films* are required to rule out structural damage. Clinical evidence of root or cord compression is an indication for *magnetic resonance imaging* (MRI); *computed tomography* (CT) with *myelography* can be performed if MRI is not available or if surgery is contemplated. Degenerative disease and ankylosing spondylitis may be suggested by *plain films* of the *neck*, but in early spondylitis, plain films of the *sacroiliac joints* may be needed to detect early bony changes. MRI is not indicated for the assessment of degenerative disk disease unless neurologic compromise is noted because test specificity is poor (up to half of asymptomatic persons have disk herniations on MRI). Suspected tumor requires *bone scan* or CT if bony involvement is suspected, and MRI if marrow or cord compression is of concern.

SYMPTOMATIC MANAGEMENT

Most causes of neck pain are self-limited and resolve with time. However, the discomfort can be considerable, so that symptomatic measures are necessary.

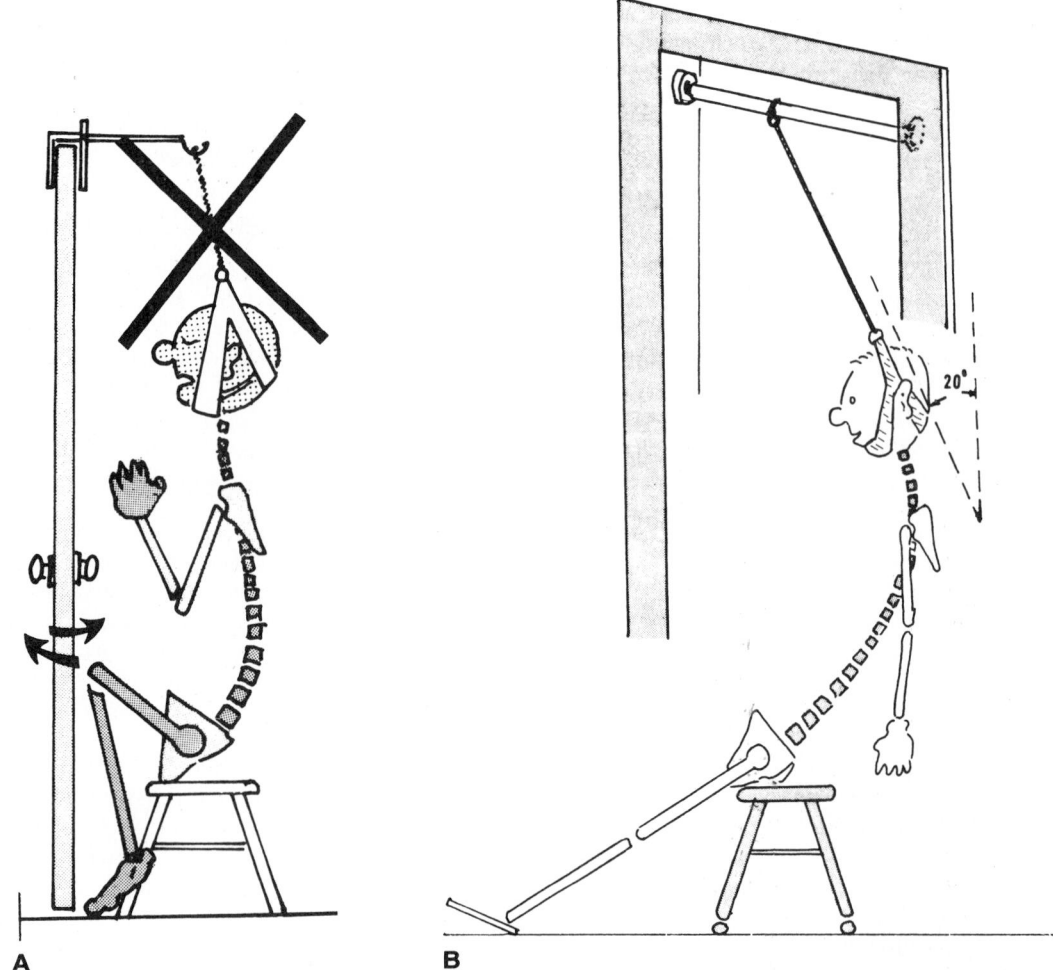

A   **B**

FIG. 148.1.   A: Ineffective home cervical traction with a door. The patient is too close to the door to obtain the correct angle for neck flexion. The door freely opens and closes and so does not permit constant traction. The patient cannot extend the legs or assume a comfortable position. This type of home traction is not recommended. **B:** Recommended home traction with a chinning bar and in the sitting position. (From Cailliet R. Soft tissue pain and disability. Philadelphia: FA Davis Co, 1977:129, with permission.)

Strain. Heat, ice, and gentle massage may ease muscle spasm. Although widely prescribed, most so-called *muscle relaxants* are actually minor tranquilizers marketed as relaxants; they are of limited value for prolonged use but can be useful on a short-term basis, especially in helping the patient to sleep. More useful and less expensive are therapeutic doses of an *NSAID* (e.g., aspirin, ibuprofen), supplemented for a few days by a small nighttime dose of a generic *benzodiazepine* (e.g., 5 mg of diazepam at bedtime). Prolonged benzodiazepine use is to be avoided (see Chapter 226). Strengthening and range-of-motion *exercises* are helpful. A soft *cervical collar* may be used to rest sore neck muscles briefly, especially at night; however, prolonged wear should be discouraged, as it may lead to muscle weakening from disuse atrophy. No good evidence has been found that injecting anesthetic into the tender body of a muscle in spasm speeds resolution of the problem; injection may actually injure the muscle.

More severe strain, such as that resulting from whiplash injury, poses a more difficult management problem. Although patients prefer wearing a cervical collar acutely because neck movement is painful, use of the collar should be limited to the period of severe pain and eliminated when pain has eased. Prolonged use of a collar actually increases the duration of pain, limits the return of neck mobility, and slows the clinical course. Emphasis should be placed on return of neck function and range of motion. A strong educational effort regarding the goals of treatment and proper neck exercises helps considerably, as does advice to settle any litigation as quickly as possible.

Spinal manipulation if often performed for patients with chronic strain, but its utility and safety and the indications for its use remain to be defined by properly designed prospective, randomized trials. Such manipulation should be avoided when neurologic compromise or nerve root or cord impingement is a possibility. *Ultrasound* and *diathermy* treatments also provide subjective improvement beyond that derived from medical management, but often no more than placebo forms of these therapies.

Degenerative Disease. In cases of disk herniation associated with radiculopathy, symptomatic therapy is aimed at countering the inflammation and root compression responsible for pain. *Nonsteroidal agents* (e.g., generic ibuprofen or naproxen) are useful to treat inflammation, and a *cervical collar* helps minimize compression. Several weeks of continuous collar use may be necessary; the collar should be worn regularly until pain disappears. After pain lessens, the collar can be worn at those times when added support may be helpful, such as at night or when riding in a motor vehicle. A properly fitting collar holds the neck in gentle flexion (the neutral position); collars that produce excessive extension are to be avoided because they may aggravate root compression.

Home cervical traction is indicated for severe, chronic, or recurrent neck pain caused by cervical spondylosis or disk herniation associated with radiculitis. Sitting cervical traction is applied at home for 20 to 30 minutes, two to four times a day, with 6 to 10 pounds of weight. The cervical traction apparatus must be carefully aligned and pull slightly forward at an angle of about 20 degrees to follow the natural line in the neck (Fig. 148.1). Proper technique is essential for effective and safe use. *Spinal manipulation* is contraindicated because of its potential to worsen root or cord compression. Ultrasound and diathermy treatments are harmless but of little proven benefit and probably no better than other means of delivering local heat to an area of concurrent muscle spasm. *Surgical management* may be required in refractory disease, especially when neurologic compromise is present.

INDICATIONS FOR ADMISSION AND REFERRAL

Meningeal signs are an obvious indication for urgent hospitalization. If significant weakness in the upper extremity or evidence of cord pressure is noted, then neurosurgical referral is indicated. Any signs suggestive of cord injury (hyperreflexia, upturned toe, incontinence or retention, bilateral neurologic deficits) are an indication for urgent neurosurgical consultation because the outcome is best when surgical treatment is early and definitive. If the patient has intractable chronic pain that is unresponsive to conservative measures, then consultation with a neurologist before the neurosurgical or orthopedic referral can sometimes be beneficial, especially to review the findings and discuss treatment options.

The patient with persistent neck pain is likely to request or ask about physiotherapy (e.g., diathermy, ultrasound, spinal manipulation). Careful review of the available data on these procedures with the patient can lead to an informed choice that is mutually satisfactory and minimizes risk and unnecessary expense. More beneficial to outcomes might be referral to a skilled physical therapist who, in a few sessions, can teach proper neck care and range-of-motion and neck-strengthening exercises.

A.H.G.

ANNOTATED BIBLIOGRAPHY

Aker PD, Gross AR, Goldsmith CH, et al. Conservative management of mechanical neck pain: systemic overview and meta-analysis. BMJ 1996:313:1291. (*Best review of the evidence regarding what works and what does not.*)

Bland JH. Disorders of the cervical spine: diagnosis and medical management. Philadelphia: WB Saunders, 1987. (*Excellent monograph for the nonsurgical reader.*)

Koes BW, Assendelft WJ, van der Heijde GJ, et al. Spinal manipulation and mobilization for back and neck pain: a blinded review. BMJ 1991;303:1298. (*A critical review; delineates the important design flaws in manipulation studies.*)

Koes BW, Bouter LM, van Mameren H, et al. The effectiveness of manual therapy, physiotherapy, and treatment by the general practitioner for nonspecific back and neck complaints. Spine 1992;17:28. (*A 3-month randomized, single-blinded, placebo-controlled trial of patients with nonspecific neck or back pain; spinal manipulation, physiotherapy, and placebo physiotherapy were superior to medical management by the general practitioner.*)

Lehto IJ, Tertti MO, Komu ME, et al. Age-related MRI changes at 0.1 T in cervical discs in asymptomatic subjects. Neuroradiology 1994;36:49. (*More than 50% over the age of 50 have evidence of disk herniation on MRI.*)

Spitzer WO, et al. Scientific monograph of the Quebec Task Force on whiplash-associated disorders: redefining "whiplash" and its management. Spine 1990;20[Suppl 8]:1S. (*Includes data on lack of efficacy of prolonged cervical collar use.*)

149
Approach to the Patient with Muscle Cramps

Muscle cramps are prolonged, involuntary muscle contractions that can be painful and difficult to manage but rarely reflect serious underlying disease. True cramps must be differentiated from ischemic pain, contracture, tetany, and dystonia. Fluid and electrolyte disorders, medication, and endocrinologic disorders must be considered in the evaluation, although they are uncommon precipitants. Patients come in requesting symptomatic relief from these painful episodes, which can be temporarily disabling.

PATHOPHYSIOLOGY AND CLINICAL PRESENTATION

True Cramps

True muscle cramping represents motor unit hyperactivity leading to prolonged, involuntary muscle contraction. Precipitants include unopposed contraction, electrolyte and volume shifts, and lower motor neuron disease. *Ordinary cramps* most commonly occur in the gastrocnemius muscle and the intrinsic muscles of the sole of the foot. Their *nocturnal* predilection appears to be related to unopposed plantar flexion of the foot in bed, which places the muscles of the calves and feet in their most shortened and therefore most vulnerable position. Without modulation by opposing muscles, the sustained contraction produces a cramp, which is experienced as sudden, severe calf pain; often, the muscle is palpable or visibly hardened. In many instances, a voluntary contraction triggers the cramp. Passive stretching relieves it.

True cramps may be precipitated by *volume* and *electrolyte shifts*, which accounts for the fact that they frequently occur during hemodialysis and can be relieved with administration of hypertonic dextrose. *Heat cramps* that occur during activity are a consequence of dehydration and sodium loss and respond to replenishment. *Hyponatremia* is a consistent feature of fluid-based muscle cramps, but hypokalemia is not, contrary to common belief. Cramps attributable to potassium-wasting diuretics are actually uncommon. Ordinary cramps are often a part of symptomatic *hypoglycemia*.

Muscle cramps are sometimes *drug-induced*, as may occur with nifedipine, β-agonists, and occasionally heavy alcohol use.

The cramp is a neural or electrical phenomenon, not primarily muscular. Electromyography shows fasciculations preceding the cramp. Cramps accompanied by clinically evident fasciculations are characteristic of *lower motor neuron diseases*, such as polio in the recovery phase, peripheral nerve injury, nerve root compression, and amyotrophic lateral sclerosis.

Other Forms of Muscle Cramping

Contractures also represent involuntary muscle contractions, but they are electrically silent and characteristically occur during exertion, not rest. They develop in persons who have inherited metabolic defects that impair the formation of adenosine triphosphate, which is needed for muscle relaxation. Most patients have McArdle's disease. Both hyperthyroid and hypothyroid disease may cause cramping. Exertional cramping has been seen in hyperthyroidism. In hypothyroidism, impaired muscle relaxation produces the "hung-up" reflexes that characterize the condition.

Tetany is a state of both motor and sensory hyperactivity, associated with muscle spasm and paresthesias. The muscles of the mouth, hands, and lower extremities are typically involved, and carpopedal spasm is a characteristic manifestation, as are Chvostek's and Trousseau's signs. Hypocalcemia, hypomagnesemia, respiratory alkalosis, and hypokalemia are known precipitants. In severe cases, seizures may ensue if the condition goes uncorrected.

Occupational cramp is a form of dystonia in which muscle contractures occur in persons engaging in fine motor activities that have taken years to perfect. The typical patient is a writer or pianist whose hands curl involuntarily when writing or playing is attempted.

DIFFERENTIAL DIAGNOSIS

See Table 149.1 for information on the differential diagnosis of muscle cramps.

WORKUP

History. A detailed description of the cramping is essential and should include the setting in which the episodes occur. Those that develop at night or in the context of hemodialysis,

Table 149.1.   Differential Diagnosis of Muscle Cramps

True Cramps
  Ordinary (nocturnal)
  Heat-induced (volume depletion, hyponatremia)
  Hemodialysis (volume and electrolyte shifts)
  Lower motor neuron
  Drug-induced (nifedipine, β-agonists)

Dystonia
  Occupational (writer's cramp)

Tetany
  Hypocalcemia
  Hypomagnesemia
  Respiratory alkalosis
  Hypokalemia

Contracture
  McArdle's disease
  Thyroid disease

Adapted from McGee SR. Muscle cramps. Arch Intern Med 1990;150:511, with permission.

hypoglycemia, or heavy sweating during prolonged exertion are likely to be true cramps, as are those coincident with use of calcium channel blockers or β-agonists. Dystonic cramping is suggested by onset with occupation-related fine motor activity, and contracture by a lifelong onset with exercise. Associated symptoms should be reviewed for the paresthesias and carpopedal spasm of tetany, the weakness and fasciculations of lower motor neuron disease, and the cold or heat intolerance, skin changes, and related symptoms of thyroid disease (see Chapters 103 and 104). The location of the cramping is a less specific finding, but if calf pain is reported, one should include intermittent claudication in the differential diagnosis, particularly if pain is brought on by walking. A review of medications is always useful, but use of a potassium-wasting diuretic is not tantamount to an etiologic diagnosis because hypokalemia is rarely responsible for true cramps (although it should be considered in the differential diagnosis of tetany). Also potentially pertinent in suspected tetany is any distant history of thyroidectomy (with coincident removal of the parathyroid glands).

Physical Examination. If dehydration is suspected, the physical examination begins with a check of postural signs for a drop in blood pressure and rise in pulse. The skin is examined for signs of thyroid disease (see Chapters 103 and 104); the neck for evidence of thyroidectomy; the lower extremities for diminished or absent pulses, muscle wasting, and fasciculations; and the nervous system for focal weakness and absent or abnormal deep tendon reflexes. If tetany is a consideration, one can try to elicit the facial spasm of Trousseau's sign by tapping the facial nerve or the carpal spasm of Chvostek's sign by inflating the arm cuff above systolic pressure.

Laboratory Determinations can be of very limited value. For the majority of people who present with a clinical story of nocturnal muscle cramps, laboratory testing is unlikely to provide additional information. Other situations do require a few simple tests. If the patient with ordinary cramps is diabetic and taking insulin, then testing for hypoglycemia is indicated (see Chapter 102). If severe dehydration and hyponatremia are suspected, then determinations of serum sodium, blood urea nitrogen, and creatinine levels can guide assessment and treatment. In the patient with possible tetany, levels of sodium, potassium, calcium, albumin (to interpret the calcium level), and magnesium must be checked. Consideration of thyroid disease is best pursued by obtaining a serum thyrotropin (TSH) determination. For the patient with fasciculations and possible lower motor neuron disease, a nerve conduction study may be required.

PRINCIPLES OF MANAGEMENT AND INDICATIONS FOR ADMISSION

Ordinary Cramps. To relieve an established cramp, one must passively stretch the contracting muscle and gradually contract the opposing one. In some cases, this can be accomplished by simply walking around, which produces a relative dorsiflexion of the foot.

Massage of the involved muscle sometimes helps. Conscious dorsiflexion at the first sign of a leg or foot cramp may abort it. Prophylactic stretching can also prevent attacks (see Chapter 18 for stretching exercise), as may positions in bed that prevent foot dorsiflexion. Swimming-induced cramps can be avoided by sacrificing the ideal kicking position of plantar flexion and maintaining a more neutral foot position.

Patients who have repeated attacks of nocturnal leg cramps seek a reduction in the frequency and severity of episodes. *Quinine sulfate* has been prescribed for decades for this purpose, but only recently have randomized, double-blind, controlled clinical trials been performed to assess its efficacy. Studies have shown that regimens with low to moderate doses (200 to 300 mg daily at bedtime) provide less benefit than those with higher doses (200 mg at supper, 300 mg at bedtime). This pattern suggests that response rates are related to the serum level attained, which can vary greatly with age of the patient and preparation used. The risk for serious side effects is quite small but increases with dose and serum level. Cinchonism (nausea, vomiting, tinnitus, hearing loss), visual impairment, and ventricular arrhythmias are the most important of these adverse effects and appear when serum levels exceed two to five times the average serum concentration. An immune thrombocytopenia, occasionally fatal, has also been reported.

Recently, a randomized, placebo-controlled, parallel-group trial, with more than 100 participants, demonstrated a substantial reduction in number of cramps and number of cramp-days with daily administration of 300 mg of *hydroquinine*. Side effects were mild and were noted by fewer than 10% of participants, and the treatment effect was sustained beyond the 2-week treatment period. The small but real risk for serious toxicity should temper one's uncritical use of quinine for this otherwise benign condition. However, for patients who are truly bothered by their symptoms, the evidence now justifies confidence in the effectiveness of quinine and its derivatives. A careful trial of quinine may be useful after the risks and benefits have been reviewed with the patient. Starting with small doses (200 to 300 mg daily at bedtime) is best, and the platelet count should be monitored periodically. Because of the evidence for a sustained effect, it is reasonable to interrupt treatment and reassess after 2 to 4 weeks.

Other drugs shown to be of some benefit include methocarbamol and chloroquine. Vitamin E is promoted in health food stores for the treatment of nocturnal cramps, but it has been found to be no better than placebo when tested in double-blind, placebo-controlled fashion. It may be found in combination with quinine. The calcium channel blocker verapamil has shown promise in preliminary study.

Patients with ordinary cramps related to dehydration and sodium depletion respond well to replacement therapy. Those with cramps as a consequence of hemodialysis are best treated with rapid volume expansion (infusion of hypertonic dextrose or saline solution). If hypoglycemia is responsible, then adjustment of the insulin regimen is needed (see Chapter 102). Altering the medication program may be necessary in cases in which β-agonists or calcium channel blockers are thought to be responsible.

Occupational Cramps are difficult to treat. Rest and occupational aids can be helpful; psychotherapy is not. Minor tranquilizers provide some short-term relief but little sustained benefit. Injection of botulinum toxin has been tried with some success.

Tetany requires urgent hospital admission and careful parenteral correction of the underlying electrolyte disturbances. For patients bothered by occasional muscle cramps, medication is not a serious consideration. For those who have frequent or prolonged cramps, prophylactic medication should be considered.

A.H.G.

ANNOTATED BIBLIOGRAPHY

Baltodano N, Gallo BV, Weidler DJ. Verapamil versus quinine in recumbent nocturnal leg cramps in the elderly. Arch Intern Med 1988;148:1969. (*In an open-label trial, eight elderly patients whose condition was refractory to treatment with quinine showed noteworthy improvement.*)

Connolly PS, Shirley EA, Wasson JH, et al. Treatment of nocturnal leg cramps. Arch Intern Med 1992;152:1877. (*Quinine but not vitamin E was effective; a program of 500 mg/d relieved cramps within 3 to 5 days.*)

Freiman JP. Fatal quinine-induced thrombocytopenia. Ann Intern Med 1990;112:308. (*A Food and Drug Administration report of two previously well patients in whom quinine-induced thrombocytopenia was fatal.*)

Fung MC, Holbrook JH. Placebo-controlled trial of quinine therapy for nocturnal leg cramps. West J Med 1989;151:42. (*A small but well-designed study; quinine produced a statistically significant reduction in the number and severity of cramps.*)

Jansen PHP, Veenhuizen KCW, Wesseling AIM, et al. Randomized controlled trial of hydroquinone in muscle cramps. Lancet 1997;349:528. (*This randomized trial, the largest, demonstrated a significant reduction in number of cramps and cramp-days, with more than two thirds of patients having a 50% or greater reduction in cramps. Side effects were mild and infrequent.*)

Man-Son-Hing M, Wells G. Meta-analysis of efficacy of quinine for treatment of nocturnal leg cramps in elderly people. BMJ 1995;310:13. (*Quinine significantly reduced the number of cramps and the number of nights with cramps, the former by 43% and the latter by 27%.*)

Man-Son-Hing M, Wells G, Lau A. Quinine for nocturnal leg cramps: a meta-analysis including unpublished data. J Gen Intern Med 1998;13:600. (*Still effective, but the relative reduction in number of cramps fell from 43% to 21% when unpublished data were added.*)

McGee SR. Muscle cramps. Arch Intern Med 1990;150:511. (*A comprehensive review; 170 references.*)

Naylor JR, Young JB. A general population survey of rest cramps. Age Ageing 1994;23:418. (*Documents a high incidence in the general population.*)

150
Approach to the Patient with Shoulder Pain

JESSE B. JUPITER
DAVID RING

The shoulder is a complex joint integrating three bones, four joints, and more than 15 muscles. The mobility of the shoulder exceeds that of all other joints, subjecting it to a wide range of stresses, both in normal activity and in occupational and recreational pursuits. Shoulder pain and dysfunction are among the more common musculoskeletal complaints encountered in office practice. Successful treatment necessitates an accurate diagnosis; common nonspecific diagnoses such as "bursitis" and "tendinitis" can be misleading and delay appropriate therapeutic measures. Besides being capable of identifying the cause of shoulder pain, the primary physician needs to know how and when to utilize exercises, antiinflammatory agents, and joint injection to provide safe and effective symptomatic relief.

PATHOPHYSIOLOGY AND CLINICAL PRESENTATION

Injury or degenerative change in the rotator cuff, bicipital tendon, or acromioclavicular joint can produce pain localized to the shoulder joint. Characteristically, focal tenderness is present and pain is aggravated during shoulder movement. Patients report difficulty in dressing, combing their hair, or reaching up. Degenerative disease of the glenohumeral joint is uncommon; symptoms include mild stiffness, crepitus, and low-grade, aching discomfort related to vigorous or sustained use. Pain originating in or about the shoulder may be referred to the upper arm or radiate to the neck, elbow, or forearm; it does not follow a specific cervical root distribution. Although pain originating in the neck may radiate to the shoulder, it is brought on by neck motion rather than by shoulder movement and is usually not affected by shoulder position. However, poorly localized sensitivity to touch extending into the shoulder may vaguely simulate shoulder disease (see Chapter 148).

Rotator Cuff Problems are the single most common source of shoulder pain seen in a primary care practice, particularly among older patients. The tendons of the cuff are subjected to considerable mechanical stress. Degenerative and attritional changes taking place over time in the tendons lead to structural weakening. The role of "impingement" of the rotator cuff between the greater tuberosity and acromion is debated. Early on during this process, the tendons become inflamed and the diagnosis of rotator cuff tendinitis is appropriate. As the degenerative process advances, failure of the tendons near their insertion into the proximal humerus may result in a *tear*. Such tears are not usually associated with specific traumatic events—they are the result of cumulative degenerative failure of the tendon. It is important to identify large tears of the rotator cuff promptly. Fatty degeneration of retracted rotator cuff muscles that occurs within a few months of a large tear makes the results of repair much less predictable.

The diagnosis of *rotator cuff tendinitis* should be applied with caution to patients younger than 40 years of age. In younger patients, rotator cuff tendinitis is usually secondary to some other process, such as instability. A tear of the rotator cuff tendon in a younger person—most commonly a tear of the *subscapularis tendon*—is typically a high-energy injury. Such tears are rare but should not be missed. Careful physical examination can verify that the rotator cuff is intact. Any doubt merits referral to an experienced shoulder surgeon.

Most patients with rotator cuff problems are older than age 40. Pain over the deltoid, especially during overhead activities and internal rotation, plus weakness of shoulder elevation and external rotation, are diagnostic features. It is very common for pain from the rotator cuff to be referred to the lateral arm. Superior shoulder pain suggests acromioclavicular joint problems. Muscle atrophy suggests a large tear.

Biceps tendinitis of the shoulder is a diagnosis that is now rarely made in isolation. Inflammation of the tendon of the long head of the biceps is a common component of rotator cuff degeneration.

Glenohumeral Joint Problems. The glenohumeral joint has little inherent stability; stability is heavily dependent on static capsuloligamentous and dynamic musculotendinous restraints. Two general categories of glenohumeral instability comprise the majority of such problems: traumatic unidirectional instability and atraumatic multidirectional instability.

Traumatic dislocation of the glenohumeral articulation almost always results in anterior dislocation of the humeral head from the glenoid articular surface of the scapula. Posterior glenohumeral dislocations are rare and are usually related to a seizure or electric shock injury. Traumatic posterior dislocations are often fracture dislocations of the glenoid articular surface.

Traumatic anterior dislocation nearly always disrupts the anterior attachment of the glenoid labrum to the glenoid articular surface (Bankart lesion). The labrum is a ring of fibrous cartilage that helps deepen the relatively shallow glenoid articular surface and is the site of attachment of the all-important glenohumeral ligaments. The likelihood that a patient who has had one traumatic anterior dislocation of the shoulder will have recurrent dislocations is related to the age of the patient at the time of the first dislocation. Of patients younger than 20 years at the time of first diagnosis, as many as 80% will have another dislocation. Older patients are less likely to have a recurrent dislocation, but tearing of the rotator cuff is common and must be identified. Recurrent anterior dislocation usually requires surgical treatment consisting of reattachment of the anterior portion of the labrum to the glenoid margin in addition to tightening of any redundant anterior capsule.

Atraumatic instability is usually related to laxity of a number of capsular restraints. In many cases, the patient may have a connective tissue disorder. Other patients, such as competitive swimmers, have multidirectional instability as a result of repetitive microtrauma. This type of instability usually responds to a program of specific exercises intended to strengthen the dynamic muscular stabilizers of the shoulder. Athletes may also need to modify their technique; a good coach or trainer can be useful in this regard.

Patients who can actively and voluntarily dislocate their shoulder should be approached with caution. Often, a subtle underlying psychiatric condition is present. Cases in which the voluntary dislocation is habitual—often, the patient has derived some attention or reward from the ability to dislocate a shoulder—can be difficult to manage. This should be distinguished from situations in which the voluntary dislocation is positional—the patient can reproduce the instability by placing the arm in certain position but is averse to doing so.

Adhesive capsulitis, or *frozen shoulder syndrome*, is a characteristic symptom complex of pain and tenderness located diffusely about the anterior and posterior regions of the shoulder joint capsule. Active and passive motions of the glenohumeral joint are limited to a small, pain-free arc. Glenohumeral motion slowly decreases during several weeks. The condition is often refractory to most forms of treatment, yet motion usually improves with time. The challenge for the clinician is to rule out the presence of an underlying rotator cuff, instability, or neurologic problem.

Osteoarthritis of the glenohumeral joint is very uncommon. It causes symptoms at rest that are exacerbated by shoulder use. The patient may note a "grinding" sound with motion. Muscle atrophy, "bone-on-bone" crepitation, and diminished motion are noted on examination. Rheumatoid arthritis frequently involves the glenohumeral joint and usually gives a picture of symmetrical bilateral inflammatory changes.

Acromioclavicular Degenerative Lesions. Degenerative changes are seen in patients who do heavy labor or engage in contact sports. Pain arises with activities above and in front of the body and localizes to the acromioclavicular joint; tenderness is maximal over the joint and does not radiate.

Infection. The patient with a shoulder joint contaminated by an improperly performed injection presents with marked swelling, redness, and fever.

Referred Pain. Shoulder–hand syndrome (also referred to as *reflex sympathetic dystrophy* or *sympathetic maintained pain*) follows myocardial infarction, stroke, trauma, and a host of other events. The characteristic features are the persistent burning pain of "causalgia," diffuse tenderness, immobilization of the shoulder, and vasomotor changes in the hands. *Gallbladder disease* is suggested by pain at the tip of the scapula in conjunction with upper abdominal pain and tenderness. With *diaphragmatic irritation*, pain may be referred to the trapezius area running from the shoulder to the lateral aspect of the neck.

DIFFERENTIAL DIAGNOSIS

The causes of shoulder pain can be considered in terms of the structures that comprise the shoulder (Table 150.1). The

Table 150.1.   Important Causes of Shoulder Pain

Rotator Cuff
  Calcific tendinitis
  Subacromial impingement
  Biceps tendinitis
  Tear
  Adhesive capsulitis

Glenohumeral Joint
  Instability
  Dislocation
  Arthritis
  Infection

Acromioclavicular Joint
  Arthritis

Referred
  Cervical spondylosis
  Myocardial ischemia
  Shoulder–hand syndrome (reflex sympathetic dystrophy)
  Diaphragmatic irritation
  Thoracic outlet syndrome
  Gallbladder disease

vast majority of nontraumatic shoulder complaints are related to tendinitis.

WORKUP

History

One should inquire about previous trauma or an inciting event, location and radiation of pain, specific limitations of movement, associated neurologic deficits, aggravating and alleviating factors, previous history of shoulder problems, and therapies utilized. It is important to be sure that no symptoms suggestive of angina, gallbladder disease, or diaphragmatic irritation are present. Pain resulting from myocardial ischemia usually originates in the precordial region but may present as shoulder or neck pain radiating into the arm. Relief with rest or administration of nitroglycerine supports the diagnosis. An occupational history is occasionally revealing, especially if the patient has engaged in heavy labor or sports.

Patients with symptoms suggestive of shoulder disease describe a combination of pain, loss of mobility, and weakness. Pain associated with activities above the horizontal level suggests subacromial impingement or acromioclavicular joint arthritis. Pain occurring at night when the patient attempts to sleep with the arm overhead is characteristic of rotator cuff problems. Calcific tendinitis can be a cause of severe acute shoulder pain.

Overuse syndromes are commonly associated with sporting activities involving throwing or use of a racquet or an occupational history of wallpapering, painting, or carpentry. A past history of shoulder dislocations might suggest glenohumeral instability.

General Physical Examination

Before proceeding to the examination of the shoulder, it is important that the physician carefully check the neck, chest, heart, and abdomen for sources of referred pain. Cervical disease is often mistaken for a shoulder problem. Cervical root compression is readily distinguished from intrinsic shoulder disease by the elicitation and reproduction of pain on neck motion to the side of the complaint. Brachial plexus injury causing shoulder pain is associated with tenderness on deep pressure over the neurovascular bundle and scalene muscles of the supraclavicular fossa. The chest is checked for effusion, pleural rub, and poor diaphragmatic movement. If the heart is examined while the patient is in pain, one can listen for transient auscultatory signs of ischemia (e.g., fourth heart sound, single second sound, mitral regurgitant murmur from papillary muscle dysfunction). The abdomen is palpated for tenderness in the right or left upper quadrant, which may signal subdiaphragmatic disease.

Shoulder Examination

The patient is comfortably seated and sufficiently disrobed to permit evaluation and comparison of both shoulders. Close *inspection* from both front and back may demonstrate asymmetry or deformity. For example, supraspinatus muscle atrophy would suggest either a rotator cuff tear or suprascapular nerve disease. The patient is instructed to place the involved shoulder *actively* through a *full range of motion*, along with similar movements of the contralateral limb for comparison. This includes forward flexion, extension, abduction, and internal and external rotation. Internal rotation is best recorded as the level at which the patient can reach posteriorly, such as the buttock or thoracolumbar junction. The scapula is observed as the patient flexes the shoulder forward against resistance. Winging of the scapula can be the result of serratus anterior muscle palsy.

The patient is instructed to point out specific *sites of tenderness* (Fig. 150.1). Palpation by the examiner routinely should include the anterior aspect of the acromion, the acromioclavicular joint, the bicipital groove (which is best palpated

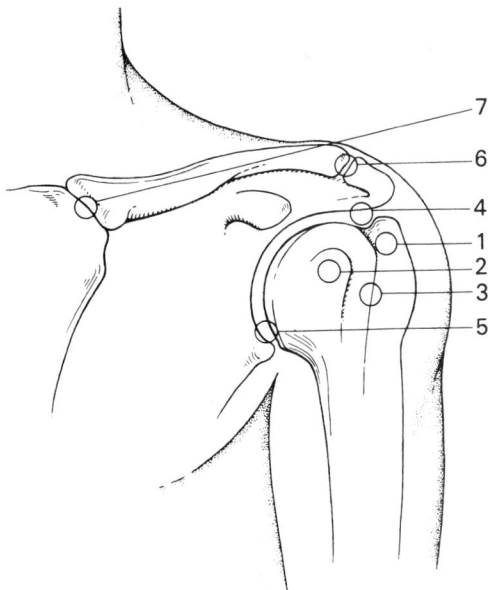

FIG. 150.1. Trigger points. Palpable "trigger points" during the examination reveal the site of disease, corroborate the history, and indicate the type of therapy. *1,* The greater tuberosity and site of supraspinatus tendon insertion. *2,* Lesser tuberosity, site of subscapularis muscle insertion. *3,* Bicipital groove, in which the bicipital tendon glides. *4,* Site of the subdeltoid bursa. *5,* Glenohumeral joint space. *6,* Acromioclavicular joint. *7,* Sternoclavicular joint. (Redrawn from Cailliet R. Shoulder pain. Philadelphia: FA Davis Co, 1973, with permission.)

with the humerus in about 10 degrees of internal rotation), the greater tuberosity, and the cervical spine. With the examiner's hand on the joint, the shoulder is passively put through a *range of motion* (Fig. 150.2). Limitations are noted, in addition to any palpable crepitation.

A manual *muscle test* is helpful, in particular for comparison with the uninvolved shoulder. Inability to "shrug" the shoulder suggests trapezial muscle weakness, whereas weakness of forward flexion is associated with derangement of the rotator cuff (the supraspinatus, infraspinatus, and teres minor muscles). A *sensory* and *deep tendon reflex* examination of the upper extremity should be included in the routine shoulder evaluation.

Diagnostic Maneuvers

Several specific maneuvers are diagnostically helpful and provide a means of quick and reliable diagnosis in the office.

Wright's Maneuver, in which the radial pulse is evaluated at the wrist with the shoulder in external rotation and abduction, may uncover an underlying *thoracic outlet syndrome*. The result of this test is considered positive if shoulder and arm symptoms are reproduced and the radial pulse is obliterated with the shoulder in this position.

Impingement Signs. *Neer's test* is performed with the examiner standing behind the patient and bringing the involved arm to the maximum degree of forward flexion with one hand while the other functions to depress the patient's shoulder girdle. If pain is elicited in the deltoid area or beneath the acromion, inflammation of the rotator cuff tendons and *impingement* of the greater tuberosity of the humerus against the undersurface of the acromion is likely. *Hawkins' sign* tests the shoulder with internal rotation at 90 degrees of forward flexion in the plane of the scapula. Results of these tests can be confirmed if an injection of 5 mL of lidocaine (Xylocaine) into the subacromial space relieves the symptoms—the so-called *impingement test.*

Tests for Rotator Cuff Tears. Large rotator cuff tears are identified with a series of specific tests. To test the posterior portion of the rotator cuff, or infraspinatus, the arm is placed at the side with the elbow maintained against the trunk. The forearm and hand are then brought passively into maximum external rotation. The patient is asked to maintain the arm actively in this position. An external rotation lag is defined as the difference between the maximum active and passive external rotation and may indicate a tear of the infraspinatus tendon.

The integrity of the anterior cuff (subscapularis tension) can be tested in either or two ways. The *lift-off test* involves maximum passive internal rotation of the arm behind the back so that the dorsum of the hand "lifts off" from the hip/back area. If the patient cannot maintain this position actively, the subscapularis tendon may be torn. For the belly press sign, the patient is asked to place the hand flat against the abdomen with the elbow held forward in this plane. The patient is then asked to maintain the hand against the belly as the examiner pulls the hand anteriorly. A posterior swing of the elbow reflects an attempt to maintain the hand against the belly by means of extension rather than internal rotation of the shoulder, in which case a tear of the subscapularis tendon may be present.

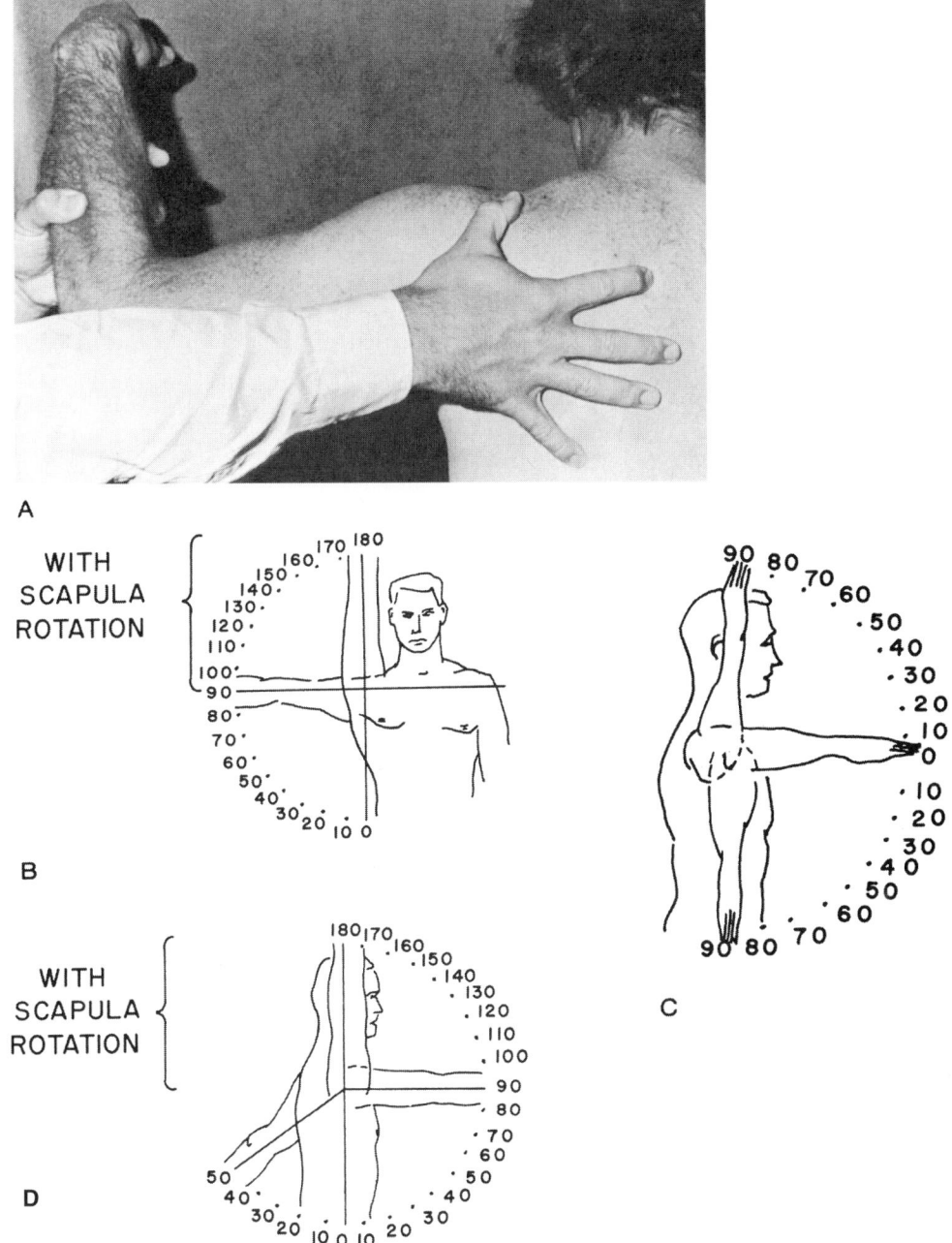

A

WITH
SCAPULA
ROTATION

B

WITH
SCAPULA
ROTATION

C

D

FIG. 150.2. **A:** Stabilization of the scapula during testing of glenohumeral joint motion. **B:** Normal range of adduction–abduction of the shoulder with and without scapular rotation. **D:** Normal range of external–internal rotation with upper arm at 90 degrees and elbow held at right angle. **D:** Normal range of flexion–extension of the shoulder with and without scapular rotation. (From Katz WA. Rheumatic diseases. Philadelphia: JB Lippincott Co, 1977.)

The supraspinatus is more difficult to isolate. Long-standing tears are associated with atrophy noted in the supraspinatus fossa of the scapula. Weakness of resisted abduction may be noted with the shoulder held in 90 degrees of abduction.

Tests for Acromioclavicular Joint Disease. In the *cross arm adduction test*, symptoms are reproduced when the patient brings the involved arm across the body so that the *hand grasps the contralateral shoulder*. The result can be confirmed by having the patient repeat the maneuver after the acromioclavicular joint has been injected with 1 mL of lidocaine; a 25-gauge needle is used to enter the joint. Patients who report a feeling of

imminent shoulder dislocation when the shoulder is positioned in 90 degrees of abduction and maximum external rotation—a *positive apprehension sign*—may have anterior shoulder instability. Confirmatory evidence is obtained by repeating the test with the patient supine and placing posterior pressure over the proximal humerus—the *relocation test*. The uncomfortable sensation of impending dislocation should be diminished if it is caused by anterior instability.

Multidirectional laxity is sought in an examination of other stabilizing structures. The patient is tested for laxity of the superior glenohumeral ligament by applying axial traction to the arm held at the side in external rotation. If the gap between the acromion and humeral head is larger than that seen during testing of the opposite side—a positive sulcus sign—the superior glenohumeral ligament may be lax. Forward flexion and posterior translation of the arm may reproduce symptoms of posterior instability. Repeating the sulcus sign in internal rotation also tests the posterior capsule.

Laboratory Studies

Radiographs of the shoulder are mandatory in the initial evaluation. A *standard anteroposterior view* is helpful in ruling out underlying bone tumor, infection, or arthritis of either the glenohumeral or acromioclavicular joint. The anteroposterior view with the shoulder in *internal* and *external rotation* can best identify calcification. Well-circumscribed, organized calcification reflects chronic calcification of degenerated tendons and is not particularly important. Patients who have acute, severe pain may be noted to have a more diffuse, disorganized pattern of calcification, which suggests acute calcific tendinitis. An *axillary view* is mandatory if dislocation is suspected; it most clearly defines the relation of the humeral head to the glenoid fossa and is also helpful in the assessment of glenohumeral arthritis. In patients with chronic or recurrent dislocations, an indentation into the humeral head (or Hill-Sachs lesion) may be apparent. Cervical spine films are needed if neck motion reproduces the shoulder pain or root compression symptoms are observed (see Chapter 148).

Shoulder arthrography has been used to identify a suspected rotator cuff tear and is still popular with some physi-cians, particularly for the diagnosis of full-thickness tears of the rotator cuff. Dye is injected directly into the glenohumeral joint, and the joint is then mobilized. Extravasation of dye from the joint into the subacromial space is highly suggestive of a complete tear of the rotator cuff.

Magnetic resonance imaging provides a noninvasive means of assessing the integrity of the rotator cuff and in some instances obviates the need for arthrography to detect a tear. It can also provide information about the size of a tear, the degree of retraction, and the status of involved muscles (i.e., whether or not they have been replaced by fat). Although useful for the assessment of a rotator cuff tear, magnetic resonance imaging is costly and is not indicated as part of the initial evaluation of shoulder pain.

If infection is suspected in the joint or joint capsule, *aspiration*, *Gram's stain*, and *culture* are urgent so that definitive therapy can be initiated without delay (see Chapter 145). If a peripheral nerve deficit is discovered on neurologic examination, *electromyography* may help to characterize the lesion better. Testing for referred pain is indicated only in the presence of a suggestive history and corroborating physical findings.

SYMPTOMATIC THERAPY

Rotator Cuff Tendinitis. If a large tear of the rotator cuff is not suspected, the tendinitis can be managed with a program consisting of avoidance of exacerbating activities, an *NSAID* (e.g., 375 mg of naproxen twice daily or 600 mg of ibuprofen

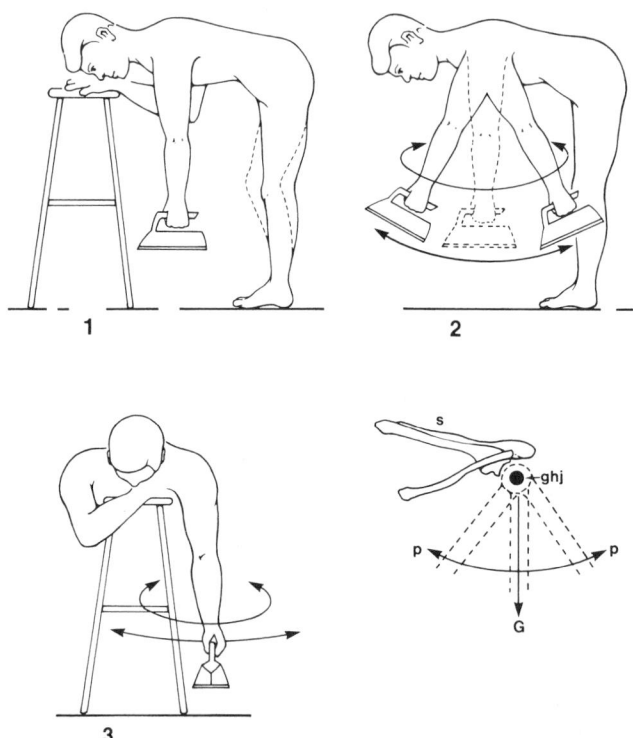

FIG. 150.3.   Active pendular glenohumeral exercise (Codman exercises). *1*, The posture to be assumed to permit the arm to "dangle" freely, with or without a weight. *2*, The arm moves in forward and backward sagittal plane, in forward and backward flexion. A circular motion in the clockwise and counterclockwise directions is also made in increasingly large circles. *3*, The front view of the exercise shows lateral pendular movement, actually in the coronal plane. The lower right diagram shows the effect of gravity, *G*, on the glenohumeral joint, *ghj*, with an immobile scapula, *s*. The *p*-to-*p* arc is the pendular movement. (Redrawn from Cailliet R. Shoulder pain. Philadelphia: FA Davis Co, 1973, with permission.)

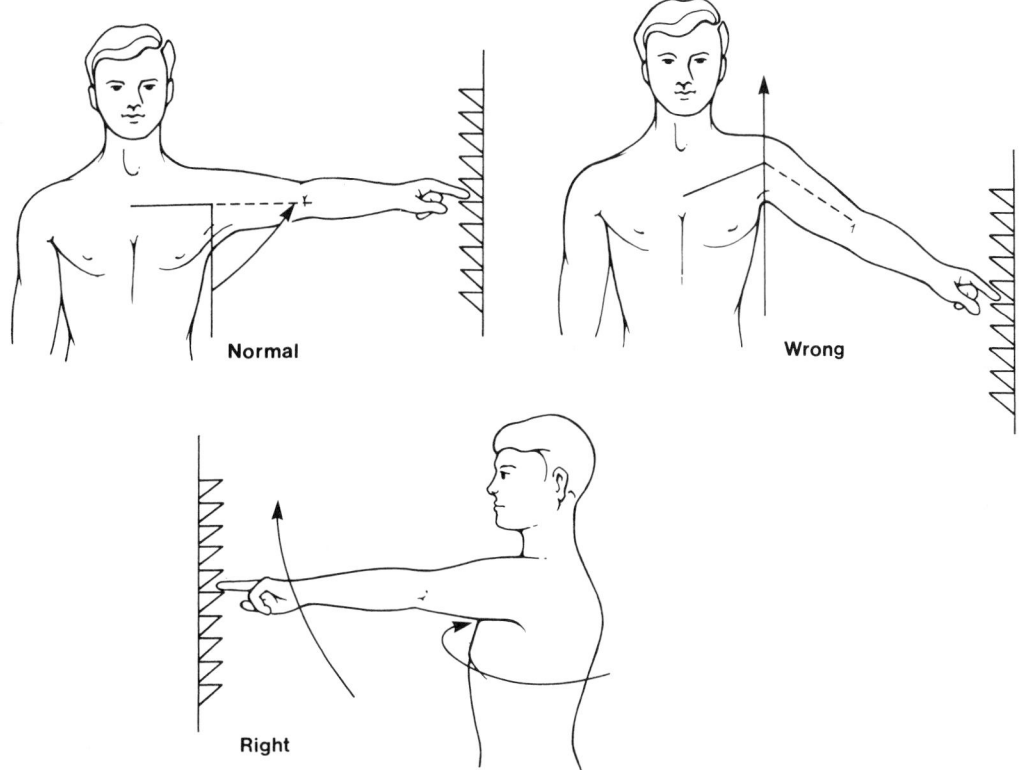

FIG. 150.4. Correct and incorrect use of "wall-climbing" exercise. The wall-climbing exercise frequently is performed improperly. The normal arm climbs with normal scapulohumeral rhythm. If a pericapsulitis is present, the wall climb in abduction is performed with "shrugging" of the scapula, and nothing is accomplished. The wall climb should be started with the patient facing the wall and gradually turning the body until at a right angle to the wall. (Redrawn from Cailliet R. Shoulder pain. Philadelphia: FA Davis Co, 1973, with permission.)

three times daily), and exercises to strengthen the rotator cuff. The exercises are best taught and supervised by a trained therapist. Commonly, a set of rubber bands providing increasing levels of resistance is used to exercise specific tendons and enhance their strength and performance.

If motion is restricted, the program should include specific exercises for restoring shoulder mobility. *Pendulum exercises* aid in maintaining joint mobility. With the patient bending forward at the waist, the arm is allowed to dangle and swing in forward-to-back, side-to-side, and circular patterns (Fig. 150.3). Additional exercises, such as "wall climbing" (Fig. 150.4), are included as the pain subsides. The patient must be counseled to expect some mild discomfort with these exercises, as they are designed specifically to stretch the joint capsule. These exercises are performed for periods of 5 to 10 minutes, three to four times each day.

When the inflammation in the tendon is so severe that exercises are not possible, or in the case of severe acute calcific tendinitis, subacromial *injection* of a *corticosteroid* and local anesthetic is often helpful. The subacromial joint can be entered by advancing the needle under the lateral edge of the acromion process. After the skin has been initially infiltrated with a few milliliters of lidocaine, the subacromial space is injected with 5 to 10 mL of lidocaine and 40 mg of methylprednisolone (Depo-Medrol, usually 1 mL) or an equivalent steroid (Fig. 150.5). Steroid injection may acutely worsen symptoms after the anesthetic wears off, but improvement is likely to follow within 48 hours. To avoid precipitating capsular atrophy, injections should be given no more often than once every 6 to 12 months

and limited to a total of three. Care must be taken not to inject into the tendon; the goal is to deliver medication into the area around it. Repeated steroid injection within a few months of the initial injection should not be attempted by the primary care physician because of the deleterious biochemical effects of glucocorticoids on connective tissue. Orthopedic referral is indicated when symptoms do not respond or when a large tear is suspected.

In patients with calcific tendinitis, pulsed *ultrasound* treatments help to reduce calcification and improve the patient's functional status and quality of life over the short term. However, the fact that no long-term benefit has been noted in comparison with placebo shows that recurrence is common if the underlying cause of tendinous injury is not alleviated.

Torn Rotator Cuff. Spontaneous healing of a torn rotator cuff is unlikely. Despite this, many patients with a partial tear or a small complete tear respond to an exercise program designed to strengthen their shoulder rotator muscles. Repetitive steroid injections have no place in this disorder because the cortisone, if anything, retards healing and accelerates the deterioration of the tendons. Large tears require prompt surgical treatment. In may not be possible to reconstruct very large or massive tears and large tears associated with retraction and degeneration of the muscle.

Adhesive Capsulitis is difficult and often frustrating to treat; the course is prolonged, and the chances for full recovery are unpredictable. The hallmark of treatment is an *active exer-*

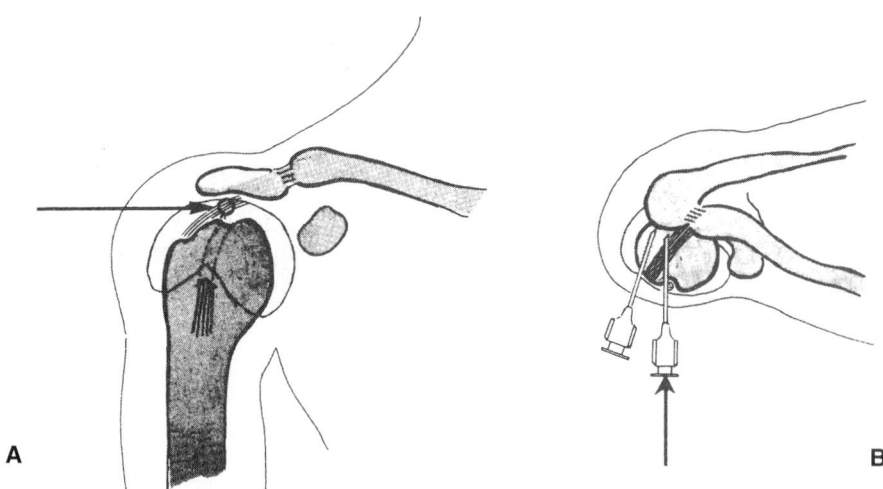

FIG. 150.5. Site of injection in acute calcific tendinitis. **A:** Region of supraspinatus insertion in the suprahumeral space. The region is palpable immediately below the overhanging acromion and over the greater tuberosity just lateral to the bicipital groove of the humerus. **B:** Insertion of needle viewed from above. Two directions of entrance are shown, with the *arrow* depicting that shown in the anterior view. (From Cailliet R. Soft tissue pain and disability. Philadelphia: FA Davis Co, 1977:161, with permission.)

cise program. The patient is instructed to precede each session with the application of local heat, either by using a heating pad or taking a warm shower, for 15 to 20 minutes. Initially, one begins by lying supine and, with the contralateral hand, bringing the involved shoulder into forward flexion. External rotation exercises are also begun; one holds a broom handle in both hands and moves from internal to external rotation. The patient should be encouraged to use the shoulder as much as possible in the normal activities of daily living. It is worthwhile for a physical therapist to keep a weekly or monthly log regarding the shoulder motion because improvement is slow and usually occurs in small increments; objective signs of improvement help to lessen patient frustration. *Forceful manipulation* of the shoulder is rarely indicated, and in fact *operative caspsulotomy* may be safer. Recently, this procedure has been performed with the arthroscope, but the indications for operative intervention are uncertain. Most people achieve a functional range of motion through a concerted, patiently applied exercise program.

Glenohumeral Arthritis. In the conservative treatment of glenohumeral arthritis, whether secondary to osteoarthritis or inflammatory arthritis, *NSAIDs* and *exercises* are used to maintain a functional range of motion. The patient can be instructed to do the same exercises as for adhesive capsulitis on a daily or twice-daily basis at home. Exercises directed at maximizing existing muscle strength are also prescribed, preferably with the supervision of a physical therapist. Improvements in total joint arthroplasty have offered a functional alternative to many patients whose condition is refractory to medical management. Cortisone injections of the glenohumeral joint also provide relief, and the number of injections that can be administered is unlimited. Injection of the glenohumeral joint can be difficult and is best performed by an orthopedic surgeon.

Acromioclavicular Arthritis. Antiinflammatory medications and modification of activity are often helpful in reducing the inflammatory component of arthritis of the acromioclavicular joint. At times, an injection of *corticosteroid* and lidocaine may

help but can be remarkably difficult to administer because of the small size and accessibility of the joint. Injection of this joint may be best left to the orthopedic specialist. Rarely, surgery is required, which consists of partial distal clavicular excision.

INDICATIONS FOR REFERRAL

Shoulder dislocation or instability, fractures about the shoulder, advanced acromioclavicular or glenohumeral joint arthritis, rotator cuff tears, and infection are best referred early to the orthopedic surgeon. Refractory rotator cuff tendinitis also is an indication for referral if resolution is not obtained with appropriate conservative treatment.

PATIENT EDUCATION

Emphasis should be placed on the importance of active participation in the treatment program. Many patients seek only relief from pain and expect oral or injectable medication to suffice. Thorough recovery entails actively performing the exercises of the treatment program, which must be carefully taught, often with the help of a physical therapist. Repeated pain and limitation of function are bound to ensue if the exercise program is not taken seriously.

ANNOTATED BIBLIOGRAPHY

American Medical Association, Council on Scientific Affairs. Musculoskeletal applications of magnetic resonance imaging. JAMA 1989;262:2420. (*Critical examination of the test and comparison with other imaging methods.*)

Cailliet R. Shoulder pain. Philadelphia: FA Davis Co, 1973. (*A clearly written and well-illustrated monograph that provides an in-depth discussion of tendinitis.*)

Ebenbichler ER, Erdogmus CB, Resch KL, et al. Ultrasound therapy for calcific tendinitis of the shoulder. N Engl J Med 1999; 340:1533. (*Well-designed study showing good short-term results.*)

Speed CA, Hazelman BL. Calcific tendinitis of the shoulder. N Engl J Med 1999;340:1582. (*Good short summary of the pathophysiology of tendinitis, plus an editorial review of the Ebenbichler article.*)

Steinfeld R, Valente RM, Stuart MJ. A common sense approach to shoulder problems. Mayo Clin Proc 1999;74:785. (*Terse, well-illustrated summary for the primary physician, with good pictures of key maneuvers.*)

Warner JJ, Allen A, Marks PH, et al. Arthroscopic release for chronic refractory adhesive capsulitis. J Bone Joint Surg Am 1996;78:1808. (*Latest surgical option for refractory disease.*)

151
Evaluation of Hip Pain
ROBERT J. BOYD

Hip pain can be a major source of misery for both patient and family. The joint is essential to locomotion and weight bearing and is frequently subject to trauma and chronic mechanical stress.

In the assessment of hip pain, the degree of pain and disability must be determined in addition to the underlying cause because surgery is now a practical therapeutic option for disabled patients whose pain is refractory to conservative measures.

PATHOPHYSIOLOGY AND CLINICAL PRESENTATION

The hip is supplied by the obturator, sciatic, and femoral nerves. Pain originating in or around the hip can be felt in the groin or buttock, with radiation to the distal thigh and anteromedial aspect of the knee. Occasionally, pain from the hip may be felt only in the thigh and knee. Pain occurs in the distribution of the L-2 and L-3 roots and rarely is referred to the lower leg or foot. Conversely, pain caused by a problem outside the hip may be referred to the hip if the lesion irritates the femoral, sciatic, or obturator nerve or the nerve roots. Problems outside the hip include herniated disks in the high lumbar region, spinal stenosis, retroperitoneal or pelvic tumor, and femoral hernia; patients who have aortoiliac insufficiency may also present with hip and buttock pain (see Chapter 147).

Hip pain may be focal or diffuse, depending on the extent to which the joint and surrounding structures are involved in the pathologic process. For example, bursitis is characterized by focal pain and tenderness over the site of the bursa; synovitis is more diffuse, involving the entire joint capsule. Stiffness, limitation of motion, limp, and crepitus are frequent accompaniments of pain. Swelling is usually not evident and is difficult to detect because the joint is buried deeply in soft tissues.

The major mechanisms of hip disease include cartilaginous degeneration, synovial inflammation, tendinitis and consequent bursitis, fracture, and ischemia.

Osteoarthritis. The hip is a major site of degenerative joint disease, with the elderly being the most affected. Obesity is also a risk factor, particularly in women. The onset is often insidious, beginning with minor aching or stiffness that may be unilateral or bilateral. Symptoms are characteristically exacerbated by prolonged standing, walking, or stair climbing. Stiffness is noted when the patient gets up after sitting for long periods. The hip begins to loosen up at first with moving about, but discomfort then worsens with continued activity. As osteoarthritis gradually progresses, it results in decreasing hip motion, increasing stiffness, and increasing pain. A limp may develop as the joint architecture is disrupted, and weight bearing becomes painful. The course of the disease is usually marked by spontaneous exacerbations and remissions.

On physical examination, the patient with substantial disease characteristically holds the hip in flexion, external rotation, and adduction. An antalgic gait, Trendelenburg's sign (buttock falls when the patient stands on the opposite foot), which is indicative of abductor weakness), and limitation of hip motion with or without crepitus may be present. Pain, muscle spasm, and guarding occur when the examiner attempts to take the hip through the full range of motion. Buttock atrophy may involve the gluteus maximus posteriorly and the gluteus medius more laterally. With severe degenerative arthritis of the hip, a marked flexion deformity may develop, and pain may be felt in the hip joint even at rest (see also Chapter 157).

Rheumatoid Arthritis. The hips are rarely affected in rheumatoid disease until other joints have become involved. Pain is characteristically bilateral and associated with morning stiffness, which lessens with activity. During flares of the disease, the hip joint is tender to palpation, and capsular fullness and thickening may be felt if effusion or chronic synovitis is present. Flexion contractures occur in advanced cases (see also Chapter 156).

Ankylosing Spondylitis is unique among the spondyloarthropathies in that the hip is sometimes affected. Concurrent sacroiliac and spinal involvement is usually present and in itself may cause pain radiating into the hip or buttock (see also Chapters 146 and 147).

Hip Fracture. At greatest risk is the frail, elderly person with a history of frequent falls and osteoporosis. The femoral neck and intertrochanteric region are common fracture sites. Loss of normal surface architecture may be associated with acute joint deformity, severe pain, guarding, and restriction of flexion and external rotation. Active straight leg raising is impaired. Competitive long-distance runners are at risk for stress fracture of the femoral neck.

Septic Arthritis. Joint infection in the hip most often follows hematogenous seeding (see Chapter 145). Because the joint is deep-seated, the ordinary signs of infection may not be readily evident. Fever, hip or knee pain (caused by referral of pain), and inability to bear weight are early symptoms. The thigh is often held in flexion, and a bulging, tender joint capsule may be palpable.

Idiopathic Avascular Necrosis. Also referred to as "aseptic" necrosis of the femoral head, this condition has an ischemic pathophysiology. It occurs in patients who take high daily doses of glucocorticoids, alcoholics, patients with hemoglobinopathies, and those who work under conditions of increased atmospheric pressure. The mechanism of steroid-induced disease involves the proliferation of intramedullary fat, tissue hypertension, and compromised perfusion of bone. Patients report the gradual onset of focal pain and limitation of movement. Diagnostic radiographic changes include wedge-shaped areas of increased density and segmental collapse of the femoral head.

Bursitis. Inflammation of the bursa occurs as a consequence of trauma or spread of an inflammatory process. Focal pain with tenderness develops over the bursa. *Trochanteric bursitis* is felt on the lateral aspect of the hip, posterior to the trochanter. Symptoms are increased by direct pressure or hip flexion and internal rotation. Pain may worsen at night and radiate down the leg to the knee. It may occur in runners who jog on uneven surfaces and those with one leg slightly shorter than the other. *Iliopectineal bursitis* causes pain on flexion and tenderness localized to the lateral border of Scarpa's triangle. *Ischiogluteal bursitis* presents with buttock pain that is worse during prolonged sitting, occurs at night, and occasionally radiates down the leg posteriorly, simulating sciatica.

Polymyalgia Rheumatica. A disease of the elderly that is often mistaken for depression, arthritis, or bursitis, polymyalgia is characterized by bilateral aching of the hips, thighs, and shoulders in conjunction with a very high sedimentation rate. It has a strong association with cranial arteritis (see Chapter 161). Joint structures and passive range of joint motion are usually preserved.

Pigmented Villonodular Synovitis. This uncommon granulomatous disease of the synovium presents with slowly progressive pain and limitation of movement. Radiographic films show large cystic areas about the hip joint, which distinguish the condition from degenerative joint disease.

Referred Pain. Any pelvic, abdominal, or retroperitoneal process irritating the obturator muscle can cause pain that is referred to the hip. Such pain is worsened by internal rotation of the hip joint.

DIFFERENTIAL DIAGNOSIS

Hip pain is usually caused by degenerative joint disease. Other important causes include joint infection, avascular necrosis of the femoral head, bursitis, polymyalgia rheumatica, and rheumatoid arthritis. On occasion, ankylosing spondylitis or villonodular synovitis is responsible. Pain may be referred to the hip from a lumbar or pelvic problem, such as a herniated disk in the high lumbar region, retroperitoneal tumor or abscess, or obturator or femoral hernia. Aortoiliac insufficiency may present with exercise-induced hip and buttock pain.

WORKUP

History. One should ascertain the onset, location, and radiation of the pain in addition to inciting and alleviating factors and the presence of numbness or weakness. It is particularly important to inquire directly about trauma, involvement of other joints, morning stiffness, relation of pain to activity, response to rest, steroid or alcohol use, and current infection or fever. A few pitfalls regarding the history should be mentioned. For example, stiffness by itself is a nonspecific finding because it may occur both with degenerative disease and with rheumatoid involvement of the hip. The response to continued activity may be of more help diagnostically; stiffness usually worsens in degenerative disease and lessens in rheumatoid arthritis. Bilateral cramping hip and buttock pain that comes on with walking and is relieved by rest may actually be a sign of vascular insufficiency rather than of joint disease.

Physical Examination. The hip should be examined for deformities such as flexion or adduction contractures, which are seen with rheumatoid disease, and for fixed external rotation, which suggests a fracture of the femoral neck. Gait is also important to check. The hip is then put through the full range of passive motion to detect crepitus, limitation of movement, flexion contracture, muscle spasm, or guarding. The normal range of hip flexion–extension is from -20 to 90 degrees with the knee straight and from 0 to 120 degrees with the knee flexed. Normal adduction–abduction is from -20 to 90 degrees; normal internal–external rotation is from -50 to +50 degrees. One of the first movements to be limited in hip disease is internal rotation with the hip hyperextended. Palpation of the joint and individual bursae for focal tenderness and swelling is important for detecting a localized inflammatory process.

The circumference of the thigh should be measured at a fixed distance from a bony reference point, such as the tibial tubercle of the knee, the anterior superior iliac spine, or the midpatella. Atrophy is suggestive of intrinsic hip disease.

Femoral pulses should be palpated for diminution and auscultated for bruits. Pelvic and rectal examinations are helpful in searching for tumors, which may cause referred pain. The back should be examined for evidence of L1-2 or L2-3 disk herniation (see Chapter 147). Neurologic assessment of the lower extremities is needed to test for weakness, sensory loss, and reflexes.

Laboratory Studies. Hip *radiography* is essential in the assessment of hip pain. Radiography may be diagnostic of degenerative joint disease, rheumatoid arthritis, avascular necrosis, or fracture. Weight-bearing films help one judge the severity of degenerative hip disease by disclosing the extent of joint space narrowing. Sacroiliac and spine films are indicated if ankylosing spondylitis is under consideration (see Chapters 146 and 147). *Magnetic resonance imaging* is the most sensitive test for avascular necrosis of the femoral head, showing expansion of intramedullary fat before bony changes become visible. It also is more sensitive than standard radiography in the detection of stress fracture of the femoral neck.

A complete blood cell count, determination of the *sedimentation rate*, and *rheumatoid factor* analysis may be useful if a rheumatoid disease is being considered (see Chapter 146). If a septic joint is suspected, aspiration for cell count, Gram's stain, and culture is urgent (see Chapter 145).

SYMPTOMATIC THERAPY AND INDICATIONS FOR REFERRAL

Degenerative Disease. Simple treatment measures for relief of an acute exacerbation include daily periods of bed rest, analgesics (e.g., 500 mg of *acetaminophen* four times daily), limitation of sitting, and crutch or cane support. *NSAIDs* offer little benefit over pure analgesics when no signs of concurrent synovial inflammation are present. Moreover, NSAIDs increase both cost and the risk for NSAID-induced gastric injury, and may even speed the rate of joint degeneration. *Glucosamine* is heavily promoted for osteoarthritis, but evidence of efficacy from properly designed trials is lacking (see also Chapter 157).

After acute symptoms lessen, the patient can begin a program to improve functional capacity. It should include avoidance of activities that specifically aggravate pain, daily mild exercise (walking short distances as tolerated) preceded by acetaminophen, cane support if necessary, weight reduction if obese, and specific daily range-of-motion and strengthening exercises, preferably taught by a physical therapist. Rest periods of 1 hour twice daily with local heat applied to the hip may be helpful if discomfort occurs after exercise. Even modest degrees of weight reduction can be remarkably helpful in alleviating pain and disability.

If conservative measures fail to control symptoms and the patient is active, *surgery* may be needed. Because results of *hip reconstructive* procedures are now quite good and the procedure entails a relatively low risk, referral for consideration of surgery need not be delayed indefinitely if symptoms are disabling and not well controlled by conservative measures. The need for reconstructive surgery must be a joint decision of patient, primary physician, and orthopedic surgeon. Despite the relative safety of surgery, expectations for outcomes need to be realistic and the amount of rehabilitative work necessary must be clearly understood (see also Chapter 157).

Bursitis. NSAID therapy (e.g., 500 mg of naproxen twice daily for 1 to 2 weeks), in conjunction with reduced activity, often suffices. The jogger who has been running on uneven surfaces should change to another running surface. A *heel lift* may help the person whose legs are not the same length. If pain does not respond and if tenderness is well localized to the bursa overlying the bony prominence of the greater trochanter, a *local steroid injection* into the bursa can be attempted to provide relief. The bursa and trochanter are identified by having the patient lie in the lateral decubitus position with the involved hip exposed; the physician palpates for focal tenderness over the bony prominence of the greater trochanter. After 2 mL of 2% lidocaine has been mixed with 1 mL (40 mg/mL) of methylprednisolone (Depo-Medrol), 1 to 2 mL of the mixture is injected into the tender area overlying the bony prominence with a 25-gauge needle, inserted until it just touches the periosteal surface of the bone and then drawn back ever so slightly for the injection. Primary physicians who are unfamiliar with the technique of injecting a hip bursa should refer the patient to an orthopedist or rheumatologist.

Rheumatoid Disease. Polymyalgia rheumatica responds dramatically to low-dose steroids (see Chapter 161), and rheumatoid arthritis to high-dose aspirin or NSAIDs (see Chapter 156).

Hip Fracture and Septic Arthritis are indications for immediate hospitalization.

ANNOTATED BIBLIOGRAPHY

American Medical Association, Council on Scientific Affairs. Musculoskeletal applications of magnetic resonance imaging. JAMA 1989;262:2420. (*Most sensitive imaging study for avascular septic necrosis of the femoral head and stress fracture of the femoral neck.*)

Barclay TS, Tsourournis C, McCart GM. Glucosamine. Ann Pharmacother 1998;32:574. (*A review of current evidence for efficacy; finds little from well-designed studies.*)

Bradley JD, Brandt KD, Katz BP, et al. Comparison of an antiinflammatory dose of ibuprofen, an analgesic dose of ibuprofen, and acetaminophen in the treatment of patients with osteoarthritis of the knee. N Engl J Med 1991;325:87. (*Pure analgesic therapy as effective as NSAIDs.*)

Burton KE, Wright V, Richards J. Patient's expectations in relation to outcome of total hip replacement surgery. Ann Rheum Dis 1979;38:471. (*A still useful article making the important point that expectations are often in excess of reality; preoperative counseling is essential.*)

Creamer P, Hochberg MC. Osteoarthritis. Lancet 1997;350:503. (*Comprehensive, well-written review that includes a discussion of hip disease.*)

Griffin MR, Brandt KD, Liang MH, et al. Practical management of osteoarthritis: integration of pharmacologic and nonpharmacologic measures. Arch Fam Med 1995;4:1049. (*Another excellent review, with especially good section on nonpharmacologic measures.*)

Hartz AJ, Fischer ME, Bril G, et al. The association of obesity with joint pain in osteoarthritis in the HANES data. J Chron Dis 1986;39:311. (*Finds obesity a predictor of pain and arthritis, especially in women.*)

Liang MH, Fortin P. Management of osteoarthritis of the hip and knee. N Engl J Med 1991;325:125. (*An overview of the approach to diagnosis and treatment.*)

Paty JG. Diagnosis and treatment of musculoskeletal running injuries. Semin Arthritis Rheum 1988;18:48. (*Includes discussion of femoral neck stress fractures and hip bursitis.*)

Pelletier JP, Martel-Pelletier J. The therapeutic effects of NSAIDs and corticosteroids in osteoarthritis: to be or not to be. J Rheumatol 1989;16:266. (*A discussion of their effects on the underlying disease process.*)

Rashad S, Revell P, Hemingway A, et al. Effect of nonsteroidal antiinflammatory drugs on the clinical course of osteoarthritis. Lancet 1989;2:519. (*Evidence that NSAIDs may speed joint deterioration in persons with advanced hip disease.*)

152
Evaluation of Knee Pain

The knee joint is frequently the site of trauma, degenerative disease, and rheumatologic conditions. Disability can be considerable because of the inability to bear weight. The primary physician is called on most often to treat minor acute injuries or chronic knee pain that limits mobility. Occasionally, an acute monoarticular arthritis is encountered. The popularity of skiing, jogging, and long-distance running has markedly increased the prevalence of acute and recurrent knee complaints.

PATHOPHYSIOLOGY AND CLINICAL PRESENTATION

Degenerative disease, trauma-induced derangements of soft tissue, and inflammatory processes are the predominant mechanisms of knee pain in the adult. The pain is characteristically worsened by weight bearing and may radiate into the anterior thigh, posterior calf, or pretibial region. An inflamed joint capsule produces diffuse pain. The site of pain is characteristic of the underlying problem (Fig. 152.1). Locking of the joint suggests a loose body or torn meniscus. Hip disease occasionally presents as knee pain (see Chapter 151).

Degenerative Disease. Changes often originate in the medial joint compartment and patellofemoral joint, related in part to mechanical stresses. The entire joint may be painful, but often the discomfort is localized to the anterior and medial portions of the knee. Prolonged standing or walking may precipitate or worsen symptoms. Mild stiffness is common on first arising in the morning and on getting up after a long period of sitting. It initially improves on moving about, but worsens with continued activity. Symptoms gradually progress but may take many years to become disabling. Considerable degenerative

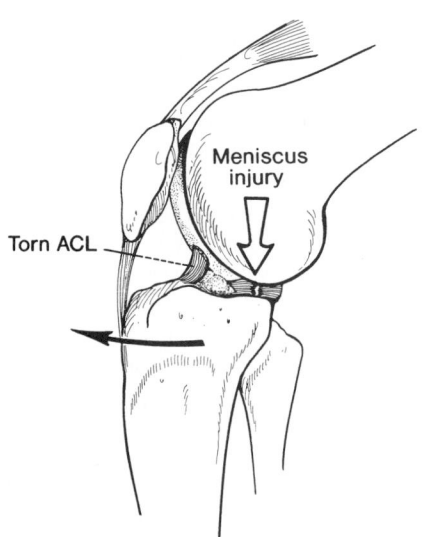

FIG. 152.1. Cruciate ligament tear with associated meniscal damage.

change and joint destruction can occur before serious knee pain develops. Small effusions may appear after prolonged weight bearing, but few other signs or symptoms of inflammation occur.

Rheumatoid Disease. Rheumatoid arthritis commonly affects the knees. Pain, swelling, and morning stiffness are characteristic. Symmetric polyarticular involvement is the rule, with joints in the hands, feet, ankles, and wrists often affected. Symptoms wax and wane; the course is chronic (see Chapter 156). Other rheumatoid diseases can produce a similar picture (see Chapter 146).

Acute Monoarticular Arthritis. The knee is a frequent site of septic arthritis, gout, pseudogout, early rheumatoid arthritis, rheumatic fever, palindromic rheumatism, and disseminated gonorrhea. Acute onset of unilateral swelling, pain, and generalized tenderness is the usual presentation (see Chapter 145). Motion is limited, and muscle spasm is prominent.

Knee Sprain. Ligamentous injury caused by excessive joint strain is extremely frequent. Sprain injuries ranging from minor tears of a few fibers to complete tears of entire ligaments result in a loss of joint stability. Mild sprains produce tenderness and local swelling without joint effusion or loss of joint stability. Moderate sprains are associated with pain when the joint is stressed, voluntary restriction of movement, some joint instability, and swelling secondary to an effusion. Severe sprains involve a total loss of integrity and immediate swelling, marked joint instability, severe pain, and a large effusion. The collateral and cruciate ligaments are frequently injured in contact sports. Ligamentous injuries are uncommon in joggers.

Tearing of the *anterior cruciate* ligament is a common sports-related knee injury; it accounts for the vast majority of sprains suffered in skiing. Typically, it occurs in the setting of sudden noncontact deceleration that causes valgus twisting of the knee. A "pop" is heard, and marked swelling ensues within a few hours because of intraarticular bleeding. The resulting subluxation of the tibia compresses the meniscus between the tibia and femur and may cause the cartilage to tear (see Fig. 152.1 and below). Initially after an anterior cruciate tear, the knee may function reasonably well, but instability develops on resumption of sports activity.

Degeneration or Tear of a Meniscus. An acute tear occurs as a consequence of excessive weight bearing, twisting, or valgus or varus stress and may be associated with the partial or complete disruption of collateral or cruciate ligaments. Usually, a history of acute trauma and immediate swelling, resulting from tissue disruption and bleeding, is elicited. A torn anterior cruciate ligament is a common precipitant of meniscal tear. If cartilaginous fragments become trapped, they cause the knee to lock. If swelling does not develop until the next day, damage is likely to be confined to the meniscus and not involve the ligament. Such swelling is caused by a reactive joint effusion. Chronic internal derangements caused by degeneration or tear of the meniscus produce recurrent pain and swelling, and a knee that gives way, catches, or locks.

Chondromalacia Patellae. Degeneration of the posterior patellar cartilage is the cause of this condition. Dessication, thinning, fissure formation, and ultimately erosion of the cartilage occur. Mechanical factors are suspected, although unproven. Chondromalacia is the most common cause of knee pain in joggers and is believed to be related to overtraining. The patient presents with retropatellar aching that is worsened by standing up, climbing stairs, or any other form of bent-knee strain. Stiffness may develop after inactivity, but usually no locking or giving way of the knee is noted. Pain is reported in the peripatellar region and lateral aspect of the knee and can be reproduced by applying pressure against the patella with the knee actively extended. Palpable grating can be elicited at the patellofemoral joint with flexion and extension of the knee. Radiographic findings are normal until late stages, when the posterior surface of the patella becomes irregular and marginal osteophytes develop.

Baker's Cyst. Rupture of one of these popliteal fossa cysts can cause acute inflammation with pain, swelling, and limitation of knee flexion. The inflammation may extend down into the calf and simulate thrombophlebitis. Baker's cysts usually communicate with the knee joint space and most commonly occur in patients with osteoarthritis or rheumatoid disease. An unruptured cyst causes only mild aching and stiffness. Trauma may initiate a rupture.

Prepatellar Bursitis results from repeated trauma—hence the name "housemaid's knee." Swelling, tenderness, and occasionally erythema over the prepatellar bursae are present. The presentations of bursitis of the suprapatellar and infrapatellar bursae are similar, with findings localized to the bursal site.

Villonodular Synovitis is a granulomatous inflammatory condition of the synovium that lines the joints, bursae, and tendon sheaths. The cause is unknown. It affects young adults, predominantly men, and presents with unilateral pain, persistent swelling, intermittent knee locking, and occasionally a palpable mass. Diagnosis requires arthroscopy or surgical exploration.

DIFFERENTIAL DIAGNOSIS

The list of conditions that can cause knee pain is extensive and includes polyarticular disease in addition to processes confined to the knee. A clinically useful classification system groups causes of knee pain according to whether the pain is acute or chronic, and whether the distribution is symmetric or asymmetric and monoarticular or polyarticular (Table 152.1).

WORKUP

History

Besides ascertaining the quality and location of pain, alleviating and aggravating factors, and associated symptoms such as swelling, redness, and warmth, the physician must determine whether the problem is acute or chronic, symmetric or asymmetric, and monoarticular or polyarticular. By combining a careful description of the problem with a characterization of its pattern and chronicity, one can quickly focus the evaluation onto a relatively limited set of conditions having similar clinical presentations (Table 152.1).

Acute Unilateral Knee Pain. One should inquire about trauma, jogging, locking, giving out, swelling, pain on climbing stairs, concurrent fever, purulent vaginal or urethral discharge, rash, recent streptococcal infection or sore throat, heart murmur, morning stiffness, and urethritis or conjunctivitis (see Chapter 145). Any prior history of gout, sickle cell disease, or hemophilia should be ascertained. When swelling is localized, it is important to determine the exact site because it may be a clue to bursitis or a Baker's cyst. A history of knee locking suggests meniscal tear with lodging of cartilaginous fragments in the joint space. Reports of the knee giving out point to anterior cruciate disruption.

Chronic Unilateral Knee Pain. Questioning should cover previous or recurrent trauma, as may occur occupationally; pain associated with prolonged walking, standing, or climbing stairs; knee locking; crepitus; focal swelling; and recurrent acute episodes or exacerbations.

Acute Bilateral Knee Pain. When both knees are involved acutely, then the focus of inquiry should be on the symptoms of rheumatoid disease (see Chapter 146) and recent trauma.

Chronic Bilateral Knee Pain. The questioning can be similar to that for chronic unilateral disease, but rheumatoid symptoms should also be considered (see Chapter 146).

Polyarticular Presentations. When other joints are also involved, inquiry into symptoms of infectious and rheumatologic conditions is essential (see Chapter 146).

Physical Examination

A complete physical examination must be performed because many systemic illnesses can present with knee pain. Skin and integument are examined for rash, clubbing, psoriatic changes, rheumatoid nodules, pallor, alopecia, and tophi. The conjunctivae are noted for erythema and petechiae, the oral cavity for aphthous ulcers, lymph nodes for enlargement, the chest for signs of consolidation and effusion, the heart for murmurs and rubs, the abdomen for organomegaly and tenderness, the pelvis for vaginal discharge and adnexal tenderness, the urethra for discharge, and the penis for balanitis. In addition, a thorough check of all joints and complete neurologic testing should be performed.

Examination of the knee should begin with a careful inspection for distortion of normal contours and irregular bony prominences at the joint margin. It is important to check for muscle atrophy. Measurements of the knee, calf, and thigh circumferences can help quantify the loss of muscle mass. The presence of an effusion needs to be determined. This is done by noting an increased knee circumference at midpatella and feeling for a distended, fluctuant capsule with a fluid wave and ballotable patella. The joint line should be palpated for localized

Table 152.1.   Differential Diagnosis of Knee Pain

| Asymmetric Involvement | | | | Symmetric Involvement | | | |
| One Knee Only | | One Knee Plus Other Joints | | Knees Only | | Symmetric Polyarthritis | |
ACUTE	CHRONIC	ACUTE	CHRONIC	ACUTE	CHRONIC	ACUTE	CHRONIC
Sprain	Osteoarthritis	See Chapters 145, 146		Rheumatoid arthritis	Osteoarthritis	See Chapter 146	
Strain	Baker's cyst			Juvenile RA	Chondromalacia patellae		
Acute gout	Chronic gout			Early phase of other rheumatoid diseases	Bursitis		
Meniscus tear	Chondromalacia patella			Trauma	Rheumatoid arthritis		
Early rheumatoid disease	Bursitis				Juvenile RA		
Gonococcal arthritis	Meniscal injuries				Chronic gout		
Septic arthritis					Neuropathic joints		
Reiter's syndrome					Hemophilia		
Bursitis							
Pseudogout							
Pallindromic rheumatism							
Ruptured Baker's cyst							
Hemophilia							
Sickle cell disease							
Rheumatic fever							

Adapted from Katz WA. Rheumatic diseases. Philadelphia, JB Lippincott Co, 1977, with permission.

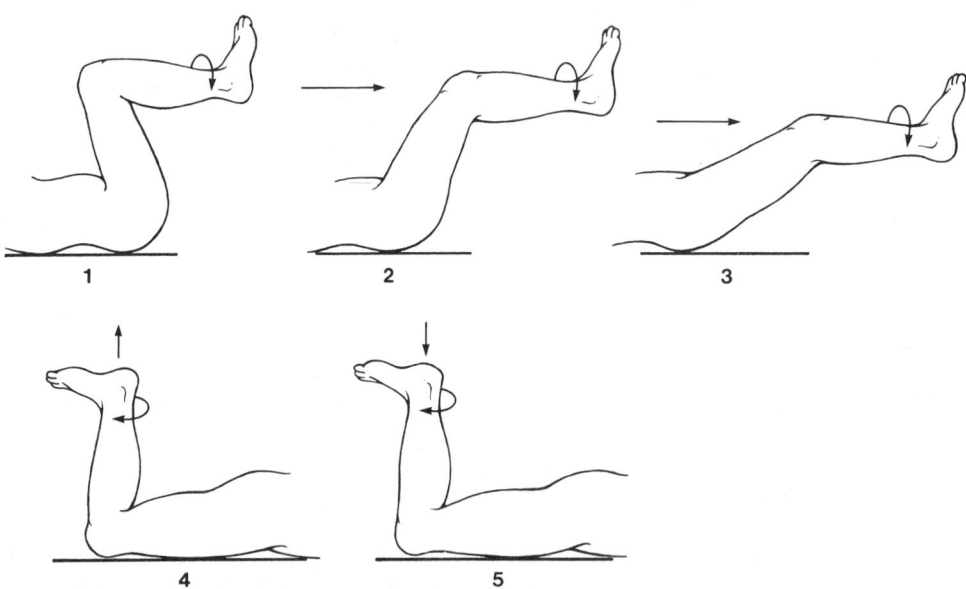

FIG. 152.2.   Meniscus signs (examination). *1,2,3,* McMurray test. The patient is supine with knee flexed, heel touching the buttocks at the start. The leg is internally rotated to test the lateral meniscus or externally rotated to test the medial meniscus. Then the knee is fully extended. A painful click occurs if a meniscus lesion is present. The test is more meaningful in the first phase of knee extension. Limited extension does not indicate a lesion of the anterior meniscus. *4,5,* Apley test. The patient is prone. The leg is internally or externally rotated with simultaneous traction. Pain indicates a capsular or ligamentous lesion. Pain caused by rotation with downward pressure indicates a meniscus lesion. (Redrawn from Cailliet R. Knee pain and disability. Philadelphia: FA Davis Co, 1973, with permission.)

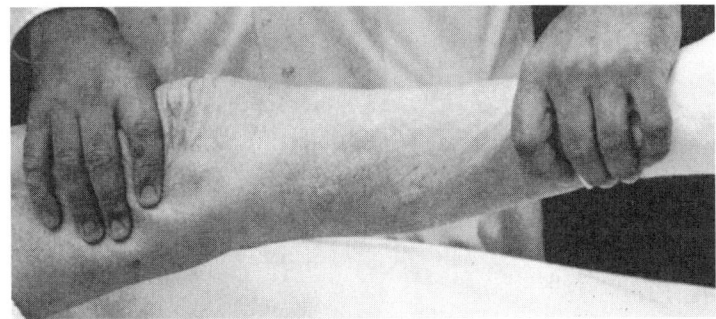

FIG. 152.3. Testing for lateral instability of the knee by fixating the lower femur with one hand and forcibly abducting and adducting the joint while grasping the leg. (From Katz WA. Rheumatic diseases. Philadelphia: JB Lippincott Co, 1977.)

joint line tenderness suggestive of a meniscal tear. The *McMurray* and *Apley tests* are performed for suspected meniscal injury (Fig. 152.2). The bursal regions should be assessed for focal tenderness and swelling indicative of bursitis.

Range of motion needs to be determined. The knees normally extend symmetrically 180 degrees and may hyperextend an additional 5 or 10 degrees. Knee flexion is also symmetric and limited to 135 to 170 degrees by contact with posterior soft-tissue or by striking of the heel against the buttock. Collateral and cruciate ligaments should be examined for stability. Collateral ligaments are tested by applying mediolateral valgus–varus strain with the knee in full extension and in 15 to 20 degrees of flexion (Fig. 152.3).

Anterior cruciate ligament stability is best assessed by the *anterior drawer test*, which is performed with the knee relaxed and flexed to about 25 degrees. One gently pulls the tibia anteriorly while the femur is held in a fixed position and notes the amount of anterior displacement of the tibia relative to the femur. Patients who describe a knee that repeatedly gives out may have anterior cruciate instability, which can be assessed by testing for pivotal shift. The validity of these tests has been confirmed by arthroscopic study. They are important parts of the examination of the injured knee.

Laboratory Studies

No set of laboratory studies is "routinely" used to assess knee pain. In cases of trauma, *radiography* is needed to rule out fracture, and stress films are indicated to determine joint stability. Knee films are also indicated for suspected degenerative or chronic rheumatoid disease. Weight-bearing films best demonstrate the degree of joint obliteration. *Magnetic resonance imaging* (MRI) has enhanced the diagnosis of disease in the soft tissues of the knee. Its sensitivity for the detection of meniscal tear exceeds 90% (better than that of arthrography), and for cruciate tear it reaches 95%. However, MRI remains expensive. The test is best reserved for instances in which the clinical findings are not sufficient to establish a diagnosis and an invasive diagnostic procedure would otherwise be necessary. *Fiberoptic arthroscopy* remains the gold standard for the diagnosis of problems in the soft tissues of the knee. Acute monoarticular effusions require prompt *arthrocentesis* for Gram's stain and cultures to rule out a septic process. Joint fluid is sent for determination of the white cell count, differential, and glucose

level and is examined for crystals (see Chapter 145). With polyarticular presentations, testing for inflammatory joint disease must be considered (see Chapter 146).

SYMPTOMATIC THERAPY AND INDICATIONS FOR REFERRAL

For the patient with a knee injury, *acute pain* responds best to restriction of weight-bearing activities and the use of crutches. A *knee brace* is applied to provide support and prevent further injury by limiting the range of motion. Only absolutely necessary walking is allowed, and kneeling, squatting, and stair climbing are forbidden. *Aspirin* may be helpful symptomatically when used in pharmacologic doses of 2 to 4 g/d. Otherwise, any one of the other *NSAIDs* is a reasonable alternative (e.g., 375 mg of naproxen twice daily or 400 mg of ibuprofen three times daily). Once swelling subsides and the full range of motion without pain returns, rehabilitation can begin. One starts with isometric *quadriceps* and *hamstring exercises*. These help prevent muscle atrophy, weakness, and thinning of ligamentous tissue. If the problem is one of acute severe injury and pain, especially if the knee gives way or locks and joint instability or internal derangement is suspected, prompt orthopedic referral is essential. Arthroscopy may be needed.

Patients who have *chronic knee pain* associated with osteoarthritis have been shown to benefit from both *aerobic exercise* and *resistance exercise* in randomized trials. In a recent trial, the benefit for aerobic exercise was modestly better than that for resistance exercise, but either was better than an education program without exercise. No evidence of more rapid disease progression was found with either form of exercise. These approaches should complement other measures for the general treatment of osteoarthritis. NSAIDs have not be shown to be superior to non-narcotic analgesics, such as acetaminophen, for providing control of chronic pain caused by osteoarthritis of the knee. Although glucosamine is popular, its effectiveness has not been demonstrated in well-designed studies; moreover, it is expensive (see also Chapter 157).

A.G.M.

ANNOTATED BIBLIOGRAPHY

Barclay TS, Tsourournis C, McCart GM. Glucosamine. Ann Pharmacother 1998;32:574. (*A review of current evidence for efficacy; finds little from well-designed studies.*)

Bradley JD, Brandt KD, Katz BP, et al. Comparison of an antiinflammatory dose of ibuprofen, an analgesic dose of ibuprofen, and acetaminophen in the treatment of patients with osteoarthritis of the knee. N Engl J Med 1991;325:87. (*Pure analgesic therapy as effective as NSAIDs.*)

Council on Scientific Affairs, American Medical Association. Musculoskeletal applications of magnetic resonance imaging. JAMA 1989;262:2420. (*Finds MRI sensitive in the diagnosis of torn cruciate ligaments and menisci.*)

Cox JS. Chondromalacia of the patella: a review and update. Contemp Orthop 1983;6:17. (*Detailed description of the problem.*)

Ettinger WH, Burns R, Messier SP, et al. A randomized trial comparing aerobic exercise and resistance exercise with a health education program in older adults with knee osteoarthritis. JAMA 1997;227:25. (*Aerobic exercise and resistance exercise responsible for 10% and 8% improvement in symptoms, respectively.*)

Hochberg MC, Altman RD, Brandt KD, et al. Guidelines for the medical management of knee osteoarthritis. Arthritis Rheum 1995; 38:1541. (*Comprehensive advice for medical approach to minimizing disability.*)

Kovar PA, Allegrante JP, MacKenzie CR, et al. Supervised fitness walking in patients with osteoarthritis of the knee. Ann Intern Med 1992;116:529. (*Pain and disability decreased while fitness increased.*)

Paty JG. Diagnosis and treatment of musculoskeletal running injuries. Semin Arthritis Rheum 1988;18:48. (*Good description of overuse syndromes.*)

Rejeski WJ, Ettinger WH, Shumaker S, et al. The evaluation of pain in patients with knee osteoarthritis: the knee pain scale. J Rheumtol 1995;22:1124. (*Addresses intensity of knee pain associated with six activities of daily living to obtain a summary pain intensity score.*)

Spector T, Harris PA, Hart DJ, et al. Risk of osteoarthritis associated with long-term weight-bearing sports. Arthritis Rheum 1996; 39:988. (*Supports hypothesis that long-term, high-intensity exercise increases risk.*)

Zarins B, Adams M. Knee injuries in sports. N Engl J Med 1988;318;950. (*Authoritative review with particularly good discussion of anterior cruciate tear and resulting meniscal injury.*)

153

Approach to Minor Orthopedic Problems of the Elbow, Wrist, and Hand

JESSE B. JUPITER
DAVID RING

As the physician of first contact, the primary care practitioner encounters a host of minor upper etremity complaints that may be causing the patient considerable discomfort. Quick recognition and proper treatment can save the patient an unnecessary referral and allow for prompt symptomatic relief.

ELBOW PAIN

The evaluation of elbow pain requires a careful correlation of the presenting symptoms with the specific anatomic site. The elbow is particularly subject to overuse syndromes, inflammatory conditions, and localized nerve entrapments. A careful history and physical examination are often all that is required to reach an accurate diagnosis and formulate a treatment plan.

Lateral Epicondylitis ("Tennis Elbow") denotes inflammation at the common tendinous origin of the extensor muscles of the forearm, in particular the extensor carpi radialis brevis, on the humeral lateral epicondyle. It is the result of repetitive overuse, as occurs when tennis players use backhand strokes or people knit. The common denominator is a strong grasp during wrist extension. The patient describes pain on the lateral aspect of the elbow. The physical examination reveals tenderness over the lateral epicondyle (Fig. 153.1), pain during resisted wrist extension with the elbow extended, and reproduction of symptoms during resisted extension of the elbow with the forearm in pronation and the wrist in palmar flexion. Radiographic findings are normal. It is often difficult to distinguish a radial nerve entrapment syndrome from lateral epicondylitis.

The management of epicondylitis consists of reducing the inflammatory component, strengthening the involved muscle, and understanding and avoiding the precipitating factors. It may take several weeks for pain to disappear. Any painful activity is best avoided, including racquet sports, handshake, forceful use of the arm in hammering or unscrewing jars, and use of a screwdriver. There is no certain way to prevent recurrences of epicondylitis related to playing tennis, but proper stroking of shots with a firm wrist and proper elbow positioning may be helpful. *Forearm bands* are often tried but usually are of limited value; however, sometimes they allow play when mild pain is present.

Systemic *antiinflammatory medication* (e.g., 375 mg of *naproxen* twice daily or 600 mg of *ibuprofen* three times daily for 1 week) often provides relief of symptoms and may help abate the process. Local steroid injection may eventually be needed, although results may not be very dramatic. Injection is best reserved for refractory cases. The area of well-localized tenderness is carefully identified and injected with 1 mL of 2% lidocaine (Xylocaine), then with 20 mg of dexamethasone. If symptoms recur after an initially successful injection, the patient may request additional injections. Repeated steroid injection incurs some risk of tendon and fascial rupture and may be associated with other problems, such as discoloration or atrophy of the overlying skin. We rarely administer more than three injections and prefer to space the injections at least 4 to 6 months apart.

Physical therapists can teach patients a set of exercises they can perform at home to stretch and condition the involved muscles. They may also recommend friction massage, ultrasound, and other modalities. Many patients obtain relief from such alternative modalities, but few data are available to support their use.

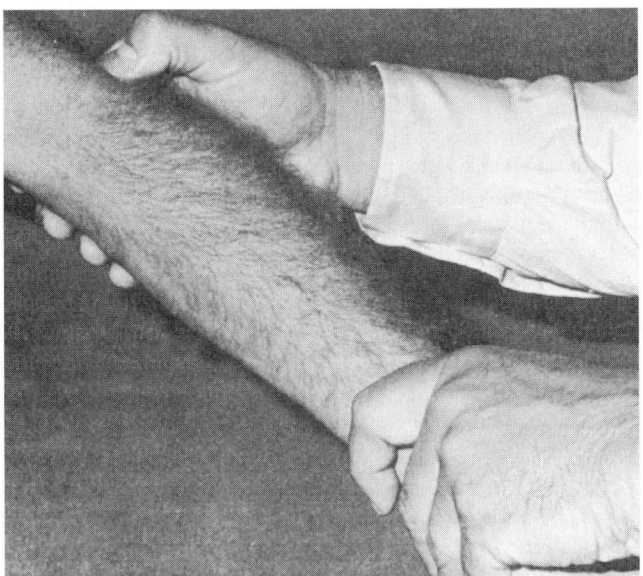

FIG. 153.1. Technique of palpating the lateral epicondyle to elicit "point" tenderness, typical of "tennis elbow." (From Katz WA. Rheumatic diseases. Philadelphia: JB Lippincott Co, 1977.)

In most cases, a program of rest, application of ice, NSAIDs, and physical therapy is successful in reducing symptoms and permitting a return to function. In the unusual recalcitrant case, operative treatment may be considered.

Medial Epicondylitis ("Golfer's Elbow") is similar to "tennis elbow" but involves the common forearm flexor origin at the humeral medial epicondyle. Occasionally seen in golfers, it more commonly is associated with certain manual or household activities. The pain is localized to the region of the medial epicondyle and is reproduced by forcefully extending the elbow against resistance with the forearm in supination and the wrist in dorsiflexion. Radiographic findings are normal. Treatment is the same as for lateral epicondylitis. The possibility of a median or ulnar nerve entrapment syndrome should be considered.

Olecranon Bursitis. The clinical presentation is a painful swelling over the posterior aspect of the elbow. The swollen bursa is usually fluctuant and can be transilluminated. Localized trauma or repetitive local pressure associated with certain occupations is the most common cause, but this bursitis can also be a manifestation of such inflammatory conditions as rheumatoid arthritis, gout, or sepsis. Patients with septic bursitis commonly report a history of antecedent trauma and cellulitis of the skin, followed by localized swelling, redness, and tenderness about the elbow. Almost all cases of septic olecranon represent spread from a contiguous soft-tissue infection. Gram's stain of the bursal fluid is positive for the causative organism in about 50% of instances. *Staphylococcus aureus* is the most common isolate, found in 80% of cases; streptococcal species account for most of the remainder. The presentation of septic bursitis in the immunocompromised patient is similar.

Unless sepsis is suspected, one should avoid aspiration or corticosteroid injection because of the possibility of introducing infection. The use of antiinflammatory medication and a sling as needed and local protection to avoid pressure are the basic treatment approaches. The presence of septic bursitis should be confirmed with needle aspiration and analysis of the fluid for cell counts, Gram's stain, culture, and sensitivities. Treatment with aspiration followed by organism-specific parenteral antibiotics is usually effective. On rare occasions, operative debridement may be required.

Nerve Entrapment Syndromes. Pain in the elbow or forearm may be secondary to compression of the ulnar nerve in the cubital tunnel, the posterior interosseous nerve in the proximal forearm, or even the median nerve in the forearm or wrist. With ulnar nerve compression, pain may be felt beneath the medial epicondyle, and the patient may experience numbness in the pinky and ring finger. Intrinsic muscle weakness is also commonly noted on examination. The presentation of posterior interosseous nerve compression is similar to that of tennis elbow, but symptoms are reproduced by extension of the middle finger against resistance (see also Chapter 167). The treatment of ulnar nerve compression can be as simple as avoidance of leaning on the elbow and nighttime use of a splint that holds the elbow in extension. Use of a protective pad may help. If entrapment is accompanied by muscle atrophy or does not respond to simple measures, referral is required.

Arthritis

The elbow is not a common site for osteoarthritis, but arthritis may be found in association with prior fracture or dislocation. In contrast, elbow involvement is common in rheumatoid arthritis. On examination, limitation of motion, swelling, and pain are common findings. Radiographs demonstrate the extent of joint space involvement. Antiinflammatory agents provide good relief (see Chapter 156).

Septic Arthritis. Most cases are the result of blood-borne infection, manifested by the rapid onset of pain, diffuse joint swelling, and erythema. Systemic symptoms are common. It is important to rule out underlying conditions such as diabetes mellitus, steroid treatment, or rheumatoid arthritis. If sepsis is suspected, arthrocentesis for Gram's stain and culture of the joint fluid is required (see Chapter 145). The differential diagnosis of an acute monoarthritis includes gout and pseudogout (calcium pyrophosphate deposition), both of which can be difficult to distinguish from infection before aspiration and fluid analysis have been performed. Treatment of confirmed infection includes operative debridement and IV administration of organism-specific antibiotics.

HAND AND WRIST PAIN

Carpal Tunnel Syndrome is an important cause of work disability and is often blamed on repetitive motion. However, such activity may be only a precipitant rather than the cause. In many cases, an underlying, often undiagnosed, medical condition renders the patient susceptible. Leading causes include hypothyroidism, inflammatory joint disease, osteoarthritis of the wrist, and recent trauma. Typically, the patient reports nocturnal symptoms, including hand and wrist pain and paresthesias that are often relieved by shaking the hand. Numbness is common, affecting the middle or three radial fingers and occasionally the thumb. A number of systemic conditions are associated with carpal tunnel syndrome, including diabetes mellitus, hypothyroidism, inflammatory arthritis, and pregnancy.

Clinical findings can be helpful in the diagnosis. With the aid of a diagram to help patients specify their hand symptoms, the history was found to have a sensitivity of 64% and a specificity of 73%. The physical examination is not much more sensitive or specific but may reveal suggestive findings. For example, altered sensibility may be noted in the thumb, index, and long fingers and the radial side of the ring finger; one may find changes only in one or two digits. Thenar (base of the thumb) muscle atrophy is present in prolonged or profound median nerve compression. *Tinel's sign*, elicited by tapping over the median nerve at the wrist crease, consists of "electric shocks" or paresthesias in the median nerve distribution. *Phelan's test* is performed by having the patient maintain the wrists in palmar flexion for 1 minute. The test result is considered positive and consistent with carpal tunnel syndrome if the patient's symptoms are reproduced. A negative result of Phelan's test or the absence of Tinel's sign does not necessarily rule out the presence of carpal tunnel syndrome. Reported sensitivities and specificities for Tinel's sign and Phelan's test range from 47% to 90%.

Definitive diagnosis can be made by *nerve conduction study* and *electromyography* (EMG). Testing is indicated if the diagnosis is unclear or if the condition persists and some numbness or weakness appears. In a patient with carpal tunnel syndrome, EMG and nerve conduction study demonstrate an increase in motor or sensory latency, which is helpful in documenting the location and degree of nerve compression. Correlating the clinical findings with the neurophysiologic test results is necessary for an accurate diagnosis because as many as 50% of asymptomatic patients may have abnormal results on nerve conduction or EMG studies.

Conservative therapy for carpal tunnel syndrome consists of wrist splinting, control of any underlying systemic metabolic disorder, and occasional local injection of corticosteroids. A firm canvas or plaster *wrist splint* worn during sleep prevents wrist positions of extreme dorsiflexion or palmar flexion, which tend to increase the local compression within the carpal tunnel. In those patients with a significant flexor tenosynovitis, an *injection of corticosteroids* (e.g., 0.5 to 1 mL of dexamethasone plus 1 to 2 mL of lidocaine) directly into the carpal tunnel may be of value. The injection is placed just proximal to the transverse retinacular ligament in the wrist. If a paresthesia is elicited, a more superficial needle placement is made to avoid injecting into the nerve. Steroid injection has been found in randomized, controlled studies to provide long-term relief to a majority of patients and obviate the need for surgery in most. *Surgical intervention* is considered if symptoms persist longer than 3 months, if an associated thenar muscle atrophy develops, or if the motor or sensory latencies on the EMG and nerve conduction studies are extremely prolonged.

De Quervain's Tenosynovitis. On the dorsal aspect of the wrist, the extensor tendons to the hand and wrist course through six well-defined compartments. The first dorsal compartment contains the abductor pollicis longus and the extensor pollicis brevis and is located just proximal and radial to the anatomic "snuff box." A relatively common disorder is a nonspecific subacute or chronic inflammation of these tendons within the first dorsal compartment. Pain is exacerbated by use of the thumb and is reproduced when the patient, with the wrist in ulnar deviation and palmar flexion, grasps the thumb with the adjacent digits (Finkelstein's test). This test differentiates tendinitis from any underlying arthritis. The usual aggravating factor is excessive repetitive work with the hand, such as needlepoint, knitting, or peeling vegetables.

Most patients respond to nonoperative treatment consisting of splinting and steroid injection. An injection preparation such as that described for carpal tunnel syndrome is carefully placed within the first dorsal extensor compartment, which has a somewhat more radial and volar location than one might think. Care is exercised to inject just above the abductor pollicis longus. A removable plaster or Orthoplast splint holding the wrist and thumb in slight dorsiflexion and radial deviation is worn for 10 to 14 days except for bathing. Oral NSAIDs may also be of use. Failure to respond should be considered an indication for surgical referral.

Trigger Finger. Tenosynovitis also commonly involves the flexor tendons to the digits or thumb at the level of the metacarpophalangeal joints just proximal to the first annular pulley of the flexor tendon sheath. Snapping of the digit (triggering) with use and locking, or the inability to extend the proximal interphalangeal joint, are the characteristic presenting symptoms. Often, the patient perceives the triggering to be at the level of the PIP joint. A palpable thickening of the flexor tendon may be felt at the level of the metacarpophalangeal joint in the palm.

Treatment consists of splinting, corticosteroid injection, and NSAIDs. The steroid–lidocaine combination is injected just proximal to the distal palmar crease, where the first annular pulley of the flexor sheath is located. Such treatment is effective in almost 90% of cases, and the risk for serious adverse reactions is minimal.

Ganglion Cysts. Ganglionic cysts are the most common mass occurring in the hand or wrist and may be found in a number of sites, including the dorsum of the wrist, where the origin is the scapholunate ligament. Another common location is on the radial volar surface of the wrist directly adjacent to (and not to be confused with) the radial artery. Ganglia are thought to be outpouchings of the wrist capsule and contain fluid very similar to joint fluid. Their origin (stalk) is in the wrist joint, which explains the high incidence of recurrence when treatment methods such as aspiration or the traditional home remedy of striking the cyst with a heavy object (e.g., a Bible!) are used.

Most ganglia require no treatment. Aspiration with a large-bore (16- or 19-gauge) needle is helpful if the diagnosis is in doubt; however, even with steroid injection, the recurrence rate is high. Surgical treatment is indicated if the cyst is painful, the appearance is unsatisfactory, or the exact nature of the mass is a concern.

Mucous Cysts, associated with degenerative arthritis of the interphalangeal joints of the digits or thumb, are outpouchings of joint fluid similar to wrist ganglia. Radiographs show joint space narrowing and, often, marginal spurs or osteophytes. Osteophytes alone are the cause of the so-called Heberden's node at the distal interphalangeal joint and Bouchard's node at the proximal interphalangeal joint.

Arthritis. Degenerative joint disease commonly affects the carpometacarpal joint at the base of the thumb (see Chapter

157). Most often affecting women, the condition is associated with localized pain, decreased dexterity, and diminished grip strength. Pain and crepitation can be elicited if the examiner grasps the thumb metacarpal and compresses it onto the trapezium (grind test). Radiographic changes may vary from mild joint space narrowing to complete joint space loss and the presence of osteophytes and loose bodies.

Once recognized, mild to moderate arthritis of the trapeziometacarpal joint of the thumb can be effectively managed with NSAIDs and a molded splint worn 4 to 6 hours daily. The splint extends beyond the metacarpophalangeal joint but leaves the wrist free (a short opponens splint). It should be custom-made by a trained occupational therapist.

The hand involvement in *rheumatoid arthritis* can vary from minimal pain and swelling to extensive deformity and joint destruction. Treatment includes pharmacologic and physical therapy (see Chapter 156). Tendon rupture is not uncommon; its occurrence should prompt early referral.

Hand Infections are potentially serious conditions, especially if they occur in a closed compartment. Presentations vary. Infection around the fingernail is termed *paronychia* and is usually caused by gram-positive organisms. Antibiotics and warm soaks suffice in mild, well-localized cases, but any spread requires referral for incision and drainage. A *felon* is a more worrisome problem because it is an infection in a closed compartment, the pulp space of the tip of the digit. The pulp is swollen, exquisitely tender, and erythematous. If not corrected, the edema can compromise arterial supply and lead to necrosis of the fingertip. Treatment includes incision, drainage, and administration of antibiotics. Early referral to a hand surgeon is essential for definitive treatment. A less troublesome infection, seen mostly in hospital personnel and children, is *herpetic infection* of the fingertip, which is characterized by the appearance of small vesicles along the pulp. It clears spontaneously, although the patient is infectious until the vesicles clear.

In *infectious flexor tenosynovitis*, the patient presents with a digit that is symmetrically swollen, painful along the entire flexor sheath, flexed, and tender on passive extension of the distal joint. Prompt recognition and, in many cases, surgical intervention are critical to preserve ultimate tendon function.

Puncture wounds, in particular human bites, may result in extremely virulent infection. Prompt and aggressive wound care, with the puncture site left open, and antibiotic treatment may abort a more serious and destructive process. Animal bites, especially from dogs and cats, can transmit *Pasteurella multocida*, which in most instances is extremely sensitive to penicillin (see Chapter 196).

SUMMARY

Localization of symptoms provides the keystone for evaluation. The examiner should attempt to determine the precise area of tenderness. A thorough functional examination (active and passive motions of the wrist, digits, and thumb; sensory testing with light touch and pinprick; determination of specific flexor and extensor tendon function) should be part of every assessment of the patient with a hand problem. Standard anteroposterior and lateral radiographs are generally advisable in most cases. EMG and a nerve conduction study are part of the workup for peripheral nerve compression.

Nonspecific tenosynovitis and mild to moderate degenerative arthritis generally respond to antiinflammatory medication and simple splinting (discussed earlier). The patient with a hand infection, fracture, nerve compression, or mass should be referred to a hand specialist.

ANNOTATED BIBLIOGRAPHY

Anderson B, Kaye S. Treatment of flexor tenosynovitis of the hand ("trigger finger") with corticosteroids. Arch Intern Med 1991;151:153. (*A prospective study; found to be safe and effective.*)

Atcheson SG, Ward JR, Lowe W. Concurrent medical disease in work-related carpal tunnel syndrome. Arch Intern Med 1998;158:1506. (*High prevalence of underlying medical disease found.*)

Atroshi I, Gummesson C, Johnsson R, et al. Prevalence of carpal tunnel syndrome in a general population. JAMA 1999;282:153. (*Large-scale epidemiologic study. The prevalence of hand complaints is high, and carpal tunnel syndrome is likely to be diagnosed in one in five symptomatic subjects after full evaluation.*)

Bernhang AM. The many causes of tennis elbow. N Y State J Med 1979;79:1363. (*Excellent overview of the subject.*)

Dammers JWHH, Veering MM, Vermeulen M. Injection with methylprednisolone proximal to the carpal tunnel: randomized double-blind trial. BMJ 1999;319:884. (*Single injection produced significant improvement in outcomes and often obviated the need for surgery.*)

Katz JN, Lew RA, Bessette L, et al. Prevalence and predictors of long-term disability due to carpal tunnel syndrome. Am J Ind Med 1998;33:543. (*Useful data applicable in determining who is at risk for long-term disability.*)

Katz JN, Larson MG, Sabra A, et al. The carpal tunnel syndrome: diagnostic utility of the history and physical examination findings. Ann Intern Med 1990;112:321. (*Sensitivities and specificities for history and physical examination analyzed.*)

Katz JN, Stirrat CR, Larson MG, et al. A self-administered hand symptom diagram for the diagnosis and epidemiologic study of carpal tunnel syndrome. J Rheumatol 1990;17:1495. (*Sensitivity of 64%, specificity of 73%.*)

Roschmann RA, Bell CL. Septic arthritis in immunocompromised patients. Am J Med 1987;83:861. (*Good description of clinical findings; presentation similar to that in immunocompetent patients.*)

154

Approach to Minor Orthopedic Problems of the Foot and Ankle

JESSE B. JUPITER
DAVID RING

Patients often consult primary physicians for advice and help regarding foot or ankle problems. Although some patients require orthopedic referral for more detailed investigation and treatment, many can be substantially helped by the nonorthopedist physician who is knowledgeable about the diagnosis and treatment of common foot and ankle complaints. Such disorders are extremely prevalent and can incapacitate a patient. The primary care physician should be familiar with the basic types of foot and ankle complaints, so as to be able to treat minor conditions effectively and refer appropriately those problems that require the skills of an orthopedic surgeon.

FOOT PROBLEMS

Foot disorders are a major cause of disability in the work force. Although often the result of normal activity, foot pain can also be precipitated by structural deformity or systemic disease. Environmental factors, such as shoe type and weight-bearing surface, add to the development and progression of symptoms.

Anatomically, the human foot has 26 bones, comprising one fourth of those in the entire skeleton, along with 100 or more ligaments, 12 extrinsic muscle insertions, and 19 intrinsic muscles. During gait, more than two times the force of body weight is borne by the foot. In normal gait, the foot assumes several roles, including that of a shock absorber, a mobile adapter to ac-

Table 154.1.   Common Causes of Foot Pain

Digital Deformities
   Hammer toe
   Claw toe
   Mallet toe

Forefoot Pain—Great Toe
   Hallux valgus (bunion)
   Hallux limitus/rigidus
   Sesamoid disorders

Forefoot Pain—Other Structures
   Tailor's bunion (bunionette)
   Metatarsalgia
   Morton's interdigital neuroma
   Metatarsal stress fracture

Hindfoot Pain—Plantar
   Plantar fasciitis
   Infracalcaneal bursitis
   Medial calcaneal nerve entrapment
   Tarsal tunnel syndrome
   Referred pain from subtalar arthritis or lumbosacral disk radiculopathy

Hindfoot Pain—Posterior
   Posterior calcaneal bursitis
   Exostosis ("pump bump")
   Achilles tendinitis
   Inflammatory arthritis

commodate uneven surfaces, and a rigid lever to propel the limb. Limitation or excess of these primary functions places the foot at risk for acquired mechanical trauma, with the prime candidates being the flat (pes planus) and high-arched (pes cavus) feet. Foot disorders are conveniently considered by anatomic zones: digits, forefoot, and hindfoot (Table 154.1). Office assessment is facilitated by familiarity with the location and manifestations of common foot problems (Fig. 154.1).

Digital Problems

Problems referable to the toes usually are related to deformities. Most digital problems present as sagittal plane deformities. The three types are *hammer toe*, *mallet toe*, and *claw toe*. Pain with or without a "corn" (clavus) is usually the primary complaint. Toe contractures develop secondary to muscle imbalances or are shoe-induced; they can be flexible or rigid. Shoes (prescription or commercial) that provide adequate room in the toe box area are the first line of treatment. If the contractures are flexible, digital splints may be helpful. In persistent or progressive disease, surgery may be necessary if foot pain compromises daily activity.

Forefoot Problems

First Metatarsophalangeal Joint. The most common deformity of this joint is the *hallux valgus*, or *bunion*. It presents as a painful swelling on the dorsomedial aspect of the first metatarsal head, associated with lateral drift of the toe. The deformity or foot–shoe incompatibility may be the presenting complaint, but just as frequently, the patient presents with secondary adjacent problems, such as hammer toes or metatarsalgia. Hyperpronation (flat feet) and inappropriate shoes (high heels, pointed toe box) contribute to the development of the painful bunion, particularly in women.

On examination, a tender bursa is often present over the inner side of the head of the first metatarsal. The great toe itself may deviate laterally and at times is not even passively reducible. Radiographs may show the underlying cause to be an increased angle between the first and second metatarsals (normal, 10 to 12 degrees). This deformity is also commonly seen in patients with rheumatoid arthritis.

Properly fitted shoes (commercial or custom-made), bunion shields, and orthotic devices can afford symptomatic relief to many patients. Surgical intervention may be required to correct the structural deformity.

Hallux limitus, or *hallux rigidus*, is characterized by limited or total loss of dorsiflexion of the first metatarsophalangeal (MTP) joint and a dorsal "bunion." The patient usually has pain while walking or problems with shoe fitting.

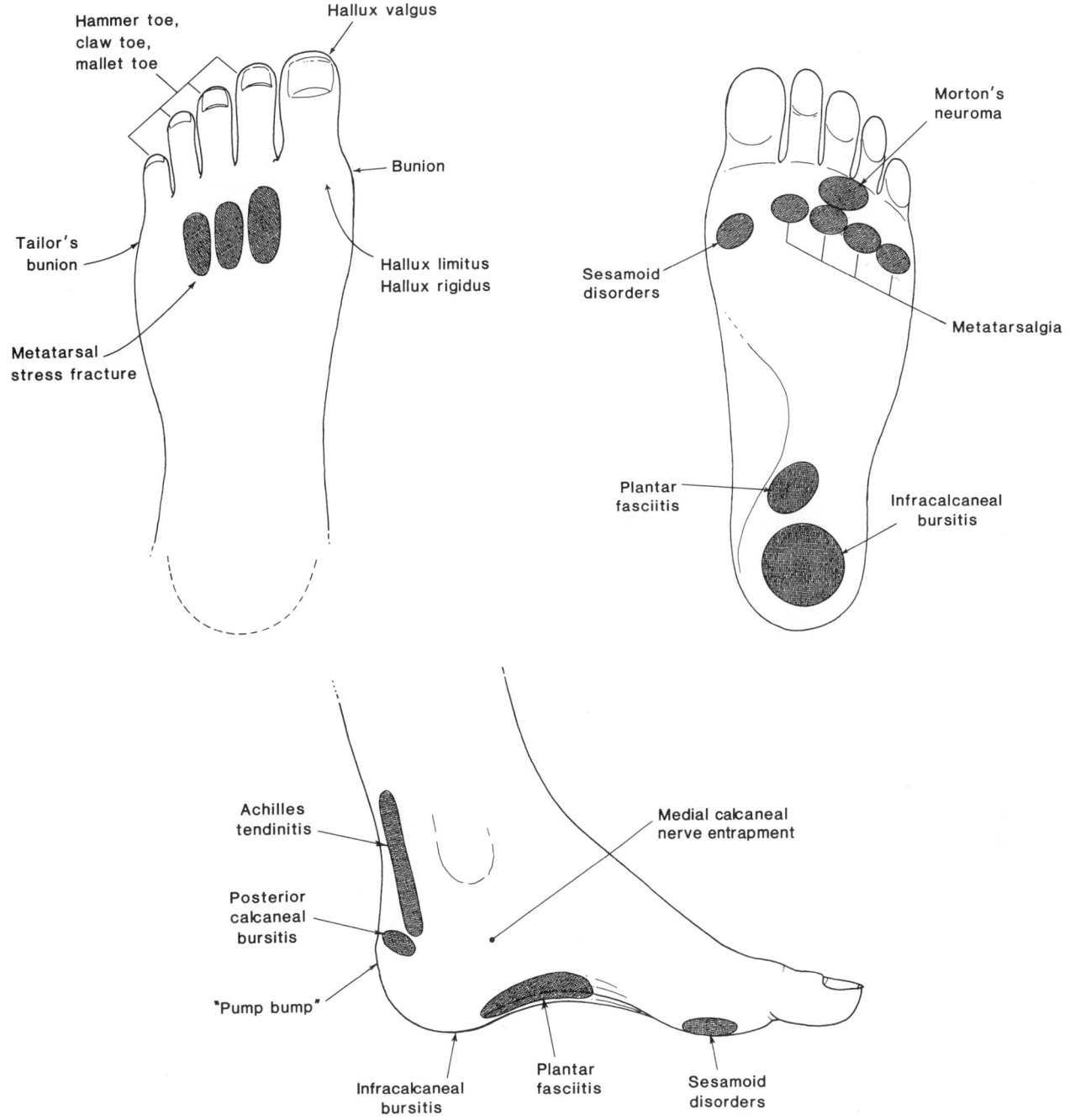

FIG. 154.1.   Sites of common foot problems.

Physical examination reveals markedly limited mobility of the first MTP joint, especially on dorsiflexion (normal, 50 to 80 degrees passively). Pain and crepitation are usually present. Radiographs reveal changes associated with degenerative joint disease, such as joint space narrowing, osteophytes, and sclerosis. Chronic gouty arthritis may resemble this condition.

The initial treatment should be directed at limiting the stresses on the joint. An orthotic device with an extension under the great toe (Morton's extension) and a shoe with extra depth should be prescribed. Limiting joint motion by stiffening the outer sole of the shoe (full-length steel shank) may also help. Surgery involving either debridement of osteophytes (so-called cheilectomy) or joint resection, replacement, or fusion is indicated if conservative treatment is unsuccessful.

Sesamoid Disorders. The first MTP joint contains two sesamoid bones (medial and lateral) that articulate on the plantar aspect with the first metatarsal and serve, to some degree, as a fulcrum in normal joint mobility. Excessive or abnormal stress about this area can lead to pain and inflammation (*sesamoiditis*), *cartilage injury*, or *sesamoid fracture*. A history of trauma may not be obvious, but sesamoid injuries are not uncommon among ballet dancers, joggers, aerobic dancers, and the like.

Localized pain and swelling are present on careful examination (plantar palpation). Radiographs should include, in addition to standard anteroposterior and lateral views, a sesamoid axial view, which is crucial for an accurate diagnosis. If a fracture is suspected, one must remember that bipartite (or multipartite) sesamoids are normal variants; a bone scan may be helpful in the diagnosis of fracture.

Treatment is directed toward providing rest and reducing the weight-bearing stresses in this area. A stiff-soled, low-heeled shoe with a full-length shank and soft innersole may be all that is required to reduce stress on the sesamoids in mild cases. Orthotic devices may be of additional help. Infrequently, excision of the involved bone is required.

Lesser Metatarsophalangeal Joints. The fifth metatarsal equivalent of the bunion is the *bunionette*, which also presents as a painful deformity and foot–shoe incompatibility. The lateral aspect of the fifth metatarsal head is tender, with a local bursal swelling. Radiographs may show the primary defect to be an excessive angle between the fourth and fifth metatarsals or an enlarged fifth metatarsal head. Alteration of shoe gear (i.e., wider or stretched) usually helps, although surgical correction may be necessary.

Metatarsalgia. True metatarsalgia is pain with weight bearing in the vicinity of the lesser metatarsal heads. Although the term is commonly used for any pain pattern in this area, it more accurately reflects an absence of other underlying conditions, such as interdigital neuroma, metatarsal stress fracture, MTP joint arthritis, or osteochondritis. The metatarsals are tender to pressure, and the plantar aspect of the foot (with the patient lying in the prone position) may reveal a protrusion in an otherwise flat forefoot surface. Hypermobility may also be found in the neighboring metatarsals. Often, a callus develops directly beneath the involved metatarsal, creating additional discomfort.

A variety of conservative methods are employed to disperse weight away from the involved metatarsal, including soft innersoles, molded shoes with innersoles, metatarsal bars, and orthotic devices. In some situations, as in deforming rheumatoid arthritis with dorsal dislocation of the MTP joints, surgical intervention (metatarsal head resection) is necessary and most rewarding.

Interdigital (Morton's) Neuroma. Burning pain and cramping, most often involving the third and fourth toes, are characteristic symptoms of this lesion. Classically, the patient is a woman who reports that symptoms are aggravated by wearing closed shoes and relieved by removal of the shoe and forefoot massage. The third intermetatarsal space is supplied by a common nerve trunk, receiving branches from both the medial and lateral plantar nerves. Compression and irritation of this trunk in a fibroosseous ring formed by the metatarsal heads, the deep transverse intermetatarsal ligament, and the plantar weight-bearing surface are implicated in this lesion.

By compressing the forefoot and pushing up in the distal third intermetatarsal space, a "click" may be felt (Mulder's sign) and the patient's symptoms reproduced. Relief is sometimes achieved through the use of wider shoes, a metatarsal bar, soft insoles, orthotic devices, NSAIDs, or local anesthetic and steroid injections. Quite often, surgical excision is required.

Metatarsal Stress Fractures. Functional overload in a lesser metatarsal (usually the second or third metatarsal) may result in a march or fatigue fracture. The onset of symptoms is sudden and often without a history of trauma. Palpation of the metatarsal shaft elicits pain over the site of injury. Between 4 and 6 weeks after injury, swelling can be palpated, reflecting the presence of a healing callus. Initially, radiographic findings are negative, but a bone scan may confirm the diagnosis early on.

Healing is uneventful if one avoids rigorous activities and wears a stiff-soled, low-heeled shoe. Occasionally, a standard wooden postoperative shoe and an Unna's boot compressive wrap are helpful in providing a more comfortable gait.

Hindfoot Problems

Plantar Heel Pain is seen in both young and old patients and can be disabling. It is often mistakenly attributed to "heel spurs," most of which are asymptomatic and unrelated to the pain.

Plantar Fasciitis classically causes pain with the initial step taken on getting out of bed in the morning. Pain often diminishes as the foot "stretches out," only to recur after periods of inactivity. Overuse syndromes, such as conditions caused by jogging, can contribute to small tears near the origin of the plantar fascia, with subsequent focal pain and localized inflammation. Characteristically, tenderness can be elicited along the medial plantar aspect of the foot, approximately three finger breadths distal to the posterior heel. Pain is increased with forced dorsiflexion of the digits during the examination. Although radiographs often demonstrate a plantar spur at the anterior inferior aspect of the calcaneus, this is usually not the cause of the symptoms.

Initial treatment focuses on tendo Achilles stretching exercises and modification of activities, application of ice, administration of NSAIDs, and use of a heel cushion to provide symptomatic relief. Patients often wonder why they should do exercises for their calf when the problem is in their foot. It must be explained that a continuous fascia sleeve extends from the calf muscles into the foot and that the stretching exercises will relieve the point of stress at the heel. If these measures are not effective, a trial of 1 to 2 months of cast immobilization can be tried—a form of enforced complete rest. Local steroid injections can be considered but should be used sparingly. Rupture of the plantar fascia can be a more difficult problem to address. Rarely, surgical release of the plantar fascia is required, but the operative results are not consistently good.

Intracalcaneal Bursitis. In contrast to plantar fasciitis, this entity presents with an aching sensation in the direct *midplantar* aspect of the calcaneus that generally increases with the duration of weight bearing. Symptoms are more pronounced as the day progresses. Examination reveals *point tenderness* directly under the midportion of the calcaneus. Localized warmth and swelling may be present. This localized lesion is most likely an inflamed bursa directly beneath the calcaneus. Therapy includes local modalities, such as ice, massage, NSAIDs, and steroid injections. A soft heel pad, heel cup, or appropriately fabricated orthotic device to relieve direct impact on this region should be added.

Neurologic Heel Pain. Local or more *proximal nerve entrapment* is an important cause of heel pain. For example, an entrapment of the medial calcaneal branch of the posterior tibial nerve in the region of the inferior calcaneus can mimic symptoms of inferior calcaneal bursitis. In this situation, however, one can elicit a proximal radiation of pain upward toward the region of the tarsal tunnel beneath the medial malleolus. The presence of Tinel's sign should be sought on examination. If local steroid injection is not effective, release of the medial calcaneal branch, or tarsal tunnel release, may be required.

As the posterior tibial nerve courses behind the medial malleolus and enters the fibroosseous tarsal tunnel, local compression of the nerve caused by local trauma (sprain, fracture), a space-occupying lesion (varicosity, lipoma), or repetitive hyperpronation can result. Symptoms include paresthesias, dysesthesias, and nocturnal pain along the plantar aspect of the foot or anywhere along the distribution of the medial or lateral plantar nerves. Results of nerve conduction studies are not consistently abnormal in this *"tarsal tunnel syndrome."* A foot surgeon should be consulted, although conservative treatment with orthotic devices and local steroid injections may preclude the need for surgical release.

Lastly, neurologically related heel pain can be the result of a *radiculopathy* secondary to a herniated lumbosacral disk. Careful examination of the low back and neurologic testing, including assessment of sensory and reflex function, should be performed, especially if the cause of the pain is not readily apparent.

Posterior Heel Pain. Two bursae are present at the posterior heel: a superficial bursa lying between the Achilles tendon and skin and a deep bursa located between the tendon and the calcaneus. *Posterior calcaneal bursitis* results from structural and functional abnormalities of the hindfoot or the wearing of inappropriate shoe gear with a firm, unyielding heel counter. Pain can be elicited by compression of the heel cord just anterior to its attachment and with passive dorsal and plantar flexion of the ankle. Several systemic inflammatory conditions (rheumatoid arthritis, ankylosing spondylitis, and Reiter's syndrome) can produce a similar clinical picture, as can a tear of the Achilles tendon and posterior calcaneal exostosis (see later discussion).

The recommended treatment of acute posterior calcaneal bursitis begins with local measures, such as application of ice in the first 24 hours, followed by moist heat, NSAID medication, and rest. With a more chronic condition, a heel lift or orthotic device to control heel motion and adjustments of the heel counter of the shoe should be considered.

Exostosis. Posterior calcaneal exostosis ("pump bump") is most commonly seen in young women, presenting as a tender enlargement about the lateral dorsal aspect of the posterior calcaneus. Pain is aggravated by a firm heel counter. A thickened bursa may overlie a true exostosis of the calcaneus, which can be seen on a lateral radiograph. The treatment of the acute, bursal inflammation parallels that for other types of heel bursitis, already described. Resection of a posterior bony exostosis is reserved only for those cases in which symptoms cannot be effectively controlled conservatively.

Achilles Tendinitis, a common affliction of athletes, reflects inflammation or small tears near the insertion of the Achilles tendon (or paratendon). Discomfort worsens during athletic activity, with subsequent swelling and stiffness. On examination, tenderness to palpation of the tendon (often extending proximally) is noted in association with a palpable fusiform

swelling. In acute cases, the first line of therapy is rest, even to the point of plaster immobilization. A heel lift, ultrasound, antiinflammatory agents, heel cord stretching, and orthotic devices are helpful in the chronic phase.

Systemically Related Foot Disorders

The foot can mirror systemic disease. Disorders of the macrovasculature or microvasculature can be the underlying cause of a variety of foot problems, including ulcers and necrosis. Neurologic disorders can compromise both form and function of the foot. Systemic or metabolic disorders, including atherosclerosis, diabetes mellitus, gout, and rheumatoid arthritis, may all have profound effects on the foot and require medical in addition to orthopedic, vascular surgical, or podiatric treatment (see Chapters 34, 102, 156, and 158).

Runner's Foot

The stress of repeated impact sustained during athletic endeavors such as jogging predisposes the foot to significant mechanical trauma. All the specific entities discussed previously occur among runners. Just as important is the biomechanical influence of the foot on the rest of the lower extremity. For example, the hyperpronated "flat" foot can cause excessive strain on the posterior tibial muscle and also increase the torque on the entire lower extremity, so that medial knee pain is felt after prolonged jogging. If one does observe significant hypermobility or hyperpronation, it is best to support the foot mechanically with a molded orthotic device. A rigid, cavus-type foot deformity prevents normal pronation with stance. When engaged in running, the foot may lose its capacity to act as a shock absorber. Increased shock is transmitted up the entire lower extremity, even to the region of the lower back. Patients with this type of foot deformity may complain of leg, knee, and hip discomfort.

ANKLE DISORDERS

Ankle Sprain. A sprain is the most common ankle injury. Lesions range from minor ligamentous damage to complete tear or avulsion of the bony attachment, fracture, and dislocation. Sprain occurs when stress is applied while the ankle is in an unstable position, causing the ligaments to overstretch. During plantar flexion, the joint is least stable and most susceptible to eversion or inversion forces. Such stresses are encountered during running or walking over uneven surfaces. Evaluation is facilitated by early presentation because the event producing injury is likely to be remembered and swelling is confined to the site of injury.

All too often, ankle sprains are considered minor injuries requiring little medical attention, even though experience has proved this concept to be misleading. Although many sprains heal with no residual disability, some do not. All reflect some degree of injury to one or several ligaments and may be classified as *first-degree* (involving stretching of ligamentous fibers), *second-degree* (involving a tear of some portion of the ligament with associated pain and swelling), and *third-degree* (involving complete ligamentous separation).

An *inversion injury*, the most common type of sprain, causes damage to the lateral ligaments. There is often a history

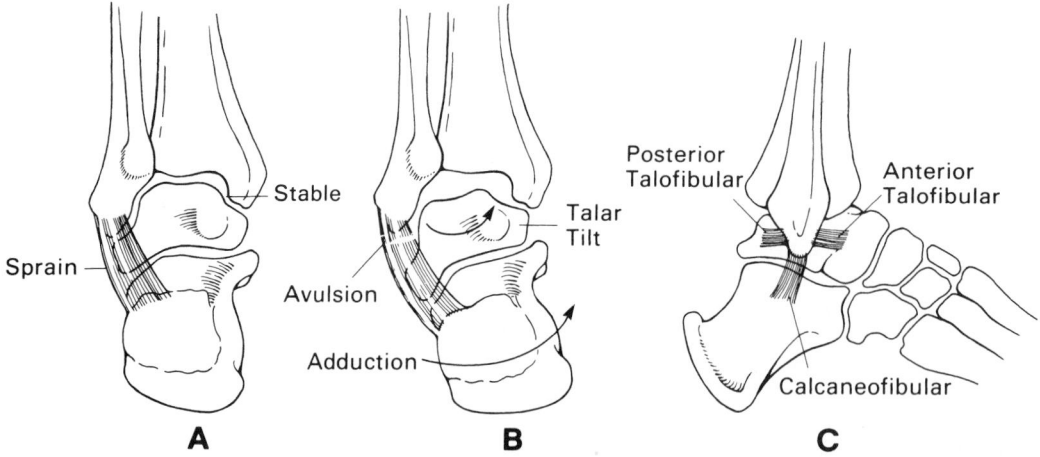

FIG. 154.2. Lateral ligamentous sprain and avulsion. **A:** Simple sprain in which the ligaments remain intact and the talus remains stable within the mortice. **B:** Avulsion of the lateral ligaments; the talus becomes unstable and tilts within the mortice when the calcaneus is adducted. **C:** Lateral ligaments of the ankle. The anterior talofibular and calcaneofibular ligaments are the ligaments most frequently involved in inversion injuries. (Redrawn form Cailliet R. Foot and ankle pain. Philadelphia: FA Davis Co, 1968, with permission.)

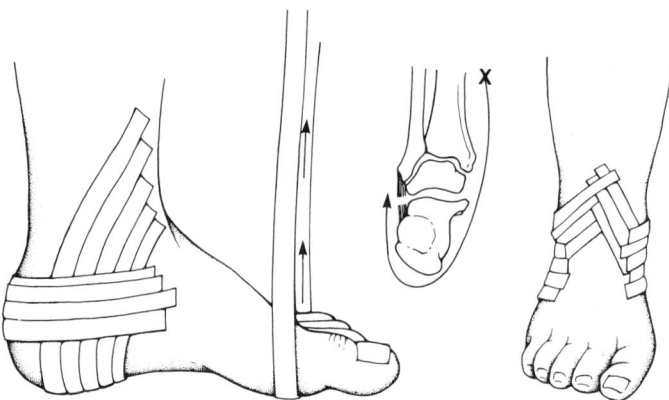

FIG. 154.3. Taping a sprained ankle. The purpose of taping the ankle is to prevent further stretching of the injured ligaments until healing has occurred. The ankle must be inverted or everted to place the strained ligament at rest. The center figure depicts an avulsed lateral ligament. The tape here begins from inside and then runs under the foot to finish on the outer leg, holding the heel everted. The horizontal strips minimize rotation of the forefoot. (Redrawn from Cailliet R. Foot and ankle pain. Philadelphia: FA Davis Co, 1968, with permission.)

of inversion during plantar flexion; a snap or tear may have been heard or felt. However, the history of injury is often inaccurate and may not be helpful in the evaluation of the extent of ligamentous damage. A careful physical examination is needed to identify the site and degree of injury, with the examiner's fingertips used to check the anterior capsule and medial and lateral ligaments (Fig. 154.2). Although significant edema commonly accompanies ligamentous injury, complete ligamentous and capsular disruption may produce remarkably little edema because of extravasation into the surrounding soft-tissue planes.

A useful indicator of significant injury is the *anterior draw sign*. The sign may be elicited by grasping the distal tibia in one hand and the calcaneus and heel in the other and sliding the entire foot forward. This is done first with the ankle in neutral position and then with 30 degrees of plantar flexion. Up to 2 mm of shift is normal. With disruption of the anterior or lateral ligaments, one sees 4 mm or more of anterior shift, as the fibers of

the anterolateral ligaments lie in an anteroposterior direction. Passive inversion of the ankle produces pain. Swelling invariably occurs, usually anterior to the lateral malleolus at the onset; ecchymoses are common. Simple strain does not result in joint instability, but with a sprain, the joint loses stability and the talus tilts if the calcaneus is adducted (Fig. 154.2), producing a gap between the talus and malleolus on the lateral aspect of the ankle. If swelling or pain interferes with evaluation, a radiographic assessment after nerve block may be needed to determine joint instability.

Radiography is useful in most cases of moderate to severe injury, helping to identify any associated skeletal injury in addition to assessing the degree of ligamentous damage. Three standard views are obtained: anteroposterior, lateral, and mortice (an anteroposterior view with the ankle in 20 to 30 degrees of internal rotation). In addition, a stress view is obtained (with the help of local anesthesia, if necessary) to check for talar tilt. A tilt of more than 15 degrees is suggestive of lateral ligament injury; more than 25 degrees of tilt is diagnostic. One must always compare the tilt of one foot with that of the other to rule out underlying ligamentous laxity.

Control of swelling is the first and immediate priority of management because effusion and hemorrhage further stretch and distend the joint and predispose to adhesions. An elastic bandage, ice water, and elevation are often helpful in controlling edema. The ankle should be placed in ice water for 15 to 20 minutes and then elevated. An ice pack can substitute for immersion. Cold application is repeated every few hours. Radiography can be performed after taping, application of ice water, and elevation. A bulky, conforming, nonconstricting soft dressing may be applied.

The soft dressing or elastic bandage is used for 1 to 2 weeks to control swelling and provide stability. When the ankle is splinted, it should be kept in neutral or slightly everted position to avoid tightening the heel cord and other posterior structures. Partial weight bearing is accomplished by use of a crutch until pain subsides. Non–weight-bearing exercises are started within 2 to 3 days of injury; these include active plantar flexion, dorsiflexion, toe flexion, inversion, and eversion.

After pain subsides and swelling resolves, full weight bearing can be resumed, often with the use of a functional plastic "sprain brace." These braces are commercially available in a number of designs; all function to support the ankle against inversion and eversion stresses while, at the same time, allowing dorsiflexion and plantar flexion of the ankle. Running should be postponed another 1 to 3 weeks depending on the severity of injury. With mild ligamentous laxity of the ankle and repeated minor sprains, proper taping to support the lateral structures is indicated for athletic activity that involves contact, running, or jumping, particularly on uneven ground. Tape strips are applied from the medial aspect to the lateral aspect of the ankle (Fig. 154.3) to hold the heel and ankle in eversion and provide support. Exercises to strengthen the ankle evertors and high-laced leather supportive shoes may also be helpful.

Ankle sprain is a serious injury; if torn ligaments result in marked ankle instability (determined by examination under anesthesia or stress radiography), cast immobilization for 4 to 8 weeks is indicated. Serious sprain requires prompt orthopedic referral to maximize chances for healing and restoration of joint stability.

ANNOTATED BIBLIOGRAPHY

Gill LL. Plantar fasciitis: diagnosis and conservative management. J Am Acad Orthop Surg 1997;5:109. (*Best for emphasis on nonsurgical management.*)

Schepsis AA, Leach RE, Gorzyca J. Plantar fasciitis: etiology, treatment, surgical results, and review of the literature. Clin Orthop 1991;266;285. (*Excellent review of literature and summary.*)

Smart GW, Taunton JE, Clement DB. Achilles tendon disorders in runners—a review. Med Sci Sports Exerc 1980;12:231. (*Good review of this common problem in runners.*)

155

Approach to the Patient with Asymptomatic Hyperuricemia

Asymptomatic hyperuricemia became commonplace when physicians began using chemistry panels that routinely included measurement of the serum uric acid. Hyperuricemia is defined as a serum uric acid concentration that exceeds the mean by at least two standard deviations. The mean (as determined by colorimetric assay, the most commonly used method) is 7.5 mg/dL for men and 6.6 mg/dL for women. By statistical definition, 2.5% of the population is hyperuricemic. The consequences of being hyperuricemic and the need for lowering the uric acid level have been subjects of debate. Some authorities have advocated prophylactic therapy in the hope of preventing acute gout, chronic tophaceous gout, stone formation, and renal failure. Others question the cost-effectiveness of such an approach and even the relationship of hyperuricemia to some of the adverse consequences attributed to it. The primary physician must decide if and when to treat the asymptomatic patient with an elevated uric acid level.

PATHOPHYSIOLOGY AND CLINICAL PRESENTATION

Uric acid is the end-product of purine metabolism. Humans have no pathway for the further breakdown of uric acid; it must be excreted by the kidneys or the serum level will rise. The pathogenesis of hyperuricemia involves either the overproduction or underexcretion of urate, or both. It is estimated that one third of hyperuricemic patients are overproducers, another third are underexcreters, and the remainder have a combined deficit.

Overproduction of uric acid is especially marked in patients undergoing treatment for myeloproliferative and lymphoproliferative malignancies and in those with severe psoriasis. Rapid cellular turnover results in the production of massive amounts of nucleic acid metabolites that are converted to uric acid. Overproduction may also develop from an increase in purine synthesis *de novo*, as occurs in patients with inborn errors of metabolism. Contrary to popular belief, excessive dietary intake of purine-rich foods is rarely responsible for hyperuricemia because dietary sources of purine make up only 10% of the uric acid pool. However, excessive intake of alcohol (>100 g of ethanol per day) results in increased urate synthesis, especially if the patient does not eat anything at the time of alcohol consumption.

Underexcretion of uric acid occurs in association with an overall decrease in the glomerular filtration or a defect in the tubular secretion of urate; uric acid is also underexcreted if another substance competes with urate for tubular secretion. A compromise in renal blood flow secondary to aging or atherosclerotic disease reduces renal urate excretion. Hyperuricemia has been noted in hypertensive patients. Although some instances may be a consequence of hypertensive renovascular injury, epidemiologic analysis suggests that most cases are caused by thiazide use. In addition to thiazides, low doses of aspirin reduce renal urate excretion. Excretion falls in patients with an increased proximal tubular reabsorption of sodium, which has been linked to hyperinsulinism and might account for the oft-noted, poorly understood relation between hyperuricemia and atherosclerotic cardiovascular disease. However, careful reexamination of the epidemiologic data linking hyperuricemia to an increased risk for cardiovascular disease reveals no independent causal relationship, but rather an association with thiazide use for the treatment of hypertension, a major cardiovascular risk factor. Fasting that results in ketosis seems to be capable of transiently reducing urate excretion and raising the serum uric acid.

Well over 90% of hyperuricemic patients present asymptomatically. Most are persons who have been subjected to multiphasic screening. Half of newly discovered patients in the Framingham study were taking thiazides, and just under 3% had elevations secondary to a concurrent illness, such as myeloproliferative disease.

PRINCIPLES OF MANAGEMENT

Prophylactic therapy might be indicated if lowering the uric acid level could prevent acute gout, chronic gouty arthritis, gouty nephropathy, or urolithiasis. For years, it was assumed that such complications are a direct result of untreated hyperuricemia, so that many clinicians treated asymptomatic hyperuricemic patients with urate-lowering drugs. The statistical relationship between hyperuricemia and atherosclerotic disease was also a concern, one that has now been eliminated.

Prevention of Acute Gouty Arthritis. Population studies (Framingham, Normative Aging, Sudbury) have confirmed that the higher the serum uric acid level, the greater the chance of an attack of acute gout; they have also confirmed that the urate concentration is the predominant determinant of risk. However, the oft-quoted 90% risk reported in the Framingham study represented a 12-year cumulative incidence figure and pertained only to 10 patients who had a uric acid level in excess of 9.0 mg/dL. More relevant is the average annual incidence, which was 4.0% in the Framingham study and 4.7% in the Normative Aging study for patients with urate concentrations in the top 2%.

To determine the utility of prophylactic therapy, one needs to consider the costs and benefits of preventing an attack of acute gout. The cost of lifelong prophylactic therapy can reach thousands of dollars because the mean age at the time of detection is 35. The prevalence of adverse drug reactions has been reported to be as high as 10% for probenecid and 25% for allopurinol. These costs appear excessive when the safety, efficacy, and minimal expense of promptly treating a single acute attack of gout with a short course of an NSAID are considered (see Chapter 158). Only if gouty attacks become disabling and frequent does the cost–benefit equation shift in favor of prophylaxis. In most instances, the intervals between recurrences of acute gout are measured in years.

Prevention of Chronic Gouty Arthritis. The issue of prophylaxis for prevention of chronic gouty arthritis is of only minor importance because almost all patients with this condition go through a stage of acute gouty attacks before chronic joint changes develop. Thus, asymptomatic patients with no evidence of clinical gout are at little if any risk for silently falling victim to chronic gouty arthritis.

Prevention of Azotemia. Despite fears to the contrary and early studies that were confounded by high exposures to lead, chronic hyperuricemia does not appear to be a significant risk factor for the development of azotemia, nor does hyperuricemia *secondary to* renal failure pose an additional threat to the kidneys. In a prospective study from Kaiser-Permanente in which 113 patients with asymptomatic hyperuricemia and 193 controls were followed for 8 years, no difference was found in the incidence of azotemia between the two groups (1.8% vs. 2.1%). In the same study, no relation between uric acid level and risk for azotemia was found in 168 patients with clinical gout followed for 10 years. In the Normative Aging study, a creatinine level above 2.0 mg/dL developed in only 0.7% of the 94 patients with a uric acid level in excess of 9.0 mg/dL during the 15 years of follow-up. One set of investigators calculated that a significant risk for renal injury from chronic hyperuricemia required that a uric acid level of 13.0 mg/dL in men and 10.0 mg/dL in women be sustained for 40 years. A 3-year prospective study of hyperuricemic patients with and without renal failure showed no change in renal function when allopurinol was used to normalize the serum urate concentration.

One group of hyperuricemic patients at risk for renal failure are those with myeloproliferative or lymphoproliferative malignancy who are undergoing chemotherapy. With each cytotoxic treatment comes a huge uric acid load that may trigger injurious urate crystal formation in the renal tubular cells. Acute oliguric renal failure may ensue. Such patients require pretreatment with allopurinol and vigorous hydration.

Prevention of Nephrolithiasis. The risk for nephrolithiasis in patients with asymptomatic hyperuricemia is very small. In the Kaiser study, renal calculi occurred in 3 (2.6%) of 113 hyperuricemic patients and in 2 (1.1%) of 193 controls. In two of the hyperuricemic patients with stones, the stone was composed of calcium. The risk for development of a stone attributable to hyperuricemia was calculated to be less than 1% annually. Among patients with gout, the control of serum uric acid was the same for those in whom stones developed and for those in whom they did not.

This minimal risk for stone development conferred by hyperuricemia alone derives from the importance of other factors in stone formation (see Chapter 135). Family history, urinary pH, and level of hydration are particularly germane. Two of the three hyperuricemic patients with stones in the Kaiser study had a family history of nephrolithiasis. Urine acidity is a critical factor because the solubility of uric acid falls precipitously as the pH falls from 8.0 to 5.0. The amount of uric acid excreted in the urine per 24 hours has also been suggested as a factor, but careful studies have shown that the level of urinary uric acid is only a weak determinant of stone formation until extreme levels are encountered. However, dehydration is a well-established precipitant.

Urolithiasis is rarely life-threatening. In a study of 1,700 patients with gout, only one patient experienced serious obstructive uropathy.

Prevention of Atherosclerotic Disease. Although a statistical relationship exists between hyperuricemia and atherosclerotic disease, it does not appear to be an etiologic one. Rather, the two conditions appear to share a common pathophysiologic link, namely thiazide therapy and hypertension. No evidence has been found that treating hyperuricemia lowers the risk for atherosclerotic disease.

THERAPEUTIC RECOMMENDATIONS

- Asymptomatic hyperuricemia is associated with an increased risk for acute gouty arthritis, but the cost of prophylactic therapy in patients who have never had an attack of gout greatly exceeds the cost of treating an acute attack symptomatically, should it occur.
- Only with the development of frequent acute gouty attacks is prophylactic therapy indicated (see Chapter 158).
- Treatment to prevent chronic tophaceous gout need not be started until clinical evidence of gout develops.
- The evidence to justify prophylaxis to prevent renal impairment is insufficient except in patients who have a myeloproliferative or lymphoproliferative disorder and are about to be treated for it. The degree of azotemia that can be attributed to hyperuricemia is mild and clinically insignificant in most other instances.
- The risk for urolithiasis is sufficiently low to justify waiting for the development of a stone before prophylactic therapy is initiated, unless the patient has a strong family history of nephrolithiasis. However, dehydration should be avoided.
- Although hyperuricemia is associated statistically with atherosclerotic disease, the relation is not etiologic, and no cardiovascular benefit is derived from lowering the serum uric acid level.

A.H.G.

ANNOTATED BIBLIOGRAPHY

Batuman V, Maesaka JK, Haddad B, et al. The role of lead in gout nephropathy. N Engl J Med 1981;304:520. (*Detected a strong relationship between lead and nephropathy in patients with gout.*)

Berger LU, Yu TF. Renal function in gout—an analysis of 524 gouty subjects including long-term follow-up studies. Am J Med 1975;59:604. (*Follow-up for 12 years showed that hyperuricemia alone has no deleterious effect on renal function in ambulatory patients with gout.*)

Brand FN, McGee DL, Kannel WB, et al. Hyperuricemia as a risk factor of coronary heart disease: the Framingham study. Am J Epidemiol 1985;121:11. (*Finds a statistical but not an etiologic relationship in atherosclerotic disease.*)

Campion EW, Glynn RJ, DeLabry LO. Asymptomatic hyperuricemia: risks and consequences in the Normative Aging Study. Am J Med 1987;82:421. (*A large study with a 15-year follow-up. Risk for gout was 4.9% annually for patients with a uric acid level above 9 mg/dL; risk for renal failure was nil.*)

Cappuccio FP, Strazzullo P, Farinaro E, et al. Uric acid metabolism and tubular sodium handling. JAMA 1993;270:354. (*Finds hyperuricemia closely linked to excessive proximal tubular reabsorption of sodium; speculates that both are manifestations of hyperinsulinemia.*)

Culleton BF, Larson MG, Kannel WB, et al. Serum uric acid and risk for cardiovascular disease and death: the Framingham Heart Study. Ann Intern Med 1999;131:7. (*Rigorous epidemiologic examination finds no evidence for a causal relationship between urate level and cardiovascular risk; previously noted link appears to be thiazide use for hypertension.*)

Faller J, Fox I. Ethanol-induced hyperuricemia. N Engl J Med 1982;307:1598. (*Ethanol increases urate synthesis.*)

Fessel JW. Renal outcomes of gout and hyperuricemia. Am J Med 1979;67:74. (*A prospective study showing that the risks for renal failure and stone formation are very small and hardly justify prophylactic therapy.*)

Hall AP, Berry PE, Dawber TR, et al. Epidemiology of gout and hyperuricemia—a long-term population study. Am J Med 1967;42:27. (*In the Framingham study, a gouty attack developed during the 12 years of follow-up in 19% of those with serum urate levels between 8 and 8.9 mg/dL and five of six patients with a uric acid level of 9 mg/dL.*)

Liang MH, Fries JF. Asymptomatic hyperuricemia: the case for conservative management. Ann Intern Med 1978;88:666. (*A well-developed approach to asymptomatic hyperuricemia.*)

MacLaughlan MJ, Rodnan GP. Effects of food, fast, and alcohol on serum uric acid and acute attacks of gout. Am J Med 1967;42:38. (*Fasting and consumption of more than 100 g/d of alcohol raised urate levels. Acute changes in levels precipitated gouty attacks.*)

Reif MC, Constantiner A, Levitt MF. Chronic gouty nephropathy: a vanishing syndrome. N Engl J Med 1981;304:535. (*An editorial summarizing the data on the lack of a relation between renal injury and most forms of hyperuricemia.*)

Singer JZ, Wallace SL. The allopurinol hypersensitivity syndrome: unnecessary morbidity and mortality. Arthritis Rheum 1986;29:82. (*High incidence of adverse reactions; the drug is not harmless for prolonged use.*)

Yu TF, Berger LU. Impaired renal function in gout. Am J Med 1982;75:95. (*Hyperuricemia alone did not affect renal function; renal insufficiency correlated best with coexisting hypertension, preexisting renal disease, and ischemic heart disease.*)

Yu TF, Gutman A. Uric acid nephrolithiasis in gout: predisposing factors. Ann Intern Med 1967;67:1133. (*In a classic study of 305 patients with gout, risk for stone formation was correlated with uric acid excretion, urine pH, serum urate level, and underlying cause.*)

156
Management of Rheumatoid Arthritis

The management of rheumatoid arthritis (RA) is a challenge because the disease is chronic, relapsing, and potentially disabling, and no completely satisfactory methods of treatment are available. The problem is common. Population surveys indicate that 3% of women and 1% of men in the United States have definite or probable RA, based on the diagnostic criteria established by the American Rheumatism Association. Prevalence increases with age, and incidence peaks in the fourth decade. The estimated annual incidence of new cases ranges from 0.5/1,000 to 3/1,000. The functional objectives of therapy are to minimize pain and stiffness and preserve range of motion and muscle strength through the use of disease-modifying agents, antiinflammatory drugs, and physical therapy measures. The primary physician needs to implement an effective program of patient education, exercise, joint rest, and symptomatic medical therapy, and to decide when referral for consideration of disease-modifying treatment is required. A trend toward earlier use of disease-modifying agents is under way, encouraged by the advent of increasingly effective new drugs. Additional tasks are to monitor closely for disease progression and treatment side effects.

PATHOPHYSIOLOGY AND CLINICAL PRESENTATION

Pathogenesis

Rheumatoid arthritis is an immunologically mediated chronic inflammatory disease of unknown etiology, manifested by synovitis and destructive arthritis of the diarthrodial joints. In genetically predisposed hosts (genotype *HLA-DRB1*04/04*), a delayed hypersensitivity reaction to an as yet unidentified stimulus (e.g., infectious agent, constituent of synovium or cartilage) appears to be the initial event. Although the precise sequence of immunologic events leading to joint injury continues to be elucidated, important cellular components of the process include CD4 helper/inducer T-cell lymphocytes, CD4 memory T cells, plasma cells, activated macrophages, and neutrophils. Cytokines (e.g., *tumor necrosis factor, interleukins, granulocyte-macrophage colony-stimulating factor*) are released and serve as important immune mediators, stimulating B- and T-cell proliferation and differentiation and activating neutrophils and monocytes. Immunoglobulin G rheumatoid factor (RF) emanating from local plasma cells may form immune complexes with articular antigens and thereby activate complement. The net result is the elaboration of prostaglandins, vasoactive amines, oxygen-derived free radicals, activated platelets, collagenases, and other lysosomal enzymes into the joint cavity, which causes direct damage to articular cartilage and bone.

Pathologically, the synovium is the principal site of initial involvement. The earliest change is immunologically mediated damage to the endothelium of the microvasculature. Small-vessel lumina become obliterated by thrombi and inflammatory cells, after which new capillary formation, synovial lining cell proliferation, edema, and leukocyte infiltration take place. Neu-

trophils migrate into the joint space. As the inflammatory process progresses, the synovium becomes more hypertrophic, edematous, hypervascular, and further infiltrated by mononuclear cells. In severe cases, the formation of *pannus* represents an invasive synovitis with proliferation of lymphocytes, plasma cells, fibroblasts, and macrophages. Pannus is capable of eroding cartilage and bone; the process typically begins at the joint margin, then spreads over the entire cartilaginous surface. Lysosomal enzymes released from within the pannus and latent collagenases are believed to contribute to the direct erosive capacity. Often, osteopenia is seen in subchondral bone adjacent to the involved joint even before pannus has denuded the cartilage.

Clinical Presentation and Course

Initially, an effusion develops, distending the joint capsule. This is followed by damage to the articular surface and weakening of the capsule and periarticular ligaments. Secondary muscle atrophy results and leads to imbalance of opposing muscle groups. The net effect is an unstable, weak, swollen, subluxated joint. The synovium of tendon sheaths and bursae may also be affected by the inflammatory process, so that tenosynovitis and bursitis develop.

The clinical onset of RA is usually insidious, often beginning with vague *arthralgias, morning stiffness,* and *fatigue.* In some patients, the onset is more acute. Signs of *articular inflammation* (swelling, pain, and warmth) soon follow. The small joints of the hands and feet—the proximal interphalangeals (PIP), metacarpophalangeals (MCP), and metatarsophalangeals (MTP)—are typically among the first to be involved, but knees, ankles, wrists, or elbows may also be affected early on. *Tenosynovitis* is common. Initially, the arthritis may be asymmetric or may even present as a monoarticular process, but the characteristic symmetric distribution supervenes in most instances.

In an occasional patient, RA is preceded by *palindromic rheumatism,* a condition characterized by repeated episodes of transient joint pain, swelling, and redness extending beyond the joint. The condition lasts a few hours to a few days, then resolves completely without causing permanent joint injury. Fingers, wrists, shoulders, and knees are most commonly affected. Typical RA develops in about 50% of these patients.

Rheumatoid nodules appear in about 25% of patients with RA, usually as the disease progresses. These subcutaneous nodules are firm, nontender, and located principally along the extensor surface of the forearm and in the olecranon bursa. Their appearance is an unfavorable prognostic sign, as is the persistence of acute disease for more than 1 year, high serum titers of RF, and age under 20 at time of presentation.

Sustained joint inflammation lasting more than a year leads to permanent *erosion* and loss of joint function. At first, the changes are partially reversible, but as cartilage and bone erode, the injury becomes permanent.

Hands and Wrists. Characteristic hand deformities include ulnar deviation of the MCP joints, boutonnière deformities of the PIP joints, and swan neck contractures of the fingers. In the wrists, a permanent loss of extension often occurs. A boggy, tender, dorsal wrist mass may result from tenosynovitis, and the median nerve can be compressed. The subsequent *carpal tunnel syndrome* is usually reversible, but nerve damage is permanent by the time wasting of the thenar eminence becomes obvious.

Feet. Erosion of the metatarsal heads can lead to ventral subluxation. Increased weight bearing on the inflamed heads and the formation of painful calluses result. Erosive disease may be silent in the MTP joints.

Hips and Knees. Involvement of these joints can be a source of much disability when weight bearing causes severe pain. Loss of internal rotation is the first change noted in the hip, followed by flexion contracture. One hip may predominate, even though the process is bilateral. In the knee, distention of the suprapatellar pouch by synovial effusion is common. If pressure rises rapidly, herniation of the synovium with formation of a popliteal *Baker's cyst* can occur, and the cyst can cause severe pain if it ruptures into the calf. Loss of full knee extension is followed by flexion contractures and gait difficulties.

Other Joints. In the *elbow*, extension may be compromised, and olecranon bursitis is often present. *Shoulder* involvement presents as a subacromial or subdeltoid bursitis or as limitation of motion. Erosion of the rotator cuff leads to painful upward subluxation of the humeral head against the acromion. In the *cervical spine*, atlantoaxial subluxation is common, but usually asymptomatic. This development is potentially serious because it can lead to direct compression of the spinal cord or of the blood supply to the brainstem; fortunately, it is a rare event. When the *temporomandibular joint* is affected, pain is felt during chewing or biting, and it is difficult to open the mouth. *Avascular necrosis of the femoral head* and *vertebral osteoporosis* and collapse are usually a consequence of corticosteroid therapy.

Radiographic Manifestations of early disease are soft-tissue swelling around the joint and periarticular osteopenia. Relatively uniform narrowing of the joint space occurs as cartilage is destroyed, a finding often noted within the first 2 years of disease. Periarticular subchondral erosion is noted at the joint margin where pannus has developed. Finally, joint architecture is lost as the joint space is obliterated and erosion of subchondral bone progresses.

Extraarticular Manifestations are most prominent in patients with persistent symptoms and high titers of RF (so-called seropositive disease), although up to 50% of patients with RA may show some form of extraarticular disease. *Pulmonary* manifestations include interstitial changes, pulmonary nodules, and pleuritis. The latter is manifested by a pleural effusion, in which the levels of *glucose* (5 to 20 mg/dL) and complement are characteristically *low*, the *leukocyte count* (5,000/mm³) is *low*, and the *lactate dehydrogenase* level is *high*. *Accompanying pleuritic pain may or may not be present. An asymptomatic pericardial effusion* also may occur. Keratoconjunctivitis sicca

(*Sjögren's syndrome*) has a strong association with RA, being found in up to 15% of patients. *Splenomegaly* is present in 5% to 10% of patients with RA, and lymphadenopathy is not unusual. The combination of RA, splenomegaly, and neutropenia (*Felty's syndrome*) is noted in an occasional patient. Neutropenia may be severe, but the arthritis is often quiescent. Other features include chronic leg ulceration, lymphadenopathy, and cryoglobulinemia. The risk for sepsis is high.

Vasculitis is believed responsible for a number of systemic manifestations, including fever, mononeuritis multiplex, Raynaud's phenomenon, chronic leg ulcers, mucosal erosions of the gastrointestinal tract, focal ischemia of the digits, and necrotizing mesarteritis. The *anemia* of chronic disease is seen in a large percentage of patients with RA.

Clinical Stages. In stage I, no symptoms or signs are present, just the presentation of the relevant antigen to an immunologically susceptible host. Stage II, in which the immune response becomes organized in the perivascular areas of the synovium, is characterized by increasing numbers of T cells, proliferation and differentiation of B cells, antibody production, synovial cell increase, and new blood vessel formation. Morning stiffness develops because fluid about the joints is increased. They are warm but not erythematous because superficial vessels are uninvolved. In stage III, the pathophysiologic processes of stage II continue, and extraarticular manifestations become evident. In stage IV, proliferating synovial membrane becomes invasive, injuring cartilage, bone, and tendons.

Clinical Course and Prognosis. The clinical course is generally one of exacerbations and remissions. About 40% of patients become disabled after 10 years, but outcomes are highly variable. Some patients experience a relatively self-limited disease, and others suffer a chronic, progressive illness. Improvements in the detection of early joint injury have provided a previously unappreciated view of how common and important early joint damage is. Nonetheless, it remains difficult at the outset to predict the course of an individual case, although the *HLA-DRB1*04/04 genotype*, a *high serum titer of RF, extraarticular manifestations*, a *large number of involved joints, age below 30, female sex*, and *systemic symptoms* all correlate with an unfavorable prognosis. Insidious onset is also an unfavorable sign. Disease that remains persistently active for more than a year is likely to lead to joint deformities and disability. Cases in which periods of activity lasting only weeks or a few months are followed by spontaneous remission have a better prognosis. The absence of RF does not necessarily portend a good prognosis. Outcome is compromised when diagnosis and treatment are delayed. Other laboratory markers of a poor prognosis include early radiologic evidence of bony injury, persistent anemia of chronic disease, and elevated levels of the C1q component of complement.

The overall mortality for patients with RA is reported to be 2.5 times that of the general population. In those with severe articular and extraarticular disease, the mortality approaches that of patients with three-vessel coronary disease or stage IV Hodgkin's disease. Much of the excess mortality derives from infection, vasculitis, and poor nutrition. Mortality from cancer is unchanged.

Most data on rates of disability derive from specialty units caring for referred patients with severe disease. Little information is available on patients seen in primary care community settings. Estimates suggest that more than 50% of these patients remain fully employed, even after 10 to 15 years of disease, with one third having only intermittent low-grade disease and another third experiencing spontaneous remission.

DIAGNOSIS

Because subclinical but important joint destruction begins early in many cases (see below), early diagnosis becomes a particularly important task for the primary physician. Delay in diagnosis is common; in a study of the problem, the time to diagnosis averaged 36 months from onset of symptoms (see Chapter 146 for a discussion of diagnostic evaluation).

PRINCIPLES OF MANAGEMENT

Management Goals and Strategy

The effective management of RA requires the design and implementation of a comprehensive treatment program that is consistent with the patient's personality and fits well into the patient's life-style and home environment. The goals are to relieve stiffness and pain, preserve muscle strength and range of motion, and minimize progressive disability and deformity. There is no cure, but *disease-modifying therapy* can reduce morbidity and mortality by slowing disease progression, preserving joint function, and limiting complications. *Early initiation* of disease-modifying therapy is increasingly encouraged to counter the important but previously unappreciated early joint destruction that characterizes RA. The early initiation of disease-modifying therapy represents a strategic shift in the pharmacologic treatment of RA, which traditionally designated the antiinflammatory agents as first-line drugs and relegated the disease-modifying agents to a second-line role. Besides early initiation, another feature of the disease-modifying strategy is the use of *multiple drug regimens*, which provide synergistic benefit and make possible a reduction in dosing and therefore a reduction in the frequency and severity of adverse drug effects. Despite the major advances in drug therapy, *nonpharmacologic measures* continue to be critically important in the maintenance of daily function and prevention of disability.

A number of factors must be considered in the design of a management program; these include the age, social and occupational responsibilities, and emotional makeup of the patient, the activity and duration of disease, and the results of prior therapies. A balanced, multifaceted approach to therapy is most likely to provide optimal results because no single drug or treatment is by itself effective. The basic components of a program must include thorough patient education, adequate rest, proper exercise, and suppression of inflammation and immune-mediated articular and vascular injury.

Nonpharmacologic Measures

The importance of nonpharmacologic measures cannot be overemphasized. Controlled trials have demonstrated that programs including such measures along with detailed patient education (see below) can provide as much benefit in terms of functional improvement as many pharmacologic therapies and reduce the costs of care by reducing the number of physician visits necessary. Thus, nonpharmacologic measures deserve considerable attention and emphasis because their implementation can be quite cost-effective.

Exercise helps to maintain range of motion and muscle strength. The goals are to strengthen supporting muscles and minimize the chances of postinflammatory contracture. Exercises that safely put involved joints through a full range of motion are taught to the patient. When pain is too severe for active exercises, isometrics can be performed, and passive exercises can be prescribed and carried out by a physical therapist. Joints with a tense effusion should be not be exercised because compression of the synovium may lead to ischemic injury. Prior application of *heat* or *cold* (either may work) will facilitate the exercise program. Hot baths, paraffin soaks, or ice packs are often efficacious in loosening stiff joints. Moist heat is also useful in relieving pain and shortening the duration of morning stiffness.

Exercises involving important muscle groups are prescribed to counteract the development of atrophy, strengthen periarticular tissues, and preserve joint stability. A judicious program of walking can play a similar role. The design and execution of an exercise program can be facilitated by the participation of a physical therapist. To protect the joint from damaging stress, the patient can be instructed in the use of implements that provide a mechanical advantage. Such "joint savers" are available commercially and are most helpful for tasks requiring use of the hands.

Rest and Splinting can be helpful, but in the patient with mild to moderate disease, complete bed rest is not only unnecessary but potentially harmful. Prolonged rest may lead to flexion contractures, osteoporosis, and muscle atrophy. Only the patient whose acute disease is severe enough to warrant hospitalization should be put to bed, in which case some benefit is derived. However, a period of rest during the day can be of considerable benefit to those patients with persistently active disease who are less ill, most of whom are usually bothered by fatigue. Selectively resting individual joints by splinting can help relieve pain and prevent contracture of severely inflamed joints, especially those too swollen to exercise. The principle is to maintain the joint in its physiologic position, especially during periods when the joint is stressed. Splinting of the wrist at night is the best example of this form of therapy. The pain of a patient with tenosynovitis of the wrist can be decreased, and flexion deformity, with its attendant loss of grip, can be prevented. A wrist splint applied at night places the joint in 10 to 15 degrees of extension. A cervical collar worn at night can provide similar relief when the cervical spine is involved. The patient with deformed feet requires specially constructed shoes.

Dietary Measures and Supplements are always appealing to patients because they offer a "natural" and presumably safe way to treat their illness. Surveys reveal that almost two thirds of patients with RA have tried dietary measures and megavitamin supplements, and about half of that group continue regular use. Although evidence of efficacy is lacking for most of these measures and supplements, an adequate *calcium* and *vitamin D* intake must be maintained because almost all patients with RA are at risk for osteoporosis, either from their disease or from its treatment. For patients taking low doses of glucocorticoids, an adequate intake of calcium and vitamin D has proved sufficient to prevent mineral loss. A total of 1.5 to 2.0 g of calcium daily and 400 IU of vitamin D daily is required and can be obtained by dietary measures and the use of low-cost supplements (see Chapter 164).

Claims for the efficacy of other dietary measures and supplements, usually put forward by commercial interests, continue to bombard patients; most are unproven. The results of well-designed, small-scale, prospective trials of high-dose γ-*linolenic acid* (an essential fatty acid and close precursor of prostaglandin E_1 with demonstrated antiinflammatory and immunoregulatory activity) have been promising. Essential fatty acids may also have an immunomodulatory effect independent of prostaglandin activity. The dihydro metabolite of γ-linolenic acid manifests such an effect, acting directly on T cells *in vitro* to suppress proliferation of interleukin-dependent T lymphocytes. The value of γ-linoleic acid remains to be established by large-scale, prospective, randomized trials.

Based on studies of *fish oil supplements*, diets high in fish and plant fatty acids and low in animal fatty acids may confer a modest degree of subjective improvement. Such fatty acids are essential for the maintenance of cell membrane structure and function.

A popular diet free of additives, preservatives, fruit, red meat, herbs, and dairy products has been advocated as a treatment for RA. The only controlled, double-blinded, randomized study of this therapy failed to show any benefit in patients with long-standing, progressive, active RA.

Alternative and Complementary Measures. A wide range of alternative measures (e.g., chiropractic manipulation, special dietary supplements, biofeedback, herbal therapies, salves, magnets, acupuncture) are tried by patients. Surveys of arthritis patients being seen by rheumatologists find that up to half have tried at least one of them in the past and that nearly a fourth continue to make regular use of at least one of them. Predictors of regular use include severe pain and a college degree. Evidence of their efficacy remains nonexistent for most, but some should soon be tested in randomized, placebo-controlled trials now that the National Institutes of Health is funding formal study of these measures.

Pharmacologic Therapy: Antiinflammatory Agents

As noted earlier, the antiinflammatory agents have traditionally been the first line of therapy, providing both analgesic and antiinflammatory effects sufficient to achieve a reasonable degree of symptomatic relief. However, they do not prevent early joint destruction or alter the course of RA. Consequently, they are increasingly relegated to a secondary role in treatment of patients with active disease, although they retain an important place in most treatment programs as a means of providing quick symptomatic relief. Among agents in this category are *aspirin*, other salicylates, and the *NSAIDs*, including the new *Cox (cyclooxygenase)-2 inhibitors.*

Aspirin remains the cornerstone of antiinflammatory pharmacologic therapy for many patients and is the best proven and least expensive agent for the treatment of RA. Its mechanism of antiinflammatory action involves inhibition of prostaglandin synthesis. In adults under age 60, serum levels of 15 to 20 mg/dL are needed to suppress the inflammation of RA effectively. No standard dose predictably achieves this level, but usually at least 3.6 to 4.8 g/d are necessary. Because of the large dose needed and the short half-life (3 to 4 hours)

of the drug, the patient must take a large number of tablets multiple times per day. The dose can be increased up to the amount at which tinnitus develops; tinnitus is a dependable and reversible sign of salicylate toxicity in adults. The most frequent adverse effect of aspirin is gastric mucosal injury, with many patients manifesting asymptomatic gastric erosions and some showing frank ulceration (see Chapter 68). Bleeding occasionally is caused by gastritis or ulceration and need not be preceded by symptoms of abdominal pain. Aspirin irreversibly inhibits platelet cyclooxygenase and impedes platelet function (see Chapter 81), causing easy bruising and a predisposition to bleeding. A single dose poisons the platelet for its entire 7-day life span.

Because regular aspirin is directly injurious to the gastric mucosa, additional aspirin preparations have been marketed as less "upsetting to the stomach." *Buffered* aspirin contains bicarbonate, but the amount is insufficient to overcome ambient acid and prevent aspirin-induced mucosal injury. Slightly better tolerated are preparations such as Ascriptin, in which aspirin is combined with a more potent antacid (magnesium hydroxide and aluminum hydroxide), but the cost is markedly increased. *Enteric coating* prevents aspirin from dissolving in the stomach and minimizes the risk for direct gastric mucosal injury; however, bioavailability is delayed, so that the onset of pain relief is slower, and again, cost is increased.

Nonacetylated Salicylates, such as *salsalate, choline magnesium salicylate,* and *sodium salicylate,* were developed to reduce the risks for gastric injury and platelet inhibition associated with aspirin yet preserve its analgesic and antiinflammatory effects. Lacking an acetyl moiety, these agents do not inhibit platelet cyclooxygenase and can be given to patients who are allergic to aspirin. However, they are still capable of causing gastric injury, and their effectiveness appears to be no better than, and in many instances less than, that of aspirin for patients with RA. The cost is much increased. *Diflunisal,* a derivative of salicylic acid, does not acetylate or break down to salicylate but does act like aspirin by virtue of its ability to inhibit prostaglandin synthesis. For patients with RA, it provides the analgesic and antiinflammatory effects of 2 to 4 g of aspirin daily, with a lower rate of gastrointestinal side effects. However, platelet inhibition does occur and can cause serious gastrointestinal bleeding. The cost of the drug is 15 times that of aspirin.

Nonsteroidal Antiinflammatory Drugs (NSAIDs). Although aspirin and its salicylate congeners are also technically NSAIDs, the term is usually reserved for the nonsalicylate NSAIDs. Because of their high cost and gastrointestinal side effects, the traditional NSAIDs should not be used until aspirin has been tried in a program sufficient to achieve therapeutic serum levels for at least 2 to 4 weeks. Only if aspirin proves inadequate or unacceptable should it be abandoned in favor of a traditional NSAID because of the high cost and associated gastrointestinal toxic effects of the latter (see below). The newer NSAIDs, which do not inhibit gastric prostaglandins, have fewer adverse gastrointestinal side effects, so that early initiation of NSAID use is reasonable in persons with a history of past or active peptic ulcer disease or gastrointestinal bleeding.

Mechanism of Action. NSAIDs derive from a host of organic acids (propionic, indolacetic, phenylacetic, enolic, mefenamic) and share the ability to inhibit *cyclooxygenase,* a key enzyme in prostaglandin synthesis. The *Cox-1* isoform is essential for renal, platelet, gastric mucosal, and vascular function; it is elaborated by the tissues it protects and is present in the serum in rather stable concentrations. The *Cox-2* isoform participates principally in inflammation, elaborating prostaglandins in response to cytokines and the action of macrophages; however, it may also be involved in the healing of gastric mucosa and some modulation of renal function. All the older NSAIDs inhibit both isoforms of cyclooxygenase and have similar side effect profiles, including significant gastrointestinal toxicity. The promise of the Cox-2–selective NSAIDs (e.g., celecoxib, rofecoxib) is antiinflammatory action without the adverse consequences of Cox-1 inhibition (see below).

Efficacy. On a milligram-per-milligram basis, NSAIDs are more potent than aspirin and longer-acting, so that a marked reduction in the number of tablets taken and the frequency of dosing becomes possible. The degree of pain relief and antiinflammatory effect achieved is equivalent to that of full-dose aspirin therapy. Although they are more convenient to use, NSAIDs, especially brand formulations can cost many times more than aspirin. See table 156.1.

No particular NSAID (including the new Cox-2 agents) has consistently proved more effective clinically than any other when used at full doses. Nonetheless, some work better for individual patients than others. NSAIDs are sometimes compared according to their values for IC_{50} (concentration that inhibits 50%), an *in vitro* measure of drug efficiency of inhibition, but the IC_{50} has little to do with clinical efficacy. Efficacy is partially a function of dose. Persons not responding to one preparation after 2 to 4 weeks often report benefit when they try another from a different class (Table 156.1). This may be a consequence of individual variations in the serum level attained by taking a given dose, but most differences in efficacy are usually a function of compliance with the drug regimen. Patients on agents that must be taken three or four times daily often fare better when they switch to preparations that require dosing only once or twice daily. No synergy is gained when more than one NSAID is used at a time; mechanisms of action are similar for all, and all bind to the same serum proteins. Although they provide relief from inflammatory symptoms, NSAIDs do not appear to alter the course of RA. Their principal role is to relieve symptoms of inflammation.

Adverse Effects. Most adverse effects are related to Cox-1 inhibition.

Gastric Ulceration and Bleeding. The integrity of the gastric mucosa depends on gastric prostaglandin activity and can be compromised by NSAIDs that inhibit Cox-1. The consequences of such inhibition include dyspepsia, abdominal pain, peptic ulceration, upper gastrointestinal bleeding, and gastric perforation. The risk for clinically important ulceration is estimated to be 1% to 4% per patient-year of NSAID therapy with a nonselective agent. The risk is significantly reduced with the use of a Cox-2–selective NSAID. Risk factors for gastrointestinal complications include previous NSAID-related gastrointestinal side effects (risk of 1.4% per year), concurrent use of prednisone (risk of 1.2% per year), advancing age (risk of 0.3% per year for every 5 years over the age of 50), and substantial disability (risk of 0.5% per year). The total annual risk for a given patient can be estimated by summing these figures. About 15% to 25% of long-term NSAID users demonstrate gastric ulceration at endoscopy; for users of a selective Cox-2 inhibitor, the figure is in the range of 5% (just slightly above that for placebo).

Risk generally increases with dose and duration of therapy, but up to one fourth of complications have been observed within the first month of therapy. There may be no warning

Table 156.1.   Nonsteroidal Antiinflammatory Drugs

CLASS	DURATION OF ACTION[a]	RELATIVE COST[b]	
		GENERIC	BRAND
Propionic Acid Derivatives			
ibuprofen	Short	.4	2.6
naproxen (generic)	Medium	8.5	6
fenoprofen	Short	N/A	4
ketoprofen (generic)	Short	12.5	16
flurbiprofen (generic)	Short	2.4	N/A
oxaprozin (generic)	Long	N/A	5.1
nabumetone	Long	N/A	8.5
Indolacetic Acid Derivatives			
indomethacin (generic)	Short	.3	6.3
indomethacin (extended-release generic)	Long	1.7	6
sulindac (generic)	Medium	1.2	8
tolmetin (generic)	Short	7.1	8
Phenylacetic and Derivatives			
diclofenac	Short	.8	13
Enolic Acid Derivatives			
piroxicam (generic)	Long	.3	10
Mefenamic and Derivatives			
meclofenamate (generic)	Short	2.4	N/A

[a]Short, up to 8 hours; tid to qid dosing.
Medium, up to 18 hours; bid dosing.
Long, 24 hours or more; once-daily dosing.
[b]Based on cost of an enteric-coated aspirin dose of 3.9 g/d. Cost of brand formulations of generic agents 5 to 40 times higher. Relative cost based on wholesale costs of NSAIDs from Drugd of Choice. Medical Letter, Inc. New Rochelle, New York, 1999. Cost to patient is likely to be 10% or more higher.

symptoms preceding severe bleeding or perforation. The risk for adverse gastrointestinal effects is similar for all nonselective NSAIDs because they all inhibit gastric prostaglandin synthesis to a significant degree. The use of a prodrug preparation (e.g., nabumetone) provides no advantage because superficial erosions are much less common than with plain aspirin. The use of NSAIDs in patients with a history of peptic ulcer disease, gastrointestinal bleeding, or abdominal pain requires careful monitoring.

Gastrointestinal risk can be reduced by the use of a selective Cox-2 inhibitor, treatment of concurrent *Helicobacter pylori* infection, use of misoprostol (a gastric prostaglandin analogue), or use of a proton pump inhibitor, such as omeprazole or lansoprazole (see Chapter 68). It is not yet clear which choice is the most cost-effective, but use of a selective Cox-2 inhibitor does significantly reduce the risk for gastric ulceration, gastritis, and gastrointestinal bleeding without any compromise in antiinflammatory efficacy. Of note, little reduction is seen in the frequency of minor gastrointestinal side effects, such as dyspepsia, mild nausea, and diarrhea, with Cox-2 drugs.

Platelet Inhibition. NSAIDs reversibly inhibit platelet cyclooxygenase. Gastrointestinal bleeding in the context of concurrent NSAID use can turn into life-threatening hemorrhage. However, unlike aspirin, NSAIDs prolong the bleeding time for only a short while; inhibition quickly ceases when drug use is stopped. The clinical effect of the Cox-2 agents on platelet function remains to be defined more fully, but the absence of platelet thromboxane inhibition may result in a relative increase in thrombus formation at the site of vascular injury.

Renal Injury. A normal, well-perfused kidney does not depend on renal prostaglandin activity to the extent that an injured, underperfused kidney does. Under situations of hemodynamic stress, prostaglandins serve as important regulators of renal blood flow. NSAID use may lead to fluid retention and diminished sodium excretion. Azotemia may worsen, and oliguria and renal shutdown have been reported in patients with preexisting renal disease. Control of hypertension may diminish with NSAID use. The risk for renal toxicity is greatest in the setting of inadequate renal perfusion (congestive heart failure, cirrhosis, dehydration, advanced age, use of potent diuretics). Renal injury may develop after only a few days of therapy but is reversible if NSAIDs are promptly stopped. Monitoring serum creatinine is advisable, especially in high-risk patients. Sulindac may be less nephrotoxic than other preparations because it has little effect on renal prostaglandin synthesis. NSAIDs may impair the action of antihypertensive agents. No nephrotoxicity has been reported with the prolonged use of high-dose aspirin.

No long-term data are yet available on the clinical effects of the Cox-2 agents with regard to renal function and blood pressure control. Available data from large-scale but relatively short-term clinical studies reveal no compromise in blood pressure control or renal function after 3 months of daily use, but fluid retention has been noted in some patients. The literature should be followed for data on the renal effects of Cox-2 agents.

Mental Impairment. The elderly are particularly susceptible. Cognitive function, mood, or personality may be altered, especially with agents that cross the blood–brain barrier (e.g., indomethacin). Confusion, poor memory, irritability, depression, lassitude, difficulty sleeping, and even paranoid behavior are among the reactions noted. Minor neurologic side effects (e.g., headache, dizziness, light-headedness) are seen in patients of all ages.

Hepatotoxicity. Mild elevation in liver enzymes is sometimes noted, but severe hepatitis is rare. Cholestatic hepatitis has been reported. Occasional monitoring of the serum aminotransferase (transaminase) will suffice; the drug is halted if levels rise above the upper limits of normal.

Selection of Nonsteroidal Antiinflammatory Drug. Because side effects are relatively similar among the traditional NSAIDs, one can use cost, frequency of dose, and response to an empiric trial (2 to 4 weeks at maximum dosage) as the basis for selection (Table 156.1). Inquiry into past experience with NSAIDs can help save time. Aspirin remains the cheapest form of antiinflammatory therapy, but frequent dosing is required and a large number of pills must be taken each day. Generic ibuprofen is the most economical of the modern NSAIDs, but dosing three times daily is required. Generic naproxen is the least expensive of the twice-daily NSAID formulations. Generic indomethacin is also inexpensive, but its utility is limited by the frequency and severity of gastrointestinal and central nervous system side effects, especially in the elderly. Piroxicam offers once-daily dosing, but at a greatly increased cost.

A Cox-2 agent is preferred in patients at increased risk for NSAID-induced peptic ulceration or its complications (e.g., prior history of peptic ulcer, bleeding, or perforation; general debility; concurrent steroid use; advanced age). The high cost of these agents is a marked disadvantage, but with declining long-term NSAID use (see below), the cost differential should be less of an issue. Moreover, some cost savings should result from the reduced frequency of stomach ulceration and its complications and from elimination of the need for concurrent proton pump or misoprostol therapy.

Corticosteroids. The principal role for corticosteroids is to provide interim symptomatic control of inflammatory symptoms and extraarticular manifestations in patients with moderate to severe disease who are waiting for disease-modifying therapy to take effect. A limited course of relatively low-dose therapy (e.g., 5 to 15 mg of prednisone per day) can provide ad-

Table 156.2. Relative Costs of Some Drugs for Rheumatoid Arthritis

DRUG AND DOSAGE	RELATIVE COST PER MONTH
Antiinflammatory Agents	
enteric-coated aspirin, 3.6 g/d	1.0
ibuprofen 800 mg tid (generic)	1.2
naproxen 500 mg bid (generic)	1.8
celecoxib 200 mg bid	9.5
rofecoxib 25 mg/d	4.8
prednisone 10 mg/d	0.4
Disease-Modifying Agents	
methotrexate 17.5 mg/wk	4.2
sulfasalazine 2 g/d	2.3
hydroxychloroquine 400 mg/d	2.4
leflunomide 20 mg/d	15.5
gold salts 50 mg/mo	1.0
cyclosporine 175 mg/d	26.3
etanercept 25 mg SQ twice weekly	63.1

Adapted from Goldring SR. JAMA 2000;283:524, with permission.

ditional symptomatic relief in those who remain very uncomfortable despite NSAID use. If evidence of vasculitis or other serious systemic complications develops, then higher glucocorticoid doses are indicated (e.g., 40 to 60 mg of prednisone per day). Low-dose prednisone started in the early stages of symptomatic RA may have a modest joint-sparing effect, but more confirmatory and longer-term data are needed before steroids can be considered a valuable disease-modifying treatment. Steroids should be tapered to the lowest effective dose once symptoms are brought under control and discontinued as soon as disease-modifying therapy takes hold.

Prolonged steroid therapy is to be avoided. Short courses of steroids that become long can produce severe *osteoporosis*, *muscle atrophy*, *ligamentous weakening*, and *aseptic necrosis* of the femoral head. Often, twice-daily administration is required to control symptoms adequately, which increases the risk for *hypothalamic–pituitary–adrenal suppression* (see Chapter 105). In extremely difficult situations, such as a disabling flare-up of joint disease, very low-dose therapy (5.0 to 7.5 mg of prednisone per day) may be restarted to tide the patient over until disease-modifying therapy takes hold. The only clear indication for parenteral high-dose steroid treatment is life-threatening extraarticular disease, such as vasculitis, pericarditis, or alveolitis. Intraarticular injection of a long-acting steroid preparation may improve functional status when one large, weight-bearing joint is disproportionately inflamed. However, repeated steroid injections into the same joint may hasten its degeneration and increase the risk for infection.

Pharmacologic Therapy: Disease-modifying Agents

Efficacy and Approach to Use. Disease-modifying therapy has become the mainstay of treatment for RA, reducing disease morbidity and mortality by nearly 30% in randomized, controlled trials. The response rates to disease-modifying therapy average about 50%; complete remissions can occur in 20% to 40% of cases but are harder to come by in more severe disease. The use of multiple drug regimens often doubles or triples response and remission rates in patients with very active disease. Initial results of adding a tumor necrosis factor (TNF) inactivator suggest that a threefold to fivefold improvement in the response rate may be possible in refractory cases.

Unlike NSAIDS, disease-modifying therapy introduced early in the course of illness can halt or slow disease progression and limit permanent joint damage. No longer is disease-modifying therapy reserved for those who fail NSAID therapy. It is now appropriately considered for all patients at the outset of symptomatic disease. Careful radiographic studies show disproportionate joint destruction early in the course of active RA and poor outcomes in patients treated solely with NSAIDs during the first 6 months of illness.

Contributing to the success of disease-modifying therapy is the use of *multiple drug regimens*. As in cancer chemotherapy, outcomes are improved without an increase in adverse effects with the combined use of agents that act at different steps in the immunopathologic sequence. The latest additions to the therapeutic armamentarium are the TNF inactivators.

The onset of action is usually slow, with 6 weeks or more passing before any effect becomes evident, and 3 to 6 months before the maximum effect is obtained. Consequently, NSAIDs and, if necessary, low-dose prednisone are started along with these agents to control symptoms. Although drug-related toxicity can be substantial and close monitoring is required to maximize safe use, the documented efficacy of disease-modifying therapy strongly argues for its early application in the management of RA. Relative cost can be high (Table 156.2).

At present, indefinite continuation of disease-modifying therapy appears to be necessary because disease activity returns when treatment is stopped. Nonetheless, certain data suggest some lasting benefit (e.g., better joint preservation) with even limited courses of treatment. More data are needed to determine the optimal duration of therapy.

Descriptions of a number of the disease-modifying agents and combinations follow:

Methotrexate is a first-line disease-modifying agent that is commonly prescribed for persons with moderate to severe disease of new onset. It is among the fastest-acting of the disease-modifying drugs, often controlling symptoms within 6 weeks. It is also quite effective and well tolerated, so that it is among the most favored agents for treatment. Low-dose therapy (7.5 mg/wk) is given orally once weekly in three doses, 12 hours apart. The liquid preparation is the least expensive. Parenteral administration is less likely to cause *gastrointestinal upset* and *stomatitis*, common side effects. Aspirin and NSAIDs should not be used concurrently because they slow the rate of methotrexate excretion and increase gastrointestinal toxicity. Renal dysfunction is a contraindication to use. Short-term, low-dose therapy is well tolerated, but bone marrow suppression, hepatocellular injury, and idiosyncratic interstitial pneumonitis can occur. The latter may lead to *pulmonary fibrosis* and is important to recognize early. Mild, nonprogressive elevations in hepatocellular enzymes are common and not a contraindication to continued therapy, although careful monitoring is required. Alcohol use is contraindicated. Folic acid supplementation (1 mg/d) reduces the risk for drug toxicity without reducing efficacy. Longer-term therapy is often given and is well tolerated, but once the cumulative dose of methotrexate exceeds 1.5 g, the risk for *hepatic fibrosis* may begin to increase. The need for liver biopsy at this point remains unresolved.

Hydroxychloroquine. Antimalarial therapy is not as effective as methotrexate but is better tolerated and therefore a reasonable selection as initial disease-modifying therapy for patients with mild disease. At least 4 to 6 weeks of therapy is needed before results are detectable; full benefit may not be evident before 3 to 4 months. The most serious toxic effect is *visual impairment* (even blindness) caused by drug accumulation in the retina; this complication is extremely rare when doses are limited to 200 to 400 mg/d. Regular (every 6 months) ophthalmologic screening is indicated for patients who have been taking hydroxychloroquine for years or who have renal insufficiency; the yield is very low in those who take less than 6.5 mg/kg per day. Tinnitus and vertigo are sometimes noted.

Sulfasalazine has a long-standing record of efficacy and safety in inflammatory bowel disease and as an alternative to hydroxychloroquine for patients with mild RA. It may be superior to hydroxychloroquine. Its safety profile makes it a popular first-line disease-modifying agent. Hypersensitivity to its sulfa moiety is common, so that its use is limited in patients allergic to sulfa. Because of occasional *hepatocellular injury* and minor degrees of *myelosuppression*, a periodic check of the complete blood cell count and aminotransferase levels is necessary. Gastrointestinal upset (anorexia, nausea, vomiting, diarrhea) is more common. Reversible oligospermia has been noted.

Combination Programs of First-line Drugs. Combining several *first-line disease-modifying agents* (e.g., methotrexate, hydroxychloroquine, and sulfasalazine) appears to provide synergistic effects, thereby improving response rates and potentially lowering the frequency of adverse effects by allowing smaller doses to be administered. Although it remains to be proved in long-term prospective studies, evidence is already accumulating that combination therapy produces significantly higher remission rates with no increase in overall risk for adverse effects. Whether combination therapy should be the initial program of choice remains a subject of debate; further study is needed. Combination programs are increasingly being instituted by rheumatologists if a patient's response to initial disease-modifying therapy with a single agent is inadequate. Combination therapy with first-line drugs may be better tolerated than therapy with a potentially more toxic second-line disease-modifying agent. Combination programs that include *second-line agents* and *anticytokine therapy* are used in more refractory disease (see below).

Leflunomide is a new pyrimidine synthesis inhibitor that interferes with the cell cycle in rapidly proliferating cells such as activated lymphocytes. In placebo-controlled comparison studies with methotrexate, it demonstrates a similar degree of disease-modifying activity but not quite the same degree of tolerability; the frequency of diarrhea and allergic skin reactions is increased.

Gold was first of the disease-modifying agents. Because of the requirement for parenteral administration, the frequency and severity of adverse effects, and the need for constant monitoring of blood and urine, gold has been relegated to a secondary role among disease-modifying agents. It is usually reserved for patients with moderate to severe disease who fail or cannot take methotrexate or combination therapy with other first-line drugs. Treatment may temporarily halt or even partially reverse articular erosion in up to 60% of cases, but fewer than 2% of patients treated have remissions that last longer than 3 years. The effects of gold are cumulative. Those who are going to respond do so by the time 1,000 mg has been given. Adverse effects are often idiosyncratic and range from *rashes* and buccal cavity *mucosal ulcers* to *bone marrow suppression*, *glomerulonephritis*, *interstitial pneumonitis*, and *exfoliative dermatitis*. Most side effects are reversible if the medication is stopped immediately.

Auranofin is an oral gold formulation usually taken twice daily. It causes fewer cases of mucocutaneous, renal, and bone marrow toxicity than parenteral gold does, but more cases of diarrhea (which is dose-related) and sometimes colitis. Often, the gastrointestinal side effects cease with continued therapy, although lowering the dose may be necessary. The efficacy is less than that of injectable gold but is still significant in placebo-controlled studies. Because of its relative safety, auranofin is worth considering to sustain remissions achieved with other agents. Monitoring is similar to that for parenteral therapy, although the frequency can be monthly rather than weekly. A low-dose regimen for 6 months is typical; if the response is inadequate, a 3-month trial at a higher dose may be considered before therapy is terminated.

Cyclosporine was developed to provide more selective inhibition of the immune mechanisms involved in autoimmune disease while leaving other immune pathways relatively unaffected. It is a selective T-cell immunosuppressor that is used as a second- or third-line agent in patients with active disease who fail combination therapy with first-line drugs. Combination with methotrexate has proved useful in refractory disease. Adverse effects include renal insufficiency, anemia, hypertension, and hirsutism, so that periodic checks of blood cell counts, renal function, and potassium levels are necessary.

Cyclophosphamide and Azathioprine are cytotoxic immunosuppressive agents that have been reserved for patients with otherwise refractory disease. Cyclophosphamide is used to treat systemic vasculitis. Both agents are contraindicated in pregnancy because they are *teratogenic*. The risk for malignancy is increased, especially with cyclophosphamide. Other adverse effects of cyclophosphamide include *hemorrhagic cystitis*, *marrow suppression*, and *sterility*. Azathioprine use is associated with gastrointestinal upset, hepatitis, and marrow depression, but the risk is low with the small doses given to patients with RA.

Penicillamine is a chelating agent that can slow aggressive disease. Adverse effects are similar to those of parenteral gold and are best mitigated by giving low doses and increasing them slowly. Fewer than 50% of patients given the drug are able to continue it for prolonged treatment. Fatal *aplastic anemia*, *leukopenia*, *agranulocytosis*, and *thrombocytopenia* can occur. Proteinuria is seen in 10% to 15% of cases and may progress to the nephrotic syndrome. Rashes and autoimmune syndromes such as myasthenia gravis have been reported. The drug is contraindicated in pregnancy. It should be reserved for those who fail to respond to all other forms of therapy and should be prescribed only under the supervision of a rheumatologist skilled in its use.

Pharmacologic Therapy: Anticytokines and Other Agents

Anticytokine Therapy: Tumor Necrosis Factor Inactivators. The agents of this class represent the first direct attempts at the use of anticytokine therapy in RA. Anticytokines bind and inactivate circulating TNF, a key inflammatory cytokine in RA. Patients previously unresponsive to first-line disease-modifying therapy demonstrate marked reductions in disease activity when one of these agents is added to the treatment program. Whether they are truly disease-modifying remains to be determined; their long-term safety and cost-effectiveness are also still unknown. The direct cost of treatment is very high (Table 156.1).

Etanercept is a fusion protein made up of two soluble TNF receptors (p75) grafted onto the Fc portion of a human immunoglobulin G1 molecule by recombinant methods. When added to methotrexate therapy in randomized, double-blinded, placebo-controlled trials, it significantly improved control in patients with active disease not adequately controlled by methotrexate alone. Response rates improved twofold to five-fold, with more than 70% of patients having at least a 20% reduction in symptoms. To date, side effects are minimal other than local discomfort at the injection site, which ceases with continuation of therapy. Theoretical concerns about increased risks for cancer and infection (TNF is part of the surveillance system of the body) have not materialized, nor have increased levels of antibody to double-stranded DNA (an early observation) been noted. Twice-weekly SQ injections are required, which can be self-administered. Antibodies to the agent have not been observed, nor are they expected, as no foreign proteins are present.

Infliximab is a monoclonal antibody that binds TNF. It is composed of a murine TNF-binding site grafted onto human immunoglobulin G. It has been used with success in Crohn's disease and is now being applied in RA. Responses in RA are similar to those for etanercept, with nearly 80% of patients showing at least a 20% improvement in symptoms within 4 weeks of a single IV dose. Antibody formation to the murine portion of the monoclonal antibody occurs in 50% of patients but does not seem to limit efficacy. Combination use with methotrexate appears to reduce antibody production and enhance response.

Minocycline is a tetracycline derivative with prominent antiinflammatory and immunosuppressive effects, including inhibition of synovial collagenase, lymphocyte proliferation, and cell division. Randomized, placebo-controlled trials in patients requiring disease-modifying therapy have provided encouraging results, although the degree of clinical benefit appears modest at best. More study is required to define its efficacy and safety in comparison with other forms of disease-modifying therapy.

Analgesics without any antiinflammatory effect have a limited role in RA. Occasionally, a narcotic analgesic is prescribed for short-term pain control. The regular use of narcotic analgesics is to be avoided because of the risk for addiction in this chronic disease.

Additional Measures

Prevention and Treatment of Osteoporosis. The risk for the development of osteoporosis is markedly increased in RA by both inactivity and the use of glucocorticoids. Preventive measures are critical and effective. Adequate dietary calcium and vitamin D are essential components of any program for osteoporosis. Hormone replacement for menopausal women and bisphosphonates (e.g., alendronate) for those taking glucocorticoids have successfully prevented or halted osteoporosis in patients with RA. A modest degree of remineralization is sometimes noted with the use of estrogens and alendronate (see Chapter 164).

Surgery. Arthroplasty is an important component of therapy in patients with destroyed joints and marked disability. Hip and knee procedures are most successful; the outcome in hand, wrist, elbow, and ankle reconstructions is less certain, but rapid progress is being made. The risk for loosening of a hip prosthesis is significant (25%), even in the absence of active disease. Conventional synovectomy is generally ineffective and results in loss of joint motion; however, arthroscopic synovectomy may permit control of particularly severe monoarticular disease involving the knee.

Total Lymphoid Irradiation and Apheresis represent desperate attempts to inhibit the immunopathology of RA. Controlled studies of irradiation suggest some benefit in extreme situations, but the risk for infection is markedly increased. The rationale behind apheresis is to remove immune complexes and other mediators of the inflammatory process. Placebo-controlled studies have failed to show significant benefit. Selective removal of lymphocytes from peripheral blood (leukopheresis) has yielded transient mild clinical improvement in refractory cases, but not of sufficient magnitude to justify the high cost. With the development of safer, more effective therapies, the demand for such measures should fade.

Monitoring

Disease activity and response to therapy are best monitored by reproducible measures, such as duration of *morning stiffness*, *sedimentation rate*, *number of tender swollen joints*, and *grip strength* (which can be measured with a blood pressure cuff). *Time required to walk 15 meters* and *ring size* are also helpful. The titer of RF does not correlate with disease activity but does decrease with gold and penicillamine therapy if the patient responds. Outcomes research has emphasized the utility of additional measures of function, such as the answers to questions regarding psychosocial functioning and the activities of daily living included in the *Health Assessment Questionnaire* and the *Arthritis Impact Measurement Scale*. The patient's self-assessment and the physician's global assessment also demonstrate validity.

Detecting early disease progression is more difficult but very important if disease-modifying therapy is to be instituted in a timely fashion. Joint space narrowing is a specific but late radiographic sign of cartilaginous erosion that may not develop until irreversible damage has already occurred. Magnetic resonance imaging has been used experimentally to detect synovial proliferation and early pannus formation, but the cost remains prohibitive for routine use. At present, one estimates the likelihood of disease progression by the duration of symptoms.

PATIENT EDUCATION AND COUNSELING

As shown in a randomized trial of the Arthritis Self-help Course (a model program of basic patient education), patient education and counseling are well worth the time invested because they help to reduce pain, disability, and frequency of physician visits. They represent a most cost-effective intervention.

Informing the Patient of the Diagnosis. With a potentially disabling disease such as RA, the act of informing the patient of the diagnosis takes on major importance. The goal is to satisfy the patient's informational needs regarding the diagnosis, prognosis, and treatment without going into an overwhelming and excessive amount of detail. Careful questioning and empathic listening are required to understand the patient's perspective, requests, and fears. Telling patients more than they are intellectually or psychologically prepared to deal with (a common practice) risks making the experience so intense as to trigger withdrawal. On the other hand, failing to address issues of importance to the patient compromises the development of trust. The patient needs to know that the primary physician understands the situation and will be available for support, advice, and therapy as the need arises. Encouraging the patient to ask questions helps to communicate interest and caring.

Discussing Prognosis and Treatment. Patients and family do best when they know what to expect and can view the illness realistically. Uncertainty contributes heavily to the "disease" of RA. Many fear crippling consequences and dependency. The most common disease manifestations should be described. Without building false hopes, the physician can point out that spontaneous remissions are frequent and that more than two thirds of patients live independently without major disability. In addition, it should be emphasized that much can be done to minimize discomfort and preserve function. A review of available therapies and their efficacy helps to overcome feelings of depression stemming from an erroneous expectation of inevitable disability. Even in patients with severe disease, guarded optimism is now appropriate, given the host of effective and well-tolerated disease-modifying treatments that are emerging. A major fear is abandonment. Patients are relieved to know that they will be followed closely by the primary physician and health care team, working in conjunction with a consulting rheumatologist and physical/occupational therapist, all of whom are committed to maximizing the patient's comfort and independence and preserving joint function.

Dealing with Misconceptions. Several common misconceptions deserve attention. A substantial proportion of patients and their families feel that they have done something to cause the illness. Explaining that there are no known controllable precipitants helps to eliminate much unnecessary guilt and self-recrimination. Dealing in an informative, evidence-based fashion with a patient who expresses interest in alternative and complementary forms of therapy can help limit expenditures on ineffective treatments. Another misconception is that a medication has to be expensive to be helpful. Aspirin, generic NSAIDs, low-dose prednisone, and the first-line disease-modifying agents are quite inexpensive (Table 156.1) yet remarkably effective, a point that bears emphasizing. The sense that one must be treated with a Cox-2 NSAID or the latest TNF inactivator can be addressed by a careful review of the overall treatment program and the proper role of such agents in the patient's plan of care. The active participation of the patient and family in the design and implementation of the therapeutic program helps to boost morale and ensure compliance, as does explaining the rationale for the therapies used.

Preserving a Sense of Self-worth. A major goal is to preserve the patient's sense of worth and independence. However, when fatigue, morning stiffness, or specific joint disease interferes with a patient's capacity to carry out the usual responsibilities at work and at home, counseling will be necessary to recommend modification of work responsibilities and perhaps retraining. With the use of occupational therapy, the treatment effort is geared to helping the patient maintain a meaningful work role within the limitations of the illness. The family plays an important part in striking the proper balance between dependence and independence. Household members should avoid overprotecting the patient (e.g., refraining from intercourse out of fear of hurting the patient) and work to sustain the patient's pride and ability to contribute to the family. Allowing the patient with RA to struggle with a task is sometimes constructive.

Supporting the Patient with Debilitating Disease. Persons with long-standing severe disease who have already sustained much irreversible joint destruction benefit from an emphasis on comfort measures, supportive counseling, and attention to minimizing further debility. Such patients need help in grieving for their disfigurement and loss of function. An accepting, unhurried, empathic manner allows the patient to express feelings. The seemingly insignificant act of touching does much to restore a sense of self-acceptance. Attending to pain with increased social support, medication, and a refocusing of attention onto function are useful. A trusting and strong patient–doctor relationship can do much to sustain a patient through times of discomfort and disability.

INDICATIONS FOR REFERRAL AND ADMISSION

The increasingly early and more aggressive use of disease-modifying drugs and the expanding armamentarium of such agents argue for prompt referral to the rheumatologist at the time of initial diagnosis. It is no longer appropriate to wait until antiinflammatory therapy proves insufficient or overt signs of joint destruction appear. The benefits of early implementation of a disease-modifying program have been sufficiently established to warrant early referral for the design and implementation of such a regimen. Patients requiring regimens associated with a high risk for serious toxicity should be periodically seen by the rheumatologist; those on programs that are better tolerated can be managed almost exclusively by the primary care physician. In all cases, a close working relationship with the rheumatologist is essential.

Patients with evidence of persistent joint inflammation should be referred back to the rheumatologist for advancement of their disease-modifying therapy, especially those with characteristics that indicate a poor prognosis (e.g., genotype *HLA-DRB1*04/04*, high serum titer of RF, extraarticular manifestations, a large number of involved joints, age less than 30, female sex, systemic symptoms).

Referral to physical and occupational therapists is greatly appreciated by patients with active disease. The emphasis should be on teaching the patient things that can be done to improve function. Well-designed exercise and self-care programs can greatly facilitate carrying out the activities of daily living and reduce discomfort and disability.

The need for surgical referral is best determined by the rheumatologist, who is well trained to judge when medical therapy is insufficient. Examples of indications for surgery include carpal tunnel syndrome that persists despite corticosteroid injection, trigger finger deformity, tendon rupture with loss of manual dexterity, and refractory dorsal wrist effusions. The patient with disabling hip or knee destruction and severe impairment of weight-bearing capacity deserves a surgical assessment regarding possible prosthetic joint replacement. Arthroscopic synovectomy may be needed for a single, very refractory joint that cannot be replaced.

When fever or other manifestations of severe extraarticular disease appear (especially signs of vasculitis or diffuse serositis), then hospital admission for workup and IV administration of steroids should be promptly considered.

THERAPEUTIC RECOMMENDATIONS

- Provide a comprehensive patient and family education program that includes psychological support and strategies for maintaining the patient's activity, independence, and self-esteem. Utilize health care team members to enhance the educational and supportive efforts.
- Consider first-line disease-modifying therapy (e.g., methotrexate, hydroxychloroquine, sulfasalazine, or any combination) at the time of initial diagnosis for all patients, especially those with very active disease or indicators of a poor prognosis (e.g., genotype *HLA-DRB1*04/04*, high serum titer of RF, extraarticular manifestations, large number of involved joints, age below 30, female sex, systemic symptoms). Obtain early rheumatologic consultation for selection of the disease-modifying regimen. Coordinate care with the rheumatologist and closely monitor the patient for response to therapy and complications of the drug program (see below).
- While waiting for disease-modifying therapy to take effect (up to 6 months may be necessary), begin antiinflammatory treatment with a generic NSAID (e.g., 3.6 g of enteric-coated aspirin daily, 800 mg of ibuprofen three times a day, or 500 mg of naproxen twice daily). Consider use of a selective Cox-2 inhibitor only if NSAIDs are not well tolerated or if the patient is at high risk for peptic ulceration and its complications. Use NSAIDs with care in patients with impaired renal perfusion; monitor blood urea nitrogen and creatinine. Also prescribe cautiously to patients with a prior history of peptic ulcer disease or gastrointestinal bleeding (see Chapter 68); monitor hematocrit and test for fecal occult blood.
- For patients with very active disease inadequately controlled by initial NSAID therapy, consider adding a small dose of corticosteroid therapy (e.g., 5 mg of prednisone per day, in split doses twice daily if necessary). Reserve daily use of systemic steroids for patients truly incapacitated by symptoms, and use only a short-term, low-dose program (e.g., 5.0 to 7.5 mg of prednisone daily until disease-modifying therapy takes hold). If steroids are to be utilized, begin a program of osteoporosis prevention that includes calcium (1.5 g/d) and vitamin D (400 to 800 IU/d) plus hormone replacement therapy, a bisphosphonate (e.g., 5 to 10 mg of alendronate per day), or both (see Chapters 144 and 164).
- Once disease-modifying therapy begins to take hold, taper and discontinue NSAIDs and corticosteroids. Continue disease-modifying program indefinitely.
- Prescribe a gentle exercise program to maintain range of motion and muscle strength, but avoid stressing a severely inflamed joint. Prior application of heat or cold (either may work) will facilitate the exercise program. Consult with a physical therapist to help design the program. Morning application of heat is particularly helpful before the patient engages in daily activity.
- Selectively rest severely inflamed individual joints that are too swollen to exercise. Maintain the joint in its physiologic position by splinting during periods when the joint is stressed (e.g., at night) to support weakened joints and prevent flexion contractures. Consult the rheumatologist if splinting appears indicated.
- Advise a daily rest period for patients bothered by generalized fatigue, but outpatients should avoid prolonged bed rest.
- Consult the rheumatologist again if the patient manifests persistently active disease. It may be necessary to advance the disease-modifying regimen or alter it. Increasingly, early rheumatologic consultation and aggressive treatment may be necessary if joint destruction is to be prevented, particularly in patients with findings suggestive of a poor prognosis.
- For patients incapacitated by one disproportionately inflamed large, weight-bearing joint, consider a single intraarticular injection of a long-acting corticosteroid (e.g., 2.5 to 10 mg of triamcinolone acetonide, depending on joint size, mixed with 1 mL of lidocaine). The knee is cleansed with iodine and alcohol and an intraarticular injection is performed under sterile conditions. Repeated injections into the same joint are to be avoided.
- Monitor disease activity and response to therapy by checking reproducible measures, such as duration of morning stiffness, sedimentation rate, number of tender swollen joints, and grip strength (have the patient squeeze a blood pressure cuff). Also monitor activities of daily living and psychosocial status.
- For patients on disease-modifying therapy, monitor for drug toxicity closely:
  - For those taking *hydroxychloroquine*, inquire regularly about visual acuity and arrange for an ophthalmologic examination every 6 months.
  - For patients taking *methotrexate*, follow the complete blood cell count, platelet count, and levels of aminotransferase, alkaline phosphatase, blood urea nitrogen, and creatinine. Inquire regularly about any pulmonary symptoms, which might be the first manifestation of interstitial pneumonitis and an indication for immediate cessation of therapy.
  - For patients taking *sulfasalazine*, monitor the complete blood cell count, inquire about gastrointestinal symptoms, and examine the skin for rashes and pruritus.

A.H.G.

ANNOTATED BIBLIOGRAPHY

American College of Rheumatology. Guidelines for monitoring drug therapy in rheumatoid arthritis. Arthritis Rheum 1996;39:723. (*A set of useful guidelines for monitoring the adverse effects of NSAIDs and disease-modifying agents.*)

Anderson JJ, Felson DT, Meenan RF, et al. Which traditional measures should be used in rheumatoid arthritis clinical trials? Arthritis Rheum 1989;32:1093. (*A critical look at measures of disease activity and function.*)

Arnett FC, Edworthy SM, Bloch DA, et al. The American Rheumatism Association 1987 revised criteria for the classification of rheumatoid arthritis. Arthritis Rheum 1988;31:315. (*Widely adopted diagnostic and classification criteria based on a collaborative study of more than 500 patients.*)

Bardwick PA, Swezey RL. Physical therapies in arthritis. Postgrad Med 1982;72:223. (*A discussion of the standard modalities of physical therapy and when to use them.*)

Bradley LA. Psychosocial factors and disease outcomes in rheumatoid arthritis. Arthritis Rheum 1989;32:1611. (*An editorial critically reviewing the role of psychological factors in outcomes.*)

Buckley LM, Seib ES, Cartularo KS, et al. Calcium and vitamin D₃ supplementation prevents bone loss in the spine secondary to low-dose corticosteroids in patients with rheumatoid arthritis. A randomized, double-blind, placebo-controlled trial. Ann Intern Med 1996;125:961. (*Evidence for efficacy in patients with RA who are taking low doses of glucocorticoids.*)

Chan FK, Sung JJ, Chung SC, et al. Randomised trial of eradication of *Helicobacter pylori* before nonsteroidal antiinflammatory drug therapy to prevent peptic ulcers. Lancet 1997;350:975. (*One means of reducing NSAID gastrointestinal risk.*)

Clive DM, Stoff JS. Renal syndromes associated with nonsteroidal antiinflammatory drugs. N Engl J Med 1984;310:563. (*Risk greatest in those with impaired renal perfusion.*)

Cryer B, Feldman M. Cyclooxygenase-1 and cyclooxygenase-2 selectivity of widely used nonsteroidal antiinflammatory drugs. Am J Med 1998;104:413. (*An in vitro study in which the serum of volunteers taking the agents was used; best data on relative effects of all the available traditional NSAIDs.*)

Fries JF, Williams CA, Morfeld D, et al. Reduction in long-term disability in patients with rheumatoid arthritis by disease-modifying antirheumatic drug-based treatment strategies. Arthritis Rheum 1996;39:616. (*Important evidence for reductions in morbidity and mortality.*)

Fuchs HA, Kaye JJ, Callahan LF, et al. Evidence of significant radiologic damage in rheumatoid arthritis within the first 2 years of disease. J Rheumatol 1989;16:585. (*Disproportionate degree of joint damage found early in the course of disease.*)

Jeurissen MEC, Boerbooms AMT, van de Putte LBA, et al. Influence of methotrexate and azathioprine on radiologic progression in rheumatoid arthritis: a randomized, double-blind study. Ann Intern Med 1991;114:999. (*Methotrexate halted disease progression and was more effective than azathioprine.*)

Kirwan JR. The effects of glucocorticoids on joint destruction in rheumatoid arthritis. N Engl J Med 1995;333:142. (*Randomized, double-blinded, controlled trial; early, low-dose prednisone significantly reduced risk for radiologically detectable joint destruction.*)

Kremer JM, Jubiz W, Michalek A, et al. Fish-oil fatty acid supplementation in active rheumatoid arthritis: a double-blinded, controlled, cross-over study. Ann Intern Med 1987;106:497. (*Subjective benefit was found, in addition to a modest reduction in leukotriene.*)

Kruger JMS, Helmick CG, Callahan LF, et al. Cost-effectiveness of the Arthritis Self-Help Course. Arch Intern Med 1998;158:1245. (*Well-documented example of the efficacy of a program emphasizing patient education to encourage proper self-care; cost-effectiveness demonstrated.*)

Leventhal LJ, Boyce EG, Zurier RB. Treatment of rheumatoid arthritis with γ-linolenic acid. Ann Intern Med 1993;119:867. (*Small-scale study, but encouraging results found with use of this dietary supplement.*)

Lorig KR, Lubeck D, Kraines RG, et al. Outcomes of self-help education for patients with arthritis. Arthritis Rheum 1985;28:680. (*Very effective; independence enhanced.*)

Maini RN, Breedbeld FC, Kalden JR, et al. Therapeutic efficacy of multiple intravenous infusions of anti–tumor necrosis factor alfa monoclonal antibody combined with low-dose weekly methotrexate in rheumatoid arthritis. Arthritis Rheum 1998;41:1552. (*Initial report; significant improvement in response noted with use of anticytokine therapy in conjunction with standard disease-modifying therapy.*)

Masi AT. Articular patterns in the early course of rheumatoid arthritis. Am J Med 1983;75:16. (*Patients with multiple joint involvement at onset have a poorer prognosis than those with more limited disease.*)

Mills JA, Pinals RA, Ropes MW, et al. Value of bed rest in patients with rheumatoid arthritis. N Engl J Med 1971;284:453. (*Classic study; minimal benefit was obtained from enforced rest.*)

Moreland LW, Baumgartner SW, Schiff MH, et al. Treatment of rheumatoid arthritis with a recombinant human tumor necrosis factor receptor (p75)-Fc fusion protein. N Engl J Med 1997;337:141 (*Original report establishing efficacy and safety of this major new approach to treatment.*)

Morgan SL, Baggott JE, Vaughn WH, et al. Supplementation with folic acid during methotrexate therapy for rheumatoid arthritis. A double-blind, placebo-controlled trial. Ann Intern Med 1994;121:833. (*Risk for toxicity significantly reduced without a compromise in efficacy.*)

Matteson EL. Current treatment strategies for rheumatoid arthritis. Mayo Clin Proc 2000;75:69. (*A useful review for the primary care physician; the strategies used by rheumatologists for treatment of RA are outlined, with an emphasis on the role of disease-modifying therapy.*)

Mottonen R, Hannonen P, Leirisalo-Repo M, et al. Comparison of combination therapy with single-drug therapy in early rheumatoid arthritis: a randomized trial. Lancet 1999;353:1568. (*Combination therapy more effective and just as safe.*)

O'Dell JR, Haire CE, Erikson N, et al. Treatment of rheumatoid arthritis with methotrexate alone, sulfasalazine and hydroxychloroquine, or a combination of all three medications. N Engl J Med 1996;333:1287. (*Carefully conducted study of aggressive use of disease-modifying therapy.*)

Pinals RS, Kaplan SB, Lawson JG, et al. Sulfasalazine in rheumatoid arthritis: a double-blind, placebo-controlled trial. Arthritis Rheum 1986;29:1427. (*Establishes its utility.*)

Rao JK, Mihaliak K, Kroenke K, et al. Use of complementary therapies for arthritis among patients of rheumatologists. Ann Intern Med 1999;131:409. (*A telephone survey study showing a high frequency of use; many patients regularly using such measures.*)

Rirestein GS, Zvaifler NJ. Anticytokine therapy in rheumatoid arthritis. N Engl J Med 1997;337:195. (*An editorial providing an overview of this new approach to the treatment of RA.*)

Rogers MP, Liang MH, Partridge AJ. Psychological care of adults with rheumatoid arthritis. Ann Intern Med 1982;96:344. (*An often overlooked area; many practical suggestions for effective personal care of both patient and family.*)

Simon LS, Weaver AL, Graham DY, et al. Antiinflammatory and upper gastrointestinal effects of celecoxib in rheumatoid arthritis. A randomized controlled trial. JAMA 1999;282:1921. (*In a large-scale, multicenter, 12-week trial that included a comparison with naproxen and endoscopic assessment, the clinical effects were equivalent, and the rate of ulcers and gastrointestinal side effects was significantly reduced.*)

Simon LS, Mills JA. Nonsteroidal antiinflammatory drugs. N Engl J Med 1980;302:1179,1237. (*Still useful basic review of the pharmacology and role of nonsteroidal agents in comparison with aspirin.*)

Tilley BC, Alarcon GS, Meyse SP, et al. Minocycline in rheumatoid arthritis: a 48-week, double-blind, placebo-controlled trial. Ann Intern Med 1995;122:81. (*Found useful for patients with moderately active disease; role in overall treatment of RA remains to be determined.*)

Tugwell P, Pincus T, Yocum D, et al. Combination therapy with cyclosporine and methotrexate in severe rheumatoid arthritis. N Engl J Med 1995;333:137. (*Randomized, double-blinded, multicenter study showing improved results with combination therapy; another example of the efficacy of aggressive treatment.*)

van der Heijde DM, Jacobs JWG, Bijlsma JWJ, et al. The effectiveness of early treatment with "second-line" antirheumatic drugs. Ann Intern Med 1996;124:699. (*In an open-label, randomized, controlled trial, disease-modifying therapy proved superior to NSAIDs for the treatment of early disease; argues for a reversal of the traditional treatment paradigm.*)

van der Heijde DM, van Riel PL, van Rijswijk MH, et al. Influence of prognostic features on the final outcome in rheumatoid arthritis: a review of the literature. Semin Arthritis Rheum 1988;17:284. (*Excellent summary of clinical and laboratory findings that help predict outcome.*)

Ward JR, Williams J, Egger MJ, et al. Comparison of auranofin, gold sodium thiomalate, and placebo in the treatment of rheumatoid arthritis. Arthritis Rheum 1982;26:1303. (*Parenteral gold was the most effective, but was also more likely to cause renal and mucocutaneous toxicity.*)

Weinblatt ME, Kremer JM, Bankhurst AD, et al. A trial of etanercept, a recombinant tumor necrosis factor receptor:Fc fusion protein, in patients with rheumatoid arthritis receiving methotrexate. N Engl J Med 1999;340:253. (*Major new treatment modality; combination with methotrexate significantly increased response without any increase in adverse effects.*)

Weyand CM, Hicok KC, Conn DL, et al. The influence of *HLA-DRB1* genes on disease severity in rheumatoid arthritis. Ann Intern Med 1992;117:801. (HLA-DRB1 *genotyping helps in the early identification of patients with a poor prognosis.*)

Wolf MM, Lichtenstein DR, Singh G. Gastrointestinal toxicity of nonsteroidal antiinflammatory drugs. N Engl J Med 1999;340:1888. (*Best review to date; includes data on the new Cox-2 inhibitors, which indicate a reduced risk for upper gastrointestinal bleeding.*)

157
Management of Osteoarthritis

Osteoarthritis (OA), the most prevalent form of arthropathy, causes symptomatic discomfort in 10% to 20% of persons over the age of 65 and accounts for somewhat more than 30% of visits to primary care practitioners. OA remains the most common cause of disability in the elderly. Most patients have primary or idiopathic disease that is strongly associated with aging. Others present with posttraumatic and hereditary forms of the disease (e.g., chondrodystrophy, hemochromatosis, inflammatory OA, chondrocalcinosis). Although many changes are irreversible, much can be done to relieve discomfort, prevent further articular damage, and keep the patient functioning independently.

PATHOPHYSIOLOGY AND CLINICAL PRESENTATION

Pathogenesis

Osteoarthritis is characterized by (a) the degeneration of articular cartilage and (b) the reactive formation of new bone. What causes the demise of the articular cartilage remains incompletely understood. The simplistic "wear-and-tear" hypothesis has been superseded by an appreciation for the role of chondrocytes in actively remodeling cartilage. Articular damage appears to be the consequence of an interplay between cartilage metabolism and mechanical stress. The synovial inflammation that is characteristic of rheumatoid disease appears to play only a minor role, if any, in most cases of OA. The significance of genetic factors has not been fully defined, but their involvement is suggested by the strong hereditary pattern of OA hand changes in women and defective collagen synthesis in some familial forms. Obesity is a major risk factor for disease affecting the knee. Poor joint alignment and trauma are other causative factors. Running *per se* is neither protective nor destructive (unless the knee has been injured, in which case running does hasten degenerative change), but excessive stress from weight bearing can be harmful in the elderly.

Histologically and biochemically, the size and aggregation of *proteoglycan* monomers are reduced with age. Proteoglycan is a critical mucopolysaccharide component of the cartilage extracellular matrix, synthesized by cartilage chondrocytes and essential for elasticity. Contributing to this reduction is increased proteolytic enzyme activity by chondrocytes. The matrix is also composed of *collagen fibrils*, which provide resiliency; these fibrils are more susceptible to damage by trauma when matrix proteoglycan declines. Synovial collagenase can penetrate damaged cartilage and further degrade its collagen. With age, bone elasticity (which provides a cushioning effect during trauma) also declines, allowing increased stress to be transmitted directly to the cartilage. Conditions that alter the mechanical relationships of joints further increase the likelihood that degenerative changes will develop.

The earliest manifestations of OA are superficial erosions of the cartilage; the response is hypertrophy and hyperplasia of chondrocytes. Early cartilaginous injury can be repaired by chondrocytes, but fissured hyaline cartilage cannot be restored. Eventually, the cartilage frays, shreds, and cracks. Underlying bone responds by remodeling, which causes trabeculae to thicken. At the joint margins, the development of hypertrophic spurs (*osteophytes*) is followed by buttressing of adjacent cortical bone (*osteosclerosis*). The joint space narrows in an irregular fashion. Cyst formation is also seen. Little synovial reaction occurs unless the degenerative process is rapid, a piece of cartilage dislodges, or calcium pyrophosphate crystals form and incite an acute inflammatory response (pseudogout).

Clinical Presentation

Radiologic evidence of OA can be found in more than 80% of adults by age 65. The subset who are symptomatic complain of deep, aching joint pain that is aggravated by motion and weight bearing. In addition, stiffness may be present that is worsened by periods of inactivity. The involved joint can be enlarged by the formation of osteophytes, but swelling is usually inconsequential because soft-tissue involvement and effusions are, in most instances, minimal. In later stages, pain occurs on motion and at rest in conjunction with stiffness. Nocturnal pain after vigorous activity is common. Patients with advanced disease have pain on weight bearing and joint instability. Examination often reveals crepitus and discomfort on movement of the joint. Occasionally, slight warmth is noted in severely affected weight-bearing joints, but erythema and marked warmth are absent. Limitation of motion, malalignment, and bony protuberances from spurs are frequent findings. The joints most commonly affected include the knees, hips, distal interphalangeal (DIP) joints of the hands, carpometacarpal joint at the base of the thumb, and the joints of the cervical and lumbosacral spine.

Knees. Symptomatic knee involvement is estimated to affect as much as 10% of the population over the age of 65. Obesity is a major risk factor. OA of the knee produces pain that is localized to the medial and/or lateral joint line and worsened by prolonged weight bearing and stair climbing. In later stages, crepitus is often marked and range of motion reduced. A very small effusion may be noted. The joint appears enlarged and feels bony. Patellofemoral joint involvement produces anterior knee pain that is exacerbated by going down stairs. On occasion, very few physical findings may be noted, although pain and radiographic changes are prominent. A skyline view of the flexed knee can reveal patellofemoral disease.

Hips. Degenerative hip disease arises in young patients with congenital dislocations or slipped femoral capital epiphyses. In the elderly, it results from wear and tear. A unilateral or asymmetric distribution is typical. The patient may describe pain that is deep in the hip and radiates into the anterior medial thigh, groin, buttock, or medial knee. The site of radiation (e.g., groin or buttock) may be the only area of reported pain. At first, pain occurs only on prolonged standing or walking, but as OA progresses, discomfort may become continuous and especially unbearable at night. The ability to engage in sexual intercourse is sometimes compromised. Loss of internal rotation during flexion is the earliest change and is as reliable as radiographic findings for diagnosis. The result of Trendelenburg's test (see Chapter 151) is positive.

Hands. Characteristic sites include the DIP joints and base of the thumb (first carpometacarpal joint); sometimes, proximal interphalangeal (PIP) joint involvement is noted. Hand disease is most common in middle-aged and elderly women, many of whom have a strongly positive family history. In some, a low-grade inflammatory response may accompany early, rapid, mucinous degenerative changes, so that the joints take on a tender, cystic inflammatory appearance. Later, osteophytes form, giving rise to characteristic bony protuberances in the DIP joints (*Heberden's nodes*) and occasionally PIP deformities (*Bouchard's nodes*) that superficially resemble those of rheumatoid disease. Eventually, all inflammatory activity resolves, and the joints are left nontender with some limitation of motion.

The base of the thumb, a site of much physical stress, is vulnerable to degenerative change. Pain develops in the region of the thenar eminence and particularly over the carpometacarpal joint. Because the thumb is so important to manual dexterity, the development of arthritis at this site may be disabling. Grip becomes impaired, and fine movements of apposition are restricted. Osteophytes are palpable and, in rare instances, may encroach on the flexor tendon sheath, causing tenosynovitis.

Cervical Spine. Degenerative changes commonly involve the posterior diarthrodial joints of the lower cervical spine (see Chapter 148). Although radiographic changes are frequent, most persons are asymptomatic. Moreover, the correlation between symptoms and radiographic findings is often poor. The patient may have pain and stiffness in the neck, but sometimes pain is reported only in the occiput, shoulder, arm, or hand. In a few instances, scapular or upper anterior chest pain is produced. Osteophytes can protrude into the foramina and impinge on nerve roots (most often C-6 and C-7), causing *radicular pain* that radiates to the shoulder, upper arms, hands, or fingers (see Chapter 167). At night, the patient may awaken with paresthesias and numbness in the arms that can be alleviated by getting up and shaking the arms.

On examination, neck motion is restricted to some extent in all directions, especially lateral flexion and extension; movement reproduces or aggravates symptoms. Reactive muscle spasm and tenderness are often present, and decreased sensation, weakness, and diminished reflexes occur when root compression is marked. However, even when symptoms of root compression are reported, neurologic findings may be scant, and their absence does not rule out the complication.

Lumbosacral Spine. Degenerative changes in the lumbosacral spine involve the intervertebral disks and the apophyseal joints. With aging, the disk nucleus becomes brittle and less elastic. Herniation posteriorly or laterally through a defect in the disk annulus may occur. Intervertebral spaces narrow and marginal osteophytes form. The apophyseal joints show typical secondary degenerative changes. Disk or osteophyte encroachment on the foramina can lead to nerve root compression. The L-4, L-5, and S-1 roots are most commonly affected. The patient reports pain across the lower back with radiation into the buttock and posterior thigh, or down into the lower leg if *root compression* has occurred. Forward flexion and extension are reduced, but lateral flexion is painless. Focal areas of tenderness are common and often caused by spasm of the paraspinous musculature. Disk or osteophyte encroachment into the spinal canal can lead to *spinal stenosis*, which affects the cauda equina and exiting nerve roots. Compression of nerve roots produces *pseudoclaudication* (pain in the buttocks or thighs during prolonged standing or walking that is relieved by sitting or bending). On examination, thigh symptoms may be brought on by 30 seconds of lumbar extension, then relieved by having the patient bend forward. In addition, the patient may have a wide-based gait and neurologic deficits in the lower extremities.

Other Sites. OA may involve the great toe at the metatarsophalangeal joint to cause bony enlargement and a valgus deformity. Crepitus and pain in the temporomandibular joint are sometimes seen secondary to bruxism (grinding of the teeth because of anxiety or anger). Pain is reproduced by opening the mouth widely. Because OA is not a systemic disease, no extraarticular manifestations and no serum abnormalities occur; the sedimentation rate is normal, as is the synovial fluid in early disease. Radiographic findings are limited to the joints and include irregular narrowing of the joint space, sclerosis of subchondral bone, bony cysts, marginal osteophytes, and buttressing of adjacent bone.

NATURAL HISTORY OF DISEASE

In large, weight-bearing joints, OA tends to be a progressive condition causing chronic joint pain, restricted joint motion, and resultant muscle weakness that compromises mobility. Through a period of 10 to 20 years, pain at rest develops in the majority of patients with untreated symptomatic OA of the knee, and they become unable to use public transportation; disability may ensue. Early onset of symptoms and varus deformity correlate with a poor prognosis. OA of the hip may follow a similar course. Obesity is a strong risk factor for progressive disease of the hips and knees (especially in women); heavy weight-bearing exercise is associated with an increased risk for knee disease in the elderly. Weight reduction reduces the risk. The progression of OA is typically limited to a few affected joints, and the disease does not become widespread. Clinical remissions do occur, especially in the hands, neck, and back.

PRINCIPLES OF MANAGEMENT

Osteoarthritis cannot be cured, and no medications (or supplements) have been shown capable of altering the course of the disease. Nonetheless, reduction in pain and restoration of activity can be achieved with a multifaceted program. The goals are to reduce abnormal stresses imposed on affected joints, restore joint alignment, strengthen muscles, and treat pain and muscle spasm. Pain relief is a first priority for most patients. Both pharmacologic and mechanical means are used. Those with severe pain are likely also to try alternative and complementary therapies. Surgical intervention should be restricted to patients who do not respond to conservative management and are so disabled that they cannot function satisfactorily.

Analgesics. In the absence of a major inflammatory component to the disease and until etiologically acting agents become available, analgesics remain the predominant pharmacologic approach to symptom relief in OA. Because an individual patient's response to analgesics is unpredictable, it may be necessary to try several different ones. Intermittent use of analgesics sometimes suffices, but continuous therapy is often needed.

Acetaminophen. Pure analgesics, such as acetaminophen, are at least as effective as NSAIDs, without the associated adverse gastrointestinal side effects and high costs (see below). The cost of acetaminophen is low, and its long-term safety is well established. The highly publicized risk for hepatic injury is rare with regular use of doses within the therapeutic range. Liver injury typically occurs only in cases of overdose or underlying alcoholic liver disease. Long-term therapy at high doses may increase the risk for renal tubular injury, but supporting data are sparse, and the risk appears no greater than that associated with prolonged NSAID use.

NSAIDs. (See also Chapter 156.) Although widely prescribed, NSAIDs are no more effective than acetaminophen in providing symptomatic relief. Their benefit seems to derive principally from their analgesic effects; they appear to have little net direct effect on the underlying disease process (despite occasional evidence pro and con). The absence of significant inflammation in OA helps explain why low, analgesic doses of NSAIDs are no better than high, antiinflammatory doses. NSAIDs can be very expensive (at up to 30 times the cost of ac-

etaminophen), and the associated risk for gastrointestinal toxicity is high (see Chapters 68 and 156). Renal compromise may develop in persons with underlying renal insufficiency. Some elderly patients experience mental confusion while taking NSAIDs that penetrate the central nervous system (e.g., indomethacin).

The use of a *selective Cox (cyclooxygenase)-2 NSAID* preparation (e.g., *celecoxib, rofecoxib*) reduces the risk for peptic ulceration but greatly increases cost. Studies in patient with OA have found the Cox-2 drugs to be equivalent to the nonselective NSAIDs and about equal to acetaminophen in providing symptomatic relief.

Narcotic Analgesics, such as codeine and oxycodone, should be used sparingly, if at all, and only for acute disabling pain interfering with essential activity. *Propoxyphene* (Darvon), an opiate derivative, is taken by many patients with OA, but its potential for causing dependence is considerable—similar to that of codeine.

Exercise. Of the nonmedical therapies, exercise shows the most consistently beneficial results for patients with OA, especially those with disease of the knees. Restoration of favorable mechanics is essential to minimizing damage to injured joints. Strengthening the supporting muscles may help maintain proper joint alignment. *Quadriceps exercises* and a *walking program* for patients with knee involvement clearly improve exercise tolerance and decrease pain. Quadriceps exercises are among the simplest to perform; the patient extends the knee and holds the straightened leg in a horizontal position while sitting in a chair. A program of supervised graduated isometric and isotonic quadriceps exercises can decrease pain and make it possible to walk for longer distances. Isometric and active exercises for the neck improve muscle tone and may sometimes help in cases of painful cervical spine disease (see Chapter 148). Exercises for the abdominal and paraspinous musculature are useful for preventing back problems (see Chapter 147).

Aerobic exercise may provide some additional benefit over strengthening programs by enhancing overall conditioning. For patients with OA of weight-bearing joints, structured aerobic exercise programs with full or partial weight bearing can greatly enhance endurance, walking distance, and sense of well-being without aggravating the arthritis. A 2-month program of supervised fitness walking combined with patient education can improve functional status by close to 40% in patients with symptomatic knee disease. Gentle cycling and swimming also improve endurance, benefiting the muscle groups of the hips and knees. Participation in such conditioning programs also boosts morale considerably.

As beneficial as exercise may be, excessive exercise may only exacerbate pain and cause further disruption of the joint. Excessive joint strain, such as results from stair climbing, should be reduced as much as possible. Supervision and patient education are essential to a successful exercise program and far superior to simply telling the patient to get more exercise.

Rest and Assist Devices. Some relief can be obtained by partially resting a very painful joint. The objective is to reduce the mechanical stress imposed on the joint. However, joint rest should be alternated with exercise to prevent muscle atrophy and worsening joint alignment. Moreover, prolonged immobility greatly disturbs cartilage metabolism.

Assist devices can help rest or protect a diseased joint from excessive mechanical stress. The pressures on hip and knee joints generated by getting up from a toilet or low seat can be decreased by the use of hand rails, grips, and a raised toilet or chair seat. An often underutilized approach to joint rest is the use of a *cane* in the contralateral hand, which can reduce the mechanical stress on a weight-bearing joint by as much as 50%. Embarrassment and awkwardness often make patients reluctant to use a cane, but physician encouragement and a few sessions with an occupational therapist can greatly help.

A *cervical collar* can ease neck pain by supporting the spine and resting the paraspinous musculature. It may be necessary to continue use intermittently for many weeks before significant benefit is achieved. Cervical traction may also help (see Chapter 148). A *corset* or *brace* for the back may be similarly helpful, but its use should be combined with an exercise program to avoid muscle atrophy (see Chapter 147).

Orthotic devices help correct malalignment. Patients with hip disease resulting from or aggravated by differences in leg length may benefit from a heal lift that equalizes leg lengths. If abnormal foot pronation is causing varus stress on the knee joint, a shoe orthotic device may reduce pain and ligamentous strain on the knee.

Weight Reduction. Excessive weight is one of the major risk factors for OA of the knees and hips. Weight bearing puts mechanical stresses on the hip and knee joints that can be as much as five times the patient's weight. Even modest degrees of weight loss may achieve substantial reductions in such mechanical stress. Epidemiologic studies show a strong correlation between obesity and risk for symptomatic knee arthritis, and a 50% reduction in such risk with weight loss in excess of 5 kg (11 lb) over 10 years. These results suggest that half-hearted, perfunctory advice to "lose weight" is insufficient and fails to provide the patient with an important opportunity to affect outcome. A comprehensive program of mechanically sensible, supervised aerobic activity combined with detailed dietary counseling should be constructed (see Chapter 233) and carried out. An assisted, supervised program is essential because obese persons with OA are otherwise likely to feel that weight loss and exercise are beyond their capacity.

Heat. Moist heat can give symptomatic relief from muscle spasm, although it has no effect on the disease itself. *Diathermy* and *ultrasound* units are expensive ways to deliver heat to deep tissues. Although many patients report improvement, controlled trials in which sham treatments were used showed no benefit. However, some patients derive considerable psychological benefit and a sense of well-being from undergoing such therapy.

Steroid Therapy. Injection of *intraarticular steroids* is a controversial treatment. Although widely used, no controlled studies have documented its efficacy. The experimental finding of steroid suppression of cartilage catabolism has renewed interest in this form of therapy. However, repeated steroid injections may accelerate joint degeneration and weaken supporting structures. Steroid injection should be considered only when a single disabling joint, refractory to other forms of therapy, is sufficiently inflamed that a trial of intraarticular steroids is justified. Facet joint injection for back pain is not effective. Epidural injections for spinal stenosis are commonly tried, but benefit is rarely long-lasting. Systemic steroids have no place in the treatment of OA.

Surgical Intervention. *Osteotomy* to correct the mechanical imbalances caused by single-compartment disease of the knee and early disease of the hip has been popular and does seem to provide at least short-term benefit. However, no data comparing such surgical therapy with conservative management (weight loss, orthotics, exercise) are available, and results of long-term follow-up are often disappointing. The role of such surgery may be viewed as a temporizing measure used to delay total joint replacement. *Arthroscopic surgery*, entailing debridement, smoothing of joint surfaces, and washing out of debris, appears to benefit the patients who undergo the procedure, although controlled trials suggest a strong placebo effect and no long-term benefit unless a foreign body or internal derangement is the cause of symptoms. *Total joint replacement* represents the most extreme form of treatment, to be undertaken only after all other therapeutic options have been exhausted. Indications include pain at rest that interferes with sleep, inability to bear weight without severe pain, unacceptable interference with daily activity, and a requirement for narcotics to control pain.

Replacement of hip and knee joints has been particularly successful. Referral for such surgery requires comprehensive consideration of the patient's medical condition, functional status, and psychosocial state. The ability to participate physically and psychologically in a demanding program of rehabilitation is an important precondition for an optimal outcome.

New intraarticular procedures currently under study and being applied selectively hold promise as potential alternatives to joint replacement, especially of the knee. Patients with focal articular defects, particularly young persons who have sustained trauma, are being treated with *autogenous cartilage implantation* and *osteochondral grafting*. In the former, chondrocytes are grown from the patient's own cartilage and implanted. Criteria for candidacy include normal knee alignment, absence of arthritis on the corresponding tibial surface, and preserved ligamentous joint stability. Outcomes data are promising in carefully selected patients. Persons with more advanced disease are being offered *intraarticular injection* of *hyaluronic acid*. The rationale is to improve the viscosity and elasticity of synovial fluid, thereby reducing discomfort and the need for medication. Response rates to a single injection range from 50% to 90%; patients with mild disease respond best. The duration of benefit may exceed 6 months. Local irritation occurs in about 7%, and pseudogout has been reported as a complication of this otherwise reasonably well-tolerated treatment.

Treatments of Unclear or No Proven Benefit. As in the management of any common chronic condition that is difficult to treat definitively, claims of benefit have been made for a host of unproven therapies for OA. Some are widely promoted to the public as safe, "natural" means of treatment, so that they appear particularly attractive. Evidence of efficacy is often absent when such therapies can be marketed under the rubric of "dietary supplement" without Food and Drug Administration review of their safety and effectiveness. Studies of patients with arthritis reveal up to half trying alternative or complementary measures, especially if they are having severe pain.

Glucosamine. This supplement is an intermediary in mucopolysaccharide synthesis. *In vitro*, it stimulates chondrocytes to produce proteoglycans—hence, the rationale for its use in the treatment OA. The few double-blinded, controlled clinical trials of glucosamine that exist have been short (4 to 8 weeks) and limited to small numbers of patients. Although these studies suggest some modest symptomatic benefit (about the same as with ibuprofen), no long-term studies of safety or efficacy have been performed. A number of glucosamine salt preparations are sold in health food stores and pharmacies without being subject to any standards of purity or uniformity. Some are combined with *chondroitin sulfate*, a glycosaminoglycan touted to promote joint viscosity and cartilage repair. These supplements can be expensive, costing several dollars per day.

Diathermy, including Ultrasound. The rationale for delivering heat by these means before exertion is that they help to relax deep tendons and muscles. Such treatment is expensive and time-consuming. As noted above, in randomized, controlled trials that included sham treatment, diathermy provided no benefit over that derived from exercise alone.

Topical Analgesic Creams. Most nonprescription topical preparations contain methylsalicylate. When methylsalicylate is applied multiple times daily, measurable amounts of salicylate can be absorbed, which may account for any benefit obtained. No controlled trials of these preparations have been performed. One such trial, of *capsaicin* (an extract of chili peppers with topical analgesic properties), has revealed a modest benefit.

Spinal Manipulation. In careful, controlled study, a short course of chiropractic manipulation of the spine appears to provide relief of acute back pain caused by musculotendinous strain; however, such treatment has no demonstrably beneficial effect on the chronic pain and discomfort resulting from degenerative disease of the spine.

Acupuncture has produced inconsistent results in double-blinded studies—sometimes working, sometimes not. Results have not been sufficiently beneficial to warrant its inclusion in a treatment program. Well-designed studies comparing acupuncture with sham needle placement reveal only a strong placebo effect, but the number of trials is very limited and more data are needed before firmer conclusions can be drawn.

Transcutaneous Electrical Nerve Stimulation (TENS). Most of the studies are poorly designed; superficially, they suggest benefit, but most appears to be derived from a placebo effect.

Antispasmodics are without effect except for their tranquilizing action.

INDICATIONS FOR REFERRAL

Treatment of the patient with OA requires a team approach. *Physical* and *occupational therapists* are essential to the design of a successful treatment program—teaching exercises, giving suggestions on how to perform the tasks of daily living, and providing psychological support. Referral should be made early in the course of disease for education in preventive measures, and also later, when OA begins to interfere with daily activity. Early referral to the *nutritionist* is critical to the care of the obese patient. A comprehensive program of diet and exercise is needed to effect a successful weight loss effort.

Surgical consultation should be considered for the significantly disabled patient who is failing conservative management. The consultation should be explained to the patient as an opportunity to weigh treatment options, rather than as an automatic capitulation to surgical intervention. The decision to refer for surgery must be made with an understanding of the risks involved and the need to undertake a vigorous postoperative exercise program. Surgery should be considered only in patients whose limitation of motion or pain has become so severe that it prevents them from living productively. They must be mentally and physically healthy enough to tolerate surgery and sufficiently motivated to carry out the exercise program needed to ensure full rehabilitation.

PATIENT EDUCATION AND PSYCHOSOCIAL SUPPORT

Patients need to know that OA is not reversible, but also that much can be done to lessen pain, prevent further joint injury, and preserve, if not enhance, overall functioning. They appreciate knowing that degenerative disease is not a generalized, systemic illness. Moreover, those with cervical or lumbosacral disease can be given some hope for a spontaneous remission of their severe pain. The need to reduce weight and strengthen supporting muscles should be stressed, in addition to the importance of avoiding activity injurious to the joints and addictive analgesics. The teaching functions of the physical and occupational therapists and nutritionist are among the most critical components of the treatment program. It is important to avoid labeling the patient as "disabled" because active participation in the treatment program is essential to preservation of function. As noted above, surgical options should be discussed with patients who have incapacitating pain of the hips or knees.

Because a principal determinant of presenting for care is the *psychosocial state* of the OA patient, the importance of eliciting and attending to psychosocial stresses cannot be overemphasized. A careful history that includes attention to job, family, and any financial or interpersonal problems is likely to help in the design of an effective treatment program. If the patient reports being disabled yet manifests only modest mechanical dysfunction, then a search for depression and somatization disorder should be undertaken (see Chapters 227 and 230). The prognosis is heavily influenced by how well the patient is coping psychosocially. The physician's concern and support are essential. Return visits should be regularly scheduled, so that the patient can be made to feel that support and caring are being provided. A strong doctor–patient relationship helps many patients to tolerate the disease and remain active.

THERAPEUTIC RECOMMENDATIONS

- Begin a comprehensive, supervised program of exercise, weight loss, and education for patients with symptomatic disease of the hips or knees.
- Provide referrals to physical and occupational therapists for the design and implementation of exercise and activity programs that strengthen quadriceps and hip muscles, increase general conditioning, avoid excessive stress on the affected joints, and ensure the proper use of assist devices.
- Obtain the services of a nutritionist to help support the obese patient in a program of weight reduction.
- Inform the patient that regular aerobic exercise is beneficial and that gentle walking, swimming, and stationary cycling are permissible.
- Advise a short period (1 to 2 days) of joint rest if severe hip or knee pain flares up, but isometric and non–weight-bearing

exercises should be continued and more prolonged inactivity avoided. Limit joint stresses (e.g., stair climbing) and prescribe use of a cane and other assist devices (e.g., railings, hand grips, elevated toilet seat).

- Consider use of a heel lift if leg lengths are unequal and use of a shoe orthotic device if marked foot pronation is noted. Check with an orthopedist or podiatrist if uncertain.
- Advise bed rest followed by exercises to strengthen supporting musculature for patients with back pain. A corset or brace may help, but not in the absence of an exercise program (see Chapter 147).
- Prescribe a soft cervical collar to those with cervical pain. It should be worn at all times, including the night. Four weeks or more of use may be necessary. Cervical traction is also helpful (see Chapter 148).
- Begin acetaminophen for control of pain; prescribe up to 4 g/d. Consider NSAIDs (including aspirin) only for patients who fail acetaminophen after trials at full doses. If NSAID therapy is used, prescribe only low, analgesic doses (e.g., 325 mg of enteric-coated aspirin three times daily or 200 mg of ibuprofen four times daily) unless the patient's arthritis has an inflammatory component. If NSAIDs are contraindicated because of a gastrointestinal condition, consider a selective Cox-2 agent (e.g., 12.5 to 25 mg of rofecoxib daily).
- Elicit and address sources of psychosocial distress.
- Avoid use of narcotics except in the setting of an acute disabling exacerbation that is not relieved by maximal doses of non-narcotic analgesics. Under such circumstances, consider no more than 1 to 2 days' worth of therapy with codeine sulfate or oxycodone.
- Refer for surgical consideration the patient with refractory, incapacitating disease of a major weight-bearing joint, provided the patient is well motivated and sufficiently healthy to tolerate surgery and engage in a rehabilitation program.

A.H.G.

ANNOTATED BIBLIOGRAPHY

Bradley JD, Brandt KD, Katz BP, et al. Comparison of an antiinflammatory dose of ibuprofen, an analgesic dose of ibuprofen, and acetaminophen in the treatment of patients with osteoarthritis of the knee. N Engl J Med 1991;325:87. (*No advantage for short-term antiinflammatory therapy.*)

Davis MA, Ettinger WM, Neuhous JM, et al. Knee osteoarthritis and physical functioning: Evidence from the NHANES I epidemiologic follow-up study. J Rheumatol 1991;18:591. (*Correlation between severity of radiologic findings and degree of functional impairment.*)

Dieppe PA, Sathapatayavong S, Jones HE, et al. Intraarticular steroids in osteoarthritis. Rheum Rehab 1980;19:212. (*A critical look at the pluses and minuses of this controversial therapy.*)

Ettinger WH Jr, Burns R, Meissier SP, et al. Regular exercise reduced pain and disability from osteoarthritis of the knee. The Fitness Arthritis and Seniors Trial (FAST). JAMA 1997;227:25. (*Randomized, long-term trial demonstrating benefit of exercise.*)

Falconer J, Hayes KW, Chang RW. Therapeutic ultrasound in the treatment of musculoskeletal conditions. Arthritis Care Res 1990;3:85. (*No benefit in controlled trials when compared with sham treatment.*)

Felson DT, Anderson JJ, Naimark A, et al. Obesity and knee osteoarthritis: the Framingham study Ann Intern Med 1988;109:18. (*Strong relationship found, especially in women.*)

Felson DT, Shang Y, Anthony JM, et al. Weight loss reduces the risk for symptomatic knee osteoarthritis in women: the Framingham study. Ann Intern Med 1992;116:535. (*Epidemiologic data suggest that 10-pound weight loss in obese women reduces the risk for development of symptomatic knee pain by more than 50%.*)

Fries JF, Singh G, Morfeld D, et al. Running and the development of disability with age. Ann Intern Med 1994;121:502. (*Long-term, prospective, longitudinal study; markedly reduced rate of disability, but no acceleration or postponement of OA.*)

Gaw AC, Chang LW, Shaw LC. Efficacy of acupuncture on osteoarthritic pain. N Engl J Med 1975;293:375. (*A double-blinded, controlled study; variable benefit.*)

Gelber AC, Hochberg MC, Mead LA, et al. Body mass index in young men and the risk of subsequent knee and hip osteoarthritis. Am J Med 1999;107:542. (*Increased risk for OA of the knee with increased body mass index in young persons; suggests cumulative weight burden may be important.*)

Hadler NM. Knee pain is the malady—not osteoarthritis. Ann Intern Med 1992;116:598. (*Argues that psychosocial variables are the most important determinants of who presents with knee pain.*)

Hamerman D. The biology of osteoarthritis. N Engl J Med 1989;320:1322. (*Useful basic science review; 97 references.*)

Hernborg JS, Nilsson BE. The natural course of untreated osteoarthritis of the knee. Clin Orthop 1977;123:130. (*A natural history study of 94 joints in 71 patients revealing a generally unfavorable prognosis, with pain developing at rest in the majority of patients.*)

Hochberg MC, Altman RD, Brandt KD, et al. Guidelines for the medical management of osteoarthritis. Part 1. Osteoarthritis of the hip. Part 2. Osteoarthritis of the knee. American College of Rheumatology. Arthritis Rheum 1995;38:1535. (*Evidence-based consensus guidelines.*)

Katz JN, Dalgas M, Stucki G, et al. Degenerative lumbar spinal stenosis: diagnostic value of the history and physical examination. Arthritis Rheum 1995;38:1236. (*History and physical found very useful; key findings reviewed.*)

Kovar PA, Allegrante JP, MacKenzie CR, et al. Supervised fitness walking in patients with osteoarthritis of the knee: a randomized, controlled trial. Ann Intern Med 1992;116:529. (*A program of patient education and supervised walking significantly improved functional status.*)

Lane NE, Bloch DA, Hubert HB, et al. Running, osteoarthritis, and bone density: initial 2-year longitudinal study. Am J Med 1990;88:452. (*No progression of OA changes in this group of middle-aged patients.*)

LaPrade RF, Swiontkowski MF. New horizons in the treatment of osteoarthritis of the knee. JAMA 1999;281:876. (*Brief review for the general reader of autogenous cartilage implantation, osteochondral grafting, and hyaluronic acid injection.*)

Liang MH, Cullen KE. Primary total hip or knee replacement: evaluation of patients. Ann Intern Med 1982;97:735. (*Good review of indications, contraindications, and results.*)

Liang MH, Fortin P. Management of osteoarthritis of the hip and knee. N Engl J Med 1991;325:125. (*An overview of the approach to diagnosis and treatment.*)

Minor HA, Hewett JE, Webel RR, et al. Efficacy of physical conditioning exercise in patients with rheumatoid arthritis and osteoarthritis. Arthritis Rheum 1989;32:1396. (*Proved very beneficial, and can be performed without injury to involved joints.*)

Pelletier JP, Martel-Pelletier J. The therapeutic effects of NSAIDs and corticosteroids in osteoarthritis: to be or not to be. J Rheumatol 1989;16:266. (*A discussion of their effects on the underlying disease process.*)

Poss R. The role of osteotomy in the treatment of osteoarthritis of the hip. J Bone Joint Surg 1984;66:144. (*A review of indications, patient selection, and results.*)

Puett DW, Griffin MR. Published trials of nonmedicinal and noninvasive therapies for hip and knee osteoarthritis. Ann Intern Med 1994;121:133. (*Best review of the evidence and lack thereof.*)

Rao JK, Mihaliak K, Kroenke K, et al. Use of complementary therapies for arthritis among patients of rheumatologists. Ann Intern Med 1999;131:409. (*High frequency of use; predictors of use include persistent pain and a college degree.*)

Salaffi F, Cavalieri F, Nolli M, et al. Analysis of disability in knee arthritis: relationship with age and psychological variables but not with radiographic score. J Rheumatol 1991;18:1581. (*Evidence for a strong psychosocial component.*)

Simon LS, Lanza FL, Fipsky PE, et al. Preliminary study of the safety and efficacy of SC-58635, a novel cyclooxygenase-2 inhibitor. Arthritis Rheum 1998;41:1591. (*Found to have analgesic benefit similar to that of other NSAIDs, but with less risk for ulcer.*)

158
Management of Gout

Gout is among the most common causes of acute monoarticular arthritis. Estimates of prevalence in the United States range from 0.3% to 2.8% of the population. Gout is predominantly a disease of adult men. Inborn errors of purine metabolism and abnormalities of uric acid excretion account for most cases of primary gout. The expanded use of agents that decrease uric acid excretion has markedly increased the incidence of secondary gout. In the Framingham study, almost half of new cases were associated with thiazide use.

The primary physician should be able to diagnose acute gout promptly, treat it, prevent recurrences, and minimize the chances for the development of chronic gouty arthritis. Patients who present with asymptomatic hyperuricemia also require attention (see Chapter 155).

PATHOPHYSIOLOGY AND CLINICAL PRESENTATION

The majority of patients with primary gout have a hereditary renal defect in uric acid excretion that leads to chronic hyperuricemia (see Chapter 155). Acute gout usually occurs after many years of sustained asymptomatic hyperuricemia. The higher the uric acid concentration, the greater the risk for an acute attack, although the risk remains relatively low until very high urate levels are reached (see Chapter 155). The mean duration of the asymptomatic period is about 30 years. During this time, urate may be deposited in synovial lining cells and possibly also in cartilage. Acute gout develops when uric acid crystals collect in the synovial fluid as a result of precipitation from a supersaturated state or release from the synovium. Trauma, a fall in temperature or pH, dehydration, starvation, excessive intake of alcohol, emotional or physical stress, and rapid changes in the serum uric acid concentration have all been implicated in the process. The risk is increased in renal transplantation patients undergoing cyclosporine therapy and in obese patients placed on very low-calorie diets.

The pathogenesis of the inflammatory response involves phagocytosis of crystals by leukocytes in the synovial fluid, disruption of lysosomes, release of enzymatic products, activation of the complement and kallikrein systems, and release of leukocyte chemotactic factor.

Acute Gouty Arthritis. In men, the first attack is usually during the fifth decade; in women, it tends to be after age 60. The episode is typically monoarticular and abrupt in onset, often occurring at night. Symptoms and signs of inflammation become maximal within a few hours of onset and last for a few days to a few weeks. Recovery is complete. The initial attack usually involves a joint of the lower extremity. In about half of patients, the *first metatarsophalangeal joint* is the site of inflammation (*podagra*). The *tarsal joint* (located at the instep), *ankle*, and *knee* are other common sites of initial attacks. Later episodes may involve a joint of the upper extremity, such as the wrist, elbow, or finger; shoulder or hip involvement is rare. More than 80% of attacks occur in a lower extremity; 85% of patients have at least one episode of podagra.

Polyarticular involvement is noted in about 5% of acute gouty attacks and may be confined to the upper extremities. Finger joint involvement is more common in women than in men and tends to present as a *Heberden's* or *Bouchard's node*. In elderly patients with gout and osteoarthritis, almost half have such nodal inflammation as the sole or initial manifestation of gout. In elderly women, the presentation of gout may be more insidious and polyarticular; multiple hand joints may be involved, with the condition resembling active rheumatoid disease.

The joint involved in an attack of acute gout appears swollen and erythematous; periarticular involvement is also common. Low-grade fever and leukocytosis may be present. A substantial fraction of patients may be *normouricemic* at the time of the acute attack. During resolution, the skin overlying the affected joint often desquamates. The clinical presentation may simulate joint infection (see Chapter 145) or even cellulitis (see Chapter 190).

Interval (Intercritical) Gout follows the initial attack. An asymptomatic period generally lasts for several years before a second episode of acute gout takes place. The original joint or another joint may be involved in subsequent attacks. Over time, the asymptomatic intervals between acute episodes shorten. In more advanced disease, polyarticular attacks are not uncommon, and resolution may be slower and less complete. Urate crystals may remain in the joint fluid.

Chronic Gouty Arthritis (Tophaceous Gout) takes years to develop. *Tophi* are typically noted an average of 10 years after the initial attack of acute gout. The risk for chronic gout is a function of the duration and severity of hyperuricemia. Tophi represent sodium urate collections surrounded by foreign body giant cell inflammatory reactions. They can occur in a variety of sites, including the synovium, subchondral bone, olecranon bursa, Achilles tendon, and subcutaneous tissue of the extensor surfaces of the arm. Eventually, cartilage erodes, joints become deformed, and chronic arthritis ensues. The joints of the lower extremities and hands are most commonly affected. In elderly women, the fingers may be the sole site of involvement by gouty disease; the condition may be mistaken for rheumatoid disease, with morning stiffness and tenderness and swelling of the metacarpophalangeal and proximal interphalangeal joints. The process is insidious; the patient notes progressive aching and stiffness. Tumescences may develop over joints of the foot and make wearing shoes difficult. Fortunately, the incidence of tophaceous gout has declined markedly with the introduction of effective antihyperuricemic agents. Chronic gouty arthritis develops in fewer than 15% of patients with acute gout.

Complications. The incidence of *nephrolithiasis* among patients with clinical gout is small; the risk for new stone formation in a patient with new onset of gout is less than 1% per year and is unrelated to the initial serum urate concentration or degree of uric acid control. Factors other than the serum urate concentration are important in stone formation and include a family history of stone formation, urine pH, hydration status, and possibly the amount of uric acid excreted by the kidneys (see Chapter 135). Stone formation is rarely dangerous; the risk for obstructive uropathy is less than 0.02%.

Concerns about the development of *chronic renal failure* as a complication of chronic hyperuricemia have been laid to rest by long-term studies (see Chapter 155). Lead intoxication is a cause in some populations; in others, it is concurrent hypertension, diabetes, cardiovascular disease, or underlying primary renal disease. *Acute renal failure* is a risk in patients undergoing treatment for lymphoproliferative or myeloproliferative disease. Immediately following chemotherapy, a massive uric acid load is present that may precipitate in renal tubules and elsewhere in the urinary tract and lead to acute oliguria.

DIAGNOSIS

Definitive diagnosis requires joint fluid examination and the finding of characteristic, negatively birefringent crystals (see Chapter 145). When classic podagra appears in a patient with a prior history of gout, a clinical diagnosis can be made with reasonable confidence, but when an acute monoarticular arthritis occurs in a less typical site, the full range of diagnostic possibilities must be considered (see Chapter 145). A chronic active polyarticular presentation in an older woman can be confusing because it may resemble rheumatoid disease, especially if confined to the fingers. A clue is the presence of Heberden's or Bouchard's nodes; the presence of tophi is another tip-off. Joint aspiration for crystal identification is needed to confirm the diagnosis. Similarly, in interval (intercritical) gout, joint aspiration and synovial fluid analysis can help establish the diagnosis, even in the absence of an acutely inflamed joint. Aspiration can be performed on a joint that is identified by history as having been previously inflamed. The serum uric acid level is not helpful diagnostically because it can be normal in the presence of active inflammatory disease.

PRINCIPLES OF THERAPY

Acute Gouty Arthritis

Acute symptoms can be relieved by the prompt institution of antiinflammatory therapy. Without treatment, an acute attack

of gout usually resolves within 7 to 10 days, although severe episodes can last for weeks. Initiation of treatment at the very first sign of an acute attack produces a prompt and excellent therapeutic response. Delay of therapy is associated with less satisfactory results. Antiinflammatory therapy is usually continued until symptoms have resolved.

Nonsteroidal Antiinflammatory Drugs given in full doses are the treatment of choice. *Indomethacin, ibuprofen,* and *naproxen* are the best studied of the NSAIDs for use in acute gout, but almost any NSAID should suffice. Experience with the selective Cox (cyclooxygenase)-2 NSAIDs in gout is too limited at present for any conclusions about their effectiveness to be drawn, but if they prove to have a role, they may be particularly useful in older patients who are at increased risk for the adverse gastrointestinal effects of traditional NSAIDs. Peptic ulcer disease and renal insufficiency are relative contraindications to the use of nonselective NSAIDs. Some elderly patients may experience mental confusion with indomethacin (see Chapter 156).

Colchicine is an alternative for patients unable to take NSAID therapy, but its tendency to cause *gastrointestinal upset* (nausea, vomiting, diarrhea) limits patient compliance. The doses needed to treat an acute attack effectively are the very ones associated with gastrointestinal side effects. *Bone marrow suppression* and an increased risk for *myopathy* and *neuropathy* have been reported in persons with concurrent *renal* or *hepatic insufficiency.*

Glucocorticoids are being used increasingly for acute gout; they can be very effective. The best candidates are persons who cannot take or do not respond to NSAIDs or colchicine. Intraarticular injection of an acutely involved joint can provide relief within 24 hours. Alternatively, one can prescribe a short course of high-dose oral prednisone, started at up to 60 mg/d and tapered rapidly to full cessation over 7 to 10 days.

Interval Gout

Although prophylactic therapy to prevent acute gouty arthritis is not necessary or cost-effective for a patient with asymptomatic hyperuricemia or a first attack of gout (see Chapter 155), it becomes cost-effective after a patient starts having two attacks per year, particularly if the episodes are disabling. Intervals between future recurrences are likely to shorten without prophylactic treatment. Of the risk factors for recurrent gouty attacks, hyperuricemia is among the most amenable to treatment. Other importance risk factors include use of thiazides and low-dose aspirin, obesity, and excessive intake of alcohol. Options include blocking urate production with allopurinol and enhancing renal excretion with *probenecid* or *sulfinpyrazone.* The goal is to lower the uric acid concentration below 6.5 mg/dL, the level at which extracellular fluid becomes saturated with uric acid.

Allopurinol is convenient to use (once-daily dosing) and relatively well tolerated, so it is widely prescribed. It inhibits the enzyme xanthine oxidase and blocks the formation of uric acid. The half-life of allopurinol is about 3 hours, but its metabolites are biologically active for up to 30 hours. As a result, the drug need be taken only once daily. Serum urate levels fall within a week of initiation of therapy, but the risk for gouty attacks does not decline until normouricemia has been sustained for 3 to 6 months.

Of the minor side effects, *rash* and gastrointestinal upset are among the more common; about 2% experience rash. If mild, the rash quickly resolves with cessation of therapy and may not recur if the drug is restarted at a low level. However, the development of a rash is associated with an increased risk for more serious adverse effects. The cumulative reported frequency of more serious adverse reactions is relatively high, at 3.5%. They include *fever, leukopenia, vasculitis,* and *hepatocellular injury.* A *fulminant hypersensitivity* syndrome characterized by *desquamative rash, fever, hepatitis, eosinophilia,* and *renal failure* is the most worrisome adverse effect. Although uncommon (prevalence <0.25%), it is associated with a 15% to 25% mortality rate and occurs mostly in patients with concurrent renal insufficiency or diuretic use. Allopurinol should always be used with caution and in reduced doses in patients with renal insufficiency. The white cell count and renal function should be monitored regularly for the first several months of treatment. Drug–drug interactions are also important. The risk for drug rash is increased 10-fold by the concurrent use of *ampicillin,* and the activity of drugs metabolized by hepatic microsomal enzymes (e.g., warfarin, azathioprine) can be potentiated.

Although allopurinol is often preferred by patients whose urate levels must be lowered because of its convenient dosing schedule and low frequency of side effects, it should not be prescribed casually. Carefully weighing the expected prophylactic benefit against the small but serious risk for a hypersensitivity reaction helps to ensure intelligent, safe use. The drug remains expensive. Patients with interval gout who are best suited for allopurinol treatment include those who are not candidates for uricosuric therapy because of hyperexcretion of uric acid (>1,000 mg/24 h), renal insufficiency, history of nephrolithiasis, or inability to tolerate or comply with a uricosuric program. Allopurinol has no beneficial effect in acute gouty arthritis; in fact, it may precipitate an attack during the early stages of therapy (see below).

Uricosuric Agents have an excellent safety record, so they are well suited for long-term prophylactic therapy. *Probenecid* and *sulfinpyrazone* are the principal uricosuric drugs; both act to inhibit renal tubular reabsorption of uric acid. About 80% of patients excreting less than 700 mg of uric acid daily can be effectively managed by uricosuric therapy. A uricosuric agent is often preferred to allopurinol therapy in persons with interval gout who are excreting less than 700 mg of uric acid per day and whose renal function is well preserved.

Their principal disadvantages are frequent dosing and an associated risk for precipitating nephrolithiasis. Because these agents are less convenient to use, compliance tends to be less than with allopurinol. Probenecid must be taken two to three times per day; sulfinpyrazone requires dosing three or four times daily. At the onset of therapy, uric acid excretion may reach extraordinary levels and trigger nephrolithiasis; therefore, initial doses must be modest. Generous fluid intake (2 to 3 L/d) and urinary alkalinization are also necessary. *Rash, autoimmune hemolytic anemia,* and *gastrointestinal upset* are the most common side effects. Sulfinpyrazone is associated with a very small risk for *marrow suppression.*

Drug–drug interactions are common. *Thiazides, loop diuretics,* and low doses of *salicylates* inhibit uricosuric action. *Probenecid* blocks the renal excretion of penicillins and the hepatic uptake of rifampin, prolonging the half-lives of both.

Losartan, an angiotensin II receptor antagonist, has been found to have uricosuric action and may be given to hypertensive patients, both to control blood pressure and prevent recurrent gouty attacks. Its cost is high, but the drug is well tolerated and requires only once-daily dosing. It may be combined with allopurinol.

Initiation of Antihyperuricemic Therapy. All drugs that reduce the serum uric acid level can trigger an attack of acute gout during the initial 3 to 6 months of therapy. This is believed to be a consequence of the mobilization of tissue deposits of uric acid. The risk is reduced when allopurinol is started at a low dose that is increased gradually during the course of a month. Only after the uric acid level has been normal for 3 to 6 months does the risk for a gouty attack begin to decline substantially. In the interim, low-dose antiinflammatory therapy is often prescribed for concurrent use with the urate-lowering agent. Both colchicine and NSAIDs are used.

Urate-lowering therapy is instituted only after all manifestations of an acute attack have fully resolved. No definitive data are available regarding the ideal duration of concurrent antiinflammatory therapy, but most authorities recommend that it be given for 3 to 6 months, or until all visible urate deposits have disappeared.

Diet. Only 10% of circulating purine is derived from dietary sources. Consequently, it is not necessary to restrict purine intake unless dietary habits or events appear to correlate strongly with attacks. Purine-rich foods include organ meats, other meats and seafood, yeast, beer and other alcoholic beverages, legumes, oatmeal, spinach, mushrooms, asparagus, and cauliflower. Most important is reduction of excess *weight* (without fasting) and abstinence from excessive *alcohol* intake and binge drinking. Obese patients with interval gout who are on a very low-calorie diet are at increased risk for an acute attack and may require prophylactic therapy.

Chronic Gouty Arthritis

Antihyperuricemic treatment is indicated in patients with tophaceous gout to prevent progressive articular damage. Prevention or relief of chronic gouty arthritis requires normalization of the serum urate level. Being the more effective and more convenient antihyperuricemic, *allopurinol* is usually prescribed for patients with tophaceous gout. Often, tophi begin to resolve after several weeks of therapy. A uricosuric agent is a reasonable alternative, provided that renal function is normal and no nephrolithiasis or excessive excretion of uric acid has been noted. Regardless of the agent selected, concurrent antiinflammatory therapy must be given until visible urate deposits have resolved.

Renal Complications

Although the risk for a renal complication is small, attention to renal issues is required in certain instances during the management of the gouty patient.

Nephrolithiasis. The gouty patient with an established uric acid stone should be treated with allopurinol and a high fluid intake; concurrent administration of a thiazide diuretic may be necessary (see Chapter 135). Allopurinol therapy to prevent stone formation is indicated for gouty patients with a prior history of nephrolithiasis and perhaps for those with a strong family history of kidney stones. All patients should be instructed to avoid dehydration, especially if they live in a warm, dry climate. Isolated hyperuricemia *per se* does not require treatment in the absence of other risk factors for nephrolithiasis (see Chapter 155).

Renal Failure. Patients undergoing chemotherapy for lymphoproliferative or myeloproliferative disease require pretreatment with allopurinol. Prolonged urate-lowering therapy has no role in the prevention of chronic renal failure in patients with gout, but avoidance of exposure to lead is important, as is the treatment of common comorbidities such as hypertension, diabetes, and cardiovascular disease.

PATIENT EDUCATION

Patients who experience an acute gouty attack are highly motivated to undertake preventive measures and are very receptive to advice. If obese, they should be advised to avoid starvation or very low-calorie diets. Drinkers should be warned against binges. Maintenance of good hydration needs to be stressed to those at risk for nephrolithiasis. On the other hand, patients will find it comforting to know that severe dietary restrictions are unnecessary. Fasting should be avoided because it may precipitate an attack. The importance of treating an acute attack at the first sign of illness also needs to be stressed. For the patient with interval gout, a discussion of the risks and benefits of prophylactic therapy and the importance of compliance is indicated. Those taking allopurinol should be warned of the risk of a hypersensitivity reaction and advised to cease intake immediately and call the physician at the first sign of a rash, fever, or other manifestation.

THERAPEUTIC RECOMMENDATIONS

Acute Gout

- At the first sign of an attack of acute gouty arthritis, begin a nonsteroidal antiinflammatory agent (e.g., 500 mg of naproxen three times daily). Continue full-dose treatment until symptoms resolve, then taper to cessation over 72 hours. Advise the patient that delay in starting therapy may impair the response.
- For patients unable to take NSAID therapy (e.g., active peptic ulcer disease), consider colchicine (0.6 mg four times daily), but warn that diarrhea and some upper gastrointestinal upset are likely during the course of therapy; monitor blood cell count and hepatic and renal function. Avoid colchicine if underlying renal or hepatic insufficiency is present.
- For refractory cases of definite acute gout, consider a 7- to 10-day course of oral corticosteroids; start with prednisone at 20 to 40 mg/d and taper as clinically indicated. Intraarticular corticosteroid therapy is another option if oral therapy is not feasible and just one joint is involved.
- Provide an extra supply of antiinflammatory therapy so that it will be available for prompt use in a future episode.

Interval Gout

- Advise weight reduction (but not starvation diets) if the patient is obese and cessation of excess alcohol use; consider providing information on a reduced purine diet if attacks appear to be precipitated by dietary events.
- Avoid use of thiazides, loop diuretics, low-dose aspirin, and niacin to the extent possible.
- Determine with the patient if gouty attacks are sufficiently frequent and disabling to warrant prophylactic therapy. Once the patient has two attacks per year, long-term urate-lowering therapy becomes cost-effective.
- If the patient is willing to take long-term urate-lowering therapy, determine whether allopurinol or a uricosuric agent is preferred by (a) inquiring into any personal or family history of kidney stones or renal dysfunction, (b) measuring renal function (blood urea nitrogen, creatinine), and (c) determining 24-hour urinary uric acid excretion.
- For the patient who is excreting more than 1,000 mg of uric acid per day, has underlying azotemia, is at increased risk for nephrolithiasis, or is allergic to or fails uricosuric therapy, begin allopurinol (started at 100 mg/d and increased to 200 to 300 mg once daily over 4 weeks). Adjust the dose upward if the response is inadequate. Reduce the dose in the setting of renal insufficiency and use cautiously, especially when diuretics or ampicillin is being given concurrently. Stop at the earliest sign of a hypersensitivity reaction. Consider restarting at a low dose if the drug rash was mild, but monitor complete blood cell count and hepatic and renal function closely. Consider desensitization for patients who require allopurinol but who react to it with a mild drug rash.
- Begin probenecid or sulfinpyrazone if the patient has normal renal function, no risk for stone disease, and a urate excretion of less than 700 mg/d. Therapy should be initiated in small doses (e.g., 250 mg of probenecid twice daily or 50 mg of sulfinpyrazone twice daily), and at the same time fluid intake should be kept large (2 to 3 L/d) to prevent precipitation of uric acid in the urinary tract. Alkalinization of the urine to a pH of 6.6 is desirable during the first week of therapy but is difficult to achieve; gram doses of sodium bicarbonate are required, supplemented by acetazolamide (250 mg) before bed.
- Advance the uricosuric dose gradually to avoid triggering massive urate excretion. Continue high fluid intake during the early months of therapy. Maximum dose of sulfinpyrazone is 100 mg three to four times daily; for probenecid, it is 500 to 1,000 mg two to three times daily. Avoid the concurrent use of aspirin because it inhibits urate excretion.
- Monitor serum uric acid concentration and treat to achieve a level of less than 6.5 mg/dL, the point of supersaturation.
- To reduce the risk for an attack of gout during the first 3 to 6 months of urate-lowering treatment, prescribe concurrent antiinflammatory prophylactic therapy with either colchicine (0.6 mg daily or twice daily) or an intermediate-acting NSAID (e.g., 250 mg of naproxen daily or twice daily).
- Advise avoidance of precipitants such as binge drinking, fasting, and very low-calorie diets.

Chronic Gouty Arthritis

- Treat as for interval gout. Continue concurrent antiinflammatory therapy until all visible manifestations of uric acid deposits have resolved, which may take 6 to 12 months.

Renal Complications

- Pretreat cancer patients with allopurinol if a large uric acid load is likely to result from an application of chemotherapy.
- Advise a marked reduction in lead exposure (e.g., home-distilled alcohol, industrial contact).
- Treat patients with urate nephrolithiasis or a strong family history of kidney stones with allopurinol (300 mg once daily) and hydration. Long-term efforts to alkalinize the urine are impractical and need not be undertaken.
- Because the risk for chronic renal failure from chronic hyperuricemia is nil, long-term urate-lowering therapy to prevent it is unnecessary.

A.H.G.

ANNOTATED BIBLIOGRAPHY

Bautman V, Maesaka JK, Haddad B, et al. The role of lead in gouty nephropathy. N Engl J Med 1981;304:520. (*An important link between gout and renal injury.*)

Berger L, Yu TF. Renal function in gout—an analysis of 524 gouty subjects including long-term follow-up studies. Am J Med 1975;59:604. (*Important 12-year follow-up study showed that hyperuricemia alone had no deleterious effect on renal function in ambulatory patients with gout.*)

Edwards NL. Gout: clinical and laboratory features. In: Klippel JD, ed. Primer on rheumatic diseases. Atlanta: Arthritis Foundation, 1997:234. (*Excellent description of presentation and diagnostic features.*)

Fam AG, Lewtas J, Stein J, et al. Desensitization to allopurinol in patients with gout and cutaneous reactions. Am J Med 1992;93:299. (*Moderately successful in persons with mild rashes.*)

Ferraz MB, O'Brien B. A cost-effectiveness analysis of urate-lowering drugs in nontophaceous recurrent gouty arthritis. J Rheumatol 1995;22:908. (*Treatment found to be cost-effective after two or more attacks per year.*)

Fessel JW. Renal outcomes of gout and hyperuricemia. Am J Med 1979;67:74. (*Risks for renal failure and stone formation were very small.*)

Groff GD, Franck WA, Raddatz DA. Systemic steroid therapy for acute gout: a clinical trial and review of the literature. Semin Arthritis Rheum 1990;19:329. (*Good evidence for efficacy.*)

Hadler NM, Franck WA, Bress NM, et al. Acute polyarticular gout. Am J Med 1974;56:715. (*In one third of patients, the condition was confined to the upper extremities, and sometimes occurred in the setting of a normal serum uric acid level.*)

Hall AP, Berry PE, Dawber TR, et al. Epidemiology of gout and hyperuricemia—a long-term population study. Am J Med 1967;42:27. (*The oft-quoted Framingham study; risk for acute gout rose with uric acid level.*)

Hande KR, Noone RM, Stone WJ. Severe allopurinol toxicity. Am J Med 1984;76:47. (*A potentially fatal hypersensitivity syndrome described.*)

Lally EV, Zimmerman B, Ho G, et al. Urate-mediated inflammation in nodal osteoarthritis: clinical and roentgenographic correlations. Arthritis Rheum 1989;32:86. (*A Heberden's or Bouchard's node was the initial or sole manifestation of gout in almost half of elderly patients with gout and osteoarthritis.*)

Lin HY, Rocher LL, McQuillan MA, et al. Cyclosporine-induced hyperuricemia and gout. N Engl J Med 1989;321:287. (*Hyperuricemia common; gout in 7%.*)

Maclaughlan MJ, Rodnan GP. Effects of food, fast, and alcohol on serum uric acid and acute attacks of gout. Am J Med 1967;42:38. (*Fasting and consumption of more than 100 g of alcohol raised urate levels and often precipitated attacks.*)

Meyers DC, Monteagudo FSE. Gout in females: an analysis of 92 patients. Clin Exp Rheumatol 1985;3:105. (*The presentation in women may be an insidious polyarthritis rather than an acute monoarthritis.*)

National Task Force on the Prevention and Treatment of Obesity. Very low-calorie diets. JAMA 1993;270:967. (*Risk for triggering an acute gouty attack is low but increased in those with prior symptomatic gout.*)

Pascual E, Batlle-Gualda E, Martinez A, et al. Synovial fluid analysis for diagnosis of intercritical gout. Ann Intern Med 1999;131:756. (*Urate crystals found in high percentage of patients with a history suggestive of gout but with no active joint inflammation.*)

Singer JZ, Wallace SL. The allopurinol hypersensitivity syndrome. Arthritis Rheum 1986;29:82. (*High mortality risk; many cases in patients who did not need the drug.*)

Wallace SL, Singer JZ. Treatment of gout. In: Schumacher HR Jr, ed. Primer on the rheumatic diseases, 9th ed. Atlanta: Arthritis Foundation, 1988:202. (*Excellent review of drug therapy.*)

Wernick R, Winkler C, Campbell S. Tophi as the initial manifestation of gout. Arch Intern Med 1992;152:873. (*Noted in the fingers of elderly women with underlying osteoarthritis, renal insufficiency, and concurrent NSAID use.*)

Yu TF, Berger LU. Impaired renal function in gout. Am J Med 1982;75:95. (*Hyperuricemia alone did not affect renal function; renal insufficiency correlated best with coexisting hypertension, pre-existing renal disease, and ischemic heart disease.*)

Yu TF, Gutman A. Uric acid nephrolithiasis in gout: predisposing factors. Ann Intern Med 1967;67:1133. (*A classic study correlating risk for stone formation with uric acid excretion, urine pH, serum urate level, and underlying disease.*)

159
Approach to the Patient with Fibromyalgia

Patients with diffuse, chronic musculoskeletal pain but no evidence of arthritis account for a large number of office visits. Some of them have mild rheumatoid disease; in other cases, their symptoms are caused by bony pathology, neuropathy, and myopathy. When no source stands out, clinicians start wondering about somatization despite protests from the patient that the problem is "not in my head."

In recent years, a syndrome of diffuse and chronic musculoskeletal pain, stiffness, focal tenderness, disordered sleep, and fatigue has become increasingly recognized as an important clinical entity. The terms *fibromyalgia*, *fibrositis*, and *fibromyositis* have been used to designate it, although the "-itis" terminology has been discouraged because no inflammatory pathophysiology has been detected. Although the cause of the syndrome is unknown, it appears to be common and is estimated to have a prevalence as high as 5% among adult women, who account for 80% to 90% of cases.

PATHOPHYSIOLOGY, CLINICAL PRESENTATION, AND COURSE

Pathogenesis. The cause of fibromyalgia remains unknown. Although the symptoms suggest somatization, careful psychological studies reveal no relationship between symptoms and psychological status. Only an increased frequency of life stress has been found. Most patients are not depressed, and any onset of depression does not correlate with the level of pain. One of the most consistent findings is an alteration in central nervous system neurotransmitter metabolism and function, with abnormal levels of serotonin, norepinephrine, and substance P found. This has suggested to some a pathophysiologic common denominator involving the neurochemistry of sleep and pain perception. Disturbances of stage 4 (non-rapid eye movement, non-REM) sleep are related to the symptoms. Neuroendocrine changes have also been observed but are not sufficient to be considered etiologic.

Muscle biopsy findings and electromyographic data demonstrate no consistent or unique changes. A subset of patients with fibromyalgia have abnormal antibodies, but they appear to have concurrent connective tissue disease. Because of the overlapping of symptoms of chronic fatigue syndrome and those of fibromyalgia, a common pathophysiology has been surmised, but the pathogenesis remains unknown for both conditions. Other patients have serology positive for Lyme disease, but treatment for Lyme disease usually does little to alleviate their symptoms. Some of these cases are believed to represent false-positive results that can be explained by the low specificity of Lyme serology and the high prevalence of fibromyalgia. A relation between recent infection and transient fibromyalgia syndrome has been observed in some cases of clinical Lyme disease and in some instances of acute mononucleosis, but no firm data are available to link infection with chronic symptoms.

Clinical Presentation. The typical patient is a woman in her midthirties to midfifties who describes chronic and diffuse musculoskeletal pain, stiffness, and fatigue. The pain tends to be constant, aching, and concentrated in axial regions (neck, shoulders, back, pelvis). Points of tenderness may also be found in the upper and lower extremities. "Stiffness" is the term often used to describe the discomfort, which is characteristically worse in the morning and exacerbated by changes in the weather, cold, humidity, sleeplessness, and stress and helped by warmth, rest, and mild exercise. Patients awake from sleep feeling tired and unrefreshed.

Physical examination findings are normal except for multiple, reproducible points of exaggerated tenderness to palpation. The tender points tend to be symmetric and located in the occiput, neck, shoulder, ribs, elbows, buttocks, and knees. Eighteen characteristic locations have been identified (Fig. 159.1).

Clinical Course. Fibromyalgia is a chronic but nonprogressive disorder. Waxing and waning with changes in the weather, degree of situational stress, and amount of rest are characteristic. The number and location of tender points tend to be stable over time. In some patients, the condition may become disabling, at least temporarily, but the clinical course overall is one of steady but nonprogressive disease. A substantial minority of patients experience spontaneous remission, and many of those who continue to have symptoms report a general improvement with time. The degree of disability can be substantial; up to a fourth of patients receive disability payments at some time during their illness. Underlying psychosocial problems are the principal determinant of disability and health care utilization in patients with fibromyalgia.

DIFFERENTIAL DIAGNOSIS

The clinical diagnosis of fibromyalgia has been facilitated by a standardized case definition utilizing diagnostic criteria established by the American College of Rheumatology: (a) widespread pain including axial pain for at least 3 months, and (b) pain in at least 11 of 18 possible tender point sites (Table 159.1). Nonetheless, the diagnosis must not be considered established until a host of similarly presenting conditions have been ruled out, conditions that may be mistakenly labeled as fibromyalgia.

Myofascial syndromes resulting from overuse may be confused with fibromyalgia, in that tender points are characteristic of both. Unlike those of fibromyalgia, the tender points of myofascial syndrome are clustered about just one area and trigger referred pain on compression (hence the term *trigger points*). Also, symptoms are focal rather than diffuse. A history of onset after excessive activity or muscle strain is typical. No fatigue or sleep disorder is associated with myofascial syndrome.

Rheumatoid disease in its early or mild forms may cause diffuse musculoskeletal discomfort, morning stiffness, fatigue,

Table 159.1. The American College of Rheumatology 1990 Criteria
for the Classification of Fibromyalgia[a]

1. History of Widespread Pain.

Definition. Pain is considered widespread when all of the following are present: pain in the left side of the body, pain in the right side of the body, pain above the waist, and pain below the waist. In addition, axial skeletal pain (cervical spine or anterior chest or thoracic spine or low back) must be present. In this definition, shoulder and buttock pain is considered as pain for each involved side. "Low back" pain is considered lower segment pain.

2. Pain in 11 of 18 Tender Point Sites on Digital Palpation (Fig. 159.1).

Definition. Pain, on digital palpation, must be present in at least 11 of the following 18 tender point sites:

Occiput: bilateral, at the suboccipital muscle insertions.
Low cervical: bilateral, at the anterior aspects of the intertransverse spaces at C1–C7.
Trapezius: bilateral, at the midpoint of the upper border.
Supraspinatus: bilateral, at origins, above the scapula spine near the medial border.
Second rib: bilateral, at the second costochondral junctions, just lateral to the junctions on upper surfaces.
Lateral epicondyle: bilateral, 2 cm distal to the epicondyles.
Gluteal: bilateral, in upper outer quadrants of buttocks in anterior fold of muscle.
Greater trochanter: bilateral, posterior to the trochanteric prominence.
Knee: bilateral, at the medial fat pad proximal to the joint line.

Digital palpation should be performed with an approximate force of 4 kg.
For a tender point to be considered "positive," the subject must state that the palpation was painful. "Tender" is not to be considered "painful."

[a]For classification purposes, patients will be said to have fibromyalgia if both criteria are satisfied. Widespread pain must have been present for at least 3 months. The presence of a second clinical disorder does not exclude the diagnosis of fibromyalgia.

From Wolfe F, Smyth HA, Yunus MB, et al. The American College of Rheumatology 1990 criteria for the classification of fibromyalgia: the Multicenter Criteria Committee. Arthritis Rheum 1990;33:160, with permission.

and focal tenderness on physical examination. However, the tenderness appears to be less exaggerated, and results of serologic studies are abnormal. *Polymyalgia rheumatica* superficially resembles fibromyalgia, but the onset is at a much later age, symptoms are confined to the hip and shoulder girdles, few tender points are present, and the sedimentation rate is markedly elevated. *Ankylosing spondylitis* produces axial discomfort, fatigue, and focal tenderness; however, most patients with axial symptoms are men, and sacroiliitis is a defining manifestation (see Chapter 146).

Spondyloarthropathy in women can easily be mistaken for fibromyalgia because the likely symptoms are diffuse and chronic axial discomfort, focal spinal pain in multiple sites, and disordered sleep. Because it is more common in men, spondyloarthropathy is not commonly considered in women, and neck pain may be more prominent than lower back pain, further confusing the picture. Clinical findings suggestive of spondyloarthropathy include a positive family history, psoriasis, inflammatory bowel disease, risk factors for Reiter's syndrome, relief of pain with exercise, sacroiliitis, and pain or tenderness at the site of insertion of a tendon or at the Achilles tendon or plantar fascia.

Chronic fatigue syndrome has been found to share many of the clinical features of fibromyalgia, including chronic, diffuse musculoskeletal pain and tender points, so that differentiation is difficult at times because both conditions are diagnosed clinically. Pain tends to be less prominent in chronic fatigue syndrome, and not all patients have tender points. Sometimes, distinguishing between chronic fatigue syndrome and fibromyalgia is impossible because of so much clinical overlap, which is not critical functionally because the approach to management is very similar for both.

Lyme disease also enters into the differential diagnosis but is readily recognized by a history of deer tick exposure, residence in an endemic area, rash, polyarthritis, and neurologic deficits (see Chapter 160). Some patients may have a transient syndrome that temporarily resembles fibromyalgia.

Hypothyroidism may be accompanied by diffuse myalgias and fatigue that simulate fibromyalgia. Differentiating features include cold intolerance, unexplained weight gain, characteristic skin changes, goiter, muscle weakness and soreness, and an elevated thyrotropin (TSH) level. Similarly, polymyositis may produce diffuse muscle achiness, but muscles are weak and diffusely sore, and the sedimentation rate and muscle enzyme levels are markedly elevated.

Depression and *somatization disorder* certainly can cause chronic musculoskeletal pain and fatigue, but no reproducible tender points are found, and these conditions are accompanied by definite manifestations of underlying psychopathology (see Chapters 227 and 230).

The pain of *hypertrophic osteoarthropathy* may be diffuse, but tender points are minimal and clubbing provides a unique hallmark.

WORKUP

The diagnosis depends entirely on the history and physical examination (Table 159.1). Laboratory studies are ordered to help rule out other conditions.

History. A careful delineation of the location of the pain is essential and helps differentiate fibromyalgia from conditions causing more localized or regional discomfort. Inquiry into associated features such as fatigue, nonrefreshing sleep, and exacerbations associated with changes in the weather facilitate differentiation. Pertinent negatives include other somatic and affective symptoms of depression (see Chapter 227), symptoms of hypothyroidism (see Chapter 104), frank arthritis, fever, rash, muscle weakness, and prior history of muscle injury.

Physical Examination. The skin, nails, mucous membranes, fundi, joints, spine, muscles, tendons, bones, and nervous system should be examined carefully for evidence of rheumatoid disease, spondyloarthropathy, myopathy, osteoarthropathy, thy-

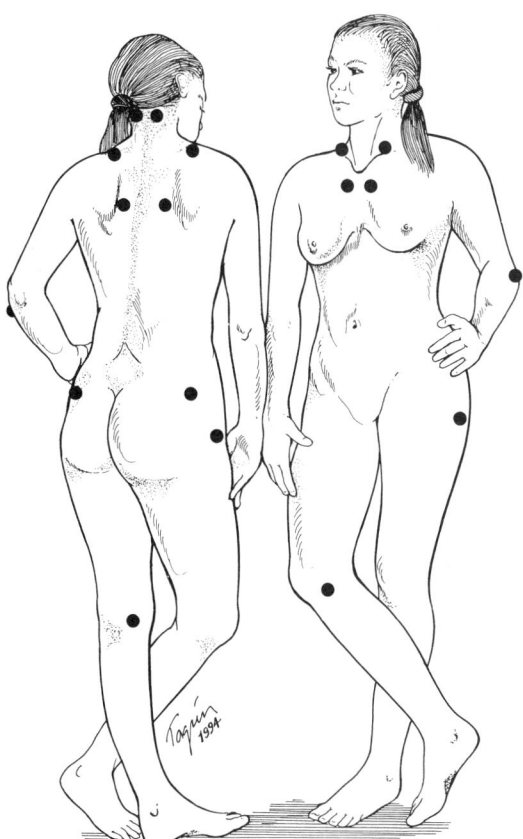

FIG. 159.1.   Tender points in fibromyalgia syndrome.

roid disease, and focal pathology (see Chapter 45 and Chapters 146 through 151). The mental status examination should be reviewed for signs of depression (see Chapter 227). If no abnormalities are found, then careful palpation of the 18 tender point sites is indicated (Fig. 159.1). Compression should be just strong enough to cause blanching of the examining fingertip. A positive response is the elicitation of exaggerated tenderness or outright pain. Tender points need to be differentiated from the trigger points of myofascial syndrome, which produce referred pain on compression. Mild discomfort during palpation is a nonspecific finding that may be elicited in a host of other musculoskeletal conditions.

Laboratory Studies. Because no diagnostic studies or characteristic laboratory findings exist, testing is conducted to rule out treatable conditions that may present in similar fashion. Among the more useful studies is an antinuclear antibody (ANA) determination; a negative result has a high negative predictive value, but a positive result has a high probability of being a false-positive if the pretest probability of lupus is low (see Chapter 146). Other parameters of use in ruling out important mimicking illness include the sedimentation rate and TSH and creatine phosphokinase levels. Obtaining Lyme titers is not indicated unless the patient has symptoms strongly suggestive of the disease (rash, arthritis, neurologic complaints, deer tick exposure, residence in an endemic area) because test specificity is very poor. When back pain is the predominant symptom, radiologic study of the spine or sacroiliac joints may have to be considered (see Chapter 147). When fatigue dominates the clin-

ical picture, more extensive evaluation may be required (see Chapter 8).

PRINCIPLES OF MANAGEMENT AND PATIENT EDUCATION

As with any incurable and chronic pain condition of unknown cause, the principal goal is maintenance and enhancement of functional capacity (see Chapter 236). Although it may be difficult to "cure" the pain, much can be done to help the patient remain active and productive. The large number of patients with fibromyalgia who are disabled represents a challenge to improve the medical care of persons with this condition. Key components of an effective treatment program include establishing the diagnosis; forming a strong patient–doctor relationship; designing a medical regimen to control pain, promote sleep, and treat any concurrent depression; and initiating a program of nonmedical therapies to enhance functional capacity. In addition, it is critical to address any underlying psychosocial problems because they are a major determinant of prognosis and response to treatment.

Establishing the Diagnosis. The value of a careful workup that can confirm the diagnosis is ranked by fibromyalgia patients as one of the most valuable components of care. Knowing what the diagnosis is puts an end to the common fear that a more serious condition with a poor prognosis is responsible for symptoms. The patient feels she is being taken seriously. Repeated requests for further evaluation are fewer, and unnecessary or inappropriate treatments (e.g., antibiotics, steroids, NSAIDs) can be avoided.

Forming an Effective Patient–Doctor Relationship. The successful care of patients with fibromyalgia requires that a trusting, understanding relationship be formed early. At the time of the initial encounter, the physician starts by eliciting the essential details of the patient's illness experience and specific concerns. Careful history taking is essential for an accurate diagnosis, and it also provides the patient with a much-needed sense of "being heard." A directed physical examination pertinent to the differential diagnosis and the patient's concerns helps to reinforce the patient's confidence and feeling of "being taken seriously." Taking time at the end of the visit for a focused but unhurried review of findings and their meaning is critical to consolidating the initial efforts to build a good working relationship.

Addressing Pain, Fatigue, and Any Concurrent Depression. Therapies that affect neurotransmitter metabolism, such as the *tricyclic antidepressants*, are among the most consistently effective in fibromyalgia. They are thought to act on the serotoninergic and adrenergic biochemistry of central pain perception, sleep, and depression. Controlled trials of tricyclic antidepressants at low doses (e.g., 25 to 50 mg of amitriptyline daily at bedtime) have repeatedly shown them to be beneficial to a significant degree, although their effect on pain seems to be the least durable. Selective serotonin reuptake inhibitors (SSRIs) have also been studied and found most helpful in the treatment of sleep disturbances and depression; their effects on pain are less demonstrable. Small doses of tricyclic antidepressants may suffice and are usually well tolerated, but larger ones are sometimes necessary and can be problematic (see Chapter 227). Improvements in all disease manifestations have been noted, but relapse commonly occurs with cessation of therapy.

Various additional therapies have been tried to reduce discomfort. Some pain control has been observed with use of the analgesic *tramadol* (see Chapter 236). The few studies examining *benzodiazepines* are of inadequate quality, but results suggest short-term improvement; however, the prolonged use that would be necessary for treatment of fibromyalgia would be inappropriate, given the risks for benzodiazepine dependency and withdrawal (see Chapter 227). *NSAIDs* and systemic *corticosteroids* have little effect on pain. *Opioids* have not been studied. Injection of tender points with topical *lidocaine* has been tried, but the large number of sites that are tender, the modest responses, and the considerable amount of pain after injection make this treatment of little consequence. *S*-adenosyl-L-methionine (*SAMe*) is a popular nonprescription derivative of methionine with purported antidepressant, analgesic, and anti-inflammatory actions. Small-scale, short studies suggest modest reductions in pain, depression, and number of tender points. *Acupuncture* may be helpful, but available studies are flawed and results are equivocal. *Biofeedback* and *hypnotherapy* have their advocates, but data are too limited to judge efficacy.

Empiric parenteral antibiotic treatment for Lyme disease has no place in the treatment of patients with fibromyalgia and positive Lyme serology. Positive serology in the absence of clinical evidence for Lyme disease is likely to represent a false-positive result. Only patients with clinical manifestations strongly suggestive of Lyme disease (rash, arthritis, heart block, or neurologic deficits) should be considered candidates for such therapy (see Chapter 160).

Enhancing Functional Capacity. As noted earlier, the goal of management is not so much the elimination of pain as the preservation and enhancement of function. Toward this end, a number of additional measures are worth considering. *Cognitive–behavioral therapy* has proved very helpful in redirecting the patient's focus away from pain and disability and toward the restoration of function and full participation in daily life. Most programs studied have been multidimensional, combining cognitive restructuring, pacing of activity, and patient and family education with aerobic exercise, relaxation training, and meditation. Results are best for those with symptoms of recent onset. Programs run from 1 to 6 months. Long-term results can be demonstrated many months after completion. *Cardiovascular fitness training* (aerobic exercise three times weekly) raises pain thresholds and global assessment scores, but sleep and fatigue levels may not improve much when training is undertaken without the implementation of other treatment modalities, and effects do not last after exercise has been stopped. No improvement has been noted with flexibility exercises only.

Refractory Complaints: Addressing Underlying Psychosocial Factors. Patients who make repeated visits and appear refractory to treatment efforts should undergo a full psychosocial assessment and be carefully evaluated for psychiatric, family, occupational, and social difficulties. Problems in these areas are the most important determinants of health care utilization and disability in patients with fibromyalgia. They have little effect on the severity of symptoms, but they do determine illness behavior. Similarly, patients who perceive their symptoms to be the consequence of an injury suffered at work or in an accident also have a poor prognosis, with disability and a poor response to treatment persisting until litigation and related issues have been settled. The first step in the management of persons with refractory disease must be a thoughtful approach that directly addresses these underlying psychosocial difficulties.

A.H.G.

ANNOTATED BIBLIOGRAPHY

Aaron LA, Bradley LA, Alarcon GS, et al. Perceived physical and emotional trauma as precipitating events in fibromyalgia: associations with health care seeking and disability status but not pain severity. Arthritis Rheum 1997;40:453. (*Evidence for the importance of psychosocial factors in prognosis.*)

Aaron LA, Bradley LA, Alarcon GS, et al. Psychiatric diagnoses in patients with fibromyalgia are related to health care–seeking behavior rather than to illness. Arthritis Rheum 1997;39:436. (*The importance of underlying psychiatric disease as a predictor of illness behavior.*)

Bennett RM. Emerging concepts in the neurobiology of chronic pain: evidence of abnormal sensory processing in fibromyalgia. Mayo Clin Proc 1999;74:385. (*A review of the conceptual basis for the chronic pain of fibromyalgia, with a focus on abnormal sensory processing.*).

Carette S, Bell MJ, Reynolds WJ, et al. Comparison of amitriptyline, cyclobenzaprine, and placebo in the treatment of fibromyalgia. A randomized, double-blind clinical trial. Arthritis Rheum 1994;37:32. (*Well-designed study showing efficacy of amitriptyline.*)

Dailey PA, Bishop GD, Russell IJ, et al. Psychological stress and the fibrositis/fibromyalgia syndrome. J Rheumatol 1990;17:1380. (*High level of life stress found.*)

Fitzcharles M-A, Esdaile JM. The overdiagnosis of fibromyalgia syndrome. Am J Med 1997;103:44. (*Spondyloarthropathies in women diagnosed as fibromyalgia.*)

Goldenberg DL. Fibromyalgia syndrome a decade later: what have we learned? Arch Intern Med 1999;159:777. (*Excellent summary of diagnosis and management for the generalist, with emphasis on the importance of underlying psychosocial factors to outcomes; 156 references.*)

Goldenberg DL, Mayskiy M, Mossey C, et al. A randomized, double-blind crossover trial of fluoxetine and amitriptyline in the treatment of fibromyalgia. Arthritis Rheum 1996;39:1852. (*The SSRI was helpful for sleep disturbances and depression but not for pain.*)

Goldenberg DL, Simms RW, Geiger A, et al. High frequency of fibromyalgia in patients with chronic fatigue seen in a primary care practice. Arthritis Rheum 1990;33:381. (*Much overlap in the two conditions.*)

Kennedy M, Felson DT. A prospective long-term study of fibromyalgia syndrome. Arthritis Rheum 1996;39:682. (*Best long-term data; study confirms chronicity of disease, but also a general trend toward improvement.*)

Leventhal LJ. Management of fibromyalgia. Ann Intern Med 1999;131:850. (*Review of the evidence for what works and what does not; excellent list of 119 references.*)

Lightfoot RW, Luft BJ, Rahn DW, et al. Empiric parenteral antibiotic treatment of patients with fibromyalgia/fatigue and a positive serologic result for Lyme disease. Ann Intern Med 1993;119:503. (*A cost-effective analysis; treatment was expensive and was associated much more with antibiotic toxicity than with clinical cures.*)

McCain GA, Bell DA, Mai FM, et al. A controlled study of the effects of a supervised cardiovascular fitness training program on the manifestations of primary fibromyalgia. Arthritis Rheum 1988;31:1135. (*Improvement achieved with cardiovascular training, but not with simple flexibility exercises.*)

Moldofsky H, Scarisbrick P, England R, et al. Musculoskeletal symptoms and non-REM sleep disturbance in patients with "fibrositis" syndrome and healthy subjects. Psychosom Med 1975;37:341. (*The original observation of disturbed sleep.*)

NIH Consensus Conference. Acupuncture. JAMA 1998;280:1518. (*Rated as "may be useful as an adjunct treatment" in the management of fibromyalgia.*)

Scudds RA, McCain GA, Rollman GB, et al. Improvements in pain responsiveness in patients with fibrositis after successful treatment with amitriptyline. J Rheumatol 1989;16:98. (*A double-blinded, crossover study; improvement in all parameters noted.*)

Simms RW, Gunderman J, Howard G, et al. The alpha-delta sleep abnormality in fibromyalgia. Arthritis Rheum 1988;31[Suppl]:S100. (*The characteristic sleep disorder of fibromyalgia.*)

Tunks E, McCain GA, Hart LE, et al. The reliability of examination for tenderness in patients with myofascial pain, chronic fibromyalgia, and controls. J Rheumatol 1995;22:944. (*Systematic study of the test; found effective for differentiation from normal controls, but some overlap with myofascial pain syndrome.*)

White KP, Nielsson WR. Cognitive behavioral treatment of fibromyalgia syndrome: a follow-up assessment. J Rheumatol 1995;22:717. (*Found effective, with benefit lasting long after treatment completed.*)

Wigers SH, Stiles TC, Vogel PA. Effects of aerobic exercise versus stress management treatment in fibromyalgia. A 4.5-year prospective study. Scand J Rheumatol 1996;25:77. (*Pain decreased; fatigue and disturbed sleep less affected.*)

Wolfe F, Smythe HA, Yunus MB, et al. The American College of Rheumatology 1990 criteria for the classification of fibromyalgia: the Multicenter Criteria Committee. Arthritis Rheum 1990;33:160. (*Consensus diagnostic criteria pending discovery of more definitive diagnostic findings.*)

Yunus MB, Ahles TA, Aldag JC, et al. Relationship of clinical features with psychological status in primary fibromyalgia. Arthritis Rheum 1991;34:15. (*Failure to find a relationship suggests that symptoms are independent of the patient's psychological status.*)

Yunus MB, Masi AT, Calabro JJ, et al. Primary fibromyalgia (fibrositis): clinical study of 50 patients with matched normal controls. Semin Arthritis Rheum 1981;11:151. (*Careful early delineation of clinical presentation and physical findings.*)

160
Approach to the Patient with Lyme Disease

Lyme disease is a treatable multisystem illness caused by infection with the tick-borne spirochete *Borrelia burgdorferi*. The condition has become the most common vector-borne disease in the United States, with more than 40,000 cases reported to the Centers for Disease Control and Prevention in the past 10 years. In most instances, the acute infection can be readily diagnosed and effectively treated. The neurologic and musculoskeletal manifestations of later stages may be more subtle and resemble those of chronic fatigue syndrome, fibromyalgia, or depression. The nonspecificity of symptoms and shortcomings of available serologic tests lead to both underdiagnosis and overdiagnosis.

The primary physician needs to be skilled in the clinical recognition of early disseminated and late disease; clinically capable of differentiating it from other acute, subacute, and chronic neurologic and musculoskeletal conditions; cognizant of the limitations of diagnostic methods; and capable of prescribing an effective antibiotic program.

EPIDEMIOLOGY, PATHOPHYSIOLOGY, AND CLINICAL PRESENTATION

Epidemiology

The spirochete causing Lyme disease is transmitted to humans by *Ixodes* ticks. Nymph-stage ticks feed on humans from May through July, transmitting the spirochete in the process. Endemic areas for species of the responsible tick include the northeastern coastal states, Wisconsin and Minnesota in the Midwest, and the coast of Oregon and northern California. Outbreaks in Europe and Asia have also been reported. In the U.S. eastern coastal regions and in the Midwest, the deer tick *I. dammini* is the principal vector. More than a third of deer ticks carry the spirochete, which accounts for outbreaks of epidemic proportion. In the western United States, the *I. pacificus* species is responsible, but the carrier rate is only 1% to 3% and human infection is much more sporadic. The condition has also been reported in Europe and Asia.

The rising frequency of Lyme disease and its geographic spread have been linked to enlarging deer populations and concurrent suburbanization. The spirochete is transmitted horizontally to field mice, which are critical to sustaining its life cycle (deer are not, but the ticks prefer them). Human infection is a biologic dead end for the spirochete.

Human babesiosis, caused by the intracellular rickettsial parasite *Babesia microti*, is endemic to many of the same areas as Lyme disease. Transmission to humans is by the same deer tick, and the same field mice serve as the animal reservoir. The shared tick vector and animal reservoir increase the risk for concurrent infection. Approximately 10% of patients with active Lyme disease are concurrently infected with *B. microti*.

Human granulocytic ehrlichiosis is yet another recently appreciated rickettsial disease that is zoonotic in the same geographic sites as babesiosis and Lyme disease. So far, no evidence of concurrent infection has been found.

Pathophysiology

The spirochete enters the bloodstream at the time of tick feeding. After a short bloodstream phase, the organism moves out of the blood and, in seemingly trophic fashion, into the skin, synovial membranes, heart, and nervous system. The means by which the spirochete damages tissue remains unclear; hypotheses range from direct injury to the production of antispirochetal antibodies that cross-react with tissue antigens. Patients with symptoms that persist after appropriate antibiotic therapy are suspected of having an exaggerated, sustained immune response. Such a response may account for the overlap in clinical manifestations with those of fibromyalgia and chronic fatigue syndrome, in which an immunologic pathophysiology is also suspected (see Chapters 8 and 159). The fact that patients who are positive for HLA-DR4 appear to be at increased risk for such chronic illness suggests that the severity and chronicity of disease may be related, in part, to cell surface antigens and genetic susceptibility.

Unlike *B. burgdorferi*, the *Babesia* organism resides predominantly in the red cells and causes mostly systemic symptoms with little localization. Infection can impair host defenses and may enhance injury caused by *B. burgdorferi*.

Clinical Presentation and Course

The biting tick is usually no larger than the size of a pencil mark and often inapparent. Shortly after the bite, the first symptoms develop. The clinical course can be divided into three stages: (a) acute, localized disease; (b) subacute, disseminated disease; and (c) chronic disease.

Stage 1: Acute Infection. In most patients, the first clinical manifestation of *B. burgdorferi* infection is a skin reaction to the organism. In about 80%, a characteristic expanding erythematous rash, *erythema migrans*, develops (Fig. 160.1). It usually begins as a red macule at the site of the tick bite and spreads out to form a large annular lesion with red secondary outer rings, an intense red outer border, and some clearing toward the center, although induration may be noted at the site of the bite. The lesion is large, averaging 15 cm. Minor constitutional *flulike symptoms* (a "summer flu") and regional *lymphadenopathy* may accompany the rash. The remaining 20% of patients have flulike symptoms without a rash or no acute-stage symptoms at all. The rash starts to fade by 3 to 4 weeks. During stage 1, the immune response is minimal.

Stage 2: Disseminated Infection. Hematogenous dissemination follows the acute phase within several days to a few weeks

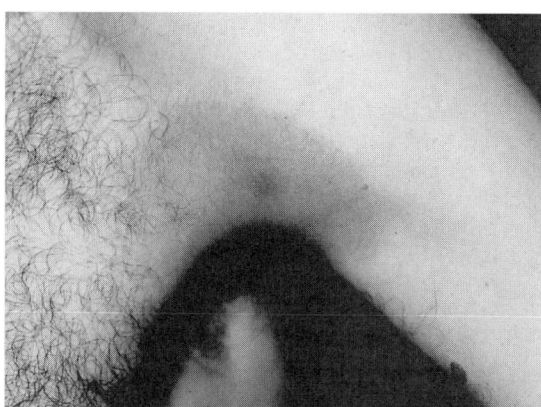

FIG. 160.1. Erythema migrans of the axcilla.

of the tick bite and leads to a host of symptoms, mostly dermatologic, musculoskeletal, and neurologic. Constitutional symptoms may be prominent, with patients complaining of generalized *malaise* and debilitating *fatigue*. Often, bouts of severe *headache* lasting a few hours may develop, accompanied by mild neck stiffness, as may *migratory arthralgias* and musculoskeletal pain.

Dermatologic Manifestations include new *annular skin lesions*, smaller and less migratory than the initial one. Malar rash, diffuse erythema, and urticaria have also been noted.

Cardiac Involvement is noted in about 5% to 10% of patients, beginning several weeks into the infection. *Transient heart block* may be a consequence, ranging from asymptomatic first-degree atrioventricular block to complete heart block with fainting. The cardiac phase lasts 3 to 6 weeks, with the most severe forms of heart block persisting for about 1 week and not requiring pacemaker placement.

Neurologic Sequestration ensues weeks to months after the initial infection, affecting 15% to 20% of untreated patients. It consists of a *lymphocytic meningitis* and cranial or peripheral neuropathy. The cerebrospinal fluid (CSF) shows a pleocytosis with about 100 lymphocytes per cubic millimeter, elevated protein and normal glucose levels, and antibodies to the spirochete. A mild *encephalopathy* may ensue and produce mood changes, somnolence, and memory disturbances. A unilateral or bilateral *Bell's palsy* is the most common cranial nerve deficit. The *peripheral neuritis* presents as motor and sensory changes of the trunk or limbs in a dermatomal distribution. These neurologic manifestations can last for weeks to months.

Musculoskeletal Symptoms evolve into frank arthritis in up to 60% of untreated patients. The onset of arthritis is variable but averages 6 months from the time of initial infection. Characteristically, self-limited attacks of acute asymmetric *monoarticular* or *oligoarticular arthritis* develop. Pain and swelling are noted in one or a few large joints. The knee is the most common site. A joint effusion may form, composed of increased numbers of neutrophils (10,000 to 25,000/mm^3). No more than three joints are usually involved in the course of the illness. Symptoms and signs last several days to a few weeks. After an attack, the joint returns to normal.

Stage 3: Chronic Infection. Following a latent period of several months and beginning a year after the time of the original infection, symptoms of chronic infection begin to appear. Bouts of arthritis may become more prolonged, and chronic neurologic deficits may ensue.

Skin Changes. Most patients in the United States do not manifest skin changes in the late phases of Lyme disease, but in Europe, a chronic atrophic form of *acrodermatitis* unique to Lyme disease has been observed.

Arthritis. The transient form of arthritis characteristic of disseminated disease is supplanted by a more persistent one that lasts months instead of weeks. The knee remains the most common site, and the pattern continues to be oligoarticular. Joint erosion is reported but uncommon and rarely leads to permanent loss of function. In a small percentage of patients, the arthritis persists even after a full course of antibiotic therapy. An immunologic mechanism is postulated. Over the years, the frequency of arthritic episodes declines.

Neurologic Impairment. Distal paresthesias, radicular pain, and memory loss comprise the principal neurologic manifestations of late disease, representing polyneuropathy and encephalopathy. Often, they occur concurrently. Tiredness may also be reported. In rare instances, a leukoencephalopathy with spastic paraparesis may develop. Two thirds of patients with neurologic symptoms have elevated levels of protein in the CSF, and half have Lyme antibodies in the CSF. In most patients, electrophysiologic study findings are abnormal, demonstrating evidence of axonal degeneration.

Natural History of Disease. Without treatment, disseminated disease develops in about 80% of patients. Attacks of oligoarthritis are common (60% to 80%) but resolve within 1 to 3 years, even without treatment. Chronic neurologic and persistent joint symptoms affect about 5% to 10% of patients. Susceptibility to late chronic disease may be genetically determined. A *"post-Lyme syndrome"* may be seen in up to a third of treated cases; it is characterized by persistence of fatigue, myalgias, and arthralgias for several more months after objective disease manifestations have resolved.

Concurrent Infection with *B. microti.* The symptoms of human *babesiosis* include fever, chills, sweats, arthralgias, headache, and lassitude. Patients with concurrent Lyme disease and babesiosis typically manifest what appears to be a more severe and prolonged case of Lyme disease. Marked fatigue, headache, sweats, chills, nausea, conjunctivitis, emotional lability, and splenomegaly occur more frequently than in patients with Lyme disease alone. Moreover, almost half remain symptomatic for more than 3 months, whereas fewer than 5% of those with Lyme disease alone remain symptomatic for that long. Similarly, patients with concurrent babesiosis and Lyme disease appear to have a more severe case of *Babesia* infection than would be typical.

DIFFERENTIAL DIAGNOSIS

Acute and Early Disseminated Stages. Lyme disease patients with acute-phase flulike symptoms, rash, and a history of tick bite may be confused with persons having *Rocky Mountain spotted fever*, which also is tick-borne and produces an acute febrile illness with rash, musculoskeletal pain, headache, and gastrointestinal upset. However, the rash of Rocky Mountain spotted fever is different; it starts within a few days of the tick bite as an outbreak of small, blanching macules on the wrists and ankles, spreads centripetally and also to the palms and soles, and then becomes generalized and petechial. As noted previously, *human babesiosis* may mimic or exacerbate the early phases of Lyme disease and should be considered when a patient with a recent tick bite in an endemic area appears to have a particularly severe set of systemic Lyme symptoms that persist beyond 3 months. *Summertime viral illnesses* enter into the differential diagnosis in patients who present with flulike symptoms but without erythema migrans or a history of tick bite.

Patients with symptoms and signs of meningeal irritation require careful evaluation. *Viral encephalitis* is among the summer viral illnesses that may present with headache, stiff neck, and mental changes. *Bacterial meningitis* must also be considered. The erythema migrans and concurrent Bell's palsy or radiculoneuritis of Lyme disease should help differentiate *B. burgdorferi* infection from other causes of meningeal irritation.

Late Disseminated and Chronic Stages. The presence of acute episodes of oligoarthritis raises the question of *gout, pseudogout,* and a *seronegative spondyloarthropathy* (e.g., Reiter's syndrome, psoriatic arthritis, ankylosing spondylitis). At the time of the initial presentation, *infectious arthritis* also enters into the differential diagnosis. Even early *rheumatoid arthritis* may present as a monoarticular or oligoarticular disease involving a large joint. The correct diagnosis can usually be made based on the associated clinical findings and the results of serologic testing and joint fluid analysis (see Chapters 145 and 146).

The subtle neurologic and joint manifestations of late Lyme disease can cause considerable diagnostic confusion. *Depression, fibromyalgia,* and *chronic fatigue syndrome* have manifestations that overlap with those of Lyme disease. Clinicians encountering patients with these difficult conditions may overdiagnose Lyme disease, especially if too much emphasis is placed on serologic testing and too little on symptoms and signs (see below and Chapters 8, 159, and 227). Adding to the confusion is the possibility that, in some instances, Lyme disease may be followed by a post-Lyme syndrome or may trigger fibromyalgia.

WORKUP

In general, the diagnosis of Lyme disease is made clinically, by recognizing the characteristic symptoms and signs within the epidemiologic context of the illness. Serologic testing for antibody against *B. burgdorferi* can supplement the clinical evaluation, particularly in persons with an intermediate pretest probability of Lyme disease, but overdiagnosis leading to overtreatment is common (see below).

Early Disease. A careful history and physical examination remain the best approach to the early diagnosis of Lyme disease. Antibody will not appear for several weeks, so that a clinical diagnosis is necessary at this stage of the illness. One asks the patient about having recently been in a wooded, brushy, or grassy area of an endemic region; tick bite; rash; and any flulike illness occurring in the spring or summer. A history of tick bite is not necessary for diagnosis. (The nymph tick is very small, and its bite is easily missed.) The presence of the characteristic annular lesion of *erythema migrans* is pathognomonic. It appears in 50% to 80% of patients. Most other clinical findings are nonspecific.

In endemic areas, patients presenting with early, nonspecific symptoms are often tested at the onset of symptoms or after a tick bite, a practice that is probably a response to patient concerns and a demand for early testing and treatment. However, it is too early to detect antibody, and the pretest probability of Lyme disease in patients with early, nonspecific symptoms is very low. Testing them at this stage maximizes the risk for false-positive and false-negative results and should be discouraged (see below). Those in an endemic area with especially severe systemic symptoms should be evaluated for concurrent babesiosis (see below).

Disseminated Disease. In disseminated disease, the principal clues to the diagnosis continue to be clinical. In addition to epidemiologic inquiry, a review of key historical features is necessary, including new erythematous lesions, palpitations, near-syncope, stiff neck, facial weakness (which may be bilateral), radicular pain, migratory musculoskeletal complaints, and later, frank oligoarticular arthritis, particularly of the knee. Physical findings of importance include the multiple annular erythematous skin lesions of *secondary erythema migrans*, irregular pulse, nuchal rigidity, facial nerve palsy, and joint swelling with effusion. Suspicion of early disseminated Lyme disease is particularly high if the lesions of secondary erythema migrans are present. Again, when patients have particularly severe and persistent systemic symptoms, concurrent babesiosis should be suspected, and they should be tested accordingly.

The diagnosis can be facilitated by obtaining serum for *antibody testing*, but only in patients with sufficient clinical evidence of Lyme disease to have an intermediate (20% to 80%) pretest probability of Lyme disease (see Table 160.1 and below). For patients with meningeal signs, lumbar puncture should be considered. The CSF is sent for antibody testing in addition to cell count, differential, and chemistries. Most patients with central nervous system involvement have detectable antibody in the CSF, a pleocytosis, and an elevated protein concentration. If a joint effusion is present, *arthrocentesis* is indicated. *Polymerase chain reaction* methods (see below) may become useful for linking *Borrelia* infection to the arthritis.

Late Disease. The diagnosis of late disease requires careful attention to the patient's musculoskeletal and neurologic symptoms. One checks for chronic oligoarticular arthritis (particularly of the knee), memory loss, spinal radicular pain, and distal paresthesias. Patients with findings suggestive of encephalopathy should undergo a *lumbar puncture* for antibody testing of the CSF, cell count, and chemistries. Peripheral polyneuropathy can be confirmed by *electrophysiologic study*, if necessary.

Differentiating Late Lyme Disease from Other Conditions. As noted earlier, *chronic fatigue syndrome* and *fibromyalgia* may be mistaken for Lyme disease. Tiredness and chronic neu-rologic and musculoskeletal symptoms are common to all three. Clinical features that help to differentiate Lyme disease from the other two include (a) oligoarticular musculoskeletal complaints that include signs of joint inflammation; (b) limited and specific neurologic deficits (memory loss, distal paresthesias, radicular pain); (c) abnormalities on CSF examination and electromyography; and (d) absence of disturbed sleep, chronic headache, depression, and tender points. Complicating differentiation are (a) the ability of Lyme disease to trigger chronic fatigue syndrome and fibromyalgia; and (b) the inadequate specificity of available diagnostic tests. Depression can also mimic some of the nonspecific manifestations of these conditions and should be considered in patients who present with fatigue and multiple nonspecific bodily complaints (see Chapters 8 and 228).

Diagnostic Studies. Laboratory confirmation of *B. burgdorferi* infection remains problematic. Antibody testing can contribute to the diagnosis, but only under carefully selected conditions and at the risk of generating false-positive results. Isolation of the spirochete is not practical, and DNA detection by polymerase chain reaction technology remains experimental. The diagnosis of Lyme disease remains predominantly a clinical one. Laboratory testing should be used only as a supplement to the clinical findings and not as the basis for the diagnosis.

Antibody Testing. Clinicians often turn to serologic testing for Lyme disease when the clinical picture is unclear or patient concerns are high. Serologic testing aims to detect immunoglobulin M and immunoglobulin G antibodies expressed against *B. burgdorferi* antigens in response to spirochete infection. Most so-called *first-step tests* utilize ELISA (enzyme-linked immunosorbent assay) technology for antibody detection. First-step antibody testing is sensitive; when performed more than 12 weeks after the onset of symptoms, its sensitivity ranges from 90% to 100%. However, the specificity is more

Table 160.1.   Pretest Probability of Lyme Disease Based on Epidemiology and Clinical Presentation

CLINICAL PRESENTATION	COMMUNITY INCIDENCE: 0.1%	COMMUNITY INCIDENCE: 1.0%	COMMUNITY INCIDENCE: 3.0%
Myalgias			
No history of rash or tick bite	0	0	0
With history of bite; no rash	0	0	0
With history of rash; no bite	0.006	0.06	0.17
With history of rash and bite	0.008	0.44	0.70
Erythema migrans only			
Typical	1.00	1.00	1.00
Atypical	0.002	0.18	0.40
Arthritis			
No history of rash or tick bite	0	0	0
History of tick bite; no rash	0	0	0
History of rash; no tick bite	0.0006	0.06	0.17

From Nichol G, Dennis DT, Steere AC, et al. Test treatment strategies for patients suspected of having Lyme disease: a cost-effectiveness analysis. Ann Intern Med 1998;128:37, with permission.

modest (70% to 90%) because some *Borrelia* antigens are shared with other microorganisms and cross-reacting antibodies are found in persons with conditions that may resemble Lyme disease (e.g., viral illnesses, other tick-borne infections, connective tissue diseases, encephalitis). Specificity can be improved by subjecting a serum sample with positive or indeterminate results by first-step assay to *Western blot testing*. This so-called *second-step test* provides enhanced specificity but is more supplementary than truly confirmatory because it detects antibodies to the same antigens as does first-step testing. Currently, 3 million serologic tests for Lyme disease are ordered annually in the United States at a cost of nearly $100 million. In untreated persons, antibody titers become detectable several weeks into *Borrelia* infection and remain positive for years. ELISA can also detect antibody in CSF. Hyperconcentration of antibody in the CSF is strong evidence for central nervous system infection.

Pitfalls. Improper use and interpretation of Lyme serology are common, often resulting in overdiagnosis, overtreatment, and the associated adverse consequences (e.g., inappropriate health care utilization, treatment-related adverse effects, disability, and depression). The Food and Drug Administration issued a public health advisory regarding the potential for the misdiagnosis of Lyme disease when commercially available antibody assays are used. The advisory and subsequent study by the Centers for Disease Control called attention to numerous shortcomings, such as lack of reproducibility of results, poor sensitivity when used in the early stages of illness, and unacceptably high false-positive rates when used in persons with a low pretest probability of disease. Moreover, Lyme antibodies usually persist for years after infection has cleared, so that the differentiation between active and previous infection is difficult. The proper use of antibody testing for Lyme disease needs to be understood by clinicians to avoid errors in diagnosis and resultant adverse outcomes.

Timing. Because it takes several weeks for immunoglobulin M and especially immunoglobulin G antibodies to be expressed in response to infection, antibody testing should not be ordered during the acute phase of illness. Such early testing maximizes the chances of a false-negative result, which can exceed 50% in the first 2 weeks after onset of symptoms. A testing strategy that utilizes acute-phase and later-phase sera does not appear to be cost-effective. False-negative test results can also occur when patients are treated during early stages of the disease.

Patient Selection. Antibody testing contributes best to clinical decision making when applied to persons with an *intermediate pretest probability* (20% to 80%) of having Lyme disease (Table 160.1 and Chapter 2). Testing persons with a high (>80%) pretest probability contributes little to diagnosis; a negative test result does not rule out the condition and a positive test result does not substantially increase the probability of disease. Patients with a low (<20%) pretest probability (Table 160.1) also do not benefit because the combination of low pretest probability together with high test sensitivity and insufficient specificity produces more false-positives than true-positives (see Chapter 2). Despite such reasons for not testing patients with a low probability of disease, many clinicians still do, often because they want to provide reassurance that the patient does not have Lyme disease. Although it is true that a negative antibody test result obtained after the acute phase of illness has passed does effectively rule out the condition, the chances of a false-positive are substantial and may only aggravate the patient's concerns and disability.

Test Selection. The Centers for Disease Control recommends a two-step testing strategy, which begins with selection of a first-step test for initial assessment followed by Western blot testing of all "indeterminate" and "positive" sera. Theoretically, this approach has the capacity to reduce false-positive results, but its cost-effectiveness remains to be proved. With more than 40 commercially available testing kits available for Lyme antibody detection, much variability in kit performance, often poor interlaboratory and intralaboratory reproducibility, and little standardization, it is essential that one use a laboratory with skill and experience in Lyme antibody testing.

DNA Detection. Better diagnostic studies are needed to differentiate active from past infection in antibody-positive patients, and to distinguish a true-positive ELISA result from a false-positive one. Short of isolating the organism (which is difficult), one can attempt to detect its DNA. Under development is use of *polymerase chain reaction* technology to detect *Borrelia* DNA sequences in bodily fluids. Preliminary studies suggest it can be used to determine active infection in arthritic joints. Further testing is needed, but if the technique proves effective, it may overcome the limitations of antibody testing.

Testing for Concurrent Babesiosis. The diagnosis can be made by identifying the parasite in red cells on *Giemsa-stained thin blood smear*, but because the parasites frequently cannot be seen, test sensitivity is greatly decreased. *Indirect immunofluorescence* is the principal antibody study available; a positive test result consists of a fourfold rise in titer and immunofluorescence persisting at a 1:32 dilution. *Polymerase chain reaction* assays are very sensitive and highly specific but not widely available.

PRINCIPLES OF MANAGEMENT

Antibiotics are effective against *B. burgdorferi*. Treatment is determined by the stage of disease and type of clinical manifestation. *Doxycycline* and *amoxicillin* are preferred for oral treatment programs, and *ceftriaxone* or *high-dose penicillin* when IV therapy is required. Optimal dose and duration of therapy continue to be the subject of study. Current recommendations are presented in Table 160.2. Response rates are excellent, but noninfectious sequelae may still develop in fully treated persons. Additional antibiotic therapy is without benefit in such persons. Patients with severe or prolonged systemic symptoms should be tested for concurrent babesiosis and treated specifically with clindamycin and quinine if the results are positive.

Stage 1: Acute Infection

The earlier antibiotic treatment is instituted, the better the outcome and the lower the risks for dissemination and chronic disease. These facts have led to the common practice of "prophylactic" therapy for all persons presenting with a tick bite in an endemic area; the practice is to be discouraged because only those with a high clinical probability of acute Lyme disease (e.g., typical erythema migrans rash, residing in or visiting an endemic area; see Table 161.1) benefit from early empiric antibiotic therapy. All others should be evaluated for the symp-

Table 160.2.   Recommendations for Antibiotic Treatment[a]

Early Lyme Disease[b]
Doxycycline, 100 mg twice orally daily for 21 to 28 days
Amoxicillin, 500 mg orally three times daily for 21 to 28 days
Cefuroxime, 500 mg orally twice daily for 21 days

Lyme Carditis
Ceftriaxone, 2 g daily IV for 14 to 21 days
Penicillin G, 20 million U IV for 14 to 21 days
Doxycycline, 100 mg orally twice daily for 14 to 28 days, may
   suffice[c] for mild disease (first degree AV block)
Amoxicillin, 500 mg orally three times daily for 14 to 21 days,
   may suffice[c] for mild disease (first degree AV block)

Neurologic Manifestations
Facial nerve paralysis
   For an isolated finding, oral regimens for early disease, used
      for at least 21 to 28 days, may suffice
   For a finding associated with other neurologic manifestations,
      IV therapy (as for meningitis if severe)
Lyme meningitis[d]
   Ceftriaxone, 2 g daily IV by single dose for 14 to 21 days
   Penicillin G, 20 million U daily IV in divided doses for 10 to 21
      days

Lyme Arthritis
Doxycycline, 100 mg orally twice daily for 30 days
Amoxicillin and probenecid, 500 mg each orally four times daily
   for 30 days
Penicillin G, 20 million U IV in divided doses daily for 14 to 28
   days
Ceftriaxone, 2 g IV daily for 14 to 28 days

In Pregnant Women
For localized early Lyme disease, amoxicillin, 500 mg orally three
   times daily for 21 days
For disseminated early Lyme disease or any manifestation of late
   disease, penicillin G, 20 million U IV daily for 14 to 21 days
For asymptomatic seropositivity, no treatment necessary

[a]These guidelines are to be modified by new findings and should always be
applied with close attention to the clinical course of individual patients.
[b]Shorter courses are reserved for disease limited to a single skin lesion.
[c]oral regimens are reserved for mild cardiac involvement (see text).
[d]Regimens for radiculoneuropathy, peripheral neuropathy, and encephalitis are
the same as those for meningitis.
Adapted from MedLett Drugs Ther. Treatment of Lyme Disease 2000;42:37.
Cefurosine (500 mg twice daily) approaches the efficacy of doxycycline.

toms and signs of Lyme disease (see above), undergo serologic testing no sooner than several weeks after the onset of symptoms (only if their pretest probability of having the disease is intermediate), and be treated if results are positive.

Doxycycline (100 mg twice daily) and *amoxicillin* (500 mg three times daily) are the agents of choice. The currently recommended duration of therapy is 21 to 28 days. Cefuroxime (500 mg twice daily) approaches the ethicasy of Doxycycline. Despite hopes that the drug azithromycin might shorten treatment for early disease, a carefully conducted multicenter study found that 7 days of azithromycin was associated with an *unacceptably high relapse rate* in comparison with 20 days of amoxicillin (16% vs. 4%).

Stage 2: Disseminated Disease

In disseminated disease, it is common for a host of organ systems to be involved, although treatment recommendations are by organ system and clinical presentation. If more than one

is involved, then the most potent antibiotic program takes precedence.

Cardiac Involvement is a potentially worrisome form of disseminated disease. Although heart block is usually self-limited, patients with a severe PR–interval in prolongation of (>0.4 seconds) are commonly treated with IV antibiotics (ceftriaxone or high-dose penicillin) to prevent significant myocardial invasion. For those with less severe PR interval prolongation oral doxycycline or amoxicillin prescribed for 21 to 28 days suffices.

Neurologic Involvement. Although most neurologic manifestations of disseminated disease eventually clear without treatment, antibiotic therapy is strongly recommended, both to shorten the duration of symptoms and to prevent sequelae.

Facial Nerve Palsy. In the absence of evidence for meningitis, treatment can be oral with doxycycline or amoxicillin for 3 to 4 weeks.

Meningitis. Antibiotic therapy produces a prompt clinical response and shortens the clinical course substantially. Both IV ceftriaxone and high-dose penicillin G are curative. Ceftriaxone is much more expensive, but its once-daily schedule makes home administration possible and obviates a prolonged hospitalization. Lumbar puncture with CSF analysis is needed to confirm the diagnosis but not to assess response to treatment. Duration of therapy is best determined by the clinical response. Most authorities recommend 2 to 4 weeks.

Polyneuropathy. Peripheral neuropathy and radiculopathy tend to occur in conjunction with meningitis and respond well to treatment of the meningitis. When no clinical or CSF evidence of meningitis is found, an oral program of either doxycycline or amoxicillin for 3 to 4 weeks is a reasonable alternative.

Arthritis. The migratory musculoskeletal pains and brief attacks of oligoarticular arthritis are typically self-limited, but antibiotic therapy is given to halt symptoms and prevent progression to chronic arthritis. The optimal antibiotic program has not been established. Because of the development of chronic arthritis that persists despite prolonged courses of antibiotics, antibiotic regimens have been made longer. Thirty days of oral doxycycline or amoxicillin (with probenecid to delay urinary excretion) is often recommended, with IV therapy reserved for more refractory chronic arthritis (see below). Intraarticular steroids are to be avoided because they increase the risk for antibiotic failure.

Stage 3: Chronic Disease

Late disease tends to be more difficult to treat, with responsiveness to antibiotics often less impressive than in disseminated disease. This has led to the use of prolonged and repeated courses of antibiotics. The inability to distinguish infectious from noninfectious sequelae has hindered the design of treatment programs. With the advent of DNA detection techniques, it should be possible to make more pathophysiologically correct treatment recommendations. It is hoped that etiologic therapy will become available to persons with noninfectious sequelae.

Arthritis. Treatment is 30 days of oral doxycycline or amoxicillin (plus probenecid) or 2 to 3 weeks of IV ceftriaxone or penicillin G. Retreatment may be necessary, but only in cases with objective evidence of persistent infection (e.g., results of polymerase chain reaction testing of synovial fluid remain positive).

Encephalopathy. Patients with Lyme disease in whom documentable memory or cognitive deficits develop in conjunction with elevations in CSF protein and antibody are candidates for antibiotic therapy. The program is identical to that for meningitis. Resolution is sometimes incomplete, and retreatment is carried out. It is unclear whether the cause in such cases is infectious or not. Polymerase chain reaction testing of the CSF may prove useful in making this distinction, but such testing remains to be evaluated.

Patients with the neuropsychiatric symptoms of chronic fatigue syndrome or fibromyalgia often request treatment for Lyme disease, especially if they test positive for antibody. Those who have no clinical evidence for Lyme disease do not respond meaningfully to antibiotic therapy, and it should not be prescribed for them, even if they are antibody-positive. Whether the occasional patient with fibromyalgia or chronic fatigue syndrome whose illness appears to have been directly precipitated by Lyme disease will respond is unclear, but it is unlikely if the mechanism is noninfectious.

Prevention

Vaccination. First-generation Lyme vaccines containing recombinant outer-surface lipoprotein A with adjuvant have been developed and approved by the Food and Drug Administration for use in high-risk settings. Administration of a three-injection program over 2 years is required to achieve maximum efficacy. At 1 year and after two injections, the reported efficacy in the prevention of symptomatic infection is 49%, and it is 76% after 2 years; for the prevention of asymptomatic infection, the rates are 83% and 100%, respectively. Vaccination interferes with current ELISA serologic testing by stimulating antibodies to outer-surface protein, which are measured by most ELISA tests. Long-term safety and required frequency of booster injections remain to be determined. Use in children has not been studied. Soreness at the injection site occurs in about 7%, and 2% have a febrile response. Because the vaccine is not fully protective, precautions still need to be taken outdoors in high-risk areas.

Avoidance Measures, Protective Clothing, Tick Removal, and Use of Repellants. Standard preventive measures begin with avoiding brushy, wooded, or grassy habitats; these include grassy dunes, but not open sandy beaches. Tucking one's pants into one's socks is also commonly suggested. Because it takes more than 24 hours of tick contact before spirochete transmission occurs, it is recommended that daily checks for ticks be performed and removal attempted if a tick is found. Proper *tick removal* is best accomplished by using a tweezers to grip the mouth parts of the tick, which is pulled straight outward with steady gentle pressure. The fingers can be used instead of a tweezers, but gloves should be worn and the hands washed afterward. Other methods (e.g., hot match tip, alcohol, petroleum jelly, nail polish) are not effective.

Diethyltoluamide (DEET)-containing repellants and acaricides such as permethrin that can be applied to clothing provide added protection to persons who cannot avoid high-risk settings. DEET-containing repellants should be used with care, especially in young children, who are quite susceptible to DEET neurotoxicity. Maximum DEET concentration in the repellant should be 15% for children and 35% for adults; use on the skin of infants, on the hands and face of young children, and on cuts, abrasions, and sunburned skin should be avoided. One should apply the repellant just once daily and wash it off with soap and water after returning indoors.

Other Management Issues

Pregnant Patients. Maternal–fetal transmission of infection with subsequent injury to the fetus has been reported. Antibiotic treatment should be instituted promptly in symptomatic patients. For localized early disease in which erythema migrans is the only symptom, the recommended treatment is oral amoxicillin for 3 weeks. For more disseminated disease, IV high-dose penicillin G is required for 2 to 3 weeks. No increased risk for fetal malformation has been found in asymptomatic women who are antibody-positive. Screening asymptomatic pregnant women for Lyme antibody and treating those who test positive is not warranted.

Patients with Concurrent Babesiosis. The program of choice is a combination of *clindamycin* and *quinine*. Treatment for concurrent disease should be carried out in consultation with an infectious disease specialist familiar with the management of tick-borne disease.

Prophylactic Therapy after a Tick Bite. The common practice of administering prophylactic antibiotics to persons in an endemic area who have been bitten by a tick should be discouraged because the risk for infection is less than the risk for an adverse drug reaction. After the tick comes in contact with the skin, it takes 24 hours for the spirochete to be transmitted. Persons who discover a tick usually do so before that much time has elapsed and remove it before transmission can occur. Under such circumstances, the risk for infection is about the same as that for an adverse or hypersensitivity drug reaction. A better approach is to follow patients for the appearance of symptoms (e.g., erythema migrans) and then treat promptly those in whom characteristic manifestations of the disease develop.

PATIENT EDUCATION AND INDICATIONS FOR REFERRAL

Patients who suspect but do not have Lyme disease require as much education about the condition as those who do. The person with depression, chronic fatigue syndrome, or fibromyalgia who insists on treatment for Lyme disease needs to know how the diagnosis is made. Those who are antibody-positive will benefit from a discussion of the minimal significance of a positive antibody test result in the absence of other defining clinical manifestations. The physician, while explaining that the probability of active Lyme disease is very low, must take care not to deny the reality and severity of the patient's symptoms. Attention should be directed to treatment of the underlying condition (see Chapters 8, 159, and 227).

Persons living in or visiting an area endemic for Lyme disease should be instructed to venture into tick-infested areas only after proper application of insect repellent (see above) and to cover skin surfaces with protective clothing. In addition, they should be taught to recognize the rash and other manifestations of early Lyme disease and the importance of early treatment. Parents of children should be taught the proper technique of tick removal (see above).

Patients with Lyme disease benefit from being informed about the excellent response of their condition to antibiotic therapy and its very favorable prognosis. However, those with protracted symptoms that do not respond to antibiotic therapy and with no evidence of persistent infection should be informed about the possibility of a noninfectious pathogenesis that is usually self-limited but slow to resolve. It is hoped that more etiologic therapy will be available for such persons in the future.

Referral is indicated when the patient with strong clinical evidence of Lyme disease fails to respond to a course of appropriate antibiotic therapy. Consultation is particularly important for those with refractory neurologic deficits, debilitating arthritis, or signs of severe cardiac involvement.

RECOMMENDATIONS

Diagnosis

- Make the diagnosis of Lyme disease predominantly according to the clinical presentation (e.g., erythema migrans, relapsing oligoarthritis, heart block, facial nerve palsy) and epidemiology (e.g., community incidence).
- Use serologic testing only as a supplement to the clinical diagnosis.
- Limit serologic testing to persons with an intermediate pretest probability of Lyme disease (based on clinical presentation).
- Avoid serologic testing early in the course of the illness because of the increased risk for false-negative results.
- Consider a two-step approach to serologic testing to reduce the false-positive rate: ELISA, followed by Western blot for sera with indeterminate or positive results by ELISA.
- Use only a high-quality laboratory that has persons skilled and experienced in performing Lyme serology.

Treatment

- Treat empirically without testing only those persons with a high clinical probability of Lyme disease (e.g., typical erythema migrans rash, endemic area).
- Treat after testing those who present with an intermediate pretest probability of Lyme disease and have a positive result on serologic testing.
- Do not treat prophylactically asymptomatic persons who report a tick bite while in an endemic area. Test such persons if sufficient symptoms and signs develop to suggest an intermediate pretest probability of Lyme disease; treat only those with positive test results.
- Do not treat empirically persons with nonspecific symptoms (e.g., flulike syndrome, chronic fatigue) who have a history of a tick bite in an endemic area but who report no characteristic rash.
- For persons with stage 1 disease (acute localized illness), prescribe amoxicillin (500 mg three times daily) doxycycline

(100 mg twice daily) for 3 weeks; do not use the 1-week azithromycin program because of an increased risk for relapse or cefuroxime (500 mg twice daily) is an effective alternative.
- For persons with stage 2 disease (acute disseminated disease), treat according to the organ(s) involved: for meningitis or severe cardiac manifestations, prescribe ceftriaxone (2 g IV once daily for 2 to 4 weeks); for peripheral neuropathy and arthritis, treat with amoxicillin (500 mg three times daily) or doxycycline (100 mg twice daily) for 3 to 4 weeks.
- For persons with stage 3 disease (chronic disease), treat the arthritis initially with the same program of amoxicillin or doxycycline as for stage 2 joint disease, but consider IV ceftriaxone if the initial program fails; treat encephalitis with ceftriaxone (2 g IV once daily for 2 to 4 weeks, the same treatment as for meningitis in stage 2 disease).

Prevention

- Teach patients the basics of avoiding tick habitats, dressing properly, using repellants safely, and removing ticks effectively.
- Consider vaccination for persons with a very high risk for infection, but only with the understanding that the vaccine is not fully protective, that it can compromise results of current serologic testing, and that long-term safety has not been established.

A.H.G.

ANNOTATED BIBLIOGRAPHY

American College of Rheumatology and the Council of the Infectious Diseases Society of America. Appropriateness of parenteral antibiotic treatment for patients with presumed Lyme disease. Ann Intern Med 1993;119;518. (*A consensus statement recommending empiric treatment for those with strong clinical evidence of Lyme disease and no treatment for those with nonspecific symptoms, even if accompanied by a positive serology.*)

Brown SL, Hansen SL, Linguine JJ. Role of serology in the diagnosis of Lyme disease. JAMA 1999;282:62. (*A review of the test performance of commercially available serologic kits. Finds great variability among tests, low reproducibility, and disappointing sensitivity and specificity under many circumstances; recommends that serologic testing be limited to those with an intermediate pretest probability of disease and that a two-step approach to testing be used.*)

Dattwyler RJ, Luft BJ, Kunkel MJ, et al. Ceftriaxone compared with doxycycline for the treatment of acute disseminated Lyme disease. N Engl J Med 1997;337:289. (*A prospective, open-label, randomized multicenter trial showing oral doxycycline to be as effective as parenteral ceftriaxone in preventing symptoms and signs of late disease.*)

Dinerman H, Steere AC. Lyme disease associated with fibromyalgia. Ann Intern Med 1992;117:281. (*Lyme disease often confused with fibromyalgia.*)

Fix AD, Strickland T, Grant J. Tick bites and Lyme disease in an endemic setting: problematic use of serologic testing and prophylactic antibiotic therapy. JAMA 1998;279:206. (*A regional surveillance study documenting the frequent use of unnecessary early serologic testing and empiric antibiotic therapy regardless of test results in persons with a low pretest probability of Lyme disease.*)

Krause PJ, Telford SR III, Spielman A, et al. Concurrent Lyme disease and babesiosis: evidence for increased severity and duration of illness. JAMA 1996;275:1657. (*A carefully conducted community-*

based serologic survey and clinic-based cohort study finding a 10% rate of concurrent infection among those with active Lyme disease; the clinical picture is one of increased severity and prolongation of systemic symptoms.)

Lightfoot RW, Luft BJ, Rahn DW, et al. Empiric parenteral antibiotic treatment of patients with fibromyalgia and fatigue and a positive serologic result for Lyme disease. Ann Intern Med 1993;119:503. (*In most instances, antibiotic therapy is not cost-effective.*)

Logigian EL, Kaplan RF, Steere AC. Chronic neurologic manifestations of Lyme disease. N Engl J Med 1990;323:1438. (*Memory loss, radiculopathy, and leukoencephalitis described.*)

Luft BJ, Dattwyler RJ, Johnson RC, et al. Azithromycin compared with amoxicillin in the treatment of erythema migrans: a double-blind, randomized, controlled trial. Ann Intern Med 1996;124:785. (*Amoxicillin was more likely to produce complete resolution and less likely to cause relapse.*)

Luft BJ, Dattwyler RJ, Johnson RC, et al. Azithromycin compared with amoxicillin in treatment of erythema migrans. Ann Intern Med 1996;124:785. (*Randomized, prospective multicenter study of 246 adults with early Lyme disease; 7-day course of azithromycin associated with a 16% relapse rate, 20 days of amoxicillin with 4%.*)

Malane MS, Grant-Kels JM, Fecer HM Jr, et al. Diagnosis of Lyme disease based on dermatologic manifestations. Ann Intern Med 1991;114:490. (*Excellent photographs and discussion of these findings, which are often pathognomonic.*)

Nocton JJ, Dressler F, Rutledge BJ, et al. Detection of *Borrelia burgdorferi* DNA by polymerase chain reaction in synovial fluid from patients with Lyme arthritis. N Engl J Med 1994;330:229. (*Use of an improved diagnostic method; suggests late arthritis is not caused by persistence of organisms in the joint.*)

Rahn DW, Malawista SE. Lyme disease: recommendations for diagnosis and treatment. Ann Intern Med 1991;114:472. (*Most useful for discussion of antibiotic programs.*)

Reid MC, Schoen RT, Evans J, et al. The consequences of overdiagnosis and overtreatment of Lyme disease: an observational study. Ann Intern Med 1998;128:354. (*Documents frequent overdiagnosis and overtreatment, which lead to inappropriate health care utilization, avoidable treatment-related adverse effects, disability, and depression.*)

Steere AC, Schoen RT, Taylor E. The clinical evolution of Lyme arthritis. Ann Intern Med 1987;107:725. (*Best study of the natural history of the disease, based on examination of untreated patients.*)

Steere AC, Taylor E, McHugh GL, et al. The overdiagnosis of Lyme disease. JAMA 1993;269:1812. (*The problem results from false-positive serology.*)

Steere AC, Sikand VK, Meurice F, et al. Vaccination against Lyme disease with recombinant *Borrelia burgdorferi* outer-surface lipoprotein A with adjuvant. N Engl J Med 1998;339:209. (*Double-blinded, randomized multicenter trial of more than 10,000 subjects; rate of infection reduced by 49% in the first year and by 76% in the second year after the third injection.*)

Tugwell P, Dennis DT, Weinstein A, et al. Laboratory evaluation in the diagnosis of Lyme disease. Ann Intern Med 1997;127:1109. (*An evidence-based clinical guideline recommending testing only for persons with an intermediate (20% to 80%) pretest probability of having the disease.*)

Wormser GP, Aguero-Rosenfeld ME, Nadelman RB. Lyme disease serology: problems and opportunities. JAMA 1999;282:79. (*An editorial review of the current state of serologic testing; suggests strategies and discusses problems involved in testing persons who have been immunized.*)

161

Approach to the Patient with Polymyalgia Rheumatica or Temporal Arteritis

Polymyalgia rheumatica (PMR) is a common nonarticular rheumatoid disease characterized by neck, shoulder-girdle, and hip-girdle complaints and an elevated erythrocyte sedimentation rate (ESR). It affects mostly Caucasian patients over the age of 50, with a 2:1 female predominance. The annual incidence in persons over age 50 is 5/10,000; the prevalence is 50/10,000. The condition is usually self-limited, but the risk for temporal arteritis (TA) is increased. Up to 40% of patients with TA have a prior history of PMR. TA (also referred to as "cranial," "giant cell," or "granulomatous" arteritis) is a vasculitic disorder of unknown origin that can cause sudden blindness and aortic aneurysm and dissection. It too is limited to persons over the age of 50. The incidence and prevalence are about one-fifth that of PMR. Women are more often affected than men.

The primary physician needs to be alert to these diseases, which can be subtle in presentation and easily dismissed as vague functional complaints or confused with other conditions. The associated risks for blindness and aortic injury make the prompt recognition and treatment of TA especially critical. Because treatment requires long-term glucocorticoid therapy, it is just as important to avoid a false-positive diagnosis.

PATHOPHYSIOLOGY, CLINICAL PRESENTATION, AND COURSE

Polymyalgia Rheumatica

The pathogenesis of PMR is unknown, but a genetic susceptibility has been suggested by an association with the HLA-DR4 allele. The onset is gradual, with the condition developing over weeks or months. Bilateral pain and stiffness of periarticular structures in the *neck* and *shoulders* is the presentation in two thirds of cases, with *hip* and *thigh* involvement accounting for the other third. Many patients have both shoulder and thigh involvement. Diffuse swelling of the *hands* occurs in some patients. *Morning stiffness* and pain with movement are highly characteristic. Synovitis have been documented histologically, and rotator cuff bursitis and synovitis can be demonstrated by magnetic resonance imaging. Muscle biopsy specimens are usually normal or show minor inflammatory infiltrates; muscle strength is unimpaired. Low-grade *fever*, *weight loss*, and *fatigue* may accompany the musculoskeletal symptoms. The *ESR* is characteristically above 40 mm/h, but an occasional patient with characteristic clinical features of PMR may have an ESR below 40 mm/h and a milder form of the disease. The ESR correlates with disease activity, as do levels of *interleukin-6* and *C-reactive protein*.

Polymyalgia rheumatica tends to be a self-limited illness with a duration of 1 to 2 years. Three subsets of patients have been described: One responds promptly to initial steroid therapy and has no flares after taper; the required course of steroids is relatively short. A second also responds satisfactorily but has repeated flares and requires a longer course of steroids. A third does not respond to the initial doses of steroids, so that higher initial amounts are necessary; also, more flares occur and a prolonged course of steroids is required. The risk for progression to TA appears low in the first group and possibly increased in the latter two. The pretreatment ESR and the response of the interleukin-6 level to treatment help to identify these subsets.

Polymyalgia rheumatica shares many of the immunologic features of TA, so that some postulate that PRM may be a *forme fruste* of arteritis. Estimates of the risk for the development of clinical TA average 10% to 15%. However, when headache, jaw claudication, cranial artery tenderness, or visual complaints develop in a patient with PMR, the probability of TA is markedly increased (see below).

Temporal Arteritis

Temporal arteritis is a vasculitic condition of unknown origin. It is characterized pathologically by histiocytic, lymphocytic, and giant cell infiltrations of the walls of medium or large arteries originating from the aortic arch. Any one of these vessels can be involved, as can the aorta, but those of the head are most often affected. The internal elastic lamina is fragmented in conjunction with proliferation. The inflammatory process tends to be segmental. Many characteristics of an autoimmune process are present, but the precise pathophysiology remains to be elucidated. The fact that TA, like PMR, is associated with HLA-DR4 suggests a genetic predisposition. Direct inflammation of the arterial wall and the resultant ischemia secondary to vasculitic narrowing account for most symptoms.

The onset is gradual. Early symptoms include headache, low-grade temperature, and the aching and stiffness of PMR. *Headache* is reported in about 70% of cases and is the initial symptom in about 35%. The pain can be piercing or throbbing, often localized to the arteries of the scalp and unlike that of any previous headache. *Polymyalgia* symptoms may be the presenting manifestation in more than 50%. *Constitutional symptoms* of fatigue, malaise, anorexia, and weight loss occur in the majority of patients. In about a fifth of patients, the presentation may be atypical, with *fever of unknown origin* (FUO) being a classic atypical presentation of TA (accounting for about 15% of cases of FUO in patients over the age of 65).

As the condition progresses, *cranial artery tenderness* and enlargement may be noted. The temporal artery is most commonly affected, but any cranial artery may become involved. Ischemic symptoms such as *masseter claudication* (jaw pain with chewing) occur in one third to one half of patients.

Visual manifestations are the consequence of vasculitis of the ophthalmic or posterior ciliary arteries. *Blindness*, the most dreaded manifestation, has an abrupt onset and irreversible course unless it is treated very aggressively and very early (see below). Vision loss is sometimes preceded by transient visual symptoms, such as amaurosis fugax, flashing lights, or field defects. In untreated patients, visual loss occurs in up to 50% of

cases. Acute *hearing loss* and *vertigo* have also been reported. An *aortic arch syndrome* may occur if the arch or a major branch vessel is involved. The risk for *aortic aneurysm* and *dissection* is increased nearly 20-fold; most often, the thoracic aorta is involved, but occasionally just the abdominal portion is affected. Granulomatous inflammation of the aortic wall is found. *Carotid* involvement may present as localized tenderness in the neck accompanied by *neurologic deficits. Subclavian* disease may cause *ischemic symptoms* in the arms (e.g., Raynaud's phenomenon, claudication); pulses are diminished, and a subclavian bruit may be heard.

A *markedly increased ESR* is characteristic of the disease; a normal sedimentation rate in the absence of strongly suggestive symptoms makes the diagnosis unlikely. A low-grade *anemia of chronic disease* and mild elevations of *serum liver enzymes* are also often present. On occasion, the anemia can be severe.

Temporal arteritis is a chronic illness that may last for years. Although it tends to be self-limited, the clinical course is highly variable. Complications of late disease are rare, but attempts to discontinue therapy often cause relapses.

DIAGNOSIS

Polymyalgia Rheumatica

The diagnosis is a clinical one. Criteria include (a) bilateral pain for at least 1 month in any two of the following: neck, shoulder girdle, hip girdle, in association with morning stiffness; (b) ESR above 40 mm/h by the Westergren method; (c) age over 50 years; (d) exclusion of other diagnoses except for TA; (e) marked clinical improvement in response to 1 week of treatment with less than 15 mg of prednisone per day. Patients meeting all criteria except an elevated ESR are usually considered to have PMR also.

Temporal Arteritis

The current American College of Rheumatology criteria for the diagnosis of giant cell (temporal) arteritis include (a) age at onset of symptoms *over 50 years*; (b) new onset or new type of localized *headache*; (c) temporal *artery tenderness* or diminished pulse; (d) *ESR above 50 mm/h* by the Westergren method; and (e) *temporal artery biopsy specimen* showing mononuclear infiltration or granulomatous infiltration with giant cells. The presence of any three criteria constitutes evidence for the diagnosis of TA (sensitivity, 93.5%; specificity, 91.2%). Some characteristic symptoms and signs have been omitted from the criteria list because of their lack of sensitivity or specificity.

Temporal Artery Biopsy is the most invasive of the diagnostic determinations and sometimes a source of concern to patients. It is performed under local anesthesia as an ambulatory procedure, and morbidity is very low. The best results are obtained when an accessible cranial artery is selected that feels tender or has a diminished pulse (not caused by atherosclerotic disease). The temporal artery is usually selected. A 2- to 4-cm specimen is optimal because the inflammatory process may be focal and may demonstrate skip areas. A single biopsy has a sensitivity of about 90%. A negative first biopsy result does not rule out the diagnosis.

Treatment with corticosteroids before biopsy may lower the test sensitivity slightly, but not by so much as to preclude immediate therapy followed by biopsy within the first 1 to 2 weeks after therapy is started. Some authorities suggest that biopsy can be omitted altogether when the clinical evidence for TA is compelling. However, most argue that histologic confirmation should be obtained before a patient is committed to such potentially morbid therapy as long-term daily corticosteroids. Biopsy is unnecessary when it will have no effect on clinical decision making. Patients with negative biopsy results and without strong clinical evidence for the diagnosis of TA have an excellent prognosis; signs of arteritis develop in fewer than 10% at a later time.

Color Duplex Ultrasonography of the temporal arteries appears promising as an alternative or complement to temporal artery biopsy. Its sensitivity for TA is 73% and its specificity is 100% when the finding of a dark halo about the vessel (believed to represent vessel wall edema) is used as the key diagnostic feature. Prospective study is necessary to validate the utility of the test, but possible applications include screening of asymptomatic patients with PMR to identify those who might need further evaluation, and confirming the diagnosis of TA without performing a biopsy in persons with clinically evident disease.

Arteriography is sensitive but nonspecific and unreliable diagnostically; however, it is helpful when an area must be chosen to sample after a first biopsy result has been negative.

PRINCIPLES OF MANAGEMENT

Polymyalgia Rheumatica

Polymyalgia rheumatica in the absence of TA characteristically responds quickly and well to modest doses of *prednisone* (e.g., 10 to 15 mg/d). Patients with severe symptoms and a very high ESR at the time of presentation may require a higher initial dose of prednisone (e.g., 20 to 30 mg/d). As the sedimentation rate falls and symptoms clear, one can begin tapering prednisone in small decrements (1 to 2.5 mg/d every 2 weeks). Therapy is titrated against symptoms and ESR. Some have suggested that following the interleukin-6 response to treatment can help predict the dose and duration of prednisone therapy. Symptomatic flares may require restarting or increasing prednisone, after which tapering is resumed. Between months and 1 to 2 years of daily low-dose steroid therapy may be required. The most prolonged therapy and the highest doses are likely to be needed by persons who manifest a markedly elevated ESR and prominent symptoms at onset and whose serum levels of interleukin-6 fail to normalize after initial steroid treatment. To minimize the adverse effects of daily steroids, the lowest possible dose of prednisone should be prescribed and taken in the morning (see Chapter 105). Osteoporosis prophylaxis is necessary if prolonged steroid therapy is required (see Chapter 146). The steroid doses required to prevent the development of TA in patients with PMR are not known, nor are the determinants of risk, but it appears that the likelihood of TA is low when disease activity is well suppressed. There is no evidence that alternate-day therapy is effective.

Temporal Arteritis

Initiation of Therapy. The first priority is to establish control of the disease quickly to limit the risk for irreversible blindness. When the patient's pretest probability of TA is high (e.g., age over 70 years, new headache, palpably enlarged and tender cra-

nial artery, jaw claudication, high ESR), it is best to begin empiric *high-dose glucocorticoid* therapy (e.g., 40 to 60 mg of prednisone per day) immediately. Biopsy confirmation of the diagnosis is necessary, but empiric therapy before biopsy is appropriate in patients manifesting characteristic clinical features. A biopsy specimen obtained within 1 to 2 weeks after onset of prednisone therapy is not likely to be altered significantly.

In most instances, the clinical response starts within 24 hours of initiation of treatment. *Daily therapy* is needed; alternate-day schedules do not control the arteritis. To minimize adrenal suppression, prednisone should be taken once daily in the morning (see Chapter 105). The initial doses can be given parenterally when visual compromise is a concern, but to be effective, parenteral treatment must be started within the first several hours of visual impairment. Ophthalmologists recommend 5 days of high-dose parenteral *methylprednisolone* (1,000 mg IV every 12 hours) under such circumstances.

Tapering. The steroid dose is titrated against symptoms and sedimentation rate. To minimize the adverse effects of prolonged daily steroid therapy (see Chapter 105), the daily prednisone dose should be tapered. Tapering can be started after clinical and laboratory manifestations have normalized; it can be steady but should not be precipitous. Rapid tapering of prednisone to less than 20 mg/d over the first 1 to 2 months is associated with a 30% relapse rate. More reasonable is tapering to a daily dose of 20 to 30 mg within the first 2 months and more slowly thereafter. The goal is a maintenance dose of less than 10 mg/d, but it may take more than a year to achieve it.

Monitoring and Termination of Therapy. As the dose is reduced, the patient must be monitored for recurrence of *symptoms* and elevation of the *sedimentation rate*. Most patients require treatment for 2 to 3 years. Relapses occur in up to 50% of patients who attempt termination of therapy before that time. Nonetheless, the risk for blindness and other serious disease-related complications is minimal late in the course of disease, and a trial of discontinuing therapy can be attempted every 6 to 12 months after the first year. The trial should be halted at the first sign of recurring symptoms or a marked rise in the ESR. Close monitoring for relapse is essential during the first 12 months that the patient is off therapy. Despite tapering efforts, many patients experience steroid-related side effects because of the prolonged duration of daily steroid therapy. Efforts to limit osteoporosis should be undertaken (see Chapter 164).

Because the risk for potentially life-threatening aortic disease is increased in TA, some have suggested that monitoring for aortic aneurysm be part of the routine follow-up. Suggestions for monitoring range from palpating the abdominal aorta for signs of enlargement (see Chapter 58) and obtaining yearly posteroanterior and lateral chest films to consideration of ultrasonographic screening. The most cost-effective approach remains to be determined.

PATIENT EDUCATION

Patients with PMR in the absence of TA can be reassured. They benefit from knowing that the risk for the development of TA is small, that the disease does not progress to disabling arthritis, and that their condition is self-limited, although it may take a few years to clear. They should be instructed to watch for symptoms of TA and report them promptly. The adverse effects of corticosteroid therapy need to be reviewed so that patients will use prednisone carefully and as directed.

Patients with TA and their families must understand the rationale for daily prednisone therapy in addition to its adverse side effects, both to ensure compliance and to provide an informed basis for long-term steroid use. Instruction in the means of minimizing steroid side effects is appreciated (see Chapter 105). Patients can be reassured that the serious complications of TA can be avoided by proper therapy.

INDICATIONS FOR REFERRAL AND ADMISSION

Prompt consultation with a rheumatologist is helpful when initiation of high-dose steroid therapy for presumed TA is being considered before a temporal artery biopsy can be performed, but therapy should not be delayed if consultation is not available immediately. Urgent ophthalmologic evaluation is needed if visual impairment is reported. If it is not available, one can proceed directly to hospitalization for immediate institution of high-dose parenteral corticosteroid therapy. Rheumatologic consultation is also indicated to consider the need for steroid therapy when cranial artery biopsy results are negative but the clinical presentation strongly suggests TA. The occasional patient with PMR or TA who does not respond adequately to steroid therapy requires a referral for reconsideration of the diagnosis and for other forms of immunosuppressive therapy (e.g., azathioprine, cyclophosphamide, dapsone).

THERAPEUTIC RECOMMENDATIONS

Polymyalgia Rheumatica

- Begin with low-dose prednisone (10 to 15 mg/d), provided no evidence of TA is found. For patients with a very high ESR and severe symptoms, consider starting prednisone at a higher dose (e.g., 20 to 30 mg/d).
- Taper in decrements of 1.0 to 2.5 mg/d every 2 weeks, titrating the dose against symptoms and ESR.
- Prescribe the lowest dose possible, to be taken in the morning.
- Continue steady tapering to full cessation of therapy if possible, monitoring symptoms and ESR for 2 years for evidence of relapse.
- Restart or increase prednisone by 5 to 10 mg/d if a flare of disease occurs; adjust the dose as needed and resume tapering as soon as remission has been achieved.
- Instruct the patient to report promptly any symptoms suggestive of TA (e.g., visual disturbances, tender cranial artery, headache, fever, jaw claudication).

Temporal Arteritis

- Begin therapy with daily high-dose glucocorticoids (e.g., 40 to 60 mg of prednisone every morning). Consider prescribing IV methylprednisolone (100 mg every 12 hours for 5 days) for patients who present with visual disturbances.
- Begin reducing the initial dose once the sedimentation rate has been normalized (<40 mm/h) and symptoms have cleared; aim for a daily prednisone dose of 20 to 30 mg after 1 to 2 months.
- Continue daily prednisone therapy, tapering slowly as tolerated over 12 to 18 months to the minimum dose sufficient to

keep the sedimentation rate normal and the patient free of symptoms; a prednisone dose of less than 10 mg/d is often sufficient.
- Monitor symptoms and the sedimentation rate to determine the rate and extent of tapering permissible. Halt tapering if the ESR rises or symptoms return.
- Continue daily steroids for 18 to 24 months; consider a trial of phasing out therapy at that time and then every 6 to 12 months.
- After cessation of therapy, continue to monitor for recurrence of symptoms and a rise in the sedimentation rate over the next 12 months.
- Watch for the development of aortic aneurysm.

A.H.G.

ANNOTATED BIBLIOGRAPHY

Achkar AA, Lie JT, Hunder GG, et al. How does previous corticosteroid treatment affect the biopsy findings in giant cell (temporal) arteritis? Ann Intern Med 1994;120:987. (*Findings not obscured by 2 weeks of prednisone.*)

Ayoub WT, Franklin CM, Torretti D. Polymyalgia rheumatica: duration of therapy and long-term outcome. Am J Med 1985;79:309. (*Some patients have a 6- to 12-month course; others require therapy for up to 2 years.*)

Casselli RJ, Hunder GG, Whisnant JP. Neurologic disease in biopsy-proven giant cell (temporal) arteritis. Neurology 1988;38:352. (*Findings include acute vertigo and hearing loss in addition to visual loss.*)

Chmelewski WL, McKnight KM, Agudelo CA, et al. Presenting features and outcomes in patients undergoing temporal artery biopsy. Arch Intern Med 1992;152:1690. (*Presenting features did not always predict biopsy results; late disease complications were rare, but prolonged therapy was required.*)

Evans JM, O'Fallon WM, Hunder GG. Increased incidence of aortic aneurysm and dissection in giant cell (temporal) arteritis. Ann Intern Med 1995;122:502. (*Markedly increased risk for aneurysm and dissection.*)

Hall S, Persellin S, Lie JT, et al. The therapeutic impact of temporal artery biopsy. Lancet 1983;2:1217. (*Helped in decision making; fewer than 10% with negative biopsy findings developed signs of arteritis or required steroid therapy.*)

Hunder GG, Bloch DA, Michel BA, et al. The American College of Rheumatology criteria for the classification of giant cell arteritis. Arthritis Rheum 1990;33:1122. (*Consensus diagnostic criteria.*)

Hunder GG, Sheps SG, Allen GL, et al. Daily and alternate-day corticosteroid regimens in the treatment of giant cell arteritis. Ann Intern Med 1975;82:613. (*Alternate-day steroids do not suffice.*)

Klein RG, Hunder GG, Stanson AW, et al. Large artery involvement in giant cell (temporal) arteritis. Ann Intern Med 1975;83:806. (*TA is not limited to the cranial arteries.*)

Kyle V, Cawston TE, Hazleman BL. Erythrocyte sedimentation rate and C-reactive protein in the assessment of polymyalgia rheumatica/giant cell arteritis on presentation and during follow-up. Ann Rheum Dis 1989;48:667. (*ESR closely parallels disease severity and activity in most cases.*)

Kyle V, Hazleman BL. Stopping steroids in polymyalgia rheumatica and giant cell arteritis: treatment usually lasts for 2 to 5 years. Br Med J 1990;300:344. (*The need for therapy can be prolonged.*)

Kyle V, Hazleman BL. Treatment of polymyalgia rheumatica and giant cell arteritis I: steroid regimens in the first 2 months. Ann Rheum Dis 1989;48:658. (*High dose required initially; then it can be reduced.*)

Layfer LF, Banner BF, Huckman MS, et al. Temporal arteriography. Arthritis Rheum 1978;21:780. (*Arteriography is highly sensitive but not specific.*)

Machado EB, Michet CJ, Ballard DJ, et al. Trends in incidence and clinical presentation of temporal arteritis in Olmstead County, Minnesota, 1950–1985. Arthritis Rheum 1988;31:745. (*Best epidemiologic data; clinical features changing; earlier detection.*)

Myklebust G, Gran JT. A prospective study of 284 patients with polymyalgia rheumatica and temporal arteritis: clinical and laboratory manifestations at onset of disease and at the time of diagnosis. Br J Rheumatol 1996;35:1161. (*Excellent data on clinical and laboratory manifestations.*)

Ponge T, Barrier JH, Grolleau JY, et al. The efficacy of selective unilateral temporal artery biopsy versus bilateral biopsies for diagnosis of giant cell arteritis. J Rheumatol 1988;15:997. (*Bilateral biopsy is sometimes necessary, but careful selection can obviate the need for routinely ordering biopsies of two sites.*)

Robb-Nicholson C, Chang RW, Anderson S, et al. Diagnostic value of the history and physical examination in giant cell arteritis. J Rheumatol 1988;15:1793. (*Clusters of symptoms had a high sensitivity, but specificity was lacking.*)

Rosenfeld SI, Kosmorsky GS, Klingele TG, et al. Treatment of temporal arteritis with ocular involvement. Am J Med 1986;80:143. (*High-dose IV steroids given acutely for 5 days offer a chance of visual recovery if started early.*)

Salvarani C, Cantini F, Olivieri I, et al. Proximal bursitis in active polymyalgia rheumatica. Ann Intern Med 1997;127:27. (*Evidence that bursitis is the cause of the shoulder pain.*)

Salvarani C, Gabriel S, Hunder GC. Distal extremity swelling with pitting edema polymyalgia rheumatica. Arthritis Rheum 1996;39:73. (*Atypical presentation, but important to note.*)

Schmidt WA, Kraft HE, Vorpahl K, et al. Color duplex ultrasonography in the diagnosis of temporal arteritis. N Engl J Med 1997;337:1336. (*Sensitivity 73%, specificity 100%; suggests a positive test result may obviate the need for biopsy.*)

Sox HC, Liang MW. The erythrocyte sedimentation rate. Ann Intern Med 1986;104:515. (*Useful for diagnosis and monitoring response to therapy.*)

Weyland CM, Fulbright JW, Evans JM, et al. Corticosteroid requirements in polymyalgia rheumatica. Arch Intern Med 1999;159:577. (*A prospective cohort study identifying three subgroups with different steroid requirements.*)

Weyland CM, Hicok KC, Hunder GC, et al. Tissue cytokine patterns in patients with polymyalgia rheumatica and giant cell arteritis. Ann Intern Med 1994;121:484. (*Many similar findings suggest a shared pathophysiology, except no production of interferon-γ in polymyalgia.*)

Wong RL, Korn JH. Temporal arteritis without an elevated sedimentation rate. Am J Med 1986;80:959. (*A normal ESR does not rule out the diagnosis when other characteristic features are present.*)

162
Management of Paget's Disease
SAMUEL R. NUSSBAUM

Paget's disease of bone, or osteitis deformans, is a focal disorder of unknown cause. It is characterized by deformity of the external contour and internal structure of bones that results from excessive resorption and rapid, disorganized formation of new bone. The incidence of Paget's disease is 3.3% in autopsy series and 0.1% to 4.0% in radiologic studies. The clinical presentation is variable. In the majority of cases, the diagnosis is made in an asymptomatic patient by the incidental discovery of an elevated alkaline phosphatase level during multiphasic screening or of the hallmark radiolucent (osteolytic) areas with compensatory new bone formation on radiographic films of the pelvis, vertebrae, or skull. Symptomatic patients report pain in the back or lower extremities, disturbances of gait, increasing head size, hearing loss, and occasionally symptoms related to high-output cardiac failure. The primary physician needs to be able to recognize the condition and know how and when to use agents that suppress osteoclastic activity.

PATHOPHYSIOLOGY AND CLINICAL PRESENTATION

The pathophysiologic hallmarks of Paget's disease are *excessive osteoclastic destruction* and resorption of bone, followed by the *unregulated osteoblastic formation of new bone*. The initial stimulus for bone resorption remains unknown, but the process culminates in an abnormal pattern of lamellar bone. Excessive local vascularity and an increase in fibrous tissue, which extends into the marrow, are characteristic. Both cortical and cancellous bone may be involved, each with several foci at different stages. The nature of the resultant bone, which is mechanically defective, distorted, and enlarged, leads to the cardinal manifestations of Paget's disease—bone pain and pathologic fractures.

Clinical Presentation. Although any bone may become involved, the common sites are *spine, pelvis, skull, femur,* and *tibia.* Most patients are asymptomatic, with Paget's disease presenting as an incidental finding on x-ray films or an isolated elevation in alkaline phosphatase. Those who are symptomatic present with bone pain, bony deformity, fracture, or a complication of increased marrow vascularity or bony encroachment on neural structures. About 15% of patients have very localized (so-called "monostotic") disease.

Bone pain may result from fracture or be independent of it. In the latter instance, it is usually located over lytic areas of bone where active osteoclastic resorption is taking place. The severity of pain does not always parallel the extent of radiographic involvement. Exacerbating factors include weight bearing, muscular activity, and cold weather.

Fractures may affect the long bones or vertebrae. The *lesser trochanter* of the femur and the upper third of the *tibia* are characteristic sites for fractures in long bones. A history of trauma can usually be elicited, but some of these fractures may occur spontaneously. Pain may result, but not always. Most vertebral fractures occur in the lumbar and sacral regions. They are usually painless but can lead to loss of height, kyphoscoliosis, and, in rare instances, spinal cord compression.

Bony deformity and *encroachment* are most notable in the *skull*, which may become visibly enlarged in the frontal and occipital regions. The overlying superficial blood vessels often become prominently dilated and visibly pulsatile. *Hearing loss* can ensue from involvement of the ossicles in the middle ear, which impinge on the eighth cranial nerve in the temporal bone. *Cerebellar* and *long-tract* signs are complications of posterior fossa encroachment. Vertebral encroachment on the *spinal cord* or *nerve roots* is rare but can cause a compression syndrome, including paraplegia. Deformity of the *long bones* is manifested as anterolateral bowing; it contributes to susceptibility to *fracture*.

Degenerative joint disease can result from hypertrophy of subchondral bone, which damages the overlying cartilage and causes joint dysfunction. Joint injury accounts for about 50% of the discomfort experienced by patients. Hip pain is a major problem in patients with long-standing subchondral bone involvement in the acetabulum and femoral head; it can lead to protrusio acetabuli. Degenerative disease of the knee joint may occur in similar fashion if the distal femur or patella becomes pagetic. Extensive and severe skeletal involvement increases the risk for *osteogenic sarcoma*, an uncommon but uniformly fatal cancer that affects fewer than 1% of pagetic patients. It is heralded by localized pain and bony enlargement and occurs more frequently in the upper extremities and skull of patients over the age of 50.

Hyperuricemia leading to gouty arthritis and *hypercalciuria* resulting in renal calculi are among the biochemical consequences of disrupted bony metabolism. *Hypercalcemia* can be precipitated by immobilization. *High-output heart failure* may occur in patients with extensive Paget's disease because of the marked increase in the vascular bed.

Laboratory and Radiographic Features. Serum *alkaline phosphatase*, produced by osteoblasts, is usually increased and correlates with the degree of new bone formation. *Urinary hydroxyproline*, a measure of bone matrix resorption, is also increased. In most patients, these parameters are complementary markers of disease activity and parallel radionuclide uptake on bone scan, the most sensitive measure of disease activity. In patients with disease localized to a single bone, results of standard serum and urine tests may be normal. The *bone-specific alkaline phosphatase* level provides a more sensitive determination of new bone formation, and the urinary level of *pyridinoline* (a specific component of bone matrix) is a better measure of bone resorption. Although these values are 50 to 100 times more expensive to obtain than the unfractionated alkaline phosphatase, they are useful indicators of disease activity in persons with involvement limited to a single bone.

Technetium *bone scan* demonstrates areas of increased uptake before diagnostic changes are visible on *standard radiography*. The first radiologic bony changes occur in the lytic phase and are well-demarcated areas of decalcification (seen best in the skull). With onset of new bone formation, areas of increased density become evident, as does expansion of bone and coarse trabeculation. In later phases, sclerosis, enlargement, and increased bone density are observed. The localized enlargement of bone that results is unique to Paget's disease and helps to distinguish it from other causes of bony sclerosis, such as prostatic cancer. Radiologic changes are most commonly evident in the pelvis, femur, and skull.

Clinical Course. Although many patients manifest slow radiologic progression, symptoms never develop in most. Others are noted to have radiologic changes that remain stable; a few have rapidly progressive disease. Although clinical remission after treatment is the rule, new complications can occur in those who do not achieve full biochemical remission (see below).

PRINCIPLES OF THERAPY

Patients with Paget's disease who are asymptomatic require no specific therapy unless the location of their disease places them at risk for a potentially serious complication (see below). Localized mild bone pain can be controlled with *analgesics* such as acetaminophen. Painful joints usually respond acutely to *acetaminophen* or an NSAID (e.g., 400 mg of *ibuprofen* three times daily or 500 mg of *naproxen* twice daily), agents commonly used for the symptomatic relief of osteoarthritis (see Chapter 157). More definitive therapy can halt the disease process by inhibiting bone resorption. The efficacy and safety of modern antipagetic therapy and the potentially disabling consequences of the disease have lowered the threshold for treatment.

The management of Paget's disease has been greatly enhanced in recent years by the development of *second-generation bisphosphonates* (e.g., *alendronate*, *risedronate*), which are well tolerated, orally effective, and capable of inhibiting osteoclast-mediated bone resorption without compromising bone mineralization. They effect radiographic, biochemical, and clinical improvement.

Indications for Disease-specific Therapy. At present, most patients are considered reasonable candidates for treatment unless they are asymptomatic and the disease is confined to areas where it is unlikely to cause complications (e.g., ribs, iliac crest, sacrum, upper limbs, scapula). Indications for immediate treatment include the following: (a) severe pain in pagetic areas; (b) compression of medulla, cauda equina, or auditory nerve with neurologic deficit; (c) high-output cardiac failure; (d) hypercalcemia secondary to immobilization; (e) marked radiographic lytic lesions in long bones and skull representing a risk for fracture or brain trauma; (f) multiple fractures; (g) prevention of disfigurement when the skull is extensively involved; (h) recurrent renal calculi secondary to hypercalciuria; and (i) severe hyperuricemia and gout. Prophylactic therapy is indicated when orthopedic surgery is planned in an involved area, and when disease is located in an area (e.g., base of skull, spine, long bones of lower extremity, hip, or knee) where progress is likely to cause a complication. Standard courses of therapy are specified, but any sign of clinical or biochemical relapse (e.g., pain, neurologic deficit, or biochemical marker >20% to 30% above normal) is an indication for repeated treatment.

Bisphosphonates, which include alendronate, risedronate, pamidronate, and etidronate, are the treatment of choice for the vast majority of patients with Paget's disease. The second-generation drugs (e.g., alendronate, risedronate) are particularly effective. After absorption, they bind primarily to bone and may persist there for months to years, which perhaps accounts for their prolonged effects long after therapy is discontinued. They markedly decrease bone turnover by inhibiting osteoclastic bone resorption. First-generation biphosphonates (e.g., etidronate) also impair bone mineralization, a distinct disadvantage. All decrease the number of osteoclasts and induce osteoclast apoptosis. The deposition of new bone proceeds in lamellar fashion rather than in the woven pattern characteristic of Paget's disease. Patients with moderate disease respond almost completely. Bone pain decreases and neurologic deficits lessen. The alkaline phosphatase level returns toward normal, and radionuclide uptake on bone scan decreases markedly. Hearing loss may not improve, but it ceases to worsen. Bony films may show some repair of lytic lesions. By turning off bone resorption, the most potent bisphosphonates may lower serum calcium, so that calcium and vitamin D supplementation becomes necessary to prevent secondary hyperparathyroidism from developing.

Alendronate is among the most effective of the available orally active bisphosphonates approved by the Food and Drug Administration. When given in full doses (40 mg/d), this second-generation bisphosphonate normalizes the alkaline phosphatase level in about half of cases and produces an overall mean reduction in the alkaline phosphatase level that approaches 75%, so that this agent is superior to etidronate and calcitonin and equal to IV pamidronate in effectiveness. Its main drawback is that is causes gastroesophageal mucosal injury that can result in ulcer; this adverse effect can be minimized by taking alendronate with a full 8-oz glass of water and remaining upright for at least 30 minutes. Because food nullifies absorption, alendronate must be taken on an empty stomach. A standard recommended course of treatment is 6 months; treatment is restarted if a relapse occurs. The remissions achieved can last from 6 months to several years. Many patients either experience a prolonged remission after a single course of therapy or respond well to repeated treatment. The remainder, who manifest more severe disease, may relapse more quickly.

Risedronate is among the latest of the second-generation bisphosphonates approved by the Food and Drug Administration. Its efficacy is similar to that reported for alendronate (73% of patients manifest biochemical remission at 6 months, and 53% at 18 months), although no direct comparison studies have been performed. The risk for gastrointestinal mucosal injury is similar to that for alendronate, so that similar precautions with use must be taken. About 10% experience flulike symptoms. The recommended duration of therapy is only 2 months; in comparison with alendronate, the cost of a course of treatment is about 10% less (i.e., the cost per tablet is much higher, but the total cost for a standard course of therapy is reduced).

Pamidronate is too injurious to the gastroesophageal mucosa for oral use to be possible, but the efficacy of IV therapy is similar to that of oral alendronate. Flulike symptoms are a common accompaniment. Pamidronate is used mostly in hospital settings when Paget's disease is complicated by important neurologic deficits, but it may also be a reasonable option when compliance with long-term oral therapy is a concern. The standard dose is 30 mg/d for 3 days. The mean duration of remission achieved is about 14 months. The inhibition of bone resorption can be sufficiently marked to lower serum calcium. Calcium and vitamin D supplementation is required to limit the risk for hypocalcemia, which can trigger the reactive secretion of parathyroid hormone. Bone mineralization is not impaired unless the cumulative dose exceeds 180 mg.

Etidronate was the first of the orally effective bisphosphonates, providing therapy that was relatively well tolerated except for some mild diarrhea. Although still available, it is less effective than alendronate or risedronate and less desirable because it can impair bone mineralization. Consequently, it is not the bisphosphonate of first choice. Patients who relapse rapidly after etidronate tend to become resistant to repeated treatment. Prolonged continuous therapy or higher doses (10 to 20 mg/kg per day) induce a mineralization defect that may lead to increased fracture rates in areas of lytic bone and a worsening bone pain. Thus, etidronate should not be used for more than 6 months consecutively, nor at a dose greater than 5 mg/kg per day. The newer bisphosphonates are more effective and do not produce mineralization defects.

Calcitonin. Before the advent of the bisphosphonates, calcitonin was the only available treatment capable of inhibiting osteoclastic activity. Biochemical and clinical remissions are achieved in one third of patients, improvement is noted in another third, and the response is minimal or unsustained in the balance of cases. Urinary hydroxyproline starts to decline within a few days of onset of therapy; after a few weeks, a reduction in alkaline phosphatase and then clinical improvement are noted. Calcitonin is used primarily in settings in which second-generation bisphosphonates are not available or cannot be used. For example, it can be given in conjunction with a slower-acting first-generation bisphosphonate, such as etidronate, to control bone pain until the effects of the latter take hold.

Synthetic salmon and human calcitonin preparations are commercially available. The salmon calcitonin preparation is the less expensive, and it differs by just one amino acid from human calcitonin. Although up to 50% of patients manifest neutralizing antibodies to synthetic salmon calcitonin, the risk for clinically important inactivation is small. Control can be reestablished by switching to human calcitonin.

The major disadvantages of calcitonin are nausea (in some patients), flushing, cost (two to three times that of bisphosphonate therapy), and the need for parenteral administration. A nasally absorbed preparation is available but is less effective and not approved by the Food and Drug Administration for use in Paget's disease. Not only is therapy expensive; it also requires patient education and the ability to learn self-injection techniques. The calcitonin dosage may be reduced when the disease is in remission. Current data suggest that a low dose needs to be continued indefinitely to prevent relapse.

Cytotoxic Agents. *Plicamycin* (formerly *mithramycin*) and *dactinomycin* are cytotoxic agents that potently suppress bone resorption. They are administered IV to patients with serious complications of Paget's disease, such as severe high-output heart failure or hypercalcemic crisis. Hospitalization and consultation are required for proper use because of the risks for acute (although reversible) renal, hepatic, and hematologic toxicities. Thrombocytopenia can be particularly severe. These agents are rarely used at present because of the availability of less toxic agents.

Surgery. Neurosurgical intervention is necessary in patients with spinal cord or nerve root compression syndromes. Orthopedic procedures such as total hip replacement and tibial or femoral osteotomy may help to restore mobility.

Monitoring Therapy. Factors found to predict the duration of remission include initial values for biochemical markers, the lowest posttreatment levels attained, and the speed of the biochemical response to the first course of therapy. These findings argue for regular monitoring of the serum *alkaline phosphatase* level, supplemented only if necessary by monitoring of the urinary *hydroxyproline* (which costs about 100 times more to perform). Two baseline alkaline phosphatase measurements should be obtained before therapy is started, followed by monthly determinations during treatment until remission is achieved. Skeletal *radiographic films* are also helpful to have at the commencement of therapy. They are not repeated routinely except when the base of the skull or a long bone of the lower extremity is involved, where disease progression can be dangerous. The technetium *bone scan* provides an alternative baseline measure. Once remission is achieved, follow-up measurement of the alkaline phosphatase level is indicated every 6 months. Patients with bone or joint pain or minor neurologic deficits benefit from an office check every 3 months while they remain symptomatic.

PATIENT EDUCATION AND INDICATIONS FOR REFERRAL

Patients should be instructed to drink at least 2 L of liquid daily, especially if they are unable to keep active, because immobilization and dehydration can precipitate hypercalcemia and renal stone formation. Patients who are candidates for calcitonin therapy require detailed teaching by a nurse in the techniques of SQ injection. Confirmation of the proper technique should be obtained before self-administration is prescribed unless another household member is going to be administering the medication.

Hospital admission and prompt neurosurgical consultation are warranted in patients who have evidence of nerve or cord compression. Admission is also indicated for severe hypercalcemia. Orthopedic surgical consultation is indicated for the person severely limited by pagetic degenerative joint disease of the hip or knee. Consultation with an endocrinologist or rheumatologist is required when initiation of specific therapy is being considered for an asymptomatic patient with radiologic or biochemical evidence of advancing disease. Referral is beneficial when standard courses of etidronate and calcitonin fail to achieve remission and when relapse occurs.

TREATMENT RECOMMENDATIONS

- Follow asymptomatic patients yearly and expectantly and as long as they have no involvement of the base of the skull, spine, hip, knee, or long bones of the lower extremity; at annual visits, assess clinically and obtain an alkaline phosphatase determination.
- For those with mild to moderate pain caused by localized bony involvement or secondary degenerative joint disease, prescribe acetaminophen (e.g., 300 mg four times daily), aspirin (325 mg three times daily), or another NSAID (e.g., 400 mg of ibuprofen up to three times daily as needed or 500 mg of naproxen up to twice daily as needed) for the short-term relief of symptoms.
- For all symptomatic patients and for those with asymptomatic disease who have bony involvement in a potentially critical area (base of the skull, spine, hip, knee, or long bone of the lower extremity), obtain baseline plain x-ray films and measurements of alkaline phosphatase and urinary hydroxyproline; then begin oral bisphosphonate therapy with a second-generation preparation (e.g., 40 mg of alendronate per day or 30 mg of risedronate per day). Specify that each dose be taken half an hour before breakfast on an empty stomach with at least 8 oz of water and without lying down.
- Continue bisphosphonate therapy for the specified standard course of treatment (e.g., 6 months for alendronate, 2 months for risedronate) or until clinical and biochemical remissions are achieved. Monitor the alkaline phosphatase monthly until remission is achieved, then every 6 months. Consider reinstituting therapy if symptoms recur or if the alkaline phosphatase level rises to 20% to 30% above the upper limit of normal.
- Consider IV pamidronate (30 mg/d) for patients with severe disease, especially those ill enough to require hospitalization.
- Consider parenteral calcitonin (100 MRC units given SQ daily) as a means of providing short-term relief for very symptomatic patients while they are waiting for bisphosphonate therapy to take effect, especially if etidronate is being used. Once clinical and biochemical remissions have been achieved, reduce the dose to 50 MRC units and continue therapy three times a week.
- Obtain two baseline measurements of the alkaline phosphatase level and a baseline skeletal roentgenogram or bone scan before therapy is started. Follow the serum alkaline phosphatase level at monthly intervals during therapy. Also monitor the serum calcium level at the outset. Routine repetition of radiologic procedures is unwarranted, but repeating radiography periodically may be helpful if the patient has a high-risk lesion (e.g., base of skull, long bone of lower extremity). If fracture is suspected, another film is essential.
- Advise the patient to avoid immobilization and dehydration. Prescribe at least 2 L of liquid per day, especially if the patient is inactive. Prescribe a total daily calcium intake of 1.5 to 2.0 g and 800 IU of vitamin D daily if the patient is on parenteral or second-generation bisphosphonate therapy. Monitor the serum calcium level if the adequacy of calcium intake is a concern.

ANNOTATED BIBLIOGRAPHY

Alvarez L, Guanabens N, Peris P, et al. Discriminative value of biochemical markers of bone turnover in assessing the activity of Paget's disease. J Bone Miner Res 1995;10:458. (*Finds bone-specific alkaline phosphatase a very sensitive marker of bone formation.*)

Bikle DD. Biochemical markers in the assessment of bone disease. Am J Med 1997;103:427. (*Excellent review that includes data on the costs of available tests in addition to their uses and shortcomings.*)

Chines A, Bekker P, Clarke P, et al. Reduction in bone pain and alkaline phosphatase in patients with severe Paget's disease of bone following treatment with risedronate. J Bone Miner Res 1996;11[Suppl 1]:S471. (*Evidence for efficacy of this new second-generation bisphosphonate.*)

Delmas PD, Meunier PJ. The management of Paget's disease of bone. N Engl J Med 1997;336:558. (*Useful review for the generalist reader; 71 references.*)

Frank WA, Bries NM, Singer FR, et al. Rheumatic manifestations of Paget's disease of bone. Am J Med 1974;56:592. (*Joint disease can be an important problem for patients with Paget's disease.*)

Krane SM. Etidronate disodium in the treatment of Paget's disease of bone. Ann Intern Med 1982;96:619. (*Classic review of the drug.*)

Liens D, Delmas PD, Meunier PJ. Long-term effects of intravenous pamidronate in fibrous dysplasia of bone. Lancet 1994;343:953. (*No impairment of bone mineralization if total dose is below 180 mg.*)

Meunier PJ, Vignot E. Therapeutic strategy in Paget's disease of bone. Bone 1995;17[Suppl]:489S. (*Long-term follow-up data and suggested approach to treatment.*)

Nagent de Deuxchaisnes, Krane SM. Paget's disease of bone: clinical and metabolic observations. Medicine (Baltimore) 1974;43:233. (*Classic review article of clinical and biochemical manifestations.*)

Patel S, Stone MD, Coupland C, et al. Determinants of remission of Paget's disease of bone. J Bone Miner Res 1993;8:1467. (*Factors found to predict duration of remission include initial values for biochemical markers, lowest posttreatment levels attained, and speed of biochemical response to first course of therapy.*)

163
Approach to the Patient with Raynaud's Phenomenon

Raynaud's phenomenon is strongly suggested when patients report bilateral blanching and discomfort in the fingers in response to cold or stress, followed by purplish discoloration and reactive erythema. For some, it is an isolated problem; for others, it may represent the first manifestation of connective tissue disease, arterial occlusion, or a hematologic problem. The primary physician needs to be able to determine what the chances are of underlying disease being present or developing, how to perform the initial workup, and how to provide symptomatic relief.

PATHOPHYSIOLOGY AND CLINICAL PRESENTATION

Alteration in dermal blood flow is a basic mechanism of thermoregulation and is also a common response to stress-induced catecholamine release. In patients with Raynaud's phenomenon, this vascular reactivity is exaggerated. It may be functional (secondary to *vasospasm*), anatomic (secondary to *arterial occlusive disease*), or rheologic (secondary to *alterations in blood viscosity or red cell deformability*). *Platelet activation* appears to play a role in patients with abnormal vascular anatomy. In many instances, the pathophysiology is multifactorial. The characteristic clinical sequence begins with a rapid onset of digital blanching (vasospastic phase), which is followed by cyanosis (venospastic phase). It ends with the restoration of flow and redness (reactive hyperemia).

Clinically, Raynaud's phenomenon is classified as "primary" or idiopathic (Raynaud's disease) if no evidence of an associated condition can be found and "secondary" if an associated condition is present. Some have objected to this designation because secondary causes (e.g., connective tissue disease) may not become clinically evident for years.

Primary Raynaud's Phenomenon: Raynaud's Disease. Patients with truly idiopathic disease appear to experience excessive vasospasm, with mild symptoms often precipitated by emotional stress. Peripheral adrenergic tone is especially high. The condition is most common in women, with onset often at menarche. Attacks may be frequent (several times daily), mild, and precipitated by emotional stress, and they may affect persons with other vasomotor problems (migraine, livedo reticu-

laris). The fingers show no edema, nail bed erythema, or ischemic changes. The prognosis is excellent in terms of ischemic injury.

A pathophysiologic relative of primary disease is is drug-induced disease. *Vasoactive drugs* used to treat migraine (β-blockers, ergotamine, methysergide) have all been implicated, as has *migraine* itself. Whether drugs can cause the problem in the absence of an underlying vasomotor disorder remains unclear.

Secondary Raynaud's Phenomenon: Underlying Disease. In many patients with seemingly isolated Raynaud's phenomenon at the time of their initial presentation, characteristic manifestations of *connective tissue disease* (especially *scleroderma* and *systemic sclerosis*) eventually develop, although sometimes not for several years. In some patients, subtle manifestations of connective tissue disease are already evident, including mild sclerodactyly, early calcinosis, telangiectasia, and presence of antinuclear antibodies. In others, they are not, but an abnormal nail fold capillary pattern is especially predictive. In comparison with primary disease, secondary Raynaud's phenomenon affects men as well as women and tends to appear later (patients in their midtwenties or older). The episodes are more severe and less likely to be precipitated by emotional stress. Loss of finger pulp and skin ulcers as a consequence of ischemia may be evident.

The chances of eventual manifestation of frank connective tissue disease (almost always systemic sclerosis) are small and likely to be much less than the reported 12.6% or 3.2/100 patient-years derived from metaanalysis of referral-based studies. The mean onset is almost 3 years from the time of diagnosis and more than 10 years after the onset of symptoms. At the time of initial presentation, the best predictors for the development of systemic sclerosis include abnormal nail bed capillary pattern, presence of antinuclear antibodies, presence of skin lesions, abnormal pulmonary function, and esophageal dysmotility. Although predictive, none of these factors has a positive predictive value in excess of 50%.

Raynaud's phenomenon is especially prevalent in patients with systemic sclerosis, occurring in more than 90% of cases. In such patients, structural narrowing of digital vessels is

Table 163.1.   Important Causes of Raynaud's Phenomenon

Vasospastic Disease
  Primary
  Drug-induced (β-blockers, ergot, methysergide)
  Migraine

Arterial Occlusive Disease (+/− platelet activation)
  Scleroderma
  Systemic sclerosis
  Systemic lupus erythematosus
  Occupational trauma (jackhammer operator)
  Atherosclerotic disease
  Compression (thoracic outlet, carpal tunnel)

Hemorrheologic Disease
  Paraproteinemia
  Polycythemia
  Cryoproteinemia

caused by intimal fibrosis. Abnormal vascular reactivity and platelet activation have been demonstrated. Symptoms may be especially severe, and the risk for digital ischemic injury is substantial. The compromise to digital blood flow is considerably less in patients with scleroderma.

A host of other conditions can cause vasoocclusive Raynaud's phenomenon, including *atherosclerotic disease*, occupational *vibratory injury* (jackhammer operators, welders, sheet-metal workers), and *neurovascular compression* syndromes (thoracic outlet, carpal tunnel). The clinical course is a function of the underlying disease, a number of which are reversible.

DIFFERENTIAL DIAGNOSIS

The causes of Raynaud's phenomenon can be grouped according to the predominant pathophysiologic mechanism (Table 163.1), although, as noted above, multiple mechanisms may be operative. About 20% of patients presenting initially with idiopathic or primary Raynaud's phenomenon prove after 2 to 3 years to have underlying connective tissue disease.

WORKUP

History and Physical Examination

Confirming the Diagnosis. The diagnosis of Raynaud's phenomenon is a clinical one, based on a history or direct observation of the characteristic changes in skin color in response to cold or stress. If the diagnosis is uncertain, one can test the patient's response to cold by immersing the hands in ice water and observing for blanching, cyanosis, and reactive hyperemia. At least two of the three characteristic skin changes must be present for the diagnosis to be confirmed.

Differentiating Primary from Secondary Disease. Because Raynaud's phenomenon is often the presenting manifestation of an underlying disease, it is important to consider such conditions in the early phase of the evaluation. Screening by history and physical examination can facilitate the selection of patients who require more detailed testing. The differentiation is facilitated by attention to age at onset, gender, frequency and severity of attacks, distribution of skin changes, ischemic skin changes, manifestations of connective tissue disease, precipitating factors, associated digital swelling, and other vasomotor phenomena, such as migraine and livedo reticularis.

Primary disease is suggested by onset in the teens, female sex, occurrence of multiple mild attacks every day, symmetric involvement, precipitation of attacks by stress, normal skin except for livedo reticularis, and migraine headaches. Secondary disease should be suspected in a male patient or in a female patient with onset in the midtwenties or later. Other clues include moderate to severe attacks not necessarily occurring every day, asymmetric presentation triggered predominantly by cold, and associated finger swelling, ischemic skin ulcers, or loss of fingertip pulp.

Further Evaluation of Suspected Secondary Disease. Patients with a presentation suggestive of secondary disease should be checked carefully for additional symptoms of connective tissue disease, such as skin rash, morning stiffness, arthralgias, joint swelling, fatigue, and fever (see Chapter 146), and of peripheral vascular disease, such as claudication, angina, and leg ulceration (see Chapter 23). Although less common, symptoms of thoracic outlet and carpal tunnel syndromes (see Chapter 167) and polycythemia (see Chapter 80) should also be sought if the diagnosis of underlying disease remains unclear. The occupational history is noted for any vibratory injury. Medications should be reviewed, and any effects of β-blockers, ergotamine, methysergide, or calcium channel blockers on symptoms noted.

The physical examination should include a thorough check for manifestations of connective tissue disease (e.g., malar flush, sclerodactyly, petechial rash, telangiectasia, calcinosis, joint redness, swelling, and effusion). The hand and arm pulses are carefully palpated, and capillary filling is noted in the digits. The fingertips are felt for loss of pulp, which is indicative of ischemia, and the skin is observed for ischemic changes. The *nail fold capillary pattern* should be examined carefully because an abnormal pattern is a prime predictor of systemic sclerosis. If available, a wide-field microscope provides excellent views of the capillary bed, but the magnification afforded by the more readily accessible hand-held ophthalmoscope may suffice. One looks at the pattern of capillary loops; asymmetry indicates dropout of capillary loops, which is characteristic and predictive of systemic sclerosis.

Laboratory Testing

Patients judged to have definite primary disease on the basis of the careful history and physical examination noted above require no additional evaluation. An antinuclear antibody test can be ordered to rule out further the risk for underlying connective tissue disease (negative predictive value of 93%), but a positive test result in the absence of other suggestive findings has a very low positive predictive value and may raise concern inappropriately. Consequently, only those with clinical evidence suggestive of connective tissue disease should be subjected to *antinuclear antibody* testing. For patients who test positive for antinuclear antibodies, an *anticentromere antibody* determination can help predict the risk for development of limited systemic sclerosis (i.e., scleroderma), but the test is expensive, and its contribution to overall clinical decision making needs to be considered before it is ordered.

Noninvasive studies of arterial flow (*plethysmography*, *Doppler ultrasonography*) can confirm anatomic vascular compromise; however, similar information can often be obtained by a careful history and physical examination, and test data usually do not help differentiate among anatomic causes of the disease.

A *complete blood cell count* and *serum globulin* determination should suffice to screen for common hematologic problems; *immunoelectrophoresis* is reserved for patients in whom myeloma is suspected (elderly, markedly elevated globulin, anemia; see Chapter 79). A *cryoprotein* determination is indicated if other manifestations suggestive of cryoglobulinemia (arthralgias, purpura, proteinuria) are present. A cold agglutinin test is worth considering for patients with anemia and splenomegaly.

MANAGEMENT

Prevention. Regardless of the underlying cause, keeping the trunk and the extremities warm on cold days is essential. Of particular importance is *truncal warmth* because any threat to the maintenance of core body temperature is a potent stimulus to reflex peripheral vasoconstriction. *Smoking cessation* and elimination of passive smoking are essential. Any drugs found to trigger episodes should be stopped or cut back.

Occupational precipitants, such as repetitive activity that leads to carpal tunnel syndrome or vibratory injury, should be reduced or eliminated. Although *pneumatic tool* operation (e.g., jackhammer) is the classic occupational association, smaller and less inertial tools that produce *high-frequency vibrations* have been found to be even more likely to cause vascular injury. Working on a vibrating or rotating tool (such as those used by welders, sheet-metal workers, carpenters, and painters) for as little as 1 to 2 hours per day can inflict vascular damage. Prevention, by limiting the number of hours such equipment is used, is the best approach but is often not feasible. Alternatively, at the first sign of symptoms, use should be markedly reduced or eliminated. Antivibration gloves and coated tool handles have not proved sufficient.

Symptomatic Relief. Because Raynaud's phenomenon has a strong vasoconstrictive component, it follows that vasodilators should provide symptomatic relief. *Calcium channel blockers* have proved symptomatically useful for patients with primary disease and for many with secondary disease. Their mechanism of action includes vasodilation plus some platelet inhibition. The resultant improvement in perfusion sometimes helps speed the healing of skin ulcers. *Nifedipine* and its congeners (*nicardipine, isradipine*, and *felodipine*) are the most potent vasodilators. However, they can produce reflex tachycardia and peripheral edema secondary to their venodilator effects; their use in persons with concurrent coronary disease or heart failure can be problematic (see Chapters 30 and 32). Occasionally, headache and flushing may be troublesome, and esophageal function may worsen in patients with scleroderma. Sustained-release preparations are convenient to use and reasonably well tolerated. There is no evidence to suggest that vasodilator therapy alters the natural history of the underlying disease.

α-Blocker therapy is also capable of providing symptomatic relief. The newer preparations such as *doxazocin* are longer-acting and appear less likely to cause first-dose syncope than older preparations such as prasozon. Postural light-headedness is still a problem, especially as the dosage is increased to above 2 to 3 mg/d.

Patients with vasospastic disease accompanied by substantial endothelial injury and platelet activation (e.g., those with systemic sclerosis) may not obtain adequate symptomatic relief with the sole use of vasodilator drugs. Painful episodes may persist, and ischemic skin ulcers may fail to heal. The addition of *aspirin* or *dipyridamole* to the treatment program has helped to heal some ulcers but has not reduced vasospastic symptoms. *Fish oil supplements* rich in omega-3 fatty acids can impair platelet activation and stimulate vasodilation through prostacyclin synthesis. Paradoxically, the best responses have been noted in patients with primary disease. IV *prostacyclin* and *iloprost* (a prostacylin analogue) are being studied; they are both vasodilators and inhibitors of platelet activation. Early results are encouraging, with effects lasting up to 3 months after a single 5-day course of therapy.

Sympathectomy has been used as a measure of last resort. Patients who respond to temporary ganglionic blockade with an injected anesthetic are the best candidates for sympathectomy.

PATIENT EDUCATION AND INDICATIONS FOR REFERRAL

The major elements of patient education are preventive (see above). For patients with occupationally induced disease, a change of job or job activities must be weighed against the risk for worsening of vascular compromise. Patients with strong features of primary disease can be reassured that the risk for underlying illness is low and that their prognosis is excellent. Those with features of secondary disease associated with a risk for development of connective tissue disease need to understand their risk, but also that it may be many years before other disease manifestations appear, if they develop at all.

Referral is indicated for those with refractory symptoms, especially if accompanied by signs of ischemia.

A.H.G.

ANNOTATED BIBLIOGRAPHY

Cherniack MG. Raynaud's phenomenon of occupational origin. Arch Intern Med 1990;150:519. (*Vibratory injury is an important and common precipitant.*)

DiGiacomo RA, Kremer JM, Shah DM. Fish-oil supplementation in patients with Raynaud's phenomenon. Am J Med 1990;86:158. (*Improved tolerance to cold exposure in patients with primary disease.*)

Fitzgerald O, Hess EV, O'Connor GT, et al. Prospective study of the evolution of Raynaud's phenomenon. Am J Med 1988;84:718. (*A connective tissue disease developed in 19% of those who presented with no obvious evidence of underlying illness; nail fold capillary pattern was predictive of systemic sclerosis.*)

Malamet R, Wise RA, Ettinger WH, et al. Nifedipine in the treatment of Raynaud's phenomenon. Am J Med 1985;78:602. (*Mechanism of action of nifedipine; some platelet inhibition suggested.*)

Minkini W, Rabhan NB. Office nail-fold capillary microscopy using ophthalmoscope. J Am Acad Dermatol 1982;7:190. (*A look at a very simple way to make this important observation.*)

O'Keeffe ST, Tsapatsaris NP, Beethan WP Jr. Increased prevalence of migraine and chest pain in patients with primary Raynaud's disease. Ann Intern Med 1992;116:985. (*Evidence for a common pathophysiology.*)

Priollet P, Vayssairet M, Housset E. How to classify Raynaud's phenomenon: long-term follow-up study of 73 patients. Am J Med

1987;83:494. (*Notes late onset of underlying disease; suggests means of early identification.*)

Sarkozi J, Bookman AAM, Lee P, et al. Significance of anticentromere antibody in idiopathic Raynaud's syndrome. Am J Med 1987;83:893. (*Predictive of scleroderma.*)

Spencer-Green G. Outcomes in primary Raynaud's phenomenon. Arch Intern Med 1998;158:595. (*A metaanalysis; risk for development of connective tissue disease approximately 12%, mostly systemic sclerosis; abnormal nail fold capillary pattern was the most predictive finding.*)

Spencer-Green G, Alter D, Welch G. Test performance in systemic sclerosis: anti-centromere and anti-Scl-70 antibodies. Am J Med

1997;103:242. (*Anticentromere antibody is reasonably sensitive for scleroderma; anti-Scl-70 is found in about half of patients with diffuse systemic sclerosis.*)

Weiner ES, Heldebrandt S, Senecal JL, et al. Prognostic significance of anti-centromere antibodies and anti-topoisomerase I antibodies in Raynaud's disease: a prospective study. Arthritis Rheum 1991;34:68. (*One of the better studies of risk for disease progression.*)

Wigley FM, Wise RA, Seibold JR, et al. Intravenous iloprost infusion in patients with Raynaud phenomenon secondary to systemic sclerosis. Ann Intern Med 1994;120:199. (*Sustained benefit achieved with this prostacyclin analogue.*)

164
Prevention and Management
of Osteoporosis

Osteoporotic fractures, particularly in aging women, represent a major health problem in industrialized nations. In the United States, more than 150,000 hip fractures occur annually in women over the age of 65, with 15% to 25% of these women experiencing excess mortality or needing long-term nursing home care. Current expenditures for hip fractures approach $10 billion yearly. Osteoporotic vertebral crush fractures, manifested by back pain, loss of height, and decreased ambulation, are present in 5% to 10% of women by age 60 and in 40% by age 80. The pathophysiologic mechanisms for postmenopausal osteoporosis are imperfectly understood, but the means to ensure maximal skeletal growth and strength, prevent loss of bone mass, and noninvasively evaluate bone mass are now available.

The primary care physician should educate women about the prevention of osteoporosis and the development of personalized strategies for maximal skeletal accretion and preservation. These tasks are facilitated by knowing how to identify high-risk patients and screen them (see Chapter 144).

PATHOPHYSIOLOGY AND CLINICAL PRESENTATION

Osteoporosis is a reduction in the mass of bone per unit volume. The World Health Organization diagnostic criterion for osteoporosis is a bone mineral density (BMD) that is 2.5 or more standard deviations below the mean for a healthy young person of the same sex (*T-score of -2.5 or less*). Because the strength of a bone is proportional to its density, the mechanical support of the skeleton is affected as bone mass declines. In contrast to osteoporosis, osteomalacia is characterized by a defect in the mineralization of the organic phase of bone.

Increased Osteoclastic Bone Resorption and Reduced New Bone Formation. The resorption and formation of bone is a continuous process throughout life. Under steady-state physiologic circumstances, the rates of these processes are equal and coupled. The explanations for the uncoupling of bone resorption and formation and the development of osteoporosis remain speculative. Estrogen receptors are present on osteoblasts, the cells that synthesize bone matrix proteins. Communication between osteoblasts and osteoclasts (which resorb bone) occurs,

but the precise mediators have not been fully identified. Cytokines in bone (e.g., interleukin-1, tumor growth factor) and skeletal growth factors may act synergistically and serve as mediators of bone formation and resorption.

With the onset of estrogen deficiency, osteoclastic bone resorption increases. Later in life, new bone formation is impaired. Fractional intestinal *absorption of calcium* in elderly persons is *decreased*. This decline in intestinal calcium absorption appears to be caused by a *decrease in the formation of 1,25-dihydroxyvitamin D*, the active form of vitamin D.

Risk Factors. Attention to risk factors is essential in estimating the probability of osteoporosis and risk for fracture, but the predictive value of most risk factors is not great. Those that seem to confer the greatest risk include *advanced age*, *low body mass index* ($<22 \ kg/m^2$), *maternal fracture*, and *current smoking*, but the strength of these associations is only moderate. Physical *inactivity* can lead to decreased bone mass, as can intense exercise that results in *amenorrhea*. A poor *lifetime intake of calcium* is a weak risk factor. Fair skin and excess alcohol consumption have been suspected but not confirmed. For osteoporotic *hip* fracture, additional risk factors are related to falling (e.g., *physical inactivity*, use of long-acting *benzodiazepines*, *impaired vision*).

Conversely, increased bone mass correlates with *increased weight*, *grip strength*, and *estrogen use for longer than 2 years*. Height and increased age at onset of menopause are also moderate predictors of increased bone mass. Increase in current calcium intake has only a minor effect on bone mass. Maintaining body weight, walking for exercise, minimizing caffeine use, and correcting impaired vision reduce the risk for hip fracture.

Medical conditions enhancing osteoporotic risk include *Cushing's syndrome*, exogenous *glucocorticoid* administration, prolonged *heparin* therapy, *thyrotoxicosis*, *hypogonadism*, *hyperprolactinemia*, *anorexia nervosa*, and *hyperparathyroidism*. However, these diseases account for a small percentage of cases of osteoporosis.

The strongest measurable determinant of risk is the *BMD*; it is necessary to measure it directly (see below and Chapter 144). The risk for osteoporotic fracture increases twofold to fourfold for every standard deviation of reduction in BMD. However, the BMD is not the only determinant of bone fragility and is an imperfect predictor of fracture risk in an individual person. A prior *history of fracture* is probably the strongest indicator of bone fragility and future fracture risk.

Clinical Presentation. Skeletal mass is usually maximal by age 35 and declines in women after age 40 and in men after age 50 when the rate of new bone formation does not equal the rate of bone resorption. The rate of decline in skeletal mass is most rapid in women *within 2 years of menopause*. The greatest loss occurs in trabecular bone in the *femoral neck* and *lumbar vertebrae*, sites where future fracture is likely.

The progressive decline in skeletal mass (which may approach 50%) becomes clinically manifest when fractures are sustained spontaneously or after minimal trauma. A *loss of height* and developing *kyphosis* generally indicate vertebral compression fracture. Fractures most commonly occur in the sacral and lumbar vertebrae, hip, humerus, and wrist. The clinical course and frequency of fractures in individual patients cannot be predicted.

Osteopenia is a radiologic term that indicates a reduced amount of bone and encompasses both osteomalacia and osteoporosis. The characteristic radiographic finding in osteoporosis is the loss of horizontal vertebral trabeculae, which accentuates the end plates and results in biconcave "codfish" vertebrae. Pseudofractures, generally occurring in weight-bearing long bones, are pathognomonic for osteomalacia.

The laboratory features of postmenopausal osteoporosis include normal serum levels of calcium, phosphate, vitamin D, parathyroid hormone, and alkaline phosphatase, although the alkaline phosphatase may be elevated in the context of a healing fracture.

WORKUP

Measurement of Bone Mineral Density. Because bone density is the principal determinant of fracture risk, its measurement is essential in diagnosis and decision making. *Dual-energy x-ray absorptiometry (DEXA)* is considered by most to be the technique of choice, representing the best combination of sensitivity, technical simplicity, reproducibility, cost, and minimization of radiation exposure. Measurement of forearm BMD provides an inexpensive approach suitable for mass screening, but separate BMD determinations in the hip and spine provide the best assessments of risk for the individual patient. The degree of osteoporotic change may be different in the hip and spine, so that separate BMD determinations are necessary. These tests are safe and acceptable to patients, and they have predictive value for the development of fractures.

The BMD measurement is expressed as the number of standard deviations from the mean for normal young adults of the same sex (*T-score*) and as the number of standard deviations from the mean for persons of the same sex and age (*Z-score*). The World Health Organization diagnostic criterion for *osteoporosis* is a *T-score below -2.5*. *Osteopenia* is defined as a *T-score between -1.0 and -2.5*. The finding of a *Z-score below -1.5* suggests a *secondary cause* of osteoporosis. The risk for osteoporotic fracture increases twofold to fourfold for every standard deviation of reduction in BMD.

If BMD measurements will affect clinical decision making, then testing should be performed. A perimenopausal woman already committed to hormonal replacement therapy need not be studied, but the untreated, newly menopausal woman at above-average risk for osteoporosis should be tested if the finding of a BMD below average would lead to the initiation of prophylactic therapy. Additionally, patients being treated for osteoporosis may require BMD measurements to determine therapeutic efficacy. Results of routine *chemistries* are normal and of little use.

Workup for Osteomalacia and Assessment for Other Secondary Causes of Osteopenia. When osteopenia is encountered radiologically or a hip fracture is noted, osteomalacia should be considered. Osteomalacia is defined as the inadequate deposition of calcium and phosphorus in bone tissue matrix. It is found in 10% to 15% of patients with hip fracture. *Vitamin D deficiency* is an important cause of osteomalacia in home-bound elderly persons, who are unlikely to eat dairy products or go out in the sun. Other causes include *impaired vitamin D metabolism*, *malabsorption*, *systemic acidosis*, and *phosphate depletion*. Osteomalacia should be suspected in patients with hypocalcemia or hypophosphatemia. Measurement of the urine pH and serum levels of 25-hydroxyvitamin D, phosphate, calcium, and bicarbonate help detect the cause. If the 24-hour urinary calcium is above 100 mg, osteomalacia is unlikely.

In the absence of pseudofractures on x-ray films, it is not possible to distinguish osteoporosis from osteomalacia radiographically. A bone biopsy is necessary for the definitive diagnosis of osteomalacia, but this is usually reserved for patients undergoing orthopedic procedures. Osteomalacia responds dramatically to treatment with *dietary vitamin D* and *calcium* and *phosphate supplements*.

The finding on DEXA determination of a Z-score below -1.5 suggests a secondary cause of osteopenia. In addition to the causes of osteomalacia noted above, other causes to be considered should include hyperthyroidism, hyperparathyroidism, anorexia nervosa, hyperprolactinemia, malignancy (e.g., myeloma, lymphoma), pernicious anemia, disease of the gastrointestinal tract (e.g., inflammatory bowel disease, chronic liver disease), rheumatoid arthritis, ankylosing spondylitis, and medications (e.g., excessive thyroid hormone, anticonvulsants, lithium, tamoxifen). Workup should be specific to the conditions suggested by the history and physical examination. In the absence of clinical clues, one might consider ordering a complete blood cell count and measurement of serum calcium and thyrotropin (TSH).

PRINCIPLES OF THERAPY

Prevention and Treatment of Osteoporosis

The goal is to reduce the risk for fracture by reducing the loss of bone mass. Prevention is more effective than treating established disease, but both require attention. Available therapies include estrogen replacement (in combination with progesterone), calcium supplementation, weight-bearing exercise, vitamin D, and bisphosphonates. If a fracture has occurred, symptomatic relief and aggressive therapy to halt further bone loss are indicated.

Estrogen. Hormone replacement therapy still remains the treatment of choice for the prevention of postmenopausal osteoporosis. Estrogen stops bone loss and can produce a modest degree of skeletal mineral accretion (on the order of 2% to 4%). Observational studies have consistently noted a 35% to 50% reduction in hip, wrist, and vertebral fractures in women who have used estrogen for at least 5 years after menopause. The risk for vertebral fracture can be reduced by up to 80%. In addition, the patient's lipid profile improves; high-density lipoprotein (HDL) cholesterol rises, low-density lipoprotein (LDL) cholesterol falls, and overall cardiovascular risk may decline. Estrogen treatment needs to be long-term, if not indefinite, for its beneficial effect on bone to last.

Preparations. Natural estrogens (estradiol, conjugated estrogens) are preferred for replacement therapy over the synthetic estrogens (ethinyl estradiol) because they are shorter-acting and less likely to cause adverse effects. *Estradiol* is the principal estrogen secreted by the ovary. It is available as *17β-estradiol* by *transdermal patch* or in a micronized *oral* preparation. The most widely used natural oral formulation, *conjugated estrogen*, is prepared from the urine of pregnant mares (hence the "marin" in the brand name). Oral preparations undergo first-pass metabolism by the liver, which converts about half of estradiol to estrone. Transdermal 17β-estradiol does not undergo hepatic first-pass metabolism, so that its duration of action is prolonged but its effect on lipid metabolism is markedly reduced.

New *synthetic conjugated estrogens,* A (Cenestin) are coming to market . They are approved only for the treatment of vasomotor symptoms, not for osteoporosis. *Phytoestrogens* (isoflavones) present in soy protein are currently very popular among women as a nonprescription or "natural estrogen" treatment for hot flashes; the estrogenic effect on bone afforded by even large quantities of dietary isoflavones appears too small to be of significance. Synthetic preparations of phytoestrogens are available, but data regarding their effect on bone are too limited at present for their role in the treatment of osteoporosis to be assessed.

Estrogen is given with *progesterone* in women with an intact uterus to avoid precipitating endometrial cancer (see below). The addition of progesterone does not cancel the positive effect of estrogen on osteoporotic bone or LDL cholesterol, but it does increase the risk for breast cancer.

Dosage and Administration. The daily dose necessary to prevent bone loss is 0.625 mg of conjugated estrogen, 1.0 mg of estradiol, or 0.05 mg of transcutaneous estrogen. Low-dose conjugated estrogen therapy (0.3 mg/d) has been found as effective as standard-dose estrogen therapy in older women (age above 65 years) when taken with calcium and vitamin D.

The estrogen and progesterone can be given cyclically or continuously. Most postmenopausal women prefer to avoid the withdrawal bleeding of cyclic therapy and opt for a *continuous program* (e.g., 0.625 mg of conjugated estrogen per day plus 2.5 to 5.0 mg of medroxyprogesterone per day). At the very onset of menopause, a *cyclic program* (e.g., daily conjugated estrogen for 28 days plus progestin for the first 14 days) may be temporarily preferred because it is less likely to precipitate excessive, unpredictable bleeding (see Chapter 118).

Initiation and Duration of Therapy. Treatment should begin at the onset of menopause if maximum prevention of bone loss is to be achieved. Once established, it is difficult to reverse the significant bone loss that occurs in the first few years of menopause. Estrogen therapy needs to be continued indefinitely because skeletal loss resumes if treatment is halted, and after several years the beneficial effects of estrogen are lost. Patients over the age of 75 not taking estrogen show little or no benefit after as many as 10 to 12 years of estrogen therapy started at the time of menopause.

Adverse Effects. For the woman with a uterus, the most serious adverse effect is a marked increase in the risk for *endometrial cancer*. The risk can be eliminated by the concurrent use of progesterone, which prevents unopposed endometrial stimulation. The effect of estrogen on the risk for *breast cancer* continues to be a matter of considerable concern among women. The magnitude of the increase in absolute risk is only a few percentage points, but the relative increase is more alarming to patients (about 35%). Estrogen and progestin use is associated with an even larger increase in breast cancer risk. Risk is a function of duration of therapy and insignificant if hormone replacement therapy is continued for less than 5 years; however, tumor growth can be stimulated by the initiation of estrogen therapy in the presence of an underlying breast cancer (see also Chapters 118 and 122).

Common side effects at the onset of therapy include transient bloating, nausea, and breast tenderness, the latter attributed to progestin use. Also attributable to progestin are irritability, depression, and headaches. Other adverse effects commonly seen with the use of synthetic estrogens include *migraine* headache (especially if estrogen is interrupted for a few days), *cholelithiasis*, worsening of *endometriosis* or fibroid tumors, and acute *thrombosis*. Smoking does not appear to increase the risk for venous thrombosis in postmenopausal women on estrogen, as it does in premenopausal women. Hormone replacement therapy does not increase blood pressure. The woman being considered for estrogen therapy requires a careful review of risk factors for breast cancer (see Chapter 106) and vascular thrombosis (see Chapters 22 and 23); breast, vascular, and pelvic examinations; a Papanicolaou test, and a mammogram before treatment is started.

Patient Selection. There is no universal agreement as to which patients should be considered for prophylactic therapy with estrogen at the time of menopause. The decision requires that not only potential skeletal benefit but also cardiovascular benefit and cancer risks be considered (see Chapter 118). From a skeletal perspective, patients with known risk factors for osteoporosis (e.g., maternal fracture, current smoker, small frame, lack of exercise, low calcium intake) are probably among the better candidates for prophylactic therapy, but these factors are not as predictive as bone density. Menopausal women who have an increased rate of decline in bone mass or a bone mass between 1.0 and 2.5 standard deviations below the mean for young adult women (i.e., a T-score between -1.0 and -2.5) should be considered for prophylactic estrogen replacement therapy. Even when osteoporosis is clinically manifested by fractures or appears radiographically as osteopenia, indicating at least a 30% to 40% loss of bone mass, it may still beneficial and important to initiate hormone replacement therapy, supplemented by calcium, vitamin D, and bisphosphonate (see below).

Selective Estrogen Receptor Modulators: Raloxifene. These so-called SERMs "designer estrogens" bind to estrogen-receptors and elicit a mix of agonist and antagonist responses that are tissue-dependent. Raloxifene inhibits bone resorption through the same mechanism as estrogen. A modest increase (1% to 2%) in bone density occurs in the spine and hip, about half the increase achieved with estrogen or alendronate. Reduction in the risk for vertebral fracture is about 50%. The risk for breast cancer is reduced by more than 50%, and raloxifene produces no stimulative effect on the postmenopausal endometrium. At the doses used for osteoporosis, no increase or decrease in the frequency of hot flashes is noted, but LDL cholesterol levels decline. The risk for thrombosis may be modestly increased, about the same as with estrogen. More data on long-term safety and efficacy are needed, but barring any major new findings, raloxifene may prove to be preferable or at least a reasonable alternative to estrogen therapy for the prevention of osteoporosis. The drug is approved by the Food and Drug Administration for the prevention of osteoporosis. Its cost is about two to three times that of estrogen and progestin therapy. *Tamoxifen* is not recommended for postmenopausal osteoporosis because its effect on bone resorption is not well defined and the risks for thrombosis and endometrial cancer are increased.

Calcium. A daily total calcium intake of 1.0 to 1.5 g is needed to help preserve cortical bone mass. Although calcium therapy does not prevent bone loss to the degree that estrogen therapy does, it does represent an essential component of all treatment programs. Its effect on bone loss falls between those of estrogen and placebo. The inadequate dietary calcium intake of most women (about 600 to 800 mg/d) and the declining fractional absorption of calcium associated with aging makes it important to ensure a total intake of 1.0 to 1.5 g/d in adolescent and young women and up to 2 g/d in older women. Serious complications such as renal stones or hypercalcemia are extremely uncommon with a daily intake of 1 to 2 g of elemental calcium.

Dietary calcium is readily available, more nutritious, and better absorbed than calcium tablets, and it is less likely to cause kidney stones (possibly by inhibiting oxalate absorption). A cup of skim milk provides 303 mg of calcium; 8 oz of low-fat yogurt provides 345 mg; a serving of canned sardines has 354 mg. Of the supplement preparations, the carbonate salt is the least costly. Chewable preparations are the best-absorbed. Splitting the daily supplement dose facilitates absorption and minimizes gastrointestinal upset. A reasonable supplemental dose of calcium is in the range of 500 to 1,500 mg/d. Larger doses, particularly in conjunction with vitamin D, may predispose the patient to hypercalcemia and hypercalciuric renal stone disease. Taking calcium with meals increases its absorption because of the favorable action of gastric acid. Concern about the solubility and gut absorption of calcium carbonate has led to the marketing of other calcium preparations (citrate, gluconate, lactate). They are often more expensive than calcium carbonate (especially the gluconate) and of little proven advantage.

Vitamin D. The principal effect of vitamin D is on gut absorption of calcium. It also directly affects osteoblasts and osteoclasts. When vitamin D is taken together with calcium, fracture rates are reduced by 30% to 70%. The benefit appears greatest in vitamin D–deficient institutionalized and homebound elderly persons, but it is also evident among those who are living independently in the community. When vitamin D supplementation is given in conjunction with calcium to otherwise healthy persons over the age of 65 with a low calcium intake, the BMD improves significantly and the risk for nonvertebral osteoporotic fracture is reduced by more than 50%. Daily dose requirements are in the range of 400 to 800 IU, with the higher dose recommended for those who get no exposure to sunlight.

Exercise. An important component of the preventive therapy of osteoporosis is ensuring the maximal development of skeletal mass. The amount of bone accumulated in *premenopausal women* may be critical to the appearance of osteoporosis later in life, as evidenced by the low incidence of osteoporosis in African-American women (and in men), who have a greater skeletal mass than white women. Exercise and physical activity have been shown to increase skeletal mass and increase total body calcium. Physical activity, in conjunction with dietary supplementation of 1,500 mg of calcium and 400 U of vitamin D daily, offers the best hope for increasing skeletal mass during skeletal growth. However, exercise programs so intensive as to induce amenorrhea and estrogen deficiency (e.g., competitive marathon running) may lead to osteoporosis.

In *postmenopausal women*, regular weight-bearing exercise (e.g., walking, low-impact aerobics, weight lifting, tennis) three times per week can substantially retard bone mineral loss (down to 0.5% of the baseline value per year), especially when combined with calcium supplementation. A more ambitious program of formal exercise training (e.g., 50 minutes of walking and jogging three times per week) in combination with calcium supplementation may have even more pronounced effects (e.g., increase in lumbar bone mineral content). Care must be taken to ensure that the exercise program in older women is safe and does not subject the patient to an increased risk for falls or other injuries.

The efficacy of a program of exercise with calcium and vitamin D supplementation suggests that it should be the core of every treatment program, be it for prophylaxis or treatment of osteoporosis. Whether it is sufficient to obviate the need for hormone replacement or other therapies remains to be established, but it can lower the doses of medication required.

Bisphosphonates. These synthetic carbon phosphate compounds, which include alendronate, etidronate, and risedronate, bind avidly to pyrophosphate in bone and inhibit bone resorption by osteoclasts. At full doses, they increase the BMD to at least the same degree as estrogen therapy and decrease the rate of fractures in the spine and hip by 30% to 50%, so that they are very useful for the treatment of established osteoporosis. Their effects are greatest in the setting of low bone density. At low doses, they provide effective prophylaxis against postmenopausal osteoporosis. Second-generation bisphosphonates (e.g., alendronate, risedronate) are more effective than first-generation agents (e.g., etidronate) and are not associated with the risk for demineralization seen when first-generation agents are taken on a daily basis. Their main drawbacks are poor intestinal absorption (uptake almost totally impaired by food intake) and *esophageal irritation and ulceration*. Careful use is essential. They must be taken on an empty stomach with a large volume of water, and the patient must remain in an upright position for a subsequent 30 minutes before food or recumbency is permitted. They should not be given to persons with active upper gastrointestinal disease or achalasia, and they must be used with caution, if at all, by those with a prior history of esophageal reflux or peptic ulceration.

The second-generation bisphosphonates appear to represent a genuine alternative to hormone therapy. Efficacy in long-term, head-to-head comparison study is equivalent to that of estrogen. A unique feature is some residual effect up to 2 years after cessation of treatment, believed to be a consequence of bisphosphonate deposition in and tight bonding to bone mineral. Alendronate is approved by the Food and Drug Administration for the prevention and treatment of osteoporosis. These agents have also demonstrated efficacy in the prevention of bone loss and fracture associated with premature menopause, corticosteroid use, and immobilization. The cost is two to three times that of estrogen and progestin treatment and about the same as that for raloxifene. Myalgias and arthralgias are sometimes reported with use. Data on long-term safety and efficacy should be forthcoming.

Calcitonin. Daily SQ injections of 100 U of salmon calcitonin or 200 IU of nasally inhaled calcitonin in combination with calcium supplementation will increase the total body calcium in postmenopausal osteoporotic women by several percentage points; this increase presumably reflects an increase in skeletal mass. The risk for vertebral fracture may decline by as much as 40%, but the risk for hip fracture is not reduced, and changes in specific bones are often too small to measure. After a year of use, no further increase in total body calcium is noted, and total body calcium declines at the same rate as in untreated control patients. Moreover, bone loss is not prevented in early menopause. The high cost and minimal sustained benefit of calcitonin make it a poor choice for long-term prophylaxis or treatment of osteoporosis. However, its initially positive effect on the risk for vertebral fracture and its coincident analgesic properties make if potentially useful as short-term therapy in elderly osteoporotic women who have sustained a painful vertebral compression fracture (see below). Nasal administration is the best-tolerated route.

Parathyroid Hormone stimulates new bone formation, increases trabecular bone, and improves the calcium balance while producing chemically and histologically normal bone without hypercalcemia. This therapeutic approach is under active investigation as one of the promising modalities with an ability to stimulate bone anabolically.

Sodium Fluoride therapy leads to a striking increase in trabecular bone density if given in doses ranging from 40 to 60 mg/d, but cortical bone density decreases, so that skeletal fragility increases. The dense fluorotic bone is abnormal both chemically and on crystallography and has undesirable mechanical properties *in vitro*. More promising results have been associated with long-term low-dose fluoride therapy (20 mg/d given as monofluorophosphate) taken in conjunction with calcium. The rate of vertebral fracture is markedly reduced without the production of any noticeable adverse bony effects. More data are needed. Fluoride is not approved by the Food and Drug Administration for use in osteoporosis.

Follow-up and Monitoring

The risk for sustaining an osteoporotic fracture is related to the severity of bone mineral loss and the chance of falling. Because compliance with therapy is often poor (50% discontinue estrogen therapy within 12 months), return visits at 6- to 12-month intervals to review and reinforce diet and exercise programs and monitor the medical regimen are warranted, especially in women with established osteoporosis. A repeated DEXA scan at 12 to 24 months is indicated to measure the BMD if the result will be useful for clinical decision making. A lack of improvement in the BMD at the time of the first repeated study may be a sign of poor compliance, but in patients taking bisphosphonate therapy, it should not be an indication to halt or switch treatment because it may also represent a statistical deviation that is likely to be corrected on the next determination. Monitoring serum bone chemistries is of no proven benefit.

Prevention of Falls

Although the prevention and treatment of osteoporosis have been the focus of this chapter, the ultimate objective is to reduce the risk for fracture. Hip fracture in the elderly can be a major source of disability and a potentially life-threatening event. Community survey reveals that about a third of community-dwelling persons over the age of 75 years report at least one recent fall. Often, many factors are involved, such as sedative use, cognitive and visual impairments, gait and balance disturbances, disabled lower extremities, and foot problems. A host of mundane but very important steps help reduce the risk for falling and sustaining a hip fracture; they correlate strongly with outcomes. Included among them are avoidance of long-acting tranquilizer use, treatment of impaired vision, and walking for exercise. Good podiatric care is essential, and physical and occupational therapy can be especially helpful in selected cases. Attention is directed toward any conditions that may impair gait or balance (see Chapter 166). Patients with a neurologic or orthopedic impairment who would benefit from using a cane or walker ought to be taught its proper use, both in the home and outside. Periodically, one should undertake a review of all medications to eliminate or reduce those that can cause postural hypotension (see Chapter 26) or sedation (see Chapters 226, 227, and 232).

Attention to the home environment is essential. Elimination of slippery surfaces and obstacle-laden paths, adequate illumination on stairways, installation of handrails in the bathroom, and the provision of seating from which it is possible to arise easily all help to ensure safety. Personal items deserve attention, such as footwear that provides good stance and stability and eyeglass prescriptions that are up to date.

Management of Vertebral Fractures

For patients who have sustained a painful osteoporotic vertebral fracture, periodic bed rest and adequate *analgesics* should be prescribed until the acute pain of the fracture subsides, often within several weeks. Thereafter, ambulation and daily exercise, such as swimming and walking, should be encouraged as tolerated. Lifting and vigorous physical activity are best avoided. Corsets and back braces, if comfortable, may facilitate ambulation in formerly bedridden patients. A course of intranasal *calcitonin* is sometimes helpful in this situation because of its analgesic effect in addition to its ability to increase bone density modestly.

Persons who have sustained a vertebral fracture should be treated for osteoporosis with aggressive antiresorptive therapy. The use of *bisphosphonates* (e.g., *alendronate* or *etidronate*) after vertebral compression fracture has been well studied and found both to increase BMD and to reduce markedly the risk for a new fracture. The few controlled studies of *estrogen* therapy in this situation also suggest a benefit, but the response to estrogen can be muted in the later phases of menopause.

Determining the efficacy of therapy can be problematic in the individual patient. Symptomatic improvement cannot be used to measure the response to therapy because fracture-free intervals may be long. The risk for fracture is not fully predictable by BMD because it is only one determinant of bone fragility. Despite these limitations, BMD measurement by DEXA can still be helpful, particularly as an objective indicator of bony response to treatment that can help guide therapy.

Preventing and Treating Steroid-induced Osteoporosis

Glucocorticoids inhibit new bone formation and calcium absorption and increase bone resorption and renal calcium excretion. Steroid-induced hypogonadism contributes to the problem in both men and women. Some degree of osteoporosis develops in more than 50% of patients on long-term steroids. Bone loss can be greatest during the first 3 to 12 months of steroid therapy; it then slows but persists for as long as steroid treatment continues. Some but not all bone mineral loss is reversible; the potential for recovery appears greatest in young persons. Patients who will be taking glucocorticoids on a daily basis for several months should be considered for prophylactic therapy. If high doses are to be used (e.g., the equivalent of >20 mg of prednisone daily), then prophylaxis should be considered even if the course of therapy will be relatively short because substantial bony changes can occur in as little as 3 months.

Prevention. The first priority should be to use the least harmful steroid program possible (i.e., lowest dose, shortest time period, alternate-day schedule; see Chapter 105). In addition, it is essential to maintain physical activity and ensure adequate daily intake of calcium and vitamin D. Sodium restriction can help improve the absorption and reduce the renal excretion of calcium. Low-dose bisphosphonate therapy (e.g., 5 mg of *alendronate* per day or 400 mg of *etidronate* per day for 2 weeks every 3 months) begun close to the outset of steroid use can increase the BMD during steroid therapy and reduce the chances for development of osteoporosis and osteoporotic fractures.

Treatment. In patients already manifesting steroid-induced osteoporosis, *bisphosphonate* therapy (e.g., 5 mg of *alendronate* per day or, if the patient is postmenopausal and not taking estrogen, 10 mg of alendronate per day) can significantly increase bone density and reduce the risk for fracture. Those who are postmenopausal or who experience steroid-induced amenorrhea (see Chapter 112) should be considered for *hormone replacement* therapy. Similarly, in men, any hypogonadism leading to loss of bone density can be countered by testosterone replacement. Hypercalciuria is an indication for *thiazide* therapy (supplemented by potassium replacement or a potassium-sparing agent). Small supplements of vitamin D can be given to those who become vitamin D–deficient, but large doses are to be avoided because of the risk for hypercalcemia.

PATIENT EDUCATION

The time spent educating the patient about osteoporosis is extremely well spent because prevention and compliance are so important to effective management. Perimenopausal women are highly concerned about osteoporosis and come in eager to discuss prevention and treatment. The full range of options should be reviewed and patient preferences elicited; failure to do so is likely to result in disappointing outcomes. One should seek to design a program that is tailored to the patient's risk profile and life-style. The decision to initiate prophylactic hormone replacement therapy requires a consideration of all risks and benefits, not just those related to osteoporosis (see Chapter 118).

THERAPEUTIC RECOMMENDATIONS

Prevention of Postmenopausal Osteoporosis

- Advise young women, especially if they are pregnant, to maintain a daily dietary intake of at least 1.0 to 1.5 g of *calcium* and 400 IU of *vitamin D*. Also encourage a program of regular physical activity. Advise against smoking and alcohol excess.
- For perimenopausal and postmenopausal women, prescribe a program of 30 minutes of *weight-bearing exercise* (e.g., walking, jogging, aerobics, dancing, tennis, weight lifting) at least three times weekly, a daily total calcium intake of 1.0 to 1.5 g, and 400 to 800 IU of vitamin D daily.
- If necessary, supplement the diet with *calcium carbonate* tablets (least expensive) or *calcium citrate* (more expensive, slightly better tolerated) to achieve the desired daily total; encourage supplement intake during meals to minimize gastrointestinal upset and risk for kidney stones, and encourage splitting the dose to maximize uptake and minimize gastrointestinal upset.
- Perform *BMD testing* (see Chapter 144).
  - Perform DEXA scan of the hip and spine at the onset of menopause in women at increased risk for osteoporosis (i.e., maternal history of osteoporotic fracture, current smoking, history of fracture as adult, body mass index below 22 kg/m^2).
  - Screen all women over the age of 65 by DEXA scan.
  - Obtain T- and Z-scores for BMD (see Chapter 144).
- **For patients with a T-score above -1.0** (i.e., BMD within one standard deviation of the mean for young women), continue calcium, vitamin D, and exercise; repeat bone density measurement in 1 to 2 years (depending on degree of osteoporosis risk).
- **For patients with a T-score between -1.0 and -2.5,** begin a more aggressive prevention program and avoid delaying the initiation of therapy because the rate of bone loss is maximal during the first few years after menopause. Choose one of the

following based on patient preferences and total health considerations (refer to Chapter 118):

- *Estrogen*: 0.625 mg of *conjugated estrogens* daily (in conjunction with 2.5 to 5.0 mg/d of *medroxyprogesterone* for the women with an intact uterus). Alternative hormone replacement regimens (e.g., transdermal estrogen patch, 50 μg/d; cyclic estrogen and progesterone) are available; careful monitoring is required (see Chapter 118); *or*
  - *Alendronate*: 5 mg every morning, taken on an empty stomach with 8 oz of water half an hour before breakfast while remaining in an upright position (to limit the risk for esophageal ulceration); *or*
  - *Raloxifene*: 60 mg/d.
  - For those who refuse or cannot take such treatment, but might be candidates if osteoporotic risk increased still further, monitor bone loss by DEXA scan every 1 to 2 years and reconsider treatment if rate of loss is marked or T-score falls below -2.5.
- Continue therapy indefinitely unless it is replaced by a therapy of nearly equal efficacy or a complication develops.
- **For patients with a T-score below -2.5,** begin a program for established postmenopausal osteoporosis (see below).

Established Postmenopausal Osteoporosis

- For asymptomatic postmenopausal patients who are found incidentally to have radiographic osteopenia or a bone densitometry T-score below -2.5, begin as follows:
- *Calcium*, *vitamin D*, and *weight-bearing exercise* (adjusted to minimize fracture risk) as detailed above; *plus*
- *Alendronate*: 10 mg every morning (as detailed above); *or*
  - *Estrogen* (as detailed above); *or*
  - *Raloxifene*: 60 mg/d; *or*
  - *Calcitonin*: 200 IU/d nasally, administered in alternating nostrils.
- Continue therapy indefinitely unless it is replaced by a therapy of nearly equal efficacy or a complication develops.

Osteoporotic Compression Fracture

- Treat initially with *bed rest* and *analgesics*. When the pain subsides, begin ambulation, followed by mild exercise such as walking or swimming. Avoid lifting and other weight-bearing stresses. Strongly consider treatment for osteoporosis.
- Consider a course of intranasal *calcitonin* (200 IU/d) for pain while marked discomfort persists.
- Begin *alendronate* (10 mg/d) and continue indefinitely to reduce the risk for recurrent fracture; *or*
- Consider *etidronate* if alendronate is not tolerated or cannot be used; prescribe 400 mg/d for 2 weeks every 3 months; no food 2 hours before intake and none for 2 hours after.
- Institute a program of *calcium* and *vitamin D* supplementation as detailed above.

Prevention of Glucocorticoid-induced Osteoporosis

- Consider a program of osteoporosis prophylaxis in persons who are going to require high-dose steroids (e.g., >20 mg of prednisone per day) for at least a few months or lesser doses for a longer period.

- Give highest priority to those at greatest risk for osteoporosis (e.g., postmenopausal women; those with prior vertebral fracture).
- Consider DEXA determination of spinal BMD at the outset of therapy to determine pretreatment risk and establish a baseline.
- For those deemed to be at increased risk (e.g., T-score below -1.0 or postmenopausal), begin as follows:
  - *Calcium* and *vitamin D* supplementation (as detailed above); *plus*
  - *Alendronate*: 5 mg every morning (as detailed above; 10 mg/d for late postmenopausal women not taking estrogen); *or*
  - *Etidronate*: 400 mg/d for 2 weeks every 3 months if alendronate not tolerated.
  - Consider *estrogen* replacement therapy if the patient is in the early menopause.

A.H.G.

ANNOTATED BIBLIOGRAPHY

Adachi JD, Bensen WG, Brown J, et al. Intermittent etidronate therapy to prevent corticosteroid-induced osteoporosis. N Engl J Med 1997;337:382. (*Prevented bone loss and reduced risk for vertebral compression fracture by 85%.*)

Aloia JF, Vaswani A, Yeh JK, et al. Calcium supplementation with and without hormone replacement therapy to prevent postmenopausal bone loss. Ann Intern Med 1994;120:97. (*Calcium produced an intermediate effect, between those of estrogen and placebo.*)

Bauer DC, Browner WS, Cauley JAA, et al. Factors associated with appendicular bone mass in older women. Ann Intern Med 1993;118:657. (*Best data on risk factors for osteoporosis.*)

Black DM, Cummings SR, Karpf DB, et al. Randomised trial of effect of alendronate on risk of fracture in women with existing vertebral fractures: Fracture Intervention Trial Research Group. Lancet 1996;348:1535. (*Major study finding a 47% reduction in rate of new fractures in comparison with placebo group.*)

Cauley JA, Seeley DG, Esrud K, et al. Estrogen replacement therapy and fractures in older women: Study of Osteoporotic Fractures Research Group. Ann Intern Med 1995;122:9. (*Relative risk for nonspinal fracture reduced by 34%.*)

Cummings SR, Palermo L, Browner W, et al. Monitoring osteoporosis therapy with bone densitometry: misleading changes and regression to the mean. JAMA 2000;283:1318. (*A provocative article suggesting that a lack of response initially may be related more to test performance than actual response to treatment; often, a very marked response is seen on follow-up determination.*)

Cummings SR, Eckert S, Krueger KA, et al. The effect of raloxifene on risk of breast cancer in postmenopausal women. JAMA 1999;281:2189. (*Risk is reduced significantly.*)

Cummings SR, Black DM, Thompson DE, et al. Effect of alendronate on risk of fracture in women with low bone density but without vertebral fractures: results from the Fracture Intervention Trial. JAMA 1998;280:2077. (*Alendronate significantly reduced risk for hip fracture.*)

Cummings SR, Nevitt MC, Browner WS, et al. Risk factors for hip fracture in white women. N Engl J Med 1995;332:767. (*Prospective cohort study; major risk factors and the means to prevent hip fracture identified.*)

Curhan GC, Willet WC, Speizer FE, et al. Comparison of dietary calcium with supplemental calcium and other nutrients as factors affecting the risk of kidney stones in women. Ann Intern Med 1997;126:497. (*From the prospective Nurses' Health Study, 12-*

year follow-up results. Dietary calcium reduces risk for stones, probably through reduction in oxalate absorption; supplemental calcium increases it.)

Dalsky GP, Stocke KS, Ehsani AA, et al. Weight-bearing exercise training and lumbar mineral content in postmenopausal women. Ann Intern Med 1988;108;824. (*Exercise for 50 minutes three times per week plus calcium supplementation produced an increase in lumbar bone mineral content.*)

Dawson-Hughes B, Harris SS, Krall EA, et al. Effect of calcium and vitamin D supplementation on bone density in men and women 65 years of age or older. N Engl J Med 1997;337:670. (*A placebo-controlled, randomized study showing a modest reduction in bone loss and significant reduction in nonvertebral fractures.*)

Dawson-Hughes B, Dallal GE, Krall KA, et al. A controlled trial of the effect of calcium supplementation on bone density in postmenopausal women. N Engl J Med 1990;323:878. (*Calcium supplementation was beneficial, mostly in older women with a low calcium intake—below 400 mg/d.*)

Delmas PD, Bjarnason NH, Mitlak BH, et al. Effects of raloxifene on bone mineral density, serum cholesterol concentrations, and uterine endometrium in postmenopausal women. N Engl J Med 1997;337:1641. (*Bone benefit intermediate, between that of standard hormone replacement therapy and placebo.*)

Eastell R. Treatment of postmenopausal osteoporosis. N Engl J Med 1998;338:736. (*A review that focuses on the evidence for efficacy of therapy.*)

Felson DT, Zhang Y, Hannan MT, et al. Effect of postmenopausal estrogen therapy on bone density in elderly women. N Engl J Med 1993;329:1141. (*Even as much as 10 years of prior treatment had a minimal effect in women over the age of 75; treatment may need to be indefinite.*)

Finklestein JS, Klibanski A, Arnold AL, et al. Prevention of estrogen deficiency–related bone loss with human parathyroid hormone: a randomized controlled trial. JAMA 1998;280:1067. (*Parathyroid hormone prevented bone loss in young women receiving pituitary suppression therapy.*)

Gregg EW, Cauley JA, Seeley DG, et al. Physical activity and osteoporotic fracture risk in older women. Ann Intern Med 1998;129:81. (*Prospective cohort study; risk for fracture of hip reduced, but not risk for fracture of spine or wrist.*)

Holmes MM, Rovner DR, Rothert ML, et al. Women's and Physicians' utilities for health outcomes in estrogen replacement therapy. J Gen Intern Med 1987;2:178. (*Prevention of fracture was more highly valued by the women; underscores the need for eliciting the patient's views.*)

Horsman A, Jones M, Francis R, et al. The effect of estrogen dose on postmenopausal bone loss. N Engl J Med 1983;309:1405. (*Dose–response relationship noted; required dose for conjugated estrogens was 0.625 mg.*)

Hosking D, Chilvers CE, Christiansen C, et al. Prevention of bone loss with alendronate in postmenopausal women under 60 years of age. Early Postmenopausal Intervention Cohort Study Group. N Engl J Med 1998;338:485. (*Results from the multicenter EPIC study; early use effective and well tolerated; dose of 5 mg better than 2.5 mg; BMD not quite as good as with hormone replacement therapy.*)

Jick H, Derby LE, Myers MW, et al. Risk of hospital admission for idiopathic venous thromboembolism among users of postmenopausal oestrogens. Lancet 1996;348:981. (*Although overall risk is increased, smoking did not exacerbate it.*)

Johnston CC Jr, Slemenda CW, Melton LJ. Clinical use of bone densitometry. N Engl J Med 1991;324:1105. (*A review of available technologies and their utility.*)

Khovidhunkit W, Shoback SM. Clinical effects of raloxifene hydrochloride in women. Ann Intern Med 1999;130:431. (*Useful review that the physician should read before prescribing the drug; 86 references.*)

Liberman UA, Weiss SR, Broll J, et al. Effects of oral alendronate on bone mineral density and the incidence of fractures in postmenopausal osteoporosis. N Engl J Med 1995;333:1437. (*Large randomized, controlled trial revealing 9% increase in BMD at spine and 6% increase at hip; 50% reduction in vertebral fracture.*)

Lufkin EG, Wahner HW, O'Fallon WM, et al. Treatment of postmenopausal osteoporosis with transdermal estrogen. Ann Intern Med 1992;117:1. (*Found effective, but lipid changes less beneficial than with oral therapy.*)

Lukert BP, Raisz LG. Glucocorticoid-induced osteoporosis: pathogenesis and management. Ann Intern Med 1990;112;352. (*Clinically relevant discussion of disease mechanisms followed by review of treatment options.*)

Osteoporosis Prevention Study Group. Alendronate prevents postmenopausal bone loss in women without osteoporosis: a double-blind, randomized, controlled trial. Ann Intern Med 1998;128:253. (*Low-dose therapy was well tolerated and effective.*)

Popcock NA, Eisman JA, Dunstan CR, et al. Recovery from steroid-induced osteoporosis. Ann Intern Med 1987;107:319. (*Reversal found in these relatively young persons.*)

Prince RL, Smith M, Dick IM, et al. Prevention of postmenopausal osteoporosis: a comparative study of exercise, calcium supplementation, and hormone replacement. N Engl J Med 1992;325:1189. (*Bone loss was slowed or prevented by exercise plus calcium and by hormone replacement.*)

Ravn P, Bidstrup M, Wasnich RD, et al. Alendronate and estrogen-progestin in the long-term prevention of bone loss: four-year results from the Early Postmenopausal Intervention Cohort Study. A randomized, controlled trial. Ann Intern Med 1999;131:935. (*Best long-term data to date; equivalent effects on bone found.*)

Recker RR, Davies M, Dowd RM, et al. The effect of low-dose continuous estrogen and progesterone therapy with calcium and vitamin D on bone in elderly women. A randomized, controlled trial. Ann Intern Med 1999;130:897. (*Low-dose therapy combined with calcium and vitamin D was as good or better than standard-dose hormone replacement therapy in this population.*)

Reginster JY, Meurmans L, Zegels B, et al. The effect of sodium monofluorophosphate plus calcium on vertebral fracture rate in postmenopausal women with moderate osteoporosis: a randomized, controlled trial. Ann Intern Med 1998;129:1. (*Additional benefit found with use of fluoride supplement.*)

Richelson LS, Wahner HW, Melton LJ, et al. Relative contributions of aging and estrogen deficiency to postmenopausal bone loss. N Engl J Med 1984;311:1273. (*Bone loss in oophorectomized women was almost as great as that in postmenopausal women, which indicates that estrogen deficiency rather than aging is the prominent cause.*)

Riggs BL, Hodgson SF, O'Fallon WM, et al. Effect of fluoride treatment on the fracture rate in postmenopausal women with osteoporosis. N Engl J Med 1990;322:802. (*Increases cancellous bone but decreases cortical bone, so that skeletal fragility is increased.*)

Saag KG, Emkey R, Schnitzer TJ, et al. Alendronate for the prevention and treatment of glucocorticoid-induced osteoporosis. N Engl J Med 1998;339:292. (*Randomized, placebo-controlled, 48-week trial found an increase in BMD with alendronate.*)

Schairer C, Lubin J, Troisi R, et al. Menopausal estrogen and estrogen-progestin replacement therapy and breast cancer risk. JAMA 2000;283:485. (*Evidence that breast cancer risk is increased and beyond that attributable to estrogen alone.*)

Sheikh MS, Santa Ana CA, Nicar MJ, et al. Gastrointestinal absorption of calcium from milk and calcium salts. N Engl J Med 1987;317:532. (*In these healthy young subjects, no significant differences were noted.*)

Tham DM, Gardner CD, Haskell WL, et al. Clinical review 97: potential health benefits of dietary phytoestrogens: a review of the clinical, epidemiological, and mechanistic evidence. J Clin Endocrinol Metab 1998;83:2223. (*Thorough review of existing evidence.*)

The Writing Group for the PEPI Trial. Effects of hormone therapy on bone mineral density. Results from the Postmenopausal Estrogen/Progestin Interventions (PEPI) Trial. JAMA 1996;276:1389. (*Randomized, double-blinded, placebo-controlled multicenter study; BMD increased at key sites with hormone replacement therapy.*)

Tilyard MW, Spears GFS, Thomson J, et al. Treatment of postmenopausal osteoporosis with calcitriol or calcium. N Engl J Med 1992;326:357. (*Continuous use reduced the rate of vertebral fractures.*)

Tinetti ME, Baker DI, McAvay G, et al. A multifactorial intervention to reduce the risk of falling among elderly people living in the community. N Engl J Med 1994;331:821. (*Because multiple factors are usually involved, treatment needs to be similarly multidimensional to be effective.*)

Watts NB, Harris ST, Genant HK, et al. Intermittent cyclic etidronate treatment of postmenopausal osteoporosis. N Engl J Med 1990;323:73. (*Increased spinal bone mass and reduced risk for new compression fracture.*)

Wimalawansa SJ. A four-year randomized, controlled trial of hormone replacement and bisphosphonate, alone or in combination, in women with postmenopausal osteoporosis. Am J Med 1998;104:219. (*Small-scale study, but an additive effect demonstrated.*)

11
Neurologic Problems

165
Approach to the Patient with Headache
AMY A. PRUITT

A complaint of headache raises numerous diagnostic possibilities. Fortunately, fewer than 1% of cases of headache that come to medical attention represent serious intracranial disease. Still, headache poses a diagnostic challenge for the primary physician, who must distinguish between the rare headache that represents a potentially life-threatening process and the vast majority, which are harmless. Both physicians and patients worry about headaches that are persistent, severe, sudden in onset, or different from a patient's usual headache. The primary physician's most immediate task is to identify efficiently by history and physical examination the occasional patient who requires aggressive workup. Additional priorities are to provide symptomatic relief and to diagnose the type of headache and its cause systematically while formulating a long-term plan for management.

Headache can be a difficult problem to evaluate and manage. Of patients who come for help, only one third claim they are satisfied with the care received. Fortunately for neurologists and primary physicians alike, recent advances in our understanding of clinical presentation and pathophysiology have greatly facilitated diagnosis and treatment.

PATHOPHYSIOLOGY AND CLINICAL PRESENTATION

Headache may originate in either intracranial or extracranial structures, with the mechanisms and presentations of pain depending on the source.

Intracranial Sources

Intracranial sources of pain referable to the head include fibers of the fifth, ninth, and tenth cranial nerves and the upper cervical nerves, the venous sinuses, parts of the dura at the base of the skull, the dural arteries (anterior and middle meningeal), and the large arteries at the base of the brain that give rise to the circle of Willis. Brain parenchyma is not pain-sensitive.

Postulated *mechanisms* include (a) *traction* resulting from direct or indirect displacement of intracranial structures; (b) *distention* of intracranial arteries; (c) *inflammation* of pain-sensitive structures; and (d) *obstruction* of cerebrospinal fluid flow by a mass lesion distorting the brain contents. If the intracranial source of pain is above the tentorium, pain is usually felt in the distribution of the fifth cranial nerve. Pain from a site in the posterior fossa is usually felt in the posterior half of the head, conveyed by the glossopharyngeal and vagus nerves and also by the upper cervical spinal roots.

Mass Lesions can cause headache by displacing a pain-sensitive structure. About one third of patients with a mass lesion have headache as an early symptom, often with the pain *localized to the side of the lesion*. Presentations vary widely, with none particularly diagnostic. The headache may be mild or severe, intermittent or persistent, aching, sharp, pressure-like, or even throbbing in quality. Characteristically, the headache remains in the *same location* but is *progressive*; increases in the duration and severity of pain over several months occur in conjunction with subtle changes in mental status or the development of focal neurologic deficits. As intracranial pressure increases, lying down may exacerbate the headache, as may straining at stool, coughing, or bending over, and a more generalized headache may develop. Nocturnal awakening is common but not diagnostic. Projectile vomiting is a late complication.

In *brain tumor*, headache may be the sole initial complaint, unaccompanied by focal neurologic deficits. However, as the condition progresses, new neurologic deficits usually ensue. *Brain abscess* may present as a mass lesion causing headache, especially in its later stages. Parenteral drug abuse, lung abscess, or parameningeal infection may serve as the source of infection. Fever and focal neurologic deficits are often absent. *Chronic subdural hematoma*, another important mass lesion, typically presents in a subtle fashion, with head trauma followed by a symptom-free interval. The injury may be forgotten, but changes in mental status and, eventually, focal neurologic deficits begin to develop.

Pseudotumor cerebri can mimic the clinical presentation of tumor. Characteristic features include onset of headache in an obese, young woman, papilledema on funduscopic examination, and compressed ventricles on computed tomography.

Nonmigrainous Cerebrovascular Sources. *Ischemic events* may be associated with acute headache. The pain most often occurs on the side of the lesion but may be frontal or diffuse. In some instances, the headache is a consequence of the ensuing cerebral edema. *Arteriovenous malformation* and berry *aneurysm* are much-feared causes of vascular intracranial headache. Acute rupture of an aneurysm produces a headache of sudden onset that reaches maximum intensity immediately and is often accompanied by meningeal irritation. In the absence of any rupture, 10% to 15% of patients with an arteriovenous malformation may experience a chronic headache characterized by unilateral (always the same side) throbbing pain. Unlike migraine, such headaches are not associated with prodromal or other symptoms. Berry aneurysms are silent until they rupture unless they are larger than 2 cm, in which case they may present with headache similar to that caused by a mass lesion.

Migraine Headache affects about 10% of adults, women three times more frequently than men. Despite the fact that migraine is associated with high rates of disability, most patients with migraine have never had their condition diagnosed by a doctor or treated with prescription medications. *Family history* is present in nearly two thirds of cases, especially in patients who have a history of migraine with aura. Migraine headaches usually begin in childhood or young adult life, although in about 16% of women afflicted by migraine, the headaches first develop at the time of menopause. The condition tends to improve in many women during pregnancy, although *oral contraceptives* have been known to precipitate migraine or convert migraine without aura to migraine with aura. In roughly one in seven women with migraine, headache occurs only during the first few days of *menses*, although many women experience an exacerbation at this time.

Mechanisms. A number of hypotheses have been advanced to explain migraine and account for its phases. The *neurogenic–inflammatory hypothesis* currently enjoys considerable support. It views migraine as a primary neuronal event, with secondary neurotransmitter-mediated changes in vasculature and blood flow. Neuropeptides are thought to act as neurotransmitters at trigeminal nerve branches, precipitating an inflammatory process with vasodilation. *Serotonin receptors* are believed to be important in mediating these events, which can be triggered by a variety of stimuli (mechanical, electrical, or chemical). The observed decrease in blood flow during migraine is now believed to be caused by a slowly spreading cortical band of decreased neuronal function elicited by such stimuli. Bidirectional influences of *depression* and migraine appear to exist. The estimated relative risk for major depression associated with prior migraine is 3.2, and the adjusted relative risk for migraine associated with prior major depression is 3.1.

Classification. Migraine formerly was designated as *"classic"* if accompanied by aural symptoms (see below) and as *"common"* if not. This taxonomy has been replaced by the more specific classifications of *migraine with aura* and *migraine without aura*. Tables 165.1 and 165.2 show the diagnostic criteria for migraine without aura and migraine with aura. Both types of migraine are accompanied by nausea and photophobia. The new classification system requires that at least two of the following be present to establish a diagnosis of migraine headache: unilateral location, pulsating quality, moderate to severe intensity, and exacerbation by physical activity. At least one of the following must accompany the headache: nausea or vomiting, photophobia, and phonophobia. Precipitants of migraine include emotional upset, menstruation, and, in some people, ingestion of tyramine- or tryptophan-rich foods (e.g., ripe cheeses, red wine, chocolate). Headache may occur shortly

Table 165.1. International Headache Society Definition of Migraine without Aura (Common Migraine)

Diagnostic Criteria
A. At least five attacks fulfilling B–D
B. Headache lasting 4 to 72 hours (untreated or unsuccessfully treated)
C. Headache with at least two of the following characteristics:
   1. Unilateral location
   2. Pulsating quality
   3. Moderate or severe intensity (inhibits or prohibits daily activities)
   4. Aggravated by walking stairs or similar routine physical activity
D. During headache, at least one of the following:
   1. Nausea and/or vomiting
   2. Photophobia and phonophobia

From Headache Classification Committee of the International Headache Society. Classification and diagnostic criteria for headache disorders, cranial neuralgias, and facial pain. Cephalalgia 1988; 8[Suppl 7]:1, with permission.

after or just before a period of psychological stress. Some patients experience a seemingly paradoxical flare-up of migraine on weekends or vacations. The risk for stroke is increased, particularly in patients who have migraine with aura.

Clinical Presentation. Attacks may comprise as many as five phases: prodrome, aura, headache, termination, and postdrome. The *prodrome* is characterized by lassitude, irritability, difficulty concentrating, and nausea. Patients with *aura* often report visual phenomena (scintillating scotomas, zigzag patterns, hemianopsia, diplopia), vertigo, aphasia, or even hemiplegia preceding the onset of the *headache*, which is typically unilateral and throbbing, although it may begin as a dull sensation and take a while to reach maximum intensity. Headache *termination* usually occurs within 24 hours but sometimes not until after 48 hours. The *postdrome* phase includes feelings of fatigue, sleepiness, or irritability. Epidemiologic studies suggest that migraineurs suffer a median of about 12 attacks per year. Many have headaches both with and without aura.

Table 165.2. International Headache Society Definition of Migraine with Aura (Classic Migraine)

Previously used terms: classic migraine; ophthalmic, hemiparesthetic, hemiplegic, or aphasic migraine

Diagnostic Criteria
A. At least two attacks fulfilling B
B. At least three of the following four characteristics:
   1. One or more fully reversible aura symptoms indicating focal cerebral cortical or brainstem dysfunction.
   2. At least one aura symptom develops gradually over more than 4 minutes, or two or more symptoms occur in succession.
   3. No aura symptom lasts more than 60 minutes. If more than one aura symptom is present, accepted duration is proportionally increased.
   4. Headache follows aura with a free interval of less than 60 minutes. (It may also begin before or simultaneously with the aura.)

From Headache Classification Committee of the International Headache Society. Classification and diagnostic criteria for headache disorders, cranial neuralgias, and facial pain. Cephalalgia 1988; 8[Suppl 7]:1, with permission.

Variants. A number of variants are seen. The most common is *migraine without aura*. Another is *acephalgic migraine*, in which a focal neurologic deficit may evolve during an aura but is not succeeded by headache. In rare instances, the symptoms of acephalgic migraine may persist for 1 to 2 days, simulating a stroke. *Basilar migraine* produces focal symptoms referable to the posterior circulation; it is more common in children.

Meningitis resulting from infection or hemorrhage produces pain that is acute in onset, severe, generalized, and constant. Symptoms may be particularly intense at the base of the skull and aggravated by forward flexion of the neck or by leg raising in conjunction with knee extension and foot dorsiflexion.

Postconcussion Headache occurs when the wrenching and displacement of pain-sensitive structures in the central nervous system during head trauma have been severe enough to cause concussion. *Postconcussion syndrome* (posttraumatic nervous instability) is a complicated, poorly characterized state manifested by chronic refractory headache, neck pain, nervousness, emotional lability, crying spells, and inability to concentrate. The symptoms are suggestive of an agitated depression following trauma; the syndrome probably represents a variant of tension-type headache. The correlation between severity of symptoms and seriousness of the injury is minimal. Often, legal proceedings and litigation are pending. Symptoms may abate once legal issues are settled.

Extracranial Sources

Extracranial sites of headache include the skin, fascia, muscles, and blood vessels of the scalp; the extracranial arteries; mucous membranes of the nasal and perinasal spaces; the external and middle ear; teeth; and muscles of the scalp and facial region. Problems involving the eyes, sinuses, cervical spine, temporal mandibular joints, or cranial nerves can be important sources of headache, although some common attributions are not always correct.

Tension-type Headache ranks among the leading types of chronic and recurrent headache. More than 90% are bilateral and are often described as a feeling of pressure or a bandlike sensation about the head. The pain is dull and steady in most instances, characteristically worsening as the day progresses and sometimes accompanied by occipital and nuchal soreness. The headache may last days, weeks, or even months. Recording of myographic potentials from head and neck muscles reveals vigorous contractions in some but not all patients with this type of headache. Vasoconstriction can also be detected and may account for the migraine-like symptoms (nausea, throbbing pain) experienced by some patients.

Precipitants include *anxiety*, *depression*, and *situational stress*. Patients with underlying psychopathology often describe their headache pain in vivid terms (e.g.,"feels like an ax" or "lightning" or "something exploding"), yet they do so without demonstrating any apparent discomfort. So psychologically engaging is the headache that many of these patients are unaware of their underlying emotional problems. Tension-type headaches may also occur secondary to muscle strain from cervical spondylosis or temporomandibular joint disease (see below).

Sinusitis. True sinusitis produces a headache that characteristically is acute in onset and worse on awakening. It gets better on arising, only to worsen again as the day progresses. The patient reports a purulent nasal discharge, and pain and skin sensitivity are predominant over the involved sinus (see Chapter 219). Many patients with other forms of headache (e.g., frontal muscle-contraction headaches) mistakenly attribute their problem to "sinusitis" and self-treat with decongestants to no avail. Because the pain of sinusitis is sometimes described as throbbing in quality and can worsen when the patient bends over, it may be mistaken for migraine or the headache of a intracranial mass lesion.

Giant Cell Arteritis, also referred to as *temporal arteritis* or *cranial arteritis*, is a disease of older persons (almost all are older than age 50). It affects medium and large arteries (especially those of the extracranial vasculature) and can cause blindness if it spreads to the ophthalmic artery. The headache may begin as a throbbing discomfort and progress to a dull, aching pain. Some patients describe burning, and others note bouts of lancinating pain. Scalp tenderness (especially when the hair is combed) localized to the involved vessel(s) is characteristic. However, the inflamed artery may not always be tender or palpable, and although the temporal artery is commonly involved, it need not be. Jaw (masticatory muscle) claudication is often part of the clinical picture, and the condition is strongly associated with *polymyalgia rheumatica* (see Chapter 161).

The most feared complication is *blindness*, which occurs when arteritis results in occlusion of the ophthalmic artery, usually about 1 to 2 months after the onset of headache. Diplopia may precede and is predictive of visual impairment (50% risk). Once visual impairment sets in, it progresses quickly over several hours to total visual loss (see Chapter 161).

Temporomandibular Joint Dysfunction. "TMJ" has received much attention in the lay press as a common, sometimes overlooked cause of chronic refractory headache. Occasionally, the problem is caused by joint changes resulting from malocclusion. However, the problem in most cases is not malocclusion, but rather tension-induced jaw clenching and nocturnal teeth grinding (*bruxism*). Such chronic involuntary oral habits lead to masticator muscle fatigue and spasm. Chronic dull, aching, unilateral discomfort may be described about the jaw, behind the eyes and the ears, and even down the neck into the shoulders. Jaw pain, clicking sounds, and difficulty opening the mouth in the morning are characteristic. Chewing may exacerbate symptoms; locking of the jaw is common. On physical examination, masticatory muscle tenderness, mandibular hypomotility, and joint clicking and deviation on opening are noted. Molar prominences may be flat from chronic grinding of the teeth (see Chapter 225).

Cluster Headache. The pathophysiology of cluster headache remains obscure, although extracerebral vasodilation appears to be a component. It occurs predominantly in middle-aged men and is the only type of headache more common in men than in women. Cluster headache is distinguished by its location, timing, and periodicity. In the most typical presentation, seen in more than 50% of cases, patients describe an intense, nonthrobbing, unilateral headache "behind the eye" that is searing, stabbing, or burning and accompanied by ipsilateral lacrimation, nasal stuffiness, and facial flushing. In 20% to 40% of cases, ipsilateral ptosis and miosis are also present. Headache typically begins a few hours after the patient goes to bed and lasts for 30 to 90 minutes. Attacks occur nightly for 2 to 3 months and then disappear, only to return several months to years later. About 10% of these patients have *chronic cluster headache*, in which attacks occur daily for 1 to 2 years; periodicity is not noted. These headaches are sometimes confused with migraine because they are unilateral and severe, but the pain is not throbbing and most of the other defining features of migraine are lacking. Stress and alcohol are believed to be precipitants, although alcohol is well tolerated between attacks.

Headaches Responsive to Indomethacin. Headaches in this group include chronic paroxysmal hemicrania, ice pick headache, and hemicrania continua. *Chronic paroxysmal hemicrania* is a rare cluster variant occurring predominantly among women and characterized by a similarly severe unilateral facial pain; unlike cluster, these headaches occur in short spasms of 10 to 20 minutes up to 20 or 30 times per day. Horner's syndrome and ipsilateral tearing are often noted. *Ice pick headache* occurs in patients suffering from migraine, although not exclusively. The headache is brief, sharp, and jabbing. *Hemicrania continua* differs from the other types in causing continuous unilateral aching discomfort, although it is accentuated by ipsilateral jabbing pain.

Systemic Infection and Fever. These conditions are among the most common causes of cranial vasodilation and diffuse, throbbing headache. The headache that frequently accompanies a *viral syndrome* is typical. Numerous *metabolic disturbances* and *drugs* may lead to vasodilation and headache. A pounding headache is a prominent symptom of early carbon monoxide poisoning and a common complaint of patients who take nitrates for angina or vasodilators for other conditions.

Hypertension. Moderate to severe *hypertension* (diastolic pressures >110 mm Hg) sometimes results in occipital headaches. The mechanism of the headache is unknown. The discomfort is worse in the morning and recedes as the day progresses. This headache resolves with correction of the hypertension. It should not be confused with the muscle-contraction and psychogenic headaches that account for most of the headaches occurring in hypertensive patients or with the headache caused by the increased intracranial pressure that accompanies malignant hypertension.

Ocular Sources. Headaches are often attributed to eye problems, especially when they are felt about the orbit. *Eyestrain* is often blamed for headaches, although in most instances the attribution is incorrect and refraction fails to improve the problem. However, in an occasional patient, astigmatism can cause difficulty when the eyes are used for close work for prolonged periods. It produces ocular muscle imbalance and sustained contraction of extraocular, frontal, and temporal muscles; aching discomfort about the orbit and the frontotemporal region results. Refraction corrects the problem. *Acute glaucoma* may produce an orbital headache of sudden onset that is accompanied by cloudy vision (see Chapters 201 and 207).

Cervical Radiculopathy. Headache is commonly the first symptom of cervical radiculopathy. The pain arises during mechanical irritation of an upper cervical root. Findings on radiography of the cervical spine are variable, ranging from normal to spondylotic. The pain is often localized to one side of the occiput or base of the skull, in conjunction with tenderness to palpation. It may start in the neck and at times even radiate to the forehead or eye. The discomfort is described as nagging or aching and is aggravated by *neck movement*. The headache tends to be worse on awakening, perhaps because of unconscious neck motion during sleep. The mechanism of pain is believed to involve entrapment of upper cervical nerve roots as they course toward the occiput through irritated nuchal ligaments and muscles. Occipital neuralgia is a particularly common variant. Patients describe sudden lancinating pain in the distribution of the greater occipital nerve, which may be precipitated by turning over in bed and is often relieved by sitting up.

Trigeminal Neuralgia (*Tic Douloureux*) is one of the most severe pain syndromes known to human beings. Paroxysms of lancinating facial or cranial pain occur in middle-aged or elderly patients; these may last only a few seconds but can be excruciating and recurrent. The jaw, gums, lips, or maxillary region may be involved. Characteristically, a trigger zone is located within the region of pain (see Chapter 176).

DIFFERENTIAL DIAGNOSIS

For differential diagnosis, headache can be divided into acute and chronic/recurrent types (Table 165.3). Of note, the International Headache Society now subdivides migraine into *migraine headache with aura* (previously called *classic migraine*) and *migraine headache without aura* (previously referred to as *common migraine*). *Tension-type headache*, with or without associated paracranial muscle spasm, has replaced the numerous

Table 165.3.   Important Causes of Headache

Acute
Meningitis
Intracranial hemorrhage (stroke, rupture of aneurysm)
Stroke
Acute increase in intracranial pressure (mostly from
    cerebral edema or hemorrhage, including hypertensive en-
    cephalopathy)
Acute glaucoma
Acute sinusitis
Acute metabolic disturbance (carbon monoxide poisoning, hypo-
    glycemia)
Acute viral illness
Initial presentation of a persistent or recurrent headache

Persistent or Recurrent
Intracranial mass lesion (neoplasm, abscess, subdural
    hematoma, large A-V malformation)
Tension-type headache
Migraine, with and without aura
Cluster headache
Indomethacin-responsive headache (ice pick, paroxysmal hemi-
    crania)
Postconcussion syndrome
Cervical spine disease
Giant cell arteritis
Trigeminal neuralgia
Hypertension
A-V malformation
Bruxism/temporomandibular joint dysfunction
Medications
Substance abuse

A-V, arteriovenous.

designations of *muscle-contraction headache, psychogenic headache,* or *tension headache* previously used.

WORKUP

As noted earlier, the first priority is to distinguish the worrisome headache from the harmless one. Headaches of concern are those that are sudden in onset, severe, or persistent. Despite the advent of elaborate imaging techniques, the history and physical examination remain indispensable.

The goal of the workup is to distinguish one of the primary headache syndromes (migraine with or without aura, cluster headache, tension-type headache) from a headache secondary to a mechanical or systemic process that would dictate a different therapy.

History

The time invested in obtaining a full description of the headache, particularly its clinical course, associated symptoms, precipitants, aggravating and alleviating factors, and patient concerns, is well worth the effort. The information obtained is often diagnostic, always critical to intelligent test selection, and essential to dealing effectively with patient worries and expectations. The medication history is also critical because a number of agents (e.g., indomethacin, nifedipine, cimetidine, captopril, nitrates, atenolol, trimethoprim/sulfamethoxazole, oral contraceptives) can trigger nonspecific headaches. Drug-related intracranial hypertension can be seen with minocycline, isoretinoin, nalidixic acid, tetracycline, trimethoprim/sulfamethoxazole, cimetidine, corticosteroids, and tamoxifen.

The history pertinent to a new headache differs slightly from that for chronic or recurrent headache.

Headache of New Onset. History should include inquiry into any *associated neurologic deficits, fever,* or *neck stiffness.* The patient unaccustomed to having headaches who presents with the sudden onset of the *"worst headache ever experienced"* deserves prompt attention, particularly if fever, neck stiffness, ataxia, alteration in mental status, focal neurologic deficit, or visual impairment is reported. Diffuse headache in conjunction with a stiff neck and fever suggests acute meningitis. When acute headache and *stiff neck* occur in conjunction with *gait ataxia* and profuse nausea and vomiting, a midline cerebellar hemorrhage must be considered. Early recognition is important because urgent surgical treatment can be life-saving. Abrupt onset of a headache that reaches maximum intensity immediately suggests rupture of a cerebral aneurysm. Hypertensive encephalopathy may be heralded by diffuse headache, nausea, vomiting, and altered mental status. Acute fever with frontal and orbital headache is suggestive of acute sinusitis. Eye pain and blurred vision raise the possibility of acute glaucoma. New onset of headache in an elderly patient requires consideration of temporal arteritis. Acute onset of a throbbing headache should trigger inquiry into migrainous epiphenomena (prodromal and aural symptoms), febrile illness, vasodilator use, carbon monoxide exposure, drug withdrawal, and hypoglycemia. A throbbing headache accompanied neurologic deficits may be migrainous, but if deficits persist beyond 12 hours, then stroke and other causes should be considered.

Recurrent or Persistent Headache. With migraine and tension-type headaches being the most common causes of chronic or recurrent headaches and brain tumor being the most feared, the history becomes critical to the evaluation. The *clinical course* can be particularly revealing. Increases in severity, frequency, or both with time raise the question of an intracranial mass lesion, whereas a headache pattern that remains constant or waxes and wanes is more typical of tension-type or migraine headache. The nightly occurrence of headache for some time followed by symptom-free intervals is among the most characteristic features of cluster headache.

In acute headache, the severity of the pain helps to identify an increased risk for serious pathology; however, in chronic or recurrent headache, the intensity of the pain is of little value. Most patients have headaches with different degrees of pain at different times. The headache of a brain tumor may begin as a relatively minor complaint, whereas the pain of a migraine, cluster, or tension-type headache may be excruciating. Careful attention to *associated symptoms* is always essential. Inquiry into migrainous epiphenomena can be diagnostic, and eliciting a report of a new neurologic deficit strongly increases the likelihood of tumor. *Location* and *quality* are sometimes helpful, although the overlap among headaches with different causes can be considerable. Whole-head, bandlike, and occipital–nuchal distributions suggest tension-type headache, as does tightness or a pressure-like quality, but such sensations may also be reported when intracranial pressure is increased. A unilateral location and throbbing are characteristic of migraine but sometimes are reported by patients with tension-type headache. Unilaterality and sameness of location suggest that the headache is caused by a mass lesion.

Associated symptoms are important for the identification of other causes of chronic or recurrent headache. Temporomandibular joint pain suggests bruxism, whereas jaw claudication and scalp vessel tenderness indicate giant cell arteritis. Concurrent shoulder and hip-girdle discomfort provide supporting evidence. Neck pain raises the question of a cervical radiculopathy. Purulent nasal discharge is indicative of sinus disease. A history of head trauma, parameningeal infection, depression, situational stress, or substance abuse and a family history of headache should always be sought, and a careful medication history must be taken. Of particular concern is *rebound headache*, a pattern of headache caused by overuse of analgesic medication, ergotamine compounds, or the serotonergic agonists known as triptans. Patients with rebound headache have fallen into a pattern of overuse of medication with consequent withdrawal headache.

Aggravating and *precipitating factors* deserve investigation. Headache worsened by straining, coughing, or bending over is characteristic of an intracranial mass lesion; bending over may also exacerbate the headache of sinusitis. Headache brought on by ingesting certain foods or beverages (chocolate, cheese, red wine) is typical of migraine, which is also exacerbated by noise, odors, and bright light. Alcohol may also trigger cluster headache during a period of disease activity. Migraine can be induced or exacerbated by a host of drugs, including cimetidine, ethinyl estradiol, atenolol, indomethacin, danazol, nifedipine, selegiline, and oral contraceptives.

Physical Examination

Acute Headache. The physical examination contributes importantly to the search for serious underlying disease. The blood pressure and temperature should be checked for elevations, the scalp for cranial artery tenderness, the sinuses for purulent discharge and tenderness, the pupils for loss of reactivity, the corneas for clouding (indicative of acute glaucoma), the disc margins for papilledema, and the neck for rigidity on anterior flexion. A neurologic examination should be performed to check for ataxia, alteration of mental status, focal deficits, and meningeal signs.

Chronic or Recurrent Headache. The physical examination begins with a check of all the areas mentioned in the evaluation of acute headache and expands into other areas based on findings from the history. For example, in a patient with a headache history that includes facial pain, the oral cavity should be examined for a trigger zone indicative of trigeminal neuralgia, the teeth for signs of bruxism, the temporomandibular joint for limitation of motion and crepitus, and the neck for signs of degenerative disease (see Chapter 148) and movements that reproduce head pain. Excessively taut muscles and focal tenderness about the shoulders, neck, and occiput are noted in many patients with tension-type headache. A careful and complete neurologic examination is essential because the finding of a fixed focal deficit is important evidence of intracranial pathology. Suspicion of a mass lesion necessitates consideration of brain abscess in addition to malignancy and subdural hematoma. Under such circumstances, the nasal cavity is examined for purulent discharge, the sinuses for tenderness, and the ears for signs of chronic otitis media (see Chapter 218). Both sinusitis and chronic otitis are potential foci for parameningeal infection that can lead to brain abscess.

Laboratory Studies

Acute Headache. Patients with acute onset of the "worst headache ever," especially if accompanied by meningeal signs or evidence of increased intracranial pressure, require prompt hospitalization. In such settings, emergency *computed tomography* is the test of choice for prompt detection of potentially life-threatening but treatable lesions (e.g., midline cerebellar hemorrhage or central nervous system mass). In patients with signs of meningeal irritation, *lumbar puncture* and examination and culture of the cerebrospinal fluid should follow computed tomography to rule out an infectious cause, provided no evidence of markedly increased intracranial pressure is found. New onset of headache in an elderly patient, especially if accompanied by cranial artery or scalp tenderness, dictates determination of the *erythrocyte sedimentation rate* to check for giant cell arteritis. In addition, a *temporal artery biopsy* should be considered (see Chapter 161).

Chronic or Recurrent Headache. Much of the controversy and discrepancies regarding the proper evaluation of headache result from the failure to differentiate patients who present with a first headache from those who have a chronic recurring headache. In the presence of normal physical examination findings and a headache history that does not suggest intracranial disease but classifies the patient's headache clearly into a recurring migrainous type, ancillary studies are not likely to be useful.

A disturbing trend toward uncritically ordering neuroimaging studies (initially *computed tomography* and now *magnetic resonance imaging*) for all patients with recurrent or chronic headache has led to escalating costs for evaluations that provide no more information than did the initial headache history and physical examination. The probability of a patient with chronic headache and normal neurologic examination findings having a positive neuroimaging study is exceedingly small. The yield is so low that in the absence of a very worrisome history or a neurologic deficit on physical examination, an imaging study is not needed. Some feel that the reassurance value of such testing can be helpful, but most patients with benign chronic headache who fear serious underlying disease can be adequately reassured if time is taken to review the clinical findings and directly address patient concerns. Such steps are essential to providing meaningful reassurance and usually obviate the need for an otherwise medically unnecessary imaging procedure.

Nonetheless, there are a few instances when a neuroimaging study might still be appropriate in the absence of abnormalities on physical and neurologic examinations. These exceptions include patients with a headache of *recent onset* (<6 months) the cause of which is still not apparent after a thorough history and physical examination. In addition, those with a persistent headache that is *worsening* with time and does not fit the pattern of a tension-type headache should be considered for imaging study. When one uncovers a history of *aura symptoms* or *loss of consciousness* suggestive of a seizure (see Chapter 170), then a search for an intracranial mass lesion is warranted. If the patient or family member reports a *persistent personality change*, a tumor of the frontal or temporal regions might be suspected. Finally, if a *change in the character* of long-standing headache is noted or if the headache fails to respond to treatment directed at a diagnosis initially suspected, such as migraine, the utility of magnetic resonance imaging or computed tomography increases.

The efforts taken to perform a careful history and physical examination are well worth the time, for these methods remain the best means available for efficient test selection and accurate diagnosis of headache.

PRINCIPLES OF MANAGEMENT

Migraine

Migraine is the one headache disorder for which relatively specific therapy currently exists; therefore, establishing its presence is extremely important to the patient. The neurogenic hypothesis has refocused attention from vasodilators to drugs designed to act on serotonin receptors. Several older drugs useful in the prophylaxis of migraine (e.g., methysergide, cyproheptadine) have been found to act as $5-HT_2$ serotonin receptor antagonists. The drugs most useful in acute migraine attacks (e.g., *ergotamine*, *triptans*) interact with the presynaptic serotonin $5-HT_{1D}$ and $5-HT_{1A}$ receptors, inhibiting the release of neurotransmitters.

For most patients, the combination of a tolerable prophylactic medication with occasional use of analgesics or abortive regimens should minimize the intrusion of this highly disabling condition into their daily lives. Because most prophylactic drugs require several weeks to several months to establish efficacy, it is particularly important to maintain a strong and sympathetic relationship with each patient being treated for migraine.

Prophylaxis. Most patients with migraine can be helped by the implementation of both prophylactic and abortive measures. Once the diagnosis is established by the criteria of the most recent classification system, the physician should ascertain the frequency of disabling headache. As a general rule, if headaches are interfering with work or other activities more than once a week, it is reasonable to consider prophylactic medication. Educating the migraine-prone patient to avoid precipitants such as certain foods (cheese, chocolates, citrus fruits, nuts, red wine—although not invariably in all patients), inadequate sleep, and prolonged fasting may help prevent some headaches. Useful information on precipitants is sometimes derived by keeping a *headache diary*.

Nonpharmacologic Measures. Prevention of attacks involves *nonpharmacologic measures* in addition to drug treatment. Because migraine may be precipitated by emotional stress or psychological conflict, it is important to investigate family, work, and social circumstances to design a program of prevention. Regular *exercise* and *relaxation techniques* (see Chapter 226) may significantly decrease the frequency and severity of headaches. These activities help reduce the impact of stress. Many patients prefer to try them before attempting other forms of therapy. Patients under significant psychological stress may benefit from informal supportive psychotherapy, which helps them to express their feelings and deal with the stress. Although extensive psychotherapy may not reduce the number of attacks, it is worth trying to pinpoint areas of stress and search with the patient for ways to resolve them. Recommending rest or a vacation may not suffice; in fact, flare-ups are common during vacations and weekends. *Biofeedback* is of unproven benefit and probably no better than relaxation exercises and other nonpharmacologic methods. The lack of adequately designed studies limits conclusions regarding biofeedback.

Pharmacologic Measures. Drug therapy should be added when nonpharmacologic measures do not suffice. Several different classes of drugs have been useful in the prophylaxis of migraine; the doses and side effects are outlined in Table 165.4. An approach of trial and error is often necessary before the appropriate medication that is most effective with the fewest side effects in any individual patient can be found. Each drug should be given at least a 2-month trial, and many patients require longer than this before full benefit is obtained. In general, a *tricyclic antidepressant* (e.g., *nortriptyline* or *amitriptyline*) is an appropriate first-line choice, especially in view of the increasingly evident relationship between migraine and major depression. *β-Blockers* are another first-line prophylactic agent, but sometimes such high doses are required that fatigue or even depression develops. Another alternative is verapamil, the most widely prescribed calcium channel blocker for migraine prophylaxis. *NSAIDs* (e.g., naproxen) have been useful, especially for patients with menstrual migraine. They are prescribed for several days before, during, and after menstruation. *Valproate*, an anticonvulsant drug that interacts with the γ-aminobutyric acid neurotransmitter system and turns off serotonergic raphe neurons, has also attracted interest, but its usefulness in patients with migraine is limited by its tendency to cause hair loss and

Table 165.4. Drugs for Migraine Headache Prophylaxis

DRUG	RECOMMENDED DOSAGES	SIDE EFFECTS, SPECIAL CONSIDERATIONS
β-Blockers		
Propranolol	40–320 mg/d	Full β-blockade required. Three months may be necessary to achieve full benefit.
Nadolol	40–240 mg/d	
Atenolol	50–150 mg/d	Contraindications: congestive heart failure, asthma.
Timolol	10–30 mg/d	Side effects: drowsiness, exercise intolerance, depression.
Tricyclic Antidepressants		
Amitriptyline	10–300 mg/d	Efficacy in headache treatment is independent of antidepressant effect and may occur earlier and with lower doses than antidepressant effect.
Nortriptyline	10–125 mg/d	
Doxepin	10–150 mg/d	Side effects: drowsiness, urinary retention, weight gain.
Calcium–Channel Blockers		
Verapamil	240–480 mg/d	May require 1 month for perceived benefit.
		Contraindications: congestive heart failure, heart block, atrial fibrillation, sick sinus syndrome.
		Side effects: hypotension atrioventricular block, headache, constipation, edema, congestive heart failure.
NSAIDs		
Naproxen	500 mg bid	Particularly useful for women with menstrual migraine, taken for several days peri-menstruation.
		Side effects: gastrointestinal upset, ulcers, worsening renal function in susceptible patients.
		Contraindications: ulcer, aspirin sensitivity, renal failure.
Anticonvulsants		
Valproate	Titration to therapeutic level from 250 mg tid	Side effects: nausea, platelet dysfunction, hair loss, hepatotoxicity, teratogenicity, neural tube defects.
Phenytoin	Adjustment to therapeutic level, usually 200-400 mg/d	Particularly useful for children. Side effects: rash, ataxia, hepatic dysfunction, gingival hypertrophy.
Serotonin Antagonist		
Methysergide	2–4 mg in divided doses; usual dose 6–8 mg/d	Idiosyncratic reaction of retroperitoneal, pulmonary, or endocardial fibrosis. Cannot be given for more than 6 months continuously. Side effects: nausea, muscle cramps, weight gain, peripheral arterial insufficiency.

weight gain and its teratogenic potential (neural tube defects). Promising results in small-scale, short-term studies suggest a possible prophylactic role for high-dose *riboflavin* (*vitamin B₂*); when given in doses of 400 mg/d, it reduces the frequency and total number of headache days. The purported mechanism is an improvement in mitochondrial function. Longer-term, larger-scale studies are needed before this treatment can be recommended.

Abortive Therapy. For the patient with only occasional migraine headaches and for patients with generally well-controlled but occasional severe breakthrough headaches, it is important to establish an effective abortive regimen. The advent of triptan therapy has greatly enhanced the ability to abort migraine attacks. However, despite the demonstrated safety and efficacy of the triptans, this class of drugs is prescribed for only about 30% of patients with migraine. Analgesics remain the most frequently prescribed remedy for migraine, even though they are not an effective treatment for this type of headache.

Treatment of Aural Symptoms. Most medicines that treat migraine episodes do not blunt aural symptoms. *NSAIDs* and prokinetic and antiemetic compounds such as *metoclopramide* and *compazine* may provide significant relief of aural symptoms. The administration of antiemetics and metoclopramide 30 minutes before analgesics improves oral absorption, combats nausea, and increases the efficacy of aspirin, acetaminophen, and caffeine-containing compounds.

Dihydroergotamine. The SQ, IM, IV, or nasal administration of ergot is highly effective. Parenteral administration in emergency department settings has helped to terminate severe, acute attacks of migraine. Although the vasoconstrictive effects of dihydroergotamine on peripheral arteries are minimal, it is contraindicated in patients with coronary disease, peripheral vascular disease, transient ischemic attacks, pregnancy, or sepsis. Nausea is a significant problem and may be minimized by prior IV administration of metoclopramide (Reglan).

Selective 5-HT₁B/₁D Agonists (Triptans) have revolutionized the management of migraine headache. Several are now on the market. The participants in the "triptan wars" are outlined in Table 165.5. Both sumatriptan and the second-generation triptans are cerebral and coronary vasoconstrictors; they act by both vasoconstriction and inhibition of neurogenic inflammation. The drugs differ in their bioavailability and half-lives. A single 6-mg SQ dose of sumatriptan has proved highly effective; it acts rapidly and is well tolerated in the treatment of severe migraine attacks. Sumatriptan is now available as an SQ autoinjection formulation, tablets, and nasal spray. In general, the second-generation triptans have better oral pharmacokinetic properties than sumatriptan does, and they last longer. Therefore, the initial relief of headache is at least as good as that with oral sumatriptan, and the recurrence rate may be lower. Recurrence may be minimized with the longer-acting triptans, such as naratriptan. A second dose of any of the triptans may be effective, but overuse of the triptans can result in a *rebound* phenomenon. The use of sumatriptan and other triptans should be restricted to no more than 1 to 2 days weekly.

Contraindications to triptan use include recent use of monoamine oxidase inhibitors, uncontrolled hypertension, coronary artery disease, and pregnancy. Patients should not take triptans during the aura phase of the migraine, and patients with complicated auras such as hemiparesis or dysphasia should not receive triptan therapy. Those on selective serotonin reuptake inhibitors may take triptans, but the dosage of both medicines should be monitored carefully.

Side effects. Sumatriptan injection is safe for large numbers of patients despite the fact up to 40% of patients report *chest-related symptoms* when specifically asked about them. The initial theoretical concerns about possible ischemia have been allayed by large-scale follow-up studies that found not a single clear incident of myocardial infarction within 24 hours of sumatriptan injection, no deaths, and no increased incidence of stroke.

Analgesics and Sedatives. In general, it is best to avoid the regular use of *analgesics* and *sedatives*. Popular combination analgesic and sedative formulations containing either acetaminophen or aspirin with butalbital and caffeine (e.g., *Fioricet* and *Fiorinal*) are often requested by patients, as they were widely prescribed in the past. Although they may be helpful for occasional use, marked caution is warranted in prescribing such combination agents because of their potential for habituation when used regularly in a chronic recurring condition such as migraine and because of the development of rebound headache

Table 165.5.   Triptans[a]

DRUG (GENERIC/BRAND)	ROUTE	DOSE[b] (mg)	BIOAVAIL-ABILITY	T₁/₂ (h)	ONSET (h)	RESPONSE RATE (RELIEF/PAIN-FREE AT 2 h)	RECURRENCE
Sumatriptan/ Imitrex	SQ PO Nasal	6[b] 25, 50,[b] 100 5, 20[b]	14%	2 2	1/6–1/4 1–1.5 1/4	87/67% 57/29% 62/33%	45% (all routes)
Zolmitripran/ Zomig	PO	2.5,[b] 5	40%	3	1	62/34%	22%
Naratriptan/ Amerge	PO	2.5[b]	63–74% men/women	6	1	68/45%	19–28%
Rizatriptan/ Maxalt Maxalt MLT	PO SL	5, 10[b] 5, 10	45%	1.5 similar to PO preparation	1	77/44%	30%
Eletriptan/ Relpax	PO	40,[b] 80	50%	4–5	1	80/37%	—

[a] All: 5-HT₁B/₁D agonists, cerebral and coronary vasoconstrictors. Variable: pharmacokinetics and lipophilicity.
[b] Preferred initial dose.

patterns. *Narcotic analgesics* are sometimes needed, but their regular use can lead to a vicious cycle of headache, narcotic intake, drug withdrawal, more headache, and more narcotic intake (see below).

Migraine and Risk for Stroke. Although the risk for ischemic stroke is low in patients who have migraine without aura, the odds ratio for stroke in patients who have migraine with aura is increased (to approximately 6). *Oral contraceptives*, even those with a low estrogen content of less than 50 μg, appear to cause an increase in ischemic stroke risk, with an odds ratio of about 2. Many neurologists discourage the use of oral contraceptives in patients who have migraine with aura and in older female patients who have migraine with other risk factors for stroke.

Cluster Headache

As with migraine, both abortive and prophylactic treatments are available. One abortive treatment for an acute attack consists of inhalation of *oxygen* (5 to 8 L/min for 10 minutes). *Ergotamine suppositories* may be effective and can be taken at bedtime during a cluster by a patient whose symptoms occur at night. *Dihydroergotamine* (IM or IV, as outlined above) is effective, as is *sumatriptan*, particularly the SQ form. A corticosteroid bolus of 8 mg of *dexamethasone* or *prednisone* started at 20 mg three times a day and tapered during 2 weeks has also been helpful in aborting a cluster.

Prophylaxis for patients with chronic cluster headaches or for those with severe frequent cluster episodes includes 360 mg of *verapamil* daily, given in divided doses. *Methysergide* at a dosage of 2 mg three times a day or *lithium* at doses achieving a therapeutic level identical to that for bipolar disease is useful. Sphenopalatine ganglion block performed by an anesthesiologist may provide significant temporary relief. A radiofrequency *trigeminal rhizotomy* is reserved for patients whose headaches are completely refractory to all the medical therapies described above.

Tension-type Headache

For the vast majority of patients with mild or occasional tension headache, mild analgesics (aspirin, acetaminophen, nonprescription doses of NSAIDs) usually suffice. Such patients usually do not consult the physician. Patients with chronic or persistent tension-type headaches are candidates for evaluation of underlying anxiety and depression (see Chapters 226 and 227). Often, definitive treatment of such headaches requires that the underlying sources of psychological distress be addressed. *Stress reduction* measures may be of considerable help for those with an anxiety state (see Appendix, Chapter 226), and *antidepressant therapy* may benefit depressed patients (see Chapter 227). Patients with chronic headache subsequent to trauma should be encouraged to conclude any pending legal proceedings.

Chronic Daily Headaches

Chronic daily headache is among the most difficult types of headache encountered by primary physicians. In some patients, a migraine syndrome evolves into a daily headache more typical of tension-type headache with superimposed migrainous events. Depression, anxiety, and drug abuse may all complicate the picture at this stage. While counseling this group of patients about precipitating factors and lifestyle modification, it is important that the physician elicit a history of analgesic and ergotamine use. Ergotamine or analgesic abuse can lead to a vicious cycle of headache, medication, and headache. As the effect of a previous dose of ergotamine or analgesic wanes, headache begins to recur and leads to further use of medication. Drug-induced sleep disturbances and psychological dependence ensue, leading to a self-sustaining rhythmic cycle of headache and medication. Thus, caution must be exerted to avoid prescribing large amounts of ergotamine or analgesics (both narcotic and non-narcotic) for a patient with migraine or tension-type headache. Total elimination of analgesics and ergotamine compounds may improve the therapeutic results of other medications chosen for the prophylaxis of headache. Hospitalization for withdrawal of medication and institution of a comprehensive program may be beneficial.

Management of Other Conditions Causing Headache

(For the treatment of temporomandibular joint dysfunction and bruxism, see Chapter 225. See Chapter 161 for the management of temporal arteritis, and Chapter 219 for the treatment of sinusitis.)

INDICATIONS FOR ADMISSION AND REFERRAL

Admission or Urgent Referral. Urgent hospitalization is indicated for the patient with acute onset of a severe headache accompanied by signs of meningeal irritation. Intracranial hemorrhage or meningeal infection may be responsible. Evidence of increased intracranial pressure is another indication for prompt admission. Severe, intractable migraine may require prompt hospital admission for one of the abortive treatments outlined above. The ophthalmologist needs to be consulted at once if acute glaucoma is thought to be the cause of an acute orbital headache.

Referral. Less urgent situations involving headache that deserve neurologic consultation include episodes of transient neurologic dysfunction, unilateral headache increasing in frequency and severity, change in personality, and new onset of progressive deficits suggestive of an evolving process or a mass lesion. Sometimes, patients with an intractable tension-type headache or severe migraine syndrome can benefit from the reassurance and suggestions provided by the neurologist. Dental consultation is indicated if temporomandibular joint problems appear refractory to conservative therapy. Surgical referral for a temporal artery biopsy may be necessary when an elderly patient is suspected of having giant cell arteritis but more definitive evidence that long-term steroid therapy is warranted is required (see Chapter 161). Ophthalmologic consultation for a vision check and assessment of the need for refraction is indicated if prolonged close work is resulting in headaches.

For patients with chronic, intractable, tension-type headache, a diagnostic consultation with a psychiatrist may serve as an important learning experience. However, many of these patients are reluctant to consider a psychological cause for their symptoms. Thus, it is important that a full medical evaluation be conducted before a psychiatric referral is suggested. This obviates any misunderstanding by patients who believe that their problem has a medical basis and who may view the referral as an inappropriate dismissal of their symptoms.

ANNOTATED BIBLIOGRAPHY

Bartleson JD. Treatment of migraine headaches. Mayo Clin Proc 1999;74:702. (*Excellent single-source review for comparison of the different triptans and other abortive and prophylactic strategies for migraine.*)

Becker WJ. Use of oral contraceptives in patients with migraine. Neurology 1999;53[Suppl 1]:S19. (*Although the risk for ischemic stroke is low in patients who have migraine without aura, the odds ratio for stroke in patients who have migraine with aura is approximately 6.*)

Breslau N, Merikangas K, Bowden CL. Comorbidity of migraine and major affective disorders. Neurology 1996;44[Suppl 7]:S17. (*This article reviews the first clear evidence of the existence of bidirectional influences of depression and migraine.*)

Frishberg BM. The utility of neuroimaging in the evaluation of headache in patients with normal neurologic examinations. Neurology 1994;44:1191. Practice parameter from the American Academy of Neurology. Neurology 1994;44:1353. (*Although they admit that the yield of diagnostic investigations in patients with primary headache syndromes and normal examination findings is very low, both documents leave open the role of clinical judgment.*)

Goadsby PJ. How do the currently used prophylactic agents work in migraine? Cephalalgia 1997;17:85. (*Here is the article to read if you want to try to tie together the various trial and error categories of medicines you have been giving your patients!*)

Headache Classification Committee of the International Headache Society. Classification and diagnostic criteria for headache disorders, cranial neuralgias, and facial pain. Cephalalgia 1988;8[Suppl 7]:1. (*The standard classification system for current headache clinical studies, updated regularly, most recently in 1996 to include chronic daily headache with and without substance abuse.*)

Katzman GL, Dagher AP, Patronas NJH. Incidental findings on brain magnetic resonance imaging from 1,000 asymptomatic volunteers. JAMA 1999;282:36. (*Although incidental lesions did occur, the vast majority of patients who had a history compatible with a primary headache syndrome and normal physical examination findings had normal results on magnetic resonance imaging.*)

Launer LJ, Terwindt GM, Ferrari MD. The prevalence and characteristics of migraine in a population-based cohort. Neurology 1999;53:537. (*In this study from the Netherlands, the lifetime prevalence of migraine in women was 33%, and in men it was 13.3%.*)

Linet MS, Cohen A. An epidemiologic study of headache among adolescents and young adults. JAMA 1989;261:2211. (*Useful information on incidence and an illustration of the use of the new classification system.*)

Lipton MS, Stewart WF. Migraine in the United States: a review of epidemiology and health care use. Neurology 1993;43[Suppl3]:S6. (*The American migraine study; best epidemiologic data.*)

Mathew NT. Cluster headache. Neurology 1992;42[Suppl 2]:22. (*Good overview.*)

O'Quinn S, Davis RL, Herman DL, et al. Prospective large-scale study of the tolerability of subcutaneous sumatriptan injection for the acute treatment of migraine. Cephalalgia 1999;19:223. (*Multicenter open-label study of 12,339 migraine patients followed for 1 year.*)

Rapoport AM. The diagnosis of migraine and tension-type headache, then and now. Neurology 1992;42[Suppl 2]:11. (*Reviews the complexities of the new classification system and offers some straightforward criteria for grouping patients and critiquing the current classification.*)

Saper JR. Daily chronic headache. Neurol Clin North Am 1990;8:891. (*A sympathetic look at the very difficult problem of daily chronic headache, with some appropriate treatment strategies.*)

Schoenen J, Jacquy J, Lenaerts M. Effectiveness of high-dose riboflavin in migraine prophylaxis: a randomized controlled trial. Neurology 1998;50:466. (*A short-term, small-scale study finding a significant reduction in frequency and number of migraine days; results promising, but confirmation by longer-term, larger-scale study needed.*)

Silberstein SD. Divalproex sodium in headache: literature review and clinical guidelines. Headache 1996;36:547. (*Depakote has been widely promoted for migraine headache, but its side effect profile and possible teratogenic effects limit its utility as a first-line agent in patients with migraine.*)

Silberstein SD, Merriam G. Sex hormones and headache 1999 (menstrual migraine). Neurology 1999;531[Suppl1]S3. (*A useful review of the often contradictory evidence about hormonal influences in migraine headache.*)

Stewart WF. Prevalence of migraine headache in the United States. JAMA 1992;267:64. (*This is likely to become a classic article dispelling many previously held tenets about the epidemiology of migraine.*)

Subcutaneous Sumatriptan International Study Group. Treatment of migraine attack with sumatriptan. N Engl J Med 1991;325:316. (*Double-blinded, randomized, controlled, parallel study demonstrating efficacy in aborting acute migraine and treating cluster headache.*)

Ziegler DK. Headache. Public health problem. Neurol Clin North Am 1990;8:781. (*Overview of the enormous impact of headache in the United States. Another analysis of this problem is presented in Hu XL, et al. Burden of migraine in the United States: disability and economic costs. Arch Intern Med 1999;159:813.*)

166
Evaluation of Dizziness
AMY A. PRUITT

Dizziness can be one of the more frustrating complaints to assess; the task is often made difficult by a vague history and a large number of possible causes, ranging from psychiatric disease and cardiovascular disorders to peripheral and central defects within the nervous system. However, with a bit of patience and careful attention to the history and physical examination findings, the primary physician can conduct a remarkably sophisticated clinical evaluation, one that will help direct further workup and treatment. With the problem of true vertigo, an additional goal of the clinical examination is at times to provide immediate bedside relief from the symptom for those patients who are found to have benign positional vertigo.

PATHOPHYSIOLOGY AND CLINICAL PRESENTATION

The patient complaining of "dizziness" may have a malfunction of virtually any organ system, including vestibular dysfunction, cardiovascular insufficiency, psychiatric illness, metabolic derangement, multiple sensory deficits, cerebellar disease, or a combination of problems.

Vestibular Disease

Patients with vestibular disease experience *true vertigo*, which is defined as a head sensation of abnormal movement or (and the distinction does not matter) abnormal movement of the environment. Descriptive terms include not only "spinning" but also "weaving," "seasickness," "ground rising and falling," "rocking," "things moving," and "merry-go-round" sensation. Nausea, vomiting, and diaphoresis accompany severe cases. Tinnitus and hearing loss indicate associated injury to the auditory component of the eighth cranial nerve. Nystagmus is frequently found on examination (see below) or can be induced.

The vestibular problem may be *central* or *peripheral*; peripheral lesions include those that are *cochlear* or *retrocochlear*. Central lesions differ from peripheral ones in that they typically present with vertigo in association with other brainstem deficits; in peripheral disease, vertigo occurs in isolation except for accompanying tinnitus or hearing loss.

Peripheral Lesions. In *benign positional vertigo*, a common problem in the elderly, vertigo is experienced only in specific positions. Onset is sudden, usually within a few seconds after the triggering position has been assumed. Symptoms cease after several minutes if the patient does not move, but they resume with further change in position. In many patients, the condition resolves within 6 months; recovery is usually complete. Head trauma sometimes results in this type of temporary vertigo. The mechanism is stimulation of the labyrinth by free-floating particulate matter in the posterior semicircular canal. A less common but more persistent cause of positional vertigo is thought to be vascular compression of the vestibular nerve. Patients with this condition have constant positional vertigo and severe nausea; it has been labeled *"disabling positional vertigo"* to distinguish it from the more common forms of positional vertiginous disease.

Ménière's disease ensues from idiopathic endolymphatic hydrops, with damage to the hair cells caused by swelling of the semicircular ducts. Patients report tinnitus, pressure in the ear, and hearing loss in conjunction with vertigo. Episodes are paroxysmal, last minutes to hours, and then decrease in frequency after multiple attacks, only to recur in several months or years. Hearing loss and tinnitus usually accompany the episodes of vertigo, and the hearing loss, although initially reversible, eventually becomes permanent.

Acute labyrinthitis develops as a consequence of viral infection involving the cochlea and labyrinth. The patient reports a viral upper respiratory syndrome followed by onset of vertigo, tinnitus, and hearing loss. Symptoms resolve entirely by 3 to 6 weeks, with no residual deficits. Vestibular neuronitis is believed to be the same illness, without any cochlear involvement; it is characterized by isolated vertigo, no hearing loss, and full clearing.

Ototoxins can injure the peripheral vestibular apparatus, although hearing impairment usually predominates. Streptomycin and gentamicin are among the toxins that are most injurious to the vestibular portion of the eighth cranial nerve.

Acoustic neuroma (Benign schwannoma of the eighth cranial nerve), the most worrisome of the peripheral lesions, is retrocochlear in location. It is distinguished from the others in that it causes the retrocochlear type of hearing loss (see below) and can produce serious brainstem compression if untreated. Symptoms start almost imperceptibly, with mild hearing loss, tinnitus, and vague dizziness, and may resemble those of other forms of peripheral vestibular disease. However, the clinical course is progressive and the hearing loss is asymmetric, which differentiates it from that associated with other peripheral lesions.

Central Lesions, as already noted, are accompanied in most instances by other brainstem symptoms. In addition, the vertigo and any accompanying nystagmus can be bidirectional or vertical, which does not occur in peripheral vestibular disease.

Multiple sclerosis associated with focal demyelination in the vestibular pathways of the brainstem is an important central cause of vertigo. Because of the often transient nature of attacks (days to weeks) and the subtlety of accompanying symptoms (slight facial numbness or huskiness of voice), multiple sclerosis may at first be mistaken for one of the self-limited peripheral causes of vertigo. Only with repeated episodes might the diagnosis become evident. The population afflicted with multiple sclerosis in general is younger than the patients (median age of 54 years) with canalithiasis as a cause of benign positional vertigo. In the aftermath of an acute attack, a central type of positional nystagmus may persist after the vertigo resolves. The vertigo has no characteristic features; attacks can be sudden, transient, recurrent, or persistent. Diagnosis depends on magnetic resonance imaging (MRI) evidence of discrete central nervous system lesions and a course of recurrent dysfunction and intervals of remission.

Vertebrobasilar insufficiency usually produces vertigo in conjunction with diplopia, sensory loss, dysarthria, dysphagia, hemiparesis, and other brainstem deficits. Self-limited episodes are manifestations of transient ischemic attacks. In about one fourth of cases, transient vertigo may be the initial and sole complaint and may indicate impending infarction in the territory of the anterior inferior cerebellar artery. A more subtle, progressive form of dizziness, usually without true vertigo, can be seen when multiple lacunar infarctions are present, particularly if the pons is involved. The MRI appearance of this socalled *ischemic pontine rarefaction* can be quite dramatic.

Migraine-associated vertigo has been diagnosed by some neurologists. The dizziness often antedates the headache phase of the syndrome and can persist in a less vivid form after the migraine headache is over. This is an atypical form of migraine with aura and may respond to migraine prophylactic medicines (see Chapter 165).

Drugs that suppress the reticular activating system of the brainstem (e.g., sedatives, anticonvulsants) can cause vertigo of a central nature, especially when taken in excess. Therapeutic doses of some drugs (e.g., phenytoin, carbamazepine) produce nystagmus.

Cardiovascular Disease

Cardiac and vascular insufficiency leading to inadequate cerebral perfusion can result in dizziness, which patients tend to describe as *"light-headedness"* or a sense of faintness (see Chapter 24). This form of dizziness is seen in patients with fixed or limited cardiac output, serious cardiac dysrhythmias, diminished vascular tone, or severe intravascular volume depletion. Symptoms typically worsen on standing and improve on lying down; postural changes in blood pressure and pulse are characteristic.

Multiple Sensory Deficits, Cerebellar Disease, and Other Causes of Disequilibrium

These neurologic problems produce sensations of *impaired balance* and *disequilibrium.* In this form of dizziness, patients report the sensation to be in the feet rather than in the head. Like light-headedness, it may come on with standing; like true vertigo, it can be aggravated by walking or turning. Multiple sensory deficits are the most common cause. Patients with multiple sensory deficits are usually elderly and have diabetes or other conditions that impair eyesight, sense of position, and motor function. Symptoms typically worsen in the dark (because of elimination of visual positional data) and improve with use of a cane or holding onto a railing. Elderly patients with disequilibrium may also have degenerative cerebellar disease, but the presence of multiple lacunar infarctions leading to ischemic pontine disease should be considered. The physical examination findings are notable for ataxia and other cerebellar signs. Acute disequilibrium may be caused by a midline cerebellar hemorrhage and present as severe dizziness, marked gait ataxia, headache, and stiff neck.

Psychiatric Illness

Patients with psychiatric difficulties complain of ill-defined dizziness ("I just feel dizzy"), constant "light-headedness," or a "foggy" feeling. *Depression, anxiety states,* and *psychosis,* in addition to the *medications* used to treat such conditions, are common precipitants. The precise mechanism of the light-headedness is unknown, but it is thought to be related to a confusional state induced by these illnesses or by the medications used to treat them. In the case of a panic attack leading to hyperventilation (see Chapter 226), the ensuing metabolic alkalosis usually causes paresthesias and light-headedness, although sometimes vertigo is reported.

Metabolic Disturbances

Alterations in central nervous system metabolic homeostasis can cause dizziness resembling that associated with inadequate cerebral perfusion. The patient describes light-headedness or feeling faint. Precipitants of acute symptoms include *hypoglycemia, hypoxia, hypocarbia, hypercarbia,* and *drugs.*

DIFFERENTIAL DIAGNOSIS

Conditions that cause dizziness can be grouped according to pathophysiologic mechanism (Table 166.1). Vestibular disease is divided into central and peripheral types. Central lesions are mostly caused by basilar artery disease and multiple sclerosis. Peripheral causes include acoustic neuroma, benign positional vertigo, vestibular neuronitis, Ménière's disease, and ototoxic drugs.

Table 166.1.   Differential Diagnosis of Dizziness

Vestibular Disease
  Benign positional vertigo
  Vestibular neuronitis and ototoxic drugs
  Ménière's disease
  Acoustic neuroma and other tumors of the cerebellopontine
    angle
  Basilar insufficiency
  Multiple sclerosis

Cardiac and Vascular Disease
  Critical aortic stenosis
  Carotid sinus hypersensitivity
  Volume depletion and severe anemia
  Autonomic insufficiency (drugs, diabetes)
  Diminished vascular reflexes of the elderly

Multiple Sensory Deficits
  Diabetes mellitus
  Cataract surgery
  Some cases of multiple sclerosis
  Cervical spondylosis
  Cerebellar disease

Psychiatric Illness
  Anxiety
  Depression
  Psychosis

Metabolic Disturbances
  Hypoxia
  Severe hypoglycemia
  Hypocapnia and hypercapnia

Cardiac and vascular diseases are a second important group. Faintness on standing may be caused by critical aortic stenosis, severe volume depletion, the use of antihypertensive drugs, autonomic insufficiency, or prolonged confinement to bed. Carotid sinus hypersensitivity results in inappropriate reduction of vascular tone.

Multiple sensory deficits are most common in diabetics and others with poor vision and peripheral neuropathies. Cervical spondylosis disturbs cervical sensory input and contributes to dizziness. Lenses used by patients following cataract surgery distort peripheral vision and can confuse their sense of position. Cerebellar dysfunction leads to a similar clinical presentation of gait unsteadiness. Less commonly, idiopathic normal pressure hydrocephalus can present with unsteadiness of gait or disequilibrium.

Psychiatric problems are often associated with light-headedness. Patients with anxiety, depression, and psychosis report feeling light-headed. At times, tranquilizers and antidepressants are responsible. Panic attacks frequently are accompanied by feelings of light-headedness or dizziness. Metabolic disturbances affecting the central nervous system have a similar presentation; hypoxia, hypoglycemia, hypocapnia, and hypercapnia are among the most important features.

In a study of 104 consecutive cases referred for evaluation of dizziness, 38% of patients had peripheral vestibular disease, 23% had hyperventilation, 13% had multiple sensory deficits, 9% had psychiatric problems, and 5% had cardiovascular or central neurologic illness. Many cases are multifactorial.

WORKUP

History

The most important initial step in the evaluation of dizziness is to obtain from the patient the best possible description of the experience and what is meant by "dizziness." A history taken without leading questions or suggested descriptions is most likely to provide meaningful clues. *True vertigo* suggests *vestibular disease*; *faintness* that is *postural* or paroxysmal implies a *cardiovascular* disorder; constant *ill-defined dizziness* or light-headedness unrelated to posture points toward a *psychogenic* cause; a feeling of *poor balance* or disequilibrium typifies *multiple sensory deficits* and *cerebellar* causes.

When the problem is light-headedness, it is worth asking if standing or turning brings on symptoms. If standing does, the use of antihypertensive, tranquilizer, or antidepressant medications should be investigated. During the examination, postural signs, carotid upstroke, and cardiac function should be evaluated, especially for signs of hemodynamically significant aortic stenosis. If turning worsens the situation, it is important to evaluate vision, search for other sensory deficits, and check for cerebellar signs (see below). If light-headedness is a constant sensation, an underlying psychiatric or metabolic disorder is likely. Anxiety and depression are frequent causes and warrant investigation (see Chapters 226 and 227).

Central versus Peripheral Disease. If the patient has *true vertigo*, then the task shifts to determining whether the lesion is *central* or *peripheral*. The most direct way of making this distinction is to inquire about brainstem symptoms (e.g., diplopia, facial numbness, weakness, hemiplegia, dysphasia). Evidence of brainstem involvement rules out a peripheral lesion. The absence of brainstem symptoms does not rule out a central lesion but does make it improbable. Even the very confusing picture of apparently isolated vertigo resulting from vertebrobasilar insufficiency or multiple sclerosis eventually becomes clearer as accompanying brainstem symptoms become more evident. The pattern of discrete central nervous system lesions and a course of recurrent episodes followed by remissions further suggest the diagnosis of multiple sclerosis (see Chapter 172). Vertebrobasilar insufficiency should be considered in the patient with multiple atherosclerotic risk factors or a prior history of cardiovascular or cerebrovascular disease.

Distinguishing among Peripheral Causes. In the patient with a suspected *peripheral lesion*, the focus turns to distinguishing *cochlear* from *retrocochlear* disease—that is, relatively benign causes from acoustic neuroma. The latter has a variable presentation and can initially mimic other peripheral types of vertigo. Episodes of vertigo, tinnitus, pressure in the ear, and hearing loss may take place, simulating Ménière's disease. However, the hearing loss is slowly and steadily progressive, rather than fluctuating or episodic. The development of brainstem symptoms (facial weakness or numbness) is a late occurrence and not very helpful for early diagnosis. When doubt still persists, physical examination and audiologic testing can be used to help make the differentiation between cochlear and retrocochlear disease (see below).

Timing and *precipitating factors* help elucidate most other peripheral causes of vertigo. If symptoms occur only on change of position and last but a few moments, the diagnosis is benign positional vertigo, a condition mostly affecting people older than age 60. It may be a recurrent problem. A single bout of severe spontaneous vertigo, sudden in onset, sometimes after a *viral illness*, is usually vestibular neuronitis. When seen in the context of inner ear infection, it is properly called *acute labyrinthitis*. Some degree of positional vertigo may remain after the acute illness resolves. Ménière's disease is suggested by acute, recurrent paroxysms of vertigo that are accompanied by *tinnitus* and temporary *hearing loss*. Tinnitus, *pressure* in the ear, and hearing loss are episodic and may precede the other symptoms. Attacks can last for hours to days; residual positional vertigo occurs in 25% of cases.

Drug History. Obtaining a thorough *drug history* is important. The ototoxic effects of the aminoglycoside antibiotics have been well documented; the diuretic ethacrynic acid also can cause injury to the eighth nerve, especially in patients with compromised renal function. Diuretics may be responsible for severe volume depletion. Vasodilators, phenothiazines, and antihypertensive agents can produce postural light-headedness. Antidepressants and minor tranquilizers cause some patients to feel dizzy.

Physical Examination

The *general appearance* of the patient can be quite informative (e.g., the anxious person will appear overly nervous and may hyperventilate or sigh frequently during the interview). *Blood pressure* and pulse should be measured, and changes between readings taken in the *supine* and *standing* positions should be noted. The skin is examined for pallor, the eyes for *nystagmus* (a few beats of nystagmus on extreme lateral gaze are normal), and the ears for tympanic membrane lesions and *hearing acuity* (see below). The carotid arteries in the neck are checked for bruits (suggestive of cerebrovascular disease) and delay in upstroke (characteristic of severe aortic stenosis). A forceful, sustained left ventricular impulse, single second heart sound, and loud ejection quality murmur on cardiac examination also support a diagnosis of significant aortic stenosis (see Chapter 21).

A thorough and careful *neurologic examination* is essential, particularly when the possibility of central vestibular disease is being considered. Most important is examination for a brainstem lesion, which suggests central pathology or extrinsic compression by an acoustic neuroma. *Cranial nerves* V, VII, and X can be affected by a large acoustic neuroma pressing at the cerebellopontine angle of the brainstem. Testing of sensory function, peripheral vision, and gait often reveals multiple defects in elderly patients troubled by dizziness. Results of the *Romberg test* (standing with feet together, eyes closed) will also be abnormal in such patients, and also in some with vestibular disease. The side to which the vertiginous patient sways helps to localize the lesion. Cerebellar testing helps to detect any ataxia.

Provocative Maneuvers designed to trigger symptoms and reproduce the patient's problem can be extremely useful. Asking the anxious patient to *hyperventilate* voluntarily for 30 to 120 seconds will often reproduce "dizziness" and associated symptoms, whereas vestibular maneuvers (see below) will not. *Standing up* from a supine position will cause the patient with cardiac or vascular disease to feel faint; it may trigger vertigo in the patient with vestibular disease. *Walking* and *turning* will cause a feeling of disequilibrium in the patient with multiple sensory deficits, cerebellar disease, or vestibular dysfunction. The *Dix-Hallpike* or *Bárány maneuver* and other forms of vestibular stimulation (see below) will trigger vertigo and associated symptoms.

Maneuvers Alleviating Symptoms are also of diagnostic use. Getting up slowly lessens the faint feeling associated with cardiovascular causes; *rebreathing into a paper bag* reduces the light, giddy feeling that follows hyperventilation; *lying still* in one position may halt positional vertigo; touching the examiner's hand or using a *cane* to walk helps the patient with sensory deficits or cerebellar dysfunction. Withholding suspected drugs may be informative.

Simple Office Tests of hearing and stimulation of the vestibular apparatus can be very helpful in distinguishing central from peripheral disease and cochlear from retrocochlear peripheral disease. The *Rinne test* (see Chapter 212) identifies which eighth cranial nerve is involved and helps differentiate between conductive and sensorineural hearing loss. Patients with a sensorineural hearing deficit may have a cochlear or a retrocochlear lesion. The distinction can be made by testing *speech discrimination*, which is easily performed in the office by whispering a series of 10 two-syllable, closely linked words (e.g., baseball, ice cream) into the patient's ear while making a sound in the other ear to limit its participation. The patient is asked to repeat each whispered word. Correctly identifying

fewer than 20% of the words is very suggestive of a retrocochlear lesion (which causes a disproportionate loss of speech discrimination); a score of 70% or better indicates that the problem is cochlear. Scores in between these are indeterminate and necessitate formal audiologic testing (see Chapter 212).

Vestibular Stimulation Testing serves both as a good provocative test for reproducing symptoms (useful when the description of dizziness remains unclear) and as a means of distinguishing peripheral from central vestibular disease. The *Dix-Hallpike (Bárány) maneuver* is the least noxious of the standard forms of vestibular stimulation. The patient starts in a sitting position on the examination table and lies down with the head extending over the edge of the table, tilted back, and turned 45 degrees to one side. The assumption of this position need not be overly abrupt, but it should be held for at least 30 seconds. The maneuver is repeated, this time with the head turned 45 degrees to the opposite side. For a final time, the test is repeated without turning the head. (Fig. 166.1)

The Dix-Hallpike maneuver provides simultaneous stimulation of all three semicircular canals. It is a useful provocative maneuver for identifying vestibular disease and potentially helpful in separating peripheral from central lesions. One asks the patient to look straight ahead and watches for onset of nystagmus (horizontal or rotatory) and reproduction of symptoms. If symptoms occur, one asks to which side things seem to be spinning; if nystagmus ensues, one notes to which side the slow phase moves. By combining these results with findings from the Romberg and Rinne tests, one can make a diagnosis of a peripheral lesion if (a) the slow phase of nystagmus moves toward the same side as the hearing loss, (b) the patient reports that the spinning is away from the side of the hearing loss, (c) the Romberg test result is positive and the patient sways toward the side of the hearing deficit. Absence of any one of these findings suggests a central lesion.

Other findings on head position testing suggestive of central vestibular disease are immediate onset of nystagmus and vertigo (peripheral disease has a latency period of 3 to 40 seconds), failure of nystagmus and vertigo to resolve (symptoms usually disappear within 30 seconds), and failure of the patient to adapt on repeated testing.

Laboratory Studies

Electronystagmography and *audiologic testing* are indicated when clinical and provocative data are insufficient to differentiate between central and peripheral causes of vertigo (see Chapter 212). An extensive battery of posturographic and other vestibular tests is reserved for those patients in whom the diagnosis is not apparent after history and initial physical examination. If acoustic neuroma is suspected, then one should consider *brainstem auditory evoked response* testing. It represents a cost-effective audiologic means of differentiating cochlear from retrocochlear disease. *MRI* of the internal auditory canal and cerebellopontine angle should follow if evidence of a retrocochlear lesion emerges from the clinical examination and audiologic testing. MRI is the most sensitive test for a small intracanalicular schwannoma. However, MRI is too often obtained simply to rule out a schwannoma in any dizzy patient. The probability of a patient with vertigo and no characteristic hearing loss having a vestibular schwannoma is less than 1 in

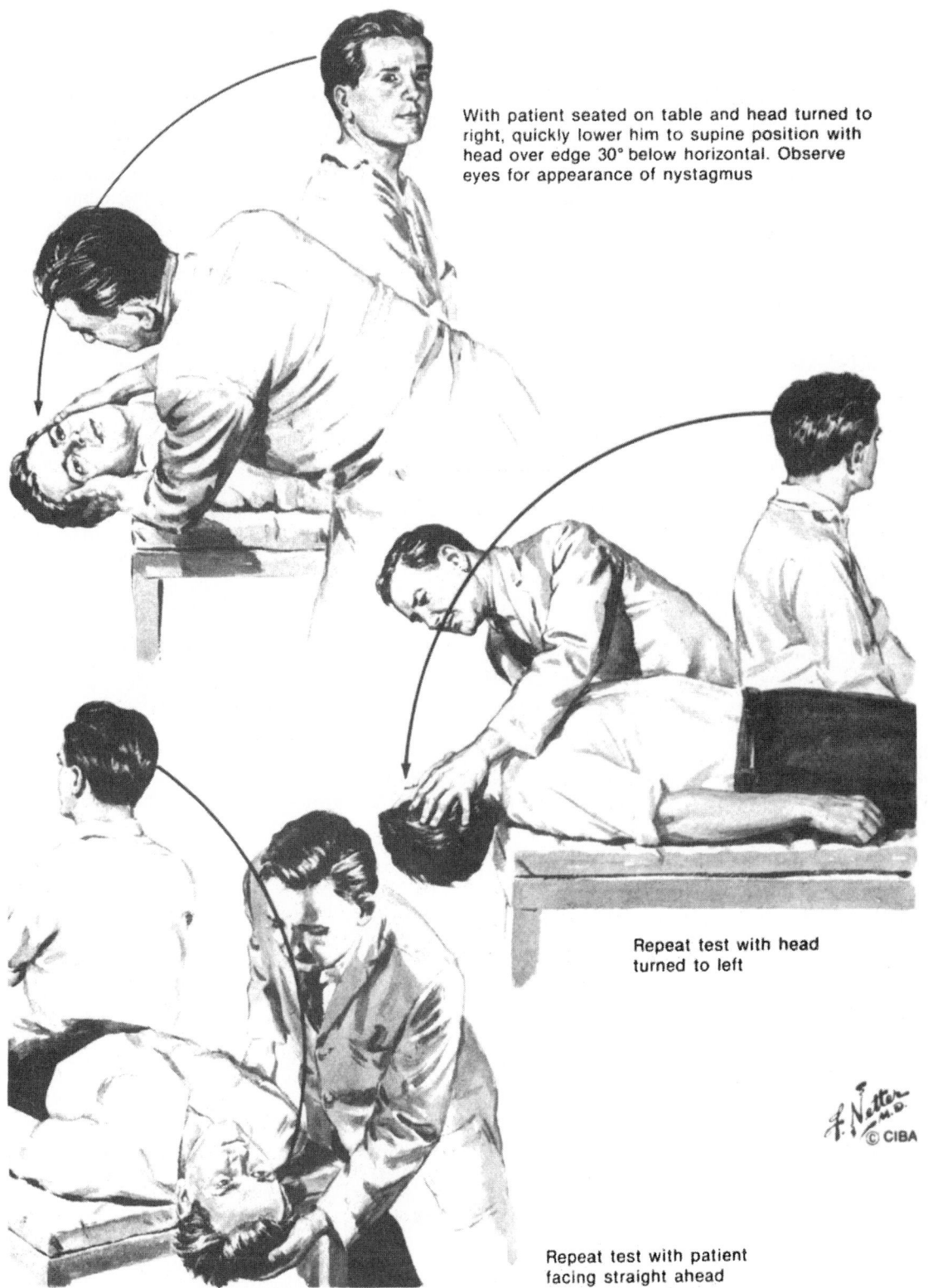

With patient seated on table and head turned to right, quickly lower him to supine position with head over edge 30° below horizontal. Observe eyes for appearance of nystagmus

Repeat test with head turned to left

Repeat test with patient facing straight ahead

FIG. 166.1. Bárány's test for vestibular disease. (©1981, Ciba Pharmaceutical Company, Division of Ciba-Geigy Corporation. Reproduced from Clinical Symposia by Frank H. Netter, M.D., with permission. All rights reserved.)

9,000; the probability increases slightly (to 1 in 600) for patients with dizziness and asymmetric hearing loss. If basilar transient ischemic attacks are suggested by transient, isolated vertiginous spells in a person with multiple atherosclerotic risk factors, then MRI with *magnetic resonance angiography* should be considered; it provides an excellent (although expensive) noninvasive means of detecting atheromatous disease of the vertebrobasilar circulation.

SYMPTOMATIC THERAPY AND PATIENT EDUCATION

Dizziness can be controlled in most instances and in some situations cured virtually at the first visit. Therapy is aimed at the underlying pathophysiology. The vast majority of people with dizziness have benign disorders. Symptomatic therapy combined with explanation and reassurance is always comforting and appreciated. In particular, patients tolerate their problems better when they know that in most instances the symptom can be controlled or will resolve on its own.

Peripheral Vestibular Disease. *Benign positional vertigo* responds to a bedside *maneuver* introduced by Epley. The maneuver relocates free-floating debris from the posterior semicircular canal into the vestibule of the vestibular labyrinth, where it no longer causes vertigo during head movement (Fig. 166.1). An 80% success rate after a single treatment is reported. The recurrence rate for a 30-month period is about 30%. Patients with a more widespread balance problem may benefit from *balance–vestibular rehabilitation therapy*. When carried out under the supervision of a trained therapist, such therapy can effectively reduce positionally provoked vertigo through vestibular "retraining " (i.e., adaptation of the central nervous system to a peripheral vestibular abnormality). The use of drugs such as *meclizine* (25 to 50 mg every 6 hours as needed) and *promethazine* (25 mg every 6 hours as needed) is now reserved for patients who have not responded satisfactorily to the Epley maneuver. Indeed, prolonged use of such vestibular suppressants may delay central adaptation. Moreover, these drugs are sedating and can cause drowsiness (which may be welcome to a patient having an acute attack but is an adverse effect in the treatment of chronic disease). Low-dose meclizine (12.5 mg three times daily) is quite sufficient in elderly patients and causes less sedation. Other drugs used to decrease acute vertigo include *dimenhydrinate* (Dramamine; 50 mg every 6 hours), which is more rapid in onset than meclizine, and the *benzodiazepines.*

Ménière's disease is usually managed with salt restriction and diuretics. Strong empiric evidence exists for restricting salt intake to the range of 1 g of sodium per day for 6 months to 1 year. Caffeine and alcohol should also be avoided. Diuretics (e.g., 250 mg of acetazolamide twice daily or 50 mg of hydrochlorothiazide twice daily) provide additional benefit.

Central Vestibular Disease. Whereas patients with peripheral causes of dizziness typically recover within months, patients with central causes of dizziness may be bothered for years.

Some patients may be helped with *lorazepam* (Ativan; 1 to 2 mg twice daily). *Gait training* and *vestibular exercises* under the supervision of a trained therapist may be beneficial. In patients with chronic vertigo, the goal is to retrain the eye and body musculature to compensate for the loss of vestibular input.

Multiple Sensory Deficits or Cerebellar Dysfunction benefits from the placement of handrails in the home, good lighting, and the use of a cane or walker. Vertigo and disequilibrium caused by lesions of the cerebellum, the area around and including the vestibular nucleus, or the floor of the fourth ventricle may be associated with persistent ataxia and nausea.

Cardiovascular Faintness also requires etiologic therapy supplemented by adequate hydration, standing up slowly, and discontinuing or reducing offending drugs (see Chapter 24). The patient with critical aortic stenosis should undergo evaluation for valve replacement (see Chapter 33).

Psychogenic Light-headedness may be refractory to symptomatic therapy, although *rebreathing into a paper bag* is effective for acute hyperventilation. Treatment with an *anxiolytic* agent may help, but it can also cause symptoms (see Chapter 226). *Antidepressant* therapy is indicated when depression is the predominant cause, although a side effect of some antidepressants is postural light-headedness (see Chapter 227).

ANNOTATED BIBLIOGRAPHY

Alexander MP. Mild traumatic brain injury: pathophysiology, natural history, and clinical management. Neurology 1995;45:1253. (*Review of postconcussive syndrome and frequency of complaints of dizziness.*)

Epley JM. Positional vertigo related to semicircular canalithiasis. Otolaryngol Head Neck Surg 1995;112:154. (*Report of postural repositioning maneuver that cures positional vertigo.*)

Fife TD. Bedside cure for benign positional vertigo. BNI Quarterly 1994;10:2. (*Another description of bedside positioning for patients with vertigo.*)

Furman JM, Cass SP. Benign paroxysmal positional vertigo. N Engl J Med 1999;341:1590. (*Good review of pathogenesis of benign positional vertigo, with discussion of examination and diagnostic criteria.*)

Gizzi M, Rosenberg ML. The diagnostic approach to the dizzy patient. Neurologist 1998;4:138. (*Audiometry, vestibular testing, and neuroimaging are discussed. If the patient is dizzy but has no abnormalities on examination and if progression of asymmetric hearing loss is not documented, neuroimaging is not recommended.*)

Kroenke K, Lucas CA, Rosenberg ML, et al. Causes of persistent dizziness: a prospective study of 100 patients in ambulatory care. Ann Intern Med 1992;117:898. (*Vestibular disease and psychiatric disorders were the most common causes.*)

Sullivan M, Clark MR, Katon WJ, et al. Psychiatric and otologic diagnoses in patients complaining of dizziness. Arch Intern Med 1993;153:1479. (*Psychiatric disease is common when vestibular disease is ruled out.*)

167

Focal Neurologic Complaints: Evaluation of Nerve Root and Peripheral Nerve Syndromes

AMY A. PRUITT

Primary physicians are frequently asked to evaluate complaints of focal numbness, tingling, weakness, pain, or some combination of these. In general, major acute neurologic disease is not at issue during an office visit. Nevertheless, the broad range of outpatient problems encountered encompasses lesions throughout the nervous system. Disorders of the nerve roots and peripheral nerves in the upper and lower extremities are especially common. The primary physician should be able to analyze several of these syndromes. The identification and localization of such problems can facilitate a thorough neurologic evaluation and accurately segregate those cases that must be referred to a neurologist.

PATHOPHYSIOLOGY AND CLINICAL PRESENTATION

Many peripheral nerves, because of their superficial location, are easily injured mechanically, and others are vulnerable because of specific anatomic variants or because of alterations in anatomy caused by degenerative disease.

Upper Extremity Syndromes

Cervical Radiculopathy and Myelopathy. Age-related loss of water and elasticity in cervical disks leads to increased stress on the vertebral bodies. Osteophytic spurs develop and may encroach on nerve roots. More serious but less common is encroachment on the spinal cord itself by progressive cervical spondylotic changes. Usually, a combination of radiculopathy involving the C-5, C-6, or C-7 roots (Figs. 167.1 and 167.2) and myelopathy is present. Cord compression resulting from spondylosis is indicated by radicular pain, variable weakness, diminished reflexes, and atrophy in the arms, with spastic weakness and hyperreflexia in the lower extremities.

It may be difficult to distinguish cervical spondylotic myelopathy from other progressive myelopathies, which include multiple sclerosis, subacute combined degeneration associated with vitamin B_{12} deficiency, spinal tumor, and syringomyelia. Suspicion of myelopathy should prompt referral to a neurologist.

Radiologic assessment usually includes *cervical spinal radiography*. Unfortunately, nearly 50% of patients older than age 50 show degenerative changes of the cervical spine on radiographic films, and these do not correlate well with the degree of abnormality found clinically in either radiculopathy or myelopathy. Nevertheless, plain films of the cervical spine with oblique views to visualize the neural foramina are often informative. *Magnetic resonance imaging* (MRI) is the best noninvasive test to assess the degree of cervical spondylosis or disk protrusion. It should be ordered when radicular pain is severe or when a motor or sensory deficit, reflex change, or myelopathic finding is present.

If the patient has only radiculopathy, a conservative trial of cervical traction is sometimes helpful (see Chapter 148). If myelopathy is suspected, myelography may be necessary to define the extent of compression, rule out neoplastic lesions, and assist the surgeon in making a decision about decompressive laminectomy.

Brachial Plexus Neuritis, a painfully disabling condition, develops in some patients after an immunization or viral infection and in others without any antecedent illness. It presents with severe pain in the shoulder and upper arm followed by weakness. Usually, the upper roots of the plexus are involved more than the lower ones. The prognosis is ultimately good, but recovery may be prolonged. Clinical examination reveals variable weakness and sensory loss in the C-5 to T-1 root distributions (Fig. 167.2), with diminished deep tendon reflexes. Because many nerve roots are involved, confusion with a cervical disk problem does not usually arise. Electromyography and nerve conduction studies help to localize the abnormality. MRI of the brachial plexus with gadolinium enhancement may be valuable in excluding neoplastic disease of the plexus.

Thoracic Outlet Syndrome. A cervical rib or bony abnormality of the first rib may cause pressure on the subclavian artery or brachial plexus as it passes through the thoracic outlet (Fig. 167.1). The diagnosis is primarily clinical and is based on the presence of pain in the arm in certain positions, color changes in the hand, and a pattern of sensory loss and weakness most pronounced in the fourth and fifth fingers. Deep tendon reflexes are usually normal. A bruit may be heard over the subclavian artery. The differential diagnosis includes Raynaud's phenomenon, ulnar nerve entrapment at the elbow, and compression of the brachial plexus by neoplasm or fibrosis resulting from radiation.

Radiography of the cervical spine is extremely important to demonstrate cervical ribs or elongated transverse processes of the seventh cervical vertebra. Results of electromyography may be entirely normal, but it will help to exclude a defect at the elbow or a carpal tunnel syndrome. Ultrasonography of the subclavian artery with the arm held in different positions may help define the extent of compression.

Most surgeons advocate removal of the potentially constricting structures (cervical rib, fascial band to first rib, or first rib). Shoulder exercises to improve posture are often advised first, and orthopedic advice should be sought in each case.

Long Thoracic Nerve Entrapment. This nerve arises from the brachial plexus and innervates the serratus anterior. It is vul-

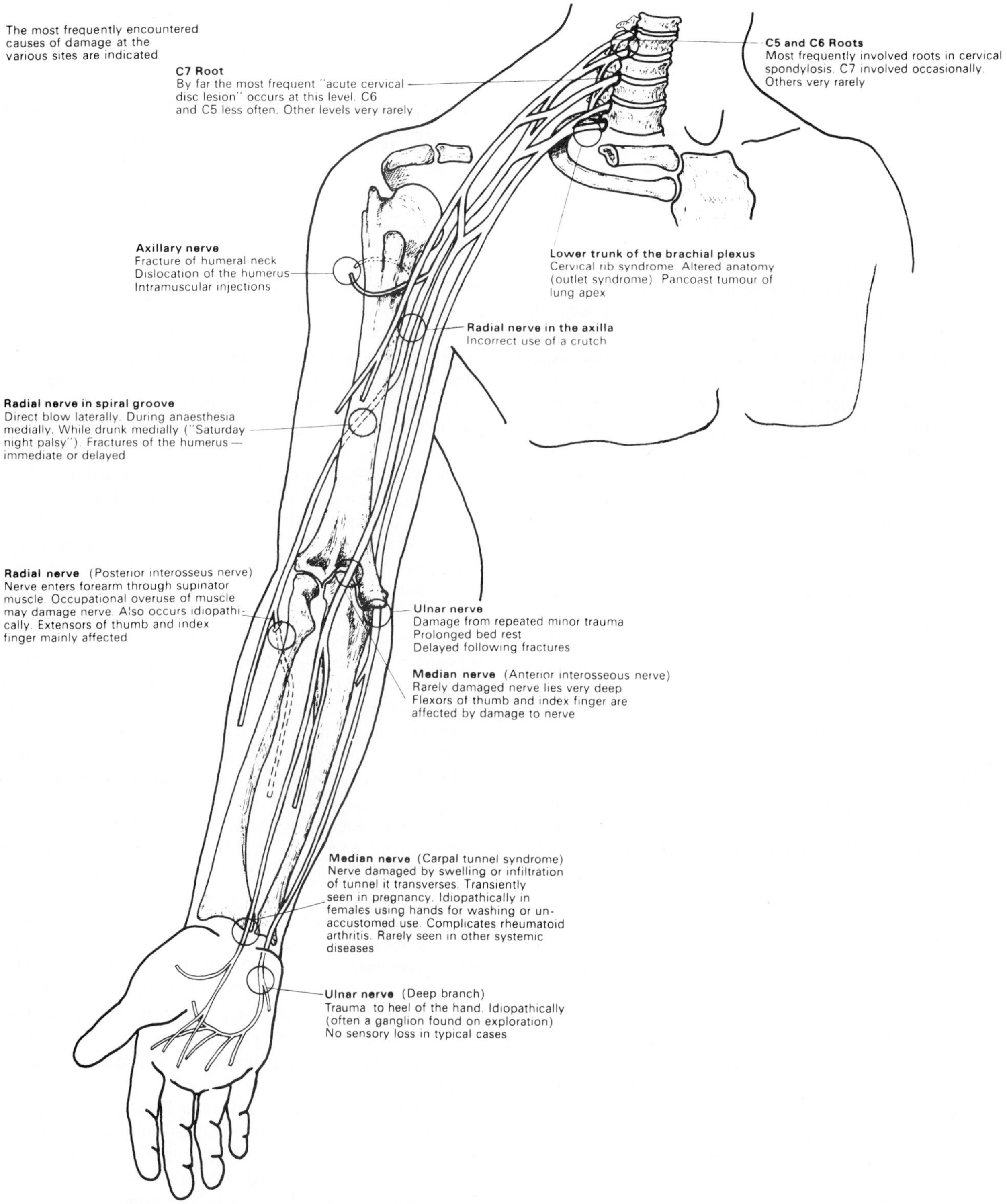

The most frequently encountered causes of damage at the various sites are indicated

C7 Root
By far the most frequent "acute cervical disc lesion" occurs at this level. C6 and C5 less often. Other levels very rarely

C5 and C6 Roots
Most frequently involved roots in cervical spondylosis. C7 involved occasionally. Others very rarely

Axillary nerve
Fracture of humeral neck
Dislocation of the humerus
Intramuscular injections

Lower trunk of the brachial plexus
Cervical rib syndrome. Altered anatomy (outlet syndrome). Pancoast tumour of lung apex

Radial nerve in the axilla
Incorrect use of a crutch

Radial nerve in spiral groove
Direct blow laterally. During anaesthesia medially. While drunk medially ("Saturday night palsy"). Fractures of the humerus — immediate or delayed

Radial nerve (Posterior interosseus nerve)
Nerve enters forearm through supinator muscle. Occupational overuse of muscle may damage nerve. Also occurs idiopathically. Extensors of thumb and index finger mainly affected

Ulnar nerve
Damage from repeated minor trauma
Prolonged bed rest
Delayed following fractures

Median nerve (Anterior interosseous nerve)
Rarely damaged nerve lies very deep
Flexors of thumb and index finger are affected by damage to nerve

Median nerve (Carpal tunnel syndrome)
Nerve damaged by swelling or infiltration of tunnel it transverses. Transiently seen in pregnancy. Idiopathically in females using hands for washing or unaccustomed use. Complicates rheumatoid arthritis. Rarely seen in other systemic diseases

Ulnar nerve (Deep branch)
Trauma to heel of the hand. Idiopathically (often a ganglion found on exploration) No sensory loss in typical cases

FIG. 167.1. Peripheral nerve distribution to the upper limb. (From Patten J. Neurological differential diagnosis. New York: Springer-Verlag, 1977, with permission.)

nerable to injury in workers who lift or push heavy loads, occurs after direct trauma from heavy backpacks, and may evolve for several months after the injury. The patient notes a change in the appearance of the shoulder, and examination reveals winging of the scapula. Most cases have a good prognosis.

Carpal Tunnel Syndrome. In this disorder, the median nerve is entrapped at the carpal tunnel (Fig. 167.1) because of pressure from ligamentous thickening. Most cases are idiopathic, but the disorder may be seen with rheumatoid arthritis, pregnancy, acromegaly, hypothyroidism, fractures of the carpal

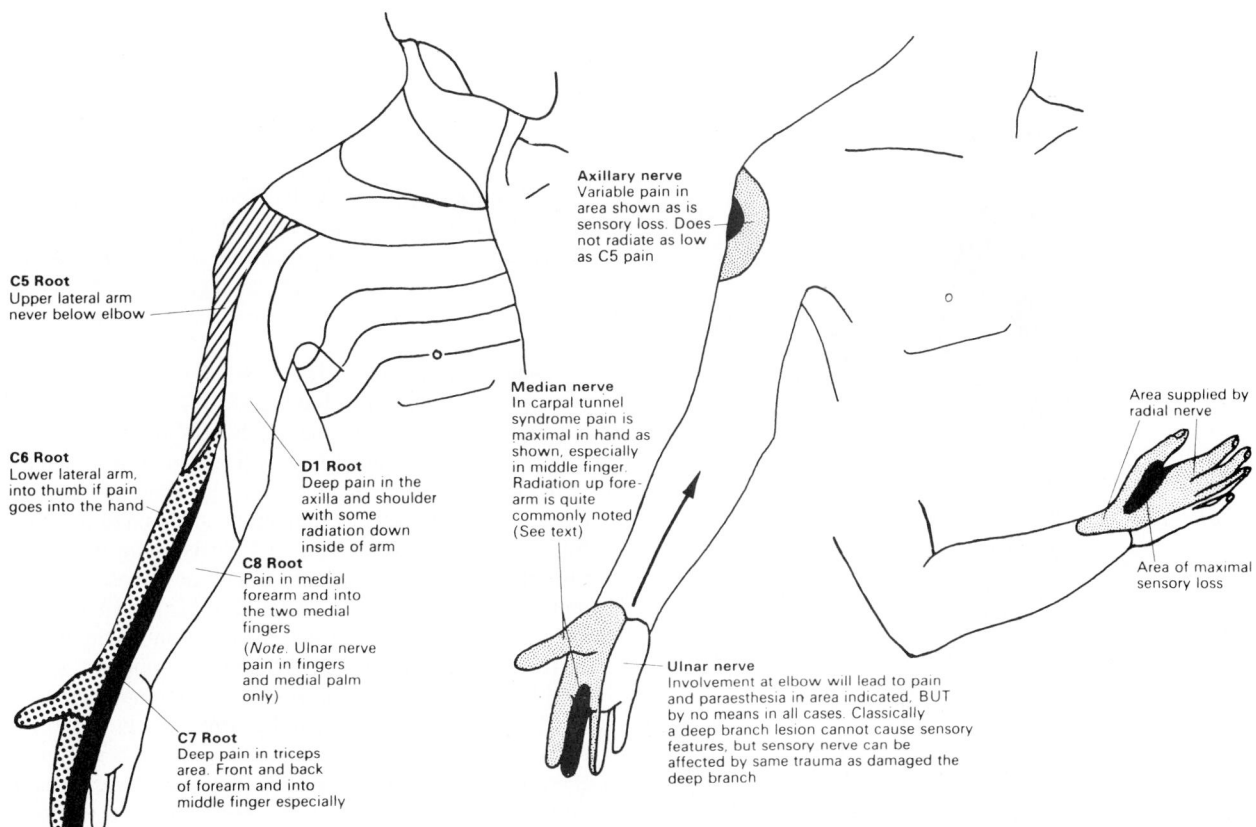

FIG. 167.2.   Left: Distribution of root pain and paresthesia. **Right:** Distribution of peripheral nerve pain and paresthesia. (From Patten J. Neurological differential diagnosis. New York: Springer-Verlag, 1977, with permission.)

bones, amyloidosis, and myeloma. Occupational causes involving repetitive traumatic actions have been implicated. A combination of pain, paresthesias, and numbness in the median nerve distribution is the earliest complaint; symptoms are often worse at night (Fig. 167.2). Later, muscle weakness (particularly of thumb abduction and apposition) occurs, and thenar atrophy may be seen. Importantly, aching pain can be felt as far up as the shoulder and should not distract the examiner's attention from the wrist. Tapping on the wrist or anywhere else along the median nerve may reproduce the pain (*Tinel's sign*).

The differential diagnosis includes radiculopathy from cervical spine disease, but the exact location of the pain should conform to the median nerve rather than to the distribution of just one nerve root. Electromyography and *nerve conduction studies* with motor and sensory conduction latencies of the median nerve provide the most useful data. Although some cases respond to conservative therapy (wrist splints, antiinflammatory medications), surgical relief is relatively easy and effective. Failure to respond to surgical therapy should prompt rechecking of the nerve conduction studies, careful reexamination, and consideration of the possibility of coexistent cervical spine disease or of median nerve compression higher in the forearm.

Ulnar Nerve Entrapment. The most common location of ulnar entrapment is the elbow (Fig. 167.1). Causes include fracture deformities, arthritis, faulty positioning of the arm during surgery, or repetitive occupational or recreational trauma (e.g.,

tennis). Sensation is usually spared in the forearm, but sensory loss occurs in the fifth finger and half of the fourth (Fig. 167.2). Wasting of the intrinsic muscles of the hand with weakness of grip occurs later. Nerve conduction studies can accurately localize the site of compression. If focal entrapment is present, repositioning of the nerve or elbow synovectomy may be necessary, but patients with trauma, diabetes, or the so-called "tardy" ulnar palsies (dysfunction developing late after injury) may not improve.

Radial Nerve Injuries. Compression of the radial nerve most often occurs in the axilla or upper arm. It may be caused by improperly used crutches, prolonged pressure during sleep (the "Saturday night" palsy), or direct injury. Wrist drop is the prominent feature. Vasomotor or atrophic changes are rarely present, and prognosis is good (recovery within 6 to 8 weeks).

Lower Extremity Syndromes

Lateral Femoral Cutaneous Nerve Compression. Also known as *meralgia paresthetica*, this syndrome involves a nerve formed by branches arising from the second and third lumbar roots. The nerve enters the thigh in close relation to the inguinal ligament, the anterior superior iliac spine, and the sartorius muscle insertion (Fig. 167.3). It is purely sensory and supplies the anterolateral and lateral aspects of the thigh almost as far as the knee (Fig. 167.4). Compression causes an extremely unpleasant, characteristic burning pain with increased

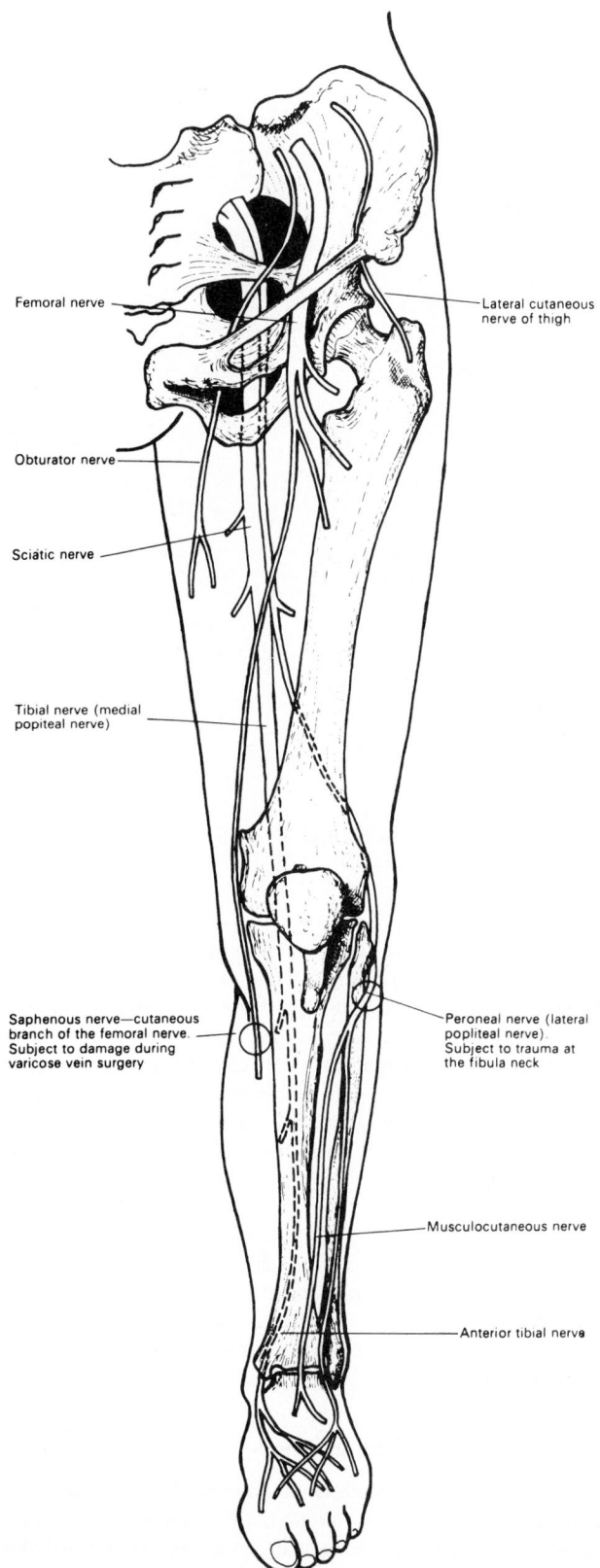

Femoral nerve

Lateral cutaneous nerve of thigh

Obturator nerve

Sciatic nerve

Tibial nerve (medial popliteal nerve)

Saphenous nerve—cutaneous branch of the femoral nerve. Subject to damage during varicose vein surgery

Peroneal nerve (lateral popliteal nerve). Subject to trauma at the fibula neck

Musculocutaneous nerve

Anterior tibial nerve

FIG. 167.3. Peripheral nerve distribution to the lower limb. (From Patten J. Neurological differential diagnosis. New York: Springer-Verlag, 1977, with permission)

cutaneous sensitivity. Sitting or lying usually provides relief, but standing or walking exacerbates the pain. The syndrome often occurs in obesity, in pregnancy, or when tight corsets are worn. It is more common in diabetics. The differential diagnosis includes a lesion of the second or third lumbar roots, usually associated with low back pain radiating into the lower leg. Sensory changes in this case will extend further down the leg and more medially, and iliopsoas or quadriceps weakness is present. Weakness and reflex changes do not occur in meralgia paresthetica. The neuropathy tends to regress spontaneously, but weight loss should be encouraged.

Femoral Neuropathy. The femoral nerve derives from the second, third, and fourth lumbar roots. Its posterior division is the major innervation to the quadriceps and terminates as the saphenous nerve, which supplies sensation to the medial aspect of the leg as far as the medial malleolus (Fig. 167.3). The onset of femoral neuropathy is frequently sudden and painful and is followed quickly by wasting and weakness in the quadriceps, loss of knee jerk, and sensory impairment over the anteromedial thigh (Fig. 167.4). If marked hip flexion weakness is also present, the site of the lesion is usually in the lumbar plexus. Sensory symptoms in the saphenous distribution are uncommon in lesions of the main trunk of the femoral nerve.

Entrapment may occur in the inguinal region and from direct retroperitoneal compression by tumor or hematoma. However, the most common cause is presumed to be nerve infarction, seen usually in diabetics. A combination of thigh pain, weakness, and sensory deficit can be a manifestation of an isolated diabetic femoral neuropathy, although electromyographically, the involvement in such cases is frequently more widespread. Although some improvement may occur, the patient is often left quite weak.

Sciatic Nerve Syndromes. The sciatic nerve arises from the lumbosacral plexus (L-4 through S-3) and terminates in the common peroneal and tibial nerves (Fig. 167.3). The tibial nerve supplies the gastrocnemius, plantaris, soleus, and popliteus muscles, and its extension into the calf, the posterior tibial nerve, supplies muscles of the calf. All these muscles are involved in plantar flexion. The common peroneal nerve divides into the superficial and deep peroneal nerves. The latter supplies the muscles of dorsiflexion of the foot and toes. The superficial peroneal nerve innervates the muscles that evert the foot.

Sciatic nerve compression may result from tumors within the pelvis or from prolonged sitting or lying on the buttocks. Gluteal abscesses and misplaced buttock injections have caused sciatic injury. Weakness of the gluteal muscles and pain in the area of the sciatic notch imply compression within the pelvis. Lesions just beyond the sciatic notch cause weakness in the hamstrings and in all the muscles of the lower leg.

Common peroneal compression usually occurs at the level of the fibular head (Fig. 167.3) and is seen in cachectic patients following prolonged bed rest, alcoholics, diabetics, and patients placed in tight casts. Injury leads to faulty dorsiflexion and eversion of the foot, which produces a characteristic foot drop with a slapping gait. Complete or partial recovery can be expected when paralysis results from transient pressure. Treatment consists of a foot brace and careful avoidance of compressive positions.

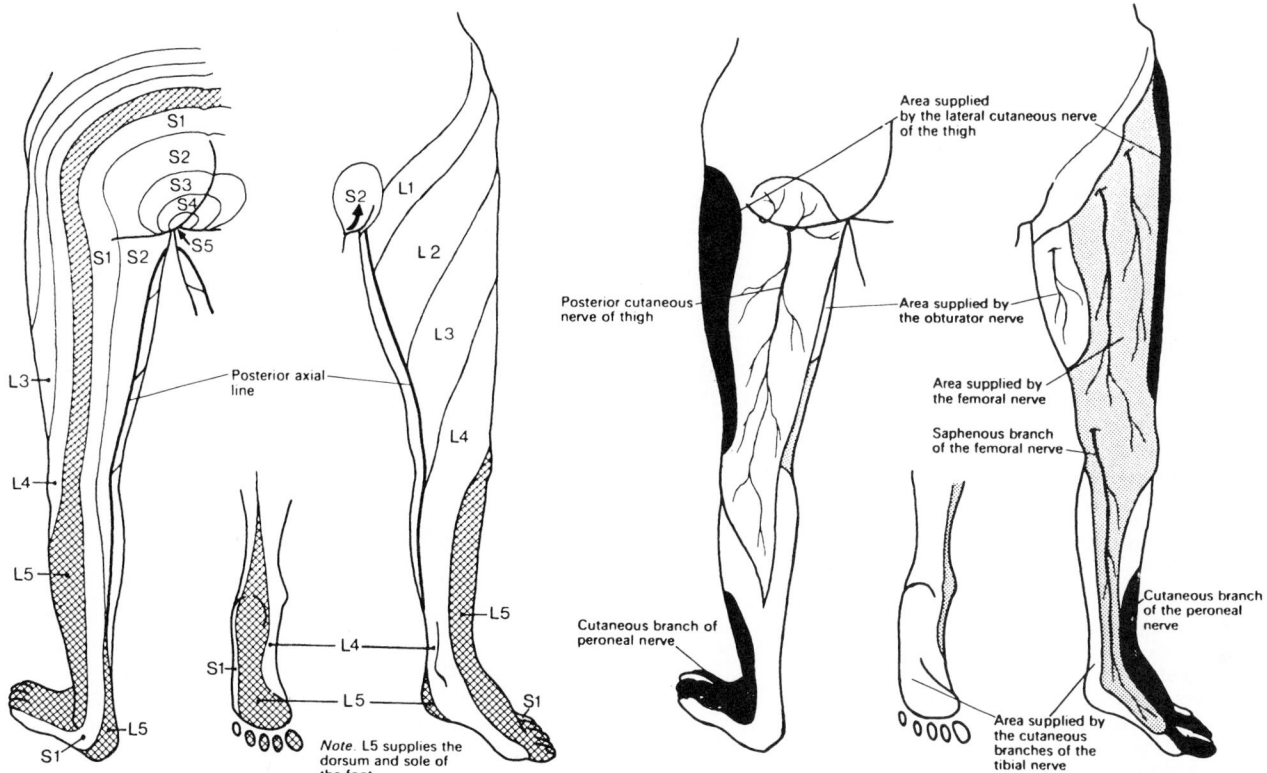

FIG. 167.4.   Left: Lumbosacral dermatomes. **Right:** Peripheral nerve distribution to the lower limb. (From Patten J. Neurological differential diagnosis. New York: Springer-Verlag, 1977, with permission.)

Lumbar Disk Syndromes. Compressive neuropathies of the lower limbs must be distinguished from the very common lumbar disk syndromes. In the lumbar region, the fourth and fifth disks are most frequently affected (i.e., the disks between the L-4 and L-5 vertebral bodies and between the L-5 and S-1 vertebrae). The most common complaint is the sudden onset of severe low back pain (see Chapter 147). The inciting event is often trivial, although heavy lifting or an acute twisting motion is sometimes reported. The pain is worsened by bending forward, sneezing, or straining.

The herniated disk can compress one or more nerve roots, but a disk herniation at a particular level generally causes a distinctive picture (see Chapter 147). *Herniation of the L4-5 disk* usually affects the L-5 root, causing pain over the sciatic notch, lateral thigh, and leg; numbness of the web of the great toe and lateral leg; weakness of dorsiflexion of the great toe and foot; and no reflex changes (Fig. 167.4). *Herniation of the disk between L-5 and S-1* catches the S-1 root, producing pain down the back of the leg to the heel; numbness in the lateral heel, foot, and toe; weakness of plantar flexion; and loss of the ankle jerk (Fig. 167.4). Once the root level is defined, the usual course is a trial of conservative therapy (see Chapter 147). However, when any combination of progressive limb weakness and numbness (especially if bilateral), uncontrollable pain, saddle anesthesia (numbness in the distribution of S-2 and S-3), and bladder and bowel dysfunction is noted, then emergent MRI examination (or myelography if MRI is not available) is needed to rule out *cauda equina syndrome.* Imaging of the spinal canal is required to detect any caudal compression and to rule out more unusual causes of lumbar radiculopathy, such as neurofibroma. MRI may also be helpful in predicting the response of a patient with disk disease to conservative therapy.

Peripheral Polyneuropathy. When patients present with distal, symmetric sensorimotor or predominantly motor symptoms and are found to have diminished sensation or motor abnormalities in a "stocking–glove" distribution with variably hypoactive deep tendon reflexes, they are likely to have a peripheral polyneuropathy. The list of causes is extensive (Table 167.1). Although most produce some degree of motor and sensory dysfunction, usually one component predominates. Sensorimotor conditions present principally with sensory deficits, although a more mixed picture develops later. Diabetes is a common source of sensorimotor polyneuropathy; symptoms respond to a tightening of glucose control (see Chapter 102). Alcoholism, deficiencies of B vitamins, renal failure, hypothyroidism, AIDS, and paraneoplastic syndromes are among the other causes. The most dramatic of the predominantly motor polyneuropathies is Guillain-Barré syndrome, an acquired autoimmune disease; the typical presentation is one of acute onset following a viral illness and rapid progression of ascending weakness over a few days in conjunction with a loss of deep tendon reflexes. Other predominantly motor polyneuropathies include those associated with monoclonal gammopathy, toxin exposure, and porphyria. A predominantly sensory polyneuropathy is seen with amyloidosis, paraneoplastic syndromes, vitamin B_6 excess, and Sjögren's syndrome.

Table 167.1. Important Peripheral Polyneuropathies

Predominantly Motor
A. Acute (days)
   1. Guillain-Barré syndrome
   2. Diphtheria
   3. Porphyria
   4. Toxin (organophosphate exposure)
B. Subacute (weeks to 1–2 years)
   1. Toxin exposure (lead poisoning, glue sniffing)
   2. Paraproteinemia
C. Chronic
   1. Hereditary (Charcot-Marie-Tooth disease)

Predominantly Sensory
A. Acute (days)
   1. None
B. Subacute (weeks to 1–2 years)
   1. Amyloidosis
   2. Drug toxicity (cisplatin, vitamin B$_6$ excess)
   3. Paraneoplastic syndrome
   4. Sjögren's syndrome
C. Chronic (years)
   1. Hereditary sensory neuropathy

Sensorimotor
A. Acute (days)
   1. Toxin exposure (arsenic)
B. Subacute (weeks to 1–2 years)
   1. Diabetes
   2. Alcohol abuse
   3. B-vitamin deficiency
   4. Renal failure
   5. Hypothyroidism
   6. Connective tissue disease
   7. Paraneoplastic syndrome
   8. Drug toxicity (isoniazid, cancer chemotherapeutic agents)
   9. AIDS
C. Chronic (years)
   1. Charcot-Marie-Tooth disease

Adapted from American College of Physicians Medical Knowledge Self-assessment Program IX, 1991, 106, with permission.

WORKUP

Peripheral Polyneuropathy

The primary physician's objective should be to discern by history and physical examination any diagnostically important variations in the peripheral polyneuropathy theme.

History includes a review of duration (years suggests a hereditary cause; weeks to months, a toxic/metabolic cause or a paraproteinemia; days, a toxin or Guillain-Barré syndrome). The distribution helps distinguish between polyneuropathy and diabetic mononeuropathy multiplex, which is more multifocal. Medication exposure is essential to review (e.g., cisplatin, isoniazid, vincristine), as are habits (alcohol abuse), diet (especially in regard to deficiencies of B vitamins), and concurrent medical illnesses (diabetes, renal failure, liver disease, cancer).

Physical Examination clarifies the relative sensory and motor components of the problem, helpful in differentiation. Signs of systemic disease may also be revealed.

Laboratory Studies should include a complete blood cell count and a determination of the erythrocyte sedimentation rate and values for blood glucose, serum liver chemistries, blood urea nitrogen, creatinine, and thyroid-stimulating hormone. Chest radiography and immunoelectrophoresis should be per-

formed. Although patients whose neuropathy is apparent from the results of the above studies (e.g., diabetic polyneuropathy) may not require *electromyography*, this procedure helps to differentiate between demyelinating disease and axonal polyneuropathy, and between root or plexus and more distal nerve trunk involvements, distinctions that are of considerable diagnostic importance. Electromyography also distinguishes upper from lower motor neuron weakness. *Nerve biopsy* is infrequently recommended; its main indication is in hereditary disorders, multifocal mononeuropathy multiplex, or asymmetric clinical syndromes, in which it can reveal such underlying conditions as vasculitis, amyloidosis, or sarcoidosis. Patients with monoclonal gammopathy may profit from tests for *antibody to myelin-associated glycoprotein* (*anti-MAG antibody*) and *anti-GM1 antibody*; these tests can identify patients who are candidates for plasmapheresis or immunosuppressive therapy.

Other Peripheral Nerve Syndromes

Identification of the nerve root or peripheral nerve syndrome and precise localization of the neurologic lesion is possible in the office setting. Assessment is facilitated by determining (a) whether the problem is peripheral (in a nerve root or peripheral nerve) or central (in the cord or above); (b) whether the problem, if peripheral, is caused by a lesion in the peripheral nerve or by nerve root injury; (c) whether evidence of cord compression (manifested by signs of myelopathy) is present, particularly in upper extremity syndromes; (d) whether evidence (in other extremities) of more widespread peripheral neuropathy is present (e.g., the diabetic patient with a femoral neuropathy who also has a diffuse peripheral neuropathy); and (e) whether weakness is caused by a muscle or nerve lesion.

The neurologic examination should be organized to address these issues and answer the following questions:

1. Is the lesion an upper motor neuron or a lower motor neuron lesion? Fasciculations, flaccidity, and a lack of reflexes indicate a lower motor neuron lesion and suggest that the disorder originates at the anterior horn cell or peripheral nerve level. Spasticity and increased reflexes are evidence for a lesion above the anterior horn cell that supplies the involved musculature. Thus, a cervical disk at the C-6 level might decrease the biceps reflex and cause biceps weakness and atrophy, while increasing reflexes and causing spasticity below that level.

2. Is the nerve dysfunction confined to one root or dermatome or to one peripheral nerve? A positive answer to this question suggests a compression neuropathy such as a radial, ulnar, or median nerve palsy. Findings of more generalized dysfunction, such as diffusely decreased deep tendon reflexes, absent vibration sense at the ankles, and a stocking–glove pattern of sensory loss, suggest a more diffuse peripheral neuropathy. Commonly seen forms of peripheral neuropathy include those associated with diabetes mellitus, excess alcohol consumption, toxin and drug exposure, and genetic conditions such as Charcot-Marie-Tooth disease. An electromyogram can localize the individual nerve abnormality and confirm the presence of a generalized neuropathy.

3. Is the weakness caused by nerve or by muscle disease? Weakness in conjunction with altered tendon reflexes and sensory loss suggests nerve disease. In primary muscle dis-

ease, reflexes and normal sensation are preserved. Characteristic patterns of muscle weakness occur in the genetically determined muscular dystrophies. The toxic and metabolic myopathies produce largely proximal muscle weakness, in contrast to almost all the primary nerve diseases, which affect distal musculature early and preferentially. Serum muscle enzyme elevations are seen in muscle disease, and some muscular disorders are associated with myotonia. The electromyogram, coupled with nerve conduction studies, can distinguish primary muscle disease from neuropathic processes.

The clinical identification of nerve root and peripheral nerve syndromes is often facilitated by the selective use of radiologic, nerve conduction, electromyographic, and serologic studies (detailed in discussions of each of the important syndromes). However, laboratory studies are usually not necessary during the initial assessment.

INDICATIONS FOR REFERRAL AND ADMISSION

Evidence of acute spinal cord or cauda equina compression is an indication for immediate neurosurgical consultation and hospitalization. The patient with symptoms and signs of a slowly progressive myelopathy requires neurologic consultation and MRI. Vitamin B_{12} deficiency, multiple sclerosis, and tumor all need to be considered in patients with a progressive myelopathy if mechanical cord compression is excluded by MRI. A root or peripheral nerve compression syndrome may require surgical repair, and the patient with such a problem will need to see a neurosurgeon or orthopedist skilled in its treatment. Nevertheless, before referral, the primary physician should have localized the problem and instituted appropriate initial therapy.

SYMPTOMATIC MANAGEMENT OF PAINFUL PERIPHERAL NEUROPATHY

The mainstay of therapy for painful peripheral neuropathy has been the *tricyclic antidepressants* (e.g., amitriptyline, nortriptyline). *Gabapentin* (Neurontin) has proved similarly effective and is reasonably well tolerated but is much more expensive than generic tricyclic therapy. Other drugs used to treat painful polyneuropathy include mexiletine and topical agents such as *capsaicin* and *lidocaine*. The treatment of painful polyneuropathy requires frequent adjustments of medication type and dose. Some patients may inquire about the efficacy of *plasmapheresis*, which is extremely useful in myasthenia gravis and chronic inflammatory demyelinating polyneuropathy. It is now administered less often in acute Guillain-Barré syndrome in part because IV immune globulin is being increasingly used to treat this condition. Plasmapheresis is also useful in monoclonal gammopathy–associated peripheral neuropathy. Patients with other peripheral neuropathic syndromes are less likely to benefit, and the primary physician should be aware of the lim-

ited value of expensive plasmapheresis in conditions other than those mentioned above.

ANNOTATED BIBLIOGRAPHY

Aids to the diagnosis of peripheral nerve injuries (Medical Research Council). London: Bailliere Tindall, 1986. (*A classic; lucid illustrations and diagrams of the function and examination of every clinically important peripheral nerve. This is a great investment and should be on the shelf of every primary care physician.*)

Asbury AK. Understanding diabetic neuropathy. N Engl J Med 1988;319:577. (*A very thorough review, with good tables, of this most common and important of peripheral neuropathies.*)

Bella I, Chad DA. Neuromuscular disorders and acute respiratory failure. Neurologic Clinics 1998;16:391. (*An excellent guide to the more emergent causes of rapidly progressive weakness, with good guidelines for respiratory management and acute triage.*)

Clark WF, Borkc GA, Buskard N, et al. Therapeutic plasma exchange: an update from the Canadian apheresis group. Ann Intern Med 1999;131:453. (*Review of data from 103,416 plasma exchanges during a 17-year period. Among the neurologic conditions for which this procedure is appropriate are myasthenia gravis, chronic inflammatory polyneuropathy, and Guillain-Barré syndrome. The use of pheresis in other polyneuropathies and most cases of multiple sclerosis is not supported by the literature.*)

Dawson DM. Entrapment neuropathies of the upper extremities. N Engl J Med 1993;329:2013. (*A nice review of carpal tunnel, ulnar, and thoracic outlet syndromes.*)

Delamonte SM. Peripheral neuropathy in the acquired immune deficiency syndrome. Ann Neurol 1988;28:485. (*This demyelinating neuropathy is being seen with increasing frequency by primary physicians and should be recognized.*)

Dyck PJ. The 10 P's: a mnemonic helpful in the characterization and differential diagnosis of peripheral neuropathy. Neurology 1992;42:14. (*It's actually a tough mnemonic, but the article is helpful in delineating the principles of classification and reviewing peripheral neuropathy.*)

Dyck PJ. Plasma exchange in polyneuropathy associated with monoclonal gammopathy of undetermined significance. N Engl J Med 1991;325:1482. (*This new treatment modality and the therapeutic efficacy of IV immune globulin are reasons for pursuing a diagnosis with immunoelectrophoresis and antibody studies.*)

Galer BS. Painful polyneuropathy. Neurol Clin 1998;16:791. (*Excellent review of clinical data supporting various oral and topical medications for polyneuropathy.*)

Morello CD, Leckband SG, Stoner CP, et al. Randomized, double-blind study comparing the efficacy of gabapentin with amitriptyline on diabetic peripheral neuropathy pain. Arch Intern Med 1999;159:1831. (*The study lacks significant power, but the results were promising, although gabapentin doses were low.*)

Sater RA, Rostami A. Treatment of Guillain-Barré syndrome with intravenous immunoglobulin. Neurology 1998;51[Suppl 5]):S9. (*Excellent summary of results with pheresis, IV immune globulin, or both.*)

Woolf CJ, Mannion RJ. Neuropathic pain: aetiology, symptoms, mechanisms, and management. Lancet 1999;353:1959. (*Excellent scholarly review emphasizing the mechanisms of action of available and investigational medicines.*)

168
Evaluation of Tremor
AMY A. PRUITT

Tremor is best defined as a regular oscillation of a body part, and it must be distinguished from other rapid, involuntary movements. Many patients assume that the development of "shakiness" is a natural concomitant of aging. The physician must determine the significance of a variety of clinically similar tremors that may have widely dissimilar diagnostic, therapeutic, and prognostic implications. Workup involves differentiating the resting tremor of early parkinsonism from essential tremor, and differentiating essential tremor from an exaggerated physiologic tremor. As new specific treatments are developed, accurate clinical distinction becomes increasingly valuable. Unfortunately, it may be difficult to differentiate tremors by clinical observation alone, and evaluation requires a working knowledge of simple electrophysiologic and pharmacologic characteristics.

PATHOPHYSIOLOGY AND CLINICAL PRESENTATION

The precise neural mechanisms of tremor remain unknown despite some clinicopathologic correlations, such as abolition of the parkinsonian and essential tremors by lesions in the ventrolateral nucleus of the thalamus. Drugs such as L-dopa, which are known to act centrally to increase catecholamines, may worsen essential tremor; this observation has led to the suggestion that β-adrenergic blockers such as propranolol may exert their therapeutic action by central antagonism of β-adrenergic receptors.

The patient most frequently reports the insidious onset of "shaking" of a limb. Very likely, the patient will have ignored the symptom initially, assuming it was a consequence of nervousness or fatigue. However, steady progression impels the patient to see the physician. Tremors can be present during maintenance of a posture, at rest, or during an action (intention tremor).

Postural or Physiologic Tremors are fine tremors with a frequency of 8 to 12 Hz; they occur normally in everyone during movement and while a fixed position is held. A true physiologic tremor is defined as one that does not produce symptoms and is within the given frequency range. The movement is usually invisible to the naked eye, but it may become exaggerated by anxiety, ingestion of coffee, or hyperthyroidism. Drugs, notably lithium and tricyclic antidepressants, may also accentuate this tremor. Amplitude and frequency vary among different people and in the same person at different times. Physiologic tremors are unaffected by propranolol or alcohol.

Intention Tremors. The major intention tremors are those labeled *"essential"* (also referred to as *"familial"* or *"senile"*). Half of cases are transmitted as an autosomal dominant trait, and half are sporadic. The condition is characterized by an intention tremor of the hands, head, voice, and sometimes legs or trunk. Typically, the tremor is most prominent when the hands or head are held outstretched in a position against gravity, and least noticeable at rest (although the tremor of early parkinsonism may also be seen best in an outstretched hand). Tremor may be accentuated by tasks that require precision, such as writing, carrying full cups of liquid (also seen in some patients with parkinsonism). Many patients report that the ingestion of a small amount of alcohol will temporarily reduce their tremor. Essential tremor may begin at any age, although early and late adult life are the most common periods of onset (which helps to differentiate the condition from parkinsonism, which typically begins in middle age).

A more dramatic action tremor is displayed by patients with *cerebellar diseases* and is characterized by progressively increasing amplitude of the tremor as the patient brings the limb toward a target. In younger patients, this is most frequently caused by multiple sclerosis, but similar clinical states may be produced by cerebellar infarction, degenerative disorders of the spinocerebellar pathways, and chronic relapsing steroid-sensitive polyneuropathy. This tremor is multiplanar, with large, irregular, and relatively slow (2 to 4 Hz) oscillations. The tremor often is worsened by alcohol. Propranolol has no effect, and no satisfactory therapy is available.

Rest Tremors. The most common rest tremor in a relaxed, supported limb is that caused by *Parkinson's disease*. It characteristically begins in the fingers and may later involve the arm and the leg. Flexion and extension of the fingers, abduction and adduction of the thumbs, and pronation and supination of the wrist produce the well-known "pill-rolling" movement. Frequently, this is the symptom that brings parkinsonian patients to the physician, and it may occur well in advance of the bradykinesia and postural difficulties characteristic of the full-blown syndrome. It is important, of course, to distinguish this tremor from essential tremor, which requires a different treatment and portends a different prognosis. The parkinsonian tremor is slow (3 to 8 Hz), and its electromyogragraphic (EMG) pattern, quite unlike that of essential tremor, shows alternating discharge in antagonistic muscle groups. This EMG activity is suppressed with voluntary movement.

A few parkinsonian patients may also have a typical action (essential) tremor, and L-dopa therapy may worsen it. Phenothiazines and haloperidol worsen the rest tremor (see Chapter 174).

Other Abnormal Movements. The definition of tremor as a regular oscillation of a body part serves to distinguish it from other rapid, intermittent movements that bespeak a different neurologic state. For diagnostic, therapeutic, and prognostic purposes, several categories of abnormal involuntary movements should be distinguished from tremor. All the following involuntary movements (and most true tremors) are greatly reduced or disappear altogether with sleep.

Tics are repetitive, coordinated, usually stereotyped movements that are seen widely in the population and increase in frequency in a given patient in response to stress. They usually involve face or hand muscles, may initially be a conscious mannerism, and usually can be suppressed by voluntary effort. *Hemifacial spasm* is a kind of oscillating movement usually beginning in a middle-aged or elderly person, localized to the facial muscles. It is thought to be caused by degenerative lesions of the facial nucleus or peripheral nerve, but the exact mechanism is unknown, and treatment is unsatisfactory.

Asterixis is an irregular contraction of skeletal muscles that results in flapping of the hands; it is electromyographically coincident with brief pauses at irregular intervals. *Chorea* is an irregular, jerking movement usually involving the fingers and often accompanied by *athetosis*, in which writhing movements of limbs or trunk may be added. *Epilepsia partialis continua* refers to a focal seizure in which continuous seizure activity may result in a somewhat rhythmic jerking of one body part. Sudden onset of the illness is the most useful distinguishing feature here.

Dyskinesias are rhythmic, involuntary movements of the orofacial musculature resulting in tongue protrusion and chewing movements. These are important to recognize because of the frequency with which they occur as early manifestations of the tardive dyskinesia syndrome caused by use of phenothiazines and other major tranquilizers.

DIFFERENTIAL DIAGNOSIS

Tremors can be divided clinically into postural, intention, and resting types. Most postural tremors are physiologic. Among the intention tremors are the essential, senile, and cerebellar varieties. Most resting tremors are caused by Parkinson's disease. Tremors must be distinguished from other voluntary movements such as dyskinesias, tics, myoclonus, and athetosis.

WORKUP

History. The clinical assessment of tremor is greatly aided by first ascertaining the circumstances under which the tremor occurs. Some tremors are present during maintenance of a posture, some during rest, and others only during an action (the intention tremors). Careful questioning will often identify the type of tremor. Common diagnostic problems include distinguishing the resting tremor of early Parkinson's disease from an essential tremor, and an essential tremor from an exaggerated physiologic tremor. All these are common, and some may in fact be present simultaneously in a given patient.

Physical Examination is directed primarily at determining whether the tremor is better or worse with activity. Patients should be asked to hold out their hands, write, perform rapid alternating movements, and touch their nose with a finger repeatedly; the objective is to detect evidence of cerebellar or extrapyramidal disease. They should be observed discretely during the history and other parts of the physical examination because calling attention to the tremor may worsen it.

Laboratory Studies. If some question remains at the end of the examination regarding whether a tremor is primarily a resting or an action tremor, a tremor recording (EMG) may be requested. Many parkinsonian patients have no other extrapyramidal signs at the time they present with tremor. The EMG can separate the two types, sometimes confirming that both tremors are present simultaneously. Thyroid function should be checked in any case of tremor.

SYMPTOMATIC MANAGEMENT

Essential Tremor. A major advance in treatment was made with the discovery of the beneficial effect of β-blockers (e.g., 120 mg of propranolol daily). Long-acting preparations are more convenient and equally effective. A decade later, the anticonvulsant drug *primidone* (Mysoline) was found to be extremely effective at reducing or eliminating essential tremor in doses far smaller than those necessary for antiepileptic activity. The mechanism of action of primidone in tremor is unknown. No consensus has been reached regarding which of these two agents is the drug of choice for tremor. Because primidone is somewhat more effective for the majority of patients, starting with a low dose of 50 mg/d and working up to as much as 250 mg/d in divided doses is a very reasonable approach to treatment. Sedation is the major side effect, but it is generally tolerated if the drug is increased slowly. Propranolol is also well tolerated in most patients, although it is relatively contraindicated in those with underlying asthma, insulin-dependent diabetes, heart block, or congestive heart failure (see Chapters 25, 32, 48, and 102). *Alprazolam* (Xanax) and other benzodiazepines have been used for essential tremor and may be effective as intermittent adjunctive agents in a patient on β-blockers or primidone.

Physiologic Tremor. Performance anxiety sometimes exaggerates an otherwise inconsequential physiologic tremor in performers (e.g., concert musicians, public speakers), and the problem can sometimes be alleviated by a small pre-performance dose of a β-blocker or a short-acting *benzodiazepine* (see Chapter 226). However, too large a dose of either can have an overly sedating effect and hinder performance. Moreover, regular use of benzodiazepines is associated with a risk for habituation (see Chapter 226), and β-blockers usually have little effect on baseline physiologic tremors.

Parkinson's Disease. The tremor of Parkinson's disease, although it does not respond as well as bradykinesia and rigidity to dopaminergic agents, may benefit from *anticholinergic therapy* (see Chapter 174).

Cerebellar Disease. The tremor of cerebellar disease is notoriously unresponsive, although β-blockers, primidone, baclofen, gabapentin, and benzodiazepines are usually tried. Wrist weights may dampen the amplitude of these tremors and make the limb more functional.

PATIENT EDUCATION AND INDICATIONS FOR REFERRAL

The cause of the tremor and the fact that it can be controlled should be discussed with the patient. Avoidance of agents that worsen symptoms must be stressed. Patients with intention tremors and cerebellar signs must be referred to a neurologist, as demyelinating or hereditary degenerative diseases may be responsible. Disabling tremors refractory to simple therapy may benefit from neurologic consultation. Neurosurgical techniques to control drug-refractory essential tremor include thalamotomy and deep brain stimulation. Patients should be referred to a center that specializes in the surgical treatment of movement disorders.

ANNOTATED BIBLIOGRAPHY

Koller WC. A new drug for treatment of essential tremor. Mayo Clin Proc 1991;66:1085. (*An editorial most useful for its review of treatment regimens.*)

Koller WC. Efficacy of primidone in the treatment of essential tremor. Neurology 1986;26:121. (*Establishes the utility of the drug in a high percentage of patients.*)

Lou JS, Jankovic J. Essential tremor: clinical correlates in 350 patients. Neurology 1991;41:234. (*Excellent description.*)

Pahwa R, Lyons KL, Wilkinson SB, et al. Bilateral thalamic stimulation for the treatment of essential tremor. Neurology 1999;53:1447. (*Thalamic stimulation was effective in reducing tremor and functional disability in essential tremor, but dysarthria was a complication.*)

169
Evaluation of Dementia
AMY A. PRUITT

Dementia is the progressive decline of intellectual ability from a previously attained level. Speech, memory, judgment, and mood may all be altered in varying proportions. The prevalence rises rapidly with age, starting at 1% at age 60 and doubling every 5 years to nearly 50% by the age of 85. At present, an estimated 600,000 persons with advanced dementia in the United States require institutional care. With the aging of the U.S. population, the social consequences of the problem are likely to be staggering if no major changes in prevention and treatment are implemented. By 2030, when nearly 20% of the U.S. population will be over the age of 65, approximately 6% will have severe dementia and an additional 10% to 15% will have mild to moderate impairment. The current annual dementia-related expense of long-term care either at home or in a nursing facility is more than $50 billion. Dementia also accounts for more admissions and hospital inpatient days than does any other geriatric psychiatric condition.

It has been estimated that more than 55 illnesses can cause dementia. Although in one sense all are treatable, at least with psychosocial intervention, the 15% of patients with significantly reversible causes or complicating conditions are depressed or exhibit drug-induced changes in mental status. When a decline in mental functioning is noted, fear of Alzheimer's disease arises in patients and their families. Each patient requires a careful workup for dementia and proper identification of the underlying cause. Primary physicians should know how to distinguish dementia from other, more specific cortical deficits (aphasia, agnosia, isolated memory deficit) and should be able to perform a screening examination for potentially reversible disease. Prompt recognition of dementia is essential, not only for the initiation of a diagnostic workup but also to protect the patient from avoidable harm, such as a fall, drug overdose, fire, or inadequate nutrition.

PATHOPHYSIOLOGY AND CLINICAL PRESENTATION

Definition and Description. Dementia is a syndrome characterized by a *generalized* and *sustained* decline in *intellectual functioning* from a previously attained level. It is a characteristically *progressive* disorder, measurable in months or years rather than days or weeks. The decline from a previously attained level of mental ability is broad-based, usually involving *memory*, *cognitive capacities*, and *adaptive behavior without alteration of consciousness*. Initially, the patient may be aware of some difficulties, but later seems mostly not to be disturbed by them. It is important, but not always possible, to distinguish the early stages of dementia from nonprogressive cognitive changes ("benign forgetfulness") that occur in normal aging.

Presentation. The onset of dementia is usually insidious, although a few conditions evolve rapidly. Patients initially may be noted to be slightly *forgetful*, with *attention* and *concentration deficits* and increasing *repetitiousness* or *inconsistencies* in their usual behavior. Later in the course of the process, patients may display increasingly impaired judgment, an inability to abstract or generalize, and *personality changes*, reacting with rigidity, perseveration, irritability, and confusion to minor changes in the environment. *Affective disturbances* or *aggressive behavior* may be prominent, and in extreme forms, patients lose all vestiges of their original personality, are unable to participate in matters of personal hygiene and nutrition, and are left helpless.

Dementia is often progressive (as in degenerative diseases), but it may be static (as in a posttraumatic brain injury state). Depending on the pathologic condition that causes dementia, indications of disease outside the areas of the brain responsible for cognitive and behavioral change may or may not be found. Concomitant disorders of extrapyramidal function are particularly common.

Some conditions that result in dementia may also cause mental retardation (e.g., Down syndrome). Patients with dementia may or may not be psychotic, and a patient with psychosis may or may not have any evidence of cognitive decline consistent with dementia.

Primary Neurologic Conditions

Alzheimer's Disease. The leading cause of dementia, Alzheimer's disease accounts for well over half of cases among the elderly and affects 15 million people worldwide. Its incidence increases with advancing age. Because many patients survive for a decade, the prevalence increases from 43% at age 65 to 47% after age 85. Most cases are *sporadic*, but a *familial autosomal dominant* form of the disease exists. Mutations in the gene for the amyloid precursor protein and the genes for presenilin 1 and 2 cause the uncommon, dominantly inherited forms of the disease that become symptomatic before the age of 60, and the *e4 variant* of *apolipoprotein E* is associated with the sporadic form and some later-onset familial forms.

No specific physical signs are characteristic, although frontal lobe release signs and secondary mild extrapyramidal features may be present. Although this disease cannot be diagnosed with certainty during life, a high probability of the diagnosis can be determined according to the criteria established by the Alzheimer's Disease and Related Disorders Work Group of 1984. Progressive worsening of memory with impairment of at least one other cognitive function is the hallmark of the disease. About two thirds of patients with moderate to severe dementia who have no other illness that can cause dementia (e.g., cerebrovascular disease, hypothyroidism) are given the diagnosis of probable Alzheimer's disease.

The diagnosis of Alzheimer's disease can be confirmed only at postmortem examination. The *brain* is *atrophied*, the *ventricles* are *enlarged*, and evidence of severe vascular disease is minimal or absent. Neuropathologic study reveals *neuronal loss*, *neurofibrillary tangles* composed of τ-protein, and *senile plaques* containing the β-amyloid peptide. Basal forebrain degeneration reduces the acetylcholine content. Loss of this transmitter correlates with memory impairment.

Dementia with Lewy Bodies. This recently appreciated but probably widespread idiopathic condition has features of Alzheimer's and Parkinson's diseases, which leads to considerable diagnostic confusion and the potential for therapeutic mismanagement. Recognition is important because these patients manifest marked sensitivity to neuroleptic drugs, which may exacerbate symptoms (see Chapter 173). The pathologic hallmarks are the widespread presence of *Lewy bodies* (intracytoplasmic inclusions) in the cortex, amygdala, hippocampus, and pars compacta of the substantia nigra and nucleus ceruleus, with loss of neuronal density in the latter areas. Unlike patients with Alzheimer's disease, these patients have only mild brain atrophy grossly and normal density of the neocortex. The initial presentation is often one of *visual hallucinations*, *episodic delirium*, *fluctuating cognitive difficulties*, and *parkinsonism* and *extrapyramidal motor symptoms* (dysarthria, poor coordination of voluntary movements). As in Alzheimer's disease, short-term memory impairment and a progressive decline in cognition interfere with social and occupational functioning. In early stages, the memory impairment may be mild, and periods of nearly normal functioning occur intermittently. Deficits in attention and visual–spatial and frontal–subcortical skills are nonetheless evident. Core features include recurrent visual hallucinations that are well formed and detailed, fluctuating consciousness, and spontaneous motor features of parkinsonism and extrapyramidal disease. Other characteristics include falls, syncope, transient loss of consciousness, hallucinations in other domains, systematized delusions, and, as noted, sensitivity to neuroleptic medications. The rate of clinical decline is generally more rapid than that of Alzheimer's disease.

Multiinfarct Dementia. "Hardening of the arteries" with cerebral hypoperfusion has been a common, although mistaken, lay view of the cause of dementia. However, multiple strokes can leave a patient with impaired cognition and produce a true dementia, often referred to as *"multiinfarct dementia."* Recent data from Scandinavia suggest that among the very elderly (over age 85), vascular dementia rivals Alzheimer's disease as the type of dementia. Although the exact contribution of vascular dementia to the overall rate of dementia remains a subject of debate, groups with a high prevalence of vascular risk factors (e.g., African-Americans, Japanese) are an increased risk. An elderly patient with hypertension, diabetes, atrial fibrillation, or known carotid disease or who smokes should be considered at risk. The clinical course may progress stepwise if discrete large-vessel occlusions occur, and is more gradual if the infarctions are primarily lacunar (see Chapter 171). Multiinfarct dementia is sometimes referred to as a *subcortical dementia* characterized by apathy, slowness, and decreased memory retrieval.

Inadequately controlled *hypertension* causing multiple cerebral infarctions is one of the more frequent and treatable conditions associated with vascular dementia. The infarctions may be large and heralded by clearly defined episodes of neurologic injury, or develop subclinically as small lacunar strokes contributing to a slow decline in intellectual function. Most patients have evidence of upper motor neuron injury (lateralized weakness, brisk reflexes, or Babinski signs.) Magnetic resonance imaging (MRI) may reveal multiple lacunar infarctions and a loss of periventricular white matter. Recent studies with positron emission tomography (PET) have shown that the degree of dementia correlates with abnormalities of cerebral glucose utilization, particularly in the frontal lobes.

Mixed Disease. As patients age, the brain becomes increasingly vulnerable to insult. Moreover, the risks for vascular and degenerative diseases increase. For this reason, it is likely that a large percentage of cases of dementia in the very elderly are of a mixed type, with both vascular disease and Alzheimer's disease as underlying conditions. The significance of this notion of mixed disease is that it focuses attention on various potential causes of dementia and the importance of controlling risk factors (e.g., improving diabetic or hypertensive control).

Normal-pressure Hydrocephalus deserves special mention, both because it is reversible and because it is generally overdiagnosed. The name of this entity denotes slow ventricular enlargement without cortical atrophy resulting from poor resorption of cerebrospinal fluid over the cerebral convexities. Most often, the precipitant is unknown, but the condition can occur when cerebrospinal fluid resorption is blocked as a consequence of remote meningeal inflammation or subarachnoid hemorrhage. *Dementia, gait disturbance*, and urinary and fecal *incontinence* comprise the classic triad. Some patients respond dramatically to ventricular–peritoneal shunting, and the diagnosis is suspected clinically and radiographically. Serial lumbar punctures with removal of large volumes (>30 mL) of cerebrospinal fluid are undertaken to try to predict which patients will respond to this maneuver.

Space-occupying Lesions such as *chronic subdural hematoma* or slowly growing *tumors* of the brain produce variable dementia depending on their size and location. When they are located on the orbital surface of the *frontal lobe* or the medial surface of the *temporal lobe*, patients may present primarily with *cognitive defects* and no other focal signs of cerebral tumor. The development of a progressive unilateral headache (see Chapter 165), a new neurologic deficit, or change in personality may provide a clue to the presence of a mass lesion.

Depression can produce the rapid onset of a true cognitive deficit that is reversible with appropriate treatment. Other symptoms of depression (hopelessness, low self-esteem, early morning awakening, fatigue, anhedonia; see Chapter 227) almost always predate the onset of the dementia and help suggest the diagnosis. Unlike patients with Alzheimer's disease, depressed patients will complain of memory loss during a mental status examination. Although depression alone can produce significant reversible cognitive impairment, severe mood disturbance may also accompany other causes of dementia, such as Alzheimer's disease or Parkinson's disease.

Other Primary Neurologic Conditions associated with dementia and specific neurologic deficits include Pick's disease, *Parkinson's* disease (see Chapter 174), *Wilson's* disease, severe *multiple sclerosis* (see Chapter 172), Creutzfeldt-Jakob disease, neurosyphilis, and *Huntington's* disease (Table 169.1). Pick's disease or frontal lobe dementia is associated with predominantly frontal and temporal lobe pathologic involvement. The cognitive deficits differ from those of Alzheimer's disease, with early impairment of executive function (the ability to modify

behavior in response to changing stimuli, solve problems, organize, think abstractly, and avoid perseveration.) Parkinson's disease and Huntington's disease are sometimes referred to as *"subcortical dementias"* because they present with significant motor dysfunction and no prominent aphasia or agnosia. Proper identification is essential to initiating effective treatment and providing accurate prognostic information.

Other Causes of Dementia

Toxins, infections, metabolic disorders, and nutritional disorders may affect the brain and result in dementia (Table 169.2). Frequently, more than one pathologic cause is present.

Intoxication. The patient with a progressive degenerative dementia may be taking an excess of a medication that is exacerbating the primary process, or the drug itself may be causing an apparent loss of cognitive abilities. Medications capable of producing dementia in patients without other underlying conditions include *opiates* and the numerous neurotropic agents available. Less obvious but frequently prescribed medications causing or aggravating dementia include the *anticholinergic preparations* used in movement disorders, *antihypertensives*, and *sedatives*. These agents are high on the list of causes of disease that can be arrested or reversed.

Infection. Any infection involving the brain can produce a picture of diffuse cognitive impairment. *Neurosyphilis*, *HIV infection* (see Chapter 13), and *cryptococcal infection* spread into

Table 169.1. Neurologic Diseases Associated with Intellectual Dysfunction

DISEASE	PHYSICAL SIGNS	CLINICAL FEATURES
Alzheimer's disease	Frontal lobe release signs; extrapyramidal signs	Enlarged ventricles *and* cortical atrophy by CT or MRI
Normal-pressure hydrocephalus	Gait disorder,[a] incontinence	Enlarged ventricles with little or no cortical atrophy
Dementia with Lewy bodies (Lewy body disease)	Visual hallucinations; periodic confusion; parkinsonism	Marked exacerbation of extrapyramidal symptoms with use of standard neuroleptics
Multiinfarct dementia	Focal deficits	Stepwise course; multiple areas of infarction, often subcortical by CT or MRI
Parkinson's disease	Extrapyramidal signs[a]	Usually present only after disease evident for several years
Intracranial tumor	Focal signs, papilledema	Often subacute evolution, seizures possible
Neurosyphilis	Frontal lobe signs, optic atrophy, Argyll-Robertson pupils	Positive serology serum and CSF
HIV infection	Variable systemic involvement	Positive HIV, cortical atrophy; dementia may be presenting symptom
Creutzfeldt-Jakob disease	Myoclonus,[a] cerebellar signs, eye movement abnormalities	Subacute course; EEG has specific abnormalities; brain biopsy diagnostic
Huntington's disease	Choreiform movements;[a] corticospinal signs	Often positive family history; caudate atrophy by CT or MRI
Multiple sclerosis	Brainstem signs, optic atrophy, corticospinal signs	Usually long-standing disease; episodic illness with remissions; often extensive white matter abnormalities by MRI
Wilson's disease	Extrapyramidal signs,[a] hepatic dysfunction, Kayser-Fleischer rings[a]	Onset in adolescence or young adult life; psychiatric disorders
Progressive supranuclear palsy	Failure of vertical downgaze[a]; extrapyramidal signs[a]	Eye movement abnormalities; differentiate from Parkinson's disease; unresponsive or only transiently responsive to levodopa

[a]Invariably present; all other physical signs are neither invariably present nor pathognomonic.

Table 169.2. Systemic Conditions Associated with Intellectual Impairment

Infectious
Syphilis with CNS involvement
HIV infection with CNS involvement
Cryptococcal infection of the CNS

Endocrine
Hypothyroidism and hyperthyroidism
Panhypopituitarism
High-dose glucocorticoid therapy

Metabolic
Vitamin B_{12} deficiency
Thiamine deficiency
Niacin deficiency (pellagra)

Chemical Poisons
Alcohol
Metals (lead, mercury)
Aniline dyes

Drug Intoxications
Barbiturates
Opiates
Anticholinergics
Lithium
Bromides
Haloperidol
Antihypertensives

the central nervous system to produce dementia, often with great regularity. Infectious agents responsible for subacute conditions like Creutzfeldt-Jakob disease and progressive multifocal leukoencephalopathy are resistant to treatment.

Endocrinologic, Metabolic, and Nutritional Disorders, including *hyperthyroidism, hypothyroidism,* and *panhypopituitarism,* and the administration of *high-dose corticosteroid therapy* can cause a generally reversible loss in cognitive abilities. The metabolic derangements resulting from advanced renal or hepatocellular failure usually cause an encephalopathic picture that differs from true dementia in that consciousness is altered. However, milder forms of metabolic disease may exacerbate an underlying dementia, as may *dehydration.* Of the hereditary metabolic diseases associated with prominent cognitive alteration, *Wilson's disease, metachromatic leukodystrophy,* and the *adrenal leukodystrophies* are among the most notable. *Nutritional disorders* may result in prominent altered mental status. *Thiamine deficiency,* if untreated, may lead to Korsakoff's dementia, which is largely irreversible. Thiamine deficiency is a preventable condition seen with alcoholism, pernicious vomiting of any cause, depression, or inadequate diet. *Pernicious anemia* can produce dementia that may be partly reversible with administration of vitamin B_{12}. *Pellagra,* uncommon in developed countries, shows a dramatic response to niacin, even when mental changes have been present for a long time.

DIFFERENTIAL DIAGNOSIS

A useful way of organizing the differential diagnosis of dementia is to divide the dementing conditions into pathologic processes that originate in the brain (Table 169.1) and those that affect the brain secondarily, such as exogenous intoxication, infections, and metabolic derangements (Table 169.2). Diseases

that are primary in the brain may be accompanied by signs of neurologic disease other than cognitive change. Diseases that affect the brain secondarily are more likely to be accompanied by signs and symptoms of medical disease and perhaps are more reversible. Among patients presenting with dementia, Alzheimer's disease accounts for some 65% of cases, vascular disease with multiple infarctions for 10% to 20%, and brain tumors for 5%; all other and unknown causes account for 10% to 15%. Among the very old (over age 85), vascular dementia and Alzheimer's disease account for the vast majority of cases.

WORKUP

The goal of the workup is to distinguish dementia from other causes of mental impairment and to identify the cause as either a primary neurologic condition or a condition that secondarily affects the brain. Differentiating among neurologic conditions is essential, not only to identify and treat reversible conditions promptly, but also to optimize the care of those with incurable disease. Not all neurologic dementia is Alzheimer's disease, and not all of these conditions respond similarly to symptomatic measures (see Chapter 173). Careful workup is essential for proper management.

History

A careful history is the most important component of the initial evaluation. The help of a family member is critical to taking an adequate history because the patient's recall may be inadequate.

Differentiating Dementia from Other Neurologic Impairments requires a description by the patient or family of the specific *cognitive, memory,* and *behavioral problems* the patient is experiencing and the *consequences* of such deficits in the patient's daily life, such as difficulties with driving, work, or family relationships. Detailed questioning should define the *temporal course* of the illness and enable the physician to ascertain whether the process is indeed chronic and progressive, stepwise, or static. A stepwise pattern in conjunction with focal deficits raises the question of a multiinfarct basis. An episode of severe hypotension followed by the onset of dementia points to hypoperfusion as the mechanism of what may be a static (nonprogressive) posthypoxic encephalopathy. A story of progressive, generalized intellectual impairment without alteration of consciousness is indicative of Alzheimer's disease and other neurodegenerative conditions, but multiple lacunar strokes may also be associated with this temporal pattern. Finally, the examiner should check for important epidemiologic *risk factors* for dementia, including a prior severe episode of *head trauma, diabetes, never having been married,* and a *low level of education.*

Identifying Treatable Causes and Differentiating among Etiologies. Once dementia is strongly suspected, the history should then focus on identifying potentially treatable causes, be they primarily neurologic or secondary. The search for neurologic disease includes inquiry into risk factors and specific neurologic accompaniments. *Cardiovascular risk factors* (e.g., smoking, hypertension, hyperlipidemia, diabetes) should be ascertained for identification of the patient at risk for vascular dementia. Questioning about *gait, incontinence,* and a prior history of *meningitis* or *subarachnoid hemorrhage* helps identify the patient at increased risk for normal-pressure hydrocephalus. A prior history of *head trauma*, unexplained onset of a *focal neurologic deficit*, and unilateral *headache* worsening over time are potential clues to a mass lesion. A history of *resting tremor* and *rigidity* are likely manifestations of Parkinson's disease. *Extrapyramidal symptoms* (dysarthria, poor coordination of voluntary movements) raise the question of Lewy body disease; if concurrent hepatocellular dysfunction is present, then Wilson's disease should be considered. Reports of vivid *visual hallucinations* suggests Lewydody disease. *High-risk sexual behavior* raises the probabilities of HIV infection and neurosyphilis. Any symptoms or prior history of *depression* need to be reviewed (see Chapter 227). A *family history* of dementia, Down syndrome, or psychiatric disorders is the basis for identifying patients at risk for one of the hereditary causes of dementia.

The history is also critical to identify non-neurologic conditions that may be causing or exacerbating a loss of mental capacity. Concurrent illnesses and precipitating factors are reviewed. For example, one asks about previous *gastric surgery* (leading to vitamin B$_{12}$ deficiency) and adequacy of *nutrition* (for thiamine, niacin, and vitamin B$_{12}$ deficiencies). A detailed review of *medications* (particularly opiates, sedative-hypnotics, analgesics, anticholinergics, anticonvulsants, corticosteroids, centrally acting antihypertensives, and psychotropics) should be elicited. *Alcohol* abuse and other forms of substance abuse are critical to rule out (see Chapters 228 and 235). It is important to check for symptoms of *hypothyroidism* (see Chapter 104) and *pituitary insufficiency* (see Chapter 101). The *occupational history* may reveal exposure to toxic substances (e.g., aniline dyes, heavy metals).

Physical Examination

Mental Status Examination. Assessment begins with a mental status examination to confirm the presence of dementia. A standardized instrument such as the Mini-Mental State Examination is easy to use and is adjusted for age and education. More detailed testing is also necessary. The complex faculties that constitute intellect are usually divided into functions, not necessarily anatomically or pathologically exclusive, that can be tested. This part of the examination should be geared both to the *detection of focal lesions* and to *signs of general brain dysfunction*. The mental status examination in the office can include immediate memory testing, with a request to remember three objects, recite digits forward and backward that are given by the examiner, and recall a short story. Remote memory testing can be approached by asking about historical events of note, family milestones, or more recent happenings in the newspaper. Language function testing should include the naming of parts of objects, following complex commands, and generating word lists. The patient should be asked to reproduce simple drawings and discern similarities among objects, a test that offers insight into categorizing ability. Judgment can be ascertained by presenting the patient with decision-requiring situations ("finding a stamped letter" or "seeing a fire in a theater"). Attention and concentration are assessed by having the patient reverse sequences, as in naming the months of the year backwards.

General Physical and Neurologic Examinations. The physician should examine the patient to help uncover evidence of any coexisting abnormalities that may be causing or contributing to the problem. One checks for physical evidence of neurovascular risk factors (see Chapter 171) and carefully palpates and auscultates the carotid arteries. In addition, the physician notes any signs of alcoholism (see Chapter 228), hepatocellular injury (see Chapter 71), renal insufficiency (see Chapter 142), and other systemic illnesses.

Specific neurologic abnormalities, such as frontal lobe release signs (grasp, suck, snout, root), visual field cut, limitation of extraocular movement, or abnormal pupillary reaction should be elicited. Nystagmus may indicate recent drug ingestion or the presence of brainstem disease. The motor examination should pay particular attention to extrapyramidal features or involuntary movements such as tardive dyskinesias, tremors, asterixis, chorea, or myoclonus. The sensory examination may reveal evidence of peripheral neuropathy or combined system disease (vitamin B$_{12}$ deficiency). Gait should be observed carefully; the small, rigid steps of frontal lobe gait apraxia can be distinguished from a wide-based cerebellar gait or the small steps associated with extrapyramidal disease.

Laboratory Studies

Diagnostic Criteria for Alzheimer's Disease. Those established by the U.S. Department of Health and Human Services require the presence of dementia "established by clinical examination and documented by the *Mini-Mental State Examination . . .* or similar examination, with evidence of deficits in two or more areas of cognition; progressive worsening of memory and other cognitive function; no disturbance of consciousness; and absence of systemic disorders or other brain disease that in and of themselves could account for the deficits." No single test will establish the presence of dementia, and a poor score on a Mini-Mental State Examination should not be the sole criterion for the diagnosis of dementia. The score should be considered clinically significant if it is corroborated by other components of the initial evaluation and history. Several clinical drug trials have confirmed what neurologic clinicians have long suspected—namely, that considerable variability in the annual Mini-Mental State Examination score is noted in patients with probable Alzheimer's disease and that variability of scores between examiners is prominent. Similarly, the existence of several different sets of criteria for vascular dementia confound both the longitudinal assessment of patients and initial diagnostic certainty. Continuing observation over time may be necessary to establish the diagnosis for some patients and to identify complicating conditions.

Screening Laboratory Studies. The laboratory tests recommended should be individualized based on the patient's history and physical and mental status examination results. Because the history and physical examination will limit the differential possibilities, the patient should be spared the inconvenience and costs of excessive testing. Undertesting is also hazardous because elderly patients in whom medical diseases may underlie nonspecific presentations of dementia comprise the usual patient population.

The guidelines specified by the National Institute of Aging Task Force on Mental Impairment in the Elderly have become the standard for investigating patients with dementia, although they are probably more appropriate for assessing an alteration in mental functioning than for detecting a treatable cause of dementia. They include determination of the following:

1. Complete blood cell count and sedimentation rate
2. Chemistry panel (electrolytes, calcium, albumin, blood urea nitrogen, creatinine, transaminase levels)
3. Thyroid-stimulating hormone level
4. VDRL (Venereal Disease Research Laboratory) test for syphilis
5. Urinalysis
6. Serum vitamin B_{12} and folate levels
7. Chest radiography
8. Electrocardiography
9. Computed tomography (CT) of the head

Because this panel was not designed to be a cost-effective workup for uncovering treatable causes of dementia, it should not be applied routinely to all patients; rather, it should be considered a menu from which tests can be selected based on the patient's clinical presentation. Some of these tests will be useful in detecting conditions that might exacerbate the mental decline of a patient with dementia. Because this list was compiled before HIV infection and AIDS were appreciated as important causes of dementia, *HIV testing* should be added to it, especially in the evaluation of younger patients with a history of high-risk activity or exposure (see Chapter 13).

The American Academy of Neurology practice parameters for the evaluation of dementia are more parsimonious than the above recommendations; they suggest that the diagnostic workup include a complete blood cell count; determination of serum electrolytes, calcium, glucose, blood urea nitrogen, and creatinine; liver function tests; thyroid function tests; determination of serum vitamin B_{12}, and syphilis serology. However, all other studies, including measurement of folate levels, chest radiography, and neuroimaging studies, are considered optional. Four clinical indicators (early onset of symptoms, noninsidious course, focal signs or symptoms, and early gait disturbance) predict the diagnostic utility of neuroimaging studies. The use of these four indicators is estimated to reduce the frequency of imaging studies by 33%, but clinically meaningful disease will be missed in 5%.

Neuroimaging of the brain by *CT* or *MRI* is appropriate in the presence of (a) a history suggestive of a mass lesion; (b) focal neurologic signs or symptoms; (c) dementia of abrupt onset; (d) a history of seizures; and (e) a history of stroke. Subdural hematomas and intracranial tumors can be readily identified, especially when contrast-enhanced studies are performed, and radiologic evidence of normal-pressure hydrocephalus also may be provided. MRI with gadolinium contrast enhancement is superior to CT for the diagnosis of multiinfarct dementia and for the elucidation of problems referable to the posterior fossa. If the clinical suspicion of tumor is high, MRI is the more sensitive test.

Other Ancillary Studies. *Lumbar puncture* may be indicated when other clinical findings suggest an active infection or vasculitis, and it is part of the evaluation of normal-pressure hydrocephalus, as described above. Sugar, protein, and gamma globulin levels, cultures, a cell count, and serology for syphilis should be obtained. Lumbar puncture for the initial evaluation of dementia is not justified. However, the primary care physician should be aware that *levels of τ-protein in the cere-*

brospinal fluid are highly sensitive and specific for differentiating Alzheimer's disease from normal aging and depression, and they may be seen early in the disease process at a time when the Mini-Mental State Examination score is above 23. Thus, it is possible that this test will be more routinely used to make the diagnosis of Alzheimer's disease earlier and offer patient access to potentially disease-modifying drug therapy.

Electroencephalographic patterns may be normal even in advanced states of dementia, or nonspecific slowing of the baseline rhythm may be found. For patients who have episodes of altered consciousness and in whom seizures may therefore be suspected, this is an indicated procedure. Occasionally, the electroencephalogram may raise suspicion of a particular disease process; focal delta slowing is seen with tumor, unilateral attenuation of voltage may suggest an extracranial mass such as subdural hematoma, and excessive beta activity may be consistent with drug ingestion. Finally, Creutzfeldt-Jakob disease has a highly specific electroencephalographic pattern.

Formal neuropsychological evaluation would be appropriate to obtain more specific information when the diagnosis is in doubt and is also helpful in providing additional information about the nature of impairment following focal brain injury. *Speech analysis* with speech therapy may improve patient and family communication. Formal *psychiatric assessment* may be desirable if depression is suspected in addition to dementia.

Studies of Limited or Uncertain Utility. Measurements of *cerebral blood flow* and *metabolism* (positron emission tomography and single-photon emission computed tomography) are not routinely used at present. Their value in predicting Huntington's disease and Alzheimer's disease is being investigated.

Brain biopsy for non-neoplastic and noninfectious diseases is rarely justified. Very occasionally, progressive multifocal leukoencephalopathy or Creutzfeldt-Jakob disease is diagnosed by this technique.

Noninvasive neurovascular studies (carotid ultrasonography, Doppler flow studies; see Chapter 171) are not of routine value in the workup of dementia unless the clinical course or physical examination findings are suggestive of cerebrovascular disease or the MRI or CT demonstrates infarction.

Genetic Testing is controversial and poses ethical issues. When the family history suggests early-onset Alzheimer's disease, tests for mutations on chromosomes 1, 14, and 21 can be considered. Clinicians can expect to be asked by patients and families about the "test for dementia" (the search for the *e4 allele* of the *gene encoding apolipoprotein E [APOE*e4]*, which is encoded on protein 19 and has been associated with Alzheimer's disease). *APOE* genotyping is not accurate enough to serve alone as a test for Alzheimer's disease, but at least one *APOE*e4* allele can be found in 65% of pathologically confirmed cases of Alzheimer's disease. When combined with clinical evaluation, *APOE* genotyping can improve diagnostic specificity, but the test lacks sufficient sensitivity to be used to rule out Alzheimer's disease. Moreover, it is not sufficiently predictive of developing dementing illness to be of prognostic value. These features of the apolipoprotein E test should be shared with patients inquiring about the "test for Alzheimer's disease." Taking a mail order test for *APOE* genotyping should be discouraged because of the shortcomings of the test and the high probability of misinterpreting the results.

MANAGEMENT

Alzheimer's Disease and Lewy Body Disease. (See Chapter 173.)

Other Causes. For the patient with vascular dementia, control of such cerebrovascular risk factors as hypertension, hyperlipidemia, smoking, and diabetes mellitus is essential (see Chapters 26, 27, 54, and 102, respectively). The question of the need for endarterectomy deserves consideration when a vascular problem is strongly suspected and a significant stenosis is found (see Chapter 171). Attention to embolic risk (see Chapters 28, 33, and 83) is also critical. Patients with dementia secondary to HIV infection may respond to intensive antiretroviral therapy (see Chapter 13), and those with Lyme disease may improve with a prolonged course of parenteral antibiotics (see Chapter 141). In cases of vitamin deficiency, correction is essential (see Chapter 82). Avoidance of toxins and discontinuation of causative drugs are the basic approaches to substance-induced disease (see Chapters 228 and 235). In those with hormonal deficiency, replacement therapy is key (see Chapters 101 and 104).

INDICATIONS FOR REFERRAL AND ADMISSION

Some families will request a neurologic consultation when a diagnostic evaluation has been completed by the primary physician and no cause is apparent other than Alzheimer's disease. Such a consultation can provide reassurance to the family that a comprehensive workup has been performed and that the diagnosis is correct. If the primary physician has conducted a thoughtful and complete examination as outlined above, the referral need not generate additional testing. If the means for conducting a full workup are not available to the primary physician, then a referral can be used to complete the evaluation. Additionally, patients suspected of having a a potentially treatable neurologic condition (Parkinson's disease, normal-pressure hydrocephalus, mass lesion, carotid artery disease) are candidates for neurologic or neurosurgical evaluation. Finally, when a suspected hereditary condition is under consideration, referral for confirmation and genetic counseling is indicated.

Admission to a hospital for behavioral management or for the treatment of intercurrent medical illness can be very stressful for patient and family. Careful attention to factors associated with the development of delirium in the hospitalized patient and use of the lowest possible doses of analgesic and sedative-hypnotic medications are essential (see also Chapter 173).

ANNOTATED BIBLIOGRAPHY

Andreasen N, Minthon L, Clarber A, et al. Sensitivity, specificity, and stability of CSF-tau in AD in a community-based patient sample. Neurology 1999;53:1488. (*Found useful in helping to differentiate patients with Alzheimer's disease from those with dementia of other causes.*)

Beal MF. Clinicopathologic conference No. 7-1998. N Engl J Med 1998;338:603. (*Lucid, case-based clinical and pathologic discussion of Lewy body disease*).

Chui HC, Mack W, Jackson JE, et al. Clinical criteria for the diagnosis of vascular dementia. Arch Neurol 2000;57:191. (*Four different clinical definitions of vascular dementia were compared for reliability between raters and were found not to be interchangeable.*)

Chui H, Zhang Q. Evaluation of dementia: a systematic study of the usefulness of the American Academy of Neurology's practice parameters. Neurology 1996;49:925. (*Found a marked reduction in cost of assessment possible and a 5% false-negative rate.*)

Clarifield AM. The reversible dementias: do they reverse? Ann Intern Med 1988;109:476. (*Most that reversed were caused by drugs or depression; comprehensive review of 32 studies.*)

Clark CM, Sheppard L, Filenbaum GG, et al. Variability in annual mini-mental state examination score in patients with probable Alzheimer disease. Arch Neurol 1999;56:857. (*Useful for screening; limited benefit for determining disease progression.*)

Inouye SK, Bogardus ST, Charpentier PA, et al. A multicomponent intervention to prevent delirium in hospitalized older patients. N Engl J Med 1999;340:669. (*Protocols for cognitive impairment, sleep deprivation, immobility, visual impairment, hearing impairment, and dehydration reduced the number and duration of episodes of delirium.*)

Mayeux R, Saunders AM, Shea S, et al. *APOE* genotype by itself was not an accurate predictor of Alzheimer disease. N Engl J Med 1998;338:506. (*At least one APOE*e4 allele was found in 65% of pathologically confirmed cases of Alzheimer's disease.*)

McKeith IG, Galasko D, Kosaka K, et al. Consensus guidelines for the clinical and pathologic diagnosis of dementia with Lewy bodies (DLB): report of the Consortium on DLB International Workshop. Neurology 1996;47:1113. (*Diagnostic criteria for this underrecognized yet important condition.*)

Mehta KM, Ott A, Kalmijn S, et al. Head trauma and risk of dementia and Alzheimer's disease. Neurology 1999;53:1959. (*No association with head trauma; no interaction between head trauma and the APOE*e4 allele.*)

Skoog I, Nilsson L, Palmertz B, et al. A population-based study of dementia in 85-year-olds. N Engl J Med 1993;328:153. (*Prevalence of vascular dementia much higher than previously suspected.*)

Woods BT. Clinicopathologic conference No. 6-1992. N Engl J Med 1992;326:397. (*Good discussion of familial dementing diseases.*)

170

Approach to the Patient with a Seizure

AMY A. PRUITT

The occurrence of a convulsion is a dramatic and frightening event. One of every 11 Americans who lives to be 80 years old has had at least one seizure. The first experience of a seizure is likely to trigger an immediate visit to an emergency department. Retrospective clarification of a "spell" is the diagnostic challenge in the office setting. In the context of evaluating an episode of lost or altered consciousness, the primary care physician needs to consider seizure (see Chapter 24). If a seizure is likely, then one should attempt to determine its type and plan to prevent future episodes while conducting a diagnostic evaluation for the underlying cause.

PATHOPHYSIOLOGY AND CLINICAL PRESENTATION

A *seizure* is a paroxysmal alteration in consciousness or other cerebral cortical function. It results from a synchronous activation of a population of neurons, either in one focal area or generally throughout the brain. The occurrence of a single seizure does *not* constitute *epilepsy*, which connotes recurrent, unprovoked seizures. Many people have a single seizure without recurrence—for example, as a consequence of a transient metabolic disturbance, such as severe hypoglycemia or hypoperfusion. Only about 1% of the U.S. population actually has epilepsy. Epileptic seizures can result from many different types of diseases, ranging from hereditary conditions to vascular, traumatic, and neoplastic causes. Seizures can be classified as *localization-related* (previously known as *partial*) or *generalized* (Table 170.1).

Localization-related Seizures may begin in one area of the brain and initially produce symptoms that are referable to the region of cortex involved. *Simple* partial seizures are focal neurologic events in which consciousness remains intact, whereas in *complex* partial seizures, consciousness is impaired. Simple seizures may evolve into complex partial seizures, and both these types of focal seizures may evolve into secondarily generalized seizures. The spread of symptoms may follow the cortical representation of body parts, beginning, for example, in the fingers and spreading up the arm or down the leg.

Symptoms of complex partial seizures are numerous and include coordinated, involuntary motor activity (automatisms), such as lip smacking or chewing, olfactory or gustatory hallucinations, and behavioral automatisms. Seizure activity typically begins in the temporal lobe or its connections. Premonitory symptoms include olfactory hallucinations, epigastric discomfort, and a sense of fear or *déjà vu*. At times, the symptoms may resemble those of a psychosis. Episodes last 1 to 3 minutes, followed by a period of confusion with consciousness

Table 170.1. International Classification of Epilepsies and Epileptic Syndromes

Localization-Related (Focal, Local, Partial) Epilepsies and Epileptic Syndromes
    Idiopathic with age-related onset
        Benign childhood epilepsy with centrotemporal spikes
        Childhood epilepsy with occipital paroxysms
        Symptomatic

Generalized Epilepsies and Epileptic Syndromes
    Idiopathic with age-related onset
        Benign neonatal epilepsy
        Childhood absence epilepsy (pyknolepsy)
        Juvenile myoclonic epilepsy (impulsive petit mal)
        Juvenile absence epilepsy with generalized tonic–clonic
            seizures on awakening
        Secondary (idiopathic or symptomatic)
        West syndrome (infantile spasms)
        Lennox-Gastaut syndrome

Symptomatic
    Nonspecific etiology (early myoclonic encephalopathy)
    Specific syndromes (epileptic seizures that may complicate
        many diseases, such as Ramsay Hunt syndrome, Unverricht's disease

usually impaired but not lost. Localization-related seizures are the most common type of epilepsy in adults, accounting for 70% of patients presenting with epilepsy after age 18. More than 50% of all patients with localization-related epilepsy have both partial and secondarily generalized tonic–clonic seizures.

Generalized Seizures are bilaterally symmetric and without focal onset. An episode may begin with a premonitory aura that is followed by a sudden loss of consciousness. A *tonic phase* of limb extension ensues, lasting 10 to 30 seconds, followed by a *clonic phase* of limb jerking of at least 30 seconds. The patient then becomes flaccid and comatose before regaining consciousness. *Postictal confusion* is characteristic and can last for hours, although 10 to 30 minutes is more typical. *Tongue biting* and *incontinence* are other characteristic features.

Important Precipitants of Seizures and Pertinent Misconceptions. A number of factors have been implicated as causes of seizures, including fever, stroke, alcohol and drug use, and head trauma. Although these factors are often important, a number of misconceptions about their role are prevalent and need to be addressed.

1. Adults rarely have convulsions with *high fever*; a temperature higher than 102°F does not suffice to explain the occurrence of a seizure in an adult.
2. Seizures are rare during the initial presentation of an *embolic stroke*, although 20% to 25% of such patients may have seizures at some time after the initial stroke.
3. *Subarachnoid hemorrhage* and *lacunar strokes* rarely have seizure activity as a sequela, although *emboli* and *cortical vein thrombosis* are more likely to lead to symptomatic epilepsy.
4. *Alcohol withdrawal* seizures occur between 7 and 48 hours after cessation of drinking, with a peak at 13 to 24 hours. Usually, only one or two convulsions occur, and status epilepticus is rare. Alcohol withdrawal is more likely to produce seizures in an epileptic patient than in a normal person, and less drinking is required to precipitate a seizure in patients with epilepsy who drink alcohol. *Other drugs* are associated with seizures, either when they are taken in overdose or when they are withdrawn (Table 170.2).
5. *Trauma* is frequently invoked as a cause for seizures. However, in two large studies, unless the trauma was severe, causing a loss of consciousness for more than a half hour or a lobar hematoma or depressed skull fracture, the incidence of posttraumatic seizures was not greater than that in the general population. With a history of closed head trauma, epilepsy usually develops within 2 years, whereas with open head trauma, seizures may develop at a longer interval after the original injury.

DIFFERENTIAL DIAGNOSIS

Conditions Mimicking Seizures. Several conditions can mimic seizures, either by causing focal deficits or producing episodic loss of consciousness. Among the former are transient ischemic attacks, migraine, and local pathology, such as nerve compression. Among the latter are syncopal attacks of any cause, including transient diminished cerebral perfusion resulting from cardiac conditions and transient ischemic attacks (see Chapter 171). Panic attacks and altered mental status during

Table 170.2.   Drugs Commonly Associated with Seizures

DRUGS	OVERDOSE SEIZURES	WITHDRAWAL SEIZURES	DOSE REQUIRED TO INDUCE SEIZURE
Alcohol	−	+	Depends on previous drinking or underlying epilepsy
Meperidine (Demerol)	+	+	2–3 g/d[a, b]
Propoxyphene (Darvon)	+	+	Variable
Pentazocine (Talwin)	−	−	May precipitate withdrawal from other opiates with as little as 100 mg
Barbiturates	−	+	>600 mg/d (short-acting)[b]
Meprobamate (Miltown)	−	+	>1.2 g/d[b]
Chlordiazepoxide, Diazepam	−	+	Unknown—may have 7- to 8-day latency period
Pheothiazines, Haloperidol	− But myoclonus may occur; may cause seizures in patients with old cortical focus	−	Variable

[a]Overdose seizure.
[b]Withdrawal seizure.
+ Occurs.
− Does not occur.

psychotic episodes may cause confusion with complex partial seizures.

Conditions Causing Seizures. The differential diagnosis of conditions responsible for a seizure is based largely on the age of the patient at the time of the first seizure and the type of seizure as determined by the history, especially that obtained from observers. *Primary* or *idiopathic epilepsy* is the most common cause of recurrent seizures in children, but it becomes increasingly rare in the young adult population. After age 30, an *underlying cause* (*secondary epilepsy*) becomes increasingly likely when a patient presents with a first seizure. Among patients with more than one documented seizure of any type, a cause becomes obvious after thorough investigation and a 10-year follow-up in only 23%. Only 15% of seizures generalized from the outset have a demonstrable cause, whereas underlying disorders can be found in more than 30% of seizures with a focal component. In the *young adult* population (ages 18 to 45), the demonstrated causes include *drugs* (usually alcohol withdrawal), *neoplasm*, and *trauma*. In the *older adult* population, underlying pathology is divided about equally among *neoplasm*, *trauma*, and *cerebrovascular disease*. A nonepileptic convulsion may occur in the context of a transient metabolic disturbance, such as cerebral hypoperfusion, hypoglycemia, a hyperosmolar state, or hyponatremia.

WORKUP

For the patient who reports a "spell," the first step is to ascertain if it was a seizure and, if so, to characterize its type. Identifying the type facilitates ascertaining whether the cause is likely to be primary (idiopathic) or secondary (underlying central nervous system pathology) (Table 170.1). Generalized seizures with no initial focus are usually primary. Such epilepsies are often inherited, age-related, and not associated with structural lesions identified by current neuroradiographic techniques. With partial or focal seizures, the prevalence of identifiable underlying disease or abnormality in the brain is much higher.

History. An effective history requires an exact description of events from both witnesses and the patient. Reports of witnesses are especially useful because the patient's consciousness and recall of the event are likely to have been compromised. Questioning should include inquiry into the presence of an aura, focal onset, loss of consciousness, and observed injury during the convulsion. Such symptoms suggest seizure rather than syncope, although it is not possible to distinguish between them absolutely on the basis of any characteristic features.

Once it has been ascertained that a seizure has occurred, it is essential to check carefully for a history of focal onset, even in patients with a history of generalized seizure. The focal onset of a witnessed seizure that later became generalized may be an important clue to an underlying lesion of the central nervous system.

History is also essential for identifying precipitants and underlying disease. It should include inquiry into drugs (e.g., alcohol, cocaine, amphetamines, antidepressants, sedatives, theophylline, insulin, diuretics), cardiac arrhythmias, valvular disease, previous malignancy, stroke, and head trauma. The examiner should check for symptoms of hyperglycemia and hypoglycemia (see Chapter 102) in addition to those of meningeal irritation (headache, stiff neck). A family history of convulsions should always be sought.

Physical Examination. The physician may have the opportunity to perform the neurologic examination shortly after the seizure. A focal residual abnormality, such as paralysis of one arm (Todd's paralysis), may suggest a focal onset even when the witnessed event was generalized. In addition to a careful neurologic examination, the physical should also include a check for postural hypotension, abnormalities in heart rate and rhythm, head trauma, carotid disease, cardiac disease, systemic infection, and signs of alcohol and drug abuse (see Chapters 228 and 235).

Laboratory Studies. It is not possible by clinical means to determine definitively whether a transient or persistent neurologic event is a seizure.

Electroencephalography is the most helpful laboratory diagnostic test in the diagnosis of a seizure disorder. An abnormal electroencephalogram (EEG) with epileptiform features such as spikes or sharp waves supports the diagnosis of seizures and may provide information about the type of seizure disorder. However, an abnormal EEG pattern is not adequate for the diagnosis of seizures, and a normal interictal EEG pattern can be found in up to 20% of patients with purely generalized seizures. The likelihood of detecting an abnormality in partial complex seizures (temporal lobe epilepsy) is increased by obtaining a *sleep EEG*. However, because the EEG concentrates on cortical disturbances, abnormalities of deep temporal lobe or diencephalic structures may not be evident on a surface EEG. Specialized units provide in-hospital telemetric monitoring of patients with suspected epilepsy. A Digitrace device allows for ambulatory EEG recording for periods of up to 72 hours. The patient records clinical events with a push-button, and the patient's experiences then can be correlated with the EEG findings.

Neuroimaging. Most neurologists would agree that *magnetic resonance imaging* (MRI) of the brain without and then with *gadolinium* contrast enhancement is an important part of the workup of a patient with a first seizure. This procedure is more sensitive than *computed tomography* (CT) and may be particularly useful in demonstrating abnormalities in the medial temporal region. *Positron emission tomography* (PET) and *single-photon emission computed tomography* (SPECT) are new methods of examining cerebral function in patients with seizures. They may confirm the presence of an organic abnormality and provide an outline of the abnormal region for which surgical treatment of epilepsy might be considered. It is unlikely that a primary physician would refer a patient for one of these studies, but the primary physician should be aware that newer methods to differentiate generalized from localization-related seizures and select patients for epilepsy surgery are available in epilepsy centers.

Other Testing. Additional laboratory studies should include blood chemistries; measurement of electrolyte, calcium, and alcohol levels and a toxic screen are important. All patients with risk factors for HIV should undergo *HIV testing* (see Chapter 7). Unless evidence of infection is found or the patient presents in status epilepticus, it is no longer common practice to perform a *lumbar puncture* for a patient with a first seizure. If fever is present or the history is compatible with systemic infection, lumbar puncture remains an essential part of the neurologic evaluation.

PRINCIPLES OF MANAGEMENT

As precise a diagnosis as possible must be made before treatment is begun. This includes both the phenotype of the seizure, the EEG findings, and the identification of any underlying cause or precipitating factors. The distinction between a single seizure and epilepsy is important. During the past 20 years, important advances have been made in the treatment of all seizure types. Monotherapy with one of the standard antiepileptic drugs (AEDs) (Table 170.3) provides adequate control in 70% of adult patients. In another 15% to 20%, seizures can be controlled with a combination regimen including one or two additional AEDs. Unsatisfactory control of the seizures of the remaining patients makes them candidates for surgery or experimental drug therapy.

The Isolated Seizure

As noted earlier, an isolated convulsion does not constitute epilepsy. When a single convulsion has occurred because of a transient metabolic disturbance or drug overdose or withdrawal, it is best treated by attending to the factors that led to the disturbance. The long-term use of drugs for seizure prophylaxis in such patients is not indicated, although a short-term

Table 170.3. Pharmacokinetic Summary of Antiepileptic Drugs

DRUG (GENERIC/BRAND)	INDICATIONS	STARTING DOSE[a] (mg/d)	MAINTENANCE DOSE (mg/d)	TIME TO STEADY-STATE ELIMINATION HALF-LIFE (h)	THERAPEUTIC STATE PLASMA CONCENTRATION[c] (d)	RANGE OF PLASMA CONCENTRATION (μg/ml)
Phenytoin (Dilantin)	T-C, CP, SP	300	200–500	10–34	7–8	10–20
Carbamazepine (Tegretol, Tegretol-XR)	T-C, CP, SP	200–400	600–1,200	14–27	3–4	4–12
Phenobarbital	T-C, CP, SP	90	90–240	46–136	14–21	10–40
Primidone (Mysoline)	T-C, CP, SP	125	750–1,500	6–18	4–7	5–12[b]
Valproic acid (Depakote)	A, M, T-C	750	1,000–4,000	6–15	1–2	40–100
Ethosuximide (Zarontin)	A	500	500–1,500	20–60	7–10	40–120
Clonazepam Klonopin)	A, AT, M	1.5	1.5–10	20–40	—	—

[a]All doses are for adults.

[b]Primidone is metabolized to phenobarbital, whose therapeutic concentrations are the same as those listed under phenobarbital. The value in this column refers to primidone concentration.

[c]This is the interval at which drug levels should be checked after any adjustment in dose.

A, absence; AT, atonic; CP, complex partial; M, myoclonic; SP, simple partial; T-C, tonic–clonic.

course may be used in the setting of alcohol or drug withdrawal (see Chapters 228 and 236). When no obvious, self-limited cause can be determined in a patient who presents with a single seizure, then prophylaxis must be considered. Social variables, such as loss of driving privileges, will influence the decision to treat. The most critical issue is to determine risk factors for recurrence. Recurrence is most common within the first 6 months after the first seizure, and more than 50% of patients who have a recurrence will have it within this period. The recurrence rate after a first unprovoked seizure varies from 36% to 77%. Risk factors for recurrence include known prior neurologic lesions, history of epilepsy in a sibling, prolonged Todd's paralysis, and EEG with generalized epileptiform discharges. The risk for recurrence after two seizures is 70%, and after a third nearly 80%.

Recurrent Epileptic Seizures

Overview of Basic Approach to Pharmacologic Treatment. The treatment of choice for recurrent epileptic seizures is the administration of a *single anticonvulsant drug* appropriate for the seizure type diagnosed (Table 170.1). Most available AEDs are used to prevent the recurrence of seizures rather than to produce any specific effect on the course of established epilepsy or to prevent the development of seizures after trauma. As a group, generalized seizures respond best to treatment, and full seizure control is possible with monotherapy for as many as 80% of patients with idiopathic epilepsy.

The drug should be used in doses sufficient to control the seizures as completely as possible. If side effects become intolerable, the drug should be replaced with another one, also used as monotherapy, until it is clear that the patient's seizures cannot be controlled with a single drug. In general, it is better initially to add rather than to substitute a second drug, and thereby provide seizure protection while the serum concentration of the second drug is rising. The first drug should then be tapered and discontinued in an attempt to continue monotherapy.

Carbamazepine and *phenytoin* remain the first-line treatments for adult patients with localization-related epilepsy. The rates for complete control of tonic–clonic seizures are similar for carbamazepine, primidone, phenobarbital, and phenytoin; carbamazepine offers better efficacy than phenobarbital and primidone for localization-related seizures and is also better tolerated. Phenytoin is approximately equally as effective as carbamazepine for localization-related epilepsy. Valproate is the first-choice drug of some neurologists for generalized epilepsy. Several studies have found no significant difference in seizure control among patients with localization-related seizures treated with phenytoin, valproate, or carbamazepine.

Side effects severe enough to necessitate a change in therapy occur in about 30% of patients treated with AEDs. Side effects and interactions of drugs may become intolerable if more than one drug is required. A second drug should not be added until it has been documented that control cannot be achieved with the first drug at a high therapeutic concentration or that the dose required to achieve control produces toxic effects.

When an AED is begun or the dosage of the drug is altered, one must wait for five drug-elimination half-lives to elapse before the effect of the change can be assessed. To achieve immediately a steady-state concentration equal to the usual maintenance concentration, it is usually necessary to give a loading dose of drug. Levels should be checked frequently while doses are adjusted (see Table 170.3 for appropriate intervals for level checks, maintenance doses, loading doses, and therapeutic levels of AEDs).

Classes of Antiepileptic Agents. Several effective drugs are available for treating each form of epilepsy, the drug of first choice being the one causing the least toxicity in any individual patient. Three types of antiepileptic drugs are available. *Type 1 drugs*, which include *carbamazepine* and *phenytoin*, block sustained repetitive firing, the rapid firing of action potentials that is produced by an applied depolarizing current and is dependent on the opening of increased numbers of sodium channels. *Type 2 drugs*, including *phenobarbital*, *valproate*, and *benzodiazepines*, have the dual actions of enhancing γ-aminobutyric acid (GABA) inhibitory transmission and blocking sustained repetitive firing. *Type 3* is represented by *ethosuximide*, an AED that has no effect on either postsynaptic GABA-ergic inhibition or sustained repetitive firing but that blocks T-calcium currents, which appear to be important in the generation of normal rhythmic activity.

Important Drug–Drug Interactions. Carbamazepine, phenobarbital, and phenytoin are *inducers* of the *hepatic microsomal cytochrome P-450 enzymes*. The production of endogenous compounds such as steroids is generally regulated by intrinsic homeostatic feedback mechanisms, but increases in dosage may be necessary for medications containing steroids, used in immunosuppression, the treatment of cerebral edema, and oral contraception. Valproate is an inhibitor of this enzyme system. Table 170.4 lists selected, clinically significant drug interactions for phenytoin that may be of relevance in primary care practice. A useful pamphlet by James Fischer summarizing many drug interactions with AEDs is published by the McMahon Publishing Group in New York and is a handy reference in the primary care office practice setting.

Phenytoin. For most seizure types occurring in adults, phenytoin is an appropriate drug choice. The proprietary formulation, Dilantin, is preferable to the generic formulation. Phenytoin is well absorbed orally and has a serum half-life of 22 to 30 hours. An initial loading dose must be administered. Dose-related side effects include nystagmus, ataxia, dysarthria, and blurred vision. The presence of nystagmus can be used as a crude guide to the adequacy of dose. Duration-related side effects include osteomalacia, peripheral neuropathy, a folate-deficiency anemia, and cerebellar degeneration. Idiosyncratic reactions include gingival hypertrophy, hypertrichosis, spiking fevers, exfoliative dermatitis, bone marrow depression, liver abnormalities, teratogenesis during the first trimester of gestation, and neonatal coagulation defects.

Carbamazepine (Tegretol) is also an excellent first-line drug for adult-onset generalized tonic–clonic seizures and for complex partial seizures. Many patients report less fatigue and better performance while on this medication than on phenytoin, but a controlled study failed to confirm that carbamazepine is clearly superior. The major disadvantages of this medication include the necessity of multiple daily dosing and the requirement for frequent blood testing during initiation of the medication to monitor for uncommon instances of *bone marrow depression*.

Valproate. For patients allergic to phenytoin or carbamazepine, valproate (Depakote) is a good choice of medication. Many neurologists would choose this as a first-line drug for spike-and-wave or generalized tonic–clonic epilepsy, even in the absence of EEG abnormalities. This drug also has to be given in multiple daily doses (Table 170.3). Major side effects

Table 170.4.   Phenytoin: Side Effects and Drug Interactions

Major Side Effects
Dose-related: nystagmus, ataxia, dysarthria, blurred vision, decrease in measured total T_4
Duration-related: osteomalacia, peripheral neuropathy, anemia, cerebellar degeneration
Idiosyncratic: gingival hypertrophy, acne, hypertrichosis, encephalopathy
Rare, toxic: high, spiking fevers; exfoliative dermatitis; bone marrow depression; pseudolymphoma and actual lymphoma; lupuslike syndrome; teratogenesis during first trimester; neonatal coagulation defects

Interactions with Commonly Prescribed Drugs
Increased phenytoin levels with
  Antimicrobials: chloramphenicol, isoniazid
  Anticoagulants: warfarin
  Amphetamines (but seizure threshold decreased)
  Disulfiram (Antabuse)
  Alcohol: acute ingestion raises phenytoin levels, but see below
  Antiinflammatory agent: phenylbutazone
  Anticonvulsants: ethosuximide; no consistent effect with simultaneous barbiturate administration
  Sedatives: chlordiazepoxide (Librium), diazepam (Valium), oxazepam (Serax), Clonazepam (Klonopin)
Decreased phenytoin levels with
  Alcohol: chronic ingestion
Phenytoin effects on levels of other drugs
  Insulin: may interfere with endogenous insulin release
  Quinidine: decreases quinidine effect at given dose
  Falsely low total T_4

T_4, thyroxine.

of valproate are nausea, weight gain, hair loss, platelet dysfunction, fetal anomalies (neural tube defects), and liver dysfunction.

Phenobarbital is no longer a first-line drug for generalized tonic–clonic seizures, although for patients allergic to the three medications described above, it provides good control, usually with acceptable side effects.

New Antiepileptic Drugs. Several new AEDs have been introduced in the past decade. These are summarized in Table 170.5. Felbamate, gabapentin, lamotrigine, topiramate, and oxazepine are effective as add-on therapy for patients with partial and secondarily generalized tonic–clonic seizures. Lamotrigine is acquiring a role as monotherapy for patients with newly diagnosed epilepsy. Felbamate carries a risk for aplastic anemia

and acute hepatic failure and is reserved for selected patients in whom the benefits outweigh the risks and in whom other AEDs have failed. Gabapentin has an excellent side effect profile and for this reason is used as add-on therapy. As a single agent, it is not sufficiently effective to control most adult forms of epilepsy.

Optimizing therapy requires selection of the AED that is most effective for the patient's epileptic syndrome and that has the most favorable safety profile. However, the tolerability and therapeutic efficacy of each AED can differ considerably among patients. Therapeutic monitoring of blood levels provides a standard for each individual patient's seizure control. Some patients require treatment with more than one agent, but alternative monotherapy should be tried first. The overall efficacy and safety of the new AEDs promises alternatives for many patients with refractory seizures. However, additional clinical trials and more widespread clinical use are at present needed to determine the exact role these drugs will play as first-line choices in epilepsy management. The older drugs remain the most cost-effective first-line drugs against localization-related and generalized epilepsy in adults.

Surgery for Epilepsy. With the advent of sophisticated monitoring techniques for the localization of epileptic foci, surgery has begun to play an increasing role in seizure management. Many neurologists would consider referral to a center specializing in epilepsy surgery for patients who have failed several standard drugs or who require more than one drug for seizure control and experience intolerable side effects of the medical regimen.

Prognosis and Duration of Therapy

The prognosis is a function of the underlying condition. The prognosis of *idiopathic epilepsy* depends on both the age at onset and type of convulsion. Patients with primary generalized seizures have the best overall prognosis. Childhood-onset seizures cease by age 20 in more than half of cases. Although statistics vary according to age at onset and type of seizure, on average, more than half of patients are seizure-free with or without medication at 10 years after diagnosis. The probability of remaining seizure-free is highest for those patients whose seizures were generalized at the outset and were diagnosed be-

Table 170.5.   New Antiepileptic Drugs

NAME	INDICATIONS	INITIAL ADULT DOSE (mg/d)	MAINTENANCE DOSE (mg/day-divided doses)	HALF-LIFE (h)	SPECIAL ISSUES
Gabapentin (Neurontin)	SP, CP, T-C	300	900–4,800	5-7, if renal function normal	Few side effects, no AED interaction
Felbamate (Felbatol)	CP, T-C, A, L-G	1,200	1,200–3,600	20	Hepatic failure, aplastic anemia
Lamotrigine (Lamictal)	CP, T-C, A, L-G	50 no VPA 25 with VPA	300–500 no VPA 100–400 with VPA	25 monotherapy 70 with VPA	Skin rash with VPA
Topiramate (Topamax)	SP, CP, T-C	50	200–600	18–30 normal renal 60 renal failure	Kidney stones, cognitive slowing
Tiagabine (Gabitril)	CP, SP, T-C	4	32–56	7–9 monotherapy 4–7 with enzyme-inducing AEDs	Dizziness, tremor
Oxcarbazepine (Trileptal)	SP, CP	150	600–1,200		

SP, simple partial; CP, complex partial; T-C, tonic–clonic; A, absence; L-G, Lennox-Gastaut; VPA, valproate; AED, antiepileptic drug.

fore age 10. Eighty percent of recurrences develop within 5 years of discontinuation of medication. The major cause of failure to control seizures is *noncompliance*, and it has been shown that as many as one third of patients do not take their medication as prescribed.

The early identification of patients with refractory epilepsy has been studied. Among patients who fail to become seizure-free with medications, those who have had many seizures before the initiation of therapy or who show an inadequate response to initial treatment with AEDs are the most likely to have refractory epilepsy. For patients with correctable structural abnormalities, surgery should be considered as soon as treatment with two first-line drugs fails. In selected groups, this approach can yield an 80% seizure-free success rate.

Discontinuing Antiepileptic Drugs. Most neurologists require a seizure-free interval of at least 2 years before considering discontinuation of medication. The EEG is of only modest help in predicting which patients may be weaned successfully from their medications; persistent EEG abnormalities would make discontinuation of medication inadvisable, but the documentation of a normal EEG does not eliminate the risk for seizure recurrence. In a large prospective study, the risk for relapse was greatest in patients who had complex partial seizures with secondary generalization, EEG abnormalities before treatment that did not change during treatment, or a requirement for valproate. According to current American Academy of Neurology recommendations, discontinuation of AEDs can be considered for a patient who has has been seizure-free for 2 to 5 years on AEDs if the patient has a single type of partial seizure, the neurologic examination findings and intelligence quotient are normal, and the EEG has normalized with treatment. For patients not meeting this profile, the risk for recurrence may be almost 40%.

INDICATIONS FOR REFERRAL AND ADMISSION

The workup of a patient with a first seizure can be accomplished by the primary care physician with a sleep-deprived EEG and MRI. Antiepileptic medication usually can be initiated in the outpatient setting, and appropriate monitoring of therapeutic levels can be planned (Table 170.3).

For the patient who fails to respond to the first-choice medication or for whom side effects are intolerable, a second drug should be tried. If it appears that the patient may require two drugs for seizure control or if the organic nature of all the witnessed spells is questionable, it is appropriate to refer the patient to a neurologic specialist experienced in drug management and the techniques of EEG and telemetry. Such a referral will also provide the patient with access to centers in which epilepsy surgery is performed and through which newer anticonvulsant medications can be obtained.

Differentiating between an epileptic attack and other systemic disorders or psychiatric conditions can be difficult. Nonepileptic attacks and epileptic seizures can coexist in patients with seizure disorders. Monitoring with telemetry for several days in the hospital may be necessary to clarify the diagnosis. However, hospitalization after a typical generalized seizure is not necessary for a patient with a known seizure disorder, unless significant trauma has occurred or it is necessary to adjust the medication program under careful monitoring.

PATIENT EDUCATION

Perhaps the most important role a physician can play in caring for an epileptic patient is that of counselor, educator, and sometimes legal advocate. A long-standing relationship must be maintained with a patient whose chronic disease is surrounded by an enormous amount of superstition, prejudice, and misunderstanding. The diagnosis of epilepsy clearly imposes certain restrictions on the patient's life, so that the certainty of the diagnosis in a healthy young person is imperative (see above).

Work. In addition to reviewing the prognosis with the patient, it is important for the physician to emphasize that even if seizures are not entirely controlled, most epileptics are able to lead productive lives. Of the nation's 4 million epileptics, 15% to 25% are unemployed, a figure higher than the national average. However, people known to have seizures are barred absolutely only from those professions that require a chauffeur's or pilot's license.

Driving. Driving laws vary from state to state, but in general, states require a *seizure-free interval* of *6 months to 1 year* before reapplication for a driver's license may be made. Continued supervision by a physician is mandatory. These laws apply both to patients with generalized epilepsy and those with localization-related seizures.

Alcohol and Caffeine. The diagnosis of epilepsy does not make absolute abstention from alcohol mandatory, although the patient should be counseled that alcohol can lower the seizure threshold and that binge drinking is contraindicated. The relationship of seizures to the ingestion of large amounts of caffeine is less clear, but the patient should be counseled to use substances containing caffeine in moderation.

Pregnancy and Contraception. Women with epilepsy face several special issues. The American Academy of Neurology recommends that during the reproductive years, monotherapy with an AED should be the aim of treatment, and that the decreased effectiveness of hormonal contraception caused by enzyme-inducing AEDs be discussed with the patient. For an epileptic woman considering *pregnancy*, folic acid supplementation should be instituted at a dosage of no less than 0.4 mg daily. The teratogenic potential of AEDs should be discussed, as should options for considering AED discontinuation before pregnancy. Women with epilepsy who take carbamazepine or valproate should be offered prenatal testing with α-fetoprotein levels at 14 to 16 weeks' gestation. Non–protein-bound AED levels should be monitored during pregnancy. The effect of pregnancy on the severity of a seizure disorder is nil in about half of women. Of the remainder, half experience a slight worsening of seizures. Ideally, with well-controlled seizures, it would be possible to taper and discontinue the patient's medication before conception. However, one does not always have such luxury, and a patient may worry about teratogenesis. The risk for fetal malformations in an epileptic woman not on medication is still roughly double that of the general population, and teratogenesis has clearly been established for phenytoin (digital and craniofacial abnormalities and some cardiac defects), valproate (neural tube defects), and carbamazepine (facial anomalies and neural tube defects). Nonetheless, women taking phenytoin still have a 94% chance of having a completely normal pregnancy outcome.

Thus, the risks of continuing AEDs must be weighed against the benefits of preventing a sustained convulsion (fetal hypoxia, mechanical injury if the mother falls). For the patient who needs to remain on AEDs during pregnancy, monthly monitoring of her drug levels is important because the combination of decreased protein binding, decreased absorption, and increased metabolism and plasma volume result in lower drug levels. Vitamin K at a dosage of 10 mg/d should be prescribed in the last trimester of pregnancy for women taking enzyme-inducing AEDs. Postpartum adjustment of the AED will be necessary for women whose dosage has been increased during pregnancy. AED dosages usually can be reduced to those given before pregnancy by 8 weeks after delivery.

Surgery. *Surgical procedures* pose no special threat to the epileptic patient as long as medications are not discontinued. Parenteral forms of phenytoin, phenobarbital, and valproate are available. Although no parenteral form of carbamazepine is available, a rectal suppository can be prepared in many hospital pharmacies.

Breast-feeding. Should the mother taking anticonvulsant therapy elect to nurse her infant, breast-feeding usually poses little problem. Some sedation in the infant is occasionally seen with phenytoin, carbamazepine, or phenobarbital. One case has been reported of an infant with thrombocytopenia and anemia, presumed to have been induced by valproate ingested through breast milk. Breast-feeding appears to be safe, without any risk for hepatic or hematologic toxicity to the infant.

Heredity of Seizures. Patients may worry considerably about the inheritance of seizures. Epilepsy is hereditary, although the precise genetics are not clear for all types. One fourth to one third of patients with idiopathic epilepsy have a family history of seizures. Seizures develop in 3% of the children of patients with idiopathic epilepsy. Febrile convulsions also appear to be more common in children who have afflicted relatives, as are posttraumatic seizures.

Teaching First Aid. Families of patients with epilepsy should know the fundamentals of emergency management of seizures. They should be instructed in the positioning that protects the airway and cautioned against use of the time-honored tongue blade. It should be emphasized to the patient's family that few seizures last long enough to impair cardiopulmonary function.

THERAPEUTIC RECOMMENDATIONS

- Establish an etiologic diagnosis and treat the underlying cause if possible. Symptomatic therapy can begin while evaluation is in progress.
- To prevent further convulsions, begin with a loading dose of a drug of choice appropriate to the seizure type identified. This can often be accomplished on an outpatient basis. A maintenance dose is then begun, and the dose is adjusted to achieve a therapeutic level, with the level checked at an interval appropriate for the drug half-life.
- If seizures persist, check the serum levels of the AED and inquire into alcohol and other drug use. Add a second drug and then taper and discontinue the first drug if the seizures cannot be controlled with the drug of first choice.

- If the seizures are controlled, have the patient continue the medication for at least 2 years. If the patient remains seizure-free, a cautious attempt to taper the medication can be made according to the guidelines explained in the preceding text.
- Teach the patient how to recognize the warning signals of a seizure and what to do to minimize injury. Instruct the patient about the role of alcohol in precipitating seizures.
- Educate the patient and family about prognosis, activity, and job precautions.

ANNOTATED BIBLIOGRAPHY

Engel J Jr. Surgery for seizures. N Engl J Med 1996;334:647. (*Advocates surgical evaluation as soon as treatment with two first-line AEDs fails.*)

First Seizure Trial Group. Randomized clinical trial on the efficacy of antiepileptic drugs in the risk of relapse after a first unprovoked tonic–clonic seizure. Neurology 1993;43:478. (*Multicenter trial of adult and pediatric patients randomized to treatment or no treatment. Cumulative risk for recurrence was 25% among treated subjects and 51% among those not treated.*)

Foldvary NO, Nashold B, Mascha E. Seizure outcome after temporal lobectomy for temporal lobe epilepsy. Neurology 2000;54:630. (*One postoperative seizure occurred in 55% of patients with a mean follow-up of 14 years; a seizure-free state at 2 years was found to be the best predictor of sustained, long-term benefit.*)

Consensus statements: medical management of epilepsy. Neurology 1998;51[Suppl 4]:S39. (*Summary of American Academy of Neurology opinions on treatment of first seizure, choice of medication, management of epilepsy during pregnancy and in the elderly, and management of status epilepticus.*)

Hauser WA, Rich SS, Lee JR, et al. Risk of recurrent seizures after two unprovoked seizures. N Engl J Med 1998;338:429. (*The risk approaches 90% in some subgroups; therefore, there is little question that a patient needs to be treated after a second unprovoked seizure.*)

Kwan P, Brodie MJ. Early identification of refractory epilepsy. N Engl J Med 2000;342:314. (*Patients who have many seizures before therapy or who have breakthrough seizures during initial treatment are likely to have refractory epilepsy.*)

Mattson RH. An overview of the new antiepileptic drugs. Neurologist 1998;S2. (*Excellent summary of felbamate, gabapentin, lamotrigine, topiramate, tiagabine, and vigabatrin. Emphasizes that extensive postmarketing study is still required to delineate optimal dosing, spectrum of efficacy, potency, and adverse effects.*)

Mattson RH. Medical management of epilepsy in adults. Neurology 1998;51[Suppl 4]:S15-20. (*Emphasizes that localization-related, or partial, epilepsy is the most common type of seizure in adults and that carbamazepine and phenytoin remain the first-line treatments for adult patients with partial seizures.*)

Meador HG. Comparative cognitive effects of anti-convulsants. Neurology 1990;43:91. (*All about equal, save for phenobarbital.*)

Tempkin NR, et al. A randomized double-blind study of phenytoin for the prevention of posttraumatic seizures. N Engl J Med 1990;32:497. (*Phenytoin does not prevent the development of posttraumatic seizures.*)

Willmore LJ. Epilepsy emergencies. The first seizure and status epilepticus. Neurology 1998;51[Suppl 4]:S34. (*Good summary of two important areas.*)

Zahn CA, Morell MJ, Collins SD, et al. Management issues for women with epilepsy. Neurology 1998;51:949. (*Along with a practice parameter advisory on management issues for women with epilepsy from the American Academy of Neurology, this article provides good guidelines for a discussion of preconception, contraception, folate repletion, teratogenesis, and vitamin K supplementation.*)

171
Management of Transient Ischemic Attack and Asymptomatic Carotid Bruit
AMY A. PRUITT

Stroke is the third leading cause of death in the United States and is the leading cause of long-term disability in the older population. Although medical and surgical therapies for stroke are improving, prevention is still the most effective strategy and a major responsibility of the primary care physician. Stroke prevention through risk factor management may be a major contributor to the rapid decline during the past two decades in death rates from stroke. The cornerstone of the preventive effort is the early identification and vigorous treatment of stroke risk factors (e.g., hypertension, diabetes, coronary artery disease, smoking; see Chapters 26, 30, 54, and 102). Atrial fibrillation, a major risk factor for embolic stroke, also requires serious attention (see Chapters 28 and 83).

Patients who present with a transient ischemic attack (TIA) or an asymptomatic carotid bruit pose the problem of stroke prevention at a more advanced stage of cerebrovascular disease. Approximately 50,000 patients with TIAs present for evaluation annually, and it is estimated that 2 million people have some degree of asymptomatic carotid stenosis. The primary physician should be able to recognize these conditions by history and physical examination, use appropriate noninvasive imaging and flow studies cost-effectively, and know when to initiate more aggressive measures, such as anticoagulant therapy or surgical intervention.

PATHOPHYSIOLOGY, CLINICAL PRESENTATION, AND COURSE

Transient Ischemic Attack

Transient ischemic attacks are defined as episodes of temporary, focal cerebral dysfunction resulting from vascular disease that last *less than 24 hours* and *usually less than 10 minutes*. TIAs are part of a spectrum that includes ischemic events lasting more than 24 hours and partially reversible, nondisabling strokes. The distinction between TIAs, cerebral infarction with transient signs (CITS), and stroke has become less clear with the advent of computed tomography (CT) and magnetic resonance imaging (MRI) because many patients whose deficits appear to resolve completely are found to have radiographic changes suggesting infarction. However, all these patients fall into a group that may be at risk for further ischemic damage.

Pathogenesis. TIAs can develop through any of several mechanisms. In the majority of cases, *emboli* of platelets and fibrin or of atheromatous material that breaks off from a vessel wall (usually the carotid) transiently occlude a cerebral or ophthalmic artery or one of its branches. Thrombus formation distal to an atherosclerotic plaque is common in tightly stenosed arteries (>75% stenosis, residual lumen <2 mm) or even in totally occluded carotid arteries, and the thrombus often serves as a source of emboli. The heart is the other important source of emboli. Cardiac lesions predisposing to cerebral embolism include mitral valve stenosis, mitral valve prolapse, calcified mitral annulus, ventricular aneurysm or dyskinesia, atrial or ventricular clot, valvular vegetation, and interatrial shunt. Atrial fibrillation greatly exacerbates the risk for cardiac embolization. Occasionally, the intracranial arteries are the source of emboli. This phenomenon occurs most frequently among male African-Americans and should be considered in patients with no extracranial vascular or cardiac source of emboli. The aortic arch may also be a source of atheromatous emboli.

Transient ischemic attacks may also develop when *transient hypotension* occurs in conjunction with a hemodynamically *significant carotid stenosis* (>75% occlusion). The resulting reduction in collateral flow to the ipsilateral carotid territory can lead to transient neurologic symptoms. The reduced blood pressure rarely results in focal symptoms unless a severely stenotic lesion is already present.

Small-vessel thrombotic or lacunar stroke may be preceded by transient, focal neurologic deficits in as many as a third of patients who go on to have a completed stroke. The clinician must be aware that the distinction between stroke mechanisms, particularly distal emboli or large-vessel origin and small-vessel thrombotic disease, may be difficult. Because management of the two types of conditions differs considerably, it is important to be aware of syndromes that commonly are associated with small-vessel disease (pure motor hemiparesis, ataxic hemiparesis, clumsy hand dysarthria syndrome).

In certain rare instances, TIAs may be attributable to one of the following: steal phenomena (e.g., subclavian steal); hyperviscosity states (e.g., polycythemia); vasculitis; coagulopathies (e.g., antiphospholipid antibody syndrome, deficiency of factor V Leiden, protein C, protein S, or antithrombin III); dissection of the carotid or vertebral artery. These underlying causes of stroke and TIA are more common in younger patients (under age 45).

Clinical Presentation. TIAs can be divided into those caused by disease in the carotid circulation and those that are a consequence of disease in the vertebrobasilar territory. Symptoms of TIA associated with *carotid disease* include transient monocular blindness; clumsiness, weakness, or numbness of the hand; and disturbed speech. Transient monocular blindness is caused by occlusion of the ophthalmic artery or branches ipsilateral to the carotid stenosis and classically is described by the patient as a "shade" or "curtain" that descends over the affected eye. In patients with symptoms suggestive of carotid disease, the detection of a carotid bruit on the same side as the symptomatic eye or cerebral hemisphere is suggestive but not diagnostic of high-grade carotid stenosis.

Symptoms of *vertebrobasilar disease* include binocular visual disturbance, vertigo, paresthesias, diplopia, ataxia, dysarthria, light-headedness, generalized weakness, loss of consciousness, and transient global amnesia. Each of these may be an isolated symptom of disease of the posterior circulation, although isolated vertigo without other brainstem symptoms is rarely caused by vertebrobasilar occlusive disease (see Chapter 166).

Certain clinical features are likely to be associated with carotid or vertebrobasilar disease, but no single feature is a consistently reliable sign. Two clinical features were found in an angiographic study to correlate with the arteriographic findings: (a) A *hemispheric attack lasting longer than 60 minutes*, whether single or multiple, was significantly associated with a *normal carotid* (attacks were most likely to be caused by emboli from the heart); (b) the *nonsimultaneous occurrence of transient hemispheric episodes* and *transient monocular blindness* correlated with an 80% incidence of carotid disease. No difference between groups with normal or diseased carotid arteries was found when the cumulative number of attacks per patient was considered. Similarly, the presence of purely ocular or purely hemispheric symptoms could not be used to distinguish between the two groups.

Clinical Course and Risk for Stroke. The interval since the most recent TIA appears to be the single most important factor in predicting the risk for stroke. Of those patients in whom stroke will develop, approximately one half will have a stroke within 1 year after the first TIA, and approximately one fifth will have a stroke during the first month after the episode. The risk for stroke cannot be predicted by the number of TIAs, duration of symptoms, or clinical phenomena. All patients with any type of TIA should be considered at risk for stroke, and those with TIA of recent onset (<1 month) should be evaluated urgently (see below). About 50% to 75% of patients with occlusive carotid disease who have a stroke have preceding TIAs.

Cardioembolic Stroke with Transient Symptoms

In patients with cardioembolic stroke who have transient symptoms, the symptoms tend to last several hours. The neurologic disorder associated with cardioembolic infarction is maximal at onset in 80% of patients, and about 75% of emboli lodge in one of the middle cerebral arteries and cause symptoms similar to those of carotid occlusive disease.

Asymptomatic Carotid Bruits

Incidental discovery on physical examination of an asymptomatic carotid bruit suggests the presence of an atherosclerotic lesion that has narrowed the lumen by at least 50%, to less than 3 mm. The pitch of the bruit increases with the severity of stenosis. Prolonged, very high-pitched bruits suggest a residual lumen of less than 1.5 mm (>75% stenosis). Most atherosclerotic lesions causing bruits tend to be located on the posterior wall of the common carotid artery at the bifurcation, compromising flow at the origin of the internal carotid. When stenosis is tight and flow is reduced, a mural thrombus may form distally in the proximal internal carotid artery, worsening occlusion and serving as a source of emboli. Plaque ulceration may also provide a nidus for mural thrombus formation.

Epidemiologic studies indicate that asymptomatic bruits are associated with an increased risk for stroke, coronary disease, and death, but not necessarily with an increased risk for stroke

on the side of the bruit. In a large, prospective study of 500 patients with asymptomatic bruit followed for an average of 2 years by clinical and Doppler examination, the overall risk for stroke in patients who remained asymptomatic was 1% at 1 year and 1.7% when those in whom TIAs developed were included. A major predictor of stroke was the severity of carotid stenosis, as was progression to high-grade stenosis (>75% stenosis, residual lumen <2 mm). Other risk factors included hypertension, preexisting heart disease, male sex, and a positive family history.

DIFFERENTIAL DIAGNOSIS

The differential diagnosis of a TIA-like episode includes any condition that causes transient symptoms in a focal distribution and is not limited to those of vascular origin. Vascular mechanisms include carotid or vertebrobasilar occlusive disease, small-vessel ischemic stroke, and occlusion by emboli originating in the heart or aortic arch. *Focal seizures* (see Chapter 170) can produce symptoms similar to those of a TIA, as can the focal aura of *migraine*, which is not always followed by headache (see Chapter 165). *Hyperventilation* can produce distal tingling and numbness. *Carpal tunnel syndrome* may present with intermittent (often nocturnal) paresthesias in a median nerve distribution. Even a protruding *cervical disk* or osteophyte may produce transient focal motor or sensory symptoms (as during manipulation of the head or neck; see Chapter 167).

WORKUP

The goals in evaluating a TIA or an asymptomatic bruit are the detection of significant vascular disease and the assessment of stroke risk. One needs to identify those patients who require aggressive intervention. In addition, if cerebrovascular disease can be ruled out as the cause, a search for other causes is required. The patient with a new onset of TIAs (<30 days) has an increased risk for stroke and should be evaluated promptly.

History. For the patient with a suspected TIA, questioning should first confirm that the transient episode was indeed a TIA, based on onset and duration. Symptoms lasting longer than 24 hours exclude TIA; cessation within 10 minutes increases the probability. An episode that lasts hours might be the consequence of an embolic event. The onset of headache during resolution of the neurologic deficit is more suggestive of a migrainous episode (see Chapter 165). A careful description of symptoms may be helpful in distinguishing vertebrobasilar involvement from carotid disease (see above). In addition, the frequency of episodes, date of first onset, and presence of underlying heart disease and cardiovascular risk factors are important to ascertain because they can help predict the clinical course. If the patient has hypertension or cardiac disease or is older (>65 years), the risk for subsequent stroke is increased. A disabling stroke is more likely to develop in patients with carotid symptoms than in those with vertebrobasilar dysfunction. The patient is at greatest risk for stroke in the first few months after the onset of TIAs.

When an apparently asymptomatic carotid bruit is found on physical examination, it is worthwhile to go back to the patient's history and check carefully for overlooked transient neurologic events. Their presence would greatly increase the significance of the physical examination finding and indicate a heightened risk for stroke.

Inquiry into a history of hypertension or heart disease and any family history of stroke further helps to determine stroke risk. Risk factors for stroke include advanced age, elevated systolic blood pressure, current smoking, and the presence of diabetes, atrial fibrillation, or coronary heart disease.

Physical Examination should be directed to the cardiovascular and nervous systems. One checks for hypertension, atrial fibrillation, and heart murmurs (see Chapters 21 and 33). Funduscopic examination at the time visual symptoms occur may reveal an embolus in one of the retinal artery branches. Neurologic examination findings are likely to be normal if the examination is conducted after the TIA has passed.

Gentle palpation and auscultation of the carotid arteries should be performed to note upstroke, volume, and the presence of a bruit. As stated above, the presence of a bruit does not invariably herald significant stenosis (a bruit can be present with hemodynamically insignificant lesions), but in as many as 70% to 80% of cases, the bruit does indicate important ipsilateral carotid disease. The pitch of the bruit and its duration should be noted because they tend to correlate with severity of stenosis.

Palpation of the facial and superficial temporal pulses with simultaneous assessment of the supratrochlear and supraorbital pulses may confirm collateral flow to the latter two vessels by way of the external carotid artery, which suggests occlusion of the internal carotid artery. Unfortunately, the vertebrobasilar circulation is not accessible to accurate physical examination.

Laboratory Studies. Initial laboratory studies should include a complete blood cell count and a determination of glucose, cholesterol, triglyceride, and electrolyte levels. Homocysteine has been independently associated with stroke risk and should be measured, along with serum folate and vitamin B_{12}. It appears that most people with low serum folate or vitamin B_{12} levels also have high homocysteine levels.

No entirely reliable noninvasive test for carotid or vertebrobasilar disease is available. In the past two decades, great strides have been made in the noninvasive evaluation of the carotid arteries and vessels of the posterior circulation. For the assessment of suspected *carotid lesions*, the combination of *Doppler* and *B-mode ultrasonography* allows a determination of lumen size and visualization of the carotid arterial lesion. In studies comparing arteriography and duplex carotid ultrasonography, a reduction in the diameter of the carotid artery of more than 60% was associated with a residual lumen at arteriography of less than 2 mm. However, in some instances, one cannot tell if the carotid artery is completely occluded or only tightly stenosed.

Magnetic resonance angiography (MRA) increasingly is being used in lieu of standard arteriography in the preoperative assessment of symptomatic carotid disease. However, most clinical studies still require the gold standard of arteriography. The use of *transcranial Doppler* techniques helps to measure flow in the ophthalmic system, assess the hemodynamic significance of the carotid stenosis, and detect any major stenosis of the intracranial vessels.

For the study of the *posterior circulation, transcranial Doppler* ultrasonography provides a relatively inexpensive means of noninvasively surveying large intracranial vessels.

The test measures the velocity of flow, which increases in the setting of stenosis. However, it does not provide direct anatomic information. *MRA* provides noninvasive visualization of the vertebrobasilar system.

To detect silent or prior infarction, unsuspected hemorrhage, or nonvascular disease, such as tumor, *CT* or *MRI* of the brain should be performed.

No entirely reliable noninvasive test for occlusive disease is available, and *arteriography* remains the definitive diagnostic procedure. Arteriography with the use of selective transfemoral catheterization or digital subtraction techniques should be performed only if the physician would proceed to endarterectomy in the instance of carotid disease or to anticoagulation in the case of vertebrobasilar disease. Thus, the procedure should lead to a critical management decision. The dye load involved in cerebrovascular angiography can be substantial and necessitates adequate hydration, particularly in patients with underlying renal disease or diabetes.

Transthoracic echocardiography makes it possible to identify cardiac lesions that predispose to embolization, but the yield is low in patients over the age of 50 without evidence of cardiac disease on physical examination (see Chapter 33). *Transesophageal echocardiography* is more sensitive and specific for detecting intracardiac and aortic sources of embolization, such as left atrial thrombus and atherosclerosis of the ascending aortic arch. It should be considered when standard echocardiography is unrevealing but clinical suspicion of embolization is strong. Ambulatory *Holter monitoring* is useful when atrial fibrillation as a precipitant of embolization is a concern and results of the *resting electrocardiogram* are normal (see Chapters 25 and 29).

Abnormalities of blood coagulation may contribute to 4% of strokes in young persons. Some authorities recommend a *coagulopathy workup* for stroke patients whose age is below 50, who have prior venous disease or a family history of abnormal clotting and no other explanation for their stroke, or whose hematocrit, platelets, prothrombin time, or partial thromboplastin time is abnormal. A full workup in the young stroke patient would require a test for anticardiolipin antibodies; measurement of protein C and protein S, antithrombin III, factor V Leiden, and homocysteine levels; an antinuclear antibody test; determination of the erythrocyte sedimentation rate; and syphilis serology.

PRINCIPLES OF MANAGEMENT

Transient Ischemic Attack

The literature on therapeutic options in TIAs is complex and often confusing. Until recently, many studies were not well controlled, and study populations were often not well defined or characterized. Recent demographic data have clarified those patients at greatest risk for stroke. As noted earlier, the interval since the most recent TIA appears to be the most important single factor in predicting the risk for stroke. Therefore, all patients with any type of TIA should be considered at risk for stroke, and those with a recent onset (<1 month) of TIA should be evaluated urgently. The physician should remember that although TIAs are predictors of stroke, myocardial infarction is still the most common cause of death in this group (annual mortality rate of 5%) and that the patient's cardiovascular status and cardiac risk factors must also be considered (see Chapter 30).

With the caveat that optimal therapy for TIAs is an evolving area and that new information is forthcoming regularly, the following guidelines for management are recommended:

Symptomatic Patients with Tight Carotid Stenosis. Patients with *more than 70% carotid stenosis*, especially those who have had *recurrent TIAs* or a TIA within 4 months of the current visit, require prompt attention and should be considered for *carotid endarterectomy*. If adequate radiologic support is available, these patients should undergo arteriography as soon as possible in addition to a careful cardiovascular evaluation (see Chapter 30). Because the risk for cardiovascular mortality and morbidity associated with noncardiac surgery is very high in this population, a careful cardiac assessment is an essential component of the determination of surgical candidacy. (Some physicians directly admit such patients to the hospital and immediately place them on IV heparin until arteriography can be performed—a practice that has been the subject of several small trials; see Annotated Bibliography).

The role of surgery has recently been clarified by the North American Symptomatic Carotid Endarterectomy Trial, published in 1991. This trial involved more than 600 *symptomatic patients* with *high-grade (70% to 99%) stenosis* of a carotid artery in the appropriate territory for their TIA. The trial was terminated early when it became clear that endarterectomy (when performed by a skilled surgical team) was significantly superior to medical management (aspirin) for patients with recent hemispheric or retinal TIA or nondisabling stroke and *ipsilateral* high-grade stenosis of the *internal carotid artery*.

Symptomatic Patients with Less Severe Carotid Stenosis. The North American Symptomatic Carotid Endarterectomy Trial also addressed the role of surgery in patients with *less severe carotid stenosis (50% to 69%)*. For those who recently have had a TIA or stroke, endarterectomy lowers the risk for stroke to a greater degree than does medical management. Patients with *less than 50% stenosis* do not benefit from surgery. These patients have a cardiovascular mortality risk from noncardiac surgery equal to that of patients with critical carotid stenosis, but a lower stroke risk. The reader is urged to watch the literature for reports from both of these multicenter trials for guidance on the best approach to the management of such patients. All patients should have a systolic blood pressure below 140 mm Hg and a diastolic blood pressure below 90 mm Hg. Smoking and excessive alcohol consumption should be stopped, coronary artery disease treated, fasting blood glucose maintained below 126 mg/dL, and a regular exercise program of 30 to 60 minutes three times per week instituted. Estrogen replacement should be maintained in postmenopausal women. Lipid-lowering therapy should be instituted in patients with elevated cholesterol.

A daily *antiplatelet agent* should be prescribed. Options include *aspirin, clopidogrel, ticlopidine*, and a combination of aspirin and extended-release dipyridamole. Aspirin (50 to 325 mg/d) is recommended as initial therapy. Ticlopidine is effective in reducing the risk for recurrent TIA or stroke in both men and women, but it may increase serum cholesterol levels and has been associated with neutropenia. Clopidogrel has a better safety profile and is a good alternative to aspirin or ticlopidine. Dipyridamole combined with aspirin (Aggrenox) is at least as effective as clopidogrel. Anticoagulant therapy with warfarin is not routinely recommended for patients with atherothrombotic TIAs. Long-term oral anticoagulation with warfarin is advised for patients with atrial fibrillation, but aspirin confers some benefit in these patients if oral anticoagulation is contraindicated (see Chapters 28 and 83).

Candidates for Medical Therapy. Medical therapy may be elected for TIA patients who are *elderly, cannot tolerate surgery*, have a *single remote TIA*, or are seen in settings where angiographic and surgical services are unavailable. The optimal medical management of TIA is *aspirin*. Several studies have evaluated the effectiveness of aspirin in different doses for patients with threatened stroke. In a Canadian Cooperative Study Group evaluation of 585 patients with TIA, a 19% overall reduced incidence of TIA, stroke, and death was shown in male patients only. The result of the U.K. study was similar, and the recent Dutch TIA trial reported that 30 mg of aspirin per day was no less effective than higher doses in preventing vascular events and caused fewer gastrointestinal side effects.

Patients with Transient Ischemic Attack and Normal Carotid Vessels should undergo a thorough cardiac evaluation to rule out an embolic source in the heart. In the absence of atrial fibrillation, valvular heart disease, or carotid disease, the proper preventive treatment for future stroke is not clear. It is common practice to place such patients on *aspirin* prophylactically (325 mg/d), and some evidence is available to recommend this practice. Although aspirin may reduce the morbidity from myocardial infarction, it is unclear whether it reduces stroke with noncarotid sources. Aspirin and warfarin have yet to be compared in a well-designed, randomized study.

Warfarin therapy is indicated for patients having TIA-like episodes believed to be caused by cardioembolic disease. Several controlled multicenter studies have demonstrated that the incidence of thromboembolic complications of *nonrheumatic atrial fibrillation* can be significantly reduced by oral anticoagulant therapy in comparison with aspirin or placebo. Warfarin anticoagulation is currently recommended, and low-intensity therapy (prothrombin time 1.2 to 1.4 times control) has proved equally efficacious and safer than standard-intensity therapy for patients with nonrheumatic atrial fibrillation (see Chapters 28 and 83).

Asymptomatic Carotid Bruit

A carotid bruit detected in an asymptomatic patient need not be considered an invariable harbinger of stroke, but it does suggest atherosclerotic carotid disease. The risk for stroke increases significantly with severity of stenosis, onset of TIAs, and progression of the lesion. The patient should undergo a thorough, noninvasive carotid evaluation (see above) to confirm the carotid origin of the bruit, the severity of stenosis, and its hemodynamic effects. Regardless of the severity of stenosis, the recognition and *prompt reporting of any TIA symptoms* should be emphasized. Previously asymptomatic patients with high-grade stenosis (70% to 99%) who subsequently experience a *TIA* are at markedly enhanced risk for stroke and should be referred promptly for consideration of *surgical intervention* (see above).

Medical Therapy. Antiplatelet therapy with low-dose aspirin (60 to 325 mg/d) is recommended; higher doses are associated with an increased risk for subarachnoid hemorrhage, especially in elderly patients with hypertension. Aggressive treatment of *cardiovascular risk factors* (i.e., *hypertension, lipids, smoking, diabetes*; see Chapters 26, 27, 54, and 102) is essential, not only because the risk for coronary events is high and can be significantly reduced (see Chapter 30), but also because the risk for stroke can be lessened. For example, clinically significant reductions in the risk for stroke and stroke mortality (12% to 23%) are associated with aggressive lipid-lowering therapy with statins, reductions in risk similar to those associated with the use of antiplatelet agents. The benefit of identifying and treating elevated *homocysteine* levels remains to be ascertained, even though such elevations appear to be associated with an increased risk for stroke.

Endarterectomy. The role of carotid endarterectomy in the asymptomatic patient with a high-grade stenosis is unresolved. The use of carotid endarterectomy is on the rise; after a 6-year decline, the number of operations rose by 94% between 1991 and 1996. The cost-effectiveness of this practice needs to be questioned in view of data from randomized trials. In the Asymptomatic Carotid Atherosclerosis Study, a 53% reduction in *relative risk* was noted, but the *absolute risk* declined by only 1% annually in a comparison with medical therapy. Sixty-seven patients would have to undergo surgery to prevent one stroke, at an additional cost of more than $1.5 million. Moreover, because patients were a select, low-risk surgical group and the surgeons and hospitals were screened for a perioperative complication rate of only 2.3%, it is difficult to extrapolate these results to practice at large. Reported perioperative complication rates in most settings are considerably higher (e.g., 6.5% for perioperative stroke and death, including a 1.8% rate of disabling stroke). Asymptomatic patients with an occluded carotid artery and asymptomatic stenosis on the other side experience a reported perioperative complication rate after endarterectomy of 12.6%. Such levels of perioperative risk appear to outweigh any benefit obtained from elective endarterectomy. To date, trials of asymptomatic persons have failed to identify a subgroup in whom prophylactic benefit clearly outweighs such operative risk. Thus, despite the temptation to conclude that these patients are at particular risk for stroke, surgery cannot yet be recommended in this asymptomatic population.

Pending definitive data on medical versus surgical therapy in the truly asymptomatic patient, some authorities recommend that endarterectomy be considered for those who demonstrate a rapid progression to hemodynamically and anatomically critical stenosis (e.g., lumen <1 mm), provided that they have no active coronary disease, are not diabetic, and have an anticipated life expectancy of more than 5 years. In support of this view is the high risk for stroke; against it is the high cardiac risk associated with surgery and the absence of proven benefit. If surgery is going to be recommended, one must have access to a skilled surgical team with a proven record of low perioperative morbidity and mortality (<2%) and be sure that a careful preoperative cardiac risk assessment is carried out (see Chapters 30 and 36).

ANNOTATED BIBLIOGRAPHY

Albers GW, Harat RG, Helmi LL, et al. Supplement to the guidelines for the management of transient ischemic attacks. Stroke 1999;30:2502. (*Consensus guidelines.*)

Albers GW, Tijssen JGP. Antiplatelet therapy: new foundations for optimal treatment decisions. Neurology 1999;53[Suppl 4]:S25. (*Good summary of safety and efficacy data for ticlopidine, clopidogrel, and aspirin/dipyridamole.*)

Barnett HJM, Haines SJ. Carotid endarterectomy for asymptomatic carotid stenosis. N Engl J Med 1993;328:267. (*Editorial arguing that benefit of endarterectomy in asymptomatic patients remains unproven.*)

Barnett HJM, Meldrum HE. Carotid endarterectomy. A neurotherapeutic advance. Arch Neurol 2000;57:40. (*A superb summary of trial results for symptomatic and asymptomatic patients with carotid disease.*)

Barnett HJM, Taylor WD, Eliasziw M, et al. Benefit of carotid endarterectomy in patients with symptomatic moderate or severe stenosis. N Engl J Med 1998;339:1415. (*The North American Symptomatic Carotid Endarterectomy Trial showed that patients with stenosis exceeding 70% had a durable benefit from endarterectomy at 8 years of follow-up.*)

Bostom AG, Rosenberg IH, Silbershatz H, et al. Nonfasting plasma total homocysteine levels and stroke incidence in elderly persons: the Framingham Study. Ann Intern Med 1999;131:352. (*Elevated homocysteine levels were independently associated with stroke incidence.*)

Bucher HC, Griffith LE, Guyatt GH. Effect of HMG CoA reductase inhibitors on stroke: a meta-analysis of randomized, controlled trials. Ann Intern Med 1998;128:89. (*Found that risk for stroke in hyperlipidemic patients treated with these agents was reduced by nearly 25%; no such result noted with use of resins or fibrates.*)

Dutch TIA Trial Study Group. Comparison of two doses of aspirin (30 mg versus 383 mg per day) in patients after a transient ischemic attack or minor ischemic stroke. N Engl J Med 1991;325:1261. (*Low-dose aspirin was as effective as higher doses in preventing stroke recurrence.*)

Executive Committee for the Asymptomatic Carotid Atherosclerosis Study. Endarterectomy for asymptomatic carotid artery stenosis. JAMA 1995;273:1421. (*The 5-year risk for ipsilateral stroke in patients with asymptomatic carotid artery stenosis of 60% or more is reduced if carotid endarterectomy is performed with less than 3% perioperative morbidity and mortality and risk factors are aggressively managed.*)

Ferguson GG, Eliasziw M, Barr HW, et al. North American Symptomatic Carotid Endarterectomy Trial: surgical results in 1,415 patients. Stroke 1999;30:1751. (*The overall stroke and death rate was 6.5%, and the rate of disabling stroke was 1.8%. Perioperative risk was not influenced by degree of stenosis, shunting, age, or vascular risk factors.*)

Gorelick PB, Born GV, A'Agostino RB, et al. Therapeutic benefit: aspirin revisited in light of the introduction of clopidogrel. Stroke 1999;30:1716-1721. (*Clopidogrel does not cause significant neutropenia, but it is 45 times more expensive than aspirin. When a combined end point of ischemic stroke, myocardial infarction, or vascular death was used, the reduction in relative risk with clopidogrel was 8.7% in comparison with aspirin.*)

Hart RG, Benavent O, McBride R, et al. Antithrombotic therapy to prevent stroke in patients with atrial fibrillation: a meta-analysis. Ann Intern Med 1999;131:492. (*Warfarin and aspirin reduce stroke in patients with atrial fibrillation. For patients with nonvalvular atrial fibrillation who cannot tolerate warfarin, aspirin does offer significant protection.*)

Hobson RW, Weiss DG, Fields WS, et al. Efficacy of carotid endarterectomy for asymptomatic carotid stenosis. N Engl J Med 1993;328:221. (*Randomized, controlled study showing reduction in rate of ipsilateral neurologic events, but not in the combined incidence of stroke and death.*)

Iso H, Hennekens CH, Stampfer MJ, et al. Prospective study of aspirin use and risk of stroke in women. Stroke 1999;30:1764. (*A 14-year follow-up in the Nurses Health Study cohort showed benefit and safety for low-dose therapy.*)

Madden KP, Karanjia PN, Adams HPJ, et al., for the TOAST investigators. Accuracy of initial stroke subtype diagnosis in the TOAST study. Neurology 1995;45:1875. [*The absence of early CT signs of infarct and the presence of pure motor hemiparesis or sensorimotor presentation involving at least two areas (e.g., arm and leg) did not always correspond to a small-vessel (lacunar) infarction.*]

North American Symptomatic Carotid Endarterectomy Trial Collaborators. Beneficial effect of carotid endarterectomy in symptomatic patients with high-grade carotid stenosis. N Engl J Med 1991;325:445. (*Major randomized multicenter study documenting the superiority of surgical over medical management in this group of patients.*)

Tu JV, Hannan EL, Anderson GM, et al. The fall and rise of carotid endarterectomy in the United States and Canada. N Engl J Med 1998;339:1441. (*The authors raise the question of whether the benefits of carotid endarterectomy in the general population are similar to those demonstrated in the clinical trials.*)

172
Management of Multiple Sclerosis
AMY A. PRUITT

Multiple sclerosis (MS) is the most common demyelinating disease of the central nervous system (CNS), affecting approximately 2.5 million young adults worldwide. Severe disability develops in approximately 30% of patients. The manifestations of the disease are protean, and its clinical course is highly variable from patient to patient. Although most patients with MS will be under the care of the neurologist during periods of marked exacerbation, they often depend on the primary physician for close monitoring, interpretation of symptoms, treatment of intercurrent infections, and decisions regarding the need for referral. Consequently, the primary physician must be familiar with the range of clinical presentations for MS, its natural history, and the available therapeutic options. Such knowledge facilitates the provision of proper primary care and ensures the optimal timing of referrals.

PATHOPHYSIOLOGY, CLINICAL PRESENTATION, AND COURSE

The etiology of multiple sclerosis remains unknown, but available research suggests an interplay of genetic susceptibility, environmental exposure(s), and defective regulation of the immune response. These factors result in a series of discrete episodes of myelin-specific *autoimmune injury* to the CNS, separated both in time and space. Acutely, an infiltrate of lymphocytes, macrophages, and plasma cells forms in areas of involvement. T cells are thought to initiate the process, and activated macrophages to damage the myelin. Localized edema and transient breakdown of the blood–brain barrier occur. The chronicity of the inflammatory process results in the formation of a plaque or glial scar, made up of proliferated astrocytes that cluster in response to inflammatory injury of the myelin sheath. Lesions occur predominantly in the white matter of the brain and spinal cord; occasionally, gray matter is involved to a minor degree.

Demyelination is characteristically focal, but axonal injury can occur early in the course of the disease. Brain atrophy also has been documented during early, clinically silent phases of the illness. Plaques are most commonly found in the optic nerves, spinal cord, brainstem, cerebellum, and periventricular areas. After an attack, some remyelination occurs, which accounts for a partial resolution of symptoms. However, partially demyelinated axons are susceptible to dysfunction, particularly under conditions of heat stress but also spontaneously. Even a hot shower may cause a temporary exacerbation.

Clinical Presentation is a function of the site of the inflammatory process. Attacks are by definition those that produce symptoms that last more than 24 hours. They average up to one per year and decrease in frequency over time. Transient *sensory deficits* are the most common initial presentation, affecting about 40% to 50% of patients. They include *paresthesias* or diminution of sensation in the upper or lower extremities. The sensory disturbance may be bilateral and symmetric, extending to involve the adjacent trunk. About 15% to 20% experience *acute monocular visual loss* because of *optic neuritis*. A central scotoma, transient pain on eye movement, and decreased pupillary reaction to light (Marcus-Gunn pupil) are characteristic features. *Diplopia* resulting from *internuclear ophthalmoplegia* or an oculomotor defect is another common symptom heralding MS. Bilateral internuclear ophthalmoplegia is very characteristic of MS and strongly suggests the diagnosis. A failure of adduction and coarse nystagmus in the abducting eye are noted. Other oculomotor functions remain intact. *Ataxia* and *intention tremor* are manifestations of cerebellar involvement. *Motor deficits* may occur acutely or insidiously, with the insidious variety particularly common in older patients. Legs are more likely to be involved than arms, initially asymmetrically. However, upturned toes are common bilaterally, even in patients with unilateral problems. *Urinary difficulties* (frequency, urgency, incontinence) are consequences of upper motor nerve injury in the spinal cord. The external sphincter fails to relax adequately, causing incomplete emptying. Such autonomic injury may also produce *constipation* and *impotence*.

Later in the course of illness, *cerebral involvement* may produce memory loss, personality change, and emotional lability. More than 60% of MS patients demonstrate abnormalities on formal neuropsychiatric testing, even if asymptomatic. *Paroxysmal symptoms* may result from dysfunction of partially demyelinated axons and simulate a transient ischemic attack or focal seizure, or produce an attack of tic douloureux (see Chapter 176). *Fatigue* may be prominent and even predate exacerbations.

Clinical Course and Prognosis. The clinical course tends to follow one of three basic patterns. Younger patients manifest a *relapsing–remitting* course, characterized by attacks followed by complete or nearly complete remission. In later years, a *secondary progressive* course, with steady gradual worsening, develops in more than 50% of patients. About 10% of patients who present with MS in later life (40 to 60 years of age at onset) have a steadily progressive course; this pattern is called *primary progressive* and tends to be associated with prominent spinal cord involvement. An uncommon form of MS, *relapsing progressive*, is diagnosed when patients have largely progressive disease exacerbated by acute attacks and little remission.

After 15 years of clinical disease, about 50% of patients are still capable of walking and 30% are able to continue working. Frequent attacks early in the course of the disease increase the chances of disability, as does late onset, a progressive course, or early cerebellar or pyramidal involvement. In about 5% to 10% of patients, the disease seems to pursue a very "benign" course, but it is difficult to predict in advance which patients safely can forego any disease-modifying therapy.

DIAGNOSIS

The diagnosis is suggested clinically by the development of symptoms and signs suggesting CNS disease separated both anatomically and in time (>1 month). At times, the symptoms suggest only a single lesion, but a careful physical examination reveals evidence of multiple lesions (upturned toes bilaterally, subtle internuclear ophthalmoplegia, mild afferent pupillary defect).

Laboratory findings help support the diagnosis, although no single test is diagnostic and clinical evidence for at least two separate neurologic lesions is still required. The most sensitive test is *magnetic resonance imaging* (MRI). Multiple periventricular plaques, presenting as areas of increased signal intensity on long TR-weighted and proton density-weighted images, are characteristic and found in more than 90% of patients with known MS. Patients with chronic progressive disease have more confluent periventricular and infratentorial lesions, but they are often most disabled by spinal cord lesions. However, the hyperintense white matter lesions seen on long TR-weighted images on MRI are nonspecific, and similar white matter lesions also occur in normal elderly persons and patients with chronic uncontrolled hypertension, advanced Lyme disease, and CNS vasculitis. The *cerebrospinal fluid* examination reveals abnormalities in 95% of MS patients. Modest increases in cell count and protein are common but nonspecific; increases in *immunoglobulin G* (IgG) and *oligoclonal IgG bands* on electrophoresis are more specific and suggest an increased risk for disseminated disease. Visual or auditory *evoked potentials* are abnormal in demyelinated tracts and may serve as additional evidence of MS when MRI results require supporting data. Exclusionary blood work in all patients suspected of having MS should include Lyme disease serology, determination of vitamin B_{12} levels and antinuclear antibody, and possibly HIV testing.

PRINCIPLES OF MANAGEMENT

The twofold goal of therapy for patients with MS is to prevent relapses and retard progressive worsening of the disease.

There is no cure for MS, but much can be done to reduce the symptoms of an acute exacerbation. A more difficult task is to improve the long-term course of the illness. Efforts to treat MS have focused on suppressing the immunologically induced inflammatory response that characterizes the condition. Disease-modifying therapy should be considered early in the course for patients with unfavorable prognostic markers, such as progressive disease from the onset, a short interval between the first two relapses, poor recovery from relapse, the presence of motor and cerebellar signs at onset, and multiple cranial lesions on long TR-weighted MRI. Since 1993, several new agents have become available to modify the course of MS. Therapeutic advances in MS depend on the conduct of clinical trials, and problems encountered in the design of such trials include the highly variable and unpredictable course of the disease and the difficulty of establishing measurements of disability.

Treatment of an Acute Attack. High-dose parenteral corticosteroids appear capable of shortening an acute attack. The best available data come from the Optic Neuritis Treatment Trial, a randomized, controlled study of patients presenting with isolated neuritis, in which 3 days of high-dose *IV methylprednisolone* followed by several weeks of oral prednisone was compared with oral prednisone alone or placebo. Patients given high-dose IV therapy demonstrated the best restoration of vision, but at 12 months, their vision was no different from that of patients given placebo. However, at 3 years, they showed a 66% reduction in relative risk for the development of definite MS. The potential significance of this finding is great, but it requires confirmation. Patients treated with oral prednisone alone did worse at 6 months than those given placebo. The worsening on oral prednisone alone is hard to explain, but oral steroids alone should not be used until more data are forthcoming. For now, a course of high-dose IV therapy is preferred. Whether it should be followed by a more prolonged course of oral prednisone remains unclear because the study did not examine such a program.

Disease-modifying Therapy. The U.S. Food and Drug Administration has approved three drugs for patients with relapsing–remitting MS. These drugs are recombinant *interferon beta-1b* (*Betaseron*), recombinant *interferon beta-1a* (*Avonex*), and *glatiramer acetate* (*Copaxone*). They have all been tested in separate placebo-controlled, double-blinded multicenter trials. Reductions in relapse rates of 33%, 37%, and 29%, respectively, were demonstrated. The interferons have also been shown to reduce the numbers of new lesions on MRI. The further indication of primary prevention has recently been added for Avonex. When Avonex was given after a single episode secondary to demyelination, fewer patients progressed to clinically definite MS. The drugs currently are available only by injection. The interferons have been associated with flulike symptoms, at times severe and persistent. Patients taking Copaxone have experienced uncommonly a systemic reaction of flushing, sweating, and palpitations.

A consensus is growing that disease-modifying therapy should be initiated early in the course of MS, before irreversible disability has developed. This opinion is supported by increased clinical and MRI evidence that the inflammatory process is active in many patients during periods of clinical remission and that irreversible axonal injury accumulates with time, even during the phase of relapsing–remitting disease. The serum of patients who continue to have clinical disease activity despite interferon therapy should be tested for neutralizing antibodies.

Treatment of Progressive Disease is more problematic. A multicenter study of interferon beta-1b was completed in Europe recently. The study found a significant delay in time to sustained progression in patients who received interferon therapy. Most neurologists offer the disease-modifying drugs to patients with secondary progressive disease. These drugs are extremely expensive and may cause several weeks of unpleasant side effects as they are started; furthermore, the patient and family must be taught how to administer them. The long-term benefits must be inferred from the results of existing studies, which have lasted only 3 to 5 years.

Patients whose disease continues to progress despite interferon or copolymer therapy may benefit from other strategies. IV immune globulin has been used monthly for 2 years in a small study that demonstrated less worsening of disability in the active treatment group. Immunosuppressive agents such as methotrexate and azathioprine have been used, but their efficacy in progressive disability is unclear. Patients with rapidly progressive disease given a course of IV *cyclophosphamide* with or without subsequent booster injections have demonstrated stabilization over 1 year. Such nonspecific immunosuppressive treatment is fraught with significant morbidity and should be reserved for patients with rapidly progressive disease who do not respond to less toxic alternatives. *Plasmapheresis*, the subject of one small, uncontrolled study, showed some benefit for patients with rapidly progressive disease. Approved in January 2000, *mitoxantrone (Novantrone)* has been shown to relieve disability significantly, improve ambulation, and reduce the relapse rate in patients with relapsing–progressive or secondary progressive disease. Data also suggest a decrease in lesions visible on gadolinium-enhanced MRI in comparison with the placebo group.

Treatment of Complications. *Paroxysmal symptoms*, such as lancinating pain or limb spasms, respond to *carbamazepine* (200 mg twice daily). Tricyclic antidepressants may help control *emotional lability* and relieve neuropathic pain. Low doses of *amitriptyline* (25 to 75 mg/d) often suffice. Higher doses of tricyclic agents are indicated for overt *depression* (see Chapter 227). *Spasticity* lessens with the use of *baclofen* in low doses (started at 5 to 10 mg three times daily), but confusion, sedation, and increased muscle weakness are limiting side effects. Diazepam and dantrolene are alternatives. When *incontinence* is problematic, an anticholinergic (e.g., 15 mg of propantheline up to four times daily as needed) or oxybutynin (Ditropan; 5 to 10 mg two or three times per day) will help if the cause is bladder spasm (frequency, urge incontinence); a cholinergic agent is best in cases of bladder atony (see Chapter 134). No specific therapy has been very useful for the debilitating fatigue accompanying this condition, but amantadine (Symmetrel; 100 mg two or three times per day) has been successful in some patients.

PATIENT EDUCATION

One of the most difficult aspects of MS is the uncertainty that accompanies the disease. If the diagnosis is in question, every effort should be made to confirm it or rule it out. Patients with MS fear becoming disabled. Providing them with as much information as possible helps them to maintain a sense of control. Even advice on handling the affairs of everyday life is greatly appreciated, such as avoiding a very hot shower that may transiently exacerbate symptoms. Although it is hard to predict a patient's future clinical course, reasonable estimates can be made based on the clinical course to date.

Patients need to know that progression to disabling disease is not inevitable, that the prognosis is highly variable, and that in many cases the disease never becomes incapacitating. Patient morale appears to be an important determinant of outcome. In randomized studies, the high frequency of remission and outright clinical improvement noted among patients randomized to placebo underscores this point. It should not be surprising that a disease of immune dysfunction such as MS might be influenced by the patient's state of mind, given the well-documented finding that the psychological state can affect T-cell function. Maintaining a hopeful perspective may have a remarkably positive effect and should not be overlooked. The value of establishing a close, supportive relationship cannot be overemphasized.

INDICATIONS FOR REFERRAL AND ADMISSION

When a diagnosis of MS is suspected on clinical grounds, a neurologic consultation can be helpful in determining the need for further diagnostic studies (MRI, lumbar puncture with immunoelectrophoresis, evoked potentials) and in selecting a treatment modality. In addition, patients experiencing an acute exacerbation of functional significance should be referred to a neurologist promptly for consideration of a course of high-dose IV glucocorticoid therapy. Neurologic consultation about the timing or appropriateness of interferon beta or copolymer treatments is important. Referral to an occupational and physical therapist can greatly facilitate the maintenance of daily functioning in patients with significant motor or sensory deficits.

ANNOTATED BIBLIOGRAPHY

Beatty WW. Cognitive and emotional disturbances in multiple sclerosis. Neurol Clin North Am 1993;11:189. (*Mild to moderate cognitive impairment is common.*)

Beck RW, Cleary PA, Trobe JD, et al. The effect of corticosteroids for acute optic neuritis on the subsequent development of multiple sclerosis. N Engl J Med 1993;329:1764. (*Treatment found to prevent the development of clinical MS.*)

Beck RW, Cleary PA, Anderson MM Jr, et al. A randomized, controlled trial of corticosteroids in the treatment of acute optic neuritis. N Engl J Med 1992;326:581. (*Best available evidence for the efficacy of high-dose steroids.*)

European Study Group on Interferon Beta-1b. Placebo-controlled multicenter randomised trial of interferon beta-1b in the treatment of secondary progressive multiple sclerosis. Lancet 1998;352:1491. (*Evidence for efficacy includes delayed progression for 9 to 12 months; reduced relapse rate and severity; fewer steroid treatments, hospital admissions, new lesions on MRI.*)

Fazekas F, Barkhof F, Filippi M, et al. The contribution of magnetic resonance imaging to the diagnosis of multiple sclerosis. Neurology 1999;53:448. (*Dynamic evolution of lesions, appearance of new lesions during apparent remissions, and effects of disease-modifying therapy have all altered the way clinicians diagnose and treat MS.*)

Hartung HP, Consett R. Mitoxantrone in progressive multiple sclerosis: a placebo-controlled, randomized, observer-blind European phase III multicenter study—clinical results. Multiple Sclerosis 1998;4:325. (*Data establish efficacy in reducing disease activity and slowing disease progression; therapy generally well tolerated, but amenorrhea, nausea, vomiting, and headache reported.*)

IFNB Multiple Sclerosis Study Group. Interferon beta-1b is effective in relapsing–remitting multiple sclerosis. Neurology 1993;43:665. (*First report that the natural history of MS can be altered.*)

Lessell S. Corticosteroid treatment of acute optic neuritis. N Engl J Med 1992;326:634. (*Editorial recommending high-dose IV therapy for acute attacks.*)

Rudick RA. Disease-modifying drugs for relapsing–remitting multiple sclerosis and future directions for multiple sclerosis therapeutics. Neurology 1999;56:1079. (*Succinct summary of data establishing efficacy for the three agents currently available, with good discussion of design and outcome measures in clinical trials.*)

Trapp BD, Peterson J, Ransonoff RM, et al. Axonal transection in the lesions of MS. N Engl J Med 1998;338:278. (*Reversing a long-held pathologic axiom, this important study demonstrates that transected axons are common in the lesions of MS and may be the pathologic correlate of irreversible neurologic impairment. This study has been used to justify early treatment with disease-modifying agents.*)

173

Management of Alzheimer's Disease and Related Dementias

M. CORNELIA CREMENS

Approximately 4 million Americans suffer from Alzheimer's disease. With the aging of the U.S. population and a doubling of the prevalence of dementia for every 5 years over the age of 65 years, the problem of caring for such patients is becoming an increasingly important medical and societal challenge. Medical care for the majority of patients with Alzheimer's disease and other dementias is usually the responsibility of the primary care physician. This role requires knowledge of the course of the illness, the best approaches to managing concomitant medical and psychiatric conditions (psychosis, anxiety, depression, behavioral disturbances), and the social services available. Skill is required in family education and counseling, appropriate application of new therapies, and cessation of life-prolonging therapy at the end of life.

CLINICAL PRESENTATION AND COURSE

Alzheimer's Disease

Early Stages. Most patients are *mildly forgetful* and complain of such memory deficits as forgetting names or where they placed household items. The patient may seem concerned but has no social or employment problems and shows no evidence of memory deficit during a clinical interview. The next stage is characterized by decreased performance in demanding work or social situations. Patients complain of *poor concentration*, difficulty in remembering words and names, more prominent memory loss, and confusion, and they may report that co-workers have noticed their relatively poor performance. Some patients present initially with *visual–spatial deficits*, whereas others may have difficulty with *speech* early in the course of the illness. Later, patients are easily disoriented and get lost when traveling to an unfamiliar location. Anxiety and depression are common, and many patients begin to deny symptoms. Changes in personality and judgment begin to cause problems with family and co-workers.

Intermediate Stages. As the illness progresses, patients become unable to travel alone and are unable to handle their personal finances. *Memory for recent events* is drastically impaired, and patients display a decreased knowledge of current events. Complex tasks are impossible, but patients remain fairly well oriented to time and person and can travel to *very* familiar places, like the corner drugstore. Many patients are aware of their deficits and are capable of understanding what is happening to them. Patients instinctively withdraw from previously challenging situations and may even have trouble with the activities of daily living. Difficulty with speech is more pronounced. *Denial* may become pronounced. Anxiety increases, along with suspiciousness and agitation. The most difficult behavior at this point is wandering and pacing, which makes it important that patients begin to wear an identification bracelet available through the Alzheimer's Association.

Late-stage Disease. Patients can no longer survive without some assistance. They are unable to recall major relevant aspects of their current lives or even the names of close friends and family members. *Delusions* and *hallucinations* are common. For example, the spouse is accused of being an impostor, or patients talk to imaginary persons or their own reflection in the mirror. *Depression, agitation,* and *violent behavior* may occur. Frequently, patients are disoriented to time or place. However, they generally remain able to eat and use the toilet without assistance, but they may have difficulty in properly choosing and putting on clothing.

Advanced Disease. In the last stages of the disease, patients become totally *incapacitated* and *disoriented*. They eventually forget their own name and may not recognize their spouse. *Incontinence* is common, with loss of bladder and bowel control. *Personality* and *emotional changes* become very pronounced, although these occasionally occur even in the earliest stages. Eventually, all verbal abilities are lost, motor skills deteriorate, and patients require total care. Total dependence on the caregiver ensues, and it is important to monitor for caregiver stress, or "burnout." Generalized cortical and focal neurologic signs and symptoms are frequently present. Death usually occurs from total debilitation or infection.

Clinical Course. The course of Alzheimer's disease from onset to death varies from 2 to 20 years. The average is about 6 to 8 years. Typically, the illness progresses at a fairly constant rate. If it has rapidly developed during the past year, it is likely to continue at that rate. A slowly progressive illness during the past 5 to 10 years suggests that the patient may survive for a number of years, especially if the patient is in otherwise good physical health. Other clinical features found to be independent predictors of more rapid progression to incapacity and death include hallucinations, paranoia, delusions, misidentification syndromes, extrapyramidal signs, and a low score on initial psychometric testing.

Dementia with Lewy Bodies

This newly identified condition has features that distinguish it from Alzheimer's disease. Accurate diagnosis is essential because of the increased sensitivity of these patients to neuroleptic agents. Because they often present initially with psychosis (usually visual hallucinations), before the onset of other characteristic features, patients who have dementia with Lewy bodies are at great risk for adverse side effects from the use of neuroleptics. Patients may present with psychiatric cognitive or parkinsonian motor symptoms, which leads to a variety of initially mistaken diagnoses. A progressive decline in cognition interferes with social or occupational functioning. Memory impairment may not be prominent in the earlier stages, but deficits in attention and visual–spatial and frontal–subcortical skills are often prominent. Core features of dementia with Lewy bodies include recurrent visual hallucinations that are well formed and detailed, fluctuating consciousness, and spontaneous motor features of parkinsonism and extrapyramidal disease. Other supportive features include falls resulting from difficulty with movement, syncope and transient loss of consciousness resulting from suspected autonomic dysfunction, hallucinations in other domains, systematized delusions, and sensitivity to neuroleptic medications. The pace of the clinical decline may be more rapid than that of Alzheimer's disease.

PRINCIPLES OF MANAGEMENT

Once treatable causes of dementia have been ruled out (see Chapter 169), the physician faces the challenge of caring for the patient with Alzheimer's disease or dementia with Lewy bodies, a person with a chronic, progressively disabling illness. Management involves the skillful interplay of medication to improve the cognitive state and functional status, psychopharmacologic therapy, and supportive care by family members (who often choose to maintain the patient at home) and community agencies. In addition to these challenges, the management of Lewy body disease requires a few unique pharmacologic considerations.

Alzheimer's Disease

Drugs for Memory Enhancement and Improvement of Cognitive Function. To date, no treatment has proved capable of markedly slowing or significantly improving the cognitive defects of Alzheimer's disease. Drugs that *enhance cholinergic transmission* have been the subject of intense study because cholinergic neuronal degeneration and a depletion of acetyl-choline-synthesizing enzyme (choline acetyltransferase) have been noted in Alzheimer's disease. Acetylcholinesterase inhibitors and cholinergic receptor agonists are being studied.

Tacrine. The first cholinesterase inhibitor on the market was tacrine (tetrahydroaminoacridine), which effected a modest but statistically significant reduction in the rate of cognitive decline. However, the improvement was not clinically meaningful (no difference in scores of global functioning), and it had to be given four times a day with monitoring of liver function, which limited its usefulness. Few patients are treated with tacrine now, and it is not recognized as an important advance in treatment.

Donepezil (Aricept) and Rivastigmine (Exelon). These newer cholinesterase inhibitors have several advantages over tacrine: less frequent dosing, improvement in behavioral as well as cognitive domains, and reasonably well-tolerated side effects (e.g., mild nausea, rare emesis, mild diarrhea, mild somnolence, occasional insomnia). Donepezil is started at 5 mg/d and increased if necessary to 10 mg/d in once-daily dosing. The drug appears safer and more effective than tacrine. Rivastigmine is started at 1.5 mg twice daily, with the dose increased to 6 to 12 mg/d. Long-term experience with rivastigmine is still limited.

Dietary Supplements (Ginkgo, Lecithin). Many dietary supplements are available and heavily promoted, but they have not proved beneficial. Ginkgo biloba demonstrated an extremely modest effect in only one study. Metaanalysis of the available data suggests modest benefit at best. Many patients and family members ask about taking herbal supplements in addition to the prescribed medications. Because the herbal agents have active ingredients, they should be used cautiously, if at all. No evidence has been found that *lecithin* has any effect or that avoidance of aluminum-containing preparations (e.g., antacids) is of any benefit, despite concerns derived from the increased deposition of aluminum in the central nervous system of patients with Alzheimer's disease.

Estrogen was in the news when epidemiologic studies suggested it as a possible link to reduced rates of Alzheimer's disease in postmenopausal women on hormone replacement. Additional studies are under way, but preliminary data are not promising. Because of speculation that *nerve growth factor* and estrogen may interact to prevent cholinergic neurons from degenerating, additional studies of such growth factors are underway.

Selegiline and Vitamin E. "Protective" therapy with antioxidants and "preventive" therapy with drugs that inhibit β-amyloid formation are under study. These approaches attempt to address the purported pathophysiologic features of Alzheimer's disease. For example, *selegiline*, a monoamine oxidase inhibitor used in Parkinson's disease, is thought to reduce neuronal oxidative injury and enhance cerebral catecholamine levels. Early evidence suggests that the administration of 10 mg/d may slow functional deterioration in persons with moderately severe disease. α-Tocopherol (vitamin E) traps free radicals and reduces cell death *in vitro* caused by exposure to β-amyloid, the protein found in Alzheimer's disease. In a recently completed randomized, controlled study, megadoses of vitamin E (2,000 IU/d) slowed disease progression and preserved function in persons with moderately severe Alzheimer's disease.

Table 173.1. Commonly Used Neuroleptics in the Elderly

POTENCY	SEDATION	ANTICHOLINERGIC EFFECT	EXTRAPYRAMIDAL EFFECT	HYPOTENSION
Low				
Thioridazine (10–50 mg)	high	high	low	high
Intermediate				
Perphenazine (0.5–5 mg)	medium	medium	medium	medium
High				
Haloperidol (0.25–2 mg)	low	low	high	low
Thiothixine (0.5–4 mg)	low	low	high	low
Atypical Antipsychotics				
Clozapine (6.25–100 mg)	high	high	low	high
Olanzapine (2.5–10 mg)	medium	medium	low	low
Quetiapine (12.5–300 mg)	medium	low	low	high
Risperidone (0.25–3 mg)	low	low	medium	medium

However, the combination of selegiline and vitamin E was no better than the use of either agent alone. Many prescribe vitamin E routinely; full benefit remains to be fully defined.

Unhelpful Treatments. Drugs found not to be helpful include cerebral vasodilators (*dihydroergotoxine*), ergoloid mesylates (*Hydergine*), central nervous system stimulants (*amphetamines*), opiate antagonists (*naloxone*), neuropeptides (*vasopressin*), and, believed to act as cerebral vasodilators, probably have some metabolic enhancer activity.

Drugs for Confusion, Agitation, and Sleep. (See also Tables 173.1 and 173.2 and Appendix.) For the safe and effective use of psychotropic medication in patients with Alzheimer's disease, adjustments in drug selection, dose, and frequency are necessary to compensate for the alterations in drug uptake and metabolism that occur in the elderly (see Appendix). Such adjustments are particularly important when neuroleptics, benzodiazepines, and sedative-hypnotics are given. In a recent study of nursing home patients, a substantial improvement was noted in many of them when psychotropic drugs, prescribed on a long-term basis, were discontinued or reduced in dose.

The long-term use of sedatives and psychoactive agents in the confused patient should be avoided unless persistent, extreme agitation hampers care. Also problematic is the regular use of sedative-hypnotic agents for sleep (see Chapter 226), as they can cause confusion amd disorientation and prolong sedation. If such therapy is contemplated, the lowest possible doses should be given for the shortest time possible. The newer atypical neuroleptics (e.g., *quetiapine* or *clozapine*) are often given

first because of their low side effect profile (Tables 173.1 and 173.2). Quetiapine is easier to prescribe because marrow suppression does not occur; weekly white cell counts are indicated with clozapine use. Patients not responsive to the atypical neuroleptics may respond to a small dose of *thioridazine* (10 to 25 mg daily at bed time). *Haloperidol* is often a first choice in the setting of delusions and hallucinations. Doses in the range of 0.5 to 1 mg two or three times a day usually suffice, but one must be careful to avoid long-term use because of the risk for inducing tardive dyskinesia. β-Blockers and anticholinergics may exacerbate confusion.

Drugs for Depression. Depression is best treated with a *selective serotonin reuptake inhibitor* (SSRI), such as citalopram, sertraline, paroxetine, or fluoxetine. Patients with depression who do not respond to the SSRIs may improve on one of the older tricyclic compounds with few anticholinergic side effects, such as *desipramine* (10 to 50 mg at bedtime) or *nortriptyline* (10 to 75 mg at bedtime), but drugs with marked anticholinergic activity (e.g., amitriptyline) may worsen memory (see Appendix, Table 173.3, and Chapter 227).

Management of Behavioral Disorders. Certain behaviors are particularly troublesome to family members. Among those cited most frequently are catastrophic reactions (including violent behavior), wakefulness, suspiciousness, and incontinence.

Catastrophic Reactions are massive emotional overresponses that are typically precipitated by task failure or minor stress. Hitting and violent resistance to care are extreme forms of such reactions. Most excessive emotional responses can be

Table 173.2. Comparison of Atypical Neuroleptics

DRUG	EXTRAPYRAMIDAL EFFECT	HYPOTENSION	SEDATION	ANTICHOLINERGIC EFFECT
Clozapine	low	high	high	high
Olanzapine	low	low	high	med
Quetiapine	low	high	med	low
Risperidone	med	med	low	low

Table 173.3. Antidepressants for Depression in the Elderly (see also Chapter 227)

DRUGS	DOSE RANGE (mg/d)	COMMENTS
TCAs		
Nortriptyline	10–150	Reliable blood levels
Desipramine	10–250	Mild anticholinergic
		Minimal orthostasis
Stimulants		
Dextroamphetamine	2.5–40	Agitation
Methylphenidate	2.5–60	Mild tachycardia
		Limited studies
SSRIs		
Fluoxetine	5–60	Akathisia
Sertraline	25–200	Anxiety/sedation
Paroxetine	10–40	Agitation
Fluvoxamine	25–300	Gastrointestinal symptoms
Citalopram	10–40	Headache
		Diarrhea/constipation
		Rash
Others		
Trazodone	25–250	Sedation
		Orthostasis
		Incontinence
		Hallucinations
		Priapism
Nefazodone	50–600	Pedal edema
		Rash
Mirtazapine	7.5–30	Sedation
		Weight gain
Venlafaxine	25–300 (slow-release available)	Increase in blood pressure Confusion
		Light-headedness
Bupropion	75–450 (slow-release available)	Seizures Less mania/cycling
		Headache/nausea

TCA, tricyclic antidepressant; SSRI, selective serotonin reuptake inhibitor.

minimized by teaching the family to avoid or remove the precipitating task or stress, to remain quiet and calm, and to change the focus of attention gently. Neuroleptic drugs, anticonvulsant drugs (e.g., valproic acid, carbamazepine, or gabapentin), or buspirone are sometimes helpful in difficult cases, but only as an adjunct to behavioral techniques (see Appendix).

Wakefulness and Night Walking often deprive the caregiver of much-needed rest. Helpful environmental interventions include placing locks on each door so that the patient will not wander out of the house at night, keeping the patient physically active during the day, and not allowing a nap. Sedative-hypnotics, such as a short-acting benzodiazepine or chloral hydrate, may be helpful (see Chapter 228). Occasionally, low doses of a neuroleptic or anticonvulsant may be needed.

Suspiciousness and accusatory behaviors are believed to result from the brain-injured person's efforts to explain misplaced possessions or misinterpreted events. If the family understands this, their frustration, hurt, and anger may be reduced. Simple interventions, such as keeping an orderly house or making a sign pointing to where an object is kept, may help. Neuroleptics may be used as a last resort.

Incontinence is typically a late manifestation of Alzheimer's disease, but when present early, it warrants a careful search for other causes, such as urinary tract infection (see Chapter 133) and other causes of dementia, such as normal-pressure hydrocephalus (see Chapter 169).

Inappropriate Sexual Behavior is very uncommon. Family members can be reassured. In the rare instances in which it occurs, self-stimulation is the usual form; Alzheimer's patients are not child molesters.

Treatment of Deterioration Caused by Concurrent Medical Illness. Patients with Alzheimer's disease deteriorate rapidly both cognitively and behaviorally when they experience a *superimposed illness*. Coexistent medical problems, such as asthma, diabetes, and congestive heart failure, should be carefully controlled. Even a minor upper respiratory tract or urinary tract infection can worsen behavior. Patients are susceptible to *medication-induced delirium*; close supervision of drug regimens is imperative.

Home Environment. As mentioned earlier, families need to be encouraged to maintain a *structured*, predictable environment for the patient. Any change can be devastating and stressful to a patient and may produce a massive emotional overresponse. A schedule in which activities such as arising, eating, taking medication, and exercise occur at the same time each day maximizes the patient's familiarity with the personal environment. At times, the use of an *orientation center* in the home, with pertinent information such as the date, time, schedule of household events, and pictures of relevant people, is very helpful.

Preventing Falls. Of particular importance to survival and quality of life is the need to reduce the risk for *falls* in the home. It has been clearly demonstrated that falls are one of the major predictors of reduced survival. Installing hand rails, encouraging the use of a walker, and eliminating throw rugs and other obstacles can be extremely important to maximizing survival and minimizing disability. In the nursing home environment, the use of both *tricyclic antidepressants* and the SSRIs has been found to increase the risk for falls. The tricyclics may decrease blood pressure and cause postural hypotension. The SSRIs do not cause orthostasis, but they may cause dizziness and increase a patient's mobility. The risk for falls is dose-related, which suggests that physicians should start some patients with doses less than the usual starting dose (see Appendix).

Driving. Frequently, patients will want to *drive* when it is clear that they are no longer safe on the roads. The family members at times will resist stopping the patient from driving, stating that the patient is a good driver. This may be true, but the patient is at great risk for becoming lost or getting into a dangerous situation. Therefore, family education is essential. If possible, it is best to avoid direct confrontation with the patient. Simple techniques such as hiding the keys, disconnecting distributor wires, or giving the patient a nonfunctional set of keys have usually been successful in discouraging patients from driving.

Firearms. Any firearms should be removed from the home for obvious reasons. In addition, smoking and cooking become potentially dangerous activities. Environmental modifications, such as removing stove knobs, having a stove cut-off switch placed in an inconspicuous place, locking rooms or closets, and locking up matches, are important for safety.

Management of the Family. Some family members may well react with dread and depression to the fact that their relative has

Alzheimer's disease. Those members who have a preexisting psychiatric illness may decompensate. Others will have suspected the diagnosis and are relieved to find an understanding physician who will be available and helpful during the course of the illness. Family members who are initially stunned and ask few questions should not have information forced on them. Careful explanation of any further tests should be provided and a follow-up appointment arranged within a week. Common questions include the following: How long will the patient live? How rapidly will the patient deteriorate? What are the chances that other family members will be affected by the disease—is it hereditary? Is there a treatment?

Most helpful for coping are the services of a social worker skilled in management of Alzheimer's disease. Within the first few weeks after the diagnosis has been made, family members should see a *social worker* who is familiar with community resources, such as visiting nurse services, delivery of meals, financial aid, and nursing homes. For the patient with very early Alzheimer's disease, this may seem premature, but family members will be reassured by the knowledge that help will be available when needed in the future. Most families read about the illness and become acutely aware of its devastating course.

Guilt, unrealistic expectations, and assumption of *excessive responsibility* are common responses of families. In discussing these and similar issues, the physician should focus on both physical realities and the family's emotional response to the patient. One frequently encountered source of difficulty is the reversal of parent–child roles that the care of an elderly person often represents. There is no one way to handle this issue; however, in the overwhelming majority of such cases, just allowing family members to discuss these and other issues will be therapeutic.

A *lack of personal time for caregivers* and *sleep disturbances* in patients are the least tolerable aspects of home care. Families do best when relatives and friends visit frequently and when provisions are made for the primary caregiver to take breaks from the responsibilities. Visiting nurses and centers that provide day care can be invaluable. Family support is the major variable in keeping the cognitively impaired elderly patient at home.

Support groups can be very helpful. Even with a compassionate and empathic physician, many families feel alone with this illness and are unable to find friends who understand. Embarrassment may make them withdraw from previous social contacts. To meet the need for communication and information, families in many areas have established *volunteer organizations* that are involved in helping each other, sharing solutions to management problems, exchanging information, supporting needed legislation and research, and educating the community. These organizations welcome members who are concerned about any of the dementing illnesses, of which Alzheimer's disease is the most common. The number of such support groups is growing rapidly, and families consistently report how helpful they are. Local volunteer organizations have established a national organization, the *Alzheimer's Association*, whose goals are family support, education, advocacy, and encouragement of research. The address of the Alzheimer's Association is 919 North Michigan Avenue, Suite 1000, Chicago, IL 60611-1672; the web address is www.alz.org; the telephone number is 800-272-3900. The national organization will give family members the addresses of local groups. Each family member should be encouraged to read one of the available lay books on Alzheimer's disease. *The 36-Hour Day* is required reading for anyone (including the physician) who is dealing with a person with a progressive dementing illness.

Nursing Home Placement and Care. It is always a difficult moment when the family considers nursing home placement. Placement represents an irrevocable loss of autonomy for the patient. The decision must be approached with careful deliberation and respect for the patient. Although the family's needs are important to consider, the physician has a special obligation to the patient. If the patient created an advance directive before becoming mentally incapacitated (see Appendix, Chapter 1), the choices set forth can be respected and followed. In the absence of such a directive, the physician needs to act as it appears the patient would have wanted. If a surrogate has been designated, this person can help in the decision making. The goal, first and foremost, is to help the patient.

Before any action is taken regarding nursing home placement, it is worth carefully reexamining the home situation to be sure all alternatives to placement have been explored. Have home health aides, senior day care, and similar supports been used to relieve the family's burden?

Only after all home care resources have been exhausted or found to be insufficient is it proper to proceed with placement. An appropriate site is one that can provide emotional support, reassurance, and security. One seeks a nursing home that preserves a sense of connection and closeness to others. The primary physician plays a critical role in ensuring that the placement is carried out well and serves the best interests of the patient.

As noted earlier, the use of psychoactive drugs in the nursing home environment can adversely affect alertness, mobility, and blood pressure. The risk of falls and the decline in overall functional status correlate with number and doses of drugs prescribed. Use should be kept to a minimum (see Appendix).

Often during advanced phases of the illness, when nutrition begins to decline because of difficulty in feeding, the question arises of the value of a *feeding tube*. The best available data show no benefit from tube feeding in regard to pressure sores, infections, cognitive function, pain, or risk for aspiration pneumonia. Moreover, survival does not appear to be prolonged. The practice of placing a feeding tube is discouraged by most authorities.

Dementia with Lewy Bodies

Although the basic principals and much of the care for this condition are identical to that for Alzheimer's disease, important exceptions exist. The most important one is the need for caution in the administration of *neuroleptics*. Because patients who have dementia with Lewy bodies may present with psychotic features (e.g., vivid visual hallucinations), physicians tend to expose them early to standard neuroleptic medications (e.g., haloperidol), often before the diagnosis is recognized. The net result is a worsening or precipitation of extrapyramidal symptoms and little improvement in mental status. Because patients with Lewy body disease are very sensitive to these medications, it is best to begin with one of the atypical neuroleptics (e.g., *quetiapine* or *clozapine*; see Table 173.2) when treatment of hallucinosis or other psychotic features is required. As noted, quetiapine is easier to prescribe because a weekly white blood cell count is not required. However, it is important to recognize that both agents cause hypotension and sedation, even at low doses. *Selegiline* (5 mg twice daily) has demonstrated some ability to slow disease progression in patients with Lewy body disease.

THERAPEUTIC RECOMMENDATIONS

- Once a progressive dementing illness has been diagnosed, the primary care physician becomes the main coordinator of the patient's care and advisor to the family. The physician should consciously decide whether to take on this responsibility or to refer the patient and family for care by a group specializing in the management of such patients.
- Family members should be apprised of the patient's diagnosis, and an open discussion should be part of the initial management.
- Early in the course of the illness, a social worker should meet with the family to help plan for care and provide emotional support.
- A predictable, well-structured home environment should be established, especially one that limits the risk for falls.
- All unnecessary medications, especially those that may cause cognitive impairment, should be stopped, or the dosage should be reduced.
- When a concomitant psychiatric problem (e.g., depression, anxiety, behavioral disorder, psychosis) develops, psychopharmacologic intervention should be considered.
- For depression, begin with a low dose of an SSRI or a well-tolerated tricyclic agent (see Table 173.3 and Chapter 227). For anxiety or difficulty with sleeping, consider a low dose of a short-acting benzodiazepine (e.g., 1.0 mg of lorazepam; see Chapter 226). For psychotic behavior or catastrophic reactions, a low dose of a neuroleptic may prove useful, with an atypical neuroleptic preferred for patients with Lewy body disease (see Tables 173.1 and 173.2). Drug treatment should be brief (except in depression), and the smallest dose possible should be given.
- Although a number of drugs are available to treat cognitive impairment, none is consistently effective, and results are modest at best. *Donepezil* (5 to 10 mg daily) or *rivastigmine* (1.5 mg twice daily) effects some improvement in cognitive function, although results are modest. These cholinesterase inhibitors may also improve behavioral problems. *Hydergine*, although widely used, is not recommended.
- Consider a trial of *selegiline* (5 mg twice daily) for patients with Lewy body disease. Every patient with memory loss or cognitive impairment should be on *vitamin E* (2,000 IU/d) to slow functional deterioration in persons with moderately severe disease.
- Family members should be advised to join the local chapter of the Alzheimer's Association and to become knowledgeable about the disease and its course by reading one of the currently available books. (*The 36-Hour Day* is an excellent resource.)
- The need for nursing home placement should be approached carefully and only after home care resources have been fully utilized. Many day care programs have been established that specialize in the care of patients with Alzheimer's disease. Emphasis is on providing for the emotional and physical needs of the patient, although family preferences also deserve consideration. The specialized care units for patients with Alzheimer's disease provide a comfortable, stimulating, and safe environment for the patient who can no longer remain at home.

ANNOTATED BIBLIOGRAPHY

Albert M. Assessment of cognitive functioning in the elderly. Psychosomatics 1984;25:310. (*Discusses the cognitive changes associated with both normal aging and dementing illness.*)

American College of Physicians. Cognitively impaired subjects. Ann Intern Med 1989;111:843. (*Position paper on ethical issues regarding care.*)

Cummings JL. Cholinesterase inhibitors: a new class of psychotropic compounds. Am J Psychiatry 2000;157:4. (*Evidenced-based use of acetylcholinestererase inhibitors for the treatment of neuropsychiatric symptoms in Alzheimer's disease.*)

Davis KL, Thal LJ, Gamzu ER, et al. A double-blind, placebo-controlled multicenter study of tacrine for Alzheimer's disease. N Engl J Med 1992;327:1253. (*Short-term study of patients who showed some response to tacrine in a preliminary phase found a statistically significant improvement in cognition, but not in global functioning or activities of daily living.*)

Drachman DA. Who may drive? Who may not? Who shall decide? Ann Neurol 1988;24:787. (*Analysis of the tricky regulation process and the physician's obligation to patients and others.*)

Finucane TE, Christmas C, Travis K. Tube feeding in patients with advanced dementia. A review of the evidence. JAMA 1999;282:1365. (*No data to suggest that tube feeding relieves pressure sores, infections, or pain, reduces the risk for aspiration pneumonia, or increases cognitive function or survival.*)

Greenberg SM, Tennis MK, Brown LB, et al. Donepezil therapy in clinical practice: a randomized crossover study. Arch Neurol 2000;57:94. (*Most recent study evaluating the effectiveness of the cholinesterase inhibitor.*)

Growdon JH. Treatment for Alzheimer's disease. N Engl J Med 1992;327:1306. (*Excellent summary of current approaches to therapy.*)

Larson EB, Kukull WA, Vuchner D, et al. Adverse drug reactions associated with global cognitive impairment in elderly persons. Ann Intern Med 1987;107:169. (*Adverse drug reactions were an important source of cognitive impairment, especially when more than four drugs were being taken.*)

Lipowski ZJ. Delirium in the elderly patient. N Engl J Med 1989;320:578. (*Short, very useful review; 32 references.*)

Mace NL, Rabins PV. The 36-hour day: a family guide to caring for persons with Alzheimer's disease, dementing illness, and memory loss in later life. Baltimore: The Johns Hopkins University Press, 1991. (*Required reading for all who care for patients with dementing illnesses. Excellent for family members.*)

Mayeux R, Sano M. Treatment of Alzheimer's disease. N Engl J Med 1999;341:1670. (*Useful review of drugs to improve cognition and treat abnormal behavior; 111 references.*)

McKeith IG, Galasko D, Kosaka K, et al. Consensus guidelines for the clinical and pathologic diagnosis of dementia with Lewy bodies. Neurology 1996;47:1113. (*Clear outline and definition of disease.*)

Meier DE, Cassel CK. Nursing home placement and the demented patient. Ann Intern Med 1986;104:98. (*A most helpful discussion of this difficult phase of care.*)

Oken BS, Stotzbach DM, Kaye JA. The efficacy of ginkgo biloba on cognitive function in Alzheimer's disease. Arch Neurol 1998;55:1400. (*In a metaanalysis of five clinical studies, a slight cognitive improvement was noted when this herbal extract was used.*)

Rojas-Fernandez OH, McKnight C. Dementia with Lewy bodies: review and pharmacotherapeutic implications. Pharmacotherapy 1999;19:795. (*Useful summary of psychopharmacologic management.*)

Sano M, Ernesto C, Thomas RG, et al. A controlled trial of selegiline, α-tocopherol or both as treatment for Alzheimer's disease. N Engl J Med 1997;336:1216. (*A double-blinded, placebo-controlled, randomized multicenter study showing that either agent can significantly slow functional deterioration in persons with moderately severe disease; no additional benefit with combination therapy.*)

Stern Y, Min-Xing T, Albert MS, et al. Predicting time to nursing home care and death in individuals with Alzheimer disease. JAMA 1997;277:806. (*A prospective cohort study with a validation component found a low psychometric test score, extrapyramidal signs, psychotic symptoms, short duration of illness, and age below 65 years at onset to be independent predictors of a poor prognosis.*)

The American Academy of Neurology Ethics and Humanities Subcommittee. Practice parameter: ethical issues in the management of the demented patient. Neurology 1996;46:1180. (*Covers aspects of the patient–physician relationship, advance directives, proxy decision making, restraints, and withdrawal of life-sustaining treatment.*)

Thompson TL, Filley CM, Mitchell WD, et al. Lack of efficacy of Hydergine in patients with Alzheimer's disease. N Engl J Med 1990;323:445. (*Hydergine had been widely prescribed but never properly studied; no benefit found in this rigorously designed, controlled study.*)

Walsh JS, Welch HG, Larson EB. Survival of outpatients with Alzheimer-type dementia. Ann Intern Med 1990;113:429. (*Length of survival is more a function of severity of disease than of duration; wandering, falling, and behavioral problems correlate with shortened survival.*)

RESOURCES

Alzheimer's Association
800-272-3900
www.alz.org
American Association of Retired Persons
800-424-3410
www.aarp.org
Eldercare Locator
800-677-1116
www.ageinfo.org/elderloc/elderb.html/
Family Caregiver Alliance
www.caregiver.org
Health Care Financing Administration
National Nursing Home Data Base
800-638-6833
www.medicaid.gov/nursing/home.asp
National Association for Incontinence
800-252-3337 (800-BLADDER)
National Caregiving Foundation
800-930-1357
www.caregivingfoundation.org
National Citizen's Coalition for Nursing Home Reform
202-332-2275
www.nccnhr.org
National Hospice Foundation
800-658-8898
National Institute on Aging
www.nih.gov/nia

National Library of Medicine
Medline
www.nlm.nih.gov/medlineplus/
Social Security Information
Retirement or Disability Benefits
800-772-1213

Appendix: Use of Psychotropic Drugs in the Elderly

MICHAEL A. JENIKE

Pharmacokinetic Changes Associated with Aging. Significant changes in drug absorption and distribution, protein binding, hepatic metabolism, and renal excretion occur in elderly patients. Gastric pH increases and splanchnic blood flow decreases, altering drug solubility and absorption. Total body fat rises from 10% of body weight at age 20 to 24% at age 60, which increases the volume of distribution for lipid-soluble drugs, such as diazepam and its metabolites, and greatly prolongs drug half-life. In addition, total body water may decrease from 25% to 18% in the same period, so that the concentrations of water-soluble drugs, such as ethanol, are higher because of decreased reservoir size. Serum albumin levels decline by 10% to 15%; as a consequence, protein-binding sites are decreased and more free active drug is released into the circulation, raising the risk for toxicity. Drug metabolism slows; the activity of hepatic cytochrome P-450 decreases, as does demethylation. The result is higher levels of unmetabolized drug. After age 40, the glomerular filtration rate and renal plasma flow decline progressively. By age 70, the reduction is about 50%, which prolongs drug action and increases the likelihood of toxicity if the dosage is not adjusted downward.

In addition to these pharmacokinetic changes, decreased levels of dopamine and acetylcholine in the central nervous system can lead to an increase in extrapyramidal and anticholinergic side effects, respectively. An increased tendency to central nervous system disinhibition in the elderly increases the likelihood of drug-associated confusion, sedation, and paradoxical reactions.

Neuroleptic Use. Violence, rage, and psychosis are common problems in patients with Alzheimer's disease. The drugs most commonly used to treat these problems are the neuroleptics (Table 173.1). Initial treatment with neuroleptics is indicated when psychotic symptoms are present, such as paranoia, delusions, and hallucinations. All the neuroleptics are equally effective in treating the above symptoms. The choice of a particular drug is based on its side effects and toxicity. The main side effects of neuroleptics are sedation, orthostatic hypotension, extrapyramidal symptoms, and anticholinergic symptoms. The newer *atypical neuroleptics* (e.g., *clozapine, quetiapine*) cause fewer side effects and may provide better treatment for these symptoms (Table 173.2).

A fairly consistent relationship is found between the potency of a neuroleptic and its side effects; as the milligram potency of a neuroleptic increases, the frequency and severity of sedation, orthostatic hypotension, and anticholinergic symptoms decrease, and extrapyramidal symptoms increase. *High-potency neuroleptics*, such as *haloperidol, thiothixene*, and *fluphenazine,* are generally safe to use in the elderly, but they should be started at very low doses (e.g., 0.5 mg of haloperidol once or twice daily). Although generally safe, these drugs are more likely than low-potency agents (e.g., chlorpromazine or thioridazine) to produce extrapyramidal symptoms in the elderly. Extrapyramidal symptoms develop in as many as 50% of all patients between the ages of 60 and 80 who are given neuroleptics, and those with brain damage, dementia, or Parkinson's disease are much more sensitive to these effects.

Sedation. Side effects can be used therapeutically. The patient who has trouble falling asleep will find sedating neuroleptics to be more helpful than nonsedating agents. Sedating neuroleptics may also be used to calm an agitated patient during the day. More commonly, however, sedation is an unwanted side effect. Daytime sedation may cause or aggravate nighttime insomnia, and sedation may also increase confusion and disorientation in the demented patient. As disorientation and confusion increase, the patient typically becomes more agitated.

Postural Hypotension. One of the most severe dangers entailed in the use of neuroleptics is the possibility of inducing *orthostatic hypotension,* which can lead to falls and fractures, stroke, or even heart attack. Hypotensive episodes are especially apt to occur at night when an elderly patient awakens and gets up to urinate.

Extrapyramidal Effects. The most troubling extrapyramidal symptoms are akathisia, parkinsonism, and akinesia. The newer atypical neuroleptics adequately treat these symptoms with fewer side effects. *Akathisia* is a feeling of motor restlessness associated with a subjective sensation of discomfort, often described as anxiety. Sleep is usually disturbed because the patient is unable to find a comfortable, motionless position. Sometimes, this restlessness is misinterpreted as an increase in psychotic symptoms and is treated with increased doses of neuroleptic dosage. A most effective treatment for akathisia is lowering the dose or switching to an atypical neuroleptic. Akathisia is also reported with the SSRIs.

Neuroleptic-induced *parkinsonism* appears to be identical to the postencephalitic or idiopathic forms. An occasional patient will be exquisitely sensitive to this side effect, and as little as one dose of a high-potency agent may precipitate the syndrome. In an effort to reduce the use of anticholinergic medications, it is best to reduce the dose and consider a switch to the newer atypical neuroleptics.

Tardive Dyskinesia, one of the unfortunately common and severe side effects of any neuroleptic agent, is manifested by a wide variety of movements, including lip smacking, sucking, jaw movements, writhing tongue movements, chorea, athetosis, dystonia, tics, and facial grimacing. In severe cases, speech, eating, walking, and even breathing can be seriously impaired. The onset is gradual, usually developing after long-term, high-dose administration, but on rare occasions it can occur with short-term or low-dose use. Advancing age correlates not only with increased prevalence but also with severity. Once tardive dyskinesia has developed, it is much less likely to reverse in an elderly patient than it is in a younger one.

The best way to *prevent* tardive dyskinesia is to avoid the use of neuroleptics. Obviously, these drugs are sometimes required, but they should not be used when indications are unclear or when less potentially toxic drugs may be as efficacious. Neuroleptics should never be used to treat simple anxiety or uncomplicated depression, nor should they be given for long periods to patients with an *acute* psychotic episode. It is important to make a baseline examination before starting a patient on neuroleptics and to note any early signs of tardive dyskinesia, such as fine vermicular movements or restlessness of the tongue, mild choreiform movements of the fingers or toes, and facial tics or frequent eye blinks. The patient should be monitored for the development of early tardive dyskinesia at least every 3 months. Currently, no consistently effective agents are available to treat tardive dyskinesia. In view of the significant risk to the elderly patient and the ineffective treatment options, physicians should avoid the use of neuroleptic drugs in elderly patients whenever possible.

Anxiolytics. (See Chapter 226.)

Hypnotics. (See Chapter 232.)

ANNOTATED BIBLIOGRPAHY

Avorn J, Soumerai SB, Everitt DE, et al. A randomized trial of a program to reduce the use of psychoactive drugs in nursing homes. N Engl J Med 1992;327:168. (*Reduction in unnecessary use of psychotropic drugs in this cohort with a high prevalence of dementia often led to improved functioning.*)

Jenike MA, Cremens MC. Geriatric psychopharmacology. Psychiatr Clin North Am 1994;1:125 (Annual of Drug Therapy). (*Monograph of medications and their use in the elderly.*)

Jenike MA. Tardive dyskinesia: special risk in the elderly. J Am Geriatr Soc 1983;31:71. (*Detailed discussion of this important complication.*)

Thapa PB, Gideon P, Cost TW, et al. Antidepressants and the risk of falls among nursing home residents. N Engl J Med 1998;339:875. (*Both tricyclics and SSRIs increased the risk for falls in dose-related fashion; although the SSRIs do not cause orthostasis, they may cause dizziness and increase mobility.*)

174

Approach to the Patient with Parkinson's Disease

AMY A. PRUITT

Of the movement disorders, the most common is Parkinson's disease, an adult-onset, neurodegenerative disease characterized by tremor at rest, rigidity, and bradykinesia. Parkinson's disease affects more than 1 million people in North America. The refinement of drug therapy for Parkinson's disease has brought relief to thousands of patients with this immobilizing condition. The recent development of therapy that may slow disease progression makes the early diagnosis and treatment of Parkinson's disease particularly critical. Proper treatment requires careful timing and skillful utilization of drugs because important difficulties are associated with pharmacologic therapy. Moreover, drug efficacy declines with time, and the therapeutic response may be blunted by improper timing or inappropriate selection of antiparkinsonian agents.

Although the "fine tuning" of Parkinson's disease is largely in the province of the neurologist, the primary care physician is in the best position to make the diagnosis, institute therapy, and monitor the often substantial side effects associated with antiparkinsonian agents.

PATHOPHYSIOLOGY, CLINICAL PRESENTATION, AND COURSE

Pathophysiology. Parkinson's disease is a *neurodegenerative* condition. Its most characteristic pathologic feature is a loss of *dopamine-containing* neurons; the nuclei of these neurons reside in the pars compacta of the *substantia nigra*, and the axons terminate in the *caudate nucleus* and *putamen* (the striatum). Other pigmented and nonpigmented nuclei in the brainstem and elsewhere are also affected. Associated with neuronal loss is the development of concentric hyalin inclusions in the cytoplasm of affected neurons, called *Lewy bodies*. Symptoms are believed related to the imbalance between dopaminergic and cholinergic influences on striatal tissue created by the loss of dopamine-containing neurons. Proper striatal function depends on this balance.

Although parkinsonism may result from substance exposures, infection, and a host of other conditions (Table 174.1), idiopathic disease remains the most common form. A possible mechanism for idiopathic disease has been suggested by the observation that symptoms of parkinsonism develop in IV drug abusers who inject MPTP (an analogue of meperidine). MPTP causes neuronal degeneration of the substantia nigra through its effects on monoamine oxidase B. Its metabolite concentrates in dopaminergic neurons, where it is bound to neuromelanin and inhibits complex 1 of the mitochondrial respiratory chain. The substantia nigra of patients with Parkinson's disease seems particularly vulnerable to *oxidative insults*. The demonstration that a toxin can produce parkinsonism has led to a thus far unfruitful search for causative environmental precipitants. A rural environment has been reported to be associated with an increased risk for Parkinson's disease, as has exposure to pesticides. Conversely, smoking has been associated with a decreased risk for the development of Parkinson's disease.

Clinical Presentation. Parkinson's disease is an affliction of middle to late adult life, although 30% of patients report recognizable symptoms before the age of 50. In another 40%, the disease develops between the ages of 50 and 60, and the remainder are more than 60 years old at the time of diagnosis. The classic syndrome of parkinsonism includes *tremor at rest, rigidity, bradykinesia, masked face, stooped posture,* and a *shuffling gait.* Although tremor is the most obvious initial finding, it is absent in 20% of patients. Parkinson's disease may begin insidiously with vague, *aching pain* in the limbs, neck, or back and with *decreased axial dexterity* before tremor is noted. *Dysarthria* may be an early feature; *dysphagia* usually occurs later. Significant *orthostatic symptoms* may predominate in some patients. Other early subtle symptoms include decreases in the caliber of *handwriting* and volume of the voice and anosmia. *Depression* is a significant component in many patients and may be a feature of the early disease. The estimated frequency of *dementia* (which usually develops late) varies widely, but cognitive impairment, including hallucinations and psychosis, develops in at least 15% to 20% of patients. However, dementia and psychosis are not inevitable, and remediable causes of changes in mental status always need to be sought.

Clinical Course. Before the introduction of levodopa, Parkinson's disease had a fairly predictable course. At 5 years after onset, 60% of patients were severely disabled, and at 10 years, nearly 80% were. The rate of progression varied widely. Death rarely was a direct consequence of parkinsonism; rather, it was a consequence of immobility (aspiration pneumonia, urinary tract infections) or of trauma. Patients with Parkinson's disease comprise several different subgroups manifesting specific clinical patterns. It is thought that patients who present primarily with tremor have a slower course than do those for whom bradykinesia is the primary symptom. Patients who present with significant instability of posture and gait are largely an older group who are more likely to have cognitive impairment and a more rapid progression of disease.

The advent of dopaminergic agents has changed the natural history of the disease significantly. The initial benefit of levodopa therapy, as mentioned above, is one of the diagnostic criteria for the disease. Although patients with idiopathic Parkinson's disease usually respond to levodopa, the initial benefits of therapy decline for as many as half of all treated patients after 2 or more years. Delay in onset of disability has been enhanced by the use of the monoamine oxidase B inhibitor deprenyl (see below).

Table 174.1. Differential Diagnosis of Parkinsonism

Idiopathic Parkinsonism (Parkinson's Disease, Lewy Body Disease)

Infectious and postinfectious
  Postencephalitic parkinsonism (von Economo's disease)
  Other viral encephalitides

Toxins
  Manganese
  Carbon monoxide
  Carbon disulfide
  Cyanide
  Methanol
  MPTP

Drugs
  Neuroleptics
  Reserpine
  Metoclopramide
  Lithium
  Amiodarone
  α-Methyldopa

Multisystem Degeneration
  Striatonigral degeneration
  Progressive supranuclear palsy
  Olivopontocerebellar degeneration
  Shy-Drager syndrome

Primary Dementing and Other Degenerative Disorders
  Alzheimer's disease
  Creutzfeldt-Jakob disease

Other CNS Disorders
  Multiple cerebral infarctions (lacunar state, Binswanger's disease)
  Hydrocephalus (normal-pressure or high-pressure)
  Posttraumatic encephalopathy (pugilistic parkinsonism)

Metabolic Conditions
  Hypoparathyroidism
  Chronic hepatocerebral degeneration
  Idiopathic calcification of basal ganglia

Hereditary Disorders
  Wilson's disease
  Juvenile Huntington's disease (rigid variant)

This list is not meant to be all-inclusive. Rather, it highlights the more common disorders that may have parkinsonism as a prominent feature.
Adapted from Koller WC. How accurately can Parkinson's disease be diagnosed? Neurology 1992;42[Suppl 1]:6, with permission.

DIAGNOSIS

The classic presentation of Parkinson's disease usually poses few diagnostic problems. However, several other presentations may be more problematic. These include isolated tremor at presentation, symptoms confined to half of the body (hemiparkinsonism), and the presence of these symptoms in younger patients. Symptomatic parkinsonism can be seen in several other disorders, such as progressive supranuclear palsy and multisystem atrophy, or as a side effect of numerous medications (Table 174.1). An extrapyramidal syndrome resembling that of parkinsonism also occurs in Alzheimer's disease and many other conditions.

The clinical diagnosis of Parkinson's disease is based on a careful examination in which the clinician looks for physical signs other than those associated with the basal ganglia, elicits a careful drug and family history, and most likely performs at least one neuroimaging study, probably magnetic resonance imaging, to exclude significant small-vessel vascular disease, which may produce a parkinsonian-like state. Table 174.2 pro-

Table 174.2. Criteria for the Diagnosis of Parkinson's Disease

INCLUSION CRITERIA	EXCLUSION CRITERIA
Presence for 1 year or more of two of the three cardial motor signs: Resting or postural tremor Bradykinesia Rigidity	Abrupt onset of symptoms Remitting or stepwise progression Neuroleptic therapy within year Exposure to drugs or toxins associated with parkinsonism History of encephalitis Oculogyric crises
Responsiveness to levodopa therapy with moderate to marked improvement and duration of improvement for 1 year or more	Supranuclear downward or lateral gaze palsy Cerebellar signs Unexplained upper motor neuron or lower motor neuron signs More than one affected relative Dementia from the onset of disease Severe autonomic symptoms

Adapted from Reich SG, DeLong M. Parkinson's disease. In: Johnson R, ed. Current Therapy in neurologic disease, 3rd ed. St. Louis: Mosby. 1990, with permission.

vides a summary of inclusion and exclusion criteria, which should help the physician in this clinical diagnosis. Among the inclusion criteria is a sustained responsiveness to levodopa therapy, with improvement lasting for 1 year or more. Many parkinsonian syndromes with other causes may show a transient response to dopaminergic agents.

PRINCIPLES OF MANAGEMENT

Parkinson's disease cannot be cured, but advances in treatment have improved prospects for patients. The goals of therapy are to delay disease progression, relieve symptoms, and preserve functional capacity. Restoring the striatal balance between dopaminergic and cholinergic activity is at the core of efforts to achieve symptomatic relief. Inhibiting oxidative injury appears helpful in retarding disease progression. The patient may be able to tolerate many of the early signs of parkinsonism, which are sufficient to prompt medical consultation but, aside from provoking psychological discomfort, are not disabling. The goal of therapy is to maintain the patient at maximum function with minimal medication.

The three categories of management strategies are preventive treatment, symptomatic relief, and regenerative therapy.

Delay of Disease Progression: Preventive Treatment

If the degeneration of dopaminergic neurons in the substantia nigra and striatum is a consequence of oxidative injury, then might it be possible to interrupt the degenerative process and slow or halt disease progression with agents that inhibit oxidative activity in the central nervous system? This hypothesis has led to the study of the monoamine oxidase B inhibitors.

Selegiline (Deprenyl). Although not universally accepted, evidence from several double-blinded, placebo-controlled studies of this monoamine oxidase B inhibitor indicates that monotherapy early in the course of disease delays the onset of disability and the need to initiate levodopa therapy. It is suspected that the mechanism of benefit is protection of striatal tissue from oxidative injury, but this theory has yet to be proved, and the major benefit may be some direct effect of relieving symptoms. Nonetheless, it seems reasonable to recommend this drug as initial treatment when Parkinson's disease is first diagnosed because it delays the requirement for levodopa therapy. It may also increase the time during which patients remain functional on levodopa and, for some patients, may decrease the levodopa requirement. This drug is given in the standard dose found to inhibit monoamine oxidase B in most patients: 5 mg given in the morning and 5 mg at noon. Side effects of tremor and dyskinesia are common when deprenyl is used in conjunction with levodopa. These are attributable to increased dopaminergic activity, which can be controlled by lowering the levodopa dose.

Other Antioxidants. In the largest and best-designed of the deprenyl studies, *tocopherol, a vitamin E analogue* with antioxidant properties, was tested. Tocopherol showed no benefit, either alone or as an enhancer of deprenyl activity. Further study of antioxidants and their prolonged effects is ongoing.

Symptomatic Relief

To restore the balance between cholinergic and dopaminergic influences requires either inhibition of cholinergic activity or enhancement of dopaminergic output. One strategy for early symptoms is to use amantadine (Symmetrel), a gluatamine antagonist that may enhance dopaminergic transmission and relieve bradykinesia; however, its effects are transient.

Anticholinergic Therapy. Anticholinergic agents were the mainstay of parkinsonian therapy for more than a century, and they have remained important. Commonly used drugs are *trihexyphenidyl* (Artane) and *benztropine* (Cogentin). These agents may be particularly beneficial for patients with tremor as a prominent symptom. Both are muscarinic blocking agents with typical anticholinergic side effects of urine retention, dry mouth, increased intraocular pressure in patients with glaucoma, and confusion (Table 174.3).

Enhancing Dopaminergic Activity: Dopamine Agonists. Treatment with one of the dopamine agonists—bromocriptine, pergolide, pramipexole, and ropinirole—is increasingly recommended as the first line of therapy for patients with mild to moderate parkinsonian symptoms. These medicines may suffice to control symptoms and delay for several years the need to prescribe levodopa. The side effects of the dopamine agonists are similar to those of levodopa, but dyskinesias and motor fluctuations tend not to occur with these medicines. Since its introduction to the U.S. market, pramipexole has become the most widely prescribed drug for early parkinsonism. Recent reports of several motor vehicle accidents in patients on pramipexole or ropinirole, as a consequence of paroxysmal attacks of sleep, have led to the recommendation that patients taking these medicines refrain from driving.

Levodopa. Eventually, most patients experience a worsening of symptoms that requires the introduction of *levodopa* (in combination with a peripheral dopa decarboxylase inhibitor). Levodopa is recommended for patients who become too symptomatic to function satisfactorily despite anticholinergic therapy with deprenyl plus a dopamine agonist. By prescribing levodopa, the physician is able to offer most parkinsonian pa-

tients much benefit, although the drug has a number of important limitations and side effects.

One limitation is the duration of action, which makes it necessary to consider carefully when to begin levodopa therapy. Weighing against early initiation of levodopa treatment is the phenomenon of a decline in its effectiveness in as many as 50% of patients after 2 years of use. This observation is the basis for the traditional view that onset of therapy should be delayed as long as possible. However, some data indicate a reduction in mortality when levodopa is started within 1 to 3 years of onset of symptoms rather than after 4 years. Clinical judgment that takes into account both of these findings is required.

Levodopa is the naturally occurring precursor of dopamine. It crosses the blood–brain barrier and enhances dopaminergic activity. However, because much of the drug is converted peripherally by a decarboxylase into dopamine (which cannot cross the blood–brain barrier), levodopa is best given in combination with a peripheral decarboxylase inhibitor, such as *carbidopa*. Combination preparations containing both agents in various strengths are commonly used. In a typical starting program, the combination preparation of 25 mg of carbidopa and 100 mg of levodopa is given (e.g., Sinemet 25-100 two or three times daily; see Table 174.3). Levodopa is rapidly absorbed after oral administration, reaches its peak effect after 30 minutes to 2 hours, and has a half-life of 1 to 3 hours. The rate of absorption is decreased by the ingestion of a protein-rich meal.

Adverse Effects. Significant adverse reactions develop in many patients; *nausea, vomiting, anorexia, hypertension, dyskinesias,* and *hallucinations* can be disturbing. The nausea can be partly overcome by taking the drug with small meals. Dyskinesias include chorea, athetosis, and dystonia. They usually occur simultaneously with peak concentrations of levodopa and are best managed by having the patient take small doses of medication at frequent intervals.

Problems in Late-stage Therapy. With disease progression, the threshold for the development of adverse central side effects appears to decline. *"Wearing off"* is the recurrence of severe symptoms hours after the most recent dose of medication and is often followed by a recurrence of rigidity and bradykinesia. A *controlled-release preparation* (Sinemet CR) relieves this problem for some patients.

As drug efficacy declines, patients may experience the *"on-off" phenomenon*, with a severe fluctuation of dose–response relations and rapid onset and termination of therapeutic and adverse effects. A study of the underlying pathophysiology has revealed impaired absorption of levodopa with meals and inhibition of levodopa transport into the brain by dietary amino acids. Treatment entails taking levodopa 1 hour before meals, adding an ergot preparation (see below), and reducing the protein content of the diet. Use of a controlled-release formulation may also help, but the development of the "on-off" state represents an advanced form of disease and a difficult one to treat. Drug "holidays" have been proposed to restore sensitivity to levodopa, but results are not impressive.

The development of a sustained-release preparation, Sinemet CR (50 mg/200 mg) has been a major therapeutic advance for patients afflicted with motor fluctuations. The controlled-release form can almost double the duration of effect to 5 to 6 hours. To match the effects of conventional levodopa preparations, a program of up to 25% more daily levodopa in the controlled-release form may be required. Doses administered after 6:00 p.m. can be given in the rapidly absorbed form

Table 174.3. Drugs Used for Parkinson's Disease

DRUG	AVAILABLE PREPARATION	DOSE (mg)	SCHEDULE	STARTING DOSE (mg)	MAINTENANCE DOSE (mg)
Anticholinergic Agents (representative examples)					
Trihexyphenidyl hydrochloride (Artane)	Scored tablets Elixir Timed-release capsule	2 mg, 5 mg 2 mg/5 mL 5 mg	3 to 4 times daily once daily	2 mg (Timed-release capsule may be substituted for regular Artane after maintenance dose is determined.)	2–10 mg
Benztropine mesylate (Cogentin)	Tablets	0.5 mg, 1 mg, 2 mg	once or twice daily	1 mg	0.5–6 mg
Dopaminergic Agents					
Carbidopa/levodopa (Sinemet)	Scored tablets 10/100 mg 25/100 mg 25/250 mg		2 to 4 times daily	50/200 mg in two divided doses	400-500 mg levodopa
Sinemet CR	50/200 mg		2 times daily	50/200 mg bid	variable
Bromocriptine (Parlodel)	Scored tablets Capsules	2.5 mg 5.0 mg	2 to 3 times daily	1.25 mg daily	7.5–30 mg
Pergolide mesylate (Permax)	Scored tablets	0.05 mg, 0.25 mg, 1.0 mg	3 times daily	0.05 mg daily	1–3 mg
Deprenyl (Eldepryl, selegiline hydrochloride)	Tablets	5.0 mg	2 times daily	5 mg daily	10 mg
Amantadine (Symmetrel)	Capsules	100 mg	2 times daily	100 mg daily	200 mg
Pramipexole (Mirapex)	Tablets	0.125 mg, 0.25 mg, 0.5 mg, 1 mg, 1.5 mg	3 times daily	0.25 mg tid	variable
Ropinirole (Requip)	Tablets	0.25 mg, 0.5 mg, 1 mg, 2 mg	3 times daily	0.25 mg tid	variable
COMT inhibitor					
Tolcapone (Tasmar)	Tablets	100 mg, 200 mg	3 times daily	100 mg tid	100 mg tid

COMT, catechol-o-methyltransferase.
Adapted from Reich SG, DeLong M. Parkinson's disease. In: Johnson R, ed. Current therapy in neurologic disease, 3rd ed. St Louis: Mosby, 1990, and Lang AE, Lozano AM. Medical progress: Parkinson's disease. N Engl J Med 1998;339:1044, 1130, with permission.

to eliminate nocturnal side effects of the medication. Other ways to manage wearing-off symptoms include administering drugs that reduce the metabolism of dopamine or levodopa. The catechol-*O*-methyltransferase (COMT) inhibitors tolcapone and entacapone have been introduced for this purpose. Tolcapone must be used with caution, as cases of fulminant hepatic failure have been reported. The physician should refer a patient requiring this therapy to a neurologist with expertise in the treatment of late-stage Parkinson's disease.

Other Dopaminergic Agents in Late-stage Disease. *Bromocriptine* and *pergolide* are direct *dopamine-receptor agonists*. These agents are used to enhance the therapeutic effects of levodopa and may be particularly helpful in late stages of the disease, when the conversion of levodopa to dopamine is inefficient in the degenerating substantia nigra. They are less likely than levodopa to cause dyskinesias and the on-off phenomenon. In addition, they may allow the use of lower doses of levodopa when given early on with levodopa as combined therapy. A small trial of gabapentin (Neurontin) has shown some efficacy for patients with advanced disease, and this drug has the advantage of causing very few side effects. Both the direct dopamine agonists and the levodopa controlled-release preparations are likely to be prescribed by neurologists, although recognition of the necessity to move to these sorts of therapies

will be in the province of the primary physician, who sees the patient most frequently.

Treatment of Psychiatric Symptoms. Nightmares, hallucinations, and increased sexual drive are disturbing psychiatric features of late-stage disease. Hallucinations and psychosis are best treated with the atypical neuroleptic clozapine. Severe depression is managed with the same medications given to patients without Parkinson's disease. However, because most of these patients are elderly, the physician must be careful of side effects of the tricyclic antidepressants. Theoretically, the combination of selegiline (deprenyl) and a selective serotonin reuptake inhibitor is problematic, and indications for this class of drug should be carefully weighed against the possibility of inducing the *serotonin syndrome* (hypertension, tachycardia, other autonomic dysfunction, and hallucinations). *Electroconvulsive therapy* may be used in depressed patients who are not confused.

Supportive Measures

Because maintaining function is a central goal of therapy, one should not forget the value of such important adjunctive measures as *physical therapy* and *psychological support*. Physical therapy can improve functioning by helping to preserve muscle strength and flexibility. Although a central component of the supportive psychological effort involves close follow-up and detailed patient education (see below), one must also be watchful for the development of depression and the need to treat it promptly and effectively (see Chapter 227).

Regenerative Therapies

As the pathophysiology of parkinsonism has become better understood, the role of functional neurosurgical procedures has grown. Surgery is reserved for disabling, medically refractory problems. In carefully selected cases, thalamotomy and deep-brain stimulation of the thalamus can control tremor. They do not help bradykinesia. When the problem is severe dyskinesia and on-off fluctuations, unilateral pallidotomy has been demonstrated to be effective. Pallidal deep-brain stimulation may be a good alternative. For the treatment of bradykinesia, *transplantation* of fetal substantia nigra tissue into the striatum relieves the signs of parkinsonism in animals with experimental lesions of the substantia nigra. Early attempts to treat humans who had Parkinson's disease with grafts of tissue, either autografts of the adrenal medulla or grafts of human fetal tissue, were disappointing, although the results with fetal tissue were better than those with the adrenal medullary grafts. Adrenal medullary grafting has been abandoned, but work on fetal tissue transplantation has continued and is producing increasingly beneficial results. Nonetheless, this method of therapy remains investigational at this time.

Other methods of therapy under development include new drugs to inhibit dopamine breakdown, synthesis of new dopamine-receptor agonists, and blockade of excitotoxic neurotransmitter receptors in the subthalamic nucleus. Small-scale, short-term study of *gabapentin*, which stimulates the striatal release of γ-aminobutyric acid (GABA), has produced promising results in patients with advanced disease. It is theorized that GABA stimulation may help overcome the loss of dopaminergic stimulation. Finally, jejunal infusion of levodopa and carbidopa has been tried in an attempt to improve levodopa absorption.

PATIENT EDUCATION

Patient and family education is essential to the success of therapy. The need for trial and error to obtain maximal benefit with minimal side effects must be explained. Frequent visits will be needed in the initiation period and later in the course of the disease. Although therapy can be proposed optimistically, the inevitable diminution in efficacy of therapy must be anticipated and discussed with patient and family so that they can be adequately prepared, both psychologically and practically. Patients are obviously concerned about their prognosis, and a frank discussion of what is known is usually appreciated. A number of helpful guidebooks are available for patients and their families.

THERAPEUTIC RECOMMENDATIONS

- After other potential causes of parkinsonism have been excluded, it is appropriate to start deprenyl (selegiline) in the early stages of disease. The daily dose is 10 mg (5 mg in the morning and 5 mg at noon). This drug may also be started in patients already taking levodopa/carbidopa (Sinemet) in an attempt to lower the amount of levodopa needed.

- If symptoms progress to impair daily functioning despite the use of deprenyl, then starting one of the dopamine agonists is appropriate. The most frequently prescribed is pramipexole (Mirapex). The initial starting dose is 0.125 mg three times daily. The dose is doubled at weekly intervals until a maintenance dose of about 1 mg three times daily is reached. As symptoms progress, the combination preparation levodopa/carbidopa (Sinemet) is indicated. Sinemet is usually begun at a dose of 25 mg/100 mg three times daily, after which the dose is adjusted according to the individual response.

- Combination treatment with anticholinergics, amantadine, and direct dopamine agonists (bromocriptine, pergolide, ropinirole) may be used to maximize effect (Table 174.3). Anticholinergics are particularly helpful for the treatment of tremor.

- Problems of long-term management and loss of efficacy include end-dose wearing off, on-off effect, drug-induced confusion, and loss of dopamine response. COMT inhibitors may be used to lessen these later problems with dopamine therapy. Appropriate consultation for adjunctive therapies can be initiated for such patients.

- The important roles of physical therapy, psychological support, and recognition and treatment of depression should not be neglected in the day-to-day management of patients with Parkinson's disease.

ANNOTATED BIBLIOGRAPHY

Diamond SG, Markham CH, Hoehn MM, et al. Multi-center study of Parkinson mortality with early versus later dopa treatment. Ann Neurol 1987;22:8. (*Mortality was less in patients treated earlier than in those treated later.*)

Duvoisin RC. Parkinson's disease: a guide for patient and family, 4th ed. New York: Raven Press, 1996. (*A sensible, very useful guide for the patient and family embarking on a course of treatment for Parkinson's disease.*)

Fahn S. Fetal-tissue transplants in Parkinson's disease. N Engl J Med 1992;327:1589. (*Progress is being made, but this is still an investigational therapy.*)

Jankovic J. New and emerging therapies for Parkinson's disease. Arch Neurol 1999;56:785. (*Good review of COMT inhibitors and research on surgical therapies.*)

Koller WC. How accurately can Parkinson's disease be diagnosed? Neurology 1992;42[suppl 1]:6. (*Entire supplement deals with the use of controlled-release Sinemet, but this chapter is a particularly lucid description of the clinical diagnosis.*)

Lang AE, Lozano AM. Medical progress: Parkinson's disease (two parts). N Engl J Med 1998;339:1044,1130. (*Superb two-part review covering pathophysiology and treatment.*)

Olson WL, Gruenthal M, Mueller ME, et al. Gabapentin for parkinsonism: a double-blind, placebo-controlled, crossover trial. Am J Med 1997;102:60. (*Small-scale, short-term study, but it shows very encouraging results in patients with advanced disease.*)

Parkinson Study Group. Effects of tocopherol and deprenyl on the progression to disability in early Parkinson's disease. N Engl J Med 1993;328:176. (*Deprenyl, but not tocopherol, effective in delaying the onset of disability and need for levodopa therapy.*)

Parkinson Study Group. Low-dose clozapine for the treatment of drug-induced psychosis in Parkinson's disease. N Engl J Med 1999;340:757. (*Very few side effects and excellent efficacy, whereas virtually all other antipsychotic agents exacerbated symptoms.*)

175

Management of Bell's Palsy (Idiopathic Facial Mononeuropathy)

AMY A. PRUITT

Bell's palsy is an idiopathic paralysis of the facial muscles innervated by the seventh cranial nerve. The condition encompasses 80% of all facial mononeuropathies. Satisfactory explanations for the condition are lacking, although serologic and DNA evidence implicates herpesvirus infection in some patients. Ischemia with subsequent edema of the facial nerve and adjacent structures has been invoked to explain facial palsy in patients with vascular risk factors. The condition shows an increasing incidence with age, is slightly more common in the winter, and is associated with pregnancy, diabetes, and hypothyroidism. In patients under the age of 50, it is more common among women, but this gender distribution reverses in patients over the age of 50.

The primary physician should be able to distinguish Bell's palsy from other, more ominous causes of facial palsy and balance therapeutic intervention against the self-limited course and favorable prognosis of the disease.

CLINICAL PRESENTATION AND COURSE

Clinical Presentation. The distinction between Bell's palsy and other facial paralyses is usually not difficult. The onset is usually acute, with maximal deficit developing within a few hours. The motor deficit is almost always unilateral and in two thirds of cases may be accompanied by pain in or behind the ear. Fever, tinnitus, and mild hearing diminution may be present during the first few hours. Symptoms may fluctuate during the first few days after onset. Voluntary and involuntary motor responses are lost. Both upper and lower parts of the face are affected, a feature that distinguishes this peripheral facial nerve lesion from a central supranuclear lesion, in which only lower facial muscles are affected. Patient symptoms include facial muscle paresis, facial asymmetry, and drooling. The palpebral fissure appears widened, the forehead is smooth, and the nasolabial fold is flattened. Bell's phenomenon (the normal upward deviation of the eye with lid closure) is exaggerated because of weakness of the orbicularis oculi. The corneal reflex may be decreased on the involved side. Lacrimation is only rarely defective, and depending on the level of the injury, loss or perversion of taste on the anterior two thirds of the tongue or hyperacusis may occur, causing altered taste, decreased tearing, decreased salivation, or altered sensitivity to sound.

Clinical Course. In 75% to 90% of cases, patients recover to a cosmetically acceptable level without treatment. Most do so within 3 weeks. Recovery is best in children; a poor prognosis has been associated with increasing age, hyperacusis, diminished taste, and severity of the initial motor deficit. The prognosis can be assessed by electromyographic testing of the involved muscles at least 72 hours after the clinical nadir. Patients with evidence of extensive axonal degeneration have a poorer prognosis. Those with partial or complete preservation of the compound muscle action potential amplitude have anatomic continuity of the facial nerve, partial axonal preservation, and a better prognosis. Electromyography is indicated only for patients with severe clinical involvement that has not improved by 7 to 10 days after onset.

Other poor outcomes in Bell's palsy result from abnormal regeneration of damaged nerve fibers. Lacrimation during eating or "crocodile tears" appear when fibers regrow and connect with lacrimal ducts instead of salivary glands. Abnormal movements (facial synkinesis) may occur if regenerating motor fibers innervate inappropriate muscles. Contracture of the involved site may be noted during voluntary movement. Seven percent of patients experience recurrent facial paralysis.

DIFFERENTIAL DIAGNOSIS

Other causes of facial paralysis involve injury to the facial nerve and include bacterial infection (from a source in the ear), herpes zoster, diabetes mellitus, sarcoidosis, Guillain-Barré syndrome, tumor (acoustic neuroma, pontine glioma, neurofibroma, cholesteatoma, parotid gland tumor, meningeal carcinomatosis), trauma (fracture of the temporal bone), and Lyme disease. Bilateral facial paralysis raises a different set of diagnostic possibilities, including Guillain-Barré syndrome (with or without HIV infection), sarcoidosis, and Lyme disease. Diseases of the neuromuscular junction such as myasthenia gravis or botulism must also be considered in the presence of bilateral facial nerve dysfunction.

WORKUP

The patient found to have a mononeuropathy of the seventh cranial nerve should be examined for evidence of an underlying cause. One checks for zosteriform lesions (see Chapter 193) on the tympanic membrane, in the external auditory canal, and behind the ear. The skin is examined for the characteristic truncal erythematous lesion of early Lyme disease (see Chapter 160) and for neurofibromas. The tympanic membrane is also checked for cholesteatoma and evidence of otitis media (see Chapter 218). The jaw is noted for tenderness and trauma to the temporal bone. The lymph nodes are palpated for enlargement, and the chest is auscultated for signs of interstitial involvement suggestive of sarcoidosis (see Chapter 51). A careful neurologic examination completes the assessment, with a focus on the detection of additional neurologic deficits.

Laboratory studies are of limited value in the assessment of this facial mononeuropathy in a patient with a characteristic history and physical findings, although they may reveal diabetes or some other medical condition associated with an increased risk for Bell's palsy. Testing for Lyme disease (see Chapter 160) may be appropriate in highly endemic areas, as suggested by a recent study in which one fourth of summertime cases of Bell's palsy demonstrated evidence of infection with the tick-borne spirochete of Lyme disease, *Borrelia burgdorferi*. The identification of Lyme disease has important consequences for management (see below and Chapter 160).

Computed tomography or magnetic resonance *imaging studies* are necessary only when a posterior fossa mass is suspected as the cause of the seventh nerve palsy. Lumbar puncture is indicated if inflammation, granuloma, or malignancy is a consideration. A mild pleocytosis of the cerebrospinal fluid has been reported in typical cases of Bell's palsy. In patients with atypical or persistent facial palsy, gadolinium-enhanced magnetic resonance imaging can help differentiate Bell's palsy from other causes. Electromyography may be used to predict recovery but is not needed for diagnosis and is most informative when at least 3 weeks have elapsed after the onset of facial paralysis.

PRINCIPLES OF MANAGEMENT

Of greatest practical importance during the acute stage of the illness is the prevention of injury to the *cornea*, which is left exposed by weakness of the orbicularis muscle. When the lid is weak, *methylcellulose drops* should be prescribed for use twice a day and at bedtime; in addition, the lid may need to be taped shut at night. If corneal abrasion is suspected because of pain, visual impairment, or other ocular symptoms (see Chapter 201), then prompt referral for ophthalmic consultation and slit-lamp examination with fluorescein is indicated.

Corticosteroids. Because the prognosis for most cases of Bell's palsy is good, little or no treatment is necessary in most instances. However, if paralysis is severe and the patient is seen within a few days of onset, a short course of *corticosteroid therapy* will increase the chances for maximal recovery. One study reported full facial recovery in 88% of a group treated with prednisone and in 64% of an untreated control group. Another study found a decrease in the frequency of chronic autonomic dysfunction (from 10% to 1%) when prednisone was administered early in the course of illness. Associated ear pain diminished more quickly when steroids were used. Nevertheless, the benefits of steroid treatment are often difficult to demonstrate because the disease has such a good prognosis. Steroid therapy seems to make a difference only in cases with poor prognostic signs. Patients with Lyme disease as the underlying cause should not receive steroids, which can worsen the situation by compromising immune function.

Therapy for Herpesvirus Infection. Based on serologic and DNA evidence that herpesvirus infection is the cause of many cases of facial paralysis, some authorities now recommend institution of appropriate therapy (e.g., 200 mg of *acyclovir* five times daily or 1,000 mg of *valacyclovir* twice daily for 7 to 10 days; see Chapter 192). Initial studies comparing prednisone therapy with and without antiviral therapy show a modest benefit from the addition of antiviral therapy. More data are needed to define the role of antiviral treatment better.

Other Treatments have been used. Based on the theory that nerve swelling contributes to the deficit, surgical decompression has been tried, but without much success. Some patients have been followed with electromyographic stimulation of the muscles to hasten particularly stubborn paralyses. The possible role of electromyographic stimulation in management is unclear; it has not been subjected to controlled study.

THERAPEUTIC RECOMMENDATIONS AND INDICATIONS FOR REFERRAL

- Ascertain that the condition is indeed Bell's palsy. Check for involvement of other cranial nerves and ear infection. Examine for zosteriform lesions on the tympanic membrane, in the external auditory canal, and behind the ear.
- In areas endemic for Lyme disease, examine the patient carefully for characteristic features and consider serologic testing (see Chapter 160).
- Explain the benign nature and good prognosis of the condition and caution the patient about corneal abrasion. Mention that altered taste, decreased tearing, decreased salivation, or altered sensitivity to sound may be experienced.
- Prescribe methylcellulose eye drops, to be used twice a day and at sleep, with taping of an especially weak lid. Tarsorrhaphy may be considered when severe lid weakness exists.
- If the patient is seen within 1 week of onset of facial weakness and if no important contraindications to corticosteroid use are found (Lyme disease would be a contraindication), then a short course of prednisone may be prescribed.
- Begin with 60 mg of prednisone every morning for 5 days. If improvement occurs or weakness does not progress during these 5 days, then taper and terminate over 10 more days. If improvement does not occur during the first 5 days, then continue the 60 mg of prednisone each morning for a total of 10 days and taper over another 10 days. If postauricular pain recurs when the dose is tapered, then reinstitute the preceding dose.
- If viral infection is suspected clinically or initial symptoms are severe, consider adding to the prednisone therapy an early course of therapy for herpesvirus infection (e.g., 200 mg of acyclovir five times daily or 100 mg of valacyclovir twice daily for 7 to 10 days; see Chapter 192).
- In the 10% of patients who do not achieve an acceptable recovery, autografting with a hypoglossal to facial anastomosis may provide reasonable cosmetic results and afford lasting protection of the eye. Patients in this category should be referred to an otolaryngologist or a neurosurgeon.

ANNOTATED BIBLIOGRAPHY

Adour KK. Diagnosis and management of facial paralysis. N Engl J Med 1982;307:348. (*A superb, succinct clinical review—not only of Bell's palsy but also of facial paralysis resulting from herpes zoster, trauma, otitis media, neoplasms, and other causes.*)

Adour KK. Bell's palsy. Results of a double-blind, placebo-controlled acyclovir–prednisone and placebo–prednisone treatment study. Br Med J 1995. (*Ninety-four patients were randomized, with a better outcome in the group receiving the combination of prednisone and acyclovir.*)

Austin JR, Peskind SP, Austin SG, et al. Idiopathic facial nerve paralysis: a randomized, double-blind, controlled study of placebo versus prednisone. Laryngoscope 1993;103:1326. (*Given preferably within 24 hours of onset of paralysis, prednisone improves cosmetic results.*)

Barringer JR. Herpes simplex virus and Bell palsy. Ann Intern Med 1995;124:63. (*A summary of the evidence for herpes virus as the etiologic agent.*)

Halperin JJ. Lyme borreliosis in Bell's palsy. Neurology 1992;42:1268. (*A very high incidence of Lyme seropositivity in patients with Bell's palsy during the summer in endemic areas.*)

Katusic SK. Incidence, clinical features, and prognosis in Bell's palsy: Rochester, MN, 1968–1982. Ann Neurol 1986;20:622. (*Best available community-based data.*)

Keane JR. Bilateral seventh nerve palsy: analysis of 43 cases and review of the literature. Neurology 1994;44:1198. (*A different set of illnesses needs to be considered, particularly Guillain-Barré syndrome and sarcoidosis.*)

Kuiper H, Devriese P, deJhongh B, et al. Absence of Lyme borreliosis among patients with presumed Bell's palsy. Arch Neurol 1992;49:940. (*In contrast to the patients in the Halperin article referenced above, almost all patients in this series had features atypical of idiopathic facial palsy and other systemic symptoms.*)

Tien R, Dillon WP, Jackler RK. Contrast-enhanced MR imaging of the facial nerve in 11 patients with Bell's palsy. Am J Neuroradiol 1990;11:735. (*Gadolinium enhancement helpful in cases with atypical or persistent facial palsy.*)

176
Management of Tic Douloureux (Trigeminal Neuralgia)

AMY A. PRUITT

Tic douloureux is among the most excruciating of pain syndromes seen in office practice. Fifteen thousand new cases occur annually in the United States; most patients are middle-aged or elderly. Some have found the pain so intolerable that they consider suicide. The primary physician needs to know how to use available medical therapies and when to send the patient for a neurosurgical consultation.

CLINICAL PRESENTATION AND NATURAL HISTORY

The illness is characterized by paroxysms of unilateral lancinating facial pain involving the jaw, gums, lips, or maxillary region (areas corresponding to branches of the trigeminal nerve). The maxillary and mandibular divisions are affected more frequently than the ophthalmic division. Minor, repeated contact with a trigger zone often precipitates an attack, setting off fierce pain that usually lasts up to a few minutes. Repeated paroxysms may continue day and night for several weeks. The disease is unilateral and unaccompanied by demonstrable sensory or motor deficits, features that distinguish it from trigeminal pain with other causes, such as tumor.

The condition can be chronic, although spontaneous remissions are not uncommon. Women are more often affected than men, and the incidence rises with age. The etiology of the condition remains unknown. Despite much speculation, no definitive evidence links it to herpes simplex virus. The pathologic lesion found in some electron micrographs appears to be a breakdown of myelin.

Although trigeminal neuralgia may be a symptom of multiple sclerosis, which should be considered in a young adult with trigeminal neuralgia, it is infrequently the initial or sole manifestation of this disease. Similarly, trigeminal neuralgia is uncommonly the isolated symptom of a cerebellopontine angle tumor. Both diseases can be demonstrated by magnetic resonance imaging (MRI), and some authors recommend MRI for all patients with trigeminal neuralgia, although the cost–benefit ratio remains to be determined.

DIFFERENTIAL DIAGNOSIS

Although few conditions absolutely mimic the lancinating pain of trigeminal neuralgia, pain referable to structures of the face may be similar. Conditions that should be excluded include dental disease, temporomandibular joint dysfunction, temporal arteritis, sphenoid sinusitis, and cluster headache. The pre-eruption pain of herpes zoster, which occurs in the distribution of the ophthalmic division of the trigeminal more frequently than in the distribution of the other two divisions, and post-herpetic neuralgia, which follows the skin eruption by a few weeks, are two other entities to be considered.

PRINCIPLES OF MANAGEMENT

Treatment is symptomatic. Because the condition may be self-limited and agents that give temporary relief are available, drug therapy should be tried before surgery is contemplated.

Carbamazepine (Tegretol) is the drug of choice; it was initially tried because anticonvulsants were believed to be helpful in causalgia. Studies have shown impressive short-term effects; most patients report marked relief of pain within 24 to 72 hours. The drug is so effective that some argue that failure to respond places the diagnosis in doubt. The starting dose is 100 to 200 mg twice daily. The maintenance dosage ranges from 400 mg to 800 mg/d and is adjusted according to serum drug levels; the therapeutic range is 5 to 12 μg/mL. An extended-release preparation of carbamazepine allows for the same total daily dose with convenient twice-daily dosing. The most common side effect is sedation.

Unfortunately, by 3 years, 30% of patients no longer obtain relief by taking carbamazepine; alternative therapy is needed. Moreover, the incidence of serious side effects (bone marrow suppression, rash, liver injury) is high (5% to 19%), so that therapy may have to be discontinued. Marrow suppression is often reversible if the drug is stopped early. Skin rash often precedes other serious side effects; it may be erythematous and pruritic. The onset of a skin rash is an early indication to halt therapy. Annoying side effects include nausea, diarrhea, ataxia, dizziness, and confusion. Neurologic reactions are reported most commonly and affect about 15% of patients. Starting carbamazepine at a dose of 200 mg daily helps to avoid many of the annoying minor side effects. During the first 2 months of therapy, a complete blood cell count and platelet count should be obtained weekly to biweekly; later, the frequency of monitoring can be reduced to monthly. It is advisable to attempt a reduction or cessation of carbamazepine therapy at least once every 2 to 3 months.

Baclofen, an agent that enhances synaptic transmission of γ-aminobutyric acid, has been used with success in a high percentage of cases. Some now consider it the drug of choice for trigeminal neuralgia. The initial dosage of 10 mg twice daily is increased slowly. The usual maintenance dosage is 50 to 60 mg/d. Sedation and nausea are the most common limiting side effects. Abrupt cessation of therapy can lead to hallucinations and seizures; therefore, discontinuation must be gradual.

Combination Therapy may be necessary because trigeminal neuralgia tends to increase in severity. Carbamazepine and baclofen in *combination* or either in conjunction with *phenytoin* can provide additional relief. The usual daily dose of phenytoin that achieves therapeutic serum levels is 300 to 400 mg (see Chapter 170). Parenteral phenytoin is sometimes used emergently for patients who are having a flurry of severe attacks and cannot take medicine orally. *Gabapentin* (Neurontin) may be prescribed if other medicines are unsuccessful, but sedation can be a limiting side effect if high doses are needed. *Narcotics* should be avoided because they are unlikely to be helpful for long-term control of pain and may lead to drug dependency.

Surgical Approaches can be considered when drug therapy proves inadequate. *Microvascular decompression* affords the best chance of long-term pain relief without sensory deficit, but because it entails more complicated surgery, it is often reserved for younger patients. The least invasive procedure producing acceptable deficits with the greatest relief of symptoms is percutaneous radio frequency rhizotomy. The small pain fibers are destroyed, whereas the more heavily myelinated touch fibers that supply the relevant zone are spared. The procedure has produced lasting relief in 90% of those treated once; only 5% have experienced an undesirable loss of sensation. The late recurrence rate is 10%, and pain relief is achieved with a repeated procedure in these patients; few need further treatment.

Formerly Used Treatment Methods include *alcohol injection* or partial section of the sensory root of the fifth cranial nerve. These techniques provided pain relief, but often only for 1 to 2 years, and at the price of unacceptable permanent sensory deficits. Total *tooth extraction* is an ineffective and erroneous treatment method.

PATIENT EDUCATION

The patient needs to be told that the condition can be controlled and is often self-limited. This knowledge can prevent a distraught sufferer from attempting suicide. The physician must keep in mind the anguish these patients may experience; they require close support. Obvious ways to prevent attacks, such as avoiding repetitive contact with the trigger zone, have usually been discovered by the patient, but they are worth mentioning. Patients treated with carbamazepine must be informed of the risk for marrow suppression and the importance of regular monitoring of the complete blood cell count.

THERAPEUTIC RECOMMENDATIONS AND INDICATIONS FOR REFERRAL

- Teach the patient to avoid repetitive contact with the trigger zone.
- Begin drug therapy for disabling and frequent episodes of pain with *carbamazepine* (100 mg twice daily, preferably in the extended-release preparation); increase the dosage by 200 mg/d until control of symptoms is achieved or a dosage of 800 to 1,000 mg/d is reached.
- During the first 2 months of carbamazepine therapy, monitor the complete blood cell and platelet counts weekly to biweekly; thereafter, monthly checks will suffice.
- Stop carbamazepine immediately if the white blood cell count falls below 3,000/mm³ or if skin rash, easy bruising, fever, mouth sores, or petechiae develop.
- An alternative to carbamazepine is *baclofen* at a dosage of 10 mg twice daily. Increase the dosage by 10 mg/d every 3 days until a response is achieved or a maximum of 60 mg/d is reached. Discontinue the medication gradually; do not withdraw it abruptly.
- If carbamazepine or baclofen alone is not sufficient to control symptoms, add *phenytoin* at a dosage of 300 mg/d.
- If the above medicines are unsuccessful, gabapentin (Neurontin) may be started at a dose of 300 mg at bedtime and then increased by 300 mg every 4 days until a total of 1,800 mg is being taken divided into three doses daily. Sedation may be a limiting side effect.
- Avoid narcotics because they are unlikely to be helpful for the long-term control of pain and may lead to drug dependency.
- Refer the patient who cannot be managed by pharmacologic measures to a neurosurgeon skilled in selective radio frequency rhizotomy or microvascular decompression.

ANNOTATED BIBLIOGRAPHY

Fromm GH, Terrence CF, Chattha AS. Baclofen in the treatment of trigeminal neuralgia: double-blind study and long-term follow-up. Ann Neurol 1984;15:240. (*Efficacy demonstrated.*)

Janetta PJ. Trigeminal neuralgia: treatment by microvascular decompression. In: Wilkins RH, Rengacharg SS, eds. Neurosurgery. New York: McGraw-Hill, 1996:3961. (*The acknowledged master of the procedure reports superb results in patients with trigeminal and glossophargyneal neuralgia and in those with hemifacial spasm.*)

Solomon S, Lipton RB. Facial pain. Neurol Clin 1992;8:913. (*Excellent review of differential diagnosis and management strategies.*)

Taha JM, Tew JM, Buncher CR. A prospective 15-year follow-up of 154 consecutive patients with trigeminal neuralgia treated by percutaneous stereotactic radio frequency thermal rhizotomy. J Neurosurg 1995;83:989. (*Report of a large neurosurgical series.*)

12

Dermatologic Problems

177

Screening for Skin Cancers
ARTHUR J. SOBER

Neoplasms of the skin are among the most common cancers in humans. It has been estimated that more than 1 million new tumors occur annually in the United States. The majority are basal cell carcinomas—relatively benign, locally mutilating tumors associated with few deaths. Squamous cell carcinoma, the second most common cutaneous malignancy, causes approximately 2,000 deaths annually. Melanoma, of which there are more than 47,000 cases annually, is responsible for approximately 7,700 deaths per year. The first two types of skin cancers derive from the epidermal keratinocytes; the third type develops from the melanocytes along the basal layer of the epidermis.

Screening for these tumors is important because they are relatively easy to diagnose in early stages, when cure is possible by simple measures. This is particularly true for melanoma, because we are in the midst of a striking, unexplained increase in its incidence. In the past decade, the incidence of melanoma in the United States has approximately doubled. Since 1960, the incidence of melanoma in the United States has increased more rapidly than that of any other cancer.

EPIDEMIOLOGY AND RISK FACTORS

Basal Cell Carcinomas are probably the most common malignancy in humans. They are distinctly sun-related, with risk proportional to total accumulated sun exposure and frequency increased in people who work outdoors (e.g., farmers, sailors). Approximately 90% occur on the head or neck. Other etiologic factors include a genetically transmitted autosomal dominant disorder, the basal cell nevus syndrome, in which multiple basal cell carcinomas occur in relatively young persons in association with palmar pits, bone cysts, and frontal bossing. Basal cell lesions can develop in persons exposed to arsenic. Scars from radiation dermatitis and thermal burns can also provide sites favorable to the development of basal cell tumors. Previously identified disease is also a risk factor.

Once a single basal cell carcinoma has developed, the chance that a second one will ensue within 1 year is 20%. After two have developed, there is a 40% likelihood that a third or more will occur within 1 year. This observation forms the basis of annual follow-up examinations after basal cell carcinoma has been detected.

Squamous Cell Carcinomas may develop from *actinic keratoses* and may also occur following arsenic ingestion or in areas of scarring from radiation dermatitis or thermal burns. Two thirds of squamous cell carcinomas occur on sun-exposed surfaces, with risk again proportional to total accumulated sun exposure. Those arising in sun-damaged skin usually behave in a less biologically aggressive fashion than do those that occur on unexposed surfaces. It is the latter group that appear to metastasize more frequently.

Melanoma, although far less common than basal cell and squamous cell cancers, accounts for 75% of skin cancer deaths. The incidence has been increasing rapidly during the past few decades and currently exceeds that for Hodgkin's disease, leukemia, pancreatic cancer, carcinoma of the thyroid, and carcinoma of the pharynx and larynx. The sex ratio for melanoma in the United States is approximately 1:1. A second primary tumor develops in up to 10% of patients; 10% have affected relatives.

Risk Factors and Precursors. Because of the rapid rise in melanoma incidence, attention has focused on melanoma risk factors and precursors. Persons with *fair skin* who tan poorly and burn easily are at greatest risk, especially those with a history of episodic, *intense sun exposure*. Blacks, Asians, and dark-skinned whites have a much lower risk.

Precursor lesions include *congenital nevi* and *dysplastic nevi* (i.e., clinically atypical moles). Although congenital nevi occur in approximately 1% of all newborns, most of these are small (≤1.5 cm in diameter). Melanoma risk has been most clearly associated with large (>20 cm) nevi. *Giant hairy nevus* (Fig. 117.1) is a form of congenital nevus associated with malignant degeneration; the overall risk for malignancy is about 6%. Melanomas may arise in these lesions at any time throughout life, but most often by age 10. Melanoma occasionally arises in smaller pigmented congenital nevi, but the exact risk is unknown.

Dysplastic nevi occur in 2% to 10% of light-skinned whites and usually are recognizable early in adolescence. Lifetime risk for melanoma is approximately 6%, or five times that of all whites in the United States. An inherited predisposition to dysplastic nevi may contribute to the 8- to 12-fold increase in

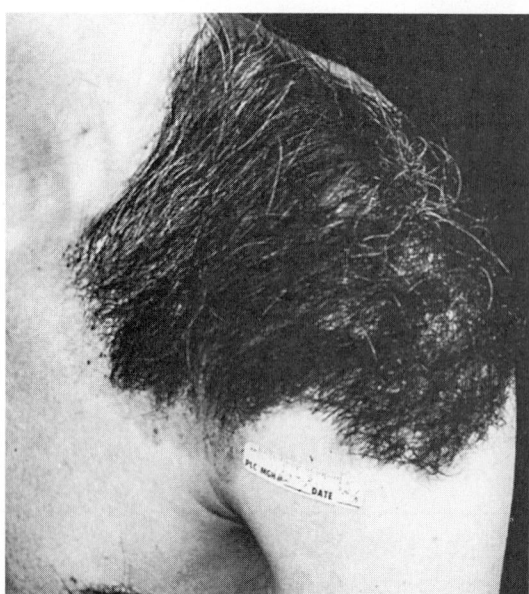

FIG. 177.1.   Giant hairy melanocytic nevus.

melanoma risk among first-degree relatives. In patients with dysplastic nevi and two or more first-degree relatives with cutaneous melanoma, the lifetime risk exceeds 50%. Patients with a large number of benign-appearing nevi may also be at increased risk.

NATURAL HISTORY OF SKIN CANCERS AND EFFECTIVENESS OF THERAPY

Basal Cell Carcinomas rarely metastasize or cause death, but they can be locally invasive and disfiguring. Metastasis is an extremely infrequent event that usually occurs in patients who have delayed therapy for many years and who have large, locally invasive, eroded lesions. The risk for other skin cancers is increased because of their shared risk factors. Population-based study raises the queston of a small but significant increase in the risk for nondermatologic cancers (e.g., testicular cancer, breast cancer, non-Hodgkin's lymphoma) in persons with basal cell cancer if basal cell disease is diagnosed before age 60. The significance of this finding remains to be elucidated.

Several effective forms of therapy exist, all yielding a cure rate of approximately 95%: *surgical excision, radiation* therapy, *electrodesiccation and curettage,* and cryotherapy with *liquid nitrogen* applied by special spray apparatus.

Treatment of the 5% of basal cell carcinomas that recur presents a greater challenge. The cure rate of a *recurrent basal cell carcinoma* is about 66% when the four modalities listed above are applied. A special form of surgery, *Mohs' micrographic surgery,* is used for difficult, recurrent, or infiltrative basal cell carcinomas. In Mohs' surgery, the excised tissue is examined directly under the microscope to determine whether the tumor has been completely removed. Additional sections of skin are removed until all the borders are histopathologically clear of tumor. With Mohs' technique, cure rates of recurrent tumors exceed 90%, and those for primary tumors are better than 98%.

The use of *5-fluorouracil* (5-FU) topically and *interferon alfa* within lesions has been advocated by some physicians for the treatment of *superficial basal cell carcinoma.* Experience has not been sufficient to permit a definition of the role of these modalities in relation to the forms of therapy that have a clearly established track record, but they may have some role in patients with multiple lesions in whom other techniques cannot be employed.

Squamous Cell Carcinomas may begin as *actinic keratoses,* of which perhaps 1 in 1,000 annually undergoes malignant change. *Bowen's disease* represents carcinoma *in situ,* which may progress to a more advanced lesion if untreated.

Actinic Keratoses. Application of *5-FU* cream or solution twice daily for 2 to 4 weeks usually results in the destruction of these lesions. Some clinically inapparent lesions will also be destroyed by this therapy. The patient must be warned about the impressive inflammation that occurs when 5-FU is used. Because 5-FU is also a photosensitizing agent, treatment in late fall or winter, when solar exposure is diminished, is preferred. Other effective modalities include cryotherapy with *liquid nitrogen* and *light desiccation.* If a cutaneous horn is present, *excisional biopsy* of the lesion may be warranted to rule out the presence of a squamous cell carcinoma. Actinic keratoses are extremely common and usually present no great threat to life.

Bowen's Disease (squamous cell carcinoma *in situ*) represents the next grade of neoplasia in the keratinocytic line; it is substantially less common than actinic keratoses. *Surgical removal* of the lesions of Bowen's disease is probably the most effective treatment. Alternatively, this tumor can be treated satisfactorily by cryotherapy with *liquid nitrogen.* A preparation of 5% 5-FU, applied two to three times daily for 6 weeks and covered by a plastic occlusive dressing, may also be used to treat Bowen's disease.

More Advanced Squamous Cell Carcinomas are treated with surgical excision or radiation; the latter is reserved for people older than 60 years.

Melanomas can be divided into four histopathologic categories, each with a characteristic natural history and clinical course.

Superficial Spreading Melanoma is the most common type in the United States, representing 70% of all melanomas diagnosed. The early lesion exists 1 to 7 years before a nodule develops, which indicates that deep penetration has occurred. Before penetration, the lesion grows superficially, and its removal during this time is associated with a 5-year survival rate approaching 100%.

Nodular Melanoma has a poorer prognosis. It may arise de novo or within a nevus as an invasive tumor from the onset. Even with early recognition, metastasis will already have occurred in a substantial proportion of patients. This type of tumor can occur on any cutaneous surface, as can superficial spreading melanoma. Nodular melanoma represents about 15% of all melanomas.

Lentigo Maligna Melanoma, the third type, accounts for about 5% of melanomas and occurs on sun-damaged skin of elderly patients. It is the least aggressive of the melanomas and may be present for 5 or more years before dermal invasion develops. Before dermal invasion, the lesion is termed *lentigo maligna.* Local excision is satisfactory in the treatment of lentigo maligna. In lentigo maligna melanoma, excision with wider margins is advocated. Surgical outcome in this type of tumor is almost uniformly favorable, although recurrence is sometimes seen. It is unusual for a patient to die of disseminated lentigo maligna melanoma.

Acral Lentiginous Melanoma occurs on palms, soles, subungual areas, and mucous membranes. This is the most common type to affect blacks and east Asians, but it may also occur in whites. The lesion begins as a flat, pigmented lesion that may be irregular in its border and pigment pattern. Early biopsy is essential to achieve cure before metastasis has occurred.

Prognosis. The most widely used system for estimating the prognosis of a patient with melanoma is that of Breslow, which utilizes *thickness* of the primary tumor as the principal determinant. Tumor thickness is measured with an ocular micrometer on a standard microscope from the granular cell layer down to the deepest tumor cell. Lesions *with a thickness of less than 0.85 mm* have a nearly uniformly favorable prognosis (5-year survival of 99%), whereas those with a thickness of more than 3.65 mm have a fairly poor prognosis (5-year survival of 42%). In between these extremes are lesions of 0.85 to 1.69 mm (5-year survival of 94%) and 1.70 to 3.64 mm (5-year survival of 78%). Ten-year survival figures follow a similar prognostic pattern according to lesion thickness (96%, 83%, 59%, and 29%, respectively).

A prognostic model that adds consideration of *age* (≤60 years vs. >60 years), *sex*, and *tumor site* (limb vs. extremity) to lesion thickness appears to improve prediction by nearly 50%, particularly for persons with lesions of intermediate thickness. The relative risk for mortality associated with a lesion on an extremity is reduced by 20% in comparison with that of a lesion on the trunk. Age below 60 years confers a 30% reduction in relative risk, and female sex lowers the relative risk by about 10%. When skin thickness alone is considered, a person with a lesion between 1.70 and 3.60 mm in thickness has a 10-year survival of 59%, but the four-variable model provides a series of predictions ranging from 89% survival (younger woman with an extremity lesion) to 24% survival (older man with a truncal lesion).

Treatment. Systems for determining prognosis are used to match treatment extent with seriousness of the lesion.

Primary Melanoma. At present, *wide local excision* is the treatment recommended for primary melanoma. The width of excision in our institution is based on primary tumor thickness. For tumors up to 1.0 mm thick, 1.0-cm margins are recommended; 2-cm margins are recommended for tumors from 1.0 to 4.0 mm thick. The therapeutic usefulness of elective regional lymph node dissection and removal is still being debated. *Sentinal lymph node biopsy* is useful as a staging procedure in high-risk patients, enabling meaningful stratification for adjuvant therapy. There is little evidence to suggest that prophylactic removal of nodes confers any more benefit than removal after the nodes have become clinically apparent.

Disseminated Melanoma. Currently, treatment remains difficult and unrewarding. With the most effective and widely used single agent, dacarbazine (dimethyl triazenoimidazole carboxamide, or DTIC), the response rate is approximately 20%. The nitrosoureas have also been utilized, with approximately the same response rate. Even patients who respond usually relapse

and die after a few months. Combinations of chemotherapy are currently being evaluated, as are new forms of immunotherapy.

Because the prognosis in disseminated melanoma is poor, attempts are being made to use *adjuvant therapy* postoperatively in patients who are at high risk for recurrence. At present, only *interferon alfa 2b* has proved beneficial in increasing disease free–survival in patients with stage III disease (nodal involvement), but increased overall survival remains to be established.

The management of giant congenital nevi is controversial. Early surgical removal is necessary to prevent malignancy. Because the risk is modest and the cosmetic consequences of surgery can be substantial, some advocate a wait-and-see approach with regular follow-up.

CLINICAL SCREENING AND DIAGNOSIS

Skin cancers are unique among cancers in their accessibility and the relative ease with which a tissue diagnosis can be made.

Basal Cell Carcinomas may take several forms. The typical appearance is that of a translucent *papule* with *telangiectases* over the surface (Fig. 177.2) that slowly enlarges, with subsequent development of a *central ulceration* (Fig. 177.3). This lesion has been termed the "rodent" ulcer. Basal cell carcinoma may also become pigmented in darker-skinned persons and be

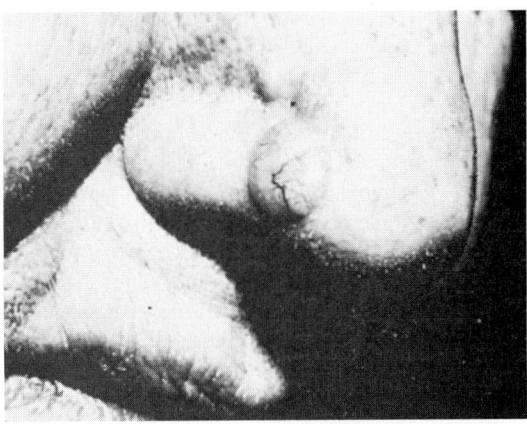

FIG. 177.2. Nodular basal cell carcinoma. Note telangiectasia.

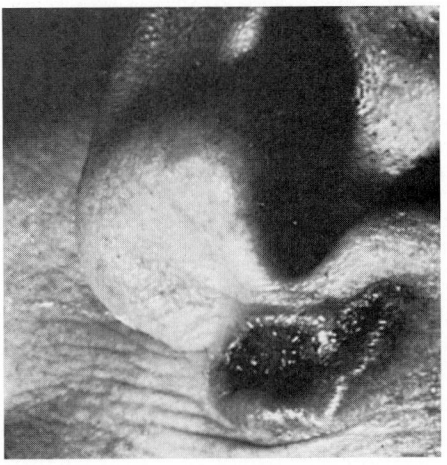

FIG. 177.3. Basal cell carcinoma—"rodent" ulcer.

confused with melanoma of the nodular or superficial spreading type. Superficial forms of basal cell carcinoma exist, most commonly on the back, that have the appearance of an *erythematous plaque*. Superficial basal cell carcinomas are also becoming more common on the legs of women. The usual presence of papular elements at the border facilitates the diagnosis. In the sclerotic form of basal cell carcinoma (morpheaform basal cell carcinoma), nests of tumor cells are interspersed within thick fibrotic bundles. This tumor is more resistant to treatment.

The differential diagnosis of basal cell carcinoma includes dermal nevi and other appendage tumors, such as *trichoepithelioma*, which can look just like a basal cell carcinoma. On histopathologic examination of a basal cell carcinoma, proliferation of basophilic cells is seen, usually in nests surrounded by discrete lacunae located in the upper dermis. This tumor is relatively easy for the pathologist to diagnose microscopically. Because basal cell carcinomas are more common in persons who have already had one, patients should be followed on an annual basis for early detection of new lesions.

Squamous Cell Carcinoma. The precursor *actinic keratosis* appears as a scaly erythematous patch that is flat to slightly raised; it may be single or multiple and occurs in sun-exposed areas (Fig. 177.4). Often, this lesion is more easily felt (a sandpaper-like texture) than observed. It appears to evolve through cycles from a macular erythematous lesion to a raised scaly lesion. In the later stages, a crusted surface, and sometimes even a horn of keratin, develop. Histopathologic examination of these lesions reveals atypical keratinocytes in the basal cell layer of the epidermis.

Bowen's disease, the carcinoma *in situ* stage, usually presents as a chronic, asymptomatic, nonhealing, slowly enlarging erythematous patch that generally has a sharp but irregular outline. It may resemble eczematous dermatitis but does not respond to topical steroid therapy (Fig. 177.5). Within the patch, areas of crusting are generally found. The sharp borders, chronicity, and lack of symptoms are clues that suggest the necessity of performing a biopsy. In dark-skinned patients, such as those of Mediterranean descent, these lesions may have a brown to blue-gray coloration. Bowen's disease can occur on

any part of the skin and on mucocutaneous sites, such as the vulva. In the vulvar area, the differential diagnosis includes lichen sclerosis et atrophicus, lichen simplex chronicus, squamous cell carcinoma, and, when the lesion is pigmented, melanoma. On histopathologic examination, atypical keratinocytes are noted throughout the epidermis but do not invade the dermis.

Invasive squamous cell carcinoma presents as a flesh-colored, asymptomatic nodule that enlarges and often undergoes ulceration and crusting (Fig. 177.6). The lesion may become keratotic and have a thickened surface. A cutaneous horn may

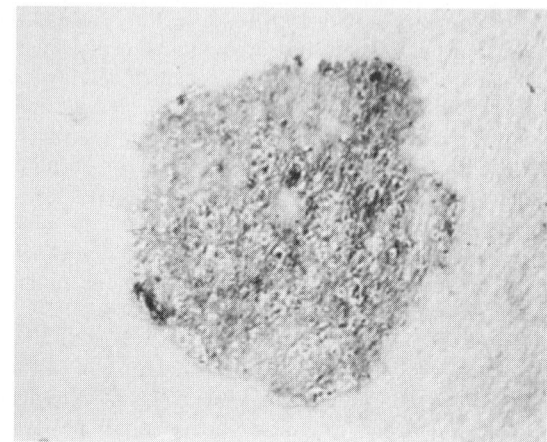

FIG. 177.5.   Bowen's disease—squamous cell carcinoma in situ.

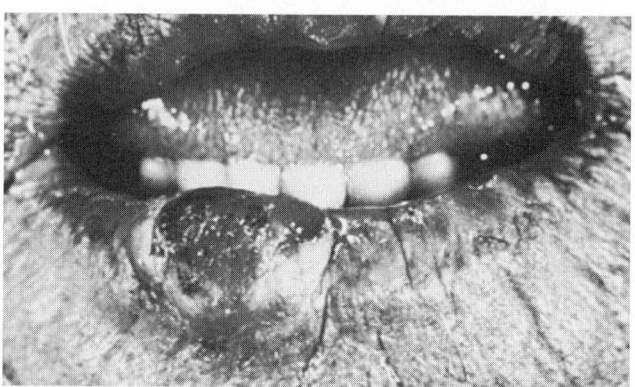

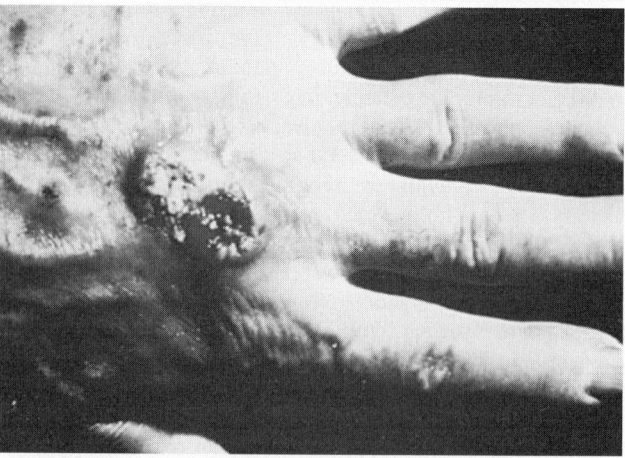

FIG. 177.6.   Squamous cell carcinoma in typical locations.

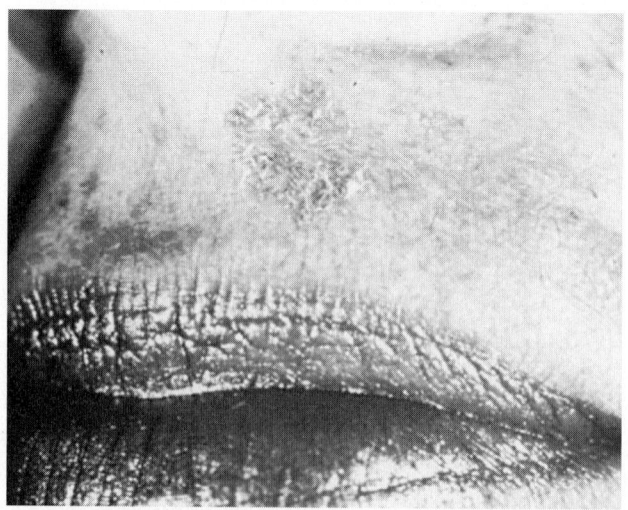

FIG. 177.4.   Actinic keratosis on the upper lip.

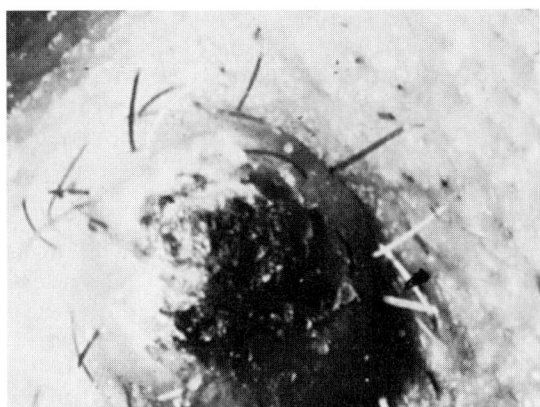

FIG. 177.7. Keratoacanthoma. Note the central keratotic plug.

be present. Excisional biopsy with close margins is the procedure of choice for the diagnosis of this lesion. Microscopically, the squamous cell carcinoma has fingers of atypical keratinocytic cells infiltrating into the dermis. The nuclei are clearly atypical; mitoses are frequently found.

Squamous cell carcinoma may sometimes be confused with a benign keratinocytic lesion, *keratoacanthoma*, which is dome-shaped and exhibits a prominent central plug (Fig. 177.7). Histopathologically, keratoacanthoma may be difficult for the pathologist to differentiate from squamous cell carcinoma. The keratoacanthoma usually exhibits more rapid growth and often regresses spontaneously.

Melanoma. The hallmarks include *asymmetry* (one half is not identical to the other) and *irregularity of the border* (sometimes a notch is present; Fig. 177.8), *variegation in the color* and *pigmentation pattern* (notably red, white, blue, and admixtures of these colors, such as grays and pinks), and *increased size* (>6 mm). The recognition of suspected pigmented lesions that may represent early disease is facilitated by use of the mnemonic *ABCD*:

A, *asymmetry* of lesion shape
B, *border irregularity*
C, *color variegation*
D, *diameter greater than 6.0 mm* (the size of a pencil eraser tip)

Use of the ABCD system has been associated with sensitivities as high as 92% and a specificity of 98%. Additional features seen in intermediate and advanced lesions include an *irregular raised surface* and *ulceration* or *bleeding* of the surface. Regardless of appearance, any pigmented lesion that undergoes change should be considered for excisional biopsy. Each type of melanoma has distinguishing features.

Superficial spreading melanomas have some irregularity in the border and some alteration in the regularity of pigment pattern and coloration (Fig. 177.8).

Nodular melanoma, which arises de novo or within nevi as an invasive tumor from the onset, has no radial growth component. It appears as a blue, blue-black, or gray nodule of varying size (Fig. 177.9). These lesions may be symmetric or have an irregular perimeter. Their borders are characteristically discrete and sharp. Most of these lesions are deeply invasive at the time of diagnosis. About 5% of nodular melanomas lack pigment (*amelanotic melanoma*).

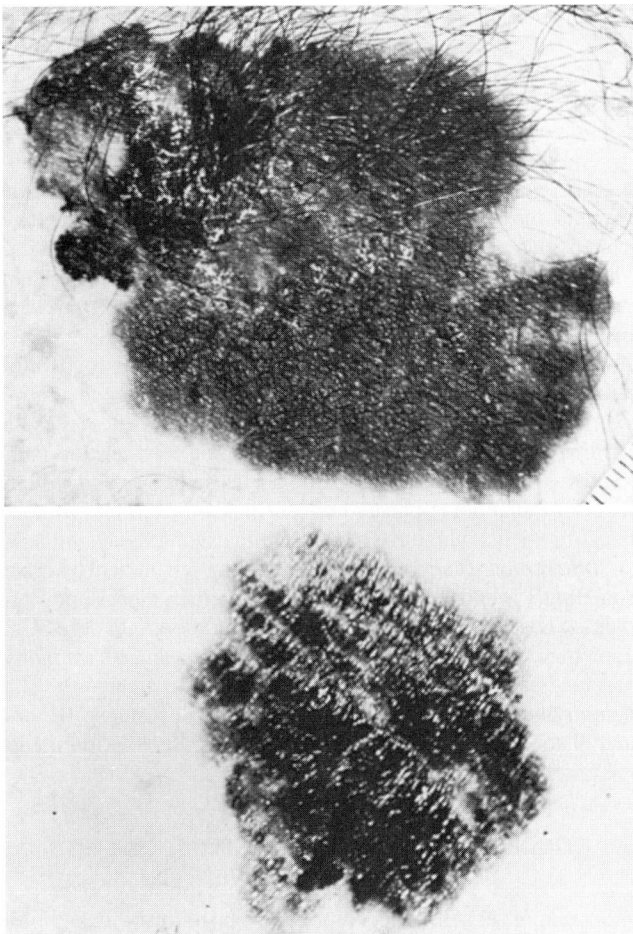

FIG. 177.8. Melanoma of the superficial spreading type. Note the irregularity of the border and prominent notch.

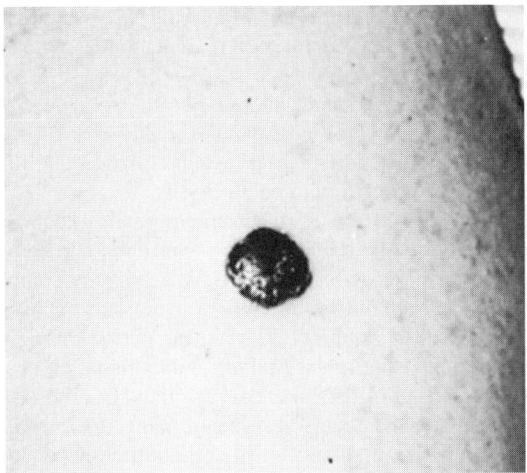

FIG. 177.9. Melanoma, nodular type.

Lentigo maligna begins as a freckle-like lesion that slowly expands. It has a markedly irregular pigmentation pattern and usually an extremely irregular border. Spontaneous regression may occur; the border may advance on one side while regressing on another, so that the lesion appears to march across the skin surface.

Acral lentiginous melanoma occurs on palms, soles, subungual areas, and mucous membranes, beginning as a flat pigmented lesion that may be irregular in its border and pigment pattern. Early biopsy is essential to achieve cure before metastasis has occurred.

The distribution of melanoma across the body surface is not uniform. In both sexes, lesions aggregate on the back. In female patients, the lower extremities are heavily affected, but they are spared in male patients, in whom the anterior torso is more likely to be involved. The bra and swim trunk areas are spared in females, and the swim trunk area and thighs are spared in males.

Because a *second primary tumor* develops in up to 10% of patients with melanoma, it is worthwhile to examine the entire skin surface to look for a second tumor on each encounter. In familial melanoma, a second primary tumor may develop in as many as 30% of patients. Because a trait favoring the development of melanoma appears to occur in families, family members of patients who have had melanoma should be examined.

Differential Diagnosis. The preceding characteristics are sometimes found in *pigmented basal cell carcinoma* and pigmented lesions of Bowen's disease. In addition, odd dermal or compound nevi, irritated seborrheic keratoses, and occasionally vascular lesions can be clinically confused with melanoma. The benign blue nevus also shares similar clinical features. Biopsy and histopathologic evaluation are warranted if a lesion meets the criteria previously noted.

CONCLUSIONS AND RECOMMENDATIONS FOR SCREENING AND PREVENTION

- Screening for skin cancer represents one of the best examples of early detection leading to an improved outcome. For example, the current 5-year survival rate for melanoma is 95% if the thickness of a lesion is less than 0.85 mm. It is estimated that with education of patients and physicians about signs of disease and the importance of early diagnosis, the overall 5-year survival rate for malignant melanoma could approach 90%.
- Every primary physician should be able to recognize the common skin cancers, and patients should be taught to avoid risk factors and report suspect lesions. In particular, the following precautions should be observed:
  - All fair-skinned persons who sunburn easily and those with evidence of solar damage or skin cancer should be warned about the hazards of continued high-intensity solar exposure. They should be advised to avoid sun exposure between 11:00 a.m. and 2:30 p.m., the period during which 70% of exposure to harmful ultraviolet radiation occurs.
  - All persons at risk for skin cancer should be advised to use a broad-spectrum sunscreen when going out into the sun. The preparation should block some ultraviolet A in addition to most ultraviolet B radiation and have a solar protection factor (SPF) of at least 15.
  - Patients with a history of exposure to arsenic or previous radiation therapy and radiation dermatitis should be watched closely for the development of cancer.
  - For nonmelanomatous skin cancer, patients should report to their physician any new, slowly growing, nodular or papular lesions that are flesh-colored or translucent, and particularly the occurrence of any bleeding, ulceration, or

horn formation. Areas of maximum solar exposure are at greatest risk.
  - For malignant melanoma, patients are asked to report to their physician any pigmented lesion with an irregular border or a variation in color, especially blue, gray, or black. Any growth in a pigmented lesion or change in color should also arouse suspicion.
  - If any doubt exists about whether a skin lesion is benign, the obligation of the primary physician is either to obtain a sample of the lesion for biopsy or to refer the patient to an experienced specialist for an opinion. If patients and physicians work together, the incidence of skin cancer and the deaths associated with it can be greatly reduced.

ANNOTATED BIBLIOGRAPHY

Alguire PC, Mathes BM. Skin biopsy technique for the internist. J Gen Intern Med 1998;13:46. (*Useful illustrated clinical review with discussion of indications and technique.*)

American Cancer Society, Massachusetts Division, 1996. Cancer manual, 9th ed. (*Practical sections on nonmelanotic and melanotic skin cancers.*)

Balch CM, Houghton AN, eds. Cutaneous melanoma, 3rd ed. St. Louis: Quality Medical Publishing, 1998. (*Comprehensive monograph.*)

Elder D, Elenitsas R, Jaworsky C, eds. Lever's histopathology of the skin, 8th ed. Philadelphia: Lippincott–Raven Publishers, 1997. (*Authoritative clinical and histopathologic description of cutaneous malignancies.*)

Epstein DS, Lange JR, Gruber SB, et al. Is physician detection associated with thinner melanomas? JAMA 1999;281:640. (*An interview survey study; physician-detected lesions were thinner and thus less advanced, evidence that screening pays off.*)

Fitzpatrick TB, Sober AJ. Sunlight and skin cancer. N Engl J Med 1985;313:818. (*An editorial reviewing the evidence for sun exposure as the principal risk factor for skin cancer.*)

Friedman RJ, eds. Cancer of the skin. Philadelphia: WB Saunders, 1991. (*A compendium on all aspects of skin cancer.*)

Frisch M, Hjalgrim H, Melbye M. Risk for subsequent cancer after diagnosis of basal-cell carcinoma: a population-based, epidemiologic study. Ann Intern Med 1996;125:815. (*A Danish population study showing an increased risk for testicular and breast cancer and non-Hodgkin's lymphoma when basal cell disease is found at a young age.*)

Friedman RJ, Rigel DS, Kopf AW. Early detection of malignant melanoma: the role of physician examination and self-examination of the skin. CA Cancer J Clin 1985;35:130. (*Reprints available from the American Cancer Society. Can be used to instruct patients in self- examination of the skin.*)

Greene MH, Clark WH, Tucker MA, et al. Acquired precursors of malignant melanoma. N Engl J Med 1985;312:91. (*An important description of the natural history of both common and dysplastic nevi, including a color atlas. An accompanying editorial provides a perspective on melanoma risk associated with dysplastic nevi.*)

Johnson T, Smith JW, Nelson BR, et al. Current therapy for cutaneous melanoma. J Am Acad Dermatol 1995;32:689. (*Through review.*)

Koh HK. Cutaneous melanoma. N Engl J Med 1991;325;171. (*Through review.*)

Luftman DB, Lowe NJ, Moy RL. Sunscreens: update and review. J Dermatol Surg Oncol 1991;17:744. (*Useful summary; helpful for advising patients.*)

Schuchter L, Schultz DJ. Synnestvedt M, et al. A prognostic model for predicting 10-year survival in patients with primary melanoma.

Ann Intern Med 1996;125:369 (*A validated model for improving prognosis; age, sex, and site of lesion, in addition to skin thickness, are readily available, independent predictors of prognosis.*)

Sober AJ, Fitzpatrick TB, Mihm MC, et al. Early recognition of cutaneous melanoma. JAMA 1979;242:2795. (*Self-assessment approach to the recognition of early lesions in this color atlas.*)

Stiller MJ, Davis JC, Shupock JL. A concise guide to topical sunscreens: state of the art. Int J Dermatol 1992;31:540. (*Includes consideration of preparations blocking ultraviolet A.*)

Thompson SC, Jolley D, Marks R. Reduction of solar keratoses by regular sunscreen use. N Engl J Med 1993;329:1147. (*Study supports value of regular sunscreen use.*)

Whited JD, Grichnik JM. Does this patient have a mole or a melanoma? JAMA 1998;279:696. (*Part of the Rational Clinical Examination series examining the accuracy and yield of the skin examination.*)

178

Evaluation of Pruritus
WILLIAM V. R. SHELLOW

Pruritus is an unpleasant cutaneous sensation that provokes the urge to scratch. It may be localized or generalized and may occur with or without skin lesions. Itching may be caused by a dermatologic condition, systemic illness, or psychological disturbance. The complaint is particularly common among the elderly. It can prove challenging when the cause remains elusive and symptoms interfere with daily functioning. The primary physician should be capable of performing a reasonably detailed evaluation and providing effective symptomatic relief.

PATHOPHYSIOLOGY AND CLINICAL PRESENTATION

Pathophysiology. The sensation of itching arises from free nerve endings of the skin. These fibers are especially concentrated in the flexor aspects of the wrist and ankles. Afferent transmission is through unmyelinated C fibers to the dorsal horn of the spinal cord, ascending to the contralateral spinothalamic tracts and terminating in the cerebral cortex. The scratch response is a spinal reflex. Many chemical mediators and modulators of itch have been suggested, including substance P, opioid and nonopioid peptides, somatostatin, neurokinin A, histamine, serotonin, kinins, and prostaglandins.

Various external stimuli decrease the threshold for itching. These include inflammation, heat, dryness, and vasodilation. Persons vary in their response to itching. The perception of itching can be influenced psychologically, which explains why a physician may experience itching after attending a patient with scabies or pediculosis.

Clinical Presentations. Pruritus may be localized or generalized and can occur with or without skin lesions. Pruritus resulting from a systemic disease can occur with or without a primary skin lesion.

Dermatologic Disease. A host of dermatologic conditions can present with itching, including pediculosis and scabies (see Chapter 195), contact dermatitis (see Chapter 184), urticaria (see Chapter 181), psoriasis (see Chapter 187), lichen planus, and dermatitis herpetiformis. Dry skin (xerosis) (see Chapter 183) is the most frequent precipitant and is particularly common in the elderly. Symptoms are worse in the winter or with use of air conditioning, which lowers indoor humidity. Tangential light reveals fine scaling and cracking. Patients with urticaria usually give a history of wheals and demonstrate dermatographism (urticaria elicited by stroking the skin with a blunt object). Scabies and dermatitis herpetiformis can have a subtle presentation, with few skin manifestations when the patient is initially seen. In dermatitis herpetiformis, vesicles are characteristic, but excoriations may obliterate them. An intense burning sensation often predates the appearance of skin lesions. Scabies is endemic in long-term care facilities. In persons with good hygiene, fewer than 10 of the characteristic burrowing-induced skin lesions (see Chapter 195) may be present. At times, the only finding may be nonspecific papules caused by an immune skin response.

Renal Disease. Pruritus may accompany severe chronic renal failure, especially in patients undergoing hemodialysis. Secondary hyperparathyroidism causing elevated levels of histamine is one suspected mechanism. Other investigations have implicated endopeptidases or kinins as substances that can accumulate in uremia.

Endocrine Disease. Generalized itching occurs among 4% to 11% of patients with Graves' disease, usually when the disease is long-standing. Increased kinin activity and slightly elevated skin temperatures are suggested mechanisms. The mechanisms for other endocrinopathies are poorly understood.

Liver Disease. Among the many disorders of the liver, obstructive cholestatic jaundice produces the greatest degree of pruritus. Itching can be especially prominent and the presenting manifestation in primary biliary cirrhosis. About 20% to 25% of patients with jaundice are plagued by itching, although it is rare in the absence of cholestasis. The pruritus of cholestasis has been linked to the release of proteases in the skin by bile salts. Itching during the last trimester of pregnancy has been reported in 1% to 3% of expectant women and is thought to be cholestatic in origin, although jaundice is uncommon.

Hematologic Disease. The itching of *polycythemia vera* affects 30% to 50% of patients and is exacerbated by a hot shower or bath. In mycosis fungoides, pruritus has been suggested as an adverse prognostic factor. *Lymphoma* and *Hodgkin's disease* may also cause pruritus; its role as a prognostic indicator is less significant than previously thought. Histamine release by an increased number of circulating basophils is postulated as the pathophysiologic mechanism. Pruritus has also been found in association with iron-deficiency anemia and with HIV infection. Mechanisms are unclear.

Psychiatric Disease. Patients with neurotic scratching report that they scratch even in the absence of itching. Itching is reported to occur more often at night, when other stimuli are lacking. Although the excoriations of this "neurodermatitis" may occur anywhere the patient can reach, they tend to be concentrated in the extremities. Depression and dsyphoric mood are particularly common among such patients, as are serious conflict and situational stress preceding the onset of pruritus.

DIFFERENTIAL DIAGNOSIS

The conditions that cause itching may be dermatologic, systemic, or psychological in origin (Table 178.1). Skin disorders account for the vast majority. The pruritus may be localized or generalized. Localized itching is usually a sign of a primary dermatologic condition, dermatophyte infection, infestation, or a psychological disorder. Generalized itching raises the possibility of a systemic condition or a psychogenic cause, although dermatologic disease still predominates. In the elderly, the most common cause of itching is xerosis. Although generalized pruritus may accompany lymphoma and other malignancies, its presence does not increase the risk for underlying or future malignancy in a person who presents with no other manifestations of malignancy.

WORKUP

A search for a primary dermatologic disease or scabies infestation is the first step in the evaluation of the pruritic patient. Often, a careful look at the skin combined with a few clues from the history suggests the diagnosis. Skin diseases associated with recognizable lesions and characteristic distribution usually do not present significant diagnostic difficulty, unless camouflaged by excoriations, lichenification, secondary eczema, or infection. Systemic illnesses require a more detailed history and a physical examination that extends beyond the skin, followed by selected laboratory studies.

History. Location, associated symptoms, precipitants, clinical course, and severity (including effect on sleep and daily activity) should be carefully elicited. A detailed description of any skin changes or rashes should be included. If the patient reports little in the way of skin findings, clues to an underlying dermatologic condition should still be sought. For example, a history of atopy, asthma, or urticaria raises the probability of an allergic origin, whereas concurrent pruritus in household members is suggestive of scabies, and worsening in winter points to dry skin. Environmental factors such as sunburn, prickly heat, the presence of cats in a household, exposure to fiberglass, and excessive drying of the skin also deserve consideration. Pharmacologic exposure is important to review because a subclinical allergic reaction may occur with almost any drug. One should also check specifically for use of opiates, amphetamines, quinidine, aspirin, B vitamins, and niacinamide.

In the setting of generalized pruritus, one should inquire about symptoms or a history of hyperthyroidism (see Chapter 103), renal failure (see Chapter 142), lymphoma (see Chapter 84), polycythemia (see Chapter 80), cholestatic liver disease (see Chapter 62), and HIV infection (see Chapter 13). Pregnancy should be suspected as the cause if the patient is a woman in her third trimester.

If the cause is not evident from the medical history, it is worth exploring psychosocial aspects of the patient's life and any relation between psychological or situational stresses and the onset of pruritus. Given the high prevalence of depression among patients with idiopathic pruritus, inquiry into symptoms of depression (see Chapter 227) may prove useful.

Physical Examination. A careful and complete inspection of the skin is essential. The presence and distribution of a rash, excoriations, lichenification, and inflammatory changes should be noted, along with any evidence of xerosis (scaling and dryness). Dry skin is especially evident on the legs; tangential lighting can help reveal the scaling.

If the complaint is localized, a more detailed look at the involved area is needed. The scalp is checked for psoriasis and seborrhea; the trunk for urticaria, scabies, and the linear lesions of contact dermatitis; the inguinal area for *Candida* infection, pediculosis, tinea, and scabies; the hands for eczema, contact dermatitis, and the telltale interdigital lesions of scabies; the

Table 178.1. Conditions Associated with Pruritus

Dermatologic
Arthropod bites and stings
Bullous pemphigoid
Dermatitis
  Atopic dermatitis
  Contact dermatitis (allergic and irritant)
  Dermatitis herpetiformis
Dermatophytosis
Infestation
  Scabies
  Pediculosis
Lichen planus
Lichen simplex chronicus
Pityriasis rosea
Psoriasis
Urticaria and dermatographism
Varicella
Xerosis

Psychological
Neurotic excoriations
Depression
Delusions of parasitosis

Systemic
Hyperthyroidism
Renal failure, chronic
Drug reaction
Hematologic disease
  Iron-deficiency anemia
  Mycosis fungoides
  Polycythemia vera
  Paraproteinemia
  Systemic mastocytosis
Hepatobiliary problems
  Intrahepatic cholestasis
  Extrahepatic obstruction
  Third trimester of pregnancy
Malignancy
  Malignant carcinoid
  Lymphoma, leukemia
  Multiple myeloma
HIV infection
Parasitosis
  Ascariasis
  Hookworm
  Onchocerciasis
  Trichinosis

legs for neurotic excoriations, stasis dermatitis, atopic dermatitis (popliteal fossa), lichen simplex (lateral malleoli), and dermatitis herpetiformis (knees); and the feet for tinea and contact dermatitis.

If the pruritus is generalized and no evidence of primary dermatologic disease can be found, a search for signs of a systemic condition is warranted. The skin is examined for jaundice and findings associated with HIV disease (see Chapter 13), the sclerae are checked for icterus, the lymph nodes for enlargement, the thyroid for goiter, and the liver and spleen for organomegaly.

Laboratory Studies. Test selection should be based on findings from the history and physical examination. Resorting initially to a "panscan" is wasteful and likely to generate false-positive results. Skin scrapings are performed to confirm a clinical diagnosis of scabies or dermatophytosis (see Chapters 195 and 191). A skin biopsy examination with special stains or direct immunofluorescence may be required to confirm a diagnosis of mastocytosis, mycosis fungoides, or one of the autoimmune bullous diseases. In the setting of suspected cholestasis, one should order a determination of serum bilirubin, alkaline phosphatase, and transaminase levels, and obtain an ultrasonogram of the biliary tree (see Chapter 62). If lymphoma or carcinoid is a concern, chest radiography or abdominal computed tomography may be indicated (see Chapters 44 and 84). HIV testing is indicated if the patient has a history of high-risk sexual behavior or IV drug use (see Chapter 13).

If the diagnosis continues to be elusive, then a complete blood cell count and measurement of blood urea nitrogen, thyroid-stimulating hormone, calcium, albumin, and globulin levels are worth considering. Pruritus *per se* is not a predictor of malignancy and need not trigger a workup for occult malignancy in the absence of other clinical evidence for cancer.

SYMPTOMATIC THERAPY AND PATIENT EDUCATION

To be most effective, the treatment of pruritus should be based on etiology if possible. However, nonspecific symptomatic measures are sometimes required, especially if the workup is still in progress and the itching is disturbing sleep and interfering with daily life. Symptomatic treatment is also indicated for refractory conditions (e.g., biliary cirrhosis). Even if little can be done for the underlying condition, relief from itching is greatly appreciated. Avoidance of provocative factors is important, complemented by simple empiric therapy of low toxicity. Teaching the patient how to overcome the itch–scratch–itch cycle is most beneficial.

Nonspecific Behavioral and Topical Measures. Patients should be told to trim their fingernails, to keep them clean to prevent excoriation or infection, and to rub with their palms rather than their fingers if they have an uncontrollable urge to scratch. If vasodilators or foods such as coffee, spices, or alcohol precipitate itching, they should be avoided. Changing one sheet at a time helps reduce the static electricity that can precipitate itching. Rough clothing, particularly wool, should be avoided. Cotton clothing that has been doubly rinsed of detergents is preferred. Humidification of the indoor environment should be maintained when an air conditioner is used and during the winter, either with humidifiers or by placing bowls of water near radiators. Frequent and prolonged showering is to be avoided because it eliminates the skin's normal oil protection and contributes to dryness. Mild soaps (Dove, Basis, Neutrogena, Purpose, Aveeno Bar) are preferred to drying, antiperspirant soap products. Use of hot water is discouraged because it worsens itching by increasing cutaneous blood flow.

Such behavioral measures can be helpful regardless of the cause of itching and often reduce or eliminate the itching without further measures. Additional topical approaches include sponging the skin with cool water and using moisturizers before bedtime. However, only lotions and creams recommended by the physician should be used. The use of simple *emollient* preparations (Moisturel, Eucerin, Lubriderm, Aveeno Lotion) is encouraged, especially after bathing. It can be useful to add Alpha-Keri or other lubricating agents to the rinse cycle when sheets are washed.

Preparations containing combinations of *menthol*, *phenol*, and *camphor* (e.g., Sarna lotion) applied several times daily may provide symptomatic relief. *Calamine* lotion may alleviate itching briefly but is drying; it is most useful on weeping lesions. *Pramoxine*-containing products (PrameGel, Prax, Pramosone) also may reduce itching, but other topical anesthetics and antihistamines should be avoided because they can be potent sensitizers. *Hydrocortisone* cream, lotion, or ointment may provide symptomatic relief of itch; however, treatment with high-potency corticosteroids should be restricted to specific steroid-responsive dermatoses because prolonged use can cause dermal atrophy.

If environmental manipulation and topical agents are not effective, then systemic medications must be considered.

Nonspecific Systemic Measures. The systemic medications most commonly used are antihistamines, sedatives, and aspirin. By occupying the histamine receptors, the *histamine$_1$-blocker antihistamines* are very effective for allergen-mediated itch. In nonallergic itch, antihistamines are no more effective than aspirin but are often worth a try. Their sedative quality makes them useful as a bedtime medication in patients who have sleep difficulties. The choice of an ideal agent is found by trial and error on the basis of the placebo, sedative, and anticholinergic effects of the drug. *Hydroxyzine* (e.g., 25 mg three times daily or 50 mg daily at bedtime) is among the most effective of these agents. It is mildly to moderately sedating and more effective than diphenhydramine or cyproheptadine, other commonly used antihistamines. The nonsedating metabolite of hydroxyzine, cetirizine (Zyrtec), is an excellent antipruritic agent when used at doses of 5 to 10 mg daily. Diphenhydramine is available without prescription and is very sedating. Nonsedating antihistamines such as astemizole (Hismanal), loratadine (Claritin), and fexofenadine (Allegra) are useful for daytime use when histamine plays a primary role, such as in urticaria, but are generally disappointing as antipruritics and do little to help the patient fall asleep.

Mild antiinflammatory agents such as *aspirin* are occasionally useful for symptomatic relief, especially if the suspected mechanism is kinin- or prostaglandin-mediated. Systemic steroids suppress itching but should not be used for symptomatic relief.

Specific Symptomatic Measures. As noted above, the most effective therapy is etiologic. A few symptomatic measures for specific causes are important to consider, especially when treatment of the underlying disease is problematic.

Hepatobiliary Disease. For extrahepatic obstruction, the treatment of choice is relieving the obstruction. For intrahepatic cholestasis, including the pruritus of pregnancy, the chelating agents *cholestyramine* and *colestipol* are used with benefit. *Ursodeoxycholic acid* has also proved useful, particularly in persons with primary biliary cirrhosis, in which pruritus can be very intense and refractory. *Ultraviolet radiation* [ultraviolet B, psoralens with ultraviolet A (PUVA)] is sometimes resorted to when the pruritus persists despite all other measures.

Psychiatric Illness. Sedatives, especially the *benzodiazepines*, can be useful in acute circumstances associated with anxiety and difficulty falling asleep, but long-term use is to be avoided because of risk for habituation (see Chapter 226). *Antidepressants* are helpful in psychogenic cases with evidence of concurrent depression. Doxepin, an antidepressant with antihistaminic properties, is particularly useful and may be given before bedtime. *Pimozide*, a neuroleptic, is effective for treating delusions of parasitosis.

HIV Infection. Pruritus may be an initial manifestation of underlying HIV infection, which is suggested when it occurs in the absence of rash or jaundice. It responds to antiretroviral therapy. Other treatable causes in HIV-infected patients include scabies (see Chapter 195), dry skin (see above), psoriasis flare (see Chapter 187), sulfa allergy associated with trimethoprim/sulfamethoxazole prophylaxis for *Pneumocystis* pneumonia (holding of drug), staphylococcal folliculitis (antibiotic therapy), and liver failure (see above).

Renal Failure. The best treatment is correction of the underlying disease, but symptomatic measures are often necessary. Recalcitrant uremic pruritus has been treated with ultraviolet photochemotherapy, IV xylocaine, activated charcoal, IV erythropoietin, exchange transfusion, and parathyroidectomy, with varying degrees of success. Topical *capsaicin* is sometimes helpful, as can be cimetidine. The opiate antagonist *naloxone* has been shown in some studies to relieve pruritus, but in others it has appeared to worsen the problem (see also Chapter 142).

INDICATIONS FOR REFERRAL

The patient with refractory or idiopathic pruritus poses a very frustrating problem that often benefits from a dermatologic consultation and consideration of skin biopsy. The consultation lets the patient know that the problem is being taken seriously and that everything is being done to address both its cause and the patient's discomfort. When pruritus represents a somatic response to psychological distress, it may be useful to consider a mental health referral with the patient.

ANNOTATED BIBLIOGRAPHY

Bernhard JD. Pruritus: advances in treatment. Adv Dermatol 1990;6:57. (*Comprehensive review of therapy.*)

Breneman DL, Cardone JS, Blumsack RF, et al. Topical capsaicin for treatment of hemodialysis-related pruritus. J Am Acad Dermatol 1992;26:91. (*Topical capsaicin four times daily relieved hemodialysis-related pruritus in 10 of 14 patients.*)

De Marchi S, Cecchin E, Villalta D, et al. Relief of pruritus and decreases in plasma histamine concentrations during erythropoietin therapy in patients with uremia. N Engl J Med 1992;326:969. (*Significantly decreased pruritus and lowered plasma histamine concentrations in 20 patients with uremia.*)

Fleischer AB Jr. Pruritus in the elderly. Adv Dermatol 1995;10:41. (*A review that considers evaluation and emphasizes the utility of the history for diagnosis.*)

Fruensgaard K. Neurotic excoriations: a controlled psychiatric examination. Acta Psychiatr Scand 1984;69[Suppl 312]:3. (*High prevalence of depression; lesions often confined to the extremities.*)

Greco PJ, Ende J. Pruritus: a practical approach. J Gen Intern Med 1992;7:340. (*Very useful evaluation strategy outlined.*)

Hagermark O, Wahlgren CF. Treatment of itch. Semin Dermatol 1995;14:320. (*A fresh look at treatment options; 62 references.*)

Kam PCA, Tan KH. Pruritus—itching for a cause and relief? Anaesthesia 1996;51:1133. (*A review of the mechanisms of pruritus and methods of providing relief.*)

Kantor GR, Bernhard JD. Investigation of the pruritic patient in daily practice. Semin Dermatol 1995;14:290. (*A practical approach to treatment, with many useful tables.*)

Khandelwal M, Malet PF. Pruritus associated with cholestasis: a review of pathogeneis and management. Dig Dis Sci 1994;39:1. (*Comprehensive look at this difficult problem.*)

Kligman AM. Water-induced itching without cutaneous sign. Arch Dermatol 1986;122:183. (*A well-characterized subset of elderly patients who had itching associated with age, dry skin, and seasonal weather conditions responded well to local measures.*)

Lober CW. Should the patient with generalized pruritus be evaluated for malignancy? J Am Acad Dermatol 1988;19:350. (*Patients with persistent pruritus do not show an increased risk for malignant disease when carefully compared with age- and sex-matched nonpruritic controls.*)

Millikan LE. Treating pruritus. What's new in safe relief of symptoms. Postgrad Med 1996;99:173. (*A practical discussion of the subject.*)

Paul R, Paul R, Jansen CT. Itch and malignancy prognosis in generalized pruritus: a 6-year follow-up of 125 patients. J Am Acad Dermatol 1987;16:1179. (*No increased risk for malignancy in persons with generalized pruritus followed for 6 years.*)

Teofoli P, Procacci P, Maresca M, et al. Itch and pain. Int J Dermatol 1996;35:159. (*An excellent review; 98 references.*)

179
Evaluation of Purpura

Purpura represents bleeding into the skin. In the office setting, patients present with easy bruising, spontaneous ecchymoses, or a petechial rash. Although many cases of purpura are caused by unappreciated trauma, patients who report easy bruising or spontaneous ecchymoses need to be evaluated for an underlying bleeding disorder (see Chapter 81). Those with petechial rashes may have a platelet problem, vasculitis, or a bacteremia. The primary physician should be able to make these distinctions and efficiently initiate the evaluation.

PATHOPHYSIOLOGY AND CLINICAL PRESENTATION

The integrity of small vessels is maintained by quantitatively and qualitatively adequate platelets and by healthy connective tissue. Normally, a break in a vessel triggers prompt formation of a platelet plug followed by a fibrin clot. Purpura occurs when the integrity of the vessel wall or the mechanisms of hemostasis are disturbed.

Purpura is divided in petechial and ecchymotic categories. *Petechiae* are red macules that measure less than 3 mm in diameter; they reflect a defect in platelets or vessel walls. When caused by disturbances of platelets, petechiae appear in dependent areas, such as the ankles and lower legs (see Chapter 81). Immune-mediated inflammation of small vessels may also produce petechial macules, which sometimes progress to palpable lesions (so-called *palpable purpura*; see below).

Ecchymoses are purpuric lesions larger than 3 mm in diameter. They may result from trauma or a clotting factor disorder as well as from a vascular or platelet problem. Clotting factor dysfunction causes delayed but more prolonged blood loss, during which continuous oozing secondary to inadequate fibrin clot formation results in ecchymoses rather than petechiae (see Chapter 81).

The mechanisms of purpura can be divided into the thrombocytopenic, thrombocytopathic, coagulopathic, vascular, connective tissue, and idiopathic varieties. The first three are discussed in detail in Chapter 81. The vascular, connective tissue, and idiopathic varieties require further elaboration here.

Vascular Defects

These range from mild disruption of the endothelium to necrotizing injury. The latter are the more important.

Small-vessel Vasculitis of a *leukocytoclastic* variety is capable of damaging vessel walls and causing palpable purpura. It usually occurs in the context of a *hypersensitivity reaction* or *rheumatoid disease*, but causes range from dysproteinemias to *Wegener's granulomatosis* (Table 179.1). In a hypersensitivity reaction, immunologically mediated, necrotizing neutrophilic infiltration of arterioles, capillaries, and venules occurs. The process can be systemic, but it is often limited to the skin. In rheumatoid disease, the postcapillary venules are the principal site of leukocytoclastic injury; systemic involvement is the rule.

The skin lesions of leukocytoclastic vasculitis typically begin as small macules that become palpable and may turn confluent or nodular. The petechial papules do not blanch; they appear in symmetric fashion and predominate in dependent areas. Urticaria, vesicles, and necrotic ulcerations may also develop. Fever, arthralgias, myalgias, arthritis, pulmonary infiltrates, effusions, pericarditis, peripheral neuropathy, abdominal pain, bleeding, and encephalopathy can occur along with the petechial rash if systemic involvement is present. The skin commonly itches, stings, or burns. Hematuria and proteinuria are often detected.

Bacteremia can lead to vascular injury and the formation of petechiae, which are sometimes palpable. Petechial lesions associated with *subacute bacterial endocarditis* are flat, do not blanch, and appear on the upper chest, neck, and extremities in addition to the mucous membranes. In *gonococcal* and *meningococcal septicemias*, petechiae develop early, become pustular, and then turn hemorrhagic and necrotic. The lower extremities are a common site for the gonococcal lesions, which resolve within 5 to 7 days. The rash of *Rocky Mountain spotted fever* begins as pink macules on the wrists, soles, ankles, and palms. The rash spreads centripetally and by the fourth day becomes petechial and papular. Hemorrhagic, ulcerated lesions may follow.

Other Forms of Vascular Injury include *stasis dermatitis*, in which petechial lesions in the legs result from capillary injury. *Scurvy* compromises the vascular endothelium, and perifollicular purpura develops because of increased capillary fragility. In *amyloidosis*, deposition of amyloid in the skin and subcutaneous tissue causes fragile vessels, with ecchymoses forming when the skin is pinched.

Connective Tissue Defects compromise vessel walls and supportive extravascular structures and lead to easy bruising. When caused by the degeneration of dermal collagen because of *age* or *corticosteroid use*, ecchymoses may develop after trivial injury and be noticed on the face, neck, dorsum of the hands, forearms, or legs. A variant is stasis or *orthostatic purpura*, which usually develops in the lower extremities of an elderly patient following a prolonged period of standing.

Idiopathic Causes include *autoerythrocyte sensitization*, a puzzling form of purpura characterized by spontaneous, painful ecchymoses surrounded by erythema and edema. Headache, nausea, and vomiting sometimes accompany the purpura. Many patients with this condition also have pronounced psychoneurotic complaints. The mechanism is unknown, but intradermal injection of autologous red cells or DNA can reproduce the clinical picture.

Purpura simplex or *easy bruising syndrome* is an idiopathic condition of young women in otherwise good health. All platelet and bleeding parameters are normal, and the risk for hemorrhage during surgery or childbirth is not increased.

Platelet and Clotting Factor Disorders

Platelet and clotting factor disorders are discussed in Chapter 81.

DIFFERENTIAL DIAGNOSIS

The causes of purpura can be divided into thrombocytopenic, thrombocytopathic, clotting factor, vascular, connective tissue, and idiopathic categories (see also Chapter 81). Purpura associated with trauma or drug-induced impairment of platelet function, benign purpura simplex, and senile purpura are the most common forms. Vasculitis is particularly troublesome because of the wide range of potentially important causes (Table 179.1).

WORKUP

The workup of the patient with purpuric lesions must emphasize the history and physical examination to avoid costly, nonproductive laboratory evaluations. The clinical findings are also essential in quickly differentiating serious hematologic, vasculitic, or infectious pathologies from more benign processes. For example, ecchymoses smaller than 6 cm, localized to such areas of trauma as the thighs, are less likely to be of pathologic significance than are larger ones; palpable purpuric lesions indicate a vasculitic process; and

Table 179.1. Important Causes of Leukocytoclastic Small-Vessel Vasculitis

ANCA-Associated
Drug-induced ANCA-associated
Wegener's granulomatosis
Microscopic polyangiitis
Churg-Strauss syndrome

Immune Complex
Rheumatoid disease (e.g., lupus, rheumatoid arthritis, Sjögren's syndrome)
Cryoglobulinemia (mixed type)
Drug-induced immune complex (penicillins, thiazides, aspirin, amphetamines)
Henoch-Schönlein purpura
Serum sickness
Goodpasture's syndrome

Inflammatory Bowel Disease
Ulcerative colitis
Primary biliary cirrhosis
Chronic active hepatitis

Paraneoplastic
Lymphoproliferative disease
Myeloproliferative disease
Carcinoma

ANCA, antineutrophil cytoplasmic autoantibody.
Adapted from Jennette JC, Falk RJ, Andrassey K, et al. Nomenclature of systemic vasculitides: proposal of an international consensus conference. Arthritis Rheum 1994,37:187, with permission.

petechial macules in dependent areas suggest a problem with platelets.

History. A careful description of the location, size, and clinical course of the purpuric lesions, along with an inquiry into associated symptoms and precipitants, comprises the essence of the history. One should quickly screen for a bleeding diathesis by inquiring about blood loss from other sites; easy bruisability; bleeding into a joint; a history of abnormally heavy bleeding with menstruation, surgery, or dental work; and a family history of a bleeding problem. A review of medications is essential, with a focus on agents that can interfere with platelet function (e.g., aspirin, NSAIDs, dipyridamole, ticlopidine, sulfinpyrazone) and those associated with hypersensitivity reactions that affect platelets (e.g., antibiotics, quinidine, phenothiazines). Any history of renal or hepatocellular failure is important to note.

Patients with an early petechial rash or palpable purpura should be carefully checked for fever, pruritus, joint pain, urticaria, dry mouth/dry eyes, morning stiffness, pleuritic pain, abdominal pain, melena, hematuria, lymphadenopathy, jaundice, symptoms of inflammatory bowel disease, chronic leg edema, and paresthesias. A recent streptococcal or staphylococcal infection may be responsible for a hypersensitivity vasculitis and should be noted. Medications to be reviewed include recent use of a penicillin, a thiazide, aspirin, or amphetamines. If fever is prominent, bacteremia must be considered, and the patient should be asked about recent purulent penile or vaginal discharge, pelvic pain, other recent infection, IV drug abuse, HIV infection, and history of a heart murmur or recent dental work.

Physical Examination begins with inspection of the skin lesions. If they appear petechial, it is useful to press a glass slide over them. Failure to blanch helps differentiate petechiae from nonpurpuric skin lesions. However, blanching lesions must not be dismissed too hastily because telangiectases and spider angiomata are signs of conditions predisposing to purpura (see Chapter 81). Shining a light tangentially to the skin is a sensitive means of detecting elevated lesions, which may be confirmed by careful palpation. The size, number, and location of purpuric lesions should be recorded and note made of whether they are palpable or macular, petechial, or ecchymotic. It is sometimes helpful to circle ecchymoses so that extension or regression can be followed objectively.

If the history suggests a bleeding problem or if the physical examination reveals petechiae in dependent areas or large ecchymoses, then the physical examination should be directed toward hematologic causes (see Chapter 81).

If palpable purpura is present, then the physical examination should include inspection for splinter hemorrhages, rheumatoid nodules, a separate malar rash, dry mucous membranes, jaundice, lymphadenopathy, pleural effusion, heart murmur, pericardial rub, hepatic abnormalities, purulent vaginal or urethral discharge, joint inflammation, and changes of stasis dermatitis.

If the history reveals only easy bruising and no evidence for hematologic or vasculitic pathology can be found, then consideration of connective tissue and idiopathic causes is in order. Does the patient appear cushingoid or have a history of long-term corticosteroid use? Is the patient elderly with multiple small ecchymotic lesions in areas of minor everyday trauma?

Are the ecchymoses tender in the absence of trauma? Is the patient an otherwise healthy young woman with easy bruising and relatively small ecchymoses?

Laboratory Studies. There is no standard battery of laboratory tests for the patient with purpura. To obtain meaningful information, the selection of studies must be based on the clinical findings.

Suspected Hematologic Disease. In patients with flat petechial rashes, the presence of platelet-related disease should be checked for with a *platelet count* and a determination of the *bleeding time* (see Chapter 81). Those with large ecchymoses may have a clotting factor problem and are best screened by measuring the *prothrombin time* and *partial thromboplastin time*. Other hematologic testing may also be in order. (See Chapter 81 for more details of the hematologic evaluation.)

Suspected Vasculitis. If palpable purpura is noted, the first priority is to rule out bacteremia. The history and physical examination often provide important clues, but two sets of *blood cultures* should be obtained at the outset, especially if fever or other manifestations of infection are noted. If rheumatoid disease is clinically suspected, one can screen by testing for *antinuclear antibodies* (ANA) and *rheumatoid factor*, although the results may be nonspecific (see Chapter 146). Patients with respiratory tract symptoms and purpura may have Wegener's granulomatosis and should undergo testing for *antineutrophil cytoplasmic autoantibodies* (ANCA) (see below). The finding of red cells on *urinalysis* or a stool positive for occult blood on *guaiac testing* may provide additional evidence for a systemic vasculitis, but the best means of confirming vasculitis is to perform a *skin biopsy* on one of the palpable, purpuric skin lesions. In addition to histologic processing, the biopsy specimen should also be cultured and a Gram's stain performed.

If a *leukocytoclastic vasculitis* is confirmed by skin biopsy, then more specific testing can be conducted if clinically indicated. The otherwise healthy patient with resolving skin lesions and nothing more than a recent history of using a potentially offending drug needs no further evaluation. If the lesions persist, more testing may be in order. Elderly persons are at risk for dysproteinemias; a serum *immunoelectrophoresis* should be considered. *Cryoprotein* and *serum complement* determinations may prove useful diagnostically in a young woman with leukocytoclastic histology. Testing for *ANCA* may help in the etiologic identification of cases presenting pathologically as small-vessel vasculitis. Consultation with a rheumatologist is advised to optimize test selection and interpretation, particularly in persons who are ANCA-positive, because more specific immunochemical testing is required to differentiate among causes.

PATIENT EDUCATION

Detailed reassurance needs to be provided to the patient with no hematologic or systemic abnormality, but only *after* a thorough evaluation has been completed. In the elderly patient with senile purpura, supportive explanation that the condition is a normal concomitant of aging is often helpful. Similarly, the young woman with a syndrome of easy bruising can be reassured. Occasionally, such patients buy and take large doses of vitamins C and K in the hope of lessening easy bruising. Such self-treatment is without any proven efficacy and adds an unnecessary expense. Avoidance of aspirin and NSAIDs is better advice.

For patients who require drugs that impair platelet function or compromise connective tissue integrity, it may be necessary to advise at least a reduction in dose; otherwise, they may have to accept the cosmetic unpleasantness of ecchymoses. It may be helpful to prepare those with palpable purpura for extended testing and the possibility of a skin biopsy.

INDICATIONS FOR ADMISSION AND REFERRAL

Any patient with fever and purpura requires prompt hospital admission because bloodstream infection and systemic vasculitis are possible causes. The person with evidence of bleeding from multiple sites is also best hospitalized, as is the patient with severe thrombocytopenia or marked prolongation of the prothrombin time or partial thromboplastin time.

As noted earlier, consultation with a rheumatologist is worthwhile to guide the evaluation of the vasculitic patient, particularly when the cause is elusive.

A.H.G.

ANNOTATED BIBLIOGRAPHY

Gibson LE, Su WPD. Cutaneous vasculitis. Rheum Dis Clin North Am 1990;16:309. (*An important cause of purpura.*)

Hunder GG, Arend WP, Bloch DA, et al. The College of Rheumatology 1990 criteria for the classification of vasculitis. Arthritis Rheum 1990;33:1065. (*Includes criteria for the leukocytoclastic variety.*)

Jennette JC, Falk RJ. Small-vessel vasculitis. N Engl J Med 1997;337:1512. (*Definitive review, with especially helpful sections on clinical presentation and diagnosis; includes discussion of the role of ANCA testing; 99 references.*)

Jennette JC, Falk RJ, Andrassey K, et al. Nomenclature of systemic vasculitides: proposal of an international consensus conference. Arthritis Rheum 1994;37:187. (*Names and definitions categorized by size of vessels involved.*)

(See also the bibliography for Chapter 81, which includes articles on clotting disorders and other hematologic causes.)

180
Evaluation of Disturbances in Pigmentation
WILLIAM V. R. SHELLOW

Disturbances in pigmentation are conspicuous and common. Patients complain about general darkening, brown spots, or depigmented areas. Pigmentary alterations may be manifestations of a genetic, endocrine, metabolic, nutritional, infectious, or neoplastic problem. Physical and chemical factors also can be important because skin color can be altered by exposure to heat, solar and ionizing radiation, trauma, drugs, and heavy metals.

PATHOPHYSIOLOGY AND CLINICAL PRESENTATION

Pigmentary changes are caused by melanin being absent, increased, decreased, or abnormally placed or distributed. Hyperpigmentation may result from an increased rate of melanosome production, an increased number of melanosomes transferred to keratinocytes, or a greater size and melanization of melanosomes. Hyperpigmentation is perceived as blue when melanin is located deeply because of the Tyndall phenomenon. The pathophysiologic mechanisms that produce hyperpigmentation through the melanocyte system include increased levels of adrenocorticotropic hormone (ACTH), which has a melanocyte-stimulating action, ultraviolet radiation, and certain drugs.

Hypomelanosis, or depigmentation, may result from the genetic loss of melanocytes or destruction by inflammation. Inflammation may be secondary to infection or burns or associated with a variety of immunologically mediated diseases.

Hyperpigmentation

Hyperpigmentation may be circumscribed or diffuse.

Circumscribed Hyperpigmentation includes freckles (ephelides), lentigines, café-au-lait spots, and melasma. *Freckles* are small, macular lesions seen on areas exposed to the sun. Freckles may become less dark in adults, but they darken after exposure to long-wave ultraviolet radiation. *Lentigines* are macular, and they are larger and darker than freckles. Histologically, the two are easily distinguishable. Senile lentigines appear on sun-exposed areas in older patients. Patients call them "liver spots" and usually do not realize that "liver" refers to the color of the lesion and not to its cause. Café-au-lait spots are light to dark brown macules ranging in size from 1 to 20 cm. They can be round or oval with smooth or irregular borders. The presence of multiple lesions is associated with neurofibromatosis and Albright's syndrome. Nevocellular nevi are also circumscribed, hyperpigmented lesions, that, if macular, may be difficult to differentiate from lentigines.

Melasma, or *chloasma*, is a blotchy hyperpigmentation that occurs on the forehead, cheeks, and upper lip, usually in women. Pregnancy, use of oral contraceptives, and other hormones contribute to its development, but exposure to sunlight appears to perpetuate the condition. During pregnancy, a physiologic darkening of the linea alba, pigmented nevi, nipples, and genitalia is caused by melanocyte-stimulating hormone (MSH) and by increased levels of estrogen and progesterone.

Diffuse Hyperpigmentation results from increased amounts of melanin in the epidermis. The color may be accentuated in sun-exposed areas, over pressure points or body folds, or in areas of trauma, such as new scars. Hyperpigmentation occurs in *Addison's disease* when the pituitary produces increased amounts of MSH and ACTH because of decreased cortisol levels.

Metabolic diseases such as Wilson's disease, von Gierke's hemochromatosis, alkaptonuria, biliary cirrhosis, and porphyria cutanea tarda may be accompanied by diffuse melanosis. On occasion, rheumatoid arthritis, Still's disease, and scleroderma have been associated with hyperpigmentation.

Drugs such as busulfan, cyclophosphamide, clofazimine, minocycline, and zidovudine can produce diffuse melanosis, as can topical nitrogen mustard. Chronic inorganic arsenic poisoning causes diffuse hyperpigmentation with normal or lighter skin areas scattered throughout, colorfully called "rain drops in the dust." Chlorpromazine, amiodarone, and antimalarial drugs tend to produce a bluish gray hyperpigmentation. Silver (argyria) and gold (chrysiasis) as well as bismuth and mercury can accumulate in the skin and cause hyperpigmentation, depending on the dose given. Bleomycin can produce hyperpigmentation in a linear, flagellate pattern. Berloque dermatitis is the name given to a type of photocontact dermatitis associated with exposure to a photosensitizer, such as oil of bergamot in perfumes and some hair preparations. A similar compound in citrus rinds causes inflammation and pigmentation in areas exposed to both the sensitizing chemical and the sun.

Diffuse melanosis may be seen during starvation, with *hepatic insufficiency*, in *malabsorption syndromes*, and with *lymphomas* and *other malignancies*. *Postinflammatory hyperpigmentation* can be caused by a number of precipitants. For example, in phytophotodermatitis, contact with photosensitizing agents present in meadow grass, citrus fruits, and edible plants is associated with an exaggerated sunburn. Hyperpigmentation follows the acute phase. Skin contact with organic dyes and aromatic compounds can lead to photosensitization followed by hyperpigmentation. Tar, pitch, and oils can induce similar changes.

Physical trauma, friction, and heat may also lead to postinflammatory pigmentary changes, as may inflammatory dermatoses that stimulate melanin formation.

Yellow discoloration is seen in jaundice, which involves the sclerae, and in carotenemia, which does not. Lycopenemia will probably be seen more frequently because lycopene in tomato products has been recommended for preventing prostate cancer. The skin color seen with excessive lycopene intake is more orange-yellow. Quinacrine, an antimalarial drug, can cause a yellowish discoloration of the skin. Other skin-yellowing drugs are phenazopyridine and canthaxanthin.

Hypopigmentation

Hypopigmentation may be hereditary or acquired. A *hereditary* disorder can be associated with a lack of or deficiency of melanin. A deficiency or lack of melanocytes accounts for the depigmented areas of partial albinism (piebaldism). A white forelock may be present. In oculocutaneous albinism, melanocytes are normal in number but unable to produce melanin secondary to defective or absent tyrosinase. Diseases involving abnormal amino acid metabolism, such as phenylketonuria and homocystinuria, are associated with hypopigmentation of the skin and hair. In tuberous sclerosis, elongated hypopigmented patches are seen. Certain cutaneous diseases lead to a loss of melanin into the dermis, which lends a gray appearance to the skin.

Vitiligo is a common, acquired disorder of hypopigmentation with an autoimmune mechanism that includes the formation of antibodies to melanocytes. It may occur in the setting of pernicious anemia, Hashimoto's thyroiditis, and a host of other autoimmune endocrine disorders. Any area of the skin can be affected. Onset is usually early in adult life. Lesions may be symmetric and occur primarily on exposed skin, intertriginous areas, and bony prominences and around orifices. In involved areas, the hair may be white. The border of the lesion is often sharp and hyperpigmented. Occasionally, vitiligo assumes a segmental or zosteriform pattern. Halo nevi—centrifugal areas of depigmentation that surround a pigmented nevus—are present in one third of cases. Premature graying of the hair occurs in about 35% of cases.

Partial repigmentation of vitiligo may occur in sun-exposed areas, but vitiliginous patches may burn because of the lack of protective pigmentation. Vitiligo has been associated with autoimmune diseases and endocrinopathies.

Depigmentation may be caused by a variety of *chemical agents*, most notably phenolic compounds that interfere with tyrosinase activity. Contact with rubber and antioxidants may also cause loss of pigment. Dermatitis may precede the loss of pigment, and areas remote from the inflamed sites may also lose pigment. The use of liquid nitrogen to treat lesions on skin types IV to VI may result in postinflammatory hypopigmentation, as can the intralesional injection of corticosteroids.

Dermatoses and Infections may result in localized areas of pigment loss. Such areas may be more noticeable in dark-skinned persons. Small, hypopigmented areas, termed *idiopathic guttate hypomelanosis*, occur on women's legs and may be related to the trauma of shaving. *Tinea versicolor*, pityriasis alba, erythema ab igne, sarcoidosis, scleroderma, cutaneous T-cell lymphoma (mycosis fungoides), and various eczematous conditions may present as areas of hypopigmentation.

DIFFERENTIAL DIAGNOSIS

Table 180.1 lists the causes of disturbances in pigmentation.

Table 180.1. Causes of Disturbances in Pigmentation

Hyperpigmentation
Circumscribed
  Freckle
  Lentigines
  Melasma–chloasma (pregnancy, estrogen, oral contraceptives)
  Postinflammatory
  Physical trauma
Diffuse
  Addison's disease
  Systemic conditions (Wilson's disease, hemochromatosis, hepatic insufficiency, biliary cirrhosis, porphyria cutanea tarda, rheumatoid arthritis, scleroderma)
  Drugs (arsenic, antimalarials, chlorpromazine, busulfan, cyclophosphamide, clofazimine, gold, silver, zidovudine)
  Nutritional (pellagra, malabsorption syndromes, starvation, folic acid deficiency)
  Malignancy (lymphomas)

Hypopigmentation
Hereditary conditions
  Partial albinism
  Phenylketonuria
  Homocysteinuria
Vitiligo (with or without concurrent autoimmune disease, including pernicious anemia, Hashimoto's thyroiditis, male hypogonadism, diabetes mellitus)
Dermatoses
  Tinea versicolor
  Pityriasis alba
  Eczema
Chemical exposure
  Rubber
  Antioxidants
  Germicides
  Phenols

WORKUP

Hyperpigmentation

Evaluation of the patient with localized hyperpigmentation requires inspection of the lesions and inquiry about previous dermatoses and the use of oral contraceptives that can produce melasma. The majority of localized hyperpigmented areas are postinflammatory and of cosmetic concern only, although they should be distinguished from more worrisome pigmented lesions, such as melanomas (see Chapter 177).

History. Diffuse hyperpigmentation necessitates a careful history that specifies the time of onset and possible sun exposure. A drug history that emphasizes agents known to produce pigmentary changes should be pursued. A general review of systems should be made, and any weakness associated with Addison's disease or any itching and hepatic dysfunction associated with biliary cirrhosis should be noted. The physician should consider the possibility of severe vitamin deficiency or malnutrition.

Physical Examination. One checks for hyperpigmentation in creases and scars (characteristic of Addison's disease) and clues to obvious underlying pathology, as may occur with malignancy, hepatic insufficiency, or malabsorption.

Laboratory Investigation is a function of the clinical findings, with biopsy a consideration if deposition of heavy metal or hemosiderosis is a diagnostic consideration.

Hypopigmentation

History. Hypopigmentation requires a careful history of approximate time of onset and possible exposure to bleaching agents, most notably phenol-containing industrial cleaners such as those used in janitorial work. Patients with vitiligo should be given a careful general review that seeks to identify associated conditions, such as pernicious anemia, thyroid disease, diabetes, or connective tissue disease.

Physical Examination. The total depigmentation of vitiligo should be differentiated from partial postinflammatory hypopigmentation. An ophthalmoscopic examination should be performed to detect retinal pigmentary changes. Persons with vitiligo should be examined for manifestations of pernicious anemia (see Chapter 79), thyroid disease (see Chapter 104), diabetes (see Chapter 102), and collagen vascular disease (see Chapter 146).

Laboratory Studies. Hypopigmented areas should be scraped and a potassium hydroxide wet mount examined microscopically to diagnose tinea versicolor. Laboratory screening to test for concurrent autoimmune disease is best undertaken according to the clinical presentation but might include evaluation for serum vitamin B_{12}, thyroid-stimulating hormone, antithyroid antibodies, random glucose, and antinuclear antibodies.

SYMPTOMATIC THERAPY AND PATIENT EDUCATION

Hyperpigmentation

In treating hyperpigmented areas, the chief symptomatic advice is strict avoidance of sunlight. Topical bleaching with *hydroquinone* cream may be effective. Strong topical corticosteroid preparations have a pigment-lightening effect, as does *retinoic acid*. A bleaching solution of 0.1% retinoic acid, 5% hydroquinone, and 0.1% dexamethasone in a hydrophilic ointment or alcohol is quite effective. Hydroquinone–sunscreen combinations such as Solaquin and Solaquin Forte are useful in treating melasma. Melanex is an alcoholic solution of hydroquinone that is cosmetically well accepted by patients. Neither agent works well in postinflammatory hyperpigmentation because the melanin is deeper. No matter what is prescribed or recommended, it is important to stress to patients that lightening of pigment that has been accomplished only after months of treatment can be undone in a single day (or less) of unprotected exposure to the sun.

Hypopigmentation

Hypopigmented areas can usually be masked by appropriate cosmetics, by bleaching normal skin, or by repigmentation with *psoralens* and *ultraviolet A radiation* (PUVA). Hundreds of treatments may be required. The primary physician must assess the desire for treatment and inform the patient of the alternatives. Age, sex, or duration of vitiligo does not affect the response. Lesions on the face and abdomen tend to become repig-

mented more rapidly than those on the hands, feet, and bony prominences. Treatment should probably be supervised by a dermatologist experienced in using these agents to achieve optimal cosmetic results. *PUVA* with both *oral* and *topical psoralens* may be effective. With oral psoralens, many months of treatment are necessary to obtain cosmetic improvements. Topical psoralen plus ultraviolet A has no systemic effects such as nausea, and eye precautions are not required. Titration is very important, however, because severe blistering can result with this method of treatment.

If careful workup reveals no accompanying hematologic or endocrinologic autoimmune disorders, the patient can be reassured that only the skin is affected. Others appreciate knowing that the condition is not contagious. The primary physician should advise the patient about cosmetic alternatives and help the patient decide on an appropriate course of treatment. Because these patients may be unhappy with their body image, psychological support and counseling can be very helpful and should not be overlooked.

ANNOTATED BIBLIOGRAPHY

Dunston GM, Halder RM. Vitiligo is associated with HLA DR4 in black patients: a preliminary report. Arch Dermatol 1990;126:56. (*Certain HLA antigens may be risk factors.*)

Hendrix JD Jr, Greer KE. Cutaneous hyperpigmentation caused by systemic drugs. Int J Dermatol 1992;31:458. (*Best listing of offending agents.*)

Kim HY, Kang KY. Epidermal grafts for treatment of stable and progressive vitiligo. J Am Acad Dermatol 1999;40:412. (*Even progressive disease was improved after epidermal grafting with a suction blister technique.*)

Kovacs SO. Vitiligo. J Am Acad Dermatol 1998;38:647. (*An encyclopedic review of the subject; 296 references.*)

Njoo MD, Spuls PI, Bos JD, Westerhof W, et al. Nonsurgical repigmentation therapies in vitiligo. Metaanalysis of the literature. Arch Dermatol 1998;134:1532. (*Class 3 corticosteroids and ultraviolet B therapy are the most effective and safest treatments for localized and generalized vitiligo, respectively.*)

Porter JR, Beuf AH, Lerner AB, et al. The effect of vitiligo on sexual relationships. J Am Acad Dermatol 1990;22:221. (*Most felt embarrassment when showing their bodies or meeting strangers.*)

Resnick S. Melasma induced by oral contraceptive drugs. JAMA 1967;199:601. (*A classic article; melasma developed in 29%.*)

Ruiz-Maldonado R, Orozco-Covarrubias ML. Post-inflammatory hypopigmentation and hyperpigmentation. Semin Cutaneous Med Surg 1997;16:36. (*Clinical examples of both types of pigmentary change are given, along with management suggestions.*)

Schwartz RA, Janniger CK. Vitiligo. Cutis 1997;60:239. (*A succinct review; 82 references.*)

Stefanato CM, Bhawan J. Diffuse hyperpigmentation of the skin: a clinicopathologic approach to diagnosis. Semin Cutaneous Med Surg 1997;16:61. (*A systematic classification based on clinical and pathologic findings is presented; 79 references.*)

Tal A, Gagel RF. The diagnostic dilemma of hyperpigmentation in patients with acquired immunodeficiency syndrome. Cutis 1991;48:153. (*Both zidovudine and adrenal insufficiency may be responsible; the presentation is similar for both.*)

181

Evaluation of Urticaria and Angioedema

Urticaria (hives) is a pruritic, often immune-mediated skin eruption of well-circumscribed wheals on an erythematous base. It is estimated that up to one fifth of the population will experience an urticarial episode, with women more likely to be affected than men (especially with regard to chronic urticaria). Angioedema is a related condition involving the deeper layers of the skin. Approximately half of patients have urticaria with angioedema, 40% have pure urticaria, and 10% have pure angioedema. If the process occurs for less than 6 weeks, it is termed acute, but if it persists beyond 6 to 8 weeks, it is termed chronic. Most chronic urticaria resolves within a year, although persistence well beyond that occurs in approximately 10% of cases. The primary physician's diagnostic responsibilities include searching for precipitants and underlying causes and distinguishing urticaria from urticarial vasculitis, a manifestation of connective tissue disease. Eliciting the cause can be difficult and is not always possible. In the absence of an identifiable and remediable precipitant, one needs to provide symptomatic relief.

PATHOPHYSIOLOGY AND CLINICAL PRESENTATION

Urticaria

Mechanisms. Urticaria is the consequence of a mast cell release of mediators that increase vascular permeability, which leads to extravasation into the skin of protein-rich fluid from small blood vessels, usually postcapillary venules. A host of mechanisms have been implicated, and much remains incompletely understood, but *mast cell activation* is usually the final common pathway. Precipitants range from physical stimuli to autoimmune mechanisms. In food-induced and some forms of drug-induced disease, ingested or infused antigens trigger mast cell activation by an *immunoglobulin E* (IgE)-mediated pathway. In other drug-induced cases (e.g., opiates, amphetamines), *direct* activation by the drug does not occur. Hyperreactivity to acetylcholine (perhaps related to inadequate production of cholinesterases) is the suspected mechanism in persons with physical urticaria. Physical urticarias may also have some degree of IgE-mediated pathophysiology. In some cases, if not a substantial proportion, idiopathic chronic urticaria may represent a form of *autoimmune* activation of mast cells.

Regardless of the initial trigger, *mast cell activation* remains the final common pathway, with release of mediators from mast cells or circulating basophils increasing vascular permeability. *Histamine* serves as a principal mediator, producing a classic wheal and flare on intracutaneous injection. Transient histamine elevations even occur in the extremities of patients with physical urticarias. Other possible mast cell-derived mediators include bradykinin, eosinophilic and high-molecular-weight neutrophilic chemotactic factors, in addition to prostaglandin D_2, leukotrienes, and platelet-activating factors. Substance P may contribute to the flare that surrounds urticarial wheals. Heat, fever, emotional stress, alcohol, and the premenstrual state can exacerbate urticaria independently of the specific pathophysiology. Additional precipitants and mediators of the urticarial reaction are constantly being identified.

Clinical Presentations. The localized accumulation of fluid produces the characteristic edematous, erythematous, well-circumscribed itchy wheals that blanch on pressure, range in size from a few millimeters to several centimeters, and manifest serpiginous borders. Individual lesions may persist for 12 to 24 hours, but most resolve spontaneously much sooner. Central clearing can lead to an annular pattern. The common final pathway for urticaria of most causes produces a rather stereotypical presentation, but each of the common types has a few distinguishing characteristics.

Food- and Drug-induced Urticarias. The attacks tend to be brief and usually do not cause chronic urticaria, but attacks may be accompanied by angioedema. The most commonly implicated foods include *eggs, shellfish, true nuts, peanuts, fish,* and *milk,* and the most common drugs are *penicillins* and *sulfa-containing agents.* IV *iodinated contrast agents, opiates,* and *amphetamines* appear to cause direct release of mediators from the mast cells. *Aspirin* and *NSAIDs* produce urticaria in a dose-related nonimmunologic manner in susceptible persons, perhaps because they have an underlying abnormality in prostaglandin synthesis, which these agents block. Patients with urticarial reactions to aspirin can tolerate sodium salicylate or choline salicylate, which do not inhibit cyclooxygenase. Chronic urticaria is often erroneously ascribed to exposure to *food additives.* Although benzoic acid derivatives (e.g., *sodium benzoate*) and several *azo food dyes* (e.g., tartrazine and sunset yellow) have been implicated, placebo-controlled trials reveal that food additives account for no more than 10% of cases. *Latex* is an increasingly important example of a contact antigen common to medical settings that may trigger urticaria, angioedema, and even anaphylaxis by an IgE-mediated pathway. The latex powder that coats latex examination gloves is especially sensitizing.

Physical Urticarias. These include dermatographism, pressure urticaria, cold urticaria, and cholinergic urticaria. In *dermatographism,* gentle stroking of the skin produces an immediate wheal and flare response. In *pressure urticaria,* application of pressure at a right angle to the skin results in a red swelling after a latent period of up to 4 hours. In *cold urticaria,* application of cold produces pruritic, erythematous eruptions within minutes. *Cholinergic* urticaria is characterized by tiny, 1- to 3-mm punctate lesions surrounded by erythema; they are intensely pruritic and triggered by *exercise* or a *hot shower.* Some exercise-induced disease may require prior ingestion of a food to which the patient is allergic. *Aquagenic urticaria* is characterized by tiny perifollicular hives that appear after contact with water. *Solar urticaria* develops in susceptible persons on exposure to ultraviolet light.

Autoimmune Mast Cell Disease. An autoimmune form of mast cell disease has been postulated and might account for many of the otherwise idiopathic cases of chronic urticaria encountered. A wheal-producing, noncytokine IgG mediator that causes mast cell release of histamine has been identified in up to half of patients with chronic urticaria. Many of these patients also have autoantibodies to thyroid antigens, which perhaps accounts for the increased frequency of urticaria in persons with active Hashimoto's thyroiditis. In studies of such patients (whether euthyroid or with clinical thyroid disease), treatment with exogenous thyroid hormone to lower the level of thyroid-stimulating hormone often resulted in resolution of urticaria. More work remains to test these hypotheses.

Infectious Diseases. The formation of antigen–antibody complexes that trigger mast cell release has been the purported mechanism of the urticaria seen in some infectious diseases. For example, in the prodromal phase of hepatitis B, symmetric arthritis of the small joints of the hands may accompany an urticarial reaction, which is thought to be complement-mediated. Some patients with chronic "idiopathic" urticaria reported that their urticaria resolved with treatment for *Helicobacter pylori* infection. These observations raise the possibility that *H. pylori* antigens may be responsible for some of the "idiopathic" disease encountered.

Angioedema

The mechanisms are basically the same as for urticaria, which accounts for the simultaneous appearance of both types of lesions. In angioedema, the extravasation of fluid occurs in deeper layers of the skin and subcutaneous tissue, especially in the periorbital, perioral, pharyngeal, palmar, and plantar surfaces of the body. The edema is more diffuse, and the overlying skin appears normal and less itchy than in urticaria. Submucosal involvement in the upper airway and gastrointestinal tract can lead to hoarseness, life-threatening airway obstruction, nausea, vomiting, and abdominal discomfort. Sometimes, the abdominal pain is severe enough to mimic an acute abdomen. Most precipitants of urticaria can also trigger angioedema, but a few causes have unique mechanisms.

Hereditary Angioedema is an autosomal dominant hereditary disease characterized by reduced or defective production of the inhibitor of the first component of complement (C1 INH). In *type I*, the most common form, C1 INH levels are markedly reduced and levels of C4 are low, whereas in *type II*, the patient has normal to elevated amounts of a dysfunctional C1 INH. Half of patients have no family history of the condition.

Acquired Angioedemas. In patients with certain malignancies (*adenocarcinoma, lymphoma, chronic lymphocytic leukemia*), autoantibodies to C1 INH may develop and lead to attacks of angioedema. C1 levels fall, as do levels of C4 and C1 INH. The angioedema that is occasionally seen with the use of *angiotensin-converting enzyme inhibitors* appears to be mediated by bradykinins. The related angiotensin II–receptor antagonists, which do not affect bradykinins, are not associated with the same risk for angioedema.

Urticarial Vasculitis

Urticarial vasculitis superficially resembles urticaria but represents a vasculitic process heralding systemic autoimmune disease (e.g., *systemic lupus, Sjögren's syndrome*). The skin lesions differ from those of urticaria in that the wheals last for longer than 24 hours and manifest a more indolent appearance that includes some central clearing, purpura, and residual pigmentation; the lesions hurt more than they itch. Patients also have systemic symptoms (e.g., fever, arthralgias, and abdominal pain) and may not obtain much relief from antihistamines. Laboratory studies may reveal an elevated sedimentation rate, the presence of antinuclear antibodies, and evidence of glomerulonephritis (microscopic hematuria, albuminuria). Biopsy demonstrates leukocytoclastic changes and extravasation of red cells, findings not seen with urticaria.

DIFFERENTIAL DIAGNOSIS

The causes of acute urticaria/angioedema are usually more straightforward, whereas the causes of chronic disease tend to be more elusive, as the relation to precipitants is often less clear (Table 181.1). Urticaria needs to be differentiated from urticarial vasculitis, a presentation of connective tissue disease.

WORKUP

The history is the most useful component of the evaluation and yields clues to an underlying cause or precipitant far more often than does the physical examination or laboratory studies. Nonetheless, the latter are essential to identify urticarial vasculitis and should not be overlooked when individual lesions persist for more than 24 hours.

History. A good description of the urticarial response is essential. Is the predominant reaction one of angioedema (suggesting possible C1 INH deficiency) or of urticaria? Do individual wheals persist for more than 24 hours (suggesting urticarial vasculitis, especially if accompanied by purpura and pigmentation), or do they clear quickly? Inquiry into illnesses, medications, foods, activities, and exposures associated with

Table 181.1. Common Causes of Urticaria and Angioedema

Acute Disease (episodes stop recurring after ,6 weeks)
Infection (viral, bacterial, fungal, parasitic)
Foods (eggs, shellfish, nuts)
Food additives (sodium benzoate, azo dyes such as tartrazine and yellow dye No. 5)
Drugs, immunologic release of mediators (penicillins, sulfa-containing agents)
Drugs, direct mediator release (IV iodinated contrast agents, opiates, amphetamines)
Drugs, prostaglandin inhibition (aspirin, other NSAIDs)
Other sensitizing antigens (e.g., latex, blood transfusion)
Insect sting
All causes of chronic urticaria

Chronic Disease (episodes continue for .6 weeks)
Idiopathic
Physical urticarias
    Cold
    Pressure
    Dermatographism
    Cholinergic (exercise, hot shower, emotional stress)
    Solar
    Vibratory
Hereditary C1 inhibitor deficiency
Acquired angioedema (lymphoma, adenocarcinoma, chronic lymphocytic leukemia)
Causes of acute urticaria

urticaria or angioedema (Table 181.1) is essential to uncovering the proximate cause, especially in cases of acute urticarial disease. Commonly overlooked is nonprescription use of NSAIDs and aspirin. Latex allergy should be considered in health care workers who present with urticaria. When a food allergy is suspected, the patient should be encouraged to keep a food diary. One should not overlook agents that may be entering through the conjunctivae, nasal mucosa, rectum, or vaginal area. Although allergy to milk and beer antigens is rare in adults, penicillin antigen may be present in dairy products and yeast in beer, factors that can precipitate urticaria in sensitized patients. It is important to determine whether exposure to pressure, cold, light, heat, or exercise precipitates lesions. A travel history may suggest a parasitic infestation. Inquiry into agents and factors that might modulate the intensity of an urticarial reaction (e.g., alcohol, NSAIDs, heat, humidity, occlusive clothing, psychological stress) can provide clinically useful information. A positive family history of angioedema is helpful, but a negative family history does not rule out C1 INH deficiency.

The review of systems should be used to check for systemic illnesses, infections, and malignancies that might present with urticaria and angioedema. Patients should be asked about night sweats, fatigue, weight loss, lymphadenopathy, recurrent peptic ulcer disease, jaundice, easy bruising, cold intolerance, dry skin, thyroid enlargement, dysuria, vaginal or sinus discharge, and pain in the teeth, joints, or sinuses.

Physical Examination. The severity of the condition and occasionally its cause are revealed by the physical examination. Dermatographism is associated with linear wheals. Small lesions with erythematous flares are typical of cholinergic urticaria. Periorbital or perioral swelling is suggestive of angioedema. Lesions that persist for more than 24 hours and are accompanied by purpura and hyperpigmentation are characteristic of urticarial vasculitis. Careful examination of the ears, pharynx, sinuses, and teeth may help uncover a focal infection. One should check for lymphadenopathy and hepatosplenomegaly, suggestive of an underlying lymphoma or hepatocellular disease. The joints are noted for swelling, effusion, and warmth, suggestive of active rheumatoid disease.

Laboratory Studies. It is usually unproductive to attempt diagnosis through the performance of an extensive panel of laboratory tests in the absence of suggestive historical and physical examination evidence. Initial studies can be limited to a *complete blood cell count* and *differential* (for infection and myeloproliferative disease) and a *sedimentation rate* (for active connective tissue disease). *Skin biopsy* is usually not necessary to diagnose urticaria but should be considered if vasculitis is suspected. The sample is taken at the margin of a lesion to include normal and involved skin. Measurement of the serum *C4 complement* level is indicated in the patient with suspected C1 INH deficiency. Checking for *antithyroid antibodies* and *thyroid-stimulating hormone* levels may provide a clue to an autoimmune pathophysiology. For the patient with clinically suspected urticarial vasculitis, an *antinuclear antibody* determination and a *urinalysis* might be ordered if the sedimentation rate is high, suggesting active disease. For the patient with idiopathic urticaria and recurrent peptic ulcer disease, *serology* for *Helicobacter* or a related test should be obtained (see Chapter 68).

A number of tests are of limited or no value. *Skin testing* is of minimal value, and the costly IgE *radioallergosorbent test* (RAST) rarely reveals a cause in elusive cases. Mean serum levels of *IgE* are usually normal. Radiologic examinations are indicated only if clinical evidence suggests a focal infection or malignancy. *Stool examination* for ova and parasites is appropriate only if recent diarrheal illness or travel to endemic areas has taken place or if peripheral eosinophilia is noted. *"Cytotoxic food allergy"* testing has no scientific validity and should be firmly discouraged.

Provocative tests can help ascertain the precipitants of physical urticarias. Placing an ice cube on the skin may induce cold urticaria, and stroking can reveal dermatographism. Cholinergic urticaria may be revealed by an intradermal injection of methacholine (0.1 mL of a 1:500 dilution). Pressure urticaria may be elicited by pressing at a right angle to the skin surface and noting whether a red swelling appears at the site after a latent period of 30 minutes to 4 hours. Placebo-controlled challenge testing for reactivity to food additives is sometimes performed by allergists, who administer capsules containing the additives in addition to placebo capsules and monitor symptoms. Such testing is not appropriate in persons with a history of asthma or airway involvement.

Therapeutic trials may be helpful in identifying a cause. An elimination diet that consists of lamb, rice, string beans, fresh peas, tea, and rye crackers excludes most common food allergens. A more limited approach would be to eliminate dairy products, beer, nuts, shellfish, berries, and food additives. It is often useful to stop all drugs or change preparations or brands to eliminate tartrazine dyes or the peculiar additives of particular toothpastes or cosmetics.

Chronic urticaria poses significant diagnostic and management challenges. Hospitalization for control of diet and observation is both expensive and low in diagnostic yield. A specific cause is identified in fewer than 10% of patients, and the idiopathic designation often applies even after extensive evaluation.

SYMPTOMATIC MANAGEMENT

The best treatment is identification and avoidance of etiologic agents, but in the many instances of chronic urticaria in which this is not possible, empiric measures for symptomatic relief are indicated. Even if an etiologic diagnosis has not been made, avoidance of substances that may aggravate symptoms (e.g., aspirin, NSAIDs, alcohol, angiotensin-converting enzyme inhibitors) should be part of any program. Half of patients with urticaria alone and 25% with associated angioedema are free of lesions within 1 year; however, 10% to 20% may experience episodes for more than 20 years.

Available Agents

Antihistamines provide excellent symptomatic control. The *histamine₁* blockers, such as *hydroxyzine* (10 to 25 mg daily at bedtime) and *diphenhydramine* (25 to 50 mg daily at bedtime), have been the mainstay of antihistamine therapy. They are inexpensive and effective but have a sedating effect. The *nonsedating H_1-blockers* (e.g., 60 mg of fexofenadine every morning) are also effective and are better tolerated for daytime use. Disadvantages are their substantial cost and, with some H_1-blockers, drug–drug interactions (see Chapter 222). It is often best to use a nonsedating antihistamine during the day and a more sedating agent at night. *Chlorpheniramine* and *diphenhydramine* are useful alternatives for nighttime use because they are available over the counter and are much less expensive; chlorpheniramine can be used in pregnancy.

In refractory cases, *H₂-blockers* (e.g., 400 mg of cimetidine three times daily) may improve control in combination with H₁-antihistamines. The rationale for the use of H₂-blockers is that 15% of the receptors in the cutaneous vasculature are H₂-receptors. *Doxepin*, a tricyclic antidepressant with H₁-blocker activity, has proved helpful in persons with urticaria complicated by anxiety or depression. Low doses (e.g., 25 mg twice daily or 25 mg daily at bedtime) may be useful. Doxepin should not be used concurrently with the H₁-blocker terfenadine.

Steroids and Other Drugs.

For severe refractory cases, oral *glucocorticosteroids* are worth considering (see below), but they must be used with care if prescribed for more than 1 to 2 weeks (see Chapter 105). Some reports suggest that the β_2-agonist *terbutaline* in fairly high doses (1.25 mg three times daily) can decrease itching and the number of episodes, but others find little benefit, whether it is used alone or in combination with antihistamines. *Nifedipine*, a calcium channel blocker, can improve the clinical appearance of lesions by interfering with mast cell activity, but overall efficacy is not impressive. *Anabolic steroids* have been used with success in hereditary angioedema (see below).

Agents of No Proven Efficacy.

Empiric trials of broad-spectrum *antibiotics* and *antifungal agents* have been advocated for the treatment of patients with idiopathic urticaria as a means of eliminating any occult infection, but there are no data to justify this hypothesis or their use. Specific treatment of infections such as sinusitis or vaginitis is appropriate only if infection is confirmed. *Topical preparations* of corticosteroids, antihistamines, and local anesthetics are expensive and without benefit in chronic urticaria.

Treatment Applications

Acute Attacks.

Mild to moderate attacks usually respond well to a full program of oral antihistamines. Severe attacks complicated by angioedema are an indication for prompt administration of SQ aqueous *epinephrine* (0.3 mL of a 1:1,000 dilution). For severe acute urticaria uncomplicated by angioedema, a short course of systemic steroids (e.g., *prednisone* started at 40 mg/d and rapidly tapered to full cessation by 1 week) can help provide symptomatic relief but should not be a substitute for a careful etiologic evaluation.

Physical Urticaria.

The physical urticarias are also treated with antihistamines. *Cyproheptadine* is an H₁-blocker that is particularly useful for aquagenic, cold-induced, and dermatographic urticaria. Topical *capsaicin* has been tried in patients with cold-induced and localized heat-induced urticaria; results are variable. Antihistamines have been useful in vibratory physical urticaria. Exercise-induced urticaria can be treated by avoiding vigorous exercise, and it is important for the patient not to exercise after eating or when taking aspirin or NSAIDs.

Chronic and Refractory Urticaria.

Controlling chronic urticaria requires empiricism and careful follow-up. One begins with an H₁-blocker, usually a nonsedating agent. If this fails, an H₂-blocker, such as cimetidine, is added. If the patient fails to respond, doxepin is substituted. In severe cases, a brief course of *systemic corticosteroids* (e.g., 20 to 40 mg of prednisone daily), with rapid taper after 10 to 14 days and a switch to alternate-day therapy with ultimate elimination by 3 to 4 weeks, is reasonable. Longer-term systemic steroid therapy usually fails to provide adequate control and is associated with adverse effects more serious than the condition for which it is being taken (see Chapter 105). Patients with chronic refractory disease who manifest antithyroid antibodies should be given a trial of exogenous *thyroid hormone* sufficient to lower the level of thyroid-stimulating hormone. The patient with idiopathic urticaria and positive *Helicobacter* serology is a reasonable candidate for consideration of *antibiotic therapy*, but antibiotics should not be administered unless evidence of active infection is present (see Chapter 68).

Hereditary Angioedema.

An acute attack that threatens airway obstruction should be treated with SQ *epinephrine* (0.3 mL of a 1:1,000 dilution). Patients with known angioedema should carry an epinephrine self-administration kit. The best treatment is prevention of attacks. Synthetic *anabolic steroids* (e.g., danazol, stanozolol) have been used in cases of frequent or severe attacks. They appear to induce synthesis of normally functioning C1 esterase inhibitor. Periodic monitoring of the C1 esterase inhibitor level and of liver function is required. A purified C1 INH is under development for prophylaxis and treatment of acute attacks.

INDICATIONS FOR REFERRAL AND ADMISSION

The management of urticaria can be frustrating, and it is often useful both for physician and patient to enlist the aid of a specialist. Allergists can help evaluate patients with repeated eruptions possibly caused by food allergies that can be detected on testing, although the probability of food allergy being the cause of chronic urticaria is low. They may also perform penicillin skin testing, particularly with minor determinants. Their experience in seeing a large number of patients with urticaria helps provides comfort and reassurance to the concerned patient. The patient with suspected urticarial vasculitis should be referred to the rheumatologist or dermatologist for skin biopsy and immunohistologic staining of the sample.

Admission for patients with acute angioedema complicated by airway symptoms or gastrointestinal symptoms may be necessary briefly for respiratory support and observation. Hospitalizations that are sometimes advocated for elimination diets are far too costly in a climate of cost containment.

PATIENT EDUCATION

It is important to educate the patient in advance of the workup that a cause is usually not found. Emphasize the variable natural history of hives and the high probability that the lesions will disappear spontaneously. Prepare the patient for the likelihood that urticaria will recur. Instruct patients to avoid exacerbating factors (e.g., aspirin, NSAIDs, heat, exertion, alcoholic beverages). Specific advice, such as the avoidance of swimming in cold water for patients with cold urticaria, can be life-saving. Reassure the patient that the medical workup will exclude serious and treatable diseases and that many options are available to shorten the process and alleviate symptoms. Eliminating unrealistic expectations can prevent the disappointment that may follow a negative workup. It is important to emphasize the overall good prognosis and the high probability that remission will occur, although it may be delayed.

A.H.G.

ANNOTATED BIBLIOGRAPHY

Casale TB, Sampson HA, Hanifin J, et al. Guide to physical urticarias. J Allergy Clin Immunol 1989;82:758. (*One of the best reviews of the topic.*)

Charlesworth EN. Uriticaria and angioedema: a clinical spectrum. Ann Allergy Asthma Immunol 1996;76:484. (*Broad overview, with especially useful section on differential diagnosis.*)

Frieri M, Madden J. Chronic steroid-resistant urticaria. Ann Allergy 1993;70:13. (*Excellent discussion of this difficult problem for both patient and physician.*)

Greaves MW. Chronic urticaria. N Engl J Med 1995;332:1767. (*Comprehensive, authoritative discussion, with good photographs, a practical algorithm for workup, and consideration of urticarial vasculitis; 59 references.*)

Kennard CD, Ellis CN. Pharmacologic therapy for urticaria. J Am Acad Dermatol 1991;25:176. (*Nonsedating antihistamines in combination with antidepressants or H_2-blockers may be useful.*)

Pollack CV Jr, Romano TJ. Outpatient management of acute urticaria: the role of prednisone. Ann Emergency Med 1995;26:5. (*Small-scale, randomized, prospective, placebo-controlled trial finding a 5-day course of prednisone effective regardless of etiology.*)

Rumbyrt JS, Katz JL, Schocket Al. Resolution of chronic urticaria in patients with thyroid autoimmunity. J Allergy Clin Immunol 1995;96:901. (*Patients with previously refractory urticaria responded to exogenous thyroid hormone.*)

Soter NA. Acute and chronic urticaria and angioedema. J Am Acad Dermatol 1991;125:146. (*History more useful than laboratory examination; half of patients with urticaria alone and 25% with associated angioedema are free of lesions within 1 year; 20% experienced episodes for more than 20 years.*)

182
Approach to the Patient with Hair Loss
WILLIAM V. R. SHELLOW

Alopecia may be described as the lack of hair in areas where it normally grows. The most noticeable area in which alopecia develops is the scalp, but a loss of body hair may also occur. Patients may seek medical care for what is perceived as excessive hair loss even when alopecia is not present. Whether the problem is genetically induced male-pattern baldness or alopecia resulting from systemic illness, the primary care physician may be the first one to whom the problem is presented and must be able to offer the patient a rational approach to diagnosis and treatment.

PATHOPHYSIOLOGY AND CLINICAL PRESENTATION

Normal Hair Growth

Hair is a product of keratinocytes in the hair bulb. The hair shaft is made of hard keratin. Synthesis results from mitoses of cells within the hair matrix. The growth of hair is cyclical, the length of the cycle varying with the location. Scalp hair grows from 3 to 10 years, involutes over 3 months, and rests for another 3 months. In healthy young persons, about 85% to 90% of all scalp hairs are in anagen, the phase of active growth. Most of the remainder are in telogen, the resting phase of the hair cycle. The number of hairs on the scalp is estimated to be 100,000. If 10% to 15% are assumed to be in the telogen phase, then an average daily loss of 100 hairs in telogen is expected.

Hairs that grow for long periods and rest briefly are the most susceptible to interruptions of the growth cycle, and variations in the ratio of growth phase to resting phase are most noticeable. The longer the growth period, the longer the hair. Scalp hair grows at the rate of approximately 0.25 mm daily, but various factors can affect the rate.

Hair Loss

The primary pathogenic mechanisms of hair loss are destruction of the hair matrix by physical agents and by infectious or immunologically mediated inflammation. Hair loss may occur when hair growth slows secondary to metabolic diseases or the administration of antimetabolites or other drugs. Physiologic alterations may also produce hair loss by altering the relation between the growing and resting phases of hair follicles. During pregnancy, fewer hairs are shed, so that fewer telogen hairs are produced. After parturition, the percentage of telogen hairs increases, and hair is lost. The process is diffuse and short-lived. This alteration in the ratio of resting hairs to the total may also develop secondary to pharmacologic changes induced by oral contraceptives. Destructive pathogenic mechanisms often produce scarring alopecia, whereas systemic illnesses and drugs usually result in nonscarring alopecia.

Alopecia can be divided into two categories, *scarring (cicatricial)* and *nonscarring (noncicatricial)*. In the latter, the hair follicles are retained and the process is potentially reversible. In the scarring type, follicles are destroyed and hair never regrows. A few conditions that begin as nonscarring alopecia may later develop into scarring alopecia as a result of chronicity.

Scarring Alopecia. An inflammatory response to injury is often present. Forms of physical trauma, such as burns, radiation, injury, and chronic traction, are commonly responsible. Traction alopecia usually results from braiding or the use of tight hair rollers. The pattern of hair loss depends on the styling. The process is initially reversible but progresses to a scarring phase with chronicity. The use of hot combs in combination with petrolatum to straighten hair may result in inflammation with consequent fibrosis and hair loss. Infections—whether bacterial (resulting in deep cellulitis), fungal (*Trichophyton schoenleinii*), or viral (e.g., recurrent herpes simplex or herpes zoster)—produce inflammatory change and alopecia. Dermatologic processes such as discoid lupus erythematosus, scleroderma, lichen planus, cutaneous neoplasms, and granulomas may produce scarring alopecia, as can factitious conditions and neurotic excoriations.

Nonscarring Alopecia. Most often, alopecia is nonscarring, with male- and female-pattern baldness accounting for most cases. *Male-pattern baldness* (androgenetic alopecia) is symmetric, usually beginning in the frontoparietal scalp. Its development is related to age, genetic predisposition, and the presence of androgenic hormones. The inheritance is probably dominant, with incomplete penetrance. The process is permanent, with pigmented scalp hairs replaced by fine, unpigmented vellus hairs.

The presence of male-pattern hair loss in a female patient should provoke concern about *androgen excess*, manifested by hirsutism in mild cases and virilization in more serious cases. Polycystic ovary disease and hyperprolactinemia are common causes of mild androgen excess and hirsutism. Frank virilization occurs with androgen-producing ovarian and adrenal tumors (see Chapter 98). Dihydrotestosterone inhibits the growth of scalp hair while it stimulates the growth of facial hair and promotes a male pattern of pubic hair growth. Laboratory investigation reveals increased levels of free testosterone, sulfated dehydroepiandrosterone (DHEA), or both.

The mechanisms of *female-pattern baldness* are similar to those of male-pattern baldness, but female-pattern baldness is more diffuse; usually, the central and frontal areas are affected, without complete baldness. Age, family tendency, and androgenic hormones are important factors. *Postpartum alopecia* resolves within 18 months, but about half of women feel they have less hair after childbirth than they did before pregnancy.

Nonscarring alopecia often is associated with systemic disease, a metabolic abnormality, or the use of certain medications. *Alopecia areata*, a condition of unknown cause in which hair is rapidly lost, usually in circular patterns, is probably the second most common form of nonscarring alopecia. *Alopecia totalis* is the loss of all scalp hair, and in *alopecia universalis*, facial and body hair are lost as well. The course of alopecia areata is unpredictable. Some persons have one episode, in which the development of one or several bald spots is followed by spontaneous regrowth. In others, new areas of baldness may develop, and they become totally bald. Onset before puberty is associated with a poorer prognosis. Most investigators believe that an autoimmune mechanism is involved and that an association with other autoimmune diseases exists.

Alopecia may follow *infectious diseases* that produce a high, persistent fever, such as typhoid or pneumonia. Secondary syphilis, superficial folliculitis, and tinea capitis also may produce nonscarring alopecia. Commonly used *medications* that can cause alopecia include β-blockers, tricyclic antidepressants, anticonvulsants, warfarin anticoagulants, allopurinol, antithyroid drugs, quinine, verapamil, indomethacin, sulfasalazine, haloperidol, and vitamin A in excessive doses. Anti-neoplastic agents such as 5-fluorouracil, paclitaxel, cyclophosphamide, and methotrexate predictably produce hair loss. Oral contraceptives, hyperandrogenism, and pregnancy are known to interfere with the relation between resting and growing hairs and cause hair loss.

Diffuse hair thinning may occur in *thyroid disease* and *iron deficiency*. Less commonly, hypopituitarism and parathyroid disease produce hair loss. Alopecia is a manifestation of *connective tissue diseases*, notably systemic lupus erythematosus and dermatomyositis. Occasionally, hair loss is self-induced, a condition known as *trichotillomania*. Such patients may not be aware that they are plucking hairs, and the condition may indicate significant psychiatric disturbance.

Hair Breakage. Hair loss must be differentiated from hair breakage, which results from physical or chemical stress to the shaft. The term *proximal trichorrhexis* is sometimes used to describe hair breakage within the first centimeter from the scalp, whereas breakage beyond this point is called *distal trichorrhexis*. Hair straightening can cause proximal trichorrhexis. Patients often recognize distal breakage as split ends; such breakage may be accelerated by exposure to sunshine or swimming in chlorinated pools.

DIFFERENTIAL DIAGNOSIS

(See Table 182.1.)

WORKUP

History. The history should begin by identifying the nature of the problem. Is the patient troubled by a specific area of hair loss or by generalized hair loss? Are symptoms of a precipitating illness, such as hypothyroidism, systemic lupus, granulomatous disease, iron deficiency, or febrile infection, present? Is there a history of physical trauma (e.g., pulling the hair; use of

Table 182.1. Differential Diagnosis of Hair Loss

Nonscarring alopecia	
Androgenic	Antidepressants
Male pattern	Anticonvulsants
Female pattern	Anticoagulants
Alopecia areata	Allopurinol, probenecid
Post febrile infection	β-Blockers
Folliculitis (mild)	Quinine
Tinea capitis (ectothrix)	High-dose vitamin A,
Hypothyroidism	isotretinoin
Iron deficiency	Oral contraceptives
Systemic lupus erythematosus	Discontinuation of
Syphilis	corticosteroids
Medications	Psychiatric
Antineoplastics	Trichotillomania
Antimetabolites	Telogen effluvium
Propylthiouracil	Crash diets
	Post pregnancy
Scarring alopecia	
Physical trauma	Discoid lupus erythematosus
Burns	Morphea
Radiation	Lichen planopilaris
Chronic traction	Pseudopelade
Infection	Neoplasms
Bacterial folliculitis (severe)	Granulomatous disease
Fungal (endothrix)	Factitial

curlers, bleaches, permanent wave lotions, straightening lotions, hot combs)? It is helpful to review the family history for male- or female-pattern baldness and to review the medication history for antimetabolites, anticonvulsants, anticoagulants, β-blockers, colchicine, antithyroid drugs, androgens, oral contraceptives, and excessive amounts of isotretinoin (Accutane) and vitamin A. Other precipitants worth noting include recent pregnancy, strenuous dieting, and the presence of skin conditions such as folliculitis and tinea.

Physical Examination. The pattern of hair loss is noted. Is it localized or diffuse? Is an androgenetic pattern present? It is essential to differentiate scarring from nonscarring alopecia. The scalp is examined carefully for areas of reduced hair growth, hair loss, and scarring. The presence of short, broken hairs suggests pulling of the hair. One examines the surrounding areas for evidence of inflammation, cellulitis, folliculitis, and fungal infection. If available, a Wood's light will produce a fluorescent glow in an area infected by some fungal organisms. Any area of inflammation should be scraped for microscopic examination (see Chapter 191) and culture.

Hair loss in women is especially troubling. It is often helpful to obtain objective evidence of hair loss to differentiate perceived from actual problems. One method is to have the patient collect the hairs lost each day in separate envelopes and count the total. Fewer than 100 hairs per day is within normal limits. Also helpful in making the differentiation between normal and excessive hair loss is the "pluck" or "pull" test. Twenty-five to 30 hairs should be grasped and extracted from the scalp by hand or with an instrument such as a hemostat. In the normal scalp, fewer than five or six telogen hairs are found.

If the circular areas characteristic of alopecia areata are seen, applying light traction to the hairs at the edge of the bald area will indicate whether disease is active at that location. If hairs come out with ease, then extension of the alopecic area is to be expected.

A *clip test* can be performed by grasping 25 to 30 hairs between the thumb and forefinger at the scalp. This sample is cut with scissors, and the portion of the hair more than 1 cm above the fingers is cut and discarded. The remaining sample is placed on a glass slide, and mounting medium and a coverslip are added. Hair shaft diameters are evaluated under the scanning objective of a microscope. In patients with resolving telogen effluvium, more than 10% of the hairs examined will have a small diameter.

Some dermatologists perform *telogen counts* by removing 100 hairs and counting how many are in the telogen phase. Telogen hair is identified by the presence of a terminal club on the hair shaft. With this procedure, the examiner can distinguish between conditions resulting from telogen excess and those resulting from broken hairs, but it may be too time-consuming to be useful to the primary physician and best reserved for the dermatologist experienced in its performance.

Evidence of systemic illness should be sought, including signs of hypothyroidism (see Chapter 104), lupus (see Chapter 146), iron deficiency (see Chapter 79), and sarcoidosis (see Chapter 51). One checks the woman with male-pattern hair loss for signs of hirsutism and virilization (see Chapter 98). It is useful to examine the nails; the presence of Beau's lines may correlate with a systemic process affecting both nail and hair growth.

Laboratory Studies. A biopsy may be helpful, particularly in cases of scarring alopecia with suspected inflammation, both to add histologic evidence and to identify areas of activity that might respond to antiinflammatory therapy. Whether to perform laboratory tests to detect systemic disease (e.g., complete blood cell count; determination of serum iron, ferritin, total iron binding capacity, thyroid-stimulating hormone, thyroxine, antinuclear antibody, androgenic hormones) depends on the history and physical findings.

PRINCIPLES OF THERAPY

The primary physician can provide the patient with reassurance, advice, and occasionally specific therapy. The treatment of alopecia depends on the identification of a probable cause. Patients with a perception of excessive hair loss that is not substantiated should be reassured, as should women with hair loss following pregnancy. Drugs associated with hair loss should be discontinued if possible and alternatives sought. Scalp infection, either bacterial or fungal, requires specific treatment (see Chapters 190 and 191), as does any underlying disease. Hair loss often resolves with successful etiologic therapy. The hair loss associated with chemotherapy is usually self-limited; it is best managed by temporarily wearing a wig or a scarf (see Chapter 88).

Symptomatic Measures

In the vast majority of cases of hair loss, the cause is either alopecia areata or androgenetic baldness, and treatment is symptomatic for those troubled by the cosmetic effects.

Alopecia Areata is often self-limited, but if the condition is severe, it may be worthwhile to consider specific medical therapy, which should be undertaken only by a dermatologist or physician skilled in its application. A traditional treatment for stimulating new hair growth is irritation with *phenol* or *ultraviolet light*. The use of *topical fluorinated corticosteroids* under occlusion may be helpful, and this may be tried by the primary physician. A superpotent corticosteroid such as clobetasol solution can be used without occlusion. *Injection* of *triamcinolone acetonide* into the scalp may be considered if topical therapy fails. When prepared as a dilute solution for injection (5 mg/mL), it is less likely to cause dermal atrophy than are other injected steroids. Small volumes are used, and multiple injections may be necessary to cover a large area. *Systemic corticosteroids* have on occasion been helpful, but their effectiveness is often lost when the drugs are discontinued, and the risks of long-term therapy (see Chapter 105) outweigh the benefits. They should be used only under exceptional circumstances and only by a dermatologist experienced in treating patients with hair problems.

Approaches under investigation include the use of agents that induce an immune-mediated hypersensitivity response, which stimulates regrowth of hair. The response rate is approximately 70%, but treatment often must be repeated, and some of the agents used are potentially mutagenic. *Anthralin*, used in the management of psoriasis, has also been used to stimulate hair growth, but it must be applied nightly and removed in the morning. Therapy with *psoralen* plus *ultraviolet A light* (PUVA) therapy has also been successful to a degree.

Despite the substantial interest in various therapies and the literature extolling them, no approach can be judged effective enough to recommend. Many experienced clinicians believe that treatment merely accelerates resolution in the approximately 50% of patients with alopecia areata in whom hair would spontaneously regrow anyway. Some argue that except in a study situation, watchful waiting is the safest and most cost-effective approach.

Male-pattern Baldness compromises the self-image and self-confidence of many young men.

Available treatments include oral *finasteride* (Propecia) and topical *minoxidil*.

Finasteride blocks the conversion of testosterone to its metabolite dihydrotestosterone, a potent androgen. In men ages 18 to 41 years, careful studies have shown that after 1 year, men treated with finasteride (1 mg daily) have higher vertex hair counts, which are maintained for up to 24 months. Fifty percent of treated men find the appearance of their hair improved. A small number of adverse events are seen, but not much more than in placebo-treated patients. These include loss of libido, erectile dysfunction, or a decrease in ejaculatory volume (occurring in about 2%). Serum levels of prostate-specific antigen are reduced by 40% to 50%, so that the values obtained must be doubled when being interpreted in prostate cancer screening. The ratio of bound to unbound (percentage of free) prostate-specific antigen is not affected by finasteride.

Minoxidil. A topical nonprescription 5% solution of the antihypertensive *minoxidil* (Rogaine) works best in younger men (<40 years) who have been bald for less than 10 years and have a balding area on the vertex that is smaller than 4 inches in diameter. The patient needs to understand that 6 months of daily treatment may be necessary before hair growth becomes apparent and that new hair persists only as long as the twice-daily applications are continued. New growth may be lost within 2 to 6 months of stopping treatment. The only side effect is local irritation, although patients with a low systolic pressure may experience postural hypotension with dizziness.

Many men use both finasteride and topical minoxidil. Both drugs may to some extent prevent further hair loss. Most patients feel that progression of their alopecia is halted by regular use of the medications. In one long-term study, hair growth tended to peak at 1 year, with a slow decline in regrowth subsequently. After 4 1/2 to 5 years of use, nonvellus hairs were maintained above the baseline counts.

Spironolactone and Dexamethasone. Women with male-pattern hair loss may have associated hirsutism. This combination suggests androgen excess and should be treated etiologically (see Chapter 98). Symptomatically, androgen excess can be treated with spironolactone (75 to 200 mg/d for at least 6 months) or dexamethasone (0.125 to 0.250 mg at bedtime for at least 6 months). The hirsutism may improve before the alopecia does.

Female-pattern Hair Loss is an increasingly common complaint, with 40% of women experiencing cosmetically significant hair loss by the sixth decade. Women whose hair is thinning, even though no baldness is apparent to the examining physician, fear that they will become bald like men with common baldness. This rarely happens, and they can be reassured concerning the prognosis. Although initially approved for use only in men, low-strength (2%) *minoxidil* can be prescribed for women, one third of whom also experience androgenetic alopecia. Some women initially experience increased hair loss, which makes them fearful of continuing minoxidil, but decreased shedding and stimulation of new hair growth within 12 months can be expected. Women should not use the 5% strength of minoxidil because hirsutism may develop on the face. Women of childbearing age must not take *finasteride*, and pregnant women should not even handle crushed or broken tablets because of the risk for development of congenital genitourinary abnormalities in male offspring. This drug may be shown safe for use in postmenopausal women, but currently it is not to be prescribed for them either.

PATIENT EDUCATION

Education can be the most important part of the primary physician's management of the patient with alopecia. Once the diagnosis is established and serious diseases are excluded, the patient can be reassured. Patients are often concerned that the hair loss will progress, and the most useful information that can be provided is the actual likelihood of progressive or total hair loss. Even men with genetic baldness are often reassured to know that they do not have a systemic disease. Success in the management of alopecia often depends on the physician's ability to help patients come to terms with their hair loss.

Hair Care. Advice on hair care is appreciated. Patients should be advised to avoid alkaline pH shampoos and excessive toweling after washing the hair. Use of a conditioner may be helpful. Combing is less injurious than brushing. If one must brush, it is useful to disentangle the hair from the brush gently and to use a brush with natural bristles or a nylon brush with rounded edges. Patients should avoid bleaching, permanent waving, straightening, use of hot combs, and excessive exposure to the sun.

Hair Weaving and Transplants. Patients are often well aware of the option of wigs but may ask the primary physician about such issues as hair weaving or hair transplants. Weaving is a relatively safe procedure performed by nonphysicians. It is successful but must be repeated periodically and so becomes expensive and a nuisance. Hair transplants are expensive and have varying rate of success. The procedure is painful and is usually not covered by insurance. Patients with coarse, dark hair are the best candidates for hair transplants. Implants of artificial hair should be discouraged because they usually fall out or elicit a chronic foreign body reaction.

ANNOTATED BIBLIOGRAPHY

Brodland DG, Muller SA. Androgenetic alopecia (common baldness). Cutis 1991;47:173. (*A review of the clinical and endocrinologic features of pattern baldness, with a discussion of therapy.*)

Fiedler VC, Alaiti S. Treatment of alopecia areata. Dermatol Clin 1996;14:733. (*Treat the entire scalp and do not change the treatment for at least 3 months; cosmetic regrowth may take a year or more to achieve.*)

Fiedler VC, Wendrow A, Szpunar GJ, et al. Treatment-resistant alopecia areata: response to combination therapy with minoxidil plus anthralin. Arch Dermatol 1990;126:756. (*The combination of two topical agents produced results in 11% of patients.*)

Hoffmann R, Happle R. Topical immunotherapy in alopecia areata. What, how and why? Dermatol Clin 1996;14:739. (*Cytokines and growth factors are involved in the pathogenesis of alopecia areata and in the therapeutic effect mediated by contact sensitizers.*)

McKinney PA, Finkenbine RD, DeVane CL. Alopecia and mood stabilizer therapy. Ann Clin Psychiatry 1996;8:183. (*Alopecia is a common side effect in patients treated with 10% lithium, 12% valproate, and 6% carbamazepine.*)

Naldi L, Parazzini F, Cainelli T, et al. Role of topical immunotherapy in the treatment of alopecia areata. J Am Acad Dermatol 1990;22:654. (*A discussion of topical immunotherapy for alopecia areata with dinitrochlorobenzene, squaric acid dibutyl ester, and diphencyprone.*)

Olsen EA. Topical minoxidil in the treatment of androgenetic alopecia in women. Cutis 1991;48:243. (*Two percent minoxidil is effective in the treatment of female pattern baldness. Five percent minoxidil cannot be used by women.*)

Olsen EA, Weiner MS, Amara IA, et al. Five-year follow-up of men with androgenetic alopecia treated with topical minoxidil. J Am Acad Dermatol 1990;22:643. (*Hair growth tended to peak at 1 year, with a slow decline in regrowth subsequently, although long-term maintainance of nonvellus hairs above baseline counts was noted.*)

Rebora A. Telogen effluvium. Dermatology 1997;195:209. (*Distinguishing acute and chronic telogen effluvium from androgenetic alopecia.*)

Roberts JL. Androgenetic alopecia in men and women: an overview of cause and treatment. Dermatol Nursing 1997;9:379. (*The selective activity of finasteride against 5α-reductase reduces levels of follicular dihydrotestosterone, the hormone that leads to miniaturization of hairs.*)

Sawaya ME. Clinical updates in hair. Dermatol Clin 1997;15:37. (*A review of androgenetic alopecia in men and women, with a discussion of the effectiveness of new drug treatments.*)

Sawaya ME. Novel agents for the treatment of alopecia. Semin Cutan Med Surg 1998;17:276. (*The role of 5% minoxidil and 1 mg of finasteride in the treatment of androgenetic alopecia.*)

Sawaya ME. Treatment options for alopecia. Cosmetic Dermatol 1998;11:25. (*This review includes investigational agents under development for androgenetic alopecia.*)

Shapiro J, Price VH. Hair regrowth. Therapeutic agents. Dermatol Clin 1998;16:341. (*Review of current therapeutic agents for androgenetic alopecia and alopecia areata.*)

Shellow WVR, Edwards JE, Koo JYM. Profile of alopecia areata: a questionnaire analysis of patient and family. Int J Dermatol 1992;31:186. (*A strong family history in 42% and an association between alopecia areata and type I diabetes.*)

Whiting DA. Chronic telogen effluvium. Dermatol Clin 1996;14:723. (*A form of diffuse hair loss in women ages 30 to 60 characterized by an abrupt onset but a self-limited course.*)

183

Disturbances of Skin Hydration: Dry Skin and Excessive Sweating

WILLIAM V. R. SHELLOW

Part 1: Management of Dry Skin

Dry skin, or simple xerosis, is commonly seen during the winter months and occurs more often in the elderly. The most common clinical presentation is mild to moderate itching (see Chapter 178). A related condition is mild irritant dermatitis or chapping. This is seen particularly on the hands and face. Fingertip fissuring is another common problem during winter months. Severe chronic dry skin can become eczematous (*asteatotic eczema*). The primary physician should recognize dry skin and use simple measures and effective patient education to relieve the symptom.

PATHOPHYSIOLOGY AND CLINICAL PRESENTATION

Although the term "dry" implies that the basic defect is a lack of water, the cause of dry skin is not fully understood. No significant differences are found in the amounts of water present in the stratum corneum of "dry" and "normal" skin. The condition is more likely related to an increase in evaporative water loss through a defective stratum corneum.

The lipids that aid in the retention of water within the stratum corneum diminish with age. Xerosis in the elderly reflects a decrease in both the number and activity of sebaceous glands and a reduced rate of perspiration. Excessive use of soap, de-

tergent, or disinfectants damages the stratum corneum and increases water loss up to 50 times the normal rate. Environmental factors such as low humidity, forced-air heat, or cold winter winds contribute to dryness. A familial tendency toward the development of dry skin remains unexplained. A variety of hygroscopic chemicals are known to retain water in the skin, including lactic acid, urea, and sodium pyrrolidine carboxylic acid. Collectively, these substances are referred to as moisturizing agents.

Dry skin is characterized by scaling and loss of suppleness and elasticity. The clinical appearance is one of fine scaling of the lower portions of the legs. In severe xerosis, loss of elasticity leads to cracking and fissuring, producing a superficial appearance of "cracked porcelain," referred to as *eczema craquelé*. Itching is a frequent concomitant and may lead to scratching and excoriation. Occasionally, dry skin is a consequence of hypovitaminosis A, drug reactions, hypothyroidism, or ichthyosis (vulgaris or acquired types).

PRINCIPLES OF THERAPY

After such systemic causes as hypothyroidism have been ruled out (see Chapter 104), treatment is largely symptomatic.

The goals are to prevent loss of water and restore hydration. The modalities available include environmental manipulations, modifications in habits, and the judicious use of agents that hold water in the skin.

Preventive Measures. It is important to humidify the indoor environment, particularly during the winter months. In cold climates, humidification can be economically achieved by leaving pails of water near radiators, but if necessary, humidifiers may be installed into forced-air heating systems.

One should teach the patient to avoid very strong soaps and detergents, which dry the skin. Many toilet bars are essentially detergents and are extremely dehydrating. Substituting a well-oiled soap is recommended. Daily bathing may also be too drying, although a brief shower is much less drying than a bath. If baths are taken, adding a bath oil is helpful. It is also wise to avoid exposure to mild irritants, such as solvents, and to wool clothing.

Restoring Hydration. The treatment of preexisting dryness requires the addition of water and the application of hydrophobic agents. The physician should instruct patients to soak affected areas several minutes and then apply a hydrophobic substance. Basically, most of the lotions and creams contain combinations of *petrolatum* (Vaseline), *mineral oil*, *lanolin*, *glycerin*, and *water* in proprietary blends. Lotions contain more water, creams have more hydrophobic ingredients, and ointments have the smallest water content. Plain petrolatum is inexpensive and effective, but it is not as pleasant to use as many proprietary preparations. Patient with an allergy to wool should avoid lanolin-based emollients.

A wide variety of agents are available, and patients are subjected to multimedia advertising for many of these products. Lubriderm and Keri lotions are light and easily applied but less occlusive than emollient creams. Lac-Hydrin Five is a 5% ammonium lactate that is available over the counter. The prescription version of Lac-Hydrin, which contains a 12% concentration, is the most potent emollient available. Aquaphor and Eucerin are greasier than the above-mentioned lotions and creams. Crisco may be the most economical emollient. To avoid the greasiness felt with petrolatum-based preparations, newer formulations such as Moisturel use esterified alcohols as emollients.

The plethora of expensive skin creams do little to retain moisture in the skin. Hygroscopic agents such as urea, α-hydroxy acids, sorbitol, and glycerol have chemical properties that retain moisture in the skin. The apparent benefit may be as much a consequence of their ability to plasticize the stratum corneum as of any real increase in moisture. Most moisturizers contain propylene glycol. If a patient experiences irritation with use of a facial moisturizer, it may be the propylene glycol that is causing the problem.

In severe cases, or to achieve immediate results, *topical corticosteroids*, often applied with an occlusive dressing, produce effective and rapid results. The use of Lac-Hydrin or Epilyt may help to relieve fissured fingertips, but sometimes a medium-potency corticosteroid ointment is required.

Occasionally, oral *antipruritic agents*, such as the antihistamines, may be required for severe, generalized itching that results from xerosis (see Chapter 178). The physician should emphasize patient education to prevent recurrence.

THERAPEUTIC RECOMMENDATIONS

- Instruct the patient about environmental modifications to increase ambient humidity. Room temperature should be kept as low as is compatible with comfort.
- Caution the patient to avoid dehydrating soaps, solvents, or disinfectants. The skin should not be scrubbed.
- Encourage the use of bath oils and well-oilated soaps. The patient should soak in the tub for 1 to 10 minutes before the bath oil is added. Warn the patient about the potential for bath oil to cause slipping.
- Emollients should be used after showering or bathing. A variety of agents can be tried, beginning with the cheapest, to find one that is acceptable. The newer emollients that use esterified alcohols or emulsifiers are the most cosmetically acceptable and also the most costly.
- Lotions or creams that contain from 2% to 20% urea or from 5% to 12% ammonium lactate help hold water in the stratum corneum and may increase the plasticity of the skin.
- In the presence of eczematous change or for a patient who insists on rapid resolution, topical corticosteroid ointments with or without occlusion may be used.
- The most important aspect of management is patient education. The physician should reinforce the adjustments that prevent the development of dryness.

ANNOTATED BIBLIOGRAPHY

Ghadially R, Halkier-Sorensen L, Elias PM. Effects of petrolatum on stratum corneum structure and function. J Am Acad Dermatol 1992;26:387. (*Petrolatum does not form or act like an impermeable membrane; rather, it permeates the interstices of the stratum corneum to allow normal barrier recovery.*)

Jennings MB, Alfieri D, Ward K, et al. Comparison of salicylic acid and urea verus ammonium lactate for the treatment of foot xerosis. A randomized, double-blind, clinical study. J Am Podiatr Med Assoc 1998;88:332. (*On the foot, both agents resulted in less severe of xerosis after 4 weeks of therapy.*)

Kempers S, Katz HI, Wildnauer R, et al. An evaluation of the effect of an α-hydroxy acid blend on moderate to severe xerosis, epidermolytic hyperkeratosis, and ichthyosis. Cutis 1998;61:347. (*α-Hydroxy acid preparations reduced the appearance and symptoms of problem dry skin.*)

Loden M. Barrier recovery and influence of irritant stimuli in skin treated with a moisturizing cream. Contact Dermatitis 1997;36:256. (*Treatment of surfactant-damaged skin with a moisturizing cream for 14 days promoted barrier recovery, as measured by water loss through the epidermis.*)

Rogers RS, Callen J, Wehr R, et al. Comparative efficacy of 12% ammonium lactate lotion and 5% lactic acid lotion in the treatment of moderate to severe xerosis. J Am Acad Dermatol 1989;21:814. (*The 12% ammonium lactate lotion Lac-Hydrin was significantly more effective than the 5% lactic acid lotion for moderate to severe xerosis.*)

Steigleder R, Raab WP. Skin protection afforded by ointments. J Invest Dermatol 1962;38:129. (*Various ointments were compared in regard to barrier effectiveness; white petrolatum proved to be the best.*)

Wehr R, Krochmal L, Bagatell F, et al. A controlled, two-center study of lactate 12% lotion and a petrolatum-based cream in patients with xerosis. Cutis 1986;37:205. (*Lac-Hydrin was significantly more effective than Eucerin Creme in reducing the severity of xerosis during treatment and thereafter.*)

Westphal SA. Unusual presentations of hypothyroidism. Am J Med Sci 1997;314:333. (*Dry skin is one of the common presentations, along with other classic signs and symptoms.*)

Part 2: Approach to Excessive Sweating

Excessive sweating (hyperhidrosis) is a common complaint, but it rarely signifies underlying pathology. Medical consultation may be sought because of abnormal wetness, a change in the pattern or amount of sweating, sweaty palms, stained clothing, or offensive odor. The amount that people sweat in response to the physiologic stimuli of heat, emotion, or eating varies greatly. The interaction of the person, the environment, and the emotions influences the amount of sweating. The primary physician must offer a scientific explanation and symptomatic management to the patient who complains of excessive sweating.

PATHOPHYSIOLOGY AND CLINICAL PRESENTATION

Sweating helps maintain temperature and fluid and electrolyte homeostasis, particularly under the environmental stresses of heat. There are two kinds of sweat glands, eccrine and apocrine. Cooling results from evaporation of eccrine sweat. Eccrine glands are concentrated on the palms and soles and are present on the face, axillae, and, to a lesser extent, the back and chest. Heat causes sweating on the face, upper chest, and back. Sweating of the palms and soles is a characteristic response to stress. Gustatory sweating occurs on the face, particularly on the upper lip, often following ingestion of spicy foods. The eccrine glands have no anatomic relation to other cutaneous appendages.

Sebaceous and apocrine glands are closely associated with hair follicles. The apocrine glands are concentrated in the axillae, areolae, groin, and perineum. Apocrine secretions consist of minuscule viscid and milky drops that produce odor after bacteria act on them.

Eccrine sweating is controlled by neural factors or a reflex. Thermal sweating is governed by the hypothalamus, and emotional sweating by the cerebral cortex. The innervation of eccrine glands is anatomically sympathetic, but for unexplained reasons, the sweat glands are under cholinergic control and are therefore mediated by acetylcholine rather than by epinephrine. Excess sweating may be induced by abnormalities of the autonomic nervous system. Autonomic overactivity of the sweat glands may occur without any identifiable cause. Sweating is associated with medical diseases that cause an increase in metabolic activity, so that heat must be dissipated. It is well-known that sweating occurs during defervescence, particularly at night. Although the eccrine glands are under cholinergic control, epinephrine stimulates excessive sweating.

Most cases of excess sweating are caused by exaggerated physiologic responses or functional variations of no pathologic consequence. Hyperhidrosis most commonly involves the palms, soles, or axillae. This may be a result of an increase in impulses from the central nervous system, or it may reflect underlying problems with the sweat glands. A relation to emotional stress is often noted, and the problem becomes disabling if it interferes with work or social interactions. Axillary hyperhidrosis is less common than palmar or plantar hyperhidrosis and makes frequent clothing changes necessary.

DIFFERENTIAL DIAGNOSIS

The most common cause of localized hyperhidrosis is the normal physiologic response to everyday stress. Menopause is the leading cause of generalized sweats. Of the pathologic causes, *fever* is the most common. Night sweats raise the possibility of underlying *infectious disease* and *malignancy*. Central neurologic injury from *stroke* or tumor may produce hyperhidrosis. *Peripheral neuropathy* involving the autonomic nerves is associated with excess sweating, as are such medical conditions as *thyrotoxicosis* and, uncommonly, *pheochromocytoma*. *Parkinson's disease* may lead to increases in both sweating and sebaceous gland activity. Various *drugs*, such as antipyretics, insulin, meperidine, emetics, alcohol, and pilocarpine, may induce sweating. Gustatory sweating, although uncommon, may be caused by compensatory diabetic neuropathy, damage to the seventh cranial nerve during parotid surgery, the rare Frey's syndrome, or injury to the sympathetic trunk following surgery.

WORKUP

History. Is the excess sweating restricted to the axillae, palms, and soles, indicative of a normal response to everyday events, or is it more generalized, suggesting an underlying medical condition? If sweating occurs primarily at night, then inquiry into fever, fatigue, adenopathy, cough, sputum production, and other symptoms of infection and malignancy should be sought (see Chapter 11). Generalized sweating should also trigger questions regarding hyperthyroidism (see Chapter 103) and menopause (see Chapter 118). Paroxysms of sweating are consistent with panic disorder (see Chapter 226) and pheochromocytoma (see Chapter 19). A careful drug history is needed, with a check for use of antipyretics, insulin, meperidine, emetics, alcohol, and pilocarpine. The physician should ask whether excess sweating began relatively recently and whether it can be correlated with stress.

Physical Examination. The degree of sweating and its location are noted. If fever or generalized night sweats are reported, careful examination for underlying infection and cancer is required (see Chapter 11). The patient should also be examined for signs of hyperthyroidism (see Chapter 103). The presence of increases in blood pressure should be noted because if the blood pressure is elevated in the setting of paroxysmal flushing and sweating, then pheochromocytoma should be considered. A careful neurologic examination is needed in patients suspected of central nervous system disease or peripheral autonomic neuropathy.

Laboratory Testing. No laboratory investigations are mandatory. Test selection is based entirely on the findings from history and physical examination. A screening "panscan" is of little use and is more likely to generate false-positive results than a true-positive one.

SYMPTOMATIC MANAGEMENT

Excessive sweating can interfere with employment and social intercourse. Many therapies have been used; several are effective, but some are associated with undesirable side effects.

Topical Therapy. The most effective topical agent for use on the hands and the axillae is a 20% alcoholic solution of *aluminum chloride hexahydrate* (Drysol). A preparation of 6.25% aluminum tetrachloride (Xerac) is a less potent alternative. A clinical improvement in axillary hyperhidrosis may be seen after one to three consecutive treatments per week. Maintenance is usually possible with only one treatment per week after dryness has been achieved. Other topical therapies include 10% *formalin compresses*, which work well but can induce allergic sensitization. Buffered *glutaraldehyde* is effective but stains the skin. *Electrical current* may be used to block sweat glands temporarily. Topical iontophoresis with either tap water or an anticholinergic agent and aluminum chloride can reduce sweating of the palms. Tap water units can be used at home. Response rates are in excess of 80% and have been reported with an average remission of about 1 month.

Systemic Therapy. *Scopolamine* and other cholinergic agents decrease sweating but can cause central nervous system side effects and precipitate glaucoma or urinary obstruction in patients with underlying prostatic hypertrophy. *Phenoxybenzamine*, an adrenergic antagonist, has been reported to be successful in several cases of generalized hyperhidrosis.

Surgery. In rare instances of genuinely incapacitating hyperhidrosis, surgery is sometimes considered. Axillary hyperhidrosis may be cured with surgical *extirpation of the eccrine glands* in the axillae. Studies suggest that liposuction of the axillae may remove the sweat glands without altering the normal architecture. Palmar sweating may respond to *sympathectomy*, which can be performed endoscopically. This is a much less invasive procedure than it once was, thanks to newer instrumentation.

Botulinum A Neurotoxin (Botox) has been used successfully for both axillary and palmar hyperhidrosis. Intradermal injection of Botox results in long-term reduction in sweating in both locations. When Botox is injected into the palm, some patients experienced reversible minor weakness in their handgrip.

PATIENT EDUCATION

Patient education is crucial to the treatment of excess sweating. Providing the patient with a scientific explanation and a firm understanding of sweating is helpful in relieving anxiety. Patients with night sweats should record their temperature so that any significant febrile illness can be identified. The application of topical agents should be well explained and carefully carried out by patients. Surgical intervention for a problem as minor as hyperhidrosis requires the patient's understanding of the risks and benefits of such a procedure and the active involvement of the primary physician in helping the patient reach a decision.

THERAPEUTIC RECOMMENDATIONS

- Reassure the patient that excess sweating is not the consequence of a pathologic condition once medical causes have been ruled out.
- For axillary sweating, recommend frequent washing and changes of clothing.
- For excess sweating of the palms or the axillae, recommend a 20% alcoholic solution of aluminum chloride hexahydrate (Drysol). An effective alternative is 6.25% aluminum tetrachloride (Xerac). It should be applied at bedtime and covered with a plastic food wrap; polyethylene or vinyl gloves can be worn if the palms are affected. In the morning, the treated areas should be washed with soap and water. Prescribe 1-3 consecutive treatments per week. Once dryness has been achieved, maintenance with one treatment per week should suffice.
- Electrical current may be used to block sweat glands temporarily. Use of the device (Drionic) daily for 1 week may relieve sweating for up to 1 month.
- Intradermal injection of botulinum toxin is gaining in popularity and should also be considered as a relatively noninvasive therapy. Liposuction techniques may also be useful.
- If topical therapy and reassurance and less invasive approaches fail, sympathectomy performed via a thoracoscope may be considered, but only if the patient's hyperhidrosis is truly incapacitating. Referral should be made to a neurosurgeon or vascular surgeon for evaluation.

ANNOTATED BIBLIOGRAPHY

Adar R, Kurchin A, Zweig A. Palmar hyperhidrosis and its surgical treatment. A report of 100 cases. Ann Surg 1977;186:34. (*Success rate of 89% with bilateral upper dorsal sympathectomy for palmar hyperhidrosis.*)

Benohanian A, Dansereau A, Bolduc C, et al. Localized hyperhidrosis treated with aluminum chloride in a salicylic acid gel base. Int J Dermatol 1998;37:701. (*Good and excellent results were achieved with the use of 20% to 30% aluminum chloride hexahydrate in a 4% salicylic acid gel base.*)

Elgart ML, Fuchs G. Tapwater iontophoresis in the treatment of hyperhidrosis. Int J Dermatol 1987;26:194. (*The device can be used at home by patients; it provides a reduction in hyperhidrosis for up to 6 weeks.*)

Payne CM, Doe PT. Liposuction for axillary hyperhidrosis. Clin Exp Dermatol 1998;23:9. (*Axillary liposuction produced a very satisfactory result in a young woman who had had hyperhidrosis for 10 years.*)

Sato K, Kang WH, Saga K, et al. Biology of sweat glands and their disorders. II. Disorders of sweat gland function. J Am Acad Dermatol 1989;20:713. (*Definitive review with comments about therapy; 117 references.*)

Schnider P, Binder M, Auff E, et al. Double-blind trial of botulinum A toxin for the treatment of focal hyperhidrosis of the palms. Br J Dermatol 1997;136:548. (*Treatment resulted in considerable improvement in comparison with saline injection in the contralateral palm.*)

Shelley WB, Talanin NY, Shelley ED. Botulinum toxin therapy for palmar hyperhidrosis. J Am Acad Dermatol 1998;38:227. (*Sweat production was significantly reduced for 4 to 12 months.*)

184
Approach to the Patient with Dermatitis
WILLIAM V. R. SHELLOW

Part 1: Atopic or Contact Dermatitis

The atopic and contact dermatitides (also referred to as *"eczema"*) are frequently encountered in medical practice and may be acute or chronic. The acute form is characterized by erythema, edema, vesiculation, oozing, crusting, and scaling. The chronic stage manifests excoriation, thickening, hyperpigmentation, and often lichenification. These conditions are defined clinically by the observable changes in the skin, which reflect a common cutaneous reaction to a variety of pathogenetic stimuli. The clinical challenges for the primary care physician are to provide symptomatic relief and identify the underlying precipitant. These tasks can be difficult, often necessitating consultation with a dermatologist.

PATHOPHYSIOLOGY AND CLINICAL PRESENTATION

Pathophysiology

Atopic Dermatitis. The pathogenesis of atopic dermatitis remains incompletely understood, but a genetic predisposition and exposure to environmental irritants are believed to be important. Certain lymphocyte subpopulations show disordered metabolism. Underactivity of thy-1 lymphocytes that produce interferon-γ and interleukin-2 (IL-2) seems to be linked with oversecretion of IL-4 and IL-5 by thy-2 lymphocytes. Elevations of immunoglobulin E are seen in 40% to 80% of patients. Two thirds of patients have family members with asthma, hay fever, or atopic dermatitis and often exhibit other forms of atopy themselves. Psychological stress may induce flares. Environmental factors also contribute. Certain fabrics, notably wool, may induce itching. Lesions are exacerbated by extremes of temperature and humidity. Defects in cell-mediated immunity have been noted, perhaps accounting for the observed increase in susceptibility to cutaneous viral infections.

Infection may also precipitate an attack. The skin of atopic persons is frequently colonized by *Staphylococcus aureus*, whereas fewer than 5% of those without atopy carry *S. aureus*. Other differences in atopic skin include the following: alteration in vascular activity, demonstrated by the formation of a white rather than a red line when the skin is stroked (white *dermatographism*); greater sweating response to acetylcholine than is seen in normal controls; deficiency of sebaceous gland lipids on the skin surface; lowered threshold for the release of histamine from basophils; and increased histamine levels in both skin and plasma.

Contact Dermatitis. The cause is exposure of the skin to a precipitant, which may have a purely irritant or an immunologic effect. Irritants penetrate and disrupt the stratum corneum, injuring the underlying epidermis and causing an inflammatory reaction. Irritant effects are universal and require no previous exposure. Strong acids, alkalis, detergents, and organic solvents are among the important irritants.

Immunologically mediated contact reactions occur only in patients who have been previously sensitized to an allergen. Important sensitizing antigens include nickel, rubber, topical anesthetics, neomycin, and the antigens of poison ivy, oak, and sumac.

Clinical Presentation

Atopic Dermatitis is characterized by intense itching that leads to scratching, eczematous change, and lichenification. In adults, the lesions characteristically involve the neck, wrists, area behind the ears, and antecubital and popliteal flexure areas. *Nummular eczema* is a variant characterized by pruritic, coin-shaped lesions on the external aspects of the extremities, the buttocks, and the posterior aspect of the trunk. The lesions may ooze, crust, and become purulent. The course varies; a few constant lesions may be present, or the number of lesions may increase gradually. The prognosis is good, with eventual clearing, although it may take years.

Contact Dermatitis can affect any area of the body. Linear patterns are pathognomonic, but almost any pattern may be seen. The distribution and location of the rash may provide clues to the irritant or allergen. Patch testing can help to identify the contactant.

Chronic Hand Dermatitis presents a diagnostic and therapeutic challenge that can frustrate the most experienced dermatologist. It may be irritant in nature (e.g., "housewives' hands"), pustular (chronic pustular eruption), or even vesicular (pompholyx or dyshidrosis). It can occur in the context of a fungal infection with "id" reaction, contact with household irritants, or dyshidrosis.

Lichen Simplex Chronicus. Regardless of the cause, chronic eczematous change may lead to *lichen simplex chronicus*. Itching can be intense, and the condition may be complicated by secondary infection. Lichen simplex chronicus can also result from localized neurodermatitis and present as a circumscribed plaque of thickened skin with increased markings, some scaling, and papulation. The occipital region is a common site. Lesions may also be seen on the wrists, thighs, or lower aspects of the legs. Women are more commonly affected. The prognosis is variable, but when scratching is stopped, lesions regress.

PRINCIPLES OF MANAGEMENT

The management of eczema embodies the fundamental principles of dermatologic therapy: precipitants should be eliminated, wet lesions dried, dry lesions hydrated, and inflammation treated with corticosteroids. Resistance to treatment should be anticipated, and if basic management fails, referral to an experienced dermatologist should be prompt. A search for precipitating factors is mandatory. Topical corticosteroids are always required.

Use of Topical Corticosteroids

Topical steroids exert antiinflammatory, antipruritic, and antiproliferative effects. Available agents vary widely in potency, as measured by vasoconstriction assays (Table 184.1). The strongest steroid is 500 times more effective in blanching the skin than is the weakest. Often, differences in potency are found between generic products and those with brand names.

Preparations and Their Selection. Preparations are categorized according to strength (Table 184.1). The halogenated preparations are the most potent, particularly those available in ointment formulation (see below). One starts with a sufficiently potent formulation to establish control of the eczematous process and then switches to a preparation with lower potency if maintenance therapy is indicated. Because of the large number of available preparations, it is recommended that the clini-

Table 184.1.   Topical Corticosteroid Preparations[a]

Group 1—Highest Potency
Betamethasone dipropionate in optimized vehicle 0.05% cream, ointment, solution (Diprolene)
Clobetasol propionate 0.05% cream, ointment, solution (Temovate)
Halobetasol propionate 0.05% cream, ointment (Ultravate)
Diflorasone diacetate 0.05% cream, ointment (Psorcon)

Group 2—High Potency
Amcinonide 0.1% ointment (Cyclocort)
Betamethasone dipropionate 0.05% ointment (Diprosone)
Desoximetasone 0.25% cream and ointment (Topicort)
Fluocinonide 0.05% cream, gel, ointment, solution (Lidex)
Halcinonide 0.1% cream, ointment (Halog)

Group 3—Medium-High Potency
Amcinonide 0.1% cream (Cyclocort)
Betamethasone dipropionate 0.05% cream (Diprosone, Maxivate)
Diflorasone diacetate 0.05% cream, ointment (Florone, Maxiflor)

Group 4—Medium Potency
Desoximetasone 0.05% cream (Topicort LP)
Flurandrenolide 0.05% ointment (Cordran)
Hydrocortisone butyrate 0.1% ointment (Locoid)
Hydrocortisone valerate 0.2% ointment (Westcort)
Mometasone furoate 0.1% cream, ointment (Elocon)
Triamcinolone acetonide 0.1% ointment (Aristocort, Kenalog)

Group 5—Low Potency
Alclometasone dipropionate 0.05% cream (Aclovate)
Betamethasone valerate 0.1% cream (Valisone)
Flurandrenolide 0.05% cream (Cordran)
Fluocinolone acetonide 0.025% cream (Synalar, Synemol, Fluonid)
Hydrocortisone butyrate 0.1% cream (Locoid)
Hydrocortisone valerate 0.2% cream (Westcort)
Triamcinolone acetonide 0.1% cream or lotion (Aristocort, Kenalog)

Group 6—Mild Potency
Desonide 0.05% cream (Tridesilon)
Fluocinolone acetonide 0.01% solution (Fluonid, Synalar)

Group 7—Lowest Potency
Dexamethasone 0.1% gel, ointment (Decadron)
Hydrocortisone 0.5%, 1%, and 2.5% cream, ointment, lotion (Hytone, Synacort, Nutracort)

[a]It is recommended that one become familiar with and use one agent from each category, making the selection on the basis of cost, cosmetic acceptability, and efficacy.

cian become familiar with one agent from each category and make the choice on the basis of cost, cosmetic acceptability, and efficacy.

Topical hydrocortisone is available over the counter in strengths that cannot exceed 1%. Mild forms of dermatitis may respond, but the patient often selects the wrong vehicle—for example, an ointment when a lotion or cream would be better.

Formulations and Application. The vehicle affects potency and cosmetic acceptability. *Ointment* formulations are more potent than *creams* and are best reserved for thick, scaling lesions. Nongreasy cream formulations are quite acceptable cosmetically and easy to use on the trunk, extremities, or face. *Gels* can be used in hairy areas and on glabrous skin, although gels are somewhat drying when used on nonhairy skin. *Lotions* are usually creamy, whereas solutions have an alcohol or propylene glycol base, but in either case, lotions are more drying than creams. Specialized formulations include aerosol *sprays*, which are used on the scalp or to cover large areas of skin in acute dermatitis.

Occlusion of the skin enhances penetration, with up to 100 times more vasoconstriction observed if a polyethylene film is used over a given formulation than if no occlusion is used. Steroid-impregnated tape (Cordran tape) provides occlusion as well, but the convenience is rarely justified by the expense. Ointments are generally not occluded because folliculitis may develop.

Topical agents are normally applied two to four times daily, but retention of corticosteroid in the stratum corneum makes one or two applications per day sufficient. Because hydration of the epidermis is salutary for healing, concomitant use of a moisturizer is beneficial.

When a topical agent is prescribed, it is helpful to estimate the quantity of topical medication that will be required. A 10-day to 2-week course of therapy applied two to three times daily requires 30 g for the face, 45 g for feet or hands, 60 g for arms or legs, 60 to 90 g for the trunk, and 120 to 150 g for the whole body.

Adverse Effects. The potent halogenated corticosteroids are the most likely to cause *atrophy*, *telangiectasia*, *purpura*, *striae*, and an *acneiform eruption*. Restrictions are recommended for the use of certain superpotent corticosteroids—no more than 45 g of medication per week for no longer than 2 weeks. Suppression of the pituitary–adrenal axis, measured by plasma cortisol levels, may be demonstrable but is rarely clinically significant. Thin-skinned areas are especially susceptible to the development of atrophy. Less potent formulations should also be used on areas such as the face, dorsum of the hands, and the scrotum. Fluorinated steroids may cause *rosacea* if used on the face. Only low-potency ophthalmic preparations should be used around the eye. Low-potency products are also preferred in the groin and axillae because of the risk for the development of striae with more potent preparations. Purpura may be seen on the dorsal aspect of the forearms and hands after prolonged use of potent topical agents.

Treatment of Specific Dermatitides

Acute Eczematous Dermatitis benefits from drying with such measures as *Burow's solution* compresses. *Systemic corticosteroids* are sometimes used on a short-term basis for generalized or incapacitating dermatitis. *Topical corticosteroids* are used in milder cases. Secondary bacterial infection may require topical mupirocin ointment three times per day, or systemic antibiotics if the condition is extensive.

Chronic Eczematous Dermatitis usually is of an irritant nature and benefits from the identification and withdrawal of possible irritants. Detergents, gasoline, polishes, and other occupational and household products should be avoided. Frequent baths or showers, exposure to hot water, and the use of drying soaps should be reduced. Although systemic corticosteroids are contraindicated in chronic eczema, *topical steroids* are helpful and are often needed for prolonged periods. Some *coal tar* preparations are useful in the treatment of chronic dermatitis.

PATIENT EDUCATION AND INDICATIONS FOR REFERRAL

Patients must be instructed about the proper use of topical steroids. They need to be warned specifically to avoid contact with the eyes and eyelids (unless a low-dose ophthalmic preparation is prescribed) and to avoid using a potent topical formulation on the face. If a brief course of oral prednisone therapy is necessary, the patient should be given a written schedule to ensure proper tapering and cessation within 10 to 14 days. For those with atopic disease, advice on substances to avoid is greatly appreciated. Simple measures such as clipping fingernails and wearing cotton gloves can reduce secondary excoriation. Early identification and treatment of eczematous exacerbations helps facilitate treatment. Patients with chronic hand dermatitis need to know that prolonged treatment may be necessary.

Chronic hand dermatitis often proves refractory to the basic measures prescribed by the primary physician. Referral to a dermatologist for more detailed identification of precipitants and advancement of the treatment program may be helpful.

THERAPEUTIC RECOMMENDATIONS

- Identify and remove potential contacts, allergens, and irritants. Treat any skin dryness (see Chapter 183). Use of rubber gloves with cotton linings may be beneficial.
- Oozing lesions should be dried with Burow's solution compresses applied two to four times a day for 10 to 30 minutes, depending on the degree of vesiculation; colloidal oatmeal baths are indicated for more generalized lesions.
- Pruritus should be suppressed, if possible, with a topical an-

tipruritic (e.g., Pramosone cream/lotion) or a systemic antihistamine (see Chapter 178).
- For acute dermatitis, begin with a fluorinated corticosteroid cream. Start with the highest-potency steroid preparation necessary and reduce potency as soon as the acute inflammation has been controlled. If the acute process is extensive and severe, begin oral prednisone at a starting dose of 1 mg/kg daily and taper rapidly to full cessation within 10 to 14 days. Alternatively, parenteral corticosteroid IM injections can be given as triamcinolone acetonide (40 mg/mL).
- For chronic lichenified eruptions, treat for prolonged periods with ointment formulations or, if unresponsive, steroid cream under occlusion. In refractory cases, intralesional injection of a diluted triamcinolone solution (2.0 to 3.0 mg/mL) by an experienced physician may be effective.
- Refer patients with refractory hand dermatitis to a dermatologist.

ANNOTATED BIBLIOGRAPHY

Brehler R, Hildebrand A, Luger TA. Recent developments in the treatment of atopic eczema. J Am Acad Dermatol 1997;36:983. (*Recently described therapies that are available or still under investigation; 154 references.*)

Cohen DE, Brancaccio RR. What is new in clinical research in contact dermatitis? Dermatol Clin 1997;15:137. (*New and clinically relevant allergens are being discovered; patch testing is important; 53 references.*)

Goa KL. Clinical pharmacology and pharmacokinetic properties of topically applied corticosteroids. A review. Drugs 1988;36:51. (*A look at absorption, potency, and side effects of these agents; 77 references.*)

Jeckler J, Larko O. Combined UVA-UVB versus UVB phototherapy for atopic dermatitis: a paired-comparison study. J Am Acad Dermatol 1990;22:49. (*Therapy with a combination of ultraviolet A and B was superior to therapy with ultraviolet B.*)

Juckett G. Plant dermatitis. Possible culprits go far beyond poison ivy. Postgrad Med 1996;100:159,167. (*An excellent discussion of plants that cause cutaneous disease.*)

Rudukoff D, Lebwohl M. Atopic dermatitis. Lancet 1998;351:1715. (*An excellent discussion of pathogenesis and treatment options; 50 references.*)

Stoughton RB, Cornell RC. Review of superpotent topical corticosteroids. Semin Dermatol 1987;6:72. (*Guidelines for safe and effective use of superpotent topical steroids.*)

Weidman AI, Sawicty HH. Nummular eczema. Review of the literature: survey of 516 case records and follow-up of 125 patients. Arch Dermatol 1956;73:58. (*Classic review and long-term evaluation of 125 patients.*)

Part 2: Management of Seborrheic Dermatitis

Seborrheic dermatitis affects almost 5% of the adult population. It is a benign but chronic inflammatory skin disease that is constitutionally determined and has no single defined cause. Its high prevalence and incurability render it a therapeutic challenge. The primary physician must be capable of treating seborrheic dermatitis and educating the patient about chronicity and the need for continued management.

PATHOPHYSIOLOGY AND CLINICAL PRESENTATION

Pathogenesis. The cause of seborrheic dermatitis remains unknown. The anatomic localization correlates with areas of sebaceous gland concentration. The quantity or composition of sebum is not the main factor necessary for its development. Hormonal influences, fatigue, and anxiety may trigger or aggravate the condition. An etiologic relation between the yeast *Pityrosporum ovale* and seborrheic dermatitis has been postulated and is supported by the finding that topical ketoconazole or other antifungal agents produce improvement or resolution in some patients. Conversely, if the number of yeast organisms increases, the problem recurs.

Clinical Presentation. Common dandruff may be the mildest expression of this disease. Seborrheic dermatitis presents as scaly patches that are occasionally slightly papular, surrounded by minimal to moderate erythema. The borders of the lesions are ill defined, and the scales may be greasy and appear yellow. The lesion is usually asymptomatic, but pruritus may occur. More extensive disease involves the forehead at the margin of the hair, eyebrows, nasal folds, and the retroauricular and presternal area. In more severe cases, intertriginous areas, the external ear canal, and the umbilicus are involved. In these areas, erythema and exudation predominate, sometimes progressing to chronic dermatitis with scaling. The scalp is most often involved, and the condition is differentiated from common dandruff by its association with erythema. At the extreme end of the spectrum, total body erythroderma may be seen. Seborrheic dermatitis can occur at any age but is most common during infancy and after the second decade of life, with the highest prevalence in the fourth and fifth decades.

Seborrheic dermatitis is associated with several conditions, such as Parkinson's disease, phenylketonuria, prior cardiac failure, zinc deficiency, and epilepsy. Cutaneous diseases such as acne vulgaris, rosacea, and psoriasis may be associated with it. Florid manifestations of seborrhea may be an early cutaneous indicator of HIV infection. The dermatitis in such patients can be very extensive and resistant to therapy.

The differential diagnosis of seborrheic dermatitis includes psoriasis vulgaris (sebopsoriasis), atopic dermatitis, contact dermatitis of the face, tinea capitis, and candidiasis.

PRINCIPLES OF MANAGEMENT

As noted earlier, the condition is chronic and persistent. The approach to treatment has evolved with the growing realization of the role of *P. ovale* in pathogenesis. Previously, treatment was strictly symptomatic, directed at removing scale, reducing oiliness and redness, and controlling itching. Currently, the approach is somewhat more etiologic and includes reducing the yeast count on the skin. Therapy is guided by severity, anatomic location, and relative degree of scale, erythema, and oiliness.

Ketoconazole (Nizoral) has proved to be very useful for topical use. It has both fungistatic and fungicidal action, depending on the concentration used. Its 3- to 9-day residual effect between applications is an added advantage. Cream and shampoo formulations are available. For mild to moderate facial or chest involvement, 2% ketoconazole cream applied to the affected areas twice a day until clearing is noted often suffices. Indefinite maintenance therapy may be required once or twice weekly. Although effective, this therapy is expensive, especially if prolonged use is required.

Shampoos to Control Scaling. Scaling can be prominent in cases of scalp involvement, and it responds well to shampoo formulations. The regular use of an over-the-counter dandruff or antiseborrheic shampoo is often sufficient. To be effective, the shampoos should generate good detergent action and be allowed to remain in contact with the scalp for at least 5 to 7 minutes. Commercially available shampoos to combat seborrhea may contain *selenium sulfide*, *zinc pyrithione*, *tar*, *salicylic acid*, and/or *sulfur*. Most preparations contain multiple agents but have one predominant active ingredient. Zinc pyrithione (Danex, DHS Zinc, Head & Shoulders, Sebulon, Zincon, and ZNP bar shampoos) and selenium sulfide (Selsun Blue and prescription Exsel and Selsun shampoos) have been classified as keratolytic agents. Their mode of action also appears to be fungicidal and cytostatic. The combination of sulfur and salicylic acid (Sebulex, Ionil, and Vanseb shampoos) has keratolytic, mild antifungal, and antiseptic effects. Coal tar is the prominent ingredient in Sebutone, Pentrax, T/Gel, and Zetar shampoos, which must be used cautiously, if at all, by people with blond or light gray hair because they can change the color of the hair.

Patients should be given a list of recommended antiseborrheic agents as a guide and advised to find one suitable to their preferences for lather, odor, and efficacy. Many patients find that a shampoo works for a period, then becomes less effective, and a new product must be chosen.

For patients with resistant seborrheic dermatitis who have tried many over-the-counter shampoos before reaching the physician, a prescription shampoo may be of benefit: 2.5% selenium sulfide shampoo (Exsel or Selsun), chloroxine shampoo (Capitrol), or 2% ketoconazole shampoo (Nizoral) may be prescribed. Heavy crusts may be softened with keratolytic lotions (Sebizon, Sebucare) or oil-based agents (DermaSmoothe F/S liquid, P & S liquid) before the hair is washed.

Topical Corticosteroids. Significant erythema requires use of a topical corticosteroid preparation. In hairy areas, a lotion, spray, or gel may be applied two to four times daily. Creams should be avoided because they cause hair to become matted. Ointments are satisfactory to use at night but make the hair greasy, so that shampooing is required again in the morning. On the scalp, a fluorinated corticosteroid is acceptable. Mild erythema on glabrous skin should be treated by washing with a mild soap twice a day, followed by application of 0.5% to 1.0% hydrocortisone cream. Hydrocortisone is relatively inexpensive and is considerably less likely to cause telangiectasia and atrophy; a 1% concentration may be used for erythematous or papular lesions.

After initial success, a period of tachyphylaxis may ensue, requiring increased concentrations of medium-potency, nonfluorinated steroids. Telangiectasia and other signs of dermal atrophy may occur with the long-term use of these products, and application on the face should be avoided. Topical ketoconazole produces no such adverse skin changes. Other over-the-counter and prescription antifungal agents may also be effective. Exudative lesions of intertriginous seborrheic dermatitis may require application of Burow's solution compresses, followed by a fluorinated corticosteroid lotion. Secondary bacterial infection may require the use of systemic antimicrobial agents.

PATIENT EDUCATION

It is reassuring for the patient to know that seborrhea is neither contagious nor progressive, but the chronic nature of the condition also needs to be emphasized. Its relation to stress may help explain flares to the patient. The patient will appreciate being provided with a list of over-the-counter preparations. If topical steroid therapy is needed, the patient should be cautioned about its potential adverse effects and instructed in proper application.

THERAPEUTIC RECOMMENDATIONS

- Provide the patient with a list of over-the-counter shampoos and suggest selecting one that meets personal preferences. For oily hair, advise daily shampooing daily for the first week; this can sometimes be decreased to two or three times a week for maintenance. For resistant cases, ketoconazole shampoo should be used every other day.
- For mild to moderate facial or chest involvement, 2% ketoconazole cream may be applied to the affected areas twice a day until clearing is noted. Maintenance therapy may be required once or twice weekly indefinitely.
- If erythema is present, prescribe a topical nonfluorinated corticosteroid preparation (e.g., 1% or 2.5% hydrocortisone cream) for the face; a fluorinated lotion is appropriate for the scalp (e.g., 0.1% betamethasone valerate lotion).
- Heavy crusts can be removed by softening with keratolytic lotions or oil-based agents before shampooing.
- Treat exudative intertriginous lesions with drying and a nonfluorinated topical steroid lotion.
- Blepharitis may be treated hygienically by gentle rubbing of the eyelashes with a washcloth and No More Tears shampoo. Occasionally, a steroid-containing eye ointment, such as Metimyd or Blephamide solution, can be used, but care must be taken not to allow prolonged use.

ANNOTATED BIBLIOGRAPHY

Faergemann J. Treatment of seborrheic dermatitis of the scalp with ketoconazole shampoo: a double-blind study. Acta Derm Venereol Suppl (Stockh) 1990;70:171. (*Ketoconazole was superior to placebo.*)

Faergemann J, Jones JC, Hettler O, et al. *Pityrosporum ovale (Malassezia furfur)* as the causative agent of seborrhoeic dermatitis: new treatment options. Br J Dermatol 1996;134[S46]:12. (*A solution of 1% terbinafine applied once daily was very effective.*)

Heng MCY, Henderson CL, Barker DC, et al. Correlation of *Pityrosporum ovale* density with clinical severity of seborrheic dermatitis as assessed by a simplified technique. J Am Acad Dermatol 1990;23:82. (*Numbers of* P. ovale *in the stratum corneum correlated with disease severity; improvement correlated with reduction in organism density.*)

Katsambas A, Antoniouu CH, Frangouli E, et al. A double-blind trial of treatment of seborrheic dermatitis with 2% ketoconazole cream compared with 1% hydrocortisone cream. Br J Dermatol 1989;121:353. (Pityrosporum *was reduced in both treatment groups, but the reduction was significantly higher in the group treated with ketoconazole.*)

Mathes BM, Douglas NC. Seborrheic dermatitis in patients with acquired immunodeficiency syndrome. J Am Acad Dermatol 1985;13:947. (*High prevalence in HIV infection; severity is greater than usual and is associated with a poor prognosis.*)

Peter RU, Barthauer U. Successful treatment and prophylaxis of scalp seborrhoeic dermatitis and dandruff with 2% ketoconazole shampoo: results of a multicentre, double-blind, placebo-controlled trial. Br J Dermatol 1995;132:441. (*An excellent response was seen in 88% of 575 patients.*)

185
Management of Acne
PAUL J. GETHNER

Acne, the most common of all skin diseases, is a polygenic, multifactorial disease that, depending on how strictly it is defined, afflicts between 50% and 100% of adolescents in the United States. It ranges in severity from a few scattered whiteheads and blackheads to disfiguring, painful, deep-seated, pus-filled and bleeding nodulocystic lesions. About 15% of surveyed patients with acne seek medical care. The primary care physician is in a unique position to identify and treat a high proportion of acne sufferers. Properly managing acne requires a thorough understanding of the development of acne in all its phases, so that therapy appropriate to the circumstances can be selected from the available modalities. Early effective treatment minimizes the physical scarring of the disease and prevents or reduces equally important psychic trauma.

PATHOPHYSIOLOGY AND CLINICAL PRESENTATION

Pathogenesis

The pathogenesis of acne involves the interaction of enzymatic, immunologic, and chemotactic effects of normal cutaneous microflora; hormonal influences; abnormal keratinization of the sebaceous follicular duct wall; increased sebum production; follicular fragility; and host responsiveness.

Acne is a disease of the sebaceous follicles. Each person has approximately 5,000 sebaceous follicles, scattered predominantly on the face and central upper back and chest. The initial event in the pathogenesis of acne is conversion of the loose, easily shed, horny layer of the epithelium lining the follicular duct wall to a self-adhering mass that gradually obstructs the follicular duct. This has been called *"retention hyperkeratosis."* It takes 1 to 2 months for the accumulated mass of keratin, sebum, and bacteria to reach visible size as a *closed comedo*, or whitehead. Whiteheads may expand the duct ("pore") opening to communicate freely with the outside. The compact, melanin-rich tip then takes on the appearance of a *blackhead*.

Chemotactic agents produced by bacteria within the duct attract leukocytes, and, in ensuing events, duct walls may rupture to release follicular contents into the surrounding dermis. This provokes a profound inflammatory response, leading to the development of papules, pustules, nodules, and suppurative nodules that are commonly, but mistakenly, termed *cysts*. These inflammatory lesions may cause permanent scarring.

Propionibacterium acnes, a normal inhabitant of the follicular canal in humans, may participate in the initiation and aggravation of inflammatory lesions by elaborating enzymes, such as lipases, that act on sebum to release potentially irritating free fatty acids. Its hyaluronidase may increase the permeability of the follicular duct wall, and its protease can damage it, which increases the leakage of materials into the surrounding dermis. In addition, *P. acnes* produces chemotactic substances that contribute to the initiation and evolution of inflammatory lesions.

Clinical Presentation

Acne can most conveniently be divided into two categories, *obstructive* and *inflammatory*. The former, resulting from the impaction of horny material, bacteria, and sebum in the dilated follicular duct wall, is characterized by *closed comedones* (whiteheads) and *open comedones* (blackheads). Leakage of intrafollicular contents from comedones produces an inflammatory response. Depending on the level of leakage into the dermis and the amount of material released, lesions vary from small, erythematous *papules* and superficial *pustules* to deeper pustules and larger, persistent, and occasionally suppurative nodules. Genetically determined immunologic factors may contribute to an exaggerated inflammatory response and more severe cystic forms of acne.

PRINCIPLES OF THERAPY

Removal of acnegenic agents is an important component of therapy. Some cosmetics, including makeup, hair sprays, oils, and moisturizing creams, are capable of producing comedones, and their use should be reduced or discontinued. The physician should advise against using acnegenic drugs as androgens, steroids, iodides, and bromides. Foods do not appear to play a role in acne. After precipitants have been eliminated, the goals of therapy shift to the treatment of existing lesions and further prevention of new lesions. The modalities employed depend on the kind of lesions present.

Obstructive Acne

The basic approach involves the use of comedolytic agents. Retinoic acid and the newer comedolytic agents are quite effective.

Retinoic Acid (Tretinoin) (Avita, Retin-A, Retin-A Micro) is the main comedolytic agent currently available. Retinoids normalize desquamation of the follicular epithelium, promote drainage of existing comedones, and prevent the formation of new comedones. Irritation is the primary adverse reaction to tretinoin. Frequency of application can be adjusted to produce minimal desquamation.

Newer Comedolytic Agents include *azelaic acid*, *adapalene*, and *tazarotene*. Azelaic acid is a naturally occurring compound that has antikeratinizing, antibacterial, and antiinflammatory properties. Adapalene is a synthetic retinoid with some of the biologic activities of tretinoin; it is highly lipophilic.

Tazarotene is also a synthetic retinoid that is used primarily for psoriasis, but it has recently been approved for use in acne.

Mild Inflammatory Acne

Mild inflammatory acne often responds to topical agents such as benzoyl peroxide and topical antibiotics.

Topical Agents. *Benzoyl peroxide* and *retinoic acid* appear to act synergistically with antibiotic therapy, possibly increasing antibiotic concentration in the follicular duct. Benzoyl peroxide is a potent bactericidal agent available in concentrations of 2.5% to 10% and in formulations that include gels, creams, lotions, and washes. *α-Hydroxy acids,* such as glycolic acid, have gained popularity in over-the-counter products and cosmetics promoted directly to patients as being helpful in the treatment of acne.

Topical Antibiotics are used in mild inflammatory acne to suppress *P. acnes* and its elaborations of harmful enzymes. This is both an active and preventive form of treatment. The topical antibiotics used for acne include *clindamycin* and *erythromycin*. These antibiotics are available in convenient roll-on dispensers, individually wrapped throw-away pledgets, and gels. Topical antibiotics are simple to use and not likely to cause the dryness and irritation associated with retinoic acid or benzoyl peroxide treatment. The efficacy of *metronidazole gel* is well-established in acne rosacea (see Chapter 186). It has been found to be equal in efficacy to systemic tetracycline when applied in conjunction with 5% benzoyl peroxide cream.

Intralesional Administration of Corticosteroids may hasten the involution of nodulocystic lesions and reduce the risk for permanent scarring. The injection of *triamcinolone acetonide* (2.0 or 2.5 mg/mL of saline solution) with a 30-gauge needle directly into specific lesions is often remarkably effective. Pseudoatrophy is a danger.

Severe Inflammatory Acne

This form of acne is characterized by large, deep papules and pustules and destructive, suppurating, nodular lesions. Systemic therapy is required. Because *P. acnes* is believed to play an important role in the pathogenesis of inflammatory acne, systemic antibiotics have become the mainstay of therapy.

Systemic Antibiotic Therapy is the best means of preventing the formation of new inflammatory lesions. When *P. acnes* is suppressed, the risk for enzymatic injury to glands is also markedly reduced. Four decades of experience with systemic antibiotic therapy, including a detailed review of the indications and hazards of such therapy by an *ad hoc* committee of the American Academy of Dermatology, has established it as rational, effective, and remarkably safe.

The usual approach to systemic antibiotic therapy is to initiate treatment with either *tetracycline* or a synthetic derivative (*doxycycline* or *minocycline*) or *erythromycin*. Response consists of clearing of old lesions and a decrease in new lesions. After a response is observed, the dosage may be gradually decreased during a period of weeks to the lowest effective maintenance dose.

Because tetracycline must be taken on an empty stomach and erythromycin often has gastrointestinal side effects, the use of the synthetic tetracyclines has gained acceptance in recent years. Although they are more expensive, they are more convenient and highly efficacious. The initial dose of doxycycline or minocycline is 100 to 200 mg daily, with gradual reduction to a maintenance dose as low as 50 mg daily or every other day.

Side Effects. In rare instances, minocycline can cause pigmentation of the mucous membranes and sun-exposed skin. Other rare adverse reactions include a lupuslike syndrome with positive findings on autoimmune blood tests, autoimmune hepatitis, and a hypersensitivity syndrome associated with pulmonary infiltrates. With the use of doxycycline or tetracycline, the development of photodermatitis on exposure to the sun is possible. Because of concern about serious side effects of minocycline, doxycycline might be a better choice if treatment is going to be prolonged. Azithromycin has been reported to be as effective as minocycline in the treatment of inflammatory acne, but it is very expensive.

Accutane (13-*cis*-retinoic acid, isotretinoin) is a powerful systemic agent for the treatment of nodulocystic inflammatory acne. It is the only agent proven to reduce sebaceous gland secretion. A 16- to 20-week course often brings severe acne under complete control, with little or no further therapy needed. However, it is essential for the physician to recognize that this is a potent *teratogen* that has caused numerous tragic birth defects. The Guidelines of Care for Acne Vulgaris, published by the American Academy of Dermatology, clearly state that 13-*cis*-retinoic acid should not be first-choice therapy; its use should be limited to patients who are unresponsive to other standard therapies. In the treatment of women of childbearing potential, it should be considered only for patients with severe, disfiguring cystic acne.

Guidelines for use in women are very well presented in a special patient use kit provided by the manufacturer. This includes a detailed informed consent protocol that must be completed by the patient. A copy is given to the patient and one is kept in the patient's record. The patient must either use two methods of contraception simultaneously or abstain totally from coitus. This program of contraception must begin at least 1 month before Accutane is started and must continue for at least 1 month after Accutane is no longer taken. The drug should not be prescribed until a negative result of a pregnancy test has been obtained within 1 week before the next menses. The patient is instructed to initiate therapy during the second or third day of the next menstrual period. She should be seen monthly or bimonthly thereafter, with suitable laboratory studies performed periodically, including a recommended monthly pregnancy test. Should a pregnancy occur, suitable counseling must be undertaken to assist the patient in deciding on the management of the pregnancy, including possible termination.

Other side effects associated with 13-*cis*-retinoic acid include hypertriglyceridemia, pseudotumor cerebri, idiopathic skeletal hyperostosis, cheilitis, nasal mucosal dryness, nosebleeds, conjunctivitis, skin fragility, the development of pyogenic granuloma-like lesions, arthralgia, headaches, and transaminase elevations, but most of these effects are reversible. A flare may be seen shortly after therapy is initiated, and the patient should be warned of the possibility.

Oral Contraceptives. Ortho Tri-Cyclen has been approved for the treatment of acne in women. However, hormone treatment introduces another dimension of possible side effects, plus the risk for a flare on introduction and a possible rebound flare on discontinuation. The possible interaction between oral antibiotics and oral contraceptives and the need for additional forms of birth control should be discussed with patients.

Spironolactone, an antiandrogen, has been prescribed empirically for women with refractory acne. Doses of 200 mg/d are effective in two thirds of women treated, but menstrual irregularities occur in 22%, and some women experience breast tenderness.

INDICATIONS FOR REFERRAL AND PATIENT EDUCATION

The treatment of acne often falls within the domain of the primary physician. The dermatologist should be consulted if basic topical and systemic therapies fail.

Patient education and cooperation are crucial to the success of therapy. Patients must understand the chronic nature of the process and not be discouraged when lesions continue to appear. Patients who unrealistically expect an immediate cure may become discouraged, uncooperative, and eventually angry.

A vast mythology about acne has developed. The patient should be assured that acne has no relation to diet, masturbation, sexual activity or inactivity, constipation, lack of cleanliness, or angry feelings. The patient should be helped to gain perspective and discouraged from self-examination in magnifying mirrors, which often produces a distorted self-image. Instructions for the use of topical and systemic agents must be precise and carefully followed. The patient should be reminded that therapeutic results are not achieved immediately, and that treatment must be continued for an extended period of time. The single most common reason for failure of therapy is lack of compliance.

THERAPEUTIC RECOMMENDATIONS

- Patient education is an essential part of treating acne, so that understanding and cooperation can be enlisted.
- Eliminate acnegenic drugs, such as steroids or androgens, exposure to oils, and habits such as rubbing the face.
- For obstructive acne, use 0.025% or 0.05% retinoic acid cream or gel. This is applied at bedtime. Sunscreens should also be recommended because tretinoin causes increased sensitivity to the sun.
- If papules or pustules are present concurrently, prescribe a topical antibiotic (e.g., erythromycin or clindamycin) in the form of a lotion, solution, or gel, topical benzoyl peroxide, or both. The topical combination preparation of erythromycin and benzoyl peroxide (Benzamycin) is a useful product in treating some patients.
- In more severe cases of inflammatory acne, prescribe a systemic antibiotic (e.g., tetracycline, doxycycline, minocycline, or erythromycin). Start with a full dose and reduce to maintenance after the acne is under control. If doxycycline is used, it should be taken with an adequate amount of liquid because it can cause esophagitis if taken with only small sips.

- For severe nodulocystic acne resistant to conventional therapy, consider systemic 13-*cis*-retinoic acid, with full awareness of its risks, especially teratogenesis, and the requirement for appropriate monitoring.

ANNOTATED BIBLIOGRAPHY

Bigby M, Stern RS. Adverse reactions to isotretinoin. J Am Acad Dermatol 1988:18:543. (*Review of the significant and less significant adverse reactions.*)

Cunliffe WJ, Poncet M, Loesche C, et al. A comparison of the efficacy and tolerability of adapalene 0.1% gel versus tretinon 0.025% gel in patients with acne vulgaris: a metaanalysis of five randomized trials. Br J Dermatol 1998;139[Suppl 52]:48. (*Adapalene is more rapidly efficacious and is better tolerated.*)

Drake LA. Guidelines of care for acne vulgaris. J Am Acad Dermatol 1990;22:676. (*A summary of the official view of the American Academy of Dermatology on the current management of acne in outline form, including guidelines for the use of 13-cis-retinoic acid.*)

Gibson JR. Rationale for the development of new topical treatments for acne vulgaris. Cutis 1996;57[1 Suppl]:13. (*The role of newer agents in the process of keratinization and their effect on stratum corneum thickness.*)

Gibson JR. Azelaic acid 20% cream (AZELEX) and the medical management of acne vulgaris. Dermatol Nursing 1997;9:339. (*The efficacy of azelaic acid is comparable with that of 0.05% tretinoin, 5% benzoyl peroxide, and 2% erythromycin, but azelaic acid is less irritating than the first two; 30 references.*)

Gruber F, Grubisic-Greblo H, Kastelan M, et al. Azithromycin compared with minocycline in the treatment of acne comedonica and papulo-pustulosa. J Chemother 1998;10:469. (*Azithromycin is as clinically effective and well tolerated as minocycline in the treatment of facial acne.*)

Humbert P, Treffel P, Chapuis JF, et al. The tetracyclines in dermatology. J Am Acad Dermatol 1991;25:691. (*A review of the tetracyclines in acne, acne rosacea, and other dermatologic conditions; 99 references.*)

Landow K. Dispelling myths about acne. Postgrad Med 1997;102:94,103,110. (*An excellent three-part review, with comments about cost effectiveness of approaches.*)

Leyden J. The role of isotretinoin in the treatment of acne: personal observations. J Am Acad Dermatol 1998;39:S45. (*Recalcitrant acne responds well to Accutane.*)

Meynadier J, Alirezai M. Systemic antibiotics for acne. Dermatology 1998;196:135. (*Review of the side effects and efficacy of commonly used oral antibiotics for acne.*)

Nielsen PG. Topical metronidazole gel use in acne vulgaris. Int J Dermatol 1991;30:662. (*Metronidazole 2% plus benzoyl peroxide cream 5% was equal to systemic tetracycline therapy.*)

Shaw JC. Antiandrogen and hormonal treatment of acne. Dermatol Clin 1996;14:803. (*A discussion of these agents in the treatment of acne in adult women.*)

Stern RS. Acne therapy: medication use and sources of care in office-based practice. Arch Dermatol 1996;132:776. (*Acne patients are seen primarily by physicians who are not dermatologists, but treatment patterns are similar.*)

Sturkenboom MC, Meier CR, Juck H, et al. Minocycline and lupuslike syndrome in acne patients. Arch Intern Med 1999;159:493. (*The risk for development of a lupuslike syndrome is increased 8.5-fold in young acne patients taking minocycline.*)

Toyoda M, Morohashi M. An overview of topical antibiotics for acne treatment. Dermatology 1998;196:130. (*Although useful for mild to moderate inflammatory acne, they are of little value in noninflammatory acne; 31 references.*)

186

Management of Rosacea and Other Acneiform Dermatoses

ALICE Y. LIU
WILLIAM V. R. SHELLOW

Acneiform lesions are seen in rosacea, perioral dermatitis, and Favre-Racouchot syndrome. Rosacea is a common condition that affects men and women between the ages of 25 and 60. Perioral dermatitis is typically seen in women between ages 20 and 40. Favre-Racouchot syndrome, or nodular elastosis with cysts and comedones, presents as periorbital comedones (blackheads) in elderly patients with actinic damage. Patients may present to the primary care physician with specific disease symptoms, or signs can be noted incidentally during examination for an unrelated diagnosis. The primary care physician should be able to identify these acneiform conditions, differentiate them from other diseases, and institute proper treatment.

PATHOPHYSIOLOGY AND CLINICAL PRESENTATION

Rosacea

Pathophysiology. Rosacea is a chronic inflammatory condition of unknown cause that involves the central face. Although rosacea can develop in persons of all races, it affects those of Irish, Scottish, and English descent more frequently. The earliest pathophysiologic change is instability of the vasculature, manifested as flushing, blushing, and eventual telangiectases. Flushing may result from a heat-regulating reflex involving the countercurrent thermal exchange between the common carotid artery and the internal jugular vein. Substance P and vasoactive peptides may also contribute. An increased prevalence of migraine headaches accompanying rosacea further suggests a background of vascular hyperreactivity. Ultraviolet damage may contribute, as dermal elastotic degeneration is noted in most patients. The role of infection is being explored. The concentration of mites (*Demodex folliculorum* and *Demodex brevis*) appears to be increased, and an increased frequency of *Helicobacter pylori* gastritis is also noted.

Clinical Presentation. Patients exhibit a spectrum of lesions, the mildest being erythema, a red face, or ruddy cheeks. Patients flush in response to triggers such as hot liquids, spicy foods, alcoholic beverages, sun exposure, vasodilator drugs, and emotional factors. Additional lesions include *papules* and *pustules* (but not comedones, the latter being more specific for acne). *Telangiectases* develop as a response to recurrent erythema and flushing. Facial edema can also result. In severe rosacea, *rhinophyma*, a thick, lobulated overgrowth of connective tissue and sebaceous glands of the nose, may ensue. Ocular complications include blepharitis, conjunctivitis, episcleritis, and, infrequently, iritis and keratitis.

Perioral Dermatitis

The cause of perioral dermatitis is unknown. Light sensitivity, rosacea, atopy, *Demodex* mite infestation, candidiasis, overgrowth of *Pityrosporum ovale*, and the use of fluoride or tartar control toothpaste have all been implicated, as have dental resins. Controversy exists as to whether the use of cosmetics and self-manipulation contribute to this disease. The condition can be replicated by prolonged use of fluorinated corticosteroid medications.

Patients present with an erythematous, scaling, papular, or papulopustular eruption around the mouth, chin, upper lip, and nasolabial folds. The lesions are usually bilateral and symmetric. Occasionally, papulopustular lesions are widespread. In the periocular variant, typical papules develop around the eyes instead of the mouth. Usually, perioral dermatitis is episodic, unlike rosacea, which tends to be chronic.

Periorbital Comedones

Favre-Racouchot syndrome presents as multiple, noninflamed, open comedones around the eyes, temples, and upper cheeks. The condition is related to a loss of elasticity in the skin of older patients. Actinically damaged follicles favor the accumulation of keratin and sebaceous materials. Comedones in the Favre-Racouchot syndrome recur more slowly than do the comedones associated with acne vulgaris.

DIFFERENTIAL DIAGNOSIS

The diagnosis is clinical. It is important to differentiate rosacea from other acneiform and erythematous diseases. Acne presents in a younger age group and features comedones in addition to papules and pustules. Rosacea can also imitate seborrheic dermatitis, *Pityrosporum* folliculitis, contact dermatitis, eczema, and drug-induced photosensitivity. Perioral dermatitis can look like rosacea, and some consider it to be a variant. Serious systemic diseases presenting similarly to rosacea include lupus erythematosus and sarcoidosis.

PRINCIPLES OF MANAGEMENT

Rosacea

Treatment involves removal of the exacerbating conditions that lead to flushing or vasodilation and the use of topical or systemic antibiotics.

Avoidance of Precipitants. Conditions to avoid include prolonged exposure to sunlight, extreme heat or cold, and ingestion of hot or spicy foods and beverages. Some medications, in-cluding vasodilators (aminophylline, hydralazine, niacin, nitroglycerine, papaverine), angiotensin-converting enzyme inhibitors, and simvastatin, have been reported to worsen rosacea. The patient should be cautioned against the use of topical fluorinated corticosteroids, which produce an initial response only to result in atrophy of skin and the development of permanent telangiectasia. Patients with rosacea should also select moisturizers or sunscreens formulated for sensitive skin. Protective ingredients such as dimethicone or cyclomethicone can help reduce irritation.

Topical Antibiotics. The mainstay of topical rosacea therapy is topical *metronidazole*. Alternatively, topical *sulfacetamide* with or without sulfur applied once daily can be of benefit. Other topical therapies, similar to those used for acne vulgaris, enhance skin turnover and restoration; these include topical *erythromycin*, *clindamycin*, *benzoyl peroxide*, and *retinoic acid*.

Systemic Therapy. Patients with papules, pustules, or ocular symptoms often need systemic treatment in addition to topical measures. The systemic antibiotics include *tetracycline*, *doxycycline*, *minocycline*, and *erythromycin*. These are initiated along with topical therapy and then tapered as the condition improves; topical therapy is continued for maintenance. For severe cases, *systemic isotretinoin* or *metronidazole* can be effective. Recent reports also detail the use of *ketoconazole* and *clarithromycin*. With all systemic therapies, side effects must be weighed against potential benefits. The tetracyclines can cause photosensitivity, and minocycline can cause pigmentation abnormalities, dizziness, and a lupuslike syndrome.

Flushing does not respond to the antiinflammatory properties of these systemic therapies and can be difficult to treat pharmacologically. Authors have mentioned the use of *anticholinergics* (e.g., glycopyrrolate), *β-blockers*, *clonidine*, and psychotropic medications to manage flushing. However, the side effects of these medications often outweigh their potential benefit.

Surgical Approaches include pulsed dye or *neodymium: yttrium-aluminum garnet* (Nd:YAG) laser for telangiectasias. Rhinophyma can be treated with *carbon dioxide laser*, *electrosurgery*, *excision*, or *dermabrasion*. Successful surgical management requires an experienced dermatologist.

Perioral Dermatitis

Patients with perioral dermatitis should avoid heavy cosmetics and topical products with a high proportion of oil. Some practitioners also advise patients to change toothpastes or mouthwashes. Topical acne preparations that increase skin turnover are useful but often inadequate if used alone. *Hydrocortisone cream* (1%) may promote rapid resolution of the dermatitis but should be discontinued promptly. Fluorinated corticosteroid creams should not be used. *Systemic tetracyclines* are consistently effective in controlling perioral dermatitis, as they are in controlling rosacea. If the tetracyclines cannot be tolerated, *erythromycin* may be used instead. Systemic treatment can be discontinued after resolution, usually within 4 to 8 weeks.

Periorbital Comedones

Periorbital comedones may be treated by *manual extraction* of the blackheads with a comedone extractor, but to avoid scarring, this must be performed by an experienced operator. Redevelopment of blackheads is somewhat slow, so that periodic extraction at 3- or 4-month intervals is adequate. Pharmacologic therapy with *retinoic acid* can aid in control of blackheads.

PATIENT EDUCATION

The major element of patient education is to explain that these conditions are common and treatable but may be chronic, with intermittent flares. Many patients are bothered by a single papule, whereas others can sustain the disfigurement of rosacea without complaint. A detailed review of aggravating factors is important for management and helps the patient to become a partner in the treatment of these stubborn conditions.

THERAPEUTIC RECOMMENDATIONS

Rosacea

- Begin oral tetracycline (500 mg twice a day) and continue for several weeks to months; the dosage is then gradually reduced to 250 mg every other day before cessation is considered. Prolonged low-dose therapy may be necessary. Alternatively, doxycycline (100 mg twice daily) or minocycline (50 mg twice daily) can be used.
- Begin topical metronidazole (0.75% twice daily or 1% once daily) along with systemic antibiotics, and maintain the patient on topical therapy after systemic therapy has been discontinued.
- If the patient cannot tolerate topical metronidazole, use topical sulfur and sodium sulfacetamide lotions twice daily.
- The patient should avoid sunlight and fluorinated steroids and limit systemic medications and foods known to exacerbate the condition.
- Consider a short-term course of a low-potency, nonfluorinated topical corticosteroid (e.g., 1% or 2.5% hydrocortisone cream twice daily) if erythema is refractory.
- Refer the patient for consideration of surgical management if rhinophyma or telangiectases are prominent.

Perioral Dermatitis

- Begin with tetracycline (500 mg twice daily) and gradually taper the dose during a period of weeks after resolution has occurred.
- The patient should avoid heavy cosmetics, creams, and fluoridated toothpastes.
- Consider a short course of hydrocortisone cream (1% or 2.5% twice daily).

Periorbital Comedones

- Refer for comedone extraction as needed.
- Initiate application of topical tretinoin (0.025% cream, 0.1% microsphere gel daily at bedtime) to the affected areas. Warn patients that tretinoin may cause irritation and that sunlight should be avoided while it is being used.
- For patients who cannot tolerate tretinoin, prescribe topical adapalene (0.1% solution or gel daily at bedtime).
- Prescribe sun protection with a noncomedogenic sunscreen.
- Consider referral for surgical approaches in severe cases.

ANNOTATED BIBLIOGRAPHY

Beacham BE, Kurgansky D, Gould WM. Circumoral dermatitis and cheilitis caused by tartar control dentifrices. J Am Acad Dermatol 1990;22:1029. (*A series of cases in 20 otherwise healthy women, ages 22 to 51 years; probably represents an irritant contact dermatitis.*)

Breneman DL, Stewart D, Hevia O, et al. A double-blind, multicenter clinical trial comparing efficacy of once-daily metronidazole 1% cream with vehicle in patients with rosacea. Cutis 1998;61:44. (*Metronidazole 1% cream daily was more effective than vehicle. However, study did not compare it with metronidazole 0.75% cream.*)

Connolly CS, Bikowski J. Recognizing rosacea's imitators. Improve your ability to differentiate acne from rosacea. Skin Aging 1999;7:34,39. (*Reviews differential diagnosis of rosacea.*)

Erbagci Z, Ozgoztasi O. The significance of *Demodex folliculorum* density in rosacea. Int J Dermatol 1998;37:421. (*Higher mite count in rosacea patients. However, no correlation of counts with severity.*)

Erdogan FG, Yurtsever P, Aksoy D, et al. Efficacy of low-dose isotretinoin in patients with treatment-resistant rosacea. Arch Dermatol 1998;134:884. (*Treatment-resistant rosacea was successfully managed with 10 mg of oral isotretinoin daily for 16 weeks. However, no follow-up data after cessation are provided.*)

Lowe NJ, Henderson T, Millikan LE, et al. Topical metronidazole for severe and recalcitrant rosacea: a prospective open trial. Cutis 1989;43:283. (*Metronidazole was as effective as systemic antibiotics in some patients.*)

Lowe NJ, Behr KL, Fitzpatrick R, et al. Flash lamp pumped dye laser for rosacea-associated telangiectasia and erythema. J Dermatol Surg Oncol 1991;17:522. (*Use of laser to remove telangiectases and reduce erythema.*)

Nelson B, Fuciarelli K. Surgical management of rhinophyma. Cutis 1998;61:313. (*Reviews surgical options, including excision, dermabrasion, skin grafting, electrosurgery, and carbon dioxide laser.*)

Nichols K, Desai N, Lebwohl MG. Effective sunscreen ingredients and cutaneous irritation in patients with rosacea. Cutis 1998;61:344. (*Least irritating formulation contained dimethicone and cyclomethicone.*)

Rebora A, Drago F, Picciotto A. *Helicobacter pylori* in patients with rosacea. Am J Gastrointerol 1994;89:1603. (*Controversial report of association of rosacea with Helicobacter pylori gastritis.*)

Torresani C. Clarithromycin: a new perspective in rosacea management. Int J Dermatol 1998;37:343. (*Suggests the use of 250 mg of clarithromycin twice daily for 4 weeks, then 250 mg daily for rosacea.*)

Veien NK, Munkvad JM, Nielsen AO, et al. Topical metronidazole in the treatment of perioral dermatitis. J Am Acad Dermatol 1991;24:258. (*Tetracycline was significantly more effective.*)

187
Management of Psoriasis
AMBER OWEN
NICHOLAS J. LOWE

Psoriasis is a chronic skin disease that affects up to 2% to 3% of the U.S. adult population. It is characterized by discrete erythematous papules and plaques covered by a silvery white scale. Pustular and erythrodermic varieties are also seen, and arthritis sometimes complicates the condition. Patients presenting to their physician express concern about the cosmetic effects of the disease and request relief from itching and pain. The type of treatment selected should be based on the type of psoriasis present, the location of the disease on the body and its severity, and the patient's age and medical history.

The primary physician should be able to treat mild and localized forms of the disease and be knowledgeable about the treatment of more severe disease to ensure appropriate referral and collaboration with the dermatologist.

PATHOPHYSIOLOGY AND CLINICAL PRESENTATION

Pathophysiology. The epidermal turnover time it takes for a cell to travel from the basal cell layer of the epidermis to the granular layer is normally 14 days. In psoriatic skin, it is reduced to 2 days. Normal cell maturation cannot take place in this short time, and subsequent keratinization is faulty. Clinically, this is seen as scaling. Histologically, the epidermis is thickened, and immature nucleated cells are seen in the stratum corneum. An accompanying dilatation of the subepidermal blood vessels and infiltration with mononuclear cells account for the characteristic erythema. Neutrophils are often seen within the stratum corneum, forming characteristic micropustules.

The exact causes of this abnormal cellular proliferation and inflammation remain unknown, but current speculation is that genetically predisposed persons experience T-cell activation in response to antigen stimulation. Affected persons have an increased incidence of several HLA antigens, including HLA-B27 in patients with psoriatic arthritis. Psoriatic plaques are rich in activated T lymphocytes, which are capable of inducing both cellular proliferation and inflammation. The search for responsible antigens is ongoing.

Drug-exacerbated psoriasis offers some insights into disease mechanisms. Lithium is believed to act by enhancing the release of inflammatory mediators from neutrophils, β-blockers by decreasing cyclic adenosine monophosphate (cAMP)-dependent protein kinase (an inhibitor of cell proliferation), and NSAIDs by causing a buildup of the inflammatory mediator arachidonic acid. Antimalarials are also associated with an exacerbation of the disease. Drug-induced exacerbations can be unpredictable and severe and may occur months after the medication is first taken.

Clinical Presentation and Course. The onset of psoriasis is usually in early adult life, but the disease may appear in childhood or old age. It typically presents with well-marginated, erythematous, elevated *papules* or *plaques*; if not previously treated, these also show thick, silvery *scaling*. Removal of the scale reveals punctate bleeding points known as *Auspitz's sign*. Nails often show punctate *pitting* and a characteristic discoloration of the surface that resembles a drop of oil. *Subungual collections* of keratotic material are also common, with distal separation of the nail from the nail bed. Mucous membranes are rarely involved. The *extensor surfaces* of the arms and legs are the most commonly affected sites; the scalp is another. Skin trauma increases the risk for involvement, but any epidermal surface can become involved, even the mucosa.

Other clinical types include *guttate psoriasis*, which presents with small, discrete, erythematous papular lesions. An *exfoliative* or *erythrodermic* form of psoriasis shows generalized erythema without any characteristic lesions of psoriasis. Localized pustular psoriasis with sterile pustules of the palms and soles may also be seen without other characteristic lesions. An uncommon but serious variant is generalized *pustular* disease, which is often accompanied by systemic symptoms and a risk for circulatory collapse. In patients with AIDS, a very extensive psoriasis may develop that is quite resistant to therapy.

The *arthritis* associated with psoriasis is often polyarticular and asymmetric, but it also may be monarticular. Classic manifestations include swelling and deformity of the distal interphalangeal joint in association with the characteristic nail changes. Juxtaarticular inflammation produces sausagelike swelling of the fingers. Radiologic features include interphalangeal joint erosion ("pencil-in-a-cup" appearance) and erosion of the distal tuft. Arthritis occurs in about 5% to 10% of patients. The skin disease usually precedes the joint disease by months to years.

The *clinical course* of psoriasis is characterized by chronicity and seasonal fluctuations, with improvement in the summer secondary to sun exposure and worsening in the winter as dry skin leads to epidermal injury.

PRINCIPLES OF MANAGEMENT

The basic approaches to therapy are direct reduction of the rate of epidermal proliferation and indirect reduction through inhibition of dermal inflammatory and immune responses. In addition, one seeks to protect the skin from drying and other forms of injury that may precipitate a flare. Approximately 75% of patients with psoriasis have relatively localized disease involving less than 20% of the body surface area. These patients are generally best managed with topical therapy as the first line of treatment. Certain overriding considerations, however, such as previous failure of topical therapy, inability to apply topical therapy, rapid relapse after previous therapy, or presence of severe psoriatic arthritis, may prompt the physician to choose systemic therapy instead.

Topical Therapies

Corticosteroids. For mild, limited plaque psoriasis, topical corticosteroids are the most commonly prescribed first-line agents because of their ease of use and convenience, short-term efficacy, broad range of potency, patient acceptability, and ready availability. A wide variety of delivery systems have been developed. Corticosteroids have antiinflammatory, antiproliferative, and immunosuppressive actions. Available formulations include ointment, cream, lotion, gel, impregnated tape, and aerosol. Factors to be considered include the anatomic site being treated, extent of involvement, age of the patient, potency of the product, application technique, duration of treatment, and any coexisting relevant conditions, such as preexisting atrophy or compromised adrenal reserve.

The classification of topical steroids is by relative potency, as determined by vasoconstrictive effect (see Chapter 184). Both the structure of the corticosteroid moiety and the type of vehicle delivery system used determine the potency and percutaneous transfer of the corticosteroid. Ointments are considered the most efficient delivery system because of the high solubility of corticosteroids in ointment bases and their relative occlusive action in comparison with other vehicles. The occlusion of localized lesions can enhance the effect of a topical corticosteroid of a given potency.

Adverse Effects and Their Prevention. Although topical corticosteroids can be highly effective in treating psoriasis, caution is advised in prescribing them because of their potential to cause local and systemic side effects. Common cutaneous side effects include *skin atrophy* and *acneiform eruptions.* Prolonged application of potent topical corticosteroids can cause *systemic steroid effects* (see Chapter 106). When potent topical therapy is discontinued, a *rebound* effect may occur, with the psoriasis becoming even more severe than the original, untreated condition. Also, a tendency toward conversion of "stable" to "unstable" (erythrodermic or pustular) disease may be noted.

To reduce the incidence of side effects, various *intermittent dosing schedules* have been developed, especially for potent topical preparations. *"Pulse therapy"* involves treating the psoriatic plaque with a superpotent steroid twice daily to initiate plaque regression; once improvement is noted, the steroid is applied on weekends only. The regimen can prolong psoriatic remissions and avoid adverse effects.

Tars

Topical *coal tar* preparations are among the oldest topical therapies for psoriasis. When used alone, they are no more effective than topical corticosteroids of low to intermediate potency, but they are effective in combination therapy. In the *Goeckerman program,* which combines topical tar with suberythemogenic *ultraviolet B* light, coal tar produces an enhanced effect. Patients with more than 10% of skin surface involvement are reasonable candidates. The treatment is associated with an 80% to 90% remission rate, and no significant evidence of an increased risk for skin cancer has been noted. Modifications of the Goeckerman program allow outpatient therapy in which less messy coal tar gels are used, followed in 2 hours by treatment with ultraviolet light. Treatment for 4 to 6 weeks is usually necessary to achieve maximum benefit.

Tar *shampoos* (Zetar, Sebutone, Pentrax, T/Gel) may be of benefit to patients with scalp psoriasis. The shampoo is massaged in thoroughly and left on for 10 minutes before water is added and the patient shampoos gently for several more minutes to remove scales. This is combined with overnight application of a moderate-strength topical steroid solution (e.g., Synalar solution) for maximum effect. Topical coal tars are messy and malodorous, which makes them inconvenient for patient use.

Anthralin

Anthralin is one of the more effective agents for topical treatment, acting to reduce epidermal inflammation and keratinocyte proliferation. Anthralin is as effective as a class II corticosteroid but causes unpleasant side effects, such as inflammation and staining of unaffected perilesional skin and clothing. These properties may make it unacceptable to patients. As a result of modifications to the once-traditional overnight anthralin therapy, the incidence of staining and side effects has decreased and application and removal have become easier, so that anthralin is now more acceptable to patients.

Short-contact application of newer anthralin cream formulations (e.g., Micanol cream) is an alternative to traditional overnight therapy. It appears that anthralin penetrates lesional skin faster than perilesional skin, so that a shortened contact time is possible without loss of efficacy in comparison with traditional therapy. The newer cream formulations cause less erythema, burning, and staining of skin and clothing and are more cosmetically acceptable than traditional anthralin, but of equal efficacy.

Vitamin D Analogues

Vitamin D analogues act via vitamin D receptors, which are members of the superfamily of steroid hormone receptors. They activate intranuclear transcription factors that bind to specific DNA sequences to modulate gene transcription activity, thereby affecting inflammation and control of epidermal growth and keratinization. Immune modulation results. The vitamin D analogues include calcitriol, calcipotriene (or calcipotriol in Europe), and talcacitol, which is not yet approved for use in the United States.

Calcipotriene (calcipotriol, Dovonex) has become a first- or second-line agent in the treatment of mild to moderate plaque psoriasis. The agent is a derivative of naturally occurring vitamin D and is highly effective in most patients for flattening plaque and decreased scale. The ointment formulation is more effective than short-contact anthralin cream in reducing psoriatic plaques, and it is more cosmetically acceptable. It also more effective than intermediate-strength topical steroids (e.g., betamethasone 17-valerate or fluocinonide ointment), with a considerably lower rate of relapse. Response begins within 2 weeks of treatment and continues to develop for 6 to 8 weeks. Patients experience improvement for up to 12 months of treatment, so that this agent is efficacious as both continuous and intermittent therapy. It is also used for intertriginous psoriasis.

Adverse Effects. The most common side effect (15% of users) is perilesional or lesional irritation and erythema. Dermatitis may also develop on the face after inadvertent transfer of the agent, so that hand washing immediately after application is necessary. *Hypercalcemia* and *hypercalciuria* can occur, especially if the topical dosage exceeds 100 g weekly, so that caution is needed, particularly when prescribing the agent for patients with renal compromise or in whom hypercalcemia or kidney stones are likely to develop. Patients with extensive psoriasis who may require a dose approaching 100 g weekly should be screened for hypercalciuria before treatment is begun.

Calcitriol (1,25-dihydroxyvitamin D_3) is a naturally occurring hormone that is a safe and effective treatment for plaque psoriasis; it reduces scale production, plaque thickness, and erythema without causing abnormalities in serum calcium levels, calciuria, or local cutaneous side effects. Compared with calcipotriene, calcitriol appears to cause only minimal irritation, even when applied to the face, and is associated with fewer changes in systemic calcium metabolism; however, it is less effective, especially when used in low doses for chronic plaque psoriasis. Higher doses are being studied for safety and efficacy.

Tazarotene

Tazarotene, a vitamin A derivative, selectively binds to retinoic acid receptors to cause negative gene regulatory effects specific to skin cells. The result is that it is less cytotoxic than other topical retinoids and produces less local irritation. Application for 2 weeks decreases keratinocyte proliferation, modulates abnormal keratinocyte differentiation, and decreases expression of inflammatory markers in the skin. The gel is effective in concentrations of both 0.05% and 0.1% applied either once or twice daily. The 0.1% tazarotene gel acts more rapidly than the 0.05% gel but is associated with a higher incidence of irritation.

Tazarotene gel (0.1% or 0.05%) applied once daily for a week is as effective as 0.05% fluocinonide cream, a topical corticosteroid, in reducing plaque elevation, but it takes longer to reduce plaque erythema. After 4 weeks of treatment, however, the overall treatment success rates are similar. Additionally, the relapse rate for 0.1% tazarotene gel is significantly lower than that for fluocinonide cream. An advantage of tazarotene over other topical agents is its sustained effect, generally within 20% of final treatment levels for up to 12 weeks after treatment. Furthermore, its onset of action is rapid, with decreased plaque elevation noticed by the first week, decreased scaling by the second week, and decreased erythema by the end of 6 weeks. Trunk and limb lesions generally respond more rapidly than thicker elbow and knee lesions. Tazarotene is also suitable for application to the face and scalp.

Combination Therapy

Because it is a chronic disease, psoriasis usually requires prolonged treatment, and although corticosteroids are often given as weekend therapy, their long-term side effects make them difficult to use as monotherapy in chronic cases. A new trend is to use combination therapy with *calcipotriene ointment* and *superpotent steroids*, such as halobetasol ointment, to induce greater improvement and reduce the side effects produced by either agent used as monotherapy. A combination of week-

end therapy with corticosteroids and weekday therapy with calcipotriene ointment increases the duration of remission of psoriasis, and a combination of morning treatment with calcipotriene ointment and evening treatment with halobetasol ointment can enhance the effect of either agent used alone. Applying the agents at different times of day is recommended because the calcipotriene molecule has been shown to be relatively unstable and is rapidly degraded when directly combined with certain corticosteroid ointments.

Another effective combination program includes topical *corticosteroids* and topical *retinoids*. A protective effect against skin atrophy is noted when 0.1% tretinoin is added to betamethasone dipropionate. A combination of *tazarotene* and an intermediate- or high-potency *corticosteroid* achieved greater reductions in the severity of psoriasis than did a combination of tazarotene and placebo cream. Tazarotene and other topical agents in combination with ultraviolet B phototherapy is another potentially useful concept that is currently under study.

Systemic Treatment of Psoriasis

Systemic treatment is indicated only for severe or incapacitating disease. Indications include *generalized pustular psoriasis*, *generalized exfoliative psoriasis*, severe *psoriatic arthropathy*, topical treatment failure, *severe uncontrolled psoriasis* (generally involving more than 20% of the body surface area), and socially incapacitating disease. An additional indication is acute *guttate psoriasis*; the use of systemic therapy may prevent this form from becoming chronic.

Photochemotherapy

Photochemotherapy combines a systemic photosensitizing agent, *psoralens*, with long-wavelength (320 to 400 nm) *ultraviolet A light* (commonly referred to as *PUVA therapy*). PUVA therapy generally produces excellent results (80% to 90% remission) in patients with otherwise recalcitrant severe psoriasis. Acute side effects of PUVA therapy may include pruritus and nausea (15% of patients), and burning may also occur. Long-term side effects include premature skin aging and carcinogenesis. The risk for skin cancer is increased with both ultraviolet A and PUVA therapies, the most common type being *squamous cell carcinoma*. However, some recent evidence suggests that patients undergoing long-term PUVA therapy are also at increased risk for the development of *melanoma*. Therefore, patients undergoing phototherapy must be given careful follow-up and regular skin checks. Patients at increased risk for skin cancer (fair skin, easily sunburned, previous radiation therapy to the skin) should not be given PUVA treatment, and PUVA treatment should be reserved for severe or recalcitrant psoriasis that is resistant to topical therapy.

Methotrexate

Methotrexate decreases the mitotic rate and DNA synthesis in the epidermis. However, it may exert part of its therapeutic effect via immunomodulation. It is effective in controlling severe disease, but the risk for serious side effects limits its use to chronic, refractory cases. Its use is also generally reserved for men and women past reproductive age because of its highly mutagenic potential. Oral regimens include either three doses at 12-hour intervals, given once weekly, or a single weekly dose. If nausea is significant, parenteral administration can be used.

Because of the potential of methotrexate to cause hematopoietic, hepatic, and renal toxicity, close monitoring and full patient compliance are essential. The patient's hematologic status and renal and liver functions should be normal before treatment is begun and monitored regularly during treatment. The monitoring program consists of weekly, followed by monthly, blood sampling. Evidence of bone marrow suppression may appear, but renal and hepatic injury are uncommon at the doses used for treatment of psoriasis. Hepatic fibrosis, however, may develop with prolonged use, so that most experts recommend consideration of pretreatment liver biopsy and repeated biopsy after a cumulative dose of 1.5 g.

Acitretin

Acitretin (Soriatane) is a systemic retinoid used in erythrodermic, pustular, and chronic plaque psoriasis. Although teratogenicity is a drawback in the use of most systemic retinoids, acitretin is rather rapidly cleared (not being lipid-bound or maintained in fat stores) and is thus safe for women of childbearing potential, provided that they use effective contraception while taking the drug and for at least 1 year after discontinuing it.

Side effects of acitretin include hyperlipidemia, dry lips, conjunctivitis, pruritus, alopecia, color blindness, and decreased night vision. The serum liver chemistries and triglyceride and cholesterol levels of patients should be evaluated before treatment is begun, and they should undergo laboratory monitoring at monthly intervals during treatment. Biopsy-proven hepatotoxicity has not been noted with long-term use of acitretin, so that the need for liver biopsy is obviated.

Acitretin and Phototherapy. Acitretin monotherapy is the preferred treatment for pustular psoriasis, whereas for plaque psoriasis, acitretin is best prescribed with adjunctive therapy, such as ultraviolet light phototherapy. The dose of acitretin and the total exposure to ultraviolet light can be reduced if they are used in combination. The dosing of ultraviolet light or PUVA, however, should be increased gradually and cautiously when patients are taking systemic retinoids because of their increased risk for ultraviolet light–induced erythema. After clearance of psoriasis has been achieved, patients can be maintained on either low doses of acitretin or PUVA alone.

Cyclosporine

Cyclosporine acts as a potent suppressor of T-cell activity and has effected significant improvement and even total clearing in more than two thirds of patients treated. However, relapse within several weeks of discontinuation of treatment is common. Moreover, hypertension, renal toxicity, hirsutism, and myalgias can occur with short-term therapy, and lymphoma with more prolonged use. Cyclosporine can be started at a low dose (2.5 mg/kg daily) and slowly increased to maintain efficacy. Once remission is achieved, the dose can be gradually decreased. There appear to be some differences in efficacy among available preparations.

PATIENT EDUCATION AND INDICATIONS FOR REFERRAL

For many, the social and psychological effects of severe or long-standing disease can be significant, leading to loneliness and depression. Regularly scheduled visits to reinforce the details of therapy and also to render support are appreciated. Knowing that disease severity can be reduced through appropriate treatment is reassuring. Informed advice about what works and what does not is essential. Concerns about contagion and genetic transmission of the disease need to be addressed. The chronic relapsing nature of psoriasis should be acknowledged, so that patient expectations will be realistic. Preventive measures should be stressed, such as keeping the skin well hydrated and avoiding sunburn and other forms of skin trauma. The safety and efficacy of most psoriatic regimens depend on strong patient compliance. Careful teaching that includes the rationale for a given practice is helpful, as are written instructions.

Patients with extensive, refractory, or acute pustular disease should be referred to a dermatologist for consideration of phototherapy, retinoids, antimetabolites, and immunosuppressive therapy. The development of generalized disease, especially if erythrodermal or pustular, requires hospitalization.

THERAPEUTIC RECOMMENDATIONS

- Treat localized, mild to moderate disease topically. Refer patients with more extensive (>20% of skin area involved) or refractory disease to a dermatologist.
- Emphasize the importance of keeping the skin well hydrated and avoiding sunburn and other forms of skin injury.
- Allow cautious sun exposure; avoid sunburn, and do not recommend sun exposure for those at increased risk for skin cancer (fair-skinned, easily burned, history of skin irradiation).
- Review medications for potential exacerbating drugs (lithium, β-blockers, NSAIDs); reduce dose or substitute if possible.
- Prescribe a topical steroid program for control of bothersome visible lesions. Begin with a "superpotent" preparation (e.g., Diprolene, Psorcon, Temovate, Ultravate), and change to a less potent preparation for maintenance. Use only milder steroids on the face and skin folds.
- Consider calcipotriene or tazarotene as alternatives to topical steroids.
- Recommend an ointment preparation for lesions with considerable scale, although a cream may be more acceptable for daytime use and suffice for plaques with minimal scale. A twice-daily regimen of steroid application achieves best results.
- For patients with excessive scale, recommend gentle removal by warm bathing.
- For mild scalp involvement, recommend nightly use of a tar shampoo. It is rubbed in gently, left on for 10 minutes, and then rinsed out gently. For more severe scalp disease, use of the tar shampoo is followed by gentle application of a topical steroid lotion (e.g., Synalar). Patients with marked scalp involvement may benefit from covering their head with a shower cap after steroid application and use of a superpotent topical steroid lotion (e.g., Diprolene), anthralin scalp preparation, Dovonex scalp lotion, or Tazorac gel.

- Refer patients who fail to respond and those with extensive disease to a dermatologist for consideration of methotrexate or other systemic therapies. Promptly admit to the hospital if generalized pustular or erythrodermal disease develops.

ANNOTATED BIBLIOGRAPHY

Bleiker TO, Bourke JF, Mumford R, et al. Long-term outcome of severe chronic plaque psoriasis following treatment with high-dose topical calcipotriol. Br J Dermatol 1998;139:285. (*Demonstrates long-term safety and efficacy.*)

Chuang T-Y, Heinrich LA, Schultz MD, et al. PUVA and skin cancer: a historical cohort study of 492 patients. J Am Acad Dermatol 1992;26:173. (*High-dose therapy associated with increased rates of squamous cell carcinoma but not of basal cell cancers.*)

Farber EM, Rein G, Lanigan SW. Stress and psoriasis: psychoneuroimmunologic mechanisms. Int J Dermatol 1991;30:8. (*Stress is associated with exacerbations; possible mechanisms are reviewed.*)

Gilbertson EO, Spellman MC, Piacquadio DJ, et al. Superpotent topical corticosteroid use associated with adrenal suppression: clinical considerations. J Am Acad Dermatol 1998;38:318. (*Discussion of adrenal suppression with various doses of topical corticosteroids.*)

Katz HI. Topical corticosteroids. Dermatol Clin 1995;13:805. (*A thorough review of these commonly prescribed medications.*)

Krueger GG, Drake LA, Elias PM, et al. The safety and efficacy of tazarotene gel, a topical acetylenic retinoid, in the treatment of psoriasis. Arch Dermatol 1998;134:57. (*Safety and efficacy of this topical agent are discussed.*)

Lebwohl M. Topical application of calcipotriene and corticosteroids: combination regimens. J Am Acad Dermatol 1997;37:S55. (*Using superpotent corticosteroids with calcipotriene results in greater improvement with fewer side effects.*)

Lebwohl MG, Breneman DL, Goffe BS, et al. Tazarotene 0.1% gel plus corticosteroid cream in the treatment of plaque psoriasis. J Am Acad Dermatol 1998;39:590. (*Tazarotene combined with topical corticosteroids increased efficacy and reduced adverse events.*)

Liem WH, McCullough JL, Weinstein GD. Effectiveness of topical therapy for psoriasis: results of a national survey. Cutis 1995;55:306. (*Treatment with high-potency corticosteroids is preferred by dermatologists.*)

Lowe NJ, Prystowsky J, Bourget T, et al. Acitretin plus UVB phototherapy for psoriasis. J Am Acad Dermatol 1991;24:591. (*More clearing occurred with the combination than with either agent used alone.*)

Muller SA, Perry HO. The Goeckerman treatment in psoriasis: six decades of experience at the Mayo Clinic. Cutis 1984;34:265. (*The standard with which new regimens must be compared.*)

Ramsay B, O'Reagan M. A survey of the social and psychological effects of psoriasis. Br J Dermatol 1988;118:195. (*The effects can be marked.*)

Roegnigk H, Averback R, Maibach HI. Methotrexate in psoriasis: revised guidelines. J Am Acad Dermatol 1988;19:145. (*Authoritative guidelines.*)

Wolverton SE. Systemic drug therapy for psoriasis. The most critical issues. Arch Dermatol 1991;127:565. (*A thoughtful editorial review.*)

188

Management of Intertrigo and Intertriginous Dermatoses
WILLIAM V. R. SHELLOW

Intertrigo is an inflammatory condition of body folds that presents as a moist lesion with erythema and scaling. It is more common in obese people and is exacerbated by warm weather. The areas of involvement are the axillary, inguinal, and inframammary folds and the toe webs. The primary physician should be capable of distinguishing intertrigo from other eruptions of the body folds, such as erythrasma, seborrheic dermatitis, psoriasis, and dermatophyte infections, and of rendering appropriate treatment.

PATHOPHYSIOLOGY AND CLINICAL PRESENTATION

Intertrigo presents as an erythematous exudative inflammation in the body folds. Patients may have soreness and itching, and with secondary infection, overt purulence may occur. The pathogenic mechanism is mechanical. Heat, moisture, and the retention of sweat produce maceration and irritation, an environment that promotes bacterial infection.

Early intertrigo is characterized by slight maceration and erythema. The moisture initially comes from eccrine sweat that cannot evaporate in the intertriginous areas because of reduced circulation of air. With time, redness becomes more intense, and the epidermis becomes eroded or even denuded. Subsequent inflammation causes exudation of serous fluid. Increased moisture may lead to bacterial colonization, which accounts for the odor that is sometimes associated with intertrigo. The groin and intergluteal areas may be colonized by gram-negative organisms. Incontinence of urine or feces may exacerbate maceration in the groin and gluteal areas.

DIFFERENTIAL DIAGNOSIS

Intertrigo in the Groin must be differentiated from *tinea cruris* and *candidiasis*. Tinea cruris is a fungal infection characterized by red, scaly patches. The lesions form circinate plaques with scaly or vesicular borders and central clearing. After scales are scraped and 20% potassium hydroxide solution is added, the finding of hyphae in specimens under low microscopic power serves to differentiate tinea cruris from intertrigo. Candidiasis produces deep, beefy red lesions with characteristic satellite vesicopustules outside the border of the primary lesion. Involvement of the scrotum is common, whereas in tinea the scrotum is usually spared.

The groin may be affected by sexually transmitted diseases such as *condyloma, herpes, scabies,* or *pediculosis.* These cause an erythematous and pruritic eruption with characteristics that point to the underlying diagnosis (see Chapters 141, 192, 193, and 195). In severe cases of intertrigo, an underlying disease such as lichen sclerosus et atrophicus should be considered. Long-standing intertrigo with scratching often leads to the development of lichen simplex chronicus.

Intertrigo in the Axilla needs to be differentiated from *candidiasis, tinea, erythrasma,* and *contact dermatitis. Candidal infection* presents with an erythematous eruption; tinea corporis in the axilla demonstrates an active border with scale; erythrasma has a reddish brown discoloration, and contact dermatitis usually spares the axillary vault. Erythrasma, caused by *Corynebacterium minutissimum,* will demonstrate coral red fluorescence under the Wood's light. A condition known as benign *familial pemphigus* should also be considered. If an axillary lesion is nodular or raised, Fox-Fordyce disease and *hidradenitis suppurativa* enter the differential.

Intertrigo of the Inframammary Region can occur with or without *candidal infection.*

PRINCIPLES OF THERAPY

Correcting Precipitants. The first principle of therapy is to alter the conditions that cause maceration and irritation of closely apposed skin. The goal is to *promote drying,* which can be accomplished by exposing the intertriginous areas to air. The use of a fan or electric bulb can promote drying. A hand-held hair dryer set to a cool setting is very effective. Addition of a nonmedicated *absorbent powder* that does not contain cornstarch is helpful. Zeasorb powder, made from corncobs, is useful. (Cornstarch is to be avoided because it serves as a food source and stimulates the growth of local bacteria). The patient should be instructed to wear loose-fitting cotton clothing. Bras that provide good support are also helpful. Hot, humid environments and clothing made of wool, nylon, or synthetic fibers can precipitate or worsen intertrigo. Nylon panty hose are a common offender. Men with groin involvement should be encouraged to wear boxer shorts rather than briefs, and women should wear cotton rather than nylon panties. Ointments and greasy preparations retain moisture and exacerbate the condition. Exudative lesions should be treated by the application of *compresses containing Burow's solution,* prepared by adding one package or tablet to a pint of water.

Treating Secondary Infection. Any secondary infection should be treated. Pustules or scales should be examined microscopically and cultured for evidence of bacteria, yeast, and dermatophytes, after which appropriate therapy should be instituted (see Chapters 190 and 191). There is no evidence that antibacterial soaps are more effective than ordinary toilet soaps. Medicated powders should not be used.

Topical Corticosteroids. As long as the area of intertriginous disease is uninfected, topical corticosteroids may be added to reduce inflammation. The strength of the preparation should match the severity of the condition. *Hydrocortisone cream* is an effective, safe, low-cost therapy for patients with mild to moderate inflammation. Fluorinated topical corticosteroids are useful when inflammation is more severe, but these should be applied only for short periods because intertriginous striae and atrophy are common complications of more prolonged use.

Combination Preparations. Some steroid preparations promoted for use in intertrigo contain an *antifungal agent* (nystatin or clotrimazole) in addition to *corticosteroid.* The rationale is concurrent treatment or prevention of secondary candidal or dermatophyte infection. Mycolog-II cream is a combination of triamcinolone (a low-potency corticosteroid) and nystatin. Its original formulation also contained sensitizing antibacterial agents and preservatives. In a randomized, controlled study comparing it with hydrocortisone, no difference in outcome was noted. Lotrisone combines medium-potency betamethasone with clotrimazole. Lotions with an alcohol base are quite drying and may sting. The popular combination formulations Vioform-Hydrocortisone (which contains the antifungal agent clioquinol) and Vytone (iodoquinol and hydrocortisone) stain clothing yellow.

Topical medication should be used sparingly to avoid retention of moisture. Concurrent medical conditions such as diabetes or obesity should be treated.

PATIENT EDUCATION

The patient must understand the mechanical effects of skin occluding skin and be encouraged to dress accordingly to ensure adequate aeration and absorption of moisture. Women with large or pendulous breasts might benefit from use of a support bra and the placement of soft cotton cloths, gauze pads, or lamb's wool between the breasts and the chest wall. The patient should be taught to inspect intertriginous zones to detect the development of erythema and maceration so that effective therapy can be instituted early. In elderly, immobile patients, the physician should educate the family or a friend to inspect intertriginous areas to prevent maceration and secondary infection.

THERAPEUTIC RECOMMENDATIONS

- Eliminate precipitating conditions. Carefully dry the area that separates folds with absorbent material, dust with drying powders, and recommend loose, absorbent clothing. In exudative lesions, a drying agent such as Burow's solution should be used as a compress.
- Advise avoidance of potential contactants in axillary eruptions.
- Treat areas with mild to moderate inflammation with topical hydrocortisone. For more severe cases, use a low- to medium-potency fluorinated topical corticosteroid for short periods only.
- Treat any secondary bacterial or fungal infection with appropriate agents (see Chapters 190 and 191).

ANNOTATED BIBLIOGRAPHY

Bray GA. Health hazards of obesity. Endocrinol Metab Clin North Am 1996;25:907. (*Intertrigo, striae, hirsutism, acanthosis nigricans, and multiple papillomas are associated with obesity.*)

Brophy MC, Dunagin WG. Intertriginous dermatoses. Postgrad Med 1985;78:105. (*An excellent review of differential diagnosis.*)

Epstein NN, Epstein WL, Epstein JH. Atrophic striae in patients with intertrigo. Arch Dermatol 1963;87:450. (*Original report of the hazard of treating intertrigo with potent topical corticosteroids.*)

Hedley K, Tooley P, Williams H. Problems with clinical trials in general practice—a double-blind comparison of cream containing mi-conazole and hydrocortisone with hydrocortisone alone in the treatment of intertrigo. Br J Clin Pract 1990;4:131. (*A well-designed study showing no difference.*)

Sarkany I, Taplin D, Blank H. Incidence and bacteriology of erythrasma. Arch Dermatol 1962;85:578. (*Concise classic discussion of the disease and its causes.*)

189
Management of Corns and Calluses
WILLIAM V. R. SHELLOW

Corns and calluses are common, vexing lesions that can interfere with daily functioning. They may not be a presenting complaint, but the primary care physician is frequently asked about them. The tasks in the primary care setting are to provide diagnosis, simple therapy, advice on prevention, and timely referral if symptoms are refractory or disabling.

PATHOPHYSIOLOGY AND CLINICAL PRESENTATION

Corns (helomata, clavi) and calluses (tylomata) have a common pathologic origin. Friction and pressure on the skin overlying bony prominences lead to hyperemia, hypertrophy of dermal papillae, and proliferation of keratin. Corns often have a central, hard core that is painful if the lesion is pressed. Ill-fitting shoes are the most common cause, and the pressure of shoes on a corn may produce pain during walking. The most common locations are on the lateral aspect of the small toe and over the metatarsal heads on the plantar aspect of the foot. Hard corns have a translucent, cone-shaped avascular core with interruption of normal skin markings. Soft corns appear as macerated white or gray lesions that may resemble dermatophytosis, but they are tender. The fourth and first interdigital web spaces are favored sites. Calluses, but usually not corns, may develop in persons who do not wear shoes. Calluses do not contain a central core and tend to occur across the area of the metatarsal heads; normal skin markings are preserved. Women are two and a half times more likely to be bothered by corns and calluses than are men.

DIFFERENTIAL DIAGNOSIS

Calluses are skin-colored or yellowish elevated, thickened plaques that are seen in areas of friction. Calluses can be confused with plantar warts but can be distinguished from them by the preservation of normal skin markings; with verrucae, these markings are interrupted. When corns are pared down with a scalpel, one does not see the small, dark brown to black dots that represent thrombosed capillaries and are characteristic of warts.

PRINCIPLES OF THERAPY

The primary physician's major contribution to therapy is to encourage *prevention* through *patient education*. The elimination of friction and pressure is the essence of prevention. Shoes must fit correctly, and pressure over the toes must be evenly distributed. Softer shoe materials and sandals are often helpful. Stockings must fit properly and should cushion the foot. Keeping the feet dry by using powder and changing shoes daily also reduces friction. Careful explanation of the rationale for such measures is essential to ensuring patient compliance.

Symptomatic relief of calluses can be achieved by *paring* hyperkeratotic lesions with a No. 10 or 15 scalpel blade. Keratin should be shaved off with the blade held parallel to the skin. Repeated strokes of the blade should be made in a direction least likely to cause penetration should the patient move suddenly. Proximal to distal movement is best. After a callus is removed, it is essential that previous weight-bearing trauma not be continued, or the callus will recur.

Patients can treat corns and calluses themselves by intermittent debridement with *keratolytic agents*. Salicylic and lactic acid combinations and 40% salicylic acid plasters are used to reduce the thickness of tissue. The patient should cut a piece of 40% salicylic acid plaster that is smaller than the lesion and apply it to the skin. It may be left on overnight or for as long as several days. The dressing should be removed and the foot soaked. The softened and macerated skin can be removed with a BufPed or pumice stone. The plaster may be carefully reapplied as often as necessary to keep the lesions flat and asymptomatic.

The treatment of soft corns involves reducing excess perspiration. Use of absorbent *lamb's wool*, soaking the foot in potassium permanganate (1:4,000 solution), and cauterization with silver nitrate have all been successful.

Intrinsic bone problems subject the foot to uneven pressure. Any pronation, flat foot, or medial or lateral imbalance should be treated. Padding of lesions with felt moleskin or lamb's wool may prevent uneven distribution of external pressure. If the lesion is surrounded with foam rubber, pressure is distributed around the lesion rather than directly on it. If underlying bony abnormalities are suspected, x-ray films of the foot should be obtained.

One investigational technique is the injection of medical-grade silicone under corns to cushion the skin from underlying bone. The technique has been one of the few approved uses for injectable silicone, but it is confined to a few investigators. Other investigators have injected cross-linked collagen between the corn and the bone.

INDICATIONS FOR REFERRAL

Referral to a podiatrist or orthopedic surgeon is indicated if simple measures and advice fail to reduce symptoms or recurrences. Latex, plastic, or silicone molds can be individually adapted to prevent localized pressure from producing corns or calluses. Shoes can be constructed by a podiatrist to redistribute weight and pressure. Occasionally, surgical removal of a subjacent bony prominence eliminates the source of abnormal pressure on the skin. Diabetics and others with impaired vascular systems should receive foot care from a podiatrist.

THERAPEUTIC RECOMMENDATIONS

- Advise the patient to avoid tight shoes with pointed toes, to wear shoes that fit properly, and to change them frequently. Socks should cushion the sensitive area.
- Corns and calluses may be treated by the patient with proprietary plasters. The physician or patient can apply a keratolytic agent to the lesion in the form of a 40% salicylic acid plaster for several days. After the lesion has improved, the use of circular pads may prevent recurrence.
- Consider paring down a large lesion. Patients can perform this procedure themselves, but instruct them never to pull loose skin. Protect the tender area with moleskin after paring.
- After the lesions have been removed or pared down, ensure that the foot is not subjected to the same pressures that originally produced the problem.

- Patients with refractory lesions and lesions caused by underlying orthopedic disease should be referred to a podiatrist or orthopedist for definitive treatment of the structural problem. A molded shoe insert device may be prescribed. Diabetics and others with an insufficient vascular supply to the foot should receive regular foot care from a podiatrist.

ANNOTATED BIBLIOGRAPHY

Brainard BJ. Managing corns and plantar calluses. Physician Sports Med 1991;19:61. (*Corns and calluses arise from foot or ankle abnormalities, poorly fitting footwear, and overuse.*)

Collagen Podiatric Investigation Group. Subdermal collagen injections for the treatment of hyperkeratotic lesions. J Am Podiatr Med Assoc 1986;76:445. (*Discusses injectable collagen.*)

Holmes GB Jr, Timmerman L. A quantitative assessment of the effect of metatarsal pads on plantar pressures. Foot Ankle 1990;11:141. (*Orthotic devices such as a metatarsal pad can be an inexpensive and effective method of reducing metatarsal pressure.*)

Montgomery RM. Relieving painful feet. Geriatrics 1974;29:137. (*Practical tips useful in the office.*)

Sheard C. Simple management of plantar clavi. Cutis 1992;50:138. (*Freezing with liquid nitrogen to induce a blister followed by shaving of the crust in 3 to 4 weeks should eliminate the corn.*)

Singh D, Bentley G, Trevino SG. Callosities, corns and calluses. BMJ 1996;312:1403. (*An excellent review of the differences in these lesions and how to provide symptomatic relief to the patient.*)

190
Approach to Bacterial Skin Infections
WILLIAM V. R. SHELLOW

Part 1: Cellulitis

Cellulitis represents bacterial infection of the skin that involves the deeper subcutaneous layers. It must be differentiated from inflammatory skin changes caused by vascular insufficiency and phlebitis. Once cellulitis is identified, the primary physician has to decide who can be managed at home on oral antibiotics and who requires hospitalization.

PATHOPHYSIOLOGY AND CLINICAL PRESENTATION

Pathogenesis. Any process that causes a break in the integrity of the skin allows normal skin bacteria to invade the underlying subcutaneous tissue and initiate an inflammatory response. Trauma, stasis ulceration, ischemia, and chronic edema are common precipitants. Contiguous or hematogenous spread from other sites occurs uncommonly.

The organisms most commonly producing cellulitis are normal skin flora, with *Streptococcus* and *Staphylococcus aureus* predominating. Staphylococci produce disease through their ability to multiply and produce a host of extracellular enzymes, including α- and β-hemolysin, leukocidin, coagulase, hyaluronidase, and lipases. Streptococci produce more than 20 extracellular enzymes.

Conditions that impair the host response may predispose to skin infection by opportunistic organisms such as *gram-negative bacteria*. Skin infections with *Escherichia coli*, *Pseudomonas*, and *Klebsiella* are seen in immunosuppressed patients, diabetics, and alcoholics. Cellulitis in the perineum may be caused by enteric aerobic and anaerobic bacteria. Injury to mucosal surfaces predisposes to infection with *anaerobic organisms*. Anaerobic bacteria can produce hyaluronidase, proteases, neuraminidase, and extracellular enzymes, and they act synergistically with aerobic bacteria. Anaerobes play an important role in diabetic foot ulcers, abscesses, and traumatic wounds. Anaerobic infection also occurs in the setting of crush injuries. The degree of pain may be disproportionate to skin findings. A mixture of aerobic and anaerobic streptococci can cause fasciitis and cellulitis. Once connective tissue is involved, infection spreads along fascial planes.

In certain settings, cellulitis is caused by unusual organisms. In persons who handle fish, poultry, or meat, cellulitic infection with *Erysipelothrix rhusiopathiae* may occur. In patients with water-related injury and sometimes in those with immunosuppression, *Aeromonas hydrophila* can cause cellulitis. Animal bites or scratches, especially from cats, are associated with cellulitis caused by a *Pasteurella multocida* organism. *Vibrio* species have been implicated in salt water-related injuries. Arthropod bites are portals of entry for conventional streptococcal or staphylococcal species, but one must also consider the unusual spreading cellulitis, a reaction to the toxin of a *brown recluse spider* or a *fire ant*. Another unusual cause of cellulitis simulating a septic thrombophlebitis is *Campylobacter* infection, often in the context of a concurrent enteritis.

Clinical Presentation. Cellulitis presents with local redness, heat, swelling, and tenderness that develops over a few days. Fever, chills, and rigors herald possible bacteremia. The clinical presentation does not allow delineation of the specific microbial etiology. Red streaks extending proximally in conjunction with tender lymph nodes indicate an associated *lymphangitis*. Crepitus indicates gas production and suggests anaerobic involvement.

Invasive strains of *group A streptococci* (M-types 1 and 3) cause not only the usual forms of invasive streptococcal disease (scarlet fever, erysipelas, necrotizing fasciitis, myositis) but also a toxic shock–like syndrome associated with mucosal or cutaneous infection. Mortality is as high as 30%. Onset is abrupt, with fever, diarrhea, rigors, and scattered pains. Bacteremia may be detected in 60%; hematogenous spread is common.

WORKUP

Cellulitis first needs to be distinguished from other causes of focal erythema, swelling, and tenderness. *Superficial thrombophlebitis* may present similarly, but the inflammatory response is usually centered in the involved vein, which is tender and palpable. The dependent rubor of *arterial insufficiency* is generalized, nontender, and associated with diminished or absent pulses and a cold extremity. *Erythema nodosum* is indicated by lesions that are typically multiple, exquisitely tender, and often pretibial in location. It is a secondary phenomenon, and the cause needs to be ascertained. It should be remembered that cellulitis may occur concurrently with phlebitis or arterial insufficiency.

History. Once it is established that cellulitis is present, predisposing factors should be identified. A history is obtained for diabetes, congestive failure, recent trauma, leg edema, claudication, previous infection, tinea pedis, and loss of sensation. One should ask about IV drug use, occupational exposure, and any recent bites and stings. A history of fever with rigors suggests bacteremia.

Physical Examination. Note is made of the temperature, area(s) of skin involved, lymphangitic streaking, proximal lymphadenopathy, heart murmur, peripheral edema, diminished peripheral pulses, decreased sensation, and any breaks in the skin, ulceration, or atrophy. Marking the borders of the lesion with an indelible pen allows objective and rapid assessment of progression and resolution. Crepitus or foul odor is suggestive of anaerobic infection. One palpates for fluctuance and inspects the viability of surrounding tissue. Any tinea, dermatitis, venous insufficiency, or previous injury should be noted.

Laboratory Studies. A *complete blood cell count* and *differential* are always helpful in gauging the severity of infection and the hematologic response. Because most cases of cellulitis

are caused by streptococci or staphylococci, *bacterial culture of the skin* is not routinely performed. Moreover, it is difficult to culture the offending organism from unbroken skin. There is no evidence that aspiration from the advancing margin is superior to sampling from any other area of involved skin. Culture is indicated in patients who have open, weeping *wounds* or infection in unusual areas, such as the *perineum*. Material from such areas should be cultured both anaerobically and aerobically.

When rigors, fever, heart murmur, or lymphangitic spread is present or the patient is immunocompromised, two separate sets of *blood cultures* should be obtained before any antibiotics are administered. Blood cultures are positive in only 5% to 10% of cellulitis cases. If crepitus, fluctuance, or devitalization is present, obtain an x-ray film to look for gas production in soft tissue, which is indicative of gangrene. In diabetic or immunocompromised patients, or in situations of previous injury, radiography is important to be sure that osteomyelitis does not lurk beneath the cellulitis.

PRINCIPLES OF MANAGEMENT

The majority of patients can be treated as outpatients with oral antibiotics and supportive measures. Patients who are afebrile and in whom adenopathy and lymphangitis are absent may not even require antibiotics, but antibiotics are usually prescribed.

Antibiotics. The drugs of choice are either *penicillin* or a penicillinase-resistant *semisynthetic penicillin* preparation. There is little definitive evidence on which to base antibiotic selection. The high prevalence of streptococci, the sensitivity of some community-acquired staphylococci to penicillin, and the low cost of penicillin make it a reasonable choice. If after 24 to 48 hours the patient is still febrile or not improving, a penicillinase-resistant preparation can be substituted. The addition of probenecid as a morning dose can increase blood levels of oral penicillin. Antibiotic therapy should continue for 10 to 14 days, depending on the rate of clinical resolution.

Supportive Measures include *elevation* of the affected part and scrupulous prevention of new trauma. *Heat* may help to resolve cellulitis by promoting blood flow to the area. In patients with underlying conditions such as congestive heart failure, stasis dermatitis, and vascular insufficiency, *control of edema* and maintenance of *skin moisturization* helps prevent recurrent episodes.

In patients with open wounds, the risk for tetanus should be considered. If a booster of *tetanus toxoid* has not been obtained within 5 years, it should be given. Patients who have not had an initial tetanus series should receive both tetanus toxoid and tetanus immune globulin (see Chapter 6).

INDICATIONS FOR REFERRAL AND ADMISSION

Abscesses should be drained and necrotic tissues should be debrided, so prompt surgical referral is necessary. Hospitalization and IV antibiotics are indicated for compromised hosts who are at risk for hematogenous spread of infection (e.g., patients with poorly controlled diabetes, alcoholics, IV drug abusers, HIV-infected persons). Other indications for prompt hospital admission and IV antibiotics include rapidly progressive or recurrent infection, cellulitis caused by group A streptococci, the presence of subcutaneous gas or necrotizing fasciitis, and cellulitis of the orbit, face, or perineum, especially when accompanied by fever and lymphangitis. Clinical signs that suggest a need for IV therapy include high fever, systemic symptoms, and pain more severe than the clinical appearance would indicate. In cases of progression despite the administration of oral antibiotics, the outpatient approach to treatment must be reconsidered. When patients appear unreliable and unable to care for themselves at home, admission is also indicated. Services that allow home administration of IV antibiotics and professional monitoring can help shorten a hospital stay.

PATIENT EDUCATION

When a lower extremity is involved, the patient should be instructed to rest in bed and elevate the limb. Getting up to go to the bathroom is allowed, but bed rest is mandatory. Exercises and anticoagulation may be needed to reduce the possibility of thrombophlebitis in patients at increased risk (see Chapter 35). It is crucial to protect the affected area and insist that the patient not scratch the involved skin. The importance of taking antibiotic therapy as instructed should be emphasized. The patient should be asked to report progress by telephone and to call if cellulitis fails to resolve within 5 to 7 days.

THERAPEUTIC RECOMMENDATIONS

- Hospitalize patients unable to care for themselves reliably at home, and also anyone with high fever, rigors, lymphangitis, rapid progression, compromised host defenses, or involvement of the face, orbit, or perineum.
- Treat the patient with mild, uncomplicated illness on an ambulatory basis. Begin with 500 mg of oral *phenoxymethyl penicillin* four times daily (1 hour before meals and at bedtime), and monitor closely during the next 48 hours.
- If inflammation and fever do not begin to resolve after 48 hours or if close monitoring is not possible, prescribe a penicillinase-resistant penicillin (e.g., 500 mg of *dicloxacillin* four times daily).
- For patients markedly allergic to penicillin (type I hypersensitivity), prescribe 500 mg of *erythromycin* four times daily. Cephalosporins, such as *cephalexin*, may be substituted if the allergy to penicillin is not well documented and was not anaphylactoid. The fluoroquinolones, such as *ciprofloxacin*, are effective against gram-negative cellulitis; however, they have only moderate antistreptococcal and antistaphylococcal activity in vitro and should be used cautiously in cellulitis.
- If anaerobes are suspected, then a fluoroquinolone plus *clindamycin* or *metronidazole* is indicated.
- Patients with an open wound but without a recent tetanus booster in the past 10 years should be given 0.5 mL of tetanus toxoid IM.

ANNOTATED BIBLIOGRAPHY

Brook I, Frazier EH. Aerobic and anaerobic microbiology of infection after trauma. Am J Emerg Med 1998;16:585. (*Only anaerobic bacteria were isolated in 32%; the predominant organisms were Bacteroides fragilis, Peptostreptococcus, and Clostridium. Only aerobic bacteria were isolated in 16%; the predominant organisms were E. coli, S. aureus, Streptococcus, and Klebsiella. Mixed aerobic and anaerobic organisms were isolated in 52%.*)

Brook I, Frazier EH. Aerobic and anaerobic infection associated with malignancy. Support Care Cancer 1998;6:125. (*Only anaerobic organisms were isolated in 30%, only aerobic organisms in 34%, and mixed aerobic and anaerobic organisms in 35%. The organisms were similar to those listed in the above citation.*)

File TM Jr, Tan JS, DiPersio JR. Group A streptococcal necrotizing fasciitis. Diagnosis and treating the "flesh-eating bacteria syndrome." Cleve Clin J Med 1998;65:241. (*During the past decade, the incidence of this condition has increased. Appropriate management requires prompt recognition, immediate antibiotic therapy, and surgical debridement or excision; 40 references.*)

Goldstein EJ, Citron DM, Nesbit CA. Diabetic foot infections. Bacteriology and activity of 10 oral antimicrobial agents against bacteria isolated from consecutive cases. Diabetes Care 1996;19:638. (*S. aureus was isolated from 76% of patients. Streptococci, enterococci, Enterobacteriaceae, and anaerobes were also present in about 40%. Sparfloxacin and levofloxacin were the most active agents tested.*)

Hauser AR. Another toxic shock syndrome. Streptococcal infection is even more dangerous than the staphylococcal form. Postgrad Med 1998;104:31,39,43. (*Hypotension, confusion, or unexplained renal insufficiency are clues to streptococcal toxic shock syndrome. Even with aggressive therapy, mortality can exceed 50%.*)

Hook EW III, Hooton TM, Horton CA, et al. Microbiologic evaluation of cutaneous cellulitis in adults. Arch Intern Med 1986;146:295. (*Efficacy of leading margin aspirates examined; 25% positive culture rate.*)

Leder K, Turnidge JD, Grayson ML. Home-based treatment of cellulitis with twice-daily cefazolin. Med J Aust 1998;169:5192. (*Eighty-nine percent of patients with moderate to severe cellulitis were cured with 2 g of cefazolin given twice daily IV at home; the median number of doses was 11, with a range of 3 to 27.*)

Lewis RT. Soft-tissue infections. World J Surg 1998;22:146. (*Classification of soft-tissue infections is based on the degree of localization and the presence of tissue necrosis.*)

Majeski J, Majeski E. Necrotizing fasciitis: improved survival with early recognition by tissue biopsy and aggressive surgical treatment. South Med J 1997;90:1065. (*During a 15-year period, 43 patients underwent bedside biopsy with local anesthesia, which was followed immediately by frozen-section evaluation. Twelve were found to have necrotizing fasciitis and were treated appropriately, and all survived. No gangrene developed in those with negative biopsy findings.*)

Schmid MR, Kossmann T, Duewell S. Differentiation of necrotizing fasciitis and cellulitis using MR imaging. AJR Am J Roentgenol 1998;170;615. (*When no deep fascial involvement is seen with magnetic resonance imaging, necrotizing fasciitis can be excluded.*)

Part 2: Management of Pyoderma

The common cutaneous bacterial infections include impetigo, ecthyma, folliculitis, furunculosis, and erysipelas. They must be recognized promptly by the primary physician and treated effectively with antibiotics.

PATHOPHYSIOLOGY AND CLINICAL PRESENTATION

The clinical manifestations are a function of the causative organism, environmental factors, area of skin involved, and host resistance. Primary cutaneous bacterial infections develop on normal skin and are usually initiated by a single organism, such as coagulase-positive staphylococci or β-hemolytic streptococci. Secondary bacterial infection is infection superimposed on diseased skin. Cutaneous bacterial infections may also be classified according to the depth of infection and the propensity for scarring.

Impetigo, a common condition caused primarily by *S. aureus*, begins as a small, erythematous macular lesion that evolves into a vesicle beneath the stratum corneum. The thin-roofed collection of fluid ruptures easily, leaving denuded, oozing areas. A honey-colored crust forms as the fluid dries and collects. Intense erythema at the base of the pustule suggests a β-hemolytic streptococcal component to the condition. New lesions appear in the same location, and they coalesce. When the honey-colored crusts are removed, the skin appears raw. Individual lesions usually do not exceed 2 cm in size. Impetigo is seen most frequently in children, but it also occurs in adults, especially those with poor hygiene. In adults, the condition is not as contagious as it is among infants. The face is the most common site of involvement. Ordinary lesions do not produce scarring but may leave erythematous marks for some time. Untreated infections may last for weeks.

Ecthyma is a deeper version of impetigo, usually caused by *streptococci*, but it is sometimes a sign of gram-negative sepsis or fungal infection. Erosion of the epidermis creates ulcerative, crusted lesions. The heaped-up crust conceals the underlying erosion. Healing is accompanied by some scarring because of the depth of the lesions. The legs are commonly involved, and children are more susceptible than are adults. Antecedent conditions include eczema, scabies, arthropod bites, trauma, and living in a hot, humid climate. The *brown recluse spider bite*, characterized by necrotizing ulcer and spreading ecthyma, is important to recognize because it requires specific therapy with dapsone.

Folliculitis is infection of the hair follicles, usually caused by coagulase-positive *staphylococci*, and may be divided into superficial and deep types. Superficial folliculitis consists of a small pustule pierced by the hair shaft. It may be seen on the scalp or other hairy portions of the body. Occupational exposure to cutting oils and the use of coal tar products or topical corticosteroids under occlusive dressings may precipitate folliculitis. Fungal folliculitis caused by *Pityrosporum ovale* may resemble bacterial folliculitis, but it is refractory to treatment with antibiotics. The diagnosis is made by the finding of yeast-like organisms on a potassium hydroxide wet mount, but a skin biopsy specimen stained for fungi is sometimes required. Rarely, small pustules with surrounding erythema caused by *Propionibacterium acnes* may develop around the occiput in male patients. *Pseudomonas folliculitis* has been described in association with bathing in hot tubs.

Furuncles and Carbuncles may develop from a preceding folliculitis and are limited to hairy areas. The erythematous lesions usually become fluctuant after 4 days. A yellowish, pointed area may be seen on the surface, and, if the lesion ruptures spontaneously, pus and necrotic tissue are extruded. The buttocks, axillae, neck, face, and waist areas are common sites of involvement. Predisposing systemic factors include diabetes,

malnutrition, obesity, and hematologic disorders. Carbuncles are a coalescence of deep furuncles with multiple points of drainage.

Erysipelas, caused by *β-hemolytic streptococci* (mainly group A, but also groups G, C, and B), is characterized by a peripherally spreading, infiltrated, erythematous, sharply circumscribed plaque. The lesion is warm to the touch. The face, scalp, hands, and genitals are frequently involved. Rapid evolution of the lesions is seen, and some patients have constitutional symptoms such as fever and malaise. Poor hygiene and lowered resistance promote infection. Trauma may elicit infection, and recurrent erysipelas may lead to brawny edema and lymphostasis (*elephantiasis verrucosa nostra*) in the lower extremities.

DIAGNOSIS

Lesions are usually diagnosed and treated on the basis of clinical appearance, but microscopic examination of Gram's-stained material is a quick and inexpensive way to confirm a diagnosis. Culture and sensitivity testing are usually not necessary for superficial infections but are needed for more destructive lesions or cases that fail to improve.

PRINCIPLES OF THERAPY

Physical measures are used to enhance resolution and make the skin surface less amenable to colonization by bacteria, and antibiotics are given to treat responsible pathogens and prevent recolonization.

Physical Measures. The physical measures employed differ with the pyoderma being treated. The crusts of impetigo must be debrided to expose the skin surface where bacteria are present. The use of a washcloth for this purpose is recommended. Furuncles and carbuncles are treated with hot compresses to enhance drainage. Fluctuant lesions usually require incision and drainage. Sometimes, packing of the wound is necessary. With exudative lesions, drying compresses are required to remove detritus and desiccate the lesion. Saline solution, tap water, or Burow's solution may be applied for 10 to 20 minutes three to four times a day. Dehydration improves the appearance of the skin and destroys many organisms.

Antibiotics. *Topical antibiotics* are usually sufficient for impetigo and folliculitis, particularly when combined with cleansing and debridement. Most cases of pyoderma are caused by gram-positive organisms and respond to topical *erythromycin* or *bacitracin*. *Mupirocin* (Bactroban), a creamy antibiotic ointment, is so effective that it has supplanted the use of systemic antibiotics in many cases. It is cosmetically well tolerated, although it appears slightly shiny on the skin. Washing with *chlorhexidine* (Hibiclens) is a valuable adjunct because of its bactericidal properties. Patients should wash the areas with the liquid two or three times daily before mupirocin is applied. Antibiotic creams and ointments containing *neomycin* can be used, although neomycin is a known contact sensitizer. However, sensitization usually develops only after long-term use on areas that are denuded.

Reducing colonization is particularly important in the treatment of recurrent furunculosis. Frequent cleansing with soap, particularly chlorhexidine, is useful. Nails should be clipped and vigorously scrubbed. *Mupirocin* ointment should be instilled into the anterior nares. It can be used on a long-term basis to reduce bacterial carriage in the nares of patients in whom pyoderma repeatedly develops. Additional preventive measures include soaking the beard with hot water for 5 minutes before shaving, and discarding blades after each use. Alternatively reusable razor blades can be soaked in rubbing alcohol. Separate towels, sheets, and clothing should be used, and frequently laundered and changed. If vigorous reduction of colonization is unsuccessful, consideration should be given to replacement of pathogenic staphylococci with a less pathogenic strain.

Systemic antibiotics are indicated when constitutional symptoms are present or if the patient is uncooperative. Phenoxymethyl *penicillin* is sufficient for streptococcal infection; oral *erythromycin* is effective against most staphylococcal and streptococcal species that cause pyoderma. Azithromycin is a good alternative. Resistant staphylococcal species may require *dicloxacillin* or *cephalexin*. There is no evidence that antibiotic therapy prevents poststreptococcal glomerulonephritis. As noted, antibiotic selection may be based on clinical appearance, but microscopic examination of Gram's-stained material is quick and inexpensive. Culture and sensitivity testing are reserved for more destructive lesions or cases that fail to improve.

PATIENT EDUCATION AND INDICATIONS FOR REFERRAL

A primary consideration in the therapy of all cases of pyoderma is patient education. Teaching aggressive and regular use of cleansing and debridement is central to the successful resolution of the infection. In addition, careful review of preventive measures and antibiotic use is essential.

If aggressive hygienic measures and attempts to eliminate the staphylococcal carrier state fail to prevent recurrent infection, consider referral for replacement with nonpathogenic staphylococci or treatment with rifampin, which is effective for eradicating nasal carriage of pathogenic staphylococci.

THERAPEUTIC RECOMMENDATIONS

Impetigo

- Apply compresses soaked in Burow's solution for 20 minutes two to four times daily, then debride gently with a washcloth and cleanse with a chlorhexidine-containing agent.
- Lightly apply mupirocin to the area after drying. A nighttime application is also advised.
- Advise the patient not to cover the lesions and the family to avoid using the same towel or washcloth; keep children away from the patient with impetigo.

Folliculitis

- Treat with debridement and topical antibiotics, as for impetigo.

Furuncles and Carbuncles

- Treat with hot compresses until the lesions are fluctuant and spontaneous drainage occurs. Larger lesions may require re-

moval of the core with a 4-mm biopsy punch to facilitate drainage.
- Treat furuncles or carbuncles that are associated with cellulitis or fever or that are located on the face with oral anti-staphylococcal antibiotics, either erythromycin (333 mg three times daily for 10 days) or dicloxacillin (250 mg four times daily for 10 days).
- Treat recurrent infection with a 10- to 14-day course of a systemic antibiotic and remove bacteria from potential sources, such as the skin, nares, nails, and razors and other fomites.

Erysipelas

- Treat with cool compresses and phenoxymethyl penicillin (500 mg four times daily) for 7 to 10 days.

Recurrent Pyoderma

- Eradicate the staphylococcal nasal carrier state. Prescribe oral dicloxacillin (500 mg four times daily for 10 to 14 days) in combination with topical mupirocin applied twice daily for at least 5 days.

ANNOTATED BIBLIOGRAPHY

Bisno AL, Stevens DL. Streptococcal infections of skin and soft tissues. N Engl J Med 1996;334:240. (*Current concepts in the range of infections caused by this organism.*)

Bisno AL. Cutaneous infections: microbiologic and epidemiologic considerations. Am J Med 1984;76:172. (*Important review.*)

Carroll JA. Common bacterial pyodermas. Taking aim against the most likely pathogens. Postgrad Med 1996;100:311,317. (*Recommended antibiotic treatment for all common cutaneous infections.*)

Duncan WC, Dodge BG, Knox JM. Prevention of superficial pyogenic skin infections. Arch Dermatol 1969;99:465. (*The regular use of an antibacterial soap reduced the incidence of superficial bacterial infections.*)

Heskel NS, Siepman NC, Pichotta PJ, et al. Erythromycin versus cefadroxil in the treatment of skin infections. Int J Dermatol 1992;31:131. (*The two antibiotics were equally effective.*)

McLinn S. A bacteriologically controlled, randomized study comparing the efficacy of 2% mupirocin (Bactroban) with oral erythromycin in the treatment of patients with impetigo. J Am Acad Dermatol 1990;22:883. (*Two percent mupirocin was as effective as oral erythromycin.*)

Odell ML. Skin and wound infections: an overview. Am Fam Physician 1998;57:2424. (*A practical review of common infections.*)

Reagan DR, Doebbeling BN, Pfaller MA, et al. Elimination of coincident *Staphylococcus aureus* nasal and hand carriage with intranasal application of mupirocin calcium ointment. Ann Intern Med 1991;114:101. (*At 3 months, 71% of subjects remained free of nasal staphylococci; hand cultures positive for organisms were reduced to 2.9%.*)

Sadick NS. Current aspects of bacterial infections of the skin. Dermatol Clin 1997;15:341. (*A very practical review with specific recommendations; 50 references.*)

Shriner DL, Schwartz RA, Janniger CK. Impetigo. Cutis 1995;56:30. (*A discussion of bullous and nonbullous varieties, with differential diagnoses*).

191

Management of Superficial Fungal Infections

WILLIAM V. R. SHELLOW

Although they are neither dangerous nor life-threatening, superficial fungal infections are prevalent, irritating, and often recurrent. They are easily diagnosed but commonly confused with nonfungal dermatoses such as impetigo (see Chapter 184). The primary physician should be capable of providing a definitive diagnosis, cost-effective therapy, and patient education for prevention.

PATHOPHYSIOLOGY AND CLINICAL PRESENTATION

Why some people resist these ubiquitous pathogens while others cannot remains unknown. Sometimes, a systemic disease such as diabetes is responsible. Hereditary factors may be involved. Dampness, darkness, and friction leading to skin maceration are important local precipitants.

Fungal infection occurs when one of these ubiquitous organisms invades the superficial layers of the skin. Dermatophytes do not invade below the level of keratin because a potent antifungal factor prevents deeper infection. Candidal infection produces inflammatory change through elaboration of an endotoxin-like substance.

Dermatophytic and candidal infections produce scaly, erythematous lesions with defined margins; these occur in characteristic areas of the body that promote the growth of fungi.

Tinea Versicolor (Pityriasis Versicolor) is characterized by brown, pink, red, or white scaly patches on the chest, back, and shoulders. During the summer, it may present as hypopigmented areas that are sometimes erroneously interpreted as vitiligo. The organism appears to prevent pigment transfer from melanocytes to epidermal cells. The diagnosis can be suspected if scratching a macular area raises a small amount of fine scale. Examination of the skin with a Wood's light reveals gold or orange-brown fluorescence. The infection is confirmed by scraping a scaly lesion and examining it with a drop of 20% potassium hydroxide for characteristic short hyphae and spores, sometimes referred to as *"spaghetti and meatballs."*

Dermatophyte Infections are defined by the area of the body they affect. The most common is *tinea cruris*, which involves the groin and inner thighs and sometimes even extends onto the abdomen and buttocks. *Tinea pedis* is characterized by blisters and inflammation on the soles and interdigital areas of the feet. *Tinea corporis* affects other areas of the body, including the trunk and extremities. If the face is involved, the condition may be called *tinea faciei*. *Tinea capitis*, or scalp ringworm, occurs almost exclusively in children. *Tinea barbae*, involving the bearded area, has become very uncommon and therefore might be missed in the differential diagnosis of a facial rash. *Onychomycosis* is characterized by the accumulation of subungual keratin, which produces a thickened, distorted, crumbling nail. *Trichophyton rubrum*, *Trichophyton mentagrophytes*, and *Epidermophyton floccosum* are the most common infecting organisms. *Microsporum canis*, which is acquired by contact with infected pet cats and dogs, is another common pathogenic fungus.

Candida Infections of the skin occur principally in *intertriginous* locations, such as the axillae, groin, intergluteal folds, inframammary area, and interdigital web spaces. Crusted involvement of the labial commissures, known as *perlèche*, and involvement of the *glans penis* also occur. The presence of erythema on the glans penis and scrotum suggests a candidal rather than a dermatophyte infection. Lesions are pustular and thin-walled, located on a red base, and often produce burning and itching. Candidiasis may be clinically suspected in the presence of characteristic *satellite pustules* outside the margin of the primary lesion.

DIAGNOSIS

The finding of scaly, erythematous lesions with defined margins in characteristic areas of the body that promote the growth of fungi should raise suspicion of a superficial fungal infection. Satellite pustules suggest a candidal involvement. In intertriginous areas, fungal infection must be differentiated from intertrigo and erythrasma. Asymptomatic, slightly erythematous to light brown, finely scaling patches in the groin and upper thigh with little or no central clearing are characteristic of erythrasma (a corynebacterial infection). Early intertrigo is characterized by slight maceration and erythema. With time, the redness becomes more intense, and the epidermis becomes eroded or even denuded.

Potassium Hydroxide Preparation. When dermatophyte infection is suspected, microscopic examination of scrapings from an involved area of skin is required. To prepare a specimen for microscopic examination, the border of the lesion is scraped lightly with a No. 15 scalpel blade or the edge of a microscope slide. The scale is collected onto a clean microscope slide, and a coverslip is used to push all the scale into a small mound. One or, at most, two drops of 20% potassium hydroxide solution or potassium hydroxide with dimethyl sulfoxide (DMSO) are placed in the center of the mound of scale, and a coverslip is laid over it. If the potassium hydroxide solution does not contain DMSO, the slide must be heated lightly to improve "clearing" of the epithelial cells. If DMSO is present, heating is not required.

Under a magnification of 40× with reduced light, threadlike hyphae can be seen crossing cell walls. If budding spores and pseudohyphae are found, the diagnosis is candidal infection.

The presence of branched, septate hyphae can be confirmed by using higher power (100x). This second step is necessary to make sure that artifacts are not being mistaken for hyphae. The wet mount should be examined within a few hours. Especially if potassium hydroxide with DMSO is used, the hyphae will dissolve after a period of time. Occasionally, a scraping must be planted on Sabouraud's dextrose agar for culturing to identify the fungal infection.

If candidal infection is identified or topical fungal infection is recurrent or extensive, one should check for conditions associated with immune compromise (e.g., HIV infection, diabetes, cirrhosis, lymphoma, steroid use, chemotherapy).

PRINCIPLES OF MANAGEMENT

Effective management requires attention to predisposing factors and proper use of antifungal agents. For example, systemically, diabetes control should be tightened and the use of immunosuppressive agents cut back. Locally, the *elimination of moisture* and *prevention of maceration* are priorities (see below and Chapter 188). Further drying of inflammatory or weeping lesions can be achieved with the application of compresses containing an astringent such as aluminum acetate, available as *Burow's* tablets or packets.

After predisposing factors have been reduced and the lesions dried, specific antifungal medication is appropriate. A host of effective agents are available. One should identify and use the least expensive, most effective agent that produces the fewest side effects. Patients with fungal infections have invariably tried over-the-counter remedies before they visit the physician. It is important to find out what they have used before prescribing the same product in its prescription version.

Antifungal Agents

Topical Agents. Four classes of topical antifungal agents are currently available (azoles, ethanolamines, allylamines, and polyene antibiotics). The over-the-counter preparations are the least expensive (although not necessarily inexpensive). New topical antifungal agents appear regularly and are usually the most costly (e.g., butenafine, terbinafine). Claims of unique efficacy are made for each one, but most within a given class provide similar cure rates. Most topical agents provide a cure rate of better than 85% for acute infections, but the rate is much lower for chronic infections. Topical lotions are more drying, less messy, and more useful for daytime application; a cream should be used at night.

Azoles comprise the largest class of topical antifungal agents; the older ones (*miconazole, clotrimazole, tolnaftate*) are available without prescription. Others include *econazole* (Spectazole), *oxiconazole* (Oxistat), *sulconazole* (Exelderm), and *ketoconazole* (Nizoral). In general, these are slightly less effective than the allylamines for the treatment of tinea pedis, but the nonprescription preparations are considerably less expensive.

Ethanolamines. This class of agents is represented solely by *ciclopirox olamine* (Loprox). The drug is best at penetrating the nail plate, which makes it useful as an adjunct topical treatment of onychomycosis.

Allylamines. These agents include *naftifine* (Naftin) and *terbinafine* (Lamisil). *Butenafine* (Mentax) has a structure similar to that of the allylamines. The allylamines are unique in that they are both fungicidal and fungistatic. Cure rates are slightly better with these agents, but cost tends to be substantially higher.

Polyene Antibiotics. Topical *amphotericin* and *nystatin* represent this class of antifungals. They are primarily anticandidal.

Combination Therapy. If marked improvement of clinical lesions and symptoms is not seen within 3 weeks, it may help to try *combination therapy*, with an antifungal agent from one class used during the day and another from a different class applied at night.

Oral Drugs. Orally administered systemic therapy may deserve consideration if a patient's condition appears to be refractory to topical therapy and discomfort from the superficial fungal infection is sufficiently severe. The risks and benefits must be weighed carefully. Such therapy is most likely to be appropriate for patients who are immunocompromised (e.g., those with HIV infection, lymphoma, chemotherapy, cirrhosis). However, the systemic antifungal agents are potentially toxic to bone marrow and liver and must be used with care, especially if prolonged courses of therapy are needed. Rapid clearing of dermatophyte infection is likely to follow, but relapses are common and recurrent courses of therapy may be necessary. An awareness of the risks associated with the commonly used oral therapies helps inform clinical decision making.

Itraconazole (Sporanox) is an orally active azole. Common side effects include nausea and abdominal discomfort; hepatitis has been reported. The potential for important *drug–drug interactions* is considerable because itraconazole *inhibits hepatic microsomal cytochrome systems*. The concentrations of many hepatically metabolized drugs are increased substantially, including digoxin, terfenadine, astemizole, triazolam, sulfonylureas, cisapride, felodipine, and quinidine. *Fatal cardiac arrhythmias* (torsades de pointes) have occurred in patients taking *terfenadine* or *cisapride* concurrently. When itraconazole is taken concurrently with *oral hypoglycemics*, the risk for severe, prolonged *hypoglycemia* is increased. High doses can cause hypokalemia and hypertension, and thrombocytopenia and leukopenia have been reported.

Terbinafine (Lamisil), an allylamine also approved for oral use in onychomycosis, causes fewer drug–drug interactions than itraconazole does, but rare instances of serious *skin reactions* (e.g., Stevens-Johnson syndrome), symptomatic *hepatobiliary dysfunction*, and *ocular lens* and *retinal changes* have been reported. The drug is cleared by the liver, and clearance is reduced by concurrent use of cimetidine or terfenadine. Common side effects include headache (13% of patients), gastrointestinal upset (16%), rash (6%), liver enzyme abnormalities (3%), and taste disturbances (3%). Liver enzymes should be measured before treatment is begun and again after 6 weeks if a longer treatment course is contemplated. The complete blood cell count should also be monitored because of reported instances of severe but reversible neutropenia.

Griseofulvin, the original oral antifungal for onychomycosis, can cause leukopenia, so that periodic blood cell counts are necessary. Liver function also must be monitored because of the risk for hepatocellular injury. Bone marrow suppression and serious hepatocellular toxicity are uncommon complications.

Headache, nausea, and abdominal discomfort are common side effects.

Ketoconazole (Nizoral). Immunocompromised patients with superficial fungal infection too widespread to be managed with topical therapy are candidates for systemic *ketoconazole*. For best results, ketoconazole should be taken with an acidic fruit juice to enhance absorption. Side effects include itching, rash, and dizziness. Serum testosterone is reduced, which may lead to gynecomastia in men and menstrual irregularities in women. Mild hepatocellar injury is common; severe impairment is rare. The risk for fatal idiosyncratic hepatotoxicity is nil when ketoconazole is taken for less than 2 weeks, but the drug should be stopped immediately whenever symptomatic hepatocellular dysfunction appears.

Fluconazole (Diflucan) is well tolerated and useful for candidal infections, but it can be teratogenic and in rare instances is associated with hepatic necrosis, Stevens-Johnson syndrome, and anaphylaxis. Gastrointestinal upset and rash are common. A few drug–drug interactions have been noted, including potentiation of phenytoin, anti-HIV agents (zidovudine, indinavir), warfarin, and sulfonylureas.

Treatment of Specific Conditions

Tinea Versicolor. For effectiveness, convenience, and least expense, a 2.5% suspension of *selenium sulfide* (Selsun) or a *pyrithione zinc* shampoo (Zincon, Head & Shoulders) can be applied with a rough washcloth. It should be allowed to remain on the affected areas for 10 minutes and then rinsed off. Daily application for 1 week is recommended. An 87% success rate at the end of 4 weeks was found with use of this program. In refractory cases, selenium sulfide suspension can be left on the skin overnight, with care taken to avoid the scrotal area. The topical antifungal agents are much more expensive but are useful in treating recalcitrant involvement of small areas. *Ketoconazole shampoo* is quite effective for treating tinea versicolor.

After treatment, patients should be reexamined for continued scaling, which suggests persistent activity. Patients with no signs of persistence or relapse should be advised that depigmentation may persist until they go back into the sun.

For immunocompromised patients with infection too widespread to be managed with topical therapy, systemic *ketoconazole* is worth consideration. A dose of 200 mg is prescribed daily for 7 to 10 days. For best results, ketoconazole should be taken with an acidic fruit juice. An alternative method is to take 400 mg once, then exercise to induce sweating. The patient is advised not to shower until the next day. This regimen is repeated 1 week later and can also be repeated monthly to prevent recurrence.

Other Diffuse Forms of Tinea. In moist intertriginous areas, the patient should dry oozing lesions by applying compresses soaked in *Burow's solution* for 30 to 60 minutes one to three times daily. A nonmedicated or antifungal *powder* may be used to absorb moisture. With very inflamed pruritic lesions of the groin and other intertriginous areas, the addition of a *topical corticosteroid* can help relieve the inflammatory component, and a topical corticosteroid is often prescribed in conjunction with topical antifungal therapy (see Chapter 188). Topical treatment suffices when glabrous skin is involved, but systemic drugs should be considered if hair sheaths are involved, involvement is widespread, or folliculitis develops.

Tinea Pedis. Athlete's foot is sometimes difficult to treat. The patient must be instructed to wear nonocclusive leather footwear or sandals and absorbent cotton socks, and to dry the feet frequently without rubbing, perhaps by using a hair dryer. *Topical antifungals* alone often suffice. The allylamines are more effective than the azoles, but they are much more expensive than the nonprescription azoles and might be reserved for refractory cases. Naftifine cream used once daily is effective for tinea pedis and may yield better results than clotrimazole used twice daily. If widespread scaling with hyperkeratosis occurs ("moccasin-type" tinea pedis), *keratolytic agents* are required. The nightly application of Keralyt gel (6% salicylic acid) under occlusion, with antifungal creams used two to three times daily, may successfully treat this difficult problem.

Onychomycosis. Nail involvement by fungus is extremely refractory to treatment, although fingernail infections usually respond better than do toenail infections. Most topical agents cannot penetrate the nail plate, but *topical ciclopirox* (Loprox) may, and it can be tried nightly with applications under occlusion. Weeks to months of treatment may be necessary before improvement is noted. Often, topical therapy is insufficient, and the question of employing systemic antifungal therapy comes up. The value of the cosmetic benefit must be weighed against the cost and risks of prolonged systemic treatment. Even with successful therapy, relapse is common.

Itraconazole (Sporanox) is aggressively promoted for the systemic treatment of onychomycosis. Dosing can be continuous (200 mg daily for 6 weeks for fingernail infections and 12 weeks for toenail infections) or intermittent (pulsed). In pulsed dosing, 200 mg of itraconazole is given twice daily for 1 week each month. Fingernail infections are treated with two pulses and toenails with three to four. Clinical cure rates of 93% have been reported with pulsed dosing, versus only 80% with continuous therapy. In trials comparing itraconazole with terbinafine, another antifungal agent used to treat onychomycosis (see below), mycologic cure rates approached 65% with a 3-month course of once-daily therapy. The drug remains in the nails for up to 9 months after discontinuation of treatment. The nails will probably not be clear when the drug is stopped, and the patient must be told that continued clearing is to be expected during the next several months.

Terbinafine (Lamisil) is another heavily promoted agent for the treatment of onychomycosis. Mycologic cure rates of 75% to 90% at 1 year have been noted. In blinded comparison studies, results have been superior to those for itraconazole at 1 year. However, relapse rates are still in the range of 15%. This drug is taken once daily (250 mg) for 6 weeks for fingernail infections and for 12 weeks for toenail infections. As noted above, in comparison with itraconazole, terbinafine causes fewer drug–drug interactions, but the complete blood cell count and liver enzymes should be monitored periodically because of the potential for bone marrow and liver injury.

Griseofulvin used to be the only available systemic treatment for onychomycosis. Treatment (250 mg two to four times daily) must be continued for 6 to 12 months until the infected portion of the nail has grown out to the end. Sometimes, it is necessary to remove the affected nail. Use has declined with the advent of safer, better-tolerated oral antifungal agents. Even if a cure is obtained, reinfection is common.

Ketoconazole was formerly used to treat patients with severe disease who did not respond to griseofulvin or who could not tolerate it, but because the risk for hepatotoxicity is greatly increased during prolonged treatment, some authorities no longer recommend that it be used for this condition, especially now that less toxic alternatives are available (see above). Baseline liver function should be documented with testing and laboratory studies repeated at least monthly.

Fluconazole is an effective systemic antifungal agent. To date, it has not yet been approved for use in onychomycosis. Based on clinical trails, the expected dosing schedule will be 300 mg once a week for up to 9 months.

Cost. The oral antifungal agents used to treat onychomycosis of the toenails can be compared by cost. According to the average wholesale prices given in the 1999 Costs and Comparisons (red book), a 12-month course of Gris-PEG (250 mg four times daily) would cost $1,577, and a course of Fulvicin P/G (330 mg three times daily) would cost $1,467. Sporanox given as four pulses would cost $876; three pulses would cost $657. Twelve weeks of Lamisil would cost $613. Because these are wholesale prices, the patient would have to pay more.

Summary. The cosmetic effects of fungal nail infection and the enhanced efficacy of available systemic agents should be weighed against the considerable expense of such therapy, its potentially serious side effects, and the need for careful monitoring and frequent blood testing. Many patients will choose to live with their fungal nail infection, especially when it is limited to the toenails (use of separate nail clippers helps to prevent spread). Many women find that they can substantially reduce cosmetic unsightliness by filing down the hyperkeratotic nail and covering it with nail polish.

Candidal Infections. Treatment begins with attention to predisposing factors, such as the use of systemic corticosteroids, birth control pills, tetracycline, and other antibiotics and the presence of diabetes, Cushing's syndrome, and HIV infection. One proceeds to meticulous drying of the area, adequate exposure to air, and specific anticandidal therapy. Gentian violet or Castellani's paint are time-proven but quite messy remedies and have largely been abandoned. Imidazole creams or lotions (e.g., *clotrimazole cream*) should be used two or three times daily, but ointments should be avoided because they maintain a moist local environment. In highly inflamed infections, initiating therapy with the combination of a topical *corticosteroid* cream and a light application of *clotrimazole* (Lotrisone) is useful. *Fluconazole* (Diflucan) is an effective oral anticandidal agent for extensive or refractory infection.

Paronychial Infection is difficult to treat. Therapy consists of avoiding exposure to water and using rubber gloves with a cotton lining whenever contact with water is unavoidable. *Nystatin lotion* or amphotericin B (Fungizone) lotion should be applied two to four times daily to the affected area. In highly inflamed conditions, nystatin or clotrimazole with steroids may be applied overnight under a fingercot. Nails grow out normally after the paronychia has healed. Fluconazole should be given orally if local therapy fails but is quite costly for the patient.

Angular Cheilitis (Perlèche) requires combined treatment, including correction of the primary oral abnormality to prevent leakage of saliva through the corners of the mouth and treatment of a possible secondary infection. The combination of *nystatin* and *triamcinolone* acetonide as an ointment formulation is the most effective topical agent. It should be used sparingly three times daily. Dental procedures should be directed at restoring the seal at the angles of the mouth. For persistent cases, the depth of the grooves of the angles may be reduced with collagen implants. *Fluconazole* may be of value in treating persistent episodes.

INDICATIONS FOR REFERRAL

Referral to the dermatologist should be considered if a fungal infection proves refractory to conventional topical treatment and prolonged or repeated systemic therapy is being contemplated. Consultation for consideration of the risks and benefits can be quite worthwhile, as can a second look at the problem. Short courses of systemic therapy (2 weeks) entail little risk and often do not require dermatologic referral.

PATIENT EDUCATION

At the time of the first incident, patients with fungal infection should be instructed about appropriate measures to prevent recurrence.

Maintaining Dryness. Instructing the patient about how to keep the skin dry and prevent maceration is critical to both successful treatment and prophylaxis. Dryness is particularly important in tinea pedis, tinea cruris, and candidal infections. Preventive measures should be taken in areas that have shown a tendency to become infected. In addition, the patient should be told to apply powder liberally to naturally moist areas of the body and to wear cotton clothing and loose-fitting underwear. Also, patients with tinea pedis should always wear socks and avoid sneakers and rubber-soled shoes, and the physician should encourage exposure of the feet to the air as often as possible. Lastly, people who sweat profusely should change their clothing more frequently, shower, and apply nonmedicated talcum powder.

Other Advice. Fungal infections may be slow to clear. To ensure compliance, it is essential to instruct the patient carefully about appropriate application and duration of treatment. Patients should be told to call at the first sign of recurrence and to institute appropriate drying measures and specific therapy after physician consultation.

THERAPEUTIC RECOMMENDATIONS

- Prescribe a topical preparation approved for once-a-day use. This is cost-effective and is also likely to improve patient compliance.
- Avoid prescribing creams for intertriginous areas because patients may use too much medication and thereby increase maceration. Prescribe a lotion or solution instead.

- If clearing is incomplete after 2 to 3 weeks, the short-term use of a systemic antifungal should be considered.
- For patients with onychomycosis, the expense and potential for serious adverse effects of systemic agents should be carefully weighed against the cosmetic consequences of living with the untreated condition.

ANNOTATED BIBLIOGRAPHY

Abraham AG, Kulp-Shorten CL, Callen JP. Remember to consider dermatophyte infection when dealing with recalcitrant dermatoses. South Med J 1998;91:359. (*Cutaneous fungal infections can be mistaken for other dermatoses; an examination with potassium hydroxide can confirm the diagnosis.*)

Borelli D, Jacobs PH, Nall L. Tinea versicolor: epidemiologic, clinical and therapeutic aspects. J Am Acad Dermatol 1991;25:300. (*An in-depth discussion of tinea versicolor, with emphasis on treatment considerations.*)

Brautigam M. Terbinafine versus itraconazole: a controlled clinical comparison in onychomycosis of the toenails. J Am Acad Dermatol 1998;38:S53. (*At 52 weeks, mycologic cure rates, determined by findings on culture and microscopy, were 81% for the terbinafine-treated patients and 63% for the itraconazole-treated patients.*)

Brodell RT, Elewski B. Superficial fungal infections. Errors to avoid in diagnosis and treatment. Postgrad Med 1997;101:279. (*Common errors in diagnosis and treatment are discussed in the form of short vignettes.*)

Gupta AK, De Docker P, Scher RK, et al. Itraconazole for the treatment of onychomycosis. Int J Dermatol 1998;37:303. (*Both continuous and pulse regimens are safe, with few adverse effects. Pulse therapy is more cost-effective.*)

Gupta AK, Einarson TR, Summerbell RC, et al. An overview of topical antifungal therapy in dermatomycoses. A North American perspective. Drugs 1998;55:645. (*A comprehensive review of topical therapy; 447 references.*)

Hart R, Bell-Syer EM, Crawford F, et al. Systematic review of topical treatments for fungal infections of the skin and nails of the feet. BMJ 1999;319:79. (*A formal, systematic review; allylamines, azoles, and undecenoic acid are all effective in placebo-controlled trials; the allylamines are slightly more effective than the azoles in head-to-head trials for tinea pedis but are much more expensive, and they should be reserved for refractory cases.*)

Hay RJ, Logan RA, Moore MK, et al. A comparative study of terbinafine versus griseofulvin in "dry-type" dermatophyte infections. J Am Acad Dermatol 1991;24:243. (*After 12 weeks of therapy, 100% of the terbinafine-treated group were clear, compared with only 45% of the group treated with griseofulvin.*)

Kovacs SO, Hruza LL. Superficial fungal infections. Getting rid of lesions that don't want to go away. Postgrad Med 1995;98:61,68,73. (*Emphasis on differential diagnosis and treatment options.*)

Macura AB. Fungal resistance to antimycotic drugs: a growing problem. Int J Dermatol 1991;30:181. (*Some antifungal agents are only fungistatic at lower concentrations; at high concentrations, they are fungicidal.*)

Sanchez JL, Torres VM. Double-blind efficacy study of selenium sulfide in tinea versicolor. J Am Acad Dermatol 1984;11:235. (*Daily 10-minute application of 2.5% selenium sulfide for 1 week proved an effective, convenient treatment, with an 87% success rate at the end of 4 weeks.*)

Smith EB, Wiss K, Hanifin JM, et al. Comparison of once- and twice-daily naftifine cream regimens with twice-daily clotrimazole in the treatment of tinea pedis. J Am Acad Dermatol 1990;22:1116. (*Naftifine cream used once daily for tinea pedis is effective and may be more effective than clotrimazole used twice daily.*)

192

Management of Cutaneous and Genital Herpes Simplex

Herpes simplex virus is a ubiquitous virus that clinically affects humans. *Herpes simplex virus type 1* (HSV-1) is the prototypical infectious agent in cutaneous disease of the upper body; *herpes simplex virus type 2* (HSV-2) generally infects the genitals and lower body, but the two types share 50% of their genetic material and may be interchangeable clinically. They differ slightly in sensitivity to antiviral drugs and in their proclivity to cause specific disease in other organs. Serologic studies indicate a 22% prevalence for HSV-2 infection among adults in the United States.

Many patients seek confirmation of a suspected herpes infection or treatment of frequent and recurrent rashes and symptoms. The primary care physician must know how to obtain a prompt diagnosis, utilize the current approaches to prevention and treatment, and address the patient's concerns and negative social stigmata that often accompany genital infection.

PATHOPHYSIOLOGY AND CLINICAL PRESENTATION

The severity and duration of symptoms are a function of the patient's state of immunity to HSV. In primary infection, preexisting antibody protection is lacking, and symptoms tend to be more severe and longer-lasting than at other stages of the illness. With time, the frequency and severity of recurrences tend to decline, especially with HSV-1 infection. Some cross-type antibody protection is also afforded, so that when a person with a prior history of HSV infection of one type contracts HSV infection of another type (i.e., first episode of nonprimary herpes), the resulting clinical presentation is less severe than that of primary disease. Because of their inability to mount effective antibody responses, immunocompromised patients are at great risk for severe, sustained outbreaks (see Chapter 13).

Primary Infection

Primary infection is usually the most dramatic form of HSV disease, but the spectrum of presentations is wide, ranging from asymptomatic disease to a florid outbreak with systemic symptoms. The characteristic lesions are *erythematous papules* that evolve during 2 to 3 days to *vesicles* with clear fluid, then progress to *pustules* that erode and leave superficial, tender *ulcerations*, especially in moist areas. Healing occurs within 2 to 6 weeks. *Systemic symptoms* develop in one third of men and two thirds of women; fever, malaise, nausea, headache, and myalgias are all reported. *Meningeal irritation*, manifested by headache, stiff neck, and photophobia, can occur. *Regional lymphadenopathy* is characteristic of primary infection; the nodes are enlarged, firm, and tender.

Primary HSV-1 Infection usually goes unnoticed but may present as severe *exudative pharyngitis* or *gingivostomatitis*, with high fevers and tender lymphadenopathy. The illness often is mistaken for streptococcal disease, other bacterial infections of the oropharynx, or mononucleosis. Systemic manifestations of the illness may be more prominent than local symptoms. HSV-1 infection may also present as painful *genital lesions*, a consequence of oral–genital sexual activity and an unappreciated risk factor for neonatal herpes.

Primary HSV-2 Infection also may be missed or misdiagnosed. In its most overt form, an exudative, painful bilateral *vulvovaginitis* is seen in female patients and painful *penile ulceration* with tender inguinal nodes in male patients. The genital lesions are painful in 95% of men and 99% of women. *Cervicitis* develops in nearly three fourths of women with primary infection, manifested by vaginal discharge and intermenstrual spotting. Local symptoms increase during the first 6 to 7 days of illness and peak between days 8 and 10, gradually decreasing during the next week. Lymph nodes are enlarged, firm, and tender. Although suppurative lymphadenopathy does not occur, superimposed bacterial infections can produce this finding.

Primary genital infection usually takes place in adolescence, but it may be contracted at the time of birth. Fever and malaise occur in 67% of patients, dysuria (resulting from urethral involvement or urinary irritation of ulcers) in 63%, and tender adenopathy in 80%. In 20%, extragenital lesions appear on the hands or in the oropharynx. Complications include secondary *yeast infection* in 11%, *aseptic meningitis* in 8%, and *sacral autonomic neuropathy* leading to bladder or bowel dysfunction in 2%. *Cervical cancer* is strongly associated with HSV-2 antibodies or the presence of HSV-2, although no study or series has directly found HSV genetic material within these cancer cells. The association of HSV infection with cervical cancer may be epidemiologic rather than etiologic.

Uncommon Presentations of Herpes Simplex Viral Infection. An unusual form of primary infection results from implantation of virus into broken skin; this produces a *herpetic whitlow* characterized by pain, swelling, and erythema of the fingers with pronounced adenopathy. In wrestlers, *herpes gladiatorum*, a primary herpes infection, may develop on exposed parts of the body that are inoculated during the rough activity of wrestling.

First Episode of Nonprimary Disease

In most cases, a first episode of nonprimary disease represents new infection with HSV-2 in persons with clinical and serologic evidence of HSV-1 exposure earlier in life. Patients with a past history of fever blisters or cold sores note a new onset of painful genital lesions. The severity and duration of symptoms are characteristically intermediate between those of primary infection and recurrent disease—lesions are fewer in number, and healing takes place within 1 to 3 weeks. Cervicitis, urethritis, adenopathy, and systemic symptoms are minimal, if present at all.

Recurrent Infection

After primary infection, latent disease develops in all patients, with the virus residing in the associated dorsal root ganglion and circulating along the endoneural sheath to the skin if host defenses break down. Emotional or physical stress, sunburn, and skin trauma are among the reported precipitants. The result is a localized, self-limited form of illness with fewer lesions that resolve more quickly than in primary infection. Recurrent infection may begin with a prodrome of tingling or discomfort in the skin, and sometimes mild systemic symptoms are present, although they are not as severe as in primary disease. Genital disease may recur in a nongenital area (e.g., legs or buttocks) in about 10% of cases. If both genital and nongenital lesions are present at the time of primary infection, the chance of a nongenital recurrence is close to 50%.

Although pain without rash develops in some symptomatic patients, most patients experience the characteristic *maculopapular–vesicular* eruption. The lesions become turbid as interferon is produced in the vesicles and as lymphocytes stimulated by interleukin-2, interleukin-6, and other cytokines begin controlling the infection. During the initial 3 to 4 days, some patients inoculate themselves in other areas (hands, eyes, periorbital areas), but secondary infections are usually brief, mild, and self-limited, and disease is not established in new regions. Infections can recur in different distributions along the same ganglia, and heterogeneity characterizes the illness.

Eventually, reepithelialization of the skin occurs, usually without scarring. Secondary bacterial infections (caused by streptococci or staphylococci) can lead to cellulitis and lymphangitis and must be anticipated. The risk for transmission is greatest in the first 96 hours after the appearance of the rash. Even without evidence of disease, silent shedding occurs in 2% to 5% of patients, particularly those with recurrent genital disease.

Complications of local recurrent infections are few but can be clinically important, such as *hemorrhagic cystitis*, *dyspareunia*, and *sacral radiculopathy* (which leads to difficulty in voiding, fecal soilage, or both). Sacral disease is also associated with a risk for recurrent *aseptic meningitis*. Perirectal disease can cause *proctitis*. Disseminated disease is rare, even in immunocompromised patients, but lesions of autoinoculation may occur on the fingers or about the eyes. Recurrent disease sometimes takes the form of *erythema multiforme* without evidence of vesicles. In atopic persons, HSV can produce a devastating generalized *eczema herpeticum*. Chronic pain syndromes associated with infection but without lesions are being identified more frequently. *Post-herpetic neuralgia* caused by HSV-1 is described as a recurrent syndrome without clinical evidence of skin lesions. Vulvar burning alone may be an expression of HSV-2 infection. *Elsberg's syndrome* with radiculomyelopathy and acute urinary retention may also be secondary to clinically inapparent disease. HSV has been associated with an acute *retinal necrosis* syndrome presenting as eye pain and visual loss.

Asymptomatic Disease

Most recurrences of genital herpes present as asymptomatic disease that is overlooked by both patient and physician, either because symptoms are very mild or atypical or because the only manifestation is truly asymptomatic shedding of virus. It is in this stage that the disease is most likely to be transmitted to sexual partners.

Neonatal Herpes

Neonatal HSV is most often the consequence of direct contact between the infant and HSV (both type 1 and type 2) during passage through the birth canal of an asymptomatic mother with active genital infection. Risk is estimated at 10% in women with recurrent or primary infection at 32 weeks and is several times higher if infection is present at term in the absence of antibody production. Congenital HSV infection frequently leads to death or severe neurodevelopmental problems. Acquisition of HSV infection early in pregnancy followed by a normal antibody response does not appear to compromise the outcome of pregnancy, but infection in the last trimester may not leave enough time for type-specific antibodies to form, so that the infant is at risk.

DIFFERENTIAL DIAGNOSIS

The differential diagnosis of genital ulceration in conjunction with inguinal lymphadenopathy includes *syphilis* and *chancroid* (see Chapter 141). Ulcerations may also be associated with noninfectious conditions, such as Behçet's syndrome and inflammatory bowel disease, or may simply represent excoriation and secondary bacterial infection caused by vigorous sexual activity. Syphilis serology should always be obtained in the setting of a genital ulcer, even one that is painful. Approximately 50% of ulcerative lesions in the genital area prove to be herpetic.

WORKUP

History. In most instances, the diagnosis is a clinical one, based on finding the characteristic lesions. However, atypical disease is common, particularly in the genital area, so that quick diagnosis is difficult. A detailed sexual history is essential (see Chapter 229) and must include inquiry about oral—genital sexual activity, as HSV-1 can also be a source of genital infection. Any history of genital redness, spotting, fissures, pain, and paresthesias, even in the absence of skin lesions, should raise suspicion of genital herpes. Any prior history of fever blisters or cold sores should also be noted because it indicates prior HSV infection and helps to identify patients with a first episode of nonprimary disease.

Physical Examination. Besides helping to identify early vesicular lesions as herpetic ("dew drop on a rose petal"), the physical examination is especially important for differentiating HSV infection from other causes of genital ulcer. Unlike the very tender ulcer of HSV infection, the ulcer (chancre) of primary syphilis is indurated and painless or only minimally uncomfortable. As in genital herpes, the base is clean, and tender, firm, nonfluctuant inguinal adenopathy may be present. These findings contrast with those of chancroid, which are characterized by very tender, soft, purulent ulcerations in conjunction with sore, fluctuant lymph nodes and erythema of the overlying skin.

Laboratory Studies. Unroofing a vesicle and performing a *Tzanck test* (see Chapter 193) can be helpful, but this is less specific than *viral culture*, which is also the most sensitive of the commonly available tests. The results (including typing) can be available within 2 to 3 days, which makes it of practical value. The best time to culture is within 48 hours after the onset of symptoms; the highest-yielding lesions are intact vesicles, pustules, and early moist ulcers. *Antigen detection* (by direct fluorescent antibody testing) is of limited sensitivity, and false-negative rates are high when it is used in populations with a low prevalence of HSV infection. Typing is not achieved. Only when used in settings of high HSV prevalence does the predictive value of a positive test result rise sufficiently to warrant its use. *DNA probes* are under development to provide a more sensitive, specific, and rapid approach to viral detection and typing. The use of *polymerase chain reaction* assays to detect the presence of specific DNA or RNA sequences offers the most sensitive and specific means for diagnosing active disease; cost is a consideration, but once these tests become widely available commercially, their cost should decrease, and they are likely to become the test of choice. Promising monoclonal and oligoclonal detection methods are also under development.

Serology can confirm prior infection, but such information is less useful in the evaluation of an ongoing episode because titers often do not rise sufficiently, and cross-reactivity between HSV-1 and HSV-2 occurs. *Western blot* assay promises to provide sensitive and specific type-specific antibody testing, but it is not yet widely available. Most commercial laboratories are presently unable to provide reliable type-specific antibody testing. Serology also has the disadvantage of not producing data while the patient is clinically affected, and patients, once exposed, carry titers forever, whether or not their infection becomes reactivated. Antibody testing could be used to identify persons at increased risk for primary infection (i.e., pregnant women with no antibody titers).

Genital herpes is a major cause of types II and III abnormalities on Papanicolaou smear and should be routinely sought if these changes are seen. It is important to differentiate this benign inflammatory abnormality from real metaplastic or anaplastic disease (see Chapter 107).

PRINCIPLES OF THERAPY

Because HSV infection is incurable and characterized by self-limited symptomatic recurrences and asymptomatic recurrences in which virus is shed, the goals of therapy center on reducing the duration of symptoms, the frequency and severity of recurrences, and the risk for transmission. Because treatment is either symptomatic or prophylactic, decisions regarding the use of antiviral therapy are customized to the physical and psychosocial needs of the patient. Treatment of symptomatic recurrences is most effective when initiated at the first sign of a relapse (during the prodromal phase); half of outbreaks can be prevented with an early start to antiviral therapy. Initiation of therapy after skin lesions have appeared is less effective, shortening the course of illness by little more than a day. Suppressive therapy can be offered to persons bothered by frequent recurrences and to those who want to decrease asymptomatic viral shedding and risk for transmission, especially to an antibody-negative partner.

The nucleoside analogues (acyclovir, valacyclovir, and famciclovir) are the principal antiviral agents available for use against HSV. They are effective for symptomatic treatment of primary and recurrent disease and can prevent recurrences and shedding of virus; however, they do not cure HSV infection. Emergence of resistant strains is very rare when antiviral therapy is used in immunocompetent persons, but it has been observed in those who are immunocompromised and take these agents for prolonged periods.

Acyclovir, the first of the nucleoside analogues, acts as a purine analogue substrate for viral thymidine kinase, which is uniquely activated in cells that are infected with HSV. Acyclovir is effective against both types of HSV, although HSV-1 is more sensitive. Oral acyclovir shortens viral shedding time and reduces the time to healing and crusting of lesions. The earlier the treatment is instituted, the better. Continuous use of acyclovir in patients with frequent recurrences reduces the number and severity of repeated episodes. Unfortunately, once the drug is discontinued, its effect on recurrence ceases. Long-term use is associated with slow adaptation of the virus to the drug, but clinically important resistance has not been reported. Cessation of use results in reversion to original sensitivity. One can readily treat for 12 months at a time without adverse consequences. Side effects include *nausea, headache,* and *vomiting*. Elimination is renal, and downward dose adjustment is required in the setting of azotemia. Half-life is less than 4 hours, so that frequent dosing is necessary.

The use of acyclovir for genital herpes in *pregnancy* appears to decrease dramatically the chance of fetal transmission in the last trimester, but safety remains to be established. Often, a cesarean section is advocated in these cases. IV acyclovir is indicated in *immunocompromised hosts* and in persons with disseminated disease, such as meningoencephalitis. IV acyclovir produces higher, more consistent blood levels than does oral acyclovir, which is only 15% absorbed. The oral vehicle is acceptable for mucocutaneous manifestations in immunocompetent hosts.

Topical acyclovir is of little use, although it has some limited efficacy in primary infection. Topical acyclovir is also of little use in keratoconjunctivitis, a dangerous illness; trifluorothymidine ointment plus oral or IV acyclovir should be used.

Famciclovir was developed to improve the absorption and effective half-life of acyclovir, so that higher serum levels could be obtained with less frequent dosing. Famciclovir is a nucleoside prodrug that is stable and well absorbed in the gastrointestinal tract and converted in the small bowel and liver to penciclovir, the active agent. The drug is effective in treating and suppressing recurrent infection and has also been used successfully for treating primary genital infection. No head-to-head studies have compared this agent with acyclovir. Adverse effects include nausea, dizziness, and headache. Drug–drug in-

teractions are possible because the conversion of famciclovir requires hepatic oxidative metabolism. Elimination is by renal tubular excretion, so that dose reduction is necessary in the setting of renal insufficiency and the concurrent use of such drugs as probenecid. No interactions with cimetidine have been observed.

Valacyclovir, a prodrug of acyclovir, is rapidly absorbed and converted to acyclovir in its first pass through the intestines and liver. Higher serum levels of acyclovir are attained than with oral administration of acyclovir. A regimen of 250 mg of valacyclovir four times daily provides the same serum levels as 800 mg of acyclovir five times daily. Efficacy is similar to or better than that of acyclovir and famciclovir. Side effects are nausea, vomiting, diarrhea, and headache. Interactions with cimetidine and probenecid are possible. The efficacy and safety of valacyclovir have not been established in immunocompromised patients and those with disseminated disease; thrombotic thrombocytopenic purpura and hemolytic/uremic syndrome have been reported in association with valacyclovir treatment in patients with advanced AIDS.

Adjuncts. Good local skin care and the use of drying agents to speed the transition from active vesicle to crusting are the essence of adjunctive therapy. Topical surfactants such as ether and chloroform seem to provide some additional relief. Some have advocated, with little evidence, the use of cimetidine because of research evidence suggesting that histamine$_2$ antagonists have antiherpes activity. Vidarabine, ribavirin, bromodeoxyuridine, and ganciclovir sodium have shown some promise of antiviral activity. Care of skin lesions is especially important in the immunocompromised or eczematous host, in whom dissemination and autoinoculation can lead to serious consequences.

Some clinicians use *topical corticosteroids* to abort the progression of herpetic lesions. This empiric approach often works, although scientific evidence is lacking and there is a theoretical concern about spread. However, no evidence has been published to document this danger.

Over-the-counter preparations such as Blistex, Campho-Phenique, and Anbesol may provide minimal symptomatic relief but do not affect the course of the eruption. Considering the long history of ineffective therapy, physicians should remain skeptical about new remedies offered.

Vaccines. Evidence is growing that benign latency can be maintained by long-term modulation of the immune system with vaccines. Of particular interest is a vaccine against HSV-2 to reduce the risks for genital herpes and associated neonatal disease. Initial results were encouraging, but further studies have been less so. Work is ongoing.

PATIENT EDUCATION

Genital Herpes. Reassurance of the frightened patient with genital herpes (and partner) is critical. The primary care physician can help reduce the shame and suspicion that often accompany confirmation of the diagnosis. Herpes has acquired an unjustifiably vicious reputation in the media, not only as a risk factor for neonatal tragedy but also as a sign of sexual infidelity. Patients need to understand that genital herpes could have been acquired decades ago and that asymptomatic shedding of virus is the most likely mode of transmission. Guilt can be assuaged by providing approaches to the prevention of transmission (e.g., safe sexual practices, suppressive therapy). Women of childbearing age appreciate knowing how neonatal herpes can be avoided and what they and their obstetrician can do to contribute to a safe delivery.

In educating patients about transmissibility, it is important to inform them about what constitutes a high-risk situation (e.g., unprotected sexual intercourse; oral–genital sexual activity between an infected patient and an antibody-negative partner, especially one who is pregnant). The concept of asymptomatic shedding must be appreciated by the patient. Transmission is less likely with the use of *condoms* but is still possible. If the presence of antibody in a sexual partner is confirmed, anxiety surrounding sexual relations can be reduced.

Pamphlets about the disease are available through the Centers for Disease Control and Prevention, the National Institutes of Health, and the American Social Health Association. These sources of information are superior to many of the lay-initiated hotlines, which tend to overplay the emotional problems. It should be emphasized that recurrent infection is far less likely to produce discomfort or pain than primary infection.

Facial Involvement. Facial lesions are always annoying and are embarrassing to some. Protection from sunburn and trauma should be urged, as should good local care, with use of drying agents to speed the transition from active vesicle to crusting. Patients are reassured by knowing that the risk for scarring is very small and that effective oral therapy is available for shortening severe episodes and reducing the risk for recurrence.

INDICATIONS FOR REFERRAL AND ADMISSION

Consult with an obstetrician regarding the safety and advisability of antiviral treatment in the third trimester versus cesarean section at the time of delivery to prevent HSV transmission to the fetus. Patients with suspected eye involvement should be referred urgently to an ophthalmologist for eye examination and treatment with trifluorothymidine and acyclovir. The immunocompromised person in whom disease appears to be disseminating requires prompt admission for IV therapy.

THERAPEUTIC RECOMMENDATIONS

Primary Infection and Nonprimary Initial Genital Disease

- Begin a 7- to 10-day course of oral acyclovir (200 mg five times daily), valacyclovir (1,000 mg twice daily), or famciclovir (250 mg three times daily). Titrate the dose according to response to treatment. Continue therapy until lesions have healed. Reduce dose for patients with renal failure. Provide a supply for use during recurrences, which are likely to develop several times in the first year after initial infection.

Recurrent Disease

- Treat bothersome symptomatic recurrences for 5 days with either acyclovir (200 mg five times daily or 400 mg three times daily), famciclovir (125 mg twice daily), or valacyclovir (500 mg twice daily). Begin treatment at the first sign of illness, preferably during the prodromal phase before skin lesions emerge.
- Consider long-term suppressive therapy for patients who have more than six to eight recurrences per year, want to minimize the risk for asymptomatic viral transmission, or are immunocompromised. Prescribe either acyclovir (400 mg twice daily), famciclovir (250 mg twice daily), or valacyclovir (500 to 1,000 mg daily). Titrate the prophylactic dose to the lowest level possible without reactivation and continue for up to 12 months at a time.
- After 12 months, halt suppressive therapy and reassess the need for continuation.

Additional Measures for All Patients

- Educate patients about the transmissibility of genital herpes, including the risk for genital infection associated with oral–genital sexual activity and with asymptomatic viral shedding; recommend the use of condoms when one partner is antibody-negative.
- Help the patient to keep the problem in perspective and address common misconceptions regarding the meaning of the infection.
- Watch for secondary bacterial infection and disseminated HSV disease. In patients who are immunosuppressed, dissemination may present as gangrenous ulcers or deep-seated eschars.
- Follow genital infections closely during pregnancy; consider monitoring antibody status in the latter part of pregnancy to determine susceptibility to primary infection and the need for extra precautions or the use of suppressive therapy in an infected male partner.

A.H.G.

ANNOTATED BIBLIOGRAPHY

Benedetti JK, Zeh J, Selke S, et al. Frequency and reactivation of nongenital lesions among patients with genital herpes simplex virus. Am J Med 1995;98:237. (*About 10% had nongenital lesions initially; a similar percentage had recurrences at a nongenital site.*)

Bierman SM. Recurrent genital herpes simplex infection. A trivial disorder. Arch Dermatol 1985;121:173. (*A good normative statement placing this illness in perspective.*)

Brown ZA, Selke S, Zeh J, et al. The acquisition of herpes simplex virus during pregnancy. N Engl J Med 1997;337:509. (*The neonates of antibody-negative patients who became infected in the later stages of pregnancy were at greatest risk for herpes.*)

Dahm C, Elgas M, Kuhn JE, et al. The diagnostic significance of the polymerase chain reaction and isoelectric focusing in herpes simplex virus encephalitis. J Med Virol 1992;36:147. (*Use of polymerase chain reaction for diagnosis of HSV infection.*)

Diaz-Mitoma F, Sibbalk G, Shafran SD, et al. Oral famciclovir for the suppression of recurrent genital herpes: a randomized, controlled trial. JAMA 1998;280:887. (*Large-scale, multicenter European study; drug found effective and safe for suppression in persons with frequent recurrences.*)

Douglas JM, Critchlow C, Benedetti J, et al. A double-blind study of oral acyclovir for suppression of recurrences of genital herpes simplex virus infection. N Engl J Med 1984;310:1551. (*Oral acyclovir given for 4 months markedly reduced but did not eliminate recurrences. The natural history of recurrences was not affected.*)

Gonzales GR. Post-herpes simplex type 1 neuralgia simulating post-herpetic neuralgia. J Pain Symptom Manage 1992;7:320. (*Gives evidence of HSV neuralgia presenting much like the post-herpetic neuralgia associated with herpes zoster.*)

Koutsky LA, Stevens CE, Holmes KK, et al. Underdiagnosis of genital herpes by current clinical and viral-isolation procedures. N Engl J Med 1992;326:1533. (*Sensitivity is low; new strategies for diagnosis reviewed.*)

Luby ED, Klinge V. Genital herpes: a pervasive psychosocial disorder. Arch Dermatol 1985;121:494. (*An article emphasizing the adverse effect of herpes on intimate sexual relationships.*)

Maccato ML, Kaufman RH. Herpes genitalis. Dermatol Clin 1992; 10:415. (*Review of genital HSV infection, with attention to silent shedding.*)

Mckay M. Vulvodynia. Diagnostic patterns. Dermatol Clin 1992;10: 423. (*Defines multiple causes, including HSV infection, of vulvar burning.*)

Mertz GJ, Critchlow CW, Benedetti J, et al. Double-blind placebo-controlled trial of oral acyclovir in first-episode genital herpes simplex virus infection. JAMA 1984;252:1147. (*One of the original controlled trials of efficacy; a course of acyclovir treatment shortened the duration of viral shedding, symptoms, and lesions but did not reduce subsequent recurrences.*)

Solomon A, Rasmussen JE, Varani J. The Tzanck smear in the diagnosis of cutaneous herpes simplex. JAMA 1984;251:633. (*Viral culture was superior, but the Tzanck preparation is still a useful, cost-effective aid in early diagnosis.*)

Spruance SL, Tyring SK, De Gregorio B, et al. A large-scale, placebo-controlled, dose-ranging trial of peroral valacyclovir for episodic treatment of recurrent herpes genitalis. Arch Intern Med 1996;156:1729. (*Treatment in the prodromal phase was most effective and prevented outbreaks in nearly half of cases.*)

Wald A, Zeh J, Barnum G, et al. Suppression of subclinical shedding of herpes simplex virus type 2 with acyclovir. Ann Intern Med 1996;12:8. (*Reduction of 90% in subclinical viral shedding achieved with a standard suppressive dose of acyclovir.*)

193

Management of Herpes Zoster

Herpes zoster (shingles) is a common viral cutaneous eruption estimated to affect 300,000 persons a year in the United States. Most cases represent reactivation of the varicella-zoster virus (VZV). The incidence increases with age and degree of host immunosuppression. A community-based study found 100 cases per 100,000 person-years between the ages of 15 to 35, with a rise each decade to 450 cases per 100,000 by age 75. The seasonal variation seen with varicella does not occur with zoster; shingles is rarely an epidemic illness. Shingles may present as a pain syndrome without vesicles and pose a diagnostic problem. The primary physician must recognize zoster, make the patient comfortable, and prevent complications.

PATHOPHYSIOLOGY AND CLINICAL PRESENTATION

Varicella, or chickenpox, usually affects people early in life; the virus then lies dormant in a nerve ganglion in a genomic state until reactivation occurs. The nerve root changes consist of necrosis and sometimes cyst formation. A decrease in *cellular immunity* may allow the latent virus to reactivate and spread along the nerve; clinical zoster is the result. Helper T cells and several lymphokines produced by other T-cell subsets usually protect the host from reactivation. The disorder occurs with increased frequency among immunocompromised patients and the elderly, probably as a consequence of defects in cellular immunity. Humoral immunity does not appear to be an important factor; even severely infected patients show significantly elevated antibody titers to zoster, and fewer than 5% of persons born in the United States do not possess varicella antibody. It has been suggested that every person who has had chickenpox harbors latent virus, that 50% of all people who live to the age of 85 will have an attack of zoster, and that approximately 10% will have at least two attacks. Occa-

sional outbreaks may result from trauma to a nerve in which the virus is latent.

There is no evidence of an increased *risk of latent cancer* in persons with herpes zoster. The relative cancer risk is only 1.1 times that of the general population, although a tenuous suggestion of a somewhat higher-than-average risk for colon cancer has been noted. The *risk for transmission* is low despite the fact that zoster skin lesions contain large amounts of virus. However, immunosuppressed patients and those who have never had chickenpox are at risk for transmission from persons with zoster. Reactivation on exposure to zoster has even been observed in a few patients with a previous history of chickenpox.

Clinical Presentation is one of radicular pain followed by the appearance of tense, grouped vesicles on an erythematous base ("dew drops on a rose petal") in a dermatomal distribution. The pain too is dermatomal and may begin as an itch or tenderness that precedes the cutaneous lesion by 1 to 7 days. Patients describe sensations of burning, tingling, and sharp, knife-like pricking, or of deep, boring discomfort. More than half of patients have a unilateral involvement of one or more thoracic dermatomes. The cranial dermatomes account for approximately 15% of cases, and cervical and lumbar dermatomes each account for approximately 10%. Vesicles on the tip of the nose were formerly thought to indicate nasociliary involvement (putting the eye at risk), but a recent review of ophthalmic zoster does not confirm the validity of this clinical saw.

The cutaneous eruption becomes pustular within a few days; crusting and healing then follow during 14 to 21 days. The crust is often dark, almost black. Scarring and atrophy can occur if the lesions are deep.

Malaise, low-grade fever, and adenopathy accompany severe eruptions. The total length of the course is related to the duration of new vesicle development; vesicle formation for several days usually predicts a 2- to 4-week course, whereas vesicle formation persisting for more than a week predicts a longer course.

About one in eight patients experiences at least one complication. Major complications include post-herpetic neuralgia, uveitis, motor deficits, infection, and systemic involvement, such as meningoencephalitis, pneumonia, deafness, or dissemination. *Post-herpetic neuralgia* occurs most frequently in patients older than age 50. The pain is often excruciating and does not respond well to conventional methods of pain control.

The presence of more than 10 lesions outside a single dermatome of distribution is early evidence of *dissemination*. Patients with AIDS may have VZV infection as part of the AIDS-related complex. In most cases, VZV infection presents as a typical dermatomal illness; occasionally, it is disseminated and can be complicated by hepatitis, pneumonia, meningitis, or proctitis. In immunocompromised hosts, VZV and herpes simplex infections may present in similar and atypical fashion, sometimes without vesicles or in unusual distributions.

DIAGNOSIS

The diagnosis is generally not difficult if the characteristic dermatomal rash and pain are present. The most serious diagnostic problem occurs during the prodromal phase, when patients present with a pain syndrome. Periorbital headache, unexplained back pain, or chest wall pain may represent the prodromal period of herpes zoster. Prodromal zoster pain has been mistaken for myocardial infarction, cholecystitis, and appendicitis. The characteristic eruption may not appear until 2 to 5 days later.

In patients with the characteristic rash, a *Tzanck preparation* demonstrating the presence of *multinucleated giant cells* provides strong supportive evidence of zoster. The Tzanck preparation has proved superior to viral isolation in the diagnosis of early lesions. Culture, although slow, allows for confirmation. The diagnosis can also be confirmed by demonstration of a *rising antibody titer*, which requires two separate determinations, or by immunofluorescence. More rapid diagnosis is afforded by *polymerase chain reaction assays*, which detect DNA sequences of VZV. Herpes zoster can also be identified by host T-cell recognition of an immediate early integument protein (IE62) or glycoprotein I of VZV. Such rapid molecular diagnostic assays are expensive and best reserved for prompt diagnosis in severely ill persons who present with acute but nonspecific symptoms (e.g., meningeal infection).

PRINCIPLES OF THERAPY

The goals of therapy are to dry the vesicles, relieve pain, and prevent secondary infection and complications. Lesions are kept clean and dry by the application of a wet-to-dry compress soaked with *Burow's solution* three to four times a day. If purulence or erythema suggestive of secondary infection develops, antibiotics are indicated. No data are available to support the use of prophylactic antibiotics.

Relief of Discomfort. Pain relief can usually be achieved with a mild analgesic such as *aspirin* or *acetaminophen*, but one should not hesitate to use *codeine* if need be. Antiviral therapy (see below) often reduces pain within 72 hours and frequently alleviates the need for stronger pain relief measures. The pain of thoracic zoster can be reduced by splinting the affected area with a *tight wrap*. Trunk lesions are covered with a nonadherent dressing, and then the area is wrapped with an elastic bandage. Malaise reflects viremia and should be treated with rest. Severe local pain can be relieved with *intralesional* injections of *triamcinolone* (2 mg/mL) in lidocaine. There is little evidence to suggest that pain can be relieved or the rate of healing hastened by the use of *systemic corticosteroids*; however, such treatment may reduce the incidence of post-herpetic neuralgia (see below). Pruritus may be relieved by oral *antihistamines* (see Chapter 178) or by *calamine lotion*, which both reduces itching and dries the rash. *Topical capsaicin* has been tried, but with only minimal success. *Peripheral nerve block* is an invasive approach to reducing acute pain that does not respond to antiviral therapy; *sympathetic blockade* has also been tried in this setting with a modicum of success.

Shortening Clinical Course and Reducing Risk for Post-herpetic Neuralgia. The nucleoside antiviral agents *acyclovir*, *famciclovir*, and *valacyclovir* can reduce acute pain, shorten the course of illness, and reduce the risk for post-herpetic neuralgia. To be maximally effective, antiviral therapy must begin as early as possible and preferably no later than 72 hours after the onset of rash. Those who benefit most from antiviral therapy are persons who present early with severe pain, are older than 50 years, or have ophthalmic involvement. Because VZV is much more resistant to acyclovir than herpes simplex virus is, double-dose therapy is required (e.g., 800 mg of acyclovir five times daily for 10 days). The newer cyclovirs offer dosing regimens more convenient than those of acyclovir (e.g., 500 to 750 mg of famciclovir three times daily for 7 days; 1 g of valacyclovir three times daily for 7 days), cause fewer central nervous system side effects in the elderly (see Chapter 192), and demonstrate equal or better efficacy, often at lower cost. Response, manifested by a reduction in pain, typically occurs within 72 hours. For immunocompetent patients, valacyclovir is the least costly and most effective of these agents, but valacyclovir treatment in patients with disseminated VZV infection and advanced HIV disease has been associated with case reports of thrombotic thrombocytopenic purpura and hemolytic/uremic syndrome, so that it must not be given to immunocompromised persons.

Because of the severity of post-herpetic neuralgia, its refractoriness to treatment, and reports of responsiveness to early use of *systemic glucocorticosteroids*, steroids have been prescribed prophylactically in conjunction with antiviral therapy, particularly in patients older than 50 years. Data regarding efficacy are limited, but recent randomized trials suggest that early therapy with high doses for a brief period is associated with a shorter duration of pain and a twofold to threefold reduction in the development of chronic pain. Steroid therapy is started at the same time as antiviral treatment. The best-studied regimen is a 3-week program of *prednisone*, in which 60 mg is given daily for the first week; the dose is then tapered to 30 mg/d during week 2 and to 15 mg/d during week 3. To minimize adverse effects, prednisone is taken in the morning with food (see Chapter 105). Persons over the age of 50 who present with severe pain and a large number of herpetic lesions are at greatest risk for post-herpetic neuralgia and are the best candidates for combination therapy.

Trials of several varicella *vaccines* have been completed, and vaccines should soon be available for adults who have not had chickenpox and for those at high risk for reactivation. It is hoped that the vaccine will stimulate T-cell subsets and cytotoxic killer T cells and make reactivation less likely. In studies of immunosuppressed persons, *interferon* and *vidarabine* have proved promising.

Treatment of Post-herpetic Neuralgia. *Tricyclic antidepressants* remain the first line of treatment (e.g., *amitriptyline* at a starting dose of 25 mg daily at bedtime); they provide significant benefit to about 50% of patients. Recently, the anticonvulsant *gabapentin* has been found to be similarly effective as a first-line agent (begun at 900 mg/d and titrated up to 3,600 mg/d) and better tolerated (dizziness and somnolence are the main adverse effects). The anticonvulsive drug *carbamazepine* has been used as a second-line agent. *Narcotics* are not well studied for long-term use in post-herpetic neuralgia, but they are often added if a first-line drug proves insufficient. Combination therapy has not been well studied but may prove useful if the agents utilized work by different pathways. Topical therapies are less effective; *capsaicin* is among the best, but efficacy is modest and a burning sensation may ensue with prolonged use.

INDICATIONS FOR REFERRAL

If any suggestion of visual compromise or other ocular involvement is present, prompt ophthalmologic consultation for herpetic eye care is essential to avoid scarring and permanent visual impairment. *Otic* involvement can lead to severe pain and otic nerve damage, so that referral to an ear, nose, and throat specialist is important. The patient with herpetic skin lesions and signs of meningeal irritation requires prompt hospitalization.

A.H.G.

ANNOTATED BIBLIOGRAPHY

Balfour HH Jr. Acyclovir therapy for herpes zoster: advantages and adverse effects. JAMA 1986;255:387. (*An editorial position on the use of acyclovir for zoster.*)

Crooks RJ, Jones DA, Fiddian AP. Zoster-associated chronic pain: an overview of clinical trials with acyclovir. Scand J Infect Dis Suppl 1991;80:62. (*Evidence suggests benefit.*)

Eaglestein WH, Katz R, Brown JS. The effects of early corticosteroid therapy on the skin eruption and pain of herpes zoster. JAMA 1970;211:1681. (*The duration of post-herpetic neuralgia was decreased by oral triamcinolone therapy begun early in the disease course.*)

Gershon AA, LaRussa P, Hardy I, et al. Varicella vaccine: the American experience. J Infect Dis 1992;166[Suppl 1]:S63. (*Use of varicella vaccines in healthy and immunocompromised hosts.*)

Jackson JL, Gibbons R, Meyer G, et al. The effect of treating herpes zoster with oral acyclovir in preventing post-herpetic neuralgia. Arch Intern Med 1997;157:909. (*A metaanalysis finding a 46% reduction in risk for this complication.*)

Kost RG, Straus DB, Coombs FP. Post-herpetic neuralgia: pathogenesis, treatment and prevention. N Engl J Med 1996;335:32. (*One of the best reviews.*)

Liesegang TJ. The varicella-zoster virus: systemic and ocular features. J Am Acad Dermatol 1984;11:165. (*A superb review, with emphasis on ophthalmic disease.*)

Ragozzino MW, Melton LJ, Kurland LT, et al. Risk of cancer after herpes zoster. N Engl J Med 1982;307:393. (*No increased risk found.*)

Rowbotham M, Harden N, Stacey B, et al. Gabapentin for the treatment of post-herpetic neuralgia. JAMA 1998;280:1837. (*A multicenter, randomized, controlled trial demonstrating a significant reduction in pain and significant improvements in sleep and quality of life.*)

Solomon AR, Rasmussen JE, Weiss JS. A comparison of the Tzanck smear and viral isolation in varicella-herpes zoster. Arch Dermatol 1986;122:282. (*Tzanck preparation was superior to viral isolation in diagnosing early lesions.*)

Watson CP, Tyler KL, Bickers DR, et al. A randomized vehicle-controlled trial of topical capsaicin in the treatment of post-herpetic neuralgia. Clin Ther 1993;15:510. (*A modest reduction in pain was achieved, but placebo effect is hard to rule out.*)

Weller TH. Varicella and herpes zoster. N Engl J Med 1983;309:1362,1434. (*A two-part review, best for epidemiology and natural history.*)

Whitley RJ, Weiss H, Gnann JW Jr, et al. Acyclovir with and without prednisone for the treatment of herpes zoster: a randomized, placebo-controlled trial. Ann Intern Med 1996;125:376. (*A 3-week program of acyclovir plus high-dose prednisone not only sped healing but also reduced pain and improved quality of life more than either drug given separately.*)

194
Management of Warts
WILLIAM V. R. SHELLOW

Warts result from skin infection with human papillomavirus (HPV). Although a relatively harmless affliction, warts can be cosmetically bothersome and occasionally a source of pain. The primary care physician should be able to distinguish warts from other skin tumors, select effective treatment, and educate the patient in proper self-care and prevention.

PATHOPHYSIOLOGY, CLINICAL PRESENTATION, AND COURSE

Human papillomavirus is a DNA virus, with more than 80 types identified. It is epitheliotropic and causes tumors of the epidermis. At least five types are potentially oncogenic, with two implicated in cervical carcinoma (see Chapter 107) and three in squamous cell carcinoma (see Chapter 177). Warts can be transmitted by direct contact or by autoinoculation. Young people have a high frequency of warts. Healing can occur spontaneously, presumably through immunologic mechanisms. Approximately two thirds of warts disappear spontaneously within 2 years of their appearance, but if they are left untreated, additional warts may develop from the original ones.

Clinical Presentations vary according to site and viral strain involved. Morphologically, nongenital warts appear in three forms: the keratotic common wart, the filiform wart, and the flat wart. Most warts are asymptomatic; however, a plantar wart can be the source of considerable foot pain, acting as a foreign body during weight bearing. Anogenital warts may become friable, bleed, and cause discomfort. Periungual lesions may become fissured.

The Common Wart (Verruca Vulgaris) is associated with HPV-2 and HPV-4 infection. It appears flesh-colored or grayish white with a papillate, hyperkeratotic surface. The wart may be punctuated with black dots that represent thrombosed superficial capillaries, which are present in large numbers. The common wart may be seen anywhere but frequently affects the elbows, knees, fingers, and palms. The filiform wart is more delicate and threadlike. The *flat wart* (*verruca plana*), caused by HPV-3, is smaller than the common wart. Flat warts are tan to flesh-colored, slightly raised papules with a relatively smooth surface. Great numbers of them may appear on the hands, in bearded areas, and on the shaved legs of women.

The Plantar Wart (Verruca Plantaris) results from infection of the plantar surface of the foot with HPV-1 or HPV-4. It appears as a small skin nodule that produces grayish or yellow interruptions in the skin lines (dermatoglyphics) of the foot. It is less elevated than other warts because weight bearing presses it inward. These warts may be solitary, multiple, or confluent; if confluent, the term *mosaic wart* is used.

Genital Warts. In the genital area, four clinical morphologic types are seen: the cauliflower variety (*condyloma acuminatum*); smooth, flesh-colored papular lesions; flat warts; and keratotic genital warts, which can mimic seborrheic keratosis. *Anogenital warts* result from the sexual transmission of HPV-6, HPV-11, HPV-16, and HPV-18 and grow on mucous membranes. They range in appearance from pinpoint to cauliflower-like. Experienced clinicians have been able to correlate the elevated, lobulated papular lesions with HPV-6 and HPV-11, whereas the flat, hyperpigmented types are high-risk lesions associated with HPV-16 and HPV-18. Coexistent sexually transmitted diseases are common. Mucocutaneous warts may become refractory to appropriate therapy.

DIFFERENTIAL DIAGNOSIS

Common warts should be differentiated from *squamous cell carcinoma*, *seborrheic keratosis*, and from a *cutaneous horn* arising from an actinic keratosis (see Chapter 177). The differential diagnosis also includes *Gottron's papules* (seen on the dorsal aspect of the fingers in dermatomyositis), *granuloma annulare*, *lichen planus*, *molluscum contagiosum*, *skin tags*, and *lichen nitidus*. Multiple flat warts on the face should be differentiated from trichoepithelioma, syringoma, and the cutaneous lesions of sarcoidosis. Anogenital warts must be differentiated from the *condyloma latum* of syphilis and from *squamous cell carcinoma*. The differential diagnosis also includes *pearly penile papules*, *ectopic sebaceous glands*, and *nevi*. Bowenoid papulosis (associated with HPV-16) appears as pigmented wart-like lesions on the male and female genitalia and is a form of carcinoma in situ, although it has little biologic tendency to behave aggressively.

WORKUP

The appearance is usually sufficient to indicate the diagnosis, but early genital warts can be difficult to identify. Typically, a patient comes for evaluation because warts have been found in a sexual partner. In a male patient, the penis and upper portion of the scrotum should be carefully examined under magnification. If no visible lesions are present, acetic acid can be used. Soaking the penis for 5 minutes with a gauze moistened with 5% acetic acid (white vinegar) demonstrates early lesions not readily evident under hand lens magnification, but magnification alone usually suffices. For the gynecologic examination, early warts are best demonstrated when they are made white with acetic acid. The colposcope provides still higher magnification. However, one must remember that the use of acetic acid is very nonspecific; any disease or lesion that alters the stratum corneum will turn white with acetic acid.

PRINCIPLES OF MANAGEMENT

Not all warts need to be removed. The primary care physician should keep in mind the basic principle that warts are benign tumors that often regress spontaneously. Treatment should not be so aggressive as to produce permanent scarring. Simple and safe treatments should be employed.

Location, discomfort, cosmetic effect, and therapies available influence the decision to treat. Larger, long-standing warts and those involving the plantar, perianal, or periungual area are the most difficult to treat but among those that patients most want to have removed. The patient's occupation, skin pigmentation, and body area should be considered when therapy is designed. The goal is to destroy the epidermal tumor while minimizing damage to the underlying dermis. The greater the dermal injury, the greater is the risk for scar formation. Only minimal scarring should be expected or considered acceptable.

A host of measures are available; choice is based on efficacy, patient acceptability, and scarring potential of the therapy and on location, size, and type of lesion. Physicians will most likely be seeing a self-selected group of patients for whom over-the-counter remedies have failed.

Common Warts. Freezing the lesion with *liquid nitrogen* applied on a cotton swab is convenient, well tolerated, often effective, and associated with a low risk for serious scarring. Solid freezing of the lesion is usually achieved by the repeated application of liquid nitrogen with a cotton swab dipped into a Styrofoam cup containing the supercold liquid. It may be useful to watch for a 30-second thaw time. For larger lesions, a repeated freeze–thaw cycle may interfere with efficacy. The freezing injury separates the wart from the underlying dermis. The successfully treated wart then falls off within 2 weeks. Before freezing, the thickened keratin should be pared off, but care should be taken not to cut into the profuse collection of capillaries within the wart. It is best to freeze a few millimeters of the surrounding normal tissue to facilitate separation from the underlying dermis. The patient should be warned that the area may hurt for several hours after treatment, and occasionally hemorrhagic blistering develops, especially with vigorous treatment.

If not completely gone, the wart can be treated again within 2 to 3 weeks. In difficult areas or with large lesions, several treatments may be necessary. Cures are related to the total number of treatments and not to the interval between. Treatment with liquid nitrogen has the advantage of being quick, bloodless, and not too painful, but the liquefied gas evaporates quickly and requires storage in special containers. Commercial kits generating sticks of "dry ice" from compressed carbon dioxide gas are available, but because the sticks are not as cold as liquid nitrogen, they are not as effective and require the application of more pressure for a longer time.

Curettage with or without *electrodesiccation* is effective but time-consuming, and substantial scarring can result if treatment is too vigorous. Some practitioners worry about the presence of virus in the smoke caused by the electrodesiccation. *Chemical cautery* with *nitric acid* or *monochloroacetic, bichloroacetic,* or *trichloroacetic acid* is an older alternative to liquid nitrogen.

Plantar Warts. Nonsurgical methods are preferred to surgical removal because scarring in this location can cause permanent discomfort. The lesion should be pared and then treated with the application of 40% *salicylic acid plasters*; these are taped in place for 1 to 3 days, after which the macerated skin is scraped off. This procedure is used for 2 to 3 weeks and can be performed by the patient. A salicylic acid preparation suspended in a karaya gum that promotes absorption (TransVerSal) is a convenient way to apply the medication. The pad containing the suspension is cut to size after the wart is pared down with an emery board. A drop of water is placed on the wart and the pad is applied and left in place for 8 hours each day. A larger salicylic acid patch (Trans Plantar) is indicated for treating large plantar warts. The convenience of this method is offset by the expense, but it is appreciated by some patients. *Liquid nitrogen* can be used on plantar warts in non–weight-bearing areas.

Daily 10% *formalin* or 25% *glutaraldehyde compresses* are sometimes used for mosaic plantar warts. Occlusal-HP is a prescription salicylic acid–lactic acid combination that contains salicylic acid in a polyacrylic vehicle. It is quite effective for plantar warts and has also been used successfully for warts on the hands.

Flat Warts. Topical *5-fluorouracil* cream or solution and *retinoic acid* cream or gel are used effectively for flat warts, especially those on the face. With both of these topical agents, patients will probably experience irritation characterized by erythema, scaling, and burning. Patients must be counseled that irritation will occur. Men should switch to an electric razor if they are using a blade razor, as cutting facial warts spreads them throughout the beard area. Similarly, women with flat warts on their legs must switch to an electric razor or use depilatory creams. Alternatively, 6% salicylic acid gel (Keralyt) is sometimes effective in treating multiple flat warts on the legs.

Genital Warts. A preparation of 20% to 40% *podophyllin* in compound tincture of benzoin is used to treat *macerated genital warts*. It must be applied sparingly, only to the wart, and allowed to dry thoroughly before the patient dresses. The medication is washed off by the patient 1 to 4 hours after application. Repeated treatment is the rule. Podophyllin is contraindicated in pregnancy. *Podofilox* 0.2% (Condylox) solution and gel are available for the treatment of external genital warts in both men and women. Podofilox is a purified fraction of podophyllin resins and is the first prescription product for the treatment of warts that is safe for self-application at home. It is applied for 3 days consecutively, followed by 4 days of no treatment; treatment is repeated if the warts persist.

Heat has been reported to be useful in treating stubborn warts. The temperature needs to be 43°C. The patient can use a candy thermometer to determine the temperature of the water. The wart should be soaked for 15 minutes twice daily. *Imiquimod 5% cream (Aldara)* can be quite effective in the treatment of anogenital warts. The drug is an immune response modulator that is applied by the patient overnight three times weekly for up to 16 weeks until the warts clear. It is very expensive, but for patients with refractory anogenital lesions, it should be considered.

The *carbon dioxide laser* is quite useful in destroying large numbers of warts in the vagina or around the anus. The procedure is carried out in an operating room environment. Postoperative morbidity is much less than when conventional methods are used.

As noted earlier, evaluation for concurrent venereal disease is mandatory in patients presenting with genital warts (see Chapters 125 and 126).

Refractory Warts. Sublesional *bleomycin,* diluted to 10 U/mL, has a distinct role in the treatment of refractory warts, both those on the hands and the plantar variety. Usually, 1 or 2 U injected beneath the wart is sufficient. Blanching occurs immediately, followed by blackening of the wart with subsequent clean sloughing. This treatment is less painful than liquid nitrogen for the most part, and causes no systemic effects.

Interferon alfa (both type 2a and type 2b) has been approved for the treatment of refractory genital warts. Intralesional injection is performed three times a week for 3 weeks. Lesions clear in fewer than 50% of patients, and this treatment has the disadvantages of being painful and expensive.

Immunostimulation is sometimes tried. *Dinitrochlorobenzene* (DNCB) sensitization followed by repeated applications of diluted DNCB has been used to treat resistant warts. This form of immunotherapy is sometimes effective, but DNCB has been shown to be a potential carcinogen in some studies. Autogenous wart *vaccines* appear no more effective than placebo.

The *carbon dioxide laser* has become an increasingly popular method for treating warts, although in many instances it is little more than an expensive method of causing tissue destruction. It is best reserved for certain situations, such as extensive vaginal or anal warts or refractory periungual lesions.

PATIENT EDUCATION

Prevention entails avoiding others with warts and having warts removed so that the viral reservoir is reduced. Although warts may initially have been acquired during contact with others, biting and picking at warts may result in the formation of additional lesions. Patients with periungual warts should be cautioned that biting the warts or pulling hangnails may result in the spread of lesions. Patients with genital warts can be reassured that warts do not develop in everyone who is exposed, but condom use should be urged.

The treatment of warts can be both time-consuming and expensive. Recurrences are seen in about one third of instances. The patient must be made to understand that warts are caused by a virus and that treatment usually does not eliminate the virus. Nonetheless, the patient can be reassured that in most instances the immune system will eventually prevent HPV from causing warts despite the continued presence of the virus. The length of treatment, cost, discomfort, risk for scarring, and possible failure of therapy should be candidly discussed before treatment is initiated.

INDICATIONS FOR REFERRAL

A Papanicolaou smear showing cervical dysplasia and evidence of HPV requires referral to a gynecologist for consideration of cervical biopsy. Women with extensive involvement by vaginal warts are also candidates for gynecologic consultation and possible laser therapy. Patients with truly refractory lesions who still insist on their removal may benefit from a dermatologic or surgical consultation. If topical treatment proves ineffective, electrocoagulation or surgical excision deserves consideration. Excision of large venereal warts that do not respond to podophyllin is indicated to rule out malignancy.

THERAPEUTIC RECOMMENDATIONS

- Use liquid nitrogen for initial treatment of common warts. Apply with a cotton swab to an area that includes a small rim of surrounding skin.
- Treat plantar warts by first paring them down carefully with a scalpel and then applying a piece of 40% salicylic acid plaster cut in the shape of, but slightly smaller than, the wart. Cover with occlusive adhesive tape and leave in place for 24 to 72 hours. Continue treatment at home, with gentle paring and reapplication of salicylic acid plaster as needed. Check progress regularly.
- Treat flat warts with topical 5-fluorouracil, retinoic acid, or Keralyt, a 6% salicylic acid gel.
- Treat moist anogenital warts with topical podophyllin; remind the patient to remove the medication after 4 to 6 hours. Consider topical podofilox for patient administration at home if repeated treatment is needed.
- Consider the use of imiquimod for anogenital lesions that do not respond to less expensive therapy.
- If these topical treatments prove ineffective or if the patient has extensive anal or genital involvement, then refer for con-

sultation and consideration of more aggressive therapy, such as carbon dioxide laser treatment.

ANNOTATED BIBLIOGRAPHY

Bart BJ, Biglow J, Vance JC, et al. Salicylic acid in karaya gum patch as treatment for verruca vulgaris. J Am Acad Dermatol 1989;20:74. (*A 69% cure rate achieved.*)

Beutner KR, Ferenczy A. Therapeutic approaches to genital warts. Am J Med 1997;102:28. (*An excellent review of conventional and investigational therapies.*)

Beutner KR, Tyring SK, Trofatter KF Jr, et al. Imiquimod, a patient-applied immune-response modifier for treatment of external genital warts. Antimicrob Agents Chemother 1998;42:789. (*Fifty-two percent of warts cleared, with a recurrence rate of 19%.*)

Bourke JF, Berth-Jones J, Hutchinson PE. Cryotherapy of common viral warts at intervals of 1, 2 and 3 weeks. Br J Dermatol 1995;132:433. (*Cure was related to the number of treatments and independent of the interval between treatments.*)

Carne CA, Dockerty G. Genital warts: need to screen for coinfection. BMJ 1990;300:459. (*High percentage of cases with coexisting venereal disease.*)

Cobb MW. Human papillomavirus infection. J Am Acad Dermatol 1990;22:547. (*Comprehensive review covering virology, epidemiology, pathogenesis, immunology, clinical manifestations, and treatment; 138 references.*)

Crum CP, Ikenberg H, Richart RM, et al. Human papillomavirus type 16 and early cervical neoplasia. N Engl J Med 1984;310:880. (*Association of type 16 subtype of papillomavirus with cervical neoplasia.*)

Dvoretzky I. Hyperthermia therapy for warts utilizing a self-administered exothermic patch. Review of two cases. Dermatol Surg 1996;22:1035. (*A new exothermic patch providing long-lasting, continuous heating of the skin surface to between 42° and 43°C for at least 2 hours was very successful.*)

Landow K. Nongenital warts. When is treatment warranted? Postgrad Med 1996;99:24549. (*A balanced discussion of various types of treatments.*)

Ling MR. Therapy of genital human papillomavirus infections. Int J Dermatol 1992;31:682,769. (*Excellent two-part review including rationale and methods for treatment; 96 references.*)

Ordoukhanian E, Lane AT. Warts and molluscum contagiosum. Beware of treatments worse than the disease. Postgrad Med 1997;101:223. (*A discussion of etiology, natural course, and treatment options.*)

Street ML, Roenigk RK. Recalcitrant periungual verrucae: the role of carbon dioxide laser vaporization. J Am Acad Dermatol 1990;23:115. (*Seventy-one percent cured after one or two treatments.*)

Tyring S, Edwards L, Cherry LK, et al. Safety and efficacy of 0.5% podofilox gel in the treatment of anogenital warts. Arch Dermatol 1998;134:33. (*Thirty-seven percent of patients treated with the podofilox gel had complete clearing of their warts after 4 weeks, and additional clearing after 8 weeks of treatment.*)

195
Management of Scabies and Pediculosis

ALICE Y. LIU
WILLIAM V. R. SHELLOW

Scabies and pediculosis are two arthropod parasitic skin diseases commonly seen in the primary care setting. Although accurate diagnosis, effective treatment, and preventive measures are available, infestations with scabies and lice are pandemic, affecting millions of patients worldwide. The primary physician should learn to recognize the manifestations of infestation quickly, and should be able to treat infestations effectively.

PATHOPHYSIOLOGY AND CLINICAL PRESENTATION

Scabies

Infestation with the human skin mite *Sarcoptes scabiei var hominis* leads to the disease scabies. Transmission is through prolonged close personal contact, either sexual or nonsexual. Persons of all socioeconomic levels, both sexes, and all age groups can be affected. Once contracted, scabies usually persists until specific therapy is instituted.

The scabies mite is an obligate arachnid human parasite, unable to live independently of its host. The mite measures 1/60 inch in length. The adult female attaches to and burrows into the horny layer of the skin. Copulation with a wandering male renders the female fertile for life. The female mite remains within her burrow for the rest of her 1-month life, laying two or three eggs a day. These eggs hatch within 3 to 4 days. Mature adults develop during the next 10 to 14 days. While in her burrow, the female feeds on epidermal cells. The average number of female mites on the body is 11.

Patients usually present with intense *pruritus*, which is often severe during the night. Pruritus also occurs when patients remove their clothing or become overheated. Eighty-five percent of infested persons have *burrows* on the fingers, interdigital areas, and wrists; these appear as linear marks a few millimeters in length, often with a dark dot at one end, which represents the female mite. Other common sites for burrows are the elbows, feet, ankles, penis, scrotum, buttocks, and axillae. Vigorous scratching may lead to excoriations, eczematous plaques, crusted papules, or secondary infection. In healthy adults, infestation is usually confined to skin below the neck. However, elderly or immunosuppressed patients may also present with head and neck lesions.

The mite is not necessarily found in all the cutaneous lesions. The rash and accompanying pruritus reflect a sensitivity reaction to the mite, eggs, or scybala (fecal droppings). In patients who have never been infested, the pruritic rash develops after a 2- to 4-week initial asymptomatic phase of infestation. In previously sensitized patients, the eruption can occur within a few days. Antiscabetic treatment kills the mite and ova but does not remove the sensitizing dead organisms or scybala from the burrow. Thus, pruritus may continue for a few weeks after treatment, until the contents of the burrow are shed with the natural turnover of skin. Persistent postscabetic papules may occur, especially on the penis, which may require intralesional injection of corticosteroids.

Crusted (Norwegian) scabies is an infrequent variant of the disease in which patients harbor a high mite load and present with hundreds of thick, keratotic papules. This form often affects patients with a decreased host defense, such as those with *HIV infection*, or without the ability to scratch, such those who have had a stroke. Crusted scabies is highly contagious because of the myriad of mites in the exfoliating scales.

Pediculosis

Human lice, which are obligate human insect parasites, are responsible for the diseases pediculosis capitis, pediculosis corporis, and pediculosis pubis. Transmission is through contact with infested humans, clothing, combs, or bedding. Body lice are most commonly found in people with poor personal hygiene or in indigent populations. Head lice are a public health problem among school children. Pubic lice are predominantly transmitted sexually. Human lice are the vectors for the transmission of typhus and trench fever.

The two species of these wingless, dorsoventrally flattened, blood-sucking insects are *Pediculus humanus* (subspecies *capitis* and *corporis*), which infests the head and clothing, and *Phthirus pubis* (crab louse), which infests the pubic area. These insects measure 3 to 4 mm in length, *Phthirus pubis* demonstrating a more rounded body in comparison with *Pediculus humanus*. Adult lice require a blood meal every 3 to 6 hours. The female insect lives 1 month and lays 7 to 10 eggs (nits) a day, which in turn hatch in about 8 to 10 days. The head louse lives on the scalp and lays eggs that are cemented onto hairs about 1 cm from the scalp. Body lice live and lay eggs in clothing, often in the seams. The crab louse prefers axillary, eyebrow, eyelash, beard, pubic, limb, and trunk hairs and lays its eggs on these hairs. Lice may be able to survive off the human host for 24 hours.

The head louse typically infests the occipital portion of the *scalp* and sometimes the postauricular region. Although few adults are present, many oval nits can be found cemented to the hair. Patients often complain of scalp *pruritus*. Cervical adenopathy may be present. Body lice cause pruritus, often representing a sensitivity reaction to lice excretions. Patients can have multiple excoriations over the trunk, and vertical excoriations are characteristic of infestation. Body lice and eggs can be seen in clothing. Pubic lice cause pruritus, often *nocturnal*. Characteristic asymptomatic, macular, blue discolorations called maculae ceruleae are sometimes seen on the trunk and thighs. Lice can be seen grasping pubic hairs, and specks of brownish feces can sometimes be seen.

DIAGNOSIS

Scabies

The diagnosis is suggested by finding the characteristic *burrows*. They should be sought on the hands, wrists, ankles, and genital areas, where the recovery rate is highest. A *scraping* is performed by shaving off the roof of the burrow with a scalpel, scraping the base to remove the contents, and placing the material on a microscope slide. Next, a drop of light mineral oil and a cover slip are added. The lowest-power objective should be used to view the specimen under a light microscope. The presence of adult mites, immature mites, ova, or tan-brown scybala confirms the diagnosis. In mineral oil, but not in potassium hydroxide, movement of the mite may be seen. In the absence of a scraping, presumptive diagnosis can be made based on the symptoms, appearance of the rash, and the history of contacts who also have symptoms of itching.

Pediculosis

The diagnosis is made by direct examination of the involved area. Few adult lice are found at the bases of the hairs, but many nits are typically seen. Both are usually visible to the naked eye, but a hand lens and bright light may help. Nits appear as gray or white specks attached to the hair. The examination should be performed with gloves to avoid infestation. The detection of head lice is facilitated by plucking a few hairs and identifying the full or empty egg cases about 7 to 10 mm up the hair shaft. Organisms may be found at the nape and behind the ears. Pyoderma of the nape or the occiput requires that pediculosis capitis be ruled out. Vertical excoriations on the trunk are a cardinal sign of body lice. The underwear of a patient infected with pubic lice is often speckled with blood.

PRINCIPLES OF MANAGEMENT

Elimination of the infestation and relief of pruritus are the goals of treatment.

Scabies

Because infestation is from person to person, close contacts of a scabies patient should be treated even if free of symptoms. After the mites and ova have died, but before they are shed from the skin, pruritus may continue for a few weeks following treatment. During this time, it may be necessary to use topical corticosteroids and oral antihistamines to help control the sensitivity rash and pruritus. Occasionally, systemic steroids are required (see Chapter 105). *Permethrin 5% cream*, which is synthetically derived from the natural compound pyrethrin, is currently the first-line treatment for scabies. Its toxicity in mammals is low because it is minimally absorbed and quickly reduced to inactive metabolites. Permethrin acts on the parasite nerve cell membranes and leads to paralysis. The 5% formulation is available with prescription in the United States.

Lindane (γ-benzene hexachloride) lotion was formerly the agent of choice for the treatment of scabies. Because of reports of organism resistance and neurotoxicity in infants and persons with an extensively compromised epidermal barrier, lindane has been relegated to alternative-treatment status. It should not be used in children under 2 years of age, or in pregnant or lactating women.

Crotamiton 10% lotion is antipruritic but is usually less successful as a scabicide than is permethrin. The cure rate after five consecutive days of therapy is only about 55%. Malathion lotion is no longer available in the United States.

Ivermectin. The off-label use of ivermectin, a new antiparasitic medication, has been gaining popularity since it was introduced in the United States for the treatment of *Strongyloides* infestation. This macrocyclic lactone preferentially inhibits glutamate-gated chloride ion channels in invertebrate nerve and muscle. Its affinity for human channels is low, and penetration of the blood–brain barrier is minimal. Typically, a single dose of 200 μg/kg is given orally, and this has been reported to be extremely successful in treating infestation. Compliance is high because of the simplicity of treatment. Topical formulation is not yet available. Although many practitioners feel that one or two doses of ivermectin are safe, increased mortality of elderly patients treated with the medication has been reported. At the present time, it should not be administered to the elderly.

Although theoretically the scabies mite should not be able to live without its human host, most recommend that bed linens and underwear of all household members be washed thoroughly in hot water with detergent or dry cleaned to prevent reinfestation. Treatment of scabies is generally effective provided that all close contacts are treated simultaneously.

Pediculosis

Permethrin 1% cream rinse shampoo is the first-line treatment for pediculosis. The 1% strength is available without a prescription in the United States. Less than 2% is absorbed, and the drug is quickly reduced to inactive metabolites. The 1% preparation is effective for the treatment of pediculosis capitis. Most other nonprescription treatments for pediculosis combine the compound *pyrethrin*, a natural extract of chrysanthemum flowers, and a synergistic compound, *piperonyl butoxide*. The synergized pyrethrins have a wide safety margin because they are minimally absorbed through the skin. Because the nits have an undeveloped nervous system, none of these neurotoxic chemicals are completely ovicidal. Only permethrin has activity against eggs because it retains residual activity for 2 weeks and remains on the hair for 14 days after treatment. Thus, eggs that hatch after treatment can be killed. Some physicians still recommend that a second permethrin treatment be given 1 week after the first, for maximum cure rate.

Reports of resistance to standard treatment with 1% permethrin have engendered alternative strategies, including 5% permethrin cream overnight under a shower cap, ivermectin as described for scabies, oral trimethoprim/sulfamethoxazole, or physical methods such as *petrolatum* application. Eyelash involvement may be treated with petrolatum, which is nonirritating and nontoxic; the lice either suffocate or slip off the greased hairs.

To prevent reinfestation, *asymptomatic close contacts* should be treated simultaneously. Sheets and all clothing worn in the past 3 days should be laundered in hot soapy water or dry cleaned. Brushes and combs should be washed in hot water for 10 to 20 minutes. Floors, furniture, and play areas should be thoroughly vacuumed to remove hairs that may have been shed with viable eggs attached.

On occasion, secondary bacterial infection may occur, which can be treated with the application of topical mupirocin 2% ointment three times daily or the administration of appropriate oral antibiotics. As in scabies treatment, the use of *lindane* for the treatment of lice is no longer considered the first choice.

PATIENT EDUCATION

Patient education is essential. Treatment failure is usually the result of poor patient compliance. Written instructions are helpful. Review of the preventive measures outlined above is very important.

THERAPEUTIC RECOMMENDATIONS

Scabies

- Prescribe 5% permethrin cream, to be applied from the neck down (including all body folds and creases) and left on overnight for 8 to 12 hours. About 30 g is sufficient for the average adult. One treatment is usually adequate. Some practitioners are recommending application to the scalp also. Application beneath the nails may prevent reinfestation.
- Advise changing and cleaning of underwear and bed linen.
- Treat all household members.
- Only if reinfestation has occurred should a second course of treatment be necessary.
- Prescribe topical corticosteroids and oral antihistamines if rash and pruritus are bothersome; if severe, oral steroids can be considered.
- For crusted scabies, the use of a keratolytic agent (10% salicylic acid or 20% urea) can hasten shedding of the affected horny layer of skin. Subungual areas should be carefully coated with permethrin cream.

Pediculosis Capitis

- Have the patient routinely shampoo without medication and thoroughly dry hair. Excess water slows the neural activity of the insect, protecting it from the neurotoxic effects of permethrin. Sufficient permethrin 1% cream rinse should be applied to wet the hair thoroughly. It is left on for 10 minutes and then rinsed out.
- Alternatively, recommend a synergized pyrethrins shampoo, to be applied undiluted until the infested areas are entirely

wet. After 10 minutes, the areas are washed thoroughly with warm water and then dried. Because it is less effective as an ovicide, this treatment should be repeated in 7 to 10 days to kill any newly hatched lice.
- Advise drying the hair with a clean towel after treatment with a pediculicide and removing any remaining nits with a fine-toothed comb. Nit removal is believed to reduce the chance of reinfestation.
- Recommend that combs, clothing, and bed linens be washed.

Pediculosis Corporis and Pediculosis Pubis

- Treatment is similar to treatment for pediculosis capitis. Permethrin 1% cream rinse or 1% cream can be applied to the body for 10 minutes before being washed off.
- The sexual partners of patients with pediculosis pubis need to be treated.
- Treat eyelash involvement with the application of petrolatum jelly up to five times a day for 5 to 7 days. Alternately, recommend physostigmine ophthalmic ointment 0.25%, applied to the lashes four times daily for three consecutive days.
- Clothing and bed linens need to be washed.

ANNOTATED BIBLIOGRAPHY

Barkwell R, Shields S. Deaths associated with ivermectin treatment of scabies. Lancet 1997;349:1144. (*Increased deaths during 6-month period following ivermectin dose delivered to nursing home residents.*)

Burkhart CG, Burkhart CN, Burkhart KM. An assessment of topical and oral prescription and over-the-counter treatments for head lice. J Am Acad Dermatol 1998;38:979. (*Reviews permethrin, pyrethrin with piperonyl butoxide, lindane, crotamiton, ivermectin.*)

Burkhart CG. Scabies: an epidemiologic reassessment. Ann Intern Med 1983;98:498. (*Reviews epidemiology, clinical manifestations, treatment, and prevention.*)

Lewis EJ, Connolly SB, Crutchfield CE, et al. Localized crusted scabies of the scalp and feet. Cutis 1998;61:87. (*Atypical scabies with AIDS.*)

Meinking T, Taplin D, Kalter DC, et al. Comparative efficacy of treatment for pediculosis capitis infestations. Arch Dermatol 1986;122:267. (*Evaluates various treatments for pediculosis and questions widespread use of lindane.*)

Meinking TL, Taplin D, Hermida JL, et al. The treatment of scabies with ivermectin. N Engl J Med 1995;333:26. (*Reports the use of a single oral 200-μg per kilogram dose of ivermectin to treat scabies in healthy and HIV-infected adults.*)

Schachner LA. Treatment-resistant head lice: alternative therapeutic approaches. Pediatr Dermatol 1997;14:409. (*Describes treatment with 5% permethrin, ivermectin, trimethoprim/sulfamethoxazole, petrolatum.*)

196
Management of Skin Trauma: Bites and Burns

Part 1: Animal and Human Bites
ELLIE J. C. GOLDSTEIN

Five million animal bites, leading to 800,000 medical encounters, occur in the United States each year. Patients often present to the primary physician for advice and therapy. Patients may appear shortly after injury concerned about rabies, tetanus, or repair of a disfiguring tear. Sometimes they delay seeking care, only to present later with infection. The primary physician must provide first aid and tetanus prophylaxis, decide whether antibiotics are necessary, and estimate the risk for rabies. Human bites are less common but potentially more serious. Particularly treacherous are clenched-fist injuries, which result from striking the teeth. Occlusional bites and paronychial injuries may also result in infection.

PATHOPHYSIOLOGY AND CLINICAL PRESENTATIONS

Most bites result in minor trauma. Approximately 80% of patients neither need nor seek medical care. Bite wounds that produce a break in the skin allow the inoculation of bacteria that normally inhabit the skin or, more usually, the oral cavity of the biting animal. Conditions favoring infection include prior splenectomy, liver disease, immune compromise, crush injury, edema, wounds to the hand, and multiple punctures. Patients with established infection usually present more than 8 hours after having sustained an injury. Patients with preexisting edema (e.g., persons with congestive heart failure or chronic venous insufficiency, women who have undergone radical or modified mastectomy) are at risk for more severe infection.

Human bites, especially *clenched-fist injuries*, in which damage is inflicted while the tendons and other tissues of the exterior area of the finger are stretched to full length, the skin is broken, and the tendon and possibly the joint are exposed, are serious. As the fingers are straightened, the damaged parts relax, and infecting organisms are carried into the tissues, producing infection in wounds that may initially appear minor. If the joint capsule is penetrated, septic arthritis or osteomyelitis is a risk.

Bacteriology. In animal bites, the infecting organisms are usually the normal oral flora of the biting animal. *Pasteurella* species, including *P. multocida*, are present in 50% of animal oral cavities and in 50% of dog and 75% of cat bite wounds. Cat bites are more prone to infection than are dog bites and may lead to severe cellulitis. Cat-scratch disease is caused by *Bartonella henselae* and *B. quintana*, fastidious gram-negative rods; it often presents with fever and lymphadenopathy and is more frequently seen during the cold weather months. Any patient who has undergone splenectomy or has alcoholic liver disease is prone to sepsis with *Capnocytophaga canimorsus* (formerly DF-2).

The oral flora of humans is more abundant than in most animals and includes *Streptococcus viridans*, *Haemophilus influenzae*, *Eikenella corrodens*, *Prevotella* species, *Porphyromonas* species, anaerobic diphtheroids, fusobacteria, and spirochetes. Wounds may also be infected by *skin flora*, such as a group A β-hemolytic streptococci (*Streptococcus pyogenes*) or staphylococci (*Staphylococcus aureus*). If anaerobic bacteria are present, the infection is more severe and may lead to abscess formation. Human bites are responsible for most severe bite wound infections.

PRINCIPLES OF THERAPY

Principles of therapy include characterization of the injury, vigorous cleansing, elevation, tetanus prophylaxis, and administration of appropriate antibiotics.

Animal Bites

It is important to elicit a history of the circumstances surrounding the injury. If an animal bite occurred, the type of animal and its behavior need to be detailed, as well as whether the animal had been vaccinated, and whether the attack was provoked or unprovoked. The wound should be diagrammed in the chart, with proximity to bones or joints noted. Minor animal puncture wounds should be cleansed with *soap and water* and treated expectantly without antibiotics. Copious *irrigation* of wounds with normal saline solution is an important therapeutic adjunct. Animal puncture wounds that are small and clean require no other treatment.

Rabies. Since 1967, only one or two cases of rabies in humans have been documented each year in the United States. No cases of rabies have occurred in New York City or Los Angeles for many years. Raccoon rabies is epidemic in all states along the entire eastern seaboard. In most other states, skunks and bats are the most common rabid animals. Rabies is more prevalent in cats than in dogs in the United States. Rabies is a concern if the attack is unprovoked, occurs in a rural setting, or involves a raccoon, a bat, a skunk, or an animal that is behaving in a peculiar manner. The local health department provides data regarding the local incidence of rabies and should be notified for follow-up and documentation. If rabies is considered a possibility, *human diploid cell vaccine* should be given along with *rabies immune globulin* without delay (see Chapter 6). If a person is bitten by a pet, the animal should be watched at home by the owner for 2 weeks and the bite reported to the local health department.

Tetanus. It is important to determine whether the patient has had an initial series of tetanus shots and a booster within the past 10 years. Those who have not had an initial series should be given both *tetanus toxoid* and *tetanus immune globulin* (see

Chapter 6). For persons who have had the initial series but no booster in 10 years, 0.5 mL of *tetanus toxoid* should be administered IM.

Tear Wounds. Therapy for tear wounds is problematic. No controlled trials of closure versus nonclosure, with or without antibiotics, have been undertaken. The principles of therapy are to cleanse and debride the wound cautiously. After the wound has been left open for 24 hours, the edges can be approximated with adhesive strips or sutured; 500 mg of *amoxicillin/ clavulanate* is then given three times a day for 3 to 5 days. Secondary closures can be performed if it is apparent that no infection is present. Facial wounds may be closed and antibiotics given. It is useful to refer these patients to a plastic surgeon.

Infected Wounds. Patients who present with infection should receive debridement, drainage, cleansing, and antibiotics. *Penicillin/amoxicillin* can be used; the combination is often effective against *P. multocida*, streptococci, anaerobes, and *E. corrodens* but is ineffective against *S. aureus*. In penicillin-allergic patients, *doxycycline* is preferred because *P. multocida* is often resistant to erythromycin and cephalexin. *Amoxicillin/ clavulanic acid* is an effective but more expensive alternative. Only in vitro and anecdotal clinical data exist regarding the use of quinolones or oral second-generation cephalosporins for animal bites.

Human Bites

Human bites are usually located on an extremity. Wounds of the hand are the most serious. The same principles of cleansing, drainage, and debridement apply. Human bites should not be closed primarily, although edges can be approximated if the tear is severe. Antibiotics should be instituted after wound cultures are taken. *Penicillin* plus a *penicillinase-resistant penicillin* or *amoxicillin/clavulanic acid* should be administered pending culture results to cover β-lactamase–producing oral anaerobes and gram-positive cocci, particularly *S. aureus*. Infrequently, the presence of a gram-negative organism necessitates a change in antibiotic regimen. All patients previously immunized who have not had a booster in 5 years should be given 0.5 mL of *tetanus toxoid*. Follow-up is essential because of the potential for late serious infection. A small risk exists for the transmission of viral pathogens such as hepatitis A, B, and C viruses and HIV.

Clenched-fist Injuries usually require specialized care. Radiographs should be taken to rule out fractures and provide a baseline for future assessment of osteomyelitis. Extension and flexion of digits should be carefully checked and sensation tested. The third metacarpophalangeal joint is most often affected. The integrity of the joint capsule must be determined, and this may require an experienced surgeon. If the capsule is intact, the hand is cleaned, debrided, immobilized, and elevated. *Penicillin* plus a *penicillinase-resistant penicillin* or *ampicillin/sulbactam* or *cefoxitin* is started and *tetanus toxoid* administered. Patients seen within 8 hours of injury with intact joint capsules can be managed as outpatients with careful follow-up. Those with torn capsules need to be admitted for surgery and treatment with IV antibiotics. Patients who present

after 8 hours should be admitted for observation to determine whether the capsule is intact or interrupted.

THERAPEUTIC RECOMMENDATIONS AND PATIENT EDUCATION

- Clean all wounds vigorously with soap and water. Copiously irrigate with normal saline solution. A needle and syringe can be used to generate a high-pressure jet to cleanse puncture wounds.
- Immunize patients who have previously been immunized but have not had a booster in the past 5 years against tetanus with 0.5 mL of IM tetanus toxoid.

Animal Bites

- Animal puncture wounds that are trivial and clean, without crush injury and not involving the hand, often require no other treatment.
- Treat moderate or severe fresh, *uninfected* animal tear wounds with cleansing, debridement, and *phenoxymethyl penicillin* (250 mg four times daily), followed by secondary closure in 24 to 48 hours if no signs of infection are present.
- Treat *infected* animal bite wounds with debridement, drainage, and cleansing. Culture the wound, delay wound closure until infection subsides, and begin *penicillin* (500 mg four times daily). Add a penicillinase-resistant penicillin (e.g., 500 mg of *dicloxacillin* four times daily) if erythema appears to be spreading or if *S. aureus* is suspected. *Amoxicillin/clavulanic acid* (875/125 mg twice daily) may be used as a single agent, as may *cefuroxime* (500 mg twice daily), especially for an infected cat bite. If the patient is allergic to penicillin, use *doxycycline* (100 mg twice daily) for initial antibiotic therapy.
- Treat for 7 to 10 days for an uncomplicated cellulitis.

Human Bites

- Treat all human bites initially with both penicillin and a penicillinase-resistant agent (e.g., *dicloxacillin*). Delay closure of the wound.
- Elevate affected limb until the swelling declines, usually after 3 to 5 days.
- Immobilize clenched-fist injuries and obtain hand surgery consultation promptly.
- Instruct the patient to watch the wound for signs of infection, such as pain, redness, warmth, swelling, or purulent exudate.

ANNOTATED BIBLIOGRAPHY

Chuinard RG, D'Ambrosia RD. Human bite infections of the hand. J Bone Joint Surg 1977;59:416. (*A classic article outlining early and aggressive surgical management; stresses the need to determine capsule integrity.*)

Fallouji MA. Traumatic love bites. Br J Surg 1990;77:100. (*The underreported problem of "love" bites.*)

Goldstein EJC. Bite wounds and infection. Clin Infect Dis 1992; 14:633. (*A review of the current literature and a guide to proper management.*)

Goldstein EJC, Citron DM, Richwald GA. Lack of *in vitro* efficacy of oral forms of certain cephalosporins, erythromycin, and oxacillin against *Pasteurella multocida*. Antimicrob Agents Chemother 1988;32:213. (*Many strains of* P. multocida *isolated from infected bite wounds are resistant to cephalexin, erythromycin, and oxacillin.*)

Mann RJ, Hoffeld TA, Farmer CB. Human bites of the hand: 20 years of experience. J Hand Surg 1977;2:97. (S. viridans *was the most common aerobic pathogen; 44% of wounds had* S. aureus. *The use of penicillinase-resistant penicillin is recommended.*)

Sacks JJ, Kresnow M, Houston B. Dog bites: how big a problem? Injury Prev 1996;2:52. (*A review of the epidemiology and incidence of dog bites.*)

Talan DA, DM Citron, FA Abrahamian, et al., and the Emergency Medicine Animal Bite Infection Study Group. The bacteriology and management of dog and cat bite wound infections presenting to emergency departments. N Engl J Med 1999;340:85. (*The bacteriology of dog and cat bite wounds and their urgent care.*)

Taylor GA. Management of human bite injuries of the hand. Can Med Assoc J 1985;133:191. (*A well-conceived approach.*)

Weber DJ, Wolfson JS, Swarz MN, et al. *Pasteurella multocida* infections: report of 34 cases and review of the literature. Medicine (Baltimore) 1984;63:133. (*Comprehensive review.*)

Part 2: Management of Minor Burns

Accidental minor burns are common. The majority of the estimated 2 million annual burn victims can be treated as outpatients. The primary physician is often asked for advice about immediate care and should render definitive treatment for localized, partial-thickness burns.

PATHOPHYSIOLOGY AND CLINICAL PRESENTATION

Burns represent direct thermal injury to the cells of the skin and underlying structures. The clinical presentation depends on the degree of damage, which is a direct function of the intensity of heat and duration of exposure.

First-degree Burns involve just the superficial layers of the epidermis. The skin is painful, red, and swollen. It blanches with pressure and shows little or no edema. Ultraviolet radiation, scalding, low-intensity exposure to steam, or brief contact with a hot object are common causes. Complete recovery usually occurs within a week, often with peeling and sometimes with postinflammatory hyperpigmentation.

Second-degree Burns involve the epidermis and dermis; a broad distinction is made between superficial and deep burns, based on the amount of dermis involved. Deep second-degree burns involve the entire papillary dermis, with penetration to some or all of the reticular dermis. Second-degree burns present as painful red blisters or broken epidermis exposing a weeping, edematous surface. They are most often caused by scalds or brief exposure to a flame. Recovery requires 2 to 3 weeks; sometimes scarring occurs.

Third-degree Burns involve all layers of the epidermis and dermis, with penetration into underlying fat and muscle. They usually result from prolonged contact with steam, hot objects, or flames and present with ulceration and tissue necrosis. They are painless because nerve tissue in the area has been destroyed. Deep tissue destruction can occur in electrical or chemical burns that may not become evident for several days.

Sunburn and Photosensitivity Reactions. Sunburn is one of the most common types of burn seen by the office-based physician. It represents ultraviolet injury to the skin. There are two phases: an immediate, initial, erythematous phase, which generally fades within 30 minutes after exposure, and a delayed response—what patients call sunburn—that occurs 3 to 6 hours after the exposure to the sun and peaks in 12 to 24 hours. Sunburn is characterized by erythema, pruritus, and tenderness but may proceed to edema, vesiculation, and even blistering. Repeated severe sunburns at an early age increase the risk for melanoma and other skin cancers later in life (see Chapter 177). Long-term excessive exposure to ultraviolet light leads to sustained elevations in skin matrix metalloproteinases, which can degrade skin collagen and contribute to premature skin aging.

Sun-related eruptions may also occur as a result of photosensitizing medications. The primary culprits are thiazide diuretics, sulfa-containing agents, tetracyclines (particularly demeclocycline), griseofulvin, phenothiazines, and nalidixic acid. Topical substances, particularly furocoumarins (found in parsley, celery, carrots, certain perfumes, and aftershave lotions as is St. John's wort) are also photosensitizing.

PRINCIPLES OF THERAPY

The first task is to assess the depth and extent of injury. Treatment of burn wounds is based on the depth and surface area of skin involved. The surface area of burns has traditionally been based on the "rule of nines." Each arm is considered to be 9% of the body surface area, each leg is 18%, the anterior and the posterior trunk are each 18%, the head is 9%, and the perineum and genitalia are 1%.

With the use of these classifications, the treatment of burns can proceed in an organized fashion. All second-degree burns involving more than 5% to 10% of the body surface, all third-degree burns, any burns associated with an electric current, and all burns of the ears, eyes, face, hands, feet, or perineum should be treated immediately at a major hospital familiar with burn care. A history of prolonged contact with scalding liquids, flaming clothing, or high-voltage electric current portends full-thickness damage and the need for referral, as does dry, parchment-like skin with a loss of hair follicles and sensation.

First-degree burns and second-degree burns involving less than 5% of the body surface can be treated on an outpatient basis by the primary physician with adequate wound care and follow-up, provided the patient is reliable and the home situation amenable.

The goals of therapy are to reduce inflammation, prevent infection, relieve pain, and promote healing.

First-degree Burns

First aid to minor burns involves immediate application of *ice packs* or *cold compresses* of water, milk, or oatmeal. Cold reduces discomfort, edema, and hyperemia and may diminish the extent of injury. The application of cold should continue until the burn is pain-free. *No dressing* is required, just skin lubricant and instructions to return if blistering occurs. Prophylactic antibiotics appear to have little or no effect.

Pain can usually be relieved with aspirin or acetaminophen. Aspirin has the advantage of suppressing inflammation and is particularly helpful in sunburn.

In cases of extensive sunburn, a topical corticosteroid lotion or spray may provide symptomatic relief. Systemic corticosteroids do not reduce the edema associated with sunburn and are not indicated.

Second-degree Burns

If the skin is broken, the wound requires protection so that healing can occur without infection. This involves gently *washing* the area of the burn with water and a mild antiseptic soap, such as one containing chlorhexidine. Washing is followed by gentle *irrigation* with sterile isotonic saline solution and application of a sterile *occlusive dressing*. With chemical burns, the involved area is placed under running water for at least 15 to 30 minutes before cleansing or debridement is started. A syringe or water pick can be used to help irrigate and remove embedded debris. Devitalized tissue should be debrided (see appendix to section 12). Patients complaining of pain or who appear anxious should be given an analgesic or a sedative before the injured area is manipulated. Adherent tar can be removed after being hardened by the application of ice or softened with a topical antibiotic such as polysporin or mupirocin (Bactroban) ointment. *Tetanus prophylaxis* is indicated and includes administration of tetanus toxoid booster to previously immunized patients (see Chapter 6).

Management of Blisters is somewhat controversial. Some argue that blisters provide an excellent burn dressing and protective barrier, but others suggest that the trapped fluid can become a culture medium for bacteria. Small, thick-walled blisters probably should be left intact, whereas those that are larger, thin-walled, located on hairy skin that is prone to infection, or located in areas where movement is likely to cause rupture should be removed. Removal should be complete because needle aspiration simply negates the protective barrier while retaining the potential culture medium for infection.

Prophylaxis against Infection is provided by the topical antibiotic preparation *silver sulfadiazine* (Silvadene). The cream is easy to apply and provides softening in addition to an antibacterial effect. It is contraindicated in persons allergic to sulfa and in pregnant and nursing women. The agent should be applied with a tongue depressor or glove in a layer thick enough to prevent the burn from being visible. Pain can be minimized by keeping the cream refrigerated. Silver sulfadiazine should be removed daily or every other day and reapplied. *Systemic antibiotics* are indicated only for established infection and are not appropriate for prophylaxis or outpatient use.

Dressings are prepared by applying a nonadherent, fine mesh gauze soaked in sterile saline solution to the burn. This is then covered with a bulky dressing into which fluid can drain without passing through (see appendix to section 12). The patient should be examined in 2 days for pain, adenopathy, and fever, and the dressing should be checked. If no evidence of infection is seen, the dressing may remain for 5 to 7 days, after which the area is reexamined to determine the need for a dressing change.

Pain Relief is an essential part of management, and usually aspirin or a nonsteroidal agent such as ibuprofen suffices. Short courses of agents containing codeine or oxycodone are appropriate for painful burns. Topical anesthetics may provide symptomatic relief but are not justified because of the risk for sensitization. In cases of extensive sunburn, topical corticosteroid sprays may provide modest symptomatic relief, but a short course of systemic steroids may be more effective.

Moisturization is important but often overlooked. After the burn heals, the new epithelial layer tends to dry and crack, and this problem can be reduced by the application of a moisturizing cream such as Eucerin or aloe vera for 4 to 8 weeks after apparent resolution.

INDICATIONS FOR REFERRAL AND ADMISSION

Referral for surgical consultation and hospitalization is indicated if burns exceed 10% to 15% of body area or full-thickness burns exceed 3%. Prompt admission and surgical consultation should be considered for circumferential or full-thickness burns; involvement of the eyes, ears, other organs of sensation, hands, or perineum; evidence of inhalation injury; or serious concurrent medical conditions such as diabetes and immunosuppression. Patients who are unreliable or unable to care for themselves may also require inpatient treatment.

PATIENT EDUCATION

Patient education is critical to successful recovery from a burn. The patient and caretaker should be instructed to keep the wound clean and note erythema or inflammation, which are signs of infection. Instruct the patient to note numbness, tingling, or a change in skin color or temperature, which may suggest that the dressing is too tight and circulation is being impaired. Explicit (often written) instructions on the removal of dressings, cleansing of the wound, reapplication of topical sulfadiazine, and treatment of dried skin are important. Patients with healed burns should be instructed to avoid exposure to direct sunlight because of increased sensitivity during the year following a burn injury. A burn provides a good opportunity to reinforce the importance of sunscreen use and to educate the patient about the warning signs of skin cancer (see Chapter 177).

The occurrence of a burn, even a minor one, is a good opportunity to reinstruct patients on the importance of burn prevention. The obvious caveats are not to smoke and to keep flammable material and matches away from children. Specific instructions on the use of pot holders, careful puncturing and removal of plastic wraps from food heated in the microwave oven, and controlling the temperature of hot tap water are all helpful. Reminders about the importance of smoke detectors and maintaining an approved fire extinguisher are important. A written burn prevention checklist is a useful aid.

THERAPEUTIC RECOMMENDATIONS

- For first-degree burns, immediately apply cold and keep the area cold until it remains free of pain even when the cold is withdrawn.
- If the skin is broken, cleanse with a mild soap and water before applying cold water or ice.
- No dressing or antibiotic is indicated for first-degree burns. Emollients such as Eucerin or aloe vera should be used if blistering does not occur after several days.
- For severe sunburn, prescribe a gentle topical corticosteroid lotion for symptomatic relief. Aspirin or ibuprofen provides analgesia and helps limit inflammation. Consider a brief course of systemic steroids for extensive sunburn.
- For second-degree burns, spread silver sulfadiazine (Silvadene) over the involved area in a thickness sufficient to prevent the burn from showing through. Refrigerating the sulfadiazine minimizes pain. Wrap the area with six or seven layers of gauze for protection.
- Prescribe systemic antibiotics, usually dicloxacillin, for any secondary cellulitis. Prophylactic oral antibiotics should not be used for fear of selecting out resistant gram-negative organisms.

ANNOTATED BIBLIOGRAPHY

Deitch EA. The management of burns. N Engl J Med 1990;323:1249. (*A comprehensive discussion, including the approach to more serious burns.*)

Fisher GJ, Wang ZQ, Datta SC, et al. Pathophysiology of premature skin aging induced by ultraviolet light. N Engl J Med 1997;337:1419. (*Best discussion of the mechanisms of sun-induced skin damage and the implications for treatment.*)

Herbert K, Lawrence JC. Chemical burns. Burns 1989;15:381. (*A good review of this important category of burn injury.*)

Peate WF. Outpatient management of burns. Am Fam Physician 1992;45:1321. (*Well-referenced discussion of outpatient management.*)

Rockwell WB, Ehrlich HP. Should burn blister fluid be evacuated? J Burn Care Rehabil 1990;11:93. (*The authors argue for removal of even intact blisters because the fluid can be a good culture medium for bacteria.*)

Waymack JP, Pruitt BA Jr. Burn wound care. Adv Surg 1990;23:261. (*Focuses on surgical management and indications for admission.*)

197
Management of Skin Ulceration
WILLIAM V. R. SHELLOW

Skin ulceration can be a troublesome, disabling, and potentially dangerous problem. Cutaneous ulcers commonly encountered in medical practice include leg and pressure ulcerations. Approximately 1% of the population is affected by venous leg ulcers. Diabetics and others with arterial insufficiency are at increased risk for ischemic ulceration and limb-threatening infection. About 20% of geriatric patients have pressure ulcers, with an associated fourfold increase in mortality. The primary physician who recognizes and effectively treats early skin changes can prevent many of the debilitating consequences.

PATHOPHYSIOLOGY AND CLINICAL PRESENTATION

Skin ulceration most commonly results from venous or arterial insufficiency or from prolonged, excessive pressure. Infectious and malignant causes are also encountered, especially in immunocompromised persons.

Venous Insufficiency. The initial manifestation of venous insufficiency is edema, usually absent on arising and severe at the end of the day. Incompetent venous valves can be associated with age, thrombophlebitis, or a hereditary tendency to the development of venous varicosities. In all three conditions, abnormally high venous pressure during ambulation causes fibrinogen to leak from the engorged capillary bed. A precapillary fibrin layer develops and interferes with oxygen and nutrient exchange. Pigmentation, induration, dermatitis (*stasis dermatitis*), and finally ulceration may develop. The rupture of delicate venules releases hemoglobin, which changes to hemosiderin, producing pigmentation. Scaling and oozing develop when the skin is scratched. Vesicles may indicate a contact dermatitis caused by a topical medication. Secondary bacterial invasion occurs and may lead to cellulitis.

Stasis ulcerations develop within areas of dermatitis or indurated cellulitis. They occur most often above the medial malleolus because of its poor vascular supply and sparse subcutaneous tissue. Minor trauma can precipitate ulceration. The stasis ulcers vary in size from small erosions to an ulcer that encircles the ankle. They may or may not be painful. The base of the ulcer is usually moist, with exuberant granulation tissue. Purulence indicates secondary infection.

Arterial Insufficiency. The most common cause of arterial insufficiency is *atherosclerotic disease.* The leg is cold and appears pale or cyanotic (although dependent rubor may be present), and peripheral pulses are lost or reduced. The ulcers are initially small, punctate, and superficial, but with worsening ischemia, they become larger and deeper. Typically, they occur on the sides of the feet, the heels, the toes, and the nail beds.

Ischemic ulcers are also associated with *hypertensive disease* and *vasculitis.* Those occurring in the context of hypertension characteristically develop over the lateral malleoli. They begin as painful, blue-red plaques that soon ulcerate. A purpuric halo may surround the ulceration. Vasculitic ulcers occur in the context of connective tissue disease, hematologic and malignant conditions, and hypersensitivity reactions, beginning as palpable purpuric lesions or hemorrhagic vesicles (see Chapter 179).

Decubitus Ulcer

The pressure sore or decubitus ulcer is common in bedridden or semiambulatory patients. It may present as nonblanchable erythema, soft-tissue loss, blisters, or eschar over bony prominences. Pressure ulcer severity is reflected by the stage of the lesion. Stage 1 lesions are manifested by nonblanchable erythema of intact skin. Stage 2 ulcers involve only the epidermis and dermis. Stage 3 ulcers extend into the subcutaneous tissues and undermine the surrounding skin. Stage 4 lesions extend through deep fascia to involve muscle and may extend to the bone.

Factors contributing to the development of pressure sores include shearing forces, friction, and moisture. Decubitus ulcers usually occur over bony prominences. The pressure gradient occludes lymphatic vessels and overloads the microvascular system, so that waste products accumulate and ultimately necrosis ensues. The lower part of the body and sacrococcygeal area are the predominant sites, with the hip, malleolus, and heel being other important areas.

Pressure sores can lead to cellulitis, bacteremia, osteomyelitis, and even meningitis. The microbiology of decubitus ulcers is polymicrobial, and the organisms that cause the most problems, including life-threatening bacteremias, are *group A streptococci, Staphylococcus aureus, Escherichia coli,* and *Bacteroides fragilis.*

PRINCIPLES OF MANAGEMENT

Many of the principles of ulcer management are similar, regardless of cause or location. Important objectives are to restore circulation (see Chapters 34 and 35), improve local factors, reduce pressure, remove necrotic tissue, maintain cleanliness, and prevent further injury.

Leg Ulcers

Regardless of cause, treatment of the leg ulcer begins with washing the leg and ankle with a mild soap. Emollients are used to prevent drying (xerosis). In leg ulcers with a clean base, application of an Unna's paste boot or an occlusive wound dressing may encourage healing and reepithelialization. An *Unna's boot* is a flesh-colored gauze roll bandage impregnated with zinc oxide, calamine, glycerin, and gelatin. Topical enzymes and hydrophilic beads are sometimes useful adjunctive agents in leg ulcers or pressure ulcers.

The bewildering array of commercially available *occlusive wound dressings* includes polyurethane films (Opsite, Tegaderm, Bioclusive), polyethylene oxide hydrogel (Vigilon, Spenco 2nd Skin), foam dressings (Lyofoam, Allevyn), laminate dressings (Biobrane), alginate dressings (Sorbsan, Kaltostat), and hydrocolloid dressings (DuoDerm). The dressing is replaced every 3 to 7 days, or sooner if it begins to leak. The patient must be warned to expect an unpleasant odor, caused by a buildup of fluid, when the dressing is removed. The optimal occlusive dressing for wound healing remains to be developed. DuoDerm is readily available and convenient to use.

Occlusive dressings are promoted as being capable of shortening the healing time, although they often prove no better than simple *wet-to-wet dressings.* Wet-to-wet dressings, along with cleaning and gentle debridement with gauze sponges several times daily, are useful. Dilute hydrogen peroxide can be used to clean the ulcerated area. Occlusive dressings do offer greater convenience and some pain relief. Occlusive dressings should not be used on wounds complicated by cellulitis.

Treatment of Stasis Dermatitis. Stasis dermatitis of any degree should be attended to because it can lead to further ulceration. Venous insufficiency and edema should be treated (see Chapter 35). *Topical corticosteroids,* creams or ointments, are useful to reduce the inflammatory component and itching. Corticosteroids should not be applied within an ulcer because they may delay wound healing. Oozing dermatitis requires wet dressings (compresses) and bed rest with leg elevation. Acute exudative dermatitis can be soothed and dried with cool *Burow's compresses.* Scratching, use of over-the-counter medications, and placement of adhesive tape on involved areas should be avoided and prohibited.

Secondarily infected dermatitis should be treated with *oral antibiotics* active against staphylococcal infection, such as dicloxacillin, amoxicillin/clavulanate (Augmentin), or erythromycin. *Topical antibiotics* may be used in mild cases. Topical mupirocin is effective against a wide range of staphylococci, including methicillin-resistant organisms, and appears to be nonsensitizing. However, its use should not be continued beyond 14 days because of the risk for emergence of resistant species with longer use. Preparations containing neomycin should be avoided because of its tendency to induce contact sensitization and dermatitis. Even the dual antibiotic ointments containing polymyxin and bacitracin have induced contact dermatitis.

External *compressive bandages* or *stockings* should be used to reduce venous pressure in the lower extremities, and compression has been shown to promote healing. Graduated compressive surgical stockings are expensive but can be helpful (see Chapter 35). The patient should apply the compression in the morning before getting out of bed. Prolonged standing should be avoided, weight loss emphasized, and periods of leg elevation encouraged. Intermittent pneumatic compression has been used successfully as an alternative to elastic compression in refractory cases to speed ulcer healing.

Decubitus Ulcer

Nutritional repletion is important to reverse catabolism and to correct all factors that affect the oxygenation of tissue, such as anemia, edema, and vascular problems. *Reducing pressure on the affected area is critical.* In some cases, an alternating-pressure air mattress may be indicated. The basic principle of debridement is to use *wet-to-wet dressings* or an occlusive dressing. A variety of biochemical agents that dissolve debris are purported to promote healing, although double-blind evidence of their efficacy is generally lacking. Occasionally, grafts are required to close the ulceration.

If decubitus ulcers are complicated by infection, the antibiotic program should include anaerobic in addition to aerobic coverage. Even a shallow ulcer may hide a deep infective sinus or a tunnel to an osteomyelitis. A roentgenogram may be useful to detect chronic osteomyelitis.

Further measures include the use of laser sterilization, growth factors, allografts, and platelet aggregation inhibitors. The best treatment remains primary prevention.

PATIENT EDUCATION

With most ulcers, prevention is the key. Patients and family must be educated to look for pre-ulcerative changes in stasis dermatitis and use compensatory measures before ulceration occurs. In patients with chronic vascular disease, advice about cutting nails, treating sores early, and seeking medical care at the first sign of a break in skin is important. For people confined to bed or a chair, the family should be educated about preventing prolonged pressure on a bony prominence.

INDICATIONS FOR REFERRAL AND ADMISISON

Failure of ulcers to heal despite good management and a compliant patient indicates the need for surgical consultation. Surgical debridement and split-thickness or full-thickness skin grafting may be necessary. If fever or other signs of bacteremia develop, then IV antibiotics and prompt hospitalization are needed. Mortality risk is high, especially with associated anemia and hypoalbuminemia.

THERAPEUTIC RECOMMENDATIONS

Venous Insufficiency and Stasis Dermatitis

- In all patients with changes of stasis, control edema with rest, elevation, diuretics, avoidance of dependency, and external compression with stockings or bandages.
- Treat any concurrent nutritional deficiency, hypertension, diabetes, or congestive heart failure.
- Treat pruritus with intermediate-potency topical corticosteroids (e.g., 0.1% triamcinolone acetonide). Ointments are indicated if the area is dry and scaly, and creams should be used if the area is moist. Avoid application near or on an ulcer because corticosteroids may delay wound healing.
- Treat acute exudative dermatitis with cool Burow's compresses (1:40 dilution) two to three times daily for 30 to 60 minutes.
- Scratching and use of over-the-counter medicaments should be discouraged.

Cutaneous Ulceration

- Prescribe application of wet-to-wet dressings, followed by cleaning and gentle debridement with gauze sponges several times daily. Dilute hydrogen peroxide can be used to clean the ulcerated area.
- Occlusive dressings are worth a trial because they may ease pain, debride ulcers, and lead to healing without the need for surgical intervention.
- In the clinical setting of secondary infection, culture for aerobic and anaerobic bacteria, and treat accordingly with oral or IV antibiotics.
- In cases of mild skin infection, topical antibiotic creams such as mupirocin can be considered for short-term use (<2 weeks), but preparations that contain neomycin should be avoided.
- In cases of persistent deep ulcers, underlying osteomyelitis should be considered. A roentgenogram may be useful.
- Refer for surgical consultation patients whose ulcers prove refractory to proper conservative management. Pinch grafting is a relatively simple approach that can be performed in the office. Culture-derived human skin-equivalent grafts (Apligraf) have been quite successful but are very expensive. Becaplermin (recombinant human platelet-derived growth factor BB) gel (Regranex) has been shown to be clinically effective in healing ulcers but is also very expensive to prescribe.
- Surgical debridement and split-thickness or full-thickness skin grafting may be necessary.
- Alternative medicine has been shown to be of some value in the healing of wounds.

ANNOTATED BIBLIOGRAPHY

Ahnlide I, Bjellerup M. Efficacy of pinch grafting in leg ulcers of different aetiolgies. Acta Derm Venereol 1997;77:144. (*Of 145 therapy-resistant leg ulcers, 36% healed after pinch grafting; 22% of these were venous ulcers, and 50% were arterial ulcers.*)

Allman RM. Pressure ulcers among the elderly. N Engl J Med 1989;320:850. (*Good discussion of risk factors.*)

Angle N, Bergan J. Chronic venous ulcer. Br Med J 1997;314:1019. (*A succinct review of mechanisms by which venous ulcers develop and ways to heal them.*)

Alvarez OM, Fahey CB, Auletta MJ, et al. A novel treatment for venous ulcers. J Foot Ankle Surg 1998;37:319. (*The efficacy of using culture-derived human skin-equivalent grafts to heal venous leg ulcers is documented.*)

Falanga V. Occlusive wound dressings. Arch Dermatol 1988;124:872. (*Reviews commercially available occlusive dressings.*)

Falanga V, Eaglestein WH. A therapeutic approach to venous ulcers. J Am Acad Dermatol 1986;14:777. (*A systematic approach emphasizing the usefulness of newer and more effective occlusive dressings.*)

Fletcher A, Cullum N, Sheldon TA. A systematic review of compression treatment for venous leg ulcers. BMJ 1997;315:576. (*Compression systems improve the healing of venous leg ulcers and should be used routinely.*)

Hofman D, Ryan TJ, Arnold F, et al. Pain in venous leg ulcers. J Wound Care 1997;6:2224. (*A prospective study of 140 patients to assess the prevalence, severity, and diagnostic utility of pain caused by venous leg ulcers.*)

Mol MAE, Nanninga PB, van Eendenburg JP, et al. Grafting of venous leg ulcers. J Am Acad Dermatol 1991;24:77. (*Indications and success of skin grafting of leg ulcers.*)

Papantonio C. Alternative medicine and wound healing. Ostomy Wound Management 1998;44:44. (*Acupuncture, energy healing, guided imagery, hypnosis, prayer, and relaxation techniques may offer benefits.*)

Phillips TJ, Dover JS. Leg ulcers. J Am Acad Dermatol 1991;25:965. (*Comprehensive review; 211 references.*)

Yarkony GM, Kirk PM, Carlson C, et al. Classification of pressure ulcers. Arch Dermatol 1990;126:1218. (*Pathophysiology and updated classification of pressure ulcers.*)

Appendix to Section 12
Minor Surgical Office Procedures for Skin Problems

ERIC KORTZ
CHARLES J. McCABE

SIMPLE LACERATIONS

Treatment of simple lacerations is one of the most commonly performed outpatient surgical procedures. All lacerations should be evaluated for the extent of injury to surrounding structures, particularly nerves. This is most important with lacerations of the face, hand, and wrist. All injuries involving peripheral nerves should be referred to an emergency room; digital nerve branches can be approximated with excellent long-term benefit. All tendon injuries should receive the attention of a hand surgeon. Those lacerations complicated by bone fracture should be treated by an orthopedic surgeon.

In uncomplicated wounds, foreign material around and within the wound, including devitalized tissue, should be removed before definitive closure.

The following materials are used to treat simple lacerations:

Anesthetic
1. 1% or 2% Xylocaine without epinephrine
2. 5-mL to 10-mL syringes
3. 19-G to 22-G needles

Prep Solution
1. Gentle soap solution
2. Betadine
3. Normal saline

Drapes
1. Three or four sterile towels

Instruments
1. Adson forceps
2. Needle holders (plastic)
3. Hemostat
4. Irrigation bulb syringe
5. Suture scissors
6. Suture material (Table 1)
7. Six to 12 sterile gauze pads
8. Sterile gloves

Dressings
1. Xeroform gauze
2. Two gauze pads
3. Tape or gauze roll

Anesthesia
- Infiltration of the wound edges may either precede or follow wound cleansing and debridement, depending on the patient and the wound.
- The path of the injecting needle should proceed from clean, prepped areas to deeper tissue levels. The interior of the wound should be avoided.
- Aspiration should precede infiltration of anesthetic to prevent intravascular injection.

Skin-Wound Preparation and Draping
- Copiously irrigate the wound with normal saline under moderate pressure. Foreign material and devitalized tissue are removed at this time. The wound and surrounding skin are then cleansed with a gentle detergent, followed by an antiseptic such as Betadine applied to the surrounding skin only.
- Sterile drapes are placed to isolate the wound completely, including enough surrounding skin to allow easy approach and a working surface area.

Wound Closure
- Hemostasis is obtained. Bleeding is usually minimal. Closure proceeds in one or several layers, depending on the depth of the wound. Subcutaneous sutures are of the absorbable type, either 3-0 or 4-0 Dexon or chromic. These sutures should be simple, interrupted stitches secured with minimal tension.
- Skin closure for minor lacerations is best achieved with a nonabsorbable monofilament suture. Nylon is an inexpensive and excellent choice. The suture placement technique should

Table 1.   Suture Selection and Removal Time

LOCATION	SUTURES	REMOVAL TIME (DAYS)
Scalp	3-0	10–14
Face	5-0, 6-0	4–5
Neck	3-0, 4-0	7–10
Trunk	3-0	7–10
Extremities	3-0	8–12
Hands	4-0, 5-0	8–12
Feet	3-0, 4-0	8–12
Oral mucosa	4-0, 3-0 chromic	10–14

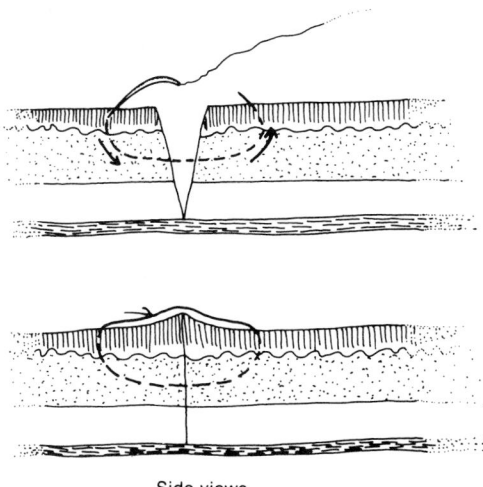

Side views

Figure 1. Simple interrupted stitch for skin closure. Notice the path of the needle; the needle enters and leaves the skin at acute angles, which allows eversion of the skin edges. (Grossman JA: Minor Injuries and Disorders: Surgical and Medical Care, p 52. Philadelphia, JB Lippincott, 1984)

be simple, interrupted, and allow for approximation of the wound edges without inducing ischemia. As Figure 1 demonstrates, the curved needle should enter the skin at an acute angle. Advancement is then with the natural curve of the needle and includes all layers (epidermis, dermis, and the upper subcutaneous tissue). Care should be taken to maintain equal depth and width from the wound edge with each stitch. A good technique is to sequentially divide the wound in half. The first stitch is placed directly in the center of the laceration. Subsequent sutures subdivide the remaining open surface. Corresponding parts of an irregular wound should be approximated first.

Dressings

- After the entire wound is closed, normal saline or a gauze sponge can be used to clean the skin of dried blood and Betadine.
- The wound is then covered with a strip of xeroform gauze and dry sterile dressing.
- Lacerations involving the fingers, palm, or wrist should be immobilized.
- Follow-up for patients with minor lacerations can be done at the time of suture removal. A convenient schedule for suture removal is presented in Table 1.

SIMPLE PARONYCHIA

Paronychia (Fig. 2) represents a soft tissue infection and abscess formation along the nail border. The patient usually complains of pain, and the area surrounding the nail base is red, swollen, and tender.

The following materials are used to treat simple paronychia:

Anesthetic

1. 1% or 2% Xylocaine without epinephrine
2. 5-mL to 10-mL syringes
3. 19-G to 22-G needles

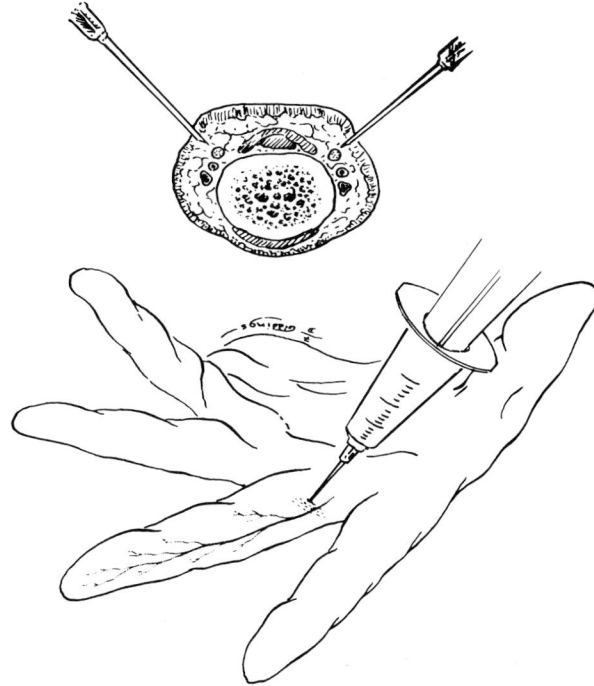

Figure 2. Metacarpal block. Entrance of needle is at the palmar base of finger, medial and lateral. The needle path is then toward the palmar metacarpal head. (Van Way CW III, Buerk CA (eds): Surgical Skills in Patient Care, p 55. St Louis, CV Mosby, 1978)

Prep Solution

1. Gentle soap solution
2. Betadine or alcohol
3. Normal saline

Drapes

1. Three or four sterile towels

Instruments

1. Adson forceps
2. Pediatric suture scissors
3. Kelly clamps
4. No. 15 scalpel blade
5. Scalpel handle
6. Sterile gloves

Dressings

1. Nu-Gauze $1/4$ inch
2. Two gauze pads
3. Tape or gauze roll

Anesthesia

Complete anesthesia of the finger may be accomplished with a metacarpal block (Fig. 3). After alcohol preparation of the skin over the metacarpophalangeal joint is performed, points for needle entrance are selected on the medial and lateral palmar surface of the metacarpal head. Care is taken to aspirate each time before the infiltration of 1 to 2 mL of Xylocaine.

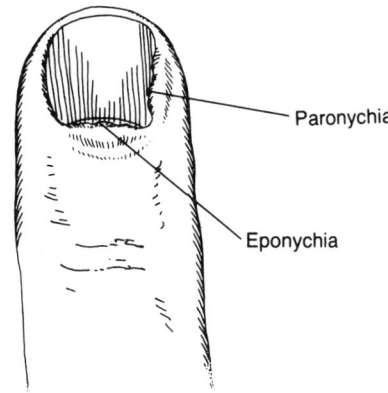

Figure 3. Simple paronychia. (Grossman JA: Minor Injuries and Disorders: Surgical and Medical Care, p 253. Philadelphia, JB Lippincott, 1984)

Preparation of Skin

The entire digit, including the metacarpal head, may be washed with a gentle soap solution, followed by application of a uniform layer of Betadine.

Draping

Placement of sterile towels must achieve isolation of the digit involved and exposure of the metacarpal area. Additional anesthesia is sometimes necessary.

Incision and Drainage

Treatment of the laterally based infection (see Figure 2) involves incising the skin along the lateral edge of the nail; a small incision is made directly over the swollen, fluctuant area. After drainage of purulent material, a wick is used to prevent premature wound closure. The wick is removed after 24 to 36 hours and soaking of the digit is begun on a twice-daily schedule.

Occasionally, a portion of the nail must be removed to establish adequate drainage, particularly if the infection has established penetration of the subungual space. A small scissors is used to separate the nail from the underlying matrix. This dissection is carried out from the tip of the nail to the base in a vertical strip involving $1/6$ to $1/4$ inch of the nail surface. The nail is then incised with a No. 15 blade or a scissors along this vertical line. A Kelly clamp is then used to grasp the portion of nail to be removed and tease the nail from beneath the eponychium.

Dressing

Xeroform or Vaseline-impregnated gauze is placed within the wound created by nail removal, taking care to place a layer between the matrix and the eponychium to ensure that nail growth can occur in the area of resection. A gauze pad covers this dressing, which is secured in place. Routine administration of antibiotics is unnecessary; however, those patients with diabetes should be placed on antistreptococcal and antistaphylococcal coverage for 7 days.

ABSCESS

A subcutaneous abscess is often seen. The patient usually complains of pain and swelling. Abscesses commonly occur in the perianal region. If fluctuance is present, incision and drainage should be preformed.

The following materials are used to treat abscesses:

Anesthetics
1. 1% to 2% Xylocaine without epinephrine
2. 5-mL to 10-mL syringes
3. 19-G to 22-G needles

Prep Solution
1. Betadine

Drapes
1. Three or four sterile towels

Instruments
1. No. 11 or 15 scalpel blade
2. Scalpel handle
3. Kelly clamps
4. Adson forceps
5. Five or six gauze pads
6. Sterile gloves

Dressing
1. $1/4$- to $1/2$-inch Nu-Gauze strip

Anesthesia

After alcohol preparation of the skin, superficial skin infiltration is carried out in a linear course across the abscess. A second linear course is then traversed directly perpendicular to the first. Care is taken to remain superficial to the abscess cavity.

Skin Preparation

A single layer of Betadine is applied to the abscess and sufficient surrounding skin for adequate exposure.

Drapes

Placement of drapes ensures isolation of the abscess and the prepared surrounding skin.

Incision and Drainage

A linear incision is made through the skin, entering the abscess cavity. The cavity is opened widely across the entire abscess dimension. If more drainage is desired, a second incision is made perpendicular to the first, forming a cruciate design.

Dressing

After complete drainage of the cavity, placement of strip gauze within the wound is necessary to maintain drainage and ensure secondary healing of the wound. Although antibiotics are not necessary for most, those patients with diabetes or accompanying cellulitis may benefit from 24 to 48 hours of gram-positive coverage. Continued packing of the wound should proceed with daily changes until healthy closure of the defect occurs.

BURNS

Burns of the skin can result from many sources: flame, steam, scald, electrical, and chemical. These agents cause variable cellular damage to the layers of epidermis, dermis, and subcutaneous fat, depending on the depth. Classification, and therefore treatment, of burn wounds is based on the depth and surface area of skin involved. *First-degree burns* are those that involve just the superficial layers of the epidermis (Fig. 4). *Second-degree burns* involve the epidermis and dermis; a broad distinction is made between superficial and deep burns, based on the amount of dermis involved. Deep second-degree burns involve the entire papillary dermis, with penetration to some or all of the reticular dermis. *Third-degree burns* involve all layers of the epidermis and dermis, with penetration into underlying fat and muscle.

The surface area of burns has traditionally been based on the rule of nines. Each arm is considered 9 percent of the body surface area, each leg is 18 percent, the anterior and the posterior trunk are each 18 percent, the head is 9 percent, and perineum/genitalia is 1 percent.

Using these classifications, the treatment of burns can proceed in an organized fashion. All second-degree burns covering more than 5 percent to 10 percent of the body, all third-degree burns, any burns associated with electrical current, and all burns of the ears, eyes, face, hands, feet, or perineum should be immediately referred to a major hospital familiar with burn care. The remaining first-degree burns and second-degree burns covering less than 5 percent of the body can be cared for on an outpatient basis with adequate wound care and follow-up.

The following materials are used to treat burns:

Prep Solution
1. pHisoHex, gentle soap
2. Normal saline

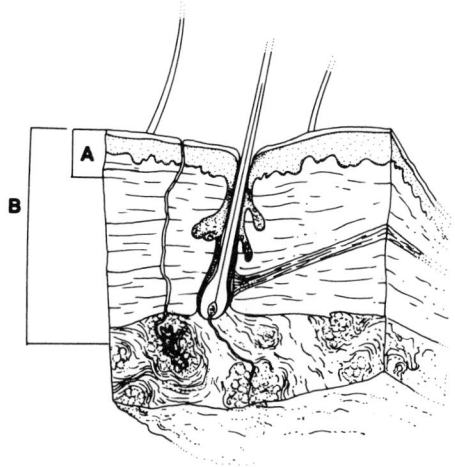

Figure 4. Anatomy of the skin demonstrating (A) epidermis. (B) epidermis and dermis (ie, full thickness). (Grossman JA: Minor Injuries and Disorders: Surgical and Medical Care, p 71. Philadelphia, JB Lippincott, 1984)

Drapes
1. Three or four sterile drapes

Instruments
1. Adson forceps
2. Suture scissors
3. Silvadene cream
4. Sterile gloves

Dressings
1. Sterile gauze pads
2. Roll gauze

Skin Preparation

Chemical burns should first receive generous lavage with normal saline to dilute the irritant. First- and second-degree burns should be washed with a gentle soap solution. For second-degree burns with ruptured bullae, all free skin should be debrided.

Draping

The cleansed, debrided area of a burn is isolated on a sterile field.

Dressing

Silvadene cream is applied to the surface of the burn in a thin, even layer. Application with a tongue depressor works nicely. Silvadene is subsequently covered with dry gauze pads, which are secured with rolled gauze. Complete dressing change should then be done twice daily, with complete cleansing of the wound before a new dressing is applied. Healing for first-degree burns can be expected in 3 to 4 days; second-degree burns require 10 to 20 days. Although controversial, treatment with oral penicillin at moderate dosages, 250 mg four times a day for 3 days, may help to prevent deepening of the burn wound secondary to strep infection.

SKIN BIOPSY

The following materials are used in skin biopsies:

Anesthesia
1. 1% to 2% Xylocaine without epinephrine
2. 5-mL syringe
3. 22-G needle

Prep Solutions
1. Gentle soap solution
2. Betadine

Drapes
1. Three or four drapes

Instruments
1. No. 15 scalpel blade and handle
2. Sterile skin biopsy punch
3. Adson forceps
4. Suture scissors

5. Needle holders
6. Nylon suture
7. Five or six sterile gauze pads
8. Pathology specimen container
9. Sterile gloves

Dressings
1. Xeroform gauze
2. Gauze pad
3. Tape or gauze roll

Anesthesia

After alcohol preparation of the skin is done, complete superficial skin infiltration is accomplished, including the lesion of interest.

Skin Preparation

After the area is cleansed with a gentle soap, a single layer of Betadine is applied.

Draping

The entire prepared area is isolated from surrounding skin and environment.

Biopsy

If a scalpel blade is to be used, an ellipse, surrounding the lesion in question, is created. The entire depth of the epidermis and dermis should be penetrated. Care is taken in the creation of the ellipse to ensure sufficient local skin mobility to allow edge approximation after skin excision has been done. Skin excision is accomplished by elevating one of the corners and sharply separating it from underlying subcutaneous tissue with sharp scissors. Hemostasis is easily obtained by gentle pressure for 1 to 2 minutes. Wound closure then follows, as described for lacerations.

Alternatively, skin biopsy can be performed by using a skin punch. After anesthesia and skin preparation, the circular punch is pressed against the skin, and cutting is achieved with a gentle twisting motion. Once the entire depth of skin has been traversed, it is separated from underlying subcutaneous tissue with sharp scissors. Wound closure is accomplished with several simple sutures. The specimen is then placed in the proper pathology container and solution.

Dressing

The sutured wound should be covered with a strip of Vaseline-impregnated gauze. A dry sterile gauze pad is placed and held securely with tape or gauze roll.

13

Ophthalmic Problems

198
Screening for Open-angle Glaucoma
CLAUDIA U. RICHTER

Open-angle glaucoma affects approximately 2.25 million Americans aged 45 years or older and is the third leading cause of blindness worldwide, causing 3 million people to be bilaterally blind. The condition represents a group of diseases characterized by optic neuropathy with characteristic optic nerve findings and visual field loss. Among adults, primary open-angle glaucoma is the most frequent type, presenting asymptomatically until visual loss is advanced. Although the underlying disease process is neither preventable nor curable, visual loss can be prevented or minimized if the patient is identified early and the intraocular pressure is controlled.

EPIDEMIOLOGY AND RISK FACTORS

The prevalence of glaucoma increases with age, with whites aged 70 and older having a prevalence of 3.5% and African-Americans, 12%. Population-based surveys have demonstrated that African-Americans have a prevalence of glaucoma three to four times that of whites.

The strong risk factors for the development of glaucoma include elevated intraocular pressure, age, African descent, and family history. Other risk factors that are less strongly correlated are myopia, diabetes, and migraine and vasospasm.

Elevated intraocular pressure is one of the most important risk factors and is currently the only modifiable risk factor. Additionally, studies have demonstrated that lowering intraocular pressure can stop or slow the progression of glaucomatous damage.

PATHOPHYSIOLOGY, NATURAL HISTORY, AND EFFECTIVENESS OF EARLY THERAPY

The essential pathophysiologic feature of glaucoma is loss of ganglion cell axons with the development of optic nerve cupping and visual field loss. The exact mechanism of optic nerve damage has not been established and is probably a combination of factors. Ischemia of the optic nerve, caused by elevated intraocular pressure and increased vascular resistance or small blood vessel disease, can result in loss of ganglion cell axons. Increased intraocular pressure can also interfere with axoplasmic flow in the ganglion cell axons, causing cell dysfunction and death. The lamina cribrosa, the sievelike structure through which axons pass when leaving the eye, may lose support for the ganglion cell axons, resulting in interference with axonal function. Apoptosis may also play a role in the development of glaucoma. These different mechanisms of axonal damage, and others still unelucidated, are of variable importance in different patients, but the final result is loss of ganglion cells and their axons, optic nerve cupping, and visual field loss.

The relationship between intraocular pressure and visual loss (as manifested by field defects) is highly variable among individuals. The mean duration of intraocular pressure elevation before development of field defects has been estimated to be 18 years. The incidence of glaucomatous field defects among patients with ocular hypertension is 5 to 10 per 1,000 per year.

Glaucomatous visual field loss is irreversible. Although incurable, optic nerve damage and visual field loss can be delayed or prevented by lowering intraocular pressure. Early diagnosis and treatment are important because the optic nerve becomes increasingly vulnerable to further damage once initial damage has occurred.

SCREENING METHODS

Tonometry. Tonometry has been the most widely used screening test for glaucoma, with 21 mm Hg the cutoff point for referral. However, half or more of those patients with glaucoma will have screening intraocular pressures below this value (low sensitivity). Conversely, many individuals with intraocular pressure repeatedly more than 21 mm Hg do not have and may never develop glaucomatous damage. Elevated intraocular pressure repeatedly measured in the high twenties or higher has been demonstrated to be a strong risk factor for the development of glaucomatous damage. However, there is no level of intraocular pressure above which damage to the optic nerve and visual loss always occurs or below which glaucomatous damage never occurs.

Ophthalmoscopy. Changes in the contour of the optic cup in the center of the optic disc provide the first definitive evidence of glaucomatous damage. The usual cup has a round regular contour. The cup in early glaucoma becomes notched on the superotemporal or inferotemporal rim. Later changes include an increase in the depth and width of the physiologic cup, nasal displacement of the central retinal vessels, and progressive pallor of the optic nerve head. Other disc changes associated with glaucoma are asymmetric discs and disc hemorrhages. The preferred technique for optic nerve evaluation involves magnified stereoscopic visualization (as with a slit-lamp biomicroscope) through a dilated pupil.

The value of ophthalmoscopy for screening is not clear. Even among acknowledged glaucoma specialists, there is wide variability and poor agreement in the assessment of optic nerve status. The need for highly trained personnel and the possible need to dilate the pupils to allow adequate visualization are additional drawbacks. The use of sophisticated techniques such as computer-assisted optical imaging of the optic nerve may improve on the validity and reliability of traditional cup-to-disc ratio estimates, but expense, immobility, and complexity of use make these techniques inappropriate for mass population screenings.

Visual Field Testing. Visual field testing is inadequate for mass glaucoma screening because of the time and technical difficulty in performing an adequate examination and the low sensitivity of manual visual field techniques and the low specificity of automated visual field methods.

Nerve Fiber Layer Analysis. Computer-assisted nerve fiber layer analysis may detect glaucomatous optic nerve damage before optic nerve cupping is visible or visual field defects are detectable. However, nerve fiber layer analysis has a high rate of false-positives and false-negatives for glaucomatous damage and is expensive and immobile and therefore not currently practical for screening examinations.

CONCLUSIONS AND RECOMMENDATIONS

- Glaucoma is highly prevalent in the older adult population and is a major cause of blindness.
- Risk factors for glaucomatous visual loss include elevated intraocular pressure, a family history of glaucoma, advancing age, and African-American heritage.
- Treatment early in the course of the disease is more effective and more likely to prevent visual loss than that which is de-

layed until onset of symptoms. Early treatment necessitates detection of the asymptomatic patient.
- Frequency of screening depends on the risk factors of each patient. Asymptomatic African-Americans should be screened every 3 to 5 years between the ages of 20 and 39, every 2 to 4 years between ages 40 and 64, and every 1 to 2 years at age 65 and after. Other asymptomatic patients need to be screened less than every 3 to 5 years between ages 20 and 39, every 2 to 4 years between ages 40 and 64, and every 1 to 2 years at age 65 and after.
- Screening for ocular hypertension by a Schiotz tonometer by the primary physician has not been demonstrated to have adequate specificity or sensitivity in detecting glaucoma to be valuable.
- Funduscopic examination, with attention to the appearance of the optic cup, is an important component of the screening evaluation and should be performed by all primary care physicians.
- Automated perimetry or nerve fiber layer analysis may be a valuable screening adjunct in the future, but cost is too great, false-positives too frequent, and the equipment too immobile to recommend these at present.

ANNOTATED BIBLIOGRAPHY

Eddy DM, Sanders LE, Eddy JF. The value of screening for glaucoma with tonometry. Surv Ophthalmol 1983;28:194. (*Nine percent of adults will have elevated intraocular pressure on single Schiotz tonometry screening, and 1 of 50 of these will be found to have glaucoma; tonometry will miss half of all patients with glaucoma because they do not have elevated intraocular pressure at the time of the test.*)

Levi L, Schwartz B. Glaucoma screening in the health care setting. Surv Ophthalmol 1983;28:164. (*A review of available data concluding that physicians should use ophthalmoscopy in screening.*)

Margolis KL, Money BE, Kopietz LA, et al. Physician recognition of ophthalmoscopic signs of open-angle glaucoma. J Gen Intern Med 1989;4:296. (*An educational program that includes good photographs of the key findings.*)

Mundorf TK, Zimmerman TJ, Nardin GF, et al. Automated perimetry, tonometry, and questionnaire in glaucoma screening. Am J Ophthalmol 1989;108:505. (*Tonometry alone is much less sensitive than perimetry.*)

Tielsch JM, Katz J, Singh K, et al. A population-based evaluation of glaucoma screening: the Baltimore Eye Survey. Am J Epidemiol 1991;134:1102. (*Glaucoma is more prevalent with increasing age and in African-Americans.*)

199

Evaluation of the Red Eye
ROGER F. STEINERT

The red eye is the most common eye problem encountered by the primary care physician. Most cases represent benign self-limited disorders that can be expeditiously diagnosed and treated by the primary physician; however, because redness of the eye may signal serious disease that threatens vision, the physician must be aware of the differential diagnosis and conduct a proper initial evaluation.

PATHOPHYSIOLOGY AND CLINICAL PRESENTATION

Redness of the eye and the periocular tissues reflects *inflammation* or *hemorrhage*. Causes of inflammation include bacterial, viral, chlamydial, and fungal infections; allergic responses; immune disorders; elevated intraocular pressure; environmental and pharmacologic irritants; foreign bodies; and trauma. Hemorrhage may be due to laceration, contusion, coagulopathy, or concomitant infection. Much less commonly, eyelid redness may be the presenting sign of benign or malignant eyelid *neoplasms* or be due to local dermatoses or systemic immunologic disease.

The pattern of conjunctival injection provides important clues in differential diagnosis. Corneal or intraocular inflammation produces "*ciliary flush*," dilatation of the fine capillaries around the corneal border producing a red-violet halo. Larger deep episcleral vessels may also be engorged. Primary conjunctivitis induces diffuse vessel engorgement on the palpebral and bulbar conjunctiva, without a ciliary flush. The clinical presentations of various causes of red eye are distinctive (Table 199.1).

A red eye may be due to pathology in the conjunctiva, cornea, uveal tract, eyelids, or orbit.

Conjunctival Pathology

Conjunctivitis is the most common cause of a red eye. Discharge, conjunctival erythema (especially of the peripheral bulbar segment), normal vision, lids stuck together in the morning, and absence of photophobia are the major manifestations. The etiology may be infectious, allergic, or chemical.

Bacterial conjunctivitis is characterized by a mucopurulent discharge and usually occurs unilaterally without preauricular adenopathy. The eyelids have a thick crust on them after a night's sleep. *Pneumococcus* is most commonly the infectious agent in temperate zones and *Haemophilus aegyptius* in tropical climates. Grossly purulent conjunctivitis suggests *Neisseria infection*, which may scar or perforate the cornea or lead to systemic dissemination. Chronic conjunctivitis is often due to *Staphylococ-*

Table 199.1. Some Important Causes of Red Eye

Conjunctival Disease
  Infection (bacterial, viral, chlamydial)
  Allergy
  Foreign body
  Subconjunctival hemorrhage
  Pinguecula
  Pterygium
  Episcleritis
  Scleritis
  Abrasion

Corneal Disease
  Herpes simplex
  Adenovirus
  Herpes zoster
  Keratoconjunctivitis sicca
  Exposure keratopathy
  Chemical trauma
  Corneal ulceration (with or without concomitant infection)

Uveal Tract Disease
  Primary iritis and choroiditis
  Secondary iritis (infection, trauma)
  Systemic diseases (collagen vascular)

Diseases of the Eyelid and Orbit
  Blepharitis
  Chalazion
  Hordeolum
  Dacryocystitis
  Cellulitis
  Hemorrhage

Intraocular Disease
  Acute glaucoma

---

cus aureus or *Moraxella lacunata*. Concomitant sterile marginal corneal ulcers are common with chronic staph infection.

Chlamydial conjunctivitis, transmitted from the genitourinary tract, occurs as bilateral "inclusion conjunctivitis" in sexually active young adults. Exudate is profuse, and preauricular adenopathy is common.

Trachoma is a major cause of blindness worldwide but is rare in the United States except among Native Americans in the Southwest. However, the rapidly increasing rate of chlamydial cervicitis (see Chapter 115) among young women raises the risk of trachoma in a much wider population of newborns.

Viral conjunctivitis is characterized by watery sometimes mucoid discharge, often beginning in one eye but spreading to the other eye several days later. Preauricular adenopathy is common. It may be associated with fever and pharyngitis (pharyngoconjunctival fever), particularly in children. Epidemic keratoconjunctivitis is a highly contagious adenoviral infection that may be accompanied by corneal epithelial defects in the first week and subepithelial infiltrates in the second week, with some diminution of vision. Pseudomembranes or scarring of the conjunctiva may occur and sometimes is painful.

Allergic conjunctivitis may be associated with seasonal allergies and atopic dermatitis and is characterized by bilateral itching and clear tears. Vernal keratoconjunctivitis is a chronic recurrent hypersensitivity reaction that may lead to the formation of corneal ulcers.

Bilateral sterile conjunctival inflammation occurs in acne rosacea, Reiter's syndrome, and Stevens-Johnson syndrome.

Hypersensitivity to eye medications may cause erythema of the external lids, especially at the lateral canthus. *Angioneurotic edema* of the lids may occur bilaterally as an allergic response to a systemic allergen, often food, or unilaterally secondary to exposure to local allergens such as topical chemicals, poison ivy, and insect bites; it develops rapidly and resolves in 1 to 2 days. Edema without erythema suggests allergy.

Pinguecula is a yellow harmless nodule of the scleral conjunctiva, usually found on the nasal side, causing only mild discoloration. However, a related disorder, *pterygium*, is vascularized. It causes redness and encroaches on the cornea. The condition is most common in patients heavily exposed to strong sunlight.

Subconjunctival hemorrhage usually occurs secondary to trauma, although the patient may be unaware of the minor trauma involved. In patients receiving anticoagulant medications, spontaneous subconjunctival hemorrhage may be a sign of overdosage. Massive subconjunctival hemorrhage accompanied by proptosis and limited extraocular movements, usually after trauma, signals orbital hemorrhage, which may compromise the optic nerve and retinal circulation.

Foreign body on the bulbar conjunctiva or under either the upper or lower lid may result in copious tearing, conjunctival injection, and a sensation that something has gotten "into" the eye. On occasion, the foreign body may be well tolerated, with the eye remaining white and quiet.

Episcleritis is usually a benign inflammation of superficial episcleral vessels. The conjunctiva manifests areas of circumscribed nodular inflammation, seen in association with collagen disease, gout, allergic conditions, and such skin diseases as psoriasis. The patient complains of tender irritated eyes. Vision and lids are normal, the corneas are clear, and the conjunctivae show local raised areas of redness.

Scleritis, often associated with rheumatoid arthritis and other immune disorders, is a potentially destructive inflammation of the collagen in the deep episcleral vessels and the sclera. The eye is sometimes painful. Fortunately, scleritis is rare. An experienced observer is required to make the diagnosis.

Corneal Disease

Keratitis presents with a perilimbal ciliary flush, accompanied by clear tears and photophobia. Corneal ulcers detected by fluorescein staining may be sterile or caused by bacteria, viruses, or fungi. Particularly distinctive is the "dendritic" figure of herpes simplex keratitis, in which the epithelium stains in a fine branching pattern. Herpes simplex and zoster may also cause broader "geographic" defects. *S. aureus* may cause a sterile infiltrate in the corneal limbus.

Corneal abrasions stain with fluorescein but have no infiltrate unless they are untreated for several days. *Hyphema* (blood layering in the anterior chamber) indicates severe trauma and requires ophthalmologic consultation. *Recurrent erosion* presents as an epithelial defect at the site of an abrasion that occurred months or years before and was often caused by organic material (e.g., tree branch, fingernail). It may also occur in corneal dystrophies. In both instances, it is due to a defect in epithelial adherence to the underlying stroma. A *corneal foreign body* may cause tearing and hyperemia with little sensation of a foreign body. This is particularly true of rust rings left by ferrous foreign bodies. Dry eyes can cause intense reactions secondary to superficial keratitis, as does overwearing of contact lenses (corneal hypoxia) and ultraviolet keratitis. *Corneal laceration* with perforation is suggested by a shallow or absent anterior chamber, markedly decreased intraocular pressure, and eccentric pupil with iris prolapse into the wound.

Chemical keratoconjunctivitis is a common industrial injury due to a splash of an irritant solution. The conjunctiva is uniformly red, the pupil constricted, vision decreased, the cornea hazy, and the eye painful because of spasm of the iris.

Uveal Tract Disease

Uveitis refers to inflammation of the uveal tract, including the iris, ciliary body, and choroid. The diagnosis is suggested by pain, photophobia, redness, and ciliary flush. Iritis presents with eye pain, photophobia, redness, and pupillary contraction. It may be unilateral or bilateral; if unilateral, the pupil is smaller than that of the other eye because of spasm. Flashlight examination shows a slightly cloudy anterior chamber. Slit-lamp examination discloses cells in the anterior chamber and "flare," representing increased aqueous humor protein. Inflammatory cells, called "keratic precipitates," may collect in clusters on the posterior cornea.

Iritis and uveitis are usually idiopathic but may be associated with a large number of systemic and ocular diseases. *Ankylosing spondylitis, sprue, granulomatous colitis, tuberculosis, sarcoidosis,* and *juvenile rheumatoid arthritis* are sometimes associated with uveitis. The HLA-B27 tissue antigen is strongly associated with iritis, often accompanied by ankylosing spondylitis or *Beháet's disease.* Secondary iritis occurs in response to blunt trauma or corneal inflammation.

Table 199.2.   Other Causes of Eyelid Inflammation

CONDITION	CAUSE
Bacterial infection	Impetigo
	Erysipelas
Viral infection	Herpes simplex
	Molluscum contagiosum
	Varicella zoster
	Papillomavirus
Parasitic infection	Pthirus pubis
Immunologic skin condition	Atopic dermatitis
	Contact dermatitis
	Erythema multiforme
	Pemphigus foliaceus
	Connective tissue disorders
	Lupus erythematosus
	Dermatomyositis
Dermatoses	Psoriasis
	Ichthyosis
	Exfoliative
	Erythroderma
Benign eyelid tumors	Pseudoepitheliomatous hyperplasia
	Actinic keratosis
	Squamous cell papilloma
	Sebaceous gland hyperplasia
	Hemangioma
	Pyogenic granuloma
Malignant eyelid tumors	Basal cell carcinoma
	Squamous cell carcinoma
	Sebaceous cell carcinoma
	Melanoma
	Kaposi's sarcoma
Other	Neurofibromatosis
	Sarcoidosis
	Down syndrome

Eyelid and Orbital Disease

Blepharitis connotes inflammation involving the structures of the lid margin with redness, scaling, and crusting. Examination of the lid margin may reveal inspissated sebaceous ma-terial. *Staphylococcal blepharitis* causes anterior lid margin findings, including dry scales, lash loss, and sometimesconjunctivitis and corneal limbal infiltrates. *Seborrheic blepharitis* is associated with anteriorly located greasy scales. Meibomian gland dysfunction is characterized by dilated vessels at the posterior eyelid margins, blocked and pouting meibomian glands, and abnormal meibomian secretions. *Meibomian gland dysfunction* is frequently associated with seborrheic dermatitis and acne rosacea. Blepharitis tends to be chronic with acute flare-ups and is more common in fair-skinned people. Table 199.2 lists other causes of eyelid inflammation.

Hordeolum is an acute staphylococcal infection of the meibomian glands (internal hordeolum) or of the glands of Zeis or Moll around the lashes (external hordeolum or sty). It may present as diffuse redness, tenderness, and edema, localized only by an inspissated meibomian gland. An internal hordeolum may point either to the skin or conjunctival side of the lid, whereas an external hordeolum always points to the skin. Hordeolum may produce a diffuse superficial lid infection known as "preseptal cellulitis."

Chalazion is a sterile granulomatous inflammation of the meibomian gland, which may be tender and mildly inflamed or a quiet discrete mass.

Acute dacryocystitis is a tender, warm, localized infection of the tear ducts over the lateral nose; purulent material may be expressed from the tear duct on the application of pressure.

Hemorrhage in the lids or forehead, either spontaneous or traumatic, may rapidly dissect along the tissue planes of the lids and cause an impressive generalized ecchymosis, greatly alarming the patient.

Orbital cellulitis is usually caused by gram-positive organisms that enter the orbit either directly from the sinuses or through venous channels. It presents as swollen red eyelids with chemosis, exophthalmos, pain, fever, and leukocytosis. If it progresses, it may lead to paresis of the third, fourth, and sixth cranial nerves or the ophthalmic division of the fifth, signs of the very serious complication *cavernous sinus thrombosis.*

Intraocular Disease

Acute glaucoma is an ocular emergency that presents as a painful red eye with prominent ciliary flush. The pupil is mid-dilated and fixed, and the cornea is cloudy secondary to edema. Intraocular pressure exceeds 40 mm Hg and may reach 70 to 80 mm Hg. The patient reports cloudy vision, colored rings around lights (due to corneal edema), and unilateral headache, often accompanied by nausea and vomiting, occasionally leading the physician to consider an acute abdomen. Acute glaucoma is usually due to closure in eyes with narrow angles but may be due to inflammatory cells or red blood cells in the anterior chamber, neovascularization of the iris (rubeosis iridis), or peripheral anterior synechiae.

DIFFERENTIAL DIAGNOSIS

The causes of red eye can be divided anatomically into the categories of conjunctival, corneal, uveal, eyelid-orbital, and intraocular disease (Table 199.1). Differentiation can usually be made on clinical grounds (Table 199.3).

WORKUP

History is directed toward ascertaining the duration of redness, rapidity of onset, the patient's activity at the time, and the degree and quality of symptoms. Ophthalmologic history and medications should be noted. Key symptoms include visual changes, pain, itching, crusting in the morning, tearing, mucoid or purulent discharge, photophobia, and foreign body sensation. Although usually helpful, the history can be misleading, because viral conjunctivitis may be accompanied by itching or a foreign body sensation or the patient may ascribe the symptoms of herpes simplex keratitis to a "chemical in the eye" because the symptoms were first noted after, for example, a home hair permanent.

Physical Examination. Accurate measurement of visual acuity, preferably at a distance, is essential. If it is abnormal, it is important to check for uncorrected optical abnormality by use of a pinhole. Any patient with reduced vision not readily explained by a preexisting or obviously harmless condition needs to be immediately referred to an ophthalmologist. Mucus and tearing may reduce vision one or two lines at most. Corneal lesions may further reduce vision, with only partial improvement on pinhole testing; a central epithelial abrasion typically maintains vision at about 20/100 or better. Preauricular nodes should be palpated. A complete examination of the eye and fundus is important. The lid margins should be inspected for crusting, ulceration, inspissations, and masses and the conjunctiva for distribution of redness, ciliary flush, foreign bodies (including lid eversion), and, if a slit-lamp is available, follicles and papillae. Corneal clarity is noted with a flashlight, and a direct ophthalmoscope set at about +15 diopters can be used to magnify corneal details.

If *fluorescein stain* is available, it can be used in conjunction with a blue filter to visualize the cornea for infection and other injury. However, if there is any suspicion of corneal injury, referral is needed quickly for slit-lamp examination.

Intraocular pressure should be determined if glaucoma is suspected. Depth of the anterior chamber of the other eye can be assessed by a flashlight aimed parallel to the iris (coronal

Table 199.3. The Red Eye

	Conjunctivitis			Corneal injury or infection	Iritis	Acute glaucoma
	Bacterial	**Viral**	**Allergic**			
Vision	−	−	−	↓ or ↓↓	↓	↓↓
Pain	−	−	−	+	+	+++
Photophobia	−	±	−	+	++	−
Foreign body sensation	−	±	±	+	−	−
Itch	±	±	++	−	−	−
Tearing	+	++	+	++	+	−
Discharge	Mucopurulent	Mucoid	−	−	−	−
Preauricular adenopathy	−	+	−	[a]	−	−
Pupils	−	−	−	NL or small[b]	Small	Mid-dilated and fixed
Conjunctival hyperemia	Diffuse	Diffuse	Diffuse	Diffuse and ciliary flush	Ciliary flush	Diffuse and ciliary flush
Cornea	Clear	Sometimes faint punctate staining or infiltrates	Clear	Depends on disorder	Clear or lightly cloudy	Cloudy
Intraocular pressure	NL	NL	NL	NL[c]	↓, NL, or ↑	↑↑

[a]In herpes keratitis.

[b]Indicates secondary iritis.

[c]Very low in perforating trauma.

NL; normal

plane) from the temporal side. A shallow anterior chamber is usually convex and will cast a shadow on the nasal iris.

Laboratory studies are usually the responsibility of an ophthalmologist. The primary practitioner may attempt *conjunctival smears*, which show polymorphonuclear leukocytes in acute bacterial conjunctivitis, lymphocytes in viral or late bacterial conjunctivitis, and eosinophils in allergic reactions. This is time consuming and generally not necessary. Purulent discharges should be *cultured* on blood agar and, if *Neisseria* is suspected, plated on chocolate agar and Gram stained. Scrapings for inclusion bodies in suspected chlamydial and viral disease are usually unrewarding, and scraping and culture of an infected corneal ulcer require an ophthalmologist.

White blood cell and differential counts are indicated, as are *blood cultures*, in suspected cellulitis. Clotting studies for subconjunctival hemorrhage are not indicated unless other evidence of coagulopathy is present (see Chapter 81) or the patient is being treated with anticoagulants (see Chapter 83).

PRINCIPLES OF MANAGEMENT AND INDICATIONS FOR REFERRAL

Red eye problems associated with eye pain, visual disturbance, or corneal damage require immediate referral, as does acute glaucoma. In most other situations, the primary physician can provide symptomatic relief or at least first aid. A nonophthalmologist should never prescribe topical steroid or steroid–antibiotic combination drops, because infection may worsen and a corneal ulcer may rapidly form and cause perforation.

Conjunctival Disease. Conjunctivitis, in the absence of photophobia, eye pain, or change in visual acuity, can be managed by the primary physician.

Viral Conjunctivitis is contagious, and live virus is shed in the tears for up to 2 weeks. The patient should be instructed to refrain from rubbing the eye and transmitting infection to the other eye or to another person. Treatment is expectant, because the condition is self-limited, usually clearing within 2 to 3 weeks. Cases that fail to improve spontaneously should be referred to the ophthalmologist.

Bacterial Conjunctivitis responds well to *erythromycin ophthalmic ointment* (prescribed four times a day) or *polymyxin/trimethoprim (Polytrim) drops* (prescribed four times a day). Improvement is usually noted in several days. Bacitracin ophthalmic ointment and sodium sulfacetamide are alternative antibiotics. Neomycin causes allergic keratitis in 5% of patients treated topically and should be avoided if possible. More potent topical antibiotics such as the aminoglycosides and fluoroquinolones are not recommended for routine conjunctivitis.

Allergic Conjunctivitis in seasonal allergies is relieved by *cool compresses* and *decongestant–antihistamine drops* (Vasocon-A, Naphcon-A, Albalon-A), antihistamine (Livostin), and mast-cell–stabilizing topical medications (Opticrom, Patanol, and others) up to four times daily. Long-term use of decongestant drops is not recommended, because marked rebound vasodilation may develop. *Acular (ketorolac) ophthalmic drops* (a nonsteroidal antiinflammatory agent) may also help alleviate allergic symptoms. Oral *antihistamines* are another alternative. Severe allergic conditions may require *topical*

steroid therapy; management of topical steroids by an ophthalmologist is mandatory because of the risks of steroid-induced glaucoma and cataract.

Subconjunctival Hemorrhage usually requires only reassurance. Compresses (initially cool, then warm) and erythromycin ophthalmic ointment or a lubricating ointment may reduce discomfort in cases with marked swelling.

Conjunctival Foreign Bodies are usually easily removed with a cotton swab or fine forceps; erythromycin ointment three times a day for 2 days is adequate for healing.

Eye Lid and Orbital Disease. Topical therapies are often helpful, at times supplemented by oral antibiotics.

Blepharitis usually responds to lid hygiene measures and topical antibiotics. One can instruct the patient to dilute Johnson's *baby shampoo* 50:50 with water and use a cotton ball to scrub the lids well with the eyes closed. After rinsing with water, a hot compress is applied to the closed lids for 5 to 10 minutes and then *erythromycin* or *bacitracin ophthalmic ointment* is instilled in the inferior fornix. The excess is rubbed into the eyelash base. Carrying out this procedure as many as three to four times daily will improve most cases. After improvement is obtained, the lids can be maintained by nightly lid hygiene and warm compresses. An occasional stubborn case will require nightly antibiotic ointment as prophylaxis.

Chronic blepharitis and meibomian gland inflammatory disease may be due to acne rosacea. In addition to topical therapy, institution of systemic treatment for the rosacea is indicated. Traditionally, this has consisted of long-term suppressive therapy with a *low-dose tetracycline*-family antibiotic (e.g., tetracycline 250 mg, doxycycline 50 or 100 mg, or minocycline 50 mg once daily). Recent evidence implicating *Helicobacter pylori* in the pathogenesis of acne rosacea has led to a therapeutic regimen of a 7- to 14-day course of double- or triple-antibiotic therapy (e.g., amoxicillin, metronidazole, bismuth subsalicylate; see Chapter 68).

A Hordeolum may respond to this treatment or, like chalazia, may require incision and curettage by an ophthalmologist.

Mild cellulitis of the lid margin (preseptal cellulitis) responds to topical treatment plus oral antibiotics. *Dicloxacillin* (250 mg four times a day) is a good first choice. *Erythromycin* (250 to 500 mg orally three times a day) is an effective alternative for patients who are penicillin allergic. *Orbital cellulitis* and orbital cellulitis complicated by *cavernous sinus thrombosis* are medical emergencies that require immediate hospitalization for intravenous antibiotics.

Acute Dacryocystitis. Warm *compresses* and oral antibiotics are also indicated, but persistent localized abscess requires *incision* and *drainage* by an ophthalmologist.

Mild Hypersensitivity Reactions of the lids respond rapidly to discontinuation of the offending agent and application of cool compresses. Systemic antihistamines are useful in moderate reactions, and steroids are useful in severe reactions.

Traumatic Lid Ecchymoses are minimized by cool compresses and ice packs applied early. Later, warm compresses speed resolution.

Corneal Disease. The prompt attention of the ophthalmologist is usually required, but a number of conditions can be treated by the primary physician in the initial stages.

Corneal Ulcers require intensive emergency evaluation and treatment by an ophthalmologist. Patients with typical herpes simplex dendritic keratitis may be started on Viroptic drops up to nine times a day or Vira-A ointment five times daily and erythromycin ointment twice daily if an ophthalmologist is not available.

Corneal Abrasions heal rapidly with *erythromycin ointment* and a tight *sterile patch* that prevents lid motion for 24 to 48 hours. If the initial abrasion was sizable (roughly 25% of the cornea or more), healing should be checked after removal of the patch. Lesions of this size also require cycloplegia for relief of painful secondary iritis during healing (see iritis treatment). After reepithelialization occurs, ointment applied three times daily for 4 days helps complete the healing process.

Foreign Bodies are treated with vigorous *irrigation*. Rust rings are treated like abrasions once the foreign body has been washed away. Foreign bodies that do not wash away with irrigation can be removed with a *cotton swab*, a sterile "golf stick," or an 18-gauge needle with a syringe as a handle, but such removal should not be attempted by the nonophthalmologist unless specifically trained to do so. Rust on the surface is easily debrided, but scraping is prohibited because it will damage Bowman's membrane and cause permanent scarring. Left untreated, rust may be irritating but will surface and slough in 1 or 2 weeks.

Contact Lens Overwear and Ultraviolet Keratitis respond to brief cycloplegia, erythromycin ointment, and sterile pressure patching for 24 hours. The associated pain often requires codeine.

Suspected Corneal Laceration and Perforation are ophthalmic emergencies. A protective metal shield ("Fox shield") should be placed over the eye; no medication should be instilled.

Uveal Tract Disease. An ophthalmologist must evaluate and treat *primary iritis*, but initial cycloplegia by tropicamide 1% four times a day or cyclopentolate 1% four times a day will prevent posterior synechia formation and relieve pain. *Iritis* secondary to corneal abrasion may be treated with these medications, or in an eye that will be patched for 1 or 2 days, several drops of scopolamine 0.25% will provide longer cycloplegia. The nonophthalmologist should avoid atropine because its effects persist for 1 to 2 weeks.

Intraocular Disease. *Acute glaucoma* should be treated by immediate administration of acetazolamide, 500 mg intravenously, and glycerol, 120 mL orally in orange juice. Pilocarpine 2% should be begun with instillation as frequently as every 15 minutes to break the attack. Immediate attention by an ophthalmologist is necessary because the only definitive treatment is laser or surgical iridotomy.

ANNOTATED BIBLIOGRAPHY

Bienfang DC, Kelly LD, Nicholson DH, et al. Ophthalmology. N Engl J Med 1990;323:956. *(Excellent review and overview for the general reader; 115 references.)*

Frucht-Pery J, Sagi E, Hemo I, et al. Efficacy of doxycycline and tetracycline in ocular rosacea. Am J Ophthalmol 1993;116:88. *(Addresses the issues of systemic treatment of this common and undertreated disorder.)*

Gigliotti F. Acute conjunctivitis of childhood. Pediatr Ann 1993; 22:353. *(An accessible review of this common disease group.)*

Isenberg SJ, Apt L, Wood M. A controlled trial of povidone-iodine as prophylaxis against ophthalmia neonatorum. N Engl J Med 1995;332:562. *(Explains the basis for the change in accepted practice patterns to avoid this dreadful disease.)*

Margo CE, Mulla ZD. Malignant tumors of the eyelid: a population-bases study of non-basal cell and non-squamous cell malignant neoplasms. Arch Ophthalmol 1998;116:195. *(Excellent review of less common malignancies.)*

Shingleton BJ, Hersh PS, Kenyon KR. Eye trauma. Philadelphia: Mosby, 1991. *(The definitive text on the subject; includes detailed sections on management of foreign bodies and abrasions.)*

Steinert RF. Current therapy for bacterial ketatitis and bacterial conjunctivitis. Am J Ophthalmol 1991;112:10S. *(Treatment options and indications.)*

Vaughan D, Asbury T. General ophthalmology, 12th ed. Los Alto: Lange, 1989. *(A practical and inexpensive reference that includes useful photographs of conditions causing a red eye.)*

200
Evaluation of Impaired Vision
CLAUDIA U. RICHTER

Patients with decreasing or blurred vision often refer themselves directly to an eye specialist, but at times they first present to their primary physician. Sudden visual loss is a medical emergency. Gradual diminution of sight raises the specter of eventual blindness and inability to function independently. Paradoxically, some elderly patients may not volunteer that their vision is decreasing because they consider it a natural part of aging. Consequently, the primary physician needs to screen elderly patients for treatable causes of decreased vision. In addition, one should be capable of distinguishing visual impairment due to refractive error, cataracts, glaucoma, retinal disease, and trauma to provide proper initial care and appropriate and timely referral.

PATHOPHYSIOLOGY AND CLINICAL PRESENTATION

Vision is impaired when there is a change in the refracting surfaces of the eye, opacification of the transparent ocular media, damage to the photoreceptor cells of the retina, or a lesion of the optic nerve, its radiations, or the visual cortex. Anatomic orientation provides a framework for considering the pathophysiology of visual difficulties, beginning with the cornea and working inward.

Refractive error is the most common cause of decreased visual acuity. It results from the inability of the eye to focus light precisely on the retina and may be due to an abnormality in the cornea, lens, or size of the globe. Myopic patients commonly present during their teens and early twenties. Patients in their forties may report decreased visual acuity but in fact simply cannot accommodate to near distances and require reading glasses. Early cataracts can increase myopia before they opacify and block transmission of light. Uncontrolled diabetes mellitus can produce swelling of the lens and myopia, which resolves with control of the blood sugar. Sulfonamides, thiazides, and anticholinergic agents may induce myopia causing blurred vision.

Eyelid Disease. Occasionally, sudden visual loss results from eyelids being closed by swelling due to trauma, insect bites, cellulitis, or angioneurotic edema. Acute blepharospasm secondary to ocular surface pain may be described as inability to see.

Corneal Disease. The cornea is the major refracting surface of the eye, and any change in it can lead to visual disturbances. A corneal abrasion, herpes simplex virus keratitis, or ulcer causes irregularity of the corneal epithelium and opacification of the normally clear cornea. Acute glaucoma causes sudden visual loss by producing corneal edema. Corneal dystrophies or degenerations result in a more gradual reduction in visual acuity, often progressing over a period of years.

Anterior Chamber Disease. The anterior chamber may be opacified by inflammatory cells resulting from *iritis* or red blood cells resulting from a *hyphema*. *Cataracts*, opacifications of the lens, are a leading cause of gradual vision loss in older patients. The usual history is one of a painless slow deterioration of eyesight. However, a traumatic cataract may develop over a period of hours to days.

Vitreous opacification occurs most often from hemorrhage and less commonly from inflammation or infection. Proliferative diabetic retinopathy, a retinal hole or detachment, trauma, sickle cell retinopathy, hypertension, and clotting abnormalities may cause vitreous hemorrhage. A *vitreous floater* may transiently blur vision or may be called a blind spot.

Glaucoma may damage nerve fibers at the optic disk and cause visual field defects. Most visual loss due to glaucoma is gradual and progressive (see Chapter 207). Four types of visual field defects occur: paracentral scotomas occurring along the distribution of the arcuate nerve fiber bundle, arcuate scotomata, sector-shaped defects, and nasal steps. As the disease progresses, these visual field defects enlarge. Central vision remains intact until late in the disease, but even this may be lost. The optic cup becomes enlarged and irregular (see Chapter 198). Acute angle-closure glaucoma produces a red eye, fixed pupil, hazy cornea, eye pain, and acute impairment of vision. Acute angle-closure glaucoma accounts for less than 5% of all glaucoma cases.

Retinal Disease. Degeneration, inflammation, trauma, detachment, or ischemia may compromise the retina, causing visual loss.

Age related macular degeneration occurs in patients over age 55 and is a leading cause of legal blindness. Central vision is impaired, whereas peripheral vision remains intact. Funduscopic examination may show loss of the foveal reflex, macular drusen, atrophy of the retinal pigment epithelium with promi-nent choroidal vessels, subretinal edema or hemorrhage, or a central fibrous scar. Some 15% of patients with senile macular degeneration have treatable disease, presenting with early visual symptoms and a subretinal neovascular net that can be obliterated with laser photocoagulation. They need to be seen promptly to maximize their chances of effective treatment. Those at particular risk of developing exudative senile macular degeneration have drusen or a disciform scar in one macula. They should screen their central vision daily with an Amsler grid (see Chapter 206).

A host of other retinal problems may lead to loss of vision. *Central serous retinopathy* is an idiopathic spontaneous detachment of the retina in the macular area. Patients range in age from 20 to 50 years old. Central vision is reduced, but recovery is usually spontaneous within a few months.

Retinal inflammation of the retina and choroid, such as histoplasmosis, toxoplasmosis, cytomegalovirus, or herpes virus infections, can involve the macula or produce a vitritis, decreasing vision. *Cytomegalovirus retinitis* is of concern in HIV-infected patients and important to recognize because it is treatable. Patients with CD4 counts less than 200 are at significantly increased risk of developing cytomegalovirus retinitis. Spread to the eye is hematogenous. Ocular symptoms include new floaters and loss of vision. Funduscopic manifestations include perivascular yellow-white retinal lesions presenting as a focal white granular infiltrate with or without hemorrhage, expanding in a "brushfire" pattern.

Trauma may cause decreased visual acuity by producing *macular edema* or a *choroidal* rupture. *Macular edema* resolves within a few days and visual acuity improves. A choroidal *rupture* causes permanent decreased visual acuity.

Retinal detachment may cause decreased visual acuity when it is extensive or may be noted as a minor field defect when it is small. Flashing lights and a shower of vitreous floaters may presage a retinal detachment. As a detachment extends, the patient may note that the visual field defect progresses like a shade being drawn. A detached retina appears ballooned forward with undulating folds.

Systemic diseases may involve the retina and cause decreased vision. Vascular injury is the most common mechanism, as occurs with hypertension, diabetes mellitus, and systemic lupus erythematosus. Infiltrative disease may also affect the retina.

Vascular Disease. The vasculature of the retina or optic nerve may be compromised, leading to sudden visual loss. The vascular diseases involving the arteries include central retinal artery occlusion, giant cell arteritis, and anterior ischemic optic neuropathy. In *central retinal artery occlusion*, there is sudden painless loss of ability to perceive light or hand movements. The patient may have had previous episodes of amaurosis fugax with fleeting blindness lasting 10 to 15 minutes. Ophthalmoscopy reveals a pale optic disc, attenuated arterioles, "boxcar" veins, hazy edematous retina, and a cherry-red spot in the macula. Occasionally, an embolus may be seen at a bifurcation of a retinal arteriole. The most common embolic sources are an atheromatous plaque in the ipsilateral carotid artery or a vegetation from a cardiac valve leaflet.

Giant cell or temporal arteritis, a granulomatous inflammation of the medium and large arteries in elderly people, may cause sudden visual loss (see Chapter 161). These patients may have premonitory visual symptoms similar to amaurosis fugax and may have symptoms of polymyalgia rheumatica. The fundus examination may reveal a swollen optic disc, a normal optic disc, or a central retinal artery occlusion.

Anterior ischemic optic neuropathy is produced by ischemia to the anterior portion of the optic nerve. The patient notes decreased visual acuity or a visual field defect, usually involving the superior or inferior visual field and the macula. The optic disc initially appears edematous, sometimes in just one portion, with a few flame-shaped hemorrhages. Optic atrophy follows the disc edema. The most common etiology is thrombosis of an arteriosclerotic vessel. The patients tend to be younger than those affected by giant cell arteritis and have hypertension or diabetes mellitus.

Central or branch retinal vein occlusions cause a sudden painless decrease in visual acuity. In central retinal vein occlusion, the fundus has a classic "blood and thunder" appearance: The veins are tortuous and dilated and the retina is edematous and covered with flame-shaped hemorrhages. The optic disc margin is blurred. The fundus changes in branch retinal vein occlusion are similar but limited to the distribution of the involved vein. Decreased visual acuity is due to macular edema and ischemia. In central retinal vein occlusion, 20% of patients have preexisting chronic open-angle glaucoma and 50% of men have preexisting hypertension. In branch retinal vein occlusion, 75% of patients have preexisting hypertension.

Optic Nerve Disease. *Optic neuritis*, inflammation of the optic nerve, presents with a relatively acute impairment of vision in young persons (ages 15 to 40). It is usually idiopathic, but 20% to 50% eventually develop clinical *multiple sclerosis*. Clinically, there is progressive loss of vision over hours to days, typically unilateral with pain on eye motion, and improved visual function in the second to third week. Examination reveals an afferent pupillary defect, globe tenderness, visual field defects, and impairment of color vision. The optic nerve may appear normal.

Infiltrative or compressive lesions of the optic nerve, such as pituitary adenomas, meningiomas, gliomas, or internal carotid artery aneurysms, cause gradual visual field loss. It is unusual for lesions posterior to the optic chiasm to present with decreased visual acuity because of the decussation of fibers in the optic chiasm. Unilateral lesions, such as a tumor or a cerebrovascular accident, cause a homonymous hemianopsia or related visual field defect. Bilateral central nervous system lesions may cause profound visual loss.

Many patients complain of blurred vision at night. Rarely, these patients may be found to have true *night blindness* caused by *retinitis pigmentosa or vitamin A deficiency*. More commonly, no etiology is found; a slight decrease in visual acuity at night is common and normal.

Psychogenic pathology sometimes presents as visual loss or compromise. Characteristically, the eye examination and objective measures of visual function that do not require the patient's report are intact. Hysteria and malingering account for most psychogenic cases.

DIFFERENTIAL DIAGNOSIS

The causes of visual impairment can be logically considered in terms of anatomic site affected (Table 200.1). The leading causes of blindness include cataracts, open-angle glaucoma, and macular degeneration.

Table 200.1. Causes of Impaired Vision

Eyelids
  Edema
  Blepharospasm

Cornea
  Abrasion
  Infection
  Edema
  Degeneration

Anterior chamber
  Inflammatory cells (from iritis)
  Hyphema

Lens
  Cataract
  Swelling (e.g., poorly controlled diabetes)

Vitreous
  Hemorrhage
  Floaters

Retina
  Age related macular degeneration
  Central serous retinopathy
  Inflammation
  Trauma
  Detachment
  Diabetes
  Hypertension

Vasculature
  Central retinal artery occlusion
  Giant cell (cranial or temporal) arteritis
  Anterior ischemic optic neuropathy
  Retinal vein occlusion

Optic nerve
  Compression (glaucoma, tumor)

Psychiatric
  Hysteria
  Malingering

Refractive error

WORKUP

History. A thorough history is most important in evaluating a complaint of visual loss. It is essential to establish the onset, duration, clinical course, and pattern of visual loss. Any associated visual phenomena should be ascertained, as well as any pain. The presence of premonitory symptoms is helpful. Acute loss is suggestive of a vascular event or retinal detachment. Preceding episodes of amaurosis fugax indicate central retinal artery occlusion or giant cell arteritis. A sudden flurry of flashes of light (photopsia) and vitreous floaters may herald a retinal detachment. Scintillating scotomata may herald migraine. Progressive visual loss points to a chronic disturbance, such as cataract, macular degeneration, or glaucoma. Previous episodes of decreased visual acuity with halos around lights and pain indicate angle-closure glaucoma. A foreign body sensation indicates a corneal abrasion, foreign body, or herpes simplex keratitis. The presence of other diseases such as diabetes mellitus, hypertension, heart disease, or sickle cell anemia may be contributory. A history of trauma is important to note, as is smoking, an important independent risk factor for age-related macular degeneration.

Physical Examination and Laboratory Studies. *Visual acuity* testing should be done formally, one eye at a time. If the patient complains of pain, a topical anesthetic such as proparacaine should be used to allow testing. If the lids are tightly swollen, it may be necessary to pry them apart forcibly. The patient should wear his or her distance glasses. A *Snellen eye chart* with its standardized letter sizes is most convenient. If letters cannot be read, the distance at which the patient can accurately count fingers or identify hand motions is noted. If targets cannot be seen, it is important to determine whether the eye can perceive light. Vision is rechecked with the patient looking through a pinhole to eliminate any residual refractive error.

The *pupils* should be examined carefully, noting size, direct and consensual reactions to light, and presence of any afferent pupillary defect. An afferent pupillary defect may be found in optic neuritis, central retinal artery occlusion, giant cell arteritis, and extensive retinal diseases. A fixed pupil in conjunction with a red eye is indicative of acute angle-closure glaucoma.

The *conjunctiva* is examined to determine whether the eye is red and inflamed or white and quiet. With the exception of trauma, acute glaucoma, and infection, the diseases that cause sudden visual loss do not cause a red eye (see Chapter 199). The cornea normally is clear with a crisp light reflex and no fluorescein stain. If a tonometer is available, the intraocular pressure should be measured.

Ophthalmoscopy is important; it should first be noted whether the fundus can be visualized or if a dense cataract or vitreous opacity is present. If the fundus can be visualized, the *optic disc* is examined for papilledema or atrophy. The *macula* is examined, looking for a cherry-red spot, hemorrhages, and scars. The *retinal vessels* are examined, with attention paid to the caliber and the presence of visible emboli. Patients over age 50 with sudden visual loss should have a careful check for temporal arteritis, which includes palpation of the *cranial arteries* for tenderness, enlargement, and loss of pulsation and determination of the *erythrocyte sedimentation rate* for marked elevation (see Chapter 161).

If a patient is a malingerer or hysterical, the examination of the eye will be normal, including opticokinetic responses, stereoscopic vision, and visual fields. One can quickly check opticokinetic responses by passing the front page of a newspaper before the eyes of the patient.

Vision Screening in Primary Care Practice. Adults with gradual onset of visual impairment often do not recognize or complain of their deficit. In addition, many patients being cared for by primary care physicians (especially hypertensives, diabetics, and the elderly) are at increased risk for potentially serious eye disease that may compromise vision. Yield for detection of important eye pathology can be high when persons at increased risk are screened by a brief ophthalmologic history complemented by Snellen chart testing of visual acuity. Findings indicative of benefit from ophthalmologic referral include age over 65 years; history of diabetes, glaucoma, eye trauma, eye infection, or other eye problem; and vision worse than 20/40 by Snellen testing or a difference of greater than two Snellen lines between eyes. Diabetics are particularly well served by referral for a screening ophthalmologic examination.

SYMPTOMATIC MANAGEMENT

Patients with sudden visual loss need immediate ophthalmologic consultation. If an ophthalmologist is not immedi-

ately available, appropriate emergency measures should be taken.

If a *central retinal artery occlusion* exists that is less than 24 hours old, it is reasonable to attempt heroic measures to salvage vision. The goal is to encourage the embolus to break apart or at least to move distally. First, one can gently massage the globe with the fingers to attempt to dislodge the embolus. Next, have the patient breathe a mixture of 5% CO_2 and 95% O_2; this will cause the retinal vessels to vasodilate and allow delivery of a high Po_2 to any viable retinal cells. If this mixture is not available, have the patient breathe into a paper bag. Next, give the patient 500-mg intravenous acetazolamide to decrease the production of aqueous humor and to lower intraocular pressure.

If *giant cell arteritis* is suspected, the patient should be started at once on high-dose glucocorticosteroids (e.g., prednisone 60 mg/d) and considered for temporal artery biopsy. Some vision may be salvaged in the affected eye, and the other eye is protected (see Chapter 161).

Acute angle-closure glaucoma should be treated at once with topical pilocarpine 2% in both eyes and acetazolamide 500 mg intravenously. The pilocarpine acts therapeutically in the involved eye and prophylactically in the uninvolved eye. Other topical medications that may help lower intraocular pressure include topical beta-blockers (timolol, betaxolol, levobunolol, etc.), α-agonists (brimonidine, apraclonidine), and carbonic anhydrase inhibitors (dorzolamide, brinzolamide). Pain medication and antiemetics are appropriate. If available, osmotic agents such as intravenous *mannitol* or oral *glycerol* should be used. All patients with acute angle-closure glaucoma need a laser iridotomy or peripheral iridectomy to prevent further attacks.

INDICATIONS FOR REFERRAL

All patients with acute loss of vision should be seen immediately by an ophthalmologist. Individuals suspected of having glaucoma, macular degeneration, retinal vein occlusion, or an infectious etiology and those in whom the cause of impaired vision is unclear should have early ophthalmologic consultation. Diabetics should be referred, even if asymptomatic, because screening and early diagnosis and treatment can prevent vision loss. Type 1 diabetics require annual ophthalmologic examination starting 5 years after onset of disease. At the time of diagnosis, type 2 diabetics should be referred for a detailed retinal examination and then annually. Patients with refractive error should be referred to an eye specialist for proper refraction. Refractive surgery may be considered for patients who have difficulty with glasses and/or contact lenses.

ANNOTATED BIBLIOGRAPHY

Bienfang DC, Kelly LD, Nicholson DH, et al. Ophthalmology. N Engl J Med 1990;323:956. *(Good overview for the general reader.)*

Bloom JN, Palestine AG. The diagnosis of cytomegalovirus retinitis. Ann Intern Med 1988;109:963. *(Required reading for those caring for HIV patients.)*

Christen WG, Glynn RJ, Manson JE, et al. A prospective study of cigarette smoking and risk of age-related macular degeneration in men. JAMA 1996;276:1174. *(Prospective cohort study of 12 years' follow-up showing smoking to be an independent risk factor.)*

Margolis KL, Money BE, Kopietz LA, et al. Physician recognition of ophthalmoscopic signs of open-angle glaucoma. J Gen Intern Med 1989;4:296. *(An educational program that includes good photographs of the key findings.)*

Seddon JM, Willett WC, Speizer FE, et al. A prospective study of cigarette smoking and age-related macular degeneration in women. JAMA 1996;276:1141. *(Prospective cohort study of 12 years' duration; smoking proved to be an independent risk factor.)*

Singer DE, Nathan DM, Fogel HA, et al. Screening for diabetic retinopathy. Ann Intern Med 1992;116:660. *(Finds screening beneficial.)*

Strahlman E, Ford D, Whelton P, et al. Vision screening in a primary care practice. Arch Intern Med 1990;150:2159. *(High yield in high-risk persons.)*

Tielsch JM, Javitt JC, Coleman A, et al. The prevalence of blindness and visual impairment among nursing home residents in Baltimore. N Engl J Med 1995;332:1205. *(The high prevalence argues for screening in primary care practice.)*

Tielsch JM, Sommer A, Witt K, et al. Blindness and visual impairment in an American urban population. Arch Ophthalmol 1990;108:286. *(Important epidemiologic data.)*

201
Evaluation of Eye Pain
ROGER F. STEINERT

Pain in the eye is most often produced by conditions that do not threaten vision. However, at times the discomfort may result from corneal or intraocular pathology that is capable of compromising eyesight. The first responsibility of the primary physician is to determine promptly if there is an immediate threat to vision that requires urgent therapy or quick referral to the ophthalmologist; minor problems can be treated symptomatically in the office.

Ocular pain is usually not the only presentation of injury or disease. Several distinct pain categories can be identified that, when combined with assessment of inflammation (see Chapter 199) and vision (see Chapter 200), allow the primary physician to categorize the nature of the problem and make appropriate disposition.

PATHOPHYSIOLOGY AND CLINICAL PRESENTATION

The external ocular surfaces (lid, conjunctiva, and cornea) and the uveal tract are richly innervated to detect pain. Localization within these structures is relatively less precise. The orbit and sinuses may give rise to pain localized to the eye. Pathology confined to the vitreous, retina, or optic nerve is rarely a source of pain.

Eyelids. Inflammation of the eyelid causes tenderness and foreign body sensation. Common causes are hordeolum (stye), trichiasis (inturned lashes), and tarsal foreign bodies. Redness and edema may accompany the pain.

Conjunctiva. Viral and bacterial conjunctivitis cause mild burning and foreign body sensation, whereas allergic conjunctivitis primarily elicits itching (see Chapter 199). Toxic, chemical, and mechanical injuries are commonly responsible for unilateral disease.

Cornea. The cornea is densely innervated by pain fibers, so that even a minor injury may result in considerable discomfort. Pain arises from exposure of nerve endings in the epithelium; the patient complains of a burning or foreign body sensation. Reflex photophobic lacrimation may accompany the discomfort. Blinking exacerbates the pain, which is generally relieved by a pressure patch holding the lid shut.

Keratitis (inflammation of the cornea) occurs with trauma, infection, exposure, vascular disease, or decreased lacrimation.

Contact lens use has become an important source of microbial keratitis. Cellular infiltration and loss of corneal luster ensue. If blood vessels invade the normally avascular corneal stroma, vision may become cloudy. Severe pain is a prominent symptom; movement of the lid typically exacerbates symptoms. Fluorescein stain reveals the epithelial defects quite well and allows identification with a penlight.

Sclera. Compared with disease of the eyelids, scleral problems are more likely to cause dull deep pain. If the condition involves the anterior sclera, it may be readily visible as an area of redness. The blood supply to the sclera is not extensive, and its metabolism is relatively inactive. Consequently, inflammatory conditions of the sclera tend to be rather torpid; many are associated with connective tissue disease.

Uveal Tract. Anterior uveitis or iritis is accompanied by a dull ache and photophobia due to the irritative spasm of the pupillary sphincter. Posterior uveitis without anterior involvement may be painless or cause deep-seated aching. Profound ocular and orbital pain radiating to the frontal and temporal regions accompanies sudden elevation of pressure, as in acute angle-closure glaucoma. Vagal stimulation with high pressure may result in nausea and vomiting. Often the patient gives a history of mild intermittent episodes of blurred vision preceding the onset of an attack of throbbing pain, nausea, vomiting, and decreased visual acuity; halos about lights are sometimes noted. A fixed midposition pupil, redness, and a hazy cornea may be present (see Chapter 207).

Orbit. Inflammation and rapidly expanding mass lesions may cause deep pain. Displacement of the globe and diplopia may ensue. One important etiology is *optic neuritis*, a condition of younger patients (aged 15 to 40 years). Onset is acute. Eye movement may cause sharp pain due to meningeal inflammation (the extraocular rectus muscles insert along the dura of the nerve sheath at the orbital apex). Most cases are idiopathic, but 10% to 15% are associated with multiple sclerosis and as many as 20% to 50% eventually develop multiple sclerosis. Symptoms include pain on eye movement, abnormal color vision, and some loss of central vision. In most instances, the optic disk appears normal, but occasionally there is edema. A central scotoma may be found.

Sinusitis may also cause secondary orbital inflammation and tenderness on extremes of eye movement. In orbital cellulitis there is proptosis, limitation of extraocular movement, injection, and diminished vision.

Other Sources. Mild headache referred to the orbit is associated with refractive error, ocular muscle imbalance, sinusitis, and other causes of nonocular headache, such as tension headache, temporal arteritis, and the prodromal phase of herpes zoster. Severe aches in the eye cannot be attributed to refractive error, nor can aches about the eye that are noted on awakening in the morning.

DIFFERENTIAL DIAGNOSIS

The causes of eye pain can be considered anatomically (Table 201.1).

WORKUP

The initial task is to ensure there is no threat to vision. Most intraocular conditions that cause eye pain may compromise vision and should be carefully checked for, as should corneal injuries.

History. The quality of the pain needs to be considered. Deep pain is suggestive of an intraocular problem; a foreign body sensation makes it likely that the problem is on the surface of the eye. The patient should be asked about any change in visual acuity or color vision, because any report of deteriorating vision requires urgent ophthalmologic consultation. A history of diplopia and displacement of the eye raises the possibility of an orbital problem. Ascertaining the aggravating and alleviating factors can aid diagnosis. Pain exacerbated by lid movement and relieved by cessation of lid motion is suggestive of a foreign body or corneal lesion. Pain worsened by eye motion may be due to retrobulbar optic neuritis, especially if accompanied by loss of central vision and a normal-appearing optic disc. Photophobia is often prominent in acute anterior uveitis. Localization of a extraocular lesion by history is often difficult, because most of the time the foreign body sensation is felt in the outer portion of the upper lid, regardless of the lesion's location. In considering causes of conjunctival irritation, it is important to ask about occupational exposures, trauma, sun, sun lamp, and other forms of ultraviolet radiation (e.g., arc welding), as well as foreign body contact. History of sinusitis and headaches should be noted.

Physical Examination. An ophthalmoscope, penlight, ability to perform lid eversion, and use of fluorescein stain can be very helpful for assessment. First, visual acuity, color vision, and extraocular movements should be tested and recorded. The eye, lid, and conjunctiva are inspected for masses and redness, the pupil for reactivity, the cornea for clarity, and the fundus for any abnormalities of the disc. A *cloudy cornea* in conjunction with a fixed midposition pupil is consistent with acute glaucoma; the eye may be red. A *constricted pupil* in the presence of an eye that is tearing excessively suggests anterior uveitis; in severe cases, the eye also may be reddened and the anterior chamber hazy. Finding a *central scotoma* should raise suspicion of retrobulbar neuritis; a normal-appearing disk supports the diagnosis. The upper lid should be inverted with a cotton-tipped

Table 201.1.   Important Causes of Eye Pain

Extraocular Causes
Lid
  Hordeolum (a small abscess of the lid)
  Acute dacryocystitis
  Cellulitis
  Chalazion
Conjunctival
  Irritant exposure (prolonged sun exposure, pollution, occupational irritants, aerosol propellants, wind, dust)
  Infection (viral or bacterial)
  Lack of sleep
Corneal
  Incipient zoster
  Abrasions
  Foreign bodies
  Ulcers
  Ingrown lashes
  Contact lens abuse
  Excessive exposure to sun or other forms of ultraviolet radiation
  Infection (bacterial or viral)
Scleral
  Episcleritis
  Scleritis (connective tissue disease)

Intraocular Conditions
Anterior eye
  Acute angle-closure glaucoma
  Acute anterior uveitis (idiopathic, connective tissue disease, sarcoidosis, inflammatory bowel disease)
  Refractive error (mild pain only)
Posterior eye
  Posterior uveitis

Orbital Disease
Tumor
Inflammatory disease
Retrobulbar optic neuritis

Referred Pain from Extraocular Sources
Sinusitis
Tooth abscess
Tension headache
Temporal arteritis
Prodrome of herpes zoster
Ocular muscle imbalance

applicator to check for a foreign body or chalazion. The penlight can then be used to survey the cornea for gross injury; examination is facilitated by use of a small hand lens. The iris should be examined for evidence of dilated vessels around the limbus; this *ciliary flush* is characteristic of intraocular inflammation and occurs in anterior uveitis. Often the flush cannot be seen without the aid of a slit lamp.

Fluorescein Staining. All but very small corneal epithelial lesions can be detected without the use of a slit lamp if fluorescein staining and a cobalt blue filtered light are used in the eye examination. Because of the ease of bacterial (particularly pseudomonal) contamination of the fluorescein, it must be instilled by means of either a single-dose container or sterile fluorescein strips wetted with sterile saline. The strip is touched to the inferior cul de sac while the patient looks upward; the patient is then asked to blink once. The fluorescein stains into denuded areas of corneal epithelium, producing a bright green color when viewed by normal light. The intensity of staining is enhanced if the eye is illuminated with a cobalt blue light. Among the lesions that can be identified by fluorescein staining are the dendritic ulcers of herpes keratitis, abrasions, small foreign bodies, and punctate defects caused by irradiation.

Intraocular Pressure. If pain is not clearly related to the external eye or adnexa, the intraocular pressure should be measured to rule out glaucoma, provided there is no infection and the globe is intact without external or penetrating foreign bodies.

INDICATIONS FOR REFERRAL

Significant loss of vision always requires prompt ophthalmic evaluation. Progressive pain, redness, or discharge that fails to respond to conservative treatment must be evaluated. Care must be taken not to mistake penetrating trauma for a simple abrasion. An eccentric pupil or shallow chamber may indicate loss of aqueous humor. One should never instill antibiotic ointment if there is a possibility of a perforation. Under such circumstances, patch the eye with a metal or plastic shield, which protects the eye, and arrange referral; do not place any pressure on the globe.

SYMPTOMATIC MANAGEMENT

Most serious causes of eye pain require prompt ophthalmologic referral, but some foreign bodies and abrasions can be managed in the office setting.

Foreign Bodies. Irrigation with normal saline from a squirt bottle, syringe without a needle, or intravenous tubing may flush out foreign material. If irrigation fails, no further attempt should be made by the nonophthalmologist to remove the foreign body if it is firmly embedded in the cornea. Use of a dry cotton-tipped applicator will only remove much normal corneal epithelium. Use of a cotton-tipped applicator or needle for foreign body removal requires topical anesthesia, good visualization, and specific training.

Abrasions. Superficial epithelial abrasions usually heal well with prophylactic antibiotic medication (e.g., erythromycin ointment) and a tight pressure patch for 24 to 48 hours.

For management of conjunctivitis and glaucoma, see Chapters 199 and 207, respectively.

ANNOTATED BIBLIOGRAPHY

Bienfang DC, Kelly LD, Nicholson DH, et al. Ophthalmology. N Engl J Med 1990;323:956. (*Excellent review and overview for the general reader; 115 references.*)

Shingleton BJ, Hersh PS, Kenyon KR. Eye trauma. Philadelphia: Mosby, 1991. (*The definitive text on the subject; includes detailed sections on management of foreign bodies and abrasions.*)

202
Evaluation of Dry Eyes
DAVID A. GREENBERG

The normal tear film provides important protection to the eye. Defects in tear production are uncommon but often occur in conjunction with systemic disease. The primary physician must decide if systemic disease does exist, provide symptomatic relief, and know when referral is needed.

PATHOPHYSIOLOGY AND CLINICAL PRESENTATION

The ocular tear film performs a host of functions, including maintenance of the corneal and conjunctival epithelium, lubrication of lid motion, delivery of oxygen and uptake of CO_2 from the cornea, carriage of antimicrobial defenses, clearance of foreign matter and tissue debris, and smoothing of the anterior ocular surface for clear vision. The tear film is inherently unstable, depending on the interaction of its three components for stability.

The outermost layer of the tear film is lipid, excreted by the lid meibomian glands. This layer retards evaporation and counters gravitational forces on the aqueous layer. The middle layer is aqueous, secreted by the lacrimal glands and accounting for most of the tear film. The innermost layer is mucinous, primarily secreted by conjunctival goblet cells and attaching to the corneal epithelium. This converts the corneal surface from a hydrophobic to a hydrophilic one. Each blink redistributes and replenishes the tear film. Dry eyes ensue from a defect in maintenance of the tear film.

Aqueous Deficiency. A defect in production of the aqueous phase by lacrimal glands causes dry eyes or *keratoconjunctivi-*
tis sicca. The condition most often occurs as a physiologic consequence of *aging,* commonly exacerbated by the desiccating effect of dry environmental conditions. It also may develop in the setting of *connective tissue disease, anticholinergic drug* use (e.g., phenothiazines, tricyclic antidepressants, antihistamines), and neurologic disease.

In *Sjögren's syndrome,* the lacrimal glands become involved in immune-mediated inflammation. The condition may occur in the context of other rheumatoid diseases or as an isolated event. Women outnumber men by 9:1. Onset is typically after age 50. The condition may present as an isolated focal problem (*primary disease*) or in the context of ongoing rheumatoid disease (*secondary disease*). Characteristic features of focal disease include dry eyes and dry mouth. Patients complain first of burning eyes and a sandy, gritty, foreign body sensation, particularly later in the day. Increased eye debris and mucus are noted. Secondary bacterial infection develops in severe cases. There also may be facial telangiectasias, parotid enlargement, altered taste, lip fissures, dental caries, and difficulty with phonation. Secondary disease manifestations include polyarthritis, fatigue, Raynaud's phenomenon, and a vasculitic rash (see Chapter 146). A seronegative form of the condition has been described in males with AIDS.

Mucin Deficiency. Mucin production may decline in the setting of *vitamin A deficiency,* which causes primary goblet cell deficiency. When this is combined with protein deficiency (as occurs in underdeveloped parts of the world), *ker-*

atomalacia results. Secondary loss of goblet cells and mucin deficiency follows chemical *burns*, benign ocular *pemphigoid*, and *trachoma*. With loss of main and accessory lacrimal production, a combined mucin-aqueous deficiency ensues. Dry eyes linked to problems in mucin production have been noted in patients using the antiacne preparation *isotretinoin* (Accutane).

Eyelid Defects. Compromised lid function may affect the entire tear film because of impaired rewetting. Incomplete blinking, fifth or seventh cranial nerve palsy, exophthalmos, and exposure during sleep are among the conditions that result in drying of the inferior interpalpebral cornea. Lid movement may also be hindered by scar formation.

Neurogenic hyposecretion is a potential consequence of such uncommon conditions as basal skull fracture or the Ramsay-Hunt syndrome.

Patients with dry eyes are more likely to report grittiness, itching, burning, soreness, difficulty in moving the eyelids, or the sensation of a foreign body present with that complaint. When ocular irritation stimulates excess reflex tearing, the patient may present paradoxically with watery eyes. In rare instances, a corneal ulcer or red eye may ensue.

DIFFERENTIAL DIAGNOSIS

The differential diagnosis of dry eyes can be organized pathophysiologically (Table 202.1). As noted, the most common cause is the generalized diminution of lacrimal secretion associated with aging, followed by systemic conditions and anticholinergic drugs. Keratoconjunctivitis sicca secondary to a mucin or lipid abnormality is less common. Environmental factors contribute. In a population-based assessment of the elderly, medication side effects proved to be the predominant etiology, accounting for 62% of cases. Risk was particularly high when three or more drugs with known drying side effects were used concurrently (e.g., tricyclics, anxiolytics, antihypertensives).

Table 202.1. Principal Causes of Dry Eyes

Lacrimal Gland Dysfunction
Age
Systemic disease (Sjögren's syndrome, sarcoidosis, Hodgkin's disease)
Anticholinergic drugs (atropine, antihistamines, tricyclics)

Compromised Eyelid Function
Fifth or seventh nerve palsy
Exophthalmos
Scar formation

Mucin Deficiency
Chemical burns
Hypovitaminosis A
Isotretinoin (Accutane)
Benign ocular pemphigoid
Trachoma

Environmental Factors
Excessive dryness
Excessive exposure (e.g., exophthalmos, Bell's palsy)

Lipid Abnormalities
Chronic blepharitis
Meibomitis

WORKUP

History. The workup should begin by noting the duration and frequency of symptoms and particularly if onset is related to dry environmental conditions. Symptoms of keratoconjunctivitis sicca are usually more pronounced as the day progresses and are frequently exacerbated by tobacco smoke. The physician should ask if tears are produced with crying and if the patient finds strands of mucus from the inner canthi on awakening (a very suggestive symptom). It is important to note any associated dry mouth, joint pains, prior ocular disease, infection, or surgery. A detailed drug history is essential, especially in the elderly, who may be taking several drugs that together may be the source of the patient's difficulty (e.g., tricyclics, anxiolytics, antihypertensives). Any prior history of rheumatoid disease or its symptoms should be sought.

Physical Examination. Attention is paid to frequency and completeness of blinking and note taken of any lid pathology. Blepharitis and meibomitis are evident as lid margin crusting and engorgement of the meibomian glands, respectively. Other physical findings may include thick yellow mucous strands in the lower fornix, hyperemic and edematous bulbar conjunctiva, and corneal dullness. It is mandatory to check for completeness of lid closure and position of eyelashes. The corneal reflex is checked if there is concern about a neuroparalytic keratitis or facial nerve palsy. Skin and joints should be examined for signs of rheumatoid disease (see Chapter 146).

Studies. The *Schirmer test* diagnoses aqueous deficiency by measuring the wetting of a filter paper strip (Whatman No. 41 filter paper, 5×35 mm). A folded end is hooked over the lower lid temporally and the patient is instructed to keep the eyes lightly closed during the test. In the Schirmer I test, wetting is measured after 5 minutes; less than 5 mm is usually abnormal. A basal Schirmer test using topical anesthetic to prevent reflex tearing caused by the paper strip is no longer performed.

Testing for Sjögren's Syndrome. Evidence by history or physical examination of *Sjögren's syndrome* or rheumatoid disease should trigger serologic testing that begins with an *antinuclear antibody* determination (95% sensitive in Sjögren's; specificity low) and a *rheumatoid factor* (75% sensitive; specificity low). If these screening serologic tests are positive, then follow-up testing for the more specific *anti-Ro* and *anti-La* antibodies (60% to 70% sensitivity, more than 90% specificity) is worth considering; see Chapter 146). *Lip biopsy* is the definitive test but often not necessary in the context of characteristic clinical and serologic findings.

SYMPTOMATIC MANAGEMENT AND INDICATIONS FOR REFERRAL

As long as there are no signs of ocular disease, the primary physician may attempt symptomatic relief. The first steps are to eliminate any unnecessary medications that may be contributing and reduce any environmental dryness that exacerbates the aqueous deficiency of aging. Often this can be accomplished by use of a room humidifier. A 2-week trial of one of the many commercially available *artificial tear substitutes* may also be helpful. Of the commercially available preparations, methylcellulose (Visulose, 0.5% or 1%), polyvinyl alcohol (Liquifilm Tears, 1.4%, or Liquifilm Forte, 3%), and hydroxypropyl methylcellulose, 1% (Ultra Tears, Tears Naturale, and Adsorbotear) have been used successfully. These nonprescription drops are soothing and, through a variety of formulations, provide aqueous replacement and sometimes mucomimetic substances.

Drops may be instilled as often as desired. Topical application of one to two drops, four times a day, is a useful starting dosage. The patient may increase the frequency of application to as often as hourly to achieve comfort; a bland ointment can be used at night. Toxicity is uncommon, but topical sensitivity or corneal epithelial damage may occur. More severe cases may warrant *punctal plugs,* which have proven superior to methylcellulose inserts (Lacrisert); acceptance of these has been limited. Steroids and antibiotics should not be prescribed for uncomplicated disease.

The patient should be instructed to seek immediate ophthalmologic attention in the event of a red eye, visual disturbance, or eye pain. An eye specialist should be consulted when simple symptomatic treatment does not give rapid relief.

PATIENT EDUCATION

It is critical for the primary physician to be certain that the patient knows how to instill the drops into the eye. Instructions should include the careful instillation of the drop into the lower fornix without contact occurring between the dropper and the eye and the utilization of digital pressure in the punctal or inner region of the lower lid to reduce drainage and prolong contact. The patient should also be educated that the instillation of more than one drop at a time exceeds the physical capacity of the inferior fornix and is wasteful.

ANNOTATED BIBLIOGRAPHY

Barsam PC, Sampson WG, Feldman GL, et al. Treatment of the dry eye and related problems. Ann Ophthalmol 1972;4:122. *(Subjective relief provided by artificial tear substitute in patients with idiopathic ocular discomfort and dry eye.)*

Holly FJ, Lemp MA. Tear physiology and dry eyes. Surv Ophthalmol 1977;22:69. *(Classic review.)*

Jones DB. Prospects in the management of tear deficiency states. Trans Am Acad Ophthalmol Otolaryngol 1977;83:OP692. *(Includes comprehensive listing of the causes by mechanism.)*

Schein OD, Hochberg MC, Munoz B, et al. Dry eye and dry mouth in the elderly: a population-based assessment. Arch Intern Med 1999;159:1359. *(Medications were the most common cause, accounting for the vast majority of cases; autoimmune disease was not a major factor.)*

Sjögren H, Block KJ. Keratoconjunctivitis sicca and Sjögren's syndrome. Surv Ophthalmol 1971;16:143. *(Classic paper.)*

Slater CA, Davis RB, Shmerling RH. Antinuclear antibody testing: a clinical study of utility. Arch Intern Med 1996;156:1421. *(Critical look at the test, finding sensitivity high but specificity low.)*

203

Evaluation of Common Visual Disturbances: Flashing Lights, Floaters, and Other Transient Phenomena
CLAUDIA U. RICHTER

Flashes of light, floaters, specks, distortions, halos, and discolorations are among the transient visual phenomena reported by patients. Flashes of light (*photopsia*) and dark moving lines and specks (*floaters*) are particularly common occurrences that are usually benign but may signal a retinal tear or detachment. Visual distortion (*metamorphopsia*) can be the presenting symptom of age-related macular degeneration. Other short-lived disturbances accompany such diverse conditions as migraine, digitalis toxicity, and acute glaucoma. The primary physician needs to know the significance of these visual phenomena and when they presage a serious ophthalmologic or systemic event that requires prompt ophthalmologic attention.

PATHOPHYSIOLOGY AND CLINICAL PRESENTATION

Floaters are vitreous opacities that cast a shadow on the retina. They can be single or multiple, characteristically moving across the visual field and transiently blurring vision if they cross the macula. Their presence is most notable when gazing at a clear blue sky or blank white wall. New onset of floaters may occur as a consequence of *vitreous detachment, a retinal tear or detachment,* or an intraocular hemorrhage.

Vitreoretinal traction is the principal cause of retinal tears and detachments, which can lead to sudden onset of flashes and floaters. As the vitreous gel liquefies with age, its fibrous matrix contracts and pulls away from the retina. Because the vitreous is attached to the retina at several sites, any traction can cause tearing that leads to a retinal hole. Detachment may develop by flow of fluid from the vitreous through the hole and beneath the retina. If the tearing involves a superficial retinal vessel, hemorrhage into the vitreous may occur.

Acute or chronic intraocular inflammation and/or infection are sometimes the cause, as in the immunocompromised patient with *cytomegalovirus (CMV) retinitis*. The sudden appearance of one or more floaters suggests onset of serious underlying pathology. Floaters that are multiple and long-standing are associated with *myopia* and *aging* with or without a vitreous detachment.

Flashes (photopsia) are perceptions of bright small flickering lights or lightning-like flashes of light. They are most vividly seen in the dark and usually occur with mechanical stimulation of the retina. They account for "seeing stars" when one suffers head trauma or coughs very hard. New onset may be a consequence of vitreous traction on the retina, leading to *retinal tear* or *detachment*. Just rubbing the eyes can cause sim-

Table 203.1. Causes of Floaters and Flashing Lights

Floaters
  Myopia
  Aging
  Vitreous detachment
  Retinal tear
  Retinal detachment
  Intraocular inflammation (uveitis, retinitis)
  Vitreous hemorrhage
Flashing Lights
  Vitreoretinal traction
  Retinal detachment
  Mechanical stimulation (cough, rubbing the eyes, head trauma)
  Classic migraine
  Seizure activity in the visual cortex (static light, colored flashes)

ilar symptoms. *Migraine* pathophysiology accounts for recurrent episodes, which are more complex and longer lasting (*scintillating scotoma*).

Distortion (metamorphopsia) refers to the curvilinear distortion of straight lines or patterns. This visual disturbance is the consequence of an altered shape of the retinal surface, either from collection of fluid beneath the retina or scarring on the surface. Metamorphopsia is seen with age-related *macular degeneration*, epiretinal fibrosis, and a variety of ocular diseases that cause traction on the retinal surface and/or retinal scarring.

Zigzag Lines. *Migraine* can produce a complex set of prodromal visual phenomena that include *zigzag lines* (sometimes referred to as *fortification phenomena*) and flashes of light with transient blind spots (*scintillating scotoma*). These may present with or without a subsequent headache. Typically, the zigzag lines occur adjacent to a gray area of shaded darkness. Both the gray area and the zigzag lines slowly expand. The visual phenomena typically end in 20 to 30 minutes with or without the onset of the headache and leave no residual visual deficit (see Chapter 165).

Halos, Discolorations, and Visual Hallucinations. The first clinical manifestations of *digitalis toxicity* may be visual (see Chapter 32) and include lightning flashes, yellow discoloration, halos, and the appearance of frost over objects. *Acute glaucoma* (see Chapter 207) also produces colored halos around lights but not lightning flashes. Visual hallucinations caused by *seizure* activity in the occipital cortex and the adjacent association area produce static light and stars. Hallucinations from the parastriate area 18 cause luminous sensations or colored flashes and rings.

DIFFERENTIAL DIAGNOSIS

The sudden onset of a visual phenomenon may be the first sign of important underlying ophthalmic or systemic pathology. Causes can be listed according to clinical presentation (Table 203.1).

WORKUP

History. A complete and detailed description of the visual disturbance uninfluenced by leading questions is the most important part of the history, followed by information re-

garding their onset, course, and presence of any associated symptoms (e.g., headache, decreased visual acuity). The sudden onset of flashing lights and/or floaters is highly suggestive of vitreoretinal traction, possibly in association with a vitreous detachment, retinal tear, or retinal detachment. New onset in an immunocompromised patient should suggest CMV retinitis. Flashes of light on waking and rubbing the eyes are usually harmless, as are floaters that have been present for an extended time without marked increase in number. The patient who complains of halos needs to be checked for glaucoma (see Chapter 198). A report of lightning flashes, yellow discoloration, or frost over objects in a patient taking a digitalis preparation requires consideration of digitalis toxicity. Visual distortion should lead to a search for subretinal fluid accumulation.

Physical Examination. Visual acuity testing, measurement of the intraocular pressure (see Chapter 198), and careful examination of the fundus should be included. One looks for hemorrhage in the vitreous, a ballooning white area suggestive of a retinal detachment, areas of retinal inflammation, and abnormalities in the appearance of the macula suggestive of macular degenerative disease. In the immunocompromised patient, funduscopic examination should include a look for the manifestations of CMV retinitis (e.g., focal, granular, perivascular yellow-white lesions with or without hemorrhage in a "brushfire" pattern). Detection of retinal tears and small retinal detachments requires indirect ophthalmoscopy or diagnostic contact lens examination performed by the ophthalmologist. Patients with migraine will have a normal ophthalmologic examination.

Studies. The most important study in patients with new flashes and/or floaters is *indirect ophthalmoscopy* and scleral depression done by the ophthalmologist. Patients with metamorphopsia need *fluorescein angiography*. The patient with halos needs to be checked for glaucoma by measurement of *intraocular pressure* (see Chapter 198). The patient taking a digitalis preparation who reports visual disturbances should have a serum drug level measured (see Chapter 32).

PATIENT EDUCATION AND INDICATIONS FOR REFERRAL

New onset of unexplained flashes or floaters requires urgent referral to an ophthalmologist because of the possibility of a retinal tear, retinal detachment, or an inflammatory/infectious process (e.g., CMV retinitis). Vision is best preserved when treatment of such conditions is prompt. If the patient or examiner detects a field loss, referral is even more urgent. Metamorphopsia is also an indication for urgent referral, because age-related macular degeneration has a better visual prognosis when subretinal neovascularization is treated with early macular photocoagulation. A report of halos should lead to referral for evaluation of glaucoma. Visual hallucinations require workup for seizure activity and visual cortex pathology.

Patients with chronic flashes and floaters should have a complete ophthalmologic examination, including indirect ophthalmoscopy, but it is not urgent. All patients with flashes and floaters need to be warned that a sudden onset of new floaters or flashes or the appearance of a peripheral visual field defect may represent a retinal hole or detachment necessitating prompt ophthalmologic attention. The patient with chronic floaters in the absence of ocular disease can be reassured; prognosis is excellent, as it is for the person with visual phenomena associated with migraine. Flashes that occur with minor mechanical stimulation (cough, rubbing of the eyes) require only reassurance and explanation, as long as there is no evidence of more serious pathology.

ANNOTATED BIBLIOGRAPHY

Aring CD. The scintillating scotoma. JAMA 1972;220:519. (*A detailed discussion of these migrainous visual phenomena.*)

Bienfang DC, Kelly LD, Nicholson DH, et al. Ophthalmology. N Engl J Med 1990;323;956. (*A succinct review of recent improvements in ophthalmologic care, including CMV retinitis.*)

Morris PH, Scheie HG, Aminlari A. Light flashes as a clue to retinal disease. Arch Ophthalmol 1974;91:179. (*In this series, 23% had demonstrable vitreoretinal disease; of these, 16% had retinal breaks.*)

204
Evaluation of Exophthalmos
CLAUDIA U. RICHTER

Exophthalmos is defined as protrusion or proptosis of the eye. It may be a variation of normal physiognomy or a sign of systemic or orbital disease. The primary physician must be able to recognize it and evaluate the patient for a possible endocrinologic, neoplastic, or vascular cause and decide on the need for further study or referral.

PATHOPHYSIOLOGY AND CLINICAL PRESENTATION

Pathologic forms of exophthalmos may result from inflammation, infiltration, a mass lesion, or a vascular abnormality.

Graves' Disease. The ophthalmopathy of Graves' disease occurs as a consequence of an autoimmune inflammatory process leading to infiltration of the soft tissues of the orbit. Risk factors include cigarette smoking, radioiodine therapy, persistent hyperthyroidism, and recurrence of hyperthyroidism after withdrawal of antithyroid drug therapy. Administration of prednisone at the time of radioiodine therapy can prevent treatment-induced ophthalmopathy. Pathologically, there is an inflammatory infiltrate of lymphocytes, mucopolysaccharides, and edema, followed by proliferation of fibroblasts and increase in the volume of orbital connective tissue. The proliferation of orbital fibroblasts and their fibrotic restriction of extraocular muscle movement account for the clinical picture of Graves' ophthalmopathy.

In its mildest form, there is minor lid retraction, stare, lid lag, and mild protrusion of the eye (proptosis). A particularly severe form, "malignant" exophthalmos, causes edema of the lids and conjunctiva, marked proptosis, limitation of extraocular movements, exposure keratopathy, and optic nerve compression. Although it is usually a bilateral disease, it may present unilaterally or asymmetrically.

The relatively close clinical relationship between ophthalmopathy of Graves' disease, pretibial dermopathy, and hyperthyroidism suggests a common pathophysiologic mechanism. However, the ophthalmopathy can occur in the absence of thyroid dysfunction or pretibial dermopathy. The precise pathophysiology remains to be elucidated. It may be triggered by antibodies to circulating thyroid antigen, accounting for the exacerbation seen with some treatments for thyrotoxicosis. Its precise mechanism(s) continues to be elucidated (see Chapter 103).

Primary orbital neoplasms, such as *meningiomas,* produce exophthalmos by mass effect. Some vascular lesions, such as *hemangiomas,* produce only a mass effect, whereas a *carotid-cavernous sinus fistula* may present with a diffusely congested orbit with exophthalmos, prominent episcleral vessels, and elevated intraocular pressure. Mass lesions and vascular abnormalities are unilateral processes. They may lead to diplopia, ocular irritation, and photophobia (secondary to corneal exposure). Stretching or compression of the optic nerve can impair visual acuity.

Orbital cellulitis is an extremely serious, although rare, cause of proptosis. Because the orbit is bordered on three sides by paranasal sinuses, orbital infection can result from sinusitis extending directly through the lamina papyracea. Lid edema, ptosis, proptosis, chemosis, and diminished ocular movements make for a dramatic clinical presentation. Retrograde extension can lead to cavernous sinus thrombosis.

DIFFERENTIAL DIAGNOSIS

Bilateral exophthalmos is usually caused by Graves' disease, but occasionally it occurs with Cushing's syndrome, acromegaly, lithium ingestion, metastatic tumor, and orbital lymphoma.

Unilateral exophthalmos may be caused by tumor, inflammatory and infectious diseases, vascular abnormalities, and skeletal abnormalities. Common orbital tumors include hemangioma, meningioma, and optic nerve glioma. Tumors extending into the orbit include those originating in the eye, lids, and paranasal sinuses. Orbital pseudotumor is an inflammatory lesion that can mimic a mass lesion. Inflammatory etiologies include sarcoidosis, foreign body, orbital thrombophlebitis, and ruptured dermoid cyst. Hemangioma, aneurysm, varices, carotid-cavernous fistula, and cavernous sinus thrombosis constitute important vascular etiologies. Skeletal abnormalities such as Paget's disease may also produce exophthalmos. Asymmetry of the orbits, severe unilateral myopia, facial nerve paresis, eyelid retraction, and congenital glaucoma may give the appearance of exophthalmos. Ptosis or enophthalmos of the opposite eye can mimic exophthalmos.

WORKUP

The first task is to determine if the condition is unilateral or bilateral. Bilateral disease has a limited differential diagnosis, with

Graves' disease accounting for most cases. Attention is directed toward its confirmation (see Chapter 103). The broader differential of unilateral disease necessitates a more extensive workup.

History should include inquiry into the time course of the exophthalmos. Old photographs are helpful in determining if the problem is of new onset or simply a long-standing anatomic variant. Associated symptoms are also important to note. Visual acuity changes, diplopia, pain, excessive lacrimation, photophobia, and foreign body sensation are indications of adverse effects from the exophthalmos. A prior history or current symptoms of trauma to the orbit, thyroid disease, cancer, severe sinus infection, or worsening headache should be noted.

Physical examination begins with documenting the degree of exophthalmos by exophthalmoscopy. The distance to be measured is from the lateral orbital rim to the apex of the cornea with the patient looking straight ahead. The upper limit of normal is 21 to 22 mm; a difference between both eyes of 2 mm is also considered significant. Visual acuity, intraocular pressure, and extraocular muscle function should also be tested. The conjunctiva and cornea are observed for signs of drying, aided by fluorescein or rose bengal dye if available. Color vision, pupillary reactivity, and visual fields are assessed to investigate possible optic nerve compression, which may produce a pale or swollen optic nerve head on ophthalmoscopic examination. The globe and orbit need to be auscultated for bruits and pulsation suggestive of vascular fistula. The sinuses must be checked for tenderness and discharge. In the setting of bilateral disease, the neck should be checked for goiter and bruit, the pretibial region for dermopathy, and the remainder of the examination for signs of thyroid hormone excess (see Chapter 103).

Laboratory Studies. *Thyroid indices* (e.g., thyroid-stimulating hormone, total T_3, free T_4 index) should be ordered in the patient with bilateral disease, but the absence of hyperthyroidism does not rule out Graves' disease. Even in patients without evidence of thyrotoxicosis, *antibodies to thyrotropin receptors* and *peroxidase* can be detected (see Chapter 103).

Patients with unilateral exophthalmos are candidates for orbital imaging. At present, axial and coronal *computed tomography* is the study of choice in the evaluation of orbital abnormalities. It provides good definition of both bony and soft orbital tissues. *Ultrasound* is sometimes used to screen for a mass lesion. Orbital *magnetic resonance imaging* may be helpful in the noninvasive evaluation of certain vascular and neoplastic disorders. Invasive study is the province of the ophthalmologist.

SYMPTOMATIC MANAGEMENT, PATIENT EDUCATION, AND INDICATIONS FOR REFERRAL

Symptomatic Management and Prevention. The primary physician must be cognizant of potential ocular complications of exophthalmos and give advice for relief of minor symptoms. Periorbital and lid edema may be reduced by *elevating the head of the bed* at night. Exposure keratopathy causes a foreign body sensation, which can be relieved by use of *artificial tear lubricants* and *taping* the *eyelids* closed at night. If such simple measures are inadequate, referral to the ophthalmologist for consideration of eyelid or orbital surgery may be necessary.

Graves' Disease. Preventive measures include complete *cessation of smoking* and effective treatment of the underlying hyperthyroidism. Treatment of the underlying Graves' disease must be done carefully in the setting of eye involvement. As noted, ophthalmopathy can worsen with some forms of therapy, perhaps due to increased release of thyroid antigen. Some authorities suggest use of *antithyroid drugs* to minimize such release; others add high-dose corticosteroids to the program (e.g., *prednisone*, 0.5 mg/kg for 1 month, beginning a few days after radioiodine administration; see Chapter 103).

Specific treatment of Graves' ophthalmopathy is undertaken only when symptoms become severe or vision is threatened. Likelihood of progression is hard to determine, and available therapies have their own adverse effects. Nonetheless, inflammatory symptoms such as periorbital edema and ocular discomfort are treated with *corticosteroids* or *orbital radiation* in conjunction with total cessation of any smoking (smoking decreases their efficacy). Such therapy may inhibit the cytokines, which perpetuate the inflammatory reaction.

Referral and Admission. Ophthalmologic consultation should be obtained early in unilateral, severe, or unexplained exophthalmos. Exophthalmos due to neoplasm requires a team approach that includes the ophthalmologist, oncologist, and radiation therapist. A suspected vascular etiology is also grounds for referral. Endocrinologic consultation is indicated for managing the ophthalmopathy of Graves' disease. Emergency admission is needed if orbital cellulitis is encountered.

Patient Education. Patients with Graves' disease need to know that their eye symptoms may persist or progress despite appropriate systemic therapy for the underlying disease but also that there are approaches to limiting risk (e.g., smoking cessation, effective control of the hyperthyroidism, steroid therapy in conjunction with radioiodine). Patients with Graves' disease need to know the adverse consequences of smoking and undergo an aggressive smoking cessation program (see Chapter 54). Home measures to lessen eye discomfort and prevent eye injury, such as *elevating the head of the bed,* use of *artificial tear lubricants,* and *taping* the *eyelids* closed at night, are important to review with the exophthalmic patient, as are symptoms warranting prompt evaluation (e.g., change in vision, ocular pain, eye injection, diplopia).

ANNOTATED BIBLIOGRAPHY

Bahn RS, Heufelder AE. Pathogenesis of Graves' ophthalmopathy. N Engl J Med 1993;329:1468. *(Clinically useful review of disease mechanisms and their relation to clinical presentation and treatment.)*

Bartalena L, Marcocci C, Bogazzi F, et al. Relation between therapy for hyperthyroidism and the course of Graves' ophthalmopathy. N Engl J Med 1998;338:73. *(Prospective randomized trial demonstrating increased risk of exophthalmos with radioiodine therapy but not with methimazole; prednisone eliminated the risk.)*

Bartalena L, Marcocci C, Tanda ML, et al. Cigarette smoking and treatment outcomes in Graves' ophthalmopathy. Ann Intern Med 1998;129:632. *(Randomized single-blinded study showing that cigarette smoking increased risk of progression of exophthalmos and decreased efficacy of treatment.)*

Tallstedt L, Lundell G, Torring O, et al. Occurrence of ophthalmopathy after treatment of Graves' hyperthyroidism. N Engl J Med 1992;326:1733. *(Some treatments may actually exacerbate the ophthalmopathy.)*

Utiger RD. Treatment of Graves' ophthalmopathy. N Engl J Med 1989;321:1405. *(An editorial critically reviewing treatment options.)*

205

Evaluation of Excessive Tearing

ROGER F. STEINERT

The presence of watery eyes reflects an increased production of tears or a decreased ability to drain them. Patients complain of watery eyes or may actually describe tears overflowing and running down their cheeks, a condition called *epiphora*. The primary physician must decide if structural pathology exists or if reassurance is the appropriate treatment.

PATHOPHYSIOLOGY AND CLINICAL PRESENTATION

Normal Tear Production and Drainage. Tears are produced by the main and accessory lacrimal glands. They flow out through upper and lower puncta, which open into canaliculi. These, in turn, drain into the lacrimal sac and then into the nasolacrimal duct, which opens under the inferior turbinate in the nose. Tears do not flow down the drainage system merely by gravity but rather are pumped by lid motion.

Hypersecretion of Tears. Epiphora most often results from hypersecretion. Common stimulants are *blepharitis* and *keratitis* of any etiology (e.g., infections, foreign body), *atopy,* and *sinusitis.* Excessive moisture may be the complaint in a patient who has one of these inflammatory processes. *Pseudoepiphora* is reflex tearing in the presence of dry eyes (see Chapter 202). Aberrant regeneration of the seventh nerve may result in *gustatory lacrimation* ("crocodile tears").

Impaired Lacrimal Drainage. Tear film movement may be *obstructed* by eyelid-margin lesions or conjunctival redundancy or folds. The pumping function of the lid may be impaired by *seventh nerve palsy* or conditions stiffening the lids, such as scars or scleroderma, or by laxity of the lids from aging. The puncta must be properly positioned. *Ectropion* prevents tears from gaining access to the canaliculus. *Senile ectropion* is the most common cause in the elderly and is characterized by a sagging lower lid. The punctum or the canaliculus may be occluded congenitally, by chemical or thermal injury, or by neoplasms. In addition, canalicular *infections* may cause occlusion. The most common of these are *Actinomyces israeli (Streptothrix)* and *Candida.* Finally, obstruction of the lacrimal sac and nasolacrimal duct may be idiopathic, congenital, or caused by neoplasms, ethmoiditis, and turbinate disease.

The more distal the obstruction, the more likely that the epiphora will be accompanied by purulent discharge or *dacryocystitis,* as the stagnant tears become infected. Digital pressure may express purulent material from the puncta.

DIFFERENTIAL DIAGNOSIS

The most common causes of watery eye are senile ectropion and increased physiologic tearing. The differential can be organized according to causes of increased production and impaired drainage (Table 205.1).

WORKUP

History. The physician should determine if tears actually run down the cheek and, if so, how frequently. Overflowing tears in the absence of environmental irritants suggests structural pathology. Watery eyes noted on exposure to cold, air conditioning, or a dry environment may be due to exaggerated physiologic tearing.

Inquiry into whether the problem is unilateral or bilateral can be helpful. Unilateral tearing is more often obstructive, but stenosis can be bilateral; environmental irritants should cause bilateral epiphora. Any sinus disease, facial fractures, infections, and surgery should be noted as possible etiologic factors, as should symptoms suggestive of Sjögren's syndrome (see Chapter 146).

Physical Examination. Lid structure and motion should be observed. Patency of the puncta is visualized under low magnification. Gentle pressure is applied over the lacrimal sac on the side of the nose and over the canaliculi to attempt to express purulent material for examination and culture. Examination for signs of dry eye (see Chapter 202) is needed to rule out paradoxical tearing, which requires an entirely different therapeutic approach.

Studies. The ophthalmologist may also evaluate the lacrimal drainage system in several ways. *Fluorescein dye* instilled in the conjunctival sac should make its way to the nose (Jones test). *Saline irrigation* and *probing* may prove patency or localize an obstruction. *Dacryocystography* (radiocontrast dye injection) may dramatically outline the obstruction and the proximal lacrimal system. Dacryoscintigraphy, in which aqueous radioactive tracer is introduced into the tear film and fol-

Table 205.1. Causes of Watery Eyes

Excessive Tear Production
  Keratitis
  Blepharitis
  Conjunctivitis
  Atopy
  Sinusitis
  Facial palsies
  Reflex tearing of dry eyes

Impaired Tear Drainage
  Dacryocystitis
  Punctal obstruction (tumor, burn, senile atresia, infection)
  Ectropion
  Sagging of the lower lid
  Obstruction of the lacrimal sac and nasolacrimal duct (idiopathic, congenital, neoplasms, ethmoiditis, and turbinate disease)

lowed during blinking, may demonstrate functional impairment (pump failure).

SYMPTOMATIC MANAGEMENT AND INDICATIONS FOR REFERRAL

Irritants must be eliminated. Sicca is treated with appropriate *lubricants* (see Chapter 202). Dacryocystitis is treated with *hot compresses* at least four times a day and systemic *antibiotics* (usually erythromycin 250 mg four times a day or dicloxacillin 250 mg four times a day directed against staphylococcal species). Patients without infection can be reassured the condition is not harmful.

Unresponsive patients are properly referred to an ophthalmologist for further evaluation and treatment. In symptomatic cases, lid surgery to correct malposition or dacryocystorhinostomy to relieve nasolacrimal obstruction may be indicated.

ANNOTATED BIBLIOGRAPHY

Jones LT, Linn ML. The diagnosis of the causes of epiphora. Am J Ophthalmol 1969;67:751. *(The classic paper on the workup of epiphora.)*

Pflugfelder SC, Tseng SC, Sanabria O, et al. Evaluation of subjective assessments and objective diagnostic tests for diagnosing tear-film disorders known to cause ocular irritation. Cornea 1998; 17:38. *(A comprehensive review of the evaluation of eye moisture disorders.)*

Schein OD, Tielsch JM, Munoz B, et al. Relation between signs and symptoms of dry eye in the elderly. A population-based perspective. Ophthalmology 1997;104:1395. *(Helpful explanation of the complex presentation of dry and wet eye complaints.)*

206

Management of the Patient with Age-Related Macular Degeneration

Age-related macular degeneration is a major cause of vision loss in the elderly. The age-related form affects an estimated 30% of persons over the age of 75. Proper geriatric eye care includes early recognition of macular degeneration so that ophthalmologic referral can be timely and the risk of visual impairment minimized.

PATHOPHYSIOLOGY AND CLINICAL PRESENTATION

Mechanisms. The retinal pigmented epithelium is critical to the maintenance of healthy retinal photoreceptors. Any compromise to the former can lead to a decline in receptor cells and loss of vision. In macular degeneration, the retinal pigmented epithelium begins to degenerate or at least change its biochemical relation with photoreceptor cells. The mechanism(s) remains poorly understood. There is a *genetic* propensity, but as of yet no specific genes have been identified. Suspected risk factors include *cardiovascular disease, atherosclerotic* risk factors, *dietary* factors (e.g., *lack of antioxidants, zinc*), and *sun* exposure. Most data supporting these hypotheses are too limited to draw conclusions, but data from two major prospective epidemiologic studies (The Nurses' Health Study and The Physicians' Health Study) revealed *cigarette smoking* to be a potent independent risk factor, with a dose-response relationship, particularly in women.

Pathologic Changes. Deposits of debris called *drusen* accumulate between the epithelial cell and the underlying basement membrane (Bruch's membrane). Although not the cause of visual loss, drusen serve as an important clinical marker of the processes that lead to it.

Hard or nodular drusen are pinhead-sized yellow-white lesions visible ophthalmoscopically in the macular region. They represent focal degenerative change. *Soft or granular drusen* are larger, have less distinct edges, and represent more widespread epithelial dysfunction. The development of *diffuse or confluent drusen* coincides with still more advanced degenerative disease and heralds detachment of the pigmented epithelium from Bruch's membrane.

Detachment of the retinal epithelium is a consequence of the degenerative process that both weakens and thickens Bruch's membrane. Detachment leads to visual loss as the overlying photoreceptor cells atrophy. In addition, new blood vessels may form (*neovascularization*) in response to the degenerative changes in Bruch's membrane. The fragile new vessels tend to leak and sometimes bleed, producing serous or hemorrhagic detachment of the pigmented epithelium from the neurosensory retina and detachment of the pigmented epithelium. If there is bleeding, fibrovascular scarring may ensue. Such complications of neovascularization exacerbate the extent and speed of visual loss. Fortunately, fewer than 20% of persons with age-related macular degeneration have neovascularization.

Clinical Presentation and Course. Because the degenerative process is concentrated in the macula, central visual acuity is most affected. Patients may complain of a loss of visual acuity that is not corrected by eyeglasses. In patients without neovascularization, the loss of visual acuity tends to be gradual and limited. Macular examination of such persons may reveal all forms of drusen, but there is no neovascularization or evidence of its consequences. The presentation without neovascularization is sometimes referred to as "*dry*" or *neovascularization* macular degeneration. It accounts for about 90% of all cases.

Those with *neovascularization* are labeled as having "*wet*" or *exudative* disease. Close to 90% of persons who lose central vision have the exudative type. With neovascularization present, vision loss may be acute and more extensive. *Distorted vision* (metamorphopsia) may herald the onset of serous retinal detachment. In addition to drusen, macular examination may show serous and hemorrhagic effusions and disk-shaped scarring.

DIAGNOSIS

Suggestive historical features include gradual or sudden loss of central visual acuity or distorted vision (metamorphopsia) in an elderly person. The latter suggests the degenerative process has progressed sufficiently to cause serous retinal detachment due to neovascularization. Characteristic ophthalmoscopic findings are concentrated in the macular region and include drusen, irregularities in macular pigmentation, hemorrhage, and discoid scarring.

Finding defects in central visual acuity further supports the diagnosis of macular degeneration. Such changes can be detected with the aid of an *Amsler grid*, a 10 × 10-cm card with a black background on which is printed a criss-crossed grid of vertical and horizontal white lines every 5 mm. In the center, there is a white dot. The patient is asked to focus on the dot and note if any of the lines appear wavy or distorted or if any of the boxes formed by the intersecting lines are missing. Each eye is tested separately with any prescribed corrective lenses worn and the grid held at a comfortable reading distance.

PRINCIPLES OF MANAGEMENT

Prevention. *Cessation of smoking* is essential. Smoking is the only known modifiable risk factor. Ongoing smoking is particularly harmful. Its identification as an independent risk factor with a dose-dependent effect makes smoking cessation a top priority (see Chapter 54). Despite occasional hints from uncontrolled studies that high doses of *zinc* or *antioxidant vitamins* (e.g., C, E, and beta-carotene) may be preventive, there are no data from ongoing prospective randomized trials that confirm these hypotheses. Although many patients with macular degeneration often take high doses of these substances on their own, there is no evidence to warrant encouraging the practice. Besides smoking cessation, there are no other known medical interventions for preventing degeneration of the pigmented retinal epithelium. However, the approach to preventing loss of visual acuity depends on whether the macular degeneration is accompanied by neovascularization.

Exudative Disease: Neovascularization Present. For the 10% of macular degeneration patients with neovascularization, the prognosis for preservation of central vision is poor but can be improved at least modestly with argon laser *photocoagulation* therapy. Candidates for laser photocoagulation therapy are those with neovascularization not unexceptably close to the fovea. Laser treatment of neovascularization close to the fovea risks destroying its intense concentration of photoreceptor cells. Other approaches, such as *surgical removal* of subretinal hemorrhage or choroidal neovascular membranes, have not been confirmed in prospective randomized trials.

To maximize benefit from laser therapy, early clinical detection of neovascularization is critical. Macular degeneration patients are instructed to watch for and promptly report any distortion of vision. Daily home use of an *Amsler grid* is an excellent and simple means of early detection. Any new defects or distortions in central vision require prompt reporting to the ophthalmologist and consideration of urgent laser treatment. Such treatment can reduce the frequency of vision loss from 60% to 25% in patients with exudative disease.

Nonexudative Disease: No Neovascularization. Although their prognosis is much better than for those with untreated exudative disease, patients without neovascularization have no definitive treatment options at the present time. For the 10% of macular degeneration patients who suffer central vision loss due to neovascularization disease, optical devices known as *low-vision aids* can be used.

PATIENT EDUCATION

No matter how severe the macular degeneration, patients can be reassured that they will not go blind because peripheral vision is largely unaffected. Such information is reassuring and greatly appreciated. The importance of early detection of neovascularization needs to be emphasized, as well as the clinical warning symptoms (e.g., distorted vision). Proper use of the *Amsler grid* should be taught so that daily self-monitoring can be performed at home. Most importantly, patient education regarding the role of *smoking* and approaches to cessation (see Chapter 54) should be a top priority for those with macular degeneration who continue to smoke.

INDICATIONS FOR REFERRAL

Any elderly patient suspected on the basis of history or physical examination to have macular degeneration should be referred to the ophthalmologist. Promptness is critical if there is distorted vision, because it may herald early serous retinal detachment and neovascularization.

A.H.G.

ANNOTATED BIBLIOGRAPHY

Christen WG, Glynn RJ, Manson JE, et al. A prospective study of cigarette smoking and risk of age-related macular degeneration in men. JAMA 1996;276:1147. *(Data from the Physicians' Health Study showing a significant increase in risk with smoking.)*

Macular Photocoagulation Study Group. Argon laser photocoagulation for senile macular degeneration: results of a randomized clinical trial. Arch Ophthalmol 1982;100:912. *(Initial report from the above group; laser therapy reduced frequency of vision loss in persons with exudative disease from 60% to 25%.)*

Macular Photocoagulation Study Group. Laser photocoagulation of subfoveal neovascular lesions of age-related macular degeneration: updated findings from two clinical trials. Arch Ophthalmol 1993;111:1200. *(Long-term results from a major randomized prospective study: laser treatment delays onset of severe vision loss in only a small percentage of eyes with exudative disease.)*

Mares-Perlman JA, Klein R, Klein BEK, et al. Association of dietary intake of zinc and antioxidant nutrients with age-related macular degeneration. Arch Ophthalmol 1996;114:991. *(A look at the epidemiologic data addressing the question; they are not consistent.)*

Newsome DA, Swartz M, Theone NC, et al. Oral zinc in macular degeneration. Arch Ophthalmol 1988;106:192. *(The small initial trial suggesting a benefit; yet to be confirmed.)*

Seddon JM, Willet WC, Speizer FE, et al. A prospective study of cigarette smoking and age-related macular degeneration in women. JAMA 1996;276:1141. *(Prospective epidemiologic data from the Nurses' Health Study finding smoking to be a strong independent risk factor.)*

Watzke RC, et al. The macular symposium: aging macular degeneration. Ophthalmology 1985;92:593. *(Detailed review.)*

207
Management of Glaucoma
CLAUDIA U. RICHTER

Glaucoma is an optic neuropathy characterized by optic nerve cupping and visual field loss. It is the leading cause of permanent blindness. The types of glaucoma include *open-angle glaucoma* (both primary and secondary types), *angle-closure glaucoma*, and *congenital glaucoma*. Although the primary physician is not responsible for the definitive diagnosis or treatment of glaucoma, one needs to identify patients at risk (see Chapter 198), recognize early stages of optic nerve damage, and understand both the systemic effects of glaucoma medications and the effects of systemic medications on intraocular pressure.

PATHOPHYSIOLOGY AND CLINICAL PRESENTATION

The intraocular pressure is maintained by the dynamic equilibrium of aqueous production and outflow. The iris divides the anterior portion of the eye into anterior and posterior chambers that communicate through the pupil. Aqueous humor, produced by the ciliary body, fills the posterior chamber, flows through the pupil into the anterior chamber, and leaves the eye through the *trabecular meshwork*, a connective tissue filter at the angle between iris and cornea. The aqueous passes through the trabecular meshwork into Schlemm's canal and into the episcleral venous system.

Pathophysiology. Although *elevated intraocular pressure* is not part of the definition of glaucoma, intraocular pressure is the only modifiable risk factor. Increased intraocular pressure is caused by *obstruction to outflow*. In open-angle glaucoma, obstruction exists at a microscopic level in the trabecular meshwork. In angle-closure glaucoma, the iris obstructs the trabecular meshwork. An anatomic variation of the anterior segment of the eye results in pupillary block and obstruction of the trabecular meshwork by the iris.

Increased intraocular pressure increases vascular resistance, causing decreased vascular perfusion of the optic nerve and ischemia. The increased pressure can interfere with axoplasmic flow in the ganglion cell axons, causing cell dysfunction and death, and it can compress the lamina cribrosa, the sievelike structure through which axons pass when leaving the eye. The altered supporting structure may then interfere with axonal function. These different mechanisms of axonal damage are of variable importance in different patients, but the final result is loss of ganglion cells and their axons, increased optic nerve cupping, and visual field loss.

Clinical Presentation. *Open-angle glaucoma*, which accounts for more than 90% of glaucoma cases, has multiple risk factors, including elevated ocular pressure, older age (more than 50 years), African-American race, and family history of glaucoma. Characteristic changes in the optic nerve and nerve fiber layer (see below) suggest early glaucomatous injury and facilitate diagnosis as does asymptomatic elevated intraocular pressure. Open-angle glaucoma is frequently called the "silent blinder" because extensive damage may occur before the patient is aware of visual field loss.

Acute angle-closure glaucoma presents with a *painful red eye*. The physical findings include decreased visual acuity, markedly elevated intraocular pressure, redness, fixed and nonreactive pupil in mid-dilation, and corneal haziness. Occasionally, the principal symptoms are nausea and vomiting, and the patient may be thought to have abdominal or coronary disease. Patients with acute angle-closure glaucoma require emergency treatment to lower intraocular pressure, and immediate referral to an ophthalmologist. *Subacute* attacks of angle-closure glaucoma may present with intermittent episodes of *halos* around lights or of *painful blurred vision*. Patients susceptible to angle-closure can be identified by shining a light parallel to the iris plane from the temporal side of the globe: eyes with narrow angles will have a shadow fall on the nasal iris.

DIAGNOSIS

Ophthalmoscopy. *Cupping* of the optic nerve is the pathognomonic finding of glaucoma. Changes in the contour of the optic cup in the center of the optic disc provide the first definitive evidence of glaucomatous damage. The usual cup has a round regular contour. The cup in early glaucoma becomes notched on the superotemporal or inferotemporal rim. Later changes include an increase in the depth and width of the physiologic cup, nasal displacement of the central retinal vessels, and progressive pallor of the optic nerve head. Other disc changes associated with glaucoma are asymmetric discs and disc hemorrhages. There is some disagreement about the value of ophthalmoscopy in detecting early glaucoma. Assessment of disc pathology is not as simple as measurement of intraocular pressure. It requires greater skill, but it improves sensitivity to as much as 85%, which is especially helpful in detection of early disease. Performing pupillary dilation greatly facilitates the evaluation. Such specificity is unattainable by other screening methods before the onset of manifest visual field defects.

Measurement of Intraocular Pressure. Because *ocular hypertension* precedes optic nerve injury and is easier to perform than ophthalmoscopy, the measurement of intraocular pressure is the screening test of choice (see Chapter 198). Presence of elevated intraocular pressure (more than 21 mm Hg) in the absence of cupping indicates ocular hypertension but not glaucoma.

Visual Field Testing. When cupping is noted, formal visual field testing is indicated to check for the characteristic peripheral field deficits.

PRINCIPLES OF THERAPY

Although there is no direct treatment for the optic nerve injury of glaucoma, it is possible to prevent further optic nerve damage and visual field loss by lowering intraocular pressure. Intraocular pressure is the only modifiable risk factor in glaucoma, and several prospective long-term randomized placebo-controlled trials have demonstrated that lowering intraocular pressure protects the optic nerve.

Chronic Open-angle Glaucoma

Treatment to achieve and maintain the target pressure involves in escalating order: topical medications, laser trabeculoplasty, and glaucoma surgery. Most patients are first treated topically with a beta-blocker, α agonist, topical carbonic anhydrase inhibitor, and/or prostaglandin analogue singly or in combination to reach the target pressure. Intraocular pressure, optic nerve appearance, visual field, and nerve fiber layer are monitored to watch for disease progression.

Topical β-Adrenergic Antagonists decrease aqueous humor production. Ophthalmic preparations include *carteolol, levobunolol, metipranolol, timolol,* and *betaxolol* (β_1-selective). Beta-blockers need to be administered once or twice daily and are well tolerated topically. However, they can have significant systemic side effects including lethargy, depression, bronchospasm, bradycardia, hypotension, worsening of congestive heart failure, heart block, and syncope. Betaxolol, the β_1-selective blocker, is less likely to trigger bronchospasm but is also slightly less efficacious in controlling glaucoma.

α2-Selective Adrenergic Agonists represent new alternatives to beta-blockers and include *apraclonidine* and *brimonidine.* The α2-selective medications decrease intraocular pressure by reducing aqueous humor production. Topical side effects of these medications include topical hyperemia and allergic conjunctivitis. Systemic side effects of α2-selective agonists include lethargy, fatigue, drowsiness, dry mouth, and decreased blood pressure.

Nonselective Adrenergic Agonists, Epinephrine and its prodrug *dipivefrin,* initially reduce aqueous humor production and later increase aqueous humor outflow. Systemic side effects of epinephrine include headaches, hypertension, and tachycardia.

Carbonic Anhydrase Inhibitors decrease intraocular pressure by reducing aqueous humor production. Carbonic anhydrase inhibitors are now available topically (*brinzolamide, dorzolamide*) and orally (*acetazolamide, dichlorphenamide,* and *methazolamide*). The topical carbonic anhydrase inhibitors have largely displaced the oral medications and are better tolerated. The oral carbonic anhydrase inhibitors are associated with significant systemic side effects including anorexia and weight loss, fatigue, malaise, paresthesias of fingers and toes, depression, diarrhea, metallic taste, nephrolithiasis, agranulocytosis, and aplastic anemia. The blood dyscrasias are not dose dependent and may also occur with the topical drugs. Some patients report the drops cause a bitter taste in their mouths.

Prostaglandin Analogues lower intraocular pressure by increasing uveoscleral outflow. They represent a new class of drugs for treatment of glaucoma and rival beta-blockers in efficacy. *Latanoprost* is the first available prostaglandin analogue for use in glaucoma. The drug is administered topically once daily. It appears well tolerated but may cause darkening of the iris. Systemic side effects (e.g., muscle and joint pains and allergic reactions of the skin) are uncommon.

Cholinergic Agonists reduce intraocular pressure by increasing aqueous outflow through the trabecular meshwork. Both *direct-acting* agonists (*carbachol* and *pilocarpine*) and *cholinesterase inhibitors* (*demecarium, echothiophate,* and *physostigmine*) are available. The ocular effects include small pupils with dimming of vision, induced myopia with blurring of vision, cataract, and retinal detachment. Systemic side effects include headache, tremor, salivation, bronchospasm, pulmonary edema, hypertension, hypotension, bradycardia, diarrhea, nausea and vomiting, and, with cholinesterase inhibitors, prolonged respiratory paralysis when given with succinylcholine.

Laser and Surgical Therapies. Laser trabeculoplasty effectively lowers intraocular pressure in many patients and is usually performed on patients whose glaucoma is uncontrolled by topical medication, although some ophthalmologists may perform it as initial therapy. Trabeculoplasty's effectiveness appears to be due to an alteration of the biology of the trabecular meshwork and improved aqueous outflow. Approximately 75% of laser-treated patients have a sufficient decrease in intraocular pressure to avoid glaucoma surgery, at least in the short term; pressure remains under control after 4 years in 50%.

Surgery is indicated when medical therapy and laser trabeculoplasty do not lower the intraocular pressure to a level protective of the optic nerve and visual field. The usual procedure is a *trabeculectomy,* which forms a drainage route from the anterior chamber to the subconjunctival space. If filtering surgery fails or cannot be performed, an aqueous tube shunt implant may be placed or laser cycloablation to the ciliary body performed.

Acute Angle-closure Glaucoma

Proper management requires prompt recognition, immediate treatment to lower intraocular pressure, and urgent referral to an ophthalmologist. Topical antiglaucomatous medications such as a beta-blocker, α agonist, and/or carbonic anhydrase inhibitor are administered. *Topical pilocarpine* 2% is administered to facilitate breaking the pupillary block. Acetazolamide may be administered orally or intravenously. Laser or surgical iridectomy is performed to prevent recurrent attacks and is indicated prophylactically in the other eye.

Prevention

Several drugs commonly used in internal medicine may increase the risk of developing glaucoma or precipitate an attack. Long-term high-dose use of nasal or inhaled *glucocorticosteroids* is associated with an increased risk of glaucoma, especially in the elderly. Such therapy should be administered only in conjunction with a plan for glaucoma screening. Drugs with *anticholinergic effects* (e.g., tricyclic antidepressants) may precipitate angle-closure glaucoma in patients with narrow angles and should be used with care. Persons with *systemic hypertension* and coincident ocular hypertension should have their systemic pressure reduced gradually. Reports exist of hypotensive optic neuropathy after precipitous lowering of systemic blood pressure. Treatment should be carried out in conjunction with the guidance of an ophthalmologist.

PATIENT EDUCATION

The first priority is to teach the patient the importance of careful follow-up examinations and compliance with the treatment regimen to preservation of vision. Reviewing technique for proper use of topical medications helps to maximize delivery of effective doses and minimize systemic absorption. Topical drug solutions are concentrated to facilitate absorption. If excess drug runs into the lacrimal duct and down into the nose, then systemic absorption through the nasal mucosa will occur. To avoid this, the patient should be taught to occlude the lacrimal duct either by direct pressure when applying drops or by closing the eyelids for 5 minutes after applying the drops. Patients should be advised about the ocular side effects of systemic drugs and the systemic effects of their glaucoma treatments.

RECOMMENDATIONS

- Have all persons over the age of 40 years screened for increased intraocular pressure (see Chapter 198).
- Take note of any cupping of the optic nerve during routine ophthalmoscopy.
- Refer promptly for treatment any persons with ocular hypertension or suspected optic nerve cupping.
- Refer urgently any person with suspected acute angle-closure glaucoma (e.g., painful red eye, decreased visual acuity, markedly elevated intraocular pressure, redness, fixed and nonreactive pupil in mid-dilation, and corneal haziness).
- Treatment begins with a topical beta-blocker, α agonist, topical carbonic anhydrase inhibitor, and/or prostaglandin analogue singly or in combination to reach the target pressure. If medical therapy proves inadequate or intolerable, laser trabeculoplasty or surgery may be indicated.
- Patients taking drops require instruction in occlusion of nasal lacrimal ducts to minimize risk of systemic absorption through the nasal mucosa.
- Have intraocular pressure, optic nerve appearance, visual field, and nerve fiber layer monitored by an ophthalmologist to watch for disease progression.
- Know the patient's ocular medications and their systemic side effects.
- Monitor intraocular pressure carefully in persons (especially the elderly) taking high-dose nasal or inhaled steroids.

ANNOTATED BIBLIOGRAPHY

Alward WLM. Medical management of glaucoma. N Engl J Med 1998;339:1298. *(Detailed review of diagnosis and medical therapy of glaucoma; 118 references.)*

Garbe E, LeLorier J, Boivin J-F, et al. Inhaled and nasal glucocorticoids and the risks of ocular hypertension or open-angle glaucoma. JAMA 1997;277:722. *(A case-control study finding that prolonged [more than 3 months] daily uses of high doses was associated with an odds ratio of 1.44 for risk of ocular hypertension or open-angle glaucoma.)*

Margolis KL, Money BE, Kopietz LA, et al. Physician recognition of ophthalmoscopic signs of open-angle glaucoma. J Gen Intern Med 1989;4:296. *(An educational program that includes good photographs of the key findings.)*

Shingleton BJ, Richter CU, Bellows AR, et al. Long-term efficacy of argon laser trabeculoplasty. Ophthalmology 1987;94:1513. *(Laser therapy effective in 50% of patients treated after 4 years.)*

Stewart WC, Garrison PM. Beta-blocker-induced complications and the patient with glaucoma: newer treatments to help reduced systemic adverse effects. Arch Intern Med 1998;158:221. *(Good review of adverse effects and new topical alternatives, such as prostaglandin analogues, α2-blockers, and topical carbonic anhydrase inhibitors.)*

Watson P, Stjernschantz J, Latanoprost Study Group. A six-month, randomized, double-masked study comparing latanoprost and timolol in patients with open-angle glaucoma and ocular hypertension. Ophthalmology 1996;103:126. *(Well-designed prospective controlled trial establishing effectiveness and safety of this prostaglandin analogue in lowering intraocular pressure.)*

208
Management of Cataracts
ROGER F. STEINERT

Cataracts are opacifications of the crystalline lens of the eye. They are unusual in young patients, but the incidence rises sharply in later years, such that virtually all elderly patients have some degree of cataract. Because of the implications of this diagnosis, the term *cataract* is best reserved for opacities resulting in functional impairment. The primary care physician should be able to detect cataract formation, monitor its progression, advise the patient on when to seek ophthalmologic consultation, help the ophthalmologist assess medical candidacy for surgery, and support the patient in the perioperative and rehabilitation phases.

PATHOPHYSIOLOGY AND CLINICAL PRESENTATION

Most cataracts occur in the elderly and reflect *senescent change*; occasionally, they ensue from systemic disease and are also frequently associated with intraocular inflammation and glaucoma. *Cigarette smoking* and *glucocorticosteroid use* have been linked epidemiologically to cataract formation. Presenile and senile cataract formation are painless and generally progress over months or years. Those found during the early years of life are either congenital or the consequence of *diabetes, Wilson's disease, Down syndrome*, and other metabolic diseases. *Trauma* is an important precipitant.

Senile Cataract. In the age-related *nuclear cataract*, the lens opacity results from protein denaturation and hydration. Sodium and calcium concentrations increase, potassium and ascorbate levels diminish, and glutathione disappears. The underlying metabolic changes leading to senile cataract are unknown. In diabetes mellitus, excess sugar is diverted to the sorbitol pathway. An insoluble alcohol accumulates, and this osmotic load causes the protein to hydrate.

As the human lens ages, the nucleus hardens (*nuclear sclerosis*). The first visual event may be a shift toward nearsightedness because of the increased refractive index and thickness of the sclerotic nucleus. As a result, the patient may temporarily experience enhanced reading vision without glasses ("*second sight*"), and a change in spectacles may be the only treatment needed. Eventually, the nucleus acquires a yellow-brown coloration ("brunescent cataract") and becomes progressively more opaque. Only a few patients are aware of the gradual spectral change, with a yellow cast to the visual world; they usually acknowledge it only after the cataract is removed. Visual impairment initially is more marked at distance than near, and a patient may fail a driver's license examination and still be able to read a newspaper. Loss of contrast sensitivity may cause a functional impairment out of proportion to the results of a standard high-contrast visual acuity test.

Presenile Cataract. Posterior *subcapsular cataracts* form at the back of the lens, usually centrally. This type of cataract is often responsible for the "presenile" cataract in the 40- to 50-year-old age group. It may be spontaneous but is often associated with prolonged use of topical, inhaled, or systemic *steroids* and with *diabetes mellitus*. The central location of the opacity causes the vision to worsen when the pupil becomes small, as in reading or on bright days. The refractile nature of the opacity commonly causes severe difficulty with glare, such as driving at night. Pupillary dilatation by mydriatic or cycloplegic drops or use of subdued light improves vision in such cases, as more light is allowed to enter the eye.

Traumatic Cataract. These most commonly result from intraocular foreign bodies that perforate the lens capsule, allowing the lens protein to hydrate and thereby denature and opacify. Occasionally, a lens will opacify after severe blunt nonpenetrating trauma. Electric shock and high-dose ionizing radiation may lead to lens opacification. Prolonged exposure to *ultraviolet B*, as occurs with unprotected *sun exposure*, is an important risk factor for cortical cataract formation; risk of nuclear cataract is not significantly increased.

WORKUP

Initial evaluation by the primary physician includes *visual acuity* determination both near and at distance. The lenticular opacity can be appreciated with the *direct ophthalmoscope* while attempting to visualize the fundus. If the angle is not shallow, dilation with one drop of 2.5% phenylephrine or 1% tropicamide is helpful. With the ophthalmoscope lens set at zero and standing about 12 inches from the patient, a bright red reflex is seen in the normal eye. Cataract formation is clearly seen by the *disruption of the red reflex*. Plus power (black numbers) in the ophthalmoscope of about 15 or 20 diopters will put the lens of the eye in focus as the physician approaches the eye. The fundus should be examined for retinal abnormalities, particularly macular degeneration (manifested by hemorrhage, scarring, and drusen), which can cause loss of vision symptomatically similar to that from cataract. In all cases of visual impairment, an ophthalmic consultation is indicated.

PRINCIPLES OF MANAGEMENT

Conservative Measures and Indications for Surgery. The only definitive treatment for cataract is surgery, and in some instances (e.g., traumatic cataracts and very advanced senile cataracts that cause inflammation and glaucoma), emergency surgery is mandatory. However, most cataract surgery is elec-

tive and reserved for unacceptable visual impairment not improved by conservative measures. In early nuclear sclerosis, an *eyeglasses prescription* may sufficiently improve vision to defer surgery. Sometimes chronic *pupillary dilation* will suffice for a patient with posterior subcapsular cataract. When such measures no longer suffice and the patient believes visual dysfunction is impairing the quality of life, then cataract surgery can be discussed as a treatment option.

Patient Selection for Surgery. In addition to marked visual impairment, other considerations help in patient selection for surgery and approach to anesthesia. Cataract surgery is often performed under local anesthesia (block or topical) with mild sedation; however, because any patient movement during surgery may be disastrous, general anesthesia may be necessary. The primary physician can assist the ophthalmologist in assessing whether age, mental status, or medical condition make general anesthesia appropriate.

Surgical Approaches. There are several options for cataract surgery. The most common is *phacoemulsification*, which uses ultrasonic energy to break up the hard nucleus and aspirate it through a small opening (about 3 mm). The small phacoemulsification wound can be constructed as a self-sealing valve, often not requiring sutures, which allows the patient rapid return to full physical activity. Although most cataract extractions in the United States use the standard phacoemulsification technique, specific circumstances may cause the surgeon to use *extracapsular extraction*, in which the lens capsule is opened and the nucleus is removed in one piece through a large wound (about 10 mm).

Postoperatively, the surgeon will prescribe topical medications. Final visual correction may be given as soon as 1 to 2 weeks postoperatively.

Visual Rehabilitation. Three methods of *visual rehabilitation* are available: eyeglasses, contact lenses, and lens implants.

Cataract spectacles used to be the only approach to correcting vision after surgery. They must be powerful to compensate for the absence of the crystalline lens. In addition to thickness and weight, these spectacles magnify vision by approximately 25%, which precludes use of a cataract lens for only one eye, because a double image would result. The spectacle thickness also severely limits side vision, producing a midperipheral blind spot. Such difficulties make adjustment to cataract glasses problematic at best, and some patients find ambulation nearly impossible with these spectacles. Cataract spectacles are now used only in highly unusual circumstances.

Contact lenses are optically superior to eyeglasses. Because the lens power is so much closer to the eye than with eyeglass lenses, magnification is only 5% to 7%, and most patients will not perceive diplopia with a contact lens, although stereoscopic acuity will be reduced. Peripheral vision will be normal. Many elderly patients have difficulty handling contact lenses, but extended wear lenses (usually soft) may facilitate use because they may be worn for weeks to months between removals for cleaning. Use of these lenses is not without difficulty, however. Lens deposits, damage, and loss may result in frequent visits to the ophthalmologist, with high cost and time lost. Devastating infectious corneal ulcers are much more common in elderly patients with extended-wear contact lenses.

Intraocular lens implantation is standard practice where not specifically contraindicated. At the time of cataract extraction (and occasionally as a secondary procedure in cases of spectacle and contact lens intolerance), the surgeon implants a delicate plastic device with optical power to replace the cataractous lens. The implant is permanent, requires no care, and restores normal optics without magnification. Although once controversial, with advances in manufacturing and surgical technique there is minimal extra risk to the implant. The implant is contraindicated in some conditions, such as chronic uveitis, which is assessed by the ophthalmologist preoperatively.

Intraocular lenses continue to improve. When the optical portion is made of a flexible material such as solid silicone elastomer, acrylic, or hydrogel, the lens can be folded during insertion so that only a small wound is needed. Multifocal lenses are now available; they may allow patients nearly total freedom from bifocals and reading glasses.

Prevention of cataract formation is important and often overlooked. *Protective eyewear* are the best means of reducing risk of cortical cataract formation due to ultraviolet B radiation from the sun. Sunglasses need to be specially treated to fully prevent penetration of ultraviolet radiation, although wearing a hat with a brim and sunglasses with plastic untreated lenses does reduce exposure. However, the darkness of a lens's tint is not necessarily a measure of protective capacity. Dark unprotective sunglasses may actually exacerbate exposure by blocking visible light transmission, causing pupillary dilation, and thus increasing penetration of ultraviolet radiation. Outdoor workers are at particularly high risk and should wear close-fitting protective sunglasses.

Smoking cessation and *limitation of steroid use* to lowest dose and minimum strength necessary (particularly in the elderly) are other potentially important preventive measures. The use of nutritional supplements such as *antioxidants* has not yet been proven to slow the rate of cataract progression despite the theoretical potential benefit.

PATIENT EDUCATION AND INDICATIONS FOR REFERRAL

Preventive measures should be taught to all patients, with an emphasis on use of *protective eyewear* (especially for those with much sun exposure), *smoking cessation*, and *limitation* in dose and duration of *steroid use*.

For elderly patients with age-related nuclear cataracts, the primary physician should help explain the condition and outline treatment options. Patients appreciate knowing that cataract formation is not a "growth" and that it poses no harm to the eye. Patients also need to understand that although surgical correction is highly successful in up to 99% of patients, it is not risk free. Occasionally, complications do occur. When vision is good in one eye and there are no important functional limitations, a conservative approach may be preferable to surgery. The degree of interference with daily activities (e.g., driving, reading, watching television) should be reviewed to help in decision making.

Those with cataracts that significantly impair daily living (e.g., causing falls, prohibiting reading, or interfering with driving) should be referred for consideration of microsurgical cataract extraction with intraocular lens implantation, which has a high likelihood of dramatically improving quality of life.

ANNOTATED BIBLIOGRAPHY

Cataract in Adults: Management of Functional Impairment. U.S. Department of Health and Human Services, Agency for Health Care Policy and Research. Clinical Practice Guideline, Number 4. February 1993. *(A guideline for care based on comprehensive review of the available evidence.)*

Garbe E, Suissa S, LeLorier J. Association of inhaled corticosteroid use with cataract extraction in elderly patients. JAMA 1998;280:539. *(Case-control epidemiologic study finding a threefold increase in risk of cataract extraction with long-term high-dose inhaled steroid use.)*

Grisso JA, Kelsey JL, Strom BL, et al. Risk factors for falls as a cause of hip fracture in women. N Engl J Med 1991;324:1326. *(Impaired vision raises the risk of hip fracture fivefold.)*

Rosenthal FS, Fakalian AE, Taylor HR. The effect of prescription eyewear on ocular exposure to ultraviolet radiation. Am J Public Health 1986;76:1216. *(Means of cutting down on ultraviolet exposure.)*

Steinert RF, ed. Cataract: evaluation, surgery, and complications. Philadelphia: W.B. Saunders, 1995. *(Comprehensive reference text.)*

Taylor HR, West SK, Rosenthal FS, et al. Effect of ultraviolet radiation on cataract formation. N Engl J Med 1988;319:1429. *(Significant relationship found between ultraviolet B exposure and cortical cataract formation; argues for wearing protective eyewear in the sun.)*

209
Management of Diabetic Retinopathy
CLAUDIA U. RICHTER

Diabetic retinopathy is a leading cause of blindness in the United States in people under age 65 years. Its incidence has increased with improved long-term survival of diabetics. The prevalence increases with duration of disease and is greatest in older age groups. Effective treatment is available not only to prevent many of the most serious complications of retinopathy, but also to reduce the risk of developing retinopathy. Therapy is most effective when rendered promptly. It is of great importance for the primary physician to know when to check for retinopathy and when to refer to the ophthalmologist for more detailed evaluation and consideration of treatment. Diabetes can also cause other eye problems, including refractive changes, cataracts, glaucoma, and reversible cranial nerve palsies (see Chapters 102, 200, 207, and 208).

PATHOPHYSIOLOGY, CLINICAL PRESENTATION, AND COURSE

Two types of diabetic retinopathy can be recognized ophthalmoscopically: nonproliferative and proliferative.

Nonproliferative retinopathy is generally the early form and consists of intraretinal vascular damage. Loss of capillary pericytes, thickening of basement membranes, swelling and proliferation of endothelial cells, and intravascular thrombosis occur. This results in both dilation of small vessels and vascular closure, leading to ischemia. In addition, there is abnormal endothelial permeability with breakdown of the normal blood–retina barrier. Retinal capillaries become permeable to water, lipids, and large molecules, which are not adequately removed by the usual cellular pump mechanism of the adjacent retinal pigment epithelium.

Clinically, this process results in *microaneurysms, intraretinal hemorrhages, cotton-wool infarctions,* and lipid and serous exudation with *retinal edema.* Microaneurysms are dilated capillaries that sometimes thrombose. They appear as red dots in the retina, similar to the small blot intraretinal hemorrhages, which result from bleeding in the deep layers of the retina. Flame-shaped hemorrhages occur in the striated superficial ganglion cell layer. White-centered hemorrhages represent hemorrhagic infarcts. Cotton-wool infarcts, also known by the misnomer soft exudates, are nerve fiber layer infarctions. The swollen axons become ophthalmoscopically visible as white, feathery, soft lesions. Hard exudates are true exudations of the intravascular lipid into the retina, leading to yellow, glistening, spherical aggregates of lipid, sometimes arranged in a circular pattern or circinate ring around leaking blood vessels. Retinal edema is more difficult to see. Accumulation of serous fluid in the intercellular spaces of the retina results in retinal thickening.

Patients with nonproliferative retinopathy are asymptomatic unless retinal edema or ischemia involves the central macula. Macular edema causes blurring or distortion followed by loss of central vision. Macular edema is the leading cause of visual loss in diabetics, especially older type II patients. Hypertension and fluid retention tend to adversely affect vascular exudation and macular edema.

Proliferative retinopathy consists of vascular pathology that extends from the retina into the vitreous cavity. This form of retinopathy generally occurs at a later stage than nonproliferative retinopathy and tends to have a worse visual prognosis without prompt treatment. Advancing capillary and arteriolar closure with more widespread retinal ischemia herald the onset and are manifested by an increase in the number of cotton-wool spots, larger intraretinal hemorrhages, venous beading, and small networks of weblike intraretinal vessels. There is a correlation between duration and degree of hyperglycemia and progression of retinopathy. Tight control (hemoglobin A1c less than 7.0%) slows the onset and severity of retinopathy and other microvascular complications of diabetes (see Chapter 102).

The retina responds to advancing ischemia with *neovascularization,* the hallmark of proliferative retinopathy, by forming networks of new vessels that extend from existing retinal vessels anteriorly into the vitreous cavity. These vessels first appear as a fine network of small vessels proliferating from the optic disc, the major retinal vessels, or from areas adjacent to retinal ischemia. As neovascularization progresses, dense, white, fibrotic tissue forms and adheres to the posterior vitreous. Such fibrosis can cause the vitreous to contract and pull anteriorly, rupturing the fragile network of vessels growing into the vitreous and producing a vitreous hemorrhage that fills the eye and compromises vision. *Retinal detachment* can also occur, either from tractional forces on the retina or in combination with retinal holes forming. The iris may also be involved with neovascularization, leading to *glaucoma* from obstruction of the trabecular meshwork.

Proliferative retinopathy can present with small floating specks or cobwebs in the visual field, representing a small vitreous hemorrhage. Sudden profound loss of vision, sometimes associated with flashing lights, may signify retinal detachment or severe vitreous hemorrhage.

Clinical Course. The *clinical course* of diabetic retinopathy does not appear until 3 to 5 years after the onset of type I diabetes. Onset in type II diabetes is probably similar but more difficult to pinpoint because of difficulty establishing onset of the underlying disease. Type I diabetics tend to progress more rapidly to proliferative retinopathy, with an incidence of 50% after 15 years. Older type II diabetics have a higher incidence of macular edema–induced vision loss.

Pregnancy poses an additional vision risk for diabetics because retinal pathology can progress with unanticipated speed and may require laser treatment sooner than expected. Close monitoring by an ophthalmologist is necessary.

WORKUP

Screening Ophthalmoscopy. Screening asymptomatic diabetic patients for retinopathy is an essential part of effective diabetic care. Available screening methods for detecting diabetic retinopathy include *nondilated ophthalmoscopy, dilated ophthalmoscopy* performed by the ophthalmologist, and *stereoscopic fundus photography.* Stereophotography is the most sensitive and nondilated ophthalmoscopy the least. Dilated ophthalmoscopy has a sensitivity of about 80% and a specificity of 99% for detection of proliferative retinopathy. Pending less costly stereophotographic methods, dilated ophthalmoscopy by an ophthalmologist is required. Dilation allows examination of the more peripheral retina and stereoscopic biomicroscopy to evaluate macular edema. Examination of the nondilated eye with a hand-held ophthalmoscope is inadequate for screening, especially when performed by the nonophthalmologic physician.

The natural history of diabetic retinopathy dictates the proper *screening schedule.* Current screening guidelines for diabetic retinopathy jointly adopted by the American College of Physicians, the American Diabetes Association, and the American Academy of Ophthalmology include the following:

- *For type I diabetes,* screen annually beginning 5 years after the onset of diabetes, generally not before the onset of puberty.
- *For type II diabetes,* screen initially at the time of diagnosis and then annually. If the initial examination uses stereo fundus photography and is found to be normal, then the next examination need not occur for 4 years. After that, annual screening is required, regardless of method used.
- *For pregnant* diabetic women, have dilated ophthalmoscopy performed during the first trimester and close follow-up throughout pregnancy. When planning pregnancy, the dia-

betic woman should be counseled on the risk of developing or worsening retinopathy. No screening is needed for women with gestational diabetes.

Such screening does not obviate ophthalmoscopic examination by the primary physician, who might be able to detect an important lesion in the interval between screening examinations, but nondilated ophthalmoscopy by the primary physician is no substitute for a formal eye examination by the ophthalmologist.

PRINCIPLES OF MANAGEMENT

Prevention. Both primary and secondary prevention are achievable by tightly controlling serum glucose, as demonstrated in the two landmark multicenter, randomized, prospective controlled trials of diabetes management: the *Diabetes Control and Complications Trial* (DCCT) for type I disease and the *United Kingdom Prospective Diabetes Study* (UKPDS) for type II disease.

In the DCCT trial, type I patients treated with intensive insulin therapy to normalize the blood glucose experienced a reduction in the risk of developing retinopathy of 76%; in those with preexisting retinopathy, the risk of progression was reduced by 54%. Transient worsening of existing retinopathy occurs during the first year of intensive treatment in about one fourth of patients and consists of soft exudates and intraretinal microvascular changes. Such changes usually disappear by 18 months with continued intensive insulin therapy, and reduction in long-term risk of progression is the same as for patients without early progression. The DCCT study was confined to patients with type I diabetes who had either no retinopathy or mild retinopathy. Whether similar results can be achieved in patients with more severe retinopathy remains to be demonstrated. In *type II diabetes*, the UKPDS similarly revealed that tight control (hemoglobin A1c less than 7%) significantly reduced both the risk of developing retinopathy and its progression. Evolving strategies for normalization of hyperglycemia have made tight control safer and more achievable (see Chapter 102).

The risk of accelerated progression of retinopathy may be greater in patients with proliferative or severe nonproliferative retinal disease, making close ophthalmologic follow-up essential. Other measures that may be helpful in preventing progression of retinopathy include good *control of hypertension* and *cessation of smoking*. Neither the use of aspirin to reduce platelet aggregation nor the use of clofibrate to decrease lipid exudates has proven effective.

Treatment. Once retinopathy is detected, its treatment is the province of the retinal specialist. Laser photocoagulation reduces the rate of vision-threatening complications from both forms of retinopathy.

Nonproliferative Retinopathy. The treatment of choice for clinically significant macular edema is *focal laser* treatment of the macular region, which reduces the rate of severe vision loss by over 50%. Vision loss from macular ischemia is not treatable.

Proliferative Retinopathy. The primary therapeutic modality outside the macular area is *panretinal photocoagulation.* The stimulus to form new vessels is reduced, and risk of severe

vision loss is reduced by 50% to 65%. Potential complications include mild reduction in vision, decreased night vision, loss of peripheral vision, inadvertent burns to the central macula, and hemorrhage and exudative detachment of the retina or choroid, leading to angle-closure glaucoma.

When a vitreous hemorrhage will not spontaneously clear or when dense fibrovascular proliferation affects the macula and causes severe vision loss, *surgery* is necessary. Vitrectomy may also allow more aggressive laser photocoagulation (either intraoperatively or postoperatively) of proliferative retinopathy.

Other Hyperglycemia-related Complications. A myopic shift in refractive error can occur due to hyperglycemia-induced osmotic swelling of the lens. Reestablishment of glycemic control can reverse this refractive shift. Diplopia due to localized demyelination of the third, fourth, or sixth cranial nerve usually recovers within 1 to 3 months. Cataracts may also form (see Chapter 208).

PATIENT EDUCATION AND INDICATIONS FOR REFERRAL

Patient education by the primary physician is essential to prevention, early detection, and prompt treatment of retinopathy. Reviewing the benefits of tight glycemic control can be a potent motivating force that improves patient behavior. The importance of smoking cessation, hypertension control, regular ophthalmologic examinations, and immediate reporting of eye symptoms needs to be stressed in conjunction with the good news that effective treatment to prevent vision loss is available.

Ophthalmologic referral is indicated for screening (see above) and is urgent when there is

- Change in vision, new appearance of floaters, or complaint of eye pain;
- Discovery of retinopathy (particularly if abnormal vessels are seen suggestive of neovascularization due to proliferative retinopathy, if there are symptoms or signs of macular edema, or signs of moderate to severe nonproliferative retinopathy);
- Loss of ability to visualize the fundus.

Treatment decisions regarding diabetic retinopathy should be made by the ophthalmologist skilled in management of retinal disease.

ANNOTATED BIBLIOGRAPHY

American College of Physicians, American Diabetes Association, and American Academy of Ophthalmology. Screening guidelines for diabetic retinopathy. Ann Intern Med 1992;116:683. *(Consensus recommendations for screening.)*

Chew EY, Mills JL, Metzger BE, et al. Metabolic control and progression of retinopathy. The Diabetes in Early Pregnancy Study. Diabetes Care 1995;18:631. *(Glycemic control reduces risk of progression.)*

The Diabetes Control and Complications Trial Research Group. The effect of intensive treatment of diabetes on the development and progression of long-term complications in insulin-dependent diabetes mellitus. N Engl J Med 1993;329:977. *(Tight glycemic control reduced risks for development and progression of retinopathy in type I diabetics.)*

The Diabetes Control and Complications Trial Research Group. The relationship of glycemic exposure (HbA_{1C}) to the risk of development and progression of retinopathy in the Diabetes Control and Complications Trial. Diabetes 1995;44:968. *(Mean HbA1c was the dominant predictor of retinopathy progression.)*

The Diabetes Control and Complications Trial Research Group. The effect of intensive diabetes treatment on the progression of diabetic retinopathy in insulin-dependent diabetes mellitus. Arch Ophthalmol 1995;113:36. *(Randomized trial demonstrated retinopathy progression in 54.1% with conventional treatment, 11.5% with intensive treatment.)*

The Diabetic Retinopathy Study Research Group. Photocoagulation treatment of proliferative diabetic retinopathy. Ophthalmology 1978;85:82. *(Classic paper; established the role of photocoagulation in treatment of proliferative diabetic retinopathy.)*

The Diabetic Retinopathy Vitrectomy Study Research Group. Early vitrectomy for severe vitreous hemorrhage in diabetic retinopathy. Arch Ophthalmol 1985;103:1644. *(Early vitrectomy improved outcome in type I diabetics.)*

The Early Treatment Diabetic Retinopathy Study Research Group. Photocoagulation for diabetic macular edema. Arch Ophthalmol 1985;103:1796. *(Focal photocoagulation of macular edema reduced the risk of visual loss.)*

Ferris FL III, Davis MD, Aiello LM. Treatment of diabetic retinopathy. N Engl J Med 1999;341:667. *(Excellent review for general reader with good photographs of eye changes and an comprehensive list of references.)*

Paetkau MD, Boyd TAS, Winship B, et al. Cigarette smoking and diabetic retinopathy. Diabetes 1977;26:46. *(Risk of proliferative retinopathy rose with increasing tobacco consumption.)*

UK Prospective Diabetes Study (UKPDS) Group. Intensive blood-glucose control with sulphonylureas or insulin compared with conventional treatment and risk of complications in patients with type 2 diabetes (UKPDS 33). Lancet 1998;352:837. *(Landmark 20-year, prospective, randomized, controlled trial of diet, sulfonylurea, insulin, and later metformin in patients with type II disease confirming that, like type I disease, risk of microvascular complications reduced by tight control; identifies HgbA1c less than 7.0% as the level necessary to minimize microvascular risk.)*

210

Correction of Vision

Part 1: Contact Lenses

ELIZABETH S. GOULD

Over 24 million Americans wear contact lenses. With proper prescription and safe use, they provide excellent correction of vision and convenience. Primary physicians are sometimes asked about the relative merits of various types of contact lenses and may be the first physician consulted when a problem with their use develops. Knowing the basics about contact lens use and the complications that may ensue can facilitate optimal eye care.

Types of Contact Lenses, Advantages, and Disadvantages

Hard and Rigid Contact Lenses. *Hard contact lenses* were the first to be developed and were fabricated from polymethyl methacrylate. The very low oxygen permeability of such lenses limited their use to daytime wear and frequently caused corneal edema. *Rigid gas-permeable lenses*, allowing greater oxygen permeability, have replaced the original hard design and provide improved comfort and longer wearing times. Rigid lenses require longer initial adaptation and may dislodge more frequently than soft contact lenses. However, rigid gas-permeable lenses provide excellent vision, especially with astigmatic patients. They are relatively easy to clean and can last for several years if cared for properly. Long-term tolerance is good, and the risk of corneal ulcerations, corneal neovascularization, and infection is low. Rigid gas-permeable lenses require advance skill and knowledge by the practitioner in fitting and designing the lenses, much more so than soft lenses.

Soft lenses were developed in the early 1960s and represent most current contact lens fittings. The primary clinical advantage of soft contact lenses is the good initial comfort and tolerance. They can be worn for longer periods, do not dislodge eas-ily, and allow the patient to switch easily between contacts and glasses, because there is less molding effect on the cornea. The disadvantages include less effective astigmatic correction of vision compared with rigid lenses, need for more frequent thorough cleaning and disinfection, and more frequent replacement. In addition, there is increased risk of ulcerative keratitis, neovascularization, and contact lens intolerance.

Disposable soft lenses represent an attempt to further enhance convenience and long-term comfort. Disposable lenses are available as single use, weekly, bimonthly, monthly, and quarterly. *Daily wear* soft contact lenses are removed for sleep and are cleaned and disinfected before insertion the following day. Daily contact lens wear does not significantly alter the mucosal defenses of the outer eye that function to prevent infection. *Extended wear* soft lenses were developed with the goal of allowing the patient to sleep with their lenses for one or more nights.

The first extended wear lenses were approved by the U.S. Food and Drug Administration (FDA) in 1979. In the mid-1980s, at the peak of popularity of extended wear lenses, it was estimated that 30% of new patient lens fittings were for extended wear. Although most patients did well, practitioners became concerned with changes in ocular tissues, including corneal microcysts, stromal edema, endothelial polymegathism, infiltrates, neovascularization, and increased risk for ulcerative keratitis.

Risk of Ulcerative Keratitis

Ulcerative keratitis (epithelial defect over a stromal infiltrate) is an infrequent but serious complication of contact lens wear. It can occur with soft or rigid gas-permeable lenses worn on a daily or extended-wear basis. The relative risk is 10 to 15 times greater with extended-wear use of lenses. *Pseudomonas aeruginosa*, a common sight-threatening pathogen, can quickly invade the injured cornea, resulting in permanent vision loss by destroying the corneal stroma. Prompt ophthalmologic referral is indicated. Response to antibiotics is usually good. The best treatment is prevention. The FDA has restricted approved use of extended-wear lenses to no more than 7 continuous days. Practitioners and patients need to be informed about the increased relative risk of overnight lens use. It is estimated that 49% to 74% of cases of contact lens–associated ulcerative keratitis could be prevented by eliminating overnight wear.

ANNOTATED BIBLIOGRAPHY

Bennett ES, Weismann BA. Clinical contact lens practice. Philadelphia: J.B. Lippincott, 1991;33:1 *(The authoritative reference.)*

McLellan KA, Cripps AW, Clancy RL, et al. The effect of successful contact lens wear on mucosal immunity of the eye. Ophthalmology 1998;105:1471. *(Daily contact lens wear does not significantly alter the mucosal defenses of the outer eye that prevent infection.)*

Soft contact lenses. Medical Letter Drugs Ther 1990;32:69-70. *(Terse summary for the generalist.)*

Schein OD, Beuhler PO, Stamler VF, et al. The impact of overnight wear on the risk of contact lens-associated ulcerative keratitis. Arch Ophthalmol 1994;112:186. *(Most cases of contact lens–associated ulcerative keratitis could be prevented by eliminating overnight wear.)*

Schein OD, Glynn RJ, Poggio EC, et al. The relative risk of ulcerative keratitis among users of daily-wear and extended-wear soft contact lenses. N Engl J Med 1989;321:773. *(Relative risk is 10 to 15 greater with extended-wear use of lenses.)*

Smith RE, MacRae SM. Contact lenses—convenience and complications. N Engl J Med 1989;321:824. *(A review of the pluses and minuses.)*

Part 2: Refractive Surgery

ROGER F. STEINERT
ELIZABETH S. GOULD

Patients with refractive errors have traditionally relied on external devices—glasses and contact lenses—to obtain clear vision. Refractive surgery offers patients a method to reduce or eliminate their dependence on these prostheses. Laser *in situ* keratomileusis (LASIK) is currently the most advanced and predictable refractive procedure available. Intense interest in this field is stimulating rapid technologic advances. Patients often ask their primary physicians for advice regarding the advisability of proceeding with such surgery, necessitating some basic knowledge about the procedures, their efficacy, and safety and criteria for patient selection.

Radial Keratotomy. Until 1990, radial keratotomy for myopia (nearsightedness) was the most commonly performed refractive surgery. Deep radial incisions placed in the cornea from the periphery toward the pupil cause the central curvature to flatten, optically compensating for myopia. Problems inherent in the procedure include unstable correction, fluctuation during the day, a tendency in some patients for a long-term drift toward hyperopia (farsightedness), vulnerability to rupture from a severe blow to the eye, irregular astigmatism, and halos from the radial scars.

Laser Vision Correction: Photorefractive Keratectomy and Laser *In Situ* Keratomileusis. Laser vision correction uses ophthalmic lasers to correct myopia, hyperopia, and astigmatism by reshaping the cornea. The most common forms of laser vision correction are photorefractive keratectomy (PRK) and *LASIK*, both using the excimer laser. Pulses from the argon fluoride 193-nm excimer laser precisely remove collagen from the corneal stroma, allowing controlled reshaping of the cornea and correction of refractive errors.

Photorefractive Keratectomy. In PRK, the epithelial surface is first removed. The excimer laser then is applied to the surface. Each laser pulse removes a fraction of a micron of tissue.

In the correction of myopia, a greater amount of tissue is removed from the center of the cornea and progressively less toward the periphery, achieving a flatter corneal contour. In hyperopic correction, the pattern is reversed, to steepen the cornea. In astigmatism correction, more tissue is removed on the steeper meridian. Postoperatively, the epithelium heals across the recontoured anterior corneal stromal surface.

Laser In Situ Keratomileusis. In LASIK, the excimer laser energy is used in essentially the same manner as in PRK. The difference is that the surgeon first creates a flap of anterior corneal tissue, typically about 30% deep, using a device known as the microkeratome. The reshaping laser pulses are applied to the exposed stromal surface, after which the flap is replaced. As a result, the corneal surface is disrupted much less than in PRK. Return of vision is faster, the patient experiences minimal pain, and the risk of anterior corneal scarring is eliminated. Patient acceptance of LASIK has been enthusiastic. Because of the minimal wound-healing response, LASIK can treat a broader range of refractive error than PRK, but LASIK requires higher surgical skills because of the necessity to create a flap with the microkeratome. Several brands of excimer lasers for PRK have been approved by the FDA for relatively mild to moderate cases of myopia and astigmatism.

Results. In the clinical trials, 66% of patients could see 20/20 or better with no glasses and 95% could see 20/40 or better. Retreatments can be performed within several months after LASIK and 6 or more months after PRK if the refractive error is not acceptably corrected. Depending on specific patient variables, LASIK can generally treat myopia up to −14 diopters, hyperopia up to +4 diopters, and up to 5 diopters of astigmatism. Presbyopic patients need to be educated that the surgery will not eliminate their need for reading glasses.

Complications. Flap complications decrease with surgeon experience and rarely lead to a decrease in visual acuity. After LASIK, patients may experience glare, halos, monocular diplopia, and dry eyes. These are generally transient and typically decrease over the first several months.

Patient Selection. Candidates for PRK and LASIK are usually at least 21 years of age and have a relatively stable refractive error. Presbyopic patients will still need reading glasses. Some patients elect surgically induced monovision, leaving one eye with low myopia for near vision. Relative contraindications include patients with an ocular history of herpes simplex keratitis, irregular astigmatism, keratoconus, corneal scars, and exposure keratitis. General health contraindications include patients with autoimmune disease disorders that could alter wound healing. Absolute contraindications for PRK, but not necessarily LASIK, include rheumatoid arthritis, lupus, immunocompromised patients, and systemic illness that affects wound healing such as keloid formers.

Intrastromal Corneal Ring Segments. Intrastromal corneal ring segments are small transparent ring segments that are implanted into the nonseeing periphery of the cornea. The procedure currently is able to correct only myopia up to −3 diopters and no astigmatism. The two main advantages of the intrastromal corneal ring segments are that they preserve the central corneal visual zone and are removable, allowing the cornea to return to its original state. Deposits around the implants have been reported in 57% to 100% of eyes treated. Corneal instability has been reported, resulting in a diurnal variation with a myopic shift at the end of the day.

Intraocular Lenses. The surgical correction of myopia with an intraocular lens implanted in the phakic eye is in early investigation. Compared with corneal refractive surgery, the refractive result with phakic intraocular lenses is more predictable, the range of correction is higher, and the quality of vision is improved by decreasing optical aberrations by moving the optical correction to the intraocular plane. Serious potential complications include endothelial cell loss leading to corneal edema, iritis, cataract development, and glaucoma. Long-term follow-up of patients in controlled studies is necessary to confirm the adequacy of the elective surgical procedure. Currently, this procedure is usually reserved for higher levels of myopia and hyperopia than can be treated by other corrective surgeries. Surgical removal of the clear lens is occasionally considered, because it uses current highly refined and reliable cataract surgical technology. Risks are similar to cataract surgery, however.

Thermokeratoplasty. The cornea can be reshaped by heat, which causes contraction of collagen. Past attempts at this concept failed due to instability of the induced corneal shape. More precision in the level of heating, with the goal of creating stable permanent cross-linking of the corneal collagen, has recently been demonstrated by the infrared holmium laser. Externally applied laser pulses may achieve the ability to correct for low to moderate hyperopia, offering technical simplicity and nearly immediate useful vision. Approval of these procedures by the FDA is pending.

ANNOTATED BIBLIOGRAPHY

Alrod L, De la Hoz F, Perez-Santonja JJ. Phakic anterior chamber lenses for the correction of myopia. Ophthalmology 1999;106:458. *(Long-term follow-up of patients in controlled studies is necessary to confirm these initially encouraging results.)*

Baikoff G, Maia N, Poulhalec D. Diurnal variations in keratometry and refraction with corneal ring segments. J Cataract Refract Surg 1999;25:1056. *(Finds corneal instability resulting in a diurnal variation with a myopic shift at the end of the day.)*

El-Maghraby E, Salah T, Waring GO, et al. Randomized bilateral comparison of excimer laser in situ keratomileusis and keratectomy for 2.50 to 8.00 diopters of myopia. Ophthalmology 1999;106:447. *(Because of the minimal wound healing response, LASIK can treat a broader range of refractive error than PRK.)*

Gurwood AS, Cohen BM. Current concepts in refractive surgery. Br J Optom Dispens 1999;7:45. *(Includes a useful discussion of complications of radial keratotomy.)*

Lin RL, Maloney RK. Flap complications associated with lamellar refractive surgery. Am J Ophthalmol 1999;127:129. *(LASIK requires higher surgical skills because of the necessity to create a flap with the microkeratome.)*

Stulting RD, Carr JD, Thompson KP, et al. Complications of laser in situ keratomileusis for the correction of myopia. Ophthalmology 1999;106:13. *(Flap complications decrease with surgeon experience and rarely lead to a decrease in visual acuity.)*

Wu H, Thompson V, Steinert RF, et al. Refractive surgery. New York: Thieme, 1998. *(Useful general reading on the subject.)*

14

Ear, Nose, and Throat Problems

211
Screening for Oral Cancer
JOHN P. KELLY

There are over 30,000 new cases of oral cancer each year in the United States, representing 4% of cancer cases in men and 2% in women. Over 9,000 deaths result from oral cancer yearly. Despite the ready accessibility of the oral cavity to inspection by physicians, dentists, and patients themselves, 50% of oral cancers already have metastasized at the time of diagnosis. Perhaps that is because pain, a manifestation of advanced disease, is the symptom that most commonly leads patients to seek medical attention. When detected early, oral cancer has a very good prognosis. The primary physician has an important role in early detection. Prevention is another responsibility, given the relation of oral cancer to use of tobacco and alcohol.

EPIDEMIOLOGY AND RISK FACTORS

The peak incidence of oral carcinoma is in the sixth decade for women and is equally frequent in each decade after the age of 50 for men. However, the appearance of the disease in the third and fourth decades is not rare and must not be overlooked.

Use of *tobacco* in all its forms is highly correlated with the risk of oral cancer. The frequency of oral cancer of the cheek and gum rises 50-fold among long-term users of *smokeless tobacco*. Use has reached epidemic proportions among teenage boys, causing the Surgeon General's Report to warn against it. Such tobacco products contain multiple carcinogens in addition to tobacco, including nitrosamines, aromatic hydrocarbons, and polonium. Pipe smokers are at increased risk for cancer of the lip. Squamous cell or epidermoid carcinoma of the lower lip also has a particularly high incidence among fair-skinned people whose occupation or residence subjects them to prolonged sun exposure.

Risk of oral cancer is high among those with heavy *alcohol* consumption. Whether this is due to a direct effect of alcohol on the oral mucosa or to associated smoking or vitamin deficiency remains to be fully elucidated.

Cancer of the tongue is highly correlated with the atrophic glossitis seen with tertiary syphilis. Cancer of the tongue is more common among nonsmokers. Mucosal atrophy from other causes is also associated with an increased incidence of oral cancers. Most notably, *chronic iron deficiency* leading to Plummer-Vinson syndrome is known to alter mucosal tissues, and this change may be related to the increased incidence of oral carcinoma. *Epstein-Barr virus* and *papilloma virus* have been found in cells of the tongue manifesting oral hairy leukoplakia, a hyperplastic change found in patients with AIDS.

Chronic irritation of the oral mucosa by ill-fitting dentures, poorly restored teeth, or particularly spicy diets has often been mentioned as contributing to the development of oral carcinoma. However, no epidemiologic data support this view.

The precise etiology of oral cancer is unknown. The etiologic factors mentioned above probably act as cocarcinogens, effecting malignant change in concert with some primary agent not yet elucidated. Increased chromosomal fragility has been found in nonsmokers who develop oral cancers.

NATURAL HISTORY

In considering the natural history of oral cancer, it is important to address premalignant and malignant disease.

Premalignant Disease

Leukoplakia, a "white patch" on the oral mucosa, is of interest because in about 10% of instances it represents premalignant change with dysplastic features on biopsy. Clinically, it ranges from slightly raised white translucent areas to dense white opaque plaques, with or without adjacent ulceration. It is difficult to differentiate completely benign from premalignant leukoplakia, except by *biopsy*. However, patients demonstrating a speckled pattern interspersed with areas of ulceration or erosion are more likely to have dysplastic disease. Lesions may occur anywhere on the oral mucosa, but those on the tongue have the greatest risk of malignant transformation. Such transformation may take anywhere from 1 to 20 years. In addition to premalignant dysplasias and squamous cell carcinoma, the differential diagnosis of oral leukoplakia includes traumatic irritation (from malposed teeth or ill-fitting dentures), chemical "burns" (typically from aspirin dissolved in the oral cavity), viral infection (so-called hairy leukoplakia seen in HIV infection), lichen planus, oral candidiasis, discoid lupus, and pemphigus vulgaris.

Erythroplasia, a red hyperplastic area of mucosa, is highly suggestive of an early carcinoma. Although most cancer screening protocols have emphasized a search for white lesions, the predominant color in premalignant or early lesions is red, not white. In fact, whereas some white lesions may only be "premalignant," the red lesions must be considered to be true malignancies unless proven otherwise by biopsy.

Malignant Disease

The average 5-year survival rate for localized oral cancer exceeds 65% but barely reaches 30% for patients with metastatic disease. When untreated, oral carcinoma metastasizes to the regional lymph nodes of the neck, ultimately leading to respiratory embarrassment or involvement of the great vessels. Ipsilateral node involvement is most common, but metastasis to the contralateral side—especially from primary lesions of the tongue or floor of the mouth—occurs with such frequency that treatment for control of metastatic disease is difficult. Hence, early diagnosis and control of the primary lesion are important. The lungs are the most frequently involved extranodal metastatic site.

Local recurrence is common. Many instances may actually represent new primary disease, suggesting a susceptibility of the entire oral mucosa to malignant change in affected patients. As many as one patient in five may be expected to develop a second primary oropharyngeal cancer, with smokers who do not quit incurring the greatest risk.

Other Oral Lesions

Other oral lesions appear black, blue, or brown. Benign conditions such as *vascular malformations, heavy metal ingestion, amalgam tattooing,* pigmented *nevi,* and the pigmentations associated with such systemic conditions as neurofibromatosis, intestinal polyposis, and Addison's disease must be differentiated from the blue-black lesion of *malignant melanoma* (see Chapter 177). Biopsy is essential if this diagnosis is suggested by the appearance of the lesion.

SCREENING AND DIAGNOSTIC PROCEDURES

The challenge to primary care physicians is to recognize premalignant and early malignant lesions of the oral cavity. The greatest hope for improved outcome is detection before the appearance of grossly invasive disease. The ready accessibility of the oral cavity to *inspection* and the appearance of premalignant mucosal changes facilitate early detection. *Biopsy* of suspicious lesions should follow. Leukoplakia and erythroplasia are the most potentially important mucosal changes.

Initial evaluation of a suspicious lesion begins with eliciting appropriate historical data to eliminate such relatively harmless lesions as the acute aspirin burn. Irritative lesions can be identified by removing or repairing jagged teeth and poorly fitting or protruding dental prostheses and following the clinical healing of the mucosal wound over a short period of time. Mucosal ulceration that fails to heal within a week or two after elimination of a presumed mechanical irritation must be biopsied. In any patient with a suspicious lesion, use of a noxious agent such as tobacco must be eliminated at the outset.

Any red or white lesion that persists for 2 weeks after initial recognition and elimination of irritating agents requires referral for biopsy. High-risk patients, specifically those with histories of smoking and drinking, should be referred for biopsy promptly, as should any patient with a deeply ulcerative or fungating lesion. Exfoliative cytology and **in vivo** staining with toluidine blue, although sometimes suggested as noninvasive diagnostic methods, do not provide sufficient sensitivity or specificity to take the place of incisional biopsy.

Any swelling beneath a normal-appearing oral mucosa must be evaluated as well. Such lesions are commonly benign and are the result of infection, bony exostosis, or mucus retention phenomena, but they may represent neoplasms of the minor salivary glands or other submucosal structures.

RECOMMENDATIONS

- A thorough visual and manual examination of the lips and oral cavity should be a part of every patient's evaluation; mucosal patches that are either red or white are sought.
- A high index of suspicion must be maintained for patients with a history of smoking, drinking, and heavy exposure to sunlight.
- Atrophic or hyperplastic areas of the oral mucosa must be viewed with suspicion, particularly if they are red or white (erythroplasia or leukoplakia) and last more than 2 weeks after cessation of smoking, drinking, and exposure to irritants.
- Referral for definitive biopsy is indicated for persistent lesions.

ANNOTATED BIBLIOGRAPHY

Connolly GN, Winn DL, Hecht SS, et al. The reemergence of smokeless tobacco. N Engl J Med 1986;314:1020. (*An extensive review documents health risks and points out alarming rise in popularity. An editorial by the Surgeon General reinforces the message.*)

Decker J, Goldstein JC. Risk factors in head and neck cancer. N Engl J Med 1982;306:1151. (*Reviews the epidemiology of oral malignancy emphasizing the importance of smoking, alcohol, and poor oral hygiene.*)

Greene JC, Louie R, Wycoff SJ. Preventive dentistry. II. Periodontal diseases, malocclusion, trauma, and oral cancer. JAMA 1990; 262:421. (*The recommendations of the U.S. Preventive Services Task Force.*)

Jacobs C. The internist in the management of head and neck cancer. Ann Intern Med 1990;113:771. (*Prevention can be achieved by cessation of tobacco use and reduction in alcohol intake; early detection greatly improves prognosis and response to therapy.*)

Mashberg A. Erythroplasia: the earliest sign of asymptomatic oral cancer. J Am Dent Assoc 1978;96:615. (*Good illustration and description of this early malignant lesion.*)

Shklar G. Oral leukoplakia. N Engl J Med 1986;315:1544. (*An editorial regarding its significance.*)

212
Evaluation of Hearing Loss
A. JULIANNA GULYA

It is estimated that more than 10% of the population of the United States has a hearing problem. The problem is particularly common among the elderly and can impair quality of life. People with seriously impaired hearing often become withdrawn or appear confused. Subtle hearing loss may go unrecognized. Patients with hearing loss often can be greatly helped, particularly if the loss is due to a conductive problem. The primary physician has the responsibility to detect hearing loss, to search for an etiology, and to decide when referral to an otolaryngologist is indicated.

PATHOPHYSIOLOGY AND CLINICAL PRESENTATION

Pathophysiology

Basic Mechanisms of Hearing and Their Impairment. Impaired hearing may result from an interference with the conduction of sound, its conversion to electrical impulses, or its transmission through the nervous system. Hearing involves an acoustic stage during which sound waves cause the tympanic membrane to vibrate. Ossicles amplify the sound, and the oscillation of the footplate of the stapes in the oval window transmits the sound waves to the perilymph of the inner ear. The endolymph of the scala media (or cochlear duct) is wedged between the perilymph of the scala vestibuli and scala tympani. Displacement of the basilar membrane stimulates the hair cells, converting sound waves to neural impulses, which are conveyed to the temporal lobes.

Molecularly, during the reception of sound, potassium ions flow through the upper surface of the cochlear hair cells; the ions then recycle by flowing down to the base and supporting cells and into the endolymph. *Connexin,* the "gap protein" that allows small molecules to pass from one cell to the next, facilitates this potassium flow. It is synthesized by the cells surrounding the sensory hair cells of the cochlea and by the fibrocytes of the cochlear duct.

Interference with mechanical reception or amplification of sound, as occurs with disease of the auditory canal, tympanic membrane, or ossicles, creates *conductive hearing loss.* Degeneration or destruction of hair cells or the acoustic nerve produces *sensorineural hearing loss,* as do defects in the synthesis of connexin. Genetic studies have facilitated uncovering a molecular basis for hearing loss. Mutations in the gene that codes for connexin are associated with nonsyndromic hearing loss, both early in life and with aging (see below). Congenital malformations of the inner ear, not necessarily hereditary, may also compromise hearing.

Conductive Hearing Loss

Conductive loss presents with diminished perception of sound, particularly for low-frequency tones and vowels. There is often a history of previous ear disease. In the Weber test, the tuning fork is perceived more loudly in the ear with a conductive hearing loss. The Rinne test shows that bone conduction is better than air conduction. Obstruction of the auditory canal by severely impacted cerumen, a foreign body, exostoses, external otitis, otitis media with effusion, or scarring or perforation of the drum due to chronic otitis may be present.

Otosclerosis, a surgically remediable cause of conductive hearing loss, is a disorder of the bony labyrinth that fixes the footplate of the stapes in the oval window. Clinical otosclerosis has an estimated prevalence of about 1% among whites and 0.1% among blacks. Two thirds of the cases are seen in women. There appears to be an association between pregnancy and otosclerotic hearing loss. The condition is thought to be inherited in an autosomal dominant fashion, with varying clinical expressivity. It generally presents in the second or third decade of life.

Exostoses are bony excrescences of the external auditory canal. They are characteristically located in the anterior, posterior, and superior quadrants of the canal. Nearly always bilaterally symmetric, their occurrence seems to be related to repetitive exposure to cold water (e.g., as in ocean swimming). They can cause symptoms by blockage of the external auditory canal, resulting in conductive hearing loss, or by sequestration of debris with subsequent infection.

Glomus Tumors or paragangliomas are benign highly vascular tumors derived from normally occurring glomus formations of the middle ear and jugular bulb. Presenting symptoms include conductive hearing loss (from middle ear mass effect); spontaneous hemorrhage from the canal; and paralysis of the ninth, tenth and eleventh cranial nerves (the jugular foramen syndrome). With progression, they may involve the intracranial space or cause bony destruction of the base of the skull.

Sensorineural Hearing Loss

Sensorineural loss arises from dysfunction of the cochlear sensorineural elements and/or of the cochlear nerve. Patients may complain that they can hear people speaking but have difficulty deciphering words because speech discrimination is poor. Shouting may only exacerbate the problem. The patient with high-frequency loss may have difficulty hearing doorbells, telephones, or a ticking watch and may note more difficulty in hearing the higher pitched female or child's voice. Recruitment, an abnormally rapid increase in perceived loudness with increased sound intensity, may be present and indicates cochlear dysfunction. With Rinne testing, air conduction is reported better than bone conduction. Tinnitus is often a concomitant complaint.

Presbycusis is hearing loss associated with aging and is the most common cause of diminished hearing in the elderly. There are four types of presbycusis, distinguished according to the correlated pathologic changes in the cochlea. Hair cell loss and cochlear neuron degeneration are the most widely recognized changes. The hearing loss is bilaterally symmetric and gradual in

Frequency (cps)

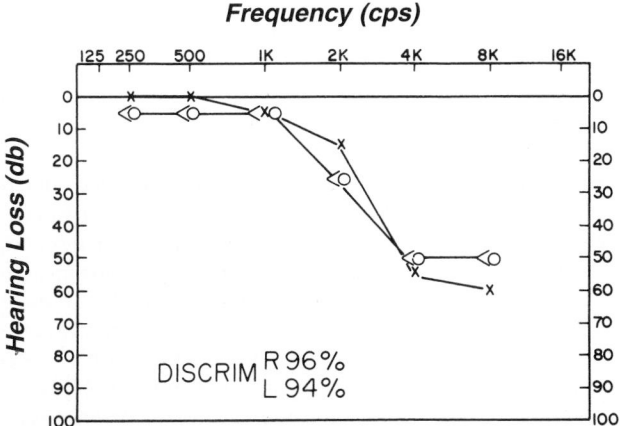

Fig. 212.1. Presbycusis due to hair cell loss. Note good hearing thresholds at the speech frequencies of 250 to 2,000 c/s. X = L ear, air; O = R ear, air; < = R ear bone.

onset. Most cases begin with a loss of the high frequencies with slow progression. Eventually, middle and low-frequency sounds also become difficult to perceive (Figs. 212.1 and 212.2).

Noise-induced hearing loss is of major epidemiologic and economic significance. Chronic exposure to sound levels in excess of 85 to 90 dB causes hearing loss, particularly in the frequency range around 4,000 Hz. The patient may be unaware of the problem because the speech frequencies (500 to 4,000 Hz) are initially unaffected. At first, there may be a temporary threshold shift in which there is a reversible elevation in the threshold for sound perception. The ear may feel full, or the patient may complain of a sense of pressure. If loud noise exposure ceases at this point, hearing returns to its previous level. If exposure persists, however, a permanent threshold shift ensues. The term *acoustic trauma* more specifically relates to a particular single noise event (e.g., a shotgun blast) that induces an immediate irreversible hearing loss.

Drug-Induced Hearing Loss. The aminoglycoside antibiotics, such as gentamicin, are representative of ototoxic drugs. An early sign of gentamicin ototoxicity is disequilibrium. Monitoring antibiotic blood levels is the best, but not perfect, way to avoid such problems, adjusting dose according to peak serum levels. Restricting dosing to once daily and duration of therapy to less than 1 week also help reduce risk. Other potentially ototoxic drugs, including those causing symmetric sensorineural hearing loss, include furosemide, ethacrynic acid, cisplatin, quinidine, and aspirin. Aspirin doses averaging 6 to 8 g/d predictably cause tinnitus and completely reversible hearing impairment.

Ménière's disease manifests with a unilateral, fluctuating, low-frequency, sensorineural hearing loss, usually associated with tinnitus, a sensation of fullness in the ear, and intermittent episodes of vertigo. Vertigo may be the presenting symptom of Ménière's disease, with later onset of fluctuating hearing loss. Progression of hearing loss may occur, eventually encompassing the higher frequencies as well.

Acoustic neuromas, benign tumors of the eighth cranial nerve, are rare but important considerations in the evaluation of

asymmetric sensorineural hearing loss, often in conjunction with disequilibrium (see Chapter 166). Speech discrimination is much worse than predicted by the pure-tone hearing loss. Symptoms progress in relentless progressive fashion.

Sudden sensorineural hearing loss can be due to head trauma or can appear without obvious cause or warning. In *idiopathic* sudden sensorineural hearing loss, recovery appears to be predicted by the pattern of hearing loss sustained, age (greater or less than 40), presence or absence of vertigo, and electronystagmogram pattern. The etiology of the idiopathic variant is still a matter of debate, but viral infection seems to be the most likely cause. Uncommonly, an acoustic neuroma may present with sudden hearing loss. Sudden hearing loss demands expeditious referral to an otolaryngologist for further evaluation and possible therapy with corticosteroids and antiviral agents.

Hereditary sensorineural hearing loss is generally bilaterally symmetric. Many syndromes have been identified in which hereditary hearing loss is associated with anomalies in other organ systems, but nonsyndromic hereditary hearing loss is also recognized. Among persons with isolated ("nonsyndromic") hearing loss, there is a high frequency of mutations in the gene *GJB2*, which codes for synthesis of *connexin*. Mutations in this gene are found not only among congenitally nonsyndromic deaf children, who are usually homozygous for the mutation, but also in the carrier state among adults with late-onset isolated hearing loss. The frequency can be as high as 3% across many different populations. It is suspected that the carrier state may predispose to hearing loss later in life and account for some if not many cases of age-related hearing loss that are commonly encountered. More work is needed to confirm these intriguing and potentially important findings. Although screening for mutations of this gene is not difficult, the degree of hearing loss and its time of onset cannot yet be predicted.

Injury to the inner ear or cochlear nerve may produce an asymmetric sensorineural hearing loss. Skull fracture, meningitis, and mumps are major etiologic factors. Trauma may also cause conductive hearing loss, for example, hemotympanum, tympanic membrane perforation, or ossicular dislocation.

Frequency (CPS)

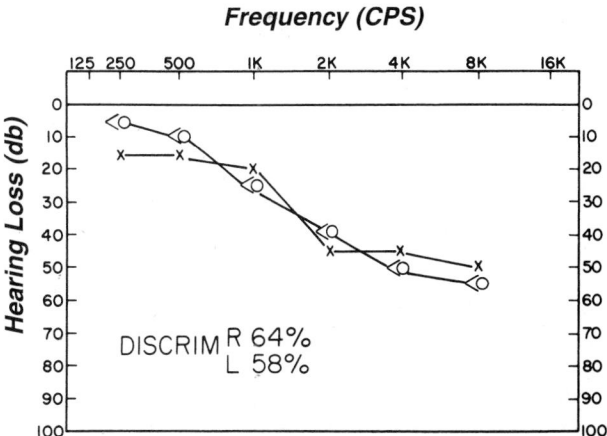

Fig. 212.2. Late presbycusis due to loss of cochlear neurons. Note poor discrimination. X = L ear, air; O = R ear, air; < = L ear bone.

Table 212.1. Common and Important Causes
of Impaired Hearing

CONDUCTIVE	SENSORINEURAL
Impacted cerumen	Presbycusis
Foreign body	Noise-induced deafness
Occlusive edema of auditory canal	Drugs (aminoglycosides, loop diuretics, quinidine, aspirin)
Perforation of tympanic membrane	Meniére's disease
	Acoustic neuroma
Chronic otitis media	Hypothyroidism (mild loss)
Serous otitis media	Idiopathic sudden deafness
External otitis	Congenital syphilis
Otosclerosis	Diabetes
Exostoses	Perilymph leak
Developmental defects	Multiple sclerosis
Glomus tumors	

Other Etiologies. *Congenital syphilis* may produce adult-onset sensorineural hearing loss. One or both ears may be affected; the course can be variable, with remissions and exacerbations. Vertigo is sometimes present as well, producing a symptom complex mimicking Ménière's disease.

Multiple Sclerosis should be considered when a young woman shows discrimination scores reduced out of proportion to the pure tone thresholds (similar to the pattern seen with acoustic neuromas). The site of the lesion is retrocochlear (often in the brainstem), and there may be an associated history of optic neuritis and/or vertigo.

Perilymph Leaks or Fistulas may cause hearing loss, with or without vertigo, in individuals who have had inner ear surgery (e.g., stapedectomy), have sustained head trauma, or have congenital inner ear anomalies. The round and/or oval windows may be involved, and it is theorized that there is intracochlear membrane rupture as well. Surgical repair may be required.

DIFFERENTIAL DIAGNOSIS

The causes of hearing loss can be grouped according to whether the problem is conductive or sensorineural (Table 212.1). The categorization is of practical use because the conductive defects lend themselves to correction in many instances.

WORKUP

History. Evaluation of the patient with hearing loss should focus on detection of the site of lesion. This search is aided by identifying whether the impairment is conductive or sensorineural. History is of substantial importance. It is worth trying to find out the sounds or situations in which the patient has most trouble hearing. Difficulty understanding spoken words suggests sensorineural hearing loss. Inquiry into drug use is essential, focusing on aminoglycosides, quinine derivatives, salicylates, chemotherapeutics, and the loop diuretics furosemide and ethacrynic acid. A history of otitis, noise exposure (both recreational and work related), or head trauma should be noted.

Inquiry into acoustic trauma is important, especially the details of occupational exposure. Family history is no less important, particularly in the consideration of gene mutations, otosclerosis, and acoustic neuromas (associated with von Recklinghausen's disease).

Physical Examination. The external auditory canal should be inspected for obstruction by impacted cerumen, a foreign body, external otitis, or exostoses. The tympanic membranes are examined for inflammation, perforation, and scarring. One notes any fluid in middle ear. A reddish mass visible through the intact tympanic membrane may indicate a high-riding jugular bulb, an aberrant internal carotid artery, or a glomus tumor. Pneumatic otoscopy assesses tympanic membrane mobility.

Nasopharyngeal examination is indicated in patients with persisting serous otitis media, particularly if it is unilateral. If there is vertigo or suspicion of a glomus or acoustic tumor, cranial nerve examination is performed to assess central nervous system involvement (see Chapter 166).

Testing Hearing. The *watch tick* was an easy, although crude, method of detecting high-frequency impairment when ticking watches were common. *Whispering*, gradually increasing the intensity of the whisper, is readily performed. One asks the patient to repeat a number of words whispered into the tested ear while masking the contralateral ear (e.g., with a Barany noise box). The best words are familiar bisyllabic ones in which both syllables are equally accented (e.g., pancake, hot dog). With practice, one can roughly estimate the patient's hearing thresholds.

Tuning forks can be used both to detect hearing loss and to differentiate conductive from sensorineural hearing losses (*Weber* and *Rinne* testing). A tuning fork that vibrates at a frequency of 512 Hz is acceptable; the 128-Hz tuning fork used for testing vibratory sensation is not. Testing is done to establish the threshold of perception by striking it against the heel of the hand and withdrawing it at 1 foot per second starting 1 inch from the ear until it becomes imperceptible. The distance is noted.

Differentiating Conductive from Sensorineural Hearing Loss. The *Weber* test is helpful. The normal response to a fork vibrating from a tap of the knee and placed midline on the skull is equal loudness in both ears. If there is a conductive loss, the sound will be heard more clearly in the ear with the loss. If there is a sensorineural loss in one ear, sound will be perceived as being heard in the better ear.

The *Rinne test* complements Weber testing. When the vibrating fork is placed on the mastoid process, it is heard for a period of time and then dies away. It is heard again if the same fork is promptly moved without any reactivation to the external auditory canal. Normally, sound conducted by air is heard about twice as long as a sound conducted by bone, because of the greater sound transmission efficiency of the middle ear apparatus.

Alternatively, with firm application of the tuning fork against the mastoid process for a few seconds and immediate transfer to the external auditory canal, the sound should be perceived as "louder" in front of the canal when compared with the mastoid position. With a substantial (generally 25 dB or greater) conductive loss, the ratio reverses. With lesser degrees of impairment, the ratio approaches 1:1. The normal ratio is preserved in sensorineural losses.

The *Schwabach test* compares the examiner's hearing by bone conduction with that of the patient's. The vibrating tuning fork is alternately placed on the mastoid process of examiner and patient. If the examiner's hearing is normal, he or she will perceive the sound for a longer time than the patient with a sensorineural deficit and for a shorter time than the patient with a conductive problem.

Laboratory Studies. An *audiogram* is an essential component of the evaluation of the patient with hearing loss. The pattern of threshold loss has considerable diagnostic and therapeutic importance, helping to establish the type of hearing loss and to localize the site of lesion. Interpretation usually requires the joint efforts of an otolaryngologist and an audiologist, but a few common patterns are useful for the primary physician to recognize (see the Appendix-audiometer).

Expensive imaging technology should be used sparingly but can be helpful in carefully selected patients. *Computed tomography* is used in the evaluation of certain middle ear and mastoid disorders, such as chronic infection and glomus tumors. *Magnetic resonance imaging*, particularly with gadolinium enhancement, has assumed a preeminent role in the evaluation of the patient with suspected retrocochlear disease (e.g., acoustic neuroma or multiple sclerosis).

Auditory brainstem response testing has also been found useful in the site-of-lesion testing, as has *electronystagmography* (see Chapter 166). Both tests require expert performance and interpretation and should be ordered only in consultation with consultants experienced in their use and interpretation.

Otoacoustic emissions, particularly those evoked by sound stimuli, are used to test the integrity of the outer hair cells of the cochlea, from which they are believed to emanate. Otoacoustic emissions show promise as a screening test for assessing auditory function in infants and other difficult-to-test patients.

Screening for Hearing Loss. An important aspect of geriatric care is assessment for hearing loss. In support of screening for hearing loss are the major impact hearing loss can have on quality of life, the availability of effective means to detect and correct hearing loss, and the ability to screen adequately in the primary care setting. The U.S. Preventive Services Task Force recommends periodic hearing assessment of all elderly persons.

The best screening methods and the optimal interval are the subjects of ongoing study. The American Academy of Otolaryngology–Head and Neck Surgery has developed a simple one-page "test" that the individual patient can self-administer to see if a hearing evaluation by an otolaryngologist is warranted.

Screening for Hearing Loss Gene Mutations. Screening for hearing loss gene mutations is technically feasible because of the frequency of mutations in *GJB2* and the ease with which these can be detected (gene size is small). However, the meaning of the findings remains unclear, making proper use of the information problematic. Further study is needed, and the reader should watch the literature closely because this is a rapidly evolving aspect of hearing loss research.

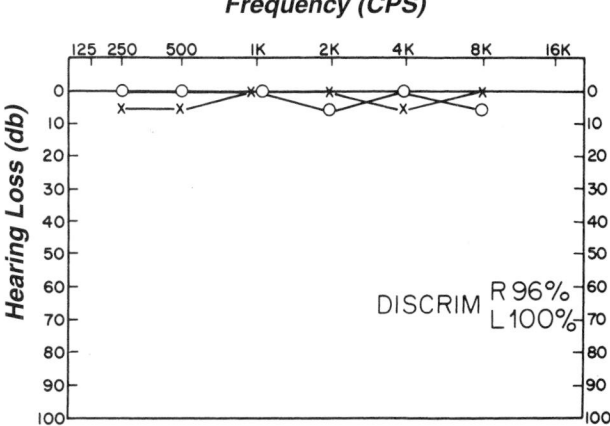

Fig. 212.3. Normal pure tone air audiogram. O = R ear, air; X = left ear, air.

SYMPTOMATIC MANAGEMENT, PATIENT EDUCATION, AND INDICATIONS FOR REFERRAL

The primary physician's role in the treatment of hearing loss is relatively limited, but simple advice and support are much appreciated. Elders report that cupping the hand behind the ear can be of help both in actual hearing and alerting others to speak more clearly or louder. Speech reading (interpreting what is being said by extrapolating from the words heard and the facial expressions) may also help and is facilitated by good lighting. Clear enunciation, not merely elevated volume of speech, along with directly facing the presbycusic patient while engaged in conversation optimizes verbal communication. Removal of impacted cerumen or other obstruction, cessation of ototoxic drugs, and treatment of otitis media (see Chapter 218) should not be overlooked. Advising patients exposed to occupational or recreational noise to use ear protection when in a noisy environment and to avoid further exposure is important.

Cerumen removal may be accomplished by gentle body temperature water irrigation using a syringe or an irrigation jet. Removal of wax, as well as some foreign bodies, may be performed using a cerumen spoon or forceps under direct visualization provided by headlight and speculum. Insects are better exterminated first by instillation of mineral oil into the canal before removal is attempted.

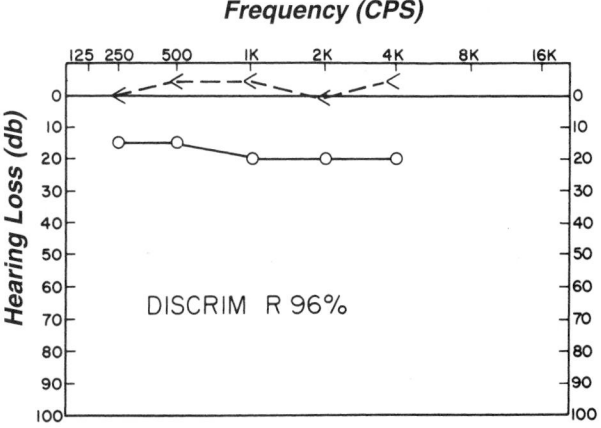

Fig. 212.4. Air–bone gap. O = R ear, air; < = R ear, bone.

Referral to an otolaryngologist for further evaluation and treatment is indicated when a conductive etiology or acoustic neuroma is suspected or when simple symptomatic measures do not suffice. The otolaryngologist needs to determine whether the patient is a candidate for medical or surgical therapy and whether a hearing aid is appropriate. A true sudden hearing loss demands immediate otolaryngologic referral.

A great variety of hearing aids is available on the market. Patients with sensorineural hearing losses—especially those with a flat threshold and good discrimination—benefit from amplification and deserve as much consideration as those patients with conductive hearing losses. Even those patients with steeply sloping high-frequency sensorineural hearing loss with poor discrimination may find amplification useful. Only an adequate trial, after careful otolaryngologic evaluation and competent hearing aid fitting, can allow one to make a decision regarding the helpfulness of amplification.

ANNOTATED BIBLIOGRAPHY

Consensus Conference. Noise and hearing loss. JAMA 1990;263:3185. *(Recommends several steps to limit noise-induced hearing loss.)*

Koike KJ, Hurst MK, Wetmore SJ. Correlation between the American Academy of Otolaryngology–Head and Neck Surgery five-minute hearing test and standard audiologic data. Otolaryngol Head Neck Surg 1994;111:625. *(Evaluates the sensitivity and specificity of a hearing screen proposed by the American Academy of Otolaryngology–Head & Neck Surgery and proposes modification of the "cutoff score".)*

Lonsbury-Martin BL, Martin GK, McCoy MJ, et al. New approaches to the evaluation of the auditory system and a current analysis of otoacoustic emissions. Otolaryngol Head Neck Surg 1995;112:50. *(Review of otoacoustic emissions and their uses in auditory evaluation.)*

Morell RJ, Kim HJ, Hood LJ, et al. Mutations in the connexin 26 gene (GJB2) among Ashkenazi Jews with nonsyndromic recessive deafness. N Engl J Med 1998;339:1500. *(Mutations in the connexin gene found in high frequency; authors estimate that the prevalence of the carrier state could account for most of the nonsyndromic age-related hearing loss in this population.)*

Paterson DL, Robson JMB, Wagener MM, et al. Risk factors for toxicity in elderly patients given aminoglycosides once daily. J Gen Intern Med 1998;13:735. *(A prospective observational study in patients over the age of 70; multivariate analysis reveals that limiting the duration of therapy to less than one week can reduce the risk of toxicity.)*

Steel KP. A new era in the genetics of deafness. N Engl J Med 1998;339:1545. *(An editorial summarizing the rapid progress being made in research on the genetic basis for hearing loss; includes excellent summary of connexin.)*

Appendix: Audiometry

Audiometry helps to classify a hearing loss as conductive or sensorineural and subclassify according to the pattern detected. The basic audiogram consists of pure-tone air and bone conduction testing with evaluation of speech reception threshold and speech discrimination. The minimal intensity (decibel) at which the patient perceives each tone is charted as the threshold for that frequency. The responses are recorded as indicated in Fig. 212.3. The pure-tone air threshold curve measures both conductive and sensorineural hearing. To appreciate a conductive component to a hearing loss, bone conduction thresholds are obtained. The bone conduction audiogram bypasses the conduction system and measures cochlear/cochlear nerve capacity. In bone conduction testing, the mastoid process of each ear is directly stimulated with an oscillator or vibrator over a similar frequency spectrum and results are graphically recorded. A discrepancy between air conduction thresholds and those for bone-conducted sounds, the so-called air–bone gap, is indicative of a conductive hearing loss (Fig. 212.4)

Additional testing includes *speech reception threshold* (SRT) and *speech discrimination testing*. The SRT is defined as the lowest intensity at which the patient can correctly identify 50% of presented words. The SRT should match, within a few decibels, the average of the pure-tone thresholds. Discrimination testing evaluates speech understanding using standardized word lists. Speech discrimination that is diminished out of proportion to the measured hearing loss is suggestive of cochlear nerve pathology. Ordinarily, patients with good pure-tone thresholds should also understand speech well.

213
Approach to Epistaxis
WILLIAM R. WILSON

Most spontaneous nosebleeds are self-limited. Patients present for medical care when the bleeding becomes unusually brisk, will not stop, or episodes become frequent. Severe or recurrent bleeding necessitates evaluation for nasal pathology and, less commonly, an underlying generalized disorder. The immediate therapeutic objective is control of bleeding.

PATHOPHYSIOLOGY AND CLINICAL PRESENTATION

Etiologies. The primary mechanism of epistaxis is disruption of the nasal mucosa, primarily caused by *trauma*. In patients with deviated septum or septal spurs in the anterior portion of the nose, trauma occurs easily, either from the drying effects of poorly humidified air or secondary to probing in or bumps on the nose. Picking, rubbing, or forceful blowing may also trigger bleeding when the nasal mucosa is inflamed from a viral, bacterial, or allergic cause.

Ulcerations, which tend to form over septal deviations and spurs, bleed easily. Repeated mucosal exposure to cocaine leads to anoxic tissue necrosis from drug-induced intense vasospasm; perforation may result from cocaine use and cause chronic crusting and bleeding. Collagen diseases such as lupus are occasionally responsible for ulceration.

Table 213.1. Major Causes of Epistaxis

LOCAL DISEASE	SYSTEMIC DISEASE
Dry indoor environment	Granulomatous disease (Wegener's, sarcoidosis)
Upper respiratory infection	
Chronic sinusitis	Hereditary hemorrhagic telangiectasia
Trauma (nose picking, forceful blowing)	
Occupational exposure to irritants	Infection (chickenpox, influenza)
Cocaine abuse	
Angiomas	Bleeding diathesis
Allergies	Malignant hypertension
Lack of humidification	
Malignancy	

Bleeding diatheses sometimes present as epistaxis (see Chapter 81). Nosebleeds are the most common initial presentation of *hereditary hemorrhagic telangiectasia* (Osler-Weber-Rendu syndrome) and its most frequent bleeding complication. Characteristic features include telangiectasias on the nasal mucosa, lips, and tongue; a positive family history; and onset of repeated bleeding episodes by the third or fourth decade. Adolescent boys with a nasopharyngeal angiofibroma experience brisk posterior epistaxis. Sinus x-rays demonstrate a nasopharyngeal mass.

Wegener's granulomatosis, midline granuloma, and *nasal malignancy* share a presentation of epistaxis, unremitting sinus infection, and opacified sinuses on x-ray. Posterior epistaxis, bleeding from the sphenopalatine plexus deep in the nose, is commonly attributed to hypertension, but epidemiologic studies show that few hypertensives experience nosebleeds.

Site of Bleeding. Regardless of etiology, the site of bleeding has distinguishing clinical characteristics. Active *anterior epistaxis* usually presents as unilateral, continuous, moderate bleeding from the septum. Recurrent episodes of bleeding, lasting a few minutes to half an hour over the preceding few days and controlled by pinching the anterior nose, are characteristic. Most adult cases and almost all spontaneous nasal hemorrhage in children occur on the anterior aspect of the nasal septum. Most are venous, but an arterial source becomes more common with advancing age because of mucosal and vascular atrophy.

Posterior epistaxis is associated with intermittent very brisk arterial bleeding, with blood flowing into the pharynx unless the patient is leaning forward. When the patient is leaning forward, the blood may run from one or both sides of the nose. Spontaneous posterior hemorrhage is more common in the older age groups and after severe facial trauma. The vessel rupture is usually just superior or inferior to the posterior tip of the inferior turbinate on the lateral nasal wall.

DIFFERENTIAL DIAGNOSIS

The differential diagnosis of nosebleeds can be divided into local and systemic disorders (Table 213.1). The local causes are most commonly inflammatory or traumatic. More than 90% of bleeds are related to local irritation; most occur in the absence of a specific underlying anatomic lesion.

WORKUP

History should begin with inquiry into the amount of bleeding, duration, and frequency. After the bleeding is under control, the patient can be questioned about easy bruising, hematuria, melena, heavy menstrual periods, family history of bleeding disorders, the use of oral anticoagulants or drugs with antiplatelet effects (aspirin and so forth), occupational exposure to irritating chemicals or dust, dry home, chronic cocaine use, and repeated nose-blowing or picking.

Physical examination should be performed with the patient sitting and leaning forward so that the blood flows from the nose. This allows the physician to assess the rate and site of bleeding and to prevent the swallowing of blood, which will quickly lead to emesis. The pulse and blood pressure should be taken, and the skin, mucous membranes, and conjunctiva should be checked for rash, pallor, purpura, petechiae, and telangiectasias. Lymph nodes should be examined for enlargement, suggesting sarcoidosis, tuberculosis, or malignancy. The sinuses are percussed for evidence of sinusitis, which would make Wegener's, midline granuloma, and nasal tumor considerations.

Laboratory studies are best ordered on the basis of findings from the history and physical examination. Patients suspected of a bleeding diathesis should have a prothrombin time test, partial thromboplastin time test, bleeding time, blood smear, and platelet count obtained (see Chapter 81). Sinus films are appropriate to evaluate the patient with recurrent bouts of sinus pain, tenderness, and bleeding.

PRINCIPLES OF MANAGEMENT

The first objective is to stop the bleeding. The approach depends on whether the source is anterior or posterior.

Anterior Septal Bleeding A few simple first-aid measures suffice for most cases. The patient should *sit up* (this reduces venous pressure) and *lean forward* (which prevents the swallowing of blood if the bleeding is anterior). A small piece of cotton or cotton balls soaked in 1:1,000 epinephrine or a vasoconstricting nosedrop such as *phenylephrine* (Neo-Synephrine) or *oxymetazoline* (Afrin) is placed in the vestibule of the nose and pressed against the bleeding site for 10 to 15 minutes. It is then removed to observe for rebleeding. This will stop almost all venous types of anterior nosebleeds. Humidification and a lubricant such as petrolatum ointment promote healing.

If these remedies fail, the mucous membrane can be anesthetized by applying cotton soaked with 4% cocaine or 4% lidocaine for 5 minutes. A *silver nitrate stick* can then be applied to the bleeding site and to any prominent vessels.

Occasionally, a small artery in the septal mucous membrane will either fail to stop bleeding or rebleed a short time later. These episodes can usually be controlled by anesthetizing and recauterizing the area. This is followed by placing a small amount of *oxidized regenerated cellulose* (Surgicel) against the bleeding artery or a small *packing of petroleum gauze* strip or Merocel sponge soaked with oxymetazoline and/or thrombin solution that is left in the nasal vestibule for 24 hours.

Patients with bleeding disorders require especially careful treatment to prevent abrading the mucous membrane. Therapy involves use of humidity, copious lubricants, and soft cotton tamponades wetted with long-acting vasoconstricting drops (oxymetazoline 0.05% Afrin nasal solution). Packing should be avoided at all costs but, if unavoidable, can be accomplished with a piece of oxidized cellulose, which does not require removal. Further treatment is best directed at the underlying bleeding disorder.

Posterior epistaxis constitutes an inherently more serious problem, because of the relative rapidity of blood loss and the relatively inaccessible and poorly visualized bleeding site in the posterior nose. Initial efforts should be made to bring the bleeding under control while awaiting an otolaryngologic consult. Hematocrit, blood pressure, and pulse should be immediately obtained, and, if necessary, a sample should be sent for type and crossmatch. The patient should be instructed to *sit up* and *lean forward*, and if there has been a temporary interruption in the bleeding, no treatment other than spraying the nose with a topical anesthetic and vasoconstricting substance, such as *4% cocaine* or oxymetazoline 0.05%, should be attempted. The nose should be suctioned or blown clear only when the medical personnel present are prepared to deal with brisk epistaxis. If the patient's blood pressure permits, a parenteral analgesic such as Demerol 50 or 100 mg intramuscularly should be given before the surgeon's *electrocautery* of the posterior nose or the placement of *compressing* balloons, packs, or tampons.

PATIENT EDUCATION

Prevention of Recurrences. Once septal bleeding is controlled in the office or emergency ward, several measures to prevent recurrences should be instituted:

- Instruct the patient on the need to avoid traumatizing the mucosa. Specifically, warn against habitual nose picking, constant rubbing with a handkerchief, and excessively forceful blowing. The fingernails of children should be trimmed short.
- Have the patient keep the septum well coated with petrolatum-based ointment such as zinc oxide, A and D ointment, or an antibiotic ointment until healed, usually in 3 to 5 days.
- Teach control of minor recurrent bleeding by the patient's use of cotton pledgets soaked in a vasoconstricting solution (e.g., 1:1,000 epinephrine) or a vasoconstricting nosedrop (e.g., *phenylephrine* [Neo-Synephrine] or *oxymetazoline* [Afrin]) and pressed against the bleeding site.
- Explain the importance of humidifying the home environment; have the patient keep a few windows partially open, place containers of water near radiators or stoves, or install a humidifier.
- Consider patient application of a water-based lubricant applied to the rims of the nostrils to maintain mucosal moisture.

First Aid. Few patients understand the proper treatment for care of minor nosebleeds at home; simple telephone instruction may obviate the need for an office or emergency room visit.

- Instruct the patient to *sit up* and remain calm, *lean forward* and *pinch the side* of the nostral against the septum on the side that is bleeding to tamponade the flow.
- Then have the patient spray the nose with any of the over-the-counter nasal sprays that contain *phenylephrine* (e.g., Neo-Synephrine) or oxymetazoline (e.g., Afrin).
- Follow with use of a small *pledget of cotton* lightly soaked with the spray and pressed against the bleeding portion of the septum. After 10 minutes, most nosebleeds will have stopped.
- Have the patient apply a *petrolatum-based ointment*, such as zinc oxide or Bacitracin, to the septum to prevent further drying and abrasion of the septum. It should is left in for a few days.
- Instruct the patient to limit heavy lifting, other forms of straining, bending over, intake of spicy or hot foods, hot showers, and medications that might impair hemostasis (see Chapter 81).

Reassure the patient when the nosebleed is purely a local phenomenon; many people attribute nosebleeds to hypertension and fear cerebral hemorrhage.

INDICATIONS FOR REFERRAL AND ADMISSION

Patients with *active posterior bleeding* should be admitted to the hospital immediately for emergency treatment to control the bleeding. All patients who undergo extensive posterior nasal packing need to be closely observed for signs of hypoxia and hypercarbia, because posterior packing can cause airway obstruction, particularly in elderly patients, due to downward displacement of the soft palate and subsequent palatal edema and swelling or slipped packing. Unfortunately, packs must be left in place for a minimum of 5 days to be effective. Posterior packing is associated with a great deal of discomfort. Patients generally require intravenous hydration because of poor oral intake due to painful swallowing. Additional needs include antibiotics to prevent sinusitis, pain medications, and careful observation by the nursing staff for impending airway obstruction. Packing can often be avoided, or removed earlier, if the patient undergoes an endoscopic nasal examination, and the site is visualized and electrocauterized directly, usually in the operation room. Failing this, where available, arterial embolization of the involved internal maxillary-sphenopalatine artery system can be used in life-threatening situations.

ANNOTATED BIBLIOGRAPHY

Hallberg OE. Severe nosebleed and its treatment. JAMA 1952; 148:355. (*A classic article that is still very useful.*)

Kirchner JA. Epistaxis. N Engl J Med 1982;307:1126. (*A review of anatomy, etiology, and therapy.*)

Perry WH. Clinical spectrum of hereditary hemorrhagic telangiectasia (Osler-Weber-Rendu disease). Am J Med 1987;82:989. (*Detailed review of clinical presentation; nosebleeds are major feature.*)

214
Evaluation of Facial Pain and Swelling
JOHN P. KELLY

The primary care physician often encounters patients whose presenting complaint of facial pain or swelling is related to the masticatory apparatus (teeth, gums, jaws, muscles) or salivary glands. Dental decay is the most prevalent disease in the United States and a major cause of conditions leading to facial pain and swelling. Because symptoms may be referred to nondental structures and because an odontogenic infection may involve areas of the head and neck seemingly unrelated to the teeth, the patient may first seek the advice of a physician rather than of a dentist. Prompt recognition and effective initial treatment may well prevent development of a serious complication such as abscess formation.

PATHOPHYSIOLOGY AND CLINICAL PRESENTATION

Odontogenic Infection. Dental decay is a multifactorial disease that encompasses dietary factors (most notably, refined carbohydrates), environmental factors (such as inavailability of fluoride ion during the production of the enamel of the teeth), and various host factors (not the least of which is the patient's oral hygiene habits). Oral bacteria use dietary carbohydrates to form plaque on the enamel of the teeth. Susceptible enamel is then decalcified, resulting in a "cavity" or carious lesion.

Tooth Decay and Inflammation of the Pulp. In its initial stages, tooth decay is asymptomatic. However, when the dentin beneath the enamel is exposed, the patient may complain of aching pain when the affected tooth comes into contact with hot, cold, or sweet substances. The frequent finding of referred pain may make localization of the offending tooth difficult and is one reason why a patient may first consult the physician rather than the dentist.

Progressive decay of the tooth will result in inflammation of the pulp (*pulpitis*). The symptoms will be unchanged until the dental pulp becomes necrotic and, eventually, suppurative. The cardinal symptom becomes deep throbbing pain on exposure to hot foods or drinks. The pain is abruptly relieved by ice or cold water. This symptom complex is distinct from the paroxysmal lancinating pain of trigeminal neuralgia, which has no relationship to extremes of temperature but may be related to eating because of the presence of trigger zones in the oral cavity (see Chapter 176).

Tooth Abscess. Simple dental decay, pulpitis, and pulpal necrosis are not associated with fever, swelling, or leukocytosis. However, when the infection of the pulp spreads beyond the confines of the tooth to involve the periodontal ligament and the adjacent alveolar bone, an acute *alveolar abscess* may ensue. In this condition, the affected tooth is tender to percussion or to masticatory forces and is mobile. The adjacent soft tissues begin to show edema, erythema, heat, and tenderness. The location of the involved tooth will determine the location of the swelling. Abscessed maxillary teeth will produce labial or infraorbital edema; an infected mandibular tooth will produce submandibular edema. Lymphadenopathy of the cervical chain can be seen in either maxillary or mandibular infection.

Complications. A facial cellulitis may result, causing fever and leukocytosis. Typically, the history reveals a preceding toothache with pain suggestive of pulpitis, followed by spontaneous regression and an asymptomatic period, corresponding to pulpal necrosis. Swelling and pain develop when the necrotic pulp becomes infected and the process spreads to adjacent anatomic structures. Further spread of infection along fascial planes or by hematogenous routes can result in life-threatening complications, such as *cavernous sinus thrombosis, meningitis, Ludwig's angina,* or *mediastinitis.* Although uncommon, such devastating complications are still seen today, even with the availability of antibiotics.

Periodontal Infection. Acute bacterial infection of the periodontal tissues is most often localized to the gingiva or mucosa adjacent to the involved tooth. The typical patient will complain of a "gum boil," and examination will reveal a discrete fluctuant swelling, which may drain easily on manual palpation.

In the late adolescent years, infection of the soft tissue surrounding erupting third molars or wisdom teeth (periocoronitis) is common. Low-grade chronic infection may be accompanied by symptoms described as "teething"; acute infection will result in pain, swelling, and difficulty in opening the mouth (trismus) as the adjacent masticator space becomes involved.

Salivary Gland Swelling. Acute infection of the major salivary glands (parotid, submandibular, and sublingual) may be either viral or bacterial. *Viral parotitis* (mumps) occurs most frequently in school-aged children and appears either unilaterally or bilaterally. The efficacy of immunization programs has made this disease a relative rarity. Viral lymphadenopathy in the preauricular area, such as that seen in infectious mononucleosis and in cat-scratch disease, may masquerade as parotid swelling and must be considered.

Sialadenitis, bacterial infection of the salivary glands, commonly affects a single gland. The infection is generally an ascending infection in which bacteria gain access to a gland made susceptible to infection by stasis of saliva. Obstruction of the salivary duct by a stone or mucinous plug is the usual inciting event, but any low-flow state can lead to sialadenitis. The condition is frequently seen in elderly, debilitated, or postoperative patients in whom dehydration may lead to decreased salivary flow and consequent infection. The parotid gland is the usual target; involvement is more often unilateral than bilateral. Purulent drainage can be obtained from the duct orifice. Previous episodes of parotitis or congenital abnormality of the acinar structure of the parotid gland may produce sialoangiectasis, which facilitates pooling and stasis of saliva within the gland and increases the patient's susceptibility to episodes of acute infection.

Systemic Conditions. Noninfectious salivary swelling may occur with diabetes mellitus, uremia, Laennec's cirrhosis,

Table 214.1. Important Causes of Facial Pain or Swelling

Odontogenic Pain
  Caries
  Pulpitis
  Periapical abscess
  Alveolar abscess

Nonodontogenic Pain
  Trigeminal neuralgia
  Temporomandibular joint dysfunction
  Myocardial ischemia (referred jaw pain)
  Giant cell arteritis (masseter claudication)

Salivary Pain and Swelling
  Viral infection (mumps)
  Bacterial infection
  Ductal obstruction
  Sjögren's syndrome
  Lymphoproliferative disease
  Tumor
  Chemical irritant

chronic alcoholism, and malnutrition. A toxic reaction to a variety of drugs, such as iodine, mercury, and guanethidine, causes a painless bilateral parotid gland swelling. A specific triad of keratoconjunctivitis sicca, salivary gland swelling, and rheumatoid arthritis is known as *Sjögren's syndrome*. The syndrome has also been related to other chronic autoimmune connective tissue disorders, such as rheumatoid arthritis, systemic lupus erythematosus, and polyarteritis nodosa. Sjögren's syndrome may initially present without apparent systemic disease. Lymphoma may develop in a patient with long-standing Sjögren's syndrome.

Lymphoproliferative Disease. Both major and minor salivary glands may become infiltrated by a lymphoproliferative process and enlarge. Lymphoma, tuberculosis, and sarcoidosis (uveoparotid fever) have all been first diagnosed from salivary gland enlargement.

DIFFERENTIAL DIAGNOSIS

The causes of facial pain or swelling can be divided into odontogenic, nonodontogenic, and salivary gland etiologies (Table 214.1).

WORKUP

History. Evaluation of facial pain and swelling requires thorough consideration of the pain's onset, severity, quality, location, radiation, aggravating or ameliorating factors, and duration. The various stages of dental infection can be characterized by specific pain histories. For example, pain brought on by contact with hot, cold, or sweet substances is indicative of dental caries, whereas aggravation by heat and relief by cold suggest a periapical abscess. If fever and swelling ensue, an alveolar abscess must be considered. Lancinating pain precipitated by contact with a trigger zone is typical of trigeminal neuralgia; it can be distinguished by history from abscess formation because symptoms are unrelated to the temperature of the contacting substance and swelling is absent.

In the patient who complains of salivary gland enlargement, it is important to inquire about site(s) of involvement, presence of fever or tenderness, history of chronic illness, malignancy,

toxin or drug exposure, and symptoms of rheumatologic disease or sicca syndrome (dry eyes, dry mouth). Unilateral painful swelling of acute onset suggests sialadenitis, especially when seen in an elderly, debilitated, or postoperative patient. A unilaterally enlarged painless parotid may be due to tumor, particularly if there is a history of progressive increase in size and extension beyond the gland. Bilateral involvement requires consideration of lymphoma and sarcoidosis and Sjögren's syndrome (which is bilateral in about half of cases).

It is important to keep in mind that episodic jaw pain may be a manifestation of coronary ischemia (see Chapter 20).

Physical Examination. A semisitting position will usually allow both patient comfort and examiner access. Although a flashlight can be used, a lighting fixture that can illuminate the oral cavity and leave the examiner with both hands free is preferable.

Inspection of the mouth for fractured, decayed, or heavily restored teeth and for heavy deposits of debris and calculus ("tartar") on the teeth and gingiva requires little experience and will direct the examiner's attention to odontogenic disease as a likely source of the pain or swelling. A dental mirror or a short-handled laryngoscopy mirror serves as a better retractor than does a wooden tongue blade. Palpation of the teeth to determine tenderness or mobility will help to identify an abscessed tooth. The soft tissues should be palpated to detect the presence of indurated or fluctuant swelling adjacent to a suspicious tooth. Tenderness to percussion of a tooth, using a short sharp tap with the dental mirror handle, is diagnostic of an abscessed tooth. The salivary glands are palpated bimanually intraorally and extraorally; the salivary duct orifices should be observed for salivary flow or purulent drainage during palpation of the individual glands. Cervical lymph nodes should be checked for enlargement and tenderness.

Laboratory Studies. Suspicion of dental caries can be confirmed by x-ray, as can abscess formation. Most other conditions produce few radiologic changes. White blood count in the potentially toxic patient or blood sugar in the diabetic patient may aid in subsequent management. Suspicion of Sjögren's syndrome can be confirmed by *lip biopsy* and followed by serum *antinuclear antibody* testing to screen for underlying rheumatologic disease. Any purulent drainage should be sent for Gram's stain, culture, and sensitivity testing.

SYMPTOMATIC MANAGEMENT AND PATIENT EDUCATION

Tooth or Periodontal Abscess. While awaiting dental evaluation, the very uncomfortable patient may require strong analgesia (e.g., ibuprofen, 600 mg, or codeine sulfate, 30 mg every 4 to 6 hours) or local anesthetic block with 2% lidocaine. Antibiotics are indicated when swelling and signs of infection are present in addition to pain. *Penicillin* remains the primary antibiotic of choice in treatment of odontogenic infection. Initiation of an oral penicillin-VK regimen of 250 to 500 mg every 6 hours is appropriate at the first recognition of swelling associated with an infected tooth or periodontal tissue.

Before certain dental work, *endocarditis prophylaxis* should be considered in patients with valvular heart disease (see Chapter 16). A single 2.0-g oral dose of *amoxicillin* 1 hour before dental procedures associated with bacteremia is the current recommendation of the American Heart Association. No postprocedure antibiotic treatment is deemed necessary. *Erythromycin* is no longer recommended for patients allergic to penicillin. The currently preferred alternatives to penicillin are *clindamycin* (600 mg), *cephalexin* (2.0 g), or *azithromycin* (500 mg) taken orally 1 hour before the procedure.

Referral of the patient to an oral surgeon for definitive drainage of the infection at the earliest opportunity is indicated and should be made simultaneously with the prescribing of antibiotics.

Sialadenitis. Acute swelling of a salivary gland, accompanied by purulent or inspissated saliva from the involved duct, requires antibiotic treatment. Stimulation of salivary flow with sour candies and warm compresses is a helpful local measure. The submandibular gland tends to be infected with the same flora as is found in odontogenic infections. Hence, *penicillin* is the drug of choice for *submandibular sialadenitis*. Acute *bacterial parotitis*, on the other hand, is associated with staphylococcal species, and one of the penicillinase-resistant antibiotics, such as *dicloxacillin*, is preferred. Antibiotic treatment for other infections that may have preceded the onset of the salivary infection can alter the oral flora and produce infection of the salivary system by unusual organisms, such as *Escherichia coli*. Thus, culturing of the purulent saliva is suggested.

Prevention. The U.S. Preventive Services Task Force has underscored the important role of the primary physician in promoting prevention of dental caries and gum disease. During the health maintenance examination, one should inquire into the time of last dental examination, examine the teeth and gums for plaque and gingival disease, urge regular brushing with a fluoride-containing dentifrice and flossing, and recommend yearly dental examination and plaque removal. Knowledge of the fluoridation status of the local public water supply is essential before the prescription of fluoride-containing vitamin preparations by the primary caregivers of the pediatric population.

INDICATIONS FOR REFERRAL

Early recognition of *dental decay* and *gingival inflammation* with consequent referral to a general dentist for complete evaluation and treatment is the most effective means of preventing infection. Referral to the dentist is especially important for patients who may have their mouth *hygiene compromised* by bulimia, Sjögren's syndrome, HIV infection, or upcoming treatment for cancer (e.g., head and neck irradiation, chemotherapy). In the patient with *valvular heart disease*, full dental evaluation on a periodic basis is mandatory and is particularly indicated before consideration of a valvular prosthesis so that potential sources of dental sepsis may be eliminated. Adequate antibiotic prophylaxis for subacute bacterial endocarditis must be provided for such patients at the time dental procedures are performed (see below and Chapter 16).

When physical examination indicates no other source of *facial pain*, referral for dental evaluation is indicated. Abscess formation necessitates prompt referral for definitive drainage. When the patient's clinical appearance demonstrates involvement of deep fascial spaces, as evidenced by fever, trismus, elevation of the tongue, or ophthalmoplegia, referral to an oral surgeon and admission to the hospital for parenteral antibiotics are urgent.

The patient with *acute salivary swelling* should be seen by an oral surgeon for radiographic examination to detect any obstructing sialoliths. Gentle dilatation of the duct may help to relieve the obstruction; in some cases, surgery is necessary to remove the stone. Sialography, or examination of the salivary system with radiographic contrast injections, is contraindicated in the acute period of infection, but noninvasive imaging with computed tomography or magnetic resonance imaging has largely taken the place of sialography in nearly all cases of salivary swelling, both acute and chronic.

When salivary swelling is chronic in nature, no antibiotics are indicated. If the differential diagnosis includes Sjögren's syndrome, sarcoidosis, or lymphoma, a biopsy of one of the minor salivary glands of the lower lip will usually confirm the diagnosis, without necessitating a more complex parotid biopsy.

ANNOTATED BIBLIOGRAPHY

Chow AW, Roser SM, Brady FA. Orofacial odontogenic infections. Ann Intern Med 1978;88:392. (*A comprehensive review of pertinent oral microbiology, surgical anatomy of the spread of infection, and the signs and symptoms of patients with odontogenic infection.*)

Dajani AS, Taubert KA, Wilson W, et al. Prevention of bacterial endocarditis: recommendations by the American Heart Association. JAMA 1997;277:1794. (*The most recent consensus recommendations for SBE prophylaxis; many important new changes.*)

Greene JC, Louie R, Wycoff SJ. Preventive dentistry: dental caries. JAMA 1989;262:3459. (*Recommendations from the U.S. Preventive Services Task Force.*)

215

Evaluation of Smell and Taste Disturbances

Impairment of taste and smell, in addition to being intrinsically unpleasant, is annoying because it interferes with the ability to derive pleasure from food. Moreover, a diminished ability to detect noxious agents in the environment leaves the patient vulnerable to them. Patients may complain of total loss, attenuation, or perversion of these senses. Problems of smell are often reported as alterations of taste because much of the awareness of taste is olfactory. The primary physician should be capable of recognizing taste and smell disturbances that are manifestations of serious illness requiring detailed evaluation and simple forms in which symptomatic relief will suffice.

PATHOPHYSIOLOGY AND CLINICAL PRESENTATION

Smell. The olfactory area is located high in the nasal vault above the superior turbinate. The neurons of the first cranial nerve penetrate the cribriform plate and travel to the cortex at the base of the frontal lobe on top of the cribriform plate. The most common mechanism of anosmia or hyposmia is *nasal obstruction* that prevents air from reaching olfactory areas high in the nose. Food is tasteless while the problem persists. In most instances, such as those related to the common cold or allergic rhinitis, the process is fully reversible, but sometimes more lasting damage is done. *Chronic infection* may lead to partial replacement of olfactory mucosa with respiratory epithelium. *Influenza* is known for its ability to cause permanent destruction of the nasal receptors; the onset is often acute. Another mechanism of acute anosmia is *head trauma*, in which the nerve filaments coming through the cribriform plate are damaged.

More gradual onset of reduced smell is typical of an expanding *mass lesion* at the base of the frontal lobe. Meningiomas and aneurysms of the anterior cerebral circulation are the most important sources of this problem. Upward extension of mass lesion into the frontal lobe is manifested by lack of initiative, personality change, and forgetfulness; posterior extension may involve the optic chiasm.

Perversion of smell (parosmia) can result from local nasal pathology such as *empyema* of the nasal sinuses, or ozena, a chronic rhinitis of unknown etiology causing thick greenish discharge and crusting (see Chapter 219). *Klebsiella* and *Pseudomonas* are often cultured from the discharge. Olfactory hallucinations are central in origin and may present as the aura of a seizure. The responsible lesion is typically found in the area of the uncus. *Olfactory delusions* are reported by schizophrenic patients while their sense of smell remains intact.

Many disorders of smell are of unknown cause. The mechanisms of reduced smell associated with *hypothyroidism, hypogonadism, and hepatitis* are not understood. Speculation has centered on the influence of various trace metals, particularly copper and zinc, but replacement therapy has been disappointing.

Taste. The tongue, seventh and ninth cranial nerves, and the hippocampal region of the cerebral cortex make up the taste apparatus. The front of the tongue detects sweet and salty tastes, the sides sense sour tastes, and the large papillae in the back detect bitter tastes. The pharynx also has the ability to sense taste. The taste buds are concentrated in the anterior two thirds of the tongue, which is innervated by the chorda tympani branch of the seventh cranial nerve. The posterior third of the tongue and palate are supplied by the glossopharyngeal nerve.

The most frequent source of diminished fine taste is *impairment of smell*. In addition, the taste buds may be directly injured by *alcohol and smoking*. The common observation that food tastes better after these habits are terminated is due to improvement in both the olfactory receptors and the taste buds. *Aging* results in small but measurable changes in acuity for salty and bitter tastes but not for sweet or sour ones. Elderly men differ from elderly women in that men selectively lose sensitivity to

Table 215.1. Some Important Causes of Impaired Taste

A. **Disturbances in Smell**
B. **Injury to Taste Buds**
  1. Age
  2. Smoking
  3. Hot liquids
  4. Dental disease
  5. Sjögren's syndrome
  6. Idiopathic conditions
C. **Cranial Nerve Lesions (seventh or ninth, partial loss only)**
  1. Ear surgery
  2. Bell's palsy
  3. Ramsay-Hunt syndrome (herpes zoster infection of the geniculate ganglion)
  4. Cholesteatoma
  5. Cerebellopontine angle tumors (advanced disease)
D. **Central Lesions**
  1. Head trauma
  2. Tumors (rare)
E. **Psychiatric Disorders**
  1. Depression
F. **Drugs**
  1. Captopril
  2. Imipramine (and other tricyclic agents)
  3. Clofibrate
  4. Lithium
  5. L-dopa
  6. Acetazolamide
  7. Metronidazole
  8. Glipizide
  9. Iron
  10. Tetracycline
  11. Allopurinol
G. **Metabolic–Endocrine Conditions**
  1. Hypogonadism
  2. Uremia
  3. Hypothyroidism
  4. Hepatitis
  5. Pregnancy

low concentrations of salt, whereas women have a more progressive loss of salt sensitivity.

Diseases and drugs that dry the mouth, for example, *Sjögren's syndrome* and *tricyclic antidepressants*, reduce the threshold for taste. Chorda tympani and seventh nerve lesions are rarely bilateral and therefore do not produce a complete loss of taste. Cerebral mass lesions usually do not involve the hippocampal gyrus. Depression, endocrinopathies, and a host of drugs are associated with complaints of altered taste. The mechanisms are unknown, but in many instances the primary disturbance seems to be, in part, an alteration of smell.

DIFFERENTIAL DIAGNOSIS

Most of the conditions that disrupt taste are annoying but not life threatening (Table 215.1). However, a disturbance in the sense of smell may be a sign of more serious illness (Table 215.2).

WORKUP

Smell

History. A primary objective is to distinguish local nasal pathology from a central or cranial nerve lesion. History of head trauma, worsening headaches, olfactory hallucinations, change in personality, unexplained forgetfulness, visual disturbances, gradual onset, or steady progression of symptoms sug-

Table 215.2. Causes of Disturbances in Smell

A. Nasal
   1. Upper respiratory tract infection
   2. Polyps
   3. Ozena
   4. Chronic sinusitis
   5. Allergic rhinitis
   6. Influenza and other virus
   7. Chemical injury (e.g., tar, formaldehyde)

B. Cranial Nerve
   1. Trauma
   2. Meningioma
   3. Cerebral aneurysm

C. Cerebral Cortex
   1. Seizure disorder
   2. Meningioma
   3. Aneurysm
   4. Schizophrenia

D. Metabolic-Endocrine
   1. Hypothyroidism
   2. Hypogonadism
   3. Liver disease

gests disease beyond the nasal cavity. History of head congestion, nasal discharge, allergies, sinus problems, influenza, chemical exposure, or a recent cold suggests the nose as the source of difficulty. Inquiry into symptoms of hepatocellular failure (see Chapter 71) and hypothyroidism (see Chapter 104) may uncover a metabolic–endocrine etiology. A careful psychiatric history is needed when there is description of abnormal smells in the absence of any other pathology.

Physical Examination. One can document the disorder by challenging each nostril with a representative sample of each primary odor: pungent, floral, mint, and putrid. Smell is most accurately assessed by the use of chemicals, such as pyridine, garlic-like odor, nitrobenzene, bitter almond, thiophene, and burnt rubber odor. Kits are available that contain these substances. Ammonia, which will produce a response by irritation even in the absence of olfactory powers, should be avoided.

On physical examination, the head is assessed for trauma and the nares are inspected for polyps, deviated septum, mucosal inflammation, and discharge. The sinuses are transilluminated to look for evidence of sinusitis. Fundi are checked for blurring of the disc margins, and the visual fields are tested by confrontation for evidence of optic chiasm compression. The skin, thyroid, and ankle jerks are examined for signs of hypothyroidism (see Chapter 104), and the hair, voice, muscles, and testes are examined for hypogonadism. Any jaundice, hepatomegaly, ascites, or asterixis should be noted.

Laboratory Studies. *Sinus films* should be reserved for patients with clinical evidence of sinusitis (see Chapter 219). *Neuroimaging studies* (computed tomography or magnetic resonance imaging) should be considered only if there is a history of recent head trauma or symptoms and signs suggestive of a mass lesion (see Chapters 100, 101, and 165). The same principle pertains to the ordering of liver, thyroid, and gonadotropin studies (see Chapters 71, 104, and 120).

Taste

History. The initial objective of the evaluation is to localize the problem. Intracranial disease is distinctly rare, so assessment can be concentrated on disease in the mouth, in the area of chorda tympani, and seventh nerve. Alcohol abuse, smoking, dental disease, and severe mouth dryness suggest a buccal cavity source. Facial palsy, herpes zoster rash about the ear, recent ear surgery, hearing problems, vertigo, and tinnitus are clues to diseases that may injure the seventh nerve. Drug use and concurrent metabolic or endocrinologic problems (see Table 215.1 and above) deserve exploration. Isolated reduction in taste requires inquiry into smell impairment and concurrent depression. Dry eyes in conjunction with dry mouth suggest Sjögren's syndrome, especially if rheumatoid arthritis is present.

Physical Examination. Careful examination of the nose, ears, oral cavity, tongue, and teeth is essential. The condition of the gums and teeth is worth noting. Taste should be assessed by challenging the withdrawn tongue with sweet, salty, bitter, and sour stimuli on each side and asking the patient to indicate what he or she tastes. Lateralizing the defect suggests a lesion of the seventh nerve. Examination of the cranial nerves needs to concentrate on testing of olfaction, hearing, and facial motor functions.

Laboratory Studies. If history or physical examination suggests hypothyroidism, a thyroid-stimulating hormone level should be obtained; likewise a blood urea nitrogen and creatinine should be obtained if renal disease is suspected. Sjögren's syndrome can be confirmed by lip biopsy. Suspicion of a cerebellopontine angle tumor is an indication for computed tomography.

SYMPTOMATIC MANAGEMENT

Smell. Local nasal pathology is often self-limited, but when chronic sinusitis or allergic rhinitis persists, definitive therapy is indicated (see Chapters 219 and 222). Avoidance of toxic fumes (e.g., formaldehyde) and removal of nasal polyps should also help. When influenza has caused sudden, complete, and permanent loss of smell, little can be done. Ozena sometimes requires local or even systemic antibiotic therapy; saline irrigations to remove obstructing crusts are helpful (see Chapter 222). Correction of hypothyroidism improves smell. A literature has developed suggesting that zinc salts will restore normal olfaction and taste, although double-blind controlled study finds zinc to be no better than placebo.

Table 215.3. Some Important Pathologic Causes of Halitosis

Oral cavity: poorly fitting dental work, periodontal disease, sialadenitis, abscess

Posterior pharynx: tonsillitis, diverticulum, tumor

Sinus: sinusitis, tumor, necrotic disease

Esophagus: reflux, diverticulum, motor dysfunction

Lungs: abscess

Metabolic: renal or hepatic failure; ketoacidosis

Psychiatric: psychosis (self-perception only)

Taste. Regardless of the cause of reduced taste, the patient should be encouraged to stop smoking and reduce alcohol consumption; often the development of a disability such as altered taste is sufficient motivation to get the patient to stop (see Chapter 54). If possible, medications that may impair taste should be stopped or reduced to determine what contribution, if any, they make to the taste disturbance. Any dental disease of consequence should be corrected. The same pertains to hypothyroidism (see Chapter 104). Concurrent depression may respond to a tricyclic antidepressant, but the drug may impair taste by causing a dry mouth (see Chapter 227); forewarning the patient can prevent side effects from becoming an unpleasant surprise. Disease related to the brainstem, chorda tympani, and inner ear requires referral for treatment.

INDICATIONS FOR REFERRAL

Olfactory hallucinations, change in personality, visual field defects, and impairment of memory in conjunction with disorders of smell and multiple cranial nerve defects, vertigo, and tinnitus in conjunction with altered taste are indications for neurologic consultation. Psychiatric consultation is worth considering when olfactory hallucinations are accompanied by other evidence of a thought disorder. Patients with ozena, nasal polyps, deviated nasal septum, refractory sinusitis, or a chorda tympani lesion may benefit from evaluation by the otolaryngologist.

A.H.G.

ANNOTATED BIBLIOGRAPHY

Rollin H. Drug-related gustatory disorders. Ann Otol Rhinol Laryngol 1978;87:1. (*A review of drugs that alter taste.*)

Schiffman SS. Taste and smell in disease. N Engl J Med 1983;308:1275. (*A two-part comprehensive review with an excellent set of references.*)

Weiffenbach Gordon RS. Variation in taste thresholds with human aging. JAMA 1982;247:775. (*Taste acuity declines selectively, not globally.*)

Appendix: Halitosis

Halitosis is defined as a foul breath odor arising from a person's oral cavity or nasal passages. It differs from disorders of taste and smell in that the condition is typically not noticeable to the patient. The condition may be physiologic or a manifestation of oral–nasal or systemic pathology.

Pathophysiology. The most common physiologic cause is so-called morning breath. The universal condition derives from the cessation of regular salivary flow with sleep. Its marked reduction and resulting buccal cavity stasis allow mouth flora an opportunity to feed on remaining food particles, sloughed epithelial cells, and stagnant saliva. The byproducts of bacterial metabolism cause the foul odor. Pathologic halitosis may derive from impairment of normal salivary flow (e.g., parotid disease, Sjögren's syndrome), increased presentation of bacterial substrate (periodontitis, sinusitis), or a metabolic derangement (renal or hepatic failure; Table 215.3). In rare instances, the patient is the only one to note the condition, strongly suggesting a hallucination of psychiatric or epileptic origin.

Workup. Similar to that described above for disorders of taste and smell, more attention should be paid to possible oral cavity pathology. It helps to begin the assessment by directly confirming the reported odor. Differentiating an oral source from a nasal one can be done by pinching the nares closed while exhaling and exhaling through the nose with the mouth closed. Esophageal and gastric etiologies may require eructation for detection. If the mouth is believed to harbor the suspected source, then the oral cavity should be examined carefully for poorly fitting dental work, periodontal disease, glossitis, tooth abscess, and tonsillar disease. The salivary glands should be checked for free flow of clear saliva in adequate volumes. Pulmonary disease and metabolic dysfunction are important to consider when the oral cavity and sinus tracts appear normal. Patients who have no objective findings but are convinced of halitosis derived from an internal source have a high probability of a hypochondriacal psychosis and need psychiatric referral.

Treatment. Treatment should be etiologic. Trying to mask the odor is far less effective than addressing its etiology. Mouthwashes are a poor substitute for good oral hygiene. Despite advertisements to the contrary, mouthwashes do little to suppress oral flora. Oral hygiene is particularly important in the elderly. Patients should be encouraged to floss and brush regularly, which help remove trapped food particles and promote healthy gums. Regular dental checkups are essential to recommend, although often overlooked.

ANNOTATED BIBLIOGRAPHY

Johnson BE. Halitosis, or the meaning of bad breath. J Gen Intern Med 1992;7:649. (*Thoughtful review of this very mundane problem; 55 references.*)

216
Approach to the Patient with Hoarseness
WILLIAM R. WILSON

Hoarseness is a symptom of laryngeal disease. Most acute episodes are self-limited and due to viral upper respiratory tract infection or voice abuse. However, the patient bothered by persistent hoarseness requires careful assessment, because carcinoma of the larynx, tumor-associated damage to the recurrent laryngeal nerve, and other serious conditions may be responsible. Prompt evaluation maximizes the chances of detecting an early lesion and achieving a cure.

PATHOPHYSIOLOGY AND CLINICAL PRESENTATION

Pathophysiology of Hoarseness

Vocal quality is determined by complex factors, including the distance between vocal cords, tenseness of the cords, and the rapidity of vibration. Hoarseness results from interference with normal apposition of the cords. Inflammatory, traumatic, and neoplastic lesions cause hoarseness by altering cord structure and function. Often the quality of the voice disturbance reflects the underlying pathophysiology.

A *"breathy"* voice occurs when the vocal cords do not approximate completely, allowing air to escape during vocalization. The cords may be kept apart by tumor, polyps, or nodules. A similar presentation occurs when the cords fail to approximate due to unilateral or bilateral cord paralysis. Patients with hysterical aphonia purposefully hold the cords apart while speaking.

A *"raspy"* or harsh voice ensues from cord thickening due to edema or inflammation. This is the voice quality characteristic of many heavy smokers. The voice is of lowered pitch and poor clarity. Associated inspiratory or expiratory cervical stridor results from laryngeal obstruction.

A high *"shaky"* voice or a low, soft, vibrating vocalization (vocal fry) often are consequences of decreased respiratory force (phonasthenia). These voices characterize elderly or debilitated patients who may complain of additional voice difficulties, such as change in voice pitch or poor vocal projection.

A *"muffled"* voice is characteristic of epiglottitis, causing airway obstruction. Although not truly "hoarseness," this cause of altered voice originates as a sore throat usually due to *Hemophilus influenzae* and may be accompanied by painful dysphagia and dyspnea.

Clinical Presentation

Acute hoarseness is associated with etiologies of acute vocal cord edema and erythema, such as *viral infection, voice abuse*, sudden excessive *smoking*, inhalation of *irritant gases, aspiration*, and occasionally *allergy* (hay fever). Vocal cord nodules may develop when edematous cords are used excessively. Fibrous tissue begins to collect at the junction of the anterior one third and the posterior two thirds of the cord. This results in a lowered breathy voice, which can harm a singing or speaking career.

Acute laryngeal edema may present as part of a generalized edematous allergic response involving the lips, tongue, and other hypopharyngeal tissues. Foods are important precipitants, especially seafoods and nuts; medications (especially angiotensin-converting enzyme inhibitors) can have a similar effect. Rarely, edema can develop from hereditary deficiency of C1 esterase inhibitor as occurs in hereditary angioneurotic edema.

Mechanical Trauma. Swelling forms in response to mechanical trauma, such as dental surgery or intubation for general anesthesia.

Croup and Epiglottitis. In the pediatric population, *subglottic* edema from viral laryngotracheal bronchitis (*croup*) can obstruct the airway. In adults, acute *epiglottitis* has been noted with increasing frequency. As noted above, it is associated with risk of airway obstruction, especially in the setting of *H. influenzae* infection. Symptoms include severe sore throat, dysphagia, dyspnea, and muffled voice.

Chronic Hoarseness. *Chronic laryngitis* causes a low raspy voice, a nonproductive cough, and a "dry throat" sensation. There is little or no pain. The voice waxes and wanes, worsening as the day progresses. *Gastroesophageal reflux disease* has been recognized as a common contributing factor. Another typical patient is a *heavy smoker* who continually talks, subjecting oneself to a combination of chemical irritation and vocal abuse. In rare instances, an infectious or chronic inflammatory condition (e.g., tuberculosis or sarcoidosis) may produce a similar picture.

Chronic Laryngeal Edema with development of dependent polyps represents another form of chronic laryngitis; it may arise in the setting of hypothyroidism, radiation therapy to the neck, or chronic sinusitis with persistent drainage and cough. Patients with this condition speak in a lowered gravelly voice with short phonation time.

Leukoplakia, another form of chronic laryngitis, is the term for the white scalelike appearance of hyperkeratotic changes involving the vocal cords. It occurs secondary to chemical irritation, especially from tobacco smoke and alcohol. Symptoms include hoarseness but no pain. Leukoplakia, which may be a premalignant state, cannot be distinguished visually from squamous cell carcinoma in situ or early invasive cancer.

Contact Ulcers of the larynx occur on the posterior third of the vocal cords where the arytenoid cartilage is covered only by a thin layer of mucosa. Once this mucosa is abraded, an ulcer often forms. Symptoms are painful phonation and a weakened breathy voice. Chronic ulcerations may in time develop into granulations that hold the cords apart, and at times these may become large enough to cause some respiratory obstruction. The ulcerations and subsequent granulations result most commonly from acute or chronic laryngeal intubation but classically are the result of vocal abuse by orators who misuse their larynx attempting to lower the pitch of their voices when speaking forcefully.

Vocal Cord Paralysis occurs with nerve injury. Usually just one cord is paralyzed (except in patients with severe central nervous system disease), causing a weak breathy voice. The position of the cord is affected by the amount of time that has elapsed since injury, because paralyzed cords tend to move toward the midline. The degree of paralysis and the clinical presentation depend on where the neural injury is located. Injury to a vagus nerve results in the loss of all ipsilateral laryngeal muscle function and sensation, leading to aspiration and a weak breathy voice. A more peripheral injury of the recurrent laryngeal nerve leads to little if any aspiration and a voice that is hoarse and somewhat weak, but less breathy. Viral neuritis is the most common cause; function usually returns in 6 to 9 months.

Laryngeal Carcinoma usually occurs in patients with a history of smoking and drinking. If the vocal cords are involved, progressive hoarseness is an early sign, but if the tumor arises on the epiglottis, hypopharynx, or false cords, hoarseness may be a late development. Pain secondary to ulceration is also a late symptom and is often perceived as referred otologic pain, especially when swallowing. These patients may have a mildly fetid breath. Patients with a hypopharyngeal or laryngeal cancer can present with an unexplained lymph node in the neck.

DIFFERENTIAL DIAGNOSIS

The causes of hoarseness are best considered in terms of acute and chronic etiologies (Table 216.1).

Table 216.1. Important Causes of Hoarseness

ACUTE HOARSENESS	CHRONIC HOARSENESS
Acute Laryngitis	Chronic laryngitis
Viral infection	Chronic or recurrent vocal abuse
Vocal abuse	Smoking
Toxic fumes	Allergy
Allergy (seasonal)	Persistent irritant exposure
Acute Laryngeal Edema	Carcinoma of larynx
Angioneurotic edema	Intrinsic to vocal cords
Infection	Extrinsic to vocal cords
Direct injury	
Nephritis	Vocal cord lesions
	Polyps
Acute Epiglottitis	Leukoplakia
	Contact ulcer and granuloma
	Vocal nodule (see vocal abuse)
	Benign tumors
	Vocal cord paralysis
	Laryngeal nerve injury (tumor, neck
	surgery, aortic aneurysm)
	Brainstem lesion
	Vocal cord trauma
	Chronic intubation
	Systemic disorders
	Hypothyroidism
	Rheumatoid arthritis
	Virilization
	Psychogenic

WORKUP

History. The evaluation of hoarseness depends on the chronicity of the condition. One needs to determine whether the onset was sudden or gradual and the course self-limited or progressive. Difficulty in breathing or stridor suggests obstruction and is an indication for emergency hospital admission. It is helpful to find out if hoarseness is exacerbated by talking, whether the voice completely disappeared, and, if so, for how long. Any recent upper respiratory tract infection, sore throat, fever, chills, sputum, or myalgias should be noted, as well as excessive voice use. Exposure to dust, fire, smoke, or irritant fumes should be documented, as should tobacco and alcohol intake. A history of neck mass, neck surgery, intubation, or lung tumor may provide important clues to etiology. Symptoms of hypothyroidism (see Chapter 104) are worth checking for when the etiology is not readily evident.

Physical Examination. There are two rules of thumb regarding patients with hoarseness. First, hoarseness of more than 2 to 3 weeks duration requires an examination of the larynx. Second, this examination will provide, in most cases, an immediate diagnosis.

Indirect Laryngoscopy. A good view of the hypopharynx and larynx is somewhat difficult to obtain, but the primary physician is encouraged to try and with practice can master the technique. Indirect laryngoscopy with a head light and warmed laryngeal mirror is a time-honored method and still provides the best and most rapidly obtained view of the area. For the gagging patient, premedication with 10 mg of diazepam orally and an analgesic throat spray (Cetacaine or

Xylocaine spray) are of benefit. For patients with uncontrollable gag reflexes, referral for examination with a fiberoptic laryngoscope will be necessary. This instrument is introduced through the nose, requiring pretreatment of the nasal passages with 4% cocaine or combination xylocaine–oxymetazoline solution for vasoconstriction and anesthesia. It is rare when a good laryngeal view cannot be obtained in this manner.

Even if laryngoscopy cannot be carried out, some clues as to etiology can be gleaned by a careful physical examination and noting voice quality. One needs to examine the oropharynx and carefully palpate the thyroid and cervical lymph nodes. The hoarse patient with an unexplained neck mass or lymph node requires a thorough check of the nose, paranasal sinuses, and nasopharynx. A breathy voice suggests poor cord apposition, which may be due to tumor, polyp, or nodule. A raspy voice is indicative of cord thickening due to edema or inflammation, as with chemical irritation, vocal abuse, and infection. The patient with a high shaky voice or a very soft one is having trouble mounting adequate respiratory force. Dyspnea is an indication for laryngoscopy.

Laboratory Studies. In most instances, the selection of studies depends on the findings at laryngoscopy and should be done in conjunction with the otolaryngologist. The patient with unilateral paresis of the left vocal cord may have a recurrent laryngeal nerve syndrome secondary to a tumor involving the nerve in the chest most commonly or at the skull base or neck necessitating radiologic evaluation of the chest and, if negative, skull base and neck. Pancoast tumors and carcinoma of the thyroid are unusual causes of vocal cord paralysis. If the cords appear chronically edematous and there is clinical suspicion of hypothyroidism, a check of a serum thyroid-stimulating hormone is indicated. Patients with a suspected carcinoma involving the larynx or with an unexplained neck node and hoarseness need a thorough evaluation of the aerodigestive tract before biopsy. Small-needle biopsies have circumvented the need for some open biopsies, which should be done only under select circumstances. The patient with recurrent edematous episodes and a positive family history might have angioneurotic edema; a check of the C1 esterase inhibitor level is indicated. Soft tissue films may be of use in the dyspneic patient.

PRINCIPLES OF MANAGEMENT AND THERAPEUTIC RECOMMENDATIONS

Regardless of causes, all patients with hoarseness should be strongly advised to *quit smoking* immediately (see Chapter 54). It is often in the setting of an associated medical problem that a smoker will finally decide to quit. Other measures are a function of the underlying etiology.

Acute Laryngitis. The best treatment is voice rest. When it is necessary to speak, the patient should use a moderate voice and not whisper. Warm sialogogues, such as *hot tea with sugar and lemon*, may be helpful. Antibiotics are not indicated unless there is documented bacterial infection. Cough suppressants, particularly with mucolytic agents, may be helpful. Also, *humidity* is of benefit. Inhalation of *steam* in a hot shower or breathing through a moist hot towel will provide immediate partial relief. When hay fever is the cause, a *topical steroid spray* such as dexamethasone or flunisolide helps provide symptomatic relief, but steroids should not be used unless there is an allergic etiology.

Professional singers or speakers should be advised to rest their voice when they become hoarse (especially during upper respiratory infections) to prevent permanent injury to the vocal cords. A vasoconstricting spray and analgesics are used by professionals when use of their voice is absolutely necessary. Occasionally, professional singers may be given a short course of topical or oral steroids to get through a singing commitment, but further cord injury may ensue.

Acute laryngeal edema represents a medical emergency; hospitalization is urgent. Treatment is based on the degree of swelling and subsequent airway compromise. An emergency airway is established if necessary; 0.3 mL of adrenaline 1 to 1,000 is administered subcutaneously, and steroids such as dexamethasone (Decadron 12 mg) may be given intravenously.

Vocal cord nodules should be treated early because often they respond to voice rest and vocal therapy. Nodules that do not respond to conservative therapy can be removed; use of an atraumatic technique (microlaryngeal surgery, carbon dioxide laser) is mandatory.

Angioneurotic edema does not respond to epinephrine or glucocorticosteroids. In an acute situation, intubation or tracheotomy may be required to maintain an airway. If available, infusion of *C1 esterase inhibitor* can be given. Otherwise, treatment is prophylactic, using anabolic steroids with attenuated androgenic effect (e.g., *danazol* and *stanozolol*) to stimulate synthesis of C1 esterase inhibitor. Such prophylaxis may be given for several days before planned surgery.

Temporary unilateral vocal cord paralysis can be treated symptomatically by the otolaryngologist through injection of collagen paste into the musculature of the paralyzed cord, moving it to the midline for 3 to 6 months. This permits the functioning cord to better approximate, thereby improving vocal quality. For permanent vocal cord paralysis, thyroplasty and arytenoid adduction procedures move the paralyzed vocal cord to the midline permanently and provide excellent results. As yet, no satisfactory procedure has been developed for bilateral vocal cord paralysis.

Carcinoma of the larynx can be cured, if detected in its early stages (T1N0). *Surgery, laser,* and *radiation* are all capable of achieving a 90% cure rate. Selection of modality depends on the type of expertise available locally and the location of the lesion. A better voice is usually obtained with irradiation. Metastases and a poor prognosis usually do not occur until the vocal cord cancer becomes larger (T3 to T4) and extends beyond the true cords. Early supraglottic carcinomas arising above the true cords can be cured in about 75% of patients with radiation therapy, partial laryngectomy, or a combination of the two. Larger lesions require combined induction chemotherapy and radiation with surgery for salvage, thereby sparing many larynges that otherwise might be resected. Prevention remains the best treatment; all smokers must be told to quit.

Leukoplakia is treated by vocal cord stripping under microscopic control. Regular follow-up examinations of the larynx are necessary. Repeated vocal cord stripping may be needed once or twice a year, particularly if the patient fails to limit use of irritants.

Dependent polyps are removed by microsurgery.

INDICATIONS FOR REFERRAL AND ADMISSION

Referral. If the primary care physician does not feel competent to visualize the vocal cords, a decision must be made about whether to refer the patient to an otolaryngologist. Hoarseness of greater than *3 weeks duration*, particularly when there has not been a history of an acute infectious process, requires referral. In those who have a resolving process and are at low risk for malignancy (young, nonsmoker, nondrinker), a complete otolaryngologic examination may be deferred pending full resolution.

Among patients who do undergo indirect laryngoscopy by the primary care physician, any patient with a *cord nodule, thickening,* or *paralysis* by indirect laryngoscopy requires referral, as does the patient with persistent unexplained hoarseness of more than 2 to 3 weeks duration and inability to tolerate indirect laryngoscopy.

Referral for *voice therapy* can help foster healthful vocal habits and is indicated for patients who experience repeated vocal trauma or who have organic disease and are in need of voice rehabilitation.

Admission. Any patient with concurrent *dyspnea* should be immediately hospitalized.

ANNOTATED BIBLIOGRAPHY

Frantz TD, Rasgon BM, Quesenberry CP Jr. Acute epiglottitis in adults: analysis of 129 cases. JAMA 1994;272:1358. *(The most common symptoms were sore throat and painful swallowing; muffled voice and pharyngeal erythema were the key signs; dyspnea was uncommon but important not to miss.)*

Vaughan CW. Diagnosis and treatment of organic voice disorders. N Engl J Med 1983;307:863. *(Still one of the best reviews for the general reader.)*

217
Evaluation of Tinnitus

A. JULIANNA GULYA

Tinnitus is an important but nonspecific symptom of otologic disease. "Ringing," "buzzing," or "roaring" are terms used to describe the sensation, which can be extremely annoying and a source of concern. The occurrence of tinnitus requires assessment for serious and treatable otologic problems. In the absence of a specifically treatable etiology, it is still important to provide the patient with some symptomatic relief, especially at night when tinnitus tends to be most bothersome.

PATHOPHYSIOLOGY AND CLINICAL PRESENTATION

Tinnitus remains very poorly understood. It appears to be a nonspecific manifestation of disease in the ear, cochlear nerve, or central auditory apparatus and is often accompanied by hearing loss.

External and Middle Ear Conditions. Tinnitus may result from *impacted cerumen, perforation* of the tympanic membrane, or fluid in the middle ear. The sensation is commonly described as low-pitched, intermittent, and accompanied by muffled hearing and a change in the sound of one's own voice. In *otosclerosis*, tinnitus is constant but may disappear as the disease progresses. *Acute otitis media* sometimes produces a pulsating type of tinnitus that resolves as inflammation subsides. Pulsatile tinnitus is also associated with *glomus tumors* and posttraumatic *arteriovenous fistulas*.

Inner Ear and Cochlear Nerve Disease. *Presbycusis, noise-induced hearing loss,* and *acoustic trauma* can give rise to a high-pitched tinnitus that is near the frequency of greatest hearing loss. Transient tinnitus that follows acute noise exposure is a forerunner of hearing loss and a warning sign to avoid repeated exposure. *Ototoxic drugs*, such as the aminoglycoside antibiotics, may produce high-pitched tinnitus and hearing loss that often persist after cessation of drug use. Salicylates are frequently responsible for reversible dose-related tinnitus. *Ménière's disease* results in transient low-pitched tinnitus that varies with the intensity of the condition's other symptoms, often worsening when vertigo and hearing loss are imminent. An *acoustic neuroma* produces a similar set of symptoms, but usually the clinical course is progressive, with unilateral or asymmetric tinnitus frequently preceding other symptoms, such as vertigo (see Chapter 166).

Other Sources. When ambient noise is reduced, all people will notice some head sounds. These may stem from a variety of events, ranging from the rushing of blood (most severe is aortic insufficiency) to contraction of auditory muscles. Loss of hearing due to conductive defects may accentuate the perception of tinnitus. *Tinnitus cerebri* is described as a roaring in the head and is believed to be vascular or neurologic in origin. A *cerebral aneurysm* with an audible bruit, a jugular megabulb anomaly, *palatal myoclonus* with audible muscle contraction, and an unusually patent *eustachian tube* that transmits respiratory sounds are examples of "objective" tinnitus in which the sounds can be heard by the examiner. Tinnitus may also be associated with temporomandibular joint dysfunction (Costen's syndrome).

Depressed and neurotic individuals may have less tolerance for normal head sounds and complain of them when in quiet settings. The ability to withstand tinnitus is also subject to much individual variation. Tolerance is lessened by fatigue and emotional stress.

DIFFERENTIAL DIAGNOSIS

Most tinnitus results from the same conditions that cause hearing loss, whether conductive or sensorineural, peripheral or central (see Chapter 212). Subjective complaints of ear or head noise in the absence of otologic pathology may be a concomitant of psychogenic disease. Objective tinnitus suggests cerebrovascular pathology, palatal myoclonus, or a patulous eustachian tube.

There are few data on the frequency of the various conditions responsible for tinnitus. Of interest is the fact that reports from otologic practice list as many as 50% of cases being of unknown etiology.

WORKUP

The diagnostic assessment of tinnitus follows the same pattern as that for hearing loss (see Chapter 212). A few additional points follow.

History. The pitch of the tinnitus is, unfortunately, of limited use in diagnosis, although some conditions are more likely than others to be associated with tinnitus of a certain pitch. Distinguishing pulsatile, nonpulsatile, subjective, and objective tinnitus may be more helpful. Any association of the sound with respiration, drug use, vertigo, noise trauma, or ear infection should be checked. A history of head trauma should be sought, because it may be associated with an arteriovenous fistula or an aneurysm of the intrapetrous portion of the internal carotid artery. When the problem is present only at night, it suggests increased awareness of normal head sounds. Most patients with tinnitus of otologic origin have an associated hearing defect or soon develop one, whereas those without other signs of ear disease may have vascular lesion or an accentuated awareness of normal head noises.

Physical Examination. One inspects the external ear and tympanic membrane for cerumen impaction, foreign bodies, perforation, signs of otitis media (see Chapter 218), and abnormal middle ear masses. Weber and Rinne testing should be performed to determine sensorineural or conductive hearing loss (see Chapter 212). The cranial nerves are examined for evidence of neuropathy or for signs of an acoustic neuroma or a glomus tumor. Testing for nystagmus (see Chapter 166) is worthwhile if vertigo is reported. The skull should be auscultated for a bruit if the origin of the problem remains obscure. Compression of the ipsilateral jugular vein will abolish the objective tinnitus of a jugular megabulb anomaly.

Laboratory Studies. An audiogram can help to identify and localize the site of lesion underlying the hearing loss. Neuroimaging studies (e.g., computed tomographic or magnetic resonance imaging) may be indicated but should not be done without first consulting an otolaryngologist to ensure proper test selection, performance, and interpretation. Gadolinium-enhanced magnetic resonance imaging may be recommended, especially in evaluation of unilateral or asymmetric tinnitus with or without hearing loss.

INDICATIONS FOR REFERRAL

Referral is essential when a conductive hearing loss is discovered because many of these lesions are correctable. Suspicion of an acoustic neuroma, glomus tumor, or cerebrovascular abnormality is also an indication for consultation, especially before embarking on an expensive workup. Referral to the otolaryngologist may be necessary to satisfy the anxious patient that everything has been explored and that there is no serious or correctable underlying condition.

SYMPTOMATIC MANAGEMENT AND PATIENT EDUCATION

For many patients, the priority is relief from the constant ringing, which can be very disturbing, especially at night. Drugs of all types have been tried, including nicotinic acid, vasodilators, tranquilizers, antidepressants, and seizure medications. None has proven superior to placebo. Nighttime use of a clock radio that shuts off after a half hour of playing background music often allows the patient to fall asleep. Keeping a radio on during the day when the patient has to work in a quiet room is also helpful. Many devices are promoted that one wears like a hearing aid (tinnitus maskers) to help mask tinnitus; they are of questionable value. Biofeedback may help in certain cases in which the tinnitus is related to stress.

ANNOTATED BIBLIOGRAPHY

Jastreboff PJ, Gray WC, Gold SL. Neurophysiologic approach to tinnitus patients. Am J Otolaryngol 1996;17:236. *(A description of the basis for the treatment protocol used at the University of Maryland Tinnitus Treatment Center consisting of counseling and the use of sound generators.)*

Levine RA. Tinnitus. Curr Opin Otolaryngol Head Neck Surg 1994; 2:171. *(A review from the neurologist's perspective of the components involved in the genesis of tinnitus.)*

Moller AR. Similarities between chronic pain and tinnitus. Am J Otolaryngol 1997;18:577. *(A review of the current understanding of the mechanisms underlying chronic pain and their relevance to tinnitus.)*

218

Approach to the Patient with Otitis

A. JULIANNA GULYA

Ear discomfort from otitis media accompanying an upper respiratory tract infection is one of the more common complaints encountered in primary care practice, particularly in pediatric settings. Adults are less susceptible but no less uncomfortable when otitis sets in. Symptoms range from vague fullness to frank pain and may be accompanied by diminution in hearing. Patients may present out of concern about the safety of upcoming air travel or underwater activities, especially if over-the-counter remedies have not brought improvement. The primary care physician should be able to effectively manage most cases. Knowing the roles of antibiotics and decongestants in the treatment of otitis media is essential. Discomfort referable to the ear may also be a consequence of otitis externa. Inspection often reveals signs of otitis media or external otitis. The primary care provider should know how to recognize and treat these common conditions.

PATHOPHYSIOLOGY AND CLINICAL PRESENTATION

Acute otitis media may be the consequence of abnormal *eustachian tube reflux* or *obstruction* that permits nasopharyngeal bacteria to infect the middle ear, which is normally free of organisms. Obstruction can result from mucosal edema and/or excessive mucus due to allergic or infectious etiologies. Viral nasopharyngitis is the most common cause, especially in the winter. It may produce little more than a *serous otitis*, which is generally "*sterile*". If there is bacterial invasion, a *purulent otitis media* may ensue. Of the bacterial species that can be isolated, the most common are *Streptococcus pneumoniae, Haemophilus influenzae*, and *Moraxella catarrhalis*. Viruses, *Staphylococcus aureus, Streptococcus pyogenes*, and other less-virulent organisms are less frequently etiologic.

The principal clinical findings are ear *pain, hearing loss*, and mild to moderate *fever*. The tympanic membrane appears bulging, and an *opaque effusion* may be noted behind the drum if a purulent exudate develops in the middle ear. If pressure builds excessively, the tympanic membrane may perforate with consequent otorrhea. A translucent *effusion* is characteristic of *serous otitis*; one may also observe apparent foreshortening of the manubrium, enhanced whiteness of the stria mallearis, and retraction of the tympanic membrane in the attic region. Most patients make a full recovery. In some patients, recurrent purulent otitis, sustained hearing loss, chronic serous otitis, or chronic otitis media may ensue.

External otitis develops in the setting of skin breakdown in the external auditory canal, leading to inflammation of the surrounding tissues. Skin breakdown is a common denominator, be it from trauma (e.g., from finger nail or cotton swab), excessive moisture (e.g., swimmer's ear), infection of a hair follicle, or chronic eczema. Itching, crusting, pain, redness, and/or discharge may be reported. Movement of the pinna is characteristically painful. Gram-positives, gram-negatives, and fungi can be variably isolated as infectious agents.

Malignant (necrotizing) external otitis is seen in immunocompromised patients and older diabetics. It develops deep in the external canal and usually represents as a pseudomonas cellulitis of the canal and adjacent tissues. Characteristics include purulent discharge, severe ear pain, and temporomandibular joint pain. Signs of facial nerve involvement may follow.

Chronic otitis media is a consequence of untreated or recurrent acute otitis media. Bony destruction or sclerosis of mastoid air cells may result, and the tympanic membrane is often perforated, draining purulent fluid. (Marginal and attic perforations may be associated with invasive cholesteatoma.) Both aerobes and anaerobes can be cultured from the drainage, including *Staphylococcus, Streptococcus, Pseudomonas*, enteric gram-negative organisms, and *Bacteroides*. Patients report little pain or fever, except during exacerbation, but hearing loss and chronic foul otorrhea are common. Radiologic evaluation may reveal the extent of disease.

DIAGNOSIS

Acute Otitis Media. The cornerstone of the clinical diagnosis of acute purulent otitis media is the finding of a *bulging tympanic membrane* with impaired mobility and loss of the bony landmarks. With serous otitis media, fever and pain are absent, and although fluid is present in the middle ear, it is translucent; the tympanic membrane is retracted and the bony landmarks are present. Cultures obtained from the nasopharynx are generally not helpful in defining the infectious agent of an acute otitis media. Needle aspiration of the middle ear is occasionally used to confirm the diagnosis and to identify the causative organism; usually such *diagnostic tympanocentesis* is reserved for those cases unresponsive to appropriate antibiotic therapy or in cases involving immunocompromised individuals.

Chronic Otitis Media and Otitis Externa. Diagnosis of chronic otitis media is suggested by presence of a *perforated drum and discharge. Pain on movement of the pinna,* erythema, and discharge in the external auditory canal are diagnostic of otitis externa. On occasion, a seemingly recurrent external otitis may reflect an unrecognized tympanic membrane perforation and chronic otitis media. Accordingly, careful otoscopic examination after resolution of the acute infection is important.

PRINCIPLES OF MANAGEMENT AND THERAPEUTIC RECOMMENDATIONS

Acute Purulent Otitis Media. Treatment includes use of analgesics, decongestants, and antibiotics. *Amoxicillin* is often the drug of choice. Because resistant strains of *Hemophilus influenzae* have been isolated in a substantial proportion of cases and because *M. catarrhalis* may be responsible for other cases, the combination preparation *amoxicillin–clavulanate* (Augmentin) is a reasonable alternative, particularly when an initial course of amoxicillin does not suffice. For penicillin-allergic persons, *trimethoprim-sulfa* or *erythromycin* may be substituted. A *sympathomimetic decongestant* (e.g., *pseudoephedrine*) may help when the otitis occurs in the setting of an upper respiratory tract infection and eustachian tube obstruction. *Myringotomy,* although not considered therapeutic, is indicated for patients with intractable pain, progressive hearing loss, or acute mastoiditis and in those who have had a poor response to medical therapy. Antihistamines are usually contraindicated, because their drying effect may lead to inspissated secretions.

Acute Serous Otitis Media. Cases secondary to eustachian tube obstruction from allergy or upper respiratory infection may improve with use of sympathomimetic *decongestants* (see Chapter 222). When allergy is suspected, some physicians add an *antihistamine,* but definitive evidence for efficacy is lacking, and, as just noted above, antihistamines may thicken secretions, impeding their clearance.

Chronic Otitis Media. The mainstay of therapy of chronic otitis media is careful aural toilet, with 1.5% *acetic acid irrigation* and *topical antibiotics* (ophthalmic drops tend to be less irritating). The acetic acid irrigation gently debrides accumulated debris and restores the normal acid pH of the external auditory canal. Despite maximal medical therapy, surgery is often re-

quired. Patients should be watched for complications such as intracranial suppuration, facial paralysis, sensorineural hearing loss, and vertigo. Persistent fever and headache are ominous in the setting of otitis media (either acute or chronic) and mandate expeditious referral to an otolaryngologist.

Otitis externa is treated with *topical antibiotics,* for example eardrops containing *polymyxin, hydrocortisone, neomycin,* and analgesics. Four drops are applied four times daily for a week, in combination with preventing water contamination (a cotton ball coated with petrolatum ointment usually suffices). Neomycin-containing eardrops, such as Cortisporin, can cause allergic skin reactions. A simple patch test will identify a sensitized patient. More severe cases of external otitis in which the canal is obstructed by edema or purulent material require referral to an otolaryngologist for suction aspiration of debris and insertion of a wick to promote antibiotic penetration.

Cellulitis/malignant external otitis requires systemic antibiotic treatment that includes coverage against *Pseudomonas aeruginosa.* The infection can be a life threatening in diabetics and immunocompromised hosts, necessitating prompt hospitalization, initiation of parenteral antibiotics, and referral to an otolaryngologist for consideration of need for debridement.

INDICATIONS FOR REFERRAL

An otolaryngologist should be consulted if acute otitis media fails to respond to medical therapy or if a complication such as tympanic membrane perforation, recurrent acute otitis, chronic serous otitis, or chronic otitis media develops. The onset of persistent fever, headache, facial nerve paralysis (or other cranial neuropathy), vertigo, or sensorineural hearing loss in the setting of otologic infection mandates emergency otolaryngologic referral. As noted above, hospitalization for parenteral antibiotic therapy is indicated if cellulitis of the external ear develops.

PATIENT EDUCATION

The pain of acute otitis media almost always leads the patient to seek prompt medical attention. Patients who have active external otitis or chronic otitis media with perforation of the eardrum should be instructed to avoid swimming and water entering the ear. As already noted, a cotton ball coated with petrolatum ointment provides a simple yet effective barrier to water entry.

Airplane Travel. Patients with serous otitis or eustachian tube dysfunction who must travel by air without delay should use oral and intranasal *decongestants* (see Chapter 222), especially in anticipation of descent for landing when the risk of barotrauma is greatest. *Self-inflation* of the eustachian tubes can provide symptomatic relief. The patient is instructed to pinch the nose shut, inhale deeply, close the mouth, and try to blow the nose while keeping it pinched shut.

ANNOTATED BIBLIOGRAPHY

Berman S. Current concepts: otitis media in children. N Engl J Med 1995;332:1560. *(A broad overview of the topic with a flow chart of treatment options.)*

Bluestone CD, Klein JO. Clinical practice guidelines on otitis media with effusion in young children: strengths and weaknesses [editorial]. Otolaryngol Head Neck Surg 1995;112:507. *(A critique of the U.S. Department of Health and Human Services clinical practice guideline.)*

Bluestone CD, Klein JO, Gates GA. "Appropriateness" of tympanostomy tubes: setting the record straight. Arch Otolaryngol Head Neck Surg 1994;120:1051. *(A summary of the indications for tympanostomy tube insertion.)*

Celin SE, Bluestone CD, Stephenson J, et al. Bacteriology of acute otitis media in adults. JAMA 1991;226:2249. *(H. influenzae and S. pneumoniae were the leading causes, and antibiotics against β-lactamase–producing organisms were not necessary in most instances.)*

Post JC, Preston RA, Aul JJ, et al. Molecular analysis of bacterial pathogens in otitis media with effusion. JAMA 1995;273:1598. *(Polymerase chain reaction analysis of pediatric middle ear effusions detects bacterial DNA in a significant percentage of culture-negative middle ear effusions.)*

Rubin J, Yu VL. Malignant external otitis: insights into pathogenesis, clinical manifestations, diagnosis, and therapy. Am J Med 1988;85:39. *(Still the most comprehensive review in the general medicine literature.)*

Stool SE, Berg AO, Berman S, et al. Otitis media with effusion in young children. Clinical Practice Guideline No. 12. AHCPR Publication No. 94-0622. Rockville, MD: Agency for Health Care Policy and Research, Public Health Service, U.S. Department of Health and Human Services, July 1994. *(Evidence-based consensus panel recommendations.)*

219
Approach to the Patient with Sinusitis
WILLIAM A. KORMOS

Sinusitis is an inflammation of one or more of the five paired paranasal sinuses surrounding the eyes. It is an extremely common, but likely overdiagnosed, condition, with over 30 million Americans treated for acute sinusitis annually. Many patients with nasal and sinus symptoms have self-limited viral infections or allergic conditions; the physician must distinguish these patients from the patient with a bacterial infection who may require antibiotics. Although acute sinusitis is often self-limited, there is significant morbidity associated with sinusitis. Extension of infection into the central nervous system and bone may be life threatening, and patients who develop chronic sinusitis rate their quality of life similar to patients with congestive heart failure or chronic obstructive pulmonary disease.

PATHOPHYSIOLOGY AND CLINICAL PRESENTATION

The normal sinuses are sterile structures lined with ciliated epithelium. Mucous is cleared from the sinus in a directed manner toward the ostia, or openings, which drain into the nasal cavity at the superior meatus and middle meatus. The superior meatus drains the posterior ethmoid and sphenoid sinuses, and the middle meatus drains the frontal, maxillary, and anterior ethmoid sinuses. Occlusion of these ostiomeatal complexes can lead to dysfunction of the normal sinus epithelium and bacterial infection. Although any sinus can become occluded through viral infection, anatomic abnormalities (including septal deviation, tumors, and polyps) or allergies can predispose to infection.

Acute Sinusitis. The *common cold* is actually a rhinosinusitis that frequently involves the paranasal sinuses. Computed tomographic study of patients with the common cold reveals that over 85% have a self-limited paranasal sinusitis that resolves without treatment. The maxillary sinuses are the most common site (87%), followed by ethmoidal (65%), sphenoidal (39%), and frontal (32%) involvement. Rhinorrhea and nasal stuffiness are the typical symptoms. In about 0.5% to 2% of cases, bacterial infection of the sinuses occurs, resulting in acute purulent bacterial sinusitis. It is characterized by nasal congestion, purulent nasal discharge, facial pain (that typically increases when the patient stoops forward), fever, fatigue, and other constitutional symptoms.

Bacteriology. In most cases, a single organism accounts for the infection; in about 25%, two organisms are present in high density. In over three fourths of cases, the causative organism proves to be either *Streptococcus pneumoniae* or *Haemophilus influenzae*. Other potentially etiologic organisms include *Moraxella catarrhalis, Streptococcus pyogenes,* and anaerobes *(Fusobacterium, Bacteroides, Peptostreptococcus)*. Anaerobes account for about 6% of all cases of sinusitis and usually occur in the setting of dental infections or chronic sinusitis, especially after recurrent courses of antibiotics. *Staphylococcus aureus* can be found on nasal culture, but only very infrequently is it isolated from sinus aspirates in acute sinusitis. *Viruses,* especially rhinovirus and influenza virus, have been isolated alone or in combination with bacteria in 15% to 20% of patients. This may represent true causation of the sinusitis or a preceding viral infection, leading to the bacterial superinfection. *Mycoplasma pneumoniae* and *Chlamydia pneumoniae* are not believed to be important etiologies for most patients. Patients who are immunosuppressed or immunocompromised are at risk for fungal infection, most commonly from *Aspergillus.*

Clinical Presentation. Sinus *pain* or *pressure* and *purulent nasal discharge* are the defining clinical features of acute sinusitis; fever is present in about half the cases. The location of the discomfort depends on the sinuses involved. *Maxillary sinusitis* is the most common and produces pain and tenderness over the *cheeks.* The pain is referred to the teeth in some patients. *Frontal sinusitis* produces pain and tenderness over the lower *forehead. Ethmoid sinusitis* results in *retroorbital* pain and may have tenderness over the upper *lateral aspect of the nose.* Isolated *sphenoid sinusitis* is uncommon but can present as retroorbital, frontal, or facial pain. Purulent nasal discharge may be visualized in the middle meatus if the frontal, maxillary, or anterior ethmoid sinuses are involved.

Chronic Sinusitis. Symptoms of chronic sinusitis include *nasal congestion* and *purulent discharge*, but pain and headache are usually mild or absent, and fever is uncommon. By definition, symptoms should be present for at least *2 to 3 months.* The predominant organisms are *S. aureus* and anaerobic organisms, such as anaerobic *streptococci and Bacteroides* species. *H. influenzae* and pneumococcus are less important etiologies in chronic infection. The pathologic importance of anaerobes in chronic sinusitis is reflected by the predominance of anaerobes in brain abscesses of sinus origin. Rarely, fungi such as *mucor, Rhizopus,* and *Aspergillus* species can produce invasive sinusitis in poorly controlled diabetics or leukemics. *Gram-negative bacilli* may cause sinusitis in hospitalized patients who are nasotracheally intubated or immunocompromised.

Complications of sinusitis are uncommon in the setting of antibiotic use but can be life threatening. Frontal sinusitis can lead to *osteomyelitis of the frontal bones*, especially in children. Patients present with headache, fever, and a characteristic doughy edema over the involved bone, which is termed "Pott's puffy tumor." The organisms involved are the same as those responsible for the underlying sinusitis except that *S. aureus* may also be involved. *Osteomyelitis of the maxilla* is an infrequent complication of maxillary sinusitis. *Orbital cellulitis* is most frequently a complication of ethmoid sinusitis due to direct extension of infection through the lamina papyracea. It usually begins with edema of the eyelids and rapidly progresses to ptosis, proptosis, chemosis, and diminished extraocular movements. Patients are usually febrile and acutely ill. Pressure on the optic nerve can lead to visual loss, which can be permanent, and retrograde spread of infection can lead to intracranial infection.

Retrograde extension of infection along venous channels from the orbit, ethmoid or frontal sinuses, or nose can produce septic *cavernous sinus thrombophlebitis*. These patients are highly febrile and appear "toxic." Lid edema, proptosis, and chemosis are present, but unlike uncomplicated orbital cellulitis, third, fourth, and sixth cranial nerve palsies are prominent; the pupil may be fixed and dilated; and funduscopic examination may reveal venous engorgement and papilledema. Although the process is usually unilateral at first, spread across the anterior and posterior intercavernous sinuses results in bilateral involvement. Patients may exhibit alterations of consciousness.

Finally, sinusitis can lead to *intracranial suppuration* either by direct spread through bone or via venous channels. A great variety of syndromes can result, including epidural abscess, subdural empyema, meningitis, and brain abscess. Clinical findings vary greatly, ranging from subtle personality changes with frontal lobe abscesses to headache, symptoms of elevated intracranial pressure, alterations of consciousness, visual symptoms, focal neurologic deficits, seizures, and, ultimately, coma and death.

DIFFERENTIAL DIAGNOSIS

The *common cold* and *allergic* or *vasomotor rhinitis* are by far the most common causes of "sinus" symptoms, but *polyps, tumors, cysts, foreign bodies*, and *vasculitides* such as Wegener's granulomatosis occasionally produce symptoms resembling sinusitis (see Chapter 222).

WORKUP

Clinical findings can be very helpful in diagnosis of sinusitis, especially when findings are considered in combination. In a prospective study comparing historical and physical findings with sinus films, no single feature had a likelihood ratio of more than 2.5 in predicting a positive x-ray, but when five individually predictive findings (see below) were considered together, the likelihood ratio rose to 6.4 if all were present and fell to 0.1 if none was found.

History. The diagnosis of sinusitis is entertained in the patient with symptoms of nasal congestion and discharge that persist beyond the expected 7 to 10 days of the common cold. The classic symptom of frontal, maxillary, retroorbital, or vertex pain that worsens on bending forward has not been found to independently predict radiographic sinusitis in several studies. A history of *purulent rhinorrhea*, however, has been associated with sinusitis in several studies (positive likelihood ratios of 1.5 to 3.5). In addition, prospective study in the primary care setting comparing clinical findings and radiographs in adult males presenting with symptoms suggestive of sinusitis also revealed that maxillary toothache and poor response to decongestants were useful predictors of radiologically confirmed sinusitis (positive likelihood ratios, 2.5 and 2.1, respectively). In a study from ear, nose, and throat practice using maxillary aspiration of purulent material for diagnosis, unilateral sinus pain also correlated with outcome. Finally, the symptom of *"double sickening"* (upper respiratory infection symptoms with initial improvement followed by increasing nasal symptoms) had a positive likelihood ratio of 2.8 in one primary care study.

Risk factors such as nasal polyps, deviated nasal septum, trauma, foreign bodies, and rapid changes in altitude should be inquired about. Special attention is paid to toxic symptoms of high fever and rigors in association with complaints suggestive of extension of infection, such as edema of the eyelids and diplopia.

Physical Examination. One should examine the nasal cavity for purulent discharge draining from one of the turbinates and transilluminate the maxillary sinuses for impaired light transmission. Transillumination must be performed in a completely darkened room with a strong light source. In a few patients, tapping the maxillary teeth may reveal a dental source of maxillary sinus infection. In the prospective study alluded to above, the best independent physical examination predictors of sinusitis were *impaired transillumination* (positive likelihood ratio, 1.6) and *mucopurulent nasal discharge* (likelihood ratio, 2.1). Other studies have found transillumination either more or less useful, which is partly explained by observer experience with transillumination. Palpation over the maxillary and frontal sinuses is often performed to elicit *sinus tenderness.* Although physicians often use this as a criterion to diagnose sinusitis, it does not appear to reliably distinguish between patients with and without sinusitis.

Laboratory Studies. As noted, the diagnosis of sinusitis remains a clinical one, albeit imprecise. The gold standard of a positive culture on sinus aspiration is too difficult and too invasive to be performed routinely for this predominantly self-limited condition. Additional testing may be appropriate in confusing cases, patients who fail to improve, patients with a suspected complication, or in patients with frequent recurrences. Some studies have suggested that an elevated erythrocyte sedimentation rate is useful in diagnosing sinusitis (likelihood ratio, 2.0); however, it is not common practice to obtain this test.

Sinus Films. Confirmation of sinusitis can be achieved by finding mucosal thickening, sinus opacification, or air–fluid levels on conventional sinus x-rays. For those with air–fluid levels or complete opacification, the positive predictive value is 80% to 100%; however, such findings are present only in 60%, reducing their sensitivity. Mucosal thickening has a sensitivity of 90%, but specificity is poor. Normal sinus x-rays in a person presenting with suspected sinusitis rules out maxillary and frontal disease (negative predictive value, 90% to 100%); ethmoidal involvement is harder to exclude. For the maxillary sinusitis, a single occipitomental (Waters') view is acceptable to examine the sinuses. Bone erosion can be present in chronic sinusitis.

Computed Tomography and Magnetic Resonance Imaging. Sensitivity of computed tomography (CT) is extremely high, so high that specificity is compromised (almost half of asymptomatic persons undergoing head CT for nonsinus reasons show mucosal abnormalities). CT is best reserved for complicated disease and search for occult ethmoidal disease in patients with refractory symptoms and negative conventional x-ray studies. It has also been most useful to delineate anatomy before endoscopic surgery. Magnetic resonance imaging has proven useful for differentiating mucosal inflammation from tumor. Neither study is appropriate for patients with routine sinus infection.

Ultrasound has been used in the diagnosis of sinusitis. Sensitivity is lower than for sinus x-rays, but specificity is higher. Expertise is not widely available.

Sinus and Nasal Cultures. Although used as the gold standard for research purposes, a culture of the aspirate from the maxillary sinus is negative in up to 40% of patients who undergo aspiration for suspected sinusitis. Cultures obtained from nasal swabs and even protected endoscopes are invariably contaminated with nasal flora and cannot be relied on. False-positive isolates of staphylococcal species are common.

PRINCIPLES OF MANAGEMENT AND THERAPEUTIC RECOMMENDATIONS

Acute Purulent Sinusitis. The optimal treatment remains controversial. The inaccuracy of the diagnosis of sinusitis and self-limited nature of the disease has led to a discordance between microbiologic and clinical outcomes. Although sinus-aspirate studies clearly document efficacy of antibiotics in eradication of bacteria from infected sinuses, randomized placebo-controlled trials find 70% rates of clearing among patients treated with nothing more than placebo. Furthermore, although many causative organisms demonstrate increasing degrees of antibiotic resistant, randomized controlled trials show no benefit for powerful broad-spectrum antibiotics over the traditional narrow-spectrum β-lactams and sulfas. Although clear evidence is lacking, perhaps elimination of underlying ostial obstruction through use of decongestants is just as important as effective antibiosis.

Decongestants are available in both topical and systemic preparations. The mixed adrenergic agonist *pseudoephedrine* is reasonably effective and can be administered by mouth. Popular sympathomimetic nasal sprays include *phenylephrine* (Neo-Synephrine) and *oxymetazoline* (Afrin), which is the longest acting of the topical decongestants. Patients should be instructed to spray each nostril once and then wait a minute to allow the anterior nasal mucosa to shrink. A repeat spray will then reach the upper and posterior mucosa, including the nasal turbinates and sinus ostia. This procedure can be repeated as needed every 4 hours with phenylephrine and every 12 hours with oxymetazoline for up to 3 days. Tachyphylaxis and irritation develops with prolonged topical use, but risk is minimal with short-term administration (1 to 3 days).

When there is an underlying allergic component to the nasal obstruction, one needs to consider *antihistamines, nasal steroids,* and *sympathomimetic decongestants* (see Chapter 222). Antihistamines are not for routine use, because in the absence of an allergic process, they may thicken secretions and worsen sinus outflow obstruction. Even in the setting of allergy-induced acute sinusitis, their use may prove problematic if too drying. Nasal steroids may be worth a trial if there is concurrent allergic rhinitis, but theoretically they could impede the response to infection, necessitating close monitoring of such therapy. Local application of heat may be soothing. Inhalation of *steam* or water and *nasal irrigation* with saline can help relieve symptoms of congestion.

Antibiotics. Patients with mild acute sinusitis may respond sufficiently well to decongestants so as to not require antibiotics, but in more severe cases of acute purulent sinusitis, antibiotics are commonly used. In the few randomized controlled studies that exist, antibiotics do demonstrate some benefit over decongestants alone, but cure rates without antibiotics remain high (approaching 70%). Nevertheless, many physicians administer antibiotics routinely to patients with sinusitis, often in response to patient demands. In a randomized trial of patients recruited from primary care practices with radiographic sinusitis, 80% of all patients, including those treated with placebo and those treated with amoxicillin, had no or few symptoms after 2 weeks. There were no significant differences between the groups in symptom improvement or in relapse rates over the following year.

Choice of Agent. Effective treatment does *not* require starting with a very expensive, broad-spectrum, penicillinase-resistant antibiotic. *Amoxicillin* (500 mg orally three times a day) and *trimethoprim-sulfamethoxazole* (TMS-DS, 160/800 mg twice daily) still remain the best options for initial treatment. *Doxycycline* has reasonable activity against known pathogens and may be used if the patient is allergic to penicillins and sulfa drugs.

Concern about rising prevalences of *multidrug-resistant S. pneumoniae* and β-lactamase–producing strains of *H. influenzae* (up to 40%) and *Moraxella* (100%) has stimulated use of such broad-spectrum penicillinase-resistant antibiotic agents as *amoxicillin-clavulanate, cefuroxime, loracarbef, azithromycin, clarithromycin, and levofloxacin* for initial treatment of acute sinusitis. However, randomized controlled trials and a recent meta-analysis have failed to demonstrate any advantage for such antibiotics over *amoxicillin* or *TMS*, suggesting that β-lactamase–producing strains and multidrug resistance may not be as clinically significant as feared. Furthermore, although intermediate penicillin resistance may be present in up to 25% of pneumococci in some communities, standard full doses of amoxicillin (e.g., 500 mg three to four times a day), but not TMS or the macrolides remain effective in achieving high rates of clinical cure. The popular second-generation macrolides such as clarithromycin and azithromycin may be less effective against the penicillin-resistant pneumococcus than previously thought, further eroding the rationale for their frequent use. The frequency of acute sinusitis and the common practice of unnecessary use of very expensive very broad-spectrum antibiotics have serious adverse implications not only for cost (10 to 20 times more costly), but also for promotion of antibiotic resistance in the community. Such agents should be relegated to a second-line role, reserved for patients who fail to respond to amoxicillin or TMS.

Knowledge of the prevalence of resistant strains in one's community can help guide initial antibiotic selection and identify when an exception to the rule to start simply is appropriate. The strong presence of a very highly clinically resistant organism in the community makes it reasonable to consider starting with a broader spectrum penicillinase-resistant agent. Alternatively, if the organism is *S. pneumoniae*, increasing the dose of a β-lactam antibiotic may suffice.

Duration of Therapy. Although the proper duration of therapy has not been identified, it is typical to treat with antibiotics and decongestants for 7 to 10 days, depending on severity and response. Partial responses and early relapses can be treated with another week of the same program. Patients who remain unchanged after 2 full weeks of therapy or deteriorate sooner should have sinus films obtained and a penicillinase-resistant drug should be prescribed. Further failure to respond is an indication for ear, nose, and throat referral.

Surgery. Surgical intervention should be avoided in acute sinusitis unless patients fail to respond to medical therapy and complications are present.

Recurrent and Chronic Sinusitis. Recurrent sinusitis is usually due to underlying allergic disease or an anatomic lesion and requires treatment of the underlying pathophysiology (see Chapter 222). Chronic sinusitis (persisting for more than 3 months) has a different bacteriology (see above) necessitating consideration of broader spectrum antibiotic coverage (e.g., *amoxicillin-clavulanate*). Treatment may need to be prolonged for several weeks. Attention also needs to be directed at underlying precipitants. Sinus irrigation or surgical drainage may be necessary.

INDICATIONS FOR ADMISSION AND REFERRAL

Admission. Any patient who appears *toxic* or has clinical evidence suggestive of *extension* to the orbit, bone, brain, or cavernous sinus requires urgent admission for emergency assessment and high-dose intravenous antibiotics. Warning symptoms include high fever, rigors, lid edema, diplopia, pupillary abnormalities, ptosis, and palsies of extraocular movements. The patient should be seen by both an otolaryngologist and infectious disease consultant. Antibiotic coverage is directed against both staphylococci and gram-negative rods. Surgical drainage may be urgently needed.

Referral to an otolaryngologist should be considered for patients who fail treatment with two courses of antibiotics, have anatomic abnormalities that predispose to sinusitis, or have frequent recurrences (greater than three per year). Functional endoscopic sinus surgery has provided a less invasive technique aimed at restoring normal anatomic drainage in the sinuses while preserving mucosal integrity.

PATIENT EDUCATION

Patients should understand that nasal congestion and frontal headaches are much more commonly caused by viral upper respiratory infections and allergic or vasomotor rhinitis than by true sinusitis. Nevertheless, decongestants are indicated in all these conditions to promote sinus drainage and prevent purulent sinusitis. The patient with recurrent symptoms should learn to recognize them and begin decongestant therapy, but the decision to begin antibiotics should be reserved by the physician. When antibiotics are prescribed, patients must be instructed to complete the entire course of therapy, because partial treatment will encourage the development of resistant organisms.

TREATMENT RECOMMENDATIONS

Acute Sinusitis

- Attend to any underlying etiologies, such as *allergic rhinitis* (see Chapter 222).
- Begin antibiotic treatment with *amoxicillin* (500 mg orally three times a day) or *TMS* (TMS-DS, 160/800 mg twice daily) unless the patient is immunocompromised or there is a known highly clinically resistant organism in high prevalence in the community. If the patient is allergic to both penicillin and sulfa, consider doxycycline.
- Consider concurrent use of a sympathomimetic decongestant (e.g., sustained-release *pseudoephedrine* 120 mg twice daily). Avoid routine use of decongestants that contain antihistamines because of their drying effect, which thickens secretions and risks aggravating obstruction.
- Treat with antibiotics for 7 to 14 days, supplemented by decongestants and systemic and topical hydration (e.g., humidification, isotonic saline nasal spray). Continue program for an additional 5 to 7 days if response is not complete.
- Consider a broad-spectrum penicillinase-resistant antibiotic agent (e.g., *amoxicillin-clavulanate, 500/125 mg three times a day; cefuroxime, 250 to 500 mg twice daily; loracarbef, 200 to 400 mg twice daily; azithromycin 500 mg day 1 followed by 250 mg every day on days 2 through 5; clarithromycin 500 mg twice daily; levofloxacin 500 mg/d*) only if there is a known highly clinically resistant organism in high prevalence in the community or if the patient fails an initial 2-week course of first-line antibiotic therapy with amoxicillin or TMS.
- Consider referral to an otolaryngologist when the patient fails two courses of antibiotics, has a suspected anatomic abnor-

mality that predisposes to sinusitis, or has frequent recurrences (more than three per year).

- Obtain dental referral when there is suspicion of an eroding tooth abscess and add anaerobic antibiotic coverage (e.g., clindamycin or metronidazole).

Chronic Sinusitis

- Refer to ear, nose, and throat specialist for identification and definitive correction of the causative pathology.
- In the meantime, treat with a broad-spectrum penicillinase-resistant antibiotic (e.g., amoxicillin/clavulanate 875/125 mg twice daily).

ANNOTATED BIBLIOGRAPHY

deFerranti SD, Ioannidis P, Lau J, et al. Are amoxicillin and folate inhibitors as effective as other antibiotics for acute sinusitis? A meta-analysis. BMJ 1998;317:632. *(An analysis of 27 controlled trials with over 2,700 patients total. No difference in clinical cure rate was apparent between amoxicillin or TMS and newer broad-spectrum antibiotics.)*

Gwaltney JM Jr, Phillips CD, Millers RD, et al. Computed tomographic study of the common cold. N Engl J Med 1994;330:25. *(Transient occlusion of the paranasal sinuses occurs in most patients with a common cold and clears without antibiotics.)*

Gwaltney JM Jr, Scheld WM, Sande MA, et al. The microbial etiology and antimicrobial therapy of adults with acute community-acquired sinusitis. J Allergy Clin Immunol 1992;90:457. *(Data on the bacteriology of community-acquired disease, including amoxicillin-resistant H. influenzae.)*

Hueston WJ, Ebertein C, Johnson D, et al. Criteria used by clinicians to differentiate sinusitis from upper viral respiratory infection. J Fam Pract 1998;46:487. *(Subjects depended on clinical features that are neither sensitive nor specific for sinusitis.)*

Poole MD. A focus on acute sinusitis in adults: changes in disease management. Am J Med 1999;106:38S. *(A concise review of diagnosis and treatment, advocating initial empiric treatment with amoxicillin or TMS.)*

van Buchem FL, Knotterus JA, Schrijnemaekers VJJ, et al. Primary-care-based randomised placebo-controlled trial of antibiotic treatment in acute maxillary sinusitis. Lancet 1997;349:683. *(A convincing large randomized trial of amoxicillin showing that about 80% of patients in both placebo and treatment groups improved at 2 weeks.)*

Williams JW Jr, Simel DL. Does this patient have sinusitis? Diagnosing acute sinusitis by history and physical examination. JAMA 1993;270:1242. *(A critical review of the clinical features used to make the diagnosis.)*

Williams JW Jr, Simel DL, Roberts L, et al. Clinical evaluation for sinusitis: making the diagnosis by history and physical examination. Ann Intern Med 1992;117:705. *(A study of adult men; five findings of predictive value.)*

220
Approach to the Patient with Pharyngitis
WILLIAM A. KORMOS

A wide variety of organisms may be responsible for pharyngitis, ranging from viruses and streptococci to gonococci and candida. The most common concern is infection due to group A β-hemolytic strep, *Streptococcus pyogenes*, because of the associated yet totally preventable risk of rheumatic fever (see Chapter 17). Because there is no single clinical feature pathognomonic for β-hemolytic strep infection, diagnosis requires attention to a host of clinical parameters complemented by timely judicious testing. The objectives are to promptly identify and treat patients with *S. pyogenes* infection and to avoid delay of therapy, inconvenience, expense, and unnecessary antibiotic exposure. Effective management of sore throat also requires an awareness of the full spectrum of etiologies and possible complications.

PATHOPHYSIOLOGY AND CLINICAL PRESENTATION

Respiratory viruses, chlamydia, mycoplasma, and streptococci account for most sore throats in adults. A host of other bacteria, viruses, fungi, and spirochetes have also been identified as etiologic agents. Allergy, inhalation of irritant gases, gastroesophageal reflux, and sleep apnea are among the noninfectious causes.

Group A β-Hemolytic Strep Infection. *S. pyogenes* infection accounts for 5% to 38% of sore throats in adults who are subjected to throat culture. The onset of discomfort is typically acute, with difficulty swallowing often noted. Pharyngeal erythema, exudate, cervical adenopathy, and fever greater than 101°F (38.3°C) are common but by no means pathognomonic. Children with "strep throat" exhibit exudate and high fever with greater frequency than do adults with the same disease. Cough, rhinorrhea, and other symptoms of upper respiratory infection are reported in less than 25% and suggest the presence of another etiology. About one fourth of adult patients give a history of recent exposure to streptococcal infection. The pharyngitis is self-limited; symptoms usually resolve within 7 to 10 days. Antibiotic therapy decreases severity and duration of symptoms.

Complications. Suppurative complications of streptococcal pharyngitis are uncommon in the setting of antibiotic use, but they are important and require attention. In *peritonsillar cellulitis*, the tonsils become edematous and inflamed. One or both tonsils may be involved. A grayish white exudate forms in conjunction with high fever, rigors, and leukocytosis. *Peritonsillar abscess* may ensue, with a fluctuant mass palpable. Other suppurative complications include retropharyngeal and parapharyngeal space infections. *Scarlet fever* is a rare complication of strep infection in adults. It results from infection with a toxigenic strain of *S. pyogenes*.

Acute rheumatic fever is the most important nonsuppurative complication. Although its incidence has declined dramatically over the past 40 years, recent epidemics in the 1980s have raised concern about the reemergence of this disease. The complication appears most frequently among children aged

5 to 15, but about 15% of hospitalized patients with rheumatic fever are over the age of 18. The chances of developing rheumatic fever increase with length of time that the organism persists in the pharynx and with the intensity of the immunologic response.

Acute glomerulonephritis is another nonsuppurative complication. Unlike rheumatic fever, it does not seem to be preventable by means of antibiotic therapy.

Other Streptococci. Groups C and G streptococci can cause pharyngitis, in some populations with a frequency approaching that of group A strep. Suppurative complications are rare, and rheumatic fever and glomerulonephritis never follow.

Viruses. Respiratory viruses, including adenovirus, parainfluenza virus, and rhinovirus, are the most common causes of sore throat. Pharyngitis can be the only manifestation of illness or may be accompanied by conjunctivitis, cough, sputum production, rhinitis, and systemic symptoms. Pharyngeal erythema, exudates, tonsillar enlargement, and cervical adenopathy are often present but with less frequency than in streptococcal disease.

Epstein-Barr virus is the agent responsible for *infectious mononucleosis* and is the cause of sore throat in 5% to 10% of young adults. Prodromal symptoms include malaise, headache, and fatigue followed by fever, sore throat, and cervical lymphadenopathy. Sore throat is the most common feature. The pharynx shows lymphoid hyperplasia, erythema, and edema. About half of patients develop tonsillar exudates, and about a third of patients will have petechiae at the junction of the hard and soft palate. Both anterior and posterior cervical adenopathy may develop; generalized adenopathy often follows. Splenomegaly is noted in about half of cases, and hepatomegaly and tenderness are present in about 10%. Clinical hepatitis sometimes ensues. A faint maculopapular rash and transient supraorbital edema occasionally appear. IgM antibody is the first to appear, followed by IgG antibody. Despite a transient flurry of interest about the possibility of Epstein-Barr virus infection causing chronic fatigue syndrome, confirmatory evidence failed to materialize (see Chapter 8).

Herpes simplex Virus and Coxsackie A Virus are other causes of pharyngitis. Herpes infection may mimic streptococcal infection with an exudative pharyngitis; shallow ulcers on the palate are characteristic. Coxsackie A infection (herpangina) is characterized by vesicles and ulcers on the tonsillar pillars and soft palate.

Other Organisms. In patients engaging in orogenital sexual activity, *gonococci* can lead to sore throat, pharyngeal exudate, and lymphadenopathy but more often results in asymptomatic colonization of the pharynx. In rare instances, bacteremia may result (see Chapter 137). *Haemophilus influenzae* is a rare cause of pharyngitis in adults, but the infection can be extremely painful and complicated by epiglottitis with life-threatening airway obstruction.

Chlamydia pneumoniae and Mycoplasma pneumoniae may account for a surprising percentage of patients presenting with pharyngitis, based on serologic evidence of infection, although the clinical significance of this finding remains unclear. The diagnosis of *M. pneumoniae* is rarely made clinically in the absence of pneumonitis.

Corynebacterium hemolyticum can cause pharyngitis and scarletiniform rash, particularly in teenagers and young adults. Administration of penicillin or erythromycin produces rapid improvement.

Meningococci are found in the pharynx in 5% to 15% of healthy people. Although sore throat may be a prodromal symptom of meningococcemia, isolated pharyngitis due to meningococcal infection is rare. Most instances of positive pharyngeal cultures for meningococcus represent asymptomatic colonization.

Corynebacterium diphtheriae causes outbreaks of diphtheria in unimmunized populations. The infection is characterized by development of an adherent whitish blue pharyngeal exudate ("pseudomembrane") that covers the pharynx and causes bleeding if removal is attempted.

Pneumococci and Staphylococci commonly reside in the nasopharynx and can cause severe disease in other parts of the respiratory tract. However, they do not cause pharyngitis except under the most unusual circumstances. When these bacterial species are cultured from the pharynx in both symptomatic and asymptomatic individuals, colonization, not causation, by these organisms should be suspected. However, mixed infections with normal mouth flora do occur in debilitated patients.

Fusobacteria and *spirochetes* can cause gingivitis ("trenchmouth") or necrotic tonsillar ulcers ("Vincent's angina"). Patients present with foul breath, pain, pharyngeal exudate, and a dirty gray membranous inflammation, which bleeds easily. A similar combination of bacteria and spirochetes can produce an extremely serious invasive gangrene of the mouth known as cancrum oris. This process occurs only in malnourished infants or patients with advanced malignancy and immunosuppression and is, fortunately, rare. *Treponema pallidum* can cause pharyngitis as part of primary or secondary syphilis. The diagnosis requires a high index of suspicion and serologic confirmation.

Yersinia enterocolitica infection typically presents as enterocolitis, but occasionally in adults it presents as pharyngitis in the absence of enteritis. Fatalities have been reported.

Candida albicans, present in the normal mouth flora, can produce pharyngitis if antibiotics, immunosuppressive agents, or debilitating illness upsets microbial interactions or host defenses. Oropharyngeal moniliasis (thrush) can be painful and is characterized by a cheesy white exudate, which can be scraped off to demonstrate yeast forms by smear and culture. Oral moniliasis may be the first symptomatic manifestation of HIV infection (see Chapter 13).

WORKUP

The first task is to attempt a clinical estimate of the risk of *S. pyogenes* infection. Often, this is done in a preliminary way over the telephone, which places a premium on risk stratification by historical features.

History. No single symptom or historical feature is diagnostic of group A β-hemolytic strep infection. Consequently, investigators have sought to identify symptoms that are at least independent predictors of strep infection and to see how clusters of such symptoms perform for triaging.

One such triaging cluster uses presence of *fever* and *difficulty swallowing* in support of the diagnosis of strep infection and *cough* as a negating factor. A score is assigned to each factor based on severity (0 through 3). The final score is derived by subtracting the score for cough from those for fever and difficulty swallowing. Designating a score of 2 or more as "positive" for a diagnosis of *S. pyogenes* infection, the system has a sensitivity of 85% and a specificity of 41.5%. In a pharyngitis population with the usual prevalence of strep (10% of sore throats due to *S. pyogenes*), a score of 6 (the highest possible score) would produce a positive predictive value of 34% for strep infection; a score of −3 (the lowest possible score) would reduce the risk to 1%. In a pharyngitis population with a high strep prevalence (prevalence, 34%), a score of 6 would indicate a 70% chance of strep infection; a score of −3 would reduce the risk to 3%. Although far from perfect, such a scheme may help in deciding who should come in for further evaluation.

History can help determine prevalence and risk from strep infection by inquiring into *exposure* to family members with current documented strep pharyngitis and any history of prior *rheumatic fever*. Other factors found predictive of strep infection that might be elicited over the telephone include *positive throat culture* in the preceding year, tender anterior cervical *adenopathy, temperature* higher than 101°F, and absence of rhinorrhea and itchy eyes.

Regarding other sore throat etiologies and complications, one should ask about orogenital sexual contact, concurrent steroid or immunosuppressive therapy, and any dyspnea.

Physical Examination. Several physical findings when considered collectively can help assess probability of group A β-hemolytic streptococcal infection. The cluster of marked *tonsillar exudate*, anterior *cervical adenopathy*, and temperature greater than *101°F* provides a positive predictive value of about 30% in pharyngitis populations with 10% prevalence of strep infection. The absence of these three features in addition to the presence of cough reduces the probability to 3%.

Examination of the pharynx is useful for identifying a less common cause of pharyngitis such as thrush, characterized by its white cheesy exudate; gingivitis or necrotic tonsillar ulcers suggest fusobacteria and spirochetes. Associated physical findings, such as a viral exanthem, conjunctivitis, petechiae, generalized lymphadenopathy, splenomegaly, or hepatic tenderness, may provide important clues to etiology. A "sandpaper" erythematous rash with accentuation in the groin and axillae is associated with scarlet fever. Patients with severe dysphagia or dyspnea require urgent evaluation to exclude airway obstruction. If epiglottitis is suspected, the airway should not be instrumented.

Laboratory Study for Suspected Strep Pharyngitis. Prompt diagnosis and treatment of *S. pyogenes* infection has been greatly facilitated by the advent of rapid strep-antigen testing. Throat culture has been relegated to a secondary role.

Rapid Strep-Antigen Testing. Office identification of group A streptococcal pharyngitis can be achieved by taking a swab of the posterior pharynx and subjecting the specimen to rapid strep-antigen testing. For most commercially available preparations, sensitivity ranges from 85% to 90% and specificity from 95% to 99%. Small numbers of organisms are less likely to be detected. Technique for obtaining the sample is similar to that for a throat culture and includes swabbing both tonsils and posterior pharynx.

Decision-analysis study finds that rapid strep-antigen testing followed by treatment is the optimal approach to workup

when the patient's pretest probability for strep infection is between 1% and 50% (which is the case for most patients). Pharyngitis patients at high risk for rheumatic fever (i.e., those with a history of rheumatic fever) and those with a very high probability of strep infection (e.g., persons in a closed population experiencing an epidemic of streptococcal pharyngitis) can forgo testing and be treated directly.

Throat Culture. Culturing a retropharyngeal swab remains the standard for identification of streptococcal pharyngitis and has a high sensitivity (90% to 95%) when performed correctly. A culture should be obtained when rapid antigen testing is negative yet clinical suspicion remains high. Patients with typical symptoms and signs of a viral upper respiratory infection and no historical or physical examination evidence suggestive of streptococcal infection do not need a throat culture.

Repeat culture after antibiotic treatment is not indicated because most positive cultures after treatment represent streptococcal carriers and not true infection. However, repeat culture should be performed in the patient with a history of rheumatic fever and may be considered during outbreaks of strep throat, especially when reinfection by close contacts is suspected.

In addition to the time required to obtain a result, an important shortcoming of throat culture is difficulty differentiating infection from colonization. As many as 20% to 30% of patients may be carriers. Definitive identification of significant infection with risk of rheumatic fever necessitates *serologic testing* for an antibody response. Such testing is of little practical use because results do not become available in time to be of help.

Laboratory Study for Other Etiologies. Laboratory testing is indicated when the result will have an impact on management. For example, viral pharyngitis due to respiratory pathogens is essentially a clinical diagnosis and requires no laboratory investigation. On the other hand, the patient with sore throat and diffuse lymphadenopathy, splenomegaly, and pharyngeal petechiae deserves evaluation for infectious mononucleosis. A *heterophile antibody* is a useful confirmatory test, provided there is no prior history of infectious mononucleosis. It may take as long as 3 weeks for the heterophile to become positive, necessitating a repeat test in a few weeks if it is initially negative. Alternatively, one can check serology for antibodies to Epstein-Barr virus. IgM antibodies can be demonstrated during the second week of illness, replaced later by IgG antibodies. Heterophile-negative mononucleosis may be due to cytomegalovirus infection.

The patient with a history of orogenital contact who is suspected of having possible gonococcal infection should have a throat swab plated onto *Thayer-Martin media* (see Chapter 137). Suspected candidal infection can be confirmed by scraping off the exudate and examining a *KOH prep* for yeast forms.

PRINCIPLES OF MANAGEMENT AND THERAPEUTIC RECOMMENDATIONS
Suspected S. pyogenes Infection
Rationale for Treatment. The reasons for treating strep infection are to speed symptomatic relief and prevent rheumatic fever, peritonsillar or retropharyngeal abscess, and spread of streptococcal infection. Rheumatic fever can be prevented by prompt eradication of *S. pyogenes* from the throat. The attack rate for rheumatic fever is reduced by over 90% if antibiotic

therapy is instituted within a week of the onset of sore throat. However, the efficacy of prophylactic therapy is substantially reduced if there is a marked delay in initiating treatment. Starting antibiotics 2 weeks after sore throat is first noted is associated with a reduction in attack rate of only 67%, and delaying treatment until 3 weeks into the illness provides no more than a 40% reduction in attack rate.

Treatment Strategies. There are several approaches to treatment of pharyngitis. The choice depends on the probability of strep infection, the likelihood of patient compliance, the chance of an adverse reaction to antibiotics, and the benefits of treating immediately versus waiting for culture results.

Immediate Treatment without Prior Testing. Pharyngitis patients with a *history of rheumatic fever* and those who are symptomatic and have a *household member* with a documented group A β-streptococcal infection should receive immediate treatment without need for prior testing or even an office visit. High-risk patients who have a prior history of rheumatic fever might already be on prophylactic therapy (see Chapter 17). Patients with a strongly suggestive clinical presentation (e.g., exudative pharyngitis, temperature higher than 101°F, tender bilateral anterior cervical adenopathy, and no rhinorrhea or cough) might also be candidates for empiric antibiotic therapy.

Antigen Testing Followed by Treatment of Positives. In most pharyngitis patients with a low to intermediate probability of strep infection, the preferred approach, as noted above, is rapid strep-antigen testing followed by treatment of positives. Throat culturing followed by treatment of a positive result is reserved for the patient with a good clinical story (two or more predictive factors) but a negative rapid antigen test.

Antibiotic Program. To be effective, antibiotic therapy must completely eradicate the streptococcus from the pharynx. This can be achieved by a single intramuscular injection of 1.2 million units of *benzathine penicillin* or a 10-day course of oral *phenoxymethyl penicillin* (250 mg three or four times a day). The advantages of the intramuscular route are the certainty of full treatment and convenience. Its major disadvantage is a 5- to 10-fold increase in the incidence of serious allergic reactions to penicillin. In the patient allergic to penicillin, oral *erythromycin* (250 mg four times a day for 10 days) is an effective alternative.

Recurrent Infection. The patient who returns with recurrent pharyngitis and a positive strep culture should be examined for alternative possibilities besides reinfection. The patient may have been *noncompliant* with oral antibiotics, and benzathine penicillin may be an appropriate option. Alternatively, the patient may be a carrier for group A streptococcus and have a concurrent *noninfectious etiology* for a sore throat, such as allergic rhinitis. Appropriate treatment depends on the underlying etiology. Tonsillectomy, once quite popular in children, remains unproven in adults to reduce recurrent infections or symptoms. Consultation with an ear, nose, and throat specialist may be considered for recalcitrant cases.

Other Types of Pharyngitis

The Meningococcal Carrier State sometimes presents a therapeutic dilemma in terms of both selecting patients who actually need treatment and in choosing antibiotics. Carriers should be treated only when there is evidence of active meningococcal disease in household or dormitory contacts. Penicillin will not eradicate the meningococcal carrier state, and because many strains are now sulfonamide resistant, rifampin should be used.

In Gonococcal Pharyngitis, the usual treatment with ceftriaxone 250 mg intramuscularly is effective (see Chapter 137). Ciprofloxacin and azithromycin have also demonstrated high cure rates. In the case of *diphtheria, antitoxin* is necessary to prevent myocarditis and peripheral neuritis and is the mainstay of therapy. Both erythromycin and penicillin can eliminate the organism from the upper respiratory tract. In *epiglottitis,* hospitalization is needed. *Necrotizing pharyngitis* due to fusobacterial infection responds to *penicillin* and good nutrition. In other bacterial etiologies of pharyngitis (*Chlamydia, Mycoplasma*), antibiotics have not been shown to improve clinical outcome.

Pharyngeal Candidiasis in the immunocompromised patient may benefit from gargling with oral *nystatin* suspension (100,000 U/mL), 15 mL swish-and-swallow six times per day, or from using a 10-mg *clotrimazole troche* held in the mouth for 15 to 30 minutes three times each day.

Viral Sore Throats are treated symptomatically. Voice rest, humidification, and lozenges or hard candy provide some relief; saline gargling and aspirin or acetaminophen also help.

PATIENT EDUCATION

Many pharyngitis patients telephone in requesting empiric antibiotic therapy for sore throat. They assume antibiotics are effective against most pathogens, desire prompt symptomatic relief, want to avoid the time and expense of testing, and have little fear of an adverse reaction to antibiotics. Much of the unnecessary antibiotic exposure associated with management of pharyngitis is probably due as much to patient insistence as to the physician's desire to do something. However, studies demonstrate that patient satisfaction is not associated with receiving antibiotics but instead correlates with addressing patient concerns and communicating a diagnosis. Unwarranted antibiotic prescriptions also run the risk of "medicalizing" the sore throat, resulting in increased patient visits for future episodes. When the probability of strep infection is deemed too low to warrant testing or treatment (see above), patients should be reassured that the risk is nil and that antibiotics are unlikely to provide any benefit. For the insistent person and the one with an intermediate risk by triage history, an invitation to come in for rapid antigen testing is the most reasonable advice.

The patient who proves to have *S. pyogenes* infection and elects oral antibiotic therapy should be carefully instructed on the risk of rheumatic fever and the importance of completing a full 10-day course of antibiotics. Otherwise, many patients will stop taking the medication when symptoms resolve.

Patients with recurrent strep infections and intact tonsils will ask about tonsillectomy. Reviewing the risks and benefits of tonsillectomy over medical therapy may help them to choose the treatment that best meets their needs.

ANNOTATED BIBLIOGRAPHY

Bisno AL, Gerber MA, Gwaltney JM, et al. Diagnosis and management of group A streptococcal pharyngitis: a practice guideline. Clin Infect Dis 1997;25:574. (*Evidence-based guideline from Infectious Disease Society of America.*)

Clancy CM, Centor RM, Campbell MS, et al. Rational decision making based on history: adult sore throats. J Gen Intern Med 1988; 3:213. (*Uses fever, difficulty swallowing, and cough to generate a score that predicts the probability of a positive rapid strep-antigen test.*)

Gerber MA, Tanz RR, Kabat W, et al. Optical immunoassay test for group A beta-hemolytic streptococcal pharyngitis. JAMA 1997; 277:899. (*In over 2,000 pediatric patients, a newer antigen detection test was more sensitive than standard blood agar culture and 84% sensitive compared with a gold standard broth-enhanced culture.*)

Hillner BE, Centor RM. What a difference a day makes: a decision analysis of adult streptococcal pharyngitis. J Gen Intern Med 1987;2:242. (*Recommends rapid strep-antigen testing for most adults with suspected strep pharyngitis.*)

Huovinen P, Lahtonen R, Ziegler T, et al. Pharyngitis in adults: the presence and coexistence of viruses and bacterial organisms. Ann Intern Med 1989;110:612. (*A wide variety of organisms found, including group C strep,* M. pneumoniae, *and* C. pneumoniae.)

Komaroff AL, Pass TM, Aronson MD, et al. The prediction of streptococcal pharyngitis in adults. J Gen Intern Med 1986;1:1. (*A clinical decision rule to identify* S. pyogenes *infection.*)

Krober MS, Bass JW, Michels GN. Streptococcal pharyngitis: clinical response to penicillin therapy. JAMA 1985;253:1271. (*Early penicillin therapy significantly ameliorates symptoms and shortens their duration.*)

Little P, Gould C, Williamson I, et al. Reattendance and complications in a randomized trial of prescribing strategies for sore throat: the medicalising effect of prescribing antibiotics. BMJ 1997;315:350. (*Patients empirically prescribed antibiotics for sore throat had a higher rate of return to the clinic for sore throat at 1 year compared with patients treated without antibiotics or with a delayed prescription.*)

McIsaac WJ, White D, Tannenbaum D, et al. A clinical score to reduce unnecessary antibiotic use in patients with sore throat. Can Med Assoc J 1998;158:75. (*A validated predictive model for* S. pyogenes *infection that includes age over 45 as a negating factor. The suggested algorithm would result in a 48% reduction in antibiotic use in the family practice site studied.*)

Ophir D, Bawnik J, Poria Y, et al. Peritonsillar abscess: a prospective evaluation of outpatient management by needle aspiration. Arch Otolaryngol Head Neck Surg 1988;114:661. (*Needle aspiration can allow outpatient management of selected patients.*)

Paradise JL, Bluestone CD, Bachman RZ, et al. Efficacy of tonsillectomy in recurrent throat infection in severely affected children. N Engl J Med 1984;310:674. (*Rates of recurrent infection decreased in both medically and surgically treated children, with surgery producing the greater reduction.*)

Shapiro J, Eavey RD, Baker AS. Adult supraglottis: a prospective study. JAMA 1988;259:563. (*A review of this life-threatening but uncommon* H. influenzae *infection.*)

Weisner PJ, Tronen E, Bonin P, et al. Clinical spectrum of pharyngeal gonococcal infection. N Engl J Med 1973;288:181. (*Describes the incidence, clinical features, and management of gonococcal pharyngitis.*)

221
Approach to the Patient with Hiccups

Hiccup is usually a transient innocuous symptom but when persistent it may become an exhausting and disabling problem. Intractable hiccup has been attributed to a host of metabolic, peridiaphragmatic, neurologic, and psychogenic conditions, but many cases are of unknown etiology. The primary physician should be able to offer the exasperated patient symptomatic relief while conducting a judicious evaluation to determine the source of difficulty.

PATHOPHYSIOLOGY AND CLINICAL PRESENTATIONS

No useful function has been found for the hiccup, which occurs as a result of synchronous clonic spasm of intercostal muscles and diaphragm that causes sudden inspiration followed by prompt closure of the glottis and inhibition of respiratory activity. It is believed to be a reflex. There is debate about whether it is centrally mediated. The afferent pathway is from T10 to T12, and the efferent limb is along the phrenic nerve. During the hiccup, the glottis is closed. Some investigators believe the hiccup is related more to gastrointestinal than to respiratory function. Current understanding of pathophysiology does not yet permit an explanation of how the presumptive etiologies operate to produce the hiccup, although the classic explanation is that it is due to stimulation of the phrenic nerve.

It is often unclear whether the reported causes of hiccup are etiologies or only associations. In a series of 220 cases seen at the Mayo Clinic, men outnumbered women by five to one, and most were in their sixties. Over 90% of the women had no concurrent illness other than an emotional problem, whereas only 7% of men were labeled as having a psychogenic disorder. About 20% of men who experienced hiccup did so after undergoing intraabdominal, intrathoracic, or neurologic surgery. About 25% had a diaphragmatic hernia, another 20% had cerebrovascular disease or another central nervous system (CNS) problem, 5% had a metabolic illness, and in 10% no associated disease or psychiatric problem was identified.

DIFFERENTIAL DIAGNOSIS

The causes of persistent hiccup typically listed are clinical associations and cannot be considered proven etiologies (Table 221.1).

WORKUP

Persistent hiccup that proves refractory to simple measures is an indication for further investigation. Extensive workup is usually not productive, but a check for a previously unsuspected metabolic or subdiaphragmatic process is sometimes rewarding.

History. Questioning should include inquiry into recent abdominal, thoracic, or neurologic surgery, abdominal pain (espe-

Table 221.1.   Conditions Associated with Persistent Hiccup[a]

A. Structural Pathology
1. Pericarditis
2. Tumor
3. Subdiaphragmatic abscess
4. Pneumonia
5. Pleuritis
6. Myocardial infarction
7. Hiatus hernia
8. Peritonitis
9. Gastric dilatation
10. Pancreatitis
11. Biliary tract disease
12. Tympanic membrane irritation
13. Aortic aneurysm

B. Metabolic Disturbances
1. Uremia
2. Diabetes
3. Alcoholism

C. Central Nervous System Disease
1. Tumor
2. Infection
3. Surgery

D. Psychogenic Disease
1. Hysteria
2. Anorexia nervosa
3. Anxiety

[a]These are not proven etiologies.

cially that which radiates to the tip of the shoulder or is worsened by respiration), prior renal disease, excess consumption of alcohol, fever, cough, diabetes, and emotional problems. Also of help is reviewing the various methods that the patient has tried for relief of symptoms. Any neurologic complaints should be noted.

Physical Examination. A temperature determination, a check of the tympanic membranes, percussion of the lungs for evidence of reduced diaphragmatic excursion, and auscultation for signs of an infiltrate, effusion, or pleuritis should be included. The abdomen is examined for distention, organomegaly, upper abdominal tenderness, and signs of peritonitis. A careful neurologic examination is needed if there is a history of neurologic difficulties.

Laboratory Studies. Patients with an acute bout of hiccups need no laboratory studies, but those with *refractory hiccups* that persist for days need to be evaluated for a pharyngeal, thoracic, diaphragmatic, intraabdominal, CNS, or metabolic/pharmacologic etiology. If a careful physical examination that includes a check of the tympanic membranes, pharynx, chest, heart, abdomen, and CNS is unrevealing, one should obtain a chest x-ray, serum sodium, creatinine, and blood urea nitrogen determinations, and consider a computed tomography of the abdomen, concentrating on the subdiaphragmatic region. If CNS disease is suspected by history or physical examination, a computed tomography or magnetic resonance image may help detect the lesion. Treatment of the underlying etiology is the best means of curing refractory hiccups.

SYMPTOMATIC THERAPY
AND INDICATION FOR REFERRAL

For patients with *self-limited* causes of hiccuping, several home remedies are capable of interrupting the reflex arc; oth-

ers simply suppress it temporarily. *Breathholding* and breathing into a *paper bag* will decrease the frequency of hiccups, but if the underlying stimulus has not disappeared, they usually return after these maneuvers are terminated. Swallowing a teaspoonful of *granulated sugar* works by irritating the pharynx sufficiently to inhibit further hiccuping. A more noxious maneuver is to have the patient put his or her finger into the back of the pharynx and *stimulate the gag reflex*. Drinking from the wrong side of the glass is another gag reflex stimulant. Rubbing the nasopharynx with a cotton swab is sometimes effective. Passage of a *nasogastric tube* causing hypopharyngeal stimulation will usually work if other methods have failed.

When symptoms are *persistent* and the cause remains undiagnosed or untreatable, symptomatic relief becomes an important goal. *Chlorpromazine* in doses of 25 to 50 mg intravenously will often terminate refractory hiccups and can be followed by oral maintenance therapy of 25 mg four times a day. *Metoclopramide* given intravenously, followed by oral therapy (10 mg three times a day), has also proven effective. Atropine and quinidine have been used but with less success. *Phenytoin* and *carbamazepine* are helpful in patients with a CNS etiology.

When all other measures have failed and the hiccups remain disabling, consideration of surgical *infiltration of the phrenic nerve* is appropriate. Fluoroscopy is needed to see if one leaf of the diaphragm is responsible and can be singled out for treatment. In addition, one needs to be sure one leaf is not already paralyzed, a circumstance that would rule out this therapeutic option. The phrenic nerve serving the offending diaphragm is infiltrated with a long-acting anesthetic; if it works but the hiccups return, reinfiltration with alcohol or *crushing* may be necessary. If both leaves of the diaphragm are involved, one phrenic nerve is treated.

In most instances, hiccups will resolve spontaneously or respond at least partially to one of these therapeutic maneuvers.

A.H.G.

ANNOTATED BIBLIOGRAPHY

Editorial. Hiccup. Br Med J 1971;1:235. (*A terse review of pathophysiology and the significance of the hiccup.*)

Engleman EG, Lankton J, Leakton B. Granulated sugar as treatment for hiccups in conscious patients. N Engl J Med 1971;285:1489. (*A letter reported successful relief of hiccups in 19 of 20 patients after swallowing a teaspoon of ordinary dry white sugar.*)

Salem MR, Baraka A, Rattenborg CC, et al. Treatment of hiccups by pharyngeal stimulation in anesthetized and conscious subjects. JAMA 1967;202:321. (*Therapeutic success in 84 of 86 patients by introduction of a catheter through the nose and stimulating the pharynx at the level of C2-3.*)

Samuels L. Hiccup: a ten-year review of anatomy, etiology, and treatment. Can Med Assoc J 1952;67:315. (*The classic paper on hiccups with differential diagnosis.*)

Souadjian JV, et al. Intractable hiccup: etiologic factors in 220 patients. Postgrad Med 1968;43:72. (*A classic review of 220 patients from the Mayo Clinic presenting probable causes.*)

Williamson BWA, MacIntyre JMC. Management of intractable hiccup. Br Med J 1977;2:501. (*A succinct review of therapeutic approaches, finding chlorpromazine and metoclopramide the most effective drugs; 39 references.*)

222
Approach to the Patient with Chronic Nasal Congestion and Discharge

It is estimated that 15% to 20% of the population suffer from chronic or recurrent nasal congestion. Allergic rhinitis accounts for most such cases; vasomotor rhinitis, mechanical obstruction, drugs, and abuse of decongestants contribute to others. Much discomfort, absenteeism, and expense result. The primary physician needs to distinguish an allergic etiology from obstruction, inflammation, or vasomotor instability. Proper utilization of allergy testing and effective use of antihistamines, decongestants, and topical corticosteroids are required.

PATHOPHYSIOLOGY AND CLINICAL PRESENTATION

Allergic Rhinitis. In atopic patients, antigen exposure stimulates production of allergen-specific IgE. This IgE attaches to mucosal mast cells. Subsequent exposure to the allergen leads to formation of antigen–IgE complexes on mast cells and basophils. The formation of antigen–antibody complexes triggers an acute-phase *degranulation* reaction, with release of histamine, kinins, prostaglandins, and esterases in concentrations proportional to the intensity of the antigen challenge. Hours later, a late-phase response can be demonstrated in persons with more severe disease, manifested by re-release of mediators (minus prostaglandins); an influx of leukocytes, eosinophils, and mononuclear cells; and increased responsiveness to antigenic and nonantigenic stimuli. With continued allergen exposure, there is heightened mucosal responsiveness due to an increase in the population of mast cells.

In addition to environmental stimuli, genetic factors play a role. Antigen-specific responses are controlled by regulatory genes, and allergic rhinitis is much more common in persons with a positive family history. The relation of allergic rhinitis to reactive lower airway disease (asthma) remains a subject of debate, but it appears that allergic rhinitis is neither a cause nor consequence of it.

Clinical Presentation. Nasal congestion, sneezing, and profuse watery discharge dominate the initial clinical presentation. Itching of the nose, throat, and eyes is common, as is postnasal drip, tearing, and conjunctival injection. Often the nasal mucosa appears pale and edematous. Symptoms typically vary over the course of the day. They are most severe on arising in the morning, lessen in the afternoon, and may worsen again by evening. With continued allergen exposure, there is increased sensitivity both to allergens and to nonallergenic stimuli.

Onset of allergic rhinitis is usually during childhood but may occur at any age. Childhood cases frequently continue into adulthood. Often, the condition improves with time. The condition is *seasonal* when the antigen is a pollen ("hay fever") and *perennial* when the allergens are dusts, molds, or animal danders. Patients living in the northern half of the United States who are sensitive to tree pollen will become symptomatic in late March and early April and those sensitive to grasses, in

mid-May to late June. Patients affected by ragweed and other summer weeds experience difficulty in late August until the first frost. Patients with seasonal allergic rhinitis outnumber those with perennial complaints by a ratio of about 10 to 1. Individuals may be allergic to a number of antigens.

In some instances, the patient has all the earmarks of allergic rhinitis but no evidence of IgE mediation, and skin tests for inhaled allergens are negative. Such patients have been designated as having *nonallergic rhinitis*, even though their nasal secretions often contain large numbers of eosinophils and they respond to corticosteroids.

Vasomotor Rhinitis. The pathophysiology is poorly understood but believed to involve abnormal autonomic responsiveness and vascular dilatation of the submucosal vessels. IgE levels are normal, and the number of eosinophils in nasal secretions is usually, but not always, normal. Abnormal autonomic reactivity is believed to account for the nasal stuffiness or rhinorrhea sometimes occurring with *emotional upset* and *sexual arousal*.

The condition may mimic perennial allergic rhinitis and is believed by some clinicians to be a diagnosis of exclusion when no allergen is identified. Others consider the condition a readily distinguishable entity characterized by a normal-appearing nasal mucosa and persistent nasal stuffiness without itching that is worsened by changes in ambient temperature and humidity. Although congestion is the most prominent symptom, a discharge may also be present. Sneezing is relatively absent.

Drugs. Overuse of topical *nasal decongestants* (e.g., oxymetazoline, phenylpropanolamine, pseudoephedrine) can result in a worsening of symptoms (*rhinitis medicamentosa*). After more than 3 days of continuous use, response to these agents becomes blunted (tachyphylaxis), leading to increased use, often on an hourly basis. Cessation results in severe rebound nasal congestion presumably due to marked reflex vasodilatation. The nasal mucosa appears erythematous. The problem resolves in 2 to 3 weeks if topical decongestants are stopped. α-Adrenergic blockers can aggravate preexisting rhinitis and cause mild nasal congestion in normal patients.

Cocaine abuse is another important cause of drug-induced nasal congestion and discharge. Being a potent sympathomimetic, the pathophysiology is analogous to that of nasal decongestant abuse. Recurrent nasal use leads to ischemic mucosal injury, atrophy, and tell-tale septal perforation.

Hormonal Etiologies. *Hypothyroidism* and *pregnancy* may cause the turbinates to become pale and edematous, leading to nasal congestion. Hypothyroidism may otherwise be subclinical save for the chronic nasal obstruction. Symptoms resolve with correction of the hypothyroidism or with delivery.

Mechanical Obstruction. Unilateral congestion, discharge, and recurrent episodes of sinusitis are characteristic of mechanical obstruction due to tumor, polyp, or deviated septum. *Neoplasm* is rare but is suggested by a blood-tinged discharge. *Polyps* can occur in association with allergic and vasomotor rhinitis, chronic sinusitis, aspirin-induced asthma, cystic fibrosis, and drug use. The mechanism of formation is unknown. Polyps move freely because they are pedunculated and nontender and appear as soft, pale gray, smooth structures. Patients with asthma and nasal polyps are often hypersensitive to aspirin. Polyps do not regress spontaneously and may become large or multiple, causing considerable obstruction. A *deviated septum* is sometimes the source of obstructive symptoms. Most are developmental and not traumatic in origin. Associated sinus occlusion is rare.

Obstruction due to crusting is seen with *atrophic rhinitis.* The condition is of unknown etiology, appears mostly in women, and is characterized by dry atrophic nasal turbinates, mucosal crusts, and a foul or fetid greenish discharge referred to as ozena. The purulent discharge is believed due to secondary infection.

Chronic Inflammatory Disease. *Midline granuloma,* an uncommon illness of unknown etiology, causes ulcerative destruction of upper respiratory tract structures and may present as nasal stuffiness, crusting, and granulations. Steady progression leads to ulcers of the nasal septum. Most patients are over 50, many with a history of allergic rhinitis. *Wegener's granulomatosis,* an immune-mediated disease of middle-aged persons, may have a similar insidious presentation with nasal obstruction, rhinorrhea, or chronic sinusitis. Necrotizing granulomatous lesions and vasculitis are found in the upper and lower airway. *Sarcoidosis* may present as bilateral nasal obstruction (see Chapter 51).

DIFFERENTIAL DIAGNOSIS

The causes of nasal congestion and discharge can be organized pathophysiologically and are listed in Table 222.1.

WORKUP

Although it is important to rule out mechanical obstruction, chronic inflammatory disease, and drug-induced illness, the most common diagnostic task is to distinguish allergic from vasomotor disease.

History. The *timing* of symptoms can be helpful diagnostically. Nasal congestion that coincides with periods of pollination is virtually diagnostic of seasonal allergic rhinitis. Continuous waxing and waning of symptoms throughout the year, with exacerbations during the hay fever season, suggest a combination of perennial and seasonal allergic disease. When symptoms occur chronically without respect to seasons, one may be dealing with vasomotor rhinitis, perennial allergy, mechanical obstruction, or a chronic inflammatory condition. Perennial rhinitis is a possibility when the patient reports frequent "colds."

Aggravating and alleviating factors should be noted. Patients bothered by dusts are generally atopic, whereas those whose symptoms are aggravated by quick changes in tempera-

Table 222.1. Important Causes of Chronic or Recurrent Nasal Congestion

A. Allergic
 1. Seasonal allergic rhinitis (pollens)
 2. Perennial allergic rhinitis (dusts, molds)

B. Vasomotor
 1. Idiopathic (vasomotor rhinitis)
 2. Abuse of nose drops
 3. Drugs (reserpine, guanethidine, prazosin, cocaine abuse)
 4. Psychologic stimulation (anger, sexual arousal)

C. Mechanical
 1. Polyps
 2. Tumor
 3. Deviated septum
 4. Crusting (as in atrophic rhinitis)
 5. Hypertrophied turbinates (chronic vasomotor rhinitis)
 6. Foreign body (usually in children)

D. Chronic Inflammatory
 1. Sarcoidosis
 2. Wegener's granulomatosis
 3. Midline granuloma

E. Infectious
 1. Atrophic rhinitis (secondary infection)

F. Hormonal
 1. Pregnancy
 2. Hypothyroidism

ture, emotion, or drugs fall into the vasomotor category. Use of antihypertensive agents and topical nasal decongestants needs to be explored, as does exposure to fur-bearing animals, feathers, other possible sources of animal danders, or chemical irritants. Pollutants are often more irritating to allergic patients but may also cause symptoms in nonatopic people.

Associated symptoms of potential importance include fever and a purulent nasal discharge, suggestive of an infectious etiology. A cold is the most likely cause of acute discharge, but chronic discharge that is fetid, foul smelling, and accompanied by crusting indicates secondary infection as in atrophic rhinitis, Wegener's granulomatosis, and midline granuloma. Bloody discharge and unilateral obstruction suggest tumor. Mechanical obstructions are often unilateral as well. The presence of asthma or aspirin sensitivity increases the likelihood of nasal polyps. Sneezing and postnasal drip are nonspecific and of little help in distinguishing among etiologies, but associated itching of the eyes, tearing, and conjunctival redness suggest an allergic mechanism.

Epidemiologic data need to be considered. Onset in childhood is typical of allergic disease, but onset of symptoms during adulthood does not rule out atopy. When chronic progressive nasal congestion develops in a middle-aged patient, particularly a woman, one must consider atrophic rhinitis or one of the necrotizing inflammatory diseases. The allergy histories of the patient's parents should be ascertained, because a positive family history strongly suggests allergic disease.

Drug use and *concurrent conditions* are important to review, including abuse of cocaine or nasal decongestants, hypothyroidism, sarcoidosis, and pregnancy.

Physical Examination. The nasal mucous membranes are inspected for erythema, pallor, atrophy, edema, crusting, and discharge. The presence of polyps, erosions, and septal perforations or deviations should be noted. A nasal speculum markedly improves visualization of the nasal cavity and should be used in every examination. Some findings are nonspecific. For example, a pale boggy appearance to the mucosa is allegedly a classic sign of allergic disease, but erythema sometimes occurs in allergy and its presence certainly does not rule it out.

Examination of the eyes for conjunctival erythema, tearing, photophobia, and papillary edema of the lids provides supportive evidence of an allergic mechanism. Transillumination and palpation of the sinuses, pharyngeal examination for erythema and discharge, a look in the ears for evidence of otitis, cervical node examination for adenopathy, and auscultation of the chest for wheezes complete the physical examination.

Laboratory Studies. Antigen challenge is sometimes helpful when the differentiation between allergic and nonallergic disease remains difficult. In vivo and in vitro methods are used. When history provides ready identification of allergens, there is little need for skin testing, but if drastic environmental measures are being contemplated, documentation of the specific allergens is indicated.

In Vivo Testing for Allergen-specific IgE (Skin Prick Testing). The procedure of choice for detection of allergen-specific IgE continues to be skin testing. For environmental allergens, an *epicutaneous (needle prick)* test is used. (*Intradermal* injection should not be used because it generates a high frequency of false-positives and risks severe systemic reactions.) Preparations of commonly inhaled allergens (dusts, molds, animal danders, and local pollens) are introduced by needle prick into the skin. A positive test is a wheal and flare reaction within 20 minutes. A positive reaction does not prove causation, only that there is sensitization to the allergen and allergen-specific IgE present. Correlation with history and physical examination is needed to establish an etiologic role for the antigen.

Antihistamines must be omitted for 12 to 24 hours before testing to avoid a false-negative result. Dermatographism is a common cause of false-positive results, occurring in 15% to 20% of the population and necessitating use of a saline control injection. Eczema and concurrent use of antipsychotic drugs can also interfere with interpretation. The size of the wheal and flare correlates well with the level of allergen-specific IgE. However, allergen preparations remain to be standardized, to avoid impairing interpretation and comparison of results.

Although many of the allergens tested by skin prick are inhaled, *inhalation challenge* remains predominantly a research method, used to evaluate nasal resistance after mucosal exposure.

In Vitro Testing for IgE and Other Markers of Allergy. When skin prick testing is not available, serum tests can contribute to diagnosis. Determination of total *serum IgE* is helpful if the level is markedly elevated, but test sensitivity is low because some cases of allergic rhinitis are not associated with high serum concentrations. The same is true for the *total eosinophil count.* A count at the time of an exacerbation that is in excess of 500 cells/mm³ is suggestive of an allergic etiology, but the absence of peripheral eosinophilia does not rule out allergic rhinitis. *Radio allergoabsorbent testing* (RAST) is an in vitro means of identifying and quantitating an allergen-specific IgE. The test involves adding the patient's serum to a purified allergen absorbed to an inert particle. If the serum contains high concentrations of specific IgE antibodies to the allergen, it will give a positive test. The shortcomings of radioallergosorbent testing are its expense and only modest sensitivity (less than that of skin testing); however, specificity is high. The test is best reserved for patients whose skin tests are equivocal and for those who cannot undergo skin testing. *IgE immunoassays* represent an alternative in vitro means of testing for specific IgE antibodies; a positive test that correlates with symptoms on natural exposure is often sufficient grounds for initiating environmental therapy.

Other Studies. Examining *smears of nasal secretions* for eosinophils is of limited specificity because eosinophils may be present in both vasomotor and allergic rhinitis, but an abundance is more suggestive of an allergic etiology. The smears can be informative if infection is in question, because neutrophils should be present in large numbers. *Sinus films* are sometimes helpful if purulent discharge, sinus opacification, or tenderness suggests an accompanying sinusitis; however, a clinical diagnosis is usually sufficient for initiating therapy (see Chapter 219).

PRINCIPLES OF MANAGEMENT AND PATIENT EDUCATION

Allergic Rhinitis

The major components of the treatment include avoidance of responsible allergens (so-called environmental therapy), antihistamines and sympathomimetics for quick symptomatic relief, topical corticosteroids or cromolyn for improved prophylaxis and control, and immunotherapy for control and prophylaxis in refractory cases.

Avoidance (Environmental) Measures. The appropriate avoidance procedures are a function of the responsible allergens and differ for seasonal and perennial disease.

Seasonal Allergic Rhinitis. Avoidance of long walks in the woods during the pollination period and staying indoors with the windows closed when symptoms are severe and the pollen count is high (e.g., hot, windy, sunny days) helps reduce allergen exposure. Some patients find air conditioners helpful, but its filter does little to remove pollen from the air. Air conditioning simply makes it more tolerable to stay indoors with the windows closed on a hot day. The outside air intake on the air conditioner should be kept closed to avoid bringing in more pollinated air. If ragweed is a problem, daisies, dahlias, and chrysanthemums should not be kept indoors. Preventing accumulation of excess dust in the bedroom and avoiding irritants such as tobacco smoke, chemical vapors, and strong perfumes lessen symptoms.

Perennial Allergic Rhinitis. Control of perennial disease requires particular attention to allergens in the home, but recommendations should be practical. Cleaning the house and especially the bedroom with a damp mop two to three times a week will reduce dust. Feather pillows should be replaced by Dacron or polyester ones, and mattresses should be covered with an elastic fabric casing. Areas where mold can collect, such as piles of old newspapers or furniture in a damp basement, should be cleaned up. A dehumidifier may prevent mold growth. Throwing out carpets and draperies is excessive, but new furnishings made of synthetic fabrics are preferable to cotton and wool to minimize dust collection. Humidification of air in winter also helps reduce dusts. Patients allergic to molds should

Table 222.2   Cost and Convenience of Drugs for Allergic Rhinitis

PREPARATION	DOSE	SCHEDULE	RELATIVE COST[a]
First-generation antihistamines			
Clorpheniramine (generic)	4 mg	qid	1.0
Long–acting	12 mg	bid	1.7
Brompheniramine (generic)	4 mg	qid	1.0
Diphenhydramine (generic)	25 mg	qid	1.5
Celmastine (Tavist)	1 mg	bid	8.2
Second-generation antihistamines			
Fexofenadine (Allegra)	60 mg	bid	20
Loratadine (Claritin)	10 mg	qd to bid	45
Cetirizine (Zyrtec)	5–10 mg	qd	37
Inhaled antihistamines			
Azelastine (Asteline spray)	137 μg	bid	19
Combination preparations			
Chlorpheniramine/pseudoephedrine	8 mg/120 mg	bid	10
Loratadine/pseudoephedrine	5 mg/60 mg	bid	28
Topical corticosteroids			
Beclomethasone			
Beconase (also AQ)	42 μg	1-bid	8
Vancenase	42 μg	1-bid	8
Vancenase AQ	84 μg	1-qd	8
Budesonide (Rhinocort)	32 μg	2-bid	14
Flunisolide (Nasalide)	25 μg	2-bid	16
Fluticasone (Flonase)	50 μg	2-bid	16
Mometasone (Nasonex)	50 μg	2-qd	18
Triamcinolone (Nasacort AQ)	55 μg	2-qd	12
Mast cell stabilizers			
Cromolyn	5.2 mg	1-tid	5

[a]Relative average wholesale price for 30-day supply of lowest starting dose.

avoid having African violets and geraniums in the home. No new fur-bearing pets should be obtained. Most pets usually have to be removed from the home entirely if symptoms are disabling. Simply keeping the pet out of the bedroom does not help sufficiently because the dander circulates in the air throughout the house.

Pharmacotherapy. Patients who find allergen avoidance impractical or ineffective often request medication. The commonly used agents include oral antihistamines, which block mast-cell activation and the effects of histamine on end organs; inhaled cromolyn sodium and its analogues, which block degranulation of mast cells and basophils; topical corticosteroids, which inhibit cytokine production, mast-cell proliferation, and other inflammatory mediators; and sympathomimetics, which decongest by means of vasoconstriction.

Antihistamines. The *first-generation* H_1-blockers (e.g., *chlorpheniramine, diphenhydramine, clemastine*) provide adequate control of mild-to-moderate symptoms, with itching, sneezing, rhinorrhea, and conjunctival irritation responding best, but nasal congestion often persisting. Bothersome sedation can be a problem in up to 15% of users, and some degree of psychomotor impairment can be demonstrated in most. *Second-generation* H_1-blockers (e.g., *loratadine, fexofenadine*) are less sedating and less inhibitory of psychomotor function because their protein-bound lipophobic structure prevents their crossing the blood–brain barrier. They also have little anticholinergic activity and thus avoid the annoying side effects of dry mouth and constipation sometimes associated with the use of first-generation agents. However, they are no more effective than first-generation antihistamines.

Rapid *absorption* occurs after oral intake on an empty stomach, with onset of action within 1 to 2 hours. Intake with food may slow absorption substantially. *Duration* of action ranges from 3 to 4 hours for nonsustained formulations of first-generation preparations to 12 hours for sustained-release preparations and 12 to 24 hours for second-generation H_1-blockers.

Antihistamine *cost* has become a major concern in an era of rapidly rising medical expenses. The second-generation antihistamines are extremely expensive, costing 20 to 45 times more than chlorpheniramine and as much as 7 times more than nasal steroids (Table 222.2). Demand for second-generation H_1-blockers has been greatly stimulated by direct advertising to patients. Approaches to *cost containment* in treatment of allergic rhinitis include

- Starting with a first-generation antihistamine and switching to a nonsedating preparation only if daytime sedation becomes a problem (tolerance to sedation commonly develops);
- Substituting an inexpensive first-generation preparation for the nighttime dose of a twice daily second-generation preparation;
- Prescribing the least expensive second-generation preparation (providing a 20% reduction in cost);
- Prescribing a nasal steroid preparation instead (see below).

Aside from sedation and anticholinergic effects, the first-generation H_1-blockers are well tolerated, as are most second-generation H_1-blockers. When prescribing daytime use of a first-generation agent, it is important to keep in mind that some degree of *psychomotor impairment* may occur even without noticeable *sedation*, an especially important consideration in persons who operate a motor vehicle, heavy equipment, or machinery. Reports of fatal *ventricular arrhythmias* (e.g., torsades de pointes) emerged with use of two second-generation agents (*terfenadine and astemizole*), leading to their withdrawal from the market. The episodes were related to drug-induced QT interval prolongation and occurred in situations that exacerbate prolongation of the QT interval (e.g., use of quinidine, disopyramide, or class IC antiarrhythmics; hypomagnesemia, hypokalemia) or interfere with hepatic antihistamine metabolism (e.g., concurrent use of antifungals or macrolide antibiotics). Fexofenadine, cetirizine, and loratadine do not appear to confer the same degree of risk for QT prolongation and ventricular dysrhythmias.

A topically active antihistamine (*azelastine*) has been developed for use as a *nasal spray*. About 40% of the nasal spray is absorbed systemically. Although similar in efficacy to other antihistamines, the drug's side effects (somnolence, bitter taste) and high cost make it less desirable than oral nonsedating antihistamines and inhaled steroids.

Sympathomimetics. Patients still bothered by marked nasal congestion despite antihistamine use may benefit from concurrent treatment with an oral sympathomimetic (e.g., pseudoephedrine). The vasoconstrictive action of adrenergic agents can help reduce edema and secretions and counter the sedative action of antihistamines. These properties make oral sympathomimetics a useful component in over-the-counter decongestant formulations, often in combination with an antihistamine such as chlorpheniramine. All sympathomimetics are effective decongestants, but those with some β activity in addition to their vasoconstrictor α-adrenergic action (e.g., *ephedrine, pseudoephedrine*) are preferred when drowsiness is a problem. *Phenylpropanolamine* has predominantly α activity. A typical regimen is pseudoephedrine, 60 mg, every 4-6 hours; lower doses may suffice in mild cases.

The addition of sympathomimetic therapy may provoke bothersome side effects (*headache, palpitations, nervousness*) or trigger harmful cardiovascular effects (e.g., *elevated blood pressure, increased heart rate*). Use, especially if continuous, in patients with hypertension, coronary artery disease, or heart failure is inadvisable. Empirical trials of various antihistamines and decongestants are often necessary to select the best agent(s) and dose(s). Combination preparations are convenient if the fixed doses match the doses needed; these preparations should not be used as initial therapy. Combination preparations containing a first-generation antihistamine and a sympathomimetic are available without prescription and popular with many patients, who find the combination less sedating and more effective than the antihistamine alone. Second-generation antihistamines are also available in combination with a sympathomimetic. Compared with single-agent therapy, the cost of combination preparations can be high.

Topical sympathomimetic decongestant sprays have a limited role because of the risks of tachyphylaxis and rebound nasal congestion. They are best used for keeping the eustachian tubes patent in patients during airplane travel (see Chapter 219). A topical application of *phenylephrine* (Neo-Synephrine) or *oxymetazoline* (Afrin) spray every 3 to 4 hours while the patient is airborne should suffice, especially when preceded by an oral decongestant an hour before flight time. Rebound congestion may occur if sprays are used repeatedly for more than 3 days in a row.

Topical Corticosteroids. For patients with persistent symptoms of seasonal or perennial allergic rhinitis, regular use of a nonabsorbable topically active *intranasal corticosteroid* preparation (e.g., *flunisolide, budesonide, beclomethasone, fluticasone, triamcinolone, mometasone*) is becoming the treatment of choice. Nasal steroid therapy in such patients has proven to be clinically more effective and more cost effective than chronic use of oral antihistamines. Only symptoms of allergic conjunctivitis are better controlled by antihistamines. No significant benefit is afforded by combination therapy. Once and twice daily nasal steroid preparations are available; cost and convenience are the principal determinants of choice (Table 222.2). Patients with dryness and crusting of the mucosa may prefer a liquid formulation rather than a powdered one. Side-effect profiles and efficacies appear comparable, although some claims of enhanced safety (e.g., less hypothalamic-pituitary-adrenal suppression with mometasone) remain to be confirmed.

At recommended doses and frequencies, significant adrenal suppression does not occur with these topical corticosteroids, even when used chronically. No adverse effects on adult bone metabolism have been documented, although concerns about growth retardation in children remain. Unresolved is the effect of long-term nasal-steroid use on risk of developing cataracts and glaucoma, an association found in the elderly exposed to long-term high-dose use of inhaled and systemic glucocorticosteroids (see Chapters 105 and 208). Other adverse effects include mucosal irritation and friability, leading to an occasional *nosebleed*. Mucosal ulceration is rare. Application of the spray can cause transient burning and sneezing. Atrophic rhinitis is a risk of chronic use. Colonization of the nose with *Candida* has been reported.

Cromolyn Sodium has been found moderately effective, making it a reasonable nonsteroidal choice in persons with less severe disease. The agent is administered either as an inhaled powder or as a dissolved liquid up to six times per day. It works by preventing degranulation of mast cells and is most effective when used prophylactically before an anticipated allergen exposure. It benefits both the immediate and late phases of the allergic reaction and can diminish the severity of an ongoing allergic episode. Nasal congestion is reduced. Patients with very high IgE levels are most responsive; many others are not. The agent is very safe and well tolerated, which has led to its being approved for over-the-counter use.

Nedocromil is a newer topically active mast-cell stabilizer, structurally different from cromolyn and possessing antiinflammatory activity as well. Nonetheless, clinical efficacy in allergic rhinitis is similar to that of cromolyn, but only twice daily administration is required.

Immunotherapy (Hyposensitization) is indicated as a last resort in patients who face prolonged (more than 6 weeks) exposure to a known allergen and who remain incapacitated despite a year's trial of a full program of pharmacotherapy and environmental measures. Hyposensitization reduces IgE production and stimulates synthesis of IgG *blocking antibody*. It may also induce IgE suppressor lymphocyte activity or reduce mast cell and basophil responsiveness. Prevention of local reaction to pollens, cat dander, and dust mites has been demonstrated in patients with allergic rhinitis. Hyposensitization involves cutaneous administration of incremental doses of allergen extract, initially at intervals of 1 to 2 weeks, progressing to intervals of 3 to 6 weeks after several months of treatment.

Immunotherapy should be considered a complement to a medical therapy, because most responses are not dramatic. Skin testing for definitive identification of the causative allergen(s) is required, and frequent visits over a prolonged period mean considerable patient inconvenience and high cost. Assessment of response to immunotherapy (improvement in symptoms, reduction in medication requirements) should be made every 6 months, and therapy should be discontinued if substantial benefit is not evident after 12 to 18 months.

Recommended Approach to Treatment. Although the heavily promoted nonsedating H₁-blockers are very popular because they are well tolerated and reasonably effective in persons with mild to moderate disease, their uncritical chronic use violates most tenets of rational cost-effective prescribing. A more cost-effective approach would be to

- Implement avoidance and environmental measures.
- Start with a trial of a first-generation antihistamine, beginning with a twice daily dose of a long-acting preparation (e.g., sustained-release chlorpheniramine 8 to 12 mg). Add a small daytime dose of a shorter acting preparation (e.g., 4 mg chlorpheniramine) if needed and continue if well tolerated, but exert caution in persons whose work requires unimpaired psychomotor performance (e.g., those operating machinery, heavy equipment, or a motor vehicle).
- If sedation is a problem and short-term treatment will suffice, then consider short-term addition of a sympathomimetic (e.g., pseudoephedrine 60 mg); avoid if there is hypertension or underlying heart disease.
- If sedation is a problem and longer term therapy is needed for mild-to-moderate disease, then begin the least costly twice daily nonsedating antihistamine preparation (e.g., fexofenadine 60 mg every morning only); for nighttime use, recommend a nonprescription first-generation antihistamine.
- If control is inadequate, proceed to daily sustained use of a topically active, nonabsorbable, nasal steroid preparation (e.g., beclomethasone one to two puffs twice daily) or cromolyn.
- Consider immunotherapy only for those who have failed a year of all the above measures and in whom chronic unavoidable exposure to the offending allergen(s) is expected in the future.

Vasomotor Rhinitis

Vasomotor rhinitis is difficult to treat. Avoidance of tobacco smoke, rapid changes in temperature or humidity, and irritant chemical vapors is helpful. Humidification of the home in winter is also worthwhile. Cessation of nasal spray use is essential. A change in antihypertensive medications may be needed. A mild adrenergic agent with some α activity (e.g., pseudoephedrine) sometimes provides partial improvement. Addition of an antihistamine for its nonspecific drying effect may give some extra relief but is ineffective by itself. A reactive depression is common in such patients; use of an antidepressant with anticholinergic activity (e.g., amitriptyline) may be considering, both for its antidepressant and drying effects.

Immunotherapy and steroids are of no proven benefit. Patients severely bothered by nasal obstruction may benefit from cryosurgical treatment of the inferior and middle turbinates; profuse rhinorrhea is occasionally treated by sectioning the parasympathetic nerve supply to the nose. Consideration of surgical approaches should be reserved only for patients whose lives are seriously impaired by their symptoms, because chances of success are limited and risk of complications is substantial.

INDICATIONS FOR REFERRAL

For the patient with allergic rhinitis whose condition is inadequately controlled on a well-designed medical regimen, referral to an allergist for skin testing and consideration of immunotherapy is a reasonable step. An allergist can also be of help when an allergic etiology cannot be distinguished from vasomotor rhinitis and when the antigen(s) must be identified for management purposes. Referral to an ear, nose, and throat specialist is indicated for removal of polyps or foreign bodies, management of a suspected tumor, necrotizing inflammatory condition, or atrophic rhinitis and for correction of deviated septa. Referral might also be worthwhile for patients with incapacitating vasomotor rhinitis.

A.H.G.

ANNOTATED BIBLIOGRAPHY

Aaronson D. Comparative efficacy of H1 antihistamines. Ann Allergy 1991;67:541. (*All are equally effective for seasonal allergic rhinitis.*)

Guerin B, Watson RD. Skin tests. Clin Rev Allerg 1988;6:211. (*Good review for the practicing physician.*)

Juniper EF, Kline PA, Hargreave FE, et al. Comparison of beclomethasone dipropionate aqueous nasal spray, astemizole, and the combination in the prophylactic treatment of ragweed pollen-induced rhinoconjunctivitis. J Allerg Clin Immunol 1989;83:627. (*Nasal steroids superior except for conjunctival irritation; no synergy from combination therapy.*)

Metzger E. Comparative safety of H₁-antihistamines. Ann Allergy 1991;67:625. (*Discussion of sedation and psychomotor impairment.*)

Naclerio RM. Understanding the pathogenesis of allergic rhinitis. J Respir Dis 1991;12[Suppl]:S13. (*Describes both immediate and delayed responses to allergen change, with the late ones part of an inflammatory process.*)

Ownby DR. Allergy testing: in vivo versus in vitro. Pediatr Clin North Am 1988;55:995. (*Detailed discussion of their relative merits.*)

Pipkorn U, Pround D, Lichtenstein LM, et al. Inhibition of mediator release in allergic rhinitis by pretreatment with topical glucocorticosteroids. N Engl J Med 1987;316:1506. (*Blocks both immediate and late-phase responses.*)

Racklin RE. Clinical and immunologic aspects of allergen-specific immunotherapy in patients with seasonal allergic rhinitis and/or allergic asthma. J Allerg Clin Immunol 1983;72:323. (*A review of immunotherapy, its procedures, and its efficacy.*)

Weiner JM, Abramson MJ, Puy RM. Intranasal corticosteroids versus oral H₁-receptor antagonists in allergic rhinitis: systematic review of randomised controlled trials. BMJ 1998;317:1624. (*Best summation of the best studies; intranasal corticosteroids superior to oral antihistamines as the first line of treatment for allergic rhinitis.*)

Wolthers OD, Pederson S. Knemometric assessment of systemic activity of once-daily intranasal dry-powder budesonide in children. Allergy 1994;49:96. (*Evidence of potential for growth inhibition in children, even in the absence of HPA suppression.*)

223
Approach to the Patient with Excessive Snoring

Snoring is essentially a lay term for soft tissue airway obstruction during sleep. The complaint almost always originates from a spouse or household member whose sleep is being disturbed. Snoring may be an annoying but medically trivial problem, but when associated with daytime sleepiness and witnessed apneic episodes, it may be a manifestation of sleep apnea (see Chapter 46).

PATHOPHYSIOLOGY AND CLINICAL PRESENTATION

Pharyngeal size in snorers and patients with obstructive sleep apnea is reduced compared with that in nonsnorers, with sleep apnea patients having the smallest cross-sectional pharyngeal area. The sound of snoring originates in the collapsible portion of the airway, the soft tissue between the choanae and the epiglottis. Tone in the lingual and pharyngeal muscles may be inadequate due to use of sedatives or alcohol. Structural abnormalities may contribute and include redundant or thickened lateral pharyngeal musculature, a long uvula, thickened pharyngeal folds, and flaccid tonsillar pillars. Large tonsils, cysts, or neoplasms sometimes may obstruct the airway. Mild maxillomandibular abnormalities, such as a small chin, overbite, and high hard palate, have been found important in women. Obstructing nasal abnormalities (e.g., severely deviated septum, polyps, sinusitis, neoplasm) may create excessive negative pressure and cause collapse of the airway during inspiration.

Severe airway obstruction may lead to *sleep apnea*. Full obstruction interrupts ventilation and, if sufficiently prolonged, results in hypercarbia and hypoxemia. Restoration of breathing usually requires arousal from sleep. The nightly occurrence of multiple apneic episodes and disturbed sleep pattern causes daytime tiredness and hypersomnolence. Uncorrected, the condition may lead to cor pulmonale from chronic arterial desaturation. The condition is most common in obese patients but not restricted to them (see Chapter 46).

WORKUP

The history is most important, especially for recognition of sleep apnea. Habitual snoring, daytime sleepiness, history of motor vehicle accidents caused by falling asleep at the wheel, or witnessed apneas should trigger concern about sleep apnea. Although the condition is most common in men, women with sleep apnea often go unrecognized. Delay in diagnosis of sleep apnea is common, especially in women because symptoms are often ignored or the presentation may be atypical (fatigue, no associated obesity or daytime sleepiness, mild maxillomandibular abnormalities).

A careful examination of the mouth and upper airway is needed to search for obstructing anatomy. Referral for formal ear, nose, and throat evaluation may be helpful. For the patient with suspected sleep apnea, consideration of nocturnal oxygen saturation monitoring and a formal sleep study are indicated (see Chapter 46).

MANAGEMENT

The patient with annoying but physiologically benign snoring can sometimes be helped by simple advice. Loss of excess *weight* and avoidance of *alcohol* and *sedatives* may prove beneficial. Sleeping on one's side rather than on the back sometimes helps minimize upper airway collapse (an old trick is to tape a marble to the patient's back to discourage lying supine). Avoidance of the excessive *neck flexion* that comes from sleeping supine on several pillows can be achieved by limiting the patient to a cervical pillow placed under the nape of the neck or by elevating the entire head of the bed (as in management of reflux esophagitis). Any nasal obstruction from chronic rhinitis should be fully treated (see Chapter 222); anatomic obstruction may benefit from a trial of an external nasal dilator (e.g., a Breath Right Strip).

For patients with disturbingly refractory snoring, a more aggressive approach is to consider use of a continuous positive airway pressure (CPAP) device. The apparatus delivers CPAP through the nose and is usually reserved for those with sleep apnea (see Chapter 46), but may be worth a try in households where marital harmony and restful sleep are threatened by excessive snoring. The devices are sometimes awkward to use and not always acceptable but newer ones are more comfortable. Consideration of dental orthosis has proven useful in preliminary studies and may be worth a referral in cases where there is an overbite or other maxillomandibular pathology. Pulmonary consultation is indicated when there is concern about sleep apnea (daytime sleepiness, nocturnal apnea; see Chapter 46). An ear, nose, and throat consultation may prove useful when snoring proves intractable and appears associated with anatomic oropharyngeal pathology.

A.H.G.

ANNOTATED BIBLIOGRAPHY

American Sleep Disorders Association. Practice parameters for the treatment of obstructive sleep apnea in adults: the efficacy of surgical modification of the upper airway. Sleep 1996:19:152. *(An evidence-based set of guidelines in those who failed or refused noninvasive treatment but have no obvious anatomic obstruction.)*

Bradley TD, Brown IG, Grossman RF, et al. Pharyngeal size in snorers, nonsnorers, and patients with obstructive sleep apnea. N Engl J Med 1986;315:1327. *(Snorers have a reduced cross-sectional area; those with sleep apnea have the smallest area.)*

Guilleminault C, Stoohs R, Kim Y, et al. Upper airway sleep-disordered breathing in women. Ann Intern Med 1995;122:493. *(Fatigue, premenopausal status, maxillomandibular abnormalities, and little obesity were among the prominent clinical features in this group.)*

Jennett S. Snoring and its treatment. BMJ 1984;289:335. *(A somewhat dated summary, but useful for its practical suggestions.)*

Kuna ST, Sant'Ambrogio G. Pathophysiology of upper airway closures during sleep. JAMA 1991;266:1384. *(Excellent review of mechanisms of upper airway obstruction.)*

Schmidt-Nowara WW, Meade TE, Hays MD, et al. Treatment of snoring and obstructive sleep apnea with a dental orthosis. Chest 1991; 99:1378. *(A promising but preliminary report of some improvement.)*

Schwab RJ, Gupta KB, Gefter WB, et al. Upper airway and soft tissue anatomy in normal subjects and patients with sleep-disordered breathing: significance of the lateral pharyngeal walls. Am J Respir Crit Care Med 1995;152:1673. *(A magnetic resonance imaging study of snorers, normals, and those with sleep apnea finding thickened lateral pharyngeal muscles more important than fat.)*

224
Management of Aphthous Stomatitis

Aphthous stomatitis (canker sores) is a common self-limited ulcerative condition of the oral mucosa. About 20% of the population is affected at one time or another. The lesions can be disturbing in appearance and very painful. The primary physician should be able to differentiate them from more serious pathology and provide symptomatic relief.

PATHOPHYSIOLOGY, CLINICAL PRESENTATION, AND COURSE

Pathogenesis remains incompletely understood, but a heightened immunologic response to oral mucosal antigens appears to play an important role. There is a genetic predisposition and an increased prevalence among patients with such autoimmune diseases as Crohn's disease, chronic ulcerative colitis, Behçet's syndrome, and Reiter's syndrome. Contributing factors include deficiencies of iron, folate, and vitamin B_{12}; psychological stress; generalized physical debility; and trauma. In some women, flares occur premenstrually. Regardless of etiology, once mucosal breakdown has occurred, the lesions are invaded by mouth flora and become secondarily infected.

Clinical Presentation Aphthous stomatitis develops in four clinical stages:

1. *Premonitory*—tingling, burning, or hyperesthetic sensation, lasting up to 24 hours;
2. *Preulcerative*—lasting from 18 hours to 3 days, characterized by moderately painful erythematous macules or papules with erythematous halos;
3. *Ulcerative*—lasting 1 to 16 days, characterized by painful discrete ulcers 2 to 10 mm in diameter, occurring singly or in groups, covered by gray yellow membrane with a dusky erythematous halo; pain ceases during this stage;
4. *Healing*—usually without scarring unless lesions are very large, averages 2 weeks (range from 4 to 5 weeks).

Aphthous ulcers are classified according to size. Most are *minor* (i.e., less than 1 cm in diameter) and appear in crops of four or five. *Major lesions* are greater than 1 cm, solitary, indolent, and, as noted, may scar as they heal. Lesions are painful and may occur anywhere within the oral cavity. In two thirds of patients, recurrent lesions do not develop, but in one third, recurrences continue for up to 40 years.

DIFFERENTIAL DIAGNOSIS

Other causes of oral mucosal ulceration include pemphigus, herpes simplex, Behçet's syndrome, and hand-foot-and-mouth disease. *Pemphigus* is suggested by the presence of bullous lesions elsewhere on the body (although oral lesions may precede others by years) and a Tzanck smear from the base of the lesion showing acantholytic cells. Immunofluorescence studies may be necessary if there is recurrent disease. The ulcerated mucosal lesions of *herpes simplex* infection are limited to mucosal surfaces attached to bone, whereas aphthous ulcers may occur anywhere in the oral cavity. The Tzanck preparation shows multinucleated giant cells. The ulcers of *Behçet's syndrome* are identical to those of aphthous stomatitis; genital ulceration and eye involvement help differentiate the condition from simple aphthous disease. In *hand-foot-and-mouth disease*, papulovesicular lesions with an erythematous halo appear on the hands, feet, and lips in addition to the mouth. The lesions ulcerate and then heal over 7 to 10 days. Because the condition is due to an enterovirus, the mucosal findings may be preceded by viral gastrointestinal symptoms.

PRINCIPLES OF MANAGEMENT

When the chief reason for seeking medical care is concern, reassurance that the lesions will heal spontaneously and that they do not represent more serious pathology will often suffice. For patients with large lesions and those bothered badly by the discomfort, additional measures are reasonable. In the presence of extremely painful lesions, use of a topical anesthetic agent (e.g., viscous lidocaine) before meals may allow the patient to eat. Avoidance of abrasive foods also helps. *Tetracycline liquid* (250 mg four times a day) used as a mouthwash that is held in the mouth for several minutes before expectorating is easy to use. *Topical corticosteroids* impregnated into a paste vehicle (e.g., Orabase) help apply the steroid to the mucous membrane and may provide some added relief. *Carbamide peroxide* gel is an oxidizing agent that has some bactericidal effect against many mouth organisms and is a mild debriding agent. In the presence of extremely painful lesions, use of *topical anesthetic agents* (e.g., viscous lidocaine) before meals may allow the patient to eat. Avoidance of abrasive foods also helps. *Levamisole*, which stimulates immune response, has been used experimentally and reported efficacious in about two thirds of cases, but the unknown long-term safety of this agent limits its use for this self-limited condition. Topical use of sucralfate liquid may provide some mucosal protection.

Women with a definite premenstrual flare may be helped by estrogen-dominated oral contraceptives. Identification and correction of an existing deficiency of folate, vitamin B12, or iron may cure aphthous stomatitis. For lesions precipitated by emotional stress, attention to the underlying problem may help (see Chapter 226). Chemical cauterization by means of silver nitrate sticks (AgNO₃) is used by some practitioners to treat acute lesions, but this involves the distinct possibility of destroying normal tissue and should not ordinarily be used.

PATIENT EDUCATION

Besides reassurance, patient education should include recommendations for avoiding mucosal trauma and maintaining good nutrition and oral hygiene. Use of a soft-bristled tooth-brush and avoidance of foods with sharp surfaces, salt, and talking while chewing can be helpful. Patients with vitamin or mineral deficiencies can be prescribed a supplement. The possibility of recurrence in one third of patients should be explained.

A.H.G.

ANNOTATED BIBLIOGRAPHY

Antoon JM, Miller RL. Aphthous ulcer: a review of the literature on etiology, pathogenesis, diagnosis, and treatment. JAMA 1980; 201:803. (*Somewhat dated but still the best review.*)

Bell GF, Rogers RS III. Observations on the diagnosis of recurrent aphthous stomatitis. Mayo Clin Proc 1982;297. (*A discussion of four cases and the key diagnostic issues they raise.*)

Graykowski EA. Aphthous stomatitis is linked to mechanical injuries, iron and vitamin deficiencies, and certain HLA types. JAMA 1982;247:774. (*A summary of findings from studies by National Institutes of Health investigators.*)

225
Management of Temporomandibular Joint Dysfunction

Temporomandibular joint (TMJ) dysfunction has received much attention in the lay press as a cause of chronic headache and facial pain (see Chapter 165). Although severe cases may require dental or oral surgical intervention, most can be managed conservatively by the primary physician.

PATHOPHYSIOLOGY AND CLINICAL PRESENTATION

Most TMJ dysfunction is psychophysiologic in origin, the consequence of chronic *bruxism* (nocturnal jaw clenching and teeth grinding). This tension-relieving oral habit develops in response to situational and intrapsychic stresses and can lead to masticatory muscle fatigue and spasm. In most instances, the problem remains *extracapsular*, with little or no internal derangement of the TMJ. However, severe prolonged bruxism may cause *intracapsular* joint derangement, resulting in degenerative disease of the joint. *Sinovitis* from connective tissue disease, infection, or trauma is another form of intracapsular pathology.

Symptoms of TMJ dysfunction include chronic, dull, aching unilateral discomfort about the jaw, behind the eyes and ears, and even down the neck into the shoulders. Jaw pain, clicking sounds, and difficulty opening the mouth widely, especially in the morning, are characteristic. Chewing may exacerbate symptoms. Locking of the jaw is common. Masticatory muscle tenderness, mandibular hypomotility, clicking, and joint deviation on opening are noted on physical examination. Molar prominences may be flat from chronic grinding. A subset of patients with symptoms referable to the TMJs also experience pain and dysfunction that extend far beyond the TMJs.

A subset of patients with TMJ complaints exhibit features characteristic of patients suffering from a chronic pain syndrome (see Chapter 236). They present to multiple doctors with refractory pain complaints, often extending beyond the TMJs. Not only is health care utilization high as such patients search repeatedly for a "cure," but physician frustration is also high as nothing seems to work. Any suggestion by the physician of a "psychological" cause clashes with the patient's etiologic view and leads to a dissonant doctor–patient relationship. Such patients often seek the comfort "TMJ" support groups.

DIAGNOSIS

The hallmark of TMJ dysfunction is chronic unilateral jaw or facial pain exacerbated by jaw movement. Other causes of jaw pain worsened by jaw movement include *acute otitis media* and *parotitis*. These are distinguished by their acute onset and associated inflammatory manifestations. More subtle is the jaw claudication from *temporal arteritis* (see Chapter 161). Intracapsular TMJ disease may be differentiated clinically from extracapsular dysfunction by the presence of markedly limited jaw movement, jaw deviation on opening of the mouth, and presence of crepitus and clicking on jaw movement. However, there is much overlap of symptoms between internal and extracapsular TMJ disease; jaw clicking may even be noted in normal persons.

Confirmation of internal derangement requires radiologic study. *Magnetic resonance imaging* (MRI) of the TMJ provides the best visualization of bony and soft tissue structures. It has become the test of choice, being more sensitive than conventional or computed tomography and free of radiation exposure. MRI test expense can be reduced substantially by imaging only the TMJ. Imaging is indicated only when internal derangement is suspected, conservative measures have failed, and more aggressive therapy is being considered.

Patients with refractory TMJ complaints that extend well beyond the TMJs and disproportionately interfere with daily functioning should have the possibility of an underlying chronic pain syndrome explored (see Chapter 236).

PRINCIPLES OF MANAGEMENT

Nonsurgical Measures. Because TMJ dysfunction is largely a psychophysiologic condition, treatment may begin with the primary physician inquiring into sources of stress and tension and offering counseling. Often, *cognitive/behavioral therapy* is more effective than insight-oriented approaches to psychotherapy (see Chapter 226). Most persons improve without formal psychiatric care. Less etiologic but helpful symptomatic measures include dietary advice, local physiotherapy, analgesics, minor tranquilizers, and sometimes antidepressants.

Dietary advice includes cutting food into small pieces and using a diet that minimizes hard repetitive chewing (e.g., no chewing gum or biting into big submarine sandwiches). *Physiotherapy* in the form of local heat and massage to the muscles of mastication helps relieve muscle spasm and the accompanying pain. Some persons achieve relief with application of *ultrasound* of *cold packs*. Analgesics such as aspirin and low doses of nonsteroidal antiinflammatory agents are also helpful when pain is prominent. Short-term use of a *minor tranquilizer* at bedtime (e.g., 2 mg of diazepam as needed for 35 days) can help reduce nocturnal muscle spasm and complement analgesic therapy. However, long-term tranquilizer use should be avoided due to the risk of dependence (see Chapter 226). The so-called muscle relaxants (e.g., Robaxin, Soma) are of no proven advantage. Patients with more refractory pain may respond to a trial of a sedating *tricyclic antidepressant* (e.g., nortriptyline 25 mg as needed). Patients with severe grinding may benefit from nighttime use of a custommade *splint* or bite guard.

A regimen that incorporates all these measures into a comprehensive treatment program has a success rate of over 75%. Patients who report refractory pain may have suffered joint damage and require consideration for regrinding or surgical intervention. When the clinical presentation is one of refractory pain accompanied by more global musculoskeletal dysfunction and disproportionately little evidence of TMJ destruction, then approaching the condition as a chronic pain syndrome may be the wisest course (see Chapter 236).

Regrinding and Surgical Therapies. Only the patient with severe malocclusion leading to marked joint trauma is a candidate for regrinding of the teeth. It is a therapy of limited efficacy, requiring careful patient selection. Many patients without objective malocclusion and significant joint injury are subjected needlessly to regrinding or surgical therapy. Surgical intervention is a consideration only when conservative measures have failed to provide relief *and* there is clinical evidence of internal joint derangement and secondary degenerative arthritis (see above). Under these circumstances, an MRI of the TMJs should be obtained and referral made if important degenerative changes are found.

Incapacitated patients refractory to conservative therapy yet found to have marked degenerative changes clearly linked to symptoms are potential candidates for surgery. They should be referred for consultation to an oral surgeon experienced in treating TMJ disease. There are almost no large-scale, prospective, randomized studies to guide choice of surgery for TMJ disease. Arthroscopic approaches appear promising. They are reported to provide significant symptomatic relief, are minimally invasive, and have a low incidence of complications; however, long-term benefit remains to be established.

A.H.G.

ANNOTATED BIBLIOGRAPHY

Clark GT, Delcanho RE, Goulet JP. The utility and validity of current diagnostic procedures for defining temporomandibular disorder patients. Adv Dent Res 1993;7:97. (*Excellent critical review of diagnostic measures.*)

Feinmann C, Harris M, Crawley R. Psychogenic facial pain: presentation and treatment. BMJ 1984:228:436. (*A terse review of approaches to the psychological dimension of TMJ dysfunction.*)

Garro LC, Stephenson KA, Good BJ. Chronic illness of the temporomandibular joints as experienced by support-group members. J Gen Intern Med 1994;9:372. (*A study exploring the perspective of patients with chronic TMJ complaints, many of whom have symptoms that extend beyond the TMJs and exhibit marked health care utilization.*)

Guralnick W, Kaban LB, Merrill RG. Temporomandibular joint afflictions. N Engl J Med 1978;299:123. (*Classic review, especially of pathophysiology.*)

Kumar KL, Cooney TG. Temporomandibular disorders. J Gen Intern Med 1994;9:106. (*Excellent summary for the generalist reader, with particularly helpful suggestions for workup and conservative management; 36 references.*)

McCain JP, Sanders B, Koslin MG, et al. Temporomandibular joint arthroscopy: a six-year multicenter retrospective study of 4,831 joints. J Oral Maxillofacial Surg 1992;50:926. (*Promising results, but data are retrospective and nonrandomized.*)

15

Psychiatric and Behavioral Problems

226

Approach to the Patient with Anxiety

JOHN J. WORTHINGTON III
SCOTT L. RAUCH

Anxiety disorders are prevalent (estimated lifetime prevalence of 25% in the general population) and a frequent precipitant of visits to the nonpsychiatric physician. Evaluation and management can be challenging because patients present with feelings of distress and concern about disease in the absence of objective evidence. Suffering no less from the subjective nature of their ailment, they fear something is amiss with their bodies and persistently seek an acceptable explanation and relief. The autonomic arousal accompanying anxiety may affect many organ systems and imitate physical disease. Moreover, anxiety and anxiety-like symptoms may be consequent to a variety of medical ailments and their treatments.

Anxiousness is a normal human affect. Distinguishing it from pathologic anxiety and anxiety disorders often requires systematic evaluation and a thorough understanding of the individual patient's physical and psychological status. Unrecognized and untreated, anxiety disorders increase the cost of medical care and render patients vulnerable to further morbidity, including demoralization, hypochondriasis, depression, and varying degrees of disability. A comprehensive and empathic assessment of the anxious patient by the primary care physician permits a reasoned and often therapeutically effective approach to the difficult problems presented.

PATHOPHYSIOLOGY AND CLINICAL PRESENTATION

Definitions. *Anxiety* is the distressing experience of dread, foreboding, or panic accompanied by a variety of autonomic—primarily sympathetic—bodily symptoms. The distress, therefore, is both psychic and physical. Patients vary considerably in their tolerance to it. The new onset or exacerbation of anxiety often occurs in response to emotional or physiologic stimuli. Most persons meet the challenge of universally anxiety-provoking situations with their own personal strengths and styles of coping. When a patient's capacity for coping is overwhelmed, excessive anxiety may emerge. *Pathologic anxiety* is distinguished from the normal by its occurrence in the absence of an appropriate stimulus and by its duration or intensity.

Neurotransmitter Mechanisms. Several monoamine and neuropeptide neurotransmitters are implicated in the neurobiology of anxiety. *Norepinephrine* plays a prominent role in mediating anxiety states centrally. The locus ceruleus of the pons serves as the chief noradrenergic nucleus. Abnormal firing patterns in the locus ceruleus have been implicated in the pathophysiology of some anxiety conditions, such as panic disorder. In contrast, the inhibitory neurotransmitter *gamma-aminobutyric acid*, ubiquitous throughout the brain, is implicated as serving an anxiolytic function within the limbic system. The resultant somatic manifestations of anxiety are principally mediated by the *sympathetic nervous system*.

Classification and Basic Components of the Clinical Presentation. The classification of anxiety disorders is largely based on clinical features (Table 226.1). In both its normal and pathologic forms, anxiety's manifestations consist of affective, cognitive, behavioral, and somatic components. The *affective component* is characterized by the experience of dread, foreboding, or panic countered by *cognitions* that make sense of or seek to neutralize the distress. A variety of *behaviors* reflect the anxious state or evolve in response to it (e.g., avoidance). Typical psychological presentations might include complaints of apprehension, motor tension or agitation (restlessness, edginess, jitteriness), and heightened arousal (including hypervigilance, distractibility, impaired concentration, and insomnia). The *somatic complaints* are mostly those of autonomic hyperactivity and include systemic, cardiopulmonary, gastrointestinal, urinary, and neurologic symptoms (Table 226.2).

Adjustment Disorder with Anxious Mood. Most presentations of anxiety within the medical setting are normal reactions to anxiety-provoking situations. For a limited time period, a patient may suffer symptoms similar to those of a generalized anxiety disorder (see below). When a patient's capacity for coping is overwhelmed, excessive anxiety may transiently emerge until the patient is able to adjust. This state is termed *adjustment disorder with anxious mood* and typically resolves in less than 6 months. Adjustment disorders may likewise be heralded by other manifestations, including depressed mood and misconduct.

Generalized Anxiety Disorder. This common condition is characterized by anxiety lasting longer than 6 months and worry extending beyond a specific subject. Typically, the patient is ruminating with worries over a variety of concerns and may have been this way for several years with a waxing and

Table 226.1. Anxiety Disorders and Defining Features

Generalized Anxiety Disorder
Chronic anxiety lasting at least 6 months.
Concern over at least two different issues (usually many).
Panic attacks may be present.

Panic Disorder
Episodic extreme anxiety consistent with panic attacks.
At least one of the attacks being followed by at least one month
of one of the following:
Persistent concern about having additional attacks,
Worry about the implications of the attack or its consequences
(e.g., losing control, having a heart attack), or
A significant change in behavior related to the attacks.

Specific Phobia
Irrational fear associated with a particular stimulus.

Social Phobia
Anxiety associated with scrutiny by others.

Obsessive-Compulsive Disorder
Obsessions (intrusive unwanted bizarre thoughts) and/or compulsions (repetitive behaviors performed in a ritualistic or
stereotypical fashion).

Posttraumatic Stress Disorder
History of severe traumatic exposure.
Subsequent anxiety symptoms lasting at least 1 month.
Reexperiencing of the trauma (e.g., flashbacks), avoidance of
stimuli associated with the trauma, and increased arousal.
Syndrome may occur with delayed onset (greater than 6 months
after original trauma).

Adjustment Disorder with Anxious Mood[a]
Anxiety develops as a maladaptive response to an identifiable
stressor.
Symptoms last less than 6 months.

[a]Categorized with adjustment disorders rather than anxiety disorders in Diagnostic and Statistical Manual, 4th edition.

Table 226.2. Somatic Symptoms of Anxiety

TYPE	SPECIFIC SYMPTOMS
General	Fatigue, weakness, diaphoresis, insomnia, flushing, chills
Neurologic	Dizziness, paresthesias, derealization, near-syncope, tremulousness, restlessness
Cardiac	Palpitations, chest pain, tachycardia
Respiratory	Dyspnea, hyperventilation, choking
Gastrointestinal	Dry mouth, diarrhea, nausea, vomiting
Urinary	Frequency, urgency

waning course. Generalized anxiety disorder also includes an array of physical concomitants, including restlessness, fatigability, poor concentration, irritability, muscle tension, and insomnia. In addition to the persistent anxious state, the patient may describe more discrete episodes of acute anxiety.

When sudden spells of extreme anxiety occur with prominent symptoms of sympathetic activation, they may be accompanied by feelings of impending doom, fear of dying, the sensation of panic, and the impulse to flee. Such symptoms characterize *panic attacks*, which may occasionally be experienced by patients with generalized anxiety disorder, although they are a more prominent feature in panic disorder.

Panic Disorder. This anxiety disorder is characterized by *recurrent unexpected panic attacks*, with at least one attack followed by no less than a month of persistent concern about having additional attacks, worry about the implications of the attack or its consequences (e.g., losing control, having a heart attack), or a significant change in behavior related to the attacks. Panic disorder is more common in females and in those with a positive family history of panic. Emergence of anxiety symptoms early in life, including a history of separation difficulties during childhood, also represent risk factors for panic disorder.

Many patients become disabled by anticipatory fear of subsequent panic attacks and by phobic *avoidant behavior* patterns. They avoid places with restricted escape (e.g., crowds, theaters, tunnels, elevators), fearful of being trapped during an attack. In its most extreme form, *agoraphobia* (literally, "fear of the market place"), avoidant behavior may reach the point where a patient is afraid to leave the safety of the home or to be left alone. In rare situations, agoraphobia has also been reported to occur in the absence of panic disorder. (More commonly, the patient whose family describes them as "never leaving the house" has depression with loss of interest in doing their activities as a prominent symptom.)

The course of panic disorder includes times of frequent panic attacks interspersed with periods of less frequent episodes, complicated by phobic avoidance and anticipatory anxiety. The paroxysmal nature of panic attacks and the prominence of autonomic symptoms may mimic cardiac or neurologic disease, causing some patients to become hypervigilant, convinced of a serious underlying medical disorder, and "doctor shoppers" in search of such a diagnosis. Such persons may become demoralized, depressed, and debilitated. Suicide risk appears to be increased in panic disorder, especially in patients with concurrent depression.

Specific Phobias. A phobia is an irrational fear related to a specific stimulus. On exposure to that stimulus, the patient almost invariably manifests an anxiety response. A patient may suffer from a specific phobia of any specific stimulus. Although specific phobias commonly generate circumscribed symptoms, they may interfere with some aspect of a patient's functioning due to avoidance of the phobic stimulus or perseverance in the face of great discomfort (e.g., fear of flying leading to difficulty with travel).

Social Phobia (Social Anxiety Disorder). Patients with social phobia develop anxiety in situations where they are the focus of attention or might be scrutinized publicly. The individual fears they will act in a way (or show anxiety symptoms) that will be humiliating or embarrassing. Such patients may experience *performance anxiety* or "stage fright" but also exhibit distress in more ordinary social settings. In the generalized type, the fear includes *most social situations* (participating in small groups, dating, initiating or maintaining conversations, speaking to authority figures, attending parties, etc.). Social phobia is to be distinguished from the more limited form of normal performance anxiety, which occurs in universally acknowledged anxiety-provoking situational settings (e.g., performing in front of a very large audience or as part of a very important event).

Obsessive-Compulsive Disorder. More common than previously recognized, obsessive-compulsive disorder (OCD) affects up to 3% of the population. It is characterized by obsessions and/or compulsions that are sufficiently severe to cause patients substantial distress or impair their ability to function.

Obsessions are unwanted intrusive thoughts of a bizarre, senseless, or extreme nature. The subject of obsessions typically includes sexual or violent themes that are very distressing to patients and may lead them to fear that they are "going crazy." The recurrent and persistent thoughts, impulses, or images themselves become a source of anxiety.

Compulsions refer to repetitive behaviors that are performed in a stereotypical or ritualized fashion, usually in response to obsessions, sometimes in an effort to neutralize them. Resisting the drive to perform compulsions causes escalating anxiety, whereas succumbing and performing them is accompanied by feelings of transient relief, followed by feelings of shame. Characteristic compulsions include hand washing (to neutralize contamination obsessions), checking behaviors (e.g., doorlocks and stove burners to counteract obsessions of uncertainty), and counting (to neutralize anxiety associated with other obsessions).

The relationship between the compulsions and obsessions may also be nonsensical or irrational. Usually patients retain insight regarding the nonsensical or extreme nature of their thoughts and behaviors, distinguishing them from psychotic persons.

Because of the *shame* associated with the symptoms of OCD, it is not uncommon for patients to hide the disorder from friends, family, and doctors. OCD may come to the attention of primary care physicians when patients' obsessions involve preoccupations with their bodily functions (e.g., urinary or bowel obsessions) or susceptibility to disease (e.g., obsessions with contamination or fear of AIDS). Rarely, the compulsions may be performed to such extreme as to pose medical risk or sequellae (e.g., dermatologic complications of hand washing).

The *onset* of OCD is variable, with a bimodal distribution of age at onset, a peak in the preteen years, and another peak in the third decade of life. There is a disproportionate representation of males in the early peak and a disproportionate representation of females in the later peak. The *clinical course* is similarly variable; symptoms may arise at any age, wax and wane, and become exacerbated in times of stress.

The etiology and underlying pathophysiology of OCD are poorly understood. It has been related genetically to Tourette's disorder and commonly occurs with *depression*. Associated disorders include *body dysmorphic disorder* (i.e., preoccupation with a defective body image) and *trichotillomania* (compulsive hair pulling).

Posttraumatic Stress Disorder. Hours to months after a traumatic exposure (e.g., combat experience, natural disaster, physical assault, rape), the posttraumatic stress disorder (PTSD) patient reports *persistent reexperiencing* of the traumatic event, via intrusive thoughts, vivid dreams, or "flashbacks." Other requisite characteristics include *avoidance* of stimuli associated with the trauma, *hyperarousal* (e.g., increased startle response), and persistence of symptoms for more than 1 month. In many cases, the symptoms may continue for years. Rarely, the syndrome emerges more than 6 months after the traumatic exposure and in such cases is designated *"PTSD with delayed onset."*

Patients may present for medical assistance with primary complaints of anxiety or with concerns and questions regarding the neurologic underpinnings of their symptoms. Alternatively, PTSD may develop as a consequence of medical illness or procedures (e.g., amputation), which by their nature represent profound trauma. Medical settings may serve to trigger reexperiencing phenomena. It is important to be aware of the entity and sensitive to the needs of its sufferers.

Substance Abuse. Anxiety is often poorly tolerated, leading some patients to seek relief through use or abuse of anxiolytic substances. A patient's reliance on *alcohol, benzodiazepines* (BZDs), or any other sedating medication may reflect an unrecognized underlying anxiety disorder. Chronic use of sedating substances can lead to neural irritability and can cause or exacerbate anxiety after withdrawal. It often becomes difficult to differentiate the cause and effect relationship between substance abuse and anxiety. Patients with anxiety disorders are 50% more likely to be alcoholic, and similarly, the prevalence of anxiety disorders is 50% higher in alcoholics.

DIFFERENTIAL DIAGNOSIS

The medical differential diagnosis of the symptoms and signs associated with anxiety includes many conditions in which there is stimulation of the sympathetic nervous system (Table 226.3). Some reports suggest that undiagnosed medical ailments are responsible for a significant number of psychiatric referrals for "anxiety." Unrecognized arrhythmias, endocrinopathies, and medication reactions may mimic anxiety disorders and vice versa.

Among the psychiatric disorders to be considered in the differential diagnosis of anxiety are the *depressive disorders*. They are among the most critical to recognize, because they are common, treatable, carry a high risk of morbidity and mortality when untreated, and frequently coexist with symptoms of anxiety (see Chapter 227). Other psychiatric conditions presenting with anxiety as a prominent component include *psychosis, dementias, and drug-related disorders*.

WORKUP

The primary care physician's evaluation of anxiety needs to include assessment for medical causes and psychiatric diagnoses.

Assessment for Medical Causes. The list of possible medical causes is much too extensive to enable a workup that includes every possibility. A reasonable alternative is to focus on any medical conditions for which the patient is already under treatment. This includes a review of the patient's concerns, fears, and ongoing therapies. In addition, attention is directed toward the most important disorders commonly linked with anxiety, such as dysrhythmias (see Chapter 25), hyperthyroidism (see Chapter 103), and drug reactions or withdrawal (see Chapters 229 and 235). If the patient has a single prominent symptom or constellation of symptoms that implicate a single organ system, it is worthwhile to medically evaluate that focus in detail. However, the presence of multiple physical symptoms (six or more), high patient rating of symptom severity, low patient rating of health status, physician perception of

Table 226.3.   Medical Causes of Anxiousness

TYPE OF CAUSE	SPECIFIC CAUSE
Cardiovascular	Angina pectoris, arrhythmias, congestive heart failure, hypertension, hypovolemia, myocardial infarction, syncope (of multiple causes), valvular disease, vascular collapse (shock)
Dietary	Caffeinism, monosodium glutamate (Chinese-restaurant syndrome), vitamin-deficiency diseases
Drug related	Akathisia (secondary to antipsychotic drugs), anticholinergic toxicity, digitalis toxicity, hallucinogens, hypotensive agents, stimulants (amphetamines, cocaine, and related drugs), withdrawal syndromes (alcohol or sedative-hypnotics)
Hematologic	Anemias
Immunologic	Anaphylaxis, systemic lupus erythematosus
Metabolic	Hyperadrenalism (Cushing's disease), hyperkalemia, hyperthermia, hyperthyroidism, hypocalcemia, hypoglycemia, hyponatremia, hypothyroidism, menopause, porphyria (acute intermittent)
Neurologic	Encephalopathies (infectious, metabolic, and toxic), essential tremor, intracranial mass lesions, postconcussion syndrome, seizure disorders (especially of the temporal lobe), vertigo
Respiratory	Asthma, chronic obstructive pulmonary disease, pneumonia, pneumothorax, pulmonary edema, pulmonary embolism
Secreting tumors	Carcinoid, insulinoma, pheochromocytoma

the patient encounter as difficult, and age less than 50 years are important clues for an underlying anxiety or depressive disorder. Such easily identified clinical features have been shown to be independent predictors of underlying psychopathology in patients presenting to primary physicians with bodily symptoms. Because there are effective treatments for anxiety disorders, a diagnostic trial of an antianxiety therapy might help resolve a difficult diagnostic situation, but suppression of anxiety symptoms does not rule out a medical disorder and may even worsen it (e.g., use of BZDs for anxiety accompanying a severe asthma attack).

Assessment for Psychiatric Disorders. The physician should recall that anxiety symptoms are typically conceptualized in three dimensions: psychological, somatic, and behavioral.

Psychological. Patients suffering from an anxiety disorder may complain of somatic manifestations of anxiety but may omit history pertaining to the psychological experience. Therefore, it is important to inquire specifically about psychic manifestations such as fear, panic, the sensation of impending doom, or the impulse to flee. Reviewing the features of the various anxiety disorders sometimes helps the patient to construct a clearer clinical picture, but care must be taken not to prejudice the patient's responses or appear too eager to make a psychiatric diagnosis.

Somatic. One also needs to determine the *onset, quality, intensity, and duration* of symptoms, being certain to include a compassionate inquiry into recent life events and situational stressors present at the time that symptoms emerged.

Behavioral. Identifiable *stimuli or exacerbating factors* should be noted and settings that create apprehension. Development of *avoidant behaviors* should be ascertained. If a particular precipitant is identified, it is helpful to inquire into its origin (e.g., a phobia of dogs arising from a remote history of a dog bite or avoidance of elevators as a consequence of having had a panic attack in one). Often, symptoms may have arisen spontaneously, contributing to the sense that they are autonomous (as in panic disorder or OCD).

Also useful is inquiry into *strategies* used to alleviate the symptoms. This may uncover additional history about substance use, avoidance, or compulsive behaviors. *Family history* is reviewed for similar symptoms, known anxiety disorders, and related disorders such as depression or substance abuse. *Past history* of childhood school phobia or early patterns of timidity may be informative. Finally, a thorough physical examination is essential, checking for undisclosed sequelae of repetitive behaviors.

PRINCIPLES OF MANAGEMENT

The treatment strategies for anxiety include psychotherapeutic and pharmacologic interventions; a combined approach yields the best results.

Psychotherapy

Psychotherapeutic treatments for anxiety help to alleviate symptoms through insight, education, support, and the reconditioning of behavioral patterns. Supportive, insight-oriented, and behavioral psychotherapies may be used individually or jointly.

Supportive Psychotherapy. The hallmark of this approach is empathic listening, education, reassurance, encouragement, and guidance. The primary care practitioner frequently performs these functions, whether or not the intervention is labeled as supportive psychotherapy. In the case of anxiety, *empathic listening* helps patients to feel that another human being can appreciate their suffering and, as importantly, not judge them harshly because of their condition. Patients with anxiety often feel ashamed, characterizing themselves as "weak" or "silly" because of their fears and behaviors. Empathy helps to cut through the shame and loneliness. Listening and encouraging them to relate their histories can have a cathartic effect. Many patients with anxiety disorders have hidden some or all of their suffering for years.

In addition to empathic listening, *patient education* is crucial. It begins by informing the patient of the diagnosis and explaining its origins, prognosis, and treatment plan. Increased knowledge and understanding is empowering because it promotes a sense of command and confidence while reducing feelings of uncertainty, helplessness, and isolation. Such changes themselves are anxiolytic. Fears of serious somatic illness, "going crazy," and incurable disease are alleviated.

Reassurance in the form of "there is nothing serious," even if given in a sympathetic nonpatronizing manner, will be demoralizing and disappointing if offered perfunctorily. Although a negative medical workup may be reassuring to some patients, the patient with an anxiety disorder is often not relieved, because he or she is still experiencing distinctive, intrusive, and distressing symptoms. Reassurance serves to heal only when it addresses what is wrong and what can be done. It must be offered in concert with true empathy and education.

Once a strategy has been developed to manage the patient's anxiety, *guidance and encouragement* are helpful to the patient in negotiating treatment trials and supervening situational stresses.

Insight-oriented Psychotherapy. The objective is to guide the patient to an understanding of the association between circumstances, emotions, and symptoms. By exploring feelings, relationships, and actions (both past and present), the patient may develop new insights into his or her inner emotional makeup. This can help reduce the symptoms of anxiety and reframe the meaning of anxiety symptoms when they do occur. Insight therapy typically requires frequent and lengthy sessions for optimal results and the skill of a good psychotherapist.

Behavioral therapy is especially effective for anxiety patients. It consists of reconditioning or modifying patients' behaviors or the association between a stimulus and response. Techniques include general relaxation-response training (for tolerating anxiety symptoms), *in vivo* exposure and desensitization (for phobias and avoidant behaviors), cognitive therapy (for panic and obsessions), and exposure-response prevention (for OCD). The effectiveness of each of these behavioral techniques is augmented if the patient's anxiety can be held in check. For this reason, the behavioral therapies may be particularly well suited for combination with pharmacotherapies. As with insight-oriented psychotherapy, behavioral therapy is best conducted by professionals specially trained in this approach.

Relaxation techniques are of benefit to almost anyone who suffers from anxiety. Deep muscle relaxation, autogenic exercises, and diaphragmatic breathing are taught (see Appendix). Together, these techniques help to minimize the escalating anxiety that results from autonomic dyscontrol. Their use allows patients to better tolerate moderate anxiety states, abort panic episodes and use more aggressive behavioral techniques.

Exposure and desensitization entail gradual *reconditioning* of patients by exposing them to feared stimuli in controlled settings that minimize and allow habituation to their anxiety response. In this way, the feared stimuli become better tolerated and avoidant behaviors are eradicated, as the association with the anxiety response is weakened. Similarly, the exposure-response prevention paradigm is used in treating OCD patients. After being exposed to a provocative stimulus, they are helped to resist the urge to perform their compulsions in response to that stimulus. Although tolerating the anxiety, they may use sanctioned relaxation techniques. Gradually, the compulsions are reduced.

Cognitive-behavioral therapy. Preoccupation with physical symptoms and misinterpretation of their meaning characterize persons with panic disorder and hypochondriasis. Cognitive-behavioral therapy consists of addressing and correcting the patient's beliefs in conjunction with teaching behavioral techniques to help patients cope with their anxiety. The approach has been particularly successful when applied in the setting of noncardiac chest pain. Referral should be directed to therapists experienced in this method, because considerable skill is required to implement it successfully.

Pharmacotherapy

Treatment outcomes for psychotherapy are often enhanced when pharmacotherapy is incorporated into the program. The primary goal of drug therapy is sufficient diminution of symptoms to enable performance of tasks previously impaired by anxiety, including an enhanced ability to benefit from behavioral therapy. Patients should be informed that treatment will be of limited duration and will reduce their symptoms but not eradicate them. BZDs are the most widely used of anxiolytics. Antidepressants, β-adrenergic blocking agents, buspirone, and neuroleptics are also used.

Benzodiazepines. For rapid specific relief of anxiety symptoms, the BZDs are regarded as the anxiolytic of choice, superior in efficacy and safety to the barbiturates and the nonbarbiturate sedatives such as meprobamate, ethchlorvynol, and glutethimide. For some patients, BZDs offer substantial or complete relief of anxiety symptoms. For others, they attenuate severe anxiety pending response to other antianxiety therapies. There is wide individual variation in clinical response, plasma levels, and dosage requirements.

Ensuring Proper Use. Overuse and drug seeking from multiple sources occur in a small percentage of patients, although rarely with the intensity and risks associated with opiates, barbiturates, and other sedatives. Nevertheless, the physician should know the patient well before prescribing BZDs and be alert for signs of concurrent alcohol or drug dependence (see Chapters 228 and 235). The efficacy of treatment should be evaluated regularly by follow-up visits, with special attention to proper use. The physician should avoid prescribing by phone, calculate exact quantities required, and remain wary of "lost prescriptions" or other signs of medication misuse. To justify continued treatment, the patient should demonstrate a decrement in anxiety, with enhanced performance or decreased avoidant behavior. Requiring the patient to be seen in person for an appointment at least every 3 months is a good guideline, as is stopping the prescription of the BZD if there is a problem with compliance (e.g., attendance at appointments). BZD overuse is uncommon in the absence of a past history of alcohol or drug abuse but can be a serious problem, at times a consequence of careless prescribing practices and inadequate patient education about proper drug use. If dose requirements escalate, especially if accompanied by addictive behaviors, referral is advised to the specialist experienced in treating this problem.

Side Effects, Tolerance, and Dependence. Side effects include *sedation* (especially in combination with alcohol or other sedative agents), *impaired memory* acquisition (including amnesia reported with single-dose triazolam use), and, rarely, *disinhibition* characterized by increased hostility or aggression. Alcohol and cimetidine slow hepatic BZD metabolism and increase risk of toxicity.

Daily use of BZDs over time leads to receptor adaptation (*tolerance*) and the development of *physical dependence*. Physical dependence does not, however, imply misuse, abuse, or even loss of benefit. Rather, dependence denotes that a discontinuation syndrome will follow abrupt cessation of therapy. *Withdrawal* is usually accompanied by only mild symptoms but may include rebound anxiety, involuntary movements, insomnia, psychomotor restlessness, and perceptual changes.

Severe withdrawal symptoms are unlikely unless high doses or a high-potency preparation (especially a short-acting one) has been used daily for a prolonged time period and then halted abruptly. In such cases, a *delirium tremens*–like syndrome may develop. *Seizures* have been reported after sudden discontinuation of alprazolam after as short a time as 1 to 2 months of maintenance therapy. For less potent or long-acting BZDs, the risk of a severe abstinence syndrome is less. Chronic daily treatment is best discontinued by tapering doses over several weeks.

Selection of Agent. The available BZDs appear equally effective for the management of generalized anxiety symptoms when equipotent doses are used. In the future, one may see new BZDs with greater treatment specificity, because heterogeneity of brain BZD receptors has been demonstrated. For now, the essential differences among BZDs are in potency and pharmacokinetics (Table 226.4). These factors determine suitability for single-dose and maintenance use and risk of physical dependence and withdrawal.

For *single-dose use*, the desirable pharmacokinetic properties are rapid rate of onset and offset. Speed of absorption from the gastrointestinal tract is the most important factor determining onset. Capacity to traverse the blood–brain barrier is also a factor; the more lipophilic, the more quickly the drug enters the central nervous system. Lipophilicity also governs rate of clinical offset by determining how rapidly the drug is redistributed into lipid stores after a single dose. Serum half-life is not relevant to duration of action of single-dose use. *Diazepam* is rapidly absorbed and very lipid soluble, giving rapid onset and offset when used in single-dose fashion. Relatively rapid onset is usually desirable in situations in which single-dose use is prescribed.

For *maintenance use*, a drug's serum half-life is the pertinent parameter, affected by liver function and whether hepatic metabolites are active or inactive. Drugs with a short half-life are simply converted to water-soluble glucuronides and rapidly cleared by the kidneys. Their disadvantage is the potential for anxiousness and even mild withdrawal symptoms between doses. The longer half-life agents are more likely to accumulate. However, because of the development of drug tolerance, there is little additional risk of clinically important central ner-

vous system suppression among most users of long-acting agents. The exceptions are the elderly and those with hepatocellular disease, in whom use of long-acting agents can lead to overwhelming drug accumulation that causes excessive sedation, drowsiness, and psychomotor impairment.

Determination of Dosage. Dosage must ultimately be determined empirically on a case-by-case basis. It is most prudent to begin with low doses and titrate up as necessary. Most patients suffering from anxiety of lesser intensity than panic will not benefit from doses greater than 8 mg/d of lorazepam or its equivalent. Starting doses should typically not exceed the equivalent of 4 mg/d of lorazepam in young otherwise healthy adults who are BZD naive. In the elderly, starting and maximum doses should be approximately halved (see below). Steady state takes longer to achieve using drugs with a long half-life, an important consideration when deciding how often to adjust dose. A clinically useful rule of thumb is that steady state is 90% achieved after five drug half-lives.

Antidepressants. *Serotonin selective reuptake inhibitors* (SSRIs) are often used as first-line agents in the treatment of anxiety. They are among the most effective agents at eradicating the core symptoms of such anxiety conditions as *panic disorder, social phobia, generalized anxiety disorder, PTSD, and OCD*. As in depression, their beneficial effects are usually delayed for several weeks (see Chapter 227). *Tricyclic antidepressants* (TCAs) and the *monoamine oxidase inhibitors* (MAOIs) are generally used in the treatment of refractory patients.

Initiation of Therapy. Although the antidepressants are "first line" in terms of their efficacy, therapy is often initiated with BZDs to offer some immediate relief. Concurrently, or after anxiety symptoms are attenuated, antidepressant medication may be added. Once the antidepressant agent has become effective, some patients become entirely asymptomatic. In such instances, the BZD may be tapered down and even discontinued. In anxiety disorders, antidepressants are initiated with low doses (e.g., imipramine, 10 mg/d; fluoxetine, 10 mg/d), because brief symptom exacerbation may occur in some patients. Full antidepressant doses, if tolerated, are usually necessary. The recommended dose, for example, of paroxetine in the treatment of panic disorder is 40 mg/d.

Use in Specific Conditions. Two SSRIs (*sertraline and paroxetine*) have received U.S. Food and Drug Administration (FDA) indications for the treatment of *panic disorder*. There is a growing body of evidence supporting the use of the other SSRIs as well. *TCAs and MAOIs* have a long history of effec-

Table 226.4.   Pharmacokinetic Properties of Commonly Used Benzodiazepines

DRUG	APPROXIMATE DOSE EQUIVALENCE (mg)	RELATIVE RAPIDITY OF EFFECT	HALF-LIFE (hr)
Alprazolam (Xanax)	0.5	Fast/intermediate	12–15
Chlordiazepoxide (Librium)	10	Intermediate	5–30
Clonazepam (Klonopin)	0.25	Fast/intermediate	15–50
Clorazepate (Tranxene)	7.5	Fast	30–200
Diazepam (Valium)	5	Fastest	20–100
Lorazepam (Ativan)	1	Intermediate	10–20
Oxazepam (Serax)	15	Slower	5–15

tiveness in panic disorder. SSRIs may also be of utility in the treatment of *generalized anxiety disorder,* especially if panic attacks are present. Patients with *PTSD* respond best to initial use of antidepressants, with continuation based on treatment response and the constellation of symptoms. *OCD* patients respond especially well to SSRIs. There is some suggestion that the obsessions respond preferentially, whereas compulsions are best addressed through behavioral interventions combined with medications. Like the other anxiety disorders, *social phobia* has been shown to be effectively treated by most of the SSRIs, with several in the process of becoming FDA approved. Again, MAOIs have a long history of being particularly effective for social phobia, although their safety and side-effect profile restrict their use to treatment-resistant cases.

Buspirone is a non-BZD anxiolytic that acts as a partial serotonergic agonist and has mild anxiolytic and antidepressant effects. Because of its benign side-effect profile (nonaddicting and no withdrawal), buspirone is a reasonable alternative to BZDs in cases where *chronic anxiolysis* is required, especially when substance abuse or noncompliance is a concern. Risk from overdose is low, and the drug is well tolerated. Its anxiolytic effects are modest compared with those of the BZDs, and onset of action may take weeks, rendering the drug ineffective for single-dose use and of little help to patients with severe symptoms. Some efficacy has been reported in OCD. As a mild anxiolytic that may be taken frequently and safely, it may benefit patients with mild generalized anxiety or adjustment disorders. Treatment is initiated at doses of 5 mg three times a day and adjusted weekly in dose increments of 5 mg/d. In patients requiring more than 20 mg three times a day, referral to a specialist is recommended.

Beta-Blockers. β-Adrenergic blocking agents blunt the peripheral catecholamine-mediated manifestations of anxiety. As such, they are very useful on a short-term as-needed basis for *performance anxiety* and stage fright (e.g., propranolol 10 to 20 mg as needed). In the case of a special performance, it is suggested that the patient try a test dose a few days earlier to determine both efficacy and side effects. Large doses may blunt psychomotor responses. For generally anxious patients with prominent somatic manifestations of adrenergic excess (e.g., tremor, palpitations), longer acting beta-blockers (e.g., atenolol 50 mg/d) facilitate symptom control when used alone or in combination with BZDs. They should be used with caution, if at all, in patients with asthma, heart failure, or heart block (see Chapters 32 and 48). Moreover, they may worsen symptoms if there is an underlying depression (see Chapter 227).

Anxiolytic Pharmacotherapy in the Elderly. Because drug metabolism is slowed in the elderly, excessive sedation is a risk with anxiolytic therapy, especially with use of long-acting agents.

Benzodiazepines. In most instances, nighttime use of a short-acting agent that has no active metabolites and in patients whose metabolism is relatively unaffected by aging is preferred. *Lorazepam and oxazepam* fulfill these requirements. Their elimination by hepatic conjugation to a water-soluble glucuronide for renal excretion changes little with age. Lorazepam is the faster in onset; oxazepam's onset is gradual. Their disadvantages include the need for frequent dosing if

continuous anxiolysis is desired and rebound anxiety and insomnia if discontinued abruptly after prolonged use. Initial oxazepam dose is 10 mg; for lorazepam, it is 0.5 mg. Both are usually given before bed. Intake should be limited to short (5- to 10-day) courses or occasional as-needed use.

For more sustained anxiolysis, a BZD with a longer effective half-life may be required (Table 226.4). However, elimination of active drug metabolites lengthens with age, markedly prolonging drug half-life (e.g., from 20 to 90 hours for diazepam). Accumulation of active metabolites can cause diminished alertness and impair memory acquisition, mimicking dementia. Excessive sedation may cause a fall with serious injury—risk of hip fracture rises markedly with use of long-acting BZDs in the elderly. Initial doses should be small (e.g., the equivalent of 2 to 5 mg/d of diazepam) and increased slowly and cautiously. It may take up to 2 weeks to achieve steady-state levels after a change in dosage.

Antipsychotics. In the elderly, anxiety accompanied by agitation or specific psychotic manifestations may require short-term antipsychotic therapy. The *atypical antipsychotics* have become first-line agents, including *olanzapine* (Zyprexa), *risperidone* (Risperdal), *quetiapine* (Seroquel) and *clozapine* (Clozaril). A small dose of a high-potency typical antipsychotic such as *haloperidol* (Haldol) or *fluphenazine* (Prolixin) is another option. Lower potency agents (e.g., chlorpromazine, thioridazine, perphenazine) necessitate use of higher doses and increase the risk of hypotensive, cardiovascular, and anticholinergic side effects.

Antidepressants. Of the antidepressants, SSRIs are the best tolerated (see Chapter 227). Of the TCAs with anxiolytic activity, those with low anticholinergic and antiadrenergic side effects (e.g., nortriptyline) are preferred. Because antidepressant metabolism slows with age, one should start with half the usual dose and titrate up slowly.

Beta-Blockers. Beta-blocker use requires particular caution, given the prevalence of congestive heart failure, heart block, and obstructive lung disease in the elderly and their susceptibility to such side effects as cognitive blunting, nightmares, and depression.

THERAPEUTIC RECOMMENDATIONS AND INDICATIONS FOR REFERRAL

General Guidelines

- Begin with supportive psychotherapy that includes explanation, empathic listening, meaningful reassurance, guidance, and encouragement.
- Teach relaxation techniques for the patient willing to use them (see Appendix).
- Consider referral for insight-oriented therapy when there is emotional upheaval or disabling symptoms.
- Supplement psychotherapeutic measures with anxiolytic drug therapy to improve the patient's ability to perform daily activities previously impaired by anxiety. In most instances, use only in an adjunctive role for a limited duration. If BZD therapy is used, advise of the risk of physical dependence. Inform that drug treatment is likely to reduce symptoms but not eradicate them.
- Refer if there is evidence of substance abuse, either as an etiologic factor or as a mode of self-treatment.

Situational Anxiety and Adjustment Disorder

- Initiate supportive psychotherapy and behavioral therapy, including identification of specific provocative stressors and their association with the onset of symptoms.
- If distress from anxiety impairs daily functioning, begin a short course (up to 5 days) of BZD therapy (e.g., clonazepam 0.5 mg twice daily).
- If the distress represents one of many such episodes in a pattern of emotional upheaval, refer for insight-oriented therapy. Also refer if symptoms endure beyond the stressful period or worsen despite treatment.

Generalized Anxiety Disorder

- Initiate supportive psychotherapy and consider insight-oriented therapy to help diminish the role of psychosocial stressors.
- Consider a short course of BZD therapy for periods of exacerbation (e.g., alprazolam 0.5 mg three times a day for up to 5 days).
- Prescribe an SSRI if there is a history of associated panic attacks or depression (e.g., begin with venlafaxine–extended release [Effexor-XR] 37.5 mg twice daily and advance dose as tolerated to 150 mg twice daily).
- Avoid chronic BZD therapy due to risk of dependency. If the patient is coming off long-term therapy, taper over several weeks according to the patient's ability to tolerate decreases. Monitor for any withdrawal symptoms (e.g., tinnitus, perceptual changes, involuntary movements).
- Consider a trial of buspirone if chronic anxiolytic therapy is desired. Begin with 5 mg three times a day and gradually advance to a maximum of 60 mg/d. Risks of physiologic dependence and withdrawal are nil, but potency is low and it may take weeks to notice any effect.
- Refer patients with disabling chronic anxiety for psychiatric care.

Panic Disorder

- Use pharmacologic therapy to achieve control and minimize phobic avoidance and depression.
- Screen for suicidality (see Chapter 227), especially if patient is despondent; refer urgently if there is concern. Otherwise, begin therapy with a low dose of a serotonin reuptake inhibitor (e.g., paroxetine 10 mg daily). If agitation is not increased, proceed gradually to full antidepressant doses (e.g., paroxetine 40 mg/d; sertraline 150 mg/d).
- In situations where the cost benefits of a generic TCA override the better tolerability of an SSRI, start with a small "test" dose (e.g., imipramine 10 mg q.h.s. and proceed gradually as tolerated to 100 to 200 mg q.h.s.). The added costs of cardiac monitoring and blood levels of the TCAs must be factored into the cost-benefit equation.
- Alternatively, an MAOI antidepressant may be prescribed, but dietary restriction and expertise in its use are required (see Chapter 227).
- If rapid relief is sought due to presence of disabling phobic behavior, start with a potent BZD (e.g., alprazolam 0.25 to 0.5 mg four times a day or clonazepam 0.5 mg q.h.s. or twice daily), pending onset of benefit from antidepressant therapy.

- After a period of well-being, taper BZD medication to the lowest possible maintenance dose or proceed to discontinuation.
- Weigh continued BZD use against risk of dependence. Use of potent BZDs poses risks of dependence and severe withdrawal. Taper slowly over several weeks when discontinuing therapy that has been continuous for more than 6 weeks.
- Refer patients with prominent phobic behavior and those with suicidal ideation.
- For patients requiring longer term maintenance therapy, it is important to continue the antidepressant medication at its full acute-phase dose.

Social Phobia

- Refer for behavioral therapy.
- Prescribe a BZD on an as-needed single-dose basis to help attenuate anxiety, decrease avoidance, and facilitate daily functioning and behavioral therapy.
- Prescribe a low-dose SSRI (e.g., paroxetine 10 mg q.h.s.) and proceed gradually to full antidepressant doses (paroxetine 40 mg q.h.s or fluoxetine 20 to 40 mg q.a.m.).
- For patients whose performances are compromised by ordinary "stage fright," consider a trial of a beta-blocker (e.g., propranolol 10 mg, up to 20 mg four times a day) on an as-needed basis. Give a preperformance trial dose to be sure performance is not compromised by the medication.

Specific Phobias

- Refer for behavioral therapy.
- Consider rapidly acting single-dose BZD therapy (e.g., alprazolam 0.25 to 0.5 mg or diazepam 10 mg) on an as-needed basis to provide symptomatic control in anxiety-provoking situations and to facilitate behavioral therapy.

Obsessive-Compulsive Disorder

- Refer for behavioral therapy.
- Initiate pharmacologic therapy with an SSRI.
- Refer to an experienced psychopharmacologist for further management of the drug treatment program.

Posttraumatic Stress Disorder

- Refer to a psychiatrist specializing in the treatment of such persons. Most programs begin with an SSRI. Mood stabilizers may be helpful for prominent irritability or anger. BZDs may sometimes be helpful in the short term but must be used with caution because of the risk of substance abuse in this vulnerable population of patients.
- Refer to an experienced psychotherapist. Three psychotherapy techniques—exposure therapy, cognitive therapy, and anxiety management—are considered to be the most useful in the treatment of PTSD. Expert therapists make distinctions among the techniques depending on which specific type of symptom presentation is most prominent. Insight-oriented psychotherapy helps to overcome emotional memories of the traumatic event; behavioral techniques may also be of benefit.

Treatment of the Elderly

- Reduce starting doses of medications by one half of the usual adult dose.
- When using BZDs for short-term anxiolysis, prescribe lorazepam or oxazepam. For chronic anxiolysis, use longer half-life agents with caution and at reduced doses and dose intervals.
- If antidepressants are indicated for anxiolysis, consider an SSRI (e.g., fluoxetine) or an MAOI (see Chapter 227).
- If agitation, "sundowning," or psychotic features accompany anxiety, prescribe small doses of an atypical neuroleptic (e.g., risperidone 0.5 mg once or twice daily).

ANNOTATED BIBLIOGRAPHY

American Psychiatric Association. Diagnostic and statistical manual of mental disorders, 4th ed. Washington, DC: American Psychiatric Association, 1994. (The standard for diagnosis.)

Apter JT, Allen LA. Buspirone: future directions. J Clin Psychopharm 1999;19:86. (Review of its clinical uses in psychiatric illness.)

Brown RL, Brown RL, Saunders LA, et al. Physicians' decisions to prescribe benzodiazepines for nervousness and insomnia. J Gen Intern Med 1997;12:44. (Reveals common misconceptions and pitfalls in use of BZDs.)

Bulow K. Management of psychosis and agitation in elderly patients: a primary care perspective. J Clin Psychiatry 1999;60[Suppl 13]:22. (Treatment strategies for agitation in elderly patients.)

Gorman J, Shear MK, Cowley D, et al. American Psychiatric Association. Practice guideline for the treatment of patients with panic disorder. Am J Psychiatry 1998;155[Suppl]. (Practice guideline developed by psychiatrists who coordinate the overall care of the patient with panic disorder.)

Greenberg PE, Sisitsky T, Kessler RC, et al. The economic burden of anxiety disorders in the 1990s. J Clin Psychiatry 1999;60:427. (A societal perspective on the cost of anxiety disorders.)

Kronke K, Jackson JL, Chamberlain J. Depressive and anxiety disorders in patients presenting with physical complaints: clinical predictors and outcome. Am J Med 1997;103:339. (Identifies a set of clinical clues that are independent predictors of underlying psychopathology in patients presenting with physical complaints.)

Mavissakalian M, Perel JM. Protective effects of imipramine maintenance treatment in panic disorder with agoraphobia. Am J Psychiatry 1992;149:1053. (Data confirming the need for maintenance treatment to protect against relapse.)

New frontiers in the management of social anxiety disorder: diagnosis, treatment and clinical course. J Clin Psychiatry 1999;60[Suppl 9]. (A comprehensive update.)

Roy-Byrne P, Stein M, Bystritsky A, et al. Pharmacotherapy of panic disorder: Guidelines for the family physician. J Am Board Fam Practice 1998;11:282. (Practical clinical care by the primary care physician.)

Roy-Byrne PP, Stein MB, Russo J, et al. Panic disorder in the primary care setting: comorbidity, disability, service utilization, and treatment. J Clin Psychiatry 1990;60:492. (Improved treatment interventions to decrease disability and potentially inappropriate medical service utilization.)

Stein MB, Liebowitz MR, Lydiard RB, et al. Paroxetine treatment of generalized social phobia (social anxiety disorder). JAMA 1998;280:708. (Data on the first medication ever FDA approved for the treatment of social phobia.)

Stein MB, McQuaid JR, Laffaye C, et al. Social phobia in the primary care medical setting. J Fam Pract 1999;48:514. (Underdiagnosis and undertreatment of a disorder that frequently presents to the primary care physician.)

Treatment of panic disorder: the state of the art. J Clin Psychiatry 1997;58[Suppl 2]. (An entire supplement on current psychotherapeutic and psychopharmacologic treatment options.)

Treatment of posttraumatic stress disorder: the expert consensus guideline series. J Clin Psychiatry 1999;60[Suppl 16]:1. (An entire journal volume devoted to treatment strategies.)

van Peski-Oosterbaan AS, Spinhoven P, Van Rood Y, et al. Cognitive-behavioral therapy for noncardiac chest pain: a randomized trial. Am J Med 1999;106:424. (A well-designed example of the successful application of cognitive-behavioral therapy.)

Weissman MM, Klerman GL, Markowitz JS, et al. Suicidal ideation and suicide attempts in panic disorder and attacks. N Engl J Med 1989;321:1209. (Risk increased and independent of other possible precipitants; adjusted odds ratios 2.6.)

Williams, DDR, McBride A. Benzodiazepines: time for reassessment. Br J Psychiatry 1998;173:361. (Editorial on their proper place in the treatment armamentarium.)

Appendix: Strategies for Stress Management

WILLIAM E. MINICHIELLO

Stress is not harmful when managed effectively. With the increased awareness of the impact of stress on the body has come a variety of stress-reducing techniques derived from behavior therapy. Stress management training enables the patient to condition his or her body to cope more adaptively with stress or anxiety. As part of a comprehensive treatment program, the primary care physician may choose to train the patient in one or more of the self-regulatory procedures. Relaxation training is by far the most effective of the procedures.

Before proceeding to train the patient in relaxation as a self-control procedure, the physician should advise reduction or elimination of caffeine from the patient's diet, because relaxation training is aimed at lowering the patient's autonomic arousal level and caffeine augments arousal.

Progressive deep muscle relaxation, autogenic training, and diaphragmatic breathing represent the major techniques practical for use in the primary care setting.

PROGRESSIVE DEEP MUSCLE RELAXATION

Progressive deep muscle relaxation is probably the most extensively used and most effective relaxation technique today for the treatment of anxiety and stress-related problems. A brief modified version can be taught to the patient in one session. The rationale for the technique is the view that anxiety and relaxation are mutually exclusive; that is, anxiety cannot be experienced when the muscles are relaxed.

Progressive deep muscle relaxation is a simple procedure contrasting tension with relaxation. Because a person generally has very little awareness of the sensation of relaxation, one is asked first to tense a set of muscles as hard as one can until they can feel tension in the muscles. Then one allows those muscles to relax and tries to become aware of ("to feel internally") the difference between tension and relaxation.

This relaxation technique entails the systematic focus of attention on specific gross muscle groups throughout the body. The patient is instructed to actively tense each muscle group for

Table 226.5.   Progressive Deep Muscle Relaxation Instructions to Patients:

Practice is to be done while sitting in a chair with your back straight, head on a line with your back, both feet on the floor and hands resting on your lap. Each muscle is to be tightened, held in tightened position for 15–20 seconds, and then slowly let go while studying the difference between tension and relaxation.

Forehead. Wrinkle up your forehead by arching your eyebrows and creasing your forehead, hold the tension, and then slowly let go of the tension.

Eyes. Squeeze your eyes together tightly, hold the tension, and then slowly let go of the tension.

Nose. Wrinkle up your nose and spread your nostrils, hold the tension, and then slowly let go of the tension.

Face. Put a forced smile on your face and spread your face, hold the tension, and then slowly let go of the tension.

Tongue. Push your tongue hard against the roof of your mouth, hold the tension, and then slowly let go of the tension.

Jaws. Clench your jaws together tightly, hold the tension, and then slowly let go of the tension.

Lips. Pucker up your lips and spread them, hold the tension, and then slowly let go of the tension.

Neck. Tighten the muscles of your neck by pulling your chin in and shrugging up your shoulders, hold the tension, and then slowly let go of the tension.

Right Arm. Tense your right arm and hand by stretching it out in front of you and clenching your fist tightly, hold the tension, and then slowly let go of the tension.

Left Arm. Tense your left arm and hand by stretching it out in front of you, and then slowly let go of the tension.

Right Leg. Extend your right leg in front of you (at the height of the chair seat), tense your thigh and leg by pointing your toes inward toward your face, hold the tension, and then slowly let go of the tension.

Left Leg. Extend your left leg in front of you, tense your thigh and leg by pointing your toes inward toward your face, hold the tension, and then slowly let go of the tension.

Upper Back. Tense your back muscles by sitting slightly forward in the chair, bending your elbows and trying to get them to touch each other behind your back, hold the tension, and then slowly let go of the tension.

Chest. Tense your chest muscles by pulling your stomach in and thrusting your chest upward and outward, hold the tension, and then slowly let go of the tension.

Stomach. Tense your stomach muscles, making them hard by pushing your stomach out, hold the tension, and then slowly let go of the tension.

Buttocks and Thighs. Tense your buttocks and thighs by placing your feet squarely on the floor, pointing your toes into the floor and forcing your heels to remain on the floor while pushing forward, hold the tension, and then slowly let go of the tension.

Practice should be engaged in twice daily for a period of 12–15 minutes. Mastery of the technique is after 2–4 weeks of twice daily practice.

---

10 to 15 seconds, after which they are told to let go of the tension in the muscles, observe the difference, and relax the muscles. The sequence of tensing the muscles, letting go of the tension, and noting the difference between tension and relaxation is systematically applied to a host of muscle groups starting at the head and ending at the toes (Table 226.5).

AUTOGENIC TRAINING

Autogenic training is a relaxation technique composed of a set of exercises that are intended to induce heaviness and warmth in the muscles through mental imagery.

Autogenic training typically involves the patient sitting comfortably in an armchair in a quiet room with the eyes closed. Verbal formulas are introduced (e.g., "my arm is heavy"), and the patient is instructed to visualize and feel the relaxation of the muscle being focused on while silently repeating and passively concentrating on that formula. The formulas, which consist of verbal somatic suggestions, are intended to facilitate concentration and "mental contact" with the parts of the body indicated by the formula.

Training consists of six psychophysiologic exercises, which are practiced several times a day. The training begins with the theme of heaviness (e.g., "my arm feels heavy and relaxed"). The second group of formulas involve warmth (e.g., "my arm feels warm and relaxed"). After warmth training, the patient continues with passive concentration on cardiac activity (e.g., "my heartbeat feels calm and regular"). The fourth exercise focuses on

breathing and respiration. In the next exercise, the patient focuses on warmth in the chest and abdomen, and in the last exercise the focus is passive concentration on cooling of the forehead.

In modern practice, the time and the six standard exercises have been condensed so that a whole round can be practiced in

Table 226.6.   Autogenic Training Instructions to Patients:

Practice is to be done while sitting in a soft, comfortable chair with your eyes closed. As attention is called to specific groups of muscles, try to *visualize* and *feel* the relaxation of those muscles. Try to let *happen* what is being suggested. Repeat each formula 2–3 times.

My forehead and scalp feel heavy, limp, loose, and relaxed.

My eyes and nose feel heavy, limp, loose, and relaxed.

My face and jaws feel heavy, limp, loose, and relaxed.

My neck, shoulders, and back feel heavy, limp, loose, and relaxed.

My arms and hands feel heavy, limp, loose, and relaxed.

My chest, solar plexus, and the central part of my body feel quiet, calm, comfortable, and relaxed.

My stomach feels heavy, limp, loose, and relaxed.

My buttocks, thighs, calves, ankles, and toes feel quiet, heavy, limp, loose, and relaxed.

My whole body feels quiet, heavy, limp, and relaxed.

Practice should be engaged in twice daily for a period of 6–8 minutes. Mastery of the technique is after 1–3 weeks of twice daily practice.

a very brief period of between 5 and 10 minutes. In this condensed version, the autogenic training phrases are focused primarily on the physiologic aspect used in the training, interspersed with general suggestions for relaxation. Each phrase is said slowly, allowing time for the patient to begin to feel some awareness of the effect of the suggestion (Table 226.6).

DIAPHRAGMATIC BREATHING

The quickest and simplest method of relaxation is to breathe slowly and deeply from the belly. Diaphragmatic breathing is an effective means of coping with and reducing stress.

For centuries, students of yoga and zen have been aware that a mastery of breathing could slow heart rate, lower blood pressure, and calm the body. Diaphragmatic breathing involves parasympathetic nervous system stimulation. Diaphragmatic breathing prevents the possibility of hyperventilation and, after 50 to 60 seconds of such breathing, brings a feeling of quiescence to the body and reduction in bodily symptoms of stress.

Training in diaphragmatic breathing can be done either sitting or lying down. In either position, a pillow should be placed at the small of the back to force the belly out. Breathing should begin by pushing the stomach out as inhalation takes place slowly and deeply. Care should be taken to minimize the movement of the chest with each inhalation. The word "relax" should be said silently before exhaling, and the stomach should fall with exhalation. While breathing in, the stomach should be pushed out; while breathing out, the stomach should come in (Table 226.7).

Table 226.7.   Diaphragmatic Breathing Instructions to Patients:

While sitting or lying down with a pillow at the small of your back

1. Breathe in slowly and deeply by pushing your stomach out.
2. Say the word "relax" silently to yourself prior to exhaling.
3. Exhale slowly, letting your stomach come in.
4. Repeat entire procedure 10 times consecutively, with emphasis on slow, deep breaths.

Practice should take place 5 times per day, 10 consecutive diaphragmatic breaths each sitting. Time for mastery is after 1–2 weeks of daily practice.

227

Approach to the Patient with Depression
JOHN J. WORTHINGTON III
SCOTT L. RAUCH

Most patients with depression present to primary care physicians, often complaining of somatic symptoms. The frequency, treatability, and potentially serious consequences of depression make its diagnosis and management high priorities for the primary care physician. Unfortunately, the diagnosis is not always evident because the symptoms may masquerade as a variety of psychiatric or somatic conditions. Moreover, the stigma of psychiatric diagnosis can impede recognition of depressive illness by both patients and physicians.

PATHOPHYSIOLOGY AND CLINICAL PRESENTATION

Mechanisms

The purported mechanisms of depression include psychodynamic, cognitive, genetic, neuroendocrine, and neurotransmitter determinants. Depression most likely represents a complex combination of these elements. Genetic factors and/or early childhood experiences may render persons more susceptible to depression. Neurotransmitter and neurohumoral elements probably serve as important effector pathways for development of symptoms.

Psychodynamic origins are believed to involve difficulties with formation and maintenance of self-esteem, which may occur from having hypercritical parents or being abused. In addition, growing up in an emotionally unresponsive environment may compromise learning ways to effectively cope with situational stresses. Suffering loss or failure as an adult is likely to be difficult, poorly responded to, and capable of reawakening prior painful feelings of inadequacy and worthlessness that lead to depression. Rigid dysfunctional defenses may be erected in an attempt to minimize the chances of loss or failure.

The cognitive perspective views depression as the consequence rather than as the origin of negative or distorted thinking. Subscribing to inflexible rules of conduct and unattainable goals can be a setup for failure and loss of self-esteem. Setbacks are viewed as a reflection of one's unworthiness and inadequacy.

Genetic determinants have been discovered from studies of twins, chromosomes, and pedigrees. In some pedigrees, there appears to be a dominant gene with incomplete penetrance. A family history of affective disease is commonly elicited. Major depression is up to three times more common among first-degree relatives of people with the disorder than in the general population.

Neurotransmitter basis of depression began with the finding that reserpine could induce depression and monoamine oxidase inhibitors could reverse it. This led to the identification of altered neurotransmitter metabolism as an important biochemical concomitant of depression and to the discovery of new antidepressant drugs, each increasing the availability of a major central neurotransmitter (e.g., norepinephrine, serotonin, or acetylcholine), usually by selective inhibition of reuptake.

Neuroendocrine hypotheses derive from the observation that most neurovegetative manifestations of depression (changes in appetite, libido, diurnal rhythms) involve hypothalamic functions. In addition, links between neurotransmitter release and neurohormone activity have been identified. Corticotropic-releasing hormone is believed to play an important role, resulting in hypercortisolism. Early morning awakening, reflecting an abnormal advance in circadian rhythm, may be one consequence.

Psychological and Somatic Manifestations

Depression's clinical presentation includes a host of psychological and bodily complaints.

Psychological Manifestations. Sadness is a very common symptom. Irritability, discouragement, loss of interest, worry, frustration, and decreased libido comprise the major dysphoric manifestations and may occur in the absence of overt sadness (Table 227.1). Some patients become preoccupied with physical complaints, such as pain or bowel dysfunction. Others exhibit changes in memory, concentration, or self-image. Diurnal mood variation is characteristic, with symptoms often worse in the morning and improving as the day progresses.

Depressed affect can be subtle, at times only noticed when sadness ensues from talking with the patient. As depression worsens, psychomotor abnormalities may appear. Although psychomotor retardation, with slowed speech and a long latency before the patient answers questions, has been thought of as the classic presentation of depression, in fact, anxiety is the

much more common symptom. Nearly three fourths of patients with a depressive disorder have worry, psychic anxiety, or somatic anxiety as one of their presenting symptoms.

Somatic Manifestations. Distinctive neurovegetative symptoms include *disturbed sleep* (most commonly *early morning awakening*), *lack of energy*, and *decreased appetite*. Neurovegetative symptoms are predictive of responsiveness to psychopharmacologic intervention. In what is termed an *atypical depression*, patients may exhibit *increased sleep and increased appetite* (hypersomnolence and hyperphagia).

Diagnostic Classification (Based on the Diagnostic and Statistical Manual, 4th edition)

Although no single classification system is universally accepted, the current standard of diagnosis in the United States is the American Psychiatric Association's Diagnostic and Statistical Manual, 4th edition (DSM-IV) (Table 227.2).

Major Depression (Unipolar Depression). This is the DSM-IV term for serious depression that is accompanied by neurovegetative symptoms. Lifetime risk of developing a major depression is estimated to be one in four for women and one in eight for men. Dysphoric mood typically dominates the clinical picture and is persistent. Four or more of the major neurovegetative symptoms dominate the clinical picture and are present for a minimum of 2 weeks, including appetite disturbance,

---

Table 227.1.   Clinical Presentation of Depressive Syndromes

Psychological Symptoms and Signs
Mood sad, "blue," and "down"
Depressed affect
Anxiety
Irritability or anger
Anhedonia (lack of pleasure)
Loss of interest in environment
Loss of interest in activities
Loss of interest in sex (decreased libido)
Social withdrawal
Guilt (may be delusional)
Poor self-esteem
Self-deprecatory thoughts
Poor concentration or indecisiveness
Rumination or obsessive thoughts
Feelings of helplessness or hopelessness
Recurrent thoughts of death or suicide
Psychotic symptoms (e.g., delusions or hallucinations)
Multiple physical complaints or hypochondriacal fears

Neurovegetative Symptoms and Signs
Sleep disturbance (frequently early morning awakening)
Decreased energy
Appetite disturbance (usually decreased)
Diurnal mood variation (usually worse in morning)
Psychomotor retardation or agitation

Table 227.2.   Classification of Depressive Syndromes

Major Affective Disorders
Major depression (unipolar depression)
  Severe and episodic with prominent neurovegetative signs and symptoms
  Atypical presentations may include chronic pain, hypochondriasis, or cognitive difficulties
  May be accompanied by psychotic features
  Treatment: antidepressant plus psychotherapy
Bipolar disorder (manic-depressive illness)
  Severe and episodic, with a history of a manic episode
  Depressed phase is clinically identical to major depression
  May be accompanied by psychotic features
  Treatment: mood stabilizing agent (plus possibly an antidepressant in depressed phase) plus psychotherapy

Chronic Affective Disorders
Dysthymic disorder
  Chronic and less severe, with fewer neurovegetative symptoms
  Frequently accompanied by personality disorder
  Treatment: psychotherapy plus trial of antidepressant if neurovegetative symptoms are distressing
Cyclothymic disorder
  Less severe, chronic mood swings
  Treatment: mood stabilizing agent plus psychotherapy

Organic Brain Syndrome
Organic affective disorder
  Depression or mania due to an organic cause
  Treatment: manage underlying medical problem; a trial of antidepressant if necessary

Other Conditions
Adjustment disorder with depressed mood
  Time limited, in response to identifiable precipitant, without neurovegetative symptoms sufficient for major depression
  Treatment: psychotherapy plus a trial of antidepressant if neurovegetative symptoms are distressing

sleep disturbance, psychomotor retardation or agitation, anhedonia, loss of energy, feelings of worthlessness or guilt, decreased concentration, and suicidal thoughts.

Onset is variable. Symptoms usually develop over weeks to months, but they may develop suddenly. Situational factors surrounding the onset of the illness have no bearing on the diagnosis. Historically, distinctions were made between *endogenous and reactive depression*, but an identifiable precipitant is no longer considered pertinent with respect to diagnosis. Frequency of episodes appears to increase with age. At least half of patients have recurrent episodes. A family history of a major affective disorder (major depression or bipolar disorder) is common. The relationship between alcoholism and depression remains controversial.

Major Depression with Psychotic Features. A subclassification of major depression, this disorder has the additional features of delusions, hallucinations, bizarre behavior, or disorganized thinking.

Major Depression in the Elderly. In the elderly, depression can mimic dementia. The patient may appear withdrawn, unkempt, inattentive, or even confused. The condition may be due to depression alone or to a combination of depression and dementia.

Bipolar Disorder–Depressed Phase. The presentation of a depressive episode in a bipolar (manic-depressive) patient is identical to that of major depression, except there is a history of prior manic or hypomanic episodes. *Mania* is manifested by periods of elation or expansive mood, increased energy, decreased need for sleep, inflated self-esteem, and overinvolvement in activities, accompanied by a decreased concern for the consequences. Its diagnosis requires adequate severity to substantially impair level of functioning. If the hallmark symptoms of mania exist, but the patient shows no decrement in functioning, the patient is described as *hypomanic*.

Distinguishing between unipolar and bipolar depressions is very important in determining treatment (see below).

Dysthymic Disorder. This category denotes a chronic low-grade depression, characterized by pervasive dysphoric mood for at least 2 years. Some complain of life-long feelings of depression. Symptoms are less severe than those of major depression and neurovegetative symptoms are fewer. Depression appears as an integral part of personality or their character (hence the older term *characterologic depression*). Such patients can be frustrating to treat because of chronic dysphoria, self-pity, and development of irrational patterns of negative thinking (e.g., "things always go wrong for me"). The physician typically develops feelings of helplessness and may unconsciously communicate a wish that the patient would go away.

Typically, onset is in adolescence or early adult life and accompanied by other symptoms of a *personality disorder*, such as a history of difficulty with interpersonal relationships, manipulativeness, feelings of emptiness, and lack of an identity. A subpopulation of dysthymic patients seems to have an attenuated chronic form of major depression with onset later in life after a period of good functioning. Neurovegetative symptoms may be more prominent.

Dysthymia and major depression can coexist in a given patient (so-called "*double depression*"), when a major depressive episode evolves in the context of preexisting dysthymia. However, incomplete recovery from a major depression should be described as major depression in partial remission rather than dysthymia.

Cyclothymic Disorder. This state resembles bipolar illness, but the mood swings are less severe. These patients have a chronic mood disturbance characterized by periods of depression alternating with periods of elevated mood. Neither are of sufficient severity or duration to meet the criteria for major depressive or manic episodes. Interspersed may be periods of normal mood lasting as long as several months.

Seasonal Affective Disorder. This depressive variant is distinguished by its seasonal pattern, characteristically beginning in the fall and ending about 5 months later. It has been linked to lack of light exposure and is more common in northern latitudes. Alterations in serotonin activity have also been noted. As in other forms of depression, sadness is the dominant affect, and fatigue and decreased libido are common. Atypical features include tendencies to overeat and oversleep. In the United States, women are more commonly affected than men (ratio, 3:1). Age of onset is typically in the 20s.

Adjustment Disorder with Depressed Mood. This occurs after a *significant life stress*. Patients usually present with depressed mood associated with feelings of hopelessness, helplessness, worthlessness, and anxiety. Their thoughts are often dominated by the problems that precipitated the episode. Sleep and appetite disturbances are common but are less severe and less persistent than in major depression. The condition is usually self-limited, lasting less than 6 months and improving when the stress is removed or the individual evolves a more adaptive coping mechanism. It is important to note that any patient with symptoms severe enough to meet the criteria for major depression (described above) should receive that diagnosis regardless of the history of a precipitant. The message that the primary care physician should gather from this chapter is that evaluating the depressive symptoms, regardless of a *suspected precipitant*, is crucial, and possibly life saving, in initiating antidepressant treatment.

DIFFERENTIAL DIAGNOSIS

It is important to consider organic causes of depression, including *drug-related* etiologies, which are among the most common (Table 227.3). Chronic feelings of fatigue and dysphoria are nonspecific symptoms common to multiple medical conditions whose differential diagnosis includes *chronic fatigue syndrome, Lyme disease, fibromyalgia, rheumatoid disease, and endocrinopathies* (see Chapter 8). Patients experiencing domestic violence may present with frank major depression or multiple bodily complaints (e.g., headache, gastrointestinal symptoms, premenstrual difficulties, sexual dysfunction) mimicking depression. In addition, several psychiatric disorders can masquerade as depression.

Uncomplicated Bereavement. Symptoms of normal grief may initially be identical to those of depression. The question

Table 227.3.   Organic Etiologies of Depression

Drug induced: alpha-methyldopa, antiarrhythmics, benzodiazepines, barbiturates and other CNS depressants, β-blockers, cholinergic drugs, corticosteroids, digoxin, H₂-blockers, and reserpine.

Substance-abuse related: alcohol abuse, sedative-hypnotic abuse, cocaine and other psychostimulant withdrawal.

Toxic-metabolic disorders: hypothyroidism or hyperthyroidism (especially in elderly), Cushing's syndrome, hypercalcemia, hyponatremia, and diabetes mellitus.

Neurologic disorders: stroke, subdural hematoma, multiple sclerosis, brain tumor, Parkinson's disease, Huntington's disease, epilepsy, and dementias.

Infectious disorders: viral infections (especially mononucleosis and influenza), HIV with or without AIDS, and syphilis.

Nutritional disorders: vitamin B₁₂ deficiency and pellagra.

Other: carcinomas (especially pancreatic carcinoma) and postsurgically (especially cardiac surgery).

CNS, central nervous system.

of a superimposed depression should be raised if mourning continues for more than 6 months, if neurovegetative symptoms are particularly severe, if there is severe impairment in the patient's ability to function, or if psychotic symptoms emerge.

Alcoholism and Drug Dependence. Many alcoholic patients appear depressed. It is not possible to delineate which symptoms are due to alcohol and which, if any, might be due to a primary affective disorder until the patient has been fully detoxified. Other substance abuse disorders may mimic depression, especially abuse of sedative-hypnotics or withdrawal from psychostimulants.

Personality Disorders. These patients frequently complain of depressive symptoms, with periods of severe dysphoria, but their affective symptoms often fluctuate markedly with environmental changes (especially with changes in interpersonal relationships). Poor impulse control, histories of unstable relationships, and a striking quality of manipulativeness or entitlement are other clues to primarily characterologic pathology.

WORKUP

The possibility of depression should always be considered in patients who present with fatigue, poor sleep, appetite disturbances, multiple bodily complaints, and expresses feelings of hopelessness or poor self-esteem. The onset of depressive symptoms and signs in patients with chronic debilitating disorders or chronic pain can be slow and subtle and should not be overlooked. When depression is suspected, specific inquiry into its manifestations is needed. However, before proceeding with the inquiry, it is useful to complete a detailed medical history for "organic" etiologies (including elicitation of specific patient concerns) and to follow later with a detailed physical examination, especially in patients who present complaining of somatic symptomatology. Not to do so risks alienating the patient, who wants his or her medical complaints taken seriously. Also useful are a few words to explain the rationale for considering depression (e.g., "it's a serious treatable condition and listed as

one of the important causes of the symptoms bothering you"). These few simple measures facilitate patient understanding and impart a sense of seriousness and thoroughness to the workup. In addition, they help reduce the stigma of considering a psychiatric diagnosis.

History

Strategy. The dimensions to explore include neurovegetative symptoms, multiple bodily complaints, psychosocial history, and past psychiatric history of patient and family. It is helpful and often less threatening to ask first about neurovegetative symptoms such as sleep, appetite, and energy. If the responses are suggestive of depression, one can proceed to inquire about mood and any loss of interest in sex, family, job, and other sources of interest or pleasure. In addition, the patient should be queried about self-opinion and any self-critical feelings. With every depressed patient, it is critical to ask about suicidal thoughts and intentions (see below). Also useful in the exploration of multiple bodily complaints is consideration of systemic illness that might mimic depression.

Screening for Neurovegetative Symptoms. Specific inquiry into these characteristic symptoms is facilitated by the mnemonic *SIG E CAPS* ("prescribe an energy capsule"):

S—Is your *sleep* disturbed?

I—Have you noted a loss of libido or *interest* in your usual activities?

G—Are you feeling *guilty* or having self-deprecatory thoughts?

E—Have you noticed a decrease in your *energy* level?

C—Have you been having trouble *concentrating*?

A—Have you experienced changes in your *appetite* and weight?

P—Have been physically slowed down or sped up (i.e., experienced *psychomotor* abnormalities)?

S—Have you had thoughts of *suicide*, feelings of hopelessness, or preoccupation with issues related to death? (See below for more detail.)

Checking for Multiple Bodily Complaints and Ruling Out Organicity. Patients with low energy, dysphoria, and multiple bodily complaints out of proportion to physical findings are likely to have depression, but, as noted earlier, they still require careful consideration of conditions that may present in similar fashion, such as *chronic fatigue syndrome, Lyme disease, fibromyalgia, rheumatoid disease, vasculitis, and endocrinopathies* (see Chapter 8 for details of workup). In addition, depression or multiple bodily complaints may be the clinical presentation of *domestic violence*. Screening for this condition can be as straightforward as asking: "At any time, has a partner ever hit you, kicked you, or otherwise physically hurt you?"

Confusion and alterations in level of consciousness strongly suggest organicity, although they are not always present. When they are, drug-induced etiologies are important to consider. Onset is usually temporally related to medication use and should be sought. Worth noting are any use of *antiarrhythmics, antihypertensives, sedative-hypnotics, and corticosteroids*, as well as over-the-counter agents and substances of abuse. The relation of *beta-blockers* to depression remains inconclusive, but risk appears greatest for those that are lipophilic and readily cross the blood–brain barrier. The elderly are particularly susceptible to adverse central nervous system (CNS) effects from drugs that cross the blood–brain barrier.

Primary neuropathology should be sought when depression is accompanied by an alteration of neurologic function. *Left frontal lobe* involvement by a *mass lesion or stroke* may trigger a depressive syndrome. Inquiry into focal signs and symptoms help to differentiate a structural lesion from a functional affective disorder.

In some medical illnesses, depression may dominate the early clinical picture. *Pancreatic cancer* is the archetypal example. Important associated findings should be sought, including profound weight loss, vague upper abdominal discomfort, and onset of painless jaundice (see Chapter 58). *HIV infection* and emergence of *AIDS* are frequently associated with depression. In such cases, the diagnosis may be obscured by comorbid medical illness (see Chapter 13). Also, depressive features may mistakenly be conceptualized as normal grief in response to the medical diagnosis and surrounding tragedy.

Psychosocial History. This should focus on the patient's current home environment and means of financial and emotional support. Does the patient live alone? If not, is the family environment accepting or, conversely, contributing to the patient's discomfort? The availability of responsible family members to observe and supervise the patient might mean the difference between outpatient treatment and hospitalization if the patient is very depressed or debilitated. What are the patient's daily responsibilities and what secondary stressors arise if the patient cannot meet these obligations?

Psychiatric History of the Patient and Family. Once the issue of medical etiologies has been put to rest, one should return to eliciting a past psychiatric history. Given depression's tendency to recur, the patient should always be asked about similar episodes in the past. If there is a history of depressive or manic disease, it is important to obtain the details of treatment and treatment response. A history of prior psychosis or suicidality is also important to elicit, because of their risks for recurrence.

Family history can be difficult to elicit because of shame about any mental illness in the family. It helps to explain that depression is thought to run in families because of hereditary biochemical factors, not defects in character. A family history of major depression, bipolar disorder, or suicide supports a diagnosis of depression in the patient. The genetic predispositions for unipolar depression and bipolar illness are distinct.

A family history of other psychiatric diagnoses must be interpreted in the context of changing nomenclature and diagnostic criteria. In the past, mania was frequently misdiagnosed as schizophrenia. "Nervous breakdown" or "going insane" were common nonspecific terms. If family psychiatric history is present, it is worth reviewing symptoms and attempting a tentative retrospective diagnosis.

Physical Examination

The importance of a careful and detailed physical examination cannot be overemphasized, especially because most depressed patients presenting to primary physicians harbor concerns about medical illness. Specific patient concerns elicited during the history should be explicitly checked for during the physical examination to facilitate the provision of meaningful reassurance. (See Chapter 8 for description of the pertinent physical examination.)

Mental Status Examination. Much of the mental status examination can be performed by taking note of the patient's appearance, affect, behavior, and responses during the history. Has the patient's condition interfered with grooming and self-care? Is there sadness, tearfulness, despondency, apathy, irritability, anxiety, or anger? Is there psychomotor retardation or agitation? Does the patient offer anything spontaneously, or is there a long period of hesitation before answering (i.e., speech latency)? Is the speech slow? Is normal inflection present?

The patient should also be asked explicitly to describe his or her *mood*. Thought is assessed for form and content. Is the patient's thought pattern clear and coherent or is it tangential, circumstantial, or nonsensical? Are there ideas of worthlessness, helplessness, hopelessness, guilt, suicidal thought, or homicidality?

Is the patient able to maintain *attention*? Distractibility may occur in depression, delirium, dementia, or severe anxiety and will interfere with the patient's overall cognitive performance. Any inattention is worth documenting by testing ability to recall a series of random numbers (digit span). Patients should be able to repeat a series of at least five to seven numbers without error. "I don't know" answers are reflective of apathy or lack of energy associated with depression. Tests of memory, calculation, abstractions, and other higher cortical functions should be performed.

Although psychotic depression is uncommon in primary care settings, it is important not to miss this very serious condition. It should be noted whether the patient appears guarded or expresses paranoid thoughts or delusions. Inquiry into any unusual experiences, such as hearing voices or seeing things that other people do not see, provide further evidence of a thought disorder. However, unusual smells, tastes, and tactile experiences suggest an organic brain syndrome.

Evaluation for Suicidality. Depression is a potentially fatal illness. Assessment of suicide risk is an integral part of the workup of every depressed patient. About 15% of patients with major affective disorders take their lives; diagnosing and treating depression can be a life-saving medical intervention by the primary care physician. With proper intervention, most suicides can be prevented. Concurrent conditions that increase the risk of suicide include chronic alcoholism, personality disorders, and both functional and drug-induced psychoses; delusional beliefs or hallucinations may lead to self-destruction. Predicting a suicide attempt is difficult, even among patients who complain of suicidal thoughts. Assessment of risk is facilitated by specific inquiry.

Technique. Assessing risk of suicide requires attention to the patient's *thoughts* (ideas, wishes, motives), *intent* (the degree to which the patient intends to act on the thoughts), and *plans*. Inquiry necessitates a calm empathic approach that allows expression of feelings and is free of any implied criticism. On any expression of hopelessness, helplessness, or suffering, one might begin with a rather indirect query (e.g., "Are you feeling so badly that sometimes you would prefer not to go on living?"). A positive response is followed by more direct questions about self-destructive thoughts and plans. A well worked out, realistic, and potentially lethal plan suggests great risk, as does the act of putting one's affairs in order.

Asking patients about suicide does not put the idea into their heads. Pitfalls include failure to ask specifically about suicidal

Table 227.4.   Risk Factors for Suicide

History of prior attempts

Depression

Psychotic features present (especially command hallucinations)

Substance abuse

Positive family history of suicide

Living alone

Age: in males, risk increased with age peaking at 75; in females, the peak for completed suicide is 55–65.

Sex: females attempt suicide three to four times more often than males, but males are successful two to three times more often than females.

Marital status: at great risk are those who never married; are widowed, separated, or divorced; or married without children; those married with children are at least risk.

Employment: unemployed are at greater risk than employed; unskilled are at greater risk than skilled.

Physical illness: 50% of all patients who attempt suicide have a physical illness. At highest risk are those with chronic pain, diagnosed chronic disease, recent surgery, or a terminal illness.

thoughts and feelings and premature interruption of the patient who mentions suicide. Any mention of suicide must be taken seriously, and *every* depressed patient must be asked about suicide. It is an error to avoid the subject for fear of doing so. Truly suicidal patients usually are relieved to be asked about it.

Mental status, especially the patient's ability to resist suicidal thoughts, is important to consider. An extremely impulsive, psychotic, or intoxicated patient has no meaningful internal controls and will require hospitalization.

Assessment of Risk. There is no simple formula for precisely assessing suicide risk. Attention to thoughts, intent, and plans is essential, facilitated by consideration of mental status and pertinent psychosocial and demographic predictors (Table 227.4). Patients expressing suicidal thoughts, especially if accompanied by intent and plans, or who lack reliable internal controls to resist suicidal impulses require emergency psychiatric consultation. Such patients should be closely supervised and not allowed to transport themselves. Patients with severe or worsening depression who have thought about suicide but steadfastly deny intent or plans should be given a prompt confirmed appointment with a psychiatrist. Depressed patients with no suicidal thoughts, intent, or plans; a normal mental status examination; and external social supports can be treated by the primary care physician, as long as frequent visits can be arranged and the depression responds to treatment. Patients with suicide potential should never be given more than 1 g or a week's supply of a tricyclic antidepressant (see below).

Laboratory Studies and Use of Diagnostic Instruments

There are no laboratory tests for depression. For a time there was interest in urinary catecholamine metabolites and the overnight dexamethasone suppression test, but shortcomings in sensitivity and specificity compromised clinical utility. Depression remains a clinical diagnosis. Nonetheless, medical causes of depressed mood and neurovegetative symptoms must be ruled out (see Chapter 8).

Written Diagnostic Instruments for In-Office Evaluation. Validated diagnostic instruments are sometimes useful supplements to the clinical evaluation. The *Beck Depression Inventory* and the *Hamilton Depression Scale* (HAM-D) help to assess severity and can be used to follow response to therapy and clinical course. The Beck Depression Inventory is a 21-item self-administered questionnaire. The Hamilton Depression Scale is a 21-item instrument that must be clinician administered. Both take approximately 15 minutes to complete and score. The higher the score, the more severe the distress.

PRINCIPLES OF MANAGEMENT

Overall Strategy

Depression is a potentially life threatening yet treatable condition. Most depressed patients (particularly those with major depression) can be treated as outpatients by their primary care physician. *Antidepressants and psychotherapy* represent the basic treatment modalities, adapted to the specific type of depressive order encountered. *Psychiatric referral* should be considered in severe cases and in those with psychotic, bipolar, or characterologic qualities.

Major Depression. The cornerstone of treatment for major depression (unipolar depression) is antidepressant medication. Psychotherapy plays a very important adjunctive role.

Bipolar Disease. Psychiatric referral is required for management of bipolar disease, which responds well to a combination of a mood-stabilizing agent and antidepressant therapy.

Psychotic Depression. Neuroleptics are required as well as psychiatric consultation. If there is an organic cause (*secondary depression*), one treats the causative medical illness and discontinues potentially offending medications. Only if the medical condition responds slowly or is intractable are trials of an antidepressant or supportive psychotherapy indicated.

Characterologic Depression/Dysthymic Disorder. A characterologic depression responds best to psychotherapy, but, when neurovegetative symptoms are prominent, a trial of antidepressants would be helpful. Dysthymia has recently been shown to be responsive to selective serotonin reuptake inhibitors (SSRIs). A patient with untreated dysthymia is five times more likely to subsequently develop an episode of major depression.

Adjustment Disorder with Depressed Mood. This can be treated by the primary care physician with supportive psychotherapy. If moderate sleep and appetite disturbances are present (as they commonly are), an antidepressant can provide symptomatic relief.

Management of major depression has two facets, psychotherapeutic and medical. The primary care physician needs to become skilled in providing supportive psychotherapy and using first-line antidepressants.

Psychotherapy

Treatment begins with establishing a strong patient–physician relationship (see Chapter 1) and providing psychological support. More intensive psychotherapy may also be beneficial. The addition of antidepressant medication improves prognosis. Psychotherapy and medication are often synergistic.

Psychological Management (Supportive Psychotherapy). Patients with major depression benefit from supportive psychotherapy, much of which can be provided by the primary care physician. A clear, empathic, hopeful manner helps to forge a therapeutic alliance and facilitates treatment. A detailed explanation of the diagnosis combined with reassurance that depression is eminently treatable do much to calm a fearful patient and family. When patients feel hopeless or undeserving, it is useful to point out that these are the characteristic symptoms of depression and they will gradually improve.

While conveying hope and optimism, the physician must take care not to dismiss as insignificant the patient's fears, pains, and negative feelings. Many feel overwhelmed by life stresses. It is important to identify these stresses. Empathic listening and thoughtful comment can help the patient devise strategies for coping. At the outset of treatment one should see the patient every 1 to 2 weeks for about half an hour. Appointments can then be spaced out according to the patient's needs. If a patient becomes severely depressed, agitated, or psychotic, emergency psychiatric referral should be made.

Cognitive-behavioral therapy has shown promise in depressed patients with medical problems, helping to reduce the depression accompanying the problem and improving control of the underlying medical condition through improved compliance.

Social and Environmental Interventions. A caring family willing to monitor the severely depressed patient can make the difference between outpatient management and hospitalization. Members can ensure medication compliance and follow-up appointments and minimize social isolation. Also helpful is identifying stressful elements in the patient's environment so that they might be modified. Worries about the consequences of taking time off from work and issues of confidentiality must be addressed. Helping the patient deal with these important concerns is essential and greatly appreciated.

Psychopharmacologic Therapy

The SSRIs serve as first-line antidepressants. Tricyclic antidepressants (TCAs) can be effective in patients who do not respond to initial trials of SSRIs. The monoamine oxidase inhibitors (MAOIs) and lithium are reserved for special situations.

Selective Serotonin Reuptake Inhibitors. As their name implies, the SSRIs (e.g., *fluoxetine [Prozac], sertraline [Zoloft], paroxetine [Paxil], fluvoxamine [Luvox], and citalopram [Celexa]*) affect CNS serotonin metabolism. All require 3 to 4 weeks of continuous use before clinical improvement becomes evident. For mild to moderate depression, they appear to be equal in efficacy to the TCAs and better tolerated. For severe depression, there has been controversy as to whether the SSRIs are as effective as the TCAs. Unlike the TCAs, many of which are sedating, many SSRIs have *energizing* or "activating" side effects, a factor favoring their selection in patients suffering anergy, apathy, and psychomotor retardation. They have become the antidepressant of first choice, especially in circumstances where avoidance of tricyclic side effects is desired.

Side Effects. These activating agents can exacerbate agitation, anxiety, and insomnia, making them problematic for depressed patients already troubled by such symptoms. The motor *restlessness* (including tremor), initial *anxiety*, and *agitation* with insomnia can be the most distressing side effects of SSRIs. Concerns about exacerbation of suicidality with SSRI use proved unfounded after detailed investigation. Nonetheless, it is always crucial to remain vigilant and inquire specifically about suicidal thoughts, even as patients begin to show improvement (see below).

Paradoxically, up to 20% experience some *sedation.* Unlike the TCAs, with their associated anticholinergic and alpha-blocking activity, there is little risk of orthostatic hypotension, tachycardia, heart block, blurred vision, or dry mouth. *Sexual dysfunction* has been reported, including impotence in men and decreased lubrication in women. Decreased libido and anorgasmia may occur in both men and women. These effects are reversible. Some weight gain from appetite stimulation may occur, but not to the extent associated with TCAs. *Headache, nausea, and diarrhea* have also been reported. All SSRIs can cause a life-threatening reaction if taken concurrently with an *MAOI.* At least 2 weeks should pass before starting an MAOI after SSRI use and 5 weeks after fluoxetine use.

Some SSRIs (fluoxetine, paroxetine, and fluvoxamine) *inhibit liver cytochrome P-450 enzymes,* slowing hepatic drug metabolism and prolonging the effects of warfarin, phenytoin, and other drugs that are hepatically metabolized. Although SSRI use in *pregnancy* does not increase the risk of birth defects or retard development of intelligence, there is some increase in risk of perinatal complications when treatment is continued during the third trimester.

Dosage. Fluoxetine is available in 10- and 20-mg capsules. Some patients with prominent anxiety symptoms do better to start with the lower dose. A liquid form enables even smaller starting doses. In nonelderly patients, fluoxetine can be initiated at 20 mg daily. Dosage may be advanced by 10 to 20 mg/d every 4 weeks. Usually, 20 or 40 mg/d suffices. The Physicians' Desk Reference maximum dose is 80 mg/d, although higher doses are used to treat obsessive-compulsive disorder (see Chapter 226). Because of the drug's long serum half-life (2 to 3 days), less frequent dosing is possible for elderly persons needing less than 20 mg daily (e.g., 20 mg every 2 to 4 days).

Sertraline is started at 50 mg/d and gradually increased to therapeutic dosages in the range of 100 to 250 mg/d. *Fluvoxamine* is also started at 50 mg/d and gradually increased to therapeutic dosages in the range of 100 to 250 mg/d. *Citalopram and paroxetine* are administered in doses comparable with those of fluoxetine. All other SSRIs have shorter half-lives than fluoxetine, but dosing is still once daily. Paroxetine is also available in a liquid form.

Tricyclic Antidepressants. The TCAs are a reasonable choice for antidepressant therapy in selected persons who fail SSRI treatment. The low cost per tablet of the generic formulations weighs in their favor (although brand formulations are very expensive) (Table 227.5). When use in properly selected patients, TCA therapy can reduce the cost of therapy by an order of magnitude, but only when used in persons who can readily tolerate the side effects. Primary care physicians should become comfortable with using at least one sedating and one

Table 227.5.   Antidepressants

GENERIC NAME	BRAND NAME	CUSTOMARY INITIAL DOSE	TITRATE DOSE UP TO	RELATIVE COST
Selective Serotonin Reuptake Inhibitors				
Citalopram	Celexa	20 mg/d	20–40 mg/d	1.0
Fluoxetine	Prozac	20 mg/d	20–40 mg/d	1.25
Fluvoxamine	Luvox	50 mg/d	100–250 mg/d	1.25
Paroxetine	Paxil	20 mg/d	20–60 mg/d	1.25
Sertraline	Zoloft	50 mg/d	100–250 mg/d	1.1
Atypical Antidepressants				
Bupropion (sustained release)	Bupropion-SR	150 mg SR qam	150–200 mg bid	1.9
Mirtazapine	Remeron	15 mg qhs	30–45 mg qhs	1.1
Nefazodone	Serzone	50 mg bid	150–300 mg bid	0.8
Trazodone	Desyrel	50–100 mg qhs	200–600 mg/d	3.6
	Generic			0.2
Venlafaxine (extended release)	Effexor-XR	37.5 mg XR bid	75–150 mg bid	1.1
Tricyclic Antidepressants				
Amitriptyline	Elavil	25 mg qhs	150–300 mg qhs	1.1
	Generic			0.03
Clomipramine	Anafranil	25 mg qhs	150–200 mg qhs	1.3
Desipramine	Norpramin	25 mg qam	150–300 mg qam	1.9
	Generic			0.3
Doxepin	Adapin	25 mg qhs	150–300 gm qhs	
Imipramine	Tofranil	25 mg qhs	150–300 mg qhs	1.5
	Generic			0.03
Nortriptyline	Pamelor	10 mg qhs	50–150 mg qhs	1.8
	Generic			0.2
Protriptyline	Vivactil	10 mg qam	30–60 mg qam	0.35
Trimipramine	Surmontil	25 mg qhs	150–250 mg qhs	0.36
Monoamine Oxidase Inhibitors				
Phenelzine	Nardil	15 mg bid	45–90 mg/d	0.44
Tranylcypromine	Parnate	10 mg bid	40–80 mg/d	0.53
L-Deprenyl	Eldepryl	10 mg bid	30–40 mg/d	2.2

nonsedating TCA compound. These agents appear to act predominantly on norepinephrine metabolism, inhibiting reuptake at CNS synapses. Some TCAs also affect serotonin and, to a lesser extent, dopamine metabolism. A large number of tricyclics are available. All are equally effective. The major differences are in the degree of *anticholinergic and sedative side effects*. All require 3 to 4 weeks of continuous use before clinical improvement becomes evident. Drug choice for a given patient is determined by attention to the side effects of available agents (Table 227.5). Patient comfort and compliance are facilitated by avoiding drugs with marked anticholinergic activity.

Selecting Among Tricyclics. In general, the TCAs tend to be sedating. Patients with severe *insomnia* might do best with a strongly sedating drug, such as *doxepin* (Adapin or Sinequan) given at bedtime. The very sedating drug *amitriptyline* (Elavil) has long been popular with physicians, but because of its strong anticholinergic side effects, it is probably not an optimal first-choice agent unless low doses suffice. The elderly and those with prostatic hypertrophy do best with a nonsedating tricyclic that has relatively mild anticholinergic activity (e.g., *desipramine* [Norpramin] or *nortriptyline* [Aventyl or Pamelor]). Nortriptyline has the advantage among tricyclics of causing the least postural hypotension. Persons bothered by anergy and psychomotor retardation are best treated with a nonsedating slightly activating TCA (e.g., desipramine) or an SSRI (as per above).

The prescribing of a *fixed combination* preparation containing a tricyclic plus a *neuroleptic* (e.g., Triavil) or a *benzodiazepine* (e.g., Limbitrol) is irrational and should be avoided.

Combinations make it difficult to achieve therapeutic levels of the tricyclic without administering too much of the other compound. Moreover, except for the depressed patient with psychotic symptoms, *typical antipsychotics* have no place in the treatment of depression. Occasionally, *atypical antipsychotics* are used for augmentation purposes in treatment-refractory patients.

Adverse Effects. Tricyclics can have *lethal* cardiovascular toxicity when taken in overdose due to severe cumulative *anticholinergic and alpha-blocking* effects. One should never write a prescription that dispenses more than 1 g of a tricyclic to a potentially suicidal patient or to a patient one does not know well. At therapeutic doses, *postural hypotension* can occur, especially in the elderly, leading to falls, fractures, and head injury. If postural hypotension is a problem, nortriptyline or an SSRI should be used. If the hypotension is always worse in the morning, it may be useful to give the nortriptyline in three divided doses. Patients should be instructed to be careful when rising from recumbency or sitting.

Before benefit is noted, patients may want to stop TCA therapy because of *dry mouth, lassitude, constipation, or mental clouding.* Such symptoms are common with use of TCAs but may also result from depression. They often pass or abate with continued therapy, a reassuring fact that helps patients to continue TCA treatment. *Weight gain* is another complaint. It results from TCA-associated stimulation of appetite.

Rarely, more severe dose-related anticholinergic symptoms occur, especially in the elderly. These include *ileus, urinary retention, and dysrhythmias.* In all patients over 40, it is good practice to obtain a baseline electrocardiogram before starting a tricyclic. At therapeutic levels, tricyclics exert anticholinergic effects on the heart, which could cause a *rise in heart rate and conduction delay*. In patients with bundle branch block, atrioventricular block, or sinus node disease, there is an increased risk of higher degrees of heart block. In patients without underlying conduction system disease, tricyclics rarely cause conduction problems.

Very rarely, a full *anticholinergic syndrome* develops in patients taking TCAs, characterized by agitation, delirium, and fever. The most common precipitant is simultaneous use of more than one anticholinergic drug. Most often implicated is concurrent use of thioridazine (Mellaril), anticholinergic antiparkinsonian drugs, antihistamines, antispasmodics, and over-the-counter sleep medications containing antihistamines. The number of anticholinergic compounds should be closely monitored, especially in the elderly.

Dosage. Tricyclics are started at a low dose with gradual increases until the therapeutic dose-range is achieved (Table 227.5). After that, trial and error is often required. Drug *serum levels* can be used to determine compliance and achievement of therapeutic serum concentrations in nonresponders. Blood levels vary widely among patients for any given oral dose due to individual differences in drug absorption and metabolism. Therapeutic serum levels have been established for imipramine, desipramine, amitriptyline, and nortriptyline (Table 227.5). For other TCAs, serum levels are useful only to ascertain compliance. Many clinical laboratories are unreliable in measuring these compounds. One should seek an experienced laboratory.

The most common cause of treatment failure is inadequate dosage. In healthy nonelderly adults, a typical *starting dose* is the equivalent of 50 mg of desipramine. (Nortriptyline has twice the milligram potency of most tricyclics; thus its starting dose is 25 mg.) The daily dose is best taken at bedtime to facilitate compliance and minimize side effects. Dosage can be increased by 50 mg every 3 to 4 days to a dose of 150 to 200 mg at bedtime. Dosages are reduced by 50% in the elderly (see below). The final dosage chosen is one that provides a therapeutic response without intolerable side effects. The usual *maximum dosage* is 300 mg of desipramine or the equivalent (150 mg for nortriptyline). This is easier said than done. In recent reviews, relatively few patients whose depression was diagnosed received a therapeutic dose of a TCA.

Atypical Antidepressants. These agents have slightly different mechanisms of action than those of the first-line SSRIs, providing them with potential benefits in selected circumstances where SSRIs do not suffice. They are mostly the province of the psychiatrist, and unless familiar with their use, the primary physician should not prescribe one of these agents in preference to a first-line drug. However, some knowledge of their characteristics is helpful when managing patients who have been prescribed an atypical antidepressant.

Venlafaxine (Effexor) is a selective inhibitor of both serotonin and norepinephrine. It is typically started at 37.5 mg twice daily (due to its short half-life) and gradually tapered up to therapeutic dosages in the range of 75 to 150 mg twice daily. At its higher doses, it has more effect on norepinephrine uptake inhibition, and some studies have suggested that it has a higher response rate.

Nefazodone (Serzone) inhibits serotonin reuptake, it is unique in blocking 5-HT$_2$ receptors and mediating 5-HT-1A transmission. It is usually started at 50 mg twice daily and gradually tapered up to therapeutic dosages in the range of 150 to 300 mg twice daily.

Mirtazapine (Remeron) is associated with an increased release of both serotonin and norepinephrine. By mediating 5-HT-1A transmission and blocking 5-HT$_2$ and 5-HT$_3$ receptors, it may account for its antidepressant and *anxiolytic* effects. It is usually started at 15 mg q.h.s. and gradually tapered up to therapeutic dosages in the range of 30 to 45 mg q.h.s.

Bupropion (Wellbutrin) appears to work by downregulating postsynaptic β-noradrenergic receptors. Unlike the SSRIs, there is no adverse effect on sexual functioning. It may be especially helpful in patients who do not respond to the SSRIs. It is now available in a sustained release form, reducing its risk of seizure to that of other antidepressants. However, even the sustained release form is still contraindicated in patients with a known seizure disorder or eating disorder. It is usually started at 150 mg SR q.a.m. and gradually tapered up to therapeutic dosages in the range of 150 to 200 mg SR twice daily.

Trazodone (Desyrel) is a nontricyclic with efficacy similar to the TCAs but generally better tolerated. The drug is sedating and particularly helpful for those who cannot sleep or tolerate anticholinergic side effects. *Postural hypotension* can be a problem in the elderly. Other common side effects include indigestion, nausea, and headaches. *Priapism*, a painful medical emergency, has been reported. Males prescribed trazodone must be warned that a sustained painful erection requires immediate medical attention. Trazodone is usually started at 50 to 100 mg q.h.s. as a sleep inducer. To be used as an antidepressant, it needs to be gradually tapered up to therapeutic dosages in the range of 200 to 600 mg q.h.s.

Monoamine Oxidase Inhibitors. MAOIs are quite useful in treating the elderly (see below), being well tolerated by virtue of their lack of anticholinergic side effects. However, they do have other side effects that bear noting.

Side Effects. The primary ones are *hypotension and insomnia*. Hypotension is unrelated to dose and may occur up to a month after starting the drug. It rarely necessitates stopping the drug. Insomnia can be minimized by giving the last daily dose no later than 4 p.m. *Hypertensive crisis* is the most serious adverse effect, caused by ingesting a large amount of tyramine. Dietary and drug precautions must be given. A *low-tyramine diet* is required, necessitating avoidance of foods such as fermented cheese, large amounts of yogurt, excessive caffeine, and chocolate, beer, and red wine. Patients can drink white wine, vodka, gin, and whiskey. A blanket warning to avoid all alcohol is not only unwarranted but may also compromise compliance. *Sympathomimetics* should be avoided. They are found in many over-the-counter medications including combination cold tablets, nasal decongestants, and appetite suppressants. *Amphetamines* are also not permitted. Treatment of a hypertensive crisis involves prompt cessation of MAOI use and initiation of antihypertensive therapy with an alpha-blocker or a direct vasodilator. (*Phentolamine*, 5 mg given slowly intravenously, is recommended.) Fever is managed by means of external cooling. Severe life-threatening reactions can also occur as a consequence of interactions between MAOIs and SSRIs or *narcotic analgesics*. A several week period between cessation of SSRI therapy and initiation of MAOI use is required, as is consultation before starting the MAOI.

Tranylcypromine (Parnate) is the preferred MAOI in the elderly because its effects last no more than 24 hours. Starting dose is 10 mg once or twice daily and gradually increased as needed over a few weeks. Usually 20 to 30 mg daily will suffice, but occasional patients require as much as 80 mg/d.

Other Agents. The benzodiazepine *alprazolam* (Xanax) has excellent antianxiety effects and *mild* antidepressant action. However, prolonged use is associated with significant risk of dependency (see Chapter 226). *Buspirone* (BuSpar) is similarly purported to have combined anxiolytic and *mild* antidepressant effects and has the advantage of a more benign side effect profile, without risk of physiologic dependence (see Chapter 226). These agents are reasonable in cases of adjustment disorders with depressive and anxiety features, but they are not indicated for the treatment of major depression.

Some nontricyclic second-generation antidepressants have fallen from use because of severe adverse effects (e.g., seizures with *maprotiline*; tardive dyskinesias with *amoxapine*). These agents are of limited safety and should be avoided.

Selection of Antidepressant for Major Depression. Choice is best made by taking into account disease severity, age, degree of psychomotor retardation and sleep disturbance, and ability to tolerate anticholinergic, cardiac, and postural side effects. *Costs* should also be considered, because these drugs are likely to be used for prolonged periods of time. The newer antidepressants are quite expensive, but so are brand-name TCA formulations (Table 227.5). Although the generic TCAs are less costly on a pill per pill basis, their requirements of cardiac monitoring, blood levels, and possibly more frequent office visits to manage their side effects can all contribute to a higher total cost in patients especially vulnerable to their side effects.

In the elderly and others with cardiac disease, prostatic hypertrophy, postural hypotension, or glaucoma, the SSRIs may be better tolerated. Some clinicians believe the SSRIs are not as effective as the TCAs for severe depression. When sedation without anticholinergic activity is desired, trazodone is a reasonable choice, particularly in the elderly. For anergic, hypersomnic, or motor-retarded patients, an activating agent is best (e.g., an SSRI or bupropion-SR or desipramine). For patients with a mixture of neurovegetative symptoms, nortriptyline is reasonable, being well tolerated and free of excessive sedating, activating, anticholinergic, or antiadrenergic effects.

Monitoring and Duration of Therapy; Failure to Respond. Monitoring response to therapy can be readily accomplished by carefully reviewing symptoms and activity level. The questionnaire instruments used for assessment of disease severity (see above) can also be used. If a patient shows little or no response to antidepressant therapy after 4 weeks at full dosage (which may be 6 weeks from initiation of therapy), then the drug trial should be considered a failure. If there is doubt as to adequacy of dosage or compliance, a serum drug level can be obtained. Failure to respond is an indication for psychopharmacologic consultation to explore whether augmentation therapy (i.e., adding a second agent, usually from a different class) or switching to another agent is the best approach. Sometimes augmen-

tation can be the more rapid approach to achieving control, but consultation is advised.

It may also be important to reassess the patient's use of alcohol. It has long been known that patients who meet criteria for alcohol abuse or dependence are less likely to respond to antidepressant treatment. In a recent report, it was shown that a group of depressed outpatients who drank an average of 1.0 ounces of alcohol per day had a lower rate of response to an 8-week course of fluoxetine. This mild to moderate level of alcohol use was enough to decrease their chance of acutely responding to their antidepressant. Thus, patients should be encouraged to either abstain from drinking alcohol while on their antidepressant or limiting their alcohol use as much as possible.

If the response to initial therapy was promising but limited by intolerance to drug side effects, then switching to another agent in the same class with a more favorable side effect profile might suffice (e.g., switching from amitriptyline to nortriptyline for postural hypotension).

If depression successfully remits, antidepressant medication is maintained for at least 6 to 9 months. Continuation-phase medication should be maintained at the same dosage as was used in the acute-phase treatment. After 6 to 9 months, the dosage can be slowly tapered over a period of 4 weeks while watching for the reemergence of depressive symptoms. Should symptoms recur, the dosage is returned to its prior level and maintained for at least another 6 to 9 months. Major depression is a medical illness with a high rate of recurrence. After a single episode, 50% of patients subsequently have a second episode. After two episodes, the chance of having a third is approximately 80%. For patients with two or more episodes, maintenance therapy for probably 3 to 5 years is indicated. Patients with a family history of depression or bipolar disorder should also be closely evaluated for long term maintenance therapy.

Prevention of Suicide

The best prevention is proper screening for suicidality and prompt referral at the time of initial evaluation. However, some patients are at greatest risk for suicide at the time when they are initially responding to antidepressant medication. Dysphoria may still persist as energy lifts, perhaps giving the patient with suicidal thoughts adequate energy to formulate a plan and follow it through. Continuous vigilance is required, as well as care in choice and amount of antidepressant prescribed. If there is a question of suicide risk, either a nontricyclic should be selected or no more than 1 g of a tricyclic dispensed at a time.

Treatment of Depression in the Elderly

Depression is the most common psychiatric disorder of the elderly, affecting close to one million older Americans. Primary treatment modalities include antidepressants and, for severely affected patients, electroconvulsive therapy (ECT). Age-related changes in drug metabolism and susceptibility to drug side effects must be taken into account in the design of the treatment program.

Choice of Antidepressant. When anergy and psychomotor retardation predominate, the activating effects of *SSRIs* make them attractive. Similarly, SSRIs are an excellent first choice if there is heart block, a dysrhythmia, or postural hypotension. Of the SSRIs, sertraline and citalopram are the least likely to interfere with hepatic drug metabolism and preferred in patients taking drugs that are metabolized by the liver (e.g., digoxin, warfarin, phenytoin). The sedating, anticholinergic, cardiac, and postural side effects of many *TCAs* make their use in the elderly especially problematic. Before starting therapy, postural signs and an electrocardiogram should be performed and particular note taken of the patient's somatic symptoms and degree of psychomotor retardation. *Amitriptyline and imipramine* are among the most difficult to use; *nortriptyline and desipramine* are better tolerated. If sedation is desired, *trazodone* is a reasonable choice, being free of anticholinergic activity.

Initiating and Monitoring Therapy. One starts with a *very low dose* of medication (e.g., 10 mg of fluoxetine, 25 mg of desipramine, 10 mg of nortriptyline, or 50 mg of trazodone). The dosage can be raised slowly every 5 to 7 days, while monitoring subjective response and heart rate and watching for anticholinergic, cardiovascular, and CNS side effects. One slows the increase in dose if tachycardia, excessive sedation, agitation, or orthostatic hypotension develops.

Often the patient is the last to recognize improvement, and family members commonly report that the patient is sleeping and eating better before the dysphoria resolves. An adequate trial may take twice as long in the elderly as in younger patients. Several studies have demonstrated elderly patients not showing their response until 8 to 10 weeks.

Failure to Respond. If there is little improvement after a reasonable trial at therapeutic doses, consultation is warranted to consider use of an alternative antidepressant (e.g., MAOI) or ECT.

Use of a Monoamine Oxidase Inhibitor. MAOIs have been used sparingly in the elderly because of concern for adverse reactions. Actually, MAOIs have no anticholinergic activity and are relatively well tolerated. Many older patients who do not respond to other antidepressants improve with MAOIs. MAOI therapy should be selected and started by a psychopharmacologic consultant, but management can then shift to the primary care physician, who needs to be familiar with drug actions and side effects (see above).

Use of Electroconvulsive Therapy. Elderly patients who are psychotically depressed, severely incapacitated, refractory or unable to take drug therapy, or in need of a rapid response should be referred for consideration of ECT. The best predictors of response are psychomotor retardation and delusions. Efficacy and safety have been well documented. Attainment of generalized seizure activity is required to achieve benefit. Customizing electrical dose to the patient's seizure threshold may help maximize efficacy and minimize adverse effects. Electrode placement appears to be more important than electrical dose as regards amnesia, with unilateral electrode placement associated with a lower risk. Amnesia occurs for events just before and up to a few weeks after treatment. More long-term cognitive functioning is no different than that for patients treated with antidepressants. Relapses occur with high frequency, making ECT an acute treatment. Maintenance ECT is not uncommon these days. Quite often an SSRI or TCA is prescribed for life-long maintenance treatment in an elderly patient.

Treatment of Seasonal Affective Disorder

Light therapy is the first line of treatment. Exposure to 10,000 lux of ordinary white fluorescent light for 30 to 45 minutes at a time once or twice a day is effective. Improvement often occurs within the first week or two of therapy. Patients typically sit about 50 cm from a light box and read for the period of treatment, with the light coming in at a 45-degree angle. Improvement has been noted both with morning and nighttime treatments, though the latter may cause insomnia. Elaborate forms of lighting that more closely simulate the spectrum of sunlight are no more effective than light from a standard white fluorescent source. The intensity of light appears to be the key determinant of efficacy. SSRIs are probably as effective as light therapy. Some clinicians use both. Efficacy of prophylactic therapy early in the winter is under study.

INDICATIONS FOR REFERRAL AND ADMISSION

Patients who should be referred for psychiatric consultation include those with refractory or disabling major depression, bipolar illness, psychosis, or substantial risk for suicide. Patients who fail to respond after 1 to 2 months of appropriate antidepressant treatment should have a psychiatric consultation. Many of these patients can be referred back to their primary care physician for follow-up after one or two psychiatric appointments.

Psychiatric hospitalization is indicated for high suicide risk, lack of reliable social supports (if the depression is severe), history of previously poor response to treatment, or symptoms that are so severe that the patient requires constant observation or nursing care.

PATIENT EDUCATION

Detailed patient education is a central component of supportive psychotherapy (see above). Patients who come from backgrounds that stigmatize mental illness or oppose psychotropic medication are comforted by learning of depression's "organic" pathophysiology, which helps them to comply with treatment. Compliance with antidepressant therapy is often compromised by side effects or mistaken attributions. Some stop their medication after only a few days if they do not notice an immediate improvement or use it only "as needed." Before initiating therapy, it is critical to review likely side effects and delayed onset of improvement. The importance of prolonged regular use must be emphasized. If the patient already has a tendency toward constipation, the prescription of a stool softener may make a tricyclic more tolerable. Patients should be instructed to report side effects rather than stopping the medication on their own and to call promptly if suicidal thoughts develop or if depression markedly worsens.

The educational process should include family and other household members. Enlisting their help in decreasing stress at home is helpful. With elderly or severely depressed patients, the family should be taught about the proper use of antidepressants and asked to monitor compliance.

THERAPEUTIC RECOMMENDATIONS

- If a depressive syndrome is identified, try to make a specific diagnosis and assess suicide risk.

- If the patient appears to be at risk for suicide, has psychotic symptoms, severe depression with no social supports, or is unable to care for him or herself, arrange prompt psychiatric consultation with a view to possible hospitalization.
- For other patients, begin supportive psychotherapy and make any social and environmental interventions that may help. Especially with elderly or severely depressed patients, involve the family in the treatment.
- For patients who have major depression (or patients with other subtypes who have neurovegetative symptoms), antidepressant medication is indicated.
- For elderly patients and those with suspected cardiac disease, obtain a baseline electrocardiogram to rule out conduction system abnormalities and check for postural hypotension prior to initiation of therapy.
- SSRIs have become the first-line treatment for depression. The rationale includes their safety during overdose and generally good tolerability. The most common side effects of the SSRIs are nausea, headache, insomnia, sedation, lack of appetite, and sexual dysfunction.
- Choice of SSRI can be based on cost when when minor differences in side effect profiles are not clinically important. Chosing a generic TCA is the least costly on a per-pill basis, but cost of monitoring and side effects can add substantially to cost.
- Patients who fail a 4- to 6-week trial of an adequate dose of an SSRI should be considered for referral to a psychiatrist.
- Initial doses of antidepressants in the elderly should be half to one third the standard starting doses noted here.
- If the patient responds to the antidepressant, it should be continued for at least 6 to 9 months and then slowly tapered.
- Never prescribe more than a week's supply or a total of 1 g of a tricyclic if there is suicidal risk.
- Explain to patients that antidepressants must be taken regularly, that they may take 4 weeks to work, and that there may be mild side effects that do not warrant discontinuation of the drug.
- Prescribe a generic formulation.

ANNOTATED BIBLIOGRAPHY

Agency for Health Care Policy and Research. Public Health Service. U.S. Department of Health and Human Services. Depression in primary care: detection, diagnosis and treatment, 1993. *(Formal consensus guidelines for the management of depression.)*

American Psychiatric Association. Diagnostic and statistical manual of mental disorders, 4th ed. Washington, DC: American Psychiatric Association, 1994. *(The standard for diagnosis.)*

Brody DS, Thompson TL II, Larson DB, et al. Strategies for counseling depressed patients by primary care physicians. J Gen Intern Med 1994;9:569. *(Reviews counseling techniques and adapts them for use by primary care physicians.)*

Brown JT, Stoudemire GA. Normal and pathological grief. JAMA 1983;250:378. *(A succinct description of normal grief and guidelines for recognition and management of pathologic reactions.)*

Candilis P. The use of screening tests for detection of psychiatric disorders. In: Stern TA, Herman JB, Slavin PL, eds. MGH guide to psychiatry in primary care. New York: McGraw-Hill, 1998. *(Chapter describing available instruments for screening in a primary care setting.)*

Chambers CD, Johnson KA, Dick LM, et al. Birth outcomes in pregnant women taking fluoxetine. N Engl J Med 1996;335:1010. *(No increased risk of pregnancy loss or major fetal anomalies but increased risk of perinatal complications.)*

Crawford MJ, Prince M, Menezes P, et al. The recognition and treatment of depression in older people in primary care. Int J Geriatr Psychiatry 1998;13:172. *(Diagnosis and management from the primary care perspective.)*

Fawcett J, Kravitz HM. Anxiety syndromes and their relationship to depressive illness. J Clin Psychiatry 1988;44:8. *(Clarifies patterns of comorbidity.)*

Frank E, Kupfer DJ, Perel JM, et al. Three-year outcomes for maintenance therapies in recurrent depression. Arch Gen Psychiatry 1990;47:1093. *(Prophylactic benefits found from maintenance treatment with imipramine and interpersonal psychotherapy.)*

Freund KM, Bak SM, Blackhail L. Identifying domestic violence in primary care practice. J Gen Intern Med 1996;11:44. *(Depression and multiple bodily complaints were among the presenting complaints in persons who admitted to domestic violence.)*

Hays RD, Wells KB, Sherbourne CD, et al. Functioning and well-being outcomes of patients with depression compared with chronic general medical illnesses. Arch Gen Psychiatry 1995;52:11. *(Patients with depressive symptoms tended to function worse than those with other chronic medical conditions.)*

Keller MB, Kocsis JH, Thase ME, et al. Maintenance phase efficacy of sertraline for chronic depression: a randomized trial. JAMA 1998;280:1665. *(Well-tolerated and effective in preventing relapse and recurrence.)*

Kinon BJ. The routine use of atypical antipsychotic agents: maintenance treatment. J Clin Psychiatry 1998;59[Suppl 19]:18. *(Guidelines for long-term management with this new generation of antipsychotics.)*

Kupfer DJ, Frank E, Perel JM, et al. Five-year outcome for maintenance therapies in recurrent depression. Arch Gen Psych 1992;49:769. *(Long-term therapy effective and required in those who have recurrences.)*

Lagomasino IT, Stern TA. Approach to the suicidal patient. In: Stern TA, Herman JB, Slavin PL, eds. MGH guide to psychiatry in primary care. New York: McGraw-Hill, 1998. *(A chapter devoted to evaluating and treating this serious problem.)*

Livingston MG, Livingston HM. New antidepressants for old people? The evidence that newer drugs are much better than the old is thin. BMJ 1999;318:1640. *(An editorial that tersely sums up the evidence.)*

Lustman PJ, Griffith LS, Freedland KE, et al. Cognitive behavior therapy for depression in type 2 diabetes mellitus: a randomized, controlled trial. Ann Intern Med 1998;129:613. *(Evidence for efficacy in persons with depression accompanying a major medical illness.)*

Mulchahey JJ, Malik MS, Sabai M, et al. Serotonin-selective reuptake inhibitors in the treatment of geriatric depression and related disorders. Int J Neuropsychopharm 1999;2:121. *(Review of the use of SSRIs in elderly depression.)*

Potter WZ, Rudorfer MV. Electroconvulsive therapy—a modern medical procedure. N Engl J Med 1993;328:882. *(An editorial emphasizing the important role of ECT in treatment of severe depression.)*

Quitkin FM, Stewart JW, McGrath PJ, et al. Columbia atypical depression: a subgroup of depressives with better response to MAOI than to tricyclic antidepressants or placebo. Br J Psychiatry 1993;163[Suppl 21]:30. *(Demonstrates differential responses among the antidepressants.)*

Roose SP, Laghrissi-Thode F, Kennedy JS, et al. Comparison of paroxetine and nortriptyline in depressed patients with ischemic heart disease. JAMA 1998;279:287. *(The SSRI was the better tolerated; the TCA was associated with a significantly higher rate of adverse cardiac events.)*

Rosenthal NE. Diagnosis and treatment of seasonal affective disorder. JAMA 1993;270;2717. *(Short but inclusive review; 44 references.)*

Schlager D, Froom J, Jaffe A. Winter depression and functional impairment among ambulatory primary care patients. Compr Psychiatry 1995;36:18. *(Winter-seasonal pain may be a common presenting symptom in seasonal affective disorder.)*

Scholle SH, Rost KM, Golding JM. Physical abuse among depressed women. J Gen Intern Med 1998;13:607. *(Very high incidence found; almost all presented to their primary physicians rather than to mental health professionals.)*

Scientific expert meeting: antidepressants in clinical practice. J Clin Psychiatry 1999;60[Suppl 17]. *(An entire supplement devoted to the broad use of available antidepressants.)*

Smoller JW, Pollack MH, Lee DK. Management of antidepressant-induced side effects. In: Stern TA, Herman JB, Slavin PL, eds. MGH guide to psychiatry in primary care. New York: McGraw-Hill, 1998. *(A practical review of side effects and methods for managing them.)*

Suttor B, Rummans TA, Jowsey SG, et al. Major depression in medically ill patients. Mayo Clin Proc 1998;73:329. *(Useful review of depression as a comorbid condition, including recognition and treatment.)*

Von Korff M, Katon W, Bush T, et al. Treatment costs, cost offset, and cost-effectiveness of collaborative management of depression. Psychosom Med 1998;60:143. *(Collaborative treatment reduces use of specialty mental health visits.)*

Worthington J, Fava M, Agustin C, et al. Consumption of alcohol, nicotine, and caffeine among depressed outpatients: relationship with response to treatment. Psychosomatics 1996;37:518. *(Demonstrates lower response in patients who drink alcohol mildly.)*

The WPA Dysthymia Working Group. Dysthymia in clinical practice. Br J Psychiatry 1995;166:174. *(Improved knowledge of this disorder has led to a more positive approach to treatment, in which antidepressants can usefully be complemented by psychosocial measures.)*

228

Approach to the Patient with Alcohol Abuse

ELEANOR Z. HANNA

The primary care physician is uniquely positioned to detect and treat harmful patterns of alcohol use and to prevent alcohol-use disorders and a host of related medical and social problems. Timely recognition is critical. Alcoholism encompasses two distinct conditions: *alcohol abuse* and *alcohol dependence*. Abuse is formally defined as a maladaptive pattern of use leading to impairment in one of several sociobehavioral domains for a 1-year period. Dependence is formally defined as a maladaptive pattern of use characterized by at least three of seven symptoms that include tolerance, withdrawal, preoccupation with and recurrent use of alcohol despite adverse consequences in important areas of life. Most problem drinkers are employed, employable, or in families, indicating that the scope of the problem extends far beyond those who meet formal diagnostic criteria.

National surveys suggest a very high prevalence of alcohol abuse, dependence, or both, approaching 8% or nearly 14 million adults. Alcohol use among youth aged 12 to 17 has increased dramatically, and the rates of abuse and dependence in persons 18 to 29 years are twice those for the nation as a whole. The overall estimated societal costs in terms of health problems, lost productivity, crime, accidental deaths, and fire are staggering (in excess of $165 billion). The estimated direct cost of treatment for alcohol problems and medical consequences approaches $20 billion, with more than $15 billion for medical care alone.

Screening for alcohol problems long before they become disabling and more difficult to manage should be a routine part of every primary care practice. One first identifies and then helps the patient understand and acknowledge the consequences of drinking, the presence of a problem, and the need for intervention. The objective then shifts to negotiating and carrying out an acceptable treatment plan, one that is personalized and multifaceted.

CAUSES OF ALCOHOL ABUSE

The etiology of alcohol abuse remains incompletely understood but is clearly multifactorial. Biogenetic, sociocultural, psychologic, and behavioral elements have been elucidated. No single model accounts for all manifestations, but each is helpful in understanding the problem.

Biogenetic Model. Genetic factors appear to influence the metabolism of alcohol and the effects of alcohol on neurotransmitters, receptors, and cell membranes. The A1 allele at the D_2 dopamine receptor gene and the G1 allele of the GABAA$_A$ receptor β3 have been identified as independent contributors, with a more robust risk for disease when combined. Alcohol abuse is clearly multigenetic in origin and more genetic risk factors are likely to be characterized.

Sociocultural Model. External factors such as poverty, socialization patterns, and cultural differences in the rules governing alcohol use are emphasized. Parental and peer values, attitudes, and behaviors regarding alcohol all contribute. This model may explain the increasing use of alcohol among women and youth and use patterns of ethnic minorities, despite an overall national decline in consumption.

Psychologic-Psychodynamic Model. In this model, underlying psychopathology (e.g., dependency conflict, depression, excessive need for power or sensation seeking, gender identification problems) is viewed as predisposing a person to drink excessively, either to mask or solve a psychologic problem. Drinking is viewed merely as a symptom.

Learning Theory/Behavioral Model. Alcoholism is seen as a learned behavior that is reversible, time limited, on a continuum with normal drinking behavior and established by a series of learning and reinforcement experiences. Social interactions, emotional stress, guilty or negative thoughts, and need for sleep or pain relief serve as precipitants and maintainers of drinking behavior. Any of these precipitants coupled with learned expectations about the effects of alcohol or deficits in social skills will initiate and maintain the drinking behavior.

CLINICAL PRESENTATION AND COURSE

Use of alcohol in moderation is characterized by varying consumption and beverage according to internal cues and external circumstances. If one chooses to drink, one does so in drinking-appropriate circumstances and rarely exceeds one or two drinks. The moderate drinker is neither likely to drive under the influence (might have a drink on arrival at a party and switch to something nonalcoholic later) nor likely to drink in order to deal with problems, escape, or get drunk.

With the caveats that a given dose of alcohol affects different people differently and that average daily consumption neglects the pattern of drinking, drinking in moderation may be defined quantitatively as two or less drinks per day for men and one or less for women and the elderly. The figure is lower in women and the elderly because they experience a higher blood alcohol level per drink due to smaller volume of distribution and decreased first-pass metabolism of alcohol. (A standard drink is assumed to contain roughly 12 g, 15 mL, or 0.5 oz of alcohol, which is the approximate content of 12 oz of beer, 5 oz of wine, or 1.5 oz of liquor.)

Alcohol misuse ranges from social drinking with a tendency for occasional excess to constant intoxication. Orderly progression is not assumed. The most commonly encountered presentations include

- The *social drinker*, who consumes alcohol in amounts and circumstances that appear socially acceptable but may develop a serious alcohol problem if there is a propensity to overindulge or to occasionally use alcohol to cope with stress.
- The *heavy social drinker*, who drinks in socially appropriate circumstances but actively seeks a life of occasions for drinking (through job or social life); has more than two drinks every day, continuously seeks out situations in which to drink, and may often overconsume but not exceeding the consumption of peers; and may never appear drunk or seem affected in social or work routines, but as drinking escalates, it becomes increasingly tied to seeking physical or psychological relief. Problem drinkers emerge from this population. Neither the person nor acquaintances suspect an alcohol abuse problem.
- The *problem drinker*, who meets the criteria for heavy social drinking, gets drunk on occasion and also exhibits medical, legal, social, or psychologic consequences of excessive alcohol consumption; makes or thinks of making attempts at cutting down or quitting; functioning may vary from seemingly intact behavior to difficulty coping; may deny a drinking problem and attribute blame to external events or persons; denial is common even among those with multiple arrests for drunk driving.

- The *alcohol-dependent patient* who tries to consume the same excessive amount of alcohol regardless of mood or situation, although external circumstances might constrain drinking for a time. Most continue to work; some even in high positions. Alcohol is given top priority in all situations (e.g., one goes to a party to drink, not to socialize). Tolerance to alcohol develops, and withdrawal symptoms (mood disturbance, tremor, nausea, sweats) may be noted during the work day when the blood alcohol level drops. Drinking at lunch and cocktail hour are needed to relieve symptoms. The patient is aware of the compulsion to drink but is difficult to reach unless family or employer notes a problem or serious medical complications develop.
- The *severely deteriorated patient* who maintains a constant state of intoxication, having no care for his or her person or surroundings; undergoes periodic hospitalizations for detoxification and for medical care necessary after alcohol-related trauma or organ damage.

Groups at increased risk include professionals; executives; young people; women, especially those of childbearing age; and the elderly as are those presenting with depression, other drug use, or a family history positive for alcoholism. Seemingly high functioning *executives and professionals* who manage their own schedules have ready access to both alcohol and drugs, the use and consequences of which remain hidden until serious sequellae become obvious. Eighty percent of *young people* drink as high school seniors and 24% binge drink, a pattern that continues and increases to 34% among college students. Adults who began drinking or smoking regularly in their early teens suffer the most serious alcohol, drug, and psychiatric problems and often manifest the greatest proportion of familial alcohol problems. *Women*, as a result of social change, are consulting clinics at double the former rates. *Elderly* patients may begin to use alcohol excessively for stress, especially in reaction to loss of a loved one or because of sleep difficulties. A peak period for onset for new alcohol-related problems is 65 to 74 years of age.

Natural History and Clinical Course. There is considerable individual variation. Onset ranges from an initial phase of social drinking to immediate heavy drinking. Prognosis remains relatively favorable until dependence sets in. Once the addiction becomes psychologic or physiologic, it is difficult to break in the absence of treatment and the clinical course is often progressive. (This makes it imperative to detect alcohol misuse long before the patient meets formal criteria for diagnosis of alcohol abuse.) At the point of addiction, continued drinking may punctuated by periods of abstinence or controlled drinking but followed by relapse and progression, especially if there is no expert intervention. Controversy continues regarding whether or not total abstinence is required to halt progression.

Medical Complications. The risk of organ damage is related in part to the dose and duration of alcohol exposure, with some conditions (e.g., *alcoholic cardiomyopathy, fatty liver*) manifesting reversibility with abstinence, and others (e.g., *cirrhosis*) seeming to progress inexorably once severe hepatocellular damage has occurred. Risk appears to be a function of a genetic predisposition and alcohol dosage and chronicity of exposure. Although cardiovascular benefits may accrue from up to two drinks a day in white men (one in women and black men), con-

Table 228.1. Criteria for Substance Abuse and Dependence according to DSM-IV

Substance Abuse
A. A maladaptive pattern of substance use leading to clinically significant impairment or distress, as manifested by at least one of the following occurring within the same 12-month period.
  1. Recurrent substance use resulting in a failure to fulfill major role obligations at work, school, or home.
  2. Recurrent substance use in situations in which it is physically hazardous.
  3. Recurrent substance-related legal problems.
  4. Continued substance use despite having persistent or recurrent social or interpersonal problems caused or exacerbated by the effects of the substance.
B. The symptoms have never met the criteria for Substance Dependence for this class of drugs.

Substance Dependence
A maladaptive pattern of substance use, leading to clinically significant impairment or distress, as manifested by at least three of the following occurring in the same 12 month time period.
1. Tolerance, as defined by either of the following:
  a. A need for markedly increased amounts of the substance to achieve intoxication or desired effect.
  b. Markedly diminished effect with continued use of the same amount of the substance.
2. Withdrawal as manifested by either of the following:
  a. The characteristics withdrawal syndrome for the substance.
  b. The same (or closely related) substance is taken to relieve or avoid withdrawal symptoms.
3. The substance is often taken in larger amounts or over a longer period that was intended.
4. There is a persistent desire or unsuccessful efforts to cut down or control substance use.
5. A great deal of time is spent in activities necessary to obtain the substance, use the substance, or recover from its effects.
6. Important social, occupational, or recreational activities are given up or reduced because of substance use.
7. The substance use is continued despite knowledge of having a persistent or recurrent physical or psychological problem that is caused or exacerbated by the substance use.
Specify if
  1. With physiological dependence if either tolerance or withdrawal is present.
  2. Without physiological dependence if neither is present.

sumption of more than three drinks a day is associated with increased risk for hypertension, among other risk factors for more serious disease.

Persistent *impotence* and *loss of libido* reflect impaired gonadotropin release and accelerated testosterone metabolism that occur as consequences of chronic alcohol excess; they predate end-stage liver disease. *Alcoholic hepatitis, pancreatitis, and gastritis* may follow binge drinking. *Fatty liver and esophagitis* ensue from chronic use. Late-stage complications include *cirrhosis, oral cancers, cardiomyopathy, Wernicke's encephalopathy, and Korsakoff's dementia.*

Fetal alcohol syndrome occurs in infants born to mothers who drink heavily during pregnancy. Features include permanently stunted growth, mental retardation, musculoskeletal abnormalities, poor coordination, and cardiac malformations. Incidence approaches 33% among pregnant women who drink more than 150 g (6.25 oz) of alcohol per day. Another third of children born to such women will have mental retardation or severe behavior disorders. Serious maternal and infant health problems and increased infant and fetal deaths accrue among women who report drinking even as little as one drink a week during pregnancy.

DIAGNOSIS

The Diagnostic and Statistical Manual of Psychiatric Disease, 4th edition (DSM-IV), specifies the most widely used criteria for the formal diagnoses of alcohol abuse and alcohol dependence (Table 228.1).

WORKUP

Formal diagnosis involves identification of excessive quantity and duration of consumption, physiologic manifestations of ethanol addiction, loss of control over drinking, and chronic

Table 228-2. The CAGE Test

Have you ever felt the need to **C**ut down on drinking?
   Have you ever felt **A**nnoyed by criticism of drinking?
   Have you ever had **G**uilty feelings about drinking?
Have you ever taken a morning **E**ye opener?

(Mayfield D, McLead G, Hall P. The CAGE questionnaire. Am J Psychiatry 1974;131:1121.)

damage to physical health and social functioning. In late stages of illness, these clinical findings are readily evident. *Detection before marked abuse or dependence has developed remains the major diagnostic challenge.*

The high prevalence of alcohol abuse, its serious consequences, and good response to early intervention argue for routinely screening all adolescents and adults who come for primary care. In addition, a high index of suspicion for alcoholism is indicated for the patient who presents with a family history positive for alcoholism, anxiety, insomnia, recurrent infection, an illness that is potentially alcohol related, child abuse, domestic violence, multiple psychosomatic problems, suicidality, depression, inability to articulate feelings, or interpersonal, occupational, financial, or legal problems.

Screening. For the patient in whom there is no clinical evidence or suspicion of alcohol abuse, the *CAGE questions* (Table 228.2) are the screening test of choice. In primary care settings, sensitivity for a score of 2 (the standard cutoff) ranges from 70% to 85% and specificity from 85% to 91%. In the *elderly*, where prevalence of alcoholism is increased but clinical presentation may be harder to ascertain, sensitivity falls to 50%, whereas specificity remains above 90%. Including questions on the quantity and frequency of drinking improves detection in the elderly.

A 10-item self-administered questionnaire, the *Alcohol Dependence Scale* is another popular research and screening tool

Table 228.3.   The Michigan Alcoholism Screening Test (MAST)

1.	Do you feel you are a normal drinker?	(No 2)	Yes
2.	Have you ever awakened in the morning after some drinking the night before and found that you could not remember part of the evening?	(Yes 2)	No
3.	Does your wife (or husband or parents) ever worry or complain about your drinking?	(Yes 1)	No
4.	Can you stop drinking without a struggle after one or two drinks?	(No 2)	Yes
5.	Do you ever feel badly about your drinking?	(Yes 2)	No
6.	Do you ever try to limit your drinking to certain times of day or to certain places?	(Yes 0)	No
7.	Do your friends or relatives think that you are a normal drinker?	(No 2)	Yes
8.	Are you always able to stop when you want to?	(No 2)	Yes
9.	Have you ever attended a meeting of Alcoholics Anonymous?	(Yes 5)	No
10.	Have you gotten into fights when drinking?	(Yes 1)	No
11.	Has drinking ever created problems with you and your wife (husband)?	(Yes 2)	No
12.	Has your wife (husband or other family member) ever gone to anyone for help about your drinking?	(Yes 2)	No
13.	Have you ever lost friends or girlfriends/boyfriends because of drinking?	(Yes 2)	No
14.	Have you ever gotten into trouble at work because of drinking?	(Yes 2)	No
15.	Have you ever lost a job because of drinking?	(Yes 2)	No
16.	Have you ever neglected your obligations, your family or your work for two days or more in a row because of drinking?	(Yes 2)	No
17.	Do you ever drink before noon?	(Yes 1)	No
18.	Have you ever been told you have liver trouble?	(Yes 2)	No
19.	Have you ever had DTs (delerium tremens), severe shaking, heard voices or seen things that weren't there after heavy drinking?	(Yes 2)	No
20.	Have you ever gone to anyone for help about your drinking?	(Yes 5)	No
21.	Have you ever been in a hospital because of drinking?	(Yes 5)	No
22.	Have you ever been a patient in a psychiatric hospital or on a psychiatric ward of a general hospital where drinking was part of the problem?	(Yes 2)	No
23.	Have you ever been seen at a psychiatric or mental health clinic, or gone to a doctor or clergyman for help with an emotional problem in which drinking has played a part?	(Yes 2)	No
24.	Have you ever been arrested, even for a few hours, because of drunken behavior?	(Yes 2)	No
25.	Have you ever been arrested for drunk driving or driving after drinking?	(Yes 2)	No

A score of three points or less is considered nonalcoholic; a score of four points is suggestive, and a score of five points or more indicates alcoholism.

(Selzer ML. The Michigan Alcoholism Screening Test. Am J Psychiatry 1971; 127:1653.)

in clinical settings. It can be incorporated into a previsit lifestyle screen to assess severity. Its benefits are high reliability and validity. A cutoff score of 5 will identify patients suitable for brief intervention in the physician's office. Other popular tests used in clinical and research settings are the *Michigan Alcohol Screening Test* (Table 228.3) and the *Alcohol Use Disorders Inventory*.

A detailed drinking history is in order for all patients suspected of having an alcohol problem on the basis of any of the following:

- A positive Alcohol Dependence Scale, CAGE, or Michigan Alcohol Screening Test test;
- A family complaint or a history of alcoholism in the family;
- A daily drinking pattern of two to three drinks accompanied by seemingly innocuous complaints that might be related to drinking (e.g., frequent nonspecific illness, accidents);
- A life-style that will perpetuate increased prolonged drinking, including tobacco or drug use;
- The occurrence of intrapsychic or interpersonal problems or actual changes in life events;

- Suggestive manifestations on physical examination, such as alcohol on the breath, spider angiomata, plethoric facies, tremor, ecchymoses;
- Abnormal liver function tests; macrocytic anemia.

Taking an Alcohol History. Except under overwhelming circumstances, patients do not volunteer drinking problems and request help. Denial is likely to be strong. Consequently, one has to use an interview technique that is kind and supportive yet firm and even confrontational when there are serious clinical concerns, especially when there is question about ability to function. Where indicated, family members, friends, and even the employer may facilitate both history taking and therapy.

The Drinking Profile. In taking a drinking history, it is critical that one go beyond issues of quantity, frequency, and development of tolerance. A profile of the patient's drinking behavior over a given time period will prove most useful and should include attention to

- Setting: time, place, and occasion for drinking;
- Social network: the people involved with the drinking and their relationship to the patient;

- Consumption: quantity, frequency, and rate of consumption as it relates to that of others in the drinking context and as it relates to the patient's expected consumption;
- Pressures (internal or external) to drink;
- Other activities related to drinking.

The physician should suspect anyone *who drinks* and is in a *drinking context on a regular basis*—that means most patients. Not only will a drinking profile help characterize an alcohol abuser or alcoholic, it will also identify those not suspected of having a problem. The profile is an effective tool for confronting the resistant patient, treating a willing patient, and educating a person with a potential problem. It also permits one to make any standard manualized treatment approach personal, and thus more effective, with patient-specific examples.

Causes for Missing the Diagnosis. These include subtlety of presentation, use of definitions of alcoholism that do not encompass early manifestations, the view that the patient is normal so long as he or she can perform daily activities, societal acceptance of dangerous levels of alcohol intake, and general expectations of alcohol consumption at most social occasions. There may be unintentional collusion with the patient in denying the problem, especially if the patient is of similar or higher social status, has similar habits and life-style, or is attractive, verbal, and intelligent.

PRINCIPLES OF MANAGEMENT

Management is most successful when it is multifaceted, personalized, and long term. Often, the primary care physician remains the one constant medical figure and the most trusted person in the patient's life. Whether one intends to personally care for the alcohol abusing patient or refer them to a specialist, the primary physician has the important initial task of assisting the patient in acknowledging the drinking problem and accepting a treatment program.

Getting Started

Dealing with Denial. One should first listen carefully to how the patient explains the findings. If the problem appears likely to be accepted internally, but the patient does not want to reveal it externally, then it is best to help the patient discover the problem for him or herself. One might suggest keeping a journal or weekly log of drinking events for reviewing links between drinking and particular environmental, interpersonal, or psychologic precipitants. This also helps determine exactly how much the patient drinks without direct confrontation and, in itself, constitutes a brief intervention.

The same technique, with some additions, can be used for the patient who is hiding the problem from him or herself. Here, one reviews the evidence on how alcohol directly affects the patient's health. Use of screening instruments (see above) and presenting the findings in terms of a specific diagnostic classification system sometimes helps to objectify the diagnosis. If the patient continues to resist, then one can bring in family, friends, or employer to present the patient with their evidence of how destructive the drinking is to him or herself and them. Again, these sessions should be factual nonjudgmental discussions of the relationship of alcohol to the patient's health and behavior and its impact on those important to him or her.

Dealing with Resistance to Treatment. Patients who agree they have a problem yet continue to refuse help or to relinquish alcohol should be handled similarly, but with more focus on their fears and resistance. The hostile or belligerent patient should be dealt with firmly, but in a manner that enhances ability to objectify and control anger (e.g., by identifying the sources of anger).

Often those who resist treatment must first fear the loss of something very important (e.g., spouse, job) before seeking help. The so-called *tough love approach*, in which loss is seriously threatened or actually carried out unless the patient goes for treatment, must be sustained for an indefinite and prolonged period because many patients return to old habits once danger of losing a loved one or job passes. The approach is not always effective and should therefore be used sparingly. It is pointless to force the patient into treatment when no medical emergency exists. It is better to present the options available, continue exploring the issue, and provide health education while treating the patient's medical problems and awaiting willingness to undergo treatment.

Should the patient agree to seek treatment, it is important to keep the waiting period brief and helpful to remind the patient a day or two ahead of the appointment.

Patient Selection for Management by the Primary Physician. The doctor–patient relationship can be used to change life-style, identify and restructure destructive patterns, and learn new coping skills. Effective care requires being available on a regular basis to provide the necessary monitoring, instruction, and support. If such support is beyond the scope of the individual primary physician or a trained assistant in the practice, then a proper and smooth referral for specialized care is indicated. Brief physician office interventions have proved effective in reducing the alcohol consumption of nondependent patients.

Long-term management by the primary care physician is best for those patients with

- Medical complications as the foremost concern;
- A strong personal tie to the primary physician;
- Good social stability;
- Only minor psychopathology;
- Intelligence and pragmatism;
- Great faith in physicians;
- An intact and supportive social network.

It is important to remember that the treatment will be long and arduous and that the patient's behavior is sick and often will be directed at the primary physician or therapist in either a covert or overtly hostile manner. The ultimate goal is to help the patient gain self-control, regulation, and a sense of responsibility. One must not counterattack.

If and when the physician finds him or herself unable to cope, the patient should be referred to a specialist, with the primary physician remaining as the coordinator of care.

Determinants of Successful Treatment. *Early detection and prompt initiation* of treatment are essential to success, with success rates of 50% to 90% attained in patients abusing alcohol but without physical or social impairment. Success rates also depend on the *length of time* a person stays in treatment, *patient involvement* in goal setting and treatment planning, and continued attachment to *family* or an integrated *social network*. Very brief *physician interventions* have also proved effective, with the key being continued health care provided by the physician serving as the advisor/monitor.

Involving family members or significant others in the confrontation and treatment assists and supports the life-style changes that must be made, particularly when the problem drinker is a woman or young person. This ensures that the patient goes for and remains in treatment.

Other determinants of successful treatment include use of a *personalized multifaceted* plan, an *active role* for the patient, and continuous *review*. Controversy continues regarding whether or not *total abstinence* is required to halt progression. Cessation certainly is necessary to halt many of the medical complications.

Treatment Modalities

Therapies can be classified as biological, psychological, behavioral, or sociocultural. Selection is best done on an individualized basis to meet the patient's specific needs. Most programs use a combination of modalities. The biologic approach includes use of drugs. In general, drug therapy plays a supportive role in the outpatient care of the alcoholic patient, mainly providing a temporary respite from alcohol consumption sufficient to enable the patient to engage in a more comprehensive and durable treatment program.

Drugs to Decrease Alcohol Consumption and Prevent Relapse. Pharmacologic agents are prescribed to reduce the urge to drink, to blunt withdrawal symptoms, and to treat underlying psychiatric problems that may be contributing to alcohol abuse. As noted, the goal is to provide the patient with time to organize the supports necessary for achievement of long-term abstinence.

Disulfiram (Antabuse) is an aversive therapy. It achieves short-term improvement in alcohol consumption when used in a supervised comprehensive outpatient program that includes other rehabilitative measures. Success requires careful compliance and a stable life-style. Patients best suited are those who seek total abstinence, request the drug; have no underlying cardiovascular, depressive, or schizophrenic disease; and are willing to return monthly for evaluation of therapy.

The drug sensitizes the patient to the effects of alcohol by inhibiting hepatic aldehyde-NAD oxidoreductase. Within minutes of taking as little as 1 ounce of alcohol, the patient experiences an increase in serum acetaldehyde concentration that leads to palpitations, flushing, tachypnea, tachycardia, and shortness of breath. Nausea, vomiting, and headache develop if a greater amount of alcohol is taken. Symptoms last about 90 minutes and usually are self-limited. Occasionally, marked hypotension or a cardiac arrhythmia may occur. Fatalities from myocardial infarction and stroke have been reported. The agent can worsen depression and schizophrenia. Candidates require careful medical and psychiatric evaluation before initiating therapy.

Side effects include drowsiness and lethargy, which are countered by administering the drug before bed. The standard dose is 250 mg at bedtime. Important drug–drug interactions occur with antihypertensive agents (potentiation of hypotensive effect with intake of alcohol), benzodiazepines (BZDs; reduced intensity of the disulfiram reaction), tricyclic antidepressants and phenothiazines (potentiation of central nervous system ef-

fects), and drugs metabolized by hepatic microsomes (prolongation of their half-lives).

Disulfiram should not be considered an option for chronic use. *Duration* of therapy is individualized. Treatment should be terminated if the patient fails to keep appointments, resumes drinking, becomes pregnant or depressed, or develops abnormalities in liver function tests or cardiovascular status.

Naltrexone (Trexan), an opioid antagonist that appears to blunt the pleasurable effects of alcohol, is U.S. Food and Drug Administration–approved to reduce cravings and provides a new approach to pharmacologic therapy. In placebo-controlled randomized trials that include a program of concurrent comprehensive care, the drug significantly increases the abstinence rate to over 50%. Like other drugs for alcoholism, its role is as an adjunct. Recommended dosage is 50 mg/d for up to 12 weeks. The drug is well tolerated, with self-limited nausea and headache as the common side effects. High doses may cause hepatocellular injury, necessitating the monitoring of liver enzymes with use. It appears to work best in persons who describe intense cravings. Contraindications include opiate use and hepatocellular disease.

Acamprosate (calcium acetylhomotaurinate), which has specificity for NMDA and GABA receptors, is a competitive antagonist that reduces cravings. It is currently used abroad but is now under study in the United States.

Psychoactive Drugs. Pharmacologic treatment of underlying psychopathology has been proposed as a means of cutting down on drinking. Anxiolytic agents such as the BZDs have been used with a modicum of success in patients who drink because of an anxiety disorder. There is no evidence for long-term efficacy in reduction of alcohol use, but some data suggest a short-term reduction in anxiety that could enable a patient to engage in more comprehensive forms of therapy. BZDs have also been proposed as a means of reducing the desire to drink that might emanate from a postulated chronic withdrawal syndrome. Supporting data for both the syndrome and the efficacy of long-term drug treatment are minimal. *Buspirone* has been effective in short trials as a treatment for severely anxious patients, but more work is required to clarify its effectiveness. *TCAs and selective serotonin reuptake inhibitors* may be effective when there is an underlying depression, especially when it is accompanied by neurovegetative symptoms (see Chapter 227). *Lithium* has been tried with lesser success.

Drugs for Withdrawal. The acute withdrawal syndrome (tachycardia, elevation in blood pressure, tremor, hyperreflexia, increased irritability) and its severest manifestations and complications (seizures, hallucinations, and delirium tremens) are best prevented and treated by use of BZDs. The determinants for drug treatment of withdrawal include severity of symptoms, past history of withdrawal, and any comorbid medical conditions. The *Clinical Institute Withdrawal Assessment-Alcohol, revised* (CIWA-Ar), is the most validated instrument for objective assessment of withdrawal severity and risk (Table 228.4). It use is common in inpatient settings but may also be helpful in the office. A rough clinical estimate of severity must suffice in its absence. For those with mild symptoms (e.g., CIWA-Ar score less than 8), no treatment is necessary other than continued monitoring unless there is a history of severe withdrawal or comorbid disease, in which case pharmacologic therapy is needed. Patients with moderate symptoms (e.g., CIWA-Ar

Table 228-4. Treatment Regimens for Alcohol Withdrawal

SEVERITY OF WITHDRAWAL SYNDROME	REGIMEN
Mild (CIWA-Ar score <8)	Monitor ever 4-8 hours until no worsening for 24 hrs; treat as for moderate or severe disease if prior history of severe withdrawal or if there is serious concurrent illness
Moderate (CIWA-Ar score 8-15)	Begin diazepam 10 mg q6h for 4 doses, then 5mg q6h for 8 doses, or chlordiazepoxide 50 mg q6h for 4 doses then 25 mg q6h for 8 doses; then halt and allow drug metabolism to achieve tapering
	For persons with concurrent liver disease, begin lorazepam 2 mg q6h for 4 doses, then 1 mg q6h for 8 doses
	Provide additional medication PRN when symptoms are not controlled
Severe (CIWA-Ar score >15)	Admit to inpatient facility and begin symptom-triggered regimen with hourly administration of diazepam 10-20 mg, chlordiazepoxide 50-100 mg, or lorazepam 2-4 mg and reassess hourly, repeating the dose if CIWA score >8-10

*After Mayo-Smith MF, et al. JAMA 1997;278:144.

score of 8 to 15) benefit symptomatically from treatment; those with severe symptoms (scores higher than 15) require pharmacologic therapy because risk of seizures is very high.

The long-acting BZDs (e.g., diazepam, chlordiazepoxide) appear more effective in preventing withdrawal seizures and in achieving a smoother withdrawal with fewer rebound symptoms than the *short-acting agents*; however, they are more likely to cause sedation, particularly in the elderly and those with liver disease. The nonhepatically metabolized BZDs (*lorazepam, oxazepam*) are indicated for use in persons with hepatocellular disease, but they are shorter acting and necessitate close monitoring of the patient. Fixed-dose, loading-dose, and symptom-triggered BZD regimens have been developed and are effective when used as intended. Fixed-dose regimens are the standard approach to treatment. *Loading-dose programs* use a large dose of a long-acting agent (e.g., diazepam 20 mg) given at the outset and repeated until the patient is sedated. Normal drug metabolism results in tapering. *Symptom-triggered* therapy using chlordiazepoxide has been shown to decrease mean duration of therapy and amount of drug required compared with fixed-dose treatment, but it requires close monitoring of the patient, usually feasible only in the inpatient setting.

Beta-blockers (e.g., atenolol, 50 to 100 mg/d) can help control adrenergic symptoms and reduce BZD requirements, but they are not sufficient as monotherapy, because they do not prevent seizures, hallucinations, or delirium tremens. *Clonidine*, a centrally acting inhibitor of noradrenergic activity, is an effective alternative to BZDs in mild to moderate withdrawal syndrome when used in a tapered program.

Outpatient administration is appropriate for those with mild symptoms of withdrawal; inpatient supervision is indicated for those with more severe symptoms or a prior history of severe withdrawal.

Inpatient versus Outpatient Programs. As noted, inpatient care may be necessary for detoxification and treatment of withdrawal. For achieving long-term abstinence, randomized studies show no overall advantage for residential over nonresidential treatment programs. As a result, expensive long-term inpatient care is no longer the standard for treatment of alcoholism. Only one methodologically sound randomized trial has demonstrated an advantage for inpatient care, and this one was part of an employee assistance program, which is itself a well-recognized determinant of success.

The net result is the current emphasis on outpatient care, except for treatment of severe acute withdrawal syndrome. Inpatient care remains an option for people who have failed all other forms of treatment and who will not deal with the problems so long as they are in environments that maintain destructive drinking. It is a costly approach and should be used as a last recourse. For most patients, an outpatient program that combines psychotherapy and behavioral-cognitive approaches can be offered in primary care practices by the physician and/or staff after some training. A national randomized controlled clinical trial of a brief alcohol intervention program tailored to patients in a medical setting resulted in significant and increasing reductions in alcohol consumption between patients in the treatment and control groups over a 2-year period.

Outpatient psychotherapy places emphasis on psychic restructuring and removal of the presumed underlying psychopathology. Such treatment is important for the person whose interpersonal or psychologic problems outweigh the alcohol abuse. The best candidates are socially intact, intellectually curious, and eager to be involved in the process. If concurrent treatment of the drinking is included, this can be a successful approach to patients with comorbid psychiatric disorders.

Alcoholism is associated with special needs that require the therapist to take a much more active role than is typical in insight-oriented psychotherapy. One must provide structure, guidance, support, nurturance, and instruction in helping the patient control drinking while working on the underlying conflicts and dysfunctional defense mechanisms.

Behavioral-cognitive therapies are based on the notion that alcoholism is a learned behavior that can be extinguished and reshaped, with controlled drinking a possible outcome. For patients who are rigid or seek treatments with defined tangible end points, behavioral therapy is often useful, as it is helpful in dealing with problems involving role changes and behaviors in specific situations. *Aversive conditioning* is designed to either eliminate alcohol use or train patients to drink in moderation only. Alternative behaviors are taught via operant conditioning.

Cognitive therapy focuses on the observables of the drinking behavior (frequency, duration, quantity, time, place, activity, age, sex, and role-appropriate drinking behaviors). It attempts to identify the precipitants to abuse and the factors that maintain and perpetuate it. This method can be incorporated effectively into brief physician-based interventions.

Table 228-5.   Blood Alcohol Level*

TIME ELAPSED SINCE FIRST DRINK (IN HOURS)	NUMBER OF DRINKS†									
	1	2	3	4	5	6	7	8	9	10
1	0.01	0.03	0.05	0.08	0.10	0.13	0.15	0.17	0.20	0.22
2	0.00	0.02	0.04	0.06	0.09	0.11	0.14	0.16	0.19	0.21
3	0.00	0.005	0.02	0.05	0.07	0.10	0.12	0.14	0.17	0.19
4	0.00	0.00	0.01	0.03	0.06	0.08	0.11	0.13	0.15	0.18
5	0.00	0.00	0.00	0.02	0.04	0.07	0.09	0.11	0.14	0.18

*Determined by the number of drinks consumed in a circumscribed time period by a presumably normal 150-lb male. Females, because they are affected more quickly, require less alcohol to achieve these levels.
†Blood alcohol levels as a function of weight, time, and number of drinks consumed:

One drink = 1.5 oz 80-proof spirits (40% alcohol)
          3.0 oz fortified wine (20% alcohol)
          5.0 oz table wine (12% alcohol)
          12.0 oz beer (4.5% alcohol)

Sociocultural treatment emphasizes altering external factors. It includes *residential care, halfway houses*, and direct social manipulation, such as *finding jobs*, helping with *shelter and money*, and removing a person from his family. This is a treatment appropriate for homeless, jobless, unstable persons whose social functioning is impaired; for repeated treatment failures; for young people; and for others with severe family problems. Any of these approaches and the community services that follow can be used as adjuncts to other treatments wherever necessary.

Community Services. *Alcoholics Anonymous* provides the critical elements of social support, caring, and structure, which are essential to many patients. The program has a quasireligious orientation, making it particularly useful to the religious person. Relatively superficial involvement (e.g., two to four meetings per month) is usually not effective as the sole means of therapy but can serve as a useful adjunct to other forms of treatment. However, the person willing to dedicate oneself to a lifetime of sobriety can achieve the goal in this carefully delineated manner. *Al-Anon and Al-Ateen* assist family members of the alcoholic. Other popular self-help groups are Women for Sobriety, which stresses individual responsibility to boost self-esteem, and Rational Recovery, which stresses using reason rather than spirituality.

Employee assistance programs can be very useful, because motivation is often high. Most large companies offer such programs, and their counselors can work in tandem with physicians. They may also offer family, marital, and financial help, as may programs available through social service agencies, community guidance centers, and even state or federal agencies. *Clergy and church organizations* can be very helpful to religious persons.

Prevention

Prevention involves more than warning people of the health hazards of alcohol abuse. It requires screening for early detection of alcohol abuse (see above) and providing patient-specific information. By taking a brief drinking history at the time of the yearly checkup, the primary physician can educate the patient and provide suitable guidelines for drinking behavior, just as one does for exercise and diet. A number of very brief physician interventions or trials of advice qualify as prevention or

Table 228-6.   Behavior Expected at Various Blood Alcohol Levels (BAL)

BAL	BEHAVIORAL EFFECTS
0.05	Relaxation; possibility of thought, judgment, and self-control being affected
0.10	Obvious impairment of voluntary motor action; legally drunk in most states
0.20	Considerable motor impairment and loss of emotional control; definite intoxication
0.40-0.50	Unconsciousness and probable death resulting from respiratory failure

early intervention programs that can be easily offered in medical practice. Randomized trials have proved this an effective method in reducing harmful levels of alcohol consumption.

People who do drink need to know how alcohol can affect them, how to behave responsibly when drinking (especially in regard to driving), and how to drink to prevent drunkenness (Tables 228.5 and 228.6). Individuals should know that their attitudes and behaviors will affect how their children/spouses drink. All should be cautioned that drinking is a dangerous way to deal with insomnia and emotional problems.

Waiting-room literature and hospital and community health-education programs can complement instruction. National campaigns focus on alcohol-related accidents, crime, concomitants of abuse, and birth defects.

INDICATIONS FOR ADMISSION AND REFERRAL

The patient who has medically decompensated because of a complication of alcohol abuse (e.g., heart failure, pancreatitis, gastrointestinal bleeding, and hepatitis) clearly requires prompt hospital admission. Other candidates include persons with evidence of severe withdrawal (tremor, agitation, hallucinations, seizures) and those unable to tolerate a severe withdrawal syndrome (prior history of severe withdrawal, concurrent medical or psychiatric illness, chronic and severe alcohol-related illness). A free-standing detoxification center may suffice for the otherwise uncomplicated patient.

Patients with major psychopathology, poor ties to the physician, or a disintegrated social network have serious drawbacks to successful treatment by even the most willing primary care physician. Such patients should be referred in a coordinated way for specialized care, ensuring continuity and a personalized treatment program. The primary physician can perform a major service for these patients by understanding available specialized referral resources in one's community and matching them to the patient's needs.

RECOMMENDATIONS

- First establish rapport. Let the patient know you accept and understand them by approaching the problem in a respectful and comfortable manner.
- Offer appropriate and sufficient instruction and explanation as you go along, always engaging the patient in establishing realistic goals and not pushing beyond limits.
- Maintain a proper balance of support, caring, and limit setting; remain flexible and adaptable to the patient's needs.
- Think of treatment as a series of short-term programs to develop and increase the patient's sense of mastery.
- Never insist on immediate abstinence. This is a goal to be negotiated and accomplished in the context of harm reduction when there is resistance to abstinence. Only if all else fails should there be confrontation and control in this area.
- If serious health problems will result from any alcohol intake and you must ask the patient to abstain, do it in the context of a supportive educational-advice session to ensure their return.
- If a patient comes to a session drunk, kindly and calmly explain why it would be pointless to have a session and reschedule the appointment. If this behavior continues, the treatment agreement should be renegotiated to include rules about it.
- Keep motivation high, not only by using the patient's fear of losing his or her health, something, or someone very important, but by getting him or her to seek and define his or her own reinforcers.
- Help the patient to identify, objectify, and deal with anger and other emotions to enhance emotional control.
- When the patient is ready, help pinpoint the actual behaviors to be changed and work on them progressively. One may need to provide information, modeling, practice, feedback, and homework as the patient learns to handle feelings and to develop new social skills, the tools necessary to assess and modify behavior.
- Encourage self-monitoring of drinking behavior via logs, teaching the patient to detect causes, consequences, and maintaining factors and thus helping to learn alternate ways of coping with the people, places, situations, and feelings associated with heavy drinking.
- Select those components of available specialized treatment programs that match to the patient's needs, wants, and ability to cope. The standard formula of detoxification—disulfiram and Alcoholics Anonymous—is no longer either the recommended or the most acceptable treatment for alcoholism.
- For spree and binge-drinking patients, whose interpersonal and psychologic problems are likely to be predominant, consider outpatient psychotherapy if they are socially intact, intellectually curious, and psychologically minded.
- For patients strongly motivated to attain total abstinence and specifically requesting disulfiram therapy, begin 250 mg qhs and renew on a monthly basis, reevaluating the need for continued drug therapy while working on psychosocial interventions that will sustain long-term abstinence. Treatment is contraindicated in those with underlying psychiatric illness or cardiovascular disease. Consider naltrexone 50 mg/d for those who relapse because of intense craving for alcohol. Use drug treatment only as a complement to and a means of participating effectively in a comprehensive program of care.
- For patients who are rigid, repressed, and resistant to open-ended therapies, consider behavioral-cognitive methods. Brief physician intervention that is personalized can be effective.
- For patients willing to dedicate themselves to a lifetime of sobriety or who will benefit from peer counseling, consider Alcoholics Anonymous, especially if there is a religious interest.
- For patients who are homeless, jobless, or have other serious social problems, refer to a community social service agency for direct aid.
- For patients who have failed outpatient treatments, can afford the time, and need to be taken out of their environment to cease drinking, consider an inpatient alcohol program.
- For treatment of withdrawal, consider outpatient management if the patient is reliable, has no or only mild symptoms, no active underlying medical illnesses, no prior history of severe withdrawal and who has a supportive family that can provide supervision. Prescribe a long-acting BZD (e.g., a fixed-schedule program of diazepam 10 mg every 6 hours for four doses, then 5 mg every 6 hours for eight doses); achieve tapering by normal drug metabolism. Unstable patients and those with other medical conditions or with symptoms suggesting potentially severe withdrawal (e.g., tachycardia, tremor, hallucinations, increased irritability) should be promptly admitted for treatment.

ANNOTATED BIBLIOGRAPHY

American Psychiatric Association. Diagnostic and Statistical Manual of Mental Disorders, 4th edition. Washington DC: American Psychiatric Association, 1997. (*Provides diagnostic criteria for alcohol abuse and alcohol dependence.*)

Buck KJ. Recent progress toward the identification of genes related to risk for alcoholism. Mammalian Genome 1998;9:927. (*Current state of the art, a brief overview of several very specific research areas covered in the same journal issue.*)

Cushman WC, Cutler JA, Hanna, EZ, et al. Prevention and treatment of hypertension study (PATHS): effects of an alcohol treatment program on blood pressure. Arch Intern Med 1998;158:1197. (*Increasing and significant reductions in alcohol consumption over a 2-year period; small, but probably most realistic, effect on blood pressure. Plethora of valuable references of use in research and practice*).

Fleming MF, Barry KL, Manwell LB, et al. Brief physician advice for problem drinkers: a randomized controlled trial in community-based primary care practices. JAMA 1997;277:1039 (*Supports screening, assessment and brief intervention for all primary care patients.*)

Frezza M, di Padova C, Pozzato G, et al. High blood alcohol levels in women: the role of decreased gastric alcohol dehydrogenase activity and first-pass metabolism. N Engl J Med 1990;322:95. (*The reason why women are more susceptible to the effects of alcohol.*)

Goldberg HI, Mullen M, Ries RK, et al. Alcohol counseling in a general medicine clinic: a randomized controlled trial of strategies to improve referral and show rates. Med Care 1991;29:JS49. (*Formal screening raised referral rates fivefold.*)

Hanna EZ. Attitudes toward problem drinkers revisited: patient-therapist factors contributing to the differential referral of patients with alcohol problems. Alcohol Clin Exp Res 1991;15:927. *(Elucidates how stereotypes interact with patient characteristics to influence professional behavior and patient compliance.)*

Hanna EZ, Faden VB, Dufour MC. The effects of substance use during gestation on birth outcome, infant and maternal health. J Substance Abuse 1997;9:111. *(Depression and substance use account for many adverse consequences; identifies high-risk groups.)*

Hanna EZ, Grant BF. Parallels to early onset alcohol use in the relationship of early onset smoking with drug use and DSM-IV drug and depressive disorders: findings from the National Longitudinal Epidemiologic Survey. Alcohol Clin Exp Res 1999. *(Covers issues of youth, comorbidity severity of illness and familial transmission.)*

McIntosh MC, Leigh G, Baldwin NJ. Reducing alcohol consumption: comparing three brief methods in family practice. Can Fam Physician 1997;43:1959. *(The answer is they all work equally well.)*

Mayo-Smith MF. Pharmacological management of alcohol withdrawal. JAMA 1997;278:144. *(Protocol of American Society of Addiction Medicine; all commonly used regimens reviewed and evidence-based treatment programs specified.)*

Mendelson J, Babor T, Mello N, et al. Alcoholism and prevalence of medical and psychiatric disorders. J Stud Alcohol 1986;47:361. *(High prevalence of significant medical and psychiatric problems.)*

Morse RM, Flavin DK. Joint Committee of the National Council on Alcoholism and Drug Dependence and the American Society of Addiction Medicine to Study the Definition and Criteria for the Diagnosis of Alcoholism. JAMA 1992;268:1012. *(Consensus definition and criteria.)*

Nace EP. The role of craving in the treatment of alcoholism. National Assoc Prev Pub Health J 1982;13:27. *(A guide to mastery over and understanding of wish/need to drink, leading to greater self-control.)*

Noble EP, Zhang X, Ritchie T, et al. D_2 dopamine receptor and GABAA receptor $\beta3$ subunit genes and alcoholism. Psychiatry Res 1998;81:133. *(Genetic risk factors identified.)*

O'Connor PG, Farren CK, Rounsaville BJ, et al. A preliminary investigation of the management of alcohol dependence with naltrexone by primary care providers. Am J Med 1997;103:477. *(Finds that naltrexone complements a program of psychological care provided in the primary care setting.)*

Parker E, Noble E. Alcohol consumption and cognitive functioning in social drinkers. J Stud Alcohol 1977;38:1224. *(Details the effects of drinking on abstracting and adaptive abilities of social drinkers.)*

Shaffer A, Naranjo CA. Recommended drug treatment strategies for the alcoholic patient. Drugs 1998;56:571. *(An up-to-date consideration of pharmacotherapies for alcohol use disorders, singly and comorbid with psychiatric disorders, with caveat that they only serve as adjuncts to other treatment.)*

Skinner HA, Allen BA. Alcohol dependence syndrome: measurement and validation. J Abn Psychol 1982;91:199. *(Original paper on this highly reliable and valid research and clinical tool predictive of DSM diagnoses and available as part of a computerized life-style questionnaire from the Addiction Research Foundation, Toronto, Canada.)*

Soderstrom CA, Smith GS, Kufera JA, et al. The accuracy of the CAGE, the BMAST and the AUDIT in screening trauma center patients for alcoholism. J Trauma 1997;43:962. *(Performance characteristics on these popularly used tests in a clinical setting.)*

Tournier R. Alcoholics Anonymous as treatment and ideology. J Stud Alcohol 1979;40:230. *(A critique of Alcoholics Anonymous; comments by other authorities starting on page 318 of the same issue.)*

Turner RC, Lichstein PR, Peden JG, et al. Alcohol withdrawal syndromes: a review of pathophysiology, clinical presentation, and treatment. J Gen Intern Med 1989;4:432. *(Comprehensive approach for the primary physician.)*

U.S. DHHS. Alcohol and Health, ninth special report to Congress, NIH Publication No. 97-4017, June 1997. *(Most complete source of information on every important aspect of this subject, includes latest national data. Useful as reference in practice and research.)*

U.S. DHHS. The economic costs of alcohol and drug abuse in the United States 1992, NIH publication No. 98-4237, September 1998. *(Most recent national report on health care costs, productivity losses, societal impact of accidents, crime, fire, and social welfare.)*

Walsh DC, Hingson RW, Merrigan DM, et al. A randomized trial of treatment options for alcohol-abusing workers. N Engl J Med 1991;325:775. *(The best data in support of inpatient treatment; a job-related program.)*

Wechsler H, Davenport A, Dowdall H, et al. Health and behavioral consequences of binge drinking in college: a national survey of students at 140 campuses. JAMA 1994;272:1672. *(Among the most significant challenges to the nation's resources.)*

Wright C, Moore RD. Disulfiram treatment of alcoholism. Am J Med 1990;88:647. *(Comprehensive literature review; 103 references.)*

Resource Materials

National Institute on Alcohol Abuse and Alcoholism, 6000 Executive Blvd. MSC7003, Bethesda, MD 20892-7003 (niaaa@willco.nih.gov). *(An excellent resource for every possible professional need. Ongoing publication of latest findings and policy positions plus resource materials for medical education and health education.)*

229

Approach to the Patient with Sexual Dysfunction

LINDA C. SHAFER

There is an important relationship between one's sexual life and emotional and physical well-being. With the advent of sildenafil (Viagra) to treat erectile dysfunction and the increased interest in pharmacologic agents to treat female sexual disorders, the frequency of sexual dysfunction complaints in primary care care practice has risen to nearly 15% to 20% of visits. However, the incidence of sexual problems in any medical practice is a function of the frequency with which physicians take a sexual history. Approximately 43% of women and 31% of men report some specific sexual dysfunction when questioned. Therefore, the primary care physician needs to know how to take a sexual history, perform an appropriate medical evaluation (see Chapters 115 and 132), and carry out basic types of sexual counseling and supportive therapy. Over 80% of sexual complaints can be treated successfully in the primary care setting.

DEFINITIONS

Disorders are classified as "*primary*" when there has never been a period of satisfactory functioning and "*secondary*" when the difficulty occurs after adequate functioning had been obtained.

Male Disorders

Erectile dysfunction (impotence) is defined as the inability of a male to maintain an erection sufficient to engage in intercourse and is considered a problem if it occurs in over 25% of attempts. Premature ejaculation is the loss of voluntary control of the ejaculatory reflex. Masters and Johnson have defined the condition in terms of the inability to satisfy the female partner at least 50% of the time. However, this presupposes that the female has no problem with orgasm. *Premature ejaculation* is most often defined as ejaculation that occurs in less than 2 minutes after penetration or on fewer than 10 thrusts. *Retarded ejaculation* is the inhibition of the ejaculatory reflex. There is a persistent failure to ejaculate in the presence of a satisfactory erection. *Retrograde ejaculation* is a physical impairment of internal vesical sphincter activity.

Female Disorders

Frigidity is a term applied to a wide variety of conditions in the female, from complete lack of any sexual response to various inadequacies in orgasmic response. Because it is nonspecific and has a derogatory connotation, the term has been eliminated from most recent classifications. It has been replaced by two more precise terms: *female sexual arousal disorder (excitement phase dysfunction)* and *orgasmic dysfunction.* Female sexual arousal disorder (excitement phase dysfunction) is defined as the inability to respond to sexual stimulation with lubrication and genital vasocongestion. Orgasmic dysfunction refers to the inability to release the orgastic reflex and have an orgasm, despite ability to enjoy sexual intercourse and have normal sexual desire. There is no distinction between "healthy" vaginal and "infantile" clitoral orgasm. Some women who can have orgasm with direct clitoral stimulation find it impossible to reach orgasm during intercourse. This is a normal variant of sensitivity requiring the pairing of direct clitoral contact with intercourse. Vaginismus is an involuntary spasm of the musculature of the outer third of the vagina, making penile penetration impossible.

Both Sexes

Dyspareunia is a condition defined as painful intercourse leading to avoidance of sexual contact. *Hypoactive sexual desire disorder (low libido)* is defined as an absence of sexual fantasies and lack of desire to engage in sexual activity. *Sexual aversion disorder* is defined as an active avoidance of genital sexual contact with a sexual partner.

PSYCHOLOGICAL MECHANISMS AND CLINICAL PRESENTATIONS

Organic conditions are responsible for between 50% and 85% of sexual problems in both sexes (see Chapters 115 and 132). This figure represents a dramatic shift in the understanding of the causes of sexual disorders that were once thought to be primarily of psychogenic origin. Organically based sexual dysfunctions are usually compounded by psychologic issues. *Depression* as a cause of or result of sexual dysfunction must be ruled out in every case. Although there are no rigid correlations between developmental factors and dysfunctional syndromes, sexual disorders can be related to *prior experiences.* Early sexual attitudes may be negatively shaped by parental communication that sex is bad, dirty, or sinful; by inadequate information about sex; or by myths and misconceptions such as the ever-ready penis or mutual climax. Other negative experiences range from unpleasant sexual encounters to childhood sexual abuse and rape. *Intrapsychic conflicts* extend from fear of sexual failure to concerns about sexual identity and profound depression.

Interpersonal issues of a sexual and nonsexual nature sometimes interfere with sexual functioning, especially in the setting of inadequate communication and lack of cooperation between partners. Sexual problems may develop from such nonsexual factors as *situational stress and financial pressures.* Finally, sexual difficulty may occur in the context of the anxiety generated by an organic illness, such as fear of death after a heart attack.

Once a sexual problem ensues, regardless of the cause, a vicious cycle of fear of failure, anxiety, and guilt is likely to ensue and remain self-perpetuating.

Clinical presentations can be quite complex. In addition to sexual dysfunction, there may be somatic complaints with no apparent medical cause (e.g., headache, low back pain, urinary symptoms, generalized pelvic pain, vulvar pruritus).

Erectile Dysfunction. Most normal men experience occasional erectile failure due to fatigue, too much alcohol, or any number of transient unfavorable circumstances. In the United States, it is estimated that 10 to 20 million men have erectile dysfunction. True impotence has an incidence that ranges from 1% in men under 35, to 40% of men over 60, to 73% of men over age 80, with the age-related increase mostly due to physiologic factors. Prolonged impotence and primary impotence are much more likely to be associated with medical disorders or more serious psychologic issues, such as fears of intimacy, feelings of intense hostility toward women, and gender identity questions.

Premature ejaculation is the most common male sexual disorder, occurring in 30% to 40% of adult men. The psychologic causes of the disorder range from early conditioning to ambivalence and hostility toward women. Its increasing frequency has been associated with women wanting more sexual satisfaction, particularly orgasm. Once premature ejaculation occurs, it can easily be reinforced by the negative attitudes expressed by the partner. In addition, prolonged periods of no sexual experience seem to make the problem worse. If premature ejaculation occurs over a long period of time and remains untreated, secondary impotence may result. It is often easily treated in the context of a good relationship and has a very good prognosis.

Retarded ejaculation occurs most often in younger less sexually experienced men. The lifetime prevalence is 2%. Its milder form is often related to anxiety-provoking situations and has an excellent prognosis. When long-standing, the condition often signifies deeper seated psychopathology, such as significant fears of rejection involved with letting go. Issues of control and commitment may be involved as well as unconscious conflicts regarding female genitals or pregnancy.

Female Sexual Arousal Disorder. These women present with a complete avoidance of sexual activity or an aversion to sex, which is stoically endured. There is often a deep-seated conflict about sexuality, which makes the outcome less favorable. Concomitant depression and interpersonal problems and a history of medications or pelvic pathology (see Chapter 115) are other important factors.

Orgasmic dysfunction is among the most frequent female sexual complaint and occurs more often during the early years of sexual activity. The capacity for orgasm appears to increase with sexual experience and that includes the aging female. Again, the psychologic factors involved are variable and the prognosis for the condition is a function of which factors are responsible. These range from fears of loss of control and unrealistic expectations about sexual performance to poor partner communication. Depression must not be overlooked.

Vaginismus is associated with a high incidence of pelvic pathology (see Chapter 115). A careful gynecologic examination is always warranted and, in fact, is the only definitive way to make a diagnosis. Vaginismus is one cause of *dyspareunia*. When related to psychologic factors, vaginismus can be considered a conditioned response and treated behaviorally. There is often confusion about sexual anatomy and physiology, leading to fears of penetration and concerns about femininity. If the condition is long-standing, partners of these women can become seriously affected, developing secondary impotence. This disorder has been at the center of many cases of unconsummated marriages of long duration.

Dyspareunia. The overall prevalence for this condition is 20% (15% of women and 5% of men). Patients seek out medical treatment, but the physical exam is often unremarkable, with no genital abnormalities. The condition is usually chronic and results in avoidance of sex.

Hypoactive Sexual Desire Disorder. The prevalence of this condition is 40% for women and 30% for men. Low libido in one partner may reflect an excessive need for sexual expression in the other partner. Depression should be ruled out in all cases. Medical conditions causing pain, weakness, disturbance of body image, and concerns of survival may be important triggers.

Sexual Aversion Disorder. The exact incidence is unknown, but this is a common disorder. Primary sexual aversion is higher in men, and secondary sexual aversion is higher in women. About 25% of patients meet the criteria for panic disorder. These individuals may have marital problems and may avoid sexual situations by covert strategies such as going to sleep early, traveling, neglecting personal appearance, using substances, or being overly involved at work.

WORKUP

Sexual History. The sexual history should be an integral part of every medical evaluation, given the importance of sexual function to overall health, the central role that sexual dysfunction might play in somatic complaints and quality of life, and the need to review safer sexual practices. The history is most easily obtained in conjunction with performing the gynecologic and menstrual review of systems in women and the genitourinary review in men. In this way, sexual practices and concerns can be comfortably elicited in the context of routine history taking, especially if the physician displays an open, nonjudgmental, unembarrassed, and accepting attitude. One needs to take into account differences in social values, class, and age.

Helpful *screening questions* include "Does your present sexual functioning meet your expectations?" "Has there been a change in your sexual functioning?" "Would you like to change anything about your sexual functioning?" Additional routine questions to ask during the AIDS era are "Have you been sexually active (or involved) with a partner in the past 6 months? (With women, men, or both?)" "Do you practice safe sex?" Failure to ask AIDS screening questions may result in criticism of inadequate treatment or even lead to a malpractice suit.

If a sexual problem is uncovered, the chief complaint should be explored in detail. Ask patients to describe the problem in their own words, noting its duration, circumstances, possible precipitating and alleviating factors, and severity. A thorough description sometimes helps to distinguish an organic from a functional etiology (see Chapters 115 and 132). For example, in the impotent male, preservation of erectile function on awakening suggests a psychologic cause as does erection with attempts at masturbation.

Also try to elicit what type of treatment is viewed as potentially helpful, be it medicine, information, or support. Anything that tends to alleviate the problem, even if only temporarily, should be sought.

Physical Examination and Laboratory Studies. With improved understanding of the pathophysiology of sexual function and more sophisticated diagnostic testing, many sexual problems once thought to be purely psychogenic have been found to have an organic component as well. Take special note of sexual dysfunction as a common side effect of selective serotonin reuptake inhibitors, occurring in more than 30% of patients taking the medication. Even when psychological or interpersonal problems are believed to be the principal cause of sexual dysfunction, a careful medical evaluation that includes a detailed physical examination in conjunction with a few pertinent laboratory studies is always indicated (see Chapters 115 and 132).

PRINCIPLES OF TREATMENT

The primary care physician is often the first person consulted by a patient with a sexual problem. Even the physician without formal training in sex therapy can help many patients deal effectively with their sexual difficulties. When the problem stems from guilt and misinformation, the physician can use his or her position as an authority figure to give *permission and reassurance,* relabeling as "neutral" or "positive" sexual activities that the patient might fear are "bad" or "sinful."

Educating patients and correcting misinformation is a function that should not be overlooked or underestimated. Giving permission or providing information may be all that is necessary to help many patients. An essential part of modern sexual counseling is the teaching of safer sexual practices and review of risk factors for HIV infection (see Chapters 7 and 13).

Behavioral Methods and Medication. When the problem goes beyond misinformation, a trial of *behavioral methods* with specific suggestions to patient and partner can be helpful and is an appropriate next step. The objectives are to increase communication between partners, decrease performance anxiety and "spectatoring," change the goal of sexual activity toward feeling good and away from emphasis on erection or orgasm, and relieve the pressure to perform at each sexual encounter. A trial of such therapy is reasonable when there is no evidence of organic illness or significant underlying psychopathology.

Oral medication prescribed for specific sexual complaints of various etiologies may be given instead of or in conjunction with behavioral techniques. *Sildenafil* (Viagra) has revolutionized the treatment of erectile dysfunction and is effective in 46% to 73% of men. *Phentolamine* (Vasomax) and apomorphine also are efficacious in the treatment of erectile disorders and are currently under U.S. Food and Drug Administration review.

Premature ejaculation can be therapeutically treated with *antidepressant* medication, specifically clomipramine (Anafranil) and *selective serotonin reuptake inhibitors,* including fluoxetine (Prozac) and sertraline (Zoloft), which are associated with delayed ejaculation. Low libido or orgasmic dysfunction in postmenopausal women may respond to estrogen/testosterone compounds. The effectiveness of sildenafil in women to treat orgasmic dysfunction and arousal disorder is currently being studied. Topical impotence medication, including alprostadil cream (Topiglan), minoxidil solution, and nitroglycerine ointment, are under investigation. The steps described above will often lead to improved sexual function without the need for referral.

Although sildenafil (Viagra) is easy to prescribe, effective, and well tolerated, both physicians and patients must address the high cost of this drug (in excess of $10/pill). Insurance companies call for physicians to document why patients require this drug, setting strict payment guidelines and refusing payment when the drug is used only to enhance the quality of life. Similar issues may arise with other pharmacologic agents used to treat sexual dysfunction that are currently under investigation. How we spend our limited health care dollars is a matter of public health policy. Yet the physical and emotional suffering of people with sexual problems should not be underestimated or downplayed. Early studies suggest that patients with sexual disorders who are treated pharmacologically respond with increased self-esteem and greater marital happiness.

TREATMENT RECOMMENDATIONS: BEHAVIORAL TECHNIQUES

Erectile Dysfunction

- First educate the patient as to his ability to satisfy his partner without having penile-vaginal intercourse.

- Then begin "sensate focus" exercises, which start with non-genital massage and progress to genital massage. There should be a prohibition against intercourse, even if erections occur.
- After erection is obtained by genital massage, progress to attempting intercourse. In the female-superior position (female on top of male), the female may manually stimulate the penis, and if erection is obtained, she may insert it into her vagina in a slow nondemanding fashion, relieving the male of any responsibility for insertion. This may also be done with a partial erection. Gradual movement is begun. There is an emphasis on the pleasures of vaginal containment.

Premature Ejaculation

- Educate the patient that his condition has little to do with the sensitivity of the penis but is usually the result of previous conditioning and anxiety.
- Suggest an increase in the frequency of sexual activity.
- Teach the Masters and Johnson "squeeze" technique. In this technique, the female manually stimulates the penis. When ejaculation is approaching the point of inevitability, as indicated by the male, the female squeezes the penis with her thumb on the frenulum, her index finger placed above, and her middle finger below the coronal ridge on the dorsal side of the penis. The pressure is applied until the male no longer feels the urgency to ejaculate (15 to 60 seconds). The squeeze technique should be repeated two or three times before ejaculation is allowed to occur.
- Once there are good results with the squeeze technique, the couple can try intercourse. In the female-superior position, the female remains motionless to accustom the male to vaginal containment. Gradual thrusting begins, using the squeeze technique as excitement intensifies.
- An alternative to the squeeze technique is the "stop-start" method. The female stimulates the male to the point of ejaculation, at which time she stops the stimulation. The erection may or may not subside. She then resumes stimulating the penis. After several stop-start procedures, the male may ejaculate.

Retarded Ejaculation (During Intercourse)

- The female stimulates the penis, asking for directions (verbal and physical) to enhance the feeling.
- Extravaginal ejaculation is obtained by continued stimulation. In the male's mind, the female should become associated with ejaculatory release.
- The female stimulates the penis manually until orgasm becomes inevitable. The penis is then inserted and the female thrusts demandingly. Manual stimulation is repeated if there is no successful ejaculation.

Female Sexual Arousal Disorder (Excitement Phase Disorder)

This disorder often results from more severe psychopathology and usually requires referral for treatment. However, on the practical side, suggestions regarding the supplemental use of lubrication such as saliva or KY jelly should be made.

Orgasmic Dysfunction

- Change the goal of sexual activity away from orgasm toward enjoyment of the experience.
- Give permission to the female to express sexual feelings.
- Begin sensate focus exercises, nongenital massage to genital massage. Use the back-protected position (male in a seated position with female between his legs with her back against his chest) with female in control to alleviate self-consciousness or spectatoring.
- Instruct the male in stimulative technique: He should not force responsivity but rather seek to accommodate desires; he should not approach the clitoris directly because of sensitivity.
- After success in manual genital stimulation, controlled intercourse in the female-superior position with the male making no demands comes next. This is followed by a lateral position that allows for mutual freedom of pelvic movement.
- For women who have never experienced orgasm, suggestions regarding self-stimulation are appropriate. The use of fantasy material is most helpful.
- For women who do have orgasms with masturbation but not intercourse, the "bridge technique" may be useful. After insertion of the penis, the male can stimulate the female (clitorally) manually or with a vibrator. This pairing can be helpful in achieving orgasm, and often after the female experiences orgasm in this way, the need for supplementary stimulation disappears.

Vaginismus

- Explain to the patient and her partner that this condition is involuntary and not willfully caused. Physical demonstration of the involuntary vaginal spasm may be done by inserting a gloved finger into the vaginal entrance.
- The couple is asked to refrain from intercourse during the early treatment.
- In a stepwise gradual fashion, the woman is encouraged to accept larger and larger objects into the vagina. This may be accomplished with the use of graduated Hegar dilators to be used in the office and at home or the woman may begin by using her fingers, first one and then several approximately the size of the penis. She may use her partner's fingers. Syringe containers of different sizes make good dilators.
- In the female-superior position, the woman gradually inserts the penis.

INDICATIONS FOR REFERRAL

Psychiatric Referral. After trying these medications and/or behavioral techniques, the patient's condition may still not be improved. This is often a sign that a referral to a psychiatrist or other mental professional trained in dealing with sexual problems is indicated and that the patient needs more intensive therapy. Often, direct referral to the specialist is indicated for patients with chronic psychopathology, such as those with *"primary" sexual dysfunctions, gender identity questions or homosexual conflicts, marked personality disorders* or significant past psychiatric history (especially of psychosis), or overt evidence of a clinical *depression* underlying the sexual complaint. Moreover, chronic severe problems in the relationship with one's partner signal the need for a referral.

Urologic Referral. For both organically based impotence and impotence refractory to psychologic treatment, it is appropriate to refer patients to urology. Treatments include a consideration of an intensive pharmacologic erection program, such as the injection of alprostadil (Caverject) into the base of the penis, the transurethral insertion of alprostadil (i.e., penile suppository) external vacuum pump therapy, and surgical penile implant (see Chapter 132). The success of any such treatment requires close collaboration between the urologist and the psychiatrist. On a case by case basis, referral to gynecology, endocrinology, and/or neurology may be warranted.

PATIENT EDUCATION

Early in one's practice, it becomes clear that patients have many sexual questions and concerns. Inadequate or inaccurate information about sexual anatomy, physiology, and practices is the basis for many sexual problems. Therefore, sex education should not be overlooked. Patients can sometimes obtain supplemental information from suggested reading material. Several time-honored books include *For Yourself: The Fulfillment of Female Sexuality* by Lonnie Garfield Barbach (New York, Doubleday, 1975); *Becoming Orgasmic: A Sexual and Personal Growth Program for Women* by Julia Heiman and Joseph LoPiccolo (Englewood Cliffs, NJ, Prentice-Hall, 1988); *The New Male Sexuality* by Bernie Zilbergeld (Boston, Little, Brown, 1992); *How to Overcome Premature Ejaculation* by Helen Singer Kaplan (New York, Brunner/Mazel, 1989); *The Illustrated Manual of Sex Therapy, 2nd edition,* by Helen Singer Kaplan (New York, Brunner/Mazel, 1987); and *The Joy of Sex,* edited by Alex Comfort (New York, Simon and Schuster, 1989). A visit to answer questions that come up in the context of reading is always appreciated.

Lack of knowledge regarding *safe sex practices* is a major contributor to the spread of HIV infection. Concern about HIV infection can also interfere with enjoyment of sexual activity. Detailed review of safe sex practices is essential, including benefits of using condoms and spermicides containing nonoxynol-9 (see Chapters 7 and 13). Condom use is critical for those with multiple sexual partners and for monogamous partners in whom HIV status is unknown. With prudent precautions and a little creativity (e.g., making condom application an early part of foreplay), a safe and enjoyable sexual life can still be attained.

ANNOTATED BIBLIOGRAPHY

Crenshaw TL, Goldberg JP. Sexual Pharmacology. New York: W.W. Norton & Co., 1996. *(Comprehensive reference on sexual side effects of drugs.)*

Davis S. The clinical use of androgens in female sexual disorders. J Sex Marital Ther 1998;23:153. *(Risks and benefits of androgen use for female sexual dysfunction.)*

Feldman H, Goldstein I, Hatzichristou D, et al. Impotence and its medical and psychosocial correlates: results of the Massachusetts Male Aging Study. J Urol 1994;151:54. *(Data on the prevalence of impotence in the aging population.)*

Goldstein I, Lue, T, Padma-Nathan H, et al. Oral sildenafil in the treatment of erectile dysfunction. N Engl J Med 1998;338:1397. *(Original randomized prospective controlled trial.)*

Laumann E, Paik A, Rosen R. Sexual dysfunction in the United States. JAMA 1999;281:537. *(Up-to-date statistical analysis of the incidence of sexual disorders in the United States.)*

Leiblum SR, Rosen RC. Principles and practice of sex therapy, 2nd edition. Update for the 1990s. New York: Guilford Press, 1989. *(Comprehensive review of sex therapy, including aspects related to HIV disease.)*

Maurice W. Sexual medicine in primary care. New York: Mosby, 1999. *(An excellent up-to-date summary of all aspects of the diagnosis and treatment of sexual disorders.)*

NIH Consensus Conference. NIH Consensus Development Panel on Impotence. JAMA 1993;270:83. *(A detailed consensus report that includes recommendations on methods of treatment.)*

Risen C. A guide to taking a sexual history. Psychiatr Clin North Am 1995;18:39. *(Framework for taking a good sexual history.)*

Shafer L. Approach to the patient with sexual dysfunction. In: Stern T, Herman J, Slavin P, eds. The MGH guide to psychiatry in primary care. New York: McGraw-Hill, 1998:271.

Shafer L. Approach to the patient with impotence. In: Stern T, Herman J, Slavin P, eds. The MGH guide to psychiatry in primary care. New York: McGraw-Hill, 1998:281. *(Easy to read outline for diagnosis and treatment of sexual disorders.)*

230

Approach to the Somatizing Patient
ARTHUR J. BARSKY, III

The somatizing patient presents with bodily complaints or disability out of proportion to any demonstrable organic pathology. Included in this category are anxious and depressed patients, hypochondriacs, chronic pain patients, and malingerers. These people are among the most frustrating and troublesome encountered in primary care, but they can be evaluated and managed successfully. Attention to the causative psychopathology helps to render symptoms understandable, enables the physician to distinguish them from those due to organic pathology, and facilitates management.

PSYCHOLOGICAL MECHANISMS AND CLINICAL PRESENTATIONS

Hypochondriasis. Hypochondriacal patients are people for whom illness, invalidism, and pursuit of medical care have become a way of life. Illness and medical treatment furnish them with a vocabulary for communicating with other people, a way of responding to stress, and a means for expressing their psychological needs. They are preoccupied with their bodies and their health, convinced that they have some occult serious medical disease. At the same time, they fear disease intensely. Their concern about being ill is remarkably persistent, and it is not assuaged by reassurance or a thorough medical evaluation. Although they have had extensive medical care, they have found it disappointing, failing to provide a cure or even relief of symptoms.

Clinical Presentation. Their symptoms shift and fluctuate over time, are often nonspecific and ambiguous, and are frequently similar to the transient sensations experienced by healthy individuals. When interviewed, such patients talk mainly about their illnesses and medical care and little about friends, work, or hobbies. Often, they seem as concerned with establishing the authenticity of their complaints as with obtaining relief. They adamantly deny any emotional contribution to their symptoms (in contrast to many patients with serious physical disease, who are willing to consider the possibility that anxiety and depression make their symptoms worse).

Explanatory Models. Hypochondriasis has been understood as a cognitive and perceptual process, an interpersonal communication, and an unconscious intrapsychic mechanism.

The *cognitive/perceptual* model suggests that hypochondriasis is a self-validating and self-perpetuating disorder of symptom amplification. Hypochondriacal patients are unusually sensitive to visceral and somatic sensation and are therefore bothered by normal physiologic sensations and minor discomforts that nonhypochondriacs ignore, dismiss, or are completely unaware of. Because bodily sensation seems so intense, noxious, and disturbing, they readily misattribute it to disease. Once the individual believes him/herself to be sick, it alters subsequent bodily perception, and a process of symptom amplification begins. The belief that one is sick makes preexisting symptoms more intense because they are now subject to closer scrutiny. This apparent worsening of their condition makes these patients even more firmly convinced they are sick. They become hypervigilant for other symptoms that confirm their suspicions and ignore contradictory information indicating that they are not in fact sick. For example, an individual may notice breathlessness after climbing a flight of stairs and wonder if this signifies the onset of heart or lung disease. With this suspicion in mind, the patient now notices that his face seems unusually pale in the mirror when he next shaves. This too seems to provide further evidence of disease progression. Thus, a self-validating and self-perpetuating cycle of cognitive and perceptual amplification has been set in motion.

In the *interpersonal communication model*, hypochondriasis emerges as a nonverbal way of saying something to the important people in the patient's life. The hypochondriacal patient is using a bodily pantomime to tell others that he is facing a seemingly insurmountable life problem which he cannot solve or cope with. He is asking to take "time out," saying to others (in a nonverbal language) "I am in a desperate situation and so I need special care and attention, unusual assistance and support at this time." Hypochondriacal patients have unwittingly learned that illness behaviors can be used to negotiate stressful circumstances, secure support, and solicit care. It is crucial to reemphasize that hypochondriacal patients do have the symptoms they report; they are not malingering or feigning disease. Rather, they have learned over the course of their lives that assuming the sick role can help them to postpone or avoid a crisis or challenge they face.

In the *intrapsychic model,* observers have emphasized the unconscious meaning and gratification of pain and discomfort. Bodily complaints may be amplified by a deprived and needy person who has only experienced caring and attention when sick or in pain. Suffering and illness can thus become ways to express and gratify yearnings for contact, comfort, and support. Other hypochondriacal individuals are angry and hostile, feeling rejected or wronged in some way. For them, physical symptoms offer a nonverbal way of expressing their anger, recrimination, and blame by reproaching and belaboring others with their suffering. Finally, symptoms and illness can unconsciously serve to distract some individuals from an even more painful sense of themselves as fundamentally worthless and defective as people. They can thus attribute their failures, disappointments, and rejections to a physical incapacity rather than to any personal inadequacy.

Anxiety (see Chapter 226). Individuals suffering from *chronic anxiety* focus on and become alarmed by normal bodily sensations. They report headache, gastrointestinal disturbance, or musculoskeletal pain. *Panic anxiety* has somatic manifestations that include palpitations, chest pain, tachycardia, dyspnea, choking sensations, diarrhea, cramps, sweating, and fainting.

Depression (see Chapter 227). Depression's *neurovegetative symptoms* may overshadow the characteristic affective, cognitive, and behavioral changes that are part of the depressive syndrome. As many as one half of somatizing ambulatory medical patients over age 40 are depressed. The chief complaint may be headache, constipation, weakness, fatigue, abdominal pain, insomnia, anorexia, or weight loss. Depressed patients worry about and focus attention on their bodies. A positive review of systems, chronic pain, or complaints involving multiple organ systems typify the clinical presentation, and symptoms often recur with the periodicity characteristic of depressions.

Conversion reactions are acute physical dysfunctions that suggest medical disorder but which are actually the expression of a psychological need or conflict. The emotional distress is thought of as being "converted" into, or expressed as, physical distress. The process is entirely unconscious. Symptoms are either sensory or neuromuscular (e.g., weakness, paralysis, ataxia, blindness, aphasia, deafness, anesthesia, paresthesias, or seizures) and generally of short duration. Other features include a prior history of similar reactions, major emotional stress before onset, and apparent symbolic meaning of the symptom (e.g., paralysis after losing control and striking someone or blindness after viewing a horrifying event). Other significant psychopathology is often, but invariably, present.

Somatic delusions are seen in schizophrenia, severe affective disorders, and organic brain syndromes. These are false fixed ideas that are often vivid, bizarre, or highly personalized. Unlike hypochondriacal concerns, they do not fluctuate. The individual may believe some extraordinary change has occurred in his body, for example, that his organs are shriveling up, that body parts are deformed or missing, or that foreign objects are inside an orifice or organ.

Some patients suffer from *body dysmorphic disorder,* a fixed circumscribed delusion that they are physically deformed, although their appearance is actually unremarkable. A facial feature is often the focus. The condition is extremely disabling, chronic, and can be quite difficult to treat.

Malingering differs from the abovementioned conditions in that the patient is not actually experiencing the symptoms reported and is consciously simulating or feigning disease. Malingering occurs in situations in which illness confers some obvious benefit, such as among prisoners, drug addicts, or in individuals under some legal threat. Symptoms are exaggerated, and the subject's description of them may vary with each interview. When the patient is unaware that she is being observed, she may relax the simulation and thus betray herself. Such individuals are frequently sociopaths or drug addicts. Some may have worked in a medically related field.

DIFFERENTIAL DIAGNOSIS

The differential diagnosis of somatizing includes anxiety, depression, conversion reaction, hypochondriasis, schizophrenia, and malingering. Somatizing patients, of course, have the same propensity for medical illness as their nonsomatizing counterparts. Thus, one must take care to rule out organic causes of the patient's symptoms, just as with any other medical patient. Medical disorders that affect multiple organ systems and produce transient or recurrent nonspecific complaints (e.g., multiple sclerosis, systemic lupus, polymyalgia rheumatica, Lyme disease, myasthenia gravis, hyperparathyroidism) pose the greatest diagnostic difficulty.

WORKUP

History: Differentiating Somatization from Organic Disease. The task is not always easy (see Chapters 8, 226, and 227), but the quality, timing, and precipitants of symptoms, as well as the patient's response to illness, attitude, and choice of words, can be of considerable help.

Quality of Symptoms. A complaint whose characteristics are inconsistent with known pathophysiology is likely to be psychogenic in origin. Psychogenic sensory complaints often involve combinations of sensory modalities that are neurologically impossible (e.g., a patient reporting loss of position and vibratory sense can nonetheless walk normally; see Chapter 167). Conversion seizures do not involve incontinence or tongue biting, and the patient with conversion blindness exhibits a withdrawal or startle reflex when a hand is flashed before the face. With conversion paralysis of the upper extremity, the patient's arm avoids the face after being held above it and released. In conversion paralysis of one lower extremity, the patient's attempts to move the afflicted leg do not invoke contraction of the other leg, as is the case in neurologic disease.

Psychogenic symptoms are more likely to resemble a symptom that has afflicted someone important to the patient (a so-called *figure of identity*) or to be excessively vague or overly detailed. Diffuse inconsistent descriptions and vivid, elaborate, highly personalized, or idiosyncratic complaints are very suggestive. Psychological factors may be revealed in the choice of words (e.g., "pain in the neck" or "not having a leg to stand on").

Timing and Precipitants. Psychogenic pain is typically unaffected by activity or by the passage of time, and the patient often seems even more concerned with the physician's accepting the authenticity of the pain than with relieving it. Although both physical and psychological illness can be precipitated by stress, the onset of psychogenic complaints is often closely associated with *significant emotional stress*, such as the loss of a loved one or the onset of a major interpersonal conflict or sexual problem. Functional complaints are also prone to occur on the *anniversary* of a psychologically meaningful event, such as the death of a loved one.

Attitude Toward Symptoms. When the patient is unconcerned, inappropriately calm, or more concerned with establishing authenticity than with obtaining relief, one should suspect a strong emotional component. It must be emphasized, however, that stoical and stolid patients may remain very unemotional when afflicted with serious organic disease. As noted, patients with psychogenic complaints who unconsciously derive considerable gain from their illness are often reluctant to consider an emotional cause for their symptoms.

History: Defining the Underlying Psychopathology. Once a psychogenic etiology is suspected on the basis of the clinical presentation, evaluation should proceed to define the underlying psychopathology. Inquiry into precipitants, response to illness, and personality can be helpful.

Precipitants and Response to Illness. The history is searched for ongoing psychological stress, pending litigation or disability proceedings, prior medical complaints without a demonstrable physical cause, depression, or anxiety disorder. Details of previous medical care experiences can be revealing. A history of consulting many physicians for the same complaints or of the immediate replacement of a treated symptom with a new one help in the diagnosis of psychogenic illness.

Personality. It is important to determine if illness, discomfort, and disability have become a way of life and to what extent they are used to deal with emotional discomfort, interpersonal difficulties, and environmental stress. Does the patient see herself as a suffering and unfortunate person whose life is filled with disappointment, "bad luck," and defeat, as well as with illness? Anger and hostility may be expressed indirectly, as in cynicism, sarcasm, and uncooperativeness. The individual feels deprived and put upon and therefore reproaches, accuses, and blames others for her state. Finally, excessive dependence on others may be a feature of her personality. One senses an overpowering desire for care, attention, sympathy, and human contact, and the patient's attitude toward the physician may have a clinging and hungry quality.

Personal Significance and Secondary Gain. What personal significance does the patient attach to his symptoms or to the suspected illness? Are there possible secondary gains, such as receiving sympathy, attention, and support (including financial support) from family and friends; being excused from duties, challenges, and responsibilities; and acquiring the power to influence and manipulate others by virtue of being sick?

Physical Examination and Laboratory Studies. A thorough physical examination and a careful mental status examination are essential. Not only may unexpected evidence of organic illness turn up, but a normal examination is a prerequisite for effective reassurance and the avoidance of unnecessary labora-

tory testing. Unless there is evidence that is strongly suggestive of organic pathology, elaborate and, particularly, invasive studies should be avoided. Performing a test in the hope that it will reassure the patient is usually futile; patients who are highly anxious about their health often find some further source of concern when the result is negative, and the likelihood of a false-positive result is higher when the pretest probability of organic pathology is low (see Chapter 2).

PRINCIPLES OF MANAGEMENT

Support. Management must be directed at the underlying psychopathology and at the presenting bodily complaints. The first step is to put the complaint in perspective, while still recognizing that the patient has come because of physical symptoms. When the results of the workup are presented, the reality of the symptoms should not be denied, nor should it be implied that they are imaginary. The patient can be told that serious damaging organic disease has been ruled out and that stress can amplify real bodily sensations and disrupt normal function. It is important to avoid saying "there is nothing wrong," because this contradicts the patient's experience and may make him or her feel foolish or angry. The presence of symptoms is an indication of considerable distress, which the patient should be encouraged to discuss. The patient needs to know that the relationship with his or her physician will not be terminated because the medical workup is "negative."

Additional visits should be scheduled on a regular basis to provide time to further discuss personal and situational problems. By offering the patient a long-term relationship that is not contingent on organic symptoms, one may remove a major stimulus for their development. Refractory cases may benefit from referral to a psychiatrist, if the patient is willing to seek such a consultation.

Role of Drug Therapy. Nonspecific attempts to suppress somatization pharmacologically should be avoided. All too often, patients are told that their symptoms are due to their "nerves" and sent away with a prescription for a minor tranquilizer. Such an approach to therapy usually fails and often alienates the patient. However, if a pharmacologically responsive psychiatric disorder is present, treatment with the appropriate agent should be initiated. It is especially important to recognize depression because of its high prevalence, subtle manifestations, and good response to pharmacotherapy. Depression responds well to medication (see Chapter 227), panic disorder is helped by the use of antipanic medication, and generalized anxiety may respond to cognitive and behavioral interventions (see Chapter 226).

Treatment of Personality Disorders. Because the best treatment is supportive, most patients with somatization due to a personality disturbance can be managed by the primary physician. Medical intervention should be minimized when possible. Major diagnostic workups for equivocal or questionable findings should be avoided (as long as it is medically responsible to do so), as should pain medication and tranquilizers. Even though medication is often requested, these patients generally do not respond to it and tend to be especially prone to development of troublesome side effects and adverse reactions.

To avoid struggles, the patient, especially if hostile and angry, should be involved as much as possible in therapeutic and diagnostic decisions. The physician ought to make it clear that his or her role is to help the patient tolerate discomfort rather than to eliminate it. Therapeutic suggestions should be made with the caveat that although they may be of moderate palliative value, they will probably not completely eliminate the problem.

The situational or psychological need to remain distressed and symptomatic must be recognized. No surgical procedure can excise, no oral medication can cure, the need to be ill. Consequently, the physician must not expect cure. The patient's self-esteem needs to be bolstered. Acknowledging her strength to endure suffering, tolerate discomfort, and survive hardship and misfortune is particularly gratifying to her. These are qualities the patient values most in herself and are a source of what little self-esteem she has.

Treatment of Conversion Reactions.   There are two aspects to the treatment of hysterical conversion reactions: symptom remission and management of the precipitating stress, internal conflict, or secondary gain to avoid recurrence or chronicity. The first is done through education, reassurance, and use of suggestion to reduce the patient's anxiety (these patients are often exceptionally suggestible). The patient should be assured that the disorder is self-limited and that the symptoms will gradually improve and finally vanish. Conversion symptoms may recur, however, unless psychotherapy is arranged to alter the psychological forces at work.

Approach to Malingering.   Malingering, once firmly established, must be dealt with by confronting the patient with the physician's conclusions. Diagnostic and therapeutic procedures should be avoided when possible because they reinforce the patient's behavior. Any abnormal laboratory tests or physical findings are suspect.

INDICATIONS FOR REFERRAL

Most somatizing patients can be managed by the primary physician. Referral is indicated when a patient has accepted a psychological explanation of his or her symptoms and wants to see a psychiatrist; when a conversion reaction, serious anxiety disorder, or psychosis is present; or when the primary physician has such a negative reaction to the patient with a personality disorder that he or she cannot serve that patient well.

TREATMENT RECOMMENDATIONS

- Explain the results of the medical workup without denying the reality of the patient's discomfort.
- Encourage discussion of psychosocial problems and set up a regular schedule of appointments for further elaboration and supportive therapy. Make it clear to the patient that physical symptoms do not need to be present to see the doctor. Avoid as-needed appointments when possible.

- Treat the underlying psychological problem specifically; do not attempt the nonspecific suppression of symptoms with tranquilizers.
- Do not try to remove or cure symptoms in the patient with a somatizing personality disorder. Acknowledge the suffering and provide support. Avoid the use of medication and the extensive workup of vague symptoms. Make adaptation to chronic discomfort the goal of care.

ANNOTATED BIBLIOGRAPHY

Barsky AJ. Clinical crossroads: a 37 year-old man with multiple somatic complaints. JAMA 1997;278:673. *(This is an extended discussion of a clinical case. The emphasis is on medical management strategies, but there is also a discussion of psychiatric consultation and referral).*

Barsky AJ, Wyshak G, Latham KS, et al. The relationship between hypochondriasis and medical illness. Arch Intern Med 1991; 151:84. *(Hypochondriacs have the same degree of organic illness as their nonhypochondriacal counterparts.)*

Barsky AJ, Wyshak G, Latham KS, et al. Hypochondriacal patients, their physicians, and their medical care. J Gen Intern Med 1991;6:413. *Hypochondriasis causes physician frustration and impaired recognition of anxiety and depression.)*

Ford CV. The somatizing disorders. Illness as a way of life. New York: Elsevier Biomedical, 1983. *(Concise lucid chapters cover the sick role, the doctor–patient relationship, the psychosocial dimensions of medical illness, disability, and malingering and the somatoform disorders.)*

Hahn SR, Kroenke K, Spitzer RL, et al. The difficult patient: prevalence, psychopathology, and functional impairment. J Gen Intern Med 1996;11:1. *(High prevalence of underlying psychopathology, with multisomatoform disorder accounting for about half of difficult cases and significant functional impairment common.)*

Kaplan C, Lipkin M Jr, Gordon GH. Somatization in primary care: patients with unexplained and vexing medical complaints. J Gen Intern Med 1988;3:177. *(A detailed review for the primary care physician that covers both theoretical and practical issues; 92 references.)*

Kroenke K, Mangelsdorff AD. Common symptoms in ambulatory care: incidence, evaluation, therapy and outcome. Am J Med 1989;86:262. *(A study of patients presenting with new somatic symptoms or with recurrent symptoms prompting a new diagnostic workup. In only 16% of the cases was an organic cause for the symptom ever definitively established.)*

Lazare A. Conversion symptoms. N Engl J Med 1981;305:745. *(Tersely considers incidence, etiology, diagnosis, prognosis, and treatment.)*

Lipsitt DR. Medical and psychological characteristics of "crocks." Psychiatry Med 1970;1:15. *(A classic paper; helps one understand and manage the chronic somatizer.)*

Monson RA, Smith GR Jr. Somatization disorder in primary care. N Engl J Med 1983;308:1464. *(Stresses the importance of a long-term physician–patient relationship and provides strategies for management.)*

Rosen G, Kleinman A, Katon W. Somatization in family practice: a biopsychosocial approach. J Fam Pract 1982;14:493. *(Emphasizes the role of the family and sociocultural forces.)*

231
Approach to the Angry Patient
ARTHUR J. BARSKY, III

Patients often become angry in response to the suffering and disability caused by disease, adverse life events, or the psychologic threats inherent in being a patient. When faced with an angry patient, the primary care physician needs to be able to recognize the source of the patient's anger, prevent it from interfering with therapeutic efforts, and help the patient to cope.

PSYCHOLOGICAL MECHANISMS

Threat from Illness. People become angry when they feel threatened or when their wishes and aims are frustrated. Disease often causes anger because it presents the threats of disfigurement, pain, lost opportunity, abandonment, and even death. Some patients are particularly enraged by the helplessness, lack of control, and enforced passivity that illness confers.

Threat of Dependency. Other patients are uncomfortable in the doctor–patient relationship because it represents the threat of dependence on the physician—of allowing someone powerful to take control of, take care of, and be responsible for them. They use anger to defend themselves against the intimacy and closeness that might develop with the doctor in the course of their relationship. Anger, then, can be an attempt to drive the physician away and allay the threat of dependency or intimacy inherent in the doctor–patient relationship.

Threats or Conflicts Elsewhere in Life. Patients commonly besiege their clinicians with anger derived from threats and stresses they are encountering elsewhere in their lives. In such instances, the animosity and hostility seem inappropriate to the situation and disproportionate to any provocation the doctor can think of. This usually occurs when patients are in conflict with important people in their lives to whom they cannot express their anger, such as an employer or a close family member.

Borderline Personality Disorder. Other patients appear to live a life permeated by a quick temper, chronic resentments, and long-standing dissatisfactions and resentments. The physician is little more than a screen onto which they project hostility garnered elsewhere. Some of these globally angry patients have a borderline personality organization. Both in their relationships with physicians and with other people, they appear explosive, stormy, and generally ungrateful. These patients relate to physicians and others in a dependent yet demanding fashion, exhibiting hostility toward and devaluation of the very people on whom they depend so desperately. Their anger expresses their expectation that people will generally be uncaring and unsympathetic. It also reflects their disappointment and feeling that they have been let down and not received the help they feel they need and deserve.

RECOGNIZING THE ANGRY PATIENT

Verbal and Nonverbal Manifestations. Anger may be expressed verbally in direct statements that convey demands, annoyance, and resentment, and in personal histories of temper outbursts and undirected violence (e.g., slamming doors). It may also be expressed more obliquely through cynicism, sarcasm, negativism, and behavior that, although superficially compliant and cooperative, is actually obstructive (i.e., passive-aggressive). Anger also finds expression in self-destructive behaviors, for example, failing to adhere to a medical regimen, keep appointments, or give up habits that are harmful to one's health.

Helpful nonverbal clues may be observed during the interview. The angry patient clenches the fists and jaws or knits their forehead in a frown. The palpebral fissures are narrowed, lips compressed, and nostrils widened. Gestures may be abrupt and gait may be jerky.

Emotional Response to Patient. Finally, the interviewer's own subjective emotional response to the patient during the interview may contain important diagnostic clues. Whenever the interviewer is aware of feeling irritated or bored with a patient, he or she should question whether these feelings are an unconscious response to anger and hostility on the part of the patient.

It is important not only to recognize that the patient is angry but also to learn what he or she is angry about. During the interview, the physician should note the subject matter that brings out irritation, annoyance, or hostility. The themes that seem to evoke anger point to the issues that are troubling the patient.

Recognizing the Boderline Patient. The globally angry patient with a borderline personality organization can be recognized by a few clinical characteristics: interpersonal relationships are either superficial or very dependent and manipulative; emotions are intense and labile, and extreme emptiness and anger predominate; social and intellectual skills may be well developed, but the patient's life is marked by lack of fulfillment and frequent failures; and impulsive, manipulative, and self-destructive behavior is present.

PRINCIPLES OF MANAGEMENT

Acknowledging the Patient's Feelings. Once the physician has recognized that the patient is angry and has defined some specific threats or frustrations that are fueling the anger, he or she can proceed to acknowledge the patient's feelings and reassure him that they will not destroy their relationship. This often helps bring about a more open give-and-take discussion between doctor and patient. The physician need not agree that the patient's feeling is justified, but he or she should acknowledge its existence by explicitly presenting the patient with observations and the reasons for concluding that the patient is angry. Such discussion introduces a quality of openness, honesty, frankness, and sensitivity into the therapeutic relationship. The physician should convey neither fear or rejection of the patient's feelings but rather interest in trying to understand them in order to be helpful.

Setting Limits. If the patient's hostility interferes with communication, the therapeutic regimen, or coping with illness, this should be pointed out in a noncondemnatory and nonjudgmental fashion. The physician needs to indicate that although he or she recognizes and acknowledges the patient's anger, it nonetheless represents a problem because it is self-destructive, interfering with the patient's care or recovery. One need not be bullied by the globally angry patient. It is possible and necessary to set limits on the patient's behavior while making it clear that there will be no counterattack in retribution.

Exploring the Causes and Responding Appropriately. Having identified the specific frustrations and threats the patient is facing, the physician should be able to approach the patient more effectively. For the patient who is angry about being ill, detailed investigation of exact fears and sources of despair is helpful. For the patient who is angry about being thrust into the patient role, one might try to structure the relationship so as to minimize those aspects that most threaten the patient. For example, if the patient most fears dependency, the physician should assume a somewhat cool, reserved, and business-like stance, while still conveying support and sympathy. Finally, if the anger seems to be displaced on the physician from some other situation or relationship, this may be pointed out, without encouraging the patient to vent the hostility on its actual source.

Avoiding Retaliation. The physician should take care to not react with hostility and subtly retaliate against the angry and provocative patient. Maintaining a clinical distance on the situation will help the physician to see the patient's anger not as a criticism of the doctor but rather a response to the patient's own inner torment of fears, threats, and frustrated wishes. By doing so, one is in a good position to help the angry patient, preserve the therapeutic relationship, and more effectively carry out medical care.

INDICATIONS FOR REFERRAL

Caring for the patient with a suspected borderline personality disorder is often quite vexing. Psychiatric referral for confirmation of the diagnosis and management suggestions can be helpful, especially if the primary care physician finds it increasingly difficult to care for the patient. Before suggesting the referral to the patient, a "curbside" consult with a psychiatric colleague can facilitate formulating a strategy for raising the issue of consultation with the patient and successfully arranging the referral.

ANNOTATED BIBLIOGRAPHY

Adler G. Valuing and devaluing in the psychotherapeutic process. Arch Gen Psychiatry 1970;22:454. *(The psychodynamics of patient anger; a classic paper.)*

Crutcher JE, Bass MJ. The difficult patient and the troubled physician. J Fam Pract 1980;11:933. *(Empirical research on the types of patients and patient problems that irritate and dismay physicians.)*

Gerrard TJ, Riddell JD. Difficult patients: black holes and secrets. Br Med J 1988;297:530. *(Descriptions of patients who are especially difficult to care for and helpful, specific suggestions for dealing with them.)*

Groves JE. Taking care of the hateful patient. N Engl J Med 1978; 298:883. *(Discussion includes the physician's own emotional responses to patients, and ways to use these responses constructively; a very valuable and helpful paper.)*

Gunderson J, Singer M. Defining borderline patients. Am J Psychol 1975;132:1. *(An excellent review identifying basic characteristics of such patients, including intense, often hostile affect.)*

Hahn SR, Kroenke K, Spitzer RL, et al. The difficult patient: prevalence, psychopathology, and functional impairment. J Gen Intern Med 1996;11:1. *(High prevalence of underlying psychopathology and much functional impairment.)*

Kahana RJ, Bibring GL. Personality types in medical management. In: Zinberg N, ed. Psychiatry and medical practice in a general hospital. New York: International University Press, 1965. *(A classic chapter that discusses the range of emotional meanings and responses to illness.)*

Lin EH, Katon W, Von Korff M, et al. Frustrating patients: physician and patient perspectives among distressed high users of medical services. J Gen Intern Med 1991;6:241. *(Physicians feel frustrated most by psychologically distressed high users of care; frustration stems from discordant views; the patients believe their problems are bodily, the physicians see them as psychosocial.)*

232
Approach to the Patient with Insomnia
JEFFREY B. WEILBURG

Approximately 40% of the general population experiences intermittent or chronic insomnia at least once. Epidemiologic studies find that between 10% and 17% of the population have some kind of insomnia at any given point in time and approximately 7% of the population have insomnia (persistent difficulty falling or staying asleep that compromises daytime functioning) of sufficient severity to warrant formal diagnosis and treatment. Insomnia affects patients of all ages and backgrounds but is especially prevalent in the elderly and in people of lower socioeconomic status.

The consequences of insomnia are significant, including impairment of work and social function, increased risk of motor vehicle accidents, and disturbance of mood. The cost of these problems combined with the cost of medication and other treatments has been estimated to exceed $100 billion/yr. The primary care physician needs to be skilled in the assessment and initial therapy of insomnia.

PATHOPHYSIOLOGY AND CLINICAL PRESENTATION

Sleep physiology is examined by using the polysomnogram, a continuous all-night recording of respiration, eye movements, electroencephalogram (EEG), muscle tone, blood oxygen saturation, and electrocardiogram.

Normal Sleep versus Insomnia. *Normal sleep* can be divided into two basic phases: *rapid eye movement sleep (REM) and non-REM (NREM)*. REM is a state of mental and physical activation. Pulse and respiration are increased but muscle tone is diminished, so little body movement occurs. The brain is active, and the EEG shows a pattern similar to that seen during waking. Most dreaming occurs during REM. In contrast, NREM is a time of deep rest. Pulse, respiration, and EEG all slow, and the patient goes from light sleep, called stages 1 and 2, to deep or delta sleep, called stages 3 and 4. REM and NREM normally cycle in a reciprocal pattern, giving a typical "architecture" to the polysomnogram. The entire cycle lasts about 90 minutes and is repeated smoothly four or five times during the night.

Insomnia is best regarded as a symptom, or complaint, which may be produced by a variety of underlying pathophysiologic processes. Therefore, insomnia has no single or pathognomonic polysomnographic pattern. Some insomniacs have slightly shorter than normal sleep times, some have less stages 3 and 4 sleep, but most have normal-appearing polysomnograms. Slight disruptions of the normal smooth cycling caused by frequent brief arousals may be related to subjectively unsatisfying sleep. Psychologic variables appear to strongly influence an insomniac's perceptions of restfulness and sleep.

Finding the underlying problem (often there are multiple problems operating simultaneously) producing the complaint is the key to effective management of insomnia.

Psychiatric Disorders appear to be the underlying cause in about half of all cases. Among patients presenting to primary care physicians, insomnia may be the initial manifestation of depression. Patients with *major depression* complain of either difficulty falling asleep or of waking in the early morning and being unable to return to sleep. Diurnal variation of mood is often noted. Severe depression with agitation may lead to markedly diminished total sleep and overall exhaustion (see Chapter 227). Patients in the manic phase of a *bipolar affective disorder* may report difficulty falling asleep or staying asleep, but they do not report feeling tired during waking times.

Patients suffering from *dysthymic disorder* (a variant of depression; see Chapter 227) typically complain of feeling tired, irritable, have difficulty falling asleep, and report that they cannot get enough sleep to feel rested. Sometimes they deny feeling sad or depressed and focus only on their physical complaints. Insomnia may be their major presenting complaint.

Patients with *anxiety and obsessive disorders* frequently have great difficulty falling asleep because they lie in bed and ruminate. *Character disorders* make up about 40% of the other psychiatrically based insomnias. Patients with narcissistic or borderline character disorders characteristically feel angry or

entitled and may have difficulty falling asleep. They lie in bed, furiously trying to make themselves sleep. Such patients may use their insomnia as a justification for their inability to function or to get ahead in life. Their lack of sleep is viewed as the source of all their troubles. Some even use it as a rationale for their inability to comply with the treatment of the insomnia itself.

Active psychosis of any type (e.g., schizophrenia) produces disturbed sleep and accounts for the other 10% of psychiatric insomnia. Hallucinations, delusions, and other signs and symptoms of psychotic illness present with the insomnia, facilitating recognition.

Drugs and Substance Abuse. Drugs and alcohol account for about 10% to 15% of all cases. *Alcohol* induces sedation, but the resulting sleep is often shallow, fragmented, and not restorative. Alcoholics can have prematurely "aged" sleep (i.e., shallow and short) during and for months after cessation of drinking.

Sedatives, especially barbiturates, when used on a regular long-term basis lead to shallow fragmented sleep. *Rebound insomnia* and rebound anxiety prompt reuse, and tolerance leads to dose escalation, so patients get caught in a vicious cycle. Sedatives and alcohol depress respiratory function, which can lead to very poor quality sleep in patients with sleep apnea.

Stimulant drugs such as amphetamine, pemoline, or methylphenidate; activating antidepressants (e.g., fluoxetine, sertraline, venlafaxine, desipramine, bupropion, phenelzine, protriptyline); and the phenylpropanolamine found in many over-the-counter decongestant, cold, and diet remedies can induce significant difficulty falling asleep. The caffeine and other stimulant xanthines found in tea, coffee, cola drinks, and chocolate are well recognized and often used for their ability to keep one awake. In those who are sensitive, even small amounts will prevent sleep. Nicotine and other substances found in cigarette smoke disrupt sleep induction and continuity. Bronchodilators such as aminophylline and β-agonists can make sleep difficult when given before bed.

Medical Problems are responsible in approximately 10% of cases. *Chronic pain* is a leading, though often overlooked, factor (e.g., that experienced by elderly persons with degenerative joint disease). *Delirium* is another important cause in the elderly, resulting from unrecognized infection or medication toxicity (as from anticholinergic agents used in over-the-counter sleep remedies). *Cardiopulmonary dysfunction* may contribute by causing orthopnea, paroxysmal nocturnal dyspnea, or nocturnal angina.

Sleep apnea is a disorder characterized by repeated apneic periods due to soft tissue upper airway obstruction followed by disruption of sleep. In severe cases, behavioral changes, pulmonary hypertension, cardiac arrhythmias, and death can occur. Patients are unaware of how disrupted their sleep is, though spouses may be kept awake by loud snoring and frightened by the apneic periods. Patients complain of marked daytime sleepiness (see Chapter 46).

Urinary frequency due to infection, prostatism, diabetes, or poor timing of diuretic use are among other important disrupters of sleep. Often, it is the nocturia and disturbed sleep that causes the patient with prostatism to finally seek definitive therapy.

Primary Sleep Disorders make up another 10% of insomnia cases. In primary or idiopathic insomnia, patients have objectively verified difficulty initiating or maintaining sleep in the absence of any identifiable underlying pathology. Such patients may need more, rather than less, sensory input to fall asleep, rather like hyperactive children who require stimulants to control their activity. Others have a persistent complaint of insomnia with *no objective evidence*. Although they believe they awaken, their polysomnographic studies reveal that they are actually sleeping. There is sleep state misperception. Their polysomnographic studies are entirely normal. A final group have poorly understood *polysomnographic aberrations*, such as the intrusion of alpha EEG into delta sleep.

In *conditioned or "psychophysiologic" insomnia*, patients begin to associate bedtime with frustration, anxiety, and sleep-preventing behaviors. In this learned disorder, they typically sleep very well while away from their usual bedroom (e.g., while on vacation or on the living room couch).

Circadian rhythm disorders may present with insomnia. In the *delayed sleep-phase syndrome*, the patient falls asleep later than the usual bedtime, sleeps well, and gets up later than is socially acceptable. This common disturbance often presents in adolescents. Other common forms are due to alternating shift work or jet travel across time zones *("jet lag")*, in which the inability to rapidly reset one's diurnal rhythm to local time leads to insomnia. For travel westward across time zones, the typical experience is awakening in the middle of night local time (morning at home) and being unable to fall back to sleep despite feeling tired. Restful sleep is not achieved. Moreover, there is marked afternoon or early evening sleepiness (bedtime at home). The inability to attain restful sleep culminates in exhaustion and the patient requests help for insomnia. Endogenous disruptions of the brain's internal circadian rhythm setter can produce a similar picture.

Nocturnal myoclonus can produce poor quality sleep and lead to the complaint of "insomnia." It is characterized by repetitive twitching of the legs, which is often unrecognized by the patient.

DIFFERENTIAL DIAGNOSIS

The most recent official version of the psychiatric diagnostic system—the Diagnostic and Statistical Manual of American Psychiatric Association, 4th edition (revised)—classifies insomnia as primary (idiopathic) and secondary (related to a primary psychiatric, medical, or substance abuse disorder). Table 232.1 provides a listing useful for primary care practice based on these categories.

It is important to note that not all persons who sleep less than average each night have insomnia. There are *natural "short sleepers,"* persons who regularly have less than 7 hours of well-maintained sleep yet suffer no problems other than too much time on their hands at night. Those who have a brief *time-limited disturbance* of sleep related to stressful events in their lives are not regarded as having a sleep disturbance. The same pertains to normal elderly patients who experience as part of the natural *aging* process a decline in total sleep time, depth, and continuity.

Table 232.1.   Causes of Insomnia

I. Psychiatric Disorders
A. Affective disorders: depression (major depression, dysthymia, bipolar disorder)
  1. Stimulating antidepressants (direct stimulant effect, production of periodic leg movements of sleep): desipramine, imipramine, buproprion, fluoxetine, sertraline
B. Substance abuse
  1. Sedative abuse and withdrawal: alcohol, narcotics, benzodiazepines
  2. Stimulant abuse and withdrawal: amphetamines, cocaine, PCP
  3. Cigarette and nicotine dependence and withdrawal
C. Character disorders
D. Psychosis
  1. Antipsychotic agent production of periodic leg movements of sleep

II. Medical/Surgical Problems
A. Musculoskeletal: arthritic pain
B. Cardiovascular: nocturnal angina, orthopnea, PND; medications: quinidine, propranolol, atenolol, pindolol, clonidine, methyldopa
C. Respiratory: COPD, asthma; medications: terbutaline, albuterol, salmeterol, metaproterenol, phenylpropanolamine, pseudoephedrine, pheylephrine
D. Endocrine: hyperthyroidism; medications: OCPs, cortisone and related steroids, progesterone, thyroid hormone
E. Neuropsychiatric: delerium

III. Primary Sleep Problems
A. Sleep apnea
B. Circadian rhythm disturbance
  1. Jet lag
  2. Shift work
  3. Delayed sleep phase syndrome
C. Periodic leg movements of sleep
  1. nocturnal myoclonus
  2. restless leg syndrome

IV. Miscellaneous
A. Caffeine
B. OTCs
C. "Diet pills"
D. Environmental factors: noise, temperature

WORKUP

When the complaint is persistent, when the sleep latency (the time between lights out and falling asleep) is consistently greater than 60 minutes, and when the insomnia is associated with compromised daytime functioning, a search for an underlying etiology should be undertaken.

History. A full description of the problem is essential and facilitated by having the patient keep a *sleep log* or diary, which includes time in bed, estimate of time asleep, any awakenings, time of morning arousal, estimate of sleep quality, and comments on unusual events and any associated symptoms (e.g., orthopnea, urinary frequency, pain, palpitations). Entries are recorded by the patient directly on getting up each morning. Close attention must also be given to use of sedatives, hypnotics (including over-the-counter preparations), and stimulants. Screening for abuse of alcohol and other substances is essential (see Chapters 228 and 235). It is most important to listen carefully for and inquire directly about symptoms of depression, bipolar disease, anxiety disorder, and psychosis (see Chapters 226 and 227). Occupational and travel patterns should be noted. Whenever possible, interviewing the spouse, bed partner, or family member is of great value, particularly for symptoms suggestive of sleep apnea (e.g., excessive snoring, apneic episodes, disturbed sleep). Past and family medical and psychiatric histories are sometimes revealing.

Physical Examination. The pertinent physical examination is a function of the history. One checks for upper airway soft tissue obstruction in the patient with suspected sleep apnea; for jugular venous distention, rales, wheezes, heaves, and gallops when there is concern about a cardiopulmonary etiology; for moist skin, tachycardia, proptosis, goiter, and tremor when hyperthyroidism is under consideration; and for prostatic enlargement in the elderly male with sleep-disturbing nocturia. Any reported sources of pain should be evaluated and confirmed by physical examination. A careful mental status examination helps in the detection of psychiatric disease (see Chapters 226 and 227).

Laboratory Testing. Testing should be limited, selective, and based on evidence from the history and physical examination (e.g., thyroid-stimulating hormone for suspected hyperthyroidism, chest x-ray for cardiopulmonary disease, toxic screen for substance abuse). Immediate referral to the sleep laboratory is indicated only if a primary sleep disorder, such as central sleep apnea or nocturnal myoclonus, is suspected. Testing is very expensive and time consuming. Home monitoring for apnea and oxygen desaturation may prove a cost-effective screening alternative to the sleep laboratory for patients with suspected obstructive sleep apnea (see Chapter 46). Psychiatric evaluation is indicated only when character problems interfere with diagnosis or management or if the nature of a suspected mental or emotional problem is obscure.

PRINCIPLES OF MANAGEMENT

For a problem with as broad a spectrum of etiologies as insomnia, the best treatment is etiologic. Nonspecific measures are unlikely to be of much help and can be harmful. Careless use of sedative/hypnotics can be especially dangerous (e.g., giving the patient with sleep apnea or alcohol abuse a benzodiazepine). Precise diagnostic assessment allows for maximally safe and effective management. For those with substance abuse, proper withdrawal and complete abstinence from drugs and alcohol are critical (see Chapters 228 and 235).

Depression and Other Affective Disorders. All *antidepressants* are equally effective for the treatment of depression. Although the evidence is still incomplete, it has been suggested that patients with affective disorders who present with insomnia may benefit from a trial of a relatively sedating antidepressant, such as *mirtazepine, paroxetine, citalopram, nefazodone, or nortriptyline.* Full doses of antidepressants should be used if affective symptoms remain after insomnia resolves (see Chapter 227). When insomnia is due to use of an activating antidepressant, such as desipramine or a fluoxetine, adding a small amount of *trazodone* (50 mg qhs) or *clonazepam* (0.5 to 1.0 mg qhs) may be helpful. Antidepressant therapy can be started at a modest dose but should be advanced to adequately treat the underlying depression (that is the cause of the sleep disturbance).

Anxiety Disorders. Transient insomnia due to situational stress is a common nonthreatening problem, which by definition resolves on its own and often responds well to *support, reassurance,* and simple behavioral advice (see below). For anxiety disorders and character disorders complicated by insomnia, *benzodiazepines* can be used safely and effectively (see Chapters 226 and 227). *Zaleplon and zolpidem* are nonbenzodiazepines that act at the benzodiazepine receptor complex and behave clinically similar to the benzodiazepines without producing some of their undesirable side effects (see below). The use of benzodiazepines for anxiety-related depression has declined relative to the use of small doses of sedating antidepressants (e.g., nortriptyline 25 to 50 mg qhs) or *trazodone* (25 to 100 mg qhs). The efficacy and safety of this practice has yet to be fully established.

Pharmacologic Therapy: Short-term versus Chronic. There is controversy as to the proper frequency and duration of therapy when insomnia due to a long-standing anxiety disorder or characterologic disturbance is chronic. Most believe it is best to treat such insomnia with a short (1-week) course of benzodiazepine therapy to help reestablish a more normal sleep pattern and then to stop. However, an occasional patient requires a program of benzodiazepine use two to three times per week over much longer periods. If chronic benzodiazepine therapy is contemplated, one first needs to review with the patient the importance of assiduous compliance, the risks of tolerance and withdrawal, and the possibility of physical dependence if the medication is not taken as prescribed (see Chapter 226). In addition, one must screen carefully for contraindications (e.g., sleep apnea, substance abuse). Concurrent use of alcohol and other sedatives must be prohibited because of the risk of oversedation.

For patients requiring prolonged therapy, careful monitoring is essential to ascertain efficacy, check for adverse effects, and ensure proper dosage and frequency. Drug holidays and attempts at alternative treatment are important components of any therapeutic program that involves prolonged benzodiazepine intake. The risks of tolerance and withdrawal should be reviewed with the patient before initiating such therapy. Withdrawal symptoms may develop within 3 to 20 days after cessation of chronic benzodiazepine use, especially if abrupt. It is best to taper therapy slowly over several weeks in patients with a history of prolonged intake (see Chapter 226).

Choice of Agent. Debate continues on the drug of choice for sleep. The benzodiazepines and benzodiazepine-like agents are preferred. The optimal agent would have a rapid onset yet short (48-hour) duration of action and would cause no rebound insomnia or mental problems such as hangover, motor incoordination, or memory disturbance. There are now several agents marketed for the treatment of insomnia, but none has been clearly shown to be significantly superior to any other, and all have some problems associated with their use (see Chapter 226).

The benzodiazepines used for insomnia can be divided into the short-, intermediate-, and long-acting agents. The *short-acting drugs* (e.g., triazolam, estazololam, zaleplon) are best prescribed for those whose primary problem is *falling asleep.* Triazolam should be used in the lowest possible doses (not to exceed 0.125 mg/d in the elderly) and should be tapered to avoid *rebound insomnia and anxiety. Zaleplon* may have somewhat lower propensity to produce rebound effects, but more experience with this new agent is required to confirm this.

The *intermediate-acting agents such as temazepam and quazepam* may be useful for those patients who complain of problems with *sleep continuity*. The possible increased receptor selectivity of quazepam has not been shown to be clearly clinically relevant. *Zolpidem* fits into the intermediate-acting group; lorazepam and diazepam may be recommended as lower cost generic alternatives. *Long-acting agents* (e.g., *flurazepam, clonazepam*) are considered when *daytime anxiety* compounds the discomfort.

Sedating *tricyclic antidepressants such as nortriptyline* (10 to 25 mg qhs) may help some patients with generalized anxiety and insomnia, as may *buspirone* (10 to 30 mg qhs) or *trazodone* (25 to 50 mg qhs). Antipsychotic agents can relieve insomnia and agitation in psychotic or delirious patients.

In rare instances where benzodiazepines are contraindicated (e.g., history of drug or alcohol dependence) and sedating antidepressants have not helped, antihistamines such as diphenhydramine may be used. However, the elderly and very young may experience delirium or paradoxical excitation from such drugs. Chloral hydrate should rarely be used, and there is almost never a place for treating new cases of insomnia with barbiturates, meprobamate, or over-the-counter remedies.

Psychotherapy and behavioral therapies may be used quite effectively in conjunction with medications for patients with psychiatric or stress-related problems. Cognitive and behavioral approaches, including education and support, stimulus control (attention to sleep hygiene), and sleep restriction therapy (gradual matching of time in bed to time asleep) can be combined with, and may be superior to, medication, especially in the elderly. Relaxation and biofeedback produce more modest improvements in sleep.

Jet Lag. *Melatonin* use is associated with some beneficial effects when prescribed to treat jet lag. In a placebo-controlled study of flight crews, use at bedtime on return from overseas flying and nightly thereafter for several days proved superior to placebo in minimizing the symptoms of jet lag. Proper dosage and mechanism of action (hypnotic effect versus resynchronization of circadian rhythm) remain to be established. Until there is standardization and quality control of preparations (some is derived from pineal glands of cows) and until there are reliable data on optimal dosing and side effects, it is advisable to defer melatonin use. Case reports of depression, gynecomastia, vasoconstriction, and low sperm counts argue for caution in use.

Treatment of Insomnia in the Elderly. The importance of cause-specific treatment is most poignantly experienced in caring for elderly persons with insomnia. In instances where the underlying cause is minor, emphasis on sleep hygiene (see below) and empathetic support are often the best course. Explanation on how the normal aging process affects sleep is appreciated by those wondering why they seem to sleep less. Sedatives should be used in reduced dose and with caution, if at all (see Chapter 226). Falls with catastrophic consequences (hip fracture, pulmonary embolization, disability, and death) are a major risk with sedative use in the elderly. The newer short-acting sedatives (see above) may be less likely to produce falls from motor incoordination or cognitive impairment during arousals than the older agents. When depression presents as difficulty sleeping, treatment should be etiologic and tailored to the special needs of older persons (see Chapter 227). Use of melatonin for chronic insomnia in the elderly has not been well studied, although the substance is widely used by patients because it can be obtained without prescription. The importance of adequate treatment of pain and any underlying medical problems cannot be overemphasized. Chronic pain should be addressed and effectively treated (see Chapter 236).

PATIENT EDUCATION

The overall promotion of good *"sleep hygiene"* is useful for many patients. Establishing a regular bed and wake time, avoiding any and all naps, having regular exercise (although not at night), using bed only for sleeping or lovemaking (rather than reading or watching TV), and getting in bed only when ready for sleep (leaving bed if sleep is not forthcoming) are useful suggestions. Avoidance of caffeinated foods, stimulants, cigarettes, and alcohol are necessary for some sensitive patients.

Instructing patients about these basic rules of sleep hygiene and helping them to avoid trying too hard to fall asleep are often useful. Disabusing patients of the myth that everyone must have 8 hours of sleep every night makes many people feel relieved. Also, informing patients that much of the time they spend in bed believing they are "only drowsy" is time actually spent in the lighter stages of sleep can ameliorate some patients' frustration.

THERAPEUTIC RECOMMENDATIONS

- If the insomnia is related to an underlying affective disorder, begin a sedating tricyclic antidepressant, such as nortriptyline (10 mg) or a selective serotonin reuptake inhibitor such as paroxetine 20 mg or mirtazepine 20 mg, taken an hour before bedtime every night for 2 weeks. See the patient frequently until symptoms resolve and increase the dose as needed to fully treat the depression.
- If the insomnia is related to an anxiety disorder, use triazolam, starting at 0.125 mg qhs or zolpidem 10 mg when the main problem is falling asleep, or clonazepam (0.5 mg) or flurazepam (15 mg) at bedtime if daytime anxiety is present.
- If symptoms recur after 2 weeks of treatment for anxiety-related insomnia, institute behavioral and relaxation therapies (see Chapter 226) and consider psychiatric consultation.
- If the insomnia is related to a character disorder, seek psychiatric consultation, require close adherence to good sleep hygiene, and use benzodiazepines only with caution.
- Make sure that a complete history of alcohol and substance use, including cigarettes, caffeine, nonprescription drugs, and stimulants, is obtained on every patient. Interview family members and obtain toxic screens of urine or blood when there is a doubt. Do not prescribe benzodiazepines for patients with current or past alcohol or drug use. Supervise withdrawal and abstinence, and seek psychiatric consultation when withdrawal symptoms or maintenance of abstinence is problematic.
- Treat pain and underlying medical problems aggressively; a short course of benzodiazepines may help reestablish a normal sleep pattern in some patients.
- Offer education and support to an elderly patient who has normal daytime function but who is lonely or upset as their sleep goes through the changes of normal aging.

ANNOTATED BIBLIOGRAPHY

Brzezinski A. Melatonin in humans. N Engl J Med 1997;336:186. *(Comprehensive review that includes basic science review of melatonin's contribution to sleep and the pharmacology of exogenous intake and its use.)*

King AC, Oman RF, Brassington GS, et al. Moderate-intensity exercise and self-rated quality of sleep in older adults: a randomized controlled trial. JAMA 1997;227:32. *(Evidence for exercise improving the quality of sleep.)*

Kupfer DJ, Reynolds CF. Management of insomnia. N Engl J Med 1997;336:341. *(Comprehensive review with excellent list of references.)*

Lamberg L. Melatonin potentially useful but safety, efficacy remain uncertain. JAMA 1996;276:1011. *(Review of its clinical use; cautionary note.)*

Morin DM, Colecchi C, Steve J, et al. Behavioral and pharmacologic therapy for late life insomnia. JAMA 1999;281:991. *(Good review of the data on treating insomnia in the elderly.)*

NIH Technology Assessment Panel. Integration of behavioral and relaxation approaches into the treatment of chronic pain and insomnia. JAMA 1996:276:313. *(Relaxation and biofeedback were found to be of only modest benefit for insomnia.)*

Nowell PD, Mazumdar S, Buysse DJ, et al. Benzodiazepines and zolpidem for chronic insomnia: a meta-analysis of treatment efficacy. JAMA 1997;278:2170. *(Both found to be effective given the data on hand, but available studies are limited in scope and duration.)*

Reite M. Insomnia. In: Schatzberg AF, Nemeroff CH, eds. The American Psychiatric Press textbook of psychopharmacology, 2nd ed. Washington DC: APA Press, 1998. *(Authoritative reference.)*

233
Management of Obesity
CAROLYN J. CRIMMINS-HINTLIAN

Obesity is a major health problem in industrialized societies. Health risk increases when weight gain results in moderate to severe obesity. Mortality rates (all-cause, cardiovascular, and cancer-related) closely parallel increases in the body mass index once levels of obesity are reached. One third of Americans are overweight, and one fifth are on some kind of weight loss program at any given time. Weight loss is not a cure for obesity, as evidenced by patients who go from one fad diet to another, sometimes jeopardizing their health in the process (mortality appears greatest in those with the greatest fluctuations in weight). Many such patients turn to their physician with requests for pharmacotherapy. However, the majority of patients who lose weight, with or without drugs, regain lost pounds and often more within the first year.

Effective management of obesity starts with a careful workup for underlying illness that may be the cause (e.g., hypothyroidism, psychosocial or behavioral problems) or the consequence (e.g., diabetes mellitus, hypertension, osteoarthritis) of obesity (see Chapter 10). A major goal is to achieve the best weight possible in the context of overall health. Biopsychosocial and behavioral dimensions of the problem require attention. Therapy should include a customized program of patient education and physical activity (see Chapter 18). Knowledge of the rationale, safety, and effectiveness of popular diets and weight loss programs, in addition to available community resources, helps guide patients through an often confusing environment of claims and products.

PRINCIPLES OF MANAGEMENT

When a treatable etiologic factor is identified, it should be addressed directly. Weight loss should not be the only attainable goal for patients embarking on a weight reduction program. The correction of a poor image of oneself and one's body, distorted eating patterns, and the physical, social, and life-style consequences of obesity is also important. Recent appreciation of the molecular mechanisms that underlie obesity has altered the approach to therapy. Although new optimism has arisen concerning the eventual development of specific drugs for specific metabolic defects, the current best approaches to treatment still require a lifelong commitment to a *change* in *life-style*, *behavior*, and *dietary practices*. As noted, the effort begins with identifying the major precipitants of the patient's weight problem (see Chapter 10). The decision to lose weight may be part of a complex decision to improve the conduct of one's life. Consequently, the physician should be aware that patients coming for treatment are likely to be highly motivated and asking for permission to also make interpersonal, environmental, or life-style changes. Once the patient's agenda and preferences are clarified, the physician can help select the most appropriate method of weight management.

No single approach is effective for all persons. Knowledge of the strengths and weaknesses of individual weight loss modalities is essential to the design of an intelligent program. Treatment modalities can be divided into dietary, behavioral, psychosocial, pharmacologic, exercise, and surgical categories.

Dietary Approaches

"Going on a diet" is the typical first step in weight reduction, but the word "diet" implies that one is making only a temporary change in one's eating habits and patterns. Quite the contrary! The most effective diet is not a diet at all but rather a weight management program that focuses on the implementation of gradual, permanent changes in eating habits and exercise that can be followed for a lifetime.

Determining Daily Caloric Intake. The desired daily caloric intake needs to be determined. One starts by estimating the number of calories necessary to maintain an obese person's weight:

- Obese female patient: 8 to 10 calories times present weight in pounds
- Obese male patient: 10 to 12 calories times present weight in pounds (the lower number in the range is for the sedentary person)

From this figure, one subtracts 500 kcal/d for every pound per week that should be lost (a deficit of 3,500 calories equals a weight loss of 1 lb). All weight reduction programs should be nutritionally adequate except for calories and should include a variety of foods. Most fad diets are neither nutritionally sound nor based on proven scientific evidence (Table 233.1). Extravagant claims that a particular food or class of foods dramatically alters weight, appetite, or calorigenesis are unfounded. The cornerstones of efficacy and safety are a reduction in calories and nutritional balance. Nutrient content and the timing and number of meals and snacks are important determinants for short-term and long-term appetite control. Limiting fat calories is critical to decreasing body fat and maintaining weight loss.

When following a prescribed dietary regimen, the patient must realize that initial rapid weight loss may occur because of a negative fluid balance. After 2 to 3 weeks, the rate of weight loss slows down. Most subsequent loss reflects the catabolism of fat. Loss of fat is directly proportional to the size and duration of the energy deficit. Patients often become discouraged when they enter the slower phase. Some adjust to caloric restriction by unknowingly diminishing their expenditure of energy, one reason why an exercise program is such an important adjunct (see below).

Dietary Counseling is an essential step in the educational process. It begins with the physician's endorsement (an essential component that is often overlooked). Patients need to achieve a basic understanding of the caloric and nutritional contents of foods to be able to choose intelligently. The patient also must be presented with an approach that focuses on the connections between the body, brain, and appetite. Some of the factors that control appetite include food that is emotionally satisfying, management of stress, and exercise that suppresses hunger. The services of a registered dietitian can be helpful in this regard because such persons are specifically trained in assessing nutritional requirements and counseling food selection and preparation. In addition, the registered dietitian attempts to help people assess and change their attitudes and behaviors toward food and eating. An assessment is made that integrates medical concerns with the patient's individual and family lifestyle, economic status, learning ability, and psychological needs. A weight control plan must be individualized to each patient's needs and food preferences. Dietary changes must be gradually implemented to ensure lifelong positive eating habits. Nutrition counseling is likely to increase patient adherence to a dietary regimen and improve outcome.

Weight Loss Programs. Many commercial and self-help programs are available (Table 233.1). Some provide menus and a line of foods to buy; others include individual or group support. Those that just sell products are of little long-term benefit. Integrated approaches that include moderate diet modification,

an exercise program, and a behavioral approach are more effective, especially for mildly to moderately overweight persons. Noncommercial self-help groups offer a low-cost alternative for those who seek the benefit of group support, but often little professional guidance is provided.

Fat Substitutes and Low-fat Foods. Intensive research and development by food companies into substances that taste and satisfy like fat without providing any of the calories continues.

Olestra, a nonabsorbable mixture of sucrose esters, has recently been approved for use in food by the Food and Drug Administration. The first products are fat-free snack foods such as potato chips. Concerns about diarrhea and cramping with intake have not materialized when fat substitutes are used in small amounts (e.g., a 1-oz bag of potato chips), but the larger concern is the potential to induce fat malabsorption and deficiencies in lipid-soluble vitamins (A, D, E, K) when intake is on a daily basis and in larger quantities (potential for use in many foods as a fat substitute). The role of such substitutes remains to be defined, but use in a snack food as an occasional treat for the person who craves a bit of the "junk food" taste is probably harmless.

"Low-fat, low-cholesterol" processed foods are popular substitutes for foods high in fat, but often they are almost as high in caloric value as the foods they replace by virtue of having a very high sugar content. Even those food preparations that truly have fewer calories and less fat may provide just as much total fat and caloric intake if eaten in excess—a very common phenomenon, especially with low-fat ice cream, frozen yogurt, and baked goods. Persons consuming diets rich in these foods may experience an undesirable decline in high-density lipoprotein cholesterol if nonatherogenic essential fatty acids and monounsaturated fats are displaced from the diet (see Chapter 27). When patients substitute large quantities of "low-fat, low-cholesterol" snack foods for cholesterol-laden foods, they are likely to derive just as many calories from fat because animal fat is simply replaced in these products by partially hydrogenated vegetable or tropical oils (which are just as atherogenic and no lower in calories; see Chapter 27).

Behavior Modification

Behavior modification programs grew out of studies suggesting that obese persons overeat because they are stimulus-bound. Behavioral treatment is directed toward the mildly to moderately obese. Operant conditioning techniques appear to be somewhat more effective than aversive ones. Obese patients appear especially prone to respond to external cues for eating. The triggering stimuli may be situational, physiologic, or emotional. The aim of the behavioral approach is to substitute an alternative eating behavior that is practical and leads to a decreased caloric intake.

Behavior modification includes four components:

1. *Describing the behavior to be controlled.* Patients are instructed to keep records of all eating behaviors, including daily weight, time and place of eating, stimuli preceding eating that the patient is aware of, and a description of surroundings.
2. *Modifying and controlling stimuli.* Food shopping, food preparation, and food storage habits are changed, in addition to visual cues.

3. *Controlling the act of eating.* The patient is taught to eat more slowly, not skip meals, and not take snacks.
4. *Promptly reinforcing behaviors that delay and control eating.* Patients are advised to eat only in one room (cue elimination), have company while eating (cue supervision), develop methods of making diet food attractive (cue strengthening), arrange for deviations from the diet, and arrange for positive feedback if they comply with exercise and diet programs.

In addition, distracting activities such as watching television or reading while eating are discouraged. Eating behavior is made to be associated with highly specific stimuli.

Both individual and group behavioral programs are available. The average length of treatment is 18 weeks. The average weight loss is 20 lb, and at 52 weeks of follow-up, almost two thirds of patients maintain that weight loss, a very positive result. Behavior modification may prove to be most helpful in helping people maintain weight loss regardless of how it was achieved.

Exercise

An exercise or physical fitness component should be included in every weight loss program. Most obese persons are less active than lean people, but it is not known whether this is a cause or consequence of obesity. Energy expenditure and basal metabolic rate decrease with weight loss on calorically restricted diets. Exercise, in conjunction with a low-calorie diet, increases the metabolic rate. Increased physical activity for many obese people can promote weight loss and decrease body fat. Lean body mass is preserved when exercise and diet are combined. Obese persons use more energy and burn more body fat for the same amount of activity than persons of normal weight because the energy cost of most exercise is proportional to body weight. The amount of exercise needed to decrease body fat is related to its duration, intensity, and frequency. Exercise may also benefit the dieter by increasing feelings of self-control, reducing stress, improving appearance, and alleviating depression. Cardiovascular morbidity and mortality may be reduced.

The Exercise Prescription. A specific exercise prescription is essential. To tell a sedentary obese person to "get more exercise" is insufficient. Moreover, the dropout rate is high. Thirty percent or more of obese patients terminate physical training programs within several weeks of initiation, and as few as a third continue for up to 1 year. To ensure compliance, the program has to be physically realistic and capable of being incorporated into the patient's daily routine. The importance of physician input and encouragement is considerable. To ensure safety, obese patients with multiple cardiac risk factors and a sedentary life-style may benefit from electrocardiographic stress testing before an exercise program is initiated (see Chapter 18).

General guidelines for implementing a realistic exercise plan include the following:

1. Begin at the patient's level of current activity. Walking for 10 minutes a day may be a lot for a sedentary person. Encourage routine activity (e.g., park some distance from destination, use stairs instead of elevators).

2. Prescribe exercise at 60% to 80% of the patient's age-adjusted maximum heart rate. (The maximum heart rate is approximated by the formula of 200 beats/min minus the person's age.) Those who have been sedentary should start at the low end of this range.
3. Encourage the patient to exercise regularly at a specific time of the day (early morning, lunch hour, after work).
4. Emphasize the need to exercise regularly. Patients should work toward a 30-minute session four or five times a week.
5. Encourage the use of a diary to chart progress. Self-monitoring reinforces effort.
6. Encourage activity with a friend, co-worker, or family member. Referral to a credible group exercise facility may be indicated.
7. Walking should be the initial activity. When an activity other than walking is undertaken, it must be easily accessible and fit the patient's life-style.

For weight to be kept off once it has been lost, exercise must become a permanent component of a person's life-style (see also Chapter 18).

Pharmacologic Treatment

Drug therapy for weight loss continues to play a minor although much-hoped-for role in the management of obesity. Although often sought, especially by persons frustrated with other weight loss efforts, medical therapy has always been and continues to be problematic. Periodic flurries of interest followed by disappointment are characteristic. In the 1950s and 1960s, the prescription of amphetamines was commonplace, but it fell out of favor when the risks of tolerance and dependence became fully appreciated. In the 1990s, the combination of fenfluramine and dexfenfluramine was very popular until its use became linked to valvular cardiac injury.

Appetite suppression is the basic goal of pharmacotherapy and is targeted by catecholaminergic stimulants (e.g., amphetamines, phentermine, diethylpropion, phenylpropanolamine, sibutramine) and serotoninergic agents (e.g., fenfluramine, dexfenfluramine, and the selective serotonin reuptake inhibitors). The evolving appreciation for the role of leptin in natural appetite suppression is the focus of much current research, with the hope of providing safer, more effective drug therapy.

Fenfluramine and Phentermine ("Fen–Phen"). A burst of interest in pharmacotherapy followed publications reporting weight loss efficacy for the combination of extended-release *fenfluramine* and *phentermine*. Combination therapy provided synergy by acting on different neurotransmitters (central nervous system stimulation for phentermine and sedation for fenfluramine); this allowed lower doses to be used and minimized side effects. In addition, the dextro form of fenfluramine, *dexfenfluramine*, proved useful as monotherapy. Dexfenfluramine added to a calorie-restricted diet resulted in greater weight loss than diet plus placebo. In general, approximately 2 to 10 kg of weight loss could be attributed to drug therapy. However, the response was highly variable and difficult to predict. Moreover, reports of *heart valve injury* began to appear in persons taking fen–phen or dexfenfluramine for more than a few months. These reports prompted the Food and Drug Administration to *withdraw* both products from the market. Pa-

Table 233.1. Noncommercial, Commercial, and Clinical Weight Loss Programs

PROGRAM	APPROACH/METHOD	CLIENTS	STAFF
Registered Dietitians in Private Practice	Dietitians design individual diet program according to client's life-style and caloric needs. Individual or group counseling may include sessions on nutrition, food preparation and recipe modification, behavior modification, and exercise.	All ages, men and women.	Registered dietitians (RD).
Non-commercial			
Take Off Pounds Sensibly	TOPS is an international nonprofit, noncommercial weight loss support group. Members obtain an exercise and food plan and goal weight from their personal physicians. TOPS provides a supportive environment in which individuals can make slow, steady, permanent life-style changes necessary to reach and maintain their personal goals. The program recognizes that each person has different health conditions and weight loss goals; it helps people meet their individual needs through group support. TOPS has programs and addresses issues related to the maintenance of healthy life-styles. Patients who have achieved their goal are an integral part of helping others in TOPS to do so. TOPS members who have reached and maintained goal weight are called KOPS (Keep Off Pounds Sensibly) and are honored accordingly.	Chapters are run on a local level by members who elect a volunteer leader. Each chapter varies in its approach according to the needs of its members, but all chapters address the complex issues involved in weight loss efforts.	Chapters frequently invite health professionals to speak at their meetings. Chapters are supported by trained field staff. Headquarters provide educational materials and a monthly magazine. A strong incentive plan with awards and recognition are woven into the program at all levels. Activities include special rallies, workshops, and recognition days as well as low-cost week-long retreats.
Overeaters Anonymous	Nonprofit international organization that provides volunteer support groups worldwide patterned after a 12-step Alcoholic Anonymous program. Members are encouraged to seek professional help for individualized diet/nutrition plan and for emotional or physical problems.	Individuals who define themselves as compulsive overeaters.	Non-professional volunteers, who meet specific criteria, lead meetings, sit on the board, and conduct activities.
Commercial			
Diet Workshop	Program consists of diet, exercise, and behavior modification. Diets range from between 1,600 and 2,600 calories and 27 to 40 g of fat per day. Menus follow the Food Guide Pyramid. The purchase of special foods is optional.	Mostly female (80%) and range in age from 25 to 65 years.	The weight loss program was developed by a team of registered dietitians, a registered nurse, a physician, and a licensed psychologist. The program is delivered by Diet Workshop graduates. Leaders must complete a 3-week training program, which covers nutrition, weight loss dynamics, customer service, and presentation. Ongoing training for the staff involves 96 to 100 hours each year.

EXPECTED WEIGHT LOSS/ LENGTH OF PROGRAM	HEALTHY LIFESTYLE COMPONENT	COMMENTS	AVAILABILITY/COST	HEADQUARTERS
Varies on an individual basis.	Individual and/or group counseling.	Offers individualized personalized approach to weight loss. To contact a registered dietitian in private practice, contact the American Dietetic Association (or the local state dietetic association).	Nationally. Professional organization. Usually hourly rates that vary according to the region, ranging from $85 to $150.	American Dietetic Association, Chicago, IL. http://www.eatright.org
There is no set timetable to reach a goal. When a personally meaningful weight goal is achieved, the focus changes to maintaining that goal. Members are invited and encouraged to remain a part of TOPS as long as they need the support.	TOPS offers programs and addresses issues related to maintaining healthy life-styles. People who have achieved their goal are an integral part of helping those in TOPS who are trying to do so.	TOPS is run by a nine-member board of directors. A medical advisor is consulted. Annual membership is $20.00 in the U.S., $25.00 in Canada. This includes the monthly magazine. Local chapters charge a small weekly fee, usually no more than $5 a month. For more information about local chapters, call toll-free **1-800-932-8677.**	Almost 300,000 members meet weekly in 11,700 meetings in the United States, Canada, and military bases around the world.	Milwaukee, WI. http://www.tops.org
Make no claims for weight loss.	Recommends emotional, spiritual, and physical recovery changes. No exercise or food recommendations.	Inexpensive. Provides group support. No need to follow a specific diet plan to participate. Minimal organization at the group level, so groups vary in approach. No health care providers on staff.	Nine thousand groups in 52 countries.	Rio Rancho, NM. (505) 891-2664 http://www.overeaters anonymous.org
A weight loss of 1 to 2 pounds per week. Length of program is determined by the amount of weight that the client needs to lose. A minimum of 3 months is required to participate in the program.	Program involves exercise and behavior modification component. Group and individual counseling are available.	Vitamin and mineral supplements are optional.	Ten thousand clients are served weekly at 15 franchises with 100 locations in the northeast U.S. Three-month behavior-modification program costs $169. A 1- to 3-month program is available for $49 per month. There is no charge for a maintenance program.	50 Cummings Parkway, Woburn, MA 01801. (800) 488-3438 http://www.dietwork shop.com

Table 233.1. CONT.   Noncommercial, Commercial, and Clinical Weight Loss Programs

PROGRAM	APPROACH/METHOD	CLIENTS	STAFF
Jenny Craig, Inc.	Hypocaloric diet, exercise, and life-style modification. Menu plans range from 1,000 to 2,300 calories, depending on the energy needs of the client. All menus are based on the Food Guide Pyramid. Jenny Craig food purchases are required at first and are gradually eliminated as client transitions to self-planned menus.	Mostly females (90%) over age 18. Adolescent program available for ages 13 to 17 (with parental permission).	Program developed by on-staff dietitians and reviewed and approved by Medical Advisory Board consisting of physicians, psychologists, and an exercise physiologist. All programs are delivered by trained employees who complete 56 hours of prior training. Staff also participate in weekly meetings and monthly continuing education sessions.
The Solution	Family systems approach involving developmental skills for the mind, body, and spirit: nurturing (emotional therapy), limit setting (cognitive therapy), body pride (body image), good health, mastery eating, mastery living. The program encourages 30 minutes or more of exercise each day. Participants are educated about eating for health. No set calorie limit is recommended.	Mostly female (80%) ages 19 years or older.	The program was developed and written by a master's level registered dietitian with input from health professionals in the fields of dietetics and nutrition, medicine, mental health, exercise, and education. The program delivery team consists of registered dietitians and licensed mental health professionals (psychologist, family therapist, social worker, and psychiatrist). All staff must complete 20 hours of training to become certified to deliver the program. Orientation is to train those who are already certified or licensed professionals. Periodic "tune-up" training is available at annual workshops and meetings.
Weight Watchers	Hypocaloric diet, exercise, and life-style modification. Diets range from 1,225 to 1,745 calories and are individualized for the client's energy needs for weight loss. Commercially sold Weight Watchers foods can be purchased but are optional for program participation.	Mostly female (95%) ages 10 years and older.	The program was developed by registered dietitians and exercise physiologists. Leaders (who are Lifetime Members) deliver the program. Initial training requires 46 hours of classroom instruction.
Clinical weight loss			
Health Management Resources	Medically supervised program for high-risk or non-medically supervised for moderate weight loss patients combines a nutritionally complete diet with intensive life-style education. Options include a very low-calorie diet (VLCD) under medical supervision (520 to 800 calories per day) and *Healthy Solutions,* a weight loss option that includes the use of regular foods (1,000 to 1,600 calories per day). Both diets include the use of meal replacements. Either option is available with or without adjunctive drug therapy. Mandatory weekly 90-minute group classes focus on teaching specific skills for overall health management. Health Risk Appraisal is available for every client. A long-term maintenance program and individual counseling are also available.	Contraindications: pregnancy, lactation, and acute substance abuse. VLCD requires physician's written approval for patients with comorbidities.	Program developed by MDs RDs, RNs, and psychologists. Each location has at least one MD, RN, and health educator on staff. Participants assigned "personal coaches" (RDs, exercise physiologists, health educators) who help dieters learn and practice weight management skills. Dieters on VLCD see MD or RN weekly.

EXPECTED WEIGHT LOSS/ LENGTH OF PROGRAM	HEALTHY LIFESTYLE COMPONENT	COMMENTS	AVAILABILITY/COST	HEADQUARTERS
Anticipated weight loss is about 1% of body weight or 1 to 2 pounds per week. The length of the program is determined by the amount of weight that the client wants to lose.	Individual consultations are available. Information is provided on healthful eating, stress management, and building an active life-style. Exercise is encouraged to aid in weight loss and maintenance. Behavior modification is part of the overall goal of the program structure.	Vitamin and mineral supplements are available.	Serves approximately 65,000 clients weekly in 660 U.S. Centres (46 states), Canada, Australia, New Zealand, and Puerto Rico. Prices vary. Programs require a one-time enrollment fee plus approximately $72 per week for food, which decreases during program term as fewer food purchases are made.	1135 N. Torrey Pines Road, LaJolla, CA 92037. (800)29-JENNY Program information also available at Jenny Craig's website: http://www.jenny craig.com Email: info@jenny craignews.com
No more than a 1-pound weight loss per week is recommended. Each session is 12 weeks for 2 hours per week. Participants can elect to continue for more than the 12-week session.	Counseling sessions are designed for eight to 12 clients; the group forms a community and members provide telephone support to practice methods between sessions. Positive behavior changes are emphasized in the program structure.	In the maintenance program, clients can return for 12-week sessions any time they desire. Every 3 months, a Saturday afternoon maintenance session for all program graduates is held.	One hundred fifty groups meet all over the U.S. For weight loss, $275 to $300 for 12 weeks, including cost of materials. There is no charge for maintenance.	University of California, San Francisco Department of Family and Community Medicine, AC-9, Box 0900, San Francisco, CA 94143-0900. (415) 457-3331 http://ww/weight solution.com
The length of the program is determined by the individual client. Individuals must enter the maintenance program when BMI reaches 20. Expected weight loss is up to 2 pounds per week.	Program includes group counseling sessions (individual counseling in limited areas). Information on both aerobic and resistance training exercise is provided, and exercise is encouraged to aid in weight loss and maintenance. Life-style modification is a component of the overall program structure.	Vitamin and mineral supplements are available.	Six hundred thousand clients are served in North America per week. There are 19,000 weekly meetings. For weight loss, there is a one-time registration fee of $16 to $20 and a weekly fee of $10 to $14. For maintenance, $10 to $14 weekly for about 6 weeks until Lifetime Member status is reached. There is no fee for Lifetime Members.	175 Crossways Park West, Woodbury, NY 11797-2055. (800) 651-6000 http://www.weight watchers.com
Averages 1 to 5 pounds weekly. Reducing phase varies according to weight loss goals but averages 12 to 20 weeks. Maintenance program recommended for up to 18 months. Most recent published data showed average weight loss of 65 pounds (22 weeks) in VLCD program. Current Health Solutions average weight loss is 20 to 25 pounds.	Health Risk Appraisals are available for each client. Recommends clients burn a minimum of 2,000 calories in physical activity weekly. Advocates consuming a diet with no more than 30% of calories from fat per week. Decreased decision making about food choices in the weight loss phase improves compliance. All options include meal replacements.	Emphasizes exercise as a means for weight loss and control. Few decisions about what to eat. Supervised by a health professional. Requires a strong commitment to physical activity. Side effects of VLCD include intolerance to cold, constipation, dizziness, dry skin, and headaches. All options include meal replacements; diet is very high in protein, even at lower calorie levels.	More than two hundred hospitals and medical settings nationwide.	Boston, MA. (617) 357-9876 or (800) 418-1367 http://www.yourbetter health.com

Table 233.1. CONT.   Noncommercial, Commercial, and Clinical Weight Loss Programs

PROGRAM	APPROACH/METHOD	CLIENTS	STAFF
New Directions	The New Directions system has been treating patients nationally for over 10 years. New Directions offers two program methods: a medically supervised Low-Calorie Diet, comprising fortified meal replacements of 600 to 800 calories per day, and the Outlook Program, which provides 1,000 to 1,500 calories per day and includes fortified nutritional bars and beverages as well as traditional foods. This is for people moderately overweight, 15 to 40 pounds. All operations materials and patient materials are included as part of the program. The goal of the New Directions program is to give complete support (nutrition, behavioral, life-style, and educational) to the patient.	Contraindications to the New Directions program: individuals less than 18 years of age, pregnant and lactating women, and those with conditions such as insulin-dependent diabetes (type 1), metastatic cancer, recent myocardial infarction, liver disease requiring protein restriction, and renal insufficiency.	RDs, master's level behavioral therapists, and exercise physiologist. Outlook Programs are led by health professionals knowledgeable in dietetics, exercise, and behavior. One-on-one interaction is part of each program. Each system is headed by a physician who serves as medical director.
Medifast	Medifast is a physician-supervised very low-calorie diet program of fortified meal replacement containing 450 to 500 calories per day. *Life-styles—the Medifast Program of Patient Support* prepares patients to maintain their goal weight after completing the VLCD. Medifast provides a low-calorie diet of approximately 860 calories per day for those not selected for the VLCD. Medifast also offers *Take Shape,* a product line that can be used as part of a weight loss or weight maintenance program.	Contraindications: Those who are not at least 30% above ideal body weight, those who have not reached sexual and physical maturation, pregnant and lactating women, recent cerebrovascular accident, bulimia, unstable angina, insulin-dependent diabetes, thrombophlebitis, active cancer, and uncompensated renal or hepatic disease.	Program supervised by a physician. At the corporate level, a medical advisory board of MDs, PhDs, and RDs is consulted on program and product development.

From Guidance for the treatment of adult obesity. Bethesda, MD: Shape Up America, 1996, with permission.

tients who took either of these drugs should be examined clinically for evidence of heart valve dysfunction, first by auscultation and then by cardiac ultrasonography if abnormalities are detected on physical examination.

Other adverse effects of these agents were also demonstrated. Diarrhea, polyuria, sleep disturbances, and sedation can occur with either fenfluramine or dexfenfluramine. Reversible short-term memory loss was reported in more than 10% of patients taking fenfluramine and phentermine in combination. The most serious adverse effect was an increased risk for reversible and irreversible *primary pulmonary hypertension* among patients taking either fenfluramine or dexfenfluramine for 3 months or more. Despite a 10- to 20-fold increase in relative risk, the absolute risk for this complication remains quite small. Contraindications included glaucoma and the use of monoamine oxidase inhibitors. Depression was a relative contraindication.

Orlistat, approved by the Food and Drug Administration, binds to and blocks the topical activity of pancreatic and gastric lipases and inhibits about 30% of gut dietary fat absorption. Randomized, double-blinded, placebo-controlled study lasting 2 years have demonstrated significant weight loss (up to 10%), a reduction in weight gain, and improvements in lipid profile and insulin levels. However, about 80% of patients experience some adverse gastrointestinal effects of the ensuing malabsorption/maldigestion (e.g., abdominal cramping, bloating, oily and greasy stools, diarrhea). The cost is high, at several dollars a day, when this agent is used three times daily, as recommended by the manufacturer. Lipid-soluble vitamin supplementation (especially vitamin D, but also vitamins A and E and β-carotene) may be necessary. Longer-term data from very large samples of patients are not yet available to characterize the risks associated with prolonged therapy, nor are data available on outcomes of cardiovascular events and other pertinent end points.

EXPECTED WEIGHT LOSS/ LENGTH OF PROGRAM	HEALTHY LIFESTYLE COMPONENT	COMMENTS	AVAILABILITY/COST	HEADQUARTERS
In the New Directions Low-Calorie Diet Program, the average weight loss is 3 pounds per week, while the Outlook Program weight loss rates vary with each individual. Length of the program participation for the Low-Calorie Program: 12 to 16 weeks in reducing, 5 to 10 weeks in adapting (transition to regular food), and 6 to 12 months in sustaining (maintenance). Ongoing participation in each phase is strongly encouraged with each patient.	Weekly classes concentrate on problem solving, life-style development, nutrition education, and a dieter-friendly light exercise program.	Each program emphasizes individualized care and consistent contact with health professionals. Program support includes a comprehensive treatment approach that is easy for patients to understand and to follow. Patients make few decisions about what to eat, which affords the opportunity to learn and practice effective skills to help make permanent life-style changes that translate into long-term success. The Outlook includes regular food with strong emphasis on life-style modification. These programs are medically monitored by an MD on a weekly or biweekly basis depending on patient's needs. The medical portion is usually covered by insurance.	The amount of weight necessary to lose, program choice, and medical conditions determine the cost of the program. Prices average from $110 to $120 per week. Medical monitoring is about $45 to $60 of the fee and is usually covered by insurance.	Robard Corporation, Medical Nutrition Division, Mt. Laurel, NJ. (800) 222-9201
Physician and patient arrive at individualized goal weight. Metropolitan Life Insurance Company tables, Dietary Guidelines for Americans, and BMI charts used as guides. Weight loss varies with individual; average weight loss is 3 to 5 pounds per week. Weight Reduction Phase lasts 16 weeks and Realignment lasts 4 to 6 weeks. Maintenance is strongly encouraged for up to 1 year.	The Medifast program includes a comprehensive education program called *Life-styles* that includes behavior modification, a recommended physical activity program, and nutrition education. Instruction booklets and patient guides provided, including a quarterly newsletter to patients.	Close contact with one or more health professionals. Low calorie level promotes rapid weight loss. Extensive product line. Must rely on company products during Reducing Phase. Maintenance program assists with transition to regular foods. Company products and regular foods are incorporated into the diet when VLCD is not recommended for the client.	Fifteen thousand physicians nationwide, primarily in office-based settings, and in six foreign countries. Costs for office visits, laboratory test, and Medifast products vary by individual physician. The program ranges from $65 to $85 per week. Insurance may cover the cost of lab work and office visits.	Healthrite, Inc., Owings Mills, MD. (800) 638-7867

Sibutramine (Meridia). At present, this is the only other agent approved by the Food and Drug Administration for the treatment of obesity. Structurally resembling amphetamines, it inhibits the reuptake of norepinephrine and serotonin to cause an increase in their central nervous system concentrations. The drug is rapidly absorbed and reaches its peak effect in 3 to 4 hours; the half-life is about 14 hours. A dose-related effect on weight loss has been noted; peak doses are associated with about 12 to 15 pounds of weight loss over 6 months; the effect appears to persist for up to 12 months with continued use. The most common side effects are dry mouth, insomnia, headache, and constipation. Other effects include an increase in blood pressure and heart rate. It is recommended that sibutramine not be used in conjunction with other agents that affect serotonin activity, such as the selective serotonin reuptake inhibitors used to treat depression, the serotonin agonists used for migraine (e.g., sumatriptan), lithium, and some analgesics (e.g., meperi-dine, fentanyl, dextromethorphan, pentazocine). The use of sibutramine within 2 weeks of use of a monoamine oxidase inhibitor is also to be avoided. The cost is high, at several dollars per day. The starting dosage is 10 mg/d. Because published data on safety and efficacy are limited, as is experience with long-term administration, most authorities do not recommend use of this agent. Moreover, concerns about the risk for valvular injury, found with the use of other agents that affect serotonin metabolism (see above), remain unanswered. Because of its similarity in structure to amphetamine, sibutramine is classified as a schedule IV drug by the Drug Enforcement Agency.

Over-The-Counter Diet Pills usually contain *phenylpro-panolamine*, *benzocaine*, or both, often in combination with vitamins or caffeine. They came into use after a few reports purported to show small degrees of weight loss associated with their intake. Phenylpropanolamine, a common decongestant sympathomimetic, is promoted as an appetite suppressant and is found in a number of over-the-counter diet pills (e.g., Dexatrim, Appedrine, Dietac, Dex-A-Diet, Prolamine). There is no compelling evidence to prove its efficacy in weight control, and it can be dangerous. Adverse reactions include hypertension, hypertensive crisis, renal failure, cardiac arrhythmias, acute psychotic episodes, and death. Although probably not as dangerous to dieters as phenylpropanolamine, benzocaine, a topical anesthetic, is also promoted as a diet aid and sold in candy and gum form. The use of such nonprescription agents should be discouraged.

Antidepressants may stimulate the appetite, which can be troublesome. Many *tricyclics* are problematic in this regard. Switching to a serotonin reuptake inhibitor that does not stimulate the appetite (e.g., *sertraline*) may solve the problem (see Chapter 227).

Phenytoin. In the rare instance of abnormal food preoccupation and binge eating in association with electroencephalographic abnormalities, phenytoin may help. More commonly, binge eaters have primitive, impulsive characters that are often diagnosed as borderline states. With successful psychotherapy, these regressive episodes tend to disappear as healthier defenses and a less chaotic life-style emerge.

Herbal Therapies and Commercial Products. Although considerable claims are made for herbal therapies, there is no evidence of their efficacy, and no consistent listing of ingredients or standardization of preparations is available. Most preparations appear to contain harmless ingredients, but not always. In Europe, one preparation containing *Stephania tetrandra* was inadvertently replaced by another containing *Aristolochia fangchi*, which caused renal injury and renal failure in more than 100 persons.

Garcinia cambogia, an herb found in plants native to India, is claimed to lower body weight and reduce fat in humans. It is a source of hydroxycitric acid, which inhibits a citrate cleavage enzyme believed to play a role in lipogenesis. Although extracts of this herb and preparations containing hydroxycitric acid are promoted and sold commercially for weight loss, there is no evidence they are effective. In a rigorous randomized, placebo-controlled study of a concentrated extract of the herb, it failed to produce any significant weight loss or evidence of fat mobilization.

Commercial food preparations and *dietary supplements* are heavily promoted and marketed, often as part of a comprehensive weight loss program (Table 233.1).

New Agents. The *leptins* are substances of the central nervous system believed important in neurotransmission of a sense of satiation, at least in animals. These and other central nervous system substances are the subject of intensive study for use in obesity.

Extreme Measures

Very Low-calorie Diets severely limit calories to between 400 and 800 per day. They achieve the more rapid and sustained rate of weight reduction associated with complete starvation while avoiding the inherent risks of starvation. These diets should be restricted to patients who are more than 30% to 40% above their ideal weight, and an initial cardiac evaluation and close medical supervision are required because of the risk for life-threatening arrhythmias. They are not do-it-yourself regimens. Goals include an optimal nitrogen balance and sparing of muscle tissue. With a very low-calorie diet, a patient can achieve a weight loss of more than 75% fat and a concomitant decrease in waist-to-hip and waist-to-thigh ratios.

These diets consist of 1.5 g of protein per kilogram of ideal body weight per day in the form of lean meat, fish, or fowl; noncaloric beverages; a multivitamin and mineral supplement containing folic acid; 1,500 mL of fluid per day; 25 mEq of potassium; and a calcium supplement. The combination of a very low-calorie diet and behavior modification appears promising. Average weight losses on the diet are 45 lb in fasting periods that last approximately 12 weeks.

The very low-calorie diet is not recommended for persons who are moderately overweight or for children, adolescents, pregnant or lactating women, or the elderly. Also, it should be avoided by patients with cardiovascular disease, essential hypertension, insulin-dependent diabetes mellitus, severe renal or hepatic impairment, active cancer, or a severe psychological disturbance. High dropout rates and poor long-term maintenance are discouraging aspects of this form of treatment.

Surgical Treatment continues to be an option for the control of morbid obesity, defined as "100 lb overweight" or over 200% of desirable weight as defined by the Metropolitan Life Insurance Company tables (see Chapter 10). Although the prevalence of morbid obesity is only 0.5% of the obese population, physicians often encounter these people in clinical practice. Their already high rates of morbidity and mortality accelerate rapidly as overweight becomes increasingly severe. Medical treatments are often ineffective.

Surgical intervention should be considered only after a comprehensive program of nonsurgical therapy has been fully tried and proven ineffective. Selection should be limited to highly motivated, morbidly obese patients free of other serious medical and psychosocial problems. Adequate financial support should be available because of the frequent need for repeated hospitalizations.

Jejunoileal Bypass was one of the first of the surgical treatments. It has been discontinued because of its high rate of serious complications, including intractable diarrhea, hypokalemia, hypocalcemia, formation of oxalate-containing kidney stones, liver failure, and protein malnutrition.

Gastric Reduction Procedures involve the construction of a small, 15- to 50-mL pouch connected through a small stoma to an outflow tract. This class of operations has emerged as the surgical approach of choice for morbid obesity. In the gastric bypass type, food passes first into the pouch and then into the jejunum. In the gastroplasty type (gastric stapling), food passes into the distal stomach and duodenum. Gastric bypass appears more effective in promoting weight loss, but gastroplasty is associated with fewer complications. Surgical mortality ranges from 0 to 4%. After surgery, patients must be instructed to eat small amounts, eat slowly, chew carefully, avoid eating when not hungry, and take no liquids with meals. Results are impressive, with an average of 50% of excess weight lost in the first 12 months, although it is not clear whether the cause is early satiety or aversive conditioning, a consequence of the development of epigastric pain and vomiting when too much is eaten at one time.

Complications include outlet obstruction, vitamin deficiencies (thiamine, B_{12}, and folate), partial temporary hair loss believed to be a result of inadequate protein intake, and an increased incidence of gallstones and gastric ulcers. Benefits include improvement in glucose intolerance, reduction in blood pressure for hypertensive patients, reversal of cardiorespiratory impairment, and reduction of serum cholesterol. Psychosocial benefits depend on the degree of weight loss and are independent of side effects and complications. Patients who lose significant amounts of weight become more employable and more physically active, show improvement in their sex life and self-esteem, and acquire a more gregarious outlook on life.

Suction Lipectomy (Liposuction), the very popular cosmetic procedure for removal of localized fat accumulations, has produced variable results. It has become the most frequently performed cosmetic operation in the United States, with more than 150,000 procedures performed annually. It is initiated with an SQ infusion of normal saline solution mixed with 1,000 mg of lidocaine and 1 mg of epinephrine per liter to provide local anesthesia and control of bleeding. SQ fat is then removed by suction. Several liters of infusate may be needed to remove 1 to 2 L of fat. Cosmetic success depends on the elastic properties of the overlying skin. Temporary loss of skin sensation, a wavy contour, and blood loss are commonly experienced. Other adverse effects include infection, extensive bruising for 2 to 3 weeks, and edema for 3 to 6 weeks. Anecdotal reports of death after liposuction are common. Well-documented reports of fatalities caused by lidocaine toxicity, drug–drug interactions, and venous thrombosis of the lower extremities have been published. Careful patient selection and full disclosure of the risks involved are required to help patients choose wisely.

Jaw Wiring, as the term implies, involves wiring the jaw shut for as long as 6 to 9 months to prevent the ingestion of solid food. The intake of high-calorie shakes and soft drinks will eliminate the benefits of surgery.

PATIENT EDUCATION

Motivation and patient education are key factors for successful weight control. Realistic goals and expectations are critical, as is the physician's support and encouragement. The patient must be willing to alter exercise and eating patterns permanently. A number of persons will be interested in commercial or nonprofit programs and appreciate reliable information regarding their effectiveness, safety, and appropriateness (Table 233.1). Although rapid weight loss programs are popular, patients need to be informed about their inadequacies for achieving long-term weight loss. Major obstacles to success need to be explored and addressed, including poor self-image, erratic eating patterns, inadequate exercise, loneliness, boredom, anger, and depression. If drug therapy is used, expectations should be realistic. Reduction to average body weight is not a realistic goal. As noted earlier, knowledge must be provided about the basic principles of nutrition, such as caloric value of foods and practical methods for changing eating habits.

Behavioral techniques are also very helpful and should include several types of action:

- Recording food intake
- Eating in only one place; using a smaller plate; not engaging in another activity while eating; keeping food otherwise out of sight
- Planning meals by shopping from a list; having low-calorie foods available; taking a brown-bag lunch; having a strategy before dining out; at parties, positioning oneself away from the food table
- Substituting an alternate activity for eating
- Increasing physical activity

INDICATIONS FOR REFERRAL

Although the interest, involvement, and encouragement of the primary physician are critical, the implementation of a comprehensive and personalized weight loss program is often best achieved with a multidisciplinary approach. Referral to a registered dietitian is enormously helpful in providing the patient with essential nutritional information and initiating a behavioral program for alteration of eating habits. Familiarity with community and commercial resources and their level of professional supervision is helpful when a patient requests a group approach. Before an exercise program is begun, it may be useful to refer the poorly conditioned, markedly obese patient for an electrocardiographic stress test (see Chapter 18). When emotional problems are too great for the primary physician and registered dietitian to handle, psychiatric referral should be considered. Surgical consultation should be considered only when the patient is so morbidly obese and so refractory to medical therapy that the risks associated with the surgery are less than those of remaining morbidly obese.

MANAGEMENT RECOMMENDATIONS

- Identify and treat specifically any etiologic factors (see Chapter 10).
- Prescribe a comprehensive approach to weight management that includes a low-fat diet, dietary counseling, behavior modification, and an exercise program (see Chapter 18).
- Avoid and discourage gimmicky food programs and appetite suppressants until safe and effective agents become available. Check any patients who have been prescribed fenfluramine or dexfenfluramine in the past for evidence of valvular cardiac injury by auscultation (and cardiac ultrasonography if valvular injury is suspected by examination).
- Individualize changes in eating and exercise patterns; make them gradual to maximize the potential for long-term compliance.
- Recommend a weight loss group to those who seek the benefit of group support; suggest one that is under professional supervision.
- Advise a dietitian-supervised weight management program for patients who continually go from one fad diet to another. Warn against diets based on unsubstantiated medical claims, which may have popular appeal but are ineffective for long-term weight control.
- Restrict the use of very-low calorie diets to patients more than 30% to 40% above their ideal weight; require medical supervision.

- Consider pharmacologic intervention only for persons at very high risk for cardiovascular, metabolic, or orthopedic morbidity.
- Consider referral for surgical therapy for only those patients with life-threatening obesity who have failed all other measures.

ANNOTATED BIBLIOGRAPHY

Abenhaim L, Moride Y, Brenot F, et al. Appetite-suppressant drugs and the risk of primary pulmonary hypertension. N Engl J Med 1996;335:609. (*Case–control study showing a sixfold risk for primary pulmonary hypertension with any use of appetite suppressants and more than a 20-fold risk with more than 3 months of use.*)

American Dietetic Association. Position of the American Dietetic Association: weight management. J Am Diet Assoc 1997;97:71. (*Defines the goals of weight management, which means achieving the best weight possible in the context of overall health.*)

Blair SN. Evidence for success of exercise in weight loss and control. Ann Intern Med 1993;119[Part 2]:702. (*Enhances weight loss, may reduce morbidity and mortality, and facilitates maintenance of weight loss.*)

Blair SN, Shaten J, Brownell K, et al. Body-weight change, all-cause mortality, and cause-specific mortality in the Multiple Risk Factor Intervention Trial. Ann Intern Med 1993;119[Part 2]:749. (*Highest mortality in those with the most extreme changes in weight.*)

Bray GA. Use and abuse of appetite-suppressant drugs in the treatment of obesity. Ann Intern Med 1993;119[Part 2]:707. (*A review of available studies; finds evidence of short-term efficacy and low risk for dependence with proper use of nonamphetamine preparations; 79 references.*)

Brolin BE. Critical analysis of results: weight loss and quality of data. Am J Clin Nutr 1992;55:577S. (*A critique of the data regarding surgical results.*)

Brownell KD. Managing patient expectations for weight loss. In: St. Geor FT, ed. New multidisciplinary strategies in obesity management. Clark, NJ: Health Learning Systems, 1997:10. (*Emphasis on realistic goal setting for patients in weight loss programs.*)

Calle EA, Thun MJ, Petrelli JM, et al. Body mass index and mortality in a prospective cohort of U.S. adults. N Engl J Med 1999;341:1097. (*The rise in all-cause mortality and mortality linked to heart disease and cancer parallels moderate to severe increases in body mass index.*)

Cheskin LJ, Miday R, Zorich N, et al. Gastrointestinal symptoms following consumption of olestra or regular triglyceride potato chips. JAMA 1998;279:150. (*A randomized, controlled trial of a single large serving found no difference in gastrointestinal side effects.*)

Consensus Development Conference Panel. Gastrointestinal surgery for severe obesity. Ann Intern Med 1991;115:956. (*Reviews efficacy and specifies criteria for selection of patients and procedures.*)

Davidson MH, Hauptman J, DiGirolamo M, et al. Weight control and risk factor reduction in obese subjects treated for 2 years with orlistat. JAMA 1999;281:235. (*A randomized, double-blinded, placebo-controlled study demonstrating significant weight loss, reduction in weight gain, and improvement in lipid profile and insulin levels.*)

Devereux RB. Appetite suppressants and valvular heart disease. N Engl J Med 1998;339:765. (*A summary of the evidence and recommendations regarding cardiac evaluation of users.*)

Everhart JE. Contributions of obesity and weight loss to gallstone disease. Ann Intern Med 1993;119:1029. (*Risk is acutely increased during weight loss in obese persons.*)

Foreyt JP, Goodrick GK. Evidence for success of behavioral modification in weight loss and control. Ann Intern Med 1993;119[Part 2]:698. (*Average weight loss is close to 20 lb, and two thirds of patients retain the loss at 1 year.*)

Heymsfield SB, Allison DB, Vasselli JR, et al. Garcinia cambogia (hydroxycitric acid) as a potential antiobesity agent: a randomized controlled trial. JAMA 1998;280:1596. (*Well-designed study failing to show evidence of efficacy.*)

Hill JO, Drougas H, Peters JC. Obesity treatment: can diet composition play a role? Ann Intern Med 1993;119[Part 2]:694. (*During active weight loss, calories are more important; during maintenance, low-fat composition is helpful.*)

Institute of Medicine. Weighing the options: criteria for evaluating weight management programs. Washington, DC: National Academy Press, 1995. (*Appropriate patients have demonstrated improved outcomes with advances in pharmacotherapy and gastric surgery.*)

Khan MA, Herzog CA, St. Peter JV, et al. The prevalence of cardiac valvular insufficiency assessed by transthoracic echocardiography in obese patients treated with appetite-suppressant drugs. N Engl J Med 1998;339:713. (*Case–control study finding a significant increase in valvular insufficiency in persons taking fen–phen or its constituent agents in comparison with matched controls.*)

Lichtman SW, Pisarsak K, Berman ER, et al. Discrepancy between self-reported and actual caloric intake and exercise in obese subjects. N Engl J Med 1992;327:1893. (*Actual caloric intake greater and exercise less than reported.*)

National Institutes of Health. Clinical guidelines on the identification, evaluation, and treatment of overweight and obesity in adults. Bethesda, MD: National Institutes of Health, June 1998. (*A definitive review of the issue that provides evidence for the effects of treatment on overweight and obesity; essential reading for all primary physicians.*)

National Task Force on the Prevention and Treatment of Obesity. Very low-calorie diets. JAMA 1993;270:967. (*Found effective and safe for short-term use under close medical supervision; means of improving outcome discussed; 124 references.*)

National Task Force on the Prevention and Treatment of Obesity. Long-term pharmacotherapy in the management of obesity. JAMA 1996;276:1907. (*An extensive review of the evidence for both benefits and risks.*)

Pawlak L. Weight matters. Appetite: the brain–body connection. Berkeley, CA: Biomed, 1998. (*Excellent review of factors affecting appetite control. Focus on brain chemistry, composition of foods, and exercise.*)

Rao RB, Ely SF, Hoffman RS. Deaths related to liposuction. N Engl J Med 1999;340:1471. (*Well-documented cases from the files of the New York State medical examiner; lidocaine-related adverse effects and thrombosis were found responsible.*)

Rosenbaum M, Leibel RL. The role of leptin in human physiology. N Engl J Med 1999;341:913. (*An editorial tersely summarizing current knowledge.*)

Senekal M, Albertse EC, Momberg DJ, et al. A multidimensional weight management program for woman. J Am Diet Assoc 1999;99:1257. (*Presents a multidimensional model for weight management that focuses on all aspects of prevention, treatment, and management of weight-related problems.*)

Serdula MK, Mokdad AH, Williamson DF, et al. Prevalence of attempting weight loss and strategies for controlling weight. JAMA 1999;282:1353. (*Report detailing the prevalence of attempted weight loss in the United States. Many people are making unsuccessful attempts at weight loss and weight maintenance because of inactivity and increased availability of "fast foods."*)

Shape Up America, American Obesity Association. Guidance for the treatment of adult obesity. Bethesda, MD: Shape Up America, 1996:1. (*Excellent educational resource for physicians that provides comprehensive medical guidance on the treatment of obesity.*)

Williamson DF, Pamuk ER. The association between weight loss and increased longevity. Ann Intern Med 1993;119[Part 2]:731. (*A review of available evidence; conclusions difficult, and reasons discussed.*)

Willet WC, Dietz WH, Colditz GA. Primary care: guidelines for healthy weight. N Engl J Med 1999;341:427. (*An excellent review article on body weight.*)

Wood PD, Stefanick ML, Dreon DM, et al. Changes in plasma lipids and lipoproteins in overweight men during weight loss through dieting as compared with exercise. N Engl J Med 1988;319:1173. (*Both produced comparable and favorable changes in lipids.*)

234

Approach to Eating Disorders
NANCY A. RIGOTTI

Anorexia nervosa, bulimia nervosa (the binge–purge syndrome), and binge-eating disorder are the principal eating disturbances of adolescents and adults. Both anorexia and bulimia are considerably more common in women and usually develop during adolescence or early adulthood. About 40% of cases of binge-eating disorder occur among boys and men. The prevalence of anorexia approaches 1 in 200 among female adolescents in Western countries, whereas bulimia may affect up to 15% of college women. These disturbances of eating behavior are psychiatric disorders that can have serious medical consequences. They extend beyond racial and socioeconomic boundaries. Because patients with these conditions often hide their problem, a high index of suspicion is required for diagnosis. Primary care physicians need to be able to recognize these disorders, evaluate and treat their medical complications, arrange and coordinate a comprehensive multidisciplinary treatment program, assist in ambulatory monitoring, and determine when a patient requires hospitalization.

PATHOPHYSIOLOGY, CLINICAL PRESENTATION, AND COURSE

Anorexia Nervosa

Anorexia nervosa is a syndrome characterized by severe weight loss (*body weight <85% of expected*, or *body mass index <17.5 kg/m²*) resulting from inadequate food intake by persons with no medical reason to lose weight. A *distorted body image* and an *intense fear of weight gain* lead to the relentless pursuit of an unreasonable and unhealthy thinness. Weight is lost in two ways. Patients with restrictive anorexia *starve* themselves. Others, with coexistent bulimia, lose weight by *purging* after eating, usually by vomiting or taking laxatives. Those with bulimic anorexia have a graver prognosis and more medical problems. Originally more prevalent among persons of high socioeconomic status, anorexia is now becoming more evenly distributed among social classes.

Pathogenesis. The precise pathogenesis of anorexia remains unknown but appears to be multifactorial. Abnormalities in central neurotransmitter activity are suggested by alterations in serotonin metabolism. Neuroendocrine abnormalities are well documented (see below), but these appear to be the consequence, not the cause, of the starvation. Psychological and psychosocial factors are important. Onset frequently coincides with a time of separation from home or the loss of a loved one. The clinical features of the condition and its association with loss cause some to view it as a variant of depression. Others attribute anorexia to problems in emotional development and disturbed family interactions. Psychological studies find these patients to be bright, compulsive perfectionists who perform well at school and work. The prevalence of obsessive–compulsive disorder is increased among patients with anorexia. Societal pressure to be thin, communicated in the media, is also believed to contribute to the problem.

Pathophysiology. Restrictive anorexia nervosa is similar to *starvation* and can be fatal. Diets are deficient in carbohydrates and total calories, but protein and vitamin intake is relatively preserved. Consequently, vitamin deficiencies are unusual. However, inadequate nutrient intake results in a profound loss of weight, fat, and muscle mass, followed by cardiac, metabolic and endocrine, hematologic, and gastrointestinal disturbances.

Cardiac Consequences. Cardiac muscle atrophy is associated with a reduction in left ventricular wall thickness and cardiac output, but congestive failure does not occur. *Arrhythmias* and electrocardiographic changes, primarily low-voltage ST-segment depression and T-wave flattening, have been documented, as have prolonged QT intervals. Autopsies of some patients performed after sudden death have shown a degeneration of myocardial cells, which may predispose to arrhythmias.

Endocrine and Metabolic Consequences. Extreme weight loss produces a number of adverse endocrine and metabolic changes. Thyroid hormone metabolism is altered, with thyroxine preferentially converted to the *inactive reverse T_3 instead of active T_3*. A compensatory rise in thyrotropin (TSH) does not occur because the hypothalamic–pituitary response is blunted (*"sick thyroid" syndrome*). Clinical features of *hypothyroidism* (see Chapter 104) may ensue. Starvation also produces reversible hypothalamic–pituitary dysfunction that can lead to *hypothalamic amenorrhea* and *estrogen deficiency* (see Chapter 112). Besides weight loss, other factors (perhaps leptin), yet to be identified, may contribute to hypothalamic dysfunction because menstruation ceases in up to 25% of female patients with anorexia before weight loss becomes significant, and amenorrhea may persist after weight is regained. In those with long-standing estrogen deficiency, very poor nutrition, and vitamin deficiencies, significant degrees of *osteoporosis* and vertebral compression fractures may develop.

Posterior pituitary function is also disrupted; a decline in vasopressin secretion leads to *central diabetes insipidus* and polyuria (see Chapter 102). In anorexia, the hypothalamus defends core temperature poorly in the face of changes in environmental temperature, so that *hypothermia* results. Many people with anorexia have *elevated plasma cortisol* levels that do not respond to an overnight dexamethasone suppression test. However, cortisol excess is not manifested clinically, perhaps because fatty or carbohydrate substrates are lacking.

Acquired defects in lipoprotein metabolism may increase serum *cholesterol* and *carotene* levels. Blood levels of glucose, protein, amino acids, and insulin are normal or mildly reduced. Severe hypoglycemia and coma have been reported when starvation is very advanced.

Gastrointestinal Consequences. Refeeding may be followed by gastric dilatation, ileus, and transient elevations of serum liver enzymes caused by *fatty liver. Delayed gastric emptying* explains some of the symptoms of abdominal bloating. The combination of slowed peristalsis and the meager dietary intake results in constipation.

Volume Changes. Refeeding frequently leads to *fluid retention*, especially in the bulimic anorectic patient, who purges and is volume-depleted. Fluid retention complicates the interpretation of weight changes and frightens the patient. If fluid retention is severe, congestive heart failure may develop as the increase in intravascular volume exceeds the capacity of the weakened heart.

Hematologic Consequences. Reversible bone marrow depression is noted. Although *mild anemia* is common, it is rarely a consequence of iron, folate, or B_{12} deficiency. The anemia may be masked in the setting of concurrent volume depletion and may not appear until rehydration is implemented. Despite *leukopenia*, the patient's susceptibility to infection is not increased. Thrombocytopenia is unusual.

Clinical Presentation. Characteristically, the patient denies she is ill, but her emaciation attracts attention. The presentation is remarkable for the lack of complaints. The patient typically claims to feel well and appears *unconcerned* about her emaciation. Hunger is not a complaint, but patients may report difficulty sleeping, abdominal discomfort and bloating after eating, constipation, cold intolerance, and polyuria. Amenorrhea is almost uniformly present in female patients. Unlike other persons who are starving, those with anorexia are not fatigued until malnutrition becomes very severe. Most are restless and physically active, and some exercise to excess. Listlessness is an ominous sign. The patient may present bundled in clothing because of cold intolerance.

On examination, the patient typically appears extremely thin, if not emaciated, but animated. Vital signs may reveal bradycardia, postural hypotension, and hypothermia. The skin may appear dry, pale or yellow-tinged (a consequence of carotenemia), and covered by fine downy hair (lanugo) over the face and arms. Often, the extremities are cold and cyanotic. In women, the female pattern of fat distribution disappears, but axillary and pubic hair is preserved.

Natural History. About 5% of patients with anorexia nervosa die. Most deaths are sudden, apparently caused by cardiac arrhythmias. Fatal hypoglycemic coma has also been reported. The risk for death appears to be higher in patients whose weight loss exceeds 40% of premorbid weight (or 30% if it has occurred within 3 months). Bulimic anorectic patients with metabolic abnormalities are probably at higher risk. The risk for suicide is also increased. The mortality rate is 12 times that of age-matched normal persons.

More than 75% of patients with anorexia regain weight to near-normal levels, and menstruation resumes in the majority, but abnormal eating habits and psychosocial problems often persist. Some become bulimic. A chronic syndrome develops in about 15%, and 5% become obese. Bulimic symptoms, lower weight, and older age at presentation are associated with poor outcome.

Bulimia (Bulimia Nervosa)

This eating disorder is driven by excessive *concern* about *body weight* or *shape* and characterized by *repeated episodes* of *binge eating* (at least two times per week for 3 months), during which large amounts of high-calorie foods are consumed, usually in secrecy. The binge is followed by self-deprecating thoughts and *purging, excessive exercise*, or *fasting* (at least two times per week for 3 months) to prevent weight gain. Most bulimic patients purge by inducing vomiting or using laxatives, but some use diuretics or exercise excessively. They fear losing control of their eating behavior and are ashamed when it happens. Binges may be repeated several times daily. At other times, people with bulimia may diet rigorously or take diet pills. In severe cases, the patient may have no regular eating pattern. The result of this behavior is frequent weight fluctuations but not severe weight loss.

In contrast to persons with anorexia, those with bulimia are aware that their behavior is abnormal but often conceal the illness because of embarrassment. The bulimic patient's near-normal weight permits the illness to be hidden. Detection of surreptitious vomiting or laxative abuse can be a challenge (see below).

Pathogenesis. The high prevalence of alcohol and drug abuse among patients with bulimia has led some to postulate that bulimia is part of an impulse control disorder. Depression has also been proposed as a precipitant. Changes in neurotransmitter metabolism and a response to antidepressant medication suggest a biochemical component to the condition. Cultural pressure to be thin probably contributes. People with bulimia commonly report that a diet preceded their disease. The bingeing sometimes observed when experimentally starved normal persons resume eating has led to speculation that strict dieting contributes to the onset of bulimia.

Complications. The medical consequences of bulimia depend on the specific behaviors present.

Of Bingeing. Bingeing has few complications, although *abdominal pain* from distention is common. Acute gastric dilation and rupture are rare.

Of Chronic Induced Emesis. Repeated regurgitation of stomach contents produces *volume depletion* and a *hypochloremic metabolic alkalosis*. Dizziness, syncope, thirst, orthostatic changes in vital signs, and an elevated blood urea nitrogen occur in the volume-depleted patient. Renal compensation for the alkalosis and volume depletion causes *potassium* *depletion* and *hypokalemia*, which may predispose to cardiac arrhythmias, muscle cramps and weakness, paresthesias, polyuria, and constipation. T-wave flattening and U waves are seen on the electrocardiogram. Serum and urine chloride levels are low.

Reversible, painless *parotid swelling* can develop with chronic vomiting and is often accompanied by *hyperamylasemia*. Irreversible dental problems also occur. Repeated exposure of the teeth to stomach acid causes *enamel decalcification* and *erosion*. Teeth diminish in size and become discolored and sensitive to temperature changes. Many vomiters have symptoms of *reflux esophagitis*. Sore throat caused by mucosal trauma sustained during induced vomiting is common, but hematemesis is unusual. Some patients use *emetine* (ipecac) to induce vomiting. Prolonged use may cause a reversible proximal *myopathy* and a potentially fatal cardiomyopathy.

Of Laxative Abuse. Laxative abuse is a common and potentially dangerous form of purging. It may begin as a response to constipation and continue because of the temporary weight loss induced through *volume depletion*. Stimulant laxatives are used most often. The resultant increase in colonic motility produces *abdominal cramps*, and electrolytes are lost in a *watery diarrhea*. Volume depletion, *hyponatremia*, *hypokalemia*, and either *metabolic acidosis* or *alkalosis* may result. Calcium and magnesium depletion have also been reported. The irritation of intestinal mucosa or development of hemorrhoids as a result of rapid fecal transit may cause *rectal bleeding*, and rectal *prolapse* can occur. When laxative abuse stops, transient fluid retention, edema, and constipation are common.

Of Diuretic Abuse. Patients use diuretics more often to prevent fluid retention than to induce weight loss. Use contributes to a *hypochloremic metabolic alkalosis*, *hypokalemia*, and *volume depletion*. Dilutional *hyponatremia* may also occur. In contrast to vomiters and laxative abusers, patients who use diuretics do not have low urinary levels of sodium and chloride. Fluid retention transiently develops when diuretics are stopped.

Natural History and Clinical Course. Little is known about the mortality and natural history of bulimia, but the behaviors can persist for decades. About half of patients achieve full recovery, another 30% experience partial recovery, and 20% show no improvement.

Binge-eating Disorder

This condition, an important cause of obesity, is characterized by recurrent binge eating (at least 2 days weekly for 6 months) and marked distress associated with eating alone, too rapidly, when not hungry, or until uncomfortably full. The patient has feelings of guilt or disgust after a binge, but does not purge, exercise excessively, or fast. Of the several eating disorders, this is the most common among male patients and is prevalent among the obese.

DIFFERENTIAL DIAGNOSIS

The differential diagnosis spans the array of conditions that may cause unexplained weight loss (see Chapter 9), secondary amenorrhea (see Chapter 112), electrolyte disturbances with volume depletion (see Chapters 59 and 64), and osteoporosis (see Chapter 164). Among them are malignancy, chronic infec-

tion, intestinal disorders (malabsorption, inflammatory bowel disease, or hepatitis), and endocrinopathies (e.g., hyperthyroidism, panhypopituitarism, adrenal insufficiency, diabetes mellitus). Tumors of the central nervous system mimic anorexia nervosa in rare cases. Psychiatric illnesses that can be confused with anorexia include depression, schizophrenia, and obsessive–compulsive neurosis (see Chapters 226, 227, and 230). Binge eating may be a manifestation of depression and, rarely, of an organic brain syndrome.

WORKUP

The diagnoses of anorexia nervosa and bulimia are based exclusively on clinical findings (Table 234.1). Laboratory studies help in the detection of complications (see below) and in ruling out other causes of weight loss (see Chapter 9).

Anorexia Nervosa

History. The history should explore the patient's attitudes toward weight loss, desired weight, and eating habits. A 24-hour dietary recall is more revealing than the answers to general questions about diet. Detailed weight and menstrual histories should be obtained, including the date and circumstances at the onset of weight loss, minimum and maximum weights, recent weight changes, and last normal menstrual period. One needs to ask all patients about bingeing, vomiting, and the use of laxatives, diuretics, diet pills, and emetics, and to quantify daily exercise (excessive exercise may be a variant of anorexia). Also important is inquiry into symptoms of malnutrition (fatigue, skin or hair changes), dehydration (light-headedness, syncope, thirst), hypokalemia (cramps, weakness, paresthesias, polyuria, palpitations), and other problems common to purgers (e.g., heartburn, abdominal pain, rectal bleeding). Because the risk

Table 234.1. American Psychiatric Association Diagnostic Criteria for Eating Disorders

Anorexia Nervosa
Low body weight (<85% of expected or BMI <17.5 kg/m²)
Inaccurate perception of own body size, weight, or shape
Intense fear of weight gain
Amenorrhea (if female)

Bulimia Nervosa
Excessive concern about body weight or shape
Recurrent binge eating (at least twice weekly for 3 months)
Recurrent purging, excessive exercise, or fasting (at least twice weekly for 3 months)
Absence of anorexia nervosa

Binge Eating Disorder
Recurrent binge eating (at least twice weekly for 6 months)
Marked distress with at least three of the following:
    Eating very rapidly
    Eating until uncomfortably full
    Eating when not hungry
    Eating alone
No recurrent purging, excessive exercise, or fasting
Absence of anorexia nervosa

BMI, body mass index.

Adapted from Becker AE, Grinspoon SK, Klibanski A, et al. Eating disorders. N Engl J Med 1999;340:1092, with permission, and based on the criteria specified in the Diagnostic and Statistical Manual of Mental Disorders, 4th ed. Washington, DC: American Psychiatric Association, 1994:539,729.

for suicide is increased in patients with an eating disorder, one must *screen for suicidality* during the initial visit (see Chapter 227). Likewise, because of the increased prevalence of depression, anxiety, and personality disorders among these patients, the history should be reviewed for suggestive symptoms (see Chapters 226, 227, and 230). Exploring the psychosocial history can provide information important not only to diagnosis but also to planning initial management.

Physical Examination. Important objectives are to assess the severity of malnutrition and dehydration and check for the development of complications. One should specifically take note of the general state of nutrition and hydration and follow with measurement of the height and weight (without street clothing). The blood pressure and pulse are checked for significant postural changes and the temperature noted for hypothermia. The skin is examined for pallor and the hair changes of lanugo, the chest for rales, and the extremities for edema and signs of peripheral vasoconstriction. Auscultation of the apical pulse may help detect an arrhythmia, rectal examination may reveal blood from laxative abuse, and eliciting the deep tendon reflexes for delayed relaxation can help detect secondary hypothyroidism.

In addition to these measures, a detailed physical examination is essential to rule out other causes of weight loss (see Chapter 9).

Laboratory Studies. Because serious volume, electrolyte, and cardiac rhythm disturbances may complicate anorexia nervosa, especially if the patient is bulimic, one needs to obtain a full set of serum *electrolytes*, plus *blood urea nitrogen, creatinine,* and *electrocardiogram* with rhythm strip. The finding of hyponatremia suggests excess water intake or inappropriate antidiuretic hormone secretion. Determination of the serum *calcium* (plus albumin) and magnesium is needed if a dysrhythmia is noted or laxative abuse is suspected. A *complete blood cell count* and measurement of *TSH, glucose, alkaline phosphatase, gonadotropins,* and serum *estrogens* (see Chapter 112) may be helpful in the initial testing for complications of starvation, such as anemia, leukopenia, secondary hypothyroidism, hypoglycemia, fatty liver, and hypothalamic amenorrhea. If amenorrhea is persistent, weight loss marked, and nutrition poor, then one should obtain a *bone mineral density* measurement to check for resultant osteoporosis (see Chapters 144 and 164). Unexplained weight loss may necessitate additional laboratory and imaging studies (see Chapter 9).

Bulimia

History. The diagnosis of bulimia requires a high index of suspicion because bingeing and purging may be concealed and no physical signs are characteristic. Clues include a preoccupation with weight and food, a history of frequent weight fluctuations, and problems common to patients who purge and become dehydrated (dizziness, thirst, syncope) or hypokalemic (muscle cramps or weakness, paresthesias, polyuria). In addition, vomiters may describe hematemesis or heartburn, and laxative abusers may complain of constipation, rectal bleeding, and fluid retention. When the diagnosis is suspected, the physician should ask directly about bingeing and purging and

should order a determination of serum electrolytes. A direct inquiry may elicit the history from a patient seeking help but ashamed to volunteer the information.

Physical Examination should include a check of postural signs for evidence of volume depletion, and any salivary gland enlargement or scars on the dorsum of the hand, suggestive of chronic self-induced vomiting, should be noted. The teeth are examined for erosion and discoloration. A careful neurologic examination is also indicated to rule out any focal abnormalities indicative of a central nervous system tumor or seizure disorder, which, in rare instances, can mimic bulimia.

Laboratory Studies. Most useful are the *serum* and *urine electrolytes, blood urea nitrogen,* and *creatinine,* and the *electrocardiogram. Calcium* and *magnesium* should be measured in laxative abusers. The pattern of serum and urine electrolytes helps to determine the mode of purging. *Hypokalemic alkalosis* suggests frequent vomiting or diuretic use. A *non–anion gap acidosis* suggests laxative abuse. Some patients who vomit deny that it is voluntary. Organic causes of chronic vomiting should be excluded in these cases (see Chapter 59).

Binge-Eating Disorder

The workup focuses on the history because physical examination and laboratory findings are almost always normal, except for obese patients (see Chapter 10). Most important is to explore the patient's experiences with eating because distress characterizes the syndrome, as do feelings of disgust and guilt after a binge.

PRINCIPLES OF MANAGEMENT AND PATIENT EDUCATION

Once it has been determined that hospitalization is not required (no suicidality, no major electrolyte or cardiac disturbances; see below), then design of the outpatient management program can proceed. The multidimensional nature of eating disorders necessitates a *multidisciplinary approach* that combines medical, nutritional, psychological, and pharmacologic measures. A *team approach* is often helpful. It can be coordinated by either the primary physician or a medical specialist experienced in treating eating disorders. Close coordination and communication are essential. A set of overall treatment goals should be collectively developed, agreed upon, and consistently communicated to the patient. Teamwork also helps ease the burden of treating these patients, who can be difficult when they deny the seriousness of their illness or exhibit deceptive, manipulative, angry, or distrusting behavior. There is *no single treatment of choice* for anorexia, bulimia, or binge eating. Several therapies produce short-term weight gain in patients with anorexia, but relapse is common, so that a comprehensive, multidimensional approach is necessary.

The immediate management tasks for the primary care physician are to identify and correct any potentially dangerous metabolic disturbances, set a few basic agreed-upon goals, initiate a few simple behavioral measures, and arrange timely referral to persons expert in the management of eating disorders. Given the potentially life-threatening nature of some eating disorders, one should proceed with referral as quickly as possible.

Outpatient Monitoring and Treatment of Metabolic Disturbances. One monitors the *weight* and *vital signs* regularly. In bulimic patients or anorectic patients who purge, it is especially important to check *postural signs*, *cardiac rhythm*, and *serum electrolytes* at each visit. If the QT interval was prolonged on the electrocardiogram at the time of the first visit, then a *repeated electrocardiogram* is warranted, especially before any tricyclic antidepressant therapy is instituted.

The hypokalemic patient who is judged safe to manage on an outpatient basis (see below) is instructed to eat potassium-rich foods (see Chapter 32). Maintaining normal electrolyte levels should be a condition of continued outpatient treatment. If the potassium level falls below normal despite dietary measures, supplemental potassium is indicated. This must be given as *potassium chloride* to correct the metabolic alkalosis that maintains the hypokalemia. Patients should be instructed to take the supplement at a time when purging will not occur; often, this is at bedtime. Patients not able to maintain a normal potassium level with supplements require hospitalization.

Setting Goals and Implementing a Dietary Plan. Setting goals is an important component of care for patients with eating disorders. Several goals are optimally specified by the primary physician. The first goal is to halt the use of diuretics and laxatives immediately. Sometimes, gradual tapering of laxatives is necessary because of the onset of severe constipation. For patients with anorexia, a *weight goal* and a *minimum acceptable weight* below which hospitalization will be required should be specified. The minimum weight is usually set at 40% below the premorbid or ideal body weight.

The weight goal is more difficult to determine and is often a point of disagreement between physician and patient. An estimate of desirable weight for height can be derived from standard tables (see Chapter 10). The weight goal should be at least 85% of the chart weight and, for female patients, a weight at which the patient has menstruated. Unless the patient was originally obese, it is usually close to the patient's premorbid weight. The patient and all caregivers should know of and agree to these weight guidelines. A *dietitian* can be very helpful in formulating and implementing an eating plan. Weight should be regained slowly, at a rate of 1 to 2 lb weekly, to avoid precipitating congestive heart failure. *Nutritional supplements* should be added if the patient is unable to gain weight at an acceptable rate.

Treating the Complications of Refeeding and Rehydration. During a reequilibration period of several weeks, temporary constipation, fluid retention, and weight gain may occur. Patients with pedal edema can be aided by *support stockings*, *leg elevation*, mild *salt restriction*, and reassurance that the condition is temporary. Diuretics in the setting of volume depletion should be avoided even if edema is present because they may exacerbate the underlying metabolic and volume disturbances. However, congestive heart failure resulting from volume overload is treated in the conventional way (see Chapter 32). To prevent constipation, patients should increase *dietary fiber* and may benefit from fiber supplements or *stool softeners*. Irritant laxative preparations are to be avoided at all costs. In cases of severe postprandial *bloating* caused by poor gastric emptying, one may be tempted to consider a prokinetic agent (e.g., metoclopramide or cisapride), but the frequency of central nervous system side effects, drug–drug interactions, and QT prolongations associated with these agents (see Chapter 61) makes their use problematic in this setting.

Amenorrhea usually responds to an *increase in weight*. Periods return within 12 months in about 70% of those who reach 90% of their ideal weight. In those who remain amenorrheic and have low serum estrogen levels leading to documented *osteoporosis*, it may be reasonable to consider *estrogen replacement therapy*, although its effects are often disappointing. No experience has been had with bisphosphonates, but they might not be very effective if the basic problem is one of too little new bone formation (see Chapter 164). Priority should be given to restoring normal weight and good nutrition, including an adequate intake of *calcium* (1.5 g/d) and *vitamin D* (400 IU/d).

Psychological and Psychopharmacologic Treatments. Because of the complex nature of eating disorders and the increased probability of serious underlying psychopathology (not to mention suicide risk), psychiatric referral for specialized multimodality care is best. Individual or group psychotherapy, behavior modification, cognitive–behavioral therapy, and family therapy are all used. Patients with early-onset anorexia appear to respond well to family therapy. Those with bulimia respond well to cognitive–behavioral measures in conjunction with interpersonal psychotherapy; so do patients with pure binge-eating disorder.

Psychopharmacologic intervention can be helpful in carefully selected instances, such as binge eating. Medication works best as a complement to psychotherapeutic and behavioral measures. *Antidepressants* have been studied the most, on the theory that eating disorders are caused by disturbances in serotonin regulation. Results have been variable. The symptoms of anorexia nervosa do not respond to antidepressant medication, but a *selective serotonin reuptake inhibitor* (SSRI) such as *fluoxetine* (up to 60 mg/d) helps sustain recovery once weight is within 15% of normal. In contrast, fluoxetine is more effective in treating the symptoms of bulimia; it is the only drug approved by the Food and Drug Administration for use in this condition. It decreases the frequency of binge eating, even in patients without coexistent depression. *Tricyclics* have also proved useful in bulimia (e.g., desipramine and imipramine, both in dosages of up to 300 mg/d). The combination of antidepressant therapy plus cognitive–behavioral therapy or psychotherapy has been found beneficial and provides the best outcomes. In binge-eating disorder, desipramine has shown promise. Unlike mild to moderate depression, in which treatment with antidepressants by primary physicians is relatively straightforward, the eating disorders should be treated with psychopharmacologic therapy only by physicians skilled and experienced in their management. One reason is the increased risk for concurrent drug and alcohol abuse, particularly among patients with bulimia.

PATIENT EDUCATION

The physician needs to inform the patient of the seriousness of her illness and its complications. The connection between the eating disorder, symptoms, and laboratory abnormalities should be explained in detail. For anorectic patients, the consequences of starvation and the necessity of weight gain must be emphasized. Patients who purge need to understand the potential consequences of their behavior (e.g., irreversible erosion of tooth enamel, cardiac arrhythmias) and the ineffectiveness of laxative or diuretic use for achieving real weight loss. Patients who have been starving themselves or abusing laxatives or diuretics should be instructed in the likelihood of transient discomfort (e.g., edema, constipation, bloating) as they stop purging and begin to eat.

INDICATIONS FOR ADMISSION AND REFERRAL

As noted earlier, anorexia is a potentially life-threatening condition. Medical criteria for hospitalization include the following: (a) loss of more than 40% of premorbid or ideal weight (or 30% if within 3 months); (b) rapid progression of weight loss; (c) presence of cardiac arrhythmias; (d) persistent hypokalemia unresponsive to outpatient treatment; and (e) symptoms of inadequate cerebral perfusion or mentation (syncope, severe dizziness, listlessness). The patient should understand that anorexia is a life-threatening illness and that the first priority is to protect life. Psychiatric hospitalization may be required for behavior beyond the patient's control or for incapacitating depression.

When outpatient management is deemed appropriate for a patient, referrals for psychiatric care and nutritional counseling are essential. It is best to select persons with expertise in the care of patients with eating disorders because treatment can be difficult. For patients with tooth enamel erosion caused by chronic emesis, a dental consultation should be obtained.

TREATMENT RECOMMENDATIONS

Effective treatment is a multidisciplinary effort, likely to require a coordinated team approach that includes care by mental health and nutritional professionals. The guidelines that follow pertain to the role of the primary physician:

- At the time of the first visit, assess the degree of malnutrition, dehydration, and electrolyte disturbance and decide whether care should proceed on an inpatient or outpatient basis.
- Be sure other causes of weight loss and its complications have been ruled out (see Chapters 9, 25, 59, 103, and 112).
- Obtain expert psychiatric and nutritional consultations; organize and coordinate a multidisciplinary team approach to management.
- Educate the patient about the medical complications of the illness.
- Set medical guidelines for outpatient management:
  - Minimum acceptable weight
  - Weight goal
  - Weight gain of 1 to 2 lb a week for underweight patients
  - Maintenance of normal electrolytes
- Monitor weight, postural signs, cardiac rhythm, and electrolytes.
- Treat any hypokalemia with potassium chloride.
- Address and treat any endocrinologic complications (see Chapters 104 and 112).
- Hospitalize the patient in the following circumstances:
  - Weight loss is in excess of 40% (or 30% if within 3 months).
  - Weight loss is rapidly progressive.
  - Cardiac arrhythmias develop (urgent).

- Persistent hypokalemia is present and unresponsive to outpatient treatment.
- Syncope, severe dizziness, or listlessness develops (urgent).
- Severe depression develops (urgent if patient becomes suicidal).

ANNOTATED BIBLIOGRAPHY

Agras WS, Rossiter EM, Arnow B, et al. One-year follow-up of psychosocial and pharmacologic treatment for bulimia nervosa. J Clin Psychiatry 1994;55:179. (*Combination therapy found to give the best results.*)

Agras WS, Rossiter EM, Arnow B, et al. Pharmacologic and cognitive-behavioral treatment of bulimia nervosa: a controlled comparison. Am J Psychiatry 1992;149:82. (*Antidepressants found useful.*)

Becker AE, Grinspoon SK, Klibanski A, et al. Eating disorders. N Engl J Med 1999;340:1092. (*Excellent and authoritative review of current evidence; 69 references.*)

Bo-Linn GW, Santa Ana CA, Morawski SG, et al. Purging and calorie absorption in bulimic patients and normal women. Ann Intern Med 1983;99:14. (*No reduction in calories absorbed; mechanism of weight loss is fluid loss from the colon.*)

Breserton TD. Toward a unified theory of serotonin dysregulation in eating and related disorders. Psychoneuroendocrinology 1995; 20:561. (*A theoretical construct that has helped direct treatment.*)

Bruce B, Wilfley D. Binge eating among the overweight population: a serious and prevalent problem. J Am Diet Assoc 1996;96:58. (*The important contribution of binge eating to obesity documented and approaches reviewed.*)

Carlat DJ, Camargo CA. A review of bulimia nervosa in males. Am J Psychiatry 1991;148:831. (*The condition is not limited to women.*)

Crago M, Shisslak CM, Estes LS. Eating disturbances among American minority groups: a review. Int J Eat Disord 1996;19:239. (*Not just a disease of middle class whites.*)

Fava M, Copeland PM, Schweiger U, et al. Neurochemical abnormalities of anorexia nervosa and bulimia nervosa. Am J Psychiatry 1989;146:963. (*Intriguing data suggesting biochemical components to these illnesses.*)

Greenfield D, Mickey D, Quinlan DM, et al. Hypokalemia in outpatients with eating disorders. Am J Psychiatry 1995;152:60. (*Good summary; results are often normal.*)

Grinspoon S, Gulick T, Askari H, et al. Serum leptin levels in women with anorexia nervosa. J Clin Endocrinol Metab 1996;81:3861. (*A possible contender for determining restoration of menses.*)

Health and Public Policy Committee, American College of Physicians. Eating disorders: anorexia nervosa and bulimia. Ann Intern Med 1986;105:790. (*A thoughtful position paper outlining the role of the primary physician in the care of patients with eating disorders.*)

Herzog DB, Nussbaum KM, Marmor AK. Comorbidity and outcome in eating disorders. Psychiatr Clin North Am 1996;19:843. (*Lots of overlap and comorbidity among patients with eating disorders; adverse impact on prognosis.*)

Isner JM, Roberts WC, Heymsfield SB, et al. Anorexia nervosa and sudden death. Ann Intern Med 1985;102:49. (*QT intervals were prolonged on ante mortem electrocardiography in three patients who died; ventricular tachycardia was the terminal rhythm.*)

Keel PK, Mitchell JE. Outcome in bulimia nervosa. Am J Psychiatry 1997;154:313. (*Useful outcomes data; about half do very well.*)

Klibanski A, Biller BMK, Schoenfeld DA, et al. The effects of estrogen administration on trabecular bone loss in young women with anorexia nervosa. J Clin Endocrinol Metab 1995;80:898. (*The rather disappointing results suggest that other factors besides es-*

trogen deficiency are involved in the osteoporosis associated with this condition.)

Mitchell JE, Seim HC, Colon E, et al. Medical complications and medical management of bulimia. Ann Intern Med 1987;107:71. (*Emphasizes importance of attention to electrolyte disturbances.*)

Ogg EC, Millar HR, Pusztai EE, et al. General practice consultation patterns preceding diagnosis of eating disorders. Int J Eat Disord 1997;22:89. (*Symptoms often misinterpreted and the eating disorder undiagnosed.*)

Oster JR, Materson BJ, Rogers AI. Laxative abuse syndrome. Am J Gastroenterol 1980;74:451. (*Reviews medical complications of prolonged laxative use, with particular attention to the pathophysiology of electrolyte disturbances.*)

Palmer EP, Guay AT. Reversible myopathy secondary to abuse of ipecac in patients with major eating disorders. N Engl J Med 1985;313:1457. (*A diffuse, gradually reversible myopathy, characterized by proximal muscle weakness and electrocardiographic abnormalities.*)

Rigotti NA, Neer RM, Skates SJ, et al. The clinical course of osteoporosis in anorexia nervosa: a longitudinal study of cortical bone mass. JAMA 1991;265:1133. (*Women with anorexia have a lower critical bone density than do normal controls, and vertebral fractures may occur.*)

Sullivan PE. Mortality in anorexia nervosa. Am J Psychiatry 1995;152:1073. (*Rate 12 times higher than that for normals underscores the seriousness of the illness.*)

Walsh BT, Wilson GT, Loeb KL, et al. Medication and psychotherapy in the treatment of bulimia nervosa. Am J Psychiatry 1997;154:523. (*Combination therapy found to be complementary.*)

235

Approach to the Substance-abusing Patient

PATRICK L. LILLARD

Abuse of and addiction to alcohol, tobacco, and illegal drugs is one of the foremost public health problems in the United States. The direct effects of these drugs produce serious morbidity and increased mortality. By their effects on behavior, however, they produce consequences even more serious. Abuse of and dependence on alcohol and other drugs disrupt interpersonal relationships and destroy lives. They contribute to accidents, crime, family violence, and lost productivity. IV drug use contributes strongly to the spread of AIDS and other infectious diseases.

Despite the pervasive penetration of substance use problems into all aspects of our culture, the ability of health care providers to assess and intervene has lagged behind the current state of knowledge. As few as 5% of substance-abusing patients presenting for medical attention have their substance abuse problem recognized. Unfortunately, physicians frequently treat the sequelae of drug abuse without directly addressing the underlying problem. To a significant extent, this is a reflection of the belief that substance abuse and dependence represent a character flaw or moral weakness rather than a disease. "The reality," in the words of Alan I. Leshner, "based on 25 years of research, is that drug addiction is a brain disease—a disease that disrupts the mechanisms responsible for generating, modulating, and controlling our cognitive, emotional, and social behavior."

DEFINITIONS

Addiction. The term *addiction* has gained many imprecise and pejorative meanings and has come to symbolize the stigma placed on patients with these disorders. The word *addict* is commonly used in the same biased manner as the words *drunk* and *junkie*. The American Psychiatric Association therefore does not use the term *addiction* and subclassifies *substance use disorders* as *substance dependence* and *substance abuse* in its current 4th edition of the *Diagnostic and Statistical Manual* (Table 235.1). It is important to note that these diagnoses are based on the presence of behavioral abnormalities; they do not indicate just physical dependence. *Substance dependence* or *abuse* is not an appropriate diagnosis for patients who are physically dependent on appropriately prescribed psychotropic or analgesic drugs, but who exhibit no addictive behaviors whatsoever (i.e., no compulsive, out-of-control use). The confusion of dependence with *addiction* may contribute to the underprescription of narcotic analgesics by physicians, even when they are indicated for cancer pain, and the undertreatment of anxiety disorders with benzodiazepines.

Substance Abuse. As noted in Table 235.1, *abuse* does not indicate dependence. It most accurately refers to the illegal, maladaptive, or dangerous use of a substance. It must be recognized that alcohol- and drug-related harm is not only the result of dependence. For example, nondependent alcohol abusers may be responsible for nearly half of alcohol-related problems, such as drunken driving, alcohol-related violence, or drunkenness on the job. Adolescent experimentation with various substances becomes abusive when it is recurrent; it does not necessary indicate dependence. The descriptive term *addict* does not apply.

Substance Dependence. In its narrowest sense, *dependence* means that a person will experience pathologic symptoms and signs when abstaining from a substance. Until recently, it was thought that the most significant indicator of *"drug addiction"* was physical dependence, manifested by symptoms of *physical withdrawal* occurring during drug abstinence, such as tremor or elevated blood pressure. Although physical dependence may certainly be a key symptom of *substance dependence* to certain drugs (e.g., alcohol or opiates), it is neither necessary nor sufficient. Some highly addictive drugs, such as cocaine and amphetamine, do not produce physical dependence or withdrawal symptoms. Moreover, many drugs with no abuse potential, such as clonidine and propranolol, may produce physical dependence (e.g., severe rebound hypertension or angina with dis-

Table 235.1. Criteria for Substance Abuse and Dependence

Substance Abuse

1. A maladaptive pattern of substance use leading to clinically significant impairment or distress, as manifested in one (or more) of the following, occurring within a 12-month period:
   - failure to fulfill major role obligations at work, school, or home
   - recurrent use in situations in which it is physically hazardous (e.g., driving an automobile)
   - recurrent use related to legal problems
   - continued use despite persistent or recurrent social or interpersonal problems caused by substance use
2. The symptoms have never met the criteria for Substance Dependence of this class of substance

Substance Dependence

A maladaptive pattern of substance use leading to clinically significant impairment or distress, as manifested by three (or more) of the following occurring at any time in the same 12-month period:
1. Tolerance, as defined by either of the following:
   a. Need for markedly increased amounts of the substance to achieve intoxication or effect
   b. Markedly diminished effect from the same amount of substance
2. Withdrawal, as manifested by either of the following:
   a. Withdrawal syndrome for the substance
   b. The same substance taken to relieve withdrawal symptoms
3. Substance taken in larger amounts or for a longer period of time than was intended
4. Persistent desire or unsuccessful efforts to cut down or control substance use
5. A great deal of time spent in activities necessary to obtain the substance
6. Important social, occupational, or recreational activities given up because of substance use
7. The substance use continued despite knowledge of having a persistent physical or psychological problem that is likely to have been caused or exacerbated by the substance

Adapted from the diagnostic criteria specified in the Diagnostic and Statistical Manual of Mental Disorders, 4th ed. Washington, DC: American Psychiatric Association, 1994, with permission.

continuation). Indeed, because cocaine does not produce physical dependence, it was widely held until the 1980s that cocaine was not addictive—a misconception that has contributed to the recent epidemic of cocaine abuse in the United States.

PATHOPHYSIOLOGY AND CLINICAL PRESENTATION

Substance Use Disorders

Data continue to accumulate supporting the concept that substance use disorders are an acquired brain disease caused by prolonged drug exposure in a vulnerable person. Neurons in the *locus coeruleus* appear to adapt to prolonged opiate exposure and fire at abnormally high rates when opiates are abruptly withdrawn, thereby triggering much of the physical withdrawal syndrome. The *mesolimbic dopamine system* provides powerful reinforcement behaviors with important survival value (e.g., sexual activity) by producing a sense of euphoria on stimulation. The most addictive of drugs (e.g., cocaine, amphetamines, opiates, alcohol, and nicotine) are thought to tap into this "brain reward" system by mimicking or enhancing the action of endogenous neurotransmitters, such as dopamine or endorphins.

With prolonged drug exposure, the neurons in this circuit undergo molecular adaptations. It has been hypothesized that the drugs that produce these adaptive responses in the mesolimbic dopamine system cause the core symptoms of substance use

disorders; a subset also produces adaptive changes in other neurons that lead to physical dependence. When the drug is stopped, the person feels that the world is intolerable without it.

In this model, the denial and manipulativeness of the person with a substance use disorder become more understandable. The key motivational system in the person's brain has been usurped by drugs. Without the drug, the person experiences strong negative emotions, an inability to feel pleasure, and an intense craving for the drug.

Why some people become addicted during the course of drug use and others do not, and why some recover and some do not, are not well understood. Factors contributing to individual vulnerability likely include genetic components, developmental experiences, intercurrent psychiatric disorders or chronic pain, current levels of distress, and complex social factors, including family and peer relationships and the availability of valued behavioral alternatives.

The debate over the origins of substance use disorders is not simply one of semantics; the inability of people to stop using alcohol, tobacco, or other drugs baffles or angers many physicians.

Cocaine, Amphetamines, and Other Central Nervous System Stimulants

Cocaine, amphetamine, and related drugs act by increasing synaptic dopamine in mesolimbic dopamine projections. Cocaine blocks the reuptake transporter that terminates the action of dopamine in the synapse. Amphetamine acts predominantly by causing dopamine release. Enhancement of the effects of serotonin and norepinephrine likely contributes to the sympathomimetic effects of these drugs. Other psychostimulants with abuse potential include methylphenidate (Ritalin) and phenmetrazine.

Pharmacokinetics. *Cocaine hydrochloride* is rapidly absorbed when taken intranasally, but it is absorbed even more rapidly during IV administration. Free-based cocaine is generally smoked, most commonly in the form of *"crack."* Because higher brain levels are achieved more rapidly, IV administration and smoking are far more addictive than intranasal "snorting."

Amphetamines include racemic amphetamine sulfate (e.g., Benzedrine and others), dextroamphetamine (e.g., Dexedrine), and methamphetamine (Methedrine). Methamphetamine is the most potent and potentially toxic form of amphetamine. Amphetamine can be taken orally or IV. Methamphetamine is also smoked (a recent name for smoked methamphetamine is "ice"). High levels of tolerance develop in persons who use amphetamine on a regular basis, so that increasing doses of the drug become necessary. These people are at high risk for the development of a paranoid psychosis.

Perhaps the most important difference between cocaine and amphetamine derivatives is in half-life; the effects of amphetamine last longer than those of cocaine. These differences in half-life lead to different use patterns (see below).

Clinical Effects and Patterns of Abuse. Cocaine and amphetamine produce many of the same clinical effects, most importantly euphoria, which is a sense of increased energy and confidence, and sympathomimetic actions. They may also produce restlessness, anxiety, hostility, and paranoia, especially with cumulative or higher doses. Other effects include tachycardia, hypertension, fever, and tremor. With dependence, patients may exhibit jitteriness, weight loss, depression, and a lack of energy.

Because the effects of cocaine are short-lived, it is often taken in binges to maintain drug-induced euphoria. At the termination of a binge, a withdrawal syndrome is often evident, characterized by severe dysphoria, anhedonia, fatigue, and a craving for cocaine.

Amphetamine may also be used in binges, but many people take the drug orally on a daily basis. They may start amphetamine to control weight or decrease fatigue. As dosages accelerate because of tolerance, many such people become irritable and paranoid. Overdosing with cocaine or amphetamine produces tachyarrhythmias, hypertension, high fever, seizures, delirium, paranoia, psychosis, coma, and cardiovascular collapse. Stroke and myocardial infarction have been reported with crack use.

Despite their similarities, cocaine and amphetamine do not parallel each other in popularity. The United States is in the waning phase of a cocaine epidemic that has lasted for nearly two decades. The use of cocaine among the middle class has declined markedly; however, use among "hard core" cocaine-dependent persons has not decreased. In this population, crack cocaine is the most frequently used form. Amphetamine, including IV methamphetamine, was popular before the start of the recent cocaine epidemic, and in the late 1990s it seems to have made a comeback.

Opiates

The opiates produce their effects by binding to endogenous opiate receptors. The major therapeutic use of opiates is for analgesia. Less potent opiates are also used as antitussives and antidiarrheal agents. The most highly abused opiates are those that interact predominantly with μ-type opiate receptors. These include heroin; less commonly morphine or meperidine, which are generally injected IV; and oxycodone and hydromorphone, which are most often taken orally. Heroin may also be smoked.

Clinical Effects and Patterns of Abuse. Opiates produce an initial sense of euphoria (a "rush"), especially after IV injection or smoking, which is followed by a sense of tranquillity and then sleepiness. Tolerance and dependence develop, so that increasing doses are required to achieve the desired euphoria. Tolerance to the respiratory depressant effects of opiates develops approximately in parallel. Tolerance to opiate-induced pupillary constriction does not develop.

Unlike alcohol, for example, opiates do not directly produce serious organ pathology. Constipation is the major side effect of opiate use and may represent a significant problem (e.g., in patients being treated for cancer pain). However, opiates produce high levels of psychological dependence, and the widely used method of administering them (IV injection, often with shared needles) may result in hepatitis B, HIV infection, endocarditis, infection of the local injection site, and other complications of nonsterile self-injection.

Overdoses of opiates may be lethal because of respiratory depression. Overdosing is most frequent when the heroin dose is purer than what the addicted person is accustomed to, when

tolerance levels are miscalculated after detoxification, and when the user is inexperienced.

Withdrawal from opiates may be uncomfortable but is not lethal. Withdrawal from heroin may begin 6 to 12 hours after the last dose in dependent persons and is manifested by agitation, drug craving, tachycardia, hypertension, fever, muscle cramps, nausea, and rhinorrhea.

Sedative-Hypnotics

The sedative-hypnotics include the *benzodiazepines*, *barbiturates*, and the *barbiturate-like drugs* (e.g., glutethimide, ethchlorvynol). These agents enhance the inhibitory effects of γ-aminobutyric acid ($GABA_A$) receptors in the brain. Because *ethyl alcohol* similarly affects these receptors, marked sedation is associated with concurrent use. In comparison with the benzodiazepines, the barbiturates and similarly acting compounds have a greater potential for abuse, overdose, and drug–drug interactions (by inducing hepatic microsomal enzymes). They have no place in general practice except as anticonvulsants (phenobarbital).

Benzodiazepines are most commonly prescribed for the short-term treatment of insomnia and for anxiety disorders (see Chapters 226 and 232). They can cause dependence with long-term use, so that the drugs must be slowly tapered after a course of treatment. The likelihood of dependence is greater with high-potency, short-acting compounds (e.g., alprazolam, triazolam) than with low-potency, long-acting compounds (e.g., diazepam, chlordiazepoxide). Although abuse and addiction may occur, it is relatively uncommon for the benzodiazepines to produce addictive behaviors (compulsive nonmedical use) except in patients with a prior history of drug abuse. Prolonged benzodiazepine use, carefully monitored, may be necessary for patients with disabling anxiety disorders (see Chapter 226).

Clinical Effects and Patterns of Abuse. When abused, the sedative-hypnotics produce disinhibition, which appears very similar to drunkenness; disinhibition is often followed by drowsiness. *Overdosing* with barbiturates produces respiratory depression and coma and may cause death. Benzodiazepines are not likely to be lethal when taken alone in overdose, but when combined with alcohol, they can cause death from respiratory depression.

Withdrawal from sedative-hypnotic drugs produces tachycardia, hypertension, fever, tremulousness, hyperreflexia, anxiety, restlessness, insomnia, and anorexia. Seizures and delirium may occur and may be severe. Unlike opiate withdrawal, sedative-hypnotic withdrawal may be fatal.

Marijuana

Marijuana is produced from the dried leaves and flowers of the hemp plant, *Cannabis sativa*. The active ingredient, D-9-tetrahydrocannabinol (THC), acts by binding to an endogenous THC receptor in the brain, the normal function of which is unknown. During the past decade, the clonal selection of hemp plants for high THC content has markedly increased the potency of marijuana sold on the street.

Marijuana is generally smoked, although occasionally it is taken orally. It produces a feeling of relaxation, mild euphoria, and increased sociability. Physical symptoms and signs include mild tachycardia, dry mouth, and conjunctival injection. The most common short-term adverse consequence is an acute panic reaction, which may occur in inexperienced users, especially after they have smoked high-potency marijuana. Rarely, large doses of high-potency marijuana can produce hallucinations, paranoia, and delirium. Marijuana is far less addictive than cocaine, amphetamine, opiates, alcohol, nicotine, or barbiturates. Nonetheless, some habitual users appear to be dependent. Prolonged use may impair testosterone secretion and lead to gynecomastia.

Hallucinogens

The hallucinogens, or psychedelic compounds, are a group of structurally diverse compounds that appear to act by mimicking the actions of serotonin at certain of its receptor subtypes. The most widely used hallucinogens are the indolalkylamine compounds, including D-*lysergic acid diethylamide* (LSD), *dimethyltryptamine* (DMT), and *psilocybin* (which is the active ingredient in *"magic" mushrooms*), and the phenylethylamine compounds, such as the "designer" drug *MDMA* (*"ecstasy"*) and *mescaline* (derived from the peyote cactus). Compounds such as MDMA, which are structurally related to amphetamine, may also have mild agonist effects on dopamine systems and produce modest euphoric effects.

Clinical Effects and Patterns of Abuse. LSD produces both *sympathomimetic* and *perceptual* effects. The sympathomimetic effects, such as increased pulse rate, blood pressure, and mydriasis, generally precede the perceptual changes, which include visual illusions, hallucinations, confusion among sensory modalities (synesthesias), depersonalization, and altered time perception. Most LSD "trips" last 8 to 12 hours. The predominant effects of psilocybin and mescaline are similar to those of LSD. MDMA produces disinhibition and increased sociability; illusions are not prominent. MDMA also produces muscle twitching and bruxism. MDMA has recently become popular at large dancing parties called "raves"; rare deaths have been reported in such circumstances from hyperthermia caused by the combination of MDMA, many hours of intense exertion, and lack of hydration.

The most common immediate adverse effect of hallucinogen use is a *panic reaction* or "bad trip." Extreme agitation or *delirium* occurs rarely, but often as a result of exposure to additional drugs or adulterants, particularly *phencyclidine*. In such circumstances, a toxic screen should be obtained.

Patients in whom *psychotic episodes* develop after hallucinogen use are difficult to sort out. Generally, the history of psychiatric disturbance precedes the use of the hallucinogen. *Flashbacks*, which consist of brief, recurrent visual illusions or hallucinations, may occur for months or, rarely, for several years after hallucinogen use.

Hallucinogens do not appear to be physically addictive. Their major dangers relate to the state of intoxication they produce, in which judgment is markedly impaired and panic reactions possible. These predispose to accidents, violence, and suicide (which may be inadvertent). In addition, animal data demonstrate that MDMA is highly toxic to serotonin neurons in the brain. Whether MDMA produces lesions of the serotonin system in humans is not known but is a concern.

Phencyclidine

Phencyclidine, like marijuana and other hallucinogens, does not produce a physiologic withdrawal pattern in humans, but a psychological abstinence syndrome is observed that includes depression, craving, and fatigue. Most important is the variable presentation of intoxication and overdose with diverse behavioral and psychological manifestations (delirium, psychosis, catatonia, mania, depression, extreme agitation and violence) or with physiologic manifestations (nystagmus, hypertension, tachycardia, hyperreflexia that may lead to rhabdomyolysis, renal failure). The behavioral and physiologic effects can occur together or in stages that complicate the diagnosis and treatment, and they can progress to life-threatening stupor and coma in which the patient is unresponsive to pain. A careful history is mandatory, as is constant awareness in the acute setting of the possibility of phencyclidine intoxication.

Alcohol and Tobacco

(See Chapters 54 and 228.)

WORKUP: SCREENING FOR SUBSTANCE ABUSE

A principal objective of the evaluation in the office setting is to screen for substance abuse. This is important in both asymptomatic persons who come in for a checkup and those who present with suggestive historical or physical findings (Table 235.2).

History. The best means of screening is by history. Because drug use may be an emotionally charged issue, it should be addressed after some rapport with the patient has been established. It is important that the physician feel comfortable in obtaining the history, neither apologizing for asking nor suggesting blame. Apologizing ("I have to ask these questions" or "I'm sure this doesn't apply to you, but...") may actually make it more difficult for the substance-abusing patient to respond honestly. The clinician with a judgmental approach will not diagnose this disease (see below).

Physical Examination should include a check for fever, tachycardia, hypertension, skin manifestations of HIV infection (see Chapter 13) and endocarditis, icterus, needle tracks, nasal septal perforation, mucosal congestion, gynecomastia, adenopathy, heart murmur, liver enlargement, tremor, and cognitive impairment.

Laboratory. When substance abuse is strongly suspected but cannot be confirmed by history, a toxic screen with urine and blood testing may be necessary. The febrile patient requires extensive evaluation, beginning with blood cultures (see Chapter 11).

PRINCIPLES OF MANAGEMENT

Substance abuse treatment may be divided into two phases, *initiation* of abstinence in the short term and *maintenance* of abstinence in the long term. For the physician, it is useful to view drug addiction, including alcoholism, as a chronic, relapsing,

Table 235.2. Historical and Physical Findings Suggestive of Substance Abuse

SUBSTANCE	HISTORY	PHYSICAL FINDINGS
Opiates	Fever HIV infection Hepatitis B Pneumonia, tuberculosis	Needle tracks, petechiae, murmur Lymphadenopathy, rash Jaundice, hepatomegaly/tenderness Pulmonary consolidation
Sedatives	Depression Seizures Lethargy, amnesia	Psychomotor retardation, sadness Observed convulsion Cognitive impairment
Stimulants	Agitation Nasal congestion Stroke, focal deficits Chest pain, infarction Syncope, palpitations	Delirium Perforated septum; mucosal edema New neurologic deficits New S_4 gallop, single S_2 Arrhythmia, enlarged heart, S_3
Halucinogens	Psychosis, hallucinations Enlarged breasts in male patient	Disordered thinking Gynecomastia
Alcohol	(see Chapter 228)	
Any substance	Withdrawal syndrome	Tremor, tachycardia, agitation, fever

Adapted from Shine RD. The diagnosis of drug dependence by primary care providers. J Gen Intern Med 1991;6[Suppl]: S32, with permission.

progressive disease. Even after successful treatment, patients remain at high risk for relapse. Relapses should be seen not as failures of treatment but as occasions to reinstate abstinence and subsequently to redouble efforts to maintain abstinence.

Getting the Patient into Care. The best chance of successful intervention, even with severe dependence and high levels of denial, is to match the patient's Stage of Change with a treatment strategy. In the *precontemplative stage* the patient does not recognize a problem and a labeling, coercive approach will fail. The best strategy is to be empathetic in demonstrating to the patient the problems (such as liver disease, or loss of employment) that results from substance abuse. In the *contemplation stage* the patient recognizes a problem but is ambivalent about stopping, and the treatment strategy is to use the ambivalence to demonstrate the downside of the substance use. Similarly, with the *planning stage,* the treatment should be designed to help the patient and family plan concrete steps to implement to change. Then in the *action stage* with support (AA is a good example) the patient carries out behavioral changes that result in abstinence. Finally in the *maintenance stage* the strategy is relapse prevention: high risk behavior is examined and changed before a return to precontemplation. It is important to honor confidentiality, but it useful to include the family in matching the treatment with stage of change.

It is valuable to keep referral numbers close at hand to take advantage of the patient's motivation. And remember, though an intoxicated patient has impaired judgment and insight, they often remember an empathic clinician and seek help later.

Once the patient acknowledges having a problem, a decision can be made with the patient regarding a treatment plan. The physician should have referral numbers close at hand so that the patient's moment of motivation is not lost.

Unfortunately, the judgment and insight of an intoxicated patient are impaired, and the patient may not be able to understand the initial efforts to provide help. However, patients often remember an empathic, nonjudgmental clinician and return for help later.

Comprehensive Substance Abuse Treatment is best left to specialists and specialized organizations. Treatment programs

vary according to the patient and the substance, but successful programs have several characteristics in common:

1. *Evaluation* for comorbid psychiatric or medical disorders (presence of a comorbid psychiatric disorder worsens prognosis)
2. *Education* about the effects of the drug and the nature of addiction
3. Use of *mutual support groups* such as Alcoholics Anonymous or the similarly organized Narcotics Anonymous
4. *Individual psychotherapy*
5. *Family involvement* and promotion of a sense of belonging, and use of other supportive measures such as exercise, meditation, and discussion of spirituality that may include organized religion
6. Emphasis on *abstinence* and *rehabilitation*

Importance of Abstinence. Most treatment programs stress a combination of abstinence and rehabilitation. Although there have been reports of alcoholic patients returning safely to controlled drinking, it is impossible to identify such persons ahead of time. It appears that for most people who have been drug-dependent, a single use reawakens the strong positive feelings that helped produce the dependence to begin with, and also loosens restraint. Thus, complete abstinence is the best way to avoid relapse.

Medication. Drugs that produce aversive reactions (*disulfiram* for alcohol) or block pleasure (*naltrexone* for opiates) can be of value in the short term but require a very motivated patient and intensive support. Specific pharmacologic treatment to diminish craving is not available for cocaine (despite limited success with desipramine). Clear evidence now suggests that naltrexone and acamprosate (soon to be available) do decrease alcohol use by decreasing craving and interfering with the pleasure of use. For opiate addicts not ready to be detoxified, *methadone* maintenance may be very helpful in permitting them to stabilize their lives and avoid the dangers of IV drug abuse. Methadone maintenance can be administered only at specially licensed treatment centers. LAMM, a longer-acting opiate agonist, and buprenorphine, a mixed agonist/antagonist, show promise as maintenance agents. *Nicotine patches* and *bupropion* may be useful in decreasing craving in some smokers and may play a useful role in smoking cessation programs when supplemented by psychosocial measures (see Chapter 54).

Treatment of Acute Overdoses and Toxic Reactions. An overdose or toxic reaction should be treated in the emergency department setting. The details of such treatment are beyond the scope of this book, but a few highlights are included here to aid in decision making and triage:

- Cocaine: no specific cocaine antagonist. Treatment is aimed at relieving symptoms and providing cardiovascular support.
- Opiates: cardiovascular and airway supportive care. Naloxone (Narcan), an opiate antagonist, is administered IV; usual dose is 0.01 mg/kg; average person will take approximately two ampules (0.8 mg). Half-life of naloxone is shorter than half-life of heroin, so that continuous observation and possibly repeated dosing are necessary.
- Sedative-hypnotics: airway and cardiovascular support. Benzodiazepine antagonist, flumazenil, is available, but clinical experience is limited.
- Marijuana: for panic reaction, reassurance that the feeling will pass, and ensuring that the patient is in a safe environment.
- Hallucinogens: for a "bad trip," reassurance and maintenance of a safe environment; rarely, 1 to 2 mg of lorazepam PO (or its equivalent) for agitation; for extreme agitation or delirium, physical restraint and 2 mg of lorazepam every 2 hours (or the equivalent) as needed. Obtain toxic screen to search for adulterants and additional drugs. For flashbacks, reassurance is best.

INDICATIONS FOR ADMISSION AND REFERRAL

Patients who are physically dependent on sedative-hypnotics, alcoholic patients with a history of severe withdrawal symptoms, persons with serious complicating medical or psychiatric conditions, and those who have previously failed to improve with outpatient treatment should be referred for inpatient treatment. Detoxification can be safely performed on an outpatient basis in appropriate cases, but a comprehensive specialized program is required.

Opiate detoxification protocols are based on the following:

1. Substitution of a long-acting oral opiate, methadone, for short-acting injected opiates, such as heroin, with a taper during 4 days to 2 weeks depending on the setting; or
2. Use of opiate agonist/antagonist buprenorphine, which can be given IM or sublingually during a course of 4 to 5 days.

All detoxification programs must be accompanied by strong psychological and social support, education, and planning for long-term treatment that should include, whenever possible, the continued support and involvement of the primary care physician.

ANNOTATED BIBLIOGRAPHY

Allen PA, Litten RZ. Screening instruments and biochemical screening tests. In: Principles of addiction medicine, 2nd ed. American Society of Addiction Medicine, 1998:263. (*Comprehensive guide with good section on screening methods.*)

Cherubin CE, Sapira JD. The medical complications of drug addiction and the medical assessment of the intravenous drug user: 25 years later. Ann Intern Med 1993;119:1017. (*Important review for the primary care physician.*)

Gawin FH, Ellinwood EH. Cocaine and other stimulants: actions, abuse, and treatment. N Engl J Med 1988;318:1173. (*Good review.*)

Leshner AI. What we know: drug addiction is a brain disease. In: Principles of addiction medicine, 2nd ed. American Society of Addiction Medicine, 1998. (*Fine summary of pathophysiology.*)

Levine SR, Brust JCM, Frutell N, et al. Cerebrovascular complications of the use of the "crack" form of alkaloidal cocaine. N Engl J Med 1990;323:699. (*Major adverse effect not fully appreciated.*)

National Consensus Development Panel on Effective Medical Treatment of Opiate Addiction. Effective medical treatment of opiate addiction. JAMA 1998;280:1936. (*Evidence-based consensus guidelines by expert panel convened by the National Institutes of Health.*)

O'Connor PG, Oliveto AH, Shi JM, et al. A randomized trial of buprenorphine maintenance for heroin dependence in a primary care clinic for substance users versus a methadone clinic. Am J Med 1998;105:100. (*A randomized trial showing effectiveness of buprenorphine maintenance in a primary care setting.*)

O'Connor PG, Kosten TR. Rapid and ultrarapid opioid detoxification techniques. JAMA 1998;279:229. (*Expert literature review; concludes available studies are inadequate to answer the question of which is best and when.*)

O'Connor PG, Waugh ME, Carroll KM, et al. Primary care-based ambulatory opioid detoxification: results of a clinical trial. J Gen Intern Med 1995;10:255. (*Finds detoxification can be carried out safely by primary care providers using a program of clonidine and naltrexone.*)

Passaro DJ, Werner B, McGee J, et al. Wound botulism associated with black tar heroin among injecting drug users. JAMA 1998;279:859. (*Injection SQ or IM with spore-infected needles is the mode of infection and can lead to flaccid paralysis.*)

Rivara FP, Mueller BA, Somes G, et al. Alcohol and illicit drug abuse and the risk of violent death in the home. JAMA 1997;278:569 (*Documentation of the seemingly obvious fact that persons in the household of a substance abuser are also at increased risk for death.*)

Sees KL, Delucchi KL, Masson C, et al. Methadone maintenance vs. 180-day psychosocially enriched detoxification for treatment of opioid dependence: a randomized controlled trial. JAMA 2000;283:1303. (*Methadone maintenance proved to be the more effective treatment in terms of reducing heroin use and high-risk behaviors.*)

Shine D. The diagnosis of drug dependence by primary care providers. J Gen Intern Med 1991;6[Suppl]:S32. (*A useful discussion of basic approaches to recognition in the office.*)

Strain EC, Bigelow GE, Liebson IA, et al. Moderate- vs. high-dose methadone in the treatment of opioid dependence: a randomized trial. (*Both were effective, but high-dose therapy produced a significantly greater decreases in illicit opioid use.*)

Tinsley JA, Watkins DD. Over-the-counter stimulants: abuse and addiction. Mayo Clin Proc 1998;73:977. (*Good review of this often overlooked area of addiction; emphasis on abuse of ephedrine and phenylpropanolamine.*)

Volpicelli JR, O'Brien C, Alterman A, et al. Naltrexone in the treatment of alcohol dependence. Arch Gen Psychiatry 1992;49:867. (*Good review of the drug.*)

Weiss RD, Greenfield SF, Mirin SM. Intoxication and withdrawal syndromes. In: Hyman SE, Tesar GE, eds. Manual of psychiatric emergencies, 3rd ed. Boston: Little, Brown, 1994. (*Useful summary for the generalist reader.*)

236
Approach to the Patient with Chronic Nonmalignant Pain
TODD E. GORMAN

Chronic pain is a highly prevalent problem, affecting up to 17% of Americans and costing society an estimated 70 billion dollars each year. Many clinicians find chronic pain an emotional and intellectual challenge. Part of this stems from the fact that there are many myths amongst clinicians surrounding chronic pain (Table 236.1).

Unlike acute pain, chronic pain tends to be more multifactorial, less amenable to "cure," and more influenced by psychological and social factors. It typically requires continuous long-term management. These characteristics necessitate an appropriate adjustment of expectations and approach by both clinician and patient to achieve a satisfactory outcome. The principal goal is improvement in quality of life and function, rather than complete elimination of the pain.

PATHOPHYSIOLOGY AND CLINICAL PRESENTATIONS

Definition and the Biopsychosocial Model of Pain

Pain is defined by the International Association for the Study of Pain as "an unpleasant sensory and emotional experience arising from actual or potential tissue damage." Pain is an inherently subjective phenomenon, originating from a biologic source and modified by psychological and social factors. Perceptions and reports of pain and its severity rely heavily on a person's psychosocial context. For this reason, the *biopsychosocial model* proves useful in the conceptualization of pain.

Biologic Components. Pain derives from afferent signals of nociceptive fibers in the periphery, triggered by tissue damage or the threat of damage (*nociceptive pain*), or by direct neuronal activation (*neuropathic pain*). These afferent nociceptive fibers course back to the central nervous system via the spinothalamic tracts to both somatosensory and frontal cortices. *Modulation networks* from the frontal cortex and hypothalamus create a final conscious perception. These networks are the medium by which psychological factors and the psychosocial context alter the sensation of pain.

The biologic component of chronic pain is less well understood than that of acute pain. It appears that many patients suffering from chronic pain do so with a minor biologic stimulus or occasionally even without one once the process has begun. Psychological and social factors clearly play a larger role in modulating the perception and perpetuating it. Perpetuation likely occurs via *neuronal sensitization* and the above-mentioned modulation networks.

In neuronal sensitization, the threshold for activating nociceptors is lowered by repetitive stimuli. Continuous triggering of nociceptive fibers generates pain even when the stimulus is minimal. Modulatory factors include *expectation*, whereby the sensation of pain is heightened by the anticipation of its arrival. This is related to the effects of norepinephrine on sympathetic input to nociceptive fibers; it lowers their threshold for activation and even activates them directly. A well-known corollary to the modulation of pain through expectation is the *placebo effect*, which is still poorly understood but clearly decreases an individual's perception of pain via neuronal modulation.

Psychological Components. Besides modulating pain, psychological components may actually be considered as a cause (i.e., *primary*) or effect (i.e., *secondary*) of chronic pain. Primary psychological considerations include whether the patient has a major *depression* (see Chapter 227), *anxiety* disorder (see Chapter 226), *somatoform disorder* or *personality disorder* (see Chapters 227 and 230), or *substance abuse* problem (see Chapter 235), or whether the patient is malingering (Table 236.2).

Most of these disorders cause a heightened awareness of somatic sensations, a charged emotional state, and a sense of expectation. Heightened awareness results in an inability to suppress stimuli that the individual might otherwise be capable of suppressing. A charged emotional state sensitizes nociceptive fibers to stimuli, also creating an enhanced conscious perception of pain.

Secondary psychological processes like depression and anxiety are common among patients with chronic pain, as is secondary substance abuse if the patient self-medicates with alcohol or narcotics. These secondary processes may also contribute to modulating and perpetuating a sensation of pain.

Table 236.1. Myths Surrounding Chronic Pain

- Patients' complaints stem from secondary gains; they do not really suffer "pain."
- Patients with chronic pain are inherently noncompliant and manipulative.
- Patients given opiates will refer manipulative friends.
- Opiates in therapeutic doses will cause respiratory depression.
- Patients given opiates will become "addicted."
- Giving patients opiates for chronic nonmalignant pain will result in investigations by state and federal review boards.
- Chronic pain can be fixed.

Table 236.2. Psychological and Social Factors Contributing to Chronic Pain

Psychological factors	Social factors
Major depression (1° or 2°)	Domestic violence
Anxiety disorders (1° or 2°)	Daily activities causing pain
Somatoform disorders	Activities hindered by pain
Personality disorders	Work hindered by pain
Substance abuse (1° or 2°)	Work contributing to pain
Malingering	Secondary gain

Social Contributors encompass elements in the home, in the work environment, and at leisure (Table 236.2). Although the home environment may serve as a potential source of relief and support for the patient with chronic pain, more often it contributes to the presentation, as with *domestic violence*. Pain may even serve as a cause for escape from a troubled home situation to the doctor. Likewise, a person's leisure and work environments may contribute to or be hindered by pain. Social factors can drive the sensation of pain into a chronic state if secondary gain is a possibility (e.g., ongoing litigation, worker's compensation).

Categorizations of Pain

Pain can be categorized by either clinical presentation (acute vs. chronic; diffuse vs. localized) or by underlying mechanism (neuropathic vs. nociceptive; biologic vs. psychosocial).

Acute versus Chronic Pain. In general, *acute pain* emanates from an identifiable biologic stimulus, is self-limited, does not have much of a psychological component, and is more amenable to pure pharmacologic intervention. *Chronic pain* is that which lasts longer than a typically expected time for healing, or 3 to 6 months. It can be further subclassified as chronic nonmalignant pain or chronic malignant pain (see Chapter 90). Chronic nonmalignant pain, on the other hand, may or may not have an identifiable biologic stimulus, is by definition *not* self-limited, has greater psychosocial underpinnings, and is less amenable to pure pharmacologic intervention.

Diffuse versus Localized Pain. Some patients present with total body pain or pain that migrates from one site to another. These cases tend to have dominant psychosocial components. Most patients present with pain localized to a certain anatomic region, which remains consistent over time. The most common presentations include pain localized to one of five regions: head and face, nonaxial musculoskeletal structures, low back, abdomen and pelvis, and peripheral nerves.

Nociceptive versus Neuropathic Pain. *Nociceptive pain* develops from actual or potential tissue or organ damage. *Somatic* nociceptive pain is typically attributable to specific anatomic areas or structures. Patients present with pain that is well localized and stabbing, throbbing, or achy. *Visceral* nociceptive pain, being organ-based, is less well localized and typically more dull and cramping.

Neuropathic pain, on the other hand, derives from direct nerve stimulation. This may occur with or without a nociceptive component. The pain is typically characterized as burning, tingling, and lancinating, often occurring in a dermatomal distribution. A sensory deficit may accompany the pain. Sensitization can lead to the nerves firing in the absence of any peripheral stimulus. Examples of neuropathic pain include post-herpetic neuralgia, diabetic neuropathy, sciatica, trigeminal neuralgia, reflex sympathetic dystrophy, and phantom limb pain.

Predominantly Biologic versus Predominantly Psychosocial. The balance of biologic and psychosocial components may vary tremendously. Some cases have a primarily *biologic* cause with no evidence of psychiatric pathology (e.g., a func-

tional, well-adjusted octogenarian with severe osteoarthritis). Others present with the subjective report of pain but no objective findings and go on to meet formal criteria for a primary *psychiatric* disorder (e.g., a young professional suffering from hypochondriasis).

The majority of patients presenting with chronic pain are somewhere in between these two extremes, with a *combination* of both biologic and psychosocial components. Quantification of overlap has not been performed extensively in patients presenting with chronic pain, although some data exist. For example, *comorbid major depression* is found in 8% to 50% of patients presenting with chronic pain, with *dysthymia* seen in more than 75%. Likewise, *anxiety disorders* (both panic attack and generalized anxiety disorder) are seen in more than 50%.

DIFFERENTIAL DIAGNOSIS

Any differential diagnosis for chronic pain must include both biologic and psychosocial factors. The biologic causes are best considered in terms of pain location (Table 236.3). The psychosocial determinants are essential considerations in assessing factors that may trigger, sustain, or aggravate pain (Table 236.2).

WORKUP

The heterogeneity of chronic pain complaints and the variety of mechanisms and presentations necessitate exploration of both biologic and psychosocial dimensions of the problem. The workup should define the patient's psychosocial context, classify the pain process precisely, and determine the likelihood of serious underlying biologic pathology.

Defining the Psychosocial Context. All patients presenting with chronic pain must be screened carefully for depression, anxiety, evidence of a somatoform disorder or personality disorder, substance use/abuse, and possible secondary gain. Clues suggesting a primary psychological or social cause include depressed or anxious affect, history of substance abuse, multiple unrelated sites of pain, onset in adolescence, history of difficult social interactions, and absence of a clear pathophysiologic mechanism (Table 236.4). Home, work, and leisure activities should be reviewed in depth for possible precipitating and aggravating social factors (see the Appendix for a more detailed discussion of screening for domestic violence).

Classifying the Process. The classic cardinal features of pain should always be documented: onset/duration, quality/severity, location/spread, alleviating/aggravating factors, and associated symptoms. Circumstances surrounding the onset of the pain, in addition to the location of pain and associated symptoms, are all particularly helpful in determining whether or not a patient's presentation might relate to a biologically plausible process or is predominantly psychological or psychosocial in origin. These features will also help determine if the pain is acute or chronic, localized or diffuse, somatic or visceral, and nociceptive or neuropathic. Correct classification helps guide further workup and management.

Patients of different cultural backgrounds will describe pain *quality* in distinctively different terms, so that some basic cultural understanding is necessary to interpret the complaint of

Table 236.3. Differential Diagnoses of Chronic Pain Based on Location

LOCATION	DIFFERENTIAL OF REVERSIBLE ETIOLOGIES		
Headache/facial Pain (see Chapters 165 and 214)	tension migraine cluster temporal arteritis large AVM hypertension dentalgia	sinusitis chronic otitis chronic meningitis abscess subdural tumor TMJ	glaucoma medication trigeminal neuralgia post-concussive glaucoma bruxism sialadenitis
Musculoskeletal Pain (see Chapters 147–154)	fibromyalgia PMR polymyostitis dermatomyositis drug myositis hypothyroidism trauma	rheumatoid arthritis osteoarthritis gout/pseudogout SLE osteomyelitis trichinosis Lyme disease	Paget's disease tumor cramps bursitis/tendinitis reflex sympathetic dystrophy sickle cell disease secondary syphilis
Low Back Pain (see Chapter 147)	chronic disk disease sciatica vertebral osteoarthropathy	osteoporotic fracture spinal stenosis epidural abscess	tumor (bone/retroperitoneum) seronegative spondylosis
Abdominal/pelvic Pain (see Chapters 58 and 116)	irritable bowel biliary colic esophagitis pancreatitis parasitosis aortic aneurysm sickle cell medicines	IBD diverticulitis gastritis/PUD hepatitis tumor (GI/GU/GYN) abdominal angina poisoning (e.g., lead) internal hernias PMS	kidney stones chronic pyelonephritis polycystic kidney endometriosis ovarian cysts PID/TOA FMF porphyria
Peripheral Nerve Pain (see Chapter 167)	DM neuropathy HIV neuropathy paraneoplastic	B_{12} deficiency CTDz renal failure	Charcot-Marie-Tooth disease hypothyroidism poisoning (EtOH, Pt, INH)

AVM, arteriovenous malformation; TMJ, temporomandibular joint; PMR, polymyalgia rheumatica; SLE, systemic lupus erythematosus; IBD, inflammatory bowel disease; PUD, peptic ulcer disease; GI, gastrointestinal; GU, genitourinary; GYN, gynecologic; PMS, premenstrual syndrome; PID, pelvic inflammatory disease; TOA, tubo-ovarian abscess; FMF, familial Mediterranean fever; DM, diabetes mellitus; EtOH, ethanol; Pt, platinum; CTDz, connective tissue disease; INH, isoniazid.

Table 236.4. Signs That Psychosocial Factors Are Predominant in a Patient's Chronic Pain

- The patient admits *depression* or *anxiety* that predates the pain.
- The pain began in adolescence or at time of trauma (suggests *pain disorder or PTSD*).
- The patient has a history of *substance abuse.*
- There are multiple, unrelated sites of pain over time (suggests *somatization disorder*).
- There is no demonstrable pathophysiologic mechanism to explain the physical symptoms.
- There is a history of difficult social interactions to suggest a *personality disorder.*
- There is evidence of physical, sexual, or emotional *abuse.*
- There is potential for or history of the patient pursuing secondary gains, such as litigation reward or worker's compensation (suggests malingering).

PTSD, posttraumatic stress disorder.

pain properly. For example, patients of Caribbean descent often describe abdominal pain as *grippée*, whereas Southeast Asians may use temperature to describe abdominal pain, and Latinos refer to many sensations as *nervios.* Pain severity can be assessed by standard severity scales, most of which are cross-culturally reproducible. Examples include the visual analogue pain scale or 1-to-10 rating scales. These scales may also be useful when applied to stepwise pharmacologic management, so it is worth documenting severity during the workup.

Determining the Likelihood of Serious Underlying Biologic Pathology. If the pain complaint is relatively new, has little in the way of associated psychiatric symptoms, and is accompanied by constitutional or other objective findings, then the likelihood of a primary biologic process increases markedly and the workup can focus on the appropriate physical examination and laboratory testing.

PRINCIPLES OF MANAGEMENT

Basic Approach

A systematic, multidimensional approach is crucial to achieving a successful outcome for the patient with chronic pain (Fig. 236.1). Simultaneously addressing the biologic and psychosocial components helps assure the patient that the validity of the complaint is not in question; as a result, compliance with psychiatric referral is improved, should it be needed.

Early Psychiatric Referral. Early referral is essential if the initial evaluation reveals evidence for a primary psychiatric or psychosocial problem (e.g., anxiety, depression, personality disorder, domestic violence). Effective management may require formal psychiatric input, including psychopharmacologic intervention, psychotherapy, and social interventions. Patients with what appears to be a psychiatric process secondary to the chronic pain are better managed by first addressing the biologic cause of the pain rather than by psychiatric referral, as attention to biologic factors is likely to improve both processes at once.

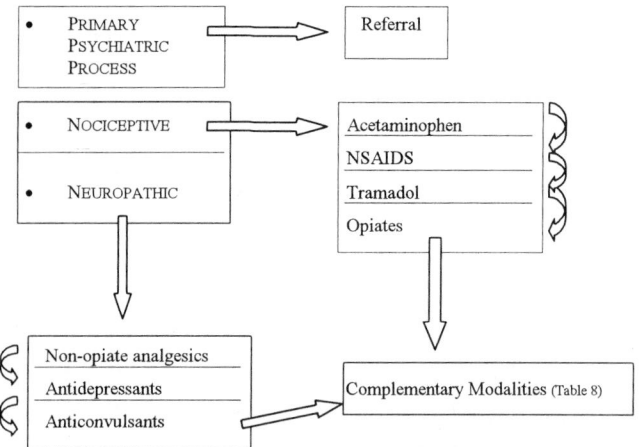

FIG. 236.1. Sample approach to the management of patients with chronic pain.

Symptomatic Relief. Early symptom relief is a priority, especially in persons with a suspected primary biologic mechanism. The intervention is usually pharmacologic, tailored to whether the pain is primarily nociceptive or neuropathic in origin. A stepwise approach is recommended, beginning with pain medications that have the greatest benefit-to-risk ratio (Table 236.5). The goal is to provide enough analgesia that daily activity can be sustained. Complementary approaches to pain control may be needed when medications do not suffice.

Nociceptive (Non-neuropathic) Pain

Treatment begins with non-narcotic analgesics and advances to narcotic agents as required. Non-narcotic analgesics are first-line treatment for nociceptive pain, with acetaminophen being the first step for most situations.

Acetaminophen. Its mechanism of action remains unknown, but it continues to be the drug of choice of the American College of Rheumatology and the National Kidney Foundation for the treatment of chronic pain. Acetaminophen in a

Table 236.5. Overview of Medications Used to Treat Pain

GENERIC NAMES	BRAND NAME	INITIAL PO DOSE (MG)	MAXIMUM PO DOSE (MG)	COMMENTS
Non-Narcotic Analgesics				
acetaminophen	Tylenol	500–1000 q4–6	1,000 qd	Reduce dose with alcohol use or known liver disease
tramadol	Ultram	50–100 q6	400/d	Nausea, vomiting, diarrhea; seizures with antidepressants
NSAIDs				
aspirin	Ectorin, Bayer	325–650 q4–6	650 q4	Dyspepsia/peptic ulcer disease
ibuprofen	Advil, Motrin, Nuprin	200–800 q6	800 q6	GI/renal
naproxen	Naprosyn, Aleve	250–500 q12	500 q12	GI/renal
etodolac	Lodine	200 q8	400 q8	GI/renal
indomethacin	Indocin	25–50 q8	50 q8	GI/renal
ketorolac	Toradol	10 q6	10 q4	GI/renal (use <5 d)
salsalate	Disalcid	500 bid	1,000 tid	GI/renal
celecoxib	Celebrex	100 bid	200 bid	Less GI toxicity
Opioid Analgesics				
codeine	In Tylenol Nos. 2–4	15 q4	60 q4	Nausea, vomiting, constipation Sedation, respiratory depression
oxycodone	In Percocet	5 q6	10 q4	(Same as codeine)
oxycodone SR	OxyContin	10 q12	30 q8	(Same as codeine)
morphine	Roxanol elixir	10 q6	30 q4	(Same as codeine), pruritus
morphine SR	MS Contin	60 q12	180 q8	(Same as codeine)
hydromorphone	Dilaudid	2 q6	2 q4	(Same as codeine)
methadone	Dolophine	20 q8	20 q4	(Same as codeine)
meperidine	Demerol	50 q4	150 q3	(Same as codeine), seizure from metabolites
fentanyl patch	Duragesic	25 μg/h q72	200 μg/h q72	(Same as codeine)
Anticonvulsants				
gabapentin	Neurontin	100 qhs	1,200 tid	Sedation
baclofen	Lioresal	5 q8	20 q6	Sedation
phenytoin	Dilantin	150 qd	300 qd (level)	(Multiple—refer to PDR); follow levels
carbamazepine	Tegretol	200 q8	400 q8 (level)	Sedation; follow levels
clonazepam	Klonopin	0.5 q6	1–5 q6	Sedation
Antidepressants				
doxepin	Sinequan	25 bid	100 q8	High sedation/low arrhythmia; anticholinergic++
amitriptyline	Elavil	25 qhs	75 bid	High sedation/high arrhythmia; anticholinergic+++
imipramine	Tofranil	75 qhs	75 bid	Moderate sedation/high arrhythmia; anticholinergic++
nortriptyline	Pamelor	25 qhs	25 q6	Moderate sedation/high arrhythmia; anticholinergic+
desipramine	Norpramin	25 qhs	150 bid	Low sedation/high arrhythmia
paroxetine	Paxil	20 qd	50 qd	GI upset, insomnia, nervousness, sedation, sexual dysfunction
fluoxetine	Prozac	20 qd	80 qd	GI upset, insomnia, nervousness, sedation, sexual dysfunction

dosage of 1,000 mg four times per day is as effective as NSAIDs. This dose of acetaminophen is safe in those patients who drink fewer than five alcoholic beverages per day and have no known hepatic dysfunction. The most common side effect is mild gastrointestinal upset.

Nonsteroidal Antiinflammatory Drugs. Diseases with a prominent inflammatory component are candidates for trials of NSAIDs if acetaminophen proves insufficient. NSAIDs are the next-most-frequently used class of agents for nociceptive pain, after non-narcotic analgesics. However, they are associated with many side effects, particularly gastrointestinal and renal. *Aspirin* is the prototypic NSAID. It also is directly analgesic, being the milligram-for-milligram equivalent of acetaminophen. However, it is not indicated for the treatment of chronic pain because of its association with gastrointestinal toxicity, which makes the long-term use of most NSAIDs problematic. The concomitant use of omeprazole or misoprostol can partly prevent gastrointestinal toxicity, but with the disadvantage of incurring the expense and side effects of another drug (see Chapter 68).

NSAIDs may differ from one another in their selectivity as inhibitors of cyclooxygenase-1 (Cox-1) or cyclooxygenase-2 (Cox-2). *Cox-2 inhibitors* (e.g., celecoxib) seem to generate fewer gastrointestinal complications in endoscopic studies, but they have been studied *in vivo* only for osteoarthritis and rheumatoid arthritis for short periods of time. The literature regarding their use as long-term therapy should be followed.

Tramadol is a centrally acting analgesic with dual effects; it acts primarily as a monoamine (norepinephrine and serotonin) reuptake inhibitor that blocks pain transmission in the spinal cord, and secondarily as a blocker of central nervous system μ-opioid receptors. It has a very low potential for abuse. Comparative studies in patients with osteoarthritis have shown it to be equivalent in analgesic effect to naproxen and propoxyphene. It is rapidly absorbed, with a peak effect at 2 hours and a half-life of 6 hours. It is metabolized by the liver, then excreted by the kidneys. Its benefits include a relative lack of potential for abuse and respiratory depression in comparison with opiates, but it still causes many side effects, including nausea, drowsiness, sweating, and constipation. Slowly titrating the dose upward can minimize the transient nausea. Tramadol might be considered as an opiate alternative once acetaminophen has failed in disease states without much objective inflammation, such as osteoarthritis.

Opiates. Opiates are the most potent class of analgesics for the treatment of chronic pain and have no ceiling for therapeutic effect. Many clinicians agonize over whether to prescribe opiates for chronic nonmalignant pain, a difficulty usually stemming from misconceptions (Table 236.1). Perhaps the most pervasive misconception is the idea that patients placed on long-term therapy with opiates will become "addicts."

Addiction, Substance Abuse, and Tolerance. Distinctions must be made between the terms *substance abuse, addiction,* and *tolerance,* as many clinicians erroneously equate them. *Substance abuse* implies the problem of dangerous use of an agent, with or without physical dependence. The term *addiction* implies compulsive substance use and an inability to control intake despite negative consequences. *Tolerance* to nar-

Table 236.6.   Criteria for Giving a Patient Opiates for Chronic Nonmalignant Pain

- Patient reports subjective chronic pain on more than one occasion consistently.
- This pain inhibits functioning and decreases quality of life.
- Reversible causes have been addressed.
- Conservative measures (including over-the-counter medications) have been tried with inadequate response.
- Patient does not meet formal criteria for substance abuse or other primary psychiatric disorder (depressive/anxiety/somatoform/personality disorders, or malingering).
- There are no other contraindications to opiates (e.g., liver disease, operator of heavy machinery, drug-tested at work).
- Patient is capable of adhering to a simple contract about appropriate follow-up and opiate use.

cotics has nothing to do with abuse or addiction; it merely implies a physical dependence in which a higher dose of an agent is required over time to achieve the same effect. It is a well-recognized phenomenon associated with long-term narcotic use.

Contracting. Patients receiving narcotics and enrolled in a chronic pain program with contracting for routine follow-up have a less than 3% chance of becoming addicts or abusers if they have not been addicts or abusers previously. A current or prior history of abuse or addiction is a relative but not an absolute contraindication to long-term narcotic use, as many such patients will adhere to the terms of a contract (Fig. 236.2). Such a contract allows for the tapering and discontinuation of a narcotic whenever a clinician fears that an abusive or addictive situation is developing. Narcotics can be prescribed for any patient who meets a few criteria for their use (Table 236.6). Opioid analgesics all affect the μ-receptor but differ in their potency, onset, duration of action, and route of administration.

Dose-related Side Effects and Dosing. Dose-related side effects tend to be similar for all opiates and include nausea, vomiting, constipation, urinary retention, pruritus, sedation, and respiratory depression (when given in toxic doses). One starts with low doses and titrates upward. The most common mistake is underdosing. In the absence of sedation, one should not hesitate to increase the dose to achieve adequate pain relief. Tolerance can develop to all opioids, and to all the various side effects. The only effect of opiates to which a patient will not develop tolerance is constipation, which should be treated preemptively.

Choice of Agent. Several narcotic preparations are best avoided. *Butorphanol* is probably best avoided because it is a combination agonist–antagonist. *Meperidine* likewise should be avoided because its metabolites tend to cause seizures. Narcotics in a *fixed combination* with cyclooxygenase inhibitors or acetaminophen should probably be avoided because of their high street value and the danger of acetaminophen overdose with dose escalations. Patients, however, should be encouraged to take maximal doses of acetaminophen simultaneously for synergy. *Oxycodone* is the long-acting agent of choice. It is formulated for oral administration and does not have the same profile of side effects as long-acting morphine—namely, there are fewer active metabolites to cause histamine release. Likewise,

Fig. 236.2.   Patient–Provider Contract for the Long-term Use of Opioids

I, _____,
realize that my provider has decided to try to relieve my suffering partly with the use of opiate analgesics (pain medicines). I recognize that these medicines have both risks and benefits, which have been explained to me by my provider, and that these medicines are only one component of my pain treatment regimen.

I understand that to receive continuing care by my provider for my chronic pain, I must adhere to the following mutual expectations:

1. Pain medicines will be used *only as directed* for my pain. I will *NOT:*
   • suddenly stop taking these medicines;
   • use them other than for treating my pain;
   • increase the dose without discussion with my provider;
   • share them with others.

2. I will receive narcotics *only from my provider* and from no one else, including ER staff.

3. I will have my prescriptions filled *at only one pharmacy* of my choice, which I have clearly specified with my provider.

4. I will ask my provider for *refills on a predetermined schedule,* asking only when I still have at least 4 days' worth of medication remaining.

5. Refills will be given *only at my provider's office.* They will not be mailed.

6. I will adhere to requests for *random drug testing* should my provider ask me.

7. It is *my responsibility* to protect my prescriptions from loss, theft, or damage. A police report will be required for any theft before my provider will consider replacing them. If a second loss, or theft or damage occurs, I realize my provider may choose to not replace them.

8. These pain medicines are only one component of my treatment strategy. I agree to *adhere to other aspects of my care* as discussed with my provider.

_____   _____
Patient signature   Date

_____   _____
Provider signature   Date

it is less frequently associated in the mind of the public with substance abuse and terminal illness.

Neuropathic Pain

Neuropathic pain is characteristically more resistant to pharmacologic interventions than is nociceptive pain. The agents generally used for neuropathic pain are *antidepressants* (tricyclics, selective serotonin reuptake inhibitors), *anticonvul-*

Table 237.7.   General Principles to Follow When Prescribing Narcotics for Chronic Pain

1. Have the patient sign a simple *contract* (Table 236.7) with a "two strikes and you're tapered to zero" approach; stick to all the terms of the contract tightly. It may be used to encourage adherence to medical advice in other important realms.

2. Treat pain *proactively* before chronic patterns and secondary psychiatric comorbidities become ingrained.

3. Use *long-acting agents* as round-the-clock treatments, avoiding short-acting medications for long-term use; use the same medication in short-acting formulation during the initial titration phase and for occasional breakthroughs.

4. Monitor *functional end points* more than analgesia, although both are important.

5. Maintain close *follow-up.*

sants (gabapentin, baclofen, carbamazepine, phenytoin), and topical *capsaicin* cream.

Antidepressants. Tricyclic antidepressants are useful in neuropathic pain. They have a rapid onset of action and vary in their side effect profiles (Table 236.5). Tricyclics have been shown in controlled trials to provide analgesia in post-herpetic neuralgia, diabetic neuropathy, tension and migraine headache, rheumatoid arthritis, and low back pain. They have also been shown to potentiate opioid analgesics and so should be used selectively in situations of nociceptive pain. The doses required for analgesia can be much lower than those needed to treat affective disorders.

Selective serotonin reuptake inhibitors have not yet been fully evaluated for most chronic pain syndromes. For tension headaches, paroxetine and fluoxetine have both been shown to provide some benefit, although citalopram did not. For migraine headaches and fibromyalgia, fluoxetine has shown conflicting results so far. For diabetic neuropathy, paroxetine and citalopram both showed some benefit but were not as effective as imipramine.

Anticonvulsants. *Phenytoin* and *carbamazepine* were first shown to relieve the pain associated with trigeminal neuralgia. Antiarrhythmic drugs followed. All these agents help by blocking the conduction of nociceptive fibers. *Gabapentin* is now the agent of choice for most neuropathic pain, especially the lancinating types (e.g., sciatica). It is well tolerated, and dosing is limited primarily by the sedating effects. Beginning with a low dose and titrating upward very gradually minimizes the side effect of sedation, so that gabapentin is useful even in the elderly. *Baclofen* is a gabapentin agonist and is also generally well tolerated. It is used primarily for painful spasticity (e.g., in patients with spinal cord injury).

Capsaicin Cream impedes afferent pain impulses by depleting substance P from sensory nerve fibers. It has been used in post-herpetic neuralgia with some success, but it must be applied several times a day to provide sufficient pain relief. It often causes severe burning at the site of application for the first 1 to 2 weeks of treatment, so that concurrent use of topical lidocaine is necessary during this period.

Table 236.8.   Overview of Complementary Approaches to the Treatment of Chronic Pain

	HEADACHE	MUSCULOSKELETAL	LOW BACK	ABDOMINAL/PELVIC	PERIPHERAL NERVE
Acupuncture	++	+++	++	+[a]	
Behavioral	+++[e]	++[b]	++[b]	+[c]	+[d]
Chiropractic			−		
Invasive		+	+	+	+[f]

[a]Menstrual cramps.
[b]Relaxation, cognitive behavior therapy.
[c]Relaxation, hypnosis.
[d]Relaxation.
[e]See text for details.
[f]Radiculopathy.

Complementary Modalities

When therapeutic goals are not achieved with initial pharmacologic and psychosocial interventions, complementary modalities can be explored. Some of the many complementary modalities available have more data behind them than do others (Table 236.8).

Acupuncture. Acupuncture has been increasing in popularity among patients and physicians during the past three decades. In the United States in 1997, more than 1 million patients made more than 5 million visits for treatment with acupuncture. Acupuncture has been applied to many conditions besides pain (e.g., asthma, depression), but its principal contribution is in pain management, the focus of a National Institutes of Health (NIH) Consensus Statement in 1998.

Mode of Action. Acupuncture stems from traditional Chinese medicine, which holds that body energy (*Qi,* pronounced "chee") becomes imbalanced to cause disease. This imbalance is thought to be corrected by manipulating specific channels, called meridians, through which energy flows. This view predates the Western approach of mind–body dualism, which emphasizes disease as a purely biologic phenomenon. The biologic mechanism of acupuncture is becoming better understood. The procedure appears to trigger serotonin release in the central nervous system and to increase circulating levels of endogenous opioids. Naloxone can block the therapeutic effects of acupuncture.

Clinical Studies of acupuncture for pain have been flawed; most are case series or case reports. The few randomized, controlled trials that have been performed lack a rigorous study design and adequate sample size and have problems with control groups. Comparisons between studies are difficult because there are many different ways of applying the needles with regard to location and manipulation. Manipulation is performed either manually, electrically, or through moxibustion (the combustion of a specific herb at the needle insertion site). Furthermore, control arms are controversial. Even "sham" acupuncture, in which needles are placed randomly, has been shown to provide pain relief, possibly through "nonspecific" opioid-releasing effects.

Evidence of Efficacy. The NIH Consensus Statement focused on studies that included either a sham or placebo control, but case series were used when necessary. The strongest evidence for the efficacy of acupuncture has been demonstrated in cases of postoperative pain and nausea related to chemotherapy or pregnancy. Ample evidence supports the efficacy of acupuncture as a therapeutic option for *myofascial pain* and nonspecific *low back pain.* Approximately half of patients in laboratory and clinical studies showed a favorable response after 10 treatments during approximately 1 month. For low back pain specifically, responses lasting to 3 months were seen; the rate of overall pain reduction was nearly 60%, with a corresponding reduction in consumption of analgesic tablets. Less convincing evidence but some positive studies support the efficacy of acupuncture in treating *headaches, osteoarthritis, fibromyalgia, carpal tunnel syndrome,* and *menstrual cramps.*

Adverse Effects. The incidence of adverse effects appears to be exceedingly low, certainly lower than that of commonly accepted pharmacologic interventions for chronic pain. Of the nearly 200 reported complications of acupuncture, *viral hepatitis* was by far the most common, stemming from a time when needles were not sterilized properly. All needles currently used by regulated providers conform to Food and Drug Administration safety regulations. Other, very rare complications include *pneumothorax* (with emphysema), *ecchymoses* (with anticoagulation), preterm induction of labor (in pregnant women), and *conduction problems* (with pacemakers when electrical stimulation of needles is used).

In the absence of clinical data, clinical judgment is critical in deciding whether or not an individual patient might benefit from a trial of acupuncture. The use of acupuncture for chronic pain will likely become more commonplace for various indications as more trials emerge and shed light on the risk–benefit ratio for specific situations. Better data will drive improved standardization of training, licensing, supervision, and reimbursement, and will help define the role of acupuncture in our treatment algorithms.

If referral of a patient to a physician acupuncturist is being considered, information can be obtained through the American Academy of Medical Acupuncture (http://www.medicalacupuncture.org). If referral to a nonphysician acupuncturist is being considered, information is available through the American Association of Oriental Medicine (http://www.aaom.org).

Behavioral Approaches. Busy primary care providers classically overlook behavioral interventions. A recent review of complementary medicine in the United States showed that millions of Americans are already using these techniques, although most of their providers remain unaware of this and are unfamiliar with the techniques. The importance of behavioral approaches in the treatment of chronic pain, however, cannot be overemphasized, as the risk is negligible and benefit has been demonstrated.

In 1996, the NIH released a Consensus Statement with regard to these modalities. Like the statement for acupuncture, this statement was prepared by a non-Federal, 12-member expert panel that reviewed the literature, presented findings to an open conference, and ultimately drafted the statement based on scientific data rather than anecdote whenever possible. The panel members focused on the four modalities most widely used and reported in the literature: *relaxation, hypnosis, cognitive behavioral therapy,* and *biofeedback* (see also Chapter 226).

Relaxation. The goal is to train patients to control their focus of conscious attention. The two components are (a) *repetitive focus* on a word, phrase, sound, prayer, body sensation, or muscular activity; and (b) adoption of a *passive attitude* toward intruding thoughts. Techniques include paced respiration, progressive muscle relaxation, concentration meditation, and movement meditation. Once patients master these techniques, they are capable of decreasing their perception of pain and level of arousal. There is strong evidence for the effectiveness of this approach in reducing chronic pain in a variety of medical conditions.

Hypnosis likewise aims at selective focus of attention but adds a suggestive phase to reinforce new responses to pain. The *presuggestion phase* involves pure focus of attention (e.g., with relaxation techniques). The *suggestive phase* is geared toward specific goals, such as analgesia. The *postsuggestive phase* involves imprinting for continued use of a new behavior. Suggestive evidence of the efficacy of hypnosis has been noted in tension headache, temporomandibular joint pain, and irritable bowel syndrome.

Cognitive Behavioral Therapy attempts to transform patterns of negative attitudes into more productive thoughts, emotions, and actions. This is accomplished by training the patient to recognize current responses and to develop healthier responses and the skills to execute them. Evidence of the efficacy of this approach has been moderate in low back pain, rheumatoid arthritis, and osteoarthritis; evidence suggests it is mildly useful for tension headache.

Biofeedback involves education about physiologic responses to painful stimuli and ways to exercise voluntary control over these responses. Measurements are made with electromyography, electroencephalography, thermometers, and cardiac monitors. These tools allow patients to see their physiologic response to pain, and they are coached on techniques to affect these responses. This leaves patients feeling more in control of their pain. Moderate evidence for the efficacy of biofeedback has been noted in the treatment of tension and migraine headaches.

Data on these behavioral techniques are currently insufficient to suggest that one technique be used over another for a particular condition. However, several metaanalyses have shown consistently positive effects of multimodal behavioral approaches, particularly for headache, joint pain, and back pain. For now, physicians should probably be capable of describing *relaxation techniques* to patients for use in the management of almost any type of chronic pain. Further instruction in any of the techniques might be pursued through psychiatric/psychologic referral.

Spinal Manipulation. Although the purported applications of spinal manipulation by chiropractors are many, low back pain accounts for the vast majority of visits. Although some evidence of its efficacy has been found in the treatment of acute back pain (see Chapter 147), little has been noted in the treatment of chronic low back pain (i.e., lasting longer than 3 months). Available data are incomparable and conflicting. The consensus expert view after review of all published studies is that it is inappropriate to refer patients with chronic low back pain for manipulation. Nonetheless, more than half of patients being treated with manipulation by chiropractors have chronic low back pain. Therefore, patients with chronic low back pain should be dissuaded from undergoing spinal manipulation, as there is currently no evidence in favor of it, the current recommendations addressing chronic low back pain weigh against it, and chiropractors do not appear to adhere to the criteria for appropriateness reliably.

Invasive Techniques

Invasive techniques gained popularity in the 1980s, after extensive studies showed them to be effective in patients with terminal cancer. Their use has now been extended to patients with nonmalignant chronic pain, based on the results of limited studies. These interventions are never used as monotherapy. They are added only when more conservative measures have been ineffective and clinical evidence is available to suggest a possible benefit, especially in the setting of neuropathic pain. Invasive techniques are performed primarily by anesthesiologists in pain centers.

Local Anesthetics (e.g., *bupivacaine*) may be given in the form of epidural or plexus blocks, and *sympathetic blocks* are performed with opioids. These techniques are primarily used for acute pain states and are rarely employed for acute flares of chronic states (e.g., reflex sympathetic dystrophy). *Neurolytic blocks* with alcohol have primarily been used in patients with chronic abdominal cancer pain, but one retrospective study has shown efficacy for lumbar sympathetic neurolytics in reducing the pain of patients with inoperable claudication.

Spinal Injection of Opioids (usually given as an intrathecal or epidural injection of morphine) has been quite effective in end-stage cancer patients who are unable to take oral opiates to therapeutic levels because of side effects. These techniques have been extended to some patients with chronic nonmalignant pain; significant reduction of pain was achieved in 60 of 80 patients under study conditions. The patients included had chronic low back pain that surgery failed to alleviate, post-herpetic neuralgia, and peripheral nerve injury. More than half of the patients had mild systemic side effects (constipation, urinary hesitancy, nausea, impotence, nightmares, pruritus); approximately 20% also had system malfunctions, and a few experienced epidural hematoma, infection (epidural abscess, pocket infection, meningitis), or cerebrospinal fluid leaks. The current recommendations are that this should remain a method of last resort, to be used only after a patient has passed a psychological evaluation and responded favorably to a 3-day test of intrathecal opiates before the pump is implanted.

Pain Centers

"Pain centers" have become increasingly numerous during the past decade as pain management has become recognized as a discipline in its own right. Centers range from small clinics offering only one type of intervention to large entities offering a multidisciplinary approach. They are directed by physicians (anesthesiologists, internists, psychiatrists) and may be staffed by nurses, physical therapists, psychologists, and social workers.

Pain specialists may be located through the American Pain Society (847-375-4715) or the American Academy of Pain Medicine (www.painmed.org). Information on more than 200 multidisciplinary centers may be found via the Rehabilitation Accreditation Commission (520-325-1044).

PATIENT EDUCATION AND INDICATIONS FOR REFERRAL

The principal objective is to redirect the patient's expectations toward a gradual improvement in *functioning* and *quality of life* rather than complete elimination of pain. Patients benefit from understanding that chronic pain has biologic and psychosocial components, which necessitates a multidisciplinary approach to therapy.

General internists should be able to manage their patients' pain medications and treat secondary psychiatric comorbidities. They must also determine the need for and coordinate appropriate referrals as follows:

- To *psychiatry* if a primary psychiatric disorder is suspected
- To a *substance abuse counseling* program if an abuse problem is uncovered
- To a *social service program* if overwhelming social factors are a factor (e.g., domestic violence)
- To *practitioners of complementary methods* (e.g., psychologists, behavioral therapists) when pharmacologic and psychotherapeutic measures prove insufficient
- To a *pain center,* primarily if complex neuropathic pain is a factor or if invasive techniques are required, which most pain centers manage (although some pain centers offer a broader range of techniques than do others)

THERAPEUTIC RECOMMMENDATIONS

- View chronic pain as a chronic disease. Treatment goals must *focus on improvement in functioning and quality of life* rather than on elimination of pain.
- Consider the *psychosocial aspects* of pain as much as the biologic aspects. Identify and address primary psychiatric processes, and treat secondary processes along with the pain.
- Classify the biologic aspect of a patient's pain as primarily *nociceptive* or *neuropathic,* localize it, and consider reversible causes of pain for the various sites.
- *Nociceptive pain* is treated stepwise with non-opiate analgesics, NSAIDs, and opiates. Tylenol remains the non-opiate of choice over tramadol. Long-term NSAID use predisposes to gastrointestinal toxicity, which is partly avoidable with concomitant omeprazole or misoprostol. The role of Cox-2 inhibitors is not yet firmly established. Do not hesitate to prescribe opiates on a long-term basis to patients who meet the criteria. Long-acting opiates should be used, with short-acting agents administered for breakthrough pain. Attempt to treat pain more proactively than reactively. Have the patient sign an opiate contract.
- *Neuropathic pain* is treated variably with antidepressants, anticonvulsants, and topical capsaicin cream where appropriate.
- A *multidisciplinary approach* to treatment is critical. This involves directed referrals to psychiatry (primary psychiatric disorders, behavioral training), pain centers (invasive techniques), and elsewhere for acupuncture when appropriate.

ANNOTATED BIBLIOGRAPHY

Backonja M, Beydoun A, Edwards KR, et al. Gabapentin for the symptomatic treatment of painful neuropathy in patients with diabetes mellitus. JAMA 1998;280:1831. (*Very convincing study, with 40% reduction in pain at 8 weeks; 23% in treatment group had somnolence and 24% had dizziness.*)

Burchman SL, Pagel PS. Implementation of a formal treatment agreement for outpatient management of chronic nonmalignant pain with opioid analgesics. J Pain Symptom Manage 1995;10:556. (*Prospective Veterans Administration study showing success of patients on contract.*)

Grant DJ, Bishop-Miller J, Winchester DM, et al. A randomized comparative trial of acupuncture vs. TENS for chronic back pain in the elderly. Pain 1999;82:93. (*One month of acupuncture decreases chronic back pain by 50% at 1 month, 60% at 3 months; pain reduction after transcutaneous electrical nerve stimulation is comparable at 1 month, but the effects wear off by 3 months.*)

Jung AC, Staiger T, Sullivan M, et al. The efficacy of SSRIs for the management of chronic pain. J Gen Intern Med 1997;12:384. (*Straightforward review of 19 randomized clinical trials.*)

Katz WA. Pharmacology and clinical experience with tramadol in OA. Drugs 1996;52S:39. (*Overview of the 20 years of experience with this agent internationally.*)

NIH Consensus Conference. Acupuncture. JAMA 1998;280:1518. (*NIH data-driven consensus recommendations on complementary therapies. Statement available through* http://consensus.nih.gov.)

NIH Panel. Integration of behavioral and relaxation approaches into the treatment of chronic pain and insomnia. JAMA 1996;276:313. (*NIH data-driven recommendations on behavioral and relaxation techniques.*)

Portenoy RK. Opioid therapy for chronic nonmalignant pain: a review of the critical issues. J Pain Symptom Manage 1996;11:203. (*Extensive but very readable overview. Synthesizes available numbers to predict risk of opiates to patients. Proposes guidelines, which should be prospectively studied.*)

Shekelle PG, Coulter I, Hurwitz EL, et al. Spinal manipulation for low back pain. Ann Intern Med 1992;117:590. (*A classic review of more than 50 trials. Data inconclusive for chronic low back pain.*)

Shekelle PG, Adams AH, Chassin MR, et al. Congruence between decisions to initiate chiropractic spinal manipulation for low back pain and appropriateness criteria in North America. Ann Intern Med 1998;129:9. (*Fifty-four percent of patients treated by chiropractors not considered "appropriate"; vast majority of these were patients with chronic low back pain.*)

Smith GR. The epidemiology and treatment of depression when it coexists with somatoform disorders, somatization or pain. Gen Hosp Psychiatry 1992;14:265. (*High overlap of pain and primary psychiatric illness.*)

Tannenbaum H, Davis P, Russell AS, et al. An evidence-based approach to prescribing NSAIDs in musculoskeletal disease: a Canadian consensus. Can Med Assoc J 1996;155:77. (*Clear overview, now somewhat dated; still recommends misoprostol over proton pump inhibitors when needed, pre-celecoxib era.*)

Turk DC, Brody MC, Okifuji EA. Physicians' attitudes and practices regarding the long-term prescribing of opioids for non-cancer pain. Pain 1994;59:201. (*Primary survey of 7,000 physicians, with 27% response rate; suggests that physicians act more on their own biases and inexperience than on germane data.*)

Winkelmuller M, Winkelmuller W, et al. Long-term effects of continuous intrathecal opioid treatment in chronic pain of non-malignant etiology. J Neurosurg 1996;85:458. (*Reduction of pain achieved in more than 50%, but complication rate of 16%.*)

Zenz M, et al. Role of invasive methods in the treatment of chronic pain. Acta Anaesthesiol Scand Suppl 1997;111:181. (*Brief overview of invasive techniques, with impressive plea for more conservative use.*)

Appendix: Screening for Domestic Violence

Domestic violence is a prevalent and potentially fatal condition that frequently goes unrecognized, especially in the office setting. Estimates of the life-time risk for battering for women range from 10% to 30%. Barriers to recognition include the reluctance of the patient to bring up the problem, time pressures, and physician discomfort in dealing with it. Moreover, the presentation may be subtle, nonspecific, or confusing. Nonetheless, the screening and timely diagnosis of domestic violence are essential tasks for the primary care physician because prompt intervention can be life-saving, not only by protecting the patient from harm by a partner but also by protecting her from self-harm (one in every four women who attempt suicide have been victims of domestic violence).

Clinical Presentation. The vast majority of victims of domestic violence are women, outnumbering men in a ratio of 9:1. The condition occurs among people of all ages (e.g., elder abuse) and sociodemographic groups. A wide range of office presentations is possible, with chronic pain or chronic gynecologic symptoms often prominent. Unexplained headache, worsening symptoms of a chronic condition, depression, anxiety, dyspareunia, severe premenstrual symptoms, irritable bowel symptoms, and alcohol abuse are among the presenting manifestations. In addition to physical harm, patients are at increased risk for somatization disorders, complications of pregnancy, sexually transmitted diseases, eating disorders, substance abuse, and noncompliance with medical regimens. Repeated visits to the emergency room for "falls" or forearm injuries (sustained during attempts at self-defense) are characteristic, as are findings such as multiple ecchymoses in various stages of healing. Other characteristics of trauma include a central distribution of injuries, involvement of the head and face, and hearing loss. Being accompanied to the office or emergency room by an overly aggressive partner is also typical.

Screening and Diagnosis. Given the frequency and importance to health of domestic violence, the problem should be screened for on a regular basis as part of the periodic health examination. A more in-depth consideration of the diagnosis is indicated when a patient reports chronic pain, unexplained worsening of a chronic condition, or one of the other typical presentations of domestic violence noted above. A *sine qua non* of the evaluation is that the patient be examined alone by a qualified health professional without the spouse, partner, family members, or friends being present. Although patients rarely present to the office complaining of domestic violence, they often demonstrate considerable relief and a willingness to discuss it once the subject is broached by the primary care physician.

A few simple screening questions preceded by a general comment about the importance of checking for domestic violence usually suffice:

Do you ever feel unsafe at home?

Has anyone at home hit you or tried to injure you in any way?

These questions have been validated for diagnostic accuracy, demonstrating a sensitivity of 71% and a specificity of 85%. Some authorities also suggest a few questions that can elicit evidence of fear of a partner's intimidating or controlling behavior:

Have you ever been afraid of your partner?

Has anyone ever threatened you or tried to control you?

Others have proposed the mnemonic SAFE to help facilitate asking questions that address **S**afety, **A**buse, **F**riend or family awareness, and **E**mergency escape plan.

If the response to any of these questions is positive, the physician should obtain a full description of the problem and perform a pertinent physical examination for any evidence of injury. Confidentiality is essential to patient safety, and all records (including telephone numbers and billing diagnoses) should be handled carefully with patient protection as the priority.

Obtaining Help. An essential component of the visit that uncovers domestic violence is to arrange for professional help. Information on local services can be obtained by calling the National Domestic Violence Hotline (1-800-799-SAFE). Patients appreciate knowing that the help to be offered is professional, typically free of charge, and designed to provide for safety and counseling. Having a member of the primary care team, preferably a trained social worker, help the patient access community services is often welcomed.

A.H.G.

ANNOTATED BIBLIOGRPAHY

Alpert EJ, Sege RD. Family violence: an overview. Acad Med 1997;72[Suppl]:S3. (*A useful overview of the scope of the problem and its manifestations across the full range of age groups.*)

Eisenstat SA, Bancroft L. Domestic violence. N Engl J Med 1999;341:886. (*Excellent and very practical review with 69 references; source of the sample questions listed above.*)

Feldhaus KM, Koziol-McLain J, Amsbury HL, et al. Accuracy of three brief screening questions for detecting partner violence in the emergency department. JAMA 1997;277:1357. (*Sensitivity and specificity data on simple screening questions.*)

Freund KM, Bak SM, Blackhall L. Identifying domestic violence in primary care practice. J Gen Intern Med 1996;11:44. (*An example of how very simple screening can greatly enhance detection.*)

Neufeld B. SAFE questions: overcoming barriers to the detection of domestic violence. Am Fam Physician 1996;53:2575. (*A suggested approach to questioning.*)

Editors' note: Given the widespread use of alternative/complementary therapies by patients and the concerns of their physicians regarding efficacy and safety, we thought a new section of this book would be helpful to readers and their patients. The goal is to provide detailed review of the available evidence pertaining to specific alternative/complementary therapies. These therapies and the sum of supporting evidence have already been considered in many of the chapters, but this section provides an opportunity for background, more in-depth analysis of the data, and recommendations. References are formally cited in the text. The section will be updated regularly in the web-based version of Primary Care Medicine. *We begin by examining some of the commonly used herbal therapies and the evidence supporting their use. We hope you find the effort useful.*

Herbal Therapies: An Evidence-Based Guide to Use

ERNIE-PAUL BARRETTE

Before 1993, herbal therapy was relatively obscure, although used by a significant number of patients. In 1993, the Food and Drug Administration proposed removing herbal therapies from the over-the-counter market, but a vigorous letter-writing campaign resulted instead in passage of the Dietary Supplement Health and Education Act (DSHEA) in 1994. DSHEA allowed the marketing of all supplements (defined broadly to include herbs, vitamins, minerals, and amino acids) to be expanded with information regarding uses based on "structure and function." Manufacturers would not be allowed to claim to treat, cure, or prevent a disease, but they could still attempt to provide the public with a considerable amount of information on when to use herbal therapies. The use of alternative medicines has dramatically increased since the passage of DSHEA. Unfortunately, DSHEA does not require any evidence of efficacy or safety, nor does it define any standards of quality. If concerns regarding the safety of a supplement are raised, it is up to the Food and Drug Administration to gather and present evidence to justify removing it from the market or limiting its availability.

STATE OF THE ART REGARDING ASSESSMENT OF HERBAL THERAPIES

The number of published clinical trials of herbal medicines is surprisingly great to those who have not reviewed this field. Unfortunately, many of the trials are in journals that are inaccessible or not published in English. Most of these studies lack adequate controls, have poorly defined inclusion criteria, and measure outcomes that are not validated or clinically relevant. Many are simply too short in duration or enroll too few subjects to provide substantive clinical information. This chapter reviews the best evidence supporting the use of several herbal therapies for specific indications. In addition, pertinent safety concerns are discussed.

In Germany, a commission was formed to evaluate the many herbs claimed to have therapeutic value. Members of the "Commission E" included physicians, pharmacists, naturopathic physicians, and scientists. They have published several hundred monographs in the German Federal Register. These monographs have been recently translated and are readily available (1). This resource represents extensive experience in Europe regarding botanical medicines. Monographs with both positive and negative recommendations are included, along with discussions of adverse effects, drug interactions, use during pregnancy and nursing, specific indications, and dosages. Unfortunately, no references are provided. Also, only a positive or negative recommendation is provided. Thus, neither the strength of the evidence nor the vigor of the recommendation can be determined.

COMMONLY USED HERBAL PREPARATIONS

Echinacea for Upper Respiratory Infections

Extracts of three species, *E. purpurea*, *E. angustifolia*, and *E. pallida*, are promoted for both treatment and prevention of upper respiratory infections. *Echinacea* was used by native Americans as an antiseptic and analgesic and was listed in the National Formulary until the introduction of synthetic antibiotics. The Commission E has recommended *Echinacea* for "supportive therapy for colds and chronic infections of the respiratory tract." Unfortunately, no standardized extract exists. Multiple species, various methods of extraction, and different parts of the plant are used, and additional herbal and homeopathic agents are frequently included with preparations of *Echinacea*. All these factors make a comparison of the literature and products very difficult.

Evidence for Efficacy. A systematic review in the Cochrane collaboration collected all the trials of *Echinacea* in the prevention or treatment of upper respiratory viral infections (2). A total of 40 controlled trials were found; 24 studies were excluded, primarily because of a lack of randomization or because a condition other than the common cold was studied. Eight trials involving 985 subjects addressed the treatment of an acute upper respiratory infection. Three different combination products and two different mono-preparations were given for 6 to 10 days in a double-blinded fashion in seven trials (single-blinded in one). Six of eight trials showed a significant benefit with *Echinacea*. However, because of the various outcome measurements and methods of presenting data, no pooling of outcomes was possible.

Five trials including 1,272 subjects tested *Echinacea* in the prevention of upper respiratory infections. Two combination products and three mono-preparations (*E. purpurea* herb, *E. purpurea* roots, and *E. angustifolia* root) were studied for 8 to 12 weeks. The incidence of upper respiratory infections was lower in the treated arms in all five studies (rate ratios of 0.51, 0.67, 0.84, 0.86, and 0.88). However, only in the first two listed trials was the result statistically significant. In the first trial listed, a large number of subjects dropped out after enrollment and were not included in the analysis. In all the studies, questions regarding the case definition of an upper respiratory infection were raised. The duration of illness was significantly shorter in one trial but unchanged in two other trials.

A recent study not included in the Cochrane review compared the fluid extract of *E. purpurea* with a placebo in 109 subjects who had a history of more than three colds in the prior year (3). The lower incidence of respiratory infections with *Echinacea* was not statistically significant (rate ratio, 0.88; 95% CI, 0.60 to 1.22). This result is similar to those of the three more rigorous trials mentioned above. It is unknown whether a much larger trial would confirm this modest benefit with a confidence interval not including one.

Safety. No serious adverse effects have been reported. Because of its immune-stimulating properties, *Echinacea* is not recommended for persons with autoimmune disorders.

Summary. Although many trials have been published, they involve many different species of *Echinacea* along with many other herbs and additives. The Cochrane reviewers felt that the quality of reporting was "insufficient" in two thirds of the trials. Because of the distinctive taste of *Echinacea*, blinding in the placebo arm in all trials is difficult. The best trials have consistently showed a nonsignificant decrease of 12% to 16% in the relative risk for respiratory infections. The substance appears well tolerated, but it should not be used by persons with autoimmune disease.

Ginkgo Biloba for Dementia

Ginkgo biloba extracts have been used in Chinese herbal medicine for many centuries. The use of ginkgo biloba has increased in Europe during the last 30 years, and it is now the most prescribed herbal medicine in Germany. It is among the top three herbal products consumed in the United States. Most products are based on a standardized extract, EGb 761, which contains 22% to 27% flavone glycosides (quercetin,

kaempferol, isorhamnetin) and 5% to 7% terpene lactones (2.8% to 3.4% ginkgolides A, B, and C; 2.6% to 3.2% bilobalide). EGb 761 is now off patent and may be used by any manufacturer. Unfortunately, another standardized extract process is also used, LI 1370. Although LI 1370 specifies 25% flavone glycosides and 6% terpenoids, the different process may result in different concentrations of individual ingredients. It is not known whether the active ingredient is a specific component or a combination. The Commission E approved ginkgo biloba for use in dementia syndromes, specifically primary degenerative dementia, vascular dementia, and mixed forms. They also approved it for intermittent claudication, vertigo, and tinnitus.

Evidence for Efficacy. The body of research regarding potential mechanisms of action is extensive; these include scavenging free radicals, blocking platelet-activating factor, increasing blood flow, stabilizing membranes, and decreasing capillary fragility, among others.

A rigorous metaanalysis has been conducted of published studies regarding the use of ginkgo biloba in Alzheimer's disease (4). Inclusion criteria for studies in the analysis were as follows: (a) well-defined patient groups with Alzheimer's disease (e.g., Diagnostic and Statistical Manual III-R definition); (b) explicit exclusion of patients with depression or other neurologic diseases or taking medications with central nervous system activity; (c) use of standardized extracts of ginkgo biloba; (d) randomized, placebo-controlled, double-blinded design; (e) objective outcome measurement of cognitive function. Remarkably, 57 articles addressing ginkgo biloba and dementia were found, mostly in German and French. However, the majority of trials used "cerebral insufficiency" as the entry criterion, which is an old imprecise term encompassing a diverse range of symptoms. After the exclusion of studies based on a criterion of "cerebral insufficiency," inadequately blinded, or lacking a placebo control, only four studies remained. An earlier metaanalysis, in which the criteria for inclusion were much less restrictive, included only 8 of the 40 trials it found (5), thus confirming the poor quality of most of the clinical studies of ginkgo biloba.

From the four good trials, a total of 424 subjects were included in the metaanalysis. Studies ranged in length from 12 to 26 weeks. All four trials used EGb 761. The analysis reported a significant effect size of 0.40 ($p <.0001$). The result was described as a modest benefit on cognitive function in Alzheimer's disease and was felt to be similar to the benefit of donepezil. The four studies reported inconsistent results in regard to noncognitive outcomes. In the only U.S. trial, which was included in the metaanalysis, improvement was noted on a functional scale, the Geriatric Evaluation by Relative's Rating Instrument (GERRI), but not on the Clinical Global Impression of Change (CGIC) Scale (6).

Safety. Because one of the known effects of gingko biloba is antagonism of platelet-activating factor, it is not surprising that several cases of severe *bleeding* during its use have been reported. These include spontaneous bilateral subdural hematomas (7), subarachnoid hemorrhage (8), subdural hematoma (9), intracerebral hemorrhage (10), and spontaneous hyphema (11). The first three patients were not taking any other medications that would have increased their risk for bleeding. The first two cases note a prolonged bleeding time.

Summary. Several adequate trials report a modest improvement in cognitive function in patients with Alzheimer's disease, similar to that seen with donepezil (see Chapter 173). Standardized extracts contain 24% flavone glycosides and 6% terpene lactones. The usual dose is 40 mg three times daily. Adverse effects are mild and rare. Case reports of severe bleeding with Ginkgo biloba suggest that it be administered with caution in all patients at risk for bleeding, especially those taking warfarin or aspirin.

Kava-Kava for Anxiety

The botanical name of kava-kava is *Piper methysticum* ("intoxicating pepper"). Kava-kava has been used in Pacific Island communities for centuries for its relaxing and tranquilizing effects (12) and was even consumed as part of a ceremony. The root was chewed (causing numbness of the tongue) and spit into a communal bowl. Later, it was ground. This macerate was mixed with water and coconut milk. After straining, the mixture was shared. Kava continues to be used in Micronesia, Melanesia, and Polynesia. Captain James Cook first reported its use to the West. The Commission E has given kava a positive rating for the "condition of nervous anxiety, stress, and restlessness."

Evidence for Efficacy. Kava was first studied by German scientists in the 19th century. Little research was performed in the early 20th century, but pharmacologic studies were restarted in Germany in the 1950s. Animal studies showed a sedative, analgesic, anticonvulsant, and muscle-relaxant effect. The active agents are felt to be the kavalactones (pyrones), primarily kawain, dihydrokawain, methysticin, and dihydromethysticin. Although the results of early studies with D,L-kawain suggested a benefit in treating anxiety, all recent trials have used an extract standardized to the content of kavalactones.

Five double-blinded, placebo-controlled trials of kava have been published. Three trials are of questionable relevance. One trial lasted for 2 days. Two trials examined kava in 40 menopausal women with poorly defined psychovegetative symptoms. The fourth trial compared kava (100 mg three times daily, the equivalent of 210 mg of kavalactones daily) with placebo for 4 weeks in 58 subjects exhibiting anxiety, tension, and agitation syndromes of nonpsychotic origin (13). Significant improvement on the Hamilton Anxiety Scale (HAMA) was noted at 1 week with kava ($p = .0039$). This benefit (compared to placebo) continued during the 4-week trial. The minimal improvement with placebo at both 1 and 4 weeks casts doubt on the validity of the blinding in this study. Another trial compared kava (210 mg of kavalactones daily) with oxazepam (15 mg daily) and bromazepam (9 mg daily) for 42 days in 172 subjects in double-blinded fashion. Similar improvements in HAMA scores were seen in all three arms (14).

The best evidence supporting the use of kava is a double-blinded, randomized, controlled multicenter trial comparing kava (100 mg three times daily, 70% kavalactones) with placebo (15). A standardized extract, WS 1490, was used that provided 210 mg of kavalactones daily. One hundred one subjects with generalized anxiety disorder, adjustment disorder with anxiety, agoraphobia, and specific phobia as defined in the Diagnostic and Statistical Manual III-R were enrolled. The trial lasted 24 weeks and used HAMA scores with an intent-to-treat analysis as the primary outcome. The HAMA score improved

in both arms, but the improvement was significantly greater with kava (30.7 to 17.1) than with placebo (31.4 to 20.3; $p = .02$) by 8 weeks. Both arms showed continued improvement for 16 weeks and then plateaued. The benefit of kava persisted from 8 weeks to the end of the trial. At 24 weeks, the HAMA scores remained improved with kava (kava, 30.7 to 9.7; placebo 31.4 to 15.2; $p < .001$). Adverse effects were minimal. Three subjects in the kava arm dropped out, two because of improvement of symptoms. Seven subjects in the placebo arm dropped out. Overall, the trial addressed concerns regarding poorly defined entry criteria and inadequate duration of follow-up.

Safety. In large, observational trials, adverse effects have been rare. In several small trials, worsening of cognitive function and coordination were seen, as expected with benzodiazepines but not with kava. Heavy, prolonged use of kava results in a well-described skin disorder characterized by dry, yellow scaling (16). Of greatest concern are the case reports of dystonic reactions in five patients, including torticollis, generalized choreoathetosis, and oral–lingual dyskinesia (17,18). A single controversial report describes a semicomatose state in a man who combined kava with alprazolam (19). Necrotizing hepatitis was seen in one woman (20).

Summary. One adequate trial suggests a benefit of kava in generalized anxiety. Sedating medications and alcohol may augment the effect of kava. Kava is contraindicated in pregnancy and nursing. Most trials used 100 mg of kava (70% kavalactones) three times daily, which provided 210 mg of kavalactones daily. However, the Commission E recommends 60 to 120 mg kavalactones daily.

Milk Thistle for Hepatitis and Cirrhosis

Milk thistle (*Silybum marianum*) has a 2,000-year history of use by herbalists. Although it was reported to relieve many conditions, it is currently promoted for liver and biliary disorders. The active ingredients are called *silymarin*, which is composed of three isomeric compounds (silibinin, silidianin, and silichristin). Twenty to forty percent of silymarin is concentrated in the bile. Milk thistle has been used in Europe for 30 years. The Commission E recommended its use as supportive treatment for chronic inflammatory liver conditions.

Evidence for Efficacy. For acute *viral hepatitis*, the evidence is inconsistent. In one double-blinded, randomized, controlled trial of 57 subjects with acute hepatitis A or B, treatment with 140 mg of silymarin three times daily for 3 to 4 weeks normalized bilirubin and AST (aspartate aminotransferase) levels more frequently did placebo ($p < .05$) (21). However, silymarin had no effect on the clearance of hepatitis B surface antigen, a more important clinical marker. In another study, of 52 nonalcoholic male patients with acute hepatitis B randomly assigned to silymarin (70 mg three times daily) or no treatment, no effect was seen on ALT (alanine aminotransferase), AST, and bilirubin levels or on clearance of hepatitis B surface antigen (22). Although milk thistle is recommended by naturopathic physicians for acute hepatitis, little evidence is available to support its use.

Many studies on milk thistle for *alcoholic hepatitis* have been published. Unfortunately, most trials either include very few subjects, are short in duration, or are poorly controlled. In a large randomized, double-blinded, controlled trial for alcoholic hepatitis, 106 men received either milk thistle (420 mg/d) or placebo (23). Subjects were enrolled after admission to a military hospital because of elevations in AST or ALT for longer than 1 month. Although alcoholism was the presumed underlying condition, 20% of the men denied alcohol use. After 4 weeks, treatment with silymarin resulted in a significant decrease in ALT and AST levels; no improvement was noted with placebo ($p < .001$). Liver biopsy also showed an improvement with treatment in comparison with placebo ($p = .022$). However, although 90 biopsies were performed at the start of the trial, only 29 were performed at 4 weeks, which may have influenced the result.

Another randomized, double-blinded, controlled trial of 116 subjects, all with histologically confirmed alcoholic hepatitis, compared silymarin (420 mg/d) with placebo (24). After 3 months, significant improvements, noted in both arms in laboratory test results and histologic findings, suggested no benefit from the addition of milk thistle to adequate supportive care. Not surprisingly, in the information prepared by supplement manufacturers, these negative trial findings are rarely discussed.

Two trials addressed the use of milk thistle in cirrhosis. In an oft-quoted European multicenter study, 170 subjects were entered in a randomized, double-blinded, controlled trial comparing silymarin (140 mg three times daily) with placebo for 2 to 6 years (mean follow-up of 41 months) (25). Cirrhosis was confirmed by biopsy in 70%. Fifty-four percent of the subjects in each arm were alcoholic. Exclusion criteria included end-stage liver disease, primary biliary cirrhosis, malignancies, and immunosuppressive therapy. Noncompliant subjects were withdrawn from the analysis. At 2 years, overall survival was trending better with silymarin (n = 105, 77% vs. 67%; $p = .07$), and at 4 years, cumulative survival was improved with silymarin (n = 29, 58% vs. 38%; $p = .036$). Survival benefit was limited to alcoholics ($p = .01$) and to those rated Child's class A on entry ($p = .03$). Unfortunately, more of the alcoholic patients receiving placebo continued to drink (73% vs. 55%), and more of the subjects rated Child's class C on entry were assigned to placebo (11% vs. 3%). Both of these factors, which favor milk thistle, may have influenced the analysis. This study represents the best evidence supporting milk thistle.

A similar European randomized, double-blinded, controlled multicenter trial compared milk thistle (150 mg three times daily) with placebo (26). Two hundred subjects with biopsy-confirmed alcoholic cirrhosis were enrolled. Exclusion criteria included other causes of cirrhosis and use of colchicine, penicillamine, or corticosteroids. One hundred twenty-five subjects completed the 2-year follow-up. Survival was not improved at 2 years or at 5 years (odds ratio, 1.01; 95% CI, 0.46 to 2.22). Retrospective testing of stored sera, which was available for 75 of the 200 entrants, showed 29 to be positive for hepatitis C. Among these 29, treatment may have been protective (silymarin deaths, 0 in 13; placebo deaths, 4 in 16; $p = .059$).

Safety. No serious adverse effects have been reported.

Summary. Results are inconclusive. The best evidence suggests a benefit in cirrhosis. Any benefit is probably limited to alcoholic persons and those rated Child's class A. The usual dosage studied is 140 mg, standardized to contain 70% to 80% silymarin, three times daily.

St. John's Wort for Depression

The history of St. John's wort (*Hypericum perforatum*) as an herbal agent dates back 2,000 years. The use of *Hypericum* for mood problems continued into the 19th century but was forgotten early in this century. During the last 30 years, Europe has produced an extensive literature. In 1984, the Commission E gave St. John's wort a positive rating for use in psychovegetative disturbances, depressive moods, and anxiety or nervous unrest. St. John's wort is the most commonly prescribed antidepressant in Germany. After press and television coverage of a metaanalysis with positive findings in 1996 (27), the sales of St. John's wort in the United States rose from $20 million to $200 million during the next 2 years. It remains one of the top three herbal remedies consumed in the United States.

Evidence for Efficacy. Evidence suggests that the active ingredients are naphthodianthrones, primarily hypericin, pseudohypericin, and protohypericin. Although monoamine oxidase inhibitor activity is seen *in vitro*, this does not appear to be clinically important. The exact mechanism of St. John's wort is not known, but the best evidence supports effects on γ-aminobutyric acid (GABA), serotonin, and norepinephrine receptors. The hypericin content of St. John's wort varies from 0.06% to 0.75%, depending on the time of harvest and quality of the plants. A standardized extract, LI 160, based on the content of hypericin has been used in most studies. However, recent studies have suggested that another component of St. John's wort, hyperforin, may be the active agent. The content of hyperforin ranges from 2% in the flowers to 4.5% in the fruit. If hyperforin is the active agent and the most commonly used standardized extract, LI 160, is titrated to hypericin, then the clinical efficacy may vary from batch to batch. Despite the extensive knowledge of the components of St. John's wort and their actions in model systems, lingering uncertainties regarding which component or components are the most clinically relevant will continue to confound efforts to standardize preparations and treatment trials.

An update of the original 1996 metaanalysis included 27 trials (28). All randomized trials comparing St. John's wort (alone or in combination with other herbal agents) with placebo or antidepressant medications in depressed patients were included. A total of 2,291 patients were included in the 27 studies. Seven trials used Diagnostic and Statistical Manual III and two trials used International Classification of Diseases 10 definitions of depression as entry criteria. In the remaining 18 studies, entry criteria were usually "neurotic depression" or "mild to moderate depressive disorders." LI 160 was tested in 11 trials. Two trials used St. John's wort with valerian. Of the 27 trials, 24 were double-blinded. However, six studies used a liquid preparation of *Hypericum*, which has a distinctive taste and is difficult to conceal. In 26 of the trials, the duration was 4 to 8 weeks. One study lasted 12 weeks but was less rigorous in design. Standard definitions of treatment responder were used. Many trials used more than one measurement, such as a Hamilton Depression Scale (HAMD) score of less than 10 or less than 50% of the baseline score (17 trials), or "much improved" on the Clinical Global Impression (CGI) Scale (12 trials).

The results from 14 of the 17 trials comparing St. John's wort with placebo were combined. The St. John's wort response rate was 56%, whereas the response rate for placebo was 25%. The pooled rate ratio confirmed a significant effect (2.47; 95% CI, 1.69 to 3.61). Ten trials compared St. John's wort with another active agent, either a tricyclic antidepressant (eight trials) or a benzodiazepine (two trials). A pooling of responder rates from these trials suggested equivalence (mono-preparations rate ratio, 1.01; 95% CI, 0.87 to 1.16; combination preparations rate ratio, 1.52; 95% CI, 0.78 to 2.94). When the analysis was limited to the four trials comparing mono-preparations of St. John's wort versus tricyclic antidepressants in patients with major depression defined according to the Diagnostic and Statistical Manual III, the results were similar. Dropouts and adverse effects were seen less with St. John's wort than with standard antidepressants (dropouts, 8.9% vs. 13.6%; any adverse effect, 26.3% vs. 44.7%).

Only one trial looked at severely depressed patients (29). In this 6-week trial comparing twice the usual dose of St. John's wort (600 mg three times daily) with imipramine (50 mg three times daily), the decrease in HAMD scores was slightly greater with imipramine (26.1 to 13.4) than with St. John's wort (25.3 to 14.4; $p < .02$).

The major criticisms of the trials published to date relate to duration and subjects. All the trials ran from 4 to 8 weeks with the one exception of a poorly designed trial lasting 12 weeks. Consequently, no data regarding the duration of response exists. The subjects entered had a baseline HAMD score in the range of 16 to 20, which is less than the usual values of 20 to 24 in most trials of antidepressants. The bulk of evidence addresses milder depression, and few subjects were more severely depressed. The comparative trials with tricyclic antidepressants used doses lower than those considered standard. Finally, the variety of commercially produced products makes comparisons difficult.

Only one recent trial comparing St John's wort with a newer antidepressant has been published. A 6-week trial comparing St. John's wort (800 mg daily) with fluoxetine (20 mg daily) enrolled 149 elderly subjects with mild to moderate depression (30). Improvement in the HAMD score was similar with both treatments (St. John's wort, 16.60 to 7.91; fluoxetine, 17.18 to 8.11).

Safety. Adverse effects, which are generally mild, include gastrointestinal upset, dizziness, sedation, restlessness, and fatigue. St. John's wort may cause photosensitivity in fair-skinned patients, which can be severe at high doses. It should not be used during pregnancy and should not be combined with other antidepressants.

Summary. St. John's wort appears to be effective in the short-term treatment of mild to moderate depression. Several studies comparing it with low-dose tricyclic antidepressants show it to be equivalent in the short term. Fewer data comparing St. John's wort with selective serotonin reuptake inhibitors are available.

Saw Palmetto for Benign Prostatic Hyperplasia

Saw palmetto (*Serenoa repens*) is a plant native to the southeastern United States. Native American Indians used the extract of the dried fruit from this dwarf palm for urinary difficulties, among other conditions. It was adopted by Naturopathic and Eclectic physicians in the 19th century and is primarily promoted as a treatment for benign prostatic hyperplasia (BPH). In Germany, 90% of prescriptions for BPH are herbal medicines. Almost all these prescriptions are for saw palmetto alone or with additional herbal agents. Saw palmetto has received a positive rating for BPH by the Commission E.

Evidence for Efficacy. One systematic review of the literature from 1966 to 1997 was able to identify 18 trials, 16 of which were double-blinded (31). Randomized, controlled trials of symptomatic BPH were included that lasted for at least 30 days. Ten trials compared saw palmetto with placebo, two trials compared saw palmetto with finasteride, and the remaining trials used products containing saw palmetto and other phytotherapeutic agents. The mean study duration was 9 weeks (range, 4 to 48 weeks), and 9.6% of subjects were lost to follow-up (range, 4% to 15%).

The results of this metaanalysis showed a modest benefit. An improvement in self-rated symptoms (risk ratio, 1.72; 95% CI, 1.21 to 2.44, favoring saw palmetto) was seen in six studies. Nocturia improved in 10 trials (weighted mean difference, -0.76 episodes per night; 95% CI, -1.22 to -0.32). Saw palmetto increased peak urine flow rates in eight trials (WMD, 1.93 mL/s; 95% CI, 0.72 to 3.14 mL/s). Because the natural history of BPH involves slow changes and some improvement in a subset of patients, the results of trials of less than 6 months' duration represent weak evidence. Also, in the large trials of pharmaceutical agents for BPH, a robust placebo response was seen. In some of the trials with saw palmetto, little change occurred with placebo. The authors of this review felt that blinding was adequate in only 9 of the 18 studies.

Two specific trials address these concerns and provide stronger evidence. A European double-blinded, randomized, controlled multicenter trial compared β-sitosterol with placebo in men who had symptomatic BPH (32). Although it is not certain, the bulk of the evidence suggests that β-sitosterol is the active ingredient in saw palmetto extract. This trial enrolled 200 men, who received 20 mg of β-sitosterol three times daily or placebo for 6 months. The self-reported symptoms measured with the International Prostate Symptom Score, a validated instrument, improved (IPSS mean change, -7.4 with treatment versus -2.1 with placebo; $p < .01$). Peak urine flow rates were significantly better with β-sitosterol (baseline 9.9 mL/s to 15.2 ml/s at 6 months) than with placebo (baseline 10.2 mL/s to 11.4 mL/s at 6 months; $p < .01$).

Another European multicenter trial compared saw palmetto with finasteride without a placebo arm (33). In this 6-month, double-blinded study, 1,098 men with symptomatic BPH were randomized either to 160 mg of saw palmetto twice daily and finasteride placebo or to 5 mg of finasteride and saw palmetto placebo. Quality-of-life scores and the IPSS improved equally with the two treatments (-37% for saw palmetto vs. -39% for finasteride), while the peak urine flow rates improved slightly more with finasteride (from 10.6 ± 2.8 to 13.3 ± 6.7 mL/s with saw palmetto, and from 10.8 ± 3.1 to 14.0 ± 7.4 mL/s with finasteride; $p = .035$). Values for prostate-specific antigen (PSA) decreased 41% with finasteride but did not change with saw palmetto. Sexual dysfunction was seen somewhat more often with finasteride.

Safety. Minimal adverse effects have been reported.

Summary. Evidence suggests a modest improvement in BPH symptoms, similar to that achieved with finasteride (little information available comparing saw palmetto with α-adrenergic blockers). The substance does not affect the PSA level. The usual dosage studied is 160 mg twice a day.

Valerian for Insomnia

Valerian (*Valeriana officinalis*) has been used for more than 100 years as a hypnotic and mild tranquilizer. With the advent of barbiturates, it was dropped from the U.S. National Formulary and U.S. Pharmacopoeia. It remains popular as a hypnotic in Europe, where it is usually combined with hops, passionflower, lemon balm, and lavender. The Commission E has given valerian a positive rating for "nervous sleep disturbances." The active components are not known, and its mechanism is poorly understood. Proposed mechanisms involve binding to GABA or serotonin receptors, and inhibiting the breakdown of GABA. The Food and Drug Administration lists valerian as GRAS (generally recognized as safe), and it is approved as a flavoring agent.

Evidence for Efficacy. Several studies suggest a benefit with valerian. However, most of the trials have serious deficiencies, such as small enrollment (n = 8, 10, 14, 12), enrollment of normal subjects rather than subjects with sleep disturbances, and use of nonvalidated symptom scores. In the largest trial, 166 volunteers received nine samples (three each of placebo, 400 mg of aqueous valerian extract, and a commercial herbal sedative containing 120 mg of valerian with 60 mg of hops) to be taken on nonconsecutive nights (34). One hundred twenty-eight subjects completed the trial (23% dropout rate). Sleep latency and sleep quality were better on the nights when valerian was taken than on placebo nights. Subset analysis showed the benefit to be limited to self-described poor sleepers. Interestingly, the commercial preparation of valerian with hops was no different from placebo.

In the most rigorous study, 121 patients with insomnia (International Classification of Diseases 10) were enrolled in a double-blinded, randomized, controlled multicenter trial comparing valerian (600 mg, 70% alcohol extract standardized to 0.4% to 0.6% valerenic acid) with placebo for 28 days (35). Those who had major depression and were taking medications were excluded. A marked placebo response suggested adequate blinding. At 14 days, a significant improvement was noted on the CGI Scale with treatment. By 28 days, valerian significantly improved sleep in comparison with placebo on three standardized scales. This study suggests that the benefit of valerian occurs slowly, during 4 weeks. If this is true, the results of earlier studies lasting 1 to 7 days are difficult to accept.

Valerian is usually standardized to the content of valerenic acid (usually 0.8%). However in the absence of a standardized extract procedure and because of uncertainty regarding the active component, different commercial products may vary in efficacy. Relative proportions of the components vary with season of harvest and species harvested. This adds further uncertainty to any comparison.

Safety. Adverse effects are rare and generally mild. A possible withdrawal reaction was reported after general anesthesia

for biopsy in a patient who had taken valerian (530 mg to 2 g) five times a day for "many years" (36). Tachycardia, high-output cardiac failure, delirium, and oliguria were noted and responded to benzodiazepine. In general, valerian should not be used with other sedating medications.

Summary. Despite its historical use as a sedative, only one adequate trial supports the use of valerian. Without a standardized extract, products likely will have very different ratios of ingredients. Valerian should not be combined with other sedatives.

REFERENCES

1. Blumenthal M, senior ed. The complete German Commission E monographs. Boston: Integrative Medicine Communications, 1998.
2. Melchart D, Linde K, Fischer P, et al. *Echinacea* for the prevention and treatment of the common cold (Cochrane Review). In: The Cochrane Library, Issue 1, 1999. Oxford: Update Software.
3. Grimm W, Müller HH. A randomized controlled trial of the effect of fluid extract of *Echinacea purpurea* on the incidence and severity of colds and respiratory infections. Am J Med 1999;106:138.
4. Oken BS, Storzbach DM, Kaye JA. The efficacy of *Ginkgo biloba* on cognitive function in Alzheimer disease. Arch Neurol 1998;55:1409.
5. Kleijnen J, Knipschild P. *Ginkgo biloba*. Lancet 1992;340:1136.
6. Le Bars PL, Katz MM, Berman N, et al. A placebo-controlled, double-blind, randomized trial of an extract of *ginkgo biloba* for dementia. JAMA 1997;278:1327.
7. Rowin J, Lewis SL. Spontaneous bilateral subdural hematomas associated with chronic *Ginkgo biloba* ingestion. Neurology 1996;46:1775.
8. Vale S. Subarachnoid haemorrhage associated with *Ginkgo biloba*. Lancet 1998;352:36.
9. Gilbert GJ. *Ginkgo biloba*. Neurology 1997;48:1137.
10. Matthews MK. Association of *Ginkgo biloba* with intracerebral hemorrhage. Neurology 1998;50:1933.
11 Rosenblatt M, Mindel J. Spontaneous hyphema associated with ingestion of *Ginkgo biloba* extract. N Engl J Med 1997;336:1108.
12. Singh YN, Blumenthal M. Kava: an overview. Herbalgram 1997;39:34.
13. Kinzler E, Krömer J, Lehmann E. Wirksamkeit eines Kava-Spezial-Extraktes bei Patienten mit Angst-, Spannungs-, und Erregungszusttänden nicht-psychotischer Genese. Arzneimittelforschung 1991;41:584.
14. Woelk H, Kapoula O, Lehrl S, et al. Behandlung von Angst-Patienten. Z Allgemeinmed 1993;69:271.
15. Volz HP, Kieser M. Kava-kava extract WS 1490 versus placebo in anxiety disorders—a randomized placebo-controlled 25-week outpatient trial. Pharmacopsychiatry 1997;30:1.
16. Norton SA, Ruze P. Kava dermopathy. J Am Acad Dermatol 1994;31:89.
17. Spillane PK, Fisher DA, Currie BJ. Neurological manifestations of kava intoxication. Med J Aust 1997;167:172.
18. Schelosky L, Raffauf C, Jendroska K, et al. Kava and dopamine antagonism. J Neurol Neurosurg Psychiatry 1995;58:639.
19. Almeida JC, Grimsley EW. Coma from the health food store: interaction between kava and alprazolam. Ann Intern Med 1996;125:940.
20. Strahl S, Ehret V, Dahm HH, et al. Necrotizing hepatitis after taking herbal remedies. Dtsch Med Wochenschr 1998;123:1410.

21. Magliulo E, Gagliardi B, Fiori GP. Zur Wirkung von Silymarin bei der Behandlung der akuten Virushepatitis. Med Klin 1978;73:1060.

22. Flisiak R, Prokopowicz D. Effect of misoprostol on the course of viral hepatitis B. Hepatogastroenterology 1997;44:1419.

23. Salmi HA, Sarna S. Effect of silymarin on chemical, functional, and morphological alterations of the liver. Scand J Gastroenterol 1982;17:517.

24. Trinchet JC, Coste T, Levy VG, et al. Traitement de l'hépatite alcoolique par la silymarine. Une étude comparative en double insu chez 116 malades. Gastroenterol Clin Biol 1989;13:120.

25. Ferenci P, Dragosics B, Dittrich H, et al. Randomized controlled trial of silymarin treatment in patients with cirrhosis of the liver. J Hepatol 1989;9:105.

26. Parés A, Planas R, Torres M, et al. Effects of silymarin in alcoholic patients with cirrhosis of the liver: results of a controlled, double-blind, randomized and multi-center trial. J Hepatol 1998; 28:615.

27. Linde K, Ramirez G, Mulrow CD, et al. St. John's wort for depression—an overview and metaanalysis of randomised clinical trials. BMJ 1996;313:253.

28. Linde K, Mulrow CD. St. John's wort for depression (Cochrane Review). In: The Cochrane Library, Issue 1, 1999. Oxford: Update Software.

29. Vorbach EU, Arnoldt KH, Hübner WD. Efficacy and tolerability of St. John's wort extract LI 160 versus imipramine in patients with severe depressive episodes according to ICD-10. Pharmacopsychiatry 1997;30[Suppl]2:81.

30. Harrer G, Schmidt U, Kuhn U, et al. Comparison of equivalence between the St. John's wort extract LoHyp-57 and fluoxetine. Arzneimittelforschung 1999;49:289.

31. Wilt TJ, Ishani A, Stark G, et al. Saw palmetto extracts for treatment of benign prostatic hyperplasia. JAMA 1998;280:1604.

32. Berges RR, Windeler J, Trampisch HJ, et al. Randomised, placebo-controlled, double-blind clinical trial of β-sitosterol in patients with benign prostatic hyperplasia. Lancet 1995;345:1529.

33. Carraro JC, Raynaud JP, Koch G, et al. Comparison of phytotherapy (Permixon) with finasteride in the treatment of benign prostate hyperplasia: a randomized international study of 1,098 patients. Prostate 1996;29:231.

34. Leathwood PD, Chauffard F, Heck E, et al. Aqueous extract of valerian root (Valeriana officinalis L.) improves sleep quality in man. Pharmacol Biochem Behav 1982;17:65.

35. Vorbach EU, Görtelmeyer R, Brünig J. Therapie von Insomnien. Baldrianpräparats: Wirksamkeit und Verträglichkeit eines Psychopharmakotherapie 1996;13:109.

36. Garges HP, Varia I, Doraiswamy PM. Cardiac complications and delirium associated with valerian root withdrawal. JAMA 1998;280:1566.

ANNOTATED BIBLIOGRAPHY

Astin JA, Marie A, Pellitier KR, et al. A review of the incorporation of complementary and alternative medicine by mainstream physicians. Arch Intern Med 1998;158:2303. (*A review of surveys performed during the past 15 years; finds referrals frequently made for acupuncture, chiropractic, and massage.*)

Eisenberg DM, Davis RB, Ettner SL, et al. Trends in alternative medicine use in the United States, 1990–1997: results of a follow-up national survey. JAMA 1998;280:1569. (*Documents the marked growth in scope and use; expenditures total in the tens of billions of dollars.*)

Eisenberg DM. Advising patients who seek alternative medical therapies. Ann Intern Med 1997;127:61. (*Excellent advice on how to discuss alternative care with patients and how to deal with those who seek it.*)

Fontanarosa PB, Lundberg GD. Alternative medicine meets science. JAMA 1998;280:1618. (*An editorial on the role of science in the assessment of alternative medicine and the standards for such assessment.*)

Kaptchuk TJ, Eisenberg DM. The persuasive appeal of alternative medicine. Ann Intern Med 1998;129:1061. (*A thoughtful discussion of why patients seek such treatment.*)

O'Hara MA, Kiefer D, Farrell K, et al. A review of 12 commonly used medicinal herbs. Arch Fam Med 1999;7:523. (*Detailed review; 112 references.*)

238
Caring for the Adolescent Patient
LAWRENCE J. RONAN

Most experts on adolescence recommend annual visits to a physician between the ages of 11 and 21 years, with a complete physical examination at least once in early adolescence (ages 11 to 14), middle adolescence (ages 15 to 17), and late adolescence (ages 18 to 21). The emphasis during the annual visits is on prevention and health promotion. Adolescent deaths are caused predominantly by accidents, homicides, and suicides. The major causes of adolescent morbidity include pregnancy, sexually transmitted diseases, substance abuse, smoking, physical violence, and depression. Because the leading causes of mortality and morbidity are unintended injury or are largely preventable, the focus of care for adolescents is on primary as well as secondary prevention. During visits, both biomedical and psychosocial issues are addressed. Adolescent care emphasizes the cultivation of healthful life-long habits to prevent heart disease and cancer. The primary care physician whose practice involves primarily adults needs to know the basics of adolescent preventive care because many adolescents present to the offices of these physicians for care.

CONSENT

In general, parents are responsible for giving consent for their children's care until the child reaches the age of 18. Adolescents, however, have a greater right than do younger children to participate in their own health care decisions. Practitioners should review their state laws regarding the specific services that minors may obtain without the consent of their parents. These services usually are related to pregnancy, birth control, abortion, the evaluation and treatment of sexually transmitted diseases (including HIV infection), substance abuse, and sexual assault. Some states also include outpatient mental health services. "Emancipated" minors have the legal right to give consent for their own care. These adolescents are married, have children, serve in the military, live apart from their parents, or are homeless. "Mature minors," adolescents who understand the risks and benefits of treatment and its alternatives, also have the legal right to give consent.

HISTORY TAKING

Adolescence is a dynamic time in the life cycle associated with rapid and dramatic changes in physical, social, and emotional development. The adolescent health history focuses on five contextual and developmental domains:

1. Social and emotional development
2. Physical development and health habits
3. Sexual development
4. Family functioning
5. School performance

The unique aspects of the five developmental domains should be explored in each stage of adolescence—early, middle, and late.

Early Adolescence: Ages 11 to 14 Years. Early adolescence heralds the start of dramatic physical changes. Girls undergo rapid spurts of growth, the development of pubic hair and breasts, and changes in the distribution of body fat. Generally, puberty begins in girls 2 to 3 years earlier than in boys. Boys acquire deeper voices, larger testicles, and pubic hair, and acne frequently develops. Early adolescents are preoccupied with looks and anxious about physical changes. Also, early teenagers move from elementary to middle school, where academic demands are higher, autonomy is greater, and socialization is increased. Their thinking, although increasingly abstract, is for the most part still concrete and oriented to the present. Early teens are focused on self, family, and peers. Sexual exploration and recreational drug experimentation begin. The profound biologic, emotional, and psychological changes experienced by early teens stress the family as they challenge limits and rules and also explore new and sometimes risky behaviors.

Middle Adolescence: Ages 15 to 17 Years. By middle adolescence, the physical development of girls is complete, and most boys are well on their way to the completion of puberty. Although the thinking of middle adolescents remains concrete, many of them are progressing from concrete to abstract, formal, operational thinking. Friends become hugely important. Middle teens, also, become aware of the larger world and social issues. The growing need for autonomy places teens in conflict with family rules. Middle teens are very aware of academic pressures and anxious about school and sports performance. They can obtain work permits and driver licenses.

Late Adolescence: Ages 18 to 21 Years. Pubertal development is complete. The late adolescent focuses on vocational and personal development. Older teens are legally responsible for themselves, often living separately from parents and struggling with decisions about further schooling, jobs, or the military. High-risk behaviors peak at this stage, including promiscuity, substance abuse, and eating disorders.

PHYSICAL EXAMINATION

Measure and plot on a standard growth chart the adolescent's height and weight. Determine the patient's body mass index. Document a blood pressure measurement at every annual visit. Evaluate for scoliosis. Look for evidence of physical abuse. Examine the adolescent's teeth for cavities, malocclusion, gingivitis, and congenital dental anomalies. Determine the Tanner stage or Sexual Maturity Rating (SMR). For girls, provide instruction in breast self-examination and inspect the external genitalia. Perform a pelvic examination with Papanicolaou smear annually for all girls who are sexually active or 18 years of age or older. Examine boys for gynecomastia and hernias. Check the testicles for abnormal masses or congenital anomalies (at high risk for testicular cancer are boys with a history of undescended testes or a single testicle). Check the skin for acne.

LABORATORY EVALUATION

Perform a random *cholesterol* determination on teen-agers who have a positive family history for early cardiovascular disease or hyperlipidemia. Adolescents who are unsure of their family history should also be screened. Girls with heavy menses, weight loss, or eating disorders, or who are extremely athletic, should have a *screening hematocrit* or hemoglobin determination.

Only adolescents at increased risk for exposure to tuberculosis require *tuberculin (purified protein derivative, or PPD) skin testing*. These risks include exposure to tuberculosis, homelessness, a history of incarceration, immigrant status, HIV infection or living with an HIV-infected person, and illicit drug use. It is reasonable to test once between 11 and 16 years if the teen-ager has no risk factors (see also Chapter 38).

Sexually active teen-agers should be screened for sexually transmitted diseases. The frequency of screening remains controversial. Usually, girls are screened during each annual pelvic examination, which should include a cervical culture for gonorrhea, immunologic testing of cervical fluid for *Chlamydia* infection, *serologic testing* for *syphilis*, and visual inspection of the genitalia and *Papanicolaou smear* for human papillomavirus. For boys, screening consists of *urine DNA* or *leukocyte esterase* analysis for *gonorrhea* and *Chlamydia* infection, serologic testing for syphilis, and visual inspection of the genitalia for human papillomavirus (see also Chapters 107, 117, 124, 125, and 136).

The clinician should offer *HIV testing* to adolescents at risk for HIV infection. Risks include the use of IV drugs, previous infection with a sexually transmitted disease, blood transfusion before 1985, exchange of sex for money or drugs, homelessness, a history of more than one sexual partner in the last 6 months, male homosexuality, or a sexual partner with any of the above risk factors for HIV infection (see also Chapter 7).

IMMUNIZATIONS

(See also Chapter 6.) Ensure that the teen-ager's immunizations are up to date at every clinical encounter. Tetanus–diphtheria (Td) toxoid; measles, mumps, and rubella (MMR) vaccine; and hepatitis B vaccine should be given to the adolescent if the previously recommended doses were missed, not documented, or given before the recommended minimum age.

(The recommended minimum age for completion of the second dose of MMR vaccination is 4 to 6 years; for varicella vaccination, 12 to 18 months; and for the third dose of hepatitis vaccine, 6 to 18 months.) By 11 to 12 years of age, the teen-ager is also due for the tetanus booster. For incompletely immunized or unimmunized adolescents (especially newly arrived immigrants), follow the recommendation of the Red Book regarding immunization schedules for adolescents. Schools routinely request documentation; make certain that your medical records regarding the patient's immunization status are kept up to date.

ANTICIPATORY GUIDANCE

Prevention of Injury and Violence. The use of seat belts reduces motor vehicle fatalities by 45% and the rate of serious injury by 50%. In 80% of road fatalities, the victim was not wearing a seat belt. Counsel adolescents to use seat belts. In addition, promote the use of other safety devices, such as bicycle and motorcycle helmets, protective gear for rollerblading and skate boarding, and appropriate athletic protective devices. Ask the teen-ager about access to weapons.

Mental Health. Screen for depression and suicidal ideation. Risk factors include poor school performance, family dysfunction, substance abuse, physical or sexual abuse, and previous suicide attempts or plans. Note that the vegetative signs associated with adult depression (e.g., sleep disturbance, lack of interest, decreased concentration) can be part of normal adolescent development. Moreover, adolescent depression may masquerade as vague somatic complaints, such as abdominal pain or headaches. Suicidal ideation requires immediate referral. Recurrent or serious depression necessitates consultation with a mental health professional.

Nutrition and Exercise. Counsel adolescents about a healthful diet, safe weight management, and regular exercise. Screen for faddist diets, anorexia and bulimia, and the use of anabolic steroids by athletes. Recommend dietary supplements of calcium (1000 mg/d) and folic acid (400 mg/d) for female adolescents.

Sexuality. Discuss sex frankly. Explore early adolescents' understanding of sexuality. Discuss responsible sexual behavior, including abstinence. Educate about birth control, stressing the use of latex condoms to prevent sexually transmitted diseases and especially HIV infection. Provide birth control and instructions on appropriate use.

Abuse of Tobacco, Alcohol, and Other Substances. Ask about smoking and the use of alcohol and other drugs during the past 6 months. Educate about the harmful effects of substance abuse. Explore family history, frequency and amount of use, and circumstances surrounding use. Encourage participation in community peer self-help groups. Determine social and psychological factors that prompt the use of drugs and refer to social services and mental health professionals as necessary.

Abuse. Screen all adolescents annually for a history of physical, emotional, and sexual abuse. Pursue aggressively any suspicion, asking about circumstances and people involved. Be aware of local reporting requirements to state offices. Involve mental health and social services professionals early in all suspected cases of abuse.

SPECIAL ISSUES AND NEED FOR REFERRAL

Scoliosis is a lateral curvature of the spine associated with rotation of the involved vertebrae. Although scoliosis may be associated with chronic illness (neurofibromatosis, cerebral palsy, Marfan syndrome, poliomyelitis), the most common type is idiopathic, generally beginning at age 8 or 10 years of age and progressing during growth through adolescence. It is classically asymptomatic. The clinician screens for scoliosis with the forward bend test and visual inspection for rib cage deformation and waistline asymmetry. A positive result on screening warrants imaging with a "scoliosis plain film series," radiography of the entire spine in both the posterior and lateral planes with the patient in the standing position. All curves greater than 15 degrees require referral to an orthopedic specialist if spinal growth is not completed. (Adolescent girls usually complete spinal growth 18 to 24 months after menarche).

Eating Disorders. Between 5% and 10% of adolescent girls and young women have an eating disorder. The diagnosis of anorexia nervosa and bulimia nervosa is made through the history. Ask about recurrent dieting, body image, interruption of menses, and physical activity. Assess for the use of laxatives and diuretics, self-induced vomiting, and starvation. Except in extreme cases, the physical examination findings and results of the laboratory evaluation are normal. In anorexia, weight loss greater than 10% of previous weight or a body mass index below the fifth percentile suggests the diagnosis. Use laboratory findings to exclude other causes of weight loss: hyperthyroidism, inflammatory bowel disease, diabetes, and connective tissue disorders (see Chapters 73, 102, 103, and 146). Once the diagnosis has been made, treatment should be carried out by a multidisciplinary team that includes the primary clinician, a psychologist or psychiatrist, and a nutritionist skilled in the management of eating disorder problems (see Chapter 234).

School Failure. Not uncommonly, an adolescent or more likely the adolescent's parent turns to the clinician for an explanation of poor academic performance. The differential diagnosis for academic failure in adolescence is broad, and more than one factor is often involved. A thorough history, physical examination, and appropriate laboratory studies should serve to identify psychological (depression, anxiety) and physical (hearing, visual) problems, chronic disease (asthma, neurologic dysfunction), learning disorders (attention deficit disorders), drug abuse, limited intellectual ability (developmental delay), and social difficulties (dysfunctional family life, poor peer relations, abuse). Coordinate with the patient's parent, teacher, and school counselor. Many school districts are mandated to provide neuropsychological testing to aid in both diagnosis and treatment strategies.

Hypertension. Definitions of normal, borderline, and high blood pressure in adolescence involve calculating the teen's percentile for age and height. Normal is below the 90th percentile, high normal is between the 90th and 95th percentiles, and high (hypertension) is a systolic or diastolic pressure equal to or greater than the 95th percentile on three separate occasions.

Consider secondary causes of hypertension, including renal disease, oral contraception, and use of drugs such as cocaine or steroids. The medical history focuses on growth and development, past illnesses (especially during the neonatal period and infancy), and family history. On physical examination, look for evidence of end-organ damage. Tailor the laboratory evaluation as the clinical situation warrants and obtain a urinalysis, values for blood urea nitrogen, creatinine, and electrolytes, and a complete blood cell count. Consider renal ultrasonography and echocardiography (see Chapters 14 and 19).

Obesity. Teen-agers with a body mass index between the 85th and 90th percentiles are at high risk for obesity and require diet assessment and counseling. Adolescents with a body mass index above the 95th percentile for age and sex require aggressive nutrition counseling and benefit from a multidisciplinary approach that involves diet, exercise, and counseling (see Chapters 10 and 233).

Gynecomastia. In the majority of male adolescents (60% to 70%), transient enlargement of one or both breasts develops during transition through Tanner stages II to III as a normal part of puberty. Type I idiopathic gynecomastia is usually unilateral (20% of cases are bilateral) and tender; it consists of a firm mass below the areola. Type II is the more generalized breast enlargement found in obese adolescents. Although more than 95% of cases of gynecomastia are idiopathic and resolve spontaneously, be alert to pathologic causes: drugs; Klinefelter's syndrome; adrenal, pituitary, and testicular tumors; hypothyroidism; and hepatic dysfunction. Most cases of gynecomastia resolve within a period of months to 2 years, and require only reassurance and support to the anxious teen. On occasion, because of severe psychological damage or a persistent problem, either pharmacologic treatment (e.g., danazol) or surgical intervention is required (see also Chapter 99).

ANNOTATED BIBLIOGRAPHY

American Academy of Pediatrics. The Red Book 2000. Report of the Committee on Infectious Diseases, 25th ed. Elk Grove Village, IL: American Academy of Pediatrics, 2000. (*Consensus guidelines.*)

American Academy of Pediatrics. Practicing adolescent medicine: a collection of resources. Elk Grove Village, IL:1998. (*Useful office resource on all aspects.*)

Becker A, Grinspoon S. Current concepts: eating disorders. N Engl J Med 1999;340:1092. (*Excellent review for the primary care physician.*)

Elster A. Guidelines for adolescent preventive services. Baltimore: Williams & Williams, 1994. (*Authoritative monograph with evidence-based guidelines.*)

Green M, ed. Bright Futures: guidelines for health supervision of infants, children, and adolescents. Arlington , VA Natl Center for Education in Maternal and Child Health, 1994. (*Resource on prevention.*)

National Heart, Lung, and Blood Institute. Update of the 1987 task force report on high blood pressure in children and adolescents: a working group report from the National High Blood Pressure Education Program. Pediatrics 1996;98:649. (*Latest iteration of the expert panel consensus guidelines.*)

National Cholesterol Education Expert Panel on Blood Cholesterol Levels in Children and Adolescents. Highlights of the report of the Expert Panel on Blood Cholesterol Levels in Children and Adolescents. Pediatrics 1992;89:495. (*Evidence-based consensus guidelines.*)

Neinstein L. Adolescent health care: a practical guide, 3rd ed. Los Angeles: University of Southern California; Baltimore: Williams & Wilkins, 1996. (*Another useful standard text in the field.*)

Websites

http://www.brightfutures.org
http://www.ama-assn.org/adolhlth/

Index

Page numbers followed by f indicate figures; page numbers followed by t indicate tabular material.